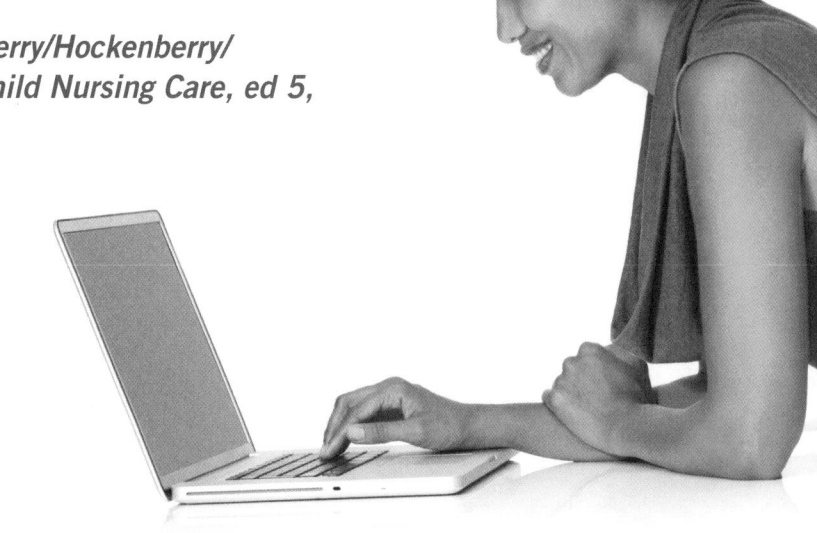

MATERNAL CHILD NURSING CARE

MATERNAL CHILD NURSING CARE

Shannon E. Perry, RN, PhD, FAAN
Professor Emerita, School of Nursing
San Francisco State University
San Francisco, California

Marilyn J. Hockenberry, PhD, RN-CS, PNP, FAAN
Bessie Baker Distinguished Professor of Nursing
Professor of Pediatrics
Chair, Duke Institutional Review Board
Duke University
Durham, North Carolina

Deitra Leonard Lowdermilk, RNC, PhD, FAAN
Clinical Professor Emerita, School of Nursing
University of North Carolina at Chapel Hill
Chapel Hill, North Carolina

David Wilson, MS, RN,C (NIC)
Staff, PALS Coordinator
Children's Hospital at Saint Francis
Tulsa, Oklahoma

FIFTH EDITION

ELSEVIER

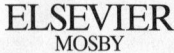

ELSEVIER
MOSBY

3251 Riverport Lane
St. Louis, Missouri 63043

Notices

Knowledge and best practice in this field are constantly changing. As new research and experience broaden our understanding, changes in research methods, professional practices, or medical treatment may become necessary.

Practitioners and researchers must always rely on their own experience and knowledge in evaluating and using any information, methods, compounds, or experiments described herein. In using such information or methods they should be mindful of their own safety and the safety of others, including parties for whom they have a professional responsibility.

With respect to any drug or pharmaceutical products identified, readers are advised to check the most current information provided (i) on procedures featured or (ii) by the manufacturer of each product to be administered, to verify the recommended dose or formula, the method and duration of administration, and contraindications. It is the responsibility of practitioners, relying on their own experience and knowledge of their patients, to make diagnoses, to determine dosages and the best treatment for each individual patient, and to take all appropriate safety precautions.

To the fullest extent of the law, neither the Publisher nor the authors, contributors, or editors, assume any liability for any injury and/or damage to persons or property as a matter of products liability, negligence or otherwise, or from any use or operation of any methods, products, instructions, or ideas contained in the material herein.

Content Manager: Laurie K. Gower
Content Development Specialist: Heather Bays
Publishing Services Manager: Deborah L. Vogel
Senior Project Manager: Jodi M. Willard
Design Direction: Karen Pauls

Printed in Canada

Last digit is the print number: 9   8   7   6   5   4   3   2   1

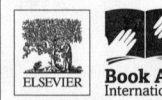

Working together
to grow libraries in
developing countries

www.elsevier.com • www.bookaid.org

ASSOCIATE EDITORS

Kitty Cashion, RN-BC, MSN
Clinical Nurse Specialist
University of Tennessee Health Science Center;
Department of Obstetrics & Gynecology
Maternal-Fetal Medicine Division
Memphis, Tennessee

Kathryn R. Alden, RN, MSN, EdD, IBCLC
Clinical Associate Professor
School of Nursing
University of North Carolina at Chapel Hill
Chapel Hill, North Carolina

CONTRIBUTORS

Pat Mahaffee Gingrich, RN-C, MSN, WHNP
Clinical Assistant Professor, School of Nursing
University of North Carolina at Chapel Hill
Chapel Hill, North Carolina

Peggy Mancuso, PhD, RN, CNM
Professor and Coordinator
Doctor of Nursing Practice Program
The Houston J. and Florence A. Doswell College of Nursing
Texas Woman's University
Dallas, Texas

Ellen F. Olshansky, PhD, RN, WHNP-BC, FAAN
Professor and Director
Program in Nursing Science
University of California, Irvine
Irvine, California

Case Studies, Evolve
Elizabeth Day, RN, MSN, CHPN
Nursing Faculty
Fresno City College & Madera Center
Fresno, California

Dusty Dix, RN, MSN
Clinical Assistant Professor
School of Nursing
University of North Carolina at Chapel Hill
Chapel Hill, North Carolina

Curriculum Guides, Powerpoint Slides, Test Bank
Barbara Pascoe, RN, BA, MA
Director
The Family Place
Concord Hospital
Concord, New Hampshire

Key Point Summaries
Joanna Cain, BSN, BA, RN
Auctorial Pursuits, Inc.
President and Founder
Austin, Texas

TEACH for Nurses
Melanie Cole, MA
Freelance Editor
Community Treatment, Inc.
University of Missouri–St. Louis
St. Louis, Missouri

Patrick F. Barrera, BS
Manager, Duke Office of Clinical Research
Duke University
Durham, North Carolina

Oliva Catolico, RN, PhD, CNL, BC
Professor
Dominican University of California
San Rafael, California

Carolyn V. Diagneau, RN, PNP-BC
Lakewood, Colorado

Amber Essman, MSN, RN, CNE
Assistant Professor
Chamberlain College of Nursing
Columbus, Ohio

Sarah Gabua, DNP(c), MSN, RN
Assistant Professor of Nursing
Rockford College
Rockford, Illinois

Shari Gould, RN, MSN
Instructor
Del Mar College
Corpus Christi, Texas

Marilyn J. Greer, MS, RN
Associate Professor of Nursing
Rockford College
Rockford, Illinois

Christina Keller, RN, MSN
Instructor
Radford University School of Nursing
RU WEST—Clinical Simulation Center
Radford, Virginia

Karen M. Lettre, RN, MSN, CEN, CPEN, EMT
Clinical Manager
Children's Medical Center Dallas Legacy Campus
Dallas, Texas

Susan K. Rice, PhD, RN, CPNP, CNS
Professor
College of Nursing
University of Toledo
Toledo, Ohio

Donna Wilsker, MSN, RN
Assistant Professor
Dishman Department of Nursing
Lamar University
Beaumont, Texas

Nancee Wozney, PhD, RN
Dean of Nursing
Minnesota State College—Southeast Technical
Winona, Minnesota

Elsevier Customer Insight Group

Debra Bacharz, RN, BSN, MSN, PhD
Associate Professor, Nursing
Cecily and John Leach College of Nursing
Saint Francis University
Joliet, Illinois

Roberta Cook, RN, MS, CPNP
Program Director, Nursing
Baker College of Auburn Hills
Auburn Hills, Michigan

Linda Macera-DiClemente, RN, BSN, BA, MSN
Nursing Faculty
Baker College of Auburn Hills
Auburn Hills, Michigan

Rita Nutt, DNP, RN
Assistant Professor, Nursing
Salisbury University
Salisbury, Maryland

Noreen Nutting, RN, BSN, MAIS
Associate Professor, Nursing
Northern Virginia Community College
Springfield, Virginia

Dana R. Sandifer, RN, BSN, MSN
Professor of Nursing
Hopkinsville Community College
Hopkinsville, Kentucky

Maridee Shogren, DNP, CNM
Clinical Instructor, Nursing
University of North Dakota
Grand Forks, North Dakota

Bridget Thompson, RN, BSN, MSN
Clinical Associate Professor, Nursing
University of North Dakota
Grand Forks, North Dakota

Barbara L. Wilson, PhD, RNC-OB
Associate Professor and Associate Dean of Academic
    Programs
College of Nursing
University of Utah
Salt Lake City, Utah

Evolve Resources

Patricia A. Floro, RN, BSN
Practical Nursing Instructor
Ohio Hi-Point Career Center
Bellefontaine, Ohio

Case Studies, Nursing Skills

Daryle Wane, PhD, ARNP-BC
Professor of Nursing
Pasco-Hernando Community College
New Port Richey, Florida

Review Questions

Christina Keller, RN, MSN
Radford University School of Nursing
RU WEST—Clinical Simulation Center
Radford, Virginia

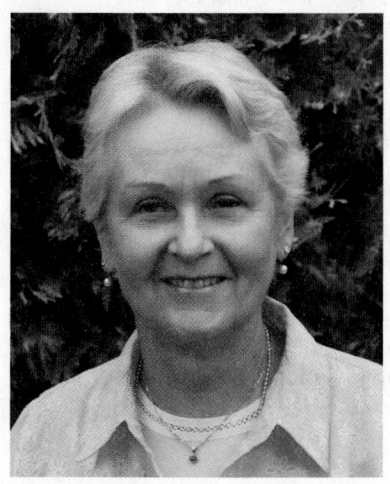

Shannon E. Perry is Professor Emerita, School of Nursing, San Francisco State University. She received her diploma in nursing from St. Joseph Hospital School of Nursing, Bloomington, Illinois; a Baccalaureate in Nursing from Marquette University; an MSN from the University of Colorado Medical Center; and a PhD in Educational Psychology with a specialty in Child Development from Arizona State University. She completed a 2-year postdoctoral fellowship in perinatal nursing at the University of California, San Francisco, as a Robert Wood Johnson Clinical Nurse Scholar.

Dr. Perry has had clinical experience as a staff nurse, head nurse, and supervisor in surgical nursing, obstetrics, pediatrics, gynecology, and neonatal nursing. She has served as an expert witness and a legal consultant. She has taught in schools of nursing in several states and was Interim Director and Director of the School of Nursing and Director of the Child and Adolescent Development Baccalaureate Program at San Francisco State University. She was Marquette University College of Nursing Alumna of the Year in 1999 and the University of Colorado School of Nursing Distinguished Alumna of the Year in 2000. She received the San Francisco State University Alumni Association Emeritus Faculty Award in 2005 and the Excellence in Education Award from the Beta Upsilon chapter of Sigma Theta Tau International in 2012.

She is co-author of *Maternity Nursing* (8th edition), *Maternity & Women's Health Care* (10th edition), and *Clinical Companion for Maternity & Newborn Nursing* (2nd edition) and has authored numerous articles on maternal-newborn topics and the legal aspects of nursing. She is a Fellow in the American Academy of Nursing and a member of the STTI Foundation Fellows Committee and the STTI International Services Task Force. Dr. Perry's experience in international nursing includes teaching international nursing courses in the United Kingdom, Ireland, Italy, Thailand, Ghana, and China and participating in health missions in Ghana, Kenya, and Honduras. For her "exemplary contributions to nursing, public service, and selfless commitment and passion in shaping the future of international health," she received the President's Award from the Global Caring Nurses Foundation, Inc, in 2008. In January 2012, she and 47 other women climbed Mt. Kilimanjaro, the highest mountain in Africa, to raise awareness of human trafficking and to raise funds to support projects to combat human trafficking.

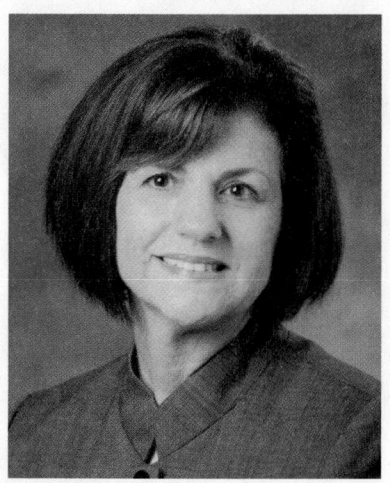

Marilyn J. Hockenberry is the Bessie Baker Distinguished Professor of Nursing and Professor of Pediatrics at Duke University. She serves as a Chair for the Duke Institutional Review Board and is Co-Chair of the Oncology Nursing Center of Excellence within the Duke Translational Nursing Institute. For over 18 years she served as the Director of the Pediatric Nurse Practitioner Program in the Texas Children's Cancer Center. Her research focuses on symptom management and treatment-related side effects experienced by children who have cancer. Dr. Hockenberry's current NIH-funded research studies are evaluating the treatment-related symptoms and neurocognitive deficits of leukemia treatment. She has authored over 80 articles and has served as the senior editor on the Wong nursing textbooks for many years.

Dr. Hockenberry completed her prenursing education at Mt. Vernon Nazarene College and received her Bachelors of Science from Capital University. She received her Masters of Science from Texas Woman's University and her PhD with distinction from the Medical College of Georgia. She is a Fellow of the American Academy of Nursing.

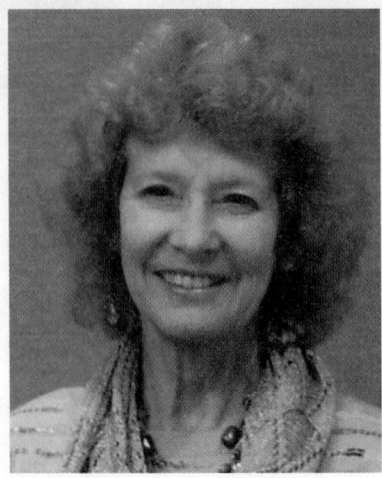

Deitra Leonard Lowdermilk is Clinical Professor Emerita, School of Nursing, University of North Carolina at Chapel Hill. She received her BSN from East Carolina University and her MEd and PhD in Education from the University of North Carolina at Chapel Hill. She is certified in In-Patient Obstetrics by the National Certification Corporation, and she is a Fellow in the American Academy of Nursing. In addition to being a nurse educator for over 34 years, Dr. Lowdermilk has clinical experience as a public health nurse and as a staff nurse in labor and delivery, postpartum, and newborn units, and she has worked in gynecologic surgery and cancer care units.

Dr. Lowdermilk has been recognized for her expertise in nursing education. She has repeatedly been selected as Classroom and Clinical Teacher of the Year by graduating seniors. She was a recipient of the Educator of the Year Award from both the District IV Association of Women's Health, Obstetric and Neonatal Nurses (AWHONN) and the North Carolina Nurses Association. She also received the 2005 AWHONN Excellence in Education Award.

She is active in AWHONN and has served as Chair of the North Carolina Section of AWHONN and as chair and member of various committees in AWHONN at the national, district, state, and local levels. She has served as guest editor for the *Journal of Obstetric, Gynecologic, and Neonatal Nursing* and served on editorial boards for other publications.

Dr. Lowdermilk's most significant contribution to nursing has been to promote excellence in nursing practice and education in women's health through integration of knowledge into practice. In 2005 she received the first Distinguished Alumni Award from East Carolina University School of Nursing for her exemplary contributions to the nursing profession in the area of maternal child care and the community. In 2011 she was inducted into the Hall of Fame for the College of Nursing at East Carolina University.

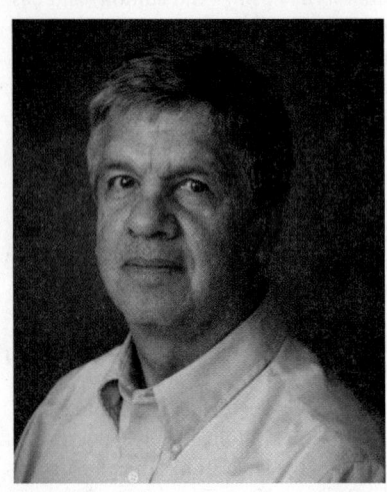

David Wilson received his BSN from Dallas Baptist College (now University) and his MSN from Texas Woman's University. He has more than 20 years of neonatal intensive care experience in Texas and Oklahoma. During his nursing career, David has worked in a number of positions, including staff nurse, neonatal educator, outreach educator, nutrition support coordinator, and BLS and Neonatal Resuscitation Program instructor. David was involved in medical missions in Costa Rica and Colombia for 2 years. David has also been nursing faculty at several universities either on a full-time or adjunct basis for 15 years. Writing for nursing publications is an endeavor he has enjoyed for many years. He has authored several articles pertaining to neonatal and pediatric nursing, has served as a reviewer for two nursing journals, and has been an author and contributor with Mosby/Elsevier since 1993. David is currently a staff nurse and PALS coordinator in the Children's Hospital at Saint Francis in Tulsa, Oklahoma.

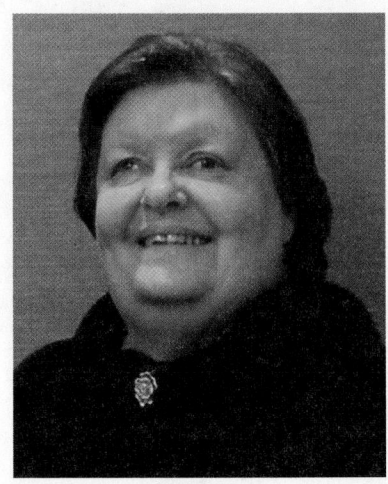

Kitty Cashion is a Clinical Nurse Specialist in the Maternal-Fetal Medicine Division at the University of Tennessee Health Science Center, Memphis, College of Medicine, Department of Obstetrics and Gynecology. She received her BSN from the University of Tennessee College of Nursing in Memphis and her MSN in Parent-Child Nursing from Vanderbilt University School of Nursing in Nashville, Tennessee. Ms. Cashion is certified as a High Risk Perinatal Nurse through the American Nurses Credentialing Center (ANCC).

Ms. Cashion's job responsibilities at the University of Tennessee include providing education regarding low and high risk obstetrics to staff nurses in West Tennessee community hospitals. In addition, she works part-time as an OB case manager at Alpha Maxx Healthcare in Memphis, Tennessee, and teaches OB clinical for nursing students at Northwest Mississippi Community College in Senatobia, Mississippi, and at Union University in Germantown, Tennessee.

Ms. Cashion has been an active AWHONN member, holding office at both the local and state levels. She is currently the Legislative Chair for the AWHONN Tennessee Section. Ms. Cashion has also served as an officer and board member of the Tennessee Perinatal Association and is an active volunteer for the Tennessee chapter of the March of Dimes Birth Defects Foundation.

Ms. Cashion has contributed to several obstetric nursing textbooks in the past and co-authored a series of Virtual Clinical Excursions workbooks to accompany four obstetric nursing textbooks published by Elsevier. More recently, she is one of the authors of *Maternity Nursing* (8th edition), *Maternity & Women's Health Care* (10th edition), and *Clinical Companion for Maternity & Newborn Nursing* (2nd edition).

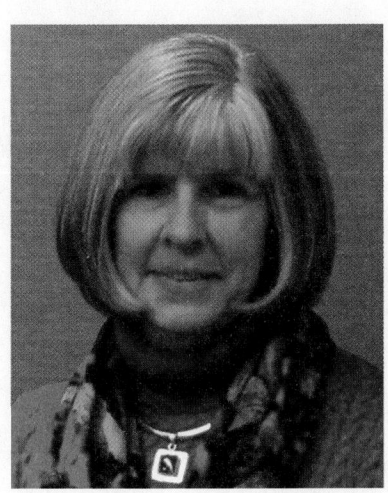

Kathryn R. Alden is Clinical Associate Professor in the School of Nursing at the University of North Carolina at Chapel Hill. She earned a bachelor's degree in nursing from UNC Charlotte, a master's degree from UNC Chapel Hill, and a doctorate in education from North Carolina State University. Dr. Alden has extensive experience as a nursing educator for baccalaureate students. At UNC Chapel Hill, she serves as course coordinator for maternal/newborn nursing and as lead academic counselor for the undergraduate nursing program. She has been recognized for her clinical teaching expertise and for her work in student counseling. Dr. Alden is an international board-certified lactation consultant who teaches prenatal breastfeeding classes for expectant parents as well as continuing education programs on breastfeeding for health care professionals.

Dr. Alden was an early adopter of human patient simulation and has been instrumental in the use of this teaching strategy with undergraduate nursing students. She has created numerous simulation scenarios, including two cases for Elsevier's *Simulation Learning System*. She has co-authored chapters on simulation for the Agency for Healthcare Research and Quality (AHRQ), the National League for Nursing, and other nursing texts. As an author, associate editor, and co-editor for Elsevier, Dr. Alden has contributed to numerous maternity textbooks.

This fifth edition of *Maternal Child Nursing Care* combines essential maternity and pediatric nursing information into one text. The text focuses on the care of women during their reproductive years and the care of children from birth through adolescence. The issues and concerns of childbearing women and the health care of children are the primary concentrations. The promotion of wellness and the management of common women's health problems and child development in the context of the family are also addressed. As we move further into the twenty-first century, this fifth edition of *Maternal Child Nursing Care* is designed to address the changing needs of women during their childbearing years and children during their developing years.

Maternal Child Nursing Care was developed to provide students with the knowledge and skills they need to become competent critical thinkers and to attain the sensitivity needed to become caring nurses. This fifth edition has been revised and refined in response to comments and suggestions from educators, clinicians, and students. It includes the most accurate, current, and clinically relevant information available.

APPROACH

Professional nursing practice continues to evolve and adapt to society's changing health priorities. The rapidly changing health care delivery system offers new opportunities for nurses to alter the practice of maternity and pediatric nursing and to improve the way care is given. Increasingly, nursing practice must be evidence based. It is incumbent on nurses to use the most up-to-date and scientifically supported information on which to base their care. To assist nurses in providing this type of care, **Evidence-Based Practice** boxes with implications for practice are included throughout the text.

Consumers of maternity and pediatric care vary in age, ethnicity, culture, language, social status, marital status, and sexual orientation. They seek care from a variety of health care providers in numerous health care settings, including the home. To meet the needs of these consumers, clinical education must offer students a variety of health care experiences in settings that include hospitals and birth centers, homes, clinics, private physicians' offices, shelters for the homeless or for women and children in need of protection, and other community-based settings.

Care Management has been used as an organizing framework for discussion in the nursing care chapters. This approach demonstrates how nursing must collaborate with other health care disciplines to provide the most comprehensive care possible to women and children. **Nursing Care Plans** reinforce the problem-solving approach to patient care. In chapters that focus on complications of childbearing, reproductive conditions, and childhood illnesses, medical interventions are included along with nursing care management. Throughout the discussion of assessment and care, we alert the nurse to signs of potential problems and provide informational boxes that highlight warning signs and emergency situations.

Patient education is an essential component of the nursing care of women and children. The chapter on women's health promotion and screening emphasizes teaching for self-care to promote wellness and to encourage preventive care. The chapter on transition to parenthood focuses on teaching for new parents and infants at home.

Special boxes highlight community care throughout the text. **Family-Centered Care** boxes incorporate family considerations important to the care of women and children. Issues concerning grandparents, siblings, and different family constellations are addressed. In the pediatric chapters, these boxes focus on the special learning needs of families. **Legal Tips** are integrated into the maternity section to emphasize issues related to the care of women and infants. **Alerts** are located throughout the text to draw attention to important information on medications, nursing care, and safety.

This fifth edition features a contemporary design with logical, easy-to-follow headings and an attractive four-color design that highlights important content and increases visual appeal. Hundreds of color photographs and drawings throughout the text, many of them new, illustrate important concepts and techniques to further enhance comprehension. To help students learn essential information quickly and efficiently, we have included numerous features that prioritize, condense, simplify, and emphasize important aspects of nursing care. In addition, the text encourages students to think critically.

SPECIAL FEATURES

- **Atraumatic Care** boxes emphasize the importance of providing competent care without creating undue physical and psychologic distress. Although many of the boxes provide suggestions for managing pain, atraumatic care also considers approaches to promoting self-esteem and preventing embarrassment.

- **Community Focus** boxes emphasize community issues, provide resources and guidance, and illustrate nursing care in a variety of settings.

- **Critical Thinking Case Studies** present students with real-life situations and encourage them to make appropriate clinical judgments. Answer guidelines are provided in *TEACH for Nurses.*

- **Cultural Competence** boxes describe beliefs and practices about pregnancy, childbirth, parenting, and women's health concerns.

- **Emergency** boxes alert students to the signs and symptoms of various emergency situations and provide interventions for immediate implementation.

- **Evidence-Based Practice** boxes are incorporated throughout the book. Findings that confirm effective practices or that identify practices with unknown, ineffective, or harmful effects are located within the narrative.

- **Family-Centered Care** boxes highlight the needs or concerns of families that should be addressed when family-centered care is provided.

- **Guidelines** boxes provide students with examples of various approaches to implementing care.

- **Home Care** boxes emphasize patient and family self-care and provide information to help students transfer learning from the hospital to the home setting.

- **Key Points** at the end of each chapter help the reader summarize major points, make connections, and synthesize information. The Key Points are expanded online and can be found on this book's Evolve site.

- **Learning Objectives** focus students' attention on the important content to be mastered.

- **Legal Tips** are integrated throughout Part 1 to provide students with relevant information to deal with important legal matters in the context of maternity nursing.

- **Medication Guide** boxes and **Medication Alerts** include key information about medications used in maternity and newborn care, including their indications, adverse effects, and nursing considerations.

- **Nursing Alerts** call the reader's attention to critical information that could lead to deteriorating or emergency situations.

- **Nursing Care Plans** are provided for many commonly encountered situations and disorders. Rationales are included for nursing interventions that might not be immediately evident to students.

- **Patient Teaching** boxes assist students to help patients and families become involved in their own care with optimal outcomes.

- **Resources,** including websites and contact information for organizations and educational resources available for the topics discussed, are listed throughout.

- **Safety Alerts** call the reader's attention to potentially dangerous situations that should be addressed by the nurse.

- During assessment, the nurse must be alert for **Signs of Potential Complications;** these are included in chapters that cover uncomplicated pregnancy and childbirth.

- A highly detailed, cross-referenced **index** allows readers to quickly access needed information.

TEACHING AND LEARNING PACKAGE

Several ancillaries for this text have been developed for instructors and students to use in classroom and clinical settings.

For Students

Evolve: Evolve is an innovative website that provides a wealth of content, resources, and state-of-the-art information on maternity and pediatric nursing. Learning resources for students include Animations, Case Studies, Content Updates, Glossary, Printable Key Points, Nursing Skills, and NCLEX-Style Review Questions.

Simulation Learning System (SLS): The Simulation Learning System (SLS) is an online toolkit that helps instructors and facilitators effectively incorporate medium- to high-fidelity simulation into their nursing curriculum. Detailed patient scenarios promote and enhance the clinical decision-making skills of students at all levels. The SLS provides detailed instructions for preparation and implementation of the simulation experience, debriefing questions that encourage critical thinking, and learning resources to reinforce student comprehension. Each scenario in the SLS complements the textbook content and helps bridge the gap between lectures and clinical practice. The SLS provides the perfect environment for students to practice what they are learning in the text for a true-to-life, hands-on learning experience.

Study Guide: This comprehensive and challenging study aid presents a variety of questions to enhance learning of key concepts and content from the text. Multiple-choice and matching questions and Critical Thinking Case Studies are included. Answers for all questions are included at the back of the study guide.

Virtual Clinical Excursions: Virtual Hospital and Workbook Companion: A Virtual Hospital and workbook package has been developed as a virtual clinical experience to expand student opportunities for critical thinking. This package guides the student through a virtual clinical environment and helps the user apply textbook content to virtual patients in that environment. Case studies are presented that allow students to use this textbook as a reference to assess, diagnose, plan, implement, and evaluate "real" patients using clinical scenarios. The state-of-the-art technologies reflected in this virtual hospital demonstrate cutting-edge learning opportunities for students and facilitate knowledge retention of the information found in the textbook. The clinical simulations and workbook represent the next generation of research-based learning tools that promote critical thinking and meaningful learning.

For Instructors

Evolve includes these teaching resources for instructors:

Electronic Test Bank in ExamView format contains more than 1850 NCLEX-style test items, including alternate-format questions. An answer key with page references to the text, rationales, and NCLEX-style coding is included.

TEACH for Nurses includes teaching strategies; in-class case studies; and links to animations, nursing skills, and nursing curriculum standards such as QSEN, concepts, and BSN Essentials.

Electronic Image Collection, containing more than 700 full-color illustrations and photographs from the text, helps instructors develop presentations and explain key concepts.

PowerPoint Slides, with lecture notes for each chapter of the text, assist in presenting materials in the classroom. *Case Studies* and *Audience Response Questions* for i-clicker are included.

A *Curriculum Guide* that includes a proposed class schedule and reading assignments for courses of varying lengths is provided. This gives educators suggestions for using the text in the most essential manner or in a more comprehensive way.

Thanks to Pat Gingrich for preparing the Evidence-Based Practice boxes in Part 1; to Julie Perry Nelson, Loveland, CO, and Cheryl Briggs, RN, Annapolis, MD, for many new photographs; and to those parents who permitted us to use photos of their infants and families. Very special thanks to Heather Bays, Jodi Willard, and Laurie Gower, whose support was crucial for the completion of this project. Thanks also to those faculty and students who provided reports and offered suggestions to ensure accuracy.

Shannon E. Perry
Deitra Leonard Lowdermilk

Special thanks to Patrick Barrera for his continued support of the Wong legacy textbooks. We are so thankful for the supportive staff at Elsevier for their continued devotion to excellence in pediatric nursing education.

Marilyn J. Hockenberry
David Wilson

The authors would like to acknowledge the following individuals for contributions to the ninth edition of *Wong's Essentials of Pediatric Nursing:* Annette L. Baker, RN, MSN, PNP; Rose Ann Urdiales Baker, PhD, PMHCNS-BC; Linda K. Ballard, CPNP, MSN; Ray Barfield, MD, PhD; Debra Brandon, PhD, RN, CCNS, FAAN; Christine A. Brosnan, DrPH, RN; Terri L. Brown, MSN, RN, CPN; Rosalind Bryant, PhD, APRN-BC, PNP; Patricia M. Conlon, RN, MS, CNS, CNP; Martha Curry, MS, RN, CPNP; Amy E. Delaney, RN, MSN, CPNP-ACIP; Sharron L. Docherty, CPNP, PhD; Quinn Franklin, MS, CCLS; Debbie Fraser, MN, RNC-NIC; Martina R. Gallagher, PhD, RN; Valerie J. Groben, RN, MSN, APRN-BC; Sarah M. Gutknecht, DNP, RN, CPNP; Eufemia Jacob, PhD, RN; Kristine C. Jordan, PhD, MPH, RD; Linda M. Kollar, RN, MSN; Deborah Suzanne Lammert, APRN-CNS, CCRN-P, MSN; Kathy McCarthy, BSN, RN; Patricia Barry McElfresh, MN, RN, PNP-BC; Tara Taneski Merck, MS, RN, CPNP; Mary A. Mondozzi, MSN, PNP-BC; Rebecca A. Monroe, MSN, RN, CPNP; Barbara Montagnino, MS, RN, CNS; Kim Mooney-Doyle, MSN, CPNP, CPON; Cynthia A. Prows, MSN, CNS, FAAN; Elizabeth Record, BSN, MSN, DNP; Robyn Rice, PhD, RN; Patricia A. Ring, MSN, RN, CPNP; Cheryl C. Rodgers, RN, PhD, CPNP, CPON; Margaret L. Schroeder, MSN, RN, PNP-BC; Jean C.K. Stansbury, RN, MSN, CNP Pediatrics; Olga A. Taylor, MPH; Cheryl Ann Thaxton, RN, MN, CPNP-PC; Sandra L. Upchurch, PhD, RN; Barbara J. Wheeler, MN, RN, IBCLC, RLC; Kristina D. Wilson, PhD, CCC-SLP.

CONTENTS

UNIT 3 PREGNANCY

UNIT 4   CHILDBIRTH

PART 2   PEDIATRIC NURSING

UNIT 7   CHILDREN, THEIR FAMILIES, AND THE NURSE

UNIT 10 SPECIAL NEEDS, ILLNESS, AND HOSPITALIZATION

UNIT 11 HEALTH PROBLEMS OF CHILDREN

21st Century Maternity Nursing

Shannon E. Perry

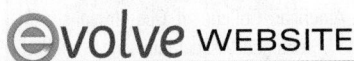 WEBSITE

http://evolve.elsevier.com/Perry/maternal

LEARNING OBJECTIVES

On completion of this chapter, the reader will be able to:
- Describe the scope of maternity nursing.
- Evaluate contemporary issues and trends in maternity nursing.
- Examine social concerns in maternity nursing.

- Explain risk management and standards of practice in the delivery of nursing care.
- Discuss legal and ethical issues in perinatal nursing.
- Examine *Healthy People 2020* goals related to maternal and infant care.

Maternity nursing encompasses care of childbearing women and their families through all stages of pregnancy and childbirth and the first 4 weeks after birth. Throughout the prenatal period nurses, nurse practitioners, and nurse-midwives provide care for women in clinics and physicians' offices and teach classes to help families prepare for childbirth. Nurses care for childbearing families during labor and birth in hospitals, in birthing centers (e.g., www.birthcenters.org), and in the home. Nurses with special training may provide intensive care for high risk neonates in special care units and high risk mothers in antepartum units, in critical care obstetric units, or in the home. Maternity nurses teach about pregnancy; the process of labor, birth, and recovery; and parenting skills. They provide continuity of care throughout the childbearing cycle.

Nurses caring for women have helped make the health care system more responsive to women's needs. They have been critically important in developing strategies to improve the well-being of women and their infants and have led the efforts to implement clinical practice guidelines and practice using an evidence-based approach. Through professional associations nurses can have a voice in setting standards and influencing health policy by actively participating in the education of the public and state and federal legislators (e.g., www.nursingworld.org; www.can-nurses.ca; www.awhonn.org; www.capwhn.ca). Some nurses hold elective office and influence policy directly. For example, Mary Wakefield, a nurse, is the administrator of the Health Resources and Services Administration, the agency that oversees approximately 7000 community clinics that serve low-income and uninsured people.

ADVANCES IN THE CARE OF MOTHERS AND INFANTS

Although tremendous advances have taken place in the care of mothers and their infants during the past 150 years (Box 1-1), serious problems exist in the United States related to the health and health care of mothers and infants. Lack of access to pre-pregnancy and pregnancy-related care for all women and the lack of reproductive health services for adolescents are major concerns. Sexually transmitted infections, including acquired immuno-deficiency syndrome (AIDS), continue to affect reproduction adversely.

EFFORTS TO REDUCE HEALTH DISPARITIES

Racial and ethnic diversity is increasing within North America. It is estimated that by the year 2050, 54% of the population will be minority, with 46% of the population European-American, 15% African-American, 30% Hispanic, 9.2% Asian-American, 2% American Indians and Alaska Natives, and 0.6% Native Hawaiian and Other Pacific Islanders (U.S. Census Bureau, 2008).

Significant disparities in morbidity and mortality rates are experienced by African-Americans, Native Americans, Hispanics, Alaska Natives, and Asian/Pacific Islanders compared to Caucasians. Shorter life expectancy, higher infant and maternal mortality rates, more birth defects, and more sexually transmitted infections are found among these ethnic and racial minority groups. The disparities are thought to result from a complex interaction among biologic factors, environment, and health behaviors. Disparities in education and income are associated with differences in morbidity and mortality.

The Health Resources and Services Administration (HRSA) Health Disparities Collaboratives are part of a national effort to eliminate disparities and improve delivery systems of health care for all people in the United States who are cared for in HRSA-supported health centers. Over 900 community health centers have implemented the collaboratives and are successful in improving quality of care (Chin, 2011). The National Institutes of Health has a commitment to improve the health of minorities and provides funding for research and training of minority researchers (www.nih.gov). The National Institute of Nursing Research includes in its strategic plan support of research that promotes health equity and eliminates health disparities.

BOX 1-1   HISTORIC OVERVIEW OF MILESTONES IN THE CARE OF MOTHERS AND INFANTS

1847—James Young Simpson in Edinburgh, Scotland used ether for an internal podalic version and birth; the first reported use of obstetric anesthesia

1861—Ignaz Semmelweis wrote *The Cause, Concept and Prophylaxis of Childbed Fever*

1906—First U.S. program for prenatal nursing care established

1908—Childbirth classes started by the American Red Cross

1909—First White House Conference on Children convened

1911—First milk bank in the United States established in Boston

1912—U.S. Children's Bureau established

1915—Radical mastectomy determined to be effective treatment for breast cancer

1916—Margaret Sanger established first American birth control clinic in Brooklyn, New York

1918—Condoms became legal in the United States

1923—First U.S. hospital center for premature infant care established at Sarah Morris Hospital in Chicago, Illinois

1929—The modern tampon (with an applicator) invented and patented

1933—Sodium pentothal used as anesthesia for childbirth; *Natural Childbirth* published by Grantly Dick-Read

1934—Dionne quintuplets born in Ontario, Canada, and survive partly due to donated breast milk

1935—Sulfonamides introduced as cure for puerperal fever

1941—Penicillin used as a treatment for infection

1941—Papanicolaou (Pap) tests introduced

1942—Premarin approved by the Food and Drug Administration (FDA) as treatment for menopausal symptoms

1953—Virginia Apgar, an anesthesiologist, published Apgar scoring system of neonatal assessment

1956—Oxygen determined to cause retrolental fibroplasia (now known as retinopathy of prematurity)

1958—Edward Hon reported on the recording of the fetal electrocardiogram (ECG) from the maternal abdomen (first commercial electronic fetal monitor produced in the late 1960s)

1958—Ian Donald, a Glasgow physician, was first to report clinical use of ultrasound to examine the fetus

1959—*Thank You, Dr. Lamaze* published by Marjorie Karmel

1959—Cytologic studies demonstrated that Down syndrome is associated with a particular form of nondisjunction now known as trisomy 21

1960—American Society for Psychoprophylaxis in Obstetrics (ASPO/Lamaze) formed

1960—International Childbirth Education Association founded

1960—Birth control pill introduced in the United States

1962—Thalidomide found to cause birth defects

1963—Title V of the Social Security Act amended to include comprehensive maternity and infant care for women who were low income and high risk

1963—Testing for PKU begun

1965—Supreme Court ruled that married people have the right to use birth control

1967—$Rh_o(D)$ immune globulin produced for treatment of Rh incompatibility

1967—Reva Rubin published article on Maternal Role Attainment

1968—Rubella vaccine became available

1969—Nurses Association of the American College of Obstetricians and Gynecologists (NAACOG) founded; renamed Association of Women's Health, Obstetric and Neonatal Nurses (AWHONN) and incorporated as a 501(c)3 organization in 1993

1969—Mammogram became available

1972—Special Supplemental Food Program for Women, Infants, and Children (WIC) started

1973—Abortion legalized in United States

1974—First standards for obstetric, gynecologic, and neonatal nursing published by NAACOG

1975—The Pregnant Patient's Bill of Rights published by the International Childbirth Education Association

1976—First home pregnancy kits approved by FDA

1978—Louise Brown, first test-tube baby, born

1987—Safe Motherhood initiative launched by World Health Organization and other international agencies

1991—Society for Advancement of Women's Health Research founded

1992—Office of Research on Women's Health authorized by U.S. Congress

1993—Female condom approved by FDA

1993—Human embryos cloned at George Washington University

1993—Family and Medical Leave Act enacted

1994—DNA sequences of BRCA1 and BRCA2 identified

1994—Zidovudine guidelines to reduce mother-to-fetus transmission of HIV published

1996—FDA mandated folic acid fortification in all breads and grains sold in United States

1998—Newborns' and Mothers' Health Act went into effect

1998—COGNN becomes AWHONN Canada

1999—First emergency contraceptive pill for pregnancy prevention (Plan B) in women who had unprotected sex approved by FDA

2000—Working draft of sequence and analysis of human genome completed

2006—HPV vaccine available

2010—Centenary of the death of Florence Nightingale

2010—Patient Protection and Affordable Care Act signed into law by President Obama

2011—AWHONN Canada becomes the Canadian Association of Perinatal and Women's Health Nurses (CAPWHN)

2012—U.S. Supreme Court upheld individual mandate but not the Medicaid expansion provisions of the Patient Protection and Affordable Care Act

2012—Scientists reported findings of the ENCODE (**Enc**yclopedia **of DNA El**ements) project showing that 80% of the human genome is active

HIV, Human immunodeficiency virus; *HPV*, human papilloma virus.

The Centers for Disease Control and Prevention (CDC) released the First Periodic Health Disparities and Inequalities Report—United States, 2011 (CDC, 2011). The report includes recent trends and variation in health disparities and inequalities in some social and health indicators and provides data against which to measure progress in eliminating disparities. Topics specific to perinatal nursing that are addressed are infant deaths, preterm births, and adolescent pregnancy and childbirth. Also in 2011 the U.S. Department of Health and Human Services (USDHHS) released an HHS Disparities Action Plan that provides a vision of "a nation free of disparities in health and health care" (USDHHS, 2011). Through this plan HHS will promote evidence-based programs, integrated approaches, and best practices to reduce disparities. The Action Plan complements the 2011 National Stakeholder Strategy for Achieving Health Equity prepared by the National Partnership for Action. This strategy proposes a comprehensive, community-driven approach to achieve health equity through collaboration and synergy (National Partnership for Action, 2011). Through these initiatives the United States is making a concerted effort to eliminate health disparities.

This chapter presents a general overview of issues and trends related to the health and health care of women and infants.

CONTEMPORARY ISSUES AND TRENDS

Healthy People 2020 Goals

Healthy People provides science-based 10-year national objectives for improving the health of all Americans. It has four overarching goals: (1) attaining high-quality, longer lives free of preventable disease, disability, injury, and premature death; (2) achieving health equity, eliminating disparities, and improving the health of all groups; (3) creating social and physical environments that promote good health for all; and (4) promoting quality of life, healthy development, and healthy behaviors across all life stages (www.healthypeople.gov/2020/about/default.aspx). The goals of *Healthy People 2020* are based on assessments of major risks to health and wellness, changes in public health priorities, and issues related to the health preparedness and prevention of our nation. Of the objectives of *Healthy People 2020*, 33 are related to maternal, infant, and child health (Box 1-2).

Millennium Development Goals

The United Nations Millennium Development Goals (MDGs) are eight goals to be achieved by 2015 that respond to the main

---

BOX 1-2   *HEALTHY PEOPLE 2020* MATERNAL, INFANT, AND CHILD HEALTH OBJECTIVES

- Reduce the rate of fetal and infant deaths.
- Reduce the 1-year mortality rate for infants with Down syndrome.
- Reduce the rate of child deaths.
- Reduce the rate of adolescent and young adult deaths.
- Reduce the rate of maternal mortality.
- Reduce maternal illness and complications caused by pregnancy (complications during hospitalized labor and delivery).
- Reduce cesarean births among low-risk (full-term, singleton, vertex presentation) women.
- Reduce low birth weight (LBW) and very low birth weight (VLBW).
- Reduce preterm births.
- Increase the proportion of pregnant women who receive early and adequate prenatal care.
- Increase abstinence from alcohol, cigarettes, and illicit drugs in pregnant women.
- Increase the proportion of pregnant women who attend a series of prepared childbirth classes.
- Increase the proportion of mothers who achieve a recommended weight gain during their pregnancies.
- Increase the proportion of women of childbearing potential with intake of at least 400 mcg of folic acid from fortified foods or dietary supplements.
- Reduce the proportion of women of childbearing potential who have low red blood cell folate concentrations.
- Increase the proportion of women delivering a live birth; increase those who receive preconception care services and practice key recommended preconception health behaviors.
- Reduce the proportion of people ages 18 to 44 years who have impaired fecundity (i.e., a physical barrier preventing pregnancy or carrying a pregnancy to term).
- Decrease postpartum relapse of smoking in women who quit smoking during pregnancy.
- Increase the proportion of women giving birth who attend a postpartum care visit with a health worker.

- Increase the proportion of infants who are put to sleep on their backs.
- Increase the proportion of infants who are breastfed.
- Increase the proportion of employers who have worksite lactation programs.
- Reduce the proportion of breastfed newborns who receive formula supplementation within the first 2 days of life.
- Increase the proportion of live births that occur in facilities that provide recommended care for lactating mothers and their babies.
- Reduce the occurrence of fetal alcohol syndrome (FAS).
- Reduce the proportion of children diagnosed with a disorder through newborn blood spot screening who experience developmental delay requiring special education services.
- Reduce the proportion of children with cerebral palsy born as LBW infants (less than 2500 g).
- Reduce occurrence of neural tube defects.
- Increase the proportion of young children with an autism spectrum disorder (ASD) and other developmental delays who are screened, evaluated, and enrolled in early intervention services in a timely manner.
- Increase the proportion of children, including those with special health care needs, who have access to a medical home.
- Increase the proportion of children with special health care needs who receive their care in family-centered, comprehensive, coordinated systems.
- Increase appropriate newborn blood-spot screening and follow-up testing.
- Increase the number of states, including the District of Columbia, that verify through linkage with vital records that all newborns are screened shortly after birth for conditions mandated by their state-sponsored screening program.
- Increase the proportion of screen-positive children who receive follow-up testing within the recommended time period.
- Increase the proportion of children with a diagnosed condition identified through newborn screening who have an annual assessment of services needed and received.
- Increase the proportion of VLBW infants born at level III hospitals or subspecialty perinatal centers.

Adapted from HealthyPeople.gov: *Maternal, infant, and child health,* 2012, www.healthypeople.gov/2020/topicsobjectives2020/objectiveslist.aspx?topicId=26.

development challenges in the world. They are drawn from the actions and targets contained in the Millennium Declaration that was adopted by 189 nations and signed by 147 heads of state and governments during the United Nations Millennium Summit in September 2000 (www.un.org/millenniumgoals/goals.html). Goals three through five of the MDGs relate specifically to women and children (Box 1-3).

Integrative Health Care

Integrative health care encompasses complementary and alternative therapies in combination with conventional Western modalities of treatment. Many popular alternative healing modalities offer human-centered care based on philosophies that recognize the value of the patient's input and honor the individual's beliefs, values, and desires. The focus of these modalities is on the whole person, not just on a disease complex. Patients often find that alternative modalities are more consistent with their own belief systems and also allow for more patient autonomy in health care decisions (Fig. 1-1). Examples of alternative modalities include acupuncture, macrobiotics, herbal medicines, massage therapy, biofeedback, meditation, yoga, and chelation therapy.

The National Center for Complementary and Alternative Medicine (NCCAM) (http://nccam.nih.gov/) is a United States government agency that supports research and evaluation of various alternative and complementary modalities and provides information to health care consumers about such modalities. It is one of the 27 institutes and centers included in the National Institutes of Health.

Problems with the U.S. Health Care System
Structure of the Health Care Delivery System
The U.S. health care delivery system is often fragmented and expensive and is inaccessible to many. Opportunities exist for nurses to alter nursing practice and improve the way care is delivered through managed care, integrated delivery systems, and redefined roles. Consumer participation in health care is increasing, and health care providers include them in decision-making; information is available on the Internet; and care is provided in a technology-intensive environment (Tiedje, Price, and You, 2008).

Reducing Medical Errors
Medical errors are a leading cause of death in the United States and result in as many as 98,000 deaths per year (Pham, Aswani, Rosen, et al., 2012). In Canada adverse events are implicated in up to 23,750 deaths per year (French, 2006). Since the Institute of Medicine

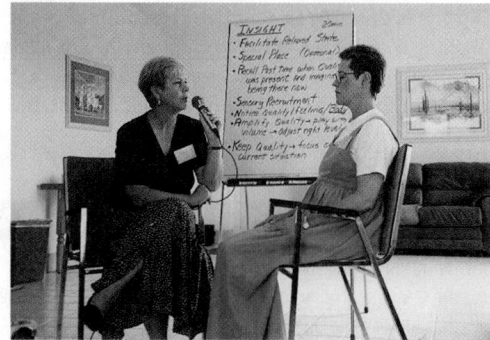

FIG 1-1 Nurse and patient during guided imagery session. (Courtesy Nurses Certificate Program in Interactive Imagery, Foster City, CA.)

(IOM) released its 1999 report, *To Err Is Human: Building a Safer Health System,* a concerted effort has been under way to analyze causes of errors and develop strategies to prevent them. Recognizing the multifaceted causes of medical errors, the Agency for Healthcare Research and Quality (AHRQ) (2000) prepared a fact sheet, *20 Tips to Help Prevent Medical Errors,* for patients and the public. Patients are encouraged to be knowledgeable consumers of health care and ask questions of providers, including physicians, midwives, nurses, and pharmacists.

In 2002 the National Quality Forum published a list of Serious Reportable Events in Healthcare. The list was updated in 2006 and again in 2011, resulting in a total of 29 events. Of these 29 events three pertain directly to maternity and newborn care (Box 1-4). The National Quality Forum published *Safe Practices for Better Healthcare* in 2003 and updated it most recently in 2010 (www.qualityforum.org). The 34 safe practices included should be used in all applicable health care settings to reduce the risk of harm that results from processes, systems, and environments of care. Table 1-1 contains a selection of practices from that document.

In August 2007 the Centers for Medicare & Medicaid Services (CMS) issued a rule that became effective October 2008 that denies payment for eight hospital-acquired conditions (O'Reilly, 2008). Five of the conditions are also on the National Quality Forum list. Conditions that might pertain to maternity nursing include a foreign object retained after surgery, air embolism, blood incompatibility, falls and trauma, and catheter-associated urinary tract infections. Almost 1300 U.S. hospitals waive (do not bill for) costs associated with serious reportable events (O'Reilly, 2008).

TABLE 1-1	SELECTED SAFE PRACTICES FOR BETTER HEALTH CARE
SAFE PRACTICE	**PRACTICE STATEMENT**
Safe Practice 2: Culture Measurement, Feedback, and Intervention	Health care organizations must measure their culture, provide feedback to leadership and staff, and undertake interventions that reduce patient safety risk.
Safe Practice 5: Informed Consent	Ask each patient or legal surrogate to "teach back" in his or her own words key information about the proposed treatments or procedures for which he or she is being asked to provide informed consent.
Safe Practice 11: Intensive Care Unit Care	All patients in general intensive care units (both adult and pediatric) should be managed by physicians who have specific training and certification in critical care medicine ("critical care certified").
Safe Practice 12: Patient Care Information	Ensure that care information is transmitted and appropriately documented in a timely manner and a clearly understandable form to patients and all of the patients' health care providers/professionals, within and between care settings, who need that information to provide continued care.
Safe Practice 19: Hand Hygiene	Comply with current Centers for Disease Control and Prevention (CDC) hand hygiene guidelines.
Safe Practice 34: Pediatric Imaging	When CT imaging studies are undertaken on children, "child-size" techniques should be used to reduce unnecessary exposure to ionizing radiation.

From National Quality Forum (NQF): *Safe practices for better healthcare—2010 update: a consensus report*, Washington, DC, 2010, NQF.
CT, Computed tomography.

High Cost of Health Care

Health care is one of the fastest-growing sectors of the U.S. economy. Currently 17.4% of the gross domestic product is spent on health care (Squires, 2012). Higher spending in the United States compared to 12 other industrialized countries is related to higher prices, readily accessible technology, and greater obesity (Squires, 2012). Most researchers agree that caring for the increased number of low-birth-weight (LBW) infants in neonatal intensive care units contributes significantly to overall health care costs.

Midwifery care has helped contain some health care costs. However, not all insurance carriers reimburse nurse practitioners and clinical nurse specialists as direct care providers. Nor do they reimburse for all services provided by nurse-midwives, a situation that continues to be a problem. Nurses must become involved in the politics of cost containment because they, as knowledgeable experts, can provide solutions to many health care problems at a relatively low cost.

Limited Access to Care

Barriers to access must be removed so pregnancy outcomes and care of children can be improved. The most significant barrier to access is the inability to pay. The number of uninsured people in the United States in 2010 was 49.9 million or 16.3% of the population (DeNavas-Walt, Proctor, and Smith, 2011). Lack of transportation and dependent child care are other barriers. In addition to a lack of insurance and high costs, a lack of providers for low-income women exists because many physicians either refuse to take Medicaid patients or take only a few such patients. This presents a serious problem because a significant proportion of births are to mothers who receive Medicaid.

Health Care Reform

In early 2010 President Obama signed into law the Patient Protection and Affordable Care Act. The Act aims to make insurance affordable, contain costs, strengthen and improve Medicare and Medicaid, and reform the insurance market. There are provisions to promote prevention and improve public health; improve the quality of care for all Americans; reduce waste, fraud, and abuse; and reform the health delivery system. There are some immediate benefits, but implementation of the act will occur over the next several years.

In 2012 26 states, several individuals, and the National Federation of Independent Business brought suit challenging the constitutionality of the individual mandate (requirement for most Americans to have minimum essential health insurance) and the Medicaid expansion (expand the scope of coverage and increase the number of individuals the states must cover). The Supreme Court upheld the individual mandate but not the Medicaid expansion (Sacks, 2012). The debate continues on how the plan will be implemented.

Health Literacy

Health literacy involves a spectrum of abilities, ranging from reading an appointment slip to interpreting medication instructions. These skills must be assessed routinely to recognize a problem and accommodate patients with limited literacy skills. Most patient education materials are written at too high a level for the average adult (Wilson, 2009). According to the National Assessment of Adult Literacy, only 12% of English-speaking adults in the United States have health literacy skills that are proficient (Kutner, Greenberg, Jin, et al., 2006). The CDC has a health literacy website (www.cdc.gov/healthliteracy) that highlights implementation of goals and strategies of the National Action Plan to Improve Health Literacy (USDHHS, Office of Disease Prevention and Health Promotion, 2010). Health literacy is part of the Patient Protection and Affordable Care Act.

As a result of the increasingly multicultural U.S. population, there is a more urgent need to address health literacy as a component of culturally and linguistically competent care. Health care providers contribute to health literacy by using simple, common words; avoiding jargon; and assessing whether the patient understands the discussion. Speaking slowly and clearly and focusing on what is important increase understanding.

Trends in Fertility and Birth Rate

Fertility trends and birth rates reflect women's needs for health care. Box 1-5 defines biostatistical terminology useful in analyzing

BOX 1-5   MATERNAL-INFANT BIOSTATISTICAL TERMINOLOGY

Abortus: An embryo or fetus that is removed or expelled from the uterus at 20 weeks of gestation or less, weighs 500 g or less, or measures 25 cm or less

Birth rate: Number of live births in 1 year per 1000 population

Fertility rate: Number of births per 1000 women between the ages of 15 and 44 years (inclusive), calculated on an annual basis

Infant mortality rate: Number of deaths of infants younger than 1 year of age per 1000 live births

Maternal mortality rate: Number of maternal deaths from births and complications of pregnancy, childbirth, and puerperium (the first 42 days after termination of the pregnancy) per 100,000 live births

Pregnancy-associated deaths: All deaths during pregnancy and within the 1 year following the end of pregnancy

Pregnancy-related deaths (subset of pregnancy-associated): Deaths that are a complication of pregnancy, an aggravation of an unrelated condition by the physiology of pregnancy, or a chain of events initiated by the pregnancy

Neonatal mortality rate: Number of deaths of infants younger than 28 days of age per 1000 live births

Perinatal mortality rate: Number of stillbirths and number of neonatal deaths per 1000 live births

Stillbirth: An infant who at birth demonstrates no signs of life such as breathing, heartbeat, or voluntary muscle movements

---

maternity health care. In 2009 the fertility rate (i.e., births per 1000 women from 15 to 44 years of age) was 66.7 (Kochanek, Kirmeyer, Martin, et al., 2012). The highest birth rates occurred among women between 25 and 29 years of age (110.5). The birth rate (i.e., number of live births in 1 year per 1000 population), was 13.5 in 2009; the teen birth rate was 39.1. In 2009 the proportion of births by unmarried women varied widely among racial groups in the United States: non-Hispanic black, 72.8%; Hispanic, 53.2%; and non-Hispanic white, 29% (Kochanek, Kirmeyer, Martin, et al., 2012).

Maternal Mortality

Worldwide approximately 800 women die each day of problems related to pregnancy or childbirth. In the United States in 2009, the annual maternal mortality rate (number of maternal deaths per 100,000 live births) was 17.8 (CDC, 2013). Although the overall number of maternal deaths is small, maternal mortality remains a significant problem because a high proportion of deaths are preventable, primarily through improving the access to and use of prenatal care services. In the United States there is significant racial disparity in the rates of maternal death: non-Hispanic black women (35.6), non-Hispanic white women (11.7), and women of other races (17.6) (CDC, 2013).

The leading causes of maternal death attributable to pregnancy differ over the world. In general three major causes have persisted for the last 50 years: hypertensive disorders, infection, and hemorrhage. Unsafe abortion is an additional factor. The three leading causes of maternal mortality in the United States today are gestational hypertension, pulmonary embolism, and hemorrhage. Factors that are strongly related to maternal death include age (younger than 20 years and 35 years or older), lack of prenatal care, low educational attainment, unmarried status, and non-Caucasian race. Worldwide strategies to reduce maternal mortality rates include improving access to skilled attendants at birth, providing postabortion care, improving family planning services, and providing adolescents with better reproductive health services (MDGs, 2008).

Maternal Morbidity

Although mortality is the traditional measure of maternal health and maternal health is often measured by neonatal outcomes, pregnancy complications are important. Currently no surveillance method is available to measure the incidence of maternal morbidity. It includes such conditions as acute renal failure, amniotic fluid embolism, cerebrovascular accident, eclampsia, pulmonary embolism, liver failure, obstetric shock, respiratory failure, septicemia, and complications of anesthesia (pulmonary, cardiac, central nervous system) (Berg, Mackay, Qin, et al., 2009). Maternal morbidity results in a high risk pregnancy. The diagnosis of high risk imposes a situational crisis on the family. The combined efforts of medical and nursing personnel are required to care for these patients, who often need the expertise of physicians and nurses trained in both critical care obstetrics and intensive care medicine or nursing.

Obesity

More than one third (36.2%) of women in the United States are obese (body mass index of 30 or greater); in Canada less than one fourth (23.9%) of women are obese. Obesity in women demonstrates significant racial disparities: in the United States 49.6% of non-Hispanic black women, 45.1% of Hispanic women, and 33.0% of non-Hispanic white women ages 20 years and older are obese (Flegal, Carroll, Ogden, et al., 2010; Shields, Carroll, and Ogden, 2011). Approximately 20% of women who give birth in the United States are obese. The two most frequently reported maternal medical risk factors are hypertension associated with pregnancy and diabetes, both of which are associated with obesity. Decreased fertility, congenital anomalies, miscarriage, and fetal death are associated with obesity. Obesity in pregnancy is associated with the use of increased health care services and longer hospital stays (Chu, Bachman, Callaghan, et al., 2008).

Regionalization of Perinatal Health Care Services

Not all facilities develop and maintain the full spectrum of services required for high risk perinatal patients. As a consequence, regionalization of hospital-based perinatal health care services occurred, and facilities within a geographic region were organized to provide different levels of care. This system of coordinated care was also applied to preconception and ambulatory prenatal care services.

Guidelines have been established regarding the level of care that can be expected at any given facility. In ambulatory settings providers must distinguish themselves by the level of care they provide. Basic care is provided by obstetricians, family practice physicians, certified nurse-midwives, and other advanced practice clinicians approved by local governance. Routine risk-oriented prenatal care, education, and support are provided. Providers offering specialty care are obstetricians who must provide fetal diagnostic testing and management of obstetric and medical complications in addition to basic care. Subspecialty care is provided by maternal-fetal medicine specialists and includes the aforementioned specialty care in addition to genetic testing, advanced fetal therapies, and management of severe maternal and fetal complications (AAP and ACOG, 2012). Collaboration among providers to meet the woman's needs is the key to reducing perinatal morbidity and mortality (AAP and ACOG, 2012).

High-Technology Care

Advances in scientific knowledge and the large number of high risk pregnancies have contributed to a health care system that emphasizes high-technology care. Maternity care has extended to preconception counseling, more and better scientific techniques to monitor the mother and fetus, more definitive tests for hypoxia and acidosis, and neonatal intensive care units. The labors of virtually all women who give birth in hospitals are monitored electronically despite the lack of evidence of efficacy of such monitoring. The numbers of assisted labors and births are increasing. Internet-based information is available to the public that enhances interactions among health care providers, families, and community providers. Point-of-care testing is available. Personal data assistants are used to enhance comprehensive care; the medical record is increasingly in electronic form.

Telehealth is an umbrella term for the use of communication technologies and electronic information to provide or support health care when the participants are separated by distance. It permits specialists, including nurses, to provide health care and consultation when distance separates them from those needing care. This technology has the potential to save billions of dollars annually for health care, but these technologic advances have also contributed to higher health care costs. In general high-technology care has flourished, whereas "health" care has become relatively neglected.

Social Media

Social media uses Internet-based technologies to allow users to create their own content and participate in dialog. The most common social media platforms are Facebook, Twitter, and LinkedIn (Duffy, 2011). Through use of these technologies, nurses can link with nurses with similar interests, share insights about patient care, and advocate for patients (Saver, 2010). However, there are pitfalls for nurses using this technology. Patient privacy and confidentiality can be violated, and institutions and colleagues can be cast in unfavorable lights with negative consequences for those posting the information. Nursing students have been expelled from school, and nurses have been fired or reprimanded by a Board of Nursing for injudicious posts. To help make nurses aware of their responsibilities when using social media, the American Nurses Association (ANA) published six principles for social networking and the nurse (Box 1-6). In addition, the National Council of State Boards of Nursing (NCSBN) issued a *White Paper: a Nurse's Guide to the Use of Social Media* (NCSBN, 2011). The paper details issues of confidentiality and privacy, possible consequences of inappropriate use of social media, common myths and misunderstandings of social media, and tips on how to avoid problems.

Community-Based Care

A shift in settings from acute care institutions to ambulatory settings, including the home, has occurred (see Chapter 2). Even childbearing women at high risk are cared for on an outpatient basis or in the home. Technology previously available only in the hospital is now found in the home. This has affected the organizational structure of care, the skills required in providing such care, and the costs to consumers.

Home health care also has a community focus. Nurses are involved in providing care for women and infants in homeless shelters and adolescents in school-based clinics and in promoting health at community sites, churches, and shopping malls. Nursing education curricula are increasingly community based.

BOX 1-6	ANA'S PRINCIPLES FOR SOCIAL NETWORKING AND THE NURSE

- Nurses must not transmit or place online individually identifiable patient information.
- Nurses must observe ethically prescribed professional patient-nurse boundaries.
- Nurses should understand that patients, colleagues, institutions, and employers may view postings.
- Nurses should take advantage of privacy settings and seek to separate personal and professional information online.
- Nurses should bring content that could harm a patient's privacy, rights, or welfare to the attention of appropriate authorities.
- Nurses should participate in developing institutional policies governing online contact.

From American Nurses Association: *Fact sheet: Navigating the world of social media*, Washington, DC, 2011, Author.

Childbirth Practices

Prenatal care can promote better pregnancy outcomes by providing early risk assessment and promoting healthy behaviors such as improved nutrition and smoking cessation. Prenatal care ideally begins before pregnancy because early decisions lay the foundation for the entire perinatal year. If at all possible, education continues in each trimester of pregnancy and extends through the early postpartum weeks. Some health care providers today promote preconception care as an important component of perinatal services. Preconception or early-pregnancy classes also emphasize health-promoting behavior and choices of care.

In 2006 69% of all women received care in the first trimester. Disparity in receiving prenatal care by race and ethnicity exists: 12.2% of Hispanic women, 11.8% of non-Hispanic blacks, and 5.2% of non-Hispanic whites received late or no prenatal care (Heron, Sutton, Xu, et al., 2010). In spite of these statistics, substantial gains have been made in the use of prenatal care since the early 1990s, which is attributed to the expansion in the 1980s of Medicaid coverage for pregnant women.

Women can choose physicians or nurse-midwives as primary care providers. In 2009 physicians (medical doctors [MDs] and doctors of osteopathy [DOs]) attended 92.1%, and certified nurse-midwives attended 7.4% of all hospital births (Martin, Hamilton, Ventura, et al., 2011) (see Critical Thinking Case Study). Home births accounted for 0.7% of U.S. births. The rate of vaginal births after cesarean (VBACs) declined, whereas cesarean births increased to 32.9% of live births in the United States in 2009 (Martin, Hamilton, Ventura, et al., 2011).

Women who choose nurse-midwives as their primary providers participate more actively in childbirth decisions and receive fewer interventions during labor. Certified nurse-midwives (CNMs) are registered nurses with education in the two disciplines of nursing and midwifery. Certified midwives (direct-entry midwives) are educated only in the discipline of midwifery. In the United States certification of midwives is through the American College of Nurse-Midwives (ACNM), the professional association for midwives. The Royal College of Midwives is the professional association for midwives in the United Kingdom. In Canada the Association of Ontario Midwives is the professional association, and the College of Midwives of Ontario is the regulatory body for midwives in Ontario;

CRITICAL THINKING CASE STUDY

Safety and Efficacy of Midwifery Care

A group of nurse-midwives is setting up practice in your hometown. They are to collaborate with one of the groups of obstetricians in the same city. A letter to the editor appeared in the local newspaper stating that the presence of midwives will jeopardize care of pregnant women in the community because midwives usually care for the poor and indigent, deliver babies at home, and therefore do not have the skills to work in hospitals and care for middle-class women who have insurance. The letter-writer urged the community to boycott the midwives to ensure safe childbirth for women in the community.

1. Evidence—Is there sufficient evidence to document the qualifications of nurse-midwives and their safety record to write a response to this letter?
2. Assumptions—Describe some assumptions about midwifery care:
   a. Education of midwives
   b. Practice sites of midwifery care
   c. Statistics about safety of midwifery care
3. What implications and priorities for education about midwifery care can be made at this time?
4. Does the evidence objectively support your conclusion?

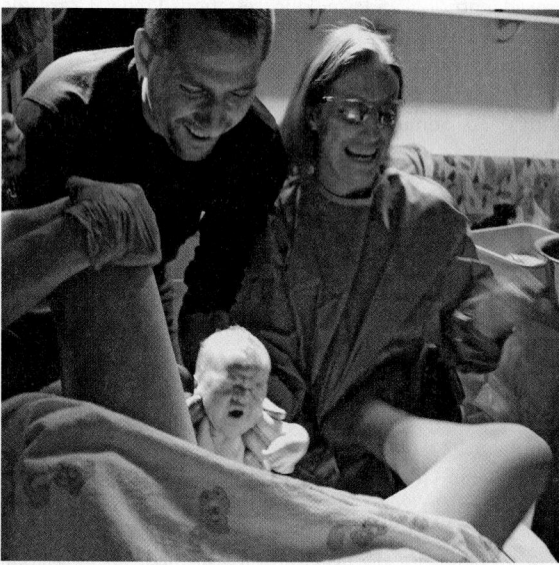

FIG 1-2 Father "catching" newborn daughter who cried before her lower body had emerged. (Courtesy Darren and Julie Nelson, Loveland, CO.)

the other provinces of Canada have similar regulatory bodies (e.g., College of Midwives of British Columbia). Many national associations belong to the International Confederation of Midwives, which comprises 97 member associations from 86 countries in the Americas and Europe, Africa, and the Asia-Pacific region.

With family-centered care, fathers, partners, grandparents, siblings, and friends may be present for labor and birth. Fathers or partners may be present for cesarean births. Fathers or partners may participate in vaginal births by "catching the baby" or cutting the umbilical cord or both (Fig. 1-2). **Doulas** (i.e., trained and experienced female labor attendants) may be present to provide a continuous, one-on-one caring presence throughout the labor and birth. Ideally newborns are placed skin-to-skin with the mother immediately after birth and encouraged to breastfeed as soon as possible. Nonseparation is common; neonates often remain in the room with their parents and may never transfer to a newborn nursery. Parents actively participate in newborn care on mother/baby units, in nurseries, and in neonatal intensive care units.

Discharge of a mother and baby within 24 hours of birth has created a growing need for follow-up or home care. In some settings discharge may occur as early as 6 hours after birth. Legislation has been enacted to ensure that mothers and babies are permitted to stay in the hospital for at least 48 hours after vaginal birth and 96 hours after cesarean birth, although they may choose to leave earlier. Focused and efficient teaching is necessary to enable the parents and infant to make the transition safely from the hospital to the home.

Involving Consumers and Promoting Self-Management

Self-management is appealing to both patients and the health care system because of its potential to reduce health care costs. Maternity care is especially suited to self-management because childbearing is primarily health focused, women are usually well when they enter the system, and visits to health care providers can present the opportunity for health and illness interventions. Measures to improve health and reduce risks associated with poor pregnancy outcomes and illness can be addressed. Topics such as nutrition education, stress management, smoking cessation, alcohol and drug treatment, prevention of violence, improvement of social supports, and parenting education are appropriate for such encounters.

International Concerns

Female genital mutilation, infibulation (surgical closure of the labia majora), genital cutting, and *circumcision* are terms used to describe procedures in which part or all of the female external genitalia is removed for cultural or nontherapeutic reasons (WHO, 2006). Worldwide many women undergo such procedures. With the growing number of immigrants from Africa and other countries where female genital mutilation is practiced, nurses in the United States and Canada will increasingly encounter women who have undergone the procedure. These women are significantly more likely to have adverse obstetric outcomes resulting in one or two additional perinatal deaths per 100 births (WHO, 2006). Ethical dilemmas arise when the woman requests that after birth the perineum be repaired as it was after infibulation and the health care provider believes that such repair is unethical. The International Council of Nurses and other health professionals have spoken out against procedures that result in mutilation as harmful to women's health. In the United States performing female genital mutilation on a person younger than 18 years is a crime (Sandy, 2011).

Human trafficking is a $32 billion business that exists in the United States and internationally (Dovydaitis, 2010). Health care professionals may interact with victims who are in captivity. This provides an opportunity to identify victims, intervene to help them obtain necessary health services, and provide information about ways to escape from their situation (see Chapter 6).

THE FUTURE OF NURSING

In 2008 the Robert Wood Johnson Foundation and the IOM initiated a 2-year process to meet the need to assess and transform the nursing profession. The IOM appointed the committee, which developed four key messages: (1) nurses should practice to the full extent of their education and training; (2) nurses should achieve higher levels of education and training through an improved education system that promotes seamless academic progression; (3) nurses should be full partners with physicians and other health care professionals in redesigning health care in the United States; and (4) effective workforce planning and policy making require better data collection and an improved information infrastructure (IOM, 2010). Throughout the United States individual states and nursing organizations are making concerted efforts to implement the recommendations of the report.

Trends in Nursing Practice

The increasing complexity of care for maternity and women's health patients has contributed to specialization of nurses working with these patients. This specialized knowledge is gained through experience, advanced degrees, and certification programs. Nurses in advanced practice (e.g., nurse practitioners and nurse-midwives) may provide primary care throughout a woman's life, including during the pregnancy cycle. In some settings the clinical nurse specialist and nurse practitioner roles are blended; and nurses deliver high-quality, comprehensive, and cost-effective care in a variety of settings. In other settings nurses educated in both critical care and high risk obstetrics are providing care in obstetric critical care units. Lactation consultants provide services in the hospital setting, in clinics and physician offices, and during home visits.

Nursing Interventions Classification

When the National IOM proposed that all patient records be computerized by the year 2000, a need for a common language to describe the contributions of nurses to patient care became evident. Nurses from the University of Iowa developed a comprehensive standardized language that describes interventions that are performed by generalist or specialist nurses. This language is included in the Nursing Interventions Classification (NIC) (Bulechek, Butcher, Dochterman, et al., 2013). Interventions commonly used by maternal-child nurses include those in Box 1-7.

Evidence-Based Practice

Evidence-based practice (i.e., providing care based on evidence gained through research and clinical trials) is emphasized increasingly. Although not all practice can be evidence based, practitioners must use the best available information on which to base their interventions. The Association of Women's Health, Obstetric and Neonatal Nurses (AWHONN) *Standards and Guidelines for Professional Nursing Practice in the Care of Women and Newborns* (AWHONN, 2009) and the *Standards for Professional Perinatal Nursing Practice and Certification in Canada* (AWHONN, 2002) include an evidence-based approach to practice. Discussion of nursing care and evidence-based practice boxes throughout this text provide examples of evidence-based practice in perinatal and women's health nursing (see Evidence-Based Practice box).

Cochrane Pregnancy and Childbirth Database

The Cochrane Pregnancy and Childbirth Database was first planned in 1976 with a small grant from the World Health Organization to Dr. Iain Chalmers and colleagues at Oxford. In 1993 the Cochrane Collaboration was formed, and the Oxford Database of Perinatal Trials became known as the Cochrane Pregnancy and Childbirth Database. The Cochrane Collaboration oversees up-to-date, systematic reviews of randomized controlled trials of health care and

---

BOX 1-7 CHILDBEARING CARE INTERVENTIONS

Level 1 Domain: Family
- Care that supports the family

Level 2 Class: Childbearing Care
- Interventions to assist in the preparation for childbirth and management of the psychologic and physiologic changes before, during, and immediately after childbirth

Level 3: Interventions
- Amnioinfusion
- Birthing
- Bleeding reduction: antepartum uterus
- Bleeding reduction: postpartum uterus
- Cesarean birth care
- Childbirth preparation
- Circumcision care
- Electronic fetal monitoring: antepartum
- Electronic fetal monitoring: intrapartum
- Environmental management: attachment process
- Family integrity promotion: childbearing family
- Family planning: contraception
- Family planning: infertility
- Family planning: unplanned pregnancy
- Fertility preservation
- Genetic counseling
- Grief work facilitation: perinatal death
- High risk pregnancy care
- Infant care: newborn
- Infant care: preterm
- Intrapartal care
- Intrapartal care: high risk delivery
- Kangaroo care
- Labor induction
- Labor suppression
- Lactation suppression
- Newborn care
- Nonnutritive sucking
- Phototherapy: neonate
- Postpartal care
- Preconception counseling
- Pregnancy termination care
- Prenatal care
- Reproductive technology management
- Resuscitation: fetus
- Resuscitation: neonate
- Risk identification: childbearing family
- Surveillance: late pregnancy
- Tube care: umbilical line
- Ultrasonography: limited obstetric

From Bulechek GM, Butcher HK, Dochterman JM, et al: *Nursing interventions classification (NIC)*, ed 6, St Louis, 2013, Mosby.

---

disseminates these reviews. The premise of the project is that these types of studies provide the most reliable evidence about the effects of care.

The evidence from these studies should encourage practitioners to implement useful measures and abandon those that are useless or harmful. Studies are ranked in six categories:

EVIDENCE-BASED PRACTICE

Seeking and Evaluating Evidence: A Necessary Competency for Quality and Safety

Throughout this text you will see Evidence-Based Practice boxes. These boxes provide examples of how a nurse might conduct an inquiry into an identified practice question. Curiosity and access to a virtual or real library are all the nurse needs to be confident that his or her practice has a sound foundation of evidence.

A literature search may reveal up to three levels of evidence. The first layer consists of primary studies. The strongest of these are randomized controlled trials. Well-designed studies, even small ones, add another piece to the puzzle.

These primary studies may be combined into the second level of evidence. In systematic analyses such as those in the Cochrane Database, the researcher uses a methodology to identify all studies relevant to a particular question. If the data are similar enough, they can be pooled into a meta-analysis. If the evidence is strong, some analyses will form the basis for recommendations for practice and to guide further inquiry.

At the tertiary level professional organizations such as the Agency for Healthcare Research and Quality (AHRQ) (www.ahrq.gov), or the National Guidelines Clearinghouse (NGC) (guideline.gov) may decide to address a broad practice question by sorting through all the available primary and secondary evidence and consulting experienced clinicians. After thoughtful review the committee of experts in the organization crafts its consensus statement. These recommendations for best practice stand on the shoulders of the systematic analysts, who stand on the many shoulders of the primary researchers.

Provided that the professional organization is well-respected and the process is rigorous, these guidelines in the consensus statement carry enormous authority. Individuals and institutions may choose to adopt them with confidence. An example of this is the Association of Women's Health, Obstetric and Neonatal Nurses(AWHONN) (www.awhonn.org) Late Preterm Infant Initiative. This initiative began in 2005 in response to the confusion that surrounded the care of infants who do not qualify for NICU admission yet require extra vigilance. Nurseries can adapt these recommendations to their specific institutions, enabling nurses to become more effective at caring for the unique problems of this population of neonates. Like AWHONN, most of the professional organizations make their guidelines available free of charge on their websites.

To develop common language and goals for nursing education, the Quality and Safety Education for Nurses (QSEN) (www.qsen.org) Project expert panel identified six competencies necessary to enable the new nurse to continuously improve the health care system: patient-centered care, teamwork and collaboration, evidence-based practice, quality improvement, safety, and informatics. Most nursing challenges require a combination of these competencies. Each competency is further defined as having targets for knowledge, skills, and attitude. The Evidence-Based Practice boxes in this textbook include examples that illustrate each of these targets specific to that competency. A mastery of QSEN competencies greatly enriches the nurse's ability to identify and improve patient and health care–system problems and communicate within the interdisciplinary team.

Pat Mahaffee Gingrich

NICU, Neonatal Intensive Care Unit.

1. Beneficial forms of care
2. Forms of care that are likely to be beneficial
3. Forms of care with a trade-off between beneficial and adverse effects
4. Forms of care with unknown effectiveness
5. Forms of care that are unlikely to be beneficial
6. Forms of care that are likely to be ineffective or harmful

Joanna Briggs Institute

Established in 1996 as an initiative of the Royal Adelaide Hospital and the University of Adelaide in Australia, the Joanna Briggs Institute (JBI) uses a collaborative approach for evaluating evidence from a range of sources (www.joannabriggs.edu.au). The JBI has formed collaborations with a variety of universities and hospitals around the world, including in the United States and Canada. In 2007 the JBI adopted the following grades of recommendation for evidence of feasibility, appropriateness, meaningfulness, and effectiveness: *A,* strong support that merits application; *B,* moderate support that warrants consideration of application; and *C,* not supported (The Joanna Briggs Institute, 2008). The JBI provides another source for perinatal nurses to access information to support evidence-based practice.

Outcomes-Oriented Practice

Outcomes of care (i.e., the effectiveness of interventions and quality of care) are receiving increased emphasis. Outcomes-oriented care measures effectiveness of care against benchmarks or standards. It is a measure of the value of nursing using quality indicators and answers the question, "Did the patient benefit or not from the care provided?" (Moorhead, Johnson, Maas, et al., 2012). The Outcome and Assessment Information Set (OASIS) is an example of an outcome system important for nursing. Its use is required by the CMS in all home health organizations that are Medicare accredited. The Nursing Outcomes Classification (NOC) is an effort to identify outcomes and related measures that can be used for evaluation of care of individuals, families, and communities across the care continuum (Moorhead, Johnson, Maas, et al., 2012). An example of outcomes classification is provided in Table 1-2.

A Global Perspective

Advances in medicine and nursing have resulted in increased knowledge and understanding in the care of mothers and infants and reduced perinatal morbidity and mortality rates. However, these advances have affected predominantly the industrialized nations. For example, approximately 3.2 million children have human immunodeficiency virus (HIV) or AIDS acquired through perinatal transmission; the majority of these children live in sub-Saharan Africa.

As the world becomes smaller because of travel and communication technologies, nurses and other health care providers are gaining a global perspective and participating in activities to improve the health and health care of people worldwide. Nurses participate in medical outreach, providing obstetric, surgical, ophthalmologic, orthopedic, or other services (Fig. 1-3); attend international meetings; conduct research; and provide international consultation. International student and faculty exchanges occur. More articles about health and health care in various countries are appearing in nursing journals. Several schools of nursing in the United States are World Health Organization Collaborating Centers.

STANDARDS OF PRACTICE AND LEGAL ISSUES IN DELIVERY OF CARE

Nursing standards of practice in perinatal and women's health nursing have been described by several organizations, including the ANA, which publishes standards for maternal-child health nursing; AWHONN, which publishes standards of practice and education for

TABLE 1-2 NURSING OUTCOMES CLASSIFICATION

Breastfeeding Establishment: Infant (1000)

Domain—Physiologic health (II)

Class—Nutrition (K)

Scale—Not adequate to totally adequate (f)

Definition: Infant attachment to and sucking from the mother's breast for nourishment during the first 3 weeks of breastfeeding

BREASTFEEDING ESTABLISHMENT: INFANT	NOT ADEQUATE	SLIGHTLY ADEQUATE	MODERATELY ADEQUATE	SUBSTANTIALLY ADEQUATE	TOTALLY ADEQUATE
	1	2	3	4	5
Indicators					
100001. Proper alignment and latch-on	1	2	3	4	5
100002. Proper areolar grasp	1	2	3	4	5
100003. Proper areolar compression	1	2	3	4	5
100004. Correct suck and tongue placement	1	2	3	4	5
100005. Audible swallow	1	2	3	4	5
100006. Swallowing a minimum of 5 to 10 minutes per breast	1	2	3	4	5
100007. Minimum 8 feedings per day	1	2	3	4	5
100008. Urinations per day appropriate for age	1	2	3	4	5
100009. Loose, yellow, seedy stools per day appropriate for age	1	2	3	4	5
100010. Appropriate weight gain for age	1	2	3	4	5
100011. Infant contentment after feeding	1	2	3	4	5

Outcome content references:
Biancuzzo M: *Breastfeeding the newborn: clinical strategies for nurses,* ed 2, St Louis, 2003, Mosby.
Henderson A, Pincombe J, Stamp G: Assisting women to establish breastfeeding: exploring midwives practices, *Breastfeeding Rev* 8(3):11–17, 2000.
Lang S: *Breastfeeding special care babies,* ed 2, London, 2002, Baillière Tindall.
Lawrence RA, Lawrence RM: *Breastfeeding: a guide for the medical professional,* ed 5, St Louis, 1999, Mosby.
Minchin M: Positioning for breastfeeding, *Birth: issues in perinatal care and education,* 16(2):67–80, 1989.
Mulford C: The mother-baby assessment (MBA): an "Apgar Score" for breastfeeding, *J Human Lactation* 8(2):79–82, 1992.
Neifert M, Seacat J: A guide to successful breastfeeding, *Contemp Pediatr* 3:1–14, 1986.
Page-Goertz S: Discharge planning for the breastfeeding dyad, *Pediatr Nurs* 15(5):543–544, 1989.
Righard L, Alade M: Sucking technique and its effect on success of breastfeeding, *Birth: Issues Perinatal Care Educ* 19(4):185–189, 1992.
Riordan J, Auerbach K: *Breastfeeding and human lactation,* ed 2, Boston, 1999, Jones & Bartlett.
Shrago L, Bocar D: The infant's contribution to breastfeeding, *J Obstet Gynecol Neonatal Nurs* 19(3):209–215, 1990.
Walker M: Functional assessment of infant breastfeeding patterns, *Birth: Issues Perinatal Care Educ* 16(3):140–147, 1989.
Moorhead S, Johnson M, Maas M, editors: *Nursing outcomes classification (NOC),* ed 3, St Louis, 2000, Mosby.

perinatal nurses (Box 1-8); American College of Nurse-Midwives (ACNM), which publishes standards of practice for midwives; and the National Association of Neonatal Nurses (NANN), which publishes standards of practice for neonatal nurses. These standards reflect current knowledge, represent levels of practice agreed on by leaders in the specialty, and can be used for clinical benchmarking.

In addition to these more formalized standards, agencies have their own policy and procedure books that outline standards to be followed in that setting. In legal terms the standard of care is that level of practice that a reasonably prudent nurse would provide in the same or similar circumstances. In determining legal negligence, the care given is compared with the standard of care. If the standard was not met and harm resulted, negligence occurred. The number of legal suits in the perinatal area typically has been high. As a consequence, malpractice insurance costs are high for physicians, nurse-midwives, and nurses who work in labor and birth settings.

LEGAL TIP: Standard of Care

When you are uncertain about how to perform a procedure, consult the agency procedure book and follow the guidelines printed therein. These guidelines are the standard of care for that agency.

Risk Management

Risk management is an evolving process that identifies risks, establishes preventive practices, develops reporting mechanisms, and

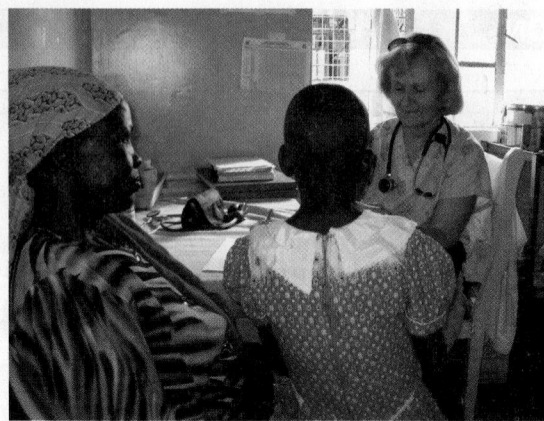

FIG 1-3 Nurse interviewing a young girl accompanied by her mother in a clinic in rural Kenya. (Courtesy Shannon Perry, Phoenix, AZ.)

delineates procedures for managing lawsuits. Nurses should be familiar with concepts of risk management and their implications for nursing practice. These concepts can be viewed as systems of checks and balances that ensure high-quality patient care from preconception until after birth. Effective risk management minimizes the risk of injury to patients and the number of lawsuits against nurses, doctors, and hospitals. Each facility or site develops site-specific risk management procedures based on accepted standards and guidelines. The procedures and guidelines must be reviewed periodically.

To decrease risk of errors in the administration of medications, The Joint Commission (TJC) (2009) developed a list of abbreviations, acronyms, and symbols *not* to use (Table 1-3). In addition, each agency must develop its own list.

Sentinel Events

TJC describes a sentinel event as "an unexpected occurrence involving death or serious physical or psychological injury, or the risk thereof. Serious injury specifically includes loss of limb or function." These events are called *sentinel* because they signal a need for an immediate investigation and response (TJC, 2010). Reportable sentinel events in perinatal nursing include any maternal death related to the process of birth, any perinatal death unrelated to a congenital condition in an infant having a birth weight greater than 2500 g, severe neonatal hyperbilirubinemia (bilirubin greater than 30 mg/dL), and infant discharge to the wrong family (TJC, 2010). Other sentinel events that may occur in perinatal nursing include hemolytic transfusion reaction involving major blood group incompatibilities, leaving a foreign body (e.g., sponge or forceps) in a patient after surgery, and falls that result in death or major permanent loss of function that is a direct result of the injuries caused by the fall. When a sentinel event occurs, there must be a root cause analysis and an action plan formulated that identifies strategies to reduce the risk of future similar events.

Failure to Rescue

Failure to rescue, that is, the failure to recognize or act on early signs of distress, was introduced in the 1990s in relation to the care of adult postsurgical patients (Beaulieu, 2009; Simpson, 2005). Mothers and babies are generally healthy, and complications leading to death in obstetrics are comparatively rare. When applying the concept of failure to rescue to the perinatal setting,

---

BOX 1-8   STANDARDS OF CARE FOR WOMEN AND NEWBORNS

Standards That Define the Nurse's Responsibility to the Patient

Assessment
- Collection of health data of the woman or newborn

Diagnosis
- Analysis of data to determine nursing diagnosis

Outcome Identification
- Identification of expected outcomes that are individualized

Planning
- Development of a plan of care

Implementation
- Performance of interventions for the plan of care

Evaluation
- Evaluation of the effectiveness of interventions in relation to expected outcomes

Standards of Professional Performance That Delineate Roles and Behaviors for Which the Professional Nurse is Accountable

Quality of Care
- Systemic evaluation of nursing practice

Performance Appraisal
- Self-evaluation in relation to professional practice standards and other regulations

Education
- Participation in ongoing educational activities to maintain knowledge for practice

Collegiality
- Contribution to the development of peers, students, and others

Ethics
- Use of American Nurses Association (ANA) Code of Ethics for Nurses with Interpretive Statements (ANA, 2001) to guide practice

Collaboration
- Involvement of patient, significant others, and other health care providers in the provision of patient care

Research
- Use of research findings in practice

Resource Utilization
- Consideration of factors related to safety, effectiveness, and costs in planning and delivering patient care

Practice Environment
- Contribution to the environment of care delivery

Accountability
- Legal and professional responsibility for practice

From Association of Women's Health, Obstetric and Neonatal Nurses (AWHONN), *Standards and guidelines for professional practice in the care of women and newborns,* ed 7, Washington, DC, 2009, Author.

TABLE 1-3 THE JOINT COMMISSION "DO NOT USE" LIST

DO NOT USE	POTENTIAL PROBLEM	USE INSTEAD
U, u (unit)	Mistaken for "0" (zero), the number "4" (four), or "cc"	Write "unit"
IU (International Unit)	Mistaken for IV (intravenous) or the number 10 (ten)	Write "International Unit"
Q.D., QD, q.d., qd (daily)	Mistaken for one another	Write "daily"
Q.O.D., QOD, q.o.d., qod (every other day)	Period after the Q mistaken for an "I" and the "O" for "I"	Write "every other day"
Trailing zero (X.0 mg)	Decimal point is missed	Write X mg
Lack of leading zero (.X mg)	Decimal point is missed	Write 0.X mg
MS	Can mean morphine sulfate or magnesium sulfate	Write "morphine sulfate"
MSO$_4$ and MgSO$_4$	Confused for one another	Write "magnesium sulfate"
Additional Abbreviations, Acronyms, and Symbols*		
> (greater than) < (less than)	Misinterpreted as the number "7" (seven) or the letter "L"; confused for one another	Write "greater than" Write "less than"
Abbreviations for drug names	Misinterpreted because of similar abbreviations for multiple drugs	Write drug names in full
Apothecary units	Unfamiliar to many practitioners Confused with metric units	Use metric units
@	Mistaken for the number "2" (two)	Write "at"
cc	Mistaken for U (units) when poorly written	Write "mL" or "ml" or "milliliters" ("mL" is preferred)
µg	Mistaken for mg (milligrams) resulting in one thousandfold overdose	Write "mcg" or "micrograms"

From The Joint Commission: *The Joint Commission "Do Not Use" list*, updated March 5, 2009. www.jointcommission.org/PatientSafety/DoNotUseList.
*For possible future inclusion in the Official "Do Not Use" List.

BOX 1-9 INSTITUTE OF MEDICINE COMPETENCIES FOR NURSING

- Patient-centered care
- Teamwork
- Collaboration
- Evidence-based practice
- Quality improvement
- Safety
- Informatics

From Institute of Medicine: *Health professions education: a bridge to quality*, Washington, DC, 2003, National Academies Press.

Simpson proposed evaluating the ability of the perinatal team to decrease the risk of adverse outcomes by measuring processes involved in common complications and emergencies in obstetrics (Simpson, 2005; 2006). Key components of failure to rescue are (1) careful surveillance and identification of complications, and (2) quick action to initiate appropriate interventions and activate a team response. For the perinatal nurse this involves careful surveillance, timely identification of complications, appropriate interventions, and activation of a team response to minimize patient harm (Beaulieu, 2009). Maternal complications that are appropriate for process measurement are placental abruption, postpartum hemorrhage, uterine rupture, eclampsia, and amniotic fluid embolism (Simpson, 2005; Simpson, 2006; Simpson, Knox, Martin, George, and Watson, 2011). Fetal complications include nonreassuring fetal heart rate and pattern, prolapsed umbilical cord, shoulder dystocia, and uterine hyperstimulation (Simpson, 2005; Simpson, 2006; Simpson, Knox, Martin, et al., 2011). Perinatal nurses can use these complications to develop a list of expectations for monitoring, timely identification, interventions, and roles of team members. The list can be used to evaluate the perinatal team's response. Promoting a culture of safety, effective communication, and team building are important in providing safe care during labor and birth (Simpson, Knox, Martin, et al., 2011).

Quality and Safety Education for Nurses

Quality and Safety Education for Nurses (QSEN) is an effort to provide nurses with the competencies to improve the quality and safety of the systems of health care in which they practice (Cronenwett, Sherwood, Barnsteiner, et al., 2007). The competencies for nursing delineated by the IOM (2003) (Box 1-9) were adapted by QSEN faculty members and defined by describing essential features of a competent and respected nurse. They then developed knowledge, skills, and attitudes (KSAs) for each competency. Incorporation of these KSAs into prelicensure education for nurses helps faculty plan learning experiences to prepare respected and qualified nurses. In this text QSEN competencies are incorporated into the evidence-based practice boxes.

Teamwork and Communication

Situation-Background-Assessment-Recommendation

The situation-background-assessment-recommendation (SBAR) technique gives a specific framework for communication among health care providers. SBAR is an easy-to-remember, useful, concrete mechanism for communicating important information that requires a clinician's immediate attention (Kaiser Permanente of Colorado, 2011) (Table 1-4). Failure to communicate is one of the major

TABLE 1-4	SAMPLE SBAR REPORT TO PHYSICIAN OR MIDWIFE ABOUT A CRITICAL SITUATION*
S	**Situation** I am calling about Mary Smith. I have just assessed her and she saturated a peripad in the last hour. Her blood pressure is 112/62, pulse 86, and respirations 18. I think she is bleeding excessively.
B	**Background** Mrs. Smith is 12 hours' postpartum after giving birth vaginally to a 9-lb, 12-oz term infant after an uncomplicated pregnancy. She had a rapid labor, just over 4 hours, and had no analgesia. She plans to bottle-feed this baby. She had an IV with 10 units of oxytocin (Pitocin), but it was completed and discontinued about 2 hours ago. This is her sixth birth. All were uncomplicated, and she had an uneventful recovery from them.
A	**Assessment** Her fundus becomes firm after massage but relaxes again. She has voided, and her bladder feels empty. I think she might have retained placenta and she needs to be examined.
R	**Recommendation** I would like you to come and examine her immediately. Do you want her IV restarted? Do you want her to have an Hb and HCT?

Hb, Hemoglobin; *HCT,* hematocrit; *IV,* intravenous infusion; SBAR, Situation-Background-Assessment-Recommendation.
*The SBAR tool was developed by Kaiser Permanente. This example was prepared by Shannon Perry.

reasons for errors in health care. The SBAR technique has the potential to serve as a means to reduce errors.

TeamSTEPPS

TeamSTEPPS was developed by the Department of Defense Patient Safety Program in collaboration with the AHRQ as a teamwork system for health professionals to provide higher-quality, safer patient care (www.teamstepps.ahrq.gov/about-2cl_3.htm). It provides an evidence base to improve communication and teamwork skills. Through this system medical teams use information, people, and resources to achieve the best possible clinical outcomes, increase team awareness and clarify roles and responsibilities of team members, resolve conflicts and improve sharing of information, and eliminate barriers to quality and safety.

ETHICAL ISSUES IN PERINATAL NURSING AND WOMEN'S HEALTH CARE

Ethical concerns and debates have multiplied with the increased use of technology and scientific advances. For example, with reproductive technology pregnancy is now possible in women who thought they would never bear children, including some who are menopausal or postmenopausal. Should scarce resources be devoted to achieving pregnancies in older women? Is giving birth to a child at an older age worth the risks involved? Should older parents be encouraged to conceive a baby when they may not live to see the child reach adulthood? Should a woman who is HIV positive have access to assisted reproduction services? Should third-party payers assume the costs of reproductive technology such as the use of induced ovulation and in vitro fertilizations? With induced ovulation and in vitro fertilization, multiple pregnancies occur, and multifetal pregnancy reduction (selectively terminating one or more fetuses) may be considered. Questions about informed consent and allocation of resources must be addressed with innovations such as intrauterine fetal surgery, fetoscopy, therapeutic insemination, genetic engineering, stem cell research, surrogate childbearing, surgery for infertility, "test tube" babies, fetal research, and treatment of very LBW (VLBW) babies. The introduction of long-acting contraceptives has created moral choices and policy dilemmas for health care providers and legislators (i.e., should some women [substance abusers, women with low incomes, or women who are HIV positive] be required to take the contraceptives?). With the potential for great good that can come from fetal tissue transplantation, what research is ethical? What are the rights of the embryo? Should cloning of humans be permitted? Discussion and debate about these issues will continue for many years. Nurses and patients, together with scientists, physicians, attorneys, lawmakers, ethicists, and clergy, must be involved in the discussions.

RESEARCH IN PERINATAL NURSING

Research plays a vital role in establishing maternity and women's health science. It can validate that nursing care makes a difference. For example, although prenatal care is clearly associated with healthier infants, no one knows exactly which nursing interventions produce this outcome. In the past medical researchers rarely included women in their studies; thus more research in this area is crucial. Many possible areas of research exist in maternity and women's health care. The clinician can identify problems in the health and health care of women and infants. Through research nurses can make a difference for these patients. Nurses should promote research funding and conduct research on maternity and women's health, especially concerning the effectiveness of nursing strategies for these patients.

Ethical Guidelines for Nursing Research

Research with perinatal patients may create ethical dilemmas for the nurse. For example, participating in research may cause additional stress to a woman concerned about outcomes of genetic testing or one who is waiting for an invasive procedure. Obtaining amniotic fluid samples or performing cordocentesis poses risks to the fetus. Nurses must protect the rights of human subjects (i.e., patients) in all of their research. For example, nurses can collect data on or care for patients who are participating in clinical trials. The nurse ensures that the participants are fully informed and aware of their rights as subjects. She or he may be involved in determining whether the benefits of research outweigh the risks to the mother and the fetus. Following the ANA ethical guidelines in the conduct, dissemination, and implementation of nursing research helps nurses ensure that research is conducted ethically.

KEY POINTS

- Maternity nursing focuses on women and their infants and families during the childbearing cycle.
- Nurses caring for women can play an active role in shaping health care systems to be responsive to the needs of contemporary women.
- Childbirth practices have changed to become more family focused and allow alternatives in care.
- Integrative medicine combines modern technology with ancient healing practices and encompasses the whole body, mind, and spirit.

- Evidence-based practice and outcomes orientation are emphasized in current practice.
- Risk management and learning from sentinel events can improve quality of care.
- *Healthy People 2020* provides an update on goals for maternal and infant health.
- Ethical concerns have multiplied with increasing use of technology and scientific advances.

REFERENCES

Agency for Healthcare Research and Quality: *20 Tips to help prevent medical errors: patient fact sheet*, 2000, www.ahqr.gov/consumer/20tips.htm.

American Academy of Pediatrics (AAP), American College of Obstetricians and Gynecologists (ACOG): *Guidelines for perinatal care*, ed 7, Washington, DC, 2012, AAP/ACOG.

American Nurses Association: *Code of Ethics for nurses with interpretive statements*, Silver Spring, MD, 2001, Author.

Association of Women's Health, Obstetric and Neonatal Nurses (AWHONN): *Standards for professional perinatal nursing practice and certification in Canada*, Washington, DC, 2002, Author.

Association of Women's Health, Obstetric and Neonatal Nurses (AWHONN): *Standards and guidelines for professional nursing practice in the care of women and newborns*, ed 7, Washington, DC, 2009, Author.

Beaulieu, MJ: Failure to rescue as a process measure to evaluate fetal safety during labor, *MCN Mater Child Nurs J* 34(1):18–23, 2009.

Berg CJ, Mackay AP, Qin C, et al: Overview of maternal morbidity during hospitalization for labor and delivery in the United States: 1993-1997 and 2001-2005, *Obstet Gynecol* 113(5):1075–1081, 2009.

Bulechek GM, Butcher HK, Dochterman JM, et al: *Nursing interventions classification (NIC)*, ed 6, St Louis, 2013, Mosby.

Centers for Disease Control and Prevention: CDC Health disparities & inequalities report—United States, 2011, *MMWR* 60(suppl):1–116, 2011.

Centers for Disease Control and Prevention: Pregnancy mortality surveillance system, 2013, http://www.cdc.gov/reproductivehealth/MaternalInfantHealth/PMSS.html.

Chin MH: Quality improvement implementation and disparities: the case of the health disparities collaborative, *Med Care* 49(suppl):S65–S71, 2011.

Chu S, Bachman D, Callaghan W, et al: Association between obesity during pregnancy and increased use of health care, *N Engl J Med* 358(14):1444–1453, 2008.

Cronenwett L, Sherwood G, Barnsteiner J, et al: Quality and safety education for nurses, *Nurs Outlook* 55(3):122–131, 2007.

DeNavas-Walt C, Proctor B, Smith J: *US Census Bureau, Current Population Reports, P60-239, Income poverty, and health insurance coverage in the United States, 2010*, Washington, DC, 2011, US Government Printing Office.

Dovydaitis T: Human trafficking: the role of the health care provider, *J Midwifery Womens Health* 55(5):462–467, 2010.

Duffy M: Facebook, Twitter, and LinkedIn, Oh My! *Am J Nurs* 111(4):56–59, 2011.

Flegal KM, Carroll MD, Ogden CL, et al: Prevalence and trends in obesity among US adults, 1999-2008, *JAMA* 303(3):235–241, 2010.

French J: Medical errors and patient safety in health care, *Can J Med Radiation Technol* 37(4):9–13, 2006.

Heron M, Sutton P, Xu J, et al: Annual summary of vital statistics, 2007, *Pediatrics* 125(1):4–15, 2010.

Institute of Medicine: *Health professions education: a bridge to quality*, Washington, DC, 2003, National Academies Press.

Institute of Medicine: *The future of nursing: leading change, advancing health*, Washington, DC, 2010, National Academy of Sciences.

Kaiser Permanente of Colorado: SBAR technique for communication: a situational briefing model, 2011, www.ihi.org/IHI/Topics/PatientSafety/SafetyGeneral/Tools/SBARTechniqueforCommunicationASituationalBriefingModel.htm.

Kochanek KD, Kirmeyer SE, Martin JA, et al: Annual summary of vital statistics, 2009, *Pediatrics* 129:338–348, 2012.

Kutner M, Greenberg E, Jin Y, et al: *The health literacy of America's adults: results from the 2003 National Assessment of Adult Literacy (NCES 2006-2483)*, Washington, DC, 2006, National Center for Education Statistics, US Department of Education.

Martin JA, Hamilton BE, Ventura MA, et al: *Births: final data for 2009, National Vital Statistics Reports*, vol 60, no 1, Hyattsville, MD, 2011, National Center for Health Statistics.

Millennium development goals (MDGs), 2008, http://siteresources.worldbank.org/DATASTATISTICS/Resources/MDGsOfficialList2008.pdf.

Moorhead S, Johnson M, Maas M, et al: *Nursing outcomes classification (NOC)*, ed 5, St Louis, 2012, Mosby.

National Council of State Boards of Nursing (NCBSN): White paper: a nurse's guide to the use of social media, 2011, www.ncsbn.org/Social_Media.pdf.

National Partnership for Action to End Health Disparities: *National stakeholder strategy for achieving health equity*, Rockville, MD, 2011, US Department of Health & Human Services, Office of Minority Health.

O'Reilly K: No pay for "never event" errors becoming standard, 2008, www.ama-assn.org/amednews/2008/01/07/prsc0107.htm.

Pham JC, Aswani MS, Rosen M, et al: Reducing medical errors and adverse events, *Annu Rev Med* 63:447–463, 2012.

Sacks M: Supreme Court health care decision: individual mandate survives, *Huff Post Politics*, 2012, available at www.huffingtonpost.com/2012/06/28/supreme-court-health-care-decision_n_1585131.html, accessed August 20, 2012.

Sandy HP: Female genital cutting: an overview, *Am J Nurse Pract* 15(1/2):53–59, 2011.

Saver C: Social responsibility: social media opportunities and pitfalls, 2010, www.news.nurse.com/article/20100809/NATIONAL01/108090045/-1/frontpage.

Shields M, Carroll MD, Ogden CL: *Adult obesity prevalence in Canada and the United States, NCHS data brief, no 56*, Hyattsville, MD, 2011, National Center for Health Statistics.

Simpson K: Failure to rescue in obstetrics, *MCN Am J Matern Child Nurs* 30(1):76, 2005.

Simpson KR: Measuring perinatal patient safety: review of current methods, *J Obstet Gynecol Neonatal Nurs* 35(3):432–442, 2006.

Simpson KR, Knox E, Martin M, et al: Michigan Health & Hospital Association Keystone Obstetrics: A statewide collaborative for perinatal patient safety in Michigan, *Joint Comm J Qual Patient Safety*, 37(12): 544–552, 2011.

Squires DA: Explaining high health care spending in the United States: an international comparison of supply, utilization, prices, and quality, *The Commonwealth Fund* 10, 2012.

The Joanna Briggs Institute: JBI grades of recommendation (2008), 2008, www.joannabriggs.edu.au.

The Joint Commission: Official "do not use" list, 2009, www.jointcommission.org/assets118Do_Not_Use_List.pdf.

The Joint Commission: Sentinel events, 2010, www.jointcommission.org/assets/1/6/2011_CAMAC_SE.pdf.

Tiedje L, Price E, You M: Childbirth is changing. What now? *MCN Am J Matern Child Nurs* 33(3):144–150, 2008.

US Census Bureau: Press release, *An older and more diverse nation by midcentury*, 2008, www.census.gov/newsroom/releases/archives/population/cb08-123.html.

US Department of Health and Human Services, Office of Disease Prevention and Health Promotion: *National action plan to improve health literacy*, Washington, DC, 2010, Author.

US Department of Health and Human Services: HHS action plan to reduce racial and ethnic health disparities, 2011, www.minorityhealth.hhs.gov/npa/files/Plans/HHS/HHS_Plan_complete.pdf.

Wilson M: Readability and patient education materials used for low-income populations, *Clin Nurse Spec* 23(1):33–40, 2009.

World Health Organization (WHO) study group on female genital mutilation and obstetric outcome (Banks E, Meirik O, Farley T, Akande O, Bathija H, Ali M): Female genital mutilation and obstetric outcome: WHO collaborative prospective study in six African countries, *Lancet* 367(9525):1835–1841, 2006.

Community Care: The Family and Culture

Shannon E. Perry

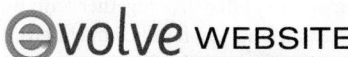

http://evolve.elsevier.com/Perry/maternal

LEARNING OBJECTIVES

On completion of this chapter, the reader will be able to:

- Describe the main characteristics of contemporary family forms.
- Identify key factors influencing family health.
- Compare theoretic approaches for working with childbearing families.
- Relate the impact of culture on childbearing families.
- Discuss cultural competence in relation to one's own nursing practice.
- Identify key components of the community assessment process.
- List indicators of community health status and their relevance to perinatal health.

- Describe data sources and methods for obtaining information about community health status.
- Identify predisposing factors and characteristics of vulnerable populations.
- List the potential advantages and disadvantages of home visits.
- Explore telephonic nursing care options in perinatal nursing.
- Describe how home fits into the maternity continuum of care.
- Discuss safety and infection control principles as they apply to the care of patients in their homes.
- Describe the nurse's role in perinatal home care.

THE FAMILY IN CULTURAL AND COMMUNITY CONTEXT

The family and its cultural context play an important role in defining the work of maternity nurses. Despite modern stresses and strains, the family forms a social network that acts as a potent support system for its members. Family care-seeking behavior and relationships with providers are all influenced by culturally related health beliefs and values. Ultimately, all of these factors have the power to affect maternal and child health outcomes. The current emphasis in working with families is on wellness and empowerment for families to achieve control over their lives. It is essential that nurses become culturally competent in order to provide the most appropriate care possible.

Defining Family

The family has traditionally been viewed as the primary unit of socialization—the basic structural unit within a community. The family plays a pivotal role in health care, representing the primary target of health care delivery for maternal and newborn nurses. As one of society's most important institutions, the family represents a primary social group that influences and is influenced by other people and institutions. A variety of family configurations exist.

Family Organization and Structure

The *nuclear family* has long represented the traditional American family in which male and female partners and their children live as an independent unit, sharing roles, responsibilities, and economic resources (Fig. 2-1). In contemporary society, this idealized family structure actually represents only a relatively small number of families, and that number is steadily decreasing.

Many nuclear families have other relatives living in the same household. These extended family members include grandparents, aunts, uncles, or other people related by blood (Fig. 2-2). For some groups, such as African-American and Latin-American, extended family is an important resource in terms of preventive health behavior. The extended family is becoming more common as American society ages.

Multigenerational families, consisting of grandparents, children, and grandchildren, are becoming increasingly common. In 2010 they made up 4.4% of all households (Lofquist, Lugaila, O'Connell, et al., 2012). This may create stress as children must care for their

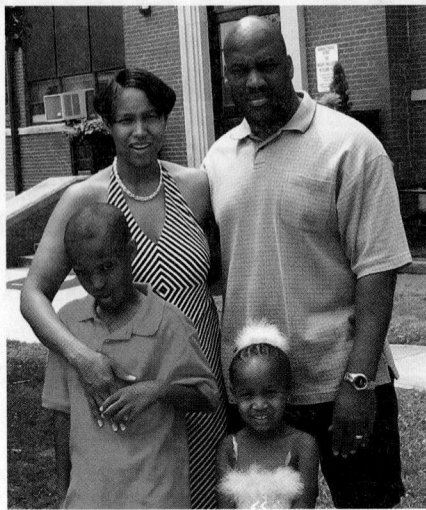

FIG 2-1 Nuclear family. (Courtesy Makeba Felton, Wake Forest, NC.)

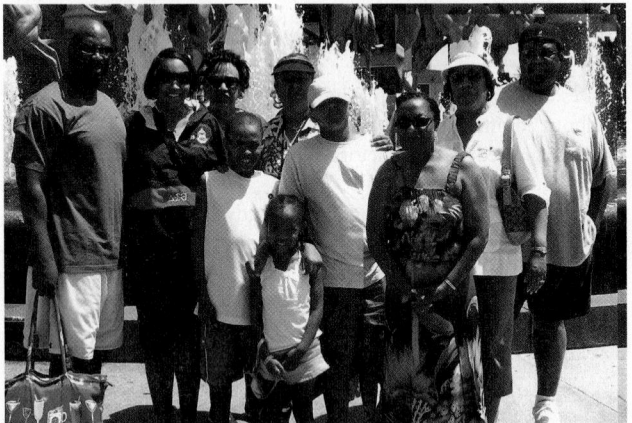

FIG 2-2 Extended family. (Courtesy Makeba Felton, Wake Forest, NC.)

parents as well as their own children. In other instances, the grandparents are supporting the children and grandchildren or are sole caregivers for the grandchildren.

No-parent families are those in which children live independently in foster or kinship care such as living with a grandparent. An estimated 5.4 million children in the United States live with grandparents (U.S. Census Bureau, 2010).

Married-parent families (biologic or adoptive parents) make up 48.4% of American families. By race and Hispanic origin, this family structure is represented as follows (Lofquist, Lugaila, O'Connell, et al., 2012):

- Caucasian: 51.1%
- Hispanic: 50.1%
- African-American: 28.5%
- Asian: 59.7%
- American Indian and Alaska Native: 40.1%
- Native Hawaiian and Pacific Islander: 51.3%

Married-blended families, those formed as a result of divorce and remarriage, consist of unrelated family members (stepparents, stepchildren, and stepsiblings) who join to create a new household.

These family groups frequently involve a biologic or adoptive parent whose spouse may or may not have adopted the child.

Cohabiting-parent families are those in which children live with two unmarried biologic parents or two adoptive parents. Hispanic children are almost twice as likely as African-American children to live in cohabiting-parent families and about four times as likely as Caucasian children to live in this kind of family arrangement (Lofquist, Lugaila, O'Connell, et al., 2012).

Single-parent families comprise an unmarried biologic or adoptive parent who may or may not be living with other adults. The single-parent family may result from the loss of a spouse by death, divorce, separation, or desertion; from either an unplanned or planned pregnancy; or from the adoption of a child by an unmarried woman or man.

The single-parent family tends to be vulnerable economically and socially, creating an unstable and deprived environment for the growth of children. This in turn affects health status, school achievement, and high risk behaviors for these children.

Homosexual families (lesbian and gay) may live together with or without children. Children in lesbian and gay families may be the offspring of previous heterosexual unions, conceived by one member of a lesbian couple through therapeutic insemination, or adopted.

The Family in Society

The social context for the family can be viewed in relation to social and demographic trends that define the population as a whole. Racial and ethnic diversity of the population has grown dramatically in the past three decades, necessitating consideration of such diversity in provision of health care.

THEORETIC APPROACHES TO UNDERSTANDING FAMILIES

Family Nursing

Family plays a pivotal role in health care, representing the primary target of health care delivery for maternal and newborn nurses. It is crucial that nurses assist families as they incorporate new additions into their family (see Nursing Care Plan). When treating the woman and family with respect and dignity, health care providers listen to and honor perspectives and choices of the woman and family. They share information with families in ways that are positive, useful, timely, complete, and accurate. The family is supported in participating in the care and decision making at the level of their choice.

Because so many variables affect ways of relating, the nurse must be aware that family members may interact and communicate with each other in ways that are distinct from those of the nurse's own family of origin. Most families will hold some beliefs about health that are different from those of the nurse. Their beliefs can conflict with principles of health care management predominant in the Western health care system.

Family Theories

A family theory can be used to describe families and how the family unit responds to events both within and outside the family. Each family theory makes certain assumptions about the family and has inherent strengths and limitations. Most nurses use a combination of theories in their work with families. A brief synopsis of several theories useful in working with families is included in Table 2-1. Application of these concepts can guide assessment and interventions for the family.

◎ NURSING CARE PLAN

Incorporating the Infant into the Family

NURSING DIAGNOSIS	EXPECTED OUTCOME	NURSING INTERVENTIONS	RATIONALES
Readiness for Enhanced Family Coping related to adaptation of family to new infant	Family members will verbalize that individual and family goals are met during a smooth transition of new family member into the home.	Assess type and amount of support available to family on daily basis during postpartum period	To facilitate adaptation of family to situation of a new member
		Encourage family to use past successful coping mechanisms.	To enhance ability to cope with new situation and promote self-esteem
		Encourage mother to use family and other support or services	To carry out daily household tasks to permit her to focus on herself and infant
		Suggest that woman take time to rest when infant sleeps	To conserve energy for healing and limit responsibility to herself and infant
		Assess family structure and relationships, including culture	To evaluate if longer period of adjustment may be expected
		Teach family about sensory needs and capabilities of infant	To motivate family to meet infant's needs and set realistic expectations for infant's capabilities
		Refer to parent support group or community agencies, as needed	To facilitate and validate ongoing positive adjustment of family to new family member
Ineffective Role Performance related to developmental challenge of addition of new family member	Each family member will verbalize realistic expectations regarding his or her role in the family and formulate a plan to incorporate the role into overall family goals.	Assess family structure, roles, and each member's perception of his or her role in family	To evaluate impact of new member on structure and roles of family as perceived by members
		Evaluate individual's perception of goals and new roles during this transition	To promote early intervention and correct any misinterpretation
		Encourage discussion of family members' thoughts and feelings regarding this transition	To promote open communication and trust
		Provide positive reinforcement for family members' actions that promote positive environment for infant	To increase self-esteem and provide encouragement
		Refer to community support groups	To provide group reinforcement and further assistance
		Give information about sibling and grandparent classes and support groups as available	To promote empowerment and self-esteem for significant others in family

Family Assessment

When selecting a family assessment framework, an appropriate model for a perinatal nurse is one that is a health-promoting rather than an illness-care model. The low risk family can be assisted in promoting a healthy pregnancy, childbirth, and integration of the newborn into the family. The high risk perinatal family has illness-care needs, and the nurse can help meet those needs while also promoting the health of the childbearing family.

A family assessment tool such as the Calgary Family Assessment Model (CFAM) (Box 2-1) can be used as a guide for assessing aspects of the family. Such an assessment is based on "the nurse's personal and professional life experiences, beliefs, and relationships with those being interviewed" (Wright and Leahy, 2009) and is not "the truth" about the family but, rather, one perspective at one point in time.

The CFAM comprises three major categories: structural, developmental, and functional. Several subcategories are within each category. The three assessment categories and the many subcategories can be conceptualized as a branching diagram (Fig. 2-3). These categories and subcategories can be used to guide the assessment that will provide data to help the nurse better understand the family and formulate a plan of care. The nurse asks questions of family members about themselves to gain understanding of the structure, development, and function of the family at this point in time. Not all questions within the subcategories should be asked at the first interview, and some questions may not be appropriate for all families. Although individuals are the ones interviewed, the focus of the assessment is on interaction of individuals within the family.

Graphic Representations of Families

A family genogram (family tree format depicting relationships of family members over at least three generations) (Fig. 2-4) provides valuable information about a family and can be placed in the nursing care plan for easy access by care providers. An ecomap, a graphic portrayal of social relationships of the woman and family, may also help the nurse understand the social environment of the family and identify support systems available to them (Fig. 2-5). Software is available to generate genograms and ecomaps (www.interpersonaluniverse.net).

TABLE 2-1 THEORIES AND MODELS RELEVANT TO FAMILY NURSING PRACTICE

THEORY	SYNOPSIS OF THEORY
Family Systems Theory (Wright and Leahy, 2009)	The family is viewed as a unit, and interactions among family members are studied rather than studying individuals. A family system is part of a larger suprasystem and is composed of many subsystems. The family as a whole is greater than the sum of its individual members. A change in one family member affects all family members. The family is able to create a balance between change and stability. Family members' behaviors are best understood from a view of circular rather than linear causality.
Family Life Cycle (Developmental) Theory (Carter and McGoldrick, 1999)	Families move through stages. The family life cycle is the context in which to examine the identity and development of the individual. Relationships among family members go through transitions. Although families have roles and functions, a family's main value is in relationships that are irreplaceable. The family involves different structures and cultures organized in various ways. Developmental stresses may disrupt the life-cycle process.
Family Stress Theory (Boss, 1996)	How families react to stressful events is the focus. Family stress can be studied within the internal and external contexts in which the family is living. The internal context involves elements that a family can change or control, such as family structure, psychologic defenses, and philosophic values and beliefs. The external context consists of the time and place in which a particular family finds itself and over which the family has no control, such as the culture of the larger society, the time in history, the economic state of society, maturity of the individuals involved, success of the family in coping with stressors, and genetic inheritance.
McGill Model of Nursing (Allen, 1997)	Strength-based approach in clinical practice with families, as opposed to a deficit approach, is the focus. Identification of family strengths and resources; provision of feedback about strengths; assistance given to family to develop and elicit strengths and use resources are key interventions.
Health Belief Model (Becker, 1974; Janz and Becker, 1984)	The goal of the model is to reduce cultural and environmental barriers that interfere with access to health care. Key elements of the Health Belief Model include the following: perceived susceptibility, perceived severity, perceived benefits, perceived barriers, cues to action, and confidence.
Human Developmental Ecology (Bronfenbrenner, 1979; 1989)	Behavior is a function of interaction of traits and abilities with the environment. Major concepts include ecosystem, niches (social roles), adaptive range, and ontogenetic development. Individuals are "embedded in a microsystem [role and relations], a mesosystem [interrelations between two or more settings], an exosystem [external settings that do not include the person], and a macrosystem [culture]" (Klein and White, 1996). Change over time is incorporated in the chronosystem.

BOX 2-1 CALGARY FAMILY ASSESSMENT MODEL

There are three major categories of the Calgary Family Assessment Model (CFAM)—structural, developmental, and functional. Each category has several subcategories. In this box, only the major categories are included. A few sample questions are included.

Structural Assessment

Determine the members of the family, relationship among family members, and context of family.

Genograms and ecomaps (see Figs. 2-4; 2-5) are useful in outlining the internal and external structures of a family.

Sample questions
- Who are the members of your family?
- Has anyone moved in or out lately?
- Are there any family members who don't live with you?

Developmental Assessment

Describe the life cycle—that is, the typical trajectory most families experience.

Sample questions
- When you think back, what do you most enjoy about your life?
- What do you regret about your life?
- Have you made plans for your care as your health declines?

Functional Assessment

Evaluate the way in which individuals behave in relation to each other in instrumental and expressive aspects. (Instrumental aspects are activities of daily living; expressive aspects include communication, problem solving, roles, etc.)

Sample questions
- Which one of the family is responsible for making sure Grandma takes her medicine?
- Whose turn is it to fix dinner for Grandma?
- How can we get Martin to help with Grandma's care?

Data from Wright LM, Leahy M: *Nurses and families: a guide to family assessment and intervention*, ed 5, Philadelphia, 2009, FA Davis.

THE FAMILY IN A CULTURAL CONTEXT

Cultural Factors Related to Family Health

Culture of an individual is influenced by religion, environment, and historic events and plays a powerful role in the individual's behavior and patterns of human interaction. Culture is not static; it is an ongoing process that influences a woman throughout her entire life, from birth to death.

Cultural knowledge includes beliefs and values about each facet of life and is passed from one generation to the next. Cultural beliefs and traditions relate to food, language, religion, art, health and healing practices, kinship relationships, and all other aspects of

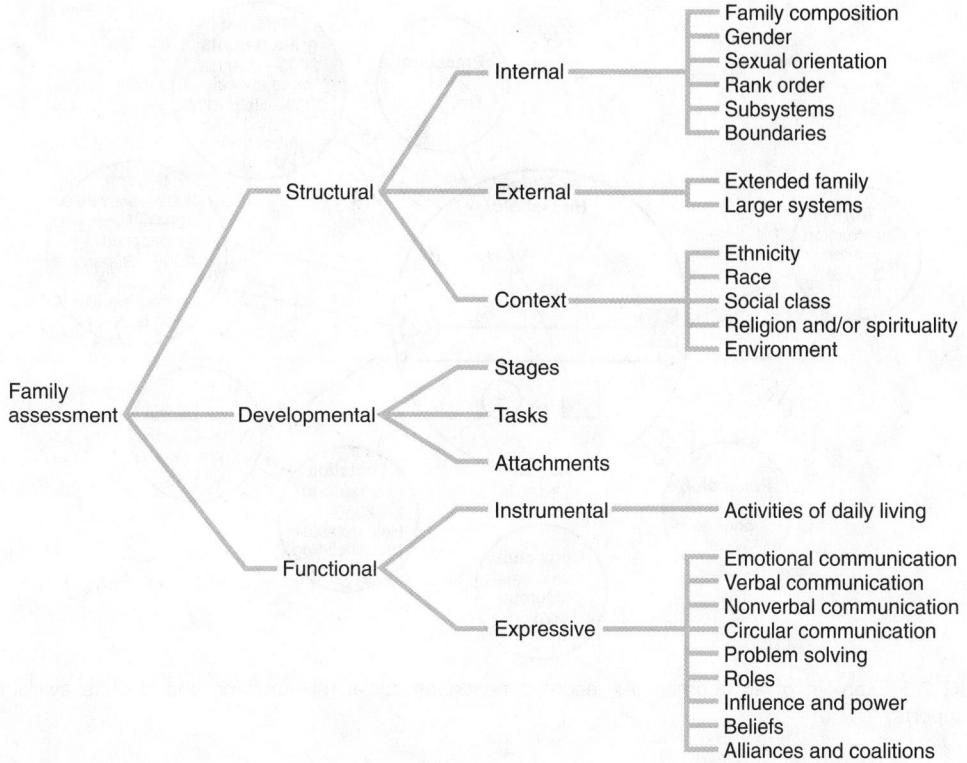

FIG 2-3 Branching diagram of Calgary Family Assessment Model (CFAM). (From Wright LM, Leahy M: *Nurses and families: a guide to family assessment and intervention,* ed 5, Philadelphia, 2009, FA Davis.)

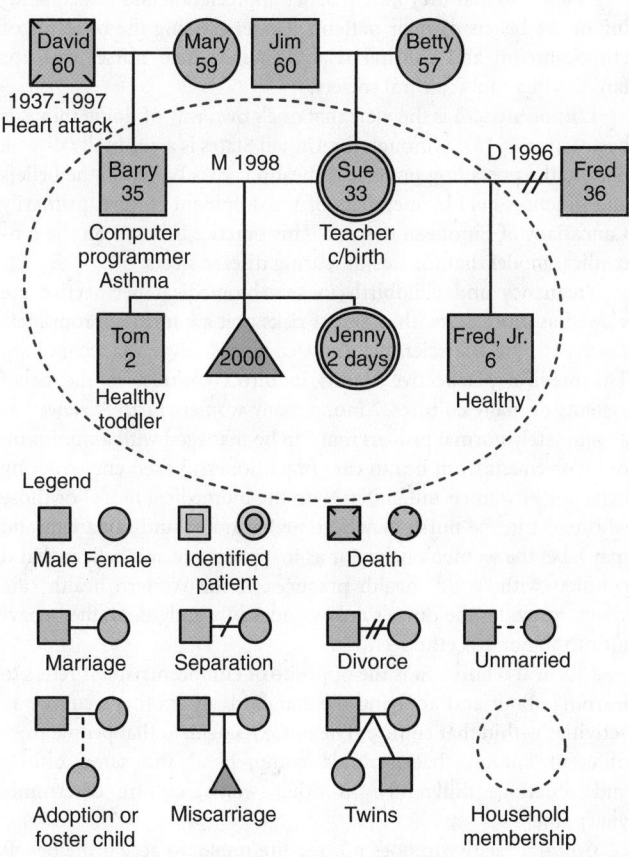

FIG 2-4 Example of a family genogram.

community, family, and individual life. Culture has also been shown to have a direct effect on health behaviors. Values, attitudes, and beliefs that are culturally acquired may influence perceptions of illness, as well as health care–seeking behavior and response to treatment. The political, social, and economic context of people's lives is also part of the cultural experience.

Culture, shared beliefs, and values of a group play a powerful role in an individual's behavior, particularly when the individual is sick. Understanding a culture can provide insight into how a person reacts to illness, pain, and invasive medical procedures, as well as patterns of human interaction and expressions of emotion. The effect of these influences must be assessed by health care professionals in providing health care and developing effective intervention strategies.

Many subcultures may be found within each culture. **Subculture** refers to a group existing within a larger cultural system that retains its own characteristics. A subculture may be an ethnic group or a group organized in other ways. For example, in the United States and Canada, many ethnic subcultures such as African-Americans, Asian-Americans, Hispanic-Americans, and Native Americans exist. It is important to note that subcultures also exist within these groups. In addition, the Caucasian population in America has multiple subcultures of its own. Because every identified cultural group has subcultures and because it is impossible to study every subculture in depth, greater differences may exist among and between groups than is generally acknowledged. It is important to be familiar with common cultural practices within these subgroups. However, it is also important to avoid the generalization that every person practices every cultural belief within a group.

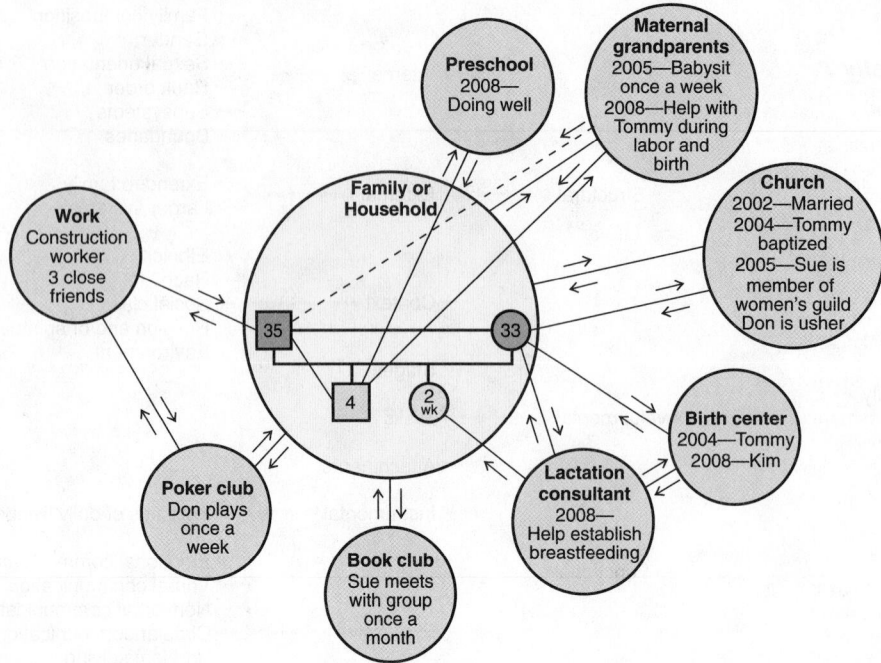

FIG 2-5 Example of an ecomap. An ecomap describes social relationships and depicts available supports.

In a multicultural society, many groups can influence traditions and practices. As cultural groups come into contact with each other, acculturation and assimilation may occur.

Acculturation refers to the changes that occur within one group or among several groups when people from different cultures come into contact with one another. People may retain some of their own culture while adopting some cultural practices of the dominant society. This familiarization among cultural groups results in overt behavioral similarity, especially in mannerisms, styles, and practices. Dress, language patterns, food choices, and health practices are often much slower to adapt to the influence of acculturation. In the United States, acculturation generally is thought to take three generations. An adult grandchild of an immigrant is usually fully Americanized.

During times of family transitions such as childbearing or during crisis or illness, a woman may rely on old cultural patterns even after she has become acculturated in many ways. This is consistent with the family developmental theory that states that during times of stress, people revert to practices and behaviors that are most comfortable and familiar.

Assimilation occurs when a cultural group loses its cultural identity and becomes part of the dominant culture. Assimilation is the process by which groups "melt" into the mainstream, thus accounting for the notion of a "melting pot," a phenomenon that has been said to occur in the United States. This is illustrated by individuals who identify themselves as being of Irish or German descent without having any remaining cultural practices or values linked specifically to that culture such as food preparation techniques, style of dress, or proficiency in the language associated with their reported cultural heritage. Spector (2013) asserts that in the United States, the melting pot, with its dream of a common culture, is a myth. Instead, a mosaic phenomenon exists in which we must accept and appreciate the differences among people.

Implications for Nursing

As our society becomes more culturally diverse, it is essential that nurses become culturally competent. Nurses must examine their own beliefs so that they have a better appreciation and understanding of the beliefs of their patients. Understanding the concepts of ethnocentrism and cultural relativism may help nurses care for families in a multicultural society.

Ethnocentrism is the view that one's own way of doing things is best (Giger, 2013). Although the United States is a culturally diverse nation, the prevailing practice of health care is based on the beliefs and practices held by members of the dominant culture, primarily Caucasians of European descent. This practice is based on the biomedical model that focuses on curing disease states.

Pregnancy and childbirth in this biomedical perspective are viewed as processes with inherent risks that are most appropriately managed by using scientific knowledge and advanced technology. The medical perspective stands in direct contrast to the belief systems of many cultures. Among many women, birth is viewed as a completely normal process that can be managed with a minimum of involvement from health care practitioners. When encountering behavior in women unfamiliar with the biomedical model or those who reject it, the nurse may become frustrated and impatient and may label the women's behavior as inappropriate and believe that it conflicts with "good" health practices. If the Western health care system provides the nurse's only standard for judgment, the behavior of the nurse is ethnocentric.

Cultural relativism is the opposite of ethnocentrism. It refers to learning about and applying the standards of another's culture to activities within that culture. The nurse recognizes that people from different cultural backgrounds comprehend the same objects and situations differently. In other words, culture determines viewpoint.

Cultural relativism does not require nurses to accept the beliefs and values of another culture. Instead, nurses recognize that the

CRITICAL THINKING CASE STUDY

Providing Culturally Appropriate Care

Elisabeth, a 22-year-old first-generation Mexican-American, comes into your office for her initial prenatal visit. You are concerned because Elisabeth's fundal height is consistent with 32 weeks of gestation and this is her first prenatal visit. Elisabeth, who lives with her husband, four children (ages 6, 4, and 3 years and 15 months), her mother, her aunt, and her uncle, states that she has been doing well this pregnancy and did not start prenatal care in her previous pregnancies until she was almost ready to give birth. She also comments that all the babies were full term with uneventful labors and births. In obtaining the history you note the presence of a safety pin in Elisabeth's shirt and wonder what this is for. You want to provide culturally competent care to this woman and her family.

1. Evidence—Is there sufficient evidence to support the components of culturally competent care for Elisabeth?
2. Assumptions—Describe an underlying assumption about culturally competent care for Elisabeth in relation to these topics:
   a. The view of pregnancy in Elisabeth's culture
   b. The role of family in Elisabeth's culture
   c. The acceptability for women of Elisabeth's age to begin having children at such young ages
   d. The religious beliefs that Elisabeth may have that affect contraception
3. What implications and priorities for nursing care can be made at this time?
4. Does the evidence objectively support your conclusion?

behavior of others may be based on a system of logic different from their own. Cultural relativism affirms the uniqueness and value of every culture.

Childbearing Beliefs and Practices

Nurses working with childbearing families care for families from many different cultures and ethnic groups. To provide culturally competent care, the nurse must assess the beliefs and practices of patients. When working with childbearing families, a nurse considers all aspects of culture including communication, space, time orientation, and family roles.

Communication often creates the most challenging obstacle for nurses working with patients from diverse cultural groups. Communication is not merely the exchange of words. Instead, it involves (1) understanding the individual's language, including subtle variations in meaning and distinctive dialects; (2) appreciating individual differences in interpersonal style; and (3) accurately interpreting the volume of speech as well as the meanings of touch and gestures. For example, members of some cultural groups tend to speak more loudly when they are excited, with great emotion and with vigorous and animated gestures; this is true whether their excitement is related to positive or negative events or emotions. It is important, therefore, for the nurse to avoid rushing to judgment regarding a person's intent when the patient is speaking, especially in a language not understood by the nurse. Instead, the nurse should withhold an interpretation of what has been expressed until it is possible to clarify the patient's intent. The nurse needs to enlist the assistance of a person who can help verify with the patient the true intent and meaning of the communication (see Critical Thinking Case Study).

Inconsistencies between the language of patients and the language of providers present a significant barrier to effective health care. For example, there are many dialects of Spanish that vary by geographic location. Because of the diversity of cultures and languages within the U.S. and Canadian populations, health care agencies are increasingly seeking the services of interpreters (of oral communication from one language to another) or translators (of written words from one language to another) to bridge these gaps and fulfill their obligation for culturally and linguistically appropriate health care (Box 2-2). Finding the best possible interpreter in the circumstance is critically important as well. Ideally, interpreters should have the same native language and be of the same religion or have the same country of origin as the patient. Interpreters should have specific health-related language skills and experience and help bridge the language and cultural barriers between the patient and the health care provider. The person interpreting also should be mature enough to be trusted with private information. However, because the nature of nursing care is not always predictable and because nursing care that is provided in a home or community setting does not always allow expert, experienced, or mature adult interpreters, ideal interpretive services sometimes are impossible to find when they are needed. In crisis or emergency situations or when family members are having extreme stress or emotional upset, it may be necessary to use relatives, neighbors, or children as interpreters. If this situation occurs, the nurse must ensure that the patient is in agreement and comfortable with using the available interpreter to assist.

When using an interpreter, the nurse respects the family by creating an atmosphere of respect and privacy. Questions should be addressed to the woman and not to the interpreter. Even though an interpreter will of necessity be exposed to sensitive and privileged information about the family, the nurse should take care to ensure that confidentiality is maintained. A quiet location free from interruptions is ideal for interpretive services to take place. Culturally and linguistically appropriate educational materials that are easy to read, with appropriate text and graphics, should be available to assist the woman and her family in understanding health care information. To ensure understanding and avoid liability issues, it is important to make certain that the material has been translated by someone who is trained appropriately.

Personal Space

Cultural traditions define the appropriate personal space for various social interactions. Although the need for personal space varies from person to person and with the situation, the actual physical dimensions of comfort zones differ from culture to culture. Actions such as touching, placing the woman in proximity to others, taking away personal possessions, and making decisions for the woman can decrease personal security and heighten anxiety. Conversely, respecting the need for distance allows the woman to maintain control over personal space and support personal autonomy, thereby increasing her sense of security. Nurses must touch patients. However, they frequently do so without any awareness of the emotional distress they may be causing patients.

Time Orientation

Time orientation is a fundamental way in which culture affects health behaviors. People in cultural groups may be relatively more oriented to past, present, or future. Those who focus on the past strive to maintain tradition or the status quo and have little motivation for formulating future goals. In contrast, individuals who focus primarily on the present neither plan for the future nor consider the

---

BOX 2-2   **WORKING WITH AN INTERPRETER**

Step 1: Before the Interview

A. Outline your statements and questions. List the key pieces of information you want/need to know.

B. Learn something about the culture so that you can converse informally with the interpreter.

Step 2: Meeting with the Interpreter

A. Introduce yourself to the interpreter and converse informally. This is the time to find out how well he or she speaks English. No matter how proficient or what age the interpreter is, be respectful. Some ways to show respect are to ask a cultural question to acknowledge that you can learn from the interpreter, or you could learn one word or phrase from the interpreter.

B. Emphasize that you do want the patient to ask questions, because some cultures consider this inappropriate behavior.

C. Make sure the interpreter is comfortable with the technical terms you need to use. If not, take some time to explain them.

Step 3: During the Interview

A. Ask your questions and explain your statements (see Step 1).

B. Make sure that the interpreter understands which parts of the interview are most important. You usually have limited time with the interpreter, and you want to have adequate time at the end for patient questions.

C. Try to get a "feel" for how much is "getting through." No matter what the language is, if in relating information to the patient, the interpreter uses far fewer or far more words than you do, something else is going on.

D. Stop now and then and ask the interpreter, "How is it going?" You may not get a totally accurate answer, but you will have emphasized to the interpreter your strong desire to focus on the task at hand. If there are

language problems, (1) speak slowly; (2) use gestures (e.g., fingers to count or point to body parts); and (3) use pictures.

E. Ask the interpreter to elicit questions. This may be difficult, but it is worth the effort.

F. Identify cultural issues that may conflict with your requests or instructions.

G. Use the interpreter to help problem solve or at least give insight into possibilities for solutions.

Step 4: After the Interview

A. Speak to the interpreter and try to get an idea of what went well and what could be improved. This will help you be more effective in the future with this or another interpreter.

B. Make notes on what you learned for your future reference or to help a colleague.

Remember

Your interview is a *collaboration* between you and the interpreter. *Listen* as well as speak.

Notes:

1. The interpreter may be a child, grandchild, or sibling of the patient. Be sensitive to the fact that the child is playing an adult role.

2. Be sensitive to cultural and situational differences (e.g., an interview with someone from urban Germany will likely be different from an interview with someone from a transitional refugee camp).

3. Younger females telling older males what to do may be a problem for both a female nurse and a female interpreter. This is not the time to pioneer new gender relations. Be aware that in some cultures it is difficult for a woman to talk about some topics with a husband or a father present.

Courtesy Elizabeth Whalley, PhD, San Francisco State University.

---

experiences of the past. These individuals do not necessarily adhere to strict schedules and are often described as "living for the moment" or "marching to their own drummer." Individuals oriented to the future maintain a focus on achieving long-term goals.

The time orientation of the childbearing family may affect nursing care. For example, talking to a family about bringing the infant to the clinic for follow-up examinations (events in the future) may be difficult for the family who is focused on the present concerns of day-to-day survival. Because a family with a future-oriented sense of time plans far in advance, thinking about the long-term consequences of present actions, they may be more likely to return as scheduled for follow-up visits. Despite the differences in time orientation, each family can be equally concerned for the well-being of its newborn.

Family Roles

Family roles involve the expectations and behaviors associated with a member's position in the larger family system (e.g., mother, father, grandparent). Social class and cultural norms also affect these roles, with distinct expectations for men and women clearly determined by social norms. For example, culture may influence whether a man actively participates in pregnancy and childbirth, yet maternity care practitioners working in the Western health care system expect fathers to be involved. This can create a significant conflict between the nurse and the role expectations of very traditional Mexican or Arab families, who usually view the birthing experience as a female

⊕ **CULTURAL COMPETENCE**

Questions to Ask to Elicit Cultural Expectations About Childbearing

1. What do you and your family think you should do to remain healthy during pregnancy?

2. What can you do to improve your health and the health of your baby?

3. What foods will help make a healthy baby?

4. Who do you want with you during your labor?

5. What can your labor support person do to help you be most comfortable during labor?

6. What actions are important for you and your family after the baby's birth?

7. What do you and your family expect from the nurse(s) caring for you?

8. How will family members participate in your pregnancy, childbirth, and parenting?

affair (see Cultural Competence box). The way that health care practitioners manage such a family's care molds its experience and perception of the Western health care system.

In maternity nursing, the nurse supports and nurtures the beliefs that promote physical or emotional adaptation to childbearing. However, if certain beliefs might be harmful, the nurse should carefully explore them with the woman and use them in the re-education

From Mattson S: Providing culturally competent care: strategies and approaches for perinatal clients, *AWHONN Lifelines* 4(5):37–39, 2000.

BOX 2-3 STRATEGIES FOR CARE DELIVERY AND PROVIDING CULTURALLY APPROPRIATE CARE

Strategies for Care Delivery

- Break down the language barriers.
- Explain your rationale and reasons for suggestions.
- Integrate folk and Western treatments.
- Enlist the family caregiver and others.
- Get consent from the right person.
- Provide language-appropriate materials.

Providing Culturally Appropriate Care

- Ask about traditional beliefs, such as the role of hot and cold.
- Be sensitive regarding interpreters and language barriers.
- Ask about important dietary practices, particularly those related to events such as childbirth.
- Ask about group practices and beliefs.
- Ask about a woman's fears and those of her family regarding an unfamiliar care setting.

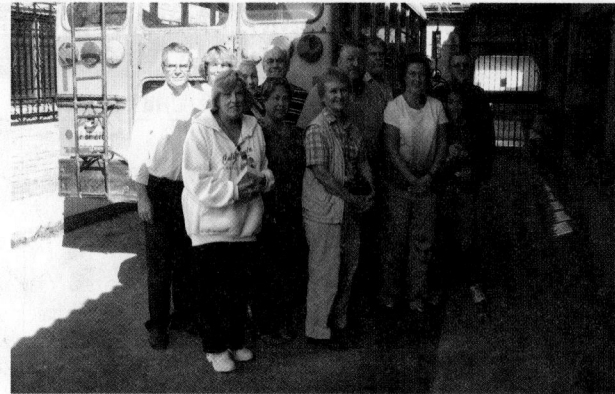

FIG 2-6 Physicians, nurses, and interpreters during a medical mission in Honduras. (Courtesy Shannon Perry, Phoenix, AZ.)

and modification process. Strategies for care delivery and providing appropriate care are presented in Box 2-3.

Table 2-2 provides examples of some cultural beliefs and practices surrounding childbearing. The cultural beliefs and customs in the table are categorized on the basis of distinct cultural traditions and are not practiced by all members of the cultural group in every part of the country. Women from these cultural and ethnic groups may adhere to a few, all, or none of the practices listed. In using this table as a guide, the nurse should take care to avoid making stereotypic assumptions about any person based on sociocultural-spiritual affiliations. Nurses should exercise sensitivity in working with every family, being careful to assess the ways in which they apply their own mixture of cultural traditions.

DEVELOPING CULTURAL COMPETENCE

Cultural competence has many names and definitions, all of which have subtle shades of difference but which are essentially the same: multiculturalism, cultural sensitivity, and intercultural effectiveness. Cultural competence involves acknowledging, respecting, and appreciating ethnic, cultural, and linguistic diversity. Culturally competent professionals act in ways that meet the needs of the patient and are respectful of ways and traditions that may be very different from their own. In today's society it is of critical importance that nurses develop more than technical skill. At every level of preparation and throughout their professional lives, nurses must engage in a continual process of developing and refining attitudes and behaviors that will promote culturally competent care (Giger, 2013).

Key components of culturally competent care include:
- Recognizing that disparity exists between one's own culture and that of the patient
- Educating and promoting healthy behaviors in a cultural context that has meaning for patients

- Taking abstract knowledge about other cultures and applying it in a practical way so that the quality of service improves and policies are enacted that meet the needs of all patients
- Communicating respectfulness for a wide range of differences, including patient use of nontraditional healing practices and alternative therapies
- Recognizing the importance of culturally different communication styles, problem-solving techniques, concepts of space and time, and desires to be involved with care decisions
- Anticipating the need to address varying degrees of language ability and literacy, as well as barriers to care and compliance with treatment

In addition to issues of preserving and promoting human dignity, the development of cultural competence is of equal importance in terms of health outcomes. Nurses who relate effectively with patients are able to motivate them in the direction of health-promoting behaviors. Provider competence to address language barriers facilitates appropriate tailoring of health messages and preventive health teaching. Cross-cultural experiences also present an opportunity for the health care professional to expand cultural sensitivity, awareness, and skills (Fig. 2-6).

COMMUNITY HEALTH PROMOTION

Best practices in community-based health initiatives involve understanding of community relationships and resources as well as participation of community leaders. The emphasis on community-based health promotion has grown in recent years, with recognition that many health issues require the collaborative efforts of a diverse community network to achieve public health goals. These efforts are particularly relevant in relation to maternal-newborn health, which is affected by multiple public health issues: lack of health insurance; recent economic challenges that include job loss; teen pregnancy; substance abuse; and the consequences of no or inadequate prenatal care.

Levels of Preventive Care

In community-based health promotion, three levels of prevention of disease exist. Primary prevention involves promoting healthy lifestyles through immunizations, encouraging exercise, and healthy nutrition. Secondary prevention involves targeting populations at risk for certain diseases. For example, women are encouraged to have

TABLE 2-2 TRADITIONAL* CULTURAL BELIEFS AND PRACTICES: CHILDBEARING AND PARENTING

PREGNANCY	CHILDBIRTH	PARENTING
Hispanic		

(Based primarily on knowledge of Mexican-Americans; members of the Hispanic community have their origins in Spain, Cuba, Central and South America, Mexico, Puerto Rico, and other Spanish-speaking countries.)

Pregnancy	*Labor*	*Newborn*
Pregnancy desired soon after marriage	Use of *partera* or lay midwife preferred in some places; may prefer presence of mother rather than husband	Breastfeeding begun after third day; colostrum may be considered "filthy" or "spoiled" or just not enough nourishment
Late prenatal care		
Expectant mother influenced strongly by mother or mother-in-law	After birth of baby, mother's legs brought together to prevent air from entering uterus	Olive oil or castor oil given to stimulate passage of meconium
Cool air in motion considered dangerous during pregnancy	Loud behavior in labor	Male infant not circumcised
Unsatisfied food cravings thought to cause a birthmark	*Postpartum*	Female infant's ears pierced
Some pica observed in the eating of ashes or dirt (not common)	Diet may be restricted after birth; for first 2 days only boiled milk and toasted tortillas permitted (special foods to restore warmth to body)	Belly band used to prevent umbilical hernia
Milk avoided because it causes large babies and difficult births		Religious medal worn by mother during pregnancy; placed around infant's neck
Many predictions about sex of baby	Bedrest for 3 days after birth	Infant protected from *mal ojo* ("evil eye")
May be unacceptable and frightening to have pelvic examination by male health care provider	Keep warm	Various remedies used to treat *mal ojo* and fallen fontanel (depressed fontanel)
	Delay bathing	
Use of herbs to treat common complaints of pregnancy	Mother's head and feet protected from cold air; bathing permitted after 14 days	
Drinking chamomile tea thought to ensure effective labor	Mother often cared for by her own mother	
	Forty-day restriction on sexual intercourse	
May wear ribbon or band around pregnant belly in belief that baby will be born healthy	Mother may want baby's first wet diaper to wipe her face in belief that it aids in making "mask of pregnancy" go away	

African-American		

(Members of the African-American community, many of whom are descendants of slaves, have different origins. Today a number of black Americans have emigrated from Africa, the West Indies, the Dominican Republic, Haiti, and Jamaica.)

Pregnancy	*Labor*	*Newborn*
Acceptance of pregnancy depends on economic status	Use of "Granny midwife" in certain parts of United States	Feeding very important:
		"Good" baby thought to eat well
Pregnancy thought to be state of "wellness," which is often the reason for delay in seeking prenatal care, especially by lower-income African-Americans	Varied emotional responses: some cry out, some display stoic behavior to avoid calling attention to selves	Early introduction of solid foods
		May breastfeed or bottle-feed; breastfeeding may be considered embarrassing
	Woman may arrive at hospital in far-advanced labor	Parents fearful of spoiling baby
Old wives' tales include beliefs that having a picture taken during pregnancy will cause stillbirth and reaching up will cause cord to strangle baby	Emotional support often provided by other women, especially the woman's own mother	Commonly call baby by nicknames
		May use excessive clothing to keep baby warm
	Postpartum	Belly band used to prevent umbilical hernia
Craving for certain foods, including chicken and greens, and nonfood substances such as clay, starch, and dirt	Vaginal bleeding seen as sign of sickness; tub baths and shampooing of hair prohibited	Abundant use of oil on baby's scalp and skin
	Sassafras tea thought to have healing power	Strong feeling of family, community, and religion
Pregnancy may be viewed by African-American men as a sign of their virility	Eating liver thought to cause heavier vaginal bleeding because of its high "blood" content	
Self-treatment for various discomforts of pregnancy, including constipation, nausea, vomiting, headache, and heartburn		

TABLE 2-2 TRADITIONAL CULTURAL BELIEFS AND PRACTICES: CHILDBEARING AND PARENTING—cont'd

PREGNANCY	CHILDBIRTH	PARENTING

Asian-American

(Typically refers to groups from China, Korea, the Philippines, Japan, Southeast Asia [particularly Thailand], Indochina, and Vietnam.)

Pregnancy	**Labor**	**Newborn**
Pregnancy considered time when mother "has happiness in her body"	Mother attended by other women, especially her own mother	Concept of family important and valued
Pregnancy seen as natural process	Father does not actively participate	Father is head of household; wife plays a subordinate role
Strong preference for female health care provider	Labor in silence	Birth of boy preferred
Belief in theory of hot and cold	Cesarean birth not desired	May delay naming child
May omit soy sauce in diet to prevent dark-skinned baby		Some groups (e.g., Vietnamese) believe colostrum is dirty; therefore they may delay breastfeeding until milk comes in
Prefer soup made with ginseng root as general strength tonic	**Postpartum**	
	Must protect self from *yin* (cold forces) for 30 days	
Milk usually excluded from diet because it causes stomach distress	Ambulation limited	
Inactivity or sleeping late may cause difficult birth	Shower and bathing prohibited	
	Warm room	
	Diet:	
	Warm fluids	
	Some women are vegetarians	
	Korean mother served seaweed soup with rice	
	Chinese diet high in hot foods	
	Chinese mother avoids fruits and vegetables	

European-American

(Members of the European-American [Caucasian] community have their origins in countries such as Ireland, Great Britain, Germany, Italy, and France.)

Pregnancy	**Labor**	**Newborn**
Pregnancy viewed as a condition that requires medical attention to ensure health	Birth is a public concern	Increased popularity of breastfeeding
Emphasis on early prenatal care	Technology dominated	Breastfeeding begins as soon as possible after childbirth
Variety of childbirth education programs available, and participation encouraged	Birthing process in institutional setting valued	
Technology driven	Involvement of father expected	**Parenting**
Emphasis on nutritional science	Physician seen as head of team	Motherhood and transition to parenting seen as stressful time
Involvement of the father valued	**Postpartum**	Nuclear family valued, although single-parenting and other forms of parenting more acceptable than in the past
Written sources of information valued	Emphasis or focus on early bonding	
	Medical interventions for dealing with discomfort	Women often deal with multiple roles
	Early ambulation and activity emphasized	Early return to prenatal activities
	Self-management valued	

Native American

(Many different tribes exist within the Native-American culture; viewpoints vary according to tribal customs and beliefs.)

Pregnancy	**Labor**	**Newborn**
Pregnancy considered a normal, natural process	Prefers female attendant, although husband, mother, or father may assist with birth	Infant not fed colostrum
Late prenatal care	Birth may be attended by whole family	Use of herbs to increase flow of milk
Avoid heavy lifting	Herbs may be used to promote uterine activity	Use of cradle boards for infant
Herb teas encouraged	Birth may occur in squatting position	Babies not handled often
	Postpartum	
	Herbal teas to stop bleeding	

Data from Amaro H: Women in the Mexican-American community: religion, culture, and reproductive attitudes and experiences, *J Comp Psychol* 16(1):6–19, 1994; Bar-Yam N: Learning about culture: a guide for birth practitioners, *Int J Childbirth Educ* 9(2):8–10, 1994; Galanti G: *Caring for patients from different cultures: case studies from American hospitals,* ed 2, Philadelphia, 1997, University of Pennsylvania Press; D'Avanzo C: *Mosby's pocket guide to cultural health assessment*, ed 4, St Louis, 2008, Mosby; Mattson S: Culturally sensitive prenatal care for Southeastern Asians, *J Obstet Gynecol Neonatal Nurs* 24(4):335–341, 1995; Spector R: *Cultural diversity in health and illness*, ed 8, Upper Saddle River, NJ, 2013, Prentice-Hall; Williams R: Issues in women's health care. In Johnson B, editor: *Psychiatric mental health nursing: adaptation and growth*, Philadelphia, 1989, JB Lippincott.

NOTE: Most of these cultural beliefs and customs reflect the traditional culture and are not universally practiced. These lists are not intended to stereotype patients but, rather, to serve as guidelines while discussing meaningful cultural beliefs with a woman and her family. Examples of other cultural beliefs and practices are found throughout this text.

*Variations in some beliefs and practices exist within subcultures of each group.

mammograms; men are encouraged to have prostate screening. Tertiary prevention focuses on rehabilitation of an individual to health as optimal as is possible in the presence of a disease or injury. For example, a person who has experienced a stroke has an optimal expectation of being able to function at his or her fullest potential. As nurses, we do what we can to ensure that this occurs.

During pregnancy, primarily primary and secondary prevention are relevant. The goal is to maintain a healthy pregnancy by preventing illness and by screening those at risk for potential illnesses or complications that could arise during pregnancy. In pregnancy, primary prevention might involve providing the influenza vaccine to women, whereas secondary prevention might involve performing an amniocentesis for a woman older than 35 years.

Promoting Family Health

Functioning within the social, cultural, environmental, and economic context of the community, the family becomes an integral component of community health-promotion efforts. For childbearing families, health promotion is focused primarily on early intervention through prenatal care and prevention of complications during the perinatal period. Often this early exposure to health information sets the stage for a successful birth and positive outcomes for mother and baby. The nurse's role in this process is focused on collaboration with the family, identifying risk factors, and providing health information to facilitate positive health behaviors. Involving expectant mothers and fathers in identification of their learning needs is an essential first step to securing their participation in the health-promotion process.

A wide variety of strategies have been used to engage families and groups in health-promoting activities or community health programs. Some are more successful than others. Generally, participant engagement in the planning process and empowerment to create internal solutions are considered key factors in effective interventions. Many communities have organized coalitions to address specific health-promotion agendas related to sharing information, educating community members, or advocating for health policies around maternal and child health issues. The benefits of partnership with faith-based organizations for community health improvement have been demonstrated in health-promotion efforts aimed at lifestyle choices, health education, and maternal-child health outcomes.

Prepared childbirth classes are a well-established mechanism for increasing awareness of healthy behaviors during pregnancy and preparing parents for the care of themselves and their newborn during the postpartum period. Mass media efforts such as those presented by the March of Dimes "Baby Your Baby" advertisements are clear consumer-friendly messages designed to reach a large target audience. Other venues include public health education in newspapers and magazines and health department programs such as the Special Supplemental Nutrition Program for Women, Infants, and Children (WIC), which offers a variety of health education and written information to mothers.

ASSESSING THE COMMUNITY

A community assessment is a tool that is used to assess the health and well-being of a community. One can define community either geographically or as having a common characteristic. For example, one can do a community assessment of people who live in a particular neighborhood or of women who have developed preterm labor. In doing the community assessment, risk factors for certain diseases, patterns of illness, cultural beliefs, religious beliefs, transportation systems, and support systems are just a few factors that are assessed to determine how these components relate to certain patterns of illness.

In a community health assessment, data are collected, analyzed, and used to educate and mobilize communities, develop priorities, garner resources, and plan actions to improve public health. Many models and frameworks of community assessment are available, but the actual process often depends on the extent and nature of the assessment to be performed, the time and resources available, and the way the information is to be used (http://assessnow.info/resources/models-of-community-health-assessment/view).

Data Collection and Sources of Community Health Data

Important measures of community health, for example, are access to care, level of provider services available, availability of transportation, and family support. Consideration of a variety of these factors helps one assess areas that may affect care so that nurses can introduce alternatives to meet the needs of patients. For example, if a woman has to work Monday through Friday, from 8 AM to 5 PM, the nurse can facilitate an after-hours appointment.

The most critical community indicators of perinatal health relate to access to care; maternal mortality; infant mortality; low birth weight; first-trimester prenatal care; and rates for mammography, Papanicolaou smears, and other similar screening tests. Nurses can use these indicators as a reflection of access, quality, and continuity of health care in a community. For women and infants, access to a consistent source of care is critical. Those with a regular source of care are more likely to use preventive services and have more positive pregnancy outcomes, but many women lack access to a usual source of care or rely primarily on emergency services.

Access to health care relates not only to the availability of health department services, hospitals, public clinics, clinic hours, or other sources of care but also to accessibility of care. In many areas where facilities and providers are available, geographic and transportation barriers render the care inaccessible for certain populations. This is particularly true in rural areas or other remote locations. Other barriers to care should also be evaluated including cultural and language barriers and lack of providers or specialty care. There is a growing trend in the United States to have walk-in clinics in grocery stores, an easily accessible location.

Health departments at the city, county, and state level are a valuable resource for annual reports of births and deaths. Local health departments also compile extensive statistics about the birth complications, causes of death, and leading causes of morbidity and mortality for each age-group. Local and state health data are compiled and reported through the Centers for Disease Control and Prevention (CDC) (www.cdc.gov) to the National Center for Health Statistics (NCHS) (www.cdc.gov/nchs). The National Health Survey published annually from this source describes national health trends. However, national data are only as accurate and reliable as the local data on which they are based, so caution is needed in interpreting the data and applying it to specific population groups.

The U.S. census provides data on population size, age ranges, sex, racial and ethnic distribution, socioeconomic status, educational level, employment, and housing characteristics. Summary data are available for most large metropolitan areas, arranged by zip code and census tract, which usually corresponds to a neighborhood comprising approximately 3000 to 6000 people. Looking at individual census tracts within a community helps identify sub-populations or aggregates whose needs may differ from those of the larger community. For example, women at high risk for inadequate prenatal care according to age, race, and ethnic or cultural group can be readily identified and outreach activities appropriately targeted.

Other sources of useful information are hospitals and voluntary health agencies. The March of Dimes Foundation, for example, has supported perinatal needs assessments in many communities across the United States (www.modimes.org). Other community health resources include health care providers or administrators, government officials, religious leaders, and representatives of voluntary health agencies. Community or county health councils exist in many areas, with oversight of specific health initiatives or programs for that region. These key informants often provide a unique perspective that may not be accessible through other sources. Community gatekeepers who address the social and health care needs of the population are also critical links to population-specific health information.

Professional associations and publications are rich and readily accessible sources of information for all nurses. Professional associations publish standards and position papers that are useful. In addition to nursing and public health journals, behavioral and social science literature offers diverse perspectives on community health status for specific populations and subgroups. The Internet has increased the availability and accessibility of national, state, and local health data as well. However, the use of Internet-based resources for health information requires caution because data reliability and validity are difficult to verify. Guidelines for evaluation of Internet health resources can be found on the "Health on the Net" website (www.hon.ch).

Data collection methods may be either qualitative (e.g., by discussion, interview, observation) or quantitative (e.g., number, mean, standard deviation, percent of data collected) and may include visual surveys that can be completed by walking through a community, participant observation, interviews, focus groups, and analysis of existing data. Potential patients and health care consumers may be asked to participate in focus groups or community forums to present their views on needed community services and programs. Formal surveys, conducted by mail, telephone, the Internet, or face-to-face interviews, can be a valuable source of information not available from national databases or other secondary sources. Several drawbacks exist with this method—surveys are generally expensive to develop and time-consuming to administer. In addition to the cost of such surveys, poor response rates often preclude a sufficiently representative response on which to base nursing interventions.

A walking survey is generally conducted by a walk-through observation of the community (Box 2-4), taking note of specific characteristics of the population, economic and social environment, transportation, health care services, and other resources. With this type of data collection, information is gathered based on what the data collector observes and is clearly objective data. Participant observation is another useful assessment method in which the nurse actively participates in the community to understand the community more fully and to validate observations. As part of the assessment process, nurses working in multiethnic and multicultural groups need an in-depth assessment of culturally based health behaviors.

Analysis and synthesis of data obtained during the assessment process help generate a comprehensive picture of the community's health status, needs, and problem areas, as well as its strengths and resources for addressing these concerns. The goal of this process is to assign priorities to community health needs and to develop a plan of action for correcting them. A comparison of community health

---

BOX 2-4   COMMUNITY WALK-THROUGH

As you observe the community, take note of the following:

- **Physical environment**—Older neighborhood or newer subdivision? Sidewalks, streets, and buildings in good or poor repair? Billboards and signs? What are they advertising? Are lawns kept up? Is there trash in the streets? Parks or playgrounds? Parking lots? Empty lots? Industries?
- **People in the area**—Old, young, homeless, children; predominant ethnicity, language? Is the population homogeneous? What signs do you see of different cultural groups?
- **Stores and services available**—Restaurants: chain, local, ethnic? Grocery stores: neighborhood or chain? Department stores, gas stations, real estate or insurance offices, travel agencies, pawn shops, liquor stores, discount or thrift stores, newspaper stands?
- **Social**—Clubs, bars, fraternal organizations (e.g., Elks, American Legion), museums?
- **Religious**—Churches, synagogues, mosques? What denominations? Do you see evidence of their use other than on religious/holy days?
- **Health services**—Drugstores, physicians' offices, clinics, dentists, mental health services, veterinarians, urgent care facilities, hospitals, shelters, nursing homes, home health agencies, public health services, traditional healers (e.g., herbalists, palmists)?
- **Transportation**—Cars, buses, taxis, light rail, sidewalks, bicycle paths, access for disabled persons?
- **Education**—Schools, before- and after-school programs, child care, libraries, bookstores? What is the reputation of the schools?
- **Government**—What is the governance structure? Is there a mayor? City council? Are meetings open to the public? Are there signs of political activity (e.g., posters, campaign signs)?
- **Safety**—How safe is the community? What is the crime rate? What types of crimes are committed? Are police visible? Is there a fire station?
- **Evaluation of the community based on your observations**—What is your impression of the community? Is the environment pleasing? Are services and transportation adequate? How difficult is it for residents to obtain needed services (i.e., how far do they have to travel)? Would you want to live in this community? Why or why not?

---

data with state and national statistics can help identify appropriate target populations and develop interventions to improve health outcomes.

Vulnerable Populations in the Community

Assessment of population health includes indicators related to diverse groups and cultures, particularly disenfranchised or "vulnerable" community members. Vulnerability in terms of health status and health outcomes may take many forms, including sociocultural, economic, and environmental risk factors that contribute to disparities in health. Health disparities are conditions that disproportionately affect certain racial, ethnic, or other groups. African-Americans, Hispanic-Americans, Native Americans, Pacific Islanders, and Asian-Americans are all considered vulnerable populations because they are more likely to have poor health and die prematurely (see Chapter 1).

Women

Women make up 51% of the U.S. population, representing a very diverse and largely at-risk, group in relation to health (U.S. Census Bureau, 2011). Although women assume leadership for health care decision making in most families, they also face significant challenges in accessing the health care system and meeting their own health needs and those of family members. Although there is no single contributing factor, the primary sources of health disparities for women fall into the areas of gender, socioeconomic status, and race or ethnicity. Significant gaps exist in the quality of care for women when compared with men.

The *National Report Card on Women's Health* describes significant deficiencies in women's health (National Women's Law Center [NWLC], 2010). States' performance in relation to 26 graded indicators was assessed; all but 3 were rated as *unsatisfactory* in relation to women's health status and policies influencing women's health. Key indicators focused on access to services, use of preventive health care and health promotion-activities, the occurrence of certain health conditions, and an assessment of the community's effect on women's health. This report suggested that one of the primary factors compromising women's health is lack of access to acceptable-quality health care, which may manifest itself in many forms: lack of health insurance, living in a medically underserved area, or an inability to obtain needed services, particularly basic services such as prenatal care. With the enactment of the Patient Protection and Affordable Care Act, many of the policy goals will be realized as the Act is implemented (NWLC, 2010).

Although many women report that they are in good to excellent health, statistics reveal significant disparities in health status of women from all age-groups and racial and ethnic backgrounds. Low levels of educational attainment (high school or lower) are also associated with lack of resources and difficulty navigating the health care system. This is particularly true of women of ethnic and racial minorities, whose limited English proficiency may compromise provider access and quality of care.

Racial and Ethnic Minorities

In addition to social, economic, and cultural barriers to optimal health, women who are in racial and ethnic minorities experience a disproportionate burden of disease, disability, and premature death. Significant health disparities continue to exist in adult women's health and the health of their infants. Although positive trends are evident, disparities persist among racial and ethnic groups in early prenatal care, an important factor in achieving healthy pregnancy outcomes.

Minority women, many of whom live in poverty, also have higher rates of chronic disease including heart disease, cancer, hepatitis, and acquired immunodeficiency syndrome (AIDS), as well as mental health issues. Women with underlying health conditions are at especially high risk for poor obstetric outcomes for themselves and their infants. They have high rates of preterm labor and gestational hypertension and often have intrauterine growth restriction resulting in the birth of infants who are small for gestational age. These are the women for whom the community-based perinatal nurse will be providing care, and their needs are complex, demanding high levels of expertise and skill.

Adolescent Girls

The adolescent population in the United States is generally considered healthy. However, adolescents participate in riskier behaviors and their health is often compromised as a result. Although adolescents are concerned about becoming pregnant, they still engage in unprotected sex. Adolescents also use a variety of sources for health information—the media, friends, and sex education—yet they are very misinformed, particularly about sexually transmitted infections (STIs) and human immunodeficiency virus (HIV) transmission.

These findings have significant implications for perinatal outcomes and emphasize the importance of aggressive prevention programs and community outreach related to sexuality, teen pregnancy, and substance abuse.

It is crucial that nurses engage adolescents in health education programs that will encourage them to make informed decisions about their sexual health. It is also vital that nurses be a resource to these young women.

Older Women

Although women have a longer life expectancy than men, they are more likely to have chronic illnesses, less likely to use preventive services, and ultimately spend more on health care. As nurses, it is important that we engage this population at all levels of prevention, from primary to tertiary.

Incarcerated Women

The number of incarcerated women in the United States has continued to climb in recent years, increasing at a significantly greater rate than for men. In 2010 there were 113,000 women incarcerated in state and federal facilities, with the highest number of these being non-Hispanic black women (Sipes, 2012). Many of these women report a history of sexual and physical abuse.

Because their relationship histories are often unstable and because they often lack the support of family, incarcerated women or those with a history of repeated incarceration frequently have difficulty providing emotional stability, secure housing, and health-promotion role modeling for their children.

The lifestyle choices of this group, including risky sexual relationships, illicit drug use, and smoking, place them at high risk for STIs, HIV, and AIDS; other chronic and communicable diseases; and complicated pregnancies.

Immigrant, Refugee, and Migrant Women

As of 2010 nearly 40 million or 13% of the population in the United States were foreign born (Grieco, Acosta, del al Cruz, et al., 2012). This accounts for a rapidly growing diverse population for which nurses will be providing care.

An immigrant is an individual who moves from one country to another in an effort to take up legal residency, whereas a refugee is an individual who is forced to leave his or her home country, often in search of a safer and more stable living environment. Both populations are often challenged with not being able to easily access health care because they are not U.S. citizens. These women often do not seek medical care for fear of deportation. Access to care is further limited by health care policies that restrict Medicaid eligibility for these groups.

Along with their profound resilience and determination, refugees and immigrants have brought rich diversity to the United States in several important dimensions including cultural heritage and customs, economic productivity, and enhanced national vitality. In general, refugees are more likely to live in poverty than are immigrants. Over time, measures of health and well-being actually decline for the immigrant population as they become part of American society. Many of the conditions or illnesses that they acquire contribute to the persistence of disparities in maternal and neonatal health outcomes for both immigrants and refugees.

Migrant workers are those who work outside their home country or migrate within their own country seeking seasonal work. Migrant laborers and their families face many problems, including financial instability, child labor, poor housing, lack of education, language and cultural barriers, and limited access to health and social services.

Poor dental health, diabetes, hypertension, malnutrition, tuberculosis, skin diseases, and parasitic infections are common health issues among migrant populations. Primary health care services are largely provided by a number of migrant health centers, of which there are more than 400 throughout the United States. In 2011 more than 862,808 seasonal and migrant farm workers and their families were served (U.S. Department of Health and Human Services [USDHHS], 2011). Routine prenatal care, as well as screening and treatment for hypertension and diabetes, is provided. Community health nurses frequently encounter the challenges of providing culturally and linguistically appropriate care while facing numerous health issues.

Numerous reproductive health issues exist for migrant women, including less consistent use of contraception and increased rates of STIs. Migrants are less likely to receive early prenatal care and have a greater incidence of inadequate weight gain during pregnancy than do other poor women (see Community Focus box).

Rural Versus Urban Community Settings

Approximately 16% of the U.S. population live in a rural area (Rural Assistance Center, 2011). Generally, rural residents are older, less educated, and in poorer health than their urban counterparts. Rural communities are disproportionately affected by poverty and poor access to health care services. Fewer physicians choose to practice in rural areas. Lack of insurance presents an additional factor for poor health in rural areas.

Rural women are especially vulnerable to financial and transportation barriers to health care. Although women in rural counties report only fair to poor health, they pay considerably more for their health care. In rural communities, women have less access to prenatal care, which contributes to higher rates of adverse pregnancy outcomes including higher rates of preterm birth, low birth weight, and infant mortality. The disproportionate distribution of poverty and of variations in race/ethnicity, age, education, and availability and access to medical resources may be the link to infant mortality in rural areas.

Homeless Women

Homelessness among women is an increasing social and health issue in the United States. Although exact numbers are unknown because of the difficulty in tracking individuals without a permanent address, it is estimated that more than 636,000 people were homeless in 2011 (Homelessness in America, 2012). Single women make up 13% of the homeless population and are often on the street to escape domestic violence (Dray, 2012). Families with children make up the fastest-growing group of the homeless. In these families, one in five children experienced food insecurity (did not have enough to eat) in 2010 (National Coalition for the Homeless, 2011).

Health issues among the homeless are numerous and result primarily from a lack of preventive care and a lack of resources in general. Health problems include chronic illness, infectious diseases, asthma, circulatory problems, diabetes, substance abuse, and mental illness. Lifestyle factors and the vulnerability resulting from being homeless contribute to health problems. Women are at increased risk for illness and injury; many have been victims of domestic abuse, assault, and rape. Although little is known about pregnancy in this population, women do become pregnant while homeless. In addition to risk factors related to inadequate nutrition, inadequate weight gain, anemia, bleeding problems, and preterm birth, homeless women face multiple barriers to prenatal care: transportation, distance, and wait times. Most of these women underutilize available prenatal services. The unsafe environment and high risk lifestyles often result in adverse perinatal outcomes (American College of Obstetricians and Gynecologists [ACOG], 2010; Richards, Merrill, and Baksh, 2011). The United States has initiated programs to address these problems. For example, the U.S. Interagency Council on Homelessness and its 19 member agencies launched *Opening Doors,* the federal strategic plan to prevent and end homelessness in 2010 and updated it in 2011 (Opening Doors, 2012).

Implications for Nursing

Working in the community or in the home with the full spectrum of family organizational styles, vulnerable populations, and cultural groups presents challenges for nurses. Whether it involves perinatal care focused on women and their newborns or women's health care directed toward treatment and prevention of other health conditions such as communicable diseases and sexually transmitted infections, nursing must exhibit a high degree of professionalism. Cultural sensitivity, compassion, and a critical awareness of family dynamics and social stressors that will affect health-related decision making are critical components in developing an effective plan of care.

Although the long-term consequences of contemporary immigration for American society are unclear, the successful incorporation of immigrant families depends on the resources, benefits, and policies that ensure their healthy development and successful social adjustment. Culturally competent health care and involvement of the immigrant community in health care programs are recommended strategies for improving the access to and effectiveness of health care for this population.

The use of camp volunteers has been effective in assisting families living in migrant worker camps to obtain prenatal, postpartum, and infant care. Working in partnership with health care professionals such as nurses, lay camp aides have been used effectively for outreach and health education; however, more strategies are needed to link traditional practices with the formal health care system. Guidance and information about other health resources are available to health care providers through the National Center for Farmworker Health, Inc. (www.ncfh.org) and the Migrant Clinicians Network (www.migrantclinician.org).

Nurses working with homeless women and families are challenged to treat them with dignity and respect to establish a **therapeutic relationship. Case management** is recommended to coordinate the services and disciplines that may be involved in meeting the complex needs of these families. Whenever possible, general screening and preventive health services must be provided

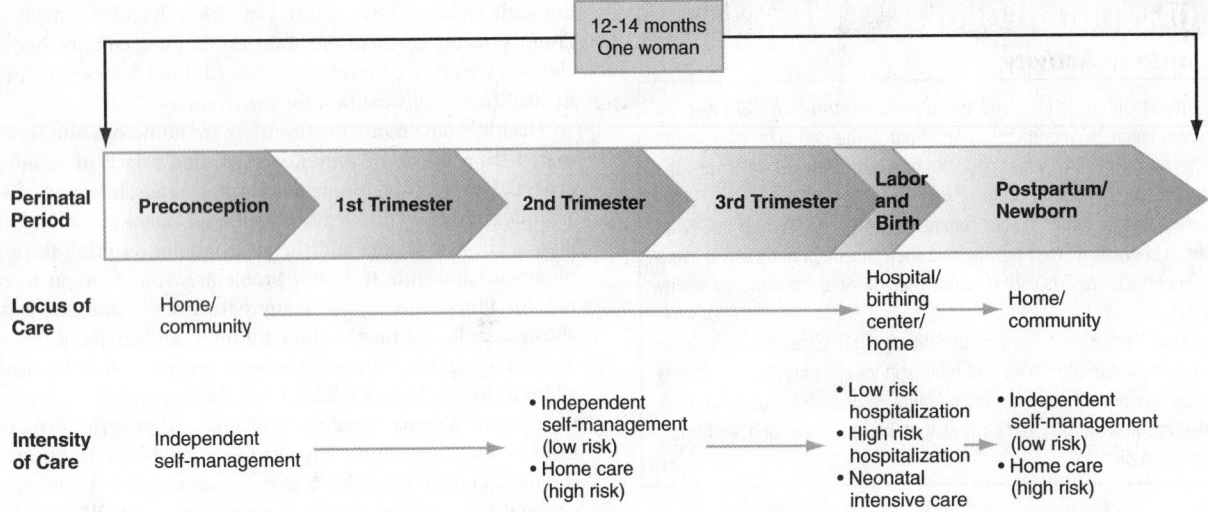

FIG 2-7 Perinatal continuum of care.

when the woman seeks treatment, because this may be the only opportunity to provide health information and intervention. Building on existing coping strategies and strengths, the health care provider helps the woman and her family reconnect with a social support system. Nurses also have an important role in advocating for funding to support health care services to the homeless and to improve access to preventive care for all homeless populations.

HOME CARE IN THE COMMUNITY

Modern home care nursing has its foundation in public health nursing, which provided comprehensive care to sick and well patients in their own homes. Specialized maternity home care nursing services began in the 1980s when public health maternity nursing services were limited and services had not kept pace with the changing practices of high risk obstetrics and emerging technology. Lengthy antepartum hospitalizations for such conditions as preterm labor and gestational hypertension created nursing care challenges for staff members of inpatient units.

Many women expressed their concern about the negative effect of antepartum hospitalizations on the family. Although clinical indications showed that a new nursing care approach was needed, home health care did not become a viable alternative until third-party payers (i.e., public or private organizations or employer groups that pay for health care) pushed for cost containment in maternity services.

In the current health care system, home care is an important component of health care delivery along the perinatal continuum of care (Fig. 2-7). The growing demand for home care is based on several factors:

- Interest in family birthing alternatives
- Shortened hospital stays
- New technologies that facilitate home-based assessments and treatments
- Reimbursement by third-party payers

As health care costs continue to rise and millions of American families lack health insurance, there is greater demand for innovative, cost-effective methods of health care delivery in the community. Large health care systems are developing clinically integrated health care delivery networks whose goals are (1) improved coordination of care and care outcomes; (2) better communication among health

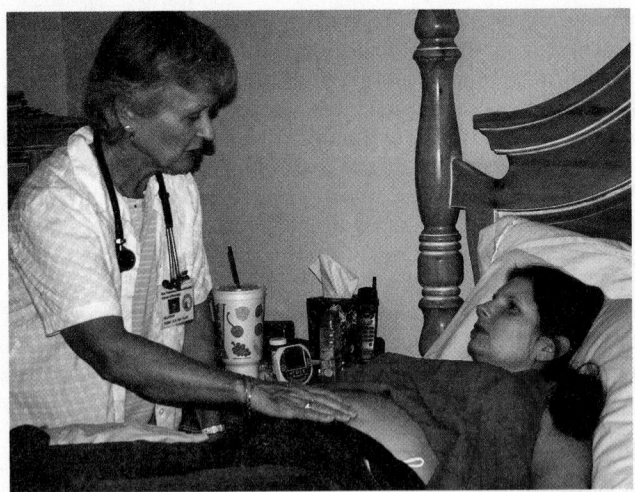

FIG 2-8 Home care nurse visits with a woman in preterm labor at home on bedrest. (Courtesy Shannon Perry, Phoenix, AZ.)

care providers; (3) increased patient, payer, and provider satisfaction; and (4) reduced cost. The integration of clinical services changes the focus of care to a continuum of services that are increasingly community based.

Communication and Technology Applications

As maternity care continues to consist of frequent and brief contacts with health care providers throughout the prenatal and postpartum periods, services that link maternity patients throughout the perinatal continuum of care have assumed increasing importance. These services include critical pathways, telephonic nursing assessments, discharge planning, specialized education programs, parent support groups, home visiting programs, nurse advice lines, and perinatal home care (Fig. 2-8). Hospitals may provide cross-training for hospital-based nurses to make postpartum home visits or to staff outpatient centers for postpartum follow-up.

Telephonic nursing care through services such as warm lines, nurse advice lines, and telephonic nursing assessments is a valuable means of managing health care problems and bridging the gaps among acute, outpatient, and home care services. Providers are using the Internet to communicate with patients who have an Internet service provider (ISP). Nursing care that occurs by telephone is interactive and responsive to immediate health care questions about particular health care needs. Warm lines are telephone lines that are offered as a community service to provide new parents with support, encouragement, and basic parenting education. Nurse advice lines, or toll-free nurse consultation services, often are supported by third-party payers or health maintenance organizations/managed care organizations (HMOs/MCOs) and are designed to provide answers to medical questions. Nurse care managers are prepared to guide callers through urgent health care situations, suggest treatment options, and provide health education. Telephonic nursing assessments or nurse consultation, assessment, and health education that take place during a telephone conversation can be added to the plan of care in conjunction with skilled nursing visits, or they may comprise a separate nursing contact for the woman. Telephonic nursing assessments are commonly used after a postpartum home care visit to reassess a woman's knowledge about the signs and symptoms of adequate hydration in breastfeeding or, after initiating home phototherapy, to assess the caregiver's knowledge regarding problems with equipment.

Guidelines for Nursing Practice

The Association of Women's Health, Obstetric, and Neonatal Nurses (AWHONN, 2009) defines home care as the provision of technical, psychologic, and other therapeutic support in the woman's home rather than in an institution. The scope of nursing care delivered in the home is necessarily limited to practices deemed safe and appropriate to be carried out in an environment that is physically separated from a health care institution and its resources. Nursing practice at home is consistent with federal and state regulations that direct home care practice. The nurse demonstrates practice competence through formalized orientation and ongoing clinical education and performance evaluation in the respective home care agency. Standards for practice from key specialty organizations such as AWHONN, the National Association of Neonatal Nurses (NANN), the ACOG, the American Academy of Pediatrics (AAP), and the Intravenous Nursing Society (INS) provide the basis for clinical protocols and pathways and organizational programs in home care practice. The Joint Commission (www.jointcommission.org) provides criteria for home care operations based on Centers for Medicare & Medicaid Services (CMS) regulations (cms.hhs.gov).

A wide range of professional health care services and products can be delivered or used in the home by means of technology and telecommunication. For example, telehealth and telemedicine make it possible for patients in the home to be interviewed and assessed by a specialist located hundreds of miles away. Home health care can be viewed as an extension of in-hospital care. Essentially, the primary difference between health care in a hospital and home care is the absence of the continuous presence of professional health care providers in a patient's home. Generally, but not always, home health care entails intermittent care by a professional who visits the patient's home for a particular reason and/or provides care onsite for fewer than 4 hours at a time. The home health care agency maintains on-call professional staff to assist home care patients who have questions about their care and for emergencies, such as equipment failure.

Perinatal Services

Home care perinatal services may be provided by hospital-based programs, independent proprietary (for-profit) agencies, or nonprofit home care agencies and by official or tax-supported agencies. Innovative programs may be supported by research grants for a period of years, but ultimately they must be sponsored by an agency with long-term funding. Home visits have advantages and disadvantages. The pregnant woman can maintain bedrest if indicated, and vulnerable neonates are not exposed to the weather or external sources of infection. The nurse can observe and interact with family members in their most natural and secure environment. Adequacy of resources and safety factors can be assessed. Teaching can be tailored to the actual home conditions, and other family members can be included. A home visit is less expensive than a day's hospitalization, but a 60- to 90-minute visit requires 2.5 to 3 hours of nursing time, including travel and documentation. Areas of challenge include limited availability of nurses with expertise in maternity care and concerns about the nurse's physical safety in the community. One alternative that is less expensive is contacting women via telephone.

Visits for outreach and health promotion are an integral part of community (or public) health nursing. In countries with national health systems, a nurse or midwife may see all women during pregnancy and after birth. In the United States, visits of this sort have been provided mainly to low-income families without health insurance and Medicaid recipients who use the clinics provided by local health departments. Until recently, private insurers did not reimburse for health-promotion visits. MCOs now recognize that anticipatory guidance can be cost-effective, but home visitation programs for the most part still target specific, high risk populations, such as adolescents and women at risk for preterm labor.

Home care agencies are subject to regulation by governmental and professional organizations and provide interdisciplinary services including social work, nutrition, and occupational and physical therapy. Increasingly, their caseloads are made up of women who require high-technology care, such as infusions or home monitoring. Although the home health nurse develops the care plan, all care must be ordered by a physician. In addition, interventions must meet the insurer's criteria for reimbursement and services are limited to registered patients. Preconception care and low risk antepartum care can usually be provided more efficiently in offices and are not currently reimbursable. High risk antepartum care can be provided by home care agencies; for example, women with hyperemesis gravidarum who require parenteral nutrition may be treated at home. Conditions requiring bedrest, such as preterm labor and hypertension, are other common indications for home care. Other conditions often managed with home care may include cardiac disease, substance abuse, and diabetes in pregnancy.

Insurers may reimburse for at least one postpartum visit to families after early discharge or in the presence of high risk factors. Phototherapy for treatment of neonatal hyperbilirubinemia can be used at home, allowing the mother and infant to be discharged to home together. Many other neonates who require long-term high-technology care are also managed with home care.

Patient Selection and Referral

The office or hospital-based nurse is often the key person in making effective referrals to home care. When considering a referral to home care, these factors are evaluated:

- Health status of mother and fetus or infant: Is the condition serious enough to warrant home care, and is it stable enough for intermittent observation to be sufficient?
- Availability of professionals to provide the needed services within the woman's community.

- Family resources, including psychosocial, social, and economic resources: Will the family be able to provide care between nursing visits? Are relationships supportive? Is third-party reimbursement available, or can it be negotiated with the insurer? Could a voluntary or tax-supported community agency provide needed care without payment?
- Cost-effectiveness: Is it more reasonable for the woman to receive these services at home or to go to a local outpatient facility to receive them?

Community referrals should not be limited to women with physiologic complications of pregnancy that require medical treatment. Women at risk (e.g., young adolescents, families with a history of abuse, members of vulnerable population groups, developmentally disabled individuals) may need follow-up care at home. As we move more and more into an interdisciplinary health care society, it is crucial that nurses communicate with social workers to tap into valuable community resources that women can use in their own communities after being discharged.

Standardized forms simplify the referral process and ensure that all needed information will be forwarded to the home health agency. The nursing assessment should include the woman's physical and psychologic status, her level of knowledge about self-management activities, her willingness to learn, the availability of caregivers and social support in the home, and her level of comfort with home care. If the referral is for a mother-and-infant home care visit, the nursing assessment should include newborn data.

High-technology home care requires additional information to be collected from the chart and consultation with the referring physician and other members of the health care team before a home care referral is made. These additional data include the medical diagnosis, medical prognosis, prescribed therapies, medication history, drug-dosing information, potential ancillary supplies, type of infusion and access device, and the available systems of social support for the woman and family. The nursing assessment and therapy data provide baseline information for the home care nurse and other health care providers involved in the care plan.

Whenever a referral is called in to a home health care agency, a member of the nursing or admissions staff determines the agency's ability to accept the woman for service. The use of telecommunication modalities such as fax machines, cellular phones, electronic files, and the Internet to transmit information has eliminated delays in initiating home care services, even in more remote rural areas.

CARE MANAGEMENT

Preparing for the Home Visit

The home care nurse reviews the available clinical data, demographic information, and completed care plan form and consults with the home care pharmacist or other health care team members who have previously contacted the woman to determine the goals of the visit. At this point, the nurse uses the medical diagnosis and the location of the case on the perinatal continuum as a starting point to organize the woman's care. The nurse reviews agency policies and procedures, professional literature about diagnosis, and community resources as part of the pre-visit preparation work (Box 2-5).

Before going on a home visit, the nurse schedules a time for the visit with the woman. It is essential that the nurse obtain clear driving directions at this time as well.

The nurse identifies herself or himself by name, title, and agency. She or he then explains who referred the woman to the agency for home care and the purpose of the home care visits. The nurse briefly explains what will occur during the visit and approximately how long the visit will last. The woman should be asked to restrain any pets during the visit. Last, the nurse asks about health supplies that may be needed for the woman's care.

First Home Care Visit

Making the first home care visit can be stressful for the nurse and the woman. The home care nurse is faced with an unknown environment controlled by the woman and her family. The woman and her family also experience feelings about the unknown, such as anxiety about the way the nurse will treat them or what the nurse will do during the visit. The challenge for the home care nurse is to establish a positive nurse-patient relationship and provide the prescribed home care services within the time provided for the initial home visit.

Implementing the following will generally make the home visit more comfortable for both the nurse and the woman: the nurse wears identification, introduces herself upon entering the home, clearly states the purpose of the visit, obtains written consent for the visit, provides privacy as desired by the woman, provides culturally sensitive care, and encourages the woman and family to become actively involved in the care provided. One of the most important roles of the home care nurse is modeling health-related behaviors for the woman and others who are in the home during the visit.

ASSESSMENT AND NURSING DIAGNOSES

The primary goals of the assessment phase are to develop a trusting relationship and collect data by various methods to obtain a comprehensive patient profile. It may not be feasible or appropriate to collect in-depth information about all areas of assessment during the first visit. However, in many instances the nurse may be limited to one visit and must obtain information pertinent to the current situation in that hour.

The major areas of the assessment are demographics, medical history, general health history, medication history, psychosocial assessment (Box 2-6), home and community environment, and physical assessment. Information can be obtained from patient records sent to the home care agency at the time of referral or from the pre-visit interview. These data will be used to develop the nursing care plan and complete the plan of care, which is required for many licensed home health care agencies.

Each plan of care has a different emphasis in the home environment. For example, women receiving infusion therapy for hyperemesis gravidarum need a safe place to store medications and infusion supplies that is out of reach of small children living in the home. The home care nurse should incorporate the agency policies and procedures for the storage and handling of infusion supplies into her walk-through inspection. During the walk-through, the home care nurse looks at the potential storage areas that are dry and clean and where the temperature can be maintained. The home care nurse should include an inspection of work areas such as countertops, tabletops, sinks, and trash areas that the woman or caregiver may use for mixing medications, changing infusion tubing, handling supplies, or disposing of used equipment and supplies.

The homes of women using electronic home health care equipment, such as phototherapy equipment or infusion pumps, require physical inspection of any electrical outlets, electrical cords, and extension cords that will be used. Homes with faulty electrical wiring may place the woman at risk for being involved in an electrical fire; faulty wiring may require inspection and repair by a

BOX 2-5   PROTOCOL FOR PERINATAL HOME VISITS

Pre-visit Interventions

1. Contact the family to arrange details for home visit.
   a. Identify self, credentials, and agency role.
   b. Review purpose of home visit follow-up.
   c. Schedule convenient time for visit.
   d. Confirm address and route to family home.
2. Review and clarify appropriate data.
   a. Review all available assessment data for mother and fetus or infant (i.e., referral forms, hospital discharge summaries, identified learning needs of the family).
   b. Review records of any previous nursing contacts.
   c. Contact other professional caregivers as necessary to clarify data (e.g., obstetrician, nurse-midwife, pediatrician, referring nurse).
3. Identify community resources and teaching materials appropriate to meet those needs already identified.
4. Plan the visit, and prepare a bag with equipment, supplies, and materials necessary for assessments of mother and fetus or infant, actual care anticipated, and teaching.

In-Home Interventions: Establishing a Relationship

1. Reintroduce yourself, and establish the purpose of the visit for mother, infant, and family; offer the family the opportunity to clarify their expectations of the contact.
2. Spend a brief time socially interacting with the family to become acquainted and establish a trusting relationship.

In-Home Interventions: Working with the Family

1. Conduct a systematic assessment of the mother and the fetus or newborn to determine their physiologic adjustment and any existing complications (see Fig. 2-8).
2. Throughout the visit, collect data to assess the emotional adjustment of individual family members to the pregnancy or birth and lifestyle changes. Note any evidence of family-newborn bonding and sibling rivalry; note relationships among mother, father, children, and grandparents.
3. Determine the adequacy of the support system.
   a. To what extent does someone help with cooking, cleaning, and other home-management tasks?
   b. To what extent is help being provided in caring for the newborn and any other children?
   c. Are support persons encouraging the new mother to care for herself and get adequate rest?
   d. Who is providing helpful information? Emotional support?
4. Throughout the visit, observe the home environment for adequacy of resources.
   a. Space: privacy, safe play of children, sleeping
   b. Overall cleanliness and state of repair

c. Number of steps pregnant woman/new mother must climb
d. Adequacy of cooking arrangements
e. Adequacy of refrigeration and other food storage areas
f. Adequacy of bathing, toilet, and laundry facilities
g. Arrangements in home for newborn: sleeping, bathing, formula preparation (if needed), layette items, and diapers

5. Throughout the visit, observe the home environment for overall state of repair and existence of safety hazards.
   a. Storage of medications, household cleaners, and other substances hazardous to children
   b. Presence of peeling paint on furniture, walls, or pipes
   c. Factors that contribute to falls, such as dim lighting, broken steps, scatter rugs
   d. Presence of vermin
   e. Use of crib or playpen that fails to meet safety guidelines
   f. Existence of emergency plan in case of fire; fire alarm or extinguisher
6. Provide care to the mother, the newborn, or both as prescribed by their respective primary care provider or in accord with agency protocol.
7. Provide teaching on the basis of previously identified needs.
8. Refer the family to appropriate community agencies or resources, such as warm lines and support groups.
9. Ensure that the woman knows potential problems to watch for and who to call if they occur.
10. Ensure that used disposable items have been handled appropriately and that reusable items are cleaned and repacked appropriately in the nurse's bag.

In-Home Interventions: Ending the Visit

1. Summarize the activities and main points of the visit.
2. Clarify future expectations, including the schedule of the next visit.
3. Review the teaching plan and provide major points in writing.
4. Provide information about reaching the nurse or agency if needed before the next scheduled visit.

Post-visit Interventions

1. Document the visit thoroughly, using the necessary agency forms to serve as a legal record of the visit and to allow third-party reimbursement, as possible.
2. Initiate the plan of care on which the next encounter with the woman and/or family will be based.
3. Communicate appropriately (e.g., by telephone, letter, progress notes, or referral form) with the primary care provider, other health care professionals, or referral agencies on behalf of the woman and family.

BOX 2-6   PSYCHOSOCIAL ASSESSMENT

Language

- Identify the primary language spoken in the home.
- Assess whether there are any language barriers to receiving support.

Community Resources/Access to Care

- Identify primary and secondary means of transportation.
- Identify community agencies family uses for health care and support.
- Assess cultural and psychosocial barriers to receiving care.

Social Support

- Determine the people living with the pregnant woman.
- Identify who assists with household chores.
- Identify who assists with child care and parenting activities.
- Identify who the pregnant woman turns to for problems or during a crisis.

Interpersonal Relationships

- Identify the way decisions are made in the family.

- Identify the family's perception of the need for home care.
- Identify roles of adults in caring for family members.

Caregiver

- Identify the primary caregiver for home care treatments.
- Identify other caregivers and their roles.
- Assess the caregiver's knowledge of treatments and the care process.
- Identify potential strain from the caregiver role.
- Identify the level of satisfaction with the caregiver role.

Stress and Coping

- Identify what the woman perceives as lifestyle changes and their effect on her and her family.
- Identify the changes she and her family have made to adjust to her health condition and home health care treatments.

professional electrician before electronic devices are used. Findings from the assessment are incorporated into the plan of care.

The nursing plan of care is developed in collaboration with the woman, based on her health care needs. Home care nurses working in home health care agencies regulated by the CMS use a plan of care that includes patient demographics, the health care provider's orders, home care goals, and the woman's level of functioning. This document is initiated at the time of referral to the home care agency and must be updated every 60 days or as specified by state regulations. The frequency of the skilled nursing visit may vary with the individual plan of care and reimbursement criteria established by the third-party payers.

Nursing Considerations

There are several areas of concern when caring for a woman in the home. In home care, the woman or family members are responsible for administration of medications in the absence of the nurse. A careful medication history should be obtained to see if the woman is taking her medications correctly and understands their desired action and potential side effects. It is important that women and

NURSING CARE PLAN

Community and Home Care

NURSING DIAGNOSIS	EXPECTED OUTCOME	NURSING INTERVENTIONS	RATIONALES
Readiness for Enhanced Family Coping related to family growth and development in new community	The family will identify at least three community groups that can serve as appropriate resources for an expectant family with small children.	Assess family structure and availability of significant others, friends, or family members to assist family with new baby and siblings	To provide database for further interventions
		Encourage family to enlist assistance of individuals who are available to help family at birth of new baby	To provide physical and emotional support
		Using therapeutic communication, assist family to assess coping strategies used in the past for new situations	To provide clarification and promote empowerment of family in new situations
		Suggest strategies to find resources available in community	To assist family during pregnancy, with new baby, and with small siblings
		Give information regarding community workshops, classes, or support groups	To promote networking, community bonding, and support
Deficient Community Health related to resettlement of refugees in the community	The community will develop programs to meet the needs of new members of the community.	Conduct needs assessment of community	To identify priority needs for new members of community
		Initiate health education programs based on topics identified in needs assessment	To meet needs of members of community
		Prepare patient education materials in a variety of languages	To enhance understanding of community members
		Identify risks in community (e.g., environmental hazards, drug sales)	To provide target for community improvement
		With community leaders, develop plan to cope with and reduce environmental hazards	To improve public health and safety
		Develop monitoring or surveillance system	To ensure that progress will continue and new problems will be identified
Ineffective Community Coping related to presence of gangs and lack of community programs to redirect activities of youth	The health status of the community will improve.	Initiate health screening programs for community members	To identify effects of environmental hazards in community
		Work with politicians and policy makers to develop community	To provide safe environment with means of economic survival for community members
		Initiate programs such as Block Watch, Safe Houses, and Neighborhood Watch	To enhance safety of environment
		Work with community leaders to develop or clean up playgrounds	To provide safe place for children to play
		With community leaders, develop community grassroots initiatives	To enable community members to take ownership in community
		Identify sites of lead exposure	To decrease potential for lead poisoning in children
		Participate in immunization or vaccination clinics	To reduce risk in community of infectious diseases
		Develop community education programs on drugs, alcohol, and tobacco	To reduce exposure of young people to these products

caregivers have a clear understanding of medication regimens and are notified when medications change in any way. Even more important is ensuring that the woman and her caregivers fully understand the information that they are provided by health care providers.

It is also important that nurses are aware of how to use and educate women on the use of all home care equipment such as infusion pumps and phototherapy lights. Nurses also have to be skilled at performing various procedures such as venipuncture and administration of intravenous medications or fluids. In addition to teaching about medications and equipment, nurses must be sure that women know how to respond in emergency situations. Women need to be able to have 24-hour access to resources in the community in emergency situations. Women and family members are also encouraged to learn how to perform cardiopulmonary resuscitation (CPR), especially for infants.

Additional patient and family education in home care includes information about the specific high risk condition(s) involved, implications for pregnancy outcome, and measures for self-monitoring. Verbal explanations should be supplemented with clearly written instructions. General information to promote well-being, such as about nutrition and common discomforts of pregnancy, should also be included. The need for preparation for childbirth can be addressed by using books or videos and supplemented by individual teaching at home. Coping with bedrest or other limitation of activity is a problem for many women with high risk pregnancies. The nurse can share strategies that others have used, help with time management, and provide information about support services. Teaching about infant care or the special needs of the preterm infant may be appropriate during the prenatal period.

Clear documentation of assessments, problems identified, treatments and interventions performed, and the woman's response is essential. Third-party payers base reimbursement on the nurse's written record of providing skilled nursing care and assessments that support the woman's continuing need for those services. The nurse must promptly inform the health care provider by telephone, facsimile, or electronic file of any significant changes. When new orders are transmitted by telephone, a written copy must be sent for the physician's signature.

Finally, as soon as home care has been provided, it is essential that the nurse document assessment findings, care provided, recommendations for change, and any patient or family teaching. Detailed documentation is necessary to justify the need for the home visit and is often crucial in obtaining reimbursement from insurance companies. The nursing care plan summarizes details to be included in caring for a woman in the home (see Nursing Care Plan).

⚡ SAFETY ALERT

In caring for the home care patient, Occupational Safety and Health Administration (OSHA) guidelines should be followed. The use of strict handwashing techniques, personal protective equipment (PPE), and proper equipment is essential in preventing the spread of disease to the care provider, the woman, and her family.

KEY POINTS

- The family is a social network that acts as an important support system for its members.
- Family theories provide nurses with useful guidelines for understanding family function.
- Family socioeconomics, response to stress, and culture are key factors influencing family health.
- The economic, religious, kinship, and political structures are embedded in the reproductive beliefs and practices of a culture.
- Nurses must develop cultural competence and integrate it into the nursing plan of care.
- Of necessity, most changes aimed at improving community health involve partnerships among community residents and health care workers.
- Methods of collecting data useful to the nurse working in the community include walking surveys, analysis of existing data, informant interviews, and participant observation.

- Vulnerable populations are groups who are at higher risk for developing physical, mental, or social health problems.
- Social and economic factors affect the scope of perinatal nursing practice.
- Perinatal home care is a unique nursing practice that incorporates knowledge from community health nursing, acute care nursing, family therapy, health promotion, and patient education.
- Perinatal home care nurses should incorporate personal safety and infection control practices in the nursing plan of care.
- Telephonic nurse advice lines, telephonic nursing assessments, and warm lines are low-cost health care services that facilitate continuous patient education, support, and health care decision making even though health care is delivered in multiple sites.

REFERENCES

Allen M: Comparative theories of the expanded role in nursing and implications for nursing practice: a working paper, *Nurs Pap* 9(2):38–45, 1997.

American College of Obstetricians and Gynecologists (ACOG): Health care for homeless women, ACOG Committee Opinion No. 454, 2012, www.acog.org/Resources_And_Publications/Committee_Opinions/Committee_on_

Health_Care_for_Underserved_Women/Health_Care_for_Homeless_Women.

Association of Women's Health, Obstetric, and Neonatal Nurses (AWHONN): *Standards for professional nursing practice in the care of women and newborns*, ed 7, Washington, DC, 2009, Author.

Becker M: The Health Belief Model and sick role behavior, *Health Educ Monogr* 2:409–419, 1974.

Boss P: *Family stress management*, ed 2, Thousand Oaks, Calif, 2002, Sage.

Bronfenbrenner U: *The ecology of human development: experiments by nature and design*, Cambridge, MA, 1979, Harvard University Press.

Bronfenbrenner U: Ecological systems theory. In Vasta R editor: Annals of child development, vol 6, Greenwich, CT, 1989, JAI, pp 187–249.

Carter B, McGoldrick M: *The expanded family life cycle: individual, family, and social perspectives*, ed 3, Boston, 1999, Allyn & Bacon.

Dray S: What are the national statistics for homelessness? 2012, www.ehow.com/about_4597051_what-national-statistics-homelessness.html.

Giger JN: *Transcultural nursing: assessment and intervention*, ed 6, St Louis, 2013, Mosby.

Grieco EM, Acosta YD, del al Cruz GP, et al: The foreign-born population in the United States: 2010, 2012, www.census.gov/prod/2012pubs/acs-19.pdf.

Homelessness in America, 2012, www.homelessnessinamerica.com.

Janz NK, Becker MH: The Health Belief Model: a decade later, *Health Educ Q* 11(1):1–47, 1984.

Klein D, White J: *Family theories: an introduction*, Newberry Park, CA, 1996, Sage.

Lofquist D, Lugaila T, O'Connell M, et al: Households and families: 2010, 2012, www.census.gov/prod/cen2010/briefs/c2010br-14.pdf.

National Coalition for the Homeless (NCFH): Hunger and food insecurity, 2011, www.nationalhomeless.org/factsheets/hunger.html.

National Women's Law Center (NWLC): Making the grade on women's health: a national and state-by-state report card, 2010, http://hrc.nwlc.org/states/national-report-card.

Opening Doors: Federal strategic plan to prevent and end homelessness: update 2011, 2012, www.usich.gov/resources/uploads/asset_library/USICH_FSPUpdate_2012_12312.pdf.

Richards R, Merrill RM, Baksh L: Health behaviors and infant health outcomes in homeless pregnant women in the United States, *Pediatrics* 128(3):438–446, 2011.

Rural Assistance Center: United States, 2011, www.raconline.org/states/unitedstates.php.

Sipes LA: Statistics on women offenders, 2012, www.corrections.com/news/article/30166-statistics-on-women-offenders.

Spector R: *Cultural diversity in health and illness*, ed 8, Upper Saddle River, NJ, 2013, Prentice-Hall.

US Census Bureau: Grandchildren characteristics: 2010 American community survey 1-year estimates, 2010, http://factfinder2.census.gov/faces/tableservices/jsf/pages/productview.xhtml?pid=ACS_10_1YR_S1001&prodType=table.

US Census Bureau: Population estimates, 2011, www.census.gov/popest/data/national/asrh/2011/index.html.

US Department of Health and Human Services (USDHHS): Primary care: the health center program, 2011, http://bphc.hrsa.gov/about.

Wright LM, Leahy M: Nurses and families: a guide to family assessment and intervention, ed 5, Philadelphia, 2009, FA Davis.

Assessment and Health Promotion

Ellen Olshansky

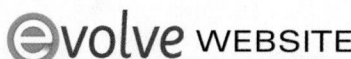 WEBSITE

http://evolve.elsevier.com/Perry/maternal

LEARNING OBJECTIVES

On completion of this chapter, the reader will be able to:

- Identify the structures and functions of the female reproductive system.
- Describe the menstrual cycle in relation to hormonal, ovarian, and endometrial responses.
- Identify the phases of the sexual response cycle.
- Identify facilitators and barriers for women to access care in the health care system.
- Analyze financial, cultural, gender, and communication barriers that may affect a woman's decision to seek and follow through with health-promoting activities.
- Describe the need for health promotion across the woman's life span.

- Analyze conditions and factors that increase health risks for women across the life span, including life stage, substance abuse, eating disorders, medical/health conditions, pregnancy, and intimate partner violence.
- Describe components of taking a woman's history and performing a physical examination.
- Review patient teaching of breast self-examination.
- Describe how the history and physical examination can be adapted for women with special needs.
- Outline the health-screening schedules for women across the life span.
- Identify the correct procedure for assisting with and collecting Papanicolaou test specimens.

Care of the well woman is focused on health promotion and illness prevention, recognizing that a woman is a bio-psycho-social-spiritual being, requiring a holistic approach to nursing care. To encourage appropriate health-promotion activities, it is important to conduct systematic health assessments and screenings. This chapter presents an overview of the nurse's role in encouraging health promotion and illness prevention in women. It provides guidelines for how to conduct a complete history and physical examination. This chapter also includes a schedule of screening tests recommended for women at different stages of their lives. As background to understanding assessment, a review of female anatomy and physiology as well as the menstrual cycle is presented. Facilitators and barriers to women to enter the health care system and risk factors for women's health across the life cycle are described. Anticipatory guidance suggestions, including nutrition and stress management, are included. Violence against women, particularly intimate partner violence (IPV) and battering of women, is discussed because it is often in the health care setting that the woman is able to acknowledge being in an abusive relationship. Examples of health-promotion efforts in the community are presented in an effort to emphasize community health approaches to care, especially since much of well woman care occurs in the community.

FEMALE REPRODUCTIVE SYSTEM

The female reproductive system consists of external structures visible from the pubis to the perineum and internal structures located in the pelvic cavity. The external and internal female reproductive structures develop and mature in response to estrogen and progesterone. This process starts in fetal life and continues through puberty and the childbearing years. Reproductive structures atrophy with age or in response to a decrease in ovarian hormone production. A complex nerve and blood supply supports the functions of these structures. The appearance of the external genitalia varies greatly among women. Heredity, age, race, and the number of children a woman has borne influence the size, shape, and color of her external organs.

External Structures

The external genital organs, or vulva, include all structures visible externally from the pubis to the perineum. These include the mons

39

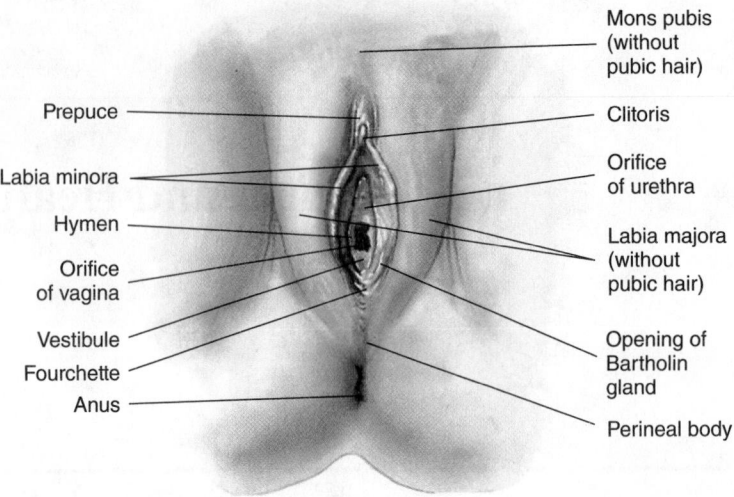

Mons pubis
(without
pubic hair)

Prepuce

Clitoris

Labia minora

Orifice
of urethra

Hymen

Labia majora
(without
pubic hair)

Orifice
of vagina

Vestibule

Fourchette

Opening of
Bartholin
gland

Anus

Perineal body

FIG 3-1 External female genitalia.

pubis, labia majora, labia minora, clitoris, vestibular glands, vaginal vestibule, vaginal orifice, and urethral opening. The external genital organs are illustrated in Fig. 3-1.

The mons pubis is a fatty pad that lies over the anterior surface of the symphysis pubis. In the postpubertal female, the mons is covered with coarse, curly hair. The labia majora are two rounded folds of fatty tissue covered with skin that extend downward and backward from the mons pubis. The labia are highly vascular structures that develop hair on the outer surfaces after puberty. They protect the inner vulvar structures. The labia minora are two flat, reddish folds of tissue visible when the labia majora are separated. There are no hair follicles on the labia minora, but many sebaceous follicles and a few sweat glands are present. The interior of the labia minora comprises connective tissue and smooth muscle and is supplied with extremely sensitive nerve endings. Anteriorly, the labia minora fuse to form the **prepuce** (the hoodlike covering of the clitoris) and the frenulum (the fold of tissue under the clitoris). The labia minora join to form a thin, flat tissue called the *fourchette* underneath the vaginal opening at midline. The clitoris is located underneath the prepuce. It is a small structure composed of erectile tissue with numerous sensory nerve endings. During sexual arousal, the clitoris increases in size.

The vaginal vestibule is an almond-shaped area enclosed by the labia minora that contains openings to the urethra, Skene glands, vagina, and Bartholin glands. The urethra is not a reproductive organ but is discussed here because of its location. It usually is found about 2.5 cm below the clitoris. Skene glands are located on each side of the urethra and produce mucus, which aids in lubrication of the vagina. The vaginal opening is in the lower portion of the vestibule and varies in shape and size. The hymen, a connective tissue membrane that surrounds the vaginal opening, can be perforated during strenuous exercise, insertion of tampons, masturbation, and vaginal intercourse. Bartholin glands lie under the constrictor muscles of the vagina and are located posteriorly on the sides of the vaginal opening, although the ductal opening usually is not visible. During sexual arousal, the glands secrete clear mucus to lubricate the vaginal introitus.

The area between the fourchette and the anus is the perineum, a skin-covered muscular area that covers the pelvic structures. The perineum forms the base of the perineal body, a wedge-shaped mass that serves as an anchor for the muscles, fascia, and ligaments of the pelvis. The muscles and ligaments form a sling that supports the pelvic organs.

Internal Structures

The internal structures include the vagina, uterus, fallopian tubes, and ovaries. The description of these structures follows.

The vagina is a fibromuscular, collapsible, tubular structure that lies between the bladder and rectum and extends from the vulva to the uterus. During the reproductive years, the mucosal lining is arranged in transverse folds called *rugae*. These rugae allow the vagina to expand during childbirth. Estrogen deprivation that occurs after childbirth, during lactation, and at menopause causes dryness and thinning of the vaginal walls and smoothing of the rugae. The vagina, particularly the lower segment, has few sensory nerve endings. Vaginal secretions are slightly acidic (pH 4 to 5) so that vaginal susceptibility to infections is limited. The vagina serves as a passageway for menstrual flow, as a female organ of copulation, and as a part of the birth canal for vaginal childbirth. The uterine cervix projects into a blind vault at the upper end of the vagina. Anterior, posterior, and lateral pockets called **fornices** (singular: *fornix*) surround the cervix. The internal pelvic organs can be palpated through the thin walls of these fornices.

The uterus is a muscular organ shaped like an upside-down pear that sits midline in the pelvic cavity between the bladder and rectum and above the vagina. Four pairs of ligaments support the uterus: cardinal, uterosacral, round, and broad. Single anterior and posterior ligaments also support the uterus. The cul-de-sac of Douglas is a deep pouch, or recess, posterior to the cervix formed by the posterior ligament.

The uterus is divided into two major parts: an upper triangular portion called the *corpus* and a lower cylindric portion called the *cervix* (Fig. 3-2). The fundus is the dome-shaped top of the uterus and is the site at which the uterine tubes (fallopian tubes) enter the uterus. The isthmus, or lower uterine segment, is a short, constricted portion that separates the corpus from the cervix.

The uterus serves for reception, implantation, retention, and nutrition of the fertilized ovum and later of the fetus during

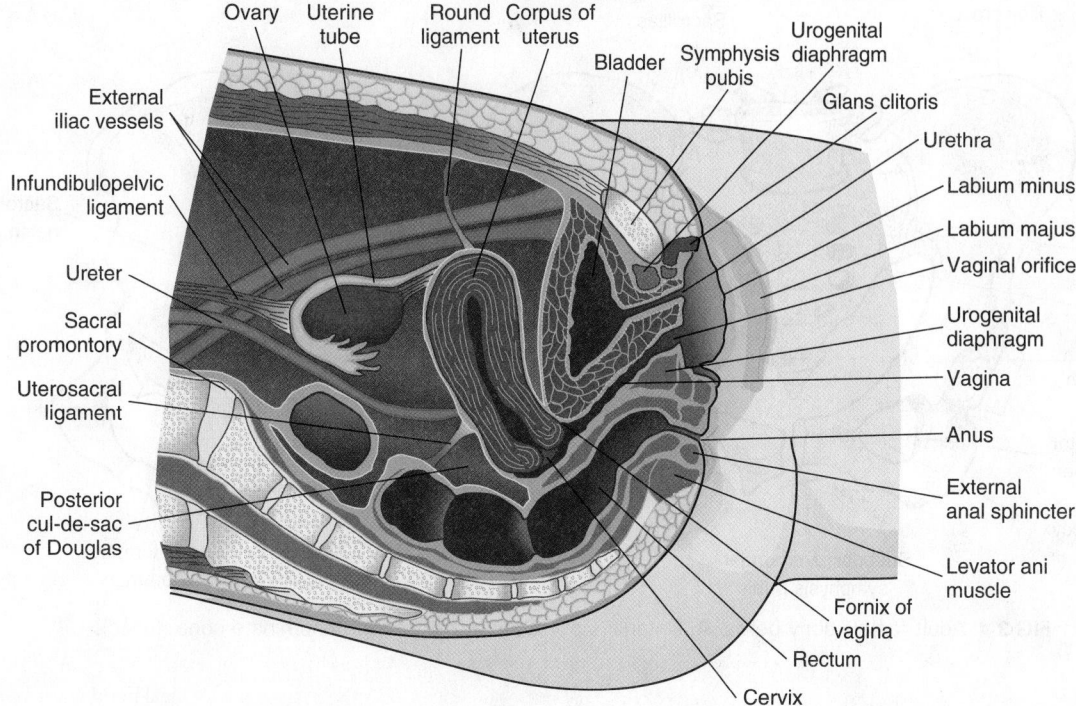

FIG 3-2 Midsagittal view of female pelvic organs with woman lying supine.

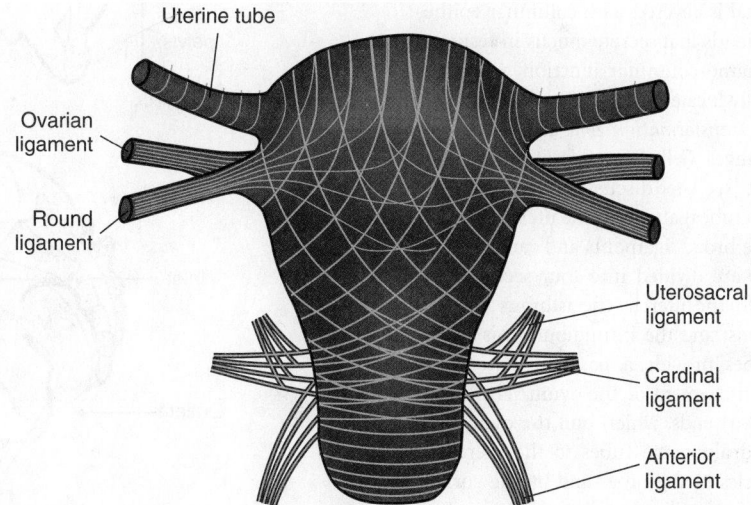

FIG 3-3 Schematic arrangement of directions of muscle fibers. Note that uterine muscle fibers are continuous with supportive ligaments of uterus.

pregnancy and for expulsion of the fetus during childbirth. It is also responsible for cyclic menstruation.

The uterine wall is made up of three layers: the **endometrium,** the myometrium, and part of the peritoneum. The endometrium is a highly vascular lining made up of three layers, the outer two of which are shed during menstruation. The myometrium is made up of layers of smooth muscles that extend in three different directions (longitudinal, transverse, and oblique) (Fig. 3-3). Longitudinal fibers of the outer myometrial layer are found mostly in the fundus, and this arrangement assists in expelling the fetus during the birth process. The middle layer contains fibers from all three directions, which form a figure-eight pattern encircling large blood vessels.

These fibers assist in ligating blood vessels after childbirth and control blood loss. Most of the circular fibers of the inner myometrial layer are around the site where the uterine tubes enter the uterus and around the internal cervical os (opening). These fibers help keep the cervix closed during pregnancy and prevent menstrual blood from flowing back into the uterine tubes during menstruation.

The cervix is made up of mostly fibrous connective tissues and elastic tissue, making it possible for the cervix to stretch during vaginal childbirth. The opening between the uterine cavity and the canal that connects the uterine cavity to the vagina (endocervical canal) is the internal os. The narrowed opening between the endocervix and the vagina is the external os, a small circular opening in

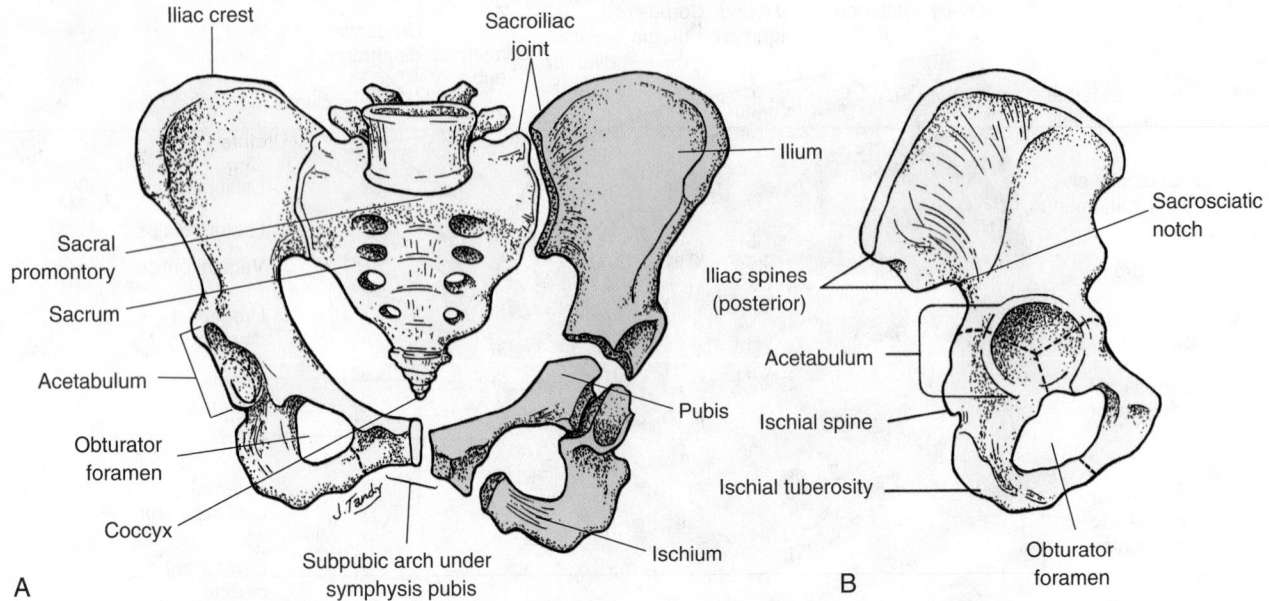

FIG 3-4 Adult female bony pelvis. **A,** Anterior view. **B,** External view of innominate bone (fused).

women who have never been pregnant. The cervix feels firm (like the end of a nose) with a dimple in the center that marks the external os.

The outer cervix is covered with a layer of squamous epithelium. The mucosa of the cervical canal is covered with columnar epithelium and contains numerous glands that secrete mucus in response to ovarian hormones. The squamo-columnar junction, where the two types of cells meet, is usually located just inside the cervical os. This junction is also called the *transformation zone* and is the most common site for neoplastic changes. Cells from this site are scraped for the Papanicolaou (Pap) test (see later discussion).

The uterine tubes (fallopian tubes) attach to the uterine fundus. The tubes are supported by the broad ligaments and range from 8 to 14 cm in length. The tubes are divided into four sections: the interstitial portion is closest to the uterus; the isthmus and the ampulla are the middle portions; and the infundibulum is closest to the ovary. The uterine tubes provide a passage between the ovaries and the uterus for the movement of the ovum. The infundibulum has fimbriated (fringed) ends, which pull the ovum into the tube. The ovum is pushed along the tubes to the uterus by rhythmic contractions of muscles of the tubes and by the current produced by the movement of the cilia that line the tubes. The ovum is usually fertilized by the sperm in the ampulla portion of one of the tubes.

The ovaries are almond-shaped organs located on each side of the uterus below and behind the uterine tubes. During the reproductive years, they are approximately 3 cm long, 2 cm wide, and 1 cm thick; they diminish in size after menopause. Before menarche, each ovary has a smooth surface; after menarche, they are nodular because of repeated ruptures of follicles at ovulation. The two functions of the ovaries are ovulation and hormone production. Ovulation is the release of a mature ovum from the ovary at intervals (usually monthly). Estrogen, progesterone, and androgen are the hormones produced by the ovaries.

The Bony Pelvis

The bony pelvis serves three primary purposes: protection of the pelvic structures, accommodation of the growing fetus during

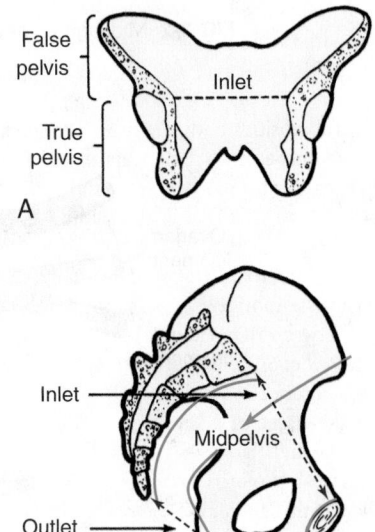

FIG 3-5 Female pelvis. **A,** Cavity of false pelvis is shallow. **B,** Cavity of true pelvis is irregularly curved canal *(arrows).*

pregnancy, and anchorage of the pelvic support structures. The two innominate (hip) bones (consisting of ilium, ischium, and pubis), the sacrum, and the coccyx make up the four bones of the pelvis (Fig. 3-4). Cartilage and ligaments form the symphysis pubis, sacrococcygeal joint, and two sacroiliac joints that separate the pelvic bones.

The pelvis is divided into two parts: the false pelvis and the true pelvis (Fig. 3-5). The false pelvis is the upper portion above the pelvic brim or inlet. The true pelvis is the lower, curved, bony canal, which includes the inlet, the cavity, and the outlet through which the fetus passes during vaginal birth. The upper portion of the outlet is at the level of the ischial spines, and the lower portion is at the

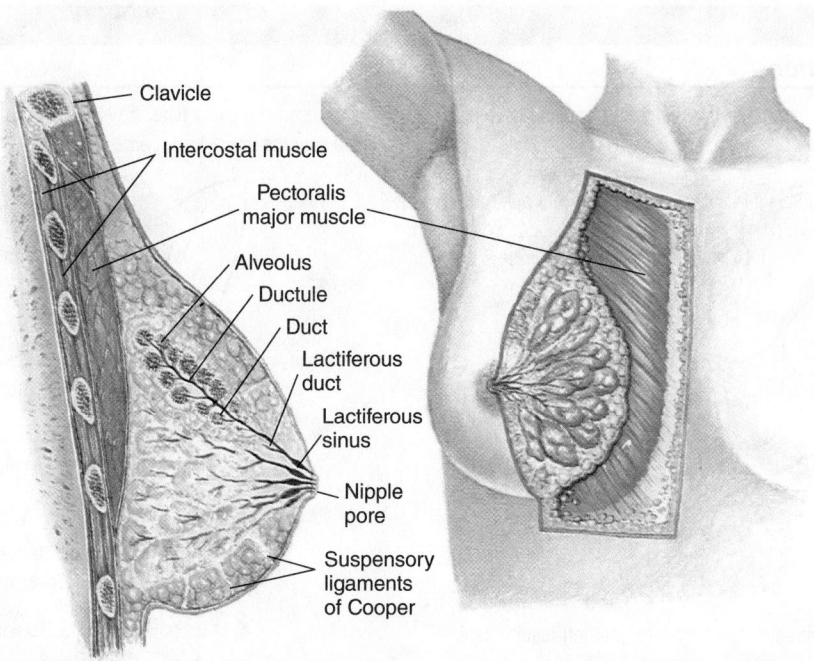

- Clavicle
- Intercostal muscle
- Pectoralis major muscle
- Alveolus
- Ductule
- Duct
- Lactiferous duct
- Lactiferous sinus
- Nipple pore
- Suspensory ligaments of Cooper

FIG 3-6 Anatomy of the breast showing position and major structures. (Adapted from Seidel H, Ball J, Dains J, et al: *Mosby's guide to physical examination,* ed 7, St Louis, 2011, Mosby.)

level of the ischial tuberosities and the pubic arch. Variations that occur in the size and shape of the pelvis are usually related to age, race, and sex. Pelvic ossification is complete at about 20 years of age.

Breasts

The breasts are paired mammary glands located between the second and sixth ribs (Fig. 3-6). About two thirds of the breast overlies the pectoralis muscle, between the sternum and midaxillary line, with an extension to the *tail of Spence.* The lower one third of the breast overlies the serratus anterior muscle. The breasts are attached to the muscles by connective tissue or fascia.

The breasts of the healthy, mature woman are approximately equal in size and shape but often are not absolutely symmetric. The size and shape vary with the woman's age, heredity, and nutrition. However, the contour should be smooth with no retractions, dimpling, or masses. Estrogen stimulates growth of the breast by inducing fat deposition in the breasts, development of stromal tissue (i.e., increase in its amount and elasticity), and growth of the extensive ductile system. Estrogen also increases the vascularity of breast tissue.

Once ovulation begins in puberty, progesterone levels increase. The increase in progesterone causes maturation of mammary gland tissue, specifically the lobules and acinar structures. During adolescence, fat deposition and growth of fibrous tissue contribute to the increase in the size of the glands. Full development of the breasts is not achieved until after the end of the first pregnancy or in the early period of lactation.

Findings from several studies using ultrasound imaging to investigate the anatomy of the breast reported differences from previous descriptions (Geddes, 2007; Love and Barsky, 2004; Ramsay, Kent, Hartmann, et al., 2005). The following description incorporates these findings. Each mammary gland is made of a number of lobes that are divided into lobules. Lobules are clusters of acini. An acinus is a saclike terminal part of a compound gland emptying

through a narrow lumen or duct. The acini are lined with epithelial cells that secrete colostrum and milk. Just below the epithelium is the myoepithelium (*myo,* or muscle), which contracts to expel milk from the acini.

The ducts from the clusters of acini that form the lobules merge to form larger ducts draining the lobes. Ducts from the lobes converge in a single nipple (mammary papilla) surrounded by an areola. The anatomy of the ducts is similar for each breast but varies among women. Protective fatty tissue surrounds the glandular structures and ducts. *Cooper's ligaments,* or fibrous suspensory, separate and support the glandular structures and ducts. Cooper's ligaments provide support to the mammary glands while permitting their mobility on the chest wall (see Fig. 3-6). The round nipple is usually slightly elevated above the breast. On each breast the nipple projects slightly upward and laterally. It contains 4 to 20 openings from the milk ducts. The nipple is surrounded by fibromuscular tissue and covered by wrinkled skin (the areola). Except during pregnancy and lactation, there is usually no discharge from the nipple.

The nipple and surrounding areola are usually more deeply pigmented than the skin of the breast. The rough appearance of the areola is caused by sebaceous glands, Montgomery tubercles, directly beneath the skin. These glands secrete a fatty substance thought to lubricate the nipple. Smooth muscle fibers in the areola contract to stiffen the nipple to make it easier for the breastfeeding infant to grasp.

The vascular supply to the mammary gland is abundant. In the nonpregnant state there is no obvious vascular pattern in the skin. The normal skin is smooth without tightness or shininess. The skin covering the breasts contains an extensive superficial lymphatic network that serves the entire chest wall and is continuous with the superficial lymphatics of the neck and abdomen. The lymphatics form a rich network in the deeper portions of the breasts. The primary deep lymphatic pathway drains laterally toward the axillae.

Breast Self-Examination

If you choose to perform a breast self-examination, the best time is when breasts are not tender or swollen.

How to examine your breasts:

1. Lie down and put a pillow under your right shoulder. Place your right arm behind your head (Fig. 1).

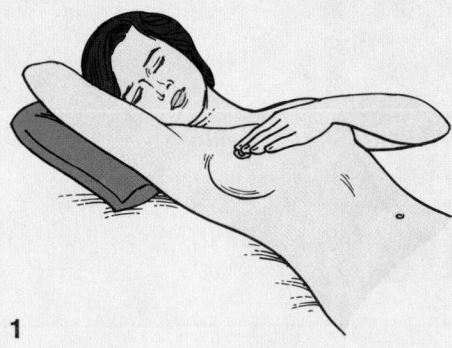

1

2. Use the finger pads of your three middle fingers on your left hand to feel for lumps or thickening. Your finger pads are the top third of each finger. Use circular motions of the finger pads to feel the breast tissue.
3. Press firmly enough to know how your breast feels. Use light pressure to feel the tissue just under the skin, medium pressure for a little deeper, and firm pressure to feel the breast tissue close to the chest and ribs. A firm ridge in the lower curve of the breast is normal.
4. Move around the breast in a set way, such as using an up-and-down or vertical line pattern (Fig. 2). Go up to the collar bone and down to the ribs and from your underarm on the side to the middle of your chest. Use the

same technique every time. It will help you to make sure that you have gone over the entire breast area and to remember how your breast feels.

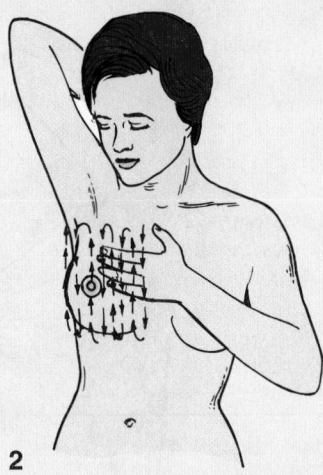

2

5. Now examine your left breast using the finger pads of your right hand.
6. You may want to check your breasts while standing in front of a mirror. See if there are any changes in the way your breasts look: dimpling of the skin, changes in the nipple, or redness or swelling.
7. Checking the area between the breast and the underarm and the underarm itself is important. Examine the area above the breast to the collarbone and to the shoulder while you are standing or sitting up with your arms slightly raised.
8. If you find any changes, see your health care provider right away.

Adapted from American Cancer Society: *Breast awareness and self-exam*, 2013, www.cancer.org.

Besides their function of lactation, breasts function as organs for sexual arousal in the mature adult female.

The breasts change in size and nodularity in response to cyclic ovarian changes throughout reproductive life. Increasing levels of both estrogen and progesterone in the 3 to 4 days before menstruation increase the vascularity of the breasts, induce growth of the ducts and acini, and promote water retention. The epithelial cells lining the ducts proliferate in number, the ducts dilate, and the lobules distend. The acini become enlarged and secretory, and lipid (fat) is deposited within their epithelial cell lining. As a result, breast swelling, tenderness, and discomfort are common symptoms just before the onset of menstruation. After menstruation, cellular proliferation begins to regress, acini begin to decrease in size, and retained water is lost. After breasts have undergone changes numerous times in response to the ovarian cycle, the proliferation and involution (regression) are not uniform throughout the breast. In time, after repeated hormonal stimulation, small, persistent areas of nodulations may develop. This normal physiologic change must be remembered when breast tissue is examined. Nodules may develop just before and during menstruation, when the breast is most active. The physiologic alternations in breast size and activity reach their minimum level about 5 to 7 days after menstruation stops. Therefore breast self-examination (BSE) (systematic palpation of breasts to detect signs of breast cancer or other changes) is best carried out during this phase of the menstrual cycle (see Guidelines box). Although monthly BSE used to be recommended to all women, the current guidelines recommend BSE as an option

(American Cancer Society, 2012b), mostly because they believe that many unnecessary biopsies and other procedures result. However, breastcancer.org (2012) continues to recommend that all women perform BSE monthly (see the Critical Thinking Case Study).

MENSTRUATION

Menarche and Puberty

Although young girls secrete small, rather constant amounts of estrogen, a marked increase occurs between 8 and 11 years of age. The term menarche denotes first menstruation. Puberty is a broader term that denotes the entire transitional stage between childhood and sexual maturity. Increasing amounts and variations in gonadotropin and estrogen secretion develop into a cyclic pattern at least a year before menarche. In North America this occurs in most girls at about 13 years of age.

Initially, menstrual periods are irregular, unpredictable, painless, and anovulatory (no ovum is released from the ovary). After 1 or more years, a hypothalamic-pituitary rhythm develops and the ovary produces adequate cyclic estrogen to make a mature ovum. Ovulatory (ovum released from the ovary) periods tend to be regular, with estrogen dominating the first half of the cycle and progesterone dominating the second half of the cycle.

Although pregnancy can occur in exceptional cases of true precocious puberty, most pregnancies in young girls occur after the normally timed menarche. All young adolescents of both sexes

Breast Self-Examination

Jessie is a 21-year-old college student who has come to the Student Health Clinic for contraception advice. During her consultation with the nurse, Jessie asks about doing breast self-examination. She said her roommate said she really needs to do them every month. What advice or counseling would you give Jessie?

1. Evidence—Is there sufficient evidence to draw conclusions about what intervention is needed?
2. Assumptions—Describe underlying assumptions about the following issues:
    a. Risk factor assessment for breast cancer
    b. Screening for breast cancer
    c. Breast self-examination practices
3. What implications and priorities for nursing care can be drawn at this time?
4. Does the evidence objectively support your conclusion?

would benefit from knowing that pregnancy can occur at any time after the onset of menses.

Menstrual Cycle

Menstruation is the periodic uterine bleeding that begins approximately 14 days after ovulation. It is controlled by a feedback system of three cycles: endometrial, hypothalamic-pituitary, and ovarian. The average length of a menstrual cycle is 28 days, but variations are normal. The first day of bleeding is designated as day 1 of the menstrual cycle, or menses (Fig. 3-7). The average duration of menstrual flow is 5 days (with a range of 3 to 6 days) and the average blood loss is 50 mL (with a range of 20 to 80 mL), but these vary greatly.

For about 50% of women, menstrual blood does not appear to clot. The menstrual blood clots within the uterus, but the clot usually liquefies before being discharged from the uterus. Uterine discharge includes mucus and epithelial cells in addition to blood.

The menstrual cycle is a complex interplay of events that occur simultaneously in the endometrium, the hypothalamus, the pituitary glands, and the ovaries. The menstrual cycle prepares the uterus for pregnancy. When pregnancy does not occur, menstruation follows. A woman's age, physical and emotional status, and environment influence the regularity of her menstrual cycles.

Endometrial Cycle

The four phases of the endometrial cycle are (1) the menstrual phase, (2) the proliferative phase, (3) the secretory phase, and (4) the ischemic phase (see Fig. 3-7). During the menstrual phase, shedding of the functional two thirds of the endometrium (the compact and spongy layers) is initiated by periodic vasoconstriction in the upper layers of the endometrium. The basal layer is always retained, and regeneration begins near the end of the cycle from cells derived from the remaining glandular remnants or stromal cells in this layer.

The proliferative phase is a period of rapid growth lasting from about the fifth day to the time of ovulation. The endometrial surface is completely restored in approximately 4 days, or slightly before bleeding ceases. From this point on, an eightfold to tenfold thickening occurs, with a leveling off of growth at ovulation. The

proliferative phase depends on estrogen stimulation derived from ovarian follicles.

The secretory phase extends from the day of ovulation to about 3 days before the next menstrual period. After ovulation, large amounts of progesterone are produced. An edematous, vascular, functional endometrium is now apparent. At the end of the secretory phase, the fully matured secretory endometrium reaches the thickness of heavy, soft velvet. It becomes luxuriant with blood and glandular secretions—a suitable protective and nutritive bed for a fertilized ovum.

Implantation of the fertilized ovum generally occurs about 7 to 10 days after ovulation. If fertilization and implantation do not occur, the corpus luteum, which secretes estrogen and progesterone, regresses. With the rapid decrease in progesterone and estrogen levels, the spiral arteries go into spasm. During the ischemic phase, the blood supply to the functional endometrium is blocked and necrosis develops. The functional layer separates from the basal layer, and menstrual bleeding begins, marking day 1 of the next cycle (see Fig. 3-7).

Hypothalamic-Pituitary Cycle

Toward the end of the normal menstrual cycle, blood levels of estrogen and progesterone decrease. Low blood levels of these ovarian hormones stimulate the hypothalamus to secrete gonadotropin-releasing hormone (GnRH). In turn, GnRH stimulates anterior pituitary secretion of follicle-stimulating hormone (FSH). FSH stimulates development of ovarian graafian follicles and their production of estrogen. Estrogen levels begin to decrease, and hypothalamic GnRH triggers the anterior pituitary to release luteinizing hormone (LH). A marked surge of LH and a smaller peak of estrogen (day 12) (see Fig. 3-7) precede the expulsion of the ovum from the graafian follicle by about 24 to 36 hours. LH peaks at about day 13 or 14 of a 28-day cycle. If fertilization and implantation of the ovum have not occurred by this time, regression of the corpus luteum follows. Levels of progesterone and estrogen decline, menstruation occurs, and the hypothalamus is once again stimulated to secrete GnRH. This process is called the *hypothalamic-pituitary cycle*.

Ovarian Cycle

The primitive graafian follicles contain immature oocytes (primordial ova). Before ovulation, from 1 to 30 follicles begin to mature in each ovary under the influence of FSH and estrogen. The preovulatory surge of LH affects a selected follicle. The oocyte matures, *ovulation* occurs, and the empty follicle begins its transformation into the corpus luteum. This follicular phase (preovulatory phase) (see Fig. 3-7) of the ovarian cycle varies in length from woman to woman. Almost all variations in ovarian cycle length are the result of variations in the length of the follicular phase. On rare occasions (i.e., 1 in 100 menstrual cycles), more than one follicle is selected and more than one oocyte matures and undergoes ovulation.

After ovulation, estrogen levels drop. For 90% of women, only a small amount of withdrawal bleeding occurs, and it goes unnoticed. In 10% of women, there is sufficient bleeding for it to be visible, resulting in what is termed midcycle bleeding.

The luteal phase begins immediately after ovulation and ends with the start of menstruation. This postovulatory phase of the ovarian cycle usually requires 14 days (range 13 to 15 days). The corpus luteum reaches its peak of functional activity 8 days after ovulation, secreting the steroids *estrogen* and *progesterone*. Coincident with this time of peak luteal functioning, the fertilized ovum is implanted in the endometrium. If no implantation occurs, the

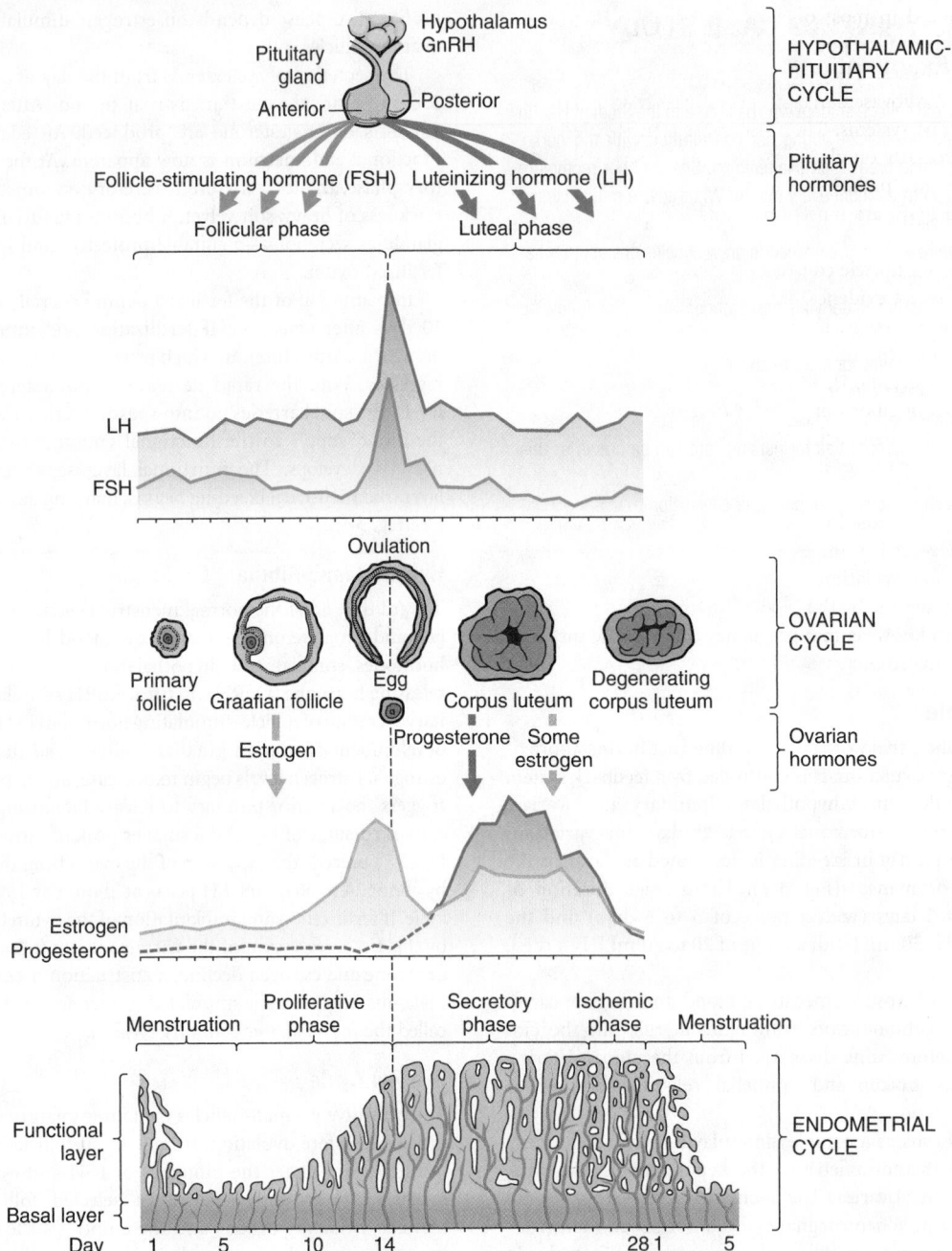

FIG 3-7 Menstrual cycle: hypothalamic-pituitary, ovarian, and endometrial. *GnRH,* Gonadotropin-releasing hormone.

corpus luteum regresses and steroid levels drop. Two weeks after ovulation, if fertilization and implantation do not occur, the functional layer of the uterine endometrium is shed through menstruation.

Other Cyclic Changes

When the hypothalamic-pituitary-ovarian axis functions properly, other tissues undergo predictable responses. Before ovulation, the woman's basal body temperature is often less than 37° C (98.6° F); after ovulation, with increasing progesterone levels, her basal body temperature rises. Changes in the cervix and cervical mucus follow a generally predictable pattern. Preovulatory and postovulatory

mucus is viscous (thick) so that sperm penetration is discouraged. At the time of ovulation, cervical mucus is thin and clear. It looks, feels, and stretches like egg white. This stretchable quality is termed spinnbarkeit. Some women have localized lower abdominal pain called mittelschmerz that coincides with ovulation. Some spotting may occur.

Prostaglandins

Prostaglandins (PGs) are oxygenated fatty acids classified as *hormones.* The different kinds of PGs are distinguished by letters (PGE and PGF), numbers (PGE_2), and letters of the Greek alphabet ($PGF_{2\alpha}$).

PGs are produced in most organs of the body, including the uterus. Menstrual blood is a potent PG source. PGs are metabolized quickly by most tissues. They are biologically active in minute amounts in the cardiovascular, gastrointestinal, respiratory, urogenital, and nervous systems. They also exert a marked effect on metabolism, particularly on glycolysis. PGs play an important role in many physiologic, pathologic, and pharmacologic reactions. $PGF_{2\alpha}$, PGE_4, and PGE_2 are most commonly used in reproductive medicine.

PGs affect smooth muscle contractility and modulation of hormonal activity. Indirect evidence indicates that PGs have an effect on ovulation, fertility, changes in the cervix and cervical mucus that affect receptivity to sperm, tubal and uterine motility, sloughing of endometrium (menstruation), onset of miscarriage and induced abortion, and onset of labor (term and preterm).

After exerting biologic actions, newly synthesized PGs are rapidly metabolized by tissues in such organs as the lungs, kidneys, and liver.

PGs may play a key role in ovulation. If PG levels do not rise along with the surge of LH, the ovum remains trapped within the graafian follicle. After ovulation, PGs may influence production of estrogen and progesterone by the corpus luteum.

The introduction of PGs into the vagina or the uterine cavity (from ejaculated semen) increases the motility of uterine musculature, which may assist the transport of sperm through the uterus and into the oviduct.

PGs produced by the woman cause regression of the corpus luteum and regression and sloughing of the endometrium, resulting in menstruation. PGs increase myometrial response to oxytocic stimulation, enhance uterine contractions, and cause cervical dilation. They may be a factor in the initiation of labor, the maintenance of labor, or both. They may also be involved in dysmenorrhea (see Chapter 4) and preeclampsia/eclampsia (see Chapter 12).

Climacteric and Menopause

The climacteric is a transitional phase during which ovarian function and hormone production decline. This phase spans the years from the onset of premenopausal ovarian decline to the postmenopausal time when symptoms stop. Menopause (from Latin *mensis*, month, and Greek *pauses*, to cease) refers only to the last menstrual period. However, unlike menarche, menopause can be dated with certainty only 1 year after menstruation ceases. The average age at natural menopause is 51.4 years, with an age range of 35 to 60 years. *Perimenopause* is a period preceding menopause that lasts about 4 years. During this time, ovarian function declines. Ova slowly diminish, and menstrual cycles may be anovulatory, resulting in irregular bleeding. The ovary stops producing estrogen, and eventually menses no longer occur.

SEXUAL RESPONSE

The hypothalamus and anterior pituitary glands in females regulate the production of FSH and LH. The target tissue for these hormones is the ovary, which produces ova and secretes estrogen and progesterone. A feedback mechanism between hormone secretion from the ovaries, the hypothalamus, and the anterior pituitary aids in the control of the production of sex cells and steroid sex hormone secretion.

Although the first outward appearance of maturing sexual development occurs at an earlier age in females, both females and males achieve physical maturity at approximately 17 years of age; however, individual development varies greatly. Anatomic and reproductive differences notwithstanding, women and men are more alike than different in their physiologic response to sexual excitement and orgasm. For example, the glans clitoris and the glans penis are embryonic homologs. Little difference exists between female and male sexual response; the physical response is essentially the same whether stimulated by coitus, fantasy, or masturbation. Physiologic sexual response can be analyzed in terms of two processes: vasocongestion and myotonia.

Sexual stimulation results in increase in circulation to circumvaginal blood vessels (lubrication in the female), causing engorgement and distention of the genitals. Venous congestion is localized primarily in the genitalia, but it also occurs to a lesser degree in the breasts and other parts of the body. Arousal is characterized by myotonia (increased muscular tension), resulting in voluntary and involuntary rhythmic contractions. Examples of sexually stimulated myotonia are pelvic thrusting, facial grimacing, and spasms of the hands and feet (carpopedal spasms).

The sexual response cycle is classically divided into four phases: excitement, plateau, orgasmic, and resolution, according to the seminal work of Masters and Johnson (1966). The four phases occur progressively, with no sharp dividing line between any two phases. The time, intensity, and duration for cyclic completion also vary for individuals and situations. Other researchers have suggested different models to explain sexual response. Leeman and Rogers (2012) emphasize the need to address sexuality and possible sexual difficulties with women in the postpartum period. Specific issues related to this period (and prior procedures such as episiotomy) must be considered in counseling to promote healthy sexuality during the postpartum period. Despite these alternate models of sexual response, it is still common to describe the classic four stages in which specific body changes take place in sequence, and this description is useful in educating and talking with women who may have concerns about possible sexual dysfunction. Table 3-1 compares male and female body changes during each of the four phases of the sexual response cycle.

BARRIERS TO ENTERING THE HEALTH CARE SYSTEM

Financial Issues

Access to care varies greatly, depending on type and size of the system, source of payment for services, private versus public programs, availability of and accessibility to providers, individual preferences, and insurance coverage or ability to pay. The existing system continues to be oriented to treatment of acute or episodic conditions rather than to the promotion of health and comprehensive care, despite the fact that people are discharged earlier from hospitals, requiring more care in homes and community settings.

In the United States, disparity among races and socioeconomic classes affects many facets of life including health. Limited finances is associated with lack of access to care, delay in seeking care, few prevention activities, and little accurate information about health and the health care system. Women use health care services more often than men but are more likely than men to have difficulty in financing the services. Many poor women have traditionally been underinsured or uninsured, but rules about health insurance and who and what are covered are undergoing a transition with the Affordable Care Act (healthcare.gov, 2012). People will not be denied insurance because of pre-existing

TABLE 3-1	FOUR PHASES OF SEXUAL RESPONSE	
REACTIONS COMMON TO BOTH SEXES	**FEMALE REACTIONS**	**MALE REACTIONS**
Excitement Phase		
Heart rate and blood pressure increase. Nipples become erect. Myotonia begins.	Clitoris increases in diameter and swells. External genitalia become congested and darken. Vaginal lubrication occurs; upper two thirds of vagina lengthens and extends. Cervix and uterus pull upward. Breast size increases.	Erection of the penis begins; penis increases in length and diameter. Scrotal skin becomes congested and thickens. Testes begin to increase in size and elevate toward the body.
Plateau Phase		
Heart rate and blood pressure continue to increase. Respirations increase. Myotonia becomes pronounced; grimacing occurs.	Clitoral head retracts under the clitoral hood. Lower one third of vagina becomes engorged. Skin color changes occur—red flush may be observed across breasts, abdomen, or other surfaces.	Head of penis may enlarge slightly. Scrotum continues to grow tense and thicken. Testes continue to elevate and enlarge. Preorgasmic emission of two or three drops of fluid appears on the head of the penis.
Orgasmic Phase		
Heart rate, blood pressure, and respirations increase to maximum levels. Involuntary muscle spasms occur. External rectal sphincter contracts.	Strong rhythmic contractions are felt in the clitoris, vagina, and uterus. Sensations of warmth spread through the pelvic area.	Testes elevate to maximum level. Point of "inevitability" occurs just before ejaculation and an awareness of fluid in the urethra. Rhythmic contractions occur in the penis. Ejaculation of semen occurs.
Resolution Phase		
Heart rate, blood pressure, and respirations return to normal. Nipple erection subsides. Myotonia subsides.	Engorgement in external genitalia and vagina resolves. Uterus descends to normal position. Cervix dips into seminal pool. Breast size decreases. Skin flush disappears.	Fifty percent of erection is lost immediately with ejaculation; penis gradually returns to normal size. Testes and scrotum return to normal size. Refractory period (time needed for erection to occur again) varies according to age and general physical condition.

conditions, and various preventive health services will be covered under health insurance. However this legislation is far from decided and its impact on the American people will not be known for years.

With a greater focus on preventive health care services and with 32 million formerly uninsured patients having access to health care, nurses, advanced practice nurses, including nurse practitioners, midwives, and clinical nurse specialists, are critical to the provision of high quality, safe, effective, and accessible health care (see the Community Focus box).

Cultural Issues

We live in a multicultural society with constantly changing demographics, and for nursing care of women to be optimal, cultural differences must be addressed with great sensitivity and competency. Nurses are in excellent positions to be responsible for providing culturally sensitive and competent health care (Escallier, Fullterton, and Messina, 2011). A variety of reasons are given to explain some of the differences in accessing care when financial barriers are adjusted. Some women experience racial discrimination or disrespectful, disillusioning, or discouraging encounters with community service providers such as social services and health care providers. Many women do not seek care from the health care system because of lack of trust (Yang, Matthews, and Hillemeier, 2011). A lack of cross-cultural communication also presents problems. Desired health outcomes are best achieved

 COMMUNITY FOCUS

Role of Nurses in Women's Health Promotion and Illness Prevention

Registered nurses work with women to promote wellness by:
- Teaching
- Encouraging
- Motivating
- Integrating various modalities of care ("integrative nurse coaching")
- Collaborating with other health care practitioners
- Providing care in the community, working with individuals, families, communities
- Working to influence health policy

Advanced practice nurses work with women to promote wellness by:
- Providing comprehensive primary care
- Coordinating care in communities (from hospitals to home to communities)
- Working with social service resources for patients in the community

when the health care provider has knowledge of and understanding about the culture, language, values, priorities, and health beliefs of those in various ethnic groups. Conversely, members of these various groups should understand the health goals to be achieved and the methods proposed to do so. Language differences can produce profound barriers between patients and providers. Even with an interpreter, misinformation can occur on both sides of the communication.

Providers must consider culturally based differences that could affect the treatment of diverse groups of women, and the women themselves must share practices and beliefs that could influence their responses to treatment or willingness to adhere to treatment. For example, women in some cultures value privacy to such an extent that they are reluctant to disrobe and, as a result, avoid physical examination unless absolutely necessary. Other women rely on their husbands to make major decisions, including those affecting the woman's health. Religious beliefs may dictate a plan of care, as with birth control measures or blood transfusions. Some cultural groups prefer folk medicine, homeopathy, or prayer to traditional Western medicine; and others attempt combinations of some or all practices. Nurses can integrate into their own practice various holistic approaches to care, in accordance with Dossey's (2010) *Theory of Integral Nursing*. It is critically important to be sensitive to cultural differences and at the same time not stereotype and assume that a woman has certain beliefs because of her ethnic background. Although the amount of health information on the Internet is increasing, information in languages other than English is limited and not all information on the Internet is accurate, making health literacy an important issue in culturally competent care.

Gender Issues

Gender influences provider-patient communication and may influence access to health care in general. Researchers have reported significant male-female differences in receipt of major diagnostic and therapeutic interventions, especially with cardiac and kidney problems. Women tend to use primary care services more often than do men and, some believe, more effectively. The gender of the provider plays a role. The concept of "gender concordance," in which the patient's gender matches the health care provider's gender, was found to be important for women seeking Pap tests (McAlearney, Oliveri, Post, et al., 2011). McAlearney et al. found that women were more comfortable having a Pap test performed by a female physician and having a female nurse present.

Sexual orientation may produce another barrier. Nurses need to understand the specific health care needs and issues related to sexual orientation (Brennan, Barnsteiner, de Leon Siantz, et al., 2012). Some lesbians may not disclose their sexual orientation to health care providers because they feel they may be at risk for hostility, inadequate health care, or breach of confidentiality. In many health care settings, heterosexuality is assumed, and the setting may be one in which the woman does not feel welcome (magazines, brochures, and environment reflect heterosexual couples, or the health care provider shows discomfort interacting with the woman). Lesbians themselves may hold beliefs that are incorrect (e.g., that they have immunity to human immunodeficiency virus [HIV], sexually transmitted infections [STIs], and certain cancers [e.g., cervical]). The perceived lack of risk can result in lesbians avoiding health care, as well as in health care providers giving incorrect advice or not providing appropriate screening for these women. Not all gynecologic cancers are related to sexual activity; lesbians who have never had children may be more at risk for breast, ovarian, and endometrial cancer. Their risk for heart disease, cancer of the lung, and colon cancer is not different from that of the heterosexual woman. To offset stereotypes, it is necessary for providers to develop an approach that does not assume that all patients are heterosexual. More content related to this issue needs to be included in nursing curricula.

CARING FOR THE WELL WOMAN ACROSS THE LIFE SPAN: THE NEED FOR HEALTH PROMOTION AND DISEASE PREVENTION

Maintaining optimal health is a goal for all women. Essential components of health maintenance are the identification of unrecognized problems and potential risks and the education and health promotion needed to reduce them. Current trends in the health care of women have expanded beyond a reproductive focus. A holistic approach to women's health care goes beyond simple reproductive needs and includes a woman's health needs throughout her lifetime, with attention to physical, mental/emotional, social, and spiritual health. Women's health is considered to be part of the primary health care delivery system with assessment and screening focusing on a multisystem evaluation that emphasizes the maintenance and enhancement of wellness. Prevention of cardiovascular disease, promotion of mental health, and prevention of cancers beyond just reproductive-related cancers are all components of well-woman care. It is important to consider all aspects of women's health, particularly in light of the fact that the leading causes of death in women in the United States include more than just reproductive health conditions (Box 3-1).

Even when focusing on reproductive health, it is critical to take a holistic approach to the health of women. This is especially important for women in their childbearing years because conditions that increase a woman's health risks are related not only to her well-being but also to the well-being of both mother and baby in the event of a pregnancy. Prenatal care is an example of prevention that is practiced after conception. However, prevention and health maintenance are needed before conception because many of the mother's risks can be identified and eliminated, or at least modified.

As a female progresses through developmental ages and stages, she is faced with conditions that are age related. An overview of conditions and circumstances that increase health risks in women across the life span is presented in the next section.

Adolescents

All teens undergo progressive development of sex characteristics. They experience the developmental tasks of adolescence such as establishing identity and sexual orientation, emancipating from family, and establishing career goals. Some of these processes can produce great stress for the adolescent, and the health care provider

BOX 3-1	TOP 10 LEADING CAUSES OF DEATH IN WOMEN IN THE UNITED STATES
1. Heart disease	6. Unintentional injury
2. Malignant neoplasm (cancer)	7. Diabetes mellitus
3. Cardiovascular disease (stroke)	8. Influenza and pneumonia
4. Chronic lower respiratory disease	9. Nephritis
5. Alzheimer's disease	10. Septicemia

Data from U.S. Department of Health and Human Services, Health Resources and Services Administration, Maternal and Child Health Bureau: *Women's health USA*, 2011, Rockville, MD; U.S. Department of Health and Human Services, 2009, mchb.hrsa.gov/whusa11.

should treat her very carefully. Female teenagers who enter the health care system usually do so for screening or because of a problem such as episodic illness or accidents. Previous guidelines recommended that young women should be screened with Pap tests at age 18 or when they become sexually active. Guidelines suggest that Pap tests begin at age 21, but controversy exists about the evidence to support these new guidelines, with some health care providers providing evidence for earlier testing (Zhao, Kalpos-Novak, and Austin, 2011). Gynecologic problems are often associated with menses (either bleeding irregularities or dysmenorrhea), vaginitis or leukorrhea, STIs, contraception, or pregnancy. The adolescent is also at risk for use of street drugs, for eating disorders, and for stress, depression, and anxiety.

Many women first enter the health care delivery system for a Pap test or for contraception. Visits to the nurse may be their only contact with the system unless they become ill. Some women postpone examination until a specific need arises such as pregnancy, infertility, pain, abnormal bleeding, or vaginal discharge. Recently the availability of the human papillomavirus (HPV) vaccine has created another reason for young women to enter the health care system (Saraiya, Rosser, and Cooper, 2012).

Teenage Pregnancy

Most young women begin having sex in the mid- to late teens. At age 15, 13% of teens have had sex, but by age 19, 70% of teens have had sexual intercourse (Guttmacher Institute, 2012). A sexually active teen who does not use contraception has a 90% chance of pregnancy within 1 year. The United States has the highest teen pregnancy rate in the industrialized world. By age 20, one third of all American girls get pregnant; most of these pregnancies are unintended (CDC, 2012).

Effective educational programs about sex and family life are imperative to control the rate of teen pregnancy and STIs (Box 3-2). The nurse can provide information regarding the need for child spacing, methods of family planning that are consistent with religious and personal preferences, non-contraceptive benefits of certain methods, the appropriate use of methods selected, and the protection of future fertility when so desired.

Pregnancy in the teenager who is 16 years of age or younger often introduces additional stress into an already stressful developmental period. The emotional level of such teens is commonly characterized by impulsiveness and self-centered behavior, and they often place primary importance on the beliefs and actions of their peers. In attempts to establish a personal and independent identity, many teens do not realize the consequence of their behavior; their thinking processes do not include planning for the future.

Teenagers usually lack the financial resources to support a pregnancy and may not have the maturity to avoid teratogens or have prenatal care and instruction or follow-up care. Children of teen mothers may be at risk for abuse or neglect because of the teen's inadequate knowledge of growth, development, and parenting. Implementation of specialized adolescent programs in schools, communities, and health care systems is demonstrating continued success in reducing the birthrate in teens.

Young and Middle Adulthood

Because women ages 20 to 40 years have a need for contraception, pelvic and breast screening, and pregnancy care, they may prefer to use their gynecologic or obstetric provider as their primary care provider. During these years the woman may be "juggling" family, home, and career responsibilities, with resulting increases in stress-related conditions. Health maintenance includes not only pelvic and breast screening but also promotion of a healthy lifestyle (i.e., good nutrition, regular exercise, no smoking, moderate or no alcohol consumption, sufficient rest, stress reduction, and referral for medical conditions and other specific problems). Common conditions requiring well-woman care include vaginitis, urinary tract infections, menstrual variations, obesity, sexual and relationship issues, and pregnancy.

Parenthood After Age 35

The woman older than 35 years does not have a different physical response to a pregnancy per se but, rather, has had health status changes as a result of time and the aging process. These changes may be responsible for age-related pregnancy conditions. For example, a woman with type 2 diabetes may not have had expression of her diabetes at age 22 years but may have full-blown disease at age 38 years. Other chronic or debilitating diseases or conditions increase in severity with time, and these in turn may predispose to increased risks during pregnancy. Of significance to women in this age-group is the risk for certain genetic anomalies (e.g., Down syndrome). The opportunity for genetic counseling should be available to all (see Chapter 6).

Late Reproductive Age

Women of later reproductive age are often experiencing change and reordering personal priorities. In general, the goals of education, career, marriage, and family have been achieved and now the woman has increased time and opportunity for new interests and activities. Divorce rates are high at this age, and children leaving home may produce an "empty nest syndrome," resulting in increased levels of depression. Chronic diseases also become more apparent. Most problems for the well woman are associated with perimenopause (e.g., bleeding irregularities and vasomotor symptoms). Health maintenance screening continues to be of importance because some conditions such as breast disease or ovarian cancer occur more often during this stage.

APPROACHES TO CARE AT SPECIFIC STAGES OF A WOMAN'S LIFE

There are certain specific approaches to care of women at different stages of their lives. Several of these approaches are described in the next section.

BOX 3-2	**CONTRACEPTIVE HEALTH PROMOTION**

- Child spacing and quality maternity care improve perinatal outcomes and health in general of mother and children.
- Achieving desired family size enables a better sharing of all resources, with attendant increases in education, health care, and other positive societal parameters.
- Contraceptives themselves may positively affect future health. For example, use of condoms may prevent acquisition of HIV infection; combined OCs may provide some protection against later development of cancer of ovary and endometrium; barrier methods decrease transmission of STIs, which can develop into pelvic inflammatory disease with resultant infertility or sterility and thus affect future childbearing capacity.

HIV, Human immunodeficiency virus; *OCs,* oral contraceptives; *STIs,* sexually transmitted infections.

Preconception Counseling and Care

Preconception health promotion provides women and their partners with information that is needed to make decisions about their reproductive future. Preconception care guides couples on how to avoid unintended pregnancies, identify and manage risk factors in their lives and their environment, and identify healthy behaviors that promote the well-being of the woman and her potential fetus. It has been estimated that 31% of pregnant women experience some complications of pregnancy, including mental health issues (mostly depression) and factors that lead to the need for cesarean birth (HealthyPeople.gov, 2012b). In addition, 12% of births result in preterm infants and 8.2% result in low-birth-weight infants (HealthyPeople.gov, 2012a).

Activities that promote healthy mothers and babies must be initiated before the period of critical fetal organ development, which is between 17 and 56 days after fertilization. By the end of the eighth week after conception and certainly by the end of the first trimester, any major structural anomalies in the fetus are already present. Because many women do not realize that they are pregnant and do not seek prenatal care until well into the first trimester, the rapidly growing fetus may be exposed to many types of intrauterine environmental hazards during this most vulnerable developmental phase. These hazards include drugs, viruses, and chemicals. In many instances, counseling can promote behavior modification before damage is done or the woman can make an informed decision about her willingness to accept potential hazards.

Preconception care is important for women who have had a problem with a previous pregnancy (e.g., miscarriage or preterm birth). Although causes are not always identifiable, in many cases problems can be discovered and treated and do not recur in subsequent pregnancies. Preconception care is also important to minimize fetal malformations. For example, the offspring of women who have type 1 diabetes mellitus have significantly more congenital anomalies than do children of mothers without diabetes. The rate of malformation is greatly reduced when the insulin-dependent woman with diabetes has excellent blood glucose control at the time she becomes pregnant and maintains euglycemia (normal blood sugar level) throughout the period of organ development in the fetus. The incidence of neural tube defects such as spina bifida and anencephaly is decreased significantly with the intake of 400 mcg of supplemental folic acid.

The components of preconception care such as health promotion, risk assessment, and interventions are outlined in Box 3-3.

Pregnancy

A woman's entry into health care is often associated with pregnancy, for either diagnosis or actual prenatal care. Early entry into prenatal care (i.e., within the first 12 weeks) allows for identification of the woman at risk for complications and initiation of measures to prevent problems or treat them if they arise. The U.S. Department of Health and Human Services (2012) has emphasized the importance of early and consistent prenatal care to improve outcomes for both mother and infant. Major goals of prenatal care are listed in Box 3-4 and should be addressed in the first visit. Extensive discussion of pregnancy is found in Unit 3.

Fertility Control and Infertility

More than half of the pregnancies in the United States each year are unintended (Taylor, Levi, and Simmonds, 2010), and the majority of these occur in women who either do not use contraception or who experienced a contraceptive failure. Education is the key to

encouraging women to make family planning choices based on preference and actual benefit-to-risk ratios. Providers can influence the user's motivation and ability to use the method correctly (see Chapter 5).

Women also enter the health care system because of their desire to become pregnant. Approximately 15% of couples in the United

---

BOX 3-3 COMPONENTS OF PRECONCEPTION CARE

Health Promotion: General Teaching
- Nutrition
  - Healthy diet, including folic acid
  - Optimal weight
- Exercise and rest
- Avoidance of substance abuse (tobacco, alcohol, "recreational" drugs)
- Use of risk-reducing sex practices
- Attending to family and social needs

Risk Factor Assessment
- Chronic diseases
  - Diabetes, heart disease, hypertension, asthma, thyroid disease, kidney disease, anemia, mental illness
- Infectious diseases
  - HIV/AIDS, other sexually transmitted infections, vaccine-preventable diseases (e.g., rubella, hepatitis B, HPV)
- Reproductive history
  - Contraception
  - Pregnancies—unplanned pregnancy, pregnancy outcomes
  - Infertility
- Genetic or inherited conditions (e.g., sickle cell anemia, Down syndrome, cystic fibrosis)
- Medications and medical treatment
  - Prescription medications (especially those contraindicated in pregnancy), over-the-counter medication use, radiation exposure
- Personal behaviors and exposures
  - Smoking, alcohol consumption, illicit drug use
  - Overweight or underweight; eating disorders
  - Folic acid supplement use
  - Spouse or partner and family situation, including intimate partner violence
  - Availability of family or other support systems
  - Readiness for pregnancy (e.g., age, life goals, stress)
- Environmental (home, workplace) conditions
  - Safety hazards
  - Toxic chemicals
  - Radiation

Interventions
- Anticipatory guidance or teaching
  - Treatment of medical conditions and results
  - Medications
  - Cessation or reduction in substance use and abuse
  - Immunizations (e.g., rubella, hepatitis)
- Nutrition, diet, weight management
- Exercise
- Referral for genetic counseling
- Referral to and use of:
  - Family planning services
  - Family and social needs management

AIDS, Acquired immunodeficiency syndrome; *HIV,* human immunodeficiency virus. *HPV,* human papillomavirus.

States have some degree of infertility. Many couples have delayed starting their families until they are in their 30s or 40s, which allows more time to be exposed to factors that affect fertility negatively (including age-related infertility for the woman). In addition, STIs, which can predispose to decreased fertility, are becoming more common and many women and men are in workplaces and home settings where they may be exposed to reproductive environmental hazards.

Infertility can cause emotional pain for many couples, and the inability to produce offspring sometimes results in feelings of failure and places inordinate stress on the couple's relationship. Much time, money, and emotional investment can be used for testing and treatment in efforts to build a family.

Steps toward prevention of infertility should be undertaken as part of ongoing routine health care, and information about how women may prevent some causes of infertility is especially appropriate in preconception counseling. Primary care providers can undertake initial evaluation and counseling before couples are referred to specialists. For additional information about infertility, see Chapter 5.

Menstrual Problems

Irregularities or problems with the menstrual period are among the most common concerns of women and often cause them to seek help from the health care system. Common menstrual disorders include amenorrhea, dysmenorrhea, premenstrual syndrome, endometriosis, and menorrhagia or metrorrhagia. Simple explanation and counseling may handle the concern; however, history and examination must be completed, as well as laboratory or diagnostic tests, if indicated. Questions should never be considered inconsequential, and age-specific reading materials are recommended, especially for teenagers. See Chapter 4 for an in-depth discussion of menstrual problems.

Perimenopause

The body responds to this natural transition in a number of ways, most of which are caused by the decrease in estrogen. Most women seeking health care during the perimenopausal period do so because of irregular bleeding. Others are concerned about vasomotor symptoms (hot flashes and flushes). Although fertility is greatly reduced during this period, women are urged to maintain some method of birth control because pregnancies still can occur. All women need to have factual information, the dispelling of myths, a thorough examination, and periodic health screenings thereafter.

IDENTIFICATION OF RISK FACTORS TO WOMEN'S HEALTH

In caring for women at all stages of life, it is important to understand the various and complex risk factors that can affect a woman's health. This section describes these risk factors. A thorough and systematic health history can elicit information about risk factors that exist for each woman.

Social, Cultural, and Genetic Factors

Differences exist among people from different socioeconomic levels and ethnic groups with respect to risk for illness and distribution of disease and death. Some diseases are more common among people of selected ethnicity (e.g., sickle cell anemia in African-Americans, Tay-Sachs disease in Ashkenazi Jews, adult lactase deficiency in Chinese, β-thalassemia in Mediterranean people, and cystic fibrosis in northern Europeans). Cultural and religious influences also increase health risks because the woman and her family may have life and societal values and a view of health and illness that dictate practices different from those expected in the Judeo-Christian Western model. These may include food taboos or frequencies, methods of hygiene, effects of climate, care-seeking behaviors, willingness to undergo screening and diagnostic procedures, and conflicts in values.

Socioeconomic status affects birth outcomes. The rates of perinatal and maternal deaths, preterm births, and low-birth-weight babies are considerably higher in disadvantaged populations (Hogue and Silver, 2011). Social consequences for poor women as single parents are great because many mothers with few skills are caught in the bind of insufficient income to afford child care. These families generate fewer and fewer resources and increase their risks for health problems. Multiple roles for women in general produce overload, conflict, and stress, resulting in higher risks for psychologic illness.

Substance Use and Abuse

Use of illicit drugs and inappropriate use of prescription drugs continue to increase and are found in all ages, races, ethnic groups, and socioeconomic levels. Addiction to substances is seen as a biopsychosocial disease, with several factors leading to risk. These include biogenetic predisposition, lack of resilience to stressful life experiences, and poor social support. Women are less likely than men to abuse drugs, but the rate in women is increasing significantly. Substance-abusing pregnant women create severe problems for themselves and their offspring, including interference with optimal growth and development and addiction. In many instances the use of substances is identified through screening programs in prenatal clinics and obstetric units.

Because of the risks to the unborn children and financial concerns, pregnant women who abuse substances can now face criminal charges under expanded interpretations of child abuse and drug trafficking statutes (Guttmacher Institute, 2010). Fifteen states define substance abuse in pregnancy to be child abuse, with 3 states defining it as reason for civil commitment. Suspected drug abuse in pregnant women is reason for reporting by health care professionals in 14 states, and prenatal drug exposure testing is required in 4 states if health care providers suspect substance abuse. Although some policymakers have proposed that pregnant women who abuse substances should be jailed or placed under house arrest, no states actually criminalize prenatal drug abuse. However, some states do commit women to psychiatric hospitals (Guttmacher Institute, 2010). Screening for substance abuse in pregnancy and encouraging prenatal care, counseling, and treatment will be of greater benefit to the mother and child than will prosecution.

Prescription Drug Use

Psychotherapeutic medications such as stimulants, sleeping pills, tranquilizers, and pain relievers are used by an estimated 2% of

American women. Such medications can bring relief from undesirable conditions such as insomnia, anxiety, and pain. Because the medications have mind-altering capacity, misuse can produce psychologic and physical dependency in the same manner as illicit drugs. Risk-to-benefit ratios should be considered when such medications are used for more than a very short period. Depression and anxiety are the most common mental health problems in women (depression used to be considered the most common, but recently it is noted that depression occurs comorbidly with anxiety). Many kinds of medications are used to treat depression and anxiety. All of these psychotherapeutic drugs can have some effect on the fetus and must be monitored very carefully.

Illicit Drug Use

Marijuana. Marijuana is a substance derived from the cannabis plant. It is usually rolled into a cigarette and smoked, but it also may be mixed into food and eaten. Marijuana produces distorted perceptions, difficulty with problem solving as well as with thinking and memory, altered state of awareness, relaxation, mild euphoria, and reduced inhibition (National Institute on Drug Abuse, 2012a). Marijuana readily crosses the placenta and causes increased carbon monoxide levels in the mother's blood, which reduces the oxygen supply to the fetus. Research findings regarding the effects of marijuana demonstrate adverse outcomes on the fetus and infant (Hayatbakhsh, Flenady, Gibbons, et al., 2012).

Cocaine. Cocaine is a powerful central nervous system stimulant that is addictive because of the tremendous sense of euphoria that it creates. It can be snorted, smoked, or injected. Crack or rock cocaine is a form of the drug that is exceedingly potent and even more highly addictive. (Some say that an individual is "hooked" after the first use or at least after two or three "hits"). After ingestion of cocaine, an intensely pleasurable high results that is followed by an uncomfortable low; this increases the urge to repeat the drug.

Predisposing factors and problems associated with cocaine use in pregnancy are polydrug use; poor nutrition; poverty; STIs; hepatitis B infection; dysfunctional family systems; employment difficulties; stress; anger; poor self-esteem; and previous or present physical, emotional, and sexual abuse. Cocaine use is especially concentrated among poor women of color.

Cocaine affects all of the major body systems. Among other complications, it produces cardiovascular stress (including tachycardia and hypertension) that can lead to heart attack or stroke, liver disease, central nervous system simulation that can cause seizures, and even perforation of the nasal septum. Needle-borne diseases such as hepatitis B and acquired immunodeficiency syndrome (AIDS) are common among cocaine users. If the user is pregnant, there is an increased incidence of miscarriage, preterm labor, small-for-gestational age babies, abruption of placenta, and stillbirth. Anomalies have been reported.

One of the promising treatments for cocaine abuse in pregnancy is acupuncture. A component of traditional Chinese medicine, acupuncture is used to redirect energy flow (chi) within the body, reduce cravings, and enhance well-being. Acupuncture has been studied and shown to be effective in detoxification in people addicted to many different drugs (Schaub and Burt, 2013).

Opiates. The opiates include opium, heroin, meperidine, morphine, codeine, and methadone. Heroin is one of the most commonly abused drugs of this class. It is usually taken by intravenous injection but can be smoked or "snorted." The signs and symptoms of heroin use are euphoria, relaxation, relief from pain, "nodding out" (apathy, detachment from reality, impaired judgment, and drowsiness), constricted pupils, nausea, constipation, slurred speech, and respiratory depression.

The incidence of heroin use among pregnant women is unknown because women with a dependency on heroin often use multiple drugs. Women who use opiates during pregnancy have a 6-times higher risk for problem outcomes (Keegan, Parva, Finnegan, et al., 2010). The recommended treatment is methadone maintenance, ideally done by stabilizing the treatment before as well as during pregnancy (Peles, Schreiber, Bloch, et al., 2012). This treatment must be closely monitored because, in pregnancy, methadone is metabolized more rapidly, leading to withdrawal symptoms in less than 24 hours in many women. Withdrawal symptoms can include fetal hyperactivity and, if severe, preterm labor or fetal death. Women may resort to heroin to alleviate the uncomfortable symptoms.

Methamphetamine. Methamphetamine is a relatively cheap and highly addictive stimulant. Over the past few years, use of this dangerous drug has decreased. In 2006 it was estimated that there were 731,000 methamphetamine users per month, decreasing in 2008 to 314,000 users per month (National Institute on Drug Abuse, 2012b). Methamphetamine makes many users feel hypersexual and uninhibited, leading to more sex and less protection from pregnancy and STIs.

The active metabolite of methamphetamine is amphetamine, a central nervous system stimulant known as both "speed" and "meth." The crystalline form, which is smoked, is known as "ice." Methamphetamine causes a person to experience an elevated mood state and pleasure as well as increased energy and creates addiction within a short period. It can lead to cardiac problems, including irregular heartbeat and hypertension and, over time, can create cognitive and mental as well as dental problems (Medline Plus, 2012). Most of the effects of amphetamines are similar to those of cocaine. Although fewer maternal and neonatal complications have been attributed to this class of substances than to cocaine, the rates of preterm births and intrauterine growth restriction with smaller head circumference are higher in methamphetamine-exposed pregnant women than in pregnant women who abuse other substances.

Phencyclidine. Phencyclidine (PCP) is a synthetic drug known by various names ("peace pill," "elephant," "angel dust," "hog"). At least 1% of 12th graders in the United States have abused PCP (National Institute on Drug Abuse, 2012c). PCP causes a person to experience dissociative symptoms that include distorted perceptions and detached feelings, delusions, hallucinations, extreme anxiety, and disordered thinking (National Institute on Drug Abuse, 2012c). Because some effects mimic the signs and symptoms of schizophrenia, a user may be admitted to a psychiatric unit. The major concerns regarding PCP use in pregnant women are its association with polydrug abuse and the neurobehavioral effects on the neonate.

Other Illicit Drugs. A number of street drugs pose risk to users. A few are derived from organic materials, but more and more are produced synthetically in laboratories. Sedatives such as "downers," "yellow jackets," or "red devils" are used to come off of "highs." Hallucinogens alter perceptions and body function. PCP ("angel dust") and lysergic acid diethylamide (LSD) produce vivid changes in sensation, often with agitation, euphoria, paranoia, and a tendency toward antisocial behavior. Their use may lead to flashbacks, chronic psychosis, and violent behavior. Hallucinogens taken during pregnancy may have negative neurobehavioral effects on the newborn.

Alcohol Consumption

Women ages 35 to 49 have the highest rates of chronic alcoholism, but women ages 21 to 34 have the highest rates of specific alcohol-related problems. About one third of alcoholics are women, and many relate the onset of their drinking problem to stressful events. Women who are problem drinkers are often depressed, have more motor vehicle injuries, and have a higher incidence of attempted suicide than do women in the general population. They are also at risk for alcohol-related liver damage. Early case finding and treatment are important in alcoholism for both the ill individual and family members.

Prenatal alcohol exposure has been found to increase the chance of birth defects significantly, with one study reporting a fourfold increase (O'Leary, Nassar, Kurinczuk, et al., 2011). Although fetal alcohol syndrome (FAS) is a known consequence of prenatal alcohol intake, studies also indicate that other consequences include increased risk for miscarriage, stillbirth, preterm birth, and sudden infant death syndrome (SIDS). Clearly, alcohol consumption during pregnancy has wide-reaching effects (Bailey and Sokol, 2011). A 2020 national health objective is to have 98.3% of pregnant women abstain from alcohol use (HealthyPeople.gov, 2012c.)

Alcohol use during pregnancy can lead to fetal alcohol spectrum disorder (FASD), which includes FAS, fetal alcohol effects, and alcohol-related neurologic developmental disabilities. Approximately 40,000 babies per year are born with FASD; however, recent research reveals that multivitamin supplement use during pregnancy may lessen the effects of prenatal alcohol exposure in the children of women who are unable or unwilling to curtail their alcohol abuse when pregnant (Avalos, Kaskutas, Block, et al., 2011). Low birth weight, intellectual disability, behavioral problems, and learning and physical problems are some of the symptoms of FAS babies (see Chapter 25). Severe facial deformities of FAS occur at day 20 of conception when women may not even suspect that they are pregnant.

Cigarette Smoking

Tobacco use is the leading cause of preventable death and illness. Smoking is linked to cardiovascular disease, various types of cancers (especially lung and cervical), chronic lung disease, and negative pregnancy outcomes. Premature death is estimated to occur in 443,000 people annually because of either smoking or being exposed to secondhand smoke, and 8.6 million people are estimated to be seriously ill as a result of smoking. However, it is also estimated that 46.6 million adults in the United States smoke; 17.3% of women are smokers (Centers for Disease Control and Prevention, 2011). Tobacco contains nicotine, which is an addictive substance that creates physical and psychologic dependence. Smoking in pregnancy is known to cause a decrease in placental perfusion and is one cause of low birth weight in infants.

Cigarette smoking impairs fertility in both women and men, may reduce the age for menopause, and increases the risk for osteoporosis after menopause. Passive, or secondhand, smoke (environmental tobacco smoke) contains similar hazards and presents additional problems for the smoker and harm for the nonsmoker. Box 3-5 describes an intervention, referred to as the "Five A's" to encourage smoking cessation.

Caffeine

Caffeine is found in society's most popular drinks: coffee, tea, and soft drinks. It is a stimulant that can affect mood and interrupt body functions by producing anxiety and sleep interruptions. Heart dysrhythmias may be made worse by caffeine, and there can

---

BOX 3-5   INTERVENTIONS FOR SMOKING CESSATION: THE FIVE A'S

Ask
- What was her age when she started smoking?
- How many cigarettes does she smoke a day? When was her last cigarette?
- Has she tried to quit?
- Does she want to quit?

Advise
- Give her information about the effects of smoking on pregnancy and her fetus, on her own future health, and on the members of her household.

Assess
- What were her reasons for not being able to quit before, or what made her start again?
- Does she have anyone who can help her?
- Does anyone else smoke at home?
- Does she have friends or family who have quit successfully?

Assist
- Provide support; give self-help materials.
- Encourage her to set a quit date.
- Refer to a smoking cessation program, or provide information about nicotine replacement products (not recommended during pregnancy) if she is interested.
- Teach and encourage use of stress-reduction activities.
- Provide for follow-up with a phone call, letter, or clinic visit.

Arrange Follow-Up
- Arrange to follow the woman to find out about smoking-cessation status.
- Make a phone call around the time of her quit date. Assess her status at every prenatal visit.
- Congratulate her on her success, or provide support for her if she relapses.
- Referral to intensive treatment may be necessary.

From Fiore MC, Jaen CR, Baker TB, et al: *Treating tobacco use and dependence: 2008 update: Clinical Practice Guideline,* Rockville, MD, 2008, US Department of Health and Human Services, Public Health Service, http://www.surgeongeneral.gov/tobacco/treating_tobacco_use08.pdf (pg. 39).

---

be interactions with certain medications such as lithium. Birth defects have not been related to caffeine consumption; however, high intake has been related to a slight decrease in birth weight and may also increase risk for miscarriage. The March of Dimes (2010) recommends that until more is known about the effects of caffeine during pregnancy, especially in regard to miscarriage, that pregnant women limit their caffeine intake to no more that 200 mg/day (an 8-ounce cup of brewed coffee has approximately 137 mg of caffeine).

Nutrition Problems and Eating Disorders

Good nutrition is essential for optimal health. A well-balanced diet helps prevent illness and also is used to treat certain health problems. Conversely, poor eating habits, eating disorders, and obesity are linked to disease and debility. *Dietary Guidelines for Americans* (U.S. Department of Agriculture, 2010) provides evidence-based recommendations to promote health and reduce risks for chronic diseases through diet and physical activity. This guide contains resources for health professionals and consumers on dietary guidelines. Recently the Food Guide Pyramid has been replaced by MyPlate, a guide to healthy eating recommended by the *Dietary Guidelines for Americans* (HealthyPeople.gov, 2012b).

In addition to specific guidelines for healthy eating, environmental factors play an important role in nutrition. Dubowitz, Ghosh-Dastidar, Eibner, et al. (2012) presented data from the Women's Health Initiative Clinical Trial (WHI CT) that indicated availability of healthy food was correlated with decreased obesity in women. These data suggest that social conditions and access to nutritious food are important contributors to women's health.

Nutritional Deficiencies

Overt disease caused by a lack of certain nutrients is rarely seen in the United States. However, insufficient amounts or imbalances of nutrients do pose problems for individuals and families. Overweight or underweight status, malabsorption, listlessness, fatigue, frequent colds and other minor infections, constipation, dull hair and nails, and dental caries are examples of problems that can be related to nutrition and indicate the need for further nutritional assessment. Poor nutrition, especially related to obesity and high fat and cholesterol intake, may lead to more serious conditions and contribute to 4 of the 10 leading causes of death in the United States: heart diseases, malignant neoplasms, cerebrovascular diseases, and diabetes.

Other dietary extremes also produce risk. For example, insufficient amounts of calcium can lead to osteoporosis, too much sodium can aggravate hypertension, and megadoses of vitamins can cause adverse effects in several body systems. Fad weight-loss programs and yo-yo dieting (repeated and cyclic weight gain and weight loss) result in nutritional imbalances and, in some instances, medical problems. Such diets and programs are not appropriate for weight maintenance. Adolescent pregnancy produces special nutritional requirements because the metabolic needs of pregnancy are superimposed on the teen's own needs for growth and maturation at a time when eating habits are not ideal. Neural tube defects are more common in infants born to women with a diet poor in folate. In their childbearing years, women should ingest at least 0.4 mg (400 mcg) of folic acid daily in additional to consuming a diet rich in folate-containing foods.

Obesity

During the past 20 years, obesity has increased dramatically in the United States. More than one third of women in the United States are obese (body mass index [BMI] of 30 or greater), with adults ages 40 to 59 having the highest prevalence. The BMI is defined as a measure of an adult's weight in relation to his or her height, specifically the adult's weight in kilograms divided by the square of his or her height in meters (Box 3-6). It is estimated that one third of adults and one sixth of children and adolescents are in the obese range (HealthyPeople.gov, 2012b). Overweight and obesity are known risk factors for premature death, diabetes, heart disease, stroke, hypertension, type 2 diabetes, gallbladder disease, diverticular disease, some anemias, oral disease, constipation, osteoarthritis, gout, osteoporosis, respiratory dysfunction, sleep apnea, and some types of cancer (uterine, breast, colorectal, kidney, and gallbladder) (American Cancer Society, 2012a). In addition, obesity is associated with high cholesterol, menstrual irregularities, hirsutism (excess body/facial hair), stress incontinence, depression, complications of pregnancy, increased surgical risk, and shortened life span. Pregnant women who are morbidly obese are at increased risk for hyperten-

BOX 3-6	IDEAL BODY WEIGHT WITH BODY MASS INDEX

BMI 18.5 or less—Underweight
BMI 18.5 to 24.9—Normal weight
BMI 25.0 to 29.9—Overweight
BMI 30.0 to 34.5—Obese
BMI 35.0 to 40—Very obese

sion, diabetes, gallbladder disease, postterm pregnancy, and musculoskeletal problems.

Eating Disorders

Anorexia nervosa and bulimia are two forms of eating disorders, although there are additional forms, such as subclinical eating disorders. Some women, especially adolescents, do not have symptoms that lend themselves to a diagnosis of anorexia nervosa or bulimia. These women are diagnosed as having a subclinical eating disorder, which is usually associated with disorders of mood and anxiety and requires accurate diagnosis and prompt treatment (Touchette, Henegar, Godart, et al., 2011). Recent research suggests that eating disorders are often associated with difficulties in intimate relationships, and interpersonal psychotherapy has been considered as an approach to treatment of women with eating disorders (Murphy, Straebler, Basden, et al., 2012).

It is important to assess for and treat women with eating disorders early because they are at increased risk for serious physical problems as well as diminished quality of life (Vallance, Latner, and Gleaves, 2011). Eating disorders during pregnancy are also associated with increased risk to the pregnant woman and her fetus (Pasternak, Weintraub, Shoham-Vardi, et al., 2012).

Anorexia Nervosa. Some women have a distorted view of their bodies and, no matter what their weight, perceive themselves to be much too heavy. As a result, they undertake strict and severe diets and rigorous extreme exercise. This chronic eating disorder is known as anorexia nervosa. Women can carry this condition to the point of starvation, with resulting endocrine and metabolic abnormalities. If not corrected, significant complications of dysrhythmias, amenorrhea, cardiomyopathy, and heart failure occur and, in the extreme, can lead to death. The condition commonly begins during adolescence in young women who have some degree of personality disorder. They gradually lose weight over several months, have amenorrhea, and are abnormally concerned with body image. A coexisting depression usually accompanies anorexia.

There are no specific tests to diagnose anorexia nervosa. A medical history, physical examination, and screening tests help identify women at risk for eating disorders. Several tools are available to use in primary care settings. The SCOFF questionnaire, developed by Morgan, Reid, and Lacey (1999) is easy to administer and can help the nurse decide whether an eating disorder is likely and whether the woman needs further assessment and possibly psychiatric and medical intervention. More recently, Hautala, Junnila, Alin, et al. (2009) provided further evidence for the validity and usefulness of the SCOFF. See Box 3-7 for a description of the SCOFF.

Bulimia Nervosa. Bulimia refers to secret, uncontrolled binge eating alternating with methods to prevent weight gain: self-induced vomiting, laxatives or diuretics, strict diets, fasting, and rigorous exercise. During a binge episode, a large number of calories are consumed, usually consisting of sweets and "junk foods." Binges

BOX 3-7   SCREENING FOR EATING DISORDERS: SCOFF QUESTIONS

Each question scores 1 point. A score of 2 or more indicates the person may have anorexia nervosa or bulimia.

1. Do you make yourself Sick (i.e., induce vomiting) because you feel too full?
2. Do you worry about loss of Control over the amount you eat?
3. Have you recently lost more than One stone (6.4 kg [14 lbs]) in a 3-month period?
4. Do you think you are too Fat even if others think you are too thin?
5. Does Food dominate your life?

From Morgan J, Reid F, Lacey J: The SCOFF questionnaire: assessment of a new screening tool for eating disorders, *BMJ* 319(7223):1467–1468, 1999.

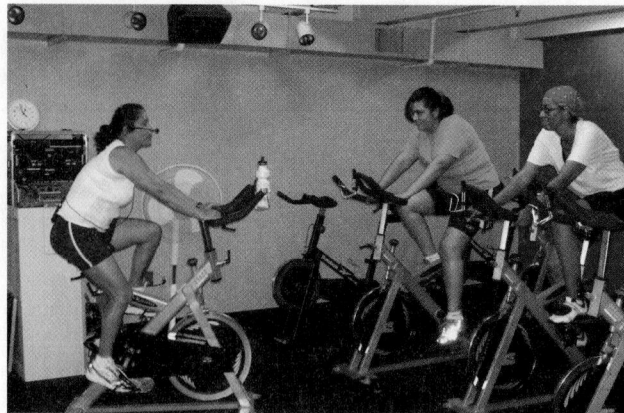

FIG 3-8 Exercise should be part of one's regular health routine. A cycle class is fun and provides moderate to vigorous exercise. (Courtesy Shari Rivera Sharpe, Chapel Hill, NC.)

occur at least twice per week. Bulimia usually begins in early adulthood (ages 18 to 25 years) and is found primarily in females. Complications can include dehydration and electrolyte imbalance, gastrointestinal abnormalities, and cardiac dysrhythmias. Bulimia is somewhat similar to anorexia in that it is an eating disorder and usually involves some degree of depression (Skinner, Haines, Austin, et al., 2012). Unlike those with anorexia, individuals with bulimia may feel shame or disgust about their disorder and tend to seek help earlier. The SCOFF screening assessment also can be used to assess patients with bulimia (see Box 3-7).

Lack of Exercise

Exercise contributes to good health by lowering risks for a variety of conditions that are influenced by obesity and a sedentary lifestyle. It is effective in the prevention of cardiovascular disease and in the management of chronic conditions such as hypertension, arthritis, diabetes, respiratory disorders, and osteoporosis (Fig. 3-8). Exercise also contributes to stress reduction and weight maintenance. Women report that engaging in regular exercise improves their body image and self-esteem and acts as a mood enhancer. Aerobic exercise produces cardiovascular involvement because an increased amount of oxygen is delivered to working muscles. Anaerobic exercise such as weight training improves individual muscle mass without stress on the cardiovascular system. Because women are concerned about both cardiovascular and bone health, weight-bearing aerobic exercises such as walking, running, racket sport, and dancing are preferred. However, excessive or strenuous exercise can lead to hormone imbalances, resulting in amenorrhea and its consequences. Physical injury is also a potential risk.

One particular exercise that is important for women is *Kegel exercise*, or pelvic muscle exercise. This exercise is used to strengthen the muscles that support the pelvic floor and should be practiced regularly. Instructions for this exercise are in presented in the Guidelines box.

Physical activity and exercise counseling for persons of all ages should be undertaken at schools, work sites, and primary care settings. Specific recommendations include 20 to 30 minutes of moderate activity at least 3 times per week. Few Americans exercise this often, and physical inactivity increases with age, especially during adolescence and early adulthood. Even small increases in activity can be beneficial. During pregnancy, an ongoing exercise regimen can be continued but intensity and duration should be decreased. Sedentary women should obtain medical clearance to initiate exercise during pregnancy and should begin with low-intensity and low-impact workouts.

Stress

The modern woman faces increasing levels of stress and, as a result, is prone to a variety of stress-induced complaints and illnesses. Stress often occurs because of multiple roles in which coping with job and financial responsibilities conflicts with parenting and duties at home. To add to this burden, women are socialized to be caregivers, which is emotionally draining, creating additional stress. They also may find themselves in positions of minimal power that do not allow them control over their everyday environments. Some stress is normal and contributes to positive outcomes. Many women thrive in busy surroundings. However, excessive or high levels of ongoing stress trigger physical reactions such as rapid heart rate, elevated blood pressure, slowed digestion, release of additional neurotransmitters and hormones, muscle tenseness, and a weakened immune system. Consequently, constant stress can contribute to clinical illnesses such as flare-ups of arthritis or asthma, frequent colds or infections, gastrointestinal upsets, cardiovascular problems, and infertility. Box 3-8 lists symptoms that may be related to chronic or extreme stress. Psychologic symptoms such as anxiety, irritability, eating disorders, depression, insomnia, and substance abuse have also been associated with stress.

Because it is neither possible nor desirable to avoid all stress, women must learn how to manage it. The nurse should assess each woman for signs of stress, using therapeutic communication skills to determine risk factors and the woman's ability to function. Some women must be referred for counseling or other mental health therapy. Women are twice as likely as men to suffer from depression, anxiety, or panic attacks. Nurses must be alert to the symptoms of serious mental disorders such as depression and anxiety and make referrals to mental health practitioners when necessary. Women experiencing major life changes such as separation and divorce, bereavement, serious illness, and unemployment also need special attention.

Many centers offer support groups to help women prevent or manage stress. Social support and good coping skills can improve a woman's self-esteem and give her a sense of mastery. Anticipatory guidance for developmental or expected situational crises can help her plan strategies for dealing with potentially stressful events. Role playing, relaxation techniques, biofeedback, meditation,

GUIDELINES

Kegel Exercises

Description and Rationale

Kegel exercises, or pelvic muscle exercise, is a technique used to strengthen the muscles that support the pelvic floor. This exercise involves regularly tightening (contracting) and relaxing the muscles that support the bladder and urethra. By strengthening these pelvic muscles, a woman can prevent or reduce accidental urine loss.

Technique

The woman needs to learn how to target the muscles for training and how to contract them correctly. One suggestion for teaching is to have the woman pretend she is trying to prevent the passage of intestinal gas. Have her use this tightening motion on the muscles around her vagina and the upper pelvis. She should feel these muscles drawing inward and upward. Other suggested techniques are to have the woman pretend she is trying to stop the flow of urine in midstream or to have her think about how her vagina is able to contract around and move up the length of the penis during intercourse.

The woman should avoid straining or bearing-down motions while performing the exercise. She should be taught how bearing down feels by having her take a breath, hold it, and push down with her abdominal muscles as though she were trying to have a bowel movement. Then the woman can be taught how to avoid straining down by exhaling gently and keeping her mouth open each time she contracts her pelvic muscles.

Specific Instructions

1. Each contraction should be as intense as possible without contracting the abdomen, thighs, or buttocks.
2. Contractions should be held for at least 10 seconds. The woman may have to start with as little as 2 seconds per contraction until her muscles get stronger.
3. The woman should rest for 10 seconds or more between contractions so that the muscles have time to recover and each contraction can be as strong as the woman can make it.
4. The woman should feel the pulling up over the three muscle layers so that the contraction reaches the highest level of her pelvis.

Data from Sampselle C: Behavior interventions in young and middle-aged women: Simple interventions to combat a complex problem, *American Journal of Nursing* 103(Suppl):9–19, 2003; Sampselle C: Behavioral interventions for urinary incontinence in women: Evidence for practice, *Journal of Midwifery & Women's Health* 45(2):94–103, 2000; Sampselle C, Wyman J, Thomas K, et al: Continence for women: a test of AWHONN's evidence-based protocol, *Journal of Obstetric, Gynecologic, and Neonatal Nursing* 29(1):312–317, 2000.

BOX 3-8 STRESS SYMPTOMS

Physical
- Perspiration/sweaty hands
- Increased heart rate
- Trembling
- Nervous tics
- Dryness of throat and mouth
- Tiring easily
- Urinating frequently
- Sleeping problems
- Diarrhea, indigestion, vomiting
- Butterflies in stomach
- Headaches
- Premenstrual tension
- Pain in neck and lower back
- Loss of appetite or overeating
- Susceptibility to illness

Behavioral
- Stuttering and other speech difficulties
- Crying for no apparent reason
- Acting impulsively
- Startling easily
- Laughing in a high-pitched and nervous tone of voice
- Grinding teeth
- Increasing smoking
- Increasing use of drugs and alcohol
- Being accident prone

Psychologic
- Feeling anxious
- Feeling scared
- Feeling irritable
- Feeling moody
- Having low self-esteem
- Being afraid of failure
- Being unable to concentrate
- Embarrassing easily
- Worrying about the future
- Being preoccupied with thoughts or tasks
- Forgetful

Adapted from State University of New York Counseling Center: *Stress management*, Buffalo, NY, 2002, University of Buffalo, State University of New York.

---

addition to depression and anxiety, women experience other mental health disorders, such as bipolar disease.

Sleep Disorders

Many women suffer from sleep disorders, including difficulty initiating sleep or staying asleep and experiencing nonrestorative sleep (Zender and Olshansky, 2009). Restless leg syndrome may be a cause of sleep disorders or a comorbid condition. Sleep disorders are correlated with physical and mental health problems, including depression, pain, and fibromyalgia. Mong, Baker, Mahoney, et al. (2011) presented a review of studies conducted on gender differences related to sleep, suggesting that, while further research is needed, women experience insomnia significantly more than do men. It is important that the nurse talk with the woman about her sleep patterns and discuss ways to improve sleep, such as avoiding alcohol before going to sleep and sleeping in a regular pattern.

Environmental and Workplace Hazards

Environmental hazards in the home, the workplace, and the community can contribute to poor health at all ages. Categories and examples of health-damaging hazards include the following: (1) pathogenic agents (viruses, bacteria, fungi, parasites); (2) natural and synthetic chemicals (natural toxins from animals, insects, and plants; consumer and industrial products such as pesticides and hydrocarbon gases; medical and diagnostic devices; tobacco; fuels; and drug and alcohol abuse); (3) radiation (radon, heat waves, sound waves); (4) food substances (added

---

desensitization, imagery, assertiveness training, yoga, diet, exercise, and weight control are all techniques nurses can include in their repertoire of helping skills.

Depression, Anxiety, and Other Mental Health Conditions

Women experience depression and/or anxiety frequently. In addition, depression is sometimes described as a co-traveler because it is exists comorbidly with other physical conditions. Depression and/or anxiety create difficulties for quality of life and, at the extreme, create a risk for suicide. Recent research (Berecki-Gisolf, McKenzie, Dobson, et al., 2012) suggests that women with comorbid anxiety and depression are at greater risk for developing cardiac disease. In

components that are not necessary for nutrition); and (5) physical objects (moving vehicles, machinery, weapons, water, and building materials).

Environmental hazards can affect fertility, fetal development, live birth, and the child's future mental and physical development. Children are at special risk for poisoning from lead found in paint and soil. Everyone is at risk from air pollutants such as tobacco smoke, carbon monoxide, smog, suspended particles (dust, ash, and asbestos), and cleaning solvents; noise pollution; pesticides; chemical additives; and poor preparation of food. Workers also face safety and health risks caused by ergonomically poor work stations and stress. It is important that risk assessments continue to be in effect to identify and understand environmental problems in public health. The March of Dimes (2011) has published a helpful resource that summarizes the various risks posed in the environment to pregnant women and their fetuses.

Risky Sexual Practices

Potential risks related to sexual activity include undesired pregnancy and STIs. The risks are particularly high for adolescents and young adults who engage in sexual intercourse at earlier and earlier ages. Adolescents report many reasons for wanting to be sexually active: peer pressure, desire to love and be loved, experimentation, to enhance self-esteem, and to have fun. However, many teens do not have the decision-making or values-clarification skills needed to take this important step. They may also lack knowledge about contraception and STIs. Many do not believe that becoming pregnant or getting an STI will happen to them.

Although some STIs can be cured with antibiotics, many cause significant problems. Possible sequelae include infertility, ectopic pregnancy, neonatal morbidity and mortality, genital cancers, AIDS, and even death. The incidence of STIs is increasing rapidly and reaching epidemic proportion. Choice of contraception has an impact on the risk for contracting an STI. No method of contraception offers complete protection. (See Chapter 4 for a discussion of STIs and Chapter 5 for a discussion of contraception.)

Prevention of STIs is predicated on the reduction of high risk behaviors by educating toward a behavioral change. Behaviors of concern include multiple and casual sexual partners and unsafe sexual practices. Specific self-management measures to prevent STIs are listed in Box 3-9. The abuse of alcohol and drugs is a high risk behavior, resulting in impaired judgment and thoughtless acts. Behavioral changes must come from within; therefore the nurse must provide sufficient information for the individual or group to "buy into" the need for change. Education is a powerful tool in health promotion and prevention of STIs and pregnancy. However, it works best when delivered in a way that considers the language, culture, and lifestyle of the intended listener.

Risk for Certain Medical Conditions

Most women of reproductive age are relatively healthy. Heart disease; lung, breast, colon, and other nongynecologic cancers; chronic lung disease; and diabetes are all concerns for adult women because they are among the leading causes of death in women. Certain medical conditions present during pregnancy can have deleterious effects on both the woman and the fetus. Of particular concern are risks from all forms of diabetes, urinary tract disorders, thyroid disease, hypertensive disorders of pregnancy, cardiac disease, and seizure disorders. Effects on the fetus vary and include intrauterine growth restriction, macrosomia, anemia, prematurity, immaturity, and stillbirth. Effects on the woman also can be severe. These conditions are discussed in later chapters.

BOX 3-9   STI AND HIV PREVENTION

- Prevention of STIs and HIV is possible only if there is no oral, genital, or rectal exchange of body fluids or if a person is in a long-term, mutually monogamous relationship with an uninfected partner.
- Correct use of latex condoms, although greatly reducing risk, is not exclusively protective.
- Sexual partners should be selected with great care.
- Partners should be asked about history of STIs.
- Preexposure vaccination is one of the most effective methods for preventing transmission of some STIs (hepatitis A and hepatitis B, human papillomavirus).
- A new condom should be used for each act of sexual intercourse.
- Abstinence from sexual intercourse is encouraged for persons who are being treated for an STI or whose partners are being treated.

Adapted from Centers for Disease Control and Prevention: Sexually transmitted diseases treatment guidelines 2010, *MMWR* 59(RR-12):11094, 2010.
STI, Sexually transmitted infection; *HIV,* human immunodeficiency virus.

Risk for Certain Gynecologic Conditions

Women are at risk throughout their reproductive years for pelvic inflammatory disease, endometriosis, STIs and other vaginal infections (see Chapter 4), uterine fibroids, uterine deformities such as bicornuate uterus, ovarian cysts, interstitial cystitis, and urinary incontinence related to pelvic relaxation. These gynecologic conditions may contribute negatively to pregnancy by causing infertility, miscarriage, preterm labor, and fetal and neonatal problems. Gynecologic cancers also affect women's health, although the risk for most cancers is low in pregnancy. Risk factors depend on the type of cancer. The impact of developing a gynecologic problem or cancer on women and their families is shaped by a number of factors, including the specific type of problem or cancer, the implications of the diagnosis for the woman and her family, and the timing of the occurrence in the woman's and the family's lives.

Female Genital Mutilation

Female genital mutilation is practiced in more than 45 countries, with the majority of these countries being in Africa. As emigrants from these countries arrive in North America, nurses in the United States and Canada will see patients who have had such procedures performed (see Cultural Competence box).

Violence Against Women

Intimate partner violence (IPV) is the most common form of violence experienced by women worldwide, with a reported incidence of one of every six women having been a victim of domestic violence. In the United States, IPV is a significant social problem and a major health care problem that affects millions of women and men each year and costs millions of dollars in annual medical costs. Statistics from the U.S. Department of Justice, Office of Violence Against Women (2012) reported that one in four women in the United States have experienced severe physical violence by a current or former intimate partner. In addition, 5.2 million women were victimized by stalkers. It is estimated that 1.3 million women are raped in the United States annually.

Although *IPV* is the preferred term, *wife battering, spouse abuse,* and *domestic* or *family violence* are also terms that may be applied to a pattern of assaultive and coercive behaviors inflicted by a male partner in a marriage or other heterosexual, significant, intimate

Female Genital Mutilation

Defined by the World Health Organization (WHO), female genital mutilation (FGM) is "all procedures that involve partial or total removal of the external female genitalia, or other injury to the female genital organs for non-medical reasons" (WHO, 2012). This includes female circumcision and is an attempt to control women through controlling their sexuality. FGM is supposed to remove sexual desire so that the girl will not become sexually active until married (McGargill, 2009).

Female circumcision occurs in women of many different ethnic, cultural, and religious backgrounds. Although circumcision is usually performed during childhood, some communities circumcise infants or older females. The procedure involves the removal of a portion of the clitoris but may extend to the removal of the entire clitoris and labia minora. In addition, the labia majora, which are often stitched together over the urethral and vaginal openings, may be affected.

The extent of the circumcision site affects the seriousness of complications. Common complications include bleeding, pain, local scarring, keloid or cyst formation, and infection. Impaired drainage of urine and menstrual blood may lead to chronic pelvic infections, pelvic and back pain, and chronic urinary tract infections. Some women may require surgery before vaginal examination, intercourse, or childbirth if the vaginal opening is obstructed.

FGM is illegal in the United States and punishable by fines, prison, and deportation. An obstetrician may incise the closed labia to deliver a baby or remove cysts but may not sew the labia back to its previous state of reinfibulation. If performed on a minor, FGM is considered child abuse in the United States. "The practice also violates the rights to health, security and physical integrity of the person, the right to be free from torture and cruel, inhuman or degrading treatment, and the right to life when the procedure results in death" (WHO, 2012).

Nurses are providing care to a growing number of women who have emigrated from the Middle East, Asia, and Africa, where female circumcision is more common. Nurses must be sensitive to the unique needs of these patients, especially if these women have concerns about maintaining or restoring the intactness of the circumcision after childbirth.

Data from McGargill P: Female genital mutilation, *On the Edge* 15(2 Summer), 2009, www.cinahl.com/cgi-bin/refsvc?jid =29638accno-2010331425; World Health Organization (2012 February). Female genital mutilation, www.who.int/mediacentre/factsheet/fs241/en/print.html.

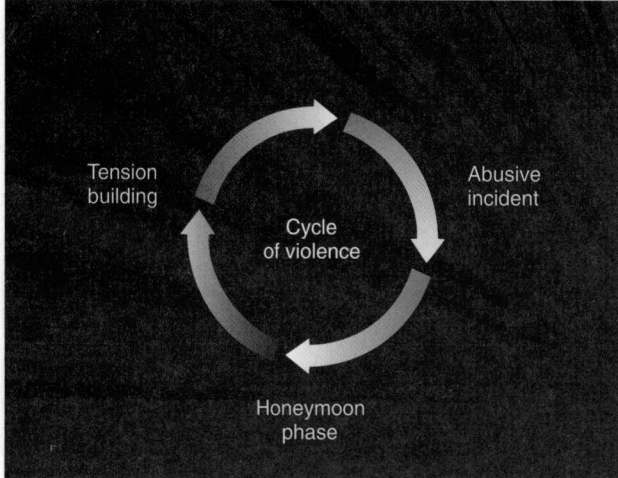

FIG 3-9 Cycle of violence.

behavior and pleas for forgiveness. This honeymoon phase lasts until stress or other factors cause conflict and tension to mount again toward another episode of battering. Over time, the tension and battering phases last longer and the calm phase becomes shorter until there is no honeymoon phase.

Because violence against women crosses all ethnic, educational, religious, and socioeconomic backgrounds and there are often misconceptions regarding who is at risk for being abused, it is important to differentiate myths from facts about this serious and often devastating condition. Table 3-2 presents myths and facts about IPV.

All women entering the health care system should be assessed for potential abuse. An abuse assessment screening tool can be used as part of the interview or written history. If a male partner is present, he should be asked to leave the room because the woman may not disclose experiences of abuse in his presence or he may try to answer questions for her to protect himself. The same procedure applies to partners of lesbians or the adult children of older women. At present there is no universally accepted screening tool for all populations (Rabin, Jennings, Campbell, et al., 2009). However, the American College of Obstetricians and Gynecologists [ACOG] and the Nursing Research Consortium on Violence and Abuse have each suggested questions that give a woman permission to disclose sensitive information. Fig. 3-10 presents a modification and combination of questions suggested by these two organizations.

It also is important that the nurse be alert to any indication from the woman that she is being abused, despite the fact that she may not have specifically stated that she is in an abusive relationship. Box 3-10 provides a list of signs of IPV.

Futures Without Violence (which was previously called the *Family Violence Prevention Fund*) collaborated with the Avon Foundation to explore ways to prevent violence on college campuses. They published a document referred to as *Beyond Title IX: Guidelines for Preventing and Responding to Gender-Based Violence in Higher Education* (Fleck-Henderson, Costello, Raghu, et al., 2012), which provides guidelines for college campuses in being vigilant to the possibility of gender-based violence.

A therapeutic relationship and skillful interviewing help women disclose and describe their abuse. Language is important when talking with women. For example, using the term *victim* connotes powerlessness and hopelessness; a more empowering term is *survivor*. Women who have identified their abuse may appear passive, hostile, anxious, depressed, or hysterical because they may think

relationship (and sometimes the man is the victim of violence). It is also important to note that not all violence against women is caused by an intimate partner; non-IPV also occurs. Montero, Escriba, Ruiz-Perez, et al. (2011) studied both IPV and non-IPV, noting that violence in general has negative effects on women's health and recommending that routine assessment of violence against women be included in primary care histories. Common elements of IPV are physical abuse; psychologic or emotional abuse; sexual assault; isolation; and controlling all aspects of the victim's life, including money, shelter, time, and food.

Battering is neither random nor constant; rather, it occurs in repeated cycles. Health care providers often refer to the "cycle of violence" (Fig. 3-9). A three-phase includes a period of increasing tension leading to the battery. The battery consists of slaps, punches to the face and head, kicking, stomping, punching, choking, pushing, breaking of bones, burns from irons, and mutilations from knives and guns. The honeymoon phase is characterized by a period of calm and remorse in which the male partner displays kind, loving

TABLE 3-2	MYTHS AND FACTS ABOUT INTIMATE PARTNER VIOLENCE
MYTHS	**FACTS**
Battering occurs in a small percentage of the population.	One fourth of all women experience battering by an intimate partner.
Being pregnant protects the woman from battering.	From 4% to 8% of all women who are battered are battered during pregnancy. Battering frequently begins or escalates in frequency and intensity during pregnancy. Pregnancy may be the result of forced sex or of the man's control of contraception.
Battering occurs only in "problem" or lower-class families.	Intimate partner violence can occur in any family. Although lower-income families have a higher reported incidence of battering, it also occurs in middle- and upper-income families. Incidence is not accurately known because of the tendency of middle- and upper-income families to hide their battering.
Battered women like to be beaten and deliberately provoke the attack. They are masochistic.	Women are terrified of their assailants and go to great lengths to avoid a confrontation. In some cases, the woman may provoke her partner to release tension that, if left unchecked, might lead to a more severe beating and possible death.
Only men with psychologic problems abuse women.	Many batterers are successful professionals, including politicians, ministers, physicians, and lawyers. Research indicates that only a small number of abusers have psychologic problems.
Only people who come from abusive families end up in abusive relationships.	Most battered women report that their partners were the first person to beat them.
Alcohol and drug abuse cause battering.	Although alcohol may be involved in abusive incidents, it is not the cause. Many batterers use alcohol as an excuse to batter and shift the blame to the alcohol.
Women would leave the relationship if the abuse were really that bad.	Women who stay in the relationship do so out of fear and financial dependence. Shelters have long waiting lists.
Batterers and battered women cannot change.	Counseling may effectively help both batterers and battered women.

Data from Gelles R: *Intimate violence in families*, ed 3, Thousand Oaks, CA: 1997, Sage; National Institute on Alcohol Abuse and Alcoholism: Alcohol, violence, and aggression, *Alcohol Alert*, 38:1–6, 1997; National Women's Health Information Center: Violence against women, 2013, www.4woman.gov/violence/index.cfm.

they are at the mercy of the man's temper or that he is "out of control." In addition, they may be embarrassed, afraid, angry, sad, and shocked. Box 3-11 summarizes guidelines for communicating with abused women.

It is imperative that the woman has knowledge of resources available to her and a plan of action if she stays with the battering partner. First, the nurse should provide services and telephone numbers of a hotline and the battered women's shelter or other safe haven. The woman can be offered use of a telephone to call the shelter if this is an option she chooses. If she chooses to go back to the abuser, a safety plan includes necessities for a quick escape: a bag packed with personal items for an overnight stay (can be hidden or left with a neighbor), money or a checkbook, an extra set of car keys, and any legal documents for identification. Legal options such as those for restraining orders or arrest of the perpetrator also are important aspects of the safety plan. A restraining order can be obtained from the county court or police department 24 hours a day. Shelters also can be helpful with assistance in obtaining orders of protection. If the woman chooses not to act in the middle of a violent episode, she may use the hotline or shelter for some counseling when the threat of harm is no longer present.

Nurses should screen all women entering the health care system for abuse. Abuse is a life-threatening public health problem that affects millions of women and their children. The risk for intimate partner violence increases during pregnancy and after separation or divorce. Help for the woman may depend on the sensitivity with which the nurse screens for abuse, the discovery of abuse, and subsequent intervention. The nurse must be familiar with the laws governing abuse in the state in which she or he practices.

Pocket cards listing emergency numbers (abuse counseling, legal protection, and emergency shelter) can be obtained from local police departments, women's shelters, or emergency departments. It is helpful to have these on hand in the setting where screening is done.

Battering During Pregnancy

Estimates of prevalence of battering in pregnancy vary, ranging from 4% to 8% to as high as 20%. Most women abused before pregnancy will be abused during pregnancy, and the incidence may escalate. Abuse also may happen for the first time during pregnancy. Pregnant adolescents are abused at higher rates than are adult women; thus they should be considered at high risk. Battering during pregnancy in teenagers constitutes a particularly difficult situation. Adolescents may be more trapped in the abusive relationship than adult women because of their inexperience. They may ignore the violence because the jealous and controlling behavior is interpreted as love and devotion. Because pregnancy in young adolescent girls is frequently the result of sexual abuse, feelings about the pregnancy should be assessed.

During pregnancy the nurse should assess for abuse at each prenatal visit and on admission to labor. Battering episodes initiate or increase in pregnancy for a variety of reasons: (1) the biopsychosocial stresses of pregnancy may strain the relationship beyond the couple's ability to cope, and frustration is followed by violence; (2) the man may be jealous of the fetus, resenting the intrusion into the couple's relationship and the woman's displacement of attention; (3) the man may be angry at the unborn child or the woman; and (4) the beating may be the man's conscious or subconscious attempt to end the pregnancy. After birth, the mother may be so physically and emotionally drained that she may have difficulty bonding with her infant. She may be at risk for becoming an abusive mother whether or not she remains in the abusive relationship.

A pregnant woman is often accompanied by her husband to the prenatal appointment, especially if the woman does not speak English and the husband does. Unless an interpreter is available, it is difficult to interview the woman alone; in addition, asking questions about abuse through an interpreter is more difficult unless the interpreter is a woman and can communicate the nurse's sensitivity and concern accurately.

ABUSE ASSESSMENT SCREEN

- Are you with a spouse or partner who threatens or physically hurts you?
  - ○ Yes _____   No _____

- Are you with a spouse or partner who emotionally hurts you?
  - ○ Yes _____   No _____

- Within the past year or in this pregnancy (if the woman is pregnant) has anyone hit, slapped, kicked, or otherwise hurt you?
  - ○ Yes _____   No _____
  - ○ If yes, by whom _____
  - ○ Number of times _____
  - ○ Mark the area of injury on the body map.

- Has anyone forced you to have sexual activities that made you uncomfortable?
  - ○ Yes _____   No _____
  - ○ If yes, by whom _____
  - ○ Number of times _____

- Are you afraid of your partner or anyone you listed above?
  - ○ Yes _____   No _____

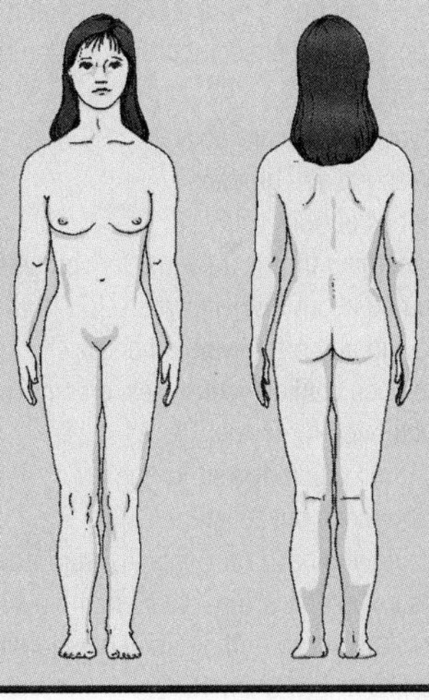

FIG 3-10 Screening for intimate partner violence. (Adapted from American College of Obstetricians and Gynecologists [ACOG] [2012]. Are you being abused? Screening tool for domestic violence. www.acog.org/About_ACOG/ACOG_Departments/Violence_Against_Women/Are_you_being_abused; Nursing Research Consortium on Violence and Abuse [1991].)

BOX 3-10   SIGNS OF INTIMATE PARTNER VIOLENCE

- Overuse of health services
- Vague, nonspecific complaints
- Missed appointments
- Unexplainable injuries
- Untreated serious injuries
- Injuries not matching the description
- Intimate partner never leaving the patient's side
- Intimate partner insisting on telling the story of the injury

Data from Krieger CL: Intimate partner violence: a review for nurses, *Nurs Women's Health* 12(3):224–234, 2008.

LEGAL TIP: Reporting Requirements for Domestic Violence

Domestic violence is considered a crime in all states, but it varies between misdemeanor and felony offenses, the majority being misdemeanors. Forty states and the District of Columbia have laws that mandate reporting by health care providers in situations in which the woman has an injury that may be caused by a deadly weapon. Some states also require reports when there is a reason to believe that the woman's injury may have resulted from an illegal act or act of violence. Because of the wide variation from state to state in mandatory reporting, nurses must be knowledgeable about the reporting requirements of the state in which they practice.

BOX 3-11   GUIDELINES FOR COMMUNICATING WITH ABUSED WOMEN

What *Not* to Say
1. Do not ask "why." This question "revictimizes" and blames the victim.
2. Do not talk negatively about the abuser to the victim. She may become defensive and stop talking.
3. Do not talk directly to the abuser about your suspicions of abuse. The abuser will assume the victim told you, and the victim risks retaliation.

What to Say
1. "I'm afraid for your safety (and the safety of your children)."
2. "I believe you."
3. "It is progressive and will only get worse."
4. "You deserve better than this. You deserve to be treated with respect."
5. "You are not alone."
6. "It is a crime."
7. "I'm here for you."

What to Do
1. Empower the victim.
2. Sit down with her.
3. Assure her of total privacy and confidentiality (but only if you can).
4. Use your best listening skills.
5. Call 911 and report any incident of imminent danger.
6. Give the woman the telephone number of the nearest battered women's shelter.

BOX 3-12 SPIRITUAL WELLNESS SELF-ASSESSMENT

The more questions for which you have an answer other than "I don't know," the higher the level of spiritual wellness.

1. What is your purpose in life?
2. What activities do you do regularly that bring you joy?
3. Do you believe in a higher power?
4. Who can you count on for encouragement and/or support?
5. To whom do you give encouragement and/or support?
6. Who loves you?
7. Whom do you love or care about?
8. In what areas are you growing?
9. What activities nurture you?
10. Is there something that you do just for yourself every day?
11. How do you go about forgiving yourself?
12. How do you go about forgiving others?
13. To whom do you confide your hopes, dreams, and pain?
14. What do you hope for in the future?
15. What do you do regularly just for fun?
16. When do you reach out to people?
17. What goals do you have for 6 months from now?
18. What goals do you have for 2 years from now?
19. Do you look forward to getting up in the morning?
20. Would you like to live to be 100?

Data from Condon M: Women's health: Body, mind, spirit: an integrated approach to wellness and illness, Upper Saddle River, NJ, 2004, Prentice-Hall.

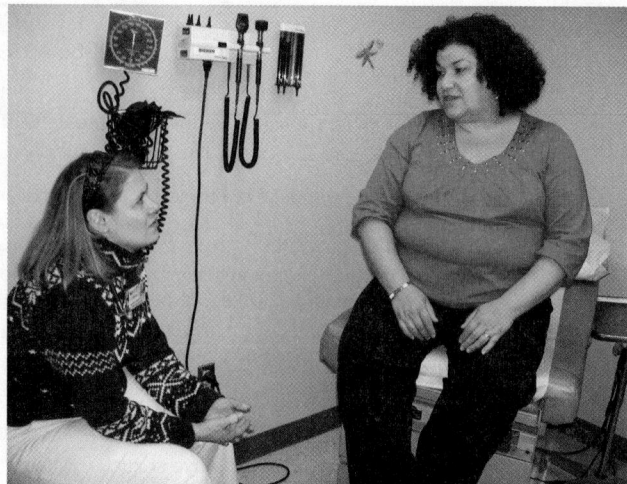

FIG 3-11 Nurse interviews a woman as part of routine history and physical examination. (Courtesy Ed Lowdermilk, Chapel Hill, NC.)

SPIRITUAL APPROACHES TO WOMEN'S HEALTH PROMOTION

Many women find that spirituality is helpful in maintaining wellness as well as coping with illness. Spirituality refers to the essence of our being and humanity, reflected in a connection to a Sacred Source (Burkhardt and Nagai-Jacobson, 2013). The concept of Sacred Source is experienced in different ways, with some experiencing it as a person, some as a presence, and some as a non-describable mystery (Burkhardt and Nagai-Jacobson, 2013). The idea of connection is important, and experiencing this connection in a sacred space is central to spirituality. Spirituality may be experienced within a context of organized religion. Nurses, taking a holistic approach to women's wellness, must be sensitive and nonjudgmental to the spiritual aspect of their patients. In an optimal healing approach to care, nurses can facilitate and encourage the patient to express her spirituality in a way that is comfortable for the patient. Box 3-12 presents a spiritual wellness self-assessment guide.

ASSESSMENT OF THE WOMAN: HISTORY AND PHYSICAL EXAMINATION

Trends in women's health have expanded beyond a reproductive focus to include a holistic approach to health care across the life span and place women's health within the scope of primary care. Women's health assessment and screening focus on a systems evaluation that begins with a careful history and physical examination. During assessment and evaluation, the responsibility for self-management, health promotion, and enhancement of wellness is emphasized.

In a market-driven system such as managed care, specific guidelines may be provided for health screening by the insurer or the managed care organization. A nurse often takes the history, orders diagnostic tests, interprets test results, makes referrals, coordinates care, and directs attention to problems requiring medical intervention. Advanced practice nurses who have specialized in women's health such as nurse practitioners, clinical nurse specialists, and nurse-midwives perform complete physical examinations, including gynecologic examinations.

History

Contact with the woman usually begins with an interview, which is an integral part of the history. This interview should be conducted in a private, comfortable, and relaxed setting (Fig. 3-11). The nurse is seated and makes sure that the woman is comfortable. The woman is addressed by her title and name (e.g., Mrs. Martinez), and the nurse introduces herself or himself using name and title. It is important to phrase questions in a sensitive and nonjudgmental manner. Body language should match oral communication. The nurse is aware of a woman's vulnerability and assures her of strict confidentiality. For many women, fear, anxiety, and modesty make the examination a dreaded and stressful experience. Many women are uninformed, misguided by myths, or afraid they will appear ignorant by asking questions about sexual or reproductive functioning. The woman is assured that no question is irrelevant.

The history begins with an open-ended question such as "What brings you into the office/clinic/hospital today?" and is furthered by other questions such as "Anything else?" and "Tell me about it." Additional ways to encourage women to share information include:

- **Facilitation:** Using a word or posture that communicates interest such as leaning forward, making eye contact, or saying "Mm-hmmm" or "Go on"
- **Reflection:** Repeating a word or phrase that a woman has used
- **Clarification:** Asking the woman what is meant by a stated word or phrase
- **Empathic Responses:** Acknowledging the feelings of a woman by statements such as "That must have been frightening"

- **Confrontation**: Identifying something about the woman's behavior or feelings not expressed verbally or apparently inconsistent with her history
- **Interpretation**: Putting into words what you infer about the woman's feelings or about the meaning of her symptoms, events, or other matters

Nurses need to develop rapport and trust with their patients as they take a history; because communication within a caring context is core to nursing practice, nurses are well suited to taking a comprehensive patient history. Nurses should ask questions incrementally to build a comprehensive understanding. They should also share insights with the woman by eliciting her concerns or thoughts as well as offering clarification to her (Fawcett and Rhynas, 2012).

At a woman's first visit, she is often expected to fill out a form with biographic and historical data before meeting with the examiner. This form aids the health care provider in completing the history during the interview. Most forms include information about these categories:

- Biographic data
- Reason for seeking care
- Present health or history of present illness
- Past health
- Family history
- Screening for abuse
- Review of systems
- Functional assessment (activities of daily living)

Box 3-13 describes a complete health history based on the categories just mentioned.

Physical Examination

In preparation for the physical examination, the woman is instructed to undress and she is given a gown to wear during the examination. She is usually given the opportunity to undress privately. Objective data are recorded by system or location. A general statement of overall health status is a good way to start. Findings are described in detail.

- **General appearance**: age, race, sex, state of health, posture, height, weight, development, dress, hygiene, affect, alertness, orientation, cooperativeness, and communication skills
- **Vital signs**: temperature, pulse, respiration, blood pressure
- **Skin**: color; integrity; texture; hydration; temperature; edema; excessive perspiration; unusual odor; presence and description of lesions; hair texture and distribution; nail configuration, color, texture, and condition; presence of nail clubbing
- **Head**: size, shape, trauma, masses, scars, rashes, or scaling; facial symmetry; presence of edema or puffiness
- **Eyes**: pupil size, shape, reactivity, conjunctival injection, scleral icterus, fundal papilledema, hemorrhage, lids, extraocular movements, visual fields and acuity
- **Ears**: shape and symmetry, tenderness, discharge, external canal, and tympanic membranes; hearing—Weber should be midline (loudness of sound equal in both ears) and Rinne negative (no conductive or sensorineural hearing loss); should be able to hear whisper at 3 feet
- **Nose**: symmetry, tenderness, discharge, mucosa, turbinate inflammation, frontal or maxillary sinus tenderness; discrimination of odors
- **Mouth and throat**: hygiene; condition of teeth; dentures; appearance of lips, tongue, buccal and oral mucosa; erythema; edema; exudate; tonsillar enlargement; palate; uvula; gag reflex; ulcers

- **Neck**: mobility, masses, range of motion, tracheal deviation, thyroid size, carotid bruits
- **Lymphatic**: cervical, intraclavicular, axillary, trochlear, or inguinal adenopathy; size, shape, tenderness, and consistency
- **Breasts**: skin changes, dimpling, symmetry, scars, tenderness, discharge, masses; characteristics of nipples and areolae
- **Heart**: rate, rhythm, murmurs, rubs, gallops, clicks, heaves, or precordial movements
- **Peripheral vascular**: jugular vein distention, bruits, edema, swelling, vein distention, Homans' sign, or tenderness of extremities
- **Lungs**: chest symmetry with respirations, wheezes, crackles, rhonchi, vocal fremitus, whispered pectoriloquy, percussion, and diaphragmatic excursion; breath sounds equal and clear bilaterally
- **Abdomen**: shape, scars, bowel sounds, consistency, tenderness, rebound, masses, guarding, organomegaly, liver span, percussion (tympany, shifting, dullness), or costovertebral angel tenderness
- **Extremities**: edema, ulceration, tenderness, varicosities, erythema, tremor, or deformity
- **Genitourinary**: external genitalia, perineum, vaginal mucosa, cervix; inflammation, tenderness, discharge, bleeding, ulcers, nodules, or masses; internal vaginal support, bimanual and rectovaginal palpation of cervix, uterus, and adnexa
- **Rectal**: sphincter tone, masses, hemorrhoids, rectal wall contour, tenderness, and stool for occult blood
- **Musculoskeletal**: posture, symmetry of muscle mass, muscle atrophy, weakness, appearance of joints, tenderness or crepitus, joint range of motion, instability, redness, swelling, or spinal deviation
- **Neurologic**: mental status, orientation, memory, mood, speech clarity and comprehension, cranial nerves II to XII, sensation, strength, deep tendon and superficial reflexes, gait, balance, and coordination with rapid alternating motions

Cultural Considerations and Communication Variations in the History and Physical

Recognizing signs and symptoms of disease and deciding to seek treatment are influenced by cultural perceptions. Culture evolves over time and is a system of symbols that are learned, shared, and passed on through generations of a social group. In recognizing the value of these differences, the nurse can modify the plan of care to meet the needs of each woman. Modifications may be necessary for the physical examination. In many cultures a woman examiner is preferred. In some cultures it may be considered inappropriate for the woman to disrobe completely for the physical examination.

Communication may be hindered by different beliefs, even when the nurse and woman speak the same language. Examples of communication variations are listed in the Cultural Competence box.

History and Physical Examination in Women with Disabilities

Women with emotional or physical disorders have special needs. Women who have vision, hearing, emotional, or physical disabilities should be respected and involved in the assessment and physical examination to the full extent of their capabilities. The nurse should communicate openly, directly, and with sensitivity. It is often helpful to learn about the disability directly from the woman

BOX 3-13 HEALTH HISTORY AND REVIEW OF SYSTEMS

Identifying data: Name, age, race, sex, marital status, occupation, religion, and ethnicity

Reason for seeking care: A response to the question, "What problem or symptom brought you here today?" More than one reason? Focus on the one she thinks is most important.

Present health: Current health status is described with attention to the following:

- *Use of safety measures:* seat belts, bicycle helmets, designated driver
- Exercise and leisure activities: regularity
- *Sleep patterns:* length and quality
- *Sexuality:* Is she sexually active? With men, women, or both? Risk-reducing sex practices?
- Diet, *including beverages:* 24-hour dietary recall
- *Nicotine, alcohol, illicit or recreational drug use:* type, amount, frequency, duration, and reactions
- *Environmental and chemical hazards:* home, school, work, and leisure setting; exposure to extreme heat or cold, noise, industrial toxins such as asbestos or lead, pesticides, radiation, cat feces, or cigarette smoke

History of present illness: A chronologic narrative of the problem that includes a description of the following—Location, quality or character, quantity or severity, timing (onset, duration, frequency), setting, factors that aggravate or relieve, associated factors, and woman's perception of the meaning of the symptom

Past health:

- *Infectious diseases:* e.g., measles, mumps, rubella, tuberculosis (TB), hepatitis, sexually transmitted infections (STIs)
- *Chronic disease and system disorders:* e.g., arthritis, cancer, diabetes, heart, lung, kidney
- *Adult injuries, accidents*
- *Hospitalizations, operations, blood transfusions*
- *Obstetric history*
- *Allergies:* medications, previous transfusion reactions, environmental allergies
- *Immunizations:* e.g., diphtheria, pertussis, tetanus, mumps, rubella, influenza
- *Last date of screening tests:* e.g., Pap test, mammogram, cholesterol test
- *Current medications:* name, dose, frequency, duration, reason for taking, and compliance with prescription medications; home remedies, over-the-counter drugs, vitamin and mineral or herbal supplements used

Family history: Information about the ages and health of family members. Check for history of diabetes, heart disease, or other chronic disorders.

Screen for abuse: Has she ever been hit, kicked, slapped, or forced to have sex against her wishes? Verbally or emotionally abused? History of childhood sexual abuse? If yes, has she received counseling or does she need referral?

Review of systems: It is probable that all questions in each system will not be included every time a history is taken. The essential areas to be explored are listed in the following head-to-toe sequence. If a woman gives a positive response to a question about an essential area, more detailed questions should be asked.

- *General:* weight change, fatigue, weakness, fever, chills, or night sweats
- *Skin:* skin, hair, and nail changes; itching, bruising, bleeding, rashes, sores, lumps, or moles
- *Lymph nodes:* enlargement, inflammation, pain, or drainage
- *Head:* trauma, vertigo (dizziness), convulsive disorder, syncope (fainting); headache: location, frequency, pain type, nausea and vomiting, or visual symptoms present
- *Eyes:* glasses, contact lenses, blurriness, tearing, itching, photophobia, diplopia, inflammation, trauma, cataracts, glaucoma, or acute visual loss
- *Ears:* hearing loss, tinnitus (ringing), vertigo, discharge, pain, fullness, recurrent infections, or mastoiditis
- *Nose and sinuses:* trauma, rhinitis, nasal discharge, epistaxis, obstruction, sneezing, itching, allergy, or smelling impairment
- *Mouth, throat, and neck:* hoarseness, voice changes, soreness, ulcers, bleeding gums, goiter, swelling, or enlarged nodes
- *Breasts:* masses, pain, lumps, dimpling, nipple discharge, fibrocystic changes, or implants; breast self-examination practice
- *Respiratory:* shortness of breath, wheezing, cough, sputum, hemoptysis
- *Cardiovascular:* hypertension, rheumatic fever, murmurs, angina, palpitations, dyspnea, tachycardia, orthopnea, edema, chest pain, cough, cyanosis, cold extremities, ascites, phlebitis, or skin color changes
- *Gastrointestinal:* appetite, nausea, vomiting, indigestion, dysphagia, abdominal pain, ulcers, bleeding with stools or black, tarry stools, diarrhea, constipation, bowel movement frequency, food intolerance, hemorrhoids, jaundice, or hepatitis
- *Genitourinary:* frequency, hesitancy, urgency, polyuria, dysuria, hematuria, nocturia, incontinence, stones, infection, or urethral discharge; menstrual history, dyspareunia, discharge, sores, itching
- *Sexual health and sexual activity:* with men, women, or both; contraceptive use; sexually transmitted infections
- *Peripheral vascular:* coldness, numbness and tingling, leg edema, varicose veins, thromboses, or emboli
- *Endocrine:* heat and cold intolerance, dry skin, excessive sweating, polyuria, polydipsia, polyphagia, thyroid problems, diabetes, or secondary sex characteristic changes
- *Hematologic:* anemia, easy bruising, bleeding, petechiae, purpura, or transfusions
- *Musculoskeletal:* muscle weakness, pain, joint stiffness, scoliosis, lordosis, kyphosis, range-of-motion, instability, redness, swelling, arthritis, or gout
- *Neurologic:* loss of sensation, numbness, tingling, tremors, weakness, vertigo, paralysis, fainting, twitching, blackouts, seizures, convulsions, loss of consciousness or memory
- *Mental status:* moodiness, depression, anxiety, obsessions, delusions, illusions, or hallucinations
- *Functional assessment:* ability to care for self

---

while maintaining eye contact. Family and significant others should be relied on only when necessary. The assessment and physical examination can be adapted to each woman's individual needs.

Communication with a woman who is hearing-impaired can be accomplished without difficulty. Many of these women can read lips, write, or both. The interviewer who speaks and enunciates each word slowly and in full view may be easily understood. If a woman is not comfortable with lip reading, she may use an interpreter. In this case it is important to continue to address the woman directly, avoiding the temptation to speak directly with the interpreter.

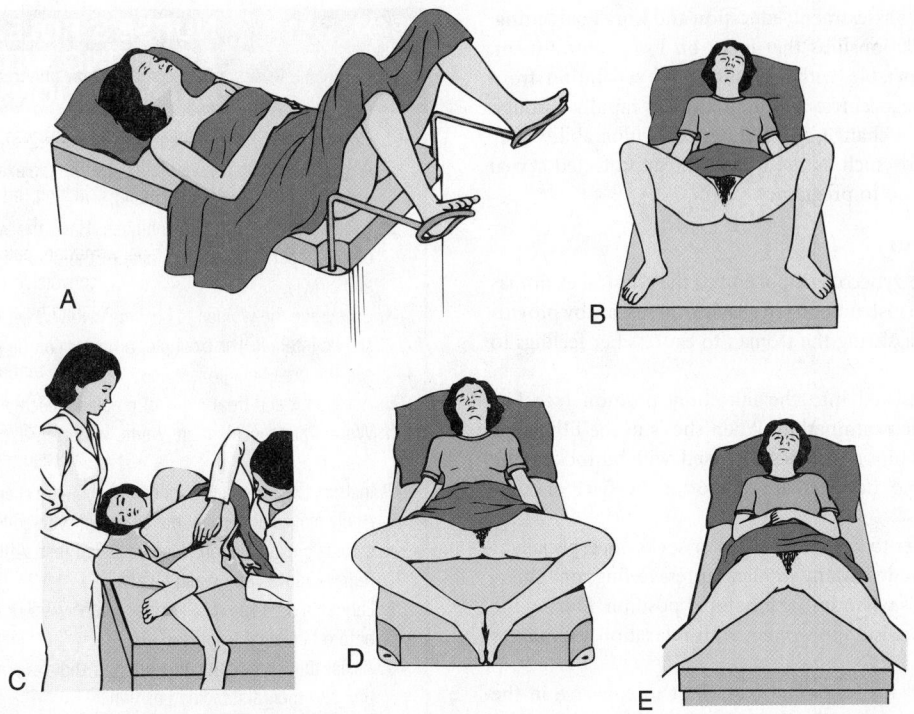

FIG 3-12 Lithotomy and variable positions for women who have a disability. **A,** Lithotomy position. **B,** M-shaped position. **C,** Side-lying position. **D,** Diamond-shaped position. **E,** V-shaped position.

🌐 CULTURAL COMPETENCE

Communication Variations

- Conversational style and pacing: Silence may show respect or acknowledgment that the listener has heard. In cultures in which a direct "no" is considered rude, silence may mean no. Repetition or loudness may mean emphasis or anger.
- Personal space: Cultural conceptions of personal space differ. Based on one's culture, for example, someone may be perceived as distant for backing off when approached or aggressive for standing too close.
- Eye contact: Eye contact varies among cultures from intense to fleeting. Consistent with the effort to refrain from invading personal space, avoiding direct eye contact may be a sign of respect.
- Touch: The norms about how people should touch each other vary among cultures. In some cultures, physical contact with the same sex (embracing, walking hand in hand) is more appropriate than that with an unrelated person of the opposite sex.
- Time orientation: In some cultures, involvement with people is more valued than being "on time." In other cultures, life is scheduled and paced according to clock time, which is valued over personal time.

Data from Galanti G: *Caring for patients from different cultures*, ed 4. Philadelphia, 2008, University of Pennsylvania Press; Mattson S: Striving for cultural competence: providing care for the changing face of the US, *AWHONN Lifelines* 4(3):48–52, 2000.

The visually impaired woman needs to be oriented to the examination room and may have her guide dog with her. As with all patients, the visually impaired woman needs a full explanation of what the examination entails before proceeding. Before touching her, the nurse explains, "Now I am going to take your blood pressure. I am going to place the cuff on your right arm." The woman can be asked if she would like to touch each of the items that will be used in the examination to reduce her anxiety.

Many women with physical disabilities cannot comfortably lie in the lithotomy position for the pelvic examination. Several alternative positions may be used, including a lateral (side-lying) position, a V-shaped position, a diamond-shaped position, and an M-shaped position (Fig. 3-12). The woman can be asked what has worked best for her previously. If she has never had a pelvic examination or has never had a comfortable pelvic examination, the nurse proceeds slowly by showing her a picture of various positions and asking her which one she prefers. The nurse's support and reassurance can help the woman relax, which will make the examination go more smoothly.

History and Physical Examination in Adolescent Girls (Ages 13 to 19)

As a young woman matures, she should be asked the same questions that are included in any history. Particular attention should be paid to hints about risky behaviors, eating disorders, and depression. Sexual activity is addressed after rapport has been established. It is best to talk to a teen with the parent (or partner or friend) out of the room. The nurse should engage with the patient in a sensitive manner, using active listening and conveying a nonjudgmental stance.

Injury prevention should be a part of the counseling at routine health examinations, with special attention to seat belts, helmets, firearms, recreational hazards, and sports involvement. The use of drugs and alcohol and the nonuse of seat belts contribute to motor vehicle injuries, accounting for the greatest proportion of accidental deaths in women. Contraceptives/STI prevention information may be needed for teens who are sexually active.

To provide developmentally appropriate care, it is important to review the major tasks for women in this stage of life. Major tasks for teens include values assessment; education and work goal setting; formation of peer relationships that focus on love, commitment, and becoming comfortable with sexuality; and separation from parents. The teen is egocentric as she progresses rapidly through emotional and physical change. Her feelings of invulnerability may lead to misconceptions such as the belief that unprotected sexual intercourse will not lead to pregnancy.

Pelvic Examination

Many women fear the gynecologic portion of the physical examination. The nurse can be instrumental in allaying these fears by providing information and assisting the woman to express her feelings to the examiner.

The woman is assisted into the lithotomy position (see Fig. 3-12, *A*) for the pelvic examination. When she is in the lithotomy position, the woman's hips and knees are flexed, with buttocks at the edge of the table, and her feet are supported by heel or knee stirrups.

Some women prefer to keep their shoes or socks on, especially if the stirrups are not padded. Many women express feelings of vulnerability and strangeness when in the lithotomy position. During the procedure the nurse assists the woman with relaxation techniques (Box 3-14).

Many women find it distressing to attempt to converse in the lithotomy position. Most women appreciate an explanation of the procedure as it unfolds, as well as coaching for the type of sensations they may expect. Generally, however, women prefer not to have to respond to questions until they are again upright and at eye level with the examiner. Being asked questions during the procedure, especially if they cannot see their questioner's eyes, may make women tense.

A teen's first speculum examination is the most important because she will develop perceptions that will remain with her for future examinations. What the examination entails should be discussed with the teen while she is dressed. Models or illustrations can be used to show exactly what will happen. All of the necessary equipment should be assembled so there are no interruptions. Pediatric specula that are 1 to 1.5 cm wide can be inserted with minimal discomfort. If the teen is sexually active, a small adult speculum may be used.

External Inspection

The examiner wears gloves and sits at the foot of the table for the inspection of the external genitalia and the speculum examination. In good lighting, external genitalia are inspected for sexual maturity, clitoris, labia, perineum, and lesions indicative of STIs. After childbirth or other trauma, healed scars may be present.

External Palpation

Before touching the woman, the examiner explains what is going to be done and what the woman should expect to feel (e.g., pressure). The examiner may touch the woman in a less sensitive area such as the inner thigh to alert her that the genitalia examination is beginning. This gesture may put the woman more at ease. The labia are spread apart to expose the structures in the vestibule: urinary meatus, Skene glands, vaginal orifice, and Bartholin glands (Fig. 3-13). To assess Skene glands, the examiner inserts one finger into the vagina and "milks" the area of the urethra. Any exudate from the urethra or the Skene glands is cultured. Masses and erythema of either structure are assessed further. Ordinarily the openings to the Skene glands are not visible; prominent openings may be seen if the glands are infected (e.g., with gonorrhea). During the examination

---

BOX 3-14 NURSE'S ROLE IN ASSISTING WITH PELVIC EXAMINATIONS

1. Wash hands. Assemble equipment (see illustration below).
2. Ask woman to empty her bladder before the examination (obtain clean-catch urine specimen as needed).
3. Assist with relaxation techniques. Have the woman place her hands on her chest at about the level of the diaphragm and breathe deeply and slowly.
4. Encourage the woman to become involved with the examination if she shows interest. For example, a mirror can be placed so that she can see the area being examined.
5. Assess for and treat signs of problems such as supine hypotension.
6. Warm the speculum in warm water if a prewarmed one is not available.
7. Instruct the woman to bear down when the speculum is being inserted.
8. Apply gloves and assist the examiner with collection of specimens for cytologic examination, such as a Pap test. After handling specimens, remove gloves and wash hands.
9. Lubricate the examiner's fingers with water or water-soluble lubricant before bimanual examination.
10. Assist the woman at completion of the examination to a sitting position and then a standing position.
11. Provide tissues to wipe lubricant from perineum.
12. Provide privacy for the woman while she is dressing.

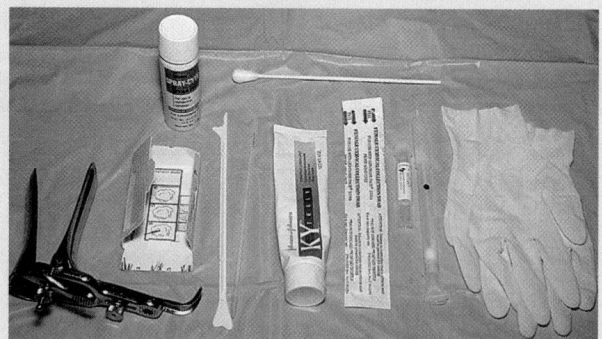

Equipment used for pelvic examination. (Courtesy Michael S. Clement, MD, Mesa, AZ.)

---

the examiner keeps in mind the data from the review of systems such as history of burning on urination.

The vaginal orifice is examined. Hymenal tags are normal findings. With one finger still in the vagina, the examiner repositions the index finger near the posterior part of the orifice. With the thumb outside the posterior part of the labia majora, the examiner compresses the area of Bartholin glands located at the 8 o'clock and 4 o'clock positions and looks for swelling, discharge, and pain.

The support of the anterior and posterior vaginal wall is assessed. The examiner spreads the labia with the index and middle finger and asks the woman to strain down. Any bulge from the anterior wall (urethrocele or cystocele) or posterior wall (rectocele) is noted and compared with the history, such as difficulty starting the stream of urine or constipation.

The perineum (area between the vagina and anus) is assessed for scars from old lacerations or episiotomies, thinning, fistulas, masses, lesions, and inflammation. The anus is assessed for hemorrhoids, hemorrhoidal tags, and integrity of the anal sphincter. The anal area is also assessed for lesions, masses, abscesses, and tumors. If there is

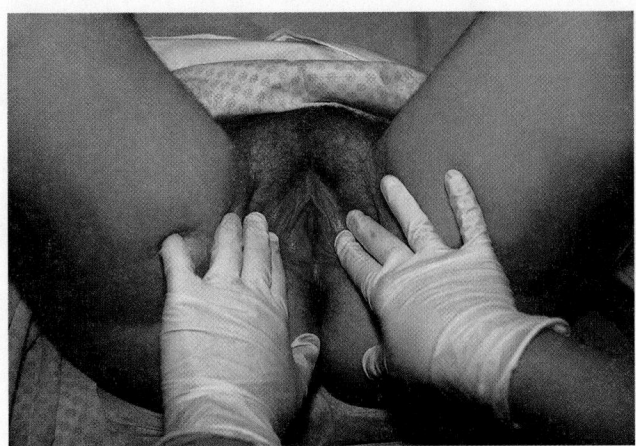

FIG 3-13 External examination: separation of the labia. (From Wilson SF, Giddens JF: *Health assessment for nursing practice*, ed 5, St Louis, 2013, Mosby.)

a history of STI, the examiner may want to obtain a culture specimen from the anal canal at this time. Throughout the genital examination the examiner notes any odor, which may indicate infection or poor hygiene.

Vulvar Self-Examination. The pelvic examination provides a good opportunity for the practitioner to emphasize the need for regular *vulvar self-examination (VSE)* and to teach this procedure. Because there has been a dramatic increase in cancerous and precancerous conditions of the vulva in recent years, VSE should be an integral part of preventive health care for all women who are sexually active or 18 years of age or older. VSE should be performed monthly between menses or more often if there are symptoms or a history of serious vulvar disease. Most lesions, including malignancy, condyloma acuminatum (wartlike growth), and Bartholin cysts, can be seen or palpated and are easily treated if diagnosed early.

The VSE can be performed by the practitioner and woman together by using a mirror. A simple diagram of the anatomy of the vulva can be given to the woman, with instructions to perform the examination herself that evening to reinforce what she has learned. She does the examination in a sitting position with adequate lighting, holding a mirror in one hand and using the other hand to expose the tissues surrounding the vaginal introitus. She then systematically examines the mons pubis, clitoris, urethra, labia majora, perineum, and perianal area and palpates the vulva, noting any changes in appearance or abnormalities such as ulcers, lumps, warts, and changes in pigmentation.

Internal Examination

A vaginal speculum consists of two blades and a handle. Specula come in a variety of types and styles. A vaginal speculum is used to view the vaginal vault and cervix. The speculum is gently placed into the vagina and inserted to the back of the vaginal vault. The blades are opened to reveal the cervix and are locked into the open position. The cervix is inspected for position and appearance of the os: color, lesions, bleeding, and discharge (Fig. 3-14, *A-D*). Cervical findings that are not within normal limits include ulcerations, masses, inflammation, and excessive protrusion into the vaginal vault. Anomalies such as a cockscomb (a protrusion over the cervix that looks like a rooster's comb), a hooded or collared cervix (seen in diethylstilbestrol [DES] daughters), or polyps are noted.

Collection of Specimens. The collection of specimens for cytologic examination is an important part of the gynecologic examination. Infection can be diagnosed by examination of specimens collected during the pelvic examination. These infections include candidiasis, trichomoniasis, bacterial vaginosis, group B streptococcus, gonorrhea, chlamydia, and herpes simplex virus. Once the diagnoses have been made, treatment can be instituted.

Papanicolaou Test. Carcinogenic conditions, whether potential or actual, can be determined by examination of cells from the cervix collected during the pelvic examination (i.e., a Pap test) (Box 3-15).

Vaginal Wall Examination. After the specimens are obtained, the vagina is viewed when the speculum is rotated. The speculum blades are unlocked and partially closed. As the speculum is withdrawn, it is rotated; the vaginal walls are inspected for color, lesions, rugae, fistulas, and bulging.

Bimanual Palpation

The examiner stands for this part of the examination. A small amount of lubricant is placed on the first and second fingers of the gloved hand for the internal examination. To avoid tissue trauma and contamination, the thumb is abducted, and the ring and little fingers are flexed into the palm (Fig. 3-15).

The vagina is palpated for distensibility, lesions, and tenderness. The cervix is examined for position, shape, consistency, motility, and lesions. The fornix around the cervix is palpated.

The other hand is placed on the abdomen halfway between the umbilicus and symphysis pubis and exerts pressure downward toward the pelvic hand. Upward pressure from the pelvic hand traps reproductive structures for assessment by palpation. The uterus is assessed for position, size, shape, consistency, regularity, motility, masses, and tenderness.

With the abdominal hand moving to the right lower quadrant and the fingers of the pelvic hand in the right lateral fornix, the adnexa is assessed for position, size, tenderness, and masses. The examination is repeated on the woman's left side.

Just before the intravaginal fingers are withdrawn, the woman is asked to tighten her vagina around the fingers as much as she can. If the muscle response is weak, the woman is assessed for her knowledge about Kegel exercises.

Rectovaginal Palpation

To prevent contamination of the rectum from organisms in the vagina (e.g., *Neisseria gonorrhoeae*), it is necessary to change gloves, add fresh lubricant, and then reinsert the index finger into the vagina and the middle finger into the rectum (Fig. 3-16). Insertion is facilitated if the woman strains down. The maneuvers of the abdominovaginal examination are repeated. The rectovaginal examination permits assessment of the rectovaginal septum, the posterior surface of the uterus, and the region behind the cervix and the adnexa. The vaginal finger is removed and folded into the palm, leaving the middle finger free to rotate 360 degrees. The rectum is palpated for rectal tenderness and masses.

After the rectal examination the woman is assisted into a sitting position, given tissues or wipes to cleanse herself, and afforded privacy to dress. The examiner returns after the woman is dressed to discuss findings and the plan of care.

Pelvic Examination During Pregnancy

The pelvic examination during pregnancy is done in the same way as it is during a routine examination on a nonpregnant woman. Pelvic measurements are completed, and uterine size is estimated. A Pap test may be done initially and cytologic specimens collected to test for gonorrhea, chlamydia, human papillomavirus, herpes simplex virus, and group B streptococcus. As the pregnancy

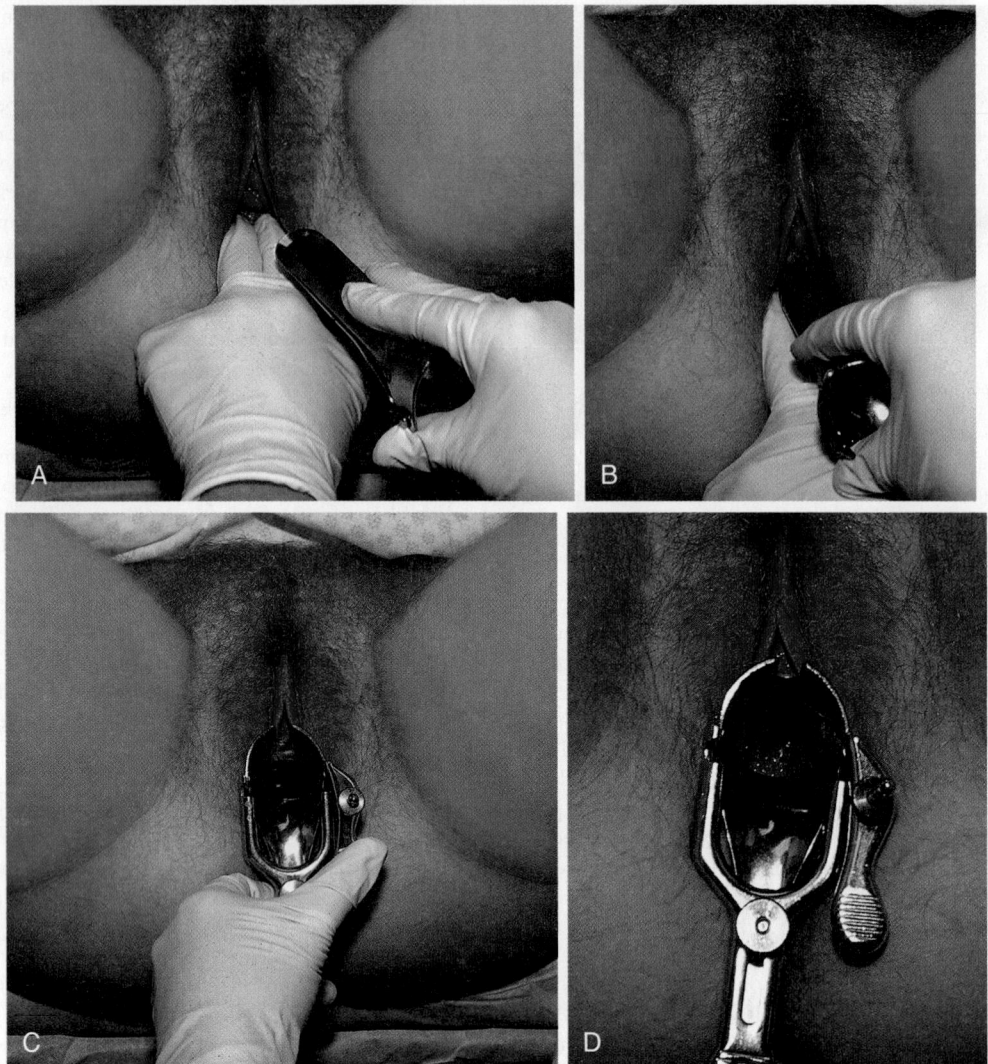

FIG 3-14 Insertion of speculum for vaginal examination. **A,** Opening of the introitus. **B,** Oblique insertion of the speculum. **C,** Final insertion of the speculum. **D,** Opening of the speculum blades. (From Wilson SF, Giddens JF: *Health assessment for nursing practice*, ed 5, St Louis, 2013, Mosby.)

progresses, the nurse inspects the woman's abdomen, palpates fetal size and position, auscultates fetal heart tones, and measures fundal height at each visit.

While the pregnant woman is in lithotomy position, the nurse must watch for supine hypotension (decrease in blood pressure) caused by the weight of the uterus pressing on the vena cava and aorta. Symptoms of supine hypotension include pallor, dizziness, faintness, breathlessness, tachycardia, nausea, clammy skin, and sweating. The woman should be positioned on her side until symptoms resolve and vital signs stabilize. The vaginal examination can be done with the woman in lateral position.

Pelvic Examination After Hysterectomy

The pelvic examination after hysterectomy is done much as it is done on a woman with a uterus. Vaginal screening using the Pap test is not recommended in women who have had a total hysterectomy with removal of the cervix for benign disease. Because of the epidemic of human papillomavirus, which causes vaginal intraepithelial neoplasia, sampling of the vaginal walls after hysterectomy may still be practiced, with schedules varying from every year to every 2 to 3 years.

Laboratory and Diagnostic Procedures

The following laboratory and diagnostic procedures are ordered at the discretion of the clinician, considering the patient and family history: hemoglobin, fasting blood glucose, total blood cholesterol, lipid profile, urinalysis, syphilis serology (Venereal Disease Research Laboratories [VDRL] or rapid plasma reagent [RPR]) and other screening tests for STIs, mammogram, tuberculosis skin testing, hearing, visual acuity, electrocardiogram, chest x-ray, pulmonary function, fecal occult blood, flexible sigmoidoscopy, and bone mineral density (dual energy x-ray absorptiometry [DEXA] scan). Results of these tests may be reported in person, by phone call, or by letter. Tests for HIV, hepatitis B, and drug screening may be offered with informed consent in high risk populations. These test results are usually reported in person.

Health Screening for Women Across the Life Span

To promote wellness and prevent illness, it is imperative that women adhere to specific screening guidelines to detect conditions that, if found early, are amenable to treatment and/or cure. Table 3-3 summarizes the screening procedures for women across the life span.

BOX 3-15   PAPANICOLAOU TEST

- In preparation, make sure the woman has not douched, used vaginal medications, or had sexual intercourse for 24 to 48 hours before the procedure. Reschedule the test if the woman is menstruating. Midcycle is the best time for the test.
- Explain to the woman the purpose of the test and what sensations she will feel as the specimen is obtained (e.g., pressure but not pain).
- The woman is assisted into a lithotomy position. A speculum is inserted into the vagina.
- The cytologic specimen is obtained before any digital examination of the vagina is made or endocervical bacteriologic specimens are taken. A cotton swab may be used to remove excess cervical discharge before the specimen is collected.

- The specimen is obtained by using an endocervical sampling device (Cytobrush, Cervex-brush, spatula, or broom) (see Figs. *A* and *B*). If the two-sample method of obtaining cells is used, the Cytobrush is inserted into the canal and rotated 90 to 180 degrees, followed by a gentle smear of the entire transformation zone by using a spatula. Broom devices are inserted and rotated 360 degrees five times. They obtain endocervical and ectocervical samples at the same time. If the patient has had a hysterectomy, the vaginal cuff is sampled. Areas that appear abnormal on visualization will require colposcopy and biopsy. If using a one-slide technique, the spatula sample is smeared first. This is followed by applying the Cytobrush sample (rolling the brush in the opposite direction from which it was obtained), which is less subject to drying artifact; then the slide is sprayed with preservative within 5 seconds.

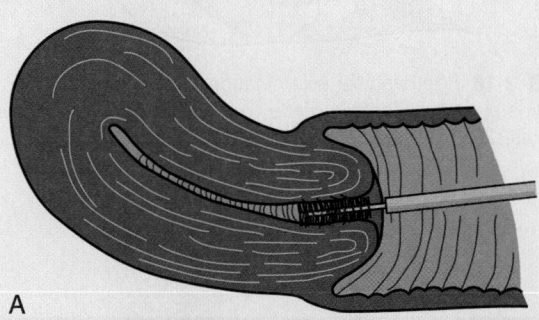 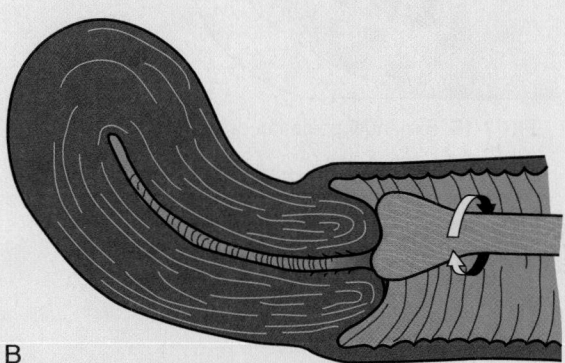

A   B

A, Collecting cells from endocervix using a Cytobrush. **B,** Obtaining cells from the transformation zone using a wooden spatula. (From Lentz GM, Lobo RA, Gershenson DM, et al: *Comprehensive gynecology*, ed 6, St Louis, 2012, Mosby.)

- The ThinPrep or SurePath Pap Test is a liquid-based method of preserving cells that reduces blood, mucus, and inflammation. The Pap specimen is obtained in the manner described above except that the cervix is not swabbed before collection of the sample. The collection device (brush, spatula, or broom) is rinsed in a vial of preserving solution that is provided by the laboratory. The sealed vial with solution is sent off to the appropriate laboratory. A special processing device filters the contents, and a thin layer of cervical cells is deposited on a slide, which is then examined microscopically. The AutoPap and Papnet tests are similar to the ThinPrep test. If cytology is abnormal, liquid-based methods allow follow-up testing for human papillomavirus (HPV) DNA with the same sample.
- Label the slides or vial with the woman's name and site. Include on the form to accompany the specimens the woman's name, age, parity, and chief complaint or reason for taking the cytologic specimens.
- Send specimens to the pathology laboratory promptly for staining, evaluation, and a written report, with special reference to abnormal elements, including cancer cells.
- Advise the woman that repeated tests may be necessary if the specimen is not adequate.
- Instruct the woman concerning routine checkups for cervical and vaginal cancer. Women vaccinated against HPV should follow the same screening guidelines as unvaccinated women. Current recommendations of the U.S. Preventive Services Task Force (USPSTF) (2012) and the American Cancer

Society (ACS) (2012) for Pap tests are that women ages 21 through 65 be screened every 3 years, or for women ages 30 through 65 every 5 years (if they had a pap test plus HPV test that were both negative). These guidelines recommend no screening in women younger than 21, although if a girl becomes sexually active, the guidelines recommend that she get a Pap test within 3 years of initiating sexual activity or at age 21—whichever comes first. Women with high risk factors such as exposure to diethylstilbestrol (DES) in utero, those treated for cervical intraepithelial neoplasia (CIN) 2, CIN 3, cervical cancer, or human immunodeficiency virus (HIV) may need more frequent screening.
- Young women who have been treated with excisional procedures for dysplasia have had an increase in premature births. A large majority of the cervical dysplasias in adolescents caused by HPV resolve on their own without treatment. It is important to avoid unnecessary instrumentation and procedures that negatively affect the cervix. Women who have had a complete hysterectomy for noncancerous reasons who have no history of high-grade CIN may have routine cervical cytology testing discontinued. Women who are older than 65 years who have not had serious cervical precancer or cancer in the past 20 years may discontinue cervical cancer screening (American Cancer Society, 2012).
- Record the examination date on the woman's record.
- Communicate findings to the woman per agency protocol.

Adapted from American Cancer Society: *Chronological history of ACS recommendations for early detection of cancer in asymptomatic people,* 2012, www.cancer.org; U.S. Preventive Services Task Force: *Screening for cervical cancer,* March 2012, www.preventiveservicestaskforce.org/uspstf/uspscerv.htm.

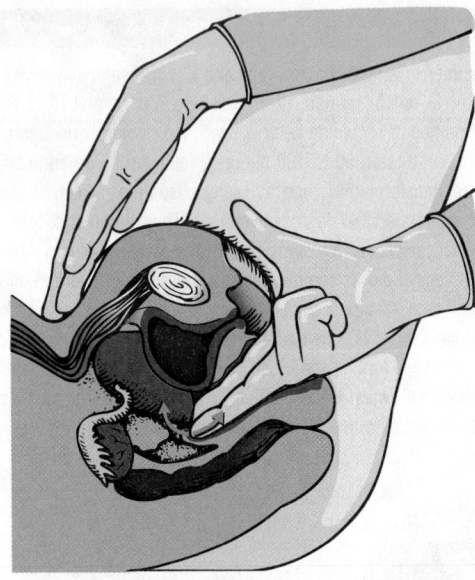

FIG 3-15 Bimanual palpation of the uterus.

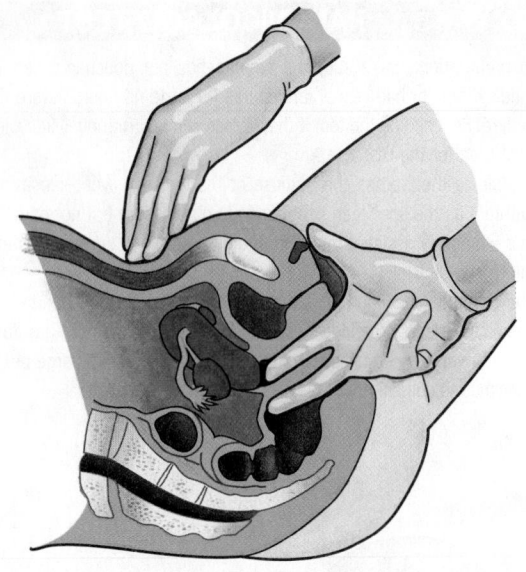

FIG 3-16 Rectovaginal examination. (From Seidel HM, Ball J, Dains J, et al: *Mosby's guide to physical examination*, ed 7, St Louis, 2011, Mosby.)

TABLE 3-3	HEALTH SCREENING GUIDELINES AND IMMUNIZATION RECOMMENDATIONS FOR WOMEN AGES 18 YEARS AND OLDER
INTERVENTION	**RECOMMENDATION***
Physical Examination	
Blood pressure	Every visit, but at least every 2 years
Height and weight	Every visit, but at least every 2 years
Pelvic examination	Annually until age 70; recommended for any woman who has ever been sexually active
Breast Examination	
Clinical examination	Every 3 years, ages 20 to 39; after age 40 with periodic examination, preferably annually
High risk	Annually after age 18 with history of premenopausal breast cancer in first-degree relative
Risk Groups	
Skin examination	Family history of skin cancer or increased exposure to sunlight every 3 years between ages 20 and 40; annually after age 40; monthly mole self-examinations also recommended
Oral cavity examination	History of mouth lesions or exposure to tobacco or excessive alcohol at least annually
Laboratory and Diagnostic Tests	
Blood cholesterol (fasting lipoprotein analysis)	Between ages 20 and 45 only if high risk; Beginning at age 45 if level is within normal limits, every 5 years; more often if abnormal levels or have risk factors for coronary artery disease
Papanicolaou (Pap) test	Between ages 21 and 65—every 3 years with Pap test done Between ages 30 and 65—every 5 years if Pap test plus human papillomavirus (HPV) test done After age 65 and 3 negative tests and no risks and after total hysterectomy for benign disease—women may choose to stop screening
Mammography†	Every 1 to 2 years between ages 40 and 49 or earlier if at high risk Annually after age 40 Annually after age 50 Biennially, ages 50 to 74 After age 75, discuss with your health care provider

Continued

TABLE 3-3   HEALTH SCREENING GUIDELINES AND IMMUNIZATION RECOMMENDATIONS FOR WOMEN AGES 18 YEARS AND OLDER—cont'd

INTERVENTION	RECOMMENDATION*
Colon cancer screening	Use 1 of these 3 methods: • Fecal occult blood test annually ages 50 to 74 • Flexible sigmoidoscopy every 5 years ages 50 to 74 • Colonoscopy every 10 years ages 50 to 74 Screen more often if family history of colon cancer or polyps After age 75, discuss with your health care provider
Hearing screen	Starting at age 18, then every 10 years until 49 Every 3 years after age 50 Annually with exposure to excessive noise or when loss is suspected
Vision screen	At least once between ages 20 and 29; at least twice between ages 30 and 39; Every 2 to 4 years between ages 40 and 64; every 1 to 2 years after age 65
Risk Groups	
Fasting blood sugar	Annually with family history of diabetes or gestational diabetes or if significantly obese; every 3 to 5 years for all women older than 45 years
Thyroid-stimulating hormone (TSH) test	As determined by the health care provider
Sexually transmitted infection test (e.g., gonorrhea, syphilis, herpes)	As needed if sexually active with multiple partners and engaging in risky sexual behaviors
Chlamydia test	If sexually active, yearly until age 25; after age 25, test as needed when sexually active with new or multiple partners
Human immunodeficiency virus (HIV) test	At least once between ages 18 and 64 to determine HIV status; test if there is a high risk for HIV infection
Tuberculin skin test	Annually with exposure to persons with tuberculosis or in risk categories for close contact with the disease
Endometrial biopsy	At menopause for women at risk for endometrial cancer; repeat as needed
Bone mineral density testing	All women age 65 and older at least once; repeat testing as needed; younger women with risk for osteoporosis may need periodic screenings
Immunizations	
Tetanus-diphtheria-pertussis (Td/Tdap)	Tdap vaccine once; then booster is given every 10 years
Measles, mumps, rubella	Once if born after 1956 and no evidence of immunity
Hepatitis A	Primary series of two injections for all who are in risk categories
Hepatitis B	Primary series of three injections for all who are in risk categories
Influenza	Annually
Pneumococcal	1-2 doses between ages 19 and 64; 1 dose after age 65
Herpes zoster (shingles)	One dose at age 65
Human papillomavirus (HPV) vaccine	Primary series of three injections for girls ages 9 to women 26 years old; intended for those not previously exposed to HPV

Data from American Cancer Society (ACS): *Cancer prevention and early detection facts and figures,* Atlanta, 2012, Author; Centers for Disease Control and Prevention (CDC) Advisory Committee on Immunization Practices: *Recommended adult immunization schedule, United States,* 2012, www.cdc.gov/vaccines; Centers for Disease Control and Prevention (CDC): Sexually transmitted diseases treatment guidelines, *MMWR Recomm Rep* 59(RR12):1–109, 2010; National Women's Health Information Center: *Screenings tests for women,* 2012, www.4woman.gov; U.S. Preventive Services Task Force: *Screening for cervical cancer,* 2012, www.preventiveservicestaskforce.org/uspstf/uspscerv.htm.

*The information in this table is only a guide; health care providers will individualize the timing of tests and immunizations for each woman.

†Note: No consensus has been reached regarding mammograms for women between 40 and 49 years of age; therefore various recommendations are listed. Women are urged to discuss circumstances with their health care providers.

KEY POINTS

- Normal feedback regulation of the menstrual cycle depends on an intact hypothalamic-pituitary-gonadal mechanism.
- The female's reproductive tract structures and breasts respond predictably to changing levels of sex steroids across her life span.
- The myometrium of the uterus is uniquely designed to expel the fetus and promote hemostasis after birth.
- Periodic health screening, including history, physical examination, and diagnostic and laboratory tests, provides the basis for overall health promotion, prevention of illness, early diagnosis of problems, and referral for management.
- Culture, religion, socioeconomic status, personal circumstances, the uniqueness of the individual, and the stage of development influence a person's recognition of need for care and the response to the health care system and therapy.
- Preconception counseling allows identification and possible remediation of potentially harmful personal and social condi-

tions, medical and psychologic conditions, environmental conditions, and barriers to care before pregnancy occurs.
- Conditions that increase a woman's health risks also increase risks for her offspring.
- Effective educational programs about sex and family life are imperative to control the rate of teen pregnancy and STIs.
- Health promotion and prevention of illness assist women to actualize health potential by increasing motivation, providing information, and suggesting how to access specific resources.
- IPV against women is a major social and health care problem in the United States and includes physical, sexual, emotional, psychologic, and economic abuse.
- Battering affects all races; all socioeconomic, educational, and religious groups; and many pregnant women.

REFERENCES

American Cancer Society: *Body weight and cancer risk*, 2012a, www.cancer.org.

American Cancer Society: *Breast cancer: early detection*, 2012b, www.cancer.org.

Avalos LA, Kaskutas L, Block G, et al: Does lack of multinutrient supplementation during early pregnancy increase vulnerability to alcohol-related preterm or small-for-gestational-age births? *Matern Child Health J* 15(8):1324–1332, 2011.

Bailey BA, Sokol RJ: Prenatal alcohol exposure and miscarriage, stillbirth, preterm delivery, and sudden infant death syndrome, *Alcohol Res Health* 34(1):86–91, 2011.

Berecki-Gisolf J, McKenzie SJ, Dobson AJ, et al: A history of co-morbid depression and anxiety predicts new onset of heart disease, *J Behav Med*, epub ahead of print, 2012.

breastcancer.org: Breast self-exam, 2012, www.breastcancer.org/symptoms/testing/types/self_exam/.

Brennan AMW, Barnsteiner J, de Leon Siantz ML, et al: Lesbian, gay, bisexual, transgendered, or intersexed content for nursing curricula, *J Prof Nurs* 28(2):96–104, 2012.

Burkhardt MA, Nagai-Jacobson MG: Spirituality and health. In Dossey BM, Keegan L, editors: *Holistic nursing: a handbook for practice*, ed 6, Burlington, MA, 2013, Jones & Bartlett, pp 721–749.

Centers for Disease Control and Prevention: Prepregnancy contraceptive use among teens with unintended pregnancies resulting in live birth: pregnancy risk assessment monitoring system (PRAMS), 2004-2008, *Morbid Mortal Week Rep (MMWR)* 61(02), 25–29, 2012.

Centers for Disease Control and Prevention: *Chronic disease prevention and health promotion: tobacco use*, 2011, www.cdc.gov/chronicdisease/resources/publications/aag/osh.htm.

Dossey BM: Theory of integral nursing. In Parker ME, Smith MC, editors: *Nursing*

theories and nursing practice, ed 3, Philadelphia, 2010, FA Davis, pp 3–57.

Dubowitz T, Ghosh-Dastidar M, Eibner C, et al: The women's health initiative: the food environment, neighborhood socioeconomic status, BMI, and blood pressure, *Obesity* 20(4):862–871, 2012.

Escallier LA, Fullterton JT, Messina BAM: Cultural competence outcomes assessment: a strategy and model, *Int J Nurs Midwifery* 3(3):35–42, 2011.

Fawcet, T, Rhynas S: Taking a patient history: the role of the nurse, *Nurs Stand* 26(24):41–46, 2012.

Fleck-Henderson A, Costello P, Raghu M, et al: *Beyond title IX: guidelines for preventing and responding to gender-based violence in higher education*, 2012, www.futureswithoutviolence.org.

Geddes DT: Inside the lactating breast: the latest anatomy research, *J Midwifery Womens Health* 52(6):556–563, 2007.

Guttmacher Institute: *Substance abuse during pregnancy*, Washington, DC, 2010, www.ncjrs.gov/App/Publications/abstract.aspx?ID=252886.

Guttmacher Institute: *Facts on American teens sexual and reproductive health*, 2012, New York, NY, www.guttmacher.org/pubs/FB-ATSRH.html.

Hautala L, Junnila J, Alin J, et al: Uncovering hidden eating disorders using the SCOFF questionnaire: cross-sectional survey of adolescents and comparison with nurse assessments, *Int J Nurs Stud* 46(11):1439–1447, 2009.

Hayatbakhsh MR, Flenady VJ, Gibbons KS, et al: Birth outcomes associated with cannabis use before and during pregnancy, *Pediatr Res* 71(2):215–219, 2012.

Healthcare.gov: *Women and the affordable care act*, 2012, www.healthcare.gov/news/factsheets/2011/08/women.html.

HealthyPeople.gov: *Maternal, infant, and child health*, 2012a, www.healthypeople.gov/2020/LHI/micHealth.aspx.

HealthyPeople.gov: *Nutrition, physical activity, and obesity*, 2012b, http://healthypeople.gov/2020/LHI/nutrition.aspx.

HealthyPeople.gov: *Pregnancy health and behaviors*. In Maternal, infant, and child health, 2012c, www.healthypeople.gov/2020/topicsobjectives2020/objectiveslist.aspx?topicid=26.

Hogue CJR, Silver RM: Racial and ethnic disparities in the United States—stillbirth rates: trends, risk factors, and research needs, *Semin Perinatol* 35(4):221–233, 2011.

Keegan J, Parva M, Finnegan M, et al: Addiction in pregnancy, *J Addict Dis* 29(2):175–191, 2010.

Leeman, LM, Rogers RC: Sex after childbirth: postpartum sexual function, *Obstet Gynecol* 119(3):647–655, 2012.

Love S, Barsky S: Anatomy of the nipple and breast ducts revisited, *Cancer* 101(9):1947–1957, 2004.

March of Dimes: *Eating and nutrition*, 2010, www.marchofdimes.com/pregnancy/nutrition_caffeine.html.

March of Dimes: *Environmental risks and pregnancy*, 2011, www.marchofdimes.com/pregnancy/stayingsafe_indepth.html.

Masters W, Johnson V: *Human sexual response*, New York, 1966, Bantam Books.

McAlearney AS, Oliveri JM, Post DM, et al: Trust and distrust among Appalachian women regarding cervical cancer screening: a qualitative study, *Patient Educ Couns* 86(1):120–126, 2011.

Medline Plus: *Methamphetamine*, 2012, U.S. National Library of Medicine, National Institutes of Health, www.nlm.nih.gov/medlineplus/methamphetamine.html.

Mong JA, Baker FC, Mahoney MM, et al: Sleep, rhythms, and the endocrine brain: influence of sex and gonadal hormones, *J Neurosci* 31(45):16107–16116, 2011.

Montero I, Escriba V, Ruiz-Perez I, et al: Interpersonal violence and women's psychological well-being, *J Womens Health* 20(2):295–301, 2011.

Morgan J, Reid F, Lacey J: The SCOFF questionnaire: assessment of a new screening tool for eating disorders, *BMJ* 319(7223):1467–1468, 1999.

Murphy R, Straebler S, Basden S, et al: Interpersonal psychotherapy for eating disorders, *Clin Psychol Psychother* 19(2):150–158, 2012.

National Institute on Drug Abuse: *Drug facts: marijuana*, 2012a, www.drugabuse.gov/publications/drugfacts/marijuana.

National Institute on Drug Abuse: *Drug facts: methamphetamine*, 2012b, www.drugabuse.gov/publications/drugfacts/methamphetamine.

National Institute on Drug Abuse: *PCP/phencyclidine*, 2012c, www.drugabuse.gov/drugs-abuse/pcpphencyclidine.

O'Leary C, Nassar N, Kurinczuk JJ, et al: Prenatal alcohol exposure and risk of birth defects, *Obstet Gynecol Surv* 66(2):88–90, 2011.

Pasternak Y, Weintraub AY, Shoham-Vardi I, et al: Obstetric and perinatal outcomes in women with eating disorders, *J Womens Health* 21(1):61–65, 2012.

Peles E, Schreiber S, Bloch M, et al: Duration of methadone maintenance treatment during pregnancy and pregnancy outcome parameters in women with opiate addiction, *J Addict Med* 6(1):18–23, 2012.

Rabin RF, Jennings JM, Campbell JC, et al: Intimate partner violence screening tools: a systematic review, *Am J Prev Med* 36(5):439–445, 2009.

Ramsay D, Kent J, Hartmann R, et al: Anatomy of the lactating breast redefined with ultrasound imaging, *J Anat* 206(6):525–534, 2005.

Saraiya M, Rosser JI, Cooper CP: Cancers that U.S. physicians believe the HPV vaccine prevents: findings from a physician survey, 2009, *J Womens Health* 21(2):111–117, 2012.

Schaub BG, Burt MM: Addiction and recovery counseling. In Dossey BM, Kegan L, editors: *Holistic nursing: a handbook for practice*, ed 6, Burlington, MA, 2013, Jones & Bartlett, pp 539–562.

Skinner HH, Haines J, Austin B, et al: A prospective study of overeating, binge eating, and depressive symptoms among adolescent and young adult women, *J Adolesc Health* 50(5):478–483, 2012.

Taylor D, Levi A, Simmonds K: Reframing unintended pregnancy prevention: a public health model, *Contraception* 81(5):363–366, 2010.

Touchette E, Henegar A, Godart NT, et al: Subclinical eating disorders and their comorbidity with mood and anxiety disorders in adolescent girls, *Psychiatry Res* 185(1):185–192, 2011.

US Department of Agriculture, Center for Nutrition and Policy Promotion: *Dietary guidelines for Americans*, 2010, www.cnpp.usda.gov/DietaryGuidelines.htm.

US Department of Health and Human Services: *Performance indicators.1.C.3*, 2012, www.hhs.gov/secretary/about/appendixb_goal1.html.

US Department of Justice: *Office on violence against women*, 2012, www.ovw.usdoj.gov/.

Vallance JK, Latner JD, Gleaves DH: The relationship between eating disorder psychopathology and health-related quality of life within a community sample, *Qual Life Res* 20(5):675–682, 2011.

Yang TS, Matthews SA, Hillemeier MM: Effect of health care system distrust on breast and cervical cancer screening in Philadelphia, Pennsylvania, *Am J Public Health* 101(7):1297–1305, 2011.

Zender R, Olshansky E: Promoting wellness in women across the lifespan, *Nurs Clin North Am* 44(3):281–291, 2009.

Zhao C, Kalpos-Novak P, Austin M: Follow-up findings in young females with high-grade squamous intraepithelial lesion Papanicolaou test results, *Arch Pathol Lab Med* 135(3):361–364, 2011.

Reproductive System Concerns

Deitra Leonard Lowdermilk

℮volve WEBSITE

http://evolve.elsevier.com/Perry/maternal

LEARNING OBJECTIVES

On completion of this chapter, the reader will be able to:

- Differentiate among the signs and symptoms of common menstrual disorders.
- Develop a nursing care plan for the woman with primary dysmenorrhea.
- Outline patient teaching about premenstrual syndrome.
- Relate the pathophysiology of endometriosis to associated symptoms.
- Evaluate the use of alternative therapies for menstrual disorders.
- Describe prevention and treatment of sexually transmitted infections in women.

- Summarize the care of women with selected viral infections (i.e., human immunodeficiency virus and hepatitis B virus).
- Differentiate signs, symptoms, and management of selected vaginal infections.
- Review principles of infection control for human immunodeficiency virus and bloodborne pathogens.
- Discuss the pathophysiology and emotional effects of selected benign breast conditions and malignant neoplasms of the breasts found in women.

Problems may occur at any point in the menstrual cycle. Many factors, including anatomic abnormalities, physiologic imbalances, and lifestyle, can affect the menstrual cycle. The average woman is likely to have some concerns related to her menstrual and gynecologic health at some point in her life and will experience bleeding, pain, discharge, or infections associated with her reproductive organs or functions. This chapter provides information on common menstrual problems, sexually transmitted infections, and selected other infections that can affect reproductive functions. Benign breast conditions are also discussed. Breast cancer is included because it is the most common reproductive cancer occurring in women.

MENSTRUAL DISORDERS

Once a cyclic, predictable pattern of monthly bleeding is established, women may worry about any deviation from that pattern or from what they have been told is normal for all menstruating women. A woman may be concerned about her ability to conceive and bear children or believe that she is not really a woman without monthly evidence. A sign such as amenorrhea or excess menstrual bleeding can be a source of severe distress and concern for a woman.

Amenorrhea

Amenorrhea, the absence of menstrual flow, is a clinical sign of a variety of disorders. Generally the following circumstances should be evaluated: (1) the absence of both menarche and secondary sexual characteristics by age 13 years; (2) the absence of menses by age 16.5 years, regardless of normal growth and development (primary amenorrhea); or (3) a 6-month or more cessation of menses after a period of menstruation (secondary amenorrhea) (Lobo, 2012d).

A moderately obese girl (20% to 30% above ideal weight) may have early-onset menstruation, whereas delay of onset is known to be related to malnutrition (starvation such as that with anorexia). Girls who exercise strenuously before menarche can have delayed onset of menstruation until about age 18 (Lobo, 2012d).

Although amenorrhea is not a disease, it is often a sign of disease. It may occur from any defect or interruption in the hypothalamic-pituitary-ovarian-uterine axis. It may also result from anatomic abnormalities, other endocrine disorders such as hypothyroidism or hyperthyroidism, chronic diseases such as type 1 diabetes, medications such as phenytoin (Dilantin), illicit drug abuse (opiates, marijuana, cocaine), eating disorders, strenuous exercise, emotional stress, and oral contraceptive use. Secondary amenorrhea is commonly the result of pregnancy.

Hypogonadotropic Amenorrhea

Hypogonadotropic amenorrhea reflects a problem in the central hypothalamic-pituitary axis. In rare instances a pituitary lesion or genetic inability to produce follicle-stimulating hormone (FSH) and luteinizing hormone (LH) is at fault.

Hypogonadotropic amenorrhea often results from hypothalamic suppression as a result of stress (in the home, school, or workplace) or a sudden and severe weight loss, eating disorders, strenuous exercise, or mental illness (Wambach and Alexander, 2012). Research on the interaction between nervous system or neurotransmitter functions and hormone regulation throughout the body has demonstrated a biologic basis for the relation of stress to physiologic processes. Women who are more than 20% underweight for height or who have had rapid weight loss and women with eating disorders such as anorexia nervosa may report amenorrhea. Amenorrhea is one of the classic signs of anorexia nervosa; and the interrelation of disordered eating, amenorrhea, and premature osteoporosis has been described as the female athlete triad (George, Leonard, and Hutchinson, 2011) (www.femaleathletetriad.org). A loss of calcium from the bone, comparable to that seen in postmenopausal women, may occur with this type of amenorrhea.

Exercise-associated amenorrhea can occur in women undergoing vigorous physical and athletic training and is thought to be associated with many factors, including body composition (height, weight, and percentage of body fat); type, intensity, and frequency of exercise; nutritional status; and presence of emotional or physical stressors. Women who participate in sports emphasizing low body weight are at greatest risk, including the following:

- Sports in which performance is subjectively scored (e.g., dance, gymnastics)
- Endurance sports favoring participants with low body weight (e.g., distance running, cycling)
- Sports in which body contour–revealing clothing is worn (e.g., swimming, diving, volleyball)
- Sports with weight categories for participation (e.g., rowing, martial arts)
- Sports in which prepubertal body shape favors success (e.g., gymnastics, figure skating).

Assessment of amenorrhea begins with a thorough history and physical examination. Specific components of the assessment process depend on a patient's age—adolescent, young adult, or perimenopausal—and whether she has menstruated previously.

An important initial step, often overlooked, is to be sure that the woman is not pregnant. Once pregnancy has been ruled out by a β-human chorionic gonadotropin (hCG) pregnancy test, diagnostic tests may include FSH level, thyroid-stimulating hormone (TSH) and prolactin levels, radiographic or computed tomography (CT) scan of the sella turcica, and a progestational challenge (Lobo, 2012d).

Management. When amenorrhea is caused by hypothalamic disturbances, the nurse is an ideal health professional to assist women because many of the causes are potentially reversible (e.g., stress, weight loss for nonorganic reasons). Counseling and education are primary interventions and appropriate nursing roles. When a stressor known to predispose a woman to hypothalamic amenorrhea is identified, initial management involves addressing the stressor. Together the woman and nurse plan how the woman can decrease or discontinue medications known to affect menstruation, correct weight loss, deal more effectively with psychologic stress, address emotional distress, and alter exercise routine.

The nurse works with the woman to help her identify, cope with, and eliminate sources of stress in her life. Deep-breathing exercises and relaxation techniques are simple yet effective stress-reduction measures. Referral for biofeedback or massage therapy also may be useful. In some instances referrals for psychotherapy may be indicated.

If a woman's exercise program is thought to contribute to her amenorrhea, several options exist for management. She may decide to decrease the intensity or duration of her training or modify her diet to include the appropriate nutrition for her age. Accepting the former alternative may be difficult for one who is committed to a strenuous exercise regimen. The woman and nurse may have several sessions before the woman elects to try exercise reduction. Many young female athletes may not understand the consequences of low bone density or osteoporosis; nurses can point out the connection between low bone density and stress fractures. The nurse and woman should also investigate other factors that may be contributing to the amenorrhea and develop plans for altering lifestyle and decreasing stress.

Although research on effectiveness is inconclusive, a daily calcium intake of 1200 to 1500 mg plus 400 to 800 International Units of vitamin D and 60 to 90 mg of potassium are recommended for women experiencing amenorrhea associated with the female athlete triad. Oral contraceptives have a positive effect on bone density in amenorrheic women but are usually not used in young women with amenorrhea associated with female athlete triad unless the woman is not willing to comply with dietary and exercise recommendations or she continues to be amenorrheic even with compliance (Joy, 2012).

Dysmenorrhea

Dysmenorrhea, pain during or shortly before menstruation, is one of the most common gynecologic problems in women of all ages. Many adolescents have dysmenorrhea in the first 3 years after menarche. Young adult women ages 17 to 24 years are most likely to report painful menses. Approximately 75% of women report some level of discomfort associated with menses, and approximately 15% report severe dysmenorrhea (Lentz, 2012); however, the amount of disruption in women's lives is difficult to determine. Researchers have estimated that as many as 10% of women with dysmenorrhea have severe enough pain to interfere with their functioning for 1 to 3 days a month. Menstrual problems, including dysmenorrhea, are relatively more common in women who smoke and are obese. Severe dysmenorrhea is also associated with early menarche, nulliparity, and stress (Lentz, 2012). Traditionally dysmenorrhea is differentiated as primary or secondary. Symptoms usually begin with menstruation, although some women have discomfort several hours before onset of flow. The range and severity of symptoms are different from woman to woman and from cycle to cycle in the same woman. Symptoms of dysmenorrhea may last several hours or several days.

Pain is usually located in the suprapubic area or lower abdomen. Women describe the pain as sharp, cramping, or gripping or as a steady dull ache. For some women pain radiates to the lower back or upper thighs.

Primary Dysmenorrhea

Primary dysmenorrhea is a condition associated with ovulatory cycles. Research has shown that primary dysmenorrhea has a

? CRITICAL THINKING CASE STUDY

Management of Dysmenorrhea

Cheri, 16, has come to the adolescent health clinic for a checkup. She reports that she has "really bad cramps" for the first 2 days of her period. She has been taking Midol Menstrual Complete but says that it does not help "a lot." She wants to know if anything else can be done to relieve her pain. How should the nurse respond?

1. Evidence—Is evidence sufficient to draw conclusions about what advice the nurse should give?
2. Assumptions—Describe underlying assumptions about the following issues:
   a. Causes and symptoms of primary dysmenorrhea
   b. Cyclic perimenstrual pain and discomfort
   c. Self-help strategies (e.g., comfort measures, medications)
3. What implications and priorities for nursing care can be drawn at this time?
4. Does the evidence objectively support your conclusion?

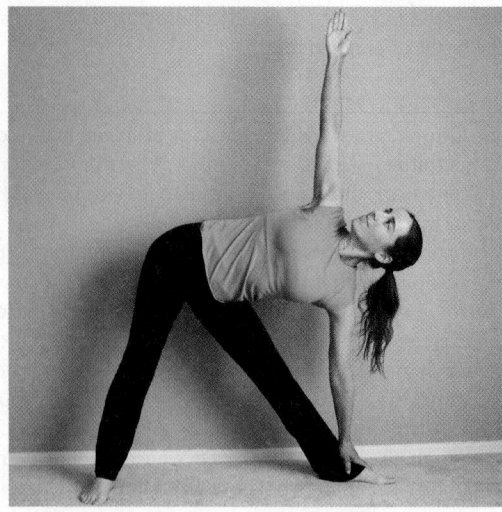

FIG 4-1 Yoga asana: triangle pose. Helpful for assisting digestion and stretching and strengthening the spine; also used for dysmenorrheal and pelvic congestion. (Courtesy Julie Perry Nelson, Loveland, CO.)

biochemical basis and arises from the release of prostaglandins with menses. During the luteal phase and subsequent menstrual flow, prostaglandin F$_2$-alpha (PGF$_{2\alpha}$) is secreted. Excessive release of PGF$_{2\alpha}$ increases the amplitude and frequency of uterine contractions and causes vasospasm of the uterine arterioles, resulting in ischemia and cyclic lower abdominal cramps. Systemic responses to PGF$_{2\alpha}$ include backache, weakness, sweats, gastrointestinal symptoms (anorexia, nausea, vomiting, and diarrhea), and central nervous system symptoms (dizziness, syncope, headache, and poor concentration). Pain usually begins at the onset of menstruation and lasts 8 to 48 hours (Lentz, 2012).

Primary dysmenorrhea usually appears 6 to 12 months after menarche when ovulation is established. Anovulatory bleeding, common in the few months or years after menarche, is painless. Because both estrogen and progesterone are necessary for primary dysmenorrhea to occur, it is experienced only with ovulatory cycles. This problem is more common among women in their late teens and early twenties than in women in older age-groups; the incidence declines with age. Psychogenic factors may influence symptoms, but symptoms are definitely related to ovulation and do not occur when ovulation is suppressed.

Management. Management of primary dysmenorrhea depends on the severity of the problem and the individual woman's response to various treatments. Important components of nursing care are information and support. Because menstruation is so closely linked to reproduction and sexuality, menstrual problems such as dysmenorrhea can have a negative influence on sexuality and self-worth. Nurses can correct myths and misinformation about menstruation and dysmenorrhea by providing facts about what is normal. Women need support to foster their feelings of positive sexuality and self-worth.

Often you can offer more than one alternative for alleviating menstrual discomfort and dysmenorrhea, which gives women options to try to decide which works best for them (see Critical Thinking Case Study).

Heat (heating pad or hot bath) minimizes cramping by increasing vasodilation and muscle relaxation and minimizing uterine ischemia. Massaging the lower back can reduce pain by relaxing paravertebral muscles and increasing the pelvic blood supply. Soft, rhythmic rubbing of the abdomen (effleurage) is useful because it provides a distraction and an alternative focal point. Biofeedback, transcutaneous electrical nerve stimulation (TENS), progressive relaxation, Hatha yoga, acupuncture, and meditation are also used to decrease menstrual discomfort, although evidence is insufficient to determine their effectiveness (Lentz, 2012) (Fig. 4-1).

Exercise helps relieve menstrual discomfort through increased vasodilation and subsequent decreased ischemia. It also releases endogenous opiates (specifically beta-endorphins), suppresses prostaglandins, and shunts blood flow away from the viscera, resulting in reduced pelvic congestion. One specific exercise that nurses can suggest is pelvic rocking.

In addition to maintaining good nutrition at all times, specific dietary changes are helpful in decreasing some of the systemic symptoms associated with dysmenorrhea. Decreased salt and refined sugar intake 7 to 10 days before expected menses may reduce fluid retention. Natural diuretics such as asparagus, cranberry juice, peaches, parsley, or watermelon may help reduce edema and related discomforts. A low-fat vegetarian diet may also help minimize dysmenorrheal symptoms (Lentz, 2012).

Medications used to treat primary dysmenorrhea include prostaglandin synthesis inhibitors, primarily nonsteroidal antiinflammatory drugs (NSAIDs) (Lentz, 2012) (Table 4-1). NSAIDs are most effective if started several days before menses or at least by the onset of bleeding. All NSAIDs have potential gastrointestinal side effects, including nausea, vomiting, and indigestion. Warn all women taking them to report dark-colored stool because this may be an indication of gastrointestinal bleeding.

! NURSING ALERT

If one NSAID is ineffective, often a different one may be effective. If the second drug is unsuccessful after a 6-month trial, combined oral contraceptive pills (OCPs) may be used. Women with a history of aspirin sensitivity or allergy should avoid all NSAIDs.

TABLE 4-1	NONSTEROIDAL ANTIINFLAMMATORY AGENTS USED TO TREAT DYSMENORRHEA				
DRUG	**BRAND NAME AND STATUS**	**RECOMMENDED DOSAGE (ORAL)***	**COMMON SIDE EFFECTS†**	**COMMENTS**	**CONTRAINDICATIONS**
Diclofenac	Cataflam Rx	50 mg tid or 100 mg initially, then 50 mg tid up to 150 mg/day	Nausea, diarrhea, constipation, abdominal distress, dyspepsia, heartburn, flatulence, dizziness, tinnitus, itching, rash	Enteric coated; immediate release	For all NSAIDs: Do not give if woman has hemophilia or bleeding ulcers; do not give if woman has had an allergic or anaphylactic reaction to aspirin or another NSAID; do not give if woman is taking anticoagulant medication
Ibuprofen	Motrin Rx, Advil OTC, Nuprin OTC, Motrin IB OTC	400 mg q 6-8 hr, 200 mg q 4-6 hr up to 1200 mg/day	See diclofenac	If GI upset occurs, take with food, milk, or antacids; avoid alcoholic beverages; do not take with aspirin; stop taking and call care provider if rash occurs	
Ketoprofen	Orudis Rx	25-50 mg q 6-8 hr up to 300 mg/day	See diclofenac	See ibuprofen	
	Orudis KT OTC, Actron OTC	12.5 mg q 6-8 hr up to 75 mg/day			
Meclofenamate	Meclomen Rx	100 mg tid up to 300 mg	See diclofenac	See ibuprofen	
Mefenamic acid	Ponstel Rx	500 mg initially, then 250 mg q 6 hr/day	See diclofenac	Very potent and effective prostaglandin-synthesis inhibitor; antagonizes already formed prostaglandins; increased incidence of adverse GI side effects	
Naproxen	Naprosyn Rx	500 mg initially, then 250 mg q 6-8 hr up to 1250 mg/day	See diclofenac	See ibuprofen	
Naproxen sodium	Anaprox Rx	550 mg initially, then 275 mg q 6-8 hr or 550 mg q 12 hr up to 1375 mg/day	See diclofenac	See ibuprofen	
	Aleve OTC	440 mg initially, then 220 mg q 6-8 hr up to 660 mg/day			
Celecoxib	Celebrex	400 mg initially, then 200 mg bid	See diclofenac	See ibuprofen	

Data from Facts and Comparisons: *Nonsteroidal antiinflammatory drugs,* 2012, www.factsandcomparisons.com; Lentz GM: Primary and secondary dysmenorrhea, premenstrual syndrome, and premenstrual dysphoric disorder: etiology, diagnosis, and management. In Lentz GM, Lobo RA, Gershenson DM, et al, editors: *Comprehensive gynecology,* ed 6, Philadelphia, 2012, Mosby; US Department of Health and Human Services, US Food and Drug Administration: *Medication guide for nonsteroidal antiinflammatory drugs (NSAIDs),* 2008, www.fda.gov/CDER/drug/infopage/COX2/NSAIDmedguide.htm.
GI, Gastrointestinal; *NSAID,* nonsteroidal antiinflammatory drug; *OTC,* over the counter.

OCPs are a reasonable choice for women who want to use a contraceptive agent. The benefits of their use are attributed to decreased prostaglandin synthesis associated with an atrophic decidualized endometrium (Lentz, 2012). OCPs are effective in relieving symptoms of primary dysmenorrhea for approximately 90% of women. No single OCP has been shown to be superior to another for the relief of primary dysmenorrheal, including low-dose and extended-cycle OCPS (Lentz, 2012). OCPs are a particularly good choice for therapy because they combine contraception with a positive effect on dysmenorrhea, menstrual flow, and menstrual

TABLE 4-2	HERBAL MEDICINALS TAKEN ORALLY FOR MENSTRUAL DISORDERS	
SYMPTOMS OR INDICATIONS	**HERBAL THERAPY***	**ACTION**
Menstrual cramping, dysmenorrhea	Black haw	Uterine antispasmodic
	Fennel	Uterotonic
	Catnip	Uterine antispasmodic
	Dong quai	Uterotonic; antiinflammatory
	Ginger	Antiinflammatory
	Motherwort	Uterotonic
	Wild yam	Uterine antispasmodic
	Valerian	Uterine antispasmodic
Premenstrual discomfort, tension	Black cohosh root	Estrogen-like luteinizing hormone suppressant; binds to estrogen receptors
	Chamomile	Antispasmodic
Breast pain	Chaste tree fruit	Decreases prolactin levels
	Bugleweed	Antigonadotropic; decreases prolactin levels
Menorrhea, metrorrhagia	Lady's mantle	Uterotonic
	Raspberry	Uterotonic
	Shepherd's purse	Uterotonic

Data from Annie's Remedy: *Herbal remedies for dysmenorrhea*, 2012, www.anniesremedy.com; National Center for Complementary and Alternative Medicine: *Herbs at a glance*, 2010, www.nccam.nih.gov.
*Many women's herbs do not have rigorous scientific studies backing their use; most uses and properties of herbs have not been validated by the US Food and Drug Administration,.

irregularities. Adolescents may benefit from use of the long-acting injectable contraceptive (depot medroxyprogesterone), but more research is needed. Since OCPs have side effects, women may not wish to use them for dysmenorrhea. They may be contraindicated for some women. (See Chapter 5 for a complete discussion of OCPs.)

Over-the-counter (OTC) preparations that are indicated for primary dysmenorrhea contain the same active ingredients (e.g., ibuprofen or naproxen sodium) as prescription preparations. However, the labeled recommended dose may be subtherapeutic. Preparations containing acetaminophen are even less effective because acetaminophen does not have the antiprostaglandin properties of NSAIDs.

Alternative and complementary therapies are increasingly popular and used in developed countries. Therapies such as acupuncture, acupressure, biofeedback, desensitization, hypnosis, massage, reiki, relaxation exercises, and therapeutic touch have been used to treat pelvic pain. Herbal preparations have long been used for managing menstrual problems, including dysmenorrhea (Table 4-2). Herbal medicines may be valuable in treating dysmenorrhea. However, it is essential that women understand that these therapies are not without potential toxicity and may cause drug interactions.

Secondary Dysmenorrhea

Secondary dysmenorrhea is menstrual pain that develops later in life than primary dysmenorrhea, typically after age 25. It is associated with pelvic pathology such as adenomyosis, endometriosis, pelvic inflammatory disease, endometrial polyps, or submucous or interstitial myomas (fibroids). Women with secondary dysmenorrhea often have other symptoms that may suggest the underlying cause. For example, heavy menstrual flow with dysmenorrhea suggests a diagnosis of leiomyomata, adenomyosis, or endometrial polyps. Pain associated with endometriosis often begins a few days before menses but can be present at ovulation and continue through the first days of menses or start after menstrual flow has begun. In contrast to primary dysmenorrhea, the pain of secondary dysmenorrhea is often characterized by dull, lower abdominal aching that radiates to the back or thighs. Often women experience feelings of bloating or pelvic fullness. In addition to a physical examination with a careful pelvic examination, diagnosis may be assisted by ultrasound examination, dilation and curettage (D&C), endometrial biopsy, or laparoscopy. Treatment is directed toward removal of the underlying pathology. Many of the measures described for pain relief of primary dysmenorrhea are also helpful for women with secondary dysmenorrhea.

Premenstrual Syndrome

Approximately 30% to 80% of women experience mood or somatic symptoms (or both) that occur with their menstrual cycles (Lentz, 2012). Establishing a universal definition of premenstrual syndrome (PMS) is difficult, given that so many symptoms have been associated with the condition and at least two different syndromes have been recognized: PMS and premenstrual dysphoric disorder (PMDD).

PMS is a complex, poorly understood condition that includes one or more of a large number (more than 150) of physical and psychologic symptoms beginning in the luteal phase of the menstrual cycle, occurring to such a degree that lifestyle or work is affected, and followed by a symptom-free period. Symptoms include fluid retention (abdominal bloating, pelvic fullness, edema of the lower extremities, breast tenderness, and weight gain), behavioral or emotional changes (depression, crying spells, irritability, panic attacks, and impaired ability to concentrate), premenstrual cravings (sweets, salt, increased appetite, and food binges), and headache, fatigue, and backache.

All age-groups are affected, with women in their 20s and 30s most frequently reporting symptoms. Ovarian function is necessary for the condition to occur because it does not occur before puberty, after menopause, or during pregnancy. The condition is not dependent on the presence of monthly menses: women who have had a hysterectomy without bilateral salpingo-oophorectomy (BSO) still can have cyclic symptoms.

PMDD is a more severe variant of PMS in which 3% to 8% of women have marked irritability, dysphoria, mood lability, anxiety, fatigue, appetite changes, and a sense of feeling overwhelmed (Lentz, 2012). The most common symptoms are those associated with mood disturbances.

A diagnosis of PMS is made when the following criteria are met (American College of Obstetricians and Gynecologists [ACOG], 2000):

- Symptoms consistent with PMS occur in the luteal phase and resolve within a few days of menses onset.
- Symptom-free period occurs in the follicular phase.
- Symptoms are recurrent.
- Symptoms have a negative effect on some aspect of a woman's life.
- Other diagnoses that better explain the symptoms have been excluded.

For a diagnosis of PMDD, the following criteria must be met (American Psychiatric Association [APA], 2000):

- Five or more affective and physical symptoms are present in the week before menses and absent in the follicular phase of the menstrual cycle.
- At least one of the symptoms is irritability, depressed mood, anxiety, or emotional lability.
- Symptoms interfere markedly with work or interpersonal relationships.
- Symptoms are not caused by an exacerbation of another condition or disorder.

These criteria must be confirmed by prospective daily ratings for at least two menstrual cycles.

The causes of PMS and PMDD continue to be investigated, but there is general agreement that they are distinct psychiatric and medical syndromes rather than an exacerbation of an underlying psychiatric disorder. They do not occur if there is no ovarian function. A number of biologic and neuroendocrine etiologies have been suggested; however, none have been conclusively substantiated as the causative factor. It is likely that biologic, psychosocial, and sociocultural factors contribute to PMS and PMDD (Lentz, 2012).

Management

There is little agreement on management. A careful, detailed history and daily log of symptoms and mood fluctuations spanning several cycles may give direction to a plan of management. Any changes that help a woman with PMS exert control over her life have a positive effect. For this reason, lifestyle changes are often effective in its treatment.

Education is an important component of the management of PMS. Nurses can advise women that self-help modalities often result in significant symptom improvement. Women have found a number of complementary and alternative therapies to be useful in managing the symptoms of PMS. Diet and exercise changes can provide symptom relief for some women. Nurses can suggest that women not smoke and limit their consumption of refined sugar, salt, red meat, alcohol, and caffeinated beverages. Women can be encouraged to include whole grains, legumes, seeds, nuts, vegetables, fruits, and vegetable oils in their diet. Three small to moderate-size meals and three small snacks a day that are rich in complex carbohydrates and fiber have been reported to relieve symptoms (American College of Obstetricians and Gynecologists [ACOG] 2011; Lentz, 2012). Use of natural diuretics (see section on dysmenorrhea management on pp. 76-78) may also help reduce fluid retention. Nutritional supplements may assist in symptom relief. Calcium (1200 mg daily) and vitamin B_6 have been shown to be moderately effective in relieving symptoms, to have few side effects, and to be safe. Daily supplements of evening primrose oil are reportedly useful in relieving breast symptoms with minimal side effects, but research reports are conflicting (Biggs and Demuth, 2011; Lentz, 2012). Other herbal therapies have long been used to treat PMS; however, research on effectiveness is lacking, or studies are flawed (Dante and Facchinetti, 2011).

Regular exercise (aerobic exercise three or four times a week), especially in the luteal phase, is widely recommended for relief of PMS symptoms (Lentz, 2012). A monthly program that varies in intensity and type of exercise according to PMS symptoms is best. Women who exercise regularly seem to have less premenstrual anxiety than do nonathletic women. Researchers believe aerobic exercise increases beta-endorphin levels to offset symptoms of depression and elevate mood.

Yoga, acupuncture, hypnosis, light therapy, chiropractic therapy, and massage therapy have all been reported to have a beneficial effect on PMS. Further research is needed for all of these therapies.

Nurses can explain the relation between cyclic estrogen fluctuation and changes in serotonin levels, that serotonin is one of the brain chemicals that assist in coping with normal life stresses, and the ways in which the different management strategies recommended help maintain serotonin levels. Support groups or individual or couples counseling may be helpful. Stress-reduction techniques also may help with symptom management (Lentz, 2012).

If these strategies do not provide significant symptom relief in 1 to 2 months, medication is often added. Many medications have been used in treatment of PMS, but no single medication alleviates all PMS symptoms. Medications often used in the treatment of PMS include diuretics, prostaglandin inhibitors (NSAIDs), progesterone, and OCPs. These have been used mainly for the physical symptoms. Studies of progesterone have not shown that it is an effective treatment (Ford, Lethaby, Roberts, et al., 2012). Serotonergic-activating agents, including the selective serotonin reuptake inhibitors (SSRIs) such as fluoxetine (Prozac or Sarafem), sertraline (Zoloft), citalopram (Celexa), escitalopram (Lexapro), and paroxetine (Paxil CR) are approved by the U.S. Food and Drug Administration (FDA) as agents for PMS and are first-line pharmacologic therapy. Use of these medications during the luteal phase of the menstrual cycle results in a decrease in emotional premenstrual symptoms, especially depression (Biggs and Demuth, 2011; Lentz, 2012). Common side effects are headaches, sleep disturbances, dizziness, weight gain, dry mouth, and decreased libido.

Endometriosis

Endometriosis is characterized by the presence and growth of endometrial tissue outside of the uterus. The tissue may be implanted on the ovaries; anterior and posterior cul-de-sac; broad, uterosacral, and round ligaments; rectovaginal septum; sigmoid colon; appendix; pelvic peritoneum; cervix; and inguinal area (Fig. 4-2). Endometrial lesions have been found in the vagina and surgical scars and on the vulva, perineum, and bladder. They have also been found on sites far from the pelvic area such as the thoracic cavity, gallbladder, and heart. A cystic lesion of endometriosis found in the ovary is sometimes described as a chocolate cyst because of the dark coloring of the contents of the cyst caused by the presence of old blood.

Endometrial tissue contains glands and stoma and responds to cyclic hormone stimulation in the same way that the uterine endometrium does but often out of phase with it. The tissue grows during the proliferative and secretory phases of the cycle. During or immediately after menstruation the tissue bleeds, resulting in an inflammatory response with subsequent fibrosis and adhesions to adjacent organs.

The overall incidence of endometriosis is 5% to 15% in reproductive-age women, 30% to 45% in infertile women, and 33% in women with chronic pelvic pain (Lobo, 2012b). Although the

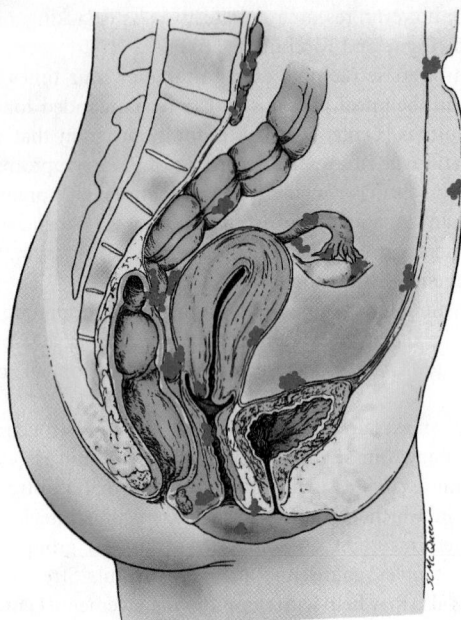

FIG 4-2 Common sites of endometriosis. (From Lentz GM, Lobo RA, Gershenson DM, et al, editors: *Comprehensive gynecology,* ed 6, Philadelphia, 2012, Mosby.)

condition usually develops in the third or fourth decade of life, endometriosis has been found in adolescents with disabling pelvic pain or abnormal vaginal bleeding. Endometriosis may worsen with repeated cycles, or it may remain asymptomatic and undiagnosed, eventually disappearing after menopause. However, it has been reported to occur in about 5% of postmenopausal women receiving menopausal hormone therapy. There appears to be a familial tendency to develop endometriosis; the condition is 7 times more prevalent in women who have a first-degree relative with endometriosis as compared to the general population (Lobo, 2012b).

Several theories concerning the cause of endometriosis have been suggested. However, the etiology and pathology of this condition continue to be poorly understood. One of the most widely accepted theories is transplantation or retrograde menstruation. According to this theory, endometrial tissue is refluxed through the uterine tubes during menstruation into the peritoneal cavity, where it implants on the ovaries and other organs. Retrograde menstruation has been documented in a number of surgical studies and is estimated to occur in 90% of menstruating women. For most women endometrial tissue outside the uterus is destroyed before it can implant or seed in the peritoneal cavity or elsewhere. Other theories include genetic disposition, immunologic changes, and hormonal influences (Lobo, 2012b).

Symptoms from nonexistent to incapacitating vary among women. Severity of symptoms can change over time and may not reflect the extent of the disease. The major symptoms of endometriosis are pelvic pain, dysmenorrhea, and dyspareunia (painful intercourse). Women may also have chronic noncyclic pelvic pain, pelvic heaviness, or pain radiating into the thighs. Many women report bowel symptoms such as diarrhea, pain with defecation, and constipation caused by avoiding defecation because of the pain. Less common symptoms include abnormal bleeding (hypermenorrhea, menorrhagia, or premenstrual staining) and pain during exercise as a result of adhesions (Lobo, 2012b).

Impaired fertility may result from adhesions around the uterus that pull the uterus into a fixed, retroverted position. Adhesions

around the uterine tubes may block the fimbriated ends or prevent the spontaneous movement that carries the ovum to the uterus.

Management

Treatment is based on the severity of symptoms and the goals of the woman or couple. Women without pain who do not want to become pregnant need no treatment. In women with mild pain who may desire a future pregnancy, treatment may be limited to use of NSAIDs during menstruation (see earlier discussion of these medications).

Suppression of endogenous estrogen production and subsequent endometrial lesion growth is the cornerstone of management of the disease. Two main classes of medications are used to suppress endogenous estrogen levels: gonadotropin-releasing hormone (GnRH) agonists and androgen derivatives. GnRH agonist therapy (leuprolide [Lupron], nafarelin acetate [Synarel], goserelin acetate [Zoladex]) acts by suppressing pituitary gonadotropin secretion. FSH and LH stimulation of the ovary declines markedly, and ovarian function decreases significantly. A medically induced menopause develops, resulting in anovulation and amenorrhea. Shrinkage of already established endometrial tissue, significant pain relief, and interruption in further lesion development follow. The hypoestrogenism results in hot flashes in almost all women. Trabecular bone loss is common, although most loss is reversible within 12 to 24 months after the medication is stopped (Lobo, 2012b).

Leuprolide (3.75 mg intramuscular injection given once a month), nafarelin (200 mg administered twice daily by nasal spray), and goserelin 3.6 mg every 28 days by subcutaneous implant are effective and well tolerated. These medications reduce endometrial lesions and pelvic pain associated with endometriosis and have posttreatment pregnancy rates similar to that of danazol (Danocrine) therapy (Lobo, 2012b). Common side effects of these drugs are those of natural menopause—hot flashes and vaginal dryness. Occasionally women report headaches and muscle aches. Treatment is usually limited to 6 months to minimize bone loss. Although unlikely, it is possible for a woman to become pregnant while taking a GnRH agonist. Because the potential teratogenicity of this drug is unclear, women should use a barrier contraceptive during treatment.

Danazol, a mildly androgenic synthetic steroid, suppresses FSH and LH secretion, thus producing anovulation and hypogonadotropism. This results in decreased secretion of estrogen and progesterone and regression of endometrial tissue. Danazol can produce side effects severe enough to cause a woman to discontinue the drug, including masculinizing traits (weight gain, edema, decreased breast size, oily skin, hirsutism, and deepening of the voice), all of which often disappear when treatment is discontinued. Other side effects are amenorrhea, hot flashes, vaginal dryness, insomnia, and decreased libido. Migraine headaches, dizziness, fatigue, and depression are also reported. Danazol treatment has been reported to adversely affect lipids, with a decrease in high-density lipoprotein levels and an increase in low-density lipoprotein levels. Danazol should never be prescribed when pregnancy is suspected, and barrier contraception should be used with it because ovulation may not be suppressed. Danazol can produce pseudohermaphroditism in female fetuses. The medication is contraindicated in women with liver disease and should be used with caution in women with cardiac and renal disease. Danazol is less frequently used to treat endometriosis than other medical therapies (Lobo, 2012b).

Women who have early symptomatic disease and who can postpone pregnancy may be treated with continuous OCPs that have a

◎ NURSING CARE PLAN

Woman with Endometriosis

NURSING DIAGNOSIS	EXPECTED PATIENT OUTCOMES	NURSING INTERVENTIONS	RATIONALE
Acute Pain related to menstruation secondary to endometriosis	Woman will verbalize a decrease in intensity and frequency of pain during each menstrual cycle.	Assess location, type, and duration of pain and history of discomfort. Administer analgesics. Administer hormone-altering medications if ordered. Provide nonpharmacologic methods such as heat.	To determine severity of dysmenorrhea To assist with pain relief To suppress ovulation To increase blood flow to the pelvic region
Deficient Knowledge related to unfamiliarity with treatment, as evidenced by woman's statements	Woman will verbalize correct understanding of the use of self-care methods and prescribed therapies.	Assess woman's current understanding of the disorder and related therapies. Give information to woman regarding the disorder and treatment regimen.	To validate the accuracy of knowledge base To empower the woman to become a partner in her own care
Situational Low Self-Esteem related to infertility as evidenced by woman's statements of decreased self-worth	Woman will verbalize positive feelings of self-worth.	Provide therapeutic communication. Refer to support group.	To validate feelings and provide support To enhance feelings of self-worth through group communication
Anxiety related to possible invasive surgical procedure as evidenced by woman's verbal report	Woman will report a decreased number of anxious feelings. Reinforce information provided to keep expectations realistic and dispel myths or inaccuracies	Provide opportunity to discuss feelings. Provide emotional support.	To identify source of anxiety To encourage verbalization of feelings
Risk for Injury related to disease progression	Woman will report any changes in health status to health care provider	Teach woman to report any changes in health status. Review side effects of medications. Encourage ongoing communication with health care provider.	To initiate prompt treatment To recognize possible causes for changes in health status To promote trust and comfort

low estrogen-to-progestin ratio to shrink endometrial tissue. Any low-dose OCPs can be used if taken for 15 weeks, followed by 1 week of withdrawal. This therapy is associated with minimal side effects and can be taken for extended periods (Lobo, 2012b). Limited data exist on the effectiveness of progestogen-only medications for treating pain related to endometriosis (Brown, Kives, and Akhtar, 2012).

Continuous combined hormone therapy (OCPs, estrogen/progestin patch, estrogen/progestin vaginal ring) for menstrual suppression and administration of NSAIDs are the usual treatment for adolescents under the age of 16 who have endometriosis. GnRH agonist therapy for severe symptoms may have possible adverse effects on bone mineralization in adolescents, and bone mineral density should be carefully monitored (Laufer, 2008).

Surgical intervention is often needed for severe, acute, or incapacitating symptoms. Decisions regarding the extent and type of surgery are influenced by a woman's age, desire for children, and location of the disease. For women who do not want to preserve their ability to have children, the only definite cure is total abdominal hysterectomy with BSO (TAH with BSO). In women who want children and in whom the disease does not prevent bearing children, reproductive capacity should be retained through careful removal by laparoscopic surgery or laser therapy (coagulation, vaporization, or resection) of all endometrial tissue possible with retention of ovarian function (Lobo, 2012b).

Regardless of the type of treatment (short of TAH with BSO), endometriosis recurs in approximately 40% of women. Thus for many women endometriosis is a chronic disease with conditions such as chronic pain or infertility. Counseling and education are critical components of nursing care for women with endometriosis. Women need an honest discussion of treatment options, with review of the potential risks and benefits of each option. Because pelvic pain is a subjective, personal experience that can be frightening, support is important. Sexual dysfunction resulting from dyspareunia is common and may necessitate referral for counseling. Support groups for women with endometriosis may be found in some locations. Resolve (www.resolve.org), an organization for infertile couples, or the Endometriosis Association (www.ivf.com/endohtml.html) may also be helpful. The nursing care discussed in the previous section on dysmenorrhea is appropriate for managing chronic pelvic pain and dysmenorrhea experienced by women with endometriosis (see Nursing Care Plan).

Alterations in Cyclic Bleeding

Women often experience changes in amount, duration, interval, or regularity of menstrual cycle bleeding. Commonly women worry about menstruation that is infrequent (oligomenorrhea), is scanty at normal intervals (hypomenorrhea), is excessive (menorrhagia), or occurs between periods (metrorrhagia).

Treatment depends on the cause and may include education and reassurance. For example, tell women that OCPs can cause scanty menstrual flow and midcycle spotting. Progestin intramuscular injections and implants can also cause midcycle bleeding. A single episode of heavy bleeding may signal an early pregnancy loss such as a miscarriage or ectopic pregnancy. This type of bleeding is often thought to be a period that is heavier than usual, perhaps delayed, and is associated with abdominal pain or pelvic discomfort. When early pregnancy loss is suspected, hematocrit and pregnancy tests are indicated.

Uterine leiomyomas (fibroids or myomas) are a common cause of menorrhagia. Fibroids are benign tumors of the smooth muscle of the uterus with an unknown cause. Fibroids occur in approximately one fourth of women of reproductive age; their incidence is higher in African-American women than in Caucasian, Asian, or in Hispanic women (Katz, 2012). Other uterine growths ranging from endometrial polyps to adenocarcinoma and endometrial cancer are common causes of heavy menstrual bleeding and intermenstrual bleeding.

> **! NURSING ALERT**
>
> If the woman herself considers the amount or duration of bleeding to be excessive, the problem should be investigated.

Treatment for menorrhagia depends on the cause of the bleeding. If the bleeding is related to contraceptive method (e.g., an intrauterine device [IUD]), provide factual information and reassurance and discuss other contraceptive options.

If there is no known cause for the bleeding and anatomic causes have been rules out, therapy is aimed at reducing the amount of heavy bleeding. Current options for treatment include OCPs and NSAIDs (non–Food and Drug Administration [FDA] approved for this use) and FDA-approved therapies: the levonorgestrel-releasing IUD and antifibrinolytic agents (e.g., tranexamic acid) (Lobo, 2012a, Wilton, 2012).

If bleeding is related to the presence of fibroids, the degree of disability and discomfort associated with the fibroids and the woman's plans for childbearing influence treatment decisions. Treatment options include medical and surgical management. Most fibroids can be monitored by frequent examinations to judge growth, if any, and correction of anemia if present. Warn women with metrorrhagia to avoid using aspirin because of its tendency to increase bleeding. Medical treatment is directed toward temporarily reducing symptoms, shrinking the myoma, and reducing its blood supply (Katz, 2012). This reduction is often accomplished with the use of a GnRH agonist. However, usually after cessation of this treatment, the myomas return to their pretreatment size (Katz, 2012). If the woman wishes to retain childbearing potential, a myomectomy may be performed. Myomectomy, or removal of the tumors only by laparoscopic or hysteroscopic resection or laser surgery, is particularly difficult if multiple myomas must be removed. One in four women will have a hysterectomy performed within 20 years of having a myomectomy. If the woman does not want to preserve her childbearing function or if she has severe symptoms (severe anemia, severe pain, considerable disruption of lifestyle), uterine artery embolization (UAE) (procedure that blocks blood supply to fibroid), or hysterectomy (removal of uterus) may be performed. After UAE

20% to 30% of women will undergo a hysterectomy within 5 years (Katz, 2012).

Important nursing roles include reassurance, counseling, education, and support.

Dysfunctional Uterine Bleeding

Abnormal uterine bleeding (AUB) is any form of uterine bleeding that is irregular in amount, duration, or timing and is not related to regular menstrual bleeding. Box 4-1 lists possible causes of AUB. Although often used interchangeably, the terms AUB and dysfunctional uterine bleeding (DUB) are not synonymous. AUB can have

---

BOX 4-1   POSSIBLE CAUSES OF ABNORMAL UTERINE BLEEDING

Pregnancy-Related Conditions
- Threatened or spontaneous miscarriage
- Retained products of conception after elective abortion
- Ectopic pregnancy
- Placenta previa/placenta abruptio
- Trophoblastic disease

Lower Reproductive Tract Infections
- Cervicitis
- Endometritis
- Myometritis
- Salpingitis

Benign Anatomic Abnormalities
- Adenomyosis
- Leiomyomata
- Polyps of the cervix or endometrium

Neoplasms
- Endometrial hyperplasia
- Cancer of cervix and endometrium
- Hormonally active tumors (rare)
- Vaginal tumors (rare)

Malignant Lesions
- Cervical squamous cell carcinoma
- Endometrial adenocarcinoma
- Estrogen-producing ovarian tumors
- Testosterone-producing ovarian tumors
- Leiomyosarcoma

Trauma
- Genital injury (accidental, coital trauma, sexual abuse)
- Foreign body
- Lacerations

Systemic Conditions
- Adrenal hyperplasia and Cushing's disease
- Blood dyscrasias
- Coagulopathies
- Hypothalamic suppression (from stress, weight loss, excessive exercise)
- Polycystic ovary disease
- Thyroid disease
- Pituitary adenoma or hyperprolactinemia
- Severe organ disease (renal or liver failure)

Iatrogenic Causes
- Medications with estrogenic activity
- Anticoagulants
- Exogenous hormone use (oral contraceptives, menopausal hormone therapy)
- Selective serotonin reuptake inhibitors
- Tamoxifen
- Intrauterine devices
- Herbal preparation (ginseng)

Modified from Albers JR, Hull SK, Wesley RM: Abnormal uterine bleeding, *Am Fam Physician* 69:1915–1926; 1931–1932, 2004.

organic causes such as systemic diseases, reproductive tract disease, or DUB that is usually hormonally related.

DUB can be anovulatory or ovulatory but is most commonly caused by anovulation. When no surge of LH occurs or if insufficient progesterone is produced by the corpus luteum to support the endometrium, it will begin to involute and shed. This process most often occurs at the extremes of a woman's reproductive years, when the menstrual cycle is just becoming established at menarche or when it draws to a close at menopause. DUB also occurs with any condition that gives rise to chronic anovulation associated with continuous estrogen production. Such conditions include obesity, hyperthyroidism and hypothyroidism, polycystic ovarian syndrome, and any of the endocrine conditions discussed in the sections on amenorrhea oligomenorrhea. A diagnosis of DUB is made only after ruling out all other causes of abnormal menstrual bleeding (Lobo, 2012a).

Management. The most effective medical treatment of acute bleeding episodes of DUB is administration of oral or intravenous estrogen. D&C may be done if the bleeding has not stopped in 12 to 24 hours. An oral conjugated estrogen and progestin regimen is usually given for at least 3 months after the acute phase has passed. Such long-term treatment will help prevent recurrence of the pattern of DUB and hemorrhage. If the woman wants contraception, she should continue to take OCPs. If she has no need for contraception, the treatment may be stopped to assess the woman's bleeding pattern. If her menses does not resume, a progestin regimen (e.g., medroxyprogesterone, 10 mg each day for 10 days before the expected date of her menstrual period) may be prescribed after ruling out pregnancy. This is done to prevent persistent anovulation with chronic unopposed endogenous estrogen hyperstimulation of the endometrium, which can result in eventual atypical tissue changes (Lobo, 2012a).

If the recurrent, heavy bleeding is not controlled by hormone therapy or D&C, ablation of the endometrium through laser treatment may be performed. Nursing roles include informing patients of their options, counseling and education as indicated, and referring to the appropriate specialists and health care services.

CARE MANAGEMENT

Nursing assessments for women who have a menstrual disorder include:
- Taking a thorough menstrual, obstetric, sexual, and contraceptive history.
- Exploring the woman's perceptions of her condition, cultural or ethnic influences, lifestyle, and patterns of coping.
- Evaluating the amount of pain or bleeding experienced and its effect on daily activities.
- Noting any home remedies and prescriptions to relieve discomfort. A symptom diary, in which the woman records emotions, behaviors, physical symptoms, diet, and exercise and rest patterns, is a useful diagnostic tool.

Possible nursing diagnoses include:
- Risk for Ineffective Individual Coping related to:
    Insufficient knowledge of the cause of the disorder
    Emotional and physiologic effects of the disorder
- Deficient Knowledge related to:
    Self-management
    Available therapy for the disorder
- Risk for Disturbed Body Image related to:
    Menstrual disorder
    Sexual dysfunction

- Risk for Situational Low Self-Esteem related to:
    Others' perception of her discomfort
    Inability to conceive
- Acute or Chronic Pain related to:
    Menstrual disorder

Expected outcomes for the woman are that she will do the following:
- Verbalize her understanding of reproductive anatomy, cause of her disorder, medication regimen, and diary use.
- Verbalize her understanding and accept her emotional and physical responses to her menstrual cycle.
- Develop personal goals that benefit her emotionally and physically.
- Choose appropriate therapeutic measures for her menstrual problems.
- Adapt successfully to the condition if cure is not possible.

In addition to the medical, surgical, and nursing interventions discussed with each problem, additional nursing interventions may include:
- Accepting the woman's symptoms as valid.
- Correlating data from the daily diary of emotional status, subjective feelings, and physical state with physiologic changes.
- Encouraging the woman to express her feelings about her symptoms.
- Providing information about therapeutic options (pharmacologic and nonpharmacologic) so the woman (couple) makes (make) choices considered best for her (them).
- Providing information about local support groups.

Care has been effective when the woman reports improvement in the quality of her life, skill in self-management, and a positive self-concept and body image.

INFECTIONS

Infections of the reproductive tract can occur throughout a woman's life and are often the cause of significant reproductive morbidity, including ectopic pregnancy and tubal factor infertility. The direct economic costs of these infections can be substantial, and the indirect cost is equally overwhelming. Some consequences of maternal infection such as infertility last a lifetime. The emotional costs may include damaged relationships and lowered self-esteem.

Sexually Transmitted Infections

Sexually transmitted infections (STIs) are infections or infectious disease syndromes transmitted primarily by sexual contact. The term sexually transmitted infection includes more than 25 infectious organisms that are transmitted through sexual activity and the dozens of clinical syndromes that they cause (Box 4-2). STIs are among the most common health problems in the United States today, with an estimated 19 million people in the United States being infected with STIs every year (CDC, 2010a). The following discussion focuses on the most common STIs in women. Chapter 25 discusses neonatal effects.

Prevention

Preventing infection (primary prevention) is the most effective way of reducing the adverse consequences of STIs for women. Prompt diagnosis and treatment of current infections (secondary prevention) also can prevent personal complications and

BOX 4-2	**SEXUALLY TRANSMITTED INFECTIONS**

Bacteria
- Chlamydia
- Gonorrhea
- Syphilis
- Chancroid
- Lymphogranuloma venereum
- Genital mycoplasmas
- Group B streptococci

Viruses
- Human immunodeficiency virus
- Herpes simplex virus, types 1 and 2
- Cytomegalovirus
- Viral hepatitis A and B
- Human papillomavirus

Protozoa
- Trichomoniasis

Parasites
- Pediculosis (may or may not be sexually transmitted)
- Scabies (may or may not be sexually transmitted)

BOX 4-3	**ASSESSING SEXUALLY TRANSMITTED INFECTION AND HUMAN IMMUNODEFICIENCY VIRUS RISK BEHAVIORS**

Sexual Risk
- Are you sexually active now?
- If no, have you had sex in the past?
- Ever had an oral, vaginal, or anal sexual experience with another person?
- With how many different people? 1? 2 or 3? 4 to 10? More than 10?
- Have your partners been men, women, both?
- Ever thought that a sex partner put you at risk for AIDS or an STI (IV drug user, bisexual)?
- Ever had an STI (herpes, gonorrhea, genital warts, chlamydia)?
- Ever had sex against your will?
- What do you do to protect yourself from HIV and STIs?
- Do you use male condoms? Female condoms? Other barriers?

Drug Use–Related Risk
- Ever injected drugs using shared equipment, including street drugs, steroids?
- Ever had sex with a person who uses and shares?
- Ever had sex while so stoned, high, or drunk that you can't remember the details?
- Ever exchanged sex for drugs, money, shelter?

Blood-Related Risks
- Ever had a blood transfusion?
- Ever had sex with a person who had a blood transfusion?
- Ever had sex with a person with hemophilia?
- Ever received donor semen, egg, transplanted organ or tissue?
- Ever shared equipment for tattoo, body piercing?

Other
- Ever had a test for HIV?
- Ever worried about AIDS and would like to talk with someone about it?

Data from Marrazzo JM, Cates W: Reproductive tract infections, including HIV and other sexually transmitted infections. In Hatcher RA, Trussell J, Nelson AL, et al., editors, *Contraceptive technology*, ed 21, Atlanta, 2011, Ardent Media.
AIDS, Acquired immunodeficiency syndrome; *HIV*, human immunodeficiency virus; *IV*, intravenous; *STI*, sexually transmitted infection.

transmission to others. Preventing the spread of STIs requires that women at risk for transmitting or acquiring infections change their behavior. A critical first step is to include questions about a woman's sexual history, sexual risk behaviors, and drug-related risky behaviors as a part of her assessment (Box 4-3). When you identify risk factors or risky behaviors, you have an opportunity to provide prevention counseling. Techniques that are effective in providing prevention counseling include using open-ended questions, using understandable language, and reassuring the woman that treatment will be provided regardless of consideration such as ability to pay, language spoken, or lifestyle (CDC, 2010a; Fantasia, Fontenot, Sutherland, et al., 2011). Prevention messages should include descriptions of specific actions to prevent contracting or transmitting STIs (e.g., refraining from sexual activity when STI-related symptoms are present) and should be individualized for each woman, giving attention to her specific risk factors.

To be motivated to take preventive actions, a woman must believe that acquiring a disease will be serious for her and that she is at risk for infection. Most individuals tend to underestimate their personal risk of infection in a given situation. Thus many women may not perceive themselves as being at risk for contracting an STI, and telling them that they should carry condoms may not be well received. Although levels of awareness of STIs are generally high, widespread misconceptions or specific gaps in knowledge also exist. Therefore nurses have a responsibility to ensure that their patients have accurate, complete knowledge about transmission and symptoms of STIs and the behaviors that place them at risk for contracting an infection.

Primary preventive measures are individual activities aimed at avoiding infection. Risk-free options include complete abstinence from sexual activities that transmit semen, blood, or other body fluids or that allow for skin-to-skin contact (CDC, 2010a). Involvement in a mutually monogamous relationship with an uninfected partner also eliminates risk of contracting STIs.

Sexually Transmitted Infections/Human Immunodeficiency Virus Prevention Strategies. An essential component of primary prevention is counseling the woman regarding sexual practices so she can avoid acquiring or transmitting STIs, including attaining knowledge of her partner, reducing her number of partners, practicing low risk sex, avoiding the exchange of body fluids, and vaccination.

Reducing the number of partners and avoiding partners who have had many previous sexual partners decrease a woman's chances of contracting an STI. Discussing each new partner's previous sexual history and exposure to STIs augments other efforts to reduce risk; however, sexual partners are not always truthful about their sexual history.

Women should be taught low risk sexual practices and which sexual practices to avoid. Sexual fantasizing is safe, as are caressing, hugging, body rubbing, and massage. Mutual masturbation is low risk as long as there is no contact with a partner's semen or vaginal secretions. All sexual activities are safe when both partners are monogamous, trustworthy, and known (by testing) to be free of disease. Anal-genital intercourse, anal-oral contact, and anal-digital activity are high risk sexual behaviors and should be avoided.

🏠 COMMUNITY FOCUS

Sexually Transmitted Infections

Interview a nurse working in a clinic about sexually transmitted infections commonly seen there.

- What are the most common infections seen in the clinic?
- Has the incidence of infections changed over the last 5 years? Which infections have increased, and which have decreased in incidence during that time?
- Are adolescents seen in the clinic? Is there a special clinic for adolescents?
- How much independence does the nurse have in diagnosing and treating sexually transmitted infections?
- What patient teaching guidelines are available in the clinic? Are the guidelines available in languages other than English?

The physical barrier promoted for the prevention of sexual transmission of human immunodeficiency virus (HIV) and other STIs is the latex male condom. The nurse should remind women to use a condom with every sexual encounter; to use latex or plastic male condoms rather than natural skin condoms for STI protection; to use a condom with a current expiration date; to use each one only once; and to handle it carefully to avoid damaging it with fingernails, teeth, or other sharp objects. Condoms should be stored away from high heat. Although it is not ideal, women may choose to safely carry condoms in wallets, shoes, or inside a bra. They can be taught the differences among condoms: price ranges, sizes, and where they can be purchased. Explicit instructions for how to apply a male condom are included in Chapter 5.

The female condom (i.e., a lubricated polyurethane sheath with a ring on each end that is inserted into the vagina) has been shown in laboratory studies to be an effective mechanical barrier to viruses, including HIV. Studies suggest that the female condom is at least as effective as male condoms in preventing transmission of STIs (CDC, 2010a). What is important and should be stressed by nurses is the consistent use of condoms for every act of sexual intimacy when there is the possibility of transmission of disease.

Evidence has shown that vaginal spermicides do not protect against certain STIs (e.g., chlamydia, cervical gonorrhea) and that frequent use of spermicides containing nonoxynol-9 has been associated with genital lesions and may increase HIV transmission. Condoms lubricated with nonoxynol-9 are not recommended (CDC, 2010a).

Vaccination is an effective method for the prevention of some STIs such as hepatitis B and human papillomavirus (HPV). Hepatitis B vaccine is recommended for women at high risk for STIs. A vaccine is available for HPV types 6, 11, 16, and 18 for girls and women 9 to 26 years of age (CDC, 2010a) (see later discussion).

Counsel women to watch out for situations that make it hard to talk about and practice risk reduction. These situations include romantic times when condoms are not available and when alcohol or drugs make it difficult to make wise decisions (see Community Focus box).

Sexually Transmitted Bacterial Infections
Chlamydia

Chlamydia trachomatis is the most frequently reported infectious disease in the United States, yet most cases are still undiagnosed (CDC, 2010a). These infections are often silent and highly destructive; their sequelae and complications are very serious. In women chlamydial infections are difficult to diagnose; the symptoms, if present, are nonspecific, and the organism is expensive to culture.

Acute salpingitis, or pelvic inflammatory disease, is the most serious complication of chlamydial infections. Past chlamydial infections are associated with an increased risk of ectopic pregnancy and tubal factor infertility. Furthermore, chlamydial infection of the cervix causes inflammation, resulting in microscopic cervical ulcerations that may increase risk of acquiring HIV infection. More than half of infants born to mothers with chlamydia will develop conjunctivitis or pneumonia after perinatal exposure to the mother's infected cervix. *C. trachomatis* is the most common infectious cause of ophthalmia neonatorum.

Sexually active women younger than 20 years are the ones most likely to become infected with chlamydia, with the highest rates in African-American women ages 15 to 19 years (CDC, 2010a). Women older than age 30 have the lowest rate of infection. Risky behaviors, including multiple partners and not using barrier methods of birth control, increase a woman's risk of chlamydial infection.

Screening and Diagnosis. In addition to obtaining information regarding the presence of risk factors (e.g., women younger than 25 years old, older women who do not use barrier contraceptives, women with new or multiple partners), inquire about the presence of any symptoms (CDC, 2010a). Although infection is usually asymptomatic, some women may experience spotting or postcoital bleeding, mucoid or purulent cervical discharge, or dysuria. Bleeding results from inflammation and erosion of the cervical columnar epithelium.

Laboratory diagnosis of chlamydia is by culture (expensive and labor intensive), DNA probe (relatively less expensive but less sensitive), enzyme immunoassay (also relatively less expensive but less sensitive), and nucleic acid amplification tests (NAATs) (expensive but have relatively higher sensitivity) of urine specimens or specimens from the endocervix/vagina (CDC, 2010a; Fantasia, Fontenot, Sutherland et al., 2011). All pregnant women should have cervical cultures for chlamydia at the first prenatal visit. Screening late in the third trimester (36 weeks) may be carried out if the woman was positive previously or if she is younger than 25 years, has a new sex partner, or has multiple sex partners.

Management. The CDC (2010a) recommendations for the treatment of chlamydial infections include doxycycline or azithromycin (Table 4-3). Azithromycin is often prescribed when compliance is a problem because only one dose is needed. Because chlamydia is often asymptomatic, caution the woman to take all medication prescribed. All exposed sexual partners should be treated. Woman treated with doxycycline or azithromycin do not need to be retested unless symptoms continue (CDC, 2010a).

Gonorrhea

Gonorrhea is probably the oldest communicable disease in the United States. An estimated 300,000 American men and women contract gonorrhea each year (CDC, 2010a). The incidence of drug-resistant cases of gonorrhea, in particular penicillinase-producing *Neisseria gonorrhoeae*, is increasing dramatically in the United States.

Gonorrhea is caused by the aerobic, gram-negative diplococci *N. gonorrhoeae*. It is almost exclusively transmitted by sexual contact. The principal means of transmission is genital-to-genital contact during sexual activity; however, it is also spread by oral-genital and anal-genital contact. There is also evidence that infection may spread in females from vagina to rectum. Although the organism has been recovered from inanimate objects artificially inoculated with the bacteria, there is no evidence that natural transmission occurs this way.

TABLE 4-3   SEXUALLY TRANSMITTED INFECTIONS AND DRUG THERAPIES FOR WOMEN*

DISEASE	NONPREGNANT WOMEN (13-17 YR)	NONPREGNANT WOMEN (>18 YR)	PREGNANT WOMEN	LACTATING WOMEN†
Chlamydia	*Recommended:* Azithromycin, 1 g orally once *or* Doxycycline, 100 mg orally bid for 7 days	*Recommended:* Azithromycin, 1 g orally once *or* Doxycycline, 100 mg orally bid for 7 days	*Recommended:* Azithromycin, 1 g orally once *or* Amoxicillin, 500 mg orally tid for 7 days	*Recommended:* Azithromycin, 1 g orally once *or* Amoxicillin, 500 mg orally tid for 7 days
Gonorrhea	*Recommended:* Ceftriaxone, 125 mg IM once (adolescents who weigh >45 kg can be treated with any regimen recommended for adults) Plus treatment for chlamydia as above	*Recommended:* Ceftriaxone, 250 mg IM once Plus treatment for chlamydia as above	*Recommended:* Ceftriaxone, 250 mg IM once Plus treatment for chlamydia as above	*Recommended:* Ceftriaxone, 250 mg IM once Plus treatment for chlamydia as above
Syphilis	**Primary, secondary, early-latent disease:** *Recommended:* Benzathine penicillin G, 2.4 million units IM once **Late-latent or unknown-duration disease:** *Recommended:* Benzathine penicillin G, 7.2 million units total, administered as three doses, 2.4 million units each, at 1-wk intervals **Penicillin allergy:** Doxycycline, 100 mg orally qid for 14 days *or* Tetracycline, 500 mg orally qid for 14 days	**Primary, secondary, early-latent disease:** *Recommended:* Benzathine penicillin G, 2.4 million units IM once **Late-latent or unknown-duration disease:** *Recommended:* Benzathine penicillin G, 7.2 million units total, administered as three doses, 2.4 million units each, at 1-wk intervals **Penicillin allergy:** Doxycycline, 100 mg orally qid for 14 days *or* Tetracycline, 500 mg orally qid for 14 days	**Primary, secondary, early-latent disease:** *Recommended:* Benzathine penicillin G, 2.4 million units IM once (some experts recommend a second dose of benzathine penicillin, 2.4 million units, 1 wk later) **Late-latent or unknown-duration disease:** *Recommended:* Benzathine penicillin G, 7.2 million units total, administered as three doses, 2.4 million units each, at 1-wk intervals No proven alternatives to penicillin in pregnancy Pregnant women who have a history of allergy to penicillin should be desensitized and treated with penicillin	**Primary, secondary, early-latent disease:** *Recommended:* Benzathine penicillin G, 2.4 million units IM once
Human papillomavirus	*Recommended for external genital warts:* **Patient-applied:** Podofilox, 0.5% solution, or gel to wart bid for 3 days followed by 4-day rest for ≤4 cycles *or* Imiquimod, 5% cream, at hs 3 times a week for ≤16 wk *or* Sinecatechins 15% oint tid for ≤16 wk **Provider-applied:** Cryotherapy with liquid nitrogen or cryoprobe *or* Podophyllin resin, 10%-25% in tincture of benzoin compound weekly (wash off in 1-4 hr). Repeat weekly as necessary *or* Trichloracetic acid (TCA) or bichloracetic acid (BCA) 80%-90% weekly	*Recommended for external genital warts:* **Patient-applied:** Podofilox, 0.5% solution, or gel to wart bid for 3 days followed by 4-day rest for ≤4 cycles *or* Imiquimod, 5% cream, at hs 3 times a week for ≤16 wk *or* Sinecatechins 15% oint tid for ≤16 wk **Provider-applied:** Cryotherapy with liquid nitrogen or cryoprobe *or* Podophyllin resin, 10%-25% in tincture of benzoin compound weekly (wash off in 1-4 hr). Repeat weekly as necessary *or* TCA or BCA 80%-90% weekly	*Recommended for external genital warts:* **Provider applied:** Cryotherapy with liquid nitrogen or cryoprobe *or* TCA or BCA 80%-90% weekly Imiquimod, podophyllin (Podocon-25), sinecatechins, and podofilox should not be used in pregnancy	*Recommended for external genital warts:* **Provider applied:** Cryotherapy with liquid nitrogen or cryoprobe *or* TCA or BCA 80%-90% weekly Imiquimod, podophyllin, sinecatechins, and podofilox should not be used during lactation

TABLE 4-3	SEXUALLY TRANSMITTED INFECTIONS AND DRUG THERAPIES FOR WOMEN*—cont'd			
DISEASE	**NONPREGNANT WOMEN (13-17 YR)**	**NONPREGNANT WOMEN (>18 YR)**	**PREGNANT WOMEN**	**LACTATING WOMEN†**
Genital herpes simplex virus (HSV-1 or HSV-2)	**Primary infection:** Acyclovir, 400 mg orally tid for 7-10 days *or* Acyclovir, 200 mg orally 5 times a day for 7-10 days *or* Famciclovir, 250 mg orally tid for 7-10 days *or* Valacyclovir, 1 g orally bid for 7-10 days **Recurrent infection:** Acyclovir, 400 mg orally tid for 5 days *or* Acyclovir, 800 mg orally bid for 5 days *or* Acyclovir, 800 mg orally tid for 2 days *or* Famciclovir, 125 mg orally bid for 5 days *or* Famciclovir 1000 mg orally bid for 1 day *or* Famciclovir, 500 mg once, then 250 mg bid for 2 days *or* Valacyclovir, 500 mg orally bid for 3 days *or* Valacyclovir, 1 g orally once a day for 5 days **Suppression therapy:** *Take daily for 1 year or more:* Acyclovir, 400 mg orally bid *or* Famciclovir, 250 mg orally bid *or* Valacyclovir, 500 mg orally once a day *or* Valacyclovir, 1 g orally once a day	**Primary infection:** Acyclovir, 400 mg orally tid for 7-10 days *or* Acyclovir, 200 mg orally 5 times a day for 7-10 days *or* Famciclovir, 250 mg orally tid for 7-10 days *or* Valacyclovir, 1 g orally bid for 7-10 days **Recurrent infection:** Acyclovir, 400 mg orally tid for 5 days *or* Acyclovir, 800 mg orally bid for 5 days *or* Acyclovir, 800 mg orally tid for 2 days *or* Famciclovir, 125 mg orally bid for 5 days *or* Famciclovir, 1000 mg orally bid for 1 day *or* Famciclovir 500 mg once, then 250 mg bid for 2 days *or* Valacyclovir, 500 mg orally bid for 3 days *or* Valacyclovir, 1 g orally once a day for 5 days **Suppression therapy:** *Take daily for 1 year or more:* Acyclovir, 400 mg orally bid *or* Famciclovir, 250 mg orally bid *or* Valacyclovir, 500 mg orally once a day *or* Valacyclovir, 1 g orally once a day	No increase in birth defects beyond the general population has been found with acyclovir use in pregnancy Acyclovir, 400 mg orally tid for 7 days for first episode or severe recurrent infection; may be given IV if infection is severe Suppression therapy 4 weeks before the birth for women with recurrent infections can reduce the need for a cesarean birth	Acyclovir usually is considered compatible with breastfeeding Acyclovir, 400 mg tid for 7 days

Data from American Academy of Pediatrics Committee on Drugs: The transfer of drugs and other chemicals into human milk, *Pediatrics* 108(3):776–789, 2002; Centers for Disease Control and Prevention: Sexually transmitted diseases treatment guidelines 2010, *MMWR Morbidity and Mortality Weekly Report,* 59(RR-12):1–109, 2010; Centers for Disease Control and Prevention (CDC): Update to CDC's sexually transmitted diseases treatment guidelines, 2010: oral cephalosporins no longer recommended for gonococcal infections, *MMWR Morbidity and Mortality Report* 61(31):590–594, 2012.
*List is not inclusive of all drugs that may be used as alternatives.
†These medications are usually compatible with breastfeeding.
bid, Twice daily; *hs,* bedtime; *HSV,* herpes simplex virus; *IM,* intramuscularly; *IV,* intravenously; *qid,* four times daily; *tid,* three times daily.

Age is probably the most important risk factor associated with gonorrhea. In the United States the highest reported rates of infection are among sexually active teenagers, young adults, and African-Americans. The majority of those contracting gonorrhea are younger than 20 years of age and engage in sexual activities with multiple partners (CDC, 2010a).

Women are often asymptomatic; but, when they are symptomatic, they may have a greenish-yellow purulent endocervical discharge or may experience menstrual irregularities. Women may complain of pain (i.e., chronic or acute severe pelvic or lower abdominal pain) or menses that last longer or are more painful than normal. Gonococcal rectal infection may occur in women after anal intercourse. Individuals with rectal gonorrhea may be completely asymptomatic or conversely may experience severe symptoms with profuse purulent anal discharge, rectal pain, and blood in the stool. Rectal itching, fullness, pressure, and pain are also common symptoms, as is diarrhea. A diffuse vaginitis with vulvitis is the most common form of gonococcal infection in prepubertal girls. There may be few signs of infection; or vaginal discharge, dysuria, or swollen, reddened labia are sometimes present.

Gonococcal infections in pregnancy potentially affect both mother and infant. Women with cervical gonorrhea may develop salpingitis in the first trimester. Perinatal complications of gonococcal infection include premature rupture of the membranes, preterm birth, chorioamnionitis, neonatal sepsis, intrauterine growth restriction, and maternal postpartum sepsis. Amniotic infection syndrome—manifested by placental, fetal, and umbilical cord inflammation following premature rupture of the membranes—may result from gonorrheal infection during pregnancy.

Screening and Diagnosis. Because gonococcal infections in women are often asymptomatic, the CDC recommends screening all women at risk for gonorrhea (CDC, 2010a). All pregnant women should be screened at the first prenatal visit, and infected women and those identified with risky behaviors rescreened at 36 weeks of gestation. Gonococcal infection cannot be diagnosed reliably by clinical signs and symptoms alone. Individuals may have "classic" symptoms, vague symptoms that may be attributed to a number of conditions, or no symptoms at all. Cultures should be obtained from the endocervix, the rectum, and when indicated the pharynx. Thayer-Martin cultures are recommended to diagnose gonorrhea in women. Because coinfection is common, any woman suspected of having gonorrhea should have a chlamydial culture and serologic test for syphilis unless one has been done within the past 2 months.

Management. Management of gonorrhea is becoming more challenging as drug-resistant strains are increasing. The treatment of choice for uncomplicated urethral, endocervical, and rectal infections in pregnant and nonpregnant women is ceftriaxone given intramuscularly once. The CDC also recommends concomitant treatment for chlamydia because coinfection is common (CDC, 2010a) (see Table 4-3). All women with both gonorrhea and syphilis should also be treated for syphilis according to CDC guidelines (see discussion of syphilis later in this chapter).

Gonorrhea is highly communicable. Recent (past 30 days) sexual partners should be examined, cultured, and treated with appropriate regimens. Most treatment failures result from reinfection. The woman needs to be informed of this and of the consequences of reinfection in terms of chronicity, complications, and potential infertility. Women are counseled to use condoms. All women with gonorrhea should be offered confidential counseling and testing for HIV infection.

> **LEGAL TIP: Reporting a Communicable Disease**
>
> Gonorrhea is a reportable communicable disease. Health care providers are legally responsible for reporting all cases of gonorrhea to health authorities, usually the local health department in the patient's county of residence. Women should be informed that the case will be reported, told why, and informed of the possibility of being contacted by a health department epidemiologist.

Syphilis

Syphilis, one of the earliest described STIs, is caused by *Treponema pallidum,* a motile spirochete. Transmission is thought to be by entry through microscopic abrasions in the subcutaneous tissue, which can occur during sexual intercourse. The disease can also be transmitted through kissing, biting, or oral-genital sex. Transplacental transmission may occur at any time during pregnancy; the degree of risk is related to the quantity of spirochetes in the maternal bloodstream.

Syphilis rates decreased in women in 2010. The rates for African-American women account for almost one-half of the cases (CDC, 2011b).

Syphilis is a complex disease that can lead to serious systemic disease and even death when untreated. Infection manifests itself in distinct stages with different symptoms and clinical manifestations. Primary syphilis is characterized by a primary lesion, the chancre, which appears 5 to 90 days after infection (Fig. 4-3, *A*). This lesion

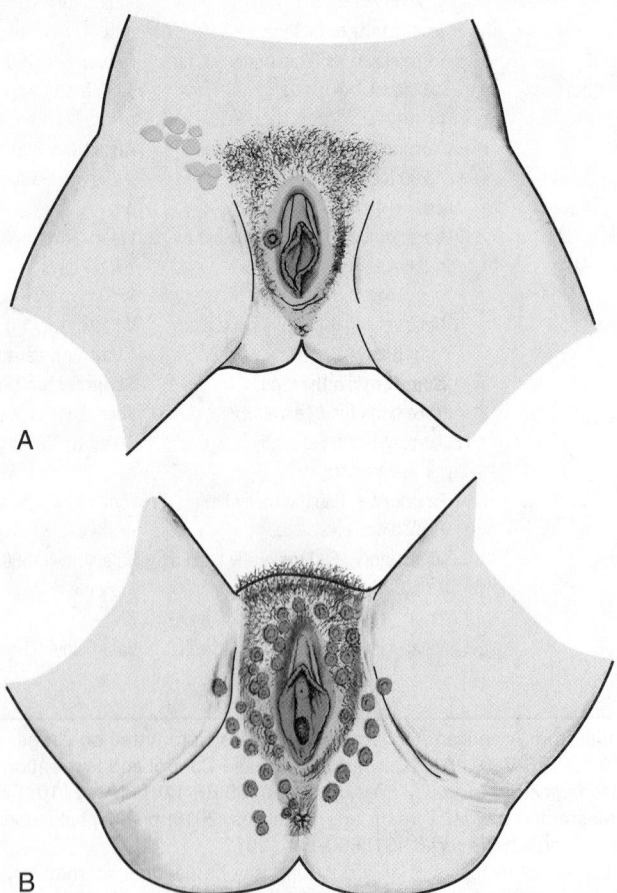

FIG 4-3 Syphilis. **A,** Primary stage: chancre with inguinal adenopathy. **B,** Secondary stage: condylomata lata.

often begins as a painless papule at the site of inoculation and erodes to form a nontender, shallow, indurated, clean ulcer several millimeters to centimeters in size. Secondary syphilis occurs 6 weeks to 6 months after the appearance of the chancre. It is characterized by a widespread, symmetric, maculopapular rash on the palms and soles and generalized lymphadenopathy. The infected individual also may experience fever, headache, and malaise. Condylomata lata (broad, painless, pink-gray, wartlike infectious lesions) may develop on the vulva, perineum, or anus (see Fig. 4-3, *B*). If the woman is untreated, she enters a latent phase that is asymptomatic for the majority of individuals. Left untreated, about one third of these women will develop tertiary syphilis. Neurologic, cardiovascular, musculoskeletal, or multiorgan system complications can develop in the third stage.

Screening and Diagnosis. All women who are diagnosed with another STI or with HIV should be screened for syphilis. All pregnant women should be screened for syphilis at the first prenatal visit, again in the late third trimester, and at the time of giving birth if high risk (CDC, 2010a). Diagnosis depends on microscopic examination of primary and secondary lesion tissue and serology during latency and late infection. A test for antibodies may not be reactive in the presence of active infection because it takes time for the immune system of the body to develop antibodies to any antigens. Up to one third of people in early primary syphilis may have nonreactive serologic tests. Two types of serologic tests are used: nontreponemal and treponemal. Nontreponemal antibody tests such as Venereal Disease Research Laboratories (VDRL) and rapid plasma reagin (RPR) are used as screening tests. False-positive results are not unusual, particularly when conditions such as acute infection, autoimmune disorders, malignancy, pregnancy, and drug addiction exist and after immunization or vaccination. The treponemal tests, fluorescent treponemal antibody absorbed, and microhemagglutination assays for antibody to *T. pallidum* are used to confirm positive results. Test results in patients with early primary or incubating syphilis may be negative. Seroconversion usually takes place 6 to 8 weeks after exposure; thus testing should be repeated in 1 to 2 months when a suggestive genital lesion exists.

Tests (e.g., wet preparations and cultures) for concomitant STIs (e.g., chlamydia and gonorrhea) should be done, and HIV testing offered if indicated.

Management. Penicillin G is the preferred drug for treating patients with all stages of syphilis, including pregnant women (see Table 4-3). Although doxycycline, tetracycline, and erythromycin are alternative treatments for penicillin-allergic patients, both tetracycline and doxycycline are contraindicated in pregnancy, and erythromycin is unlikely to cure a fetal infection. Therefore if necessary pregnant women should receive skin testing and be treated with penicillin or be desensitized (CDC, 2010a). Specific protocols are recommended by the CDC.

> **! NURSING ALERT**
>
> Patients treated for syphilis may experience a Jarisch-Herxheimer reaction. This is an acute febrile reaction often accompanied by headache, myalgias, and arthralgias that develop within the first 24 hours of treatment. The reaction may be treated symptomatically with analgesics and antipyretics. If treatment precipitates this reaction in the second half of pregnancy, women are at risk for preterm labor and birth. They should be advised to contact their health care provider if they notice any change in fetal movement or have any contractions.

Monthly follow-up is mandatory so repeated treatment may be given if needed. The nurse should emphasize the necessity of long-term serologic testing even in the absence of symptoms. The woman should be advised to practice sexual abstinence until treatment is completed, all evidence of primary and secondary syphilis is gone, and serologic evidence of a cure is demonstrated. Women should be told to notify all partners who may have been exposed. They should be informed that the disease is reportable. Preventive measures should be discussed.

Pelvic Inflammatory Disease

Pelvic inflammatory disease (PID) is an infectious process that most commonly involves the uterine tubes, causing salpingitis; the uterus, causing endometritis; and, more rarely, the ovaries and peritoneal surfaces. Multiple organisms have been found to cause PID; most cases are associated with more than one organism. In the past the most common causative agent was thought to be *N. gonorrhoeae*; however, *C. trachomatis* is now estimated to cause one half of all cases. In addition to gonorrhea and chlamydia, a wide variety of anaerobic and aerobic bacteria cause PID. It encompasses a wide variety of pathologic processes; the infection can be acute, subacute, or chronic and can have a wide range of symptoms.

Most PID results from the ascending spread of microorganisms from the vagina and endocervix to the upper genital tract. This spread most commonly happens at the end of or just after menses following reception of an infectious agent. During the menstrual period several factors facilitate the development of an infection: the cervical os is slightly open, the cervical mucus barrier is absent, and menstrual blood is an excellent medium for growth. PID also may develop after a miscarriage or an induced abortion, pelvic surgery, or childbirth.

Risk factors for acquiring PID are those associated with the risk of contracting an STI, including young age, multiple partners, high rate of new partners, and a history of STIs. Women who use IUDs may be at increased risk for PID if they have more than one sexual partner or if the partner has other sexual partners because they are at higher risk for acquiring an STI. Most of this risk occurs in the 3 weeks after IUD insertion (Eckert and Lentz, 2012). PID tends to recur.

Women who have had PID are at increased risk for ectopic pregnancy, infertility, and chronic pelvic pain. After a single episode of PID, a woman's risk for ectopic pregnancy increases sevenfold compared with the risk for women who have never had it. Other problems associated with PID include dyspareunia, pyosalpinx (pus in the uterine tubes), tubo-ovarian abscess, and pelvic adhesions.

The symptoms of PID vary, depending on whether the infection is acute, subacute, or chronic; however, pain is common to all types of infection. It may be dull, cramping, intermittent (subacute) or severe, persistent, and incapacitating (acute). Women may also report one or more of the following: fever, chills, nausea and vomiting, increased vaginal discharge, symptoms of a urinary tract infection, and irregular bleeding. Abdominal pain is usually present (Eckert and Lentz, 2012).

Screening and Diagnosis. PID is difficult to diagnose because of the accompanying wide variety of symptoms. The CDC recommends treatment for PID in all sexually active young women and others at risk for STIs if the following criteria are present and no other cause or causes of the illness are found: lower abdominal tenderness, bilateral adnexal tenderness, and cervical motion tenderness. Other criteria for diagnosing PID include an oral temperature of 38.3° C or above, abnormal cervical or vaginal discharge, elevated erythrocyte sedimentation rate, elevated C-reactive protein, and laboratory documentation of cervical infection with *N. gonor-rhoeae* or *C. trachomatis* (CDC, 2010a).

Management. Perhaps the most important nursing intervention is prevention counseling. Primary prevention includes education in avoiding contracting STIs; secondary prevention involves preventing a lower genital tract infection from ascending to the upper genital tract. Instructing women in self-protective behaviors such as practices to avoid contracting STIs and using barrier methods is critical. Women using hormonal contraception or an IUD and those who have chosen tubal ligation must be reminded to use a condom with intercourse when indicated. Also important is the detection of asymptomatic gonorrheal and chlamydial infections through routine screening of women who practice risky behaviors or have specific risk factors such as age.

Although treatment regimens vary with the infecting organism, generally a broad-spectrum antibiotic is used (CDC, 2010a). Treatment for mild-to–moderately severe PID may be oral (e.g., ceftriaxone plus doxycycline with or without metronidazole) or parenteral (e.g., cefotetan or cefoxitin plus doxycycline [oral]), and regimens can be administered in inpatient or outpatient settings. Pregnant women should be hospitalized and given parenteral antibiotics (CDC, 2010a).

The woman with acute PID should be on bed rest in a semi-Fowler's position. Comfort measures include analgesics for pain and all other nursing measures applicable to a patient confined to bed. Few pelvic examinations should be done during the acute phase of the disease. During the recovery phase the woman should restrict her activity and make every effort to get adequate rest and a nutritionally sound diet. Follow-up laboratory work after treatment should include endocervical cultures for a test of cure.

Health education is central to effective management of PID. Nurses should explain the nature of the disease to women and encourage them to comply with all therapy and prevention recommendations, emphasizing the need to take all medication, even if symptoms disappear. Any potential problems (such as a lack of money for prescriptions or a lack of transportation to return for follow-up appointments) that would prevent a woman from completing a course of treatment should be identified, referrals made for assistance as needed, and the importance of follow-up visits stressed. Women should be counseled to refrain from sexual intercourse until their treatment is completed. Contraceptive counseling, including information on barrier methods such as condoms, the contraceptive sponge, and the diaphragm, should be provided.

The potential or actual loss of reproductive capabilities can be devastating and can adversely affect the woman's self-concept. Part of the nurse's role is to help the woman adjust her self-concept to fit reality and accept alterations in a way that promotes health. Because PID is so closely tied to sexuality, body image, and self-concept, the woman diagnosed with it needs supportive care. Her feelings should be discussed, and her partner(s) included when appropriate.

Sexually Transmitted Viral Infections
Human Papillomavirus
Human papillomavirus (HPV) infection, also known as *condylomata acuminata*, or *genital warts,* is the most common viral STI seen in ambulatory health care settings. An estimated 20 million Americans are infected with HPV, and about 6.2 million new infections occur every year (CDC, 2012a). HPV, a double-stranded DNA virus, has more than 30 serotypes that can be sexually transmitted, 5 of which are known to cause genital wart formation, and 8 of which

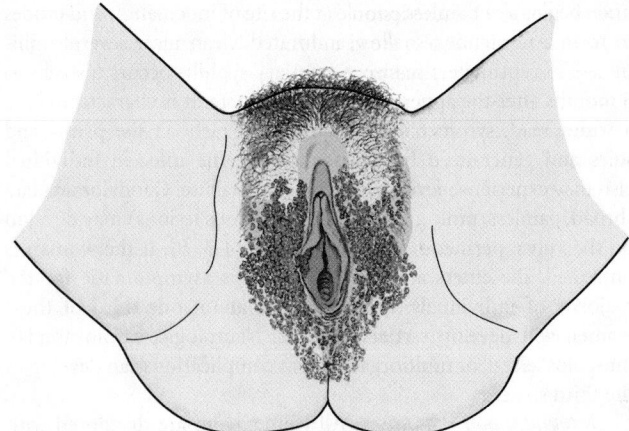

FIG 4-4 Human papillomavirus infection. Genital warts or condylomata acuminata.

are currently thought to have oncogenic potential (CDC, 2010a). HPV is the primary cause of cervical neoplasia (ACS, 2012).

In women HPV lesions are most commonly seen in the posterior part of the introitus. Lesions also are found on the buttocks, vulva, vagina, anus, and cervix (Fig. 4-4). Typically the lesions are small (2 to 3 mm in diameter and 10 to 15 mm in height), soft, papillary swellings occurring singly or in clusters on the genital and anal-rectal region. Infections of long duration may appear as a cauliflower-like mass. In moist areas such as the vaginal introitus, the lesions may appear to have multiple fine, fingerlike projections. Vaginal lesions are often multiple. Flat-topped papules, 1 to 4 mm in diameter, are seen most often on the cervix. Often these lesions are visualized only under magnification. Warts are usually flesh colored or slightly darker on Caucasian women, black on African-American women, and brownish on Asian women. The lesions are usually painless; but they may be uncomfortable, particularly when very large, inflamed, or ulcerated. Chronic vaginal discharge, pruritus, or dyspareunia can occur.

HPV infections are thought to be more common in pregnant than in nonpregnant women, with an increase in incidence from the first trimester to the third. Furthermore, a significant proportion of preexisting HPV lesions enlarge greatly during pregnancy, a proliferation presumably resulting from the relative state of immunosuppression present during this period. Lesions may become so large during pregnancy that they affect urination, defecation, mobility, and fetal descent, although birth by cesarean is rarely necessary. Cesarean birth may be performed when extensive growths are present. Initial observation of large growths can be misleading, suggesting that the entire vagina is involved. However, all of the growth may derive from one stalk; and in such cases it may be possible to push the large mass to the side, allowing the baby to pass through.

Screening and Diagnosis. A woman with HPV lesions may complain of symptoms such as a profuse, irritating vaginal discharge; itching; dyspareunia; or postcoital bleeding. She also may report "bumps" on her vulva or labia. History of a known exposure is important; however, because of the potentially long latency period and the possibility of subclinical infections in men, the lack of a history of known exposure cannot be used to exclude a diagnosis of HPV infection.

Physical inspection of the vulva, the perineum, the anus, the vagina, and the cervix is essential whenever HPV lesions are suspected or seen in one area. Because speculum examination of the vagina may block some lesions, it is important to rotate the speculum blades until all areas are visualized. When lesions are visible, the characteristic appearance previously described is considered diagnostic. However, in many instances cervical lesions are not visible, and some vaginal or vulvar lesions also may be unobservable to the naked eye. Because of the potential spread of vulvar or vaginal lesions to the anus, gloves should be changed between vaginal and rectal examinations.

Viral screening and typing for HPV are available but not standard practice. History, evaluation of signs and symptoms, Papanicolaou (Pap) test, and physical examination are used in making a diagnosis. The HPV-DNA test can be used in women older than the age of 30 in combination with the Pap test to screen for types of HPV that are likely to cause cancer or in women with abnormal Pap test results (ACS, 2012). The only definitive diagnostic test for presence of HPV is histologic evaluation of a biopsy specimen.

Management. Untreated warts may resolve on their own in young women since their immune systems may be strong enough to fight the HPV infection. Treatment of genital warts, if needed, is often difficult. No therapy has been shown to eradicate HPV. Therefore the goal of treatment is removal of warts and relief of signs and symptoms. The patient often must make multiple office visits; frequently many different treatment modalities will be used.

Treatment of genital warts should be guided by preference of the woman, available resources, and experience of the health care provider. No one of the treatments is superior to all other treatments, and no one treatment is ideal for all warts (CDC, 2010a). Imiquimod, podophyllin, and podofilox are common treatments but should not be used during pregnancy (see Table 4-3). Because the lesions can proliferate and become friable during pregnancy, many experts recommend their removal using cryotherapy or various surgical techniques (CDC, 2010a).

Women who have discomfort associated with genital warts may find that bathing with an oatmeal solution and drying the area with cool air from a hair dryer provides some relief. Keeping the area clean and dry also decreases the growth of the warts. Cotton underwear and loose-fitting clothes that decrease friction and irritation may lessen discomfort. Women should be advised to maintain a healthy lifestyle to aid the immune system and be counseled regarding diet, rest, stress reduction, and exercise.

Patient counseling is essential. Women must understand the virus, how it is transmitted, that no immunity is conferred with infection, and that reinfection is likely with repeated contact (Royer and Falk, 2012). Encourage all sexually active women with multiple partners or a history of HPV to use latex condoms for intercourse to decrease acquisition or transmission of the infection. Semiannual or annual health examinations are recommended to assess disease recurrence and screening for cervical cancer. Women who have been treated for HPV infections should have at least annual Pap tests (CDC, 2010a).

Prevention. Preventive strategies that have been suggested include abstinence from all sexual activity, staying in a long-term monogamous relationship, and prophylactic vaccination (CDC, 2010a). Two vaccines, Cervarix and Gardasil, are available; and other vaccines continue to be investigated. Cervarix prevents infection from HPV viruses 16 and 18, whereas Gardasil prevents infection from viruses 6, 11, 16, and 18. Both can be administered to girls and women ages 9 to 26. The three-dose vaccines are most effective if given before the woman has her first sexual contact (CDC, 2012a). Practitioners should stay current with results of these clinical trials and make recommendations about vaccination based on the outcomes of the research.

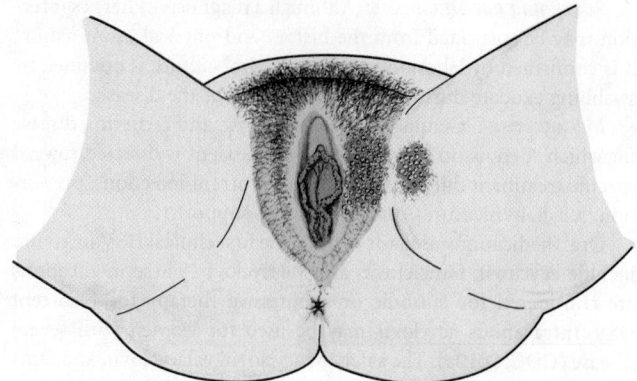

FIG 4-5 Herpes genitalis.

Herpes Simplex Virus

Unknown until the middle of the twentieth century, herpes simplex virus (HSV) infection is now widespread in the United States, especially in women. It results in painful, recurrent ulcers. It is caused by two different antigen subtypes of HSV: HSV type 1 (HSV-1) and HSV type 2 (HSV-2). HSV-2 is usually transmitted sexually, and HSV-1 nonsexually. Although HSV-1 is more commonly associated with gingivostomatitis and oral labial ulcers (fever blisters) and HSV-2 with genital lesions, neither type is exclusively associated with the respective sites.

Although HSV infection is not a reportable disease, it is estimated that about 50 million people in the United States are infected with genital herpes (CDC, 2010a). Women between the ages of 15 and 34 are most likely to become infected, especially if they have multiple partners. Recurrent HSV infections are much more common. Most persons infected with HSV-2 have not been diagnosed, and most infections are transmitted by persons unaware that they are infected.

An initial HSV genital infection is characterized by multiple painful lesions, fever, chills, malaise, and severe dysuria and may last 2 to 3 weeks. Women generally have a more severe clinical course than do men. Women with primary genital herpes have many lesions that progress from macules to papules; they then progress to form vesicles, pustules, and ulcers that crust and heal without scarring (Fig. 4-5). These ulcers are extremely tender, and primary infections may be bilateral. Women also may have itching, inguinal tenderness, and lymphadenopathy. Severe vulvar edema may develop, and women may have difficulty sitting. HSV cervicitis is common with initial HSV-2 infections. The cervix may appear normal or be friable, reddened, ulcerated, or necrotic. A heavy, watery-to-purulent vaginal discharge is common. Extragenital lesions may be present because of autoinoculation. Urinary retention and dysuria may occur secondary to autonomic involvement of the sacral nerve root.

Women with recurrent episodes of HSV infections commonly have only local symptoms that are usually less severe than those associated with the initial infection. Systemic symptoms are usually absent, although the characteristic prodromal genital tingling is common. Recurrent lesions are unilateral, are less severe, and usually last 5 to 7 days. Lesions begin as vesicles and progress rapidly to ulcers. Few women with recurrent disease have cervicitis.

During pregnancy maternal infection with HSV-2 can have adverse effects on both the mother and fetus. Viremia occurs during the primary infection, and congenital infection is possible although rare. Primary infections during the first trimester have been associated with increased miscarriage rates (CDC, 2010a).

Screening and Diagnosis. Although a diagnosis of herpes infection may be suspected from the history and physical examination, it is confirmed by laboratory studies. A viral culture is obtained by swabbing exudate during the vesicular stage of the disease.

Management. Genital herpes is a chronic and recurring disease for which there is no known cure. Management is directed toward specific treatment during primary and recurrent infections, prevention, self-help measures, and psychologic support.

Oral medications used for treating the first clinical HSV infection include acyclovir, famciclovir, and valacyclovir. These medications are considered for episodic or suppressive therapy for recurrent HSV. Intravenous acyclovir may be used for women with severe disease (CDC, 2010a). The safety of acyclovir, valacyclovir, and famciclovir therapy during pregnancy has not been established; however, acyclovir may be used to reduce the symptoms of HSV if the benefits to the woman outweigh the potential harm to the fetus (CDC, 2010a). Continued investigation of HSV therapy with these medications during pregnancy is needed.

Cleaning lesions twice a day with saline helps prevent secondary infection. Bacterial infection must be treated with appropriate antibiotics. Measures that may increase comfort for women when lesions are active include warm sitz baths with baking soda; keeping lesions dry by using cool air from a hair dryer or patting dry with a soft towel; wearing cotton underwear and loose clothing; using drying aids such as hydrogen peroxide, Burow's solution, or oatmeal baths; and applying cool, wet, black tea bags to lesions. Women can also apply compresses with an infusion of cloves or peppermint oil and clove oil to lesions.

Oral analgesics such as aspirin or ibuprofen may be used to relieve pain and systemic symptoms associated with initial infections. Because the mucous membranes affected by herpes are extremely sensitive, any topical agents should be used with caution. Nonantiviral ointments, especially those containing cortisone, should be avoided. A thin layer of lidocaine ointment or an antiseptic spray may be applied to decrease discomfort, especially if walking is difficult.

Counseling and education are critical components of the nursing care of women with herpes infections. Information regarding the etiology, signs and symptoms, transmission, and treatment should be provided. The nurse should explain that each woman is unique in her response to herpes and emphasize the variability of symptoms. Women should be helped to understand when viral shedding and thus transmission to a partner are most likely. They should be counseled to refrain from sexual contact from the onset of prodrome until complete healing of lesions.

Some authorities recommend consistent use of condoms for all persons with genital herpes. Condoms may not prevent transmission, particularly male-to-female transmission; however, this does not mean that the partners should avoid all intimacy. Women can be encouraged to maintain close contact with their partners while avoiding contact with lesions. They should be taught how to look for herpetic lesions using a mirror and good light source and a wet cloth or finger covered with a finger cot to rub lightly over the labia. The nurse should ensure that women understand that, when lesions are active, sharing intimate articles (e.g., washcloths or wet towels) that come into contact with the lesions should be avoided. Only plain soap and water are needed to clean hands that have come in contact with herpetic lesions; isolation is neither necessary nor appropriate.

Stress, menstruation, trauma, febrile illnesses, chronic illness, and ultraviolet light have all been found to trigger genital herpes. Women may wish to keep a diary to identify stressors that seem to be associated with recurrent herpes attacks so they can avoid these stressors when possible. The role of exercise in reducing stress can be discussed. Referral for stress-reduction therapy, yoga, or meditation classes may be indicated. Avoiding excessive heat, sun, and hot baths and using a lubricant during sexual intercourse to reduce friction also may be helpful. Women in their childbearing years should be counseled regarding the risk of herpes infection during pregnancy. They should be instructed to use condoms if there is any risk of contracting an STI from a sexual partner. If they become pregnant while taking acyclovir, the risk of birth defects does not appear to be higher than for the general population; however, continued use should be based on whether the benefits for the woman outweigh the possible risks to the fetus. Acyclovir does enter breast milk, but the amount of medication ingested during breastfeeding is very low and usually not a health concern (Weiner and Buhimschi, 2009).

Because neonatal HSV infection is such a devastating disease, prevention is critical. Current recommendations include carefully examining and questioning all women about symptoms at onset of labor (CDC, 2010a). If visible lesions are not present at onset of labor, vaginal birth is acceptable. Cesarean birth within 4 hours after labor begins or membranes rupture is recommended if visible lesions are present. Infants who are born through an infected vagina should be observed carefully and cultured. Some experts recommend presumptive treatment of infants who were exposed to HSV during birth. Because HSV infection may be associated with cervical dysplasia, women must be encouraged to have annual Pap tests and gynecologic examinations.

The emotional effect of contracting an incurable STI such as herpes is considerable. At diagnosis many emotions may surface— helplessness, anger, denial, guilt, anxiety, shame, or inadequacy. Women need the opportunity to discuss their feelings and help in learning to live with the disease. Herpes can affect a woman's sexuality, her sexual practices, and her current and future relationships. She may need help in raising the issue with her partner or future partners.

Hepatitis

Five different viruses (hepatitis viruses A, B, C, D, and E) account for almost all cases of viral hepatitis in humans. Hepatitis viruses A, B, and C are discussed here. Hepatitis D and E viruses, common among users of intravenous drugs and recipients of multiple blood transfusions, are not included in this discussion.

Hepatitis A. Hepatitis A virus (HAV) infection is acquired primarily through a fecal-oral route by ingestion of contaminated food, particularly milk, shellfish, or polluted water, or via person-to-person contact. Influenza-like symptoms with malaise, fatigue, anorexia, nausea, pruritus, fever, and upper–right quadrant pain characterize HAV infection. Serologic testing to detect the immunoglobulin M (IgM) antibody confirms acute infections. Because HAV infection is self-limited and does not result in chronic infection or chronic liver disease, treatment is usually supportive. Women who become dehydrated from nausea and vomiting or who have fulminating hepatitis A may need to be hospitalized. Medications that might cause liver damage or that are metabolized in the liver should be used with caution. No specific diet or activity restrictions are necessary. Hepatitis A vaccine and immunoglobulin (IG) for intramuscular administration are effective in preventing most hepatitis A infections (CDC, 2010a).

Hepatitis B. Hepatitis B virus (HBV) infection is an STI and is the virus most threatening to the fetus and neonate. It is caused by a large DNA virus and is associated with three antigens and their antibodies: hepatitis B surface antigen (HBsAg), HBV antigen (HBeAg), HBV core antigen (HBcAg), antibody to HBsAg (anti-HBs), antibody to HBeAg (anti-HBe), and antibody to HBcAg (anti-HBc). Screening for active or chronic disease or disease immunity is based on testing for these antigens and their antibodies.

Populations at risk include women of Asian, Pacific Island (Polynesian, Micronesian, Melanesian), or Alaskan-Eskimo descent and those born in Haiti or sub-Saharan Africa. Women who have a history of acute or chronic liver disease, who work or receive treatment in a dialysis unit, or who have household or sexual contact with a hemodialysis patient are at greater risk. Women who work or live in institutions for the mentally handicapped are considered to be at risk, as are those with a history of multiple blood transfusions. Health care workers and public safety workers exposed to blood in the workplace are at risk. Behaviors such as multiple sexual partners and a history of intravenous drug use increase the risk of contracting HBV infections.

HBsAg has been found in blood, saliva, sweat, tears, vaginal secretions, and semen. Drug abusers who share needles are at risk, as are health care workers who are exposed to blood and needlesticks. Perinatal transmission most often occurs in infants of mothers who have acute hepatitis infection late in the third trimester or during the intrapartum or postpartum periods from exposure to HBsAg-positive vaginal secretions, blood, amniotic fluid, saliva, and breast milk. HBV has also been transmitted by artificial insemination. Although it can be transmitted by blood transfusion, the incidence of such infections has decreased significantly since testing of blood for HBsAg became routine.

HBV infection is a disease of the liver and is often a silent infection. In the adult its course can be fulminating, and the outcome fatal. Symptoms of HBV infection are similar to those of hepatitis A: arthralgias, arthritis, lassitude, anorexia, nausea, vomiting, headache, fever, and mild abdominal pain. Later the woman may have clay-colored stools, dark urine, increased abdominal pain, and jaundice. Between 5% and 10% of individuals with HBV have persistent HBsAg and become chronic hepatitis B carriers.

Screening and Diagnosis. All women at high risk for contracting HBV should be screened on a regular basis. However, screening only individuals at high risk may not identify up to 50% of HBsAg-positive women. Screening for the presence of HBsAg is recommended on all pregnant women at the first prenatal visit, regardless of whether they have been tested previously; screening should be done on admission for labor and birth for women at high risk for infection during pregnancy or if prenatal test results are not available (CDC, 2012b, USPSTF, 2009).

The HBsAg screening test is usually performed, given that a rise in HBsAg occurs at the onset of clinical symptoms and usually indicates an active infection. If HBsAg persists in the blood, the woman is identified as a carrier. If the HBsAg test result is positive, further laboratory studies may be ordered: anti-HBe, anti-HBc, serum glutamic-oxaloacetic transaminase (SGOT), alkaline phosphatase, and liver panel.

Management. There is no specific treatment for hepatitis B. Recovery is usually spontaneous in 3 to 16 weeks. Pregnancies complicated by acute viral hepatitis are managed on an outpatient basis. Women should be advised to increase bed rest; eat a high-protein, low-fat diet; and increase their fluid intake. They should avoid medications metabolized in the liver and alcohol. Pregnant women with a definite exposure to HBV should be given HBIG and begin the hepatitis B vaccine series within 14 days of the most recent contact to prevent infection (CDC, 2010a). Vaccination during pregnancy is not thought to pose risks to the fetus.

All nonimmune women at high or moderate risk of hepatitis should be informed of the availability of hepatitis B vaccine. Vaccination is recommended for all individuals who have had multiple sex partners within the past 6 months (CDC, 2010a). In addition, intravenous drug users, residents of correctional or long-term care facilities, persons seeking care for an STI, prostitutes, women whose partners are intravenous drug users or bisexual, and women whose occupation exposes them to high risk should be vaccinated. The vaccine is given in a series of three (four if rapid protection is needed) doses over a 6-month period, with the first two doses given at least 1 month apart. The vaccine is given in the deltoid muscle (CDC, 2010a).

Patient education includes explaining the meaning of hepatitis B infection, including transmission, state of infectivity, and sequelae. The nurse also should explain the need for immunoprophylaxis for household members and sexual contacts. To decrease transmission of the virus, women with hepatitis B or those who test positive for HBV should be advised to maintain a high level of personal hygiene (e.g., wash hands after using the toilet; carefully dispose of tampons, pads, and bandages in plastic bags; not to share razor blades, toothbrushes, needles, or manicure implements; have male partner use a condom if unvaccinated and without hepatitis; avoid sharing saliva through kissing or sharing silverware or dishes; and wipe up blood spills immediately with soap and water). They should inform all health care providers of their carrier state. Postpartum women should be reassured that breastfeeding is not contraindicated if their infants received prophylaxis at birth and are currently on the immunization schedule.

Hepatitis C. Hepatitis C virus (HCV) infection is approximately the most common chronic bloodborne infection in the United States and is responsible for nearly 50% of the cases of chronic viral hepatitis (CDC, 2010a). The most common risk factor for pregnant women is a history of intravenous drug use. Other risk factors include STIs such as HBV and HIV, multiple sexual partners, and a history of blood transfusions. HCV is readily transmitted through exposure to blood.

Most patients with HCV are asymptomatic or have general flu-like symptoms similar to those of HAV. HCV infection is confirmed by the presence of anti-C antibody during laboratory testing. Interferon alfa alone or with ribavirin for 6 to 12 months is the main treatment for HCV infection, although effectiveness of this treatment varies (CDC, 2010a). Currently there is no vaccine to prevent HCV. Its transmission through breastfeeding has not been reported.

Human Immunodeficiency Virus

An estimated 34,247 new HIV infections occur in the United States each year (CDC, 2011a). An estimated 23% of these new infections occur in women. African-American women are estimated to have 57% of these infections, Caucasian women 17%, Hispanic women 14%, and Native American women less than 1% (CDC, 2011a).

Severe depression of the cellular immune system associated with HIV infection characterizes acquired immunodeficiency syndrome (AIDS). Although behaviors that place women at risk have been well documented, all women should be assessed for the possibility of HIV exposure. The most commonly reported opportunistic diseases are *Pneumocystis (jirovecii)* pneumonia (PCP), *Candida* esophagitis, and wasting syndrome. Other viral infections such as HSV and cytomegalovirus infections seem to be more prevalent in women than men (CDC, 2010a). PID is often more severe in HIV-infected women than in the general population, and rates of HPV and cervical dysplasia are sometimes higher in non–HIV-infected women (Eckert and Lentz, 2012). The clinical course of HPV infection in women with HIV infection is accelerated, and recurrence is more frequent in non–HIV-infected women.

Once HIV enters the body, seroconversion to HIV positivity usually occurs within 6 to 12 weeks. Although HIV seroconversion may be totally asymptomatic, it usually is accompanied by a viremic, influenza-like response. Symptoms include fever, headache, night sweats, malaise, generalized lymphadenopathy, myalgias, nausea, diarrhea, weight loss, sore throat, and rash.

Laboratory studies may reveal leukopenia, thrombocytopenia, anemia, and an elevated erythrocyte sedimentation rate. HIV has a strong affinity for surface-marker proteins on T lymphocytes. This affinity leads to significant T-cell destruction. Both clinical and epidemiologic studies have shown that declining CD4 levels are strongly associated with increased incidence of AIDS-related diseases and death in many different groups of HIV-infected persons.

Transmission of the virus from mother to infant can occur throughout the perinatal period. Exposure may occur to the fetus through the maternal circulation as early as the first trimester of pregnancy, to the infant during labor and birth by inoculation or ingestion of maternal blood and other infected fluids, or to the infant through breast milk.

Screening and Diagnosis. Screening, teaching, and counseling regarding HIV risk factors; indications for being tested; and testing are major roles for nurses caring for women today. A number of behaviors place women at risk for HIV infection, including intravenous drug use, high risk sex partners, multiple sex partners, and a previous history of multiple STIs. HIV infection is usually diagnosed by using HIV-1 and HIV-2 antibody tests. Antibody testing is done first with a sensitive screening test such as the enzyme immunoassay. Reactive screening tests must be confirmed by an additional test such as the Western blot or an immunofluorescence assay. If a positive antibody test is confirmed by a supplemental test, it means that a woman is infected with HIV and is capable of infecting others. HIV antibodies are detectable in at least 95% of patients within 3 months after infection. Although a negative antibody test usually indicates that a person is not infected, antibody tests cannot exclude recent infection. Because HIV antibody crosses the placenta, definite diagnosis of HIV in children younger than 18 months is based on laboratory evidence of HIV in blood or tissues by culture, nucleic acid, or antigen detection (CDC, 2010a).

The FDA has approved six methods of rapid testing for HIV, variously using a blood sample obtained by fingerstick or venipuncture, serum, or plasma or an oral fluid sample. The tests have accuracy rates of 98% to 99%. If the results are reactive, further testing is done (CDC, Division of HIV/AIDS prevention, 2008a; USFDA, 2008). Quick results mean that patients don't have to make extra visits for follow-up standard tests, and the oral test provides an option for patients who do not want to have a blood test.

The CDC (2010a) recommends offering HIV testing to all women whose behavior places them at risk for HIV infection. It may be useful to allow women to self-select for HIV testing. On entry to the health care system, a woman can be handed written information about the risk factors for the AIDS virus and asked to inform the nurse if she believes she is at risk. She should be told that she does not have to say why she may be at risk, only that she thinks she might be.

Counseling for HIV Testing. Counseling before and after HIV testing is standard nursing practice today. It is a nursing responsibility to assess a woman's understanding of the information such a test would provide and to be sure the woman thoroughly understands the emotional, legal, and medical implications of a positive or negative test before she is ready to take it.

> ### ! NURSING ALERT
>
> Counseling associated with HIV testing has two components: pretest and posttest. During pretest counseling, a personalized risk assessment is conducted, the meaning of positive and negative test results is explained, informed consent for HIV testing is obtained, and women are helped to develop a realistic plan for reducing risk and preventing infection. Posttest counseling includes informing the patient of the test results, reviewing the meaning of the results, and reinforcing prevention messages. All pretest and posttest counseling should be documented.

Given the strong social stigma attached to HIV infection, nurses must consider the issue of confidentiality and documentation before providing counseling and offering HIV testing to patients.

> ### LEGAL TIP: HIV Testing
>
> If HIV test results are placed in the patient's chart—the appropriate place for all health information—they are available to all who have access to the chart. Inform the woman of this availability before testing. Informed consent must be obtained before an HIV test is performed. In some states written consent is mandated. In many sites HIV testing is performed unless patients decline (i.e., opt-out testing). Nurses must know which procedures are being used for informed consent in their facility.

Unless rapid testing is done, there is generally a 1- to 3-week waiting period after testing for HIV; this can be a very anxious time for the woman. It is helpful if the nurse informs her that this time period between blood drawing and test results is routine. Test results must always be communicated in person, and women should be informed in advance that this is the procedure. Whenever possible, the person who provided the pretest counseling should also tell the woman her test results.

When some women are informed of negative results, they may escalate risk behaviors because they equate negativity with immunity. Others may believe that negative means "bad" and positive means "good." The woman's reaction to a negative test should be explored by asking, "How do you feel?" Counseling sessions for women with an HIV-negative result are another opportunity to provide education. Emphasis can be placed on ways in which a woman can remain HIV free. She should be reminded that, if she has been exposed to HIV in the past 6 months, she should be retested, and that she should have ongoing testing if she continues high risk behaviors.

In posttest counseling of an HIV-positive woman, privacy with no interruptions is essential. Adequate time for the counseling sessions also should be provided. The nurse should make sure that the woman understands what a positive test means and review the reliability of the test results. Risk reduction practices should be reemphasized. Referral for appropriate medical evaluation and follow-up should be made, and the need or desire for psychosocial or psychiatric referrals should be assessed.

The importance of early medical evaluation so a baseline assessment can be made and prophylactic medication begun should be stressed. If possible, the nurse should make a referral or appointment for the woman at the posttest counseling session.

Management. During the initial contact with an HIV-infected woman, the nurse should establish what the woman knows about HIV infection and that she is being cared for by a medical practitioner or facility with expertise in caring for persons with HIV infections, including AIDS. Psychologic referral also may be indicated. Resources such as counseling for financial assistance, legal advocacy, suicide prevention, and death and dying may be appropriate. All women who are drug users should be referred to a substance-abuse program. A major focus of counseling is prevention of transmission of HIV to partners.

Nurses counseling seropositive women wishing contraceptive information can recommend oral contraceptives and latex condoms or tubal sterilization or vasectomy and latex condoms. Suggest female condoms or abstinence to women whose male partners refuse to use condoms.

No cure is available for HIV infections at this time. Rare and unusual diseases are characteristic of HIV infections. Opportunistic infections and concurrent diseases are managed vigorously with treatment specific to the infection or disease. Routine gynecologic care for HIV-positive women should include a pelvic examination every 6 months. Thorough Pap screening is essential because of the greatly increased incidence of abnormal findings on examination (CDC, 2010a). In addition, HIV-positive women should be screened for syphilis, gonorrhea, chlamydia, and other vaginal infections and treated if infections are present. General prevention strategies are an important part of care (e.g., smoking cessation, sound nutrition) as is antiretroviral therapy. Discussion of the medical care of HIV-positive women or women with AIDS is beyond the scope of this chapter because of the rapidly changing recommendations. The reader is referred to the CDC (www.cdc.gov), AIDS hotlines (800-342-2437), and Internet websites such as HIV/AIDS Treatment Information Service (www.hivatis.org) for the current information and recommendations.

Pregnancy and Human Immunodeficiency Virus. HIV counseling and testing should be offered to all women at their initial entry into prenatal care as part of routine prenatal testing unless the woman opts out of the screening (CDC, 2010a). Universal testing versus selective testing for maternal HIV is recommended because it results in a greater number of women being screened and treated and can reduce the likelihood of perinatal transmission and maintain the health of the woman (CDC, 2010a). The CDC also recommends retesting in the third trimester for women known to be at high risk for HIV and rapid HIV testing in labor for women with unknown HIV status.

Perinatal transmission of HIV has decreased significantly in the past decade because of the administration of antiretroviral prophylaxis (e.g., zidovudine) to pregnant women in the prenatal and the perinatal periods. Treatment of HIV-infected women with the triple-drug antiviral therapy or highly active antiretroviral therapy (HAART) during pregnancy has been reported to decrease the mother-to-child transmission to 1% to 2% (CDC, 2010a). All HIV-infected women should be treated with a combination of antiretroviral drugs (e.g., HAART) during pregnancy, regardless of their CD4 cell counts (Panel on Treatment of HIV-Infected Pregnant Women and Prevention of Perinatal Transmission, 2010). Data are insufficient to support or refute the teratogenic risk of antiretroviral medications given for prophylaxis in the first 10 weeks or pregnancy. Current research does not support major teratogenic effects for most of the antiretroviral agents (Panel on Treatment of HIV-Infected Pregnant Women and Prevention of Perinatal Transmission, 2010). Women who are infected with HIV and need treatment for their own health should start the therapy as soon as possible, even in the first trimester. Women who are taking the therapy as prophylaxis usually start therapy after the first trimester (Panel on Treatment of HIV-Infected Pregnant Women and Prevention of Perinatal Transmission, 2010).

Antiviral therapy is administered orally and continued throughout pregnancy. The major side effect of this therapy is bone marrow suppression. Periodic hematocrit, white blood cell count, and platelet count assessments should be performed (Panel on Treatment of HIV-Infected Pregnant Women and Prevention of Perinatal Transmission, 2010). Women who are HIV positive should also be vaccinated against hepatitis B, pneumococcal infection, *Haemophilus influenzae* type B, and viral influenza. To support any pregnant woman's immune system, appropriate counseling is provided about optimal nutrition, sleep, rest, exercise, and stress reduction. Use of condoms is encouraged to minimize further exposure to HIV if her partner is the source.

In the intrapartum period antiretroviral therapy and cesarean birth are recommended to prevent vertical transmission of HIV (Panel on Treatment of HIV-Infected Pregnant Women and Prevention of Perinatal Transmission, 2010). The Panel recommends a scheduled cesarean birth at 38 weeks of gestation for women with a viral load of more than 1000 copies/mL. A vaginal birth may be an option for HIV-infected women who have a viral load of less than 1000 copies/mL at 36 weeks, if a woman has ruptured membranes and labor is progressing rapidly, or if she declines a cesarean birth. Intravenous zidovudine is recommended for all HIV-infected pregnant women during the intrapartum period. The drug is administered 3 hours before a scheduled cesarean birth and continued until the baby is born. It should be given during labor if the woman is having a vaginal birth (Panel on Treatment of HIV-Infected Pregnant Women and Prevention of Perinatal Transmission, 2010). Fetal scalp electrode and scalp pH sampling should be avoided because these procedures may result in inoculation of the virus into the fetus. Similarly the use of forceps or vacuum extractor should be avoided when possible. Infants should receive oral zidovudine for 6 weeks after birth. Avoidance of breastfeeding is recommended in the United States and most developed countries (American Academy of Pediatrics Committee on Pediatric AIDS, 2008).

Women who have HIV but who are without symptoms may have an unremarkable postpartum course. Immunosuppressed women with symptoms may be at increased risk for postpartum urinary tract infections (UTIs), vaginitis, postpartum endometritis, and poor wound healing. Good perineal hygiene should be stressed. Women who are HIV positive but who were not on antiretroviral drugs before pregnancy should be tested in the postpartum period to determine whether therapy that was initiated in pregnancy should be continued (Panel on Treatment of HIV-Infected Pregnant Women and Prevention of Perinatal Transmission, 2010). After the initial bath the newborn can be with the mother. In planning for discharge, comprehensive care and support services need to be arranged. After discharge the woman and her infant are referred to physicians who are experienced in the treatment of HIV and AIDS and associated conditions for intensive monitoring and follow-up (Panel on Treatment of HIV-Infected Pregnant Women and Prevention of Perinatal Transmission, 2010).

Vaginal Infections

Vaginal discharge and itching of the vulva and vagina are among the most common reasons a woman seeks help from a health care provider. More women complain of vaginal discharge than any other gynecologic symptom. Women who have adequate endogenous or exogenous estrogen have vaginal secretions. Vaginal discharge resulting from infection must be distinguished from normal secretions. Normal vaginal secretions (or leukorrhea) are clear to cloudy in appearance. The discharge may turn yellow after drying; is slightly slimy; is nonirritating; and has a mild, inoffensive odor. Normal vaginal secretions are acidic, with a pH range of 4 to 5. The amount of leukorrhea differs with phases of the menstrual cycle, with greater amounts occurring at ovulation and just before menses. Leukorrhea is also increased during pregnancy. Normal vaginal secretions contain lactobacilli and epithelial cells.

Vaginitis, or abnormal vaginal discharge, is an infection caused by a microorganism. The most common vaginal infections are bacterial vaginosis (BV), candidiasis, and trichomoniasis. Although streptococcus B is considered normal vaginal flora, it may also cause infection. Vulvovaginitis (i.e., inflammation of the vulva and vagina) may be caused by vaginal infection; copious leukorrhea, which can cause maceration of tissues; and chemical irritants, allergens, and foreign bodies, which may produce inflammatory reactions.

Bacterial Vaginosis

BV, formerly called *nonspecific vaginitis, Haemophilus vaginitis,* or *Gardnerella,* is the most common type of symptomatic vaginitis today (Eckert and Lentz, 2012). It is associated with preterm labor and birth. The exact cause of BV is unknown. It is a syndrome in which normal, hydrogen peroxide–producing lactobacilli are replaced with high concentrations of anaerobic bacteria (e.g., *Gardnerella, Mobiluncus*). With the increase of anaerobes, the level of vaginal amines is raised, and the normal acidic pH of the vagina is altered. Epithelial cells slough, and numerous bacteria attach to their surfaces (clue cells). When the amines are volatilized, the characteristic odor of BV occurs.

Many women with BV complain of a characteristic "fishy odor." The odor may be noticed by the woman or her partner after heterosexual intercourse because semen releases the vaginal amines. When present, the BV discharge is usually profuse; thin; and white, gray, or milky in appearance. Some women also may experience mild irritation or pruritus.

Screening and Diagnosis. A focused history may help distinguish BV from other vaginal infections if the woman is symptomatic. Reports of fishy odor and increased thin vaginal discharge are most significant, and a report of increased odor after intercourse is also suggestive of BV. You should question women with previous occurrence of similar symptoms, diagnosis, and treatment because women with BV often have been treated incorrectly because of misdiagnosis.

Microscopic examination of vaginal secretions is always performed (Table 4-4). Both normal saline and 10% potassium hydroxide (KOH) smears are made. The presence of clue cells (vaginal epithelial cells coated with bacteria) on wet saline smear is highly diagnostic because the phenomenon is specific to BV. Test vaginal secretions for pH and amine odor. Nitrazine paper is sensitive enough to detect a pH of 4.5 or greater. The fishy odor of BV will be released when KOH is added to vaginal secretions on the lip of the withdrawn speculum.

Management. Treatment of BV with oral metronidazole (Flagyl) is most effective (CDC, 2010a), although vaginal preparations (e.g., metronidazole gel, clindamycin cream) are also used. Side effects of metronidazole are numerous, including sharp, unpleasant metallic taste in the mouth; furry tongue; central nervous system reactions; and urinary tract disturbances. When the woman is taking oral metronidazole, advise her to avoid drinking alcoholic beverages or she will experience the severe side effects of abdominal distress, nausea, vomiting, and headache. Gastrointestinal symptoms are common whether alcohol is consumed or not. Treatment of sexual partners is not recommended routinely (CDC, 2010a).

TABLE 4-4	**WET SMEAR TESTS FOR VAGINAL INFECTIONS**	
INFECTION	**TEST**	**POSITIVE FINDINGS**
Trichomoniasis	Saline wet smear (vaginal secretions mixed with normal saline on a glass slide)	Presence of many white blood cell protozoa
Candidiasis	Potassium hydroxide (KOH) preparation (vaginal secretions mixed with KOH on a glass slide)	Presence of hyphae and pseudohyphae (buds and branches of yeast cells)
Bacterial vaginosis	Normal saline smear	Presence of clue cells (vaginal epithelial cells coated with bacteria)
	Whiff test (vaginal secretions mixed with KOH)	Release of fishy odor

Several adverse outcomes are associated with BV during pregnancy: preterm labor and birth, premature rupture of the membranes, intraamniotic infection, and postpartum endometritis. Therefore pregnant women should be treated to relieve vaginal symptoms and the signs of infection (CDC, 2010a).

Metronidazole is not recommended if the woman is breastfeeding. If it is necessary to prescribe it, she can suspend breastfeeding temporarily (pump and discard milk to maintain supply) and resume it 12 to 24 hours after taking the last dose.

Candidiasis

Vulvovaginal candidiasis, or yeast infection, is the second most common type of vaginal infection in the United States. Although vaginal candidiasis infections are common in healthy women, those seen in women with HIV infection are often more severe and persistent. Genital candidiasis lesions may be painful, and coalescing ulcerations necessitate continuous prophylactic therapy.

The most common organism is *Candida albicans.* It is estimated that 90% of yeast infections in women are caused by this organism. However, in the past 10 years the incidence of non–*C. albicans* infections has increased steadily. Women with chronic or recurrent infections often are infected with a higher percentage of non–*C. albicans* species than are women with their first infection or who have few recurrences (Eckert and Lentz, 2012).

Numerous factors have been identified as predisposing a woman to yeast infections. These include antibiotic therapy, particularly broad-spectrum antibiotics such as ampicillin, tetracycline, cephalosporins, and metronidazole; diabetes, especially when uncontrolled; pregnancy; obesity; diets high in refined sugars or artificial sweeteners; use of corticosteroids and exogenous hormones; and immunosuppressed states. Clinical observations and research have suggested that tight-fitting clothing and underwear or pantyhose made of nonabsorbent materials create an environment in which a vaginal fungus can grow.

The most common symptom of yeast infection is vulvar and possibly vaginal pruritus. The itching may be mild or intense, interfere with rest and activities, and occur during or after intercourse. Some women report a feeling of dryness. Others may have painful urination as the urine flows over the vulva. The latter usually occurs in women who have excoriations resulting from scratching. Most often the discharge is thick, white, lumpy, and cottage cheese like. The discharge may be found in patches on the vaginal walls, cervix, and labia. Commonly the vulva is red and swollen, as are the labial folds, vagina, and cervix. Although there is no odor characteristic of yeast infections, sometimes a yeasty or musty smell is noted.

Screening and Diagnosis. In addition to noting the woman's symptoms, their onset, and their course, the history is a valuable screening tool for identifying predisposing risk factors. Physical examination should include a thorough inspection of the vulva and vagina. A speculum examination is always done. Commonly saline and KOH wet smear and vaginal pH are obtained (see Table 4-4). Vaginal pH is normal (less than 4.5) with a yeast infection. The characteristic pseudohypha (bud or branching of a fungus) may be seen on a wet smear done with normal saline; however, they may be confused with other cells and artifacts (CDC, 2010a).

Management. A number of antifungal preparations are available for the treatment of *C. albicans*. Many of these medications (e.g., miconazole [Monistat] and clotrimazole [Gyne-Lotrimin]) are available as over-the-counter (OTC) agents. Exogenous lactobacillus (in the form of dairy products [yogurt] or powder, tablet, capsule, or suppository supplements) and garlic have been suggested for prevention and treatment of vulvovaginal candidiasis; but research is inconclusive, and no recommendations have been developed for use in practice (Eckert and Lentz, 2012). The first time a woman suspects that she may have a yeast infection, she should see a health care provider for confirmation of the diagnosis and treatment recommendation. If she has another infection, she may wish to purchase an OTC preparation and self-treat. If she elects to do this, she should always be counseled to seek care for numerous recurrent or chronic yeast infections. If vaginal discharge is extremely thick and copious, vaginal debridement with a cotton swab followed by application of vaginal medication may be effective.

Women who have extensive irritation, swelling, and discomfort of the labia and vulva may find sitz baths helpful in decreasing inflammation and increasing comfort. Adding colloidal oatmeal powder to the bath may also increase the woman's comfort. Not wearing underpants to bed may help decrease symptoms and prevent recurrences. Completing the full course of treatment prescribed is essential to removing the pathogen. Medication should be continued even during menstruation. Women should be counseled not to use tampons during menses because the medication will be absorbed by the tampon. If possible, intercourse is avoided during treatment; if this is not feasible, the woman's partner should use a condom to prevent introduction of more organisms. Suggested measures to prevent genital tract infections are in the Patient Teaching box.

Trichomoniasis

Trichomonas vaginalis is almost always an STI and is also a common cause of vaginal infection (5% to 50% of all vaginitis) and discharge (Eckert and Lentz, 2012).

Trichomoniasis is caused by *T. vaginalis,* an anaerobic, one-celled protozoan with characteristic flagella. Although trichomoniasis may be asymptomatic, women commonly experience characteristically yellowish-to-greenish, frothy, mucopurulent, copious, malodorous discharge. Inflammation of the vulva, vagina, or both may be present; and the woman may complain of irritation and pruritus.

PATIENT TEACHING

Prevention of Genital Tract Infections in Women

- Practice genital hygiene.
- Choose underwear or hosiery with a cotton crotch.
- Avoid tight-fitting clothing (especially tight jeans).
- Select cloth car seat covers instead of vinyl.
- Limit the time spent in damp exercise clothes (especially swimsuits, leotards, and tights).
- Limit exposure to bath salts or bubble bath.
- Avoid colored or scented toilet tissue.
- If sensitive, discontinue use of feminine hygiene deodorant sprays.
- Use condoms.
- Void before and after intercourse.
- Decrease dietary sugar.
- Drink yeast-active milk and eat yogurt (with lactobacilli).
- Do not douche.

Dysuria and dyspareunia are often present. Typically the discharge worsens during and after menstruation. The cervix and vaginal walls demonstrate characteristic "strawberry spots" or tiny petechiae in less than 10% of women, and the cervix may bleed on contact. In severe infections the vaginal walls, the cervix, and occasionally the vulva are acutely inflamed.

Screening and Diagnosis. In addition to obtaining a history of current symptoms, obtain a thorough sexual history. Note any history of similar symptoms in the past and treatment used. Determine whether the woman's partner or partners were treated and if she has had subsequent relations with new partners.

A speculum examination is always performed, even though it may be uncomfortable for the woman. Any of the classic signs may or may not be seen on physical examination. The typical one-celled flagellate trichomonads are easily distinguished on a normal saline wet preparation (see Table 4-4). The pH of the discharge is greater than 5.0. Because trichomoniasis is an STI, once diagnosis is confirmed, the appropriate laboratory studies for other STIs should be carried out.

Management. The recommended treatment is metronidazole or tinidazole orally in a single dose (CDC, 2010a). Although the male partner is usually asymptomatic, he should receive treatment also because he often harbors the trichomonads in the urethra or prostate. Nurses need to discuss the importance of partner treatment with their patients. If partners are not treated, the infection will likely recur.

Women with trichomoniasis need to understand the sexual transmission of this disease. The woman should know that the organism can be present without symptoms, perhaps for several months, and that determining when she became infected is impossible.

Group B Streptococcus

Group B streptococcus (GBS) may be considered a normal vaginal flora in a woman who is not pregnant. It is present in 9% to 23% of healthy pregnant women. However, GBS infection is associated with poor pregnancy outcomes. These infections are an important factor in perinatal and neonatal morbidity and mortality, usually resulting from vertical transmission from the birth canal of the infected mother to the infant during birth (Cunningham, Leveno, Bloom, et al., 2010).

Risk factors for neonatal GBS infection include positive prenatal culture for GBS in the current pregnancy; preterm birth of less than 37 weeks of gestation; premature rupture of membranes for longer than 18 hours; intrapartum maternal fever higher than 38° C (100.4° F); and a positive history for early-onset neonatal GBS (Cunningham, Leveno, Bloom, et al., 2010).

To decrease the risk of neonatal GBS infection, it is recommended that all women be screened at 35 to 37 weeks of gestation for GBS using a rectovaginal culture and that intravenous antibiotic prophylaxis (IAP) be offered to all who test positive. If a culture is not available at onset of labor or if risk factors are present, IAP is also offered. It is not recommended before a cesarean birth if labor or rupture of membranes has not occurred. The recommended treatment is penicillin G, 5 million units in an intravenous loading dose, and then 2.5 million units intravenously every 4 hours during labor. Ampicillin, 2 g intravenous loading dose, followed by 1 g intravenously every 4 hours, is an alternative therapy (CDC, 2010b).

Effects of Sexually Transmitted Infections on Pregnancy and the Fetus

STIs in pregnancy are responsible for significant morbidity and mortality. Some consequences of maternal infection such as infertility and sterility last a lifetime. Congenitally acquired infection may affect a child's length and quality of life. Table 4-5 describes the effects of several common STIs on pregnancy and the fetus. It is difficult to predict these effects with certainty. Factors such as co-infection with other STIs and at what point in pregnancy the infection was treated can affect outcomes.

Infection Control

Infection control measures are essential to protect care providers and prevent nosocomial infection of patients, regardless of the infectious agent. The risk for occupational transmission varies with the disease. Even when the risk is low as with HIV, the existence of any risk warrants reasonable precautions. Precautions against airborne disease transmission are available in all health care agencies. Standard Precautions (precautions to use in care of all persons for infection control) are listed in Box 4-4.

PROBLEMS OF THE BREAST

Benign Problems

Fibrocystic Changes

Approximately 50% of women experience a breast problem at some point in their adult life. The most common benign breast problem is fibrocystic changes (Katz and Dotters, 2012). Fibrocystic changes occur in varying degrees in breasts of healthy women. The etiologic agent responsible for these changes has not been found. One theory is that estrogen excess and progesterone deficiency in the luteal phase of the menstrual cycle may cause changes in breast tissue.

Fibrocystic changes are characterized by lumpiness, with or without tenderness, in both breasts. Single simple cysts can also occur. Symptoms usually develop approximately a week before menstruation begins and subside approximately a week after menstruation ends. Symptoms include dull heavy pain and a sense of fullness and tenderness often in the upper outer quadrants of the breasts. Physical examination may reveal excessive nodularity that many describe as feeling similar to a "plateful of peas" (Katz and Dotters, 2012). Larger cysts are often described as feeling like water-filled balloons. Women in their twenties report the most severe pain.

TABLE 4-5	PREGNANCY AND FETAL EFFECTS OF COMMON SEXUALLY TRANSMITTED INFECTIONS	
INFECTION	**MATERNAL EFFECTS**	**FETAL EFFECTS**
Chlamydia	Premature rupture of membranes Preterm labor Postpartum endometritis	Low birth weight
Gonorrhea	Miscarriage Preterm labor Amniotic infection syndrome Chorioamnionitis Postpartum endometritis Postpartum sepsis Premature rupture of membranes	Preterm birth IUGR
Group B streptococci	Urinary tract infection Chorioamnionitis Postpartum endometritis Sepsis Meningitis (rare)	Preterm birth
Herpes simplex virus	Intrauterine infection (rare)	Congenital infection (rare)
Human papillomavirus (HPV)	Dystocia from large lesions Excessive bleeding from lesions after birth trauma	
Syphilis	Miscarriage Preterm labor	IUGR Preterm birth Stillbirth Congenital infection

Data from Gilbert E: *Manual of high risk pregnancy and delivery*, ed 5, St Louis, 2011, Mosby; Duff P, Sweet R, Edwards R: Maternal and fetal infections. In Creasy RK, Resnik R, Iams JD, et al, editors: *Creasy and Resnik's maternal-fetal medicine: Principles and practice*, ed 6, Philadelphia, 2009, Saunders.
IUGR, Intrauterine growth restriction.

Women in their thirties have premenstrual pain and tenderness; small multiple nodules are usually present. Women in their forties usually do not report severe pain, but cysts are tender and often regress in size (Katz and Dotters, 2012).

Steps in the workup of a breast lump may begin with ultrasonography to determine whether it is fluid filled or solid. Fluid-filled cysts are aspirated, and the woman is monitored on a routine basis for the development of other cysts. If the lump is solid, a mammogram is obtained if the woman is older than age 50 years. A fine-needle aspiration (FNA) is performed, regardless of the woman's age, to determine the nature of the lump (Katz and Dotters, 2012).

Management depends on the severity of the symptoms. Women who have severe cyclic breast pain may find relief with eating dietary flaxseed (Chase, Wells, and Eley, 2011). Although research findings are contradictory, some practitioners advocate reducing consumption or eliminating methylxanthines (e.g., colas, coffee, tea,

BOX 4-4   STANDARD PRECAUTIONS

Medical history and examination cannot reliably identify all persons infected with human immunodeficiency virus (HIV) or other bloodborne pathogens. Therefore Standard Precautions should be used consistently in the care of all persons. These precautions apply to blood; body fluids; and all secretions and excretions, except sweat, nonintact skin, and mucous membranes. The following infection-control practices should be applied during the delivery of health care to reduce the risk of transmission of microorganisms from known and unknown sources of infection (Seigel, Rhinehart, Jackson, et al., and the Healthcare Infection Control Practices Advisory Committee, 2007):

1. *Hand hygiene.* During the delivery of health care, avoid unnecessary touching of surfaces in close proximity to the patient to prevent both contamination of clean hands from environmental surfaces and transmission of pathogens from contaminated hands to surfaces. Wash dirty or contaminated hands with either a nonantimicrobial or an antimicrobial soap and water. If hands are not visibly soiled, decontaminate them with an alcohol-based hand rub, or they may be washed with an antimicrobial soap and water. Perform hand hygiene (1) before having direct contact with patients; (2) after contact with blood, body fluids, excretions, mucous membranes, nonintact skin, or wound dressings; (3) after contact with a patient's intact skin (e.g., when taking a pulse or blood pressure or lifting a patient); (4) if hands will be moving from a contaminated to a clean body site during patient care; (5) after contact with inanimate objects (including medical equipment) in the immediate vicinity of the patient; and (6) after removing gloves. Wash hands with nonantimicrobial soap and water or with antimicrobial soap and water if contact with spores (e.g., *Clostridium difficile* or *Bacillus anthracis*) is likely to have occurred. The physical action of washing and rinsing hands under such circumstances is recommended because alcohols, chlorhexidine, iodophors, and other antiseptic agents have poor activity against spores. Do not wear artificial fingernails or extenders if duties include direct contact with patients at high risk for infection and associated adverse outcomes.

2. *Personal protective equipment (PPE).* Observe the following principles of use:
   - *Gloves.* Wear gloves when a reasonably anticipated possibility exists that contact with blood or other potentially infectious materials, mucous membranes, nonintact skin, or potentially contaminated intact skin (e.g., of a patient incontinent of stool or urine) might occur. Gloves should be worn during infant eye prophylaxis, care of the umbilical cord, circumcision site, parenteral procedures, diaper changes, contact with colostrum, and postpartum assessments. Wear gloves with fit and durability appropriate to the task. Remove gloves after contact with a patient or the surrounding environment (including medical equipment), using proper technique to prevent hand contamination. Do not wear the same pair of gloves for the care of more than one patient. Change gloves during patient care if the hands will move from a contaminated (e.g., perineal area) to a clean (e.g., face) body site.

   - *Gowns.* Wear a gown that is appropriate to the task to protect the skin and prevent soiling or contamination of clothing during procedures and patient-care activities when contact with blood, body fluids, secretions, or excretions is anticipated. Remove the gown and perform hand hygiene before leaving the patient's environment. Do not reuse gowns, even for repeated contacts with the same patient. Routine donning of gowns on entrance into a high risk unit (e.g., intensive care unit [ICU], neonatal intensive care unit [NICU]) is not indicated.

   - *Mouth, nose, eye protection.* Use PPE to protect the mucous membranes of the eyes, nose, and mouth during procedures and patient-care activities that are likely to generate splashes or sprays of blood, body fluids, secretions, and excretions. Select masks, goggles, face shields, and combinations of each according to the need anticipated by the task performed.

   - *Respiratory hygiene and cough etiquette.* Post signs at entrances and in strategic places (e.g., elevators, cafeterias) within ambulatory and inpatient settings with instructions to patients and other persons with symptoms of a respiratory infection to cover their mouth and nose when coughing or sneezing, use and dispose of tissues, and perform hand hygiene after hands have been in contact with respiratory secretions. Provide tissues and no-touch receptacles (e.g., foot pedal–operated lid or open, plastic-lined wastebasket) for disposal of tissues. Provide resources and instructions for performing hand hygiene in or near waiting areas in ambulatory and inpatient settings; provide conveniently located dispensers of alcohol-based hand rubs and, where sinks are available, supplies for handwashing. During periods of increased prevalence of respiratory infections in the community, offer masks to coughing patients and other symptomatic persons (e.g., persons who accompany ill patients) on entry into the facility and encourage them to maintain special separation, ideally a distance of at least 3 feet, from others in common waiting areas.

3. *Safe injection practices.* The following recommendations apply to the use of needles, cannulas that replace needles, and, where applicable, intravenous delivery systems:
   - Use aseptic technique to prevent contamination of sterile injection equipment. Needles, cannulas, and syringes are sterile, single-use items; they should not be reused for another patient. Use fluid infusion and administration sets (i.e., intravenous bags, tubing, and connectors) for one patient only and dispose appropriately after use. Use single-dose vials for parenteral medications whenever possible. If multidose vials must be used, both the needle (or cannula) and the syringe used to access the multidose vial must be sterile. Do not keep multidose vials in the immediate patient treatment area and store in accordance with manufacturer recommendations; discard if sterility is compromised or questionable.

Data from Siegel JD, Rhinehart E, Jackson M, et al, and the Healthcare Infection Control Practices Advisory Committee: *Guideline for isolation precautions: preventing transmission of infectious agents in healthcare settings,* 2007, www.cdc.gov/ncidod/dhqp/pdf/isolation2007.pdf.

chocolate) and tobacco (Chase, Wells, and Eley, 2011; Katz and Dotters, 2012).

Women may report decreased symptoms with such measures as eating a low-fat diet, decreasing sodium intake, or taking mild diuretics shortly before menses; but supporting evidence is lacking (Chase, Wells, and Eley, 2011). Other pain-relief measures that include taking analgesics or NSAIDs, wearing a supportive bra, and applying heat or cold to the breasts are supported by research (Katz and Dotters, 2012).

Evening primrose oil and vitamin E supplements may be effective for some women, although more research is needed (Chase, Wells, and Eley, 2011). Oral contraceptives, danazol, bromocriptine, and tamoxifen have also been used with varying degrees of success (Katz and Dotters, 2012).

TABLE 4-6	COMPARISON OF COMMON MANIFESTATIONS OF BENIGN BREAST MASSES			
FIBROCYSTIC CHANGES	**FIBROADENOMA**	**LIPOMA**	**INTRADUCTAL PAPILLOMA**	**MAMMARY DUCT ECTASIA**
Multiple lumps	Single lump	Single lump	Single or multiple	Mass behind nipple
Nodular	Well delineated	Well delineated	Not well delineated	Not well delineated
Palpable	Palpable	Palpable	Nonpalpable	Palpable
Movable	Movable	Movable	Nonmobile	Nonmobile
Round, smooth	Round, lobular	Round, lobular	Small, ball-like	Irregular
Firm or soft	Firm	Soft	Firm or soft	Firm
Tenderness influenced by menstrual cycle	Usually asymptomatic	Nontender	Usually nontender	Painful, burning, itching
Bilateral	Unilateral	Unilateral	Unilateral	Unilateral
May or may not have nipple discharge	No nipple discharge	No nipple discharge	Serous or bloody nipple discharge	Thick, sticky nipple discharge

Fibroadenoma

The next most common benign neoplasm of the breast is a fibroadenoma. It is the single most common type of tumor seen in the adolescent population, although it can also occur in women in their thirties. Fibroadenomas are discrete, usually solitary lumps averaging 2.5 cm in diameter (Katz and Dotters, 2012). Occasionally the woman with a fibroadenoma experiences tenderness in the tumor during the menstrual cycle. Fibroadenomas do not increase in size in response to the menstrual cycle as cysts do. They increase in size during pregnancy and decrease in size as the woman ages. The cause of fibroadenomas is unknown.

Diagnosis is made by reviewing patient history and physical examination. Mammography, ultrasound, or magnetic resonance imaging (MRI) helps determine the type of lesion. FNA may be used to determine underlying pathologic conditions. Surgical excision may be necessary if the lump is suspicious or if the symptoms are severe. Periodic observation of masses by professional physical examination or mammography may be all that is necessary for masses not needing surgical intervention (Katz and Dotters, 2012). Breast self-examination can be practiced by the woman between professional examinations (see Chapter 3).

Nipple Discharge

Nipple discharge is a common occurrence that concerns many women. Although most nipple discharge is physiologic, evaluate each woman who has this problem thoroughly because a small percentage will be found to have a serious endocrine disorder or malignancy. Most nipple discharge is elicited (i.e., discharge is a result of the breast being compressed or stimulated) and is usually not a concern unless the woman is postmenopausal or a mass is present in the breast (Lobo, 2012c).

Another form of breast discharge not related to malignancy is galactorrhea, a bilaterally spontaneous, milky, sticky discharge. It is a normal finding in pregnancy. It can also occur as the result of elevated prolactin levels caused by a thyroid disorder, pituitary tumor, or chest wall surgery or trauma. Obtaining a complete medication history on each woman is essential. Some tranquilizers (e.g., tricyclic antidepressants), narcotics, antihypertensive medications, and oral contraceptives can precipitate galactorrhea in some women (Lobo, 2012c).

Diagnostic tests that may be indicated include a prolactin level, a microscopic analysis of the discharge from each breast, a thyroid profile, a pregnancy test, and a mammogram (Lobo, 2012c).

Mammary Duct Ectasia

Mammary duct ectasia is an inflammation of the ducts behind the nipple. It occurs most often in perimenopausal women. In mammary duct ectasia nipple discharge is thick; sticky; and colored white, brown, green, or purple. The woman frequently experiences a burning pain, an itching, or a palpable mass behind the nipple.

The workup includes a mammogram and aspiration and culture of fluid. Treatment is usually symptomatic; mild pain relievers, warm compresses applied to the breast, or wearing a supportive bra may provide relief. If a mass is present or an abscess occurs, treatment may include a local excision of the affected duct or ducts, provided that the woman has no future plans to breastfeed (Mayo Foundation for Medical Education and Research, 2012).

Intraductal Papilloma

Intraductal papilloma is a rare benign condition that develops within the terminal nipple ducts. The cause is unknown. It usually occurs in women between ages 30 and 50. The papilloma is usually too small to be palpated, and the characteristic sign is spontaneous unilateral nipple discharge that is serous, serosanguineous, or bloody. After eliminating the possibility of malignancy, the affected segments of the ducts and breasts are surgically excised (Katz and Dotters, 2012). Table 4-6 compares manifestations of benign breast diseases.

Collaborative Care

The history should focus on risk factors for breast diseases, events related to the breast mass, and health maintenance practices. Risk factors for breast cancer are discussed later in this chapter. Information related to the breast mass should include how, when, and by whom the mass was discovered. The following patient information is documented: presence of pain, whether symptoms increase with menses, dietary habits, smoking habits, and use of oral contraceptives. The woman's emotional status, including her stress level, fears, and concerns and her ability to cope, also should be assessed.

Physical examination may include assessment of the breasts for symmetry, masses (size, number, consistency, mobility), and nipple discharge.

Nursing actions might include the following:

- Discuss the intervals for and facets of breast screening, including professional examination and mammography (see Table 3-3). Women with breast implants may need special views of the breast, and precautions might have to be taken to prevent rupturing the implant during mammography.
- Provide written educational materials.
- Encourage the verbalization of fears and concerns about treatment and prognosis.
- Provide specific information regarding the woman's condition and treatment, including dietary changes, drug therapy, comfort measures, stress management, and surgery.
- Demonstrate correct breast self-examination technique if the woman desires to practice it (see Chapter 3, p. 44).
- Describe pain-relieving strategies in detail and collaborate with the primary health care provider to ensure effective pain control.
- Encourage discussion of feelings about body image.
- Refer to a support group or stress-management resource if needed to cope with long-term consequences of benign breast conditions.

Cancer of the Breast

The United States has one of the highest rates of carcinoma in the world. After skin cancer, breast cancer is the most diagnosed cancer and the leading cause of cancer deaths in women (ACS, 2012). One in eight American women will develop breast cancer in her lifetime (National Cancer Institute, 2012). No clear method for prevention has been formulated. The prognosis for and survival of the woman are improved with early detection. Therefore women must be educated about risk factors, early detection, and screening.

Although the exact cause of breast cancer is still unknown, researchers have identified certain factors that increase a woman's risk for developing a malignancy. Box 4-5 lists these factors. The most important predictor for breast cancer is age; the risk increases as the woman ages.

Much discussion has taken place about possible links between breast cancer and hormone therapy; several large research studies, including the Women's Health Initiative, have found that the risk of breast cancer increases when a woman is taking combined estrogen and progesterone but declines quickly once therapy is stopped. No consensus about possible links has been reached (Katz and Dotters, 2012).

Studies that include a long-term study of breast implant patients implemented by the National Cancer Institute concluded that silicone breast implants did not increase the risk of breast cancer (Katz and Dotters, 2012).

Although most breast cancers are not related to genetic factors, the identification of the BRCA1 and BRCA2 genes has demonstrated the role of heredity and genetic mutations in this disease. Only approximately 5% to 10% of all breast cancers are attributed to heredity. Women who have abnormalities in the BRCA1 and BRCA2 genes have up to an 80% chance of developing breast cancer (ACS, 2012). Other genetic mutations that can cause breast cancer include mutations of the ataxia telangiectasia mutated (ATM) gene, the p53 tumor suppressor gene, the phosphatase and tensin homolog (PTEN) gene, and the checkpoint kinase 2 (CHEK2) gene (ACS, 2012).

BOX 4-5 RISK FACTORS FOR BREAST CANCER*

Risks that are not modifiable:

- Age—risk increases with age
- Previous history of breast cancer
- Family history of breast cancer, especially a mother or sister (particularly significant if premenopausal)
- Inherited genetic mutations in BRCA1 and BRCA2 genes
- Previous history of ovarian, endometrial, colon, or thyroid cancer
- High breast tissue density
- Early menarche (before age 12)
- Late menopause (after age 55)
- Previous history of benign breast disease with epithelial hyperplasia
- Race (Caucasian women have highest incidence)

Lifestyle and modifiable risks:

- Nulliparity or first pregnancy after age 30
- Not breastfeeding
- Postmenopausal use of combined estrogen-progestin replacement therapy
- Obesity after menopause
- Alcohol consumption of more than one drink per day
- Sedentary lifestyle
- Vitamin D—low levels increase risk

Data from American Cancer Society (ACS): *Breast cancer 2011*, www.cancer.org; American Cancer Society (ACS): *Cancer facts and figures*, Atlanta, 2012, American Cancer Society.
*Risk factors are cumulative (i.e., the more risk factors that are present, the greater is the likelihood of breast cancer occurring).

BOX 4-6 RISK FACTORS INCLUDED IN THE BREAST CANCER RISK ASSESSMENT TOOL

- Woman's age
- Number of first-degree relatives affected
- Age of woman at menarche
- Age of woman at first live birth
- Number of breast biopsies
- History of atypical hyperplasia in biopsy specimens

Information about breast cancer risks can be confusing, and women can overestimate or underestimate their risks. Women and health professionals can use the Breast Cancer Risk Assessment Tool to calculate risk. This tool was developed and verified by the National Cancer Institute (NCI) to predict the risk of breast cancer in 5 years and over the lifetime (to age 90) of a woman. The risk factors used are in Box 4-6. The tool is available at www.nci.nih.gov/bcrisktool/. Although the clinical applicability of risk factors has limits, screen women at increased risk at frequent intervals and help them consider changing risk factors that can be changed such as losing weight if obese and limiting alcohol intake (ACS, 2012).

Prevention

Chemoprevention is the use of medications to reduce cancer risk. Tamoxifen and raloxifene block the effect of estrogen on breast tissue. Studies have shown that these two drugs can reduce the risk of breast cancer, and the FDA has approved them for such use (ACS,

MEDICATION GUIDE

Tamoxifen (Nolvadex)

Action

Antiestrogenic effects; attaches to hormone receptors on cancer cells and prevents natural hormones from attaching to the receptors

Indications

For treatment of advanced-stage or metastatic breast cancer; for treatment of early-stage breast cancer after breast cancer surgery and radiation therapy; to reduce the incidence of breast cancer in women at high risk

Dosage

20 mg orally daily

Adverse Reactions

Common side effects include hot flashes, night sweats, nausea, vaginal bleeding or discharge, and mood swings. Hair loss is an uncommon effect. Serious side effects include deep vein thrombosis, increased risk of endometrial cancer, and stroke.

Nursing Considerations

The medication may be taken on an empty stomach or with food. Missed doses should be taken as soon as possible, but taking two doses at once is not recommended. A barrier or nonhormonal form of contraception is recommended in premenopausal women because tamoxifen may be harmful to the fetus if pregnancy should occur.

MEDICATION GUIDE

Raloxifene Hydrochloride (Evista)

Action

A selective estrogen receptor modulator, serving as an agonist and antagonist to estrogen receptor sites

Indications

Treatment and prevention of osteoporosis; reduction in the risk of invasive breast cancer in postmenopausal women with osteoporosis; and reduction of risk of invasive breast cancer in postmenopausal women at high risk for invasive breast cancer

Dosage

60 mg orally daily

Adverse Reactions

Common side effects include hot flashes, nausea, peripheral edema, joint pain, leg cramps, flu-like symptoms, sweating. Serious and life-threatening side effects can occur from existing condition. Women who have had or are at risk for a heart attack have increased risk of dying from a stroke. Risk of blood clots in the legs and lungs is increased. Raloxifene is contraindicated in women with an active or past history of venous thromboembolism.

Nursing Considerations

The medication may be taken on an empty stomach or with food. Missed doses should be taken as soon as possible, but taking two doses at once is not recommended. Counsel woman to contact her health care provider if leg pain or feeling of warmth in lower legs, swelling of hands and feet, sudden chest pain or shortness of breath, or sudden changes in vision occur. Calcium 1500 mg plus vitamin D 400 to 800 International Units daily are recommended.

2011) (see Medication Guides). The role of aromatase inhibitors (e.g., anastrozole) also is being examined to see if these drugs are effective for prevention.

Surgical prophylaxis (bilateral mastectomy, oophorectomy) can reduce the risk of breast cancer, but it should be considered only for people at very high risk (Katz and Dotters, 2012).

Screening and Diagnosis

Breast cancer in its earliest form can be detected by a mammogram before it is felt by a woman. However, estimates indicate that women detect 90% of all breast lumps. Of this 90%, only 20% to 25% are malignant. More than half of all lumps are discovered in the upper outer quadrant of the breast. The most common presenting symptom is a lump or thickening of the breast. The lump may feel hard and fixed or soft and spongy. It may have well-defined or irregular borders. It may be fixed to the skin, thereby causing dimpling to occur. A nipple discharge that is bloody or clear also may be present.

Early detection and diagnosis reduce the risk of mortality because cancer is found when it is smaller, lesions are more localized, and the tendency is to have a lower percentage of positive nodes. However, cultural factors may influence a woman's decision to participate in breast cancer screening. Knowledge of these factors and use of culturally sensitive messages and materials that appeal to the unique concerns, beliefs, and reading abilities of target groups assist the nurse in helping women overcome barriers to seeking care. For example, the ACS (2012) reported that women who are African-American, Hispanic, or Native American were less likely to get mammograms than Caucasian or Asian-American women.

Other barriers to breast cancer screening include older age, expense, lack of health insurance, fear, ignorance, and organizational barriers such as scheduling problems and lack of available services.

Clinical examination by a qualified health care provider and screening mammography (x-ray film examination of the breast) (Fig. 4-6) may aid in the early detection of breast cancers. A diagnostic mammogram is performed when a screening mammogram identifies something that needs further inspection or when the woman or examiner finds a breast symptom that is new.

When a suspicious finding on a mammogram is noted or a lump is detected, the diagnosis is confirmed by needle aspiration, a core needle biopsy, or surgical excision (Fig. 4-7). Ultrasound may also be used to assess a specific area of abnormality found during a mammogram procedure (ACS, 2012). Women need specific information regarding advantages and disadvantages of these procedures in making a decision about which one is most appropriate for them.

Laboratory examination of breast tissue determines if cancer is present and, if so, the extent. Other tests performed to determine the spread of the cancer include chest x-ray film examination, bone scan, CT, MRI, and positron emission tomography (PET scan) (ACS, 2012).

An important step in evaluating a breast cancer is to test for the presence of estrogen and progesterone receptors in the biopsied tissue. Cancer cells may contain one, both, or neither of these receptors. Breast cancers that contain estrogen receptors are often called *ER-positive* cancers, whereas those containing progesterone receptors are called *PR-positive* cancers. Women with hormone-positive tumors tend to respond better to treatment and have higher survival rates than the general population (Katz and Dotters, 2012).

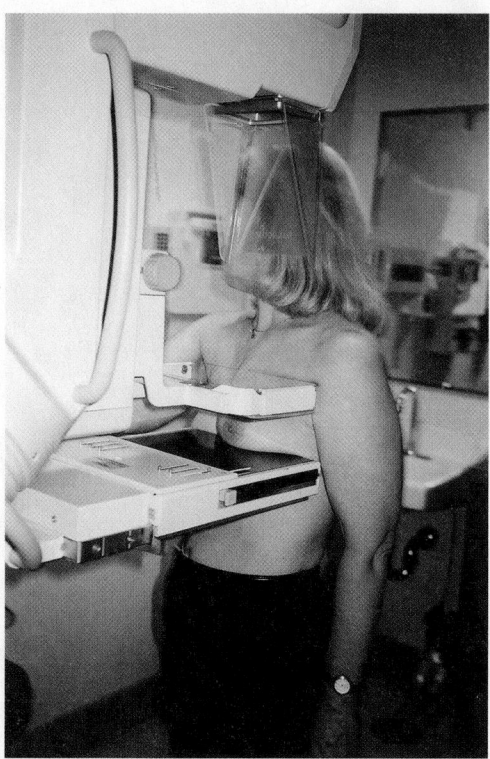

FIG 4-6 Patient undergoing mammography. (Courtesy Shannon Perry, Phoenix, AZ.)

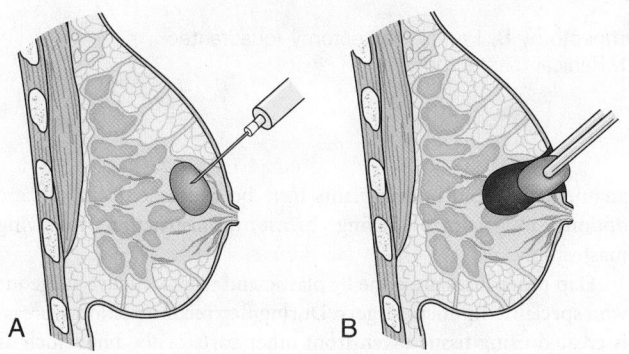

FIG 4-7 Diagnosis. **A,** Needle aspiration. **B,** Open biopsy. (Redrawn from National Women's Health Resource Center: Breast health, *Natl Womens Health Rep* 13(5):3, 1995.)

An HER2/neu test also may be performed on the biopsied breast tissue. HER2/neu is a growth-promoting hormone; and in approximately 15% to 30% of breast cancers, excessive amounts of the hormone are present, causing the cancer to be more aggressive in spreading than other types of breast cancer (ACS, 2011).

CARE MANAGEMENT

Medical Management. Controversy continues regarding the best treatment for breast cancer. Nodal involvement, tumor size, receptor status, and aggressiveness are important variables for treatment selection. Medical management of breast cancer includes surgery, breast reconstruction, radiation therapy, adjuvant hormone

therapy, biologic targeted therapy, and chemotherapy. Many women face difficult decisions about the various treatment options. Box 4-7 lists questions that must be addressed in decision making.

Most health care providers recommend that the malignant mass and the axillary nodes, specifically the sentinel node, be removed for staging purposes (Katz and Dotters, 2012). The treatment can be conservative or more radical. The most frequently recommended surgical approaches for the treatment of breast cancer are lumpectomy and total simple mastectomy. Breast-conserving surgery such as a **lumpectomy** (Fig. 4-8, *A*) or partial mastectomy (e.g., quadrantectomy, wide excision) (Fig. 4-8, *B*) is the removal of the breast tumor and a small amount of surrounding tissue. Sampling of axillary lymph nodes usually occurs through a separate incision at the time of these procedures, and the surgery is usually followed by radiation therapy to the remaining breast tissue (Katz and Dotters, 2012). These procedures are for the primary treatment of women with early-stage (I or II) breast cancer. Lumpectomy offers survival equivalent to that with modified radical mastectomy.

A total **simple mastectomy** (Fig. 4-8, *C*) is the removal of the breast containing the tumor. A **modified radical mastectomy** is the removal of the breast tissue, skin, and fascia of the pectoralis muscle and dissection of the axillary nodes. A **radical mastectomy** (Fig. 4-8, *D*), although rarely performed, is the removal of the breast and underlying pectoralis muscles and complete axillary node dissection. After surgery follow-up treatment may include radiation, chemotherapy, or hormone therapy (Katz and Dotters, 2012). The decision to include follow-up therapy is based on the stage of disease, age and menopausal status of the woman, the woman's preference, and her hormone receptor status. Follow-up treatment is usually initiated to decrease the risk of recurrence in women who have no evidence of metastasis.

Radiation is usually recommended as follow-up therapy for women who have stage I or II cancer. Radiation can be external for 5 to 6 weeks or as short as 3 weeks. Internal radiation is in the form of needles, seeds, wires, or catheters filled with a radioactive substance that is inserted into the breast near the tumor. Hormone therapy with tamoxifen, an estrogen agonist, is recommended for women over the age of 50 for at least 5 years (see Medication Guide [tamoxifen]).

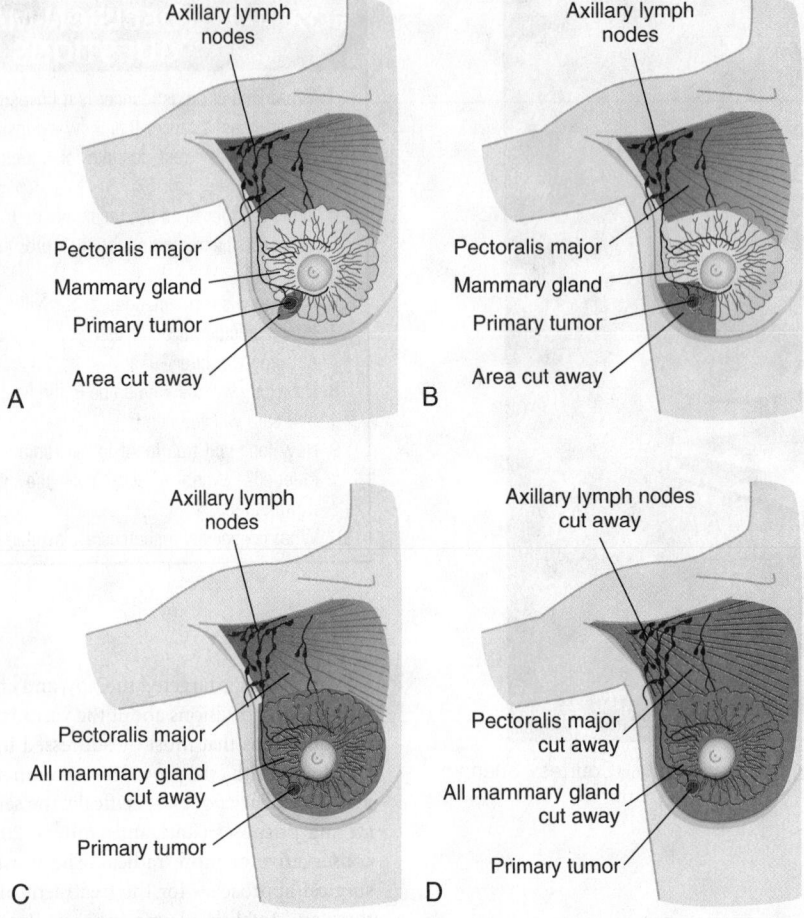

FIG 4-8 Surgical alternatives for breast cancer. **A,** Lumpectomy **B,** Partial mastectomy (quadrantectomy, wide excision). **C,** Total (simple) mastectomy. **D,** Radical mastectomy.

Aromatase inhibitors markedly suppress plasma estrogen levels in postmenopausal women by inhibiting or inactivating aromatase, the enzyme responsible for synthesizing estrogens from androgenic substrates. Aromatase inhibitors such as anastrozole, letrozole, and exemestane have shown to be effective agents in hormone therapy for breast cancer. In early-stage breast cancer, adjuvant therapy with anastrozole appears to be superior to adjuvant therapy with tamoxifen in reducing recurrence in postmenopausal women (see Medication Guide). The aromatase inhibitors appear to be well tolerated, with a lower incidence of adverse effects compared to tamoxifen (ACS, 2011).

Chemotherapy is often given to premenopausal women who have positive nodes. Therapy for more advanced tumors usually includes surgery followed by chemotherapy, radiation, or both (Katz and Dotters, 2012).

The goals of surgical breast reconstruction are achievement of symmetry and preservation of body image. Surgical reconstruction can be done immediately or at a later date. Immediate reconstruction at the time of mastectomy does not change survival rates or interfere with therapy or the treatment of recurrent disease.

The types of surgical option for breast reconstruction include implants and flap procedures. Implants are made of silicone or saline or a combination of both and can be inserted at the same time as a mastectomy or later. They are placed underneath the chest muscle versus on top of it, as in the case of breast augmentation. Silicone implants have been deemed safe and are options for women having breast reconstruction following mastectomy.

Flap procedures are done by plastic and reconstructive surgeons who specialize in microsurgery. During flap reconstruction a breast is created using tissue taken from other parts of the body such as the abdomen, back, or buttocks, or thighs, which is then transplanted to the chest by reconnecting the blood vessels to new ones in the chest region.

After a woman has recovered from initial reconstructive surgery, she may choose to have nipple and areolar reconstruction. Nipple reconstruction is achieved by using an autologous skin graft to construct a nipple, either from tissue from the remaining nipple or from a donor site (Katz and Dotters, 2012).

Nursing Care. Surgery may be performed in an outpatient surgical setting or as an inpatient procedure, depending on which type of surgery is being performed. Nursing care and teaching are focused on the perioperative period. Before surgery assess the woman's psychologic readiness, specific teaching needs related to the procedure, and what to expect after surgery. A visit from a woman who has had a similar experience may be beneficial before and after surgery.

Discuss reconstruction surgery, including the risks and benefits before the surgery if appropriate. A discussion of partial and full external prostheses also may be appropriate, including where to purchase one and the types of bras that may be worn. Local ACS

MEDICATION GUIDE

Anastrozole (Arimidex)

Action

An aromatase inhibitor; inhibits the conversion of androgens to estrogen

Indication

For adjuvant treatment of early breast cancer in postmenopausal women who have received 5 years of tamoxifen therapy; first-line treatment of postmenopausal women with hormone receptor–positive or hormone receptor–unknown locally advanced or metastatic cancer; adjuvant treatment of postmenopausal women with hormone receptor–positive early breast cancer

Dosage and Route

1 mg once a day by mouth

Adverse Reactions

Common side effects include hot flashes, nausea, increased sweating, joint or muscle pain, fluid retention, vaginal dryness, constipation, dizziness, fatigue, headache; severe side effects include severe allergic reactions (e.g., rash, hives, difficulty breathing), vomiting, chest pain, severe bone pain, calf pain or tenderness

Nursing Considerations

The medication may be taken on an empty stomach or with food. The woman should use caution if driving or using machinery because this medication may cause drowsiness or dizziness. Advise her that the medicine may decrease bone strength, increase her risk for fractures, and increase cholesterol.

---

units can provide sources, and volunteers of Reach to Recovery can offer hints and suggestions for wearing apparel and coping with prostheses.

Postoperative nursing care focuses on recovery. Women who had surgery in an outpatient setting usually go home within a few hours after surgery. A 24- to 48-hour stay is usual after modified radical mastectomy.

! NURSING ALERT

Avoid taking blood pressure, giving injections, or taking blood from the arm on the affected side.

The woman may have drainage tubes from the incision site that you will need to assess and drain. Incision care may include dressing changes. If postoperative arm exercises are appropriate, initiate these during the early postoperative period (Box 4-8). The woman is usually discharged to home after being given self-management instructions. Because teaching time is short, providing printed information gives the woman and her family something to refer to at home (see Patient Teaching box).

Concerns about appearance after breast surgery may affect the woman's self-concept. Before surgery the woman and her partner need information about the woman's postoperative appearance. They need to be able to discuss feelings and concerns about accepting the changes. Nurses can help the couple communicate these feelings and concerns. Information about community resources and support groups such as Reach to Recovery are often beneficial (see Community Focus box).

PATIENT TEACHING

After a Mastectomy Without Reconstruction

- Wash hands well before and after touching incision area or drains.
- Empty surgical drains twice a day and as needed, recording the date, time, drain sites (if more than one drain is present), and amount of drainage in milliliters in the diary that you will take to each surgical checkup until your drains are removed. (Before discharge you may receive a graduated container for emptying drains and measuring drainage.)
- Avoid driving, lifting more than 10 pounds, or reaching above your head until given permission by the surgeon.
- Take medications for pain as soon as pain begins.
- Perform arm exercises as directed.
- Call health care provider if inflammation of incision or swelling of the incision or the arm occurs.
- Avoid tight clothing, tight jewelry, and other causes of decreased circulation in the affected arm.
- Until drains are removed, wear loose-fitting underwear (camisole or half-slip) and clothes, pinning surgical drains inside of clothing. (You will be taught how to do this safely.)
- After drains are removed and surgical sites are healing and still tender, wear a mastectomy bra or camisole with a cotton-filled, muslin temporary prosthesis. Temporary prostheses of this type are often available from Reach to Recovery.
- Avoid depilatory creams; strong deodorants; and shaving of affected chest area, axilla, and arm.
- Sponge bathe for the first 48 hours; then you may shower. Thoroughly dry yourself afterward and reapply fresh dressings.
- Return to the surgeon's office for incision check, drain inspection, and possible drain removal as directed.
- Contact Reach to Recovery or a breast center nursing staff member for assistance in obtaining external prosthesis and lingerie when dressings, drains, and staples are removed and wound is healing and nontender.
- Contact insurance company for information about coverage of prosthesis and wig if needed. Obtain prescriptions for prosthesis and wig to submit with receipts of purchase for these items to the insurance company. If insurance does not pay for these items, contact hospital or agency social worker or local American Cancer Society for assistance.
- Practice BSE of unaffected side and affected surgical site and axilla.
- Keep follow-up visits for professional examination, mammography, and testing to detect recurrent breast cancer.
- Expect decreased sensation and tingling at incision sites and in the affected arm for weeks to months after surgery.
- Resume sexual activities as desired.
- Participate in breast cancer survivor support group if desired.
- Encourage mother, sisters, and daughters (if applicable) to learn and practice BSE and have annual professional breast examinations and mammography (if appropriate).

Additional Nursing Care for Women Undergoing Mastectomy with Reconstruction

- Apply no tight compression of the reconstructed breasts until approved by the plastic surgeon.
- Wear loosely fitting garments for first 3 to 4 weeks.
- Know that surgery is still a work in progress and that final cosmetic result of reconstruction takes many weeks.
- Assess skin for potential of poor peripheral circulation that may cause skin necrosis and report any skin changes immediately.
- See drain care instructions under axillary dissection section.

BSE, Breast self-examination.

BOX 4-8   EXERCISES AFTER BREAST SURGERY

It is important to talk to your physician before starting any exercises. A physical or occupational therapist can help design an exercise program for you.

Exercises in Lying Position

These exercises should be performed on a bed or the floor while lying on your back with your knees and hips bent, feet flat.

Wand Exercise

This exercise helps increase the forward motion of the shoulders. You will need a broom handle, yardstick, or other similar object to perform it.

- Hold the wand in both hands with palms facing up.
- Lift the wand up over your head (as far as you can), using your unaffected arm to help lift it until you feel a stretch in your affected arm.
- Hold for 5 seconds.
- Lower arms and repeat 5 to 7 times.

Elbow Winging

This exercise helps increase the mobility of the front of your chest and shoulder. It may take several weeks of regular exercise before your elbows will get close to the bed (or floor).

- Clasp your hands behind your neck with your elbows pointing toward the ceiling.
- Move your elbows apart and down toward the bed (or floor).
- Repeat 5 to 7 times

Exercises in Sitting Position
Shoulder Blade Stretch

This exercise helps increase the mobility of the shoulder blades.

- Sit in a chair very close to a table with your back against the chair back.
- Place the unaffected arm on the table with your elbow bent and palm down. Do not move this arm during the exercise.
- Place the affected arm on the table, palm down with your elbow straight.
- Without moving your trunk, slide the affected arm toward the opposite side of the table. You should feel your shoulder blade move as you do this.
- Relax your arm and repeat 5 to 7 times.

Shoulder Blade Squeeze

This exercise also helps increase the mobility of the shoulder blade.

- Facing straight ahead, sit in a chair in front of a mirror without resting on the back of the chair.
- Arms should be at your sides with elbows bent.
- Squeeze shoulder blades together, bringing your elbows behind you. Keep your shoulders level as you do this exercise. Do not lift them up toward your ears.
- Return to the starting position and repeat 5 to 7 times.

Side Bending

This exercise helps increase the mobility of the trunk/body.

- Clasp your hands together in front of you and lift your arms slowly over your head, straightening your arms.
- When your arms are over your head, bend your trunk to the right while bending at the waist and keeping your arms overhead.
- Return to the starting position and bend to the left.
- Repeat 5 to 7 times.

Exercises in Standing Position
Chest Wall Stretch

This exercise helps stretch the chest wall.

- Stand facing a corner with toes approximately 8 to 10 inches from the corner.
- Bend your elbows and place forearms on the wall, one on each side of the corner. Your elbows should be as close to shoulder height as possible.
- Keep your arms and feet in position and move your chest toward the corner. You will feel a stretch across your chest and shoulders.
- Return to starting position and repeat 5 to 7 times.

Shoulder Stretch

This exercise helps increase the mobility in the shoulder.

- Stand facing the wall with your toes approximately 8 to 10 inches from it.
- Place your hands on the wall. Use your fingers to "climb the wall," reaching as high as you can until you feel a stretch.
- Return to starting position and repeat 5 to 7 times.

Modified from American Cancer Society: *Exercises after breast surgery*, 2010, www.cancer.org/docroot/CRI/content/CRI_2_6x_Exercises_After_Breast_Surgery.asp?sitearea=CRI&viewmode=print&.

🏠 COMMUNITY FOCUS

Reach to Recovery

Check the Internet for the American Cancer Society's (*www.cancer.org*) Reach to Recovery program. Identify the services provided by the program and the requirements to become a volunteer. Visit the women's clinic in a local community health agency. Are materials about the Reach to Recovery program visible in the waiting areas? Talk to one of the nurses who works in the clinic (make an appointment for this conversation). What does she know about Reach to Recovery? Does she refer her patients to this program? What is her evaluation of the program? Has she met any of the volunteers? Do her patients have positive things to say about the program?

KEY POINTS

- Menstrual disorders diminish the quality of life for affected women and their families.
- Primary dysmenorrhea is a condition associated with ovulatory cycles and is related to the release of prostaglandins with menses.
- PMS is a disorder that begins in the luteal phase of the menstrual cycle and resolves with the onset of menses.
- PMS is a disorder with both psychologic and physiologic characteristics.
- Endometriosis is characterized by dysmenorrhea; infertility; and, less often, alterations in menstrual cycle bleeding and dyspareunia.
- Reduced risky sexual practices are key STI prevention strategies.

- HIV is transmitted through body fluids, primarily blood, semen, and vaginal secretions.
- Prevention of mother-to-newborn HIV transmission is most effective when the woman receives antiretroviral drugs during pregnancy and labor and birth and the infant also receives the drugs after the birth.
- HPV is the most common viral STI.
- Syphilis has reemerged as a common STI, affecting more African-American women than any other ethnic group.
- Chlamydia is the most common STI in U.S. women and the most common cause of PID.
- Young sexually active women who do not practice reduced-risk sexual behaviors and have multiple partners are at greatest risk for STIs and HIV infection.

- STIs are responsible for substantial morbidity and mortality, personal suffering, and a heavy economic burden in the United States.
- The development of breast neoplasms, whether benign or malignant, can have a significant physical and emotional effect on the woman and her family.
- The risk of U.S. women developing breast cancer is one in eight.
- Clinical breast examinations by a health care provider and routine screening mammograms are recommended for early detection of breast cancer.
- The primary therapy for most women with stage I or II breast cancer is breast-conserving surgery with axillary or sentinel lymph node sampling followed by radiation therapy.
- Tamoxifen is a common adjuvant therapy for breast cancers that are estrogen-receptor positive.

REFERENCES

American Academy of Pediatrics Committee on Pediatric AIDS: HIV testing and prophylaxis to prevent mother-to-child transmission in the United States, *Pediatrics* 122(5):1127–1134, 2008.

American Cancer Society (ACS): *Breast cancer facts & figures 2011-2012*, Atlanta, 2011, ACS.

American Cancer Society (ACS): *Cancer facts and figures 2012*, Atlanta, 2012, ACS.

American College of Obstetricians and Gynecologists (ACOG): *Premenstrual syndrome*, ACOG Practice Bulletin No 15, Washington, DC, 2000, ACOG.

American College of Obstetricians and Gynecologists (ACOG): *Frequently asked questions—premenstrual syndrome FAQ057*, 2011, www.acog.org.

American Psychiatric Association (APA): *Diagnostic and statistical manual of mental disorders*, ed 4, text revision, Washington, DC, 2000, APA Press.

Biggs WS, Demuth RH: Premenstrual syndrome and premenstrual dysphoric disorder, *Am Fam Physician* 84(8):918–924, 2011.

Brown J, Kives S, Akhtar M: Progestagens and anti-progestagens for pain associated with endometriosis, *Cochrane Database Syst Rev* 3:CD002122, 2012.

Centers for Disease Control and Prevention (CDC): *FDA-approved rapid HIV antibody screening tests*, 2008a, www.cdc.gov/hiv/topics/testing.

Centers for Disease Control and Prevention (CDC): Sexually transmitted diseases treatment guidelines, *MMWR* 59(RR12):1–109, 2010a.

Centers for Disease Control and Prevention (CDC): 2010 guidelines for the prevention of perinatal group b streptococcal disease, *MMWR* 59(RR10):1–32, 2010b.

Centers for Disease Control and Prevention (CDC): *HIV among women*, 2011a, www.cdc.gov/hiv/topics/women/index.htm.

Centers for Disease Control and Prevention (CDC): *STD trends in the United States: 2010 national data for gonorrhea, chlamydia, and syphilis*, 2011b, www.cdc.gov/std/stats10/trends.htm.

Centers for Disease Control and Prevention (CDC): *ABCs of hepatitis*, 2012a, www.cdc.gov/hepatits/resources/professionals/PDFs/ABCTable-bw.pdf.

Centers for Disease Control and Prevention (CDC): *Genital HPV infection—fact sheet*, 2012b, www.cdc.gov/std/HPV/STDFact-HPV.htm.

Chase C, Wells J, Eley S: Caffeine and breast pain: revisiting the connection, *Nurs Womens Health* 15(4):286–294, 2011.

Cunningham F, Leveno K, Bloom S, et al: *Williams obstetrics*, ed 23, New York, 2010, McGraw-Hill.

Dante G, Facchinetti F: Herbal treatments for alleviating premenstrual symptoms: a systematic review, *J Psychosom Obstet Gynaecol* 32(1):42–51, 2011.

Eckert LO, Lentz GM: Infections of the lower and upper genital tract: Vulva, vagina, cervix, toxic shock syndrome, endometritis, and salpingitis. In Lentz GM, Lobo RA, Gershenson DM, et al, editors: *Comprehensive gynecology*, ed 6, Philadelphia, 2012, Mosby, pp 519–559.

Fantasia HC, Fontenot HB, Sutherland M, et al: Sexually transmitted infections in women, *Nurs Womens Health* 15(1):47–57, 2011.

Ford O, Lethaby A, Roberts H, et al: Progesterone for premenstrual syndrome, *Cochrane Database Syst Rev* 3:CD003415, 2012.

George CA, Leonard JP, Hutchinson MR: The female athlete triad: a current concepts review, *S Afr J Sports Med* 23(2):50–56, 2011.

Joy E: Invited commentary: is the pill the answer for patients with female athlete triad? *Curr Sports Med* 11(2):54–55, 2012.

Katz VL: Benign gynecologic lesions. Vulva, vagina, cervix, uterus, oviduct, ovary, ultrasound imaging of pelvic structures. In Lentz GM, Lobo RA, Gershenson DM, et al, editors: *Comprehensive gynecology*, ed 6, Philadelphia, 2012, Mosby, pp 383–432.

Katz VL, Dotters D: Breast disease: diagnosis and treatment of benign and malignant disease. In Lentz GM, Lobo RA, Gershenson DM, et al, editors: *Comprehensive gynecology*, ed 6, Philadelphia, 2012, Mosby, pp 301–334.

Laufer MR: Current approaches to optimizing the treatment of endometriosis in adolescents, *Gynecol Obstet Invest* 66(suppl 1):19–27 2008.

Lentz GM: (2012). Primary and secondary dysmenorrheal, premenstrual syndrome, and premenstrual dysphoric disorder. In Lentz GM, Lobo RA, Gershenson DM, et al, editors: *Comprehensive gynecology*, ed 6, Philadelphia, 2012, Mosby, pp 791–803.

Lobo RA: Abnormal uterine bleeding: ovulatory and anovulatory dysfunctional uterine bleeding: management of acute and chronic excessive bleeding. In Lentz GM, Lobo RA, Gershenson DM, et al, editors: *Comprehensive gynecology*, ed 6, Philadelphia, 2012a, Mosby, pp 805–814.

Lobo RA: Endometriosis. Etiology, pathology, diagnosis, management. In Lentz GM, Lobo RA, Gershenson DM, et al, editors: *Comprehensive gynecology*, ed 6, Philadelphia, 2012b, Mosby, pp 433–452.

Lobo RA: Hyperprolactinemia, galactorrhea, and pituitary adenomas: Etiology, differential diagnosis, natural history, management. In Lentz GM, Lobo RA, Gershenson DM, et al, editors: *Comprehensive gynecology*, ed 6, Philadelphia, 2012c, Mosby, pp 837–848.

Lobo RA: Primary and secondary amenorrhea and precocious puberty. In Lentz GM, Lobo RA, Gershenson DM, et al, editors: *Comprehensive gynecology*, ed 6, Philadelphia, 2012d, Mosby, pp 815–836.

Mayo Foundation for Medical Education and Research: *Mammary duct ectasia*, 2012, www.mayoclinic.com/health/mammary-duct-ectasia/DS00751.

National Cancer Institute: Cancer of the breast-SEER stat fact sheets, 2012, www.seer/cancer.gov.

Panel on Treatment of HIV-Infected Pregnant Women and Prevention of Perinatal Transmission: *Recommendations for use of antiretroviral drugs in pregnant HIV-1-infected women for maternal health and interventions to reduce perinatal HIV transmission in the United States*, 2010, pp 1–117, http://aidsinfo.nih.gov/ContentFiles/PerinatalGL.pdf.

Royer HR, Falk EC: Young women's beliefs regarding human papillomavirus,

J Obstet Gynecol Neonatal Nurs 4 (1):92–102, 2012.

US Food and Drug Administration (USFDA): *HIV testing*, 2008, www.fda.gov/oashi/aids/test.html.

US Preventive Services Task Force (USPSTF): *Screening for hepatitis B virus infection in pregnancy: guide to clinical preventive services, 2009: recommendations of the US Preventive Services Task Force*, Rockville, MD, 2009, Agency for Healthcare Research and Quality.

Wambach CM, Alexander CJ: Menstrual disorders. In DiSaia PJ, Chaudhuri G, Giudice LC, et al: *Women's health review: a clinical update in obstetrics-gynecology*, Philadelphia, 2012, Saunders.

Weiner C, Buhimschi C: *Drugs for pregnant and lactating women*, ed 2, Philadelphia, 2009, Saunders.

Wilton JM: Tranexamine acid: a new option for heavy menstrual bleeding, *Nurs Womens Health* 16(2):146–150, 2012.

Infertility, Contraception, and Abortion

Peggy Mancuso

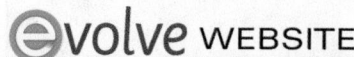 WEBSITE

http://evolve.elsevier.com/Perry/maternal

LEARNING OBJECTIVES

On completion of this chapter, the reader will be able to:
- List common causes of infertility.
- Discuss the psychologic impact of infertility.
- Describe common diagnoses and treatments for infertility.
- Compare reproductive alternatives for couples experiencing infertility.
- Identify the advantages and disadvantages of the following methods of contraception: fertility awareness methods, barrier methods, hormonal methods, intrauterine devices, and sterilization.
- Explain common nursing interventions that facilitate contraceptive use.
- Describe the techniques used for medical and surgical interruption of pregnancy.
- Recognize ethical, legal, cultural, and religious considerations of infertility, contraception, and elective abortion.

INFERTILITY

Incidence

Infertility is a serious concern that affects quality of life of 10% to 15% of reproductive-age couples (American Society for Reproductive Medicine [ASRM], 2012). Commonly infertility is considered to be a diagnosis for couples who have not achieved pregnancy after 1 year of regular, unprotected intercourse when the woman is less than 35 years of age or after 6 months when the woman is older than 35 (Practice Committee of the ASRM, 2008). Fecundity is the term used to describe the chance of achieving pregnancy and subsequent live birth within one menstrual cycle. Fecundity averages 20% in couples who are not experiencing reproductive problems.

The prevalence of infertility is relatively stable among the overall population; although, as the U.S. population ages, the numbers of infertile women will decline with the decrease in numbers of reproductive-age women. Infertility increases with the age of the woman, with fertility rates in women ages 40 to 45 being 95% lower than women ages 20 to 24. Probable causes of infertility include the trend toward delaying pregnancy until later in life, a time when fertility decreases naturally and the prevalence of diseases such as endometriosis and ovulatory dysfunction increases. Questions exist regarding whether there has been an increase in male infertility or whether male infertility is more readily identified because of improvements in diagnosis.

For the couple experiencing infertility, diagnosis and treatment strategies require considerable physical, emotional, and financial investment over an extended period of time. Feelings connected with infertility are many and complex. The origins of some of these feelings are myths, superstitions, misinformation, or magical thinking about the causes of infertility. Other feelings of anxiety and helplessness arise from the need to undergo many tests and examinations and from a perception of being "different" from others (RESOLVE, 2012). Nurses who care for infertile couples should consider the following four goals:
- Provide the couple with accurate information about human reproduction, infertility treatments, and prognosis for pregnancy. Dispel any myths or inaccuracies from friends or the mass media that the couple may believe to be true.
- Help the couple and the health care team accurately identify and treat possible causes of infertility.
- Provide emotional support. The couple may benefit from anticipatory guidance, counseling, and support group meetings, either face-to-face or online. The organization RESOLVE (www.resolve.org) provides online support, advocacy, and education about infertility for both the infertility community and health care providers.
- Guide and educate those who fail to conceive biologically as a couple about other forms of treatment such as in vitro fertilization (IVF), donor eggs or semen, surrogate

motherhood, and adoption. Support the couple in their decisions regarding their future family.

Nurses should also remember that among healthy women and men promotion of normal reproduction and prevention of infertility can be achieved if both partners maintain a normal body mass index (BMI) and avoid sexually transmitted infections (STIs) and exposures to substances or habits (such as smoking) that impair reproductive ability. As they make plans for their future family, adults should also know that realistically fertility decreases with age.

Factors Associated with Infertility

Although exact percentages vary somewhat with populations, approximately 80% of couples have an identifiable cause of infertility, with about 40% of these causes related to factors in the female partner, 40% related to factors in the male partner, and 20% related to factors in both partners. About 20% or more couples will experience unexplained or idiopathic causes of infertility (ASRM, 2012). Nevertheless the focus of infertility treatment has shifted from attempting to correct a specific pathology to recommending and initiating the treatment that is most effective in achieving pregnancy for this unique couple at this time in their reproductive life span. Assisted reproductive technologies (ARTs) have proven to be effective, even in couples who experience unexplained infertility.

Unassisted human conception requires a normally developed reproductive tract in both the male and female partners. For simplification, each live birth necessitates synchronization of the following:

- The male must deposit semen with sperm that has the capacity to fertilize an egg close to the cervix at the time of ovulation. The sperm must be able to ascend through the uterus and fallopian tubes (male factor).
- The cervix must be sufficiently open to allow semen to enter the uterus and provide a nurturing environment for sperm (cervical factor).
- The fallopian tubes must be able to capture the ovum, transport semen to the ovum, and transport the fertilized embryo to the uterus (tubal factor).
- Ovulation of a healthy oocyte must occur, ideally within the parameters of a regular, predictable menstrual cycle (ovarian factor).
- The uterus must be receptive to implantation of the embryo and capable of nourishing the growth and development of the fetus throughout the normal duration of pregnancy (uterine factor).

An alteration in one or more of these structures, functions, or processes results in some degree of impaired fertility. Boxes 5-1 and 5-2 list factors affecting female and male infertility.

For ovulation to occur, both partners must have normal, intact hypothalamic-pituitary-gonadal hormonal axes that support the formation of sperm in the male and ova in the female. Sperm can remain viable within a woman's reproductive tract for at least 3 days and for as long as 5 days. The oocyte can only be successfully fertilized for 12 to 24 hours after ovulation (Fritz and Speroff, 2011c). The couple seeking pregnancy should be taught about the menstrual cycle and ways to detect ovulation (see Chapter 3). They should be counseled to have intercourse 2 to 3 times a week; or, if timed intercourse does not increase anxiety, they should be encouraged to engage in intercourse the day before and the day of ovulation. Fertility decreases markedly 24 hours after ovulation.

BOX 5-1 FACTORS AFFECTING FEMALE FERTILITY

Ovarian Factors
- Developmental anomalies
- Anovulation—primary
  - Pituitary or hypothalamic hormone disorders
  - Adrenal gland disorders (rare)
  - Congenital adrenal hyperplasia (rare)
- Anovulation—secondary
  - Disruption of hypothalamic-pituitary-ovarian axis
  - Anorexia
  - Insufficient body fat in athletic women
  - Increased prolactin levels
  - Thyroid disorders
  - Premature ovarian failure
  - Polycystic ovarian disorder
- Medications
  - Oral contraceptives
  - Progestins
  - Antidepressant and antipsychotic drugs
  - Corticosteroids
  - Chemotherapy

Tubal/Peritoneal Factors
- Developmental anomalies of the tubes (see Fig. 5-1)
- Reduced tubal motility
- Inflammation within the tube
- Tubal adhesions
- Disruption caused by tubal pregnancy
- Endometriosis

Uterine Factors
- Developmental anomalies of the uterus (see Fig. 5-1)
- Endometrial and myometrial fibroid tumors
- Asherman's syndrome (uterine adhesions or scar tissue)

Vaginal-Cervical Factors
- Vaginal-cervical infections
- Cervical mucus inadequate
- Isoimmunization (development of sperm antibodies)

Other Factors
- Nutritional deficiencies
- Obesity
- Thyroid dysfunction (hyperthyroidism and hypothyroidism)
- Idiopathic conditions

CARE MANAGEMENT

The nurse assists in the assessment and education of the infertile couple. As part of the assessment process he or she obtains information from the couple through interview and physical examination, including if this couple's situation is one of primary (never experienced pregnancy) or secondary (previous pregnancy) infertility. Religious, cultural, and ethnic data may place restrictions on use of available treatments. Box 5-3 describes some of the concerns related to religion that may affect the couple's choices regarding infertility treatment. The Cultural Competence box notes cultural rituals and beliefs regarding fertility. In addition, the nurse obtains and monitors results of diagnostic testing. Some of the information and data needed to investigate impaired fertility are of a sensitive, personal

BOX 5-2 FACTORS AFFECTING MALE FERTILITY

Hormonal Disorders
- Congenital disorders
- Tumors of the pituitary and hypothalamus
- Trauma to the pituitary or hypothalamus
- Hyperprolactinemia
- Excess of androgens, estrogen, cortisol
- Drugs and substance abuse (recreational and prescribed drugs)
- Chronic illnesses
- Nutritional deficiencies
- Obesity
- Endocrine disorders (e.g., diabetes)

Testicular Factors
- Congenital disorders
- Undescended testes
- Hypospadias
- Varicocele
- Viral infections (e.g., mumps)
- Sexually transmitted infections (gonorrhea, chlamydial infection)
- Obstructive lesions of the epididymis and vas deferens
- Environmental toxins
- Trauma
- Torsion
- Castration
- Systemic illnesses
- Changes in sperm from cigarette smoking or use of heroin, marijuana, amyl nitrate, butyl nitrate, ethyl chloride, or methaqualone
- Decrease in libido from use of heroin, methadone, selective serotonin reuptake inhibitors, or barbiturates
- Impotence from use of alcohol or antihypertensive medications
- Antisperm antibodies

Factors Associated with Sperm Transport
- Drugs
- Sexually transmitted infections of the epididymis
- Ejaculatory dysfunction
- Premature ejaculation

Idiopathic Male Infertility

BOX 5-3 RELIGIOUS CONSIDERATIONS CONCERNING INFERTILITY

The health care provider must always be aware of civil laws and religious proscriptions about sexual activities. Conservative and reform Jewish couples accept most infertility treatment; however, the Orthodox Jewish husband and wife may face problems in infertility investigation and management because of religious laws that govern marital relations. For example, according to Jewish law the Orthodox couple may not engage in marital relations during menstruation and through the following seven "preparatory days." The wife then is immersed in a ritual bath *(Mikvah)* before relations can resume. Fertility problems can arise when the woman has a short cycle (i.e., a cycle of 24 days or fewer, when ovulation would occur on day 10 or earlier).

The Roman Catholic Church regards the embryo as a human being from the first moment of existence. Therefore technical procedures such as in vitro fertilization (IVF), therapeutic donor insemination, and freezing embryos are not accepted or endorsed.

Other religious groups may have ethical concerns about infertility tests and treatments. For example, most Protestant denominations and Muslims usually support infertility management as long as IVF is done with the husband's sperm, there is no reduction of fertilized embryos after implantation, and insemination is done with the husband's sperm. These groups are less supportive of surrogacy and use of donor sperm and eggs. Christian Scientists do not permit surgical procedures or IVF but do permit insemination with husband and donor sperm.

Care providers should seek to understand the woman's spirituality and how beliefs affect her perception of health care, especially in relation to infertility. Women may wish to seek infertility treatment but have questions about proposed diagnostic and therapeutic procedures because of religious proscriptions. These women are encouraged to consult their minister, rabbi, priest, or other spiritual leader for advice.

Data from D'Avanzo C: *Mosby's pocket guide to cultural health assessment*, ed 4, St Louis, 2008, Mosby.

BOX 5-4 INSURANCE COVERAGE FOR INFERTILITY

As of October 2012, only 15 states had mandated some form of insurance coverage for infertility. These mandates included in vitro fertilization in some states, whereas others only covered some diagnostic tests. Some states require health maintenance organizations (HMOs) to cover some costs, whereas in others HMOs are exempt. Patients need information about what they can expect from their insurers. For questions about an individual state, call the state Insurance Commissioner's office. The website for the American Society for Reproductive Medicine (www.asrm.org) has more complete information.

nature. The couple may experience feelings of invasion of privacy, and the nurse must exercise tact and express concern for their well-being throughout the interview. The tests and examinations associated with infertility diagnosis and treatment are occasionally painful and often intrusive. The couple's intimacy and feelings of romantic attachment are often impaired as they engage in this process. A high level of motivation is needed to endure the investigation and subsequent treatment. Because multiple factors involving both partners are common, the investigation of impaired fertility is conducted systematically and simultaneously for both male and female partners (see Cultural Competence box). Both partners must be interested in the solution to the problem. The medical investigation requires time (3 to 4 months) and considerable financial expense. Box 5-4 describes the status of insurance coverage for infertility treatment.

Assessment of Female Infertility

Evaluation for infertility should be offered to couples who have failed to become pregnant after 1 year of regular intercourse or after 6 months if the woman is over 35. Investigation of impaired fertility begins for the woman with a complete history and physical examination. A complete general physical examination should include height and weight and estimation of BMI. Both obesity and being underweight are associated with anovulation disorders. Signs and symptoms of androgen excess such as excess body hair or pigmentation changes should be noted. The general physical examination is followed by a specific assessment of the reproductive tract. A history of infections of the genitourinary tract and any signs of infections, especially STIs that could impair tubal patency, should be assessed.

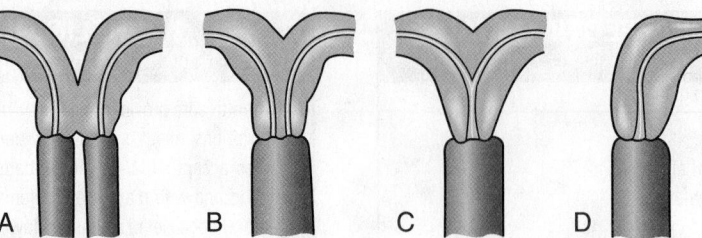

FIG 5-1 Abnormal uterus. **A,** Complete bicornuate uterus with vagina divided by a septum. **B,** Complete bicornuate uterus with normal vagina. **C,** Partial bicornuate uterus with normal vagina. **D,** Unicornuate uterus.

⊕ CULTURAL COMPETENCE

Fertility and Infertility

Worldwide cultures continue to use symbols and rites that celebrate fertility. One fertility rite that persists today is the custom of throwing rice at the bride and groom. Other fertility symbols and rites include passing out congratulatory cigars, candy, or pencils by a new father and baby showers held in anticipation of a child's birth.

In many cultures the responsibility for infertility is usually attributed to the woman. A woman's inability to conceive may be caused by previous sins, evil spirits, or personal inadequacies. In some cultures male virility remains in question until a man demonstrates his ability to reproduce by having at least one child (D'Avanzo, 2008).

Bimanual examination of internal organs may reveal lack of mobility of the uterus or abnormal contours of the uterus and tubes. A woman may have an abnormal uterus and tubes (Fig. 5-1) as a result of congenital abnormalities during fetal development). These uterine abnormalities increase risk for early pregnancy loss.

Laboratory data, including routine urine and blood tests, are collected. The initial clinic visit serves as a preconceptual visit and as initial assessment of possible causes of infertility. The woman should be taking folic acid supplements, and all immunizations should be current to prepare for possible pregnancy.

Diagnostic Testing. The basic infertility survey of the female involves evaluation of the cervix, uterus, tubes, and peritoneum; detection of ovulation; and hormone analysis. Timing and descriptions of common tests are presented in Table 5-1. Previous status regarding ovulation can be evaluated through menstrual history, serum hormone studies, and use of an ovulation predictor kit. If the woman is over age 35, the clinician may choose to assess "ovarian reserve" or how many potential ova remain within the ovaries. A common evaluation of ovarian reserve is measurement of follicle-stimulating hormone (FSH) levels on the third day of the menstrual cycle. The uterus and fallopian tubes can be visualized for abnormalities and tubal patency through hysterosalpingogram (x-ray film examination of the uterine cavity and tubes after instillation of radiopaque contrast material through the cervix). If the woman is at risk for endometriosis (implants of endometrial tissue outside of the uterus) or adhesions, diagnostic laparoscopy may be indicated. Test findings favorable for fertility are summarized in Box 5-5.

Assessment of Male Infertility

The systematic investigation of infertility in the male patient begins with a thorough history and physical examination. Assessment of the male patient proceeds in a manner similar to that of the female patient, starting with noninvasive tests.

Diagnostic Testing and Semen Analysis. The basic test for male infertility is semen analysis. A complete semen analysis, study of the effects of cervical mucus on sperm forward motility and survival, and evaluation of the ability of the sperm to penetrate an ovum provide basic information. Sperm counts vary from day to day and depend on emotional and physical status and sexual activity. Therefore a single analysis may be inconclusive. A minimum of two analyses must be performed several weeks apart to assess male fertility.

Semen is collected by ejaculation into a clean container or a plastic sheath that does not contain a spermicidal agent. The specimen is usually collected by masturbation following 2 to 7 days of abstinence from ejaculation. The semen is examined at the collection site or taken to the laboratory in a sealed container within 2 hours of ejaculation. Exposure to excessive heat or cold is avoided. Commonly accepted values for semen characteristics are given in Box 5-6. If results are in the fertile range, no further sperm evaluation is necessary. If results are not within this range, the test is repeated. If subsequent results are still in the subfertile range, further evaluation is needed to identify the problem.

Hormone analyses are done for testosterone, gonadotropin, FSH, and luteinizing hormone (LH). The sperm penetration assay and other alternative tests can be used to evaluate the ability of sperm to penetrate an egg. Testicular biopsy may be warranted. Scrotal ultrasound can be used to examine the testes for presence of varicoceles and identify abnormalities in the scrotum and spermatic cord. Transrectal ultrasound is used to evaluate the ejaculatory ducts, seminal vesicles, and vas deferens.

Psychosocial Considerations

Infertility is recognized as a major life stressor that can affect self-esteem; relations with the spouse, family, and friends; and careers. Psychologic responses to the diagnosis of infertility may tax a couple's capacity for giving and receiving physical and sexual closeness. The prescriptions and proscriptions for achieving conception may add tension to a couple's sexual functioning. They may report decreased desire for intercourse, orgasmic dysfunction, or midcycle erectile disorders.

To be able to deal comfortably with a couple's sexuality, nurses must be comfortable with their own sexuality so they can better help couples understand why aspects of a private act, lovemaking, need to be shared with health care professionals. Nurses need current factual knowledge about human sexual practices and must be accepting of the preferences and activities of others without being judgmental. They must be skilled in interviewing and therapeutic use of self, sensitive to the nonverbal cues of others, and

TABLE 5-1 GENERAL TESTS FOR IMPAIRED FERTILITY

TEST OR EXAMINATION	TIMING (MENSTRUAL CYCLE DAYS)	RATIONALE
Hysterosalpingogram (HSG) (uterine abnormalities, tubal patency)	7-10	Late follicular, early proliferative phase; will not disrupt a fertilized ovum; may open uterine tubes before time of ovulation
Chlamydia immunoglobulin G antibodies (tubal patency)	Variable	Negative antibody test may indicate tubal patency assessment (HSG); not needed in low risk women
Hysterosalpingo-contrast sonography (uterine abnormalities, tubal patency)	7-10	Late follicular, early proliferative phase; will not disrupt a fertilized ovum; evaluates tubal patency, uterine cavity, and myometrium
Serum progesterone (ovulation)	7 days before expected menses	Midluteal-phase progesterone levels; check adequacy of corpus luteum progesterone production
Assessment of cervical mucus (ovulation)	Variable, ovulation	Cervical mucus should have low viscosity, high spinnbarkeit (ability to stretch) during ovulation
Basal body temperature (ovulation)	Chart entire cycle	Elevation occurs in response to progesterone; documents ovulation
Urinary ovulation predictor kit (ovulation)	Variable, ovulation	Detects timing of lutein hormone surge before ovulation
Semen analysis (male factor)	2 to 7 days after abstinence	Detects ability of sperm to fertilize egg
Sperm penetration assay (male factor)	After 2 days but ≤1 wk of abstinence	Evaluation of ability of sperm to penetrate egg
Follicle-stimulating hormone (FSH) level (ovarian reserve)	Day 3	High FSH levels (>20) indicate that pregnancy will not occur with woman's own eggs; value <10 indicates adequate ovarian reserve
Clomiphene citrate challenge test (CCCT) (ovarian reserve)	Administer clomiphene 100 mg days 3 through 10	Assess FSH on days 3 and 10 in presence of clomiphene stimulation; high FSH levels (>20) indicate that pregnancy will not occur with woman's own eggs; FSH <15 suggestive of adequate ovarian reserve

BOX 5-5 SUMMARY OF FINDINGS FAVORABLE TO FERTILITY

1. Follicular development, ovulation, and luteal development are supportive of pregnancy:
   a. Basal body temperature (presumptive evidence of ovulatory cycles) is biphasic, with temperature elevation that persists for 12 to 14 days before menstruation.
   b. Cervical mucus characteristics change appropriately during phases of the menstrual cycle.
   c. Days 3 to 10 follicle-stimulating hormone (FSH) levels are low enough to verify presence of adequate ovarian follicles.
   d. Day 3 estradiol levels are low enough to verify presence of adequate ovarian follicles.
   e. Woman reports a history of regular, predictable menses with consistent premenstrual and menstrual symptoms.
2. The luteal phase is supportive of pregnancy:
   a. Levels of plasma progesterone are adequate to indicate ovulation.
   b. Luteal phase of menstrual cycle is of sufficient duration to support pregnancy.
3. Cervical factors are receptive to sperm during expected time of ovulation:
   a. Cervical os is open.
   b. Cervical mucus is clear, watery, abundant, and slippery and demonstrates good spinnbarkeit and arborization (fern pattern) at time of ovulation.
   c. Cervical examination reveals no lesions or infections.

4. The uterus and uterine tubes support pregnancy:
   a. Uterine and tubal patency are documented by (1) spillage of dye into the peritoneal cavity, and (2) outlines of uterine and tubal cavities of adequate size and shape with no abnormalities.
   b. Laparoscopic examination verifies normal development of internal genitals and absence of adhesions, infections, endometriosis, and other lesions.
5. The male partner's reproductive structures are normal:
   a. There is no evidence of developmental anomalies of penis, testicular atrophy, or varicocele (varicose veins on the spermatic vein in the groin).
   b. There is no evidence of infection in prostate, seminal vesicles, and urethra.
   c. Testes are more than 4 cm in largest diameter.
6. Semen is supportive of pregnancy:
   a. Sperm (number per milliliter) are adequate in ejaculate.
   b. Most sperm show normal morphology.
   c. Most sperm are motile, forward moving.
   d. No autoimmunity exists.
   e. Seminal fluid is normal.

BOX 5-6 **SEMEN ANALYSIS**

- Semen volume at least 1.5 L
- Semen pH 7.2 or higher
- Sperm density greater than 15 million/mL
- Total sperm count greater than 39 million per ejaculate
- Normal morphologic features greater than 4% (normal oval)
- Motility (important consideration in sperm evaluation)—percentage of forward-moving sperm estimated with respect to abnormally motile and nonmotile sperm, 40%
- Liquification—usually within 15 minutes but no longer than 60 minutes

Source: World Health Organization (WHO): *Laboratory manual for the examination of human semen*, ed 5, Geneva, 2010, WHO.
NOTE: These values are not absolute but are only relative to final evaluation of the couple as a single reproductive unit. Values also differ according to source used as a reference.

? CRITICAL THINKING CASE STUDY

Infertility

Diane is a 39-year-old accountant who has recently married for the first time. Charles is 41 and has two children from a previous marriage. Diane has a history of amenorrhea when she was in college and a member of the track team. Currently her menstrual periods are irregular. She wants to have a baby "before it's too late," and she and Charles have been having unprotected sex for almost a year. They have come to the fertility clinic today for an evaluation. Diane tells the nurse that she has heard a lot about the success of in vitro fertilization (IVF) and wants to know if she will be able to have it performed. How should the nurse respond to Diane's comments and questions?

1. Evidence—Is evidence sufficient to draw conclusions about what response the nurse should give?
2. Assumptions—Describe underlying assumptions about the following issues:
   a. Age and fertility
   b. Infertility as a major life stressor
   c. Success rates for IVF pregnancy and birth
   d. Causes of female infertility
3. What implications and priorities for nursing care can be drawn at this time?
4. Does the evidence objectively support your conclusion?

---

knowledgeable regarding each couple's sociocultural and religious beliefs (see Critical Thinking Case Study).

The couple facing infertility exhibit behaviors of the grieving process such as those associated with other types of loss. The loss of one's genetic continuity with the generations to come can provoke decreased self-esteem, a sense of inadequacy as a woman or a man, and feelings of loss of control over personal destiny. Infertile individuals can perceive greater dissatisfaction with their marriages. Not all people have all the reactions described, nor can it be predicted how long any reaction will last for an individual.

If the couple does not conceive, they should be assessed regarding their desire to be referred for help with adoption, donor eggs or semen, surrogacy, or other reproductive alternatives. The couple may choose to continue in a childfree state. Both health care providers and patients should have a list of agencies, support groups, and

other resources within their community such as the ASRM (www.asrm.org) and RESOLVE (www.resolve.org).

Nonmedical Treatments

Both men and women can benefit from healthy lifestyle changes that result in a BMI within the normal range; moderate daily exercise; and abstinence from alcohol, nicotine, and recreational drugs. For the woman with a BMI >27 and polycystic ovary syndrome, losing just 5% to 10% of body weight can restore ovulation within 6 months. Anovulatory women with a BMI <17 who have eating disorders or intense exercise regimens benefit from weight gain. Nevertheless, this population sometimes is reluctant to alter their behaviors, and counseling should be advised.

Simple changes in lifestyle may be effective in the treatment of subfertile men. Only water-soluble lubricants should be used during intercourse because many commonly used lubricants contain spermicides or have spermicidal properties. High scrotal temperatures can be caused by daily hot tub baths or saunas that keep the testes at temperatures too high for efficient spermatogenesis. These conditions lead to only lessened fertility and should not be used as a means of contraception.

Most herbal remedies have not been proven clinically to promote fertility or to be safe in early pregnancy and should be taken by the woman only as prescribed by a physician or nurse-midwife who has expertise in herbology. Relaxation, osteopathy, stress management (e.g., aromatherapy, yoga), and nutritional and exercise counseling have been reported to increase pregnancy rates in some women. Herbs to avoid while trying to conceive include licorice root, yarrow, wormwood, ephedra, fennel, goldenseal, lavender, juniper, flaxseed, pennyroyal, passionflower, wild cherry, cascara, sage, thyme, and periwinkle. All supplements or herbs should be purchased from trusted sources to ensure that they do not contain contaminants.

Medical Therapy

One goal of infertility assessment and treatment is to determine which couples could respond to conventional therapies in a timely manner. Another goal is to refer couples who will need ARTs to conceive early in the process. In general, any fertility treatment is more likely to result in a live birth in women who are younger than age 35, with successful outcomes decreasing for women over age 40.

Pharmacologic therapy for female infertility is often directed at treating ovulatory dysfunction by either stimulating or enhancing ovulation so more oocytes mature. These medications include (a) clomiphene citrate as initial therapy for many women with intermittent anovulation; (b) a combination of clomiphene and metformin for women with anovulation and insulin resistance; (c) human menopausal gonadotropin (HMG), FSH, and recombinant FSH (rFSH) to stimulate follicle formation in women who do not respond to clomiphene therapies; (d) human chorionic gonadotropin to induce ovulation when follicles are ripe, (e) gonadotropin-releasing hormone (GnRH) agonists at the beginning of a cycle to sequence HMG therapies, (f) progesterone to support the luteal phase of the cycle, and (g) bromocriptine (Parlodel) for women who have excess prolactin (see Medication Guide).

Treatment of certain medical conditions can result in improved fertility. The woman who is hypothyroid benefits from thyroid hormone supplementation. Treatment of endometriosis could include trials of danazol, progesterone, continuous combined oral contraceptives, or GnRH agonists to suppress menstruation and shrink endometrial implants. This regimen would be followed by

MEDICATION GUIDE

Selected Infertility Medications

DRUG	INDICATION	MECHANISM OF ACTION	DOSAGE	COMMON SIDE EFFECTS
Clomiphene citrate	Ovulation induction, treatment of luteal-phase inadequacy	Thought to bind to estrogen receptors in the pituitary, blocking them from detecting estrogen	Tablets, starting with 50 mg/day by mouth for 5 days beginning on fifth day of menses; if ovulation does not occur, may increase dose next cycle; variable dosage	Vasomotor flushes, abdominal discomfort, nausea and vomiting, breast tenderness, ovarian enlargement
Menotropins (human menopausal gonadotropins)	Ovarian follicular growth and maturation	LH and FSH in 1:1 ratio, direct stimulation of ovarian follicle; given sequentially with hCG to induce ovulation	IM injections; dosage regimen variable based on ovarian response. Initial dose is 75 International Units of FSH and 75 International Units of LH (1 ampule) daily for 7-12 days followed by 10,000 International Units hCG	Ovarian enlargement, ovarian hyperstimulation, local irritation at injection site, multifetal gestations
Follitropins (purified FSH)	Treatment of polycystic ovarian disease; follicle stimulation for assisted reproductive techniques	Direct action on ovarian follicle	Subcutaneous or IM injections; dosage regimen variable	Ovarian enlargement, ovarian hyperstimulation, local irritation at injection site, multifetal gestations
Human chorionic gonadotropin (hCG)	Ovulation induction	Direct action on ovarian follicle to stimulate meiosis and rupture of the follicle	5000-10,000 International Units IM 1 day after last dose of menotropins; dosage regimen variable	Local irritation at injection site; headaches, irritability, edema, depression, fatigue
GnRH agonists (nafarelin acetate, leuprolide acetate)	Treatment of endometriosis, uterine fibroids	Desensitization and downward regulation of GnRH receptors of pituitary, resulting in suppression of LH, FSH, and ovarian function	Nafarelin, 200 mcg (1 spray) intranasally twice daily for 6 months; leuprolide acetate 3.75 mg IM every month for 3 to 6 months	Nafarelin—irritation, nosebleeds. Both nafarelin and leuprolide—hot flashes, vaginal dryness, myalgia and arthralgia, headaches, mild bone loss (usually reversible within 12-18 months after treatment)
Progesterone	Treatment of luteal-phase inadequacy	Direct stimulation of endometrium	Vaginal gel 8%, 1 prefilled applicator per day; after ovulation induction, continue through 10-12 weeks of pregnancy	Breast tenderness, local irritation, headaches
GnRH antagonists (ganirelix acetate, cetrorelix acetate)	Controlled ovarian stimulation for infertility treatment	Suppress gonadotropin secretion, inhibit premature LH surges in women undergoing ovarian hyperstimulation	250 mcg daily subcutaneously, usually in the early to midfollicular phase of the menstrual cycle; usually followed by hCG administration	Abdominal pain, headache, vaginal bleeding, irritation at the injection site
Metformin	Restores cyclic ovulation and menses in many women with polycystic ovary disease	Induces ovulation through reducing insulin resistance, thus affecting gonadotropins and androgens; simulates the ovary	Initial dose is 500 mg and titrated up over several weeks to 1500 mg/day; administered orally	Nausea, vomiting, diarrhea, lactic acidosis, liver dysfunction
Letrozole	Ovulation induction	Aromatase inhibitor that inhibits E_2 production, which causes an increase in LH:FHS ratio	2.5- to 5-mg tablets administered orally for 5 days beginning on cycle day 3 to 5	Hot flashes, headaches, breast tenderness; may increase risk of congenital anomalies

Data from American Society for Reproductive Medicine (ASRM). *Medications for inducing ovulation: A patient guide, 2012,* www.asrm.org/Factsheetsandbooklets/; Facts and Comparisons. *A to Z drug facts,* 2013, www.factsandcomparisons.com; and Lobo, R: Infertility: Etiology, diagnostic evaluation, management, prognosis. In Lentz G, Lobo R, Gershenson D, Katz V, editors: *Comprehensive gynecology,* ed 6, Philadelphia, 2012, Mosby.

ovulation induction. Adrenal hyperplasia is treated with prednisone. Any infections present in the infertile couple should be treated with appropriate antimicrobial formulations.

Clomiphene citrate (with the possible addition of metformin) is often the initial pharmacologic treatment of the infertile woman because it is inexpensive and the side effect profile is less than other medications that induce ovulation. There is an increased risk of twins with clomiphene therapy.

The more powerful medications used to induce ovulation include GnRH agonists followed by gonadotropin therapy. These medications are extremely potent and require daily ovarian ultrasonography and monitoring of estradiol levels to prevent hyperstimulation of the ovaries. The incidence of multiple pregnancies with the use of these medications is greater than 25%. Combinations of these medications are used with ART to stimulate ovulation before harvesting eggs.

Drug therapy may be indicated for male infertility. As with women, problems with the thyroid or adrenal glands are corrected with appropriate medications. Infections are identified and treated with antimicrobials. FSH, HMG, and clomiphene may be used to stimulate spermatogenesis in men with hypogonadism. Men who do not respond to these therapies are candidates for intracytoplasmic sperm injection (ICSI), which is a procedure that injects sperm directly into the egg as part of IVF. ICSI has enabled men with very low sperm counts to achieve biologic reproduction.

The primary care provider is responsible for fully informing patients about the prescribed medications. The nurse must be ready to answer patients' questions and confirm their understanding of the drug, its administration, potential side effects, and expected outcomes. Because information varies with each drug, the nurse must consult the medication package inserts, pharmacology references, health care provider, and pharmacist as necessary. The nurse should also provide anticipatory guidance regarding the time given for a medication trial before referral to a specialist in ART would be indicated if the couple wants to continue to attempt to become pregnant.

Surgical Therapies

A number of surgical procedures can be used for problems causing female infertility. Ovarian tumors must be excised. Whenever possible, functional ovarian tissue is left intact. Scar tissue adhesions caused by chronic infections may cover much of the ovary. These adhesions usually necessitate surgery to free and expose the ovary so ovulation can occur.

Hysterosalpingography is useful for identification of tubal obstruction and also for the release of blockage as demonstrated in Fig. 5-2. During laparoscopy delicate adhesions may be divided and removed, and endometrial implants may be destroyed by electrocoagulation or laser, as illustrated in Fig. 5-3. Laparotomy and microsurgery may be required for extensive repair of the damaged tube. Prognosis depends on the degree to which tubal patency and function can be restored. In general laparoscopic surgery for tubal patency is most effective in younger women with distal tubal damage. Older women or those with significant proximal disease should be referred for ARTs that bypass the fallopian tube.

In women with uterine abnormalities reconstructive surgery (e.g., the unification operation for bicornuate uterus) can improve the ability to conceive and carry a fetus to term. Surgical removal of tumors or fibroids involving the endometrium or muscular walls of the uterus could also improve the woman's chance of conceiving and maintaining a pregnancy to viability, depending on the location and size of the fibroid or tumor. Surgical treatment of uterine tumors or

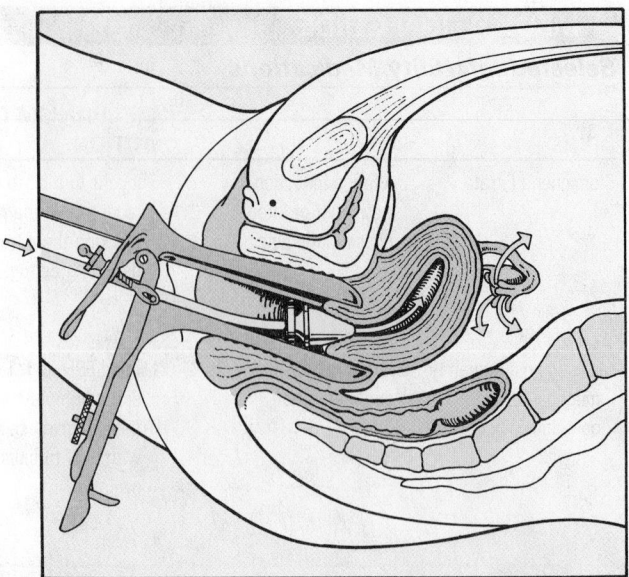

FIG 5-2 Hysterosalpingography. Note that the contrast medium flows through the intrauterine cannula and out through the uterine tubes.

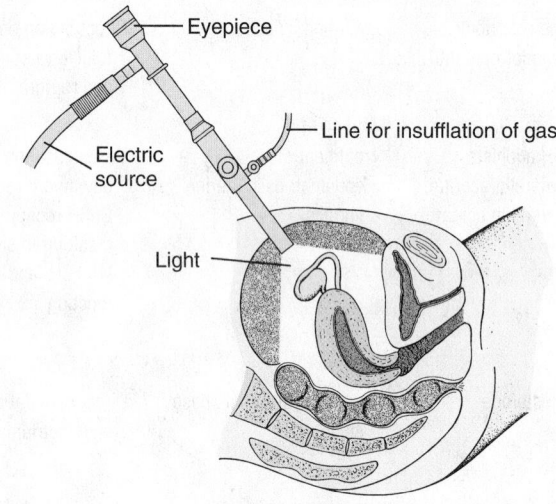

FIG 5-3 Laparoscopy.

maldevelopment that results in successful pregnancy usually necessitates birth by cesarean surgery near term gestation because the enlarging uterus can rupture as a result of weakness in the area of reconstructive surgery.

Chronic inflammation and infection can be eliminated by radial chemocautery (destruction of tissue with chemicals) or thermocautery (destruction of tissue with heat, usually electrical) of the cervix, cryosurgery (destruction of tissue by application of extreme cold, usually liquid nitrogen), or conization (excision of a cone-shaped piece of tissue from the endocervix). When the cervix has been deeply cauterized or frozen or when extensive conization has been performed, the cervix may produce less mucus. Therefore the absence of a mucus bridge from the vagina to the uterus can make sperm migration difficult or impossible. Therapeutic intrauterine insemination may be necessary to carry the sperm directly through the internal os of the cervix.

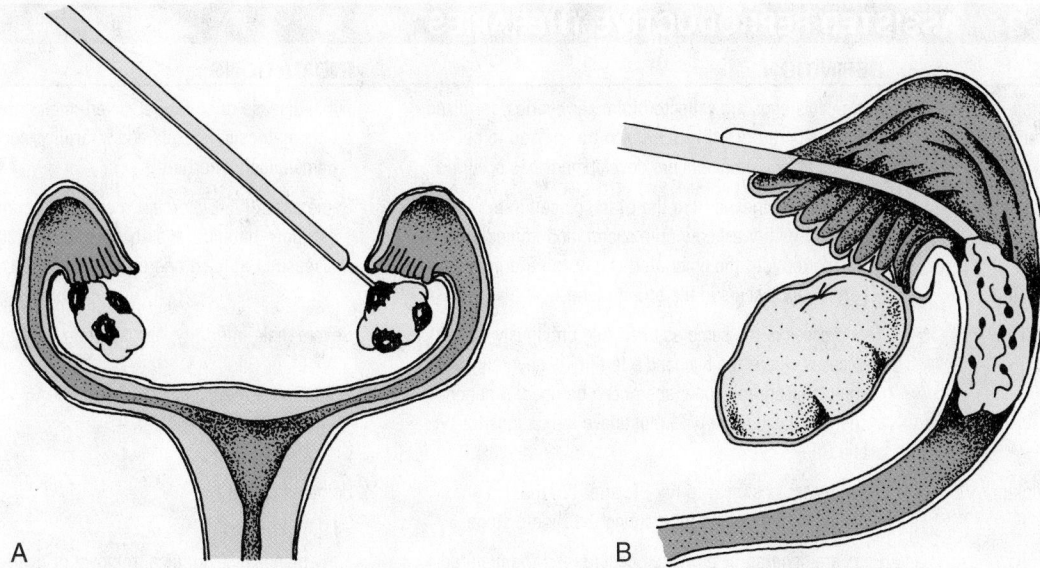

FIG 5-4 Gamete intrafallopian transfer (GIFT). **A,** Through laparoscopy a ripe follicle is located, and fluid containing the egg is removed. **B,** The sperm and egg are placed separately in the uterine tube, where fertilization occurs.

Surgical procedures may also be used for problems causing male infertility. Surgical repair of varicocele has been relatively successful in increasing sperm count but not fertility rates. Microsurgery to reanastomose (restore tubal continuity) the sperm ducts after vasectomy can restore fertility.

Assisted Reproductive Therapies

The Centers for Disease Control and Prevention (CDC) (2012) defines assisted reproductive technology (ART) as fertility treatments in which both eggs and sperm are handled. In general these treatments involve removing the eggs from the woman, fertilizing the eggs in the laboratory, and returning the embryo or embryos to the woman or surrogate carrier. The CDC reported that in 2010 there were approximately 147,260 ART cycles with 47,090 births and 61,564 infants (some multiple births) from these cycles. Although the use of ART is still relatively rare compared to the potential demand, its use has doubled over the past decade. Births that were conceived through ART comprise over 1% of all infants born in the United States every year.

Some of the ARTs for treatment of infertility include in vitro fertilization–embryo transfer (IVF-ET), gamete intrafallopian transfer (GIFT) (Fig. 5-4), zygote intrafallopian transfer (ZIFT), ovum transfer (oocyte donation), embryo adoption, embryo hosting and surrogate motherhood, therapeutic donor insemination (TDI), intracytoplasmic sperm injection (ICSI), assisted embryo hatching, and preimplantation genetic diagnosis (PGD). Table 5-2 describes these procedures and the possible indications for ARTs. Donor sperm and donor eggs can be used with ARTs. In addition, surrogates may carry the couple's biologic child. ARTs are associated with many ethical and legal issues (Box 5-7).

The lack of or misleading information about success rates and the risks and benefits of treatment alternatives prevent couples from making informed decisions. Nurses can provide information so couples have an accurate understanding of their chances for a successful pregnancy and live birth. Nurses also can provide anticipatory guidance about the moral and ethical dilemmas regarding the use of ARTs. If a couple is fortunate enough to have multiple embryos available, they may choose to preserve these for later implantation, which could have legal implications.

> **LEGAL TIP: Cryopreservation of Human Embryos**
> Couples who have excess embryos frozen for later transfer must be fully informed before consenting to the procedure and make decisions regarding the disposal of embryos in the event of death or divorce and a decision at a later time if they no longer want the embryos.

Complications

Other than the established risks associated with laparoscopy and general anesthesia, few risks are associated with IVF-ET, GIFT, and ZIFT. The more common transvaginal needle aspiration requires only local or intravenous analgesia. Congenital anomalies occur no more frequently than among naturally conceived embryos. Multiple gestations are more likely and are associated with increased risks for both the mother and fetuses. Nevertheless, ectopic pregnancies do occur more often and pose significant maternal risk. There is no increase in maternal or perinatal complications with TDI and the same frequencies of anomalies (about 5%) and obstetric complications (between 5% and 10%) that accompany natural insemination (through sexual intercourse).

Preimplantation Genetic Diagnosis

PGD is a form of early genetic testing designed to eliminate embryos with serious genetic diseases before implantation through one of the ARTs and to avoid future termination of pregnancy for genetic reasons. Micromanipulation allows removal of a single cell from a multicellular embryo for genetic study (i.e., embryo biopsy) (Fritz and Speroff, 2011c). PGD is used clinically in over 20 centers around the world. Couples must be counseled about their options and choices and the implications of their choices when genetic analysis is considered.

TABLE 5-2 ASSISTED REPRODUCTIVE THERAPIES

PROCEDURE	DEFINITION	INDICATIONS
In vitro fertilization–embryo transfer (IVF-ET)	A woman's eggs are collected from her ovaries, fertilized in the laboratory with sperm, and transferred to her uterus after normal embryo development has occurred.	Tubal disease or blockage; severe male infertility; endometriosis; unexplained infertility; cervical factor; immunologic infertility
Gamete intrafallopian transfer (GIFT)	Oocytes are retrieved from the ovary, placed in a catheter with washed motile sperm, and immediately transferred into the fimbriated end of the uterine tube. Fertilization occurs in the uterine tube.	Same as for IVF-ET, except there must be normal tubal anatomy, patency, and absence of previous tubal disease in at least one uterine tube
IVF-ET and GIFT with donor sperm	This process is the same as described previously except in cases where the husband's fertility is severely compromised and donor sperm can be used; if donor sperm are used, the wife must have indications for IVF and GIFT.	Severe male infertility; azoospermia; indications for IVF-ET or GIFT
Zygote intrafallopian transfer (ZIFT)	This process is similar to IVF-ET; after IVF the ova are placed in one uterine tube during the zygote stage.	Same as for GIFT
Donor oocyte	Eggs are donated by an IVF procedure, and the donated eggs are inseminated. The embryos are transferred into the recipient's uterus, which is hormonally prepared with estrogen/progesterone therapy.	Early menopause; surgical removal of ovaries; congenitally absent ovaries; autosomal or sex-linked disorders; lack of fertilization in repeated IVF attempts because of subtle oocyte abnormalities or defects in oocyte-spermatozoa interaction
Donor embryo (embryo adoption)	A donated embryo is transferred to the uterus of an infertile woman at the appropriate time (normal or induced) of the menstrual cycle.	Infertility not resolved by less aggressive forms of therapy; absence of ovaries; male partner azoospermic or severely compromised
Gestational carrier (embryo host); surrogate mother	A couple undertakes an IVF cycle, and the embryo(s) is/are transferred to another woman's uterus (the carrier), who has contracted with the couple to carry the baby to term. The carrier has no genetic investment in the child. Surrogate motherhood is a process by which a woman is inseminated with semen from the infertile woman's partner and then carries the baby until birth.	Congenital absence or surgical removal of uterus; reproductively impaired uterus, myomas, uterine adhesions, or other congenital abnormalities; medical condition that might be life threatening during pregnancy (e.g., diabetes; immunologic problems; or severe heart, kidney, or liver disease)
Therapeutic donor insemination (TDI)	Donor sperm are used to inseminate the female partner.	Male partner is azoospermic or has very low sperm count; couple has genetic defect; male partner has antisperm antibodies
Intracytoplasmic sperm injection	One sperm cell is selected to be injected directly into the egg to achieve fertilization. It is used with IVF.	Same as TDI
Assisted hatching	The zona pellucida is penetrated chemically or manually to create an opening for the dividing embryo to hatch and implant into the uterine wall.	Recurrent miscarriages; to improve implantation rate in women with previously unsuccessful IVF attempts; advanced age

Data from American Society for Reproductive Medicine: *Assisted reproductive technologies,* 2011, www.asrm.org.

BOX 5-7 ISSUES TO BE ADDRESSED BY INFERTILE COUPLES BEFORE TREATMENT

- Risks of multiple gestation
- Possible need for multifetal reduction
- Possible need for donor oocytes, sperm, or embryos or for gestational carrier (surrogate mother)
- Whether or how to disclose facts of conception to offspring
- Freezing embryos for later use
- Possible risks of long-term effects of medications and treatment on women, children, and families

Adoption

Couples may choose to build their family by adopting children who are not their own biologically. With increased availability of birth control and abortion and an increase in single mothers who choose to keep their babies, the availability of healthy newborn infants in the United States is limited. Infants with diverse ethnic and racial heritages, infants with special needs, older children, and foreign adoptions are other options (Fig. 5-5).

Couples who decide to adopt a child have decided that being a parent is more important than the actual process of birthing the child. The birth process is a very small aspect of having a baby and becoming a parent. So much emphasis is placed on being pregnant and having a child composed of one's own genetic makeup that the

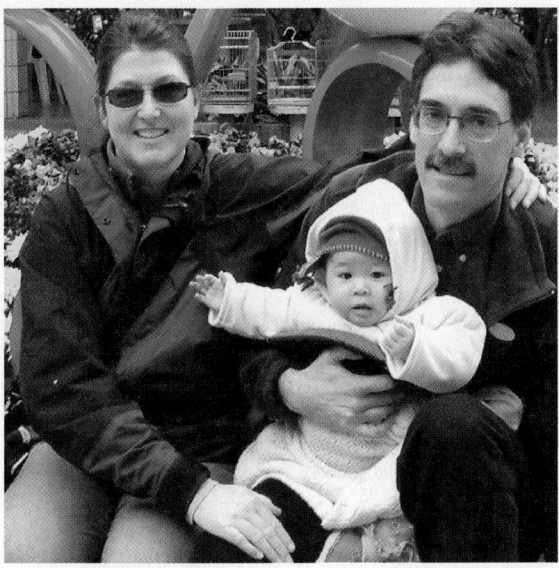

FIG 5-5 After two miscarriages this couple chose foreign adoption. (Courtesy Shannon Perry, Phoenix, AZ.)

COMMUNITY FOCUS

Education for Contraceptive Use

Nurses provide discharge planning after childbirth; they commonly staff family planning clinics and provide contraceptive information to those patients and others in the community. Education concerning contraceptive use in the postpartum period is a common component of discharge planning in many countries, with wide variation among health care delivery systems. Education at this time assumes women's receptiveness to information about contraception and that education or receptiveness to such information could be less at a later period. However, clinical trials have not demonstrated that education in the immediate postpartum period is effective. When assessing effectiveness of contraceptive education, attendance at family planning clinics, cessation of breastfeeding, knowledge about contraception, unplanned pregnancies, and satisfaction with care are factors that should be included. The content, timing, and organization of contraceptive education offered in the postpartum period and throughout the couple's lifetime need to be addressed.

focus of the reason to have a child is not clear. The question to be answered by couples who want to adopt is, "Do you want to give birth to a baby, or do you want to become parents?"

CONTRACEPTION

The CDC noted that the capability of Americans to engage in effective family planning as a result of the modern era of contraception was one of the 10 greatest public health achievements of the 20th century. Nevertheless, nearly half of all U.S. pregnancies are not planned (Finer and Zolna, 2011). Among adolescent women approximately 80% of those who became pregnant did not intend to do so (Fritz and Speroff, 2011b). The nurse can play a vital role in preventing unwanted pregnancy through counseling and education regarding family planning, contraception, and effective birth control. Family planning is the conscious decision about when to conceive or to avoid pregnancy throughout the reproductive years. Contraception is defined as the intentional prevention of pregnancy during sexual intercourse. Birth control is the device and/or practice used to decrease the risk of conceiving or bearing offspring.

With the wide assortment of birth control options available, it is possible for a woman to use several different contraceptive methods at various stages throughout her fertile years. Nurses interact with the couple to compare and contrast available contraceptive options. Factors to consider include reliability, relative cost of the method, any protection from STIs, the individual's comfort level with the method, and the partner's willingness to use a particular birth control method. Those who use contraception can still be at risk for pregnancy if their choice of contraceptive method results in a method that is not used correctly. Providing adequate instruction about how to use a contraceptive method, when to use a backup method, and when to use emergency contraception (EC) can decrease the risk of unintended pregnancy. The Community Focus box presents information about contraceptive education.

CARE MANAGEMENT

A multidisciplinary approach may help a woman choose and correctly use an appropriate contraceptive method. Nurses,

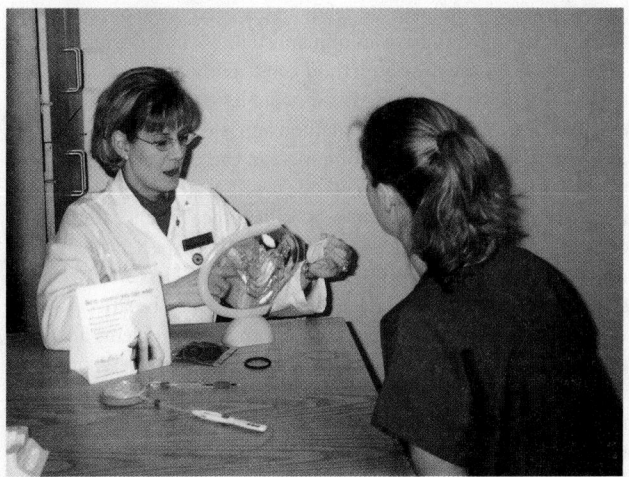

FIG 5-6 Nurse counseling woman about contraceptive methods. (Courtesy Dee Lowdermilk, Chapel Hill, NC.)

nurse-midwives, nurse practitioners, other advanced practice nurses, and physicians have the knowledge and expertise to help a woman make decisions about contraception that will satisfy her personal, social, cultural, and interpersonal needs.

Assessment for the couple desiring contraception involves assessment of the woman's reproductive history (menstrual, obstetric, gynecologic, contraceptive), physical examination, and sometimes current laboratory tests. The nurse must determine the woman's knowledge about reproduction, contraception, and STIs and her sexual partner's commitment to any particular method. Fig. 5-6 illustrates contraceptive counseling. The nurse obtains information about the frequency of coitus, number of sexual partners (present and past), and any objections that she or her partner might have about specific birth control methods. In addition, the nurse must determine a woman's willingness to touch her genitals. Religious and cultural factors may influence a couple's choice regarding a particular contraceptive method. The couple may believe in certain reproductive myths. For example, 30% of all adolescent pregnancies were in women who engaged in unprotected intercourse because of the perception that they could not get pregnant. Unbiased patient

BOX 5-8 FACTORS AFFECTING CONTRACEPTIVE METHOD EFFECTIVENESS

- Frequency of intercourse
- Motivation to prevent pregnancy
- Understanding of how to use the method
- Adherence to the method
- Provision of short- or long-term protection
- Likelihood of pregnancy for the individual woman
- Consistent use of the method

---

teaching is fundamental to initiating and maintaining any form of contraception. The nurse counters myths with facts, clarifies misinformation, and fills in gaps in knowledge. The ideal contraceptive should be safe, easily available, economical, acceptable, simple to use, and promptly reversible. Although no method may ever achieve all of these objectives, significant advances in the development of new contraceptive technologies have occurred over the past 30 years.

Contraceptive failure rate refers to the percentage of contraceptive users expected to have an unplanned pregnancy during the first year even when they use a method consistently and correctly. Contraceptive effectiveness varies from couple to couple and depends on both the properties of the method and the characteristics of the user (Box 5-8). Effectiveness of a method can be expressed as theoretic (i.e., how effective the method is with perfect use) and typical (i.e., how effective the method is with typical use). Failure rates decrease over time, either because a user gains experience with and uses a method more appropriately or because the less effective users stop using the method. Safety of a method may be affected by a woman's medical history (e.g., thromboembolic problems and contraceptive methods containing estrogen). Nevertheless, in most instances pregnancy would be more dangerous to the woman with medical problems than a particular contraceptive method. In addition, many contraceptive methods have health promotion effects. Barrier methods such as the male condom offer some protection from acquiring STIs, and oral contraceptives lower the incidence of ovarian and endometrial cancer.

Following assessment and analysis, the couple determines possible contraceptive methods that are appropriate for their unique situation. Factors to consider when determining a contraceptive method are effectiveness, convenience, affordability, duration of action of method, reversibility of method, time of return to fertility, effects on uterine bleeding patterns, side effects, adverse events, health promotion effects of methods, effect of method on transmission of STIs, and medical contraindications for use.

The most effective reversible contraceptive methods at preventing pregnancy are the long–acting, reversible contraceptive (LARC) methods (e.g., contraceptive implants, intrauterine contraception). With these methods theoretic and typical pregnancy rates are the same because the method requires no user intervention after correct insertion. Effective methods include those that prevent pregnancy through exogenous hormones (estrogen and/or progestins) such as contraceptive injections, oral contraceptive pills, contraceptive patches, and vaginal rings. Each of these methods involves user interventions; thus typical-use pregnancy rates are higher than pregnancy rates with perfect use. The least effective contraceptive methods include the barrier methods and natural family planning. Examples include condoms, diaphragms, cervical caps, spermicides, withdrawal, and periodic abstinence during perceived ovulation.

Contraception for Adolescents

Maria is a 16-year-old Hispanic female who comes to the family planning clinic seeking contraception. She has recently become sexually active and tells the nurse that she is concerned that her mother will find out. She also has many questions about the type of contraception to use. She seeks the nurse's advice to help in her decision making.

1. Evidence—Is there sufficient evidence to draw conclusions about what advice to give Maria?
2. Assumptions—What assumptions can be made about contraception for adolescents:
   a. Types of contraception
   b. Legal issues
   c. Implications of culture on choice
3. What implications and priorities for nursing care can be drawn at this time?
4. Does the evidence objectively support your conclusion?

Effectiveness rates for these methods vary from user to user, depending on correct application of the method and consistency of use.

Expected outcomes related to contraceptive counseling are that the couple will verbalize understanding about appropriate contraceptive methods, state they are satisfied with the method chosen, use the method correctly and consistently, experience no adverse sequelae as a result of the chosen contraceptive method, and prevent unplanned pregnancy. The nurse assists with obtaining appropriate informed consent concerning contraception or sterilization, provides appropriate education to the couple, and documents the couple's understanding of the contraceptive method chosen. Evaluation involves achievement of patient-centered outcomes when the couple engage in effective use of the chosen contraceptive device, experience no adverse sequelae, and achieve pregnancy only when they desire to do so.

Methods of Contraception

The following discussion of contraceptive methods provides the nurse with information needed for patient teaching. After implementing the appropriate teaching for contraceptive use, the nurse supervises return demonstrations and practice to assess patient understanding (see Critical Thinking Case Study). The couple is given written instructions, telephone numbers, and/or email contact information for questions. If the woman has difficulty understanding written instructions, she and her partner, if available, are offered graphic material, a telephone number to call as necessary, and an opportunity to return for further instruction.

Coitus Interruptus

Coitus interruptus (withdrawal) involves the male partner withdrawing his penis from the woman's vagina before he ejaculates. Although coitus interruptus has been criticized as being an ineffective method of contraception, it is a good choice for couples who do not have another contraceptive available. Effectiveness is similar to barrier methods and depends on the man's ability to withdraw his penis before ejaculation. The percentage of women who experience an unintended pregnancy within the first year of typical use (failure rate) of withdrawal is about 27% (Kowal, 2011). Coitus interruptus does not protect against STIs or human immunodeficiency virus (HIV) infection.

Fertility Awareness Methods

Fertility awareness methods (FAMs) of contraception depend on identifying the beginning and end of the fertile period of the menstrual cycle. When women who want to use FAMs are educated about the menstrual cycle, three phases are identified:

1. Infertile phase: Before ovulation
2. Fertile phase: About 5 to 7 days around the middle of the cycle, including several days before and during ovulation and the day after ovulation
3. Infertile phase: After ovulation

Although ovulation can be unpredictable in many women, teaching the woman about how she can directly observe her fertility patterns is an empowering tool. In addition, knowledge about the signs and symptoms of ovulation can be very helpful when the couple desires pregnancy. There are nearly a dozen categories of FAMs. To prevent pregnancy each one uses a combination of charts, records, calculations, tools, observations, and either abstinence (natural family planning [NFP]) or barrier methods of birth control during the fertile period of the menstrual cycle. The charts and calculations associated with these methods can also be used to increase the likelihood of detecting the optimal timing of intercourse to achieve conception.

Advantages of these methods include low-to-no cost, absence of chemicals and hormones, and lack of alteration in the menstrual flow pattern. Disadvantages of FAMs include adherence needed for strict record keeping, unintentional interference from external influences that may alter the woman's core body temperature and vaginal secretions, decreased effectiveness in women with irregular cycles (particularly adolescents who have not established regular patterns of ovulation), decreased spontaneity of coitus, and the necessity of attending possibly time-consuming training sessions by qualified instructors. The typical failure rate for most FAMs is 24% during the first year of use (Trussell and Guthrie, 2011). FAMs do not protect against STIs or HIV infection.

FAMs involve several techniques to identify high risk, fertile days. The following discussion includes the most common techniques.

Natural Family Planning (Periodic Abstinence). Natural family planning (NFP), or periodic abstinence, provides contraception by using methods that rely on avoiding intercourse during fertile days. NFP methods are the only methods of contraception acceptable to the Roman Catholic Church. Signs and symptoms of fertility awareness most commonly used with abstinence are menstrual bleeding, cervical mucus, and basal body temperature. Development and marketing of ovulation predictor kits have also been very helpful for couples who choose NFP. Several application products have been developed for smart phones, which make FAM record tracking convenient and portable.

The human ovum can be fertilized no later than 16 to 24 hours after ovulation. Motile sperm have been recovered from the uterus and oviducts as long as 7 days after coitus. However, their ability to fertilize the ovum probably lasts no longer than 24 hours. Pregnancy is unlikely to occur if a couple abstains from intercourse for 4 days before and 3 or 4 days after ovulation (fertile period). Unprotected intercourse on the other days of the cycle (safe period) should not result in pregnancy. Nevertheless the exact time of ovulation cannot be predicted accurately, and couples may find it difficult to abstain from sexual intercourse for several days before and after ovulation. Women with irregular menstrual periods have the greatest risk of failure with this form of contraception.

Calendar Rhythm Method. Practice of the calendar rhythm method is based on the number of days in each cycle, counting from the first day of the menstrual cycle (first day of menstrual vaginal

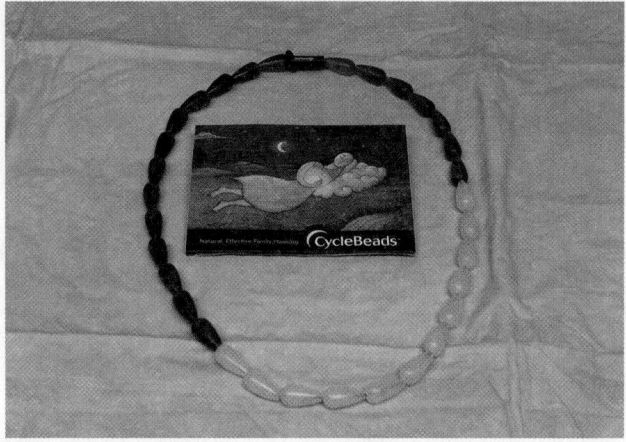

FIG 5-7 CycleBeads. *Red bead* marks the first day of the menstrual cycle. *White beads* mark days that are likely to be fertile days; therefore unprotected intercourse should be avoided. *Brown beads* are days when pregnancy is unlikely and unprotected intercourse is permitted. (Courtesy Dee Lowdermilk, Chapel Hill, NC.)

bleeding). The fertile period is determined after accurately recording the lengths of menstrual cycles for 6 months. The beginning of the fertile period is estimated by subtracting 18 days from the length of the shortest cycle. The end of the fertile period is determined by subtracting 11 days from the length of the longest cycle. If the shortest cycle is 24 days and the longest is 30 days, application of the formula to calculate the fertile period is as follows:

$$\text{Shortest cycle, } 24 - 18 = \text{day } 6$$

$$\text{Longest cycle, } 30 - 11 = \text{day } 19$$

To avoid conception the couple would abstain during the fertile period, days 6 through 19.

If the woman has very regular cycles of 28 days each, the formula indicates the fertile days to be as follows:

$$\text{Shortest cycle, } 28 - 18 = \text{day } 10$$

$$\text{Longest cycle, } 38 - 11 = \text{day } 17$$

To avoid conception the couple would abstain from days 10 through 17 because ovulation occurs on day 14 ± 2 days. A major drawback of the calendar method is that the couple is attempting to predict future events with past data. The unpredictability of the menstrual cycle is also not taken into consideration. The calendar rhythm method is most useful as an adjunct to the basal body temperature or cervical mucus method.

Standard Days Method. The standard days method (SDM) is essentially a modified form of the calendar rhythm method that has a "fixed" number of days of fertility for each cycle (i.e., days 8 to 19). A CycleBeads necklace (i.e., a color-coded string of beads) can be purchased as a concrete tool to track fertility (Fig. 5-7) or as a smart phone application. Day 1 of the menstrual flow is counted as the first day to begin counting. Women who use this device are taught to avoid unprotected intercourse on days 8 to 19 (white beads on CycleBeads necklace). Although this method is useful to women whose cycles are 26 to 32 days long, it is unreliable for those who have longer or shorter cycles (CycleBeads, 2012).

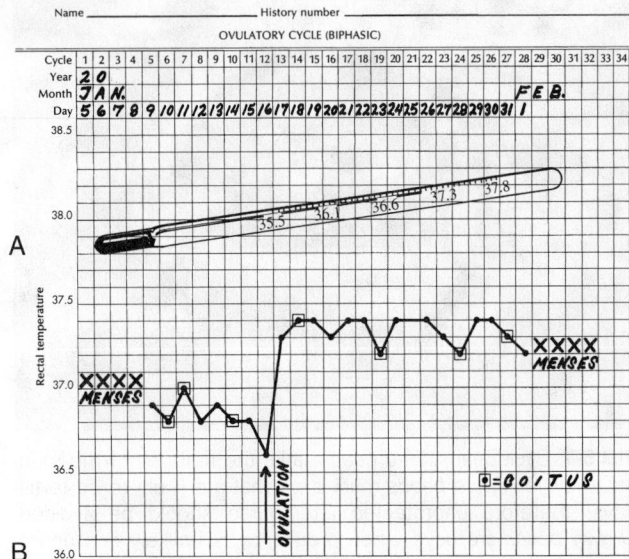

FIG 5-8 A, Special thermometer for recording basal body temperature, marked in tenths to enable person to read more easily. **B,** Basal temperature record shows decrease and sharp increase at time of ovulation. Biphasic curve indicates ovulatory cycle. A digital thermometer may also be used.

Basal Body Temperature Method. The basal body temperature (BBT) is the lowest body temperature of a healthy person, taken immediately after waking and before getting out of bed. The BBT usually varies from 36.2° to 36.3° C during menses and for approximately 5 to 7 days afterward (Fig. 5-8).

About the time of ovulation a slight drop in temperature (approximately 0.5° C) may occur in some women, but others may have no decrease at all. After ovulation, in concert with the increasing progesterone levels of the early luteal phase of the cycle, the BBT increases slightly (approximately 0.4° to 0.8° C). The temperature remains on an elevated plateau until 2 to 4 days before menstruation. Then BBT decreases to the low levels recorded during the previous cycle unless pregnancy has occurred. In pregnant women the temperature remains elevated. If ovulation fails to occur, the pattern of lower body temperature continues throughout the cycle.

To use this method the fertile period is defined as the day of first temperature drop, or first elevation, through 3 consecutive days of elevated temperature. Abstinence begins the first day of menstrual bleeding and lasts through 3 consecutive days of sustained temperature rise (at least 0.2° C). The decrease and subsequent increase in temperature are referred to as the thermal shift. When the temperatures of the entire month are recorded on a graph, the pattern described is more apparent. It is more difficult to perceive day-to-day variations without the entire picture (see Guidelines box). Either a glass mercury thermometer or a digital thermometer may be used for BBT, but the thermometer must measure the temperature within one tenth of a degree. The glass mercury thermometer needs no batteries but is fragile and can break. A digital thermometer requires batteries but may have a history recall function and an audible beep when the temperature assessment is finished. Digital thermometers that monitor temperature throughout the day combined with an accelerometer to monitor movement have been cleared for use by the Food and Drug Administration (FDA). These devices can be wirelessly uploaded to a computer through a companion device. Their use in FAM needs further research.

GUIDELINES

Basal Body Temperature

- Discuss basal body temperature (BBT) with the woman.
- Show the woman a diagram depicting the phases of the menstrual cycle.
- Discuss the hormones in the woman's body that are responsible for her menstrual cycle and ovulation. Leave time for questions.
- Show the woman a sample BBT graph (see Fig. 5-8) and the biphasic line seen in ovulatory cycles.
- Show the woman the BBT thermometer and how it is calibrated.
- Provide a demonstration.
- Encourage the woman to demonstrate taking and reading the thermometer and graphing the temperature while the nurse watches.
- Encourage the woman to start a log to keep track of any other activity that might interfere with her true BBT.

Infection, fatigue, less than 3 hours of sleep per night, awakening late, and anxiety may cause temperature fluctuations and alter the expected pattern. If a new BBT thermometer is purchased, this fact is noted on the chart because the readings may vary slightly. Jet lag, alcohol taken the evening before, or sleeping in a heated waterbed must also be noted on the chart because each affects the BBT. Therefore the BBT alone is not a reliable method of predicting ovulation.

Cervical Mucus Ovulation-Detection Method. The cervical mucus ovulation-detection method (i.e., Billings method or Creighton model ovulation method) requires that the woman recognize and interpret the cyclic changes in the amount and consistency of cervical mucus that characterize her own unique pattern of changes at the time of ovulation. Cervical mucus changes before and during ovulation to facilitate and promote the viability and motility of sperm. Without adequate cervical mucus, coitus does not result in conception. This method requires that a woman check the quantity and character of mucus on the vulva or introitus with her fingers or tissue paper each day for several months. This way she can learn how her cervical mucus responds to ovulation during her menstrual cycles. To ensure an accurate assessment of changes, the cervical mucus should be free from semen, contraceptive gels or foams, and blood or discharge from vaginal infections for at least one full cycle. Other factors that create difficulty in identifying mucus changes include douches and vaginal deodorants, being in the sexually aroused state (which thins the mucus), and taking medications such as antihistamines (which dry the mucus). Intercourse is considered safe without restriction beginning the fourth day after the last day of wet, clear, slippery mucus, which would indicate that ovulation has occurred 2 to 3 days previously.

Some women find this method unacceptable if they are uncomfortable touching their genitals. Whether or not a woman wants to use this method for contraception, it is to her advantage to learn to recognize mucus characteristics at ovulation (see Guidelines box). Self-evaluation of cervical mucus can be highly accurate and useful diagnostically for any of the following purposes:

- To alert the couple to the reestablishment of ovulation while breastfeeding and after discontinuation of oral contraception
- To note anovulatory cycles at any time and at the beginning of menopause
- To help couples plan a pregnancy

GUIDELINES

Cervical Mucus Characteristics

Setting the Stage

- Show charts of the menstrual cycle along with changes in the cervical mucus.
- Have the woman practice assessing mucus using raw egg white.
- Supply her with a basal body temperature (BBT) log and graph if she does not already have one.
- Explain that the assessment of cervical mucus characteristics is best when mucus is not mixed with semen, contraceptive jellies or foams, or discharge from infections.

Content Related to Cervical Mucus

- Explain to the woman (or couple) how cervical mucus changes throughout the menstrual cycle.
- Right before ovulation the watery, thin, clear mucus becomes more abundant and thick. It feels like a lubricant and can be stretched approximately

5 cm between the thumb and forefinger; this is called *spinnbarkeit*. This characteristic indicates the period of maximum fertility. Sperm deposited in this type of mucus can survive until ovulation occurs.

Assessment Technique

- Stress that good hand washing is imperative to begin and end all self-assessment.
- Start observation from last day of menstrual flow.
- Assess cervical mucus several times a day for several cycles. Mucus can be obtained from vaginal introitus; there is no need to reach into vagina to cervix.
- Record findings on the same record on which her BBT is entered.

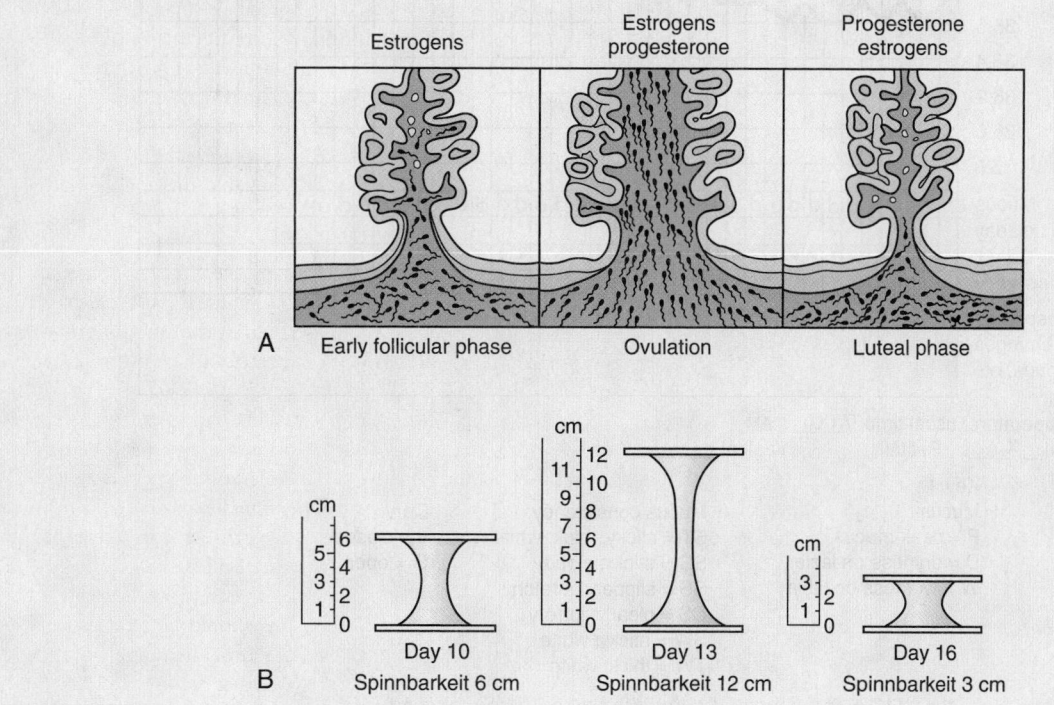

Symptothermal Method. The symptothermal method combines the BBT and cervical mucus methods with awareness of secondary phase–related symptoms of menstrual cycle. The woman gains fertility awareness as she learns the psychologic and physiologic symptoms that mark the phases of her cycle. Secondary symptoms include increased libido, midcycle spotting, mittelschmerz (cramplike pain before ovulation), pelvic fullness or tenderness, and vulvar fullness.

The woman is taught to palpate her cervix to assess for changes indicating ovulation: the cervical os dilates slightly, the cervix softens and rises in the vagina, and cervical mucus is copious and slippery. The woman notes days on which coitus, changes in routine, illness, and other changes that might affect BBT have occurred (Fig. 5-9). Calendar calculations and cervical mucus changes are used to estimate the onset of the fertile period; changes

in cervical mucus or the BBT are used to estimate the end of the fertile period.

TwoDay Method of Family Planning. Based on monitoring and the recording of cervical secretions, an algorithm for identifying the fertile window has been developed by the Institute for Reproductive Health at Georgetown University (Institute for Reproductive Health Georgetown University, 2012; Jennings and Burke, 2011). The TwoDay algorithm appears to be simpler to teach, learn, and use than other natural methods. Results suggest that the algorithm can be an effective alternative for low-literacy populations or for programs that find current NFP methods too time consuming or otherwise not feasible to incorporate within their services. Two questions are posed. Each day the woman is to ask herself, (1) "Did I note secretions today?" and (2) "Did I note secretions yesterday?" If the answer to either question is yes, she should avoid coitus or use a backup

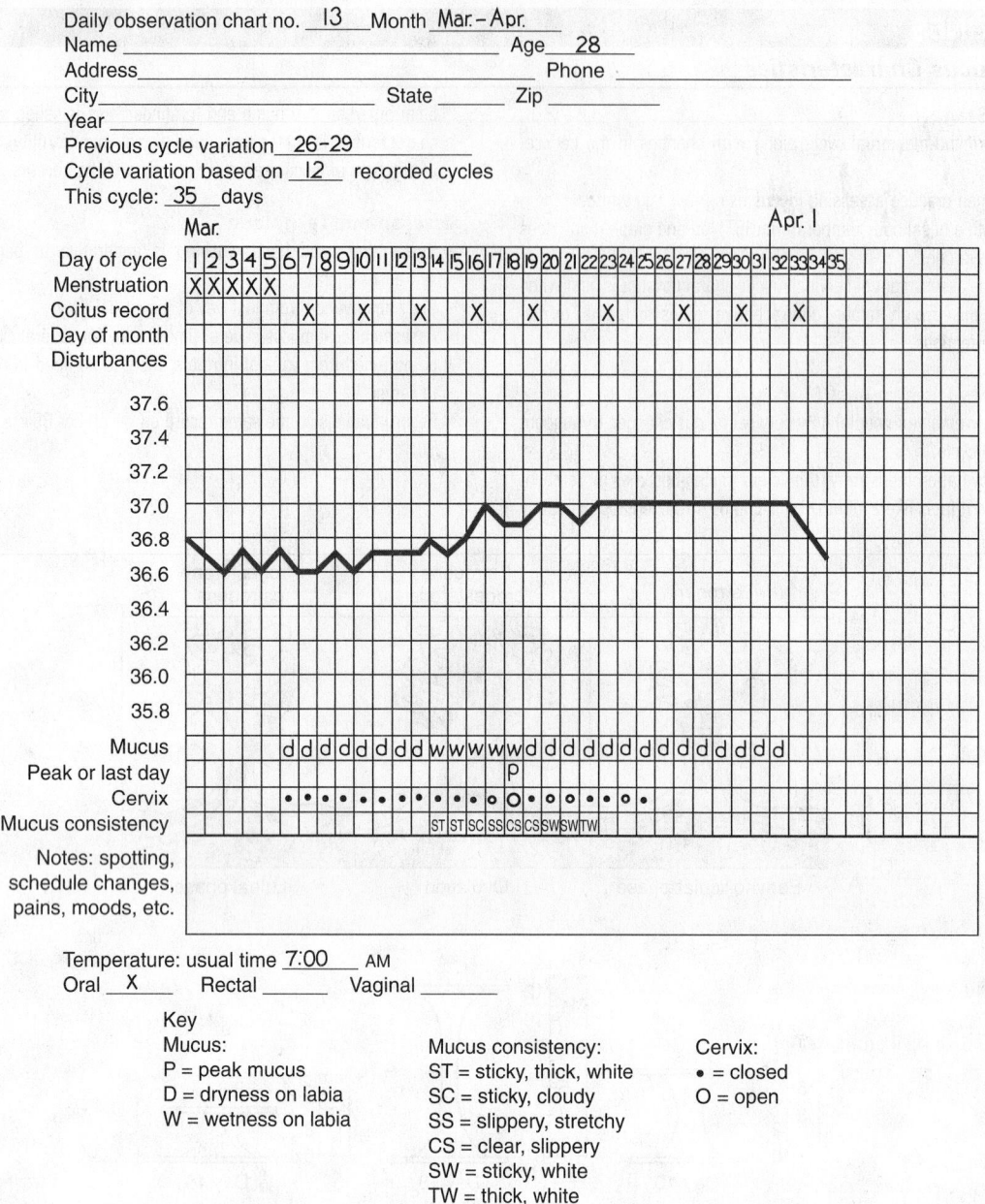

Daily observation chart no. __13__ Month __Mar.-Apr.__
Name _____ Age __28__
Address_____ Phone _____
City_____ State _____ Zip _____
Year _____
Previous cycle variation __26-29__
Cycle variation based on __12__ recorded cycles
This cycle: __35__ days

Temperature: usual time __7:00__ AM
Oral __X__   Rectal _____   Vaginal _____

Key
Mucus:
P = peak mucus
D = dryness on labia
W = wetness on labia

Mucus consistency:
ST = sticky, thick, white
SC = sticky, cloudy
SS = slippery, stretchy
CS = clear, slippery
SW = sticky, white
TW = thick, white

Cervix:
• = closed
O = open

FIG 5-9 Example of completed symptothermal chart.

method of birth control. If the answer to both questions is no, her probability of getting pregnant is low. Further studies are needed to determine the efficacy of the TwoDay algorithm in avoiding pregnancy and to assess its acceptability to users and providers.

Home Predictor Test Kits for Ovulation. Although the methods previously discussed are characteristic of ovulation, they do not prove that ovulation actually occurred or indicate the exact timing. The urine predictor test for ovulation is a major addition to the NFP and fertility-awareness methods to help women who want to plan the time of their pregnancies and for those who are trying to conceive (Fig. 5-10). The urine predictor test for ovulation detects the sudden surge of LH that occurs approximately 12 to 24 hours before ovulation. Unlike BBT, this test is not affected by illness, emotions, or physical activity. For home use a test kit contains sufficient

material for several days' testing during each cycle. A positive response indicating an LH surge is noted by a color change that is easy to interpret. Directions for use of urine predictor test kits vary with the manufacturer.

The Marquette Model. The Marquette Model (MM) is a natural family planning method that was developed through the Marquette University College of Nursing Institute for Natural Family Planning (Fehring, Schneider, and Barron, 2008). The MM uses cervical monitoring along with the ClearPlan Easy Fertility Monitor. The ClearPlan monitor is a handheld device that uses test strips to measure urinary metabolites of estrogen and LH. The monitor provides the user with "low," "high," and "peak" fertility readings. The MM incorporates the use of the monitor as an aid to learning NFP and fertility awareness.

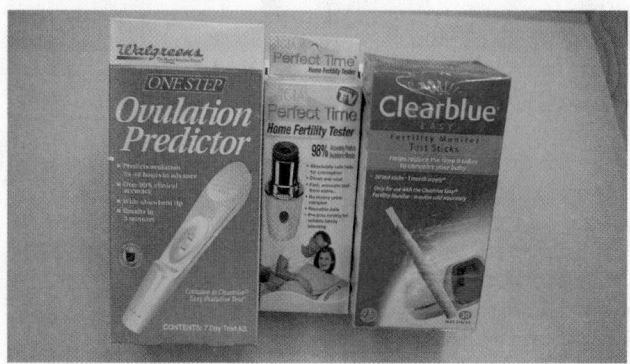

FIG 5-10 Examples of ovulation predictor tests. (Courtesy Shannon Perry, Phoenix, AZ.)

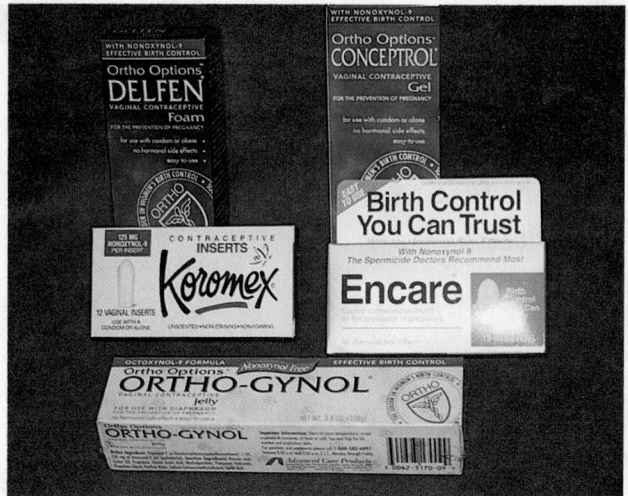

FIG 5-11 Spermicides. (Courtesy Marjorie Pyle, RNC, Life Circle, Costa Mesa, CA.)

Research continues on the efficacy of available home test kits and devices for the prevention of pregnancy (Jennings and Burke, 2011).

Breastfeeding: Lactational Amenorrhea Method. Lactational amenorrhea method (LAM) can be a highly effective, *temporary* method of birth control. LAM is more popular in underdeveloped countries and traditional societies in which breastfeeding is used to prolong birth intervals. The method has seen limited use in the United States because most American women do not establish breastfeeding patterns that provide maximum protection against pregnancy (Kennedy and Trussell, 2011a).

When the infant suckles at the mother's breast, a surge of prolactin is released. Prolactin inhibits estrogen production and suppresses ovulation and the return of menses. LAM works best if the mother is exclusively breastfeeding, if she has not had a menstrual flow since birth, and if the infant is under 6 months of age. Effectiveness is enhanced by frequent feedings at intervals of less than 4 hours during the day and no more than 6 hours during the night, long duration of each feeding, and no bottle supplementation. The woman should be counseled that disruption of the breastfeeding pattern or formula supplementation can increase the risk of pregnancy. The typical failure rate is 2% (Kennedy and Trussell, 2011b).

Barrier Methods

Barrier contraceptives have gained in popularity not only as a contraceptive method but also as protection against the spread of STIs such as human papilloma virus and herpes simplex virus (HSV). Some male condoms and female vaginal methods provide a physical barrier to several STIs, and some male condoms provide protection against HIV. Spermicides serve as chemical barriers against semen and inhibit the ability of sperm to fertilize the ovum.

The nurse should remember that any user of a barrier method of contraception must also be aware of emergency contraception (EC) options in case there is a failure of the method. An example of a barrier method failure would be if a condom broke during intercourse. In this instance EC would be indicated to prevent unplanned pregnancy.

Spermicides. Spermicides such as nonoxynol-9 (N-9) work by reducing the mobility of the sperm. The chemicals attack the sperm flagella and body, thereby preventing the sperm from reaching the cervical os. N-9, the most commonly used spermicidal chemical in the United States, is a surfactant that destroys the sperm cell membrane. Results from data analyses now suggest that frequent use

(more than 2 times a day) of N-9 or the use of N-9 as a lubricant during anal intercourse may increase the transmission of HIV and can cause lesions (Trussell and Guthrie, 2011). There is no evidence that the addition of spermicides to male condoms decreases the risk of subsequent pregnancy. Women with high risk behaviors that increase their likelihood of contracting HIV and other STIs are advised to avoid the use of spermicidal products containing N-9, including lubricated condoms, diaphragms, and cervical caps to which N-9 is added.

Intravaginal spermicides are marketed and sold without prescriptions as aerosol foams, tablets, suppositories, creams, films, and gels (Fig. 5-11). Preloaded, single-dose applicators small enough to be carried in a small purse are available. Effectiveness of spermicides depends on consistent and accurate use. Not more than 1 hour before sexual intercourse, the spermicide should be inserted high into the vagina so it makes contact with the cervix. Spermicide must be reapplied for each additional act of intercourse, even if a barrier method is used. Studies have shown varying effectiveness rates for spermicidal use alone. Typical failure rate in the first year of spermicidal use alone is 29% (Trussell and Guthrie, 2011). Some female barrier methods (e.g., diaphragm, cervical caps) offer more effective protection against pregnancy with the addition of spermicides.

Condoms. The male condom is a thin, stretchable sheath that covers the penis before genital, oral, or anal contact and is removed when the penis is withdrawn from the partner's orifice after ejaculation. Condoms are made of latex rubber, which provides a barrier to sperm and STIs (including HIV); polyurethane (strong, thin plastic); or natural membranes (animal tissue). In addition to providing a physical barrier for sperm, nonspermicidal latex condoms also provide a barrier for STIs (particularly gonorrhea, chlamydia, and trichomonas) and HIV transmission. Condoms lubricated with N-9 are not recommended for preventing STIs or HIV and do not increase protection against pregnancy. Latex condoms break down with oil-based lubricants (e.g., petroleum jelly and suntan oil) and should be used only with water-based or silicone lubricants. Because of the growing number of people with latex allergies, condom manufacturers have begun using polyurethane, which is thinner and stronger than latex.

BOX 5-9   MALE CONDOMS

Mechanism of Action

Sheath is applied over the erect penis before insertion or loss of preejaculatory drops of semen. Used correctly, condoms prevent sperm from entering the cervix. Spermicide-coated condoms cause ejaculated sperm to be immobilized rapidly, thus increasing contraceptive effectiveness.

Failure Rate

- Typical users, 18%
- Correct and consistent users, 2%

Advantages

- Safe
- No side effects
- Readily available
- Premalignant changes in cervix can be prevented or ameliorated in women whose partners use condoms
- Method of male nonsurgical contraception

Disadvantages

- Lovemaking must be interrupted to apply sheath.
- Sensation may be altered.
- If used improperly, spillage of sperm can result in pregnancy.
- Condoms occasionally may tear during intercourse.

Sexually Transmitted Infection Protection

If a condom is used throughout the act of intercourse and there is no unprotected contact with female genitals, a latex rubber condom, which is impermeable to viruses, can act as a protective measure against sexually transmitted infections.

Nursing Considerations

Teach man to do the following:

- Use a new condom (check expiration date) for each act of sexual intercourse or other acts between partners that involve contact with the penis.

- Place the condom after the penis is erect and before intimate contact.
- Place the condom on the head of the penis (A) and unroll it all the way to the base (B).
- Leave an empty space at the tip (A); remove any air remaining in the tip by gently pressing air out toward the base of the penis.
- If a lubricant is desired, use water-based products such as K-Y lubricating jelly. Do not use petroleum-based products because they can cause the condom to break.
- After ejaculation carefully withdraw the still-erect penis from the vagina, holding onto the condom rim; remove and discard the condom.
- Store unused condoms in a cool, dry place.
- Do not use condoms that are sticky, brittle, or obviously damaged.

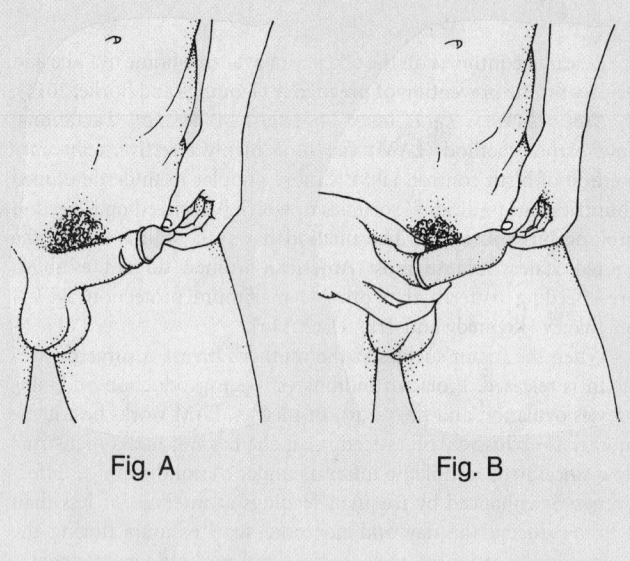

Fig. A   Fig. B

Although polyurethane condoms are as effective for STI prevention as latex condoms, they are more likely to slip or lose contour when compared to latex condoms. Therefore with perfect use latex condoms offer better protection against pregnancy. Polyurethane condoms do offer pregnancy protection equivalent to that of most barrier products. A small percentage of condoms are made from lamb cecum (natural skin). Natural skin condoms do not provide the same protection against STIs and HIV infection as latex condoms. Natural skin condoms contain small pores that could allow passage of viruses such as hepatitis B, HSV, and HIV and are not generally recommended.

A functional difference in condom shape is the presence or absence of a sperm reservoir tip. To enhance vaginal stimulation, some condoms are contoured and rippled or have ribbed or roughened surfaces. Thinner construction increases heat transmission and sensitivity; a variety of colors increases condom acceptability and attractiveness. A wet jelly or dry powder lubricates some condoms. Typical failure rate for the first year of use of the male condom is 18%. Effective condom use is a skill that must be taught.

! NURSING ALERT

It is a false assumption that everyone knows how to use condoms. To prevent unintended pregnancy and the spread of STIs, it is essential for condoms be used correctly. Proper instruction in use must be provided. The sheath is applied over the erect penis before insertion and before the loss of preejaculatory drops of semen (see Box 5-9). All types of condoms must be discarded after each single use. Condoms are available without prescription from a variety of sources, including vending machines.

Box 5-9 summarizes advantages and disadvantages of male condoms.

The female condom is a vaginal sheath made of nitrile, a nonlatex, synthetic rubber and has flexible rings at both ends (Fig. 5-12, A). The closed end of the pouch is inserted into the vagina and anchored around the cervix; the open ring covers the labia. A woman whose partner will not wear a male condom can use this device as a protective mechanical barrier. Rewetting drops or oil- or water-based lubricants can be used to help decrease the distracting noise that is produced while penile thrusting occurs. The female condom is available in one size, is intended for single use only, and is sold over the counter. Male condoms should not be used concurrently because the friction from both sheaths can increase the likelihood of either or both tearing (Female Health Company, 2012). Typical failure rate in the first year of female condom use is 21% (Trussell and Guthrie, 2011).

Diaphragm. The contraceptive **diaphragm** is a shallow, dome-shaped, latex or silicone device with a flexible rim that covers the cervix. The diaphragm is a mechanical barrier to the meeting of sperm with the ovum. By holding spermicide in place against the cervix for the 6 hours it takes to destroy the sperm, the diaphragm also provides a chemical barrier to pregnancy. Diaphragms are available in a wide range of diameters (50 to 95 mm) and differ in the inner construction of the circular rim. The types of rims are coil spring, arcing spring, and wide-seal rim. The diaphragm should be the largest size the woman can wear without being aware of its presence. Typical failure rate of the diaphragm combined with spermicide is 12% in the first year of use (Trussell and Guthrie, 2011).

Nursing Considerations. The woman using a diaphragm needs an annual gynecologic examination to assess its fit (Fritz and Speroff, 2011a). The device may need to be refitted after a 20% weight loss or gain, term birth, or second-trimester miscarriage and after any abdominal or pelvic surgery. Because various types of diaphragms are on the market, the nurse uses the package insert when teaching the woman how to use and care for the diaphragm (see Home Care box).

Disadvantages of diaphragm use include the reluctance of some women to insert and remove it. Although it can be inserted up to 6 hours before intercourse, a cold diaphragm and a cold gel temporarily reduce vaginal response to sexual stimulation if insertion occurs immediately before intercourse. Some women or couples object to the messiness of the spermicide. These annoyances associated with diaphragm use, along with failure to insert the device once foreplay

has begun, are the most common reasons for failures of this method. Side effects may include irritation of tissues related to contact with spermicides.

The diaphragm is not a good option for women with poor vaginal muscle tone or recurrent urinary tract infections. For proper placement the diaphragm must rest behind the pubic symphysis and completely cover the cervix. To decrease the chance of exerting urethral pressure, the woman should be reminded to empty her bladder before diaphragm insertion and immediately after intercourse. Diaphragms are contraindicated for women with pelvic relaxation (uterine prolapse) or a large cystocele. Women with a latex allergy should not use latex diaphragms.

Although reported in very small numbers, **toxic shock syndrome (TSS)** can occur in association with the use of the contraceptive diaphragm and cervical caps. The nurse should instruct the woman about ways to reduce her risk for TSS. These measures include prompt removal 6 to 8 hours after intercourse, not using the diaphragm or cervical caps during menses, and learning and watching for danger signs of TSS.

> ### ! NURSING ALERT
>
> The nurse should alert the woman who uses a diaphragm or cervical cap as a contraceptive method for signs of TSS. The most common signs include a sunburn type of rash, diarrhea, dizziness, faintness, weakness, sore throat, aching muscles and joints, sudden high fever, and vomiting.

Cervical Cap. The FemCap is the only type of cervical cap available in the United States (see Fig. 5-12, *B*). It comes in three sizes and is made of silicone rubber. The cap fits snugly around the base of the cervix close to the junction of the cervix and vaginal fornices. It is recommended that the cap remain in place no less than 6 hours and no more than 48 hours at a time. It is left in place at least 6 hours after the last act of intercourse. The seal provides a physical barrier to sperm; spermicide inside the cap adds a chemical barrier.

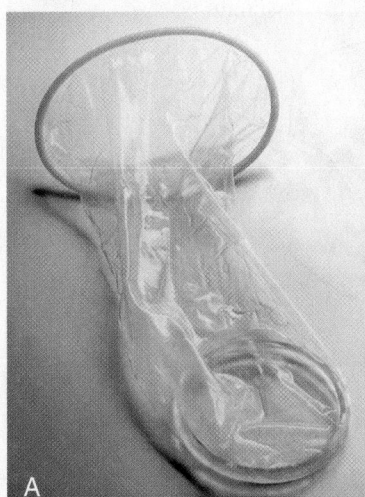 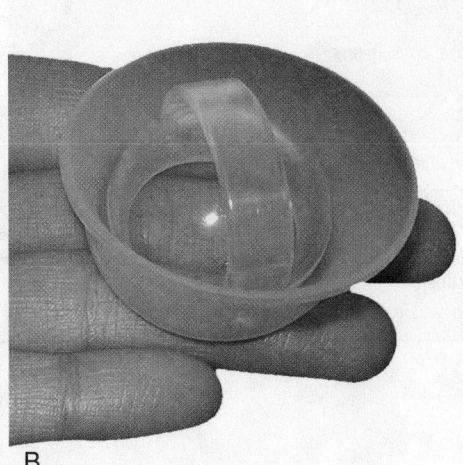 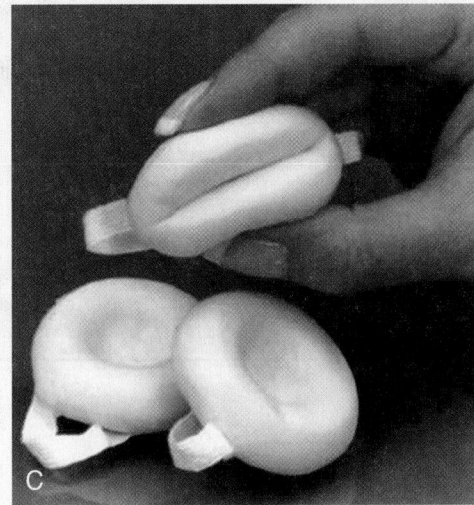

FIG 5-12 Barrier methods. **A,** Female condom (FC2). **B,** FemCap. **C,** Contraceptive sponge. (*A* Courtesy The Female Health Company, Chicago, IL. *B* Courtesy FemCap, Del Mar, CA. *C* Courtesy Allendale Pharmaceuticals, Allendale, NJ.)

HOME CARE

Use and Care of the Diaphragm

Positions for Insertion of Diaphragm

Squatting
* Squatting is the most commonly used position, and most women find it satisfactory.

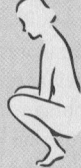

Leg-Up Method
* Another position is to raise the left foot (if right hand is used for insertion) on a low stool and, while in a bending position, insert the diaphragm.

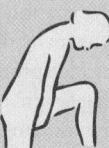

Chair Method
* Another practical method for diaphragm insertion is to sit far forward on the edge of a chair.

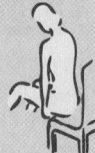

Reclining
* You may prefer to insert the diaphragm while in a semireclining position in bed.

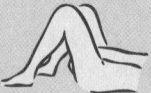

Inspection of Diaphragm

Your diaphragm must be inspected carefully before each use. The best way to do this is:

* Hold the diaphragm up to a light source. Carefully stretch it at the area of the rim, on all sides, to make sure that there are no holes. Remember, it is possible to puncture the diaphragm with sharp fingernails.
* Another way to check for pinholes is to carefully fill the diaphragm with water. If there is any problem, it will be seen immediately.
* If your diaphragm is puckered, especially near the rim, this could mean thin spots.
* The diaphragm should not be used if you see any of these; consult your health care provider.

Preparation of Diaphragm

* Rinse off cornstarch. Your diaphragm must always be used with a spermicidal lubricant to be effective. Pregnancy cannot be prevented effectively by the diaphragm alone.
* Always empty your bladder before inserting the diaphragm. Place about 2 tsp of contraceptive jelly or contraceptive cream on the side of the diaphragm that will rest against the cervix (or whichever way you have been instructed). Spread it around to coat the surface and the rim. This aids in insertion and offers a more complete seal. Many women also spread some jelly or cream on the other side of the diaphragm (Fig. A).

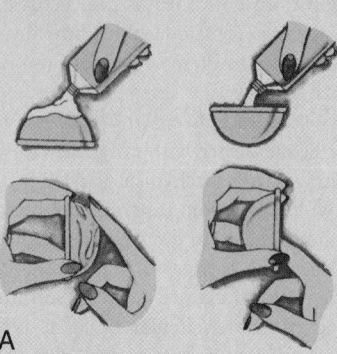

A

Insertion of Diaphragm

* The diaphragm can be inserted as long as 6 hours before intercourse. Hold it between your thumb and fingers. The dome can be either up or down, as directed by your health care provider. Place your index finger on the outer rim of the compressed diaphragm (Fig. B).

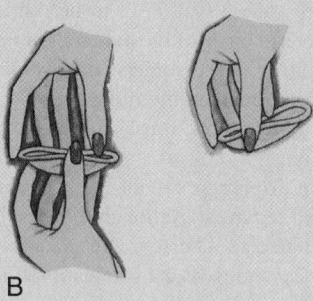

B

* Use the fingers of the other hand to spread the labia (lips of the vagina). This will aid in guiding the diaphragm into place.
* Insert the diaphragm into the vagina. Direct it inward and downward as far as it will go to the space behind and below the cervix (Fig. C).

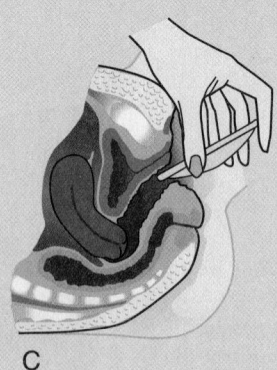

C

HOME CARE

Use and Care of the Diaphragm—cont'd

- Tuck the front of the rim of the diaphragm behind the pubic bone so the rubber hugs the front wall of the vagina (Fig. D).

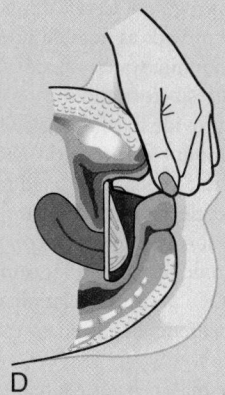

D

- Feel for your cervix through the diaphragm to be certain that it is placed properly and covered securely by the rubber dome (Fig. E).

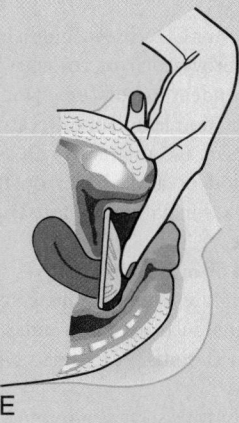

E

General Information

- Regardless of the time of the month, you must use your diaphragm every time intercourse takes place. It must be left in place for at least 6 hours after the last intercourse. If you remove it before the 6-hour period, your chance of becoming pregnant could be greatly increased. If you have repeated acts of intercourse, you must add more spermicide for each act.

Removal of Diaphragm

- The only proper way to remove the diaphragm is to insert your forefinger up and over the top side of the diaphragm and slightly to the side.
- Next turn the palm of your hand downward and backward, hooking the forefinger firmly on top of the inside of the upper rim of the diaphragm, breaking the suction.
- Pull the diaphragm down and out. This avoids the possibility of tearing it with the fingernails. You should not remove it by trying to catch the rim from below the dome (Fig. F).

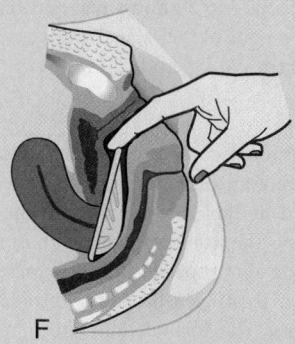

F

Care of Diaphragm

- When using a vaginal diaphragm, avoid using oil-based products such as certain body lubricants, mineral oil, baby oil, vaginal lubricants, or vaginitis preparations. These products can weaken the rubber.
- A little care means longer wear for your diaphragm. After each use wash it in warm water and mild soap. Do not use detergent soaps, cold-cream soaps, deodorant soaps, and soaps containing oil products because they can weaken the rubber.
- After washing dry the diaphragm thoroughly. All water and moisture should be removed with a towel. Dust the diaphragm with cornstarch. Scented talc, body powder, baby powder, and the like should not be used because they can weaken the rubber.
- To clean the introducer (if one is used), wash with mild soap and warm water, rinse, and dry thoroughly.
- Place the diaphragm back in the plastic case for storage. Do not store it near a radiator or heat source or exposed to light for an extended period.

The extended period of wear may be an added convenience for women.

Instructions for the actual insertion and use of the cervical cap closely resemble the instructions for use of the contraceptive diaphragm. Some of the differences are that the cervical cap can be inserted hours before sexual intercourse without a later need for additional spermicide, the cervical cap requires less spermicide than the diaphragm when initially inserted, and no additional spermicide is required for repeated acts of intercourse. Effectiveness of the first-generation FemCap has been found to be less than that of the diaphragm (Fritz and Speroff, 2011a).

Nursing Considerations. The angle of the uterus, the vaginal muscle tone, and the shape of the cervix may interfere with the

ease of fitting and use of the cervical cap. Correct fitting requires time, effort, and skill of both the woman and the clinician, although the FemCap may be easier to fit than previous types of cervical caps.

Because of the potential risk of TSS associated with the use of the cervical cap, another form of birth control is recommended for use during menstrual bleeding and up to at least 6 weeks after birth. The cap should be refitted after any gynecologic surgery or birth and after major weight losses or gains. Otherwise the size should be checked at least once a year.

Women who are not good candidates for wearing the cervical cap include those with abnormal Papanicolaou (Pap) test results, those who cannot be fitted properly with the existing cap sizes or who find the insertion and removal of the device too difficult, those with a history of TSS or with vaginal or cervical infections, and those who experience allergic responses to the cap or to spermicide.

Contraceptive Sponge. The vaginal sponge is a small, round, polyurethane sponge that contains N-9 spermicide (see Fig. 5-12, C). It is designed to fit over the cervix (one size fits all). The side that is placed next to the cervix is concave for better fit. The opposite side has a woven polyester loop to be used for removal of the sponge.

The sponge must be moistened with water before it is inserted into the vagina to cover the cervix. It provides protection for up to 24 hours and for repeated instances of sexual intercourse. It should be left in place for at least 6 hours after the last act of intercourse. Wearing it longer than 24 to 30 hours may put the woman at risk for TSS. Typical failure rate of the vaginal sponge is greater than that of the diaphragm (Fritz and Speroff, 2011a).

Hormonal Methods

Many different hormonal contraception therapies using different delivery methods are available in the United States today. General classes are described in Table 5-3. Because of the wide variety of preparations available, the woman and nurse must read the package insert for information about specific products prescribed. Formulations include combined estrogen-progestin steroidal medications or progestational agents. The formulations are administered orally, transdermally, vaginally, by implantation, or by injection.

Combined Estrogen-Progestin Contraceptives

Oral Contraceptives. The normal menstrual cycle is maintained through hormonal feedback mechanisms. FSH and LH are secreted in response to fluctuating levels of ovarian estrogen and progesterone. Regular ingestion of combined oral contraceptive pills (COCs) suppresses the action of the hypothalamus and anterior pituitary, leading to insufficient secretion of FSH and LH; therefore follicles do not mature, and ovulation is inhibited.

Other contraceptive effects are induced by the combined steroids. Maturation of the endometrium is altered, making the uterine

lining a less favorable site for implantation. COCs also have a direct effect on the endometrium; thus from 1 to 4 days after the last COC is taken the endometrium sloughs and bleeds as a result of hormone withdrawal. The withdrawal bleeding is usually less profuse than that of normal menstruation and may last only 2 to 3 days. Some women have no bleeding at all. The cervical mucus remains thick from the effect of the progestin. Cervical mucus under the effect of progesterone does not provide as suitable an environment for sperm penetration as does the thin, watery mucus that the healthy reproductive woman produces before and during ovulation.

Monophasic pills provide fixed dosages of estrogen and progestin. They alter the amount of progestin and sometimes estrogen within each cycle. These preparations reduce the total dosage of hormones in a single cycle without sacrificing contraceptive efficacy. To maintain adequate hormone levels for contraception and enhance compliance, COCs should be taken at the same time each day. Taken exactly as directed, COCs prevent ovulation, and pregnancy cannot occur. The overall theoretic effectiveness rate of COCs is almost 100%.

Because taking the pill does not relate directly to the sexual act, COC acceptability may be increased. Improvement in sexual response may occur once the possibility of pregnancy is not an issue. For many women it is convenient to know when to expect the next menstrual flow.

Contraindications for COC use include a history of thromboembolic disorders, cerebrovascular or coronary artery disease, breast cancer, estrogen-dependent tumors, pregnancy, impaired liver function, liver tumor, lactation less than 6 weeks postpartum, smoking if older than 35 years of age, migraine with aura, surgery with prolonged immobilization or any surgery on the legs, hypertension (160/100), and diabetes mellitus (of more than 20 years' duration) with vascular disease.

The effectiveness of oral contraceptives is decreased when the following medications are taken simultaneously:

- Anticonvulsants such as barbiturates, oxcarbazepine, phenytoin, phenobarbital, carbamazepine, primidone, and topiramate
- Systemic antifungals such as griseofulvin
- Antituberculosis drugs such as rifampicin and rifabutin
- Anti-HIV protease inhibitors such as nelfinavir and amprenavir

After discontinuing oral contraception fertility usually returns quickly, but fertility rates may be slightly lower the first 3 to 12 months after discontinuation.

Nursing Considerations. Many different preparations of oral hormonal contraceptives are available. Because of these wide variations in pills, each woman must be clear about the unique dosage regimen for the preparation prescribed for her and follow directions on the package insert. Directions for care after missing one or two tablets also vary. Fig. 5-13 illustrates a standard approach to missed pills. A simpler recommendation is to implement EC after two missed pills, regardless of dose. Signs of potential complications associated with the use of oral contraceptives must be reviewed with the woman, as noted in Box 5-10. Oral contraceptives do not protect a woman against STIs. Male condoms used in combination with COCs provide protection against STIs, and this combination gives excellent protection against unplanned pregnancy.

Transdermal Contraceptive System. The contraceptive patch delivers continuous levels of progesterone and ethynyl estradiol. The patch can be applied to the lower abdomen, upper outer arm, buttock, or upper torso (except the breasts). Application is on the

TABLE 5-3	HORMONAL CONTRACEPTION	
COMPOSITION	**ROUTE OF ADMINISTRATION**	**DURATION OF EFFECT**
Combination estrogen and progestin (synthetic estrogens and progestins in varying doses and formulations)	Oral	24 hours (extended cycle possible with daily pill for 12 weeks)
	Transdermal patch	7 days
	Vaginal ring insertion	3 weeks
Progestin only		
• Norethindrone, norgestrel	Oral	24 hours
• Medroxyprogesterone acetate	Intramuscular or subcutaneous injection	3 months
• Etonogestrel	Subdermal implant	Up to 3 years
• Levonorgestrel	Intrauterine device	1 year

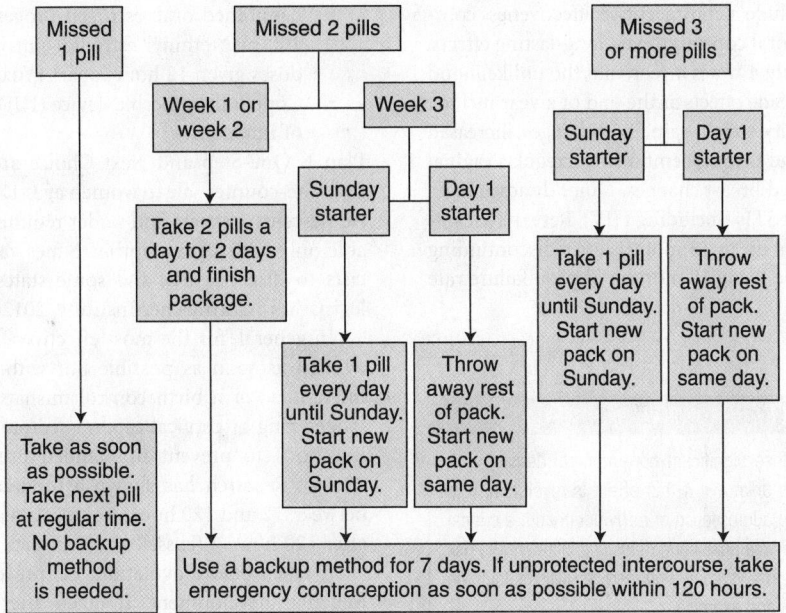

FIG 5-13 Flowchart for missed contraceptive pills. (Courtesy Patsy Huff, PharmD, Chapel Hill, NC.)

same day once a week for 3 weeks but not at the same site, followed by a week without the patch. Withdrawal bleeding occurs during the "no patch" week. Mechanisms of action, contraindications, and side effects are similar to those of COCs. The typical failure rate during the first year of use is under 2% in women weighing less than 198 lbs.

Vaginal Contraceptive Ring. The vaginal ring (made of ethylene vinyl acetate co-polymer) delivers continuous levels of progesterone and ethynyl estradiol. Mechanisms of action, contraindications, and side effects are similar to those of COCs. One vaginal ring is worn for 3 weeks, followed by a week without the ring. Withdrawal bleeding occurs during the "no ring" week. The ring can be inserted by the woman and does not have to be fitted. Some wearers may experience vaginal discomfort, usually related to increased vaginal discharge; but other wearers report that the ring alleviates symptoms of vaginitis. Some couples say that the ring can be felt during intercourse. Although it is not recommended that the ring be removed

for intercourse, contraceptive effectiveness would not decrease if it were replaced within 3 hours. The typical failure rate of the vaginal contraceptive ring is under 2% during the first year of use.

Progestin-Only Contraception. Progestin-only methods impair fertility by inhibiting ovulation, thickening and decreasing the amount of cervical mucus, thinning the endometrium, and altering cilia in the uterine tubes. Because progestin-only methods do not contain estrogen, they may be used in certain instances such as lactation, when estrogen would not be recommended.

Oral Progestins (Minipill). Progestin-only pills are less effective than COCs. Because minipills contain such a low dose of progestin, they must be taken at the same time every day. If the pill is taken more than 3 hours late (27 hours after the last pill), a backup contraceptive method must be initiated. Much of the contraceptive effectiveness of the minipill depends on progestin-induced changes in cervical mucus, and this effect lasts about 24 hours after oral ingestion of the pill. Users often complain of irregular vaginal bleeding. The failure rate for typical users of the minipill is approximately 8% during the first year of use. Effectiveness is increased if minipills are taken correctly. There are two instances in which the minipill is quite effective: in lactating women and women over 40. The reduced fecundity of lactation and the perimenopause period enhance the contraceptive effects of the minipill.

Injectable Progestins. Depot medroxyprogesterone acetate (DMPA; Depo-Provera) is given subcutaneously or intramuscularly in the deltoid or gluteus maximus muscle. It should be initiated during the first 5 days of the menstrual cycle and administered every 11 to 13 weeks.

! NURSING ALERT

When administering an injection of progestin (e.g., DMPA), the site should not be massaged after the injection because this action can hasten the absorption and shorten the period of effectiveness.

Advantages of DMPA include a contraceptive effectiveness comparable to that of combined oral contraceptives, long-lasting effects, requirement of injections only 4 times a year, and the unlikelihood of lactation being impaired. Side effects at the end of a year include decreased bone mineral density, weight gain, lipid changes, increased risk of venous thrombosis and thromboembolism, irregular vaginal spotting, decreased libido, and breast changes. Other disadvantages include no protection against STIs (including HIV). Return to fertility may be delayed as long as up to 18 months after discontinuing DMPA, with the median time being 10 months. Typical failure rate is 3% in the first year of use.

> ### ! NURSING ALERT
>
> Women who use DMPA may lose significant bone mineral density with increasing duration of use. It is unknown if this effect is reversible. It is unknown if use of DMPA during adolescence or early adulthood, a critical period of bone accretion, will reduce peak bone mass and increase the risk of osteoporotic fracture in later life. Women who receive DMPA should be counseled about calcium intake and exercise.

Implantable Progestins. Contraceptive implants consist of one or more nonbiodegradable flexible tubes or rods that are inserted under the skin of a woman's arm. These implants contain a progestin hormone and are effective for contraception for at least 3 years. They must be removed at the end of the recommended time. The FDA has approved two devices for use in the United States, a two-rod subdermal levonorgestrel implant (Jadelle) and a single-rod etonogestrel implant (Implanon, Nexplanon). Jadelle is unavailable in the United States (Raymond, 2011).

Insertion and removal of the single-rod etonogestrel capsule are minor surgical procedures involving a local anesthetic, a small incision, and no sutures. The capsule is placed subdermally in the inner aspect of the nondominant upper arm. The progestin prevents some, but not all, ovulatory cycles and thickens cervical mucus. Other advantages of the single-rod implant are that it provides long-term continuous contraception that is not related to frequency of coitus and is quickly reversible. The single-rod implant can be inserted immediately after the birth in breastfeeding women without affecting lactation. Irregular menstrual bleeding is the most common side effect. Less common side effects include headaches, nervousness, nausea, skin changes, and vertigo. The implant does not protect against STIs. As in other hormonal contraception methods, condoms should be used for protection against STIs. Typical failure rates for the first year of use are 0.05% (Trussell and Guthrie, 2011).

Emergency Contraception

EC offers protection against pregnancy after intercourse occurs in instances such as broken condoms, sexual assault, dislodged cervical cap, disruption of use of any other method, or any other case of unprotected intercourse. Methods that are available in the United States that could provide postcoital contraception include:

- Ella (Ulipristal): single 30-mg pill containing an antiprogestin
- Plan B One-Step: single progestin-only pill containing 1.5 mg levonorgestrel
- Next Choice: two levonorgestrel 0.75-mg tablets taken orally 12 hours apart or both together
- Combined oral: estrogen-progestin contraceptive pills (e.g., 100-mcg ethinyl estradiol plus 0.5 mg levonorgestrel); two doses given 12 hours apart (Yuzpe regimen)
- Copper intrauterine device (IUD) insertion within 120 hours of intercourse

Plan B One-Step and Next Choice are approved by the FDA for over-the-counter sale to women ages 17 and older with proof of age. Adolescents 16 years and under require a prescription. Ella is available only with a prescription. States vary in the ability of pharmacists to dispense EC, and some states have implemented refusal legislation (Guttmacher Institute, 2012b).

In general, for the most effectiveness, EC should be taken by a woman as soon as possible but within 72 hours of unprotected intercourse or a birth control mishap (e.g., broken condom, dislodged ring or cervical cap, missed oral contraceptive pills, late for injection) to prevent unintended pregnancy (Fritz and Speroff, 2011a). Research has shown a moderate amount of effectiveness between 72 and 120 hours but no data are available for effectiveness after 120 hours (Trussell and Schwartz, 2011).

If taken before ovulation, EC prevents ovulation by inhibiting follicular development. If taken after ovulation occurs, there is little effect on ovarian hormone production or the endometrium. To minimize the side effect of nausea that occurs with high doses of estrogen and progestin (Yuzpe regimen), the woman can be advised to take an over-the-counter antiemetic 1 hour before each dose. Nausea is not as common with the Plan B (One-Step, Next Choice) regimen. Women with contraindications for estrogen use should use progestin-only EC. No medical contraindications for EC exist, except pregnancy and undiagnosed abnormal vaginal bleeding (Trussell and Schwarz, 2011).If the woman does not begin menstruation within 21 days after taking the pills, she should be evaluated for pregnancy (Trussell and Schwarz, 2011). EC is ineffective if the woman is pregnant since the pills do not disturb an implanted pregnancy. Risk of pregnancy is reduced by as much as 75% and 89% if the woman takes EC pills (Trussell and Schwarz, 2011).

> ### ! NURSING ALERT
>
> EC will not protect the woman against pregnancy if she engages in unprotected intercourse in the days or weeks that follow treatment. Because ingestion of EC pills may delay ovulation, caution the woman that she needs to establish a reliable form of birth control to prevent unintended pregnancy (Trussell and Schwarz, 2011). Information about EC method options and access to providers is available on the Internet at www.NOT-2-LATE.com or by calling 888-NOT-2-LATE.

IUDs containing copper (see later discussion) provide another EC option. The IUD should be inserted within 8 days of unprotected intercourse (Trussell and Schwarz, 2011). This method is suggested only for women who wish to have the benefit of long-term contraception. The risk of pregnancy is reduced by as much as 99% with emergency insertion of the copper-releasing IUD.

Contraceptive counseling should be provided to all women requesting EC, including a discussion of modification of risky sexual behaviors to prevent STIs and unwanted pregnancy.

Intrauterine Devices

An intrauterine device (IUD) is a small T-shaped device with bendable arms for insertion through the cervix into the uterine

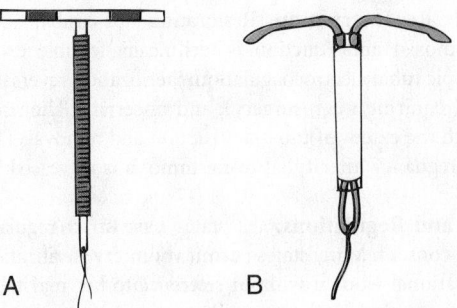

FIG 5-14 Intrauterine devices. **A,** Copper T380A. **B,** Levonorgestrel-releasing intrauterine device.

BOX 5-11 SIGNS OF POTENTIAL COMPLICATIONS: INTRAUTERINE DEVICES

Signs of potential complications related to intrauterine devices can be remembered using the *pains* mnemonic:

P   Period late, abnormal spotting or bleeding
A   Abdominal pain, pain with intercourse
I   Infection exposure, abnormal vaginal discharge
N   Not feeling well, fever, or chills
S   String missing: shorter or longer

cavity. Two strings hang from the base of the stem through the cervix and protrude into the vagina for the woman to feel for assurance that the device has not been dislodged (Fig. 5-14). There are two FDA-approved IUDs. The Copper T380A (Paragard) IUD is made of radiopaque polyethylene and fine solid copper and is approved for 10 years of use. The copper primarily serves as a spermicide and inflames the endometrium, preventing fertilization. Sometimes women experience an increase in bleeding and cramping within the first year after insertion, but nonsteroidal antiinflammatory drugs (NSAIDs) can provide pain relief. The typical failure rate in the first year of use of the copper IUD is 0.8% (Dean and Schwarz, 2011).

The levonorgestrel intrauterine system (IUS) (Mirena) releases levonorgestrel from its vertical reservoir. Effective for up to 5 years, it impairs sperm motility, irritates the lining of the uterus, and has some anovulatory effects. Uterine cramping and uterine bleeding are usually decreased with this device, although irregular spotting is common in the first few months following insertion. The typical failure rate in the first year of use is 0.2% (Dean and Schwarz, 2011).

IUDs offer constant contraception without the need to remember to take pills each day or engage in other manipulation before or between coital acts. If pregnancy can be excluded, either device (the Copper T380A or the levonorgestrel intrauterine system) can be placed at any time during the menstrual cycle. These devices may be inserted immediately after childbirth or following a first-trimester abortion. The contraceptive effects are reversible. When pregnancy is desired, the health care provider removes the device.

Disadvantages of IUD use include increased risk of pelvic inflammatory disease within the first 20 days after insertion, especially if infection is present at the time of insertion. There is also a slight risk of uterine perforation. Neither the Copper T380A nor the levonorgestrel intrauterine system offers protection against STIs or HIV. The Copper T380A is more likely to be associated with regular menses that may have heavier flow. Women who have the levonorgestrel intrauterine system are more likely to experience scant, irregular episodes of vaginal bleeding or amenorrhea.

Nursing Considerations. The woman should be taught to check for the presence of the IUD thread after menstruation to rule out expulsion of the device. If pregnancy occurs with the IUD in place, the IUD should be removed immediately in the first trimester if the strings are visible. Later in pregnancy ultrasound examination should be used to localize the IUD and rule out placenta previa. Retention of the IUD during pregnancy increases the risk of septic miscarriage and ectopic pregnancy. Some women allergic to copper

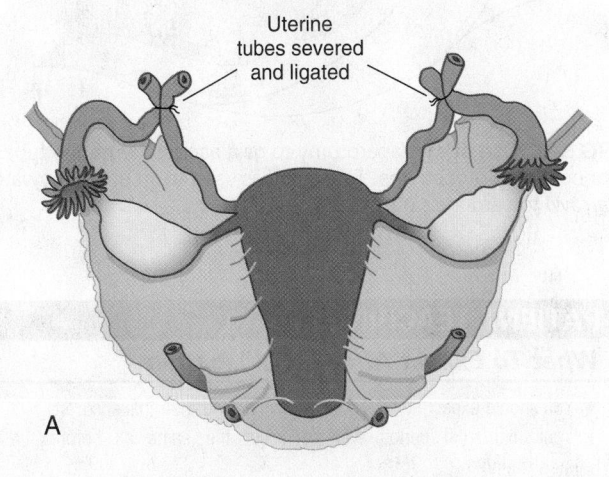

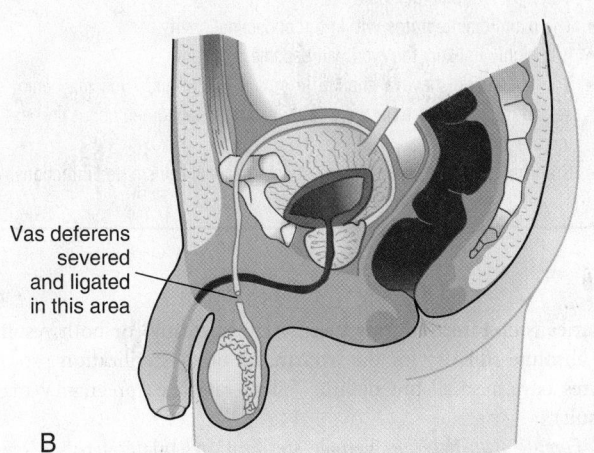

FIG 5-15 Sterilization. **A,** Uterine tubes ligated and severed (tubal ligation). **B,** Sperm duct ligated and severed (vasectomy).

develop a rash, necessitating removal of the copper-bearing IUD. Signs of potential complications of intrauterine contraception are listed in Box 5-11.

Sterilization

Sterilization refers to surgical procedures intended to render the person infertile. Most procedures involve the occlusion of the passageways for the ova and sperm (Fig. 5-15). For the woman the oviducts (uterine tubes) are occluded; for the man the sperm ducts (vas deferens) are occluded. Only surgical removal of the

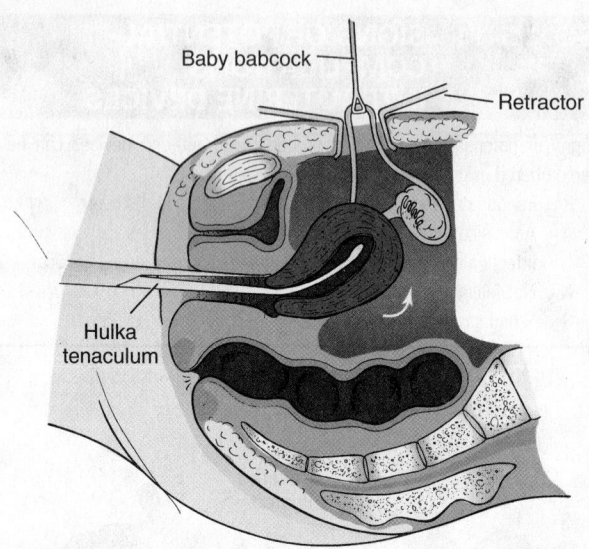

Baby babcock

Retractor

Hulka tenaculum

FIG 5-16 Use of minilaparotomy to gain access to uterine tubes for occlusion procedures. Tenaculum is used to lift uterus upward *(arrow)* toward incision.

PATIENT TEACHING

What To Expect After Tubal Ligation

- You should expect no change in hormones and their influence.
- Your menstrual period will be about the same as before the sterilization.
- You may feel pain at ovulation.
- The ovum disintegrates within the abdominal cavity.
- It is highly unlikely that you will become pregnant.
- You should not have a change in sexual functioning; you may enjoy sexual relations more because you will not be concerned about becoming pregnant.
- Sterilization offers no protection against sexually transmitted infections. Therefore you may need to use condoms.

ovaries (oophorectomy) or uterus (hysterectomy) or both results in absolute sterility for the woman. All other sterilization procedures have a small but definite failure rate (i.e., pregnancy may result).

Female Sterilization. Female sterilization (bilateral tubal ligation) may be done immediately after giving birth (within 24 to 48 hours), concomitantly with abortion, or as an interval procedure (during any phase of the menstrual cycle). Half of all female sterilization procedures are performed immediately after a pregnancy. Sterilization procedures can be done safely on an outpatient basis. Failure rate for methods of female sterilization vary by the method and the woman's age, but the average is 0.5% (Roncari and Hou, 2011).

Tubal Occlusion. A laparoscopic approach or a minilaparotomy may be used for tubal ligation (Fig. 5-16), tubal electrocoagulation, or the application of bands or clips. Electrocoagulation and ligation are considered to be permanent methods. Use of the bands or clips has the theoretic advantage of possible removal and return of tubal patency (see Patient Teaching box).

Tubal Reconstruction. Restoration of tubal continuity (reanastomosis) and function is technically feasible except after laparoscopic tubal electrocoagulation. Sterilization reversal is costly, difficult (requiring microsurgery), and uncertain. The success rate varies with the extent of tubal destruction and removal. The risk of ectopic pregnancy after tubal reanastomosis is increased by 2% to 12.5%.

Laws and Regulations. All states have strict regulations for informed consent. Many states permit voluntary sterilization of any mature, rational woman without reference to her marital or pregnancy status. Although the partner's consent is not required by law, the woman is encouraged to discuss the situation with her partner, and health care providers may request the partner's consent. Sterilization of minors or mentally incompetent individuals is restricted by most states and often requires the approval of a board of eugenicists or other court-appointed individuals.

LEGAL TIP: Sterilization

If federal funds are used for sterilization, the person must be at least 21 years of age. Informed consent must include an explanation of the risks, benefits, and alternatives; a statement that describes sterilization as a permanent, irreversible method of birth control; and a statement that mandates a 30-day waiting period between giving consent and the sterilization. Informed consent must be in the person's native language, or an interpreter must be provided to read the consent form to the person.

Male Sterilization. Vasectomy is the sealing, tying, or cutting of a man's vas deferens so the sperm cannot travel from the testes to the penis. Vasectomy is the easiest and most commonly used operation for male sterilization. The surgery can be performed with local anesthesia on an outpatient basis. Pain, bleeding, infection, and other postsurgical complications are considered to be possible disadvantages to the surgical procedure.

Two methods are used for scrotal entry: conventional and no-scalpel vasectomy. The surgeon identifies and immobilizes the vas deferens through the scrotum. Then the vas is ligated or cauterized (see Fig. 5-15, *B*). Surgeons vary in their techniques to occlude the vas deferens: ligation with sutures, division, cautery, application of clips, excision of a segment of the vas, fascial interposition, or some combination of these methods.

Vasectomy has no effect on potency (ability to achieve and maintain erection) or volume of ejaculate. Endocrine production of testosterone continues so secondary sex characteristics are not affected. Sperm production continues, but sperm are unable to leave the epididymis and are lysed by the immune system. Vasectomy does not change the man's transmission of the HIV virus if he is infected. He will need to be instructed to engage in a number of ejaculations until there are no viable sperm remaining above the area of the surgery. Until this occurs, as documented by semen analysis, the couple should use back-up contraception.

Complications after bilateral vasectomy are uncommon and usually not serious. They include bleeding (usually external), suture reaction, and reaction to the anesthetic agent. Men occasionally develop a hematoma, infection, or epididymitis. Less common are painful granulomas from accumulation of sperm. The failure rate for male sterilization is 0.15% (Roncari and Hou, 2011).

Tubal Reconstruction. Microsurgery to reanastomose (restore tubal continuity) the sperm ducts can be accomplished successfully (i.e., sperm in the ejaculate) in more than 90% of cases; however, the fertility rate following reanastomosis is only about 50%. The rate of success decreases as the time since the procedure was initially performed increases. The vasectomy may result in permanent changes in the testes that leave men unable to father children. The changes are those ordinarily seen only in the elderly (e.g., interstitial fibrosis [scar tissue between the seminiferous tubules]). In addition some men develop antibodies against their own sperm (autoimmunization).

Nursing Considerations. The nurse plays an important role in helping people make decisions so all requirements for informed consent are met. The nurse also provides information about alternatives to sterilization such as contraception.

Information must be given about what is entailed in the various procedures, how much discomfort or pain can be expected, and what type of care is needed. Many individuals fear sterilization procedures because of imagined effects on sexual functioning. They need reassurance concerning the hormonal and psychologic basis of sexual functioning. The fact that uterine tube occlusion or vasectomy has no biologic sequelae in terms of sexual adequacy needs to be communicated and reinforced.

Preoperative care includes health assessment, which includes a psychologic assessment, physical examination, and laboratory tests. The nurse confirms that the individual understands printed instructions. Ambivalence and extreme fear of the procedure should be reported to the physician.

Postoperative care depends on the procedure performed (e.g., laparoscopy, laparotomy for tubal occlusion, or vasectomy). General care includes recovery after anesthesia, vital signs, fluid-electrolyte balance (intake and output, laboratory values), prevention of or early identification and treatment of infection or hemorrhage, control of discomfort, and assessment of emotional response to the procedure and recovery.

Discharge planning depends on the type of procedure performed. In general the patient is given written instructions about observing for and reporting symptoms and signs of complications, the type of recovery to be expected, and the date and time for a follow-up appointment.

ABORTION

Induced abortion is the purposeful interruption of a pregnancy before 20 weeks of gestation. (Spontaneous abortion or miscarriage is discussed in Chapter 12.) If the abortion is performed at the woman's request, the term elective abortion is usually used; if performed for reasons of maternal or fetal health or disease, the term therapeutic abortion applies. Many factors contribute to a woman's decision to have an abortion. Indications include (1) preservation of the life or health of the mother, (2) genetic disorders of the fetus, (3) rape or incest, and (4) the pregnant woman's request. The control of birth, dealing as it does with human sexuality and the question of life and death, is one of the most emotional components of health care. It has been the most controversial social issue in the last half of the twentieth century and continues to be so today. Regulations exist to protect the mother from the complications of abortion.

Abortion is regulated in most countries, including the United States. Before 1970 legal abortion was not widely available in the United States. However, in January 1973 the U.S. Supreme Court set aside previous antiabortion laws and legalized it. This decision established a trimester approach to abortion.

Following the U.S. Supreme Court ruling in 1973 in the case of Roe versus Wade, the decision of first-trimester abortion was deemed to be between the pregnant woman and her health care provider, and state laws determining abortion to be illegal were struck down. During the second trimester abortion is left to the discretion of the individual states to regulate procedures as long as these regulations are reasonably related to the woman's health. In the third trimester abortions may be limited or even prohibited by state regulation unless the restriction interferes with the life or health of the pregnant woman (*Roe v. Wade,* 1973). Hospitals maintained by Roman Catholics and some of those maintained by strict fundamentalists forbid abortion (and often sterilization) despite legal challenges.

Currently 39 states legislate that abortion be performed by a licensed physician. Nurse practitioners can perform abortions (if the practice is within their scope of practice) in the states of California, Montana, Vermont, New Hampshire, and Rhode Island. Congress has legislated that Medicaid funds can only be used to pay for abortion when a woman's life is endangered. States vary on the financing of abortions, with 17 states using their own funds to pay for them, depending on the circumstances surrounding the procedure. States also vary regarding parental notification and/or consent regarding abortion, with 37 states providing legislation for some type of parental involvement in the abortion of a pregnant daughter who is a minor. Individual health care providers may refuse to participate in abortion in 46 states (Guttmacher Institute, 2012a).

In 2008 in the United States there were approximately 6.5 million pregnancies, and approximately 19% of these pregnancies ended in termination (Sedgh, Singh, Shah, et al., 2012). The number of abortions in the United States has decreased from 1.31 million in 2000 to 1.21 million in 2008 (Guttmacher Institute, 2012a). Most terminations were performed in women who were unmarried (84%). Non-Hispanic Caucasian women comprised 36% of those who experienced elective abortion. Non-Hispanic African-American women comprised 30% of those who experienced elective abortions, Hispanic women accounted for 25% of elective abortions, and women of other races accounted for 9% of abortions (Guttmacher Institute, 2012a). Most abortions occur in women who already have children, and abortion rates tend to be higher in women whose income is below the poverty level.

The Association of Women's Health, Obstetric and Neonatal Nurses (AWHONN, 2009) supports a nurse's right to choose whether to participate in abortion procedures in keeping with her or his "personal, moral, ethical, or religious beliefs." AWHONN also advocates that "nurses have a professional obligation to inform their employers, at the time of employment, of any attitudes and beliefs that may interfere with essential job functions."

Rates of biologic complications after abortions such as ectopic pregnancy, infection, or hemorrhage tend to be low if the woman aborts during the first trimester. Psychologic sequelae of induced abortion are uncommon and may be related to circumstances and support systems surrounding the pregnant woman such as the attitudes reflected by friends, family, and health care workers. The woman facing an abortion is pregnant and exhibits the emotional responses shared by all pregnant women, including the possibility of depression.

Nurses and other health care providers often struggle with the same values and moral convictions as those of the pregnant woman.

BOX 5-12 SELECTED NURSING DIAGNOSES FOR WOMEN HAVING ELECTIVE ABORTION

- Decisional conflict related to
  - Value system
- Fear related to
  - Abortion procedure
  - Potential complications
  - Implications for future pregnancies
  - What others might think
- Grieving related to
  - Distress at loss or feelings of guilt
- Risk for infection related to
  - Effects of the procedure
  - Lack of understanding of preoperative and postoperative self-care
- Acute pain related to
  - Effects of the procedure or postoperative events

The conflicts and doubts of the nurse can be readily communicated to women who are already anxious. Regardless of personal views on abortion, nurses who provide care to women seeking abortion have an ethical responsibility to counsel women about their options and make appropriate referrals.

LEGAL TIP: Institutional Policies for Nurses' Rights and Responsibilities Related to Abortion

Nurses' rights and responsibilities related to caring for abortion patients should be protected through policies that describe how the institution accommodates the nurse's ethical or moral beliefs and what the nurse should do to avoid patient abandonment in such situations. Nurses should know what policies are in place in their institutions and encourage such policies to be written.

CARE MANAGEMENT

A thorough assessment is conducted through history, physical examination, and laboratory tests. The length of pregnancy and the condition of the woman must be determined to select the appropriate type of abortion procedure. An ultrasound examination should be performed before a second-trimester abortion is done. If the woman is Rh-negative, she is a candidate for prophylaxis against Rh isoimmunization. She should receive $Rh_o(D)$ immune globulin within 72 hours after the abortion if she is D-negative and if Coombs' test results are negative (if the woman is unsensitized or isoimmunization has not developed).

The woman's understanding of alternatives, the types of abortions, and expected recovery is assessed. Misinformation and gaps in knowledge are identified and corrected. The record is reviewed for the signed informed consent, and the woman's understanding is verified. General preoperative, operative, and postoperative assessments are performed.

Analysis of data leads to identification of the appropriate nursing diagnoses for the woman undergoing elective abortion. Potential nursing diagnoses are listed in Box 5-12. Counseling about abortion includes helping the woman identify how she perceives the pregnancy, providing information about the choices available (i.e.,

---

❓ CRITICAL THINKING CASE STUDY
Termination of Pregnancy

Angelica is a 19-year-old single woman whose contraceptive failed. She is 6 weeks' pregnant and is seeking termination of the pregnancy. She has many questions for the nurse in the family planning clinic: Which procedure is most likely to be chosen at this gestation? What are the risks associated with the procedure? Should her boyfriend be involved in the decision to terminate the pregnancy?

1. Evidence—Is there sufficient evidence to draw conclusions about what information the nurse should provide Angelica?
2. Assumptions—What assumptions can be made about Angelica's reaction to termination of the pregnancy?
   a. Psychologic/emotional reaction and sequelae
   b. Physical response
   c. Future childbearing
   d. Relationship with her boyfriend
3. What implications and priorities for nursing care can be drawn at this time?
4. Does the evidence objectively support your conclusion?

---

having an abortion or carrying the pregnancy to term and then either keeping the infant or placing the baby for adoption), and informing about the types of abortion procedures (see Critical Thinking Case Study).

First-Trimester Abortion

Methods for performing early elective abortion (less than 9 weeks of gestation) include surgical (aspiration) and medical methods (mifepristone with prostaglandin and methotrexate with misoprostol). About 90% of abortions in the United States are performed during the first trimester, with more than 60% performed by 8 weeks after the last menstrual period (Paul and Stein, 2011).

Surgical (Aspiration) Abortion

Aspiration (vacuum or suction curettage) is the most common procedure in the first trimester. Aspiration abortion is usually performed under local anesthesia in a physician's office, a clinic, or a hospital. The ideal time for performing this procedure is 8 to 12 weeks after the last menstrual period. The suction procedure for performing an early elective abortion usually requires less than 5 minutes.

A bimanual examination is done before the procedure to assess uterine size and position. A speculum is inserted, and the cervix is anesthetized with a local anesthetic agent. The cervix is dilated if necessary, and a cannula connected to suction is inserted into the uterine cavity. The products of conception are evacuated from the uterus.

During the procedure the woman is kept informed about what to expect next (e.g., menstrual-like cramping and sounds of the suction machine). The nurse assesses the woman's vital signs. The aspirated uterine contents must be inspected carefully to ascertain whether all fetal parts and adequate placental tissue have been evacuated. After the abortion the woman rests on the table until she is ready to stand. She remains in the recovery area or waiting room for 1 to 3 hours for detection of excessive cramping or bleeding; then she is discharged.

Bleeding after the operation is normally about the equivalent of a heavy menstrual period, and cramps are rarely severe. Excessive vaginal bleeding and infection such as endometritis or salpingitis are the most common complications of induced abortion. Retained products of conception are the primary cause of vaginal bleeding. Evacuation of the uterus, uterine massage, and administration of oxytocin or methylergonovine (Methergine) may be necessary to decrease vaginal bleeding (Paul and Stein, 2011). Prophylactic antibiotics to decrease the risk of infection are commonly prescribed. Generally postabortion pain can be relieved with NSAIDs such as ibuprofen.

Nursing Interventions. Instructions following a surgical abortion differ among health care providers (e.g., tampons should not be used for at least 3 days or should be avoided for up to 3 weeks, and resumption of sexual intercourse may be permitted within 1 week or discouraged for 2 weeks). The woman may shower daily. Instruction is given to watch for excessive bleeding and other signs of complications and to avoid douches of any type. The woman can expect her menstrual period to resume 4 to 6 weeks after the day of the procedure. The nurse offers information about the birth control method the woman prefers if contraceptive counseling has not been done during the counseling interview that usually precedes the decision to have an abortion. The woman must be strongly encouraged to return for her follow-up visit so complications can be detected and an acceptable contraceptive method prescribed. A pregnancy test may also be performed to determine if the pregnancy has been terminated successfully.

⚡ SAFETY ALERT

The woman who has an induced abortion should be given clear instructions to return immediately to the health care facility or emergency department for any of the following symptoms:
- Fever greater than 38° C (100.4° F)
- Chills
- Bleeding greater than two saturated pads in 2 hours or heavy bleeding lasting a few days
- Foul-smelling vaginal discharge
- Severe abdominal pain, cramping, or backache
- Abdominal tenderness (when pressure applied)

Source: Paul M, Stein T: Abortion. In Hatcher RA, Trussell J, Nelson AL, editors: *Contraceptive technology*, ed 20, Atlanta 2011, Ardent Media.

Medical Abortion

Early abortion using medication rather than surgery has been popular in Canada and Europe for more than 15 years, but medical abortion is a relatively new procedure in the United States. Medical abortions are available for use in the United States for up to 9 weeks after the last menstrual period. Methotrexate, misoprostol, and mifepristone are the drugs used in the current regimens to induce early abortion. About 17% of all reported abortion procedures in 2008 were medical procedures (Guttmacher Institute, 2012a).

Methotrexate is a cytotoxic drug that causes early abortion by blocking folic acid in fetal cells so they cannot divide. Misoprostol (Cytotec) is a prostaglandin analog that acts directly on the cervix to soften and dilate and on the uterine muscle to stimulate contractions. Mifepristone, formerly known as RU 486, was approved by the FDA in 2000. It works by binding to progesterone receptors and blocking the action of progesterone, which is necessary for maintaining pregnancy (Paul and Stein, 2011).

Methotrexate and Misoprostol. Methotrexate can be given intramuscularly or orally (usually mixed with orange juice). Vaginal placement of misoprostol follows in 3 to 7 days. Women commonly have nausea, vomiting, and cramping after the misoprostol insertion. The woman returns for a follow-up visit to confirm the abortion is complete. If abortion does not occur, misoprostol is repeated, or vacuum aspiration is performed to remove the products of conception (Paul and Stein, 2011).

Mifepristone and Misoprostol. Mifepristone can be taken up to 7 weeks after the last menstrual period. The FDA-approved regimen is that the woman takes 600 mg of mifepristone orally; 48 hours later she returns to the office and takes 400 mcg of misoprostol orally (unless abortion has already occurred and been confirmed). Two weeks after the administration of mifepristone, the woman must return to the office for a clinical examination or ultrasound to confirm that the pregnancy has been terminated. In 1% to 5% of cases the drugs do not work, and surgical abortion (aspiration) is needed (Paul and Stein, 2011).

With any medical abortion regimen, the woman usually experiences bleeding and cramping. Side effects of the medications include nausea, vomiting, diarrhea, headache, dizziness, fever, and chills. These are attributed to misoprostol and usually subside in a few hours after administration (Paul and Stein, 2011).

Second-Trimester Abortion

Because the great majority of induced abortions in the United States occur in the first trimester, only about 10% are performed in the second trimester. Second-trimester abortion is associated with more complications and costs than first-trimester abortions. Dilation and evacuation (D&E) accounts for almost all procedures performed in the United States. In general medical administration of second-trimester abortions involves the same drugs (misoprostol and mifepristone) used in medical termination of pregnancy during the first trimester. The D&E procedure is generally preferred by patients because it is less expensive and better tolerated than medical abortion during the second trimester (Fritz and Speroff, 2011b).

Dilation and Evacuation

D&E can be performed at any point up to 20 weeks of gestation, although it is more often performed between 13 and 16 weeks (Paul and Stein, 2011). The cervix requires more dilation because the products of conception are larger. Often laminaria are inserted several hours or several days before the procedure, or misoprostol can be applied to the cervix to soften the tissue. The procedure is similar to that of vaginal aspiration, except that a larger cannula is used and other instruments may be needed to remove the fetus and placenta. Nursing care includes monitoring vital signs, providing emotional support, administering analgesics, and postoperative monitoring. Disadvantages of D&E include possible long-term harmful effects on the cervix.

Nursing Considerations

The woman considering an abortion will need help to explore the meaning of the various alternatives for elective abortion and consequences to herself and her significant others. It is often difficult for a woman to express her true feelings (e.g., what abortion means to her now and in the future and what support or regret her friends and peers may demonstrate). A calm, matter-of-fact approach on the part of the nurse can be helpful. Clarifying, restating, and reflecting statements; open-ended questions; and feedback are communication techniques that can be used to maintain a realistic focus on the situation and bring the woman's problems into the open. If family or friends cannot be involved, scheduling time for nursing personnel to give the necessary support is an essential component of the care plan.

Information about alternatives to abortion such as referral to adoption agencies or support services if the woman chooses to keep her baby is provided. If a decision is made to have an abortion, the woman must be assured of continued support. Information about what is entailed in various procedures, how much discomfort or pain can be expected, and what type of care is needed must be given. A discussion of the various feelings, including depression, guilt, regret, and relief, that the woman might experience after the abortion is needed. Information about community resources for postabortion counseling may be needed.

After the abortion studies have indicated that most women report relief, but some have temporary distress or mixed emotions. Evidence of long-term depression after elective abortion has been inconclusive. Guilt and anxiety may occur more with young women, women with poor social support, multiparous women, and women with a history of psychiatric illness. Women having second-trimester abortions may have more emotional distress than women having abortions in the first trimester. Because symptoms can vary among women who have had abortions, nurses must assess women for grief reactions and facilitate the grieving process through active listening and nonjudgmental support and care.

KEY POINTS

- Infertility is the inability to conceive and carry a fetus to term gestation at a time the couple has chosen to do so.
- Infertility increases in women older than 35 years of age.
- In the United States about 40% of infertility is related to female causes, 40% is related to male causes, and 20% of infertility causes are unexplained.
- Common etiologic factors associated with infertility include decreased sperm production, ovulation disorders, tubal occlusion, and endometriosis.
- Reproductive alternatives for family building include IVF-ET, GIFT, ZIFT, oocyte donation, embryo donation, TDI, surrogate motherhood, and adoption.
- A variety of contraceptive methods with various effectiveness rates, advantages, and disadvantages are available.
- Women and their partners should choose the contraceptive method(s) best suited to them.
- Effective contraceptives are available through both prescription and nonprescription sources.
- Proper use of latex condoms provides protection against STIs.
- Tubal ligations and vasectomies are permanent sterilization methods used by increasing numbers of women and men.
- Emergency contraception pills should be taken as soon as possible after unprotected intercourse but no later than 120 hours.
- Induced abortion performed in the first trimester is safer and less complex than an abortion performed in the second trimester.
- The most common complications of induced abortion include infection, retained products of conception, and excessive vaginal bleeding.

REFERENCES

American Society for Reproductive Medicine [ASRM]: *Infertility: an overview*, 2012, asrm.org/awards/detail. aspx?id=9516&terms=(+%40Publish_ To+Both+Sites+or+%40Publish_To+ASRM +Only+)+and+infertility+diagnosis.

Association of Women's Health, Obstetric and Neonatal Nurses: Ethical decision making in the clinical setting: Nurses' rights and responsibilities, 2009, http://www.awhonn. org/awhonn/binary.content. do?name=Resources/Documents/pdf/ 5_Ethics.pdf.

Centers for Disease Control and Prevention (CDC): *Most recent ART data*, 2012, www.cdc.gov/ART/index.htm

CycleBeads: *The original family planning tool identifies fertile days using the standard days method*, 2012, www.cyclebeads.com/ cyclebeads.

D'Avanzo C: *Mosby's pocket guide to cultural health assessment*, ed 4, St Louis, 2008, Mosby.

Dean G, Schwarz E: Intrauterine contraceptives (IUCs). In Fritz M, Speroff L, editors: *Clinical gynecologic endocrinology and infertility*, ed 8, Philadelphia, 2011, Lippincott Williams & Wilkins.

Fehring RJ, Schneider M, Barron ML: Efficacy of the Marquette method of natural family planning, *MCN The American Journal of Maternal/Child Nursing* 33(6), 348–354, 2008.

Female Health Company: FC2 FAQs, 2012, www.fc2femalecondom.com/images/ FC2_FAQs.pdf.

Finer LB, Zolna MR: Unintended pregnancy in the United States: incidence and disparities, 2006, *Contraception* (84):478– 485, 2011.

Fritz M, Speroff L: Barrier methods of contraception and withdrawal. In Fritz M, Speroff L, editors: *Clinical gynecologic endocrinology and infertility*, ed 8, Philadelphia, 2011a, Lippincott Williams & Wilkins.

Fritz M, Speroff L: Family planning, sterilization and abortion. In Fritz M, Speroff L, editors: *Clinical gynecologic endocrinology and infertility*, ed 8, Philadelphia, 2011b, Lippincott Williams & Wilkins.

Fritz M, Speroff L: Sperm and egg transport, fertilization, and implantation. In Fritz M, Speroff L, editors: *Clinical gynecologic endocrinology and infertility*, ed 8,

Philadelphia, 2011c, Lippincott Williams & Wilkins.

Guttmacher Institute: An overview of abortion laws, 2012a, http://www.guttmacher.org/ statecenter/spibs/spib_OAL.pdf.

Guttmacher Institute: Emergency contraception, 2012b, www.guttmacher.org/statecenter/ spibs/spib_EC.pdf.

Institute for Reproductive Health Georgetown University: TwoDay method fact sheet, 2012, www.irh.org/sites/default/files/TDM%20 Fact%20Sheet.pdf.

Jennings VH, Burke AE: Fertility awareness-based methods. In Hatcher RA, Trussell J, Nelson AL, editors: *Contraceptive technology*, Atlanta, 2011, Ardent Media.

Kennedy K, Trussell J: Postpartum contraception and lactation. In Hatcher RA, Trussell J, Nelson AL, editors: *Contraceptive technology*, Atlanta, 2011a, Ardent Media.

Kennedy K, Trussell J: Contraceptive efficacy. In Hatcher RA, Trussell J, Nelson AL, editors: *Contraceptive technology*, Atlanta, 2011b, Ardent Media.

Kowal D: Coitus interruptus. In Hatcher RA, Trussell J, Nelson AL, editors: *Contraceptive technology*, Atlanta, 2011, Ardent Media.

Paul M, Stein T: Abortion. In Hatcher RA, Trussell J, Nelson AL, editors: *Contraceptive technology*, Atlanta, 2011, Ardent Media.

Practice Committee of the American Society for Reproductive Medicine: *Effectiveness and treatment for unexplained infertility*, 2008, asrm.org/uploadedFiles/ASRM_Content/News_and_Publications/Practice_Guidelines/Educational_Bulletins/effectiveness_and_treatment_for_unexplained_infertility(1).pdf.

Raymond E: Contraceptive implants. In Hatcher RA, Trussell J, Nelson AL, editors: *Contraceptive technology*, Atlanta, 2011, Ardent Media.

RESOLVE: *Emotional aspects of infertility*, 2012, www.resolve.org/support-and-services/Managing-Infertility-Stress/emotional-aspects.html.

Roe v. Wade: 410 US 113, 154, 1973.

Roncari D, Hou M: Female and male sterilization. In Fritz M, Speroff L, editors: *Clinical gynecologic endocrinology and infertility*, ed 8, Philadelphia, 2011, Lippincott Williams & Wilkins.

Sedgh G, Singh S, Shah IH, et al: Induced abortion: incidence and trends worldwide from 1995 to 2008, *Lancet* 379(9816):625–632, 2012.

Trussell J, Guthrie K: Choosing a contraceptive: efficacy, safety, and personal considerations. In Hatcher RA, Trussell J, Nelson AL, editors: *Contraceptive technology*, Atlanta, 2011, Ardent Media.

Trussell J, Schwarz E: Emergency contraception. In Hatcher RA, Trussell J, Nelson AL, editors: *Contraceptive technology*, Atlanta, 2011, Ardent Media.

6

Genetics, Conception, and Fetal Development

Shannon E. Perry

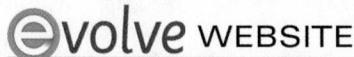 **WEBSITE**

http://evolve.elsevier.com/Perry/maternal

LEARNING OBJECTIVES

On completion of this chapter, the reader will be able to:
- Explain the key concepts of basic human genetics.
- Explore how recent advances in genetics have changed the field of health care.
- Discuss key findings and the ethical, legal, and social implications of the Human Genome Project.
- Describe expanded roles for nurses in genetics and genetic counseling.
- Identify genetic disorders commonly tested for in maternity and newborn nursing.
- Discuss the current status of gene therapy.

- Summarize the process of fertilization.
- Describe the development, structure, and functions of the placenta.
- Describe the composition and functions of the amniotic fluid.
- Identify three organs or tissues arising from each of the three primary germ layers.
- Summarize the significant changes in growth and development of the embryo and fetus.
- Identify the potential effects of teratogens during vulnerable periods of embryonic and fetal development.

This chapter presents a brief discussion of genetics and the role of the nurse in genetics. It also provides an overview of the process of fertilization and of the development of the normal embryo and fetus.

GENETICS

Recent advances in molecular biology and genomics have revolutionized the field of health care by providing the tools needed to determine the hereditary component of many diseases as well as improve our ability to predict susceptibility to disease, onset and progression of disease, and response to medications (Guttmacher, McGuire, Ponder, et al., 2010). This increase in genetic knowledge has resulted in a gradual shift from genetics to genomics. Genetics is the study of individual genes and their effect on relatively rare single-gene disorders, whereas genomics is the study of all the genes in the human genome together, including their interactions with each other, the environment, and the influence of other psychosocial factors and cultural factors. Genes are basic physical units of inheritance that are passed from parents to offspring and contain the information needed to specify traits. The genome is the entire set of genetic instructions found in each cell. For these and other definitions of genetic terms, visit the *Talking Glossary of Genetic Terms* (www.genome.gov/Glossary).

Genetic services are rapidly becoming an integral part of routine health care as a result of:
- Growing public interest in personalized genomic information (information about much or all of a person's genome)
- Increasing development of practice guidelines
- Mounting commercial pressures
- Ever-increasing opportunities for individuals, families, and communities to participate in the direction and design of their genomic health care (Guttmacher, McGuire, Ponder, et al., 2010)

Moreover, many individuals and families have participated in direct-to-consumer genetic testing (testing marketed directly to consumers through television, print advertisements, and websites for companies such as DNA Direct [www.dnadirect.com/web], 23 and Me [www.23andme.com], and DeCODEme [www.decodeme.com]). Although much of the information provided by direct-to-consumer testing companies is recreational (e.g., ancestry information, information about type of ear wax, bitter taste perception), some of it is health related and could be interpreted as diagnosis (Evans and Green, 2009). Because of this, direct-to-consumer testing that is provided without the involvement of competent health care professionals may be not only unhelpful but even harmful (Guttmacher, McGuire, Ponder, et al., 2010; McGuire and Burke, 2010).

Genetic disorders affect people of all ages, from all socioeconomic levels, and from all racial and ethnic backgrounds. Genetic disorders affect not only individuals but also families, communities, and society. Advances in genetic testing and genetically based treatments have altered the care provided to affected individuals. Improvements in diagnostic capability have resulted in earlier diagnosis and enabled individuals who previously would have died in childhood to survive into adulthood. However, for most genetic conditions, therapeutic or preventive measures do not exist or are very limited. Consequently, the most useful means of reducing the incidence of these disorders is by preventing their transmission. It is standard practice to assess all pregnant women for heritable disorders to identify potential problems.

Nursing Expertise in Genetics and Genomics

Genetic disorders span every clinical practice specialty and site, including schools, clinics, offices, hospitals, mental health agencies, and community health settings. Because the potential impact on families and the community is significant, genetic information, technology, and testing must be incorporated into health care services. Genetics must be integrated into nursing education and practice.

Expanded roles for nurses with expertise in genetics and genomics are developing in many areas of maternity and women's health nursing. These areas include but are not limited to:

- Preconception counseling and testing
- Neonatal genetic screening and testing
- Palliative care for infants with life-threatening genetic conditions and their families
- The identification and care of individuals with genetic conditions and their families
- The care of women with genetic conditions who require specialized care during pregnancy, such as women with congenital heart disease, cystic fibrosis, and factor V Leiden.

Essential Competencies in Genetics and Genomics for All Nurses

Nearly 50 organizations, including the Association of Women's Health, Obstetric and Neonatal Nurses (AWHONN) and the National Association of Neonatal Nurses (NANN), have endorsed the *Essentials of Genetic and Genomic Nursing: Competencies, Curricula Guidelines, and Outcome Indicators* (ed 2) (Consensus Panel on Genetic/Genomic Nursing Competencies, 2009). The competencies in the document reflect the minimum amount of genetic and genomic competency expected of all nurses. The competencies are not intended to replace or recreate current standards of practice. The document is available at www.genome.gov/Pages/Careers/HealthProfessionalEducation/geneticscompetency.pdf. Some of the competencies most relevant to nurses in maternity nursing include:

- Constructs a pedigree from collected family history information using standardized symbols and terminology
- Develops a plan of care that incorporates genetic and genomic assessment information
- Provides patients with credible, accurate, appropriate, and current genetic and genomic information, resources, services, and/or technologies that facilitate decision making
- Recognizes when one's own attitudes and values related to genetic and genomic science may affect care provided to patients
- Facilitates referrals for specialized genetic and genomic services for patients as needed

- Evaluates impact and effectiveness of genetic and genomic technology, information, interventions, and treatments on patients' outcome

Human Genome Project and Implications for Clinical Practice

The Human Genome Project was a publicly funded international effort coordinated by the National Institutes of Health (NIH) and the U.S. Department of Energy (www.doegenomes.org). When the Human Genome Project was initiated in 1990, the ultimate goal of the project was to map the human genome (the complete set of genetic instructions in the nucleus of each human cell) by 2005. Considering that the human genome consists of approximately 3 billion base pairs of DNA, many people regarded this as an impossible task. However, by 2003 a substantially complete version of the human genome was announced.

Two key findings from the Human Genome Project were that (1) all human beings are 99.9% identical at the DNA level and (2) there are approximately 20,500 genes in the human genome. The finding that human beings are 99.9% identical at the DNA level should help discourage the use of science as a justification for drawing precise racial boundaries around certain groups of people. Originally scientists had estimated that there were 50,000 to 140,000 genes in the human genome.

A more recent effort by the National Human Genome Research Institute (NHGRI) called the **Enc**yclopedia of **DNA E**lements, or ENCODE, was organized to identify the genome's functional elements. By 2012 researchers "linked more than 80% of the human genome sequence to a specific biological function and mapped more than 4 million regulatory regions where proteins specifically interact with the DNA" (ENCODE, 2012). This made clearer the active genome in which genes are turned on and off by proteins using sites that may be at a great distance from the genes. Identification of regulatory regions will help explain different functions of different types of cells (www.genome.gov/pfv.cfm?pageID=27549810).

Importance of Family History

Completion of the Human Genome Project and the resultant identification of the inherited causes for many diseases have created a renewed interest in family history. Although it is easy to be impressed by the 1900 genetic tests currently available, family history will most likely continue to be the single most cost-effective piece of genetic information. A complete three-generation family history that includes ethnicity information concerning both sides of the family is the best genetic "test" applicable to preconception care. When nurses and other clinicians conduct a family history, they can gain not only valuable information about the structure of the family and diseases that affect various individuals in the family but also a rich understanding of family relationships, social context, occupations, lifestyle, and health habits. The process of collecting this information often facilitates the development of a relationship between the patient/family and the clinician. In 2004 the United States Department of Health and Human Services (USDHHS) launched the Family History Initiative by designating Thanksgiving Day as National Family History Day. The U.S. Surgeon General encouraged families to use their family gatherings as a time to talk about and collect important family health history. A number of family history tools are available free of charge online. One of the most widely used is the *My Family Health Portrait* (https://familyhistory.hhs.gov). Another family health history tool—*Does it run in the family?*—was developed by the Genetic Alliance (www.doesitruninthefamily.org).

Gene Identification and Testing

Initial efforts to sequence and analyze the human genome have proven invaluable in the identification of genes involved in disease and in the development of genetic tests. Hundreds of genes involved in diseases such as breast cancer, colorectal cancer, Alzheimer's disease, and cystic fibrosis (CF) have been identified. The number of commercially available genetic tests continues to increase and can be found on GeneTests, a publicly funded genetics information resource for clinicians (www.ncbi.nlm.nih.gov/sites/GeneTests/).

Genetic testing involves the analysis of human DNA, ribonucleic acid (RNA), chromosomes (threadlike packages of genes and other DNA in the nucleus of a cell), or proteins to detect abnormalities related to an inherited condition. Genetic tests can be used to examine directly the DNA and RNA that make up a gene (direct or molecular testing), look at markers that are coinherited with a gene that causes a genetic condition (linkage analysis), examine the protein products of genes (biochemical testing), or examine chromosomes (cytogenetic testing).

Most of the genetic tests now being offered in clinical practice are tests for single-gene disorders in patients with clinical symptoms or who have a family history of a genetic disease. Some of these genetic tests are prenatal tests or tests used to identify the genetic status of a pregnancy at risk for a genetic condition. Current prenatal testing options include:

- Maternal serum screening (a blood test used to see if a pregnant woman is at increased risk for carrying a fetus with a neural tube defect or chromosomal abnormalities such as Down syndrome, trisomy 18, and trisomy 13)
- Fetal ultrasound or sonogram (an imaging technique using high-frequency sound waves to produce images of the fetus inside the uterus)
- Invasive procedures (amniocentesis and chorionic villus sampling)

(See Chapter 10 for discussion of these tests.) Other tests are carrier screening tests used to identify individuals who have a gene mutation for a genetic condition but do not show symptoms of the condition because it is an autosomal recessive condition (e.g., CF, sickle cell disease, Tay-Sachs disease).

Another type of genetic testing is predictive testing, which is used to clarify the genetic status of asymptomatic family members. The two types of predictive testing are presymptomatic and predispositional. Mutation analysis for Huntington's disease (HD), a neurodegenerative disorder, is an example of presymptomatic testing. If the gene mutation for HD is present, symptoms of HD are certain to appear if the individual lives long enough. Testing for a BRCA1 gene mutation to determine breast cancer susceptibility is an example of predispositional testing. Predispositional testing differs from presymptomatic testing in that a positive result (indicating that a BRCA1 mutation is present) does not indicate a 100% risk for developing the condition (breast cancer).

In addition to using genetic tests for single-gene disorders in patients with clinical symptoms or with a family history of a genetic disease, genetic tests are being used for population-based screening. For example, newborn screening for phenylketonuria (PKU) and other inborn errors of metabolism (IEMs) has been going on in the United States and many other countries for decades (Guttmacher, McGuire, Ponder, et al., 2010). Initially, state-mandated newborn screening in the United States was concerned with only a few conditions. With the advent of tandem mass spectrometry, the number of conditions tested for during newborn screening grew rapidly. Currently, most states use blood spots collected from newborns to test for at least 30 different metabolic and genetic diseases. The conditions most commonly tested for are PKU, congenital hypothyroidism, galactosemia, and sickle cell disease and other hemoglobinopathies. A complete list of conditions tested for in each state is available on the National Newborn Screening and Genetics Resource website (genes-r-us.uthscsa.edu).

Genetic tests are also used to determine paternity, identify victims of war and other tragedies, and profile criminals (www.genetests.org).

Pharmacogenomics

One of most promising clinical applications of the Human Genome Project has been pharmacogenomic testing (the use of genetic information to individualize drug therapy). Associations between genetic variation and drug effect have been observed for a number of commonly used drugs. One of these drugs is warfarin, an anticoagulant commonly used to reduce the risk for thromboembolic events in patients with a history of deep vein thrombosis, pulmonary embolism, myocardial infarction, or atrial fibrillation (Meckley, Gudgeon, Anderson, et al., 2010). There is mounting evidence that genotype-guided warfarin dosing may not only help reduce the serious adverse drug reactions commonly associated with warfarin but also increase dosing accuracy, shorten the time to dose stabilization, and help identify individuals who may require more frequent monitoring.

Gene Therapy

The aim of gene therapy is to correct defective genes that are responsible for disease development. Generally, gene therapy involves inserting a healthy copy of the defective gene into the somatic cells (any cell of the body except sperm and egg cells) of the affected individual. Although the early optimism about gene therapy was probably never fully justified, gene therapy has now moved from preclinical to clinical studies for many diseases. These diseases range from hemophilia and other single-gene disorders to complex disorders such as cancer, HIV, and cardiovascular disorders. Major challenges to gene therapy include determining how to target the right gene to the right location in the right cells, expressing the transferred gene at the right time, and minimizing adverse reactions.

Ethical, Legal, and Social Implications

Because of widespread concern about misuse of the information gained through genetics research, 5% of the Human Genome Project budget was designated for the study of the ethical, legal, and social implications (ELSI) of human genome research. Two large ELSI programs were created to identify, analyze, and address the ELSIs of human genome research at the same time that the basic science issues were being studied. During the past decade, issues of high priority for these programs have been:

- Privacy and fairness in the use and interpretation of genetic information
- Clinical integration of new genetics technologies
- Issues surrounding genetics research, such as possible discrimination and stigmatization
- Education for professionals and the general public about genetics, genetics health care, and ELSI of human genome research

Both ELSI programs have excellent websites that include much educational information, as well as links to other informative sites (www.genome.gov/10001618; www.ornl.gov/sci/techresources/Human_Genome/elsi/elsi.shtml).

The major risk associated with genetic testing concerns what happens with the information gained through testing—it may result in increased anxiety and altered family relationships; it may be difficult to keep confidential; and it may result in discrimination and stigmatization. More important, there is a large gap between the ability to test for a genetic condition and the ability to treat that same condition. Informed consent is difficult to ensure when some of the outcomes, benefits, and risks of genetic testing remain unknown.

Factors Influencing the Decision to Undergo Genetic Testing

The decision to undergo genetic testing is seldom autonomous and based solely on the needs and preferences of the individual being tested. Instead, it is often a decision based on feelings of responsibility and commitment to others. For example, a woman who is receiving treatment for breast cancer may undergo BRCA1/BRCA2 mutation testing not because she wants to find out if she carries a BRCA1 or BRCA2 mutation but, instead, because her two unaffected sisters have asked her to be tested and she feels a sense of responsibility and commitment to them. A female airline pilot with a family history of HD, who has no desire to find out if she has the gene mutation associated with HD, may undergo mutation analysis for HD because she feels she has an obligation to her family, her employer, and the people who fly with her.

Decisions about genetic testing are shaped and, in many instances, constrained by factors such as social norms where care is received and socioeconomic status. Most pregnant women in the United States now have at least one ultrasound examination, many undergo some type of multiple-marker screening, and a growing number undergo other types of prenatal testing. The range of prenatal testing options available to a pregnant woman and her family may vary significantly, based on where the pregnant woman receives prenatal care and her socioeconomic status. Certain types of prenatal testing may not be available in smaller communities and rural settings (e.g., chorionic villus sampling and fluorescent in situ hybridization [FISH] analysis). In addition, certain types of genetic testing may not be offered in conservative medical communities (e.g., preimplantation diagnosis). Some types of genetic testing are expensive and typically not covered by health insurance. Because of this, these tests may be available only to a relatively small number of individuals and families—those who can afford to pay for them.

Cultural and ethnic differences also have a significant impact on decisions about genetic testing. When prenatal diagnosis was first introduced, the principal constituency was a self-selected group of Caucasian, well-informed, middle- to upper-class women. Today the widespread use of genetic testing has introduced prenatal testing to new groups of women, women who had not previously considered genetics services. The fact that many of the women currently undergoing prenatal testing may not share mainstream U.S. views about the role of medicine and prenatal care, the meaning of disability, or how to respond to scientific risks and uncertainties further amplifies the complexity of ethical issues associated with prenatal testing.

Clinical Genetics
Genetic Transmission

Human development is a complicated process that depends on the systematic unraveling of instructions found in the genetic material of the egg and the sperm. Development from conception to birth of a normal, healthy baby occurs without incident in most cases; occasionally, however, some anomaly in the genetic code of the embryo creates a birth defect or disorder.

Genes and Chromosomes

The hereditary material carried in the nucleus of each of the somatic cells determines an individual's characteristics. This material, called *DNA* (deoxyribonucleic acid), forms threadlike strands known as *chromosomes.* Each chromosome is composed of many smaller segments of DNA referred to as *genes.* Genes or combinations of genes contain coded information that determines an individual's unique characteristics. The code is found in the specific linear order of the molecules that combine to form the strands of DNA. Genes control both the types of proteins that are made and the rate at which they are produced. Genes never act in isolation; they always interact with other genes and the environment.

All normal human somatic cells contain 46 chromosomes arranged as 23 pairs of homologous (matched) chromosomes; one chromosome of each pair is inherited from each parent. There are 22 pairs of *autosomes,* which control most traits in the body, and one pair of sex chromosomes. The larger female chromosome is called the *X;* the smaller male chromosome is the *Y.* Whereas the Y chromosome is primarily concerned with sex determination, the X chromosome contains genes that are involved in much more than sex determination. Generally, the presence of a Y chromosome causes an embryo to develop as a male; in the absence of a Y chromosome, the individual develops as a female. Thus in a normal female, the homologous pair of sex chromosomes are XX, and in a normal male, the homologous pair are XY.

Homologous chromosomes (except the X and Y chromosomes in males) have the same number and arrangement of genes. In other words, if one chromosome has a gene for hair color, its partner chromosome also will have a gene for hair color and these hair-color genes will have the same loci or be located in the same place on the two chromosomes. Although both genes code for hair color, they may not code for the same hair color. Genes at corresponding loci on homologous chromosomes that code for different forms or variations of the same trait are called alleles. An individual having two copies of the same allele for a given trait is said to be homozygous for that trait. With two different alleles, the person is heterozygous for the trait.

The term genotype typically is used to refer to the genetic makeup of an individual when discussing a specific gene pair, but at times, genotype is used to refer to an individual's entire genetic makeup or all the genes that the individual can pass on to future generations. Phenotype refers to the observable expression of an individual's genotype, such as physical features, a biochemical or molecular trait, and even a psychologic trait. A trait or disorder is considered *dominant* if it is expressed or phenotypically apparent when only one copy of the gene is present. It is considered *recessive* if it is expressed only when two copies of the alleles associated with the trait are present.

As more is learned about genetics and genomics, the concepts of dominance and recessivity have become more complex, especially in X-linked disorders. For example, traits considered to be recessive may be expressed even when only one copy of a gene located on the X chromosome is present. This occurs frequently in males because males have only one X chromosome; thus they have only one copy of the genes located on the X chromosome. Whichever gene is present on the one X chromosome determines which trait is expressed. Females, conversely, have two X chromosomes, so they have two copies of the genes located on the X chromosome. However, in any female somatic cell, only one X chromosome is functioning (otherwise there would be inequality in gene dosage between males and females). This process, known as *X-inactivation* or the *Lyon hypothesis,* is generally a random occurrence. That is, there is a 50-50

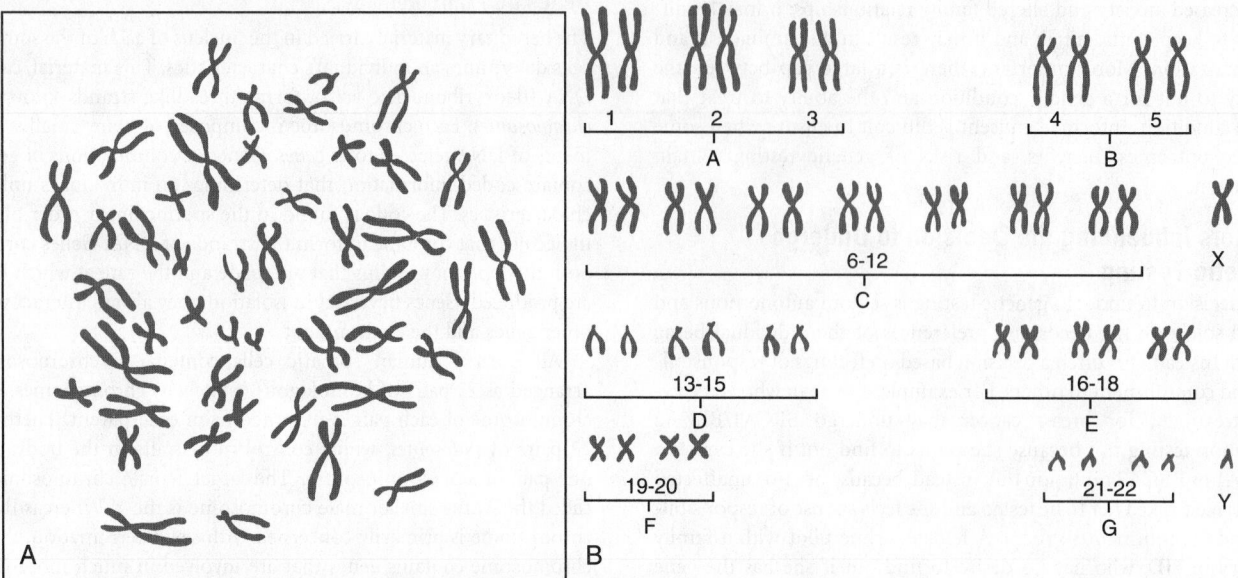

FIG 6-1 Chromosomes during cell division. **A,** Example of photomicrograph. **B,** Chromosomes arranged in karyotype; female and male sex-determining chromosomes.

chance as to whether the maternal X or the paternal X is inactivated. Occasionally the percentage of cells that have the X with an abnormal or mutant gene is very high. This helps explain why hemophilia, an X-linked recessive disorder, can clinically manifest itself in a female known to be a heterozygous carrier (a female who has only one copy of the gene mutation). It also helps explain why traditional methods of carrier detection are less effective for X-linked recessive disorders; the possible range for enzyme activity values can vary greatly, depending on which X chromosome is inactivated.

Chromosomal Abnormalities

Chromosomal abnormalities are a major cause of reproductive loss, congenital problems, and gynecologic disorders. The incidence of abnormalities is approximately 0.6% in newborns, 6% in stillbirths, and 60% in spontaneous abortions (Martin, 2008). Errors resulting in chromosomal abnormalities can occur in mitosis (cell division occurring in somatic cells that results in two identical daughter cells containing a diploid number of chromosomes) or meiosis (division of a sex cell into two and four haploid cells). These errors can occur in either the autosomes or the sex chromosomes. Even without the presence of obvious structural malformations, small deviations in chromosomes can cause problems in fetal development.

The pictorial analysis of the number, form, and size of an individual's chromosomes is known as a karyotype. Cells from any nucleated, replicating body tissue (not red blood cells, nerves, or muscles) can be used. The most commonly used tissues are white blood cells and fetal cells in amniotic fluid. The cells are grown in a culture and arrested when they are in metaphase (during metaphase, the chromosomes are condensed and visible with a light microscope), and then the cells are dropped onto a slide. This breaks the cell membranes and spreads the chromosomes, making them easier to visualize. Next, the cells are stained with special stains (e.g., Giemsa stain) that create striping or "banding" patterns. These patterns aid in the analysis because they are consistent from person to person. Once the chromosome spreads are photographed or scanned by a computer, they are cut out and arranged in a specific numeric order according to their length and shape. The chromosomes are numbered from largest to smallest, 1 to 22, and the sex chromosomes are designated by the letter X or Y. Each chromosome is divided into two "arms" designated by p (short arm) and q (long arm). A female karyotype is designated as 46,XX and a male karyotype is designated as 46,XY. Fig. 6-1 illustrates the chromosomes in a body cell and a karyotype.

Autosomal Abnormalities

Autosomal abnormalities involve differences in the number or structure of autosome chromosomes (pairs 1 through 22). They result from unequal distribution of the genetic material during gamete (egg and sperm) formation.

Abnormalities of Chromosome Number. A euploid cell is a cell with the correct or normal number of chromosomes within the cell. Because most gametes are haploid (1N, 23 chromosomes) and most somatic cells are diploid (2N, 46 chromosomes), they are both considered euploid cells. Deviations from the correct number of chromosomes per cell can be one of two types: (1) polyploidy, in which the deviation is an exact multiple of the haploid number of chromosomes or one chromosome set (23 chromosomes); or (2) aneuploidy, in which the numeric deviation is not an exact multiple of the haploid set. A triploid (3N) cell is an example of a polyploidy. It has 69 chromosomes. A tetraploid (4N) cell, also an example of a polyploidy, has 92 chromosomes.

Aneuploidy is the most commonly identified chromosome abnormality in humans and the leading genetic cause of intellectual disability. A monosomy is the product of the union between a normal gamete and a gamete that is missing a chromosome. Monosomic individuals have only 45 chromosomes in each of their cells. The product of the union of a normal gamete with a gamete containing an extra chromosome is a trisomy. The most common autosomal aneuploid conditions involve trisomies. Trisomic individuals have 47 chromosomes in most or all of their cells.

The vast majority of trisomies occur during oogenesis (the process by which a premeiotic female germ cell divides into a mature egg); the incidence of these types of chromosomal errors increases exponentially with advancing maternal age. Although variation exists among trisomies with regard to the parent and stage of origin of the extra chromosome, most trisomies are maternal meiosis I (MI) errors. This means that most trisomies are caused by nondisjunction during the first meiotic division. The first meiotic division involves the segregation of homologous or similar chromosomes. One pair of chromosomes fails to separate. One resulting cell contains both chromosomes, and the other contains none. The fact that most trisomies are maternal MI errors is not that surprising, because maternal MI occurs over a long time span. It is initiated in precursor cells during fetal development, but it is not completed until the time those cells undergo ovulation after menarche.

The most common trisomy abnormality is Down syndrome (DS). Approximately one in every 691 newborns has DS; there are over 400,000 individuals with DS living in the United States (www.ndss.org). Ninety-five percent of individuals with DS have trisomy 21 (nondisjunction) or an extra chromosome 21 (47,XX+21, female with DS; or 47,XY+21, male with DS). Another type of DS, translocation, occurs when extra chromosome 21 material is present in every cell of the individual but it is attached to another chromosome. In the third type of DS, mosaicism, extra chromosome 21 material is found in some but not all of the cells.

Although the risk for having a child with DS increases with maternal age (incidence is approximately 1 in 1200 for a 25-year-old woman; 1 in 350 for a 35-year-old woman; and 1 in 30 for a 45-year-old woman), children with Down syndrome can be born to mothers of any age (www.ndss.org). Eighty percent of children with Down syndrome are born to mothers younger than 35 years. The risk for a mother having a second child with Down syndrome is about 1% when the cause of the Down syndrome is trisomy 21.

Other autosomal trisomies that maternity nurses might see are trisomy 18 (Edwards syndrome) and trisomy 13 (Patau syndrome). Trisomy 18 is more common than trisomy 13; it occurs in about 1 of 3000 live births versus 1 of 10,000 live births for trisomy 13. Infants with trisomy 18 and trisomy 13 usually have severe to profound intellectual disabilities. Although both conditions have a poor prognosis, with the vast majority of affected infants dying before they reach their first birthday, a growing number of infants with these trisomies are living longer and a small number are actually living into their 40s and 50s.

Nondisjunction can also occur during mitosis. If this occurs early in development, when cell lines are forming, the individual has a mixture of cells, some with a normal number of chromosomes and others either missing a chromosome or containing an extra chromosome. This condition is known as *mosaicism*. The most common form of mosaicism in autosomes is mosaic Down syndrome.

Abnormalities of Chromosome Structure. Structural abnormalities can occur in any chromosome. Types of structural abnormalities include translocation, duplication, deletion, microdeletion, and inversion. Translocation results when there is an exchange of chromosomal material between two chromosomes. Exposure to certain drugs, viruses, and radiation can cause translocations, but often they arise for no apparent reason.

The two major types of translocation are reciprocal and robertsonian. Reciprocal translocations are the most common. In a reciprocal translocation, either the parts of the two chromosomes are exchanged equally (balanced translocation) or a part of a chromosome is transferred to a different chromosome, creating an unbalanced translocation because there is extra chromosomal material—extra of one chromosome but correct amount or deficient amount of the other chromosome. In a balanced translocation, the individual is phenotypically normal because there is no extra chromosome material; it is just rearranged. In an unbalanced trans-

location, the individual will be both genotypically and phenotypically abnormal.

In a robertsonian translocation, the short arms (p arms) of two different acrocentric chromosomes (chromosomes with very short p arms) break, leaving sticky ends that then cause the two long arms (q arms) to stick together. This forms a new, large chromosome that is made of the two long arms. The individual with a balanced robertsonian translocation has 45 chromosomes. Because the short arm of acrocentric chromosomes contains genes for ribosomal RNA and these genes are represented elsewhere, the individual usually does not show any symptoms. The individual may produce an unbalanced gamete (sperm or egg with too many or two few genes). This can lead to reproductive difficulties such as miscarriages or birth defects.

In duplication, there is an extra chromosomal segment within the same homologous or another nonhomologous chromosome. Clinical findings are highly variable and depend on which of the chromosomal segments are involved.

Deletions result in the loss of chromosomal material and partial monosomy for the chromosome involved. Microdeletions are deletions too small to be detected by standard cytogenetic techniques. Whenever a portion of a chromosome is deleted from one chromosome and added to another, the gamete produced may have either extra copies of genes or too few copies. The clinical effects produced may be mild or severe depending on the amount of genetic material involved. Two of the more common conditions are the deletion of the short arm of chromosome 5 (cri du chat syndrome) and the deletion of the long arm of chromosome 18.

Inversions are deviations in which a portion of the chromosome has been rearranged in reverse order. Few birth defects have been attributed to the presence of inversions, but it is suspected that inversions may be responsible for problems with infertility and miscarriages. More than 40% of inversions involve chromosome 9.

Sex Chromosome Abnormalities

Several sex chromosome abnormalities are caused by nondisjunction during gametogenesis in either parent. The most common deviation in females is *Turner syndrome,* or monosomy X (45,X). The affected female exhibits juvenile external genitalia with undeveloped ovaries. She is short in stature and often has webbing of the neck, a low hairline in the back, low-set ears, and lymphedema of her hands and feet. Intelligence may be impaired. Most affected embryos miscarry spontaneously. In most cases of Turner syndrome, it is the paternal X or Y that is lost.

The most common deviation in males is *Klinefelter syndrome,* or trisomy XXY. The affected male has poorly developed secondary sexual characteristics and small testes. He is infertile, usually tall, and effeminate and may be slow to learn (www.genetic.org). Males who have mosaic Klinefelter syndrome may be fertile.

Patterns of Genetic Transmission

Heritable characteristics are those that can be passed on to offspring. The patterns by which genetic material is transmitted to the next generation are affected by the number of genes involved in the expression of the trait. Many phenotypic characteristics result from two or more genes on different chromosomes acting together (referred to as *multifactorial inheritance);* others are controlled by a single gene *(unifactorial inheritance).* Specialists in genetics (e.g., geneticists, genetic counselors, and nurses with advanced expertise in genetics) predict the probability of the presence of an abnormal gene from the known occurrence of the trait in the individual's family and the known patterns by which the trait is inherited.

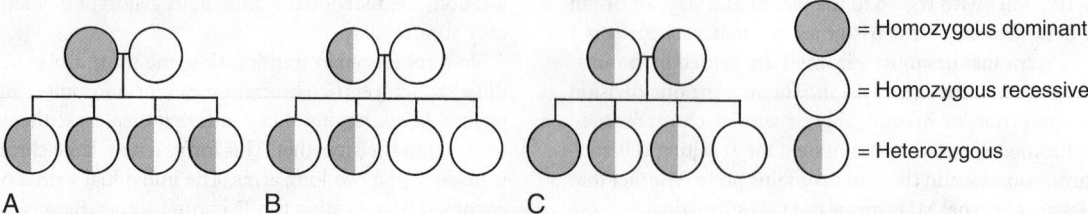

FIG 6-2 Possible offspring in three types of matings. **A,** Homozygous-dominant parent and homozygous-recessive parent. Children: all heterozygous, displaying dominant trait. **B,** Heterozygous parent and homozygous-recessive parent. Children: 50% heterozygous, displaying dominant trait; 50% homozygous, displaying recessive trait. **C,** Both parents heterozygous. Children: 25% homozygous, displaying dominant trait; 25% homozygous, displaying recessive trait; 50% heterozygous, displaying dominant trait.

Multifactorial Inheritance

Most common congenital malformations result from multifactorial inheritance, a combination of genetic and environmental factors. Examples are cleft lip, cleft palate, congenital heart disease, neural tube defects, and pyloric stenosis. Each malformation can range from mild to severe, depending on the number of genes for the defect present or the amount of environmental influence. A neural tube defect may range from spina bifida (a bony defect in the lumbar region of the vertebrae with little or no neurologic impairment) to anencephaly (absence of brain development, which is always fatal). Some malformations occur more often in one sex. For example, pyloric stenosis and cleft lip are more common in males, and cleft palate is more common in females.

Unifactorial Inheritance

If a single gene controls a particular trait or disorder, its pattern of inheritance is referred to as *unifactorial mendelian* or *single-gene inheritance.* The number of single-gene disorders far exceeds the number of chromosomal abnormalities. Potential patterns of inheritance for single-gene disorders include autosomal dominant, autosomal recessive, and X-linked dominant and recessive modes of inheritance (Fig. 6-2).

Autosomal Dominant Inheritance. Autosomal dominant inheritance disorders are those in which only one copy of a variant allele is needed for phenotypic expression. The variant allele may be a result of a mutation—a spontaneous and permanent change in the normal gene structure in which case the disorder occurs for the first time in the family. Usually an affected individual comes from multiple generations having the disorder. An affected parent who is heterozygous for the trait has a 50% chance of passing the variant allele to each offspring (see Fig. 6-2, *B* and *C*). There is a vertical pattern of inheritance (i.e., there is no skipping of generations; if an individual has an autosomal dominant disorder such as HD, so must one of his or her parents). Males and females are equally affected.

Autosomal dominant disorders are not always expressed with the same severity of symptoms. For example, a woman who has an autosomal dominant disorder may show few symptoms and may not become aware of her diagnosis until after she gives birth to a severely affected child. Predicting whether an offspring will have a minor or severe abnormality is not possible. Examples of autosomal dominant disorders are HD, Marfan syndrome, neurofibromatosis, myotonic dystrophy, Stickler syndrome, Treacher Collins syndrome, and achondroplasia (dwarfism).

Autosomal Recessive Inheritance. Autosomal recessive inheritance disorders are those in which both genes of a pair associated with the disorder must be abnormal for the disorder to be expressed. Heterozygous individuals have only one variant allele and are unaffected clinically because their normal gene overshadows the variant allele. They are known as *carriers* of the recessive trait. Because these recessive traits are inherited by generations of the same family, an increased incidence of the disorder occurs in consanguineous matings (closely related parents). For the trait to be expressed, two carriers must each contribute a variant allele to the offspring (see Fig. 6-2, *C*). The chance of the trait occurring in each child is 25%. A clinically normal offspring may be a carrier of the gene. Autosomal recessive disorders have a horizontal pattern of inheritance rather than the vertical pattern seen with autosomal dominant disorders. That is, autosomal recessive disorders are usually observed in one or more siblings but not in earlier generations. Males and females are equally affected. Most inborn errors of metabolism (IEMs), such as phenylketonuria, galactosemia, maple syrup urine disease, Tay-Sachs disease, sickle cell anemia, and cystic fibrosis, are autosomal recessive inherited disorders.

Inborn Errors of Metabolism. More than 350 *inborn errors of metabolism* have been recognized (Jorde, Carey, and Bamshad, 2010). Individually, IEMs are relatively rare, but collectively, they are common (1 in 5000 live births). Most IEMs are inherited in an autosomal recessive pattern. IEMs occur when a gene mutation reduces the efficiency of encoded enzymes to a level at which normal metabolism cannot occur. Defective enzyme action interrupts the normal series of chemical reactions from the affected point onward. The result may be an accumulation of a damaging product, such as phenylalanine in PKU, or the absence of a necessary product, such as the lack of melanin in albinism caused by lack of tyrosinase. Diagnostic and carrier testing is available for a growing number of IEMs. In addition, many states in the United States have started screening for specific IEMs as part of their expanded newborn screening programs using tandem mass spectrometry. However, many of the deaths caused by IEMs are the result of enzyme variants not currently screened for in many of the newborn screening programs (Jorde, Carey, and Bamshad, 2010). (See discussion of IEMs in Chapter 25.)

X-Linked Dominant Inheritance. X-linked dominant inheritance disorders occur in males and heterozygous females, but because of X inactivation, affected females are usually less severely affected than affected males and they are more likely to transmit the variant allele to their offspring. Heterozygous females (females who have one wild-type allele and one variant allele) have a 50% chance of transmitting the variant allele to each offspring. The variant allele is often lethal in affected males since, unlike affected females, they have no normal gene (wild-type allele). Mating of an affected male and an unaffected female is uncommon as a result of the tendency for the variant allele to be lethal in affected males. Relatively few X-linked dominant disorders have been identified. Two examples are vitamin D–resistant rickets and Rett syndrome.

X-Linked Recessive Inheritance. Abnormal genes for X-linked recessive inheritance disorders are carried on the X chromosome. Females may be heterozygous or homozygous for traits carried on the X chromosome because they have two X chromosomes. Males are hemizygous because they have only one X chromosome, which carries genes with no alleles on the Y chromosome. Therefore X-linked recessive disorders are most commonly manifested in the male with the abnormal gene on his single X chromosome. Hemophilia, color blindness, and Duchenne muscular dystrophy are X-linked recessive disorders.

The male with an X-linked recessive disorder receives the disease-associated allele from his carrier mother on her affected X chromosome. Female carriers (those heterozygous for the trait) have a 50% probability of transmitting the disease-associated allele to each offspring. An affected male can pass the disease-associated allele to his daughters but not to his sons. The daughters will be carriers of the trait if they receive a normal gene on the X chromosome from their mother. They will be affected only if they receive a disease-associated allele on the X chromosome from both their mother and their father.

GENETIC COUNSELING

It is standard practice in obstetrics to determine whether a heritable disorder exists in a couple or in anyone in either of their families. The goal of screening is to detect or define risk for disease in low risk populations and identify those for whom diagnostic testing may be appropriate. A nurse can obtain a genetics history using a questionnaire or checklist such as the one in Fig. 6-3.

Genetic counseling is a professional service that provides genetics information, education, and support to individuals and families with ongoing or potential genetic health concerns. It is typically provided by a team of genetics specialists that includes clinical geneticists (physicians), medical geneticists with a PhD, genetics fellows, genetics counselors, and, in a growing number of cases, advanced practice genetics nurse specialists. Cytogeneticists, biochemical geneticists, and molecular geneticists support the clinical genetics team by providing laboratory expertise that helps with the diagnosis and management of individuals and families affected by genetic conditions.

Genetic counseling occurs in regional genetics centers, major medical centers, outreach or satellite genetics clinics, public health clinics, some community hospitals, and now that genetics has entered the mainstream of health care, in a wide variety of other settings. These include but are not limited to managed health care organizations, commercial facilities, and private practices. A number of specialized groups provide genetics education and counseling for individuals and families affected by specific genetic disorders, such as DS, CF, diabetes, muscular dystrophy, HD, and cancer. Genetic counseling also is offered over the Internet.

Individuals and families seek out or are referred for genetic counseling for a wide variety of reasons and at all stages of their lives. Some seek preconception or prenatal information; others are referred after the birth of a child with a birth defect or a suspected genetic condition; still others seek information because they have a family history of a genetic condition. Regardless of the setting or the individual's and family's stage of life, genetic counseling should be offered and available to all individuals and families who have

questions about genetics and their health. However, there is a shortage of appropriately trained genetics professionals who can provide genetic counseling. This means that many individuals and families will not be offered genetic counseling when they undergo genetic testing. Moreover, some of the genetics education and counseling that is provided will be inadequate (see Community Focus box).

Existing genetics resources include:
- Centers for Disease Control and Prevention (www.cdc.gov/genetics/activities/ogdp.htm)
- Genetic Alliance (www.geneticalliance.org/)
- National Coalition for Health Professional Education in Genetics (www.nchpeg.org/)
- Genetics Education Program for Nurses at Cincinnati Children's Hospital Medical Center (www.cincinnatichildrens.org/ed/clinical/gpnf/default.htm)
- NHGRI Education (www.genome.gov/Education/)
- National Center for Biotechnology Information (www.ncbi.nlm.nih.gov/)
- Other websites, such as www.hsl.unc.edu/Services/Guides/focusonclingen.cfm

Some of these resources may be in health care professionals' own communities, but others are regional, national, and international resources.

Estimation of Risk

Most families with a history of genetic disease want an answer to the following question: What is the chance that our future children will have this disease? Because the answer to this question may have profound implications for individual family members and the family as a whole, health care professionals must be able to answer this question as accurately as they can in a timely manner. In some cases, estimation of risk is rather straightforward; in other cases, it is complicated.

If a couple has not yet had children but they are known to be at risk for having children with a genetic disease, they will be given an occurrence risk. Once the mating of a couple has produced one or more children with a genetic disease, the couple will be given a recurrence risk. Both occurrence and recurrence risks are determined by the mode of inheritance for the genetic disease in question. For genetic diseases caused by a factor that segregates during cell division (genes and chromosomes), risk can be estimated with a high degree of accuracy by application of mendelian principles.

In an autosomal dominant disorder, both the occurrence and recurrence risk is 50%, or one in two, that a subsequent offspring will be affected when one parent is affected and the other is not. The

Risk Factors for Genetic Disorders

Answer the following questions about risk factors. If you answer "yes" to any of them, you may be at increased risk for having a baby with a genetic disorder.

_____ Will you be age 35 years or older when your baby is due?

_____ Will the baby's father be age 50 years or older when your baby is due?

_____ If you or the baby's father are of Mediterranean or Asian descent, do either of you or does anyone in your families have thalassemia?

_____ Is there a family history of neural tube defects?

_____ Have you or the baby's father ever had a child with a neural tube defect?

_____ Is there a family history of congenital heart defects?

_____ Is there a family history of Down syndrome?

_____ Have you or the baby's father ever had a child with Down syndrome?

_____ If you or the baby's father are of Eastern European Jewish, French Canadian, or Cajun descent, is there a family history of Tay-Sachs disease?

_____ If you or your partner are of Eastern European Jewish descent, is there a family history of Canavan disease or any other genetic disorders?

_____ If you or your partner are African-American, is there a family history of sickle cell disease or sickle cell trait?

_____ Is there a family history of hemophilia?

_____ Is there a family history of muscular dystrophy?

_____ Is there a family history of cystic fibrosis?

_____ Is there a family history of Huntington's disease?

_____ Does anyone in your family or the family of the baby's father have cystic fibrosis?

_____ Is anyone in your family or the family of the baby's father's mentally retarded?

_____ If so, was that person tested for fragile X syndrome?

_____ Do you, the baby's father, anyone in your families, or any of your children have any other genetic diseases, chromosomal disorders, or birth defects?

_____ Do you have a metabolic disorder such as diabetes or phenylketonuria?

_____ Do you have a history of pregnancy issues (miscarriage or stillbirth)?

FIG 6-3 Questionnaire for identifying couples having increased risk for offspring with genetic disorders. (Courtesy American College of Obstetricians and Gynecologists: _Your pregnancy and childbirth month to month_, ed 5, Washington, DC, 2010, Author.)

recurrence risk for autosomal recessive disorders is 25%, or one in four, if both parents are carriers (they each have one recessive disease gene and one normal gene). Occasionally an individual homozygous for a recessive disease gene mates with an individual who is a carrier of the same recessive gene. In this case, the recurrence risk is 50%, or one in two. If two individuals affected by an autosomal recessive disorder mate, all of their children will be affected. For X-linked disorders, recurrence risk is related to the sex of the child. Translocation chromosomes have a high risk for recurrence.

A number of autosomal disorders display fairly complex patterns of inheritance, making estimation of risk somewhat difficult. For example, if a child is born with a genetic disease and there has been no history of the disease in the family, the disease may have been caused by a new mutation (this is more likely if the disease in question is an autosomal dominant disorder, such as achondroplasia). If the child's genetic disease has been caused by a new mutation, the recurrence risk for the parents' subsequent children is low (1% to 2%), but it is not as low as that for the general population. Offspring of the affected child may have a substantially elevated occurrence risk.

The risk for recurrence for multifactorial conditions can be estimated empirically. An empiric risk is based not on genetics theory but, rather, on experience and observation of the disorder in other families. Recurrence risks are determined by applying the frequency of a similar disorder in other families to the case under consideration.

An important concept to be emphasized to individuals and families during a genetic counseling session is that *each pregnancy is an independent event*. For example, in monogenic disorders in which the risk factor is one in four that the child will be affected, the risk remains the same no matter how many affected children are already in the family. Families may maintain the erroneous assumption that the presence of one affected child ensures that the next three will be free of the disorder. However, "chance has no memory." The risk is one in four for each pregnancy. Conversely, in a family with a child who has a disorder with multifactorial causes, the risk increases with each subsequent child born with the disorder.

Interpretation of Risk

The guiding principle for genetics counselors has traditionally been nondirectiveness. According to the principle of nondirectiveness, the individual who is providing genetic counseling respects the right of the individual or family being counseled to make autonomous decisions. Counselors using a nondirective approach avoid making recommendations, and they try to communicate genetics information in an unbiased manner. The first step in providing nondirective counseling is becoming aware of one's own values and beliefs. Another important step is recognizing how one's values and beliefs can influence or interfere with the communication of genetics information.

If the individual who is providing genetic counseling has difficulty being nonjudgmental and objective, he or she may either intentionally or unintentionally influence the decision-making process. Individuals and families also may pressure the counselor to make decisions for them with questions such as "What would you do if you were me?" Families and individuals need education, guidance, and support throughout the counseling process. They should be given the facts and possible consequences as well as all of the assistance they need in problem solving, but the final decision regarding a course of action must be their own.

Multiple Roles for Nurses in Genetics

Nurses play many roles in genetics. Some nurses play a key role in the identification of families in need of genetic counseling, and they collaborate with other health care professionals to make referrals to specialists in genetics. Other nurses take a more active role in genetic counseling.

Probably the most important of all nursing functions is to provide emotional support during all aspects of the counseling process. Feelings that are generated under the real or imagined threat posed by a genetic disorder are as varied as the people being counseled. Responses may include a variety of stress reactions, such as apathy, denial, anger, hostility, fear, embarrassment, grief, and loss of self-esteem. Guilt and self-blame are universal reactions. Many look on the disorder as a stigma, especially if the disorder is visible to others. Old wives' tales, superstitions, and long-held misconceptions may influence a family's reaction to a genetic disorder.

Nurses are ideally positioned to help individuals and families maximize the benefits of the genetics revolution, but first, nurses need (1) a working knowledge of human genetics, (2) an awareness of recent advances in genetics and genomics, and (3) an understanding of the potential effects of genomic discoveries on individual and family well-being. More research is needed concerning the family experience of genetic testing. Nurses must understand why individuals and families decide to undergo or to forgo genetic testing. Nurses also need to be aware of how individuals and families define and manage ethical, legal, and social issues that emerge during the genetic testing experience.

CONCEPTION

Cell Division

Cells are reproduced by two different methods: mitosis and meiosis. In mitosis, the body cells replicate to yield two cells with the same genetic makeup as the parent cell. First the cell makes a copy of its DNA, and then it divides. Each daughter cell receives one copy of the genetic material. Mitotic division facilitates growth and development or cell replacement.

Meiosis, the process by which germ cells divide and decrease their chromosomal number by half, produces gametes (eggs and sperm). Each homologous pair of chromosomes contains one chromosome received from the mother and one from the father; thus meiosis results in cells that contain one of each of the 23 pairs of chromosomes. Because these germ cells contain 23 single chromosomes, half of the genetic material of a normal somatic cell, they are called *haploid*. This halving of the genetic material is accomplished by replicating the DNA once and then dividing twice. When the female gamete (egg or ovum) and the male gamete (spermatozoon) unite to form the zygote, the diploid number of human chromosomes (46, or 23 pairs) is restored.

The process of DNA replication and cell division in meiosis allows different alleles (genes on corresponding loci that code for variations of the same trait) for genes to be distributed at random by each parent and then rearranged on the paired chromosomes. The chromosomes then separate and proceed to different gametes. Because the two parents have genotypes derived from four different grandparents, many combinations of genes on each chromosome are possible. This random mixing of alleles accounts for the variation of traits seen in the offspring of the same two parents.

Gametogenesis

Oogenesis, the process of egg (ovum) formation, begins during fetal life of the female. All the cells that may undergo meiosis in a woman's lifetime are contained in her ovaries at birth. The majority of the estimated 2 million primary oocytes (the cells that undergo the first meiotic division) degenerate spontaneously. Only 400 to 500 ova will mature during the approximately 35 years of a woman's reproductive life. The primary oocytes begin the first meiotic division (i.e., they replicate their DNA) during fetal life, but they remain suspended at this stage until puberty (Fig. 6-4, *A*). Then, usually monthly, one primary oocyte matures and completes the first meiotic division, yielding two unequal cells: the secondary oocyte and a small polar body. Both contain 22 autosomes and one X sex chromosome.

At ovulation the second meiotic division begins. However, the ovum does not complete the second meiotic division unless fertilization occurs. At fertilization, when the sperm is united with the mature ovum, a second polar body and the zygote (the united egg and sperm) are produced (see Fig. 6-4, *C*). The three polar bodies degenerate.

When a male reaches puberty, his testes begin the process of spermatogenesis. The cells that undergo meiosis in the male are called *spermatocytes*. The primary spermatocyte, which undergoes the first meiotic division, contains the diploid number of chromosomes. The cell has already copied its DNA before division, so four alleles for each gene are present. The cell is still considered diploid because the copies are bound together (i.e., one allele plus its copy on each chromosome).

During the first meiotic division, two haploid secondary spermatocytes are formed. Each secondary spermatocyte contains 22

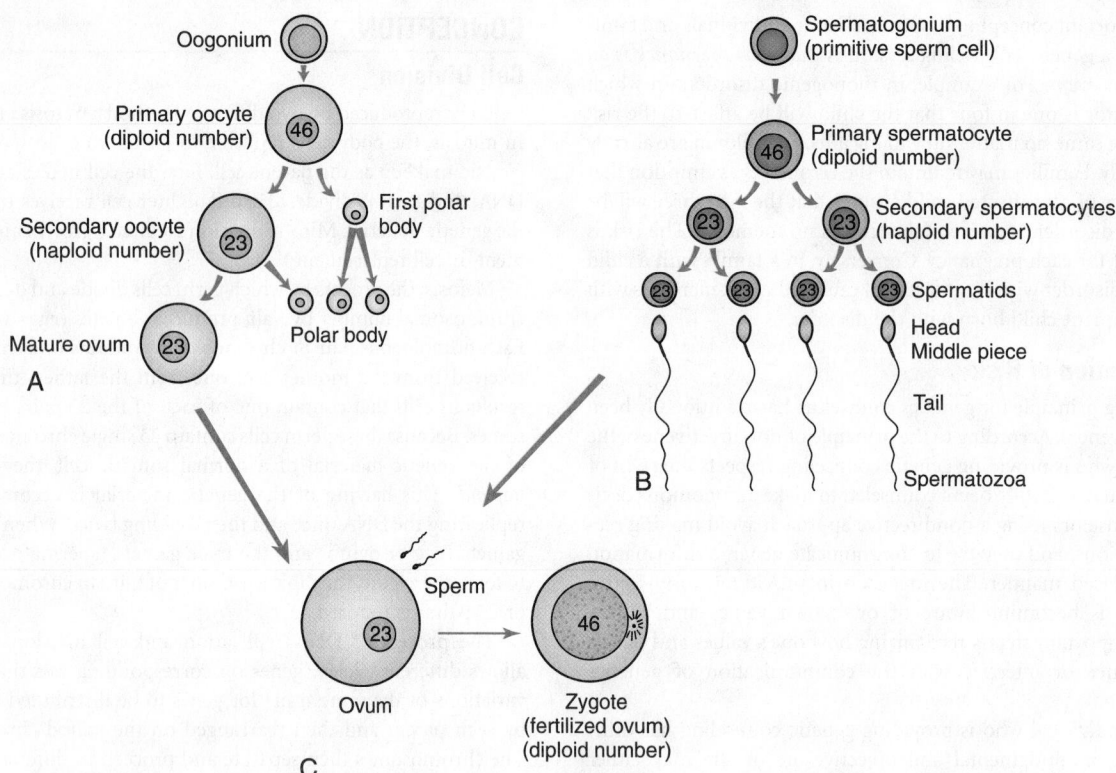

FIG 6-4 Gametogenesis and fertilization. **A,** Oogenesis. Gametogenesis in the female produces one mature ovum and three polar bodies. Note relative difference in overall size between ovum and sperm. **B,** Spermatogenesis. Gametogenesis in the male produces four mature gametes, the sperm. **C,** Fertilization results in the single-cell zygote and restoration of the diploid number of chromosomes.

autosomes and one sex chromosome; one contains the X chromosome (plus its copy) and the other, the Y chromosome (plus its copy). During the second meiotic division, the male produces two gametes with an X chromosome and two gametes with a Y chromosome, all of which will develop into viable sperm (see Fig. 6-4, *B*).

Conception

Conception, defined as the union of a single egg and sperm, marks the beginning of a pregnancy. Conception occurs not as an isolated event but as part of a sequential process. This sequential process includes gamete (egg and sperm) formation, ovulation (release of the egg), union of the gametes (which results in an embryo), and implantation in the uterus.

Ovum

Meiosis occurs in the female in the ovarian follicles and produces an egg, or ovum. Each month one ovum matures with a host of surrounding supportive cells. At ovulation the ovum is released from the ruptured ovarian follicle. High estrogen levels increase the motility of the uterine tubes so that their cilia can capture the ovum and propel it through the tube toward the uterine cavity. An ovum cannot move by itself.

Two protective layers surround the ovum (Fig. 6-5). The inner layer is a thick, acellular layer called the *zona pellucida*. The outer layer, called the *corona radiata*, is composed of elongated cells.

Ova are considered fertile for about 24 hours after ovulation. If unfertilized by a sperm, the ovum degenerates and is resorbed.

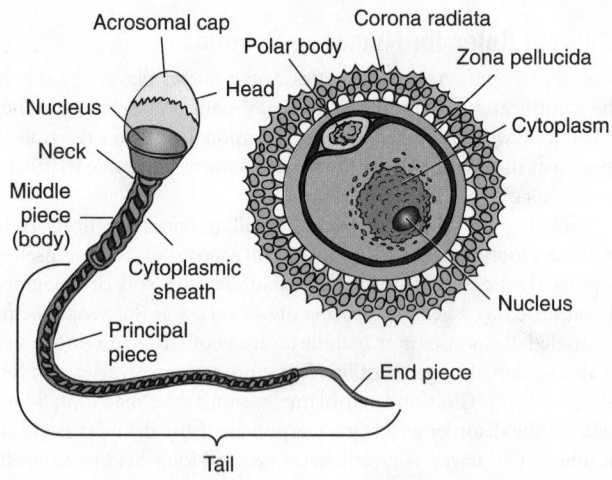

FIG 6-5 Ovum and sperm.

Sperm

Ejaculation during sexual intercourse normally propels about a teaspoon of semen containing as many as 200 to 500 million sperm into the vagina. The sperm swim by means of the flagellar movement of their tails. Some sperm can reach the site of fertilization within 5 minutes, but average transit time is 4 to 6 hours. Sperm remain viable within the woman's reproductive system for an average of 2 to 3 days. Most sperm are lost in the vagina, within the

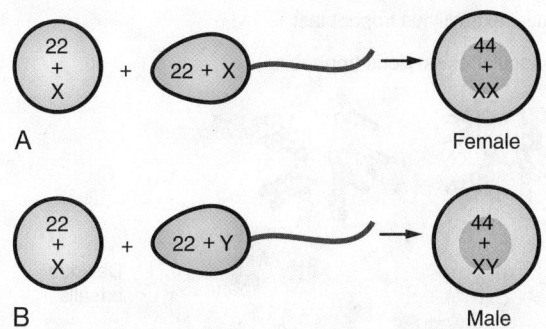

FIG 6-6 Fertilization. **A,** Ovum fertilized by X-bearing sperm to form female zygote. **B,** Ovum fertilized by Y-bearing sperm to form male zygote.

cervical mucus, or in the endometrium; or they enter the tube that contains no ovum.

As sperm travel through the female reproductive tract, enzymes are produced to aid in their capacitation. *Capacitation* is a physiologic change that removes the protective coating from the heads of the sperm. Small perforations then form in the acrosome (a cap on the sperm) and allow enzymes (e.g., hyaluronidase) to escape (see Fig. 6-5). These enzymes are necessary for the sperm to penetrate the protective layers of the ovum before fertilization.

Fertilization

Fertilization takes place in the ampulla (the outer third) of the uterine tube. When a sperm successfully penetrates the membrane surrounding the ovum, both sperm and ovum are enclosed within the membrane and the membrane becomes impenetrable to other sperm; this process is termed the zona reaction. The second meiotic division of the secondary oocyte is then completed, and the nucleus of the ovum becomes the female pronucleus. The head of the sperm enlarges to become the male pronucleus, and the tail degenerates. The nuclei fuse and the chromosomes combine, restoring the diploid number (46) (Fig. 6-6). Conception, the formation of the zygote (the first cell of the new individual), has been achieved.

Mitotic cellular replication, called *cleavage*, begins as the zygote travels the length of the uterine tube into the uterus. This voyage takes 3 to 4 days. Because the fertilized egg divides rapidly with no increase in size, successively smaller cells, called *blastomeres*, are formed with each division. A 16-cell morula, a solid ball of cells, is produced within 3 days and is still surrounded by the protective zona pellucida (Fig. 6-7, *A*). Further development occurs as the morula floats freely within the uterus. Fluid passes through the zona pellucida into the intercellular spaces between the blastomeres, separating them into two parts: the trophoblast (which gives rise to the placenta) and the embryoblast (which gives rise to the embryo). A cavity forms within the cell mass as the spaces come together, forming a structure called the *blastocyst cavity*. When the cavity becomes recognizable, the whole structure of the developing embryo is known as the *blastocyst*. Stem cells are derived from the inner cell mass of the blastocyst. The outer layer of cells surrounding the cavity is the trophoblast. The trophoblast differentiates into villous and extravillous trophoblast (Fig. 6-8).

Implantation

The zona pellucida degenerates, the trophoblast cells displace endometrial cells at the implantation site, and the blastocyst embeds in the endometrium, usually in the anterior or posterior fundal region. Between 6 and 10 days after conception, the trophoblast secretes

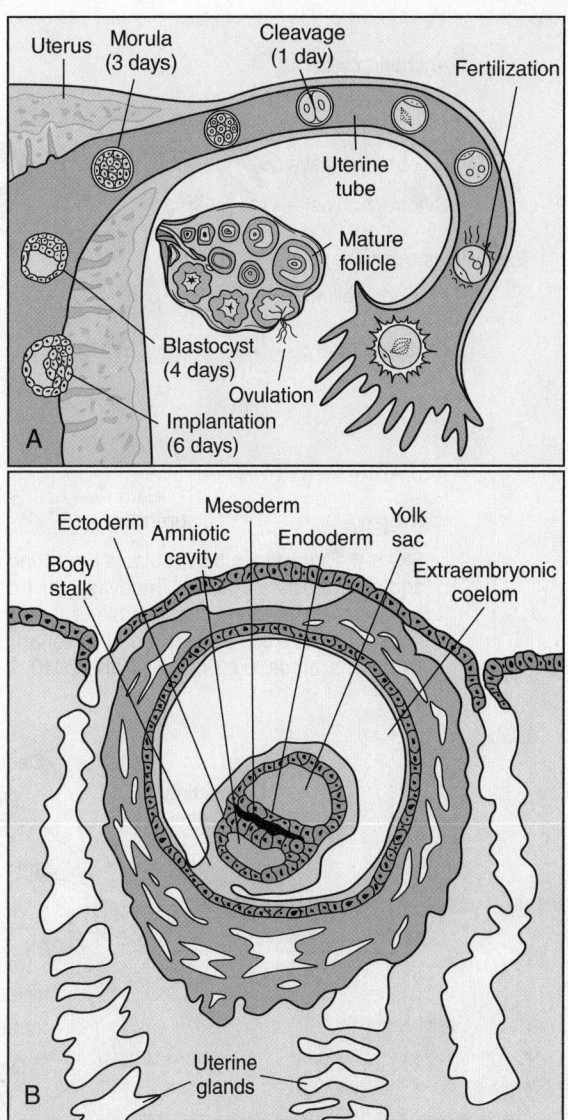

FIG 6-7 First weeks of human development. **A,** Follicular development in ovary, ovulation, fertilization, and transport of early embryo down uterine tube and into uterus, where implantation occurs. **B,** Blastocyst embedded in endometrium. Germ layers forming. (*A,* From Carlson BM: *Human embryology and developmental biology,* ed 5, St Louis, 2013, Mosby; *B,* Adapted from Langley LL, Telford IR, Christensen, JB: *Dynamic human anatomy and physiology,* ed 5, New York, 1980, McGraw-Hill.)

enzymes that enable it to burrow into the endometrium until the entire blastocyst is covered. This is known as *implantation.* Endometrial blood vessels erode, and some women have implantation bleeding (slight spotting and bleeding at the time of the first missed menstrual period). Chorionic villi, fingerlike projections, develop out of the trophoblast and extend into the blood-filled spaces of the endometrium. These villi are vascular processes that obtain oxygen and nutrients from the maternal bloodstream and dispose of carbon dioxide and waste products into the maternal blood.

After implantation, the endometrium is called the decidua. The portion directly under the blastocyst, where the chorionic villi tap into the maternal blood vessels, is the decidua basalis. The portion covering the blastocyst is the decidua capsularis, and the portion lining the rest of the uterus is the decidua vera (Fig. 6-9).

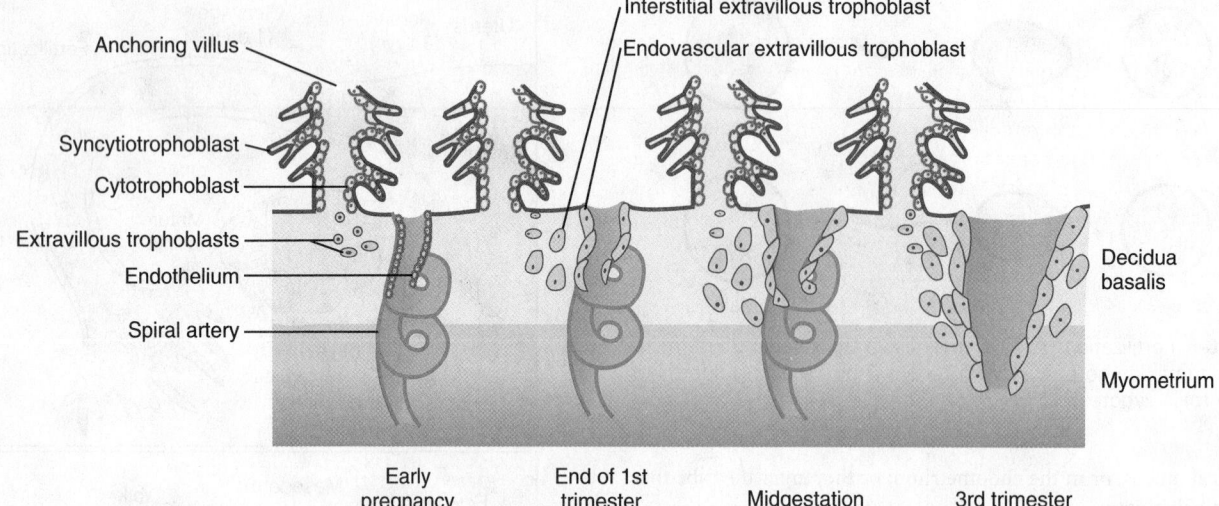

FIG 6-8 Extravillous trophoblasts are found outside the villus and can be subdivided into endovascular and interstitial categories. Endovascular trophoblasts invade and transform spiral arteries during pregnancy to create low-resistance blood flow that is characteristic of the placenta. Interstitial trophoblasts invade the decidua and surround spiral arteries. (From Cunningham F, Leveno K, Bloom S, et al: *Williams obstetrics*, ed 23, New York, 2010, McGraw-Hill.)

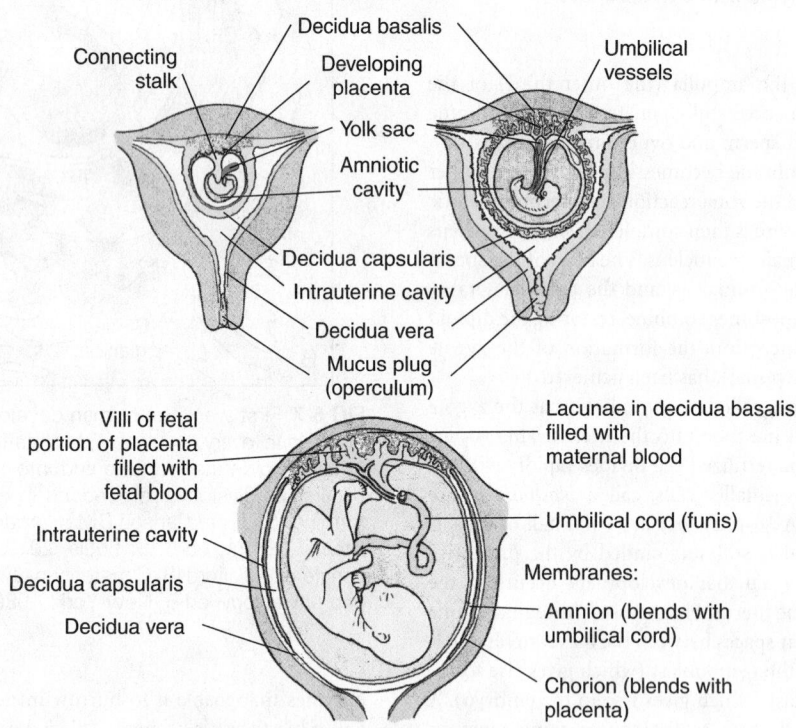

FIG 6-9 Development of fetal membranes. Note gradual obliteration of intrauterine cavity as decidua capsularis and decidua vera meet. Also note thinning of uterine wall. Chorionic and amnionic membranes are in apposition to each other but may be peeled apart.

THE EMBRYO AND FETUS

Pregnancy lasts approximately 10 lunar months, 9 calendar months, 40 weeks, or 280 days. Length of pregnancy is computed from the first day of the last menstrual period (LMP) until the day of birth. However, conception occurs approximately 2 weeks after the first day of the LMP. Thus the postconception age of the fetus is 2 weeks less, for a total of 266 days or 38 weeks. Postconception age is used in the discussion of fetal development.

Intrauterine development is divided into three stages: ovum or preembryonic, embryo, and fetus (see Fig. 6-19). The stage of the ovum lasts from conception until day 14. This period covers cellular replication, blastocyst formation, initial development of the embryonic membranes, and establishment of the primary germ layers.

Primary Germ Layers

During the third week after conception, the embryonic disk differentiates into three primary germ layers: the ectoderm, the mesoderm, and the endoderm (or entoderm) (see Fig. 6-7, B). All tissues and organs of the embryo develop from these three layers.

The ectoderm, the upper layer of the embryonic disk, gives rise to the epidermis, glands (anterior pituitary, cutaneous, and mammary), nails and hair, central and peripheral nervous systems, lens of the eyes, tooth enamel, and floor of the amniotic cavity.

The mesoderm, the middle layer, develops into the bones and teeth, muscles (skeletal, smooth, and cardiac), dermis and connective tissue, cardiovascular system and spleen, and urogenital system.

The endoderm, the lower layer, gives rise to the epithelium lining the respiratory tract and digestive tract, including the oropharynx, liver and pancreas, urethra, bladder, and vagina. The endoderm forms the roof of the yolk sac.

Development of the Embryo

The stage of the embryo lasts from day 15 until approximately 8 weeks after conception, when the embryo measures approximately 3 cm from crown to rump. The embryonic stage is the most critical time in the development of the organ systems and the main external features. Developing areas with rapid cell division are the most vulnerable to malformation caused by environmental teratogens (substances or exposure that causes abnormal development). At the end of the eighth week, all organ systems and external structures are present and the embryo is unmistakably human (see Fig. 6-19 and Visible Embryo, www.visembryo.com, for a pictorial view of normal and abnormal development).

Membranes

At the time of implantation, two fetal membranes that will surround the developing embryo begin to form. The chorion develops from the trophoblast and contains the chorionic villi on its surface. The villi burrow into the decidua basalis and increase in size and complexity as the vascular processes develop into the placenta. The chorion becomes the covering of the fetal side of the placenta. It contains the major umbilical blood vessels that branch out over the surface of the placenta. As the embryo grows, the decidua capsularis stretches. The chorionic villi on this side atrophy and degenerate, leaving a smooth chorionic membrane.

The inner cell membrane, the amnion, develops from the interior cells of the blastocyst. The cavity that develops between this inner cell mass and the outer layer of cells (trophoblast) is the amniotic cavity (see Fig. 6-7, B). As it grows larger, the amnion forms on the side opposite the developing blastocyst (see Fig. 6-7, B, and Fig. 6-9). The developing embryo draws the amnion around itself to form a fluid-filled sac. The amnion becomes the covering of the umbilical cord and covers the chorion on the fetal surface of the placenta. As the embryo grows larger, the amnion enlarges to accommodate the embryo/fetus and the surrounding amniotic fluid. The amnion eventually comes in contact with the chorion surrounding the fetus (see the Critical Thinking Case Study).

Amniotic Fluid

The amniotic cavity initially derives its fluid by diffusion from the maternal blood. Fluid secreted by the respiratory and gastrointestinal tracts of the fetus also enters the amniotic cavity (Moore, Persaud, and Torchia, 2013). The amount of fluid increases weekly, and 700 to 1000 mL of transparent liquid is normally present at term. The volume of amniotic fluid changes constantly. The fetus swallows fluid, and fluid flows into and out of the fetal lungs.

CRITICAL THINKING CASE STUDY

Ultrasound Dating of Pregnancy

Sandra believes she is 8 weeks pregnant, but her obstetrician believes she is closer to 12 weeks of gestation. Sandra has come to the clinic for an ultrasound examination for dating. She has many questions for the nurse: How can they tell what gestation she is? What would the fetus look like at this time if she is 8 weeks of gestation? If she is 12 weeks of gestation? What fetal structures would be apparent on ultrasound if she is 8 weeks pregnant? If she is 12 weeks pregnant? Would any structural anomalies be apparent at 8 weeks? At 12 weeks? Why is it important to date a pregnancy accurately?

What information should the nurse provide Sandra?

1. Evidence—Is there sufficient evidence to draw conclusions about what information the nurse should provide Sandra?
2. Assumptions—Describe an underlying assumption about the following factors:
   a. Sandra's motivation to learn about fetal development
   b. Sandra's understanding of fetal development
   c. Sandra's knowledge about ultrasound examinations
   d. Why dating the pregnancy is important
3. What implications and priorities for nursing care can be drawn at this time?
4. Does the evidence objectively support your conclusion?

Beginning in week 11, the fetus urinates into the fluid, increasing its volume.

Amniotic fluid serves many functions. It helps maintain a constant body temperature. It serves as a source of oral fluid and as a repository for waste and assists in maintenance of fluid and electrolyte homeostasis. It cushions the fetus from trauma by blunting and dispersing outside forces. It allows freedom of movement for musculoskeletal development. It acts as a barrier to infection and allows fetal lung development (Moore, Persaud, and Torchia, 2013). The fluid keeps the embryo from tangling with the membranes, facilitating symmetric growth. If the embryo does become tangled with the membranes, amputations of extremities or other deformities can occur from constricting amniotic bands.

The volume of amniotic fluid is an important factor in assessing fetal well-being. Having less than 300 mL of amniotic fluid (oligohydramnios) is associated with fetal renal abnormalities. Having more than 2 L of amniotic fluid (hydramnios) is associated with gastrointestinal and other malformations.

Amniotic fluid contains albumin, urea, uric acid, creatinine, lecithin, sphingomyelin, bilirubin, fructose, fat, leukocytes, proteins, epithelial cells, enzymes, and lanugo hair. Study of fetal cells in amniotic fluid through amniocentesis yields much information about the fetus. Genetic studies (karyotyping) provide knowledge about the sex and the number and structure of chromosomes. Other studies such as the lecithin/sphingomyelin (L/S) ratio determine the health or maturity of the fetus (see Chapter 10).

Yolk Sac

When the amniotic cavity and amnion are forming, another blastocyst cavity forms on the other side of the developing embryonic disk (see Fig. 6-7, B). This cavity becomes surrounded by a membrane, forming the yolk sac. The yolk sac aids in transferring maternal nutrients and oxygen, which have diffused through the chorion, to the embryo. Blood vessels form to aid transport. Blood cells and plasma are manufactured in the yolk sac during the second and third weeks while uteroplacental circulation is being established and is forming primitive blood cells until hematopoietic activity begins. At the end of the third week, the primitive heart begins to beat and circulate the blood through the embryo, the connecting stalk, the chorion, and the yolk sac.

The folding in of the embryo during the fourth week results in incorporation of part of the yolk sac into the embryo's body as the primitive digestive system. Primordial germ cells arise in the yolk sac and move into the embryo. The shrinking remains of the yolk sac degenerate (see Fig. 6-7, *B*), and by the fifth or sixth week, the remnant has separated from the embryo.

Umbilical Cord

By day 14 after conception, the embryonic disk, the amniotic sac, and the yolk sac are attached to the chorionic villi by the connecting stalk. During the third week, the blood vessels develop to supply the embryo with maternal nutrients and oxygen. During the fifth week, the embryo has curved inward on itself from both ends, bringing the connecting stalk to the ventral side of the embryo. The connecting stalk becomes compressed from both sides by the amnion and forms the narrower umbilical cord (see Fig. 6-7). Two arteries carry blood from the embryo to the chorionic villi, and one vein returns blood to the embryo. Approximately 1% of umbilical cords contain only two vessels: one artery and one vein. This occurrence is sometimes associated with congenital malformations.

The cord rapidly increases in length. At term the cord is 2 cm in diameter and ranges from 30 to 90 cm in length (with an average of 55 cm. It twists spirally on itself and loops around the embryo/fetus. A true knot is rare, but false knots occur as folds or kinks in the cord and may jeopardize circulation to the fetus. Connective tissue called *Wharton's jelly* prevents compression of the blood vessels and ensures continued nourishment of the embryo/fetus. Compression can occur if the cord lies between the fetal head and the pelvis or is twisted around the fetal body. When the cord is wrapped around the fetal neck, it is called a nuchal cord.

Because the placenta develops from the chorionic villi, the umbilical cord is usually located centrally. A peripheral location is less common and is known as a *battledore placenta*. The blood vessels are arrayed out from the center to all parts of the placenta (Fig. 6-10).

Placenta
Structure

The placenta begins to form at implantation. During the third week after conception, the trophoblast cells of the chorionic villi continue to invade the decidua basalis. As the uterine capillaries are tapped, the endometrial spiral arteries fill with maternal blood. The chorionic villi grow into the spaces with two layers of cells: the outer syncytium and the inner cytotrophoblast. A third layer develops into anchoring septa, dividing the projecting decidua into separate areas called *cotyledons*. In each of the 15 to 20 cotyledons, the chorionic villi branch out and a complex system of fetal blood vessels forms. Each cotyledon is a functional unit. The whole structure is the placenta (see Fig. 6-10).

The maternal-placental-embryonic circulation is in place by day 17, when the embryonic heart starts beating. By the end of the third week, embryonic blood is circulating between the embryo and the chorionic villi. In the intervillous spaces, maternal blood supplies oxygen and nutrients to the embryonic capillaries in the villi (Fig. 6-11). Waste products and carbon dioxide diffuse into the maternal blood.

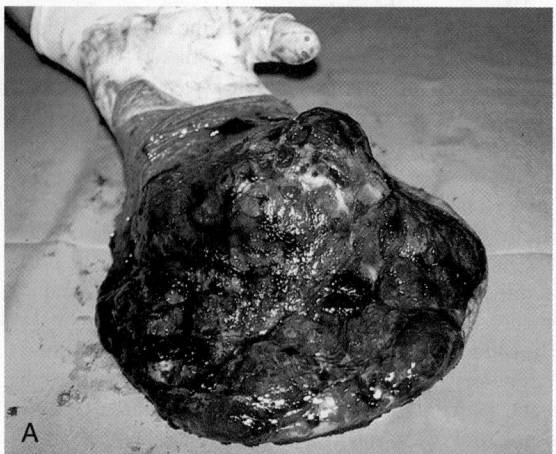

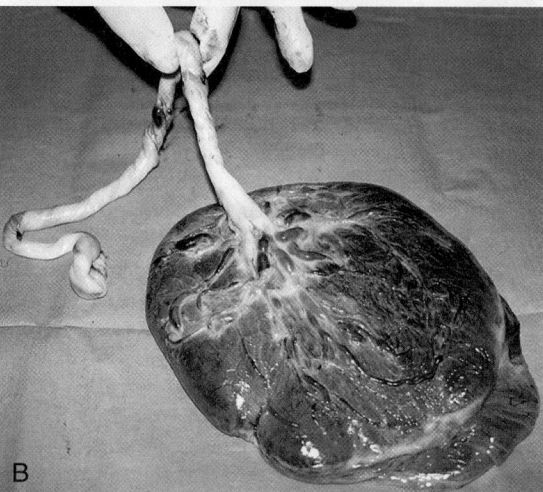

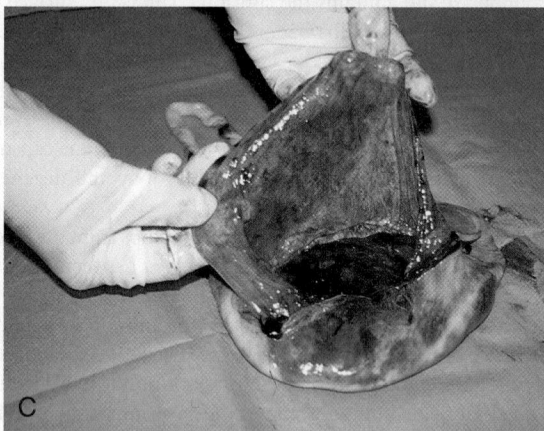

FIG 6-10 Term placenta. **A,** Maternal (or uterine) surface, showing cotyledons and grooves. **B,** Fetal (or amniotic) surface, showing blood vessels running under amnion and converging to form umbilical vessels at attachment of umbilical cord. **C,** Amnion and smooth chorion are arranged to show that they are (1) fused and (2) continuous with margins of placenta. (Courtesy Marjorie Pyle, RNC, Lifecircle, Costa Mesa, CA.)

The placenta functions as a means of metabolic exchange. Exchange is minimal at this time because the two cell layers of the villous membrane are too thick. Permeability increases as the cytotrophoblast thins and disappears; by the fifth month, only the single layer of syncytium is left between the maternal blood and the fetal

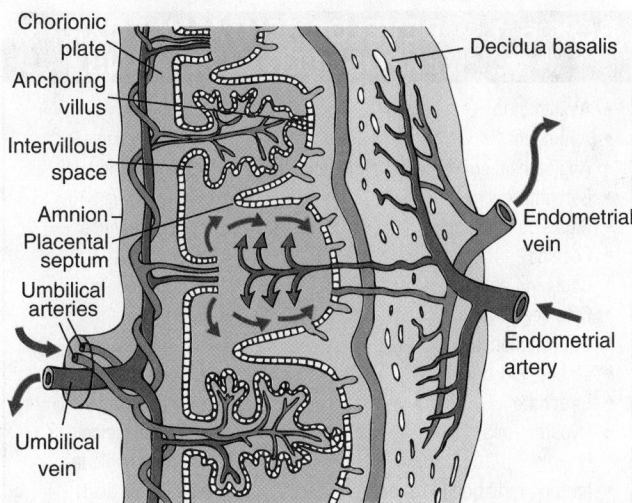

FIG 6-11 Schematic drawing of placenta illustrating how it supplies oxygen and nutrition to embryo and removes its waste products. Deoxygenated blood leaves fetus through the umbilical arteries and enters placenta, where it is oxygenated. Oxygenated blood leaves placenta through the umbilical vein, which enters the fetus via the umbilical cord.

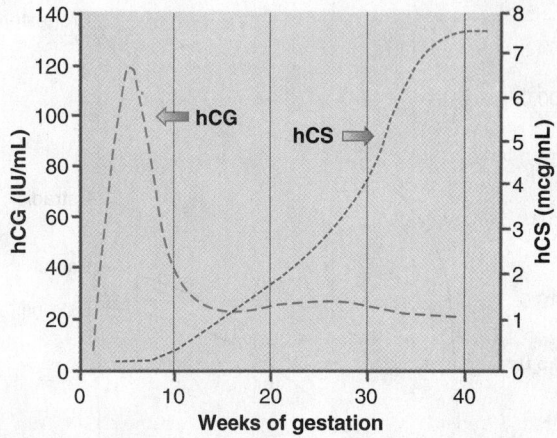

FIG 6-12 Distinct profile for the concentrations of human chorionic gonadotropin (hCG) and human chorionic somatomammotropin (hCS) in serum of women through normal pregnancy. *IU,* International units. (Adapted from Cunningham F, Leveno K, Bloom S, et al: *Williams obstetrics,* ed 23, New York, 2010, McGraw-Hill.)

capillaries. The syncytium is the functional layer of the placenta. By the eighth week, genetic testing may be done on a sample of chorionic villi obtained by aspiration biopsy; however, limb defects have been associated with chorionic villi sampling done before 10 weeks. The structure of the placenta is complete by the twelfth week. The placenta continues to grow wider until 20 weeks, when it covers about half of the uterine surface. It then continues to grow thicker. The branching villi continue to develop within the body of the placenta, increasing the functional surface area.

Functions

One of the early functions of the placenta is as an endocrine gland that produces four hormones necessary to maintain the pregnancy and support the embryo/fetus. The hormones are produced in the syncytium.

The protein hormone *human chorionic gonadotropin* (hCG) can be detected in the maternal serum by 8 to 10 days after conception, shortly after implantation. This hormone is the basis for pregnancy tests. The hCG preserves the function of the ovarian corpus luteum, ensuring a continued supply of estrogen and progesterone needed to maintain the pregnancy. Miscarriage occurs if the corpus luteum stops functioning before the placenta can produce sufficient estrogen and progesterone. The hCG reaches its maximum level at 50 to 70 days and then begins to decrease.

The other protein hormone produced by the placenta is *human chorionic somatomammotropin* (hCS) or *human placental lactogen* (hPL). This substance is similar to a growth hormone and stimulates maternal metabolism to supply needed nutrients for fetal growth. hCS increases the resistance to insulin, facilitates glucose transport across the placental membrane, and stimulates breast development to prepare for lactation (Fig. 6-12).

The placenta eventually produces more of the steroid hormone *progesterone* than the corpus luteum does during the first few months of pregnancy. Progesterone maintains the endometrium, decreases the contractility of the uterus, and stimulates maternal metabolism and development of breast alveoli.

By 7 weeks after fertilization, the placenta is producing most of the maternal estrogens, which are steroid hormones. The major estrogen secreted by the placenta is estriol, whereas the ovaries produce mostly estradiol. Estriol levels may be measured to determine placental functioning. Estrogen stimulates uterine growth and uteroplacental blood flow. It causes a proliferation of the breast glandular tissue and stimulates myometrial contractility. Placental estrogen production increases greatly toward the end of pregnancy. One theory for the cause of the onset of labor is the decrease in circulating levels of progesterone and the increased levels of estrogen (Fig. 6-13).

The metabolic functions of the placenta are respiration, nutrition, excretion, and storage. Oxygen diffuses from the maternal blood across the placental membrane into the fetal blood, and carbon dioxide diffuses in the opposite direction. In this way the placenta functions as lungs for the fetus.

Carbohydrates, proteins, calcium, and iron are stored in the placenta for ready access to meet fetal needs. Water, inorganic salts, carbohydrates, proteins, fats, and vitamins pass from the maternal blood supply across the placental membrane into the fetal blood, supplying nutrition. Water and most electrolytes with a molecular weight less than 500 readily diffuse through the membrane. Hydrostatic and osmotic pressures aid in the flow of water and some solutions. Facilitated and active transport assist in the transfer of glucose, amino acids, calcium, iron, and substances with higher molecular weights. Amino acids and calcium are transported against the concentration gradient between the maternal blood and fetal blood.

The fetal concentration of glucose is lower than the glucose level in the maternal blood because of its rapid metabolism by the fetus. This fetal requirement demands larger concentrations of glucose than simple diffusion can provide. Therefore maternal glucose moves into the fetal circulation by active transport.

Pinocytosis is a mechanism used for transferring large molecules, such as albumin and gamma globulins, across the placental membrane. This mechanism conveys the maternal immunoglobulins that provide early passive immunity to the fetus.

Metabolic waste products of the fetus cross the placental membrane from the fetal blood into the maternal blood. The maternal

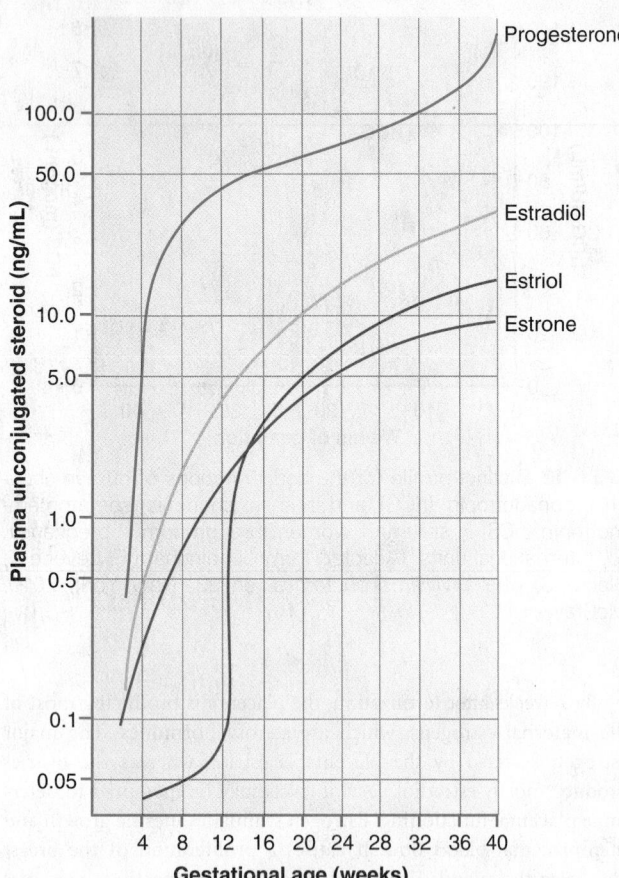

FIG 6-13 Plasma levels of progesterone, estradiol, estrone, and estriol in women during the course of gestation. (From Cunningham F, Leveno K, Bloom S, et al: *Williams obstetrics*, ed 23, New York, 2010, McGraw-Hill.)

kidneys then excrete them. Many viruses can cross the placental membrane and infect the fetus. Some bacteria and protozoa first infect the placenta and then infect the fetus. Drugs can also cross the placental membrane and may harm the fetus. Caffeine, alcohol, nicotine, carbon monoxide and other toxic substances in cigarette smoke, and prescription and recreational drugs (e.g., marijuana, cocaine) readily cross the placenta (Box 6-1).

Although no direct link exists between the fetal blood in the vessels of the chorionic villi and the maternal blood in the intervillous spaces, only one cell layer separates them. Breaks occasionally occur in the placental membrane. Fetal erythrocytes then leak into the maternal circulation, and the mother may develop antibodies to the fetal red blood cells. This is often the way the Rh-negative mother becomes sensitized to the erythrocytes of her Rh-positive fetus (see the discussion of isoimmunization in Chapter 19).

Although the placenta and fetus are analogous to living tissue transplants, they are not destroyed by the host mother (Mor and Abrahams, 2009). Either the placental hormones suppress the immunologic response, or the tissue evokes no response.

Placental function depends on the maternal blood pressure supplying the circulation. Maternal arterial blood, under pressure in the small uterine spiral arteries, spurts into the intervillous spaces (see Fig. 6-11). As long as rich arterial blood continues to be supplied, pressure is exerted on the blood already in the intervillous spaces, pushing it toward drainage by the low-pressure uterine veins. At term gestation, 10% of the maternal cardiac output goes to the uterus.

If there is interference with the circulation to the placenta, the placenta cannot supply the embryo or fetus. Vasoconstriction, such as that caused by hypertension or cocaine use, diminishes uterine blood flow. Decreased maternal blood pressure or decreased cardiac output also diminishes uterine blood flow.

When a woman lies on her back with the pressure of the uterus compressing the vena cava, blood return to the right atrium is diminished (see Fig. 16-5) and the discussion of supine hypotension in Chapter 16. Excessive maternal exercise that diverts blood to the muscles away from the uterus compromises placental circulation. Optimum circulation is achieved when the woman is lying at rest on her side. Decreased uterine circulation may lead to intrauterine growth restriction of the fetus and infants who are small for gestational age.

Braxton Hicks contractions seem to enhance the movement of blood through the intervillous spaces, aiding placental circulation. However, prolonged contractions or intervals that are too short between contractions during labor can reduce the blood flow to the placenta.

Fetal Maturation

The stage of the fetus lasts from 9 weeks (when the fetus becomes recognizable as a human being) until the pregnancy ends. Changes during the fetal period are not as dramatic, because refinement of structure and function is taking place. The fetus is less vulnerable to teratogens except for those that affect central nervous system functioning.

Viability refers to the capability of the fetus to survive outside the uterus. With modern technology and advances in maternal and neonatal care, infants who are 22 to 25 weeks of gestation are now considered to be on the threshold of viability (Cunningham, Leveno, Bloom, et al., 2010). The limitations on survival outside the uterus when an infant is born at this early stage are based on central nervous system function and oxygenation capability of the lungs.

Fetal Circulatory System

The cardiovascular system is the first organ system to function in the developing human. Blood vessel and blood cell formation begins

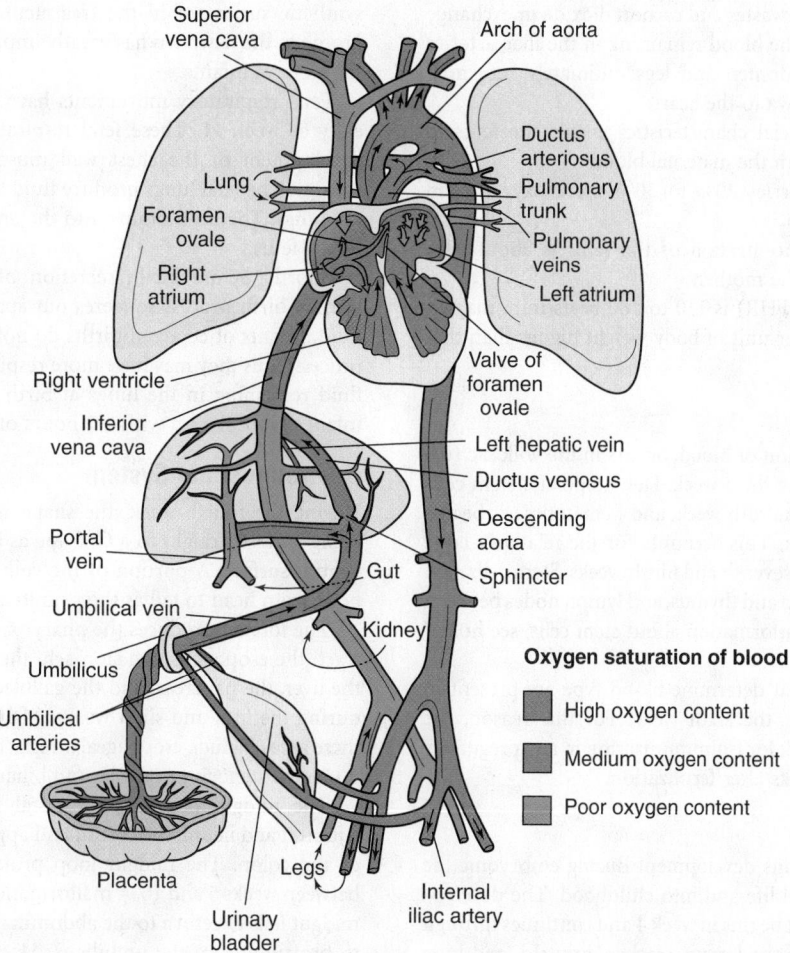

Superior
vena cava

Arch of aorta

Ductus
arteriosus

Pulmonary
trunk

Pulmonary
veins

Left atrium

Lung

Foramen
ovale

Right
atrium

Valve of
foramen
ovale

Right ventricle

Left hepatic vein

Inferior
vena cava

Ductus venosus

Portal
vein

Descending
aorta

Gut

Sphincter

Umbilical vein

Kidney

Umbilicus

Oxygen saturation of blood

Umbilical
arteries

High oxygen content

Medium oxygen content

Poor oxygen content

Placenta

Legs

Urinary
bladder

Internal
iliac artery

FIG 6-14 Schematic illustration of fetal circulation. The *colors* indicate the oxygen saturation of the blood, and the *arrows* show the course of the blood from the placenta to the heart. The organs are not drawn to scale. Observe that three shunts permit most of the blood to bypass the liver and lungs: (1) ductus venosus, (2) foramen ovale, and (3) ductus arteriosus. A small amount of highly oxygenated blood from the inferior vena cava remains in the right atrium and mixes with poorly oxygenated blood from the superior vena cava. This medium oxygenated blood then passes into the right ventricle. The poorly oxygenated blood returns to the placenta for oxygen and nutrients through the umbilical arteries. (From Moore KL, Persaud TVN, Torchia MG: *Before we are born: essentials of embryology and birth defects*, ed 8, Philadelphia, 2013, Saunders.)

in the third week and supplies the embryo with oxygen and nutrients from the mother. By the end of the third week, the tubular heart begins to beat and the primitive cardiovascular system links the embryo, connecting stalk, chorion, and yolk sac. During the fourth and fifth weeks, the heart develops into a four-chambered organ. By the end of the embryonic stage, the heart is developmentally complete.

The fetal lungs do not function for respiratory gas exchange, so a special circulatory pathway, the ductus arteriosus, bypasses the lungs. Oxygen-rich blood from the placenta flows rapidly through the umbilical vein into the fetal abdomen (Fig. 6-14). When the umbilical vein reaches the liver, it divides into two branches; one branch circulates some oxygenated blood through the liver. Most of the blood passes through the ductus venosus into the inferior vena cava. There it mixes with the deoxygenated blood from the fetal legs and abdomen on its way to the right atrium. Most of this blood passes straight through the right atrium and through the foramen ovale, an opening into the left atrium. There it mixes with the small

amount of deoxygenated blood returning from the fetal lungs through the pulmonary veins.

The blood flows into the left ventricle and is squeezed out into the aorta, where the arteries supplying the heart, head, neck, and arms receive most of the oxygen-rich blood. This pattern of supplying the highest levels of oxygen and nutrients to the head, neck, and arms enhances the cephalocaudal (head-to-rump) development of the embryo/fetus.

Deoxygenated blood returning from the head and arms enters the right atrium through the superior vena cava. This blood is directed downward into the right ventricle, where it is squeezed into the pulmonary artery. A small amount of blood circulates through the resistant lung tissue, but the majority follows the path with less resistance through the ductus arteriosus into the aorta, distal to the point of exit of the arteries supplying the head and arms with oxygenated blood. The oxygen-poor blood flows through the abdominal aorta into the internal iliac arteries, where the umbilical arteries direct most of it back through the umbilical cord to the placenta.

There the blood gives up its wastes and carbon dioxide in exchange for nutrients and oxygen. The blood remaining in the iliac arteries flows through the fetal abdomen and legs, ultimately returning through the inferior vena cava to the heart.

The following three special characteristics enable the fetus to obtain sufficient oxygen from the maternal blood:

- Fetal hemoglobin carries 20% to 30% more oxygen than maternal hemoglobin.
- The hemoglobin concentration of the fetus is about 50% greater than that of the mother.
- The fetal heart rate (FHR) is 110 to 160 beats/min, making the cardiac output per unit of body weight higher than that of an adult.

Hematopoietic System

Hematopoiesis, the formation of blood, occurs in the yolk sac (see Fig. 6-7, *B*) beginning in the third week. Hematopoietic stem cells seed the fetal liver during the fifth week, and hematopoiesis begins there during the sixth week. This accounts for the relatively large size of the liver between the seventh and ninth weeks. Stem cells seed the fetal bone marrow, spleen and thymus, and lymph nodes between weeks 8 and 11 (for more information about stem cells, see http:// stemcells.nih.gov/index.asp).

The antigenic factors that determine blood type are present in the erythrocytes soon after the sixth week. For this reason, the Rh-negative woman is at risk for isoimmunization in any pregnancy that lasts longer than 6 weeks after fertilization.

Respiratory System

The respiratory system begins development during embryonic life and continues through fetal life and into childhood. The development of the respiratory tract begins in week 4 and continues through week 17 with formation of the larynx, trachea, bronchi, and lung buds. Between 16 and 24 weeks, the bronchi and terminal bronchioles enlarge and vascular structures and primitive alveoli are formed. Between 24 weeks and term birth, more alveoli form. Specialized alveolar cells, type I and type II cells, secrete pulmonary surfactants to line the interior of the alveoli. After 32 weeks, sufficient surfactant is present in developed alveoli to provide infants with a good chance of survival.

Pulmonary Surfactants

The detection of the presence of pulmonary surfactants, surface-active phospholipids, in amniotic fluid has been used to determine the degree of fetal lung maturity, or the ability of the lungs to function after birth. Lecithin (L) is the most critical alveolar surfactant required for postnatal lung expansion. It is detectable at approximately 21 weeks and increases in amount after week 24. Another pulmonary phospholipid, sphingomyelin (S), remains constant in amount. Thus the measure of lecithin in relation to sphingomyelin, or the L/S ratio, is used to determine fetal lung maturity. When the L/S ratio reaches 2:1, the infant's lungs are considered to be mature. This occurs at approximately 35 weeks of gestation (Mercer, 2009).

Certain maternal conditions that cause decreased maternal placental blood flow, such as maternal hypertension, placental dysfunction, infection, or corticosteroid use, accelerate lung maturity. This apparently is caused by the resulting fetal hypoxia, which stresses the fetus and increases the blood levels of corticosteroids that accelerate alveolar and surfactant development.

Conditions such as gestational diabetes and chronic glomerulonephritis can retard fetal lung maturity. The use of intrabronchial synthetic surfactant in the treatment of respiratory distress syndrome in the newborn has greatly improved the chances of survival for preterm infants.

Fetal respiratory movements have been seen on ultrasound as early as week 11. These fetal respiratory movements may aid in development of the chest wall muscles and regulate lung fluid volume. The fetal lungs produce fluid that expands the air spaces in the lungs. The fluid drains into the amniotic fluid or is swallowed by the fetus.

Shortly before birth, secretion of lung fluid decreases. The normal birth process squeezes out approximately one third of the fluid. Infants of cesarean births do not benefit from this squeezing process; thus they may have more respiratory difficulty at birth. The fluid remaining in the lungs at birth is usually resorbed into the infant's bloodstream within 2 hours of birth.

Gastrointestinal System

During the fourth week, the shape of the embryo changes from being almost straight to a **C** shape as both ends fold in toward the ventral surface. A portion of the yolk sac is incorporated into the body from head to tail as the primitive gut (digestive system).

The foregut produces the pharynx, part of the lower respiratory tract, the esophagus, the stomach, the first half of the duodenum, the liver, the pancreas, and the gallbladder. These structures evolve during the fifth and sixth weeks. Malformations that can occur in these areas include esophageal atresia, hypertrophic pyloric stenosis, duodenal stenosis or atresia, and biliary atresia (see Chapter 41).

The midgut becomes the distal half of the duodenum, the jejunum and ileum, the cecum and appendix, and the proximal half of the colon. The midgut loop projects into the umbilical cord between weeks 5 and 10. A malformation, omphalocele, results if the midgut fails to return to the abdominal cavity, causing the intestines to protrude from the umbilicus. Meckel diverticulum is the most common malformation of the midgut. It occurs when a remnant of the yolk stalk that failed to degenerate attaches to the ileum, leaving a blind sac.

The hindgut develops into the distal half of the colon, the rectum and parts of the anal canal, the urinary bladder, and the urethra. Anorectal malformations are the most common abnormalities of the digestive system.

The fetus swallows amniotic fluid beginning in the fifth month. Gastric emptying and intestinal peristalsis occur. Fetal nutrition and elimination needs are taken care of by the placenta. As the fetus nears term, fetal waste products accumulate in the intestines as dark-green to black, tarry meconium. Normally this substance is passed through the rectum within 24 hours of birth. Sometimes with a breech presentation or fetal hypoxia, meconium is passed in utero into the amniotic fluid. The failure to pass meconium after birth may indicate atresia somewhere in the digestive tract; an imperforate anus (Fig. 6-15); or meconium ileus, in which a firm meconium plug blocks passage (seen in infants with cystic fibrosis).

The metabolic rate of the fetus is relatively low, but the infant has great growth and development needs. Beginning in week 9, the fetus synthesizes glycogen for storage in the liver. Between 26 and 30 weeks, the fetus begins to lay down stores of brown fat in preparation for extrauterine cold stress. Thermoregulation in the neonate requires increased metabolism and adequate oxygenation.

The gastrointestinal system is mature by 36 weeks. Digestive enzymes (except pancreatic amylase and lipase) are present in sufficient quantity to facilitate digestion. The neonate cannot digest starches or fats efficiently. Little saliva is produced.

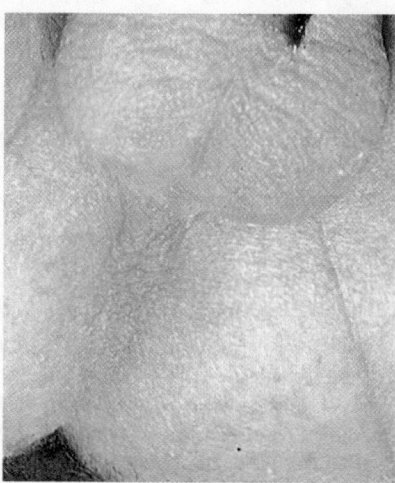

FIG 6-15 Anorectal malformation (imperforate anus). (From Chessell GSJ, Jamieson MJ, Morton RA, et al: *Diagnostic picture tests in clinical medicine* (vol 2), St Louis, 1984, Mosby.)

Hepatic System

The liver and biliary tract develop from the foregut during the fourth week of gestation. Hematopoiesis begins during the sixth week and requires that the liver be large. The embryonic liver is prominent, occupying most of the abdominal cavity. Bile, a constituent of meconium, begins to form in the twelfth week.

Glycogen is stored in the fetal liver beginning at week 9 or 10. At term, glycogen stores are twice those of the adult. Glycogen is the major source of energy for the fetus and for the neonate stressed by in utero hypoxia, extrauterine loss of the maternal glucose supply, the work of breathing, or cold stress.

Iron is also stored in the fetal liver. If maternal intake is sufficient, the fetus can store enough iron to last for 5 months after birth.

During fetal life, the liver does not have to conjugate bilirubin for excretion because the unconjugated bilirubin is cleared by the placenta. Therefore the glucuronyl transferase enzyme needed for conjugation is present in the fetal liver in amounts less than those required after birth. This predisposes the neonate, especially the preterm infant, to hyperbilirubinemia.

Coagulation factors II, VII, IX, and X cannot be synthesized in the fetal liver because of the lack of vitamin K synthesis in the sterile fetal gut. This coagulation deficiency persists after birth for several days and is the rationale for the prophylactic administration of vitamin K to the newborn.

Renal System

The kidneys form during the fifth week and begin to function approximately 4 weeks later. Urine is excreted into the amniotic fluid and forms a major part of the amniotic fluid volume. Oligohydramnios is indicative of renal dysfunction. Because the placenta acts as the organ of excretion and maintains fetal water and electrolyte balance, the fetus does not need functioning kidneys while in utero. At birth, however, the kidneys are required immediately for excretory and acid-base regulatory functions.

A fetal renal malformation can be diagnosed in utero. Corrective or palliative fetal surgery may treat the malformation successfully, or plans can be made for treatment immediately after birth.

At term, the fetus has fully developed kidneys. However, the glomerular filtration rate (GFR) is low, and the kidneys lack the ability to concentrate urine. This makes the newborn more susceptible to both overhydration and dehydration.

Neurologic System

The nervous system originates from the ectoderm during the third week after fertilization. The open neural tube forms during the fourth week. It initially closes at what will be the junction of the brain and spinal cord, leaving both ends open. The embryo folds in on itself lengthwise at this time, forming a head fold in the neural tube at this junction. The cranial end of the neural tube closes, and then the caudal end closes. During week 5, different growth rates cause more flexures in the neural tube, delineating three brain areas: the forebrain, the midbrain, and the hindbrain.

The forebrain develops into the eyes (cranial nerve II) and cerebral hemispheres. The development of all areas of the cerebral cortex continues throughout fetal life and into childhood. The olfactory system (cranial nerve I) and thalamus also develop from the forebrain. Cranial nerves III and IV (oculomotor and trochlear) form from the midbrain. The hindbrain forms the medulla, the pons, the cerebellum, and the remainder of the cranial nerves. Brain waves can be recorded on an electroencephalogram by week 8.

The spinal cord develops from the long end of the neural tube. Another ectodermal structure, the neural crest, develops into the peripheral nervous system. By the eighth week, nerve fibers traverse throughout the body. By week 11 or 12 the fetus makes respiratory movements, moves all extremities, and changes position in utero. The fetus can suck his or her thumb, swim in the amniotic fluid pool, and turn somersaults and can occasionally tie a knot in the umbilical cord.

At term, the fetal brain is approximately one-fourth the size of an adult brain. Neurologic development continues. Stressors on the fetus and neonate (e.g., chronic poor nutrition or hypoxia, drugs, environmental toxins, trauma, disease) damage the central nervous system long after the vulnerable embryonic time for malformations in other organ systems. Neurologic insult can result in cerebral palsy, neuromuscular impairment, intellectual disability, and learning disabilities.

Sensory Awareness

Purposeful movements of the fetus have been demonstrated in response to a firm touch transmitted through the mother's abdomen. Because it can feel, the fetus requires anesthesia when invasive procedures are done.

Fetuses respond to sound by 24 weeks. Different types of music evoke different movements. The fetus can be soothed by the sound of the mother's voice. Acoustic stimulation can be used to evoke a fetal heart rate response. The fetus becomes accustomed (habituates) to noises heard repeatedly. Hearing is fully developed at birth.

The fetus is able to distinguish taste. By the fifth month, when the fetus is swallowing amniotic fluid, a sweetener added to the fluid causes the fetus to swallow faster. The fetus also reacts to temperature changes. A cold solution placed into the amniotic fluid can cause fetal hiccups.

The fetus can see. Eyes have both rods and cones in the retina by the seventh month. A bright light shone on the mother's abdomen in late pregnancy causes abrupt fetal movements. During sleep time, rapid eye movements (REMs) have been observed similar to those occurring in children and adults while dreaming.

Endocrine System

The thyroid gland develops along with structures in the head and neck during the third and fourth weeks. The secretion of thyroxine begins during the eighth week. Maternal thyroxine does not readily cross the placenta; therefore the fetus that does not produce thyroid hormones will be born with congenital hypothyroidism. If untreated, hypothyroidism can result in severe intellectual disability. Screening for hypothyroidism is typically included in newborn screening after birth.

The adrenal cortex is formed during the sixth week and produces hormones by the eighth or ninth week. As term approaches, the fetus produces more cortisol. This is believed to aid in initiation of labor by decreasing the maternal progesterone and stimulating production of prostaglandins.

The pancreas forms from the foregut during the fifth through eighth weeks. The islets of Langerhans develop during the twelfth week. Insulin is produced by week 20. In fetuses of mothers with uncontrolled diabetes, maternal hyperglycemia produces fetal hyperglycemia, stimulating hyperinsulinemia and islet cell hyperplasia. This results in a macrosomic (large) fetus. The hyperinsulinemia also blocks lung maturation, placing the neonate at risk for respiratory distress and hypoglycemia when the maternal glucose source is lost at birth. Control of the maternal glucose level before and during pregnancy minimizes problems for the fetus and infant.

Reproductive System

Sex differentiation begins in the embryo during the seventh week. Female and male external genitalia are indistinguishable until after the ninth week. Distinguishing characteristics appear around the ninth week and are fully differentiated by the twelfth week. When a Y chromosome is present, testes are formed. By the end of the embryonic period, testosterone is being secreted and causes formation of the male genitalia. By week 28, the testes begin descending into the scrotum. After birth, low levels of testosterone continue to be secreted until the pubertal surge.

The female, with two X chromosomes, forms ovaries and female external genitalia. By the sixteenth week, oogenesis has been established. At birth, the ovaries contain the female's lifetime supply of ova. Most female hormone production is delayed until puberty. However, the fetal endometrium responds to maternal hormones, and withdrawal bleeding or vaginal discharge (pseudomenstruation) may occur at birth when these hormones are lost. The high level of maternal estrogen also stimulates mammary engorgement and secretion of fluid ("witch's milk") in newborn infants of both sexes.

Musculoskeletal System

Bones and muscles develop from the mesoderm by the fourth week of embryonic development. At that time, the cardiac muscle is already beating. The mesoderm next to the neural tube forms the vertebral column and ribs. The parts of the vertebral column grow toward each other to enclose the developing spinal cord. Ossification, or bone formation, begins. If there is a defect in the bony fusion, various forms of spina bifida can occur. A large defect affecting several vertebrae may allow the membranes and spinal cord to pouch out from the back, producing neurologic deficits and skeletal deformity.

The flat bones of the skull develop during the embryonic period, and ossification continues throughout childhood. At birth, connective tissue sutures exist where the bones of the skull meet. The areas where more than two bones meet (called fontanels) are especially prominent. The sutures and fontanels allow the bones of the skull to mold, or move during birth, enabling the head to pass through the birth canal.

The bones of the shoulders, arms, hips, and legs appear in the sixth week as a continuous skeleton with no joints. Differentiation occurs, producing separate bones and joints. Ossification will continue through childhood to allow growth. Beginning in the seventh week, muscles contract spontaneously. Arm and leg movements are visible on ultrasound examination although the mother does not perceive them until sometime between 16 and 20 weeks.

Integumentary System

The epidermis begins as a single layer of cells derived from the ectoderm at 4 weeks. By the seventh week, there are two layers of cells. The cells of the superficial layer are sloughed and become mixed with the sebaceous gland secretions to form the white, cheesy vernix caseosa, the material that protects the skin of the fetus. The vernix is thick at 24 weeks but becomes scant by term.

The basal layer of the epidermis is the germinal layer, which replaces lost cells. Until 17 weeks, the skin is thin and wrinkled, with blood vessels visible underneath. The skin thickens, and all layers are present at term. After 32 weeks, as subcutaneous fat is deposited under the dermis, the skin becomes less wrinkled and red in appearance.

By 16 weeks, the epidermal ridges are present on the palms of the hands, the fingers, the bottom of the feet, and the toes. These handprints and footprints are unique to that infant.

Hairs form from hair bulbs in the epidermis that project into the dermis. Cells in the hair bulb keratinize to form the hair shaft. As the cells at the base of the hair shaft proliferate, the hair grows to the surface of the epithelium. Very fine hairs, called lanugo, appear first at 12 weeks on the eyebrows and upper lip. By 20 weeks, they cover the entire body. At this time, the eyelashes, eyebrows, and scalp hair are beginning to grow. By 28 weeks, the scalp hair is longer than the lanugo, which thins and may disappear by term gestation.

Fingernails and toenails develop from thickened epidermis at the tips of the digits beginning during the tenth week. They grow slowly. Fingernails usually reach the fingertips by 32 weeks, and toenails reach toe tips by 36 weeks.

Immunologic System

During the third trimester, albumin and globulin are present in the fetus. The only immunoglobulin (Ig) that crosses the placenta, IgG, provides passive acquired immunity to specific bacterial toxins. The fetus produces IgM by the end of the first trimester. This is produced in response to blood group antigens, gram-negative enteric organisms, and some viruses. IgA is not produced by the fetus; however, colostrum, the precursor to breast milk, contains large amounts of IgA and can provide passive immunity to the neonate who is breastfed.

The normal term neonate can fight infection but not as effectively as an older child. The preterm infant is at much greater risk for infection.

Table 6-1 summarizes embryonic and fetal development.

MULTIFETAL PREGNANCY

Twins

The incidence of twinning is 1 in 43 pregnancies. There has been a steady rise in multiple births since 1973 (Benirschke, 2009). This is partly attributed to the availability of assisted reproductive technologies and the increasing age at which women give birth (Malone and D'Alton, 2009).

TABLE 6-1	MILESTONES IN HUMAN DEVELOPMENT BEFORE BIRTH SINCE LAST MENSTRUAL PERIOD (LMP)	
4 WEEKS	**8 WEEKS**	**12 WEEKS**
External Appearance		
Body flexed, **C** shaped; arm and leg buds present; head at right angles to body	Body fairly well formed; nose flat, eyes far apart; digits well formed; head elevating; tail almost disappeared; eyes, ears, nose, and mouth recognizable	Nails appearing; resembles a human; head erect but disproportionately large; skin pink, delicate
Crown-to-Rump Measurement; Weight		
0.4 to 0.5 cm; 0.4 g	2.5 to 3 cm; 2 g	6 to 9 cm; 19 g
Gastrointestinal System		
Stomach at midline and fusiform; conspicuous liver; esophagus short; intestine a short tube	Intestinal villi developing; small intestines coil within umbilical cord; palatal folds present; liver very large	Bile secreted; palatal fusion complete; intestines have withdrawn from cord and assume characteristic positions
Musculoskeletal System		
All somites present	First indication of ossification—occiput, mandible, and humerus; fetus capable of some movement; definitive muscles of trunk, limbs, and head well represented	Some bones well outlined, ossification spreading; upper cervical to lower sacral arches and bodies ossify; smooth muscle layers indicated in hollow viscera
Circulatory System		
Heart develops, double chambers visible, begins to beat; aortic arch and major veins completed	Main blood vessels assume final plan; enucleated red cells predominate in blood	Blood forming in marrow
Respiratory System		
Primary lung buds appear	Pleural and pericardial cavities forming; branching bronchioles; nostrils closed by epithelial plugs	Lungs acquire definite shape; vocal cords appear
Renal System		
Rudimentary ureteral buds appear	Earliest secretory tubules differentiating; bladder-urethra separates from rectum	Kidneys able to secrete urine; bladder expands as a sac
Nervous System		
Well-marked midbrain flexure; no hindbrain or cervical flexures; neural groove closed	Cerebral cortex begins to acquire typical cells; differentiation of cerebral cortex, meninges, ventricular foramina, cerebrospinal fluid circulation; spinal cord extends entire length of spine	Brain structural configuration almost complete; cord shows cervical and lumbar enlargements; fourth ventricle foramina are developed; sucking present
Sensory Organs		
Eye and ear appearing as optic vessel and otocyst	Primordial choroid plexuses develop; ventricles large relative to cortex; development progressing; eyes converging rapidly; internal ears developing	Earliest taste buds indicated; characteristic organization of eyes attained
Genital System		
Genital ridge appears (fifth week)	Testes and ovaries distinguishable; external genitalia sexless but begin to differentiate	Sex recognizable; internal and external sex organs specific

Continued

TABLE 6-1   MILESTONES IN HUMAN DEVELOPMENT BEFORE BIRTH SINCE LAST MENSTRUAL PERIOD (LMP)—cont'd

16 WEEKS	20 WEEKS	24 WEEKS
External Appearance		
Head still dominant; face looks human; eyes, ears, and nose approach typical appearance on gross examination; arm/leg ratio proportionate; scalp hair appears	Vernix caseosa appears; lanugo appears; legs lengthen considerably; sebaceous glands appear	Body lean but fairly well proportioned; skin red and wrinkled; vernix caseosa present; sweat glands forming
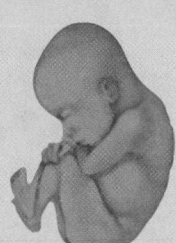	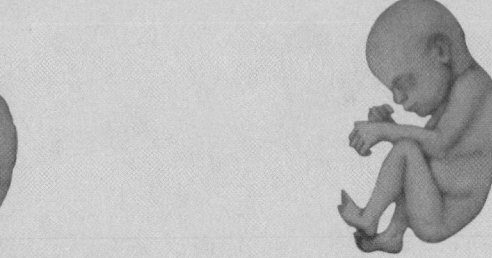	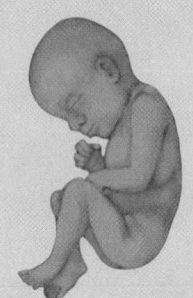
Crown-to-Rump Measurement; Weight		
11.5 to 13.5 cm; 100 g	16 to 18.5 cm; 300 g	23 cm; 600 g
Gastrointestinal System		
Meconium in bowel; some enzyme secretion; anus open	Enamel and dentine depositing; ascending colon recognizable	
Musculoskeletal System		
Most bones distinctly indicated throughout body; joint cavities appear; muscular movements can be detected	Sternum ossifies; fetal movements strong enough for mother to feel	
Circulatory System		
Heart muscle well developed; blood formation active in spleen		Blood formation increases in bone marrow and decreases in liver
Respiratory System		
Elastic fibers appear in lungs; terminal and respiratory bronchioles appear	Nostrils reopen; primitive respiratory-like movements begin	Alveolar ducts and sacs present; lecithin begins to appear in amniotic fluid (weeks 26 to 27)
Renal System		
Kidneys in position; attain typical shape		
Nervous System		
Cerebral lobes delineated; cerebellum assumes some prominence	Brain grossly formed; cord myelination begins; spinal cord ends at level of first sacral vertebra (S-1)	Cerebral cortex layered typically; neuronal proliferation in cerebral cortex ends
Sensory Organs		
General sense organs differentiated	Nose and ears ossify	Can hear
Genital System		
Testes in position for descent into scrotum; vagina open		Testes at inguinal ring in descent to scrotum

TABLE 6-1	MILESTONES IN HUMAN DEVELOPMENT BEFORE BIRTH SINCE LAST MENSTRUAL PERIOD (LMP)—cont'd	
28 WEEKS	**30-31 WEEKS**	**36 AND 40 WEEKS**
External Appearance		**36 Weeks**
Lean body, less wrinkled and red; nails appear	Subcutaneous fat beginning to collect; more rounded appearance; skin pink and smooth; has assumed birth position	Skin pink, body rounded; general lanugo disappearing; body usually plump
	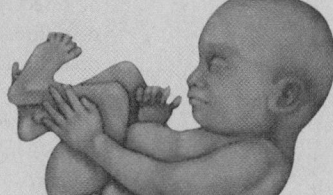	**40 Weeks**
		Skin smooth and pink; scant vernix caseosa; moderate to profuse hair; lanugo on shoulders and upper body only; nasal and alar cartilage apparent
Crown-to-Rump Measurement; Weight		**36 Weeks**
27 cm; 1100 g	31 cm; 1800 to 2100 g	35 cm; 2200 to 2900 g
		40 Weeks
		40 cm; 3200+ g
Musculoskeletal System		**36 Weeks**
Astragalus (talus, ankle bone) ossifies; weak, fleeting movements, minimum tone	Middle fourth phalanxes ossify; permanent teeth primordia seen; can turn head to side	Distal femoral ossification centers present; sustained, definite movements; fair tone; can turn and elevate head
		40 Weeks
		Active, sustained movement; good tone; may lift head
Respiratory System		**36 Weeks**
Lecithin forming on alveolar surfaces	L/S ratio = 1.2:1	L/S ratio ≥2:1
		40 Weeks
		Pulmonary branching only two-thirds complete
Renal System		**36 Weeks**
		Formation of new nephrons ceases
Nervous System		**36 Weeks**
Appearance of cerebral fissures, convolutions rapidly appearing; indefinite sleep-wake cycle; cry weak or absent; weak suck reflex		End of spinal cord at level of third lumbar vertebra (L-3); definite sleep-wake cycle
		40 Weeks
		Myelination of brain begins; patterned sleep-wake cycle with alert periods; cries when hungry or uncomfortable; strong suck reflex
Sensory Organs		
Eyelids reopen; retinal layers completed, light receptive; pupils capable of reacting to light	Sense of taste present; aware of sounds outside mother's body	
Genital System		**40 Weeks**
	Testes descending to scrotum	Testes in scrotum; labia majora well developed

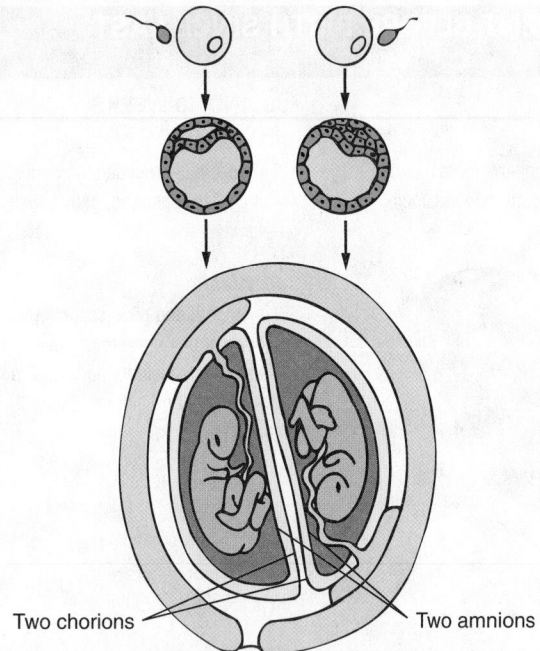

FIG 6-16 Formation of dizygotic twins. There is fertilization of two ova, two implantations, two placentas, two chorions, and two amnions.

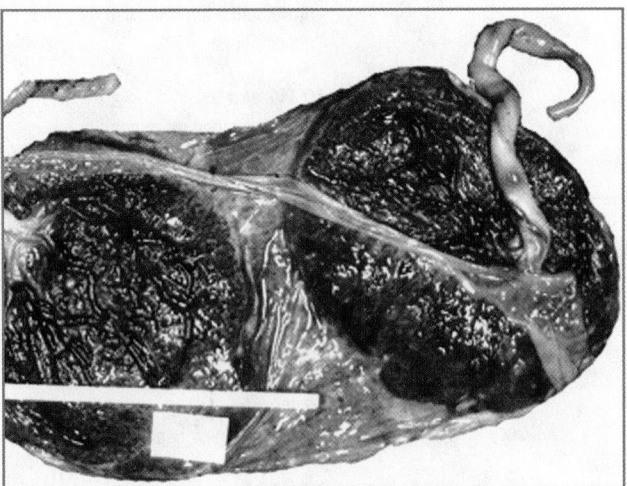

FIG 6-17 Diamniotic dichorionic (separate) twin placentas. (From Benirschke K: Multiple gestation: the biology of twinning. In Creasy R, Resnik R, Iams J, et al, editors: *Creasy & Resnik's maternal-fetal medicine: principles and practice*, ed 6, Philadelphia, 2009, Saunders.)

Dizygotic Twins

When two mature ova are produced in one ovarian cycle, both have the potential to be fertilized by separate sperm. This results in two zygotes, or dizygotic twins (Fig. 6-16). There are always two amnions, two chorions, and two placentas that may be fused (Fig. 6-17). These dizygotic or fraternal twins may be the same sex or different sexes and are genetically no more alike than siblings born at different times. Dizygotic twinning occurs in families with a history of twinning, more often among African-American women than Caucasian

women, and least often among Asian-American women. Dizygotic twinning increases in frequency with maternal age up to 35 years, with parity, and with the use of fertility drugs.

Monozygotic Twins

Identical or monozygotic twins develop from one fertilized ovum, which then divides (Fig. 6-18). They are the same sex and have the same genotype. If division occurs soon after fertilization, two embryos, two amnions, two chorions, and two placentas that may be fused will develop. Most often, division occurs between 4 and 8 days after fertilization, and there are two embryos, two amnions, one chorion, and one placenta. Rarely, division occurs after the eighth day after fertilization. In this case, there are two embryos within a common amnion and a common chorion with one placenta. This often causes circulatory problems because the umbilical cords may tangle together and one or both fetuses may die. If division occurs very late, cleavage may not be complete and conjoined or "Siamese" twins could result. Monozygotic twinning occurs in approximately 3.5 to 4 per 1000 births (Benirschke, 2009). There is no association with race, heredity, maternal age, or parity. Fertility drugs increase the incidence of monozygotic twinning.

Conjoined Twins

Conjoined twins are a type of monozygotic twins in which there is incomplete embryonic division at 13 to 15 days postconception (see Fig. 6-18). The estimated frequency is 1 in 50,000 births (Malone and D'Alton, 2009). Prenatal diagnosis is possible with three-dimensional ultrasonography. Cesarean birth minimizes trauma to mother and fetuses.

Other Multifetal Pregnancies

The occurrence of multifetal pregnancies with three or more fetuses has increased with the use of fertility drugs and in vitro fertilization. Triplets occur in about 1 of 1341 pregnancies (Benirschke, 2009). They can occur from the division of one zygote into two, with one of the two dividing again, producing identical triplets. Triplets can also be produced (1) from two zygotes, one dividing into a set of identical twins and the second zygote a single fraternal sibling or (2) from three zygotes. Quadruplets, quintuplets, sextuplets, and so on have similar possible derivations.

NONGENETIC FACTORS INFLUENCING DEVELOPMENT

Congenital disorders may be inherited or may be caused by environmental factors or by inadequate maternal nutrition. *Congenital* means that the condition was present at birth. Some congenital malformations may be the result of teratogens, that is, environmental substances or exposures that result in functional or structural disability. In contrast to other forms of developmental disabilities, disabilities caused by teratogens are theoretically totally preventable. Known human teratogens are drugs and chemicals, infections, exposure to radiation, and certain maternal conditions such as diabetes and PKU (Box 6-2). A teratogen has the greatest effect on the organs and parts of an embryo during its periods of rapid growth and differentiation. This occurs during the embryonic period, specifically from days 15 to 60. During the first 2 weeks of development, teratogens either have no effect on the embryo or have effects so severe that they cause miscarriage. Brain

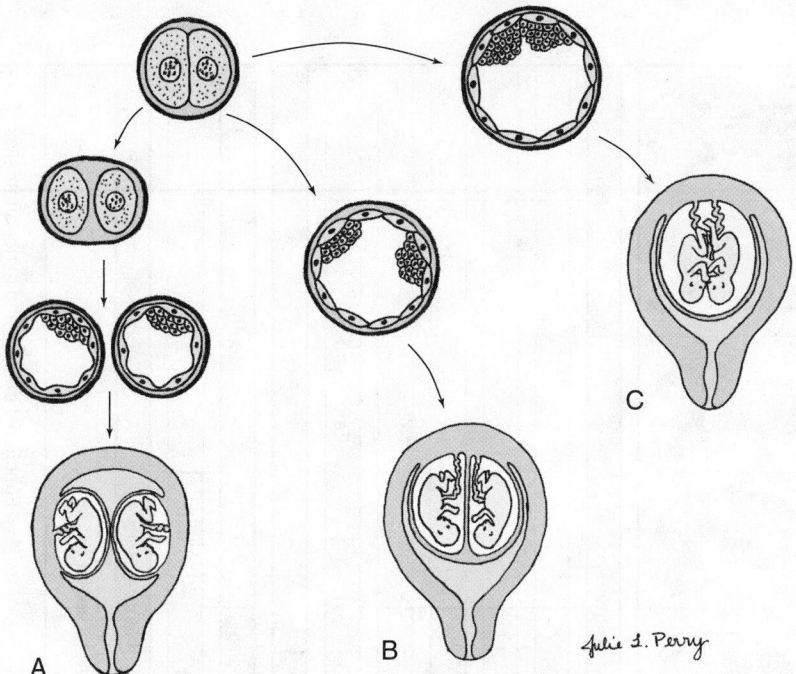

FIG 6-18 Formation of monozygotic twins. **A,** One fertilization: blastomeres separate, resulting in two implantations, two placentas, and two sets of membranes. **B,** One blastomere with two inner cell masses, one fused placenta, one chorion, and separate amnions. **C,** One blastomere with incomplete separation of cell mass resulting in conjoined twins.

BOX 6-2	**ETIOLOGY OF HUMAN MALFORMATIONS**

Environmental
- Maternal conditions
  - Alcoholism, diabetes, endocrinopathies, phenylketonuria, smoking, nutritional problems
- Infectious agents
  - Rubella, toxoplasmosis, syphilis, herpes simplex, cytomegalic inclusion disease, varicella, Venezuelan equine encephalitis
- Mechanical problems (deformations)
  - Amniotic band constrictions, umbilical cord constraint, disparity in uterine size and uterine contents
- Chemicals, drugs, radiation, hyperthermia

Genetic
- Single-gene disorders
- Chromosomal abnormalities

Unknown
- Polygenic/multifactorial (gene-environment interactions)
- "Spontaneous" errors of development
- Other unknowns

Adapted from Parikh AS, Wiesner GL: Congenital anomalies. In Martin RJ, Fanaroff AA, Walsh MC, editors: *Fanaroff and Martin's neonatal-perinatal medicine: diseases of the fetus and infant,* ed 9, Philadelphia, 2011, Mosby.

---

growth and development continue during the fetal period, and teratogens can severely affect mental development throughout gestation (Fig. 6-19).

In addition to genetic makeup and the influence of teratogens, the adequacy of maternal nutrition influences development. The embryo and fetus must obtain the nutrients they need from the mother's diet; they cannot tap the maternal reserves. Malnutrition during pregnancy produces low-birth-weight newborns who are susceptible to infection. Malnutrition also affects brain development during the latter half of gestation and can result in learning disabilities in the child. Inadequate folic acid is associated with neural tube defects.

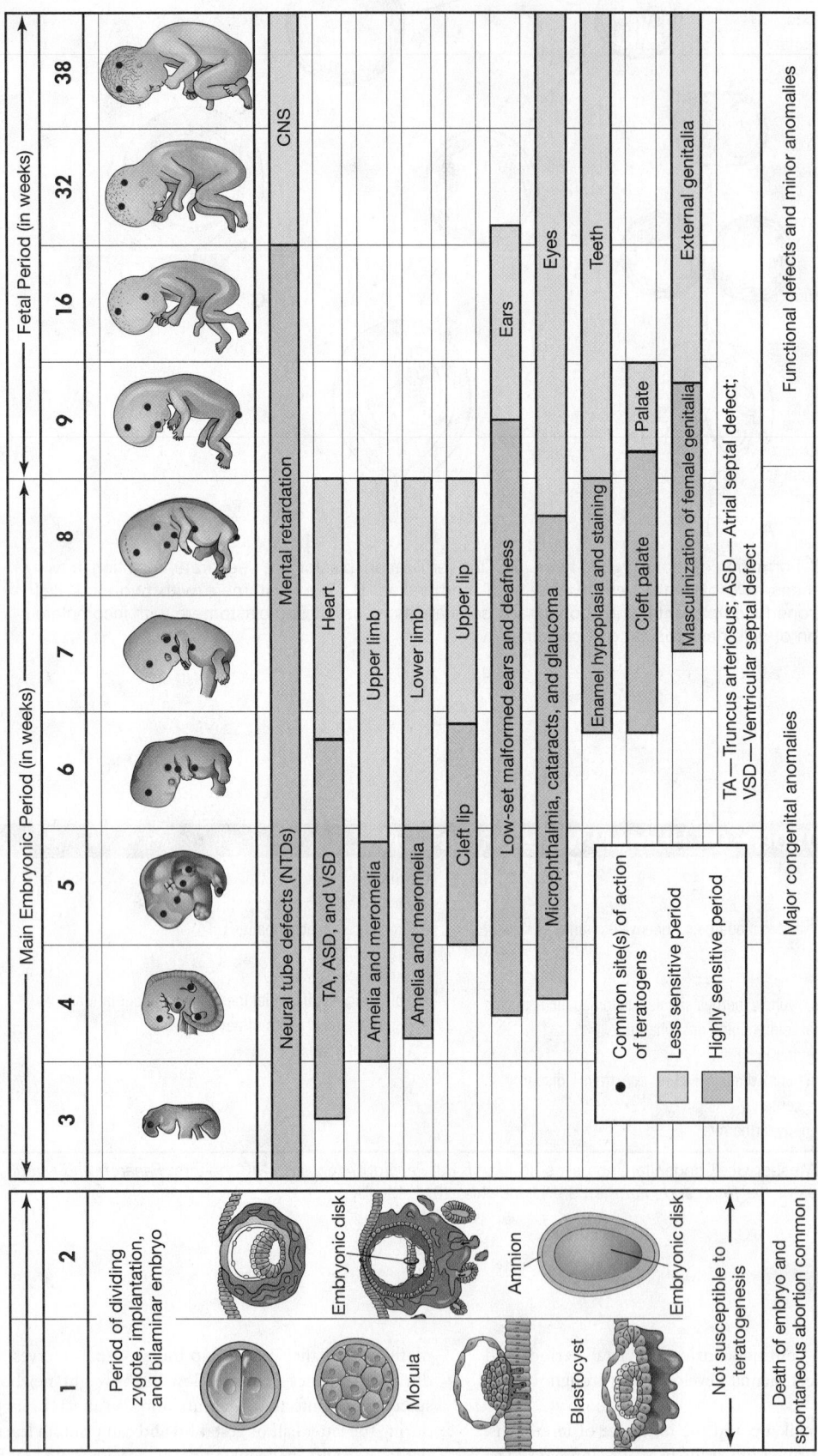

FIG 6-19 Critical periods in human development. *Dark color* denotes highly sensitive periods; *light color* indicates stages that are less sensitive to teratogens. *CNS,* Central nervous system. (From Moore KL, Persaud TVN, Torchia MG: *Before we are born: essentials of embryology and birth defects,* ed 8, Philadelphia, 2013, Saunders.)

KEY POINTS

- Genetic disease affects people of all ages, from all socioeconomic levels, and from all racial and ethnic backgrounds.
- Nurses in all clinical specialties with advanced preparation are assuming important roles in genetic counseling.
- Pharmacogenomics will probably be the most immediate clinical application of the Human Genome Project.
- Genes are the basic units of heredity responsible for all human characteristics. They comprise 23 pairs of chromosomes: 22 pairs of autosomes and one pair of sex chromosomes.
- Chromosomal abnormalities occur in both autosomes and sex chromosomes.
- Multifactorial inheritance includes both genetic and environmental contributions.

- Human gestation is approximately 280 days after the LMP or 266 days after conception.
- Fertilization occurs in the uterine tube within 24 hours of ovulation. The zygote undergoes mitotic divisions, creating a 16-cell morula.
- The organ systems and external features develop during the embryonic period, that is, the third to the eighth week after fertilization.
- During critical periods in human development, the embryo and fetus are vulnerable to environmental teratogens.
- There has been a steady rise in the incidence of multifetal pregnancies, which is partly due to ART and the increasing age at which women give birth.

REFERENCES

Benirschke K: Multiple gestation: the biology of twinning. In Creasy R, Resnik R, Iams J, et al, editors: *Creasy & Resnik's maternal-fetal medicine: principles and practice*, ed 6, Philadelphia, 2009, Saunders.

Consensus Panel on Genetic/Genomic Nursing Competencies: *Essentials of genetic and genomic nursing: competencies, curricula guidelines, and outcome indicators*, ed 2, Silver Spring, MD, 2009, American Nurses Association.

Cunningham F, Leveno K, Bloom S, et al: *Williams obstetrics*, ed 23, New York, 2010, McGraw-Hill.

ENCODE data describes function of human genome, September 5, 2012, www.genome.gov/pfv.cfm?pageID=27549810.

Evans J, Green R: Direct to consumer genetic testing: avoiding a culture war, *Genet Med* 11(8):568–569, 2009.

Guttmacher A, McGuire A, Ponder B, et al: Personalized genomic information: preparing for the future of genetic medicine, *Nat Rev Genet* 11(2):161–165, 2010.

Jorde L, Carey J, Bamshad M: *Medical genetics*, ed 4, St Louis, 2010, Mosby.

Malone F, D'Alton M: Multiple gestation: clinical characteristics and management. In Creasy R, Resnik R, Iams J, et al, editors: *Creasy & Resnik's maternal-fetal medicine: principles and practice*, ed 6, Philadelphia, 2009, Saunders.

Martin R: Meiotic errors in human oogenesis and spermatogenesis, *Reprod Biomed Online* 16(4):523–531, 2008.

McGuire A, Burke W: An unwelcome side effect of direct-to-consumer personal genome testing, *JAMA* 300(22):2669–2671, 2010.

Meckley L, Gudgeon J, Anderson J, et al: A policy model to evaluate the benefits, risks, and costs of warfarin pharmacogenetic testing, *Pharmacogenomics* 28(1):61–74, 2010.

Mercer B: Assessment and induction of fetal pulmonary maturity. In Creasy R, Resnik R, Iams J, et al, editors: *Creasy and Resnik's maternal-fetal medicine: principles and practice*, ed 6, Philadelphia, 2009, Saunders.

Moore KL, Persaud TVN, Torchia MG: *Before we are born: essentials of embryology and birth defects*, ed 8, Philadelphia, 2013, Saunders.

Mor G, Abrahams V: The immunology of pregnancy. In Creasy R, Resnik R, Iams J, et al, editors: *Creasy and Resnik's maternal-fetal medicine: principles and practice*, ed 6, Philadelphia, 2009, Saunders.

Anatomy and Physiology of Pregnancy

Kathryn R. Alden

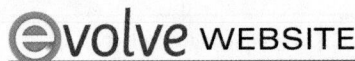 WEBSITE

http://evolve.elsevier.com/Perry/maternal

LEARNING OBJECTIVES

On completion of this chapter, the reader will be able to:

- Determine gravidity and parity using the two- and five-digit systems.
- Describe the various types of pregnancy tests, including the timing of tests and interpretation of results.
- Explain the expected maternal anatomic and physiologic adaptations to pregnancy.

- Differentiate among presumptive, probable, and positive signs of pregnancy.
- Identify maternal hormones produced during pregnancy, their target organs, and their major effects on pregnancy.
- Compare the characteristics of the abdomen, vulva, and cervix of the nullipara and multipara.

The goal of maternity care is a healthy pregnancy with a physically safe and emotionally satisfying outcome for mother, infant, and family. Consistent health supervision and surveillance are of utmost importance. However, many maternal adaptations are unfamiliar to pregnant women and their families. Helping the pregnant woman recognize the relationship between her physical status and the plan for her care assists her in making decisions and encourages her to participate in her own care.

GRAVIDITY AND PARITY

An understanding of the following terms used to describe pregnancy and the pregnant woman (Cunningham, Leveno, Bloom, et al., 2010) is essential to the study of maternity care:

Gravida—A woman who is pregnant

Gravidity—Pregnancy

Multigravida—A woman who has had two or more pregnancies

Multipara—A woman who has completed two or more pregnancies to 20 weeks of gestation or more

Nulligravida—A woman who has never been pregnant and is not currently pregnant

Nullipara—A woman who has not completed a pregnancy with a fetus or fetuses beyond 20 weeks of gestation

Parity—The number of pregnancies in which the fetus or fetuses have reached 20 weeks of gestation, not the number of fetuses (e.g., twins) born. Parity is not affected by whether the fetus

is born alive or is stillborn (i.e., showing no signs of life at birth).

Postdate or postterm—A pregnancy that goes beyond 42 weeks of gestation

Preterm—A pregnancy that has reached 20 weeks of gestation but ends before completion of 37 weeks of gestation

Primigravida—A woman who is pregnant for the first time

Primipara—A woman who has completed one pregnancy with a fetus or fetuses who have reached 20 weeks of gestation

Term—A pregnancy from the beginning of week 38 of gestation to the end of week 42 of gestation

Viability—The capacity to live outside the uterus; there are no clear limits of gestational age or weight. Infants born at 22 to 25 weeks of gestation are considered to be on the threshold of viability and are especially vulnerable to brain injury if they survive.

Gravidity and parity information is obtained during history-taking interviews. Obtaining and documenting this information accurately is important in planning care for the pregnant woman.

> **! NURSING ALERT**
>
> Information may be recorded in patient records in a variety of ways because no one standardized system exists. It is important that the nurse understand the documentation system used by the health care facility.

Two commonly used systems of summarizing the obstetric history are discussed here. Gravidity and parity can be described with only two digits: the first digit indicates the number of pregnancies the woman has had, including the present one, and parity the number of pregnancies that have reached 20 weeks of gestation. For example, the abbreviation gravida 1 para 0 (1/0) means that a woman is pregnant for the first time (primigravida) and has not carried a pregnancy to 20 weeks (nullipara). If a woman had twins at 36 weeks with her first pregnancy, she would also be gravida 1, para 1 (remember that para refers to pregnancies, not fetuses) (Cunningham, Leveno, Bloom, et al., 2010).

Another system, consisting of five digits separated by hyphens, is commonly used in maternity centers. This system provides more information about the woman's obstetric history, although it may not provide accurate information about parity since it provides information about births and not pregnancies reaching 20 weeks of gestation (Beebe, 2005). The first digit represents gravidity; the second digit represents the total number of term births; the third indicates the number of preterm births; the fourth identifies the number of abortions (miscarriage or elective termination of pregnancy); and the fifth is the number of children currently living. The acronym *GTPAL* (gravidity, term, preterm, abortions, living children) may be helpful in remembering this system of notation. For example, if a woman pregnant only once gives birth at week 35 and the infant survives, the abbreviation that represents this information is "1-0-1-0-1." During her next pregnancy the abbreviation is "2-0-1-0-1." Additional examples are in Table 7-1.

PREGNANCY TESTS

Early detection of pregnancy allows for early initiation of care. Human chorionic gonadotropin (hCG) is the earliest biologic marker for pregnancy. Pregnancy tests are based on the recognition of hCG or a beta (β) subunit of hCG. Production of β-hCG begins as early as the day of implantation and can be detected in maternal serum or urine as early as 7 to 8 days after ovulation. The level of hCG rises until it peaks at 60 to 70 days and then declines until about 16 weeks. Plasma levels of hCG remain at this lower level for the remainder of the pregnancy. Higher-than-normal levels of hCG are associated with abnormal gestation (e.g., fetus with Down syndrome, gestational trophoblastic disease) or multiple gestation. Abnormally slow increase in hCG or lower levels can indicate impending miscarriage or ectopic pregnancy (Cunningham, Leveno, Bloom, et al., 2010).

Serum and urine pregnancy tests are performed in clinics, offices, women's health centers, and laboratory settings. Urine pregnancy tests may be performed at home (see Community Focus box). Both serum and urine tests can provide accurate results. A 7- to 10-mL sample of venous blood is collected for serum testing. Most urine tests require a first-voided morning urine specimen because it contains levels of hCG approximately the same as those in serum. Random urine samples usually have lower levels. Urine tests are less expensive and provide more immediate results than serum tests.

Many different pregnancy tests are available (Fig. 7-1). The wide variety of tests precludes discussion of each. The nurse should read the manufacturer's directions for the test to be used and determine if the woman understands the directions. A study by Wallace, Zite, and Homewood (2009) reported that instructions for most home pregnancy tests do not comply with the recommended guidelines for use of plain language and that most instructions were written at a seventh-grade level or above.

Enzyme-linked immunosorbent assay (ELISA) testing is the most popular method of testing for pregnancy. It uses a specific monoclonal antibody (anti-hCG) with enzymes that bond with hCG in urine. ELISA technology is the basis for most over-the-counter home pregnancy tests. With these one-step tests, the woman usually applies urine to a strip or absorbent-tipped applicator and reads the results. The test kits come with directions for collection of the specimen, the testing procedure, and reading of results. A positive test result is indicated by a simple color change reaction or a digital reading. Most manufacturers of the kits provide a toll-free telephone number to call if users have concerns and questions about

🏠 COMMUNITY FOCUS

Home Pregnancy Test Kits

Visit a pharmacy in your neighborhood. How many different types of home pregnancy test kits are available in the pharmacy? Read the labels on three different types of home pregnancy test kits. Do the kits include material for more than one test? Are the directions printed in more than one language? After reading the directions, do you have questions about how to perform the test or how to interpret the results? If so, what does that say about the likelihood that the tests will be used correctly?

TABLE 7-1 OBSTETRIC HISTORY USING FIVE-DIGIT AND TWO-DIGIT SYSTEM

	FIVE-DIGIT SYSTEM					TWO-DIGIT SYSTEM
	G	T	P	A	L	G/P
CONDITION	**GRAVIDITY**	**TERM BIRTH**	**PRETERM BIRTHS**	**ABORTIONS AND MISCARRIAGES**	**LIVING CHILDREN**	**GRAVIDITY/PARITY**
Olivia is pregnant for the first time.	1	0	0	0	0	1/0
She carries the pregnancy to term, and the neonate survives.	1	1	0	0	1	1/1
She is pregnant again.	2	1	0	0	1	2/1
Her second pregnancy ends in miscarriage at 10 wk.	2	1	0	1	1	2/1
During her third pregnancy, she gives birth at 36 wk to twins.	3	1	2	1	3	3/2

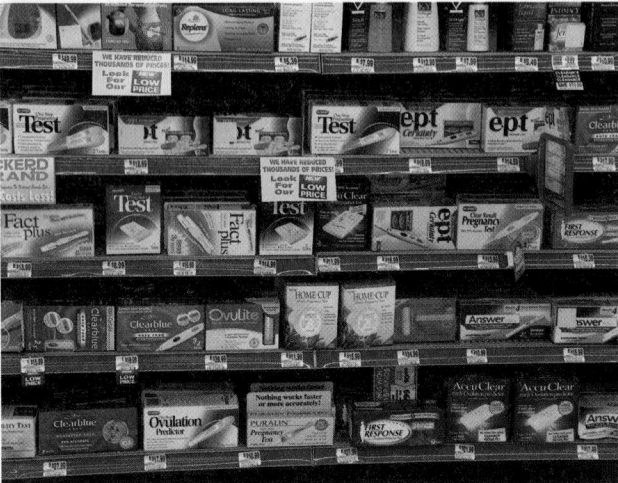

FIG 7-1 Many pregnancy test products are available over the counter. (Courtesy Dee Lowdermilk, Chapel Hill, NC.)

PATIENT TEACHING

Home Pregnancy Testing

1. Follow the manufacturer's instructions carefully. Do not omit steps.
2. Review the manufacturer's list of foods, medications, and other substances that can affect the test results.
3. Use a first-voided morning urine specimen.
4. If the test done at the time of your missed period is negative, repeat the test in 1 week if you still have not had a period.
5. If you have questions about the test, contact the manufacturer.
6. Contact your health care provider for follow-up if the test result is positive or if the test result is negative and you still have not had a period.

test procedures or results. A common error in performing home pregnancy tests is doing the test too early in pregnancy before a significant rise in hCG level; this can cause a false negative result (Pagana and Pagana, 2011).

Interpreting the results of pregnancy tests requires some judgment. The type of pregnancy test and its degree of sensitivity (the ability to detect low levels of a substance) and specificity (the ability to discern the absence of a substance) must be considered in conjunction with the woman's history. This includes the date of her last normal menstrual period, her usual cycle length, and results of previous pregnancy tests. It is important to know if the woman abuses substances and what medications she is taking. Medications such as anticonvulsants and tranquilizers can cause false-positive results, whereas diuretics and promethazine can cause false-negative results (Pagana and Pagana, 2011). Improper collection of the specimen, hormone-producing tumors, and laboratory errors can also cause inaccurate results.

Women who use a home pregnancy test should be advised about the variations in accuracy and to use caution when interpreting results. Whenever there is any question, further evaluation or retesting may be appropriate (see Patient Teaching box).

ADAPTATIONS TO PREGNANCY

Maternal physiologic adaptations are attributed to the hormones of pregnancy and to mechanical pressures arising from the enlarging uterus and other tissues. These adaptations protect the woman's

? CRITICAL THINKING CASE STUDY

Awareness of Physiologic Changes of Pregnancy

Marlys is pregnant with her first child, and Janice is pregnant with her third child. They are both at approximately 18 weeks of gestation and have come to a prenatal appointment. While they are in the waiting room, you overhear Marlys asking Janice about some "old wives' tales" that she has heard:

- If she raises her arms above her head, the cord will wrap around the baby's neck.
- Putting a knife under the bed while she is laboring will "cut" the pain.
- If she dangles a needle in front of her abdomen, she will be able to tell if the baby is a boy or a girl.
- A rapid fetal heartbeat means that the baby will be a boy.

Marlys says that she has not felt her baby move yet, whereas Janice says that she has been feeling fetal movement for over 2 weeks. Marlys also has questions about some of the changes in her body that she has experienced or expects to experience. Janice bases her responses on her own experience. Based on the conversation you have overheard, you identify a need to spend some time with Marlys and Janice discussing physiologic changes of pregnancy.

1. Evidence—Is there sufficient evidence to draw conclusions about the normal physiologic changes in pregnancy in primigravidas and multiparas that the nurse should discuss with Marlys and Janice?
2. Assumptions—Describe an underlying assumption about each of the following topics:
   a. Differences in the normal physiologic changes in pregnancy between primigravidas and multiparas
   b. Reversibility of these physiologic changes in pregnancy
   c. Information provided by the health care provider
   d. Deviations from normal in the physiologic changes of pregnancy
3. What implications and priorities for nursing care can be drawn at this time?
4. Does the evidence objectively support your conclusion?

normal physiologic functioning, meet the metabolic demands that pregnancy imposes on her body, and provide a nurturing environment for fetal development and growth (see Critical Thinking Case Study). Although pregnancy is a normal phenomenon, problems can occur.

Signs of Pregnancy

Some physiologic adaptations are recognized as the signs and symptoms of pregnancy. Three commonly used categories of these signs and symptoms are:

- Presumptive—those changes felt by the woman (e.g., amenorrhea, fatigue, breast changes)
- Probable—those changes observed by an examiner (e.g., Hegar sign, ballottement, pregnancy tests)
- Positive—those signs attributed only to the presence of the fetus (e.g., hearing fetal heart tones, visualizing the fetus, palpating fetal movements)

Table 7-2 summarizes these signs of pregnancy in relation to when they might occur and gives other possible causes for their occurrence.

Reproductive System and Breasts
Uterus

Changes in Size, Shape, and Position. High levels of estrogen and progesterone stimulate phenomenal uterine growth in the first

TABLE 7-2	SIGNS OF PREGNANCY	
TIME OF OCCURRENCE (GESTATIONAL AGE)	**SIGN**	**OTHER POSSIBLE CAUSE**
Presumptive		
3-4 wk	Breast changes	Premenstrual changes, oral contraceptives
4 wk	Amenorrhea	Stress, vigorous exercise, early menopause, endocrine problems, malnutrition
4-14 wk	Nausea, vomiting	Gastrointestinal virus, food poisoning
6-12 wk	Urinary frequency	Infection, pelvic tumors
12 wk	Fatigue	Stress, illness
16-20 wk	Quickening	Gas, peristalsis
Probable		
5 wk	Goodell sign	Pelvic congestion
6-8 wk	Chadwick sign	Pelvic congestion
6-12 wk	Hegar sign	Pelvic congestion
4-12 wk	Positive pregnancy test (serum)	Hydatidiform mole, choriocarcinoma
6-12 wk	Positive pregnancy test (urine)	False-positive result may be caused by pelvic infection, tumors
16 wk	Braxton Hicks contractions	Myomas, other tumors
16-28 wk	Ballottement	Tumors, cervical polyps
Positive		
5-6 wk	Visualization of fetus by real-time ultrasound examination	No other causes
6 wk	Fetal heart tones detected by ultrasound	No other causes
16 wk	Visualization of fetus by radiographic study	No other causes
8-17 wk	Fetal heart tones detected by Doppler ultrasound stethoscope	No other causes
17-19 wk	Fetal heart tones detected by fetal stethoscope	No other causes
19-22 wk	Fetal movements palpated	No other causes
Late pregnancy	Fetal movements visible	No other causes

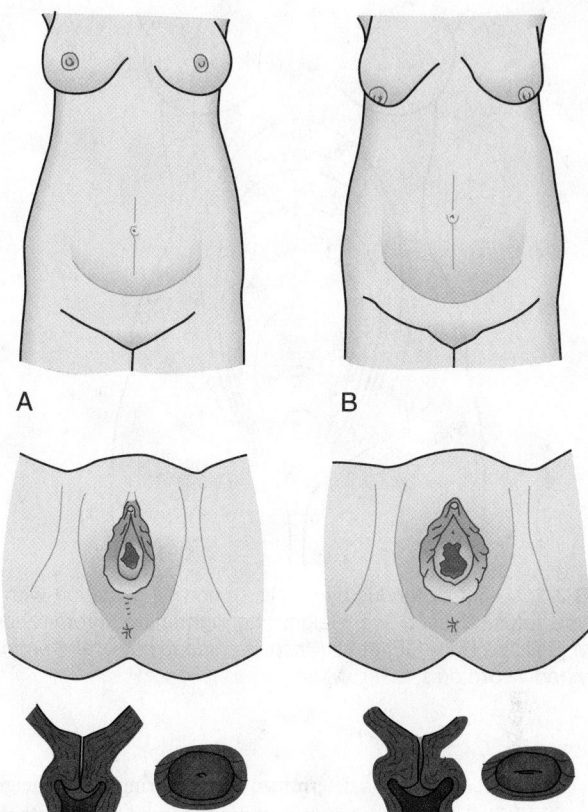

FIG 7-2 Comparison of abdomen, vulva, and cervix in **A,** nullipara, and **B,** multipara, at the same stage of pregnancy.

trimester. Early uterine enlargement results from increased vascularity and dilation of blood vessels, hyperplasia (production of new muscle fibers and fibroelastic tissue) and hypertrophy (enlargement of preexisting muscle fibers and fibroelastic tissue), and development of the decidua. By 7 weeks of gestation, the uterus is the size of a large hen's egg; by 10 weeks, it is the size of an orange (twice its nonpregnant size); and by 12 weeks, it is the size of a grapefruit. After the third month, uterine enlargement is primarily the result of mechanical pressure of the growing fetus.

As the uterus enlarges, it also changes in shape and position. At conception, the uterus is shaped like an upside-down pear. During the second trimester, as the muscular walls strengthen and become more elastic, the uterus becomes spherical or globular. Later, as the fetus lengthens, the uterus becomes larger and more ovoid and rises out of the pelvis into the abdominal cavity.

The pregnancy may "show" after the fourteenth week, although this depends to some degree on the woman's height and weight. Abdominal enlargement may be less apparent in the nullipara with good abdominal muscle tone (Fig. 7-2). Posture also influences the type and degree of abdominal enlargement that occurs. In normal pregnancies, the uterus enlarges at a predictable rate.

As the uterus grows, it may be palpated above the symphysis pubis sometime between the twelfth and fourteenth weeks of pregnancy (Fig. 7-3). The uterus rises gradually to the level of the umbilicus at 22 to 24 weeks of gestation and nearly reaches the xiphoid process at term. Between weeks 38 and 40, fundal height decreases as the fetus begins to descend and engage in the pelvis (lightening) (see Fig. 7-3, *dashed line*). Generally, lightening occurs in the nullipara about 2 weeks before the onset of labor and in the multipara at the start of labor.

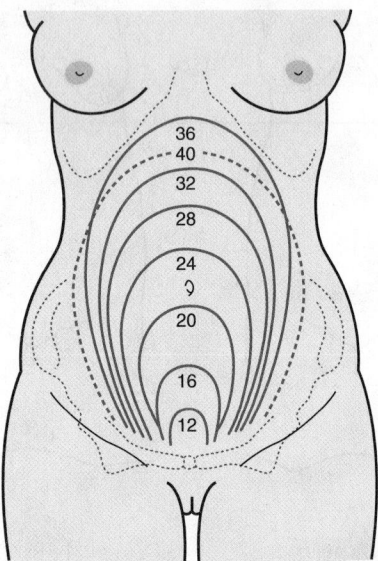

FIG 7-3 Height of fundus by weeks of normal gestation with a single fetus. *Dashed line,* Height after lightening. (From Seidel HM, Ball JW, Dains JE, et al: *Mosby's guide to physical examination,* ed 7, St Louis, 2011, Mosby.)

Uterine enlargement is determined by measuring fundal height (see Fig. 8-7). This measurement is commonly used to estimate the duration of pregnancy. However, variation in the position of the fundus or the fetus, variations in the amount of amniotic fluid present, the presence of more than one fetus, maternal obesity, and variation in examiner technique can reduce the accuracy of this estimation.

Generally the uterus rotates to the right as it elevates, probably because of the presence of the rectosigmoid colon on the left side. However, the extensive hypertrophy (enlargement) of the round ligaments keeps the uterus in the midline. Eventually the growing uterus touches the anterior abdominal wall and displaces the intestines to either side of the abdomen (Fig. 7-4). When a pregnant woman is standing, most of her uterus rests against the anterior abdominal wall and contributes to altering her center of gravity.

At approximately 6 weeks of gestation, softening and compressibility of the lower uterine segment (uterine isthmus) occurs (Hegar sign) (Fig. 7-5). This results in exaggerated uterine anteflexion during the first 3 months of pregnancy. In this position, the uterine fundus presses on the urinary bladder, causing the woman to have urinary frequency.

Changes in Contractility. Soon after the fourth month of pregnancy, uterine contractions can be felt through the abdominal wall. These contractions are referred to as Braxton Hicks contractions. Braxton Hicks contractions are irregular and painless contractions that occur intermittently throughout pregnancy. Although Braxton Hicks contractions are not painful, some women complain that they are annoying. After the twenty-eighth week, these contractions become more definite but they usually cease with walking or exercise. Braxton Hicks contractions can be mistaken for true labor; however, they do not increase in intensity or duration or cause cervical dilation. Conversely, premature labor contractions can be mistaken for Braxton Hicks contractions and lead to a delay in seeking treatment.

Uteroplacental Blood Flow. Placental perfusion depends on the maternal blood flow to the uterus. Blood flow increases rapidly as the uterus increases in size. Although uterine blood flow increases twentyfold, the fetoplacental unit grows even more rapidly. Consequently, more oxygen is extracted from the uterine blood during the latter part of pregnancy (Cunningham, Leveno, Bloom, et al., 2010). In a normal term pregnancy, one sixth of the total maternal blood volume is within the uterine vascular system. The rate of blood flow through the uterus averages 450 to 650 mL/min at term, and oxygen consumption of the gravid uterus increases to meet fetal needs. Three factors known to decrease uterine blood flow are low maternal arterial pressure, contractions of the uterus, and maternal supine position. Estrogen stimulation may increase uterine blood flow. Doppler ultrasound examination can be used to measure uterine blood flow velocity, especially in pregnancies at risk because of conditions associated with decreased placental perfusion (e.g., hypertension, intrauterine growth restriction, diabetes mellitus, multiple gestation) (Blackburn, 2013).

Using an ultrasound device or a fetal stethoscope, the examiner may hear the uterine souffle or bruit, a rushing or blowing sound of maternal blood flowing through uterine arteries to the placenta that is synchronous with the maternal pulse. The funic souffle, which is synchronous with the fetal heart rate and is caused by fetal blood coursing through the umbilical cord, may also be heard, as well as the actual heartbeat of the fetus (see Fig. 8-8).

Cervical Changes. In a normal, unscarred cervix, softening of the cervical tip may be observed about the beginning of the sixth week. This probable sign of pregnancy, Goodell sign, is brought about by increased vascularity, slight hypertrophy, and hyperplasia (increase in number of cells). The muscle and its collagen-rich connective tissue become loose, edematous, highly elastic, and increased in volume. The glands near the external os proliferate beneath the stratified squamous epithelium, giving the cervix the velvety appearance characteristic of pregnancy. Friability (tissue is easily damaged) is increased and can result in slight bleeding after vaginal examination or after coitus with deep penetration.

Pregnancy can also cause the squamocolumnar junction, the site for obtaining cells for cervical cancer screening, to be located away from the cervix. Because of these changes, evaluation of abnormal Papanicolaou (Pap) tests during pregnancy can be complicated. However, careful assessment of all pregnant women is important because approximately 3% of all invasive cervical cancers occur during pregnancy (Salani, Eisenhauer, and Copeland, 2012). The cervix of the nullipara is rounded. Lacerations of the cervix almost always occur during the birth process. After childbirth, with or without lacerations, the cervix becomes more oval in the horizontal plane and the external os appears as a transverse slit (see Fig. 7-2).

Changes Related to the Presence of the Fetus. Passive movement of the unengaged fetus is called ballottement and can be identified generally between the sixteenth and eighteenth week. Ballottement is a technique of palpating a floating structure by bouncing it gently and feeling it rebound. To palpate the fetus, the examiner places a finger within the vagina and taps gently upward on the cervix, causing the fetus to rise. The fetus then sinks, and a gentle tap is felt on the finger.

The first recognition of fetal movements, or "feeling life," by the multiparous woman may occur as early as 14 to 16 weeks. The nulliparous woman may not notice these sensations until the eighteenth week or later. Quickening is commonly described as a flutter and is difficult to distinguish from peristalsis. Fetal movements gradually increase in intensity and frequency as pregnancy progresses. The week in which quickening occurs provides a tentative clue in dating the duration of gestation.

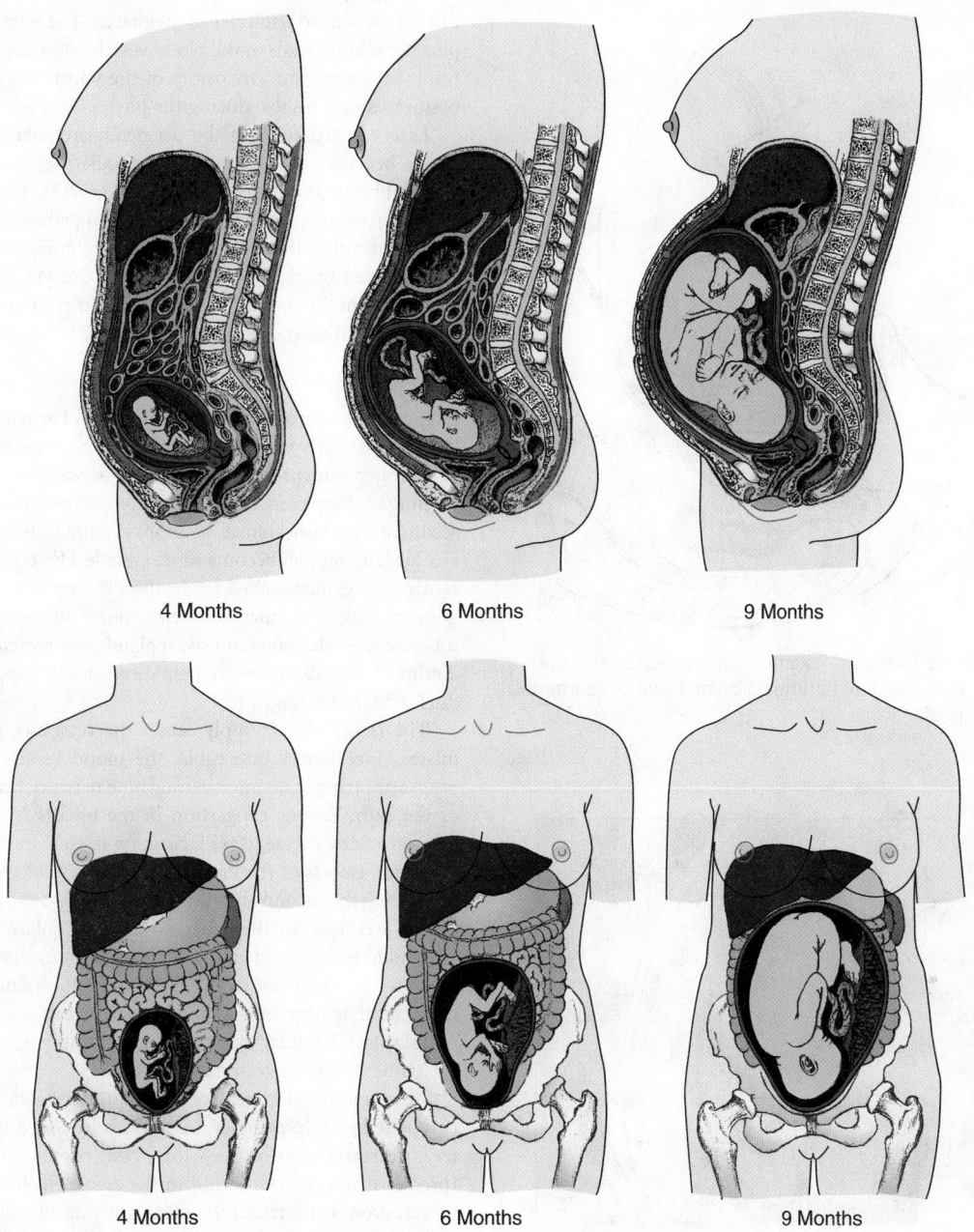

FIG 7-4 Displacement of internal abdominal structures and diaphragm by the enlarging uterus at 4, 6, and 9 months of gestation.

Vagina and Vulva

Pregnancy hormones prepare the vagina for stretching during labor and birth by causing the vaginal mucosa to thicken, the connective tissue to loosen, the smooth muscle to hypertrophy, and the vaginal vault to lengthen. Increased vascularity results in a violet-bluish color of the vaginal mucosa and cervix. The deepened color, termed Chadwick sign, can be evident as early as the sixth week but is easily noted by the eighth week of pregnancy (Blackburn, 2013).

Leukorrhea is a white or slightly gray mucoid discharge with a faint musty odor. This copious mucoid fluid occurs in response to cervical stimulation by estrogen and progesterone. The fluid is whitish because of the presence of many exfoliated vaginal epithelial cells caused by the hyperplasia of normal pregnancy. This vaginal discharge is never pruritic or blood stained. The mucus fills the endocervical canal, resulting in the formation of the mucus plug (operculum) (Fig. 7-6). The operculum acts as a barrier against bacterial invasion during pregnancy.

During pregnancy, the pH of vaginal secretions is more acidic, ranging from about 3.5 to about 6.0 (nonpregnant, 4.0 to 5.0), because of increased production of lactic acid (Cunningham, Leveno, Bloom, et al., 2010). Although this acidic environment provides more protection from some organisms, the pregnant woman is more vulnerable to other infections, especially yeast infections, because the glycogen-rich environment of the vagina is more susceptible to *Candida albicans* (Duff, Sweet, and Edwards, 2009).

The increased vascularity of the vagina and other pelvic viscera results in a marked increase in sensitivity. The increased sensitivity may lead to a high degree of sexual interest and arousal, especially

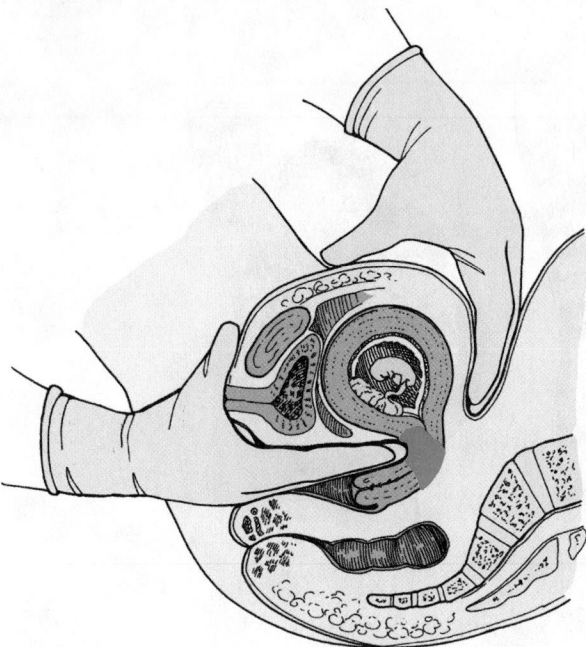

FIG 7-5 Hegar sign. Bimanual examination for assessing compressibility and softening of isthmus (lower uterine segment) while the cervix is still firm.

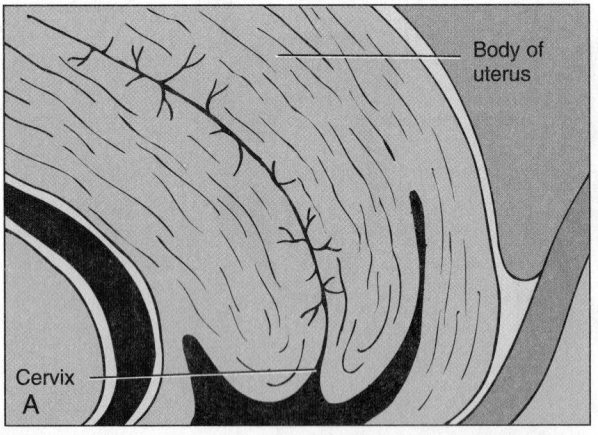

Body of uterus

Cervix

A

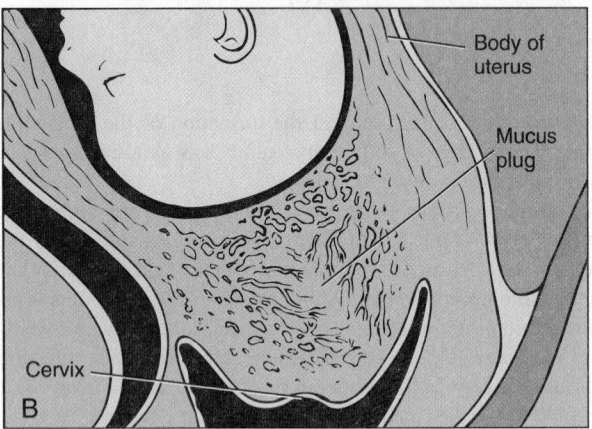

Body of uterus

Mucus plug

Cervix

B

FIG 7-6 A, Cervix in nonpregnant woman. **B,** Cervix during pregnancy.

during the second trimester of pregnancy. The increased congestion, plus the relaxed walls of the blood vessels and the heavy uterus, may result in edema and varicosities of the vulva. The edema and varicosities usually resolve during the postpartum period.

External structures of the perineum are enlarged during pregnancy because of an increase in vasculature, hypertrophy of the perineal body, and deposition of fat (Fig. 7-7). The labia majora of nullipara women approximate (come together) and obscure the vaginal introitus; those of the parous woman separate and gape after childbirth and perineal or vaginal injury. See Fig. 7-2 for a comparison of the nullipara and the multipara in relation to the pregnant abdomen, vulva, and cervix.

Breasts

Fullness, heightened sensitivity, tingling, and heaviness of the breasts begin in the early weeks of gestation in response to increased levels of estrogen and progesterone. Breast sensitivity varies from mild tingling to sharp pain. Nipples and areolae become more pigmented; secondary pinkish areolae develop, extending beyond the primary areolae; and nipples become more erectile. Hypertrophy of the sebaceous (oil) glands embedded in the primary areolae, called Montgomery tubercles, may be seen around the nipples. Within the tubercles are sebaceous and sweat glands that secrete lubricating and antiinfective substances to help protect the nipples and areolae during breastfeeding.

The richer blood supply causes the vessels beneath the skin to dilate. Once barely noticeable, the blood vessels become visible, often appearing in an intertwining blue network beneath the surface of the skin. Venous congestion in the breasts is more obvious in primigravidas. Striae gravidarum, or stretch marks, can appear at the outer aspects of the breasts.

During the second and third trimesters, growth of the mammary glands accounts for the progressive breast enlargement (Fig. 7-8). The high levels of luteal and placental hormones in pregnancy promote proliferation of the lactiferous ducts and lobule-alveolar tissue so that palpation of the breasts reveals a generalized coarse nodularity. Glandular tissue displaces connective tissue, resulting in the tissue becoming softer and looser.

Although development of the mammary glands is functionally complete by midpregnancy, lactation is inhibited until the estrogen level decreases after birth. A thin, clear, viscous secretory material (precolostrum) can be found in the acini cells by the third month of gestation. Colostrum, the creamy, white-to-yellowish-to-orange premilk fluid secreted during the second trimester may be expressed from the nipples as early as 16 weeks of gestation (Lawrence and Lawrence, 2011). See Chapter 24 for a discussion of lactation.

General Body Systems
Cardiovascular System

Maternal adjustments to pregnancy involve extensive anatomic and physiologic changes in the cardiovascular system. Cardiovascular adaptations protect the woman's normal physiologic functioning, meet the metabolic demands pregnancy imposes on her body, and provide for fetal developmental and growth needs.

Slight cardiac hypertrophy (enlargement) is probably secondary to increased blood volume and cardiac output that occur in pregnancy. The heart returns to its normal size after childbirth. As the diaphragm is displaced upward by the enlarging uterus, the heart is elevated upward and rotated forward to the left (Fig. 7-9). The apical impulse, point of maximal intensity, is shifted upward and laterally about 1 to 1.5 cm (0.4 to 0.6 cm). The degree of shift depends on the duration of pregnancy and the size and position of the uterus.

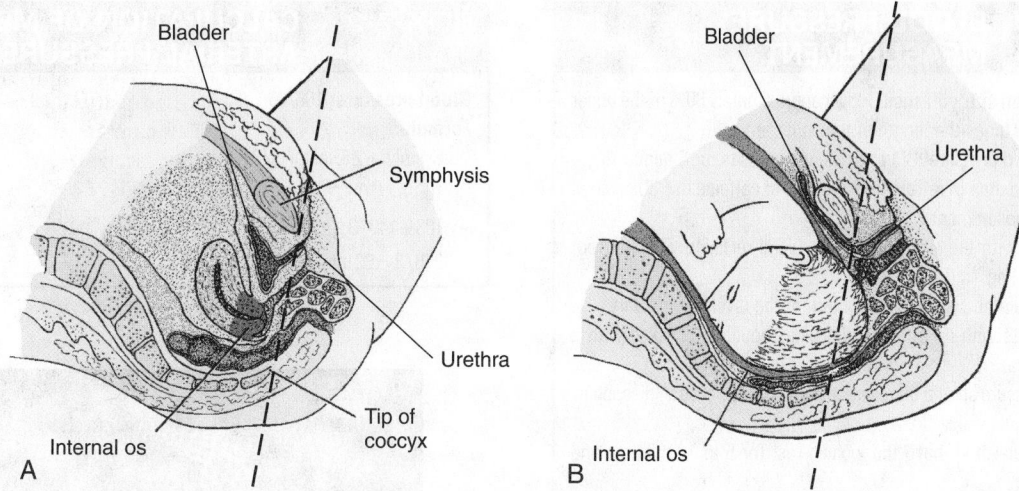

FIG 7-7 A, Pelvic floor in nonpregnant woman. **B,** Pelvic floor at end of pregnancy. Note marked hypertrophy and hyperplasia below *dotted line* joining tip of coccyx and inferior margin of symphysis. Note elongation of bladder and urethra as a result of compression. Fat deposits are increased.

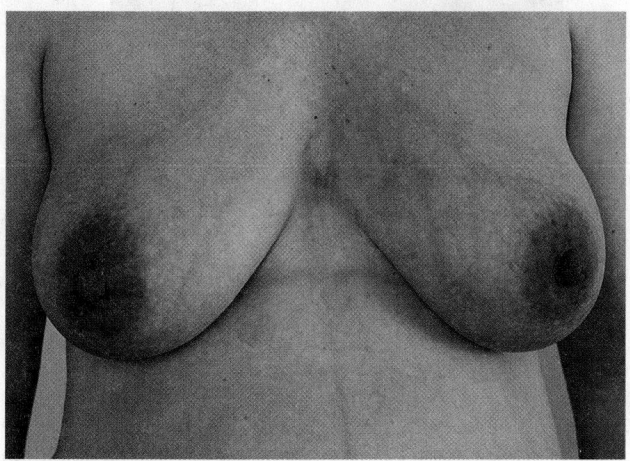

FIG 7-8 Enlarged breasts in pregnancy with venous network and darkened areolae and nipples. (From Seidel HM, Ball JW, Dains JE, et al: *Mosby's guide to physical examination*, ed 7, St Louis, 2011, Mosby.)

The changes in heart size and position and the increases in blood volume and cardiac output contribute to auscultatory changes common in pregnancy. There is more audible splitting of S_1 and S_2, and S_3 may be readily heard after 20 weeks of gestation. In addition, systolic and diastolic murmurs may be heard over the pulmonic area. These changes are transient and disappear in most women shortly after they give birth (Cunningham, Leveno, Bloom, et al., 2010).

Between 14 and 20 weeks of gestation, the pulse increases about 10 to 15 beats/min, and this persists to term. Palpitations may occur. In twin gestations, the maternal heart rate increases significantly in the third trimester (Blackburn, 2013).

The cardiac rhythm may be disturbed. The pregnant woman may experience sinus dysrhythmia, premature atrial contractions, and premature ventricular systole. In the healthy woman with no underlying heart disease, no therapy is needed. Women with pre-existing heart disease need close medical and obstetric supervision during pregnancy (see Chapter 11).

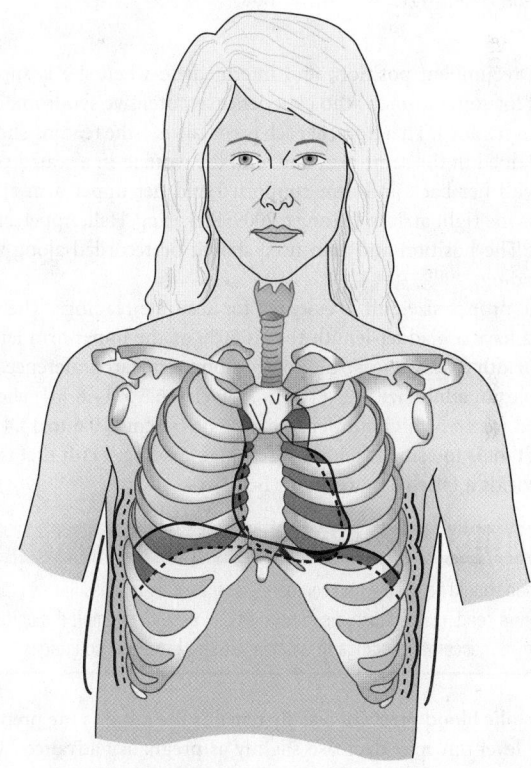

FIG 7-9 Changes in position of heart, lungs, and thoracic cage in pregnancy. *Broken line,* Nonpregnant state; *solid line,* change that occurs in pregnancy.

Blood Pressure. Arterial blood pressure (brachial artery) varies with age, activity level, presence of health problem, circadian rhythm, use of alcohol, smoking, and pain. Additional factors to consider during pregnancy include maternal position and type of blood pressure apparatus. Maternal anxiety can elevate readings. If an elevated reading is found, the woman is given time to rest and the reading is repeated.

Maternal position affects readings. Brachial blood pressure is highest when the woman is sitting; lowest when she is lying in the

BOX 7-1   BLOOD PRESSURE MEASUREMENT

1. Use correct cuff size; cuff should cover approximately 80% of the upper arm or be 1.5 times the length of the upper arm.
2. Measure blood pressure (BP) after the woman sits for 5 minutes.
3. Instruct the woman to refrain from tobacco or caffeine use 30 minutes before BP measurement.
4. Measure BP with the woman sitting or semi-reclining with her feet flat, not dangling.
5. The arm should be supported on a desk at the level of the heart.
6. Measurements with an automated device should be checked with a manual device.
7. Diastolic pressure should be recorded at Korotkoff phase V (disappearance of sound).
8. If the BP is elevated, have the woman rest for 5 to 10 minutes and then retake it.
9. BP may vary by >10 mm Hg from one arm to the other; record the higher reading.
10. Take the average of two readings at least 1 minute apart.

Data from Peters R: High blood pressure in pregnancy, *Nurs Womens Health* 12(5):412–421, 2008.

BOX 7-2   CALCULATION OF MEAN ARTERIAL PRESSURE

Blood pressure: 106/70
Formula:

Systolic + 2 (Diastolic)/3

106 + 2 (70)/3

106 + 140/3

246/3 = 82 mm Hg

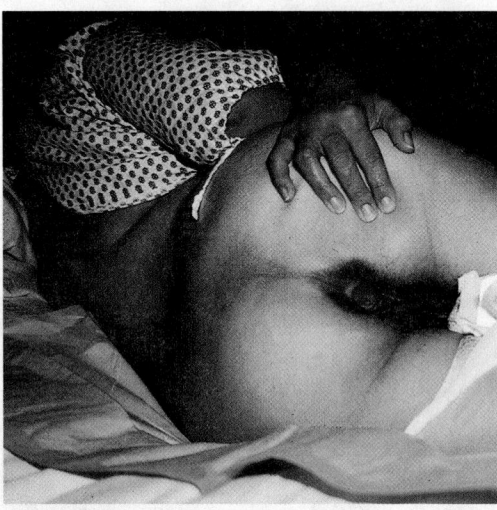

FIG 7-10 Hemorrhoids. (Courtesy Marjorie Pyle, RNC, Lifecircle, Costa Mesa, CA.)

lateral recumbent position; and intermediate when she is supine, except for some women who experience hypotensive syndrome (see later discussion). Therefore, at each prenatal visit, the reading should be obtained in the same arm and with the woman in a seated position with her back and arm supported and her upper arm at the level of the right atrium (Monga, 2009; Pickering, Hall, Appel, et al., 2005). The position and arm used should be recorded along with the reading.

The proper-size cuff is essential for accurate readings. The cuff should have a bladder length that is 80% of the upper arm length and a width that is at least 40% of the upper arm circumference. For example, an adult-size cuff (16 cm × 30 cm [6.3 × 11.8 in]) should be used for an arm circumference of 27 to 34 cm (10.6 to 13.4 in). A cuff that is too small yields a falsely high reading; a cuff that is too large yields a falsely low reading (Box 7-1).

! NURSING ALERT

Caution should be used when comparing auscultatory and oscillatory blood pressure readings because discrepancies can occur. Automated monitors can give inaccurate readings in women with hypertensive conditions.

Systolic blood pressure usually remains the same as the prepregnancy level but may decrease slightly as pregnancy advances. Diastolic blood pressure begins to decrease in the first trimester, continues to drop until 24 to 32 weeks, and gradually increases and returns to prepregnancy levels by term (Blackburn, 2013).

Calculating the mean arterial pressure (MAP) (mean of the blood pressure in the arterial circulation) can increase the diagnostic value of the findings. Normal MAP readings in the nonpregnant woman are 86 ± 7.5 mm Hg. MAP readings for a pregnant woman at term are slightly higher at 90 ± 5.8 (Cunningham, Leveno, Bloom, et al., 2010). Box 7-2 illustrates one way to calculate MAP.

Some degree of compression of the vena cava occurs in all women who lie on their back during the second half of pregnancy. Some women experience a fall of more than 30 mm Hg in their systolic pressure. After 4 to 5 minutes, a reflex bradycardia is noted, cardiac output is reduced by half, and the woman feels faint. This condition is called supine hypotensive syndrome (Cunningham, Leveno, Bloom, et al., 2010).

Compression of the iliac veins and inferior vena cava by the uterus causes increased venous pressure and reduced blood flow in the legs, except when the woman is in the lateral position. These alterations contribute to the dependent edema, varicose veins in the legs and vulva, and hemorrhoids that develop in the latter part of term pregnancy (Fig. 7-10).

Blood Volume and Composition. The degree of blood volume expansion varies considerably. Blood volume increases by approximately 1500 mL, or 40% to 50% above nonpregnancy levels (Cunningham, Leveno, Bloom, et al., 2010). This increase consists of 1000 mL of plasma plus 450 mL of red blood cells (RBCs). The increase in volume starts at weeks 10 to 12, peaks at weeks 32 to 34, and decreases slightly at week 40. The volume in a multiple gestation increases above that for a single fetus (Blackburn, 2013). Increased blood volume is a protective mechanism. It is essential for meeting the blood volume needs of the hypertrophied vascular system of the enlarged uterus, for adequately hydrating fetal and maternal tissues when the woman assumes an erect or supine position, and for providing a fluid reserve to compensate for blood loss during birth and postpartum. Peripheral vasodilation allows for a normal blood pressure despite the increased blood volume in pregnancy.

During pregnancy, there is an accelerated production of RBCs (nonpregnant, 4.2 to 5.4 million/mm³). The percentage of increase depends on the amount of iron available. The RBC mass increases by 20% to 30% (Blackburn, 2013).

Because the plasma increase is greater than the increase in RBC production, there is a decrease in normal hemoglobin values (12 to 16 g/dL blood) and hematocrit values (37% to 47%). This state of hemodilution is referred to as physiologic anemia. The decrease is more noticeable during the second trimester, when rapid expansion of blood volume occurs faster than RBC production. If the hemoglobin value drops to 11 g/dL or less during the first or third trimester or less than 10.5 g/dL during the second trimester or if the hematocrit decreases to 32% or less, the woman is considered anemic (Hark and Catalano, 2012).

The total white blood cell count increases during the second trimester and peaks during the third trimester. This increase is primarily in the granulocytes; the lymphocyte count stays about the same throughout pregnancy. See Table 7-3 for laboratory values during pregnancy.

Cardiac Output. Cardiac output increases from 30% to 50% over the nonpregnant rate by week 32 of pregnancy; it declines to about a 20% increase at 40 weeks of gestation. This elevated cardiac output is largely a result of increased stroke volume and heart rate and occurs in response to increased tissue demands for oxygen (Monga, 2009).

Cardiac output in late pregnancy is appreciably higher when the woman is in the lateral recumbent position than when she is supine. In the supine position, the large, heavy uterus often impedes venous return to the heart and affects blood pressure. Cardiac output increases with any exertion such as labor and birth. Table 7-4 summarizes cardiovascular changes in pregnancy.

Circulation and Coagulation Times. The circulation time decreases slightly by week 32. It returns to near normal by term. There is a greater tendency for blood to coagulate (clot) during pregnancy because of increases in various clotting factors (i.e.,

TABLE 7-3   LABORATORY VALUES FOR PREGNANT AND NONPREGNANT WOMEN

VALUES	NONPREGNANT	PREGNANT
Hematologic		
Complete Blood Count		
Hemoglobin, g/dL	12-16*	>11*
Hematocrit, packed cell volume, %	37-47	>33*
RBC volume, per mL	1400	1650
Plasma volume, per mL	2400	40%-60% increase
RBC count, million/mm³	4.2-5.4	5-6.25
White blood cells, total per mm³	5000-10,000	5000-15,000
Neutrophils, %	55-70	60-85
Lymphocytes, %	20-40	15-40
Erythrocyte sedimentation rate, mm/hr	20	Elevated in second and third trimesters
Mean corpuscular hemoglobin concentration, g/dL packed RBCs	32-36	No change
Mean corpuscular hemoglobin, pg	27-31	No change
Mean corpuscular volume per mm³	80-95	No change
Blood Coagulation and Fibrinolytic Activity†		
Factor VII	65-140	Increases in pregnancy, returns to normal in early puerperium
Factor VIII	55-145	Increases during pregnancy and immediately after birth
Factor IX	60-140	Same as factor VII
Factor X	45-155	Same as factor VII
Factor XI	65-135	Decreases in pregnancy
Factor XII	50-150	Same as factor VII
Prothrombin time, sec	11-12.5	Decreases slightly in pregnancy
Partial thromboplastin time, sec	60-70	Decreases slightly in pregnancy and decreases during second and third stages of labor (indicates clotting at placental site)
Bleeding time, min	1-9 (Ivy method)	No appreciable change
Coagulation time, min	6-10 (Lee-White method)	No appreciable change
Platelets, per mm³	150,000-400,000	No significant change until 3-5 days after birth and then increases rapidly (may predispose woman to thrombosis) and gradually returns to normal
Fibrinolytic activity		Decreases in pregnancy and then abruptly returns to normal (protection against thromboembolism)
Fibrinogen, mg/dL	200-400	Levels increase late in pregnancy

Continued

TABLE 7-3   LABORATORY VALUES FOR PREGNANT AND NONPREGNANT WOMEN—cont'd

VALUES	NONPREGNANT	PREGNANT
Hematologic—cont'd		
Mineral/Vitamin Concentrations		
Vitamin B_{12}, folic acid, ascorbic acid	Normal	Moderate decrease
Serum Proteins		
Total, g/dL	6.4-8.3	5.5-7.5
Albumin, g/dL	3.5-5	Slight increase
Globulin, total, g/dL	2.3-3.4	3.0-4.0
Blood Glucose		
Fasting, mg/dL	70-105	Decreases
2-hr postprandial, mg/dL	<140	<140 after a 100-g carbohydrate meal is considered normal
Acid-Base Values in Arterial Blood		
PO_2, mm Hg	80-100	104-108 (increased)
PCO_2, mm Hg	35-45	27-32 (decreased)
Sodium bicarbonate (HCO_3), mEq/L	21-28	18-31 (decreased)
Blood pH	7.35-7.45	7.40-7.45 (slightly increased, more alkaline)
Hepatic		
Bilirubin, total, mg/dL	≤1	Unchanged
Serum cholesterol, mg/dL	120-200	Increases from 16-32 wk of pregnancy; remains at this level until after birth
Serum alkaline phosphatase, units/L	30-120	Increases from wk 12 of pregnancy to 6 wk after birth
Serum albumin, g/dL	3.5-5	Increases slightly
Renal		
Bladder capacity, mL	1300	1500
Renal plasma flow, mL/min	490-700	Increases by 25%-30%
Glomerular filtration rate, mL/min	88-128	Increases by 30%-50%
Nonprotein nitrogen, mg/dL	25-40	Decreases
Blood urea nitrogen, mg/dL	10-20	Decreases
Serum creatinine, mg/dL	0.5-1.1	Decreases
Serum uric acid, mg/dL	2.7-7.3	Decreases but returns to prepregnancy level by end of pregnancy
Urine glucose	Negative	Present in 20% of pregnant women
Intravenous pyelogram	Normal	Slight to moderate hydroureter and hydronephrosis; right kidney larger than left kidney

Data from Blackburn S: *Maternal, fetal, & neonatal physiology: a clinical perspective,* ed 4, St Louis, 2013, Saunders; Gordon M: Maternal physiology. In Gabbe SG, Niebyl JR, Simpson JL, et al, editors: *Obstetrics: normal and problem pregnancies,* ed 6, Philadelphia, 2012, Saunders; Pagana KD, Pagana TJ: *Mosby's diagnostic and laboratory test reference,* ed 10, St Louis, 2011, Mosby; Samuels P: Hematology complications of pregnancy. In Gabbe SG, Niebyl JR, Simpson JL, et al, editors: *Obstetrics: normal and problem pregnancies,* ed 6, Philadelphia, 2012, Saunders.
ng, Nanogram; *PCV,* packed cell volume; *pg,* picogram; *RBC,* red blood cell.
NOTE: Abbreviations should not be used in practice.
*At sea level. Permanent residents of higher levels (e.g., Denver) require higher levels of hemoglobin.
†Pregnancy represents a hypercoagulable state.

factors VII, VIII, IX, X, and fibrinogen). This tendency, combined with the fact that fibrinolytic activity (the splitting up or dissolving of a clot) is depressed during pregnancy and the postpartum period, provides a protective function to decrease the chance of bleeding but also makes the woman more vulnerable to thrombosis, especially after cesarean birth.

Respiratory System

Structural and ventilatory adaptations occur during pregnancy to provide for maternal and fetal needs. Maternal oxygen requirements increase in response to the acceleration in metabolic rate and the need to add to the tissue mass in the uterus and breasts. In addition, the fetus requires oxygen and a way to eliminate carbon dioxide.

TABLE 7-4	CARDIOVASCULAR CHANGES IN PREGNANCY
PARAMETER	**CHANGE**
Heart rate	Increases 10-15 beats/min
Blood pressure	
Systolic	Slight or no decrease from prepregnancy levels
Diastolic	Slight decrease to midpregnancy (24-32 wk) and gradual return to prepregnancy levels by end of pregnancy
Blood volume	Increases by 1500 mL or 40%-50% above prepregnancy level
Red blood cell mass	Increases 17%
Hemoglobin	Decreases
Hematocrit	Decreases
White blood cell count	Increases in second and third trimesters
Cardiac output	Increases 30%-50%

Data from Gordon M: Maternal physiology. In Gabbe SG, Niebyl JR, Simpson JL, et al, editors: *Obstetrics: normal and problem pregnancies,* ed 6, Philadelphia, 2012, Saunders.

TABLE 7-5	RESPIRATORY CHANGES IN PREGNANCY
PARAMETER	**CHANGE**
Respiratory rate	Unchanged or slightly increased
Tidal volume	Increased 30%-40%
Vital capacity	Unchanged
Inspiratory capacity	Increased
Expiratory reserve volume	Decreased
Total lung capacity	Unchanged to slightly decreased
Oxygen consumption	Increased 20%-40%

Data from Gordon M: Maternal physiology. In Gabbe SG, Niebyl JR, Simpson JL, et al, editors: *Obstetrics: normal and problem pregnancies,* ed 6, Philadelphia, 2012, Saunders.

Elevated levels of estrogen cause the ligaments of the rib cage to relax, permitting increased chest expansion (see Fig. 7-9). The transverse diameter of the thoracic cage increases by about 2 cm (0.8 in) and the circumference by 6 cm (2.4 in) (Cunningham, Leveno, Bloom, et al., 2010). The costal angle increases, and the lower rib cage appears to flare out. The chest may not return to its prepregnant state after birth (Seidel, Ball, Dains, et al., 2011).

The diaphragm is displaced by as much as 4 cm (1.6 in) during pregnancy. With advancing pregnancy, chest breathing replaces abdominal breathing and it becomes less possible for the diaphragm to descend with inspiration. Thoracic breathing is accomplished primarily by the diaphragm rather than by the costal muscles (Blackburn, 2013).

The upper respiratory tract becomes more vascular in response to elevated levels of estrogen. As the capillaries become engorged, edema and hyperemia develop within the nose, pharynx, larynx, trachea, and bronchi. This congestion within the tissues of the respiratory tract gives rise to several conditions commonly seen during pregnancy, including nasal and sinus stuffiness, epistaxis (nosebleed), changes in the voice, and marked inflammatory response to even a mild upper respiratory infection.

Increased vascularity of the upper respiratory tract also can cause the tympanic membranes and eustachian tubes to swell, giving rise to symptoms of impaired hearing, earaches, or a sense of fullness in the ears.

Pulmonary Function. Respiratory changes in pregnancy are related to the elevation of the diaphragm and changes in the chest wall. Changes in the respiratory center result in a lowered threshold for carbon dioxide. The actions of progesterone and estrogen are presumed to be responsible for the increased sensitivity of the respiratory center to carbon dioxide. See Table 7-5 for respiratory changes in pregnancy. Although pulmonary function is not impaired by pregnancy, diseases of the respiratory tract can be more serious during this time (Cunningham, Leveno, Bloom, et al., 2010). One important factor responsible for this can be the increase in oxygen requirements.

Basal Metabolic Rate. The basal metabolic rate (BMR) increases during pregnancy. The elevation in BMR reflects increased oxygen demands of the uterine-placental-fetal unit and greater oxygen consumption because of increased maternal cardiac work. This increase varies considerably, depending on the prepregnancy nutritional status of the woman and fetal growth. By the third trimester, the BMR is increased by 10% to 20% over the nonpregnant state (Cunningham, Leveno, Bloom, et al., 2010). The BMR returns to nonpregnant levels by 5 to 6 days after birth. Peripheral vasodilation and acceleration of sweat gland activity help dissipate the excess heat resulting from the increased BMR during pregnancy. Pregnant women may experience heat intolerance. Lassitude and fatigability after only slight exertion are experienced by many women in early pregnancy. These feelings, along with a greater need for sleep, may persist and may be caused in part by the increased metabolic activity.

Acid-Base Balance. By about the tenth week of pregnancy, there is a decrease of about 5 mm Hg in the partial pressure of carbon dioxide (PCO_2). Progesterone may be responsible for increasing the sensitivity of the respiratory center receptors so that tidal volume increases and PCO_2 decreases, the base excess (HCO_3, or bicarbonate) decreases, and pH increases slightly (Cunningham, Leveno, Bloom, et al., 2010). These alterations in acid-base balance indicate that pregnancy is a state of respiratory alkalosis (Gordon, 2012) (see Table 7-3). These changes also facilitate the transport of CO_2 from the fetus and O_2 release from the mother to the fetus.

Renal System

The kidneys are responsible for maintaining electrolyte and acid-base balance, regulating extracellular fluid volume, excreting waste products, and conserving essential nutrients.

Anatomic Changes. Changes in renal structure result from hormonal activity (estrogen and progesterone), pressure from an enlarging uterus, and an increase in blood volume. As early as the tenth week of pregnancy, the renal pelves and the ureters dilate. Dilation of the ureters is more pronounced above the pelvic brim, in part because they are compressed between the uterus and the pelvic brim. In most women, the ureters below the pelvic brim are normal size. The smooth-muscle walls of the ureters undergo hyperplasia and hypertrophy and muscle tone relaxation. The ureters elongate, become tortuous, and form single or double curves. In the latter part of pregnancy, the renal pelvis and ureter dilate more on the right side than on the left because the heavy uterus is displaced to the right by the sigmoid colon.

Because of these changes, a larger volume of urine is held in the pelves and ureters and urine flow rate is slowed. Urinary stasis or stagnation has several consequences:

- A lag occurs between the time urine is formed and when it reaches the bladder. Therefore clearance test results may reflect substances contained in glomerular filtrate several hours before.
- Stagnated urine is an excellent medium for the growth of microorganisms. In addition, the urine of pregnant women contains more nutrients, including glucose, that increase the pH (making the urine more alkaline). This makes pregnant women more susceptible to urinary tract infection.

Bladder irritability, nocturia, and urinary frequency and urgency (without dysuria) are commonly reported in early pregnancy. These bladder symptoms may return near term, especially after lightening occurs.

Urinary frequency results initially from increased bladder sensitivity and later from compression of the bladder (see Fig. 7-7). In the second trimester, the bladder is pulled up out of the true pelvis into the abdomen. The urethra lengthens to 7.5 cm (3 in) as the bladder is displaced upward. The pelvic congestion that occurs in pregnancy is reflected in hyperemia of the bladder and urethra. This increased vascularity causes the bladder mucosa to be easily traumatized. Bladder tone may decrease, which increases the bladder capacity to 1500 mL. At the same time, the bladder is compressed by the enlarging uterus, resulting in the urge to void even if the bladder contains only a small amount of urine.

Functional Changes. In normal pregnancy, renal function is altered considerably. Glomerular filtration rate (GFR) and renal plasma flow increase early in pregnancy (Monga, 2009). These changes are caused by pregnancy hormones; an increase in blood volume; and the woman's posture, physical activity, and nutritional intake. The woman's kidneys must manage the increased metabolic and circulatory demands of the maternal body as well as the excretion of fetal waste products.

Renal function is most efficient when the woman lies in the lateral recumbent position and least efficient when the woman assumes a supine position. A side-lying position increases renal perfusion, which increases urine output and decreases edema. When the pregnant woman is lying supine, the heavy uterus compresses the vena cava and the aorta and cardiac output decreases. As a result, blood flow to the brain and heart is continued at the expense of other organs, including the kidneys and uterus.

Fluid and Electrolyte Balance. Selective renal tubular reabsorption maintains sodium and water balance, regardless of changes in dietary intake and losses through sweat, vomitus, or diarrhea. About 900 mEq of sodium is normally retained during pregnancy to meet fetal needs, although maternal serum levels of sodium decrease by 3 to 4 mmol/L (Gordon, 2012). To prevent excessive sodium depletion, the maternal kidneys undergo a significant adaptation by increasing tubular reabsorption. Because of the need for increased maternal intravascular and extracellular fluid volume, additional sodium is needed to expand fluid volume and maintain an isotonic state. As efficient as the renal system is, it can be overstressed by excessive dietary sodium intake or restriction or by use of diuretics. Severe hypovolemia and reduced placental perfusion are two consequences of using diuretics during pregnancy.

The capacity of the kidneys to excrete water is more efficient during the early weeks than later in pregnancy. As a result, some women feel thirsty in early pregnancy because of the greater amount of water loss. The pooling of fluid in the legs in the latter part of pregnancy decreases renal blood flow and GFR. This pooling is sometimes referred to as physiologic or dependent edema and requires no treatment. The normal diuretic response to the water load is triggered when the woman lies down, preferably on her side, and the pooled fluid reenters general circulation.

Normally the kidney reabsorbs almost all the glucose and other nutrients from the plasma filtrate. However, in pregnant women, tubular reabsorption of glucose is impaired, causing glucosuria to occur at varying times and to varying degrees. Normal values range from 0 to 20 mg/dL, meaning that during any day, the urine is sometimes positive and sometimes negative for glucose. In nonpregnant women, blood glucose levels must be at 160 to 180 mg/dL before glucose is "spilled" into the urine (not resorbed). During pregnancy, glucosuria occurs when maternal glucose levels are lower than 160 mg/dL. Why glucose, as well as other nutrients such as amino acids, is wasted during pregnancy is not understood, nor has the exact mechanism been discovered. Although glucosuria may be found in normal pregnancies (2+ levels can be seen with increased anxiety states), the possibility of diabetes mellitus and gestational diabetes must be considered.

Proteinuria does not usually occur in normal pregnancy except during labor or after birth (Cunningham, Leveno, Bloom, et al., 2010). However, the increased amounts of amino acids that must be filtered may exceed the capacity of the renal tubules to absorb them, and small amounts of protein may be lost in the urine. The amount of protein excreted is not an indication of the severity of renal disease, nor does an increase in protein excretion in a pregnant woman with known renal disease necessarily indicate a progression in her disease. However, a pregnant woman with hypertension and proteinuria must be evaluated carefully because she may be at greater risk for an adverse pregnancy outcome (Gordon, 2012).

Integumentary System

Alterations in hormone balance and mechanical stretching are responsible for several changes in the integumentary system during pregnancy. Hyperpigmentation is stimulated by the anterior pituitary hormone *melanotropin,* which is increased during pregnancy. Darkening of the nipples, areolae, axillae, and vulva occurs at about the sixteenth week of gestation. Melasma (also called chloasma or mask of pregnancy) is a blotchy, brownish hyperpigmentation of the skin over the cheeks, nose, and forehead, especially in pregnant women with dark complexions. Melasma appears in 50% to 70% of pregnant women, beginning after the sixteenth week and increasing gradually until term. The sun intensifies this pigmentation in susceptible women. Melasma caused by normal pregnancy usually fades after birth but often recurs with oral contraceptive use or subsequent pregnancies (Kroumpouzos, 2012).

The linea nigra (Fig. 7-11) is a pigmented line extending from the symphysis pubis to the top of the fundus in the midline. This line is known as the linea alba before hormone-induced pigmentation. In primigravidas, the extension of the linea nigra, beginning in the third month, keeps pace with the rising height of the fundus; in multigravidas, the entire line often appears earlier than the third month. Not all pregnant women develop linea nigra, and some women notice hair growth along the line with or without the change in pigmentation.

Striae gravidarum, or "stretch marks," (seen over the lower abdomen in Fig. 7-11) appear in 50% to 90% of pregnant women

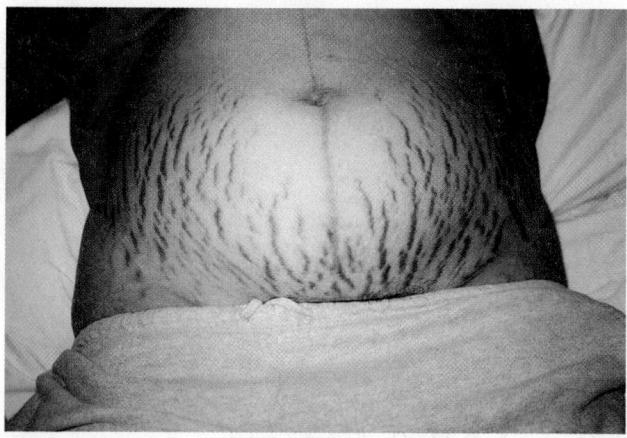

FIG 7-11 Striae gravidarum and linea nigra in a dark-skinned person. (Courtesy Shannon Perry, Phoenix, AZ.)

Mild pruritus is a relatively common dermatologic symptom during pregnancy. The goal of management is to relieve the itching; this is done through the use of oral antihistamines and topical corticosteroid creams. The problem usually resolves during the postpartum period (Cunningham, Leveno, Bloom, et al., 2010). Systemic diseases can also cause pruritus, but these causes are uncommon or rare. Pre-existing skin diseases can complicate pregnancy or can improve during pregnancy.

> **! NURSING ALERT**
>
> The effect of pregnancy on acne is unpredictable, although in some women, acne improves during pregnancy. Women with severe acne taking isotretinoin (Accutane) should avoid pregnancy while receiving the treatment because it is teratogenic and associated with major fetal malformations.

during the second half of pregnancy. These may be caused by the action of adrenocorticosteroids. Striae reflect separation within the underlying connective (collagen) tissue of the skin. These slightly depressed streaks tend to occur over areas of maximum stretch (the abdomen, thighs, and breasts). The stretching sometimes causes a sensation that resembles itching. The tendency to develop striae may be familial. After birth, they usually fade, although they never disappear completely. Color of striae varies, depending on the pregnant woman's skin color. The striae appear pinkish on a woman with light skin and are lighter than the surrounding skin in dark-skinned women. In the multipara, in addition to the striae of the present pregnancy, glistening silvery lines (in light-skinned women) or purplish lines (in dark-skinned women) are commonly seen. These represent the scars of striae from previous pregnancies.

Angiomas are commonly referred to as vascular spiders. These tiny, star-shaped or branched, slightly raised, and pulsating end-arterioles are usually found on the neck, thorax, face, and arms. They occur as a result of elevated levels of circulating estrogens. The spiders are bluish in color and do not blanch with pressure. Vascular spiders appear during the second to fifth month of pregnancy in about 65% of Caucasian women and 10% of African-American women. The spiders usually disappear after birth (Blackburn, 2013).

Pinkish red, diffusely mottled, or well-defined blotches are seen over the palmar surfaces of the hands in about two thirds of Caucasian women and one third of African-American women during pregnancy (Cunningham, Leveno, Bloom, et al., 2010). These color changes, called *palmar erythema,* are related primarily to increased estrogen levels.

> **! NURSING ALERT**
>
> Integumentary system changes vary greatly among women of different racial backgrounds. Therefore, when performing physical assessments, the color of a woman's skin should be noted along with any changes that may be attributed to pregnancy.

Some dermatologic conditions have been identified as unique to pregnancy or as having an increased incidence during pregnancy.

Gum hypertrophy may occur. An **epulis** (gingival granuloma gravidarum) is a red, raised nodule on the gums that bleeds easily. This lesion may develop around the third month and usually continues to enlarge as pregnancy progresses. It is usually managed by avoiding trauma to the gums (e.g., using a soft toothbrush). An epulis usually regresses spontaneously after birth.

Nail growth may be accelerated. Some women may notice thinning and softening of the nails. Oily skin and acne vulgaris may occur during pregnancy. In some women, the skin clears and looks radiant. Hirsutism, the excessive growth of hair or growth of hair in unusual places, is commonly reported. An increase in fine hair growth may occur but tends to disappear after pregnancy. However, growth of coarse or bristly hair does not usually disappear after pregnancy. The rate of scalp hair loss slows during pregnancy; increased hair loss may be noted in the postpartum period.

Increased blood supply to the skin leads to increased perspiration. Women feel hotter during pregnancy, possibly related to a progesterone-induced increase in body temperature and the increased BMR.

Musculoskeletal System

The gradually changing body and increasing weight of the pregnant woman usually cause noticeable changes in her posture (Fig. 7-12). The great abdominal distention gives the pelvis a forward tilt, decreased abdominal muscle tone, and increased weight bearing. The woman's center of gravity shifts forward, requiring a realignment of the spinal curvatures. An increase in the normal lumbosacral curve (lordosis) develops, and a compensatory curvature in the cervicodorsal region (exaggerated anterior flexion of the head) develops to help her maintain balance. Aching, numbness, and weakness of the upper extremities may result. Large breasts and a stoop-shouldered stance further accentuate the lumbar and dorsal curves. The ligamentous and muscular structures of the middle and lower spine may be severely stressed. These and related changes often cause musculoskeletal discomfort, especially in older women or those with a back disorder or a faulty sense of balance.

Slight relaxation and increased mobility of the pelvic joints are normal during pregnancy. These adaptations permit enlargement of pelvic dimensions to facilitate labor and birth. The degree of relaxation varies, but considerable separation of the symphysis pubis and the instability of the sacroiliac joints may cause pain and difficulty

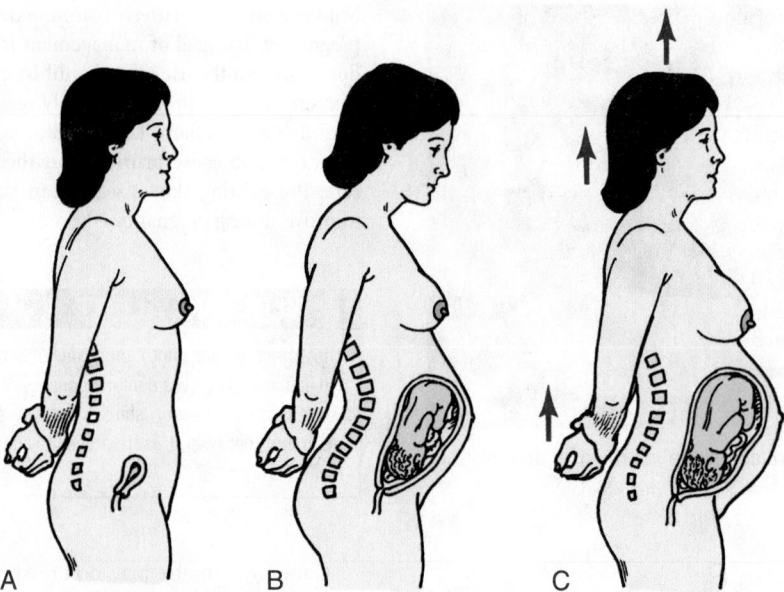

FIG 7-12 Postural changes during pregnancy. **A,** Nonpregnant. **B,** Incorrect posture during pregnancy. **C,** Correct posture during pregnancy.

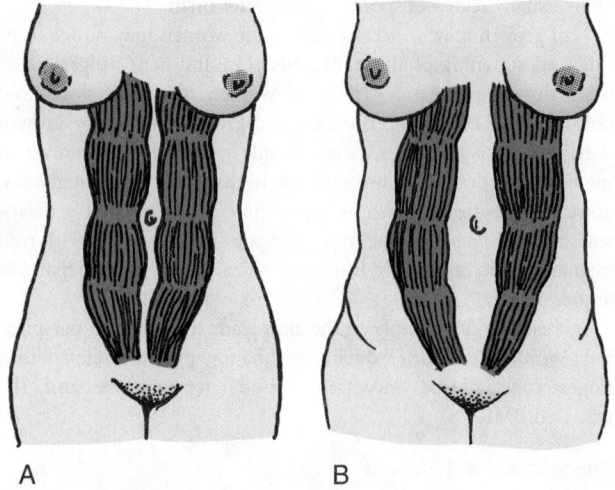

FIG 7-13 Possible change in rectus abdominis muscles during pregnancy. **A,** Normal position in nonpregnant woman. **B,** Diastasis recti abdominis in pregnant woman.

in walking. A waddling gait is common. Obesity or multifetal pregnancy tends to increase the pelvic instability. Peripheral joint laxity also increases as pregnancy progresses, but the cause is not known (Murray and Hassall, 2009).

The muscles of the abdominal wall stretch and ultimately lose some tone. During the third trimester, the rectus abdominis muscles may separate (Fig. 7-13), allowing abdominal contents to protrude at the midline. The umbilicus flattens or protrudes. After birth, the muscles gradually regain tone. However, separation of the muscles (diastasis recti abdominis) may persist.

Neurologic System

Little is known regarding specific alterations in function of the neurologic system during pregnancy aside from hypothalamic-pituitary neurohormonal changes. Specific physiologic alterations resulting from pregnancy may cause the following neurologic or neuromuscular symptoms:

- Compression of pelvic nerves or vascular stasis caused by enlargement of the uterus may result in sensory changes in the legs.
- Dorsolumbar lordosis may cause pain because of traction on nerves or compression of nerve roots.
- Edema involving the peripheral nerves may result in carpal tunnel syndrome during the last trimester. The syndrome is characterized by paresthesia (abnormal sensation such as burning or tingling) and pain in the hand, radiating to the elbow. The sensations are caused by edema that compresses the median nerve beneath the carpal ligament of the wrist. Smoking and alcohol consumption can impair the microcirculation and may worsen the symptoms. The dominant hand is usually affected most, although many women report symptoms in both hands. Symptoms usually regress after pregnancy. In some cases, surgical treatment is necessary (Cunningham, Leveno, Bloom, et al., 2010).
- Acroesthesia (numbness and tingling of the hands) is caused by the stoop-shouldered stance (see Fig. 7-12, *B*) assumed by some women during pregnancy. The condition is associated with traction on segments of the brachial plexus.
- Tension headache is common when anxiety or uncertainty complicates pregnancy. However, vision problems such as refractive errors, sinusitis, or migraine may also be responsible for headaches.
- "Light-headedness," faintness, and even syncope (fainting) are common during early pregnancy. Vasomotor instability, postural hypotension, or hypoglycemia may be responsible.
- Hypocalcemia can cause neuromuscular problems such as muscle cramps or tetany.

Gastrointestinal System

Appetite. During pregnancy, the woman's appetite and food intake fluctuate. Early in pregnancy, some women have nausea with or without vomiting (morning sickness), possibly in response to increasing levels of hCG and altered carbohydrate metabolism. Morning sickness or nausea and vomiting of pregnancy (NVP) appears at about 4 to 6 weeks of gestation and usually subsides by the end of the third month (first trimester) of pregnancy (see Chapter 8). Severity varies from mild distaste for certain foods to more severe vomiting. The condition may be triggered by the sight or odor of various foods. By the end of the second trimester, the appetite increases in response to increasing metabolic needs. Rarely does NVP have harmful effects on the embryo, the fetus, or the woman. Whenever the vomiting is severe or persists beyond the first trimester or when it is accompanied by fever, pain, or weight loss, further evaluation is necessary and medical intervention is likely.

Women may have changes in their sense of taste, leading to cravings and changes in dietary intake. Some women have nonfood cravings (**pica**) such as for ice, clay, and laundry starch. Pica is often a manifestation of iron deficiency (Kilpatrick, 2009). Usually the subjects of these cravings, if consumed in moderation, are not harmful to the pregnancy if the woman has adequate nutrition with appropriate weight gain. (Cunningham, Leveno, Bloom, et al., 2010). See Chapter 9 for a discussion of nutrition in pregnancy.

Mouth. The gums become hyperemic, spongy, and swollen during pregnancy. They tend to bleed easily because the increasing levels of estrogen cause selective increased vascularity and connective tissue proliferation (a nonspecific gingivitis). Epulis (discussed in the section on the integumentary system) may develop at the gum line. Some pregnant women complain of **ptyalism** (excessive salivation), which may be caused by the unconscious decrease in swallowing by the woman when nauseated or caused by stimulation of salivary glands by eating starch (Cunningham, Leveno, Bloom, et al., 2010).

Esophagus, Stomach, and Intestines. Increased progesterone production causes decreased tone and motility of smooth muscles, resulting in esophageal regurgitation (reflux), slower emptying time of the stomach, and reverse peristalsis. As a result, the woman may experience "acid indigestion" or heartburn (**pyrosis**) beginning as early as the first trimester and intensifying through the third trimester.

The incidence of hiatal hernia is increased during pregnancy as a result of the upward displacement of the stomach by the enlarging uterus, which causes a widening of the hiatus of the diaphragm. Hiatal hernia occurs more often in multiparas and older or obese women.

Increased estrogen production causes decreased secretion of hydrochloric acid. This is associated with a decreased incidence of peptic ulcer disease (PUD) during pregnancy. Existing PUD tends to improve during pregnancy (Kelly and Savides, 2012).

In response to increased needs during pregnancy, iron is absorbed more readily in the small intestine. Even when the woman is deficient in iron, it will continue to be absorbed in sufficient amounts for the fetus to have a normal hemoglobin level.

Smooth muscle relaxation and reduced peristalsis caused by increased progesterone result in an increase in water absorption from the colon and may cause constipation. Constipation can also result from food choices, lack of fluids, iron supplementation, decreased activity level, abdominal distention by the pregnant uterus, and displacement and compression of the intestines. If the pregnant woman has hemorrhoids (see Fig. 7-10) and is constipated, the hemorrhoids can evert or bleed during straining at stool.

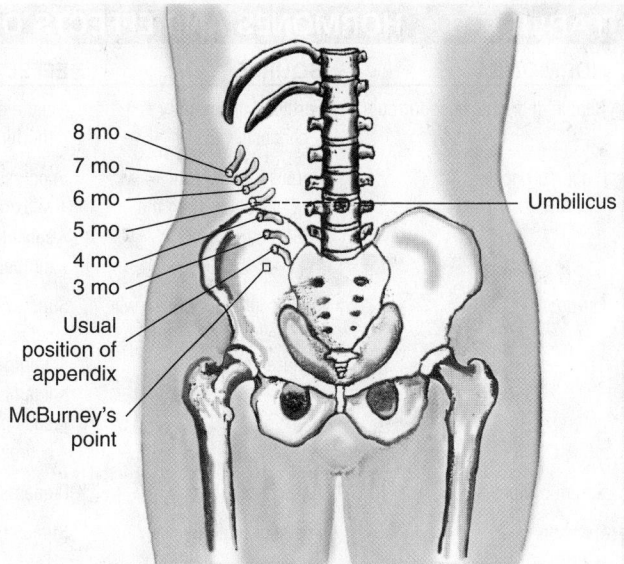

FIG 7-14 Change in position of appendix in pregnancy. Note McBurney's point.

Gallbladder and Liver. The gallbladder is often distended because of its decreased muscle tone during pregnancy. Increased emptying time and thickening of bile caused by prolonged retention are typical changes. These features, together with slight hypercholesterolemia from increased progesterone levels, may account for the development of gallstones during pregnancy.

Hepatic function is difficult to appraise during pregnancy. However, only minor changes in liver function develop. Occasionally, intrahepatic cholestasis (retention and accumulation of bile in the liver caused by factors within the liver) occurs late in pregnancy in response to placental steroids. It may result in **pruritus gravidarum** (severe itching) with or without jaundice. These distressing symptoms are difficult to treat during pregnancy and may be associated with fetal risk. However, symptoms subside after birth (Williamson and Mackillop, 2009).

Abdominal Discomfort. Intraabdominal alterations that can cause discomfort include pelvic heaviness or pressure, round ligament tension, flatulence, distention and bowel cramping, and uterine contractions. In addition to displacement of intestines, pressure from the expanding uterus causes an increase in venous pressure in the pelvic organs. Although most abdominal discomfort is a consequence of normal maternal alterations, the health care provider must be constantly alert to the possibility of disorders such as bowel obstruction or an inflammatory process.

Appendicitis may be difficult to diagnose in pregnancy because the appendix is displaced upward and laterally, high and to the right, away from McBurney's point (Fig. 7-14).

Endocrine System

Profound endocrine changes are essential for pregnancy maintenance, normal fetal growth, and postpartum recovery. Hormones, their sources, and their effects on the pregnancy are presented in Table 7-6.

TABLE 7-6	HORMONES AND EFFECTS OF CHANGES DURING PREGNANCY	
HORMONE	**SOURCE**	**EFFECTS OF CHANGES DURING PREGNANCY**
Human chorionic gonadotropin	Fertilized ovum and chorionic villi	Maintains corpus luteum production of estrogen and progesterone until placenta takes over the function
Progesterone	Corpus luteum until 14 wk of gestation, then the placenta	Suppresses secretion of FSH and LH by the anterior pituitary; maintains pregnancy by relaxing smooth muscles, decreasing uterine contractility; causes fat to deposit in subcutaneous tissues over the maternal abdomen, back, and upper thighs; decreases mother's ability to use insulin
Estrogen	Corpus luteum until 14 wk of gestation, then the placenta	Suppresses secretion of FSH and LH by the anterior pituitary; causes fat to deposit in subcutaneous tissues over the maternal abdomen, back, and upper thighs; promotes enlargement of genitals, uterus, and breasts; increases vascularity; relaxes pelvic ligaments and joints; interferes with folic acid metabolism; increases the level of total body proteins; promotes retention of sodium and water; decreases secretion of hydrochloric acid and pepsin; decreases mother's ability to use insulin
Serum prolactin	Anterior pituitary	Prepares breasts for lactation
Oxytocin	Posterior pituitary	Stimulates uterine contractions; stimulates milk ejection from breasts
Human chorionic somatomammotropin (previously called *human placental lactogen*)	Placenta	Acts as a growth hormone; contributes to breast development; decreases maternal metabolism of glucose; increases the amount of fatty acids for metabolic needs
Thyroxine-binding globulin, thyroxine, triiodothyronine	Thyroid	Causes moderate enlargement of the thyroid gland but woman remains euthyroid; possibly plays role in early neural development of the fetus
Parathyroid	Parathyroid	Controls calcium and magnesium metabolism
Insulin	Pancreas	Increases production of insulin to compensate for insulin antagonism caused by placental hormones; effect of insulin antagonists is to decrease tissue sensitivity to insulin or ability to use insulin
Cortisol	Adrenal glands	Stimulates production of insulin; increases peripheral resistance to insulin
Aldosterone	Adrenal glands	Stimulates reabsorption of excess sodium from the renal tubules

FSH, Follicle-stimulating hormone; *LH,* luteinizing hormone.

KEY POINTS

- The biochemical, physiologic, and anatomic adaptations that occur during pregnancy are profound and revert to the nonpregnant state after birth and lactation.
- Maternal adaptations are attributed to the hormones of pregnancy and to mechanical pressures arising from the enlarging uterus and other tissues.
- Adaptations to pregnancy protect the woman's normal physiologic functioning, meet the metabolic demands that pregnancy imposes, and provide for fetal developmental and growth needs.
- ELISA testing, with monoclonal antibody technology, is the most popular method of pregnancy testing and is the basis for most over-the-counter home pregnancy tests.
- Presumptive, probable, and positive signs of pregnancy aid in the diagnosis of pregnancy; only positive signs (identification of a fetal heart tone, verification of fetal movements, and visualization of the fetus) can establish the diagnosis of pregnancy.
- Although the pH of the pregnant woman's vaginal secretions is more acidic than in the nonpregnant state, she is more vulnerable to some vaginal infections, especially yeast infections.
- Increased vascularity and sensitivity of the vagina and other pelvic viscera may lead to a high degree of sexual interest and arousal.
- Some adaptations to pregnancy result in discomforts such as fatigue, urinary frequency, nausea, constipation, and breast sensitivity.
- Balance and coordination are affected by changes in joints and in the woman's center of gravity as pregnancy progresses.

REFERENCES

Beebe K: The perplexing parity puzzle, *AWHONN Lifelines* 9(5):394–399, 2005.

Blackburn S: *Maternal, fetal, & neonatal physiology: a clinical perspective,* ed 4, St Louis, 2013, Saunders.

Cunningham F, Leveno K, Bloom S, et al: *Williams obstetrics,* ed 23, New York, 2010, McGraw-Hill.

Duff W, Sweet R, Edwards RK: Maternal and fetal infections. In Creasy RK, Resnik R, Iams JD, et al, editors: *Creasy & Resnik's maternal-fetal medicine: principles and practice,* ed 6, Philadelphia, 2009, Saunders.

Gordon M: Maternal physiology. In Gabbe SG, Niebyl JR, Simpson JL, et al, editors: *Obstetrics: normal and problem pregnancies,* ed 6, Philadelphia, 2012, Saunders.

Hark L, Catalano PM: Nutritional management during pregnancy. In Gabbe SG, Niebyl JR, Simpson JL, et al, editors: *Obstetrics: normal and problem pregnancies*, ed 6, Philadelphia, 2012, Saunders.

Kelly TF, Savides TJ: Gastrointestinal disease in pregnancy. In Gabbe SG, Niebyl JR, Simpson JL, et al, editors: *Obstetrics: normal and problem pregnancies*, ed 6, Philadelphia, 2012, Saunders.

Kilpatrick SJ: Anemia and pregnancy. In Creasy RK, Resnik R, Iams JD, et al, editors: *Creasy & Resnik's maternal-fetal medicine: principles and practice*, ed 6, Philadelphia, 2009, Saunders.

Kroumpouzos G: Skin disease in pregnancy and puerperium. In Gabbe SG, Niebyl JR, Simpson JL, et al, editors: *Obstetrics: normal and problem pregnancies*, ed 6, Philadelphia, 2012, Saunders.

Lawrence RA, Lawrence RM: *Breastfeeding: a guide for the medical profession*, ed 7, St Louis, 2011, Mosby.

Monga M: Maternal cardiovascular, respiratory, and renal adaptations to pregnancy. In Creasy RK, Resnik R, Iams JD, et al, editors: *Creasy & Resnik's maternal-fetal medicine: principles and practice*, ed 6, Philadelphia, 2009, Saunders.

Murray I, Hassall J: Change and adaptation in pregnancy. In Fraser D, Cooper M, editors: *Myles textbook for midwives*, ed 15, Edinburgh, 2009, Churchill Livingstone.

Pagana KD, Pagana TJ: *Mosby's diagnostic and laboratory test reference*, ed 10, St Louis, 2011, Mosby.

Pickering TG, Hall JE, Appel LJ, et al: Recommendations for blood pressure measurement in humans and experimental animals, Part 1: Blood pressure measurement in humans—a statement for professionals from the Subcommittee of Professional and Public Education of the American Heart Association Council on High Blood Pressure Research, *Hypertension* 45(1):142–161, 2005 (epub Dec. 20, 2004).

Salani R, Eisenhauer E, Copeland L: Malignant diseases and pregnancy. In Gabbe SG, Niebyl JR, Simpson JL, et al, editors: *Obstetrics: normal and problem pregnancies*, ed 6, Philadelphia, 2012, Saunders.

Seidel HM, Ball JW, Dains JE, et al: *Mosby's guide to physical examination*, ed 7, St Louis, 2011, Mosby.

Wallace L, Zite N, Homewood V: Making sense of home pregnancy instructions, *J Womens Health* 18(3):363–368, 2009.

Williamson C, Mackillop L: Diseases of the liver, biliary system, and pancreas. In Creasy RK, Resnik R, Iams JD, et al, editors: *Creasy & Resnik's maternal-fetal medicine: principles and practice*, ed 6, Philadelphia, 2009, Saunders.

Nursing Care of the Family During Pregnancy

Kathryn R. Alden

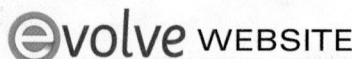 WEBSITE

http://evolve.elsevier.com/Perry/maternal

LEARNING OBJECTIVES

On completion of this chapter, the reader will be able to:

- Describe the processes of confirming pregnancy and estimating the date of birth.
- Summarize the physical, psychosocial, and behavioral changes that usually occur as the mother and other family members adapt to pregnancy.
- Evaluate the benefits of prenatal care and problems of accessibility for some women.
- Outline the patterns of health care used to assess maternal and fetal health status at the initial visit and follow-up visits during pregnancy.
- Conceptualize common nursing assessments, diagnoses, interventions, and methods of evaluation in providing care for the pregnant woman.

- Plan education needed by pregnant women to understand physical discomforts related to pregnancy and to recognize the signs and symptoms of potential complications.
- Examine the effect of culture, age, parity, and number of fetuses on the response of the family to the pregnancy and on the prenatal care provided.
- Determine the scope of childbirth and perinatal education in the community.
- Compare philosophies underlying maternal choices for childbirth.
- Describe the available options for health care providers and birth setting choices.

The prenatal period is a time of physical and psychologic preparation for birth and parenthood. Becoming a parent is one of the maturational milestones of adult life. It is a time of intense learning for parents and those close to them. The prenatal period provides a unique opportunity for nurses and other members of the health care team to influence family health. During this period, essentially healthy women seek regular care and guidance. The nurse's health-promotion interventions can affect the well-being of the woman, her unborn child, and the rest of her family for many years.

Regular prenatal visits, ideally beginning soon after the first missed menstrual period, offer opportunities to optimize the health of the expectant mother and her fetus. Prenatal health care permits diagnosis and treatment of preexisting maternal disorders and those that may develop during the pregnancy. Care is designed to monitor the growth and development of the fetus and identify abnormalities that can interfere with the course of normal labor and birth. The woman and her family can seek support to reduce stress and learn parenting skills.

In recent years, the concept of preconception care has been recognized as an important contributor to good pregnancy outcomes (see Chapter 3). If women can be taught healthy lifestyle behaviors and then practice them before conception—specifically, good nutrition, entering pregnancy with as healthy a weight as possible, adequate intake of folic acid, avoidance of alcohol and tobacco use, prevention of sexually transmitted infections (STIs) and other health hazards—a healthier pregnancy may result. Likewise, women who have health problems related to chronic diseases such as diabetes mellitus can be counseled regarding their special needs with the intent to minimize maternal and fetal complications.

Pregnancy spans 9 calendar months. However, health care providers use the concept of lunar months, which last 28 days (or 4 weeks), to describe the duration of pregnancy or gestational age. Thus normal pregnancy lasts about 10 lunar months, that is, 40 weeks, or 280 days. Pregnancy is divided into three 3-month periods, or trimesters. The first trimester covers weeks 1 through 13; the second, weeks 14 through 26; and the third, weeks 27 through term gestation (38 to 40 weeks). The focus of this chapter is on working with the expectant family to promote a healthy pregnancy that culminates in the birth of a healthy baby.

DIAGNOSIS OF PREGNANCY

Women often suspect pregnancy when they miss a menstrual period. Many women come to the first visit after a positive home pregnancy test; however, the clinical diagnosis of pregnancy before the second missed period can be difficult in some women. Physical variations, obesity, or tumors, for example, can confound even the experienced examiner. Accuracy is important because emotional, social, medical, or legal consequences related to an inaccurate diagnosis, either positive or negative, can be extremely serious. A correct date for the first day of the last (normal) menstrual period (LMP), the date of intercourse, and a basal body temperature record can be of great value in the accurate diagnosis of pregnancy (see Chapter 5).

Signs and Symptoms

Great variability is possible in the subjective symptoms and objective signs of pregnancy. Therefore the diagnosis of pregnancy may be uncertain for a time. It is based on signs and symptoms that are reported during history taking or found during physical examination. These signs and symptoms are classified as *presumptive, probable,* and *positive* (see Table 8-2).

Estimating Date of Birth

When pregnancy is confirmed, the woman's first question usually concerns when she will give birth. This date has traditionally been called the *estimated date of confinement* or *estimated date of delivery.* However, to promote a more positive perception of both pregnancy and birth, the term *estimated date of birth (EDB)* is now used. Accurate dating of pregnancy and calculation of the EDB have implications for timing of specific prenatal screening tests, assessing fetal growth, and making critical decisions for managing pregnancy complications. Ultrasound dating of gestational age is accurate, especially during the first half of pregnancy (ACOG, 2009).

Because the exact date of conception is usually unknown, several formulas have been suggested for calculating the EDB. None of these guides are infallible, but **Nägele's rule** is reasonably accurate and a commonly used method.

Nägele's rule is as follows: after determining the first day of the LMP, subtract 3 months, add 7 days and 1 year; or add 7 days to the LMP and count forward 9 months. For example, if the first day of the LMP was September 10, 2014, the EDB is June 17, 2015.

Nägele's rule assumes that the woman has a 28-day menstrual cycle and that the pregnancy occurred on the fourteenth day of the cycle. An adjustment is in order if the cycle is longer or shorter than 28 days. Only about 5% of pregnant women give birth spontaneously on the EDB as determined by Nägele's rule. Most women give birth during the period extending from 7 days before to 7 days after the EDB.

ADAPTATION TO PREGNANCY

Pregnancy affects all family members, and each family member must adapt to the pregnancy and interpret its meaning in light of his or her own needs. This process of family adaptation to pregnancy takes place within a cultural environment influenced by societal trends. Dramatic changes have occurred in Western society in recent years, and the nurse must be prepared to support not only traditional families but also single-parent families, reconstituted families, dual-career families, and alternative families.

Much of the research on family dynamics in pregnancy in the United States and Canada has been done with Caucasian, middle-class nuclear families. Therefore findings may not apply to families who do not fit the traditional North American model. Adaptation of terms is appropriate to avoid offense to the family and embarrassment to the nurse. Additional research is needed on a variety of families to determine if study findings generated in traditional families are applicable to others.

Maternal Adaptation

Women of all ages use the months of pregnancy to adapt to the maternal role—a complex process of social and cognitive learning.

Pregnancy is a maturational milestone that can be stressful but also rewarding as the woman prepares for a new level of caring and responsibility. Her self-concept changes in readiness for parenthood as she prepares for her new role. She moves gradually from being self-contained and independent to being committed to a lifelong concern for another human being. This growth requires mastery of certain developmental tasks: accepting the pregnancy, identifying with the role of mother, reordering the relationships between herself and her mother and between herself and her partner, establishing a relationship with the unborn child, and preparing for the birth experience. The partner's presence and emotional support are important factors in the successful accomplishment of these developmental tasks. Single women with limited support may have difficulty making this adaptation.

Accepting the Pregnancy

The first step in adapting to the maternal role is accepting the idea of pregnancy and assimilating the pregnant state into the woman's way of life. Mercer (1995) described this process as *cognitive restructuring* and credited Rubin (1975, 1984) as the nurse theorist who pioneered our understanding of maternal role attainment.

The degree of acceptance is reflected in the woman's emotional responses. Initially, many women are dismayed at finding themselves pregnant, especially if the pregnancy is unplanned or unintended. Eventual acceptance of pregnancy parallels the growing acceptance of the reality of a child. Nonacceptance of the pregnancy should not be equated with rejection of the child. A woman may dislike being pregnant but feel love for the child to be born.

Women who are happy and pleased about their pregnancy have high self-esteem and tend to be confident about outcomes for themselves, their babies, and other family members. Despite a general feeling of well-being, many pregnant women are surprised to experience *emotional lability,* that is, rapid and unpredictable changes in mood. These swings in emotions and increased sensitivity to others are disconcerting to the expectant mother and those around her. Increased irritability, explosions of tears and anger, and feelings of great joy and cheerfulness alternate, apparently with little or no provocation. Profound hormonal changes that are part of the maternal response to pregnancy may be responsible for mood changes.

Most women have ambivalent feelings during pregnancy, whether or not the pregnancy was intended. Ambivalence—having conflicting feelings at the same time—is considered a normal response for people preparing for a new role. For example, during pregnancy, women may feel great pleasure that they are fulfilling a lifelong dream but they also may feel great regret that life as they now know it is ending.

Even women who are pleased to be pregnant may experience feelings of hostility toward the pregnancy or the unborn child from time to time. Such incidents as a partner's chance remark about the attractiveness of a slim, nonpregnant woman or news of a colleague's promotion can give rise to ambivalent feelings. Body sensations, feelings of dependence, or the realization of the responsibilities of child care also can generate such feelings.

Intense feelings of ambivalence that persist through the third trimester can indicate an unresolved conflict with the motherhood role (Mercer, 1995). After the birth of a healthy child, memories of these ambivalent feelings usually are dismissed. If the child is born with a defect, a woman may look back at the times when she did not want the pregnancy and feel intense guilt. She may believe that her ambivalence caused the birth defect. She will then need reassurance that her feelings were not responsible for the problem.

Identifying with the Mother Role

The process of identifying with the mother role begins early in each woman's life when she is being mothered as a child. Her cultural and social group's perception of what constitutes the feminine role can subsequently influence her toward choosing between motherhood or a career, being married or single, being independent rather than interdependent, or being able to manage multiple roles. Practice roles such as playing with dolls, baby-sitting, and taking care of siblings may increase her understanding of what being a mother entails.

Many women have always wanted a baby; they enjoy children and look forward to motherhood. Their high motivation to become a parent promotes acceptance of pregnancy and eventual prenatal and parental adaptation. Other women apparently have not considered in any detail what motherhood means to them. During pregnancy, these women must resolve conflicts such as not wanting the pregnancy and child-related or career-related decisions.

Reordering Personal Relationships

Close relationships of the pregnant woman undergo change as she prepares emotionally for the new role of mother. As family members learn their new roles, periods of tension and conflict can occur. Promoting effective communication patterns between the expectant mother and her own mother and between the expectant mother and her partner are common nursing interventions provided during the prenatal visits.

The woman's relationship with her mother is significant in adapting to pregnancy and motherhood. Important components in the pregnant woman's relationship with her mother are the mother's availability (past and present), her reactions to the daughter's pregnancy, respect for her daughter's autonomy, and the willingness to reminisce (Mercer, 1995).

The mother's reaction to the daughter's pregnancy signifies her acceptance of the grandchild and of her daughter. If the mother is supportive, the daughter has an opportunity to discuss pregnancy and labor and her feelings of joy or ambivalence with a knowledgeable and accepting woman (Fig. 8-1). Reminiscing about the pregnant woman's early childhood and sharing the prospective grandmother's account of her childbirth experience help the daughter anticipate and prepare for labor and birth.

Although the woman's relationship with her mother is significant in considering her adaptation in pregnancy, the most important person to the pregnant woman is usually the father of her child. Women express two major needs within this relationship during pregnancy: feeling loved and valued and having the child accepted by the partner (Fig. 8-2).

The marital or committed relationship is not static but, instead, evolves over time. The addition of a child changes forever the nature of the bond between partners. This can be a time when couples grow closer and the pregnancy has a maturing effect on the partners' relationship as they assume new roles and discover new aspects of one another. Partners who trust and support each other are able to share mutual dependency needs (Mercer, 1995).

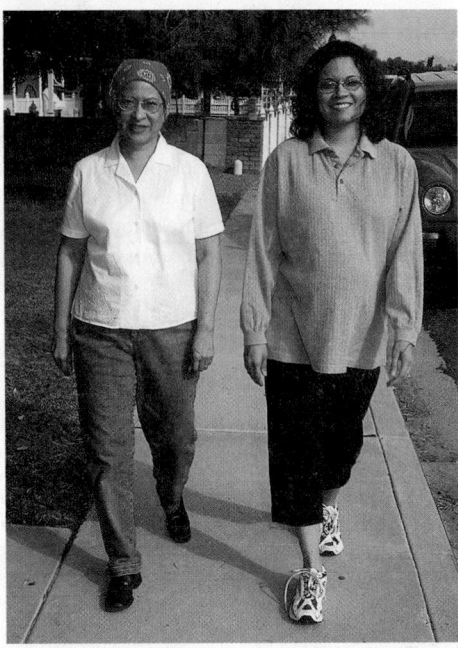

FIG 8-1 Pregnant woman and her mother enjoying a walk together. (Courtesy Michael S. Clement, MD, Mesa, AZ.)

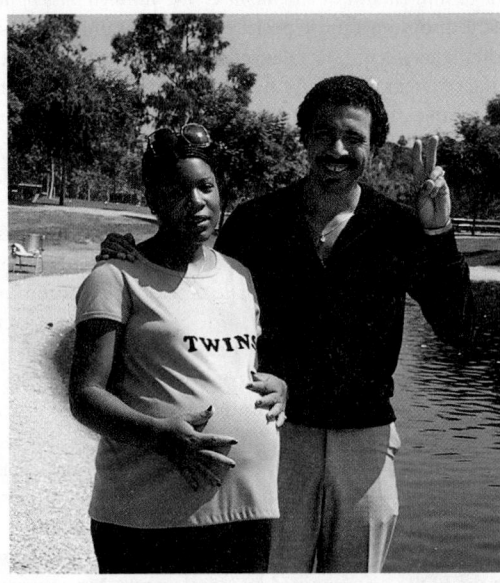

FIG 8-2 Prospective mother and father walk together. Women respond positively to their partner's interest and concern. (Courtesy Marjorie Pyle, RNC, Lifecircle, Costa Mesa, CA.)

Sexual expression during pregnancy is highly individual. The sexual relationship is affected by physical, emotional, and interactional factors, including misinformation about sex during pregnancy, sexual dysfunction, and physical changes in the woman. An individual may inaccurately attribute anomalies, intellectual disability, and other injuries to the fetus and mother to sexual relations during pregnancy. Some couples fear that the woman's genitalia will be drastically changed by the birth process. Couples may not express their concerns to the health care provider because of embarrassment or because they do not want to appear foolish.

As pregnancy progresses, changes in body shape, body image, and levels of discomfort influence both partners' desire for sexual expression. During the first trimester, the woman's sexual desire may decrease, especially if she has breast tenderness, nausea, or fatigue. As she progresses into the second trimester, her sense of well-being, combined with the increased pelvic congestion that occurs at this time, may increase her desire for sexual release. In the third trimester, somatic complaints and physical bulkiness may increase her physical discomfort and diminish her interest in sex. Partners need to feel free to discuss their sexual responses during pregnancy with each other and with their health care provider (see later discussion).

Establishing a Relationship with the Fetus

Emotional attachment—feelings of being tied by affection or love—begins during the prenatal period as women use fantasizing and daydreaming to prepare themselves for motherhood (Rubin, 1975). They think of themselves as mothers and imagine maternal qualities they would like to possess. Expectant parents desire to be warm, loving, and close to their child. They try to anticipate changes that the child will bring in their lives and wonder how they will react to noise, disorder, reduced freedom, and caregiving activities. The mother-child relationship progresses through pregnancy as a developmental process that unfolds in three phases.

In phase 1, the woman accepts the biologic fact of pregnancy. She needs to be able to state, "I am pregnant." In phase 2, the woman accepts the growing fetus as distinct from herself and as a person to nurture. She can now say, "I am going to have a baby." Attachment by a mother to her child is enhanced by experiencing a planned pregnancy, and it increases when ultrasound examination and quickening confirm the reality of the fetus. During phase 3, the woman prepares realistically for the birth and parenting of the child. She expresses the thought "I am going to be a mother" and defines the nature and characteristics of the child. For example, she may speculate about the child's sex (if she has not had an ultrasound that confirms the sex) and personality traits based on patterns of fetal activity.

Although the mother alone experiences the child within, both parents and siblings believe the unborn child responds in a very individualized, personal manner. Family members may interact with the unborn child by talking to the fetus and stroking the mother's abdomen, especially when the fetus shifts position. They may sing to, play music for, or read to the fetus. The fetus may have a nickname used by family members.

Parents may occasionally show or voice disappointment over the sex of the child. The parents may experience grief and a sense of loss at birth as they release their fantasized image of the child and begin to accept the real child. However, these negative responses are usually temporary. Providing an accepting environment for parental reactions facilitates the parents' ability to move beyond disappointment to acceptance.

Preparing for Childbirth

Many women actively prepare for birth. They read books and information on various websites, view films, attend parenting classes, and talk to other women. They seek the best caregiver possible for advice, monitoring, and caring. The multipara has her own history of labor and birth, which influences her approach to preparation for this childbirth experience.

Anxiety can arise from concern about safe passage for herself and her child during the birth process (Mercer, 1995; Rubin, 1975). This concern may not be expressed overtly, but cues are given as the nurse listens to plans women make for care of the new baby and other children in case "anything should happen." These feelings persist despite statistical evidence about the safe outcome of pregnancy for mothers and their infants. Many women fear the pain of childbirth or mutilation because they do not understand anatomy and the birth process. Education by the nurse can alleviate many of these fears.

Toward the end of the third trimester, breathing is difficult and fetal movements become vigorous enough to disturb the mother's sleep. Backaches, frequency and urgency of urination, constipation, and varicose veins can become troublesome. The bulkiness and awkwardness of her body interfere with the woman's ability to care for other children, perform routine work-related duties, and assume a comfortable position for sleep and rest. A strong desire to see the end of pregnancy, to be over and done with it, makes women at this stage ready to move on to childbirth.

Paternal Adaptation

The father's beliefs and feelings about the ideal mother and father and his cultural expectation of appropriate behavior during pregnancy affect his response to his partner's need for him. One man may engage in nurturing behavior; another may feel lonely and alienated as the woman becomes physically and emotionally engrossed in the unborn child. The man may seek comfort and understanding outside the home or become interested in a new hobby or involved with his work. Some men view pregnancy as a proof of their masculinity and their dominant role. To others, pregnancy has no meaning in terms of responsibility to either mother or child. However, for most men, pregnancy is a time of preparation for the parental role, fantasy, great pleasure, and intense learning.

Accepting the Pregnancy

The ways fathers adjust to the parental role have been the subject of considerable research. In older societies, the man enacted the ritual couvade; that is, he behaved in specific ways and respected taboos associated with pregnancy and giving birth. In this way, the man's new status was recognized and endorsed. Now some men experience pregnancy-like symptoms, such as nausea, weight gain, and other physical symptoms. This phenomenon is known as the couvade syndrome. Changing cultural and professional attitudes have encouraged fathers' participation in the birth experience.

The man's emotional response to becoming a father, his concerns, and his informational needs change during the course of pregnancy. Phases of the developmental pattern become apparent. May (1982) described three phases characterizing the developmental tasks experienced by the expectant father:

- The *announcement phase* may last from a few hours to a few weeks. The developmental task is to accept the biologic fact of pregnancy. Men react to the confirmation of pregnancy with joy or dismay, depending on whether the pregnancy is desired, unplanned, or unwanted. Ambivalence in the early stages of pregnancy is common. If pregnancy is unplanned or unwanted, some men find the alterations in life plans and lifestyles difficult to accept. Some men engage in extramarital affairs for the first time during their partner's pregnancy. Others batter their wives for the first time or escalate the frequency of battering episodes.
- The second phase, the *moratorium phase*, is the period when he adjusts to the reality of pregnancy. The developmental task is to accept the pregnancy. Men appear to put conscious thought of the pregnancy aside for a time. They become more introspective and engage in many discussions about their philosophy of life, religion, childbearing, and childrearing practices and their relationships with family members,

particularly with their father. Depending on the man's readiness for the pregnancy, this phase may be relatively short or persist until the last trimester.

- The third phase, the *focusing phase*, begins in the last trimester and is characterized by the father's active involvement in both the pregnancy and his relationship with his child. The developmental task is to negotiate with his partner the role he is to play in labor and to prepare for parenthood. In this phase, the man concentrates on his experience of the pregnancy and begins to think of himself as a father.

Identifying with the Father Role

Each man brings to pregnancy attitudes that affect the way in which he adjusts to the pregnancy and parental role. His memories of the fathering he received from his own father, the experiences he has had with child care, and the perceptions of the male and father roles within his social group guide his selection of the tasks and responsibilities he will assume. Some men are highly motivated to nurture and love a child. They may be excited and pleased about the anticipated role of father. Others may be more detached or even hostile to the idea of fatherhood.

Reordering Personal Relationships

The partner's main role in pregnancy is to nurture the pregnant woman and to respond supportively to her feelings of vulnerability. The partner also must deal with the reality of the pregnancy. The partner's support indicates involvement in the pregnancy and preparation for attachment to the child.

Some aspects of a partner's behavior indicate rivalry. Direct rivalry with the fetus may be evident, especially during sexual activity. Men may protest that fetal movements prevent sexual gratification or that the fetus is watching them during sexual activity. Feelings of rivalry may be unconscious and not verbalized but expressed in subtle behaviors.

The woman's increased introspection may cause her partner to feel uneasy as she becomes preoccupied with thoughts of the child and of motherhood, with her growing dependence on her physician or midwife, and with her reevaluation of the couple's relationship.

Establishing a Relationship with the Fetus

The father-child attachment can be as strong as the mother-child relationship, and fathers can be as competent as mothers in nurturing their infants. The father-child attachment also begins in pregnancy. A father may rub or kiss the maternal abdomen; try to listen, talk, or sing to the fetus; or play with the fetus as he notes fetal movement. Calling the unborn child by name or nickname helps confirm the reality of pregnancy and promote attachment.

Men prepare for fatherhood in many of the same ways that women prepare for motherhood (i.e., by reading and fantasizing about the baby). Daydreaming about their role as father is common in the last weeks before the birth; men rarely describe their thoughts unless they are reassured that such daydreams are normal. They may adjust work commitments or plan vacations so that they can spend time with their new family.

Nurses can help fathers identify concerns and prepare for the reality of a baby by asking questions such as:

- What do you expect the baby to look and act like?
- What do you think being a father will be like?
- Have you thought about the baby's crying? Changing diapers? Burping the baby? Being awakened at night? Sharing your partner with the baby?

Some fathers may not wish to answer such questions when they are asked but may need time to think them through or discuss them with their partners.

As the birth date approaches, fathers have more questions about fetal and newborn behaviors. Some fathers are shocked or amazed at the small size of the clothes and furniture for the baby. The nurse can tell the father about the unborn child's ability to respond to light, sound, and touch and encourage him to feel and talk to the fetus. A tour of the birthing facility and an opportunity to see newborn infants or have discussions with new fathers, as in childbirth classes, may be welcomed.

Some men become involved by choosing the child's name and anticipating the child's sex if it is not already known. Some couples select the name of the child as early as the first month of pregnancy. Family tradition, religious customs, and the continuation of the parent's name or names of relatives or friends are important in the selection process.

Preparing for Childbirth

The days and weeks immediately before the expected day of birth are characterized by anticipation and anxiety. Boredom and restlessness are common as the couple focuses on the birth process; however, during the last 2 months of pregnancy, many expectant fathers experience a surge of creative energy at home and on the job. They can become dissatisfied with their present living space. When possible, they tend to act on the need to alter the environment (e.g., remodeling, painting). This activity can be overt evidence of their sharing in the childbearing experience. They are able to channel the anxiety and other feelings experienced during the final weeks before birth into productive activities. This behavior earns recognition and compliments from friends, relatives, and their partners.

Major concerns for the man are getting the mother to the birthing facility in time for the birth and not appearing ignorant. Many men want to be able to recognize labor and determine when it is appropriate to leave for the hospital or call the physician or midwife. They fantasize different situations and plan what they will do in response to them; they may rehearse taking various routes to the hospital, timing each route at different times of the day.

Some prospective fathers have questions about the labor suite's furniture, nursing staff, and location, as well as the availability of the physician and anesthesiologist. Others want to know what is expected of them when their partners are in labor. The man may have fears concerning safe passage of his partner and the mutilation or death of his partner or child. It is important that he verbalizes these fears; otherwise he cannot help his mate deal with her unspoken or overt apprehension.

With the exception of childbirth preparation classes, a man has few opportunities to learn ways to be an involved and active partner in this rite of passage into parenthood. The tensions and apprehensions of the unprepared, unsupportive father are readily transmitted to the mother and may increase her fears.

The same fears, questions, and concerns may affect birth partners who are not the biologic fathers. Birth partners need to be kept informed, supported, and included in all activities in which the mother desires their participation. The nurse can do much to promote pregnancy and birth as a family experience.

Sibling Adaptation

Sharing the spotlight with a new brother or sister may be the first major crisis for a child. The older child often experiences a sense of loss or feels jealous at being "replaced" by the new baby. Some of the factors that influence the child's response are age, the parents'

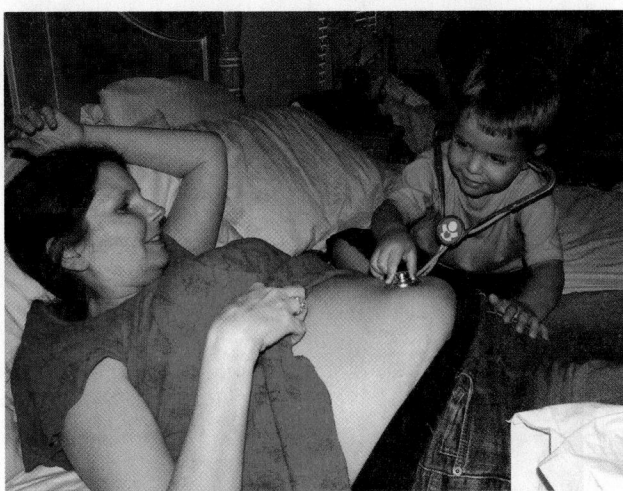

FIG 8-3 Four-year-old likes to examine the pregnant abdomen of his mother. (Courtesy Kara George, Phoenix, AZ.)

attitudes, the father's role, the length of separation from the mother, the hospital's visitation policy, and how the child has been prepared for the change.

A mother with other children must devote time and energy to reorganizing her relationships with these children. She needs to prepare siblings for the birth of the baby (Fig. 8-3 and Box 8-1). She can begin the process of role transition in the family by including the children in the pregnancy and being sympathetic to older children's concerns about losing their places in the family hierarchy. No child willingly gives up a familiar position.

Sibling responses to pregnancy vary with age and dependency needs. The 1-year-old infant seems largely unaware of the process, but the 2-year-old child notices the change in the mother's appearance and may comment, "Mommy's fat." The 2-year-old child's need for sameness in the environment makes the child aware of any change. Toddlers may exhibit more clinging behavior and revert to dependent behaviors in toilet training or eating.

By age 3 or 4 years, children like to be told the story of their own beginning and accept its being compared to the present pregnancy. They like to listen to heartbeats and feel the baby moving in utero (see Fig. 8-3). Sometimes they worry about how the baby is being fed and what it wears.

School-age children take a more clinical interest in their mother's pregnancy. They may want to know in more detail "How did the baby get in there?" and "How will it get out?" Children in this age-group notice pregnant women in stores, churches, and schools and sometimes seem shy if they need to approach a pregnant woman directly. On the whole, they look forward to the new baby, see themselves as "mothers" or "fathers," and enjoy buying baby supplies and readying a place for the baby. Because they still think in concrete terms and base judgments on the here and now, they respond positively to their mother's current good health.

Early and middle adolescents preoccupied with the establishment of their own sexual identity may have difficulty accepting the overwhelming evidence of the sexual activity of their parents. They reason that if they are too young for such activity, certainly their parents are too old. They seem to take on a critical parental role and may ask, "What will people think?" or "How can you let yourself get so fat?" Many pregnant women with teenage children confess that their teenagers are the most difficult factor in their current pregnancy.

BOX 8-1   TIPS FOR SIBLING PREPARATION

Prenatal
- Adjust the timing and content of information about the expected infant to the age and understanding of the older child.
- Take your child on a prenatal visit. Let the child listen to the fetal heartbeat and feel the baby move.
- Involve the child in preparations for the baby such as helping decorate the baby's room.
- Move the child to a bed (if still sleeping in a crib) at least 2 months before the baby is due.
- Read books, show videos, or take child to sibling preparation classes (Fig. 8-4), including a hospital tour.
- Answer your child's questions about the coming birth, what babies are like, and any other questions.
- Take your child to the homes of friends who have babies so that the child has realistic expectations of what babies are like.

During the Hospital Stay
- Have someone bring the child to the hospital to visit you and the baby (unless you plan to have the child attend the birth).
- Make sure you are not holding the new baby when the child arrives.
- Don't force interactions between the child and the baby. Often the child will be more interested in seeing you and being reassured of your love.
- Help the child explore the infant by showing how and where to touch the baby.
- Give the child a gift (from you or from you, your partner, and the baby).

Going Home
- Leave the child at home with a relative or baby-sitter.
- Have someone else carry the baby from the car so that you can hug the child first.

Adjustment After the Baby Is Home
- Arrange for a special time for the child to be alone with each parent.
- Don't exclude the child during infant feeding times. The child can sit with you and the baby and feed a doll or drink juice or milk with you or sit quietly with a game.
- Prepare small gifts for the child so that, when the baby receives gifts, the sibling won't feel left out. The child can also help open the baby gifts.
- Praise the child for acting age appropriately (so that being a baby does not seem better than being older).

Late adolescents do not appear to be unduly disturbed. They realize that they soon will be gone from home. Parents usually report that late adolescents are comforting and act more like other adults than children.

Grandparent Adaptation

Every pregnancy affects all family relationships. For expectant grandparents, a first pregnancy in a child is undeniable evidence that they are growing older. Many think of a grandparent as old, white-haired, and becoming feeble of mind and body; however, some people face grandparenthood while still in their 30s or 40s. A mother-to-be announcing her pregnancy to her mother may be greeted by a negative response that indicates she is not ready to be a grandmother. Both daughter and mother may be startled and hurt by the response.

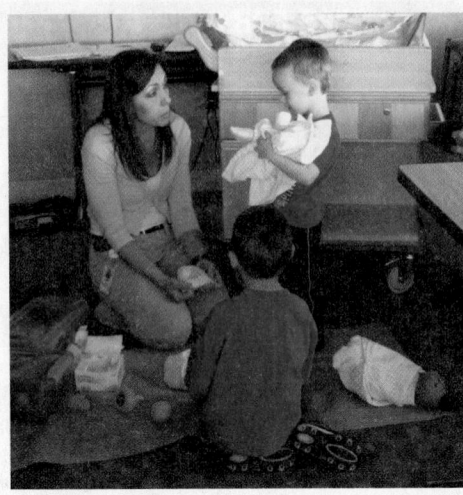

FIG 8-4 Preschoolers in a sibling class learn about childbirth and infant care using dolls and a bunny. (Courtesy Julie and Darren Nelson, Loveland, CO.)

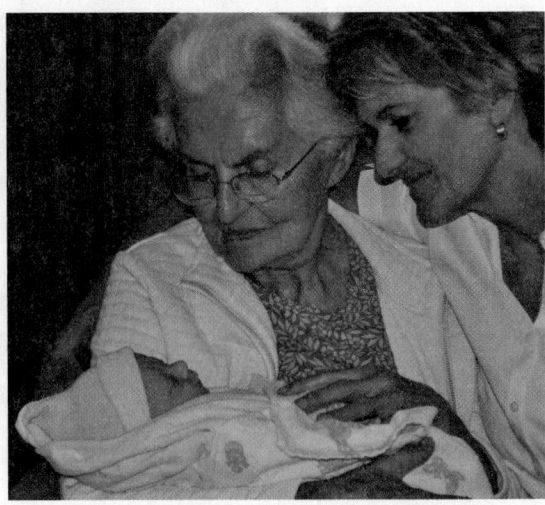

FIG 8-5 Great-grandmother and grandmother admiring new baby. (Courtesy Barbara Wilson, West Jordan, UT.)

In some family units, expectant grandparents are nonsupportive and may inadvertently decrease the self-esteem of the parents-to-be. Mothers may talk about their terrible pregnancies; fathers may discuss the endless cost of rearing children; and mothers-in-law may complain that their sons are neglecting them because their concern is now directed toward the pregnant daughters-in-law.

However, most grandparents are delighted with the prospect of a new baby in the family. It reawakens their feelings of their own youth, the excitement of giving birth, and their delight in the behavior of the parents-to-be when they were infants. They set up a memory store of their child's first smiles, first words, and first steps that can be used later for "claiming" the newborn as a member of the family. Their satisfaction and that of the parents come with the realization that continuity between past and present is guaranteed.

The grandparent is the historian who transmits the family history, a resource person who shares knowledge based on experience, a role model, and a support person. The grandparent's presence and support can strengthen family systems by widening the circle of support and nurturance (Fig. 8-5). Other sources of information cannot replace the unique contribution that grandparents make (www.grandparents.com; www.grandparenting.org).

CARE MANAGEMENT

The goal of prenatal care is to promote the health and well-being of the pregnant woman, her fetus, the newborn, and the family (Gregory, Niebyl, and Johnson, 2012). Major emphasis is placed on preventive aspects of care, primarily to motivate the pregnant woman to practice optimal self-management and report unusual changes early so that problems can be minimized or prevented. In holistic care, nurses provide information and guidance about not only the physical changes but also the psychosocial impact of pregnancy on the woman and members of her family. Therefore the goals of prenatal nursing care are to promote positive pregnancy outcomes, to foster a safe birth for the infant and mother, and to promote satisfaction of the mother and family with the pregnancy and birth experience.

According to the National Center for Health Statistics, based on data from 27 states and Puerto Rice, 71% of women received prenatal care in the first trimester. Only 7% of women started prenatal care late (during third trimester) or had no prenatal care. The subgroups most likely to receive late or no prenatal care were American Indian, Alaska Native, African-American, and Hispanic (Osterman, Martin, Mathews, et al., 2011). Although women of middle or high socioeconomic status routinely seek prenatal care, women living in poverty or those who lack health insurance are not always able to use public health care services or gain access to private care. Lack of culturally sensitive care providers and barriers in communication caused by differences in language also interfere with access to care. Immigrant women from cultures in which prenatal care is not emphasized may not know to seek routine prenatal care. Thus birth outcomes in these populations are less positive, with higher rates of maternal and fetal or newborn complications. In particular, problems with low birth weight (LBW) (less than 2500 g [5.5 lb]) and infant mortality have been associated with inadequate prenatal care (Cunningham, Leveno, Bloom, et al., 2010).

Barriers to obtaining health care during pregnancy include a lack of motivation to seek care, especially for unintended pregnancies; inadequate finances; lack of transportation; unpleasant clinic personnel, facilities, or procedures; inconvenient clinic hours; child care problems; and personal attitudes (Novick, 2009; Phillippi, 2009). The availability and accessibility of prenatal care may be improved by increasing the use of advanced practice nurses in collaborative practice with physicians or midwives. A regular schedule of home visits by nurses aids in reducing barriers to care and contributes to improved maternal and infant outcomes (Agency for Healthcare Research and Quality [AHRQ] Healthcare Innovations Exchange, 2012).

The traditional model for provision of prenatal care has been used for more than a century. The initial visit usually occurs in the first trimester, with monthly visits through week 28 of pregnancy. Thereafter, visits are scheduled every 2 weeks until week 36 and then every week until birth. More recently, the trend is toward individualizing the schedule of care. Women with low-risk pregnancies may have fewer routine prenatal visits, whereas those at risk for complications may be seen more frequently than the traditional schedule (American Academy of Pediatrics [AAP] Committee on Fetus and Newborn and American College of Obstetricians and Gynecologists [ACOG] Committee on Obstetric Practice, 2012).

Group prenatal care is an alternative model to traditional care during pregnancy. In group prenatal care, authority is shifted from the provider to the woman and other women who have similar due dates. The model creates an atmosphere that facilitates learning, encourages discussion, and develops mutual support. Centering-Pregnancy (https://www.centeringhealthcare.org/) is a well-known model of group prenatal care that involves three components: health care assessment, education, and peer support. Most care takes place in the group setting after the initial visit and continues for ten 2-hour sessions that begin at about 16 weeks. At each meeting, the first 30 to 40 minutes consists of assessments (by the woman herself and by the health care provider) and the remaining 60 to 75 minutes is spent in group discussion of specific issues such as discomforts of pregnancy and preparation for labor and birth. Families and partners are encouraged to participate. Benefits associated with group prenatal care include improved birth outcomes such as lower rates of preterm birth, increased knowledge, improved satisfaction, and higher breastfeeding initiation rates (Herrman, Rogers, and Ehrenthal, 2012; Picklesimer, Billings, Hale, et al., 2012; Rotundo, 2011; Robertson, Aycock, and Darnell, 2009).

Prenatal care is ideally a multidisciplinary activity in which nurses work with nurse-midwives, nutritionists, physicians, social workers, and others. Collaboration among these individuals is necessary to provide holistic care. The case management model, which makes use of care maps and critical pathways, is one system that promotes comprehensive care with limited overlap in services. To emphasize the nursing role, care management for the initial visit and follow-up visits is organized around the central elements of the nursing process: assessment, nursing diagnoses, expected outcomes, plan of care and interventions, and evaluation.

In recent years, the concept of preconception care has been recognized as an important contributor to good pregnancy outcomes (see Chapter 3). If women can be taught healthy lifestyle behaviors and then practice them before conception—specifically, good nutrition, entering pregnancy with as healthy a weight as possible, adequate intake of folic acid, avoidance of alcohol and tobacco use, prevention of sexually transmitted infections (STIs) and other health hazards—a healthier pregnancy may result. Likewise, women who have health problems related to chronic diseases such as diabetes mellitus can be counseled regarding their special needs with the intent to minimize maternal and fetal complications.

Initial Visit

Once the pregnancy is confirmed and the woman's desire to continue the pregnancy has been validated, prenatal care is begun. The assessment process begins at the initial visit and is continued throughout the pregnancy. Assessment techniques include the interview, physical examination, and laboratory tests. Because the initial visit and follow-up visits are distinctly different in content and process, they are described separately.

Interview

The pregnant woman and her partner or family members who may be present should be told that the first prenatal visit is longer and more detailed than future visits. The initial evaluation includes a comprehensive health history emphasizing the current pregnancy, previous pregnancies, the family, a psychosocial profile, a physical assessment, diagnostic testing, and an overall risk assessment.

The therapeutic relationship between the nurse and the woman is established during the initial assessment interview. Two types of data are collected: the woman's subjective appraisal of her health status and the nurse's objective observations.

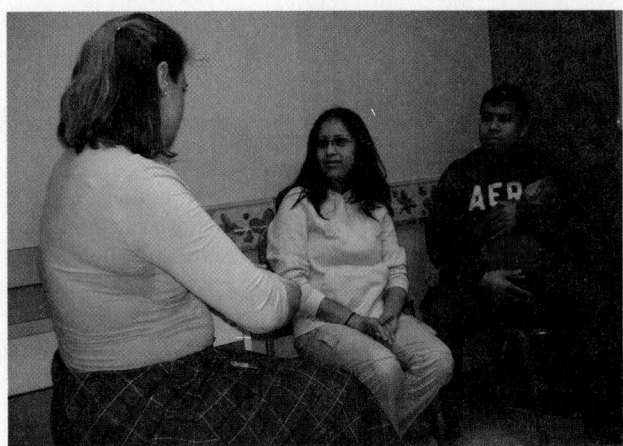

FIG 8-6 Prenatal interview. (Courtesy Dee Lowdermilk, Chapel Hill, NC.)

With the woman's permission, include persons accompanying her in the initial prenatal interview (Fig. 8-6). Observations and information about the woman's partner and/or family are then included in the database. For example, if the woman has small children with her, the nurse can ask about her plans for child care during the time of labor and birth. Note any special needs at this time (e.g., wheelchair access, assistance in getting on and off the examining table, and cognitive deficits).

Reason for Seeking Care

Although pregnant women are scheduled for "routine" prenatal visits, they often come to the health care provider seeking information or reassurance about a particular concern. When the woman is asked a broad, open-ended question such as "How have you been feeling?" she may reveal problems that could otherwise be overlooked. The woman's chief concerns should be recorded in her own words to alert other personnel to the priority of needs identified by her. At the initial visit, a typical desire is for information about the normal course of pregnancy.

Current Pregnancy

The presumptive signs of pregnancy, such as nausea and vomiting, may be of great concern to the woman. A review of symptoms she is experiencing and how she is coping with them helps establish a database to develop a plan of care. Some early teaching may be provided at this time.

Childbearing and Female Reproductive System History

Data are gathered on the woman's age at menarche; menstrual history; contraceptive history; history of infertility or gynecologic conditions; history of any STIs; her sexual history; and a detailed history of all her pregnancies, including the present one, and their outcomes. The date of the last Papanicolaou (Pap) test and the result are noted. The date of her LMP is obtained to establish the EDB.

Health History

The health history includes those physical or surgical procedures that can affect the pregnancy or that can be affected by the pregnancy. For example, a pregnant woman who has diabetes or epilepsy requires special care. Because most women are anxious during the initial interview, the nurse's reference to cues such as a MedicAlert bracelet prompts the woman to explain allergies; chronic diseases;

or medications being taken such as cortisone, insulin, or anticonvulsants.

The woman should also describe any previous surgical procedures. If a woman has had uterine surgery or extensive repair of the pelvic floor, a cesarean birth may be necessary; previous appendectomy rules out appendicitis as a cause of right lower quadrant pain in pregnancy; spinal surgery may contraindicate the use of spinal or epidural anesthesia; and breast augmentation or reduction procedures may influence the ability to breastfeed. Note any injury involving the pelvis.

Women may forget to mention chronic or handicapping conditions during the initial assessment because they have adapted to them. Special shoes or a limp may indicate the existence of a pelvic structural defect—an important consideration in pregnant women. The nurse who observes these special characteristics and sensitively inquires about them can obtain individualized data that will provide the basis for a comprehensive nursing care plan to help optimize pregnancy outcomes (Signore, Spong, Krotoski, et al., 2011). Observations are a vital component of the interview process because they prompt the nurse and the woman to focus on the specific needs of the woman and her family.

Nutritional History

The nutritional status of a pregnant woman has a direct effect on the growth and development of the fetus. A dietary assessment can reveal special diet practices, food allergies, eating behaviors, the practice of pica, and other factors related to her nutritional status (see Box 9-7). Pregnant women are usually motivated to learn about good nutrition and respond well to nutritional advice generated by this assessment.

It is essential that obese women receive counseling about weight gain, nutrition, and food choices. They should also be advised about their risk for complications for themselves and increased risk for congenital abnormalities (Davies, Maxwell, McLeod, et al., 2010). Women with a history of bariatric surgery are nutritionally at risk and should be followed closely throughout pregnancy to promote maternal and fetal well-being (Magdaleno, Pereira, Chaim, et al., 2012).

History of Use of Drugs and Herbal Preparations

A woman's past and present use of drugs, both legal (over-the-counter [OTC], prescription, and herbal drugs; caffeine; alcohol; nicotine) and illegal (marijuana, cocaine, heroin), must be assessed because many substances cross the placenta and can harm the developing fetus. See Chapter 11 for discussion of substance abuse during pregnancy. Increasing numbers of individuals are using herbal preparations, and this includes pregnant women. Therefore it is important for health care providers to question pregnant women regarding the use of herbal preparations and document their responses.

> **LEGAL TIP: Testing for Drug Use**
> Health care providers must obtain informed consent from a pregnant woman before she can be tested for drug use (Wong, Ordean, and Kahan, 2011).

Family History

The family history provides information about the woman's family, including parents, grandparents, siblings, and children. These data help identify familial or genetic disorders or conditions that could affect the present health status of the woman or her fetus.

Social, Experiential, and Occupational History

Situational factors such as the family's ethnic and cultural background and socioeconomic status are assessed while the history is obtained. The following information may be obtained over several encounters. The woman's perception of this pregnancy is explored by asking her such questions as:
- Is this pregnancy planned or unintended?
- Is the woman/couple pleased or displeased, accepting or nonaccepting?
- What problems related to finances, career, or living accommodations may arise as a result of the pregnancy?

The family support system is determined by asking her such questions as:
- Who is her primary support?
- Which roles does she expect her significant other or father of the baby to play?
- Are changes needed to promote adequate support?
- What are the existing relationships among mother, father/partner, siblings, and in-laws?
- What preparations are being made for her care and that of dependent family members during labor and for the care of the infant after birth?
- Is financial, educational, or other support needed from the community?
- What are the woman's ideas about childbearing, her expectations of the infant's behavior, and her outlook on life and the female role?

Other questions that should be asked include:
- What does the woman think it will be like to have a baby in the home?
- How is her life going to change by having a baby?
- What plans are interrupted by having a baby at this time?

During interviews throughout the pregnancy, the nurse should remain alert for the appearance of potential parenting problems such as depression, lack of family support, and inadequate living conditions. The nurse must assess the woman's attitude toward health care, particularly during childbearing; her expectations of health care providers; and her view of the relationship between herself and the nurse.

Coping mechanisms and patterns of interacting are identified. Early in the pregnancy, the nurse should determine the woman's knowledge of pregnancy, maternal changes, fetal growth, self-management, and care of the newborn, including feeding. It is important to ask about attitudes toward unmedicated or medicated childbirth and about her knowledge of the availability of parenting skills classes. Before planning for nursing care, the nurse needs information about the woman's decision-making abilities and living habits (e.g., exercise, sleep, diet, diversional interests, personal hygiene, clothing). Common stressors during childbearing include the baby's welfare, the labor and birth process, the behaviors of the newborn, the relationship with the baby's father or partner and her family, changes in body image, and physical symptoms.

Explore attitudes concerning the range of acceptable sexual behavior during pregnancy by asking, for example, What has your family (partner, friends) told you about sex during pregnancy? The woman's sexual self-concept is given emphasis by asking such questions as: How do you feel about the changes in your appearance? How does your partner feel about your body now? How do you feel about wearing maternity clothes?

Women should be questioned regarding their occupation, past and present, since this may adversely affect maternal and fetal health. For some women, heavy lifting and exposure to chemicals and radiation may be part of their daily work, and these activities can negatively affect the pregnancy. For others, long hours of sitting at a desk working on a computer can contribute to carpal tunnel syndrome or circulatory stasis in the legs.

History of Physical Abuse

All women should be assessed for a history of or risk for physical abuse, particularly because the likelihood of intimate partner violence (IPV) increases during pregnancy (see Chapter 3). This screening should be done at the first prenatal visit, at least once each trimester, and at the postpartum visit (American College of Obstetricians and Gynecologists Committee on Health Care for Underserved Women, 2012a). It is essential that the screening is done in a safe, private setting with the woman alone. Nurses can ask the woman screening questions with routine assessments during pregnancy. Examples of questions that might be asked include:

- Are you with a spouse or partner who threatens or physically hurts you? If yes, who?
- Within the past year or in this pregnancy, has anyone hit, slapped, kicked, or otherwise hurt you? If yes, who? Are you currently with that person?
- Has anyone forced you to have sexual activities that made you uncomfortable? If yes, who? Are you currently with that person?

Although visual cues from the woman's appearance or behavior may suggest the possibility of abuse, no one profile of the battered woman exists. Identification of abuse and immediate clinical intervention that includes information about safety can result in behavior that may prevent future abuse and increase the safety and well-being of the woman and her infant. During pregnancy, the target body parts change during abusive episodes. Women report physical blows directed to the head, breasts, abdomen, and genitalia. Sexual assault is common.

Battering and pregnancy in teenagers constitutes a particularly difficult situation. Adolescents may be trapped in the abusive relationship because of their inexperience. Routine screening for abuse and sexual assault is recommended for pregnant adolescents. Because pregnancy in young adolescent girls is commonly the result of sexual abuse, the nurse should assess the girl's desire to maintain the pregnancy.

Nurses should be aware that victims of human trafficking may be seen in prenatal settings because of unintended pregnancy. These women or young girls are forced or deceived into commercial sex acts (prostitution) with little or no pay. They are under strict control by their traffickers. Similar to victims of IPV, these women are likely to exhibit signs of physical abuse or neglect such as scars, bruises, burns, unusual bald patches, or tattoos that may be a sign of branding. They are likely to be accompanied by someone who never leaves them alone and speaks for them. They may not speak English and may lack identification documents. If the woman is alone, she may have her cell phone on and in speaker mode so that the person on the other end can hear everything that is said during the visit. Nurses and other health care providers must be creative in getting the woman alone for questioning. Strategies might include sending the other person to the front desk to fill out paperwork, interviewing the woman in the restroom, or telling her she needs to go for testing and cannot take her cell phone. With the consent of suspected or confirmed victims of human trafficking, intervention plans can be developed. An excellent resource is the National Human Trafficking Resource Center (1-888-373-7888) (Dovydaitis, 2010; Tracy and Konstantopoulos, 2012).

Review of Systems

During the review of systems, ask the woman to identify and describe pre-existing or concurrent problems in any of the body systems and assess her mental status. Question the woman about physical symptoms she has experienced such as shortness of breath or pain. Pregnancy affects and is affected by all body systems; therefore information on the present status of body systems is important in planning care. For each sign or symptom described, the following additional data should be obtained: body location, quality, quantity, chronology, aggravating or alleviating factors, and associated manifestations (onset, character, and course) (Seidel, Ball, Dains, et al., 2011).

Physical Examination

The initial physical examination provides the baseline for assessing subsequent changes. The examiner should determine the woman's needs for basic information regarding reproductive anatomy and provide this information, along with a demonstration of the equipment that may be used during the examination and an explanation of the procedure itself. The interaction requires an unhurried, sensitive, and gentle approach with a matter-of-fact attitude.

The physical examination begins with assessment of vital signs, including blood pressure (BP), height, and weight (for calculation of body mass index [BMI]) (see Chapter 9). The bladder should be empty before pelvic examination.

Each examiner develops a routine for proceeding with the physical examination; most choose the head-to-toe progression. Heart and lung sounds are evaluated, and extremities are examined. The skin is assessed for changes in pigmentation, rashes, and edema. Distribution, amount, and quality of body hair are of particular importance because the findings reflect nutritional status, endocrine function, and attention to hygiene. The thyroid gland is assessed carefully, as are the breasts and abdomen. The height of the fundus is noted if the first examination occurs after the first trimester of pregnancy. During the examination, the examiner must remain alert to the woman's cues that give direction to the remainder of the assessment and that indicate imminent untoward response, such as feeling lightheaded or dizzy. See Chapter 3 for a detailed description of the physical examination.

Whenever a pelvic examination is performed, the tone of the pelvic musculature and the woman's knowledge of Kegel exercises are assessed. Particular attention is paid to the size of the uterus because this is an indication of the duration of gestation. The nurse present during the examination can coach the woman at this time in breathing and relaxation techniques as needed. One vaginal examination during pregnancy is recommended; another is usually not done unless indicated for medical reasons.

Laboratory Tests

The data yielded by laboratory examination of specimens obtained during the examination add important information concerning the symptoms of pregnancy and the woman's health status.

Specimens are collected at the initial visit so that any abnormal findings can be treated. Blood is drawn for a variety of tests (Table 8-1). A sickle cell screen is recommended for women of African, Asian, or Middle Eastern heritage. Testing for antibody to the human immunodeficiency virus (HIV) is strongly recommended for all pregnant women; this testing must be voluntary and without coercion (ACOG Committee on Obstetric Practice, 2011a; Centers for Disease Control and Prevention [CDC], 2010) (Box 8-2). The folate level is measured when indicated. Cystic fibrosis (CF) carrier screening tests should be offered to all pregnant women; if the woman is a CF carrier, the father of the baby should be tested. Concurrent testing is recommended if there are time constraints related to prenatal diagnostic evaluation (ACOG Committee on Genetics, 2011).

TABLE 8-1 LABORATORY TESTS IN THE PRENATAL PERIOD

LABORATORY TEST	PURPOSE
Hemoglobin, hematocrit/WBC, differential	Detects anemia/detects infection
Hemoglobin electrophoresis	Identifies women with hemoglobinopathies (e.g., sickle cell anemia, thalassemia)
Blood type, Rh, and irregular antibody	Identifies fetuses at risk for developing erythroblastosis fetalis or hyperbilirubinemia in neonatal period
Rubella titer	Determines immunity to rubella
Tuberculin skin testing; chest film after 20 wk of gestation in women with reactive tuberculin tests	Screens for exposure to tuberculosis
Urinalysis, including microscopic examination of urinary sediment; pH, specific gravity, color, glucose, albumin, protein, RBCs, WBCs, casts, acetone; hCG	Identifies women with glycosuria, renal disease, hypertensive disease of pregnancy; infection; occult hematuria
Urine culture	Identifies women with asymptomatic bacteriuria
Renal function tests: BUN, creatinine, electrolytes, creatinine clearance, total protein excretion	Evaluates level of possible renal compromise in women with a history of diabetes, hypertension, or renal disease
Papanicolaou test	Screens for cervical intraepithelial neoplasia; if a liquid-based test is used, may also screen for HPV
Vaginal or rectal smear for *Neisseria gonorrhoeae*, chlamydia, HPV, GBS	Screens high risk population for asymptomatic infection; GBS done at 35-37 wk
RPR/VDRL/FTA-ABS	Identifies women with untreated syphilis
HIV antibody,* hepatitis B surface antigen, toxoplasmosis	Screens for the specific infection
1-hr glucose tolerance	Screens for gestational diabetes; done at initial visit for women with risk factors; done at 24-28 wk for pregnant women at risk whose initial screen was negative; women with low risk usually not tested
3-hr glucose tolerance	Screens for diabetes in women with elevated glucose level after 1-hr test; must have two elevated readings for diagnosis
Cardiac evaluation: ECG, chest x-ray film, and echocardiogram	Evaluates cardiac function in women with a history of hypertension or cardiac disease

BUN, Blood urea nitrogen; *ECG,* electrocardiogram; *FTA-ABS,* fluorescent treponemal antibody absorption test; *GBS,* group B streptococcus; *hCG,* human chorionic gonadotropin; *HIV,* human immunodeficiency virus; *HPV,* human papilloma virus; *RBC,* red blood cell; *RPR,* rapid plasma reagin; *VDRL,* Venereal Disease Research Laboratories; *WBC,* white blood cell.
*With patient permission.

A urine specimen is collected for cultures and metabolic function tests. A purified protein derivative tuberculin test may be administered to assess exposure to tuberculosis. During the pelvic examination, cervical and vaginal smears can be obtained for cytologic studies and for diagnosis of infection (e.g., chlamydia, gonorrhea).

Recognition of risk factors during pregnancy may indicate the need to repeat some tests at other times. For example, exposure to tuberculosis or an STI would necessitate repeat testing. STIs are common in pregnancy and may have negative effects on mother and fetus (see Table 4-5 on p. 98). Careful assessment and thorough screening are essential.

Follow-Up Visits

Monthly visits are scheduled routinely during the first and second trimesters, although additional appointments may be made as the need arises. During the third trimester, the possibility for complications increases and closer monitoring is necessary. Starting with week 28, visits are scheduled every 2 weeks until week 36; then visits are scheduled every week until birth unless the health care provider individualizes the schedule. Individual needs, complications, and risks of the pregnant woman may warrant visits more or less often. The pattern of interviewing the woman first and then assessing physical changes and performing laboratory tests is maintained.

In prenatal care models that use a reduced-frequency screening schedule or in group prenatal care models such as CenteringPregnancy, the timing of follow-up visits will be different but assessments and care will be similar.

Interview

Follow-up visits are less intensive than the initial prenatal visit. At each of these follow-up visits, the woman is asked to summarize relevant events that have occurred since the previous visit. She is asked about her general emotional and physical well-being, complaints or problems, and questions she may have. Personal and family needs are identified and explored.

A woman's emotional state can affect her and her family's general well-being. Therefore the nurse asks whether the woman has had any mood swings, reactions to changes in her body image, bad dreams, or worries. Positive feelings (her own and those of her family) are also noted. The reactions of family members to the pregnancy and the woman's progression through the developmental tasks of pregnancy are also assessed and recorded.

During the third trimester, current family situations and their effect on the woman are assessed (e.g., the response of partner, siblings, and grandparents to the pregnancy and the coming child). The nurse needs to assess the parents' understanding of the following: the warning signs that indicate emergencies such as bleeding

<table>
<tr><td colspan="2">

BOX 8-2   **HUMAN IMMUNODEFICIENCY VIRUS SCREENING**

</td></tr>
</table>

- Pregnant women are ethically obligated to seek reasonable care during pregnancy and to avoid causing harm to the fetus. Women's health nurses should be advocates for the fetus while accepting of the pregnant woman's decision regarding testing and/or treatment for HIV.
- The incidence of perinatal transmission from an HIV-positive mother to her fetus ranges from 16% to 25%. Triple drug antiviral or highly active antiretroviral therapy (HAART) during pregnancy decreases perinatal transmission to as low as 1% to 2% (Burr, 2011).
- The CDC (2010) recommends testing for HIV infections for all pregnant women as early as possible in pregnancy and a second test in the third trimester, ideally before 36 weeks. This is especially important for women known to be at high risk for HIV infection.
- Testing has the potential to identify HIV-positive women who can then be treated. Health care providers have an obligation to ensure that pregnant women are well informed about HIV symptoms, testing, and methods of decreasing maternal-fetal transmission. The Centers for Disease Control and Prevention (CDC) and the American College of Obstetricians and Gynecologists (ACOG) recommend universal opt-out screening, which means that all pregnant women are offered HIV screening but have the opportunity to opt out if desired (ACOG Committee on Obstetric Practice, 2011; CDC, 2010). The Association of Women's Health, Obstetric and Neonatal Nurses (AWHONN, 2008) supports this system of HIV screening that allows all pregnant women to be offered screening.

Data from American College of Obstetricians and Gynecologists Committee on Obstetric Practice: Committee opinion no. 418: prenatal and perinatal human immunodeficiency virus testing—expanded recommendations, *Obstet Gynecol* 104(5 Part 1):1119–1124, 2011; AWHONN: *HIV screening procedures for pregnant women and newborns—policy position statement*, Washington, DC, 2008, Author; Burr C: Reducing maternal-infant HIV transmission. In Coffey S, editor: *Guide for HIV/AIDS clinical care*, Rockville, MD, 2011, US Department of Health and Human Services, Health Resources and Services Administration, http://hab.hrsa.gov/deliverhivaidscare/clinicalguide11/cg-402_pmtct.html; Centers for Disease Control and Prevention: Sexually transmitted diseases treatment guidelines, *Morb Mortal Wkly Rep* 59(RR12):1–110, 2010.

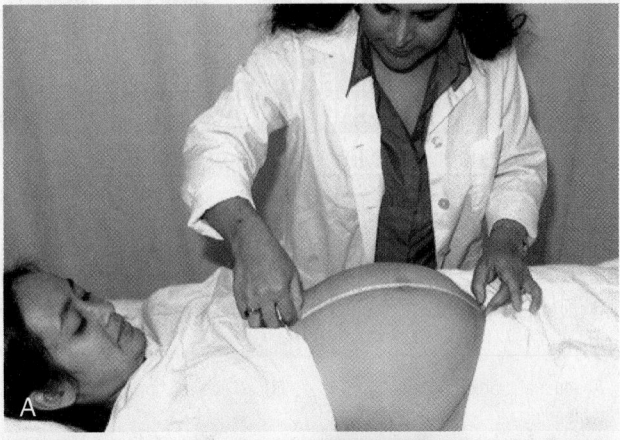
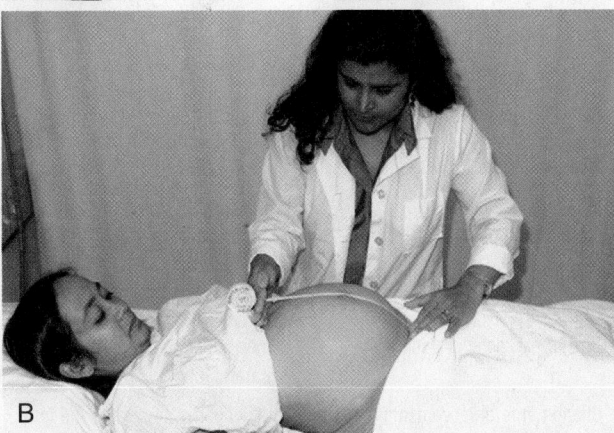

FIG 8-7 Measurement of fundal height from symphysis that **A,** includes the upper curve of the fundus and **B,** does not include the upper curve of the fundus. Note position of hands and measuring tape. (Courtesy Chris Rozales, San Francisco, CA.)

✚ EMERGENCY

Supine Hypotension

Signs and Symptoms
- Pallor
- Dizziness, faintness, breathlessness
- Tachycardia
- Nausea
- Clammy (damp, cool) skin; sweating

Intervention
- Position woman on her side until her signs and symptoms subside and vital signs stabilize within normal limits.

and abdominal pain, the signs of preterm and term labor, the labor process and anxieties about labor, fetal development, and methods to assess fetal well-being. The nurse should ascertain whether the woman is planning to attend childbirth preparation classes and what she knows about the control of discomfort during labor. If she is having a home birth, she should be queried as to whether all the necessary supplies have been obtained.

A review of the woman's physical systems is appropriate at each visit, and any suggestive signs or symptoms are assessed in depth. Discomforts reflecting adaptations to pregnancy are identified. Special inquiries are made about possible infections (e.g., genitourinary tract, respiratory tract). The woman's knowledge of and success with self-management measures are assessed, as well as outcomes of prescribed therapy.

Physical Examination

Reevaluation is a constant aspect of a pregnant woman's care. Each woman reacts differently to pregnancy. As a result, careful monitoring of the pregnancy and her reactions to care is vital. Physiologic changes are documented as the pregnancy progresses and reviewed for possible deviations.

At each visit, physical parameters are measured. BP is taken at every visit, using the same arm and with the woman seated. Her weight is measured, and the appropriateness of the weight gain is evaluated in relation to her BMI. The woman is asked to empty her bladder. Urine may be checked by dipstick. The presence and degree of edema are noted. For examination of the abdomen, the woman lies on her back with her arms by her side and head supported by a pillow; a small wedge should be placed under her right hip to prevent supine hypotension. Supine hypotension can occur when the woman lies on her back and the weight of the abdominal contents compresses the vena cava and aorta, causing a decrease in BP and a feeling of faintness (see Emergency box). Abdominal inspection is followed by measurement of the height of the fundus (Fig. 8-7).

TABLE 8-2	SIGNS OF POTENTIAL COMPLICATIONS DURING THE FIRST, SECOND, AND THIRD TRIMESTERS

SIGNS AND SYMPTOMS	POSSIBLE CAUSES
First Trimester	
Severe vomiting	Hyperemesis gravidarum
Chills, fever	Infection
Burning on urination	Infection
Diarrhea	Infection
Abdominal cramping; vaginal bleeding	Miscarriage, ectopic pregnancy
Second and Third Trimesters	
Persistent, severe vomiting	Hyperemesis gravidarum, hypertension, preeclampsia
Sudden discharge of fluid from vagina before 37 weeks	Premature rupture of membranes
Vaginal bleeding, severe abdominal pain	Miscarriage, placenta previa, abruptio placentae
Chills, fever, burning on urination, diarrhea	Infection
Severe backache or flank pain	Kidney infection or stones; preterm labor
Change in fetal movements: absence of fetal movements after quickening, any unusual change in pattern or amount	Fetal jeopardy or intrauterine fetal death
Uterine contractions; pressure; cramping before 37 weeks	Preterm labor
Visual disturbances: blurring, double vision, or spots	Hypertensive conditions, preeclampsia
Swelling of face or fingers and over sacrum	Hypertensive conditions, preeclampsia
Headaches: severe, frequent, or continuous	Hypertensive conditions, preeclampsia
Muscular irritability or convulsions	Hypertensive conditions, preeclampsia
Epigastric or abdominal pain (perceived as severe stomachache)	Hypertensive conditions, preeclampsia, abruptio placentae
Glycosuria, positive glucose tolerance test reaction	Gestational diabetes mellitus

The information provided during the interview and physical examination reflects the status of maternal adaptations. When any of the findings is suspicious, an in-depth examination is performed. For example, careful interpretation of BP is important in the risk factor analysis of all pregnant women. BP is evaluated on the basis of absolute values and the length of gestation and is interpreted in the light of modifying factors. See Chapter 12 for an in-depth discussion of problems associated with hypertension. Signs and symptoms other than hypertension also may be present that indicate potential complications (Table 8-2).

Fetal Assessment

Toward the end of the first trimester, before the uterus is an abdominal organ, the fetal heart tones (FHTs) can be heard with an ultrasound fetoscope or an ultrasound stethoscope (Fig. 8-8). To hear the FHTs, place the instrument in the midline just above the symphysis pubis and apply firm pressure. The woman and her family should be offered the opportunity to listen to the FHTs. The health status of the fetus is assessed at each visit for the remainder of the pregnancy.

Fundal Height. During the second trimester, the uterus becomes an abdominal organ. The fundal height, or measurement of the height of the uterus above the symphysis pubis, is used as one indicator of fetal growth.

The measurement also provides a gross estimate of the duration of pregnancy. From gestational weeks (GW) 18 to 32, the height of the fundus in centimeters is approximately the same as the number of weeks of gestation (±2 GW) if the woman's bladder is empty at the time of measurement. As much as a 3-cm variation is possible if the bladder is full (Cunningham, Leveno, Bloom, et al., 2010). For example, the fundal height of a woman of 28 weeks of gestation with an empty bladder would measure from 26 to 30 cm. In addition, the fundal height measurement may aid in the identification of risk factors. A stable or decreased fundal height may indicate the presence of intrauterine growth restriction (IUGR); an excessive increase could indicate the presence of multifetal gestation (more than one fetus) or polyhydramnios (excessive amniotic fluid).

A disposable paper metric tape measure is preferred for measuring fundal height. To increase the reliability of the measurement, the same person examines the pregnant woman at each of her prenatal visits; however, often this is not possible. All clinicians who examine a particular pregnant woman should be consistent in their measurement technique. Ideally, each prenatal setting should establish a protocol for fundal height measurement that specifies the woman's position on the examining table, the measuring device, and the technique to be used. Fig. 8-7 presents two methods of measuring fundal height.

Gestational Age. In an uncomplicated pregnancy, fetal gestational age is estimated after the duration of pregnancy and the EDB are determined. Fetal gestational age is determined from the menstrual history, contraceptive history, pregnancy test results, and the following findings obtained from the clinical evaluation:

- First uterine evaluation: date, size
- Fetal heart first heard: date, method (Doppler stethoscope, fetoscope)
- Date of quickening
- Current fundal height, estimated fetal weight
- Current week of gestation by history of LMP or ultrasound examination (or both)
- Ultrasound examination: date, week of gestation, biparietal diameter
- Reliability of dates

Quickening ("feeling life") refers to the mother's first perception of fetal movement. It usually occurs between weeks 16 and 20 of gestation and is initially experienced as a fluttering sensation. The mother's report should be recorded. Multiparas often perceive fetal movement earlier than do primigravidas.

The use of ultrasound examination (also called a *sonogram*) in early pregnancy has become routine, and many health care providers have this equipment available in the office. This procedure can be used to establish the duration of pregnancy if the woman cannot give a precise date for her LMP or if the size of the uterus does not conform to the EDB as calculated by Nägele's rule. Ultrasound

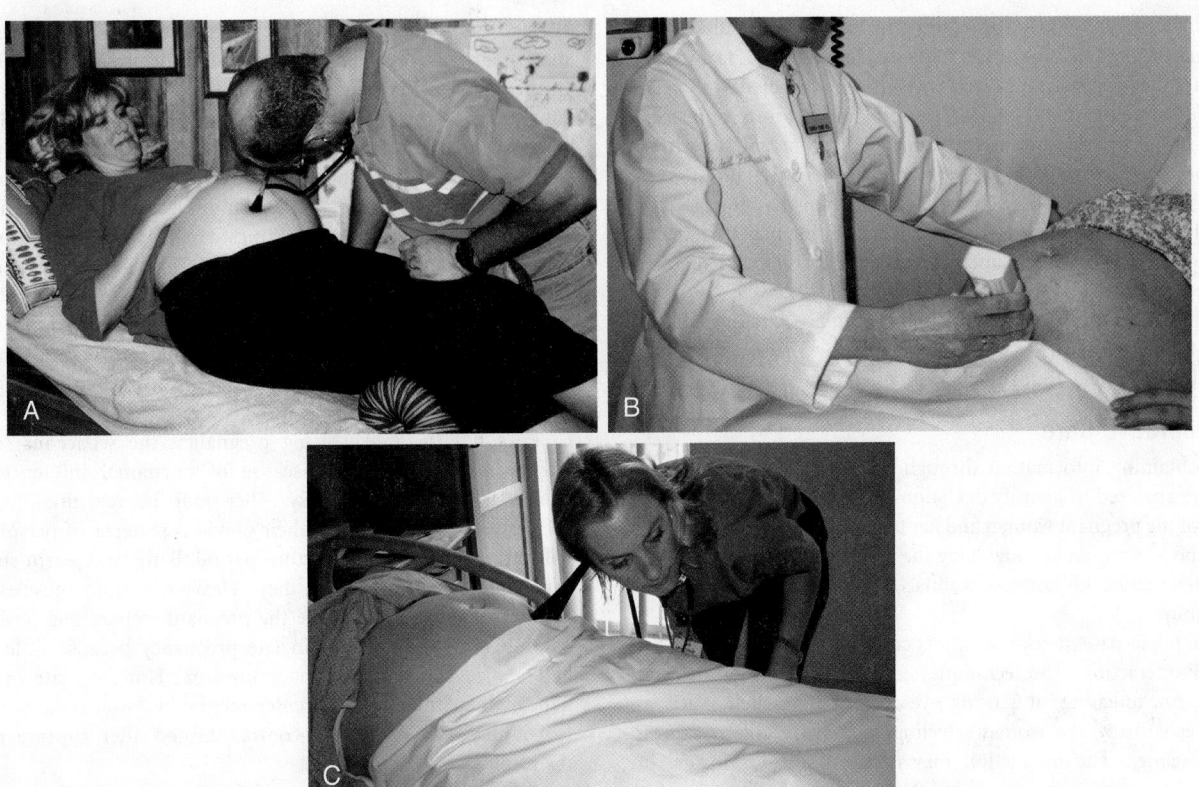

FIG 8-8 Detecting fetal heartbeat. **A,** Father can listen to the fetal heart with a fetoscope (first detectable at 18 to 20 weeks with a fetoscope). **B,** Doppler ultrasound stethoscope (fetal heartbeat detectable at 12 weeks). **C,** Pinard stethoscope. **NOTE:** Hands should not touch stethoscope while nurse is listening. (*A,* Courtesy Shannon Perry, Phoenix, AZ. *B,* Courtesy Dee Lowdermilk, Chapel Hill, NC. *C,* Courtesy Julie Perry Nelson, Loveland, CO.)

also provides information about the well-being of the fetus (see Chapter 10).

Health Status. The assessment of fetal health status includes consideration of fetal movement. The mother is instructed to note the extent and timing of fetal movements and report immediately if the pattern changes or movement ceases. Regular movement is a reliable indicator of fetal health (Cunningham, Leveno, Bloom, et al., 2010).

The fetal heart rate (FHR) is checked on routine visits once it has been heard (see Fig. 8-8). Early in the second trimester, the heartbeat may be heard with the Doppler stethoscope (see Fig. 8-8, *B*). To detect the heartbeat before the fetal position can be palpated by Leopold maneuvers (see Box 16-6), the scope is moved around the abdomen until the heartbeat is audible. The heartbeat is counted for 1 minute, and the quality and rhythm are noted. Later in the second trimester, the FHR can be determined with the fetoscope or Pinard fetoscope (see Fig. 8-8, *A* and *C*). A normal rate and rhythm are other good indicators of fetal health. Once the heartbeat is noted, its absence is cause for immediate investigation.

Intensive investigation of fetal health status is initiated if any maternal or fetal complications arise (e.g., maternal hypertension, IUGR, premature rupture of membranes [PROM], irregular or absent FHR, absence of fetal movements after quickening). Careful, precise, and concise recording of patient responses and laboratory results contributes to the ongoing evaluation of maternal and fetal well-being.

Laboratory Tests. The number of routine laboratory tests done during follow-up visits in pregnancy is limited. A clean-catch urine specimen is obtained to test for levels of glucose, protein, nitrites, and leukocytes at each visit. When indicated, urine specimens for culture and sensitivity are obtained and cervical and vaginal smears and blood tests are repeated.

First-trimester screening for chromosomal abnormalities is offered as an option between 11 and 14 weeks. This multiple marker screen includes ultrasound evaluation of nuchal translucency (NT) and biochemical markers—pregnancy-associated placental protein (PAPP-A) and free beta-human chorionic gonadotropin (β-hCG). Between 15 and 20 weeks, maternal serum alpha-fetoprotein (MSAFP) screening, the QUAD test (alpha-fetoprotein, hCG, estriol, and inhibin A), or Penta Screen (components of QUAD test plus invasive trophoblast antigen [ITA]) can be done to screen for neural tube defects (NTDs) and other chromosomal abnormalities. Women who had first-trimester screening need MSAFP testing after 15 weeks for NTD screening (Gregory, Niebyl, and Johnson, 2012).

An ultrasound is often done at 18 to 24 weeks to survey fetal anatomy. At the same time, assessment of cervical length may be done as a screening tool for preterm labor risk. If cervical length is determined to be short, a transvaginal ultrasound should be done (Society for Maternal-Fetal Medicine Publications Committee, 2012). If the cervix is confirmed to be short, further assessment for preterm birth risk factors should occur and management options should be considered.

If not done earlier in pregnancy, a glucose screen is obtained between 24 and 28 weeks of gestation for women at high risk for gestational diabetes. Group B strep (GBS) testing is done between 35 and 37 weeks of gestation; cultures collected earlier will not accurately predict GBS status at time of birth. Other cultures for STIs may be obtained in the last trimester, based on risk factors and geographic prevalence rates. Tests that are often repeated at 28 weeks include hemoglobin and hematocrit, serologic test for syphilis, and HIV testing. In addition, at 28 weeks, an Rh type and screen for antibodies is performed. If the woman is Rh negative and unsensitized, she should receive 300 mcg of Rh immune globulin (RhIG) (see Medication Guide, p. 503). Hematocrit testing may be repeated at 36 weeks in women with anemia and those at risk for peripartum hemorrhage (Gregory, Niebyl, and Johnson, 2012).

Other diagnostic tests, such as amniocentesis, are available to assess the health status of both the pregnant woman and the fetus (see Chapters 9 and 15 for further discussion).

Collaborative Care

After obtaining information through the assessment process, the data are analyzed to identify deviations from the norm and unique needs of the pregnant woman and her family. Care is optimized with a collaborative approach involving the physician or midwife, nurse, other relevant health care professionals, the woman, her partner, and her family.

The nurse-patient relationship is critical in setting the tone for further interaction. The techniques of listening with an attentive expression, touching, and using eye contact have their place, as does recognizing the woman's feelings and her right to express these feelings. The interaction may occur in various formal or informal settings. A clinical setting, home visits, or telephone conversations all provide opportunities for contact and can be used effectively.

Education About Maternal and Fetal Changes

Expectant parents typically are curious about the growth and development of the fetus and the consequent changes that occur in the mother's body. Mothers may be more tolerant of the discomforts related to the continuing pregnancy if they understand the underlying causes. Educational literature (printed, electronic, or web-based materials) that describes fetal and maternal changes is available and can be used to explain changes as they occur. Couples can track the development of their growing fetus through websites such as www.babycenter.com/fetal-development or www.parents.com/pregnancy/stages/fetal-development/. To be most effective, the material should be appropriate for the pregnant woman's or couple's ethnicity, culture, and literacy level and the agency's resources.

Education for Self-Management

The expectant mother needs information on many topics. The nurse who is observant, listens, and is familiar with typical concerns of expectant parents can anticipate the questions that will be asked and can encourage mothers and their partners to discuss what is on their minds. Printed literature can be given to supplement the individualized teaching the nurse provides; women often avidly read books, pamphlets, and web information related to their own experience. When nurses read the literature before they distribute it, they have an opportunity to point out areas that may not correspond with local health care practices. Nurses who work with expectant parents should be aware of popular web-based resources and programs related to pregnancy.

Pregnant women who receive conflicting advice or instruction are likely to grow increasingly frustrated with members of the health care team and the care provided. Several topics that may cause concern for pregnant women are discussed in the following sections.

Nutrition. Good nutrition is important in the maintenance of maternal health during pregnancy and in the provision of adequate nutrients for embryonic and fetal development. Assessing a woman's nutritional status and weight gain and providing information on nutrition are part of the nurse's responsibilities in providing prenatal care. Teaching may include discussion about foods high in iron, encouragement to take prenatal vitamins, and recommendations to limit caffeine intake. In some settings, a registered dietitian conducts classes for pregnant women about nutrition during pregnancy or interviews them to assess their knowledge of these topics. Nurses can refer women to a registered dietitian if a need is identified during the nursing assessment. (For detailed information concerning maternal and fetal nutritional needs and related nursing care, see Chapter 9.)

Personal Hygiene. During pregnancy, the sebaceous (sweat) glands are highly active because of hormonal influences and women often perspire freely. They may be reassured that the increase is normal and that their previous patterns of perspiration will return after the postpartum period. Baths and warm showers can be therapeutic because they relax tense, tired muscles; help counter insomnia; and make the pregnant woman feel fresh. Tub bathing is permitted even in late pregnancy because little water enters the vagina unless under pressure. However, late in pregnancy, when the woman's center of gravity lowers, she is at risk for falling. Tub bathing is contraindicated after rupture of the membranes.

Prevention of Urinary Tract Infection. Because of physiologic changes that occur in the renal system during pregnancy (see Chapter 7), infections of the lower urinary tract (acute urethritis, acute cystitis) are common. *Escherichia coli (E. coli)* is the most common causative organism for urinary tract infection (UTI) in pregnant women (Duff, 2012). Although UTIs can be asymptomatic, typical symptoms include frequency, urgency, dysuria, dribbling, and hesitancy; gross hematuria may occur. Women should be instructed to inform their health care provider promptly if they experience these symptoms. Urinary tract infections pose a risk to the mother and fetus; thus their prevention or early treatment is essential. Oral antibiotics are commonly prescribed.

The nurse can assess the woman's understanding of appropriate hand hygiene techniques to use before and after urinating and the importance of wiping the perineum from front to back. Soft, absorbent toilet tissue, preferably white and unscented, should be used; harsh, scented, or printed toilet paper may cause irritation. Bubble bath or other bath oils should be avoided because these can irritate the urethra. Women should wear underpants and panty hose with a cotton crotch and avoid wearing tight-fitting slacks or jeans for long periods. Anything that allows a buildup of heat and moisture in the genital area can foster the growth of bacteria.

Some women do not consume enough fluid. After exploring the woman's fluid preferences, the nurse should advise her to drink at least 2 liters (L) (eight glasses) of liquid a day to maintain an adequate fluid intake that ensures frequent urination. Pregnant women should not limit fluids in an effort to reduce the frequency of urination. Women need to know that if urine looks dark (concentrated), they must increase their fluid intake. The consumption of yogurt and acidophilus milk can help prevent urinary tract and vaginal infections. Although drinking cranberry juice is often recommended, there is conflicting evidence regarding its effectiveness and, in particular, the effective dose needed to prevent urinary tract infections.

The nurse should review healthy urination practices with the woman. Women should be told not to ignore the urge to urinate, because holding urine lengthens the time bacteria are in the bladder and allows them to multiply. Women should plan ahead when faced with situations that may normally require them to delay urination (e.g., a long car ride). They should always urinate before going to bed at night. Bacteria also can be introduced during intercourse. It is helpful to wash the genital area with warm water before sex, to urinate before and after intercourse, and then to drink a large glass of water to promote additional urination.

Kegel Exercises. Kegel exercises—deliberate contraction and relaxation of the pubococcygeus muscle—strengthen the muscles around the reproductive organs and improve muscle tone. Many women are not aware of the muscles of the pelvic floor until it is pointed out that these are the muscles used during urination and sexual intercourse and that they can be consciously controlled. The pelvic floor muscles encircle the vaginal outlet, and they need to be exercised. An exercised muscle can stretch and contract readily at birth. Practice of pelvic muscle exercise during pregnancy also results in fewer complaints of urinary incontinence in late pregnancy and postpartum.

Preparation for Breastfeeding the Newborn. Pregnant women are usually eager to discuss their plans for feeding the newborn. The American Academy of Pediatrics (AAP) recommends exclusive breastfeeding for the first 6 months, continued breastfeeding as complementary feedings are introduced, and breastfeeding for at least 1 year and beyond as desired by the mother and infant (AAP Section on Breastfeeding, 2012). In the mother, medical contraindications to breastfeeding are uncommon and include untreated active tuberculosis (until treated for 2 weeks and deemed noninfectious), active herpes simplex lesions on the breast, human T-cell lymphotropic virus type I or II, and untreated brucellosis. Women on antimetabolite medications (chemotherapy) should not breastfeed, but they can pump and discard their milk temporarily; this is also true for radiopharmaceuticals and a few other medications (AAP Section on Breastfeeding, 2012; Lawrence and Lawrence, 2011). In developed countries, breastfeeding is discouraged in women who are HIV positive because of the risk for HIV transmission; however, in developing countries, breastfeeding is recommended because the advantages of breastfeeding for infants outweigh the risk for HIV transmission (Lawrence and Lawrence, 2011). Although hepatitis B antigen has not been shown to be transmitted through breast milk, as an added precaution it is recommended that infants born to hepatitis B antigen–positive women receive hepatitis B vaccine and hepatitis B immune globulin immediately after birth (Lawrence and Lawrence, 2011). Most women who choose to breastfeed do so because they are aware of the numerous benefits. Lack of knowledge about the benefits of breastfeeding and perceived personal and social disadvantages to breastfeeding can influence a woman not to breastfeed. Modesty issues, lack of support by the partner and family, incompatibility with lifestyle, and lack of confidence are among the reasons cited by women who decide to formula-feed their infants (Lawrence and Lawrence, 2011; Nelson, 2012).

A woman's decision about the method of infant feeding is usually made before pregnancy; thus it is essential to educate women of childbearing age about the benefits of breastfeeding. The woman and her partner are encouraged to decide what method of feeding is suitable for them; however, the benefits of breastfeeding should be emphasized. Once the couple has been given information about the advantages and disadvantages of breastfeeding and bottle-feeding, they can make an informed choice. Health care providers support these decisions and provide any needed assistance.

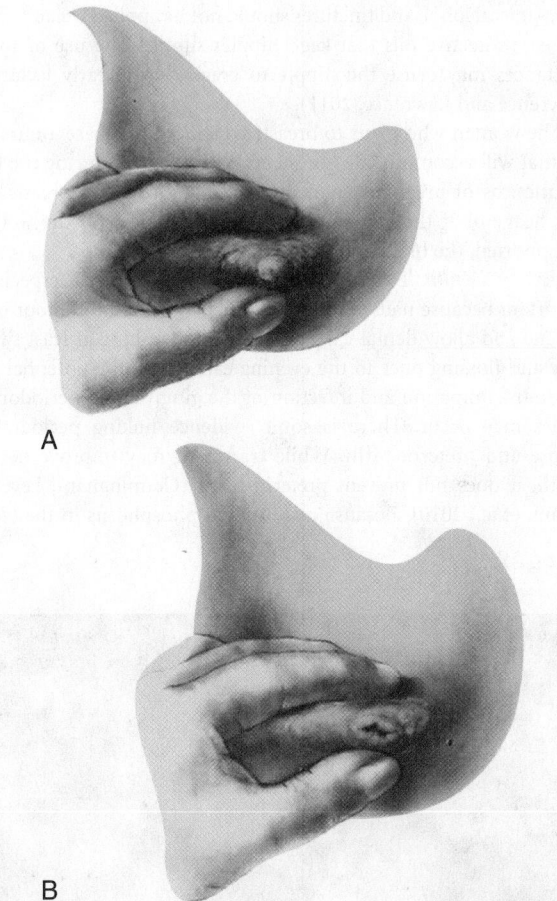

A

B

FIG 8-9 Test for inverted nipples **A,** Normal nipple everts with gentle pressure. **B,** Inverted nipple inverts with gentle pressure. (Adapted from Lawrence RA, Lawrence RM: *Breastfeeding: a guide for the medical profession,* ed 7, St Louis, 2011, Mosby.)

Assessment of breasts during the prenatal period may reveal potential concerns related to breastfeeding. Scars on the breast may indicate previous breast reduction surgery, which can impact milk production. The woman may have breast implants; this may or may not affect successful breastfeeding. Examination of the breasts may reveal flat or inverted nipples, which can affect the baby's ability to successfully latch on to the breast. To determine if nipples are inverted, a woman can perform a test on her nipples to determine freedom of protrusion (Fig. 8-9). The woman places her thumb and forefinger on her areola and presses inward gently. A normal nipple will evert or stand erect while an inverted nipple will appear to withdraw (Lawrence and Lawrence, 2011).

Exercises to break the adhesions that cause the nipple to invert do not work and may cause uterine contractions (Lawrence and Lawrence, 2011). Some clinicians recommend the prenatal use of breast shells (Fig. 8-10) during the last trimester for women with flat or inverted nipples, although evidence to support their effectiveness is lacking (Lawrence and Lawrence, 2011). They can be uncomfortable and cause irritation to the nipple or areola. Breast stimulation is contraindicated in women at risk for preterm labor; therefore the decision to suggest the use of breast shells to women with flat or inverted nipples must be made judiciously (Lawrence and Lawrence, 2011; Walker, 2010).

The woman is taught to cleanse the nipples with warm water to prevent blocking of the ducts with dried colostrum. Soap, ointments, alcohol, and tinctures should not be applied because they remove protective oils that keep nipples supple. The use of these substances may cause the nipple to crack during early lactation (Lawrence and Lawrence, 2011).

The woman who plans to breastfeed should purchase a nursing bra that will accommodate her increased breast size during the last few months of pregnancy and during lactation. If her breasts are very heavy or if the woman feels uncomfortable with the weight unsupported, the bra can be worn day and night.

Dental Health. Dental care during pregnancy is especially important because nausea during pregnancy may lead to poor oral hygiene and allow dental caries to develop. Brushing at least twice daily and flossing once in the evening can reduce the potential for caries. Inflammation and infection of the gingival and periodontal tissues may occur. There is some evidence linking periodontal disease and preterm birth. While treatment may improve dental health, it does not prevent preterm birth (Cunningham, Leveno, Bloom, et al., 2010). Because calcium and phosphorus in the teeth

are fixed in enamel, the old adage "for every child a tooth" is not true. Diagnosis and treatment of oral health problems, including necessary dental x-rays, are safe during pregnancy (Cunningham, Leveno, Bloom, et al., 2010; Kumar and Samelson, 2009). Dental care and nonemergent procedures are best scheduled during the second trimester when the woman is past the stage of feeling nauseous and can sit comfortably in the dental chair. To avoid supine hypotension during dental procedures, the pregnant woman in her second or third trimester is positioned in the dental chair with a small pillow under her right hip (Kumar and Samelson, 2009).

Physical Activity. Physical activity promotes a feeling of well-being and can help reduce anxiety in the pregnant woman (see Evidence-Based Practice box). It improves circulation, promotes relaxation and rest, and counteracts boredom, as it does in the non-pregnant woman. The U.S. Department of Health and Human Services (USDHHS) recommends 150 minutes of moderate exercise each week during pregnancy for women who are not already active or engaging in moderate exercise. Women who are highly active or engage in vigorous aerobic exercise can continue during pregnancy if they remain healthy and discuss with their health care provider about adjusting activity over time as needed (USDHHS, 2008). Detailed exercise tips for pregnancy are presented in the Home Care box.

Exercises that help relieve the low back pain that often arises during the second trimester because of the increased weight of the fetus are demonstrated in Fig. 8-11.

Posture and Body Mechanics. Skeletal, musculature, and hormonal changes in pregnancy can predispose the woman to backache and possible injury. As pregnancy progresses, the pregnant woman's center of gravity changes, pelvic joints soften and relax, and stress is placed on abdominal musculature. Poor posture and body mechanics contribute to the discomfort and potential for injury (see Patient Teaching box). To minimize these problems, women can learn good body posture and body mechanics (Fig. 8-12). The activities described in the Home Care box can also promote greater physical comfort.

Rest and Relaxation. The pregnant woman is encouraged to plan regular rest periods, particularly as pregnancy advances. The side-lying position is recommended to promote uterine perfusion and fetoplacental oxygenation by eliminating pressure on the

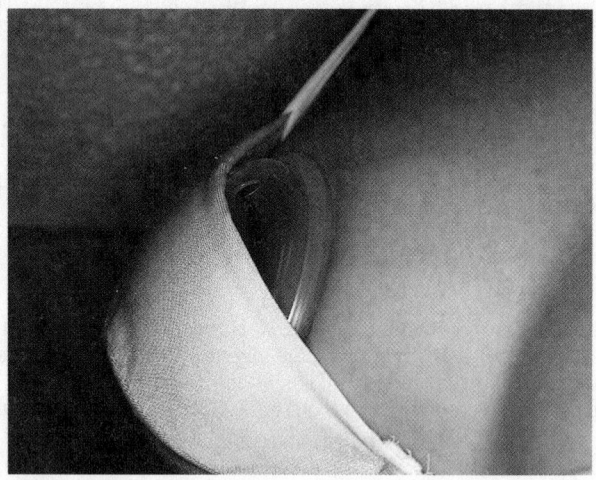

FIG 8-10 Breast shell in place inside bra; sometimes recommended for flat or inverted nipples. (Courtesy Michael S. Clement, MD, Mesa, AZ.)

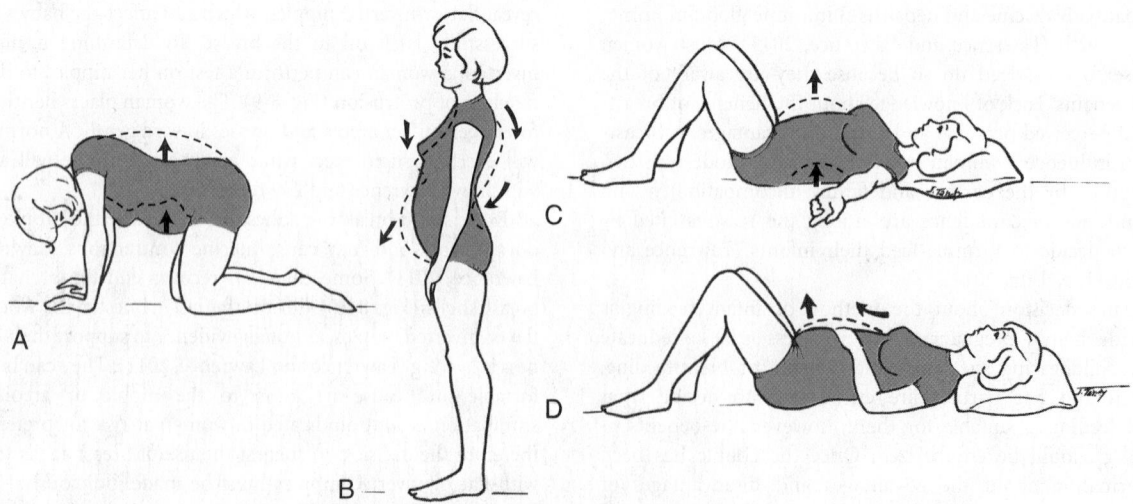

FIG 8-11 Exercises. **A, B,** and **C,** Pelvic rocking relieves low backache (excellent for relief of menstrual cramps as well). **D,** Abdominal breathing aids relaxation and lifts abdominal wall off uterus.

ascending vena cava and descending aorta, which can lead to supine hypotension (Fig. 8-13). The woman should also be shown the way to rise slowly from a side-lying position to prevent placing strain on the back and minimize the orthostatic hypotension caused by changes in position common in the latter part of pregnancy.

To stretch and rest back muscles at home or at work, the nurse can suggest that the woman do the following exercises:
- While standing behind a chair, the woman supports and balances herself using the back of the chair (Fig. 8-14). She squats for 30 seconds and then stands for 15 seconds. She should repeat 6 times, in several sets per day, as needed.

EVIDENCE-BASED PRACTICE

Nonpharmacologic Mind-Body Support Interventions for Healthy Pregnancy

Ask the Question
For pregnant women at risk for anxiety and depression, can antenatal support interventions improve health and birth outcomes?

Search for the Evidence
Search Strategies
English research–based publications on pregnancy support, anxiety, prenatal depression, and postpartum depression were included.

Databases Used
Cochrane Collaborative Database, National Guideline Clearinghouse (AHRQ), PubMed, UpToDate, CINAHL, and the professional website for AWHONN.

Critically Analyze the Evidence
- A systematic review finds that pregnant women who were taught guided imagery and who practice relaxation techniques experience less anxiety during labor and decreased anxiety and depression in the immediate post-partum period (Marc, Toureche, Ernst, et al., 2011).
- For women with prenatal depression, being randomized to regular yoga or massage therapy improved scores for depression, anxiety, back and leg pain, and relationship over controls randomized to standard prenatal care. Additional benefits included greater gestational age and birth weight (Field, Diego, Hernandez-Reif, et al., 2012).
- Even brief antenatal group interventions focusing on stress management and coping skills for depressed women can reduce the risk of postpartum depression as much as 18%. In addition, the group intervention reduced depression in women with poor partner support and in women experiencing unplanned pregnancy (Kozinszky, Dudas, Devosa, et al., 2012).
- For women at risk for low-birth-weight babies, additional antenatal social support did not change the birth weights, but it did reduce admissions to hospitals for pregnancy complications and cesarean birth (Hodnett, Fredericks, and Weston, 2010).
- Exercise is a strongly recommended intervention for mental and physical well-being and weight control in pregnancy, especially for at-risk populations. Qualitative research finds that barriers to exercise for low-income African-Americans include poor motivation, misinformation, lack of affordable nearby facilities, and sociocultural barriers. Women exercised more when they were part of a group exercise class and when safe, low-cost facilities were present in their communities (Krans and Chang, 2011).

Apply the Evidence: Nursing Implications
- Women at risk for anxiety or depression may be especially vulnerable during pregnancy, when medication may not be advisable. Teaching stress management, guided imagery, and relaxation may help them cope with the changes of pregnancy and parenthood. Regular yoga and massage therapy may also provide additional benefits.
- All pregnant women benefit from social support. Some obstetric practices have adopted group prenatal appointments to try to facilitate group support. It is important that these not only include nurse-led patient education, but also allow time for social bonding and dialogue. Women at risk for depression and anxiety may benefit the most.

- The nurse can also assess the community for safe, low-cost exercise opportunities and make this information readily available to local pregnant women, along with information about the benefits of exercise. Initiating a regular walking club or encouraging daily walking partners provides a low-cost, safer, and social activity that can improve overall pregnancy well-being. In the bigger picture, advocating for safer communities decreases stress and improves health for all.

Quality and Safety Competencies: Evidence-Based Practice*
Knowledge
Describe EBP to include the components of research evidence, clinical expertise, and patient/family values.
Describe the strong evidence from systematic reviews, relevant information from single randomized controlled trials, and the ideas suggested by qualitative research.

Skills
Locate evidence reports related to clinical practice topics and guidelines.
Look for patterns and ideas that can be translated to nursing care.

Attitudes
Appreciate strengths and weaknesses of scientific bases for practice.
Value EBP that embraces both information that lends itself to randomized control trials, as well as qualitative research whose rich data may foster novel solutions.

References
Field T, Diego M, Hernandez-Reif, M, et al: Yoga and massage therapy reduce prenatal depression and prematurity, *J Bodyw Mov Ther* 16(2):204–209, 2012.

Hodnett E, Fredericks S, Weston J: Support during pregnancy for women at increased risk of low birthweight babies. In *The Cochrane Database of Systematic Reviews* 2010, Issue 6, Chichester, UK, 2010, John Wiley & Sons. DOI: 10.1002/14651858.CD000198.pub2.

Kozinszky Z, Dudas RB, Devosa I, et al: Can a brief antepartum preventive group intervention help reduce postpartum depressive symptomatology? *Psychother Psychosom* 81(2):98–107, 2012.

Krans E, Chang J: A will without a way: barriers and facilitators to exercise during pregnancy for low-income African American women, *Women Health* 51(8):777–794, 2011.

Marc I, Toureche N, Ernst E, et al: Mind-body interventions during pregnancy for preventing or treating women's anxiety. In *The Cochrane Database of Systematic Reviews* 2011, Issue 7, Chichester, UK, 2011, John Wiley & Sons. DOI: 10.1002/14651858.CD007559.pub2.

Pat Mahaffee Gingrich

*Adapted from QSEN at www.qsen.org/

HOME CARE

Exercise Tips for Pregnant Women

- *Consult your health care provider* when you know or suspect that you are pregnant. Discuss your medical and obstetric history, your current exercise regimen, and the exercises you would like to continue throughout pregnancy.
- *Seek help in determining an exercise routine* that is well within your limit of tolerance, especially if you have not been exercising regularly.
- *Consider decreasing weight-bearing exercises* (jogging, running) as pregnancy progresses and concentrating on non–weight bearing activities such as swimming, cycling, or stretching. If you are a runner, starting in your seventh month you may wish to walk instead.
- *Avoid risky activities* such as surfing, mountain climbing, skydiving, and racquetball because such activities that require precise balance and coordination may be dangerous. Avoid activities that require holding your breath and bearing down (Valsalva maneuver). Jerky, bouncy motions also should be avoided.
- *Exercise regularly* at least three times a week, as long as you are healthy, to improve muscle tone and increase or maintain your stamina. If you exercise sporadically, this may put undue strain on your muscles. Limit activity to shorter intervals. Exercise for 10 to 15 minutes, rest for 2 to 3 minutes, and then exercise for another 10 to 15 minutes.
- *Decrease your exercise level* as your pregnancy progresses. The normal alterations of advancing pregnancy such as decreased cardiac reserve and increased respiratory effort may produce physiologic stress if you exercise strenuously for a long time.
- *Take your pulse* every 10 to 15 minutes while you are exercising. If it is more than 140 beats/min, slow down until it returns to a maximum of 90 beats/min. You should be able to converse easily while exercising. If you cannot, you need to slow down.
- *Avoid becoming overheated* for extended periods. It is best not to exercise for more than 35 minutes, especially in hot, humid weather. As your body temperature rises, the heat is transmitted to your fetus. Prolonged or repeated elevation of fetal temperature may result in birth defects, especially during the first 3 months. Your temperature should not exceed 38° C (100° F).
- *Do not use hot tubs and saunas.*
- *Perform warm-up and stretching exercises* to prepare your joints for more strenuous exercise and lessen the likelihood of strain or injury to your joints. After the fourth month of gestation, you should not perform exercises flat on your back.
- *Include a cool-down period* of mild activity involving your legs after an exercise period to help bring your respiration, heart, and metabolic rates back to normal and prevent the pooling of blood in the exercised muscles.
- *Rest for 10 minutes after exercising*, lying on your side. As the uterus grows, it puts pressure on a major vein in your abdomen, which carries blood to your heart. Lying on your side removes the pressure and promotes return circulation from your extremities and muscles to your heart, thereby increasing blood flow to your placenta and fetus. You should rise gradually from the floor to prevent dizziness or fainting (orthostatic hypotension).
- *Stay hydrated.* Drink two or three 8-oz glasses of water after you exercise to replace the body fluids lost through perspiration. While exercising, drink water whenever you feel the need.
- *Increase your caloric intake* to replace the calories burned during exercise and provide the extra energy needs of pregnancy. Choose high-protein foods such as fish, milk, cheese, eggs, or meat.
- *Take your time.* This is not the time to be competitive or train for activities requiring speed or long endurance.
- *Wear a supportive bra.* Your increased breast weight may cause changes in posture and put pressure on the ulnar nerve.
- *Wear supportive shoes.* As your uterus grows, your center of gravity shifts and you compensate for this by arching your back. These natural changes may make you feel off balance and more likely to fall.
- *Stop exercising immediately* and consult your health care provider if you experience shortness of breath, dizziness, numbness, tingling, pain of any kind, more than four uterine contractions per hour, decreased fetal activity, or vaginal bleeding, and consult your health care provider.
- *Recognize signs of danger, including* vaginal bleeding*; blurred vision*; nausea; dizziness; fainting*; breathlessness; heart palpitations; increased swelling in your hands, feet, and ankles; sharp pain in the abdomen and chest*; and sudden change in body temperature.
- *Avoid the following exercises during pregnancy:* downhill snow skiing because the center of gravity changes and there is risk for falls; contact sports such as ice hockey, soccer, and basketball; and scuba diving because the pressure from the water could put the baby at risk for decompression sickness.

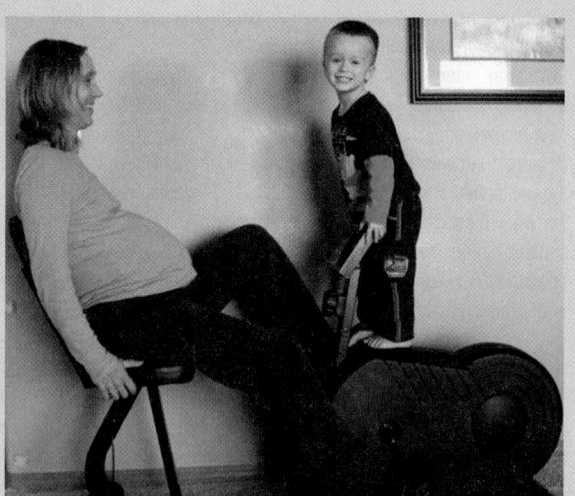

Riding recumbent bicycle provides exercise while supplying back support. Big brother becomes involved. (Courtesy Julie Perry Nelson, Loveland, CO.)

Data from American College of Obstetricians and Gynecologists Committee on Obstetric Practice: Committee opinion no. 267: *Exercise during pregnancy and the postpartum period*, 2009, www.acog.org/~/media/Committee%20Opinions/Committee%20on%20Obstetric%20Practice/co267.pdf?dmc=1&ts=20120814T2219033404; American College of Obstetricians and Gynecologists: *Exercise during pregnancy* (FAQ 0119), 2011, www.acog.org/~/media/For%20Patients/faq119.pdf?dmc=1&ts=20120814T2219033424; American Pregnancy Association: *Top recommended exercises*, 2008, www.americanpregnancy.org/pregnancyhealth/toprecommendedexercises.html.
*If you experience any of these signs, contact your physician or midwife immediately.

PATIENT TEACHING

Safety During Pregnancy

Changes in the body caused by pregnancy include relaxation of joints, alteration to center of gravity, faintness, and discomforts. Problems with coordination and balance are common. Therefore the woman should follow these guidelines:
- Use good body mechanics.
- Use safety features on tools/vehicles (safety seat belts, shoulder harnesses, headrests, goggles, helmets) as specified.
- Avoid activities requiring coordination, balance, and concentration.
- Take rest periods; reschedule daily activities to meet rest and relaxation needs.

The developing embryo and fetus are vulnerable to environmental teratogens. Many potentially dangerous chemicals are present in the home, yard, and workplace: cleaning agents, paints, sprays, herbicides, and pesticides. The soil and water supply may be unsafe. Therefore the woman should follow these guidelines:
- Read all labels for ingredients and proper use of product.
- Ensure adequate ventilation with clean air.
- Dispose of wastes appropriately.
- Wear gloves when handling chemicals.
- Change job assignments or workplace as necessary.

HOME CARE

Posture and Body Mechanics

To Prevent or Relieve Backache
Do pelvic tilt:
- Pelvic tilt (rock) on hands and knees (see Fig. 8-11, *A*) and while sitting in straight-back chair.
- Pelvic tilt (rock) in standing position against a wall or lying on floor (see Fig. 8-11, *B* and *C*).
- Perform abdominal muscle contractions during pelvic tilt while standing, lying, or sitting to help strengthen rectus abdominis muscle (see Fig. 8-11, *D*).

Use good body mechanics.
- Use leg muscles to reach objects on or near floor. Bend at the knees, not the back. Knees are bent to lower body to squatting position. Feet are kept 12 to 18 inches apart to provide a solid base to maintain balance (see Fig. 8-12, *A*).
- Lift with the legs. To lift a heavy object (e.g., young child), one foot is placed slightly in front of the other and kept flat as the woman lowers herself onto one knee. She lifts the weight, holding it close to her body and never higher than the chest. To stand up or sit down, one leg is placed slightly behind the other as she raises or lowers herself (see Fig. 8-12, *B*).

To Restrict the Lumbar Curve
- For prolonged standing (e.g., ironing or because of employment), place one foot on low footstool or box; change positions often.
- Move car seat forward so that knees are bent and higher than hips. If needed, use a small pillow to support low back area.
- Sit in chairs low enough to allow both feet to be placed on floor, preferably with knees higher than hips.

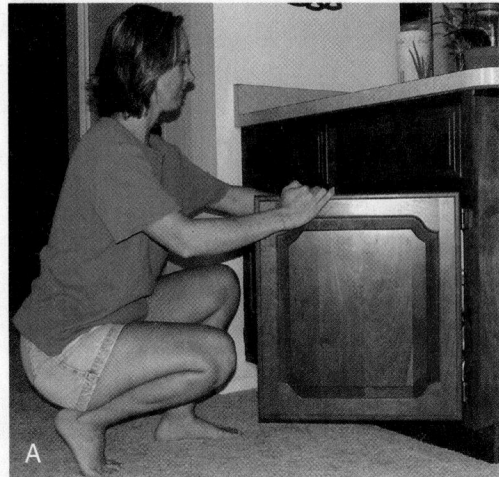

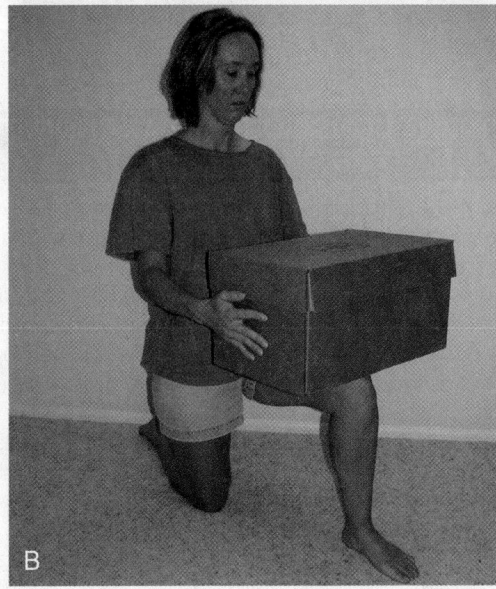

FIG 8-12 Correct body mechanics. **A,** Squatting. **B,** Lifting. (Courtesy Julie Perry Nelson, Loveland, CO.)

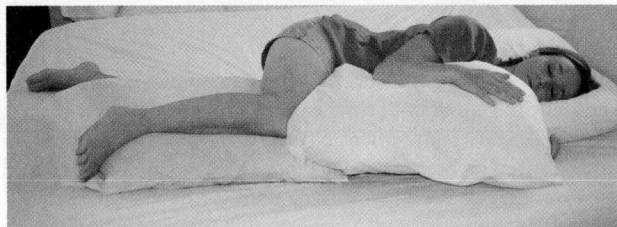

FIG 8-13 Side-lying position for rest and relaxation. (Courtesy Julie Perry Nelson, Loveland, CO.)

- While sitting in a chair, the woman lowers her head to her knees for 30 seconds, then raises her head. She repeats this 6 times, several times per day, as needed.

Conscious relaxation is the process of releasing tension from the mind and body through deliberate effort and practice. The ability to relax consciously and intentionally can be beneficial for the following reasons:
- To relieve the normal discomforts related to pregnancy
- To reduce stress and diminish pain perception during the childbearing cycle
- To heighten self-awareness and trust in one's own ability to control responses and functions
- To help cope with stress in everyday life situations, whether or not the woman is pregnant

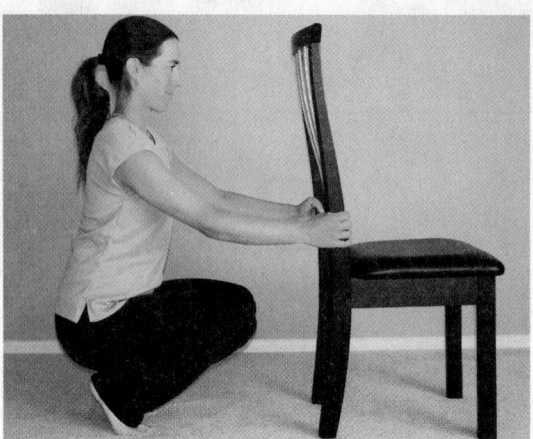

FIG 8-14 Squatting for muscle relaxation and strengthening and for keeping leg and hip joints flexible. (Courtesy Julie Perry Nelson, Loveland, CO.)

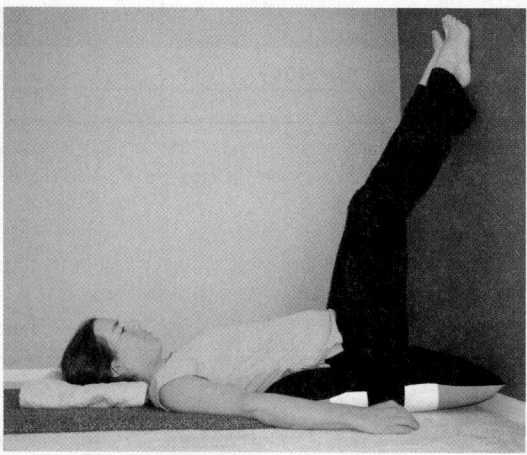

FIG 8-15 Position for resting legs and reducing edema and varicosities. Encourage the woman with vulvar varicosities to include a pillow under her hips. (Courtesy Julie Perry Nelson, Loveland, CO.)

BOX 8-3 **CONSCIOUS RELAXATION TIPS**

Preparation—Loosen clothing, assume a comfortable sitting or side-lying position with all parts of your body well supported with pillows. The use of soothing music is optional.

Beginning—Allow yourself to feel warm and comfortable. Inhale and exhale slowly and imagine peaceful relaxation coming over each part of your body, starting with the neck and working down to the toes. People who learn conscious relaxation often speak of feeling relaxed even if some discomfort is present.

Maintenance—Use imagery (fantasy or daydream) to maintain the state of relaxation. Using *active imagery*, imagine yourself moving or doing some activity and experiencing its sensations. Using *passive imagery*, imagine yourself watching a scene such as a lovely sunset.

Awakening—Return to the wakeful state gradually. Slowly begin to take in stimuli from the surrounding environment.

Further retention and development of the skill—Practice regularly for some periods each day (e.g., at the same hour for 10 to 15 minutes each day to feel refreshed, revitalized, and invigorated).

The techniques for conscious relaxation are numerous and varied. The guidelines given in Box 8-3 can be used by anyone.

Employment. Employment of pregnant women usually has no adverse effects on pregnancy outcomes. Unless complications occur, most women can continue working until the onset of labor (AAP Committee on Fetus and Newborn and ACOG Committee on Obstetric Practice, 2012). Pregnant women should not perform any job that subjects them to severe physical strain or exposes them to harmful substances (Cunningham, Leveno, Bloom, et al., 2010).

Job discrimination that is based solely on pregnancy is illegal. However, some job environments pose potential risk to the fetus (e.g., dry cleaning plants, chemical laboratories, and parking garages). Excessive fatigue is usually the deciding factor in the termination of employment. Strategies to improve safety during pregnancy are described in the Patient Teaching box on p. 205.

Women in sedentary jobs need to walk around at intervals to counter the sluggish circulation in the legs. They should neither sit nor stand in one position for long periods. They should avoid crossing their legs at the knees because all of these activities can foster

the development of varices and thrombophlebitis. Standing for long periods also increases the risk for preterm labor. The pregnant woman's chair should provide adequate back support. Use of a footstool can prevent pressure on veins, relieve strain on varicosities, minimize swelling of feet, and prevent backache.

Clothing. Some women continue to wear their usual clothes during pregnancy as long as they fit and feel comfortable. If maternity clothing is needed, outfits may be purchased new or found in good condition at thrift shops or garage sales. Comfortable, loose clothing is best. Tight bras and belts, stretch pants, garters, tight-top knee socks, body shapers, and other constrictive clothing should be avoided, because tight clothing over the perineum encourages vaginitis and miliaria (heat rash) and impaired circulation in the legs can cause varicosities.

Maternity bras are constructed to accommodate the increased breast weight, chest circumference, and size of breast tail tissue (under the arm). These bras have drop-flaps over the nipples to facilitate breastfeeding. A good bra can help prevent neck ache and backache.

Maternity support (compression) hose give considerable comfort and promote greater venous emptying in women with large varicose veins. Ideally, support stockings should be put on before the woman gets out of bed in the morning. Fig. 8-15 demonstrates a position to rest the legs and reduce swelling.

Comfortable shoes that provide firm support and promote good posture and balance are advisable. Very high heels and platform shoes are not recommended because of the woman's changed center of gravity, which can cause her to lose her balance. In addition, the woman's pelvis tilts forward in the third trimester, increasing her lumbar curve. The resulting leg aches and cramps will be aggravated by shoes that do not provide good support. Fig. 8-16 shows exercises to relieve leg cramps.

Travel. Travel is not contraindicated for low risk pregnant women. Women with high risk pregnancies are advised to avoid long-distance travel after fetal viability has been reached to avert the economic and psychologic consequences of giving birth to a preterm infant far from home. Travel to areas where medical care is poor, water is untreated, or malaria is prevalent should be avoided if possible. Women who contemplate foreign travel should be aware that many health insurance carriers do not cover birth in a foreign setting

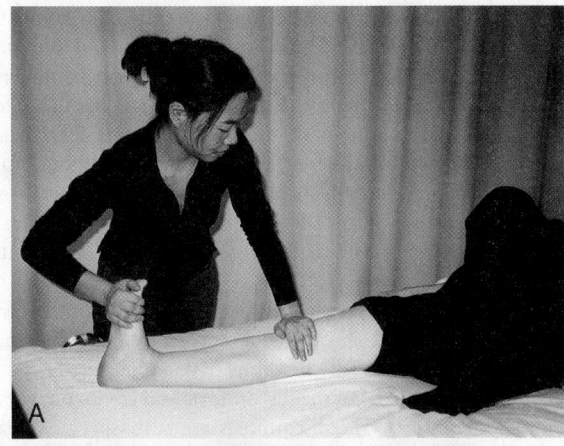

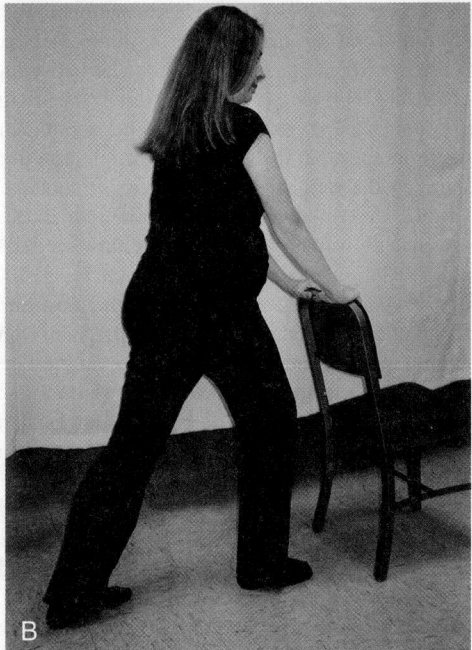

FIG 8-16 Relief of muscle spasm (leg cramps). **A,** Another person dorsiflexes foot with knee extended. **B,** Woman stands and leans forward, thereby dorsiflexing foot of affected leg. (Courtesy Shannon Perry, Phoenix, AZ.)

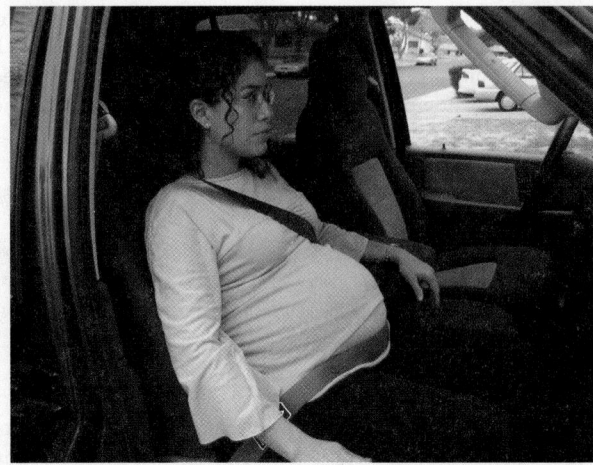

FIG 8-17 Proper use of seat belt and headrest. (Courtesy Brian and Mayannyn Sallee, Anchorage, AK.)

or even hospitalization for preterm labor. In addition, vaccinations for foreign travel may be contraindicated during pregnancy.

Pregnant women who travel long distances should schedule periods of activity and rest. While sitting, the woman can practice deep breathing, foot circling, and alternately contracting and relaxing different muscle groups. She should avoid becoming fatigued. Although travel in itself is not a cause of adverse outcomes such as miscarriage or preterm labor, certain precautions are recommended when traveling in a car. For example, women riding in a car should wear automobile restraints and stop to walk every hour.

Maternal death as a result of injury is the most common cause of fetal death. The next most common cause is placental separation (abruptio placentae) that occurs because body contours change in reaction to the force of a motor vehicle collision. The uterus as a muscular organ can adapt its shape to that of the body, but the placenta is not resilient. At the impact of collision, placental separation can occur. A combination lap belt and shoulder harness is the most effective automobile restraint, and both should be used. The lap belt should be worn low across the hip bones and as snug as is comfortable (Fig. 8-17). The shoulder harness should be worn above the gravid uterus and below the neck to prevent chafing. The pregnant woman should sit upright. The headrest should be used to avoid whiplash injury. Airbags if present should remain engaged, but the steering wheel should be tilted upward away from the abdomen and the seat moved back away from the steering wheel as much as possible.

Air travel in large commercial jets usually poses little risk to the pregnant woman, but policies vary from airline to airline. The pregnant woman is advised to inquire about restrictions or recommendations from her carrier. Most health care providers allow air travel up to 36 weeks of gestation in women without medical or pregnancy complications. Air travel is not recommended for women with severe anemia, sickle cell disease or trait, history of thrombophlebitis, or placental abnormalities. Women at risk for preterm labor should avoid air travel (Sutton, 2012). Magnetometers (metal detectors) used at airport security checkpoints are not harmful to the fetus. The 8% humidity at which cabins are maintained in commercial airlines may result in some water loss; hydration (with water) should be maintained under these conditions. Sitting in the cramped seat of an airliner for prolonged periods may increase the risk for superficial and deep thrombophlebitis. A pregnant woman is encouraged to take a 15-minute walk around the aircraft during each hour of travel to minimize this risk.

Medications and Herbal Preparations. Although much has been learned in recent years about fetal drug toxicity, the possible teratogenicity of many prescription and OTC drugs is still unknown. This is especially true for new medications and combinations of medications. Moreover, certain subclinical errors or deficiencies in intermediate metabolism in the fetus may cause an otherwise harmless drug to be converted into a hazardous one. The greatest danger of drug-caused developmental defects in the fetus extends from the time of fertilization through the first trimester, a time when the woman may not realize she is pregnant. Self-treatment must be discouraged. The use of all drugs, including OTC medications, herbs, and vitamins, should be limited; and a careful record should be kept of all therapeutic and nontherapeutic agents used.

The use of complementary and alternative medicine by pregnant women is widespread and is based primarily on historical use and anecdotal information. There is limited research evidence about the safety of herbal preparations, especially during pregnancy. While the use of complementary and alternative therapies is consistent with the holistic, woman-centered approach to care, caution is warranted in their use because of the lack of evidence (Hall, McKenna, and Griffiths, 2010).

> ### ⚡ SAFETY ALERT
>
> Although some complementary and alternative medicine (CAM) may benefit the woman during pregnancy, some practices should be avoided because they may increase risk for complications. It is important to ask the woman about all medications she is taking, including OTC and herbal preparations.

Immunizations. Some concern has been raised over the safety of various immunization practices during pregnancy. Immunization with live or attenuated live virus or live bacterial vaccines is generally contraindicated during pregnancy (CDC, 2013). Live virus vaccines include those for measles (rubeola and rubella), chickenpox (varicella), and the Sabin (oral) poliomyelitis vaccine (no longer used in the United States). Human papilloma virus (HPV) vaccine is not recommended during pregnancy. Vaccines consisting of killed viruses that may be administered during pregnancy include tetanus, diphtheria, recombinant hepatitis B, and influenza vaccines (CDC, 2013).

The Centers for Disease Control and Prevention (CDC, 2013) recommends routine administration of the tetanus, diphtheria, and acellular pertussis (Tdap) vaccine during each pregnancy. The optimal timing for the vaccine is between 27 and 36 weeks of gestation.

> ### ⚡ SAFETY ALERT
>
> Pregnant women who become ill with seasonal respiratory influenza (flu) are more likely than other persons to develop serious complications, such as pneumonia. All women whose pregnancy will take place from November through March should be offered an influenza vaccination.

Alcohol, Cigarette Smoke, Caffeine, and Drugs. Ethanol (alcohol) is a powerful teratogen that can have devastating effects on the developing fetus (e.g., fetal alcohol syndrome). Women who are pregnant or considering pregnancy should totally abstain from alcohol (Cunningham, Leveno, Bloom, et al., 2010). Cigarette smoking or continued exposure to secondhand smoke (even if the mother does not smoke) is associated with IUGR and an increase in perinatal and infant morbidity and mortality. Smoking can affect fertility and may lead to a greater risk for ectopic pregnancy. Smoking is associated with an increased incidence of spontaneous abortion, ectopic pregnancy, preterm birth, PROM, abruptio placentae, placenta previa, and fetal death (Cunningham, Leveno, Bloom, et al., 2010; Sidransky, Norman, McCarthy, et al., 2010). Smoking cessation activities should be incorporated into routine prenatal care. All women who smoke should be strongly encouraged to quit or at least reduce the number of cigarettes they smoke. In addition, pregnant women should be told about the negative effects of secondhand smoke on the fetus and encouraged to avoid such environments.

Research findings suggest that caffeine intake less than 200 mg per day during pregnancy does not appear to be a major contributing factor to miscarriage or preterm birth. The relationship between maternal caffeine intake and low birth weight has not been substantiated by research (ACOG, 2010). The March of Dimes (2010) recommends that pregnant women limit their daily caffeine to less than 200 mg per day. Women should be aware of the caffeine content of foods, drinks, and certain OTC medications and should intentionally limit their intake as recommended. Any drug or environmental agent that enters the pregnant woman's bloodstream has the potential to cross the placenta and harm the fetus. Marijuana, heroin, and cocaine are common examples of such substances. Although substance abuse in pregnancy is a major public health concern and comprehensive care of drug-addicted women improves maternal and neonatal outcomes, few facilities are available for treatment of these women (see Chapter 11).

Normal Discomforts. Pregnant women are confronted with symptoms that would be considered abnormal in the nonpregnant state. Women pregnant for the first time have an increased need for explanations of the causes of the discomforts and advice on ways to relieve the discomforts. The discomforts are fairly specific to each trimester of pregnancy. Table 8-3 provides information about the physiology, prevention, and self-management of discomforts experienced during the three trimesters. Box 8-4 lists alternative therapies used in pregnancy. Nurses can do much to allay a first-time mother's anxiety about such symptoms by telling her about them in advance, using terminology that the woman (or couple) can understand. Understanding the rationale for treatment promotes their participation in their care. Interventions should be individualized, with attention given to the woman's lifestyle and culture (see Nursing Care Plan).

Recognizing Potential Complications. One of the most important responsibilities of care providers is to alert the pregnant woman to signs and symptoms that indicate a potential complication of pregnancy. The woman needs to know how and to whom to report such warning signs (see Table 8-2). The woman and her family should receive a printed list of warning signs, written at the appropriate literacy level, that warrant a call to the health care provider (HCP) or clinic; phone numbers for the HCP or clinic should be listed. The nurse must answer questions honestly as they arise during pregnancy. Pregnant women often have difficulty deciding when to report signs and symptoms. The mother is encouraged to refer to the printed list of potential complications and to listen to her body. If she senses that something is wrong, she should call her care provider immediately. Several signs and symptoms must be discussed more extensively. These include vaginal bleeding,

Text continued on p. 213

> ## BOX 8-4 ALTERNATIVE THERAPIES USED IN PREGNANCY
>
> **Touch and Energetic Therapies**
> - Massage
> - Acupressure
> - Therapeutic touch
> - Healing touch
> - Mind-body healing
> - Imagery
> - Meditation, prayer, reflection
> - Biofeedback
> - Aromatherapy
> - Other modalities that may fall outside of nurse practice guidelines unless the nurse has completed additional training or certification:
>   - Herbs
>   - Homeopathy
>   - Traditional Chinese medicine

TABLE 8-3	**DISCOMFORTS RELATED TO PREGNANCY**	
DISCOMFORT	**PHYSIOLOGY**	**EDUCATION FOR SELF-MANAGEMENT**
First Trimester		
Breast changes, enlargement; pain, tingling, tenderness	Hypertrophy of mammary glandular tissue and increased vascularization, pigmentation, and size and prominence of nipples and areolae caused by hormonal stimulation	Wear supportive maternity bras with pads to absorb discharge (may be worn at night); wash with warm water and keep dry; breast tenderness may interfere with sexual expression/foreplay but is temporary
Urgency and frequency of urination	Vascular engorgement and altered bladder function caused by hormones; bladder capacity reduced by enlarging uterus and fetal presenting part	Empty bladder regularly; perform Kegel exercises; limit fluid intake before bedtime; wear perineal pad; report pain or burning sensation to primary health care provider
Languor and malaise; fatigue (early pregnancy, most commonly)	Unexplained; may be caused by increasing levels of estrogen, progesterone, and hCG or by elevated BBT; psychologic response to pregnancy and its required physical and psychologic adaptations	Rest as needed; eat well-balanced diet to prevent anemia
Nausea and vomiting, morning sickness—occurs in 50%-75% of pregnant women; starts between first and second missed periods and lasts until about fourth missed period; may occur any time during day; fathers also may have symptoms	Cause unknown; may result from hormonal changes, possibly hCG; may be partly emotional, related to ambivalence about or rejection of pregnant state	Avoid empty or overloaded stomach; maintain good posture—give stomach ample room; stop smoking; eat dry carbohydrate on awakening; remain in bed until feeling subsides or alternate dry carbohydrate 1 hr with fluids such as hot herbal decaffeinated tea, milk, or clear coffee the next hour until feeling subsides; eat five to six small meals per day; avoid fried, odorous, spicy, greasy, or gas-forming foods; acupressure, wristbands, ginger, vitamin B_6 alone or with doxylamine may be helpful; consult primary health care provider if intractable vomiting occurs
Ptyalism (excessive salivation) may occur starting 2-3 wk after first missed period	Possibly caused by elevated estrogen levels; may be related to reluctance to swallow because of nausea	Use astringent mouthwash, chew gum, eat hard candy as comfort measures
Gingivitis and epulis (hyperemia, hypertrophy, bleeding, tenderness); condition disappears spontaneously 1-2 mo after birth	Increased vascularity and proliferation of connective tissue from estrogen stimulation	Eat well-balanced diet, with adequate protein and fresh fruits and vegetables; brush teeth gently and observe good dental hygiene; avoid infection; see dentist
Nasal stuffiness; epistaxis (nosebleed)	Hyperemia of mucous membranes related to high estrogen levels	Use humidifier; avoid trauma; normal saline nose drops or spray may be used
Leukorrhea: often noted throughout pregnancy	Hormonally stimulated cervix becomes hypertrophic and hyperactive, producing abundant amount of mucus	Not preventable; do not douche; wear perineal pads; perform hygienic practices such as wiping front to back; report to primary health care provider if accompanied by pruritus, foul odor, or change in character or color
Psychosocial dynamics, mood swings, mixed feelings	Hormonal and metabolic adaptations; feelings about female role, sexuality, timing of pregnancy, and resultant changes in life and lifestyle	Participate in pregnancy support group; communicate concerns to partner, family, and others; request referral for supportive services if needed (financial assistance)
Second Trimester		
Pigmentation deepens, acne, oily skin	Melanocyte-stimulating hormone (from anterior pituitary)	Not preventable; it usually resolves during puerperium
Spider nevi (angiomas) appear over neck, thorax, face, and arms during second or third trimester	Focal networks of dilated arterioles (end-arteries) from increased concentration of estrogens	Not preventable; they fade slowly during late puerperium but rarely disappear completely
Palmar erythema occurs in 50% of pregnant women; may accompany spider nevi	Diffuse reddish mottling over palms and suffused skin over thenar eminences and fingertips; may be caused by genetic predisposition or hyperestrogenism	Not preventable; condition fades within 1 wk after giving birth

Continued

TABLE 8-3   DISCOMFORTS RELATED TO PREGNANCY—cont'd

DISCOMFORT	PHYSIOLOGY	EDUCATION FOR SELF-MANAGEMENT
Pruritus (noninflammatory)	Unknown cause; various types as follows: nonpapular; closely aggregated pruritic papules Increased excretory function of skin and stretching of skin possible factors	Keep fingernails short and clean; contact primary health care provider for diagnosis of cause Not preventable; symptomatic; can be managed with emollient baths, mild sedation, distraction, tepid baths with sodium bicarbonate or oatmeal added to water, lotions and oils, change of soaps or reduction in use of soap, loose clothing
Palpitations	Unknown; should not be accompanied by persistent cardiac irregularity	Not preventable; contact primary health care provider if accompanied by symptoms of cardiac decompensation
Supine hypotension (vena cava syndrome) and bradycardia	Induced by pressure of gravid uterus on ascending vena cava when woman is supine; reduces uteroplacental and renal perfusion	Assume side-lying position or semisitting posture, with knees slightly flexed (see also Emergency box, p. 197)
Faintness and, rarely, syncope (orthostatic hypotension); may persist throughout pregnancy	Vasomotor lability or postural hypotension from hormones; in late pregnancy, may be caused by venous stasis in lower extremities	Exercise moderately (deep breathing, vigorous leg movements); avoid sudden changes in position* and warm crowded areas; move slowly and deliberately; keep environment cool; avoid hypoglycemia by eating five or six small meals per day; wear compression hose; sit as necessary; if symptoms are serious, contact primary health care provider
Food cravings	Cause unknown; craving determined by culture or geographic area	Not preventable; satisfy craving unless it interferes with well-balanced diet; report unusual cravings to primary health care provider
Heartburn (pyrosis or acid indigestion): burning sensation, occasionally with burping and regurgitation of a little sour-tasting fluid	Progesterone slows GI tract motility and digestion, reverses peristalsis, relaxes cardiac sphincter, and delays emptying time of stomach; stomach displaced upward and compressed by enlarging uterus	Limit or avoid gas-producing or fatty foods and large meals; maintain good posture; sip milk for temporary relief; drink hot herbal tea; primary health care provider may prescribe antacid between meals; contact primary health care provider for persistent symptoms
Constipation	GI tract motility slowed because of progesterone, resulting in increased reabsorption of water and drying of stool; intestines compressed by enlarging uterus; predisposition to constipation because of oral iron supplementation	Drink six to eight glasses of water per day; include roughage in diet; exercise moderately; maintain regular schedule for bowel movements; use relaxation techniques and deep breathing; do not take stool softener, laxatives, mineral oil, other drugs, or enemas without first consulting primary health care provider
Flatulence with bloating and belching	Reduced GI motility because of hormones, allowing time for bacterial action that produces gas; swallowing air	Chew foods slowly and thoroughly; avoid gas-producing foods, fatty foods, large meals; exercise, maintain regular bowel habits
Varicose veins (varicosities): may be associated with aching legs and tenderness; may be present in legs and vulva; hemorrhoids are varicosities in perianal area	Hereditary predisposition; relaxation of smooth muscle walls of veins because of hormones, causing tortuous, dilated veins in legs and pelvic vasocongestion; condition aggravated by enlarging uterus, gravity, and bearing down for bowel movements; thrombi from leg varices rare but may be produced by hemorrhoids	Avoid lengthy standing or sitting, constrictive clothing, and constipation and bearing down with bowel movements; exercise moderately; rest with legs and hips elevated (see Fig. 8-15); wear compression hose; thrombosed hemorrhoid may be evacuated; relieve swelling and pain with warm sitz baths; apply astringent compresses locally
Leukorrhea: often noted throughout pregnancy	Hormonally stimulated cervix becomes hypertrophic and hyperactive, producing abundant amount of mucus	Not preventable; do not douche; maintain good hygiene; wear perineal pads; report to primary health care provider if accompanied by pruritus, foul odor, or change in character or color
Headaches (through wk 26)	Emotional tension (more common than vascular migraine headache); eye strain (refractory errors); vascular engorgement and congestion of sinuses resulting from hormone stimulation	Conscious relaxation; rest, massage, application of heat or cold; OTC analgesics (check with provider); contact primary health care provider for constant "splitting" headache to assess for preeclampsia

TABLE 8-3   DISCOMFORTS RELATED TO PREGNANCY—cont'd

DISCOMFORT	PHYSIOLOGY	EDUCATION FOR SELF-MANAGEMENT
Carpal tunnel syndrome (involves thumb, second and third fingers, lateral side of little finger)	Compression of median nerve resulting from changes in surrounding tissues; pain, numbness, tingling, burning; loss of skilled movements (typing); dropping of objects	Not preventable; elevate affected arms; splinting of affected hand may help; regressive after pregnancy; surgery is curative
Periodic numbness, tingling of fingers (acrodysesthesia) occurs in 5% of pregnant women	Brachial plexus traction syndrome resulting from drooping of shoulders during pregnancy (occurs especially at night and early morning)	Maintain good posture; wear supportive maternity bra; condition will disappear if lifting and carrying baby does not aggravate it
Round ligament pain (tenderness)	Stretching of ligament caused by enlarging uterus	Not preventable; rest, maintain good body mechanics to avoid overstretching ligament; relieve cramping by squatting or bringing knees to chest; sometimes heat helps
Joint pain, backache, and pelvic pressure; hypermobility of joints	Relaxation of symphyseal and sacroiliac joints because of hormones, resulting in unstable pelvis; exaggerated lumbar and cervicothoracic curves caused by change in center of gravity resulting from enlarging abdomen	Maintain good posture and body mechanics; avoid fatigue; wear low-heeled shoes; abdominal supports may be useful; practice conscious relaxation; sleep on firm mattress; apply local heat or ice; get back rubs; do pelvic rock exercise; rest; condition disappears 6-8 wk after birth

Third Trimester

DISCOMFORT	PHYSIOLOGY	EDUCATION FOR SELF-MANAGEMENT
Shortness of breath and dyspnea: occur in 60% of pregnant women	Expansion of diaphragm limited by enlarging uterus; diaphragm elevated about 4 cm; some relief after lightening	Maintain good posture; sleep with extra pillows; avoid overloading stomach; stop smoking; contact health care provider if symptoms worsen to rule out anemia, emphysema, and asthma
Insomnia (later weeks of pregnancy)	Fetal movements, muscle cramping, urinary frequency, shortness of breath, or other discomforts	Reassurance, conscious relaxation, back massage or effleurage, support of body parts with pillows, and warm milk or warm shower before retiring are helpful
Psychosocial responses: mood swings, mixed feelings, increased anxiety	Hormonal and metabolic adaptations; feelings about impending labor, birth, and parenthood	Reassurance and support from significant other and nurse and improved communication with partner, family, and others are helpful
Gingivitis and epulis (hyperemia, hypertrophy, bleeding, tenderness): condition disappears spontaneously 1-2 mo after birth	Increased vascularity and proliferation of connective tissue from estrogen stimulation	Eat a well-balanced diet with adequate protein and fresh fruits and vegetables; gently brush teeth and practice good dental hygiene; avoid infection; see dentist for teeth cleaning
Urinary frequency and urgency return	Vascular engorgement and altered bladder function caused by hormones; bladder capacity reduced by enlarging uterus and fetal presenting part	Empty bladder regularly, do Kegel exercises; limit fluid intake before bedtime; reassurance is helpful; wear perineal pad; contact health care provider for pain or burning sensation
Perineal discomfort and pressure	Pressure from enlarging uterus, especially when standing or walking; multifetal gestation	Rest, conscious relaxation, and good posture are helpful; contact health care provider for assessment and treatment if pain is present
Leg cramps (gastrocnemius spasm), especially when reclining	Compression of nerves supplying lower extremities because of enlarging uterus; reduced level of diffusible serum calcium or elevation of serum phosphorus; aggravating factors: fatigue, poor peripheral circulation, pointing toes when stretching legs or when walking, drinking more than 1 L (1 qt) of milk per day	Dorsiflex foot until spasm relaxes (see Fig. 8-16, A); apply heat over affected muscle; stand on cold surface; supplement orally with magnesium lactate or citrate; aluminum hydroxide antacid removes phosphorus by absorbing it
Ankle edema (nonpitting) to lower extremities	Edema aggravated by prolonged standing, sitting, poor posture, lack of exercise, constrictive clothing (e.g., garters), or hot weather	Intake ample fluid for natural diuretic effect; put on support stockings before arising; rest periodically with legs and hips elevated (see Fig. 8-15); exercise moderately; contact health care provider if generalized edema develops; *diuretics are contraindicated*

BBT, Basal body temperature; *GI*, gastrointestinal; *hCG*, human chorionic gonadotropin; *OTC*, over-the-counter.
*Caution woman to rise slowly and sit on edge of bed or to assume hands-and-knees posture before rising and to get up slowly after sitting or squatting.

◎ **NURSING CARE PLAN**

Discomforts of Pregnancy and Warning Signs

NURSING DIAGNOSIS	EXPECTED OUTCOME	NURSING INTERVENTIONS	RATIONALES
First Trimester			
Anxiety related to deficient knowledge about schedule of prenatal visits throughout pregnancy as evidenced by woman's questions and concerns	Woman will verbalize correct appointment schedule for duration of pregnancy and feelings of being "in control."	Provide information regarding schedule of visits, tests, and other assessments and interventions that will be provided throughout pregnancy	To empower woman to function in collaboration with caregiver and diminish anxiety
		Allow woman time to describe level of anxiety	To establish basis for care
		Provide information to woman regarding prenatal classes and labor area tours	To decrease feelings of anxiety about unknown
Imbalanced Nutrition: Less Than Body Requirements related to nausea and vomiting as evidenced by woman's report and weight loss	Woman will gain 1 to 2.5 kg during first trimester.	Verify prepregnant weight	To plan realistic diet according to individual woman's nutritional needs
		Obtain diet history	To identify current meal patterns and foods that may be implicated in nausea
		Advise woman to consume small, frequent meals and avoid having empty stomach	To avoid further nausea episodes
		Suggest that woman eat a simple carbohydrate such as dry crackers before arising in morning	To avoid empty stomach and decrease incidence of nausea and vomiting
		Advise woman to call health care provider if vomiting is persistent and severe	To identify possible incidence of hyperemesis gravidarum
Fatigue related to hormonal changes in first trimester as evidenced by woman's complaints	Woman will report decreased number of episodes of fatigue	Advise woman to rest as needed	To avoid increasing feeling of fatigue
		Advise woman to eat well-balanced diet	To meet increased metabolic demands and avoid anemia
		Discuss use of support systems to help with household responsibilities	To decrease workload at home and decrease fatigue
		Reinforce to woman the transitory nature of first trimester fatigue	To provide emotional support
		Explore with woman a variety of techniques to prioritize roles	To decrease family expectations
Second Trimester			
Constipation related to progesterone influence on gastrointestinal (GI) tract as evidenced by woman's report of altered patterns of elimination	Woman will report return to normal bowel elimination pattern after implementation of interventions.	Provide information to woman regarding pregnancy-related causes: progesterone slowing GI motility, growing uterus compressing intestines, and influence of iron supplementation	To provide basic information for self-management during pregnancy
		Assist woman to plan diet that will promote regular bowel movements, such as increasing amount of oral fluid intake to at least 6 to 8 glasses of water a day, increasing the amount of fiber in daily diet, and maintaining moderate exercise program	To promote self-management care
		Reinforce for woman that she should not take any laxatives, stool softeners, or enemas without first consulting the health care provider	To prevent any injuries to woman or fetus
Anxiety related to deficient knowledge about course of first pregnancy as evidenced by woman's questions regarding possible complications of second and third trimesters	Woman will correctly list signs of potential complications that can occur during second and third trimesters and exhibit no overt signs of stress.	Provide information concerning potential complications or warning signs that can occur during second and third trimesters, including possible causes of signs and importance of calling health care provider immediately	To ensure identification and treatment of problems in timely manner
		Provide a written list of complications	To have a reference list for emergencies

◎ **NURSING CARE PLAN**

Discomforts of Pregnancy and Warning Signs—cont'd

NURSING DIAGNOSIS	EXPECTED OUTCOME	NURSING INTERVENTIONS	RATIONALES
Third Trimester			
Fear related to deficient knowledge regarding onset of labor and processes of labor related to inexperience as evidenced by woman's questions and statement of concerns	Woman will verbalize basic understanding of signs of labor onset and when to call health care provider, identify resources for childbirth education, and express increasing confidence in readiness to cope with labor.	Provide information regarding signs of labor onset and when to call health care provider; give written information regarding local childbirth education classes	To empower and promote self-management
		Promote ongoing effective communication with health care provider	To promote trust and decrease fear of unknown
		Provide woman with decision-making opportunities	To promote effective coping
		Provide opportunity for woman to verbalize fears regarding childbirth	To assist in decreasing fear through discussion
Disturbed Sleep Pattern related to discomforts or insomnia of third trimester as evidenced by woman's report of inadequate rest	Woman will report improvement of quality and quantity of rest and sleep.	Assess current sleep pattern, and review need for increased requirement during pregnancy	To identify need for change in sleep patterns
		Suggest change of position to side-lying with pillows between legs or to semi-Fowler's position	To increase support and decrease any problems with dyspnea or heartburn
		Reinforce possibility of use of various sleep aids such as relaxation techniques, reading, and decreased activity before bedtime	To decrease possibility of anxiety or physical discomforts before bedtime
Ineffective Sexuality Pattern related to changes in comfort level and fatigue	Woman will verbalize feelings regarding changes in sexual desire, and woman and her partner will express satisfaction with sexual activities.	Assess couple's usual sexuality patterns	To determine how patterns have been altered by pregnancy
		Provide information regarding expected changes in sexuality patterns during pregnancy	To correct any misconceptions
		Allow couple to express feelings in nonjudgmental atmosphere	To promote trust
		Refer couple for counseling as appropriate	To assist couple to cope with sexuality pattern changes
		Suggest alternative sexual positions	To decrease pressure on enlarging abdomen of woman and increase sexual comfort and satisfaction of couple

alteration in fetal movements, symptoms of preeclampsia, rupture of membranes, and preterm labor.

Recognizing Preterm Labor. Teaching each expectant mother to recognize preterm labor is necessary for early diagnosis and treatment. Preterm labor occurs after the twentieth week but before the thirty-seventh week of pregnancy. It consists of uterine contractions that, if untreated, cause the cervix to dilate and efface earlier than normal, resulting in preterm birth (see Chapter 17).

Warning signs and symptoms of preterm labor are listed in the Home Care box. Fig. 8-18 shows where in the body the signs and symptoms of preterm labor may be located.

Sexual Counseling

Sexual counseling of expectant couples includes countering misinformation, providing reassurance of normality, and suggesting alternative behaviors. The uniqueness of each couple is considered within a biopsychosocial framework (see Home Care box). Nurses can initiate discussion about sexual adaptations that must be made during pregnancy. They need a sound knowledge base about the

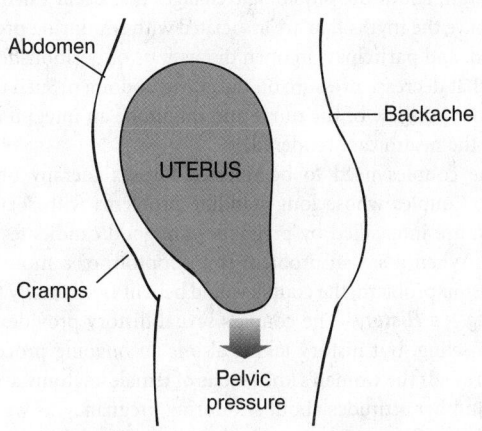

FIG 8-18 Symptoms of preterm labor.

HOME CARE
How to Recognize Preterm Labor

- Because the onset of preterm labor is subtle and often hard to recognize, it is important to know how to feel your abdomen for uterine contractions. You can feel for contractions in the following way. While lying down, place your fingertips on the top of your uterus. A contraction is the periodic tightening or hardening of your uterus. If your uterus is contracting, you will actually feel your abdomen get tight or hard and then feel it relax or soften when the contraction is over.
- If you think you are having any of the other signs and symptoms of preterm labor, empty your bladder, drink three to four glasses of water for hydration, lie down tilted toward your side, and place a pillow at your back for support.
- Check for contractions for 1 hour. To tell how often contractions are occurring, check the minutes that elapse from the beginning of one contraction to the beginning of the next.
- It is *not normal* to have frequent uterine contractions (every 10 minutes or more often for 1 hour).
- Contractions of labor are regular, frequent, and hard. They also may be felt as a tightening of the abdomen or a backache. This type of contraction causes the cervix to efface and dilate.
- Call your doctor, nurse-midwife, clinic, or labor and birth unit or go to the hospital if any of the following signs occur:
  - You have uterine contractions every 10 minutes or more often for 1 hour *or*
  - You have any of the other signs and symptoms for 1 hour *or*
  - You have any bloody spotting or leaking of fluid from your vagina
- It is often difficult to identify preterm labor. Accurate diagnosis requires assessment by the health care provider, usually in the hospital or clinic.
- Post these instructions where they can be seen by everyone in the family.

HOME CARE
Sexuality in Pregnancy

- Be aware that maternal physiologic changes such as breast enlargement, nausea, fatigue, abdominal changes, perineal enlargement, leukorrhea, pelvic vasocongestion, and orgasmic responses may affect sexuality and sexual expression.
- Discuss responses to pregnancy with your partner.
- Keep in mind that cultural prescriptions (do's) and proscriptions (don'ts) may affect your responses.
- Although your libido may be depressed during the first trimester, it often increases during the second trimester.
- Discuss and explore the following with your partner:
  - Alternative behaviors (e.g., mutual masturbation, foot massage, cuddling).
  - Alternative positions (e.g., female superior, side-lying) for sexual intercourse.
- Intercourse is safe as long as it is not uncomfortable. There is no correlation between intercourse and miscarriage, but observe the following precautions:
  - Abstain from intercourse if you experience uterine cramping or vaginal bleeding; report event to your health care provider as soon as possible.
  - Abstain from intercourse (or any activity that results in orgasm) if you have a history of premature dilation of the cervix until the problem is corrected.
- Continue to use risk-reduction behaviors. Women at risk for acquiring or conveying sexually transmitted infections are encouraged to use condoms during sexual intercourse throughout pregnancy.

physical, social, and emotional responses to sex during pregnancy. Not all maternity nurses are comfortable dealing with the sexual concerns of their patients. Be aware of your personal strengths and limitations in dealing with sexual content, and be prepared to make referrals if necessary.

Many women merely need permission to be sexually active during pregnancy. Many other women, however, need to be given information about the physiologic changes that occur during pregnancy, have the myths that are associated with sex during pregnancy dispelled, and participate in open discussions of positions for intercourse that decrease pressure on the gravid abdomen. Such tasks are within the purview of the nurse and should be an integral component of the health care rendered.

Some couples need to be referred for sex therapy or family therapy. Couples whose long-standing problems with sexual dysfunction are intensified by pregnancy are good candidates for sex therapy. When a sexual problem is a symptom of a more serious relationship problem, the couple would benefit from family therapy.

Using the History. The couple's sexual history provides a basis for counseling, but history taking also is an ongoing process. The history reveals the woman's knowledge of female anatomy and physiology and her attitudes about sex during pregnancy, as well as her perceptions of the pregnancy, the health status of the couple, and the quality of their relationship.

Countering Misinformation. Many myths and much of the misinformation related to sex and pregnancy are masked by seemingly unrelated issues. For example, a discussion about the baby's ability

to hear and see in utero may be prompted by questions about the baby being an "unseen observer" of sexual activities. The nurse must be extremely sensitive to the issues behind such questions when counseling in this highly charged emotional area.

Suggesting Alternative Behaviors. Research has not demonstrated that coitus and orgasm are contraindicated at any time during pregnancy for the obstetrically and medically healthy woman (Cunningham, Leveno, Bloom, et al., 2010). However, a history of more than one miscarriage; a threatened miscarriage in the first trimester; impending miscarriage in the second trimester; and PROM, bleeding, or abdominal pain during the third trimester warrant caution regarding coitus and orgasm.

Solitary and mutual masturbation and oral-genital intercourse may be used by couples as alternatives to penile-vaginal intercourse. Partners who enjoy cunnilingus (oral stimulation of the clitoris or vagina) may feel "turned off" by the normal increase in amount and odor of vaginal discharge during pregnancy. Couples who practice cunnilingus should be cautioned against the blowing of air into the vagina, particularly during the last few weeks of pregnancy when the cervix may be slightly open. An air embolism can occur if air is forced between the uterine wall and fetal membranes and enters the maternal vascular system through the placenta.

Showing the woman or couple illustrations of the possible variations of coital position is helpful (Fig. 8-19). The female-superior, side-by-side, rear-entry, and facing-each-other positions are alternatives to the traditional male-superior position. The woman astride (superior position) allows her to control the angle and depth of penile penetration, as well as protect her breasts and abdomen. During the third trimester, the side-by-side position or any position

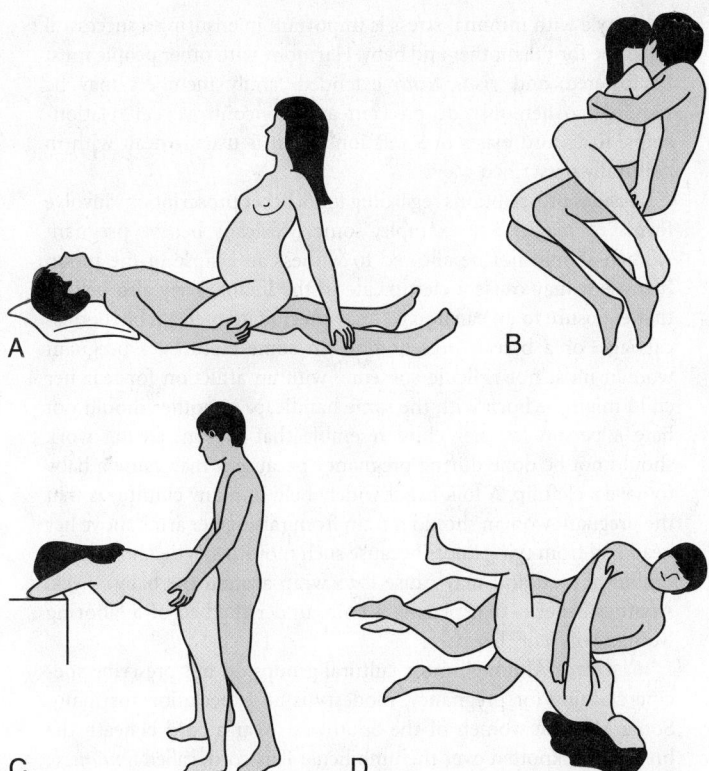

FIG 8-19 Positions for sexual intercourse during pregnancy. **A,** Female superior. **B,** Side by side. **C,** Rear entry. **D,** Facing each other.

that places less pressure on the pregnant abdomen and requires less energy may be preferred.

Multiparous women sometimes have significant breast tenderness in the first trimester. A coital position that avoids direct pressure on the woman's breasts and decreased breast fondling can be recommended to such couples. The woman should also be reassured that this condition is normal and temporary.

Some women complain of lower abdominal cramping and backache after orgasm during the first and third trimesters. A back rub can often relieve some of the discomfort and provide a pleasant experience. A tonic uterine contraction, often lasting up to a minute, replaces the rhythmic contractions of orgasm during the third trimester. Changes in FHR without fetal distress have also been reported.

The objective of risk reduction is to provide prophylaxis against the acquisition and transmission of sexually transmitted infections (STIs) (e.g., herpes simplex virus, human papilloma virus, and HIV). Because these diseases may be transmitted to the woman and her fetus, the use of condoms is recommended throughout pregnancy if the woman is at risk for acquiring an STI.

There is a lack of evidence regarding the safety of the use of sex toys during pregnancy. Popular pregnancy websites suggest that it is generally safe to use these devices in low-risk pregnancies (e.g., www.baby.com; www.parents.com). However, safety practices should be followed. Sex toys must be carefully cleaned. Sex toys inserted into the anus should never be inserted into the vagina. If a vibrator or other device is made of a material that is firmer than human flesh, force should not be used when inserting it into the vagina. The use of sex toys should be discontinued if pain occurs (Quilliam, 2010). Safer sex practices to reduce the risk of STIs

include using condoms and avoiding the sharing of sex toys (ACOG Committee on Health Care for Underserved Women, 2012b).

Well-informed nurses who are comfortable with their own sexuality and the sex counseling needs of expectant couples can offer information and advice in this valuable but often neglected area. They can establish an open environment in which couples can feel free to introduce their concerns about sexual adjustment and seek support and guidance. This intervention is as important for lesbian women and their partners as it is for women partnered with men.

Psychosocial Support

Esteem, affection, trust, concern, consideration of cultural and religious responses, and listening are all components of the emotional support given to the pregnant woman and her family. The woman's satisfaction with her relationships and support, her feeling of competence, and her sense of being in control are important issues to be addressed in the third trimester. A discussion of fetal responses to stimuli such as sound, light, maternal posture, and tension, as well as patterns of sleeping and waking, can be helpful. Other issues of concern that can arise for the pregnant woman and couple include fear of pain, loss of control, and possible birth of the infant before reaching the hospital. Parental concerns about the responsibilities and tasks of parenthood; the safety of the mother and unborn child; siblings and their acceptance of the new baby; social and economic responsibilities; and possible conflicts in cultural, religious, or personal value systems are addressed. The father's or partner's commitment to the pregnancy, the couple's relationship, and their concerns about sexuality and sexual expression can emerge as issues for many expectant parents.

Providing the prospective mother and father with opportunities to discuss their concerns and validating the normality of their responses can meet their needs to some degree. Nurses must also recognize that men feel more vulnerable during their partner's pregnancy. Female partners may also have these feelings. Anticipatory guidance and health promotion strategies can help partners cope with their concerns. Nursing intervention may help them deal with such concerns either directly through counseling or indirectly through the education of the mothers. Health care providers can stimulate and encourage open dialog between the couple.

Variations in Prenatal Care

The course of prenatal care described thus far can seem to suggest that the experiences of childbearing women are similar and that nursing interventions are uniform across all populations. Although typical patterns of response to pregnancy are easily recognized and many aspects of prenatal care indeed are consistent, pregnant women enter the health care system with individual concerns and needs. The nurse's ability to assess unique needs and tailor interventions to the individual is the hallmark of expertise in providing care. Variations that influence prenatal care include culture, age, and number of fetuses.

Cultural Influences

Prenatal care as we know it is a phenomenon of Western medicine. In the U.S. biomedical model of care, women are encouraged to seek prenatal care as early as possible in their pregnancy by visiting a physician and/or a nurse-midwife. This model not only is unfamiliar but also seems strange to women of other cultures.

Many cultural variations are found in prenatal care. Even if the prenatal care described is familiar to a woman, some practices may conflict with the beliefs and practices of a subculture group to which she belongs. Because of these and other factors, such as lack of money, lack of transportation, and language barriers, women from diverse cultures may not participate in the prenatal care system, for instance, by not keeping prenatal appointments. Such behavior may be misinterpreted by nurses as uncaring, lazy, or ignorant.

A concern for modesty is a deterrent to many women seeking prenatal care. For some women, exposing body parts, especially to a man, is considered a major violation of their modesty. For many women, invasive procedures, such as a vaginal examination, may be so threatening that they cannot be discussed even with their own husbands; therefore many women prefer a female health care provider. Too often, health care providers assume that women lose this modesty during pregnancy and labor, but most women value and appreciate efforts to maintain their modesty.

For many cultural groups, a physician is deemed appropriate only in times of illness. Because pregnancy is considered a normal process and the woman is in a state of health, the services of a physician are considered inappropriate. Western medicine's view of problems in pregnancy may differ from that of members of other cultural groups.

Although pregnancy is considered normal by many, certain practices are expected of women of all cultures to ensure a good outcome. *Cultural prescriptions* tell women what to do, and *cultural proscriptions* establish taboos. The purposes of these practices are to prevent maternal illness caused by a pregnancy-induced imbalanced state and to protect the vulnerable fetus. Prescriptions and proscriptions regulate the woman's emotional response, clothing, physical activity and rest, sexual activity, and dietary practices. Exploration of the woman's beliefs, perceptions of the meaning of childbearing, and health care practices may help health care providers foster her self-actualization, promote attainment of the maternal role, and positively influence her relationship with her spouse.

To provide culturally sensitive care, the nurse must be knowledgeable about practices and customs. Although it is not possible to know everything about every culture and subculture or the many lifestyles that exist, it is important to learn about the varied cultures in the setting in which a nurse practices. When exploring cultural beliefs and practices related to childbearing, the nurse can support and nurture the beliefs that promote physical or emotional adaptation (Fig. 8-20). However, if potentially harmful beliefs or activities are identified, the nurse should sensitively provide education and propose modifications.

Emotional Response. Virtually all cultures emphasize the importance of maintaining a socially harmonious and agreeable environment for the pregnant woman (see Community Focus box).

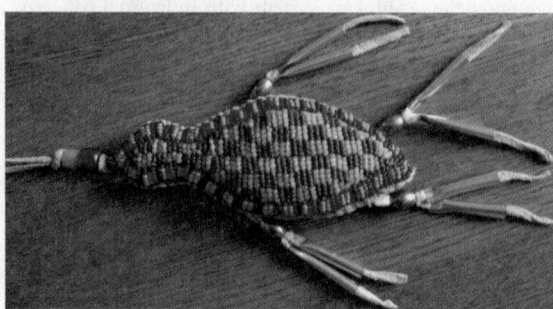

FIG 8-20 Umbilical amulet. Northern Plains tribes of Native Americans made amulets to hold the umbilical cord of a newborn child. The parents protected the child by ensuring that it was carried or worn by the child. (Courtesy Shannon Perry, Phoenix, AZ.)

A lifestyle with minimal stress is important in ensuring a successful outcome for the mother and baby. Harmony with other people must be fostered, and visits from extended family members may be required to demonstrate pleasant and noncontroversial relationships. If discord exists in a relationship, it is usually dealt with in culturally prescribed ways.

Besides proscriptions regarding food, other proscriptions involve forms of magic. For example, some Mexicans believe pregnant women should not be allowed to witness an eclipse of the moon because it may cause a cleft palate in the infant. They also believe that exposure to an earthquake may precipitate preterm birth, miscarriage, or a breech presentation. In some cultures, a pregnant woman must not ridicule someone with an affliction for fear her child might be born with the same handicap. A mother should not hate a person lest her child resemble that person. Dental work should not be done during pregnancy because it may cause a baby to have a cleft lip. A folk belief widely held in many cultures is that the pregnant woman should refrain from raising her arms above her head and from tying knots because such movements tie knots in the umbilical cord and may cause it to wrap around the baby's neck. Another belief is that placing a knife under the bed of a laboring woman will "cut" her pain.

Clothing. Although most cultural groups do not prescribe specific clothing for pregnancy, modesty is an expectation for many. Some Mexican women of the Southwest wear a cord beneath the breasts and knotted over the umbilicus. This cord, called a *muñeco,* is thought to prevent morning sickness and ensure a safe birth. Amulets, medals, and beads also may be worn to ward off evil spirits.

Physical Activity and Rest. Norms that regulate physical activity of mothers during pregnancy vary tremendously. Many groups, including Native Americans and some Asian groups, encourage women to be active, to walk, and to engage in normal although not strenuous activities to ensure that the baby is healthy and not too large. Other groups such as Filipinos believe that any activity is dangerous, and others willingly take over the work of the pregnant woman. Some Filipinos believe that this inactivity protects the mother and child. The mother is encouraged simply to produce the succeeding generation. If health care providers do not know of this belief, they could misinterpret this behavior as laziness or noncompliance with the desired prenatal health care regimen. It is important for the nurse to find out the way each pregnant woman views activity and rest.

Sexual Activity. In most cultures, sexual activity is not prohibited until the end of pregnancy. Some Latinos view sexual activity as necessary to keep the birth canal lubricated. Conversely, some Vietnamese have definite proscriptions about sexual intercourse,

COMMUNITY FOCUS
Culture and Childbirth Beliefs and Practices

Select an immigrant or other minority group in your community and identify childbirth-related beliefs and practices that are unique to that group. Are there stores in the area that sell items that meet the needs of that group? Does the community center have activities or classes that are directed toward that group? Are childbirth education programs available that provide essential information while incorporating cultural patterns? Are childbirth classes available in languages other than English? What could you, as a nurse, contribute to the community that would help meet the needs of that group?

requiring abstinence throughout the pregnancy because it is thought that sexual intercourse may harm the mother and the fetus.

Nutrition. Nutritional information given by Western health care providers may be a source of conflict for many cultural groups. Such a conflict commonly is not known by health care providers unless they understand the dietary beliefs and practices of the particular people for whom they are caring. For example, Muslims have strict regulations regarding preparation of food, and if meat cannot be prepared as prescribed, they may omit it from their diets. Many cultures permit pregnant women to eat only warm foods.

Age Differences

The age of the childbearing couple may have a significant influence on their physical and psychosocial adaptation to pregnancy. Normal developmental processes that occur in both very young and older mothers are interrupted by pregnancy and require a different type of adaptation to pregnancy from that of the woman of typical childbearing age. Although the individuality of each pregnant woman is recognized, special needs of expectant mothers 15 years of age or younger or those 35 years of age or older are summarized here.

Adolescents. Teenage pregnancy is a worldwide problem. The United States has one of the highest teen birth rates among industrialized nations. However, the rate of teen births has declined in the United States since the 1950s. From 2009 to 2010, the teen birth rate decreased 9% to the historic low of 34.3%. In 2010, there were 367,752 births to teens from ages 15 to 19 years, which is 43% lower than the highest number recorded in 1970 (644,708) (Hamilton and Ventura, 2012). Hispanic adolescents have the highest birth rate, although the rate for African-American adolescents also is high. Most of these young women are unmarried, and many are not ready for the emotional, psychosocial, and financial responsibilities of parenthood.

Numerous adolescent pregnancy-prevention programs have had varying degrees of success. Characteristics of programs that make a difference are those that have sustained commitment to adolescents over a long period, involve the parents and other adults in the community, promote abstinence and personal responsibility, and assist adolescents to develop a clear strategy for reaching future goals such as a college education or a career.

When adolescents become pregnant and decide to give birth, they are much less likely than older women to receive adequate prenatal care, with many receiving no care at all. These young women also are more likely to smoke and less likely to gain adequate weight during pregnancy. As a result of these and other factors, babies born to adolescents are at greatly increased risk for LBW, neglect and abuse, serious and long-term disability, and dying during the first year of life.

Delayed entry into prenatal care may be the result of late recognition of pregnancy, denial of pregnancy, or confusion about the services that are available. Such a delay in care may leave inadequate time before birth to attend to correctable problems. The very young pregnant adolescent is at higher risk for each of the confounding variables associated with poor pregnancy outcomes (e.g., socioeconomic factors) and for the conditions associated with a first pregnancy, regardless of age (e.g., gestational hypertension). However, when prenatal care is initiated early and consistently and confounding variables are controlled, very young pregnant adolescents are at no greater risk (nor are their infants) for an adverse outcome than older pregnant women. Thus the role of the nurse in reducing the risks and consequences of adolescent pregnancy is to encourage early and continued prenatal care; to provide early and ongoing education about pregnancy, birth, and parenting (Fig. 8-21); and to

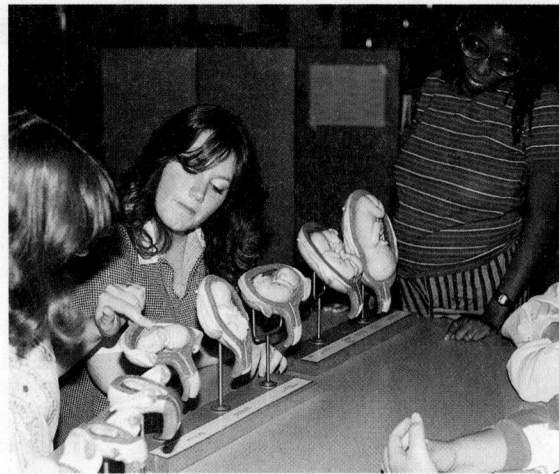

FIG 8-21 Pregnant adolescents review fetal development. (Courtesy Marjorie Pyle, RNC, Lifecircle, Costa Mesa, CA).

refer the adolescent, if necessary, for appropriate social support services, which can help reverse the effects of a negative socioeconomic environment (see Nursing Care Plan).

Women Older Than 35 Years. Two groups of older parents have emerged in the population of women having a child late in their childbearing years. One group consists of women who have many children or who have an additional child during the menopausal period. The other group consists of women who have deliberately delayed childbearing until their late 30s or early 40s.

The U.S. birth rate for women who are 40 to 44 years of age was 10.2 births per 1000 women, which is the highest rate since 1967. The birth rate for women 45 to 49 years of age is stable at 0.7 births per 1000 women (Hamilton, Martin, and Ventura, 2011).

Multiparous Women. Multiparous women may have never used contraceptives because of personal choice or a lack of knowledge concerning contraceptives. They also may be women who have used contraceptives successfully during the childbearing years but, as menopause approaches, cease menstruating regularly or stop using contraception and subsequently become pregnant. The older multiparous woman may believe that pregnancy separates her from her peer group and that her age is a hindrance to close associations with young mothers. Other parents welcome the unexpected infant as evidence of continuing maternal and paternal roles.

Primiparous Women. The number of first-time pregnancies in U.S. women between ages 35 and 40 years has increased significantly over the past three decades (Heron, Sutton, Xu, et al., 2010) to 10.5 per 1000 births (Hamilton, Martin, and Ventura, 2011). Seeing women in their late 30s or 40s during their first pregnancy is no longer unusual for health care providers. Reasons for delaying pregnancy include a desire to obtain advanced education, career priorities, and use of better contraceptive measures. Women who are infertile do not delay pregnancy deliberately but may become pregnant at a later age as a result of fertility studies and therapies.

These women choose parenthood. They often are established in a career and a lifestyle with a partner that includes time for self-attention, the establishment of a home with accumulated possessions, and freedom to travel. When asked the reason they chose pregnancy later in life, many reply, "Because time is running out."

The dilemma of choice includes recognition that being a parent will have both positive and negative consequences. Couples need to discuss the consequences of childbearing and childrearing before

◎ **NURSING CARE PLAN**

Adolescent Pregnancy

NURSING DIAGNOSIS	EXPECTED OUTCOMES	INTERVENTIONS	RATIONALES
Imbalanced Nutrition: Less Than Body Requirements related to intake insufficient to meet metabolic needs of fetus and adolescent patient	Adolescent will gain weight as prescribed by age, take prenatal vitamins/iron as prescribed, and maintain normal hematocrit and hemoglobin.	Assess current diet history/intake	To determine prescriptions for additions or changes in present dietary pattern
		Compare prepregnancy weight with current weight	To determine if pattern of weight gain is consistent with appropriate fetal growth and development
		Provide information concerning food prescriptions for appropriate weight gain, considering preferences for "fast food" and peer influences	To correct any misconceptions and increase chances for compliance with diet
		Include adolescent's immediate family or support system during instruction	To ensure that person preparing family meals receives information
Risk for Injury, maternal or fetal, related to inadequate prenatal care and screening	Adolescent will experience uncomplicated pregnancy and give birth to healthy fetus at term.	Provide information, using therapeutic communication and confidentiality	To establish relationship and build trust
		Discuss importance of ongoing prenatal care and possible risks to adolescent patient and fetus	To reinforce that ongoing assessment is crucial to health and well-being of patient and fetus, even if patient feels well. The adolescent patient is more at risk for certain complications that may be avoided or managed early if prenatal visits are maintained
		Discuss risks of alcohol, tobacco, and recreational drug use during pregnancy	To minimize risks to patient and fetus because adolescent patients have higher abuse rate than rest of pregnant population
		Assess for evidence of sexually transmitted infection (STI), and provide information regarding sexual practices	To minimize risk to patient and fetus because adolescent is more at risk for STIs
		Screen for preeclampsia on an ongoing basis	To minimize risk because adolescent population is more at risk for preeclampsia
Social Isolation related to body image changes of pregnant adolescent as evidenced by patient statements and concerns	Adolescent will identify support systems and report decreased feelings of social isolation.	Establish a therapeutic relationship	To listen objectively and establish trust
		Discuss with patient changes in relationships that have occurred as result of pregnancy	To determine extent of isolation from family, peers, and father of baby
		Provide referrals and resources appropriate for developmental stage of patient	To give information for patient support
		Provide information regarding parenting classes, breastfeeding classes, and childbirth preparation classes	To give further information and group support, which lessens social isolation
Interrupted Family Processes related to adolescent pregnancy	Adolescent will reestablish relationship with her mother and father of baby.	Encourage communication with mother	To clarify roles and relationships related to birth of infant
		Encourage communication with father of baby (if she desires continued contact)	To ascertain level of support to be expected of father of baby
		Refer to support group	To learn more effective problem-solving methods and reduce conflict within the family
Disturbed Body Image related to situational crisis of pregnancy	Adolescent will verbalize positive comments regarding her body image during pregnancy.	Assess pregnant adolescent's perception of self related to pregnancy	To provide basis for further interventions
		Give information regarding expected body changes occurring during pregnancy	To provide a realistic view of these temporary changes
		Provide opportunity to discuss personal feelings and concerns	To promote trust and support

NURSING CARE PLAN

Adolescent Pregnancy—cont'd

NURSING DIAGNOSIS	EXPECTED OUTCOMES	INTERVENTIONS	RATIONALES
Risk for Impaired Parenting related to immaturity and lack of experience in new role of adolescent mother	Parents will demonstrate parenting roles with confidence.	Provide information on growth and development	To enhance knowledge so that adolescent mother can have basis for caring for her infant
		Refer to parenting classes	To enhance knowledge and obtain support for providing appropriate care to newborn and infant
		Initiate discussion of child care	To assist adolescent in problem solving for future needs
		Assess parenting abilities of adolescent mother and father	To provide baseline for education
		Provide information on parenting classes that are appropriate for parents' developmental stage	To give opportunity to share common feelings and concerns
		Assist parents to identify pertinent support systems	To give assistance with parenting as needed

committing themselves to this lifelong venture. Partners in this group seem to share the preparation for parenthood, the planning for a family-centered birth, and the desire to be loving and competent parents. However, the reality of child care may prove difficult for them.

First-time mothers older than 35 years select the "right time" for pregnancy; this time is influenced by their awareness of the increasing possibility of infertility or of genetic defects in the infants of older women. Such women seek information about pregnancy from books, friends, and electronic resources. They actively try to prevent fetal disorders and are careful in searching for the best possible maternity care. They identify sources of stress in their lives. They have concerns about having enough energy and stamina to meet the demands of parenting and their new roles and relationships.

If older women become pregnant after treatment for infertility, they may suddenly have negative or ambivalent feelings about the pregnancy. They may experience a multifetal pregnancy that may create emotional and physical problems. Adjusting to parenting two or more infants requires adaptability and additional resources.

During pregnancy, parents explore the possibilities and responsibilities of changing identities and new roles. They must prepare a safe and nurturing environment during pregnancy and after birth. They must integrate the child into an established family system and negotiate new roles (parent, sibling, and grandparent roles) for family members.

Adverse perinatal outcomes are more common in older primiparas than in younger women, even when they receive good prenatal care. Women 35 years of age and older are more likely than younger primiparas to have infants with chromosomal abnormalities, LBW infants, preterm birth, abruptio placentae, and multiple gestation (Johnson and Tough, 2012). The incidence of malpresentation also is more common in older primiparas, and they are more likely to have a cesarean birth. In addition, in women ages 35 years or older, there is an increased risk for maternal mortality from hemorrhage, infection, embolisms, hypertensive disorders of pregnancy, cardiomyopathy, and strokes.

Multifetal Pregnancy

A multifetal pregnancy, or pregnancy with more than one fetus, places the mother and fetuses at increased risk for adverse outcomes.

The maternal blood volume is increased, resulting in an increased strain on the maternal cardiovascular system. Anemia often develops because of a greater demand for iron by the fetuses. Marked uterine distention, increased pressure on the adjacent viscera and pelvic vasculature, and diastasis of the two rectus abdominis muscles may occur (see Fig. 7-13). Placenta previa develops more commonly in multifetal pregnancies because of the large size or placement of the placentas. Premature separation of the placenta may occur before the second and any subsequent fetuses are born.

Twin pregnancies often end prematurely. Spontaneous rupture of membranes before term is common. Congenital malformations are twice as common in monozygotic twins as in singletons, although there is no increase in the incidence of congenital anomalies in dizygotic twins. Two-vessel cords (i.e., cords with a single umbilical artery) occur more often in twins than in singletons; this abnormality is most common in monozygotic twins. The most serious problem for the fetus is the local shunting of blood between placentas (twin-to-twin transfusion); this causes the recipient twin to be larger and the donor twin to be small, pallid, dehydrated, malnourished, and hypovolemic. However, the larger twin may develop congenital heart failure during the first 24 hours after birth.

The clinical diagnosis of multifetal pregnancy is accurate in about 90% of cases. The likelihood of a multifetal pregnancy is increased if any one or a combination of the following factors is noted during a careful assessment:

- History of dizygotic twins in the female lineage
- Use of fertility drugs
- More rapid uterine growth for the number of weeks of gestation
- Polyhydramnios
- Palpation of more than the expected number of small or large parts
- Asynchronous fetal heartbeats or more than one fetal electrocardiographic tracing
- Ultrasonographic evidence of more than one fetus

The diagnosis of multifetal pregnancy is a shock to many expectant parents, and they may need additional support and education to help them cope with the changes they face. The mother needs nutrition counseling so that she gains more weight than that needed for a singleton birth. She should also be counseled that maternal adaptations will probably be more uncomfortable, and she should be provided with information about the possibility of a preterm birth.

If the presence of more than three fetuses is diagnosed, the parents may face decisions regarding selective reduction of the fetuses to reduce the incidence of premature birth and improve the opportunities for the remaining fetuses to grow to term gestation (Cunningham, Leveno, Bloom, et al., 2010). This situation poses an ethical dilemma for many couples, especially those who have worked hard to overcome problems with infertility and those who harbor strong values regarding the right to life. Nurses can initiate discussions with couples to help them identify resources (e.g., a minister, priest, rabbi, or mental health counselor) to aide in the decision-making process.

Prenatal care for women with multifetal pregnancies includes changes in the pattern of care and modifications in other aspects such as the amount of weight gained and the nutritional intake necessary. For example, the prenatal visits of these mothers are scheduled at least every 2 weeks in the second trimester and weekly thereafter. Fetal growth is carefully monitored throughout pregnancy using regular ultrasound evaluations. The recommended weight gain is increased with twin gestation; women with normal prepregnancy weight should gain 17 to 25 kg (37.4 to 55 lb) (Rasmussen and Yaktine, 2009). Iron and vitamin supplements are desirable.

The considerable uterine distention involved in a multifetal pregnancy can worsen the backache commonly experienced by pregnant women. Maternity support hose may be worn to control leg varicosities. Every multifetal pregnancy is at risk for preterm labor; thus the women receive frequent ultrasound examinations, FHR monitoring, and nonstress tests. Routine bedrest is not recommended in twin pregnancies at low risk for preterm labor. Some practitioners recommend bedrest beginning at 20 weeks for women carrying triplets or more to prevent preterm labor (Newman and Unal, 2012). If bedrest is recommended, the mother needs to assume the lateral position to promote increased placental perfusion. If birth is delayed until after the thirty-sixth week, the risk for morbidity and mortality decreases for the neonates.

Multiple newborns will likely place a strain on finances, space, workload, and the mother's and family's coping abilities. Lifestyle changes may be necessary. Parents will need assistance in making realistic plans for the care of the babies (e.g., whether to breastfeed and whether to raise them as "alike" or as separate individuals). Parents can be referred to national organizations such as Mother of Twins (www.nomotc.org) and the La Leche League (www.lalecheleague.org) for further support.

CHILDBIRTH AND PERINATAL EDUCATION

The goal of childbirth and perinatal education is to assist individuals and their family members to make informed, safe decisions about pregnancy, birth, and early parenthood. It also is to assist them to comprehend the long-lasting effects that empowering birth experiences have in the lives of women and the impact of early experiences on the development of children and the family. Perinatal education ideally begins in the preconception period when women are considering pregnancy and continues throughout the prenatal period as nurses and other health care providers provide ongoing education for pregnant women and their partners during regular prenatal visits.

Contemporary perinatal education programs are an expansion of the earlier childbirth education movement that originally offered a set of classes in the third trimester of pregnancy to prepare parents for birth. Today perinatal education programs consist of a menu of class series and activities from preconception through the early months of parenting.

Health-promoting education should be provided in a context that emphasizes how a healthy body is best able to adapt to the changes that accompany pregnancy. Without this context of health, routine care and testing for risks may contribute to a mindset of families that pregnancy is a pathologic as opposed to a healthy mind-body-spirit event.

Some of the decisions the childbearing family must consider are whether to have a baby, followed by choices of a care provider and type of care (a midwifery model [natural oriented] versus a medical [intervention oriented] model); the place for birth (hospital, birthing center, home); and the type of infant feeding (breast or bottle) and infant care. If a woman previously had a cesarean birth, she may consider a trial of labor after cesarean (TOLAC) to attempt a vaginal birth. Perinatal education can provide information to help childbearing families make informed decisions about these issues.

Previous pregnancy and childbirth experiences are important elements that influence current learning needs. Other important factors include the age of the woman and her support person, their cultural background, personal philosophy with regard to childbirth, socioeconomic status, spiritual beliefs, and learning styles. The nurse considers all of these in helping the woman and her partner develop the best plan to meet their needs.

Typically, the pregnant woman is accompanied by her partner when attending childbirth education classes, although sometimes a friend, teenage daughter, or parent is the designated support person. There are also classes for grandparents and siblings to prepare them for their attendance at birth and/or the arrival of the baby. Siblings often see a film about birth and learn ways they can help welcome the baby. They also learn to cope with changes that include a reduction in parental time and attention. Grandparents learn about current child care practices and how to help their adult children adapt to parenting in a supportive way.

Perinatal Education Programs

Childbearing, when one is prepared and well supported, presents to women a unique and powerful opportunity to find their core strength in a manner that forever changes their self-perception. Expectant parents and their families have different interests and information needs as the pregnancy progresses.

A variety of approaches to childbirth education have evolved as childbirth educators attempt to meet learning needs of expectant parents. In addition to classes designed specifically for pregnant adolescents, their partners, and/or parents, classes exist for other groups with special learning needs. These include classes for first-time mothers older than 35 years, single women, adoptive parents, parents of multiples, or women with disabilities such as those who are visually impaired or deaf. Refresher classes for parents with children not only review coping techniques for labor and birth but also help couples prepare for sibling reactions and adjustments to a new baby. Cesarean birth classes are available for couples who have this kind of birth scheduled because of breech presentation or other risk factors. Other classes focus on vaginal birth after cesarean (VBAC) because many women can successfully give birth vaginally after previous cesarean birth.

Throughout the series of classes, support systems that people can use during pregnancy and after birth are discussed. Such support systems help parents function independently and effectively. During all the classes, the open expression of feelings and concerns about any aspect of pregnancy, birth, and parenting is welcomed.

Early pregnancy ("early bird") classes provide fundamental information. Classes are developed around the following areas: (1) early fetal development, (2) physiologic and emotional changes of pregnancy, (3) human sexuality, and (4) the nutritional needs of the mother and fetus. The classes often address environmental and workplace hazards. Exercises, nutrition, warning signs, drugs, and self-medication also are topics of interest and concern.

Mid-pregnancy classes emphasize the woman's participation in self-management. Classes provide information on preparation for breastfeeding and formula-feeding, infant care, basic hygiene, common complaints and simple safe remedies, infant health, parenting, and updating and refining the birth plans.

Late pregnancy classes emphasize labor and birth. There are different methods of coping with labor and birth, and these are often the basis for various prenatal classes. These include Lamaze, Bradley, and Dick-Read. These classes usually include a tour of the birthing facility. Because fear of pain in labor is a key issue for many women, preparation for childbirth classes provide information on management of discomfort during labor and birth. Topics include relaxation and breathing techniques, imagery and visualization, biofeedback, and pharmacologic interventions such as intravenous medications and epidural analgesia. Couples need information about the advantages and disadvantages of pain medication and about other techniques for coping with labor. An emphasis on non-pharmacologic pain management strategies helps couples manage the labor and birth with dignity and increased comfort. Most instructors teach a flexible approach, which helps couples learn and master many techniques to use during labor (see Chapter 14 for further discussion).

Perinatal Care Choices

Often the first decision the woman makes is who will be her primary health care provider for the pregnancy and birth. This decision is doubly important because it usually affects where the birth will take place. The nurse can provide information about the different types of health care providers and what kind of care to expect from each type. Women are encouraged to ask potential care providers a series of pertinent questions (Box 8-5).

Physicians

Physicians (obstetricians, family medicine physicians, osteopathic physicians) attended 92% of hospital births and 5% of home births in the United States in 2009 (MacDorman, Mathews, and Declercq, 2012). Family practice physicians and osteopathic physicians provide care for primarily low risk pregnant women and refer high risk patients to obstetricians. Obstetricians see low risk and high risk patients. Care often includes pharmacologic and medical management of problems as well as use of technologic procedures.

Nurse-Midwives

Certified nurse-midwives are registered nurses with education in the two disciplines of nursing and midwifery. Throughout history, midwives have held a holistic view of childbirth. In 2009, certified nurse midwives attended 7.4% of hospital births and 19% of home births (MacDorman, Mathews, and Declercq, 2012). Nurse-midwives practice with physicians or independently with an arrangement for physician backup. They usually see low risk obstetric patients. Care is often noninterventionist, and the woman and her family are encouraged to be active participants in the care. Nurse-midwives refer patients with complications to physicians.

BOX 8-5	QUESTIONS TO ASK POTENTIAL MATERNITY CARE PROVIDERS

The Coalition to Improve Maternity Services (CIMS), a group of more than 50 nursing and maternity care–oriented organizations, produced a document to assist women in selecting their perinatal care. After some explanation of choices, women are encouraged to ask potential care providers the following questions:

- Who can be with me during labor and birth?
- What happens during a normal labor and birth in your setting?
- How do you allow for differences in culture and beliefs?
- Can I walk and move around during labor? What position do you suggest for birth?
- How do you make sure everything goes smoothly when my nurse, doctor, midwife, or agency works with each other?
- What things do you normally do to a woman in labor?
- How do you help mothers stay as comfortable as they can be? Besides drugs, how do you help mothers relieve the pain of labor?
- What if my baby is born early or has special problems?
- Do you circumcise babies?
- How do you help mothers who want to breastfeed?

Adapted from Coalition to Improve Maternity Services (CIMS): *Having a baby? 10 questions to ask*, 2000, www.motherfriendly.org/Resources/Documents/Having_a_Baby-English.pdf.

Direct-Entry Midwives

Direct-entry midwives (also called *certified professional midwives*) are trained in midwifery schools or universities as a profession distinct from nursing. In the United States, their certification process is administered by the American College of Nurse-Midwives. They also refer the patients in whom problems develop to physicians. Increasing numbers of midwives in the United Kingdom and Ireland are in this category.

Independent Midwives

Independent midwives, who also may be called *lay midwives*, are nonprofessional caregivers. Their training varies greatly, from self-teaching to formal training. They manage about 1% of births in the United States. Patients who develop problems are referred to a physician. A majority of births are managed in the home setting. In many international settings, lay midwives are called *traditional birth attendants*. Births are in the home.

Doulas

A doula is professionally trained to provide labor support, including physical, emotional, and informational support, to women and their partners during labor and birth. The doula does not become involved with clinical tasks (Doulas of North America [DONA], 2008). Today many couples, no matter which type of childbirth classes they take, also employ a doula for labor support.

A doula typically meets with the woman and her partner before labor. At this meeting, the doula assesses the woman's expectations and desires for the birth experience. With this information as a guide during labor and birth, the doula focuses efforts on assisting the woman to achieve her goals. Doulas work collaboratively with other health care providers and the partner or other support persons, but their primary goal is to assist the woman. Doulas who are also trained medical interpreters can enhance the care of women with limited English proficiency (Maher, Crawford-Carr, and Neidigh, 2012).

BOX 8-6 QUESTIONS TO ASK WHEN CHOOSING A DOULA

To discover the specific training, experience, and services offered by anyone who provides labor support, potential patients, nursing supervisors, physicians, midwives, and others should ask the following questions of that person:

- What training have you had?
- Tell me about your experience with birth, both personally and as a doula.
- What is your philosophy about childbirth and supporting women and their partners through labor?
- May we meet to discuss our birth plans and the role you will play in supporting me through childbirth?
- May we call you with questions or concerns before and after the birth?
- When do you try to join women in labor? Do you come to our home or meet us at the hospital?
- Do you meet with us after the birth to review the labor and answer questions?
- Do you work with one or more backup doulas for times when you are not available? May we meet them?
- What is your fee?

Adapted from Doulas of North America: *Doulas of North America position paper: the birth doula's contribution to modern maternity care*, 2008, www.dona.org/pdfs/position_papers/BIRTH%20 Paper–%204%20page.pdf.

Doulas may be found through community contacts, other health care providers, or childbirth educators; a number of organizations offer information or referral services. It is important that the expectant mother be comfortable with the doula who will be attending her. See Box 8-6 for a list of questions to ask when arranging for a doula. Doulas of North America (DONA) is an organization that certifies doulas (www.dona.org). Although the doula role originally developed as an assistant during labor, some women and their families benefit from assistance during the postpartum period. Postpartum doulas provide assistance to the new mother as she develops competence with infant care, feeding, and other maternal tasks and to the family as they adjust to life with a new baby.

Birth Plans

The birth plan is a natural evolution of a contemporary wellness-oriented lifestyle in which patients assume a level of responsibility for their own health. The birth plan is a tool with which parents can explore their childbirth options and choose those that are most important to them. The plan must be viewed as tentative since the realities of what is feasible may change as the actual labor and birth unfold. It is understood to be a preference list based on a best-case scenario.

It is useful for the nurse in a prenatal practice setting to initiate a discussion of choices and birth planning during the first and second prenatal visits. Some maternity practices provide printed material describing available options and giving answers to commonly asked questions, and tours of the birth setting are offered by almost all birthing facilities. The nurse can provide couples with pertinent information and make them aware of the various options for care and the advantages and consequences of each so they can begin making informed decisions. Early plans can be modified as the couple learn more details in their childbirth class. Topics for the expectant parents to consider when creating a birth plan are listed in the Family-Centered Care box.

FAMILY-CENTERED CARE

Creating a Birth Plan

Topics for birth plan discussion and decision making may include any or all of the following:

Partner's participation: Attend prenatal visits? Childbirth and parent education classes? Present during labor? During birth? During cesarean birth?

Birth setting: Hospital delivery room or birthing room (if available)? A birthing center? Home?

Labor management: Walk around during labor? Use a rocking chair? Use a shower? Use a Jacuzzi, if available? Intermittent versus continuous use of an electronic fetal monitor? Have music or dimmed lighting? Have older children or other people present? Is telemetry monitoring available? Consider stimulation of labor? Consider medication—what kind?

Birth: Positions—Side-lying? On hands and knees, kneeling, or squatting? Use a birthing bed or delivery table? Will you be photographing, videotaping, or recording any of the labor or birth? Who would you like to be present—partner, older siblings, other family members, or friends? What do you know about the use of forceps? Episiotomy? Will your partner want to cut the umbilical cord? Emergency considerations/contingencies (e.g., cesarean)?

Immediately after birth: Do you want to hold the baby skin-to-skin right away? Breastfeed immediately?

Postpartum care: What kind of care do you anticipate—labor, delivery, recovery, postpartum room; mother-baby couplet care? How long does your insurance company provide coverage for you to stay? Would you like to attend self-management classes, or do you prefer to get such information from media sources? On which subjects?

The birth plan can serve as a means of open communication between the pregnant woman and her partner and also between the couple and health care providers. An early introduction to the idea of a birth plan allows the couple time to think about events or situations that could make their childbearing experience more meaningful and those they would prefer to avoid (Anderson and Kilpatrick, 2012).

Traditionally, birth plans are created prenatally and implemented upon admission to the labor and birth unit. However, when women without predesigned birth plans are admitted, nurses can use a template with simple questions about preferences for care to help them develop a simple birth plan (Anderson and Kilpatrick, 2012; Kuo, Lin, Hsu, et al., 2010). This is in accordance with the Association of Women's Health, Obstetrics and Neonatal Nurses's (AWHONN's) position statement on nursing support of laboring women, specifically creating individualized care plans for laboring women based on their needs, desires, and expectations (AWHONN, 2011).

Birth Setting Choices

With careful thought, the concept of natural, family, or woman-centered maternity care can be implemented in any setting. The three primary options for birth settings today are the hospital, birth center, and home. Women consider several factors in choosing a setting for childbirth, including the preference of their health care provider, characteristics of the birthing unit, and preference of their third-party payer. Approximately 99% of all births in the United States take place in a hospital setting (MacDorman, Mathews, and Declercq, 2012). However, the types of labor and birth services vary greatly, from the traditional labor and delivery rooms with separate

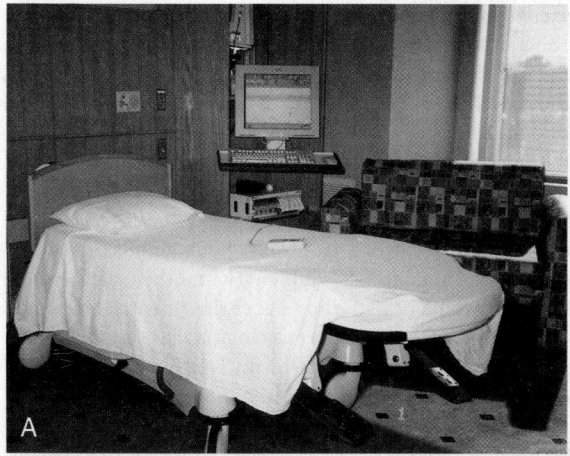

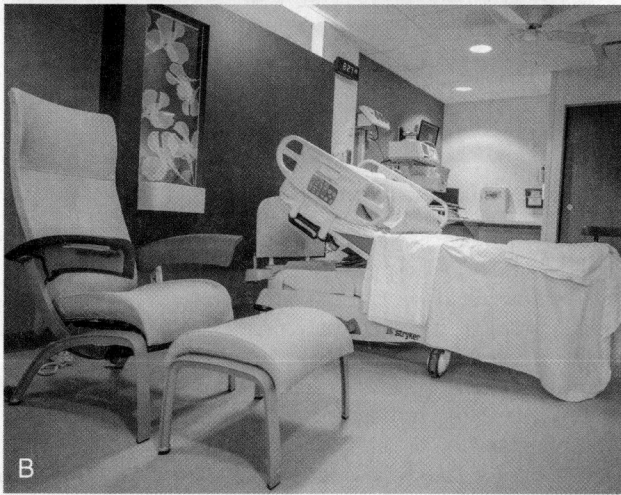

FIG 8-22 Labor, delivery, recovery, and postpartum (LDRP) units. (*A,* Courtesy Dee Lowdermilk, Chapel Hill, NC. *B,* Courtesy Mercy Hospital, St Louis, MO.)

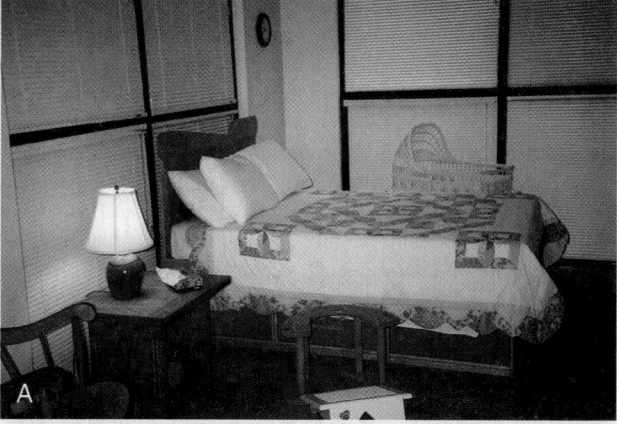

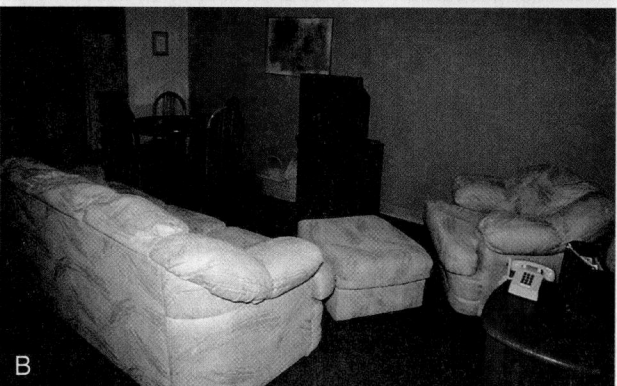

FIG 8-23 Birth center. **A,** Note double bed, baby crib, and birthing stool. **B,** Lounge and kitchen. (*A,* Courtesy Dee Lowdermilk, Chapel Hill, NC. *B,* Courtesy Michael S. Clement, MD, Mesa, AZ. Photo location: Bethany Birth Center, Phoenix, AZ.)

postpartum and newborn units to in-hospital birthing centers where all or almost all care takes place in a single unit.

Labor, Delivery, Recovery, Postpartum (Birthing) Rooms

Labor, delivery, and recovery (LDR) and labor, delivery, recovery, and postpartum (LDRP) rooms offer families a comfortable, private space for childbirth (Fig. 8-22). Women are admitted to LDR units, labor and give birth, and spend the first 1 to 2 hours postpartum there for immediate recovery and to have time with their families to bond with their newborns. After this period of recovery, the mothers and newborns are transferred to a postpartum unit and nursery or mother-baby unit for the duration of their stay. Care is provided by different nursing staff (e.g., labor and delivery nurses, postpartum nurses, nursery nurses). In some hospitals, the same nurse provides care for both mothers and newborns (mother-baby or couplet care).

In LDRP units, total care is provided from admission for labor through postpartum discharge in the same room and usually by the same nursing staff. The woman and her family may stay in this unit for 6 to 48 hours after giving birth. The units are furnished in a homelike atmosphere, similar to LDR units but have accommodations for family members to stay overnight (see Fig. 8-22, *A*).

Both units are equipped with fetal monitors, emergency resuscitation equipment for both mother and newborn, and heated cribs or warming units for the newborn. Often this equipment is out of sight in cabinets or closets when it is not being used (see Fig. 8-22, *B*).

Birth Centers

Free-standing birth centers are usually built in locations separate from the hospital but may be located nearby in case transfer of the woman or newborn is needed. These birth centers are intended to offer families an alternative to hospital or home birth, providing a third choice that is a safe and cost-effective compromise. The centers are usually staffed by nurse-midwives or physicians who also have privileges at the local hospital. Only women at low risk for complications are included for care.

Birth centers typically have homelike accommodations, including a double bed for the couple and a crib for the newborn (Fig. 8-23, *A*). Emergency equipment and drugs are available but stored out of view. Private bathroom facilities are incorporated into each birth unit. There may be an early labor lounge or a living room and small kitchen (see Fig. 8-23, *B*). The family is admitted to the birth center for labor and birth and will remain there until discharge, which often takes place within 6 hours of the birth.

Other services provided by the free-standing birth centers include those necessary for safe management during the childbearing cycle. Attendance at childbirth and parenting classes is required of all patients. Expectant families develop birth plans (i.e., the practices and procedures they would like to either include or exclude from their childbirth experience). Patients must understand that some situations require transfer to a hospital, and they must agree to abide by those guidelines.

Birth centers and hospitals with a comprehensive birthing program may have resources for parents such as a lending library that includes books and videotapes; reference files on related topics; recycled maternity clothes, baby clothes, and equipment; and supplies and reference materials for childbirth educators. The centers may also have referral files for community resources that offer services relating to childbirth and early parenting, including support groups (e.g., for single parents, postbirth support, and parents of twins), genetic counseling, women's issues, and consumer action.

When births occur in a birth center or a home setting, they should be located close to a major hospital so that quick transfer to that institution is possible when necessary. Ambulance service and emergency procedures must be readily available. Fees vary with the services provided but typically are less than or equal to those charged by local hospitals. Some base fees on the ability of the family to pay (a reduced-fee sliding scale). Several third-party payers, as well as Medicaid and the Civilian Health and Medical Programs of the Uniformed Services (TRICARE/CHAMPUS), recognize and reimburse these centers.

Home Birth

Home birth has always been popular in certain countries such as Sweden and The Netherlands. In developing countries, hospitals or adequate lying-in facilities often are unavailable to most pregnant women and home birth is a necessity. In the United States, 0.72% of births occurred in a home setting in 2009. This is a 29% increase from 0.56% in 2004 (MacDorman, Mathews, and Declercq, 2012).

Home birth remains a controversial topic in American health care (Lowe, 2009). Organizations such as the American College of Obstetricians and Gynecologists (ACOG) and the American Medical Association agree that the safest setting for birth is a hospital or birthing center that meets standards set forth by AAP and ACOG or a freestanding birth center that meets standards of the Accreditation Association for Ambulatory Health Care (ACOG Committee on Obstetric Practice, 2011b; American Medical Association, 2008). ACOG emphasizes the need to inform women considering planned home birth about risks and benefits; while they note that absolute risk may be low, they cite a twofold to threefold increased risk for neonatal death with home birth compared with planned hospital birth (ACOG Committee on Obstetric Practice, 2011b). Research findings based on cohort and observational studies do not support this stance. Large-scale studies have documented the safety of planned home birth for healthy, low risk women who are attended

by registered midwives and when there is a system in place for transfer to a hospital facility (de Jonge, van der Goes, Ravelli, et al., 2009; Hutton, Reitsma, and Kaufman, 2009; Janssen, Saxell, Page, et al., 2009; McIntyre, 2012). The National Perinatal Association (2008) and the American College of Nurse Midwives (2011) support planned home birth for carefully selected low risk women within a system that provides hospitalization as needed.

With a home birth, the family is in control of the experience and the birth may be more physiologically natural in familiar surroundings (see Critical Thinking Case Study). The mother may be more relaxed than she would be in the hospital environment. Home births are typically unmedicated (no pharmacologic analgesia). The family can assist in and be a part of the birth, and the mother-father/partner-infant (and sibling-infant) contact is immediate and sustained. Home birth may be less expensive than a hospital confinement. Serious infection may be less likely (assuming strict aseptic principles are followed) because it is usual for people to be relatively immune to the bacteria in their own home.

? CRITICAL THINKING CASE STUDY

Deciding About a Home Birth

Maxine, 37 years old and gravida 1, para 0, is interested in having a home birth. She has insulin-dependent diabetes. She is currently 14 weeks pregnant, and her pregnancy is progressing normally. According to an ultrasound examination, she has one fetus of appropriate size for gestational age with no detectable anomalies. She asks a nurse on the obstetric clinic about how to find a midwife who will attend a home birth.

1. Evidence—Is there sufficient evidence to draw conclusions about the safety of a home birth for Maxine?
2. Assumptions—Describe an underlying assumption about each of the following issues:
   a. Assessments that are necessary to identify whether it is feasible and safe for Maxine to have a home birth
   b. Supports necessary for a home birth
   c. How to identify providers who are willing to attend a home birth
   d. Ethics of the nurse assisting Maxine to find a midwife who will attend a home birth
3. What implications and priorities for nursing care can be drawn at this time?
4. Does the evidence objectively support your conclusion?

■ KEY POINTS

- The prenatal period is a preparatory one, both physically and psychologically.
- Psychosocial aspects of care may affect pregnancy, childbirth, and the adjustment of the new family.
- The pregnant woman's readiness to learn is at a high level, making this an excellent time to help her expand her self-management skills.
- Maternal physical and familial adaptations to pregnancy generate needs that the nurse can anticipate and meet.
- Even with a normal pregnancy, the nurse must remain alert to hazards such as supine hypotension, warning signs and symptoms, and signs of family maladaptations.
- Each pregnant woman needs to know how to recognize and report preterm labor.

- Parent-child, sibling-child, and grandparent-child relationships are affected by pregnancy.
- Cultural prescriptions and proscriptions influence responses to pregnancy and to the health care delivery system.
- Childbirth education teaches tuning in to the body's inner wisdom and coping strategies that enhance women's ability to know how to give birth.
- Childbirth education is a process designed to help parents make the transition from the role of expectant parents to the role and responsibilities of parents of a new baby.
- Nurses provide information that enables expectant parents to make informed choices about their health care provider and birth setting.

REFERENCES

Agency for Healthcare Research and Quality (AHRQ) Healthcare Innovations Exchange: Nurse home visits improve outcomes for low-income, first-time mothers and their children, 2012, www.innovations.ahrq.gov/content.aspx?id=2229.

American Academy of Pediatrics (AAP) Committee on Fetus and Newborn and American College of Obstetricians and Gynecologists (ACOG) Committee on Obstetric Practice: Guidelines for perinatal care, ed 7, Washington, DC, 2012, Author.

American Academy of Pediatrics (AAP) Section on Breastfeeding: Breastfeeding and the use of human milk, Pediatrics 129(3): e827–e841, 2012.

American College of Nurse Midwives: Position statement: home birth, 2011, www.midwife.org/ACNM/files/ACNMLibraryData/UPLOADFILENAME/000000000251/Home%20Birth%20Aug%202011.pdf.

American College of Obstetricians and Gynecologists (ACOG): Practice bulletin 101: ultrasonography in pregnancy, Obstet Gynecol 113(2 Pt 1): 451–461, 2009.

American College of Obstetricians and Gynecologists (ACOG) Committee on Obstetric Practice: Committee opinion no. 462: moderate caffeine consumption during pregnancy, Obstet Gynecol 116(2):467–468, 2010.

American College of Obstetricians and Gynecologists (ACOG) Committee on Genetics: Committee opinion no. 486: update on carrier screening for cystic fibrosis, Obstet Gynecol 117(4):1028–1031, 2011.

American College of Obstetricians and Gynecologists (ACOG) Committee on Health Care for Underserved Women: Committee opinion no. 518: intimate partner violence, Obstet Gynecol 119(2): 412–417, 2012a.

American College of Obstetricians and Gynecologists (ACOG) Committee on Health Care for Underserved Women: Committee opinion no. 525: Health care for lesbians and bisexual women, Obstet Gynecol 119(5):1077–1080, 2012b.

American College of Obstetricians and Gynecologists (ACOG) Committee on Obstetric Practice: Committee opinion no. 418: prenatal and perinatal human immunodeficiency virus testing—expanded recommendations, 2011a, www.acog.org/About_ACOG/ACOG_Departments/HIV/~/media/Committee%20Opinions/Committee%20on%20Obstetric%20Practice/co418.pdf.

American College of Obstetricians and Gynecologists (ACOG) Committee on Obstetric Practice: Committee opinion no. 476: planned home birth, Obstet Gynecol 117(2 Part 1):425–428, 2011b.

American Medical Association: Home deliveries, resolution no. 205, 2008, www.aolcdn.com/tmz_documents/0617_ricki_lake_wm.pdf.

Anderson CJ, Kilpatrick C: Patients' birth plans: theories, strategies, and implications for nurses, Nurs Womens Health 16(3):211–218, 2012.

Association of Women's Health, Obstetric and Neonatal Nurses (AWHONN): HIV screening procedures for pregnant women and newborns—policy position statement, Washington, DC, 2008, Author.

Association of Women's Health, Obstetric and Neonatal Nurses (AWHONN): Nursing support for laboring women, J Obstet Gynecol Neonatal Nurs 40(5):665–666, 2011.

Burr C: Reducing maternal-infant HIV transmission. In Coffey S, editor: Guide for HIV/AIDS clinical care, Rockville, MD, 2011, US Department of Health and Human Services, Health Resources and Services Administration, http://hab.hrsa.gov/deliverhivaidscare/clinicalguide11/cg-402_pmtct.html.

Centers for Disease Control and Prevention (CDC): Sexually transmitted diseases treatment guidelines, Morb Mortal Wkly Rep 59(RR12):1–110, 2010.

Centers for Disease Control and Prevention (CDC): Advisory Committee on Immunization Practices recommended immunization schedule for adults aged 19 years and older—United States, Morb Mortal Wkly Rep 62(1):9–19, 2013.

Cunningham F, Leveno K, Bloom S, et al: Williams obstetrics, ed 23, New York, 2010, McGraw-Hill.

Davies G, Maxwell C, McLeod L, et al: Obesity in pregnancy, J Obstet Gynaecol Can 32(2):165–173, 2010.

de Jonge A, van der Goes BY, Ravelli AC, et al: Perinatal mortality and morbidity in a nationwide cohort of 529,688 low-risk planned home and hospital births, BJOG 116(9):1177–1184, 2009.

Doulas of North America (DONA): Doulas of North America position paper: the birth doula's contribution to modern maternity care, 2008, www.dona.org/.

Dovydaitis T: Human trafficking: the role of the health care provider, J Midwifery Womens Health 55(5):462–467, 2010.

Duff P: Maternal and perinatal infection—bacterial. In Gabbe SG, Niebyl JR, Simpson JL, et al, editors: Obstetrics: normal and problem pregnancies, ed 6, Philadelphia, 2012, Saunders.

Gregory KD, Niebyl JR, Johnson TR: Preconception and prenatal care: part of the continuum. In Gabbe SG, Niebyl JR, Simpson JL, et al, editors: Obstetrics: normal and problem pregnancies, ed 6, Philadelphia, 2012, Saunders.

Hall H, McKenna L, Griffiths D: Complementary and alternative medicine: where's the evidence? Brit J Midwifery 18(7):350–358, 2010.

Hamilton BE, Martin JA, Ventura SJ: Births: preliminary data for 2010, Natl Vital Stat Rep 60(2):1–26, 2011.

Hamilton BE, Ventura SJ: Birth rates for US teenagers reach historic lows for all age and ethnic groups, NCHS Data Brief No. 89, Hyattsville, MD, 2012, National Center for Health Statistics.

Heron M, Sutton P, Xu J, et al: Annual summary of vital statistics, 2007, Pediatrics 125(1):4–15, 2010.

Herrman JW, Rogers S, Ehrenthal DB: Women's perceptions of CenteringPregnancy: a focus group study, MCN Am J Matern Child Nurs 37(1):19–26, 2012.

Hutton EK, Reitsma AH, Kaufman K: Outcomes associated with planned home and planned hospital births in low-risk women attended by midwives in Ontario, Canada, 2003-2006—a retrospective cohort study, Birth 36(3):180–189, 2009.

Janssen PA, Saxell L, Page L, et al: Outcomes of planned home birth with registered midwife versus planned hospital birth with midwife or physician, CMAJ 181(6-7):377–383, 2009.

Johnson JA, Tough S: Delayed child-bearing, J Obstet Gynaecol Can 34(1):80–93, 2012.

Kumar J, Samelson R: Oral health care during pregnancy: recommendations for oral health professionals, N Y State Dental J 75(6):29–33, 2009.

Kuo S, Lin K, Hsu C, et al: Evaluation of the effects of a birth plan on Taiwanese women's childbirth experiences, control and expectations fulfillment—a randomized controlled trial, Int J Nurs Studies 47(7):806–814, 2010.

Lawrence RA, Lawrence RM: Breastfeeding: a guide for the medical profession, ed 7, St Louis, 2011, Mosby.

Lowe NK: The "authorities" resolve against home birth, J Obstet Gynecol Neonatal Nurs 38(1):1–3, 2009.

MacDorman MF, Mathews TJ, Declercq E: Home births in the United States, 1990-2009, NCHS Data Brief No. 184, Hyattsville, MD, 2012, National Center for Health Statistics.

Magdaleno R, Pereira BG, Chaim EA, et al: Pregnancy after bariatric surgery: a current view of maternal, obstetrical, and perinatal challenges, Arch Gynecol Obstet 285(3):559–566, 2012.

Maher S, Crawford-Carr A, Neidigh K: The role of the interpreter/doula in the maternity setting, Nurs Womens Health, 16(6): 472–481, 2012.

March of Dimes: Caffeine in pregnancy, 2010, www.marchofdimes.com/pregnancy/nutrition_caffeine.html.

May KA: Three phases of father involvement in pregnancy, Nurs Res 31(6):337–342, 1982.

McIntyre M: Safety of non-medically led primary maternity care models: a critical review of the international literature, *Aust Health Rev* 36(2):140–147, 2012.

Mercer R: *Becoming a mother*, New York, 1995, Springer.

National Perinatal Association: Position paper: choice of birth setting, 2008, www.nationalperinatal.org/advocacy/pdf/Choice-of-Birth-Setting.pdf.

Nelson AM: A meta-synthesis related to infant feeding decision making, *MCN Am J Matern Child Nurs* 37(4):247–252, 2012.

Newman R, Unal ER: Multiple gestations. In Gabbe SG, Niebyl JR, Simpson JL, et al, editors: *Obstetrics: normal and problem pregnancies*, ed 6, Philadelphia, 2012, Saunders.

Novick G: Women's experiences of prenatal care: an integrative review, *J Midwifery Womens Health* 54(3):226–237, 2009.

Osterman MJ, Martin JA, Mathews TJ, et al: Expanded data from the new birth certificate, 2008, *Natl Vital Stat Rep* 59(7):1–28, 2011, www.cdc.gov/nchs/data/nvsr/nvsr59/nvsr59_07.pdf.

Phillippi JC: Women's perceptions of access to prenatal care in the United States: a review, *J Midwifery Womens Health* 54(3):219–225, 2009.

Picklesimer AH, Billings D, Hale N, et al: The effect of CenteringPregnancy group prenatal care on preterm birth in a low-income population, *Am J Obstet Gynecol* 206(5):415.e1–415.e7, 2012.

Quilliam S: Sex during pregnancy: yes, yes, yes! *J Fam Plann Reprod Health Care* 36(2):97–98, 2010.

Rasmussen KM, Yaktine AL, editors: *Institute of Medicine Committee to Reexamine IOM Pregnancy Weight Guidelines, Food and Nutrition Board and Board on Children, Youth, and Families: Weight gain during pregnancy: reexamining the guidelines*, Washington, DC, 2009, National Academy Press.

Robertson B, Aycock DM, Darnell LA: Comparison of CenteringPregnancy to traditional care in Hispanic mothers, *Matern Child Health J* 13(3):407–414, 2009.

Rotundo G: CenteringPregnancy: the benefits of group prenatal care, *Nurs Womens Health* 15(6):508–518, 2011.

Rubin R: Maternal tasks in pregnancy, *Matern Child Nurs J* 4(3):143–153, 1975.

Rubin R: *Maternal identity and the maternal experience*, New York, 1984, Springer.

Seidel HM, Ball JW, Dains JE, et al: *Mosby's guide to physical examination*, ed 7, St Louis, 2011, Mosby.

Sidransky D, Norman LA, McCarthy A, et al, editors: *How tobacco smoke causes disease: the biology and behavioral basis for smoking attributable disease—a report of the Surgeon General*, Rockville, MD, 2010, U.S. Dept of Health and Human Services.

Signore C, Spong CY, Krotoski D, et al: Pregnancy in women with physical disabilities, *Obstet Gynecol* 117(4):935–947, 2011.

Society for Maternal-Fetal Medicine Publications Committee: Progesterone and preterm birth prevention: translating clinical trials data into clinical practice, *Am J Obstet Gynecol* 206(5):377–386, 2012.

Sutton MY: Advising travelers with specific needs. In Brunette GW, Kozarsky PE, Magill AJ, et al, editors: *CDC health information for international travel*, New York, 2012, Oxford University Press.

Tracy EE, Konstantopoulos WM: Human trafficking: a call for heightened awareness and advocacy by obstetrician-gynecologists, *Obstet Gynecol* 119(5):1045–1047, 2012.

U.S. Department of Health and Human Services (USDHHS): *2008 physical activity guidelines for Americans summary*, Washington, DC, 2008, Author, www.health.gov/paguidelines/guidelines/summary.aspx.

Walker M: Breast pumps and other technologies. In Riordan J, Wambach K, editors: *Breastfeeding and human lactation*, Boston, 2010, Jones & Bartlett.

Wong S, Ordean A, Kahan M: Society of Obstetricians and Gynecologists of Canada (SOGC) clinical practice guidelines: substance use in pregnancy no. 256, *Int J Gynaecol Obstet* 114(2):190–202, 2011.

Maternal and Fetal Nutrition

Shannon E. Perry

evolve WEBSITE

http://evolve.elsevier.com/Perry/maternal

LEARNING OBJECTIVES

On completion of this chapter, the reader will be able to:

- Explain recommended maternal weight gain during pregnancy.
- Compare the recommended level of intake of energy sources, protein, and key vitamins and minerals during pregnancy and lactation.
- Give examples of the food sources that provide the nutrients required for optimal maternal nutrition during pregnancy and lactation.

- Examine the role of nutrition supplements during pregnancy.
- List five nutritional risk factors during pregnancy.
- Compare the dietary needs of adolescent and mature pregnant women.
- Analyze examples of eating patterns of women from two different ethnic or cultural backgrounds and identify potential dietary problems.
- Assess nutritional status during pregnancy.

Nutrition is one of the many factors that influence the outcome of pregnancy (Fig. 9-1). However, maternal nutritional status is an especially significant factor, both because it is potentially alterable and because good nutrition before and during pregnancy is an important preventive measure for a variety of problems. These problems include birth of low-birth-weight (LBW) (birth weight of 2500 g or less) and preterm infants. Evidence is growing that a mother's nutrition and lifestyle affect the long-term health of her children. Thus the importance of good nutrition must be emphasized to all women of childbearing potential. Key components of nutrition care during the preconception period and pregnancy include (Harnisch, Harnisch, and Harnisch, 2012):

- Nutrition assessment that includes appropriate weight for height and adequacy and quality of dietary intake and habits
- Diagnosis of nutrition-related problems or risk factors such as diabetes, phenylketonuria (PKU), and obesity
- Intervention based on an individual's dietary goals and plan to promote appropriate weight gain, ingestion of a variety of foods, appropriate use of dietary supplements, and physical activity
- Evaluation as an integral part of the nursing care provided to women during the preconception period and pregnancy, with referral to a nutritionist or dietitian as necessary

NUTRIENT NEEDS BEFORE CONCEPTION

The first trimester of pregnancy is a crucial one in terms of embryonic and fetal organ development. A healthful diet before conception is the best way to ensure that adequate nutrients are available for the developing fetus. Folate or folic acid intake is of particular concern in the periconception period. Folate is the form in which this vitamin is found naturally in foods, and folic acid is the form used in fortification of grain products and other foods and in vitamin supplements. Neural tube defects (failure in closure of the neural tube) are more common in infants of women with poor folic acid intake. Proper closure of the neural tube is required for normal formation of the spinal cord, and the neural tube begins to close within the first month of gestation, often before the woman realizes that she is pregnant (Box 9-1).

Maternal and fetal risks in pregnancy are increased when the mother is significantly underweight or overweight when pregnancy begins. Ideally, all women would achieve their desirable body weights before conception.

NUTRIENT NEEDS DURING PREGNANCY

Nutrient needs are determined, at least in part, by the stage of gestation. The amount of fetal growth varies during the different stages

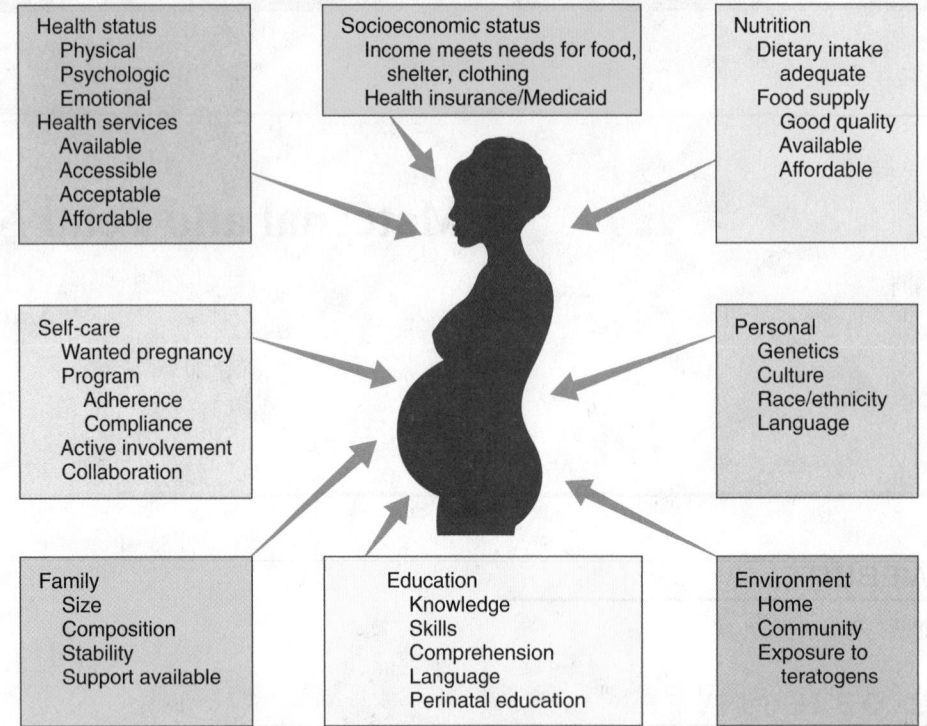

FIG 9-1 Factors that influence the outcome of pregnancy.

| BOX 9-1 | FOOD SOURCES OF FOLATE |

Foods Providing 500 mcg or More per Serving
- Liver: chicken, turkey, goose (100 g [3.5 oz])

Foods Providing 200 mcg or More per Serving
- Liver: lamb, beef, veal (100 g [3.5 oz])

Foods Providing 100 mcg or More per Serving
- Legumes, cooked (½ cup)
  - Peas: black-eyed, chickpea (garbanzo)
  - Beans: black, kidney, pinto, red, navy
  - Lentils
- Vegetables (½ cup)
  - Asparagus
  - Spinach, cooked
- Papaya (1 medium)
- Breakfast cereal, ready-to-eat ½ to 1 cup)
- Wheat germ (¼ cup)

Foods Providing 50 mcg or More per Serving
- Vegetables (½ cup)
  - Broccoli
  - Beans: lima beans, baked beans, or pork and beans
  - Greens: collards or mustard, cooked
  - Spinach, raw
- Fruits (½ cup)
  - Avocado
  - Orange or orange juice
- Pasta, cooked (1 cup)
- Rice, cooked (1 cup)

Foods Providing 20 mcg or More per Serving
- Bread (1 slice)
- Egg (1 large)
- Corn (½ cup)

when most of the fetal stores of energy sources and minerals are deposited. Thus as fetal growth progresses during the second and third trimesters, the pregnant woman's need for some nutrients increases greatly. Factors that contribute to the increase in nutrient needs include the following factors:

- The uterine-placental-fetal unit.
- Maternal blood volume and constituents: During pregnancy the total blood volume increases by about 40% to 50% over normal. The plasma volume increases by 50% in women in their first pregnancies and more than this in multifetal pregnancies. Although red blood cell (RBC) production also is stimulated, the expansion of RBC mass is not as great as that of plasma volume.
- Maternal mammary development.

Dietary Reference Intakes (DRIs) (www.iom.edu) have been established for the people of the United States and Canada and are updated regularly. The DRIs include recommendations for daily nutritional intakes that meet the needs of almost all (97% to 98%) of the healthy members of the population. They are divided into age, sex, and life-stage categories (e.g., infancy, pregnancy, and lactation), and they can be used as goals in planning the diets of individuals (Table 9-1).

Energy Needs

Energy (kilocalories [kcal]) needs are met by carbohydrate, fat, and protein in the diet. No specific recommendations exist for the amount of carbohydrate and fat in the diet of the pregnant women, but the intake of these nutrients should be adequate to support the recommended weight gain. Although protein can be used to supply energy, its primary role is to provide amino acids for the synthesis of new tissues (see discussion later in this chapter). Longitudinal assessment of weight gain during pregnancy is the best way to determine whether the kcal intake is

of pregnancy. During the first trimester, the synthesis of fetal tissues places relatively few demands on maternal nutrition. Therefore during the first trimester, when the embryo or fetus is very small, the needs are only slightly increased over those before pregnancy. In contrast, the last trimester is a period of noticeable fetal growth

TABLE 9-1 RECOMMENDATIONS FOR DAILY INTAKES OF SELECTED NUTRIENTS DURING PREGNANCY AND LACTATION

NUTRIENT (UNITS)	RECOMMENDATION FOR NONPREGNANT WOMAN*	RECOMMENDATION FOR PREGNANCY*	RECOMMENDATION FOR LACTATION*	ROLE IN RELATION TO PREGNANCY AND LACTATION	FOOD SOURCES
Energy (kilocalories [kcal] or kilojoules [kJ]†)	Variable	First trimester, same as nonpregnant; second trimester, nonpregnant needs + 340 kcal (1424 kJ); third trimester, nonpregnant needs + 452 kcal (1892 kJ)	First 6 months, nonpregnant needs + 330 kcal (1382 kJ); second 6 months, nonpregnant needs + 400 kcal (1675 kJ)	Growth of fetal and maternal tissues; milk production	Carbohydrate, fat, and protein
Protein (g)	46	First trimester, same as nonpregnant; second and third trimesters, nonpregnant needs + 25 g‡	Nonpregnant needs + 25 g	Synthesis of the products of conception; growth of maternal tissue and expansion of blood volume; secretion of milk protein during lactation	Meats, eggs, cheese, yogurt, legumes (dry beans and peas, peanuts), nuts, grains
Water (L) in food and beverages	2.7	3	3.8	Expansion of blood volume, excretion of wastes; milk secretion	Water and beverages made with water, milk, juices; all foods, especially frozen desserts, fruits, lettuce and other fresh vegetables
Fiber (g)	25	28	29	Promotes regular bowel elimination; reduces long-term risk for heart disease, diverticulosis, and diabetes	Whole grains, bran, vegetables, fruits, nuts and seeds
Minerals					
Calcium (mg)	1300/1000	1300/1000	1300/1000	Fetal skeleton and tooth formation; maintenance of maternal bone and tooth mineralization	Milk, cheese, yogurt, sardines or other fish eaten with bones left in, deep green leafy vegetables except spinach or Swiss chard, calcium-set tofu, baked beans, tortillas
Iron (mg)	15/18	30	10/9	Maternal hemoglobin formation, fetal liver iron storage	Liver, meats, whole grain or enriched breads and cereals, deep green leafy vegetables, legumes, dried fruits
Zinc (mg)	9/8	12/11	13/12	Component of numerous enzyme systems, possibly important in preventing congenital malformations	Liver, shellfish, meats, whole grains, milk

Continued

TABLE 9-1   RECOMMENDATIONS FOR DAILY INTAKES OF SELECTED NUTRIENTS DURING PREGNANCY AND LACTATION—cont'd

NUTRIENT (UNITS)	RECOMMENDATION FOR NONPREGNANT WOMAN*	RECOMMENDATION FOR PREGNANCY*	RECOMMENDATION FOR LACTATION*	ROLE IN RELATION TO PREGNANCY AND LACTATION	FOOD SOURCES
Iodine (mcg)	150	220	290	Increased maternal metabolic rate	Iodized salt, seafood, milk and milk products, commercial yeast breads, rolls, and donuts
Magnesium (mg)	360/310-320	400/350-360	360/310-320	Involved in energy and protein metabolism, tissue growth, muscle action	Nuts, legumes, cocoa, meats, whole grains
Fat-Soluble Vitamins					
A (mcg)	700	750/770	1200/1300	Essential for cell development, tooth bud formation, bone growth	Dark green leafy vegetables, dark yellow vegetables and fruits, liver, fortified margarine and butter
D (mcg)	5	5	5	Involved in absorption of calcium and phosphorus, improves mineralization	Fortified milk and breakfast cereals; salmon, tuna, and other oily fish; butter, liver
E (mg)	15	15	19	Antioxidant (protects cell membranes from damage), especially important for preventing breakdown of red blood cells (RBCs)	Vegetable oils, green leafy vegetables, whole grains, liver, nuts and seeds, cheese, fish
Water-Soluble Vitamins					
C (mg)	65/75	80/85	115/120	Tissue formation and integrity, formation of connective tissue, enhancement of iron absorption	Citrus fruits, strawberries, melons, broccoli, tomatoes, peppers, raw dark green leafy vegetables
Folate (mcg)	400	600	500	Prevention of neural tube defects, increased maternal RBC formation	Fortified ready-to-eat cereals and other grain products, green leafy vegetables, oranges, broccoli, asparagus, artichokes, liver
B_6 or pyridoxine (mg)	1.2/1.3	1.9	2	Involved in protein metabolism	Meats, liver, dark green vegetables, whole grains
B_{12} (mcg)	2.4	2.6	2.8	Production of nucleic acids and proteins, especially important in formation of RBCs and neural functioning	Milk and milk products, eggs, meats, liver, fortified soy milk

Data from Otten JJ, Helwig JP, Meyers LD, editors: *Dietary reference intakes: the essential guide to nutrient requirements*, Washington, DC, 2006, National Academies Press.

*When two values appear, separated by a diagonal slash, the first is for females younger than 19 years and the second is for those 19 to 50 years of age.

†The international metric unit of energy measurement is the joule (J). 1 kcal = 4.184 kJ.

‡Add an additional 25 g in twin pregnancies.

adequate; very underweight or active women may require more than the recommended increase in kcal to sustain the desired rate of weight gain.

Weight Gain

The desirable weight gain during pregnancy varies among women. The primary factor to consider in making a weight-gain recommendation is the appropriateness of the prepregnancy weight for the woman's height—that is, whether the woman's weight was normal before pregnancy or whether she was underweight or overweight. Whenever possible, the woman should achieve a weight in the normal range for her height before pregnancy. Maternal and fetal risks in pregnancy are increased when the mother is significantly underweight or overweight before pregnancy and when weight gain during pregnancy is either too low or too high. Severely underweight women are more likely to have preterm labor and to give birth to LBW infants. Both normal-weight and underweight women with inadequate weight gain have an increased risk for giving birth to an infant with intrauterine growth restriction (IUGR). Greater-than-expected weight gain during pregnancy may occur for many reasons, including multiple gestation, edema, gestational hypertension, and overeating. When obesity is present (either preexisting obesity or obesity that develops during pregnancy), there is an increased likelihood of macrosomia and fetopelvic disproportion; operative vaginal birth; emergency cesarean birth; postpartum hemorrhage; wound, genital tract, or urinary tract infection; birth trauma; and late fetal death. Obese women are more likely than normal-weight women to have preeclampsia and gestational diabetes.

A commonly used method of evaluating the appropriateness of weight for height is the body mass index (BMI), which is calculated by the following formula:

$$BMI = Weight \div Height^2$$

in which the weight is in kilograms and height is in meters. Thus for a woman who weighed 51 kg before pregnancy and is 1.57 m tall:

$$BMI = 51\,kg \div (1.57\,m)^2,\ or\ 20.7$$

Prepregnant BMI can be classified into the following categories: less than 18.5, underweight or low; 18.5 to 24.9, normal; 25 to 29.9, overweight or high; and greater than 30, obese (www.nhlbisupport.com/bmi). The BMI can be calculated on this website (see also Box 3-6).

At the first health care visit, the pregnant woman should be helped to establish a weight-gain goal for pregnancy that is suited to her prepregnancy weight. Progress toward this goal should be monitored at each visit.

For women with single fetuses, current recommendations are that women with normal BMI should gain 11.5 to 16 kg (25 to 35 lbs) during pregnancy (Fig. 9-2). Box 9-2 lists recommended weight gain for pregnancies with single fetuses, twin gestations, and multifetal (more than 2) gestations for women who are normal weight, underweight, and overweight.

Pattern of Weight Gain

The optimal rate of weight gain depends on the stage of pregnancy. During the first and second trimesters, growth takes place primarily in maternal tissues; during the third trimester, growth occurs primarily in fetal tissues. During the first trimester of singleton pregnancy, the average total weight gain is only 1 to 2 kg. Thereafter the recommended weight gain increases to approximately 0.5 kg per

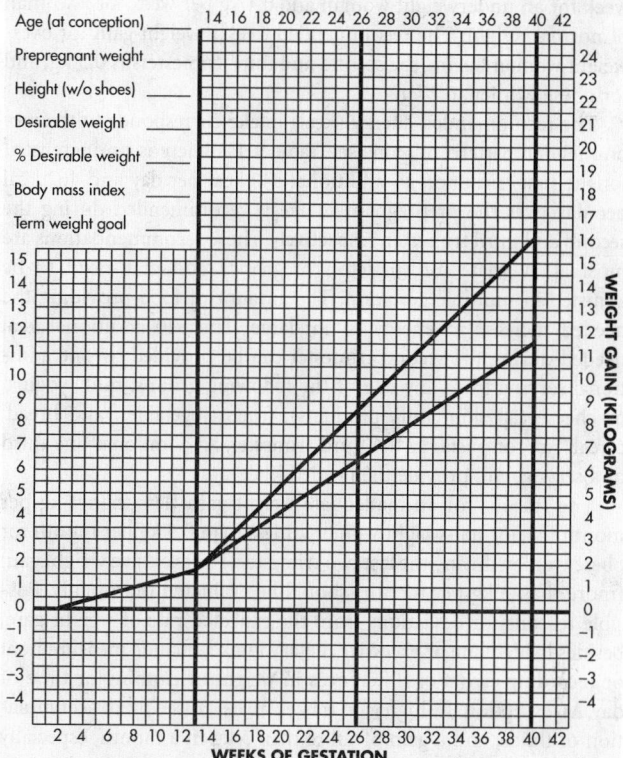

FIG 9-2 Prenatal weight-gain chart for plotting weight gain for normal-weight women.

BOX 9-2   WEIGHT GAIN DURING PREGNANCY

- Progressive weight gain during pregnancy is essential to ensure normal fetal growth and development and the deposition of maternal stores that promote successful lactation.
- Recommended weight gain during pregnancy is determined largely by prepregnancy weight for height. The recommended total weight gain is as follows: underweight women, 12.5 to 18 kg (28 to 40 lbs); normal-weight women, 11.5 to 16 kg (25 to 35 lbs); overweight women, 7 to 11.5 kg (15 to 25 lbs); and obese women 5 to 9 kg (11 to 20 lbs). For twin gestations, the recommended total weight gain is 21 to 28 kg (46 to 62 lbs) for women who are underweight before conception, 17 to 25 kg (37 to 54 lbs) for normal-weight women, 14 to 23 kg (31 to 50 lbs) for overweight women, and 11 to 19 kg (25 to 42 lbs) for obese women.
- There is not enough information available to make firm recommendations about optimal weight gain for women with more than 2 fetuses, but provisional recommendations have been made for all prepregnancy body mass index (BMI) categories except the underweight category (Institute of Medicine [IOM], 2009). The provisional recommendations for a gestation with more than 2 fetuses suggest that normal-weight women gain 17 to 25 kg, overweight women gain 14 to 23 kg, and obese women gain 11 to 19 kg.
- Weight gain should be achieved through a balanced diet of regular foods chosen from all the different food groups (see Table 9-3).
- The pattern of weight gain is important: approximately 0.5 kg per week during the second and third trimesters for underweight women, 0.4 kg per week for normal-weight women, 0.3 kg per week for overweight women, and 0.2 kg per week for obese women.

week for an underweight woman and 0.4 kg per week for a woman of normal weight. The recommended weekly weight gain for overweight women during the second and third trimesters is 0.3 kg, and for obese women, 0.2 kg.

The recommended energy (kcal) intake corresponds to the recommended pattern of gain (see Table 9-1). There is no increment for the first trimester; an additional 340 kcal per day and 462 kcal per day over the prepregnant intake is recommended during the second and third trimester, respectively. These recommendations are most appropriate for singleton pregnancy and may need to be adjusted in multiple gestation. The amount of food providing the needed increase in energy is not large. The 340 additional kcal needed during the second trimester can be provided by one additional serving from any one of the following groups: milk, yogurt, or cheese (all skim milk products); fruits; vegetables; and bread, cereal, rice, or pasta. In the third trimester, an additional one third of a serving will provide the needed kcal.

The reasons for an inadequate weight gain (less than 1 kg per month for normal-weight women or less than 0.5 kg per month for obese women during the last two trimesters) or excessive weight gain (more than 3 kg per month) should be evaluated thoroughly. Possible reasons for deviations from the expected rate of weight gain, besides inadequate or excessive dietary intake, include measurement or recording errors or differences in weight of clothing or time of day. An exceptionally high gain is likely to be caused by an accumulation of fluids, and a gain of more than 3 kg in a month, especially after the twentieth week of gestation, often indicates the development of preeclampsia.

Hazards of Restricting Adequate Weight Gain

An obsession with thinness and dieting pervades the North American culture. Figure-conscious women may find it difficult to make the transition from guarding against weight gain before pregnancy to valuing weight gain during pregnancy. In counseling these women, the nurse can emphasize the positive effects of good nutrition as well as the adverse effects of maternal malnutrition (manifested by poor weight gain) on infant growth and development. This counseling includes information on the components of weight gain during pregnancy (Table 9-2) and the amount of this weight that will be lost at birth. Because lactation can help reduce maternal energy stores gradually, this also provides an opportunity to promote breastfeeding.

TABLE 9-2	TISSUES CONTRIBUTING TO MATERNAL WEIGHT GAIN AT 40 WEEKS OF GESTATION	
TISSUE	**KILOGRAMS**	**POUNDS**
Fetus	3.2-3.9	7-8.5
Placenta	0.9-1.1	2-2.5
Amniotic fluid	0.9	2
Increase in uterine tissue	0.9	2
Breast tissue	0.5-1.8	1-4
Increased blood volume	1.8-2.3	4-5
Increased tissue fluid	1.4-2.3	3-5
Increased stores (fat)	1.8-2.7	4-6

In the United States, 20% of women who give birth are obese (www.cdc.gov/reproductivehealth/MaternalInfantHealth/PregComplications.htm). Pregnancy is not a time for a weight-reduction diet. Even overweight or obese pregnant women need to gain at least enough weight to equal the weight of the products of conception (fetus, placenta, and amniotic fluid). If they limit their energy intake to prevent weight gain, they may also excessively limit their intake of important nutrients. Moreover, dietary restriction results in catabolism of fat stores, which in turn augments the production of ketones. The long-term effects of mild ketonemia during pregnancy are not known, but ketonuria is associated with the occurrence of preterm labor. It should be stressed to obese women (and to all pregnant women) that the quality of the weight gain is important, with emphasis placed on the consumption of nutrient-dense foods and the avoidance of empty-calorie foods (see Critical Thinking Case Study).

Excessive Weight Gain

Weight gain is important, but pregnancy is not an excuse for uncontrolled dietary indulgence. The woman should place an emphasis on the quality of her food intake as she considers her needs and those of her fetus. Excessive weight gained during pregnancy may be difficult to lose after pregnancy, thus contributing to chronic overweight or obesity—an etiologic factor in a host of chronic diseases, including hypertension, diabetes mellitus, and arteriosclerotic heart disease. The woman who gains 18 kg or more is especially at risk (Box 9-3). Food energy intake and particularly intake of fat is likely to be high among pregnant women, especially low-income women (see Evidence-Based Practice box).

Protein

Protein, with its essential constituent *nitrogen,* is the nutritional element basic to growth. Adequate protein intake is essential to meet increasing demands in pregnancy.

❓ CRITICAL THINKING CASE STUDY

Nutrition and the Overweight Pregnant Woman

Tamara, age 27, of African-American and Asian heritage, is 3 months pregnant and comes to her initial appointment for diagnosis and care. She appears to be overweight for her height (5′ 6″ tall, 172 lbs [78 kg]). To provide optimal care for her, you plan to calculate her prepregnancy body mass index (BMI). When her pregnancy is confirmed, you are asked to plan a diet with Tamara that meets the minimum daily requirements and allows for growth of the pregnancy. You know that it is important to include consideration of personal preferences and cultural factors in your plan. With Tamara, identify barriers to implementing the plan.

1. Evidence—Is there sufficient evidence to draw conclusions about an appropriate nutrition plan, considering personal preferences and cultural factors?
2. Assumptions—Describe underlying assumptions about each of the following issues:
   a. Dietary Reference Intakes for pregnancy and lactation
   b. Indicators of nutritional risk in pregnancy; possibility of lactose intolerance
   c. Daily food guide for pregnancy and lactation
   d. Sources of calcium for women who do not drink milk
3. What implications and priorities for nursing care can be drawn at this time?
4. Does the evidence objectively support your conclusion?

BOX 9-3	BARIATRIC OBSTETRIC CARE

Obstetricians today are seeing more morbidly obese pregnant women—those who weigh 400, 500, and even 600 pounds. Obesity creates many risks for pregnant women, including hypertension, diabetes, and prematurity. To manage their conditions and to meet their logistical needs, a new medical subspecialty—bariatric obstetrics—has arisen. Extra-wide blood pressure cuffs, scales that can accommodate up to 880 pounds, and extra-wide surgical tables designed to hold the weight of these women are used. Special techniques for ultrasound examination and longer surgical instruments for cesarean birth are required. In the bariatric obstetric clinic at St. Louis University in St. Louis, Missouri, women are counseled to avoid gaining weight and even to lose weight during pregnancy. New evidence indicates that when obese women maintain or lose weight during pregnancy, they have fewer complications and give birth to healthier babies.

From Paul AM: Too fat and pregnant, *New York Times*, July 13, 2008.

EVIDENCE-BASED PRACTICE

Weight Management in Pregnancy

Ask the Question
For obese and overweight pregnant women, are weight-management interventions safe and beneficial to mother and baby?

Search for the Evidence
Search Strategies
- English language research-based publications on pregnancy, obesity, weight gain, diet, exercise were included.
- Exclusions included trials in developing countries with food shortages.

Databases Used
- Cochrane Collaborative Database, National Guideline Clearinghouse (Agency for Healthcare Research and Quality [AHRQ]), CINAHL, PubMed, UpToDate, and the professional website for the Association of Women's Health, Obstetric and Neonatal Nurses (AWHONN).

Critically Analyze the Evidence
- Obesity in pregnancy is associated with offspring with attention deficit hyperactivity disorder (ADHD) in childhood, eating disorders in adolescence, and psychotic disorders in adulthood (Van Lieshout, Taylor, and Boyle, 2011).
- Weight-management interventions for obese pregnant women result in significantly decreased weight gain and in significantly less preeclampsia and shoulder dystocia (Thangaratinam, Rogozinska, Jolly, et al., 2012).
- The most effective interventions were dietary resulting in decreased risk for preeclampsia, gestational hypertension, and preterm birth, with no harm to the fetus (Thangaratinam, Rogozinska, Jolly, et al., 2012).
- In a systematic review, researchers found that goal setting was a useful technique for achieving optimal weight gain. Obese women may require further counseling (Brown, Sinclair, Liddle, et al., 2012).
- Regular activity improved maternal glycemic control and fetal outcomes. Caregivers should recommend physical activity to most pregnant women as safe and beneficial (Ferraro, Gaudet, and Adamo, 2012).

Apply the Evidence: Nursing Implications
- Preconceptional counseling should include prevention of obesity, ideally from childhood. Obese women are at risk for cardiac and pulmonary diseases, gestational hypertension and diabetes, and obstructive sleep apnea. Obesity in pregnancy may result in higher risk for congenital anomalies, operative birth, and surgical complications (Davies, Maxwell, McLeod, et al., SOGC, 2010).
- Nurses are frequently the main educators for their pregnant patients. Counseling obese pregnant women about nutrition and food choices and using collaborative goal setting for weight gain can prevent pregnancy risks and avoid weight gain that may persist beyond pregnancy.

- Activity needs to be frequent, fun, and affordable. An excellent idea is encouraging the woman to walk with other pregnant women, which provides social support and increased safety. In addition, the nurse can advocate for low-cost indoor facilities in the community.

Quality and Safety Competencies: Evidence-Based Practice*
Knowledge
- Explain the role of evidence in determining best clinical practice.
- Both nutrition counseling and motivation work best for weight management in pregnancy.

Skills
- Locate evidence reports related to clinical practice topics and guidelines.
- Dietary and activity interventions are safe and beneficial in pregnancy for obese women.

Attitudes
- Appreciate the importance of regularly reading relevant professional journals.
- Systematic reviews and professional guidelines highlight interventions that have evidence of success, such as motivational goal setting for weight management.

References
Brown MJ, Sinclair M, Liddle D, et al: A systematic review investigating healthy lifestyle interventions incorporating goal setting strategies for preventing excess gestational weight gain, *PLoS One* 7(7):e39503, 2012, DOI: 10.1371/journal.pone.0039503.

Davies GA, Maxwell C, McLeod L, et al: Society of Obstetricians and Gynaecologists of Canada (SOGC): Obesity in pregnancy, *J Obstet Gynaecol Can* 32(2):165–173, 2010.

Ferraro ZM, Gaudet L, Adamo KB: The potential impact of physical activity during pregnancy on maternal and neonatal outcomes, *Obstet Gynecol Surv* 67(2):99–110, 2012.

Thangaratinam S, Rogozinska E, Jolly K, et al: Interventions to reduce or prevent obesity in pregnant women: a systematic review, *Health Technol Assess* 16(31):1–192, 2012.

Van Lieshout RJ, Taylor VH, Boyle MH: Pre-pregnancy and pregnancy obesity and neurodevelopmental outcomes in offspring: a systematic review, *Obes Rev* 12(5):e548–559, 2011, DOI: 10.1111/j.1467-789X.2010.00850.x.

Pat Mahaffee Gingrich

*Adapted from Quality and Safety Education for Nurses (QSEN) at www.qsen.org/.

These demands arise from:
- The rapid growth of the fetus
- The enlargement of the uterus and its supporting structures, the mammary glands, and the placenta
- The increase in the maternal circulating blood volume and the subsequent demand for increased amounts of plasma protein to maintain colloidal osmotic pressure
- The formation of amniotic fluid

Milk, meat, eggs, and cheese are complete protein foods with a high biologic value. Legumes (dried beans and peas), whole grains, and nuts are also valuable sources of protein. In addition, these protein-rich foods are a source of other nutrients such as calcium, iron, and B vitamins. Plant sources of protein often provide needed dietary fiber. The recommended daily food plan (Table 9-3) is a guide to the amounts of these foods that would supply the quantities of protein needed. The recommendations provide for only a modest increase in protein intake (25 g daily) over the prepregnant levels in adult women.

Protein intake in many people in the United States is relatively high; thus many women may not need to increase their protein intake at all during pregnancy. Three servings of milk, yogurt, or cheese (four for adolescents) and two servings (5 to 6 oz [140 to 168 g]) of meat, poultry, or fish would supply most of the recommended protein for a pregnant woman. Additional protein is provided by vegetables and breads, cereals, rice, or pasta. Pregnant adolescents, women from impoverished backgrounds, and women

TABLE 9-3 DAILY FOOD GUIDE FOR PREGNANCY AND LACTATION

FOOD GROUP	DAILY AMOUNT OF FOOD RECOMMENDED FOR WOMEN*	SERVING SIZE
Grains	6- to 8-ounce equivalents At least half of grain servings should be whole grains. *Whole grains* are those that contain the entire grain kernel (bran, germ, endosperm) (e.g., whole wheat or cornmeal, oatmeal, and brown rice). Refined grains have been milled to remove the bran and germ (e.g., white flour, white bread, degermed cornmeal, white rice, and corn or flour tortillas).	1-ounce equivalent = 1 slice bread, 1 cup ready-to-eat cereal, or ½ cup cooked rice or pasta or cooked cereal
Vegetables Vary the vegetables consumed to take advantage of the different nutrients they offer	2½ to 3 cups Weekly intake should include at least the following: 3 cups dark green vegetables (e.g., spinach or greens, broccoli, bok choy, romaine lettuce); 2 cups orange vegetables (e.g., carrots; acorn, butternut, or Hubbard squash; sweet potatoes); 3 cups dry beans or peas (e.g., black, navy, or kidney beans; chickpeas; black-eyed peas; split peas; lentils; soybeans; tofu); 3 cups starchy vegetables (corn, green peas, potatoes); and 6½ cups of other vegetables (e.g., artichokes, asparagus, bean sprouts, green beans, cauliflower, cucumber, tomatoes, iceberg or head lettuce).	1 cup = 2 cups raw leafy greens; 1 cup of other vegetables, raw or cooked; or 1 cup of vegetable juice
Fruits	2 cups	1 cup = 1 cup raw, frozen, or canned fruit; 1 cup 100% juice; or ½ cup dried fruit
Milk, yogurt, and cheese (milk group)	3 cups Most milk group choices should be fat free or low fat.	1 cup = 1 cup milk or yogurt; 1½ ounces natural cheese; 2 ounces processed cheese (e.g., American); 2 cups cottage cheese; 1½ cups ice cream (choose fat-free or low-fat most often)
Meat, poultry, fish, dry beans, eggs, and nuts (meat and beans† groups)	5½- to 6½-ounce equivalents Most meat and poultry choices should be lean or low fat. Fish, nuts, and seeds contain healthy oils, so choose these foods frequently instead of meat or poultry.	1 ounce-equivalent = 1 ounce (30 g) meat, poultry, or fish; ¼ cup cooked dried beans†; 1 egg; 1 tablespoon (15 mL) peanut butter; ½ ounce nuts or seeds
Oils	6 teaspoons (30 mL) Choose oils rather than solid fats. Solid fats are fats that are solid at room temperature, such as butter, shortening, stick margarine, and pork, chicken, or beef fat. Read the label: choose products with no *trans* fats, limit intake of saturated fats, and choose oils high in monounsaturated and polyunsaturated fats.	1 teaspoon = 1 teaspoon liquid oil (e.g., olive, canola, sunflower, safflower, peanut, soybean, cottonseed) or soft margarine (tub or squeeze bottle); 1 tablespoon mayonnaise or Italian salad dressing; ¾ tablespoon Thousand Island salad dressing; 8 large olives; ⅛ medium avocado; ⅓ ounce dry roasted peanuts, mixed nuts, cashews, sunflower seeds†

*These are approximate amounts based on a relatively sedentary lifestyle and should be individualized. Intake may have to be increased for women with a more active lifestyle or multiple gestation, those who are underweight before pregnancy, or those exhibiting poor gestational weight gain. Needs during lactation may also be greater than these recommendations.
†Beans are also part of the vegetable group; avocados are also part of the fruit group, and nuts and seeds are part of the meat and beans group.

adhering to unusual diets such as a macrobiotic (highly restricted vegetarian) diet are those whose protein intake is most likely to be inadequate. High-protein supplements are not recommended because they have been associated with an increased incidence of preterm births.

Pregnant and nursing women should be especially careful when choosing fish to select those that are low in mercury.

⚡ SAFETY ALERT

High levels of mercury can harm the developing nervous system of the fetus or young child, and certain fish are especially high in mercury. Women who may become pregnant, women who are pregnant or nursing, and young children need to follow some precautions: (1) avoid eating shark, swordfish, king mackerel, and tilefish; (2) check local advisories about the safety of fish caught by family and friends in local bodies of water, but if no advisory is available, limit intake of these fish to 6 ounces and eat no other fish that week; and (3) eat as much as 12 ounces a week of a variety of commercially caught fish and shellfish low in mercury, such as shrimp, salmon, pollock, catfish, and canned light tuna (but limit intake of albacore or "white" tuna and tuna steaks, which contain more mercury, to 6 ounces per week). Additional information about mercury levels in a variety of commercial fish is available at www.cfsan.fda.gov/~frf/sea-mehg.html.

Fluids

Water is the main substance of cells, blood, lymph, amniotic fluid, and other vital body fluids. It is essential during the exchange of nutrients and waste products across cell membranes. It also aids in maintaining body temperature. A good fluid intake promotes regular bowel function, which is sometimes a problem during pregnancy. The recommended daily intake is about 8 to 10 glasses (2.3 L) of fluid. Water, milk, and decaffeinated tea are good sources. Foods in the diet should supply an additional 700 mL or more of fluid. Dehydration may increase the risk for cramping, contractions, and preterm labor.

The safety of caffeine use in pregnancy is an important consideration. Some investigators (e.g., Weng, Odouli, and Li, 2008) but not others (e.g., Pollack, Louis, Sundaram, et al., 2010) found that women who consume more than 200 mg of caffeine daily (equivalent to about 12 oz of coffee) may be at increased risk for miscarriage. Data also suggest that excess caffeine intake may contribute to IUGR. In their review, Jahanfar and Sharifah (2009) found that there is insufficient evidence to determine whether caffeine has any effect on pregnancy outcome. Although the evidence about caffeine is far from conclusive, the March of Dimes recommends a daily intake of no more than 200 mg of caffeine (March of Dimes, 2010). Caffeine is found not only in coffee but also in tea, some soft drinks, and chocolate (Table 9-4).

Aspartame (NutraSweet, Equal), acesulfame potassium (Sunett), and sucralose (Splenda)—artificial sweeteners commonly used in low- or no-calorie beverages and low-calorie food products—have not been found to have adverse effects on the normal mother or fetus and therefore are approved by the U.S. Food and Drug Administration (FDA) for use during pregnancy. Aspartame, which contains phenylalanine, should be avoided by pregnant women with PKU (Box 9-4). Stevia (stevioside) is a sweetener sold as a dietary supplement; no acceptable daily intake has been established for stevia.

Minerals and Vitamins

In general, the nutrient needs of pregnant women, with perhaps the exception of folate and iron, can be met through dietary

sources. Counseling about the need for a varied diet rich in vitamins and minerals should be a part of early prenatal care of every pregnant woman and should be reinforced throughout pregnancy (see Community Focus box). It has been suggested that taking a micronutrient supplement (including vitamins and trace minerals) before and during pregnancy reduces the risk for congenital defects, LBW, and preterm birth, as well as preeclampsia. There is no conclusive evidence to support this suggestion, but further research is needed on maternal and fetal benefits of micronutrient supplementation. Supplements are especially advisable for women with known nutritional risk factors (Box 9-5). It is important that the pregnant woman understand that the use of a vitamin-mineral supplement does not lessen the need to consume a nutritious, well-balanced diet.

TABLE 9-4	CAFFEINE CONTENT OF COMMON BEVERAGES AND FOODS
BEVERAGE OR FOOD	**CAFFEINE (MG)**
Coffee (8 oz [240 mL])	95
Espresso (1 oz [30 mL])	64
Tea, black, brewed (8 oz [240 mL])	47
Tea, ready-to-drink, with lemon (12 oz [360 mL])	7
Tea, green, brewed (8 oz [240 mL])	50
Tea, white, brewed (8 oz [240 mL])	35
Energy drink, Rockstar (8 oz [240 mL])	79
Energy drink, Red Bull (8.4 oz [250 mL])	77
Energy drink, Vault (8 oz [250 mL])	68
Energy drink, AMP (8 oz [240 mL])	74
Cola beverage, regular (12 oz [360 mL])	29
Hot chocolate, homemade or from mix (8 oz [240 mL])	5
Dark chocolate bar (1 oz [30 g])	23
Candy bar, milk chocolate with almonds (1.5 oz [45 g])	7

Data from Chin J, Merves M, Goldberger B, et al: Caffeine content of brewed teas, *J Anal Toxicol* 32(8):702–704, 2008; Reissig C, Strain E, Griffiths R: Caffeinated energy drinks—a growing problem, *Drug Alcohol Depend* 99(1–3):1–10, 2009; U.S. Department of Agriculture, Agricultural Research Service: *USDA national nutrient database for standard reference, release 24*, 2011, Nutrient Data Laboratory home page, www.ars.usda.gov/ba/bhnrc/ndl.

🏠 COMMUNITY FOCUS

Nutrition Education in the Prenatal Clinic

Visit a prenatal clinic. Identify sources of nutrition education that are evident in the waiting room. Does the clinic employ a nutritionist/dietitian? Who provides nutrition counseling in the clinic? Are print materials available in multiple languages? Are interpreters available? Are there sources for free materials on nutrition that could be placed in the clinic? Identify strengths and weaknesses of nutrition education in that setting. Develop a feasible plan for improving nutrition education in the clinic.

BOX 9-4 USE OF ARTIFICIAL SWEETENERS DURING PREGNANCY

All of the following sweeteners are approved for use in all age-groups, including pregnant women, in the United States:

Acesulfame K
- Brand names: Sunett, Sweet One
- Primary uses: baked goods, frozen desserts, candies, beverages
- Sweetness: 200 times sweeter than sugar
- Shelf life: long
- Suitability for cooking: good; does not break down when heated
- Health concerns: none known

Aspartame
- Brand names: Equal, NutraSweet, NatraTaste
- Primary uses: beverages, frozen desserts, dairy products, chewing gum, breakfast cereals, tabletop sweetener
- Sweetness: 180 times sweeter than sugar
- Shelf life: relatively short (approximately 5 months in a soft drink)
- Suitability for cooking: breaks down and loses sweetness if cooked at high temperatures or for long periods
- Health concerns: contains phenylalanine, a consideration in the diets of people with phenylketonuria

Saccharin
- Brand name: Sweet'N Low
- Primary uses: fountain drinks, chewable vitamins and medications, tabletop sweetener
- Sweetness: 300 times sweeter than sugar
- Shelf life: long
- Suitability for cooking: good; does not lose sweetness during cooking
- Health concerns: linked to bladder cancer in rats

Sucralose
- Brand name: Splenda
- Primary uses: baked goods, beverages, frozen desserts, gelatins, tabletop sweetener
- Sweetness: 600 times sweeter than sugar
- Shelf life: long

- Suitability for cooking: very good; does not break down during cooking (maltodextrin is added to give products better bulk and texture)
- Health concerns: none known

Sugar Alcohols (not technically artificial sweeteners; contain almost as many calories as sugar)
- Types: sorbitol, xylitol, lactitol, mannitol, and maltitol
- Primary uses: sugar-free candy, cookies, and chewing gum
- Sweetness: most are approximately 70% as sweet as sugar; xylitol equals sugar in sweetness
- Shelf life: long
- Suitability for cooking: good
- Advantages over sugar: do not promote tooth decay and are more slowly metabolized, thus do not create a rapid peak in blood glucose
- Health concerns: diarrhea can occur with large intakes

Sugar is important for the volume and moisture of baked goods. Artificial sweeteners may produce a good-tasting product, but some sugar is necessary in many recipes to yield normal volume and texture.

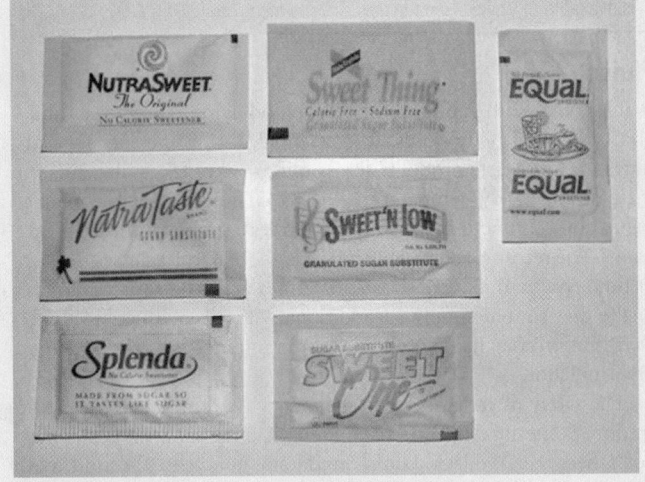

BOX 9-5 INDICATORS OF NUTRITIONAL RISK IN PREGNANCY

- Adolescence or less than 2 years postmenarche
- Frequent pregnancies: three within 2 years
- Poor fetal outcome in a previous pregnancy
- Poverty/food insecurity
- Poor diet habits with resistance to change
- Use of tobacco, alcohol, or drugs
- Weight at conception under or over normal weight
- Problems with weight gain
  - Any weight loss
  - Weight gain of less than 1 kg/month after the first trimester
  - Weight gain of more than 3 kg/month after the first trimester
- Multifetal pregnancy
- Low hemoglobin and/or hematocrit values
- Diabetes
- Chronic illness, including an eating disorder, that affects intake, absorption, or metabolism of nutrients

Iron

Iron is needed to allow transfer of adequate iron to the fetus and to permit expansion of the maternal RBC mass. Beginning in the latter part of the first trimester, the blood volume of the mother increases steadily, peaking at about 1500 mL more than that in the nonpregnant state. In twin gestations, the increase is at least 500 mL greater than that in pregnancies with single fetuses. Plasma volume increases more than RBC mass, with the difference between plasma and RBCs being greatest during the second trimester. The relative excess of plasma causes a modest decrease in the hemoglobin concentration and hematocrit, known as physiologic anemia of pregnancy. This is a normal adaptation during pregnancy.

Poor iron status, which can result in iron deficiency anemia, is relatively common among women in the childbearing years. Iron deficiency (not necessarily anemia) is estimated to affect approximately 10% of nonpregnant women in the childbearing years in the United States. Anemic women are poorly prepared to tolerate hemorrhage at the time of birth. In addition, women who have iron deficiency anemia during early pregnancy are at increased risk for preterm birth. Iron deficiency during the third trimester apparently does not carry the same risk. In the United States, anemia is most common among adolescents, African-American women, and women of lower socioeconomic status.

A supplement of 30 mg of ferrous iron daily starting by 12 weeks of gestation helps ensure an adequate iron intake. Iron supplements may be poorly tolerated during the nausea prevalent in the first trimester, and starting the supplement after this point may improve tolerance. If maternal iron deficiency anemia is present (preferably diagnosed by measurement of serum ferritin, a storage form of iron), increased dosages (60 to 120 mg daily) may be required. Certain foods taken with an iron supplement can promote or inhibit absorption of iron from the supplement. See the Patient Teaching box later in the chapter regarding iron supplementation. Even when a woman is taking an iron supplement, she should also include good food sources of iron in her daily diet (see Table 9-1).

Calcium

There is no increase in the DRI of calcium during pregnancy and lactation compared with the recommendation for the nonpregnant woman (see Table 9-1). The DRI (1000 mg daily for women 19 years and older and 1300 mg for those younger than 19 years) appears to provide sufficient calcium for fetal bone and tooth development to proceed while maintaining maternal bone mass. Milk and yogurt are especially rich sources of calcium, providing approximately 300 mg per cup (240 mL). Nevertheless, many women do not consume these foods or do not consume adequate amounts to provide the recommended intakes of calcium. One problem that can interfere with milk consumption is lactose intolerance, the inability to digest milk sugar (lactose) caused by the lack of the lactase enzyme in the small intestine. It is relatively common in adults, particularly African-Americans, Asians, Native Americans, and Inuits (Alaska Natives). Milk consumption can cause abdominal cramping, bloating, and diarrhea in such people, although many lactose-intolerant individuals can tolerate small amounts of milk without symptoms. Yogurt, sweet acidophilus milk, buttermilk, cheese, chocolate milk, and cocoa may be tolerated even when fresh fluid milk is not. Commercial lactase supplements (e.g., Lactaid) are widely available to consume with milk, and many supermarkets stock lactase-treated milk. The lactase in these products hydrolyzes, or digests, the lactose in milk, making it possible for lactose-intolerant people to drink milk.

In some cultures it is uncommon for adults to drink milk. For example, Puerto Ricans and other Hispanic people may use milk only as an additive in coffee. Pregnant women from these cultures may need to consume nondairy sources of calcium (Box 9-6). If calcium intake appears low and the woman does not change her dietary habits despite counseling, a supplement containing 600 mg of elemental calcium may be needed daily. Calcium supplements may also be recommended when a pregnant woman experiences leg cramps caused by an imbalance in the calcium-to-phosphorus ratio.

⚡ SAFETY ALERT

Bone meal, which is sometimes used as a calcium source by pregnant women, is frequently contaminated with lead. Lead freely crosses the placenta; thus regular maternal intake of bone meal may result in high levels of lead in the fetus (Shannon, 2003).

Other Minerals and Electrolytes

Magnesium. Diets of women in the childbearing years are likely to be low in magnesium, and as many as half of pregnant

---

BOX 9-6   CALCIUM SOURCES FOR WOMEN WHO DO NOT DRINK MILK

Each of the following provides approximately the same amount of calcium as 1 cup of milk:

Fish
- 3-oz can of sardines
- 4½-oz can of salmon (if bones are eaten)

Beans and Legumes
- 3 cups of cooked dried beans
- 2½ cups of refried beans
- 2 cups of baked beans with molasses
- 1 cup of tofu (calcium added in processing)

Greens
- 1 cup of collards
- 1½ cups of kale or turnip greens

Baked Products
- 3 pieces of cornbread
- 3 English muffins
- 4 slices of French toast
- 2 (7-inch diameter) waffles

Fruits
- 11 dried figs
- 1⅛ cups of orange juice with calcium added

Sauces
- 3 oz of creamy pesto sauce
- 5 oz of cheese sauce

---

and lactating women may have inadequate intakes. Adolescents and low-income women are especially at risk. Dairy products, nuts, whole grains, and green leafy vegetables are good sources of magnesium.

Sodium. During pregnancy the need for sodium increases slightly, primarily because the body water is expanding (e.g., the expanding blood volume). Sodium is essential for maintaining body water balance. In the past, dietary sodium was routinely restricted in an effort to control the peripheral edema that commonly occurs during pregnancy. It is now recognized that moderate peripheral edema is normal in pregnancy, occurring as a response to the fluid-retaining effects of elevated levels of estrogen. Sodium is not routinely restricted in pregnancy, and restriction has not proved effective in reducing the rates of preeclampsia. Severe sodium restriction may make it difficult for pregnant women to achieve an adequate diet. Grain, milk, and meat products, which are good sources of nutrients needed during pregnancy, are significant sources of sodium. In addition, sodium restriction may stress the adrenal glands and the kidneys as they attempt to retain adequate sodium. In general, sodium restriction is necessary only if the woman has a medical condition such as renal or liver failure or hypertension that warrants such a restriction.

Excessive intake of sodium is discouraged during pregnancy because it may contribute to development of hypertension in salt-sensitive individuals. An adequate sodium intake for pregnant and lactating women, as well as for nonpregnant women in the childbearing years, is estimated to be 1.5 g/day, with a recommended upper limit of intake of 2.3 g/day. Table salt (sodium chloride) is the richest source of sodium, with approximately 2.3 g of sodium contained in 1 teaspoon (5 g) of salt. Most canned foods contain added salt unless the label states otherwise. Large amounts of sodium are also found in many processed foods, including meats (e.g., smoked or cured meats, cold cuts, and corned beef), frozen entrees and meals, baked goods, mixes for casseroles or grain products, soups, and condiments. Products low in nutritive value and excessively high in sodium include pretzels, potato and other chips (except salt free), pickles, catsup, prepared mustard, steak and Worcestershire sauces, some soft drinks, and bouillon. A moderate sodium intake can usually be achieved by salting food lightly during cooking; adding no additional salt at the table; and avoiding low-nutrient, high-sodium foods.

Potassium. Diets including adequate intakes of potassium are associated with reduced risk for hypertension. Potassium has been identified as one of the nutrients most likely to be lacking in the diets of women of childbearing years. A diet including 8 to 10 servings of unprocessed fruits and vegetables daily, along with moderate amounts of low-fat meats and dairy products, has been effective in reducing sodium intake while providing adequate amounts of potassium.

Zinc. Zinc is a constituent of numerous enzymes involved in major metabolic pathways. Zinc deficiency is associated with malformations of the central nervous system in infants. When large amounts of iron and folic acid are consumed, the absorption of zinc is inhibited and the serum zinc levels are reduced as a result. Because iron and folic acid supplements are commonly prescribed during pregnancy, pregnant women should be encouraged to consume good sources of zinc daily (see Table 9-1). Women with anemia who receive high-dose iron supplements also need supplements of zinc and copper.

Fluoride. There is no evidence that prenatal fluoride supplementation reduces the child's likelihood of tooth decay during the preschool years. No increase in fluoride intake over the nonpregnant DRI is recommended during pregnancy.

Fat-Soluble Vitamins

The fat-soluble vitamins include vitamins A, D, E, and K. These are of special concern during pregnancy because vitamin E intake is among the nutrients most likely to be lacking in the diets of women of childbearing age; intake of vitamins A and D is also low in the diets of some women. Fat-soluble vitamins are stored in the body tissues; in the event of prolonged overdoses, these vitamins can reach toxic levels. Because of the high potential for toxicity, pregnant women are advised to take fat-soluble vitamin supplements only as prescribed. However, toxicity from dietary sources is very unlikely.

Vitamin E is needed for protection against oxidative stress, and pregnancy is associated with increased oxidative stress. Oxidative stress above that usually associated with pregnancy has been proposed as an explanation for the etiology of preeclampsia, although supplementation with vitamin E has not been effective in reducing rates of preeclampsia. Vegetable oils and nuts are especially good sources of vitamin E, and whole grains and green leafy vegetables are moderate sources.

Adequate intake of vitamin A is needed so that sufficient amounts of the vitamin can be stored in the fetus. A well-chosen diet, including adequate amounts of deep yellow and deep green vegetables and fruits such as leafy greens, broccoli, carrots, cantaloupe, and apricots, provides sufficient amounts of carotenes that can be converted in the body to vitamin A. Congenital malformations have occurred in infants of mothers who took excessive amounts of preformed vitamin A (from supplements) during pregnancy; thus supplements are not recommended routinely for pregnant women. Vitamin A analogs (e.g., isotretinoin [Accutane]), which are prescribed for the treatment of cystic acne, are a special concern. Isotretinoin use during early pregnancy has been associated with an increased incidence of heart malformations, facial abnormalities, cleft palate, hydrocephalus, and deafness and

blindness in the infant, as well as an increased risk for miscarriage. Topical agents such as tretinoin (Retin-A) do not appear to enter the circulation in substantial amounts, but their safety in pregnancy has not been confirmed.

Vitamin D plays an important role in absorption and metabolism of calcium. The main food sources of this vitamin are enriched or fortified foods such as milk and ready-to-eat cereals. Vitamin D is also produced in the skin by the action of ultraviolet light (in sunlight). A severe deficiency may lead to neonatal hypocalcemia and tetany, as well as to hypoplasia of the tooth enamel. Women with lactose intolerance and those who do not include milk in their diet for any reason are at risk for vitamin D deficiency. Other risk factors for deficiency are dark skin, with African-American women being at high risk for deficiency; habitual use of clothing that covers most of the skin (e.g., Moslem women with extensive body covering); and living in northern latitudes where sunlight exposure is limited, especially during the winter. Use of recommended amounts of sunscreen with a sun protection factor (SPF) rating of 15 or greater reduces skin vitamin D production by as much as 99%, thus bringing about a need for regular intake of fortified foods or a supplement.

Water-Soluble Vitamins

Body stores of water-soluble vitamins are much smaller than those of fat-soluble vitamins, and the water-soluble vitamins, in contrast to fat-soluble vitamins, are readily excreted in the urine. Therefore good sources of these vitamins must be consumed frequently. Toxicity with overdose is less likely than it is in people taking fat-soluble vitamins.

Folate/Folic Acid. Because of the increase in RBC production during pregnancy, as well as the nutritional requirements of the rapidly growing cells in the fetus and placenta, pregnant women should consume about 50% more folic acid than nonpregnant women, or about 0.6 mg (600 mcg) daily. In the United States, all enriched grain products (which include most white breads, flour, and pasta) must contain folic acid at a level of 1.4 mg/kg of flour. This level of fortification is designed to supply approximately 0.1 mg of folic acid daily in the average American diet and has significantly increased folic acid consumption in the population as a whole. All women of childbearing potential need careful counseling about including good sources of folate in their diets (see Box 9-1). Supplemental folic acid is usually prescribed to ensure that intake is adequate. Women who have borne a child with a neural tube defect are advised to consume 4 mg (4000 mcg) of folic acid daily, and a supplement is required for them to achieve this level of intake.

Pyridoxine. Pyridoxine, or vitamin B_6, is involved in protein metabolism. Although levels of a pyridoxine-containing enzyme have been reported to be low in women with preeclampsia, there is no evidence that supplementation prevents or eradicates the condition. Pyridoxine has been effective in reducing the nausea and vomiting of early pregnancy in some trials.

Vitamin C. Vitamin C, or ascorbic acid, plays an important role in tissue formation and enhances the absorption of iron. The vitamin C needs of most women are readily met by a diet that includes at least one or two daily servings of citrus fruit or juice or another good source of the vitamin (see Table 9-1), but women who smoke need more.

Vitamin B_{12}. Vitamin B_{12} is involved in production of nucleic acids and protein; it is especially important in formation of RBCs and neural functioning. It is found in milk and milk products, eggs, meats, liver, and fortified soy milk.

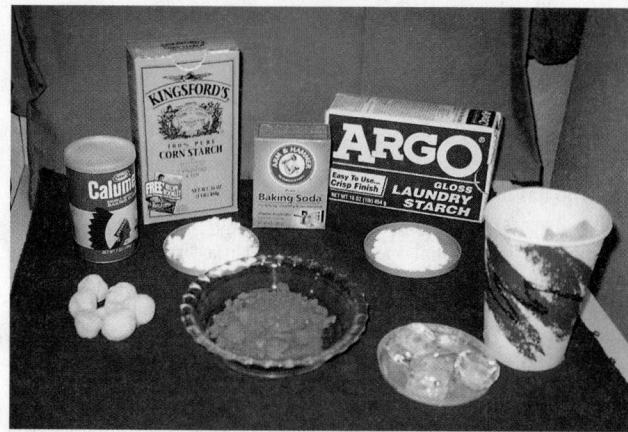

FIG 9-3 Nonfood substances consumed in pica: red clay from Georgia, nzu from East Nigeria, baking powder, cornstarch, baking soda, laundry starch, and ice. Some individuals practice *poly-pica*, consuming more than one of these or other nonfood substances. (Courtesy Shannon Perry, Phoenix, AZ.)

Other Nutritional Issues During Pregnancy

Pica and Food Cravings

Pica, which is the practice of consuming nonfood substances (e.g., clay, dirt, and laundry starch) or excessive amounts of foodstuffs low in nutritional value (e.g., cornstarch, ice or freezer frost, baking powder, or baking soda), is often influenced by the woman's cultural background (Fig. 9-3). In the United States, it appears to be most common among African-American and Hispanic women, women from rural areas, and women with a family history of pica. One problem with pica is that regular and heavy consumption of low-nutrient products may cause more nutritious foods to be displaced from the diet. As an example, cornstarch ingestion is popular among African-American women. It is a source of "empty" calories; half a cup (64 g) provides 240 kcal but almost no vitamins, minerals, or protein. Overuse of cornstarch can contribute to development of gestational diabetes. In addition, the pica items consumed may interfere with the absorption of nutrients, especially minerals. Women with pica have been found to have lower hemoglobin levels than do those without pica.

Moreover, there is a risk that nonfood items are contaminated with heavy metals or other toxic substances. Among Mexican-American women, consumption of "tierra" includes both soil and pulverized Mexican pottery. Lead contamination of soils and soil-based products has caused high levels of lead in pregnant women and their newborns. Regular household use of Mexican pottery in cooking or serving food or ingestion of ground pottery must be included in interviews or questionnaires regarding nutrition intake of pregnant women. The possibility of pica must be considered when pregnant women are found to be anemic, and the nurse should provide counseling about the health risks associated with pica.

The existence of picas, as well as details of the types and amounts of products ingested, is likely to be discovered only by the sensitive interviewer who has developed a relationship of trust with the woman. It has been proposed that pica and food cravings (e.g., the urge to have ice cream, pickles, or pizza) during pregnancy are caused by an innate drive to consume nutrients missing from the diet. However, research has not supported this hypothesis.

Adolescent Pregnancy Needs

Many adolescent females have diets that provide less than the recommended intakes of key nutrients, including calcium and iron. Pregnant adolescents and their infants are at increased risk for complications during pregnancy and parturition. Growth of the pelvis is delayed in comparison with growth in stature, and this helps explain why cephalopelvic disproportion and other mechanical problems associated with labor are common among young adolescents. Competition for nutrients between the growing adolescent and the fetus may also contribute to some of the poor outcomes apparent in teen pregnancies. Recommended weight-gain goals are not different from those of adult women. Pregnant adolescents are encouraged to choose a weight-gain goal at the upper end of the range for their BMI. BMI is calculated as for adult women (Institute of Medicine [IOM], 2009) rather than by using the adolescent BMI growth charts available from the Centers for Disease Control and Prevention (CDC) (www.cdc.gov). Adolescent females who have given birth have greater percentages of total fat and visceral fat (associated with the metabolic syndrome and cardiovascular disease) than those who have never given birth (Gunderson, Striegel-Moore, Schreiber, et al., 2009); thus the adolescent mother needs careful teaching regarding nutritional intake and physical activity to control body weight in the postpartum period.

Efforts to improve the nutritional health of pregnant adolescents focus on:

- Improving the nutrition knowledge, meal planning, and selection and food preparation skills of young women
- Promoting access to prenatal care
- Developing nutrition interventions and educational programs that are effective with adolescents
- Striving to understand the factors that create barriers to change in the adolescent population

Preeclampsia

There has been speculation that the poor intake of various nutrients might contribute to development of preeclampsia, but no definitive evidence exists. At present, a diet adequate in the recommended nutrients (see Table 9-1), along with use of a supplement that provides micronutrients both before and during pregnancy, appears to be the best means of reducing the risk for preeclampsia.

Physical Activity During Pregnancy

Moderate exercise during pregnancy yields numerous benefits, including improving muscle tone, potentially shortening the course of labor, and promoting a sense of well-being. If no medical or obstetric problems contraindicate physical activity, pregnant women should engage in a minimum of 30 minutes of moderate physical exercise on most, if not all, days of the week. Two nutritional concepts are especially important for women who choose to exercise during pregnancy. First, a liberal amount of fluid should be consumed before, during, and after exercise because dehydration can trigger premature labor. Second, the calorie intake should be sufficient to meet the increased needs of pregnancy and the demands of exercise.

NUTRIENT NEEDS DURING LACTATION

Nutritional needs during lactation are similar in many ways to those during pregnancy. Needs for energy (calories), protein, calcium, iodine, zinc, the B vitamins (thiamine, riboflavin, niacin, pyridoxine, and vitamin B_{12}), and vitamin C remain greater than nonpregnant needs. The recommendations for some of these (e.g., vitamin C, zinc, and protein) are slightly to moderately higher than during pregnancy (see Table 9-1). This allowance covers the amount of the nutrients released in the milk, as well as the needs of the mother for tissue maintenance. In the case of iron and folic acid, the recommendation during lactation is lower than that during pregnancy. Both of these nutrients are essential for RBC formation and thus for maintaining the increase in the blood volume that occurs during pregnancy. With the decrease in maternal blood volume to nonpregnant levels after birth, maternal iron and folic acid needs also decrease. Many lactating women have a delay in the return of menses, which also conserves blood cells and reduces iron and folic acid needs. It is especially important that the calcium intake be adequate; if it is not, a supplement of 600 mg of calcium per day may be needed.

The recommended energy intake for the first 6 months is an increase of 330 kcal more than the woman's nonpregnant intake. It becomes difficult to obtain adequate nutrients for maintenance of lactation if total caloric intake is less than 1800 kcal. Because of the deposition of energy stores, the woman who has gained the optimal amount of weight during pregnancy is heavier after birth than at the beginning of pregnancy. As a result of the caloric demands of lactation, the lactating mother usually experiences a gradual but steady weight loss. Most women rapidly lose several kilograms during the first month after birth, whether or not they breastfeed. After the first month, the average loss during lactation is 0.5 to 1 kg a month, and a woman who is overweight may be able to lose up to 2 kg without decreasing her milk supply.

Fluid intake must be adequate to maintain milk production, but the mother's level of thirst is the best guide to the right amount. There is no need to consume more fluids than those needed to satisfy thirst.

Smoking, alcohol intake, and excessive caffeine intake should be avoided during lactation. Smoking not only may impair milk production but also exposes the infant to the risk of passive smoking. It is speculated that the infant's psychomotor development may be affected by maternal alcohol use, and alcohol use may impair the milk-ejection reflex. Caffeine intake can lead to a reduced iron concentration in milk and consequently contribute to the development of anemia in the infant. The caffeine concentration in milk is only approximately 1% of the mother's plasma level, but caffeine levels build up in the infant. Breastfed infants of mothers who drink large amounts of coffee or caffeine-containing soft drinks may be unusually active and wakeful.

CARE MANAGEMENT

During pregnancy, nutrition plays a key role in achieving an optimal outcome for the mother and her unborn baby. The motivation to learn about nutrition is usually greater during pregnancy because parents strive to "do what's right for the baby." Optimal nutrition cannot eliminate all problems that may arise during pregnancy, but it does establish a good foundation for supporting the needs of the mother and her unborn baby.

Assessment

Ideally a nutritional assessment is performed before conception so that any recommended changes in diet, lifestyle, and weight can be undertaken before the woman becomes pregnant.

Information on nutrition and diet is obtained from an interview and review of the woman's health records, physical examination, and laboratory results.

Obstetric and Gynecologic Effects on Nutrition

Nutrition reserves may be depleted in the multiparous woman or one who has had frequent pregnancies (especially three pregnancies within 2 years). A history of preterm birth or the birth of an LBW or small-for-gestational-age (SGA) infant may indicate inadequate dietary intake. Birth of a large-for-gestational-age (LGA) infant often indicates the existence of maternal diabetes mellitus. Contraceptive methods also may affect reproductive health. Increased menstrual blood loss often occurs during the first 3 to 6 months after placement of an intrauterine contraceptive device; consequently the user may have low iron stores or even iron deficiency anemia. Oral contraceptive agents are associated with decreased menstrual losses and increased iron stores; however, oral contraceptives may interfere with folic acid metabolism.

Health History

Chronic maternal illnesses such as diabetes mellitus, renal disease, liver disease, cystic fibrosis or other malabsorptive disorders, seizure disorders and the use of anticonvulsant agents, hypertension, and PKU may affect a woman's nutritional status and dietary needs. In women with illnesses that have resulted in nutrition deficits or that require dietary treatment (e.g., diabetes mellitus, PKU), it is extremely important for nutritional care to be started and for the condition to be optimally controlled before conception. A registered dietitian can provide in-depth counseling for the woman who requires medical nutrition therapy during pregnancy and lactation.

Usual Maternal Diet

The woman's usual food and beverage intake, the adequacy of her income and other resources to meet her nutrition needs, any dietary modifications, food allergies and intolerances, and all medications and nutrition supplements being taken, as well as pica and cultural dietary requirements, should be ascertained. In addition, the presence and severity of nutrition-related discomforts of pregnancy such as morning sickness, constipation, and pyrosis (heartburn) should be determined. The nurse should be alert to any evidence of eating disorders such as anorexia nervosa, bulimia, or frequent and rigorous dieting before or during pregnancy.

The effect of food allergies and intolerances on nutritional status ranges from very important to almost nil. Lactose intolerance is of special concern in pregnant and lactating women because no other food group equals milk and milk products in terms of calcium content. If a woman has lactose intolerance, the interviewer should explore her intake of other calcium sources (see Box 9-6).

The assessment must include an evaluation of the woman's financial status and her knowledge of sound dietary practices. The quality of the diet improves with increasing socioeconomic status and educational level. Poor women may not have access to adequate refrigeration and cooking facilities and may find it difficult to obtain adequate nutritious food. Food-borne illnesses may cause adverse effects in pregnancy, and the woman's understanding of safe food-handling practices such as the following should be assessed:

- Cleansing hands, food preparation surfaces, and utensils frequently
- Avoiding contact between raw meat, fish, or poultry and other foods that will not be cooked before consumption
- Storing foods properly
- Cooking foods to a safe temperature

Box 9-7 provides a simple tool for obtaining diet history information. When potential problems are identified, they should be followed up with a careful interview.

Physical Examination

Anthropometric (body) measurements provide short-term and long-term information on a woman's nutritional status and are thus essential to the assessment. At a minimum, the woman's height and weight must be determined at the time of her first prenatal visit, and her weight should be measured at each subsequent visit (see earlier discussion of BMI).

A careful physical examination can reveal objective signs of malnutrition (Table 9-5). It is important to note, however, that some of these signs are nonspecific and that the physiologic changes of pregnancy may complicate the interpretation of physical findings. For example, lower extremity edema often occurs when calorie and protein deficiencies are present but it may also be a normal finding in the third trimester of pregnancy. The interpretation of physical findings is made easier by a thorough health history and by laboratory testing if indicated.

Laboratory Testing

The only nutrition-related laboratory testing needed by most pregnant women is a hematocrit or hemoglobin measurement to screen for the presence of anemia. Because of the physiologic anemia of pregnancy, the reference values for hemoglobin and hematocrit must be adjusted during pregnancy. The lower limit of the normal range for hemoglobin during pregnancy is 11 g/dL in the first and third trimesters and 10.5 g/dL in the second trimester (compared with 12 g/dL in the nonpregnant state). The lower limit of the normal range for hematocrit is 33% during the first and third trimesters and 32% in the second trimester (compared with 36% in the nonpregnant state). Cutoff values for anemia are higher in women who smoke or live at high altitudes because the decreased oxygen-carrying capacity of their RBCs causes them to produce more RBCs than other women produce.

A woman's history or physical findings may indicate the need for additional testing. These tests might include a complete blood cell count with a differential to identify megaloblastic or macrocytic anemia and measurement of levels of specific vitamins or minerals believed to be lacking in the diet.

Nutrition Care and Teaching

For many women with uncomplicated pregnancies, the nurse can serve as the primary source of nutrition education. The registered dietitian, who has specialized training in diet evaluation and planning, nutritional needs during illness, ethnic and cultural food patterns, as well as translating nutrient needs into food patterns, frequently serves as a consultant. Pregnant women with serious nutritional problems, those with intervening illnesses such as diabetes (either preexisting or gestational), and any others requiring in-depth dietary counseling should be referred to the dietitian. The nurse, dietitian, physician, and nurse-midwife collaborate in helping the woman achieve nutrition-related expected outcomes. Nutritional care and teaching generally involve:

- Acquainting the woman with nutritional needs during pregnancy and the characteristics of an adequate diet, if necessary
- Helping her individualize her diet so that she achieves an adequate intake while conforming to her personal, cultural, financial, and health circumstances
- Acquainting her with strategies for coping with the nutrition-related discomforts of pregnancy
- Helping her use nutrition supplements appropriately
- Consulting with and making referrals to other professionals or services as indicated

Two programs that provide nutrition services are the food stamp program and the Special Supplemental Nutrition Program for Women, Infants and Children (WIC), which provides vouchers for selected foods for pregnant and lactating women as well as for infants and children at nutritional risk (see the Nursing Care Plan). WIC foods include items such as eggs, cheese, milk, juice, and fortified cereals—foods chosen because they provide iron, protein, vitamin C, and other vitamins.

Adequate Dietary Intake

Nutrition teaching can take place in a one-on-one interview or in a group setting. In either case, teaching should emphasize the importance of choosing a varied diet composed of readily available foods (rather than specialized diet supplements). Good nutrition practices (and avoidance of poor practices such as smoking and alcohol or drug use) are essential content for prenatal classes designed for women in early pregnancy.

MyPlate (www.choosemyplate.gov) can be used as a guide to making daily food choices during pregnancy and lactation, just as it is during other stages of the life cycle. Additional individualized information and resources for professionals are available from the website. The importance of consuming adequate amounts from the milk, yogurt, and cheese group must be emphasized, especially for adolescents and women younger than 25 years, who are still actively adding calcium to their skeletons; adolescents need at least three or four servings from the milk group daily.

Pregnancy. The pregnant woman must understand what adequate weight gain during pregnancy means, recognize the reasons for its importance, and be able to evaluate her own gain in terms of the desirable pattern. Many women, particularly those who have worked hard to control their weight before pregnancy, may find it difficult to understand why the weight-gain goal is so high when a newborn infant is so small. The nurse can explain that maternal weight gain consists of increments in the weight of many tissues, not just the growing fetus (see Table 9-2).

Dietary overindulgence, which may result in excessive fat stores that persist after giving birth, should be discouraged. Nevertheless, it is best not to focus unduly on weight gain because this could result in feelings of stress and guilt in the woman who does not follow the preferred pattern of gain. Teaching regarding weight gain during pregnancy is summarized in Box 9-2.

Postpartum. An important goal of postpartum nutrition is for the woman to lose the weight gained during pregnancy. Retention of this weight can contribute to overweight/obesity and the

BOX 9-7 FOOD INTAKE QUESTIONNAIRE

Which of the following did you eat or drink yesterday? If the way you ate yesterday wasn't the way you usually eat, choose a recent day that was typical for you.

FOOD OR DRINK	NUMBER OF SERVINGS	FOOD OR DRINK	NUMBER OF SERVINGS
Beer, wine, other alcoholic drinks	_____	Orange or grapefruit juice	_____
Tea	_____	Fruit juice other than orange or grapefruit	_____
Coffee	_____	Soft drinks	_____
Caffeinated	_____	Milk	_____
Decaffeinated	_____	Cereal with milk	_____
Fruit drink	_____	Yogurt	_____
Water	_____	Pizza	_____
Cheese	_____	Melon (e.g., watermelon, cantaloupe, honeydew)	_____
Macaroni and cheese	_____	Berries (kind)	_____
Other foods with cheese (e.g., lasagna, enchiladas, cheeseburgers)	_____	Apples	_____
Orange or grapefruit	_____	Other fruit	_____
Bananas	_____	Broccoli	_____
Peaches or apricots	_____	Green beans	_____
Green salad	_____	Potatoes (other than fried)	_____
Spinach or greens	_____	Corn	_____
Green peas	_____	Other vegetables	_____
Sweet potatoes	_____	Chicken or turkey	_____
Carrots	_____	Egg	_____
Meat	_____	Nuts	_____
Fish	_____	Hot dog	_____
Peanut butter	_____	Cold cuts (e.g., bologna)	_____
Dried beans or peas	_____	Roll/bagel	_____
Bacon or sausage	_____	Noodles	_____
Bread	_____	Chips	_____
Rice	_____	Cake	_____
Spaghetti or other pasta	_____	Donut or pastry	_____
Tortillas	_____	Cookie	_____
French fries	_____	Pie	_____

Are you often bothered by any of the following? (Circle all that apply)

Nausea   Vomiting   Heartburn   Constipation

Are you on a special diet? No _____ Yes _____
    If yes, what kind?

_____

Do you try to limit the amount or kind of food you eat to control your weight?
No _____ Yes _____

Do you avoid any foods for health or religious reasons? No _____ Yes _____
    If yes, what foods?

_____

Do you take any prescribed drugs or medications? No _____ Yes _____
    If yes, what are they?

_____

Do you take any over-the-counter medications (e.g., aspirin, cold medicines, acetaminophen [Tylenol])? No _____ Yes _____
    If yes, what are they?

_____

Do you take any herbal supplements? No _____ Yes _____
    If yes, what are they?

_____

Do you ever have trouble affording the food you need? No _____ Yes _____

Do you have any help getting the food you need? No _____ Yes _____
    If yes, what kind? Food stamps _____ WIC _____ School lunch or breakfast _____
    Food from a food pantry, soup kitchen, or food bank _____ Other _____

TABLE 9-5   PHYSICAL ASSESSMENT OF NUTRITIONAL STATUS

SIGNS OF GOOD NUTRITION	SIGNS OF POOR NUTRITION
General Appearance Alert, responsive, energetic, good endurance	Listless, apathetic, cachectic, easily fatigued, looks tired
Muscles Well developed, firm, good tone, some fat under skin	Flaccid, poor tone, tender, "wasted" appearance
Gastrointestinal Function Good appetite and digestion, normal regular elimination, no palpable organs or masses	Anorexia, indigestion, constipation or diarrhea, liver or spleen enlargement
Cardiovascular Function Normal heart rate and rhythm, no murmurs, normal blood pressure for age	Rapid heart rate, enlarged heart, abnormal rhythm, elevated blood pressure
Hair Shiny, lustrous, firm, not easily plucked, healthy scalp	Stringy, dull, brittle, dry, thin and sparse, depigmented, can be easily plucked
Skin (General) Smooth, slightly moist, good color	Rough, dry, scaly, pale, pigmented, irritated, easily bruised, petechiae
Face and Neck Skin color uniform, smooth, pink, healthy appearance; no enlargement of thyroid gland; lips not chapped or swollen	Scaly, swollen, skin dark over cheeks and under eyes, lumpiness or flakiness of skin around nose and mouth; thyroid enlarged; lips swollen, angular lesions or fissures at corners of mouth
Oral Cavity Reddish pink mucous membranes and gums; no swelling or bleeding of gums; tongue healthy pink or deep reddish in appearance, not swollen or smooth, surface papillae present; teeth bright and clean, no cavities, no pain, no discoloration	Gums spongy, bleed easily, inflamed or receding; tongue swollen, scarlet and raw, magenta color, beefy, hyperemic and hypertrophic papillae, atrophic papillae; teeth with unfilled caries, absent teeth, worn surfaces, mottled
Eyes Bright, clear, shiny, no sores at corners of eyelids, membranes moist and healthy pink color, no prominent blood vessels or mound of tissue (Bitot spots) on sclera, no fatigue circles beneath	Eye membranes pale, redness of membrane, dryness, signs of infection, redness and fissuring of eyelid corners, dryness of eye membrane, dull appearance of cornea, blue sclerae
Extremities No tenderness, weakness, or swelling; nails firm and pink	Edema, tender calves, tingling, weakness; nails spoon-shaped, brittle
Skeleton No malformations	Bowlegs, knock-knees, chest deformity at diaphragm, beaded ribs, prominent scapulae

development of later health problems including the metabolic syndrome, cardiovascular disease, and diabetes.

The need for a varied diet with food from all the food groups continues throughout lactation. The lactating woman should be advised to consume at least 1800 kcal daily, and she should receive counseling if her diet appears to be inadequate in any nutrients. Special attention should be given to her zinc, vitamin B₆, and folic acid intake because the recommendations for these remain higher than for nonpregnant women (see Table 9-1). Sufficient calcium is needed to allow for both milk formation and maintenance of maternal bone mass. It may be difficult for lactating women to consume enough of these nutrients without careful meal planning.

Obese women and normal-weight women who gain more than the recommended amount of weight during pregnancy are less likely to breastfeed than normal-weight women with appropriate weight gain. Obese women who do choose to breastfeed have a statistically shorter period of lactation than normal-weight women. The woman who does not breastfeed can lose weight gradually if she consumes a balanced diet that provides slightly less than her daily energy expenditure, although overweight and obese women with excessive weight gain during pregnancy have an increased likelihood of failing to return to their prepregnancy weights (Siega-Riz, Viswanathan, Moos, et al., 2009). A reasonable weight-loss goal for nonlactating women is 0.5 to 0.9 kg per week; a loss of 1 kg per month is recommended for most lactating women. Those at risk for obesity and overweight need follow-up to ensure that they know how to make wise food choices, primarily from fruits, vegetables, whole grains, lean meats, and low-fat dairy products. An hour of moderately vigorous physical activity (e.g., walking, jogging, swimming, cycling, aerobic dance) most days of the week will improve the ability of the woman to lose weight gradually and maintain the weight loss.

◎ NURSING CARE PLAN

Nutrition During Pregnancy

NURSING DIAGNOSIS	EXPECTED OUTCOME	INTERVENTIONS	RATIONALES
Deficient Knowledge related to nutritional requirements during pregnancy	Woman will describe nutritional requirements and exhibit evidence of incorporating requirements into diet.	Review basic nutritional requirements for healthy diet by using recommended dietary guidelines and MyPlate	To provide knowledge baseline for discussion
		Discuss increased nutrient needs (calories, protein, minerals, vitamins) that occur as result of being pregnant	To increase knowledge needed for altered dietary requirements
		Discuss relation between weight gain and fetal growth	To reinforce interdependence of fetus and mother
		Calculate appropriate total weight gain range during pregnancy using woman's body mass index as guide, and discuss recommended rates of weight gain during various trimesters of pregnancy	To provide concrete measures of dietary success
		Review food preferences, cultural eating patterns or beliefs, and prepregnancy eating patterns	To enhance integration of new dietary needs
		Discuss how to fit nutritional needs into usual dietary patterns and how to alter any identified nutritional deficits or excesses	To increase chances of success with dietary alterations
		Discuss food aversions or cravings that may occur during pregnancy and strategies to deal with these if they are detrimental to fetus (e.g., pica)	To ensure well-being of fetus
		Have woman keep food diary delineating eating habits, dietary alterations, aversions, and cravings	To track eating habits and potential problem areas
Imbalanced Nutrition: Less Than Body Requirements related to inadequate intake of needed nutrients	Woman's weekly weight gain will be increased to appropriate rate using her body mass index (BMI) and recommended weight gain ranges as guidelines.	Review recent diet history (including food aversions) using food diary, 24-hour recall, or food frequency approach	To ascertain dietary inadequacies contributing to insufficient weight gain
		Review normal activity and exercise routines and discuss eating patterns and reasons that lead to decreased food intake (e.g., morning sickness, pica, fear of becoming fat, stress, boredom)	To determine level of energy expenditure and to identify habits that contribute to inadequate weight gain
		Review optimal weight gain guidelines and their rationale	To ensure that woman is knowledgeable about healthful weight gain rates
		Set target weight gains for remaining weeks of pregnancy	To establish set goals
		Review increased nutrient needs (calories, protein, minerals, vitamins) that occur as result of being pregnant	To ensure woman is knowledgeable about altered dietary requirements
		Review relation between weight gain and fetal growth	To reinforce that adequate weight gain is needed to promote fetal well-being
		Discuss with woman what changes can be made in diet, activity, and lifestyle	To enhance chances of meeting set weight gain goals and nutrient needs of mother and fetus
		If woman has fear of being fat, if symptoms of eating disorder are evident, or if problems in adjusting to changing body image surface, refer woman to appropriate mental health professional for evaluation	Because intensive treatment and follow-up may be required to ensure fetal health
Nausea related to physiologic alterations of first trimester of pregnancy	Nausea will not be so severe that it interferes with adequate nutrient intake or substantially reduces quality of life.	Assess state of hydration and assess pattern of weight gain during pregnancy	To ensure that woman does not have deficient fluid volume; to ensure that nausea is not preventing adequate energy intake
		Review nausea history (i.e., frequency of episodes of nausea, likelihood of nausea progressing to vomiting, factors precipitating or associated with nausea, and any relief measures that woman has tried)	To determine severity of problem and to begin to identify effective and ineffective measures for coping with nausea
		Review measures for prevention or relief of morning sickness	To ensure that woman is knowledgeable about measures that are often effective in alleviating morning sickness
		Discuss with woman what relief measures she will try	To determine whether she understands how to implement measures

Daily Food Guide and Menu Planning

The daily food plan (see Table 9-3) can be used as a guide for educating women about nutritional needs during pregnancy and lactation. This food plan is general enough to be used by women from a wide variety of cultures, including those who follow a vegetarian diet. One of the more helpful teaching strategies is to help the woman plan daily menus that follow the food plan and are affordable, have realistic preparation times, and are compatible with personal preferences and cultural practices. Information regarding cultural food patterns is provided later in this chapter.

Medical Nutrition Therapy

During pregnancy and lactation, the food plan for women with special medical nutrition therapy may have to be modified. The registered dietitian can instruct these women about their diets and assist them in meal planning. However, the nurse should understand the basic principles of the diet and be able to reinforce the teaching.

The nurse should be especially aware of the dietary modifications necessary for women with diabetes mellitus (either gestational or preexisting). This disease is relatively common, and fetal morbidity and mortality occur more often in pregnancies complicated by hyperglycemia or hypoglycemia (see discussion of diabetes in Chapter 11). Every effort should be made to maintain blood glucose levels in the normal range throughout pregnancy. The food plan of the woman with diabetes usually includes four to six meals and snacks daily, with the daily carbohydrate intake distributed fairly evenly among the meals and snacks. The complex carbohydrates—fibers and starches—should be well represented in the diet. To maintain strict control of the blood glucose level, the pregnant woman with diabetes usually must monitor her own blood glucose daily.

Counseling About Iron Supplementation

The nutrition supplement most commonly needed during pregnancy is iron. However, a variety of dietary factors can affect the completeness of absorption of an iron supplement. The Patient Teaching box summarizes important points regarding iron supplementation.

Coping with Nutrition-Related Discomforts of Pregnancy

The most common nutrition-related discomforts of pregnancy are nausea and vomiting (or "morning sickness"), constipation, and pyrosis.

Nausea and Vomiting. Nausea and vomiting of pregnancy (NVP) is most common during the first trimester. Usually, NVP causes only mild to moderate problems nutritionally, although it may be a source of substantial discomfort. Antiemetic medications, vitamin B$_6$, ginger, and P6 acupressure may be effective in reducing the severity of nausea, although the evidence supporting them is not strong. The pregnant woman may find the suggestions in Box 9-8 helpful in alleviating NVP.

Hyperemesis gravidarum, or severe and persistent vomiting causing weight loss, dehydration, and electrolyte abnormalities, occurs in up to 1% of pregnant women. Intravenous fluid and electrolyte replacement, enteral tube feeding, and in some instances total parenteral nutrition have been used to nourish women with hyperemesis gravidarum. There is very limited evidence that acupressure and ginger might provide some relief.

Constipation. Improved bowel function generally results from increasing the intake of fiber (e.g., bran and whole-wheat products, popcorn, and raw or lightly steamed vegetables) in the diet. Fiber helps create a bulky stool that stimulates intestinal peristalsis. The recommendation for pregnant women for fiber is 28 g daily. An adequate fluid intake (at least 50 mL/kg/day) helps hydrate the fiber and increase the bulk of the stool. Making a habit of regular physical activity that uses large muscle groups (walking, swimming, water aerobics) also helps stimulate bowel motility.

Pyrosis. Pyrosis, or heartburn, is usually caused by reflux of gastric contents into the esophagus. This condition can be

---

PATIENT TEACHING

Iron Supplementation

- A diet rich in vitamin C (in citrus fruits, tomatoes, melons, and strawberries) and **heme iron** (in meats) increases the absorption of iron supplement; therefore include these in the diet often.
- Bran, tea, coffee, milk, oxalates (in spinach and Swiss chard), and egg yolk decrease iron absorption. Avoid consuming them at the same time as the supplement.
- Iron is absorbed best if it is taken when the stomach is empty; that is, take it between meals with a beverage other than tea, coffee, or milk.
- Iron can be taken at bedtime if abdominal discomfort occurs when it is taken between meals.
- If an iron dose is missed, take it as soon as it is remembered if that is within 13 hours of the scheduled dose. Do not double up on the dose.
- Keep the supplement in a childproof container and out of the reach of any children in the household.
- The iron may cause stools to be black or dark green.
- Constipation is common with iron supplementation. A diet high in fiber with adequate fluid intake is recommended.

BOX 9-8 SUGGESTIONS FOR MANAGING NAUSEA AND VOMITING DURING PREGNANCY

- Eat dry, starchy foods such as dry toast, melba toast, or crackers on awakening in the morning and at other times when nausea occurs.
- Avoid consuming excessive amounts of fluids early in the day or when nauseated (but compensate by drinking fluids at other times).
- Eat small amounts frequently (every 2 to 3 hours), and avoid large meals that distend the stomach.
- Avoid skipping meals and thus becoming extremely hungry, which may worsen nausea. Have a snack such as cereal with milk, a small sandwich, or yogurt before bedtime.
- Avoid sudden movements. Get out of bed slowly.
- Decrease intake of fried and other fatty foods. Try high-carbohydrate foods such as toast, rice, or potatoes. Some women find high-protein meals or snacks helpful.
- Breathe fresh air to help relieve nausea. Keep the environment well ventilated (e.g., open a window), go for a walk outside, or decrease cooking odors by using an exhaust fan.
- Eat foods served at cool temperatures and foods that give off little aroma. Avoid spicy foods.
- Avoid brushing teeth immediately after eating.
- Try salty and tart foods (e.g., potato chips and lemonade) during periods of nausea. Sucking a lemon slice may help.
- Try herbal teas such as those made with raspberry leaf or peppermint to decrease nausea.

minimized by eating small, frequent meals rather than two or three larger meals daily. Because fluids increase the distention of the stomach, they should not be consumed with foods. The woman needs to drink adequate amounts between meals. Avoiding spicy foods may help alleviate the problem. Reflux can be exacerbated by lying down immediately after eating and wearing clothing that is tight across the abdomen.

Cultural Influences

Consideration of a woman's cultural food preferences enhances communication and provides a greater opportunity for following the agreed-on pattern of intake. Women in most cultures are encouraged to eat a diet typical for them. The nurse needs to be aware of what constitutes a typical diet for each cultural or ethnic group present in her patient population. However, several variations may occur within one cultural group. Thus a careful exploration of individual preferences is needed. Although ethnic and cultural food beliefs may seem at first glance to conflict with the dietary instruction provided by physicians, nurses, and dietitians, it is often possible for the empathic health care provider to identify cultural beliefs that are congruent with the modern understanding of pregnancy and fetal development. Many cultural food practices have some merit or the culture would not have survived. Food cravings during

pregnancy are considered normal by many cultures, but the kinds of cravings often are culturally specific. In most cultures, women crave acceptable foods, such as chicken, fish, and greens among African-Americans. Cultural influences on food intake usually lessen if the woman and her family become more integrated into the dominant culture. Nutritional beliefs and the practices of selected cultural groups are summarized in Table 9-6.

Vegetarian Diets

Vegetarian diets represent another cultural effect on nutritional status. Foods basic to almost all vegetarian diets are vegetables, fruits, legumes, nuts, seeds, and grains, but with many variations. Lacto-vegetarians include milk products. Lacto-ovovegetarians consume eggs and dairy products in addition to plant products. Strict vegetarians, or vegans, consume only plant products. All of these types of vegetarian diets, if they are well planned, can be nutritionally adequate for pregnant and lactating women (Craig and Mangels, 2009). Because vitamin B_{12} is found only in foods of animal origin, this diet is deficient in vitamin B_{12}. As a result, strict vegetarians should take a supplement or regularly consume vitamin B_{12}—fortified foods such as fortified soy milk two or three times a day or take a supplement. Vitamin B_{12} deficiency can result in megaloblastic anemia, glossitis (inflamed red tongue), and neurologic deficits in

TABLE 9-6	**POPULAR FOODS OF VARIOUS CULTURAL AND ETHNIC GROUPS AND THEIR PLACE IN MYPLATE**				
CULTURAL OR ETHNIC GROUP OR EATING PATTERN	**FOOD GROUPS**				
	GRAINS	**VEGETABLE**	**FRUIT**	**DAIRY**	**PROTEIN**

Mexican	Tortilla
	Taco shell
	Posole (corn soup)
	Rice
	Postres (pastries)*
		Other vegetables:
		  Chayote (Mexican squash)
		  Jicama (root vegetable)
		  Nopales (cactus leaves)
		  Tomato
		  Corn
			Avocado
			Mango
			Papaya
			Plantano (cooking banana)
			Zapote (sweet, yellowish fruit)
				Queso blanco (white Mexican cheese)
				Custard (1 cup = 1 cup milk serving)
				Leche (milk)
					Chorizo (sausage)*
					Chicken, beef, goat, or pork
					Beans, dried, cooked

African-American soul food (Southern-style cooking)	Biscuit Cornbread Grits, rice, macaroni, or noodles Hominy Crackers Hush puppies	*Dark green:* Collard, kale, mustard, or turnip greens *Orange:* Sweet potatoes *Other:* Okra Snap, pole (green), lima, and butter beans Turnips Summer squash (yellow or zucchini) Coleslaw	Blackberries Melons Muscadines (grapes) Peaches	Buttermilk	Pork (cured ham and uncured cuts), chicken, beef, fish Peas or beans (black-eyed, crowder, purple-hull, or cream)
Vegetarian	Whole-grain bread Cereal, cooked or ready-to-eat Brown rice Whole-grain pasta Bagel	All	All	Milk and cheese (lacto-vegetarians) Soy milk, calcium-fortified Soy cheese	Cooked dried beans or peas Tofu (soybean curd) or tempeh (fermented soy) Nuts or seeds Peanut butter Egg (ovovegetarians)

TABLE 9-6	POPULAR FOODS OF VARIOUS CULTURAL AND ETHNIC GROUPS AND THEIR PLACE IN MYPLATE—cont'd				
CULTURAL OR ETHNIC GROUP OR EATING PATTERN	**FOOD GROUPS**				
	GRAINS	**VEGETABLE**	**FRUIT**	**DAIRY**	**PROTEIN**
Italian	Breadsticks, breads	*Dark green:*	Berries	Cheeses (e.g., mozzarella,	Veal or beef
	Gnocchi (dumplings)	Spinach	Figs	Parmesan, Romano,	Fish
	Polenta (cornmeal	*Other:*	Pomegranate	ricotta)	Sausage*
	mush)	Artichoke		Gelato (Italian ice cream)	Luncheon meats*
	Risotto (creamy rice	Eggplant			Lentils
	dish)	Mushrooms			Squid
	Pastas	Marinara sauce			Almonds, pistachios
Chinese	Rice or millet	*Other:*	Guava	Soy milk	Pork, fish, chicken
	Rice vermicelli (thin	Pea pods	Lychee		Shrimp, crab, lobster
	rice pasta)	Yard-long beans	Persimmon		Tofu or tempeh
	Cellophane noodles	Baby corn	Pummelo		
	(bean thread)	Bamboo shoots	Kumquat		
	Steamed rolls	Straw mushrooms	Star fruit		
	Rice congee (soup)	Eggplant			
	Rice sticks	Bitter melon			
Indian (south Asia)	Breads: roti	*Dark green:*	Mango	Yogurt	Dal (lentils, mung beans,
	(chapati), naan,	Saag (mixed greens and	Dates		other dried beans)
	paratha, batura,	potatoes)	Raisins		Beef, chicken (some are
	puris, dosa, idli	Spinach	Melons		vegetarian)
	Rice or rice pilau	*Other:*	Figs		
	Pooha, upma,	Green peppers	Fruit juices and		
	sabudana	Cabbage	nectars		
		Eggplant			
		Green beans			
		Methi (fenugreek			
		leaves)			
		Cucumbers			
		Chutney or vegetable			
		pickles			
Native American†	Bread	*Orange:*	Berries		Wild game (deer, rabbit,
	Fry bread	Winter squash (hard	Cherries		elk, beaver)
	Wild rice or oats	outer shell)	Plums		Lamb
	Popcorn	*Starchy:*	Apples		Salmon and other fish
	Tortilla	Potato	Peaches		Clams, mussels
	Mush (cooked	Corn			Crab
	cereal)	*Other:*			Duck or quail
		Rhubarb			
Middle Eastern	Rice or bulgur	*Yellow:*	Apricots	Yogurt	Lamb, goat, fish
	(cracked wheat)	Pumpkin or winter	Grapes		Almonds
	Couscous	squash (butternut)	Melons		Pistachio nuts
	Bread	*Other:*	Dried fruits:		Dried beans and peas,
	Pita	Peppers	dates, raisins,		lentils
		Tomatoes	apricots		Eggs
		Grape leaves			
		Cucumbers			
		Fava beans			
		Eggplant			

*High fat, use sparingly.
†Varies widely depending on tribal grouping and locale.

the mother. Infants born to affected mothers are likely to have mega-loblastic anemia and exhibit neurodevelopmental delays. The diet should be carefully planned to include adequate minerals. Iron and zinc may not be as well absorbed from plant foods as they are from meats, and calcium intake can be low if milk products are avoided.

Plant proteins tend to be "incomplete," in that they lack one or more amino acids required for growth and the maintenance of body tissues. However, the daily consumption of a variety of different plant proteins—grains, dried beans and peas, nuts, and seeds—can provide all of the essential amino acids.

KEY POINTS

- A woman's nutritional status before, during, and after pregnancy contributes, to a significant degree, to her well-being and that of her developing fetus and newborn.
- Many physiologic changes occurring during pregnancy influence the need for additional nutrients and the efficiency with which the body uses them.
- Both the total maternal weight gain and the pattern of weight gain are important determinants of the outcome of pregnancy.
- The appropriateness of the mother's prepregnancy weight for height (BMI) is a major determinant of her recommended weight gain during pregnancy.
- Nutritional risk factors include adolescent pregnancy; abuse of nicotine, alcohol, or drugs; bizarre or faddish food habits; a low or high weight for height; and frequent pregnancies.

- Iron supplementation is usually routinely recommended during pregnancy. Other supplements may be warranted when nutritional risk factors are present.
- The nurse and the woman are influenced by cultural and personal values and beliefs during nutrition counseling.
- Pregnancy complications that may be nutrition-related include anemia, gestational hypertension, gestational diabetes, and IUGR.
- Dietary adaptation can be effective intervention for some of the common discomforts of pregnancy, including nausea and vomiting, constipation, and heartburn.

REFERENCES

Craig W, Mangels A: Position of the American Dietetic Association: vegetarian diets, *J Am Diet Assoc* 109(7):1266–1282, 2009.

Gunderson E, Striegel-Moore R, Schreiber G, et al: Longitudinal study of growth and adiposity in parous compared with nulligravid adolescents, *Arch Pediatr Adolesc Med* 163(4):349–356, 2009.

Harnisch JM, Harnisch PH, Harnisch DR: Family medicine obstetrics: pregnancy and nutrition, *Prim Care* 39(1):39–54, 2012.

Institute of Medicine (IOM): *Weight gain during pregnancy: reexamining the guidelines,*

Washington, DC, 2009, National Academies Press.

Jahanfar S, Sharifah H: Effects of restricted caffeine intake by mother on fetal, neonatal and pregnancy outcome (Cochrane Review), *The Cochrane Database of Systematic Reviews* 2:CD006965, 2009.

March of Dimes: Caffeine in pregnancy, 2010, www.marchofdimes.com/pregnancy/nutrition_caffeine.html.

Pollack A, Louis G, Sundaram R, et al: Caffeine consumption and miscarriage: a prospective cohort study, *Fertility and Sterility,* 93(1):304–306, 2010.

Shannon M: Severe lead poisoning in pregnancy, *Ambul Pediatr* 3(1):37–39, 2003.

Siega-Riz A, Viswanathan M, Moos M, et al: A systematic review of outcomes of maternal weight gain according to the Institute of Medicine recommendations: birthweight, fetal growth, and postpartum weight retention, *Am J Obst Gynecol* 201(4):339, e1–14, 2009.

Weng X, Odouli R, Li D: Maternal caffeine consumption during pregnancy and the risk of miscarriage: a prospective study, *Am J Obst Gynecol* 198(3):279, e1–e8, 2008.

Assessment of High Risk Pregnancy

Kitty Cashion

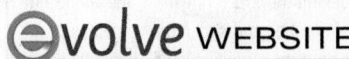 WEBSITE

http://evolve.elsevier.com/Perry/maternal

LEARNING OBJECTIVES

On completion of this chapter, the reader will be able to:
- Explore biophysical, psychosocial, sociodemographic, and environmental influences on high risk pregnancy.
- Examine risk factors identified through history, physical examination, and diagnostic techniques.
- Discuss psychologic considerations associated with a high risk pregnancy diagnosis.

- Differentiate among screening and diagnostic techniques, including when they are used in pregnancy and for what purpose.
- Develop a teaching plan to explain screening and diagnostic techniques and implications of findings to women and their families.

In 2010, the most recent year for which figures are available, four million births occurred in the United States (Martin, Hamilton, Sutton, et al., 2012). Many of these births were the result of pregnancies considered to be *high risk* because the life or health of the mother, fetus, or newborn was jeopardized by circumstances coincidental with or unique to the pregnancy. Care of these high risk patients requires the combined efforts of medical and nursing personnel. Factors associated with a diagnosis of a high risk pregnancy are identified in this chapter. Diagnostic techniques often used to monitor the maternal-fetal unit at risk are also described.

ASSESSMENT OF RISK FACTORS

Pregnancies can be designated as high risk for any of several undesirable outcomes. In the past risk factors were evaluated only from a medical standpoint. Therefore only adverse medical, obstetric, or physiologic conditions were considered to place the woman at risk. Today a more comprehensive approach to high risk pregnancy is used, and the factors associated with high risk childbearing are grouped into broad categories based on threats to health and pregnancy outcome. Categories of risk include biophysical, psychosocial, sociodemographic, and environmental (Box 10-1). Risk factors are interrelated and cumulative in their effects.

Biophysical risks include factors that originate within the mother or fetus and affect the development or functioning of either one or both. Examples include genetic disorders, nutritional and general

health status, and medical or obstetric-related illnesses. Box 10-2 lists common risk factors for several pregnancy-related problems.

Psychosocial risks consist of maternal behaviors and adverse lifestyles that have a negative effect on the health of the mother or fetus. These risks may include emotional distress, disturbed interpersonal relationships, inadequate social support, and unsafe cultural practices.

Sociodemographic risks arise from the mother and her family. These risks may place the mother and fetus at risk. Examples include lack of prenatal care, low income, marital status, and ethnicity (see Box 10-1).

Environmental factors include hazards in the workplace and the woman's general environment and may include environmental chemicals (e.g., lead, mercury), anesthetic gases, and radiation (Chambers and Weiner, 2009; Cunningham, Leveno, Bloom, et al., 2010).

PSYCHOLOGIC CONSIDERATIONS RELATED TO HIGH RISK PREGNANCY

Once a pregnancy has been identified as high risk, the pregnant woman and her fetus are monitored carefully throughout the remainder of the pregnancy. All women who undergo antepartum assessments are at risk for real and potential problems and may feel anxious. In most instances the tests are ordered because of suspected fetal compromise, deterioration of a maternal condition, or both. In the third trimester pregnant women are most concerned about

BOX 10-1   CATEGORIES OF HIGH RISK FACTORS

Biophysical Factors

- *Genetic considerations.* Genetic factors may interfere with normal fetal or neonatal development, result in congenital anomalies, or create difficulties for the mother. These factors include defective genes, transmissible inherited disorders and chromosomal anomalies, multiple pregnancy, large fetal size, and ABO incompatibility.
- *Nutritional status.* Adequate nutrition, without which fetal growth and development cannot proceed normally, is one of the most important determinants of pregnancy outcome. Conditions that influence nutritional status include the following: young age; three pregnancies in the previous 2 years; tobacco, alcohol, or drug use; inadequate dietary intake because of chronic illness or food fads; inadequate or excessive weight gain; and hematocrit value less than 33%.
- *Medical and obstetric disorders.* Complications of current and past pregnancies, obstetric-related illnesses, and pregnancy losses put the woman at risk (see Box 10-2).

Psychosocial Factors

- *Smoking.* A strong, consistent, causal relation has been established between maternal smoking and reduced birth weight. Risks include low-birth-weight infants, higher neonatal mortality rates, increased rates of miscarriage, and increased incidence of premature rupture of membranes. These risks are aggravated by low socioeconomic status, poor nutritional status, and concurrent use of alcohol.
- *Caffeine.* Birth defects in humans have not been related to caffeine consumption. However, pregnant women who consume more than 200 mg of caffeine daily (equivalent to about 12 ounces of coffee per day) may be at increased risk for miscarriage or giving birth to infants with intrauterine growth restriction.
- *Alcohol.* Although the exact effects of alcohol in pregnancy have not been quantified and its mode of action is largely unexplained, it exerts adverse effects on the fetus, resulting in fetal alcohol syndrome, fetal alcohol effects, learning disabilities, and hyperactivity.
- *Drugs.* The developing fetus may be affected adversely by drugs through several mechanisms. They can be teratogenic, cause metabolic disturbances, produce chemical effects, or cause depression or alteration of central nervous system function. This category includes medications prescribed by a health care provider or bought over the counter and commonly abused drugs such as heroin, cocaine, and marijuana. (See Chapter 11 for more information about drug and alcohol abuse.)
- *Psychologic status.* Childbearing triggers profound and complex physiologic, psychologic, and social changes, with evidence to suggest a relationship between emotional distress and birth complications. This risk factor includes conditions such as specific intrapsychic disturbances and addictive lifestyles; a history of child or spouse abuse; inadequate support systems; family disruption or dissolution; maternal role changes or conflicts; noncompliance with cultural norms; unsafe cultural, ethnic, or religious practices; and situational crises.

Sociodemographic Factors

- *Low income.* Poverty underlies many other risk factors and leads to inadequate financial resources for food and prenatal care, poor general health, increased risk of medical complications of pregnancy, and greater prevalence of adverse environmental influences.
- *Lack of prenatal care.* Failure to diagnose and treat complications early is a major risk factor arising from financial barriers or lack of access to care; depersonalization of the system resulting in long waits, routine visits, variability in health care personnel, and unpleasant physical surroundings; lack of understanding of the need for early and continued care or cultural beliefs that do not support the need; and fear of the health care system and its providers.
- *Age.* Women at both ends of the childbearing age spectrum have an increased incidence of poor outcomes; however, age may not be a risk factor in all cases. Physiologic and psychologic risks should be evaluated.
- *Adolescents.* More complications are seen in young mothers (younger than 15 years), who have a 60% higher mortality rate than those older than 20 years, and in pregnancies occurring less than 6 years after menarche. Complications include anemia, preeclampsia, prolonged labor, and contracted pelvis and cephalopelvic disproportion. Long-term social implications of early motherhood are lower educational attainment, lower income, increased dependence on government support programs, higher divorce rates, and higher parity.
- *Mature mothers.* The risks to older mothers are not from age alone but from other considerations such as number and spacing of previous pregnancies, genetic disposition of the parents, medical history, lifestyle, nutrition, and prenatal care. The increased likelihood of chronic diseases and complications that arise from more invasive medical management of a pregnancy and labor combined with demographic characteristics put an older woman at risk. Conditions more likely to be experienced by mature women include chronic hypertension and preeclampsia, diabetes, prolonged labor, cesarean birth, placenta previa, placental abruption, and death. Her fetus is at greater risk for low birth weight and macrosomia, chromosomal abnormalities, congenital malformations, and neonatal death.
- *Parity.* The number of previous pregnancies is a risk factor associated with age and includes all first pregnancies, especially a first pregnancy at either end of the childbearing age continuum. The incidence of preeclampsia and dystocia is increased with a first birth.
- *Marital status.* The increased mortality and morbidity rates for unmarried women, including an increased risk for preeclampsia, are often related to inadequate prenatal care and a young childbearing age.
- *Residence.* The availability and quality of prenatal care vary widely with geographic residence. Women in metropolitan areas have more prenatal visits than those in rural areas who have fewer opportunities for specialized care and consequently a higher incidence of maternal mortality. Health care in the inner city, where residents are usually poorer and begin childbearing earlier and continue longer, may be of lower quality than in a more affluent neighborhood.
- *Ethnicity.* Although ethnicity by itself is not a major risk, race is associated with some poor pregnancy outcomes. Non-Caucasian women are more than 3 times as likely as Caucasian women to die of pregnancy-related causes. African-American babies have the highest rates of prematurity and low birth weight, with the infant mortality rate among African-Americans being more than double that among Caucasians.

Environmental Factors

- Various environmental substances can affect fertility and fetal development, the chance of a live birth, and the child's subsequent mental and physical development. Environmental influences include infections, radiation, chemicals such as mercury and lead, therapeutic drugs, illicit drugs, industrial pollutants, cigarette smoke, stress, and diet. Paternal exposure to mutagenic agents in the workplace has been associated with an increased risk of miscarriage.

BOX 10-2   SPECIFIC PREGNANCY PROBLEMS AND RELATED RISK FACTORS

Polyhydramnios
- Poorly controlled diabetes mellitus
- Fetal congenital anomalies (e.g., gastrointestinal obstruction, twin-twin transfusion syndrome)

Intrauterine Growth Restriction
Maternal Causes
- Hypertensive disorders
- Diabetes
- Chronic renal disease
- Collagen vascular disease
- Thrombophilia
- Cyanotic heart disease
- Poor weight gain
- Smoking, alcohol use, illicit drug use
- Living at a high altitude

Fetoplacental Causes
- Chromosomal abnormalities
- Congenital malformations
- Intrauterine infection
- Genetic syndromes (e.g., trisomy 13 and trisomy 18)
- Abnormal placental development

Oligohydramnios
- Renal agenesis (Potter syndrome)
- Premature rupture of membranes
- Prolonged pregnancy
- Uteroplacental insufficiency
- Severe intrauterine growth restriction (IUGR)
- Maternal hypertensive disorders

Chromosomal Abnormalities
- Advanced maternal age
- Parental chromosomal rearrangements
- Previous pregnancy with autosomal trisomy
- Abnormal ultrasound findings during the current pregnancy (e.g., fetal structural anomalies, IUGR, amniotic fluid volume abnormalities)
- Increased risk, as calculated from noninvasive screening results (e.g., nuchal translucency and maternal serum analytes)

Data from Baschat A, Galan H, Gabbe S: Intrauterine growth restriction. In Gabbe S, Niebyl J, Simpson J, et al, editors: *Obstetrics: normal and problem pregnancies*, ed 6, Philadelphia, 2012, Saunders; Gilbert W: Amniotic fluid disorders: In Gabbe S, Niebyl J, Simpson J, et al, editors: *Obstetrics: normal and problem pregnancies*, ed 6, Philadelphia, 2012, Saunders; Simpson J, Richards D, Otano L, et al: Prenatal genetic diagnosis. In Gabbe S, Niebyl J, Simpson J, et al, editors: *Obstetrics: normal and problem pregnancies,* ed 6, Philadelphia, 2012, Saunders.

BOX 10-3   COMMON MATERNAL AND FETAL INDICATIONS FOR ANTEPARTUM TESTING

- Diabetes
- Chronic hypertension
- Preeclampsia
- Fetal growth restriction
- Multiple gestation
- Oligohydramnios
- Preterm premature rupture of membranes
- Postdates or postterm gestation
- Previous stillbirth
- Decreased fetal movement
- Systemic lupus erythematosus
- Renal disease
- Cholestasis of pregnancy

From Miller LA, Miller DA, Tucker SM: *Mosby's pocket guide to fetal monitoring: a multidisciplinary approach*, ed 7, St Louis, 2013, Mosby.

and opportunities to make as many choices as possible about the woman's care.

ANTEPARTUM TESTING

Antepartum testing has two major goals. The first is to identify fetuses at risk for injury caused by acute or chronic interruption of oxygenation so permanent injury or death might be prevented. The second goal is to identify appropriately oxygenated fetuses so unnecessary intervention can be avoided (Miller, Miller, and Tucker, 2013). In most cases monitoring begins by 32 to 34 weeks of gestation and continues regularly until birth. Assessment tests should be selected on the basis of their effectiveness, and the results must be interpreted in light of the complete clinical picture. Box 10-3 lists common maternal and fetal indications for antepartum testing that are supported by currently available evidence (Miller, Miller, and Tucker, 2013).

The remainder of this chapter describes maternal and fetal assessment tests that are often used to monitor high risk pregnancies.

BIOPHYSICAL ASSESSMENT

Daily Fetal Movement Count

Assessment of fetal activity by the mother is a simple yet valuable method for monitoring the condition of the fetus. The daily fetal movement count (DFMC) (also called *kick count*) can be assessed at home and is noninvasive, inexpensive, and simple to understand and usually does not interfere with a daily routine. It is frequently used to monitor the fetus in pregnancies complicated by conditions that may affect fetal oxygenation (see Box 10-2). The presence of movements is generally a reassuring sign of fetal health. During the third trimester the fetus makes about 30 gross body movements each hour. The mother is able to recognize 70% to 80% of these movements (Greenberg, Druzin, and Gabbe, 2012).

Several different protocols are used for counting. One recommendation is to count once a day for 60 minutes (Fig. 10-1). Fig. 10-1 is an example of a form used to record fetal kick counts. Other common recommendations are that mothers count fetal activity 2 or 3 times daily (e.g., after meals or before bedtime) for 2 hours or until 10 movements are counted or all fetal movements in a 12-hour period each day until a minimum of 10 movements are counted. Except for establishing a very low number of daily fetal movements or a trend toward decreased motion, the clinical value of the absolute number of fetal movements has not been established, other than

protecting themselves and their fetuses and consider themselves most vulnerable to outside influences. The label of *high risk* often increases this sense of vulnerability.

When a woman is diagnosed with a high risk pregnancy, she and her family will likely experience stress related to the diagnosis. The woman may exhibit various psychologic responses, including anxiety, low self-esteem, guilt, frustration, and inability to function. A high risk pregnancy can also affect parental attachment, accomplishment of the tasks of pregnancy, and family adaptation to the pregnancy. If the woman is fearful for her well-being, she may continue to feel ambivalent about the pregnancy or may not accept its reality. She may not be able to complete preparations for the baby or go to childbirth classes if she is placed on restricted activity at home or hospitalized. The family may become frustrated because they cannot engage in activities that prepare them for parenthood. The nurse can help the woman and her family regain control and balance in their lives by providing support and encouragement, information about the pregnancy problem and its management,

FETAL MOVEMENT CHART

1. This chart will help us find out how your baby is doing.

2. Carefully count the number of baby movements during the same hour every evening. (Baby moves more during the evening hours.) Example: 8-9 PM every evening.

3. If the baby has not moved for 12 hours, it is important that you notify the clinic (555-1234). If the clinic is closed, a recorded message will give you further instructions for contacting a doctor who is on-call.

4. Bring this chart with you whenever you come to the clinic or hospital.

DAILY CHART OF BABY KICKS

DAYS OF WEEK	MON	TUES	WED	THURS	FRI	SAT	SUN
DATE							
KICKS							
DATE							
KICKS							
DATE							
KICKS							
DATE							
KICKS							
DATE							
KICKS							
DATE							
KICKS							
DATE							
KICKS							
DATE							
KICKS							

X-IMR-2211 (03/C1) OTHER

FIG 10-1 Fetal movement (kick count) chart. (Courtesy St Joseph Hospital and Medical Center, Phoenix, AZ.)

in the situation in which fetal movements cease entirely for 12 hours (the so-called *fetal alarm signal*). A count of fewer than three fetal movements within 1 hour warrants further evaluation by a non-stress test or a contraction stress test and a complete or modified biophysical profile (see later discussion). Women should be taught the significance of the presence or absence of fetal movements, the procedure for counting that is to be used, how to record findings on a daily fetal movement record, and when to notify the health care provider.

! NURSING ALERT

In assessing fetal movements it is important to remember that they are usually not present during the fetal sleep cycle; they may be reduced temporarily if the woman is taking depressant medication, drinking alcohol, or smoking a cigarette. They do not decrease as the woman nears term. Obesity decreases perception of fetal movements and consequently the ability of the mother to count them.

Ultrasonography

Sound is a form of wave energy that causes small particles in a medium to oscillate. The frequency of sound, which refers to the number of peaks or waves that move over a given point per unit of time, is expressed in hertz (Hz). Sound with a frequency of one cycle, or one peak per second, has a frequency of 1 Hz. When directional beams of sound strike an object, an echo is returned. The time delay between the emission of the sound and the return and direction of the echo is noted. From these data the distance and location of an object can be calculated. Ultrasound is sound frequency higher than that detectable by humans (greater than 20,000 Hz). Ultrasound images are a reflection of the strength of the sending beam, the strength of the returning echo, and the density of the medium (e.g., muscle [uterus], bone, tissue [placenta], fluid, or blood) through which the beam is sent and returned.

Diagnostic ultrasonography is an important, safe technique in antepartum fetal surveillance. It is considered by many to be the most valuable diagnostic tool used in obstetrics (Richards, 2012). It

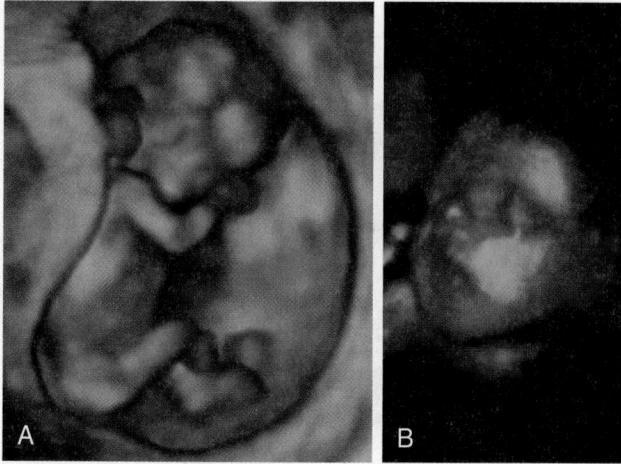

FIG 10-2 Fetus seen on three-dimensional ultrasound. **A,** Full body view of fetus at 11 weeks and 6 days of gestation. **B,** Close-up view of fetal face later in pregnancy. (*A,* Courtesy Shannon Perry, Phoenix, AZ; *B,* Courtesy Margaret Spann, New Johnsonville, TN.)

BOX 10-4   **TYPES OF ULTRASOUND SCANS**

Two-Dimensional (2D)
- This is the standard medical scan used in pregnancy.
- Sound waves are sent straight down from the ultrasound transducer.
- The image produced includes only two dimensions (length and width), so it appears flat.
- The image is viewed in black, white, or shades of gray.

Three-Dimensional (3D)
- This scan can be used for diagnostic purposes, but often the images are produced simply for the enjoyment of pregnant women and their families.
- Sound waves are sent out at different angles. The returning echoes are processed by a computer program, which adds a third dimension (depth) to the 2D scan, producing a three-dimensional image.
- The image is usually displayed in sepia tones rather than in black and white.

Four-Dimensional (4D)
- This scan adds a fourth dimension (time) to the 3D scan.
- The images produced are recorded and played back in succession. As the image is continuously updated, the fetus is viewed in real time.

---

provides critical information to health care providers regarding fetal activity and gestational age, normal versus abnormal fetal growth curves, fetal and placental anatomy, fetal well-being, and visual assistance with which invasive tests can be performed more safely (Richards, 2012; Simpson, Richards, Otano, et al., 2012).

An ultrasound examination can be performed either abdominally or transvaginally during pregnancy. Ultrasound scans produce a two- or three-dimensional view of the area being examined and can be used to create pictorial images (Fig. 10-2, *A* and *B*). Box 10-4 explains the differences in these scans and the views they produce.

Abdominal ultrasonography is more useful after the first trimester when the pregnant uterus becomes an abdominal organ. During the procedure the woman usually should have a full bladder to displace the uterus upward to provide a better image of the fetus. Transmission gel or paste is applied to the woman's abdomen to enhance the transmission and reception of the sound waves before a transducer is moved over the skin. She is positioned with small pillows under her head and knees. The display panel is positioned so the woman or her partner (or both) can observe the images on the screen if they desire.

Transvaginal ultrasonography, in which the probe is inserted into the vagina, allows pelvic anatomic features to be evaluated in greater detail and intrauterine pregnancy to be diagnosed earlier. A transvaginal ultrasound examination is well tolerated by most pregnant women because it removes the need for a full bladder. It is especially useful in obese women whose thick abdominal layers cannot be penetrated adequately with an abdominal approach. A transvaginal ultrasound may be performed with the woman in a lithotomy position or with her pelvis elevated by towels, cushions, or a folded pillow. This pelvic tilt is optimal to image the pelvic structures. A protective cover such as a condom, the finger of a clean surgical glove, or a special probe cover provided by the manufacturer is used to cover the transducer probe. The probe is lubricated with a water-soluble gel and placed in the vagina either by the examiner or by the woman herself. During the examination the position of the probe or the tilt of the examining table may be changed so the complete pelvis is in view. The procedure is not physically painful, although the woman feels pressure as the probe is moved. Transvaginal ultrasonography is optimally used in the first trimester to detect ectopic pregnancies, monitor the developing embryo, help identify abnormalities, and help establish gestational age. In some instances it may be used along with abdominal scanning to evaluate preterm labor in second- and third-trimester pregnancies.

Levels of Ultrasonography

The American College of Obstetricians and Gynecologists (ACOG, 2009) described three levels of ultrasonography. The *standard* (also called *basic*) examination is used most frequently and can be performed by ultrasonographers or other health care professionals, including nurses, who have had special training. Indications for standard ultrasonography are described in detail in the next section. In the second and third trimesters a standard ultrasound examination is used to evaluate fetal presentation, amniotic fluid volume (AFV), cardiac activity, placental position, fetal growth parameters, and number of fetuses. It is also used to perform an anatomic survey of the fetus (ACOG, 2009). *Limited* examinations are performed for specific indications such as identifying fetal presentation during labor or estimating AFV (ACOG, 2009). *Specialized* (also called *detailed*) or targeted examinations are performed if a woman is suspected of carrying an anatomically or physiologically abnormal fetus. Indications for this comprehensive examination include abnormal history or laboratory findings or the results of a previous standard or limited ultrasound examination. Specialized ultrasonography is performed by highly trained and experienced personnel (ACOG, 2009).

Indications for Use

Major indications for obstetric sonography are listed by trimester in Table 10-1. During the first trimester ultrasound examination is performed to obtain information regarding the number, size, and location of gestational sacs; the presence or absence of fetal cardiac and body movements; the presence or absence of uterine abnormalities (e.g., bicornuate uterus or fibroids) or adnexal masses (e.g., ovarian cysts or an ectopic pregnancy); and pregnancy dating.

During the second and third trimesters information regarding the following conditions is sought: fetal viability, number, position, gestational age, growth pattern, and anomalies; amniotic fluid

TABLE 10-1	MAJOR USES OF ULTRASONOGRAPHY DURING PREGNANCY	
FIRST TRIMESTER	**SECOND TRIMESTER**	**THIRD TRIMESTER**
Confirm pregnancy	Establish or confirm dates	Confirm gestational age
Confirm viability	Confirm viability	Confirm viability
Determine gestational age	Detect polyhydramnios, oligohydramnios	Detect macrosomia
Rule out ectopic pregnancy	Detect congenital anomalies	Detect congenital anomalies
Detect multiple gestation	Detect intrauterine growth restriction (IUGR)	Detect IUGR
Determine cause of vaginal bleeding	Assess placental location	Determine fetal position
Use for visualization during chorionic villus sampling	Use for visualization during amniocentesis	Detect placenta previa or placental abruption
Detect maternal abnormalities such as bicornuate uterus, ovarian cysts, fibroids		Use for visualization during amniocentesis, external version
		Biophysical profile
		Amniotic fluid volume assessment
		Doppler flow studies
		Detect placental maturity

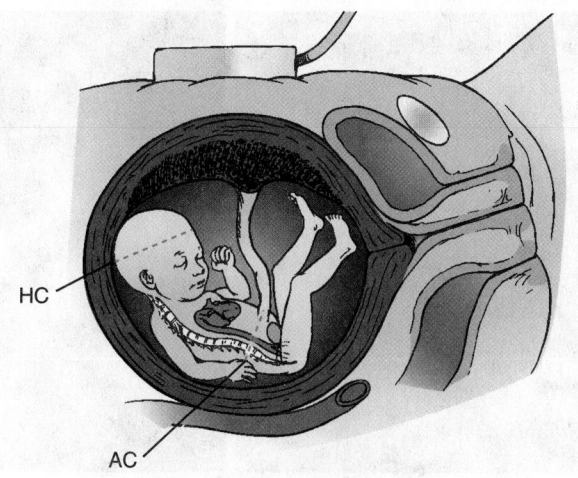

FIG 10-3 Appropriate planes of sections *(dotted lines)* for head circumference *(HC)* and abdominal circumference *(AC)*.

volume; placental location and condition; presence of uterine fibroids or anomalies; presence of adnexal masses; and cervical length.

Ultrasonography provides earlier diagnoses, allowing therapy to be instituted earlier in the pregnancy, thereby decreasing the severity and duration of morbidity, both physical and emotional, for the family. For instance, early diagnosis of a fetal anomaly gives the family choices such as intrauterine surgery or other therapy for the fetus, termination of the pregnancy, or preparation for the care of an infant with a disorder.

Fetal Heart Activity. Fetal heart activity can be demonstrated by about 6 weeks of gestation using transvaginal ultrasound. When the fetus is in a favorable position, good views of the fetal cardiac anatomy are possible in most patients at 13 weeks of gestation (Richards, 2012). Fetal death can be confirmed by lack of heart motion along with the presence of fetal scalp edema and maceration and overlap of the cranial bones.

Gestational Age. Gestational dating by ultrasonography is indicated for conditions such as uncertain dates for the last normal menstrual period, recent discontinuation of oral contraceptives, a bleeding episode during the first trimester, uterine size that does not agree with dates, and other high risk conditions. In fact, growing evidence suggests that pregnancies should be dated by an ultrasound performed before 22 weeks of gestation rather than by menstrual dates because the ultrasound dating is more accurate than even "sure" menstrual dates (Richards, 2012). A standard set of measurements has been accepted as being the most useful for determining gestational age. These measurements include the crown-rump length (after 10 weeks), the biparietal diameter (BPD) (after 12 weeks), the femur length (after 12 weeks), the head circumference, and the abdominal circumference (Fig. 10-3). An ultrasound

examination performed for pregnancy dating between 14 and 22 weeks of gestation is comparable to one performed during the first trimester in terms of accuracy. However, after that time ultrasound dating is less reliable because of variability in fetal size (Richards, 2012).

Fetal Growth. Fetal growth is determined by both intrinsic growth potential and environmental factors. Conditions that require ultrasound assessment of fetal growth include poor maternal weight gain or pattern of weight gain, previous pregnancy with intrauterine growth restriction (IUGR), chronic infections, ingestion of drugs (tobacco, alcohol, and over-the-counter and street drugs), maternal diabetes, hypertension, multifetal pregnancy, and other medical or surgical complications.

Serial evaluations of BPD, limb length, and abdominal circumference can allow differentiation among size discrepancies resulting from inaccurate dates, true IUGR, and macrosomia. IUGR may be symmetric (the fetus is small in all parameters) or asymmetric (head and body growth do not match). Symmetric IUGR reflects a chronic or long-standing insult and may be caused by low genetic growth potential, intrauterine infection, chromosomal anomaly, maternal undernutrition, or heavy smoking. Asymmetric growth suggests an acute or late-occurring deprivation such as placental insufficiency resulting from hypertension, renal disease, or cardiovascular disease. Reduced fetal growth is still one of the most frequent conditions associated with stillbirth. Macrosomic infants (those weighing 4000 g or more) are at increased risk for traumatic injury and asphyxia during birth. Macrosomia may also be characterized as symmetric or asymmetric.

Fetal Anatomy. Anatomic structures that can be identified by ultrasonography (depending on the gestational age) include the following: head (including ventricles and blood vessels), neck, spine, heart, stomach, small bowel, liver, kidneys, bladder, and limbs. Ultrasonography permits the confirmation of normal anatomy and detection of major fetal malformations. The presence of an anomaly may influence the location of birth (e.g., a subspecialty center versus a basic care center) and the method of birth (vaginal versus cesarean) to optimize neonatal outcomes. For example, plans are often made for a fetus with a condition that will require immediate surgery to be born in or near a hospital able to provide that care rather than in a small community hospital that is totally unequipped to meet the newborn's needs.

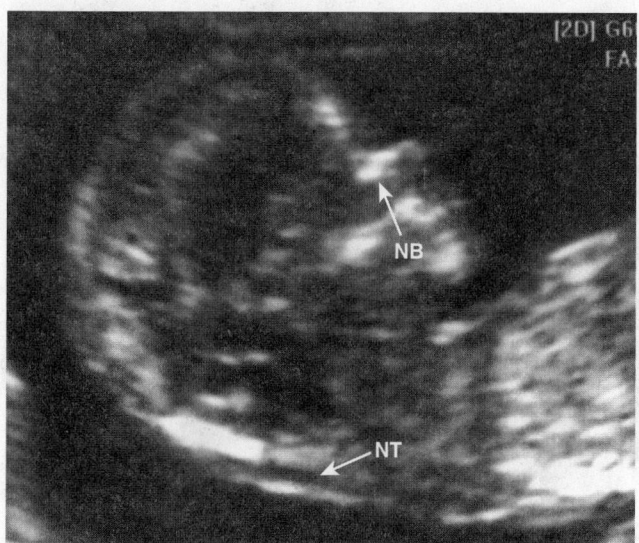

FIG 10-4 Midsagittal view of a 12-week fetus showing the nuchal translucency *(NT)* and nasal bone *(NB)*.

The number of fetuses and their presentations can be assessed by ultrasonography, allowing plans for therapy and mode of birth to be made in advance.

Fetal Genetic Disorders and Physical Anomalies. A prenatal screening technique called *nuchal translucency* (NT) screening uses ultrasound measurement of fluid in the nape of the fetal neck between 10 and 14 weeks of gestation to identify possible fetal abnormalities (Fig. 10-4). A fluid collection that is greater than 3 mm is considered abnormal. When combined with low maternal serum marker levels, elevated NT indicates a possible increased risk of certain chromosomal abnormalities in the fetus, including trisomies 13, 18, and 21. An elevated NT alone indicates an increased risk of fetal cardiac disease. If the NT is abnormal, diagnostic genetic testing is recommended (ACOG, 2009; Gilbert, 2011).

Other ultrasound findings, including the presence or absence (and length, if present) of a nasal bone, short femur or humerus, echogenic intracardiac focus, echogenic bowel, and pyelectasis (enlargement of the renal pelvis, the part of the kidney that collects urine), have been associated with trisomy 21 (Down syndrome) in the fetus. These findings are considered soft markers only; they are not diagnostic for the anomaly. Women in whom these soft markers are found who are at low risk to have a fetus with trisomy 21 should receive expert counseling about the advisability of further diagnostic testing (Simpson, Richards, Otano, et al., 2012).

Placental Position and Function. The pattern of uterine and placental growth and the fullness of the maternal bladder influence the apparent location of the placenta by ultrasonography. During the first trimester differentiation between the endometrium and small placenta is difficult. By 14 to 16 weeks the placenta is clearly defined; but, if it is seen to be low lying, its relationship to the internal cervical os can sometimes be altered dramatically by varying the fullness of the maternal bladder. In approximately 4% to 6% of all pregnancies in which ultrasound scanning is performed during the second trimester, the placenta seems to be overlying the os. However, most cases of placenta previa diagnosed during the second trimester resolve by term, primarily because of the elongation of the lower uterine segment as pregnancy advances. Therefore, if placenta previa is diagnosed during the second trimester, repeated ultrasounds should be performed as pregnancy progresses until the placenta

moves well away from the cervical os or it becomes clear that the previa will persist (Francois and Foley, 2012; Richards, 2012).

Another use for ultrasonography is grading of placental aging. Calcium and fibrin deposits in an aging placenta result in intervillous hemorrhagic infarcts. Also, as blood vessels in the placenta age and thicken, oxygen transport is affected. However, whether these placental changes adversely affect fetal outcomes in postterm pregnancies is unknown, given that most fetuses continue to grow (Gilbert, 2011).

Adjunct to Other Invasive Tests. The safety of amniocentesis is increased when the positions of the fetus, placenta, umbilical cord, and pockets of amniotic fluid can be identified accurately. Ultrasound scanning has reduced risks previously associated with amniocentesis such as fetomaternal hemorrhage from a pierced placenta. Percutaneous umbilical blood sampling and chorionic villus sampling also are guided by ultrasonography to identify the cord and chorion frondosum accurately.

Fetal Well-being. Physiologic parameters of the fetus that can be assessed with ultrasound scanning include AFV, vascular waveforms from the fetal circulation, heart motion, fetal breathing movements (FBMs), fetal urine production, and fetal limb and head movements. Assessment of these parameters, alone or in combination, yields a fairly reliable picture of fetal well-being. The significance of these findings is discussed in the following sections.

Doppler Blood Flow Analysis. One of the major advances in perinatal medicine is the ability to study blood flow noninvasively in the fetus and placenta with ultrasound. Doppler blood flow analysis is a helpful tool in the management of pregnancies at risk because of maternal hypertension and diabetes mellitus, IUGR, multiple fetuses, and preterm labor because it provides an indication of fetal adaptation and reserve.

When a sound wave is reflected from a moving target, a change occurs in the frequency of the reflected wave relative to the transmitted wave, called the *Doppler effect*. An ultrasound beam scattered by a group of red blood cells (RBCs) is an example of this effect. The velocity of the RBCs can be determined by measuring the change in the frequency of the sound wave reflected off the cells (Fig. 10-5).

The shifted frequencies can be displayed as a plot of velocity versus time, and the shape of these waveforms can be analyzed to give information about blood flow and resistance in a given circulation. Velocity waveforms from the umbilical and uterine arteries, reported as systolic/diastolic (S/D) ratios, can be first detected at 15 weeks of pregnancy. Because of the progressive decline in resistance in both the umbilical and uterine arteries, this ratio normally decreases as pregnancy advances. Findings of absent or reversed end-diastolic blood flow and S/D ratios above 3 indicate placental vascular disease. IUGR may result from this placental insufficiency. In addition to IUGR, abnormal elevations in the S/D ratio are seen in hypertensive disorders of pregnancy or other causes of uteroplacental insufficiency (UPI) (Baschat, Galan, and Gabbe, 2012; Gilbert, 2011). In postterm pregnancies evaluated by Doppler umbilical flow studies, an elevated S/D ratio indicates a poorly perfused placenta. Abnormal results also are seen with certain chromosomal abnormalities (trisomy 13 and 18) in the fetus and lupus erythematosus in the mother. Exposure to nicotine from maternal smoking also has been reported to increase the S/D ratio (see Fig. 10-5).

Amniotic Fluid Volume. Abnormalities in AFV are frequently associated with fetal disorders. Subjective determinants of oligohydramnios (decreased fluid) include the absence of fluid pockets in the uterine cavity and the impression of crowding of small fetal parts. An objective criterion of decreased AFV is met if the largest pocket of fluid measured in two perpendicular planes is less than

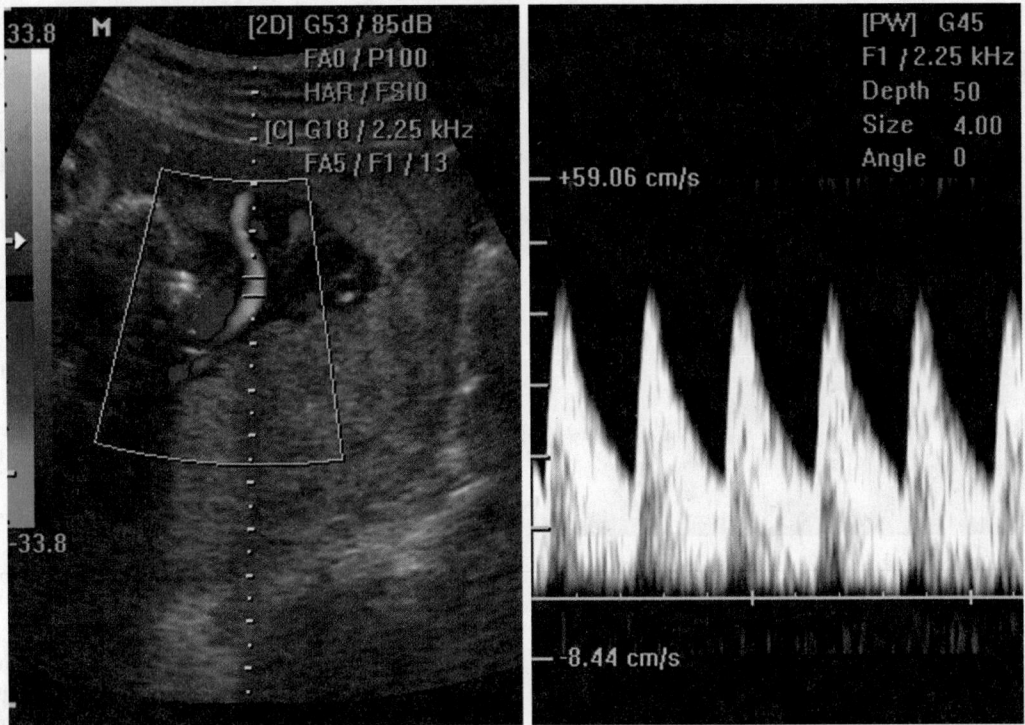

FIG 10-5 Color and spectral Doppler evaluation of the umbilical artery. In the left panel the coiling arteries and vein are shown. *Red* indicates flow toward the transducer, and *blue* is flow away. The sample gate for the pulse Doppler is superimposed. On the right is the result of the pulse Doppler, depicting a normal flow velocity waveform.

2 cm (Harman, 2009). Increased amniotic fluid is called *polyhydramnios* or sometimes just *hydramnios*. Subjective criteria for polyhydramnios include multiple large pockets of fluid, the impression of a floating fetus, and free movement of fetal limbs. Hydramnios is usually defined as pockets of amniotic fluid measuring more than 8 cm (Gilbert, 2012).

The total AFV can be evaluated by a method in which the vertical depths (in centimeters) of the largest pocket of amniotic fluid in all four quadrants surrounding the maternal umbilicus are totaled, providing an amniotic fluid index (AFI). A normal AFI is 10 cm or greater, with the upper range of normal around 25 cm. AFI values between 5 and 10 cm are considered to be low normal, whereas an AFI of less than 5 cm indicates oligohydramnios. With polyhydramnios the AFI would be above 25 cm (Miller, Miller, and Tucker, 2013). Oligohydramnios is associated with congenital anomalies (e.g., renal agenesis [Potter syndrome]), growth restriction, and an abnormal fetal heart rate pattern during labor (caused by compression of the umbilical cord due to the decreased amount of amniotic fluid). Polyhydramnios is associated with neural tube defects (NTDs), obstruction of the fetal gastrointestinal tract, multiple fetuses, and fetal hydrops.

Biophysical Profile. Real-time ultrasound permits detailed assessment of the physical and physiologic characteristics of the developing fetus and cataloging of normal and abnormal biophysical responses to stimuli. The biophysical profile (BPP) is a noninvasive dynamic assessment of a fetus that is based on acute and chronic markers of fetal disease. The BPP includes AFV, FBMs, fetal movements, and fetal tone determined by ultrasound and fetal heart rate (FHR) reactivity determined by means of the nonstress test. Therefore the BPP can be considered a physical examination of the fetus, including determination of vital signs. FHR reactivity, FBMs,

fetal movement, and fetal tone reflect current central nervous system (CNS) status, whereas the AFV demonstrates the adequacy of placental function over a longer period of time (Miller, Miller, and Tucker, 2013). BPP scoring and management are detailed in Tables 10-2 and 10-3.

The BPP is used frequently in the late second and the third trimester for antepartum fetal testing because it is a reliable predictor of fetal well-being. A BPP of 8 or 10 with a normal AFV is considered normal. Advantages of the test include excellent sensitivity and a low false-negative rate (Miller, Miller, and Tucker, 2013). One limitation of the test is that, if the fetus is in a quiet sleep state, the BPP can require a long period of observation. Also, unless the ultrasound examination is videotaped, it cannot be reviewed (Greenberg, Druzin, and Gabbe, 2012).

Modified Biophysical Profile. The modified BPP (mBPP) is being used increasingly as a way to shorten the testing time required for the complete BPP by assessing the components that are most predictive of perinatal outcome. The mBPP combines the nonstress test, which assesses the current fetal condition, with measurement of the quantity of amniotic fluid, an indicator of placental function over a longer period of time. The AFI (rather than the AFV) is often used to measure the amount of amniotic fluid present. Desired test results are a reactive nonstress test and a normal AFI. An AFI greater than 5 is generally considered normal (Greenberg, Druzin, and Gabbe, 2012; Miller, Miller, and Tucker, 2013).

Nursing Role

Although a growing number of nurses perform ultrasound scans and BPPs in certain centers, the main roles of nurses are counseling and educating women about the procedure. Ultrasound is widely used and in fact is considered a standard part of current prenatal

TABLE 10-2	SCORING THE BIOPHYSICAL PROFILE	
BIOPHYSICAL VARIABLE	**SCORE 2**	**SCORE 0**
Fetal breathing movements	At least one episode of fetal breathing movements of at least 30-second duration in a 30-minute observation	Absent fetal breathing movements or less than 30 seconds of sustained fetal breathing movements in 30 minutes
Fetal movements	At least three trunk/limb movements in 30 minutes	Fewer than three episodes of trunk/limb movements in 30 minutes
Fetal tone	At least one episode of active extension with return to flexion of fetal limb or trunk; opening and closing of hand considered normal tone	Absence of movement or slow extension/flexion
Amniotic fluid index (AFI)	AFI >5 cm or at least one pocket >2 cm	AFI ≤5 cm and no single pocket >2 cm
Nonstress test	Reactive	Nonreactive

From Miller LA, Miller DA, Tucker SM: *Mosby's pocket guide to fetal monitoring: A multidisciplinary approach*, ed 7, St Louis, 2013, Mosby.

TABLE 10-3	BIOPHYSICAL PROFILE MANAGEMENT	
SCORE	**INTERPRETATION**	**MANAGEMENT**
10	Normal; low risk for chronic asphyxia	Repeat testing at weekly to twice-weekly intervals.
8	Normal; low risk for chronic asphyxia	Repeat testing at weekly to twice-weekly intervals.
6	Suspect chronic asphyxia	If ≥36-37 weeks of gestation or <36 weeks with positive testing for fetal pulmonary maturity, consider delivery; if <36 weeks and/or fetal pulmonary maturity testing negative, repeat biophysical profile in 4 to 6 hr; deliver if oligohydramnios is present.
4	Suspect chronic asphyxia	If ≥36 weeks of gestation, deliver; if <32 weeks of gestation, repeat score.
0-2	Strongly suspect chronic asphyxia	Extend testing time to 120 min; if persistent score ≤4, deliver, regardless of gestational age.

Modified from Manning FA, Harman CR, Morrison I, et al: Fetal assessment based on fetal biophysical profile scoring, *Am J Obstet Gynecol* 162:703, 1990; and Manning FA: Biophysical profile scoring. In Nijhuis J, editor: *Fetal behaviour*, New York, 1992, Oxford University Press, p 241.

care. Unlike many diagnostic tests, most women look forward to and enjoy their prenatal ultrasound. Exposure to diagnostic ultrasonography during pregnancy appears to be safe for the fetus (Richards, 2012).

Use of Ultrasonography for Nonmedical or "Entertainment" Purposes

In recent years the use of three- and four-dimensional ultrasonography for nonmedical purposes has become increasingly popular with pregnant women and their families. Although insurance does not cover the cost, women can make appointments to have ultrasound images made of the fetus, just as professional photographs are often taken of infants and children. Both the American Institute of Ultrasound in Medicine and the ACOG have published statements that strongly discourage this practice. Although ultrasonography is considered safe, exposure of the fetus to high-frequency sound waves without a clear medical indication for doing so should be avoided. In addition, casual ultrasonography performed by people who are not qualified health care professionals could give false reassurance to women or result in the discovery of abnormalities in settings that are not conducive to discussion and follow-up of findings (ACOG, 2009; Richards, 2012).

Magnetic Resonance Imaging

Magnetic resonance imaging (MRI) is a noninvasive radiologic technique used for obstetric and gynecologic diagnosis. Similar to computed tomography (CT), MRI provides excellent pictures of soft tissue. Unlike CT, ionizing radiation is not used. Therefore vascular structures within the body can be visualized and evaluated without injecting an iodinated contrast medium, thus eliminating any known biologic risk. Similar to sonography, MRI is noninvasive and can provide images in multiple planes, but no interference occurs from skeletal, fatty, or gas-filled structures, and imaging of deep pelvic structures does not require a full bladder.

With MRI the examiner can evaluate fetal structure (CNS, thorax, abdomen, genitourinary tract, musculoskeletal system) and overall growth, the placenta (position, density, and presence of gestational trophoblastic disease), and the quantity of amniotic fluid. Maternal structures (uterus, cervix, adnexa, and pelvis), the biochemical status (pH, adenosine triphosphate content) of tissues and organs, and soft-tissue, metabolic, or functional anomalies can also be evaluated.

The woman is placed on a table in the supine position and moved into the bore of the main magnet, which is similar in appearance to a CT scanner. Depending on the reason for the study, the procedure may take from 20 to 60 minutes, during which time the woman must be perfectly still except for short respites. Because of the long time needed to produce MRIs, the fetus will probably move, which will obscure anatomic details. The only way to ensure that this problem does not occur is to administer a sedative to the mother, but this approach should be reserved for selected cases in which visualization of fetal detail is critical.

MRI has little effect on the fetus. Concerns that the FHR or fetal movement would decrease have not been supported.

BIOCHEMICAL ASSESSMENT

Biochemical assessment involves biologic examination (e.g., of chromosomes in exfoliated cells) and chemical determinations (e.g., lecithin/sphingomyelin [L/S] ratio, or surfactant/albumin [S/A] ratio [TDX FLM assay]) (Table 10-4). Procedures used to obtain the

TABLE 10-4	SUMMARY OF BIOCHEMICAL MONITORING TECHNIQUES	
TEST	**POSSIBLE FINDINGS**	**CLINICAL SIGNIFICANCE**
Maternal Blood		
Coombs' test	Titer of 1:8 and increasing	Significant Rh incompatibility
AFP	See AFP later in table	
Amniotic Fluid Analysis		
Lung profile:		Fetal lung maturity
L/S ratio	2:1	
Phosphatidylglycerol	Present	
S/A ratio (TDX FLM assay)	≥55 mg/g	
Creatinine	>2 mg/dL	Gestational age >36 weeks
Lipid cells	>10%	Gestational age >35 weeks
AFP	High levels after 15 weeks of gestation	Open neural tube or other defect
Osmolality	Declines after 20 weeks of gestation	Advancing gestational age
Genetic disorders: Sex-linked Chromosomal Metabolic	Dependent on cultured cells for karyotype and enzymatic activity	Counseling possibly required

AFP, Alpha-fetoprotein; *L/S,* lecithin/sphingomyelin; *S/A,* surfactant/albumin. *TDX FLM assay,* name of specific test used to determine S/A ratio.

BOX 10-5	FETAL RIGHTS

Amniocentesis, percutaneous umbilical blood sampling (PUBS), and chorionic villus sampling (CVS) are prenatal tests used for diagnosing fetal defects in pregnancy. They are invasive and carry risks to the mother and fetus. A consideration of induced abortion is linked to the performance of these tests because no treatment for genetically affected fetuses has been developed; therefore the issue of fetal rights is a key ethical concern in prenatal testing for fetal defects.

needed specimens include amniocentesis, percutaneous umbilical blood sampling, chorionic villus sampling, and maternal sampling (Box 10-5).

Amniocentesis

Amniocentesis is performed to obtain amniotic fluid, which contains fetal cells. Under direct ultrasonographic visualization, a needle is inserted transabdominally into the uterus, amniotic

fluid is withdrawn into a syringe, and the various assessments are performed (Fig. 10-6). Amniocentesis is possible after week 14 of pregnancy, when the uterus becomes an abdominal organ and sufficient amniotic fluid is available for testing. Indications for the procedure include prenatal diagnosis of genetic disorders or congenital anomalies (NTDs in particular), assessment of pulmonary maturity, and rarely diagnosis of fetal hemolytic disease.

Complications in the mother and fetus occur in less than 1% of cases and include the following:
- *Maternal:* Leakage of amniotic fluid, hemorrhage, fetomaternal hemorrhage with possible maternal Rh isoimmunization, infection, labor, placental abruption, inadvertent damage to the intestines or bladder, and amniotic fluid embolism (anaphylactoid syndrome of pregnancy)
- *Fetal:* Death, hemorrhage, infection (amnionitis), and direct injury from the needle

Many of the complications have been minimized or eliminated by using ultrasonography to direct the procedure.

> ⚡ **SAFETY ALERT**
>
> Because of the possibility of fetomaternal hemorrhage, administering Rh$_0$D immunoglobulin to the woman who is Rh negative is standard practice after an amniocentesis.

Indications for Use

Genetic Concerns. Historically prenatal assessment of genetic disorders focused on women older than 35 years (Box 10-6), women with a previous child with a chromosomal abnormality, or a family history of chromosomal anomalies. Inherited errors of metabolism (such as Tay-Sachs disease), hemophilia, thalassemia, and other disorders for which marker genes are known also can be detected by prenatal screening. Fetal cells can be cultured for karyotyping of chromosomes (see Chapter 6). Karyotyping also permits determination of fetal gender, which is important if an X-linked disorder (occurring almost always in a male fetus) is suspected.

Biochemical analysis of enzymes in amniotic fluid can detect inborn errors of metabolism or fetal structural anomalies. For example, alpha-fetoprotein (AFP) levels in amniotic fluid are assessed as a follow-up for elevated levels in maternal serum. High AFP levels in amniotic fluid help confirm the diagnosis of an NTD such as spina bifida or anencephaly or an abdominal wall defect such as omphalocele. The elevation results from the increased leakage of cerebrospinal or abdominal fluid into the amniotic fluid through the closure defect. AFP levels may also be elevated in a normal multifetal pregnancy and intestinal atresia, presumably caused by lack of fetal swallowing.

A concurrent test that finds the presence of acetylcholinesterase almost always indicates a fetal defect (Wapner, Jenkins, and Khalek, 2009). In such instances follow-up ultrasound examination is recommended.

Fetal Maturity. Late in pregnancy accurate assessment of fetal lung maturity is possible by examining amniotic fluid for the presence of phosphatidylglycerol (PG). Determination of the L/S ratio and the S/A ratio [TDx FLM assay] are other methods to evaluate it. The FLM assay is often used as the primary test for determining fetal lung maturity in clinical practice because it is simple to perform and accurate. FLM test results are similar to those of the PG test and the L/S ratio in terms of predicting pulmonary maturity (Mercer, 2009) (see Table 10-4).

Fetal Hemolytic Disease. In the past amniocentesis was used for identification and follow-up of fetal hemolytic disease in cases of

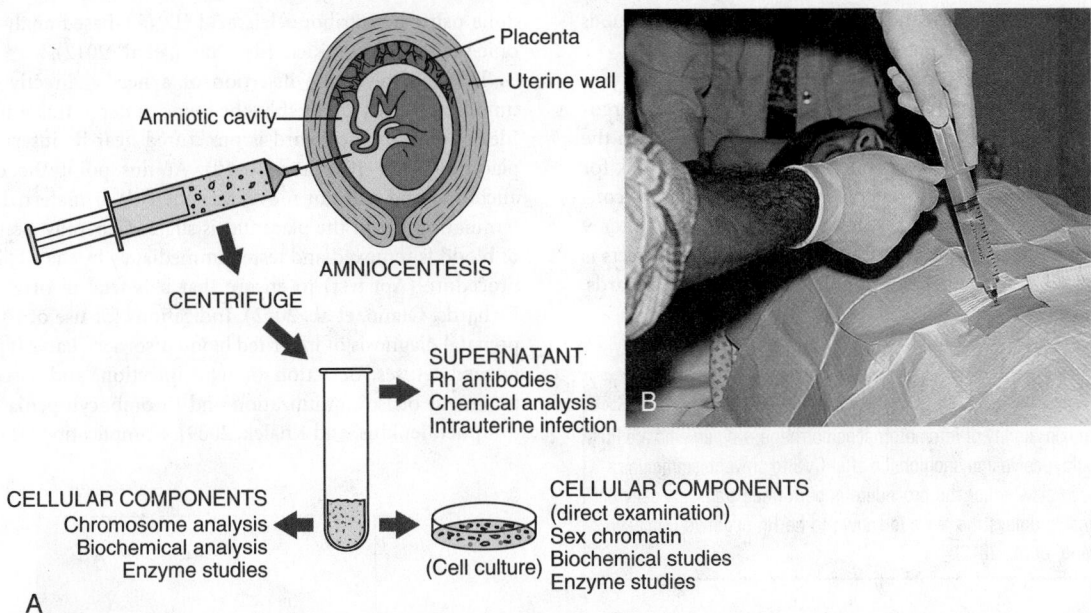

FIG 10-6 **A,** Amniocentesis and laboratory use of amniotic fluid aspirant. **B,** Transabdominal amniocentesis. (*B,* Courtesy Marjorie Pyle, RNC, Lifecircle, Costa Mesa, CA.)

BOX 10-6   ELIMINATION OF MATERNAL AGE AS AN INDICATION FOR INVASIVE PRENATAL DIAGNOSIS

Maternal age of 35 years and older has been a standard indication for invasive prenatal testing since 1979. However, because most genetically abnormal children are born to parents of varying ages who have no history of abnormality, genetic screening is now recommended for all women, regardless of age (Gilbert, 2011). The American College of Obstetricians and Gynecologists (ACOG) published new guidelines in 2007 (and reaffirmed them in 2011) stating that no specific age should be used as a threshold for invasive or noninvasive screening. Furthermore, all women, regardless of age, should have the option of invasive testing without first having screening (ACOG, 2007).

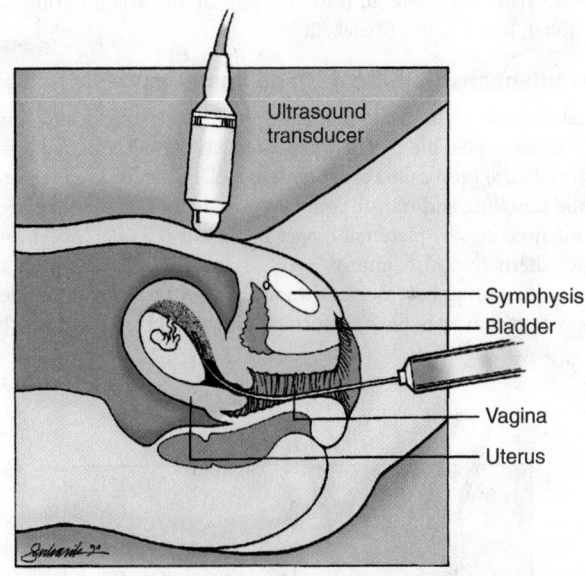

FIG 10-7 Transcervical chorionic villus sampling. (From Gabbe S, Niebyl J, Simpson J, et al, editors: *Obstetrics: normal and problem pregnancies,* ed 6, Philadelphia, 2012, Saunders.)

isoimmunization. Amniocentesis is now only performed for this reason in rare circumstances because of the availability of noninvasive testing. Doppler velocimetry of the fetal middle cerebral artery is now the method of choice to monitor accurately and noninvasively for fetal anemia in isoimmunized pregnancies (Moise, 2012).

Chorionic Villus Sampling

The combined advantages of earlier diagnosis and rapid results have made chorionic villus sampling (CVS) a popular technique for genetic studies in the first trimester. Indications for CVS are similar to those for amniocentesis, although CVS cannot be used for maternal serum marker screening because no fluid is obtained. CVS performed in the second trimester carries no greater risk of pregnancy loss than amniocentesis and is considered equal to amniocentesis in diagnostic accuracy. When performed after the first trimester, the procedure is better known as *late CVS* or *placental biopsy* (Simpson, Richards, Otano, et al., 2012).

CVS can be performed in the first or second trimester, ideally between 10 and 13 weeks of gestation, and involves the removal of a small tissue specimen from the fetal portion of the placenta

(Figs. 10-7 and 10-8). Because chorionic villi originate in the zygote, this tissue reflects the genetic makeup of the fetus (Gilbert, 2011).

CVS procedures can be accomplished transcervically or transabdominally. In transcervical sampling a sterile catheter is introduced into the cervix under continuous ultrasonographic guidance, and a small portion of the chorionic villi is aspirated with a syringe. The aspiration cannula and obturator must be placed at a suitable site, and rupture of the amniotic sac must be avoided (see Fig. 10-7). The transcervical procedure is contraindicated if a cervical infection such as chlamydia or herpes is present (Gilbert, 2011).

If the abdominal approach is used, an 18- or 20-gauge spinal needle with stylet is inserted under sterile conditions through the abdominal wall into the chorion frondosum under ultrasound guidance. The stylet is then withdrawn, and the chorionic tissue is aspirated into a syringe (see Fig. 10-8).

CVS is a relatively safe procedure. The incidence of IUGR, placental abruption, and preterm birth is no higher in women undergoing CVS than would be expected in the general population. In the early 1990s there was controversy concerning an increased risk for fetal limb reduction defects associated with CVS. However, the consensus of further studies is that, when CVS is performed after 9 completed weeks of gestation, the risk for limb reduction defects is no higher than it is in the general population (Simpson, Richards, Otano, et al., 2012).

⚡ SAFETY ALERT

Because of the possibility of fetomaternal hemorrhage, women who are Rh negative should receive immunoglobulin after CVS to prevent isoimmunization, regardless of whether the procedure is performed transcervically or transabdominally, unless the fetus is known to be Rh negative (Simpson, Richards, Otano, et al., 2012).

Use of amniocentesis and CVS is declining because of advances in noninvasive screening techniques. These techniques include measurement of NT, maternal serum screening tests in the first and second trimesters, and ultrasonography in the second trimester (Wapner, Jenkins, and Khalek, 2009).

Percutaneous Umbilical Blood Sampling

Direct access to the fetal circulation during the second and third trimesters is possible through percutaneous umbilical blood sampling (PUBS) (also called cordocentesis). PUBS can be used for fetal blood sampling and transfusion. However, PUBS has been replaced in many centers by placental biopsy because it is a safer, easier, and faster alternative. Also, improvements in cytogenetic and molecular diagnostic testing have decreased the need for fetal blood samples. Many tests that were once performed using fetal blood can now be

done using deoxyribonucleic acid (DNA)–based analysis of chorionic villi (Simpson, Richards, Otano, et al., 2012).

PUBS involves the insertion of a needle directly into a fetal umbilical vessel, preferably the vein, under ultrasound guidance. Ideally the umbilical cord is punctured near its insertion into the placenta (Figs. 10-9 and 10-10). At this point the cord is well anchored and will not move, and the risk of maternal blood contamination (from the placenta) is slight. Generally a small amount of blood is removed and tested immediately by the Kleihauer-Betke procedure (Apt test) to ensure that it is fetal in origin (Simpson, Richards, Otano, et al., 2012). Indications for use of PUBS include prenatal diagnosis of inherited blood disorders, karyotyping of malformed fetuses, detection of fetal infection, and assessment and treatment of isoimmunization and thrombocytopenia in the fetus (Wapner, Jenkins, and Khalek, 2009). Complications that can occur

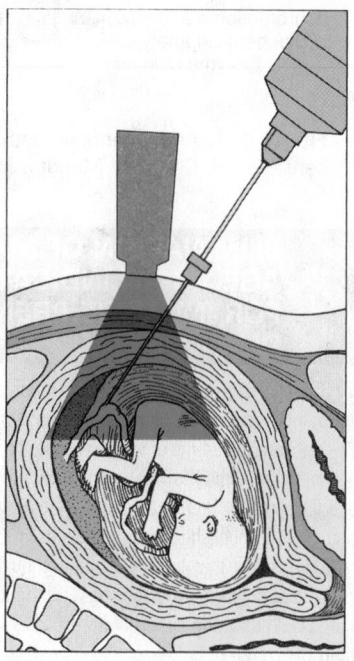

FIG 10-9 Technique for percutaneous umbilical blood sampling guided by ultrasound.

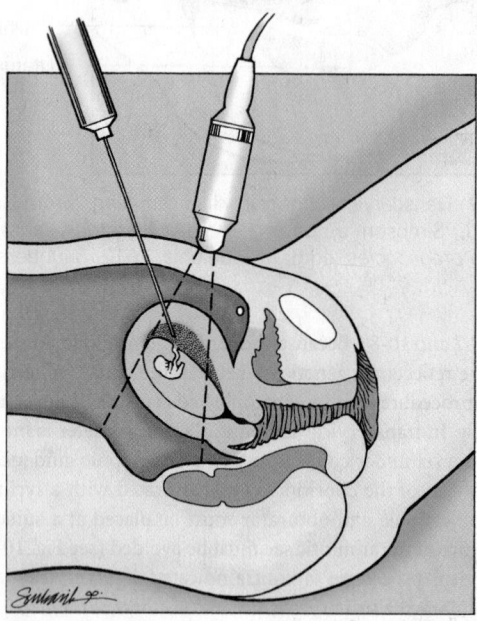

FIG 10-8 Transabdominal chorionic villus sampling. (From Gabbe S, Niebyl J, Simpson J, et al, editors: *Obstetrics: normal and problem pregnancies*, ed 6, Philadelphia, 2012, Saunders.)

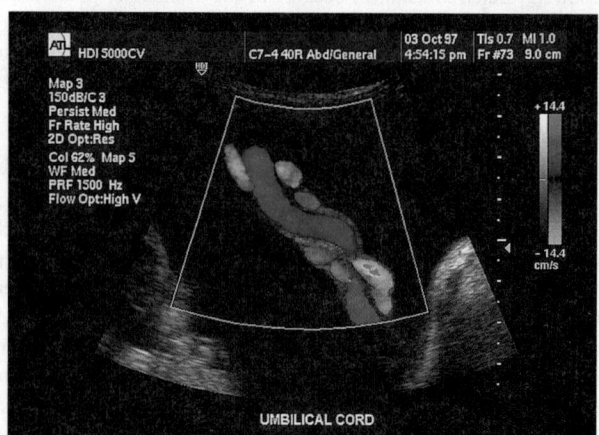

FIG 10-10 Umbilical cord as seen on ultrasound at 26 weeks of gestation. (Courtesy Advanced Technology Laboratories, Bothell, WA.)

include loss of the pregnancy, hematomas, bleeding from the puncture site in the umbilical cord, transient fetal bradycardia, and feto-maternal hemorrhage. Maternal complications are rare but include hemorrhage and transplacental hemorrhage (Simpson, Richards, Otano, et al., 2012).

In fetuses at risk for isoimmune hemolytic anemia, PUBS permits precise identification of fetal blood type and RBC count and may prevent the need for further intervention. If the fetus is positive for the presence of maternal antibodies, a direct blood test can confirm the degree of anemia resulting from hemolysis. Intrauterine transfusion of severely anemic fetuses can be performed 4 to 5 weeks earlier than through the intraperitoneal route.

Follow-up includes continuous FHR monitoring for 1 to 2 hours after the procedure. Women should also be taught to count fetal movements at home (Gilbert, 2011).

Maternal Assays
Alpha-Fetoprotein

Maternal serum alpha-fetoprotein (MSAFP) levels are used as a screening tool for NTDs in pregnancy. Through this technique approximately 80% to 85% of all open NTDs and open abdominal wall defects can be detected early. Screening is recommended for all pregnant women.

The cause of NTDs is not well understood, but 95% of all affected infants are born to women with no family history of similar anomalies (Wapner, Jenkins, and Khalek, 2009). The defect occurs in approximately 2 of 1000 births in the United States. The rate of NTDs is decreasing as a result of the use of folate preconceptionally and during early pregnancy for prevention of this condition (Manning, 2009).

AFP is produced by the fetal liver, and increasing levels are detectable in the serum of pregnant women from 14 to 34 weeks of gestation. Although amniotic fluid AFP measurement is diagnostic for NTD, MSAFP is a screening tool only and identifies candidates for the more definitive procedures of amniocentesis and ultrasound examination. MSAFP screening can be performed with reasonable reliability any time between 15 and 20 weeks of gestation (16 to 18 weeks being ideal) (Wapner, Jenkins, and Khalek, 2009).

Once the maternal level of AFP is determined, it is compared with normal values for each week of gestation. Values also should be correlated with maternal age, weight, race, presence of a multifetal pregnancy, and whether the woman has insulin-dependent diabetes. If findings are abnormal, follow-up procedures include genetic counseling for families with a history of NTD, repeated AFP, specialized ultrasound examination, and possibly amniocentesis (Cunningham, Leveno, Bloom, et al., 2010).

Multiple Marker Screens

Screening to detect fetal chromosomal abnormalities, particularly trisomy 21 (Down syndrome) is now available, beginning in the first trimester of pregnancy. This first-trimester screen is done at 11 to 14 weeks of gestation. It includes measurement of two maternal biochemical markers, pregnancy-associated placental protein (PAPP-A) and human chorionic gonadotropin (hCG) or the free beta-human chorionic gonadotropin (β-hCG) subunit, and evaluation of fetal NT, or a combination of both. In the presence of a fetus with trisomy 21, hCG levels are higher than normal in the first trimester, whereas PAPP-A levels are lower than normal. First-trimester screening using PAPP-A and hCG or β-hCG levels has been shown to be as accurate for detecting fetuses with trisomy 21 as triple screening in the second trimester (Cunningham, Leveno, Bloom, et al., 2010; Wapner, Jenkins, and Khalek, 2009).

About one third of all fetuses with an increased NT have a chromosomal abnormality; half of these are trisomy 21. Combining the serum marker and NT values results in the detection of Down syndrome in 79% to 87% of cases. These results are comparable to those obtained with quad screening in the second trimester (Cunningham, Leveno, Bloom, et al., 2010).

In the second trimester triple and quad screening are available to screen for fetuses with trisomy 21 and trisomy 18. The *triple-marker screen*, performed at 16 to 18 weeks of gestation, measures the levels of three maternal serum markers: MSAFP, unconjugated estriol, and hCG. In the presence of a fetus with trisomy 21 the MSAFP and unconjugated estriol levels are low, whereas the hCG level is elevated. Low values in all three markers are associated with trisomy 18 (Cunningham, Leveno, Bloom, et al., 2010; Gilbert, 2011).

The *quad-screen* adds an additional marker, a placental hormone called *inhibin A*, to increase the accuracy of screening for Down syndrome in women less than 35 years of age. Low inhibin A levels indicate the possibility of Down syndrome (Gilbert, 2011). The addition of inhibin A to the other three markers increases the detection rate for Down syndrome to about 75% in women who are less than 35 years of age and to more than 80% in women 35 years of age or older (Simpson, Richards, Otano, et al., 2012). Similar to triple marker screening, the optimal time to perform the quad screen is between 16 and 18 weeks of gestation (Gilbert, 2011).

The ability of multiple marker tests to detect chromosomal abnormalities depends on the accuracy of gestational age assessment. These tests are screening procedures only and are not diagnostic. A positive screening test result indicates an increased risk but is not diagnostic of trisomy 21 or another chromosome abnormality. Women with positive results should be offered diagnostic testing by amniocentesis or fetal blood sampling for fetal karyotyping (Cunningham, Leveno, Bloom, et al., 2010).

Coombs Test

The indirect Coombs test is a screening tool for Rh incompatibility. If the maternal titer for Rh antibodies is greater than 1:8, amniocentesis for determination of bilirubin in amniotic fluid is indicated to establish the severity of fetal hemolytic anemia. However, as previously discussed, middle cerebral artery Doppler studies to determine the degree of fetal hemolysis have almost entirely replaced serial amniocentesis (Moise, 2012). The Coombs test can also detect other antibodies that may place the fetus at risk for incompatibility with maternal antigens.

Cell-Free Deoxyribonucleic Acid in Maternal Blood

A new screening method for noninvasive prenatal genetic diagnosis has recently become available for use in the clinical setting. Cell-free DNA screening already provides a definitive diagnosis noninvasively for fetal Rh status, fetal gender, and certain paternally transmitted single gene disorders (Simpson, Richards, Otano, et al., 2012).

The method works by amplifying cell-free DNA. If the fetus has a normal karyotype, the amount of DNA is consistent with the known standard for the normal amount. For example, if more than the expected amount of chromosome 21 DNA is detected, it can then be assumed that the fetus is contributing the extra amount and therefore has trisomy 21. The same is true for trisomy 13 and 18. The test cannot actually distinguish fetal from maternal DNA, but it can accurately predict the fetal status by measuring the amount of DNA circulating in maternal blood and comparing it to known standards. The cell-free DNA screen in combination with ultrasound does not provide a definitive diagnosis for all cases of fetal trisomy 21. Women who have a positive cell-free circulating DNA test without confirming ultrasound findings or a negative blood screen with abnormal ultrasound findings require invasive diagnostic testing such as amniocentesis or CVS for a definitive diagnosis (Palomaki, Kloza, Lambert-Messerlian, et al., 2011).

Circulating cell-free DNA studies for the detection of fetal chromosomal abnormalities can be performed any time after 10 weeks of gestation. The test is offered to women considered to be at risk for chromosomal abnormalities, including those with advanced maternal age, screen-positive maternal serum screens, or ultrasound abnormalities. Women who have previously given birth to a child with a chromosomal abnormality are also candidates for the screen. It is simple to perform; a sample of maternal blood is obtained by venipuncture and sent to a commercial laboratory. Results are usually available in about 10 business days. The screen has been shown to be 98% effective at detecting trisomy 21 and 99% effective at detecting trisomies 13 or 18. In less than 1% of cases no result is available because not enough DNA was retrieved to perform the screen (Palomaki, Kloza, Lambert-Messerlian, et al., 2011; Palomaki, Deciu, Kloza, et al., 2012).

ANTEPARTUM ASSESSMENT USING ELECTRONIC FETAL MONITORING

Indications

First- and second-trimester antepartum assessment is directed primarily at the diagnosis of fetal anomalies. The goal of third-trimester testing is to determine whether the intrauterine environment continues to support the fetus. The testing is often used to determine the timing of childbirth for women at risk for UPI. Gradual loss of placental function results first in inadequate nutrient delivery to the fetus, leading to IUGR. Subsequently respiratory function also is compromised, resulting in fetal hypoxia. Evidence-based recommendations for condition-specific testing schemes in cases of identified risk factors have been difficult to develop and often do not exist. There is no ideal single test or testing strategy for all high risk pregnancies (Greenberg, Druzin, and Gabbe, 2012).

However, there is evidence to support antepartum assessment using electronic fetal monitoring in pregnancies complicated by the risk factors listed in Box 10-7. Currently the nonstress test and the mBPP are the primary methods used for antepartum fetal evaluation in high risk patients at most sites. The complete BPP and the contraction stress test are used for follow-up evaluation in patients

---

BOX 10-7   INDICATIONS FOR FETAL ASSESSMENT USING ELECTRONIC FETAL MONITORING

- Diabetes
- Hypertension
- Intrauterine growth restriction
- Multiple gestation
- Oligohydramnios
- Intrahepatic cholestasis
- Renal disease
- Decreased fetal movement
- Previous fetal death
- Postterm pregnancy
- Systemic lupus erythematosus

Data from Greenberg M, Druzin M, Gabbe S: Antepartum fetal evaluation. In Gabbe S, Niebyl J, Simpson J, et al, editors: *Obstetrics: Normal and problem pregnancies*, ed 6, Philadelphia, 2012, Saunders.

---

who have a persistently nonreactive nonstress test or mBPP. Traditionally testing has begun at 32 to 34 weeks of gestation, with earlier initiation of testing recommended for women with multiple high risk conditions. Testing is usually performed once or twice weekly (Greenberg, Druzin, and Gabbe, 2012).

Nonstress Test

The nonstress test (NST) is the most widely applied technique for antepartum evaluation of the fetus. The basis for the NST is that the normal fetus produces characteristic heart rate patterns in response to fetal movement, uterine contractions, or stimulation. In the term fetus, accelerations are associated with movement more than 85% of the time (Greenberg, Druzin, and Gabbe, 2012). The most common reason for the absence of FHR accelerations is the quiet fetal sleep state. However, medications such as narcotics, barbiturates, and beta-blockers; maternal smoking; and the presence of fetal malformations can also adversely affect the test (Gilbert, 2011; Greenberg, Druzin, and Gabbe, 2012). The NST can be performed easily and quickly in an outpatient setting because it is noninvasive, easy to perform and interpret, relatively inexpensive, and has no known contraindications. In most cases only 10 to 15 minutes are required to complete the test. Disadvantages include the requirement for twice-weekly testing and a high false-positive rate. The test also is slightly less sensitive in detecting fetal compromise than the contraction stress test or the BPP (Greenberg, Druzin, and Gabbe, 2012; Miller, Miller, and Tucker, 2013).

Procedure

The woman is seated in a reclining chair (or in semi-Fowler position) with a slight lateral tilt to optimize uterine perfusion and prevent supine hypotension. The FHR is recorded with a Doppler transducer, and a tocodynamometer is applied to detect uterine contractions or fetal movements. The tracing is observed for signs of fetal activity and a concurrent acceleration of FHR. If evidence of fetal movement is not apparent on the tracing, the woman may be asked to depress a button on a handheld event marker connected to the monitor when she feels fetal movement. The movement is then noted on the tracing. Because almost all accelerations are accompanied by fetal movement, the movements need not be recorded for the test to be considered reactive. The test is usually completed within 20 to 30 minutes, but more time may be required if the fetus must be awakened from a sleep state.

Care providers sometimes suggest that the woman drink orange juice or be given glucose to increase her blood sugar level and thereby stimulate fetal movements. Although this practice is common, there is no evidence that it increases fetal activity (Greenberg, Druzin, and Gabbe, 2012).

Vibroacoustic stimulation is often used to stimulate fetal activity if the initial NST result is nonreactive and thus hopefully shortens the time required to complete the test (Greenberg, Druzin, and Gabbe, 2012).

Interpretation

NST results are either reactive (Fig. 10-11) or nonreactive (Fig. 10-12). Box 10-8 lists criteria for both results.

A nonreactive test requires further evaluation. The testing period is often extended, usually for an additional 20 minutes, with the expectation that the fetal sleep state will change and the test will become reactive. During this time vibroacoustic stimulation (see later discussion) may be used to stimulate fetal activity. If the test does not meet the criteria after 40 minutes, a BPP usually will be

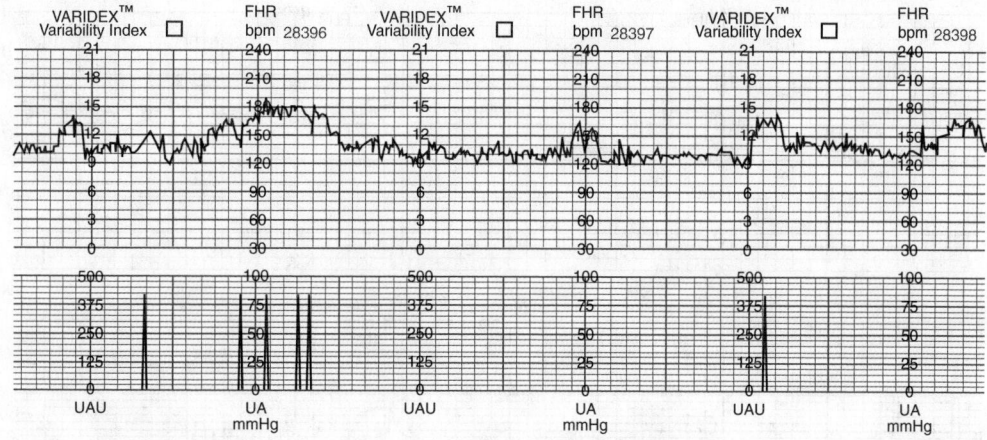

FIG 10-11 Reactive nonstress test. (From Gabbe S, Niebyl J, Simpson J, et al, editors: *Obstetrics: normal and problem pregnancies,* ed 6, Philadelphia, 2012, Saunders.)

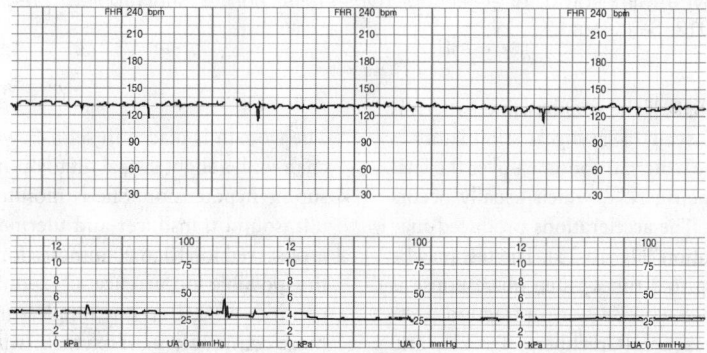

FIG 10-12 Segment of nonreactive nonstress test in term pregnancy. The lack of accelerations meeting minimum criteria continued for 40 minutes. (From Miller LA, Miller DA, Tucker SM: *Mosby's pocket guide to fetal monitoring: a multidisciplinary approach,* ed 7, St Louis, 2013, Mosby.)

performed. Once NST testing is initiated, it is usually repeated once or twice weekly for the remainder of the pregnancy (Greenberg, Druzin, and Gabbe, 2012) (see Critical Thinking Case Study).

Vibroacoustic Stimulation

Vibroacoustic stimulation (also called the *fetal acoustic stimulation test [FAST]*) is another method of testing antepartum FHR response. This test is generally performed in conjunction with the NST and uses a combination of sound and vibration to stimulate the fetus. Whether the acoustic or the vibratory component alters the fetal state is unclear. The fetus is monitored for 5 minutes before

---

BOX 10-8   INTERPRETATION OF THE NONSTRESS TEST

Reactive test: Two accelerations in a 20-minute period, each lasting at least 15 seconds and peaking at least 15 beats/min above the baseline. (Before 32 weeks of gestation, an acceleration is defined as a rise of at least 10 beats/min lasting at least 10 seconds from onset to offset) (see Fig. 10-11).

Nonreactive test: A test that does not demonstrate at least two qualifying accelerations within a 20-minute window (see Fig. 10-12).

From Miller LA, Miller DA, Tucker SM: *Mosby's pocket guide to fetal monitoring: a multidisciplinary approach,* ed 7, St Louis, 2013, Mosby.

? CRITICAL THINKING CASE STUDY

Fetal Assessment Using the Nonstress Test

LaTonya is a 30-year-old G5 T3 P0 A1 L3 who is now at 32 weeks of gestation. LaTonya was diagnosed with diabetes 4 years ago and also has chronic hypertension. Her physician has scheduled her for twice-weekly nonstress testing, and this appointment is her first. You are the nurse assigned to perform LaTonya's nonstress test (NST) today. As you help her get comfortable and attach the fetal heart rate and contraction monitors, LaTonya grumbles, "I don't see why I had to come get this test done. It was really hard to find a babysitter for my kids, and I live on the other side of town!"

1. Evidence—Is there sufficient evidence regarding the benefits of performing fetal assessment using the nonstress test during the third trimester of pregnancy in women who have preexisting diabetes and chronic hypertension?
2. Assumptions—Describe an underlying assumption about each of the following issues:
   a. The physiologic principle on which the NST is based
   b. Advantages of the NST
   c. The desired result of the NST
   d. LaTonya's understanding of why the test is necessary
3. What implications and priorities for nursing care can be drawn at this time?
4. Does the evidence objectively support your argument (conclusion)?

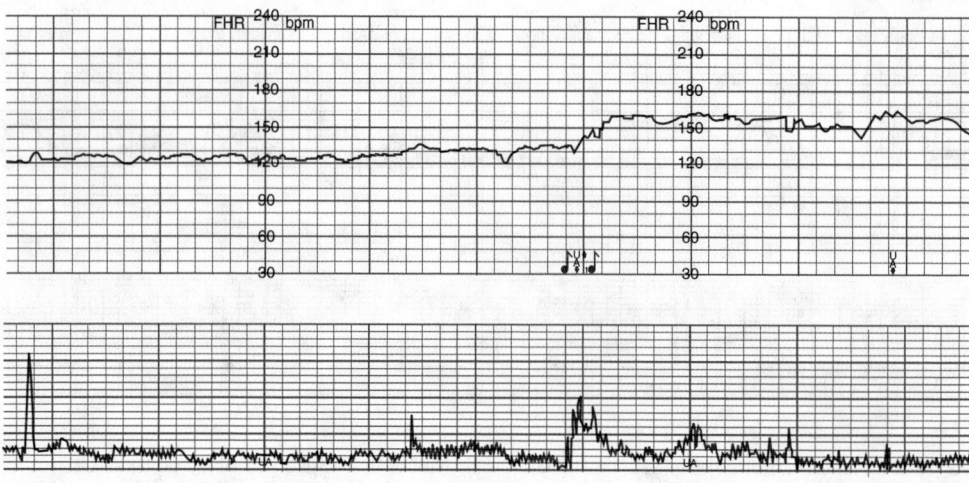

FIG 10-13 Reactive nonstress test after vibroacoustic stimulation. The stimulus was applied at the point marked by the musical notes. A sustained fetal heart rate acceleration was produced. (From Gabbe S, Niebyl J, Simpson J, et al, editors: *Obstetrics: normal and problem pregnancies,* ed 6, Philadelphia, 2012, Saunders.)

stimulation to obtain a baseline FHR. If the fetal baseline pattern is nonreactive, the sound source (usually a laryngeal stimulator) is then activated for 3 seconds on the maternal abdomen over the fetal head. The desired result is a reactive NST, which usually occurs within 3 minutes of stimulation. The accelerations produced may have a significant increase in duration (Fig. 10-13). The test may be repeated at 1-minute intervals up to 3 times when no response is noted. Further evaluation is needed with BPP or contraction stress test if the pattern is still nonreactive (Greenberg, Druzin, and Gabbe, 2012).

Contraction Stress Test

The contraction stress test (CST) or oxytocin challenge test (OCT) was the first widely used electronic fetal assessment test. It was devised as a graded stress test of the fetus, and its purpose was to identify the jeopardized fetus that was stable at rest but showed evidence of compromise after stress. Uterine contractions decrease uterine blood flow and placental perfusion. If this decrease is sufficient to produce hypoxia in the fetus, a deceleration in FHR results.

> **! NURSING ALERT**
>
> In a healthy fetoplacental unit uterine contractions do not usually produce late decelerations; whereas, if underlying UPI exists, contractions produce late decelerations.

The CST provides an earlier warning of fetal compromise than the NST and produces fewer false-positive results. However, the CST is more time consuming and expensive than the NST. It is also an invasive procedure if oxytocin stimulation is required. In general the CST cannot be performed on women who should not give birth vaginally at the time the test is done. Absolute contraindications for the CST are the following: preterm labor, placenta previa, vasa previa, reduced cervical competence, multiple gestations, and previous classic incision for cesarean birth (Miller, Miller, and Tucker, 2013). Because of these disadvantages, the CST is used infrequently.

Procedure

The woman is placed in semi-Fowler position or sits in a reclining chair with a slight lateral tilt to optimize uterine perfusion and avoid supine hypotension. She is monitored electronically with the fetal ultrasound transducer and uterine tocodynamometer. The tracing is observed for 10 to 20 minutes for baseline rate and variability and the possible occurrence of spontaneous contractions. The two methods of CST are the nipple-stimulated contraction test and the more commonly used oxytocin-stimulated contraction test.

Nipple-Stimulated Contraction Test. Several methods of nipple stimulation have been described. In one approach the woman applies warm, moist washcloths to both breasts for several minutes. She is then asked to massage one nipple for 10 minutes. Massaging the nipple causes a release of oxytocin from the posterior pituitary. An alternative approach is for her to massage one nipple through her clothes for 2 minutes, rest for 5 minutes, and repeat the cycles of massage and rest as necessary to achieve adequate uterine activity. When adequate contractions or hyperstimulation (defined as uterine contractions lasting more than 90 seconds or five or more contractions in 10 minutes) occurs, stimulation should be stopped.

Oxytocin-Stimulated Contraction Test. Exogenous oxytocin also can be used to stimulate uterine contractions. An intravenous (IV) infusion is begun, and a dilute solution of oxytocin (e.g., 30 units in 500 mL of fluid) is infused into the tubing of the main IV line through a piggyback port and delivered by an infusion pump to ensure an accurate dose. One method of oxytocin infusion is to begin at 0.5 milliunits/min and double the dose every 20 minutes until three uterine contractions of moderate intensity, each lasting 40 to 60 seconds, are observed within a 10-minute period. These criteria for contractions were selected to approximate the stress experienced by the fetus during the first stage of labor (Greenberg, Druzin, and Gabbe, 2012).

Interpretation

CST results are negative, positive, equivocal, suspicious, or unsatisfactory. If no late decelerations are observed with the contractions, the findings are considered negative (Fig. 10-14, *A*). Repetitive late decelerations render the test results positive (see Fig. 10-14, *B*). Table 10-5 lists criteria for each possible test result and the clinical significance of each.

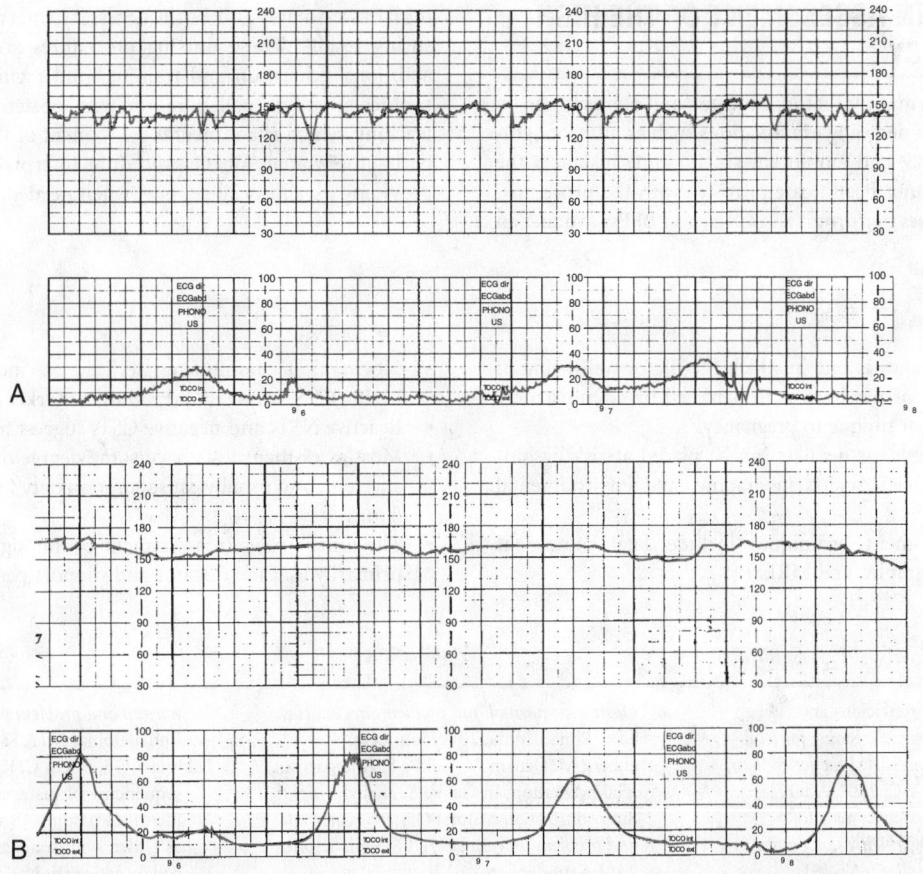

FIG 10-14 Contraction stress test (CST). **A,** Negative CST. **B,** Positive CST. (From Tucker SM: *Mosby's pocket guide to fetal monitoring: a multidisciplinary approach,* ed 5, St Louis, 2004, Mosby.)

TABLE 10-5	INTERPRETATION OF THE CONTRACTION STRESS TEST
INTERPRETATION	**CLINICAL SIGNIFICANCE**
Negative At least three uterine contractions in a 10-minute period, with no late or significant variable decelerations	Usually resume routine weekly testing schedule
Positive Late decelerations occur with 50% or more of contractions, even if there are fewer than three contractions in 10 minutes	Usually warrants hospital admission for further evaluation and/or delivery
Suspicious or Equivocal Prolonged, variable, or late decelerations occurring with less than 50% of the contractions	Repeat testing next day
Equivocal-Hyperstimulatory Decelerations that occur in the presence of contractions more frequent than every 2 min or lasting longer than 90 seconds	Repeat testing next day
Unsatisfactory Failure to produce three contractions within a 10-minute window or inability to trace the fetal heart rate	Repeat test next day

From Miller LA, Miller DA, Tucker SM: *Mosby's pocket guide to fetal monitoring: a multidisciplinary approach,* ed 7, St Louis, 2013, Mosby.

The desired CST result is negative because it has consistently been associated with good fetal outcomes. The likelihood of fetal death occurring within 1 week of a negative CST is less than 1 in 1000 (Greenberg, Druzin, and Gabbe, 2012). Positive CST results have been associated with intrauterine fetal death, late FHR decelerations in labor, IUGR, and meconium-stained amniotic fluid. A positive CST result usually leads to hospitalization for further close observation or birth. Unsatisfactory, suspicious, and equivocal tests must be repeated within 24 hours (Miller, Miller, and Tucker, 2013).

NURSES' ROLE IN ASSESSMENT OF THE HIGH RISK PREGNANCY

The nurse's role is primarily that of educator and support person when the woman is undergoing examinations such as ultrasonography, MRI, CVS, PUBS, and amniocentesis. In some instances the nurse may assist another health care provider with the procedure. In many settings nurses perform NSTs, CSTs, and BPPs; conduct an initial assessment; and begin necessary interventions for nonreassuring results. These nursing procedures are accomplished after additional education and training, under guidance of established protocols, and in collaboration with obstetric providers. Patient teaching, which is an integral component of this role, involves preparing the woman for the procedure, interpreting the findings, and providing psychosocial support when needed.

█ KEY POINTS

- A high risk pregnancy is one in which the life or well-being of the mother, fetus, or newborn is jeopardized by circumstances coincidental with or unique to pregnancy.
- The pregnancy, fetus, or neonate can be placed at risk by biophysical, psychosocial, sociodemographic, and environmental factors.
- Biophysical assessment techniques include fetal movement counts, ultrasonography, and MRI.
- Biochemical monitoring techniques include amniocentesis, PUBS, CVS, MSAFP, and multiple marker screens.
- Reactive NSTs and negative CSTs suggest fetal well-being.
- Most assessment tests have some degree of risk for the mother and fetus and usually cause some anxiety for the woman and her family.
- The nurse's roles in assessment of the high risk pregnancy are primarily that of educator and support person.

REFERENCES

American College of Obstetricians and Gynecologists (ACOG): *Screening for fetal chromosomal abnormalities, Practice Bulletin No. 77,* Washington, DC, 2007, ACOG.

American College of Obstetricians and Gynecologists (ACOG): *Ultrasonography in pregnancy. Practice Bulletin No 101,* Washington, DC, 2009, ACOG.

Baschat A, Galan H, Gabbe S: Intrauterine growth restriction. In Gabbe S, Niebyl J, Simpson J, et al, editors: *Obstetrics: normal and problem pregnancies,* ed 6, Philadelphia, 2012, Saunders.

Chambers C, Weiner C: Teratogenesis and environmental exposure. In Creasy R, Resnik R, Iams J, editors: *Creasy and Resnik's maternal-fetal medicine: principles and practice,* ed 6, Philadelphia, 2009, Saunders.

Cunningham F, Leveno K, Bloom S, et al: *Williams obstetrics,* ed 23, New York, 2010, McGraw-Hill.

Francois KE, Foley MR: Antepartum and postpartum hemorrhage. In Gabbe S, Niebyl J, Simpson J, et al, editors: *Obstetrics: normal and problem pregnancies,* ed 6, Philadelphia, 2012, Saunders.

Gilbert E: *Manual of high risk pregnancy and delivery,* ed 5, St Louis, 2011, Mosby.

Gilbert WM: Amniotic fluid disorders. In Gabbe S, Niebyl J, Simpson J, et al, editors: *Obstetrics: normal and problem pregnancies,* ed 6, Philadelphia, 2012, Saunders.

Greenberg M, Druzin M, Gabbe S: Antepartum fetal evaluation. In Gabbe S, Niebyl J, Simpson J, et al, editors: *Obstetrics: normal and problem pregnancies,* ed 6, Philadelphia, 2012, Saunders.

Harman CR: Assessment of fetal health. In Creasy R, Resnik R, Iams J, editors: *Creasy and Resnik's maternal-fetal medicine: principles and practice,* ed 6, Philadelphia, 2009, Saunders.

Manning F: Imaging in the diagnosis of fetal anomalies. In Creasy R, Resnik R, Iams J, editors: *Creasy and Resnik's maternal-fetal medicine: principles and practice,* ed 6, Philadelphia, 2009, Saunders.

Martin J, Hamilton B, Sutton P, et al: Births: final data for 2010, *Natl Vital Stat Rep* 61(1):1–100, 2012.

Mercer B: Assessment and induction of fetal pulmonary maturity. In Creasy R, Resnik R, Iams J, editors: *Creasy and Resnik's maternal-fetal medicine: principles and practice,* ed 6, Philadelphia, 2009, Saunders.

Miller L, Miller D, Tucker S: *Mosby's pocket guide to fetal monitoring: a multidisciplinary approach,* ed 7, St Louis, 2013, Mosby.

Moise K: Red cell alloimmunization. In Gabbe S, Niebyl J, Simpson J, et al, editors: *Obstetrics: normal and problem pregnancies,* ed 6, Philadelphia, 2012, Saunders.

Palomaki GE, Deciu C, Kloza EM, et al: DNA sequencing of maternal plasma reliably identifies trisomy 18 and trisomy 13 as well as Down syndrome: an international collaborative study, *Genet Med* 14(3):296–305, 2012.

Palomaki GE, Kloza EM, Lambert-Messerlian GM, et al: DNA sequencing of maternal plasma to detect Down syndrome: an international clinical validation, *Genet Med* 13(11):913–920, 2011.

Richards DS: Obstetrical ultrasound: imaging, dating, and growth. In Gabbe S, Niebyl J, Simpson J, et al, editors: *Obstetrics: normal and problem pregnancies,* ed 6, Philadelphia, 2012, Saunders.

Simpson J, Richards D, Otano L, et al: Prenatal genetic diagnosis. In Gabbe S, Niebyl J, Simpson J, et al, editors: *Obstetrics: normal and problem pregnancies,* ed 6, Philadelphia, 2012, Saunders.

Wapner RJ, Jenkins TM, Khalek N: Prenatal diagnosis of congenital disorders. In Creasy R, Resnik R, Iams J, editors: *Creasy and Resnik's maternal-fetal medicine: principles and practice,* ed 6, Philadelphia, 2009, Saunders.

High Risk Perinatal Care: Preexisting Conditions

Kitty Cashion

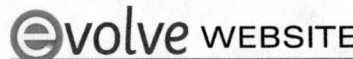

LEARNING OBJECTIVES

On completion of this chapter, the reader will be able to:

- Differentiate the types of diabetes mellitus and their respective risk factors in pregnancy.
- Compare insulin requirements during pregnancy, during the postpartum period, and with lactation.
- Identify maternal and fetal risks or complications associated with diabetes in pregnancy.
- Develop a plan of care for the pregnant woman with pregestational or gestational diabetes.
- Compare the management of a pregnant woman with hyperthyroidism with one who has hypothyroidism.

- Differentiate the management of various cardiovascular disorders in pregnant women.
- Discuss the different types of anemia and their effects during pregnancy.
- Explain the care of pregnant women with pulmonary disorders.
- Discuss the effects of neurologic disorders on pregnancy.
- Describe the care of women whose pregnancies are complicated by autoimmune disorders.
- Discuss the care of pregnant women who use, abuse, or are dependent on alcohol or illicit or prescription drugs.

For most women pregnancy represents a normal part of life. However, for some women it presents a significant risk because it is superimposed on a chronic illness. With well-motivated patients who actively participate in the treatment plan and with careful management from a multidisciplinary health care team, positive pregnancy outcomes are often possible.

Providing safe and effective care for women experiencing high risk pregnancy and their fetuses is a challenge. Although unique maternal and fetal needs prompted by these conditions exist, these women also experience many of the same pregnancy-related feelings, needs, and concerns as their "normal" counterparts. The primary objective of nursing care must be to guide and support the woman and her family in achieving optimal outcomes for both the pregnant woman and the fetus.

This chapter focuses on metabolic disorders, including diabetes mellitus and thyroid disorders; cardiovascular disorders; selected disorders of the respiratory, integumentary, and central nervous systems; and autoimmune disorders. Substance abuse is also discussed. For each disorder, management throughout the entire perinatal period (antepartum, intrapartum, and postpartum) is included in this chapter; thus all the information for each condition is located in one place in the text.

DIABETES MELLITUS

Worldwide, the incidence of diabetes mellitus is increasing at a rapid rate. In 2011 an estimated 25.8 million people in the United States (8.3% of the total population) had diabetes. Of these, 7 million were undiagnosed. If current trends continue, by 2050 one in three U.S. adults will have diabetes (National Center for Chronic Disease Prevention and Health Promotion, 2011). In the United States experts predict a marked increase in the number of women with preexisting diabetes who will become pregnant (Moore and Catalano, 2009). Diabetes mellitus is currently the most common endocrine disorder associated with pregnancy, occurring in approximately 4% to 14% of pregnant women (Gilbert, 2011). The perinatal mortality rate for well-managed diabetic pregnancies, excluding major congenital malformations, is approximately the same as for any other pregnancy (Landon, Catalano, and Gabbe, 2012). The key to an optimal pregnancy outcome is strict maternal glucose control before conception and throughout the gestational period. Consequently for women with diabetes, much emphasis is placed on preconception counseling.

Pregnancy complicated by diabetes is still considered high risk. It is most successfully managed by a multidisciplinary approach involving the obstetrician, perinatologist, internist or endocrinologist, ophthalmologist, nephrologist, neonatologist, nurse, nutritionist or dietitian, and social worker, as needed. A favorable outcome requires commitment and active participation by the pregnant woman and her family.

Pathogenesis

Diabetes mellitus refers to a group of metabolic diseases characterized by hyperglycemia resulting from defects in insulin secretion, insulin action, or both (ADA, 2009). Insulin, produced by the beta cells in the islets of Langerhans in the pancreas, regulates blood glucose levels by enabling glucose to enter adipose and muscle cells, where it is used for energy. When insulin is insufficient or ineffective in promoting glucose uptake by the muscle and adipose cells, glucose accumulates in the bloodstream, and hyperglycemia results. Hyperglycemia causes hyperosmolarity of the blood, which attracts intracellular fluid into the vascular system, resulting in cellular dehydration and expanded blood volume. Consequently the kidneys function to excrete large volumes of urine (polyuria) in an attempt to regulate excess vascular volume and excrete the unusable glucose (glycosuria). Polyuria, along with cellular dehydration, causes excessive thirst (polydipsia).

The body compensates for its inability to convert carbohydrate (glucose) into energy by burning proteins (muscle) and fats. However, the end products of this metabolism are ketones and fatty acids, which in excess quantities produce ketoacidosis and acetonuria. Weight loss occurs as a result of the breakdown of fat and muscle tissue. This tissue breakdown causes a state of starvation that compels the individual to eat excessive amounts of food (polyphagia).

Over time diabetes causes significant changes in the microvascular and macrovascular circulations. These structural changes affect a variety of organ systems, particularly the heart, eyes, kidneys, and nerves. Complications resulting from diabetes include premature atherosclerosis, retinopathy, nephropathy, and neuropathy.

Diabetes may be caused either by impaired insulin secretion, when the beta cells of the pancreas are destroyed by an autoimmune process, or by inadequate insulin action in target tissues at one or more points along the metabolic pathway. Both of these conditions are commonly present in the same person; and determining which, if either, abnormality is the primary cause of the disease is difficult (ADA, 2009). For additional information on diabetes, visit the ADA website at www.diabetes.org.

Classification

The current classification system includes four groups: type 1 diabetes, type 2 diabetes, other specific types (e.g., diabetes caused by genetic defects in beta cell function or insulin action, disease or injury of the pancreas, or drug-induced diabetes), and gestational diabetes mellitus (GDM) (ADA, 2009; Moore and Catalano, 2009).

Type 1 diabetes includes cases that are caused primarily by pancreatic islet beta cell destruction and that are prone to ketoacidosis. People with type 1 diabetes usually have an abrupt onset of illness at a young age and an absolute insulin deficiency. Type 1 diabetes includes cases thought to be caused by an autoimmune process and those for which the cause is unknown (ADA, 2009; Landon, Catalano, and Gabbe, 2012).

Type 2 diabetes is the most prevalent form of the disease and includes individuals who have insulin resistance and usually relative (rather than absolute) insulin deficiency. Specific causes of type 2 diabetes are unknown at this time. It often goes undiagnosed for years because hyperglycemia develops gradually and is often not severe enough for the person to recognize the classic signs of polyuria, polydipsia, and polyphagia. Most people who develop type 2 diabetes are obese or have an increased amount of body fat distributed primarily in the abdominal area. Other risk factors for the development of type 2 diabetes include aging, a sedentary lifestyle, family history and genetics, puberty, hypertension, and prior gestational diabetes. Type 2 diabetes often has a strong genetic predisposition (ADA, 2009; Moore and Catalano, 2009).

Pregestational diabetes mellitus is the label sometimes given to type 1 or type 2 diabetes that existed before pregnancy.

Gestational diabetes mellitus (GDM) is any degree of glucose intolerance with the onset or first recognition occurring during pregnancy. This definition is appropriate whether or not medication is used for treatment or the diabetes persists after pregnancy. It does not exclude the possibility that the glucose intolerance preceded the pregnancy or that medication might be required for optimal glucose control. Women diagnosed with gestational diabetes should be retested 6 to 12 weeks after the pregnancy ends (Landon, Catalano, and Gabbe, 2012).

White's Classification of Diabetes in Pregnancy

Dr. Priscilla White, a physician who worked with pregnant women with diabetes during the 1940s, developed a classification system specifically for use with this group of women (Table 11-1). White's system was based on age at diagnosis; duration of illness; and presence of end-organ involvement, especially eye and kidney (Landon, Catalano, and Gabbe, 2012; Moore and Catalano, 2009). Her classification system has been modified through the years but is still used frequently to assess both maternal and fetal risk. Women in classes A through C generally have positive pregnancy outcomes as long as their blood glucose levels are well controlled. However, women in classes D through T usually have poorer pregnancy outcomes because they have already developed the vascular damage that often accompanies long-standing diabetes.

TABLE 11-1	WHITE'S CLASSIFICATION OF DIABETES IN PREGNANCY (MODIFIED)
Gestational Diabetes	
Class A₁	Woman has two or more abnormal values on OGTT with normal fasting blood sugar. Blood glucose levels are diet controlled.
Class A₂	Woman was not known to have diabetes before pregnancy but requires medication for blood glucose control.
Pregestational Diabetes	
Class B	Onset of disease occurs after age 20 and duration of illness <10 years.
Class C	Onset of disease occurs between 10 and 19 years of age or duration of illness for 10 to 19 years or both.
Class D	Onset of disease occurs at <10 years of age or duration of illness >20 years or both.
Class F	Patient has developed diabetic nephropathy.
Class R	Patient has developed retinitis proliferans.
Class T	Patient has had a renal transplant.

OGTT, Oral glucose tolerance test.

Metabolic Changes Associated with Pregnancy

Normal pregnancy is characterized by complex alterations in maternal glucose metabolism, insulin production, and metabolic homeostasis. During normal pregnancy adjustments in maternal metabolism allow for adequate nutrition for the mother and the developing fetus. Glucose, the primary fuel used by the fetus, is transported across the placenta through the process of carrier-mediated facilitated diffusion, meaning that the glucose levels in the fetus are directly proportional to maternal levels. Although glucose crosses the placenta, insulin does not. Around the tenth week of gestation the fetus begins to secrete its own insulin at levels adequate to use the glucose obtained from the mother. Therefore, as maternal glucose levels rise, fetal glucose levels are increased, resulting in increased fetal insulin secretion.

During the first trimester of pregnancy the pregnant woman's metabolic status is significantly influenced by the rising levels of estrogen and progesterone. These hormones stimulate the beta cells in the pancreas to increase insulin production, which promotes increased peripheral use of glucose and decreased blood glucose, with fasting levels being reduced by approximately 10% (Fig. 11-1, *A*). At the same time an increase in tissue glycogen stores and a decrease in hepatic glucose production occur, which further encourage lower fasting glucose levels. As a result of these normal metabolic changes of pregnancy, women with insulin-dependent diabetes are prone to hypoglycemia during the first trimester.

During the second and third trimesters pregnancy exerts a "diabetogenic" effect on the maternal metabolic status. Because of the major hormonal changes, decreased tolerance to glucose, increased insulin resistance, decreased hepatic glycogen stores, and increased hepatic production of glucose occur. Rising levels of human chorionic somatomammotropin, estrogen, progesterone, prolactin, cortisol, and insulinase increase insulin resistance through their actions as insulin antagonists. Insulin resistance is a glucose-sparing mechanism that ensures an abundant supply of glucose for the fetus. Maternal insulin requirements gradually increase from approximately 18 to 24 weeks of gestation to approximately 36 weeks of

gestation. Maternal insulin requirements may double or quadruple by the end of the pregnancy (see Fig. 11-1, *B* and *C*).

At birth expulsion of the placenta prompts an abrupt drop in levels of circulating placental hormones, cortisol, and insulinase (see Fig. 11-1, *D*). Maternal tissues quickly regain their prepregnancy sensitivity to insulin. For the nonbreastfeeding mother the prepregnancy insulin-carbohydrate balance usually returns in approximately 7 to 10 days (see Fig. 11-1, *E*). Lactation uses maternal glucose; therefore the breastfeeding mother's insulin requirements remain low during lactation. On completion of weaning the mother's prepregnancy insulin requirement is reestablished (see Fig. 11-1, *F*).

PREGESTATIONAL DIABETES MELLITUS

Only about 10% of pregnancies complicated by diabetes occur in women who have preexisting disease (Landon, Catalano, and Gabbe, 2012). Women who have pregestational diabetes mellitus may have either type 1 or 2 diabetes, which may be complicated by vascular disease, retinopathy, nephropathy, or other diabetic complications. Type 2 is a more common diagnosis than type 1. Almost all women with pregestational diabetes are insulin dependent during pregnancy. According to White's classification system, these women fall into classes B through T (see Table 11-1).

The diabetogenic state of pregnancy imposed on the compromised metabolic system of the woman with pregestational diabetes has significant implications. The normal hormonal adaptations of pregnancy affect glycemic control, and pregnancy may accelerate the progress of vascular complications.

During the first trimester, when maternal blood glucose levels are normally reduced and the insulin response to glucose is enhanced, glycemic control is improved. The insulin dose for the woman with well-controlled diabetes may have to be reduced to prevent hypoglycemia. Nausea, vomiting, and cravings typical of early pregnancy result in dietary fluctuations that influence maternal glucose levels and may also necessitate a reduction in the insulin dose.

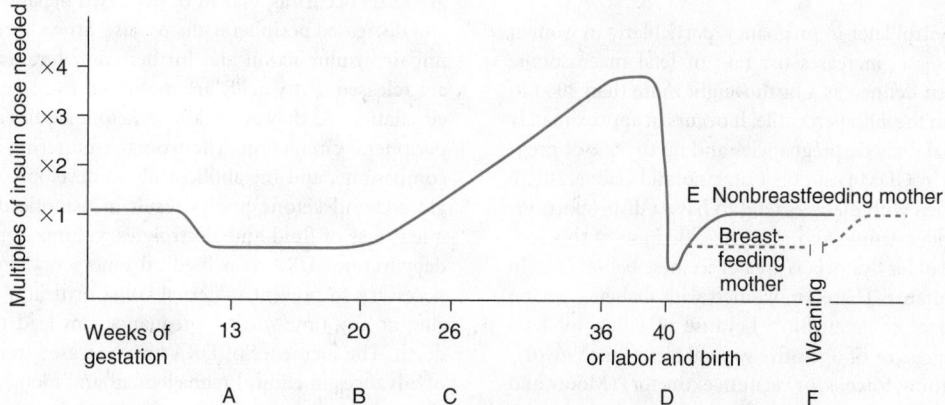

FIG 11-1 Changing insulin needs during pregnancy. **A,** First trimester: Insulin need is reduced because of increased insulin production by pancreas and increased peripheral sensitivity to insulin; nausea, vomiting, and decreased food intake by mother and glucose transfer to embryo or fetus contribute to hypoglycemia. **B,** Second trimester: Insulin needs begin to increase as placental hormones, cortisol, and insulinase act as insulin antagonists, decreasing effectiveness of insulin. **C,** Third trimester: Insulin needs may double or even quadruple but usually level off after 36 weeks of gestation. **D,** Day of birth: Maternal insulin requirements decrease drastically to approach prepregnancy levels. **E,** Breastfeeding mother maintains lower insulin requirements, as much as 25% less than those of prepregnancy; insulin needs of nonbreastfeeding mother return to prepregnancy levels in 7 to 10 days. **F,** Weaning of breastfeeding infant causes mother's insulin needs to return to prepregnancy levels.

Because insulin requirements steadily increase after the first trimester, the insulin dose must be adjusted accordingly to prevent hyperglycemia. Insulin resistance begins as early as 14 to 16 weeks of gestation and continues to rise until it stabilizes during the last few weeks of pregnancy.

Preconception Counseling

Preconception counseling is recommended for all women of reproductive age who have diabetes because it is associated with less perinatal mortality and fewer congenital anomalies (Moore and Catalano, 2009). Under ideal circumstances women with pregestational diabetes are counseled before the time of conception to plan the optimal time for pregnancy, establish glycemic control before conception, and diagnose any vascular complications of diabetes. However, estimates indicate that less than 20% of women with diabetes in the United States participate in preconception counseling (Landon, Catalano, and Gabbe, 2012).

The woman's partner should be included in the counseling to assess the couple's level of understanding related to the effects of pregnancy on the diabetic condition and the potential complications of pregnancy as a result of diabetes. The couple should also be informed of the anticipated alterations in management of diabetes during pregnancy and the need for a multidisciplinary team approach to health care. Financial implications of diabetic pregnancy and other demands related to frequent maternal and fetal surveillance should be discussed. Contraception is another important aspect of preconception counseling to help the couple plan effectively for pregnancy.

Maternal Risks and Complications

Although maternal morbidity and mortality rates have improved significantly, the pregnant woman with diabetes remains at risk for the development of complications during pregnancy. Poor glycemic control around the time of conception and in the early weeks of pregnancy is associated with an increased incidence of miscarriage. Women with good glycemic control before conception and in the first trimester are no more likely to miscarry than women who do not have diabetes (Moore and Catalano, 2009) (see Evidence-Based Practice box).

Poor glycemic control later in pregnancy, particularly in women without vascular disease, increases the rate of fetal macrosomia. Macrosomia has been defined as a birth weight more than 4000 to 4500 g or greater than the 90th percentile. It occurs in approximately 40% of pregestational diabetic pregnancies and up to 50% of pregnancies complicated by GDM (Landon, Catalano, and Gabbe, 2012). Infants born to women with diabetes tend to have a disproportionate increase in shoulder, trunk, and chest size. Because of this tendency the risk of shoulder dystocia is greater in these babies than in other macrosomic infants. Therefore women with diabetes face an increased likelihood of cesarean birth because of failure of fetal descent or labor progress or of operative vaginal birth (birth involving the use of episiotomy, forceps, or vacuum extractor) (Moore and Catalano, 2009).

Women with preexisting diabetes are at risk for several obstetric and medical complications. In general the risk of developing these complications increases with the duration and severity of the woman's diabetes. In one study the rates of preeclampsia, preterm birth, cesarean birth, and maternal mortality were much higher in women with preexisting diabetes than in women who did not have this disease. For example, approximately a third of women who have had diabetes for more than 20 years develop preeclampsia. Women with nephropathy and hypertension in addition to diabetes are also increasingly likely to develop preeclampsia. The rate of hypertensive disorders in all types of pregnancies complicated by diabetes is 15% to 30%. Chronic hypertension occurs in 10% to 20% of all pregnant women with diabetes and in up to 40% of women who have preexisting renal or retinal vascular disease (Moore and Catalano, 2009).

Hydramnios (polyhydramnios) frequently develops during the third trimester of pregnancy in women with diabetes. Its cause is unknown. One theory is that hydramnios in women with diabetes is caused by an increased glucose concentration in amniotic fluid resulting from maternal and fetal hyperglycemia. The complications most frequently associated with hydramnios (usually defined as an amniotic fluid index [AFI] greater than 24 to 25 cm) are abruptio placentae (placental abruption), uterine dysfunction, and postpartum hemorrhage (Cunningham, Leveno, Bloom, et al., 2010).

Infections are more common and more serious in pregnant women with diabetes than in those without the disease. Disorders of carbohydrate metabolism alter the normal resistance of the body to infection. The inflammatory response, leukocyte function, and vaginal pH are all affected. Vaginal infections, particularly monilial vaginitis, are more common. Urinary tract infections (UTIs) are also more prevalent. Infection is serious because it causes increased insulin resistance and may result in ketoacidosis.

Ketoacidosis (accumulation of ketones in the blood resulting from hyperglycemia and leading to metabolic acidosis) occurs most often during the second and third trimesters, when the diabetogenic effect of pregnancy is the greatest. When the maternal metabolism is stressed by illness or infection, the woman is at increased risk for diabetic ketoacidosis (DKA). DKA can also be caused by poor compliance with treatment or the onset of previously undiagnosed diabetes (Moore and Catalano, 2009). The use of beta-mimetic drugs such as terbutaline (Brethine) for tocolysis to stop preterm labor or corticosteroids given to enhance fetal lung maturation may also contribute to the risk for hyperglycemia and subsequent DKA (Cunningham, Leveno, Bloom, et al., 2010; Iams, Romero, and Creasy, 2009).

DKA may occur with blood glucose levels barely exceeding 200 mg/dL, compared with 300 to 350 mg/dL in the nonpregnant state. In response to stress factors such as infection or illness, hyperglycemia occurs as a result of increased hepatic glucose production and decreased peripheral glucose use. Stress hormones, which act to impair insulin action and further contribute to insulin deficiency, are released. Fatty acids are mobilized from fat stores to enter the circulation. As they are oxidized, ketone bodies are released into the peripheral circulation. The woman's buffering system is unable to compensate, and metabolic acidosis develops. The excessive blood glucose and ketone bodies result in osmotic diuresis with subsequent loss of fluid and electrolytes, volume depletion, and cellular dehydration. DKA is a medical emergency. Prompt treatment is necessary to prevent maternal coma or death. Ketoacidosis occurring at any time during pregnancy can lead to intrauterine fetal death. The incidence of DKA has decreased in recent years because of advances in clinical management and blood glucose monitoring (Inturrisi, Lintner, and Sorem, 2013). Currently it affects only about 1% of pregnant women with diabetes (Cunningham, Leveno, Bloom, et al., 2010). The rate of intrauterine fetal demise (IUFD) with DKA, formerly approximately 35%, is 10% or less (Moore and Catalano, 2009) (Table 11-2).

The risk of hypoglycemia (a less than normal amount of glucose in the blood) is also increased during pregnancy. Early in pregnancy, when hepatic production of glucose is diminished and peripheral use of glucose is enhanced, hypoglycemia occurs frequently, often during sleep. Later in pregnancy it may also result as insulin doses

---

EVIDENCE-BASED PRACTICE

Glycemic Control and Vitamin D for Improving Pregnancy Outcomes in Patients with Diabetes

Ask the Question

For women with diabetes, which preconception and pregnancy interventions help improve fetal and maternal outcomes?

Search for the Evidence

Search Strategies

English research-based publications on diabetes in pregnancy were included.

Databases Used

Cochrane Collaborative Database, National Guideline Clearinghouse (AHRQ), CINAHL, PubMed, UpToDate, and the professional website for AWHONN

Critically Analyze the Evidence

- Preexisting type 1 or 2 diabetes in pregnancy is a known risk for increased birth weight and perinatal loss. Loose glycemic control is associated with increased risk for preeclampsia, macrosomia, and cesarean birth. Moderate and tight glycemic controls have improved outcomes, but tight control leads to significantly more hypoglycemia and longer hospital stays. Moderate control is recommended (Middleton, Crowther and Simmonds, 2012).
- Vitamin D is a steroid hormone that is necessary for bone metabolism and vascular, immune, metabolic, and placental function. Vitamin D deficiency in pregnancy is associated with gestational diabetes, higher fasting blood sugar, and higher insulin levels (Poel, Hummel, Lips, et al., 2012; Senti, Thiele, and Anderson, 2012). Vitamin D deficiency may also be associated with preeclampsia, preterm labor, cesarean birth, and infections. Clinical recommendations for vitamin D during pregnancy are 600 international units (IU) daily (Urrutia and Thorp, 2012).
- A meta-analysis found that preconception glycemic control in women with preexisting diabetes leads to significantly lower hemoglobin A1$_c$ (HgA1$_c$) in the first trimester and fewer congenital anomalies, preterm births, perinatal mortality, and maternal complications (Wahabi, Alzeidan, Bawazeer, et al., 2010).

Apply the Evidence: Nursing Implications

- For women with diabetes who are contemplating pregnancy, preconception attention to glycemic control should be a part of patient education by the nurse. Women should know that lower HgA1$_c$ and moderate glycemic control before and during pregnancy are associated with significantly improved maternal and birth outcomes.
- All women need preconception information about vitamin D deficiency, which is associated with gestational diabetes. Vitamin D supplementation

of 600 international units daily is recommended during pregnancy. A blood test can confirm adequate vitamin D levels.

Quality and Safety Competencies: Evidence-Based Practice*

Knowledge

Differentiate clinical opinion from research and evidence summaries.

Moderate, not tight, glycemic control results in the best outcomes.

Skills

Locate evidence reports related to clinical practice topics and guidelines.

Meta-analyses show that vitamin D, 600 IU, in pregnancy is associated with less gestational diabetes.

Attitudes

Value the concept of evidence-based practice as integral to determining best clinical practice.

Attention to preconception counseling for glycemic control and vitamin D results in better pregnancy outcomes.

References

Middleton P, Crowther CA, Simmonds L: Different intensities of glycaemic control for pregnant women with pre-existing diabetes, *Cochrane Database Syst Rev* 8:CD008540.pub3. DOI: 10.1002/14651858, Chichester, UK, 2012, John Wiley and Sons.

Poel YH, Hummel P, Lips P, et al: Vitamin D and gestational diabetes: a systematic review and meta-analysis, *Eur J Intern Med* 23(5):465–469, 2012. PMID: 22726378.

Senti J, Thiele DK, Anderson CM: Maternal vitamin D status as a critical determinant in gestational diabetes, *J Obstet Gynecol Neonatal Nurs* 41(3):328–338, 2012. 2012. DOI: 10.1111/j. 1552-6909.2012.01366.x.

Urrutia RP, Thorp JM: Vitamin D in pregnancy: current concepts, *Curr Opin Obstet Gynecol* 24(2):57–64, 2012. PMID: 22327734.

Wahabi HA, Alzeidan RA, Bawazeer GA, et al: Preconception care for diabetic women for improving maternal and fetal outcomes: a systematic review and meta-analysis, *BMC Pregnancy Childbirth* 10:63, 2010. PMID: 20946676.

Pat Mahaffee Gingrich

*Adapted from QSEN at www.qsen.org/.

---

are adjusted to maintain **euglycemia** (a normal blood glucose level). Women with a prepregnancy history of severe hypoglycemia are at increased risk for severe hypoglycemia during gestation. Mild-to-moderate hypoglycemic episodes do not appear to have significant damaging effects on fetal well-being (see Table 11-2).

Fetal and Neonatal Risks and Complications

From the moment of conception the infant of a woman with diabetes faces an increased risk of complications that may occur during the antepartum, intrapartum, or neonatal periods. Infant morbidity and mortality rates associated with diabetic pregnancy are significantly reduced with strict control of maternal glucose levels before and during pregnancy.

Despite the improvements in care of pregnant women with diabetes, IUFD results in *stillbirth* and remains a major concern.

Approximately 2% to 5% of all fetal deaths occur in women whose pregnancies are complicated by preexisting diabetes. Hyperglycemia, ketoacidosis, congenital anomalies, infections, and maternal obesity are thought to be reasons for fetal death. In the third trimester fetal acidosis is the most likely cause of fetal death (Paidas and Hossain, 2009).

The most important cause of perinatal loss in diabetic pregnancy is congenital malformations, which account for 30% to 50% of all perinatal loss in pregnancies complicated by diabetes (Landon, Catalano, and Gabbe, 2012). The incidence of congenital malformations is related to the severity and duration of the diabetes. Hyperglycemia during the first trimester of pregnancy, when organs and organ systems are forming, is the main cause of diabetes-associated birth defects. Anomalies commonly seen in infants affect primarily the cardiovascular system, the central nervous system (CNS), and

TABLE 11-2 DIFFERENTIATION OF HYPOGLYCEMIA (INSULIN SHOCK) AND HYPERGLYCEMIA (DIABETIC KETOACIDOSIS)

CAUSES	ONSET	SYMPTOMS	INTERVENTIONS
Hypoglycemia (Insulin Shock)			
Excess insulin	Rapid (regular insulin)	Irritability	Check blood glucose level when symptoms first appear.
Insufficient food (delayed or missed meals)	Gradual (modified insulin or oral hypoglycemic agents)	Hunger	Eat or drink 15 g fast sugar (simple carbohydrate) immediately.
Excessive exercise or work		Sweating	
Indigestion, diarrhea, vomiting		Nervousness	Recheck blood glucose level in 15 minutes and eat or drink another 15 g fast sugar (simple carbohydrate) if glucose remains low.
		Personality change	
		Weakness	
		Fatigue	
		Blurred or double vision	
		Dizziness	Recheck blood glucose level in 15 minutes.
		Headache	
		Pallor; clammy skin	Notify primary health care provider if no change in glucose level.
		Shallow respirations	
		Rapid pulse	If woman is unconscious, administer 50% dextrose IV push, 5% to 10% dextrose in water IV drip, or 1 mg glucagon subcutaneously.
		Laboratory values	
		Urine: Negative for sugar and acetone	
		Blood glucose: ≤60 mg/dL	Obtain blood and urine specimens for laboratory testing.
Hyperglycemia (DKA)			
Insufficient insulin	Slow (hours to days)	Thirst	Notify primary health care provider.
Excess or wrong kind of food		Nausea or vomiting	Administer insulin in accordance with blood glucose levels.
Infection, injuries, illness		Abdominal pain	
Emotional stress		Constipation	Give IV fluids such as normal saline solution or one-half normal saline solution; potassium when urinary output is adequate; bicarbonate for pH <7.
Insufficient exercise		Drowsiness	
		Dim vision	
		Increased urination	
		Headache	Monitor laboratory testing of blood and urine.
		Flushed, dry skin	
		Rapid breathing	
		Weak, rapid pulse	
		Acetone (fruity) breath odor	
		Laboratory values	
		Urine: Positive for sugar and acetone	
		Blood glucose: ≥200 mg/dL	

DKA, Diabetic ketoacidosis; *IV,* intravenous.

the skeletal system (Cunningham, Leveno, Bloom, et al., 2010; Moore and Catalano, 2009) (see Chapter 25).

The fetal pancreas begins to secrete insulin at 10 to 14 weeks of gestation. The fetus responds to maternal hyperglycemia by secreting large amounts of insulin (hyperinsulinism). Insulin acts as a growth hormone, causing the fetus to produce excess stores of glycogen, protein, and adipose tissue and leading to increased fetal size, or macrosomia. Birth injuries are more common in infants born to mothers with diabetes compared with mothers who do not have diabetes, and macrosomic fetuses have the highest risk for this complication. Common birth injuries associated with diabetic pregnancies include brachial plexus palsy, facial nerve injury, humerus or clavicle fracture, and cephalhematoma. Most of these injuries are associated with difficult vaginal birth and shoulder dystocia (Moore and Catalano, 2009). Hypoglycemia at birth is also a risk for infants born to mothers with diabetes. Degree of hypoglycemia is influenced by maternal glucose control during the last half of pregnancy and during labor and birth (Landon, Catalano, and Gabbe, 2012).

(For further discussion of neonatal complications related to maternal diabetes, see Chapter 25.)

CARE MANAGEMENT

Antepartum

When a pregnant woman with diabetes initiates prenatal care, a thorough evaluation of her health status is completed. At the initial visit a complete physical examination is performed to assess the woman's health status. In addition to the routine prenatal examination, specific efforts are made to assess the effects of the diabetes, especially retinopathy, nephropathy, peripheral and autonomic neuropathy, peripheral vascular, and cardiac involvement (Gilbert, 2011).

Routine prenatal laboratory tests are performed, and baseline renal function may be assessed with a 24-hour urine collection for total protein excretion and creatinine clearance. Urinalysis and culture are performed to assess for the presence of a UTI, which is

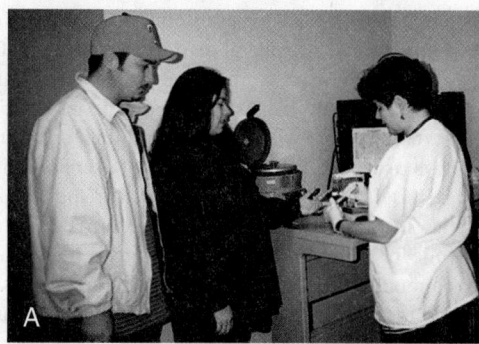 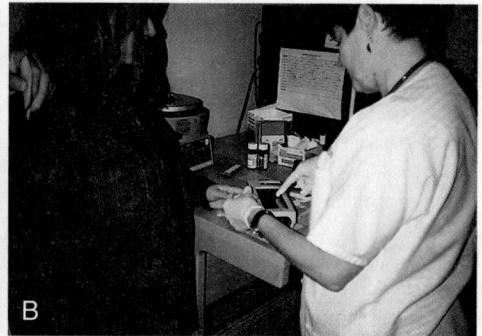

FIG 11-2 A, Clinic nurse collects blood to determine glucose level. **B,** Nurse interprets glucose value displayed by monitor. (Courtesy Dee Lowdermilk, UNC Ambulatory Care Clinics, Chapel Hill, NC.)

common in diabetic pregnancy. Because of the risk of coexisting thyroid disease, thyroid function tests may also be performed (see later discussion of thyroid disorders). The glycosylated hemoglobin A1$_c$ level may be measured to assess recent glycemic control. With prolonged hyperglycemia some of the hemoglobin remains saturated with glucose for the life of the red blood cell (RBC). Therefore a test for glycosylated hemoglobin provides a "diabetic report card," an evaluation of glycemic control over the previous 4 to 6 weeks. Hemoglobin A1$_c$ levels greater than 6 indicate elevated glucose levels during the previous 4 to 6 weeks (Gilbert, 2011). Fasting blood glucose or random (1 to 2 hours after eating) glucose levels may be assessed during antepartum visits (Fig. 11-2). Self-monitoring blood glucose records may also be reviewed.

Because of her high risk status, a woman with pregestational diabetes is monitored much more frequently and thoroughly than other pregnant women. During the first and second trimesters of pregnancy, her routine prenatal care visits are scheduled every 1 to 2 weeks. In the last trimester she will likely be seen 1 or 2 times each week. In the past routine hospitalization for management of the diabetes such as insulin dose changes was common. With the availability of improved home glucose monitoring and the growing reluctance of third-party payers to reimburse for hospitalization, pregnant women with diabetes generally are now managed as outpatients. Some patient and family education and maternal and fetal assessment may be performed in the home, depending on the woman's insurance coverage and care provider preference.

Achieving and maintaining constant euglycemia, with plasma glucose levels in the range of 65 to 95 mg/dL before meals and no higher than 130 to 140 mg/dL when measured 1 hour after a meal (Table 11-3), is the primary goal of medical therapy (Moore and Catalano, 2009). Euglycemia is achieved through a combination of diet, insulin, and exercise. Providing the woman with the knowledge, skill, and motivation she needs to achieve and maintain excellent blood glucose control is the primary nursing goal.

Achieving euglycemia requires commitment on the part of the woman and her family to make the necessary lifestyle changes, which can sometimes seem overwhelming. Maintaining tight blood glucose control necessitates that the woman follow a consistent daily schedule. She must get up and go to bed, eat, exercise, and take insulin at the same time each day. Blood glucose measurements are taken frequently to determine how well the major components of therapy (diet, insulin, and exercise) are working together to control blood glucose levels (see Community Focus box). The pregnant woman with diabetes should wear a medical identification bracelet at all times and carry insulin, syringes, and sources of fast sugar (simple carbohydrate) with her whenever she is away from home.

TABLE 11-3	**TARGET BLOOD GLUCOSE LEVELS DURING PREGNANCY**
TIME OF DAY	**TARGET PLASMA GLUCOSE LEVEL (MG/DL)**
Premeal or fasting	>65 but <95
Postmeal (1 hr)	<130-140
Postmeal (2 hr)	≤120
2 AM to 6 AM	>60

Data from Landon MB, Catalano PM, Gabbe SG: Diabetes mellitus complicating pregnancy. In Gabbe SG, Niebyl JR, Simpson JL, et al, editors: *Obstetrics: normal and problem pregnancies*, ed 6, Philadelphia, 2012, Saunders; Moore TR, Catalano PM: Diabetes in pregnancy. In Creasy RK, Resnik R, Iams JD, et al, editors: *Creasy & Resnik's maternal-fetal medicine: principles and practice*, ed 6, Philadelphia, 2009, Saunders.

🏠 COMMUNITY FOCUS
Accessibility of Diabetes Supplies

Visit your local pharmacy and examine the diabetes equipment and supplies that are available. Locate glucose meters, urine test strips, insulin syringes, and insulin pens. How much does each of these items cost? Check to see which items are covered by most types of insurance and Medicaid. Read the directions for use of each item. How easily could you follow the instructions? Could a woman with low literacy skills read and understand them? Do the directions contain illustrations? Are they written in more than one language (e.g., in Spanish or French) in addition to English? Does the pharmacy have someone who can teach women? How can you use the information you have obtained in this exercise in your patient teaching?

Because the woman with pregestational diabetes is at increased risk for infections, eye problems, and neurologic changes, foot and general skin care are important. A daily bath that includes thorough perineal and foot care is important. For dry skin lotions, creams, or oils can be applied. Tight clothing should be avoided. Shoes or slippers that fit properly should be worn at all times and are best worn with socks or stockings. Feet should be inspected regularly; toenails should be cut straight across, and professional help should be sought for any foot problems. Extremes of temperature should be avoided.

Diet. The woman with pregestational diabetes has usually had nutrition counseling regarding management of her diabetes.

PATIENT TEACHING

Dietary Management of Diabetic Pregnancy

- Follow the prescribed diet plan.
- Eat a well-balanced diet, including daily food requirements for a normal pregnancy.
- Divide daily food intake among three meals and two or three snacks, depending on individual needs.
- Eat a substantial bedtime snack to prevent a severe drop in blood glucose level during the night.
- Take daily vitamins and iron as prescribed by the health care provider.
- Avoid foods high in refined sugar.
- Eat consistently each day; never skip meals or snacks.
- Eat foods high in dietary fiber.
- Avoid alcohol, nicotine, and caffeine.

However, because pregnancy produces special nutrition concerns and needs, the woman must be educated to incorporate these changes into dietary planning. The woman who has "controlled" her diabetes for several years may find the changes in her insulin and dietary needs mandated by pregnancy to be difficult. Nutrition counseling is usually provided by a registered dietitian.

Dietary management during diabetic pregnancy must be based on blood (not urine) glucose levels. The diet is individualized to allow for increased fetal and metabolic requirements, with consideration of such factors as prepregnancy weight and dietary habits, overall health, ethnic background, lifestyle, stage of pregnancy, knowledge of nutrition, and insulin therapy. The dietary goals are to provide weight gain consistent with a normal pregnancy, prevent ketoacidosis, and minimize wide fluctuation of blood glucose levels.

For nonobese women dietary counseling based on preconception body mass index (BMI) is 30 to 35 kcal/kg/day (Cunningham, Leveno, Bloom, et al., 2010). In contrast, for obese women with a BMI greater than 30, experts recommend that the caloric intake total 25 kcal/kg/day (Moore and Catalano, 2009). The average diet includes 2200 calories (first trimester) to 2500 calories (second and third trimesters). Total calories may be distributed among three meals and one evening snack or, more commonly, three meals and two or three snacks. Meals should be eaten on time and never skipped. Going more than 4 hours without food intake increases the risk for episodes of hypoglycemia. Snacks must be planned carefully in accordance with insulin therapy to prevent fluctuations in blood glucose levels. A large bedtime snack of at least 25 g of carbohydrate with some protein or fat is recommended to help prevent hypoglycemia and starvation ketosis during the night (Moore and Catalano, 2009).

The ideal diet is composed of 55% carbohydrate, 20% protein, and 25% fat, with less than 10% as saturated fat (Cunningham, Leveno, Bloom, et al., 2010) (see Patient Teaching box). Simple carbohydrates are limited. Complex carbohydrates that are high in fiber content are recommended because the starch and protein in such foods help regulate the blood glucose level by more sustained glucose release (Gilbert, 2011; Moore and Catalano, 2009).

Exercise. Although studies have shown that exercise enhances the use of glucose and decreases insulin need in women without diabetes, data regarding exercise in women with pregestational diabetes are limited. Any prescription of exercise during pregnancy for women with diabetes should be given by the primary health care provider and monitored closely to prevent complications. Regular exercise may be contraindicated in women with diabetes who also have uncontrolled hypertension, advanced retinopathy, or severe autonomic or peripheral neuropathy (Gilbert, 2011).

When exercise is prescribed by the health care provider as part of the treatment plan, specific instructions are given to the woman. Aerobic exercise with resistance training for at least 30 minutes most days of the week is the best type of exercise (Gilbert, 2011). Other exercises that may be recommended are non–weight-bearing activities such as arm exercises or use of a recumbent bicycle. The best time for exercise is after meals, when the blood glucose level is rising. To monitor the effect of insulin on blood glucose levels the woman can measure her blood glucose before, during, and after exercise.

! NURSING ALERT

Uterine contractions may occur during exercise. The woman should be advised to stop exercising immediately if they are detected, drink two to three glasses of water, and lie down on her side for an hour. If the contractions continue, she should contact her health care provider.

Insulin Therapy. Adequate insulin is the primary factor in the maintenance of euglycemia during pregnancy, thus ensuring proper glucose metabolism of the woman and fetus. Insulin requirements during pregnancy change dramatically as the pregnancy progresses, necessitating frequent adjustments in the dose. In the first trimester, from weeks 3 to 7 of gestation, insulin requirements are increased followed by a decrease between weeks 7 and 15 of gestation. The commonly prescribed dose is 0.7 units/kg in the first trimester for women with type 1 diabetes. During the second and third trimesters, because of insulin resistance, the dose must be increased significantly to maintain target glucose levels. Insulin requirements normally plateau after 35 weeks of gestation and often drop significantly after 38 weeks (Moore and Catalano, 2009).

For the woman with type 1 pregestational diabetes who has typically been accustomed to one injection per day of intermediate-acting insulin, multiple daily injections of mixed insulin are a new experience. The woman with type 2 diabetes previously treated with oral hypoglycemics is faced with the task of learning to self-administer injections of insulin. The nurse is instrumental in the education and support of women with pregestational diabetes in regard to insulin administration and adjustment of the insulin dose to maintain euglycemia (see Patient Teaching box on p. 275 and Box 11-1).

Since 1982 most insulin preparations have been produced by inserting portions of DNA ("recombinant DNA") into special laboratory-cultivated bacteria or yeast cells. The cells then produce synthetic human insulin (Humulin), which is less likely to cause antibody formation than animal-derived (beef or pork) insulin. More recently insulin products called *insulin analogs,* in which the structure differs slightly from human insulin, have been produced. This small alteration in insulin structure results in changes in the onset and peak of action of the medication. The most commonly used insulin preparations include rapid-acting, short-acting, intermediate-acting, and long-acting (Landon, Catalano, and Gabbe, 2012) (Table 11-4). Mixtures of short- and intermediate-acting insulins in several proportions are also available.

Lispro (Humalog) and aspart (NovoLog) are commonly prescribed rapid-acting insulins with a shorter duration of action than regular insulin. They are preferred for use during pregnancy (Landon, Catalano, and Gabbe, 2012). Advantages of rapid-acting insulins include convenience because they are injected immediately before mealtime, less hyperglycemia after meals, and fewer hypoglycemic episodes in some people. Because their effects last only 3 to 5

BOX 11-1 HELPFUL HINTS FOR USING INSULIN

- The most common type of insulin used during pregnancy is a biosynthetic human insulin (Humulin) made by programming *Escherichia coli* bacteria to produce insulin.
- Insulin is classified either as rapid acting, short acting, intermediate acting, or long acting (see Table 11-4).
- Unused vials of insulin should be stored in the refrigerator until reaching their expiration date. Insulin should not be frozen. Vials currently in use can be stored at room temperature for up to a month. They should not be stored in direct sunlight.
- Regular insulin can be mixed with NPH insulin in the same syringe. Lispro insulin can also be mixed in a syringe with NPH or Ultralente insulin. Once mixed, the syringe can be used immediately or stored for future use. If it is used later, the syringe should be rotated 20 times before injection.
- Glargine insulin is administered at bedtime. It cannot be mixed with any other insulin in the same syringe. Prepared syringes are stable for 2 weeks in the refrigerator.
- Insulin may be administered by pen injector, jet injector, or insulin pump, in addition to syringe.
- The abdomen is the preferred injection site because insulin is best absorbed there. Other possible injection sites are the upper outer arm (not the deltoid area), the thighs, and the buttocks.
- Each injection should be given 1 inch from the previous injection. Each individual injection site should not be used more often than once in 30 days.

PATIENT TEACHING

Self-Administration of Insulin

Procedure for Mixing NPH (Intermediate-Acting) and Regular (Short-Acting) Insulin

- Wash hands thoroughly and gather supplies. Be sure that insulin syringe corresponds to concentration of insulin you are using.
- Check insulin bottle to be certain that it is the appropriate type and check expiration date.
- Gently rotate (do not shake) insulin vial to mix insulin.
- Wipe off rubber stopper of each vial with alcohol.
- Draw into syringe the amount of air equal to total dose.
- Inject air equal to NPH dose into NPH vial. Remove needle from vial.
- Inject air equal to regular insulin dose into regular insulin vial.
- Invert regular insulin bottle and withdraw regular insulin dose.
- Without adding more air to NPH vial, carefully withdraw NPH dose.

Procedure for Self-Injection of Insulin

- Select proper injection site.
- Injection site should be clean. No need to use alcohol. If alcohol is used, let it dry before injecting.
- Pinch skin up to form a subcutaneous pocket and, holding syringe as you would hold a pencil, puncture skin at a 45- to 90-degree angle. If a great deal of fatty tissue is at the site, spread skin taut and inject syringe at a 90-degree angle.
- Slowly inject insulin.
- As you withdraw needle, cover injection site with sterile gauze and apply gentle pressure to prevent bleeding.
- Record insulin dose and time of injection.

TABLE 11-4 COMMON INSULIN PREPARATIONS

TYPE OF INSULIN	EXAMPLES GENERIC (TRADE) NAME	ONSET OF ACTION	PEAK OF ACTION	DURATION OF ACTION
Rapid-acting	Lispro (Humalog)	15 min	30-90 min	4-5 hr
	Aspart (NovoLog)	15 min	1-3 hr	3-5 hr
Short-acting	Humulin R	30 min	2-4 hr	5-7 hr
	Novolin R	30 min	2.5-5 hr	6-8 hr
Intermediate-acting	Humulin NPH	1-2 hr	6-12 hr	18-24 hr
	Novolin N	1.5 hr	4-20 hr	24 hr
	Humulin Lente	1-3 hr	6-12 hr	18-24 hr
	Novolin L	2.5 hr	7-15 hr	22 hr
Long-acting	Humulin Ultralente	4-6 hr	8-20 hr	>36 hr
	Glargine (Lantus)	1 hr	None	24 hr

Data from Landon MB, Catalano PM, Gabbe SG: Diabetes mellitus complicating pregnancy. In Gabbe SG, Niebyl JR, Simpson JL, et al, editors: *Obstetrics: normal and problem pregnancies*, ed 6, Philadelphia, 2012, Saunders.
L, Lente; *NPH* (or *N*), neutral protamine Hagedorn; *R,* regular.

---

hours, most patients require a longer-acting insulin in addition to the rapid-acting insulin to maintain optimal blood glucose levels (Landon, Catalano, and Gabbe, 2012; Moore and Catalano, 2009) (see Table 11-4). Glargine (Lantus) is long-acting insulin lasting approximately 24 hours. Small amounts of glargine insulin are released slowly, with no pronounced peak. This preparation is most often used with women who have insulin-resistant diabetes (type 2) requiring high doses of long-acting insulin. Glargine insulin is combined with rapid-acting insulin to prevent hypoglycemia. Glargine

insulin appears to be safe for use during pregnancy. When it is administered with rapid-acting or short-acting insulin, unpredictable spikes in insulin levels and resulting hypoglycemia appear to occur less often (Landon, Catalano, and Gabbe, 2012) (see Table 11-4).

Most women with insulin-dependent diabetes are managed with two or three injections per day (Landon, Catalano, and Gabbe, 2012). Usually two thirds of the daily insulin dose, with intermediate-acting and short-acting insulin combined in a 2:1 ratio, is given

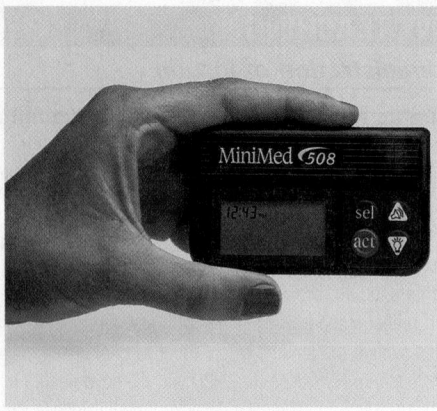

FIG 11-3 Insulin pump shows basal rate for pregnant women with diabetes. (Courtesy MiniMed, Inc., Sylmar, CA.)

before breakfast. The remaining one third is administered in the evening. It may be given as a combination of short- and intermediate-acting insulin before dinner or split, with rapid-acting insulin at dinner and intermediate-acting insulin at bedtime (Landon, Catalano, and Gabbe, 2012). An alternative insulin regimen that works well for some women is to administer short-acting insulin before each meal and longer-acting insulin at bedtime (Moore and Catalano, 2009).

Continuous subcutaneous insulin infusion (CSII) systems are used increasingly during pregnancy. The insulin pump is designed to mimic more closely the function of the pancreas in secreting insulin (Fig. 11-3). This portable battery-powered device is worn similar to a pager during most daily activities. The pump infuses rapid-acting insulin (usually lispro) (Landon, Catalano, and Gabbe, 2012) at a set basal rate and has the capacity to deliver up to four different basal rates in 24 hours. It also delivers bolus doses of insulin before meals to control postprandial blood glucose levels. A fine-gauge plastic catheter is inserted into subcutaneous tissue, usually in the abdomen, and attached to the pump syringe by connecting tubing. The subcutaneous catheter and connecting tubing are changed every 2 to 3 days, although the infusion tubing can be left in place for several weeks without local complications. Although the insulin pump is convenient and generally provides good glycemic control, complications such as pump failure, precipitation of insulin inside the pump mechanism, abscess formation, and poor uptake from the infusion site can still occur. Therefore use of the insulin pump requires a knowledgeable, motivated woman; skilled health care providers; and prompt 24-hour availability of emergency assistance (Moore and Catalano, 2009).

Monitoring Blood Glucose Levels. Blood glucose testing at home with a glucose reflectance meter is considered the standard of care for monitoring blood glucose levels during pregnancy. It provides the most important tool available to the woman to assess her degree of glycemic control. Most of the newer reflectance meters are calibrated to provide plasma (rather than whole blood) glucose values. Plasma glucose values are 10% to 15% lower than those measured in whole blood from the same sample (Moore and Catalano, 2009).

⚡ SAFETY ALERT

The nurse must be knowledgeable about the specific glucose reflectance meter that the woman uses because target glucose values depend on the type of meter used (Moore and Catalano, 2009).

PATIENT TEACHING

Self-Testing of Blood Glucose Level

- Gather supplies, check expiration date, and read instructions on testing materials. Prepare glucose reflectance meter for use according to manufacturer directions.
- Wash hands in warm water (warmth increases circulation).
- Select site on side of any finger (all fingers should be used in rotation).
- Pierce site with lancet (may use automatic spring-loaded, puncturing device). Cleaning site with alcohol is not necessary.
- Drop hand down to side; with other hand gently squeeze finger from hand to fingertip.
- Allow blood to fill entire testing area on the strip.
- Determine blood glucose value using glucose reflectance meter following manufacturer instructions.
- Record results.
- Repeat as instructed by health care provider and as needed for signs of hypoglycemia or hyperglycemia.

To perform blood glucose monitoring a drop of blood is obtained, usually by means of a fingerstick, and placed on a test strip. Some newer glucose meters allow the user to obtain the blood sample from the forearm rather than a finger. After a specified amount of time the glucose level is displayed by the meter (see Patient Teaching box). Blood glucose levels are routinely measured at various times throughout the day such as before breakfast, lunch, and dinner; 2 hours after each meal; at bedtime; and in the middle of the night. When any readjustment in the insulin dose or diet is made, more frequent measurement of blood glucose is warranted. If nausea, vomiting, or diarrhea occurs or if any infection is present, the woman is asked to monitor her blood glucose levels more closely than usual.

❗ NURSING ALERT

Hyperglycemia is most likely to be identified in 2-hour postmeal values because blood glucose levels peak approximately 2 hours after a meal.

Target levels of blood glucose during pregnancy are lower than nonpregnant values (see Table 11-3). Acceptable fasting levels are generally between 65 and 95 mg/dL, and 1-hour postmeal levels should be less than 130 to 140 mg/dL (Moore and Catalano, 2009). Two-hour postmeal levels should be 120 mg/dL or less (Landon, Catalano, and Gabbe, 2012). The woman should be told to report episodes of hypoglycemia (less than 60 mg/dL) and hyperglycemia (more than 200 mg/dL) immediately to her health care provider so adjustments in diet or insulin therapy can be made.

Pregnant women with diabetes are much more likely to develop hypoglycemia than hyperglycemia. Most episodes of mild or moderate hypoglycemia can be treated with oral intake of 15 g of simple carbohydrate (fast sugar) (see Patient Teaching box on p. 277). If severe hypoglycemia occurs, in which case the woman experiences a decrease in or loss of consciousness or an inability to swallow, she will require a parenteral injection of glucagon or intravenous (IV) glucose. Because hypoglycemia can develop rapidly and impaired judgment can be associated with even moderate episodes, family members, friends, and work colleagues must be able to recognize signs and symptoms quickly and initiate proper treatment if necessary.

Hyperglycemia is less likely than hypoglycemia to occur, although it can rapidly progress to DKA, which is associated with an increased risk of fetal death (Cunningham, Leveno, Bloom et al., 2010; Moore and Catalano, 2009). Women and family members should be particularly alert for signs and symptoms of hyperglycemia, especially when infections or other illnesses occur (see Patient Teaching box).

Urine Testing. Urine testing for glucose is not beneficial during pregnancy. Because of the lowered renal threshold for glucose, the degree of glycosuria does not accurately reflect the blood glucose level. However, urine testing for ketones continues to have a place in diabetic management. Monitoring for urine ketones may detect inadequate caloric or carbohydrate intake or skipped meals or snacks. Testing may also be performed when illness occurs or when the blood glucose level is greater than 200 mg/dL (Gilbert, 2011).

Complications Requiring Hospitalization. Occasionally hospitalization is necessary to regulate insulin therapy and stabilize glucose levels. Infection, which can lead to hyperglycemia and DKA, is an indication for hospitalization, regardless of gestational age. Hospitalization during the third trimester for close maternal and fetal observation may be indicated for women whose diabetes is poorly controlled. In addition, women with diabetes are 10% to 20% more likely than women who do not have diabetes to also have preexisting hypertension or develop preeclampsia, which may necessitate hospitalization (Moore and Catalano, 2009).

Fetal Surveillance. Diagnostic techniques for fetal surveillance are often performed to assess fetal growth and well-being. The goals of fetal surveillance are to detect fetal compromise as early as possible and prevent IUFD or unnecessary preterm birth.

Early in pregnancy the estimated date of birth is determined. A baseline sonogram is obtained during the first trimester to assess gestational age. Follow-up ultrasound examinations are usually performed during the pregnancy (as often as every 4 to 6 weeks) to monitor fetal growth; estimate fetal weight; and detect hydramnios, macrosomia, and congenital anomalies.

Because the fetus of a woman with diabetes is at increased risk for neural tube defects (e.g., spina bifida, anencephaly, microcephaly), measurement of maternal serum alpha-fetoprotein is performed between 15 and 20 weeks of gestation (ideally between 16 and 18 weeks of gestation) (Wapner, Jenkins, and Khalek, 2009). This assessment is often performed in conjunction with a detailed ultrasound study to examine the fetus for neural tube defects.

Fetal echocardiography may be performed between 20 and 22 weeks of gestation to detect cardiac anomalies, especially in women who had less-than-desirable glucose control early in pregnancy, as demonstrated by a hemoglobin A1$_c$ level above 6% at the first prenatal visit (Gilbert, 2011; Moore and Catalano, 2009). Some practitioners repeat this fetal surveillance test at 34 weeks of gestation. Doppler studies of the umbilical artery may be performed in women with vascular disease to detect placental compromise.

Most fetal surveillance measures are concentrated in the third trimester, when the risk of fetal compromise is greatest. The goals of antepartum testing during the third trimester are to prevent IUFD and maximize the opportunity for the woman to safely give birth vaginally. Pregnant women should be taught how to make daily fetal movement counts, beginning at 28 weeks of gestation (see Chapter 10) (Moore and Catalano, 2009).

The nonstress test (NST) is the preferred primary method to evaluate fetal well-being. It is usually begun by 32 weeks of gestation and performed at least twice weekly. If the NST is nonreactive, a biophysical profile or contraction stress test will be performed. Testing often begins earlier, between 28 and 32 weeks of gestation, in women who have vascular disease or poor glucose control (Landon, Catalano, and Gabbe, 2012) (see Chapter 10).

Determination of Date and Mode of Birth. The optimal time for birth is between 38.5 and 40 weeks of gestation, as long as good metabolic control is maintained and parameters of antepartum fetal surveillance remain within normal limits. Reasons to proceed with birth before this time include poor metabolic control, worsening hypertensive disorders, fetal macrosomia, or fetal growth restriction (Moore and Catalano, 2009).

Many practitioners plan for elective labor induction between 38 and 40 weeks of gestation. To confirm fetal lung maturity an amniocentesis should be performed when birth will occur before 38.5 weeks of gestation. For the pregnancy complicated by diabetes, fetal lung maturation is best predicted by the amniotic fluid phosphatidylglycerol (greater than 3%). If the fetal lungs are still immature, birth should be postponed until 40 weeks of gestation as long as fetal assessment test results remain reassuring. However, after that time the benefits of conservative management are outweighed by the increasing risk of fetal compromise if the pregnancy is allowed to continue. Despite poor fetal lung maturity, birth may be necessary when testing suggests fetal compromise or worsening maternal condition such as deteriorating renal function or severe preeclampsia (Moore and Catalano, 2009).

Although vaginal birth is expected for most women with pregestational diabetes, the cesarean rate for these women ranges from 50% to 80% (Cunningham, Leveno, Bloom, et al., 2010). The ACOG recommends that cesarean birth be considered when the estimated fetal weight is expected to be greater than 4500 g in an attempt to reduce the risk of shoulder dystocia. This recommendation appears to result in a small improvement in neonatal outcome (Moore and Catalano, 2009). Abnormal fetal status and induction failures before term also contribute to the high rate of cesarean birth in these women (Gilbert, 2011).

Intrapartum

During the intrapartum period the woman with pregestational diabetes must be monitored closely to prevent complications related to dehydration, hypoglycemia, and hyperglycemia. An IV line is inserted for infusion of a maintenance fluid. Initially this infusion may be normal saline. Once active labor begins or glucose levels fall below 70 mg/dL, the infusion is changed to one containing 5% dextrose. This fluid provides the energy (calories) necessary for the woman to accomplish the work and manage the stress of labor and birth. Most commonly insulin is administered by continuous infusion, piggybacked into the main IV line. Only regular (short-acting) insulin can be administered intravenously. Determination of blood glucose levels is made every hour, and fluids and insulin are adjusted to maintain the blood glucose level at 140 mg/dL or less. Maintaining this target glucose level is essential because hyperglycemia during labor can cause metabolic problems in the neonate, particularly hypoglycemia (Landon, Catalano, and Gabbe, 2012).

If a cesarean birth is planned, it should be scheduled in the early morning to facilitate glycemic control. Women should take their full dose of insulin the night before surgery. No morning insulin is given on the day of surgery, and the woman is given nothing by mouth. Epidural anesthesia is recommended because hypoglycemia can be detected earlier if the woman is awake. After surgery glucose levels should be monitored carefully. Generally sliding scale insulin is used to control blood glucose levels until the woman resumes a regular diet (Moore and Catalano, 2009).

Postpartum

In the immediate postpartum period insulin requirements decrease substantially because the major source of insulin resistance, the placenta, has been removed. Women may require only one third to one half of their last pregnancy insulin doses on the first postpartum day, provided that they are eating a full diet. Many women with type 2 diabetes do not require insulin at all for the first 1 to 2 days after giving birth (Landon, Catalano, and Gabbe, 2012). Women who give birth by cesarean may require an IV infusion of glucose and insulin until they resume a regular diet (Moore and Catalano, 2009). After birth, several days may be required to reestablish carbohydrate homeostasis (see Fig. 11-1, *D* and *E*). Blood glucose levels are monitored carefully in the postpartum period; the insulin dose is adjusted, often using a sliding scale (the amount of insulin to be administered is determined by the woman's blood glucose level at the time the dose is given). The woman who has insulin-dependent diabetes must realize the importance of eating on time even if the

baby needs to be fed or other pressing demands exist (Moore and Catalano, 2009).

Possible postpartum complications include preeclampsia or eclampsia, hemorrhage, and infection. Hemorrhage is a possibility if the mother's uterus was overdistended (hydramnios, macrosomic fetus) or overstimulated (oxytocin induction). Postpartum infections such as endometritis are more likely to occur in women with diabetes than in women who do not have diabetes.

Mothers are encouraged to breastfeed. In addition to the advantages of maternal satisfaction and pleasure, breastfeeding has an antidiabetogenic effect for the children of women with diabetes and women with GDM (Moore and Catalano, 2009). This effect is important because a child born to a mother with type 2 diabetes has a 70% chance of also developing type 2 diabetes later in life. In addition, children who were exposed to hyperglycemia prenatally have an increased risk for obesity in childhood (Gilbert, 2011).

Insulin requirements in breastfeeding women may be one half of prepregnancy levels because of the carbohydrate used in human milk production. Because glucose levels are lower than normal, breastfeeding women are at increased risk for hypoglycemia, especially in the early postpartum period and after breastfeeding sessions, particularly after late-night nursing (Gilbert, 2011; Moore and Catalano, 2009). Breastfeeding mothers with diabetes may be at increased risk for mastitis and yeast infections of the breast. The insulin dose, which is decreased during lactation, must be recalculated at weaning (see Fig. 11-1, *F*).

The mother may have early breastfeeding difficulties. Poor metabolic control may delay lactogenesis and contribute to decreased milk production (Moore and Catalano, 2009). Initial contact with and opportunity to breastfeed the infant may be delayed for mothers who gave birth by cesarean or if infants are placed in neonatal intensive care units or special care nurseries for observation during the first few hours after birth. Support and assistance from nursing staff and lactation specialists can facilitate the mother's early experience with breastfeeding and encourage her to continue nursing.

The new mother needs information about family planning and contraception. Although family planning is important for all women, it is essential for the woman with pregestational diabetes to safeguard her own health and promote optimal outcomes in future pregnancies. The risks and benefits of contraceptive methods should be discussed with the mother and her partner before discharge from the hospital. Barrier methods are often recommended as safe, inexpensive options that have no inherent risks for women with diabetes. The intrauterine device (IUD) may also be used without concerns about an increased risk of infection (Landon, Catalano, and Gabbe, 2012).

Use of oral contraceptives by women with diabetes is controversial because of the risk of thromboembolic and vascular complications and the effect on carbohydrate metabolism. In nonsmoking women who are younger than 35 years old and do not have vascular disease, combination low-dose oral contraceptives may be prescribed. Progestin-only oral contraceptives also may be used because they affect carbohydrate metabolism minimally if at all (Cunningham, Leveno, Bloom, et al., 2010). Close monitoring of blood pressure and lipid levels is necessary to detect complications (Landon, Catalano, and Gabbe, 2012).

Opinion is divided about the use of long-acting parenteral progestins such as medroxyprogesterone (Depo-Provera). Some health care providers recommend their use, particularly in women who are noncompliant with daily dosing oral contraceptives. In contrast, other health care providers believe that this method may adversely affect glycemic control. In addition, although Depo-Provera may lower serum triglyceride and high-density lipoprotein (HDL) cholesterol levels, it does not lower total cholesterol or low-density lipoprotein (LDL) levels. For this reason it is not recommended as a first-choice method of contraception for women with diabetes (Landon, Catalano, and Gabbe, 2012).

The transdermal (patch) and transvaginal (vaginal ring) are newer contraceptive methods, particularly effective in women who prefer weekly or every-third-week dosing, respectively. For women weighing more than 90 kg (198 lbs) the contraceptive failure rate with transdermal administration is higher than in normal-weight women. Therefore this method would be contraindicated in obese women. Women who choose the patch as their contraceptive method should have no risk factors for cardiovascular or thromboembolic disease (Cunningham, Leveno, Bloom, et al., 2010).

The risks associated with pregnancy increase with the duration and severity of diabetes. In addition, pregnancy may contribute to the vascular changes associated with diabetes. This information needs to be discussed thoroughly with the woman and her partner. Sterilization is often recommended for the woman who has completed her family, has poor metabolic control, or has significant vascular problems.

GESTATIONAL DIABETES MELLITUS

GDM complicates approximately 3% to 9% of all pregnancies (Moore and Catalano, 2009) and accounts for more than 90% of all cases of diabetic pregnancy (Landon, Catalano, and Gabbe, 2012). It occurs more often now than in the past in the United States, probably because of increasing rates of overweight and obesity (ACOG, 2011). According to White's classification system, women with GDM fall into classes A_1 and A_2 (see Table 11-1). It is more likely to occur among Hispanic, Native American, Asian, and African-American women than Caucasians and is likely to recur in future pregnancies; the risk for development of overt diabetes in later life is also increased (Moore and Catalano, 2009). This tendency is especially true of women whose GDM is diagnosed early in pregnancy (Landon, Catalano, and Gabbe, 2012). Classic risk factors for GDM include a family history of diabetes and a previous pregnancy that resulted in an unexplained stillbirth or the birth of a malformed or macrosomic fetus. Other risk factors for GDM include obesity, hypertension, glycosuria, and maternal age older than 25 years. Interestingly, more than half of all women diagnosed with GDM do not have these risk factors (Landon, Catalano, and Gabbe, 2012).

Although most women are screened for GDM between 24 and 28 weeks of gestation, those with strong risk factors should be screened earlier in pregnancy. Women with morbid obesity, a strong family history of diabetes, a history of GDM in a previous pregnancy, or a history of giving birth to a macrosomic stillborn infant or an infant weighing more than 4500 g are candidates for early screening. If the early screening results are normal, they should be rescreened at 24 to 28 weeks of gestation (Landon, Catalano, and Gabbe, 2012).

GDM is usually diagnosed during the second half of pregnancy. As fetal nutrient demands rise during the late second and the third trimesters, maternal nutrient ingestion induces greater and more sustained levels of blood glucose. At the same time maternal insulin resistance is also increasing because of the insulin-antagonistic effects of the placental hormones, cortisol, and insulinase. Consequently maternal insulin demands rise as much as threefold. Most pregnant women are capable of increasing insulin production to compensate for insulin resistance and maintain euglycemia.

However, when the pancreas is unable to produce sufficient insulin or the insulin is not used effectively, GDM can result.

Fetal Risks

No increase in the incidence of birth defects has been found among infants of women who develop GDM after the first trimester because the critical period of organ formation has already passed by that time (Moore and Catalano, 2009). However, Anderson, Waller, Canfield, et al., (2005) found that women who were obese before conception (BMI more than 30 kg/m^2) and developed GDM were at greater risk to give birth to infants with CNS defects.

Screening for Gestational Diabetes Mellitus

All pregnant women not known to have pregestational diabetes should be screened for GDM by history, clinical risk factors, or laboratory screening of blood glucose levels. Based on history and clinical risk factors, some women are at low risk for the development of GDM. Therefore glucose testing for this low risk population is not cost-effective (ADA, 2009). This group includes normal-weight women younger than 25 years of age who have no family history of diabetes, are not members of an ethnic or a racial group known to have a high prevalence of the disease, and have no history of abnormal glucose tolerance or adverse obstetric outcomes usually associated with GDM (ADA, 2009).

Two different screening methods for GDM are currently in use. In the one-step procedure a diagnostic oral glucose tolerance test is performed without prior glucose screening. In the United States a two-step screening method generally is used. The first step is a screen consisting of a 50-g oral glucose load followed by a plasma glucose measurement 1 hour later. The woman need not be fasting when the screen is done. A glucose value of 130 to 140 mg/dL is considered a positive screen. An initial positive screening result is followed by step 2, a 3-hour (100-g) oral glucose tolerance test (OGTT) (Landon, Catalano, and Gabbe, 2012). ACOG currently recommends use of the two-step screening procedure because there is no evidence at this time that the one-step method leads to clinically significant improvements in maternal or newborn outcomes. However, use of the one-step method would significantly increase health care costs (ACOG, 2011).

The OGTT is administered after an overnight fast and at least 3 days of unrestricted diet (at least 150 g of carbohydrate) and physical activity. The woman is instructed to avoid caffeine because it increases glucose levels and to abstain from smoking for 12 hours before the test. The 3-hour OGTT requires a fasting blood glucose level, which is drawn before giving a 100-g glucose load. Blood glucose levels are then drawn 1, 2, and 3 hours later. The woman is diagnosed with GDM if two or more values are met or exceeded (Moore and Catalano, 2009) (Fig. 11-4).

Nursing diagnoses and expected outcomes of care for women with GDM are basically the same as those for women with pregestational diabetes except that the time frame for planning may be shortened with GDM because the diagnosis is usually made later in pregnancy (see Nursing Care Plan).

CARE MANAGEMENT

Antepartum

When the diagnosis of GDM is made, treatment begins immediately, allowing little or no time for the woman and her family to adjust to the diagnosis before they are expected to participate in the treatment plan. With each step of the treatment plan the nurse and other health care providers should educate the woman and her family,

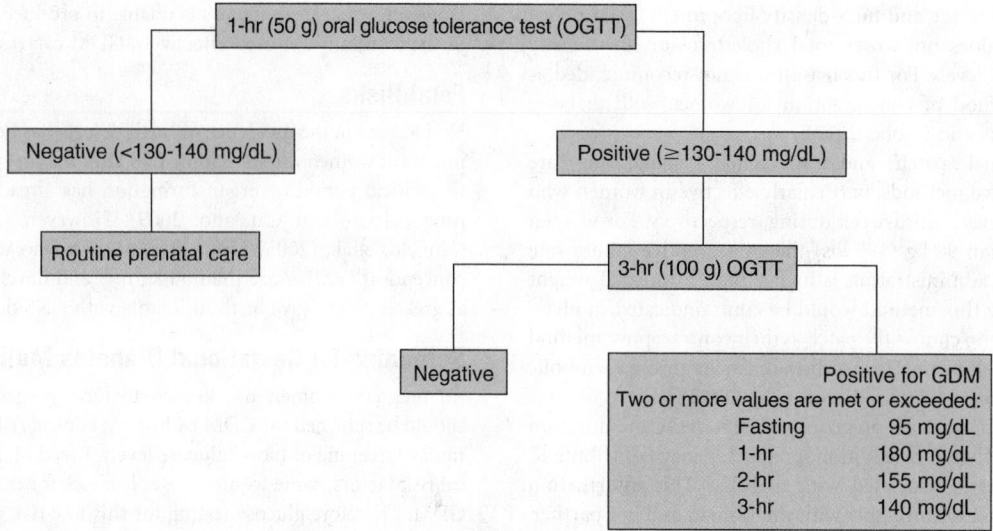

FIG 11-4 Screening and diagnosis for gestational diabetes. *GDM,* Gestational diabetes mellitus. (Data from American Diabetes Association (ADA): Position statement: diagnosis and classification of diabetes mellitus, *Diabetes Care* 32(suppl):S62–S67, 2009; Moore TR, Catalano PM: Diabetes in pregnancy. In Creasy RK, Resnik R, Iams JD, et al, editors: *Creasy & Resnik's maternal-fetal medicine: principles and practice,* ed 6, Philadelphia, 2009, Saunders.)

providing detailed and comprehensive explanations to ensure understanding, participation, and adherence to the necessary interventions. Potential complications should be discussed, and the need for maintenance of euglycemia throughout the remainder of the pregnancy reinforced. Knowing that GDM typically disappears when the pregnancy is over may be reassuring for the woman and her family.

As with pregestational diabetes, the aim of therapy in women with GDM is strict blood glucose control. Fasting blood glucose levels should range from 65 to 95 mg/dL, and 1-hour postmeal blood glucose levels should be less than 130 to 140 mg/dL (Moore and Catalano, 2009). Postmeal glucose levels at 2 hours should be less than 120 mg/dL (Landon, Catalano, and Gabbe, 2012) (see Table 11-3).

Diet. Dietary modification is the mainstay of treatment for GDM. The woman with GDM is placed on a standard diabetic diet. The usual prescription is 30 kcal/kg/day based on a normal preconception weight. For obese women the usual prescription is up to 25 kcal/kg/day, which translates into 1500 to 2000 kcal/day. Carbohydrate intake is restricted to approximately 50% of caloric intake (Moore and Catalano, 2009). Dietary counseling by a registered dietitian is recommended.

Exercise. Several studies have examined the benefits of exercise in women with GDM. Three randomized trials found that exercise improved cardiovascular fitness without improving pregnancy outcome. Another study found that exercise decreased the need for insulin in overweight women with GDM (Cunningham, Leveno, Bloom, et al., 2010).

Monitoring Blood Glucose Levels. Blood glucose monitoring is necessary to determine whether euglycemia can be maintained by diet and exercise. Women are instructed to monitor their blood sugar daily. The frequency and timing of blood glucose monitoring should be individualized for each woman. A typical schedule for monitoring blood glucose is on rising in the morning, after breakfast, before and after lunch, after dinner, and at bedtime (Moore and Catalano, 2009). Women with GDM usually perform self-monitoring at home with additional monitoring at the clinic or office visit.

Medications for Controlling Blood Glucose Levels. Approximately 25% of women with GDM require insulin during the pregnancy to maintain satisfactory blood glucose levels, despite compliance with the prescribed diet (Landon, Catalano, and Gabbe, 2012). In contrast to women with insulin-dependent diabetes, women with GDM are managed initially with diet and exercise alone. If fasting plasma glucose levels are greater than 95 mg/dL or 2-hour postmeal levels are greater than 120 mg/dL, insulin therapy is begun (Cunningham, Leveno, Bloom, et al., 2010) (see Table 11-3).

For the past several years oral hypoglycemic therapy has been used as an alternative to insulin in women with GDM who require medication in addition to diet for blood glucose control. Women who are unable or unwilling to take insulin by injection or are cognitively impaired also may be candidates for oral hypoglycemic medication.

Glyburide is the oral agent most frequently prescribed. The fact that only minimal amounts of glyburide cross the placenta to the fetus makes it a good drug for use during pregnancy (Moore and Catalano, 2009). Several studies have shown that glyburide controls blood glucose levels as well as insulin does in women with GDM. Furthermore, research revealed no increase in hypoglycemia or macrosomia in neonates whose mothers took glyburide. However, in one study neonates born to women taking glyburide were found to be more likely to experience birth injury or require phototherapy (Landon, Catalano, and Gabbe, 2012). Glyburide may not work as well in women who are obese or who had higher levels of hyperglycemia discovered early in pregnancy (Landon, Catalano, and Gabbe, 2012). Studies have shown that glyburide should be taken at least 30 minutes (preferably 1 hour) before a meal so its peak effect covers the 2-hour postmeal blood glucose level. Because episodes of hypoglycemia can occur between meals, women taking glyburide should always carry with them sources of fast sugar (Moore and Catalano, 2009).

Metformin is another oral hypoglycemic agent sometimes used in the management of GDM. Although metformin crosses the placenta, it does not appear to be teratogenic. However, glyburide may

◎ NURSING CARE PLAN

The Pregnant Woman with Gestational Diabetes

NURSING DIAGNOSIS	EXPECTED OUTCOME	INTERVENTIONS	RATIONALES
Deficient Knowledge related to gestational diabetes as evidenced by the woman's questions and concerns	Woman will be able to verbalize important information regarding gestational diabetes, its management, and potential effects on the pregnancy and fetus.	Assess woman's current knowledge base regarding the disease process, management, effects on pregnancy and fetus, and potential complications.	To provide database for further teaching
		Explain pathophysiologic aspects of diabetes, effects on pregnancy and fetus, and potential complications.	To promote compliance with treatment plan
		Explain principles of diabetic diet and have woman plan her meals for 1 day following these principles.	To promote self-management and compliance with treatment plan
		Demonstrate procedure for blood glucose monitoring and obtain return demonstration.	To establish woman's comfort and competence with procedure
		Demonstrate procedure for insulin administration, should this become necessary, and obtain return demonstration.	To establish woman's comfort and competence with procedure
		Explain importance of correctly taking oral hypoglycemic medication (right dose, right time), should this become necessary.	To promote self-management and compliance with treatment plan
		Review signs and symptoms of hypoglycemia and hyperglycemia and appropriate interventions for both.	To promote prompt recognition of complications and self-management
		Provide contact numbers for health care team for prompt interventions and answers to questions on ongoing basis.	To promote comfort
		Review expected plan of care.	To allay anxiety and enlist cooperation of woman in her care
Risk for Fetal Injury related to elevated maternal glucose levels.	The fetus will remain free of injury and be born at term in a healthy state.	Assess woman's current diabetic control.	To identify risk for fetal macrosomia
		Monitor fundal height during each prenatal visit.	To identify appropriate fetal growth
		Assess fetal movement and heart rate during each prenatal visit and perform fetal assessment tests as ordered during the third trimester.	To assess fetal well-being.
Anxiety related to threat to maternal and fetal well-being as evidenced by the woman's verbal expressions of concern	The woman will identify sources of anxiety and report feeling less anxious.	Through therapeutic communication promote open relationship with woman.	To promote trust
		Listen to woman's feelings and concerns.	To assess for any misconception or misinformation that may be contributing to anxiety
		Review potential dangers by providing factual information.	To correct any misconceptions or misinformation
		Encourage woman to share concerns with her health care team.	To promote collaboration in her care

be better than metformin at controlling blood glucose levels in women with GDM (Landon, Catalano, and Gabbe, 2012).

Fetal Surveillance. Women with GDM whose blood glucose levels are well controlled by diet are at low risk for an IUFD. Therefore antepartum fetal testing is not performed routinely in these women unless they also have hypertension, a history of a prior stillbirth, or suspected macrosomia. Women with these complications or those who require insulin for blood glucose control may have twice-weekly NSTs beginning at 32 weeks of gestation. Women with uncomplicated GDM begin fetal testing at 40 weeks of gestation. In general women with GDM can continue pregnancy until 40 weeks of gestation and the spontaneous onset of labor. However, fetal growth should be monitored carefully because the risk for

macrosomia as the pregnancy approaches 40 weeks of gestation is apparently increased (Landon, Catalano, and Gabbe, 2012).

Intrapartum

During the labor and birth process blood glucose levels are monitored hourly to maintain levels at 80 to 120 mg/dL (Moore and Catalano, 2009). Levels within this range decrease the incidence of neonatal hypoglycemia. Infusing rapid-acting insulin intravenously may be necessary during labor to maintain these levels. However, it is usually possible to maintain excellent glucose control in women with Class A$_1$ GDM during labor by simply avoiding IV fluids containing dextrose (Gilbert, 2011; Moore and Catalano, 2009). Although GDM is not an indication for cesarean birth, this procedure may be necessary in the presence of preeclampsia or macrosomia.

Postpartum

Most women with GDM return to normal glucose levels after childbirth. However, the recurrence risk for GDM in the next pregnancy is 35% to 75%. Women who have had GDM also have a 35% to 60% risk for developing type 2 diabetes mellitus within the next 20 years (Gilbert, 2011). Currently ACOG recommends assessing all women who had GDM for carbohydrate intolerance with a 75-g, 2-hr OGTT or a fasting plasma glucose level at 6 to 12 weeks after delivery. The optimal frequency of subsequent testing has not been established. However, the ADA recommends repeat testing at least every 3 years for women with a history of GDM and normal postpartum glucose testing results (Landon, Catalano, and Gabbe, 2012). Obesity is a major risk factor for the later development of diabetes. Women with a history of GDM, particularly those who are overweight, should be encouraged to make lifestyle changes that include weight loss and exercise to reduce this risk (Gilbert, 2011). Children born to women with GDM are also at risk for becoming obese in childhood or adolescence (Landon, Catalano, and Gabbe, 2012).

THYROID DISORDERS

Hyperthyroidism

Hyperthyroidism in pregnancy is rare, occurring in approximately 1 of every 1000 to 2000 pregnancies (Cunningham, Leveno, Bloom, et al., 2010). In 90% to 95% of pregnant women it is caused by Graves' disease (Nader, 2009). Clinical manifestations of hyperthyroidism include heat intolerance, diaphoresis, fatigue, anxiety, emotional lability, and tachycardia. Many of these symptoms also occur with pregnancy; thus the disorder can be difficult to diagnose. Signs that may help differentiate hyperthyroidism from normal pregnancy changes include weight loss, goiter, and a pulse rate greater than 100 beats/min (Nader, 2009). Laboratory findings include elevated free thyroxine (T_4) and triiodothyronine (T_3) levels and greatly suppressed thyroid-stimulating hormone (TSH) levels (Cunningham, Leveno, Bloom, et al., 2010; Nader, 2009). Moderate and severe hyperthyroidism must be treated during pregnancy. Untreated or inadequately treated women have an increased risk of miscarriage; preterm birth; and giving birth to stillborn infants or infants with goiter, hyperthyroidism, or hypothyroidism. However, most neonates born to women with hyperthyroidism have normal thyroid function. Women with hyperthyroidism are at increased risk for developing severe preeclampsia and heart failure (Cunningham, Leveno, Bloom, et al., 2010; Nader, 2009).

The primary treatment of hyperthyroidism during pregnancy is drug therapy. The medications most often prescribed in the United States are propylthiouracil (PTU) or methimazole (MM). Both drugs are effective at controlling symptoms, but both have potentially dangerous maternal and fetal side effects. PTU can cause hepatic toxicity serious enough to require liver transplantation. When prescribed during the first trimester of pregnancy, MM can cause choanal atresia or esophageal atresia, facial anomalies, and developmental delay in exposed fetuses. Although the likelihood of maternal and fetal side effects from both drugs is low, a panel convened by the U.S. Food and Drug Administration (FDA) and the American Thyroid Association recommended that PTU be used only in the first trimester of pregnancy. Women requiring drug therapy for hyperthyroidism should be switched to MM for the remainder of pregnancy (Mestman, 2012).

The usual starting dose of PTU is 100 to 150 mg three times a day. For MM the initial dose is generally 20 mg/day. Women usually show clinical improvement (weight gain and less tachycardia) within 2 to 6 weeks after beginning therapy. Once clinical improvement occurs, the dose of PTU or MM may be cut in half. If symptoms worsen the medication dosage is doubled (Mestman, 2012). During therapy thyroid test results are used to taper the drug to the smallest effective dose to prevent development of unnecessary fetal or neonatal hypothyroidism. In many women the medication can be discontinued by 32 to 36 weeks of gestation. PTU readily crosses the placenta and may cause fetal hypothyroidism, which is characterized by goiter, bradycardia, and intrauterine growth restriction (IUGR) (Nader, 2009).

Both medications work well in and are well tolerated by most women. The most common maternal side effects of both PTU and MM are pruritus and skin rash. Other possible side effects include drug-related fever, bronchospasm, migratory polyarthritis, a lupus-like syndrome, and cholestatic jaundice (Mestman, 2012; Nader, 2009). The most severe side effect is agranulocytosis, which occurs rarely and usually develops only in older women and in those taking high doses of the drug. Symptoms of agranulocytosis are fever and unexpected sore throat, which should be reported immediately to the health care provider; and the woman should stop taking the medication (Cunningham, Leveno, Bloom, et al., 2010; Mestman, 2012; Nader, 2009). Beta-adrenergic blockers such as propranolol (Inderal) or atenolol (Tenormin) may be used in severe hyperthyroidism to control maternal symptoms, especially heart rate. However, long-term use of these medications is not recommended because of the potential for IUGR, bradycardia, and hypoglycemia (Nader, 2009).

After birth women taking either PTU or MM who choose to breastfeed should be informed that the medications do not appear to adversely affect the neonate's thyroid function. The woman should take her antithyroid medication just after breastfeeding, thus allowing a 3- to 4-hour period before nursing again (Mestman, 2012; Nader, 2009).

Radioactive iodine must not be used in diagnosis or treatment of hyperthyroidism in pregnancy because therapeutic doses given to treat maternal thyroid disease may also destroy the fetal thyroid (Cunningham, Leveno, Bloom, et al., 2010). In severe cases surgical treatment of hyperthyroidism, subtotal thyroidectomy, can be performed during pregnancy. Surgery is best performed during the second trimester of pregnancy, although it can be done during the first or third trimester if necessary. Surgery is usually reserved for women with severe disease, those for whom drug therapy proves toxic, and those who are unable to follow the prescribed medical regimen. Risks associated with the surgery are hypoparathyroidism, recurrent laryngeal nerve paralysis, and anesthesia-related complications (Nader, 2009).

> **! NURSING ALERT**
>
> A serious but uncommon complication of undiagnosed or partially treated hyperthyroidism is thyroid storm, which can occur in response to stress such as labor and vaginal birth, infection, preeclampsia, or surgery. A woman with this emergency disorder may have fever, restlessness, tachycardia, vomiting, hypotension, or stupor. Prompt treatment is essential. IV fluids and oxygen are administered, along with high doses of PTU. After administration of PTU, iodide is given. Other medications include antipyretics, dexamethasone, and beta-blockers (Cunningham, Leveno, Bloom, et al., 2010; Nader, 2009).

Hypothyroidism

Hypothyroidism occurs in two to three pregnancies per 1000. Because severe hypothyroidism is often associated with infertility and an increased risk of miscarriage, it is not often seen during pregnancy (Cunningham, Leveno, Bloom, et al., 2010). Although iodine deficiency is rare in the United States, it is a common cause of maternal, fetal, and neonatal hypothyroidism in the rest of the world (Nader, 2009). Adult hypothyroidism is usually caused by glandular destruction by autoantibodies, most commonly because of Hashimoto's thyroiditis. Characteristic symptoms of hypothyroidism include weight gain, lethargy, decrease in exercise capacity, and cold intolerance. Women who are moderately symptomatic can also develop constipation, hoarseness, hair loss, brittle nails, and dry skin. Laboratory values in pregnancy include elevated levels of TSH, with or without low T_4 levels (Nader, 2009).

Pregnant women with untreated hypothyroidism are at increased risk for miscarriage, preeclampsia, gestational hypertension, placental abruption, preterm birth, and stillbirth. Infants born to mothers with hypothyroidism may also be of low birth weight (Cunningham, Leveno, Bloom, et al., 2010; Nader, 2009). These outcomes can be improved with early treatment (Nader, 2009).

Thyroid hormone supplements are used to treat hypothyroidism. Levothyroxine (e.g., T_4 [Synthroid]) is most often prescribed during pregnancy. The usual beginning dosage is 0.1 to 0.15 mg/day, with adjustment by 25 to 50 mcg every 4 to 6 weeks as necessary based on the maternal TSH level (Cunningham, Leveno, Bloom, et al., 2010; Nader, 2009). The aim of drug therapy is to maintain the TSH level at the lower end of the normal range for pregnant women. Women with little or no functioning thyroid tissue require higher doses of levothyroxine. In addition, as pregnancy progresses increased doses of thyroid hormone are usually required. This increased demand during pregnancy is probably related to increased estrogen levels (Cunningham, Leveno, Bloom, et al., 2010; Nader, 2009).

! NURSING ALERT

If taking iron supplementation, pregnant women should be told to take levothyroxine at a different time of day than their iron tablets because ferrous sulfate decreases absorption of T_4 (Nader, 2009).

The fetus depends on maternal thyroid hormones until approximately 18 weeks of gestation, when fetal production begins. Normal maternal T_4 levels early in pregnancy are important for proper fetal brain development. Studies have shown that even mild maternal hypothyroidism during the first trimester has been associated with long-term neuropsychologic damage in their children. More research needs to be conducted on this topic (Mestman, 2012).

CARE MANAGEMENT

Education of the pregnant woman with thyroid dysfunction is essential to promote compliance with the plan of treatment. Important points to discuss with the woman and her family include the disorder and its potential effect on her, her family, and her fetus; the medication regimen and possible side effects; the need for continuing medical supervision; and the importance of compliance.

The woman often needs the nurse's help to cope with the discomforts and frustrations associated with symptoms of the disorder. For example, the woman with hyperthyroidism who has nervousness and hyperactivity along with weakness and fatigue can benefit from suggestions to channel excess energies into quiet diversional activities such as reading or crafts. Discomfort associated with hypersensitivity to heat (hyperthyroidism) or cold intolerance (hypothyroidism) can be minimized by appropriate clothing and regulation of environmental temperatures and by avoiding temperature extremes.

Nutrition counseling with a registered dietitian may provide guidance in selecting a well-balanced diet. The woman with hyperthyroidism who has increased appetite and poor weight gain and the hypothyroid woman who has anorexia and lethargy need counseling to ensure adequate intake of nutritionally sound foods to meet both maternal and fetal needs.

MATERNAL PHENYLKETONURIA

Phenylketonuria (PKU), a recognized cause of cognitive impairment, is an inborn error of metabolism caused by an autosomal recessive trait that creates a deficiency in the enzyme phenylalanine hydrolase. Absence of this enzyme impairs the ability of the body to metabolize the amino acid phenylalanine found in all protein foods. Consequently toxic accumulation of phenylalanine in the blood occurs, which interferes with brain development and function. Individuals with this disorder also have hypopigmentation of hair, eyes, and skin because phenylalanine inhibits melanin production. PKU affects 1 in every 10,000 to 15,000 Caucasian newborns (Cunningham, Leveno, Bloom, et al., 2010).

PKU was the first inborn error of metabolism for which to be universally screened in the United States. Since 1961 all newborns have been tested soon after birth for this disorder. Prompt diagnosis and therapy with a phenylalanine-restricted diet significantly decreases the incidence of cognitive impairment (Aminoff, 2009). The special diet should be followed indefinitely because individuals who do not continue phenylalanine restriction have been reported to have significantly lower IQs (Cunningham, Leveno, Bloom, et al., 2010).

The keys to the prevention of fetal anomalies caused by PKU are the identification of women in their reproductive years with the disorder and dietary compliance for women who are diagnosed. Screening for undiagnosed homozygous maternal PKU at the first prenatal visit may be warranted, especially in individuals with a family history of the disorder, with low intelligence of uncertain origin, or who have given birth to microcephalic infants. Ideally women with PKU begin dietary phenylalanine restriction before conception and continue it throughout pregnancy (Gilbert, 2011). The dietary modification normally excludes all high-protein foods such as meat, milk, eggs, and nuts and wheat products, making it very similar to a vegan diet (Feillet and Agostoni, 2010; Gilbert, 2011). Phenylalanine levels are monitored at least once and preferably twice a week throughout pregnancy (Gilbert, 2011). Experts recommend that maternal phenylalanine levels be less than 6 mg/dL for at least 3 months before conception and range between 2 and 6 mg/dL throughout pregnancy. These levels are associated with a decrease in fetal sequelae (Cunningham, Leveno, Bloom, et al., 2010; Gilbert, 2011). High maternal phenylalanine levels are associated with microcephaly, cognitive impairment, and congenital heart defects in their children (Aminoff, 2009; Cunningham, Leveno, Bloom, et al., 2010). Ultrasound examinations are used for fetal surveillance beginning in the first trimester. A spontaneous vaginal birth is anticipated.

Women with PKU should be advised against breastfeeding because their milk will contain a high concentration of phenylalanine (Aminoff, 2009). If these women choose to breastfeed despite the risk, their phenylalanine blood levels must be monitored closely

(Lawrence and Lawrence, 2005). Infants diagnosed with PKU can usually be breastfed safely because human breast milk is a relatively low phenylalanine food (Feillet and Agostoni, 2010). If infants with PKU are breastfed, the amount of human breast milk ingested daily may be monitored so phenylalanine levels do not get too high. Another strategy that may be implemented is to alternate human breast milk feedings with products that contain little or no phenylalanine (Feillet and Agostoni, 2010).

CARDIOVASCULAR DISORDERS

During a normal pregnancy the maternal cardiovascular system undergoes many changes that place a physiologic strain on the heart. The major cardiovascular changes that occur during a normal pregnancy and affect the woman with cardiac disease are increased intravascular volume, decreased systemic vascular resistance, cardiac output changes occurring during labor and birth, and the intravascular volume changes that occur just after childbirth. The strain is present during pregnancy and continues after birth. The normal heart can compensate for the increased workload so pregnancy, labor, and birth are generally well tolerated; but the diseased heart is hemodynamically challenged.

If the cardiovascular changes are not well tolerated, cardiac failure can develop during pregnancy, labor, or the postpartum period. In addition, if myocardial disease develops, valvular disease exists, or a congenital heart defect is present, cardiac decompensation (inability of the heart to maintain a sufficient cardiac output) may occur. Fever and infection are the major causes of cardiac decompensation during pregnancy (Easterling and Stout, 2012).

From 0.5% to 4% of pregnancies are complicated by heart disease. Cardiac disorders are one of the most important nonobstetric causes of maternal mortality (Gaddipati and Troiano, 2013). The rate of rheumatic fever, once responsible for the vast majority of cardiac disease in pregnancy, is now declining (Gilbert, 2011). Currently cardiomyopathy and congenital heart disease are the major causes of cardiac disease in pregnant women (Gaddipati and Troiano, 2013). Thanks to better management of congenital heart disease in childhood, pregnancy outcomes for women with these conditions are generally positive. However, cardiac disease accounts for 15% of maternal mortality during pregnancy (Gilbert, 2011). Box 11-2 lists maternal cardiac disease risk groups and their related mortality rates. Pregnancy is not advised in women who have several cardiac conditions, including pulmonary hypertension, Marfan syndrome with aortic involvement, and Eisenmenger syndrome, because the associated maternal mortality rate is extremely high, up to 50% (Easterling and Stout, 2012; Gaddipati and Troiano, 2013).

The degree of disability experienced by the woman with cardiac disease is often more important in the treatment and prognosis during pregnancy than the diagnosis of the type of cardiovascular disease. The New York Heart Association (NYHA) functional classification of heart disease is a widely accepted standard:

- Class I: Asymptomatic without limitation of physical activity
- Class II: Symptomatic with slight limitation of activity
- Class III: Symptomatic with marked limitation of activity
- Class IV: Symptomatic with inability to carry on any physical activity without discomfort

No classification of heart disease can be considered rigid or absolute, but the NYHA classification offers a basic practical guide for treatment, assuming that frequent prenatal visits, good patient cooperation, and appropriate obstetric care occur. Medical therapy is conducted by a team approach and includes the cardiologist, the

---

BOX 11-2 MATERNAL CARDIAC DISEASE RISK GROUPS

Group I (Mortality Rate <1%)
- Atrial septal defect
- Ventricular septal defect (uncomplicated)
- Patent ductus arteriosus
- Pulmonic and tricuspid disease
- Biosynthetic valve prosthesis (porcine and human allograft)
- Tetralogy of Fallot (corrected)
- Mitral stenosis (New York Heart Association [NYHA] class I and II)

Group II (Mortality Rate 5%-15%)
- Mitral stenosis NYHA class III and IV or with atrial fibrillation
- Aortic stenosis
- Coarctation of aorta (uncomplicated)
- Uncorrected tetralogy of Fallot
- Previous myocardial infarction
- Marfan syndrome with normal aorta
- Artificial heart valve

Group III (Mortality Rate 25%-50%)
- Pulmonary hypertension
- Coarctation of the aorta (complicated)
- Endocarditis
- Marfan syndrome with aortic involvement
- Eisenmenger syndrome

Data from Gaddipati S, Troiano NH: Cardiac disorders in pregnancy. In Troiano NH, Harvey CJ, Chez BF, editors: *AWHONN's high risk and critical care obstetrics*, ed 3, Philadelphia, 2013, Lippincott Williams and Wilkins.

---

obstetrician, and nurses. The functional classification may change for the pregnant woman because of the hemodynamic changes that occur in the cardiovascular system. A 30% to 45% increase in cardiac output occurs compared with nonpregnancy resting values, with most of the increase in the first trimester and the peak at 20 to 26 weeks of gestation (Blanchard and Shabetai, 2009). The functional classification of the disease is determined at 3 months and again at 7 or 8 months of gestation. Pregnant women may progress from class I or II to class III or IV during the pregnancy as cardiac output increases and more stress is placed on the heart.

Miscarriage and stillbirth both occur more often in the pregnant woman with cardiac problems than in healthy women. In addition, IUGR is common, probably because of low oxygen pressure in the mother (Blanchard and Shabetai, 2009).

A diagnosis of cardiac disease depends on the history, physical examination, radiographic and electrocardiographic findings, Holter monitoring, echocardiography, and if indicated ultrasonographic results. Most diagnostic studies are noninvasive and can be performed safely during pregnancy. The differential diagnosis of heart disease also involves ruling out respiratory problems and other potential causes of chest pain.

Congenital Cardiac Diseases
Atrial Septal Defect

Atrial septal defect (ASD) is an abnormal opening between the atria. It is one of the causes of a left-to-right shunt and one of the most common congenital defects seen during pregnancy (Gaddipati and Troiano, 2013). This defect may go undetected because the woman is usually asymptomatic. The pregnant woman with an ASD usually has an uncomplicated pregnancy. However, some women may develop congestive heart failure or arrhythmias as the pregnancy progresses as a result of increased plasma volume. Another possible complication is the development of emboli (blood clots) (Gaddipati and Troiano, 2013).

Ventricular Septal Defect

Ventricular septal defect (VSD), an abnormal opening between the right and left ventricles, is another cause of a left-to-right shunt. It may occur as a single lesion or in combination with other cardiac anomalies such as tetralogy of Fallot. The defect is usually diagnosed and corrected early in life. As a result a VSD is not very common in pregnancy. Women with small, uncomplicated VSDs usually do not have pregnancy complications. For women with a large VSD, there is a higher risk for congestive heart failure or pulmonary hypertension. Medical management includes administration of anticoagulants if indicated, along with rest and decreased physical activity (Gaddipati and Troiano, 2013).

Coarctation of the Aorta

Coarctation of the aorta is a localized narrowing of the aorta near the insertion of the ductus. Patients with this lesion have hypertension in their upper extremities but hypotension in the lower extremities. Coarctation of the aorta is an example of an acyanotic congenital heart lesion. If at all possible, the lesion should be corrected surgically before pregnancy. However, pregnancy is usually relatively safe for the woman with uncomplicated, uncorrected coarctation. The maternal mortality rate is approximately 3% (Blanchard and Shabetai, 2009). Complications that can occur include hypertension, congestive heart failure, cerebrovascular accident (stroke), aortic dissection, and rupture of associated aneurysms (Blanchard and Shabetai, 2009; Easterling and Stout, 2012). The mainstays of treatment for uncorrected coarctation of the aorta during pregnancy are rest and antihypertensive medications, preferably beta-adrenergic blocking agents. Some authorities recommend cesarean birth to prevent blood pressure elevations during second-stage labor that could possibly lead to rupture of the aorta or cerebral blood vessels. However, vaginal birth is usually recommended, with cesarean birth performed only for obstetric indications. If bacteremia is suspected, antibiotic prophylaxis is given during labor and birth (Cunningham, Leveno, Bloom, et al., 2010).

Tetralogy of Fallot

Tetralogy of Fallot is by far the most common cyanotic heart disease observed during pregnancy (Blanchard and Shabetai, 2009). Components of tetralogy of Fallot include a VSD; pulmonary stenosis; overriding aorta; and right ventricular hypertrophy, leading to a right-to-left shunt. Women with tetralogy of Fallot are encouraged to have surgical repair preconceptionally because pregnancy does not cause a significant risk once the VSD and pulmonary stenosis have been repaired (Gaddipati and Troiano, 2013). On the other hand, women with uncorrected tetralogy of Fallot experience more right-to-left shunting during pregnancy, resulting in reduced blood flow through the pulmonary circulation and increasing hypoxemia, which can cause syncope or death (Gaddipati and Troiano, 2013). Maintenance of venous return in women with uncorrected tetralogy of Fallot is critical. Therefore the most dangerous time for these women is the late third trimester of pregnancy and the early postpartum period, when venous return is reduced by the large pregnant uterus and peripheral venous pooling after birth. Use of pressure-graded support hose is recommended. Blood loss during birth may also adversely affect venous return; thus blood volume must be

adequately maintained. Prophylactic antibiotics should be given during the intrapartum period (Blanchard and Shabetai, 2009).

Acquired Cardiac Diseases
Mitral Valve Prolapse

Mitral valve prolapse (MVP) is a fairly common, usually benign, condition. Recently more specific echocardiographic diagnostic criteria have resulted in significantly reduced prevalence estimates for MVP (perhaps 1% of the female population) than previously thought (Blanchard and Shabetai, 2009). In MVP the mitral valve leaflets prolapse into the left atrium during ventricular systole, allowing some backflow of blood. Midsystolic click and late systolic murmur are hallmarks of this syndrome. Most cases are asymptomatic. A few women have atypical chest pain (sharp and located in the left side of the chest) that occurs at rest and does not respond to nitrates. They may also have anxiety, palpitations, dyspnea on exertion, and syncope. If women are symptomatic, beta-blocking drugs are given to relieve chest pain and palpitations and reduce the risk of life-threatening arrhythmias (Cunningham, Leveno, Bloom, et al., 2010). If symptoms are unusually severe, thyroid function should also be checked (Blanchard and Shabetai, 2009). Pregnancy and its associated hemodynamic changes may change or alleviate the murmur and click of MVP and its symptoms. Pregnancy is generally well tolerated unless bacterial endocarditis occurs. Antibiotic prophylaxis is often given before birth to prevent bacterial endocarditis (Cunningham, Leveno, Bloom, et al.; Easterling and Stout, 2012).

Mitral Stenosis

Mitral stenosis is almost always caused by rheumatic heart disease (RHD), a consequence of rheumatic fever (Easterling and Stout, 2012). Rheumatic fever develops suddenly, often several symptom-free weeks after an inadequately treated group A beta-hemolytic streptococcal throat infection. Episodes of rheumatic fever create an autoimmune reaction in the heart tissue, leading to permanent damage of heart valves (usually the mitral valve) and the chordae tendineae cordis. This damage is classified as RHD. RHD may be evident during acute rheumatic fever or discovered years later. Recurrences of rheumatic fever are common, each with the potential to increase the severity of heart damage.

Mitral stenosis is a narrowing of the opening of the mitral valve caused by stiffening of valve leaflets, which obstructs blood flow from the atrium to the ventricle. As the mitral valve narrows, dyspnea worsens, occurring first on exertion and eventually at rest. A tight stenosis plus the increase in blood volume and cardiac output of normal pregnancy may cause pulmonary edema, atrial fibrillation, right-sided heart failure, infective endocarditis, pulmonary embolism, and massive hemoptysis (Blanchard and Shabetai, 2009; Cunningham, Leveno, Bloom, et al., 2010). Approximately 25% of women with mitral valve stenosis may become symptomatic for the first time during pregnancy. Maternal mortality is related to functional capacity. Almost all maternal deaths related to mitral stenosis occur in women who are classified as NYHA class III or IV (Cunningham, Leveno, Bloom, et al., 2010).

Women with a history of RHD who are at risk for exposure to streptococcal infection should receive prophylaxis with daily oral penicillin G or monthly benzathine penicillin (Bicillin) injections. Pregnant women are usually considered at high risk for exposure because they generally live around groups of children (Easterling and Stout, 2012). In addition, women with mitral stenosis may require diuretics such as furosemide (Lasix) to prevent pulmonary edema and beta blockers or calcium channel blockers to prevent tachycardia (Easterling and Stout, 2012). Cardioversion may be needed for new-onset atrial fibrillation, a complication associated with mitral stenosis. Women who have chronic atrial fibrillation may need digoxin or beta blockers to control the heart rate. In addition, anticoagulant therapy may be needed to prevent embolism (Blanchard and Shabetai, 2009).

The care of the woman with mitral stenosis is typically managed by reducing her activity, restricting dietary sodium, and increasing bed rest, in addition to the pharmacologic management discussed previously (Cunningham, Leveno, Bloom, et al., 2010). The pregnant woman with mitral stenosis should be monitored clinically for symptoms and with echocardiograms to assess the atrial and ventricular size and heart valve function. Prophylaxis for intrapartum endocarditis and pulmonary infections may be given to women at high risk (Blanchard and Shabetai, 2009; Easterling and Stout, 2012).

During labor adequate pain control is required to prevent tachycardia. Epidural analgesia for labor is preferred (Easterling and Stout, 2012). Encourage the woman to labor and give birth in the lateral decubitus position and avoid the supine and lithotomy positions. Shortening the second stage of labor by vacuum- or forceps-assisted birth is also important to decrease the cardiac workload. Cesarean birth should be performed only for obstetric indications. Aggressive diuresis is initiated immediately after birth because fluid shifts can place the woman at risk for pulmonary edema (Blanchard and Shabetai, 2009; Easterling and Stout, 2012).

For women with NYHA class III or IV cardiac disease, surgical intervention may be necessary. Valve replacement and open commissurotomy have been performed successfully during pregnancy. Currently balloon valvotomy is likely to be the procedure of choice. Surgical intervention should be considered only when symptoms cannot be controlled by medical therapy (Easterling and Stout, 2012).

Aortic Stenosis

Aortic stenosis is a narrowing of the opening of the aortic valve leading to an obstruction to left ventricular ejection. It is rarely encountered as a complication of pregnancy because most women who develop this condition do so after their childbearing years are over. In the past the maternal mortality rate was reported to be as high as 17%, but it has decreased over the last several decades (Easterling and Stout, 2012). Medical management is similar to that for mitral stenosis.

Ischemic Heart Disease
Myocardial Infarction

Myocardial infarction (MI), an acute ischemic event, rarely occurs in women of childbearing age. It is estimated to occur in only 1 of 10,000 pregnancies (Blanchard and Shabetai, 2009). However, authorities anticipate that the incidence will rise, considering the number of women who delay childbearing until later in life (Gaddipati and Troiano, 2013). Frequently women with coronary artery disease have classic risk factors such as diabetes, hypertension, cigarette smoking, hyperlipidemia, and obesity (Cunningham, Leveno, Bloom, et al., 2010). The cardiac changes that normally occur in a pregnant woman may provoke symptoms for the first time. It is also possible for women with a history of MI to become pregnant (Gaddipati and Troiano, 2013).

MI occurs most frequently in the last trimester of pregnancy and in women older than 33 years. The maternal mortality rate from an MI during pregnancy is approximately 20%. Women are most likely to die at the time of the infarction or during labor and birth (Blanchard and Shabetai, 2009). The risk of maternal death increases if women give birth within 2 weeks of an MI (Easterling and Stout, 2012).

Medical management for pregnant women with MI is the same as that for nonpregnant women and includes the administration of morphine, nitrates, lidocaine, beta blockers, aspirin, magnesium sulfate, and calcium antagonists (Easterling and Stout, 2012). Thrombolytic agents such as urokinase, streptokinase, and tissue plasminogen activator (tPA) do not appear to cross the placenta. However, their use is considered to be relatively contraindicated in pregnancy because of the risk for subsequent maternal and fetal hemorrhage (Gaddipati and Troiano, 2013). Because pain can lead to tachycardia and increased cardiac demands, pain control during labor is crucial. The side-lying position is preferred to prevent pressure on the vena cava. Vaginal birth is preferable, with avoidance of maternal pushing and a vacuum- or forceps-assisted birth (Easterling and Stout, 2012).

Other Cardiac Diseases and Conditions
Primary Pulmonary Hypertension

Women with primary pulmonary hypertension (PPH) have constriction of the arteriolar vessels in the lungs, leading to an increase in the pulmonary artery pressure. As a result of this pathology, there is right ventricular hypertension, right ventricular hypertrophy and dilation, and finally right ventricular failure with tricuspid regurgitation and systemic congestion. The major physiologic difficulty in PPH is maintaining blood flow to the lungs. Any event that significantly decreases venous return to the heart such as hypotension impairs the ability of the right ventricle to pump blood through the pulmonary vessels with their high, fixed vascular resistance. Because hypotension can occur quickly and is often unresponsive to medical therapy, it must be avoided at all costs (Blanchard and Shabetai, 2009).

Symptoms may be nonspecific such as fatigue and shortness of breath. Dyspnea on exertion is the most common symptom (Cunningham, Leveno, Bloom, et al., 2010).

PPH is diagnosed by electrocardiography. The diagnosis is confirmed by right-sided cardiac catheterization, which may be deferred during pregnancy (Cunningham, Leveno, Bloom, et al., 2010). Mortality rates reported during pregnancy are as high as 50%; thus pregnancy is not advised in women with this condition (Blanchard and Shabetai, 2009). The most dangerous times for these women are the intrapartum and early postpartum periods because of increases in cardiac output and fluid shifts.

Medical management of PPH during pregnancy includes limiting activity and avoiding supine positioning. Diuretics, supplemental oxygen, and vasodilator medications are also ordered. During labor and birth hypotension must be avoided by carefully establishing epidural analgesia and preventing blood loss (Cunningham, Leveno, Bloom, et al., 2010).

Peripartum Cardiomyopathy

Peripartum cardiomyopathy (PCM) is congestive heart failure with cardiomyopathy. The classic criteria for the diagnosis of PCM include development of congestive heart failure during the last month of pregnancy or within the first 5 postpartum months; absence of heart disease before the last month of pregnancy; a left ventricular ejection fraction of less than 45%; and, most important, lack of another cause for heart failure. The cause of the disease is unknown (Blanchard and Shabetai, 2009). Theories that have been suggested include autoimmune mechanisms or nutritional deficiencies (Easterling and Stout, 2012; Gaddipati and Troiano, 2013). At one time viral infections were considered to be a possible cause, but the prevalence of antibodies to echovirus and Coxsackie virus has not been found to be greater in women with cardiomyopathy than in those who do not have the disease (Easterling and Stout, 2012). The incidence of PCM is 1 in 1300 to 1 in 15,000 live births in the United States (Gaddipati and Troiano, 2013).

Associated risk factors include maternal age older than 30 years, multiparity, African descent, obesity, tocolytic use, preeclampsia, and chronic hypertension. Clinical findings are those of congestive heart failure (left ventricular failure). Clinical manifestations include dyspnea, fatigue, edema, and radiologic findings of cardiomegaly (Gaddipati and Troiano, 2013).

Medical management of PCM includes a regimen used for congestive heart failure: diuretics, sodium and fluid restriction, afterload-reducing agents, and digoxin. Anticoagulation may be necessary if the cardiac chambers are significantly dilated and contract poorly because of the increased risk for clot formation. Angiotensin-converting enzyme inhibitors, often prescribed to achieve afterload reduction, can be used only in the postpartum period because they are associated with fetal renal dysfunction. During labor epidural anesthesia is often used for pain control to decrease the cardiac workload and reduce tachycardia. Cesarean birth should be performed only for obstetric indications (Easterling and Stout, 2012).

In one half of all women with PCM left ventricular dysfunction resolves within 6 months. These women generally do well. However, if left ventricular dysfunction does not resolve within 6 months, approximately 85% of women with PCM will die in the next 4 to 5 years. Death is usually the result of progressive congestive heart failure, arrhythmia, or thromboembolism (Easterling and Stout, 2012). The recurrence rate for cardiomyopathy in a subsequent pregnancy is high, anywhere from 20% to 50%. The risk of recurrence is increased in women who did not completely recover left ventricular function after the initial episode of PCM (Blanchard and Shabetai, 2009).

Infective Endocarditis

Infective endocarditis, or inflammation of the innermost lining (endocardium) of the heart caused by invasion of microorganisms, is an uncommon disorder during pregnancy. It may be seen in women taking street drugs intravenously, although people who have had corrective surgery for congenital heart disease are at greatest risk to develop infective endocarditis (Cunningham, Leveno, Bloom, et al., 2010). Bacterial endocarditis, leading to incompetence of heart valves and thus congestive heart failure and cerebral emboli, can result in death. Treatment is with antibiotics.

Eisenmenger Syndrome

Eisenmenger syndrome is a right-to-left or bidirectional shunting that can be at either the atrial or the ventricular level of the heart and is combined with elevated pulmonary vascular resistance. It is associated with an underlying structural cardiac defect, either a VSD (most common) or a patent ductus arteriosus (Blanchard and Shabetai, 2009). Eisenmenger syndrome is associated with high mortality (50% in mothers and 50% in fetuses). Because of the poor pregnancy outcomes, pregnancy should be avoided by women with the syndrome. Termination may be recommended if pregnancy occurs (Gaddipati and Troiano, 2013). Although sudden death can occur at any time, the intrapartum and early postpartum periods seem to be the most dangerous (Blanchard and Shabetai, 2009). Maternal morbidity is associated with right ventricular failure and associated cardiogenic shock (Cunningham, Leveno, Bloom, et al., 2010).

In women who continue pregnancy despite the risks, management includes measures to maintain pulmonary blood flow. Physical activity is strictly limited. Other interventions include the use of pressure-graded elastic support hose and oxygen therapy. Antepartal hospitalization may be necessary to provide optimal care (Blanchard and Shabetai, 2009). During labor and birth narcotic-based regional anesthesia provides pain relief without causing excessive hemodynamic instability. Hypotension must be prevented at all costs because it results in more right-to-left shunting, thereby increasing hypoxemia, increasing pulmonary vascular resistance, and worsening the shunt. Volume overload or excessive systemic resistance must also be prevented because it further stresses the failing right side of the heart. Cesarean birth should be performed only for obstetric indications and avoided whenever possible (Easterling and Stout, 2012).

Marfan Syndrome

Marfan syndrome is an autosomal dominant disorder characterized by generalized weakness of the connective tissue, resulting in the characteristic feature of the disease, aortic root dilation. Other signs and symptoms associated with Marfan syndrome include dislocation of the optic lens, deformity of the anterior thorax, scoliosis, long limbs, joint laxity, and arachnodactyly. Diagnosis is usually based on family history and physical examination, including ocular, cardiovascular, and skeletal features (Easterling and Stout, 2012).

The majority of deaths from Marfan syndrome are caused by aortic dissection and rupture. Excruciating chest pain is the most common symptom of aortic dissection. Aortic dissection most often occurs in the third trimester of pregnancy or after birth. Overall the maternal mortality rate associated with Marfan's syndrome is greater than 50%. However, it is significantly increased if the aortic root diameter measures more than 4 cm (Easterling and Stout, 2012).

Preconception counseling for women with Marfan syndrome is essential to make women aware of the risks of pregnancy with this disease. An accurate assessment of the aortic root using noninvasive imaging with transesophageal echocardiography, computed tomography, or magnetic resonance imaging must be obtained to assess the woman's specific risk and make management recommendations. Elective repair of the aorta is recommended when the aortic root diameter measures 5.5 to 6 cm. Therefore women with an aortic root diameter greater than 5.5 cm should be counseled to have it repaired before becoming pregnant. On the other hand, women with an aortic root diameter less than 4 cm can attempt pregnancy with only modest risk (Easterling and Stout, 2012). Because the condition is inherited, each child born to a woman with Marfan syndrome has a 50% chance of having the disorder (Gaddipati and Troiano, 2013).

Management during pregnancy includes restricted activity and use of beta blockers to maintain a resting heart rate of approximately 70 beats/min. Tachycardia should also be prevented during labor. Women with aortic root diameters less than 4 cm can give birth vaginally, reserving cesarean birth for obstetric indications. Some authorities believe that women with larger aortic root diameters should give birth by elective cesarean because of concerns about increased pressure in the aorta during labor. However, data do not exist to make this a firm recommendation (Blanchard and Shabetai, 2009; Easterling and Stout, 2012).

Heart Transplantation

Increasing numbers of heart recipients are completing pregnancies successfully. Before conception the woman should be assessed for quality of ventricular function and potential rejection of the transplant. She should also be considered to be stabilized on her immunosuppressant regimen. Women who have no evidence of rejection and have normal cardiac function at the beginning of the pregnancy appear to do well during pregnancy, labor, and birth. Research has shown that the transplanted heart responds normally to pregnancy-related changes. Complications that are common in women who have had a heart transplant include hypertension and at least one episode of rejection (Cunningham, Leveno, Bloom, et al., 2010). Conception should be postponed for at least 1 year after transplantation to prevent acute rejection episodes (Blanchard and Shabetai, 2009).

CARE MANAGEMENT

The presence of cardiac disease is a significant influencing factor in the decision-making process for or against becoming pregnant. Couples planning a pregnancy must understand the risks involved in their situation. If the pregnancy is unplanned, the nurse should explore the couple's desire to continue it in light of the risks involved. Pregnancy termination is one option, depending on the severity of the cardiac defect. The family may need further information to make an informed decision regarding the future of the pregnancy.

The pregnant woman with a cardiac disorder is in a high risk situation. Her care is provided by a multidisciplinary team, including a cardiologist, obstetrician, perinatologist, and registered nurse experienced in the care of women with high risk pregnancies. If she chooses to continue the pregnancy, the woman's condition may be assessed as often as weekly. For additional information on cardiac disease, visit the American Heart Association website at www.americanheart.org.

Antepartum

Therapy for the pregnant woman with heart disease is focused on minimizing stress on the heart, which intensifies as cardiac output increases. Cardiac output begins to rise significantly early in pregnancy and probably peaks somewhere between 25 and 30 weeks of gestation (Gordon, 2012). Factors that increase the risk of cardiac decompensation are avoided. The workload of the cardiovascular system is reduced by appropriate treatment of any coexisting emotional stress, hypertension, anemia, hyperthyroidism, or obesity.

Signs and symptoms of cardiac decompensation are taught at the first prenatal visit and reviewed at each subsequent visit (Box 11-3 and Patient Teaching box).

Infections are treated promptly because respiratory, urinary, or gastrointestinal (GI) tract infections can complicate the condition by accelerating the heart rate and by direct spread of organisms (e.g., streptococci) to the heart structure. As previously mentioned, infections are a major cause of cardiac decompensation during pregnancy. The woman should notify her health care provider at the first sign of infection or exposure to an infection. Vaccination against influenza and pneumococci can be given (Easterling and Stout, 2012).

Nutrition counseling is necessary, optimally with the woman's family present. The pregnant woman needs a well-balanced diet with iron and folic acid supplementation, high protein levels, and adequate calories to gain weight. Iron supplements tend to cause constipation; thus the woman should increase her intake of fluids and fiber. A stool softener may also be prescribed. It is important that the woman with a cardiac disorder avoid straining during defecation, thus causing the Valsalva maneuver (forced expiration against a closed airway, which when released, causes blood to rush to the heart and overload the cardiac system). Sodium restriction may be necessary. The woman's intake of potassium may be monitored to prevent hypokalemia, especially if she is taking diuretics.

BOX 11-3 SIGNS OF POTENTIAL COMPLICATIONS: CARDIAC DECOMPENSATION

Pregnant Woman: Subjective Symptoms
- Increasing fatigue or difficulty breathing, or both, with her usual activities
- Feeling of smothering
- Frequent cough
- Palpitations; feeling that her heart is "racing"
- Generalized edema: Swelling of face, feet, legs, fingers (e.g., rings do not fit anymore)

Nurse: Objective Signs
- Irregular, weak, rapid pulse (≥100 beats/min)
- Progressive, generalized edema
- Crackles at base of lungs after two inspirations and exhalations that do not clear after coughing
- Orthopnea; increasing dyspnea
- Rapid respirations (≥25 breaths/min)
- Moist, frequent cough
- Cyanosis of lips and nail beds

PATIENT TEACHING

The Pregnant Woman at Risk for Cardiac Decompensation

Instruct woman to:
- Watch for and immediately report signs of cardiac decompensation or congestive heart failure: generalized edema; distention of neck veins; dyspnea; frequent, moist cough; or palpitations.
- Watch for and immediately report signs of thromboembolism: pain, redness, tenderness, or swelling in extremities or chest pain.
- Avoid constipation and thus straining with bowel movements (Valsalva maneuver) by taking in adequate fluids and fiber. A stool softener may also be helpful.

Teach importance of:
- Daily weighing. Sudden weight gain indicates fluid retention.
- Keeping all prenatal visit appointments, although they will be scheduled more frequently than for "normal" pregnant women.
- Limiting activity (depending on classification of her heart disease). Patients with class I or II cardiac disease need 10 hours of sleep every night and 30 minutes of rest after meals. Patients with class III or IV cardiac disease usually need bed rest for most of each day.

Modified from Gilbert ES: *Manual of high risk pregnancy and delivery*, ed 5, St Louis, 2011, Mosby.

Depending on the specific cardiac condition, some women may be limited in their total daily fluid intake. A referral to a registered dietitian may be necessary for a nutritional plan of care.

Cardiac medications are prescribed as needed, with attention to fetal well-being. The hemodynamic changes that occur during pregnancy such as increased plasma volume and increased renal clearance of drugs can alter the amount of medication needed to establish and maintain a therapeutic drug level (Blanchard and Shabetai, 2009). Therefore monitoring drug levels during pregnancy is crucial to maintain effective therapy for the woman while minimizing risk to the fetus.

Anticoagulant therapy may be prescribed during pregnancy for several conditions such as recurrent venous thrombosis, pulmonary embolus, RHD, prosthetic valves, or cyanotic congenital heart defects. If anticoagulant therapy is required during pregnancy, unfractionated heparin or low-molecular-weight heparin (Lovenox) is most commonly prescribed. Heparin, a large-molecule drug, is safe for use during pregnancy because it does not cross the placenta and has no teratogenic effects associated with its use. Warfarin (Coumadin), another popular anticoagulant, does cross the placenta (Gilbert, 2011). It can cause fetal bone and eye anomalies and cognitive impairment when taken early in pregnancy. Eye anomalies and cognitive impairment can occur in exposed fetuses even when the drug is taken only after the first trimester has ended (Niebyl and Simpson, 2012). Therefore warfarin is generally not prescribed during pregnancy. However, it is sometimes used from the second trimester until close to birth in women who have mechanical heart valves because of the increased risk of venous thromboembolism in these patients when heparin is used (Gilbert, 2011).

Tests for fetal maturity and well-being and placental sufficiency may be necessary. Other therapy is directly related to the functional classification of heart disease. The nurse must reinforce the need for close medical supervision.

Intrapartum

For all pregnant women the intrapartum period is the one that evokes the most apprehension in patients and caregivers. The woman with impaired cardiac function has additional reasons to be anxious because labor and giving birth place an additional burden on her already compromised cardiovascular system.

Assessments include the routine assessments for all laboring women and those for cardiac decompensation. In addition, arterial blood gases (ABGs) may be needed to assess for adequate oxygenation. A pulmonary artery catheter may be inserted to monitor hemodynamic status accurately during labor and birth. Electrocardiograph (ECG) monitoring and continuous monitoring of blood pressure and oxygen saturation (pulse oximetry) are usually instituted for the woman, and continuous fetal monitoring is used to monitor the fetus.

> **! NURSING ALERT**
>
> A pulse rate above 100 beats/min or a respiratory rate greater than 24 breaths/min, particularly when associated with dyspnea, may indicate impending ventricular failure (Cunningham, Leveno, Bloom, et al., 2010).

Nursing care during labor and birth focuses on the promotion of cardiac function. Minimize anxiety by maintaining a calm atmosphere. Provide anticipatory guidance by keeping the woman and her family informed of labor progress and events that are likely to occur and answering any questions they have. Support the woman's childbirth preparation method to the degree that it is feasible for her cardiac condition. Nursing techniques that promote comfort such as back massage are also used.

Cardiac function is supported by keeping the woman's head and shoulders elevated and body parts resting on pillows. The side-lying position usually facilitates positive hemodynamics during labor. Discomfort is relieved with medication and supportive care. Physiologically the ideal labor for a woman with heart disease is one that is short and pain free. Therefore use of epidural analgesia is encouraged, although care must be taken to avoid hypotension, a common side effect of regional anesthesia (Easterling and Stout, 2012; Gaddipati and Troiano, 2013).

Beta-adrenergic agents such as terbutaline (Brethine) are associated with various side effects, including tachycardia, irregular pulse,

myocardial ischemia, and pulmonary edema. Therefore these medications should not be used in women with known or suspected heart disease (Gilbert, 2011; Iams, Romero, and Creasy, 2009; Simhan, Iams, and Romero, 2012).

Spontaneous or induced (with a favorable cervix) labor followed by vaginal birth is preferred for women with cardiac disease. If no obstetric problems exist, vaginal birth may be accomplished with the woman in the side-lying position to facilitate uterine perfusion. The supine position should be avoided but, if it is used, place a pad under one hip to displace the uterus laterally and minimize the danger of supine hypotension. Have the woman flex her knees and place her feet flat on the bed. To prevent compression of popliteal veins and an increase in blood volume in the chest and trunk as a result of the effects of gravity, do not use stirrups. Open-glottis pushing is recommended. The woman should avoid the Valsalva maneuver when pushing in the second stage of labor because it reduces diastolic ventricular filling and obstructs left ventricular outflow. Mask oxygen is important. Episiotomy and vacuum extraction or outlet forceps are often used to decrease the length of the second stage of labor and the workload of the heart during that time. Cesarean birth is not routinely recommended for women who have cardiovascular disease because of the risks of dramatic fluid shifts, sustained hemodynamic changes, and increased blood loss.

Routine intrapartum antibiotic prophylaxis for the prevention of bacterial endocarditis is not recommended by the American Heart Association, but it is optional in high risk patients who give birth vaginally. Because bacteremia is common during both vaginal and cesarean birth, many practitioners routinely give antibiotic prophylaxis to all high risk patients. Ampicillin (vancomycin for women who are allergic to penicillin) and gentamicin are the medications recommended for prophylaxis (Easterling and Stout, 2012; Gaddipati and Troiano, 2013). Oxytocin is usually given immediately after birth to prevent hemorrhage. Ergot products (e.g., methylergonovine [Methergine]) should not be used because they increase blood pressure. Fluid balance should be maintained, and blood loss replaced. If tubal sterilization is desired, it is best to delay surgery until the woman is hemodynamically near normal, afebrile, nonanemic, and able to ambulate normally (Cunningham, Leveno, Bloom, et al., 2010).

Postpartum

Monitoring for cardiac decompensation in the postpartum period is essential. The first 24 to 48 hours after birth are the most hemodynamically difficult for the woman. Hemorrhage or infection or both may worsen the cardiac condition. The woman with a cardiac disorder may continue to require a pulmonary artery catheter and ABG monitoring.

> **! NURSING ALERT**
>
> The immediate postbirth period is hazardous for a woman whose heart function is compromised. Cardiac output increases rapidly as extravascular fluid is remobilized into the vascular compartment. At the moment of birth, intraabdominal pressure is reduced drastically; pressure on veins is removed, the splanchnic vessels engorge, and blood flow to the heart is increased.

Care in the postpartum period is tailored to the woman's functional capacity. Postpartum assessment of the woman with cardiac disease includes vital signs, oxygen saturation levels, lung and heart auscultation, presence and degree of edema, amount and character of bleeding, uterine tone and fundal height, urinary output, pain (especially chest pain), the activity-rest pattern, dietary intake, mother-infant interactions, and emotional state. The head of the bed is elevated, and the woman is encouraged to lie on her side. Bed rest may be ordered, with or without bathroom privileges. Progressive ambulation may be permitted as tolerated. The nurse or family members may need to help the woman with her grooming and hygiene needs and other activities. Bowel movements without stress or strain are promoted with stool softeners, diet, and fluids.

The woman may need a family member to help in the care of the infant. Breastfeeding is not contraindicated, but some women with heart disease (particularly those with life-threatening disease) may be unable to breastfeed. The woman who chooses to breastfeed needs the support of her family and the nursing staff to be successful. For example, she may need assistance in positioning herself and/or the infant for feeding. To further conserve the woman's energy, the infant can be brought to her and taken from her after the feeding. Most medications used to manage cardiac disorders are compatible with breastfeeding. However, thiazide diuretics may suppress lactation (Blanchard and Shabetai, 2009). Because diuretics can cause neonatal diuresis that can lead to dehydration, lactating women must be monitored closely to determine if medication doses can be reduced and still be effective. Neonatal nurses should be alerted to watch for voiding patterns and amounts and to monitor the infant closely for signs of dehydration.

If the woman is unable to breastfeed and her energies do not allow her to bottle-feed the infant, the baby can be kept at the bedside so she can look at and touch her baby to establish an emotional bond with a low expenditure of energy. The infant should be held at the mother's eye level near her lips and brought to her fingers. At the same time, involving the mother passively in her infant's care helps her feel vitally important—as she is—to the infant's well-being (e.g., "You can offer something no one else can: you can provide your baby with your sounds, touch, and rhythms that are so comforting"). Perhaps the woman can be encouraged to make a tape recording of her talking, singing, or whispering, which can be played for the baby in the nursery to help the infant feel her presence and be in contact with her voice. This also enhances maternal-infant bonding.

Preparation for discharge is planned carefully with the woman and family. Provision of help for the woman in the home by relatives, friends, and others must be addressed. If necessary, the nurse refers the family to community resources (e.g., for assistance with household activities). Rest and sleep periods, activity, and diet must be planned. The couple may need information about reestablishing sexual relations and contraception or sterilization.

Women with congenital heart disease should be offered contraceptive counseling. In general, for women with congenital heart disease the complications associated with pregnancy are usually greater than the risks associated with any form of contraception (Easterling and Stout, 2012). Women at particular risk for thromboembolism should avoid combined estrogen-progestin oral contraceptives, but progestin-only pills may be used. Parenteral progestins (e.g., medroxyprogesterone [Depo-Provera]) are safe and effective for women with cardiac disease. However, they cause irregular bleeding, which may be problematic for women on anticoagulant therapy. An IUD may be used by women with congenital heart lesions (Easterling and Stout, 2012).

Monitoring for cardiac decompensation continues through the first few weeks after birth because of hormonal shifts that affect hemodynamics. Little data are available regarding how quickly cardiac output returns to normal after giving birth. Older studies suggested that this occurred by 8 to 10 weeks postpartum. However,

a longitudinal study that followed women before, during, and after pregnancy found that both nulliparous and multiparous women had significantly higher cardiac outputs above their prepregnancy values even at 1 year after giving birth (Katz, 2012).

Men and women with a congenital heart defect are at increased risk for having children who also have a defect. The risk for affected mothers is greater, approximately 2 to more than 3 times that of affected fathers. Children born with a congenital heart defect to parents with congenital heart defects appear to inherit the risk for cardiac maldevelopment in general rather than a specific defect because they often do not have the same defect as the parent (Easterling and Stout, 2012). Therefore preconception and genetic counseling before a subsequent pregnancy are essential.

OTHER MEDICAL DISORDERS IN PREGNANCY

Anemia

Anemia is a common medical disorder of pregnancy, affecting from 20% to 60% of pregnant women (Kilpatrick, 2009). It results in a reduction of the oxygen-carrying capacity of the blood; thus the heart tries to compensate by increasing the cardiac output. This effort increases the workload of the heart and stresses ventricular function. Therefore anemia that occurs with any other complication (e.g., preeclampsia) may result in congestive heart failure.

An indirect index of the oxygen-carrying capacity is the packed RBC volume, or hematocrit level. The normal hematocrit range in nonpregnant women is 37% to 47%. However, normal values for pregnant women with adequate iron stores may be as low as 33%. According to the Centers for Disease Control and Prevention (CDC), anemia in pregnancy is defined as hemoglobin less than 11 g/dL in the first and third trimesters and less than 10.5 g/dL in the second trimester (Kilpatrick, 2009). A hemoglobin level less than 6 to 8 mg/dL is considered severe anemia (Blackburn, 2013).

When a woman has anemia during pregnancy, the loss of blood at birth, even if minimal, is not well tolerated. She is at an increased risk for requiring blood transfusions. Women with anemia have a higher incidence of postpartum complications such as infection than pregnant women with normal hematologic values.

Care of the anemic pregnant woman requires that the health care provider distinguish between the normal physiologic anemia of pregnancy and disease states. The majority of cases of anemia in pregnancy are caused by iron deficiency. The other types include a considerable variety of acquired and hereditary anemias such as folic acid deficiency, sickle cell anemia, and thalassemia.

Iron Deficiency Anemia

Iron deficiency anemia is by far the most common anemia of pregnancy, accounting for approximately 75% of cases. It is diagnosed by checking the woman's serum ferritin level in addition to her hemoglobin and hematocrit levels. The serum ferritin level reflects iron reserves (Samuels, 2012). Serum ferritin levels below 12 mcg/L along with a low hemoglobin level indicate iron deficiency anemia (Blackburn, 2013). An association appears to exist between maternal iron deficiency anemia, especially severe anemia, and preterm birth and low-birth-weight infants, although whether these poor pregnancy outcomes are caused by iron deficiency anemia is uncertain (Samuels, 2012). Usually even the fetus of an anemic woman receives adequate iron stores from the mother at the cost of further depleting the mother's iron level (Blackburn, 2013).

Generally iron deficiency anemia is preventable or easily treated with iron supplements. Because of the increased amounts of iron needed for fetal development and maternal stores, pregnant women are often encouraged to take prophylactic iron supplementation (Blackburn, 2013; Gilbert, 2011). Most women with iron deficiency anemia can absorb as much iron as they need by taking one 325-mg tablet of ferrous sulfate twice each day (Samuels, 2012). Some pregnant women cannot tolerate the prescribed oral iron because of nausea and vomiting associated with the pregnancy and as a side effect of iron therapy. In such cases the woman may receive parenteral iron therapy such as an iron-dextran complex (Imferon). This medication can be given either by intravascular or intramuscular injection, although the intramuscular injection is very painful. Women who are severely anemic may require blood transfusions (Samuels, 2012).

Teach the importance of iron supplements for preventing or treating iron deficiency anemia (see Patient Teaching box on p. 245). In addition, teach dietary ways to increase the oral intake of iron-rich foods and decrease the GI side effects of iron therapy.

Folic Acid Deficiency Anemia

Folate is a water-soluble vitamin found naturally in dark green leafy vegetables, citrus fruits, eggs, legumes, and whole grains. Even in well-nourished women, folate deficiency is common. Poor diet, cooking with large volumes of water, and increased alcohol use may contribute to folate deficiency. During pregnancy the need for folate increases, both because of fetal demands and because folate is less well absorbed from the GI tract during gestation.

Folic acid is the form of the vitamin used in vitamin supplements. The recommended daily intake of folic acid for nonpregnant women is 400 mcg. Pregnant women need 50% more, or 600 mcg/day (Otten, Helwig, and Meyers, 2006). Since 1998 the FDA has required the addition of folic acid to cereals, pasta, breads, and other food that are labeled "enriched." However, the amount added is small, and most pregnant women need a supplement. Both prescription and nonprescription prenatal vitamins contain more than the recommended daily intake of folic acid and should be sufficient to prevent and treat folate deficiency. Women at particular risk for folate deficiency include those who have significant hemoglobinopathies, take anticonvulsant medication, are pregnant with a multifetal gestation, or have frequent pregnancies. These women require larger than usual doses of folic acid (Samuels, 2012).

Folate deficiency is the most common cause of megaloblastic anemia during pregnancy, but a vitamin B_{12} deficiency must also be considered. Vitamin B_{12} deficiency in pregnant women is seen much more often now than in the past because of the increasing numbers of women who become pregnant after undergoing bariatric surgery (Samuels, 2012). Megaloblastic anemia rarely occurs before the third trimester of pregnancy (Kilpatrick, 2009; Samuels, 2012). Women with megaloblastic anemia caused by folic acid deficiency have the usual presenting symptoms and signs of anemia: pallor; fatigue; lethargy; and glossitis and skin roughness, which are associated specifically with megaloblastic anemia (Kilpatrick, 2009). Folate deficiency usually improves rapidly with folic acid therapy. It rarely occurs in the fetus and is not a significant cause of perinatal morbidity. Iron deficiency often occurs along with folate deficiency (Samuels, 2012).

Sickle Cell Hemoglobinopathy

Sickle cell hemoglobinopathy is a disease caused by the presence of abnormal hemoglobin in the blood. Sickle cell trait (SA hemoglobin pattern) is sickling of the RBCs but with a normal RBC life span. Most people with sickle cell trait are asymptomatic. Approximately 1 in 12 African-American adults in the United States have sickle cell trait (Samuels, 2012). Women with sickle cell trait require genetic counseling and partner testing to determine their risk of producing children with sickle cell trait or disease.

Women with sickle cell trait usually do well in pregnancy. However, they are at increased risk for preeclampsia, intrauterine fetal death, preterm birth and low-birth-weight infants, and postpartum endometritis. They are also at increased risk for UTIs and may be deficient in iron (Kilpatrick, 2009; Samuels, 2012).

Sickle cell anemia (sickle cell disease) is a recessive, hereditary, familial hemolytic anemia that affects persons of African or Mediterranean ancestry. These individuals usually have abnormal hemoglobin types (SS or SC). The average life span of RBCs in a person with sickle cell anemia is only 5 to 10 days compared to the 120-day life span of a normal RBC. Sickle cell anemia occurs in 1 in 708 African-Americans in the United States (Samuels, 2012). People with sickle cell anemia have recurrent attacks (crises) of fever and pain, most often in the abdomen, joints, or extremities, although virtually all organ systems can be affected. These attacks are attributed to vascular occlusion when RBCs assume a characteristic sickled shape. Crises are usually triggered by dehydration, hypoxia, or acidosis (Samuels, 2012).

Women with sickle cell anemia require genetic counseling before pregnancy. All children born to a woman with sickle cell anemia will be affected in some way by the disease. The woman's partner must be tested to determine the couple's risk of producing children with sickle cell disease rather than sickle cell trait. Women with sickle cell anemia are at risk for poor pregnancy outcomes, including miscarriage, IUGR, and stillbirth. Although maternal mortality is rare, maternal morbidity is significant and includes an increased risk for preeclampsia and infection, particularly in the urinary tract and the lungs. The frequency of painful crises also appears to be increased during pregnancy (Samuels, 2012) (see Critical Thinking Case Study).

The woman is monitored carefully during pregnancy for the development of UTI or preeclampsia. In addition, she has serial ultrasound examinations to monitor fetal growth and will likely have antepartum fetal testing performed regularly during the third trimester. Infections are treated aggressively with antibiotics. If crises occur they are managed with analgesia, oxygen, and hydration. Some authorities still recommend prophylactic transfusions, which replace the woman's sickle cells with normal RBCs, to improve oxygen-carrying capacity and suppress the synthesis of sickle

---

❓ CRITICAL THINKING CASE STUDY

Sickle Cell Hemoglobinopathy

Latasha is a 23-year-old G1 P0 with sickle cell anemia who is hospitalized with a crisis at 16 weeks of gestation. She says, "I've been in and out of the hospital all my life because of my sickle cell disease. I sure hope my baby won't have it!"

1. Evidence—Is there sufficient evidence to counsel Latasha regarding her baby's chance of having sickle cell disease?
2. Assumptions—Describe an underlying assumption about each of the following issues:
   a. The chance that Latasha's baby will inherit either sickle cell trait or sickle cell disease
   b. Pregnancy risks related to sickle cell disease
   c. Usual pregnancy management in women with sickle cell disease
3. What implications and priorities for nursing care can be drawn at this time?
4. Does the evidence objectively support your argument (conclusion)?

hemoglobin. However, most clinicians believe that prophylactic transfusions do not improve fetal or neonatal outcome and are not worth the associated risks of isosensitization, viral infection, transfusion reactions, and hemochromatosis (Samuels, 2012).

⚡ **SAFETY ALERT**

Women with sickle cell anemia are not iron deficient. Therefore routine iron supplementation, even that found in prenatal vitamins, should be avoided because these women can develop iron overload (Samuels, 2012).

If no complications occur, pregnancy can continue until term. Intrapartum women with sickle cell disease should be encouraged to labor in a side-lying position. They may require supplemental oxygen. Adequate hydration should be maintained while preventing fluid overload. Conduction anesthesia (e.g., epidural or combined spinal epidural anesthesia) is recommended because it provides excellent pain relief. Vaginal birth is preferred. Cesarean birth should be performed only for obstetric indications (Samuels, 2012).

Thalassemia

Thalassemia is a relatively common anemia in which an insufficient amount of hemoglobin is produced to fill the RBCs. It is a hereditary disorder that involves the abnormal synthesis of the alpha or beta chains of hemoglobin. Beta thalassemia is the more common variety in the United States and usually occurs in persons of Mediterranean, North African, Middle Eastern, and Asian descent (Kilpatrick, 2009).

Beta thalassemia minor is the heterozygous form of this disorder. People with heterozygous beta thalassemia are carriers of the disorder and are usually asymptomatic (Samuels, 2012). They may be mildly anemic but are usually healthy otherwise. Women whose pregnancies are complicated by beta thalassemia minor generally do not experience associated maternal or infant complications if their condition is stable (Blackburn, 2013) and do not require antepartum fetal testing (Samuels, 2012). Iron therapy should only be prescribed for women who are iron deficient, although folic acid supplementation is recommended for all women with beta thalassemia minor (Samuels, 2012).

The homozygous form of beta thalassemia is known as thalassemia major, or Cooley's anemia. Persons with this form of the disease usually have hepatosplenomegaly and bone deformities caused by massive marrow tissue expansion. These individuals usually die of infection or cardiovascular complications fairly early in life. If women live to reach childbearing age, infertility is common. If women with this disorder do become pregnant, they usually experience severe anemia and congestive heart failure, although successful full-term pregnancies have been reported. Women with beta thalassemia major are managed much like those with sickle cell anemia during pregnancy (Samuels, 2012).

Pulmonary Disorders

As pregnancy advances and the enlarged uterus presses on the thoracic cavity, any pregnant woman may experience increased respiratory difficulty. This difficulty is compounded by pulmonary disease.

Asthma

Asthma is a chronic inflammatory disorder involving the tracheobronchial airways, with increased airway responsiveness to a variety of stimuli. It is characterized by periods of exacerbations and remissions. Exacerbations are triggered by allergens, marked change in ambient temperature, or emotional tension. In many cases the actual cause may be unknown, although a family history of allergy is common. In response to stimuli, narrowing of the hyperreactive airways is widespread, causing difficulty with breathing; however, the condition is reversible. The clinical manifestations are expiratory wheezing, productive cough, thick sputum, dyspnea, or any combination.

Asthma may be the most common potentially serious medical condition to complicate pregnancy. It affects 8% of all pregnancies. The prevalence and morbidity rates are increasing, although the asthma-related mortality has dropped in recent years (Whitty and Dombrowski, 2012).

The effect of pregnancy on asthma is unpredictable. The severity of the disease is unchanged in one third, improved in one third, and worsened in one third of pregnant women. If asthma worsens, the more severe symptoms usually occur between 17 and 24 weeks of gestation (Gilbert, 2011). Asthma appears to be associated with preeclampsia, low birth weight or IUGR, preterm birth, and perinatal mortality (Whitty and Dombrowski, 2012).

The ultimate goal of asthma therapy in pregnancy is maintaining adequate oxygenation of the fetus by preventing hypoxic episodes in the mother. Achieving this goal requires monitoring lung function objectively (e.g., peak expiratory flow rate and forced expiratory volume in one second), avoiding or controlling asthma triggers (e.g., dust mites, animal dander, pollen, wood smoke), educating patients about the importance of controlling asthma during pregnancy, and drug therapy. Current drug therapy for asthma emphasizes treatment of airway inflammation to decrease airway hyperresponsiveness and prevent asthma symptoms. Decreasing airway inflammation with inhaled corticosteroids is currently the preferred treatment for managing persistent asthma during pregnancy (Whitty and Dombrowski, 2009).

During pregnancy women with moderate-to-severe, poorly controlled asthma need ultrasound examinations to assess fetal growth and date the pregnancy. Repeat ultrasound examinations should be performed after an asthma exacerbation to evaluate fetal activity and growth (Whitty and Dombrowski, 2012). Women with moderate or severe asthma will probably begin antepartum fetal testing by 32 weeks of gestation (Whitty and Dombrowski, 2009). Acute exacerbations may require albuterol, steroids, aminophylline, beta-adrenergic agents, and oxygen. Women with severe exacerbations unresponsive to treatment may require intubation and mechanical ventilation (Whitty and Dombrowski, 2012). Although asthma attacks during labor are rare, medications for asthma are continued during labor and the postpartum period. Women who have received systemic corticosteroids during the previous 4 weeks should be given stress doses of corticosteroids during labor and for the first 24 hours after birth (Whitty and Dombrowski, 2012). Pulse oximetry should be instituted during labor. Epidural anesthesia reduces oxygen consumption and is recommended for pain relief. Fentanyl, a nonhistamine-releasing narcotic, may also be used for pain control and is not associated with bronchospasm (Cunningham, Leveno, Bloom, et al., 2010; Whitty and Dombrowski, 2009).

During the postpartum period women who have asthma are at increased risk for hemorrhage. If excessive bleeding occurs, prostaglandin (PG)E_2 or E_1 can be given, although the patient's respiratory status should be monitored (Whitty and Dombrowski, 2012). Because carboprost (15-methyl $PGF_{2\alpha}$ [Hemabate]) and ergonovine and methylergonovine (Methergine) can cause bronchospasm, their use should be avoided (Cunningham, Leveno, Bloom, et al., 2010). In general, only small amounts of asthma medications enter breast milk; therefore their use is not considered a contraindication to breastfeeding. However, in sensitive individuals theophylline in breast milk can cause vomiting, feeding difficulties, jitteriness, and cardiac arrhythmias in neonates (Whitty and Dombrowski, 2012). The woman usually returns to her prepregnancy asthma status within 3 months after giving birth.

Cystic Fibrosis

Cystic fibrosis is a common autosomal recessive genetic disorder in which the exocrine glands produce excessive viscous secretions, which causes problems with both respiratory and digestive functions. Most people with cystic fibrosis have chronic obstructive pulmonary disease, pancreatic exocrine insufficiency, and elevated sweat electrolytes. Morbidity and mortality are usually caused by progressive chronic bronchial pulmonary disease (Whitty and Dombrowski, 2009).

Since the gene for cystic fibrosis was identified in 1989, data can be collected for the purposes of genetic counseling for couples regarding carrier status. In the United States approximately 4% of the Caucasian population are carriers of the cystic fibrosis gene. Cystic fibrosis occurs in 1 in 3000 live Caucasian births. People with cystic fibrosis now live much longer than they did in the past because of earlier diagnosis of the disease and advances in antibiotic therapy and nutritional support. Currently over 45% of all individuals in the United States with cystic fibrosis are more than 18 years old. Men tend to live a little longer (median age of survival is 29.6 years) compared to women, whose median age of survival is 27.3 years. Although most men with cystic fibrosis are infertile, women with the disease are often fertile and thus able to become pregnant (Whitty and Dombrowski, 2012).

In women with good nutrition, mild obstructive lung disease, and minimal lung impairment, pregnancy is tolerated well (Whitty and Dombrowski, 2012). In women with severe disease the pregnancy is often complicated by chronic hypoxemia and frequent pulmonary infections. Risk factors that may predict a poor pregnancy outcome are poor prepregnancy nutritional status, significant pulmonary disease with hypoxemia, pulmonary hypertension, liver disease, and diabetes mellitus (Whitty and Dombrowski, 2009). Increased maternal and perinatal mortality is related to severe pulmonary infection. The incidence of preterm birth, IUGR, and uteroplacental insufficiency is increased (Whitty and Dombrowski, 2009).

Care of the pregnant woman with cystic fibrosis requires a team effort. Ideally the woman should reach 90% of her ideal body weight before becoming pregnant. A weight gain of 11 to 12 kg (24 to 26 lbs) is recommended during pregnancy. Women who are unable to achieve the recommended weight gain through oral supplements may require nasogastric tube feedings at night. Pancreatic insufficiency may put the woman at risk for malnutrition because she cannot meet the increased nutritional requirements of pregnancy. If malnutrition is severe, parenteral hyperalimentation may be necessary. Fat-soluble vitamins may not be well absorbed, resulting in deficiency in those nutrients. Throughout pregnancy frequent monitoring of the woman's weight, blood glucose, hemoglobin, total protein, serum albumin, prothrombin time, and fat-soluble vitamins A and E is suggested. Pancreatic enzymes should be adjusted as necessary (Whitty and Dombrowski, 2012).

Baseline pulmonary function tests ideally should be completed before pregnancy and continued as needed during pregnancy. Inhaled recombinant human deoxyribonuclease I may be given to improve lung function by decreasing sputum viscosity. Inhaled 7% saline is also beneficial in this regard (Cunningham, Leveno, Bloom, et al., 2010). Early detection and treatment of infection are critical. Management of infection includes IV antibiotics along with chest physical therapy and bronchial drainage (Whitty and Dombrowski, 2012).

Fetal assessment is essential, given that the fetus is at risk for uteroplacental insufficiency, which can result in IUGR. Maternal nutritional status and weight gain during pregnancy significantly affect fetal growth. Fundal height should be measured routinely, and ultrasound examinations performed to evaluate fetal growth and amniotic fluid volume. Fetal movement counts are often recommended, starting at 28 weeks of gestation. NSTs should be initiated at 32 weeks of gestation or sooner if evidence of fetal compromise exists (Whitty and Dombrowski, 2012).

During labor increased cardiac output stresses the cardiovascular system and can lead to cardiopulmonary failure in the woman with pulmonary hypertension or cor pulmonale. These women are also more likely to develop right-sided heart failure. Epidural or local analgesia is the preferred analgesic for birth, with vaginal birth recommended. Cesarean birth should be reserved for obstetric indications. If general anesthesia is needed for cesarean birth, anticholinergic medications should not be given before surgery because they tend to promote airway drying (Whitty and Dombrowski, 2012).

Breastfeeding appears to be safe as long as the sodium content of the milk is not abnormal. Pumping and discarding the milk are continued until the sodium content has been determined. Milk samples should be tested periodically for sodium, chloride, and total fat; and the infant's growth pattern should be monitored (Lawrence and Lawrence, 2005).

Integumentary Disorders

Dermatologic disorders induced by pregnancy include melasma (chloasma), vascular "spiders," palmar erythema, and striae gravidarum. A number of chronic skin disorders may complicate pregnancy. These disorders may be present before pregnancy or appear for the first time during pregnancy. Their course varies during pregnancy. For example, acne may improve. Psoriasis improves in 40% of women, remains unchanged in 40% of women, and worsens in 20% of women during pregnancy. Lesions from neurofibromatosis may increase in size and number during pregnancy (Cunningham, Leveno, Bloom, et al., 2010). Explanation, reassurance, and commonsense measures should suffice for normal skin changes. In contrast, disease processes during and soon after pregnancy may be extremely difficult to diagnose and treat.

> ### ⚡ SAFETY ALERT
>
> Isotretinoin (Accutane), commonly prescribed for cystic acne, is highly teratogenic. There is a risk for craniofacial, cardiac, and CNS malformations in exposed fetuses. This drug should not be taken during pregnancy.

Pruritus is a major symptom in several pregnancy-related skin diseases. *Pruritus gravidarum*, generalized itching without the presence of a rash, develops in up to 14% of pregnant women. It is often limited to the abdomen and is usually caused by skin distention and development of striae. Pruritus gravidarum is not associated with poor perinatal outcomes. It is treated symptomatically with skin lubrication, topical antipruritics, and oral antihistamines. Ultraviolet light and careful exposure to sunlight decrease itching. Pruritus gravidarum usually disappears shortly after birth but can recur in approximately half of all subsequent pregnancies (Rapini, 2009).

Pruritic Urticarial Papules and Plaques of Pregnancy

Another common pregnancy-specific cause of pruritus is pruritic urticarial papules and plaques of pregnancy (PUPPP) (Fig. 11-5),

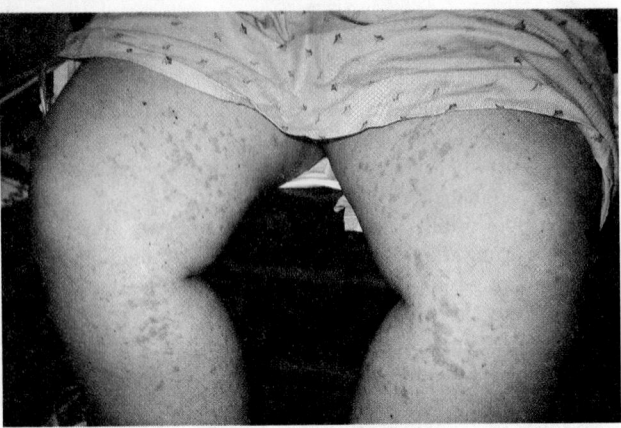

FIG 11-5 Woman with pruritic urticarial papules and plaques of pregnancy. Lesions also are present on her arms, back, abdomen, and buttocks. (Courtesy Shannon Perry, Phoenix, AZ.)

also known as *polymorphic eruption of pregnancy*. PUPPP classically appears in primigravidas during the mid to late third trimester and occurs a bit more frequently in women carrying male fetuses. The disorder is much more commonly seen in multiple gestations than in singletons (Kroumpouzos, 2012). The abdomen is usually affected, but lesions can spread to the arms, thighs, back, and buttocks. PUPPP almost always causes pruritus, and the itching is severe in 80% of cases. However, it is not associated with poor maternal or fetal outcomes. Therefore the goal of therapy is simply to relieve maternal discomfort. Antipruritic topical medications, topical steroids, and oral antihistamines usually provide relief. Women with severe symptoms may require oral prednisone. PUPPP usually resolves before birth or within several weeks after birth. However, on rare occasions it may persist or even begin after birth. PUPPP does not usually recur in subsequent pregnancies (Kroumpouzos, 2012; Rapini, 2009).

Intrahepatic Cholestasis of Pregnancy

Intrahepatic cholestasis of pregnancy (ICP) is a liver disorder unique to pregnancy that is characterized by generalized pruritus. The itching usually begins during the third trimester, most severely affects the palms and soles, and is worse at night (Cappell, 2012). ICP occurs more frequently during the winter months. A geographic variance in the prevalence of the disease has also been noted. It occurs most often in Southeast Asia, Chile, Bolivia, and Scandinavia; although it is seen less frequently now in Chile and Scandinavia than in the past (Cappell, 2012; Williamson and Mackillop, 2009).

No skin lesions are present. Women with ICP have elevated serum bile acids and liver function tests. Jaundice may or may not be present. As many as one half of women with ICP develop dark urine and light-colored stools. The cause of ICP is unknown, but approximately half of women have a family history of the disorder. Other risk factors for ICP are multiple gestations and a history of ICP in a previous pregnancy (Cappell, 2012).

Poor fetal outcomes, including meconium ileus, preterm birth, and stillbirth, are associated with ICP. The cause of these complications is likely related to increased levels of fetal serum bile levels. Treatment consists of medication, usually ursodeoxycholic acid, which effectively controls the pruritus and laboratory abnormalities associated with ICP, and continued monitoring of liver function tests and bile acids (Cappell, 2012; Williamson and Mackillop, 2009). If fetal complications do not occur, birth should

be considered at or near term after lung maturity has been documented. Symptoms generally disappear quickly after birth, and usually there are no long-term sequelae. However, postpartum hemorrhage is more likely in women who had ICP, and they are also at risk to develop cholelithiasis after birth. ICP recurs in about two thirds of subsequent pregnancies (Cappell, 2012).

Neurologic Disorders

The pregnant woman with a neurologic disorder must deal with potential teratogenic effects of prescribed medications, changes of mobility during pregnancy, and impaired ability to care for the baby. The nurse should be aware of all medications the woman is taking and the associated potential for producing congenital anomalies. As the pregnancy progresses, the woman's center of gravity shifts and causes balance and gait changes. The nurse should advise the woman of these expected changes and suggest safety measures as appropriate. Family and community resources may be needed to help provide infant care for the neurologically impaired woman.

Epilepsy

Epilepsy (often called *seizure disorder*) is a disorder of the brain that causes recurrent seizures and is the most common major neurologic disorder accompanying pregnancy. Less than 1% of all pregnant women have a seizure disorder (Aminoff, 2009). Seizure disorders are either acquired (less than 15% of all cases) or idiopathic (more than 85% of all cases), which means that a specific cause for the seizures cannot be identified. The majority of women with a seizure disorder who become pregnant have an uneventful pregnancy with an excellent outcome (Samuels and Niebyl, 2012).

Women with epilepsy should receive preconception counseling if at all possible. A detailed history of medication use and seizure frequency should be obtained. If the woman has frequent seizures before conception, she is likely to continue this pattern during pregnancy; therefore achieving effective seizure control is extremely important before conception, even if changing medications is required (Samuels and Niebyl, 2012).

Infants born to women taking anticonvulsant medications have an increased incidence of congenital anomalies, including cleft lip and palate, congenital heart disease, and neural tube defects (NTDs). These anomalies are related to the dose, type, and number of anticonvulsant medications taken, not to epilepsy itself (Samuels and Niebyl, 2012).

> ⚡ **SAFETY ALERT**
>
> Carbamazepine (Tegretol) and valproate (Depakote) should be avoided if possible during pregnancy, especially during the first trimester, because their use is associated with NTDs in the fetus.

Several new anticonvulsant medications have been developed for use within the last decade. More information is needed regarding the fetal effects of these medications. However, any anticonvulsant medication required to achieve good seizure control in a woman with epilepsy should be used, regardless of the increased risk of fetal anomalies, because the most important goal during pregnancy is the prevention of seizures (Samuels and Niebyl, 2012).

Pregnant women with epilepsy are advised to take a folic acid supplement of 4 mg daily, which may decrease the incidence of NTDs. They are also encouraged to take a prenatal vitamin containing vitamin D daily because anticonvulsant medications can interfere with production of the active form of this vitamin (Cunningham, Leveno, Bloom, et al., 2010; Samuels and Niebyl, 2012).

If possible, only one anticonvulsant medication—at the lowest dose level that is effective at keeping the woman seizure free—should be prescribed during pregnancy. The increase in plasma volume that is a normal pregnancy change can affect drug metabolism and distribution. Therefore blood levels of anticonvulsant medications should be checked, and drug dosages adjusted as necessary. With patient cooperation and close monitoring, most women with epilepsy should experience no change or even have fewer seizures during pregnancy. An increase in seizure frequency is usually related either to noncompliance with taking prescribed anticonvulsant medications or with sleep deprivation (Samuels and Niebyl, 2012). If an increase in seizure activity does occur during pregnancy, it is usually in women who had frequent seizures (more than one per month) before pregnancy (Aminoff, 2009).

In addition to congenital anomalies, the fetus of a woman with epilepsy is also at risk for IUGR. Determining an accurate gestational age as early as possible is important. This information decreases any confusion later in pregnancy regarding fetal growth issues. If the patient's weight gain and fundal height appear appropriate, serial ultrasounds for fetal weight assessment may not be necessary. Maternal serum screening around 16 weeks of gestation and ultrasound examination at 18 to 22 weeks of gestation should be performed to assess for the presence of an NTD or other fetal anomalies. Nonstress testing later in pregnancy is not necessary unless the woman has other medical or obstetric factors that increase the risk for stillbirth (Samuels and Niebyl, 2012).

Management of anticonvulsant therapy during prolonged labor is challenging. During labor absorption of medications given orally is unpredictable, especially if vomiting occurs. Women who are maintained on phenytoin (Dilantin) or phenobarbital may be given these medications parenterally during labor. No parenteral form of carbamazepine has been developed. Oral administration of carbamazepine may be attempted; but, if the woman experiences a seizure or a preseizure aura, she may be given phenytoin intravenously instead to carry her through labor. Vaginal birth is preferred (Samuels and Niebyl, 2012).

After birth the levels of anticonvulsant medications must be monitored frequently for the first few weeks because they can rise rapidly. If medication dose levels were increased during pregnancy, they need to be reduced quickly to prepregnancy levels. All of the major anticonvulsant medications are found in breast milk, but the use of these medications is not a contraindication to breastfeeding. However, topiramate has been associated with neonatal weight loss; thus it probably should not be prescribed if the woman is breastfeeding (Samuels and Niebyl, 2012).

During the neonatal period infants exposed in utero to phenobarbital, phenytoin, and primidone, which cause a vitamin K deficiency, can hemorrhage. However, infants who receive vitamin K at birth have not been shown to have an increased risk of bleeding. This problem is now rare, because most infants routinely receive an intramuscular injection of vitamin K immediately after birth. In addition, phenobarbital and primidone are almost never prescribed, and phenytoin is used to treat epilepsy much less often now than in the past (Samuels and Niebyl, 2012).

All methods of contraception can be used by women with an idiopathic seizure disorder. However, commonly prescribed anticonvulsant medications such as carbamazepine and phenytoin (also topiramate and oxcarbazepine at higher doses) reduce the effectiveness of oral contraceptives. Women taking low-dose oral contraceptives especially may have more breakthrough bleeding and be at risk for an unplanned pregnancy (Cunningham, Leveno, Bloom, et al., 2010; Samuels and Niebyl, 2012). Lamotrigine, zonisamide, gabapentin, tiagabine, valproate, and levetiracetam have not been reported to cause oral contraceptive failure (Aminoff, 2009; Samuels and Niebyl).

In terms of planning for future childbearing, couples should be informed that children born to women with a seizure disorder of unknown cause have a 4 times greater chance (risk of 2% to 4%) for an idiopathic seizure disorder compared to the general population. Epilepsy in the father does not appear to increase a child's risk for developing a seizure disorder (Samuels and Niebyl, 2012).

Multiple Sclerosis

Multiple sclerosis (MS), a patchy demyelinization of the spinal cord and CNS, may be a viral disorder. It occurs equally in men and women. Onset of symptoms, which include weakness of one or both lower extremities, visual complaints, and loss of coordination, is subtle and usually occurs between the ages of 20 and 40 years. The disease is characterized by exacerbations and remissions. Pregnancy does not seem to worsen the disease (Samuels and Niebyl, 2012).

Remissions during pregnancy are common. If an exacerbation occurs, it is more likely to do so during the third trimester of pregnancy or postpartum. Treatment may include corticosteroids and immunosuppressive agents. Several new drugs and biopharmaceuticals are available for treating MS. Their use in pregnancy has been limited; thus few data and no controlled studies are available. However, many consist of molecules that are too large to cross the placenta. Therefore they may be acceptable for use during pregnancy. They do not appear to be associated with anomalies (Samuels and Niebyl, 2012). Interferon is also sometimes used to treat MS relapses during pregnancy and postpartum. Its safety for use during pregnancy has not been established, although in theory it should not cross the placenta because of its large molecular size (Stuart and Bergstrom, 2011).

Women who have become paraplegic with MS are more likely to develop UTIs during pregnancy but may feel no symptoms. Therefore they should be screened routinely. Women who have become paraplegic or have lumbosacral lesions as a result of MS may have little pain during labor. Determining when labor begins may be difficult for them. Uterine contractions occur normally, but these women may have difficulty pushing effectively during the second stage of labor. Therefore, vacuum- or forceps-assisted birth may be necessary (Samuels and Niebyl, 2012). Epidural anesthesia can be used during labor (Stuart and Bergstrom, 2011).

Depression is common among women with MS; thus they should be assessed frequently for evidence of postpartum depression. Breastfeeding is encouraged, although medications that are Lactation Risk Category L5 should not be prescribed. IV immunoglobulin (IVIG) is considered safe for use during lactation; no adverse effects in infants have been reported. All hormonal contraceptives may be used by women with MS (Stuart and Bergstrom, 2011).

Bell Palsy

Bell palsy is an acute idiopathic facial paralysis. The cause is unknown, but it may be related to the reactivation of herpesvirus infection or acute human immunodeficiency virus type 1 (HIV-1) retroviral infections. Bell palsy occurs fairly often, especially in women of reproductive age. Women are affected 2 to 4 times more often than men (Cunningham, Leveno, Bloom, et al., 2010). An association between Bell palsy and pregnancy was first cited by Bell in 1830. Pregnant women are affected 3 to 4 times more often than nonpregnant women. The incidence usually peaks during the third trimester and the puerperium. Women who develop Bell palsy during pregnancy have an increased risk for gestational hypertension as well (Cunningham, Leveno, Bloom, et al., 2010).

The clinical manifestations of Bell palsy include the sudden development of a unilateral facial weakness, with maximum weakness within 48 hours after onset, pain surrounding the ear, difficulty closing the eye on the affected side, hyperacusis (abnormal acuteness of the sense of hearing), and occasionally a loss of taste (Aminoff, 2009; Cunningham, Leveno, Bloom, et al., 2010).

No effects of maternal Bell palsy have been observed in infants. Maternal outcome is generally good unless a complete block in nerve conduction occurs. Steroid therapy may improve outcome, although its benefits have not always been proven in past research studies. To be effective, steroids should be administered within the first 5 to 6 days after the paralysis develops (Aminoff, 2009). Supportive care includes prevention of injury to the constantly exposed cornea, facial muscle massage, careful chewing and manual removal of food from inside the affected cheek, and reassurance. Although 80% of affected men and nonpregnant women recover to a satisfactory level within a year, only approximately half of women who develop the disorder during pregnancy do so (Cunningham, Leveno, Bloom, et al., 2010).

Autoimmune Disorders

Autoimmune disorders, also called *collagen vascular diseases,* make up a large group of conditions that disrupt the function of the immune system of the body. In these types of disorders the immune system is unable to distinguish "self" from "nonself." As a result, antibodies develop that attack its normally present antigens, causing tissue damage. Autoimmune disorders can occur during pregnancy because a large percentage of women with an autoimmune disease are women of childbearing age (Gilbert, 2011). Common autoimmune diseases include systemic lupus erythematosus, myasthenia gravis, antiphospholipid syndrome, rheumatoid arthritis, and systemic sclerosis (Chin and Branch, 2012; Cunningham, Leveno, Bloom, et al., 2010).

Systemic Lupus Erythematosus

Systemic lupus erythematosus (SLE) is a chronic, multisystem inflammatory disease that affects the skin, joints, kidneys, lungs, serous membranes, nervous system, liver, and heart. The exact cause of the disease is unknown but probably involves the interaction of several factors, including immunologic, environmental, hormonal, and genetic factors. SLE is the most common serious autoimmune disease affecting women of reproductive age. It occurs 2 to 4 times more often in African-American and Hispanic women than in Caucasian women and is 7 to 15 times more common in women than in men. Most cases of SLE occur in adolescence or young adulthood. Recently the incidence of SLE has nearly tripled, probably because of increased diagnosis (Chin and Branch, 2012; Gilbert, 2011).

Common symptoms, including myalgias, fatigue, weight change, and fevers, occur in nearly all women with SLE at some time during the course of the disease. Although a diagnosis of SLE is suspected based on clinical signs and symptoms, it is confirmed by laboratory testing that demonstrates the presence of circulating autoantibodies. As is the case with other autoimmune diseases, SLE is characterized by a series of exacerbations (flares) and remissions (Chin and Branch, 2012).

Authorities have conflicting opinions as to whether pregnancy increases the likelihood of SLE flares. However, it appears that disease activity at the beginning of pregnancy is an important predictor of exacerbations during pregnancy. Therefore women are advised to wait until they have been in remission for at least 6

months before attempting to become pregnant (Chin and Branch, 2012; Gilbert, 2011). In addition to exacerbations, other maternal risks include an increased rate of miscarriage, nephritis, preeclampsia, possible need to give birth at a preterm gestation, and an increased risk of cesarean birth. Fetal risks include stillbirth, IUGR, and preterm birth (Chin and Branch, 2012).

Medical therapy during pregnancy is kept to a minimum in women who are in remission or who have a mild form of SLE. Immunosuppressive medications should be discontinued before conception. Nonsteroidal antiinflammatory drugs and aspirin are ordinarily the most commonly used antiinflammatory drugs, but they are not recommended for use during pregnancy. Aspirin should not be used after 24 weeks of gestation because of an increased risk of premature closure of the fetal ductus arteriosus (Cunningham, Leveno, Bloom, et al., 2010). Glucocorticoids such as prednisone are often used to treat SLE during pregnancy, as either maintenance therapy or short-term treatment for flares. There is a small risk for fetal cleft lip and palate if glucocorticoids are used during early pregnancy. Prolonged use of this group of medications also increases the risks for bone demineralization, gestational diabetes, preeclampsia, premature rupture of membranes (PROM) and IUGR. Given the significant risks associated with long-term glucocorticoid use, hydroxychloroquine, an antimalarial drug, may be the best medication for maintenance SLE therapy during pregnancy. It significantly reduces SLE disease activity but appears to cause no adverse effects on the fetus (Chin and Branch, 2012).

Prenatal care otherwise focuses on close monitoring to detect common pregnancy complications such as hypertension, proteinuria, and IUGR. Ultrasound examinations are performed frequently to monitor fetal growth. Fetal assessment tests, including daily fetal movement counts and weekly or twice-weekly NSTs and amniotic fluid volume assessments or biophysical profiles, likely begin at 30 to 32 weeks of gestation (see Chapter 10). More frequent ultrasound examinations and fetal testing are necessary if the woman develops an SLE flare, antiphospholipid syndrome, hypertension, proteinuria, or evidence of IUGR (Chin and Branch, 2012).

Women with SLE can develop an exacerbation during labor. Any maintenance medications should be continued throughout the intrapartum period or resumed immediately postpartum at the last pregnancy dose. Even if a flare does not occur, all women who have received chronic glucocorticoid therapy (20 mg or more of prednisone daily for at least 3 weeks) need larger (stress) doses of steroids during labor (Chin and Branch, 2012). Vaginal birth is preferred, but cesarean birth is common because of maternal and fetal complications.

Close monitoring of all women with SLE should continue after birth. Women who have more severe SLE manifestations or who had an SLE exacerbation during pregnancy are at greatest risk to experience a postpartum flare (Chin and Branch, 2012).

Women with SLE and chronic vascular or renal disease should limit their number of pregnancies because of maternal complications associated with the illness and increased adverse perinatal outcomes (Cunningham, Leveno, Bloom, et al., 2010). If desired, the safest time for tubal sterilization is during the postpartum period or when the disease is in remission. Estrogen-containing oral contraceptives may increase the risk of thromboembolism (Gilbert, 2011). Progestin-only implants and injections provide effective contraception with no known effects on lupus flares (Cunningham, Leveno, Bloom, et al., 2010). Barrier methods, in addition to progestin-only contraceptive options, are the least risky forms of contraception for women with SLE (Gilbert, 2011). Evidence does not support concerns regarding an increased risk of infection when IUDs are prescribed for women receiving immunosuppressive therapy (Cunningham, Leveno, Bloom, et al., 2010).

Myasthenia Gravis

Myasthenia gravis (MG), an autoimmune motor (muscle) end-plate disorder that involves acetylcholine use, affects the motor function at the myoneural junction. Muscle weakness, particularly of the eyes, face, tongue, neck, limbs, and respiratory muscles, results. In addition, women may experience ptosis, diplopia, and dysphagia. Women are affected twice as often as men, and the incidence peaks between the ages of 20 and 30 years (Porter and Branch, 2006). Because the greatest period of risk is during the first year after diagnosis, pregnancy should probably be avoided until symptomatic improvement occurs (Cunningham, Leveno, Bloom, et al., 2010). The response of women with MG to pregnancy is unpredictable; remission, exacerbation, or continued stability during pregnancy can occur.

Pregnancy does not appear to affect the overall course of MG, but as the uterus enlarges respirations may be compromised. In addition, the normal fatigue experienced by many pregnant women may be tolerated poorly by those with MG (Cunningham, Leveno, Bloom, et al., 2010). Treatment during pregnancy is the same as for nonpregnant women. Usual medications include glucocorticoids and acetylcholinesterase inhibitors. Monitoring blood glucose values is important because hyperglycemia may result from corticosteroid therapy. Thymectomy may result in remission of the disease but is best performed before or after pregnancy if at all possible. For severe weakness plasmapheresis or IVIG therapy may be needed.

Because MG does not affect smooth muscle, most women tolerate labor well. Vaginal birth is desired, but vacuum or forceps assistance may be required because of muscle weakness. Oxytocin may be given, but medications that cause muscular relaxation should be avoided if at all possible. Narcotics must be used cautiously because they may cause respiratory depression, and women with MG are already at risk for respiratory muscle weakness. Regional analgesia is preferred (Aminoff, 2009; Cunningham, Leveno, Bloom, et al., 2010). After birth women must be supervised carefully because relapses often occur during the puerperium.

⚡ **SAFETY ALERT**

Magnesium sulfate must not be administered to women with MG because it inhibits the release of acetylcholine and can trigger myasthenic crisis.

Approximately 10% to 15% of neonates born to women with MG develop neonatal myasthenia. This transient disorder results from the transfer of maternal antibody against acetylcholine receptors across the placenta. Symptoms, including a poor cry, respiratory difficulties, weakness in suckling, a weak Moro reflex, and feeble limb movements, usually appear within the first 72 hours after birth. Neonatal myasthenia can be treated with anticholinesterase medications and usually resolves by 6 weeks after birth (Aminoff, 2009).

SUBSTANCE ABUSE

Abuse of both legal and illegal substances (alcohol and drugs), whether by pregnant women or other people, can result in addiction. In 2011 the American Society of Addiction Medicine (ASAM) published a short definition of addiction, in which they state the following:

Addiction is a primary, chronic disease of brain reward, motivation, memory and related circuitry. Dysfunction in these circuits leads to characteristic biological, psychological, social and spiritual manifestations …. Like other chronic diseases, addiction often involves cycles of relapse and remission. Without treatment or engagement in recovery activities, addiction is progressive and can result in disability or premature death" (ASAM, 2011).

Dual diagnosis, which is very common, is the coexistence of substance abuse and another psychiatric disorder. Mood and anxiety disorders are the psychiatric disorders that are most commonly seen along with substance abuse in women. The psychiatric illness usually occurs before substance use begins (Wisner, Sit, Altemus, et al., 2012).

The damaging effects of alcohol and illicit drugs on pregnant women and their unborn babies are well documented (Gilbert, 2011; Wisner, Sit, Altemus, et al., 2012). Alcohol and other drugs easily pass from a mother to her baby through the placenta. Smoking during pregnancy has serious health risks, including bleeding complications, miscarriage, stillbirth, prematurity, low birth weight, and sudden unexplained infant death (Gilbert, 2011; Wisner, Sit, Altemus, et al., 2012). Congenital anomalies have occurred in infants of mothers who have taken drugs. With one exception the safest pregnancy is one in which the woman is drug and alcohol free. For women addicted to opioids, methadone maintenance treatment is the current standard of care during pregnancy (Wisner, Sit, Altemus, et al., 2012).

Because many pregnant women are reluctant to reveal their use of substances or the extent of their use, data on prevalence are highly variable. Approximately 15% of all pregnant women have a substance-abuse problem (Gilbert, 2011). Blinded urine drug screens conducted at hospitals across the United States revealed that similar rates of substance use during pregnancy occurred in women of different ages, races, and social classes, although the specific substances used differed by race and social class. African-American and poor women were more likely to use illicit substances, particularly cocaine, whereas Caucasian and educated women were more likely to use alcohol, although polysubstance abuse was common (Wisner, Sit, Altemus, et al., 2012).

Less than 10% of pregnant women who are substance abusers receive treatment for their addictions. Social stigma, labeling, and guilt are significant barriers (Brady and Ashley, 2005). Women often do not seek help because of the fear of losing custody of their child or children or criminal prosecution. Pregnant women who abuse substances commonly have little understanding of the ways in which these substances affect them, their pregnancies, and their babies. In many instances pregnant mothers who use psychoactive substances receive negative feedback from society and health care providers, who not only may condemn them for endangering the life of the fetus but may also even withhold support as a result. Barriers within the drug treatment system may also deter these women from receiving the help they need. Traditionally substance-abuse treatment programs have not addressed issues that affect pregnant women such as concurrent need for obstetric care and child care for other children. Long waiting lists and lack of health insurance present further barriers to treatment. Pregnant women with co-occurring substance abuse and psychiatric disorders face unique barriers because of the social stigma attached to both conditions and insufficient knowledge and training to manage coexisting disorders (Brady and Ashley, 2005).

Because of the risks to the unborn children and financial concerns, pregnant women who abuse substances can now face criminal charges under expanded interpretations of child abuse and drug trafficking statutes (Guttmacher Institute, 2010). See Chapter 3 for additional discussion of this issue.

LEGAL TIP: Drug Testing During Pregnancy

There is no requirement in the United States for a health care provider to test either the pregnant woman or the newborn for the presence of drugs. However, nurses need to know the practices of the states in which they are working. In some states a woman whose urine drug screen is positive at the time of labor and birth must be referred to child protective services. If the mother is not in a drug treatment program or is judged unable to provide care, the infant may be placed in foster care. The U.S. Supreme Court has ruled that in all states it is unlawful to test for drug use without the pregnant woman's permission (Harris and Paltrow, 2003).

CARE MANAGEMENT

Screening

Screening questions for alcohol and drug abuse should be included in the overall assessment at the first prenatal visit of all women. Information about drug use should be obtained by first asking about the woman's intake of over-the-counter and prescribed medications. Next her use of legal drugs such as caffeine, nicotine, and alcohol should be determined. Finally she should be questioned about her use of illicit drugs such as cocaine, heroin, and marijuana. The approximate frequency and amount should be documented for each drug used (Seidel, Ball, Dains, et al., 2011).

The *4 Ps Plus* is a screening tool designed specifically to identify pregnant women who need in-depth assessment (Box 11-4). It consists of five questions and takes less than a minute to complete. Because women frequently deny or greatly underreport usage when asked about drug or alcohol consumption during pregnancy, asking about substance use before pregnancy is often an effective screening method (Wisner, Sit, Altemus, et al., 2012).

Urine toxicologic testing is often performed to screen for illicit drug use. Drugs may be found in urine days to weeks after ingestion, depending on how quickly they are metabolized and excreted from the body. Meconium (from the neonate) and hair can also be analyzed to determine past drug use over a longer period (Gilbert, 2011).

Because substance-abusing pregnant women are at risk for a variety of infections and medical conditions, a comprehensive medical history should be obtained, and a complete physical examination performed. Laboratory assessments likely include screening for syphilis, hepatitis B and C, and HIV. A complete blood count and a skin test to screen for tuberculosis may also be ordered. In addition, the woman may be tested for other common sexually transmitted infections such as gonorrhea and chlamydia (Wisner, Sit, Altemus, et al., 2012). Initial and serial ultrasound studies are usually performed to determine gestational age because the woman may have had amenorrhea as a result of her drug use or have no idea when her last menstrual period occurred.

Initial Care

Intervention with the pregnant substance abuser begins with education about specific effects on pregnancy, the fetus, and the newborn for each drug used. Consequences of perinatal drug use should be clearly communicated, and abstinence recommended as the safest course of action unless the woman is abusing opioids. Women are often more receptive to making lifestyle changes during pregnancy than at any other time in their lives. The casual, experimental, or recreational drug user is frequently able to achieve and maintain sobriety when she receives education, support, and continued monitoring throughout the remainder of the pregnancy. Periodic screening throughout pregnancy of women who have admitted to drug use may help them to continue abstinence.

Treatment for substance abuse is individualized for each woman, depending on the type of drug used and the frequency and amount of use. Women are more likely to attempt to stop smoking during pregnancy than at any other time in their lives. Quitting before conception is ideal, but even quitting before 16 weeks of gestation significantly decreases the adverse risks. Smoking-cessation programs during pregnancy are effective and should be offered to all pregnant smokers. These programs should continue throughout the postpartum period as well, because many women resume smoking after the birth. Many smoking cessation resources are available, both in print and online (Gilbert, 2011; Wisner, Sit, Altemus, et al., 2012). For more information on smoking cessation, visit the American Lung Association website at www.lungusa.org or the CDC website at www.cdc.gov/tobacco/quit_smoking/index.htm. In addition, see Box 3-5 for smoking cessation resources provided by the ACOG.

Detoxification, short-term inpatient or outpatient treatment, long-term residential treatment, aftercare services, and self-help support groups are all possible options for alcohol and drug abuse. Women for Sobriety may be a more helpful organization for women than Alcoholics Anonymous or Narcotics Anonymous, which were originally developed for male substance abusers. In general long-term treatment of any sort is becoming increasingly difficult to obtain, particularly for women who lack insurance coverage. Although some programs allow a woman to keep her children with her at the treatment facility, far too few of them are available to meet the demand.

Pregnant women requiring withdrawal from alcohol should be admitted for inpatient management. Alcohol withdrawal treatment during pregnancy consists of the administration of benzodiazepines. Chlordiazepoxide (Librium), diazepam (Valium), lorazepam (Ativan), and oxazepam (Serax) are benzodiazepines that are commonly used. Disulfiram (Antabuse) is teratogenic; therefore its use in aversion therapy is contraindicated during pregnancy. Currently there are four medications approved by the FDA for the treatment of alcohol dependence, but their use during pregnancy has been very limited. Acute management of alcohol withdrawal also includes thiamine replacement and maintenance of adequate hydration and electrolyte balance (Wisner, Sit, Altemus, et al., 2012).

Methadone maintenance treatment (MMT) is currently considered the standard of care for pregnant women who are dependent on heroin or other narcotics. Buprenorphine (Subutex or Suboxone) is another medication approved for opioid addiction treatment that is being used increasingly during pregnancy. Opioid replacement therapy has been shown to decrease opioid and other drug abuse; reduce criminal activity; improve individual functioning; and decrease rates of infections such as hepatitis B and C, HIV, other sexually transmitted infections, and tuberculosis. In addition, opioid replacement therapy is associated with reduced fetal exposure to illicit drug use and improved neonatal outcomes. However, 30% to 80% of infants exposed to opioids, including methadone or buprenorphine, in utero require treatment for neonatal abstinence syndrome (NAS). Neither the incidence nor the severity of NAS correlates directly with the maternal medication dose at birth (Wisner, Sit, Altemus, et al., 2012).

Pregnant women who use cocaine should be advised to stop using immediately. These women need a great deal of assistance such as an alcohol and drug treatment program, individual or group counseling, and participation in self-help support groups to accomplish this major lifestyle change successfully.

Methamphetamines are stimulants with vasoconstrictive characteristics similar to those of cocaine and are used similarly. As is the case with cocaine users, methamphetamine users are urged to immediately stop all use during pregnancy. Unfortunately, because methamphetamine users are extremely psychologically addicted, the rate of relapse is very high.

Although substance abusers may be difficult to care for at any time, they are often particularly challenging during the intrapartum and postpartum periods because of manipulative and demanding behavior. Typically these women display poor control over their behavior and a low threshold for pain. Increased dependency needs and poor parenting skills may also be apparent.

Nurses must understand that substance abuse is an illness and that these women deserve to be treated with patience, kindness, consistency, and firmness when necessary (Box 11-5). Even women who are actively abusing drugs experience pain during labor and after giving birth and may need both pain medication and nonpharmacologic interventions. Developing a standardized plan of care so patients have limited opportunities to play staff members against one another is helpful. Mother-infant attachment should be promoted by identifying the woman's strengths and reinforcing positive maternal feelings and behaviors. Staffing should be sufficient to ensure strict surveillance of visitors and prevent unsupervised drug use.

Advice regarding breastfeeding must be individualized. Although all abused substances appear in breast milk, some in greater amounts than others (Lawrence and Lawrence, 2005), breastfeeding is definitely contraindicated in women who use amphetamines, alcohol, cocaine, heroin, or marijuana. However, methadone use is not a contraindication to breastfeeding. The baby's nutrition and safety needs are of primary importance in this consideration. For some

BOX 11-5	DEALING WITH PREGNANT SUBSTANCE ABUSERS

- Realize that the decision to become and remain sober can *only* be made by the substance abuser.
- Understand that nurses do not have the power to cure anyone. They are only cheerleaders and supporters!
- Educate yourself about the effects of drug use in general and its effect on pregnancy and the newborn specifically.
- Treat substance abusers with the same respect and consideration that you show other people.
- Become familiar with your local treatment centers. Learn which of them accept pregnant women. Keep an up-to-date list of groups meeting in your community.
- Remember that there are no "hopeless cases." It is never too late to quit!
- Practice patience and persistence. It may take months or years to see the effects of your work.

women a desire to breastfeed may provide strong motivation to achieve and maintain sobriety.

Smoking can interfere with the let-down reflex. Women who smoke in the postpartum period and breastfeed should avoid smoking for 2 hours before a feeding to minimize the nicotine in the milk and improve the let-down reflex. All smokers should be discouraged from smoking in the same room with the infant because exposure to secondhand smoke can increase the likelihood that the infant will experience behavioral and respiratory health problems (Lawrence and Lawrence, 2005).

Follow-up Care

Before a known substance abuser is discharged with her baby, the home situation must be assessed to determine that the environment is safe and that someone will be available to meet the infant's needs if the mother is unable to do so. The social services department of the hospital is usually involved in interviewing the mother before discharge to ensure that the infant's needs will be met. Family members or friends are sometimes asked to become actively involved with the mother and infant after discharge. A home care or public health nurse may be asked to make home visits to assess the mother's ability to care for the baby and provide guidance and support. If serious questions about the infant's well-being exist, the case is likely to be referred to the state child protective services agency for further action.

KEY POINTS

- Careful monitoring of blood glucose levels, insulin, or oral hypoglycemic medication administration when necessary and dietary counseling are used to create a normal intrauterine environment for fetal growth and development in the pregnancy complicated by pregestational diabetes or GDM.
- Poor maternal glycemic control before conception and during pregnancy may be responsible for fetal congenital malformations and maternal complications such as miscarriage, infection, and dystocia (difficult labor) caused by macrosomia.
- Maternal insulin requirements increase as the pregnancy progresses and may quadruple by term as a result of insulin resistance created by placental hormones, insulinase, and cortisol.

- Thyroid dysfunction during pregnancy requires close monitoring of thyroid hormone levels to regulate therapy and prevent fetal insult.
- High levels of phenylalanine in the maternal bloodstream cross the placenta and are teratogenic to the fetus. Damage can be prevented or minimized by dietary restriction of phenylalanine.
- The stress of the normal maternal adaptations to pregnancy on a heart the functions of which are already taxed may cause cardiac decompensation.
- Anemia is a common medical disorder of pregnancy, affecting at least 20% of pregnant women.

- Asthma may be the most common potentially serious medical condition to complicate pregnancy. The prevalence and morbidity rates are increasing, although the asthma-related mortality has dropped in recent years.
- A pregnant woman with epilepsy should take only one anticonvulsant medication, at the lowest dose level that is effective at keeping her seizure free if at all possible.

- Many autoimmune disorders (e.g., SLE and MG) are often diagnosed in women during their reproductive years; therefore they may occur during pregnancy.
- Support from a variety of sources, including family and friends, health care providers, and the recovery community, is needed to help perinatal substance abusers achieve and maintain sobriety.

REFERENCES

American College of Obstetricians and Gynecologists (ACOG): *Screening and diagnosis of gestational diabetes mellitus, ACOG Committee Opinion, No. 504,* Washington, DC, 2011, ACOG.

American Diabetes Association (ADA): Position statement: diagnosis and classification of diabetes mellitus, *Diabetes Care* 32(suppl):S62–S67, 2009.

American Society of Addiction Medicine (ASAM): Public policy statement: definition of addiction, 2011, www.asam.org/for-the-public/definition-of-addiction.

Aminoff MJ: Neurologic disorders. In Creasy RK, Resnik R, Iams J, et al, editors: *Creasy & Resnik's maternal-fetal medicine: principles and practice,* ed 6, Philadelphia, 2009, Saunders.

Anderson J, Waller D, Canfield M, et al: Maternal obesity, gestational diabetes, and central nervous system birth defects, *Epidemiology* 16(1):87–92, 2005.

Blackburn S: *Maternal, fetal, and neonatal physiology: a clinical perspective,* ed 4, St Louis, 2013, Mosby.

Blanchard DG, Shabetai R: Cardiac diseases. In Creasy RK, Resnik R, Iams J, et al, editors: *Creasy & Resnik's maternal-fetal medicine: principles and practice,* ed 6, Philadelphia, 2009, Saunders.

Brady T, Ashley O: *Women in substance abuse treatment: results from alcohol and drug services study (ADSS), USDHHS Publication No. SMA 04-3968 analytic series A 26,* Rockville, MD, 2005, Substance and Mental Health Services Administration, Office of Applied Studies.

Cappell M: Hepatic and gastrointestinal diseases. In Gabbe S, Niebyl J, Simpson J, et al, editors: *Obstetrics: normal and problem pregnancies,* ed 6, Philadelphia, 2012, Saunders.

Chin J, Branch D: Collagen vascular diseases. In Gabbe S, Niebyl J, Simpson J, et al, editors: *Obstetrics: normal and problem pregnancies,* ed 6, Philadelphia, 2012, Saunders.

Cunningham F, Leveno K, Bloom S, et al: *Williams obstetrics,* ed 23, New York, 2010, McGraw-Hill.

Easterling TR, Stout K: Heart disease. In Gabbe S, Niebyl J, Simpson J, et al, editors: *Obstetrics: normal and problem pregnancies,* ed 6, Philadelphia, 2012, Saunders.

Feillet F, Agostoni C: Nutritional issues in treating phenylketonuria, *J Inherited Metabol Dis* 33(6):659–664, 2010.

Gaddipati S, Troiano N: Cardiac disorders in pregnancy. In Troiano N, Harvey C, Chez B, editors: *AWHONN's high risk and critical care obstetrics,* ed 3, Philadelphia, 2013, Wolters Kluwer/Lippincott Williams & Wilkins.

Gilbert E: *Manual of high risk pregnancy and delivery,* ed 5, St Louis, 2011, Mosby.

Gordon M: Maternal physiology. In Gabbe S, Niebyl J, Simpson J, et al, editors: *Obstetrics: normal and problem pregnancies,* ed 6, Philadelphia, 2012, Saunders.

Guttmacher Institute: Substance abuse during pregnancy, 2010, Washington, DC, www.ncjrs.gov/App/Publications/abstract.aspex?ID=252886.

Harris LH, Paltrow L: The status of pregnant women and fetuses in US criminal law, *JAMA* 289(13):1697–1699, 2003.

Iams J, Romero R, Creasy R: Preterm labor and birth. In Creasy RK, Resnik R, Iams J, et al, editors: *Creasy & Resnik's maternal-fetal medicine: principles and practice,* ed 6, Philadelphia, 2009, Saunders.

Inturrisi M, Lintner, NC, Sorem K: Diabetic ketoacidosis and continuous insulin infusion management in pregnancy. In Troiano N, Harvey C, Chez B, editors: *AWHONN's high risk and critical care obstetrics,* ed 3, Philadelphia, 2013, Wolters Kluwer/Lippincott Williams & Wilkins.

Katz V: Postpartum care. In Gabbe S, Niebyl J, Simpson J, et al, editors: *Obstetrics: normal and problem pregnancies,* ed 6, Philadelphia, 2012, Saunders.

Kilpatrick SJ: Anemia and pregnancy. In Creasy RK, Resnik R, Iams J, et al, editors: *Creasy & Resnik's maternal-fetal medicine: principles and practice,* ed 6, Philadelphia, 2009, Saunders.

Kroumpouzos G: Skin disease in pregnancy and puerperium. In Gabbe S, Niebyl J, Simpson J, et al, editors: *Obstetrics: normal and problem pregnancies,* ed 6, Philadelphia, 2012, Saunders.

Landon M, Catalano P, Gabbe S: Diabetes mellitus complicating pregnancy. In Gabbe S, Niebyl J, Simpson J, et al, editors: *Obstetrics: normal and problem pregnancies,* ed 6, Philadelphia, 2012, Saunders.

Lawrence RA, Lawrence RM: *Breastfeeding: a guide for the medical profession,* ed 6, St Louis, 2005, Mosby.

Mestman JH: Thyroid and parathyroid diseases in pregnancy. In Gabbe S, Niebyl J, Simpson J, et al, editors: *Obstetrics: normal and*

problem pregnancies, ed 6, Philadelphia, 2012, Saunders.

Moore TR, Catalano P: Diabetes in pregnancy. In Creasy RK, Resnik R, Iams J, et al, editors: *Creasy & Resnik's maternal-fetal medicine: principles and practice,* ed 6, Philadelphia, 2009, Saunders.

Nader S: Thyroid disease and pregnancy. In Creasy RK, Resnik R, Iams J, et al, editors: *Creasy & Resnik's maternal-fetal medicine: principles and practice,* ed 6, Philadelphia, 2009, Saunders.

National Center for Chronic Disease Prevention and Health Promotion: Diabetes successes and opportunities for population-based prevention and control at a glance, 2011, www.cdc.gov/chronicdisease/resources/publications/AAG/ddt.htm.

Niebyl J, Simpson J: Drugs and environmental agents in pregnancy and lactation: Embryology, teratology, epidemiology. In Gabbe S, Niebyl J, Simpson J, et al, editors: *Obstetrics: normal and problem pregnancies,* ed 6, Philadelphia, 2012, Saunders.

Otten JJ, Helwig JP, Meyers LD, editors: *Dietary reference intakes: the essential guide to nutrient requirements,* Washington, DC, 2006, National Academies Press.

Paidas M, Hossain N: Embryonic and fetal demise. In Creasy RK, Resnik R, Iams J, et al, editors: *Creasy & Resnik's maternal-fetal medicine: principles and practice,* ed 6, Philadelphia, 2009, Saunders.

Porter T: Branch D: Autoimmune diseases. In James D, Steer P, Weiner C, et al, editors: *High risk pregnancy: management options,* ed 3, Philadelphia, 2006, Saunders.

Rapini R: The skin and pregnancy. In Creasy RK, Resnik R, Iams J, et al, editors: *Creasy & Resnik's maternal-fetal medicine: principles and practice,* ed 6, Philadelphia, 2009, Saunders.

Samuels P: Hematologic complications of pregnancy. In Gabbe S, Niebyl J, Simpson J, et al, editors: *Obstetrics: normal and problem pregnancies,* ed 6, Philadelphia, 2012, Saunders.

Samuels P, Niebyl JR: Neurologic disorders. In Gabbe S, Niebyl J, Simpson J, et al, editors: *Obstetrics: normal and problem pregnancies,* ed 6, Philadelphia, 2012, Saunders.

Seidel H, Ball J, Dains J, et al: *Mosby's guide to physical examination,* ed 7, St Louis, 2011, Mosby.

Simhan H, Iams J, Romero R: Preterm birth. In Gabbe S, Niebyl J, Simpson J, et al, editors:

Obstetrics: normal and problem pregnancies, ed 6, Philadelphia, 2012, Saunders.

Stuart M, Bergstrom L: Pregnancy and multiple sclerosis, *J Midwifery Women's Health* 56(1):41–47, 2011.

Wapner R, Jenkins T, Khalek N: Prenatal diagnosis of congenital disorders. In Creasy RK, Resnik R, Iams J, et al, editors: *Creasy & Resnik's maternal-fetal medicine: principles and practice,* ed 6, Philadelphia, 2009, Saunders.

Whitty JE, Dombrowski MP: Respiratory diseases in pregnancy. In Creasy RK, Resnik R, Iams J, et al, editors: *Creasy & Resnik's maternal-fetal medicine: principles and practice,* ed 6, Philadelphia, 2009, Saunders.

Whitty J, Dombrowski M: Respiratory diseases in pregnancy. In Gabbe S, Niebyl J, Simpson J, et al, editors: *Obstetrics: normal and problem pregnancies,* ed 6, Philadelphia, 2012, Saunders.

Williamson C, Mackillop L: Diseases of the liver, biliary system, and pancreas. In Creasy RK, Resnik R, Iams J, et al, editors: *Creasy & Resnik's maternal-fetal medicine: principles and practice,* ed 6, Philadelphia, 2009, Saunders.

Wisner K, Sit D, Altemus M, et al: Mental health and behavioral disorders in pregnancy. In Gabbe S, Niebyl J, Simpson J, et al, editors: *Obstetrics: normal and problem pregnancies,* ed 6, Philadelphia, 2012, Saunders.

High Risk Perinatal Care: Gestational Conditions

Kitty Cashion

evolve WEBSITE

http://evolve.elsevier.com/Perry/maternal

LEARNING OBJECTIVES

On completion of this chapter, the reader will be able to:
- Differentiate among gestational hypertension, preeclampsia, and chronic hypertension.
- Describe etiologic theories and pathophysiology of preeclampsia.
- Compare care management of women with mild gestational hypertension or preeclampsia versus severe gestational hypertension or preeclampsia.
- Discuss the preconception, antepartum, intrapartum, and postpartum management of the woman with chronic hypertension.
- Explain the effects of hyperemesis gravidarum on maternal and fetal well-being.
- Differentiate among causes, signs and symptoms, possible complications, and management of miscarriage,

ectopic pregnancy, cervical insufficiency, and hydatidiform mole.
- Compare and contrast placenta previa and placental abruption in relation to signs and symptoms, complications, and management.
- Discuss the diagnosis and management of disseminated intravascular coagulation.
- Discuss signs and symptoms, effects on pregnancy, and management of urinary tract infections.
- Explain the basic principles of care for a pregnant woman undergoing abdominal surgery.
- Discuss implications of trauma on mother and fetus during pregnancy.
- Identify priorities in assessment and stabilization measures for the pregnant trauma victim.

Some women experience significant problems during the months of gestation that can greatly affect pregnancy outcome. Some of these conditions develop as a result of the pregnant state; others are problems that can happen to anyone at any time of life but occur in this case during pregnancy. This chapter discusses a variety of disorders that did not exist before pregnancy, all of which have at least one thing in common: their occurrence in pregnancy puts the woman and fetus at risk. Hypertension in pregnancy, hyperemesis gravidarum, hemorrhagic complications of early and late pregnancy, urinary tract infection (UTI), surgery during pregnancy, and trauma are discussed. For each problem, management throughout the entire perinatal period (antepartum, intrapartum, and postpartum) is included in this chapter; thus all the information for each condition is located in one place in the text.

HYPERTENSION IN PREGNANCY

Significance and Incidence

Hypertensive disorders are some of the most common medical complications of pregnancy, occurring in approximately 5% to

10% of all pregnancies. The incidence varies among hospitals, regions, and countries. Hypertensive disorders are a major cause of maternal and perinatal morbidity and mortality worldwide (Sibai, 2012). In the United States and Canada they are one of the top causes of maternal morbidity and mortality (Harvey and Sibai, 2013). The four most common types of hypertensive disorders occurring in pregnancy are: (1) gestational hypertension, (2) preeclampsia-eclampsia, (3) chronic hypertension, and (4) preeclampsia superimposed on chronic hypertension (Gilbert, 2011; Harvey and Sibai, 2013).

Classification

The classification of hypertensive disorders in pregnancy is confusing because not all health care providers consistently use standard definitions. The classification system most commonly used in the United States is based on reports from the American College of Obstetricians and Gynecologists (ACOG, 2002) and the National High Blood Pressure Education Program (2000). This classification system is summarized in Table 12-1.

TABLE 12-1	CLASSIFICATION OF HYPERTENSIVE STATES OF PREGNANCY
TYPE	**DESCRIPTION**
Gestational Hypertensive Disorders	
Gestational hypertension	Development of hypertension after week 20 of pregnancy in previously normotensive woman without proteinuria
Preeclampsia	Development of hypertension and proteinuria in previously normotensive woman after 20 weeks of gestation or in early postpartum period; in presence of trophoblastic disease preeclampsia can develop before 20 weeks of gestation
Eclampsia	Development of convulsions or coma not attributable to other causes in preeclamptic woman
Chronic Hypertensive Disorders	
Chronic hypertension	Hypertension in pregnant woman present before pregnancy or diagnosed before 20 weeks of gestation and persistent after 12 weeks postpartum
Superimposed preeclampsia or eclampsia	In women with hypertension before 20 weeks of gestation, new-onset proteinuria In women with both hypertension and proteinuria before 20 weeks of gestation: worsening hypertension or proteinuria

Data from American College of Obstetricians and Gynecologists (ACOG): *Diagnosis and management of preeclampsia and eclampsia,* AGOG Practice Bulletin No. 33, Washington DC, 2002, ACOG; Harvey C, Sibai B: Hypertension in pregnancy. In Troiano NH, Harvey CJ, Chez BF, editors: *AWHONN's high risk and critical care obstetrics,* ed 3, Philadelphia, 2013, Lippincott Williams & Wilkins.

Gestational Hypertension

Gestational hypertension is the onset of hypertension without proteinuria after week 20 of pregnancy (ACOG, 2002; National High Blood Pressure Education Program, 2000). Hypertension is defined as a systolic blood pressure (BP) greater than 140 mm Hg or a diastolic BP greater than 90 mm Hg. The hypertension should be recorded on at least two separate occasions at least 4 to 6 hours apart but within a maximum of a 1-week period (ACOG, 2002; Harvey and Sibai, 2013; National High Blood Pressure Education Program, 2000). Only one pressure (either systolic or diastolic) needs to be elevated to meet the definition of hypertension (Harvey and Sibai, 2013). Both the National High Blood Pressure Education Program and the American Heart Association (AHA) have published extensive recommendations for accurately measuring BP (Pickering, Hall, Appel, et al., 2005; National High Blood Pressure Education Program, 2000). Box 12-1 provides detailed instructions for measurement.

Gestational hypertension is further classified as either mild or severe. The definitions of mild and severe gestational hypertension are the same as the definitions for BP readings for mild and severe preeclampsia (Table 12-2). Gestational hypertension does not persist longer than 12 weeks postpartum and usually resolves during the first postpartum week (Harvey and Sibai, 2013). Some women who

BOX 12-1	BLOOD PRESSURE MEASUREMENT

- Measure blood pressure with the woman seated (ambulatory) or in the lateral recumbent position with the arm at heart level. Neither the woman nor the health care provider should talk while the blood pressure is being measured.
- After positioning allow the woman at least 10 minutes of quiet rest before blood pressure measurement to encourage relaxation.
- Instruct the woman to refrain from tobacco or caffeine use 30 minutes before blood pressure measurement.
- Use the right arm each time.
- Support the arm in a horizontal position at heart level.
- Use the proper-size cuff (cuff should cover approximately 80% of the upper arm or be 1½ times the length of the upper arm).
- Maintain a slow, steady deflation rate.
- Take the average of two readings at least 6 hours apart to minimize recorded blood pressure variations across time.
- Use Korotkoff phase V (disappearance of sound) for recording the diastolic value.
- Use accurate equipment. The mercury sphygmomanometer is the most accurate device.
- If interchanging manual and electronic devices, use caution in interpreting different blood pressure values.

initially are thought to have gestational hypertension will eventually be diagnosed with chronic hypertension. Others will develop proteinuria, thereby changing their diagnosis to preeclampsia.

Preeclampsia

Preeclampsia is a pregnancy-specific condition in which hypertension and proteinuria develop after 20 weeks of gestation in a woman who previously had neither condition. It occurs in approximately 2% to 7% of healthy nulliparous pregnant women and much more frequently in women with multifetal gestation, a history of preeclampsia, chronic hypertension, and preexisting diabetes (Sibai, 2012). Preeclampsia is a vasospastic, systemic disorder and is usually categorized as mild or severe for purposes of management (ACOG, 2002; National High Blood Pressure Education Program, 2000). Table 12-2 lists criteria for mild and severe preeclampsia, and Table 12-3 gives common laboratory changes that occur in both.

Eclampsia

Eclampsia is the onset of seizure activity or coma in a woman with preeclampsia who has no history of preexisting pathology that can result in seizure activity (Harvey and Sibai, 2013; Roberts and Funai, 2009). Eclamptic seizures can occur before, during, or after birth. Approximately one third of eclamptic seizures occur after birth, almost always within the first 48 hours after birth (Roberts and Funai, 2009).

Chronic Hypertensive Disorders

Chronic Hypertension. Chronic hypertension is defined as hypertension that is present before the pregnancy or develops before 20 weeks of gestation. Hypertension initially diagnosed during pregnancy that persists longer than 12 weeks postpartum is also classified as chronic hypertension (Harvey and Sibai, 2013; Roberts and Funai, 2009). Chronic hypertension is further classified as mild or severe based on systolic and diastolic BPs. Most women with mild chronic hypertension experience uncomplicated pregnancies. However,

TABLE 12-2	DIFFERENTIATION BETWEEN MILD AND SEVERE PREECLAMPSIA	
	MILD PREECLAMPSIA	**SEVERE PREECLAMPSIA**
Maternal Effects		
Blood pressure (BP)	BP reading ≥140/90 mm Hg × 2, at least 4-6 hr apart but within a maximum of a 1-wk period	Rise to ≥160/110 mm Hg on two occasions at least 6 hr apart
Proteinuria		
Qualitative dipstick	≥1+ on dipstick on two random urine samples collected at least 4-6 hr apart	≥3+ on dipstick on two random urine samples collected at least 4 hr apart
Quantitative 24-hr analysis	Proteinuria of ≥300 mg in a 24-hr specimen	Proteinuria of ≥5 g in a 24-hr specimen
Urine output	≥25-30 mL/hr	<500 mL/24 hr
Headache	Absent or transient	Persistent or severe
Visual problems	Absent	Blurred, photophobia
Irritability or changes in affect	Transient	May be severe
Epigastric or right upper quadrant pain, nausea, and vomiting	Absent	May be present
Thrombocytopenia	Absent	May be present
Impaired liver function	Normal	May be present
Pulmonary edema	Absent	May be present
Fetal Effects		
Placental perfusion	Reduced	Decreased perfusion expressing as IUGR in fetus; abnormal fetal status on antepartum testing

Data from American College of Obstetricians and Gynecologists (ACOG): *Diagnosis and management of preeclampsia and eclampsia*, ACOG Practice Bulletin No. 33, Washington DC, 2002, ACOG; Harvey C, Sibai B: Hypertension in pregnancy. In Troiano NH, Harvey CJ, Chez BF, editors: *AWHONN's high risk and critical care obstetrics*, ed 3, Philadelphia, 2013, Lippincott Williams & Wilkins.
IUGR, Intrauterine growth restriction.

those with severe chronic hypertension have an increased risk of perinatal mortality (Gilbert, 2011).

Chronic Hypertension with Superimposed Preeclampsia. Women with chronic hypertension may develop superimposed preeclampsia, which increases the morbidity for mother and fetus. A diagnosis of chronic hypertension with superimposed preeclampsia is made with the following findings (Harvey and Sibai, 2013):

- In women with hypertension before 20 weeks of gestation
- New-onset proteinuria
  - In women with both hypertension and proteinuria before 20 weeks of gestation
  - Significant worsening of hypertension or proteinuria

PREECLAMPSIA

Etiology

Preeclampsia is a condition unique to human pregnancy. Signs and symptoms develop only during pregnancy and disappear soon after birth of the fetus and expulsion of the placenta. Common risk factors associated with the development of preeclampsia are listed in Box 12-2. The strongest risk factors are a first pregnancy when the woman is younger than 19 or older than 40 years of age, a first pregnancy with a new partner, and a history of severe preeclampsia (Gilbert, 2011).

The cause of preeclampsia is unknown. Many theories have been suggested to explain its etiology. Current theories that are still being considered include abnormal trophoblast invasion, immunologic response to partially foreign genetic placental and fetal tissue, stimulation of the inflammatory system by cardiovascular changes of pregnancy, various dietary deficiencies, and genetic abnormalities (Harvey and Sibai, 2013).

Pathophysiology

Preeclampsia can progress along a continuum from mild-to-severe preeclampsia to eclampsia. Current thought is that the pathologic changes that occur in the woman with preeclampsia are caused by disruptions in placental perfusion and endothelial cell dysfunction (Gilbert, 2011; Harvey and Sibai, 2013; Sibai, 2012). These changes are present long before the clinical diagnosis of preeclampsia is made (Roberts and Funai, 2009). Normally in pregnancy the spiral arteries in the uterus widen from thick-walled muscular vessels to thinner, saclike vessels with much larger diameters. This change increases the capacity of the vessels, allowing them to handle the increased blood volume of pregnancy. Because this vascular remodeling does not occur or only partially develops in women with preeclampsia, decreased placental perfusion and hypoxia result (Harvey and Sibai, 2013). Placental ischemia is thought to cause endothelial cell dysfunction by stimulating the release of a substance that is toxic to endothelial cells. This anomaly causes generalized vasospasm, which results in poor tissue perfusion in all organ systems, increased peripheral resistance and BP, and increased endothelial cell permeability, leading to intravascular protein and fluid loss and ultimately to less plasma volume. The main pathogenic factor is not an increase in BP but poor perfusion as a result of vasospasm and reduced plasma volume (Fig. 12-1) (Gilbert, 2011; Roberts and Funai, 2009). Fig. 12-2 demonstrates how endothelial cell dysfunction causes many of the common signs and symptoms of preeclampsia.

Reduced kidney perfusion decreases the glomerular filtration rate and can lead to degenerative glomerular changes and oliguria. Pathologic changes in the endothelial cells of the glomeruli (glomerular endotheliosis) are uniquely characteristic of preeclampsia. Protein, primarily albumin, is lost in the urine. Uric acid clearance is decreased, but serum uric acid levels increase. Sodium and water are retained. Acute tubular necrosis and renal failure may occur (Gilbert, 2011; Roberts and Funai, 2009).

Plasma colloid osmotic pressure decreases as serum albumin levels decrease. Intravascular volume is reduced as fluid moves out of the intravascular compartment, resulting in hemoconcentration,

TABLE 12-3 COMMON LABORATORY CHANGES IN PREECLAMPSIA

	NORMAL NONPREGNANT	PREECLAMPSIA	HELLP
Hemoglobin, hematocrit	12-16 g/dL, 37%-47%	May ↑	↓
Platelets (cells/mm³)	150,000-400,000/mm³	Unchanged or <100,000/mm³	<100,000/mm³
Prothrombin time (PT), partial thromboplastin time (PTT)	12-14 sec, 60-70 sec	Unchanged	Unchanged
Fibrinogen	200-400 mg/dL	300-600 mg/dL	↓
Fibrin split products (FSPs)	Absent	Absent or present	Present
Blood urea nitrogen (BUN)	10-20 mg/dL	↑	↑
Creatinine	0.5-1.1 mg/dL	>1.2 mg/dL	↑
Lactate dehydrogenase (LDH)*	45-90 units/L	↑	↑ (>600 units/L)
Aspartate aminotransferase (AST)	4-20 units/L	Elevated	↑ (>70 units/L)
Alanine aminotransferase (ALT)	3-21 units/L	Elevated	↑
Creatinine clearance	80-125 mL/min	130-180 mL/min	↓
Burr cells or schistocytes	Absent	Absent	Present
Uric acid	2-6.6 mg/dL	>5.9 mg/dL	>10 mg/dL
Bilirubin (total)	0.1-1 mg/dL	Unchanged or ↑	↑ (>1.2 mg/dL)

Data from American College of Obstetricians and Gynecologists (ACOG): *Diagnosis and management of preeclampsia and eclampsia,* ACOG Practice Bulletin No. 33, Washington DC, 2002, ACOG; Cunningham F, Leveno K, Bloom S, et al, editors: *Williams obstetrics,* ed 23, New York, 2010, McGraw-Hill; Dildy G: Complications of preeclampsia. In Dildy G, Belfort M, Saade G, et al, editors: *Critical care obstetrics,* ed 4, Malden, MA, 2004, Blackwell Science; Harvey C, Sibai B: Hypertension in pregnancy. In Troiano NH, Harvey CJ, Chez BF, editors: *AWHONN's high risk and critical care obstetrics,* ed 3, Philadelphia, 2013, Lippincott Williams & Wilkins.
*LDH values differ according to the test or assays being performed.

BOX 12-2 COMMON RISK FACTORS FOR PREECLAMPSIA

- Primigravida younger than 19 or older than 40 years old
- Severe preeclampsia in a previous pregnancy
- Family history (mother or sister) of preeclampsia
- Paternal history (partner previously fathered a preeclamptic pregnancy in another woman)
- African descent
- Multifetal gestation
- Maternal infection/inflammation in current pregnancy (i.e., urinary tract infection, periodontal disease)
- Preexisting medical or genetic conditions
  - Chronic hypertension
  - Renal disease
  - Pregestational diabetes mellitus
  - Connective tissue disease (i.e., systemic lupus erythematosus, rheumatoid arthritis)
  - Thrombophilia (i.e., antiphospholipid antibody syndrome, protein C or S deficiency, factor V Leiden mutation)
  - Obesity

From Gilbert ES: *Manual of high risk pregnancy and delivery,* ed 5, St Louis, 2011, Mosby; Harvey C, Sibai B: Hypertension in pregnancy. In Troiano N, Harvey C, Chez B, editors: *AWHONN's high risk and critical care obstetrics,* ed 3, Philadelphia, 2013, Lippincott Williams & Wilkins.

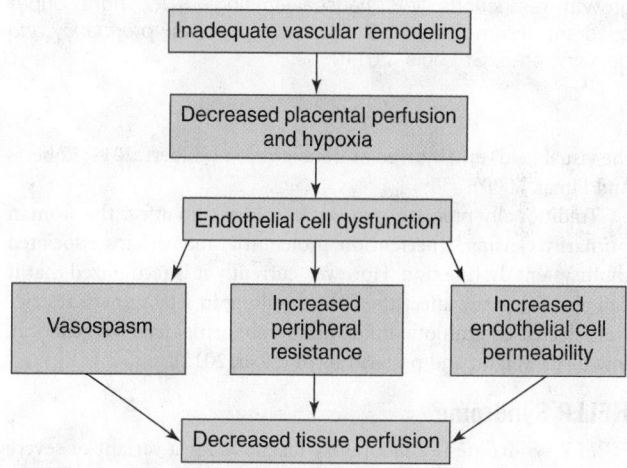

FIG 12-1 Etiology of preeclampsia: disruptions in placental perfusion and endothelial cell dysfunction.

increased blood viscosity, and tissue edema. The hematocrit value increases as fluid leaves the intravascular space. Arteriolar vasospasm can lead to endothelial damage and increased capillary permeability, predisposing the woman to pulmonary edema (see Fig. 12-2) (Gilbert, 2011; Roberts and Funai, 2009).

Decreased liver perfusion can lead to impaired liver function and elevated liver enzyme levels. If hepatic edema and subcapsular hemorrhage develop, the woman may complain of epigastric or right upper quadrant pain. Hemorrhagic necrosis in the liver can result in a subcapsular hematoma, which is a rare occurrence (Gilbert, 2011). Rupture of a subcapsular hematoma is a life-threatening complication and a surgical emergency (see Fig. 12-2).

Neurologic complications associated with preeclampsia include cerebral edema and hemorrhage and increased central nervous system (CNS) irritability. CNS irritability manifests as headaches, hyperreflexia, positive ankle clonus, and seizures. Arteriolar vasospasms and decreased blood flow to the retina can lead to visual disturbances such as scotoma (dim vision or blind or dark spots in

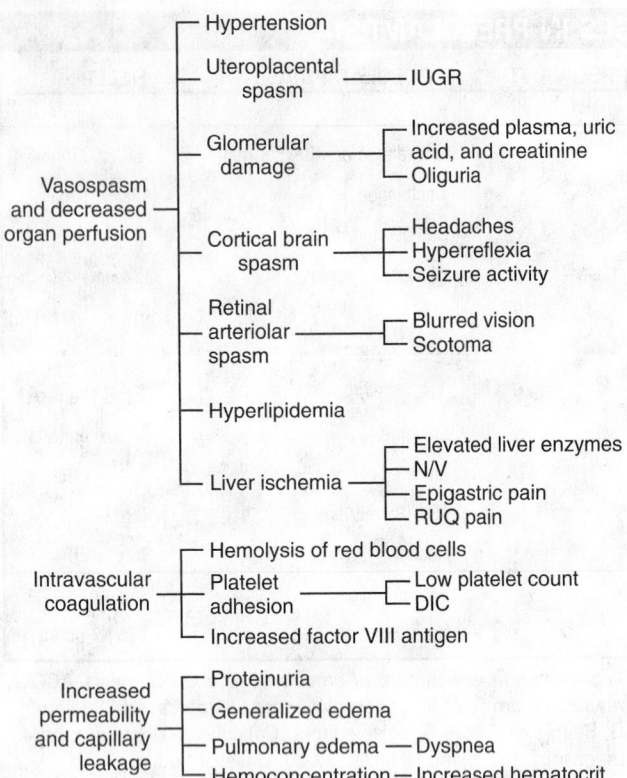

FIG 12-2 Consequences of endothelial cell dysfunction. *DIC,* Disseminated intravascular coagulation; *IUGR,* intrauterine growth restriction; *N/V,* nausea/vomiting; *RUQ,* right upper quadrant. (From Gilbert ES: *Manual of high risk pregnancy and delivery,* ed 5, St Louis, 2011.)

the visual field) and blurred or double vision (Gilbert, 2011; Roberts and Funai, 2009).

Traditionally preeclampsia was considered to affect the woman primarily, causing hypertension, proteinuria, and perhaps associated multisystem dysfunction. However, currently it is recognized that it can also primarily affect the fetus, resulting in fetal growth restriction, decreased amniotic fluid volume, abnormal fetal oxygenation, low birth weight, and preterm birth (Sibai, 2012).

HELLP Syndrome

HELLP syndrome is a laboratory diagnosis for a variant of severe preeclampsia that involves hepatic dysfunction, characterized by hemolysis *(H),* elevated liver enzymes *(EL),* and low platelet count *(LP).* It is not a separate illness. Specific laboratory findings are needed to diagnose HELLP syndrome and distinguish it from other serious diseases that share the same signs and symptoms. HELLP syndrome occurs in 0.5% to 0.9% of all pregnancies. Ten to twenty percent of women with severe preeclampsia develop it (Harvey and Sibai, 2013). Table 12-3 lists laboratory changes that occur in HELLP syndrome. Traditionally it was not diagnosed unless all three laboratory abnormalities were present. Recently, however, women who develop only one or two of the diagnostic laboratory values are being diagnosed with incomplete HELLP, partial HELLP, or the ELLP syndrome (Harvey and Sibai, 2013).

The pathophysiologic changes of HELLP syndrome occur as a result of arteriolar vasospasm, endothelial cell dysfunction with fibrin deposits, and adherence of platelets in blood vessels. Red blood cells are damaged as they pass through narrowed blood vessels and become hemolyzed, resulting in a decreased red blood cell and platelet count and hyperbilirubinemia. Endothelial damage and fibrin deposits in the liver lead to impaired liver function and can cause hemorrhagic necrosis. Liver enzymes are elevated when hepatic tissue is damaged (Gilbert, 2011).

HELLP syndrome usually develops during the antepartum period. The clinical presentation is often nonspecific. Most women with the disorder report a history of malaise, influenza-like symptoms, and epigastric or right upper quadrant abdominal pain. Symptoms tend to worsen at night and improve during the daytime. HELLP syndrome can progress rapidly (Harvey and Sibai, 2013).

> **! NURSING ALERT**
>
> An extremely important point to understand is that many women with HELLP syndrome may not have signs or symptoms of severe preeclampsia. For example, although most women have hypertension, BP may be only mildly elevated in 15% to 50% of cases. Proteinuria may be absent. As a result, women with HELLP syndrome are often misdiagnosed with a variety of other medical or surgical disorders (Sibai, 2012).

HELLP syndrome appears to occur more frequently in Caucasian women than women of other races. A diagnosis of HELLP syndrome is associated with an increased risk for maternal death and adverse perinatal outcomes, including pulmonary edema, acute renal failure, disseminated intravascular coagulopathy (DIC), placental abruption, liver hemorrhage or failure, acute respiratory distress syndrome (ARDS), sepsis, and stroke (Sibai, 2012). The reported perinatal mortality rate ranges from 7.4% to 34%, with a maternal mortality rate of approximately 1% (Sibai, 2012). The rate of preterm birth in women with HELLP syndrome is approximately 70%, with 15% of these occurring before 28 weeks of gestation. Most of the perinatal deaths occur before 28 weeks of gestation in association with placental abruption or severe fetal growth restriction (Sibai, 2012).

CARE MANAGEMENT

Identifying and Preventing Preeclampsia

Numerous clinical trials have examined various interventions to prevent preeclampsia, including protein or salt restriction; zinc, magnesium, fish oil, or vitamins C and E supplementation; use of diuretics or other antihypertensive medications; and use of heparin or low dose aspirin. All of these interventions demonstrated minimal to no benefit in preventing or reducing the severity of preeclampsia (Sibai, 2012).

No reliable test that can be used as a routine screening tool for predicting preeclampsia has yet been developed. However, the search for biomarkers that can identify individual women who will develop hypertension during pregnancy is ongoing (Harvey and Sibai, 2013). For example, the tyrosine kinase (sFLt) and serum placental growth factor (PIGF) ratio at 22 to 26 weeks of gestation was shown in one study to be highly predictive of early-onset preeclampsia (Gilbert, 2011). An abnormal uterine artery Doppler velocimetry in the first or second trimester of pregnancy has also been suggested as a good screening test to predict preeclampsia (Gilbert, 2011).

Although research offers future promise, much work remains before a screening test for preeclampsia is available for widespread clinical use. Nurses should be aware of what strategies are being studied and use the most valid results so they can counsel pregnant women about interventions that are evidence based. Meanwhile the best preeclampsia prevention methods include early prenatal care for the identification of women at risk and early detection of the disease.

Physical Examination

Accurate measurement of BP is essential in the early detection of hypertensive disorders. Personnel caring for pregnant women need to be consistent in taking and recording BP measurements in a standardized manner (see Box 12-1).

Assessment for edema is another component of the physical examination, although the presence of edema is no longer included in the definition of preeclampsia. Edema is assessed for distribution, degree, and pitting. Dependent edema is edema of the lowest or most dependent parts of the body, where hydrostatic pressure is greatest. If a pregnant woman is ambulatory, the edema may first be evident in the feet and ankles. If she is confined to bed, it is more

likely to occur in the sacral region. Pitting edema leaves a small depression or pit after finger pressure is applied to the swollen area (Fig. 12-3). The pit, which is caused by movement of fluid to adjacent tissue away from the point of pressure, normally disappears within 10 to 30 seconds. Although the amount of edema is difficult to quantify, the method shown in Fig. 12-4 may be used to record relative degrees of edema formation.

Deep tendon reflexes (DTRs) reflect the balance between the cerebral cortex and spinal cord. They are evaluated as a baseline and to detect any changes. The biceps and patellar reflexes are assessed, and the findings recorded (Fig. 12-5 and Table 12-4). To elicit the biceps reflex, the examiner strikes a downward blow over the thumb, which is situated over the biceps tendon (see Fig. 12-5, *A*). Normal response is flexion of the arm at the elbow, described as a 2+ response. The patellar reflex is elicited with the woman's legs hanging freely over the end of the examining table or with the woman lying on her side with the knee slightly flexed (see Fig. 12-5, *D*). The patellar tendon (inferior to the patella) is tapped with a percussion hammer. Normal response is the extension or kicking out of the leg.

To assess for hyperactive reflexes (clonus) at the ankle joint, the examiner supports the leg with the knee flexed (see Fig. 12-5, *F*). With one hand the examiner sharply dorsiflexes the foot, maintains

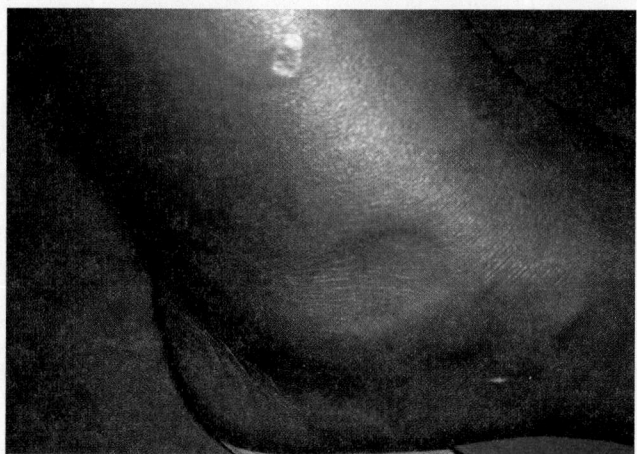

FIG 12-3 Pitting edema. (Courtesy Shannon Perry, Phoenix, AZ.)

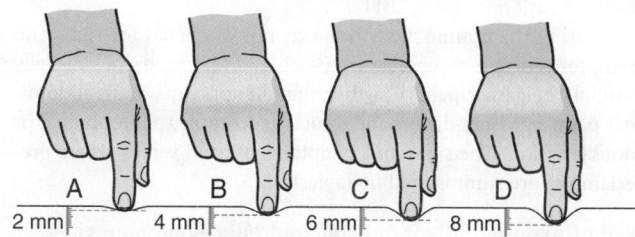

FIG 12-4 Assessment of pitting edema of lower extremities. **A,** +1; **B,** +2; **C,** +3; **D,** +4.

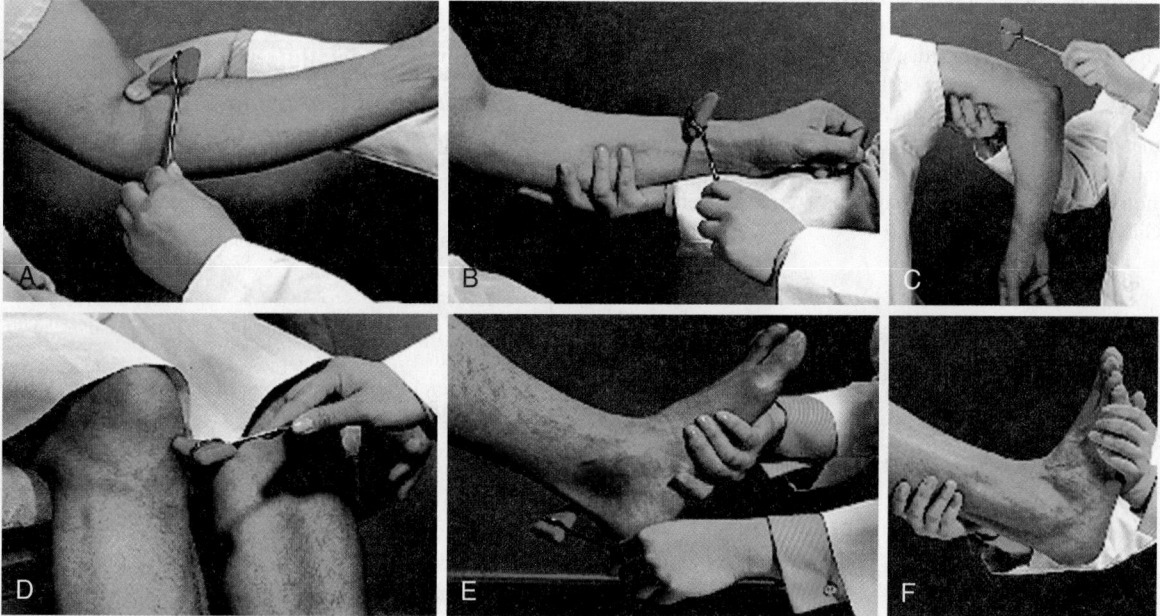

FIG 12-5 Location of tendons for evaluation of deep tendon reflexes. **A,** Biceps. **B,** Brachioradial. **C,** Triceps. **D,** Patellar. **E,** Achilles. **F,** Evaluation of ankle clonus. (From Seidel H, Ball J, Dains J, et al: *Mosby's guide to physical examination,* ed 7, St Louis, 2011, Mosby.)

the position for a moment, and then releases it. Normal (negative clonus) response is elicited when no rhythmic oscillations (jerks) are felt while the foot is held in dorsiflexion. When the foot is released, no oscillations are seen as the foot drops to the plantar-flexed position. Abnormal (positive clonus) response is recognized by rhythmic oscillations of one or more "beats" felt when the foot is in dorsiflexion and seen as the foot drops to the plantar-flexed position.

The presence of *proteinuria* is determined from dipstick testing on a clean-catch or catheterized urine specimen or evaluation of a 24-hour urine collection. Proteinuria is defined as a concentration at or greater than 30 mg/dL (≥1+ on dipstick measurement) in at least two random urine specimens collected at least 6 hours apart. In a 24-hour specimen proteinuria is defined as a concentration at or greater than 300 mg/24 hours. A diagnosis of severe preeclampsia requires a concentration of ≥5 g protein in a 24-hour urine collection or a value of ≥3+ on dipstick (Harvey and Sibai, 2013). Because a 24-hour collection to measure the quantity of protein and creatinine clearance is more reflective of true renal status, it is preferred over dipstick testing. Alkaline, concentrated, or dilute urine can yield a false reading. Urine contaminated with bacteria, blood, and amniotic fluid also can yield a false positive for proteinuria. Therefore, to ensure accurate results, proteinuria should be determined using only a urine specimen that has been collected by either a thorough clean-catch, midstream technique or catheterization (Gilbert, 2011).

During the examination the woman is evaluated for signs and symptoms of severe preeclampsia such as severe headaches (usually frontal); epigastric pain (heartburn); right upper quadrant abdominal pain; or visual disturbances such as scotoma, photophobia, or double vision. The signs and symptoms of mild versus severe preeclampsia are summarized in Table 12-2.

Mild Gestational Hypertension and Mild Preeclampsia

The goals of therapy for women with mild gestational hypertension and mild preeclampsia are to ensure maternal safety and have the woman give birth to a healthy newborn as close to term as possible. At 37 weeks or more of gestation, the plan of care for a woman with mild gestational hypertension or mild preeclampsia is most likely to be the induction of labor, preceded, if necessary, by cervical ripening (Sibai, 2012). When mild gestational hypertension or mild preeclampsia is suspected before 37 weeks of gestation, close observation of maternal and fetal status is necessary. Women with mild gestational hypertension and mild preeclampsia can be managed safely at home, provided they have frequent maternal and fetal evaluation (Gilbert, 2011; Sibai, 2012).

Criteria for home care include BP less than 150/100; proteinuria less than 500 mg/day; normal platelet count, liver enzymes, and creatinine levels; normal fetal status; no signs or symptoms of severe preeclampsia; and a reliable, compliant patient (Gilbert, 2011; Sibai, 2012). Successful home care requires the woman to be well educated about preeclampsia and highly motivated to follow the plan of care (see Patient Teaching box). All teaching should include the woman and her family; and time must be allowed for them to absorb information, ask questions, and voice concerns. Methods for enhancing learning include visual aids, DVDs or Internet videos, handouts, and demonstrations with return demonstrations. Furthermore, the effects of illness, language, age, cultural beliefs, and support systems must be considered.

Maternal and Fetal Assessment. Initial maternal laboratory evaluation includes measurement of serum creatinine, platelet count, liver enzymes, and a 24-hour urine protein assessment. Thereafter the platelet count, liver enzymes, and serum creatinine are usually assessed once each week. Women are also evaluated for signs or symptoms of worsening preeclampsia such as severe headaches, blurred or double vision, mental confusion, right upper quadrant or epigastric pain, nausea or vomiting, shortness of breath, and decreased urinary output (Sibai, 2012). Fetal evaluation generally includes daily fetal movement counts and nonstress testing or a biophysical profile (BPP) once or twice weekly until birth. (See Chapter 10 for more information on fetal assessment tests.) Ultrasound evaluation of amniotic fluid status and determination of estimated fetal weight are performed at the time mild preeclampsia is diagnosed and serially thereafter, depending on findings (Sibai, 2012).

Activity Restriction. Complete or partial bed rest for the duration of the pregnancy is still recommended frequently. However, no evidence has been found that this practice improves pregnancy outcome. Moreover, prolonged bed rest is known to increase the risk of thrombophlebitis (Sibai, 2012). Other adverse physiologic outcomes related to complete bed rest include cardiovascular deconditioning; diuresis with accompanying fluid, electrolyte, and weight loss; muscle atrophy; and psychologic stress. These changes begin

TABLE 12-4	ASSESSING DEEP TENDON REFLEXES
GRADE	DEEP TENDON REFLEX RESPONSE
0	No response
1+	Sluggish or diminished
2+	Active or expected response
3+	More brisk than expected, slightly hyperactive
4+	Brisk, hyperactive, with intermittent or transient clonus

From Seidel HM, Ball JW, Dains JE, et al: *Mosby's guide to physical examination*, ed 7, St Louis, 2011, Mosby.

PATIENT TEACHING

Assessing and Reporting Clinical Signs of Preeclampsia

- Take your blood pressure as directed. Use your right arm in a sitting position each time for consistent and accurate readings. Support the arm on a table in a horizontal position at heart level.
- Report to your health care provider immediately any increase in your blood pressure.
- Dipstick test your clean-catch urine sample as directed to assess proteinuria.
- Report to your health care provider if proteinuria is 2+ or more or if you have a decrease in urine output.
- Assess your baby's activity daily. Decreased activity (four or fewer movements per hour) may indicate fetal compromise and should be reported.
- Be sure to keep your scheduled prenatal appointments so any changes in your or your baby's condition can be detected.
- Keep a daily log or diary of your assessments for your home health care nurse or bring it with you to your next prenatal visit.
- Report to your health care provider immediately any headache, dizziness, or blurring of vision.

on the first day of bed rest and continue for the duration of therapy. Therefore restricted activity rather than complete bed rest is recommended (Sibai, 2012).

Women with mild preeclampsia generally feel reasonably well; therefore boredom from activity restriction is common. Diversionary activities, including television and computer or smart phone use, visits from friends, and creation of a comfortable and convenient environment are ways to cope with the boredom. Participation in online prenatal classes may also be possible. Gentle exercise (e.g., range-of-motion exercises, stretching, Kegel exercises, pelvic tilts) is important in maintaining muscle tone, blood flow, regularity of bowel function, and a sense of well-being (see Patient Teaching box).

A high risk pregnancy can be very stressful for the woman and her family. Family stressors include separation from family members when hospitalized, need for activity restriction, financial concerns, ability to manage the household, family activities, and child care. The family needs to use coping mechanisms and support systems to help them through this crisis. An excellent Internet-based support group for pregnant women on bed rest is Sidelines

(www.sidelines.org) (Gilbert, 2011). Relaxation techniques can also help to reduce stress and prepare the woman for labor and birth.

Diet. Women with mild preeclampsia can have a regular diet with adequate protein (60 to 70 g), calcium (1200 mg), 600 mcg of folic acid, and adequate zinc (11 to 12 mg) and sodium (1.5 g) (Gilbert, 2011; Otten, Helwig, and Meyers, 2006). Adequate fluid intake (six to eight 8-ounce glasses of water per day) is encouraged to enhance renal perfusion and bowel function (Gilbert, 2011) (see Patient Teaching box on p. 310).

Severe Gestational Hypertension and Severe Preeclampsia

Women with severe gestational hypertension are at greater risk for pregnancy complications than are women with mild preeclampsia. Therefore these women should be managed as if they have severe preeclampsia. Women diagnosed with severe gestational hypertension or severe preeclampsia should be hospitalized immediately for a thorough evaluation of maternal-fetal status (Sibai, 2012). These women are placed on magnesium sulfate on admission to prevent eclamptic seizures. Maternal assessments include monitoring BP;

PATIENT TEACHING

Coping with Activity Restriction

At Home

- Clarify with your health care provider: What is bed rest? Question your activity level, positioning, bathroom privileges, children's visits, activities, personal hygiene, mobility, diet, and visitors.
- Have your computer or smart phone available at your bedside. Both devices can be used for communication with friends, to conduct business, and to shop as necessary. Also use your computer or smart phone to communicate with Internet support groups and obtain information.
- Have a television and DVD player to watch television programs or movies and a radio, CD player, or MP3 player to listen to music.
- Delegate responsibilities to family members or friends as much as possible (i.e., attend to the laundry, pick up groceries, drop off and pick up dry cleaning, meet repair people, attend to child care, organize meals).
- Have these available for use on your bed or couch:
  - Egg crate mattress
  - Pillows and more pillows (body pillow)
- Keep a big trash basket near your bed and daytime resting place.
- Place a box or crate near the bed/sofa to store items such as:
  - Post-it notes
  - Cups with lids and flexible straws
  - Paper plates
  - Plastic forks, spoons, and knives
  - Baby monitor or walkie-talkies
  - Wet wipes
  - Notebook to record questions for providers, telephone numbers, to-do lists
  - Envelopes and stationery
  - Take-out menus
  - Reading materials
  - Books
  - Audio books
  - Magazines
- Stock mini-refrigerator or cooler with water or other beverages or healthy snacks.

- Plan for family time—visits and interaction, particularly with small children (see the Patient Teaching box: Activities for Children of Women on Activity Restriction on p. 447).
- Explore your interest in a new hobby.
  - Work crossword or jigsaw puzzles.
  - Learn to embroider, smock, crochet, or knit.
  - Do mending or sewing.
- Do craft projects; make something for the baby.
- Identify relaxation exercises and activities (music) and implement.
- Arrange to have a facial, manicure/pedicure, neck massage, or other special treat when you need a lift.

In the Hospital

- Clarify with your health care provider: What is bed rest? Question your activity level, positioning, bathroom privileges, children's visits, activities, personal hygiene, mobility, diet, and visitors.
- In addition to survival tips for the home, the following may be useful in the hospital setting:
  - Bring your own pillow, shampoo, and conditioner.
  - Have a wheelchair for outside visits or visiting other antepartal women if allowed.
  - If possible bring a laptop computer so you can watch movies or television programs if Internet access is available.
  - Ask friends to bring healthy food and snacks rather than flowers when visiting.
  - Explore your interest in handheld games.
  - Work with staff regarding scheduling (e.g., obstetric provider examinations, vital signs, nursing assessments).
  - Bring earplugs to block the hospital noise.
  - Ask for a room with a view.
  - Have a large calendar and clock for easy viewing. Record significant events on the calendar.

PATIENT TEACHING

Diet for Preeclampsia

- Eat a nutritious, balanced diet (60 to 70 g protein, 1200 mg calcium, 600 mcg of folic acid, 11 to 12 mg of zinc, and 1.5 g of sodium). Consult with registered dietitian on the diet best suited for you as an individual.
- Salt foods to taste. Limiting excessively salty foods (luncheon meats, pretzels, chips, pickles, and sauerkraut) will likely be necessary to meet the recommended sodium intake of 1.5 g/day.
- Eat foods with roughage (whole grains, raw fruits, and vegetables).
- Drink six to eight 8-ounce glasses of water per day.
- Avoid alcohol and tobacco and limit caffeine intake.

BOX 12-3 HOSPITAL PRECAUTIONARY MEASURES FOR WOMEN WITH PREECLAMPSIA

- Environment:
  - Quiet
  - Nonstimulating
  - Lighting subdued
- Seizure precautions:
  - Suction equipment tested and ready to use
  - Oxygen administration equipment tested and ready to use
  - Call button within easy reach
- Emergency medications available on the unit:
  - Hydralazine
  - Labetalol
  - Nifedipine
  - Magnesium sulfate
  - Calcium gluconate or calcium chloride
- Emergency birth pack easily accessible

---

urine output; cerebral status; and the presence of epigastric pain, tenderness, labor, or vaginal bleeding (Sibai, 2012). Laboratory evaluation includes a platelet count, liver enzymes, and serum creatinine (see Table 12-3). Fetal assessment includes continuous electronic fetal heart rate monitoring, a BPP, and ultrasound evaluation of fetal growth and amniotic fluid (Sibai, 2012).

After this initial assessment period a multidisciplinary plan of care is developed with the woman and her family. The goals of care management are to ensure maternal safety, assess the degree of maternal and fetal risk, formulate a plan for giving birth, and prevent eclampsia and other serious complications. If the pregnancy is 34 weeks of gestation or greater, birth will likely be accomplished promptly, either as cesarean or after labor induction. By 34 weeks of gestation, the risks of continuing the pregnancy are considered greater than the risks of preterm birth (Sibai, 2012).

Expectant Management

Women who are between 24 0/7 and 32 6/7 weeks of gestation and have no indication for giving birth immediately may be candidates for expectant management. These women should be hospitalized at a tertiary care facility that is able to provide both maternal and neonatal intensive care. Care-management decisions should be made in consultation with a maternal fetal medicine (perinatologist) specialist, and patient and family counseling by a neonatologist should be provided (Sibai, 2012).

Expectant management includes the use of oral antihypertensive medications as needed to maintain the systolic BP between 140 and 155 mm Hg and the diastolic BP between 90 and 105 mm Hg. Management also includes ongoing maternal and fetal assessment for indicators of worsening condition (Sibai, 2012). Corticosteroids (betamethasone) are ordered to enhance fetal lung maturation. The dose is 12.5 mg intramuscularly, repeated in 24 hours. Optimal benefit begins 24 hours after the first dose is administered and lasts for 7 days (Gilbert, 2011; Sibai, 2012). Most women managed expectantly develop a maternal or fetal indication for giving birth within 2 weeks, although some are able to continue their pregnancies safely for several more weeks. Immediate birth is indicated if eclampsia, pulmonary edema, placental abruption, DIC, or renal dysfunction develops (Sibai, 2012).

Intrapartum Care

Intrapartum nursing care is directed toward the early identification of fetal heart rate (FHR) abnormalities and the prevention of maternal complications. Continuous FHR and uterine contraction monitoring are initiated, and the woman is assessed for signs of placental abruption such as uterine tachysystole or vaginal bleeding. Maternal evaluation also includes assessment of the central nervous, cardiovascular, pulmonary, and renal systems. Vital signs and assessments are performed as ordered and per hospital policy (see Nursing Care Plan). Patient and family education and supportive measures are also initiated (Gilbert, 2011; Simpson and Creehan, 2008).

The woman with severe preeclampsia is maintained on bed rest with the side rails up in a quiet, darkened environment. Emergency drugs, oxygen, and suction equipment should be checked and readily available (Box 12-3). To reduce the risk of pulmonary edema, total intravenous (IV) and oral fluids should not exceed 125 mL/hr. Intensive hemodynamic monitoring is not a routine standard of care and is indicated only in the presence of pulmonary edema or oliguria unresponsive to fluid challenge or severe hypertension unresponsive to medications. A pulmonary artery (Swan-Ganz) catheter can be inserted to evaluate central venous and pulmonary artery pressures (Gilbert, 2011; Simpson and Creehan, 2008).

Magnesium Sulfate. Magnesium sulfate is the drug of choice in the prevention and treatment of seizure activity (eclampsia) caused by severe preeclampsia (see Evidence-Based Practice box). It is almost always administered intravenously as a secondary infusion (piggyback) by a volumetric infusion pump. Per protocol or health care provider's order, an initial loading dose of 4 to 6 g of magnesium sulfate is infused over 15 to 30 minutes. This dose is followed by a maintenance dose of magnesium sulfate that is diluted in an IV solution (e.g., 40 g of magnesium sulfate in 1000 mL of lactated Ringer's solution [1 g = 25 mL]) and administered by an infusion pump at 2 g/hr. This dose should maintain a therapeutic serum magnesium level of 4 to 7 mEq/L. After the loading dose, transient lowering of the arterial BP may occur secondary to relaxation of smooth muscle (Cunningham, Leveno, Bloom, et al., 2010; Gilbert, 2011).

Magnesium sulfate is rarely given intramuscularly because the absorption rate cannot be controlled, injections are painful, and tissue necrosis may occur. However, the intramuscular (IM) route may be used in low-resource settings or with some women who are being transported to a tertiary care center. The IM dose is a 10-g loading dose (administered as two separate injections of 5 g in each buttock). The maintenance dosage is 5 g administered every 4 hours in alternating buttocks (Harvey and Sibai, 2013). Local anesthetic can be added to the solution to reduce injection pain. The Z-track technique should be used for the deep IM injection, followed by gentle massage at the site.

◎ NURSING CARE PLAN

Severe Preeclampsia

NURSING DIAGNOSIS	EXPECTED OUTCOME	INTERVENTIONS	RATIONALES
Risk for Injury to woman and fetus related to CNS irritability (seizures)	Woman will show diminished signs of CNS irritability (e.g., DTRs ≤2+, absence of clonus) and have no seizure activity.	Establish baseline data (e.g., DTRs, clonus).	To use as basis for evaluating effectiveness of treatment
		Administer IV magnesium sulfate per physician's orders.	To decrease hyperreflexia and minimize risk of seizure activity
		Monitor maternal vital signs, level of consciousness, FHR, urine output, DTRs, IV flow rate, and serum levels of magnesium sulfate.	To assess for and prevent magnesium sulfate toxicity (e.g., drowsiness, lethargy, slurred speech, loss of DTRs, depressed respirations, cardiac arrest)
		Have calcium gluconate or calcium chloride on the unit.	To be available if needed as an antidote for magnesium sulfate toxicity
		Maintain a quiet, darkened environment.	To avoid stimuli that may precipitate seizure activity
Ineffective Tissue Perfusion related to preeclampsia secondary to arteriolar vasospasm	Woman will exhibit signs of adequate tissue perfusion (i.e., adequate urine output and normal FHR tracing).	Administer IV magnesium sulfate per physician order.	To relax vasospasms and increase renal perfusion
		Place woman on bed rest in side-lying position.	To maximize uteroplacental blood flow, reduce blood pressure, and promote diuresis
		Monitor fetal heart for rate, baseline variability, and absence of late decelerations.	To assess for evidence of adequate uteroplacental oxygenation

Other Possible Nursing Diagnoses

Risk for Excess Fluid Volume related to increased sodium retention secondary to administration of magnesium sulfate	Woman will exhibit signs of normal fluid volume (i.e., balanced intake and output, normal serum creatinine levels, normal breath sounds), adequate oxygenation (i.e., normal respirations; full orientation to person, time, and place), normal range of cardiac output (i.e., normal pulse rate and rhythm), and fetal well-being (i.e., adequate fetal movement, normal FHR).	Monitor woman for signs of fluid volume excess (increased edema, decreased urine output, elevated serum creatinine level, weight gain, dyspnea, crackles).	To detect potential complications
Risk for Impaired Gas Exchange related to pulmonary edema secondary to increased vascular resistance		Monitor woman for signs of impaired gas exchange (increased respirations, dyspnea, altered blood gases, hypoxemia).	To detect potential complications
Risk for Decreased Cardiac Output related to use of antihypertensive drugs		Monitor woman for signs of decreased cardiac output (altered pulse rate and rhythm).	To detect potential complications
Risk for Injury to Fetus related to uteroplacental insufficiency secondary to use of antihypertensive medications		Monitor fetus for abnormal signs (decreased fetal activity, abnormal FHR or pattern).	To prevent complications
		Record findings and report signs of increasing problems to physician.	To enable timely interventions

CNS, Central nervous system; *DTR*, deep tendon reflex; *FHR*, fetal heart rate; *IV*, intravenous.

❗ NURSING ALERT

High serum levels of magnesium can cause relaxation of smooth muscle such as the uterus. However, when administered as a 4- to 6-g loading dose followed by a 1- to 2-g/hr maintenance dose, magnesium sulfate has not been shown to significantly affect the need for oxytocin (Pitocin) stimulation of labor. Other than a brief period of uterine muscle relaxation during and immediately after administration of the loading dose, no evidence of decreased uterine contractility has been observed (Cunningham, Leveno, Bloom, et al., 2010).

It is unclear how magnesium sulfate works to prevent and treat eclamptic seizures. It may cause vasodilation in the peripheral and cerebral circulation, prevent or decrease cerebral edema, or function as a central anticonvulsant (Harvey and Sibai, 2013). Because magnesium is excreted in the urine, accurate recordings of maternal urine output must be obtained. If renal function declines, not all of the magnesium sulfate will be excreted adequately, resulting in magnesium toxicity. Common side effects of magnesium sulfate are a feeling of warmth, flushing, diaphoresis, and burning at the IV site. Symptoms of mild toxicity include lethargy, muscle weakness, decreased or absent DTRs, double vision, and slurred speech.

EVIDENCE-BASED PRACTICE

Common Treatments for Eclampsia and Preeclampsia

Ask the Question

For women whose pregnancies are complicated by eclampsia or preeclampsia, are the treatments commonly used today evidence based and cost-effective?

Search for the Evidence
Search Strategies

English research-based publications on preeclampsia, eclampsia, HELLP, magnesium, calcium, and corticosteroids were included.

Databases Used

Cochrane Collaborative Database, National Guideline Clearinghouse (AHRQ), CINAHL, PubMed, UpToDate, and the professional websites for AWHONN and SOGC

Critically Analyze the Evidence

- Severe preeclampsia (hypertension plus proteinuria) is an inflammatory disease of pregnancy associated with maternal risks for stroke, renal or liver failure, and clots. Eclampsia (seizure) is associated with increased risk for maternal and fetal death and preterm birth and low birth weight.
- Magnesium sulfate ($MgSO_4$) is commonly used for treatment of preeclampsia and eclampsia but not for hypertension without proteinuria. A systematic review found that using $MgSO_4$ for eclampsia was associated with lower risks for maternal death, recurrent seizure, and major morbidity (McDonald, Lutsiv, Dzaja, et al., 2012).
- A meta-analysis found that, when compared to placebo or no treatment, $MgSO_4$ given to preeclamptic women halved the risk of eclampsia, decreased the risk for placental abruption, and probably decreased maternal death (Duley, Gulmezoglu, Henderson-Smart, et al., 2010). Although the risk for cesarean birth was increased, there were no differences in severe maternal morbidity or perinatal or infant death up to 1 year.
- Calcium supplements are often recommended to prevent preeclampsia. A systematic review found that calcium supplements in pregnancy reduced the risk of preeclampsia to half that of placebo or no treatment, especially for populations with lower baseline calcium intake (Hofmeyr, Lawrie, Atallah, et al., 2010). The risk of preterm birth decreased with calcium, although overall perinatal death was unchanged. A slight paradoxical increase in the incidence of hemolysis, elevated liver enzymes, and low platelets (HELLP) was puzzling but did not change the overall recommendation for calcium supplementation in pregnancy.
- In the presence of HELLP, corticosteroids have commonly been used to decrease the inflammatory process; but a systematic analysis found that, although corticosteroid use improved platelet counts, it did not change maternal mortality or severe morbidity or perinatal death (Woudstra, Chandra, Hofmeyr, et al., 2010).

Apply the Evidence: Nursing Implications

- As a muscle relaxer $MgSO_4$ has many uses in the maternal hospital setting: the treatment of preeclampsia and eclampsia, the treatment of preterm labor, and as prophylactic neuroprotection against cerebral palsy for a fetus at risk for preterm birth. The nurse must understand the difference and be able to communicate each of these uses to the patient and family.

- $MgSO_4$ is associated with a higher cesarean birth rate and maternal adverse effects such as flushing, decreased urinary output, toxicity, respiratory depression, and hyporeflexia.
- For women at risk for preeclampsia, especially women with low baseline calcium such as low-income and lactose-intolerant populations, calcium supplements are an evidence-based preventive therapy, well accepted, readily available, and low-cost.
- Blood pressure can be expected to peak at 3 to 6 days postpartum.
- Preconception and postpartum teaching for women at greater risk for preeclampsia should include attaining and keeping a healthy body mass index, ideal pregnancy intervals of >2 years and <10 years, and monitoring for other cardiovascular risk factors.
- Corticosteroids do not appear to alter the outcomes of HELLP, although improved platelet counts may prevent excessive bleeding.

Quality and Safety Competencies:
Evidence-Based Practice*
Knowledge

Describe how the strength and relevance of available evidence influence the choice of interventions in providing patient-centered care.

Calcium supplements in pregnancy decrease the risk of preeclampsia.

Skills

Read original research and evidence reports related to area of practice.

Systematic analyses confirm the benefits of $MgSO_4$ for improving outcomes for women with eclampsia and preeclampsia.

Attitudes

Value the need for continuous improvement in clinical practice based on new knowledge.

Synthesize the best preventive evidence for patient preconception and postpartum teaching.

References

Duley L, Gulmezoglu AM, Henderson-Smart DJ, et al: Magnesium sulfate and other anticonvulsants for women with pre-eclampsia, *Cochrane Database Syst Rev* 2010 CD000025.pub2. DOI: 10.1002/14651858, Issue 11, Chichester, UK, 2010, John Wiley and Sons.

Hofmeyr GJ, Lawrie TA, Atallah AN, et al: Calcium supplementation during pregnancy for preventing hypertensive disorders and related problems, *Cochrane Database Syst Rev* 2010 CD001059.pub3. DOI:10.1002/14651858, Issue 8, Chichester, UK, 2010, John Wiley and Sons.

McDonald SD, Lutsiv O, Dzaja N, et al: A systematic review of maternal and infant outcomes following magnesium sulfate for pre-eclampsia/eclampsia in real-world use, *Int J Gynaecol Obstet* 118(2):90–96, 2012. PMID: 22703834.

Woudstra DM, Chandra S, Hofmeyr GJ, et al: Corticosteroids for HELLP (hemolysis, elevated liver enzymes, low platelets) syndrome in pregnancy, *Cochrane Database Syst Rev* 2010 CD008148.pub2. DOI: 10.1002/14651858, Issue 9, Chichester, UK, 2010, John Wiley and Sons.

Pat Mahaffee Gingrich

*Adapted from QSEN at www.qsen.org/.

BOX 12-4 CARE OF THE WOMAN WITH PREECLAMPSIA RECEIVING MAGNESIUM SULFATE

Patient and Family Teaching

- Explain technique, rationale, and reactions to expect:
  - Route and rate
  - Purpose of "piggyback" infusion
- Reasons for use:
  - Tailor information to woman's readiness to learn.
  - Explain that magnesium sulfate is used to prevent disease progression.
  - Explain that magnesium sulfate is used to prevent seizures, *not* to decrease blood pressure.
- Reactions to expect from medication:
  - Initially the woman appears flushed and feels hot, sedated, and nauseated. She may experience burning at the IV site, especially during the bolus.
  - Sedation continues.
- Monitoring to anticipate:
  - *Maternal:* Blood pressure, pulse, respiratory rate, DTRs, level of consciousness, urine output (indwelling catheter), presence of headache, visual disturbances, epigastric pain
  - *Fetal:* FHR and activity

Administration

- Verify physician's order.
- Position woman in side-lying position.
- Prepare solution and administer with an infusion control device (pump).
- Piggyback solution of 40 g of magnesium sulfate in 1000 mL lactated Ringer's solution with infusion control device at the ordered rate: loading dose—initial bolus of 4 to 6 g over 15 to 30 min; maintenance dose—2 g/hr, according to unit protocol or specific physician's order.

Maternal and Fetal Assessments

Vital signs and assessments are performed as ordered by the health care provider and per hospital protocol.

- Monitor blood pressure, pulse, respiratory rate every 15 to 30 minutes, depending on woman's condition.
- Monitor FHR and contractions continuously.
- Monitor intake and output, proteinuria, DTRs, presence of headache, visual disturbances, level of consciousness, and epigastric pain at least hourly.
- Restrict hourly fluid intake to a total of no more than 125 mL/hr; urinary output should be at least 25 to 30 mL/hr.

Reportable Conditions

- Blood pressure: systolic ≥160 mm Hg or diastolic ≥110 mm Hg
- Respiratory rate: <12 breaths/min
- Urinary output: <25 to 30 mL/hr
- Presence of headache, visual disturbances, decrease in level of consciousness, or epigastric pain
- Increasing severity or loss of DTRs, increasing edema, proteinuria
- Any abnormal laboratory values (magnesium level, platelet count, creatinine clearance, levels of uric acid, AST, ALT, prothrombin time, partial thromboplastin time, fibrinogen, fibrin split products)
- Any other significant change in maternal or fetal status

Emergency Measures

- Keep emergency drugs and intubation equipment immediately available.
- Keep side rails up.
- Keep lights dimmed and maintain a quiet environment.

Documentation

- All of the above

ALT, Alanine aminotransferase; *AST,* aspartate aminotransferase; *DTR,* deep tendon reflex; *FHR,* fetal heart rate; *IV,* intravenous.

Increasing toxicity may be indicated by maternal hypotension, bradycardia, bradypnea, and cardiac arrest (Gilbert, 2011). Blood can be drawn to determine precisely the serum magnesium level if mild or severe toxicity is suspected (Box 12-4).

MEDICATION ALERT

If magnesium toxicity is suspected, prompt actions are needed to prevent respiratory or cardiac arrest. The magnesium infusion should be discontinued immediately. Calcium gluconate or calcium chloride (antidotes for magnesium sulfate) can be given intravenously (Cunningham, Leveno, Bloom, et al., 2010).

Magnesium sulfate does not seem to affect the FHR in a healthy term fetus. Doses of magnesium sulfate that prevent maternal seizures have been determined to be safe for the fetus. Neonatal serum magnesium levels approximate the levels of the mother (Roberts and Funai, 2009).

MEDICATION ALERT

Magnesium sulfate is considered a high-alert medication because it can cause patient harm when administered incorrectly. Measures to improve the safe use of this medication include developing detailed policies, procedures, protocols, and standing orders and thorough assessment and documentation. *Never* abbreviate magnesium sulfate as MgSO₄ anywhere in the medical record (Institute for Safe Medication Practices [ISMP], 2012).

Control of Blood Pressure. Antihypertensive medications are indicated when the systolic BP exceeds 160 mm Hg or the diastolic BP exceeds 110 mm Hg. Maternal risks associated with severe hypertension include left ventricular failure, cerebral hemorrhage, and placental abruption. To maintain uteroplacental perfusion, antihypertensive therapy must not decrease the arterial pressure too much or too rapidly. Hydralazine, labetalol, and nifedipine are effective drugs for treating hypertension intrapartum. They may also be used during pregnancy or in the postpartum period for BP control (Cunningham, Leveno, Bloom, et al., 2010; Gilbert, 2011; Harvey and Sibai, 2013). Table 12-5 compares antihypertensive agents often used to treat hypertension in pregnancy.

Postpartum Care

Throughout the postpartum period the woman needs careful monitoring of her vital signs, intake and output, DTRs, and level of consciousness. The magnesium sulfate infusion is continued after birth for seizure prophylaxis as ordered, usually for 12 to 24 hours. Assessments for effects and side effects continue until the medication is discontinued. Given that magnesium sulfate potentiates the action of narcotics, CNS depressants, and calcium channel blockers, these medications must be administered with caution.

Most women with gestational hypertension become normotensive during the first week after giving birth. On the other hand, hypertension may take longer to resolve in women with preeclampsia. Women with severe gestational hypertension or severe

TABLE 12-5	PHARMACOLOGIC CONTROL OF HYPERTENSION IN PREGNANCY			
ACTION	**TARGET TISSUE**	**MATERNAL EFFECTS**	**FETAL EFFECTS**	**NURSING ACTIONS**
Hydralazine (Apresoline, Neopresol)				
Arteriolar vasodilator	Peripheral arterioles: to decrease muscle tone, decrease peripheral resistance; hypothalamus and medullary vasomotor center for minor decrease in sympathetic tone	Headache, flushing, palpitations, tachycardia, some decrease in uteroplacental blood flow, increase in heart rate and cardiac output, increase in oxygen consumption, nausea and vomiting	Tachycardia; late decelerations and bradycardia if maternal diastolic pressure <90 mm Hg	Assess for effects of medication; alert woman (family) to expected effects of medication; assess blood pressure frequently because precipitous drop can lead to shock and perhaps placental abruption; if giving multiple doses, wait at least 20 minutes after the first dose is given to administer an additional dose to allow time to assess the effects of the initial dose; assess urinary output; maintain bed rest in lateral position with side rails up; use with caution in presence of maternal tachycardia.
Labetalol Hydrochloride (Normodyne, Trandate)				
Combined alpha- and beta-blocking agent causing vasodilation without significant change in cardiac output	Peripheral arterioles (see hydralazine)	Minimal: flushing, tremulousness, orthostatic hypotension; minimal change in pulse rate	Minimal, if any	See hydralazine; less likely to cause excessive hypotension and tachycardia; less rebound hypertension than hydralazine. Do not use in women with asthma or heart failure. Do not exceed 80 mg in a single dose.
Methyldopa (Aldomet)				
Maintenance therapy if needed: 250-500 mg orally every 8 hr (α_2-receptor agonist)	Postganglionic nerve endings: interferes with chemical neurotransmission to reduce peripheral vascular resistance; causes CNS sedation	Sleepiness, postural hypotension, constipation; rare: drug-induced fever in 1% of women and positive Coombs' test result in 20% of women	After 4 months of maternal therapy, positive Coombs' test result in infant	See hydralazine.
Nifedipine (Adalat, Procardia)				
Calcium channel blocker	Arterioles: to reduce systemic vascular resistance by relaxation of arterial smooth muscle	Headache, flushing; may interfere with labor	Minimal	See hydralazine. Avoid concurrent use with magnesium sulfate because skeletal muscle blockade can result. Do not administer sublingually.

CNS, Central nervous system.

preeclampsia are frequently discharged from the hospital on an antihypertensive medication such as labetalol or nifedipine. If this is the case, the BP needs to be checked frequently either at home or at the health care provider's office. Within a few weeks after birth antihypertensive medications often can be discontinued.

Remember, too, that severe preeclampsia or severe gestational hypertension may develop for the first time after birth. The nurse should assess the postpartum woman regularly for any symptoms of preeclampsia such as headaches, visual disturbances, or epigastric pain. Women should be taught to contact their health care provider

or return to the hospital immediately if they notice any of these symptoms after discharge (Sibai, 2012).

Future Health Care

Women with severe preeclampsia have a significantly increased risk of developing severe preeclampsia in a future pregnancy. This risk is especially likely in women who initially developed it earlier (during the second trimester) in pregnancy (Sibai, 2012). Even if these women remain normotensive in a subsequent pregnancy, they may have a greater likelihood of an adverse pregnancy outcome such as preterm birth, small-for-gestational-age infant, and perinatal death (Sibai, 2012).

Women with preeclampsia (especially early-onset and severe preeclampsia) also have an increased risk of developing chronic hypertension and cardiovascular disease later in life. These women are also more likely to have underlying renal disease (Sibai, 2012). The postpartum period provides an excellent opportunity to educate women about lifestyle changes that may decrease their risk for developing future health problems (Gilbert, 2011; Sibai, 2012).

Eclampsia

Eclampsia is usually preceded by premonitory signs and symptoms, including persistent headache, blurred vision, severe epigastric or right upper quadrant abdominal pain, and altered mental status. However, convulsions can appear suddenly and without warning in a seemingly stable woman with only minimal BP elevations (Sibai, 2012). The convulsions that occur in eclampsia are frightening to observe. Tonic contraction of all body muscles (seen as arms flexed, hands clenched, legs inverted) precedes the tonic-clonic convulsion. During this stage muscles alternately relax and contract. Respirations are halted and then begin again with long, deep, stertorous inhalations. Hypotension follows; and muscular twitching, disorientation, and amnesia persist for a while after the convulsion. The woman may also vomit or be incontinent of urine or stool.

Immediate Care

Nursing actions during a convulsion are directed toward ensuring a patent airway and patient safety (see Emergency box).

It is important to note the time of onset and duration of the seizure. Call for help but do not leave the bedside. Make certain that the side rails on the bed are raised; pad them with a folded blanket or pillow if possible. Women with eclampsia have been known to sustain fractures from falling out of bed during the seizure. Immediately after the convulsion, lower the head of the bed and turn the woman onto her side. This helps prevent aspiration of vomitus (Gilbert, 2011).

Nursing actions after a convulsion are directed toward maternal stabilization. First assess the status of the woman's airway, breathing, and pulse. Suction secretions from her glottis to clear the airway, insert an oral airway, and administer oxygen at 10 L/min by nonrebreather face mask. If an IV infusion is not in place, start one with an 18-gauge needle. If an IV line was in place before the seizure, it may have infiltrated and will need to be restarted immediately. As soon as IV access is obtained, administer magnesium sulfate as ordered (Gilbert, 2011).

If eclampsia develops after initiating magnesium sulfate therapy, additional magnesium sulfate should be administered. Magnesium sulfate is the drug of choice for treating eclamptic seizures and preventing repeated seizures. One of the advantages of magnesium sulfate over other antiseizure medications such as diazepam (Valium) is that it reduces the risk of aspiration because it does not depress the gag reflex (Harvey and Sibai, 2013).

A rapid assessment of uterine activity, cervical status, and fetal status is performed after the convulsion. During a convulsion the uterus becomes hypercontractile and hypertonic. As a result, the membranes may have ruptured, or the cervix may have dilated rapidly, and birth may be imminent. The FHR tracing may demonstrate bradycardia, late decelerations, minimal baseline variability, or any combination. These findings usually resolve soon after the convulsion ends and the woman's hypoxia is corrected (Sibai, 2012). Help the woman with hygiene and a change of linens and gown if needed.

✚ EMERGENCY

Eclampsia

Tonic-Clonic Convulsion Signs
- Stage of invasion: 2-3 seconds, eyes fixed, twitching of facial muscles
- Stage of contraction: 15-20 seconds, eyes protrude and are bloodshot, all body muscles in tonic contraction
- Stage of convulsion: Muscles relax and contract alternately (clonic), respirations halted and then begin again with long, deep, stertorous inhalation; coma ensues

Intervention
- Keep airway patent: turn head to one side, place pillow under one shoulder or back if possible.
- Call for assistance. Do not leave bedside.
- Protect with padded side rails up.
- Observe and record convulsion activity.

After Convulsion
- Do not leave unattended until fully alert.
- Observe for postconvulsion confusion, coma, incontinence.
- Use suction as needed.
- Administer oxygen via nonrebreather face mask at 10 L/min.
- Start intravenous fluids and monitor for potential fluid overload.
- Give magnesium sulfate or other anticonvulsant drug as ordered.
- Insert indwelling urinary catheter.
- Monitor blood pressure, pulse, and respirations frequently until stabilized.
- Monitor fetal and uterine status.
- Expedite laboratory work as ordered to monitor kidney function, liver function, coagulation system, and drug levels.
- Provide hygiene and a quiet environment.
- Support and keep woman and family informed.
- Be prepared to assist with birth when woman is in stable condition.

❗ NURSING ALERT

Immediately after a seizure a woman may be very confused and can be combative. Restraints may be necessary temporarily. Several hours may be needed for the woman to regain her usual level of mental functioning.

After stabilization of the woman and fetus, a decision is made regarding timing and method of birth. Eclampsia alone is not an indication for immediate cesarean birth. The route of birth (induction of labor versus cesarean birth) depends on maternal and fetal condition, fetal gestational age, presence of labor, and the cervical Bishop score. Regional anesthesia is not recommended for eclamptic women with coagulopathy or a platelet count less than $50,000/mm^3$ (Sibai, 2012).

Chronic Hypertension

An increasing number of women who give birth have chronic hypertension, which affects approximately 4% to 5% of all pregnancies (Gilbert, 2011). Non-Hispanic black women are much more likely to have a pregnancy complicated by chronic hypertension than are women of other races or ethnicities. In 2010 the rate of chronic hypertension in non-Hispanic black women who gave birth (28.1) was more than double the rate of that reported in women of all races who gave birth (13.6) (Martin, Hamilton, Sutton, et al., 2012). In addition to race, other risk factors for chronic hypertension in pregnancy are older age and obesity. As more women delay childbearing and are obese, the number of pregnancies complicated by chronic hypertension can be expected to increase (Sibai, 2012).

More than 90% of women with chronic hypertension have primary or essential hypertension. In the remaining 10% the hypertension is secondary to a medical condition such as renal or collagen disease (Harvey and Sibai, 2013). Chronic hypertension in pregnancy is associated with an increased incidence of placental abruption, superimposed preeclampsia, and increased perinatal mortality (threefold or fourfold). Fetal effects include intrauterine growth restriction (IUGR) and preterm birth (Cunningham, Leveno, Bloom, et al., 2010; Sibai, 2012).

Ideally the management of chronic hypertension in pregnancy begins before conception. An evaluation is performed to assess the cause and severity of the hypertension and the presence of any target organ damage (e.g., heart, eye, and kidney). Moreover, the woman should be encouraged to make lifestyle changes before conception such as smoking and alcohol cessation, participating in aerobic exercise, and losing weight if indicated. A diet that includes a maximum of 2.4 g sodium per day is recommended (Gilbert, 2011). These lifestyle modifications should continue throughout the pregnancy.

Based on the BP and presence of target organ damage, women with chronic hypertension are classified as either high or low risk for pregnancy complications. Antihypertensive medications are frequently discontinued before pregnancy in women with low risk chronic hypertension. This decreases the risk of fetal exposure to some medications (e.g., angiotensin-converting enzyme [ACE] inhibitors) that can be teratogenic (Harvey and Sibai, 2013). Women who are high risk are managed with antihypertensive medication and frequent assessments of maternal and fetal well-being. Methyldopa (Aldomet) is most often recommended for treating chronic hypertension in pregnancy. However, because it is rarely used for treating chronic hypertension in nonpregnant women, it may not be practical to switch medications because of pregnancy. Labetalol and nifedipine are other antihypertensive medications used during pregnancy (see Table 12-5). Women who are high risk are monitored closely, and the route and timing of the birth depend on the maternal and fetal status. After giving birth the woman should be monitored closely for complications such as pulmonary edema, hypertensive encephalopathy, and renal failure. Women with chronic hypertension can breastfeed if they desire. All antihypertensive medications are present to some degree in breast milk. Levels of methyldopa in breast milk appear to be low and are considered safe. Labetalol also has a low concentration in breast milk. Little is known about the transfer of calcium channel blockers such as nifedipine in breast milk, but no apparent side effects have been noted in infants (Sibai, 2012).

HYPEREMESIS GRAVIDARUM

Nausea and vomiting complicate as many as 80% of all pregnancies, typically beginning at 4 weeks of gestation. These symptoms are usually confined to the first 20 weeks of gestation (Kelly and Savides, 2009). Although nausea and vomiting are distressing, they are typically benign, with no significant metabolic alterations or risks to the mother or fetus. The cause of nausea and vomiting in pregnancy is not well understood, although it may involve relaxation of the smooth muscle of the stomach and increasing levels of estrogen, progesterone, and human chorionic gonadotropin (hCG). Pregnancies complicated by nausea and vomiting generally have a more favorable outcome than those without these symptoms (Gordon, 2012; King and Murphy, 2009).

When vomiting during pregnancy becomes excessive enough to cause weight loss, electrolyte imbalance, nutritional deficiencies, and ketonuria, the disorder is termed hyperemesis gravidarum. This disorder occurs in approximately 0.5% of all live births. Hyperemesis gravidarum usually begins during the first trimester, but approximately 10% of women with the disorder continue to have symptoms throughout the pregnancy (Kelly and Savides, 2009). Hyperemesis gravidarum is the second most common reason for hospitalization during pregnancy in the United States (King and Murphy, 2009).

Risk factors for the condition include clinical hyperthyroid disorders, prepregnancy psychiatric diagnosis, previous pregnancy complicated by hyperemesis gravidarum, molar pregnancy, multiple gestation with a male and female fetus, diabetes, and gastrointestinal disorders (King and Murphy, 2009). For unknown reasons women carrying a female fetus are more likely than those carrying a male fetus to develop hyperemesis (Cunningham, Leveno, Bloom, et al., 2010; Kelly and Savides, 2009). A family history of hyperemesis may also be present (Gilbert, 2011; King and Murphy, 2009). Women 30 years of age and older and women who smoke have a lower risk of hyperemesis (King and Murphy, 2009).

Complications accompanying severe hyperemesis gravidarum include esophageal rupture and deficiencies of vitamin K and thiamine with resulting Wernicke encephalopathy (CNS involvement) (Cunningham, Leveno, Bloom, et al., 2010; Kelly and Savides, 2009). Fetal and neonatal complications include small-for-gestational-age fetuses, low birth weight, prematurity, and 5-minute Apgar scores less than 7 (Kelly and Savides, 2009).

Etiology

The cause of hyperemesis gravidarum remains obscure. Several theories have been proposed as to the cause, although none of them adequately explains the disorder. It may be related to high levels of estrogen or hCG or associated with transient hyperthyroidism during pregnancy. Gastric dysrhythmias, esophageal reflux, and reduced gastric motility may also contribute to the development of hyperemesis gravidarum (Kelly and Savides, 2009).

Psychosocial, cultural, and psychogenic factors may play a part in the development of hyperemesis gravidarum for some women (King and Murphy, 2009). Conflicting feelings regarding prospective motherhood, body changes, and lifestyle alterations may contribute to episodes of vomiting, particularly if these feelings are excessive or unresolved. Women with associated psychosocial factors usually improve dramatically while in the hospital but may resume vomiting after discharge (Cunningham, Leveno, Bloom, et al., 2010).

Clinical Manifestations

The woman with hyperemesis gravidarum usually has significant weight loss and dehydration. She may have dry mucous membranes, decreased BP, increased pulse rate, and poor skin turgor. Frequently she is unable to keep down even clear liquids taken by mouth. Laboratory tests may reveal electrolyte imbalances.

Management

Assessment

Whenever a pregnant woman has nausea and vomiting, the first priority is a thorough assessment to determine the severity of the problem. In most cases the woman should be told to come immediately to the health care provider's office or the emergency department because the severity of the illness is often difficult to determine by telephone conversation.

The assessment should include frequency, severity, and duration of episodes of nausea and vomiting. If the woman reports vomiting, the assessment should also include the approximate amount and color of the vomitus. Other symptoms such as diarrhea, indigestion, and abdominal pain or distention also are identified. The woman is asked to report any precipitating factors relating to the onset of her symptoms. Any pharmacologic or nonpharmacologic treatment measures used should be recorded. Prepregnancy weight and documented weight gain or loss during pregnancy are important to note.

The woman's weight and vital signs are measured; and a complete physical examination is performed, with attention to signs of fluid and electrolyte imbalance and nutritional status. The most important initial laboratory test to be obtained is a determination of ketonuria. Other laboratory tests that may be ordered are a urinalysis, a complete blood cell count, electrolytes, liver enzymes, and bilirubin levels. These tests help rule out the presence of underlying diseases such as gastroenteritis, pyelonephritis, pancreatitis, cholecystitis, peptic ulcer, and hepatitis (Cunningham, Leveno, Bloom, et al., 2010). Because of the recognized association between hyperemesis gravidarum and hyperthyroidism, thyroid levels may also be measured (Nader, 2009).

Psychosocial assessment includes asking the woman about anxiety, fears, and concerns related to her own health and the effects on pregnancy outcome. Family members should be assessed both for anxiety and their role in providing support for the woman.

Initial Care

Initially the woman who is unable to keep down clear liquids by mouth requires IV therapy for correction of fluid and electrolyte imbalances. In the past women requiring IV therapy were admitted to the hospital. However, today they may be and often are successfully managed at home, even if on enteral therapy. Medications may be used if nausea and vomiting are uncontrolled. The ACOG recommends the use of pyridoxine (vitamin B$_6$), either alone or in combination with doxylamine (Unisom) as initial medical management because these medications are considered to be safe and effective (Gordon, 2012). Other frequently prescribed drugs include promethazine (Phenergan), chlorpromazine (Thorazine), prochlorperazine (Compazine), metoclopramide (Reglan), and ondansetron (Zofran) (Gordon, 2012; Kelly and Savides, 2009). Corticosteroids (methylprednisolone [Medrol] or hydrocortisone) may be prescribed, although there is little evidence that their use is effective (Cunningham, Leveno, Bloom, et al., 2010). Finally, enteral or parenteral nutrition may be used for women who are nonresponsive to other medical therapies (Kelly and Savides, 2009). Because of potential risks, parenteral therapy should only be used after multiple medical management and enteral tube feeding attempts have been unsuccessful (Gordon, 2012).

Nursing care of the woman with hyperemesis gravidarum involves implementing the medical plan of care, whether it is given in the hospital or home setting. Interventions may include initiating and monitoring IV therapy, administering drugs and nutritional supplements, and monitoring the woman's response to interventions. The nurse observes the woman for any signs of complications such as metabolic acidosis (secondary to starvation), jaundice, or hemorrhage and alerts the health care provider should these occur. Monitoring includes assessment of the woman's nausea, retching without vomiting, and vomiting, given that these symptoms, although related, are separate. Intake and output, including the amount of emesis, should be measured accurately and recorded. Oral hygiene while the woman is receiving nothing by mouth and after episodes of vomiting helps allay associated discomforts. Assistance with positioning and providing a quiet, restful environment that is free from odors may increase the woman's comfort.

PATIENT TEACHING

Diet for Hyperemesis

- Avoid an empty stomach. Eat frequently, at least every 2 to 3 hours. Separate liquids from solids and alternate every 2 to 3 hours.
- Eat a high-protein snack at bedtime.
- Eat dry, bland, low-fat, and high-protein foods. Cold foods may be better tolerated than those served at a warm temperature.
- In general eat what sounds good to you rather than trying to balance your meals.
- Follow the salty and sweet approach; even so-called junk foods are okay.
- Eat protein after sweets.
- Dairy products may stay down more easily than other foods.
- If you vomit even when your stomach is empty, try sucking on a Popsicle.
- Try ginger tea. Peel and finely dice a knuckle-sized piece of ginger and place it in a mug of boiling water. Steep for 5 to 8 minutes and add brown sugar to taste.
- Try warm ginger ale (with sugar, not artificial sweetener) or water with a slice of lemon.
- Drink liquids from a cup with a lid.

Once the vomiting has stopped, feedings are started in small amounts at frequent intervals. In the beginning limited amounts of oral fluids and bland foods such as crackers, toast, or baked chicken are offered. The diet progresses slowly as tolerated by the woman until she is able to consume a nutritionally sound diet. Because sleep disturbances may accompany hyperemesis gravidarum, promoting adequate rest is important. The nurse can help coordinate treatment measures and periods of visitation to provide opportunity for rest periods.

Follow-up Care

Most women are able to take nourishment by mouth after several days of treatment. They should be encouraged to eat small, frequent meals and foods that sound appealing (e.g., nongreasy, dry, sweet, and salty foods). In many instances women discover that foods they normally like have no appeal at all during this time. See the Patient Teaching box for more suggestions. Many pregnant women find exposure to cooking odors nauseating. Having other family members cook may lessen the woman's nausea and vomiting, even if only temporarily. The woman is counseled to contact her health care provider immediately if the nausea and vomiting recur.

The woman with hyperemesis gravidarum needs calm, compassionate, and sympathetic care, with recognition that the manifestations of hyperemesis can be physically and emotionally debilitating to her and stressful for her family. Irritability, tearfulness, and mood changes are often consistent with this disorder. Fetal well-being is a primary concern of the woman. The nurse can provide an environment conducive to discussion of concerns and help the woman identify and mobilize sources of support. The family should be included in the plan of care whenever possible. Their participation may help alleviate some of the emotional stress associated with this disorder.

HEMORRHAGIC DISORDERS

Bleeding in pregnancy may jeopardize maternal and fetal well-being. Maternal blood loss decreases oxygen-carrying capacity, which places the woman at increased risk for hypovolemia, anemia, infection, and preterm labor and adversely affects oxygen delivery to the fetus. Fetal risks from maternal hemorrhage include blood loss or anemia, hypoxemia, hypoxia, anoxia, and preterm birth. Hemorrhagic disorders in pregnancy are medical emergencies. The incidence and type of bleeding vary by trimester. Ruptured ectopic pregnancy and abruptio placentae (placental abruption) have the highest incidence of maternal mortality. Prompt assessment and intervention by the health care team are essential to save the lives of both the woman and her fetus.

Early Pregnancy Bleeding

Bleeding during early pregnancy is alarming to the woman and of concern to health care providers. The common bleeding disorders of early pregnancy include miscarriage (spontaneous abortion), reduced cervical competence (premature dilation of the cervix), ectopic pregnancy, and hydatidiform mole (molar pregnancy).

Miscarriage (Spontaneous Abortion)

A pregnancy that ends as a result of natural causes before 20 weeks of gestation is defined as a miscarriage (spontaneous abortion). This 20-week marker is considered to be the point of viability when a fetus may survive in an extrauterine environment. A fetal weight less than 500 g also may be used to define an abortion (Cunningham, Leveno, Bloom, et al., 2010). The term *miscarriage* is used throughout this discussion because it is more appropriate than abortion to use with patients. Abortion may be perceived as an insensitive term to use with families who are grieving a pregnancy loss. Therapeutic or elective induced abortion is discussed in Chapter 5.

Incidence and Etiology. Of all clinically recognized pregnancies, 10% to 15% end in miscarriage (Simpson and Jauniaux, 2012). The

majority—more than 80% of miscarriages—are early pregnancy losses, occurring before 12 weeks of gestation (Cunningham, Leveno, Bloom, et al., 2010). Of all clinically recognized pregnancy losses, at least 50% result from chromosomal abnormalities (Cunningham, Leveno, Bloom, et al., 2010; Simpson and Jauniaux, 2012). Other possible causes of early miscarriage include endocrine imbalance (as in women who have luteal phase defects, hypothyroidism, or insulin-dependent diabetes mellitus with high blood glucose levels in the first trimester), immunologic factors (e.g., antiphospholipid antibodies), systemic disorders (e.g., lupus erythematosus), and genetic factors. Infections are not a common cause of early miscarriage (Cunningham, Leveno, Bloom, et al., 2010), but there is an increased risk for a spontaneous abortion with varicella infection in the first trimester (Gilbert, 2011).

A late miscarriage, sometimes called a *second-trimester loss*, occurs between 12 and 20 weeks of gestation. It usually results from maternal causes such as advancing maternal age and parity; premature dilation of the cervix and other anomalies of the reproductive tract; inadequate nutrition; tobacco, alcohol, and caffeine use (Cunningham, Leveno, Bloom, et al., 2010); obesity; and stressful life events (Gilbert, 2011). Little can be done to prevent genetically caused pregnancy loss, but correction of maternal disorders, a healthy lifestyle, adequate early prenatal care, and treatment of pregnancy complications can do much to prevent other causes of miscarriage.

Types. The types of miscarriage include threatened, inevitable, incomplete, complete, and missed. All types of miscarriage can recur in subsequent pregnancies. All types except the threatened miscarriage can lead to infection (Fig. 12-6).

Clinical Manifestations. Signs and symptoms of miscarriage depend on the duration of pregnancy. The presence of uterine bleeding, uterine contractions, or abdominal pain is an ominous

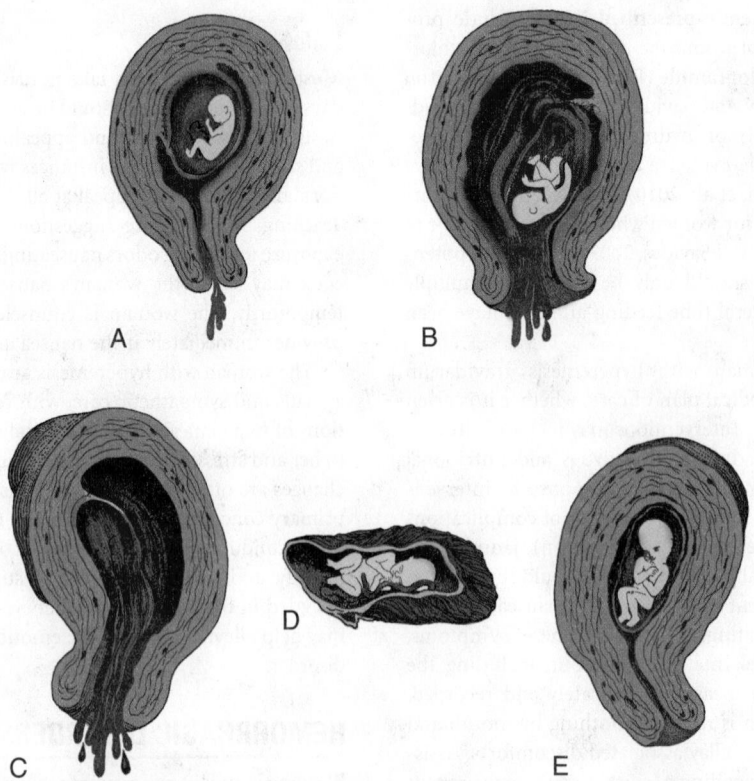

FIG 12-6 Miscarriage. **A,** Threatened. **B,** Inevitable. **C,** Incomplete. **D,** Complete. **E,** Missed.

sign during early pregnancy and must be considered a threatened miscarriage until proven otherwise.

If miscarriage occurs before the sixth week of pregnancy, the woman may report what she believes to be a heavy menstrual flow. Miscarriage that occurs between weeks 6 and 12 of pregnancy causes moderate discomfort and blood loss. After week 12 miscarriage is typified by severe pain similar to that of labor because the fetus must be expelled. Diagnosis of the type of miscarriage is based on the signs and symptoms present (Table 12-6).

Symptoms of a *threatened* miscarriage (see Fig. 12-6, *A*) include spotting of blood but with the cervical os closed. Mild uterine cramping may be present.

TABLE 12-6	ASSESSING MISCARRIAGE AND THE USUAL MANAGEMENT				
TYPE OF MISCARRIAGE	AMOUNT OF BLEEDING	UTERINE CRAMPING	PASSAGE OF TISSUE	CERVICAL DILATION	MANAGEMENT
Threatened	Slight, spotting	Mild	No	No	Bed rest is often ordered but has not proven to be effective in preventing progression to actual miscarriage. Repetitive transvaginal ultrasounds and assessment of human chorionic gonadotropin and progesterone levels may be done to determine if the fetus is still alive and in the uterus. Further treatment depends on whether progression to actual miscarriage occurs.
Inevitable	Moderate	Mild to severe	No	Yes	Bed rest if no pain, fever, or bleeding. If rupture of membranes, bleeding, pain, or fever is present, the uterus is emptied promptly, usually by dilation and curettage.
Incomplete	Heavy, profuse	Severe	Yes	Yes, with tissue in cervix	May or may not require additional cervical dilation before curettage. Suction curettage may be performed.
Complete	Slight	Mild	Yes	No (cervix has already closed after tissue passed)	No further intervention may be needed if uterine contractions are adequate to prevent hemorrhage and no infection is present. Suction curettage may be performed to ensure no retained fetal or maternal tissue.
Missed	None, spotting	None	No	No	If spontaneous evacuation of the uterus does not occur within 1 month, the uterus is emptied by a method appropriate for the gestational age. Blood clotting factors are monitored until uterus is empty. Disseminated intravascular coagulation and incoagulability of blood with uncontrolled hemorrhage may develop in cases of fetal death after the twelfth week if products of conception are retained for longer than 5 weeks. May be treated with dilation and curettage, or misoprostol (Cytotec) given orally or vaginally.
Septic	Varies, usually malodorous	Varies	Varies	Yes, usually	The uterus is immediately emptied by a method appropriate for the gestational age. Cervical culture and sensitivity studies are performed, and broad-spectrum antibiotic therapy (e.g., ampicillin) is started. Treatment for septic shock is initiated if necessary.
Recurrent (generally defined as three or more consecutive miscarriages)	Varies	Varies	Yes	Yes, usually	Varies; depends on type. Prophylactic cerclage may be performed if premature cervical dilation is the cause. Tests of value include parental cytogenetic analysis and lupus anticoagulant and anticardiolipin antibody assays on the woman.

Data from Cunningham F, Leveno K, Bloom S, et al, editors: *Williams obstetrics*, ed 23, New York, 2010, McGraw-Hill; Gilbert ES: *Manual of high risk pregnancy and delivery*, ed 5, St Louis, 2011, Mosby.

Inevitable (see Fig. 12-6, *B*) and *incomplete* (see Fig. 12-6, *C*) miscarriages involve a moderate-to-heavy amount of bleeding with an open cervical os. Tissue may be present with the bleeding. Mild-to-severe uterine cramping may be present. An inevitable miscarriage is often accompanied by rupture of membranes (ROM) and cervical dilation. Passage of the products of conception occurs. An incomplete miscarriage involves the expulsion of the fetus with retention of the placenta.

In a *complete* miscarriage (see Fig. 12-6, *D*) the cervix has already closed after all fetal tissue was expelled. Slight bleeding may occur, and mild uterine cramping may also be present.

The term *missed* miscarriage (see Fig. 12-6, *E*) refers to a pregnancy in which the fetus has died but the products of conception are retained in utero for up to several weeks. It may be diagnosed by ultrasound examination after the uterus stops increasing or even decreases in size. There may be no bleeding or cramping, and the cervical os remains closed.

Recurrent early (habitual) miscarriage is three or more spontaneous pregnancy losses before 20 weeks of gestation. The causes of recurrent miscarriage are the same as those discussed earlier in this section. Another possible cause of recurrent pregnancy loss is parental chromosomal abnormalities. The evaluation of couples experiencing recurrent pregnancy loss usually includes karyotyping of both partners, evaluating the woman's uterine cavity, and testing for antiphospholipid antibody syndrome. No cause can be identified in approximately half of all couples who experience recurrent pregnancy loss. However, 60% to 70% of these couples will go on to have a successful pregnancy with no treatment (Cunningham, Leveno, Bloom, et al., 2010).

Miscarriages can become septic, although this is uncommon. Symptoms of a septic miscarriage include fever and abdominal tenderness. Vaginal bleeding, which may be slight to heavy, is usually malodorous.

Management

Initial Care. Management depends on the classification of the miscarriage and signs and symptoms (see Table 12-6). Traditionally threatened miscarriages have been managed expectantly with supportive care. However, there are no proven effective therapies for this condition. Although bed rest is often prescribed, it does not prevent progression to actual miscarriage. Repetitive transvaginal ultrasounds and measurement of hCG and progesterone levels may be performed to determine if the fetus is alive and within the uterus (Cunningham, Leveno, Bloom, et al., 2010).

Follow-up treatment depends on whether the threatened miscarriage progresses to actual miscarriage or symptoms subside and the pregnancy remains intact. If bleeding and infection do not occur, expectant management is a reasonable option. In approximately half of all threatened miscarriages managed in this way, the pregnancy continues (Cunningham, Leveno, Bloom, et al., 2010).

Once the cervix begins to dilate, the pregnancy cannot continue, and miscarriage becomes inevitable. If all the products of conception are passed, no surgical intervention is necessary. However, if heavy bleeding, excessive cramping, or infection is present, the remaining embryonic, fetal, or placental tissue must be removed from the uterus, usually by suction curettage. In women who are clinically stable, expectant management to allow spontaneous resolution of an incomplete miscarriage is another treatment option (Cunningham, Leveno, Bloom, et al., 2010; Gilbert, 2011).

Most missed miscarriages eventually end spontaneously. Women may be offered expectant management at the time the pregnancy loss is diagnosed. Expectant management results in eventual spontaneous miscarriage in 16% to 76% of cases (Gilbert, 2011).

Medical management is another treatment option if bleeding and infection are not present. Prostaglandin medications (e.g., misoprostol [Cytotec]) may be given orally or vaginally and are usually effective in completing the miscarriage within 7 days (Cunningham, Leveno, Bloom, et al., 2010). If medical management is chosen, nursing care is similar to the care for any woman whose labor is being induced (see Chapter 17). Special care may be needed for management of side effects of prostaglandin such as nausea, vomiting, and diarrhea. If the products of conception are not passed completely, the woman may be prepared for manual or surgical evacuation of the uterus.

A third management option, and one that is often chosen, is dilation and curettage (D&C), a surgical procedure in which the cervix is dilated and a suction curette is inserted to scrape the uterine walls and remove uterine contents (Cunningham, Leveno, Bloom, et al., 2010). Before a surgical procedure is performed, a full history should be obtained, and general and pelvic examinations conducted. General preoperative and postoperative care is appropriate for the woman requiring surgical intervention for miscarriage. Analgesics and anesthesia that are appropriate to the procedure are used. The nurse reinforces explanations, answers any questions or concerns, and prepares the woman for surgery.

After evacuation of the uterus, oxytocin is often given to prevent hemorrhage. For excessive bleeding after the miscarriage, ergot products such as ergonovine (Methergine) or a prostaglandin derivative such as carboprost tromethamine (Hemabate) may be given to contract the uterus. (See the Medication Guide: Drugs Used To Manage Postpartum Hemorrhage, in Chapter 21.) Antibiotics are given as necessary. Analgesics such as antiprostaglandin agents (e.g., nonsteroidal antiinflammatory drugs [NSAIDs]) may decrease discomfort from cramping. Transfusion therapy may be required for shock or anemia. The woman who is Rh negative and is not isoimmunized is given $Rh_O(D)$ immunoglobulin (Cunningham, Leveno, Bloom, et al., 2010).

Psychosocial aspects of care focus on what the pregnancy loss means to the woman and her family. Grief from perinatal loss is complex and unique to each individual. Explanations are provided regarding the nature of the miscarriage, expected procedures, and possible future implications for childbearing.

As with other fetal or neonatal losses, the woman should be offered the option of seeing the products of conception. She may also want to know what the hospital does with the products of conception or whether she needs to make a decision about final disposition of fetal remains.

> **! NURSING ALERT**
>
> Procedures for disposition of the fetal remains vary from hospital to hospital and state to state. The nurse should know what the usual procedures are in his or her setting.

Follow-up Care. The woman will likely be discharged home within a few hours after a D&C or as soon as her vital signs are stable, vaginal bleeding remains minimal, and she has recovered from anesthesia. Discharge teaching emphasizes the need for rest. If significant blood loss has occurred, iron supplementation may be ordered. Teaching includes information about normal physical findings such as cramping, type and amount of bleeding, resumption of sexual activity, and family planning (see Patient Teaching box). Frequently the woman and her partner want to know when she should attempt to become pregnant again. Discuss with them the importance of completely resolving the loss before attempting another pregnancy (Gilbert, 2011). Follow-up care should assess the woman's physical and emotional recovery. Referrals to local support groups should be provided as needed. Share Pregnancy and Infant Loss Support, Inc. (www.nationalshare.org) is an excellent online resource for families who have experienced an early pregnancy loss.

Follow-up telephone calls after a loss are important. The woman may appreciate a telephone call on what would have been her due date. These calls provide opportunities for the woman to ask questions, seek advice, and receive information to help process her grief (see Community Focus box).

Reduced Cervical Competence (Recurrent Premature Dilation of the Cervix)

One cause of late miscarriage is reduced cervical competence (premature dilation of the cervix), which has traditionally been defined as passive and painless dilation of the cervix during the second trimester. In the past this condition was called *cervical incompetence*. This definition assumed an all-or-nothing role for the cervix: it was either competent or incompetent. However, current thinking is that cervical competence varies and exists as a continuum that is determined in part by cervical length. Other related causative factors include composition of the cervical tissue and the individual circumstances associated with the pregnancy in terms of maternal stress and lifestyle. Iams (2009) and other

---

PATIENT TEACHING

Discharge Teaching for the Woman After Early Miscarriage

- Clean the perineum after each voiding or bowel movement and change perineal pads often.
- Shower (avoid tub baths) for 2 weeks.
- Avoid tampon use, douching, and vaginal intercourse for 2 weeks.
- Notify health care provider if an elevated temperature or a foul-smelling vaginal discharge develops.
- Eat foods high in iron and protein to promote tissue repair and red blood cell replacement.
- Seek assistance from support groups, clergy, or professional counseling as needed.
- Allow yourself (and your partner) to grieve the loss before becoming pregnant again.

🏠 COMMUNITY FOCUS

Online Resources for Pregnancy-Related Bleeding Problems

- Visit the Miscarriage Support website (www.silentgrief.com), which provides assistance for families who have experienced the loss of a child by miscarriage. Review the information about the stages of grief and resources. What resources are available in your community for women who experience a perinatal loss?
- Visit the American Pregnancy Association website (www.american pregnancy.org) and go to the pregnancy complications link. Select an antepartum hemorrhagic disorder such as miscarriage, ectopic pregnancy, molar pregnancy, placental abruption, or placenta previa and evaluate the accuracy and comprehensiveness of the information regarding causes, risk factors, symptoms, diagnosis, and treatment.

---

high risk perinatal experts refer to this condition as *cervical insufficiency*.

Etiology. Etiologic factors include a history of previous cervical trauma such as lacerations during childbirth, excessive cervical dilation for curettage or biopsy, or ingestion of diethylstilbestrol (DES) by the woman's mother while pregnant with the woman. However, because DES has not been used since the early 1970s, this risk factor should soon be of only historic interest. Women who have had prior cervical surgery such as a biopsy in which a large cone specimen was removed or destroyed or who have had multiple prior cervical procedures are probably at risk for cervical insufficiency (Ludmir and Owen, 2012).

Diagnosis. Reduced cervical competence is a clinical diagnosis based on history. Short labors, recurring loss of the pregnancy at progressively earlier gestational ages, advanced cervical dilation at the time of first presentation for care, and a history of prior cervical surgery or trauma suggest reduced cervical competence (Iams, 2009). Ultrasound examination during pregnancy is used to diagnose this condition objectively. A short cervix (less than 25 mm) indicates reduced cervical competence. Often the short cervix is accompanied by cervical funneling (beaking) or effacement of the internal cervical os (Cunningham, Leveno, Bloom, et al., 2010; Iams, 2009; Ludmir and Owen, 2012).

Management. Medical management consists of bed rest, pessaries, antibiotics, antiinflammatory drugs, and progesterone supplementation (Iams, 2009). Surgical management with placement of a cervical cerclage may be chosen instead. During pregnancy the McDonald technique is often the procedure of choice. In this procedure suture is placed around the cervix beneath the mucosa to constrict the internal os of the cervix (Fig. 12-7) (Cunningham, Leveno, Bloom, et al., 2010). A cerclage may be placed prophylactically or as a rescue procedure once the cervix has been found to be effaced or dilated (Cunningham, Leveno, Bloom, et al., 2010; Gilbert, 2011).

A prophylactic cerclage is usually placed at 11 to 15 weeks of gestation. The cerclage is removed electively (usually in an office or as a clinic procedure) when the woman reaches 37 weeks of gestation, or it may be left in place until spontaneous labor begins. Occasionally the cerclage is left in place, and a cesarean birth performed. The best treatment for reduced cervical competence is uncertain at this time. Research results indicate that selective cerclage placement during pregnancy based on repeated ultrasound examination of the

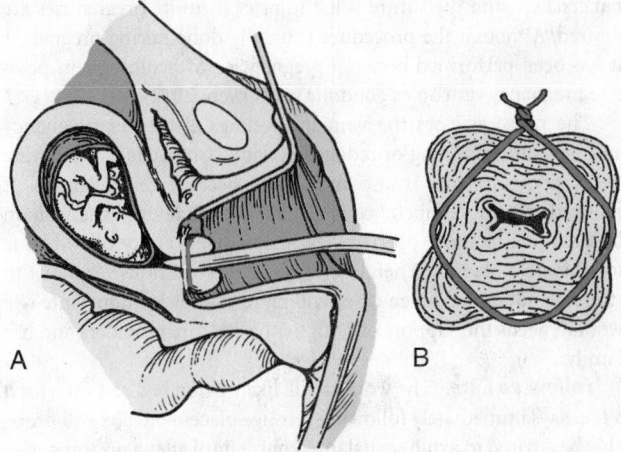

FIG 12-7 A, Cerclage correction of premature dilation of the cervical os. **B,** Cross-sectional view of closed internal os.

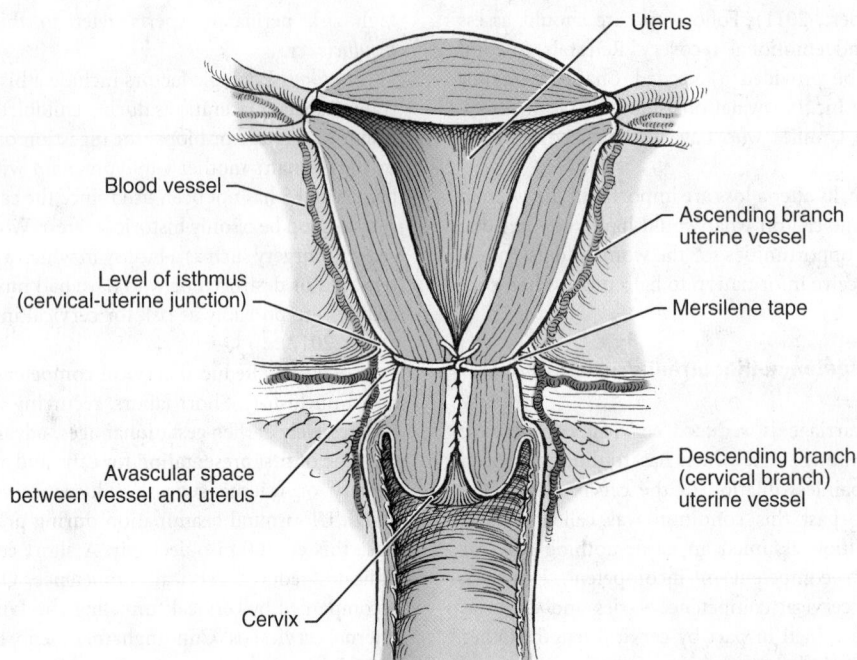

FIG 12-8 Abdominal cerclage. Surgical placement of circumferential Mersilene tape around uterine isthmus and median to uterine vessel. Knot is tied anteriorly. (From Gabbe S, Niebyl J, Simpson J, et al, editors: *Obstetrics: normal and problem pregnancies,* ed 6, Philadelphia, 2012, Saunders.)

cervix may produce pregnancy outcomes that are just as good as those obtained after prophylactic cerclage placement. Ultrasound surveillance begins at 15 to 16 weeks of gestation. Selective cerclage placement is offered if the cervical length decreases to less than 20 to 25 mm before 23 to 24 weeks (Iams, 2009). Risks of the procedure include premature ROM (PROM), preterm labor, and chorioamnionitis. Although no consensus has been reached, 24 weeks is often used as the upper gestational age limit for cerclage placement (Iams, 2009).

In women with an extremely short cervix such as those who were exposed prenatally to DES, who have a history of a large cone biopsy, or who have had a failed vaginal cerclage, an abdominal cerclage may be performed instead. This procedure is usually done at 11 to 13 weeks of gestation by means of a laparotomy. Suture (Mersilene tape) is placed at the junction of the lower uterine segment and the cervix (Fig. 12-8). Cesarean birth is necessary following an abdominal cerclage, and the suture is left in place if future pregnancies are desired. Although the procedure is usually done during pregnancy, it has been performed between pregnancies with subsequent positive pregnancy outcomes (Ludmir and Owen, 2012).

The nurse assesses the woman's feelings about her pregnancy and her understanding of reduced cervical competence. Evaluating her support systems is also important. Because the diagnosis of reduced cervical competence is usually not made until the woman has lost one or more pregnancies, she may feel guilty or to blame for this possible loss. Therefore assessing for previous reactions to stresses and appropriateness of coping responses is important. The woman needs the support of both her health care providers and her family.

Follow-up Care. The woman will likely be on bed rest for a least a few days immediately following cerclage placement. She will probably be advised to avoid sexual intercourse until after a postoperative check. Thereafter decisions about physical activity and intercourse are individualized based on the status of the woman's cervix as determined by digital and ultrasound examination (Ludmir and Owen, 2012). The woman must understand the importance of initial activity restriction at home and the need for close observation and supervision. Additional instruction includes the need to watch for and report signs of preterm labor, ROM, and infection. Finally the woman should know the signs that would warrant an immediate return to the hospital, including strong contractions less than 5 minutes apart, ROM, severe perineal pressure, and an urge to push. If management is unsuccessful and the fetus is born before viability, appropriate grief support should be provided. If the fetus is born prematurely, appropriate anticipatory guidance and support are necessary.

Ectopic Pregnancy

Incidence and Etiology. An ectopic pregnancy is one in which the fertilized ovum is implanted outside the uterine cavity (Fig. 12-9). Two percent of all first-trimester pregnancies in the United States are ectopic, and these account for 9% of all pregnancy-related maternal deaths. Women are less likely to have a successful subsequent pregnancy after an ectopic pregnancy (Cunningham, Leveno, Bloom, et al., 2010; Gilbert, 2011). Ectopic pregnancy is a leading cause of infertility.

Ectopic pregnancies are often called *tubal pregnancies* because approximately 95% are located in the uterine tube (Cunningham, Leveno, Bloom, et al., 2010). Although they are much less common, ectopic pregnancies can also occur in the abdominal cavity, on an ovary, or on the cervix. Of all tubal ectopic pregnancies, more than half (approximately 55%) are located in the ampulla, or largest portion of the tube (Gilbert, 2011).

The reported incidence of ectopic pregnancy rose through 1990 in the United States. Since then, because more cases are managed medically, reliable data on the actual number of ectopic pregnancies have not been available (Cunningham, Leveno, Bloom, et al., 2010). Some of the increased incidence is likely because of improved

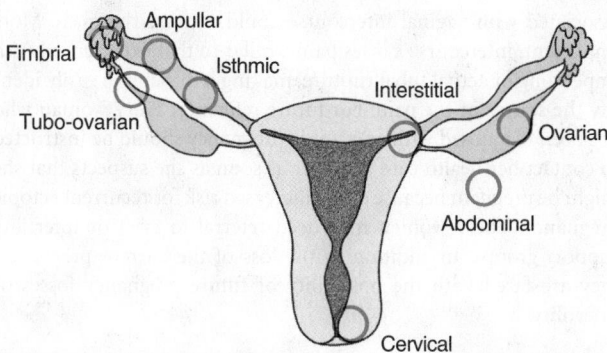

FIG 12-9 Sites of implantation of ectopic pregnancies. Order of frequency of occurrence is ampulla, isthmus, interstitium, fimbria, tubo-ovarian ligament, ovary, abdominal cavity, and cervix (external os).

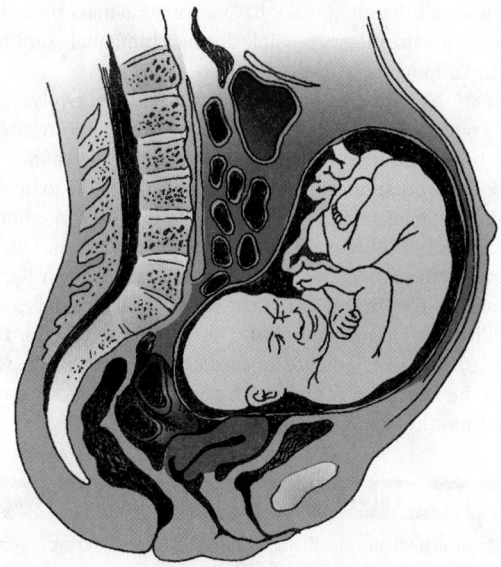

FIG 12-10 Ectopic pregnancy, abdominal.

diagnostic techniques such as more sensitive β-hCG measurement and transvaginal ultrasound, resulting in the identification of more cases. Other causes for the rise include an increased incidence of sexually transmitted infections, tubal infection and damage, popularity of contraceptive methods that predispose failures to be ectopic (e.g., the intrauterine device [IUD]), use of tubal sterilization methods that increase the chance of ectopic pregnancy, increased use of assisted reproductive techniques, and increased use of tubal surgery (Cunningham, Leveno, Bloom, et al., 2010; Gilbert, 2011).

Ectopic pregnancy is classified according to site of implantation (e.g., tubal, ovarian, or abdominal). The uterus is the only organ capable of containing and sustaining a term pregnancy. Only approximately 5% of abdominal pregnancies reach viability. However, surgery to remove the embryo or fetus is usually performed as soon as an abdominal pregnancy is identified because of the high risk for hemorrhage at any time during the pregnancy (Cunningham, Leveno, Bloom, et al., 2010; Gilbert, 2011). The chance of fetal survival in an abdominal pregnancy depends on gestational age at birth. The risk for fetal deformity in an abdominal pregnancy is high as a result of pressure deformities caused by oligohydramnios. The most common problems include facial or cranial asymmetry, various joint deformities, limb deficiency, and CNS anomalies (Fig. 12-10) (Cunningham, Leveno, Bloom, et al., 2010; Gilbert, 2011).

Clinical Manifestations. Most cases of ectopic (tubal) pregnancy are diagnosed before rupture based on the three most classic symptoms: (1) abdominal pain, (2) delayed menses, and (3) abnormal vaginal bleeding (spotting) that occurs approximately 6 to 8 weeks after the last normal menstrual period (Gilbert, 2011). Abdominal pain occurs in almost every case. It usually begins as a dull, lower-quadrant pain on one side. The discomfort can progress from a dull to a colicky pain when the tube stretches, to sharp, stabbing pain (Cunningham, Leveno, Bloom, et al., 2010; Gilbert, 2011). It progresses to a diffuse, constant, severe pain that is generalized throughout the lower abdomen (Gilbert, 2011). As many as 90% of women with an ectopic pregnancy report a period that is delayed 1 to 2 weeks or lighter than usual or an irregular period. Mild-to-moderate dark red or brown intermittent vaginal bleeding occurs in up to 80% of women (Gilbert, 2011).

If the ectopic pregnancy is not diagnosed until after rupture has occurred, referred shoulder pain may be present in addition to generalized, one-sided, or deep lower-quadrant acute abdominal pain. Referred shoulder pain results from diaphragmatic irritation caused by blood in the peritoneal cavity. The woman may exhibit signs of

shock such as faintness and dizziness related to the amount of bleeding in the abdominal cavity and not necessarily related to obvious vaginal bleeding. An ecchymotic blueness around the umbilicus (Cullen sign) indicating hematoperitoneum may also develop in an undiagnosed, ruptured intraabdominal ectopic pregnancy.

Diagnosis. The differential diagnosis of ectopic pregnancy involves consideration of numerous disorders that share many signs and symptoms. Many of these women come to the emergency department experiencing first-trimester bleeding or pain. Miscarriage, ruptured corpus luteum cyst, appendicitis, salpingitis, ovarian cysts, torsion of the ovary, and UTI are possible diagnoses. The key to early detection of ectopic pregnancy is having a high index of suspicion for this condition. *Every* woman with abdominal pain, vaginal spotting or bleeding, and a positive pregnancy test should undergo screening for ectopic pregnancy.

The most important screening tools for ectopic pregnancy are quantitative β-hCG levels and transvaginal ultrasound examination. When β-hCG levels are greater than 1500 to 2000 milli-international units/mL, a normal intrauterine pregnancy should be visible on transvaginal ultrasound. Therefore, if β-hCG levels are greater than 1500 milli-international units/mL but no intrauterine pregnancy is seen on transvaginal ultrasound, an ectopic pregnancy is very likely. β-hCG levels will probably be redrawn every 48 hours to determine if the pregnancy is viable. A transvaginal ultrasound may also be repeated to determine if the pregnancy is inside the uterus. Sometimes the location of an ectopic pregnancy is visible on transvaginal ultrasound (Cunningham, Leveno, Bloom, et al., 2010; Gilbert, 2011).

Another laboratory test that can be ordered to decide if the pregnancy is developing normally is a progesterone level. A progesterone level >25 ng/mL almost always rules out the presence of an ectopic pregnancy. However, a level <5 ng/mL suggests either an ectopic or an abnormal intrauterine pregnancy (Cunningham, Leveno, Bloom, et al., 2010).

The woman should also be assessed for the presence of active bleeding, which is associated with tubal rupture. If internal bleeding is present, assessment may reveal vertigo, shoulder pain, hypotension, and tachycardia. A vaginal examination should be performed only once and then with great caution. Approximately 20% of women with a tubal pregnancy have a palpable mass on examination. Rupturing the mass is possible during a bimanual examination; thus a gentle touch is critical.

Medical Management. Medical management involves giving methotrexate to dissolve the tubal pregnancy. Methotrexate is an antimetabolite and folic acid antagonist that destroys rapidly dividing cells. The woman must be hemodynamically stable to be eligible for medical management. The best results following methotrexate therapy are usually obtained if the mass is unruptured and measures less than 3.5 cm in diameter by ultrasound, if no fetal cardiac activity is noted on ultrasound, and if the serum β-hCG level is less than 5000 milli-international units/mL (Cunningham, Leveno, Bloom, et al., 2010). To be a candidate for medical management the woman must also be willing to comply with posttreatment lifestyle restrictions and monitoring.

> ### 💊 MEDICATION ALERT
>
> The woman on methotrexate therapy who drinks alcohol and takes vitamins containing folic acid (such as prenatal vitamins) increases her risk of having side effects of the drug or exacerbating the ectopic rupture.

Methotrexate therapy avoids surgery and is a safe, effective, and cost-effective way of managing many cases of tubal pregnancy. The woman is informed of how the medication works, possible side effects, who to call if she has concerns or if problems develop, and the importance of follow-up care (Box 12-5).

> ### ⚠ NURSING ALERT
>
> Women receiving methotrexate to treat an ectopic pregnancy should refrain from taking any analgesic stronger than acetaminophen. Stronger analgesics can mask symptoms of tubal rupture.

Surgical Management. Surgical management depends on the location and cause of the ectopic pregnancy, the extent of tissue involvement, and the woman's desires regarding future fertility. One option is removal of the entire tube (salpingectomy). If the tube has not ruptured and the woman desires future fertility, salpingostomy may be performed instead. In this procedure an incision is made over the pregnancy site in the tube, and the products of conception are gently and very carefully removed. The incision is not sutured but left to close by secondary intention, given that this method results in less scarring.

If surgery is planned, general preoperative and postoperative care is appropriate for the woman with an ectopic pregnancy. Before surgery vital signs (pulse, respirations, and BP) are assessed every 15 minutes or as needed, according to the severity of the bleeding and the woman's condition. Preoperative laboratory tests include determination of blood type and Rh status, complete blood cell count, and serum quantitative β-hCG level. Ultrasonography is used to confirm an extrauterine pregnancy. Blood replacement may be necessary. The nurse verifies the woman's Rh and antibody status and administers $Rh_o(D)$ immunoglobulin after surgery if appropriate.

Follow-up Care. The woman and her family should be encouraged to share their feelings and concerns related to the loss. Vaginal intercourse should be avoided until β-hCG levels indicate that the ectopic pregnancy has dissolved completely. This could require abstaining from sexual activity for several months. Abstinence is necessary because there is a small risk that the pelvic pressure associated with vaginal intercourse could rupture the mass. More important, intercourse causes pain similar to that experienced with impending or actual tubal rupture, making it difficult to easily identify the source of the pain. For future reference, every woman who has been diagnosed with an ectopic pregnancy should be instructed to contact her health care provider as soon as she suspects that she might be pregnant because of the increased risk for recurrent ectopic pregnancy. These women may need referral to grief or infertility support groups. In addition to the loss of the current pregnancy, they are faced with the possibility of future pregnancy losses or infertility.

BOX 12-5 NURSING CONSIDERATIONS FOR WOMEN UNDERGOING METHOTREXATE TREATMENT FOR ECTOPIC PREGNANCY

Administration

- Obtain woman's height and weight. These measurements are used to calculate the correct dose.
- Check to make sure that laboratory and diagnostic tests have been completed, including:
  - Complete blood cell count and blood type and Rh-antibody status.
  - Liver and renal function tests.
  - Serum beta–human chorionic gonadotropin (β-hCG) level (should be <5000 milli-international units/mL).
  - Transvaginal ultrasound confirming size of mass and absence of fetal cardiac activity.
- Administer methotrexate intramuscularly (IM). The usual dose is 50 mg/m^2, but it may also be ordered as 1 mg/kg.
- Administer Rho(D) immunoglobulin (150 mcg to 300 mcg IM as ordered if woman has Rh-negative blood).

Patient and Family Teaching

- Review how methotrexate works.
- Inform woman of possible side effects—gas pain, stomatitis and conjunctivitis are common; rare effects include pleuritis, gastritis, diarrhea, oral ulcers, dermatitis, alopecia, enteritis, increased liver enzymes, and bone marrow suppression.
- Advise woman to:
  - Discontinue folic acid supplements.
  - Avoid "gas-forming" foods.
  - Avoid sun exposure because the drug makes her more photosensitive.
  - Refrain from strenuous activities.
  - Avoid putting anything in her vagina—no tampons, douches, or vaginal intercourse.
  - Report to her health care provider immediately if she has severe abdominal pain, which may be a sign of impending or actual tubal rupture.

Follow-Up

- Have woman return to the clinic or office as instructed by her health care provider for measurement of β-hCG level.
- If β-hCG level does not drop appropriately, a second dose of methotrexate may be necessary.
- Advise woman that she will need to return to the clinic or office for weekly measurements of β-hCG until the level is less than 15 milli-international units/mL. Weekly follow-up visits may be required for several months until the desired β-hCG level is reached.

Hydatidiform Mole (Molar Pregnancy)

Hydatidiform mole (molar pregnancy) is a benign proliferative growth of the placental trophoblast in which the chorionic villi develop into edematous, cystic, avascular transparent vesicles that hang in a grapelike cluster. Hydatidiform mole is a **gestational trophoblastic disease (GTD).** GTD is a group of pregnancy-related trophoblastic proliferative disorders without a viable fetus that are caused by abnormal fertilization. In addition to hydatidiform mole, GTD includes invasive mole and choriocarcinoma (DiGiulio, Wiedaseck, and Monchek, 2012).

Incidence and Etiology. Hydatidiform mole occurs in 1 in 1000 pregnancies in the United States (Cohn, Ramaswamy, and Blum, 2009). The cause is unknown, although it may be related to an ovular defect or a nutritional deficiency. Women at increased risk for hydatidiform mole formation are those who have had a prior molar pregnancy and those who are in their early teens or older than 40 years of age (DiGiulio, Wiedaseck, and Monchek, 2012).

Types. A hydatidiform mole may be further categorized as a complete or partial mole. The complete mole results from fertilization of an egg in which the nucleus has been lost or inactivated (Fig. 12-11, *A*). The nucleus of a sperm (23,X) duplicates itself (resulting in the diploid number 46,XX) because the ovum has no genetic material or the material is inactive. It is also possible for an "empty" egg to be fertilized by two normal sperm, thereby producing either a 46,XX or 46,XY karyotype. The mole resembles a bunch of white grapes (see Fig. 12-11, *B*). The hydropic (fluid-filled) vesicles grow rapidly, causing the uterus to be larger than expected for the duration of the pregnancy. Usually the complete mole contains no fetus, placenta, amniotic membranes, or fluid (Fig. 12-12). Maternal blood has no placenta to receive it; therefore hemorrhage into the uterine cavity and vaginal bleeding occur. Approximately 15% to 20% of women with a complete mole have evidence of persistent GTD (Cunningham, Leveno, Bloom, et al., 2010).

For a partial mole chromosomal studies often show a karyotype of 69,XXY; 69,XXX; or rarely 69,XYY. This arrangement occurs as a result of two sperm fertilizing an apparently normal ovum (Fig. 12-13). Partial moles often have embryonic or fetal parts and an amniotic sac. Congenital anomalies are usually present. The risk of persistent GTD is much less than with a complete mole. If persistent

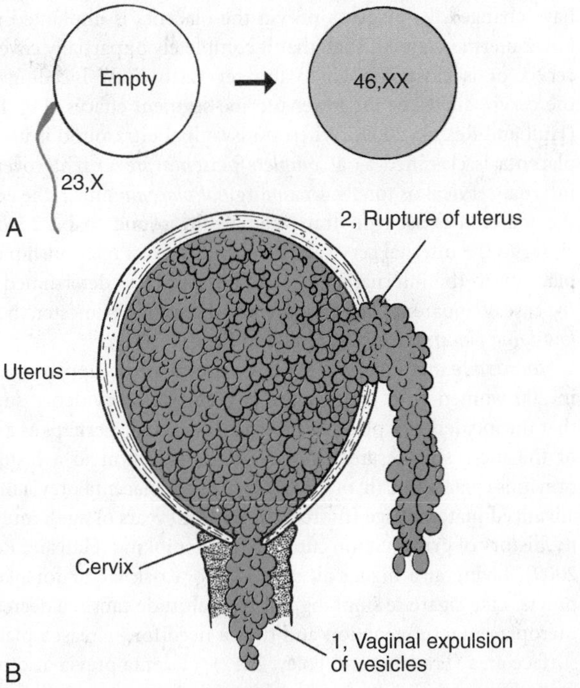

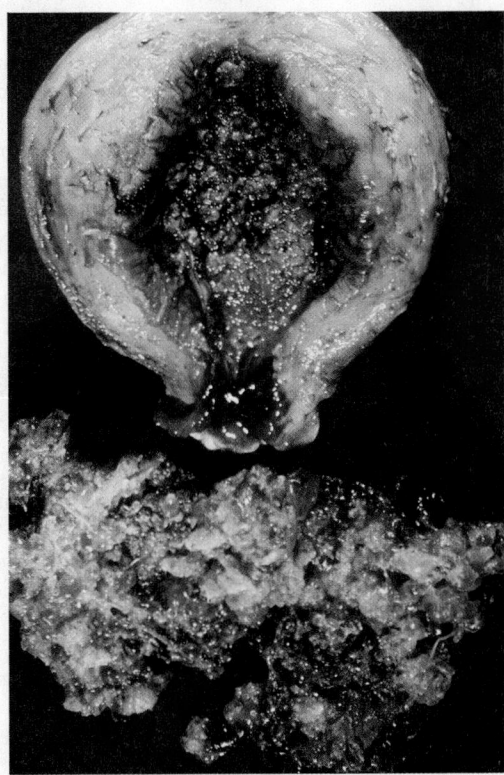

FIG 12-12 Gross specimen in a woman treated for complete hydatidiform mole with primary hysterectomy. (Courtesy John Soper, MD. From DiSaia PJ, Creasman WT: *Clinical gynecologic oncology*, ed 8, Philadelphia, 2012, Mosby.)

FIG 12-11 A, Chromosomal origin of complete mole. Single sperm *(color)* fertilizes an "empty" ovum. Reduplication of 23,X of sperm set gives completely homozygous diploid 46,XX. Similar process follows fertilization of empty ovum by two sperm with two independently drawn sets of 23,X or 23,Y; therefore both karyotypes of 46,XX and 46,XY can result. **B,** Uterine rupture with hydatidiform mole. *1,* Evacuation of mole through cervix. *2,* Rupture of uterus and spillage of mole into peritoneal cavity (rare).

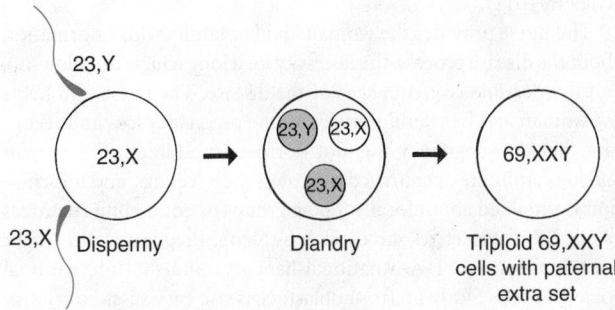

FIG 12-13 Chromosomal origin of triploid partial mole. Normal ovum with 23,X haploid set is fertilized by two sperm to give total of 69 chromosomes. Sex configuration of XXY, XXX, or XYY is possible.

GTD does occur, it is usually not a choriocarcinoma (Cunningham, Leveno, Bloom, et al., 2010).

Clinical Manifestations. In the early stages the clinical manifestations of a complete hydatidiform mole cannot be distinguished from those of normal pregnancy. Later vaginal bleeding occurs in almost 95% of cases. The vaginal discharge may be dark brown (resembling prune juice) or bright red and either scant or profuse. It may continue for only a few days or intermittently for weeks. Early in pregnancy the uterus in approximately one half of affected women is significantly larger than expected from menstrual dates. The percentage of women with an excessively enlarged uterus increases as length of time since the last menstrual period increases. Approximately 25% of affected women have a uterus smaller than would be expected from menstrual dates.

Anemia from blood loss, excessive nausea and vomiting (hyperemesis gravidarum), and abdominal cramps caused by uterine distention are relatively common findings. Women may also pass vesicles, which frequently are avascular edematous villi, from the uterus. Preeclampsia occurs in approximately 70% of women with large, rapidly growing hydatidiform moles and occurs earlier than usual in the pregnancy. If preeclampsia is diagnosed before 24 weeks of gestation, hydatidiform mole should be suspected and ruled out. Hyperthyroidism is another serious complication of hydatidiform mole. Usually treatment of the hydatidiform mole restores thyroid function to normal. Partial moles cause few of these symptoms and may be mistaken for an incomplete or missed miscarriage (Cohn, Ramaswamy, Blum, et al., 2009; DiGiulio, Wiedaseck, and Monchek, 2012; Nader, 2009; Roberts and Funai, 2009).

Diagnosis. Transvaginal ultrasound and serum hCG levels are used for diagnosis. Transvaginal ultrasound is the most accurate tool for diagnosing a hydatidiform mole. A characteristic pattern of multiple diffuse intrauterine masses, often called a *snowstorm pattern*, is seen in place of or along with an embryo or a fetus. The trophoblastic tissue secretes the hCG hormone. In a molar pregnancy hCG levels are persistently high or rising beyond 10 to 12 weeks of gestation, the time they would begin to decline in a normal pregnancy (Gilbert, 2011).

Management. Although most moles abort spontaneously, suction curettage offers a safe, rapid, and effective method of evacuating a hydatidiform mole if necessary (Cunningham, Leveno, Bloom, et al., 2010; Gilbert, 2011). Induction of labor with oxytocic agents or prostaglandin is not recommended because of the increased risk of embolization of trophoblastic tissue. Postevacuation administration of Rh$_O$(D) immunoglobulin to women who are Rh negative is necessary to prevent isoimmunization (Gilbert, 2011).

The nurse provides the woman and her family with information about the disease process, the necessity for a long course of follow-up, and the possible consequences of the disease. The nurse also helps the woman and her family cope with the pregnancy loss and recognize that the pregnancy was not normal. In addition, the woman and her family are encouraged to express their feelings, and information is provided about local support groups or counseling resources as needed. Internet resources such as Share: Pregnancy and Infant Loss Support, Inc. (www.nationalshare.org) and the International Society for the Study of Trophoblastic Disease (www.isstd.org) may also be useful. Explanations about the importance of postponing a subsequent pregnancy and contraceptive counseling are provided to emphasize the need for consistent and reliable use of the method chosen.

! NURSING ALERT

To avoid confusion regarding rising levels of hCG that are normal in pregnancy but could indicate GTD, pregnancy should be avoided during the follow-up assessment period. Any contraceptive method except an IUD is acceptable. Oral contraceptives are preferred because they are highly effective.

Follow-up Care. Follow-up care includes frequent physical and pelvic examinations along with weekly measurements of the β-hCG level until the level decreases to normal and remains normal for 3 consecutive weeks. Monthly measurements are then taken for 6 months. The follow-up assessment period usually continues for a year. During that time a rising β-hCG level and an enlarging uterus may indicate GTD (DiGiulio, Wiedaseck, and Monchek, 2012; Gilbert, 2011).

Late Pregnancy Bleeding

The major causes of bleeding in late pregnancy are placenta previa and premature separation of the placenta (abruptio placentae or placental abruption). Rapid assessment for and diagnosis of the cause of bleeding are essential to reduce maternal and perinatal morbidity and mortality (Table 12-7).

Placenta Previa

Because of advances in ultrasonography, especially transvaginal ultrasound, and an increased understanding of the changing relationship between the placenta and the internal cervical os as pregnancy progresses, definitions and classifications of placenta previa have changed. In placenta previa the placenta is implanted in the lower uterine segment such that it completely or partially covers the cervix or is close enough to the cervix to cause bleeding when the cervix dilates or the lower uterine segment effaces (Fig. 12-14) (Hull and Resnik, 2009). When transvaginal ultrasound is used, the placenta is classified as a *complete placenta previa* if it covers the internal cervical os totally. In a *marginal placenta previa* the edge of the placenta is seen on transvaginal ultrasound to be 2.5 cm or closer to the internal cervical os. When the exact relationship of the placenta to the internal cervical os has not been determined or in the case of apparent placenta previa in the second trimester, the term *low-lying placenta* is used (Hull and Resnik, 2009).

Incidence and Etiology. Placenta previa affects approximately 1 in 200 women with pregnancies at term. Some evidence suggests that the incidence of placenta previa is increasing, perhaps as a result of the increasing cesarean birth rate. In addition to a history of previous cesarean birth, other risk factors for placenta previa include advanced maternal age (more than 35 to 40 years of age), multiparity, history of prior suction curettage, and smoking (Hull and Resnik, 2009). Living at a higher altitude is also a risk factor for placenta previa. Like cigarette smoking, a higher altitude causes a decrease in uteroplacental oxygenation and thus a need for increased placental surface area (Francois and Foley, 2012). Placenta previa also occurs more frequently in women carrying male fetuses. A possible explanation for this is that placental sizes are larger in pregnancies involving male fetuses. Disagreement exists regarding an increased risk for placenta previa with multiple gestations. Some studies have found a higher incidence with twins, but others have not (Francois and Foley, 2012). Women who had placenta previa in a previous pregnancy are more likely to develop the problem in a subsequent pregnancy, perhaps as a result of a genetic predisposition. Previous cesarean birth and curettage in the past for miscarriage or induced

TABLE 12-7	SUMMARY OF FINDINGS: PLACENTAL ABRUPTION AND PLACENTA PREVIA			
	PLACENTAL ABRUPTION			
	GRADE 1 MILD SEPARATION (10%-20%)	**GRADE 2 MODERATE SEPARATION (20%-50%)**	**GRADE 3 SEVERE SEPARATION (>50%)**	**PLACENTA PREVIA**
Bleeding, external, vaginal	Minimal	Absent to moderate	Absent to moderate	Minimal to severe and life threatening
Total amount of blood loss	<500 mL	1000-1500 mL	>1500 mL	Varies
Color of blood	Dark red	Dark red	Dark red	Bright red
Shock	Rare; none	Mild shock	Common, often sudden, profound	Uncommon
Coagulopathy	Rare, none	Occasional DIC	Frequent DIC	None
Uterine tonicity	Normal	Increased, may be localized to one region or diffuse over uterus; uterus fails to relax between contractions	Tetanic, persistent uterine contractions; boardlike uterus	Normal
Tenderness (pain)	Usually absent	Present	Agonizing, unremitting uterine pain	Absent
Ultrasonographic Findings				
Location of placenta	Normal, upper uterine segment	Normal, upper uterine segment	Normal, upper uterine segment	Abnormal, lower uterine segment
Station of presenting part	Variable to engaged	Variable to engaged	Variable to engaged	High, not engaged
Fetal position	Usual distribution*	Usual distribution*	Usual distribution*	Commonly transverse, breech, or oblique
Gestational or chronic hypertension	Usual distribution*	Commonly present	Commonly present	Usual distribution*
Fetal effects	Normal fetal heart rate pattern	Abnormal fetal heart rate pattern	Abnormal fetal heart rate pattern; fetal death can occur	Normal fetal heart rate pattern

DIC, Disseminated intravascular coagulation.
*Usually refers to the expected variations of incidence seen when there is no concurrent problem.

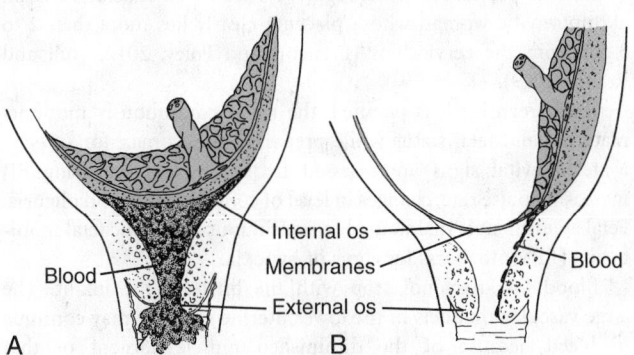

Internal os
Membranes
External os
Blood
Blood

A   B

FIG 12-14 Types of placenta previa. **A,** Complete. **B,** Marginal.

abortion are also risk factors for placenta previa because both result in endometrial damage and uterine scarring (Francois and Foley, 2012; Hull and Resnik, 2009).

Clinical Manifestations. Placenta previa is typically characterized by painless bright red vaginal bleeding during the second or third trimester. In the past placenta previa was usually diagnosed after an episode of bleeding. However, currently most cases are diagnosed by ultrasound before significant vaginal bleeding occurs. This bleeding is associated with the disruption of placental blood vessels that occurs with stretching and thinning of the lower uterine segment (Francois and Foley, 2012). The initial bleeding is usually a small amount and stops as clots form. However, it can recur at any time (Gilbert, 2011).

Vital signs may be normal, even with heavy blood loss, because a pregnant woman can lose up to 40% of her blood volume without showing signs of shock. Clinical presentation and decreasing urinary output may be better indicators of acute blood loss than vital signs alone. The FHR is normal unless a major detachment of the placenta occurs.

Abdominal examination usually reveals a soft, relaxed, nontender uterus with normal tone. The presenting part of the fetus usually remains high because the placenta occupies the lower uterine segment. Thus the fundal height is often greater than expected for gestational age. Because of the abnormally located placenta, fetal malpresentation (breech and transverse or oblique lie) is common.

Maternal and Fetal Outcomes. The major maternal complication associated with placenta previa is hemorrhage. Another serious complication is development of an abnormal placental attachment (e.g., *placenta accreta, increta,* or *percreta*) (see Chapter 21).

If excessive bleeding cannot be controlled, hysterectomy may be necessary (Cunningham, Leveno, Bloom, et al., 2010; Hull and Resnik, 2009). Because most women with placenta previa have a cesarean birth, surgery-related trauma to structures adjacent to the uterus and anesthesia complications are also possible. In addition, blood transfusion reactions, anemia, thrombophlebitis, and infection may occur.

The greatest risk of fetal death is caused by preterm birth. Other fetal risks include stillbirth, malpresentation, and fetal anemia. IUGR has also been associated with placenta previa. This association can be related to poor placental exchange (Gilbert, 2011). One study found an increased incidence of fetal anomalies in pregnancies complicated by placenta previa (Cunningham, Leveno, Bloom, et al., 2010).

Diagnosis. All women with painless vaginal bleeding after 20 weeks of gestation should be assumed to have a placenta previa until proven otherwise. A transabdominal ultrasound examination should be performed initially, followed by a transvaginal scan unless the transabdominal ultrasound clearly shows that the placenta is not located in the lower uterine segment. A transvaginal ultrasound is better than a transabdominal scan for accurately determining placental location (Hull and Resnik, 2009). If ultrasonographic scanning reveals a normally implanted placenta, a speculum examination may be performed to rule out local causes of bleeding (e.g., cervicitis, polyps, carcinoma of the cervix), and a coagulation profile is obtained to rule out other causes of bleeding.

Management. Once placenta previa has been diagnosed, a management plan is developed. The woman is managed either expectantly or actively, depending on the gestational age, amount of bleeding, and fetal condition.

Expectant Management. Expectant management (observation and bed rest) is implemented if the fetus is at less than 36 weeks of gestation and has a normal FHR tracing, the bleeding is mild (<250 mL) and stops, and the woman is not in labor. The purpose of expectant management is to allow the fetus time to mature (Gilbert, 2011). The woman initially is hospitalized in a labor and birth unit for continuous FHR and contraction monitoring. Large-bore IV access should be initiated immediately. Initial laboratory tests include hemoglobin, hematocrit, platelet count, and coagulation studies. A "type and screen" blood sample should be maintained at all times in the transfusion services department of the hospital to allow for immediate crossmatch of blood component therapy if necessary. If the woman is at less than 34 weeks of gestation, antenatal corticosteroids should be administered (Francois and Foley, 2012; Gilbert, 2011).

If the bleeding stops, the woman most likely is placed on bed rest with bathroom privileges and limited activity (able to use the bathroom, shower, and move around her hospital room for 15 to 30 minutes at a time 4 times a day). No vaginal or rectal examinations are performed, and the woman is placed on "pelvic rest" (nothing in the vagina). Ultrasound examinations may be performed every 2 to 3 weeks. Fetal surveillance may include a nonstress test (NST) or BPP once or twice weekly. Bleeding is assessed by checking the amount of bleeding on perineal pads, bed pads, and linens. Serial laboratory values are evaluated for decreasing hemoglobin and hematocrit levels and changes in coagulation values. The woman should also be monitored for signs of preterm labor. Magnesium sulfate can be given for tocolysis if uterine contractions are identified (Francois and Foley, 2012; Gilbert, 2011).

The woman with placenta previa should always be considered a potential emergency because massive blood loss with resulting hypovolemic shock can occur quickly if bleeding resumes. The possibility always exists that she will require an emergency cesarean birth. Placenta previa in a preterm gestation may be an indication for transfer to a tertiary-care perinatal center, given that a neonatal intensive care unit may be necessary for care of the preterm infant. In addition, because many community hospitals are not prepared to perform emergency surgery 24 hours per day, 7 days per week, transfer of the woman to a tertiary-care center may be necessary to ensure constant access to cesarean birth.

Home Care. Sometimes women with placenta previa are discharged from the hospital before giving birth to be managed at home. The woman's condition should be stable, and she should have experienced no vaginal bleeding for at least 48 hours before discharge (Hull and Resnik, 2009). A candidate for home care must meet other strict criteria as well. She should be willing and able to comply with activity restrictions (bed rest with bathroom privileges and pelvic rest); live within 20 minutes of the hospital; and have access to a telephone, close supervision by family or friends in the home, and constant access to transportation (Francois and Foley, 2012). If bleeding resumes, she needs to return to the hospital immediately. She must also be able to keep all appointments for fetal testing, laboratory assessments, and prenatal care. Visits by a perinatal home care nurse may be arranged.

If hospitalization or home care with activity restriction is prolonged, the woman can have concerns about her work- or family-related responsibilities or become bored with inactivity. She should be encouraged to participate in her own care and decisions about care as much as possible. Providing diversionary activities or encouraging her to participate in activities she enjoys and can perform during bed rest are necessary. Participating in a support group made up of other women on bed rest while hospitalized or online if at home may be a helpful coping mechanism (see Patient Teaching box, p. 309).

Active Management. If the woman is at or beyond 36 weeks of gestation or bleeding is excessive or persistent, immediate cesarean birth is indicated (Hull and Resnik, 2009). Expectant management is terminated as soon as the fetus is mature, if excessive bleeding develops, active labor begins, or any other obstetric reason to end the pregnancy (e.g., chorioamnionitis) develops (Gilbert, 2011). Cesarean birth is indicated in all women with ultrasound evidence of placenta previa. However, vaginal birth may be considered in an asymptomatic woman whose placenta clearly lies more than 2 to 3 cm from the cervical os (Francois and Foley, 2012; Hull and Resnik, 2009).

If cesarean birth is planned, the nurse continuously monitors maternal and fetal status while preparing the woman for surgery. Maternal vital signs are assessed frequently for decreasing BP, increasing pulse rate, changes in level of consciousness, and oliguria. Fetal assessment is maintained by continuous electronic fetal monitoring (EFM) to assess for signs of hypoxia.

Blood loss may not stop with the birth of the infant. The large vascular channels in the lower uterine segment may continue to bleed because of the diminished muscle content of that segment. The natural mechanism to control bleeding so characteristic of the upper part of the uterus (i.e., the interlacing muscle bundles, the "living ligature" contracting around open vessels) is absent in the lower part of the uterus. Therefore postpartum hemorrhage may occur even if the fundus is contracted firmly (see Chapter 21).

Emotional support for the woman and her family is extremely important. The actively bleeding woman is concerned not only for her own well-being but also for that of her fetus. All procedures should be explained, and a support person should be present. The

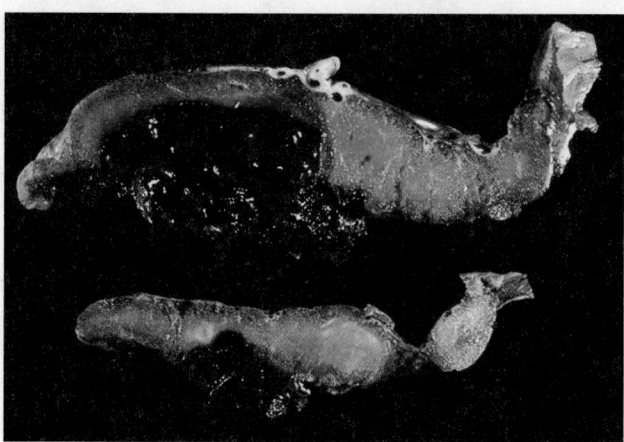

FIG 12-15 Placental abruption. Premature separation of normally implanted placenta. A large retroplacental clot is present. (From Creasy RK, Resnik R, Iams JD, et al: *Creasy and Resnik's maternal-fetal medicine: principles and practice*, ed 6, Philadelphia, 2009, Saunders.)

woman should be encouraged to express her concerns and feelings. If the woman and her support person or family desire pastoral support, the nurse can notify the hospital chaplain service or provide information about other supportive resources.

Premature Separation of Placenta (Abruptio Placentae [Placental Abruption])

Premature separation of the placenta, or abruptio placentae (placental abruption), is the detachment of part or all of a normally implanted placenta from the uterus (Fig. 12-15). Separation occurs in the area of the decidua basalis after 20 weeks of gestation and before the birth of the infant.

Incidence and Etiology. Premature separation of the placenta is a serious complication that accounts for significant maternal and fetal morbidity and mortality. Approximately 1 in 75 to 1 in 226 pregnancies is complicated by placental abruption. The range in incidence likely reflects both variable criteria for diagnosis and an increased recognition of milder forms of abruption. Approximately one third of all antepartum bleeding is caused by placental abruption (Francois and Foley, 2012) (see Critical Thinking Case Study).

Maternal hypertension, whether chronic or pregnancy related, is the most consistently identified risk factor for abruption. Cocaine use is also a risk factor because it causes vascular disruption in the placental bed. Blunt external abdominal trauma, most often the result of motor vehicle accidents (MVAs) or maternal battering, is another frequent cause of placental abruption (Cunningham, Leveno, Bloom, et al., 2010; Francois and Foley, 2012). Other risk factors include cigarette smoking, a history of abruption in a previous pregnancy, preterm PROM, and the presence of inherited or acquired thrombophilias (e.g., factor V Leiden mutation or protein C or S deficiency) (Cunningham, Leveno, Bloom, et al., 2010; Francois and Foley, 2012; Hull and Resnik, 2009; Paidas and Hossain, 2009). Abruption is more likely to occur in twin gestations than in singletons (Francois and Foley, 2012). Women who have had two previous abruptions have a recurrence risk of 25% in the next pregnancy (Hull and Resnik, 2009).

Classification. The most common classification of placental abruption is according to type and severity. This classification system is summarized in Table 12-7.

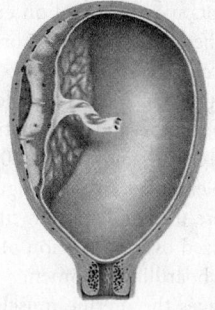
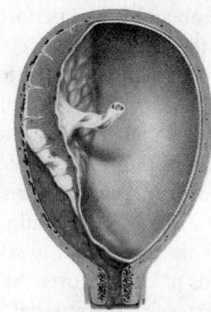

Partial separation
(concealed hemorrhage)

Partial separation
(apparent hemorrhage)

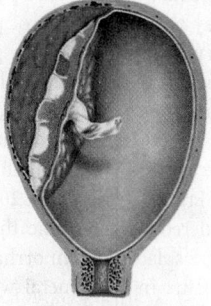

Complete separation
(concealed hemorrhage)

FIG 12-16 Placental abruption showing partial and complete placental separation.

? CRITICAL THINKING CASE STUDY

Third-Trimester Vaginal Bleeding

Ashley is a 29-year-old G6 P5 who presents to the emergency department with heavy vaginal bleeding and contractions. She has had no prenatal care but is approximately 33 weeks of gestation by her LMP. During her medical screening examination Ashley admitted to past cocaine use and reported that her boyfriend punched her in the abdomen earlier in the day.

1. Evidence—Is there sufficient evidence to determine the cause of Ashley's bleeding?
2. Assumptions—Describe an underlying assumption about each of the following issues:
   a. Possible diagnoses for Ashley
   b. Laboratory and diagnostic tests necessary to diagnose the cause of Ashley's bleeding
   c. Management options for Ashley
   d. Need for a social work consultation regarding intimate partner violence
3. What implications and priorities for nursing care can be drawn at this time?
4. Does the evidence objectively support your argument (conclusion)?

LMP, Last menstrual period.

Clinical Manifestations. The separation may be partial or complete, or only the margin of the placenta may be involved. Bleeding from the placental site may dissect (separate) the membranes from the decidua basalis and flow out through the vagina (70% to 80%), it may remain concealed (retroplacental hemorrhage) (10% to 20%), or both (Fig. 12-16) (Francois and Foley, 2012; Gilbert, 2011). Clinical symptoms vary with degree of separation (see Table 12-7).

If cesarean birth is performed, blood clots may be noted on entry into the uterus. A blood clot is often attached to the posterior surface of the placenta (referred to as a *retroplacental clot*) (see Fig. 12-15).

Classic symptoms of placental abruption include vaginal bleeding, abdominal pain, and uterine tenderness and contractions (Cunningham, Leveno, Bloom, et al., 2010; Hull and Resnik, 2009). Bleeding may result in maternal hypovolemia (i.e., shock, oliguria, anuria) and coagulopathy. Mild-to-severe uterine hypertonicity is present. Pain is mild to severe and localized over one region of the uterus or diffuses over the uterus with a boardlike abdomen.

Extensive myometrial bleeding damages the uterine muscle. If blood accumulates between the separated placenta and the uterine wall, it may produce a Couvelaire uterus. The uterus appears purple or blue rather than its usual "bubble-gum pink" color, and contractility is lost. Shock may occur and is out of proportion to apparent blood loss. Laboratory findings include a positive Apt test result (blood in the amniotic fluid); a decrease in hemoglobin and hematocrit levels, which may appear later; and a decrease in coagulation factor levels. Clotting defects (e.g., disseminated intravascular coagulation [DIC]) may be present when more than 50% of the placental surface area abrupts (Francois and Foley, 2012). A Kleihauer-Betke (KB) test may be ordered to determine the presence of fetal-to-maternal bleeding (transplacental hemorrhage), although this test appears to have no value in the general workup of women with abruption. The KB test may be useful to guide $Rh_o(D)$ immunoglobulin therapy in Rh-negative women who have had an abruption (Hull and Resnik, 2009).

Maternal and Fetal Outcomes. The mother's prognosis depends on the extent of placental detachment, overall blood loss, degree of coagulopathy present, and time between placental detachment and birth. Maternal complications are associated with the abruption or its treatment. Hemorrhage, hypovolemic shock, hypofibrinogenemia, and thrombocytopenia are associated with severe abruption. Renal failure and pituitary necrosis may result from ischemia. In rare cases women who are Rh negative can become sensitized if fetal-to-maternal hemorrhage occurs and the fetal blood type is Rh positive.

Fetal complications, which include IUGR and preterm birth, are related to the severity and timing of the hemorrhage. The size of the hemorrhage is related to fetal survival. Large (>60 mL) hemorrhages are associated with 50% or higher fetal mortality (Francois and Foley, 2012). Risks for neurologic defects, cerebral palsy, and death from sudden infant death syndrome are greater in newborns following placental abruption (Cunningham, Leveno, Bloom, et al., 2010; Francois and Foley, 2012).

Diagnosis. Placental abruption is primarily a clinical diagnosis. Although ultrasound can be used to rule out placenta previa, it cannot detect all cases of abruption. A retroplacental mass may be detected with ultrasonographic examination, but negative findings do not rule out a life-threatening abruption. In fact, at least 50% of abruptions cannot be identified on ultrasound (Hull and Resnik, 2009). Hypofibrinogenemia and evidence of DIC support the diagnosis, but many women with placental abruption do not develop coagulopathy. The diagnosis of abruption is confirmed after birth by visual inspection of the placenta. Adherent clots on the maternal surface of the placenta and depression of the underlying placental surface are usually present (see Fig. 12-15) (Francois and Foley, 2012; Gilbert, 2011).

Placental abruption should be highly suspected in the woman who experiences a sudden onset of intense, usually localized, uterine pain, with or without vaginal bleeding. Initial assessment is much the same as for placenta previa. Physical examination usually reveals abdominal pain, uterine tenderness, and contractions. The fundal height may be measured over time because an increasing fundal height indicates concealed bleeding. Approximately 60% of live fetuses exhibit abnormal FHR patterns, and elevated uterine resting tone may also be noted on the monitor tracing (Francois and Foley, 2012). Coagulopathy, as evidenced by abnormal clotting studies (fibrinogen, platelet count, partial thromboplastin time [PTT], fibrin split products), may be present if a large or complete abruption has occurred.

Management

Expectant Management. Management depends on the severity of blood loss and fetal maturity and status. If the fetus is less than 34 weeks of gestation and both the woman and fetus are stable, expectant management can be implemented. The woman is monitored closely because the abruption may extend at any time. The fetus is assessed regularly for evidence of appropriate growth because there is risk for IUGR. In addition, assessments of fetal well-being (e.g., NST and BPP) are performed regularly. See Chapter 10 for further discussion of these tests. Corticosteroids are given to accelerate fetal lung maturity (Hull and Resnik, 2009).

Active Management. Immediate birth is the management of choice if the fetus is at term gestation or the bleeding is moderate to severe and the mother or fetus is in jeopardy. At least one large-bore (16- to 18-gauge) IV line should be started. Maternal vital signs are monitored frequently to observe for signs of declining hemodynamic status such as increasing pulse rate and decreasing BP. Serial laboratory studies include hematocrit or hemoglobin determinations and clotting studies. Continuous EFM is mandatory. An indwelling catheter is inserted for continuous assessment of urine output, an excellent indirect measure of maternal organ perfusion. Blood and fluid volume replacement may be necessary, along with administration of blood products to correct any coagulation defects.

Vaginal birth is usually feasible and is desirable, especially in cases of fetal death. Labor induction or augmentation may be initiated as long as the mother and fetus are monitored closely for any evidence of compromise. Although vaginal birth is usually preferable, cesarean birth may become necessary. Cesarean birth should not be attempted when the women has severe and uncorrected coagulopathy because it can result in uncontrollable bleeding (Francois and Foley, 2012).

Nursing care of women experiencing moderate-to-severe abruption is demanding because it requires constant close monitoring of the maternal and fetal condition. Information about placental abruption, including the cause, treatment, and expected outcome, is given to the woman and her family. Emotional support is also extremely important because the woman and her family may be experiencing fetal loss in addition to the woman's critical illness.

Cord Insertion and Placental Variations

When fetal vessels lie over the cervical os, the condition is termed *vasa previa.* Usually these vessels are protected only by the fetal membranes (not by Wharton's jelly); thus they are at risk for rupture or compression. There are two variations of vasa previa. In both situations ROM or traction on the cord may rupture one or more of the fetal vessels. As a result the fetus may rapidly bleed to death. Risk factors for vasa previa include low-lying placentas, pregnancies resulting from assisted reproductive technology, and multiple gestations (Francois and Foley, 2012).

One variation of vasa previa, velamentous insertion of the cord, occurs when the cord vessels begin to branch at the membranes and then course onto the placenta (Fig. 12-17). The other variant of vasa previa occurs when the placenta has divided into two or more lobes

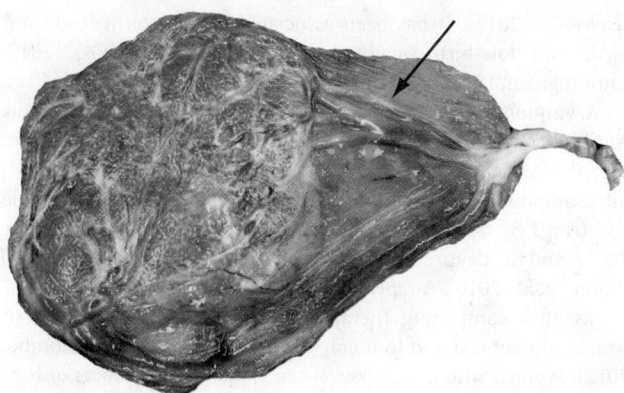

FIG 12-17 Vasa previa (velamentous insertion of cord). *Arrow* shows velamentous cord insertion in placenta. (From Creasy RK, Resnik R, Iams JD, et al: *Creasy and Resnik's maternal-fetal medicine: principles and practice*, ed 6, Philadelphia, 2009, Saunders.)

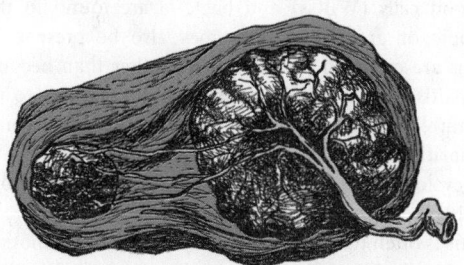

FIG 12-18 Vasa previa (succenturiate placenta).

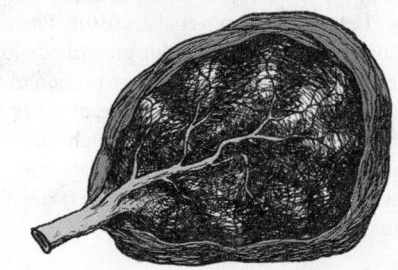

FIG 12-19 Battledore (marginal) cord insertion.

Clotting Disorders in Pregnancy
Normal Clotting
Normally a delicate balance (homeostasis) exists between the opposing hemostatic and fibrinolytic systems. The hemostatic system stops the flow of blood from injured vessels, first by a platelet plug, then by the formation of a fibrin clot. The coagulation process involves an interaction of the coagulation factors that constantly circulate in the bloodstream, in which each factor sequentially activates the factor next in line, the "cascade effect" sequence. The fibrinolytic system is the process through which the fibrin clot is split into fibrinolytic degradation products and circulation is restored.

Clotting Problems
Disseminated Intravascular Coagulation. Disseminated intravascular coagulation (DIC), or consumptive coagulopathy, is a pathologic form of clotting that is diffuse and consumes large amounts of clotting factors, causing widespread external bleeding, internal bleeding, or both, and clotting (Cunningham, Leveno, Bloom, et al., 2010). DIC is never a primary diagnosis. Instead it results from some problem that triggered the clotting cascade, either extrinsically by the release of large amounts of tissue thromboplastin or intrinsically by widespread damage to vascular integrity.

In the obstetric population DIC is most often triggered by the release of large amounts of tissue thromboplastin, which occurs in placental abruption (the most common cause of severe consumptive coagulopathy in obstetrics), the retained dead fetus syndrome, and the amniotic fluid embolus (anaphylactoid syndrome of pregnancy). Severe preeclampsia, HELLP syndrome, and gram-negative sepsis are examples of conditions that can trigger DIC because of widespread damage to vascular integrity (Cunningham, Leveno, Bloom, et al., 2010; Gilbert, 2011). DIC is an overactivation of the clotting cascade and the fibrinolytic system, resulting in depletion of platelets and clotting factors, which causes the formation of multiple fibrin clots throughout the vasculature of the body, even in the microcirculation. Blood cells are destroyed as they pass through these fibrin-choked vessels. Thus DIC results in a clinical picture of clotting, bleeding, and ischemia (Cunningham, Leveno, Bloom, et al., 2010). Clinical manifestations and laboratory test results are summarized in Box 12-6.

rather than remaining as a single mass. This is known as a *succenturiate* placenta (Fig. 12-18). Fetal vessels then run between the lobes of the placenta. The vessels collect at the periphery, and the main trunks eventually unite to form the vessels of the cord. During the third stage of labor one or more of the separate lobes may remain attached to the decidua basalis, preventing uterine contraction and increasing the risk of postpartum hemorrhage.

Another placental variation is *Battledore* (marginal) insertion of the cord (Fig. 12-19). This variation also increases the risk of fetal hemorrhage, especially after marginal separation of the placenta.

BOX 12-6 CLINICAL MANIFESTATIONS AND LABORATORY SCREENING RESULTS FOR WOMEN WITH DISSEMINATED INTRAVASCULAR COAGULATION

Possible Physical Examination Findings
- Spontaneous bleeding from gums, nose
- Oozing, excessive bleeding from venipuncture site, intravenous access site, or site of insertion of urinary catheter
- Petechiae (e.g., on arm where blood pressure cuff was placed)
- Other signs of bruising
- Hematuria
- Gastrointestinal bleeding
- Tachycardia
- Diaphoresis

Laboratory Coagulation Screening Test Results
- Platelets: Decreased
- Fibrinogen: Decreased
- Factor V (proaccelerin): Decreased
- Factor VIII (antihemolytic factor): Decreased
- Prothrombin time: Prolonged
- Partial prothrombin time: Prolonged
- Fibrin degradation products: Increased
- D-dimer test (specific fibrin degradation fragment): Increased
- Red blood smear: Fragmented red blood cells

Management. Medical management in all cases of DIC involves correction of the underlying cause (e.g., removal of the dead fetus, treatment of existing infection or of preeclampsia or eclampsia, or removal of an abrupted placenta). Volume expansion, rapid replacement of blood products and clotting factors, optimization of oxygenation, achievement of normal body temperature, and continued reassessment of laboratory parameters are the usual forms of treatment. Vitamin K administration, recombinant activated factor VIIa, fibrinogen concentrate, and hemostatic agents should be considered as additional therapies (Francois and Foley, 2012).

Nursing interventions include assessing for signs of bleeding (see Box 12-6) and complications from the administration of blood and blood products, administering fluid or blood replacement as ordered, cardiac and hemodynamic monitoring, and protecting the woman from injury. Because renal failure is one consequence of DIC, urinary output is monitored closely by using an indwelling catheter. Urinary output must be maintained at more than 30 mL/hr (Gilbert, 2011). Vital signs are assessed frequently. If DIC develops before birth, continuous EFM is necessary. The woman should be maintained in a side-lying tilt to maximize blood flow to the uterus. Oxygen may be administered through a nonrebreather face mask at 10 L/min or per hospital protocol or health care provider order. DIC usually is "cured" with the birth and as coagulation abnormalities resolve.

The woman and her family will be anxious and concerned about her condition and prognosis. The nurse offers explanations about care and provides emotional support to them through this critical time.

INFECTIONS ACQUIRED DURING PREGNANCY

Sexually Transmitted Infections

Sexually transmitted infections (STIs) in pregnancy are responsible for significant morbidity rates. Some consequences of maternal infection, such as infertility and sterility, last a lifetime. Psychosocial sequelae may include altered interpersonal relationships and lowered self-esteem. Congenitally acquired infections may affect the length and quality of a child's life. Chapter 4 discusses the diagnosis and management of STIs.

Urinary Tract Infections

UTIs are a common medical complication of pregnancy, occurring in approximately 20% of all pregnancies. They are also responsible for 10% of all hospitalizations during pregnancy (Duff, Sweet, and Edwards, 2009). UTIs include asymptomatic bacteriuria, cystitis, and pyelonephritis. They are usually caused by coliform organisms that are a normal part of the perineal flora. By far the most common cause is *Escherichia coli*, a gram-negative bacterium responsible for 85% of cases. Another gram-negative bacterium that causes UTIs is *Klebsiella pneumoniae*. The gram-positive organisms group B streptococci, enterococci, and staphylococci account for approximately 3% to 7% of all infections (Gilbert, 2011).

Asymptomatic Bacteriuria

Asymptomatic bacteriuria refers to the persistent presence of bacteria within the urinary tract of women who have no symptoms. A clean-voided urine specimen containing more than 100,000 colonies per milliliter of a single organism is diagnostic. If asymptomatic bacteriuria is not treated, up to 40% of infected women will subsequently develop symptomatic infection during the pregnancy (Colombo, 2012). Therefore the ACOG recommends that all women be screened for asymptomatic bacteriuria at their first prenatal visit

(Colombo, 2012). It has been associated with preterm labor and birth and low-birth-weight infants (AAP and ACOG, 2012; Cunningham, Leveno, Bloom, et al., 2010).

Asymptomatic bacteriuria should be treated with an antibiotic. Antibiotics that are often prescribed include amoxicillin, ampicillin, cephalexin (Keflex), ciprofloxacin (Cipro), levofloxacin (Levaquin), nitrofurantoin (Macrodantin), and trimethoprim-sulfamethoxazole (Bactrim DS). Several different regimens, including single dose or 3-, 7-, and 10-day treatment may be used (Cunningham, Leveno, Bloom, et al., 2010). A repeat urine culture is usually ordered 1 to 2 weeks after completing therapy because approximately 15% of women do not respond to therapy or have a reinfection (Colombo, 2012). Women who have persistent or frequent recurrences of bacteriuria may be placed on suppressive therapy, often nitrofurantoin, each night at bedtime for the remainder of the pregnancy (Cunningham, Leveno, Bloom, et al., 2010).

Cystitis

Cystitis (bladder infection) is characterized by dysuria, urgency, and frequency, along with lower abdominal or suprapubic pain. Usually white blood cells (WBCs) and bacteria are found in the urine. Microscopic or gross hematuria may also be present. Typically symptoms are confined to the bladder rather than becoming systemic. Cystitis is usually uncomplicated, but it may lead to ascending UTI if untreated. Approximately 40% of pregnant women with pyelonephritis experienced symptoms of bladder infection before developing pyelonephritis (Cunningham, Leveno, Bloom, et al., 2010).

Cystitis is often treated with a 3-day course of antibiotic therapy, which is usually 90% effective in curing the infection. Antibiotics often prescribed include amoxicillin, ampicillin, cephalexin (Keflex), ciprofloxacin (Cipro), levofloxacin (Levaquin), nitrofurantoin (Macrodantin), and trimethoprim-sulfamethoxazole (Bactrim DS) (Cunningham, Leveno, Bloom, et al., 2010). Phenazopyridine (Pyridium), a urinary analgesic, is often prescribed along with an antibiotic for relief of symptoms caused by irritation of the urinary tract. Although phenazopyridine is effective at relieving dysuria, urgency, and frequency, women should be taught that the medication colors urine and tears orange. Therefore they should be instructed to avoid wearing contact lenses while taking this medication and warned that it will stain underwear.

Pyelonephritis

Renal infection (pyelonephritis) is a common serious medical complication of pregnancy and the second most common nondelivery reason for hospitalization (Cunningham, Leveno, Bloom, et al., 2010). The most common maternal complications associated with pyelonephritis include anemia, septicemia, transient renal dysfunction, and pulmonary insufficiency. Women with pyelonephritis can develop urosepsis, sepsis syndrome, and renal dysfunction. In addition, pulmonary injury resembling ARDS can occur in pregnant women with acute pyelonephritis, most likely as the result of damage to alveolar tissue caused by the release of endotoxins from gram-negative bacteria (Colombo, 2012; Cunningham, Leveno, Bloom, et al., 2010). Recurrent pyelonephritis is thought to cause fetal death and IUGR. Acute pyelonephritis is associated with preterm labor (Colombo, 2012).

Pyelonephritis develops most often during the second trimester of pregnancy and is usually caused by the *E. coli* organism. Infection develops only in the right kidney in more than half of all cases. The onset of pyelonephritis is often abrupt, with fever, shaking chills, and aching in the lumbar area of the back. Anorexia and nausea and vomiting also can be present. Usually one or both costovertebral angles are tender to palpation.

Women diagnosed with pyelonephritis are admitted to the hospital immediately. Treatment with IV antibiotics is started as soon as urine and blood samples for culture and sensitivity have been collected. Ampicillin, gentamicin, cefazolin (Ancef), or ceftriaxone (Rocephin) are often ordered initially because they are broad-spectrum antibiotics that are usually effective. The woman must be monitored closely for the possible development of sepsis (Cunningham, Leveno, Bloom, et al., 2010).

Clinical symptoms generally resolve within a couple of days after antibiotic therapy is begun. The antibiotic may need to be changed based on the results of the initial culture and sensitivity testing or if the woman has not responded to therapy within 48 hours (Gilbert, 2011). Most women become afebrile within 72 hours. If no clinical improvement is seen within 48 to 72 hours, an ultrasound should be performed to assess for a urinary tract obstruction. Once the woman is afebrile, she is changed from IV to oral antibiotics (Cunningham, Leveno, Bloom, et al., 2010).

Usually oral antibiotic therapy is continued for 10 to 14 days after IV therapy has been completed (Colombo, 2012). A urine culture will likely be repeated 1 to 2 weeks after antibiotic therapy has been completed. Recurrent infection develops in 30% to 40% of women after completion of treatment for pyelonephritis. Therefore urine cultures should be obtained each trimester for the remainder of the pregnancy. Many women are maintained on a prophylactic antibiotic (often nitrofurantoin once or twice daily) for the remainder of the pregnancy (Colombo, 2012; Cunningham, Leveno, Bloom, et al., 2010).

Patient Education

Nurses are often responsible for teaching pregnant women about taking medications safely and effectively. This education is especially important in regard to antibiotics because this type of medication is so often misused by the general public. The woman should be instructed to finish the entire course of prescribed antibiotic therapy rather than stopping the medication as soon as she feels better. Failure to complete the entire course can lead to the creation of additional drug-resistant organisms. Antibiotics should be taken on time and around the clock so medication levels in the body remain constant. Finally, many women develop a yeast infection while taking antibiotics because the medication kills normal flora in the genitourinary tract as well as pathologic organisms. Therefore they should be encouraged to include yogurt, cheese, or milk containing active acidophilus cultures in their diet while on antibiotics.

The woman should also be taught simple ways to prevent future UTIs. See the Patient Teaching box on p. 97 for several suggestions.

SURGICAL EMERGENCIES DURING PREGNANCY

Approximately 1 in 500 women require nonobstetric surgery during pregnancy. However, pregnancy can make the diagnosis more difficult. An enlarged uterus and displaced internal organs can make abdominal palpation more difficult, alter the position of an affected organ, and/or change the usual signs and symptoms associated with a particular disorder. Two common nonobstetric abdominal conditions requiring surgery during pregnancy are appendicitis and symptomatic cholelithiasis (Schwartz, Adamczak, and Ludmir, 2012).

Appendicitis

The most common nonobstetric surgical emergency during pregnancy is appendicitis, occurring in about 1 in 1000 pregnancies

(Cappell, 2012). The diagnosis of appendicitis is often delayed because the usual signs and symptoms mimic some normal changes of pregnancy such as nausea and vomiting and increased WBC count. As pregnancy progresses the appendix is pushed upward and to the right from its usual anatomic location (Cunningham, Leveno, Bloom, et al., 2010). Because of these changes, rupture of the appendix and the subsequent development of peritonitis occur in up to 25% of pregnant women with appendicitis (Cappell, 2012).

The most common symptom of appendicitis in pregnant women, regardless of gestational age, is right lower-quadrant abdominal pain. Nausea and vomiting are often present, but loss of appetite is not a reliable indicator of appendicitis. Fever, tachycardia, a dry tongue, and localized abdominal tenderness are commonly found in nonpregnant people with appendicitis, but they are less likely indicators for the disorder in pregnant women. Because of the physiologic increase in WBCs that occurs in pregnancy, this test is not helpful in making the diagnosis. A urinalysis and chest x-ray should be performed to rule out UTI and right lower-lobe pneumonia, given that both of these conditions can cause lower abdominal pain (Kelly and Savides, 2009). Appendicitis can also be confused with other disorders such as cholecystitis, preterm labor, pyelonephritis, or placental abruption (Cunningham, Leveno, Bloom, et al., 2010).

Radiologic imaging is necessary if appendicitis is suspected after history, physical examination, and laboratory studies have been completed. Although computed tomography (CT) is the imaging test of choice in nonpregnant patients because it is highly accurate, the use of ultrasound during pregnancy is preferred to avoid fetal exposure to radiation from CT (Cappell, 2012). Magnetic resonance imaging (MRI) may be used if appendicitis has not been confirmed by other imaging techniques (Cappell, 2012; Kelly and Savides, 2009).

Prompt surgical intervention to remove the appendix is still the standard treatment (Kelly and Savides, 2009). Laparoscopic surgery may be performed during the first and second trimesters of pregnancy if the appendix has not ruptured or the diagnosis is uncertain. Antibiotics are often administered for uncomplicated appendicitis and are definitely necessary if rupture, abscess, or peritonitis has occurred. Clindamycin and gentamicin are often prescribed because they are considered both effective and safe. The maternal mortality rate from ruptured appendix is about 4%. The fetal mortality rate from ruptured appendix is much higher, more than 30% (Cappell, 2012).

Cholelithiasis and Cholecystitis

Cholelithiasis (the presence of gallstones in the gallbladder) occurs more often in women than in men. Its incidence increases during pregnancy, probably because of increased hormone levels and pressure from the enlarged uterus that interferes with the normal circulation and drainage of the gallbladder. Most gallstones are asymptomatic during pregnancy. Usually the first symptom of cholelithiasis is biliary colic, epigastric or right upper-quadrant pain that can radiate to the back or shoulders. Pain may occur spontaneously or after eating a high-fat meal. Approximately two thirds of patients with biliary colic have recurrent attacks (Cappell, 2012).

Cholecystitis (inflammation of the gallbladder) is usually caused when a gallstone obstructs a cystic duct. As in biliary colic that occurs with cholelithiasis, epigastric or right upper-quadrant pain is present, but the pain is usually more severe and prolonged. Nausea, vomiting, and fever may also be present. Acute cholecystitis is the third most common indication for nonobstetric surgical intervention in pregnancy, occurring in about 4 cases per 10,000 pregnancies (Cappell, 2012).

Often gallbladder surgery is postponed until the puerperium. The woman can usually be managed conservatively for the remainder of the pregnancy (see Patient Teaching box). However, women with recurrent biliary colic or acute cholecystitis generally require immediate cholecystectomy. Although the second trimester has traditionally been considered the safest time for this surgery, it is increasingly performed at any time during pregnancy because of improved surgical techniques and outcomes. Both laparoscopic and open cholecystectomy procedures are acceptable during pregnancy (Cappell, 2012; Cunningham, Leveno, Bloom, et al., 2010). Preoperative care includes IV fluids, discontinuing oral intake, analgesia, and usually antibiotics (Cappell, 2012).

Gynecologic Problems

Pregnancy predisposes a woman to ovarian problems, especially during the first trimester. Ovarian cysts and twisting (torsion) of ovarian cysts or twisting of adnexal tissues may occur. Other problems include retained or enlarged cystic corpus luteum of pregnancy and bacterial invasion of reproductive or other intraperitoneal organs. Serial ultrasounds, MRIs, and transvaginal color Doppler are used to diagnose most ovarian abnormalities (Cunningham, Leveno, Bloom, et al., 2010). Ovarian masses generally regress by 16 to 20 weeks of gestation. If they do not, elective surgery may be performed to remove masses. Laparotomy or laparoscopy may be required to discriminate between ovarian problems and early ectopic pregnancy, appendicitis, or an infectious process.

▌CARE MANAGEMENT

Initial assessment of the pregnant woman requiring surgery focuses on her presenting signs and symptoms. A thorough history and physical examination are performed. Laboratory testing includes, at a minimum, a complete blood count with differential and a urinalysis. Additional laboratory and other diagnostic tests may be necessary to reach a diagnosis. In addition, FHR and activity and uterine activity should be monitored, and constant vigilance for symptoms of impending obstetric complications maintained. The extent of preoperative assessment is determined by the immediacy of surgical intervention and the specific disorder that requires surgery.

Hospital Care

When surgery becomes necessary during pregnancy, the woman and her family are concerned about the effects of the procedure and medication on fetal well-being and the course of pregnancy. An important aspect of preoperative nursing care is encouraging the woman to express her fears, concerns, and questions.

Preoperative procedures such as preparation of the operative site and time of insertion of IV lines and urinary retention catheters vary with the physician and the facility. However, in every instance there is a total restriction of solid foods and liquids or a clear specification of the type, amount, and time at which clear liquids may be taken before surgery. Some bowel preparation such as clear liquids and laxatives may be required before surgery. Food by mouth is restricted for several hours before a scheduled procedure. Even if she has had nothing by mouth but, more important, if surgery is unexpected, the woman is in danger of vomiting and aspirating; special precautions are taken before anesthetic is administered (e.g., administering an antacid).

Intraoperatively perinatal nurses may collaborate with the surgical staff to increase their knowledge about the special needs of pregnant women undergoing surgery. One intervention to improve fetal oxygenation is positioning the woman on the operating table with a lateral tilt to avoid compression of the maternal vena cava. Continuous FHR and uterine contraction monitoring during surgery may be performed if the fetus is considered viable. Monitoring may be accomplished by using sterile Aquasonic gel and a sterile sleeve for the transducer. During abdominal surgery uterine contractions may be palpated manually. However, many practitioners simply monitor the fetus before and after the procedure.

In the immediate recovery period general observations and care pertinent to postoperative recovery are initiated. Frequent assessments are carried out for several hours after surgery. Whether the woman is cared for in the surgical postanesthesia recovery area or in a labor and birth unit, continuous fetal and uterine monitoring are likely to be initiated or resumed because of the potential risk for preterm labor. Tocolysis may be necessary if preterm labor occurs (see Chapter 17).

Home Care

Plans for the woman's return home and for convalescent care should be completed as early as possible before discharge. Depending on her insurance coverage, nursing care can be provided through a home health agency. If not, the woman and other support persons must be taught necessary skills and procedures such as wound care. Ideally the woman and other caregivers should have opportunities for supervised practice before discharge so they can feel comfortable with their knowledge and ability before being totally responsible for providing care. Box 12-7 lists information that should be included in discharge teaching for the postoperative patient. The woman also

---

PATIENT TEACHING

Nutrition Counseling for the Pregnant Woman with Cholecystitis or Cholelithiasis

- Assess your diet for foods that cause discomfort and gas and omit foods that trigger episodes.
- Reduce dietary fat intake to 40 to 50 g/day.
- Limit protein to 10% to 12% of total calories.
- Choose foods so most of the calories come from carbohydrates.
- Prepare food without adding fats or oils as much as possible.
- Avoid fried foods.

BOX 12-7 DISCHARGE TEACHING FOR HOME CARE AFTER SURGERY

- Care of incision site
- Diet and elimination related to gastrointestinal function
- Signs and symptoms of developing complications (wound infection, thrombophlebitis, pneumonia)
- Equipment needed and technique for assessing temperature
- Recommended schedule for resumption of activities of daily living
- Treatments and medications ordered
- List of resource persons and their telephone numbers
- Schedule of follow-up visits
- If birth has not occurred:
  - Assessment of fetal activity (kick counts)
  - Signs of preterm labor

may need referrals to various community agencies for evaluation of the home situation, child care, home health care, and financial or other assistance.

TRAUMA DURING PREGNANCY

Trauma remains a common complication during pregnancy because most pregnant women in the United States continue their usual activities. Approximately 30,000 pregnant women in the United States experience treatable injuries each year because of trauma (Mozurkewich and Pearlman, 2012).

Significance

Trauma is estimated to occur in approximately 5% to 15% of pregnancies (Ruth and Miller, 2013). As pregnancy progresses the risk of trauma increases, because more cases of trauma are reported in the third trimester than earlier in gestation. Most maternal injuries are a result of motor vehicle accidents (MVAs) and falls (Martin and Foley, 2009), and most maternal deaths are caused by MVAs (Ruth and Miller, 2013). Serious injuries are more likely to occur in an MVA if the woman is not wearing a seat belt with a shoulder harness and is ejected from the vehicle. Therefore, to improve chances of survival for mother and fetus, pregnant women should wear properly positioned restraints at all times when in a motor vehicle (see Fig. 8-17) (Cunningham, Leveno, Bloom, et al., 2010). Other sources of trauma include intimate partner violence, assaults, and suicide attempts (Martin and Foley, 2009).

Trauma is the leading cause of death among women of childbearing age. It is also the leading cause of nonobstetric maternal death in the United States (Ruth and Miller, 2013). Fetal morbidity and mortality are also significantly impacted by maternal trauma. In fact, trauma causes fetal death more often than maternal death (Gilbert, 2011). Fetal death rates related to maternal trauma are reported to be as high as 65% (Ruth and Miller, 2013), and this information is probably underreported (Mozurkewich and Pearlman, 2012). Fortunately most trauma injuries during pregnancy are minor and have no effect on pregnancy outcome. However, each case must be evaluated carefully because pregnancy can mask signs of severe injury.

The effect of trauma on pregnancy is influenced by the length of gestation, type and severity of the trauma, and degree of disruption of uterine and fetal physiologic features. Trauma increases the incidence of preterm labor and birth, placental abruption, and fetal or neonatal death (Martin and Foley, 2009). Other common fetal effects of trauma include PROM, fetomaternal transfusion, skull injuries, and hypoxia because of maternal respiratory compromise (Gilbert, 2011).

Special considerations for mother and fetus are necessary when trauma occurs during pregnancy because of the physiologic alterations that accompany pregnancy and because of the presence of the fetus.

Maternal Physiologic Characteristics

Optimal care for the pregnant woman after trauma depends on understanding the physiologic state of pregnancy and its effects on trauma. The pregnant woman's body exhibits responses different from those of a nonpregnant person to the same traumatic insults. Because of the different responses to injury during pregnancy, management strategies must be adapted for appropriate resuscitation, fluid therapy, positioning, assessments, and most other interventions. Significant maternal adaptations and the relation to trauma are summarized in Table 12-8.

TABLE 12-8 MATERNAL ADAPTATIONS DURING PREGNANCY AND RELATION TO TRAUMA

SYSTEM	ALTERATION	CLINICAL RESPONSES
Respiratory	↑ Oxygen consumption	↑ Risk of acidosis
	↑ Tidal volume	↑ Risk of respiratory mismanagement
	↓ Functional residual capacity	
	Chronic compensated alkalosis ↓ PaCO₂ ↓ Serum bicarbonate	↓ Blood-buffering capacity
Cardiovascular	↑ Circulating volume, 1600 mL	Can lose 1000 mL blood
	↑ CO	No signs of shock until blood loss >30% total blood volume
	↑ Heart rate	
	↓ SVR	↓ Placental perfusion in supine position
	↓ Arterial blood pressure	
	Heart displaced upward to left	Point of maximal impulse, fourth intercostal space
Renal	↑ Renal plasma flow	
	Dilation of ureters and urethra	↑ Risk of stasis, infection
	Bladder displaced forward	↑ Risk of bladder trauma
Gastrointestinal	↓ Gastric motility ↑ Hydrochloric acid production	↑ Risk of aspiration
	↓ Competency of gastroesophageal sphincter	Passive regurgitation of stomach acid if head lower than stomach
Reproductive	↑ Blood flow to organs	Source of ↑ blood loss
	Uterine enlargement	Vena caval compression in supine position
Musculoskeletal	Displacement of abdominal viscera	↑ Risk of injury, altered rebound response
	Pelvic venous congestion	Altered pain referral
	Cartilage softened	↑ Risk of pelvic fracture Center of gravity changed
	Fetal head in pelvis	↑ Risk of fetal injury
Hematologic	↑ Clotting factors	↑ Risk of thrombus formation
	↓ Fibrinolytic activity	

CO, Cardiac output; *PaCO₂,* arterial partial pressure of carbon dioxide; *SVR,* systemic vascular resistance.

The uterus and bladder are confined to the bony pelvis during the first trimester of pregnancy and are at reduced risk for injury in cases of abdominal trauma. After pregnancy progresses beyond the 14th week, the uterus becomes an abdominal organ, and the risk for injury in cases of abdominal trauma increases. During the second and third trimesters the distended bladder becomes an abdominal organ and is at increased risk for injury and rupture. Bowel injuries occur less often during pregnancy because of the protection provided by the enlarged uterus.

The elevated levels of progesterone that accompany pregnancy relax smooth muscle and profoundly affect the gastrointestinal tract. Gastrointestinal motility decreases, with a resultant increased time required for gastric emptying; whereas the production of hydrochloric acid increases in the last trimester, and the gastroesophageal sphincter relaxes (Ruth and Miller, 2013). Because of these changes, airway management of the unconscious pregnant woman is critically important.

> **! NURSING ALERT**
>
> The unconscious pregnant woman is at increased risk for regurgitation of gastric contents and aspiration whenever her head is positioned lower than her stomach or if abdominal pressure is applied.

A pregnant woman has decreased tolerance for hypoxia and apnea because of her decreased functional residual capacity and increased renal loss of bicarbonate. Acidosis develops more quickly in the pregnant than in the nonpregnant state.

Cardiac output increases 30% to 50% over prepregnancy values and is position dependent in the third trimester. Because of compression of the inferior vena cava and descending aorta by the pregnant uterus, cardiac output decreases dramatically if the woman is placed in the supine position. Therefore the supine position must be avoided, even in women with cervical spine injuries. It is a primary priority that lateral uterine displacement be accomplished without any head movement. As soon as the neck is immobilized, the stretcher should be tilted laterally (Mozurkewich and Pearlman, 2012; Ruth and Miller, 2013).

Circulating blood volume increases 40% to 50% during gestation, and pregnant women can tolerate a 1000-mL blood loss readily without demonstrating clinical signs. Hemodynamic instability that indicates the need for transfusion may not be apparent until blood loss exceeds 1500 mL (Martin and Foley, 2009).

Fetal Physiologic Characteristics

Perfusion of the uterine arteries, which provide the primary blood supply to the uteroplacental unit, depends on adequate maternal arterial pressure because these vessels lack autoregulation. Therefore maternal hypotension decreases uterine and fetal perfusion. Maternal shock results in splanchnic and uterine artery vasoconstriction, which decreases blood flow and oxygen transport to the fetus. EFM tracings can help in the evaluation of maternal status after trauma. They reflect fetal cardiac responses to hypoxia and hypoperfusion, including tachycardia or bradycardia, minimal or absent baseline variability, and/or late decelerations.

Careful monitoring of fetal status assists greatly in maternal assessment because the fetal monitor tracing works as an "oximeter" of internal maternal well-being. Hypoperfusion can be present in the pregnant woman before the onset of clinical signs of shock. The EFM tracings may show the first signs of maternal compromise (e.g., when maternal heart rate, BP, and color appear normal yet the EFM printout shows signs of fetal hypoxia) (Miller, Miller, and Tucker, 2013).

Mechanisms of Trauma

Blunt Abdominal Trauma

Blunt abdominal trauma is most commonly the result of MVAs but also may be the result of battering or falls. Maternal and fetal mortality and morbidity rates are directly correlated with whether the mother remains inside the vehicle or is ejected. Maternal death is usually the result of a head injury or exsanguination from a major vessel rupture. Serious retroperitoneal hemorrhage after lower abdominal and pelvic trauma is reported more frequently during pregnancy. Serious maternal abdominal injuries are usually the result of splenic rupture or liver or renal injury.

When the mother survives, placental abruption is the most common cause of fetal death (Gilbert, 2011). Placental separation is thought to be a result of deformation of the elastic myometrium around the relatively inelastic placenta. Shearing of the placental edge from the underlying decidua basalis results and is worsened by the increased intrauterine pressure resulting from the impact. It is critical that all pregnant victims be evaluated carefully for signs and symptoms of placental abruption after even minor blunt abdominal trauma.

> **! NURSING ALERT**
>
> Signs and symptoms of placental abruption include uterine tenderness or pain, uterine irritability, uterine contractions, vaginal bleeding, leaking of amniotic fluid, or a change in FHR characteristics.

Pelvic fracture may result from severe injury and produce bladder trauma or retroperitoneal bleeding with the two-point displacement of pelvic bones that usually occurs. One point of displacement is commonly at the symphysis pubis, and the second point is posterior because of the structure of the pelvis. Careful evaluation for clinical signs of internal hemorrhage is indicated.

Direct fetal injury as a complication of trauma during pregnancy most often involves the fetal skull and brain. Most commonly this injury accompanies maternal pelvic fracture in late gestation, after the fetal head becomes engaged. When the force of the impact is great enough to fracture the maternal pelvis, the fetus often sustains a skull fracture. Evaluation for fetal skull fracture or intracranial hemorrhage is indicated.

Uterine rupture as a result of trauma is rare, occurring in less than 1% of severe cases. Rupture is more likely to occur in a previously scarred uterus. When uterine rupture occurs, it is usually associated with a direct blow delivered with substantial force (Cunningham, Leveno, Bloom, et al., 2010). Traumatic uterine rupture almost always results in fetal death. Maternal death occurs less frequently, in about 30% of cases (Ruth and Miller, 2013).

Penetrating Abdominal Trauma

Bullet wounds are the most frequent cause of penetrating abdominal injury, followed by stab wounds. When the uterus sustains penetrating wounds, the fetus is more likely than the mother to be injured seriously. The enlarged uterus may protect other maternal organs, particularly the bowel, but the fetus is more vulnerable (Cunningham, Leveno, Bloom, et al., 2010; Martin and Foley, 2009).

Numerous factors determine the extent and severity of maternal and fetal injury from a bullet wound, including size and velocity of the bullet, anatomic region penetrated, angle of entry, path of the bullet, organs damaged, gestational age, and exit wound. Once the bullet enters the body, it may ricochet several times as it encounters organs or bone, or it may sever a large blood vessel. During the second half of pregnancy the fetus usually sustains a direct injury from the bullet. Gunshot wounds require surgical exploration to determine the extent of injury and repair damage as needed.

Stab wounds are limited by the length and width of the penetrating object and are usually confined to the pathway of the weapon. Maternal and fetal injury is less if the stab wound is located in the upper abdomen and is from movement of the penetrating object from above the head downward toward the abdomen rather than from movement from the ground upward toward the lower abdomen. Stab wounds usually require surgical exploration to clean out debris, determine extent of injury, and repair damage.

Thoracic Trauma

Thoracic trauma is reported to produce 25% of all trauma deaths. Pulmonary contusion results from nearly 75% of blunt thoracic trauma and is a potentially life-threatening condition. Pulmonary contusion can be difficult to recognize, especially if flail chest also is present or if there is no evidence of thoracic injury. Pulmonary contusion should be suspected in cases of thoracic injury, especially after blunt acceleration or deceleration trauma such as that occurring when a rapidly moving vehicle crashes into an immovable object.

Penetrating wounds into the chest can result in pneumothorax or hemothorax. This type of injury is usually caused by an MVA that results in impalement by the steering column or a loose article in the vehicle that became a projectile with the force of impact. Stab wounds into the chest also may occur as a result of violence.

Management
Immediate Stabilization

Immediate priorities for stabilization of the pregnant woman after trauma should be identical to those of the nonpregnant trauma patient. Pregnancy should not result in any restriction of the usual diagnostic, pharmacologic, or resuscitative procedures or maneuvers (AAP and ACOG, 2012). The initial response of many trauma team members when caring for the pregnant woman is to assess fetal status first because of the concern for a healthy neonate. Instead the trauma team should follow a methodic evaluation of maternal status to ensure complete assessment and stabilization of the mother. Fetal survival depends on maternal survival, and stabilization of the mother improves the chance of fetal survival.

> **NURSING ALERT**
>
> Priorities of care for the pregnant woman after trauma must be to resuscitate the woman and stabilize her condition first and then consider fetal needs.

Primary Survey

The systematic evaluation begins with a *primary survey* and the initial *CABDs* of resuscitation: *compressions, airway, breathing,* and *defibrillation.* Increased oxygen needs during gestation necessitate a rapid response. The presence of a cervical spine injury is always assumed.

> **NURSING ALERT**
>
> Hyperextension of the neck is avoided; instead jaw thrust is used to establish an airway for the trauma victim.

Once an airway is established, assessment should focus on adequacy of oxygenation. The chest wall is observed for movement. If breathing is absent, ventilations and endotracheal intubation are initiated. Supplemental oxygen should be administered with a tight-fitting, nonrebreather face mask at 10 to 12 L/min to maintain adequate oxygen availability to the fetus. The chest wall is assessed for penetrating chest wound or flail chest. Breathing with a flail chest is rapid and labored; chest wall movements are uncoordinated and asymmetric; crepitus from bony fragments may be palpated.

Rapid placement of two large-bore (14- to 16-gauge) IV lines is necessary in the majority of seriously injured women. It is important to place the lines while veins are still distended. Cardiac arrest during the immediate stabilization period is usually the result of profound hypovolemia, necessitating massive fluid resuscitation. 1 to 2 L of warmed crystalloid solutions should be infused. Ringer's solution and normal saline solution are the fluids of choice for volume resuscitation (Ruth and Miller, 2013). Because of the 50% increase in blood volume during pregnancy, published formulas for nonpregnant adults used for estimating crystalloid and blood replacement to counter blood loss must be adjusted upward.

Replacement of red blood cells and other blood components is anticipated; and blood is drawn for type, crossmatch, complete blood cell count, and platelet count. Infusion of type-specific whole blood or packed red blood cells is usually necessary to improve fetal oxygenation status and replace blood loss. During an extreme emergency type O Rh-negative blood may be administered without matching.

Administering vasopressor drugs to treat maternal hypotension should be avoided if possible. These medications may significantly reduce uterine blood flow and thus decrease oxygen delivery to the fetus. In addition, their use does not address the cause of the hypovolemia (Ruth and Miller, 2013).

After 20 weeks of gestation venous return to the heart is best accomplished by positioning the uterus to one side to eliminate the weight of the uterus compressing the inferior vena cava or the descending aorta. This facilitates efforts to establish the forward flow of blood through resuscitation and stabilization.

Cardiopulmonary Resuscitation of the Pregnant Woman. Trauma, cardiac abnormalities, embolism, magnesium overdose, sepsis, intracranial hemorrhage, anesthetic complications, eclampsia, and uterine rupture are the most common causes of cardiac arrest in a pregnant woman (Martin and Foley, 2009). Special modifications are necessary when cardiopulmonary resuscitation (CPR) is performed during the second half of pregnancy. In nonpregnant women chest compressions produce a cardiac output of only about 30% of normal. Cardiac output in pregnant women may be even less as a result of aortocaval compression caused by the gravid uterus. Therefore uterine displacement during resuscitation efforts is critical (Cunningham, Leveno, Bloom, et al., 2010). The uterus may be displaced laterally either manually or by placing a wedge, rolled blanket, or towel under one of the woman's hips. If defibrillation is needed, the paddles must be placed one rib interspace higher than usual because the heart is displaced slightly by the enlarged uterus (see Emergency box).

Complications, including laceration of the liver, rupture of the spleen or uterus, hemothorax, hemopericardium, or fracture of ribs or sternum may be associated with CPR on a pregnant woman. Fetal complications, including cardiac arrhythmia or asystole related to maternal defibrillation and medications and CNS depression related to antiarrhythmic drugs and inadequate uteroplacental perfusion, with possible fetal hypoxemia and acidemia, also may occur.

✚ EMERGENCY

Cardiopulmonary Resuscitation for the Pregnant Woman

Assessment
- Determine unresponsiveness and no breathing or no normal breathing.
- Activate emergency medical system and get AED if available.
- Return to victim and check for pulse.
- Begin chest compressions if no pulse is felt.

Compressions
- Position the woman on a flat, firm surface with her uterus displaced laterally with a wedge (e.g., a rolled towel placed under her hip) or manually or place her in a lateral position.
- Begin chest compressions at a rate of 100/min. Push hard and push fast! At the end of each compression allow chest to recoil (reexpand) completely.
  - Chest compressions may be performed slightly higher on the sternum if the uterus is enlarged enough to displace the diaphragm into a higher position.
- After five cycles of 30 compressions and two breaths (or approximately 2 min), check for a pulse. If no pulse is present, continue CPR.

Airway
- Open airway using head tilt-chin lift maneuver.

Breathing
- Deliver breaths using a face mask or bag-mask device if possible.
- Deliver each breath over 1 second, watching for chest rise.
- Deliver breaths using a ratio of 30 chest compressions to 2 breaths.

Defibrillation
- Use an AED according to standard protocol to analyze heart rhythm and deliver shock if indicated.

Data from Aufderheide TP, Cave DM, Hazinski MF, et al: Part 5: Adult Basic Life Support: 2010 American Heart Association Guidelines for Cardiopulmonary Resuscitation and Emergency Cardiovascular Care Science, *Circulation* 122(suppl 3):S685–S705. *AED,* Automated external defibrillator; *CPR,* cardiopulmonary resuscitation.

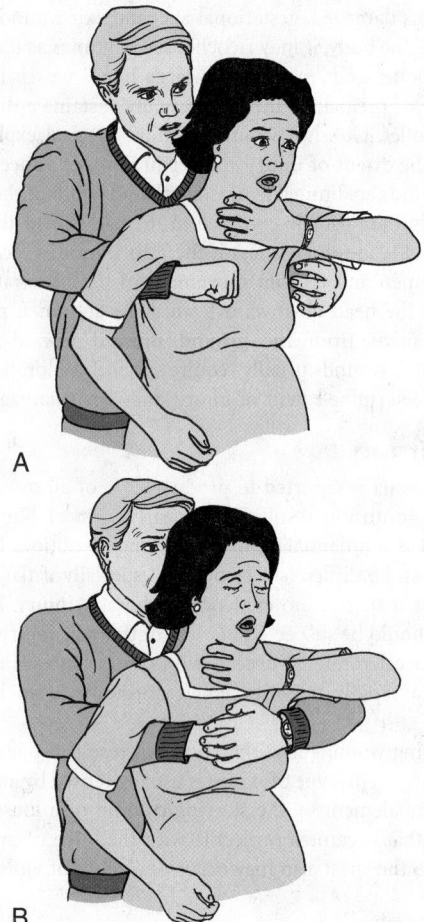

FIG 12-20 Clearing airway obstruction in woman in late stage of pregnancy. **A,** Standing behind victim, place your arms under woman's armpits and across chest. Place thumb side of your clenched fist against middle of sternum, and place other hand over fist. **B,** Perform backward chest thrusts until foreign body is expelled or woman becomes unconscious (see Emergency box below).

✚ EMERGENCY

Relief of Foreign Body Airway Obstruction

If the pregnant woman is unable to speak or cough, perform chest thrusts. Stand behind the woman and place your arms under her armpits to encircle her chest. Press backward with quick thrusts until the foreign body is expelled (see Fig. 12-20). If the woman becomes unconscious, carefully support her to the ground, immediately activate EMS, and begin CPR.

Data from Aufderheide TP, Cave DM, Hazinski MF, et al: Part 5: Adult Basic Life Support: 2010 American Heart Association Guidelines for Cardiopulmonary Resuscitation and Emergency Cardiovascular Care Science, *Circulation* 122(suppl 3):S685–S705. *EMS,* Emergency medical services; *CPR,* cardiopulmonary resuscitation.

If the resuscitation is successful, the woman must be monitored carefully afterward. She remains at increased risk for recurrent cardiac arrest and arrhythmias (e.g., ventricular tachycardia, supraventricular tachycardia, bradycardia). Therefore her cardiovascular, pulmonary, and neurologic status should be assessed continuously. If the pregnancy remains intact, uterine activity and resting tone must be monitored. Fetal status and gestational age should also be determined and used in decision making regarding the continuation of the pregnancy or the timing and route of birth.

Another common reason for performing CPR on a pregnant woman is airway obstruction caused by choking. Clearing an airway obstruction is usually accomplished by performing abdominal thrusts. However, during the second and third trimesters of pregnancy, chest thrusts rather than abdominal thrusts should be used (see Emergency box and Fig. 12-20).

Secondary Survey

After immediate resuscitation and successful stabilization measures, a more detailed *secondary survey* of the mother and fetus should be completed. A complete physical assessment, including all body systems, is performed.

The maternal abdomen should be evaluated carefully because a large percentage of serious injuries involve the uterus, intraperitoneal structures, and the retroperitoneum. The greatest clinical concern after severe abdominal trauma is placental abruption because as many as 40% of these women have an abruption. If placental abruption occurs, the associated fetal mortality rate can be as high as 50% to 80% (Mozurkewich and Pearlman, 2012). Assessments should focus on recognition of this complication, with careful evaluation of fetal monitor tracings, uterine tenderness, labor, or vaginal bleeding. Ultrasound examination may be performed to determine gestational age, viability of the fetus, and placental location. However, ultrasound studies cannot exclude placental abruption. Most cases of abruption that occur as a result of trauma are associated with relatively minor injuries (Cunningham, Leveno, Bloom, et al., 2010; Martin and Foley, 2009).

If trauma is the result of a penetrating wound, the woman should be undressed completely and examined carefully for all entrance and exit wounds. Ultrasonography and CT scan should be performed to assess for the likelihood of intraabdominal bleeding. Peritoneal lavage can be performed on hemodynamically stable women if ultrasound and CT findings do not provide a clear diagnosis. Under direct visualization the peritoneum is incised, and a peritoneal dialysis catheter is positioned. If aspiration yields free-flowing blood, the test is considered positive, and a laparotomy is warranted (Cunningham, Leveno, Bloom, et al., 2010; Martin and Foley, 2009).

Exploratory laparotomy is necessary after a gunshot wound to assess the abdominal cavity for organ damage and repair any damage, with careful examination of all organs, the entire bowel, and posterior vessels. If uterine injury is found, a careful evaluation of the risks and benefits of cesarean birth is quickly accomplished. A cesarean birth is desirable if the fetus is alive and near term and may be necessary for the preterm fetus because of the high incidence of direct fetal injury in these cases. The fetus usually tolerates surgery and anesthesia if adequate uterine perfusion and oxygenation are maintained. Tetanus prophylaxis guidelines are not changed by pregnancy.

Trauma may affect numerous systems in the maternal body and more than the pregnancy. External signs of maternal trauma should suggest the possibility of internal trauma. Back and neck pain suggest spine injury, abrasions on the chest suggest chest injury, and limb pain and malposition suggest limb fractures. If head injury results in nonresponsiveness, suspect spinal, thoracic, and abdominal injuries. Hypovolemic shock can occur with internal hemorrhage, fracture of long bones, ruptured liver or spleen, hemothorax, or arterial dissection.

All female trauma victims of childbearing age should be considered pregnant until proven otherwise. Determination of the health history and a history of the events preceding the trauma are important components of care. If the pregnant woman was involved in an MVA, it should be determined whether she was the driver or a passenger and if she was ejected from the vehicle or used a restraining device and remained within the vehicle.

Electronic Fetal Monitoring. External FHR and contraction monitoring is recommended after blunt trauma in a viable gestation for a minimum of 4 hours, regardless of injury severity. Fetal monitoring should be initiated soon after the woman is stable (Cunningham, Leveno, Bloom, et al., 2010; Martin and Foley, 2009). Continuous EFM may show early signs of placental abruption, including a change in baseline rate; loss of accelerations; or the presence of late decelerations, especially when accompanied by absent or minimal variability. The external device to monitor uterine activity, the tocodynamometer, is unable to measure pressures; the pattern made with this device shows the frequency and duration of contractions only. Palpation is required to evaluate the intensity of contractions and the uterine resting tone. It is important to palpate between contractions to verify that the uterus is well relaxed. If it

does not relax between contractions, placental abruption could be present.

The exact duration of FHR and contraction monitoring required after blunt abdominal trauma is not known. Monitoring should be continued indefinitely if uterine contractions, abnormal FHR characteristics, vaginal bleeding, uterine tenderness or irritability, serious maternal injury, or ruptured membranes are present. Most physicians recommend continuous monitoring for at least 24 hours. Most abruptions develop soon after the traumatic event, although in rare cases abruption has developed days afterward (Cunningham, Leveno, Bloom, et al., 2010; Martin and Foley, 2009).

LEGAL TIP: Care of the Pregnant Woman Involved in a Minor Trauma Situation

After minor trauma the pregnant woman may be discharged after an adequate period of EFM that demonstrates a normal (category I) tracing (see Chapter 15) and absence of uterine contractions. However, clear instructions must be given for immediate return if vaginal bleeding, leaking of amniotic fluid, decreased fetal movement, or severe abdominal pain occurs.

Fetal-Maternal Hemorrhage. The potential for fetal-maternal hemorrhage exists after trauma. Hemorrhage can lead to fetal anemia, distress, or even death. If the pregnant trauma victim is Rh negative, fetal-maternal hemorrhage can result in sensitization and hemolytic disease of the neonate. The KB assay is often performed in women following blunt abdominal trauma to estimate the amount of fetal blood within the maternal circulation. However, because most cases have less than 30 mL of hemorrhage, KB test results seldom alter management (Cunningham, Leveno, Bloom, et al., 2010; Martin and Foley, 2009). Usually the routine administration of 300 mcg of $Rh_o(D)$ immunoglobulin is sufficient to protect almost all Rh-negative pregnant trauma patients from isoimmunization (Morzurkewich and Pearlman, 2012).

Ultrasound. Ultrasound after trauma is not as sensitive as EFM for diagnosing placental abruption. It may be useful to help establish gestational age, locate the placenta, evaluate cardiac activity (to determine whether the fetus is alive), and determine amniotic fluid volume. It may also be used to evaluate the presence of intraabdominal fluid that would suggest the presence of intraabdominal hemorrhage.

Radiation Exposure. If the pregnant woman has sustained serious injuries, any necessary radiographic examination should be performed, regardless of fetal exposure. If radiographic examination would be performed for the nonpregnant trauma victim, it also should be performed for the pregnant woman. Abdominal or pelvic CT scanning can be used to visualize extraperitoneal and retroperitoneal structures and the genitourinary tract. Radiation exposure of less than 5 rads has not been associated with fetal abnormalities or pregnancy loss, and the radiation level associated with abdominal or pelvic CT scans is far below this amount (Martin and Foley, 2009). Blunt head trauma and loss of consciousness necessitate skull films and CT assessment with neurosurgical consultation. MRI can also be used safely to assess injuries because it does not produce ionizing radiation (Martin and Foley, 2009).

Perimortem Cesarean Birth

In the presence of multisystem trauma, *perimortem cesarean birth* may be indicated. Removal of the stressor of pregnancy early in the process of resuscitation may increase the chance for maternal survival. Therefore, to facilitate resuscitative efforts, a cesarean birth should be performed after 4 minutes of resuscitative efforts if there is no evidence of a maternal pulse (Martin and Foley, 2009; Mozurkewich and Pearlman, 2012; Ruth and Miller, 2013). It should be emphasized that perimortem cesarean birth is rarely successful, especially when the maternal arrest is related to trauma (Ruth and Miller, 2013).

KEY POINTS

- Hypertensive disorders during pregnancy are a leading cause of maternal and perinatal morbidity and mortality worldwide.
- The cause of preeclampsia is unknown, and there are no known reliable tests for predicting women at risk for developing preeclampsia.
- Preeclampsia is a multisystem disease, and the pathologic changes are present long before clinical manifestations such as hypertension are evident.
- HELLP syndrome, which is usually diagnosed during the third trimester, is a variant of severe preeclampsia, not a separate illness.
- Magnesium sulfate, the anticonvulsant of choice for preventing or controlling eclamptic seizures, requires careful monitoring of reflexes, respirations, and renal function.
- The intent of emergency interventions for eclampsia is to prevent self-injury, enhance oxygenation, reduce aspiration risk, and establish control with magnesium sulfate.
- The woman with hyperemesis gravidarum may have significant weight loss and dehydration; management focuses on restoring fluid and electrolyte balance and preventing recurrence of nausea and vomiting.
- Some miscarriages occur for unknown reasons, but fetal or placental maldevelopment and maternal factors account for many others.
- The type of miscarriage and signs and symptoms direct care management.
- Ectopic pregnancy is a significant cause of maternal morbidity and mortality.
- Placental abruption and placenta previa are differentiated by type of bleeding, uterine tonicity, and presence or absence of pain.
- Pyelonephritis is a serious medical complication of pregnancy and the second most common nondelivery reason for hospitalization.
- Perioperative care for a pregnant woman differs from that for a nonpregnant woman in one significant aspect: the presence of at least one other person—the fetus.
- Most maternal trauma results from MVAs and falls. Most maternal deaths are caused by MVAs.
- Fetal survival depends on maternal survival. After trauma the first priority is resuscitation and stabilization of the mother before consideration of the fetus.
- Maternal trauma can be associated with major complications for the pregnancy, including placental abruption, fetomaternal hemorrhage, preterm labor and birth, and fetal death.

REFERENCES

American Academy of Pediatrics (AAP) and American College of Obstetricians and Gynecologists (ACOG): *Guidelines for perinatal care*, ed 7, Washington, DC, 2012, ACOG.

American College of Obstetricians and Gynecologists (ACOG): *Diagnosis and management of preeclampsia and eclampsia: ACOG Practice Bulletin number 33*, Washington, DC, 2002, ACOG.

Cappell M: Hepatic and gastrointestinal diseases. In Gabbe S, Niebyl J, Simpson J, et al, editors: *Obstetrics: normal and problem pregnancies*, ed 6, Philadelphia, 2012, Saunders.

Cohn D, Ramaswamy B, Blum K: Malignancy and pregnancy. In Creasy RK, Resnik R, Iams J, et al, editors: *Creasy and Resnik's maternal-fetal medicine: principles and practice*, ed 6, Philadelphia, 2009, Saunders.

Colombo D: Renal disease. In Gabbe S. Niebyl J, Simpson J, et al, editors: *Obstetrics: normal and problem pregnancies*, ed 6, Philadelphia, 2012, Saunders.

Cunningham F, Leveno K, Bloom S, et al: *Williams obstetrics*, ed 23, New York, 2010, McGraw-Hill.

DiGiulio M, Wiedaseck S, Monchek R: Understanding hydatidiform mole, *MCN Am J Matern Child Nurs* 37(1):30–34, 2012.

Duff P, Sweet R, Edwards R: Maternal and fetal infections. In Creasy RK, Resnik R, Iams J, et al, editors: *Creasy and Resnik's maternal-fetal medicine: principles and practice*, ed 6, Philadelphia, 2009, Saunders.

Francois KE, Foley MR: Antepartum and postpartum hemorrhage. In Gabbe S, Niebyl J, Simpson J, et al, editors: *Obstetrics: normal and problem pregnancies*, ed 6, Philadelphia, 2012, Saunders.

Gilbert E: *Manual of high risk pregnancy and delivery*, ed 5, St Louis, 2011, Mosby.

Gordon MC: Maternal physiology. In Gabbe S, Niebyl J, Simpson J, et al, editors: *Obstetrics: normal and problem pregnancies*, ed 6, Philadelphia, 2012, Saunders.

Harvey C, Sibai B: Hypertension in pregnancy. In Troiano N, Harvey C, Chez B, editors: *AWHONN's high risk and critical care obstetrics*, ed 3, Philadelphia, 2013, Wolters Kluwer/Lippincott Williams & Wilkins.

Hull AD, Resnik R: Placenta previa, placenta accreta, abruptio placentae, and vasa previa. In Creasy RK, Resnik R, Iams J, et al, editors:

Creasy and Resnik's maternal-fetal medicine: principles and practice, ed 6, Philadelphia, 2009, Saunders.

Iams JD: Cervical insufficiency. In Creasy RK, Resnik R, Iams J, et al, editors: *Creasy and Resnik's maternal-fetal medicine: principles and practice*, ed 6, Philadelphia, 2009, Saunders.

Institute for Safe Medication Practices (ISMP): *ISMP's list of high-alert medications*, 2012, www.ismp.org.

Kelly TF, Savides TJ: Gastrointestinal disease in pregnancy. In Creasy RK, Resnik R, Iams J, et al, editors: *Creasy and Resnik's maternal-fetal medicine: principles and practice*, ed 6, Philadelphia, 2009, Saunders.

King TL, Murphy PA: Evidence-based approaches to managing nausea and vomiting in early pregnancy, *J Midwifery Women's Health* 54(6):430–444, 2009.

Ludmir J, Owen J: Cervical insufficiency. In Gabbe S, Niebyl J, Simpson J, et al, editors: *Obstetrics: normal and problem pregnancies*, ed 6, Philadelphia, 2012, Saunders.

Martin SR, Foley MR: Intensive care monitoring of the critically ill pregnant patient. In Creasy RK, Resnik R, Iams J, et al, editors:

Creasy and Resnik's maternal-fetal medicine: principles and practice, ed 6, Philadelphia, 2009, Saunders.

Martin J, Hamilton B, Sutton P, et al: Births: final data for 2010, *Natl Vital Stat Rep* 61(1):1–100, 2012.

Miller L, Miller D, Tucker S: *Mosby's pocket guide to fetal monitoring: a multidisciplinary approach*, ed 7, St Louis, 2013, Mosby.

Mozurkewich E, Pearlman M: Trauma and related surgery in pregnancy. In Gabbe S, Niebyl J, Simpson J, et al, editors: *Obstetrics: normal and problem pregnancies*, ed 6, Philadelphia, 2012, Saunders.

Nader S: Thyroid disease and pregnancy. In Creasy RK, Resnik R, Iams J, et al, editors: *Creasy and Resnik's maternal-fetal medicine: principles and practice*, ed 6, Saunders: Philadelphia, 2009.

National High Blood Pressure Education Program: *Working group report on high blood pressure in pregnancy*, NIH Pub No 00-3029, Bethesda, MD, 2000, National Institutes of Health, National Heart, Lung, and Blood Institute.

Otten JJ, Helwig JP, Meyers LD, editors: *Dietary reference intakes: the essential guide to nutrient requirements*, Washington, DC, 2006, National Academies Press.

Paidas M, Hossain N: Embryonic and fetal demise. In Creasy RK, Resnik R, Iams J, et al, editors: *Creasy and Resnik's maternal-fetal medicine: principles and practice*, ed 6, Philadelphia, 2009, Saunders.

Pickering T, Hall J, Appel L, et al: Recommendations for blood pressure measurement in humans and experimental animals. Part I: Blood pressure measurement in humans: a statement for professionals from the subcommittee of professional and public education of the American Heart Association Council on High Blood Pressure Research, *Hypertension* 45:142–161, 2005.

Roberts J, Funai EF: Pregnancy-related hypertension. In Creasy RK, Resnik R, Iams J, et al, editors: *Creasy and Resnik's maternal-fetal medicine: principles and practice*, ed 6, Philadelphia, 2009, Saunders.

Ruth D, Miller RS: Trauma in pregnancy. In Troiano N, Harvey C, Chez B, editors: *AWHONN's high risk and critical care obstetrics*, ed 3, Philadelphia, 2013, Wolters Kluwer/Lippincott Williams & Wilkins.

Schwartz N, Adamczak J, Ludmir J: Surgery during pregnancy. In Gabbe S, Niebyl J, Simpson J, et al, editors: *Obstetrics: normal and problem pregnancies*, ed 6, Philadelphia, 2012, Saunders.

Sibai B: Hypertension. In Gabbe S, Niebyl J, Simpson J, et al, editors: *Obstetrics: normal and problem pregnancies*, ed 6, Philadelphia, 2012, Saunders.

Simpson K, Creehan P: *AWHONN's perinatal nursing*, ed 3, Philadelphia, 2008, Lippincott Williams & Wilkins.

Simpson J, Jauniaux E: Pregnancy loss. In Gabbe S, Niebyl J, Simpson J, et al, editors: *Obstetrics: normal and problem pregnancies*, ed 6, Philadelphia, 2012, Saunders.

Labor and Birth Processes

Kitty Cashion

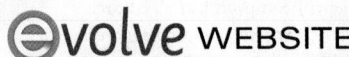 WEBSITE

http://evolve.elsevier.com/Perry/maternal

LEARNING OBJECTIVES

On completion of this chapter, the reader will be able to:
- Explain the five major factors that affect the labor process.
- Describe the anatomic structure of the bony pelvis.
- Recognize the normal measurements of the diameters of the pelvic inlet, cavity, and outlet.
- Explain the significance of the size and position of the fetal head during labor and birth.
- Summarize the cardinal movements of the mechanism of labor for a vertex presentation.
- Examine the maternal anatomic and physiologic adaptations to labor.
- Describe factors thought to contribute to the onset of labor.
- Describe fetal adaptations to labor.

During late pregnancy the woman and fetus prepare for the labor process. The fetus has grown and developed in preparation for extrauterine life. The woman has undergone various physiologic adaptations during pregnancy that prepare her for giving birth and motherhood. Labor and birth represent the end of pregnancy, the beginning of extrauterine life for the newborn, and a change in the lives of the family. This chapter discusses the factors affecting labor, the processes involved, the normal progression of events, and the adaptations made by both the woman and fetus.

FACTORS AFFECTING LABOR

At least five factors affect the process of labor and birth. These are easily remembered as the five *Ps*: *p*assenger (fetus and placenta), *p*assageway (birth canal), *p*owers (contractions), *p*osition of the mother, and *p*sychologic response. The first four factors are presented here as the basis of understanding the physiologic process of labor. The fifth factor is discussed in Chapter 16. Other factors that may be a part of the woman's labor experience may be important as well. VandeVusse (1999) identified external forces, including place of birth, preparation, type of provider (especially nurses), and procedures. Physiology (sensations) was identified as an internal force. These factors are discussed generally in Chapter 16 as they relate to nursing care during labor. Further research investigating essential forces of labor is recommended.

Passenger

The movement of the passenger, or fetus, through the birth canal is determined by several interacting factors: the size of the fetal head, fetal presentation, fetal lie, fetal attitude, and fetal position. Because the placenta also must pass through the birth canal, it can be considered a passenger along with the fetus; however, the placenta rarely impedes the process of labor in normal vaginal birth. An exception is the case of placenta previa (see Chapter 12).

Size of the Fetal Head

Because of its size and relative rigidity, the fetal head has a major effect on the birth process. The fetal skull is composed of two parietal bones, two temporal bones, the frontal bone, and the occipital bone (Fig. 13-1, *A*). These bones are united by membranous sutures: the sagittal, lambdoidal, coronal, and frontal (see Fig. 13-1, *B*). Membrane-filled spaces called *fontanels* are located where the sutures intersect. During labor after rupture of membranes, palpation of fontanels and sutures during vaginal examination reveals fetal presentation, position, and attitude.

The two most important fontanels are the anterior and posterior (see Fig. 13-1, *B*). The larger of these, the anterior fontanel, is diamond shaped, about 3 cm by 2 cm, and lies at the junction of the sagittal, coronal, and frontal sutures. It closes by 18 months after birth. The posterior fontanel lies at the junction of the sutures of the two parietal bones and the occipital bone, is triangular, and is about 1 cm by 2 cm. It closes 6 to 8 weeks after birth.

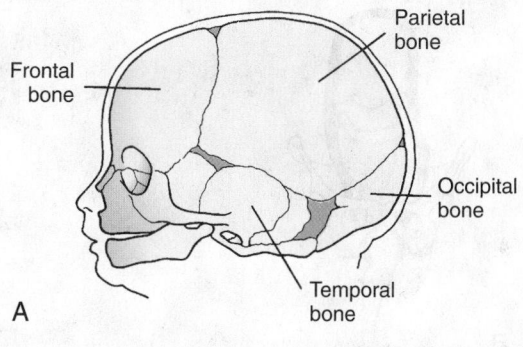

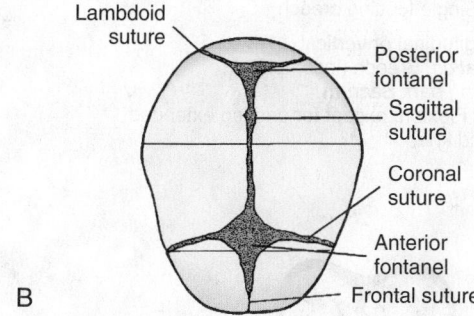

FIG 13-1 Fetal head at term. **A,** Bones. **B,** Sutures and fontanels.

Sutures and fontanels make the skull flexible to accommodate the infant brain, which continues to grow for some time after birth. However, because the bones are not firmly united, slight overlapping, or molding of the shape of the head, occurs during labor. This capacity of the bones to slide over one another also permits adaptation to the various diameters of the maternal pelvis. Molding can be extensive, but the heads of most newborns assume their normal shape within 3 days after birth.

Although the size of the fetal shoulders may affect passage, their position can be altered relatively easily during labor so one shoulder may occupy a lower level than the other. This creates a shoulder diameter that is smaller than the skull, facilitating passage through the birth canal. The circumference of the fetal hips is usually small enough to not create problems.

Fetal Presentation

Presentation refers to the part of the fetus that enters the pelvic inlet first and leads through the birth canal during labor at term. The three main presentations are *cephalic presentation* (head first), occurring in 96% of births (Fig. 13-2); *breech presentation* (buttocks, feet, or both first), occurring in 3% of births (Fig. 13-3, *A-C*); and *shoulder presentation*, seen in 1% of births (see Fig. 13-3, *D*). The presenting part is that part of the fetus that lies closest to the internal os of the cervix. It is the part of the fetal body first felt by the examining finger during a vaginal examination. In a cephalic presentation the presenting part is usually the occiput; in a breech

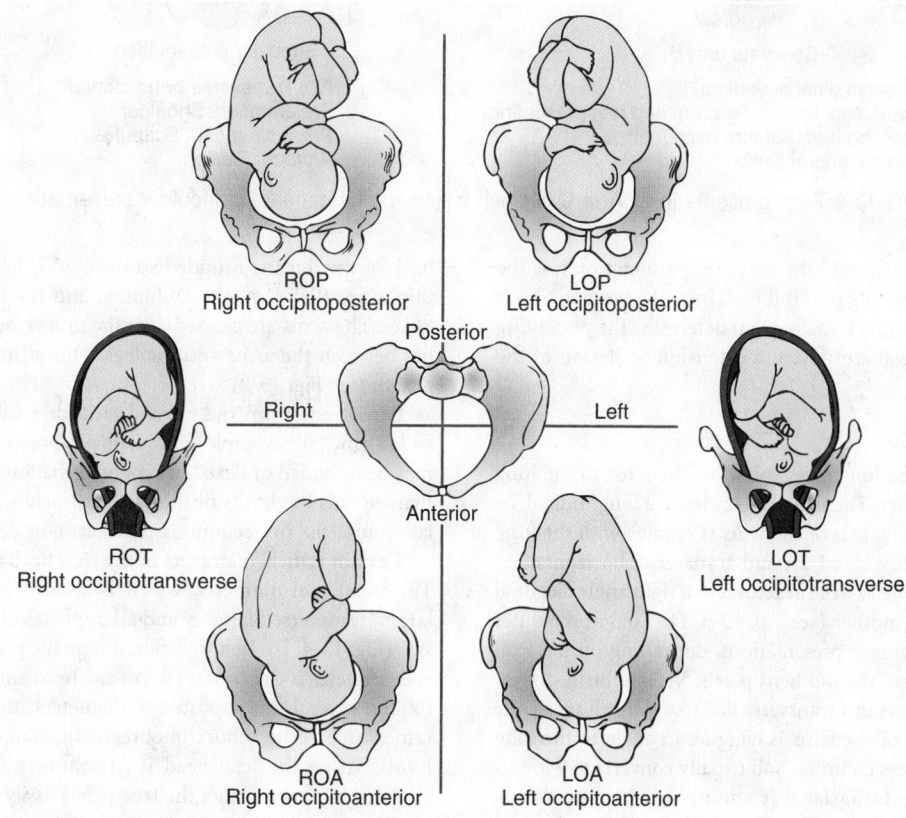

Lie: Longitudinal or vertical
Presentation: Vertex
Reference point: Occiput
Attitude: General flexion

FIG 13-2 Examples of fetal vertex (occiput) presentations in relation to front, back, or side of maternal pelvis.

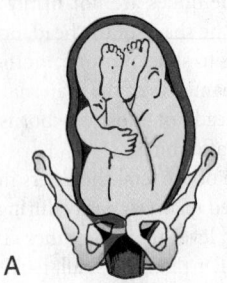

A
Frank breech

Lie: Longitudinal or vertical
Presentation: Breech (incomplete)
Presenting part: Sacrum
Attitude: Flexion, except for legs at knees

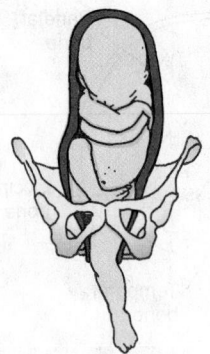

B
Single footling breech

Lie: Longitudinal or vertical
Presentation: Breech (incomplete)
Presenting part: Sacrum
Attitude: Flexion, except for one leg extended at hip and knee

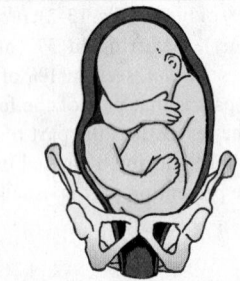

C
Complete breech

Lie: Longitudinal or vertical
Presentation: Breech (sacrum and feet presenting)
Presenting part: Sacrum (with feet)
Attitude: General flexion

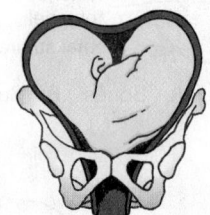

D
Shoulder presentation

Lie: Transverse or horizontal
Presentation: Shoulder
Presenting part: Scapula
Attitude: Flexion

FIG 13-3 Fetal presentations. **A** to **C,** Breech (sacral) presentation. **D,** Shoulder presentation.

presentation it is the sacrum; in the shoulder presentation it is the scapula. When the presenting part is the occiput, the presentation is noted as vertex (see Fig. 13-2). Factors that determine the presenting part include fetal lie, fetal attitude, and extension or flexion of the fetal head.

Fetal Lie

Lie is the relation of the long axis (spine) of the fetus to the long axis (spine) of the mother. The two primary lies are longitudinal, or vertical, in which the long axis of the fetus is parallel with the long axis of the mother (see Fig. 13-2); and transverse, horizontal, or oblique, in which the long axis of the fetus is at a right angle diagonal to the long axis of the mother (see Fig. 13-3, *D*). Longitudinal lies are either cephalic or breech presentations, depending on the fetal structure that first enters the mother's pelvis. Vaginal birth cannot occur when the fetus stays in a transverse lie. An oblique lie (i.e., one in which the long axis of the fetus is lying at an angle to the long axis of the mother) is less common and usually converts to a longitudinal or transverse lie during labor (Cunningham, Leveno, Bloom, et al., 2010).

Fetal Attitude

Attitude is the relation of the fetal body parts to one another. The fetus assumes a characteristic posture (attitude) in utero partly because of the mode of fetal growth and partly because of the way the fetus conforms to the shape of the uterine cavity. Normally the

back of the fetus is rounded so the chin is flexed on the chest, the thighs are flexed on the abdomen, and the legs are flexed at the knees. The arms are crossed over the thorax, and the umbilical cord lies between the arms and the legs. This attitude is termed *general flexion* (see Fig. 13-2).

Deviations from the normal attitude may cause difficulties in childbirth. For example, in a cephalic presentation the fetal head may be extended or flexed in a manner that presents a head diameter that exceeds the limits of the maternal pelvis, leading to prolonged labor, forceps- or vacuum-assisted birth, or cesarean birth.

Certain critical diameters of the fetal head are usually measured. The biparietal diameter, which is about 9.25 cm at term, is the largest transverse diameter and an important indicator of fetal head size (Fig. 13-4, *B*). In a well-flexed cephalic presentation the biparietal diameter is the widest part of the head entering the pelvic inlet. Of the several anteroposterior diameters, the smallest and most critical one is the suboccipitobregmatic diameter (about 9.5 cm at term). When the fetal head is in complete flexion, this diameter allows it to pass through the true pelvis easily (see Fig. 13-4, *A*; Fig. 13-5, *A*). As the head is more extended, the anteroposterior diameter widens, and the head may not be able to enter the true pelvis (see Fig. 13-5, *B* and *C*).

Fetal Position

The presentation or presenting part indicates the portion of the fetus that overlies the pelvic inlet. Position is the relationship of a

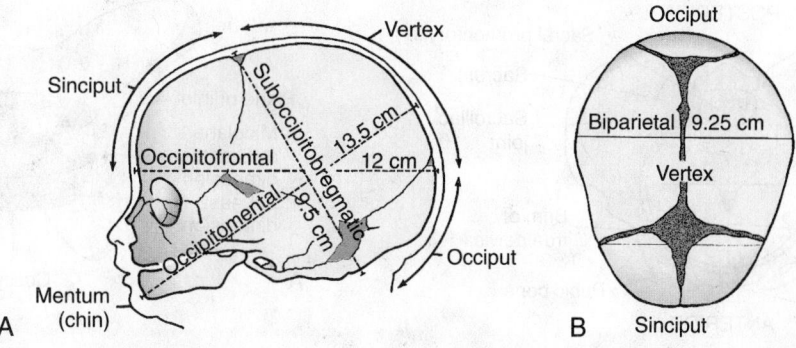

FIG 13-4 Diameters of fetal head at term. **A,** Cephalic presentations: occiput, vertex, and sinciput; and cephalic diameters: suboccipitobregmatic, occipitofrontal, and occipitomental. **B,** Biparietal diameter.

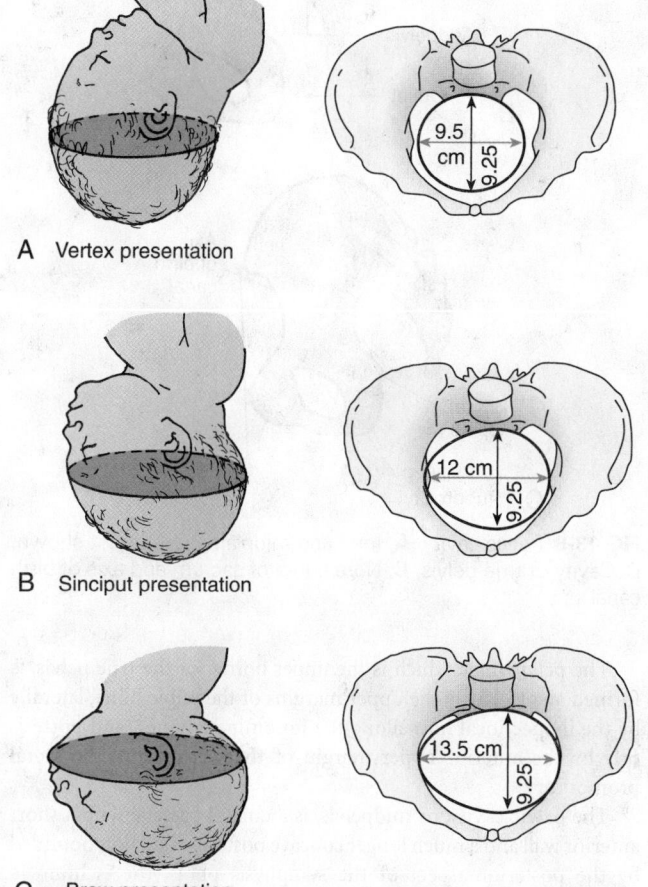

A Vertex presentation

B Sinciput presentation

C Brow presentation

FIG 13-5 Head entering pelvis. Biparietal diameter is indicated with shading (9.25 cm). **A,** Suboccipitobregmatic diameter: complete flexion of head on chest so smallest diameter enters. **B,** Occipitofrontal diameter: moderate extension (military attitude) so large diameter enters. **C,** Occipitomental diameter: marked extension (deflection) so largest diameter, which is too large to permit head to enter pelvis, is presenting.

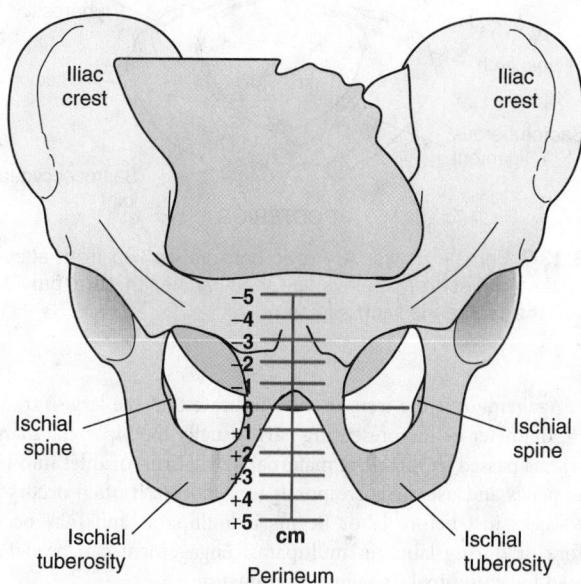

FIG 13-6 Stations of presenting part, or degree of descent. Lowermost portion of presenting part is at level of ischial spines, station 0.

reference point on the presenting part (occiput, sacrum, mentum [chin] or sinciput [deflexed vertex]) to the four quadrants of the mother's pelvis (see Fig. 13-2). Position is denoted by a three-letter abbreviation. The first letter of the abbreviation denotes the location of the presenting part in the right (R) or left (L) side of the mother's pelvis. The middle letter stands for the specific presenting part of

the fetus (O for occiput, S for sacrum, M for mentum [chin], and Sc for scapula [shoulder]). The third letter stands for the location of the presenting part in relation to the anterior (A), posterior (P), or transverse (T) portion of the maternal pelvis. For example, ROA means that the occiput is the presenting part and is located in the right anterior quadrant of the maternal pelvis (see Fig. 13-2). LSP means that the sacrum is the presenting part and is located in the left posterior quadrant of the maternal pelvis (see Fig. 13-3).

Station is the relationship of the presenting fetal part to an imaginary line drawn between the maternal ischial spines and is a measure of the degree of descent of the presenting part of the fetus through the birth canal. The placement of the presenting part is measured in centimeters above or below the ischial spines (Fig. 13-6). For example, when the lowermost portion of the presenting part is 1 cm above the spines, it is noted as being minus (−)1. At the level of the spines the station is referred to as 0 (zero). When the presenting part is 1 cm below the spines, the station is said to be plus (+)1. Birth is imminent when the presenting part is at +4 to +5 cm. The station of the presenting part should be determined when labor begins so the rate of descent of the fetus during labor can be determined accurately.

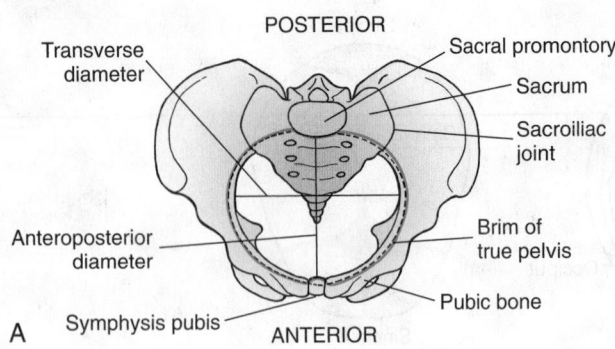

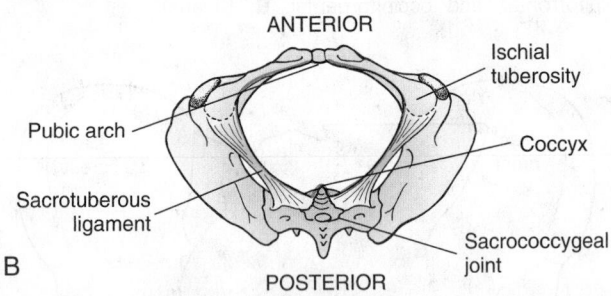

FIG 13-7 Female pelvis. **A,** Pelvic brim as viewed from above. **B,** Pelvic outlet from below, as seen by health care provider when the woman is lying supine.

Engagement is the term used to indicate that the largest transverse diameter of the presenting part (usually the biparietal diameter) has passed through the maternal pelvic brim or inlet into the true pelvis and usually corresponds to station 0. It often occurs in the weeks just before labor begins in nulliparas and may occur before or during labor in multiparas. Engagement can be determined by abdominal or vaginal examination.

Passageway

The passageway, or birth canal, is composed of the mother's rigid bony pelvis and the soft tissues of the cervix, the pelvic floor, the vagina, and the introitus (the external opening to the vagina). Although the soft tissues, particularly the muscular layers of the pelvic floor, contribute to vaginal birth of the fetus, the maternal pelvis plays a far greater role in the labor process because the fetus must successfully accommodate itself to this relatively rigid passageway. The size and shape of the pelvis can be determined at the initial prenatal visit or on admission in labor. This information can then be used in the assessment of labor progress (Thorp, 2009).

Bony Pelvis

The anatomy of the bony pelvis is described in Chapter 3. The following discussion focuses on the importance of pelvic configurations as they relate to the labor process. (It may be helpful to refer to Figs. 3-4 and 3-5.)

The bony pelvis is formed by the fusion of the ilium, ischium, pubis, and sacral bones. The four pelvic joints are the symphysis pubis, the right and left sacroiliac joints (Fig. 13-7, *A*), and the sacrococcygeal joint (Fig. 13-7, *B*). The bony pelvis is separated by the brim, or inlet, into two parts: the false and the true pelves. The false pelvis is the part above the brim and plays no part in childbearing. The true pelvis, the part involved in birth, is divided into three planes: the inlet, or brim; the midpelvis, or cavity; and the outlet.

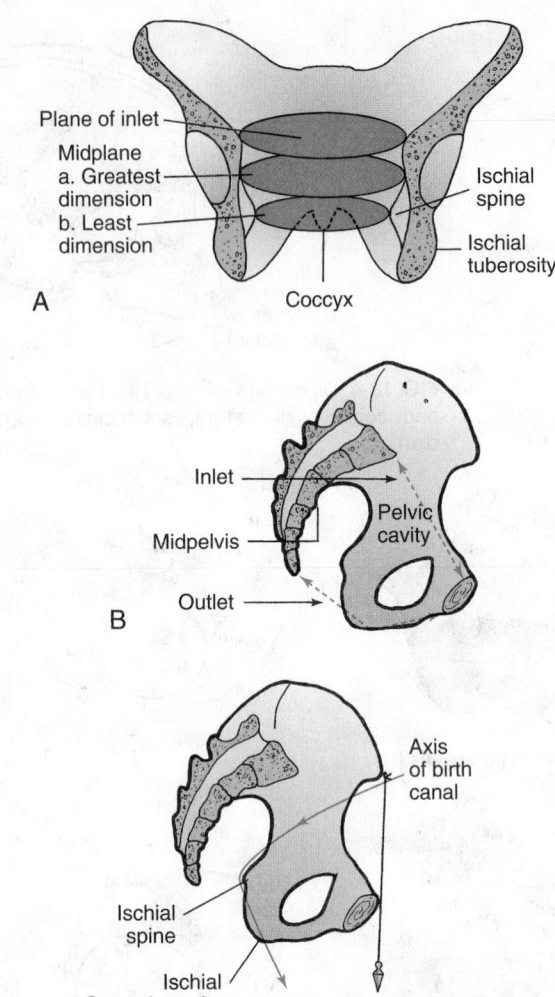

FIG 13-8 Pelvic cavity. **A,** Inlet and midplane. Outlet not shown. **B,** Cavity of true pelvis. **C,** Note curve of sacrum and axis of birth canal.

The pelvic inlet, which is the upper border of the true pelvis, is formed anteriorly by the upper margins of the pubic bone, laterally by the iliopectineal lines along the innominate bones, and posteriorly by the anterior upper margin of the sacrum and the sacral promontory.

The pelvic cavity, or midpelvis, is a curved passage with a short anterior wall and a much longer concave posterior wall. It is bounded by the posterior aspect of the symphysis pubis, the ischium, a portion of the ilium, the sacrum, and the coccyx.

The pelvic outlet is the lower border of the true pelvis. Viewed from below it is ovoid; somewhat diamond shaped; and bounded by the pubic arch anteriorly, the ischial tuberosities laterally, and the tip of the coccyx posteriorly (see Fig. 13-7, *B*). In the latter part of pregnancy the coccyx is movable unless it has been broken (e.g., in a fall during skiing or skating) and has fused to the sacrum during healing.

The pelvic canal varies in size and shape at various levels. The diameters at the plane of the pelvic inlet, midpelvis, and outlet plus the axis of the birth canal (Fig. 13-8) determine whether vaginal birth is possible and the manner by which the fetus may pass down the birth canal.

The subpubic angle, which determines the type of pubic arch, together with the length of the pubic rami and the intertuberous

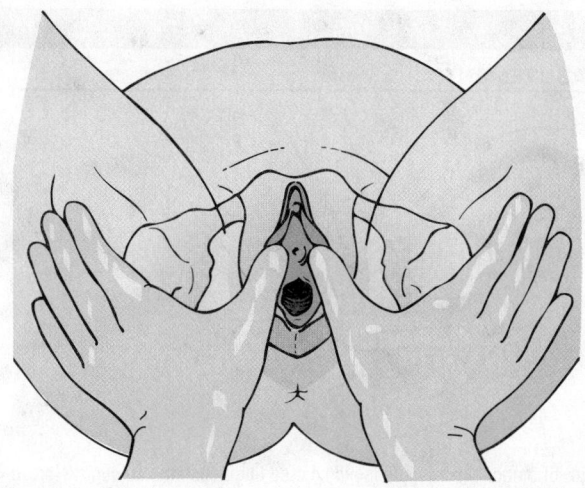

FIG 13-9 Estimation of angle of subpubic arch. With both thumbs examiner externally traces descending rami down to tuberosities. (From Barkauskas VH, Baumann LC, Darling-Fisher CS: *Health and physical assessment*, ed 3, St Louis, 2002, Mosby.)

diameter, is of great importance. Because the fetus must first pass beneath the pubic arch, a narrow subpubic angle is less accommodating than a rounded wide arch. The method of measurement of the subpubic arch is shown in Fig. 13-9. A summary of obstetric measurements is given in Table 13-1.

The four basic types of pelvis are classified as follows:

1. Gynecoid (the classic female type)
2. Android (resembling the male pelvis)
3. Anthropoid (resembling the pelvis of anthropoid apes)
4. Platypelloid (the flat pelvis)

The gynecoid pelvis is the most common, with major gynecoid pelvic features present in 50% of all women. Anthropoid and android features are less common, and platypelloid pelvic features are the least common. Mixed types of pelves are more common than are pure types (Cunningham, Leveno, Bloom, et al., 2010). Examples of pelvic variations and their effects on mode of birth are given in Table 13-2.

Assessment of the bony pelvis can be performed during the first prenatal evaluation and need not be repeated if the pelvis is of adequate size and suitable shape. In the third trimester of pregnancy the examination of the bony pelvis may be more thorough, and the results more accurate because there is relaxation and increased mobility of the pelvic joints and ligaments as a result of hormonal influences. Widening of the joint of the symphysis pubis and the resulting instability may cause pain in any or all of the pelvic joints.

Because the examiner does not have direct access to the bony structures and because the bones are covered with varying amounts of soft tissue, estimates of size and shape are approximate. Precise bony pelvis measurements can be determined by use of computed tomography, ultrasound, or x-ray films. However, radiographic examination is rarely done during pregnancy because the x-ray may damage the developing fetus.

Soft Tissues

The soft tissues of the passageway include the distensible lower uterine segment, the cervix, the pelvic floor muscles, the vagina, and the introitus. Before labor begins the uterus is composed of the uterine body (corpus) and the cervix (neck). After labor has begun,

uterine contractions cause the uterine body to have a thick and muscular upper segment and a thin-walled, passive, muscular lower segment. A *physiologic retraction ring* separates the two segments (Fig. 13-10). The lower uterine segment gradually distends to accommodate the intrauterine contents as the wall of the upper segment thickens and its accommodating capacity is reduced. The contractions of the uterine body thus exert downward pressure on the fetus, pushing it against the cervix.

The cervix effaces (thins) and dilates (opens) sufficiently to allow the first fetal portion to descend into the vagina. As the fetus descends, the cervix is actually drawn upward and over this first portion.

The pelvic floor is a muscular layer that separates the pelvic cavity above from the perineal space below. This structure helps the fetus rotate anteriorly as it passes through the birth canal. As noted earlier, the soft tissues of the vagina develop throughout pregnancy until at term the vagina can dilate to accommodate the fetus and permit its passage to the external world.

Powers

Involuntary and voluntary powers combine to expel the fetus and placenta from the uterus. Involuntary uterine contractions, called the *primary powers*, signal the beginning of labor. Once the cervix has dilated, voluntary bearing-down efforts by the woman, called the *secondary powers*, augment the force of the involuntary contractions.

Primary Powers

The involuntary contractions originate at certain pacemaker points in the thickened muscle layers of the upper uterine segment. From the pacemaker points contractions move downward over the uterus in waves, separated by short rest periods. Terms used to describe these involuntary contractions include *frequency* (the time from the beginning of one contraction to the beginning of the next), *duration* (length of contraction), and *intensity* (strength of contraction at its peak).

The primary powers are responsible for the effacement and dilation of the cervix and descent of the fetus. Effacement means the shortening and thinning of the cervix during the first stage of labor. The cervix, normally 2 to 3 cm long and about 1 cm thick, is obliterated or "taken up" by a shortening of the uterine muscle bundles during the thinning of the lower uterine segment that occurs in advancing labor. Only a thin edge of the cervix can be palpated when effacement is complete. Effacement generally is advanced in first-time term pregnancy before more than slight dilation occurs. In subsequent pregnancies effacement and dilation of the cervix tend to progress together. Degree of effacement is expressed in percentages, from 0% to 100% (e.g., a cervix is 50% effaced) (Fig. 13-11, *A* to *C*).

Dilation of the cervix is the enlargement or widening of the cervical opening and the cervical canal that occurs once labor has begun. The diameter of the cervix increases from less than 1 cm to full dilation (approximately 10 cm) to allow birth of a term fetus. When the cervix is fully dilated (and completely retracted), it can no longer be palpated (see Fig. 13-11, *D*). Full cervical dilation marks the end of the first stage of labor.

Dilation of the cervix occurs by the drawing upward of the musculofibrous components of the cervix caused by strong uterine contractions. Pressure exerted by the amniotic fluid while the membranes are intact or by the force applied by the presenting part can promote cervical dilation. Scarring of the cervix as a result of prior infection or surgery may slow cervical dilation.

TABLE 13-1   OBSTETRIC MEASUREMENTS

PLANE	DIAMETER	MEASUREMENTS
Inlet (Superior Strait)		
Conjugates		
Diagonal	12.5-13 cm	
Obstetric: measurement that determines whether presenting part can engage or enter superior strait	1.5-2 cm less than diagonal (radiographic)	
True (vera) (anteroposterior)	≥11 cm (12.5) (radiographic)	

Length of diagonal conjugate (solid colored line), obstetric conjugate (broken colored line), and true conjugate (blue line)*

Midplane		
Transverse diameter (interspinous diameter)	10.5 cm	
The midplane of the pelvis normally is its largest plane and the one of greatest diameter		

Measurement of interspinous diameter*

Outlet		
Transverse diameter (intertuberous diameter) (biischial)	≥8 cm	
The outlet presents the smallest plane of the pelvic canal		

Use of Thom's pelvimeter to measure intertuberous diameter*

*From Seidel HM, Ball JW, Dains JE, et al: *Mosby's guide to physical examination*, ed 7, St Louis, 2011, Mosby.

TABLE 13-2	COMPARISON OF PELVIC TYPES			
	GYNECOID (50% of Women)	**ANDROID** (23% of Women)	**ANTHROPOID** (24% of Women)	**PLATYPELLOID** (3% of Women)
Brim	Slightly ovoid or transversely rounded	Heart shaped, angulated	Oval, wider anteroposteriorly	Flattened anteroposteriorly, wide transversely
Shape	◯ Round	♡ Heart	◖ Oval	⬭ Flat
Depth	Moderate	Deep	Deep	Shallow
Side walls	Straight	Convergent	Straight	Straight
Ischial spines	Blunt, somewhat widely separated	Prominent, narrow interspinous diameter	Prominent, often with narrow interspinous diameter	Blunted, widely separated
Sacrum	Deep, curved	Slightly curved, terminal portion often beaked	Slightly curved	Slightly curved
Subpubic arch	Wide	Narrow	Narrow	Wide
Usual mode of birth	Vaginal Spontaneous Occipitoanterior position	Cesarean Vaginal Difficult, with forceps	Vaginal Forceps/spontaneous Spontaneous Occipitoposterior or occipitoanterior position	Vaginal Spontaneous

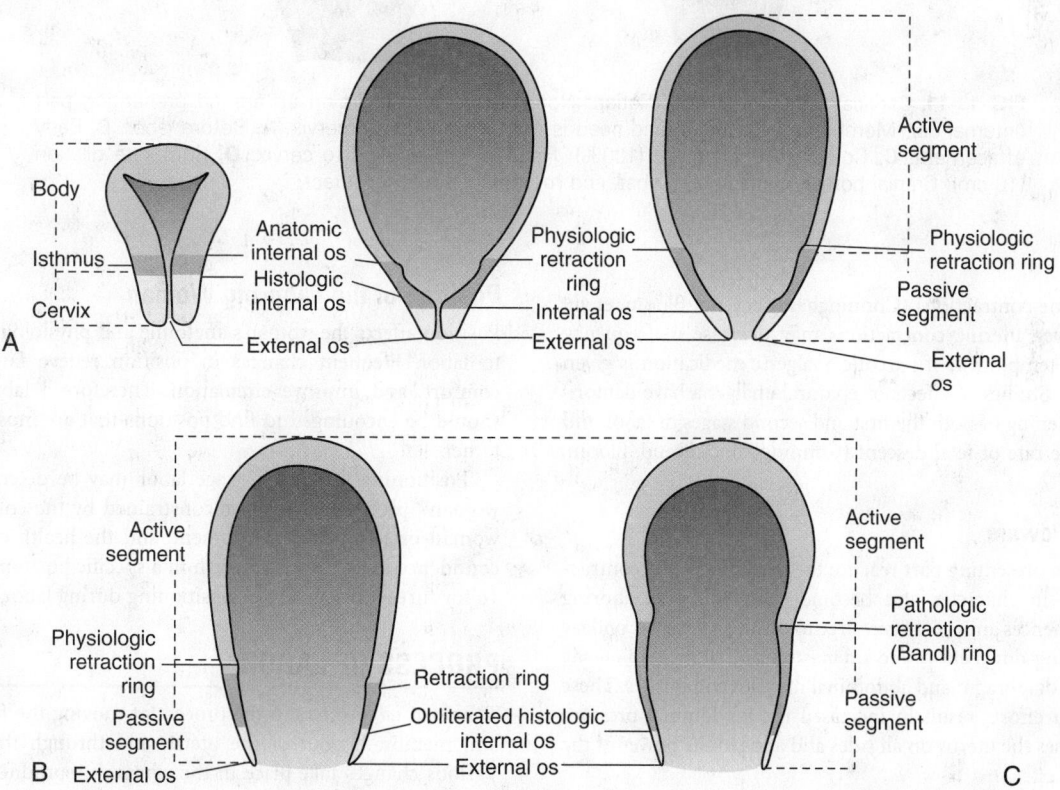

FIG 13-10 Uterus in normal labor **A,** in early first stage; and **B,** in second stage. Passive segment is derived from lower uterine segment (isthmus) and cervix, and physiologic retraction ring is derived from anatomic internal os. **C,** Uterus in abnormal labor in second-stage dystocia. Pathologic retraction (Bandl) ring that forms under abnormal conditions develops from physiologic ring.

In the first and second stages of labor increased intrauterine pressure caused by contractions exerts pressure on the descending fetus and the cervix. When the presenting part of the fetus reaches the perineal floor, mechanical stretching of the cervix occurs. Stretch receptors in the posterior vagina cause release of endogenous oxytocin that triggers the maternal urge to bear down, or the *Ferguson reflex.*

Uterine contractions are usually independent of external forces. For example, laboring women who are paralyzed because of spinal cord lesions above the twelfth thoracic vertebra have normal but

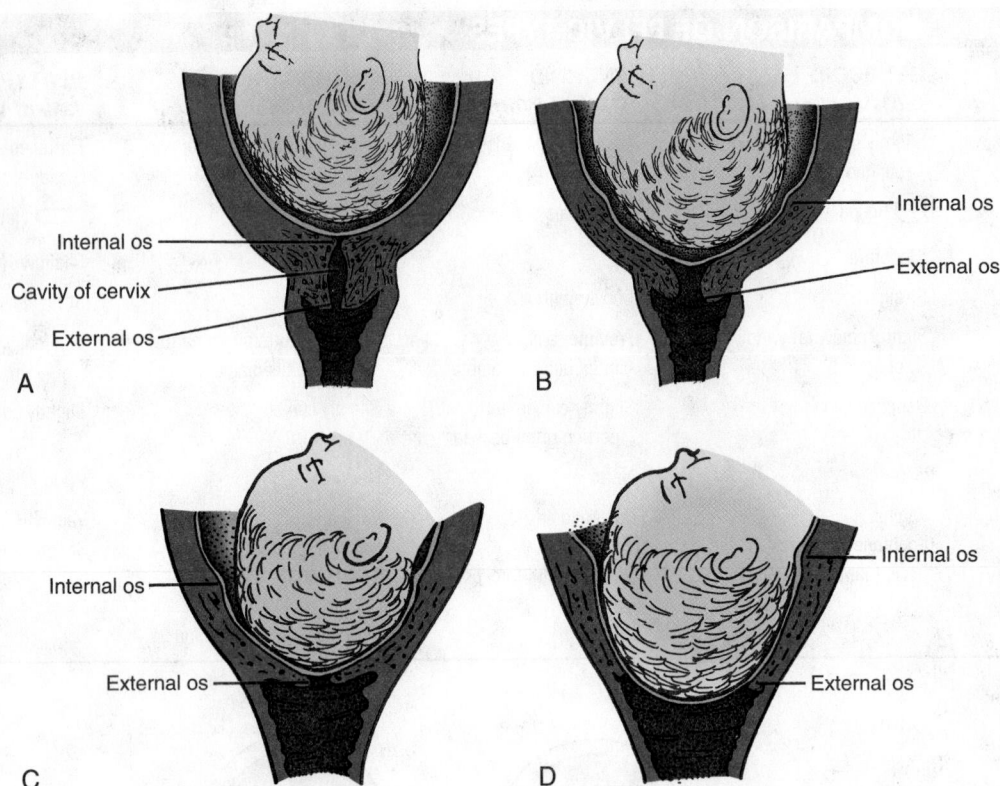

FIG 13-11 Cervical effacement and dilation. Note how cervix is drawn up around presenting part (internal os). Membranes are intact, and head is not well applied to cervix. **A,** Before labor. **B,** Early effacement. **C,** Complete effacement (100%). Head is well applied to cervix. **D,** Complete dilation (10 cm). Cranial bones overlap somewhat, and membranes are still intact.

painless uterine contractions (Cunningham, Leveno, Bloom, et al., 2010). However, uterine contractions may decrease in frequency and intensity temporarily if narcotic analgesic medication is given early in labor. Studies of effects of epidural analgesia have demonstrated lengthening of both the first and second stages of labor and slowing of the rate of fetal descent (Cunningham, Leveno, Bloom, et al., 2010).

Secondary Powers

As soon as the presenting part reaches the pelvic floor, the contractions change in character and become expulsive. The laboring woman experiences an involuntary urge to push. She uses secondary powers (bearing-down efforts) to aid in expulsion of the fetus as she contracts her diaphragm and abdominal muscles and pushes. These bearing-down efforts result in increased intraabdominal pressure that compresses the uterus on all sides and adds to the power of the expulsive forces.

The secondary powers have no effect on cervical dilation, but they are of considerable importance in the expulsion of the infant from the uterus and vagina after the cervix is fully dilated. When and how a woman pushes in the second stage of labor are much-debated topics. Continued study is needed to determine the effectiveness and appropriateness of strategies used by nurses to teach pushing techniques, the suitability and effectiveness of various pushing techniques related to abnormal fetal heart patterns, and the standards for length of pushing in terms of maternal and fetal outcomes. See Chapter 16 for further discussion regarding pushing during the second stage of labor.

Position of the Laboring Woman

Position affects the woman's anatomic and physiologic adaptations to labor. Frequent changes in position relieve fatigue, increase comfort, and improve circulation. Therefore a laboring woman should be encouraged to find positions that are most comfortable to her.

Positioning for second-stage labor may be determined by the woman's preference, but it is constrained by the condition of the woman or fetus, the environment, and the health care provider's confidence in assisting in a birth in a specific position. See Chapter 16 for further discussion of positioning during labor and birth.

PROCESS OF LABOR

The term *labor* refers to the process of moving the fetus, placenta, and membranes out of the uterus and through the birth canal. Various changes take place in the woman's reproductive system in the days and weeks before labor begins. Labor itself can be discussed in terms of the mechanisms involved in the process and the stages through which the woman moves.

Signs Preceding Labor

In first-time pregnancies the uterus sinks downward and forward about 2 weeks before term, when the presenting part of the fetus (usually the fetal head) descends into the true pelvis. This settling is called lightening, or "dropping," and usually happens gradually. After lightening women feel less congested and breathe more easily, but usually more bladder pressure results from this shift;

BOX 13-1	SIGNS PRECEDING LABOR

- Lightening
- Return of urinary frequency
- Backache
- Stronger Braxton Hicks contractions
- Weight loss of 0.5 to 1.5 kg
- Surge of energy
- Increased vaginal discharge; bloody show
- Cervical ripening
- Possible rupture of membranes

consequently there is a return of urinary frequency. In a multiparous pregnancy lightening may not take place until after uterine contractions are established and true labor is in progress.

The woman may complain of persistent low backache and sacroiliac distress as a result of relaxation of the pelvic joints. She may identify strong, frequent, but irregular uterine (Braxton Hicks) contractions.

The vaginal mucus becomes more profuse in response to the extreme congestion of the vaginal mucous membranes. Brownish or blood-tinged cervical mucus may be passed (bloody show). The cervix becomes soft (ripens) and partially effaced and may begin to dilate. The membranes may rupture spontaneously.

Other phenomena are common in the days preceding labor: (1) loss of 0.5 to 1.5 kg in weight caused by water loss resulting from electrolyte shifts that in turn are produced by changes in estrogen and progesterone levels; and (2) a surge of energy. Women speak of having a burst of energy that they often use to clean the house and put everything in order. Less commonly some women have diarrhea, nausea, vomiting, and indigestion. Box 13-1 lists signs that may precede labor.

Onset of Labor

The onset of true labor cannot be ascribed to a single cause. Many factors, including changes in the maternal uterus, cervix, and pituitary gland, are involved. Hormones produced by the normal fetal hypothalamus, pituitary, and adrenal cortex probably contribute to the onset of labor. Progressive uterine distention and increasing intrauterine pressure seem to be associated with increasing myometrial irritability. This is a result of increased concentrations of estrogen, oxytocin, and prostaglandins and decreasing progesterone levels. The mutually coordinated effects of these factors result in the occurrence of strong, regular, rhythmic uterine contractions (Blackburn, 2013; Kilpatrick and Garrison, 2012). The outcome of these factors working together is normally the birth of the fetus and the expulsion of the placenta; however, how certain alterations trigger others and the ways in which proper checks and balances are maintained are not known.

Stages of Labor

The course of labor at or near term gestation in a woman without complications and a fetus in vertex presentation consists of: (1) regular progression of uterine contractions, (2) effacement and progressive dilation of the cervix, and (3) progress in descent of the presenting part. Four stages of labor are recognized. An overview of these stages is included here. They are discussed in greater detail, along with nursing care for the laboring woman and family, in Chapter 16.

The *first stage of labor* is considered to last from the onset of regular uterine contractions to full dilation of the cervix. Commonly the onset of labor is difficult to establish because the woman may be admitted to the labor unit just before birth and the beginning of

labor may be only an estimate. The first stage is much longer than the second and third combined. However, great variability is the rule, depending on the factors discussed previously in this chapter. The first stage of labor is divided into three phases: a latent phase, an active phase, and a transition phase. During the latent phase there is more progress in effacement of the cervix and little increase in descent. During the active and transition phases there is more rapid dilation of the cervix and increased rate of descent of the presenting part.

The *second stage of labor* lasts from the time the cervix is fully dilated to the birth of the fetus. It is composed of two phases: the latent phase and the active pushing (descent) phase. During the latent phase the fetus continues to descend passively through the birth canal and rotate to an anterior position as a result of ongoing uterine contractions. The urge to bear down during this phase is not strong, and some women do not experience it at all. During the active pushing phase the woman has strong urges to bear down as the presenting part of the fetus descends and presses on the stretch receptors of the pelvic floor.

The *third stage of labor* lasts from the birth of the fetus until the placenta is delivered. The placenta normally separates with the third or fourth strong uterine contraction after the infant has been born. After it has separated, the placenta can be delivered with the next uterine contraction.

The *fourth stage of labor* arbitrarily lasts about 2 hours after delivery of the placenta. It is the period of immediate recovery when homeostasis is reestablished. The fourth stage of labor is also the time when parent-child bonding and attachment begins and breastfeeding is initiated. It is an important period of observation for complications such as abnormal bleeding (see Chapter 21).

Mechanism of Labor

As already discussed, the female pelvis has varied contours and diameters at different levels, and the presenting part of the passenger is large in proportion to the passage. Therefore for vaginal birth to occur the fetus must adapt to the birth canal during the descent. The turns and other adjustments necessary in the human birth process are termed the *mechanism of labor* (Fig. 13-12). The seven cardinal movements of the mechanism of labor that occur in a vertex presentation are engagement, descent, flexion, internal rotation, extension, external rotation (restitution), and finally birth by expulsion. Although these movements are discussed separately, in actuality a combination of movements occurs simultaneously. For example, engagement involves both descent and flexion.

Engagement

When the biparietal diameter of the head passes the pelvic inlet, the head is said to be engaged in the pelvic inlet (see Fig. 13-12, *A*). In most nulliparous pregnancies this occurs before the onset of active labor because the firmer abdominal muscles direct the presenting part into the pelvis. In multiparous pregnancies in which the abdominal musculature is more relaxed, the head often remains freely movable above the pelvic brim until labor is established.

Asynclitism. The head usually engages in the pelvis in a synclitic position (i.e., one that is parallel to the anteroposterior plane of the pelvis). Frequently asynclitism occurs (the head is deflected anteriorly or posteriorly in the pelvis), which can facilitate descent because the head is being positioned to accommodate to the pelvic cavity (Fig. 13-13). Extreme asynclitism can cause cephalopelvic

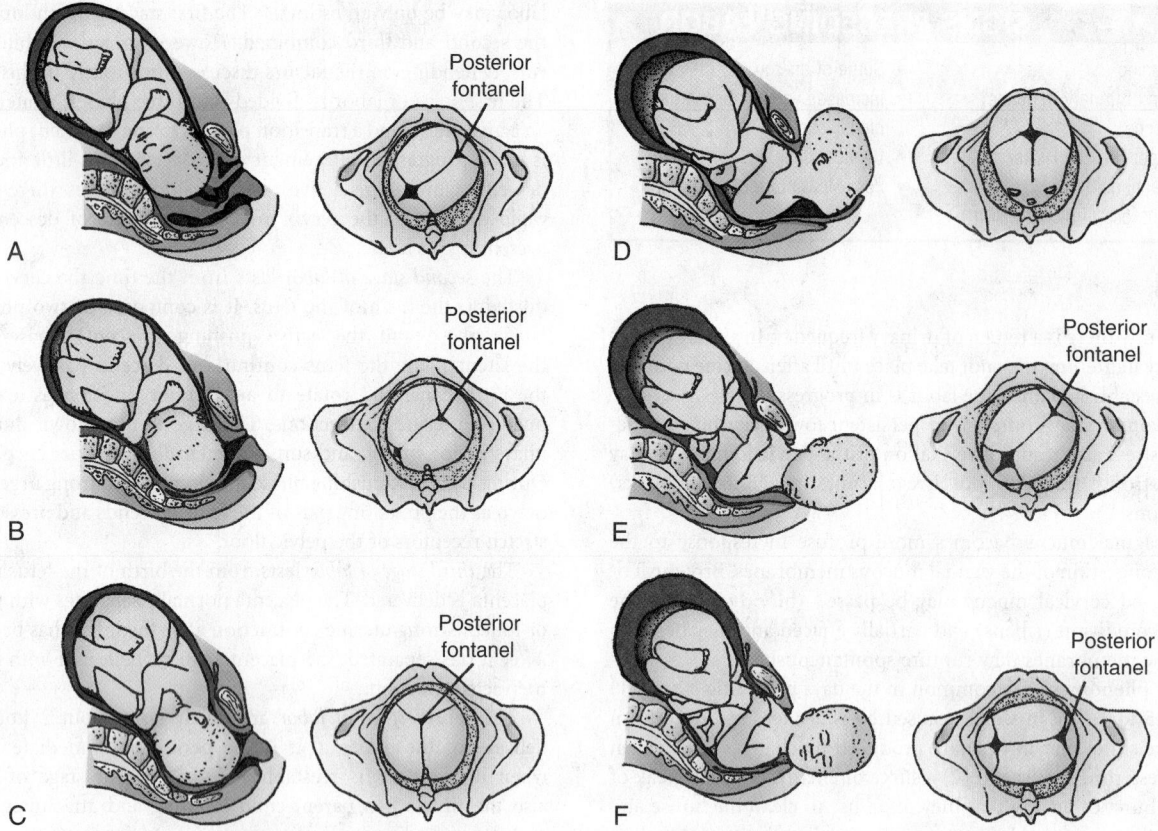

FIG 13-12 Cardinal movements of the mechanism of labor. Left occipitoanterior *(LOA)* position. Pelvic figures show position of fetal head as seen by birth attendant. **A,** Engagement and descent. **B,** Flexion. **C,** Internal rotation to occipitoanterior *(OA)* position. **D,** Extension. **E,** External rotation beginning (restitution). **F,** External rotation.

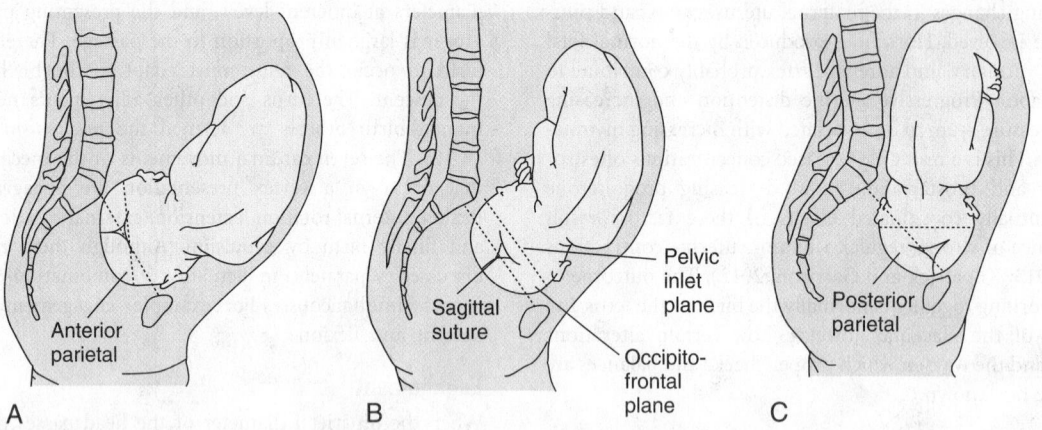

FIG 13-13 Synclitism and asynclitism. **A,** Anterior asynclitism. **B,** Normal synclitism. **C,** Posterior asynclitism.

disproportion, even in a normal-size pelvis, because the head is positioned so it cannot descend.

Descent

Descent refers to the progress of the presenting part through the pelvis. It depends on at least four forces: (1) pressure exerted by the amniotic fluid, (2) direct pressure exerted by the contracting fundus on the fetus, (3) force of the contraction of the maternal diaphragm and abdominal muscles in the second stage of labor,

and (4) extension and straightening of the fetal body. The effects of these forces are modified by the size and shape of the maternal pelvic planes and the size of the fetal head and its capacity to mold.

The degree of descent is measured by the station of the presenting part (see Fig. 13-6). As mentioned, little descent occurs during the latent phase of the first stage of labor. Descent accelerates in the active phase when the cervix has dilated to 5 to 7 cm. It is especially apparent when the membranes have ruptured.

In a first-time pregnancy descent is usually slow but steady; in subsequent pregnancies descent may be rapid. Progress in descent of the presenting part is determined by abdominal palpation and vaginal examination until the presenting part can be seen at the introitus (see Chapter 16).

Flexion

As soon as the descending head meets resistance from the cervix, pelvic wall, or pelvic floor, it normally flexes so the chin is brought into closer contact with the fetal chest (see Fig. 13-12, *B*). Flexion permits the smaller suboccipitobregmatic diameter (9.5 cm) rather than the larger diameters to present to the outlet.

Internal Rotation

The maternal pelvic inlet is widest in the transverse diameter; therefore the fetal head passes the inlet into the true pelvis in the occipitotransverse position. The outlet is widest in the anteroposterior diameter; for the fetus to exit the head must rotate. Internal rotation begins at the level of the ischial spines but is not completed until the presenting part reaches the lower pelvis. As the occiput rotates anteriorly, the face rotates posteriorly. With each contraction the fetal head is guided by the bony pelvis and the muscles of the pelvic floor. Eventually the occiput will be in the midline beneath the pubic arch. The head is almost always rotated by the time it reaches the pelvic floor (see Fig. 13-12, *C*). Both the levator ani muscles and the bony pelvis are important for achieving anterior rotation. A previous childbirth injury or regional anesthesia may compromise the function of the levator sling.

Extension

When the fetal head reaches the perineum for birth, it is deflected anteriorly by the perineum. The occiput passes under the lower border of the symphysis pubis first, and the head emerges by extension: first the occiput, then the face, and finally the chin (see Fig. 13-12, *D*).

Restitution and External Rotation

After the head is born, it rotates briefly to the position it occupied when it was engaged in the inlet. This movement is referred to as restitution (see Fig. 13-12, *E*). The 45-degree turn realigns the infant's head with her or his back and shoulders. The head can then be seen to rotate further. This external rotation occurs as the shoulders engage and descend in maneuvers similar to those of the head (see Fig. 13-12, *F*). As noted earlier, the anterior shoulder descends first. When it reaches the outlet, it rotates to the midline and is delivered from under the pubic arch. The posterior shoulder is guided over the perineum until it is free of the vaginal introitus.

Expulsion

After birth of the shoulders, the head and shoulders are lifted up toward the mother's pubic bone, and the trunk of the baby is born by flexing it laterally in the direction of the symphysis pubis. When the baby has emerged completely, birth is complete, and the second stage of labor ends.

PHYSIOLOGIC ADAPTATION TO LABOR

In addition to the maternal and fetal anatomic adaptations that occur during birth, physiologic adaptations must occur. Accurate assessment of the laboring woman and fetus requires knowledge of these expected adaptations.

Fetal Adaptation

Several important physiologic adaptations occur in the fetus. These changes occur in fetal heart rate (FHR), fetal circulation, respiratory movements, and other behaviors.

Fetal Heart Rate

FHR monitoring provides reliable and predictive information about the condition of the fetus related to oxygenation. The average FHR at term is 140 beats/min. The normal range is 110 to 160 beats/min. Earlier in gestation the FHR is higher, with an average of approximately 160 beats/min at 20 weeks of gestation. The rate decreases progressively as the maturing fetus reaches term. However, temporary accelerations and slight early decelerations of the FHR can be expected in response to spontaneous fetal movement, vaginal examination, fundal pressure, uterine contractions, abdominal palpation, and fetal head compression. Stresses to the uterofetoplacental unit result in characteristic FHR patterns (see Chapter 15 for further discussion).

Fetal Circulation

Fetal circulation can be affected by many factors, including maternal position, uterine contractions, blood pressure, and umbilical cord blood flow. Uterine contractions during labor tend to decrease circulation through the spiral arterioles and subsequent perfusion through the intervillous space. Most healthy fetuses are well able to compensate for this stress and exposure to increased pressure while moving passively through the birth canal during labor. Usually the umbilical cord moves freely in the amniotic fluid. However, it can be compressed during uterine contractions (Blackburn, 2013; Miller, Miller, and Tucker, 2013).

Fetal Respiration

Certain changes stimulate chemoreceptors in the aorta and carotid bodies to prepare the fetus for initiating respirations immediately after birth (Blackburn, 2013; Rozance and Rosenberg, 2012). These changes include the following:

- Fetal lung fluid is cleared from the air passages as the infant passes through the birth canal during labor and (vaginal) birth.
- Fetal oxygen pressure (Po_2) decreases.
- Arterial carbon dioxide pressure (Pco_2) increases.
- Arterial pH decreases.
- Bicarbonate level decreases.
- Fetal respiratory movements decrease during labor.

Maternal Adaptation

As the woman progresses through the stages of labor, various body system adaptations cause her to exhibit both objective and subjective symptoms (Box 13-2).

Cardiovascular Changes

During each contraction an average of 400 mL of blood is emptied from the uterus into the maternal vascular system. By the end of the first stage of labor cardiac output during contractions is increased by 51% above baseline pregnancy values at term. Cardiac output peaks about 10 to 30 minutes after both vaginal and cesarean birth and returns to its prelabor baseline within the first postpartum hour. A drop in maternal heart rate accompanies this increase in cardiac output (Gordon, 2012).

Changes in blood pressure also occur. In general, both systolic and diastolic pressures increase during contractions and return to baseline levels between contractions. Systolic values increase more than diastolic values (Blackburn, 2013).

BOX 13-2   MATERNAL PHYSIOLOGIC CHANGES DURING LABOR

- Cardiac output increases 10% to 15% in first stage; 30% to 50% in second stage.
- Heart rate increases slightly in first and second stages.
- Systolic blood pressure increases during uterine contractions in first stage; systolic and diastolic pressures increase during uterine contractions in second stage.
- White blood cell count increases.
- Respiratory rate increases.
- Temperature may be slightly elevated.
- Proteinuria may occur.
- Gastric motility and absorption of solid food are decreased; nausea and vomiting may occur during transition to second-stage labor.
- Blood glucose level decreases.

? CRITICAL THINKING CASE STUDY

Anxiety in a Multipara in Active Labor

Jody was admitted in active labor to an LDR room 2 hours ago. She is a 24-year-old G2 P1 at 39 weeks of gestation. She is noticeably anxious and tells you that her first pregnancy ended at term but that the labor was "terrible. It was 22 hours long. I had an epidural but had to push and push to get the baby out." Which interventions are appropriate?

1. Evidence—Is there sufficient evidence to draw any conclusions about which intervention is needed?
2. Assumptions—Describe an underlying assumption about each of the following issues:
   a. Effect of anxiety on progress in labor
   b. Effect of parity on labor
   c. Effect of epidural analgesia on length of labor
   d. Effect of epidural analgesia on ability to push
3. What implications and priorities for nursing care can be drawn at this time?
4. Does the evidence objectively support your argument (conclusion)?

LDR, Labor, delivery, and recovery.

Supine hypotension (see Fig. 16-5) occurs when the ascending vena cava and descending aorta are compressed. The laboring woman is at greater risk for supine hypotension if the uterus is particularly large because of multifetal pregnancy or polyhydramnios or if she is obese, dehydrated, or hypovolemic. In addition, anxiety, pain, and some medications can cause hypotension.

The woman should be discouraged from using the Valsalva maneuver (holding one's breath and tightening abdominal muscles) for pushing during the second stage. This activity increases intrathoracic pressure, reduces venous return, and increases venous pressure. Cardiac output and blood pressure increase, and the pulse slows temporarily. During the Valsalva maneuver fetal hypoxia may occur. The process is reversed when the woman takes a breath.

The white blood cell (WBC) count can increase (Blackburn, 2013). Although the mechanism leading to this increase in WBCs is unknown, it may be secondary to physical or emotional stress or tissue trauma. Labor is strenuous, and physical exercise alone can increase the WBC count.

Some peripheral vascular changes occur, perhaps in response to cervical dilation or compression of maternal vessels by the fetus passing through the birth canal. Flushed cheeks, hot or cold feet, and eversion of hemorrhoids may result.

Respiratory Changes

Increased physical activity with greater oxygen consumption is reflected in an increase in the respiratory rate. Hyperventilation may cause respiratory alkalosis (an increase in pH), hypoxia, and hypocapnia (decrease in carbon dioxide). In the unmedicated woman in the second stage oxygen consumption almost doubles. Anxiety also increases oxygen consumption.

Renal Changes

During labor spontaneous voiding may be difficult for various reasons: tissue edema caused by pressure from the presenting part, discomfort, analgesia, and embarrassment. Proteinuria of 1+ is a normal finding because it can occur in response to the breakdown of muscle tissue from the physical work of labor.

Integumentary Changes

The integumentary system changes are evident, especially in the great distensibility (stretching) in the area of the vaginal introitus.

The degree of distensibility varies with the individual. Despite this ability to stretch, even in the absence of episiotomy or lacerations, minute tears in the skin around the vaginal introitus occur.

Musculoskeletal Changes

The musculoskeletal system is stressed during labor. Diaphoresis, fatigue, proteinuria (1+), and possibly an increased temperature accompany the marked increase in muscle activity. Backache and joint ache (unrelated to fetal position) occur as a result of increased joint laxity at term. The labor process itself and the woman's pointing her toes can cause leg cramps.

Neurologic Changes

Sensorial changes occur as the woman moves through the phases of the first stage of labor and from one stage to the next. Initially she may be euphoric. Euphoria gives way to increased seriousness, then to amnesia between contractions during the second stage, and finally to elation or fatigue after giving birth. Endogenous endorphins (morphinelike chemicals produced naturally by the body) raise the pain threshold and produce sedation. In addition, physiologic anesthesia of perineal tissues caused by pressure of the presenting part decreases perception of pain (see Critical Thinking Case Study).

Gastrointestinal Changes

During labor gastrointestinal motility and absorption of solid foods are decreased, and stomach-emptying time is slowed. Nausea and vomiting of undigested food eaten after the onset of labor are common. Nausea and belching also occur as a reflex response to full cervical dilation. The woman may state that diarrhea accompanied the onset of labor, or the nurse may palpate the presence of hard or impacted stool in the rectum.

Endocrine Changes

The onset of labor may be triggered by decreasing levels of progesterone and increasing levels of estrogen, prostaglandins, and oxytocin (Norwitz and Lye, 2009). Metabolism increases, and blood glucose levels may decrease with the work of labor.

KEY POINTS

- Labor and birth are affected by the five Ps: *passenger, passageway, powers, position* of the woman, and *psychologic* response.
- Because of its size and relative rigidity, the fetal head is a major factor in determining the course of birth.
- The diameters at the plane of the pelvic inlet, the midpelvis, and the outlet plus the axis of the birth canal determine whether vaginal birth is possible and the manner in which the fetus passes down the birth canal.
- Involuntary uterine contractions act to expel the fetus and placenta during the first stage of labor; these are augmented by voluntary bearing-down efforts during the second stage.
- The first stage of labor lasts from the time dilation begins to the time when the cervix is fully dilated.
- The second stage of labor lasts from the time of full cervical dilation to the birth of the infant.
- The third stage of labor lasts from the infant's birth to the expulsion of the placenta.
- The fourth stage of labor is the first 2 hours after birth.
- The cardinal movements of the mechanism of labor are engagement, descent, flexion, internal rotation, extension, restitution and external rotation, and expulsion of the infant.
- Although the events precipitating the onset of labor are unknown, many factors, including changes in the maternal uterus, cervix, and pituitary gland, are thought to be involved.
- A healthy fetus with an adequate uterofetoplacental circulation is able to compensate for the stress of uterine contractions.
- As the woman progresses through labor, various body systems adapt to the birth process.

REFERENCES

Blackburn ST: *Maternal, fetal, and neonatal physiology: a clinical perspective*, ed 4, St Louis, 2013, Saunders.

Cunningham F, Leveno K, Bloom S, et al: *Williams obstetrics*, ed 23, New York, 2010, McGraw-Hill.

Gordon M: Maternal physiology. In Gabbe SG, Niebyl JR, Simpson JL, et al, editors: *Obstetrics: normal and problem pregnancies*, ed 6, Philadelphia, 2012, Saunders.

Kilpatrick S, Garrison E: Normal labor and delivery. In Gabbe SG, Niebyl JR, Simpson JL, et al, editors: *Obstetrics: normal and problem pregnancies*, ed 6, Philadelphia, 2012, Saunders.

Miller L, Miller D, Tucker SM: *Mosby's pocket guide to fetal monitoring: a multidisciplinary approach*, ed 7, St Louis, 2013, Mosby.

Norwitz E, Lye S: Biology of parturition. In Creasy R, Resnik R, Iams J, et al, editors: *Creasy & Resnik's maternal-fetal medicine: principles and practice*, ed 6, Philadelphia, 2009, Saunders.

Rozance P, Rosenberg A: The neonate. In Gabbe SG, Niebyl JR, Simpson JL, et al, editors: *Obstetrics: normal and problem pregnancies*, ed 6, Philadelphia, 2012, Saunders.

Thorp J: Clinical aspects of normal and abnormal labor. In Creasy R, Resnik R, Iams J, et al, editors: *Creasy & Resnik's maternal-fetal medicine: principles and practice*, ed 6, Philadelphia, 2009, Saunders.

VandeVusse L: The essential forces of labor revisited: 13 Ps reported in women's birth stories, *MCN Am J Matern Child Nurs* 24(4):176–184, 1999.

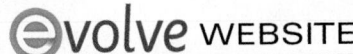 WEBSITE

http://evolve.elsevier.com/Perry/maternal

LEARNING OBJECTIVES

On completion of this chapter, the reader will be able to:

- Describe breathing and relaxation techniques used for each stage of labor.
- Identify nonpharmacologic strategies to enhance relaxation and decrease pain during labor.
- Compare pharmacologic methods used to relieve pain in different stages of labor and for vaginal or cesarean birth.
- Describe nursing responsibilities appropriate in providing care for a woman receiving analgesia and anesthesia during labor.

Pain is an unpleasant, complex, highly individualized phenomenon with sensory and emotional components. Pregnant women commonly worry about the pain they will experience during labor and birth and about how they will react to and deal with that pain. A variety of nonpharmacologic and pharmacologic methods can help the woman or the couple cope with the pain of labor. The methods selected depend on the situation, the availability, and the preferences of the woman and her health care provider. This chapter will discuss sources of intrapartum pain and factors that affect women's response to pain. It will also describe nonpharmacologic and pharmacologic methods commonly used for pain relief.

PAIN DURING LABOR AND BIRTH

Neurologic Origins

The pain and discomfort of labor have two origins—visceral and somatic. During the first stage of labor, uterine contractions cause cervical dilation and effacement. Uterine ischemia (decreased blood flow and therefore local oxygen deficit) results from compression of the arteries supplying the myometrium during uterine contractions. Pain impulses during the first stage of labor are transmitted via the T10 to T12 and L1 spinal nerve segments and accessory lower thoracic and upper lumbar sympathetic nerves. These nerves originate in the uterine body and cervix (Blackburn, 2013).

The pain from distention of the lower uterine segment, stretching of cervical tissue as it effaces and dilates, pressure and traction on adjacent structures (e.g., uterine tubes, ovaries, ligaments) and nerves, and uterine ischemia during the first stage of labor is visceral pain. It is located over the lower portion of the abdomen. Referred pain occurs when pain that originates in the uterus radiates to the abdominal wall, lumbosacral area of the back, iliac crests, gluteal area, thighs, and lower back (Blackburn, 2013; Zwelling, Johnson, and Allen, 2006).

During most of the first stage of labor, the woman usually has discomfort only during contractions and is free of pain between contractions. Some women, especially those whose fetus is in a posterior position, experience continuous contraction-related low back pain, even in the interval between contractions. As labor progresses and pain becomes more intense and persistent, women become fatigued and discouraged, often experiencing difficulty coping with contractions (Creehan, 2008; Zwelling, Johnson, and Allen, 2006).

During the second stage of labor, the woman has somatic pain, which is often described as intense, sharp, burning, and well localized. This pain results from:

- Distention and traction on the peritoneum and uterocervical supports during contractions
- Pressure against the bladder and rectum
- Stretching and distention of perineal tissues and the pelvic floor to allow passage of the fetus
- Lacerations of soft tissue (e.g., cervix, vagina, and perineum)

As women concentrate on the work of bearing down to give birth to their baby, they may report a decrease in pain intensity (Blackburn, 2013; Creehan, 2008). Pain impulses during the second stage of labor are transmitted via the pudendal nerve through S2 to S4 spinal nerve segments and the parasympathetic system (Blackburn, 2013).

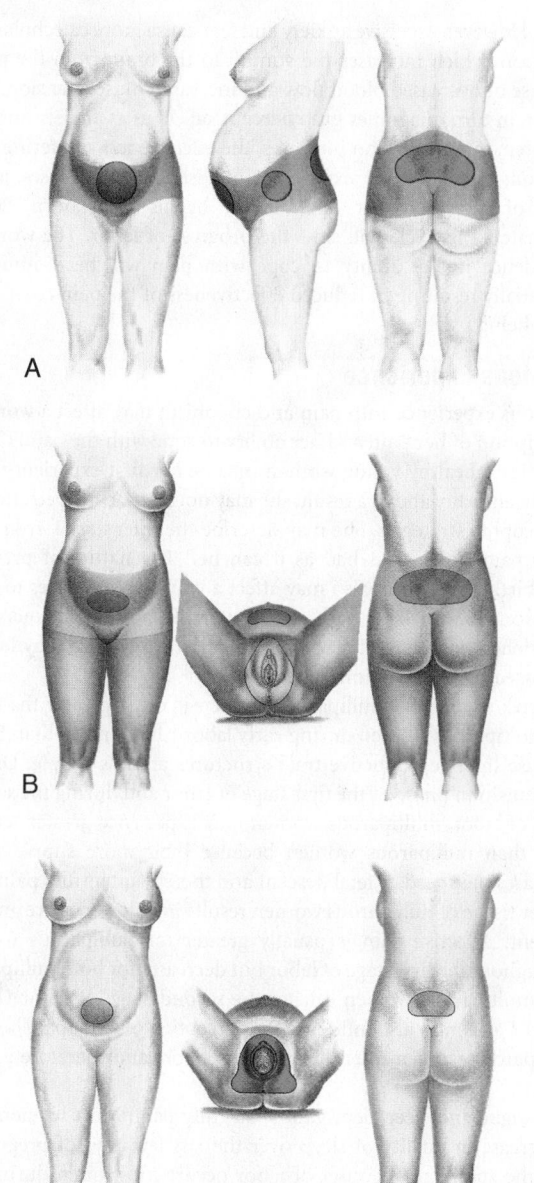

FIG 14-1 Pain during labor. **A,** Distribution of labor pain during first stage. **B,** Distribution of labor pain during transition and early phase of second stage. **C,** Distribution of pain during late second-stage and actual birth. (*Gray areas* indicate mild discomfort; *light pink areas* indicate moderate discomfort; *dark red areas* indicate intense discomfort.)

Pain experienced during the third stage of labor and the after-pains of the early postpartum period are uterine, similar to the pain experienced early in the first stage of labor. Areas of pain during labor are shown in Fig. 14-1.

Perception of Pain

Although the pain threshold is remarkably similar in everyone regardless of gender, social, ethnic, or cultural differences, these differences play a definite role in the person's perception of and behavioral responses to pain. The effects of factors such as culture, counterstimuli, and distraction in coping with pain are not fully understood. The meaning of pain and the verbal and nonverbal expressions given to pain are apparently learned from interactions within the primary social group. Cultural influences may impose certain behavioral expectations regarding acceptable and unacceptable behavior when experiencing pain.

Pain tolerance refers to the level of pain a laboring woman is willing to endure. When this level is exceeded, she will seek measures to relieve the pain. Factors that influence a woman's pain tolerance level and her request for pharmacologic pain relief measures include her desire for a natural, vaginal birth; her preparation for childbirth; the nature of her support during labor; and her willingness and ability to participate in nonpharmacologic measures for comfort (Creehan, 2008).

Expression of Pain

Pain results in physiologic effects and sensory and emotional (affective) responses. During childbirth, pain gives rise to identifiable physiologic effects. Sympathetic nervous system activity is stimulated in response to intensifying pain, resulting in increased catecholamine levels. Blood pressure and heart rate increase. Maternal respiratory patterns change in response to an increase in oxygen consumption. Hyperventilation, sometimes accompanied by respiratory alkalosis, can occur as pain intensifies and more rapid, shallow breathing techniques are used during contractions. Pallor and diaphoresis may be seen. Gastric acidity increases, and nausea and vomiting are common in the active and transition phases of the first stage of labor. Placental perfusion may decrease, and uterine activity may diminish, potentially prolonging labor and affecting fetal well-being.

Certain emotional (affective) expressions of pain often are seen. Such changes include increasing anxiety with lessened perceptual field, writhing, crying, groaning, gesturing (hand clenching and wringing), and excessive muscular excitability throughout the body.

FACTORS INFLUENCING PAIN RESPONSE

Pain during childbirth is unique to each woman. How she perceives or interprets that pain is influenced by a variety of physiologic, psychologic, emotional, social, cultural, and environmental factors (Zwelling, Johnson, and Allen, 2006).

Physiologic Factors

A variety of physiologic factors can affect the intensity of childbirth pain. Women with a history of dysmenorrhea may experience increased pain during childbirth as a result of higher prostaglandin levels. Back pain associated with menstruation also may increase the likelihood of contraction-related low back pain. Other physical factors that affect pain intensity include fatigue, the interval and duration of contractions, fetal size and position, rapidity of fetal descent, and maternal position (Zwelling, Johnson, and Allen, 2006).

Beta (β) endorphins are endogenous opioids secreted by the pituitary gland that act on the central and peripheral nervous systems to reduce pain. The level of β endorphins increases during pregnancy and birth in humans. β endorphins are associated with feelings of euphoria and analgesia. The pain threshold may rise as β endorphin levels increase, enabling women in labor to tolerate acute pain (Blackburn, 2013).

Culture

The population of pregnant women reflects the increasingly multicultural nature of society in the United States. As nurses care for women and families from a variety of cultural backgrounds, they must have knowledge and understanding of how culture mediates pain. Although all women expect to experience at least some pain and discomfort during childbirth, it is their culture and religious belief system that determines how they will perceive, interpret, and respond to and manage the pain. For example, women with strong religious beliefs often accept pain as a necessary and inevitable part of bringing a new life into the world (Callister, Khalaf, Semenic, et al., 2003). An understanding of the beliefs, values, expectations, and practices of various cultures will narrow the cultural gap and help the nurse assess the laboring woman's pain experience more accurately. The nurse can then provide appropriate, culturally sensitive care by using pain relief measures that preserve the woman's sense of control and self-confidence (see Cultural Competence box). Recognize that although a woman's behavior in response to pain may vary according to her cultural background, it may not accurately reflect the intensity of the pain she is experiencing. Assess the woman for the physiologic effects of pain, and listen to the words she uses to describe the sensory and affective qualities of her pain (see Community Focus box).

Anxiety

Anxiety is commonly associated with increased pain during labor. Mild anxiety is considered normal for a woman during labor and

🌐 CULTURAL COMPETENCE

Some Cultural Beliefs About Pain

The following examples demonstrate how women of different cultural backgrounds may react to pain. Because they are generalizations, the nurse must assess each woman experiencing pain related to childbirth.

- Chinese women may not exhibit reactions to pain, although exhibiting pain during childbirth is acceptable. They consider accepting something when it is first offered as impolite; therefore pain interventions must be offered more than once. Acupuncture may be used for pain relief.
- Arab or Middle Eastern women may be vocal in response to labor pain. They may prefer medication for pain relief.
- Japanese women may be stoic in response to labor pain, but they may request medication when pain becomes severe.
- Southeast Asian women may endure severe pain before requesting relief.
- Hispanic women may be stoic until late in labor, when they may become vocal and request pain relief.
- Native-American women may use medications or remedies made from indigenous plants. They are often stoic in response to labor pain.
- African-American women may express pain openly. Use of medication for pain relief varies.

🏠 COMMUNITY FOCUS

Culture and Pain

Talk to a man and a woman from a culture different from your own who have experienced childbirth. Ask her to describe her reactions to pain, how she sought relief of pain, the atmosphere of the childbirth setting, and the attitudes of the health care providers. Ask him if he was present for the birth and what his role in the birth was. How did his culture influence his role and reaction to childbirth? How did her culture influence her response to labor and the associated pain? What expressions of pain are "acceptable" in her culture? If he was present, how did he help her deal with the pain? What is the role of support persons in the labor process? Are the responses of the couple different from your responses to those same questions?

birth. However, excessive anxiety and fear cause more catecholamine secretion, which increases the stimuli to the brain from the pelvis because of decreased blood flow and increased muscle tension. This action, in turn, magnifies pain perception. Thus as anxiety and fear heighten, muscle tension increases, the effectiveness of uterine contractions decreases, the experience of discomfort increases, and a cycle of increased fear and anxiety begins (Blackburn, 2013). Ultimately this cycle will slow the progress of labor. The woman's confidence in her ability to cope with pain will be diminished, potentially resulting in reduced effectiveness of the pain relief measures being used.

Previous Experience

Previous experience with pain and childbirth may affect a woman's description of her pain and her ability to cope with the pain. Childbirth for a healthy young woman may be her first experience with significant pain, and as a result, she may not have developed effective pain coping strategies. She may describe the intensity of even early labor pain as pain "as bad as it can be." The nature of previous childbirth experiences also may affect a woman's responses to pain. For women who have had a difficult and painful previous birth experience, anxiety and fear from this past experience may lead to increased pain perception.

Sensory pain for nulliparous women is often greater than that for multiparous women during early labor (dilation less than 5 cm) because their reproductive tract structures are less supple. During the transition phase of the first stage of labor and during the second stage of labor, multiparous women may experience greater sensory pain than nulliparous women because their more supple tissue increases the speed of fetal descent and thereby intensifies pain. The firmer tissue of nulliparous women results in a slower, more gradual descent. Affective pain is usually greater for nulliparous women throughout the first stage of labor but decreases for both nulliparous and multiparous women during the second stage of labor (Lowe, 2002). Parity may also influence the perception of labor pain because nulliparous women often have longer labors and therefore greater fatigue.

Fatigue and sleep deprivation magnify pain. Most women have a decrease in quality of sleep over the last few days of pregnancy, and the spontaneous onset of labor occurs most often during the night (Beebe and Lee, 2007). Thus many women have an increased perception of the intensity of pain during labor.

Gate-Control Theory of Pain

Even particularly intense pain stimuli can at times be ignored. This is possible because certain nerve cell groupings within the spinal cord, brainstem, and cerebral cortex have the ability to modulate the pain impulse through a blocking mechanism. This gate-control theory of pain helps explain the way hypnosis and the pain relief techniques taught in childbirth preparation classes work to relieve the pain of labor. According to this theory, pain sensations travel along sensory nerve pathways to the brain but only a limited number of sensations, or messages, can travel through these nerve pathways at one time. Using distraction techniques such as massage or stroking, music, focal points, and imagery reduces or completely blocks the capacity of nerve pathways to transmit pain. These distractions are thought to work by closing down a hypothetic gate in the spinal cord, thus preventing pain signals from reaching the brain. The perception of pain is thereby diminished.

In addition, when the laboring woman engages in neuromuscular and motor activity, activity within the spinal cord itself further modifies the transmission of pain. Cognitive work involving

BOX 14-1   SUGGESTED MEASURES FOR SUPPORTING A WOMAN IN LABOR

- Provide companionship and reassurance.
- Offer positive reinforcement and praise for her efforts.
- Encourage participation in distracting activities and nonpharmacologic measures for comfort.
- Give nourishment (if allowed by primary health care provider).
- Assist with personal hygiene.
- Offer information and advice.
- Involve the woman in decision making regarding her care.
- Interpret the woman's wishes to other health care providers and to her support group.
- Create a relaxing environment.
- Use a calm and confident approach.
- Support and encourage the woman's family members by role modeling labor support measures and providing time for breaks.

concentration on breathing and relaxation requires selective and directed cortical activity that activates and closes the gating mechanism as well. As labor intensifies, more complex cognitive techniques are required to maintain effectiveness. The gate-control theory underscores the need for a supportive birth setting that allows the laboring woman to relax and use various higher mental activities.

Comfort

Although the predominant medical approach to labor is that it is painful and the pain must be removed, an alternative view is that labor is a natural process and women can experience comfort and transcend the discomfort or pain to reach the joyful outcome of birth. Having needs and desires met promotes a feeling of comfort. The most helpful interventions in enhancing comfort are a caring nursing approach and a supportive presence.

Support

Current evidence indicates that a woman's satisfaction with her labor and birth experience is determined by how well her personal expectations of childbirth were met and the quality of support and interaction she received from her caregivers (Box 14-1). In addition, satisfaction is influenced by the degree to which she was able to stay in control of her labor and to participate in decision making regarding her labor, including the pain relief measures to be used (Albers, 2007; Zwelling, Johnson, and Allen, 2006).

The value of the continuous supportive presence of a person (e.g., doula, childbirth educator, family member, friend, nurse, or partner) during labor who provides physical comforting, facilitates communication, and offers information and guidance to the woman in labor has long been known. Emotional support is demonstrated by giving praise and reassurance and conveying a positive, calm, and confident demeanor when caring for the woman in labor (Creehan, 2008). It is interesting to note that research findings have concluded that a more positive effect is achieved when the continuous support is provided by people who are not hospital staff members (Hodnett, Gates, Hofmeyr, et al., 2011).

Environment

The quality of the environment can influence pain perception and the laboring woman's ability to cope with her pain. Environment includes the individuals present (e.g., how they communicate, their

philosophy of care including a belief in the value of nonpharmacologic pain relief measures, practice policies, and quality of support) and the physical space in which the labor occurs (Creehan, 2008; Zwelling, Johnson, and Allen, 2006). Women usually prefer to be cared for by familiar caregivers in a comfortable, homelike setting. The environment should be safe and private, allowing a woman to feel free to be herself as she tries out different comfort measures. Stimuli such as light, noise, and temperature should be adjusted according to her preferences. The environment should have space for movement and equipment such as birth balls. Comfortable chairs, tubs, and showers should be readily available to facilitate participation in a variety of nonpharmacologic pain relief measures. The familiarity of the environment can be enhanced by bringing items from home such as pillows, objects for a focal point, music, and DVDs.

NONPHARMACOLOGIC PAIN MANAGEMENT

The alleviation of pain is important. Commonly it is not the amount of pain the woman experiences but whether she meets the goals she set for herself to cope with the pain that influences her perception of the birth experience as good or bad. The observant nurse looks for clues to the woman's desired level of control in the management of pain and its relief.

Nonpharmacologic measures are often simple and safe, have few if any major adverse reactions, are relatively inexpensive, and can be used throughout labor. In addition, they provide the woman with a sense of control over her childbirth as she makes choices about the measures that are best for her. During the prenatal period, she should explore a variety of nonpharmacologic measures. Techniques she usually finds helpful in relieving stress and enhancing relaxation (e.g., music, meditation, massage, warm baths) may be very effective as components of a plan for managing labor pain. The woman should be encouraged to communicate to her health care providers her preferences for relaxation and pain relief measures and to actively participate in their implementation.

Many of the nonpharmacologic methods for relief of discomfort are taught in different types of prenatal preparation classes, or the woman or couple may have read various books and magazine articles on the subject in advance. Many of these methods require practice for best results (e.g., hypnosis, patterned breathing and controlled relaxation techniques, biofeedback), although the nurse may use some of them successfully without the woman or couple having prior knowledge (e.g., slow-paced breathing, massage and touch, effleurage, counterpressure). Women should be encouraged to try a variety of methods. Often nonpharmacologic methods are used in combination with pharmacologic methods, particularly as labor progresses.

With the increasing use of epidural analgesia, nurses may be less likely to encourage women to use nonpharmacologic measures, in part because these methods may be viewed as more complex and time consuming than monitoring a woman receiving an epidural. In addition, new nurses may not have had the opportunity to develop skill in the implementation of these methods. It is imperative that perinatal nurses develop a commitment to and expertise in using a variety of nonpharmacologic pain relief strategies in order for women in labor to be comfortable using them. Although research data to support the effectiveness of many of these nonpharmacologic measures are limited, there are sufficient reports of their benefits from women and health care providers to recommend that nurses encourage their use (Creehan, 2008). The analgesic effect of many nonpharmacologic measures is comparable

NONPHARMACOLOGIC STRATEGIES TO ENCOURAGE RELAXATION AND RELIEVE PAIN

Cutaneous Stimulation Strategies
- Counterpressure
- Effleurage (light massage)
- Therapeutic touch and massage
- Walking
- Rocking
- Changing positions
- Application of heat or cold
- Transcutaneous electrical nerve stimulation (TENS)
- Acupressure
- Water therapy (showers, whirlpool baths)
- Intradermal water block

Sensory Stimulation Strategies
- Aromatherapy
- Breathing techniques
- Music
- Imagery
- Use of focal points

Cognitive Strategies
- Childbirth education
- Hypnosis
- Biofeedback

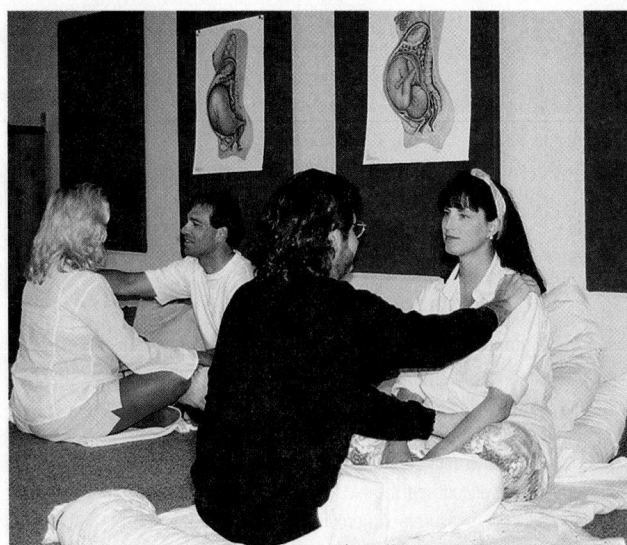

FIG 14-2 Expectant parents learning relaxation techniques. (Courtesy Marjorie Pyle, RNC, Lifecircle, Costa Mesa, CA.)

to or even superior to opioids that are administered parenterally (Box 14-2).

Childbirth Preparation Methods

The childbirth education movement began in the 1950s. Today most health care providers recommend or offer childbirth preparation classes for expectant parents. Historically, popular childbirth methods taught in the United States were the Dick-Read method, the Lamaze (psychoprophylaxis) method, and the Bradley (husband-coached childbirth) method. Although these three organizations continue to exist, they are now less focused on a "method" approach. Rather, women are assisted to develop their birth philosophy and inner knowledge and then choose from a variety of skills to use to cope with the labor process. Many childbirth educators teach a variety of techniques that originated in several different organizations or publications. Women are encouraged to choose the techniques that work best for them.

Gaining popularity are methods developed and promoted by Birthing From Within, Birthworks, Association of Labor Assistants and Childbirth Educators (ALACE), Childbirth and Postpartum Professional Association (CAPPA), and HypnoBirthing, to name a few. These methods offer classes and other services that focus on fostering a woman's confidence in her innate ability to give birth. The woman or couple are helped to recognize the uniqueness of their pregnancy and childbirth experience.

Relaxation and Breathing Techniques

Relaxation

Relaxation or reduction of body tension is a technique suggested by virtually all childbirth education organizations. Learning relaxation in childbirth education classes can help couples with the stresses of pregnancy, childbirth, and adjustment to parenting and can be a form of stress management throughout life (Fig. 14-2). Evidence suggests that relaxation may improve the management of labor pain (Jones, Othman, Dowswell, et al., 2012). Relaxation is ideally combined with activity such as walking, slow dancing, rocking, and position changes that help the baby rotate through the pelvis. Rhythmic motion stimulates mechanoreceptors in the brain, which decreases pain perception.

The nurse can assist the woman by providing a quiet and relaxed environment, offering cues as needed, and recognizing signs of tension (e.g., frowning, change in tone of voice, clenching of fists). A relaxed environment for labor is created by controlling sensory stimuli (e.g., light, noise, temperature) and reducing interruptions. Nurses should remain calm and unhurried in their approach and sit rather than stand at the bedside whenever possible (Creehan, 2008).

Imagery and Visualization

Imagery and visualization are useful techniques in preparation for birth and are often used in combination with relaxation. Although research on their use is scant, clinical reports suggest that imagery and visualization can be used to produce a sense of well-being during pregnancy, assist with cervical dilation, and decrease the experience of pain and tension during labor. Imagery involves techniques such as imagining a walk through a restful garden or breathing in light, energy, and healing color and breathing out worries and tension. A variety of skills taught in childbirth classes augment relaxation during pregnancy and labor. All can be taught as lifetime skills useful to the couple and can be used to teach their children to cope with the stresses of life.

Breathing Techniques

Different approaches to childbirth preparation stress varying breathing techniques to provide distraction, thereby reducing the perception of pain and helping the woman maintain control throughout contractions. In the first stage of labor, such breathing techniques can promote relaxation of the abdominal muscles and thereby increase the size of the abdominal cavity. This lessens discomfort generated by friction between the uterus and abdominal wall during contractions. Because the muscles of the genital area also become more relaxed, they do not interfere with fetal descent. In the second stage, breathing is used to increase abdominal pressure and thereby assist in expelling the fetus. Breathing also can be used to relax the pudendal muscles to prevent precipitate expulsion of the fetal head (Fig. 14-3).

For couples who have prepared for labor by practicing relaxing and breathing techniques, a simple review with occasional reminders may be all that is necessary to help them along. For those who

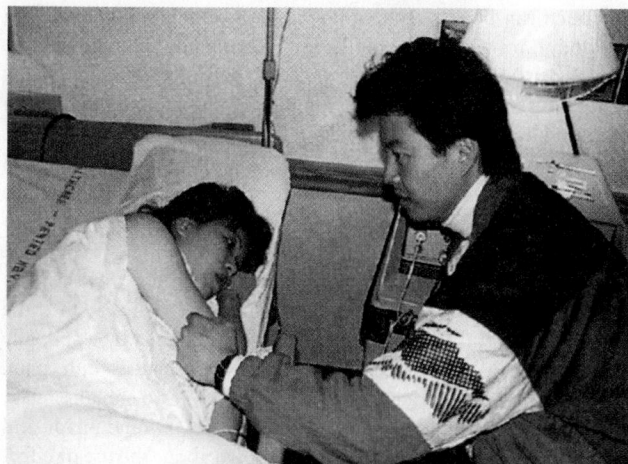

FIG 14-3 A laboring woman using breathing techniques during a uterine contraction with coaching from her partner. (Courtesy Marjorie Pyle, RNC, Lifecircle, Costa Mesa, CA.)

❓ CRITICAL THINKING CASE STUDY

Laboring Without an Epidural

Jamie is a 16-year-old G1 P0 who has been admitted with severe pre-eclampsia (HELLP syndrome) at 34 weeks of gestation. Jamie's physician plans to induce labor and anticipates a vaginal birth. Jamie has not attended any childbirth preparation classes and has been planning to have an epidural for labor and birth. Unfortunately, because her platelet count is very low (28,000), the anesthesia care provider refuses to place an epidural block. Jamie bursts into tears and says, "I can't make it through labor without an epidural! It's going to hurt too much! Help me!!"

1. Evidence—Is there sufficient evidence regarding avoiding regional anesthesia in women who have low platelet counts?
2. Assumptions—Describe an underlying assumption about each of the following nonpharmacologic or pharmacologic methods for pain relief during labor.
   a. Breathing and relaxation techniques
   b. Application of heat and cold
   c. Systemic analgesia
   d. Presence of a support person to increase effectiveness of interventions for pain
3. What implications and priorities for nursing care can be drawn at this time?
4. Does the evidence objectively support your argument (conclusion)?

HELLP, **H**emolysis, **E**levated **L**iver enzymes, **L**ow **P**latelet count.

---

have had no preparation, instruction and practice in simple breathing and relaxation techniques can be given early in labor and often is surprisingly successful. Nurses can also model breathing techniques and breathe in synchrony with the woman and her partner. Motivation is high and readiness to learn is enhanced by the reality of labor (see Critical Thinking Case Study).

Various breathing techniques can be used for controlling pain during contractions (Box 14-3). The nurse needs to determine what, if any, techniques the laboring couple know before giving them instruction. Simple patterns are more easily learned. Paced breathing is most associated with prepared childbirth and includes slow-paced, modified-paced, and patterned-paced breathing (pant-blow) techniques. Each labor is different, and nursing support includes

---

BOX 14-3   PACED BREATHING TECHNIQUES

Cleansing Breath
- Relaxed breath in through nose and out through mouth. Used at the beginning and end of each contraction.

Slow-Paced Breathing (Approximately 6 to 8 Breaths per Minute)
- Performed at approximately half the normal breathing rate (number of breaths per minute divided by 2)
- IN-2-3-4/OUT-2-3-4/IN-2-3-4/OUT-2-3-4 …

Modified-Paced Breathing (Approximately 32 to 40 Breaths per Minute)
- Performed at about twice the normal breathing rate (number of breaths per minute multiplied by 2)
- IN-OUT/IN-OUT/IN-OUT/IN-OUT …
- For more flexibility and variety, the woman may combine the slow and modified breathing by using the slow breathing for beginnings and ends of contractions and modified breathing for more intense peaks. This technique conserves energy, lessens fatigue, and reduces risk for hyperventilation.

Patterned-Paced or Pant-Blow Breathing (Same Rate as Modified)
- Enhances concentration
- 3:1 Patterned breathing IN-OUT/IN-OUT/IN-OUT/IN-BLOW (repeat through contraction)
- 4:1 Patterned breathing IN-OUT/IN-OUT/IN-OUT/IN-OUT/IN-BLOW (repeat through contraction)

Adapted from Nichols F: Paced breathing techniques. In Nichols FH, Humenick SS, editors: *Childbirth education: practice, research, and theory*, ed 2, Philadelphia, 2000, Saunders; Perinatal Education Associates: *Breathing*, 2008, www.birthsource.com/scripts/article.asp?articleid=211.

---

assisting couples to adapt breathing techniques to their individual labor experience.

All patterns begin with a deep, relaxing, cleansing breath to "greet the contraction" and end with another deep breath exhaled to "gently blow the contraction away." These deep breaths ensure adequate oxygen for mother and baby and signal that a contraction is beginning or has ended. As the breath is exhaled, respiratory and voluntary muscles relax (Creehan, 2008). In general, *slow-paced breathing* is performed at approximately half the woman's normal breathing rate and is initiated when she can no longer walk or talk through contractions. The woman should take no fewer than three or four breaths per minute. Slow-paced breathing aids in relaxation and provides optimum oxygenation. The woman should continue to use this technique for as long as it is effective in reducing the perception of pain and maintaining control. As contractions increase in frequency and intensity, the woman often needs to change to a more complex breathing technique, which is shallower and faster than her normal rate of breathing but should not exceed twice her resting respiratory rate. This *modified-paced breathing* pattern requires that she remain alert and concentrate more fully on breathing, thus blocking more painful stimuli than the simpler slow-paced breathing pattern (Perinatal Education Associates, 2008 [www.birthsource.com]).

The most difficult time to maintain control during contractions comes during the transition phase of the first stage of labor, when the cervix dilates from 8 cm to 10 cm. Even for the woman who has prepared for labor, concentration on breathing techniques is difficult to maintain. *Patterned-paced (pant-blow) breathing* is suggested during this phase. It is performed at the same rate as modified-paced breathing and consists of panting breaths combined with soft blowing breaths at regular intervals. The patterns may vary (i.e., *pant, pant, pant, pant, blow* [4:1 pattern] or *pant, pant, pant, blow* [3:1 pattern]) (Perinatal Education Associates, 2008). An undesirable reaction to this type of breathing is hyperventilation. The woman and her support person must be aware of and watch for symptoms of the resultant respiratory alkalosis: lightheadedness, dizziness, tingling of the fingers, or circumoral numbness. Respiratory alkalosis may be eliminated by having the woman breathe into a paper bag held tightly around her mouth and nose. This enables her to rebreathe carbon dioxide and replace the bicarbonate ions. The woman also can breathe into her cupped hands if no bag is available. Maintaining a breathing rate that is no more than twice the normal rate will lessen chances of hyperventilation. The partner can help the woman maintain her breathing rate with visual, tactile, or auditory cues.

As the fetal head reaches the pelvic floor, the woman may feel the urge to push and may automatically begin to exert downward pressure by contracting her abdominal muscles. During second-stage pushing, the woman should find a breathing pattern that is relaxing and feels good to her and is safe for her baby. Any regular or rhythmic breathing that avoids prolonged breath holding during pushing should maintain a good oxygen flow to the fetus (Perinatal Education Associates, 2008).

The woman can control the urge to push by taking panting breaths or by slowly exhaling through pursed lips (as though blowing out a candle or blowing up a balloon). This type of breathing can be used to overcome the urge to push when the cervix is not fully prepared (e.g., less than 8 cm dilated, not retracting) and to facilitate a slow birth of the fetal head.

Effleurage and Counterpressure

Effleurage (light massage) and counterpressure have brought relief to many women during the first stage of labor. The gate-control theory may supply the reason for the effectiveness of these measures. Effleurage is light stroking, usually of the abdomen, in rhythm with breathing during contractions. It is used to distract the woman from contraction pain. Often the presence of monitor belts makes it difficult to perform effleurage on the abdomen; therefore a thigh or the chest may be used. As labor progresses, hyperesthesia (hypersensitivity to touch) may make effleurage uncomfortable and thus less effective.

Counterpressure is steady pressure applied by a support person to the sacral area with a firm object (e.g., tennis ball) or the fist or heel of the hand. Pressure can also be applied to both hips (double hip squeeze) or to the knees (Creehan, 2008). Application of counterpressure helps the woman cope with the sensations of internal pressure and pain in the lower back. It is especially helpful when back pain is caused by pressure of the occiput against spinal nerves when the fetal head is in a posterior position. Counterpressure lifts the occiput off these nerves, thereby providing pain relief. The support person will need to be relieved occasionally because application of counterpressure is hard work.

Touch and Massage

Touch and massage have been an integral part of the traditional care process for women in labor. A variety of massage techniques have been shown to be safe and effective during labor (Gilbert, 2011; Zwelling, Johnson, and Allen, 2006).

Touch can be as simple as holding the woman's hand, stroking her body, and embracing her. When using touch to communicate caring, reassurance, and concern, it is important that the woman's preferences for touch (e.g., who can touch her, where they can touch her, and how they can touch her) and responses to touch be determined. A woman with a history of sexual abuse or certain cultural beliefs may be uncomfortable with touch. Touch also can involve very specialized techniques that require manipulation of the human energy field.

Therapeutic touch (TT) uses the concept of energy fields within the body called *prana*. Prana are thought to be deficient in some people who are in pain. TT uses laying-on of hands by a specially trained person to redirect energy fields associated with pain. Research has demonstrated the effectiveness of TT to enhance relaxation, reduce anxiety, and relieve pain (Aghabati, Mohammadi, and Pour Esmaiel, 2010); however, little is known about the use or effectiveness of TT for relieving labor pain.

Head, hand, back, and foot massage may be very effective in reducing tension and enhancing comfort. Some evidence suggests that massage may improve management of labor pain (Jones, Othman, Dowswell, et al., 2012). Hand and foot massage may be especially relaxing in advanced labor when hyperesthesia limits a woman's tolerance for touch on other parts of her body. The woman and her partner should be encouraged to experiment with different types of massage during pregnancy to determine what might feel best and be most relaxing during labor.

Application of Heat and Cold

Warmed blankets, warm compresses, heated rice bags, a warm bath or shower, or a moist heating pad can enhance relaxation and reduce pain during labor. Heat relieves muscle ischemia and increases blood flow to the area of discomfort. Heat application is effective for back pain caused by a posterior presentation or general backache from fatigue.

Cold application such as cold cloths, frozen gel packs, or ice packs applied to the back, the chest, and/or the face during labor may be effective in increasing comfort when the woman feels warm. They also may be applied to areas of musculoskeletal pain. Cooling relieves pain by reducing the muscle temperature and relieving muscle spasms (Creehan, 2008). However, a woman's culture may make the use of cold during labor unacceptable.

Heat and cold may be used alternately for a greater effect. Neither heat nor cold should be applied over ischemic or anesthetized areas because tissues can be damaged. One or two layers of cloth should be placed between the skin and a hot or cold pack to prevent damage to the underlying integument (see Critical Thinking Case Study).

Acupressure and Acupuncture

Acupressure and acupuncture can be used in pregnancy, in labor, and postpartum to relieve pain and other discomforts. Pressure, heat, or cold is applied to acupuncture points called *tsubos*. These points have an increased density of neuroreceptors and increased electrical conductivity. Acupressure is said to promote circulation of blood, the harmony of yin and yang, and the secretion of neurotransmitters, thus maintaining normal body functions and enhancing well-being (Tournaire and Theau-Yonneau, 2007). Acupressure is best applied over the skin without using lubricants. Pressure is usually applied with the heel of the hand, fist, or pads of the thumbs and fingers (Fig. 14-4). Tennis balls or other devices also may be used. Pressure is applied with contractions initially and then continuously as labor progresses to the transition phase at the end of the first stage of labor (Tournaire and Theau-Yonneau, 2007).

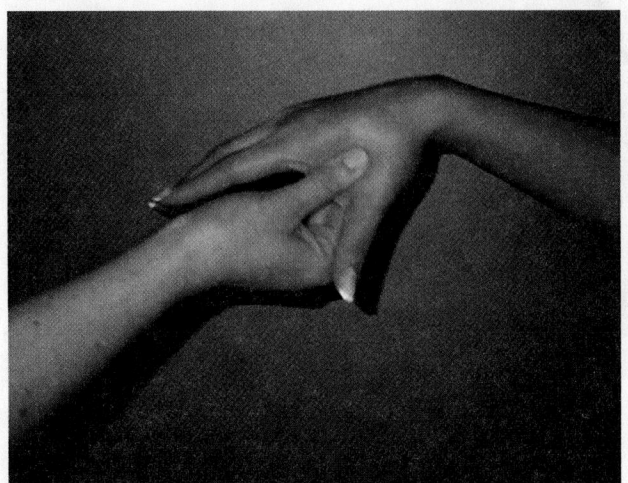

FIG 14-4 Ho-Ku acupressure point (back of hand where thumb and index finger come together) used to enhance uterine contractions without increasing pain. (Courtesy Julie Perry Nelson, Loveland, CO.)

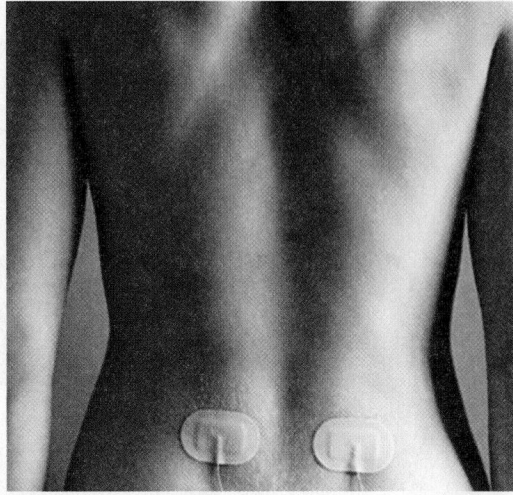

FIG 14-5 Placement of transcutaneous electrical nerve stimulation (TENS) electrodes on back for relief of labor pain.

Synchronized breathing by the caregiver and the woman is suggested for greater effectiveness. Acupressure points are found on the neck, the shoulders, the wrists, the lower back including sacral points, the hips, the area below the kneecaps, the ankles, the nails on the small toes, and the soles of the feet. Evidence is insufficient to support the effectiveness of acupressure as a method of pain relief during labor (Smith, Collins, Cyna, et al., 2006).

Acupuncture is the insertion of fine needles into specific areas of the body to restore the flow of *qi* (energy) and to decrease pain, which is thought to be obstructing the flow of energy. Effectiveness may be attributed to the alteration of chemical neurotransmitter levels in the body or to the release of endorphins as a result of hypothalamic activation. Acupuncture should be done by a trained certified therapist, and arranging to have a qualified and credentialed acupuncture provider available during labor and birth may be challenging (Hawkins and Bucklin, 2012). Current evidence indicates that acupuncture may be beneficial for relief of labor pain; however, further study is indicated (Hawkins and Bucklin, 2012; Jones, Othman, Dowswell, et al., 2012).

Transcutaneous Electrical Nerve Stimulation

Transcutaneous electrical nerve stimulation (TENS) involves the placing of two pairs of flat electrodes on either side of the woman's thoracic and sacral spine (Fig. 14-5). These electrodes provide continuous low-intensity electrical impulses or stimuli from a battery-operated device. During a contraction, the woman increases the stimulation from low to high intensity by turning control knobs on the device. High intensity should be maintained for at least 1 minute to facilitate release of endorphins. Women describe the resulting sensation as a tingling or buzzing. TENS is most useful for lower back pain during the early first stage of labor. Women tend to rate the device as helpful although its use does not decrease pain. It appears that the electrical impulses or stimuli somehow make the pain less disturbing. No serious safety concerns are associated with the use of TENS (Hawkins and Bucklin, 2012).

Water Therapy (Hydrotherapy)

Bathing, showering, and jet hydrotherapy (whirlpool baths) with warm water (e.g., at or below body temperature) are nonpharmacologic measures that can promote comfort and relaxation during labor (Fig. 14-6). The warm water stimulates the release of endorphins, relaxes fibers to close the gate on pain, promotes better circulation and oxygenation, and helps soften the perineal tissues. Most women find immersion in water to be soothing, relaxing, and comforting. While immersed, they may find it easier to let go and allow labor to take its course (Gilbert, 2011). Some evidence suggests that immersion in water may improve management of labor pain (Jones, Othman, Dowswell, et al., 2012).

Before initiating hydrotherapy measures, agency policy should be consulted to determine if the approval of the laboring woman's primary health care provider is required and if criteria need to be met in terms of the status of the maternal and fetal unit (e.g., stable vital signs and fetal heart rate [FHR] and pattern, and stage of labor). To reduce the risk of a prolonged labor, hydrotherapy is usually initiated when the woman is in active labor, at approximately 5 cm. It is at this time that she may be getting discouraged and will welcome the change that hydrotherapy offers. Remember to preserve her modesty because she may be shy about the exposure of her body when getting into a tub or shower (Creehan, 2008).

In addition to pain relief and relaxation, hydrotherapy offers other benefits. If a woman is having "back labor" as the result of an occiput posterior or transverse position, assuming a hands-and-knees or a side-lying position in the tub enhances spontaneous fetal rotation to the occiput anterior position as a result of increased buoyancy. Because less effort is needed to change positions while in the water, women are encouraged to assume upright positions and to alter positions more frequently, facilitating the progress of their labors and helping them cope with labor-associated stressors (Stark, Rudell, and Haus, 2008).

When hydrotherapy is in use, FHR monitoring is done by Doppler, fetoscope, or wireless external monitor (see Fig. 14-6, *C*). Placement of internal electrodes is contraindicated for jet hydrotherapy. There is no limit to the time women can stay in the bath, and often they are encouraged to stay in it as long as desired. However, most women use jet hydrotherapy for 30 to 60 minutes at a time. During the bath, if the woman's temperature and the FHR increase, if the labor process becomes less effective (e.g., slows or becomes too intense), or if relief of pain is reduced, the woman can come out of the bath and return at a later time. Repeated baths with

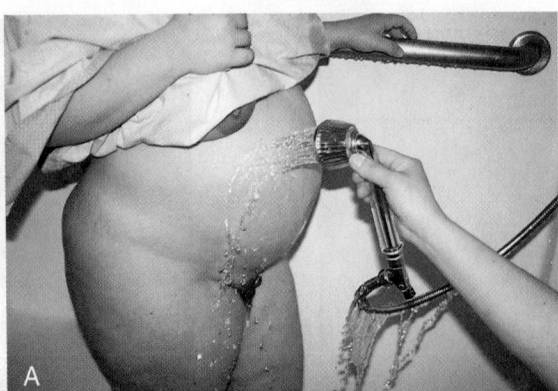
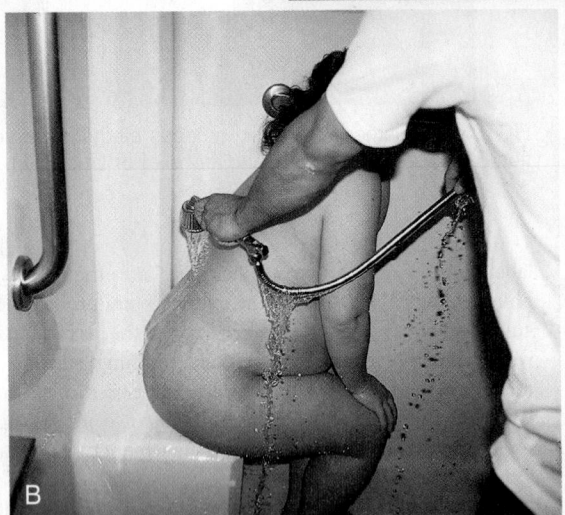
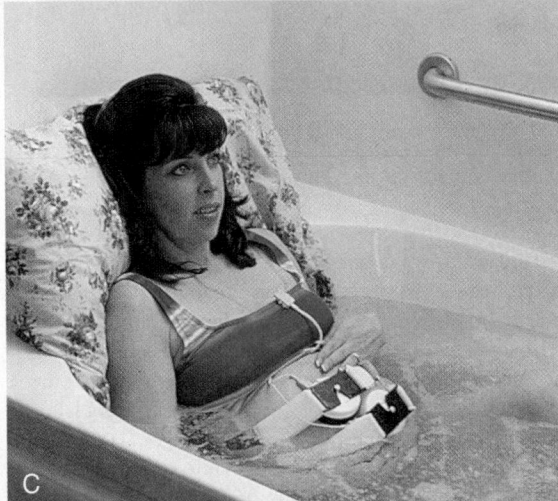

FIG 14-6 Water therapy during labor. **A,** Use of shower during labor. **B,** Woman experiencing back labor relaxes as partner sprays warm water on her back. **C,** Laboring woman relaxes in Jacuzzi. Note that fetal monitoring can continue during time in the Jacuzzi. (*A* and *B*, Courtesy Marjorie Pyle, RNC, Lifecircle, Costa Mesa, CA; *C*, courtesy Spacelabs Medical, Redmond, WA.)

occasional breaks may be more effective in relieving pain in long labors than extended amounts of time in the water. The temperature of the water should be maintained at 36° to 37°C (96.8° to 98.6°F) with the water covering the woman's abdomen to gain maximum effect from the hydrostatic pressure and buoyancy of the water. Her shoulders should remain out of the water to facilitate the dissipation of heat (Creehan, 2008).

The American Academy of Pediatrics Committee on Fetus and Newborn has expressed concerns about actual birthing in water because of the lack of research demonstrating its safety. There are rare but reported instances of asphyxia or infection that have occurred during or as a result of underwater birth. This group believes that underwater birth should be considered an experimental procedure, performed only after informed parental consent has been obtained (Hawkins and Bucklin, 2012).

Using a shower provides comfort through the application of heat as the handheld shower head is directed to areas of discomfort (see Fig. 14-6, *A* and *B*). The coach or partner can participate in this comfort measure by holding and directing the shower head.

⚡ SAFETY ALERT

Because warm water can cause dizziness, a shower stool should be used and the woman should be assisted when getting into and out of the tub.

Intradermal Water Block

An intradermal water block involves the injection of small amounts of sterile water (e.g., 0.05 to 0.1 mL) by using a fine-gauge needle (e.g., 25 gauge) into four locations on the lower back to relieve low back pain (Fig. 14-7). It is a simple procedure to perform, and there is evidence that it is effective, perhaps because of the gate-control mechanism (Hawkins and Bucklin, 2012). Other possible explanations for the effectiveness of the intradermal water block are the mechanism of counterirritation (i.e., reducing localized pain in one area by irritating the skin in an area nearby) or an increase in the level of endogenous opioids (endorphins) produced by the injections. Intense stinging will occur for about 20 to 30 seconds after injection, but relief of back pain for up to 2 hours has been reported. The procedure can be repeated although the woman may find that the stinging that occurs with administration creates too much discomfort (Creehan, 2008).

Aromatherapy

Aromatherapy uses oils distilled from plants, flowers, herbs, and trees to promote health and to treat and balance the mind, body, and spirit. These essential oils are highly concentrated, complex essences and are mixed with lotions or creams before they are applied to the skin (e.g., for a back massage). Certain essential oils can tone the uterus, encourage contractions, reduce pain, relieve tension, diminish fear and anxiety, and enhance the feeling of

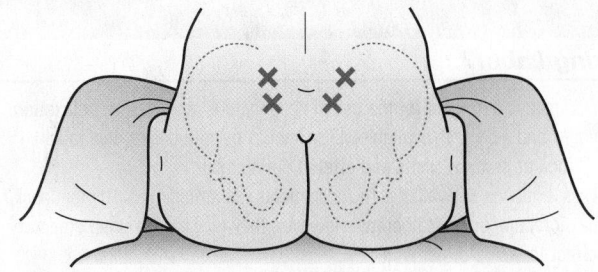

FIG 14-7 Intradermal injections of 0.1 mL of sterile water in the treatment of women with back pain during labor. Sterile water is injected into four locations on the lower back, two over each posterior superior iliac spine (PSIS) and two 3 cm below and 1 cm medial to the PSIS. The injections should raise a bleb on the skin. Simultaneous injections administered by two clinicians will decrease the pain of the injections. (From Leeman L, Fontaine P, King V, et al: The nature and management of labor pain: Part I. Nonpharmacologic pain relief, *Am Fam Physician* 68[6]:1109–1112, 2003.)

well-being. Lavender, rose, and jasmine oils can promote relaxation and reduce pain. Rose oil also acts as an antidepressant and uterine tonic, whereas jasmine oil strengthens contractions and decreases feelings of panic in addition to reducing pain. Essential oils of bergamot or rosemary can be diffused or used in a massage oil to relieve exhaustion (Gilbert, 2011; Tournaire and Theau-Yonneau, 2007; Walls, 2009). Oils may also be used by adding a few drops to a warm bath, to warm water used for soaking compresses that can be applied to the body, or to an aromatherapy lamp to vaporize a room. Drops of essential oils can be put on a pillow or on a woman's brow or palms or used as an ingredient in creating massage oil (Simkin and Bolding, 2004; Walls, 2009; Zwelling, Johnson, and Allen, 2006). Certain odors or scents can evoke pleasant memories and feelings of love and security. As a result, it would be helpful for a woman to choose the scents that she will use (Trout, 2004). There is insufficient evidence to support the effectiveness of aromatherapy for pain relief in labor although its use has elicited promising results (Jones, Othman, Dowswell, et al., 2012; Smith, Collins, Cyna, et al., 2006; Zwelling, Johnson, and Allen, 2006).

> ⚡ **SAFETY ALERT**
>
> Never apply the essential oils used for aromatherapy full strength directly to the skin. Most oils should be diluted in a vegetable oil base before use. Essential oils vary in terms of safe use during pregnancy. Inhaling vapors from the oils can lead to unpleasant side effects, including nausea or headaches.

Music

Music, recorded or live, can provide a distraction, enhance relaxation, and lift spirits during labor, thereby reducing the woman's level of stress, anxiety, and perception of pain. It can be used to promote relaxation in early labor and to stimulate movement as labor progresses. Music can help create a more relaxed atmosphere in the birth room, leading to a more relaxed approach by health care providers (Creehan, 2008; Zwelling, Johnson, and Allen, 2006). Women should be encouraged to prepare their musical preferences in advance and to bring a CD player or MP3 player (e.g., iPod) to the hospital or birthing center. They should choose familiar music that is associated with pleasant memories, which can also facilitate the process of guided imagery. Use of a headset or earphones may

increase the effectiveness of the music because other sounds will be shut out. Live music provided at the bedside by a support person may be very helpful in transmitting energy that decreases tension and elevates mood. Changing the tempo of the music to coincide with the rate and rhythm of each breathing technique may facilitate proper pacing. Evidence is insufficient to support the effectiveness of music as a method of pain relief during labor. Further research is recommended (Smith, Collins, Cyna, et al., 2006).

Hypnosis

Hypnosis is a form of deep relaxation, similar to daydreaming or meditation (see www.hypnobirthing.com). While under hypnosis, women are in a state of focused concentration and the subconscious mind can be more easily accessed. Women who attend certain childbirth preparation classes may be taught to perform self-hypnosis. Hypnosis techniques used for labor and birth place an emphasis on enhancing relaxation and diminishing fear, anxiety, and perception of pain. Women using this technique report a greater sense of control over painful contractions and a higher level of satisfaction with their childbirth experience. Because it reduces the need for pain medication, hypnosis can be helpful when used with other interventions during labor. A few negative effects of hypnosis have been reported, including mild dizziness, nausea, and headache. These negative effects seem to be associated with failure to dehypnotize the woman properly (Tournaire and Theau-Yonneau, 2007). Some current evidence suggests that hypnosis may be beneficial (Smith, Collins, Cyna, et al., 2006), although other studies have not found it to be more effective than the use of a placebo or other interventions for pain management during labor (Jones, Othman, Dowswell, et al., 2012).

Biofeedback

Biofeedback may provide another relaxation technique that can be used for labor. Biofeedback is based on the theory that if a person can recognize physical signals, certain internal physiologic events can be changed (i.e., whatever signs the woman has that are associated with her pain). For biofeedback to be effective, the woman must be educated during the prenatal period to become aware of her body and its responses and how to relax. The woman must learn how to use thinking and mental processes (e.g., focusing) to control body responses and functions. Informational biofeedback helps couples develop awareness of their bodies and use strategies to change their responses to stress. If the woman responds to pain during a contraction with tightening of muscles, frowning, moaning, and breath holding, her partner uses verbal and touch feedback to help her relax. Formal biofeedback, which uses machines to detect skin temperature, blood flow, or muscle tension, also can prepare women to intensify their relaxation responses. Using these techniques effectively requires the strong support of caregivers (Tournaire and Theau-Yonneau, 2007). Evidence is insufficient to show that biofeedback is more effective than use of a placebo or other interventions for pain management during labor (Jones, Othman, Dowswell, et al., 2012) (see Evidence-Based Practice box).

PHARMACOLOGIC PAIN MANAGEMENT

Pharmacologic measures for pain management should be implemented before pain becomes so severe that catecholamines increase and labor is prolonged. It is unacceptable for women in labor to endure severe pain when safe and effective relief measures are available (American College of Obstetricians and Gynecologists [ACOG],

EVIDENCE-BASED PRACTICE
What Nonpharmacologic Therapies Offer Pain Relief During Labor?

Ask the Question
Do women in labor have nonpharmacologic therapies that can provide safe and effective pain relief?

Search for the Evidence
Search Strategies
English research-based publications on pain, labor, nonpharmacologic pain relief, and complementary and alternative therapies were included.

Database Used
Cochrane Collaborative Database

Critically Analyze the Evidence
Many women seek alternative or complementary pain relief during labor to delay or avoid pharmacologic or invasive therapies. Evidence regarding their efficacy has been sparse, and so they have remained under-utilized. The Cochrane Database has recently published a series of systematic reviews of the evidence for several of the best-known therapies:

- Acupuncture is associated with less pain intensity, increased satisfaction of pain relief, decreased use of analgesia drugs, and fewer instrumental births than placebo control. Acupressure lessened pain intensity when compared with placebo control (Smith, Collins, Crowther, et al., 2011).
- Relaxation techniques such as meditation, visualization, and breathing decrease pain intensity and assisted birth and increase satisfaction in pain relief when compared with placebo. Yoga is associated with pain relief, increased satisfaction with pain relief and birth, and reduced length of labor (Smith, Levett, Collins, et al., 2011). Evidence for music and audio analgesia was insufficient to make recommendations.
- Massage was associated with less pain and anxiety than control during the first stage of labor (Smith, Levett, Collins, et al., 2012). Massage was more effective than music for decreasing pain. There were no reflexology studies.
- Water immersion during labor is associated with significantly decreased use of analgesia/anesthesia and shorter first-stage labor by a mean of 32 minutes (Cluett and Burns, 2009).
- Transcutaneous Electrical Nerve Stimulation (TENS), which sends an electrical impulse to the back, acupuncture sites, or the cranium, may block or compete with pain pathways and is typically controlled by the patient. In labor, women using TENS report less severe pain and would use it again for pain control (Dowswell, Bedwell, Lavender, et al., 2009). TENS had no effect on labor length, interventions, or maternal or infant well-being.
- Intracutaneous or subcutaneous sterile water, typically injected on four places on the back, creates stinging sensations that block or compete with pain pathways. Compared with normal saline controls, which do not sting, sterile water injections show a nonsignificant trend toward decreased pain but do not show any differences between groups on cesarean births, rescue analgesia, timing of birth, or Apgar scores. Women reported that they would use the method in a subsequent labor (Derry, Straube, Moore, et al., 2012).
- Biofeedback involves teaching patients to control certain body signals, which are read by a machine. Small studies using a myographic machine to measure muscle tension may show some pain relief in early labor (Loayza, Sola, and Prats, 2011).
- Aromatherapy compared with control showed no differences in groups. Evidence is insufficient to make recommendations (Smith, Collins, and Crowther, 2011).

Apply the Evidence: Nursing Implications
- Evidence is still insufficient or scanty regarding the use of various alternative or complementary therapies but suggests that they may help and they probably do not cause harm.
- Evidence is strongest for the use of acupuncture, acupressure, relaxation, yoga, and TENS. If available, they should be introduced and taught to women at prenatal visits and offered during labor.
- Less evidence is available to recommend saline injections, biofeedback, music/audio, or aromatherapy. However, they may have a complementary effect for some patients.
- Nonpharmacologic methods of pain relief may be most effective in latent or early active labor. Women's needs must be continually reevaluated, and women should know what pharmacologic choices are available. Nurses should advocate for appropriate pain relief choices during labor.

Quality and Safety Competencies:
Evidence-Based Practice*
Knowledge
Differentiate clinical opinion from research and evidence summaries.
Nurses advocate for women to have many options in pain management beyond conventional pharmacologic measures.

Skills
Question rationale for routine approaches to care that result in less-than-desired outcomes or adverse events.
Women can learn the basics for yoga, relaxation, and/or biofeedback in prenatal classes.

Attitudes
Acknowledge own limitations in knowledge and clinical expertise before determining when to deviate from evidence-based best practices.
Biases against complementary therapies may be rooted in unfamiliarity with the evidence.

References
Cluett ER, Burns E: Immersion in water in labour and birth, *Cochrane Database Syst Rev* (Issue 2), 2009, Chichester, UK, John Wiley & Sons, DOI: 10.1002/14651858.CD000111.pub3.

Derry S, Straube S, Moore RA, et al: Intracutaneous or subcutaneous sterile water injections compared with blinded controls for pain management in labour, *Cochrane Database Syst Rev* (Issue 1), 2012, Chichester, UK, John Wiley & Sons, DOI: 10.1002/14651858.CD009107.pub2.

Dowswell T, Bedwell C, Lavender T, et al: Transcutaneous electrical nerve stimulation (TENS) for pain management in labour, *Cochrane Database Syst Rev* (Issue 2), 2009, Chichester, UK, John Wiley & Sons, DOI: 10.1002/14651858.CD007214.pub2.

Loayza IMB, Sola I, Prats CJ: Biofeedback for pain management during labour, *Cochrane Database Syst Rev* (Issue 6), 2011, Chichester, UK, John Wiley & Sons, DOI: 10.1002/14651858.CD006168.pub2.

Smith CA, Collins CT, Crowther CA: Aromatherapy for pain management in labour, *Cochrane Database Syst Rev* (Issue 7), 2011, Chichester, UK, John Wiley & Sons, DOI: 10.1002/14651858.CD009215.

Smith CA, Collins CT, Crowther CA, et al: Acupuncture or acupressure for pain management in labour, *Cochrane Database Syst Rev* (Issue 7), 2011, Chichester, UK, John Wiley & Sons, DOI: 10.1002/14651858.CD009232.

Smith CA, Levett KM, Collins CT, et al: Relaxation techniques for pain management in labour, *Cochrane Database Syst Rev* (Issue 12), 2011, Chichester, UK, John Wiley & Sons. DOI: 10.1002/14651858.CD009514.

Smith CA, Levett KM, Collins CT, et al: Massage, reflexology and other manual methods of pain management during labour, *Cochrane Database Syst Rev* (Issue 2), 2012, Chichester, UK, John Wiley & Sons, DOI: 10.1002/14651858.CD009290.pub2.

Pat Mahaffee Gingrich

*Adapted from QSEN at www.qsen.org/.

2008). Pharmacologic and nonpharmacologic measures, when used together, increase the level of pain relief and create a more positive labor experience for the woman and her family. Nonpharmacologic measures can be used for relaxation and pain relief, especially in early labor. Pharmacologic measures can be implemented as labor becomes more active and discomfort and pain intensify. Less pharmacologic intervention often is required because nonpharmacologic measures enhance relaxation and potentiate the analgesic effect. However, women are increasingly using pharmacologic measures, especially epidural analgesia, to relieve their pain during labor and birth.

Sedatives

Sedatives relieve anxiety and induce sleep. They may be given to a woman experiencing a prolonged latent phase of labor when there is a need to decrease anxiety or promote sleep. They may also be given to augment analgesics and reduce nausea when an opioid is used.

Barbiturates such as secobarbital sodium (Seconal) can cause undesirable side effects including respiratory and vasomotor depression affecting the woman and newborn. Because of the potential for neonatal central nervous system (CNS) depression, barbiturates should be avoided if birth is anticipated within 12 to 24 hours. The depressant effects are increased if a barbiturate is administered with another CNS depressant such as an opioid analgesic. However, pain will be magnified if a barbiturate is given without an analgesic to women experiencing pain because normal coping mechanisms may be blunted. As a result of these disadvantages, barbiturates are seldom used during labor (Creehan, 2008).

Phenothiazines (e.g., promethazine [Phenergan]) do not relieve pain. In the past, promethazine was often given with opioids to enhance the analgesic effects of opioids, as well as to decrease anxiety and apprehension, increase sedation, and reduce nausea and vomiting. However, research has shown that promethazine actually impairs the analgesic efficacy of opioids. Metoclopramide (Reglan), an antiemetic, has been found to effectively potentiate the effects of analgesics. Therefore its use is recommended, rather than promethazine (Hawkins and Bucklin, 2012).

Benzodiazepines (e.g., diazepam [Valium], lorazepam [Ativan]), when given with an opioid analgesic, seem to enhance pain relief and reduce nausea and vomiting. A major side effect of the benzodiazepines is significant maternal amnesia. A major disadvantage of diazepam is that it disrupts thermoregulation in newborns, making them less able to maintain body temperature. Flumazenil (Romazicon) is a specific benzodiazepine antagonist, which can effectively reverse benzodiazepine-induced sedation and respiratory depression (Hawkins and Bucklin, 2012).

Analgesia and Anesthesia

The use of analgesia and anesthesia was not generally accepted as part of obstetric management until Queen Victoria used chloroform during the birth of her son in 1853. Since then, much study has gone into the development of pharmacologic measures for controlling discomfort during the birth period. The goal of researchers is to develop methods that will provide adequate pain relief to women without increasing maternal or fetal risk or affecting the progress of labor.

Nursing management of obstetric analgesia and anesthesia combines the nurse's expertise in maternity care with a knowledge and understanding of anatomy and physiology and of medications and their therapeutic effects, adverse reactions, and methods of administration.

BOX 14-4 PHARMACOLOGIC CONTROL OF DISCOMFORT BY STAGE OF LABOR AND METHOD OF BIRTH

First Stage
- Opioid agonist analgesics
- Opioid agonist-antagonist analgesics
- Epidural (block) analgesia
- Combined spinal-epidural (CSE) analgesia
- Nitrous oxide

Second Stage
- Nerve block analgesia and anesthesia
  - Local infiltration anesthesia
  - Pudendal block
  - Spinal (block) anesthesia
  - Epidural (block) analgesia
  - CSE analgesia
- Nitrous oxide

Vaginal Birth
- Local infiltration anesthesia
- Pudendal block
- Epidural (block) analgesia and anesthesia
- Spinal (block) anesthesia
- CSE analgesia and anesthesia
- Nitrous oxide

Cesarean Birth
- Spinal (block) anesthesia
- Epidural (block) anesthesia
- General anesthesia

Anesthesia encompasses analgesia, amnesia, relaxation, and reflex activity. Anesthesia abolishes pain perception by interrupting the nerve impulses to the brain. The loss of sensation may be partial or complete, sometimes with the loss of consciousness.

The term **analgesia** refers to the alleviation of the sensation of pain or the raising of the threshold for pain perception without loss of consciousness.

The type of analgesic or anesthetic chosen is determined in part by the stage of labor of the woman and by the method of birth planned (Box 14-4).

Systemic Analgesia

Systemic analgesics (opioids) can be administered in intermittent doses intravenously (IV) or intramuscularly (IM) by health care providers or by the patient herself using patient controlled analgesia (PCA). With PCA, the woman self-administers small doses of an opioid analgesic by using a pump programmed for dose and frequency. Overall, a lower total amount of analgesic is used. Women appreciate the sense of autonomy provided by this method of pain relief, as well as the elimination of treatment delays while the patient's nurse obtains and administers the medication (Hawkins and Bucklin, 2012).

Opioids provide sedation and euphoria, but their analgesic effect in labor is limited. The pain relief they provide is incomplete, temporary, and more effective in the early part of active labor (Anderson, 2011). All opioids cause side effects, the most serious of which is respiratory depression. Other undesirable opioid side effects include sedation, nausea and vomiting, dizziness, altered mental status, euphoria, decreased gastric motility, delayed gastric emptying, and urinary retention (Anderson, 2011). Prolonged gastric emptying time increases the risk for aspiration if general anesthesia becomes necessary in a woman who has received opioids (Hawkins and Bucklin, 2012). Bladder and bowel elimination can be inhibited. Because heart rate (e.g., bradycardia, tachycardia), blood pressure (e.g., hypotension), and respiratory effort (e.g., depression) can be adversely affected, opioid analgesics should be used cautiously in women with respiratory and cardiovascular disorders. Safety precautions should be taken after opioid administration, because several opioid side effects increase the risk for injury.

Opioids readily cross the placenta. Effects on the fetus and newborn can be profound, including absent or minimal FHR variability during labor and significant neonatal respiratory depression requiring treatment after birth (Hawkins and Bucklin, 2012).

⚡ SAFETY ALERT

Opioids decrease maternal heart and respiratory rate and blood pressure, which affects fetal oxygenation. Therefore maternal vital signs and FHR and pattern must be assessed and documented before and after administration of opioids for pain relief.

Classifications of analgesic drugs used to relieve the pain of childbirth include opioid (narcotic) agonists and opioid (narcotic) agonist-antagonists. Choice of which medication to use often depends on the primary health care provider's preferences and the characteristics of the laboring woman. The type of systemic analgesics used therefore often varies among obstetric units (see Critical Thinking Case Study on p. 361).

Opioid Agonist Analgesics. Opioid (narcotic) agonist analgesics commonly used in obstetrics are meperidine (Demerol) and fentanyl (Sublimaze) (Hawkins and Bucklin, 2012). As pure opioid agonists, they stimulate major opioid receptors, mu and kappa. They have no amnesic effect but create a feeling of well-being or euphoria and enhance a woman's ability to rest between contractions. Because opioids can inhibit uterine contractions, they should not be administered until labor is well established unless they are being used to enhance therapeutic rest during a prolonged latent phase of labor (Creehan, 2008).

Meperidine hydrochloride (Demerol) is a synthetic opioid that is the most widely used systemic medication for labor pain. Demerol's widespread use is probably related to its low cost, the fact that care providers are quite familiar with the drug, and studies that were done many years ago that found that meperidine caused less respiratory depression than morphine (see Medication Guide: Meperidine Hydrochloride [Demerol]). However, its use during labor is becoming more controversial because of undesirable side effects, particularly in the neonate (Anderson, 2011). Both meperidine and normeperidine, an active metabolite of meperidine, cross the placenta and cause prolonged neonatal sedation and neurobehavioral changes. These metabolite-related effects cannot be reversed with naloxone (Anderson, 2011). Because meperidine and normeperidine have long half-lives, the neonatal effects can persist for the first 2 to 3 days of life (Hawkins and Bucklin, 2012).

Fentanyl citrate (Sublimaze) is a potent short-acting opioid agonist analgesic (see Medication Guide: Fentanyl Citrate [Sublimaze]). It rapidly crosses the placenta so is present in fetal blood within 1 minute after intravenous maternal administration (Anderson, 2011). As compared with meperidine, fentanyl provides equivalent analgesia with fewer neonatal effects and less maternal sedation and nausea. Fentanyl is used as a labor analgesic because of its rapid onset of action, short half-life, and lack of a metabolite (Anderson, 2011). A disadvantage of fentanyl is that more frequent dosing is required because of its relatively short duration of action (Hawkins and Bucklin, 2012). As a result, this medication is most commonly administered by PCA pump or intrathecally or epidurally, alone or in combination with a local anesthetic agent.

Opioid (Narcotic) Agonist-Antagonist Analgesics. An agonist is an agent that activates or stimulates a receptor to act; an

💊 MEDICATION GUIDE

Meperidine Hydrochloride (Demerol)

Classification
Opioid Agonist Analgesic

Action
Synthetic opioid agonist analgesic that stimulates both mu and kappa opioid receptors to decrease the transmission of pain impulses. Meperidine 100 mg is roughly equivalent in analgesic effect to morphine 10 mg, but it is reported to cause less maternal respiratory depression. Intravenously, the onset of action begins in 5 minutes and the duration of action is 2 to 4 hours.

Indication
Moderate to severe labor pain and postoperative pain after cesarean birth

Dosage and Route
IV: 25 to 50 mg every 1 to 2 hours
PCA Pump: 15 mg every 10 minutes as needed until delivery

Adverse Effects
Tachycardia, sedation, nausea and vomiting, dizziness, altered mental status, euphoria, decreased gastric motility, delayed gastric emptying, and urinary retention

Nursing Considerations
Implement safety measures as appropriate, including use of siderails and assistance with ambulation; continue use of nonpharmacologic pain relief measures. Do not give if birth is expected to occur within 1 to 4 hours after administration, because infants born to women who received meperidine during labor may have respiratory depression, peaking at 2 to 3 hours after administration of the drug. Respiratory depression caused by normeperidine, an active metabolite of meperidine, cannot be reversed by naloxone. Both meperidine and normeperidine have long half-lives. Therefore neonates whose mothers received meperidine during labor can exhibit sedation and neurobehavioral changes for the first 2 to 3 days of life.

Sources: Anderson D: A review of systemic opioids commonly used for labor pain relief, *J Midwifery Womens Health* 56(3):222–239, 2011; Hawkins J, Bucklin B: Obstetrical anesthesia. In Gabbe S, Niebyl J, Simpson J, et al, editors: *Obstetrics: normal and problem pregnancies*, ed 6, Philadelphia, 2012, Saunders.

antagonist is an agent that blocks a receptor or a medication designed to activate a receptor. Butorphanol (Stadol) and Nalbuphine (Nubain) are commonly used opioid (narcotic) agonist-antagonist analgesics (Hawkins and Bucklin, 2012). These medications are agonists at kappa opioid receptors and either antagonists or weak agonists at mu opioid receptors. In the doses used during labor, these mixed opioids provide adequate analgesia without causing significant respiratory depression in the mother or neonate. Their major advantage is their ceiling effect for respiratory depression; higher doses do not produce additional respiratory depression. They are less likely to cause nausea and vomiting, but sedation may be as great or greater when compared with pure opioid agonists (Anderson, 2011; Hawkins and Bucklin, 2012). As a result of these effects, parenteral opioid agonist-antagonist analgesics are used more commonly during labor than the opioid agonist analgesics. Intramuscular, subcutaneous, and intravenous routes of administration can be used, but the IV route is preferred. This classification of opioid analgesics, especially nalbuphine, is not

MEDICATION GUIDE

Fentanyl Citrate (Sublimaze)

Classification
Opioid Agonist Analgesic

Action
Opioid agonist analgesic that stimulates both mu and kappa opioid receptors to decrease the transmission of pain impulses. Has a rapid onset of action with a short duration (0.5 to 1 hour IV; 1 to 2 hours IM).

Indication
Moderate to severe labor pain and postoperative pain after cesarean birth

Dosage and Route
IV: 50 to 100 mcg every hour
IM: 50 to 100 mcg every hour

Adverse Effects
Sedation, respiratory depression, nausea, and vomiting

Nursing Considerations
Assess for respiratory depression; naloxone should be available as an antidote. Implement safety measures as appropriate, including use of siderails and assistance with ambulation; continue use of nonpharmacologic pain relief measures. Because of its short duration of action, frequent dosing will be necessary when given intravenously. Maximum total dose for labor is usually 500 to 600 mcg.

Source: Anderson D: A review of systemic opioids commonly used for labor pain relief, *J Midwifery Womens Health* 56(3):222–239, 2011.

BOX 14-5 SIGNS OF POTENTIAL COMPLICATIONS: MATERNAL OPIOID ABSTINENCE SYNDROME (OPIOID/NARCOTIC WITHDRAWAL)

- Yawning, rhinorrhea (runny nose), sweating, lacrimation (tearing), mydriasis (dilation of pupils)
- Anorexia
- Irritability, restlessness, generalized anxiety
- Tremors
- Chills and hot flashes
- Piloerection ("gooseflesh" or "chill bumps")
- Violent sneezing
- Weakness, fatigue, and drowsiness
- Nausea and vomiting
- Diarrhea, abdominal cramps
- Bone and muscle pain, muscle spasms, kicking movements

MEDICATION GUIDE

Butorphanol Tartrate (Stadol)

Classification
Opioid Agonist-Antagonist Analgesic

Action
Mixed agonist-antagonist analgesic that stimulates kappa opioid receptors and blocks or weakly stimulates mu opioid receptors, resulting in good analgesia but with less respiratory depression and nausea and vomiting when compared with opioid agonist analgesics. Butorphanol produces a maternal ceiling effect on pain relief and respiratory depression. IV administration of 2 mg of butorphanol produces respiratory depression similar to that of 10 mg of morphine IV or 70 mg of meperidine IV, but 4 mg of butorphanol will produce less respiratory depression than 20 mg of morphine or 140 mg of meperidine. Whether given intravenously or intramuscularly, the drug's duration of action is 4 to 6 hours.

Indication
Moderate to severe labor pain and postoperative pain after cesarean birth

Usual Dosage and Route
IV: 1 to 2 mg every 3 to 4 hours as needed
IM: 1 to 2 mg every 3 to 4 hours as needed

Adverse Effects
Confusion, sedation, hallucinations, "floating" feeling, drowsiness, transient nonpathologic sinusoidal-like fetal heart rate pattern, respiratory depression, nausea and vomiting

Nursing Considerations
May precipitate withdrawal symptoms in opioid-dependent women and their newborns. Assess maternal vital signs, degree of pain, fetal heart rate (FHR), and uterine activity before and after administration. Observe for maternal respiratory depression, notifying primary health care provider if maternal respirations are ≤12 breaths/min. Encourage voiding every 2 hours, and palpate for bladder distention. If birth occurs within 1 to 4 hours of dose administration, observe newborn for respiratory depression. Implement safety measures as appropriate, including use of siderails and assistance with ambulation. Continue use of nonpharmacologic pain relief measures.

Source: Anderson D: A review of systemic opioids commonly used for labor pain relief, *J Midwifery Womens Health* 56(3):222–239, 2011.

newborn, or both, although the current practice of giving lower doses of opioids intravenously has reduced the incidence and severity of opioid-induced CNS depression. Opioid (narcotic) antagonists such as naloxone (Narcan) can promptly reverse the CNS depressant effects, especially respiratory depression, in most situations. As stated earlier, however, naloxone cannot reverse the effects of normeperidine, an active metabolite of meperidine. In addition, the antagonist counters the effect of the stress-induced levels of endorphins. An opioid antagonist is especially valuable if labor is more rapid than expected and birth occurs when the opioid is at its peak effect. The antagonist may be given intravenously, or it can be administered intramuscularly (see Medication Guide: Naloxone Hydrochloride [Narcan]). The woman should be told that the pain that was relieved with the use of the opioid analgesic will return with the administration of the opioid antagonist.

suitable for women with an opioid dependence, because the antagonist activity could precipitate withdrawal symptoms (abstinence syndrome) in both the mother and her newborn (Hawkins and Bucklin, 2012) (see Medication Guide: Butorphanol Tartrate [Stadol], Medication Guide: Nalbuphine Hydrochloride [Nubain], and Box 14-5).

Opioid (Narcotic) Antagonists. Opioids such as meperidine and fentanyl can cause excessive CNS depression in the mother, the

MEDICATION GUIDE

Nalbuphine Hydrochloride (Nubain)

Classification
Opioid Agonist-Antagonist Analgesic

Action
Mixed agonist-antagonist analgesic that stimulates kappa opioid receptors and blocks or weakly stimulates mu opioid receptors, resulting in good analgesia but with less respiratory depression and nausea and vomiting when compared with opioid agonist analgesics. Nalbuphine's analgesic effect is equivalent to morphine, on a milligram to milligram basis. Produces a maternal ceiling effect on pain relief and respiratory depression after 30 mg of the drug has been administered. Duration of action is 2 to 4 hours when given intravenously and 4 to 6 hours when given intramuscularly.

Indication
Moderate to severe labor pain and postoperative pain after cesarean birth

Dosage and Route
IV: 10 mg every 3 hours as needed
IM: 10 mg every 3 hours as needed

Adverse Effects
Sedation, drowsiness, nausea, vomiting, dizziness, respiratory depression, temporary absent or minimal fetal heart rate variability

Nursing Considerations
May precipitate withdrawal symptoms in opioid-dependent women and their newborns. Assess maternal vital signs, degree of pain, fetal heart rate (FHR), and uterine activity before and after administration. Observe for maternal respiratory depression, notifying primary health care provider if maternal respirations are ≤12 breaths/min. Encourage voiding every 2 hours, and palpate for bladder distention. If birth occurs within 1 to 4 hours of dose administration, observe newborn for respiratory depression. Implement safety measures as appropriate, including use of siderails and assistance with ambulation. Continue use of nonpharmacologic pain relief measures.

Source: Anderson D: A review of systemic opioids commonly used for labor pain relief, *J Midwifery Womens Health* 56(3):222–239, 2011.

MEDICATION ALERT

An opioid antagonist (e.g., naloxone [Narcan]) is contraindicated for opioid-dependent women because it may precipitate abstinence syndrome (withdrawal symptoms). For the same reason, opioid agonist-antagonist analgesics such as butorphanol (Stadol) and nalbuphine (Nubain) should not be given to opioid-dependent women (see Box 14-5 and the Critical Thinking Case Study on p. 361).

Nerve Block Analgesia and Anesthesia

A variety of local anesthetic agents are used in obstetrics to produce regional analgesia (some pain relief and motor block) and regional anesthesia (complete pain relief and motor block). Most of these agents are related chemically to cocaine and end with the suffix *-caine*. This helps identify a local anesthetic.

The principal pharmacologic effect of local anesthetics is the temporary interruption of the conduction of nerve impulses, notably pain. Examples of common agents given are bupivacaine

MEDICATION GUIDE

Naloxone Hydrochloride (Narcan)

Classification
Opioid Antagonist

Action
Blocks both mu and kappa opioid receptors from the effects of opioid agonists

Indication
Reverses opioid-induced respiratory depression in woman or newborn; may be used to reverse pruritus from epidural opioids

Dosage and Route
Adult
Opioid overdose: 0.4 to 2 mg IV, may repeat IV at 2- to 3-min intervals until a maximum of 10 mg has been given; if IV route unavailable, IM or subcutaneous administration may be used.

Newborn
Opioid-induced depression: Initial dose is 0.1 mg/kg; preferred route is IV but may be administered IM.

Adverse Effects
Maternal hypotension or hypertension, tachycardia, hyperventilation, nausea and vomiting, sweating, and tremulousness

Nursing Considerations
Woman should delay breastfeeding until medication is out of her system. Do not give to woman or the newborn if the woman is opioid dependent—may cause abrupt withdrawal in the woman and newborn. If given to woman for reversal of respiratory depression caused by opioid analgesic, pain will return suddenly. The duration of action of naloxone is shorter than that of most opioids. Therefore the patient must be monitored closely for the return of opioid depression when the effects of naloxone are gone. Additional doses of naloxone may be necessary to maintain reversal.

(Marcaine), chloroprocaine (Nesacaine), and lidocaine (Xylocaine). Rarely, people are sensitive (allergic) to one or more local anesthetics. Such a reaction may include respiratory depression, hypotension, and other serious adverse effects. Epinephrine, antihistamines, oxygen, and supportive measures should reverse these effects. Sensitivity may be identified by administering tiny amounts of the drug to test for an allergic reaction.

Local Perineal Infiltration Anesthesia. Local perineal infiltration anesthesia may be used when an episiotomy is to be performed or when lacerations must be sutured after birth in a woman who does not have regional anesthesia. Rapid anesthesia is produced by injecting approximately 5 to 15 mL of 1% lidocaine into the skin and then subcutaneously into the region to be anesthetized. Epinephrine often is added to the solution to localize and intensify the effect of the anesthesia in a region and to prevent excessive bleeding and systemic absorption by constricting local blood vessels. Injections can be repeated to keep the woman comfortable while postbirth repairs are completed.

Pudendal Nerve Block. Pudendal nerve block, administered late in the second stage of labor, is useful if an episiotomy is to be performed or if forceps or a vacuum extractor is to be used to facilitate birth. It can also be administered during the third stage of labor if an episiotomy or lacerations must be repaired (American Academy

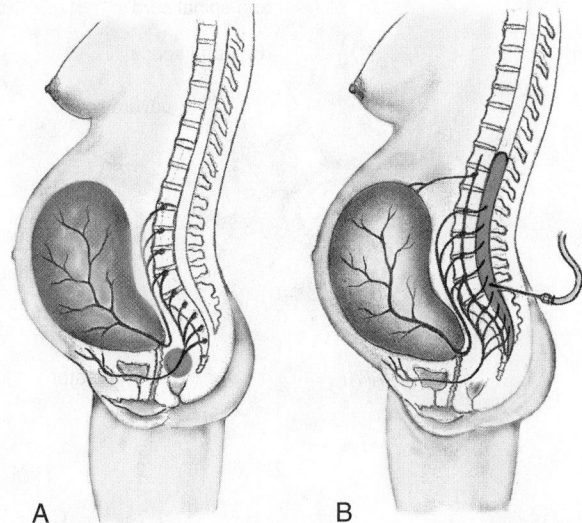

FIG 14-8 Pain pathways and sites of pharmacologic nerve blocks. **A,** Pudendal nerve block: suitable during second and third stages of labor and for repair of episiotomy or lacerations. **B,** Epidural block: suitable for all stages of labor and types of birth and for repair of episiotomy and lacerations.

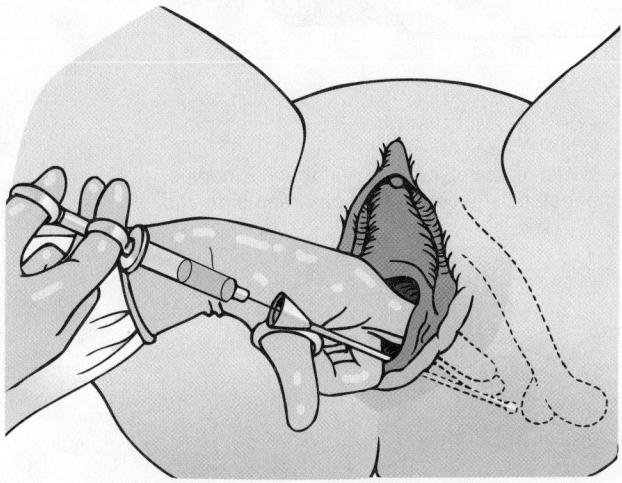

FIG 14-9 Pudendal nerve block. Use of needle guide (Iowa trumpet) and Luer-Lok syringe to inject medication.

of Pediatrics [AAP] and American College of Obstetricians and Gynecologists [ACOG], 2012). A pudendal nerve block is considered to be reasonably effective for pain relief, simple to perform, and very safe (Cunningham, Leveno, Bloom, et al., 2010; Hawkins and Bucklin, 2012). Although a pudendal nerve block does not relieve the pain from uterine contractions, it does relieve pain in the lower vagina, the vulva, and the perineum (Fig. 14-8, *A*). A pudendal nerve block should be administered 10 to 20 minutes before perineal anesthesia is needed.

The pudendal nerve traverses the sacrosciatic notch just medial to the tip of the ischial spine on each side. Injection of an anesthetic solution at or near these points anesthetizes the pudendal nerves peripherally (Fig. 14-9). The transvaginal approach is generally used because it is less painful for the woman, has a higher rate of success in blocking pain, and tends to cause fewer fetal complications. Pudendal block does not change maternal hemodynamic or

respiratory functions, vital signs, or the FHR. However, the bearing-down reflex is lessened or lost completely.

Spinal Anesthesia. In spinal anesthesia (block), an anesthetic solution containing a local anesthetic alone or in combination with an opioid agonist analgesic is injected through the third, fourth, or fifth lumbar interspace into the subarachnoid space (Fig. 14-10, *A* and *B*), where the anesthetic solution mixes with cerebrospinal fluid (CSF). Low spinal anesthesia (block) may be used for vaginal birth, but it is not suitable for labor. Spinal anesthesia (block) used for cesarean birth provides anesthesia from the nipple (T6) to the feet. If it is used for vaginal birth, the anesthesia level is from the hips (T10) to the feet (see Fig. 14-10, *C*).

For spinal anesthesia (block), the woman sits or lies on her side (e.g., modified Sims' position) with back curved to widen the intervertebral space; this position facilitates insertion of a small-gauge spinal needle and injection of the anesthetic solution into the spinal canal. The nurse supports the woman and encourages her to use breathing and relaxation techniques because she must remain still during the placement of the spinal needle. The needle is inserted and the anesthetic injected between contractions. After the anesthetic solution has been injected, the woman may be positioned upright to allow the heavier (hyperbaric) anesthetic solution to flow downward to obtain the lower level of anesthesia suitable for a vaginal birth. To obtain the higher level of anesthesia desired for cesarean birth, she will be positioned supine with head and shoulders slightly elevated. To prevent supine hypotensive syndrome, the uterus is displaced laterally by tilting the operating table or placing a wedge under one of her hips. Usually the level of the block will be complete and fixed within 5 to 10 minutes after the anesthetic solution is injected, but it can continue to creep upward for 20 minutes or longer (Hawkins and Bucklin, 2012). The anesthetic effect will last 1 to 3 hours, depending on the type and amount of agent used (Fig. 14-11).

> ⚡ **SAFETY ALERT**
>
> To reduce the risk for transmission of pathogens, it is recommended that (1) the patient's back is cleansed before the procedure and (2) during the induction of spinal and epidural anesthesia/analgesia, the anesthesia care provider removes jewelry, washes hands, and wears sterile gloves and a facemask.

Marked hypotension, impaired placental perfusion, and an ineffective breathing pattern may occur during spinal anesthesia. Before induction of the spinal anesthetic, maternal vital signs are assessed and a 20- to 30-minute electronic fetal monitoring (EFM) strip is obtained and evaluated. In addition, the woman's fluid balance is assessed. A bolus of IV fluid (usually 500 to 1000 mL of lactated Ringer's or normal saline solution) may be administered 15 to 30 minutes before induction of the anesthetic to decrease the potential for hypotension caused by sympathetic blockade (vasodilation with pooling of blood in the lower extremities decreases cardiac output). Although the practice guidelines for obstetric anesthesia published by the American Society of Anesthesiologists (2007) state that this preanesthetic fluid bolus is not required, it is still usually administered in most clinical settings. Fluid that is used for the bolus should not contain dextrose, which could contribute to neonatal hypoglycemia (Hawkins and Bucklin, 2012).

After induction of the anesthetic, maternal blood pressure, pulse, and respirations and fetal heart rate and pattern must be checked and documented every 5 to 10 minutes. If signs of serious maternal hypotension (e.g., the systolic blood pressure drops to 100 mm Hg

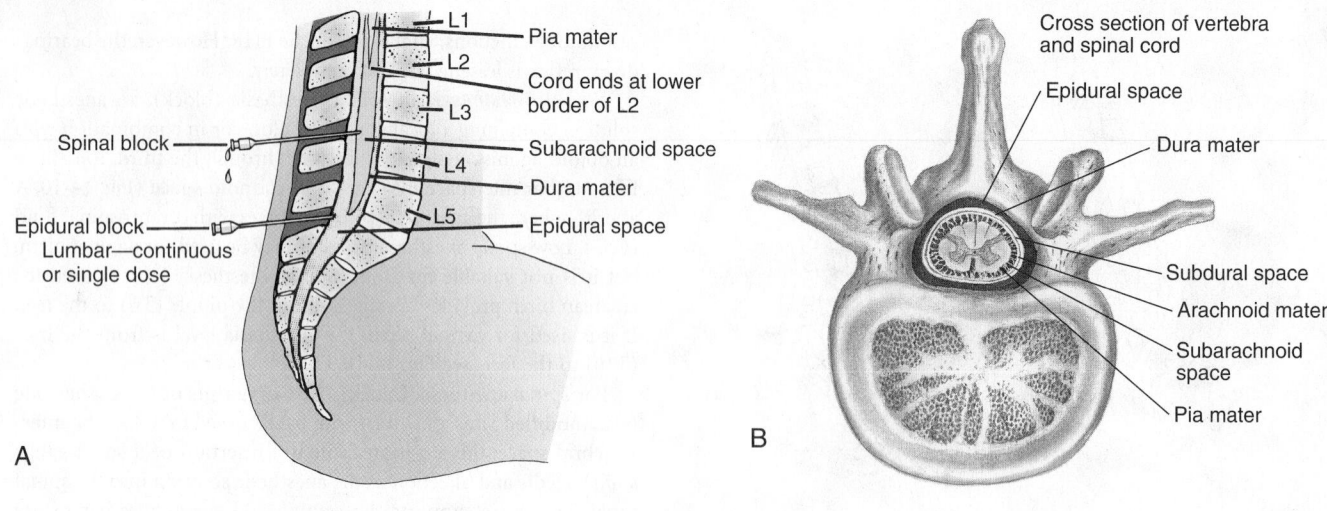

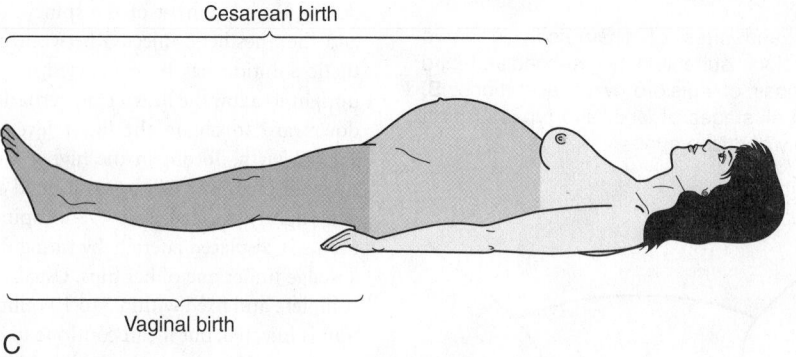

FIG 14-10 A, Membranes and spaces of spinal cord and levels of sacral, lumbar, and thoracic nerves. **B,** Cross section of vertebra and spinal cord. **C,** Level of anesthesia necessary for cesarean birth and for vaginal birth.

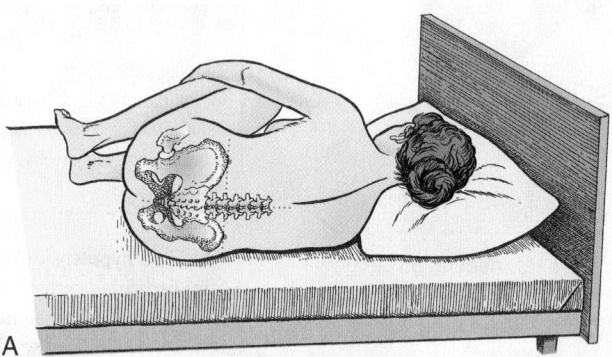

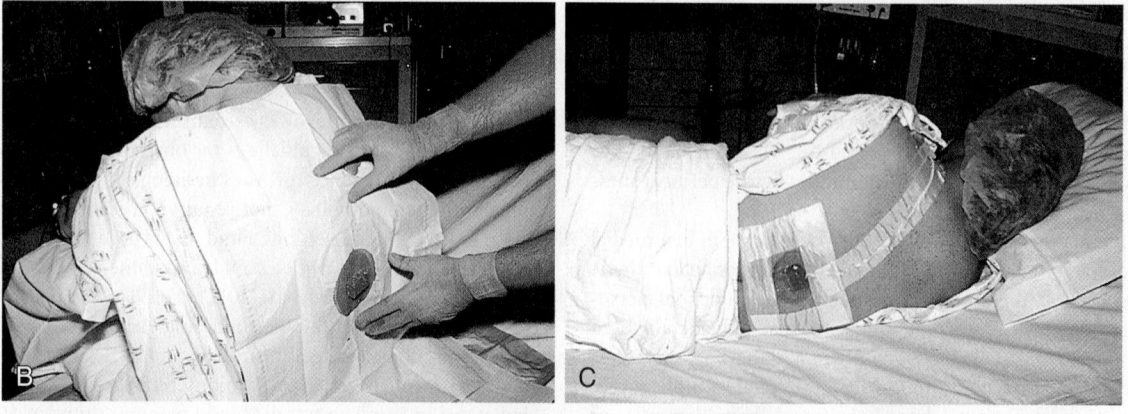

FIG 14-11 Positioning for spinal and epidural blocks. **A,** Lateral position. **B,** Upright position. **C,** Catheter for epidural is taped to woman's back with port segment located near her shoulder. (*B* and *C,* Courtesy Michael S. Clement, MD, Mesa, AZ.)

Maternal Hypotension with Decreased Placental Perfusion

Signs and Symptoms
- Maternal hypotension (20% decrease from preblock baseline level or ≤100 mm Hg systolic)
- Fetal bradycardia
- Absent or minimal fetal heart rate (FHR) variability
- Interventions
  - Turn woman to lateral position or place pillow or wedge under hip to displace uterus.
  - Maintain intravenous (IV) infusion at rate specified, or increase administration per hospital protocol.
  - Administer oxygen by nonrebreather facemask at 10 to 12 L/min or per protocol.
  - Elevate the woman's legs.
  - Notify the primary health care provider, anesthesiologist, or nurse anesthetist.
  - Administer IV vasopressor (e.g., ephedrine 5 to 10 mg or phenylephrine 50 to 100 mcg) per protocol if previous measures are ineffective.
  - Remain with woman; continue to monitor maternal blood pressure and FHR every 5 minutes until her condition is stable or per primary health care provider's order.

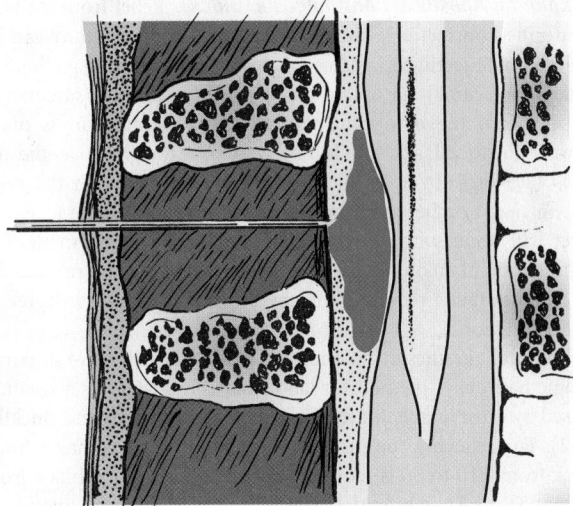

FIG 14-12 Blood-patch therapy for spinal headache.

or less or the blood pressure falls 20% or more below the baseline) or fetal distress (e.g., bradycardia, minimal or absent variability, late decelerations) develop, emergency care must be given (Creehan, 2008) (see Emergency box).

Because the woman is unable to sense her contractions, she must be instructed when to bear down during a vaginal birth. Using a combination of a local anesthetic agent and an opioid reduces the degree of motor function loss, enhancing a woman's ability to push effectively. If the birth occurs in a delivery room (rather than a labor-delivery-recovery room), the woman will need assistance in the transfer to a recovery bed after expulsion of the placenta and perineal repair if required.

Advantages of spinal anesthesia include ease of administration and absence of fetal hypoxia with maintenance of maternal blood pressure within a normal range. Maternal consciousness is maintained, excellent muscular relaxation is achieved, and blood loss is not excessive.

Disadvantages of spinal anesthesia include possible medication reactions (e.g., allergy), hypotension, and an ineffective breathing pattern; cardiopulmonary resuscitation may be needed. When a spinal anesthetic is given, the need for operative birth (e.g., episiotomy, forceps-assisted birth, or vacuum-assisted birth) tends to increase because voluntary expulsive efforts are reduced or eliminated. After birth, the incidence of bladder and uterine atony, as well as postdural puncture headache, is higher.

Leakage of CSF from the site of puncture of the dura mater (membranous covering of the spinal cord) is thought to be the major causative factor in *postdural puncture headache* (PDPH), commonly referred to as a *spinal headache*. Spinal headache is much more likely to occur when the dura is accidentally punctured during the process of administering an epidural block. The needle used for an epidural block has a much larger gauge than the one used for spinal anesthesia and thus creates a bigger opening in the dura, resulting in a greater loss of CSF (i.e., "wet tap"). Presumably,

postural changes cause the diminished volume of CSF to exert traction on pain-sensitive CNS structures. Characteristically, assuming an upright position triggers or intensifies the headache whereas assuming a supine position achieves relief (Hawkins and Bucklin, 2012). The resulting headache, auditory problems (e.g., tinnitus), and visual problems (e.g., blurred vision, photophobia) begin within 2 days of the puncture and may persist for days or weeks.

The likelihood of headache after dural puncture can be reduced if the anesthesia care provider uses a small-gauge spinal needle and avoids making multiple punctures of the meninges. Passing an epidural catheter through the dural opening at the time of puncture to provide continuous spinal anesthesia, with removal of the catheter 24 hours later, may help prevent spinal headache. Injecting preservative-free saline through the spinal catheter before removing it also may decrease the incidence of headache. Hydration and bedrest in the prone position have been recommended as preventive measures but have not been proven to be of much value (Hawkins and Bucklin, 2012).

Conservative management for a PDPH includes administration of oral analgesics and methylxanthines (e.g., caffeine or theophylline). Methylxanthines cause constriction of cerebral blood vessels and may provide symptomatic relief. An autologous epidural blood patch is the most rapid, reliable, and beneficial relief measure for PDPH. The woman's blood (i.e., 20 mL) is injected slowly into the lumbar epidural space, creating a clot that patches the tear or hole in the dura mater. Treatment with a blood patch is considered if the headache is severe or debilitating or does not resolve after conservative management. The blood patch is remarkably effective and is nearly complication free (Hawkins and Bucklin, 2012) (Fig. 14-12).

The woman should be observed for alteration in vital signs, pallor, clammy skin, and leakage of CSF for 1 to 2 hours after the blood patch is performed. If no complications occur, she may then resume normal activity. She should, however, be instructed to avoid coughing or straining for the first day after the blood patch (Hawkins and Bucklin, 2012). She is also taught to avoid analgesics that affect platelet aggregation (e.g., nonsteroidal antiinflammatory drugs [NSAIDs]) for 2 days, drink plenty of fluids, and observe for signs of infection at the site and for neurologic symptoms such as pain, numbness and tingling in the legs, and difficulty with walking or elimination.

Epidural Anesthesia or Analgesia (Block). Relief from the pain of uterine contractions and birth (vaginal and cesarean) can be achieved by injecting a suitable local anesthetic agent (e.g., bupivacaine, ropivacaine), an opioid analgesic (e.g., fentanyl, sufentanil), or both into the epidural (peridural) space. Injection is made between the fourth and fifth lumbar vertebrae for a lumbar epidural block (see Figs. 14-8, *B*, and 14-10, *A*). Depending on the type, amount, and number of medications used, an anesthetic or analgesic effect will occur with varying degrees of motor impairment. The combination of an opioid with the local anesthetic agent reduces the dose of anesthetic required, thereby preserving a greater degree of motor function.

Epidural anesthesia and analgesia is the most effective pharmacologic pain relief method for labor that is available. As a result, it is used by most women in the United States (Hawkins and Bucklin, 2012). For relieving the discomfort of labor and vaginal birth, a block from T10 to S5 is required. For cesarean birth, a block from at least T8 to S1 is essential. The diffusion of epidural anesthesia depends on the location of the catheter tip, the dose and volume of the anesthetic agent used, and the woman's position (e.g., horizontal or head-up). The woman must cooperate and maintain her position without moving during the insertion of the epidural catheter to prevent misplacement, neurologic injury, or hematoma formation.

> ### ! NURSING ALERT
> Epidural anesthesia effectively relieves the pain caused by uterine contractions. For most women, however, it does not completely remove the pressure sensations that occur as the fetus descends in the pelvis.

For the induction of an epidural block, the woman is positioned as for a spinal block. She may sit with her back curved or assume a modified Sims' position with her shoulders parallel, legs slightly flexed, and back arched. It is important to avoid severe spinal flexion because it could compress the epidural space, increasing the risk for dural puncture (Creehan, 2008) (see Fig. 14-11). A large-bore needle is inserted into the epidural space. A catheter is then threaded through the needle until its tip rests in the epidural space. The needle is then removed, and the catheter is taped in place. After the epidural catheter is inserted and secured, a small amount of medication, called a *test dose,* is injected to be sure that the catheter has not been accidentally placed in the subarachnoid (spinal) space or in a blood vessel (Hawkins and Bucklin, 2012).

Initiating epidural anesthesia may be difficult when the woman is obese. She may find it harder to assume a position necessary for catheter placement. In addition, excess adipose tissue can obscure the anatomic landmarks used to identify the location of the appropriate insertion site (Jevitt, 2009). Although epidural catheter placement can present technical challenges, use of regional anesthesia can provide adequate pain management for the obese woman during labor and birth. Placing the catheter in early labor when the woman is more comfortable and is able to fully cooperate is a recommended solution (Creehan, 2008; Saravanakumar, Rao, and Cooper, 2006). Early placement of a functioning epidural may reduce the potential complications associated with intubation during an emergent delivery. Note that epidural anesthesia presents less risk for the obese woman than does general anesthesia.

After the epidural has been initiated, the woman is positioned preferably on her side; this is done so that the uterus does not compress the ascending vena cava and descending aorta, which can impair venous return, reduce cardiac output and blood pressure, and decrease placental perfusion. Her position should be alternated from side to side every hour. Upright positions and ambulation may be possible, depending on the degree of motor impairment. Oxygen should be available if hypotension occurs despite maintenance of hydration with IV fluid and displacement of the uterus to the side. Ephedrine or phenylephrine (vasopressors used to increase maternal blood pressure) and increased IV fluid infusion may be needed (see Emergency box). The fetal heart rate and pattern, contraction pattern, and progress in labor must be monitored carefully because the woman may not be aware of changes in the strength of the uterine contractions or the descent of the presenting part.

Several methods can be used for an epidural block. An intermittent block is achieved by using repeated injections of anesthetic solution; it is the least common method. The most common method is the continuous block, achieved by using a pump to infuse the anesthetic solution through an indwelling plastic catheter. Patient-controlled epidural analgesia (PCEA) is the newest method; it uses an indwelling catheter and a programmed pump that allows the woman to control the dosing.

The advantages of an epidural block are numerous:
- The woman remains alert and is more comfortable and able to participate.
- Good relaxation is achieved.
- Airway reflexes remain intact.
- Only partial motor paralysis develops.
- Gastric emptying is not delayed.
- Blood loss is not excessive.

Fetal complications are rare but may occur in the event of rapid absorption of the medication or marked maternal hypotension. The dose, volume, type, and number of medications used can be modified (1) to allow the woman to push, to assume upright positions, and even to walk; (2) to produce perineal anesthesia; and (3) to permit forceps-assisted, vacuum-assisted, or cesarean birth if required.

The disadvantages of epidural block also are numerous. The woman's ability to move freely and to maintain control of her labor is limited, related to the use of numerous medical interventions (e.g., an intravenous infusion and electronic monitoring) and the occurrence of orthostatic hypotension and dizziness, sedation, and weakness of the legs. CNS effects (Box 14-6) can occur if a solution containing a local anesthetic agent is accidentally injected into a blood vessel or if excessive amounts of local anesthetic are given.

> ### BOX 14-6 SIDE EFFECTS OF EPIDURAL AND SPINAL ANESTHESIA
>
> - Hypotension
> - Local anesthetic toxicity
>   - Lightheadedness
>   - Dizziness
>   - Tinnitus (ringing in the ears)
>   - Metallic taste
>   - Numbness of the tongue and mouth
>   - Bizarre behavior
>   - Slurred speech
>   - Convulsions
>   - Loss of consciousness
> - High or total spinal anesthesia
> - Fever
> - Urinary retention
> - Pruritus (itching)
> - Limited movement
> - Longer second-stage labor
> - Increased use of oxytocin
> - Increased likelihood of forceps- or vacuum-assisted birth

High spinal or "total spinal" anesthesia, resulting in respiratory arrest, can occur if the relatively high dosage used with an epidural block is accidentally injected into the subarachnoid space. Women who receive an epidural have a higher rate of fever (i.e., intrapartum temperature of 38°C [100.4°F] or higher), especially when labor lasts longer than 12 hours; the temperature elevation most likely is related to thermoregulatory changes, although infection cannot be ruled out. The elevation in temperature can result in fetal tachycardia and neonatal workup for sepsis, whether or not signs of infection are present (see Box 14-6).

Hypotension as a result of sympathetic blockade can occur in about 10% to 30% of women who receive regional (spinal or epidural) analgesia during labor (Witcher and McLendon, 2013) (see Emergency box). Hypotension can result in a significant decrease in uteroplacental perfusion and oxygen delivery to the fetus. Urinary retention and stress incontinence can occur in the immediate postpartum period. This temporary difficulty in urinary elimination could be related not only to the effects of the epidural block and the need for catheterization but also to the increased duration of labor and need for forceps- or vacuum-assisted birth associated with the block. Pruritus (itching) is a side effect that often occurs with the use of an opioid, especially fentanyl. A relationship between epidural analgesia and longer second-stage labor, use of oxytocin, and forceps- or vacuum-assisted birth has been documented. Research findings have been unable to demonstrate a significant increase in cesarean birth associated with epidural analgesia (Hawkins and Bucklin, 2012). For some women, the epidural block is not effective and a second form of analgesia is required to establish effective pain relief. When women progress rapidly in labor, pain relief may not be obtained before birth occurs.

Combined Spinal-Epidural Analgesia.
In the combined spinal-epidural (CSE) analgesia technique, sometimes referred to as a "walking epidural," an epidural needle is inserted into the epidural space. Before the epidural catheter is placed, a smaller-gauge spinal needle is inserted through the bore of the epidural needle into the subarachnoid space. A small amount of opioid or combination of opioid and local anesthetic is then injected intrathecally to rapidly provide analgesia. Afterward, the epidural catheter is inserted as usual. The CSE technique is an increasingly popular approach that can be used to block pain transmission without compromising motor ability. The concentration of opioid receptors is high along the pain pathway in the spinal cord, in the brainstem, and in the thalamus. Because these receptors are highly sensitive to opioids, a small quantity of an opioid agonist analgesic produces marked pain relief lasting for several hours. If additional pain relief is needed, medication can be injected through the epidural catheter (see Fig. 14-10, A). The most common side effects of CSE are pruritus, urinary retention, immediate or delayed respiratory depression, and nausea. Naloxone can be given intravenously to manage these side effects without decreasing the degree of analgesia achieved (Cunningham, Leveno, Bloom, et al., 2010; Hawkins and Bucklin, 2012). CSE analgesia is also associated with a greater incidence of FHR abnormalities than is epidural analgesia alone, necessitating close assessment of fetal heart rate and pattern (Cunningham, Leveno, Bloom, et al., 2010).

Although women can walk (hence the term "walking epidural"), they often choose not to do so because of sedation and fatigue, abnormal sensations in and weakness of the legs, and a feeling of insecurity. Often health care providers are reluctant to encourage or assist women to ambulate for fear of injury. However, women can be assisted to change positions and use upright positions during labor and birth.

Epidural and Intrathecal (Spinal) Opioids.
Opioids also can be used alone, eliminating the effect of a local anesthetic altogether. The use of epidural or intrathecal opioids without the addition of a local anesthetic agent during labor has several advantages. Opioids administered in this manner do not cause maternal hypotension or affect vital signs. The woman feels contractions but not pain. Her ability to bear down during the second stage of labor is preserved because the pushing reflex is not lost and her motor power remains intact.

Fentanyl, sufentanil, or preservative-free morphine can be used. Fentanyl and sufentanil produce short-acting analgesia (i.e., 1.5 to 3.5 hours), and morphine can provide pain relief for 4 to 7 hours. Morphine can be combined with fentanyl or sufentanil. Using short-acting opioids with multiparous women and morphine with nulliparous women or women with a history of long labors is appropriate. Because opioids alone usually do not provide adequate analgesia, however, they are most often given in combination with a local anesthetic (Cunningham, Leveno, Bloom, et al., 2010).

A more common indication for the administration of epidural or intrathecal analgesics is for the relief of postoperative pain. For example, a woman who gives birth by cesarean can receive fentanyl or morphine through a catheter. The catheter can then be removed, and the woman is usually free of pain for 24 hours. Occasionally the catheter is left in place in the epidural space in case another dose is needed.

Women receiving epidurally administered morphine after a cesarean birth can ambulate sooner than women who do not. The early ambulation and freedom from pain also facilitate bladder emptying, enhance peristalsis, and prevent clot formation (e.g., thrombophlebitis) in the lower extremities. Women may require additional medication for breakthrough pain during the first 24 hours after surgery. If so, they will usually be given an NSAID such as ketorolac (Toradol), indomethacin (Indocin), or ibuprofen (Motrin) rather than a narcotic.

Side effects of opioids administered by the epidural and intrathecal routes include nausea, vomiting, diminished peristalsis, pruritus, urinary retention, and delayed respiratory depression. These effects are more common when morphine is administered. Antiemetics, antipruritics, and opioid antagonists are used to relieve these symptoms. For example, naloxone or metoclopramide may be administered. Hospital protocols or detailed physician orders should provide specific instructions for the treatment of these side effects. Use of epidural opioids is not without risk. Respiratory depression is a serious concern; for this reason the woman's respiratory status should be assessed and documented every hour for 24 hours or as designated by hospital protocol. Naloxone should be readily available for use if the respiratory rate decreases to less than 10 breaths per minute or if the oxygen saturation rate decreases to less than 89%. Administration of oxygen by nonrebreather facemask also can be initiated, and the anesthesia care provider should be notified.

Contraindications to Subarachnoid and Epidural Blocks.
Contraindications to epidural analgesia (Creehan, 2008; Cunningham, Leveno, Bloom, et al., 2010; Hawkins and Bucklin, 2012) include:
- Active or anticipated serious maternal hemorrhage. Acute hypovolemia leads to increased sympathetic tone to maintain the blood pressure. Any anesthetic technique that blocks the sympathetic fibers can produce significant hypotension that can endanger the mother and fetus.
- Maternal hypotension.
- Coagulopathy. If a woman is receiving anticoagulant therapy (e.g., last dose of low-molecular-weight heparin within 12

hours) or has a bleeding disorder, injury to a blood vessel may cause the formation of a hematoma that may compress the cauda equina or the spinal cord and lead to serious CNS complications.

- Infection at the needle insertion site. Infection can be spread through the peridural or subarachnoid spaces if the needle traverses an infected area.
- Increased intracranial pressure caused by a mass lesion.
- Allergy to the anesthetic drug.
- Maternal refusal or inability to cooperate.
- Some types of maternal cardiac conditions.

Epidural Block Effects on Newborn. Analgesia or anesthesia during labor and birth has little or no lasting effect on the physiologic status of the newborn. There is no evidence that the administration of maternal analgesic or anesthetic agents during labor and birth has a significant effect on the child's later mental and neurologic development (AAP and ACOG, 2012).

Nitrous Oxide for Analgesia

Nitrous oxide was used more widely for labor analgesia in the United States in the past but never as extensively as in other countries. Recently, however, interest in using nitrous oxide during labor has increased in the United States (Rooks, 2011). Nitrous oxide mixed with oxygen can be inhaled in a low concentration (50% or less) to provide analgesia during the first and second stages of labor. At the lower doses used for analgesia, it helps women relax, gives them a sense of control, and reduces their perception of pain even though they may still be aware that pain is present (Rooks, 2011).

A facemask or mouthpiece is used to self-administer the gas. The woman places the mask over her mouth and nose or inserts the mouthpiece 30 seconds before the onset of a contraction (if regular) or as soon as a contraction begins (if irregular). When she inhales, a valve opens and the gas is released. She should continue to inhale the gas slowly and deeply until the contraction starts to subside. When inhalation stops, the valve closes. Between contractions, the woman should remove the device and breathe normally (Cunningham, Leveno, Bloom, et al., 2010).

The nurse should observe the woman for nausea and vomiting, drowsiness, dizziness, hazy memory, and loss of consciousness. Loss of consciousness is more likely to occur if opioids are used with the nitrous oxide (Cunningham, Leveno, Bloom, et al., 2010). The use of nitrous oxide does not appear to depress uterine contractions or cause adverse reactions in the fetus and newborn. Its ease of use and rapid onset of action make nitrous oxide a good option for labor analgesia (Rooks, 2011).

General Anesthesia

General anesthesia rarely is used for uncomplicated vaginal birth. It is used for only about 10% of cesarean births in the United States (Hawkins and Bucklin, 2012). General anesthesia may be necessary if a spinal or epidural block is contraindicated or if indications necessitate rapid birth (vaginal or emergent cesarean) without sufficient time or available personnel to perform a block (Witcher and McLendon, 2013). In addition, being awake and aware during major surgery may be unacceptable for some women having a cesarean birth. The major risks associated with general anesthesia are difficulty with or inability to intubate and aspiration of gastric contents (Cunningham, Leveno, Bloom, et al., 2010; Hawkins and Bucklin, 2012). Anesthesia care providers are more likely to encounter difficulty with intubating morbidly obese patients, especially in an emergency situation, than women of normal weight (Witcher and McLendon, 2013).

If general anesthesia is being considered, give the woman nothing by mouth and ensure that an IV infusion is in place. If time allows, premedicate the woman with a nonparticulate (clear) oral antacid (e.g., sodium citrate/citric acid [Bicitra]) to neutralize the acidic contents of the stomach. Aspiration of highly acidic gastric contents will damage lung tissue. Some anesthesia care providers also order the administration of a histamine (H_2)-receptor blocker such as famotidine (Pepcid) or ranitidine (Zantac) to decrease the production of gastric acid and metoclopramide (Reglan) to accelerate gastric emptying (Hawkins and Bucklin, 2012). Before the anesthesia is given, a wedge should be placed under one of the woman's hips to displace the uterus. Uterine displacement prevents compression of the aorta and vena cava, which maintains cardiac output and placental perfusion (Hawkins and Bucklin, 2012).

Before the induction of anesthesia, the woman will be preoxygenated with 100% oxygen by nonrebreather facemask for 2 to 3 minutes. This is especially important in pregnant women, who are more likely than other adults to rapidly become hypoxemic if there is a delay in successful intubation. Thiopental, a short-acting barbiturate, or ketamine is administered intravenously to render the woman unconscious. Next, succinylcholine, a muscle relaxer, is administered to facilitate passage of an endotracheal tube (Cunningham, Leveno, Bloom, et al., 2010; Hawkins and Bucklin, 2012). Sometimes the nurse is asked to assist with applying cricoid pressure before intubation as the woman begins to lose consciousness. This maneuver blocks the esophagus and prevents aspiration should the woman vomit or regurgitate (Fig. 14-13). Pressure is released once the endotracheal tube is securely in place.

After the woman is intubated, nitrous oxide and oxygen in a 50:50 mixture are administered. A low concentration of a volatile halogenated agent (e.g., isoflurane) also may be administered to increase pain relief and to reduce maternal awareness and recall (Cunningham, Leveno, Bloom, et al., 2010; Hawkins and Bucklin, 2012). In low concentrations, these agents do not relax the uterus, so bleeding should not increase because of their use (Hawkins and Bucklin, 2012). In higher concentrations, isoflurane or methoxyflurane relaxes the uterus quickly and facilitates intrauterine manipulation, version, and extraction. However, at higher concentrations, these agents cross the placenta readily and can produce narcosis in the fetus and could reduce uterine tone after birth,

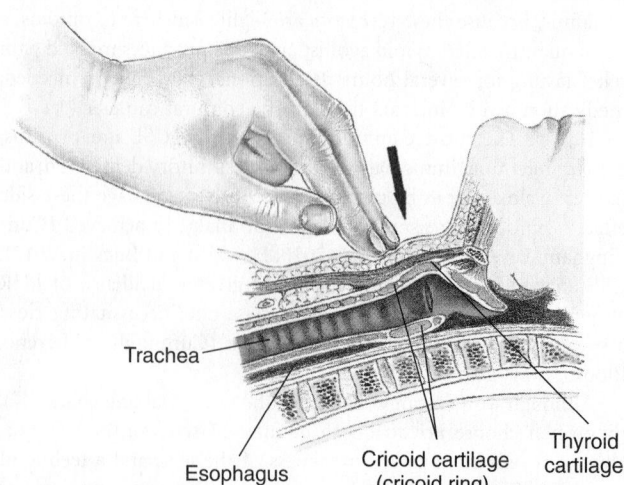

FIG 14-13 Technique of applying pressure on cricoid cartilage to occlude esophagus to prevent aspiration of gastric contents during induction of general anesthesia.

increasing the risk for hemorrhage. Because of this risk for neonatal narcosis, it is critical that the baby be delivered as soon as possible after the induction of the anesthetic to reduce the degree of fetal exposure to the anesthetic agents and the CNS depressants administered.

Priorities for recovery room care are to maintain an open airway and cardiopulmonary function and to prevent postpartum hemorrhage. Women who had surgery under general anesthesia will require pain medication soon after regaining consciousness. Routine postpartum care is organized to facilitate parent-infant attachment as soon as possible and to answer the mother's questions. When appropriate, the nurse assesses the mother's readiness to see her baby, as well as her response to the anesthesia and to the event that necessitated general anesthesia (e.g., emergency cesarean birth when vaginal birth was anticipated).

CARE MANAGEMENT

The choice of pain relief interventions depends on a combination of factors, including the woman's special needs and wishes, the availability of the desired method or methods, the knowledge and expertise in nonpharmacologic and pharmacologic methods of the health care providers involved in the woman's care, and the phase and stage of labor.

Nonpharmacologic Interventions

The nurse supports and assists the woman as she uses nonpharmacologic interventions for pain relief and relaxation. During labor, the nurse should ask the woman how she feels to evaluate the effectiveness of the specific pain management techniques used. Appropriate interventions can then be planned or continued for effective care, such as trying other nonpharmacologic methods or combining nonpharmacologic methods with medications (see Nursing Care Plan). A pain scale, where 0 represents no pain and 10 represents pain as bad as it could possibly be, is often used to evaluate a woman's pain before and after pain relief interventions are implemented. Comparing the woman's answers provides a way to objectively evaluate the effectiveness of pain relief interventions.

Pharmacologic Interventions
Informed Consent

Pregnant women have the right to be active participants in determining the best pain care approach to use during labor and birth. The primary health care provider and anesthesia care provider are responsible for fully informing women of the alternative methods of pharmacologic pain relief available in the hospital. A description of the various anesthetic techniques and what they entail is essential to informed consent, even if the woman received information about analgesia and anesthesia earlier in her pregnancy. The initial discussion of pain management options ideally should take place in the third trimester so the woman has time to consider alternatives. Nurses play a part in the informed consent by clarifying and describing procedures or by acting as the woman's advocate and asking the primary health care provider for further explanations. The three essential components of an informed consent are:

- First, the procedure and its advantages and disadvantages must be thoroughly explained.
- Second, the woman must agree with the plan of labor pain care as explained to her.
- Third, her consent must be given freely without coercion or manipulation from her health care provider.

LEGAL TIP: Informed Consent for Anesthesia

The woman receives (in an understandable manner):

- Explanation of alternative methods of anesthesia and analgesia available
- Description of the anesthetic, including its effects and the procedure for its administration
- Description of the benefits, discomforts, risks, and consequences for the mother, the fetus, and the newborn
- Explanation of how complications can be treated
- Information that the anesthetic is not always effective
- Indication that the woman may withdraw consent at any time
- Opportunity to have any question answered
- Opportunity to have components of the consent explained in the woman's own words

The consent form will:

- Be written or explained in the woman's primary language
- Have the woman's signature
- Have the date of consent
- Carry the signature of the anesthetic care provider, certifying that the woman has received and expresses understanding of the explanation

---

! NURSING ALERT

In some cultures, the husband must consent to procedures performed on the wife. Although in the United States the woman is the person who gives consent and signs any necessary forms, she may not be willing to do so unless her husband also approves.

Timing of Administration

It is often the nurse who notifies the primary health care provider that the woman is in need of pharmacologic measures to relieve her pain and discomfort. Orders are often written for the administration of pain medication as needed by the woman and based on the nurse's clinical judgment. In the past, pharmacologic measures for pain relief were usually not implemented until labor had advanced to the active phase of the first stage of labor and the cervix had dilated approximately 4 to 5 cm, to avoid suppressing the progress of labor. However, it is now known that epidural anesthesia in early labor does not increase the rate of cesarean birth. Whereas it may shorten the duration of first-stage labor in some women, epidural anesthesia lengthens it in others (Hawkins and Bucklin, 2012). It is no longer recommended that women in labor reach a certain level of cervical dilation or fetal station before receiving epidural anesthesia (AAP and ACOG, 2012; Cunningham, Leveno, Bloom, et al., 2010). It is, however, still recommended that the administration of systemic opioid analgesics be delayed until labor is well established (Creehan, 2008). Nonpharmacologic measures can be used to relieve pain and stress and enhance progress at any time in labor.

Preparation for Procedures

The methods of pain relief available to the woman are reviewed and information is clarified as necessary. The procedure and what will be expected of the woman (e.g., to maintain flexed position during insertion of epidural needle) must be explained.

The woman also can benefit from knowing the way that the medication is to be given, the interval before the medication takes effect, and the expected pain relief from the medication. Skin-preparation measures are described, and an explanation is given for the need to empty the bladder before the analgesic or anesthetic is

◎ NURSING CARE PLAN

Nonpharmacologic Pain Management

NURSING DIAGNOSIS	EXPECTED OUTCOME	INTERVENTIONS	RATIONALES
Anxiety related to lack of confidence in ability to cope effectively with pain during labor	Woman will express decrease in anxiety and experience satisfaction with her labor and birth performance.	Assess whether woman and significant other have attended childbirth classes, their knowledge of labor process, and their current level of anxiety	To plan supportive strategies that address couple's specific needs
		Encourage support person to remain with woman in labor	To provide support and increase probability of positive response to comfort measures
		Teach or review nonpharmacologic techniques available to decrease anxiety and pain during labor (e.g., focusing, relaxation and breathing techniques, effleurage, and sacral pressure)	To enhance chances of success in using techniques
		Explore other techniques that woman or significant other may have learned in childbirth classes (e.g., hypnosis, hydrotherapy, acupressure, biofeedback, therapeutic touch, aromatherapy, imaging, music)	To provide more options for coping strategies
		Explore use of transcutaneous electrical nerve stimulation if ordered by primary health care provider	To provide increased perception of control over pain and increase in release of endogenous opiates (endorphins)
		Assist woman to change positions and to use pillows	To reduce stiffness, aid circulation, and promote comfort
		Assess bladder for distention, and encourage voiding often	To avoid bladder distention, subsequent discomfort, and potential for suppression of uterine contractions
		Encourage rest between contractions	To minimize fatigue
		Keep woman and significant other informed about progress	To allay anxiety
		Guide couple through labor stages and phases, helping them use and modify comfort techniques that are appropriate to each phase	To ensure greatest effectiveness of techniques used
		Support couple if pharmacologic measures are required to increase pain relief, explaining safety and effectiveness	To reduce anxiety and maintain self-esteem and sense of control over labor process
Readiness for enhanced childbearing process related to desire for healthy outcome of labor and birth	Woman will participate in planning care for labor.	Discuss woman's birth plan and knowledge about birth process	To collect data for nursing plan of care
		Provide information about labor process	To correct any misconceptions
		Inform woman about her labor status and the fetus' well-being	To promote comfort and confidence
		Discuss rationales for all interventions	To incorporate woman into plan of care
		Incorporate nonpharmacologic interventions into plan of care	To increase woman's sense of control during labor
		Provide emotional support and ongoing positive feedback	To enhance positive coping mechanisms

administered and the reason for keeping the bladder empty. When an indwelling catheter is to be threaded into the epidural space, the woman should be told that she may have a momentary twinge down her leg, hip, or back and that this feeling is not a sign of injury (Box 14-7).

Administration of Medication

Accurate monitoring of the progress of labor forms the basis for the nurse's judgment that a woman needs pharmacologic control of pain. Knowledge of the medications used during childbirth is essential. The most effective route of administration is selected for each woman; then the medication is prepared and administered correctly.

Any medication can cause a minor or severe allergic reaction. As part of the assessment for such allergic reactions, the nurse should monitor the woman's vital signs, respiratory effort, cardiovascular status, integument, and platelet and white blood cell count. The woman is observed for side effects of drug therapy, especially

BOX 14-7   NURSING INTERVENTIONS FOR THE WOMAN RECEIVING EPIDURAL OR SPINAL ANESTHESIA

Prior to the Block
- Assist primary health care provider and/or anesthesia care provider with explaining the procedure and obtaining the woman's informed consent.
- Assess maternal vital signs, level of hydration, labor progress, and fetal heart rate (FHR) and pattern.
- Insert an intravenous (IV) line and infuse a bolus of fluid (Ringer's lactate or normal saline) if ordered (e.g., 500 to 1000 mL 15 to 30 minutes before induction of the anesthesia).
- Obtain laboratory results (hematocrit or hemoglobin level, other tests as ordered).
- Assess the woman's level of pain using a pain scale (from 0 [no pain] to 10 [pain as bad as it could possibly be]).
- Assist the woman to void.

During Initiation of the Block
- Assist the woman with assuming and maintaining proper position.
- Verbally guide the woman through the procedure, explaining sounds and sensations as she experiences them.
- Assist the anesthesia care provider with documentation of vital signs, time and amount of medications given, etc.
- Monitor maternal vital signs (especially blood pressure) and FHR as ordered.
- Have oxygen and suction readily available.
- Monitor for signs of local anesthetic toxicity (see Box 14-6) as the test dose of medication is administered.

While the Block is in Effect
- Continue to monitor maternal vital signs and FHR as ordered (continuous monitoring of maternal heart rate [electrocardiogram (ECG)] and blood pressure may be ordered to monitor for accidental intravenous injection of medication).
- Continue to assess the woman's level of pain with every check of vital signs using a pain scale (from 0 [no pain] to 10 [pain as bad as it could possibly be]).
- Monitor for bladder distention:
  - Assist with spontaneous voiding on bedpan or toilet.
  - Insert urinary catheter if necessary.
- Encourage or assist the woman to change positions from side to side every hour.
- Promote safety:
  - Keep siderails up on the bed.
  - Place telephone and call light within easy reach.
  - Instruct woman not to get out of bed without help.
  - Make sure there is no prolonged pressure on anesthetized body parts.
- Keep the epidural catheter insertion site clean and dry.
- Continue to monitor for anesthetic side effects (see Box 14-6).

While the Block Is Wearing off After Birth
- Assess regularly for the return of sensory and motor function.
- Continue to monitor maternal vital signs as ordered.
- Monitor for bladder distention:
  - Assist with spontaneous voiding on bedpan or toilet.
  - Insert urinary catheter if necessary.
- Promote safety:
  - Keep siderails up on the bed.
  - Place telephone and call light within easy reach.
  - Instruct woman not to get out of bed without help.
  - Make sure there is no prolonged pressure on anesthetized body parts.
- Keep the epidural catheter insertion site clean and dry.
- Continue to monitor for anesthetic side effects (see Box 14-6).

---

drowsiness and dyspnea. Minor reactions can consist of rash, rhinitis, fever, shortness of breath, or pruritus. Management of the less acute allergic response is not an emergency.

Severe allergic reactions (anaphylaxis) may occur suddenly and lead to shock or death. The most dramatic form of anaphylaxis is sudden, severe bronchospasm, upper airway obstruction, and/or hypotension (Brown, Mullins, and Gold, 2006). Signs of anaphylaxis are largely caused by contraction of smooth muscles and may begin with irritability, extreme weakness, nausea, and vomiting. This may lead to dyspnea, cyanosis, convulsions, and cardiac arrest. Anaphylaxis must be diagnosed and treated immediately. Initial treatment usually consists of placing the woman in a supine position, injecting epinephrine intramuscularly (IM), administering fluid intravenously (IV), supporting the airway with ventilation if necessary, and giving oxygen. If response to these measures is inadequate, intravenous epinephrine should be given (Brown, Mullins, and Gold, 2006.). Cardiopulmonary resuscitation may be necessary (see Chapter 12).

Intravenous Route. The preferred route of administration of medications such as meperidine, fentanyl, butorphanol, or nalbuphine is through IV tubing, administered into the port nearest the point of insertion of the infusion (proximal port). The medication is given slowly and in small increments during a contraction. It may be given over a period of three to five consecutive contractions if needed to complete the dose. It is given during contractions to decrease fetal exposure to the medication because uterine blood vessels are constricted during contractions and the medication stays within the maternal vascular system for several seconds before the uterine blood vessels reopen. The IV infusion is then restarted slowly to prevent a bolus of medication from being administered. With this method of injection, the amount of medication crossing the placenta to the fetus is minimized. With decreased placental transfer, the mother's degree of pain relief is maximized. The IV route has the following advantages:
- Onset of pain relief is rapid and more predictable.
- Pain relief is obtained with small doses of the drug.
- Duration of effect is more predictable.

Intramuscular Route. Although analgesics are still sometimes given IM, that is not the preferred route of administration for the woman in labor. The advantages of using the IM route are quick administration and no need to start an IV line.

Disadvantages of the IM route include:
- Onset of pain relief is delayed.
- Higher doses of medication are required.
- Medication is released at an unpredictable rate from the muscle tissue and is available for transfer across the placenta to the fetus.

The maternal medication levels (after IM injections) are unequal because of uneven distribution (maternal uptake) and metabolism. IM injections given in the upper arm (deltoid muscle) seem to result in more rapid absorption and higher blood levels of the medication than when administered in other sites (Bricker and Lavender, 2002).

If regional anesthesia is planned later in labor, the deltoid muscle is the preferred site. The autonomic blockade from the regional (e.g., epidural) anesthesia increases blood flow to the gluteal region and accelerates absorption of medication that may be sequestered there. Administration of opioids subcutaneously in the upper arm avoids this risk and, as a result, is often used as an alternative to IM injection.

Regional (Epidural or Spinal) Anesthesia. According to professional standards (Association of Women's Health, Obstetric and Neonatal Nurses [AWHONN], 2012), the nonanesthetist registered nurse is permitted to monitor the status of the woman, the fetus, and the progress of labor; replace empty infusion syringes or bags with the same medication and concentration; stop the infusion and initiate emergency measures if the need arises; and remove the catheter if properly educated to do so. Only qualified, licensed anesthesia care providers are permitted to insert a catheter and initiate epidural anesthesia, verify catheter placement, inject medication through the catheter, or alter the medication or medications, including the type, the amount, or the rate of infusion.

> ⚡ **SAFETY ALERT**
>
> Safe regional anesthesia administration requires specialized education, experience, and competence. There is potential for significant maternal and/or fetal morbidity and mortality associated with some obstetric anesthesia complications. Therefore a licensed, credentialed anesthesia care provider should manage regional anesthesia and analgesia during labor and birth and be readily available to manage obstetric anesthesia-related emergencies (AWHONN, 2012).

Because spinal nerve blocks can reduce bladder sensation, resulting in difficulty voiding, the woman should empty her bladder before the induction of the block and should be encouraged to void at least every 2 hours thereafter. The nurse should palpate for bladder distention and measure urinary output to ensure that the bladder is being completely emptied. A distended bladder can inhibit uterine contractions and fetal descent, resulting in a slowing of the progress of labor. For this reason, an indwelling urinary catheter (Foley) is often routinely inserted immediately after epidural or spinal anesthesia is initiated and left in place for the remainder of the first stage of labor.

The status of the maternal-fetal unit and the progress of labor must be established before the block is initiated. The nurse must assist the woman to assume and maintain the correct position for induction of epidural and spinal anesthesia (see Fig. 14-11, *A* and *B*).

Depending on the level of motor blockade, the woman should be assisted to remain as mobile as possible. When in bed, her position should be alternated from side to side every hour to ensure adequate distribution of the anesthetic solution and to maintain circulation to the uterus and placenta.

> ⚡ **SAFETY ALERT**
>
> After receiving an epidural block or opioid intravenously for pain, the woman should not be allowed to ambulate alone. She must either remain in bed or request assistance before attempting to get out of bed. The nurse assesses the woman for signs of orthostatic hypotension and return of sensation and motor function of the lower extremities before ambulation.

Health care providers should be aware that effective epidural anesthesia prolongs the second stage of labor by 15 to 30 minutes. A delay in the second stage of labor does not negatively affect maternal or fetal outcome, however, as long as the FHR tracing is normal, maternal hydration and analgesia are adequate, and there is ongoing progress in the descent of the fetal head. Therefore operative interventions (e.g., the use of forceps or vacuum) to hasten the birth solely because the second stage is prolonged are unnecessary. Reducing the density of the epidural block during the second stage of labor, delaying pushing until the woman feels the urge to do so, and avoiding arbitrary definitions for the "normal" duration of second-stage labor are suggested as interventions to decrease the risk of operative vaginal birth (Hawkins and Bucklin, 2012). (See Chapter 16 for a full discussion of second-stage labor management.) Box 14-7 summarizes the nursing interventions for women receiving epidural or spinal anesthesia.

Safety and General Care

The nurse monitors and records the woman's response to nonpharmacologic pain relief methods and to medication(s). This includes the degree of pain relief, the level of apprehension, the return of sensations and perception of pain, and allergic or adverse reactions (e.g., hypotension, respiratory depression, fever, pruritus, and nausea and vomiting). The nurse continues to monitor maternal vital signs and fetal heart rate and pattern at frequent intervals, the strength and frequency of uterine contractions, changes in the cervix and station of the presenting part, the presence and quality of the bearing-down reflex, bladder filling, and state of hydration. Determining the fetal response after administration of analgesia or anesthesia is vital. The woman is asked if she (or the family) has any questions. The nurse also assesses the woman's and her family's understanding of the need for ensuring her safety (e.g., keeping side rails up, calling for assistance as needed).

The time that elapses between the administration of an opioid and the baby's birth is documented. Medications given to the newborn to reverse opioid effects are recorded. After birth, the woman who has had spinal, epidural, or general anesthesia is assessed for return of sensory and motor function in addition to the usual postpartum assessments. Both the nurse and the anesthesia provider are responsible for documenting assessments and care in relation to regional (epidural or spinal) anesthesia.

▌ KEY POINTS

- Nonpharmacologic pain and stress management strategies are valuable for managing labor discomfort alone or in combination with pharmacologic methods.
- The gate-control theory of pain and the stress response are the bases for many of the nonpharmacologic methods of pain relief.
- The type of analgesic or anesthetic to be used is determined by maternal and health care provider preference, the stage of labor, and the method of birth.

- Sedatives may be appropriate for women in prolonged early labor when there is a need to decrease anxiety or promote sleep or therapeutic rest.
- Naloxone (Narcan) is an opioid (narcotic) antagonist that can reverse narcotic effects, especially respiratory depression.
- Pharmacologic control of pain during labor requires collaboration among the health care providers and the laboring woman.

- The nurse must understand medications, their expected effects, potential side effects, and methods of administration.
- Maintenance of maternal fluid balance is essential during spinal and epidural nerve blocks.
- Maternal analgesia or anesthesia potentially affects neonatal neurobehavioral response.
- The use of opioid agonist-antagonist analgesics in women with pre-existing opioid dependence may cause symptoms of abstinence syndrome (opioid withdrawal).

- Epidural anesthesia and analgesia is the most effective pharmacologic pain relief method for labor that is available. Therefore it is used by most women in the United States.
- General anesthesia is rarely used for vaginal birth but may be used for cesarean birth or whenever rapid anesthesia is needed in an emergency childbirth situation.

REFERENCES

Aghabati N, Mohammadi E, Pour Esmaiel Z: The effect of therapeutic touch on pain and fatigue of cancer patients undergoing chemotherapy, *Evid Based Complement Alternat Med* 7(3):375–381, 2010.

Albers L: The evidence for physiologic management of the active phase of the first stage of labor, *J Midwifery Womens Health* 52(3):207–215, 2007.

American Academy of Pediatrics (AAP) and American College of Obstetricians and Gynecologists (ACOG): *Guidelines for perinatal care*, ed 7, Washington, DC, 2012, ACOG.

American College of Obstetricians and Gynecologists (ACOG): *Pain relief during labor* (Committee Opinion No. 295), Washington, DC, Reaffirmed 2008, Author.

American Society of Anesthesiologists Task Force on Obstetric Anesthesia: Practice guidelines for obstetric anesthesia, *Anesthesiology* 106(4):843–863, 2007.

Anderson D: A review of systemic opioids commonly used for labor pain relief, *J Midwifery Womens Health* 56(3):222–239, 2011.

Association of Women's Health, Obstetric and Neonatal Nurses (AWHONN): Role of the registered nurse in the care of the pregnant woman receiving analgesia and anesthesia by catheter techniques: clinical position statement, *J Obstet Gynecol Neonatal Nurs* 41(3):455–457, 2012.

Beebe KR, Lee K: Sleep disturbance in late pregnancy and early labor, *J Perinat Neonatal Nurs* 21(2):103–108, 2007.

Blackburn ST: *Maternal, fetal, and neonatal physiology: a clinical perspective*, ed 4, St Louis, 2013, Saunders.

Bricker L, Lavender T: Parenteral opioids for labor pain relief: a systematic review, *Am J Obstet Gynecol* 186(5 Suppl):S94–S109, 2002.

Brown S, Mullins R, Gold M: Anaphylaxis: diagnosis and management, *Med J Aust* 185(5):283–289, 2006.

Callister L, Khalaf I, Semenic S, et al: The pain of childbirth: perceptions of culturally diverse women, *Pain Manag Nurs* 4(4):145–154, 2003.

Creehan P: Pain relief and comfort measures in labor. In Rice Simpson K, Creehan P, editors: *AWHONN's perinatal nursing*, ed 3, Philadelphia, 2008, Lippincott Williams & Wilkins.

Cunningham F, Leveno K, Bloom S, et al: *Williams obstetrics*, ed 23, New York, 2010, McGraw-Hill.

Gilbert E: *Manual of high risk pregnancy & delivery*, ed 5, St Louis, 2011, Mosby.

Hawkins J, Bucklin B: Obstetrical anesthesia. In Gabbe S, Niebyl J, Simpson J, et al, editors: *Obstetrics: normal and problem pregnancies*, ed 6, Philadelphia, 2012, Saunders.

Hodnett E, Gates S, Hofmeyr G, et al: Continuous support for women during childbirth, *Cochrane Database Syst Rev* (Issue 3), 2011, CD003766.

Jevitt C: Pregnancy complicated by obesity: midwifery management, *J Midwifery Womens Health* 54(6):445–451, 2009.

Jones L, Othman M, Dowswell T, et al: Pain management for women in labor: an overview of systematic reviews, *Cochrane Database Syst Rev* (Issue 3), 2012, CD009234.

Lowe NK: The nature of labor pain, *Am J Obstet Gynecol* 186(5 Suppl):S16–S24, 2002.

Perinatal Education Associates: Breathing, 2008, www.birthsource.com/scripts/article.asp?articleid=211.

Rooks J: Safety and risks of nitrous oxide labor analgesia: a review, *J Midwifery Womens Health* 56(6):557–565, 2011.

Saravanakumar K, Rao S, Cooper G: The challenges of obesity and obstetric anesthesia, *Curr Opin Obstet Gynecol* 18(6):631–635, 2006.

Simkin P, Bolding A: Update on nonpharmacologic approaches to relieve labor pain and prevent suffering, *J Midwifery Womens Health* 49(6):489–504, 2004.

Smith C, Collins C, Cyna A, et al: Complementary and alternative therapies for pain management in labour, *Cochrane Database Syst Rev* Issue 4, 2006 CD003521.

Stark M, Rudell B, Haus G: Observing position and movements in hydrotherapy: a pilot study, *J Obstet Gynecol Neonatal Nurs* 37(1):116–122, 2008.

Tournaire M, Theau-Yonneau A: Complementary and alternative approaches to pain relief during labor, *Evid Based Complement Alternat Med* 4(4):409–417, 2007.

Trout K: The neuromatrix theory of pain: implications for selected nonpharmacologic methods of pain relief for labor, *J Midwifery Womens Health* 49(6):482–488, 2004.

Walls D: Herbs and natural therapies for pregnancy, birth, and breastfeeding, *Int J Childbirth Educ* 24(2):29–37, 2009.

Witcher P, McLendon K: Anesthesia emergencies in the obstetric setting. In Troiano N, Harvey C, Chez B, editors: *AWHONN's high risk & critical care obstetrics*, ed 3, Philadelphia, 2013, Wolters Kluwer/Lippincott Williams & Wilkins.

Zwelling E, Johnson K, Allen J: How to implement complementary therapies for laboring women, *MCN Am J Matern Child Nurs* 31(6):364–372, 2006.

15

Fetal Assessment During Labor

Kitty Cashion

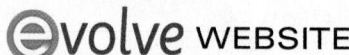 **WEBSITE**

http://evolve.elsevier.com/Perry/maternal

LEARNING OBJECTIVES

On completion of this chapter, the reader will be able to:
- Identify typical signs of normal and abnormal fetal heart rate patterns.
- Compare fetal heart rate monitoring performed by intermittent auscultation with external and internal electronic methods.
- Explain the baseline fetal heart rate and evaluate periodic changes.

- Describe nursing measures that can be used to maintain fetal heart rate patterns within normal limits.
- Differentiate among the nursing interventions used for managing specific fetal heart rate patterns, including tachycardia and bradycardia, absent or minimal variability, and late and variable decelerations.
- Review the documentation of the monitoring process necessary during labor.

The ability to assess the fetus by auscultation of the fetal heart was initially described more than 300 years ago. With the advent of the fetoscope and stethoscope after the turn of the twentieth century, the listener could hear clearly enough to count the fetal heart rate (FHR). When electronic FHR monitoring made its debut for clinical use in the early 1970s, the anticipation was that its use would result in less intrapartum asphyxia and thus fewer cases of cerebral palsy. Consequently the use of electronic fetal monitoring rapidly expanded (Garite, 2012). However, the rate of cerebral palsy has not declined since that time and is not likely to decrease because more preterm infants are surviving (Gilbert, 2011). Prematurity is the leading cause of cerebral palsy. Intrapartum asphyxia accounts for 25% of cases or less of this disorder (Garite, 2012).

Still electronic fetal monitoring (EFM) is a useful tool for visualizing FHR patterns on a monitor screen or printed tracing. It continues to be the primary mode of intrapartum fetal assessment in the United States and is the most commonly performed obstetric procedure in that country (ACOG, 2009; Miller, Miller, and Tucker, 2013). Pregnant women should be informed about the equipment and procedures used and the risks, benefits, and limitations of intermittent auscultation (IA) and EFM. This chapter discusses the basis for intrapartum fetal monitoring, the types of monitoring, and nursing assessment and management of abnormal fetal status.

BASIS FOR MONITORING

Fetal Response

Because labor is a period of physiologic stress for the fetus, frequent monitoring of fetal status is part of the nursing care during labor. The fetal oxygen supply must be maintained during labor to prevent fetal compromise and promote newborn health after birth. The fetal oxygen supply can decrease in a number of ways:
- Reduction of blood flow through the maternal vessels as a result of maternal hypertension (chronic hypertension, preeclampsia, or gestational hypertension), hypotension (caused by supine maternal position, hemorrhage, or epidural analgesia or anesthesia), or hypovolemia (caused by hemorrhage)
- Reduction of the oxygen content in the maternal blood as a result of hemorrhage or severe anemia
- Alterations in fetal circulation, occurring with compression of the umbilical cord (transient, during uterine contractions [UCs], or prolonged, resulting from cord prolapse), partial placental separation or complete abruption, or head compression (head compression causes increased intracranial pressure and vagal nerve stimulation with an accompanying decrease in the FHR)
- Reduction in blood flow to the intervillous space in the placenta secondary to uterine hypertonus (generally caused by excessive exogenous oxytocin) or secondary to deterioration

of the placental vasculature associated with maternal disorders such as hypertension or diabetes mellitus

Fetal well-being during labor can be assessed by the response of the FHR to UCs. A group of fetal monitoring experts recommended that FHR tracings demonstrating certain reassuring characteristics be described as *normal* (category I) (Box 15-1).

Uterine Activity

Table 15-1 describes normal uterine activity (UA) during labor.

Fetal Compromise

The goals of intrapartum FHR monitoring are to identify and differentiate the normal (reassuring) patterns from the abnormal (nonreassuring) patterns, which can indicate fetal compromise. Although the 2008 National Institute of Child Health and Human Development workshop (Macones, Hankins, Spong, et al., 2008) and the ACOG (2009) both recommend use of the terms *normal* and *abnormal* to describe FHR tracings, the terms *reassuring* and *nonreassuring* are still frequently used clinically.

Abnormal FHR patterns are those associated with fetal hypoxemia, which is a deficiency of oxygen in the arterial blood. If uncorrected, hypoxemia can deteriorate to severe fetal hypoxia, an inadequate supply of oxygen at the cellular level that can cause metabolic acidosis. The term asphyxia is used when fetal hypoxia results in metabolic acidosis (Garite, 2012). See Box 15-1 for examples of abnormal (category III) FHR tracings.

BOX 15-1 THREE-TIER FETAL HEART RATE CLASSIFICATION SYSTEM

Category I

Category I fetal heart rate (FHR) tracings include all of the following:

- Baseline rate 110 to 160 beats/min
- Baseline FHR variability: Moderate
- Late or variable decelerations: Absent
- Early decelerations: Either present or absent
- Accelerations: Either present or absent

Category II

Category II FHR tracings include all FHR tracings not categorized as category I or category III. Examples of category II tracings include any of the following:

- Baseline rate
  - Bradycardia not accompanied by absent baseline variability
  - Tachycardia
- Baseline FHR variability
  - Minimal baseline variability
  - Absent baseline variability not accompanied by recurrent decelerations
  - Marked baseline variability
- Accelerations
  - No acceleration produced in response to fetal stimulation
- Periodic or episodic decelerations
  - Recurrent variable decelerations accompanied by minimal or moderate baseline variability
  - Prolonged decelerations (≥2 minutes but <10 minutes)
  - Recurrent late decelerations with moderate baseline variability
  - Variable decelerations with other characteristics such as slow return to baseline, "overshoots," or "shoulders"

Category III

Category III FHR tracings include either:

- Absent baseline variability and any of the following:
  - Recurrent late decelerations
  - Recurrent variable decelerations
  - Bradycardia
- Sinusoidal pattern

From Macones GA, Hankins GD, Spong CY, et al: The 2008 National Institute of Child Health and Human Development Workshop Report on Electronic Fetal Monitoring: update on definitions, interpretation, and research guidelines, *J Obstet Gynecol Neonatal Nurs* 37(5):510–515, 2008.

TABLE 15-1 NORMAL UTERINE ACTIVITY DURING LABOR

CHARACTERISTIC	DESCRIPTION
Frequency	Contraction frequency overall generally ranges from two to five per 10 minutes during labor, with lower frequencies seen in first stage of labor and higher frequencies (up to five contractions in 10 minutes) seen during second stage of labor.
Duration	Contraction duration remains fairly stable throughout first and second stages, ranging from 45-80 seconds, not generally exceeding 90 seconds.
Strength	Uterine contractions generally range from peaking at 40-70 mm Hg in first stage of labor to over 80 mm Hg in second stage. Contractions palpated as "mild" would likely peak at less than 50 mm Hg if measured internally, whereas contractions palpated as "moderate" or greater would likely peak at 50 mm Hg or greater if measured internally.
Resting tone	Average resting tone during labor is 10 mm Hg; if using palpation, should palpate as "soft" (i.e., easily indented, no palpable resistance).
Relaxation time	Relaxation time is commonly 60 seconds or more in first stage and 45 seconds or more in second stage.
Montevideo units (MVUs)	MVUs usually range from 100-250 in first stage; may rise to 300-400 in the second stage. Contraction intensities of 40 mm Hg or more and MVUs of 80-120 are generally sufficient to initiate spontaneous labor. MVUs are used only with internal monitoring of contractions.

Data from Macones GA, Hankins GD, Spong CY, et al: The 2008 National Institute of Child Health and Human Development Workshop Report on Electronic Fetal Monitoring: update on definitions, interpretation, and research guidelines, *J Obstet Gynecol Neonatal Nurs* 37(5):510–515, 2008; Miller LA, Miller DA, Tucker SM: *Mosby's pocket guide to fetal monitoring: a multidisciplinary approach*, ed 7, St Louis, 2013, Mosby.

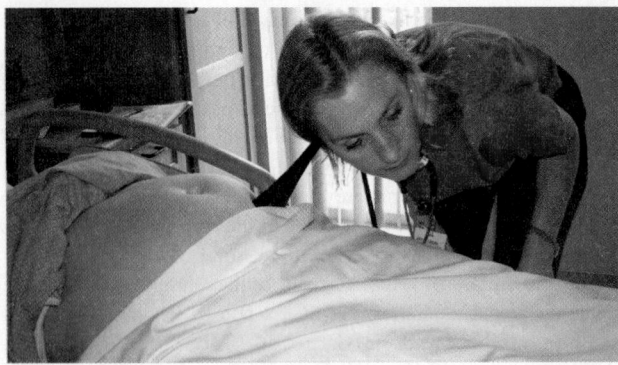

FIG 15-1 Pinard stethoscope. NOTE: Hands should not touch stethoscope while nurse is listening. (Courtesy Julie Perry Nelson, Loveland, CO.)

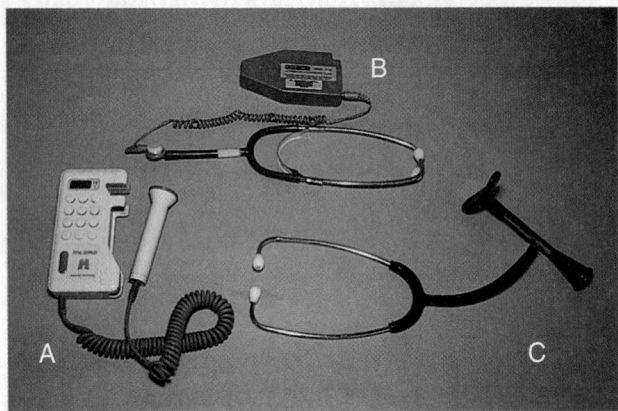

FIG 15-2 A, Ultrasound fetoscope. **B,** Ultrasound stethoscope. **C,** DeLee-Hillis fetoscope. (Courtesy Michael S. Clement, MD, Mesa, AZ.)

MONITORING TECHNIQUES

The ideal method of fetal assessment during labor continues to be debated. Research findings support the use of both IA of the FHR and EFM (Gilbert, 2011). Although IA is a high-touch, low-technology method of assessing fetal status during labor that places fewer restrictions on maternal activity, more than 85% of laboring women in the United States are monitored electronically for at least part of their labor (ACOG, 2009; Miller, Miller, and Tucker, 2013). The continued use of EFM in place of IA is thought to be because of concerns about liability and the increased nurse-patient ratio required with IA. Because all surveillance methods, including EFM, have limitations, some believe that the evidence supports a return to the use of IA for low risk laboring women (ACOG, 2009; Miller, Miller, and Tucker, 2013).

Intermittent Auscultation

Intermittent auscultation involves listening to fetal heart sounds at periodic intervals to assess the FHR. IA of the fetal heart can be performed with a Pinard stethoscope (Fig. 15-1), Doppler ultrasound (Fig. 15-2, *A*), an ultrasound stethoscope (see Fig. 15-2, *B*), or a DeLee-Hillis fetoscope (see Fig. 15-2, *C*). Doppler ultrasound and ultrasound stethoscopes transmit ultra high–frequency sound waves, reflecting movement of the fetal heart, and convert these sounds into an electronic signal that can be counted. The fetoscope is applied to the listener's forehead because bone conduction

1. Palpate maternal abdomen to identify fetal presentation and position.
2. Apply ultrasonic gel to device if using Doppler ultrasound. Place listening device (see Figs. 15-1 and 15-2) over area of maximal intensity and clarity of fetal heart sounds to obtain clearest and loudest sound, which is easiest to count. This location is usually over the fetal back. If using fetoscope, firm pressure may be needed.
3. Count maternal radial pulse while listening to FHR to differentiate it from fetal rate.
4. Palpate abdomen for presence or absence of UA to count FHR between contractions.
5. Count FHR for 30 to 60 seconds after a uterine contraction to identify auscultated baseline rate and changes (increases or decreases) in it.
6. Auscultate FHR before, during, and after contraction to identify FHR during the contraction or as a response to the contraction and to assess for absence or presence of increases or decreases in FHR.
7. When distinct discrepancies in FHR are noted during listening periods, auscultate for longer period during, after, and between contractions to identify significant changes that may indicate need for another mode of FHR monitoring.

From Miller LA, Miller DA, Tucker SM: Mosby's pocket guide to fetal monitoring: a multidisciplinary approach, ed 7, St Louis, 2013, Mosby.
FHR, Fetal heart rate; *UA,* uterine activity.

amplifies the fetal heart sounds for counting. Box 15-2 describes how to perform IA.

IA is easy to use, inexpensive, and less invasive than EFM. It is often more comfortable for the woman and gives her more freedom of movement. Other care measures such as ambulation and the use of baths or showers are easier to carry out when IA is used. However, it may be difficult to perform transabdominally in women who are obese. A transvaginal fetal Doppler probe is now available. It provides closer proximity to the uterus, making it easier to auscultate the FHR when the woman is obese or early in gestation (Miller, Miller, and Tucker, 2013). Because IA is intermittent, significant events may occur during a time when the FHR is not being auscultated. In addition, IA does not provide a permanent documented visual record of the FHR and cannot be used to assess visual patterns of the FHR variability or periodic changes (Miller, Miller, and Tucker, 2013). By using IA the nurse can assess the baseline FHR, rhythm, and increases and decreases from baseline.

The American College of Nurse-Midwives (ACNM) reviewed references from the United States, Great Britain, and Canada regarding the recommended frequency of IA in low risk women and found consistent recommendations for every 15 minutes in the active phase of the first stage of labor and every 5 minutes in the second stage of labor (Miller, Miller, and Tucker, 2013). The ACOG (2009) agrees that these time frames are acceptable for IA in low risk women. The Association of Women's Health, Obstetric and Neonatal Nurses recommends different IA frequencies: every hour in the latent phase of first-stage labor, every 30 minutes in the active phase of first-stage labor, and every 15 minutes in the second stage of labor (AWHONN, 2009). However, the optimal frequency for IA in low risk women during labor has not been determined (Nageotte and Gilstrap, 2009).

! NURSING ALERT

When the FHR is auscultated and documented, it is inappropriate to use the descriptive terms associated with EFM (e.g., moderate variability, variable deceleration) because most of the terms are visual descriptions of the patterns produced on the monitor tracing. However, terms that are numerically defined such as bradycardia and tachycardia can be used. When FHR is auscultated, it should be described as a baseline number or range and as having a regular or irregular rhythm. The presence or absence of accelerations or decelerations both during and after contractions should also be noted (AWHONN, 2009; Miller, Miller, and Tucker, 2013).

Every effort should be made to use the method of fetal assessment the woman desires if possible. However, auscultation of the FHR in accordance with the frequency guidelines suggested earlier may be difficult in today's busy labor and birth units. When used as the primary method of fetal assessment, auscultation requires a one-to-one nurse-to-patient staffing ratio. If acuity and census change so auscultation standards are no longer met, the nurse must inform the physician or nurse-midwife that continuous EFM will be used until staffing can be arranged to meet the standards.

The woman can become anxious if the examiner cannot readily count the fetal heartbeats. It often takes time for the inexperienced listener to locate the heartbeat and find the area of maximal intensity. To allay the mother's concerns, she can be told that the nurse is "finding the spot where the sounds are loudest." If it takes considerable time to locate the fetal heartbeats, the examiner can reassure the mother by offering her an opportunity to listen to them. If the examiner cannot locate the fetal heartbeat, assistance should be requested. In some cases ultrasound can be used to help locate the fetal heartbeat. Seeing the FHR on the ultrasound screen is reassuring to the mother if there was initial difficulty in locating the best area for auscultation.

When using IA, UA is assessed by palpation. The examiner should keep his or her fingertips placed over the fundus before, during, and after contractions. The contraction intensity is usually described as mild, moderate, or strong. The contraction duration is measured in seconds, from the beginning to the end of the contraction. The frequency of contractions is measured in minutes, from the beginning of one contraction to the beginning of the next. The examiner should keep his or her hand on the fundus after the contraction is over to evaluate uterine resting tone or relaxation between contractions. Resting tone between contractions is usually described as soft or relaxed (AWHONN, 2009).

Accurate and complete documentation of fetal status and UA is especially important when IA and palpation are being used because no paper tracing record or computer storage of these assessments is provided as is the case with continuous EFM. Labor flow records or computer charting systems that prompt notations of all assessments are useful for ensuring such comprehensive documentation.

Electronic Fetal Monitoring

The purpose of EFM is the ongoing assessment of fetal oxygenation. FHR tracings are analyzed for characteristic patterns that suggest fetal hypoxic events and metabolic acidosis during labor. When hypoxia or metabolic acidosis is suspected in labor, interventions to resolve the problem can be implemented in a timely manner before permanent damage or death occurs (Garite, 2012). The two modes of EFM are the external mode, which uses external transducers placed on the maternal abdomen to assess FHR and UA; and the internal mode, which uses a spiral electrode applied to the fetal

TABLE 15-2	EXTERNAL AND INTERNAL MODES OF MONITORING	
EXTERNAL MODE	**INTERNAL MODE**
Fetal Heart Rate	
Ultrasound transducer:	*Spiral electrode:*
High-frequency sound waves reflect mechanical action of fetal heart; noninvasive; does not require rupture of membranes or cervical dilation; used during both antepartum and intrapartum periods	Converts fetal ECG as obtained from presenting part to FHR via cardiotachometer; can be used only when membranes are ruptured and cervix is sufficiently dilated during intrapartum period; electrode penetrates into fetal presenting part by 1.5 mm and must be attached securely to ensure good signal
Uterine Activity	
Tocotransducer:	*Intrauterine pressure catheter (IUPC):*
Monitors frequency and duration of contractions by means of pressure-sensing device applied to maternal abdomen; used during both antepartum and intrapartum periods.	Monitors frequency, duration, and intensity of contractions; two types of IUPCs: fluid-filled system and solid catheter; both measure intrauterine pressure at catheter tip and convert pressure into millimeters of mercury on uterine activity panel of strip chart; both can be used only when membranes are ruptured and cervix is sufficiently dilated during intrapartum period

ECG, Electrocardiogram; *FHR*, fetal heart rate.

presenting part to assess the FHR and an intrauterine pressure catheter (IUPC) to assess UA and uterine resting tone. The differences between the external and internal modes of EFM are summarized in Table 15-2.

External Monitoring

Separate transducers are used to monitor the FHR and UCs (Fig. 15-3). The ultrasound transducer works by reflecting high-frequency sound waves off a moving interface, in this case the fetal heart and valves. It is sometimes difficult to reproduce a continuous and precise record of the FHR because of artifact introduced by fetal and maternal movement. Maternal obesity, occiput posterior position of the fetus, and anterior attachment of the placenta can cause weak or absent signals (AWHONN, 2009). The FHR is printed on specially formatted monitor paper. The standard paper speed used in the United States is 3 cm/min. Once the area of maximal intensity of the FHR has been located, conductive gel is applied to the surface of the ultrasound transducer, and the transducer is then positioned over this area and held securely in place using an elastic belt (see Critical Thinking Case Study).

The tocotransducer (tocodynamometer) measures UA transabdominally. The device is placed over the fundus above the umbilicus and held securely in place with an elastic belt (see Fig. 15-3, *B*). UCs or fetal movements depress a pressure-sensitive surface on the side next to the abdomen. The tocotransducer can measure and record the frequency and approximate duration of UCs but not their intensity. This method is especially valuable for measuring UA during the first stage of labor in women with intact membranes or for

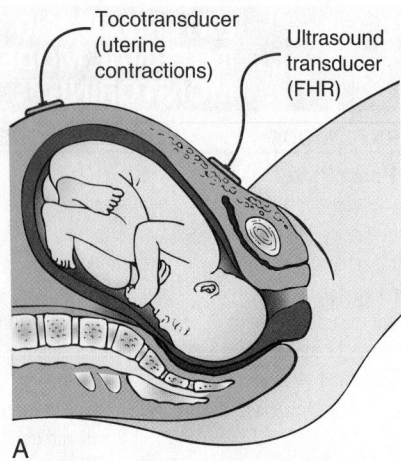
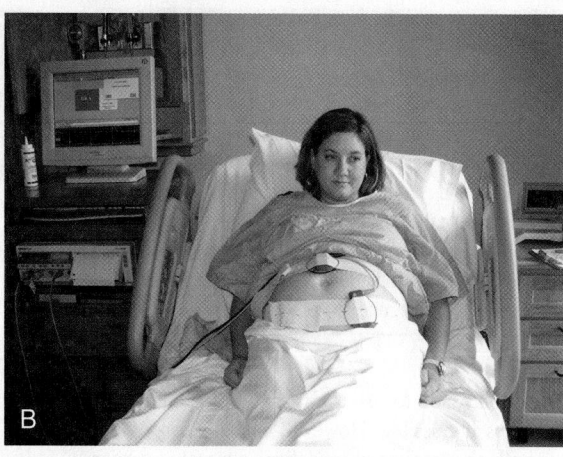

FIG 15-3 A, External noninvasive fetal monitoring with tocotransducer and ultrasound transducer. *FHR,* fetal heart rate. **B,** Ultrasound transducer is placed below umbilicus over area where fetal heart rate is best heard, and tocotransducer is placed on uterine fundus. (*B,* Courtesy Julie Perry Nelson, Loveland, CO.)

CRITICAL THINKING CASE STUDY

Fetal Heart Rate Recording

You are assigned to Lauren, a 29-year-old G1 P0 who is in the first stage of labor. She wonders why the fetal heart rate (FHR) is sometimes not being recorded on the monitor paper. She asks if there is "something wrong with the baby" when the FHR is not recording continuously. Based on your knowledge of how the external monitor works, you explain the lack of continuous recording of the FHR and how you plan to improve the tracing and document your observations.

1. Evidence—Is there sufficient evidence to draw any conclusions about what causes gaps in recording on the monitor paper and ways to improve the tracing?
2. Assumptions—Describe an underlying assumption about each of the following issues:
   a. Efficacy of FHR monitoring in improving pregnancy outcome
   b. Causes of poor quality tracings when using the external mode of FHR monitoring
   c. Signs of abnormal FHR patterns
   d. Causes of periodic and episodic changes in the FHR
3. What implications and priorities for nursing care can be drawn at this time?
4. Does the evidence objectively support your argument (conclusion)?

antepartum testing. If the woman is obese, the tocotransducer may be unable to detect the exact frequency and duration of UA.

Because the tocotransducer of most electronic fetal monitors is designed for assessing UA in the term pregnancy, it may not be sensitive enough to detect preterm UA. When monitoring the woman in preterm labor, remember that the fundus may be located below the level of the umbilicus. The nurse may need to rely on the woman to indicate when UA is occurring and to use palpation as an additional way of assessing contraction frequency and validating the monitor tracing.

The external transducers are applied easily by the nurse but often must be repositioned as the woman or fetus changes position. The woman is asked to assume a semi-Fowler's or lateral position. Use of external transducers confines the woman to bed or chair.

Portable **telemetry** monitors allow observation of the FHR and UC patterns by means of centrally located electronic display stations. These portable units permit the woman to walk around during electronic monitoring.

In 2011 an external monitor became available for use in the United States. The Monica AN24 uses abdominally obtained electronic impulses to monitor both FHR and UA (Fig. 15-4, A and B). The monitor uses five electrodes placed on the woman's abdomen to directly monitor the electrocardiogram from the maternal and fetal hearts and the electromyogram from the uterine muscle. This information is transmitted wirelessly, via Bluetooth technology, to an interface device that allows the FHR and UA data to print or display on a standard fetal monitor (Miller, Miller, and Tucker, 2013).

The Monica AN24 eliminates much of the problem caused by signal loss resulting from maternal or fetal movement or maternal obesity that often occurs with traditional external monitors. The monitor also more accurately measures the frequency, occurrence of peak, and duration of UCs than does the traditional tocotransducer, although it does not provide actual intensity measurement in millimeters of mercury (mm Hg) as an IUPC does. Other advantages of the Monica AN24 are that it eliminates the need for abdominal belts and frequent readjustment of the tocotransducer and ultrasound transducer and provides some patient mobility. The woman may move up to 50 feet away from the interface device without signal loss (Fig. 15-5, A and B). In the United States the Monica AN24 is only approved for use in pregnancies that have reached 36 completed weeks or more of gestation (Miller, Miller, and Tucker, 2013). The Monica AN24 monitor may not be readily available for use in all labor and birth settings.

Internal Monitoring

The technique of continuous internal FHR or UA monitoring provides a more accurate appraisal of fetal well-being during labor than external monitoring because it is not interrupted by fetal or maternal movement or affected by maternal size (Fig. 15-6). For this type of monitoring the membranes must be ruptured, the cervix sufficiently dilated (at least 2 to 3 cm), and the presenting part low enough to allow placement of the spiral electrode or IUPC or both. Internal and external modes of monitoring may be combined (i.e., internal FHR with external UA or external FHR with internal UA) without difficulty.

Internal monitoring of the FHR is accomplished by attaching a small spiral electrode to the presenting part. For UA to be monitored

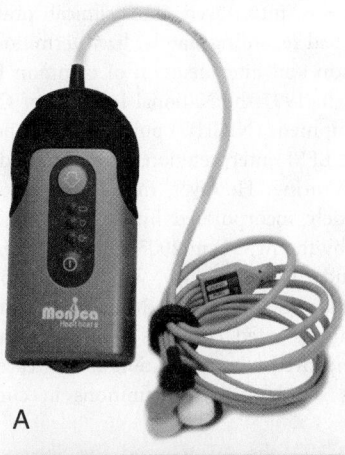

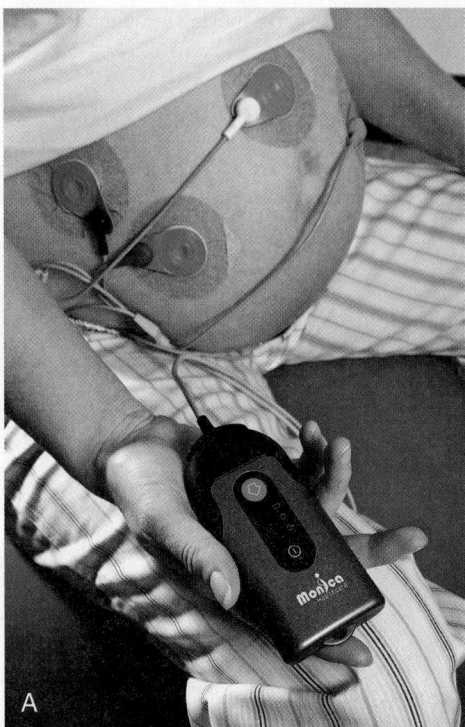

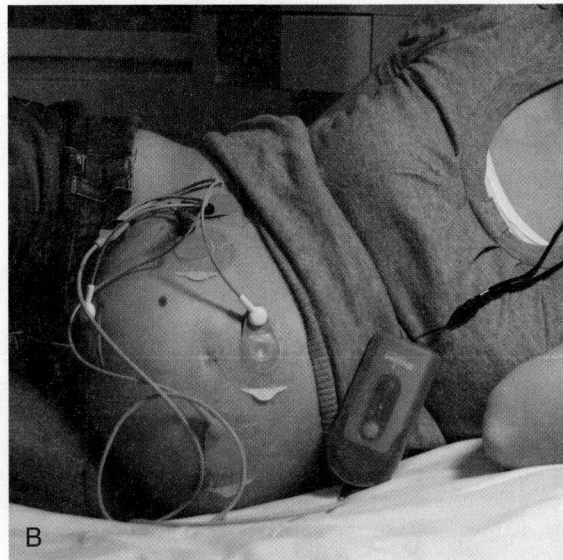

FIG 15-4 A, Monica AN24 is a wireless and beltless device that can be used with existing monitors to obtain fetal heart rate via abdominal electrocardiogram (ECG). **B,** Electrodes placed on maternal abdomen monitor ECG from fetal and maternal heart and electromyogram (EMG) from uterine muscle. (Courtesy Monica Healthcare Ltd, Nottingham, UK.)

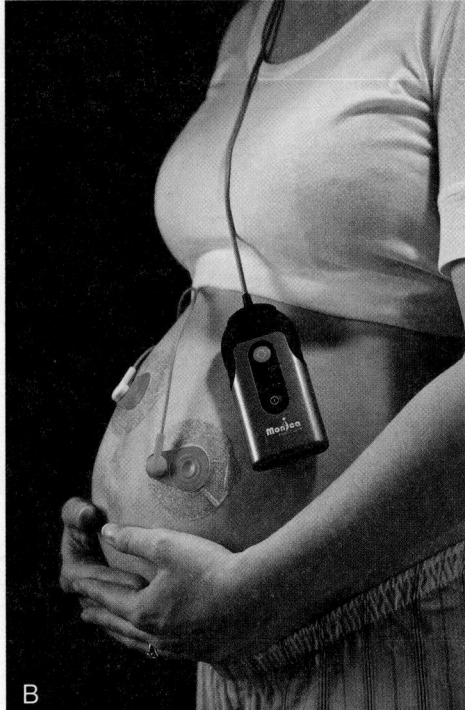

FIG 15-5 A, Woman sitting on birthing ball, and **B,** woman ambulating, both wearing Monica AN 24. (Courtesy Monica Healthcare Ltd, Nottingham, UK.)

internally an IUPC is introduced into the uterine cavity. The catheter has a pressure-sensitive tip that measures changes in intrauterine pressure. As the catheter is compressed during a contraction, pressure is placed on the pressure transducer. This pressure is then converted into a pressure reading in millimeters of mercury. The IUPC can objectively measure the frequency, duration, and intensity of UCs and uterine resting tone.

Because it can measure the intensity of individual UCs precisely, the IUPC can be used to evaluate the adequacy of UA for achieving progress in labor. **Montevideo units (MVUs)** are calculated by subtracting the baseline uterine pressure from the peak contraction pressure for each contraction that occurs in a 10-minute window and then adding together the pressures generated by each contraction that occurs during that period of time. Spontaneous labor usually begins when MVUs are between 80 and 120. Uterine activity during the first stage of normal labor rarely exceeds 250 MVUs (see Table 15-1) (Cunningham, Leveno, Bloom, et al., 2010; Miller, Miller, and Tucker, 2013).

Display

The FHR and UA are displayed on the monitor paper or computer screen, with the FHR in the upper section and UA in the lower section. Fig. 15-7 contrasts the internal and external modes of electronic monitoring. Note that each small square on the monitor paper or screen represents 10 seconds; each larger box of six squares equals 1 minute (when paper is moving through the monitor at the rate of 3 cm/min).

FETAL HEART RATE PATTERNS

Characteristic FHR patterns are associated with fetal and maternal physiologic processes and have been identified for many years.

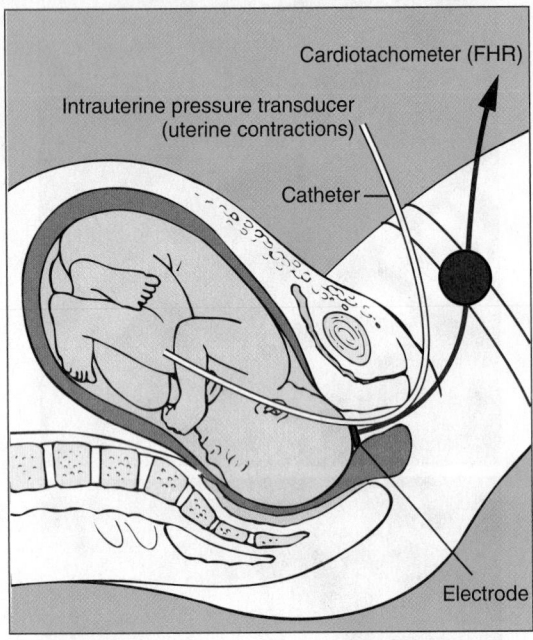

FIG 15-6 Diagrammatic representation of internal invasive fetal monitoring with intrauterine pressure catheter and spiral electrode in place (membranes ruptured and cervix dilated).

However, because EFM was introduced into clinical practice before consensus was reached regarding standardized terminology, variations in the description and interpretation of common FHR patterns were often great. In 1997 the National Institute of Child Health and Human Development (NICHD) published a proposed nomenclature system for EFM interpretation with standardized definitions for FHR monitoring. However, the NICHD recommendations were not widely incorporated into clinical practice until they were endorsed by the ACOG in 2005. Shortly thereafter use of the NICHD standard terminology was also endorsed by the AWHONN and the ACNM (Miller, Miller, and Tucker, 2013). All three organizations cited concerns regarding patient safety and the need for improved communication among caregivers as reasons for using standard EFM definitions in clinical practice.

In April 2008 the NICHD, the ACOG, and the Society for Maternal-Fetal Medicine partnered to sponsor another workshop to revisit the FHR definitions recommended by the NICHD in 1997. The 1997 FHR definitions were reaffirmed at this workshop. In addition, new definitions related to UA and a three-tier system of FHR pattern interpretation and categorization were recommended (see Box 15-1) (Macones, Hankins, Spong, et al., 2008).

Baseline Fetal Heart Rate

The intrinsic rhythmicity of the fetal heart, the central nervous system (CNS), and the fetal autonomic nervous system control the FHR. An increase in sympathetic response results in acceleration of the FHR, whereas an increase in parasympathetic response produces a slowing of the FHR. Usually a balanced increase of sympathetic and parasympathetic response occurs during contractions, with no observable change in the baseline FHR.

The baseline FHR is the average rate during a 10-minute segment that excludes periodic or episodic changes, periods of marked variability, and segments of the baseline that differ by more than 25

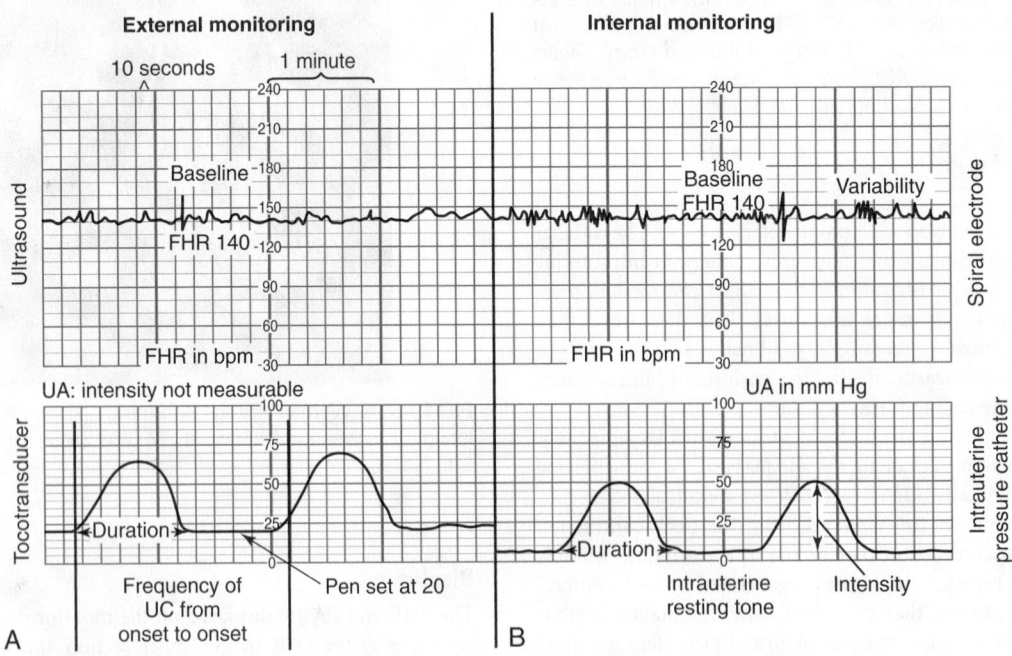

FIG 15-7 Display of fetal heart rate **(A)** and uterine activity **(B)**. *FHR,* Fetal heart rate; *UC,* uterine contraction. (From Miller LA, Miller DA, Tucker SM: *Mosby's pocket guide to fetal monitoring: a multidisciplinary approach,* ed 7, St Louis, 2013, Mosby.)

beats/min. There must be at least 2 minutes of interpretable baseline data in a 10-minute segment of tracing to determine the baseline FHR (Macones, Hankins, Spong, et al., 2008). After 10 minutes of tracing is observed, the approximate mean rate is rounded to the closest 5 beats/min interval (AWHONN, 2009). For example, if the FHR rate varies between 130 and 140 beats/min over a 10-minute period, the baseline is recorded as 135 beats/min. The normal range at term is 110 to 160 beats/min. In the preterm fetus the baseline rate is slightly higher.

Variability

Variability of the FHR can be described as irregular waves or fluctuations in the baseline FHR of two cycles per minute or greater (Macones, Hankins, Spong, et al., 2008). It is a characteristic of the baseline FHR and does not include accelerations or decelerations of the FHR. Variability is quantified in beats per minute and is measured from the peak to the trough of a single cycle. Four possible categories of variability have been identified: absent, minimal, moderate, and marked (Fig. 15-8). In the past variability was described

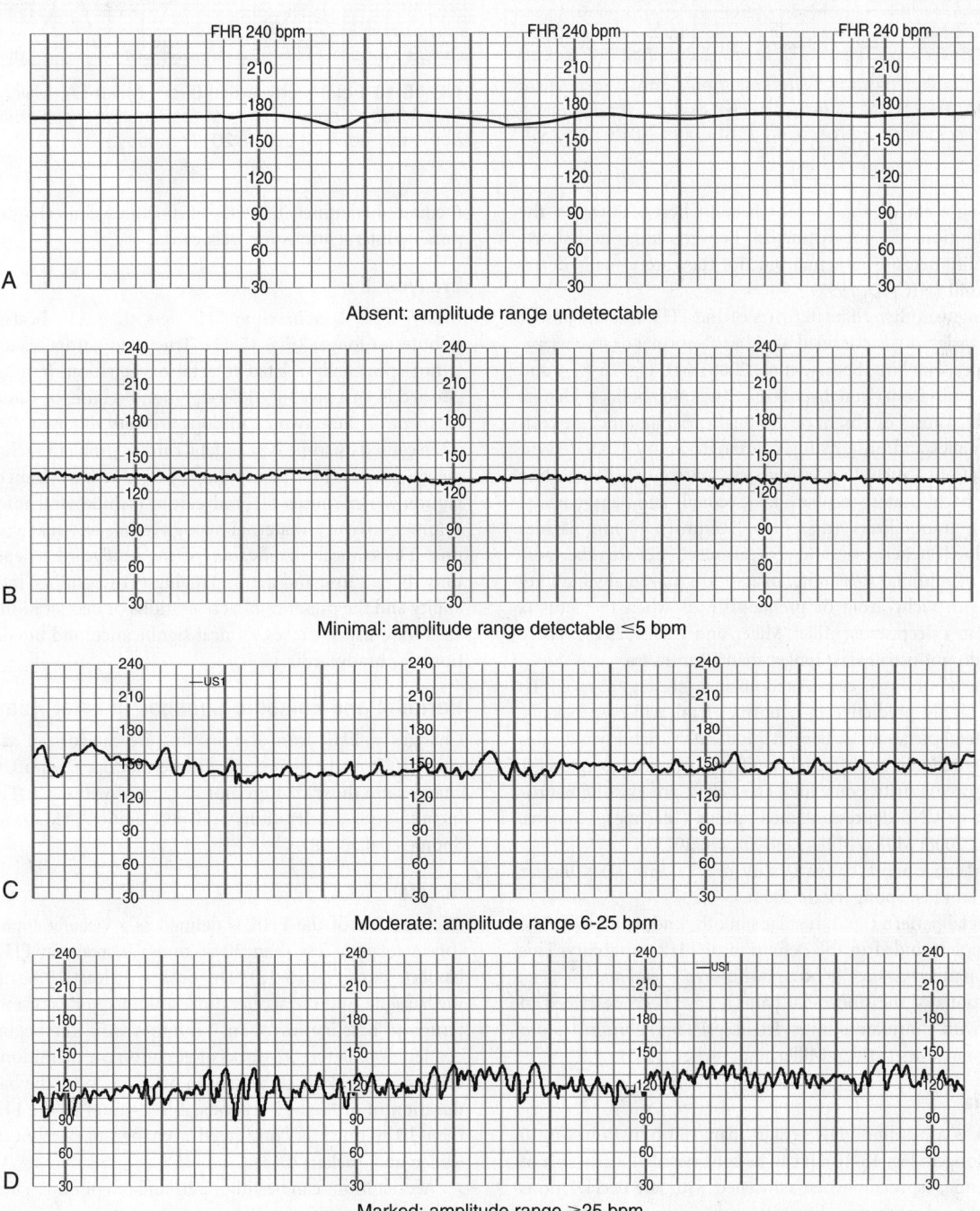

FIG 15-8 Fetal heart rate variability. **A,** Absent: amplitude range undetectable. **B,** Minimal: amplitude range detectable ≤5 beats/min. **C,** Moderate: amplitude range 6-25 beats/min. **D,** Marked: amplitude range ≥25 beats/min. *FHR,* Fetal heart rate. (From Miller LA, Miller DA, Tucker SM: *Mosby's pocket guide to fetal monitoring: a multidisciplinary approach,* ed 7, St Louis, 2013, Mosby.)

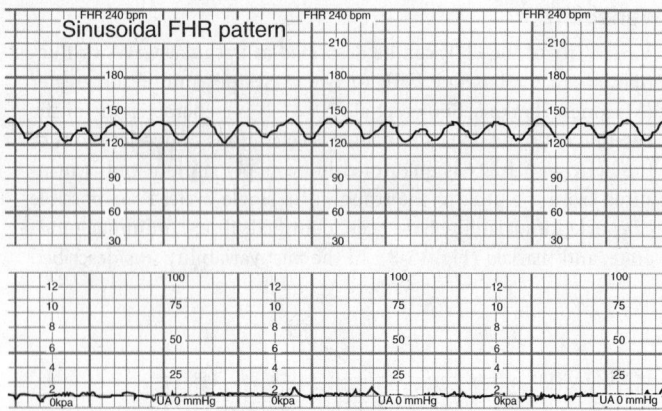

FIG 15-9 Sinusoidal pattern. *FHR,* Fetal heart rate. (From Miller LA, Miller DA, Tucker SM: *Mosby's pocket guide to fetal monitoring: a multidisciplinary approach*, ed 7, St Louis, 2013, Mosby.)

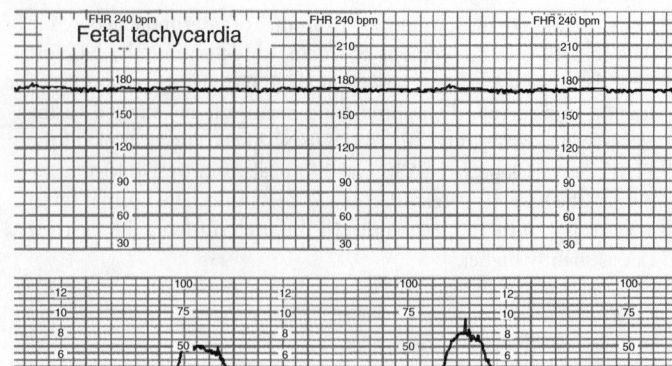

FIG 15-10 Fetal tachycardia. (From Miller LA, Miller DA, Tucker SM: *Mosby's pocket guide to fetal monitoring: a multidisciplinary approach*, ed 7, St Louis, 2013, Mosby.)

as either long term or short term (beat to beat). However, the NICHD definitions do not distinguish between long- and short-term variability because in actual practice they are visually determined as a unit (NICHD, 1997).

Depending on other characteristics of the FHR tracing, absent or minimal variability is classified as either abnormal or indeterminate (Macones, Hankins, Spong, et al., 2008) (see Fig. 15-8, *A* and *B*). It can result from fetal hypoxemia and metabolic acidemia. Other possible causes of absent or minimal variability include congenital anomalies and pre-existing neurologic injury. CNS depressant medications, including analgesics, narcotics (meperidine [Demerol]), barbiturates (secobarbital [Seconal] and pentobarbital [Nembutal]), tranquilizers (diazepam [Valium]), phenothiazines (promethazine [Phenergan]), and general anesthetics are other possible causes of minimal variability. In addition, minimal variability can occur with tachycardia or prematurity or when the fetus is temporarily in a sleep state (Miller, Miller, and Tucker, 2013). These sleep states do not usually last longer than 30 minutes.

Moderate variability is considered normal (see Fig. 15-8, *C*). Its presence is highly predictive of a normal fetal acid-base balance (absence of fetal metabolic acidemia). Moderate variability indicates that FHR regulation is not affected significantly by fetal sleep cycles, tachycardia, prematurity, congenital anomalies, pre-existing neurologic injury, or CNS depressant medications (Macones, Hankins, Spong, et al., 2008; Miller, Miller, and Tucker, 2013).

The significance of marked variability (see Fig. 15-8, *D*) is unclear (Macones, Hankins, Spong, et al., 2008).

A sinusoidal pattern (i.e., a regular smooth, undulating wavelike pattern) is not included in the definition of FHR variability. This uncommon pattern classically occurs with severe fetal anemia (Fig. 15-9). Variations of the sinusoidal pattern have been described in association with chorioamnionitis, fetal sepsis, and administration of narcotic analgesics (Miller, Miller, and Tucker, 2013).

Tachycardia

Tachycardia is a baseline FHR greater than 160 beats/min for 10 minutes or longer (Fig. 15-10). It can be considered an early sign of fetal hypoxemia, especially when associated with late decelerations and minimal or absent variability. Fetal tachycardia can result from maternal or fetal infection such as prolonged rupture of membranes with amnionitis; from maternal hyperthyroidism or fetal anemia; or in response to medications such as atropine, hydroxyzine (Vistaril), terbutaline (Brethine), or illicit drugs such as cocaine or

methamphetamines. Table 15-3 lists causes, clinical significance, and nursing interventions for tachycardia.

Bradycardia

Bradycardia is a baseline FHR less than 110 beats/min for 10 minutes or longer (Fig. 15-11). True bradycardia occurs rarely and is not specifically related to fetal oxygenation. It must be distinguished from a prolonged deceleration because the causes and management of these two conditions are very different. Bradycardia is often caused by some type of fetal cardiac problem such as structural defects involving the pacemakers or conduction system or fetal heart failure. Other causes of bradycardia include viral infections (e.g., cytomegalovirus), maternal hypoglycemia, and maternal hypothermia. The clinical significance of the bradycardia depends on the underlying cause and accompanying FHR patterns, including variability and the presence of accelerations or decelerations. (See Table 15-3 for a list of causes, clinical significance, and nursing interventions for bradycardia.)

Periodic and Episodic Changes in Fetal Heart Rate

Changes in FHR from the baseline are categorized as periodic or episodic. Periodic changes are those that occur with UCs. Episodic changes are those that are not associated with UCs. These changes include both accelerations and decelerations (Macones, Hankins, Spong, et al., 2008).

Accelerations

Acceleration of the FHR is defined as a visually apparent, abrupt (onset to peak less than 30 seconds) increase in FHR above the baseline rate (Fig. 15-12). The peak is at least 15 beats/min above the baseline, and the acceleration lasts 15 seconds or more, with the return to baseline less than 2 minutes from the beginning of the acceleration. Before 32 weeks of gestation the definition of an acceleration is a peak of 10 beats/min or more above the baseline and a duration of at least 10 seconds. Acceleration of the FHR for more than 10 minutes is considered a change in baseline rate (Miller, Miller, and Tucker, 2013).

Accelerations can be either periodic or episodic. They may occur in association with fetal movement or spontaneously. If accelerations do not occur spontaneously, they can be elicited by fetal scalp or vibroacoustic stimulation. Similar to moderate variability, accelerations are considered an indication of fetal well-being. Their presence is highly predictive of a normal fetal acid-base balance (absence

TABLE 15-3	TACHYCARDIA AND BRADYCARDIA
TACHYCARDIA	**BRADYCARDIA**
Definition	
FHR >160 beats/min lasting >10 minutes	FHR <110 beats/min lasting >10 minutes
Possible Causes	
Early fetal hypoxemia	Atrioventricular dissociation (heart block)
Fetal cardiac arrhythmias	Structural defects
Maternal fever	Viral infections (e.g., cytomegalovirus)
Infection (including chorioamnionitis)	Medications
Parasympatholytic drugs (atropine, hydroxyzine)	Fetal heart failure
β-Sympathomimetic drugs (terbutaline)	Maternal hypoglycemia
Maternal hyperthyroidism	Maternal hypothermia
Fetal anemia	
Drugs (caffeine, cocaine, methamphetamines)	
Clinical Significance	
Persistent tachycardia in absence of periodic changes does not appear serious in terms of neonatal outcome (especially true if tachycardia is associated with maternal fever); tachycardia is abnormal when associated with late decelerations, severe variable decelerations, or absent variability.	Baseline bradycardia alone is not specifically related to fetal oxygenation. Clinical significance of bradycardia depends on underlying cause and accompanying FHR patterns, including variability, accelerations, or decelerations.
Nursing Interventions	
Dependent on cause; reduce maternal fever with antipyretics as ordered and cooling measures; oxygen at 10 L/min by nonrebreather face mask may be of some value; carry out health care provider's orders based on alleviating cause	Dependent on cause

FHR, Fetal heart rate.

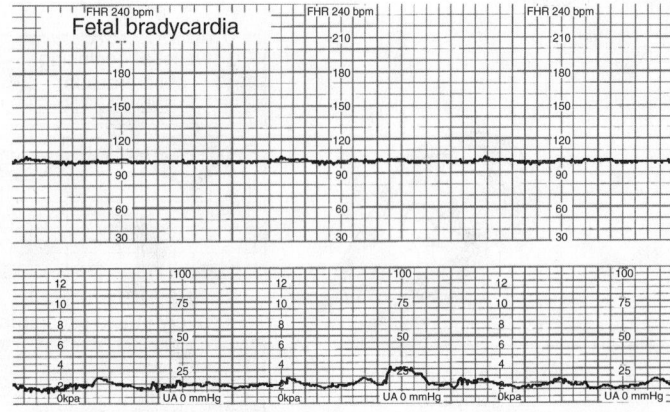

FIG 15-11 Fetal bradycardia. (From Miller LA, Miller DA, Tucker SM: *Mosby's pocket guide to fetal monitoring: a multidisciplinary approach*, ed 7, St Louis, 2013, Mosby.)

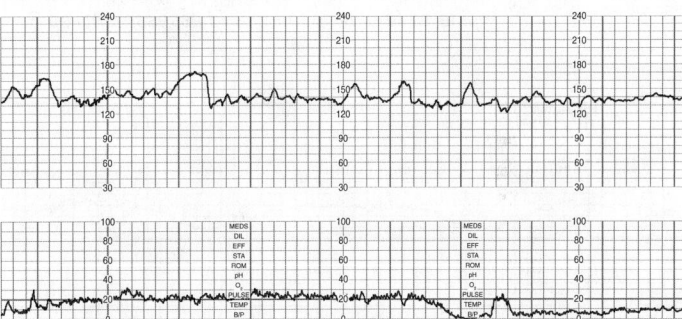

FIG 15-12 Accelerations of fetal heart rate in a term pregnancy. (From Miller LA, Miller DA, Tucker SM: *Mosby's pocket guide to fetal monitoring: a multidisciplinary approach*, ed 7, St Louis, 2013, Mosby.)

BOX 15-3	ACCELERATIONS

Causes
- Spontaneous fetal movement
- Vaginal examination
- Electrode application
- Fetal scalp stimulation
- Fetal reaction to external sounds
- Breech presentation
- Occiput posterior position
- Uterine contractions
- Fundal pressure
- Abdominal palpation

Clinical Significance
- Normal pattern: Acceleration with fetal movement signifies fetal well-being representing fetal alertness or arousal states.

Nursing Interventions
- None required

of fetal metabolic acidemia) (Miller, Miller, and Tucker, 2013). Box 15-3 lists causes, clinical significance, and nursing interventions for accelerations.

Decelerations

A deceleration (caused by dominance of a parasympathetic response) may be benign or abnormal. FHR decelerations are categorized as early, late, variable, or prolonged. They are described by their visual relation to the onset and end of a contraction and by their shape.

Early Decelerations. Early deceleration of the FHR is a visually apparent, gradual (onset to lowest point ≥30 seconds) decrease in

and return to baseline FHR associated with UCs. It is thought to be caused by transient fetal head compression and is considered a normal and benign finding (Macones, Hankins, Spong, et al., 2008; Miller, Miller, and Tucker, 2013). Generally the onset, nadir, and recovery of the deceleration correspond to the beginning, peak, and

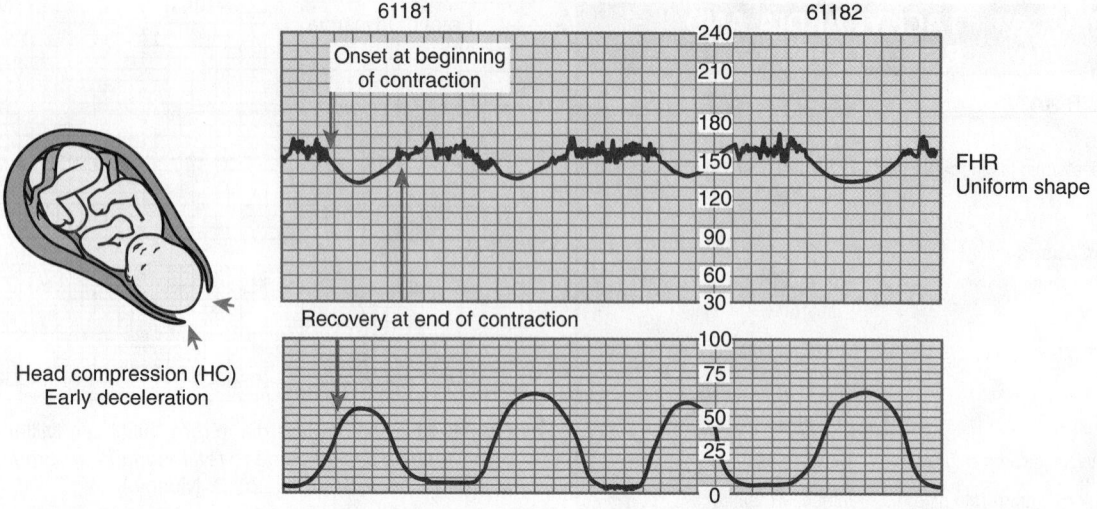

61181   61182

Onset at beginning of contraction

FHR
Uniform shape

Recovery at end of contraction

Head compression (HC)
Early deceleration

FIG 15-13 Line drawing illustrating early decelerations. *FHR,* Fetal heart rate. (From Tucker SM: *Pocket guide to fetal monitoring and assessment,* ed 5, St Louis, 2004, Mosby.)

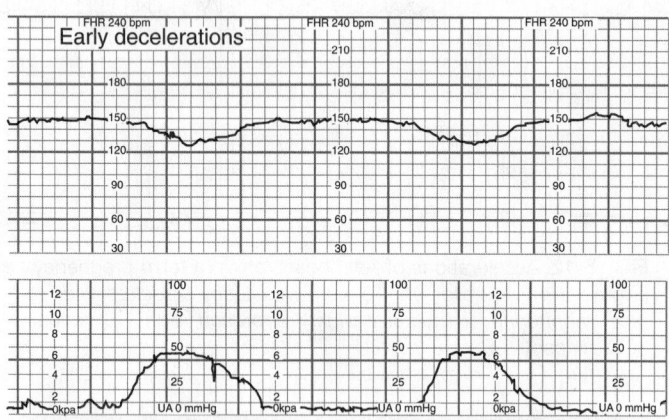

FIG 15-14 Electronic fetal monitor tracing showing early decelerations. *FHR,* Fetal heart rate; *UA,* uterine activity. (From Miller LA, Miller DA, Tucker SM: *Mosby's pocket guide to fetal monitoring: a multidisciplinary approach,* ed 7, St Louis, 2013, Mosby.)

end of the contraction (Figs. 15-13 and 15-14). For this reason an early deceleration is sometimes called the *mirror image* of a contraction.

Early decelerations may occur during UCs, during vaginal examinations, as a result of fundal pressure, and during placement of the internal mode of fetal monitoring. When present, they usually occur during the first stage of labor when the cervix is dilated 4 to 7 cm. However, they are sometimes seen during the second stage when the woman is pushing.

Because early decelerations are considered to be benign, interventions are not necessary. The value of identifying them is so they can be distinguished from late or variable decelerations, which can be abnormal and for which interventions are appropriate. Box 15-4 lists causes, clinical significance, and nursing interventions for early decelerations.

Late Decelerations. Late deceleration of the FHR is a visually apparent, gradual (onset to lowest point ≥30 seconds) decrease in and return to baseline FHR associated with UCs (Macones, Hankins, Spong, et al., 2008). The deceleration begins after the contraction has started, and the lowest point of the deceleration occurs after

BOX 15-4   EARLY DECELERATIONS

Cause
Head compression resulting from the following:
- Uterine contractions
- Vaginal examination
- Fundal pressure
- Placement of internal mode of monitoring

Clinical Significance
Normal pattern; not associated with fetal hypoxemia, acidemia, or low Apgar scores

Nursing Interventions
None required

the peak of the contraction. The deceleration usually does not return to baseline until after the contraction is over (Figs. 15-15 and 15-16).

Traditionally late decelerations have been attributed to uteroplacental insufficiency. however, in reality a number of factors can disrupt oxygen transfer to the fetus, even with mild UCs and a normally functioning placenta (Miller, Miller, and Tucker, 2013). These factors include maternal hypotension, uterine tachysystole (e.g., more than five contractions in 10 minutes averaged over a 30-minute window), preeclampsia, postdate or postterm pregnancy, amnionitis, small-for-gestational-age fetuses, maternal diabetes, placenta previa, placental abruption, conduction anesthetics, maternal cardiac disease, and maternal anemia. Rarely fetal oxygenation can be interrupted sufficiently to result in metabolic acidemia. For that reason late decelerations should be considered an ominous sign when they are associated with absent or minimal variability (Miller, Miller, and Tucker, 2013). The most common cause of late decelerations is uterine tachysystole, usually caused by oxytocin (Pitocin) administration (Garite, 2012).The clinical significance and nursing interventions for late decelerations are described in Box 15-5.

Variable Decelerations. Variable deceleration of the FHR is defined as a visually abrupt (onset to lowest point <30 seconds) and

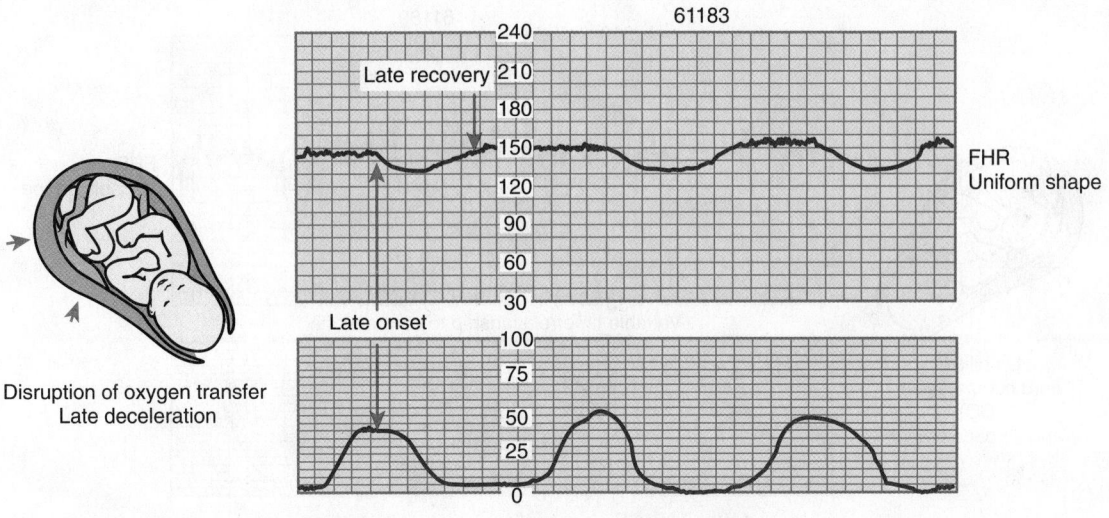

61183

FIG 15-15 Line drawing illustrating late decelerations. *FHR,* Fetal heart rate. (Modified from Tucker SM: *Pocket guide to fetal monitoring and assessment,* ed 5, St Louis, 2004, Mosby.)

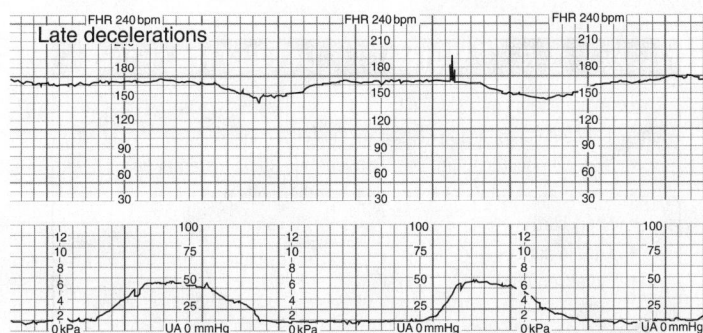

FIG 15-16 Electronic fetal monitor tracing showing late decelerations. *FHR,* Fetal heart rate; *UA,* uterine activity. (From Miller LA, Miller DA, Tucker SM: *Mosby's pocket guide to fetal monitoring: a multidisciplinary approach,* ed 7, St Louis, 2013, Mosby.)

apparent decrease in FHR below the baseline. The decrease is at least 15 beats/min or more below the baseline, lasts at least 15 seconds, and returns to baseline in less than 2 minutes from the time of onset (Macones, Hankins, Spong, et al., 2008). Variable decelerations occur any time during the UC phase and are caused by compression of the umbilical cord (Figs. 15-17 and 15-18).

The appearance of variable decelerations differs from those of early and late decelerations, which closely approximate the shape of the corresponding UC. Instead variable decelerations have a U, V, or W shape, characterized by a rapid descent and ascent to and from the nadir (lowest point) of the deceleration (see Figs. 15-17 and 15-18). Some variable decelerations are preceded and followed by brief accelerations of the FHR known as *shoulders,* which is an appropriate compensatory response to compression of the umbilical vein.

Occasional variables have little clinical significance. However, recurrent variable decelerations indicate repetitive disruption in the oxygen supply of the fetus. This can result in hypoxemia and metabolic acidemia. Variable decelerations are often noted during the transition phase of first-stage labor or the second stage of labor as a result of umbilical cord compression and stretching during fetal descent (Garite, 2012). Box 15-6 lists causes, clinical significance, and nursing interventions for variable decelerations.

BOX 15-5   LATE DECELERATIONS

Cause
Disruption of oxygen transfer from environment to fetus caused by the following:
- Uterine tachysystole
- Maternal supine hypotension
- Epidural or spinal anesthesia
- Placenta previa
- Placental abruption
- Hypertensive disorders
- Postmaturity
- Intrauterine growth restriction
- Diabetes mellitus
- Intraamniotic infection

Clinical Significance
Abnormal pattern associated with fetal hypoxemia, acidemia, and low Apgar scores; considered ominous if persistent and uncorrected, especially when associated with absent or minimal baseline variability

Nursing Interventions
The usual priority is as follows:
1. Change maternal position (lateral).
2. Correct maternal hypotension by elevating legs.
3. Increase rate of maintenance intravenous solution.
4. Palpate uterus to assess for tachysystole.
5. Discontinue oxytocin if infusing.
6. Administer oxygen at 8 to 10 L/min by nonrebreather face mask.
7. Notify physician or nurse-midwife.
8. Consider internal monitoring for more accurate fetal and uterine assessment.
9. Assist with birth (cesarean or vaginal assisted) if pattern cannot be corrected.

Prolonged Decelerations. A prolonged deceleration is a visually apparent decrease (may be either gradual or abrupt) in FHR of at least 15 beats/min below the baseline and lasting more than 2 minutes but less than 10 minutes. A deceleration lasting more than 10 minutes is considered a baseline change (Macones, Hankins, Spong, et al., 2008) (Fig. 15-19).

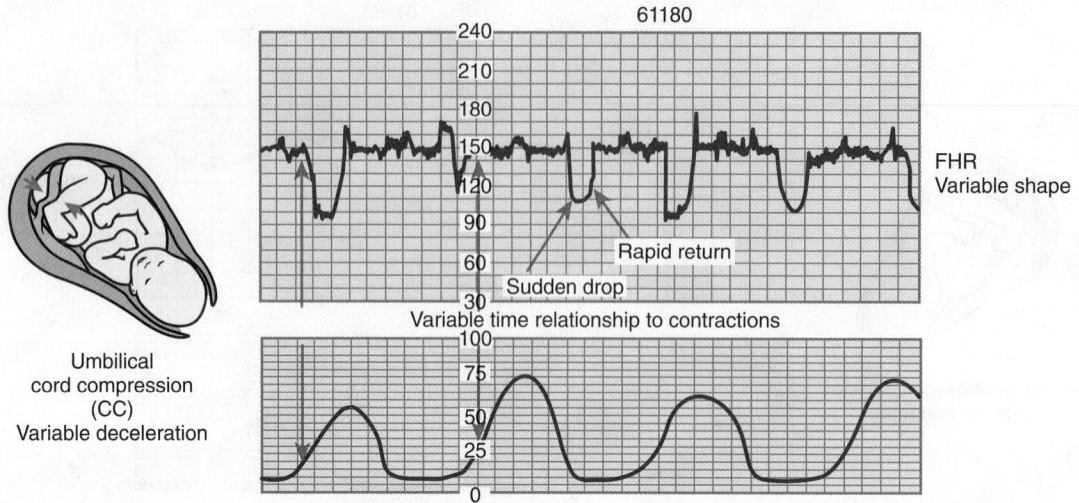

FIG 15-17 Line drawing illustrating variable decelerations. *FHR*, Fetal heart rate. (From Tucker SM: *Pocket guide to fetal monitoring and assessment*, ed 5, St Louis, 2004, Mosby.)

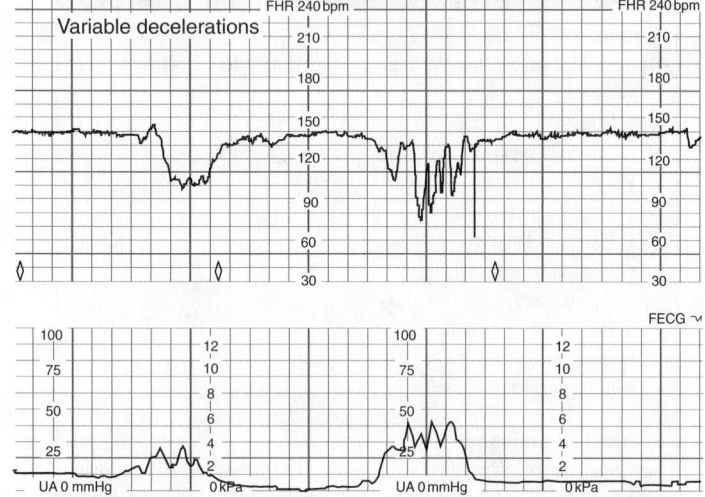

FIG 15-18 Electronic fetal monitor tracing showing variable decelerations. *FHR*, Fetal heart rate; *FECG*, fetal electrocardiogram. (From Miller LA, Miller DA, Tucker SM: *Mosby's pocket guide to fetal monitoring: a multidisciplinary approach*, ed 7, St Louis, 2013, Mosby.)

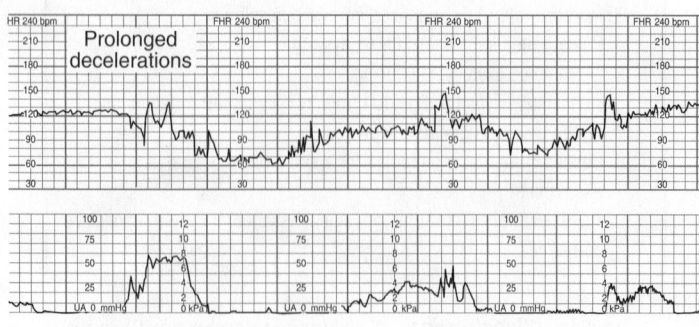

FIG 15-19 Prolonged decelerations. *FHR*, Fetal heart rate; *UA*, uterine activity. (From Miller LA, Miller DA, Tucker SM: *Mosby's pocket guide to fetal monitoring: a multidisciplinary approach*, ed 7, St Louis, 2013, Mosby.)

BOX 15-6 VARIABLE DECELERATIONS

Cause

Umbilical cord compression caused by the following:

- Maternal position with cord between fetus and maternal pelvis
- Cord around fetal neck, arm, leg, or other body part
- Short cord
- Knot in cord
- Prolapsed cord

Clinical Significance

Variable decelerations occur in approximately 50% of all labors and usually are transient and correctable

Nursing Interventions

The usual priority is as follows:

1. Change maternal position (side to side, knee chest).
2. Discontinue oxytocin if infusing.
3. Administer oxygen at 8 to 10 L/min by nonrebreather face mask.
4. Notify physician or nurse-midwife.
5. Assist with vaginal or speculum examination to assess for cord prolapse.
6. Assist with amnioinfusion if ordered.
7. Assist with birth (vaginal assisted or cesarean) if pattern cannot be corrected.

Prolonged decelerations are caused when the mechanisms responsible for late or variable decelerations last for an extended period (more than 2 minutes). Examples of conditions that can cause an interruption in the fetal oxygen supply long enough to produce a prolonged deceleration include maternal hypotension, uterine tachysystole or rupture, extreme placental insufficiency, and prolonged cord compression or prolapse (Garite, 2012; Miller, Miller, and Tucker, 2013). The presence and degree of hypoxia are thought to correlate with the depth and duration of the deceleration, how abruptly it returns to the baseline, how much variability is lost during the deceleration, and whether rebound tachycardia and loss of variability occur after the deceleration (Garite, 2012).

BOX 15-7 CHECKLIST FOR FETAL MONITORING EQUIPMENT

Preparation of Monitor

1. Is paper inserted correctly (if using paper)?
2. Are transducer cables plugged securely into appropriate port on monitor?
3. Is paper speed set to 3 cm/min?
4. Were monitor date and time verified (when using electronic documentation)?

Ultrasound Transducer

1. Has ultrasound transmission gel been applied to transducer?
2. Was fetal heart rate (FHR) tested and noted on monitor strip?
3. Was FHR compared with maternal pulse and noted?
4. Does a signal light flash or an audible beep occur with each heartbeat?
5. Is belt secure and snug but comfortable for the laboring woman?

Tocotransducer

1. Is tocotransducer firmly positioned at site of least maternal tissue?
2. Has it been applied without gel or paste?
3. Was uterine activity (UA) baseline adjusted between contractions to print at the 20 mm Hg line?
4. Is belt secure and snug but comfortable for the laboring woman?

Spiral Electrode

1. Is connector attached firmly to electrode pad (on leg plate or abdomen)?
2. Is spiral electrode attached to presenting part of fetus?
3. Is inner surface of electrode pad pregelled or covered with electrode gel?
4. Is electrode pad properly secured to woman's thigh or abdomen?

Internal Catheter or Strain Gauge

1. Is length line on catheter visible at introitus?
2. Is it noted on monitor paper that UA test or calibration was performed?
3. Has monitor been set to zero according to manufacturer directions?
4. Is intrauterine pressure catheter properly secured to woman?
5. Is baseline resting tone of uterus documented?

From Miller LA, Miller DA, Tucker SM: *Mosby's pocket guide to fetal monitoring: a multidisciplinary approach*, ed 7, St Louis, 2013, Mosby.

! NURSING ALERT

Nurses should notify the physician or nurse-midwife immediately and initiate appropriate treatment of abnormal patterns when they see a prolonged deceleration.

CARE MANAGEMENT

Care of the woman receiving EFM in labor begins with evaluation of the EFM equipment. The nurse must ensure that the monitor is recording FHR and UA accurately and that the tracing is interpretable. If external monitoring is not adequate, changing to a fetal spiral electrode or IUPC may be necessary. A checklist for fetal monitoring equipment can be used to evaluate the equipment functions (Box 15-7).

After ensuring that the monitor is recording properly, the FHR and UA tracings are evaluated regularly throughout labor. *Guidelines for Perinatal Care*, published jointly by the AAP and the ACOG

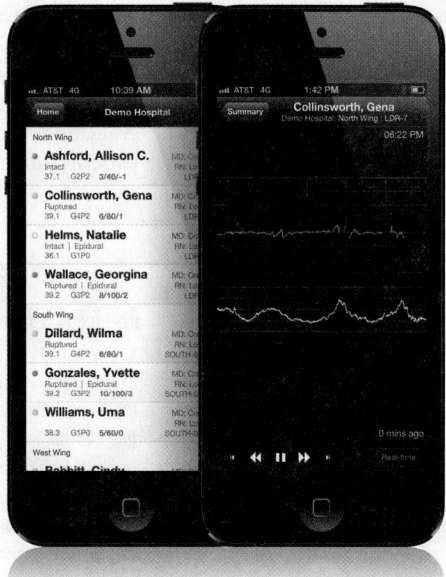

FIG 15-20 Providers can access near real-time fetal heart rate tracings and review patient data using their mobile phones. (Courtesy AirStrip Technologies, Inc., San Antonio, TX.)

(2012), recommends that the FHR tracing be evaluated at least every 30 minutes during the first stage of labor and every 15 minutes during the second stage of labor in low risk women. If risk factors are present, the FHR tracing should be evaluated more frequently: every 15 minutes in the first stage of labor and every 5 minutes in the second stage of labor.

Assessing FHR and UA patterns, implementing independent nursing interventions, documenting observations and actions according to the established standard of care, and reporting abnormal patterns to the primary care provider (e.g., physician, certified nurse-midwife) are the responsibilities of the nurse providing care to women in labor.

Current technology has made access to and communication regarding electronic FHR tracings much more convenient for health care providers. Many hospitals use central monitor displays, which provide the opportunity to view the tracings of several women at the same time at the nurses' station. Health care providers can also access the FHR tracings of one woman or several patients from remote locations, including office and home. It is even possible to access FHR tracings and other patient data using mobile phones (Fig. 15-20) (Miller, Miller, and Tucker, 2013).

Electronic Fetal Monitoring Pattern Recognition and Interpretation

Nurses must evaluate many factors to determine whether an FHR pattern is normal or abnormal. They evaluate these factors based on the presence of other obstetric complications, progress in labor, and use of analgesia or anesthesia. They also must consider the estimated time interval until birth. Therefore interventions are based on clinical judgment of a complex, integrated process.

Categorizing Fetal Heart Rate Tracings

As previously mentioned, a three-tier system of categorizing FHR tracings is recommended (see Box 15-1). Category I FHR tracings are normal and strongly predictive of normal fetal acid-base status at the time of observation. These tracings may be followed in a routine manner and do not require any specific action. Category II FHR tracings are indeterminate. This category includes all tracings that do not meet category I or category III criteria. Category II tracings require continued observation and evaluation. Category III FHR tracings are abnormal. Immediate evaluation and prompt intervention are required when these patterns are identified (Macones, Hankins, Spong, et al., 2008).

LEGAL TIP: Fetal Monitoring Standards

Nurses who care for women during childbirth are legally responsible for correctly interpreting FHR patterns, initiating appropriate nursing interventions based on those patterns, and documenting the outcomes of those interventions. Perinatal nurses are responsible for the timely notification of the physician or nurse-midwife in the event of abnormal FHR patterns. They also are responsible for initiating the institutional chain of command should differences in opinion arise among health care providers concerning the interpretation of the FHR pattern and the intervention required.

Nursing Management of Abnormal Patterns

The five essential components of the FHR tracing that must be evaluated regularly are baseline rate, baseline variability, accelerations, decelerations, and changes or trends over time. Whenever one of these five essential components is assessed as abnormal, corrective measures must be taken immediately. The purpose of these actions is to improve fetal oxygenation (Miller, Miller, and Tucker, 2013). The term *intrauterine resuscitation* is sometimes used to refer to specific interventions initiated when an abnormal FHR pattern is noted. Basic corrective measures include providing supplemental oxygen, instituting maternal position changes, and increasing intravenous fluid administration. These interventions are implemented to improve uterine and intervillous space blood flow and increase maternal oxygenation and cardiac output (Miller, Miller, and Tucker, 2013). Box 15-8 lists basic interventions to improve maternal and fetal oxygenation status.

Depending on the underlying cause of the abnormal FHR pattern, other interventions such as correcting maternal hypotension, reducing UA, and altering second-stage pushing techniques also may be instituted (Miller, Miller, and Tucker, 2013). Box 15-8 lists interventions for these specific problems. Some of the items listed are not independent nursing interventions. For example, any medications administered must be authorized either through inclusion in a unit protocol or by a verbal or written order. Some interventions are specific to the FHR pattern. (See Table 15-3 and Boxes 15-5 and 15-6 for nursing interventions for tachycardia, late decelerations, and variable decelerations.) Based on the FHR response to these interventions, the primary health care provider decides whether additional interventions should be instituted or whether immediate vaginal or cesarean birth should be performed.

Other Methods of Assessment and Intervention

A major shortcoming of EFM is its high rate of false-positive results. Even the most abnormal patterns are poorly predictive of neonatal morbidity. Therefore other methods of assessment have been developed to evaluate fetal status. Fetal scalp stimulation, vibroacoustic stimulation, and umbilical cord acid-base determination are frequently performed assessments. Fetal scalp blood sampling is another available assessment technique (see Evidence-Based Practice box). Amnioinfusion and tocolytic therapy are interventions often used in an attempt to improve abnormal FHR patterns.

BOX 15-8   MANAGEMENT OF ABNORMAL FETAL HEART RATE PATTERNS

Basic Interventions
- Administer oxygen by nonrebreather face mask at rate of 10 L/min for approximately 15 to 30 minutes.
- Assist woman to a side-lying (lateral) position.
- Increase maternal blood volume by increasing rate of primary IV infusion.

Interventions for Specific Problems
- Maternal hypotension
  - Increase rate of primary IV infusion.
  - Change to lateral or Trendelenburg positioning.
  - Administer ephedrine or phenylephrine if other measures are unsuccessful in increasing blood pressure.
- Uterine tachysystole
  - Reduce or discontinue dose of any uterine stimulants in use (e.g., oxytocin [Pitocin]).
  - Administer uterine relaxant (tocolytic) (e.g., terbutaline [Brethine]).
- Abnormal fetal heart rate pattern during second stage of labor
  - Use open-glottis pushing.
  - Use fewer pushing efforts during each contraction.
  - Make individual pushing efforts shorter.
  - Push only with every other or every third contraction.
  - Push only with perceived urge to push (in women with regional anesthesia).

IV, Intravenous.

Assessment Techniques

Fetal Scalp and Vibroacoustic Stimulation. Several research studies undertaken in the 1980s found that an FHR acceleration in response to digital or vibroacoustic stimulation was highly predictive of a normal scalp blood pH. The two methods of fetal stimulation used most often in clinical practice are scalp stimulation (using digital pressure during a vaginal examination) and vibroacoustic stimulation (using an artificial larynx or fetal acoustic stimulation device on the maternal abdomen over the fetal head continuously for 1 to 5 seconds). Another stimulation method that can be used is placing a specialized halogen light source on the maternal abdomen. The desired result of these stimulation methods is acceleration in the FHR of at least 15 beats/min for at least 15 seconds (Miller, Miller, and Tucker, 2013). FHR acceleration indicates the absence of metabolic acidemia. If the fetus does not respond to stimulation with an acceleration, fetal compromise is not necessarily indicated; however, further evaluation of fetal well-being is needed. Fetal stimulation should be performed at times when the FHR is at baseline. Neither fetal scalp nor vibroacoustic stimulation should be instituted if FHR decelerations or bradycardia is present (Miller, Miller, and Tucker, 2013).

Umbilical Cord Acid-Base Determination. In assessing the immediate condition of the newborn after birth, a sample of cord blood is a useful adjunct to the Apgar score, especially if there has been an abnormal or confusing FHR tracing during labor or neonatal depression at birth. Generally the procedure is performed by withdrawing blood from both the umbilical artery and the umbilical vein. Both samples are then tested for pH, carbon dioxide pressure (Pco_2), oxygen pressure (Po_2), and base deficit or base excess (Garite, 2012; Miller, Miller, and Tucker, 2013). Umbilical arterial values reflect fetal condition, whereas umbilical vein values indicate placental function (Miller, Miller, and Tucker, 2013).

EVIDENCE-BASED PRACTICE

Fetal Cardiac Assessment During Labor: How Are You Doing in There?

Ask the Question

For low risk women, which assessments of fetal cardiac function during labor provide better outcomes?

Search for the Evidence

Search Strategies

English research-based publications on fetal assessment, monitoring, labor, cardiotocography, auscultation, pulse oximetry, electrocardiogram, scalp pH, scalp lactate were included.

Exclusions included preterm, postterm, high risk

Databases Used

Cochrane Collaborative Database, Joanna Briggs Institute, National Guideline Clearinghouse (AHRQ), CINAHL, PubMed, UpToDate, and the professional websites for AWHONN and SOGC.

Critically Analyze the Evidence

- Intermittent auscultation of fetal heart rate can be accomplished with a fetal stethoscope, Pinard (trumpet-shaped) device, or hand-held Doppler ultrasound device. Admission electronic fetal monitoring (EFM) for 20-30 minutes is intended to identify risk for fetal distress.
  - Routine admission 20-minute EFM is associated with higher rates of continuous fetal monitoring, fetal scalp blood sampling, and a 20% higher risk for cesarean birth than intermittent auscultation. There are no significant differences in instrumental vaginal births, artificial rupture of membranes, labor augmentation, or perinatal death. These findings do not support routine admission EFM strips for low risk term laboring women because of the risk for overtreatment (Devane, Lalor, Daly, et al., 2012).
- Inadequate fetal oxygenation leads to abnormal fetal heart rate and electrocardiogram (ECG) patterns, including elevation or suppression of the ST segment. Monitoring the fetal ECG requires cervical dilation of at least 3 cm and ruptured membranes to directly access the fetal presenting part.
  - EFM plus ECG results in fewer fetal scalp blood samples, instrument-assisted births, and admissions to special care nursery units than EFM alone. However, there are no differences in cesarean births or the following neonatal conditions: severe acidosis, encephalopathy, low APGAR scores at 5 minutes, or need for intubation. The reviewers suggest that fetal ECG may be useful in decision making when contemplating continuous EFM (Neilson, 2012).
  - A poorly oxygenated fetus develops acidosis, lower pH, and increased lactate in the blood. Fetal blood sampling requires cervical dilation and ruptured membranes.
  - Fetal lactate sampling requires much less blood volume than pH, making it more successful. No differences are found in birth interventions or perinatal outcomes for the fetus between lactate versus pH sampling done in response to EFM abnormalities (East, Leader, Sheehan, et al., 2010).

Apply the Evidence: Nursing Implications

- Evidence that a routine admission EFM strip is not recommended for low risk term labor may meet resistance in institutions that have made this their practice for decades. Evaluating and communicating the evidence becomes paramount to changing long-term institutional habits.

- Overtreatment such as unnecessary cesarean births may be a result of fear of litigation and create additional risks and costs. New evidence of patient safety using intermittent auscultation should reassure caregivers and low risk laboring women.
- A limited assessment of ECG plus EFM is probably not any better than EFM alone, except in the case in which continuous EFM is being contemplated. The decision to initiate continuous EFM usually greatly decreases the mobility of laboring women and may prolong labor and increase the cascade of interventions.
- Both ECG and scalp blood sampling require rupture of membranes. If this is not spontaneous, there is debate about the benefits versus risks of artificially rupturing membranes (increased maternal contraction pain, fetal infection, fetal distress).
- Fetal lactate sampling uses a very narrow capillary tube of blood, which is collected after a small incision in the fetal scalp or presenting part. Parents will probably find this distressing and need to understand the reasons for it, the small risk for infection, and the puncture site they may notice on their newborn.

Quality and Safety Competencies: Quality Improvement*

Knowledge

Recognize that nursing and other health profession students are parts of systems of care and care processes that affect outcomes for patients and families.

Nurses can use evidence to advocate for change in institutional habits such as overtesting that leads to overtreatment.

Skills

Seek information about outcomes of care for populations served in care setting.

Seek out the highest-level evidence and demonstrate its relevance to this setting.

Attitudes

Appreciate the value of what individuals and teams can do to improve care.

Education of the whole health care team is necessary to improve buy-in for institutional change.

References

Devane D, Lalor JG, Daly S, et al: Cardiotocography versus intermittent auscultation of fetal heart on admission to labour ward for assessment of fetal wellbeing. In *Cochrane Database Syst Rev* 2:CD005122.pub4. DOI: 10.1002/14651858. Chichester, UK, 2012, John Wiley & Sons.

East CE, Leader LR, Sheehan P, et al: Intrapartum fetal scalp lactate sampling for fetal assessment in the presence of a non-reassuring fetal heart rate trace. In *Cochrane Database Syst Rev* 3:CD006174.pub2. DOI: 10.1002/14651858. Chichester, UK, 2010, John Wiley & Sons.

Neilson JP: Fetal electrocardiogram (ECG) for fetal monitoring during labour. In *Cochrane Database Syst Rev* 4:CD000116.pub3. DOI: 10.1002/14651858. Chichester, UK, 2012, John Wiley & Sons.

Pat Mahaffee Gingrich

*Adapted from QSEN at www.qsen.org/.

The ACOG (2010) suggests obtaining cord blood values in the following clinical situations: cesarean birth for fetal compromise, low 5-minute Apgar score, severe intrauterine growth restriction, abnormal FHR tracing, maternal thyroid disease, intrapartum fever, and multifetal gestation. Normal umbilical artery and vein cord blood values are listed in Table 15-4. Normal findings preclude the presence of acidemia at or immediately before birth. If acidemia is present (e.g., pH less than 7.20), the type of acidemia is determined (respiratory, metabolic, or mixed) by analyzing the blood gas values (Table 15-5) (Miller, Miller, and Tucker, 2013).

Fetal Scalp Blood Sampling. Sampling of the fetal scalp blood for pH determination was first described in the 1960s and performed extensively in the 1970s. The procedure is performed by obtaining a sample of fetal scalp blood through the dilated cervix after the membranes have ruptured. Its use is limited by many factors, including the requirement for cervical dilation and membrane rupture, technical difficulty of the procedure, need for repetitive pH determinations, and uncertainty regarding interpretation and application of results. Fetal scalp blood sampling is now seldom used in the United States but remains a common practice in many other countries (Miller, Miller, and Tucker, 2013).

Interventions

Amnioinfusion. Amnioinfusion is infusion of room-temperature isotonic fluid (usually normal saline or lactated Ringer's solution) into the uterine cavity if the volume of amniotic fluid is low. Without the buffer of amniotic fluid, the umbilical cord can easily become compressed during contractions or fetal movement, diminishing the flow of blood between the fetus and placenta. The purpose of amnioinfusion is to relieve intermittent umbilical cord compression that results in variable decelerations and transient fetal hypoxemia by restoring the amniotic fluid volume to a normal or near-normal level (Miller, Miller, and Tucker, 2013). Women with an abnormally small amount of amniotic fluid (oligohydramnios) or no amniotic fluid (anhydramnios) are candidates for this procedure. Conditions that can result in oligohydramnios or anhydramnios include uteroplacental insufficiency and premature rupture of membranes.

TABLE 15-4	**APPROXIMATE NORMAL VALUES FOR CORD BLOOD**			
VESSEL	**pH**	**Pco$_2$ (mm Hg)**	**Po$_2$ (mm Hg)**	**BASE DEFICIT (mmol/L)**
Artery	7.2-7.3	45-55	15-25	<12
Vein	7.3-7.4	35-45	25-35	<12

From Miller LA, Miller DA, Tucker SM: *Mosby's pocket guide to fetal monitoring: a multidisciplinary approach,* ed 7, St Louis, 2013, Mosby.

TABLE 15-5	**TYPES OF ACIDEMIA**		
VALUE	**RESPIRATORY**	**METABOLIC**	**MIXED**
pH	<7.20	<7.20	<7.20
Pco$_2$	Elevated	Normal	Elevated
Base deficit	<12 mmol/L	≥12 mmol/L	≥12 mmol/L

From Miller LA, Miller DA, Tucker SM: *Mosby's pocket guide to fetal monitoring: a multidisciplinary approach,* ed 7, St Louis, 2013, Mosby.

Risks of amnioinfusion are overdistention of the uterine cavity and increased uterine tone. Fluid is administered through an IUPC by either gravity flow or an infusion pump. Usually a bolus of fluid is administered over 20 to 30 minutes; then the infusion is slowed to a maintenance rate. Likely no more than 1000 mL of fluid will need to be administered. The fluid can be warmed for the preterm fetus by infusing it through a blood warmer (Miller, Miller, and Tucker, 2013).

Intensity and frequency of UCs should be assessed continually during the procedure. The recorded uterine resting tone during amnioinfusion appears higher than normal because of resistance to outflow and turbulence at the end of the catheter. Uterine resting tone should not exceed 40 mm Hg during the procedure. The amount of fluid return must be estimated and documented during amnioinfusion to prevent overdistention of the uterus. The volume of fluid returned should be approximately the same as the amount infused (Miller, Miller, and Tucker, 2013).

Tocolytic Therapy. Tocolysis (relaxation of the uterus) can be achieved through the administration of drugs that inhibit UCs. This therapy can be used as an adjunct to other interventions in the management of fetal stress when the fetus is exhibiting abnormal patterns associated with increased UA. Tocolysis improves blood flow through the placenta by inhibiting UCs. It may be implemented by the primary health care provider when other interventions to reduce UA such as maternal position change and discontinuance of an oxytocin infusion have not diminished the UCs effectively. Tocolytics are often administered when women are having excessive UCs spontaneously. They are also frequently administered after a decision for cesarean birth has been made while preparations for surgery are under way. The most commonly used tocolytic in these situations is terbutaline (Brethine) given subcutaneously. Terbutaline works quickly and has been demonstrated to improve Apgar scores and cord pH values without apparent complications such as postpartum hemorrhage (Garite, 2012). If the FHR and UC patterns improve, the woman may be allowed to continue labor; if no improvement is seen, immediate cesarean birth may be needed.

Patient and Family Teaching

Although the use of EFM can be reassuring to many parents, it can be a source of anxiety to some. Therefore the nurse must be particularly sensitive and respond appropriately to the emotional, informational, and comfort needs of the woman in labor and those of her family (Fig. 15-21; Box 15-9).

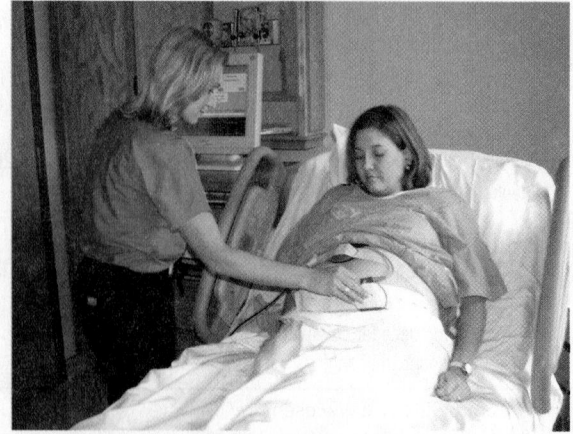

FIG 15-21 Nurse explains electronic fetal monitoring as ultrasound transducer monitors the fetal heart rate. (Courtesy Julie Perry Nelson, Loveland, CO.)

Part of the nurse's role includes acting as a partner with the woman to achieve a high-quality birthing experience. In addition to teaching and supporting the woman and her family with understanding of the laboring and birth process, breathing techniques, use of equipment, and pain-management techniques, the nurse can help with two factors that have an effect on fetal status: positioning and pushing. The nurse should enlist the woman's cooperation in avoiding the supine position. Instead the woman should be encouraged to maintain a side-lying or semi-Fowler's position with a lateral tilt to the uterus. In addition, the nurse should instruct the woman to keep her mouth and glottis open and to let air escape from her lungs as she pushes. Both of these interventions help to improve fetal oxygenation. See Chapter 16 for further discussion of maternal positioning and pushing techniques.

DOCUMENTATION

Clear and complete documentation in the woman's medical record is essential. Each FHR and UA assessment must be documented completely. More and more hospitals are moving to use of the electronic medical record and computerized charting. With computerized charting each required component usually appears on the

---

BOX 15-9   PATIENT AND FAMILY TEACHING WHEN ELECTRONIC FETAL MONITOR IS USED

The following guidelines relate to patient teaching and the functioning of the monitor.

- Explain purpose of monitoring.
- Explain each procedure.
- Provide rationale for maternal position other than supine.
- Explain that fetal status can be assessed continuously by electronic fetal monitoring (EFM), even during contractions.
- Explain that lower tracing on the monitor strip paper shows uterine activity (UA); upper tracing shows the fetal heart rate (FHR).
- Reassure woman and partner that prepared childbirth techniques can be implemented without difficulty.
- Explain that during external monitoring effleurage can be performed on sides of abdomen or upper portion of thighs.

- Explain that breathing patterns based on time and intensity of contractions can be enhanced by observing uterine activity on monitor strip, which shows the onset of contractions.
- Note peak of contraction; knowing that contraction will not get stronger and is halfway over is usually helpful.
- Note diminishing intensity.
- Coordinate with appropriate breathing and relaxation techniques.
- Reassure woman and partner that use of internal monitoring does not restrict movement, although she is confined to bed.*
- Explain that use of external monitoring usually requires woman's cooperation during positioning and movement.
- Reassure woman and partner that use of monitoring does not imply fetal jeopardy.

*Portable telemetry monitors allow FHR and uterine contraction patterns to be observed on centrally located display stations. These portable units permit ambulation during electronic monitoring.

Fetal Monitor Integration

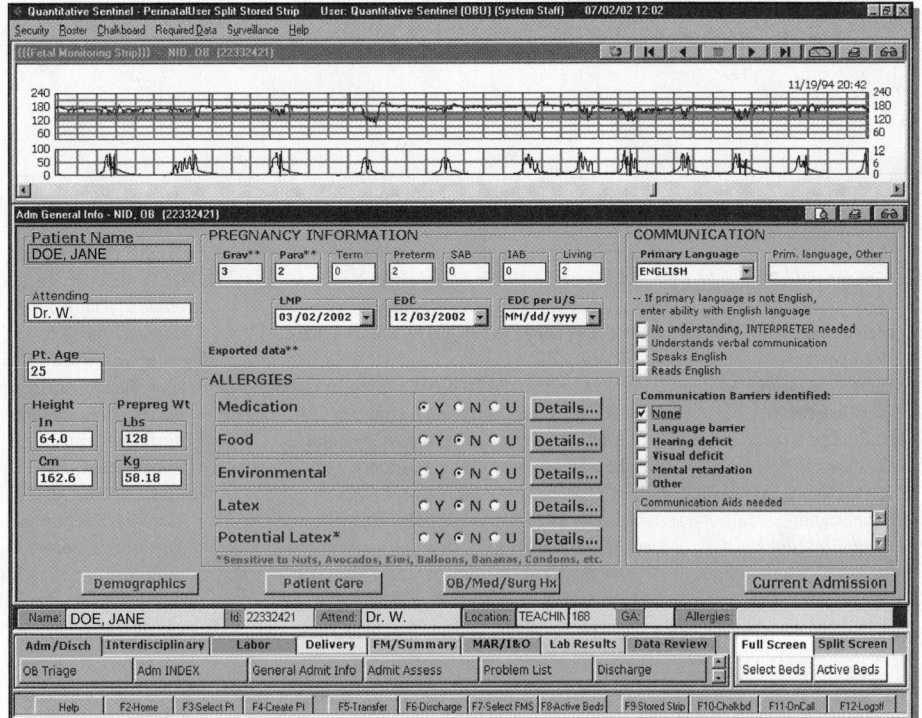

FIG 15-22 With integration of the fetal monitor tracing into the electronic medical record, the nurse can view the fetal tracing while charting. (Courtesy General Electric Healthcare Technologies, Barrington, IL.)

screen so it will be addressed routinely. Computerized charting often includes forced choices that greatly increase the use of standardized FHR terminology by all members of the health care team. In the past nurses were often encouraged to chart both on the monitor strip and in the medical record. However, charting directly on the monitor strip is unnecessary when an electronic medical record is used (Fig. 15-22). Any information that is handwritten on the monitor strip will not be recorded in the computer record. Furthermore, given that the EFM tracing is stored on computer, the paper strips are destroyed after the woman is discharged. No permanent record of the handwritten charting exists.

In institutions that still use a paper chart, documentation on the woman's monitor strip is started before the initiation of monitoring and consists of identifying information plus other relevant data. This documentation is continued and updated according to institutional protocol as monitoring continues and labor progresses.

In some institutions observations noted and interventions implemented are recorded on the monitor strip to produce a comprehensive document that chronicles the course of labor and the care rendered. In other institutions this documentation is confined to the labor flow record. Advocates of documenting on both the medical record and the EFM strip cite as advantages of this approach the ease of writing directly on the strip while at the bedside and the improved accuracy in documenting critical events and the interventions implemented. Others believe that charting on the EFM strip constitutes duplicate documentation of the same information noted in the medical record and thus it is unnecessary additional paperwork for the nurse.

A disadvantage of documenting on both the EFM strip and in the medical record is that the times noted for events and interventions on the EFM strip frequently do not correlate with what is later documented in the medical record. These inaccuracies can lead people involved in the retrospective review process carried out during litigation to infer that documentation errors have occurred. Therefore, if institutional policy mandates documentation both on the monitor strip and in the medical record, the nurse must make sure that the times and notations of events and interventions recorded in each place agree.

KEY POINTS

- Fetal well-being during labor is gauged by the response of the FHR to UCs.
- Standardized definitions for many common FHR patterns have been adopted for use in clinical practice by the ACNM, ACOG, and AWHONN.
- The five essential components of the FHR tracing are baseline rate, baseline variability, accelerations, decelerations, and changes or trends over time.
- The monitoring of fetal well-being includes FHR and UA assessment and assessment of maternal vital signs.
- The FHR can be monitored by either IA or EFM. The FHR and UA can be assessed by EFM using either the external or internal monitoring mode.

- Assessing FHR and UA patterns, implementing independent nursing interventions, and reporting abnormal patterns to the physician or nurse-midwife are the nurse's responsibilities.
- The AWHONN and ACOG have established and published health care provider standards and guidelines for FHR monitoring.
- The emotional, informational, and comfort needs of the woman and her family must be addressed when the mother and her fetus are being monitored.
- Documentation of fetal assessment is initiated and updated according to institutional protocol.

REFERENCES

American Academy of Pediatrics (AAP) and American College of Obstetricians and Gynecologists (ACOG): *Guidelines for perinatal care*, ed 7, Washington, DC, 2012, ACOG.

American College of Obstetricians and Gynecologists (ACOG): *Intrapartum fetal heart rate monitoring: nomenclature, interpretation, and general management principles*, ACOG Practice Bulletin No. 106, Washington, DC, 2009, ACOG.

American College of Obstetricians and Gynecologists (ACOG): *Umbilical cord blood gas and acid-base analysis*, ACOG Committee Opinion No. 348, Washington, DC, 2010, ACOG.

Association of Women's Health, Obstetric and Neonatal Nurses (AWHONN): *Fetal heart monitoring principles and practice*, ed 4, Dubuque, IA, 2009, Kendall/Hunt.

Cunningham F, Leveno K, Bloom S, et al: *Williams obstetrics*, ed 23, New York, 2010, McGraw-Hill.

Garite T: Intrapartum fetal evaluation. In Gabbe S, Niebyl J, Simpson J, et al, editors: *Obstetrics: normal and problem pregnancies*, ed 6, Philadelphia, 2012, Saunders.

Gilbert E: *Manual of high risk pregnancy & delivery*, ed 5, St Louis, 2011, Mosby.

Macones G, Hankins G, Spong C, et al: The 2008 National Institute of Child Health and Human Development Workshop Report on Electronic Fetal Monitoring: update on definitions, interpretation, and research guidelines, *J Obst Gynecol Neonat Nurs* 37(5):510–515, 2008.

Miller L, Miller D, Tucker SM: *Mosby's pocket guide to fetal monitoring: a multidisciplinary approach*, ed 7, St Louis, 2013, Mosby.

Nageotte M, Gilstrap L: Intrapartum fetal surveillance. In Creasy R, Resnik R, Iams J, editors: *Creasy & Resnik's maternal-fetal medicine: principles and practice*, ed 6, Philadelphia, 2009, Saunders.

National Institute of Child Health and Human Development Research Planning Workshop: Electronic fetal heart rate monitoring: research guidelines for interpretation, *Am J Obstet Gynecol* 177(6):1385–1390, 1997.

Nursing Care of the Family During Labor and Birth

Kitty Cashion

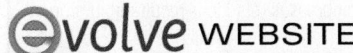 WEBSITE

http://evolve.elsevier.com/Perry/maternal

LEARNING OBJECTIVES

On completion of this chapter, the reader will be able to:
- Review the factors included in the initial assessment of the woman in labor.
- Describe the ongoing assessment of maternal progress during the first, second, third, and fourth stages of labor.
- Recognize the physical and psychosocial findings indicative of maternal progress during labor.
- Describe fetal assessment during labor.
- Identify signs of developing complications during labor and birth.
- Incorporate evidence-based nursing interventions into a comprehensive plan of care relevant to each stage of labor.

- Recognize the importance of support (family, partner, doula, nurse) in fostering maternal confidence and facilitating the progress of labor and birth.
- Analyze the influence of cultural and religious beliefs and practices on the process of labor and birth.
- Evaluate research findings on the importance of support from family, partner, doula, and nurse in facilitating maternal progress during labor and birth.
- Describe the role and responsibilities of the nurse during emergency childbirth.
- Evaluate the impact of perineal trauma on the woman's reproductive and sexual health.

The labor process is an exciting and anxious time for the woman and her significant others (support persons, family). In a relatively short period they experience one of the most profound changes in their lives. Although most women in the United States labor and give birth in a hospital under the care of a physician, others choose different settings and care providers. Available childbirth options vary greatly from place to place (see Community Focus box).

For most women labor begins with the first uterine contraction, continues with hours of hard work during cervical dilation and birth, and ends as the woman and her family begin the attachment process with the newborn. Nursing care management focuses on assessment and support of the woman and her significant others throughout labor and birth, with the goal of ensuring the best possible outcome for all involved.

FIRST STAGE OF LABOR

The **first stage of labor** begins with the onset of regular uterine contractions and ends with complete cervical effacement and dilation. The first stage of labor consists of three phases: the **latent phase** (through 3 cm of dilation), the **active phase** (4 to 7 cm of dilation), and the **transition phase** (8 to 10 cm of dilation).

CARE MANAGEMENT

Most nulliparous women seek admission to the hospital in the latent phase because they have not experienced labor before and are unsure of the "right" time to come in. Multiparous women usually do not come to the hospital until they are in the active phase. Even though no two labors are identical, women who have given birth before often are less anxious about the process unless their previous experience has been negative.

ASSESSMENT

Assessment begins at the first contact with the woman, whether by telephone or in person. Many women call the hospital or birthing center first for validation that it is all right for them to come in for evaluation or admission or that they can remain at home. However, many hospitals discourage the nurse from giving advice regarding what to do because of legal liability. Nurses are often instructed to tell women who call with questions to call their primary health care provider or to come to the hospital if they feel the need to be checked. The nature of the telephone conversation, including any

🏠 **COMMUNITY FOCUS**

Availability of Alternative Childbirth Options in the Community

Consult the yellow pages of the telephone directory and the Internet to explore options for childbearing families in your community. Is there a birthing center in your community? Are certified nurse-midwives available? Are other types of licensed midwives available? Is there an option for a home birth? For a water birth? During your clinical rotation in maternity nursing, interview a staff nurse in labor and delivery (L&D) and ascertain his or her views of midwives and home births. Interview a childbirth educator and ascertain his or her views of midwives and home births. Contrast the views of the L&D nurse and the childbirth educator. Is there a difference in their views? Prepare a patient handout listing the options for childbearing families in your community. Discuss the findings from your interview with your clinical group.

advice or instructions given, should be documented in the patient's record (Gilbert, 2011).

A pregnant woman may first call her primary care provider or come to the hospital while in false labor or early in the latent phase of the first stage of labor. She may feel discouraged, angry, or confused on learning that the contractions that feel so strong and regular to her do not indicate true labor because they are not causing cervical dilation or that they are still not strong or frequent enough for admission. During the third trimester of pregnancy women should be instructed regarding the stages of labor and the signs indicating its onset. They should be informed of the possibility that they will not be admitted if they are 3 cm or less dilated (see Patient Teaching box).

If the woman lives near the hospital and has adequate support and transportation, she may be encouraged to stay home or return home to allow labor to progress (i.e., until the uterine contractions are more frequent and intense). The ideal setting for the low risk woman at this time usually is the familiar environment of her home. However, the woman who lives at a considerable distance from the hospital, who lacks adequate support and transportation, or who has a history of rapid labors in the past may be admitted in latent labor. The same measures used by the woman at home should be offered to the hospitalized woman in early labor.

A warm shower is often relaxing during early labor. However, warm baths before labor is well established could inhibit uterine contractions and prolong the labor process (Waterbirth International, 2012). Soothing back, foot, and hand massage or a warm drink of preferred liquids such as tea or milk can help the woman rest and even sleep, especially if false or early labor is occurring at night. Diversional activities such as walking outdoors or in the house, reading, watching television, "playing" on the computer, or talking with friends can reduce the perception of early discomfort, help time pass, and reduce anxiety.

When the woman arrives at the perinatal unit, assessment is the top priority (Fig. 16-1). The nurse first performs a screening assessment by using the techniques of interview and physical assessment and reviews the laboratory and diagnostic test findings to determine the health status of the woman and her fetus and the progress of her labor. The nurse also notifies the primary health care provider; and, if the woman is admitted, a detailed systems assessment is done.

PATIENT TEACHING

How to Distinguish True Labor from False Labor

True Labor
Contractions
- Occur regularly, becoming stronger, lasting longer, and occurring closer together
- Become more intense with walking
- Are usually felt in lower back, radiating to lower portion of abdomen
- Continue despite use of comfort measures

Cervix (by vaginal examination)
- Shows progressive change (softening, effacement, and dilation signaled by appearance of bloody show)
- Moves to an increasingly anterior position

Fetus
- Presenting part usually becomes engaged in pelvis, which results in increased ease of breathing; at the same time, presenting part presses downward and compresses bladder, resulting in urinary frequency

False Labor
Contractions
- Occur irregularly or become regular only temporarily
- Often stop with walking or position change
- Can be felt in back or abdomen above navel
- Can often be stopped through use of comfort measures

Cervix (by vaginal examination)
- May be soft but with no significant change in effacement or dilation or evidence of bloody show
- Is often in posterior position

Fetus
- Presenting part is usually not engaged in pelvis

LEGAL TIP: Obstetric Triage and EMTALA

The Emergency Medical Treatment and Active Labor Act (EMTALA) is a federal regulation enacted to ensure that a woman gets emergency treatment or active labor care whenever such treatment is sought. According to the EMTALA, true labor is considered to be an emergency medical condition. Nurses working in labor and birth units must be familiar with their responsibilities according to the EMTALA regulations, which include providing services to pregnant women when they experience an urgent pregnancy problem (e.g., labor, decreased fetal movement, rupture of membranes [ROM], recent trauma) and fully documenting all relevant information (e.g., assessment findings, interventions implemented, patient responses to care measures provided). A pregnant woman presenting in an obstetric triage is considered to be in "true" labor until a qualified health care provider certifies that she is not. Agencies need to have specific policies and procedures in place so compliance with EMTALA regulations is achieved while safe and efficient care is provided (Miller, Miller, and Tucker, 2013).

When the woman is admitted, she is usually moved from an observation area to the labor room; the labor, delivery, and recovery (LDR) room; or the labor, delivery, recovery, and postpartum (LDRP) room. If she wishes, include her partner in the assessment and admission process. The nurse can direct significant others not participating in this process to the appropriate waiting area. The woman undresses and puts on her own gown or a hospital gown. The nurse places an

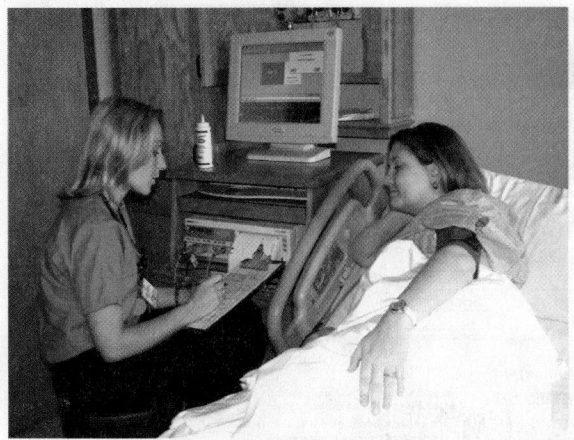

FIG 16-1 Woman being admitted. (Courtesy Julie Perry Nelson, Loveland, CO.)

identification band on the woman's wrist. Her personal belongings are put away safely or given to family members according to agency policy. Women who participate in expectant parent classes often bring a birth bag or Lamaze bag with them. The nurse then shows the woman and her partner the layout and operation of the unit and room, how to use the call light and telephone system, how to adjust lighting in the room, and the different bed positions.

The nurse reassures the woman that she is in competent, caring hands and that she and people to whom she gives permission can ask questions related to her care and status and that of her fetus at any time during labor. The nurse can minimize the woman's anxiety by explaining terms commonly used during labor. The woman's interest, response, and prior experience guide the depth and breadth of these explanations.

Most hospitals have specific forms, whether paper or electronic, that are used to obtain important assessment information when a woman in labor is being evaluated or admitted (Fig. 16-2, *A* and *B*). More and more hospitals now use an electronic medical record; almost all charting is done on computer. Sources of data include the prenatal record, initial interview, physical examination to determine baseline physiologic parameters (e.g., vital signs), laboratory and diagnostic test results, expressed psychosocial and cultural factors, and clinical evaluation of labor status.

Prenatal Data

The nurse reviews the prenatal record to identify the woman's individual needs and risks. Copies of prenatal records are generally filed in the perinatal unit at some time during the woman's pregnancy (usually in the third trimester) or accessed by computer so they are readily available on admission. If the woman has had no prenatal care or her prenatal records are unavailable, the nurse must obtain certain baseline information. If she is having discomfort, the nurse should ask questions between contractions when she can concentrate more fully on her answers. At times the partner or support person(s) may need to be secondary sources of essential information. According to the Health Insurance Portability and Accountability Act (HIPAA), the woman must give permission for other persons to be involved in the exchange of information regarding her care. This permission should be obtained during pregnancy, and a signed form included in her health records.

Knowing the woman's age is important so the nurse can individualize care to the needs of her age-group. For example, a 14-year-old girl and a 40-year-old woman have different but specific needs, and their ages place them at risk for different problems. Accurate height and weight measurements are important. A pregnancy weight gain greater than recommended may place the woman at a higher risk for cephalopelvic disproportion and cesarean birth. This is especially true for women who are petite and have gained 16 kg or more. A prepregnancy body mass index (BMI) greater than 30 is also a cause for concern. Other factors to consider are the woman's general health status, current medical conditions or allergies, respiratory status, and previous surgical procedures.

The nurse should review the woman's prenatal records carefully, taking note of her obstetric and pregnancy history, including gravidity; parity; and problems such as history of vaginal bleeding, gestational hypertension, anemia, pregestational or gestational diabetes, infections (e.g., bacterial, viral, sexually transmitted), and immunodeficiency status. In addition, the expected date of birth (EDB) should be confirmed. Other important data found in the prenatal record include patterns of maternal weight gain; physiologic measurements such as maternal vital signs (blood pressure, temperature, pulse, respirations); fundal height; baseline fetal heart rate (FHR); and laboratory and diagnostic test results. See Table 8-1 for a list of common prenatal laboratory tests. Common diagnostic and fetal assessment tests performed prenatally include amniocentesis, nonstress test (NST), biophysical profile (BPP), and ultrasound examination. See Chapter 10 for more information.

If this labor and birth experience is not the woman's first, the nurse needs to note the characteristics of her previous experiences. This information includes the duration of previous labors, the type of anesthesia used, the kind of birth (e.g., spontaneous vaginal, forceps-assisted, vacuum-assisted, or cesarean birth), and the condition of the newborn. Explore the woman's perception of her previous labor and birth experiences because this perception may influence her attitude toward her current experience.

Interview

The woman's primary reason for coming to the hospital is determined in the interview. For example, it may be that her bag of waters (BOW, amniotic membranes) ruptured with or without contractions. The woman may have come in for an obstetric check to determine if she is truly in labor. She may be admitted to the Labor and Birth Unit for a period of observation lasting up to 23 hours. If it is determined after several hours of observation that she is not in true labor, she is discharged. Admission for 23 hours of observation is much less expensive than an inpatient admission; thus it minimizes or avoids cost to the woman and her health insurance plan.

Even the experienced woman may have difficulty determining the onset of labor. She is asked to recall the events of the previous days and describe the following:

- Time and onset of contractions and progress in terms of frequency, duration, and intensity
- Location and character of discomfort from contractions (e.g., back pain, abdominal or suprapubic discomfort)
- Persistence of contractions despite changes in maternal position and activity (e.g., walking or lying down)
- Presence and character of vaginal discharge or "show"
- The status of amniotic membranes such as a gush or seepage of fluid (spontaneous rupture of membranes [SROM]). If there has been a discharge that may be amniotic fluid, she is asked the date and time the fluid was first noted and its characteristics (e.g., amount, color, unusual odor). In many instances a sterile speculum examination and a Nitrazine (pH) and fern test can confirm that the membranes are ruptured (Box 16-1).

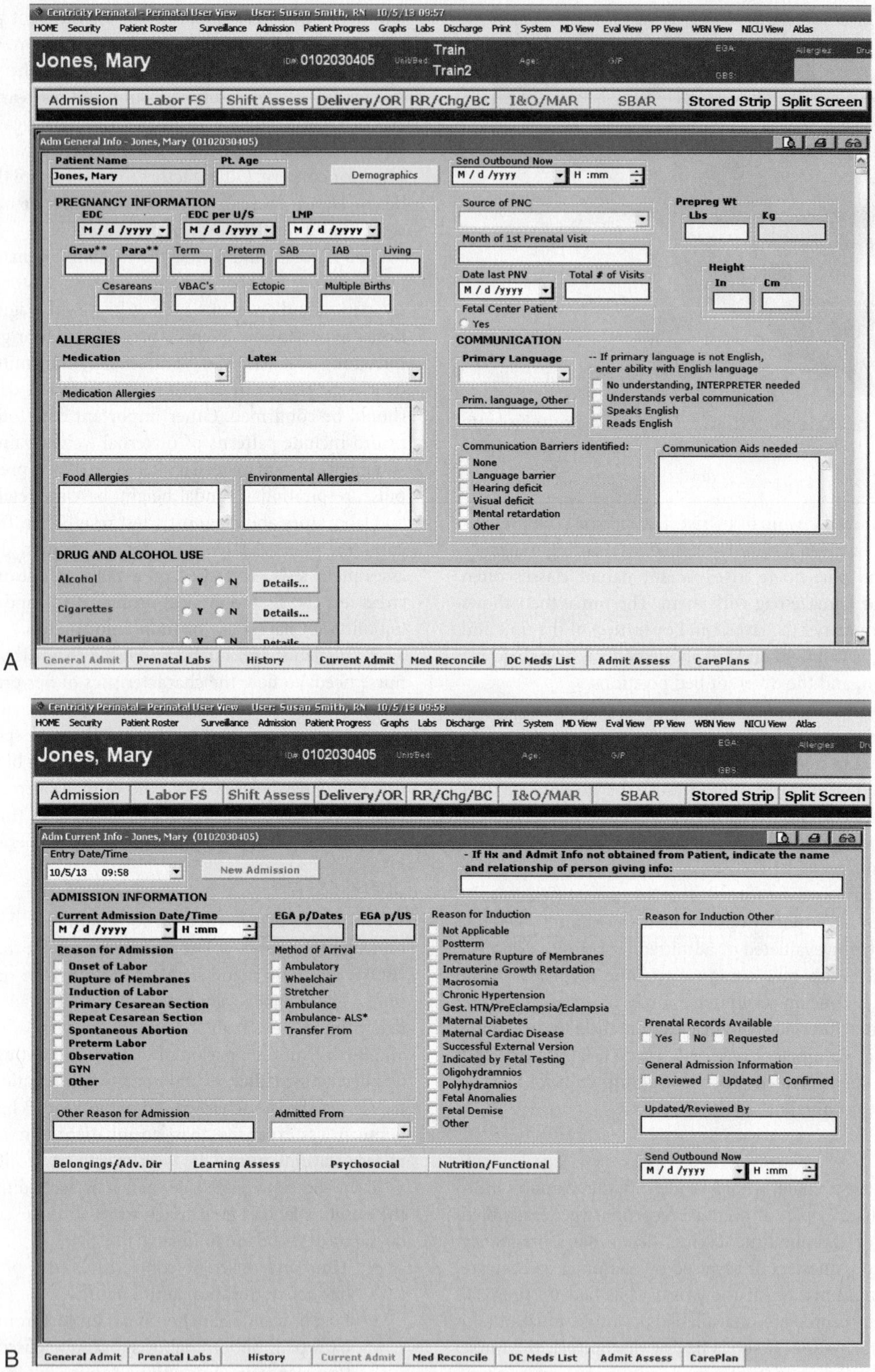

FIG 16-2 Admission screens in an electronic medical record. **A,** General admission screen. **B,** Current admission screen. (Courtesy Kitty Cashion, Memphis, TN.)

These descriptions help the nurse assess the degree of progress in the process of labor. Bloody show is distinguished from bleeding by the fact that it is pink and feels sticky because of its mucoid nature. There is very little bloody show in the beginning, but the amount increases with effacement and dilation of the cervix. A woman may report a small amount of brownish-to-bloody discharge that may be attributed to cervical trauma resulting from vaginal examination or coitus (intercourse) within the last 48 hours.

Assessing the woman's respiratory status is important in case general anesthesia is needed in an emergency. The nurse determines this status by asking the woman if she has a cold or related symptoms (e.g., "stuffy nose," sore throat, cough). The status of allergies,

BOX 16-1 PROCEDURE: TESTS FOR RUPTURE OF MEMBRANES

Nitrazine Test for pH
- Explain procedure to woman or couple.

Procedure
- Wash hands.
- Use cotton-tipped applicator impregnated with Nitrazine dye for determining pH (differentiates amniotic fluid, which is slightly alkaline, from urine and purulent material [pus], which are acidic).
- Dip cotton-tipped applicator deep into vagina to pick up fluid. (Procedure may be performed during speculum examination.)

Read Results
- Membranes probably intact: Identifies vaginal and most body fluids that are acidic:

Yellow	pH 5.0
Olive-yellow	pH 5.5
Olive-green	pH 6.0

- Membranes probably ruptured: Identifies amniotic fluid that is alkaline:

Blue-green	pH 6.5
Blue-gray	pH 7.0
Deep blue	pH 7.5

- Realize that false test results are possible because of presence of bloody show, insufficient amniotic fluid, or semen.
- Provide pericare as needed.
- Remove gloves and wash hands.

Document Results
- Results are positive or negative.

Test for Ferning or Fern Pattern
- Explain procedure to woman or couple.

Procedure
- Wash hands, apply sterile gloves, obtain specimen of fluid (usually during sterile speculum examination).
- Spread drop of fluid from vagina on clean glass slide with sterile cotton-tipped applicator.
- Allow fluid to dry.
- Examine slide under microscope; observe for appearance of ferning (a frondlike crystalline pattern) (do not confuse with cervical mucus test, when high levels of estrogen cause ferning).
- Observe for absence of ferning (alerts staff to possibility that amount of specimen was inadequate or that specimen was urine, vaginal discharge, or blood).
- Provide pericare as needed.
- Remove gloves and wash hands.

Document Results
- Results are positive or negative.

BOX 16-2 THE BIRTH PLAN

The birth plan should include the woman's or couple's preferences related to:
- Presence of birth companions such as the partner, older children, parents, friends, and doula and the role each will play.
- Presence of other persons such as students, male attendants, and interpreters.
- Clothing to be worn.
- Environmental modifications such as lighting, music, privacy, focal point, items from home such as pillows.
- Labor activities such as preferred positions for labor and for birth, ambulation, birth balls, showers and whirlpool baths, oral food and fluid intake.
- List of comfort and relaxation measures.
- Labor and birth medical interventions such as pharmacologic pain-relief measures, intravenous therapy, electronic monitoring, induction or augmentation measures, and episiotomy.
- Care and handling of the newborn immediately after birth such as cutting of the cord, eye care, and breastfeeding.
- Cultural and religious requirements related to the care of the mother, newborn, and placenta.

The childbirth website www.childbirth.org provides couples with an interactive birth plan along with examples of birth plans and descriptions of options that can be included.

nurse records the time and type of the woman's most recent solid and liquid intake.

The nurse obtains any information not found in the prenatal record during the admission assessment. Pertinent data include the birth plan (Box 16-2), the choice of infant feeding method, the type of pain management preferred, and the name of the pediatric health care provider. Obtain a patient profile that identifies the woman's preparation for childbirth, the support person or family members desired during childbirth and their availability, and ethnic or cultural expectations and needs. Determine the woman's use of alcohol, drugs, and tobacco before or during pregnancy.

The nurse reviews the birth plan. If no written plan has been prepared, he or she helps the woman formulate one by describing options available and determining the woman's wishes and preferences. As caregiver and advocate the nurse integrates the woman's desires into the nursing care plan as much as possible. She or he also prepares the woman for the possibility of change in her plan as labor progresses and assures her that the staff will provide information so she can make informed decisions. However, the woman must also realize that the longer her wish list, the greater is the likelihood that her expectations will not be met.

The nurse should discuss with the woman and her partner their plans for preserving childbirth memories through the use of photography and videotaping. Information should be provided about agency policies regarding these practices and under which circumstances they are allowed. Protection of privacy and safety and infection control are major concerns for the expecting parents and the agency. To avoid future embarrassment and distress, the nurse should clarify with the woman exactly which parts of her childbirth she wishes to have photographed and the degree of detail. Remind patients and families that pictures should not be posted on social media sites without the knowledge and consent of every person who appears in the picture. The woman's record should reflect that the childbirth was recorded. Some hospitals and health care providers

including allergies to latex and tape, and medications routinely used in obstetrics such as opioids (e.g., hydromorphone [Dilaudid], butorphanol [Stadol], fentanyl [Sublimaze], nalbuphine [Nubain]), anesthetic agents (e.g., bupivacaine, lidocaine, ropivacaine), and antiseptics (Betadine) is reviewed. Some allergic responses cause swelling of the mucous membranes of the respiratory tract, which could interfere with breathing and the administration of inhalation anesthesia. Because vomiting and subsequent aspiration into the respiratory tract can complicate an otherwise normal labor, the

TABLE 16-1 EXPECTED MATERNAL PROGRESS DURING FIRST STAGE OF LABOR

CRITERION	PHASES MARKED BY CERVICAL DILATION*		
	0-3 cm (LATENT)	4-7 cm (ACTIVE)	8-10 cm (TRANSITION)
Duration†	About 6-8 hr	About 3-6 hr	About 20-40 min
Contractions			
Strength	Mild to moderate	Moderate to strong	Strong to very strong
Rhythm	Irregular	More regular	Regular
Frequency	5-30 min apart	3-5 min apart	2-3 min apart
Duration	30-45 sec	40-70 sec	45-90 sec
Descent			
Station of presenting part	Nulliparous: 0	Varies: +1 to +2 cm	Varies: +2 to +3 cm
	Multiparous: −2 cm to 0	Varies: +1 to +2 cm	Varies: +2 to +3 cm
Show			
Color	Brownish discharge, mucus plug, or pale pink mucus	Pink-to-bloody mucus	Bloody mucus
Amount	Scant	Scant to moderate	Copious
Behavior and appearance‡	Excited; thoughts center on self, labor, and baby; may be talkative or silent, calm or tense; some apprehension; pain controlled fairly well; alert, follows directions readily; open to instructions	Becomes more serious, doubtful of pain control, more apprehensive; desires companionship and encouragement; attention more inwardly directed; fatigue evidenced; malar (cheeks) flush; has some difficulty following directions	Pain described as severe; backache common; frustration, fear of loss of control, and irritability may be voiced; expresses doubt about ability to continue; vague in communications; amnesia between contractions; writhing with contractions; nausea and vomiting, especially if hyperventilating; hyperesthesia; circumoral pallor, perspiration of forehead and upper lip; shaking tremor of thighs; feeling of need to defecate, pressure on anus

*In the nullipara effacement is often complete before dilation begins; in the multipara it occurs simultaneously with dilation.
†Duration of each phase is influenced by such factors as parity; maternal emotions; position; level of activity; and fetal size, presentation, and position. For example, the labor of a nullipara tends to last longer, on average, than the labor of a multipara. Women who ambulate and assume upright positions or change positions frequently during labor tend to experience a shorter first stage. Descent is often prolonged in breech presentations and occiput posterior positions.
‡Women who have epidural analgesia for pain relief may not demonstrate some of these behaviors.

do not allow videotaping of the birth because of concerns related to legal liability.

Psychosocial Factors

The woman's general appearance and behavior (and that of her partner) provide valuable clues to the type of supportive care she will need. However, keep in mind that general appearance and behavior may vary, depending on the stage and phase of labor (Table 16-1 and Box 16-3).

Women with a History of Sexual Abuse. Labor can trigger memories of sexual abuse, especially during intrusive procedures such as vaginal examinations. Monitors, intravenous (IV) lines, and epidurals can make the woman feel a loss of control or as if she is being confined to bed and "restrained." Being observed by students and having intense sensations in the uterus and genital area, especially at the time when she must push the baby out, can also trigger memories.

The nurse can help the abuse survivor associate the sensations she is experiencing with the process of childbirth and not with her past abuse. Help maintain her sense of control by explaining all procedures and why they are needed, validating her needs, and

paying close attention to her requests. Wait for the woman to give permission before touching her, and accept her often extreme reactions to labor (Simpson, 2008). Avoid words and phrases that can cause the woman to recall the words of her abuser (e.g., "open your legs," "relax and it won't hurt so much"). Limit the number of procedures that invade her body (e.g., vaginal examinations, urinary catheter, internal monitor, forceps or vacuum extractor) as much as possible. Encourage her to choose a person (e.g., doula, friend, family member) to be with her during labor to provide continuous support and comfort and act as her advocate. Nurses are advised to care for all laboring women in this manner because it is not unusual for a woman to choose not to reveal a history of sexual abuse. These care measures can help a woman perceive her childbirth experience in positive terms.

Stress in Labor

The way in which women and their support person or family members approach labor is related to the manner in which they have been socialized to the childbearing process. Their reactions reflect their life experiences regarding childbirth—physical, social, cultural, and religious. Society communicates its expectations regarding

BOX 16-3   PSYCHOSOCIAL ASSESSMENT OF THE LABORING WOMAN

Verbal Interactions

- Does the woman ask questions?
- Can she ask for what she needs?
- Does she talk to her support person(s)?
- Does she talk freely with the nurse or respond only to questions?

Body Language

- Does she change positions or lie rigidly still?
- What is her anxiety level?
- How does she react to being touched by the nurse or support person?
- Does she avoid eye contact?
- Does she look tired? If she appears tired, ask her how much rest she has had in the past 24 hours.

Perceptual Ability

- Is there a language barrier?
- Are repeated explanations necessary because her anxiety level interferes with her ability to comprehend?
- Can she repeat what she has been told or otherwise demonstrate her understanding?

Discomfort Level

- To what degree does the woman describe what she is experiencing, including her pain experience?
- How does she react to a contraction?
- How does she react to assessment and care measures?
- Are any nonverbal pain messages noted?
- Can she ask for comfort measures?

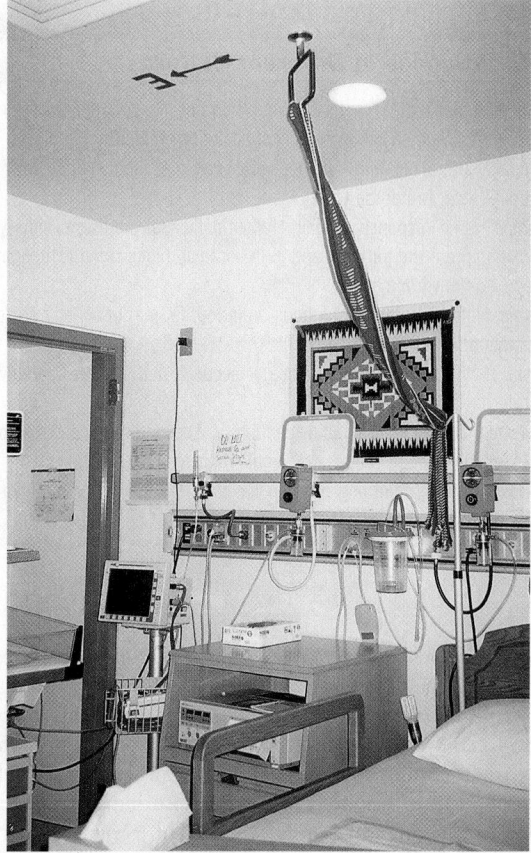

FIG 16-3 Birthing room specific to Native-American population. Note arrow pointing east, rug on wall, and rope or sash belt hanging from ceiling. (Courtesy Patricia Hess, San Francisco, CA; Chinle Comprehensive Health Care Center, Chinle, AZ.)

acceptable and unacceptable maternal behaviors during labor and birth. These expectations may be used by some women as the basis for evaluating their own actions during childbirth. An idealized perception of labor and birth may be a source of guilt and cause a sense of failure if the woman finds the process less than joyous, especially when the pregnancy is unplanned or is the product of a dysfunctional or terminated relationship. Often women have heard horror stories or have seen friends or relatives going through labors that appear anything but easy. Multiparous women often base their expectations of the present labor on their previous childbirth experiences.

Discuss the feelings that a woman has about her pregnancy and fears regarding childbirth. This discussion is especially important if the woman is a primigravida who has not attended childbirth classes or a multiparous woman who has had a previous negative childbirth experience. Women in labor usually have a variety of concerns that they will voice if asked but rarely volunteer. Major fears and concerns relate to the process and effects of childbirth, maternal and fetal well-being, and the attitude and actions of the health care staff. Unresolved fears increase a woman's stress and can slow the process of labor as a result of the inhibiting effects of catecholamines associated with the stress response on uterine contractions.

The father, coach, or significant other also experiences stress during labor. The nurse can assist and support these individuals by identifying their needs and expectations and helping to make sure that these are met. She or he can determine what role the support person intends to fulfill and whether that person is prepared for the role by making observations and asking herself or himself such questions as, "Has the couple attended childbirth classes?" "What role does this person expect to play?" "Does he or she do all the talking?" "Is she or he nervous, anxious, aggressive, or hostile?" "Does he or she look hungry, tired, worried, or confused?" "Does he or she watch television, sleep, or stay out of the room instead of paying attention to the woman?" "Where does he or she sit?" "Does he or she touch the woman; what is the character of the touch?" Be sensitive to the needs of support persons and provide teaching and support as appropriate. In many instances the support that these people provide to the laboring woman is in direct proportion to the support they receive from the nurses and other health care providers.

Cultural Factors

As the population in the United States and Canada becomes more diverse, it is increasingly important to note the woman's ethnic or cultural and religious values, beliefs, and practices to anticipate nursing interventions to add or eliminate from an individualized, mutually acceptable plan of care that provides a feeling of safety and control (Fig. 16-3). Nurses should be committed to providing culturally sensitive care and developing an appreciation and respect for cultural diversity (Callister, 2008). Encourage the woman to request specific caregiving behaviors and practices that are important to her. If a special request contradicts usual practices in that setting, the woman or the nurse can ask the woman's primary health care provider to write an order to accommodate

🌐 CULTURAL COMPETENCE

Birth Practices in Different Cultures

- *Somalia:* Because Somalis in general do not like to show any sign of weakness, women are extremely stoic during childbirth
- *Japan:* Natural childbirth methods practiced; may labor silently; may eat during labor; father may be present
- *China:* Stoic response to pain; father not usually present; side-lying position preferred for labor and birth because this position is thought to reduce infant trauma
- *India:* Natural childbirth methods preferred; father not usually present; female relatives usually present
- *Iran:* Father not present; female support and female caregivers preferred
- *Mexico:* May be stoic about discomfort until second stage, and then may request pain relief; father and female relatives may be present
- *Laos:* May use squatting position for birth; father may or may not be present; female attendants preferred

the special request. For example, in many cultures it is unacceptable to have a male caregiver examine a pregnant woman. In some cultures it is traditional to take the placenta home; in others the woman has only certain nourishments during labor. Some women believe that cutting her body, as with an episiotomy, allows her spirit to leave her body and that rupturing the membranes prolongs, not shortens, labor. It is important to explain the rationale for required care measures carefully (see Cultural Competence box).

Within cultures women may have an idea of the "right" way to behave in labor and may react to the pain experienced in that way. These behaviors can range from total silence to moaning or screaming, but they do not necessarily indicate the degree of pain. A woman who moans with contractions may not be in as much physical pain as a woman who is silent but winces during contractions. Some women believe that screaming or crying out in pain is shameful if a man is present. If the woman's support person is her mother, she may perceive the need to "behave" more strongly than if her support person is the father of the baby. She perceives herself as failing or succeeding based on her ability to follow these "standards" of behavior. Conversely a woman's behavior in response to pain may influence the support received from significant others. In some cultures women who lose control and cry out in pain may be scolded, whereas in others support persons become more helpful (D'Avanzo, 2008).

Culture and Father Participation. A companion is an important source of support, encouragement, and comfort for women during childbirth. The woman's cultural and religious background influences her choice of birth companion as do trends in the society in which she lives. For example, in Western societies the father is viewed as the ideal birth companion. For European-American couples, attending childbirth classes together has become a traditional, expected activity. Laotian (Hmong) husbands also traditionally participate actively in the labor process. In some other cultures the father may be available; but his presence in the labor room with the mother may not be considered appropriate, or he may be present but resist active involvement in her care. Such behavior could be perceived by the nursing staff to indicate a lack of concern, caring, or interest. Women from many cultures prefer female caregivers and want to have at least one female companion present during labor

and birth. They also are usually very concerned about modesty. If couples from these cultures immigrate to the United States or Canada, their roles may change. The nurse needs to talk to the woman and her support people to determine the roles they will assume.

The Non–English Speaking Woman in Labor. A woman's level of anxiety in labor increases when she does not understand what is happening to her or what is being said. Non–English speaking women often feel a complete loss of control over their situation if no health care provider is present who speaks their language. They can panic and withdraw or become physically abusive when someone tries to do something they perceive might harm them or their babies. A support person is sometimes able to serve as an interpreter. However, caution is warranted because the interpreter may not be able to convey exactly what the nurse or others are saying or what the woman is saying, which can increase the woman's stress level even more.

Ideally a bilingual nurse cares for the woman. Alternatively a hospital employee or volunteer interpreter may be contacted for assistance. Ideally the interpreter is from the woman's culture. For some women a female is more acceptable than a male interpreter. If no one in the hospital is able to interpret, call a service so interpretation can take place over the telephone. Even when the nurse has limited ability to communicate verbally with the woman, in most instances the woman appreciates his or her efforts to do so. Speaking slowly and avoiding complex words and medical terms can help a woman and her partner understand. Often the woman understands English much better than she speaks it.

Physical Examination

The initial physical examination includes a general systems assessment and an assessment of fetal status. During the examination uterine contractions are assessed, and a vaginal examination is performed. The findings of the admission physical examination serve as a baseline for assessing the woman's progress from that point. The information obtained from a complete and accurate assessment during the initial examination serves as the basis for determining whether the woman should be admitted and what her ongoing care should be. Expected maternal progress and minimal assessment guidelines during the first stage of labor are presented in Table 16-1 and Box 16-4.

Birth is a time when nurses and other health care providers are exposed to a great deal of maternal and newborn blood and body fluids. Therefore Standard Precautions should guide all assessment and care measures (Box 16-5). Hand hygiene (e.g., washing hands with soap or application of an alcohol-based antiseptic rub) before and after assessing the woman and providing care is a critical step in the prevention of infection transmission. The nurse should explain assessment findings to the woman and her partner whenever possible. Throughout labor accurate documentation following agency policy is done as soon as possible after a procedure has been performed (Fig. 16-4).

General Systems Assessment. On admission the nurse should perform a brief systems assessment. This includes an assessment of the heart, lungs, and skin and an examination to determine the presence and extent of edema of the face, hands, sacrum, and legs. It also includes testing of deep tendon reflexes and for clonus if indicated. Also note the woman's weight. Increasing numbers of women are overweight or obese. Excessive size can make nursing care during labor and birth more difficult and places the woman at risk for complications such as operative birth, infection, and blood clots. See Chapter 17 for further information.

BOX 16-4 NURSING ASSESSMENTS IN FIRST-STAGE LABOR

Latent Phase
- Perform every 30 to 60 minutes: maternal blood pressure, pulse, respirations.
- Perform every 30 to 60 minutes, depending on risk status: fetal heart rate (FHR) and pattern, uterine activity, vaginal show.
- Assess temperature every 4 hours until membranes rupture and then every 2 hours.
- Perform vaginal examination as needed to identify progress.
- Observe every 30 minutes: changes in maternal appearance, mood, affect, energy level, and condition of partner/coach.

Active Phase
- Perform every 30 minutes: maternal blood pressure, pulse, and respirations.
- Perform every 15 to 30 minutes, depending on risk status: FHR and pattern, uterine activity, vaginal show.
- Assess temperature every 4 hours until membranes rupture and then every 2 hours.
- Perform vaginal examination as needed to identify progress.
- Observe every 15 minutes: changes in maternal appearance, mood, affect, energy level, and condition of partner/coach.

Transition Phase
- Perform every 15 to 30 minutes: maternal blood pressure, pulse, and respirations.
- Perform every 15 to 30 minutes, depending on risk status: FHR and pattern.
- Assess every 10 to 15 minutes: uterine activity, vaginal show.
- Assess temperature every 4 hours until membranes rupture and then every 2 hours.
- Perform vaginal examination as needed to identify progress.
- Observe every 5 minutes: changes in maternal appearance, mood, affect, energy level, and condition of partner/coach.

BOX 16-5 STANDARD PRECAUTIONS DURING CHILDBIRTH

- Wash hands before and after putting on gloves and performing procedures; cleansing alcohol rubs can be used if hands are not visibly soiled.
- Wear gloves (clean or sterile, as appropriate) when performing procedures that require contact with the woman's genitalia and body fluids, including bloody show (e.g., during vaginal examination, amniotomy, hygienic care of the perineum, insertion of an internal scalp electrode and intrauterine pressure monitor, and urinary catheterization).
- Wear a mask that has a shield or protective eyewear and cover gown when assisting with the birth. Cap and shoe covers are worn for cesarean birth but are optional for vaginal birth in a birthing room. Gowns worn by the primary health care provider who is attending the birth should have a waterproof front and sleeves and should be sterile. Mask also should be worn during spinal puncture or insertion of an epidural catheter.
- Drape the woman with sterile towels and sheets as appropriate. Explain to the woman what can and cannot be touched.
- Help the woman's partner put on appropriate coverings for the type of birth such as cap, mask, gown, and shoe covers. Show the partner where to stand and what can and cannot be touched.
- Wear gloves and gown when handling the newborn immediately after birth.
- Use an appropriate method to suction the newborn's airway such as a bulb syringe or mechanical wall suction.

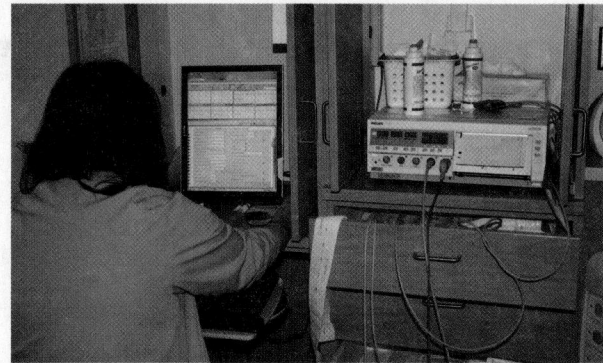

FIG 16-4 Nurse documenting assessment findings on computer in a labor, delivery, recovery, postpartum room. (Courtesy Shannon Perry, Phoenix, AZ.)

Vital Signs. Assess vital signs (temperature, pulse, respirations, and blood pressure using a correct size cuff) on admission. The initial values are used as the baseline for comparison for all future measurements. If the blood pressure is elevated, reassess it 30 minutes later between contractions to obtain a reading after the woman has relaxed. Encourage the woman to lie on her side to prevent supine hypotension and the resulting fetal hypoxemia (Fig. 16-5). Monitor her temperature so you can identify signs of infection or a fluid deficit (e.g., dehydration associated with inadequate intake of fluids).

Leopold Maneuvers (Abdominal Palpation). Leopold maneuvers are performed with the woman briefly lying on her back (Box 16-6). These maneuvers help identify the (1) number of fetuses; (2) presenting part, fetal lie, and fetal attitude; (3) degree of descent into the pelvis of the presenting part; and (4) expected location of the point of maximal intensity (PMI) of the FHR on the woman's abdomen.

Assessment of Fetal Heart Rate and Pattern. The PMI of the FHR is the location on the maternal abdomen at which the FHR is heard the loudest. It is usually directly over the fetal back. In a vertex presentation you can usually hear the FHR below the mother's umbilicus in either the right or the left lower quadrant of the abdomen. In a breech presentation you usually hear the FHR above the mother's umbilicus. Box 16-4 summarizes assessments recommended for determining fetal status. In addition, you must assess the FHR after ROM because this is the most common time for the umbilical cord to prolapse, after any change in the contraction pattern or maternal status and before and after the woman receives medication or a procedure is performed.

Assessment of Uterine Contractions. A general characteristic of effective labor is regular uterine activity (i.e., contractions becoming more frequent with increased duration), but uterine activity is not directly related to labor progress. Uterine contractions are the primary powers that act involuntarily to expel the fetus and placenta from the uterus. Several methods are used to evaluate uterine contractions, including the woman's subjective description, palpation and timing of contractions by a health care provider, and electronic monitoring.

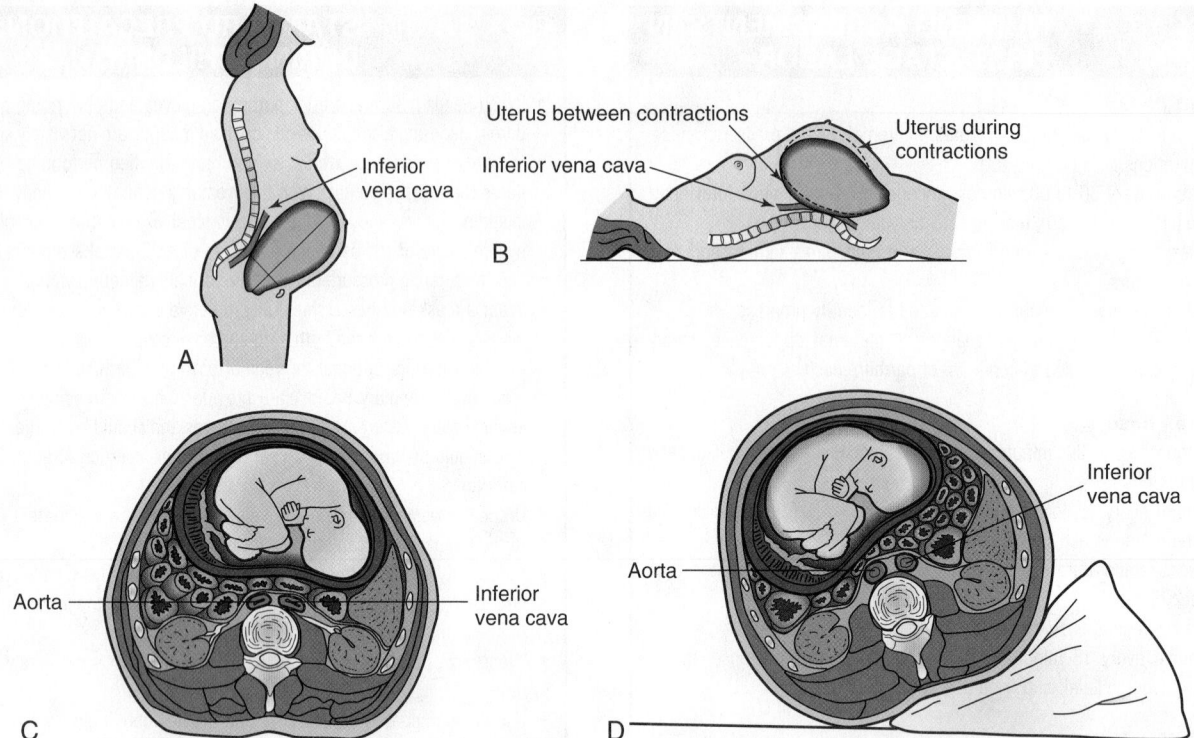

FIG 16-5 Supine hypotension. Note relationship of gravid uterus to ascending vena cava in standing posture **(A)** and supine posture **(B). C,** Compression of aorta and inferior vena cava with woman in supine position. **D,** Relieved by use of wedge pillow placed under woman's right side.

BOX 16-6 PROCEDURE: LEOPOLD MANEUVERS

- Wash hands.
- Ask woman to empty bladder.
- Position woman supine with one pillow under her head and her knees slightly flexed.
- Place small rolled towel under woman's right or left hip to displace uterus off major blood vessels (prevents supine hypotensive syndrome; see Fig. 16-5, *D*).
- If right-handed, stand on woman's right, facing her (if left-handed, stand on woman's left):
  1. Identify fetal part that occupies the fundus. The head feels round, firm, freely movable, and palpable by ballottement; the breech feels less regular and softer. This maneuver identifies fetal lie (longitudinal or transverse) and presentation (cephalic or breech) (Fig. A).
  2. Using palmar surface of one hand, locate and palpate the smooth convex contour of the fetal back and the irregularities that identify the small parts (feet, hands, elbows). This maneuver helps identify fetal presentation (Fig. B).

3. With right hand determine which fetal part is presenting over the inlet to the true pelvis. Gently grasp the lower pole of the uterus between the thumb and fingers, pressing in slightly (Fig. C). If the head is presenting and not engaged, determine the attitude of the head (flexed or extended).
4. Turn to face the woman's feet. Using both hands, outline the fetal head (Fig. D) with the palmar surface of the fingertips. When the presenting part has descended deeply, only a small portion of it may be outlined. Palpation of the cephalic prominence helps identify the attitude of the head. If the cephalic prominence is found on the same side as the small parts, this means that the head must be flexed and the vertex is presenting (see Fig. D). If the cephalic prominence is on the same side as the back, this indicates that the presenting head is extended and the face is presenting.
- Document fetal presentation, position, and lie and whether presenting part is flexed or extended, engaged, or free floating. Use agency protocol for documentation (e.g., "Vtx, LOA, floating").

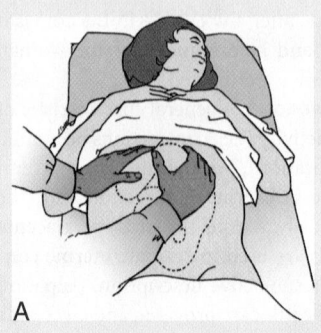
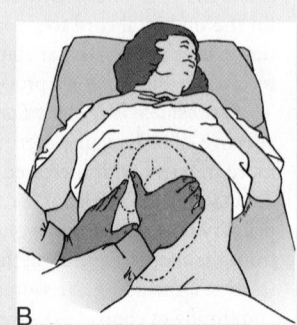
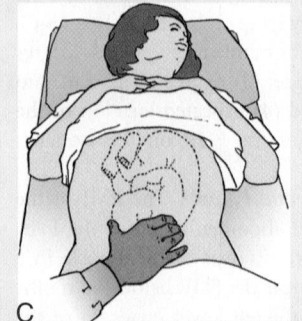
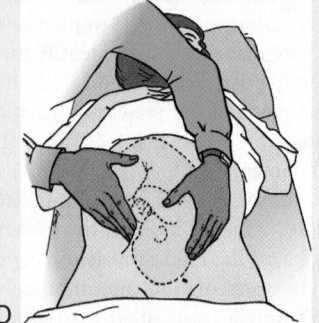

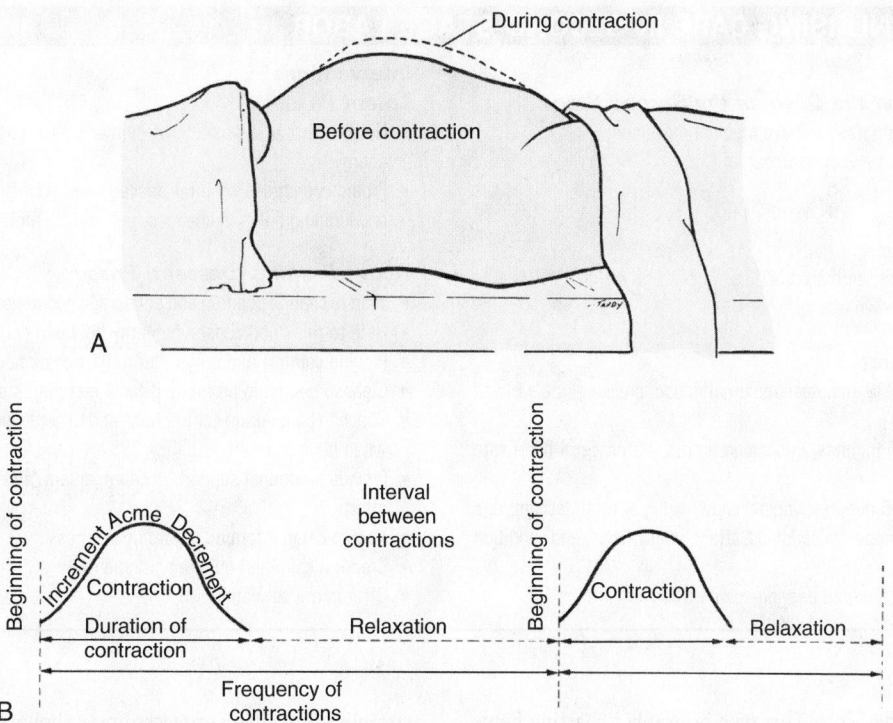

FIG 16-6 Assessment of uterine contractions. **A,** Abdominal contour before and during uterine contraction. **B,** Wavelike pattern of contractile activity.

Each contraction exhibits a wavelike pattern. It begins with a slow increment (the "building up" of a contraction from its onset), gradually reaches a peak, and diminishes rapidly (decrement, the "letting down" of the contraction). An interval of rest ends when the next contraction begins. The outward appearance of the woman's abdomen during and between contractions and the pattern of a typical uterine contraction are shown in Fig. 16-6.

A uterine contraction is described in terms of the following characteristics:

- *Frequency:* How often uterine contractions occur; the time that elapses from the beginning of one contraction to the beginning of the next
- *Intensity:* The strength of a contraction at its peak
- *Duration:* The time that elapses between the onset and end of a contraction
- *Resting tone:* The tension in the uterine muscle between contractions; relaxation of the uterus

Uterine contractions are assessed by palpation or by using an external or internal electronic monitor (see Chapter 15 for further discussion). Frequency and duration can be measured by all three methods of uterine activity monitoring. The accuracy of determining intensity and resting tone varies by the method used. The woman's description and palpation are more subjective and less precise ways of determining the intensity of uterine contractions and resting tone than is the electronic fetal monitor. The following terms describe what is felt on palpation:

- *Mild:* Slightly tense fundus that is easy to indent with fingertips (feels like touching finger to tip of nose)
- *Moderate:* Firm fundus that is difficult to indent with fingertips (feels like touching finger to chin)
- *Strong:* Rigid boardlike fundus that is almost impossible to indent with fingertips (feels like touching finger to forehead)

Women in labor tend to describe the pain of contractions in terms of the sensations they are experiencing in the lower abdomen or back, which are sometimes unrelated to the firmness of the uterine fundus. Therefore their assessment of the strength of their contractions can be less accurate than that of the health care provider, although the amount of discomfort reported is valid.

External electronic monitoring provides some information about the strength of uterine contractions when the appearance of contractions on admission is compared to those that occur later in labor. However, internal electronic monitoring with an intrauterine pressure catheter is the most accurate way of assessing the intensity of uterine contractions and resting tone.

On admission, uterine contractions and FHR and pattern are monitored electronically for at least a 20- to 30-minute period as a baseline. The minimal times for assessing uterine activity during the various phases of first- and second-stage labor are given in Box 16-4 and Box 16-7, and the findings expected as labor progresses are summarized in Tables 16-1 and Table 16-2.

> ! **NURSING ALERT**
>
> If you find the characteristics of contractions to be abnormal, either exceeding or falling below what is considered acceptable in terms of the standard characteristics, report this finding to the primary health care provider.

You must consider uterine activity in the context of its effect on cervical effacement and dilation and the degree of descent of the presenting part (see Chapter 13). You must also consider the effect on the fetus. You can verify the progress of labor effectively through the use of graphic charts (partograms) on which you plot cervical

BOX 16-7   NURSING CARE IN SECOND-STAGE LABOR

Assessment

Signs That Suggest the Onset of the Second Stage

- Urge to push or feeling need to have a bowel movement
- Sudden appearance of sweat on upper lip
- An episode of vomiting
- Increased bloody show
- Shaking of extremities
- Increased restlessness; verbalization (e.g., "I can't go on.")
- Involuntary bearing-down efforts

Physical Assessment

- Perform every 5 to 30 minutes: maternal blood pressure, pulse, and respirations.
- Assess every 5 to 15 minutes, depending on risk status: fetal heart rate and pattern
- Assess every 10 to 15 minutes: vaginal show; signs of fetal descent; and changes in maternal appearance, mood, affect, energy level, and condition of partner/coach.
- Assess every contraction and bearing-down effort.

Interventions

Latent Phase

- Help to rest in a position of comfort; encourage relaxation to conserve energy.
- Promote progress of fetal descent and onset of urge to bear down by encouraging position changes, pelvic rock, ambulation, showering.

Active Pushing (Descent) Phase

- Help to change position and encourage spontaneous bearing-down efforts.
- Help to relax and conserve energy between contractions.
- Provide comfort and pain-relief measures as needed.
- Cleanse perineum promptly if fecal material is expelled.
- Coach to pant during contractions and to gently push between contractions when head is emerging.
- Provide emotional support, encouragement, and positive reinforcement of efforts.
- Keep woman informed regarding progress.
- Create a calm and quiet environment.
- Offer mirror to watch birth.

---

dilation and station (descent). This type of graphic charting helps in early identification of deviations from expected labor patterns. Fig. 16-7 provides examples of partograms. Hospitals and birthing centers may develop their own assessment graphs that may include data not only on dilation and descent but also maternal vital signs, FHR, and uterine activity.

> **! NURSING ALERT**
>
> The nurse should recognize that active labor can actually last longer than the expected labor patterns because each woman is different. This finding is not a cause for concern unless the maternal-fetal unit exhibits signs of stress (e.g., abnormal FHR patterns, maternal fever).

Vaginal Examination. The vaginal examination reveals whether the woman is in true labor and enables the examiner to determine whether the membranes have ruptured (Fig. 16-8). Because this examination is often stressful and uncomfortable for the woman, perform it only when indicated by the status of the woman and her fetus. For example, perform a vaginal examination on admission, before administering medications (e.g., analgesics, increasing oxytocin infusion), when significant change has occurred in uterine activity, on maternal perception of perineal pressure or the urge to bear down, when membranes rupture, or when you note variable decelerations of the FHR. A full explanation of the examination and support of the woman are important in reducing the stress and discomfort associated with the examination (Simpson, 2008) (Box 16-8).

Laboratory and Diagnostic Tests

Analysis of Urine Specimen. A clean-catch urine specimen may be obtained to gather further data about the pregnant woman's health. Analysis of the specimen is a convenient and simple procedure that can provide information about her hydration status (e.g., specific gravity, color, amount); nutritional status (e.g., ketones); infection status (e.g., leukocytes); or the status of possible

complications such as preeclampsia, shown by finding protein in the urine. In most hospitals this test must be done in the laboratory rather than at the bedside, even if a urine "dipstick" is used.

Blood Tests. The blood tests performed vary with hospital protocol and the woman's health status. Currently all blood tests must be performed in the hospital laboratory rather than on the perinatal unit. Often blood samples are obtained from the hub of the catheter when an IV line is started. A hematocrit is likely ordered. More comprehensive blood assessments such as white blood cell count, red blood cell count, hemoglobin level, hematocrit, and platelet values are included in a complete blood count (CBC). A CBC may be ordered for women with a history of infection, anemia, gestational hypertension, or other disorders. Any woman whose human immunodeficiency virus (HIV) status is undocumented at the time of labor should be screened with a rapid HIV test unless she declines (opts out of) testing (CDC, Branson, Handsfield, Lampe, et al., 2006).

Most hospitals require that a "type and screen" to determine the woman's blood type and Rh status be performed on admission. Even if these tests have already been performed during pregnancy, the hospital laboratory or blood bank must verify the results in house. If the woman had no prenatal care or if her prenatal records are not available, a prenatal screen is likely drawn on admission. The prenatal screen includes laboratory tests that would normally have been drawn at the initial prenatal visit (see Table 8-1).

Other Tests. If the woman's group B streptococci status is not known, a rapid test may be done on admission. The rapid test results are usually available within an hour and determine if the woman must be given antibiotics during labor.

Assessment of Amniotic Membranes and Fluid. Labor is initiated at term by SROM in approximately 25% of pregnant women. A lag period rarely exceeding 24 hours may precede the onset of labor. Membranes (the BOW) also can rupture spontaneously any time during labor but most commonly in the transition phase of the first stage of labor. Box 16-1 explains how to determine if membranes are ruptured. If the membranes do not rupture spontaneously, the BOW will likely be ruptured artificially at some time during labor. Artificial rupture of membranes

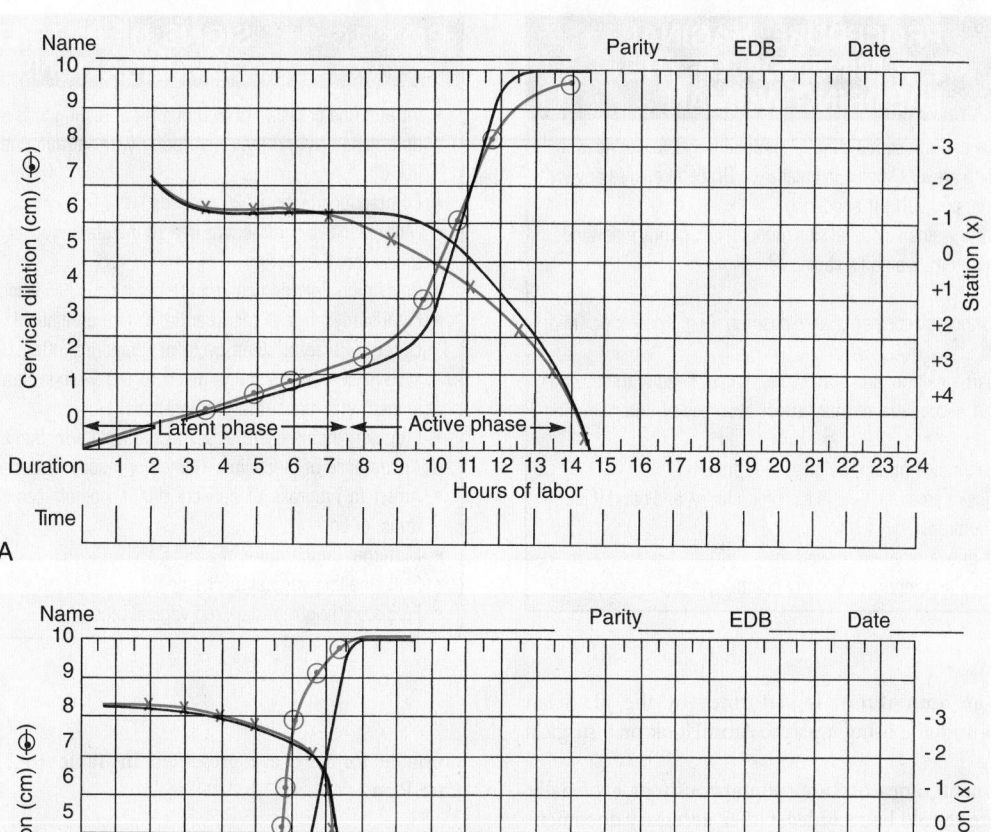

FIG 16-7 Partograms for assessment of patterns of cervical dilation and descent. Individual woman's labor patterns *(colored)* are superimposed on prepared labor graph *(black)* for comparison. **A,** Labor of a nulliparous woman. **B,** Labor of a multiparous woman. The rate of cervical dilation is plotted with the circled plot points. A line drawn through these symbols depicts the slope of the curve. Station is plotted with *X*s. A line drawn through the *X*s reveals the pattern of descent.

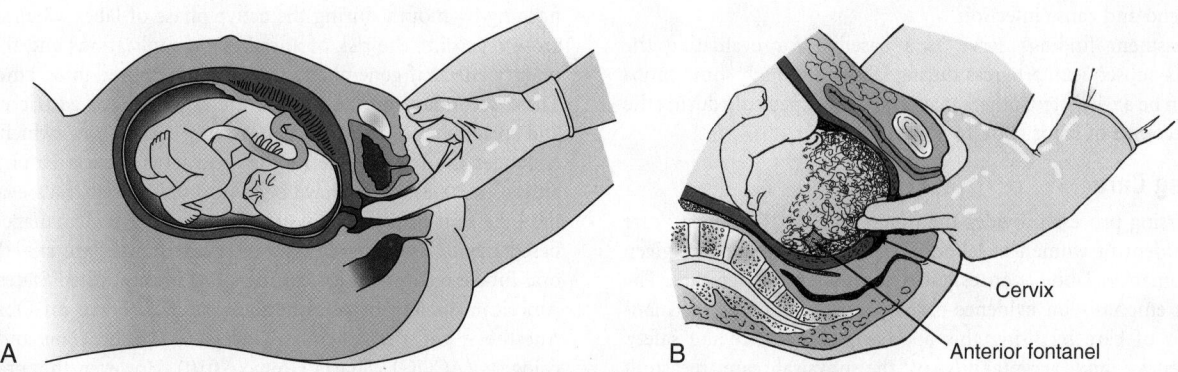

FIG 16-8 Vaginal examination. **A,** Undilated, uneffaced cervix; membranes intact. **B,** Palpation of sagittal suture line. Cervix effaced and partially dilated.

BOX 16-8 **PROCEDURE: VAGINAL EXAMINATION OF THE LABORING WOMAN**

- Use sterile glove and antiseptic solution or soluble gel for lubrication.
- Position woman to prevent supine hypotension. Drape to ensure privacy.
- Cleanse perineum and vulva if needed.
- After obtaining the woman's permission to touch her, gently insert index and middle fingers into woman's vagina.
- Determine:
  - Cervical dilation, effacement, and position (e.g., posterior, mid, anterior).
  - Presenting part, position, and station; molding of head with development of caput succedaneum (may affect accuracy of determination of station).
  - Status of membranes (intact, bulging, or ruptured).
  - Characteristics of amniotic fluid (e.g., color, clarity, and odor) if membranes are ruptured.
- Explain findings of examination to woman.
- Document findings and report to primary health care provider.

BOX 16-9 **SIGNS OF POTENTIAL COMPLICATIONS**

- Intrauterine pressure of ≥80 mm Hg or resting tone of ≥20 mm Hg (both determined by internal monitoring with intrauterine pressure catheter [IUPC])
- Contractions lasting ≥90 seconds
- More than five contractions in a 10-minute period (occur more frequently than every 2 minutes)
- Relaxation between contractions lasting <30 seconds
- Fetal bradycardia or tachycardia; absent or minimal variability not associated with fetal sleep cycle or temporary effects of central nervous system depressant drugs given to the woman; late, variable, or prolonged fetal heart rate decelerations
- Irregular fetal heart rate; suspected fetal arrhythmias
- Appearance of meconium-stained or bloody fluid from the vagina
- Arrest in progress of cervical dilation or effacement, descent of the fetus, or both
- Maternal temperature of ≥38° C
- Foul-smelling vaginal discharge
- Persistent bright or dark red vaginal bleeding

(AROM), called an **amniotomy,** is performed by the physician or certified nurse-midwife using a plastic AmniHook or a surgical clamp.

Whether the membranes rupture spontaneously or artificially, the time of rupture should be recorded. Other necessary documentation includes information regarding the color (clear or meconium-stained), estimated amount, and odor of the fluid. See Chapter 17 for additional information.

❗ NURSING ALERT

The umbilical cord may prolapse when the membranes rupture. The FHR and pattern should be monitored closely for several minutes immediately after ROM to determine fetal well-being, and the findings should be documented.

Infection. When membranes rupture, microorganisms from the vagina can then ascend into the amniotic sac, causing chorioamnionitis and placentitis to develop. For this reason assess maternal temperature and vaginal discharge frequently (at least every 2 hours) so you can quickly identify an infection developing after ROM. However, even when membranes are intact microorganisms can ascend and cause infection.

Assessment findings serve as a baseline for evaluating the woman's subsequent progress during labor. Although some problems can be anticipated, others may appear unexpectedly during the clinical course of labor (Box 16-9).

Nursing Care

The nursing process provides the framework for the nursing care management of women in labor. The physical nursing care given to a woman in labor is an essential component of her care. The current emphasis on evidence-based practice supports the management of care by using this approach to enhance the safety, effectiveness, and acceptability of the physical care measures chosen to support the woman during labor and birth (Box 16-10). The various physical needs, the necessary nursing actions, and the

rationale for care are presented in Table 16-2 and the Nursing Care Plan.

General Hygiene

Offer women in labor the use of showers or warm-water baths if they are available to enhance the feeling of well-being and minimize the discomfort of contractions. Water immersion during active labor is associated with decreases in the use of analgesia and reported maternal pain (Berghella, Baxter, and Chauhan, 2008). A recent Cochrane review suggested that immersion in water during the first stage of labor reduces the length of this stage and use of epidural or spinal anesthesia during labor (Cluett and Burns, 2009). Also encourage women to wash their hands or use cleansing foam after voiding and perform self-hygiene measures.

Change the linen if it becomes wet or stained with blood and use linen savers (Chux), changing them as needed.

Nutrient and Fluid Intake

Oral Intake. Before the 1940s women were allowed to eat and drink during labor to maintain the energy required to sustain labor and the stamina required to give birth. This practice changed, allowing the laboring woman only clear liquids or ice chips or nothing by mouth during the active phase of labor when concern arose regarding the risk of anesthesia complications and their secondary effects if general anesthesia were required in an emergency. These secondary effects include the aspiration of gastric contents and resultant compromise in oxygen perfusion, which could endanger the lives of the mother and fetus (Sharts-Hopko, 2010; Simpson, 2008). There have been no randomized trials evaluating the ingestion of solid foods in labor; thus current management is based mostly on expert opinions. Clear liquids are still the only oral intake recommended during labor in the United States by the American Society of Anesthesiologists Task Force on Obstetrical Anesthesia and the American College of Obstetricians and Gynecologists (ACOG) (Sharts-Hopko, 2010). However, this practice is being challenged by some health care providers because regional anesthesia is used more often than general anesthesia, even for

TABLE 16-2   PHYSICAL NURSING CARE DURING LABOR

NEED	NURSING ACTIONS	RATIONALE
General Hygiene		
Showers or bed baths, Jacuzzi bath	Assess for progress in labor.	Determines appropriateness of the activity
	Supervise showers closely if woman is in true labor.	Prevents injury from fall; labor may be accelerated
	Suggest allowing warm water to flow over back.	Aids relaxation; increases comfort
Perineum	Cleanse frequently, especially after rupture of membranes and when show increases.	Enhances comfort and reduces risk of infection
Oral hygiene	Offer toothbrush or mouthwash or wash teeth with ice-cold wet washcloth as needed.	Refreshes mouth; helps counteract dry, thirsty feeling
Hair	Brush, braid per woman's wishes.	Improves morale; increases comfort
Hand washing	Offer washcloths or cleansing foam before and after voiding and as needed.	Maintains cleanliness; prevents infection
Face	Offer cool washcloth.	Provides relief from diaphoresis; cools and refreshes
Gowns and linens	Change as needed.	Improves comfort; enhances relaxation
Nutrient and Fluid Intake		
Oral	Offer fluids and solid foods as ordered by primary health care provider and desired by laboring woman.	Provides hydration and calories; enhances positive emotional experience and maternal control
Intravenous (IV)	Establish and maintain IV line as ordered.	Maintains hydration; provides venous access for medications
Elimination		
Voiding	Encourage voiding at least every 2 hours.	A full bladder may impede descent of presenting part; overdistention may cause bladder atony and injury and postpartum voiding difficulty
Ambulatory woman	Allow ambulation to bathroom according to orders of primary health care provider, if:	
	Presenting part is engaged.	Reinforces normal process of urination
	Membranes are not ruptured.	Precautionary measure to protect against prolapse of umbilical cord
	Woman is not medicated.	Precautionary measure to protect against injury
Woman on bed rest	Offer bedpan	Prevents complications of bladder distention and ambulation
	Encourage upright position on bedpan, allow tap water to run; place woman's hands in warm water; pour warm water over vulva; give positive suggestion.	Encourages voiding
	Provide privacy.	Shows respect for woman
	Put up side rails on bed.	Prevents injury from fall
	Place call bell and telephone within reach.	Reinforces safe care
	Offer washcloth or cleansing foam for hands.	Maintains cleanliness; prevents infection
	Wash vulvar area.	Maintains cleanliness; enhances comfort; prevents infection
Catheterization	Catheterize according to orders of primary health care provider or hospital protocol if measures to facilitate voiding are ineffective.	Prevents complications of bladder distention
	Insert catheter between contractions.	Minimizes discomfort
	Avoid force if obstacle to insertion is noted.	"Obstacle" may be caused by compression of urethra by presenting part
Bowel elimination—sensation of rectal pressure	Perform vaginal examination.	Prevents misinterpretation of rectal pressure from presenting part as need to defecate
		Determines degree of descent of presenting part
	Help woman ambulate to bathroom or offer bedpan if rectal pressure is not from presenting part.	Reinforces normal process of bowel elimination and safe care
	Cleanse perineum immediately after passage of stool.	Reduces risk of infection and sense of embarrassment

---

BOX 16-10 **EVIDENCE-BASED CARE PRACTICES DESIGNED TO PROMOTE, PROTECT, AND SUPPORT NORMAL LABOR AND BIRTH**

- Allow labor to begin on its own: Encourage spontaneous labor rather than fostering elective labor inductions.
- Encourage freedom of movement throughout labor to facilitate the progress of labor and enhance maternal comfort and control of the labor process.
- Provide labor support beginning early in labor and continuing throughout the process of childbirth to relieve maternal anxiety and stress and decrease the risk for epidural anesthesia and cesarean birth; support should be provided by someone not employed by the hospital (e.g., doula).
- Avoid routine implementation of interventions (e.g., intravenous fluids, oral intake restrictions, continuous electronic fetal monitoring, labor augmentation measures [e.g., amniotomy, oxytocin administration], and epidural anesthesia).
- Support the practice of spontaneous, nondirected pushing in nonsupine positions (e.g., lateral, squatting, standing, kneeling, and semisitting) to facilitate the progress of fetal descent and shorten the second stage of labor.
- Avoid separation of the mother from her healthy baby after birth by encouraging skin-to-skin contact of mother and baby to keep newborn warm, prevent neonatal infection, enhance newborn's physiologic adjustment to extrauterine life, and foster early breastfeeding.

◎ NURSING CARE PLAN

Care of the Woman in Labor

NURSING DIAGNOSIS	EXPECTED OUTCOME	INTERVENTIONS	RATIONALES
Anxiety related to labor and the birthing process	Woman reports decreased anxiety level using an anxiety scale (from 0 [no anxiety] to 10 [anxiety as bad as it could possibly be]).	Orient woman and significant others to labor and birth unit and explain admission protocol	To allay initial feelings of anxiety
		Assess woman's knowledge, experience, and expectations of labor; note any signs or expressions of anxiety, nervousness, or fear	To establish baseline for intervention
		Discuss expected progression of labor and describe what to expect during process	To decrease anxiety associated with unknown
		Identify specific source(s) of anxiety	To better target interventions
		Actively involve woman in care decisions during labor, interpret sights and sounds of environment (monitor sights and sounds, unit activities), and share information on progression of labor (vital signs, fetal heart rate [FHR], dilation, effacement)	To increase her sense of control and lessen fears
Acute Pain related to increasing frequency and intensity of contractions	Woman reports decreased pain level using a pain scale (from 0 [no pain] to 10 [pain as bad as it could possibly be]).	Assess woman's level of pain and strategies that she has used to cope with it	To establish baseline for intervention
		Encourage significant other to remain as support person during labor process	To assist with support and comfort measures because measures are often more effective when delivered by familiar person
		Instruct woman and support person in use of specific techniques such as conscious relaxation, focused breathing, effleurage, massage, and application of sacral pressure	To increase relaxation, decrease intensity of contractions, and promote use of controlled thought and direction of energy
		Provide comfort measures such as frequent mouth care to prevent dry mouth, application of damp cloth to forehead, and changing of damp gown or bed covers	To relieve discomfort associated with diaphoresis
		Help woman to change position	To reduce stiffness, promote comfort, and facilitate progress of birth
		Explain which analgesics and anesthesia are available for use during labor and birth	To provide knowledge to help woman make decisions about pain control
		Administer analgesics and/or assist with regional anesthesia (e.g., epidural) as ordered or desired	To provide effective pain relief during labor and birth

⊚ **NURSING CARE PLAN**

Care of the Woman in Labor—cont'd

NURSING DIAGNOSIS	EXPECTED OUTCOME	INTERVENTIONS	RATIONALES
Risk for Impaired Urinary Elimination related to sensory impairment secondary to labor	Woman's bladder is emptied at least every 2 hours, either by spontaneous voiding or urinary catheter.	Palpate bladder superior to symphysis on frequent basis (at least every 2 hours)	To detect full bladder that occurs from increased fluid intake and inability to feel urge to void
		Encourage frequent voiding (at least every 2 hours) and catheterize if necessary	To avoid bladder distention because it impedes progress of fetus down birth canal and may result in trauma to bladder
		Help woman to bathroom or commode to void, if appropriate; provide privacy, and use techniques to stimulate voiding such as running water	To facilitate bladder emptying with an upright position (natural) and relaxation
Risk for Ineffective Individual Coping related to birthing process	Woman actively participates in birth process with no evidence of injury to her or her fetus.	Constantly monitor events of labor and birth, including physiologic responses of woman and fetus and emotional responses of woman and partner	To ensure maternal, partner, and fetal well-being
		Provide ongoing feedback to woman and partner	To decrease anxiety and enhance participation
		Continue to provide comfort measures and minimize distractions	To decrease discomfort and aid in focus on birth process
		Encourage woman to experiment with various positions	To assist downward movement of fetus
		Ensure that woman takes deep cleansing breaths before and after each contraction	To enhance gas exchange and oxygen transport to fetus
		Encourage woman to push spontaneously when urge to bear down is perceived during contraction	To aid descent and rotation of fetus
		Encourage woman to exhale, holding breath for short periods while bearing down	To avoid holding breath and triggering Valsalva maneuver, thereby increasing intrathoracic and cardiovascular pressure and decreasing perfusion of placental oxygen, placing fetus at risk
		Have woman take deep breaths and relax between contractions	To reduce fatigue and increase effectiveness of pushing efforts
		Have mother pant as fetal head crowns	To control birth of head and reduce risk for perineal trauma or fetal head injury
		Explain to woman and labor partner what is expected in the third stage of labor	To enlist cooperation
		Have woman maintain her position	To facilitate delivery of placenta
Fatigue related to energy expenditure required during labor and birth	Woman's energy levels are restored	Educate woman and partner about need for rest and help them plan strategies (e.g., restricting visitors, increasing role of support systems performing functions associated with daily routines) that allow specific times for rest and sleep	To ensure that woman can restore depleted energy levels in preparation for caring for new infant
		Monitor woman's fatigue level and amount of rest received	To ensure restoration of energy
		Group care activities as much as possible	To allow for periods of uninterrupted rest

emergency cesarean births. Women are awake during regional anesthesia and able to participate in their own care and protect their airway.

A recent Cochrane database review of this topic concluded that there is no justification for restricting food or fluid intake during labor in women at low risk for complications (Singata, Tranmer, and Gyte, 2010). Nurses should follow the orders of the woman's primary health care provider when offering the woman food or fluids during labor. However, as advocates nurses can facilitate change by informing others of the current research findings that support the safety and effectiveness of the oral intake of food and fluid during labor and initiating such research themselves.

An adequate intake of fluids and calories is required to meet the energy demands and fluid losses associated with childbirth. The progress of labor slows, with a more rapid development of hypoglycemia and ketosis if these demands are not met and fat is metabolized. Reduced energy for bearing-down efforts (pushing) increases the risk for a forceps- or vacuum-assisted birth. This is most likely to occur in women who begin to labor early in the morning after a night without caloric intake. When women are permitted to consume fluids and food freely, they typically regulate their own oral intake, eating light foods (e.g., eggs, yogurt, ice cream, dry toast and jelly, fruit) and drinking fluids during early labor and tapering off to the intake of clear fluids and sips of water or ice chips as labor intensifies and the second stage approaches(Sharts-Hopko, 2010).

Herbal teas can provide not only hydration but also other beneficial effects. Chamomile tea can enhance relaxation, lemon balm or peppermint tea can reduce nausea, and teas of ginger or ginseng root are energizing (Walls, 2009). A woman's culture may influence what she will eat and drink during labor. In addition, women who use nonpharmacologic pain-relief measures and labor at home or in birthing centers are more likely to eat and drink during labor. The amount of solid and liquid carbohydrates to offer a woman in labor is still unclear. Although it is known that energy needs increase as labor becomes prolonged, there is limited evidence regarding the effect of oral carbohydrate intake in enhancing the progress of labor and reducing the risk for dystocia (Sharts-Hopko, 2010).

Intravenous Intake. Fluids are administered intravenously to the laboring woman to maintain hydration, especially when a labor is long and the woman is unable to ingest a sufficient amount of fluid orally or if she is receiving epidural or intrathecal anesthesia. In most cases an electrolyte solution without glucose (e.g., Ringer's lactate or normal saline) is adequate and does not introduce excess glucose into the bloodstream. This is important because an excessive maternal glucose level results in fetal hyperglycemia and hyperinsulinism. After birth the neonate's high level of insulin reduces his or her glucose stores, and hypoglycemia results. Infusions containing glucose can also reduce sodium levels in the woman and fetus, leading to transient neonatal tachypnea. If maternal ketosis occurs, the primary health care provider may order an IV solution containing a small amount of dextrose to provide the glucose needed to aid in fatty acid metabolism.

! NURSING ALERT

Nurses should carefully monitor the intake and output of laboring women receiving IV fluids because they face an increased danger of hypervolemia as a result of the fluid retention that occurs during pregnancy.

Elimination

Voiding. Encourage voiding every 2 hours. A distended bladder may impede descent of the presenting part, slow or stop uterine contractions, and lead to decreased bladder tone or uterine atony after birth. Women who receive epidural analgesia or anesthesia are especially at risk for the retention of urine. Therefore the need to void should be assessed more frequently with them.

Help the woman to the bathroom to void or use a bedside commode unless any of the following apply: the primary health care provider has ordered bed rest; the woman is receiving epidural analgesia or anesthesia; internal monitoring is being used; or ambulation will compromise the status of the laboring woman or her fetus.

External monitoring can usually be interrupted long enough for the woman to go to the bathroom.

If using a bedpan is necessary, encourage spontaneous voiding by providing privacy and having the woman sit upright (as she would on a toilet). Other interventions to encourage urination, either in the bathroom or on the bedpan, are having the woman listen to the sound of water slowly running from a faucet, placing her hands in warm water, having her blow bubbles into a glass of water using a straw, or pouring warm water over the vulva and perineum with a peri bottle.

Catheterization. If the woman is unable to void and her bladder is distended, she may need to be catheterized. Many hospitals have protocols that rely on the nurse's judgment concerning the need for catheterization. Before performing the catheterization, clean the vulva and perineum because vaginal show and amniotic fluid may be present. If an obstacle that prevents advancement of the catheter is present, this obstacle is most likely the fetal presenting part. If you cannot advance the catheter, stop the procedure and notify the primary health care provider of the difficulty (see Evidence-Based Practice box).

Bowel Elimination. Most women do not have bowel movements during labor because of decreased intestinal motility. Stool that has formed in the large intestine often moves downward toward the anorectal area as a result of pressure exerted by the fetal presenting part as it descends. This stool is often expelled during second-stage pushing and birth. However, the passage of stool with bearing-down efforts increases the risk of infection and may embarrass the woman, thereby reducing the effectiveness of her pushing efforts. To prevent these problems, the nurse should immediately cleanse the perineal area to remove any stool, while reassuring the woman that the passage of stool at this time is a normal and expected event because the same muscles used to expel the baby also expel stool.

Routine use of enemas on admission for women at term has shown only modest benefits. There is a trend toward lower infection rates, and the newborns have fewer lower respiratory tract infections and less need for antibiotics. However, because enemas cause discomfort for women and increase the costs of giving birth, the small benefits do not outweigh the disadvantages of this practice (Berghella, Baxter, and Chauhan, 2008). In addition, a recent Cochrane review of this topic found that the evidence does not support the routine use of enemas during labor (Reveiz, Gaitan, and Cuervo, 2007).

When the presenting part is deep in the pelvis, even in the absence of stool in the anorectal area, the woman may feel rectal pressure and think she needs to defecate. If she expresses the urge to defecate, the nurse should perform a vaginal examination to assess cervical dilation and station. When a multiparous woman experiences the urge to defecate, this often means that birth will follow quickly.

Ambulation and Positioning

Confinement to bed is the norm for labor management in the United States. The increased use of epidurals during childbirth accompanied by multiple medical interventions (e.g., monitors, IV infusions) and reduced motor control contribute to this practice, thereby interfering with a woman's freedom of movement. However, upright positions and mobility during labor may be more pleasant for laboring women. These practices have also been associated with improved uterine contraction intensity and shorter labors, less need for pain medications, reduced rate of operative birth (e.g., cesarean birth, forceps- and vacuum-assisted birth), increased maternal

EVIDENCE-BASED PRACTICE

Reduction of Indwelling Urinary Catheters in Labor Patients with Epidural Anesthesia

Ask the Question

In a labor patient with epidural anesthesia, does allowing her to void independently or performing intermittent catheterization versus placing an indwelling urinary catheter alter the second stage of labor and the patient's perception of her labor experience and/or reduce catheter-associated urinary tract infections (CAUTIs)?

Search for the Evidence
Search Strategies

Search selection criteria included English language research-based publications on catheters, urinary catheters, labor patients, maternity patients, CAUTI, and perception of birth experience without time limitation.

Databases Used

CINAHL, UpToDate, OVID, Cochrane Database of Systematic Reviews, Joanna Briggs Institute, AHRQ

Critically Analyze the Evidence

- Indwelling urinary catheters versus intermittent catheterization did not shorten second stage of labor. Randomized controlled study of 209 labor patients resulted in shorter second stage in patients who were catheterized intermittently versus those with indwelling catheter (Evron, Dimitrochenko, Khazin, et al., 2008).
- Urinary retention is not favorably affected by the use of an indwelling catheter versus intermittent catheterization (Evron, Dimitrochenko, Khazin, et al., 2009).
- Reducing the use of urinary catheters in labor and delivery is one way to reduce CAUTIs (Srinivas, 2008).
- Hospitals will institute evidence-based practices to reduce CAUTIs (The Joint Commission, 2012).
- In a randomized, nonblinded trial of 146 women, bacterial urinary tract infections were found to be higher in those who were catheterized intermittently than in those who had an indwelling catheter (Millet, Shaha, and Bartholomew, 2012).
- Nurses should use as few interventions during labor as possible to promote normal birth experiences for their patients (Romano and Lothian, 2008).
- There is no evidence to support routine labor interventions such as intravenous fluids, augmentation of labor, epidural anesthesia, and indwelling urinary catheters. These inhibit mobility, various comfort measures, and spontaneous voiding and may increase the patient's stress levels (Romano and Lothian, 2008).
- The bladder should be assessed frequently, and the patient should be given the opportunity to void independently before catheterization. The psychologic effects of this procedure should not be taken lightly and can affect the woman's perception of her ability to participate and make decisions about her labor experience (DeSevo and Semeraro, 2010).
- A woman's perception of her birth experience can be affected by her ability to control her body and participate in decision making about her care during labor (Bryanton, Gagnon, Johnston, et al., 2008).
- Women should receive prenatal education regarding the effects of epidural anesthesia as it relates to their ability to void during labor (Walsh, 2007).

Apply the Evidence: Nursing Implications

- There is sufficient evidence to support reducing the use of indwelling urinary catheters in labor patients with epidural anesthesia (Evron, Dimitrochenko, Khazin, et al., 2009; Srinivas, 2008; The Joint Commission, 2012). Nurses must support women in their ability to make decisions about their care during labor to support the natural labor process. These decisions have been shown to make an impact on women's perception of their birth experience (Bryanton, Gagnon, Johnston, et al., 2008; Romano and Lothian, 2008).

Quality and Safety Competencies:
Evidence-Based Practice*
Knowledge

Differentiate clinical opinion from research and evidence-based summaries.

Describe reasons for reducing indwelling catheter use in laboring patients with epidural anesthesia.

Skills

Base individualized care plan on patient values, clinical expertise, and evidence.

Nurses use critical thinking skills to assess clinical situations when an indwelling catheter is an appropriate intervention.

Attitudes

Value the concept of evidence-based practice as integral to determining best clinical practice.

Value the evidence for supporting women in labor by using fewer interventions as a means of enhancing their labor experience and providing safe and high-quality care.

References

Bryanton J, Gagnon A, Johnston C, et al: Predictors of women's perceptions of the childbirth experience, *J Obstet Gynecol Neonatal Nurses* 37(1):24–34, 2008.

DeSevo M, Semeraro P: Urinary catheterization during epidural anesthesia, *Nurs Women's Health* 14(1):11–13, 2010.

Evron S, Dimitrochenko V, Khazin V, et al: The effect of intermittent versus continuous bladder catheterization on labor duration and postpartum urinary retention and infection: a randomized trial, *J Clin Anesth* 20(8):567–572, 2008.

Millet L, Shaha S, Bartholomew M: Rates of bacteriuria in laboring women with epidural analgesia: continuous vs intermittent bladder catheterization, *Am J Obstet Gynecol* 206(4):316.e1–316.e7, 2012.

Romano J, Lothian J: Promoting, protecting and supporting normal birth: a look at the evidence, *J Obstet Gynecol Neonat Nurses* 37:94–105, 2008.

Srinivas S: Intermittent versus continuous bladder catheterization during labor: does it matter? *J Clin Anesth* 20(8):565–566, 2008.

The Joint Commission: National Patient Safety Goals, Oakbrook Terrace, IL, 2012, Author, www.jointcommission.org.

Walsh D: The medicalization of bladder care, *Br J Midwifery* 15(2):1–3, 2007.

Ellen Schneiderman

*Adapted from the Quality and Safety Education for Nurses at www.qsen.org/.

autonomy and control, distraction from the discomforts of labor, and an opportunity for close interaction with the woman's partner and care provider as they help her assume upright positions and remain mobile (Lawrence, Lewis, Hofmeyr, et al., 2009; Simpson, 2008; Zwelling, 2010). No harmful effects have been observed from maternal activity and position changes.

> ⚡ **SAFETY ALERT**
>
> A woman may experience dizziness as she changes upright positions during labor. It is essential that the nurse or support person be present to provide assistance should dizziness occur.

Encourage ambulation if membranes are intact, if the fetal presenting part is engaged after ROM, and if the woman has not received medication for pain (Fig. 16-9). The woman also may find it comfortable to stand and lean forward on her partner, doula, or nurse for support at times during labor (Fig. 16-10, *A*). At times, ambulation may be contraindicated because of maternal or fetal status.

When the woman lies in bed, she usually changes her position spontaneously as labor progresses. If she does not change position every 30 to 60 minutes, encourage or help her to do so. The side-lying (lateral) position is preferred because it promotes optimal uteroplacental and renal blood flow and increases fetal oxygen saturation (Fig. 16-11, *B*). If the woman wants to lie supine, the nurse should place a pillow under one hip as a wedge to prevent the uterus from compressing the aorta and vena cava (see Fig. 16-5, *D*). Sitting is not contraindicated unless it adversely affects fetal status, which you can determine by checking the FHR and pattern. If the fetus is in the occiput posterior position, it may be helpful to encourage the woman to squat during contractions because this position increases the pelvic diameter, allowing the head to rotate to a more anterior position (see Fig. 16-11, *A*). A hands-and-knees position during contractions or a lateral position on the same side as the fetal spine also is recommended to facilitate the rotation of the fetal occiput from a posterior to an anterior position as gravity pulls the fetal back forward. These positions also provide access to the back for application of counterpressure by the partner, doula, or nurse (Hanson, 2009; Simpson, Cesario, Morin, et al., 2008; Zwelling, 2010) (see Fig. 16-10, *B*). Women with epidural anesthesia may not be able to squat or assume a hands-and-knees position, depending on the degree of motor involvement resulting from the epidural.

Much research continues to focus on acquiring a better understanding of the physiologic and psychologic effects of maternal position in labor. Box 16-11 describes a variety of positions that are commonly used and recommended.

The woman can use a birth ball (gymnastic ball, physical therapy ball) to support her body as she assumes a variety of labor and birth positions (Fig. 16-12). She can sit on the ball while leaning over the bed or lean over the ball to support her upper body and reduce stress on her arms and hands when she assumes a hands-and-knees position. The birth ball can encourage pelvic mobility and pelvic and perineal relaxation when the woman sits on the firm yet pliable ball and rocks in rhythmic movements. Warm compresses applied to the

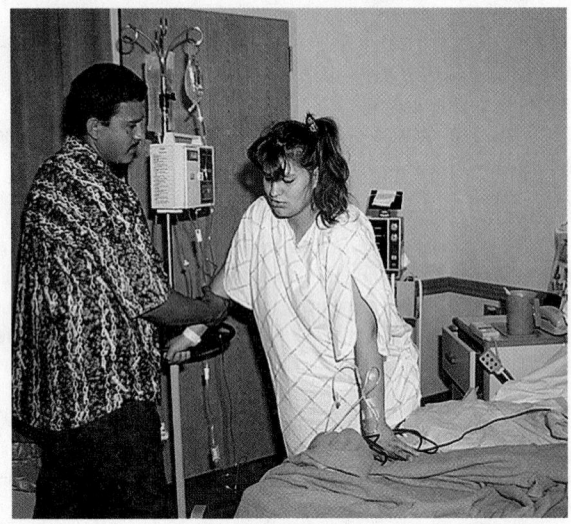

FIG 16-9 Woman preparing to walk with partner. (Courtesy Marjorie Pyle, RNC, Lifecircle, Costa Mesa, CA.)

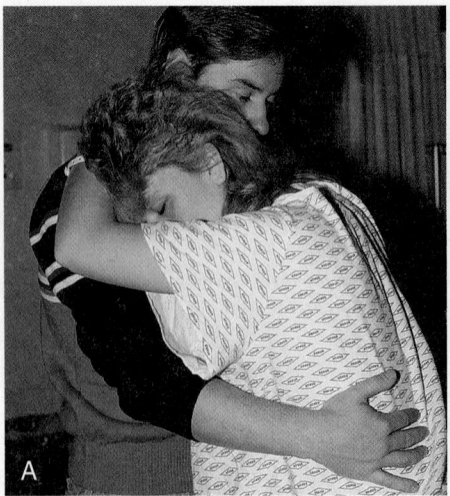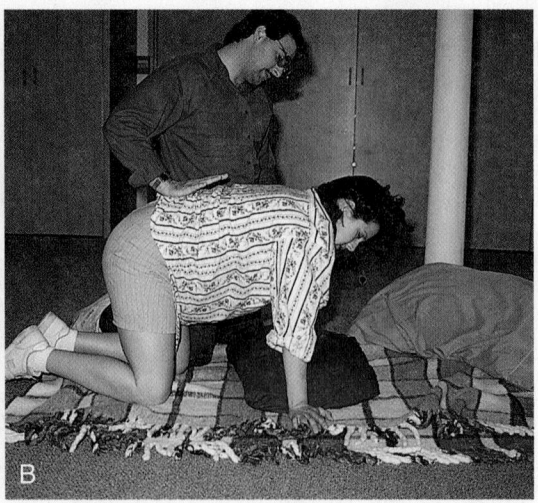

FIG 16-10 A, Woman standing and leaning forward with support. **B,** Woman in hands-and-knees position. (Courtesy Marjorie Pyle, RNC, Lifecircle, Costa Mesa, CA.)

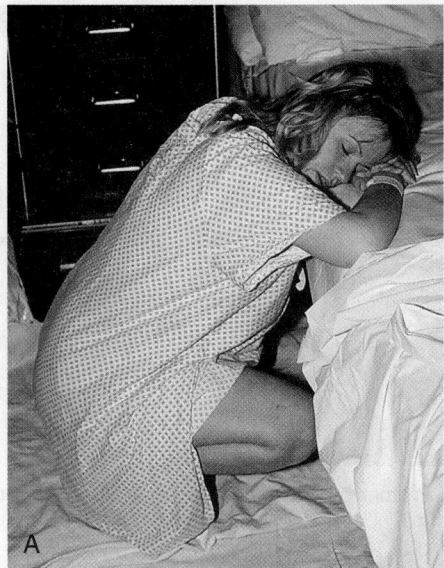

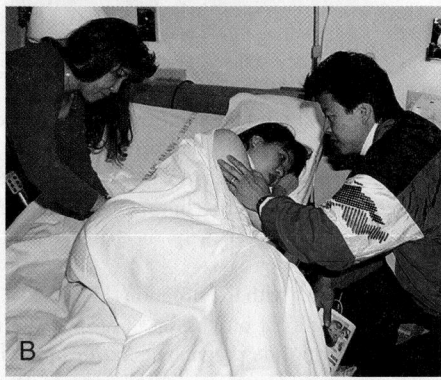

FIG 16-11 Maternal positions for labor. **A,** Squatting. **B,** Lateral position. Support person is applying sacral pressure while partner provides encouragement. (Courtesy Marjorie Pyle, RNC, Lifecircle, Costa Mesa, CA.)

perineum and lower back can maximize this relaxation and comfort effect. The birth ball should be large enough that, when the woman sits, her knees are bent at a 90-degree angle and her feet are flat on the floor and approximately 2 feet apart.

Supportive Care During Labor and Birth

Support during labor and birth involves emotional support, physical care and comfort measures, and advice and information. The value of the continuous supportive presence of a person (e.g., doula, childbirth educator, family member, friend, nurse, partner) during labor has long been known. Women who have continuous support beginning in early labor are less likely to use pain medication or epidurals, more likely to have a spontaneous vaginal birth, and less likely to report dissatisfaction with their birth experience. No harmful effects from continuous labor support have been identified. To the contrary, there is good evidence that labor support improves important health outcomes (AWHONN, 2011; Berghella, Baxter, and Chauhan, 2008; Hodnett, Gates, Hofmeyr, et al., 2011).

Labor rooms should be airy, clean, and homelike. The laboring woman should feel safe in this environment and free to be herself and use the comfort and relaxation measures she prefers. To enhance relaxation turn off bright overhead lights when not needed

---

BOX 16-11   COMMON MATERNAL POSITIONS* DURING LABOR AND BIRTH

Semirecumbent Position (see Figs. 16-14, *B*, and 16-15, *B*)

With woman sitting with her upper body elevated to at least a 30-degree angle, place wedge or small pillow under hip to prevent vena cava compression and reduce likelihood of supine hypotension (see Fig. 16-5).

- The greater the angle of elevation, the more gravity or pressure is exerted that promotes fetal descent, the progress of contractions, and the widening of pelvic dimensions.
- Position is convenient for rendering care measures and external fetal monitoring.

Lateral Position (see Figs. 16-11, *B*, and 16-14, *A*)

Have woman alternate between left and right side-lying position and provide abdominal and back support as needed for comfort.

- Removes pressure from the vena cava and back, enhances uteroplacental perfusion, and relieves backache
- Facilitates internal rotation of fetus in a posterior position to an anterior position (woman should lie on same side as fetal spine)
- Makes it easier to perform back massage or counterpressure
- Associated with less frequent but more intense contractions
- May be more difficult to obtain good external fetal monitor tracings
- May be used as a birthing position
- Takes pressure off perineum, allowing it to stretch gradually
- Reduces risk for perineal trauma

Upright Position

The gravity effect enhances the contraction cycle and fetal descent. The weight of the fetus places increasing pressure on the cervix; the cervix is pulled upward, facilitating effacement and dilation; impulses from the cervix to the pituitary gland increase, causing more oxytocin to be secreted; and contractions are intensified, thereby applying more forceful downward pressure on the fetus, but they are less painful.

- Fetus is aligned with pelvis, and pelvic diameters are widened slightly.
- Effective upright positions include:
  - Ambulation (see Fig. 16-9)
  - Standing and leaning forward with support provided by coach (see Fig. 16-10, *A*), end of bed, back of chair, or birth ball; relieves backache and facilitates application of counterpressure or back massage
  - Sitting up in bed, chair, or birthing chair or on toilet or bedside commode (see Fig. 16-14, *B*)
  - Squatting (see Fig. 16-11, *A*, and Fig. 16-15, *E*)

Hands-and-Knees Position—Position for Posterior Positions of the Presenting Part (see Figs. 16-10, *B* and 16-12)

Assume an "all fours" position or lean over an object (e.g., birth ball) while on knees in bed or on a covered floor; can also place knees on seat section of bed while leaning up over back of raised head of bed; allows for pelvic rocking.

- Relieves backache characteristic of "back labor"
- Facilitates internal rotation of the fetus by increasing mobility of the coccyx, increasing the pelvic diameters, and using gravity to turn the fetal back and rotate the head (NOTE: A side-lying position, double hip squeeze, or knee squeeze can also facilitate internal rotation.)

---

*Assess the effect of each position on the laboring woman's comfort and anxiety level, progress of labor, and fetal heart rate and pattern. Alternate positions every 30 to 60 minutes, allowing the woman to take control of her position changes.

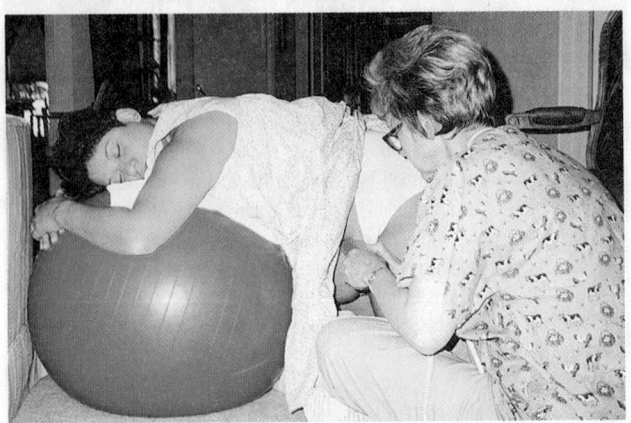

FIG 16-12 Woman laboring using birth ball. (Courtesy Polly Perez, Cutting Edge Press, Johnson, VT.)

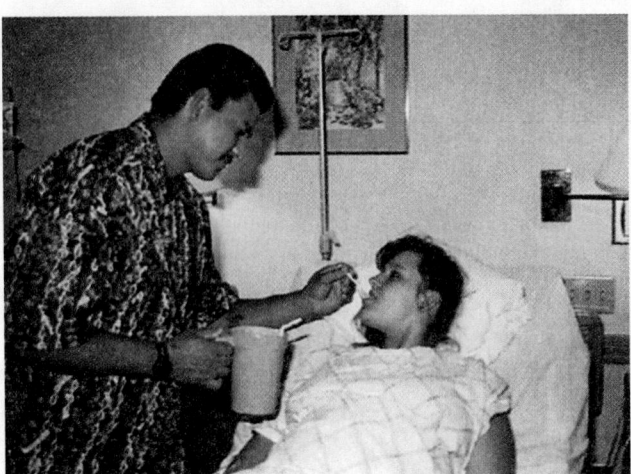

FIG 16-13 Partner providing comfort measures. (Courtesy Marjorie Pyle, RNC, Lifecircle, Costa Mesa, CA.)

and keep noise and intrusions to a minimum. Control the temperature to ensure the laboring woman's comfort. The room should be large enough to accommodate a comfortable chair for the woman's partner, the monitoring equipment, and hospital personnel. Encourage women to bring their own pillows to make the hospital surroundings more homelike and facilitate position changes. Environmental modifications should reflect the preferences of the woman, including the number of visitors and availability of a telephone, television, and music.

Labor Support by the Nurse

Supportive nursing care for a woman in labor includes:

- Helping her maintain control and participate to the extent she wishes in the birth of her infant.
- Providing continuity of care that is nonjudgmental and respectful of her cultural and religious values and beliefs.
- Meeting her expected outcomes for her labor.
- Listening to her concerns and encouraging her to express her feelings.
- Acting as her advocate, supporting her decisions and respecting her choices as appropriate and relating her wishes as needed to other health care providers.
- Helping her conserve her energy and cope effectively with her pain and discomfort by using a variety of comfort measures that are acceptable to her.
- Helping control her discomfort.
- Acknowledging her efforts during labor, including her strength and courage and those of her partner, and providing positive reinforcement.
- Protecting her privacy, modesty, and dignity.

Women who have attended childbirth education programs that teach the psychoprophylactic (Lamaze) approach know something about the labor process, coaching techniques, and comfort measures. The nurse plays a supportive role and keeps the woman and her partner informed of the labor progress. If necessary, review the methods learned in class and practiced at home because it may be difficult for the woman to use these methods and techniques effectively now that she is in labor and in an unfamiliar setting.

Even when a laboring woman has not attended childbirth classes, the nurse can teach her simple breathing and relaxation techniques during the early phase of labor. In this case the nurse provides more of the coaching and supportive care until the support person feels ready to take on a more active coaching role (see Chapter 14). The nurse can demonstrate comfort measures while encouraging the support person to assist and the laboring woman to express her needs and feelings. Observing the comforting approaches of the nurse can help the partner learn effective comfort measures.

Comfort measures vary with the situation (Fig. 16-13). The nurse can draw on the woman's list of comfort measures and relaxation techniques learned during the pregnancy and through life experiences. Such measures include maintaining a comfortable, calm, supportive atmosphere in the labor and birth area; using touch therapeutically (e.g., heat or cold applied to the lower back in the event of back labor, a cool cloth applied to the forehead, massage); providing nonpharmacologic measures to relieve discomfort (e.g., hydrotherapy); and, most important, just being there (see Table 16-1; Table 16-3). See Chapter 14 for a full discussion of pharmacologic and nonpharmacologic comfort measures.

Most women in labor respond positively to touch, but you should obtain permission before using any touching measures. Women appreciate gentle handling by staff members. Back rubs and counterpressure may be offered, especially if the woman is experiencing back labor. Teach the support person to exert counterpressure against the woman's sacrum over the occiput of the head of a fetus in a posterior position (see Fig. 16-11, *B*). Double hip or knee squeezes can also be helpful in reducing back pain. The back pain is caused by the occiput pressing on spinal nerves; counterpressure lifts the occiput off these nerves, providing some pain relief. However, the partner needs to be relieved after a while because exerting counterpressure is hard work. Hand and foot massage also can be soothing and relaxing.

The woman's perception of the soothing qualities of touch may change as labor progresses. Many women become more sensitive to touch (hyperesthesia) as labor progresses. This is a typical response during the transition phase (see Table 16-1). They may tell their coach to leave them alone or not to touch them. The partner who is unprepared for this normal response may feel rejected and react by withdrawing active support. The nurse can reassure him or her that this response is a positive indication that the first stage is ending and the second stage is approaching. Women with increased

TABLE 16-3	EXPECTED MATERNAL PROGRESS IN THE SECOND STAGE OF LABOR	
CRITERION	**LATENT PHASE (AVERAGE DURATION, 10-30 MINUTES)**	**ACTIVE PUSHING (DESCENT) PHASE (AVERAGE DURATION VARIES)***
Contractions		
Intensity	Period of physiologic lull for all criteria; period of peace and rest; "laboring down"	Significant increase becoming overwhelmingly strong and expulsive
Frequency		Every 2 to 2.5 minutes progressing to every 1 to 2 minutes
Duration		90 seconds
Descent, station	0 to +2	+2 to +4; Rate of descent increases and Ferguson reflex† is activated; fetal head becomes visible at introitus, and birth occurs
Show: color and amount		Significant increase in dark red bloody show; bloody show accompanies emergence of head
Spontaneous bearing-down efforts	Slight to absent, except at peak of strongest contractions	Increased urge to bear down; becomes stronger as fetus descends to vaginal introitus and reaches perineum
Vocalization	Quiet; concern over progress	Grunting sounds or expiratory vocalizations; announces contractions; may scream or swear
Maternal behavior	Experiences sense of relief that transition to second stage is finished	Senses increased urge to push and describes increasing pain; describes *ring of fire* (burning sensation of acute pain as vagina stretches and fetal head crowns)
	Feels fatigued and sleepy	Expresses feeling of powerlessness
	Feels a sense of accomplishment and optimism because the "worst is over"	Shows decreased ability to listen to or concentrate on anything but giving birth
	Feels in control	Alters respiratory pattern: has short 4- to 5-second breath holds with regular breaths in between, 5 to 7 times per contraction
		Frequent repositioning
		Often shows excitement immediately after birth of head

Data from Hanson L: Second-stage labor care, *J Perinat Neonatal Nurs* 23(1):31–39, 2009; Simpson K, Cesario S, Morin K, et al: *Nursing care and management of the second stage of labor: evidence-based clinical practice guideline,* ed 2, Washington, DC, 2008, Association of Women's Health, Obstetric, and Neonatal Nurses; Roberts JE: The "push" for evidence: management of the second stage, *J Midwifery Womens Health* 47(1):2–15, 2002; Simkin P, Ancheta R: *The labor progress,* Malden, MA, 2000, Blackwell Science.
*Duration of descent phase can vary, depending on maternal parity, effectiveness of bearing-down effort, and presence of spinal anesthesia or epidural analgesia.
†Pressure of presenting part on stretch receptors of pelvic floor stimulates release of oxytocin from posterior pituitary, resulting in more intense uterine contractions.

sensitivity to touch may tolerate it better on surfaces of the body where hair does not grow such as the forehead, palms of the hands, and soles of the feet.

Labor Support by the Father or Partner

Although another woman or a man other than the father may be the woman's partner, the father of the baby is frequently the support person during labor. He is often able to provide the comfort measures and touch that the laboring woman needs. When the woman becomes focused on her pain, sometimes the partner can persuade her to try nonpharmacologic variations of comfort measures. In addition, he usually is able to interpret the woman's needs and desires for staff members.

The feelings of a first-time father change as labor progresses. Although he is often calm at the onset of labor, feelings of fear and helplessness begin to dominate as labor becomes more active and the father realizes that it is more stressful than he anticipated. A study of Swedish fathers' birth experiences found that, although about three quarters of the men reported positive or very positive experiences, less positive experiences were associated with

emergency cesarean birth, assisted vaginal birth, and dissatisfaction with their partners' medical care. The interactions of health care providers with the fathers and the fathers' perception of the health care providers' competence were also related to the fathers' birth experiences (Johansson, Rubertsson, Radestad, et al., 2012). Staff members should tell the father that his presence is helpful and encourage him to be involved in the care of the woman to the extent to which he and his partner are comfortable. He should be reassured that he is not assuming the responsibility for observation and management of his partner's labor but that his responsibility is to support her as the labor progresses. The nurse can suggest alternative comfort measures when those he is using are no longer helpful or are rejected by his partner.

The first-time father may feel excluded as birth preparations begin during the transition phase. Once the second stage begins and birth nears, the father's focus changes from the woman to the baby who is about to be born. The father will be exposed to many sights and smells he may never have experienced. Therefore the nurse needs to tell him what to expect and make him comfortable about leaving the room to regain his composure should something occur

BOX 16-12	GUIDELINES FOR SUPPORTING THE FATHER/PARTNER*

- Orient him to the labor room and the unit; explain location of the cafeteria, toilet, waiting room, and nursery; give information about visiting hours; introduce personnel present by name and describe their functions.
- Inform him of sights and smells he can expect to encounter; encourage him to leave the room if necessary.
- Respect his or the couple's decision about the degree of his involvement. Offer them freedom to make decisions.
- Tell him when his presence has been helpful and continue to reinforce this throughout labor.
- Offer to teach him comfort measures; demonstrate or role model performance of these measures.
- Inform him frequently of the progress of the labor and the woman's needs. Keep him informed about procedures to be performed.
- Prepare him for changes in the woman's behavior and physical appearance.
- Remind him to eat; offer him snacks and fluids if possible.
- Relieve him of the job of support person as necessary. Offer him blankets if he is to sleep in a chair by the bedside.
- Acknowledge the stress experienced by each partner during labor and birth and identify normal responses.
- Attempt to modify or eliminate unsettling stimuli such as extra noise and extra light; create a relaxing and calm environment.

*These guidelines are appropriate for any support person or partner.

that surprises him but make sure that someone else is available to support the woman during his absence.

Nursing actions that support the father convey several important concepts: first, that he is a person of value; second, that he can be a partner in the woman's care; and third, that childbearing is a team effort. Box 16-12 details ways in which the nurse can support the father-partner. A well-informed father can make an important contribution to the health and well-being of the mother and child, their family interrelationship, and his self-esteem.

Labor Support by Doulas

Continuity of care has been cited by women as a critical component of a satisfying childbirth experience. A specially trained, experienced female labor attendant called a doula can meet this need. The doula provides a continual one-on-one caring presence throughout the labor of the woman she is attending and the birth (Simkin and Way, 2008). The primary role of the doula is to focus on the laboring woman and provide physical and emotional support by using soft, reassuring words of praise and encouragement; touching; stroking; and hugging. The doula also administers comfort measures to reduce pain and enhance relaxation and coping, walks with the woman, helps her to change positions, and coaches her bearing-down efforts. Doulas provide information about labor progress and explain procedures and events. They advocate for the woman's right to participate actively in the management of her labor.

The doula also supports the woman's partner, who often feels unqualified to be the sole labor support and may find it difficult to watch the woman when she is experiencing pain. The doula can encourage and praise the partner's efforts, create a partnership as

caregivers, and provide respite care. Doulas also facilitate communication between the laboring woman and her partner and between the couple and the health care team (Simkin and Way, 2008).

Doula support during labor is associated with decreased use of analgesia, decreased incidence of operative birth, increased incidence of spontaneous vaginal birth, and increased maternal satisfaction with the childbirth experience (Berghella, Baxter, and Chauhan, 2008; Hodnett, Gates, Hofmeyr, et al., 2011).

The roles of the nurse and the doula are complementary. They should work together as a team, recognizing and respecting the role each plays in supporting and caring for the woman and her partner during the childbirth process. The doula provides supportive nonmedical care measures, whereas the nurse focuses on monitoring the status of the maternal-fetal unit, implementing clinical care protocols (including pharmacologic interventions) and documenting assessment findings, actions, and responses (Simkin and Way, 2008).

Labor Support by Grandparents

When grandparents act as labor coaches, it is especially important to support and treat them with respect. They may have ways to deal with pain based on their experience. Grandparents should be encouraged to help as long as their actions do not compromise the status of the mother or the fetus. The nurse treats grandparents with dignity and respect by acknowledging the value of their contributions to parental support and recognizing the difficulty parents have in witnessing the woman's discomfort or crisis. If they have never witnessed a birth, the nurse may need to provide explanations of what is happening. Many of the activities used to support fathers also are appropriate for grandparents.

Siblings During Labor and Birth

Preparing siblings for acceptance of the new child helps promote the attachment process and may help the older children accept this change. The older child or children who know that they are important to the family become active participants. Rehearsal for the event before labor is essential.

The age and developmental level of children influence their responses; therefore preparation for the children to be present during labor is adjusted to meet each child's needs. (See Box 8-1.) The child younger than 2 years shows little interest in pregnancy and labor. However, for the older child such preparation may reduce fears and misconceptions. Parents need to be prepared for labor and birth themselves and feel comfortable about the process and the presence of their children. Most parents have a "feel" for their children's maturational level and their physical and emotional ability to observe and cope with the events of the labor and birth process. Preparation can include a description of the anticipated sights, events (e.g., ROM, monitors, IV infusions), smells, and sounds; a labor and birth demonstration; a tour of the birthing unit; and an opportunity to be around a real newborn (see Fig. 8-4). Storybooks about the birth process can be read to or by children to prepare them for the event. Films are available for preparing preschool and school-age children to participate in the labor and birth experience. Children must learn that their mother will be working hard during labor and birth. She will not be able to talk to them during contractions. She may groan, scream, grunt, and pant at times and say things she would not say otherwise (e.g., "I can't take this anymore," "Take this baby out of me," or "This pain is killing me"). You can tell them that labor is uncomfortable, but that their mother's body is made for the job.

Most agencies require that a specific person be designated to watch over the children who are participating in their mother's childbirth experience to provide them with support, explanations, diversions, and comfort as needed. Health care providers involved in attending women during birth must be comfortable with the presence of children and the unpredictability of their questions, comments, and behaviors.

Emergency Interventions

Emergency conditions that require immediate nursing intervention can arise with startling speed.

See Chapter 15 for information on management of abnormal FHR. Management of other emergency situations, including meconium-stained amniotic fluid, shoulder dystocia, prolapsed umbilical cord, ruptured uterus, and amniotic fluid embolus, is discussed in Chapter 17.

SECOND STAGE OF LABOR

The second stage of labor is the stage in which the infant is born. This stage begins with full cervical dilation (10 cm) and complete effacement (100%) and ends with the baby's birth. The force exerted by uterine contractions, gravity, and maternal bearing-down efforts facilitates achievement of the expected outcome of a spontaneous, uncomplicated vaginal birth. The median duration of second-stage labor is 50 to 60 minutes in nulliparous women and 20 to 30 minutes in multiparous women. In addition to parity, maternal size and fetal weight, position, and descent influence the length of this stage. The use of epidural anesthesia during labor often increases the length of the second stage of labor because the epidural blocks or reduces the woman's urge to bear down and limits her ability to attain an upright position to push. The upper limits for the duration of normal second-stage labor are (Wing and Farinelli, 2012):

- Nulliparous women:
  2 hours with no regional anesthesia
  3 hours with regional anesthesia

- Multiparous women:
  1 hour with no regional anesthesia
  2 hours with regional anesthesia

A prolonged second stage is diagnosed after these time limits are reached. A thorough assessment of the status of the maternal fetal unit and a determination regarding the likely effectiveness and safety of further bearing-down efforts should be made (Simpson et al., 2008).

The second stage of labor is composed of two phases: the latent phase and the active pushing (descent) phase. Maternal verbal and nonverbal behaviors, uterine activity, the urge to bear down, and fetal descent characterize these phases (Hanson, 2009; Simpson, Cesario, Morin, et al., 2008).

The latent phase is a period of rest and relative calm (i.e., "laboring down"). During this early phase the fetus continues to descend passively through the birth canal and rotate to an anterior position as a result of ongoing uterine contractions. The woman is quiet and often relaxes with her eyes closed between contractions. The urge to bear down is not strong, and some women do not experience it at all or only during the acme (peak) of a contraction. Delayed pushing has been shown to result in significant decreases in pushing time, significant increases in the duration of second-stage labor, and a reduction in the number of operative vaginal births. On the other hand, no differences in the number of cesarean births, perineal lacerations or episiotomies, or fetal complications have been linked to delayed pushing (Kelly, Johnson, Lee, et al., 2010). In a randomized clinical trial, allowing a woman to rest during this phase and waiting until the urge intensified to begin pushing significantly reduced the amount of time spent pushing but did not significantly increase the total length of second-stage labor. In this study maternal fatigue scores, perineal injuries, and FHR decelerations were similar in the immediate- and delayed-pushing groups (Kelly, Johnson, Lee, et al., 2010). Another study also found a significant decrease in pushing time in nulliparous women with epidural anesthesia who practiced delayed pushing during second-stage labor (Gillesby, Burns, Dempsey, et al., 2010).

Careful monitoring with assurance of normal fetal status should be used during delayed pushing. If descent is slow and the woman becomes anxious, she should be encouraged to change positions frequently or to stand by the bedside to use the advantage of gravity and movement to facilitate descent and progress to the active pushing phase signaled by a perception of the need to bear down (Hanson, 2009).

During the phase of active pushing (descent) the woman has strong urges to bear down as the Ferguson reflex is activated when the presenting part presses on the stretch receptors of the pelvic floor. At this point the fetal station is usually +1, and the position is anterior. This stimulation causes the release of oxytocin from the posterior pituitary gland, which provokes stronger expulsive uterine contractions. The woman becomes more focused on bearing-down efforts, which become rhythmic. She changes positions frequently to find a more comfortable pushing position. The woman often announces the onset of contractions and becomes more vocal as she bears down. The urge to bear down intensifies as descent progresses and the presenting part reaches the perineum. The woman may be more verbal about the pain she is experiencing; she may scream or swear and may act out of control.

The nurse encourages the woman to "listen" to her body as she progresses through the phases of the second stage of labor. When a woman listens to her body to tell her when to bear down, she is using an internal locus of control and often feels more satisfied with her efforts to give birth to her baby. This enhances her sense of self-esteem and accomplishment, and her efforts become more effective. Always encourage the woman's trust in her own body and her ability to give birth to her baby. Validate the woman's experience of pressure, stretching, and straining as normal and a signal that the descent of the fetus is progressing and her body is capable of withstanding birth. Honestly explain what is happening and describe the progress being made.

CARE MANAGEMENT

The only certain objective sign that the second stage of labor has begun is the inability to feel the cervix during vaginal examination, indicating that it is fully dilated and effaced. The precise moment that this occurs is not easily determined because it depends on when a vaginal examination is performed to validate full dilation and effacement. This makes timing of the actual duration of the second stage difficult. Other signs that suggest the onset of the second stage include the urge to push or feeling the need to have a bowel movement. These signs commonly appear at the time the cervix reaches full dilation. However, they can appear earlier in labor. Women with an epidural block may not exhibit such signs.

Women can begin to experience an irresistible urge to bear down before full dilation. For some this occurs as early as 5-cm dilation. This is most often related to the station of the presenting part below the level of the ischial spines of the maternal pelvis. This occurrence

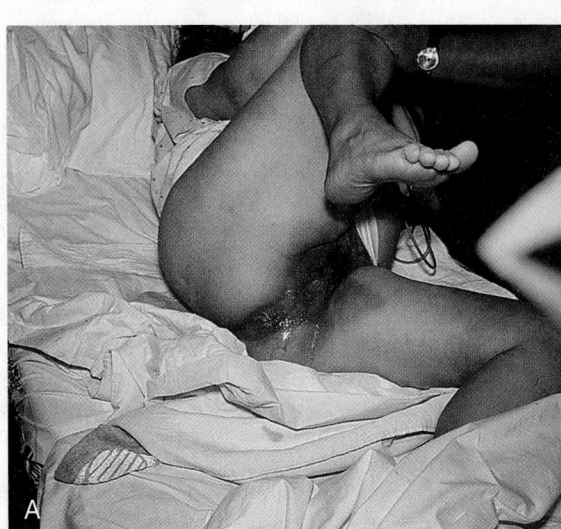 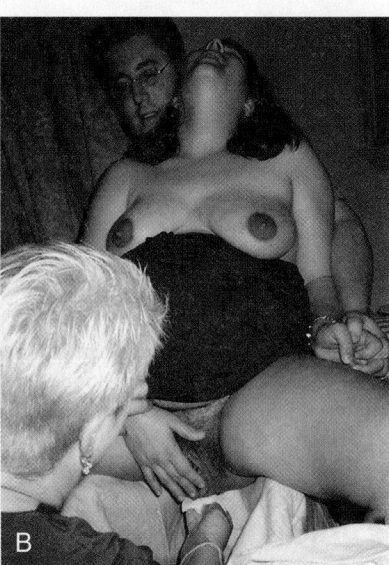

FIG 16-14 A, Pushing, side-lying position. Perineal bulging can be seen. **B,** Pushing, semisitting position. Midwife helps mother feel top of fetal head. (*A* Courtesy Michael S. Clement, MD, Mesa, AZ. *B* Courtesy Roni Wernik, Palo Alto, CA.)

creates a conflict between the woman, whose body is telling her to push, and her health care providers, who believe that pushing the fetal presenting part against an incompletely dilated cervix will result in cervical edema and lacerations and slow the labor progress. Evaluate the premature urge to bear down as a sign of labor progress, possibly indicating the onset of the second stage of labor. Base the timing of when a woman pushes in relation to whether her cervix is fully dilated on research evidence rather than on tradition or routine practice. Pushing with the urge to bear down at the acme of a contraction may be safe and effective for a woman if her cervix is soft, retracting, and 8 cm or more dilated and if the fetus is at +1 station and rotating to an anterior position (Hanson, 2009).

Assessment is continuous during the second stage of labor. Professional standards and agency policy determine the specific type and timing of assessments and the way in which findings are documented. Signs and symptoms of impending birth (see Table 16-3) may appear unexpectedly, requiring immediate action by the nurse (Box 16-13).

The nurse continues to monitor maternal-fetal status and events of the second stage and provide comfort measures for the mother. This includes helping her change position; providing mouth care; maintaining clean, dry bedding; and keeping unnecessary noise, conversation, and other distractions (e.g., laughing, talking of attending personnel in or outside the labor area) to a minimum. The woman is encouraged to indicate other support measures she would like (see Box 16-7).

In the hospital birth may occur in an LDR, LDRP, or delivery room. If the mother is to be transferred to the delivery room for birth, perform the transfer early enough to avoid rushing her. The birth area also is readied.

Preparing for Birth
Maternal Position

No single position for childbirth exists. Labor is a dynamic, interactive process involving the woman's uterus, pelvis, and voluntary muscles. In addition, angles between the baby and the woman's pelvis constantly change as the infant turns and flexes down the birth canal. The woman may want to assume various positions for childbirth. She should be encouraged to change positions frequently and assisted in attaining and maintaining her position(s) of choice (Figs. 16-14 and 16-15). Supine, semirecumbent, or lithotomy positions are still widely used in Western societies despite evidence that women prefer upright positions for their bearing-down efforts and birth.

Birth attendants play a major role in influencing a woman's choice of positions for birth, with nurse-midwives tending to advocate nonlithotomy positions (e.g., upright, lateral) for the second stage of labor. An upright position (walking, sitting, kneeling, or squatting) offers a number of advantages. Gravity can promote the descent of the fetus. Uterine contractions are generally stronger and more efficient in effacing and dilating the cervix, resulting in shorter labor (Blackburn, 2013; Lawrence, Lewis, Hofmeyr, et al., 2009; Zwelling, 2010). An upright position also is beneficial to the mother's cardiac output, thereby increasing perfusion of the uterus. The use of upright and lateral positions is also associated with less pain and perineal damage, fewer episiotomies and abnormal FHR patterns, and fewer operative vaginal births (Berghella, Baxter, and Chauhan, 2008; James, 2011; Simpson, Cesario, Morin, et al., 2008; Zwelling, 2010). The benefits of upright positions may be related to:

- Straightening of the longitudinal axis of the birth canal and improvement in the alignment of the fetus for passage through the pelvis.
- Application of gravity to direct the fetal head toward the pelvic inlet, thereby facilitating descent.
- Enlargement of pelvic dimensions and restriction of the encroachment of the sacrum and coccyx into the pelvic outlet.
- Increased uteroplacental circulation, resulting in more intense, efficient uterine contractions.
- Enhancement of the woman's ability to bear down effectively, thereby minimizing maternal exhaustion.

BOX 16-13 GUIDELINES FOR ASSISTANCE AT THE EMERGENCY BIRTH OF A FETUS IN THE VERTEX PRESENTATION

1. The woman usually assumes the position most comfortable for her. A lateral position is often recommended to facilitate a controlled birth of the head, thereby minimizing the risk for perineal trauma and neonatal head injury.
2. Reassure the woman that birth is usually uncomplicated in these situations. Use eye-to-eye contact and a calm, relaxed manner. If there is someone else available such as the partner, he or she could help support the woman in the position, assist with coaching, and provide positive reinforcement and praise of her efforts.
3. Wash your hands and put on gloves if available.
4. Place under woman's buttocks whatever clean material is available.
5. Avoid touching the vaginal area to decrease the possibility of infection.
6. As the head begins to crown, perform the following tasks:
   a. Tear the amniotic membranes if they are still intact.
   b. Instruct the woman to pant or pant-blow, thus minimizing the urge to push.
   c. Place the flat side of your hand on the exposed fetal head and apply *gentle* pressure toward the vagina to prevent the head from "popping out." The mother may participate by placing her hand under yours on the emerging head. NOTE: Rapid birth of the fetal head must be prevented because a rapid change of pressure within the molded fetal skull follows, which may result in dural or subdural tears. Rapid birth also may cause vaginal or perineal lacerations.
7. After the birth of the head, check for the umbilical cord. If the cord is around the baby's neck, try to slip it over his or her head or pull it *gently* to get some slack so you can slip it over the shoulders.
8. Support the fetal head as external rotation occurs. With one hand on each side of the baby's head, exert *gentle* pressure downward so the anterior shoulder emerges under the symphysis pubis and acts as a fulcrum; as *gentle* pressure is exerted in the opposite direction, the posterior shoulder, which has passed over the sacrum and coccyx, emerges.
9. Be alert! Hold the baby securely because the rest of the body may emerge quickly. The baby will be slippery!
10. Cradle the baby's head and back in one hand and the buttocks in the other. Keep his or her head down to drain away the mucus. If a bulb syringe is available, use it to remove mucus from the baby's mouth and then from the nose.
11. Dry the baby quickly to prevent rapid heat loss. Keep him or her at the same level as the mother's uterus until the end of the cord stops pulsating. NOTE: The baby should be kept at the same level as the mother's uterus to prevent his or her blood from flowing to or from the placenta and the resultant hypovolemia or hypervolemia. Do not "milk" the cord.
12. Place the baby on the mother's abdomen, cover him or her (remember to keep the head warm, too) with the mother's clothing, and have her cuddle the baby. Compliment her (them) on a job well done and on the baby if appropriate.

13. Wait for the placenta to separate. *Do not* tug on the cord. NOTE: Inappropriate traction may tear the cord, separate the placenta, or invert the uterus. Signs of placental separation include a slight gush of dark blood from the introitus, lengthening of the cord, and change in the uterine contour from a discoid to globular shape.
14. Instruct the mother to push to deliver the separated placenta. Gently ease out the placental membranes with an up-and-down motion until the membranes are removed. If birth occurs outside a hospital setting, to minimize complications do not cut the cord without proper clamps and a sterile cutting tool. Inspect the placenta for intactness. Place the baby on the placenta and wrap the two together for additional warmth.
15. Check the firmness of the uterus. Gently massage the fundus and demonstrate to the mother how she can massage her own fundus properly.
16. If supplies are available, clean the mother's perineal area and apply a peripad.
17. In addition to gentle massage of the fundus, the following measures can be taken to prevent or minimize hemorrhage:
    a. Put the baby to the mother's breast as soon as possible. Sucking or nuzzling and licking the nipple stimulates the release of oxytocin from the posterior pituitary. NOTE: If the baby does not or cannot nurse, manually stimulate the mother's nipples.
    b. Do not allow the mother's bladder to become distended. Assess the bladder for fullness and encourage her to void if fullness is found.
    c. Expel any clots from the mother's uterus after ensuring that the fundus is firm.
18. Comfort or reassure the mother and her family or friends. Keep the mother and the baby warm. Give her fluids if available and tolerated.
19. If this birth is multifetal, identify the infants in order of birth (e.g., using letters *A, B*).
20. Make notations regarding the following aspects of the birth:
    a. Fetal presentation and position
    b. Presence of cord around neck (nuchal cord) or other parts and number of times cord encircled part
    c. Color, character, and estimated amount of amniotic fluid if rupture of membranes occurs immediately before birth
    d. Time of birth
    e. Estimated time of determination of Apgar score (e.g., 1 and 5 minutes after birth), resuscitation efforts implemented, and ultimate condition of baby
    f. Sex of baby
    g. Time of placental expulsion and the appearance and completeness of the placenta
    h. Maternal condition: affect, behavior, and demeanor, amount of bleeding, and status of uterine tonicity
    i. Any unusual occurrences during the birth (e.g., maternal or paternal response, verbalizations, or gestures in response to birth of baby)

Squatting is highly effective in facilitating the descent and birth of the fetus. It is one of the best and most natural positions for second-stage labor and has been associated with the same benefits of other upright and lateral positions (Simpson, Cesario, Morin, et al., 2008). Women should assume a modified, supported squat until the fetal head is engaged, at which time a deep squat can be used. A firm surface is required for this position, and the woman needs side support (see Fig. 16-11, *A*). In a birthing bed a squat bar is available that she can use to help support herself (Fig. 16-15, *E*). A birth ball can also be used to help a woman maintain the squatting position. The fetus is aligned with the birth canal, and pelvic and perineal relaxation is facilitated as she sits on the ball or holds it in front of her for support as she squats (see Box 16-11).

When a woman uses the supported standing position for bearing down, her weight is borne on both femoral heads, allowing the pressure in the acetabulum to cause the transverse diameter of the pelvic outlet to increase by up to 1 cm. This can be helpful if descent of the head is delayed because the occiput has not rotated from the lateral (transverse diameter of pelvis) to the anterior position. Birthing chairs or rocking chairs may be used to provide women with a good physiologic position to enhance bearing-down efforts during childbirth (see Box 16-11), although some women feel restricted by a chair. The upright position also provides a potential psychologic advantage in that it allows the mother to see the birth as it occurs and to maintain eye contact with the attendant.

Oversized beanbag chairs and large floor pillows may be used for both labor and birth. They can mold around and support the mother in whichever position she selects. These chairs are of particular value for mothers who wish to be actively involved in the birth process. Birthing stools can be used to support the woman in an upright position similar to squatting. Some women may feel more comfortable sitting on the toilet or commode during pushing because they are concerned about stool incontinence during this stage. Encourage them to empty their bladder to avoid the effects of a distended bladder. However, the nurse must closely monitor these women and remove them from the toilet before birth becomes imminent. Because sitting on chairs, stools, toilets, or commodes can increase perineal edema and blood loss, help the woman change her position frequently (e.g., every 10 to 15 minutes).

The side-lying (lateral) position, with the upper part of the woman's leg held by the nurse or coach or placed on a pillow, is an effective position for the second stage of labor (see Fig. 16-14, *A*, and Box 16-11). Some women prefer a semisitting (semirecumbent) position instead (see Fig. 16-15, *B*, and Box 16-11). If the semirecumbent position is used, do not force the woman's legs against her abdomen as she bears down. This position increases perineal stretching and the risk for perineal trauma and spinal and lower-extremity neurologic injuries (Simpson, Cesario, Morin, et al., 2008). The hands-and-knees position is yet another effective position for birth (see Fig. 16-10, *B*, and Box 16-11).

The birthing bed commonly used can be set for different positions according to the woman's needs (Figs. 16-15 and 16-16). The woman can squat, kneel, sit, recline, or lie on her side, choosing the position most comfortable for her without having to climb into bed for the birth. At the same time the birthing bed provides excellent exposure for examinations, electrode placement, and birth. You can position the bed for the administration of anesthesia, and it is ideal to help women receiving an epidural to assume different positions to facilitate birth. You can also use the bed to transport the woman to the operating room if a cesarean birth is necessary. The woman can use squat bars, over-the-bed tables, birth balls, and pillows for support.

Bearing-Down Efforts

As the fetal head reaches the pelvic floor, most women experience the urge to bear down. Reflexively the woman begins to exert downward pressure by contracting her abdominal muscles while relaxing her pelvic floor. This bearing down is an involuntary response to the Ferguson reflex. A strong expiratory grunt or groan (vocalization) often accompanies pushing when the woman exhales as she pushes. This natural vocalization by women during open-glottis bearing-down efforts should be encouraged.

When coaching women to push, encourage them to push as they feel like pushing (instinctive, spontaneous pushing) rather than to give a prolonged push on command (directed, closed-glottis pushing). Prolonged breath-holding, or sustained, directed bearing

Delayed Pushing in Second Stage Labor

You are the nurse assigned to care for Emily, a 25-year-old G1 P0 at 39 weeks of gestation. You have just performed a vaginal examination and found that Emily's cervix is completely dilated. She has an epidural, which is working well. Currently Emily is feeling neither pressure nor pain. On learning that Emily's cervix is completely dilated, her health care provider exclaims, "Good! Get in there and help her push so we can have this baby! I'm ready to go home. I've had a long day!"

1. Evidence—Is there sufficient evidence to draw conclusions about effective management of second-stage labor?
2. Assumptions—Describe an underlying assumption about each of the following issues:
   a. Delayed pushing
   b. Positioning for pushing
   c. Spontaneous versus directed pushing efforts
3. What implications and priorities for nursing care can be drawn at this time?
4. Does the evidence objectively support your argument (conclusion)?

down is still a common practice, often beginning at 10-cm dilation and before the urge to bear down is perceived. The woman is coached to hold her breath, closing her glottis, and to push while the nurse or partner counts to 10. This method of bearing down may trigger the Valsalva maneuver, which occurs when the woman closes her glottis (closed-glottis pushing), which increases intrathoracic and cardiovascular pressure. This reduces cardiac output and decreases perfusion of the uterus and the placenta. Adverse effects associated with prolonged breath-holding and forceful pushing efforts include fetal hypoxia and subsequent acidosis, increased risk for pelvic floor damage (structural and neurogenic), and perineal trauma (Blackburn, 2013; Hanson, 2009; Simpson, Cesario, Morin, et al., 2008). The benefits of spontaneous pushing efforts rather than sustained Valsalva pushes include less fatigue and enhanced comfort. In addition, these more effective bearing-down efforts result in less time spent actively pushing (Hanson, 2009; James, 2011). Based on this evidence it is essential that perinatal nurses advocate for the practice of delayed and spontaneous bearing-down efforts with the woman in an upright or lateral position (Hanson, 2009) (see Critical Thinking Case Study).

A woman can become confused and anxious when she is being told to do something in conflict with what her body is telling her. Using phrases such as, "You are doing so well; do it again," "You're moving the baby down," and "Follow what your body is telling you," rather than "Push, push, push," encourages a woman to feel confident in her body and what she is feeling (Hanson, 2009).

Monitor the woman's breathing so she does not hold her breath for more than 6 to 8 seconds at a time followed by a slight exhale (a combination of open-glottis and voluntary closed-glottis pushing). Remind her to ventilate her lungs fully by taking deep cleansing breaths before and after each contraction. Bearing down while exhaling (open-glottis pushing) and taking breaths between bearing-down efforts help to maintain adequate oxygen levels for the mother and fetus, thus enhancing fetal well-being. The active pushing phase of the second stage of labor is considered to be the most physiologically stressful part of labor. Therefore every effort should be made to ensure that women use nondirected spontaneous pushing to conserve energy and maximize the effect of each bearing-down effort. A woman's bearing-down efforts naturally will become more

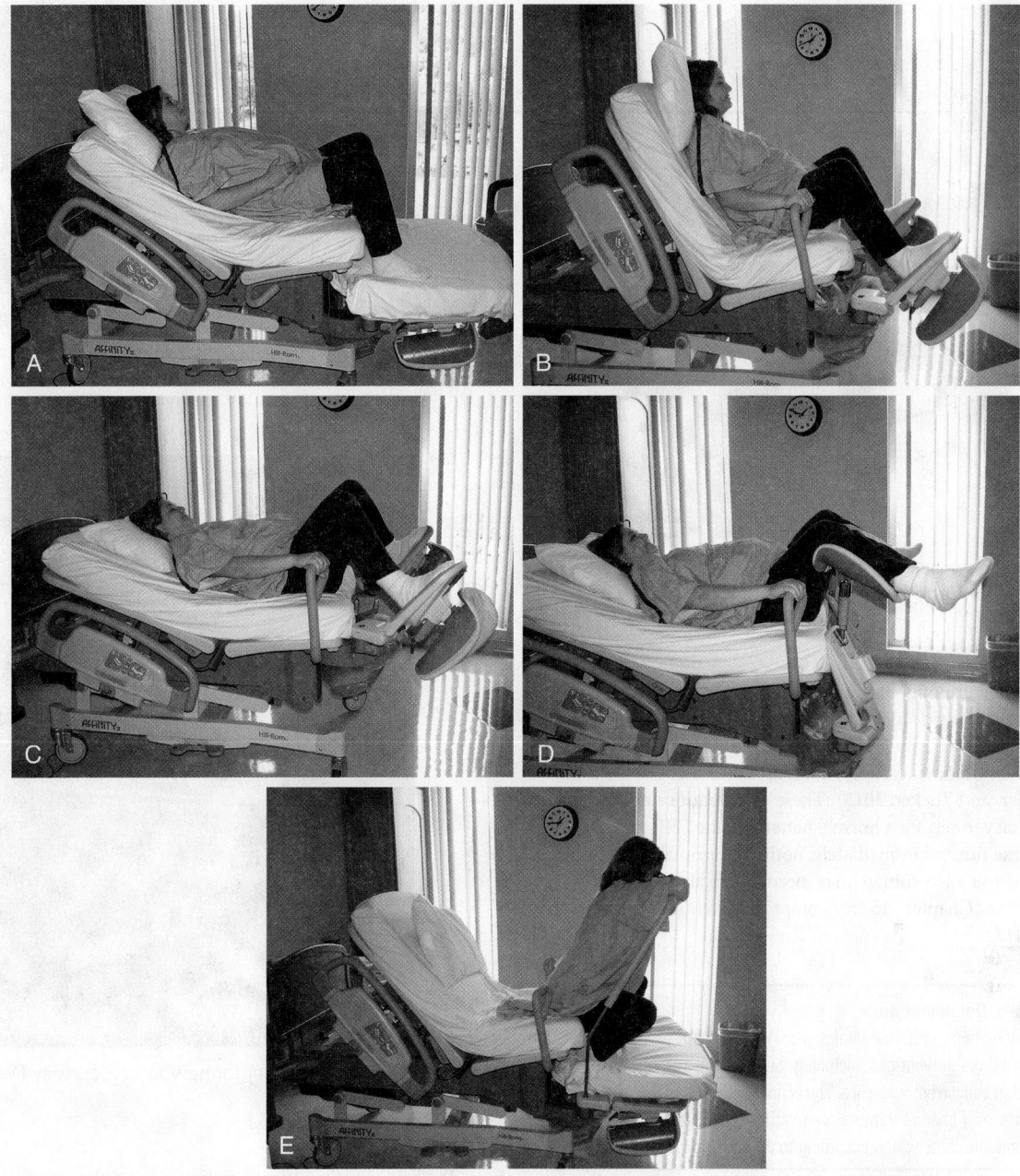

FIG 16-15 The versatility of today's birthing bed makes it practical in a variety of settings. NOTE: OB table used for lithotomy position. **A,** Labor bed. **B,** Birth chair. **C,** Birth bed. **D,** OB table. **E,** Squatting or birth bar. (Courtesy Julie Perry Nelson, Loveland, CO.)

forceful and frequent as the second stage progresses to birth (Simpson, Cesario, Morin, et al., 2008).

A woman may reach the second stage of labor and then experience a lack of readiness to complete the process and give birth to her child. She may have doubts about her readiness to be a mother or desire to wait for her support person or primary health care provider to arrive. Fear, anxiety, or embarrassment regarding unfamiliar or painful sensations and behaviors during pushing (e.g., sounds made, passage of stool) may be other inhibiting factors. Fear that the baby will be in danger once it emerges from the protective intrauterine environment also may be present. By recognizing that a woman may experience a need to hold back the birth of her baby, you can address her concerns and effectively coach her during this stage of labor.

To ensure the slow birth of the fetal head, encourage the woman to control the urge to bear down by coaching her to take panting breaths or exhale slowly through pursed lips as the baby's head crowns. At this point the woman needs simple, clear directions from one person. Amnesia between contractions often occurs in the second stage; therefore you may have to rouse the woman to get her to cooperate in the bearing-down process. Parents who have attended childbirth education classes may have devised a set of verbal cues for the laboring woman to follow.

Fetal Heart Rate and Pattern

As noted, you must check the FHR regularly (see Chapter 15 for further discussion). If the baseline rate begins to slow, if absent or minimal variability occurs, or if deceleration patterns develop (e.g.,

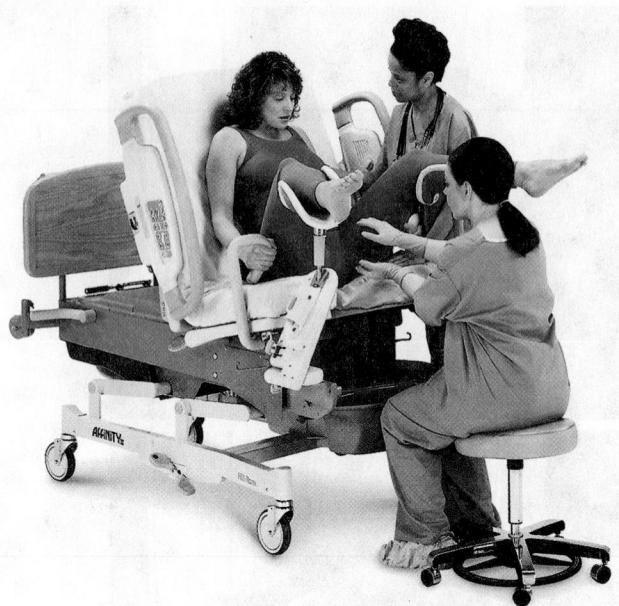

FIG 16-16 Birth bed. (Courtesy Hill-Rom, Batesville, IN.)

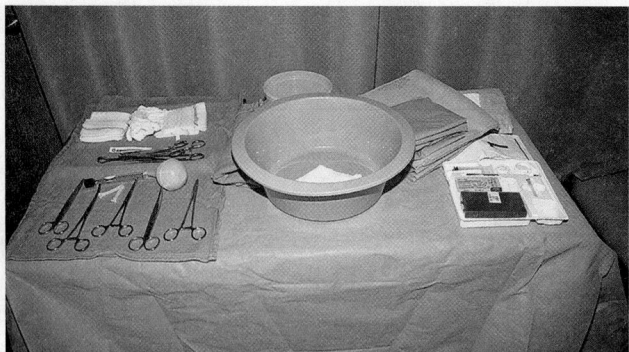

FIG 16-17 Instrument table. (Courtesy Marjorie Pyle, RNC, Life-circle, Costa Mesa, CA.)

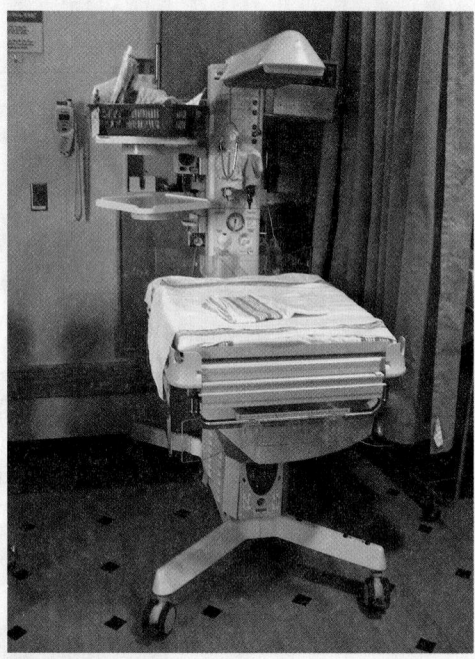

FIG 16-18 Radiant warmer for newborn. (Courtesy Dee Lowdermilk, Chapel Hill, NC.)

late, variable, or prolonged), initiate interventions promptly. Turn the woman onto her side to reduce the pressure of the uterus against the ascending vena cava and descending aorta (see Fig. 16-5). Oxygen can be administered by nonrebreather mask at 10 L/min (Miller, Miller, and Tucker, 2013). These interventions are often all that is necessary to restore a normal pattern. If the FHR and pattern do not become normal immediately, notify the primary health care provider because the woman may need medical intervention to give birth. See Chapter 15 for more interventions related to abnormal FHR.

LEGAL TIP: Documentation

All observations (e.g., maternal vital signs, FHR and pattern, progress of labor) and nursing interventions, including the woman's response, should be documented concurrent with care. The course of labor and the maternal-fetal response may change without warning. All documentation must be accurate, complete, timely, and according to agency policy.

Support of the Father or Partner

During the second stage the woman needs continuous support and coaching (see Table 16-3 and Box 16-7). Because the coaching process is often physically and emotionally tiring for support persons, the nurse offers them nourishment and fluids and encourages them to take short breaks as needed (see Box 16-12). If birth occurs in an LDR or LDRP room, the support person usually wears street clothes. Instruct the support person who attends the birth in a delivery room to put on a cover gown or scrub clothes, mask, hat, and shoe covers if required by agency policy. The nurse also specifies support measures that can be used for the laboring woman and points out areas of the room in which the partner can move freely.

Encourage partners to be present at the birth of their infants if doing so is in keeping with their cultural and personal expectations and beliefs. The presence of partners maintains the psychologic closeness of the family unit, and the partner can continue to provide the supportive care given during labor. The woman and her partner need to have an equal opportunity to initiate the attachment process with the baby.

Supplies, Instruments, and Equipment

To prepare for birth in any setting, the birthing table is usually set up during the transition phase for nulliparous women and during the active phase for multiparous women.

Prepare the birthing bed or table and arrange instruments on the instrument table or delivery cart (Fig. 16-17). Follow standard procedures for gloving, identifying and opening sterile packages, adding sterile supplies to the instrument table, unwrapping sterile instruments, and handing them to the primary health care provider. Ready the crib or radiant warmer and equipment for the support and stabilization of the infant (Fig. 16-18).

The items used for birth may vary among different facilities; therefore consult the procedure manual for each facility to determine the protocols specific to that facility.

The nurse estimates the time until the birth will occur and notifies the primary health care provider if she or he is not in the woman's room. Even the most experienced nurse can miscalculate the time left before birth occurs; therefore every nurse who attends a woman in labor must be prepared to assist with an emergency birth if the primary health care provider is not present (see Box 16-13).

Birth in a Delivery Room or Birthing Room

The woman needs assistance if she must move from the labor bed to the delivery table (Fig. 16-19). The positions assumed for birth in a delivery room are the Sims or lateral position, in which the attendant supports the upper part of the woman's leg, the dorsal position (supine position with one hip elevated), and the lithotomy position.

The lithotomy position makes dealing with complications that arise more convenient for the primary health care provider (see Fig. 16-15, *D*). To place the woman in this position, bring her buttocks to the edge of the bed or table and place her legs in stirrups. Take care to pad the stirrups, raise and place both legs simultaneously, and adjust the shanks of the stirrups so the calves of the legs are supported. No pressure should be placed on the popliteal space. Stirrups that are not the same height strain ligaments in the woman's back as she bears down, leading to considerable discomfort in the postpartum period. The lower portion of the table may be dropped down and rolled back under the table.

The maternal position for birth in a birthing room varies from a lithotomy position with the woman's legs in stirrups or with her legs held and supported by the nurse or support person; to one in

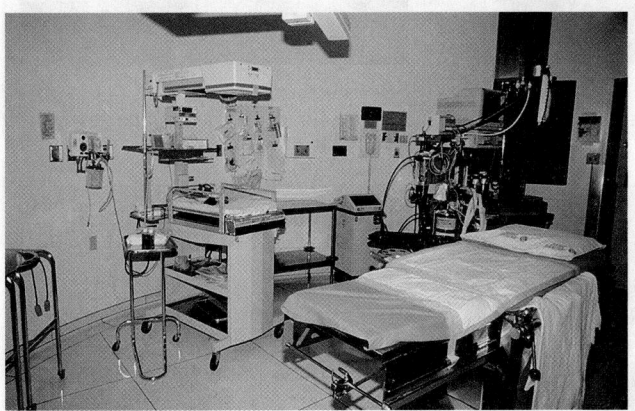

FIG 16-19 Delivery room. (Courtesy Michael S. Clement, MD, Mesa, AZ.)

which her feet rest on footrests while she holds on to a squat bar; to a side-lying position with the woman's upper leg supported by the coach, nurse, or squat bar. Once the woman is positioned, the foot of the bed is removed so the primary health care provider attending the birth can gain better perineal access for performing an episiotomy, delivering a large baby, or using forceps or vacuum extractor. Alternately the foot of the bed can be left in place and lowered slightly to form a ledge that allows access for birth and also serves as a place to lay the newborn (see Fig. 16-15, *A*).

Once the woman is positioned for birth either in a delivery room or birthing room, the vulva and perineum are cleansed. Hospital protocols and the preferences of primary health care providers for cleansing may vary.

The nurse continues to coach and encourage the woman and monitor the fetal status (see Box 16-7). Keep the primary health care provider informed of the FHR and pattern. Prepare or obtain an oxytocic medication such as oxytocin (Pitocin) so it is ready to be administered immediately after expulsion of the placenta. Always follow Standard Precautions as care is administered during the process of labor and birth (see Box 16-5).

In the delivery room the primary health care provider puts on a cap, a mask that has a shield or protective eyewear, and shoe covers. After washing hands the provider puts on a sterile gown (with waterproof front and sleeves) and sterile gloves. Nurses attending the birth also may need to wear caps, protective eyewear, masks, gowns, and gloves. The woman may then be draped with sterile drapes. In the birthing room Standard Precautions are observed, but the amount and types of protective coverings worn by those in attendance may vary.

Maintain contact with the parents by touching, verbally comforting, describing progress, explaining the reasons for care, and sharing in the parents' joy at the birth of their child.

Mechanism of Birth: Vertex Presentation

The three phases of the spontaneous birth of a fetus in a vertex presentation are (1) birth of the head, (2) birth of the shoulders, and (3) birth of the body and extremities (see Chapter 13).

With voluntary bearing-down efforts the head appears at the introitus (Fig. 16-20, *A* to *D*). **Crowning** occurs when the widest part of the head (the biparietal diameter) distends the vulva just before birth. Immediately before birth the perineal musculature becomes greatly distended. If an **episiotomy** (incision into the perineum to enlarge the vaginal outlet) is necessary, it is done at this time to minimize soft-tissue damage. A local anesthetic may be administered if necessary before performing an episiotomy. Box 16-14

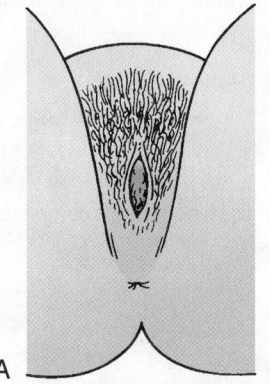
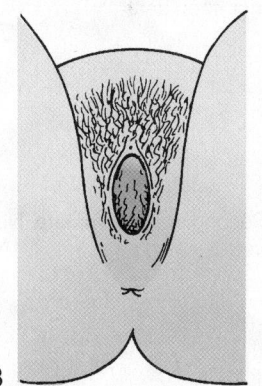
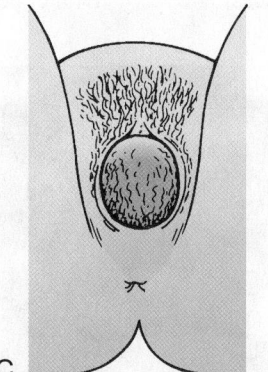
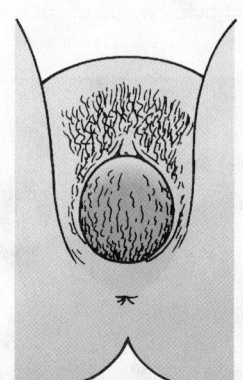

FIG 16-20 Beginning birth with vertex presenting. **A,** Anteroposterior slit. **B,** Oval opening. **C,** Circular shape. **D,** Crowning.

BOX 16-14   NORMAL VAGINAL CHILDBIRTH

First Stage

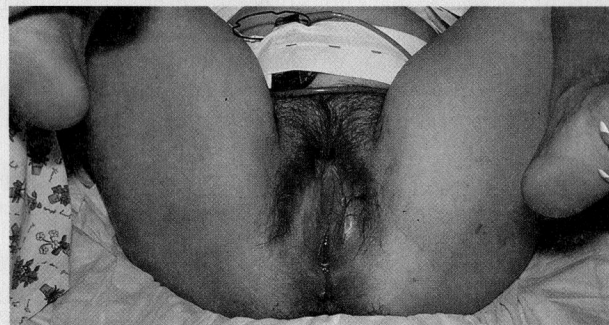

Anteroposterior slit. Vertex visible during contraction.

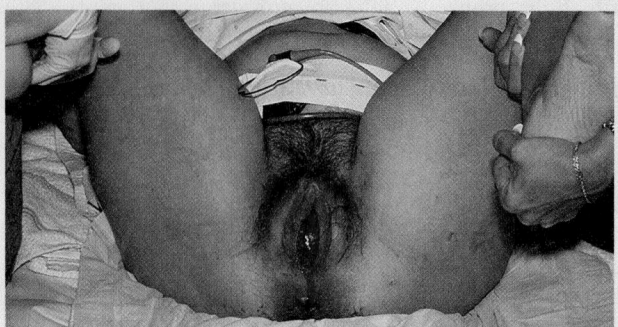

Oval opening. Vertex presenting. NOTE: Nurse *(on left)* is wearing gloves, but support person *(on right)* is not.

Second Stage

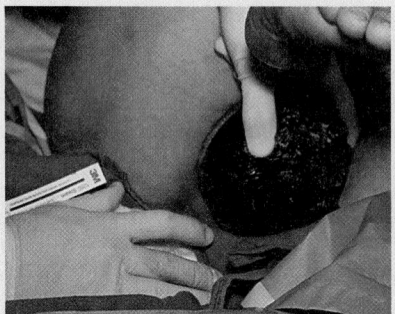

Crowning.

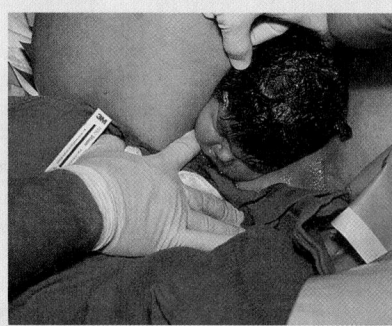

Nurse-midwife using Ritgen maneuver as head is born by extension.

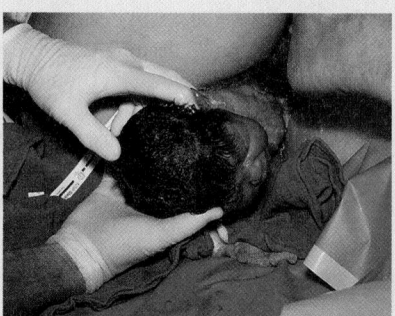

After nurse-midwife checks for nuchal cord, she supports head during external rotation and restitution.

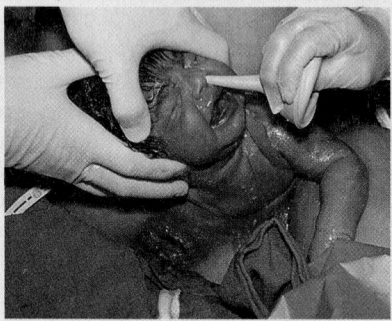

Use of bulb syringe to suction mucus.

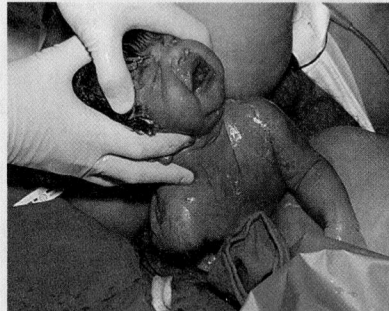

Birth of posterior shoulder.

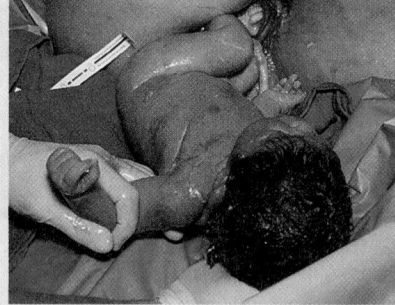

Birth of newborn by slow expulsion.

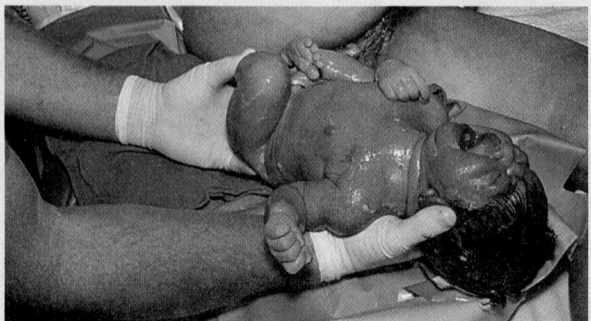

Second stage complete. Note that newborn is not completely pink yet.

BOX 16-14 NORMAL VAGINAL CHILDBIRTH—cont'd

Third Stage

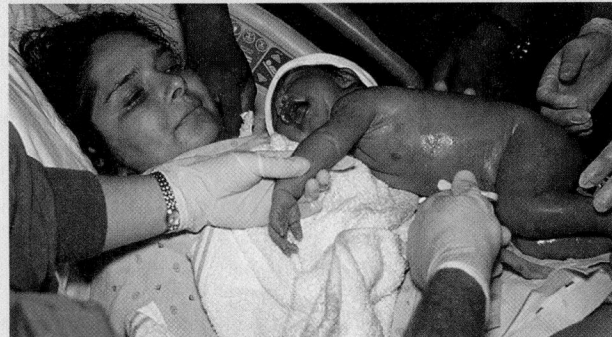

Newborn placed on mother's abdomen while cord is clamped and cut.

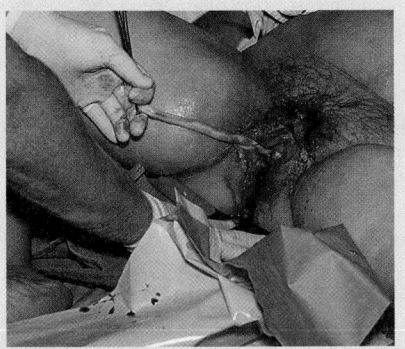

Note increased bleeding as placenta separates.

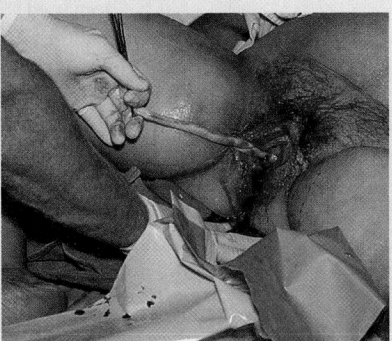

Expulsion of placenta.

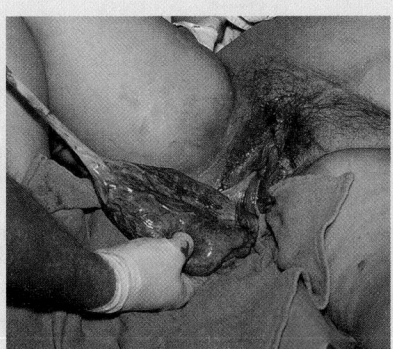

Expulsion is complete, marking end of third stage.

The Newborn

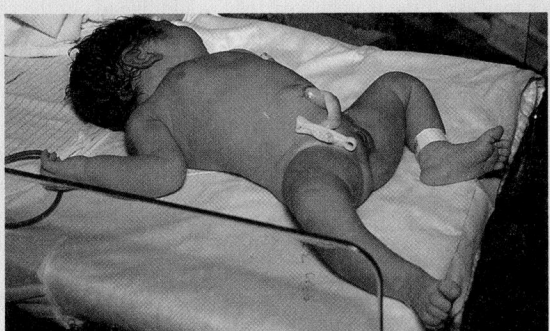

Newborn awaiting assessment. Note that color is almost completely pink.

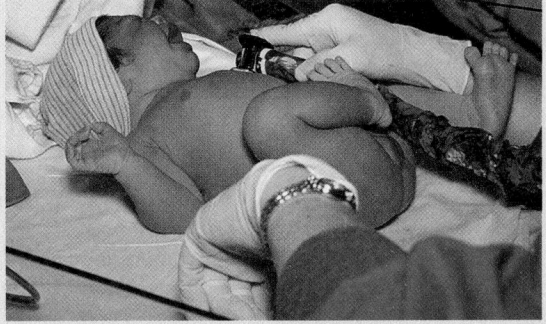

Newborn assessment under radiant warmer.

Parents admiring their newborn.

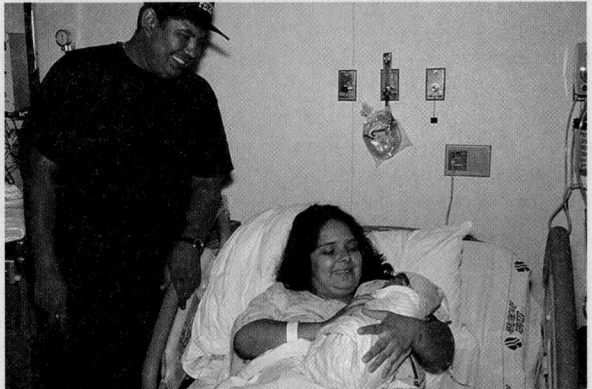

Photos courtesy Michael S. Clement, MD, Mesa, AZ.

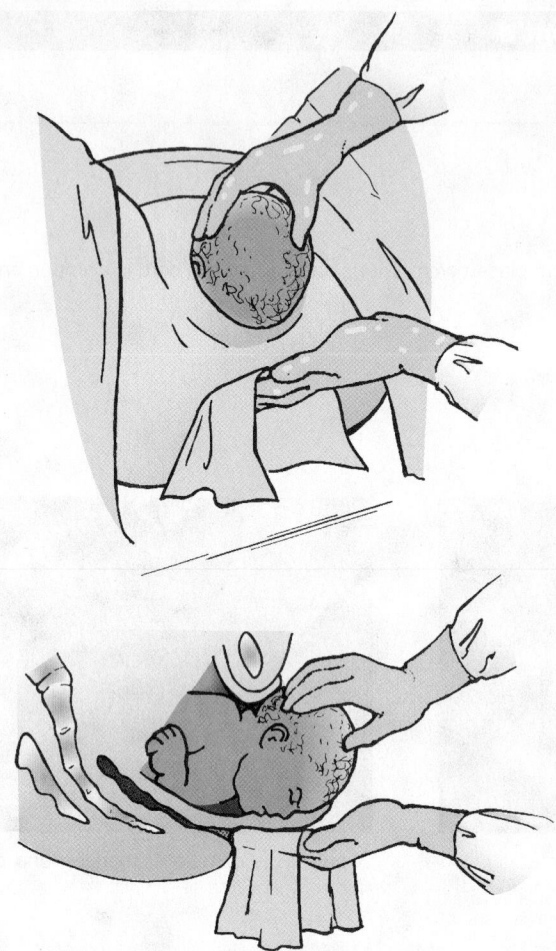

FIG 16-21 Birth of head with modified Ritgen maneuver. Note control to prevent too-rapid birth of head.

shows the process of normal vaginal childbirth using a series of photographs.

The physician or nurse-midwife may use a hands-on approach to control the birth of the head, believing that guarding the perineum results in a gradual birth that will prevent fetal intracranial injury, protect maternal tissues, and reduce postpartum perineal pain. This approach involves: (1) applying pressure against the rectum, drawing it downward to aid in flexing the head as the back of the neck catches under the symphysis pubis; (2) applying upward pressure from the coccygeal region (modified Ritgen maneuver) (Fig. 16-21) to extend the head during the actual birth, thereby protecting the musculature of the perineum; and (3) assisting the mother with voluntary control of the bearing-down efforts by coaching her to pant while letting uterine forces expel the fetus.

Some health care providers use a hands-poised (hands-off) approach when attending a birth. In this approach hands are prepared to place light pressure on the fetal head to prevent rapid expulsion. The provider does not place hands on the perineum or use them to assist with birth of the shoulders and body.

The hands-on and hands-poised approaches have similar results in terms of perineal and vaginal tears, but the hands-on technique is associated with a higher incidence of third-degree tears and episiotomies. In one study the hands-poised approach resulted in fewer third-degree tears (Berghella, Baxter, and Chauhan, 2008). However, the hands-on approach may result in less perineal pain.

The umbilical cord often encircles the neck (nuchal cord) but rarely so tightly as to cause hypoxia. After the head is born, gentle palpation is used to feel for the cord. If present, the health care provider slips it gently over the head if possible. If the loop is tight or if there is a second loop, he or she usually clamps the cord twice, cuts between the clamps, and unwinds the cord from around the neck before the birth is allowed to continue. Mucus, blood, or meconium in the nasal or oral passages may prevent the newborn from breathing. To eliminate this problem, moist gauze sponges are used to wipe the nose and mouth. A bulb syringe is inserted first into the mouth and oropharynx and then into both nares to aspirate contents.

Fundal Pressure

Fundal pressure is the application of gentle, steady pressure against the fundus of the uterus to facilitate the vaginal birth. Historically it has been used when the administration of analgesia and anesthesia decreased the woman's ability to push during the birth, in cases of shoulder dystocia, and when second-stage fetal bradycardia or other abnormal FHR patterns were present. Use of fundal pressure by nurses is not advised because there is no standard technique available for this maneuver. In addition, no current legal, professional, or regulatory standards exist for its use; and no evidence related to its effectiveness in facilitating a safe vaginal birth is available (Simpson, Cesario, Morin, et al., 2008).

Immediate Assessments and Care of the Newborn

The time of birth is the precise time when the entire body is out of the mother; this time is recorded. In the case of multiple births each birth would be noted in the same way. If the newborn's condition is not compromised, he or she may be placed on the mother's abdomen immediately after birth and covered with a warm, dry blanket. The cord may be clamped at this time, and the primary health care provider may ask if the woman's partner would like to cut the cord. If so, the partner is given a sterile pair of scissors and instructed to cut the cord 2.5 cm above the clamp.

The care given immediately after birth focuses on assessing and stabilizing the newborn. The nurse is usually the primary person responsible for care of the infant at this time because the primary health care provider is involved with the delivery of the placenta and care of the mother. The nurse must watch the infant for any signs of distress and initiate appropriate interventions should any appear.

Perform a brief assessment of the newborn immediately, even while the mother is holding the infant. This assessment includes assigning Apgar scores at 1 and 5 minutes after birth (see Table 23-1). Maintaining a patent airway, supporting respiratory effort, and preventing cold stress by drying and covering the newborn with a warmed blanket or placing him or her under a radiant warmer are the major priorities in terms of the newborn's immediate care. Postpone further examination, identification procedures, and care until later in the third stage of labor or early in the fourth stage.

Perineal Trauma Related to Childbirth

Most acute injuries and lacerations of the perineum, vagina, uterus, and their support tissues occur during childbirth. Alternative measures for perineal management such as application of warm compresses and gentle perineal massage and stretching have been suggested to lessen the degree of perineal lacerations and trauma. However, limited evidence exists for the benefit of perineal measures used during the second stage of labor. In fact, research findings are mixed; some studies indicate an increased risk for perineal trauma when using these measures; other studies indicate that they may lessen the degree of perineal lacerations (Simpson, Cesario, Morin, et al., 2008). Therefore these measures should be avoided during labor until further research can provide evidence of their benefit (Berghella, Baxter, and Chauhan, 2008).

Some degree of damage occurs to the soft tissues of the birth canal and adjacent structures during every birth. The tendency to sustain lacerations varies with each woman (i.e., the soft tissue in some women may be less distensible). Damage usually is more pronounced in nulliparous women because the tissues are firmer and more resistant than are those in multiparous women. Heredity is also a factor. For example, the tissue of light-skinned women, especially those with reddish hair, is not as readily distensible as that of darker-skinned women; and healing may be less efficient. Other risk factors associated with perineal trauma include maternal position, pelvic inadequacy (e.g., narrow subpubic arch with a constricted outlet), fetal malpresentation and position (e.g., breech presentation, occiput posterior position), large (macrosomic) infants, use of forceps or vacuum to facilitate birth, prolonged second stage of labor, and rapid labor in which there is insufficient time for the perineum to stretch.

Some injuries to the supporting tissues, whether they are acute or nonacute or were repaired or not, may lead to genitourinary and sexual problems later in life (e.g., pelvic relaxation, uterine prolapse, cystocele, rectocele, dyspareunia, urinary and bowel dysfunction). Use of Kegel exercises in the prenatal and postpartum periods improves and restores the tone and strength of the perineal muscles (see Chapter 3). Health practices, including good nutrition and appropriate hygienic measures, help maintain the integrity and suppleness of the perineal tissues, enhance healing, and prevent infection.

Perineal Lacerations

Perineal lacerations usually occur as the fetal head is being born. The extent of the laceration is defined in terms of its depth:

- *First degree:* Laceration that extends through the skin and structures superficial to muscles
- *Second degree:* Laceration that extends through muscles of the perineal body
- *Third degree:* Laceration that continues through the anal sphincter muscle
- *Fourth degree:* Laceration that also involves the anterior rectal wall

Perineal injury often is accompanied by small lacerations on the medial surfaces of the labia minora below the pubic rami and to the sides of the urethra (periurethral) and clitoris. Lacerations in this highly vascular area often result in profuse bleeding. Third- and fourth-degree lacerations must be repaired carefully so the woman retains fecal continence. Simple perineal injuries usually heal without permanent disability, regardless of whether they were repaired. However, repairing a new perineal injury to prevent future complications is easier than correcting long-term damage.

Vaginal and Urethral Lacerations

Vaginal lacerations often occur in conjunction with perineal lacerations. Vaginal lacerations tend to extend up the lateral walls (sulci) and, if deep enough, involve the levator ani muscle. Additional injury may occur high in the vaginal vault near the level of the ischial spines. Vaginal vault lacerations are often circular and may result from use of forceps to rotate the fetal head, rapid fetal descent, or precipitous birth.

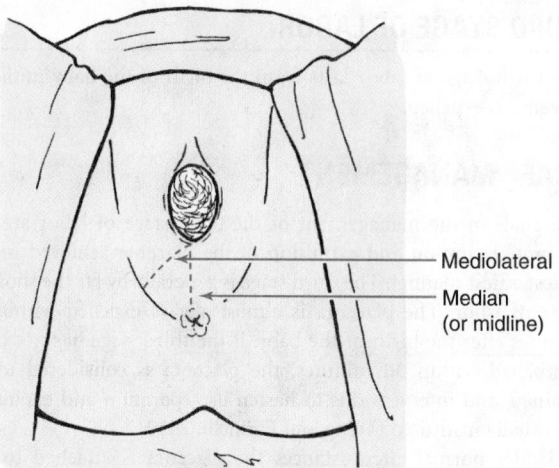

FIG 16-22 Types of episiotomies.

Cervical Injuries

Cervical injuries occur when the cervix retracts over the advancing fetal head. They occur at the lateral angles of the external os. Most lacerations are shallow, and bleeding is minimal. Larger lacerations may extend to the vaginal vault or beyond it into the lower uterine segment; serious bleeding may occur. Extensive lacerations may follow hasty attempts to enlarge the cervical opening artificially or deliver the fetus before full cervical dilation is achieved. Injuries to the cervix can have adverse effects on future pregnancies and childbirths.

Episiotomy

An episiotomy is an incision made in the perineum to enlarge the vaginal outlet (Fig. 16-22). It is performed more commonly in the United States and Canada than in Europe. The side-lying position for birth, used routinely in Europe, causes less tension on the perineum, making possible a gradual stretching of the perineum with fewer indications for episiotomies.

Different types of episiotomies are performed, depending on the site and direction of the incision (see Fig. 16-22); the type that provides the best outcome is unknown (Berghella, Baxter, and Chauhan, 2008). Midline (median) episiotomy is most commonly used in the United States. It is effective, easily repaired, and generally the least painful. However, midline episiotomies also are associated with a higher incidence of third- and fourth-degree lacerations. Sphincter tone is usually restored after primary healing and a good repair. Mediolateral episiotomy is used in operative births when the need for posterior extension is likely. Although a fourth-degree laceration may be prevented, a third-degree laceration may occur. The blood loss is also greater, and the repair more difficult and painful than with midline episiotomies. It is also more painful in the postpartum period, and the pain lasts longer.

Routine use of episiotomies has declined in the United States in recent years. The practice in many settings now is to support the perineum manually during birth and allow it to tear rather than perform an episiotomy. Tears are often smaller than an episiotomy, are repaired easily or not at all, and heal quickly. Episiotomies are associated with more posterior perineal trauma, suturing and healing complications, and later pain with intercourse. Therefore episiotomy should be avoided if at all possible (Berghella, Baxter, and Chauhan, 2008).

THIRD STAGE OF LABOR

The third stage of labor lasts from the birth of the baby until the placenta is expelled.

CARE MANAGEMENT

The goals in the management of the third stage of labor are the prompt separation and expulsion of the placenta achieved in the easiest, safest manner. The third stage is generally by far the shortest stage of labor. The placenta is almost always expelled within 15 minutes after the birth of the baby. If the third stage has not been completed within 30 minutes, the placenta is considered to be retained, and interventions to hasten its separation and expulsion are usually instituted (Wing and Farinelli, 2012).

Under normal circumstances the placenta is attached to the decidual layer of the thin endometrium of the basal plate by numerous fibrous anchor villi, much in the same way a postage stamp is attached to a sheet of postage stamps. After the birth of the fetus strong uterine contractions and the sudden decrease in uterine size cause the placental site to shrink. This causes the anchor villi to break and the placenta to separate from its attachments. Normally the first few strong contractions that occur after the baby's birth cause the placenta to shear away from the basal plate. A placenta cannot detach itself from a flaccid (relaxed) uterus because the placental site is not reduced in size.

Placental Separation and Expulsion

Depending on preference, the primary health care provider may use either a passive or an active approach to manage the third stage of labor. Passive management involves patiently watching for signs that the placenta has separated from the uterine wall spontaneously and monitoring for spontaneous expulsion. This approach is commonly practiced in the United States (Burke, 2010). Active management of third-stage labor is currently practiced in many countries around the world. Components of active management include administering an oxytocic medication (e.g., oxytocin [Pitocin]) when the anterior shoulder is birthed or immediately following the birth of the fetus, clamping and cutting the umbilical cord within 3 minutes after birth, and gently controlling cord traction following uterine contraction and separation of the placenta. Evidence-based literature and the World Health Organization now recommend active management of the third stage of labor because its use decreases the rate of postpartum hemorrhage caused by uterine atony (Burke, 2010).

To assist in the delivery of the placenta, the woman is instructed to push when signs of separation have occurred (Fig. 16-23). If possible, the woman should expel the placenta during a uterine contraction. Alternate compression and elevation of the fundus and minimal, controlled traction on the umbilical cord may also be used to facilitate delivery of the placenta and amniotic membranes. Oxytocics are usually administered after the placenta is removed because they stimulate the uterus to contract, thereby helping to prevent hemorrhage (Box 16-15).

Whether the placenta first appears by its shiny fetal surface (Schultze mechanism) or turns to show its dark roughened maternal surface first (Duncan mechanism) is of no clinical importance.

After the placenta and the amniotic membranes emerge, the primary health care provider examines them for intactness to ensure that no portion remains in the uterine cavity (i.e., no fragments of the placenta or membranes are retained) (Fig. 16-24).

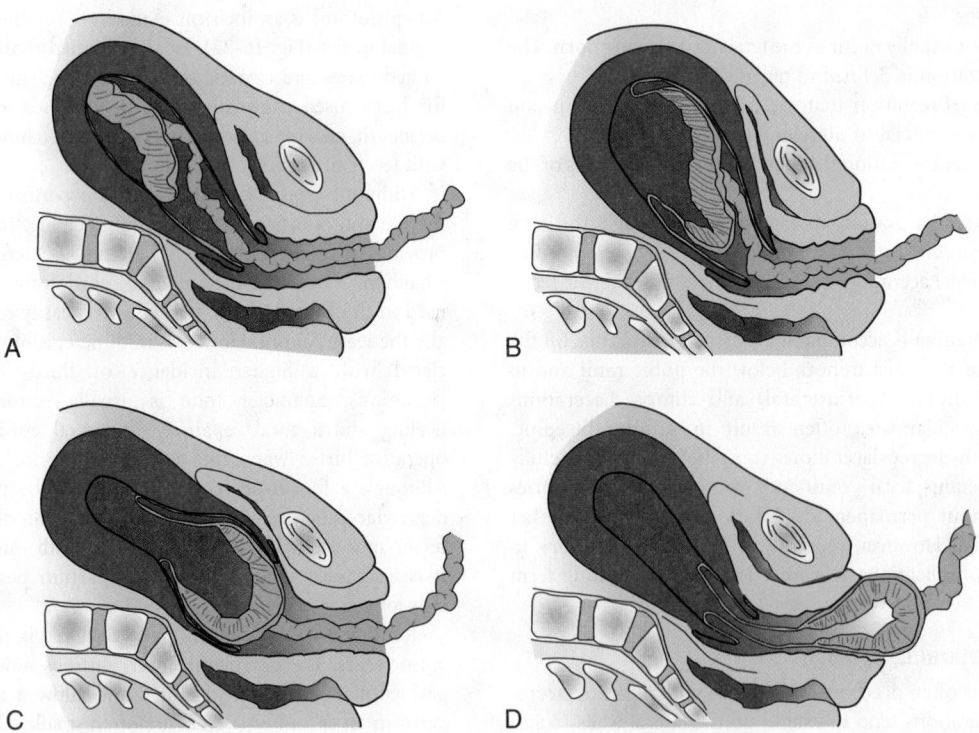

FIG 16-23 Third stage of labor. **A,** Placenta begins to separate in central portion, accompanied by retroplacental bleeding. Uterus changes from discoid to globular shape. **B,** Placenta completes separation and enters lower uterine segment. Uterus has globular shape. **C,** Placenta enters vagina, cord is seen to lengthen, and there may be an increase in bleeding. **D,** Expulsion (delivery) of placenta and completion of third stage.

BOX 16-15   NURSING CARE IN THIRD-STAGE LABOR

Assessment

Signs That Suggest the Onset of the Third Stage

- A firmly contracting fundus
- A change in the uterus from a discoid to a globular ovoid shape as the placenta moves into the lower uterine segment
- A sudden gush of dark blood from the introitus
- Apparent lengthening of the umbilical cord as the placenta descends to the introitus
- The finding of vaginal fullness (the placenta) on vaginal or rectal examination or of fetal membranes at the introitus

Physical Assessment

- Perform every 15 minutes: maternal blood pressure, pulse, and respirations.
- Assess for signs of placental separation and amount of bleeding.
- Assist with determination of Apgar score at 1 and 5 minutes after birth (see Table 23-1).
- Assess maternal and paternal response to completion of childbirth process and their reaction to the newborn.

Interventions

- Assist to bear down to facilitate expulsion of the separated placenta.
- Administer an oxytocic medication as ordered to ensure adequate contraction of the uterus, thereby preventing hemorrhage.
- Provide nonpharmacologic and pharmacologic comfort and pain-relief measures.
- Perform hygienic cleansing measures.
- Keep informed of progress of placental separation and expulsion and perineal repair if appropriate.
- Explain purpose of medications administered.
- Introduce parents to their baby and facilitate the attachment process by delaying eye prophylaxis; wrap mother and baby together for skin-to-skin contact.
- Provide private time for parents to bond with new baby; help them create memories.
- Encourage breastfeeding if desired.

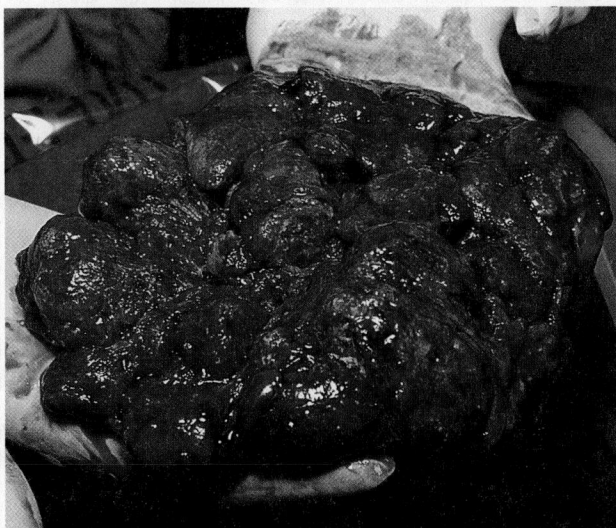

FIG 16-24 Examination of placenta. (Courtesy Michael S. Clement, MD, Mesa, AZ.)

When the third stage of labor has been completed, the primary health care provider examines the woman for any perineal, vaginal, or cervical lacerations requiring repair. If an episiotomy was performed, it is sutured. Immediate repair promotes healing, limits residual damage, and decreases the possibility of infection. The woman usually feels some discomfort while the primary health care provider carries out the postbirth vaginal examination. Help her to use breathing and relaxation or distraction techniques to assist her in dealing with the discomfort. During this time the nurse performs a quick assessment of the newborn's physical condition, weighs the baby, and places matching identification bands on baby and mother. The baby may also receive eye prophylaxis and a vitamin K injection at this time.

After any necessary repairs have been completed, cleanse the vulvar area gently with warm water or normal saline and apply a perineal pad or an ice pack to the perineum. Reposition the birthing bed or table and lower the woman's legs simultaneously from the stirrups if she gave birth in a lithotomy position. Remove any drapes and place dry linen under the woman's buttocks. Provide her with a clean gown and blanket, which is warmed if needed.

Some women and their families may have culturally based beliefs regarding the care of the placenta and the manner of its disposal after birth, viewing the care and disposal of the placenta as a way of protecting the newborn from bad luck and illness. In Spanish the placenta is referred to as *el compañero* or "the companion of the child" (Callister, 2008). A request by the woman to take the placenta home and dispose of it according to her customs sometimes conflicts with health care agency policies, especially those related to infection control and the disposal of biologic wastes. Many cultures follow specific rules regarding the disposal of the placenta in terms of method (burning, drying, burying, eating), site for disposal (in or near the home), and timing of disposal (immediately after birth, time of day, astrologic signs). Disposal rituals may vary according to the sex of the child and the length of time before another child is desired. Some cultures believe that eating the placenta is a means of restoring a woman's well-being after birth or ensuring high-quality breast milk. Health care providers can provide culturally sensitive care by encouraging women and their families to express their wishes regarding the care and disposal of the placenta and establishing a policy to fulfill these requests (D'Avanzo, 2008).

FOURTH STAGE OF LABOR

The first 1 to 2 hours after birth, sometimes called the **fourth stage of labor**, is a crucial time for mother and newborn. Both are not only recovering from the physical process of birth but are also becoming acquainted with one another and additional family members. During this time maternal organs undergo their initial readjustment to the nonpregnant state, and the functions of body systems begin to stabilize.

CARE MANAGEMENT

In most hospitals the mother remains in the labor and birth area during this recovery time. In an institution where LDR rooms are used, the woman stays in the same room where she gave birth. In traditional settings women are taken from the delivery room to a separate recovery area for observation. Arrangements for care of the newborn vary during the fourth stage of labor. In many settings the baby remains at the mother's bedside, and the labor or birth nurse cares for both of them. In other institutions the baby is taken to the nursery for several hours of observation after an initial bonding period with the parents, siblings, and perhaps other family members (Fig. 16-25).

ASSESSMENT

If the recovery nurse has not previously cared for the new mother, she begins with an oral report from the nurse who attended the woman during labor and birth and a review of the prenatal, labor, and birth records. Of primary importance are conditions that could predispose the mother to hemorrhage such as precipitous labor, a large baby, grand multiparity (i.e., having given birth to six or more viable infants), induced labor, or a magnesium infusion during

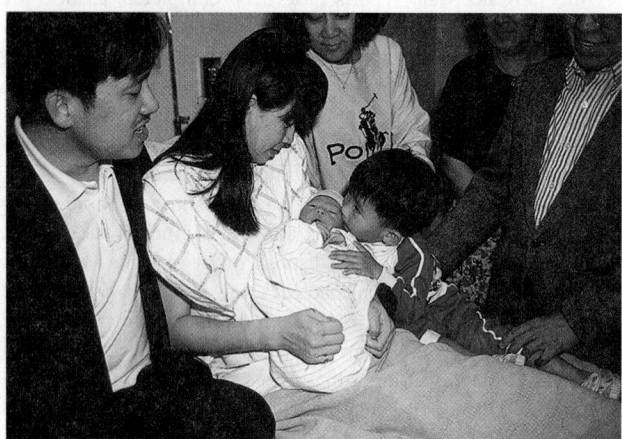

FIG 16-25 Big brother becomes acquainted with new baby sister. (Courtesy Marjorie Pyle, RNC, Lifecircle, Costa Mesa, CA.)

labor. For healthy women hemorrhage is the most dangerous potential complication during the fourth stage of labor.

During the first hour following birth the mother is assessed frequently. Box 16-16 describes the physical assessment of the mother during the fourth stage of labor. All factors except temperature are assessed every 15 minutes for 1 hour. Temperature is assessed at the beginning and after the first hour of the recovery period. After the fifth 15-minute assessment (which completes the first hour of recovery), if all parameters have stabilized within the normal range, the process is usually repeated once in the second hour.

Postanesthesia Recovery

The woman who has given birth by cesarean or received regional anesthesia for a vaginal birth requires special attention during the recovery period. Obstetric recovery areas are held to the same standard of care that would be expected of any other postanesthesia recovery (PAR) unit (AAP and ACOG, 2012). A PAR score is determined for each woman on arrival and is updated as part of every 15-minute assessment. Components of the PAR score include activity, respirations, blood pressure, level of consciousness, and color.

If the woman received general anesthesia, she should be awake and alert and oriented to time, place, and person. Her respiratory rate should be within normal limits, and her oxygen saturation level at least 95% as measured by a pulse oximeter. If the woman received epidural or spinal anesthesia, she should be able to raise her legs, extended at the knees, off the bed or flex her knees; place her feet flat on the bed; and raise her buttocks well off the bed. The numb or tingling, prickly sensation should be entirely gone from her legs. The length of time required to recover from regional anesthesia varies greatly. Often it takes several hours for these anesthetic effects to disappear completely.

BOX 16-16   ASSESSMENT DURING THE FOURTH STAGE OF LABOR

Blood Pressure
- Measure blood pressure every 15 minutes for the first hour.

Pulse
- Assess rate and regularity. Measure every 15 minutes for the first hour.

Temperature
- Determine temperature at the beginning of the recovery period and after the first hour of recovery.

Fundus
- Position woman with knees flexed and head flat.
- Just below umbilicus cup hand and press firmly into abdomen. At the same time stabilize uterus at symphysis with opposite hand (see Fig. 19-4).
- If fundus is firm (and bladder is empty), with uterus in midline, measure its position relative to woman's umbilicus. Lay fingers flat on abdomen under umbilicus; measure how many fingerbreadths (fb) or centimeters (cm) fit between umbilicus and top of fundus. Fundal height is documented according to agency guidelines. For example, if fundus is 1 fb or 1 cm above umbilicus, fundal height may be recorded as either +1, u+1, or 1/u. If fundus is 1 fb or 1 cm below umbilicus, fundal height may be recorded as either −1, u−1, or u/1.
- If fundus is not firm, massage it gently to contract and expel any clots before measuring distance from umbilicus.
- Place hands appropriately; massage gently only until firm.

- Expel clots while keeping hands placed as in Fig. 19-1. With upper hand firmly apply pressure downward toward vagina; observe perineum for amount and size of expelled clots.

Bladder
- Assess distention by noting location and firmness of uterine fundus and observing and palpating bladder. A distended bladder is seen as a suprapubic rounded bulge that is dull to percussion and fluctuates like a water-filled balloon. When bladder is distended, uterus is usually boggy in consistency, well above umbilicus, and to woman's right side.
- Help woman void spontaneously. Measure amount of urine voided.
- Catheterize as necessary.
- Reassess after voiding or catheterization to make sure that bladder is not palpable and fundus is firm and in midline.

Lochia
- Observe lochia on perineal pads and linen under the mother's buttocks. Determine amount and color; note size and number of clots; note odor.
- Observe perineum for source of bleeding (e.g., episiotomy, lacerations).

Perineum
- Ask or help woman turn on her side and flex upper leg on hip.
- Lift upper buttock.
- Observe perineum in good lighting.
- Assess episiotomy or laceration repair for redness (erythema), edema, ecchymosis (bruising), drainage, and approximation (REEDA).
- Assess for presence of hemorrhoids.

Care of the New Mother

Restriction of food and fluid intake and the loss of fluids (blood, perspiration, or emesis) during labor cause many women to be very hungry and thirsty soon after birth. In the absence of complications a woman who has given birth vaginally; has recovered from the effects of the anesthetic; and has stable vital signs, a firm uterus, and small-to-moderate lochial flow may have fluids and a regular diet as desired (AAP and ACOG, 2012). In the immediate postpartum period women who give birth by cesarean are usually restricted to clear liquids and ice chips.

As soon as they have had a chance to bond with the baby and eat, most new mothers are ready for a nap or at least a quiet period of rest. Following this rest period the woman may want to shower and change clothes. Most new mothers are capable of self-management or are helped in these activities by family members or support persons.

Care of the Family

Most parents enjoy being able to handle, hold, explore, and examine the baby immediately after birth. Both parents can help with the thorough drying of the infant. Usually the infant is wrapped in a receiving blanket and given to the mother or father/partner to hold. If skin-to-skin contact is desired, place the unwrapped infant on the woman's chest or abdomen and cover the baby with a warm blanket. Holding the newborn next to her skin helps the mother maintain the baby's body heat and provides skin-to-skin contact. Stockinette caps are often used to keep the newborn's head warm and prevent heat loss.

Many women wish to begin breastfeeding their newborns at this time to take advantage of the infant's alert state (first period of reactivity) and stimulate the production of oxytocin that promotes contraction of the uterus and prevents hemorrhage. In baby-friendly hospitals, breastfeeding is initiated within the first hour after birth. Some women prefer to wait to breastfeed until after they have had time to rest. Be aware that in some cultures (e.g., Vietnamese and Hispanic) breastfeeding is not acceptable to some women until the milk comes in.

Family-Newborn Relationships

The woman's reaction to the sight of her newborn may range from excited outbursts of laughing, talking, and even crying to apparent apathy. A polite smile and nod may be her only acknowledgment of the comments of nurses and the primary health care provider. Occasionally the reaction is one of anger or indifference; the woman turns away from the baby, concentrates on her own pain, and sometimes makes hostile comments. These varied reactions can arise from pleasure, exhaustion, or deep disappointment. When evaluating parent-newborn interactions after birth, the nurse should consider the cultural characteristics of the woman and her family and the expected behaviors of that culture. In some cultures the birth of a male child is preferred, and women may grieve when a female child is born (D'Avanzo, 2008).

Whatever the reaction and its cause, the woman needs continuing acceptance and support from all staff. Make a notation regarding the parents' reaction to the newborn in the recovery record. Assess this reaction by asking yourself such questions as, "How do the parents look?" "What do they say?" "What do they do?" Conduct further assessment of the parent-newborn relationship as you give care during the period of recovery. This assessment is especially important if you notice warning signs (e.g., passive or hostile reactions to the newborn, disappointment with the sex or appearance of the newborn, absence of eye contact, or limited interaction of parents with one another) immediately after birth. Nurses often find it helpful to discuss warning signs with the woman's primary health care provider.

Siblings who may have appeared only remotely interested in the final phases of the second stage tend to experience renewed interest and excitement when the newborn appears. They can be encouraged to hold the baby (see Fig. 16-25).

Parents usually respond to praise of their newborn. Many need to be reassured that the dusky appearance of their baby's extremities immediately after birth is normal until circulation is well established. If appropriate, explain the reason for the molding of the newborn's head. Communicate information about hospital routine. However, recognize that the cultural background of the parents may influence their expectations regarding the care and handling of their newborn immediately after birth. For example, some traditional Southeast Asians believe that the head should not be touched because it is the most sacred part of a person's body. They also believe that praise of the baby is dangerous because jealous spirits may then cause the baby harm or take him or her away (D'Avanzo, 2008). Hospital staff members can provide the environment for making this a satisfying experience for parents, family, and significant others by their interest and concern.

KEY POINTS

- The onset of labor may be difficult to determine for both nulliparous and multiparous women.
- The familiar environment of her home is most often the ideal place for a woman during the latent phase of the first stage of labor.
- The nurse assumes much of the responsibility for assessing the progress of labor and keeping the primary health care provider informed about progress in labor and deviations from expected findings.
- The FHR and pattern reveal the fetal response to the stress of the labor process.
- Assessment of the laboring woman's urinary output and bladder is critical to ensure her progress and prevent injury to the bladder.
- Regardless of the actual labor and birth experience, the woman's or couple's perception of the birth experience is most likely to be positive when events and performances are consistent with expectations, especially in terms of maintaining control and adequacy of pain relief.
- The woman's level of anxiety may increase when she does not understand what is being said to her about her labor because of the medical terminology used or because of a language barrier.
- Coaching, emotional support, and comfort measures help the woman use her energy constructively in relaxing and working with the contractions.
- The progress of labor is enhanced when a woman changes her position frequently during the first stage of labor.

- Doulas provide a continuous supportive presence during labor that can have a positive effect on the process of childbirth and its outcome.
- The cultural beliefs and practices of a woman and her significant others, including her partner, can have a profound influence on their approach to labor and birth.
- Siblings present for labor and birth need preparation and support for the event.
- Women with a history of sexual abuse often experience profound stress and anxiety during childbirth.
- Inability to palpate the cervix during vaginal examination indicates that complete effacement and full dilation have occurred and is the only certain, objective sign that the second stage has begun.
- Women may have an urge to bear down at various times during labor; for some it may be before the cervix is fully dilated, and for others it may not occur until the active phase of the second stage of labor.
- When encouraged to respond to the rhythmic nature of the second stage of labor, the woman normally changes body positions, bears down spontaneously, and vocalizes (open-glottis pushing) when she perceives the urge to push (Ferguson reflex).
- Women should bear down several times during a contraction using the open-glottis pushing method. They should avoid sustained closed-glottis pushing because this inhibits oxygen transport to the fetus.
- Nurses can use the role of advocate to prevent routine use of episiotomy and reduce the incidence of lacerations by empowering women to take an active role in their childbirth and educating health care providers about approaches to managing childbirth that reduce the incidence of perineal trauma.
- Objective signs indicate that the placenta has separated and is ready to be expelled; excessive traction (pulling) on the umbilical cord before the placenta has separated can result in maternal injury.
- During the fourth stage of labor the woman's fundal tone, lochial flow, and vital signs should be assessed frequently to ensure that she is physically recovering well after giving birth.
- Most parents/families enjoy being able to handle, hold, explore, and examine the baby immediately after the birth.

REFERENCES

American Academy of Pediatrics (AAP) and American College of Obstetricians and Gynecologists (ACOG): *Guidelines for perinatal care,* ed 7, Washington, DC, 2012, ACOG.

Association of Women's Health, Obstetric, and Neonatal Nurses (AWHONN): AWHONN Position Statement: Nursing support of laboring women, *J Obstet Gynecol Neonat Nurs* 40(5):665–666, 2011.

Berghella V, Baxter J, Chauhan S: Evidence-based labor and delivery management, *Am J Obstet Gynecol* 199(5):445–454, 2008.

Blackburn ST: *Maternal, fetal, and neonatal physiology: a clinical perspective,* ed 4, St Louis, 2013, Saunders.

Burke C: Active versus expectant management of the third stage of labor and implementation of a protocol, *J Perinat Neonat Nurs* 24(3):215–228, 2010.

Callister L: Integrating cultural beliefs and practices when caring for childbearing women and families. In Rice Simpson K, Creehan P, editors: *AWHONN's perinatal nursing,* ed 3, Philadelphia, 2008, Lippincott Williams & Wilkins.

Centers for Disease Control and Prevention (CDC), Branson B, Handsfield H, et al: Revised recommendations for HIV testing of adults, adolescents, and pregnant women in health-care settings, *MMWR Morbid Mortal Weekly Rep* 55(RR-14):1–17, 2006.

Cluett ER, Burns E: Immersion in water in labour and birth, *Cochrane Database Syst Rev* 2:CD000111.pub3. DOI: 10.1002/14651858, 2009.

D'Avanzo CE: *Mosby's pocket guide to cultural health assessment,* ed 4, St Louis, 2008, Mosby.

Gilbert E: *Manual of high risk pregnancy & delivery,* ed 5, St Louis, 2011, Mosby.

Gillesby E, Burns S, Dempsey A, et al: Comparison of delayed versus immediate pushing during second stage of labor for nulliparous women with epidural anesthesia, *J Obstet Gynecol Neonat Nurs* 39(6):635–643, 2010.

Hanson L: Second-stage labor care: challenges in spontaneous bearing down, *J Perinat Neonat Nurs* 23(1):31–39, 2009.

Hodnett E, Gates S, Hofmeyr G, et al: Continuous support for women during childbirth, *Cochrane Database Syst Rev* 3:CD003766, 2011.

James D: Routine obstetrical interventions: research agenda for the next decade, *J Perinat Neonat Nurs* 25(2):148–152, 2011.

Johansson M, Rubertsson C, Radestad I, et al: Childbirth—an emotionally demanding experience for fathers, *Sex Reprod Healthc* 3(1):11–20, 2012.

Kelly M, Johnson E, Lee V, et al: Delayed versus immediate pushing in second stage of labor, *MCN Am J Matern/Child Nurs* 35(2):81–87, 2010.

Lawrence A, Lewis L, Hofmeyr GJ, et al: Maternal positions and mobility during first stage labour, *Cochrane Database Syst Rev* 2:CD003934.pub 2. DOI: 10.1002/14651858, 2009.

Miller L, Miller D, Tucker SM: *Mosby's pocket guide to fetal monitoring: a multidisciplinary approach,* ed 7, St Louis, 2013, Mosby.

Reveiz L, Gaitan H, Cuervo L: Enemas during labour, *Cochrane Database Syst Rev* 4:CD000330, 2007.

Sharts-Hopko N: Oral intake during labor: a review of the evidence, *MCN Am J Matern/Child Nurs* 35(4):197–203, 2010.

Simkin P, Way K: Doulas of North America (DONA) International Position Paper: the birth doula's contribution to modern maternity care, 2008, www.DONA.org.

Simpson K: Labor and birth. In Rice Simpson K, Creehan P, editors: *AWHONN's perinatal nursing,* ed 3, Philadelphia, 2008, Lippincott Williams & Wilkins.

Simpson K, Cesario S, Morin K, et al: *Nursing care and management of the second stage of labor: evidence-based clinical practice guideline,* ed 2, Washington, DC, 2008, Association of Women's Health, Obstetric and Neonatal Nurses.

Singata M, Tranmer J, Gyte GML: Restricting oral fluid and food intake during labour, *Cochrane Database Syst Rev* 1:CD003930. pub2, DOI: 10.1002/14651858, 2010.

Walls D: Herbs and natural therapies for pregnancy, birth, and breastfeeding, *Int J Childbirth Educ* 24(2):29–37, 2009.

Waterbirth International: Frequently asked questions, 2012, www.waterbirth.org.

Wing D, Farinelli C: Abnormal labor and induction of labor. In Gabbe S, Niebyl J, Simpson J, et al, editors: *Obstetrics: normal and problem pregnancies,* ed 6, Philadelphia, 2012, Saunders.

Zwelling E: Overcoming the challenges: maternal movement and positioning to facilitate labor progress, *MCN Am J Matern/Child Nurs* 35(2):72–78, 2010.

Labor and Birth Complications

Kitty Cashion

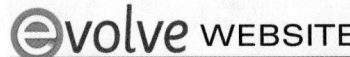 WEBSITE

http://evolve.elsevier.com/Perry/maternal

LEARNING OBJECTIVES

On completion of this chapter, the reader will be able to:

- Differentiate between preterm birth and low birth weight.
- Discuss major risk factors associated with preterm labor.
- Analyze current interventions to prevent spontaneous preterm birth.
- Discuss the use of tocolytics and antenatal glucocorticoids in preterm labor.
- Evaluate the effects of prescribed bed rest on pregnant women and their families.
- Design a nursing care plan for women with preterm premature rupture of the membranes (preterm PROM).

- Describe the care of a woman with postterm pregnancy.
- Explain the challenge of caring for obese women during labor and birth.
- Summarize the nursing care for a woman experiencing a trial of labor, induction or augmentation of labor, a forceps- or vacuum-assisted birth, a cesarean birth, or a vaginal birth after a cesarean birth (VBAC).
- Discuss obstetric emergencies and their appropriate management.

When complications arise during labor and birth, risk for perinatal morbidity and mortality increases. Some complications are anticipated, especially if the woman is identified to be at high risk during the antepartum period; other complications are unexpected or unforeseen. It is crucial for nurses to understand the normal birth process to prevent and detect deviations from normal labor and birth and to promptly implement nursing measures when complications arise. Optimal care of the laboring woman, fetus, and family experiencing complications is possible only when the nurse and other members of the obstetric team use their knowledge and skills in a concerted effort to provide competent and compassionate care. This chapter focuses on the problems of preterm labor and birth, postterm pregnancy, dystocia, obesity, and obstetric emergencies.

PRETERM LABOR AND BIRTH

Preterm labor is defined as cervical changes and uterine contractions occurring between 20 and 37 weeks of pregnancy. Preterm birth is any birth that occurs before the completion of 37 weeks of pregnancy, regardless of birth weight. Complications related to preterm birth account for more newborn and infant deaths than any other cause (Simhan, Iams, and Romero, 2012).

In 2010 the preterm birthrate for all races in the United States dropped for the fourth year in a row, to 11.99% (Martin, Hamilton, Sutton, et al., 2012). This decline was largely the result of three major practice changes: (1) improved fertility practices that reduced the risk for higher-order multiple gestations; (2) limiting scheduled births at less than 39 weeks of gestation to only those with valid indications; and (3) increased use of strategies to prevent recurrent preterm birth (Simhan, Iams, and Romero, 2012).

The World Health Organization estimates that 9.6% (almost 13 million) of all births worldwide in 2005 were preterm. The rate of preterm birth is highest in Africa and North America and lowest in Europe. In the United States, African-American women have the highest rates of preterm birth, almost twice as high as those of other racial and ethnic groups. This is particularly apparent for births that occur at less than 32 weeks of gestation (Simhan, Iams, and Romero, 2012).

About 75% of all preterm births in the United States are termed late preterm because they occur between 34 and 36 weeks of gestation. Late preterm infants are at increased risk for early death and long-term health problems when compared with infants who are born full term. Although late preterm babies do experience significant problems, the great majority of infant deaths and the most serious morbidity occur among the 16% of all preterm infants who are born before 32 weeks of gestation (very preterm birth) (Iams, Romero, and Creasy, 2009).

Preterm Birth versus Low Birth Weight

Although they have distinctly different meanings, the terms *preterm birth* or *prematurity* and *low birth weight* are often interchanged. Preterm birth describes length of gestation (i.e., less than 37 weeks regardless of the weight of the infant), whereas low birth weight describes only weight at the time of birth (i.e., 2500 g or less). Because birth weight was far easier to determine than gestational age, in many settings and publications low birth weight was used as a substitute term for preterm birth. Preterm birth, however, is a more dangerous health condition for an infant because less time in the uterus correlates with immaturity of body systems. Low-birth-weight babies can be, but are not necessarily, preterm. Low birth weight can be caused by conditions other than preterm birth, such as intrauterine growth restriction (IUGR), a condition of inadequate fetal growth not necessarily correlated with initiation of labor. Pregnant women who have various complications of pregnancy that interfere with uteroplacental perfusion, such as gestational hypertension or poor nutrition, may give birth to a baby at term who is low birth weight because of IUGR. However, infants born at a preterm gestation can weigh more than 2500 g at birth, such as infants born to women with diabetes who have poorly controlled blood glucose levels. Today, thanks to advances in pregnancy dating, outcomes related to gestational age can increasingly be distinguished from outcomes related to birth weight (Iams, Romero, and Creasy, 2009).

Spontaneous versus Indicated Preterm Birth

Preterm birth is divided into two categories: spontaneous and indicated. Spontaneous preterm birth occurs after an early initiation of the labor process and comprises nearly 75% of all preterm births in the United States. Conditions such as preterm labor with intact membranes, preterm premature rupture of membranes (preterm PROM), cervical insufficiency, or amnionitis often result in preterm birth (Iams, Romero, and Creasy, 2009).

Indicated preterm birth occurs as a means to resolve maternal or fetal risk related to continuing the pregnancy. About 25% of all preterm births in the United States are indicated because of medical or obstetric conditions that affect the mother, the fetus, or both. An increase in the number of indicated preterm births between 34 and 36 weeks of gestation accounts for much of the recent rise in late preterm births (Iams, Romero, and Creasy, 2009; Simhan, Iams, and Romero, 2012). Box 17-1 lists some common causes of indicated preterm births.

The remainder of this section deals with spontaneous preterm labor and birth.

Predicting Spontaneous Preterm Labor and Birth

Major risk factors for spontaneous preterm birth are listed in Box 17-2. Poverty, lack of education, living in a disadvantaged neighborhood, state, or region, and lack of access to prenatal care also have been identified as risk factors. In addition, the risk for preterm birth appears to be genetically related. For example, women who were themselves born prematurely have an increased risk for giving birth prematurely (Simhan, Iams, and Romero, 2012). Researchers have developed many risk scoring systems in an attempt to determine which women might go into labor prematurely. No risk scoring system has been very successful in lowering the preterm birthrate, however, because at least 50% of all women who ultimately give birth prematurely have no identifiable risk factors (Iams, Romero,

---

BOX 17-1 COMMON CAUSES OF INDICATED PRETERM BIRTH

- Pre-existing or gestational diabetes
- Chronic hypertension
- Preeclampsia
- Obstetrical disorders or risk factors in the current or a previous pregnancy
  - Previous cesarean birth via a classic uterine incision
- Placental disorders
- Medical disorders
  - Seizures
  - Thromboembolism
  - Maternal HIV or herpes infection
  - Obesity
- Advanced maternal age
- Fetal disorders
  - Chronic (IUGR) or acute (abnormal NST or BPP) fetal compromise
  - Excessive or inadequate amount of amniotic fluid
  - Birth defects

Data from Simhan H, Iams J, Romero R: Preterm birth. In Gabbe S, Niebyl J, Simpson J, et al, editors: *Obstetrics: normal and problem pregnancies*, ed 6, Philadelphia, 2012, Saunders. *BPP*, Biophysical profile; *HIV*, human immunodeficiency virus; *IUGR*, intrauterine growth restriction; *NST*, nonstress test.

BOX 17-2 RISK FACTORS FOR SPONTANEOUS PRETERM LABOR

- History of previous spontaneous preterm birth
- African-American race
- Genital tract infection
- Multifetal gestation
- Second-trimester bleeding
- Low prepregnancy weight

Data from Iams J, Romero R, Creasy R: Preterm labor and birth. In Creasy R, Resnik R, Iams J, et al, editors: *Creasy and Resnik's maternal-fetal medicine: principles and practice*, ed 6, Philadelphia, 2009, Saunders; Simhan H, Iams J, Romero R: Preterm birth. In Gabbe S, Niebyl J, Simpson J, et al, editors: *Obstetrics: normal and problem pregnancies*, ed 6, Philadelphia, 2012, Saunders.

---

and Creasy, 2009; Simhan, Iams, and Romero, 2012). Therefore it is important that all women be educated about prematurity, not only in early pregnancy but also in the preconception period. Unless all women are included in prevention efforts, a widespread reduction of preterm birthrates cannot be expected.

Fetal Fibronectin Test

Fetal fibronectin, a biochemical marker, has been studied extensively and is marketed in the United States as a diagnostic test for preterm labor. It is a glycoprotein "glue" found in plasma and produced during fetal life. Fetal fibronectin normally appears in cervical and vaginal secretions early in pregnancy and then again in late pregnancy. The test is performed by collecting fluid from the woman's vagina using a swab during a speculum examination. The presence of fetal fibronectin during the late second and early third trimesters of pregnancy may be related to placental inflammation, which is thought to be one cause of spontaneous preterm labor. However, the presence of fetal fibronectin is not very sensitive as a predictor of preterm birth. Before 35 weeks of gestation, a positive fetal fibronectin test predicts preterm birth only about 25% of the time. The test's sensitivity may be better earlier in pregnancy. In one study, the fetal fibronectin test predicted 65% of preterm births occurring before 28 weeks when it was performed between 22 and 24 weeks. Often the test is used to predict who will *not* go into preterm labor because preterm labor is very unlikely to occur in women with a negative result. Use of the fetal fibronectin test as a screening tool in women who are at low risk for preterm birth is not recommended (Iams, Romero, and Creasy, 2009).

Cervical Length

Another possible predictor of preterm labor is endocervical length. Changes in cervical length occur before uterine activity, so cervical measurement can identify women in whom the labor process has begun. However, because preterm cervical shortening occurs over a period of weeks, neither digital nor ultrasound cervical examination is very sensitive at predicting imminent preterm birth (Iams, Romero, and Creasy, 2009). Women whose cervical length is greater than 30 mm are unlikely to give birth prematurely even if they have symptoms of preterm labor (Iams, Romero, and Creasy, 2009; Simhan, Iams, and Romero, 2012).

Causes of Spontaneous Preterm Labor and Birth

Infection is definitely associated with preterm labor. Women in spontaneous preterm labor with intact membranes commonly have organisms that are normally found in the lower genital tract present in their amniotic fluid, placenta, and membranes. Clinical and laboratory evidence of infection are more common when birth occurs earlier than 30 to 32 weeks of gestation rather than closer to term. Urinary tract and intraabdominal (e.g., appendicitis) infections have also been related to preterm birth (Simhan, Iams, and Romero, 2012). Women with periodontal disease have been shown to have an increased risk for preterm birth. However, the risk is not reduced by periodontal care, suggesting that the link between periodontal disease and preterm birth is not a cause-and-effect relationship (Simhan, Iams, and Romero, 2012).

Another proposed cause of preterm labor and birth is bleeding at the site of placental implantation in the uterus in the first or second trimester of pregnancy. The resulting uteroplacental ischemia or hemorrhage at the decidual layer of the placenta may somehow activate the preterm labor process. Intrauterine inflammation is associated with infection, uterine vascular compromise, and decidual hemorrhage and may contribute to preterm labor. Maternal and fetal stress, uterine overdistention, allergic reaction, and a decrease in progesterone are other factors that may play a part in initiating preterm labor. It is becoming increasingly clear that preterm labor is caused by multiple pathologic processes that eventually result in uterine contractions, cervical changes, and membrane rupture (Iams, Romero, and Creasy, 2009; Romero and Lockwood, 2009).

CARE MANAGEMENT

Because all pregnant women must be considered at risk for preterm labor, nursing assessment for factors that contribute to this risk begins early in pregnancy and continues throughout the prenatal period. The onset of preterm labor is often insidious and can be easily mistaken for normal discomforts of pregnancy. Nursing diagnoses, expected outcomes of care, and evidence-based interventions are established for each woman based on her assessment findings (see Nursing Care Plan).

Prevention

Primary prevention strategies that address risk factors associated with preterm labor and birth are less costly in human and financial terms than the high-tech and often lifelong care required by preterm infants and their families. Programs aimed at health promotion and disease prevention that encourage healthy lifestyles for the population in general and women of childbearing age in particular should be developed. Preconception counseling and care for women, especially those with a history of preterm birth, may identify correctable risk factors and provide a means to encourage women to participate in health-promoting activities. Smoking cessation, for example, has been shown to prevent preterm labor and birth (Freda, 2006; Iams, Romero, and Creasy, 2009).

Preterm birth can be prevented in some women by administering prophylactic progesterone supplementation. Both daily vaginal suppositories or creams and weekly intramuscular injections of 17-alpha hydroxyprogesterone caproate have been shown to decrease the rate of preterm birth by about 40% in women with a history of prior preterm birth or with a short (less than 15 mm to 20 mm length) cervix before 24 weeks of gestation. Supplementation begins at 16 weeks and continues until 36 weeks of gestation. Progesterone supplementation does not affect the rate of preterm birth in women with multiple gestations. Exactly how progesterone works to prevent preterm birth is unclear (Simhan, Iams, and Romero, 2012).

Many interventions intended to prevent spontaneous preterm birth have been recommended in the past and are still often prescribed. However, some of these interventions have not been shown to reduce the rate of preterm birth. Ongoing research is needed, especially since our understanding of the pathophysiology of preterm birth is increasing (Iams, Romero, and Creasy, 2009).

Early Recognition and Diagnosis

Although preterm birth often is not preventable, early recognition of preterm labor is still essential to implement interventions that have been demonstrated to reduce neonatal and infant morbidity and mortality. These interventions include (Simhan, Iams, and Romero, 2012):

- Transferring the mother before birth to a hospital equipped to care for her preterm infant
- Giving antibiotics during labor to prevent neonatal group B streptococci infection
- Administering glucocorticoids to women in labor to prevent or reduce neonatal and infant morbidity and mortality from health problems including respiratory distress syndrome, intraventricular hemorrhage, and necrotizing enterocolitis
- Administering magnesium sulfate to women giving birth before 32 weeks of gestation to reduce the incidence of cerebral palsy in their infants

Although maternal transport helps ensure a better health outcome for the mother and the baby, it also has a downside. Women may be transported to tertiary centers far from home, making visits by family and friends difficult and increasing the anxiety levels of the woman and her family. Attention to the needs of the woman and her family before, during, and after the transport is essential to comprehensive nursing care.

Because more than half of preterm births occur in women without obvious risk factors, it is essential that all pregnant women be taught the symptoms of preterm labor (Box 17-3). The nurse caring for women in a prenatal setting should use methods that are known to be successful for teaching pregnant women about how to recognize these symptoms and then assess for these symptoms at each prenatal visit. Women also must be taught the significance of

◎ NURSING CARE PLAN

Preterm Labor

NURSING DIAGNOSIS	EXPECTED OUTCOME	NURSING INTERVENTIONS	RATIONALES
Deficient Knowledge related to recognition of preterm labor	Woman and partner describe signs and symptoms of preterm labor.	Assess what woman and partner know about preterm labor and birth and how to recognize its presence	To identify areas of deficit
		Discuss signs and symptoms that serve as warning signs of preterm labor so that woman or her partner has adequate information	To identify problems early
		Provide written supplemental materials that include list of warning signs and instructions regarding what to do if any of listed signs occur	Couple can reinforce and review learning and act swiftly and appropriately should a sign occur
		Discuss and demonstrate how to assess and time contractions	To provide needed skills to assess signs of labor
Risk for Injury (maternal/fetal) related to recurrence of preterm labor	Woman demonstrates ability to assess self for signs of recurring labor; maternal-fetal well-being is maintained.	Teach woman and partner how to monitor uterine contraction activity daily	To provide immediate evidence of worsening condition
		Have woman and partner report rupture of membranes, vaginal bleeding, cramping, pelvic pressure, or low backache to appropriate health care resource immediately	Because such symptoms can be signs of labor
		Have woman monitor her weight, diet, fluid intake, and vital signs on daily basis	To evaluate for potential problems
		Have woman limit activities to those recommended in restricted activity plan.	To decrease likelihood of onset of labor
		Encourage woman to use side-lying position when reclining	To enhance placental perfusion
		Teach woman signs and symptoms of thrombophlebitis, and encourage gentle exercise of lower extremities	Because pregnancy and limited activity increase risk for clot formation
		Counsel woman to abstain from sexual intercourse and nipple stimulation if symptoms of preterm labor occur	Because such activities may stimulate uterine contractions
		Encourage woman to practice relaxation techniques	To decrease uterine tone and decrease anxiety and stress
		Teach woman to take tocolytic or other medications per physician's orders	To inhibit uterine contractions
		Teach woman and partner about and have them report any medication side effects immediately	To prevent medication-induced complications
		Have family arrange for alternative strategies in carrying out woman's usual roles and functions	To decrease stress and limit temptations to increase activity
		If small children are part of household, encourage family to make alternative arrangements for child care	To enhance woman's adherence to her restricted activity protocol
Anxiety related to preterm labor and potentially premature neonate	Feeling and symptoms of anxiety are reduced.	Provide calm, soothing atmosphere, and encourage family to provide emotional support	To facilitate coping
		Encourage verbalization of fears	To decrease intensity of emotional response
		Involve woman and family in home management of her condition	To promote greater sense of control
		Help woman identify and use appropriate coping strategies and support systems	To reduce fear/anxiety
		Explore use of desensitization strategies such as progressive muscle relaxation, visual imagery, or thought stopping	To reduce fear-related emotions and related physical symptoms
		Provide information about online support groups	To reduce fear and anxiety

◎ NURSING CARE PLAN

Preterm Labor—cont'd

NURSING DIAGNOSIS	EXPECTED OUTCOME	NURSING INTERVENTIONS	RATIONALES
Deficient Diversional Activity related to modified bed rest	Woman will verbalize diminished feelings of boredom.	Assist woman to creatively explore personally meaningful activities that can be pursued from the bed	To ensure activities that have meaning, purpose, and value to individual
		Maintain emphasis on personal choices of woman	Because doing so promotes control and minimizes imposition of routines by others
		Evaluate support and system resources that are available in environment	To assist in providing diversional activities
		Explore ways for woman to remain active participant in home management and decision making	To promote control
		Engage support of family and friends in carrying out chosen activities and making necessary environmental alterations	To ensure success
		Encourage woman to use the Internet to communicate with other women on bed rest	To obtain support and share feelings
		Teach woman about stress management and relaxation techniques	To help manage tension of confinement

---

BOX 17-3 SIGNS AND SYMPTOMS OF PRETERM LABOR

Uterine Activity
- Uterine contractions occurring more frequently than every 10 minutes persisting for 1 hour or more
- Uterine contractions may be painful or painless

Discomfort
- Lower abdominal cramping similar to gas pains; may be accompanied by diarrhea
- Dull, intermittent low back pain (below the waist)
- Painful, menstrual-like cramps
- Suprapubic pain or pressure
- Pelvic pressure or heaviness; feeling that "baby is pushing down"
- Urinary frequency

Vaginal Discharge
- Change in character or amount of usual discharge: thicker (mucoid) or thinner (watery), bloody, brown or colorless, increased amount, odor
- Rupture of amniotic membranes

PATIENT TEACHING

What to Do If Symptoms of Preterm Labor Occur

- Empty your bladder.
- Drink two to three glasses of water or juice.
- Lie down on your side for 1 hour.
- Palpate for contractions.
- If symptoms continue, call your health care provider or go to the hospital.
- If symptoms go away, resume light activity but not what you were doing when the symptoms began.
- If symptoms return, call your health care provider or go to the hospital.
- If any of the following symptoms occur, call your health care provider or go to the hospital immediately:
  - Uterine contractions every 10 minutes or less for 1 hour or more
  - Vaginal bleeding
  - Fluid leaking from the vagina

---

these symptoms of preterm labor and what to do should they occur (see Patient Teaching box).

In particular, patient education regarding any symptoms of uterine contractions or cramping between 20 and 37 weeks of gestation must emphasize that these symptoms are not just normal discomforts of pregnancy but, rather, indications of possible preterm labor (Fig. 17-1). Waiting too long to see a health care provider could result in inevitable preterm birth without sufficient time to implement the interventions that have been shown to improve infant outcomes (see preceding discussion).

The diagnosis of preterm labor is based on three major diagnostic criteria:
- Gestational age between 20 and 37 weeks
- Uterine activity (e.g., contractions)
- Progressive cervical change (e.g., effacement of 80% or cervical dilation of 2 cm or greater)

If the presence of fetal fibronectin is used as another diagnostic criterion, a sample of cervical and vaginal secretions for testing should be obtained before an examination for cervical changes because the lubricant used to examine the cervix can reduce the accuracy of the test for fetal fibronectin. The presence of vaginal bleeding or ruptured membranes or a history of intercourse within the past 24 hours can also reduce the accuracy of the test results.

The pregnant woman at 30 weeks with an irritable uterus but no documented cervical change is not in preterm labor, although she should be carefully evaluated during follow-up care to determine whether she has progressed to active preterm labor (e.g., effacement, dilation, or both). Misdiagnosis of preterm labor can lead to inappropriate use of pharmacologic agents that can be dangerous to the health of the woman, the fetus, or both.

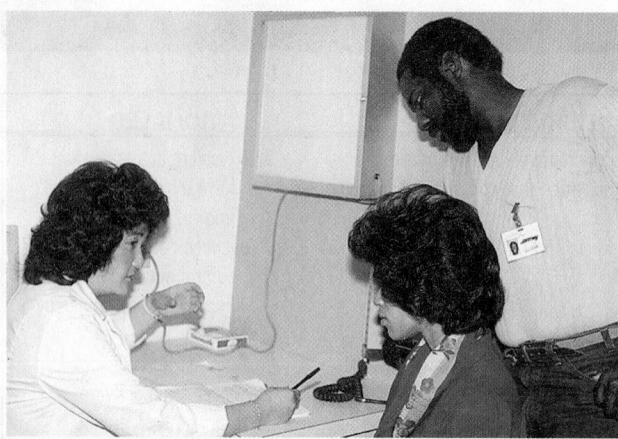

FIG 17-1 Nurse teaching a couple signs and symptoms of preterm labor. (Courtesy Marjorie Pyle, RNC, Lifecircle, Costa Mesa, CA.)

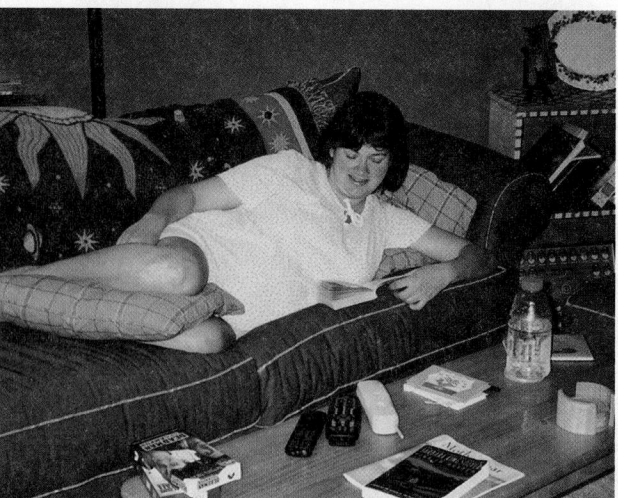

FIG 17-2 Woman at home on restricted activity for preterm labor prevention. Note how she has arranged her daytime resting area so that needed items are close at hand. (Courtesy Amy Turner, Cary, NC.)

Lifestyle Modifications

Activity Restriction. Activity restriction, including bed rest and limited work, is a commonly prescribed intervention for the prevention of preterm birth. Bed rest, however, is not a benign intervention, and no evidence has been published in the literature to support the effectiveness of this intervention in reducing preterm birthrates (Simhan, Iams, and Romero, 2012). Research indicates that bed rest causes adverse physical effects, including risk for thrombus formation, muscle atrophy, osteoporosis, and cardiovascular deconditioning. In many instances, these symptoms are not resolved by 6 weeks postpartum. In addition, bed rest affects women and their families psychologically, emotionally, socially, and financially. Box 17-4 lists adverse effects of bed rest. Many health care providers now recommend only modified bed rest.

Restriction of Sexual Activity. Restriction of sexual activity is frequently recommended for women at risk for preterm birth. This intervention has not been shown to be effective at preventing preterm birth. However, sexual abstinence has not been studied in women with specific risk factors for preterm birth, such as a short cervix. Therefore more research is indicated (Iams, Romero, and Creasy, 2009). If, however, symptoms of preterm labor occur after sexual activity, then that activity may need to be curtailed until 37 weeks of gestation.

Home Care. Home care of the woman at risk for preterm birth is still challenging for the nurse, who must assist the woman and her family in dealing with the many difficulties faced by families when one member is unable to fulfill usual role responsibilities.

The woman's environment can be modified for convenience by using tables and storage units around her bed or daytime resting place to keep essential items within reach (e.g., cell or smart phone, television, radio, MP3 player, CD player, computer with Internet access, snacks, books, magazines, newspapers, and items for hobbies) (Fig. 17-2). Ensuring that the bed or couch is near a window and the bathroom is also helpful. Covering the bed with an eggcrate mattress can relieve discomfort. Women often find that a daily schedule of smaller, more frequent meals, activities (e.g., paying bills, planning and helping with meal preparation, hobbies), limited naps, and hygiene and grooming (e.g., shower, dressing in street clothes, applying makeup) reduces boredom and helps them maintain control and normalcy. See the Patient Teaching box on p. 309 for more information.

BOX 17-4 ADVERSE EFFECTS OF BED REST

Maternal Effects (Physical)
- Weight loss; indigestion; loss of appetite
- Muscle wasting, weakness; aching muscles
- Bone demineralization and calcium loss
- Decreased plasma volume and cardiac output
- Increased clotting tendency; risk for thrombophlebitis
- Cardiac deconditioning
- Alteration in bowel function
- Sleep disturbance, fatigue
- Prolonged postpartum recovery

Maternal Effects (Psychosocial)
- Loss of control associated with role reversals
- Dysphoria—anxiety, depression, hostility, and anger
- Guilt associated with difficulty complying with activity restriction and inability to meet role responsibilities
- Boredom, loneliness
- Emotional lability (mood swings); difficulty concentrating
- Increased stress

Effects on Support System
- Stress associated with role reversals, increased responsibilities, and disruption of family routines
- Financial strain associated with loss of maternal income and cost of treatment
- Fear and anxiety regarding the well-being of the mother and fetus

---

See the Patient Teaching box on p. 447 for additional ideas and suggestions. With modified bedrest, women are usually allowed bathroom privileges for toileting and showering and can be up to the table for meals.

Suppression of Uterine Activity

Tocolytics are medications given to arrest labor after uterine contractions and cervical change have occurred. No medications that

PATIENT TEACHING

Activities for Children of Women on Activity Restriction

- Schedule brief play periods throughout the day.
- Keep a few favorite toys in a box or basket close to the bed or couch.
- Read to the children.
- Put puzzles together.
- Watch videos, play video games (remote control for television is ideal).
- Play card or board games.
- Color in coloring books.
- Cut out pictures from magazines and paste on cardboard.
- Play bed basketball with a soft (sponge) ball or rolled up sock and a trash can or empty laundry basket.

BOX 17-5 CONTRAINDICATIONS TO TOCOLYTIC THERAPY

Maternal
- Severe preeclampsia or severe gestational hypertension
- Significant vaginal bleeding
- Cardiac disease

Fetal
- Gestational age of 37 weeks or more
- Fetal demise
- Lethal fetal anomaly
- Chorioamnionitis
- Evidence of acute or chronic fetal compromise

Data from Simhan H, Iams J, & Romero R: Preterm birth. In Gabbe S, Niebyl J, Simpson J, et al, editors: *Obstetrics: normal and problem pregnancies*, ed 6, Philadelphia, 2012, Saunders.

BOX 17-6 NURSING CARE FOR THE WOMAN RECEIVING TOCOLYTIC THERAPY

- Explain to the woman and her family the purpose and side effects of the tocolytic medication(s) ordered.
- Position the woman on her side to enhance placental perfusion and reduce pressure on the cervix.
- Monitor maternal vital signs including lung sounds and respiratory effort, fetal heart rate and pattern, and labor status according to hospital protocol and professional standards.
- Assess mother and fetus for signs of adverse reactions related to the tocolytic medication(s) being administered (see Medication Guide on p. 448).
- Determine maternal fluid balance by measuring daily weight and intake and output.
- Limit fluid intake to 2500 to 3000 mL/day, especially if a beta-adrenergic agonist or magnesium sulfate is being administered.
- Provide psychosocial support and opportunities for the woman and family to express feelings and concerns.
- Offer comfort measures as needed.
- Encourage diversional activities and relaxation techniques.

MEDICATION ALERT

Because magnesium sulfate depresses function of the central nervous system (CNS), it is essential that the nurse frequently assess the woman's respiratory status, deep tendon reflexes, and level of consciousness to identify signs that the magnesium sulfate is reaching toxic serum levels.

have been approved for use as tocolytics by the United States Food and Drug Administration are currently available in the United States. Ritodrine (Yutopar) was approved but has been withdrawn from the market in the United States. However, it is still used as a tocolytic in other countries. Drugs marketed for other purposes, such as treatment of asthma or hypertension or as antiinflammatory or analgesic agents, are used on an "off-label" basis (i.e., drugs known to be effective for a specific purpose, although not specifically developed and tested for this purpose) to suppress preterm labor (Iams, Romero, and Creasy, 2009). No tocolytic has been shown to reduce the rate of preterm birth. Rather, the rationale for giving these medications is to delay birth long enough to allow time for maternal transport and for corticosteroids to reach maximum benefit to reduce neonatal morbidity and mortality. Studies of individual drugs used for tocolysis rarely contain information about whether delaying birth improved infant outcomes (Simhan, Iams, and Romero, 2012). Maternal and fetal contraindications to tocolytic therapy are listed in Box 17-5. Box 17-6 describes nursing care for women receiving tocolytic therapy.

Magnesium sulfate inhibits uterine contractions and decreases intracellular calcium levels (Simhan, Iams, and Romero, 2012). It is almost always administered intravenously but can also be given intramuscularly. Magnesium sulfate produces few serious maternal or neonatal complications, and clinicians are familiar with its use. However, although magnesium sulfate is still frequently used, a recent meta-analysis of tocolytic agents found that it is not effective when given for tocolysis (see Medication Guide on pp. 448-449) (Simhan, Iams, and Romero, 2012).

Beta$_2$-adrenergic agonists (e.g., terbutaline [Brethine]) have been widely used in the past as tocolytics. They cause many maternal and fetal side effects, however, including beta$_1$-stimulated cardiopulmonary effects (e.g., tachycardia) and beta$_2$-stimulated metabolic effects (e.g., hyperglycemia). Therefore beta$_2$-adrenergic agonists are increasingly being replaced by medications that are safer and have fewer adverse reactions. They should not be used in women with known or suspected heart disease, severe preeclampsia or eclampsia, pregestational or gestational diabetes, or hyperthyroidism (Iams, Romero, and Creasy, 2009; Simhan, Iams, and Romero, 2012). Use of beta$_2$-adrenergic agonists is also contraindicated in women with migraine headaches (Gilbert, 2011).

Terbutaline, the most commonly administered beta-adrenergic agonist used for tocolysis in the United States, works by relaxing uterine smooth muscle as a result of stimulation of beta$_2$-receptors in the uterine smooth muscle. A single dose of terbutaline given subcutaneously may help diagnose preterm labor. In one study, women whose contractions persisted or recurred after a single injection of terbutaline were more likely to actually be in preterm labor than those whose contractions ceased. Terbutaline is often given subcutaneously to facilitate maternal transfer to a tertiary center or to initiate tocolytic therapy while another agent with a slower onset of action is administered concurrently. In addition, a subcutaneous injection of 0.25 mg may be given to suppress uterine tachysystole during labor induction or augmentation or to suppress contractions before cesarean birth. Long-term oral or subcutaneous administration (e.g., terbutaline pump) as maintenance therapy to suppress preterm labor has not been proven to be effective at reducing prematurity or neonatal morbidity (Gilbert, 2011; Iams, Romero, and

MEDICATION GUIDE

Tocolytic Therapy for Preterm Labor

MEDICATION AND ACTION	DOSAGE AND ROUTE*	ADVERSE EFFECTS	NURSING CONSIDERATIONS
Magnesium Sulfate CNS depressant; relaxes smooth muscles including uterus	Intravenous fluid should contain 40 g in 1000 mL, piggyback to primary infusion, and administer using controller pump: Loading dose: 4-6 g over 20-30 min Maintenance dose: 1-4 g/hr Use for stabilization only Discontinue within 24-48 hr at the maintenance dose or if intolerable adverse effects occur	**Maternal** • Hot flushes, sweating, burning at the IV insertion site, nausea and vomiting, dry mouth, drowsiness, blurred vision, diplopia, headache, ileus, generalized muscle weakness, lethargy, dizziness • Hypocalcemia • SOB • Transient hypotension • Some reactions may subside when loading dose is completed **Intolerable** • Respiratory rate fewer than 12 breaths/min • Pulmonary edema • Absent DTRs • Chest pain • Severe hypotension • Altered level of consciousness • Extreme muscle weakness • Urine output less than 25-30 mL/hr or less than 100 mL/4 hr • Serum magnesium level of 10 mEq/L (9 mg/dL) or greater **Fetal (uncommon)** • Decreased breathing movement • Reduced FHR variability • Nonreactive NST	Assess woman and fetus to obtain baseline before beginning therapy and then before and after each incremental change; follow frequency of agency protocol. Monitor serum magnesium levels with higher doses; therapeutic range is between 4 and 7.5 mEq/L or 5-8 mg/dL. Discontinue infusion and notify physician if intolerable adverse affects occur. Ensure that calcium gluconate 1 g (10 mL of 10% solution) or calcium chloride (normal dose is 500 mg IV infused over 30 min) is available for emergency administration to reverse magnesium sulfate toxicity. Should not be given to women with myasthenia gravis. Total IV intake should be limited to 125 mL/hr.
Beta-Adrenergic Agonist (Beta-Mimetic) *Terbutaline (Brethine)* Relaxes smooth muscles, inhibiting uterine activity, and causing bronchodilation	Subcutaneous injection of 0.25 mg every 4 hr Treatment should last no longer than 24 hr Discontinue use if intolerable adverse effects occur	**Maternal (most are mild and of limited duration)** • Tachycardia, chest discomfort, palpitations, dysrhythmias • Tremors, dizziness, nervousness • Headache • Nasal congestion • Nausea and vomiting • Hypokalemia • Hyperglycemia • Hypotension **Intolerable** • Tachycardia greater than 130 beats/min • BP less than 90/60 mm Hg • Chest pain • Cardiac dysrhythmias • Myocardial infarction • Pulmonary edema	Should not be used in women with a history of cardiac disease, pregestational or gestational diabetes, severe gestational hypertension, preeclampsia or eclampsia, migraine headaches, or hyperthyroidism, or with significant hemorrhage. Myocardial infarction leading to death has been reported after use. Validate that woman is in PTL and is >20 wk and <35 wk of gestation.

MEDICATION GUIDE

Tocolytic Therapy for Preterm Labor—cont'd

MEDICATION AND ACTION	DOSAGE AND ROUTE*	ADVERSE EFFECTS	NURSING CONSIDERATIONS
Terbutaline (Brethine)—cont'd		**Fetal** • Tachycardia • Hyperinsulinemia • Hyperglycemia	Assess woman and fetus according to agency protocol, being alert for adverse effects. Assess maternal glucose and potassium levels before treatment is initiated and periodically during treatment. Significant hyperglycemia (greater than 180 mg/dL) and hypokalemia (less than 2.5 mEq/L) may occur. Notify physician if the woman exhibits: • Maternal heart rate greater than 130 beats/min; dysrhythmias, chest pain • BP less than 90/60 mm Hg • Signs of pulmonary edema (e.g., dyspnea, crackles, decreased SaO₂) • Fetal heart rate greater than 180 beats/min Hyperglycemia occurs more frequently in women who are being treated simultaneously with corticosteroids. Ensure that propranolol (Inderal) is available to reverse adverse effects related to cardiovascular function.
Prostaglandin Synthetase Inhibitors (NSAIDS) *Indomethacin (Indocin)* Relaxes uterine smooth muscle by inhibiting prostaglandins	Loading dose: 50 mg orally, then 25-50 mg orally every 6 hr for 48 hr	**Maternal (common)** • Nausea and vomiting • Heartburn **Less common, but more serious** • Gastrointestinal bleeding • Prolonged bleeding time • Thrombocytopenia • Asthma in aspirin-sensitive patients **Fetal** • Constriction of ductus arteriosus • Oligohydramnios, caused by reduced fetal urine production • Neonatal pulmonary hypertension	The long-acting formulations decrease the incidence of adverse effects. Used only if gestational age is less than 32 wk. Administer for 48 hr or less. Do not use in women with renal or hepatic disease, active peptic ulcer disease, poorly controlled hypertension, asthma, or coagulation disorders. Can mask maternal fever. Assess woman and fetus according to agency policy, being alert for adverse effects. Determine amniotic fluid volume and function of fetal ductus arteriosus before initiating therapy and within 48 hr of discontinuing therapy; assessment is critical if therapy continues for more than 48 hr. Administer with food to decrease GI distress. Monitor for signs of postpartum hemorrhage.
Calcium Channel Blockers *Nifedipine (Adalat, Procardia)* Relaxes smooth muscles including the uterus by blocking calcium entry	Initial dose: 10-20 mg orally every 3-6 hr until contractions are rare, followed by long-acting formulations of 30 or 60 mg every 8-12 hr for 48 hr while corticosteroids are being given (however, the ideal dose has not been established)	**Maternal (most effects are mild)** • Hypotension • Headache • Flushing • Dizziness • Nausea **Fetal** • Hypotension (questionable)	Avoid concurrent use with magnesium sulfate because skeletal muscle blockade can result. Should not be given simultaneously with or immediately after terbutaline because of effects on heart rate and blood pressure. Assess woman and fetus according to agency protocol, being alert for adverse effects. Do not use sublingual route of administration.

Data from Gilbert E: *Manual of high risk pregnancy & delivery*, ed 5, St Louis, 2011, Mosby; Iams J, Romero R, Creasy R: Preterm labor and birth. In Creasy R, Resnik R, Iams J, et al, editors: *Creasy and Resnik's maternal-fetal medicine: principles and practice*, ed 6, Philadelphia, 2009, Saunders; Simhan H, Iams J, Romero R: Preterm birth. In Gabbe S, Niebyl J, Simpson J, et al, editors: *Obstetrics: normal and problem pregnancies*, ed 6, Philadelphia, 2012, Saunders.

CNS, Central nervous system; *DTRs*, deep tendon reflexes; *FHR*, fetal heart rate; *GI*, gastrointestinal; *IV*, intravenous; *NSAIDs*, nonsteroidal antiinflammatory drugs; *NST*, nonstress test; *PTL*, preterm labor; *SaO₂*, arterial oxygen saturation; *SOB*, shortness of breath.

*Recommended administration protocols vary; always consult agency protocol, which should be evidence-based.

Creasy, 2009; Simhan, Iams, and Romero, 2012) (see Medication Guide on pp. 448-449).

Nifedipine (Adalat, Procardia), a calcium channel blocker, is another tocolytic agent that can suppress contractions. It works by inhibiting calcium from entering smooth muscle cells, thus reducing uterine contractions. Because of its ease of administration and low incidence of significant maternal and fetal side effects, the use of nifedipine is increasing. The drug is rapidly absorbed after oral administration. Maternal side effects, which include headache, flushing, dizziness, and nausea, are generally mild and relate primarily to the hypotension and reflex tachycardia that occur with administration. The decrease in blood pressure that occurs may be helpful for women who are also diagnosed with gestational hypertension or preeclampsia. However, at least one myocardial infarction has been reported in a healthy young woman who received a second dose of nifedipine. Concerns regarding adverse fetal effects have been lessened. Safety is achieved by following recommended dosages, avoiding concurrent use with magnesium sulfate, and maintaining maternal blood pressure, thereby preserving effective uteroplacental perfusion (Iams, Romero, and Creasy, 2009; Simhan, Iams, and Romero, 2012) (see Medication Guide on pp. 448-449).

MEDICATION ALERT

Administering both nifedipine and magnesium sulfate can cause skeletal muscle blockade. In addition, nifedipine should not be given along with or immediately following a beta$_2$-adrenergic agonist (e.g., terbutaline [Brethine]) (Iams, Romero, and Creasy, 2009; Simhan, Iams, and Romero, 2012).

⚡ SAFETY ALERT

Because using a calcium channel blocker can result in orthostatic hypotension and dizziness, it is essential to instruct women to slowly change position from supine to upright and then sit before standing until any dizziness disappears. In addition, it is important to maintain adequate fluid balance to reduce the drop in blood pressure that can occur with the drug-related vasodilation.

Indomethacin (Indocin), a nonsteroidal antiinflammatory drug (NSAID), has been shown in some trials to suppress preterm labor by blocking the production of prostaglandins. Serious maternal side effects are uncommon, and indomethacin is usually well tolerated. However, three serious fetal or neonatal side effects have caused major concerns about its use as a tocolytic. These side effects include constriction of the ductus arteriosus, oligohydramnios, and neonatal pulmonary hypertension. Therefore limiting the use of indomethacin to a short duration of treatment in women with preterm labor at less than 32 weeks of gestation is recommended (Iams, Romero, and Creasy, 2009; Simhan, Iams, and Romero, 2012) (see Medication Guide on pp. 448-449).

Promotion of Fetal Lung Maturity

Antenatal glucocorticoids are given as intramuscular injections to the mother to accelerate fetal lung maturity by stimulating fetal surfactant production. They are now considered one of the most effective and cost-efficient interventions for preventing morbidity and mortality associated with preterm labor. Antenatal glucocorticoids have been shown to significantly reduce the incidence of respiratory distress syndrome, intraventricular hemorrhage, necrotizing enterocolitis, and death in neonates without increasing the risk for

---

💊 MEDICATION GUIDE

Antenatal Glucocorticoid Therapy with Betamethasone or Dexamethasone

Action
- Stimulates fetal lung maturation by promoting release of enzymes that induce production or release of lung surfactant. **NOTE:** The U.S. Food and Drug Administration has not approved these medications for this use (i.e., this is an unlabeled use for obstetrics).

Indication
- To prevent or reduce the severity of neonatal respiratory distress syndrome by accelerating lung maturity in fetuses between 24 and 34 weeks of gestation. Infants born to women who received antenatal glucocorticoids are also less likely to experience intraventricular hemorrhage, necrotizing enterocolitis, or neonatal death.

Dosage and Route
- Betamethasone: 12 mg intramuscular (IM) for two doses 24 hours apart
- Dexamethasone: 6 mg IM for four doses 12 hours apart

Maternal Effects
- Transient (lasting 72 hours) increase in white blood cell (WBC) count
- Hyperglycemia

Fetal Effects
- Transient (lasting 72 hours) decrease in fetal breathing and body movements

Nursing Considerations
- Give deep IM in ventral gluteal or vastus lateralis muscle.
- Medication *must* be given by intramuscular injection; oral administration is *not* an acceptable alternative.
- Injection is painful.
- Medication should *not* affect maternal blood pressure.
- Assess blood glucose levels. Women with diabetes whose blood sugars have previously been well controlled may require increased insulin doses for several days.

Data from Simhan H, Iams J, Romero R: Preterm birth. In Gabbe S, Niebyl J, Simpson J, et al, editors: *Obstetrics: normal and problem pregnancies*, ed 6, Philadelphia, 2012, Saunders.

---

infection in either mothers or newborns (Mercer, 2009a). The National Institutes of Health (NIH) consensus panel recommended that all women between 24 and 34 weeks of gestation be given a single course of antenatal glucocorticoids when preterm birth is threatened unless evidence indicates that glucocorticoids will have an adverse effect on the mother or birth is imminent. In general, women who are candidates for tocolytic therapy are also candidates for antenatal glucocorticoids (Mercer, 2009a). The regimen for administration of antenatal glucocorticoids is given in the Medication Guide (above).

❗ NURSING ALERT

All women between 24 and 34 weeks of gestation who are at risk for preterm birth within 7 days should receive treatment with a single course of antenatal glucocorticoids. Because optimal benefit to the fetus begins 24 hours after the first injection, timely administration is essential (Mercer, 2009a).

Management of Inevitable Preterm Birth

When preterm birth appears inevitable, magnesium sulfate may be administered to reduce or prevent neonatal neurologic morbidity (e.g., cerebral palsy). Current recommendations are that magnesium sulfate for neuroprotection be given to women who are at least 24 but less than 32 weeks of gestation at the time birth is expected to occur. How magnesium sulfate works to provide neuroprotection is not well understood. Although it is likely that the neuroprotective effects are the result of residual concentrations of the medication in the neonate's system, data are insufficient to determine the precise maternal dose necessary to confer the benefit (Simhan, Iams, and Romero, 2012). Currently the dose of magnesium sulfate administered for neuroprotection is the same as that given for tocolysis (see Medication Guide on pp. 448-449).

Labor that has progressed to a cervical dilation of 4 cm or more is likely to lead to inevitable preterm birth. If birth appears imminent, preparations to care for a small, immature neonate should be made. Women in preterm labor may rapidly progress to birth and a very small fetus may be born through a partially dilated cervix. Also, malpresentation (e.g., breech presentation) occurs much more frequently in preterm than in term fetuses. Therefore nurses must be prepared to handle the emergency birth of a preterm infant, from either cephalic or breech presentation, without the woman's primary health care provider being present. Personnel skilled at neonatal resuscitation should be present at the time of birth. Equipment, supplies, and medications used for neonatal resuscitation should be gathered in advance and prepared for immediate use. If birth occurs in a hospital that is not prepared to provide continuing care for a preterm neonate, plans should be made for transfer of the baby to a higher level of care as soon as possible after stabilization.

Fetal and Early Neonatal Loss

Preterm birth or the presence of congenital anomalies or genetic disorders incompatible with life are major reasons for intrauterine fetal demise (stillbirth) or early neonatal death. In many of these situations, the parents will have already been told that the fetus has died or that the baby has a condition that is incompatible with life and will most likely die very soon after birth. Sometimes, however, the fetal death will be unexpected, diagnosed only after the woman has been admitted to the labor and birth unit. Whatever the case, labor and birth nurses must be prepared to provide sensitive care to these women and their families.

If fetal or early neonatal death is expected, the parents and members of the health care team need to discuss the situation before the birth and decide on a management plan that is acceptable to everyone. Despite counseling about the likelihood of a poor outcome, some parents want "everything possible," including cesarean birth for an abnormal fetal heart rate (FHR) tracing, to be done for the baby. If such intervention is not desired, usually the FHR will not be monitored during labor.

Another major decision is whether to attempt neonatal resuscitation and to what lengths resuscitation should go. Sometimes the feasibility of neonatal resuscitation cannot be determined until the baby's size and physical appearance have been assessed. If the baby is too small, too immature, or too malformed for effective resuscitation, comfort care can be provided instead. The baby is kept warm and comfortable, either at the mother's bedside or in the nursery, depending on the parents' desires, until death occurs. Parents can choose to view and hold the baby as they wish.

After the birth, the woman should be given the opportunity to decide if she wants to stay on the maternity unit or be moved to another hospital unit. She may prefer to be away from the sound of crying babies and exposure to other families who have had healthy infants. However, postpartum care and grief support may not be as good on another hospital unit where the staff is not experienced in postpartum and bereavement care.

Whether death occurs in utero or after birth, parents are faced with the same needs. See Chapter 25 for additional information on dealing with families experiencing a perinatal loss.

> ### BOX 17-7 RISK FACTORS FOR PRETERM PREMATURE RUPTURE OF MEMBRANES (PRETERM PROM)
>
> - History of prior preterm birth, especially if associated with preterm PROM
> - History of cervical conization or cerclage
> - Urinary or genital tract infection
> - Short cervical length in the second trimester
> - Preterm labor in the current pregnancy
> - Uterine overdistention
> - Second- and third-trimester bleeding
> - Pulmonary disease
> - Connective tissue disorders
> - Low socioeconomic status
> - Low body mass index
> - Nutritional deficiencies (copper and ascorbic acid)
> - Cigarette smoking

Data from Mercer B: Premature rupture of the membranes. In Gabbe S, Niebyl J, Simpson J, et al, editors: *Obstetrics: normal and problem pregnancies,* ed 6, Philadelphia, 2012, Saunders.

PREMATURE RUPTURE OF MEMBRANES

Premature rupture of membranes (PROM) is the spontaneous rupture of the amniotic sac and leakage of amniotic fluid beginning before the onset of labor at any gestational age. **Preterm premature rupture of membranes (preterm PROM)** (i.e., membranes rupture before the completion of 37 weeks of gestation) is associated with approximately 10% of all preterm births in the United States. Preterm PROM occurs twice as often in African-Americans as in other racial groups. The frequency of preterm PROM appears to have decreased over the past decade (Mercer, 2012). Preterm PROM most likely results from pathologic weakening of the amniotic membranes caused by inflammation, stress from uterine contractions, or other factors that cause increased intrauterine pressure. Infection of the urogenital tract is a major risk factor associated with preterm PROM (Mercer, 2009b; Mercer, 2012). Box 17-7 lists other risk factors. PROM or preterm PROM is diagnosed after the woman reports either a sudden gush of fluid or a slow leak of fluid from the vagina.

Chorioamnionitis is the most common maternal complication of preterm PROM, making it a major complication of pregnancy (see later discussion). Other less common but serious maternal complications include placental abruption, retained placenta and hemorrhage requiring dilation and curettage (D&C), sepsis, and death. Fetal complications from preterm PROM are related primarily to intrauterine infection, cord prolapse, umbilical cord compression associated with oligohydramnios, and placental abruption. Another possible fetal complication when preterm PROM occurs before 20 weeks of gestation is pulmonary hypoplasia (Mercer, 2009b; Mercer, 2012).

CARE MANAGEMENT

Management of PROM is determined for each woman based on an assessment of the estimated risk for maternal, fetal, and neonatal complications if pregnancy is allowed to continue or immediate labor and birth are attempted. At term, because infection is the greatest maternal, fetal, and neonatal risk, birth is the best option. Labor will most likely be induced if it does not begin spontaneously soon after PROM occurs (Mercer, 2009b; Mercer, 2012).

Preterm PROM (occurring at or after 23 weeks of gestation) is often managed expectantly or conservatively if the risks to the fetus and newborn associated with preterm birth are considered to be greater than the risks of infection. Women with preterm PROM are usually hospitalized for conservative management in an attempt to prolong the pregnancy and allow additional time for fetal maturation unless intrauterine infection, significant vaginal bleeding, placental abruption, advanced labor, or non-reassuring fetal assessment occurs (Mercer, 2012). Nursing support of the woman and her family is critical at this time. They are often anxious about the health of the baby, and the woman may fear that she was responsible in some way for the membrane rupture. The nurse can reassure the woman that in most cases the cause of PROM is unknown (Gilbert, 2011). Other nursing interventions include encouraging expression of feelings and concerns, providing information, and making referrals as needed.

Conservative management of preterm PROM includes fetal assessment by nonstress test (NST) and biophysical profile (BPP) at least daily. The woman should also be taught how to assess her fetus using daily fetal movement counts (DFMC), because a slowing of fetal movement has been shown to be a precursor to severe fetal compromise. (See Chapter 10 for further discussion of these tests.) In addition, the woman will be monitored for signs of labor, placental abruption, and the development of intrauterine infection. Antenatal glucocorticoids will be administered to women who are less than 32 weeks of gestation, because they have been proven to decrease the risk for several neonatal complications. Also, a 7-day course of broad-spectrum antibiotics (e.g., ampicillin, erythromycin) will be administered. Antibiotic treatment has been shown to prolong the time between membrane rupture and birth, decrease maternal chorioamnionitis and postpartum endometritis, and prevent sepsis, pneumonia, and intraventricular hemorrhage in the neonate (Mercer, 2012).

Vigilance for signs of infection is a major part of the nursing care and patient education after preterm PROM. The woman must be taught how to keep her genital area clean and that nothing should be introduced into her vagina. Signs of infection (e.g., fever, foul-smelling vaginal discharge, maternal and fetal tachycardia) should be reported immediately. If chorioamnionitis develops, labor will be induced. Should preterm labor occur, tocolytic medications may be administered in an attempt to gain time for transporting the woman to a hospital capable of providing care to a preterm infant or for antenatal corticosteroids or antibiotics to reach effective levels (Gilbert, 2011).

CHORIOAMNIONITIS

Chorioamnionitis, bacterial infection of the amniotic cavity, is a major cause of complications for both mothers and newborns at any gestational age. It occurs in approximately 1% to 5% of term births but in as many as 25% of preterm births (Duff, 2012). Other terms for this condition include *clinical chorioamnionitis, amnionitis, intrapartum infection, amniotic fluid infection,* and *intra-amniotic infection.* Chorioamnionitis is usually diagnosed by the clinical findings of maternal fever, maternal and fetal tachycardia, uterine tenderness, and foul odor of amniotic fluid (Duff, Sweet, and Edwards, 2009).

Chorioamnionitis most often occurs after membranes rupture or labor begins, as organisms that are part of the normal vaginal flora ascend into the amniotic cavity. Many of the risk factors for chorioamnionitis are associated with a long labor, such as prolonged membrane rupture, multiple vaginal examinations, and use of internal FHR and contraction monitoring modes (Duff, Sweet, and Edwards, 2009). Other risk factors include young maternal age, low socioeconomic status, nulliparity, and preexisting infections of the lower genital tract (Duff, 2012).

Women with chorioamnionitis can develop bacteremia. They are also more likely to have dysfunctional labor, which can result in the need for cesarean birth (see later discussion). If cesarean birth is necessary, wound infection or pelvic abscess is a possible complication. Neonatal risks include pneumonia, bacteremia, and sepsis. Death is more likely to occur in preterm than in term infants (Duff, 2012; Duff, Sweet, and Edwards, 2009). An association between chorioamnionitis and long-term neurologic development in the newborn, including cerebral palsy, has been reported (Duff, Sweet, and Edwards, 2009).

To prevent maternal and neonatal complications, prompt treatment with intravenous broad-spectrum antibiotics and birth of the fetus are necessary. Ampicillin or penicillin and gentamicin are the antibiotics most often used to treat chorioamnionitis during labor. After cesarean birth, an antibiotic that provides coverage for anaerobic organisms, such as clindamycin (Cleocin) or metronidazole (Flagyl) should be added. Antibiotics can usually be discontinued soon after birth (Duff, 2012).

The increased use of intrapartum antibiotic prophylaxis during labor in women who are group B streptococci positive has decreased the incidence of chorioamnionitis. Other measures that have proven to be effective in decreasing the frequency of chorioamnionitis are active management of labor (see later discussion) and induction of labor, rather than expectant management, after rupture of membranes at term (Duff, Sweet, and Edwards, 2009).

POSTTERM PREGNANCY, LABOR, AND BIRTH

A **postterm pregnancy** (also sometimes referred to as a *postdate* or *prolonged pregnancy*) is one that extends beyond the end of week 42 of gestation, or 294 days from the first day of the last menstrual period (LMP). The incidence of postterm pregnancy is estimated to be between 2% and 13%, depending on the population studied (Rampersad and Macones, 2012). Many pregnancies are misdiagnosed as prolonged. The use of first-trimester ultrasound for pregnancy dating has confirmed that the first day of the LMP, traditionally used for pregnancy dating, is much less reliable as a predictor of true gestational age. Therefore use of the LMP alone for pregnancy dating tends to greatly overestimate the number of postterm gestations (Rampersad and Macones, 2012; Resnik and Resnik, 2009).

The exact cause of true postterm pregnancy is still unknown. However, it is clear that the timing of labor is determined by complex interactions among the fetus, the placenta and membranes, the uterine myometrium, and the cervix. For example, congenital primary fetal adrenal hypoplasia and placental sulfatase deficiency cause low estrogen production. Low levels of estrogen may result in a decrease in prostaglandin precursors, thereby preventing normal cervical ripening, reducing the formation of oxytocin receptors in the myometrium, and delaying the onset of labor. Although postterm pregnancy is more common in primiparous women, a woman who experiences one postterm pregnancy is more likely to experience it again in subsequent pregnancies (Rampersad and Macones, 2012; Resnik and Resnik, 2009).

Clinical manifestations of postterm pregnancy include maternal weight loss (more than 3 lbs/wk) and decreased uterine size (related to decreased amniotic fluid), meconium in the amniotic fluid, and advanced bone maturation of the fetal skeleton with an exceptionally hard fetal skull (Gilbert, 2011).

Maternal and Fetal Risks

Maternal risks are often related to dysfunctional labor, such as increased risk for perineal injury related to fetal macrosomia. Risk for hemorrhage and infection is higher. Interventions such as induction of labor with prostaglandins or oxytocin, forceps- or vacuum-assisted birth, and cesarean birth are more likely to be necessary. Each of these interventions, of course, carries its own set of risks. The woman also may experience fatigue, physical discomfort, and psychologic reactions such as depression, frustration, and feelings of inadequacy as she passes her estimated date of birth. Relationships with close friends and family members may become strained, and the woman's negative feelings about herself may be projected as feelings of resentment toward the fetus (Gilbert, 2011).

Another complication associated with postterm pregnancy is abnormal fetal growth. Although the risk for having a small-for-gestational-age infant is increased, only 10% to 20% of postterm fetuses are undernourished. Macrosomia (birth weight more than 4000 g) occurs far more often. Macrosomia occurs when the placenta continues to provide adequate nutrients to support fetal growth after 40 weeks of gestation. Macrosomic infants have an increased risk for birth injuries caused by difficult forceps-assisted births and shoulder dystocia (Resnik and Resnik, 2009).

Other fetal risks associated with postterm gestation are related to the intrauterine environment. After 43 to 44 weeks of gestation, the placenta begins to age. Enlarging areas of infarction and increased deposition of calcium and fibrin in its tissue decrease the placenta's reserve and may affect its ability to oxygenate the fetus. Decreased amniotic fluid (less than 400 mL), oligohydramnios, is the complication most frequently associated with postterm pregnancy. Because of the decreased amount of amniotic fluid, there is a potential for cord compression and resulting hypoxemia (Gilbert, 2011). Other potential complications include meconium-stained amniotic fluid, increased chance of meconium aspiration, and low Apgar scores. Oligohydramnios magnifies the effect of meconium staining. Having less than the normal amount of amniotic fluid available to dilute it makes the meconium thicker and stickier than it would otherwise be (Resnik and Resnik, 2009).

Postmaturity syndrome occurs in about 20% of neonates born after postterm pregnancies. Postmaturity syndrome is characterized by dry, cracked, peeling skin; long nails; meconium staining of skin, nails, and umbilical cord; and perhaps loss of subcutaneous fat and muscle mass (Gilbert, 2011).

CARE MANAGEMENT

The management of postterm pregnancy is still controversial. However, because perinatal morbidity and mortality increase greatly after 42 weeks of gestation, pregnancies are usually not allowed to continue after this time. In the United States, most physicians induce labor at 41 weeks of gestation. An alternative approach is to initiate twice-weekly fetal testing at 41 weeks of gestation. The

---

testing generally consists of either a BPP or a NST along with an assessment of amniotic fluid volume (modified BPP) (see Chapter 10 for discussion of these tests). Evidence is insufficient to determine which of the two management approaches is better (Resnik and Resnik, 2009).

During the postterm period, the woman is encouraged to assess fetal activity daily, assess for signs of labor, and keep appointments with her primary health care provider (see Patient Teaching box). The woman and her family should be encouraged to express their feelings (e.g., frustration, anger, impatience, fear) about the prolonged pregnancy and helped to realize that these feelings are normal. At times, the emotional and physical strain of a postterm pregnancy may seem overwhelming. Referral to a support group or another supportive resource may be needed.

During labor, the fetus of a woman with a postterm pregnancy should be continuously monitored electronically for a more accurate assessment of the FHR and pattern. Inadequate fluid volume can lead to compression of the umbilical cord, which results in fetal hypoxia that is reflected in variable or prolonged deceleration patterns. If oligohydramnios is present, an amnioinfusion may be performed to restore amniotic fluid volume to maintain a cushioning of the cord. See Chapter 15 for additional information on amnioinfusion (see Evidence-Based Practice box).

DYSFUNCTIONAL LABOR (DYSTOCIA)

Dysfunctional labor (dystocia) is defined as a long, difficult, or abnormal labor caused by various conditions associated with the five factors affecting labor. It is estimated that dysfunctional labor occurs in approximately 8% to 11% of all births, and it is the most common indication for cesarean birth (Gilbert, 2011). Dysfunctional labor is responsible for approximately 60% of all primary cesarean births in the United States (Cunningham, Leveno, Bloom, et al., 2010). It can be caused by any of the following factors:

- Ineffective uterine contractions or maternal bearing-down efforts (the powers)
- Alterations in the pelvic structure (the passage)
- Fetal causes, including abnormal presentation or position, anomalies, excessive size, and number of fetuses (the passenger)
- Maternal position during labor and birth
- Psychologic responses of the mother to labor related to past experiences, preparation, culture and heritage, and support system

These five factors are interdependent. In assessing the woman for an abnormal labor pattern, the nurse must consider the ways in which these factors interact and influence labor progress. Dysfunctional labor is suspected when there is an alteration in the characteristics of uterine contractions, a lack of progress in the rate of cervical dilation, or a lack of progress in fetal descent and expulsion.

EVIDENCE-BASED PRACTICE

Amnioinfusion in Labor

Ask the Question

Is amnioinfusion a safe and effective intervention and/or treatment for certain complications of labor?

Search for the Evidence

Search Strategies

English research-based publications on amnioinfusion, labor, labour, meconium, oligohydramnios, rupture of membranes were included.

Databases Used

Cochrane Collaborative Database, National Guideline Clearinghouse (AHRQ), CINAHL, PubMed, UpToDate, and the professional website for AWHONN.

Critically Analyze the Evidence

- Oligohydramnios, or low amniotic fluid level, may occur as a result of ruptured membranes or fetal abnormality. Some fetuses show signs of distress, which may be caused by pressure on the umbilical cord leading to fetal hypoxia and acidosis. This stress may lead to fetal passing of meconium, increasing the risk for meconium aspiration and respiratory distress at birth.
- Amnioinfusion is the instillation of normal saline or lactated Ringer's solution into the uterus via the cervix or transabdominally to relieve the pressure on the fetus and cord. For potential or suspected cord compression, amnioinfusion is associated with fewer cesarean births, fewer 5-minute Apgar scores less than 7, less meconium below the vocal cords, less postpartum maternal endometritis, improved pH, and decreased hospital stay (Hofmeyr and Lawrie, 2012).
- The American College of Obstetricians and Gynecologists (ACOG) states that the highest level of evidence recommends amnioinfusion as a treatment for category III fetal heart rate (FHR) tracing of absent or minimal variability and recurrent variable decelerations (ACOG, 2010).
- Another possible benefit of amnioinfusion is the dilution of meconium. Amnioinfusion is associated with decreased cesarean birth, decreased meconium aspiration syndrome, less meconium below the vocal cords, reduced neonatal ventilation, fewer NICU admissions, and a trend toward lower perinatal mortality (Hofmeyr and Xu, 2010). It is not clear if the benefits are from the relief of oligohydramnios or dilution of meconium. Amnioinfusion is recommended for facilities where babies are at risk because of limited fetal monitoring.
- In the case of preterm premature rupture of membranes, four small trials show improved umbilical arterial pH, decreased persistent variable decelerations for transcervical amnioinfusion, and decreased perinatal death, decreased neonatal sepsis, and decreased pulmonary hypoplasia (small lungs) and less maternal sepsis with transabdominal amnioinfusion (Hofmeyr, Essilfie-Appiah, and Lawrie, 2011). However, the evidence is too small to recommend amnioinfusion routinely for this purpose.

Apply the Evidence: Nursing Implications

- In labor, it is usually the nurses who will be monitoring the electronic fetal heart rate and patterns. Category III FHR patterns include absent baseline variability plus recurrent late or recurrent variable decelerations,

bradycardia, or sinusoidal pattern, which require consultation with the medical team.
- A known rupture of membranes or oligohydramnios demonstrated by an ultrasound amniotic fluid index of less than 5 cm, plus FHR evidence of fetal distress, requires medical decision making regarding improving fetal well-being. An order for amnioinfusion may be one of the interventions. The nurse is often responsible for setting this up, as well as communicating with the patient and family.
- Other supportive nursing therapy that can increase uteroplacental oxygenation includes maternal repositioning, oxygen, and intravenous access for increasing fluids. Modifying or stopping oxytocin in the presence of fetal distress is also a nursing judgment.
- Any sign of meconium staining in amniotic fluid requires planning for specialized attention to the newborn at birth to prevent as much as possible the complications of meconium aspiration.

Quality and Safety Competencies: Evidence-Based Practice*

Knowledge

Describe Reliable Sources for Locating Evidence Reports and Clinical Practice Guidelines.

The nurse will understand the evidence-based clinical usefulness of amnioinfusion.

Skills

Locate Evidence Reports Related to Clinical Practice Topics and Guidelines.

The nurse can locate the highest-level evidence about ongoing research and evaluate its applicability.

Attitudes

Appreciate the Importance of Regularly Reading Relevant Professional Journals.

The nurse follows clinical recommendations as they are updated and strengthened with newer evidence.

References

American College of Obstetricians and Gynecologists (ACOG): *Management of intrapartum fetal heart rate tracings* (ACOG Practice Bulletin No. 16), 2010, National Guidelines Clearinghouse, NGC: 008177.

Hofmeyr GJ, Essilfie-Appiah G, Lawrie TA: Amnioinfusion for preterm premature rupture of membranes, *Cochrane Database Syst Rev* (12), 2011, Chichester, UK, John Wiley & Sons, DOI: 10.1002/14651858.CD000942.pub2.

Hofmeyr GJ, Lawrie TA: Amnioinfusion for potential or suspected umbilical cord compression in labor, *Cochrane Database Syst Rev* (1), 2012, Chichester, UK, John Wiley & Sons, DOI: 10.1002/14651858.CD000013.pub2.

Hofmeyr GJ, Xu H: Amnioinfusion for meconium-stained liquor in labour, *Cochrane Database Syst Rev* (1), 2010, Chichester, UK, John Wiley & Sons, DOI: 10.1002/14651858.CD000014.pub3.

Pat Mahaffee Gingrich

NICU, Neonatal intensive care unit.
*Adapted from QSEN at www.qsen.org/.

Gilbert (2011) cited several factors that seem to increase a woman's risk for dysfunctional labor including:

- Overweight
- Short stature
- Advanced maternal age
- Infertility difficulties
- Prior version
- Masculine characteristics
- Uterine abnormalities (e.g., congenital malformations; overdistention, as with multiple gestation; or polyhydramnios)

- Malpresentations and positions of the fetus
- Cephalopelvic disproportion (CPD) (or fetopelvic disproportion [FPD])
- Uterine overstimulation with oxytocin
- Maternal fatigue, dehydration and electrolyte imbalance, and fear
- Administration of an analgesic medication too early in labor or use of continuous epidural analgesia

Abnormal Uterine Activity

Abnormal uterine activity can be further described as being *hypertonic* or *hypotonic.*

Hypertonic Uterine Dysfunction

The woman experiencing hypertonic uterine dysfunction, or primary dysfunctional labor, often is an anxious first-time mother who is having painful and frequent contractions that are ineffective in causing cervical dilation or effacement to progress. These contractions usually occur in the latent phase of first-stage labor (cervical dilation of less than 4 cm) and are usually uncoordinated. The force of the contractions may be in the midsection of the uterus rather than in the fundus; therefore the uterus cannot apply downward pressure to push the presenting part against the cervix. The uterus may not relax completely between contractions.

Women with hypertonic uterine dysfunction may be exhausted and express concern about loss of control because of the intense pain they are experiencing and the lack of progress. Therapeutic rest (achieved with a warm bath or shower and the administration of an analgesic such as morphine, to inhibit uterine contractions, reduce pain, and encourage sleep) is usually prescribed to manage hypertonic uterine dysfunction. In the absence of pain, zolpidem (Ambien) may be used to facilitate rest and sleep. After a 4- to 6-hour rest, these women are likely to awaken in active labor with a normal uterine contraction pattern (Gilbert, 2011; Wing and Farinelli, 2012).

Hypotonic Uterine Dysfunction

The second and more common type of uterine dysfunction is hypotonic uterine dysfunction, or secondary uterine inertia. The woman initially makes normal progress into the active phase of first-stage labor, but then the contractions become weak and inefficient or stop altogether. The uterus is easily indented, even at the peak of contractions. Intrauterine pressure (IUP) during the contraction (usually less than 25 mm Hg) is insufficient for progress of cervical effacement and dilation. CPD and malposition are common causes of this type of uterine dysfunction.

A woman with hypotonic uterine dysfunction may become exhausted and be at increased risk for infection. Management usually consists of ruling out CPD and assessing the FHR and pattern, characteristics of the amniotic fluid if the membranes are ruptured, and maternal well-being. An intrauterine pressure catheter (IUPC) may be inserted to evaluate uterine activity accurately. If findings are normal, labor augmentation measures may be implemented (e.g., ambulation, hydrotherapy, rupture of membranes, nipple stimulation, oxytocin infusion).

Secondary Powers

Secondary powers, or bearing-down efforts, are compromised when large amounts of analgesic medications are given. Anesthesia may also block the bearing-down reflex and, as a result, alter the effectiveness of voluntary bearing-down efforts. Exhaustion resulting from lack of sleep or long labor and fatigue resulting from inadequate hydration and food intake reduce the effectiveness of the woman's voluntary bearing-down efforts. Maternal position can work against the forces of gravity and decrease the strength and efficiency of the contractions. Table 17-1 summarizes the characteristics of dysfunctional labor.

Abnormal Labor Patterns

Six abnormal labor patterns were identified and classified by Friedman (1989) according to the nature of the cervical dilation and fetal descent. These patterns are (1) prolonged latent phase, (2) protracted active-phase dilation, (3) secondary arrest: no change, (4) protracted descent, (5) arrest of descent, and (6) failure of descent. Table 17-2 further describes these abnormal labor patterns. These patterns may result from a variety of causes, including ineffective uterine contractions, pelvic contractures, CPD, abnormal fetal presentation or position, early use of analgesics, nerve block analgesia or anesthesia, and anxiety and stress. Progress in either the first or the second stage of labor can be protracted (prolonged) or arrested (stopped). Abnormal progress can be identified by plotting cervical dilation and fetal descent on a labor graph (partogram) at various intervals after the onset of labor and comparing the resulting curve with the expected labor curve for a nulliparous or multiparous labor. If a woman exhibits an abnormal labor pattern, the primary health care provider should be notified.

Maternal morbidity and mortality from uterine rupture, infection, severe dehydration, and postpartum hemorrhage are higher for women experiencing dysfunctional labor. The fetus is at increased risk for hypoxia. A long and difficult labor also can have an adverse psychologic effect on the mother, father, and family.

Precipitous Labor

Precipitous labor is defined as labor that lasts less than 3 hours from the onset of contractions to the time of birth. This abnormal labor pattern occurs in approximately 2% of all births in the United States. Precipitous birth alone is usually not associated with significant maternal or infant morbidity or mortality (Wing and Farinelli, 2012).

Precipitous labor may result from hypertonic uterine contractions that are tetanic in intensity. Conditions often associated with this type of uterine contractions include placental abruption, uterine tachysystole, and recent cocaine use (Wing and Farinelli, 2012). Maternal complications can include uterine rupture, lacerations of the birth canal, amniotic fluid embolus (anaphylactoid syndrome of pregnancy), and postpartum hemorrhage. Fetal complications include shoulder dystocia (Wing and Farinelli, 2012), hypoxia caused by decreased periods of uterine relaxation between contractions, and, in rare instances, intracranial trauma related to rapid birth (Cunningham, Leveno, Bloom, et al., 2010).

Women who have experienced precipitous labor often describe feelings of disbelief that their labor began so quickly, alarm that their labor progressed so rapidly, panic about the possibility they would not make it to the hospital in time to give birth, and finally, relief when they arrived at the hospital. In addition, women have expressed frustration when nurses did not believe them when they reported their readiness to push. Progress can be so rapid in some women that they may have difficulty remembering the details of their childbirth. They should be provided with an opportunity to discuss their labor and birth with caregivers who were present.

Alterations in Pelvic Structure
Pelvic Dystocia

Pelvic dystocia can occur whenever contractures of the pelvic diameters exist that reduce the capacity of the bony pelvis, including the

TABLE 17-1   DYSFUNCTIONAL LABOR: PRIMARY AND SECONDARY POWERS

PRIMARY POWERS (ABNORMAL UTERINE ACTIVITY)		SECONDARY POWERS
HYPERTONIC UTERINE DYSFUNCTION	**HYPOTONIC UTERINE DYSFUNCTION**	**INADEQUATE VOLUNTARY EXPULSIVE FORCES**
Description		
Usually occurs before 4 cm dilation; cause unknown, may be related to fear and tension	Cause is usually cephalopelvic disproportion or fetal malposition	Involves abdominal and levator ani muscles Occurs in second stage of labor; cause may be related to nerve block anesthetic, analgesia, exhaustion
Change in Pattern of Progress		
Pain out of proportion to intensity of contractions and to effectiveness of contractions in effacing and dilating the cervix Contractions increase in frequency and are uncoordinated Uterus is contracted between contractions, cannot be indented	Contractions decrease in frequency and intensity Uterus easily indented even at peak of contractions Uterus relaxed between contractions (normal)	No voluntary urge to push or bear down or inadequate or ineffective pushing
Potential Maternal Effects		
Loss of control related to intensity of pain and lack of progress Exhaustion Fear regarding unexpected nature of labor	Infection Exhaustion Stress regarding change in progress	Spontaneous vaginal birth prevented; assisted birth likely
Potential Fetal Effects		
Fetal asphyxia with meconium aspiration	Fetal infection Fetal and neonatal death	Fetal asphyxia
Care Management		
Initiate therapeutic rest measures Administer analgesic (e.g., morphine) if membranes are intact and pelvic adequacy is confirmed Relieve pain to permit mother to rest Assist with measures to enhance rest and relaxation (e.g., hydrotherapy, massage, music, distracting activities)	Rule out cephalopelvic disproportion Augment labor with oxytocin (Pitocin) Perform amniotomy Assist with measures to enhance the progress of labor (e.g., position changes, ambulation, hydrotherapy)	Coach mother in bearing down with contractions; assist with relaxation between contractions Position mother in favorable position for pushing Reduce epidural infusion rate Assist with forceps- or vacuum-assisted birth Prepare for cesarean birth if abnormal fetal status occurs

TABLE 17-2   ABNORMAL LABOR PATTERNS

PATTERN	NULLIPARAS	MULTIPARAS
Prolonged latent phase	>20 hr	>14 hr
Protracted active phase dilation	<1.2 cm/hr	<1.5 cm/hr
Secondary arrest: no change	≥2 hr	≥2 hr
Protracted descent	<1 cm/hr	<2 cm/hr
Arrest of descent	≥1 hr	≥½ hr
Failure of descent	No change during deceleration phase and second stage	
Precipitous labor	>5 cm/hr	10 cm/hr

inlet, the midpelvis, the outlet, or any combination of these planes. Pelvic contractures may be caused by congenital abnormalities, maternal malnutrition, neoplasms, or lower spinal disorders. An immature pelvic size predisposes some adolescent mothers to pelvic dystocia. Pelvic deformities also may be the result of automobile or other accidents or trauma.

Soft-Tissue Dystocia

Soft-tissue dystocia results from obstruction of the birth passage by an anatomic abnormality other than that involving the bony pelvis. The obstruction may result from placenta previa (low-lying placenta) that partially or completely obstructs the internal cervical os. Other causes, such as leiomyomas (uterine fibroids) in the lower uterine segment, ovarian tumors, and a full bladder or rectum, may prevent the fetus from entering the pelvis. Occasionally cervical edema occurs during labor when the cervix is caught between the presenting part and the symphysis pubis or when the woman begins bearing-down efforts prematurely, thereby inhibiting complete dilation. Sexually transmitted infections (e.g., human papillomavirus) can alter cervical tissue integrity and thus interfere with adequate effacement and dilation.

Fetal Causes

Dystocia of fetal origin may be caused by anomalies, excessive fetal size (macrosomia), malpresentation, malposition, or multifetal pregnancy. Complications associated with dystocia of fetal origin include neonatal asphyxia, fetal injuries or fractures, and maternal vaginal lacerations. Although spontaneous vaginal birth is possible in these instances, a forceps-assisted, vacuum-assisted, or cesarean birth often is necessary.

Anomalies

Gross ascites, large tumors, open neural tube defects (e.g., myelo-meningocele), and hydrocephalus are examples of fetal anomalies that can cause dystocia. The anomalies affect the relationship of the fetal anatomy to the maternal pelvic capacity, with the result that the fetus cannot descend through the birth canal.

Cephalopelvic Disproportion

Cephalopelvic disproportion (CPD), also called *fetopelvic disproportion (FPD)*, is disproportion between the size of the fetus and the size of the mother's pelvis. With CPD, the fetus cannot fit through the maternal pelvis to be born vaginally. Although CPD is often related to excessive fetal size, or macrosomia (i.e., 4000 g or more), the problem in many cases is malposition of the fetal presenting part rather than true CPD (Wing and Farinelli, 2012). Fetal macrosomia is associated with maternal diabetes mellitus, obesity, multiparity, or the large size of one or both parents. If the maternal pelvis is too small, abnormally shaped, or deformed, CPD may be of maternal origin. In this case, the fetus may be of average size or even smaller. CPD cannot be accurately predicted (Wing and Farinelli, 2012).

Malposition

The most common fetal malposition is persistent occipitoposterior position (i.e., right occipitoposterior [ROP] or left occipitoposterior [LOP]; see Chapter 13), occurring in approximately 15% of all labors during the latent phase of the first stage of labor. About 5% of all fetuses are in this position at birth (Gilbert, 2011). Labor, especially the second stage, is prolonged. The woman typically complains of severe back pain from the pressure of the fetal head (occiput) pressing against her sacrum. See Box 16-11 for suggested positions to relieve back pain and encourage rotation of the fetal occiput to an anterior position, which will facilitate birth.

Malpresentation

Malpresentation (the fetal presentation is something other than cephalic or head first) is another commonly reported complication of labor and birth. Breech presentation is the most common form of malpresentation, occurring in 3% to 4% of all labors (Lanni and Seeds, 2012). The three types of breech presentation are (Gilbert, 2011) (Fig. 17-3):
- Frank breech (hips flexed, knees extended)
- Complete breech (hips and knees flexed)
- Footling breech (when one foot [single footling] or both feet [double footling] present before the buttocks)

Breech presentations are associated with multifetal gestation, preterm birth, fetal and maternal anomalies, hydramnios, and oligohydramnios. High rates of breech presentation are also noted in fetuses with certain genetic disorders (e.g., trisomies 13, 18, and 21; Potter's syndrome [renal agenesis]; and myotonic dystrophy). Fetuses with neuromuscular disorders have a high rate of breech presentation, perhaps because they are less capable of movement within the uterus. Abnormal amniotic fluid volume (both increased and decreased) also contributes to more breech presentations

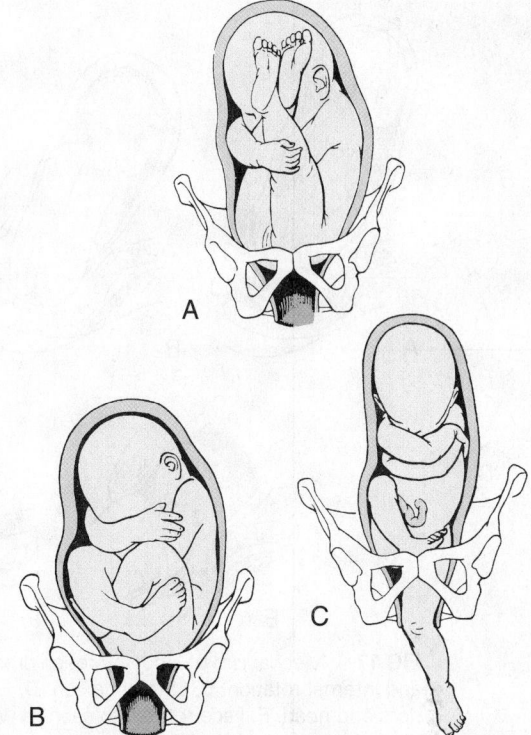

FIG 17-3 Breech presentation. **A,** Frank breech. **B,** Complete breech. **C,** Single footling breech. (From Gilbert E: *Manual of high risk pregnancy & delivery*, ed 5, St Louis, 2011, Mosby.

because it affects fetal mobility. Breech presentation is diagnosed by abdominal palpation (e.g., Leopold maneuvers) and vaginal examination and usually confirmed by ultrasound scan (Lanni and Seeds, 2012; Thorp, 2009).

During labor, the descent of the fetus in a breech presentation may be slow because the breech is not as effective a dilating wedge as is the fetal head. There is risk for prolapse of the cord if the membranes rupture in early labor. The presence of meconium in amniotic fluid is not necessarily a sign of fetal distress because it results from pressure on the fetal abdominal wall as it traverses the birth canal. Assessment of FHR and pattern should be used to determine whether the passage of meconium is an expected finding associated with breech presentation or is an abnormal sign associated with fetal hypoxia. The heart tones of fetuses (fetal heart tones [FHTs]) in a breech position are best heard at or above the umbilicus.

Vaginal birth is accomplished by mechanisms of labor that manipulate the buttocks and lower extremities as they emerge from the birth canal (Fig. 17-4). Risks associated with vaginal birth from a breech presentation include prolapse of the umbilical cord (especially in single or double footling breech presentations) and trapping of the after-coming fetal head (especially with preterm infants). Safe vaginal birth from a breech presentation largely depends on the experience, judgment, and skill of the health care provider who assists the birth. Criteria for attempting a vaginal birth from a breech presentation are (Thorp, 2009):
- Frank or complete breech presentation
- Estimated fetal weight between 2000 and 3800 g
- Normal (gynecoid) maternal pelvis
- Flexed fetal head

External cephalic version (ECV) (see later discussion) may be tried to turn the fetus to a vertex presentation. If the attempt at ECV is unsuccessful, the woman usually gives birth by cesarean (Gilbert, 2011).

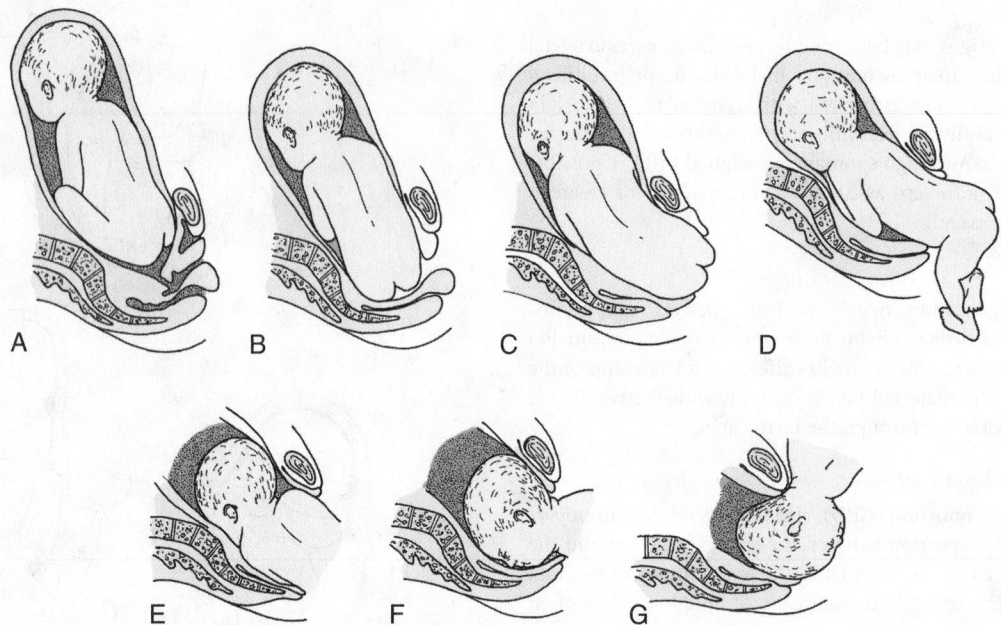

FIG 17-4 Mechanism of labor in breech presentation. **A,** Breech before onset of labor. **B,** Engagement and internal rotation. **C,** Lateral flexion. **D,** External rotation or restitution. **E,** Internal rotation of shoulders and head. **F,** Face rotates to sacrum when occiput is anterior. **G,** Head is born by gradual flexion during elevation of fetal body.

Face and brow presentations are uncommon and are associated with fetal anomalies, pelvic contractures, and CPD. Spontaneous vaginal birth is possible if the fetus flexes to a vertex presentation, although forceps often are used. Cesarean birth is indicated if the presentation persists, if fetal distress occurs, or if labor stops progressing.

Cesarean birth is usually necessary for a fetus in a transverse lie (i.e., shoulder) presentation, although ECV may be attempted after 36 to 37 weeks of gestation (Thorp, 2009).

Multifetal Pregnancy

Multifetal pregnancy is the gestation of twins, triplets, quadruplets, or more infants. Multiple gestations now account for more than 3% of all live births in the United States (Malone and D'Alton, 2009). The increasing number of twin gestations has been attributed to the use of fertility-enhancing medications and procedures and the older age of childbearing women. When compared with younger women, those ages 35 years and older are naturally more likely to have a multifetal pregnancy. The rate of triplet and higher-order multiple pregnancies has been steadily declining since the all-time high rate of 193.5 per 100,000 in 1998. This decrease has been attributed to refinements in the treatments used for infertility, particularly limiting the number of embryos transferred during in vitro fertilization (IVF) procedures (Malone and D'Alton, 2009; Newman and Unal, 2012).

Multiple births are associated with more complications (e.g., dysfunctional labor) than single births. The higher incidence of fetal and newborn complications and higher risk for perinatal mortality stem primarily from the birth of low-birth-weight infants resulting from preterm birth or IUGR (or both), in part related to placental dysfunction and twin-to-twin transfusion. Fetuses can experience distress and asphyxia during the birth process as a result of cord prolapse and the onset of placental separation with the birth of the first fetus. As a result, the risk for long-term problems such as cerebral palsy is higher among infants who were part of a multiple birth.

In addition, fetal complications such as congenital anomalies and abnormal presentations can result in dysfunctional labor and an increased incidence of cesarean birth. For example, in only 40% to 45% of all twin pregnancies do both fetuses present in the vertex position, the most favorable for vaginal birth. In 35% to 40% of the pregnancies, one twin may present in the vertex position and the other in a breech or transverse lie presentation (Malone and D'Alton, 2009).

The health status of the mother may be compromised by an increased risk for hypertension, anemia, and hemorrhage associated with uterine atony, placental abruption, and multiple or adherent placentas. Duration of the phases and stages of labor may vary from the duration experienced with singleton births.

Teamwork and planning are essential components of the management of childbirth in multiple pregnancies, especially those of higher-order multiples. The nurse plays a key role in coordinating the activities of many highly skilled health care professionals. Early detection and management of the maternal, fetal, and newborn complications associated with multiple births are essential to achieve a positive outcome for mother and babies. Maternal positioning and active support are used to enhance labor progress and placental perfusion. Stimulation of labor with oxytocin, epidural anesthesia, internal or external version, and forceps and vacuum assistance may be used to accomplish the vaginal birth of twins. Cesarean birth is almost always performed with higher-order multiple births. Each infant will have its own team of health care providers present at the birth. Emotional support that includes expression of feelings and full explanations of events as they occur and of the status of the mother and the fetuses and newborns is important to reduce the anxiety and stress the mother and her family experience.

Position of the Woman

The functional relationship among the uterine contractions, the fetus, and the mother's pelvis are altered by the maternal position. In addition, the position can provide a mechanical advantage or disadvantage to the mechanisms of labor by altering the effects of gravity and the body-part relationships that are important to the progress of labor. See Box 16-11 for suggested positions to enhance fetal descent.

Discouraging maternal movement or restricting labor to the recumbent or lithotomy position may compromise progress. The incidence of dysfunctional labor in women confined to these positions is increased, resulting in a greater need for augmentation of labor or forceps-assisted, vacuum-assisted, or cesarean birth.

Psychologic Responses

Hormones and neurotransmitters released in response to stress (e.g., catecholamines) can cause dysfunctional labor. Sources of stress vary for each woman, but pain and the absence of a support person are two factors often related to dysfunctional labor. Confinement to bed and restriction of maternal movement can be a source of psychologic stress that compounds the physiologic stress caused by immobility in the unmedicated laboring woman. When anxiety is excessive, it can inhibit cervical dilation and result in prolonged labor and increased pain perception. Anxiety also causes increased levels of stress-related hormones (e.g., beta-endorphin, adrenocorticotropic hormone, cortisol, and epinephrine). These hormones act on the smooth muscles of the uterus. Increased levels can cause dysfunctional labor by reducing uterine contractility.

Management

Risk assessment is a continuous process in the laboring woman. By reviewing the woman's past labor or labors and observing her physical and psychologic responses to the current labor, any factors that might contribute to dysfunctional labor should be identified. Nursing diagnoses, expected outcomes of care, and interventions are then established for each woman based on assessment findings. Many interventions for dysfunctional labor (e.g., ECV, cervical ripening, induction or augmentation of labor, and operative procedures [forceps- or vacuum-assisted birth, cesarean birth]) are implemented collaboratively with other members of the health care team. Commonly performed interventions are discussed in detail in the Obstetric Procedures section.

When providing care for a woman who is experiencing labor or birth complications, all members of the health care team are responsible for complying with professional standards of care.

LEGAL TIP: Standard of Care—Labor and Birth Complications
- Document all assessment findings, interventions, and the woman's responses in the medical record according to unit protocols, procedures, and policies and professional standards.
- Assess whether the woman (and her family, if appropriate) is fully informed about the procedures for which she is consenting.
- Provide full explanations regarding what is happening and what needs to be done to help her and her baby.
- Maintain safety in administering medications and treatments correctly.
- Have telephone orders signed as soon as possible.
- Provide care at the acceptable standard (e.g., according to unit protocols and professional standards).
- If short staffing occurs in the unit and the nurse is assigned additional patients, the nurse should document that rejecting this additional assignment would have placed these patients in danger as a result of abandonment.
- Continue maternal and fetal monitoring until birth according to the policies, procedures, and protocols of the birthing facility, even after a decision to carry out cesarean birth is made.

OBESITY

Excessive weight is an increasingly serious problem for children, adolescents, and adults living in affluent nations, including the United States, and pregnant women are no exception. The body mass index (BMI) is used to define obesity. Persons with a BMI of 25 or greater kg/m^2 are categorized as overweight, whereas those with a BMI of 30 or greater kg/m^2 are considered obese. Individuals with a BMI of 40 kg/m^2 or greater are classified as severely obese (Picklesimer and Dorman, 2013).

Obese women are likely to begin pregnancy with pre-existing medical conditions such as chronic hypertension and type 2 diabetes. While pregnant, they may develop pregnancy-associated hypertensive disorders or gestational diabetes may be diagnosed. Obese women also have an increased incidence of postdates pregnancy. All of these risk factors make them more likely to undergo labor induction (Picklesimer and Dorman, 2013). In addition to an increased risk for cesarean birth in general, obese women are also more likely to require emergency cesarean birth. As the woman's BMI increases, the risk for developing these complications also rises (Cunningham, Leveno, Bloom, et al., 2010; Walters and Taylor, 2009/2010). During the postpartum period, obese women are at risk for thromboembolism and wound disruption and infection after cesarean birth (Picklesimer and Dorman, 2013).

CARE MANAGEMENT

Nursing care of obese women during labor and birth is challenging for a number of reasons. Sometimes standard furniture such as beds, chairs, and operating tables is simply not large enough to accommodate the woman's size. Extra-large furniture may not fit through a standard doorway, so room renovation may be necessary. Some hospitals have created rooms specifically designed to accommodate obese patients (Fig. 17-5). Continuous external FHR and contraction monitoring may be extremely difficult if not impossible to perform. Special equipment, such as extra-large blood pressure cuffs, is necessary to properly assess the woman's condition.

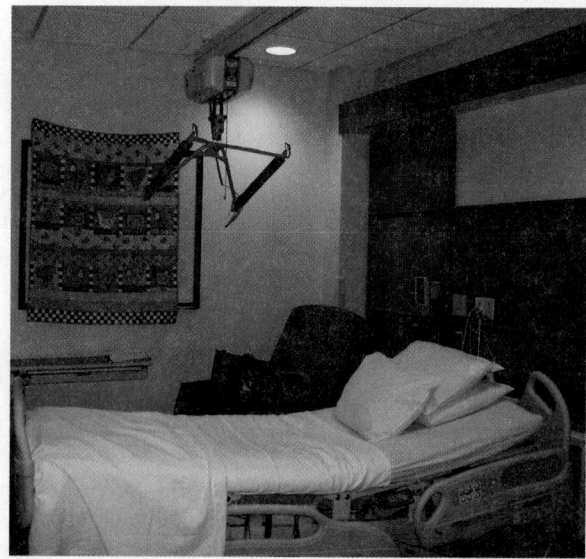

FIG 17-5 Room specifically designed to accommodate obese pregnant patients. Note lift attached to ceiling for use in transferring women from the bed to chairs or stretchers. (Courtesy Dee Lowdermilk, Chapel Hill, NC.)

Even routine procedures will require more time and effort to accomplish when a woman is obese. This is extremely worrisome, given that obesity is a risk factor for emergency cesarean birth when time is often of the essence. Establishing intravenous access, for example, may require multiple attempts, sometimes by multiple persons. Mobility is often a problem. Moving the woman from a labor room to the operating room and transferring her from a bed to the operating table may require the assistance of additional personnel or special equipment, especially if regional anesthesia is already in effect. If it is not, surgery may be further delayed by anesthetic complications, such as difficulty establishing an epidural or spinal block or accomplishing endotracheal intubation.

Postoperatively, obese women are at increased risk for blood clot formation. In the immediate recovery period, use of thromboembolic deterrent anti-embolism stockings (TED hose) and sequential compression devices (SCD boots) help decrease the chance for clot formation. Some women may also be given heparin prophylactically for clot prevention (Cunningham, Leveno, Bloom, et al., 2010). Women should also be encouraged to get out of bed and begin ambulating as soon as possible.

Keeping the incision clean and dry to prevent wound infection and promote healing is another postoperative challenge. Many obese women have a *pannus* (large roll of abdominal fat) that overlies a lower abdominal transverse skin incision made just above the pubic area. The pannus causes the area to remain moist, which encourages infection development. Women should be taught to wash the incision with soap and water several times a day, thoroughly drying the area afterward. Using a handheld hair dryer on a low setting works well for this purpose. Sutures or staples used to close the skin incision are generally left in place longer than usual to avoid possible wound disruption when they are removed. Sometimes the skin and subcutaneous layers of the incision are left open to heal by secondary intention to avoid possible dehiscence. If this course of action is chosen, the woman and other family members must be taught to do dressing changes and wound care.

OBSTETRIC PROCEDURES

Version

Version is the turning of the fetus from one presentation to another. It may be performed externally or internally by the physician.

External Cephalic Version

External cephalic version (ECV) is used in an attempt to turn the fetus from a breech or shoulder presentation to a vertex presentation for birth. It may be attempted in a labor and birth setting after 37 weeks of gestation. ECV is accomplished by the exertion of gentle, constant pressure on the abdomen (Fig. 17-6). Before ECV is attempted, ultrasound scanning is done to:

- Determine the fetal position
- Locate the umbilical cord
- Rule out placenta previa
- Evaluate the adequacy of the maternal pelvis
- Assess the amount of amniotic fluid, the gestational age, and the presence of any anomalies

An NST is performed to confirm fetal well-being, or the FHR and pattern are monitored for a period of time (i.e., 10 to 20 minutes). Informed consent is obtained. A tocolytic agent such as terbutaline often is given to relax the uterus and facilitate the maneuver. ECV is sometimes performed under regional anesthesia (Lanni and Seeds, 2012; Thorp, 2009). Contraindications to ECV include (Thorp, 2009):

- Uterine anomalies
- Third-trimester bleeding
- Multiple gestation
- Oligohydramnios
- Evidence of uteroplacental insufficiency
- A nuchal cord (identified by ultrasound)
- Previous cesarean birth or other significant uterine surgery
- Obvious CPD

ECV is most successful in a multiparous woman who has a normal amount of amniotic fluid and whose fetus is not yet engaged in the pelvis (Cunningham, Leveno, Bloom, et al., 2010). If ECV is not successful, the American College of Obstetricians and Gynecologists (ACOG) recommends that the woman undergo planned cesarean birth (Thorp, 2009).

During an attempted ECV, the nurse continuously monitors the FHR and pattern, especially for bradycardia and variable decelerations; checks the maternal vital signs; and assesses the woman's level of comfort because the procedure may cause discomfort. After the procedure is completed, the nurse continues to monitor maternal vital signs and uterine activity and to assess for vaginal bleeding until the woman's condition is determined to be stable. FHR and pattern monitoring should continue for at least 1 hour. Women who are Rh negative should receive Rh immune globulin because the manipulation can cause fetomaternal bleeding (Thorp, 2009).

Internal Version

With internal version, the fetus is turned by the physician, who inserts a hand into the uterus and changes the presentation to cephalic (head) or podalic (foot). Internal version is rarely used, most often in twin gestations to assist with the birth of the second fetus. The safety of this procedure has not been documented; maternal and fetal injury are possible. Cesarean birth is the usual method for managing malpresentation in multifetal pregnancies. The nurse's role is to monitor the status of the fetus and to provide support to the woman.

Induction of Labor

Induction of labor is the chemical or mechanical initiation of uterine contractions before their spontaneous onset for the purpose of bringing about birth. Labor may be induced either electively or for indicated reasons. Induction of labor is one of the most commonly performed obstetrical procedures in the United States. Approximately 24% of term births (infants born between 37 and 41 weeks of gestation) result from labors that were induced (Hill and Harvey, 2013). The rate of labor induction for all births more than

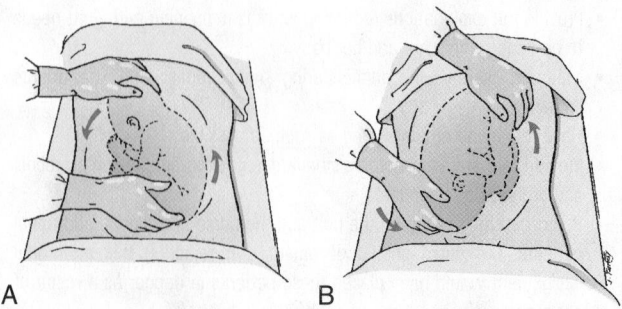

FIG 17-6 External version of fetus from breech to vertex presentation. This must be achieved without force. **A,** Breech is pushed up out of pelvic inlet while head is pulled toward inlet. **B,** Head is pushed toward inlet while breech is pulled upward.

doubled between 1990 and 2010, reaching a rate of 23.4% in 2010 (Martin, Hamilton, Sutton, et al., 2012). It is likely that the rate of elective inductions is increasing more rapidly than the rate of indicated inductions. Also, there is concern that elective inductions may increase the risk for cesarean birth especially among primigravid women and particularly those older than 35 years (Martin, Hamilton, Sutton, et al., 2012; Thorp, 2009; Wing and Farinelli, 2012).

Induction of labor is indicated if continuing the pregnancy could be dangerous for either the woman or the fetus and if no contraindications exist to artificial rupture of the membranes (amniotomy) or augmenting uterine contractions with oxytocin. Before labor induction, gestational age should be determined and any potential risks to mother or fetus evaluated. Women must be fully counseled regarding risks, benefits, and alternatives of labor stimulation methods as part of the process for informed consent (ACOG, 2009; Thorp, 2009). Box 17-8 lists indications and contraindications for labor induction.

Elective Induction of Labor

An elective induction is one in which labor is initiated without a medical indication. Methods to ripen the cervix (e.g., application of

---

BOX 17-8   INDICATIONS AND CONTRAINDICATIONS FOR LABOR INDUCTION

Indications
- Hypertensive complications of pregnancy: gestational hypertension, preeclampsia, eclampsia
- Fetal death
- Chorioamnionitis
- Maternal medical conditions: diabetes mellitus, renal disease, cardiopulmonary conditions, chronic hypertension, antiphospholipid syndrome
- Postterm pregnancy, especially when oligohydramnios is present
- Fetal compromise: intrauterine growth restriction, isoimmunization
- Premature rupture of membranes with established fetal maturity

Contraindications
- Acute, severe fetal distress
- Shoulder presentation (transverse lie)
- Floating fetal presenting part
- Uncontrolled hemorrhage
- Umbilical cord prolapse
- Active genital herpes infection
- Placenta previa
- Previous uterine incision that prohibits a trial of labor

Relative Contraindications
- Grand multiparity (≥5 pregnancies that ended after 20 weeks of gestation)
- Multiple gestation
- Suspected cephalopelvic disproportion
- Breech presentations
- Inability to adequately monitor fetal heart rate (FHR) or contractions (or both) throughout labor

Data from American College of Obstetricians and Gynecologists (ACOG): *Induction of labor* (ACOG Practice Bulletin No. 107), Washington, DC, 2009, Author; Thorp JM: Clinical aspects of normal and abnormal labor. In Creasy R, Resnik R, Iams J, et al, editors: *Creasy and Resnik's maternal-fetal medicine: principles and practice,* ed 6, Philadelphia, 2009, Saunders.

---

prostaglandins or intracervical insertion of a balloon catheter) enhance the likelihood of successful induction. Therefore they have been a factor in the use of elective induction as an option for managing childbirth rather than waiting for labor to begin spontaneously. Many of these elective inductions are purely for the convenience of the woman or her primary health care provider. At times, however, labor may be electively induced to allay maternal fears and anxieties associated with prior perinatal losses or to ensure that experienced multispecialty personnel are available to handle anticipated maternal or neonatal complications immediately after birth (Moleti, 2009; Wing and Farinelli, 2012).

The major risks associated with elective labor induction at term are increased rates of cesarean birth, neonatal morbidity, and cost (Wing and Farinelli; 2012). ACOG and the American Academy of Pediatrics (AAP) have for many years recommended that elective induction of labor not be initiated until the woman reaches 39 weeks or more of gestation (Simpson, 2011). Both the National Quality Forum and The Joint Commission have also developed perinatal quality measures to monitor appropriate gestational age for elective birth (Simpson, 2011). The March of Dimes and the Association of Women's Health, Obstetric and Neonatal Nurses (AWHONN) have created informational campaigns to educate pregnant women and their families about the dangers of early term births (visit their websites at www.gothefull40.com and www.marchofdimes.com/pregnancy/getready_atleast39weeks.html) (Craighead, 2012). Birth data from the United States for 2010, the most recent data available, indicate that births at 37 to 38 weeks of gestation have declined, while births at 39 weeks of gestation or more are increasing (Martin, Hamilton, Sutton, et al., 2012) (see Community Focus box).

Chemical, mechanical, physical, and alternative methods are used to ripen the cervix and induce labor. Intravenous oxytocin (Pitocin) and amniotomy are the most common methods used in the United States. Success rates for induction of labor are higher when the condition of the cervix is favorable, or inducible. Cervical ripeness is the most important predictor of successful induction. A rating system such as the Bishop score (Table 17-3) can be used to evaluate inducibility. For example, a score of 8 or more on this 13-point scale indicates that the cervix is soft, anterior, 50% or more effaced, and dilated 2 cm or more and that the presenting part is engaged. When the Bishop score totals 8 or more, induction of labor is usually successful (ACOG, 2009; Gilbert, 2011; Moleti, 2009). The Bishop score should be documented before the use of methods to ripen the cervix or induce labor.

Cervical Ripening Methods

Chemical Agents. Preparations of prostaglandins E_1 (PGE_1) and E_2 (PGE_2) have been shown to be effective when used before induction to "ripen" (soften and thin) the cervix (see Medication Guides on pp. 462 and 463) (Hill and Harvey, 2013). In some cases, women

---

🏠 COMMUNITY FOCUS

Elective Induction of Labor

Visit the March of Dimes website (www.marchofdimes.com) and download patient teaching materials regarding the importance of avoiding an elective early term birth by waiting until at least 39 weeks of gestation for labor induction. Then talk with a woman who is 36 to 38 weeks pregnant. Ask if she wants to have her labor induced immediately. If so, what are her reasons? Share the information you obtained from the March of Dimes website with her. Were you able to change her mind?

MEDICATION GUIDE

Prostaglandin E₁ (PGE₁): Misoprostol (Cytotec)

Action
- PGE₁ ripens the cervix, making it softer and causing it to begin to dilate and efface; it stimulates uterine contractions.

Indications
- PGE₁ is used for preinduction cervical ripening (ripen the cervix before oxytocin induction of labor when the Bishop score is 4 or less) and for inducement of labor or abortion (abortifacient agent); it has not yet been approved by the FDA for cervical ripening or labor induction (i.e., this is an unlabeled use for obstetrics).
- It should not be used if the woman has a history of previous cesarean birth or other major uterine surgery.

Dosage and Administration
- Misoprostol is available either as a 100-mcg or a 200-mcg tablet. Therefore tablets must be broken to prepare the correct dose. This preparation should take place in the pharmacy to ensure accurate doses.
- Recommended initial dose is 25 mcg. Insert intravaginally into the posterior vaginal fornix using the tips of index and middle fingers without the use of a lubricant. Repeat every 3 to 6 hours up to 6 doses in a 24-hour period or until an effective contraction pattern is established (three or more uterine contractions in 10 minutes), the cervix ripens (Bishop score of 8 or greater), or significant adverse effects occur.

Adverse Effects
- Higher doses (e.g., 50 mcg every 6 hours) are more likely to result in adverse reactions such as nausea and vomiting, diarrhea, fever, uterine tachysystole with or without an abnormal FHR and pattern, or fetal passage of meconium. The risk for adverse reactions is reduced with lower dosages and longer intervals between doses.

Nursing Considerations
- Explain the procedure to the woman and her family; ensure that an informed consent has been obtained as per agency policy.
- Assess the woman and fetus before each insertion and during treatment following agency protocol for frequency. Assess maternal vital signs and health status, FHR and pattern, and status of pregnancy, including indications for cervical ripening or induction of labor, signs of labor or impending labor, and the Bishop score. Recognize that an abnormal FHR and pattern; maternal fever, infection, vaginal bleeding, or hypersensitivity; and regular, progressive uterine contractions contraindicate the use of misoprostol.
- Avoid giving aluminum hydroxide and magnesium-containing antacids along with misoprostol.
- Use with caution in women with renal failure because the medication is eliminated through the kidneys.
- Have the woman void before insertion.
- Assist the woman to maintain a supine position with a lateral tilt or a side-lying position for 30 to 40 minutes after insertion.
- Prepare to (1) swab the vagina to remove unabsorbed medication using a saline-soaked gauze wrapped around fingers or (2) administer terbutaline 0.25 mg subcutaneously if significant adverse effects occur.
- Initiate oxytocin for induction of labor no sooner than 4 hours after the last dose of misoprostol was administered, following agency protocol, if ripening has occurred and labor has not begun.
- Document all assessment findings and administration procedures.

Data from Hill W, Harvey C: Induction of labor. In Troiano N, Harvey C, Chez B, editors: *AWHONN's high risk & critical care obstetrics*, ed 3, Philadelphia, 2013, Wolters Kluwer/Lippincott Williams & Wilkins; Moleti C: Trends and controversies in labor induction, *MCN Am J Matern Child Nurs* 34(1):40–47, 2009; Thorp JM: Clinical aspects of normal and abnormal labor. In Creasy R, Resnik R, Iams J, et al, editors: *Creasy and Resnik's maternal-fetal medicine: principles and practice*, ed 6, Philadelphia, 2009, Saunders.
FDA, Food and Drug Administration; *FHR*, fetal heart rate.

TABLE 17-3   BISHOP SCORE

	SCORE			
	0	**1**	**2**	**3**
Dilation (cm)	0	1-2	3-4	≥5
Effacement (%)	0-30	40-50	60-70	≥80
Station (cm)	−3	−2	−1, 0	+1, +2
Cervical consistency	Firm	Medium	Soft	Soft
Cervical position	Posterior	Midposition	Anterior	Anterior

spontaneously begin laboring after the administration of prostaglandin, thereby eliminating the need to administer oxytocin to induce labor. Additional advantages of prostaglandin use for cervical ripening include decreased oxytocin induction time and a decrease in the amount of oxytocin required for successful induction (Gilbert, 2011). PGE₁, although much less expensive and more effective than PGE₂ for inducing labor and birth, is associated with a higher risk for uterine tachysystole with abnormal fetal heart rate and pattern changes and passage of meconium into the aminotic fluid. Most of these adverse outcomes are associated with higher dose protocols

(ACOG, 2009; Wing and Farinelli, 2012). Although the drug's manufacturer has acknowledged for several years that PGE₁ is effective for cervical ripening and labor induction, it has not yet been approved by the Food and Drug Administration (FDA) for these uses (Thorp, 2009). PGE₂ in the form of a vaginal insert (dinoprostone [Cervidil]), although more expensive than PGE₁, has the major advantage of easy removal should adverse reactions, including uterine tachysystole, occur (Moleti, 2009).

Mechanical and Physical Methods. Mechanical dilators ripen the cervix by stimulating the release of endogenous prostaglandins. Balloon catheters (e.g., Foley catheter) can be inserted through the intracervical canal to ripen and dilate the cervix. The catheter balloon is inflated above the internal cervical os with 30 to 50 mL of sterile water. This process results in pressure and stretching of the lower uterine segment and the cervix, as well as the release of endogenous prostaglandins. It is especially helpful for women who cannot receive exogenous prostaglandins for cervical ripening. The balloon will fall out when cervical dilation reaches approximately 3 cm in about 8 to 12 hours after it is inserted. Evidence supports the insertion of a balloon catheter as a cervical ripening method because of its low cost compared with prostaglandins, stability at room temperature, and reduced risk for uterine tachysystole with or without fetal heart rate changes (ACOG, 2009; Hill and Harvey, 2013; Simpson, 2008).

MEDICATION GUIDE

Prostaglandin E₂ (PGE₂): Dinoprostone (Cervidil Insert; Prepidil Gel)

Action

- PGE₂ ripens the cervix, making it softer and causing it to begin to dilate and efface; it stimulates uterine contractions. Dinoprostone is the only FDA-approved medication for cervical ripening or labor induction.

Indications

- PGE₂ is used for preinduction cervical ripening (ripen the cervix before oxytocin induction of labor when the Bishop score is 4 or less) and for inducement of labor or abortion (abortifacient agent).
- It is not recommended for use if the woman has a history of previous cesarean birth or other major uterine surgery.

Dosage and Route

Cervidil Insert:

- Dosage is 10 mg of dinoprostone designed to be gradually released (approximately 0.3 mg/hr) over 12 hours. Insert is placed transvaginally into the posterior fornix of the vagina. The insert is removed after 12 hours or at the onset of active labor or earlier if tachysystole or abnormal FHR and patterns occur.

Prepidil Gel:

- Dosage is 0.5 mg of dinoprostone in a 2.5-mL syringe. Gel is administered through a catheter attached to the syringe into the cervical canal just below the internal cervical os. Dose may be repeated every 6 hours as needed for cervical ripening up to a maximum cumulative dose of 1.5 mg (3 doses) in a 24-hour period.

Adverse Effects

- Potential adverse effects include headache, nausea and vomiting, diarrhea, fever, hypotension, uterine tachysystole with or without an abnormal FHR and pattern, or fetal passage of meconium.

Nursing Considerations

- Explain the procedure to the woman and her family. Ensure that an informed consent has been obtained as per agency policy.

- Assess the woman and fetus before each insertion and during treatment following agency protocol for frequency. Assess maternal vital signs and health status, FHR and pattern, and status of pregnancy, including indications for cervical ripening or induction of labor, signs of labor or impending labor, and the Bishop score. Recognize that an abnormal FHR and pattern; maternal fever, infection, vaginal bleeding, or hypersensitivity; and regular, progressive uterine contractions contraindicate the use of dinoprostone.
- Avoid use in women with asthma, glaucoma, and hypotension or hypertension.
- Use with caution if the woman has cardiac, renal, or hepatic disease, anemia, jaundice, diabetes, epilepsy, or genitourinary (GU) infections.
- Bring the gel to room temperature just before administration. Do not force the warming process by using a warm-water bath or other source of external heat such as microwave because heat may cause inactivation.
- Keep the insert frozen until just before insertion. No warming is needed.
- Have the woman void before insertion.
- Assist the woman to maintain a supine position with a lateral tilt or a side-lying position for at least 30 minutes after insertion of the gel or for 2 hours after placement of the insert.
- Allow the woman to ambulate after the recommended period of bed rest and observation.
- Prepare to pull the string to remove the insert and to administer terbutaline 0.25 mg subcutaneously if significant adverse effects occur. There is no effective way to remove the gel from the vagina if uterine tachysystole or abnormal FHR and patterns occur.
- Delay the initiation of oxytocin for induction of labor for 6 to 12 hours after the last instillation of the gel or for 30 to 60 minutes after removal of the insert, or follow agency protocol for induction if ripening has occurred but labor has not begun.
- Document all assessment findings and administration procedures.

Data from Hill W, Harvey C: Induction of labor. In Troiano N, Harvey C, Chez B, editors: *AWHONN's high risk & critical care obstetrics*, ed 3, Philadelphia, 2013, Wolters Kluwer/Lippincott Williams & Wilkins; Moleti C: Trends and controversies in labor induction, *MCN Am J Matern Child Nurs* 34(1):40–47, 2009.
FDA, Food and Drug Administration; *FHR*, fetal heart rate.

Hydroscopic dilators (substances that absorb fluid from surrounding tissues and then enlarge) also can be used for cervical ripening. Laminaria tents (natural cervical dilators made from desiccated seaweed) and synthetic dilators containing magnesium sulfate (Lamicel) are inserted into the endocervix without rupturing the membranes. As they absorb fluid, they expand and cause cervical dilation and the release of endogenous prostaglandins. These dilators are left in place for 6 to 12 hours before being removed to assess cervical dilation. Fresh dilators are inserted if further cervical dilation is necessary. Synthetic dilators swell faster than natural dilators and become larger with less discomfort. When compared with prostaglandins, these mechanical methods achieved a lower rate of birth within 24 hours but caused no change in the cesarean birthrate. Also, they were less likely to cause uterine tachysystole with or without changes in the fetal heart rate (ACOG, 2009; Thorp, 2009).

Hydroscopic dilators compare favorably with prostaglandins in terms of their effectiveness in ripening the cervix but are associated with increased discomfort at insertion and during expansion and with a higher incidence of postpartum maternal and newborn infections. They are a reliable alternative when prostaglandins are contraindicated or are unavailable. Nursing responsibilities for women who have dilators inserted include (Gilbert, 2011):

- Documenting the number of dilators and sponges inserted during the procedure, as well as the number removed
- Assessing for urinary retention, rupture of membranes, uterine tenderness or pain, contractions, vaginal bleeding, infection, and fetal distress

Amniotic membrane stripping or sweeping is a method of inducing labor through the release of prostaglandins and oxytocin. The procedure involves separation of the membrane from the wall of the cervix and lower uterine segment by inserting a finger into the internal cervical os and rotating it 360 degrees. Membrane stripping seems to work best when the woman is a primigravida at term with an unripe cervix and with the vertex well applied to the cervix. The procedure is uncomfortable and increases the risk for infection, rupture of membranes, bleeding, and precipitous labor and birth (Simpson, 2008; Wing and Farinelli, 2012).

Routine membrane stripping is not recommended because there is no evidence that this practice improves maternal or fetal outcome. However, weekly membrane stripping at term shortens the time interval to the onset of spontaneous labor and may decrease the need for labor induction using chemical or mechanical methods. Therefore membrane stripping may be offered after 39 weeks of gestation to women who wish to hasten the onset of spontaneous labor (Wing and Farinelli, 2012).

Physical methods such as sexual intercourse (prostaglandins in the semen and stimulation of contractions with orgasm), nipple stimulation (release of endogenous oxytocin from the pituitary gland), and walking (gravity applies pressure to the cervix, which stimulates the secretion of endogenous oxytocin) may be used by women to "self-induce" labor in an effort to "get it over with." Breast (nipple) stimulation has been shown to initiate or enhance labor, especially the latent phase of labor. Although orgasm does stimulate uterine contractions, there is inadequate evidence to support the belief that sexual intercourse enhances cervical ripening (Gilbert, 2011). Ambulation is an effective measure to augment labor (Moleti, 2009).

Alternative Methods. A variety of alternative methods have been used by women to stimulate cervical ripening and the onset of labor. For example, blue cohosh and castor oil can be used for their labor stimulation effects and black cohosh and evening primrose oil can ripen the cervix. Nurses must be knowledgeable about these preparations and ask about their use when assessing women during prenatal visits and on admission during labor. Women may accidentally take too much of the preparation or use it incorrectly. Also, these preparations may potentiate the effect of pharmacologic methods to stimulate cervical ripening and uterine contractions, thereby increasing the potential for tachysystole and precipitous labor and birth (Gilbert, 2011; Moleti, 2009).

Acupuncture has been used effectively to induce labor and has been found, in several studies, to reduce the duration of labor, the use of oxytocin, and the rate of cesarean birth. Specific points have been identified to stimulate uterine contractions or to facilitate cervical dilation. More than one treatment may be required to establish labor (Gilbert, 2011; Moleti, 2009).

Amniotomy. Amniotomy (i.e., artificial rupture of membranes [AROM]) can be used to induce labor when the condition of the cervix is favorable (ripe) or to augment labor if progress begins to slow. Labor usually begins within 12 hours of the rupture. Amniotomy can decrease the duration of labor by up to 2 hours, even without oxytocin administration. However, if amniotomy does not stimulate labor, the resulting prolonged rupture may lead to intraamniotic infection. Variable FHR deceleration patterns can occur as a result of cord compression associated with umbilical cord prolapse or decreased amniotic fluid. Once an amniotomy is performed, the woman is committed to labor with an unknown outcome for how and when she will give birth. For this reason, amniotomy often is used in combination with oxytocin induction.

Before the procedure, the woman should be told what to expect. She also should be assured that the actual rupture of the membranes is painless for her and the fetus, although she may experience some discomfort when the Amnihook or other sharp instrument is inserted through the vagina and cervix (Box 17-9). The presenting part of the fetus should be engaged and well applied to the cervix before the procedure to prevent cord prolapse (Wing and Farinelli, 2012). The woman should also be free of active infection of the genital tract (e.g., herpes) and should be human immunodeficiency virus (HIV) negative or have a viral load low enough that vaginal birth is acceptable. After rupture, the amniotic fluid is allowed to

---

BOX 17-9 **PROCEDURE: ASSISTING WITH AMNIOTOMY**

Procedure
- Explain to the woman what will be done.
- Assess fetal heart rate (FHR) and pattern before procedure begins to obtain a baseline reading.
- Place several underpads under the woman's buttocks to absorb the fluid.
- Position the woman on a padded bedpan, fracture pan, or rolled-up towel to elevate her hips.
- Assist the health care provider who is performing the procedure by providing sterile gloves and lubricant for the vaginal examination.
- Unwrap the sterile package containing an Amnihook or Allis clamp and pass the instrument to the primary health care provider, who inserts it alongside the fingers and then hooks and tears the membranes.
- Reassess the FHR and pattern.
- Assess the color, consistency, and odor of the fluid.
- Assess the woman's temperature every 2 hours or per protocol.
- Evaluate the woman for signs and symptoms of infection.

Documentation
- Record the following:
  - FHR and pattern before and after the procedure
  - Time of rupture
  - Color, odor, and consistency of the fluid
  - Maternal status (how well procedure was tolerated)

---

drain slowly. The color, odor, and consistency of the fluid are assessed (i.e., for the presence or absence of meconium or blood). The time of rupture and characteristics of the fluid are recorded.

> **⚠ NURSING ALERT**
>
> The FHR is assessed before and immediately after the amniotomy to detect any changes (e.g., transient tachycardia is common, but bradycardia and variable decelerations are not) that may indicate cord compression or prolapse.

The woman's temperature should be checked at least every 2 hours after rupture of membranes and more frequently if signs or symptoms of infection are noted. If her temperature is 38° C (100.4° F) or higher, notify the primary health care provider. The nurse assesses for other signs and symptoms of infection, such as maternal chills, uterine tenderness on palpation, foul-smelling vaginal drainage, and fetal tachycardia. Comfort measures, such as frequently changing the woman's underpads and perineal cleansing, are implemented.

> **LEGAL TIP: Performing Amniotomy**
>
> Performing amniotomy is outside the scope of practice of nurses. In some locations, however, nurses have been asked to perform this procedure. A policy that is consistent with professional standards of care and clearly explains the nurse's role in amniotomy should be in place in all labor and birth areas.

Oxytocin

Oxytocin is a hormone normally produced by the posterior pituitary gland. It stimulates uterine contractions and aids in milk let-down. Synthetic oxytocin (Pitocin) may be used either to induce labor or to augment a labor that is progressing slowly because of inadequate uterine contractions. Oxytocin is used in the majority of all births in the United States. It is also the drug most commonly associated with adverse events during childbirth. The most common errors involving oxytocin administration during labor are dose related (Clark, Simpson, Knox, et al., 2009; Mahlmeister, 2008; Simpson and Knox, 2009).

Oxytocin use can present hazards to the mother and fetus. Maternal hazards include placental abruption, uterine rupture, unnecessary cesarean birth because of abnormal FHR and patterns, postpartum hemorrhage, and infection. When placental perfusion is diminished by contractions that are too frequent or prolonged, the fetus can experience hypoxemia and acidemia, which eventually results in late decelerations and minimal or absent baseline variability. The goal of oxytocin use is to produce contractions of normal intensity, duration, and frequency while using the lowest dose of medication possible (Simpson and Knox, 2009).

The primary health care provider writes the order for the induction or augmentation of labor with oxytocin. The nurse implements the order by initiating the primary intravenous infusion and administering the oxytocin solution through a secondary line. The nurse's actions related to assessment and care of a woman whose labor is being induced are guided by hospital protocol and professional standards (see Fig. 17-7 and Medication Guide).

The recommended protocol for administering oxytocin is to begin with a starting dose of 1 milliunit/min and to increase by 1 to 2 milliunits/min no more frequently than every 30 to 60 minutes (Simpson, 2011; Simpson and Knox, 2009). This recommendation is based on research findings related to the pharmacokinetics of oxytocin. The uterus responds to oxytocin within 3 to 5 minutes of intravenous administration. The half-life of oxytocin (the time required to metabolize and eliminate half the dose) is approximately 10 to 12 minutes. Approximately 40 minutes is required to reach a steady state of oxytocin (the point in time when the rate of oxytocin administered intravenously equals the rate of oxytocin elimination) and for the full effect of a dosage increment to be reflected in more intense, frequent, and longer contractions (Mahlmeister, 2008; Hill and Harvey, 2013) (see Medication Guide on p. 466 and Fig. 17-7). Low-dose (physiologic) protocols such as the one described result in decreased risk for oxytocin-induced tachysystole and unnecessary cesarean birth because of abnormal FHR or patterns (Simpson, 2011). High-dose protocols, in which the initial dose of oxytocin is larger and the dosage is increased more rapidly, have been found to result in shorter labors, less forceps-assisted births, fewer cesarean births because of dystocia, less chorioamnionitis, and less neonatal sepsis (Wing and Farinelli, 2012). However, high-dose protocols have been associated with more uterine tachysystole and more cesarean births related to fetal stress (Wing and Farinelli, 2012). Some practitioners administer oxytocin in 8- to 10-minute pulsed infusions rather than as a continuous infusion. This method, which is more like endogenous secretion of oxytocin than the other approaches, is reported to be effective for labor induction and requires significantly less oxytocin administration (Gilbert, 2011; Wing and Farinelli, 2012).

Nursing Considerations. An evidence-based written protocol for the preparation and administration of oxytocin should be established by the obstetric department (physicians, nurses) in each institution. Other safety measures recommended for use of this high-alert drug are using a standard concentration of oxytocin and a standard definition of uterine tachysystole that does not include an abnormal FHR or pattern or the woman's perception of pain. In addition, standardized treatment of oxytocin-induced uterine tachysystole is recommended (Simpson, 2011) (see Emergency box on p. 467).

There has existed a need for standardizing the definition of excessive uterine contractions. The Eunice Kennedy Shriver National Institute of Child Health and Human Development along with the ACOG and the Society for Maternal-Fetal Medicine sponsored a workshop in April 2008 to review definition, interpretation, and research recommendations for intrapartum fetal monitoring. Workshop participants also recommended standardizing definitions regarding uterine contractions for use in clinical practice. This group defined uterine tachysystole as more than five contractions in 10 minutes, averaged over a 30-minute window. The term *tachysystole* applies to both spontaneous and stimulated labor. Participants also recommended that use of the terms *hyperstimulation* and *hyperactivity* be abandoned because they are not defined (Macones, Hankins, Spong, et al., 2008).

Augmentation of Labor

Augmentation of labor is the stimulation of uterine contractions after labor has started spontaneously but progress is unsatisfactory. Augmentation is usually implemented for the management of hypotonic uterine dysfunction, resulting in a slowing of the labor process (protracted active phase). Common augmentation methods include oxytocin infusion and amniotomy. Noninvasive methods such as emptying the bladder, ambulation and position changes, relaxation measures, nourishment and hydration, and hydrotherapy should be attempted before initiating invasive interventions. The administration procedure and nursing assessment

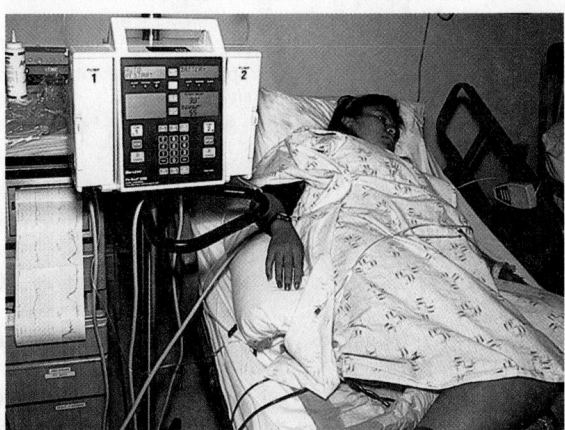

FIG 17-7 Woman in side-lying position receiving oxytocin. (Courtesy Michael S. Clement, MD, Mesa, AZ.)

MEDICATION GUIDE

Oxytocin (Pitocin)

Action

- Oxytocin is a hormone produced in the posterior pituitary gland that stimulates uterine contractions and aids in milk let-down. Pitocin is a synthetic form of this hormone.

Indications

- Oxytocin is used primarily for labor induction and augmentation. It is also used to control postpartum bleeding.

Dosage

- The intravenous solution containing oxytocin should be mixed in a standard concentration. Concentrations often used are 10 units in 1000 mL of fluid, 20 units in 1000 mL of fluid, or 30 units in 500 mL of fluid.
- Use isotonic intravenous solutions (e.g., 0.9% sodium chloride, lactated Ringer's [LR]) to avoid electrolyte imbalance.
- Oxytocin is administered intravenously through a secondary line connected to the main line at the proximal port (connection closest to the intravenous insertion site). Oxytocin is always administered by pump.
- Begin oxytocin administration at 1 milliunit/min. Increase the rate by 1 to 2 milliunits/min, no more frequently than every 30 to 60 minutes based on the response of the woman and fetus and the progress of labor.
- The goal of oxytocin administration is to produce acceptable uterine contractions as evidenced by:
  - Consistent achievement of 200 to 220 MVUs *or*
  - A consistent pattern of one contraction every 2 to 3 minutes, lasting 80 to 90 seconds, and strong to palpation

Adverse Effects

- Possible maternal adverse effects include uterine tachysystole, placental abruption, uterine rupture, unnecessary cesarean birth caused by abnormal FHR and patterns, postpartum hemorrhage, infection, and death from water intoxication (e.g., severe hyponatremia).
- Possible fetal adverse effects include hypoxemia and acidosis, eventually resulting in abnormal FHR and patterns.

Nursing Considerations

- Patient and partner teaching and support:
  - Reasons for use of oxytocin (e.g., start or improve labor)
  - Reactions to expect concerning the nature of contractions: the intensity of the contraction increases more rapidly, holds the peak longer, and ends more quickly; contractions will come regularly and more often
  - Monitoring to anticipate
- Continue to keep woman and her partner informed regarding progress.
- Remember that women vary greatly in their response to oxytocin; some require only very small amounts of medication to produce adequate contractions, whereas others need larger doses.
- Assessment
  - Fetal status using electronic fetal monitoring; evaluate tracing every 15 minutes and with every change in dose during the first stage of labor and every 5 minutes during the active pushing phase of the second stage of labor.
  - Monitor the contraction pattern and uterine resting tone every 15 minutes and with every change in dose during the first stage of labor and every 5 minutes during the second stage of labor.
  - Monitor blood pressure, pulse, and respirations every 30 to 60 minutes and with every change in dose.
  - Assess intake and output; limit IV intake to 1000 mL in 8 hours; urine output should be 120 mL or more every 4 hours.
  - Perform vaginal examination as indicated.
  - Monitor for side effects, including nausea, vomiting, headache, hypotension.
  - Observe emotional responses of woman and her partner.
- Use a standard definition for uterine tachysystole that does not include an abnormal FHR and pattern or the woman's perception of pain (see the Emergency Box on p. 467).
- The rate of oxytocin infusion should be continually titrated to the lowest dose that achieves acceptable labor progress. Usually the oxytocin dose can be decreased or discontinued after rupture of membranes and in the active phase of first-stage labor.
- Documentation
  - The time the oxytocin infusion is begun, and each time the infusion is increased, decreased, or discontinued
  - Assessment data as described above
  - Interventions for uterine tachysystole and abnormal FHR and patterns and the response to the interventions
  - Notification of the primary health care provider and that person's response

Data from American College of Obstetricians and Gynecologists (ACOG): *Induction of labor* (ACOG Practice Bulletin No. 107), Washington, DC, 2009, Author; Clark S, Simpson K, Knox G, et al: Oxytocin: new perspectives on an old drug, *Am J Obstet Gynecol* 200(1):35, e1–e6, 2009; Hill W, Harvey C: Induction of labor. In Troiano N, Harvey C, Chez B, editors: *AWHONN's high risk & critical care obstetrics*, ed 3, Philadelphia, 2013, Wolters Kluwer/Lippincott Williams & Wilkins; Mahlmeister L: Best practices in perinatal care: evidence-based management of oxytocin induction and augmentation of labor, *J Perinat Neonatal Nurs* 22(4):259–263, 2008; Simpson K: Labor and birth. In Simpson K, Creehan P, editors: *AWHONN's perinatal nursing*, ed 3, Philadelphia, 2008, Lippincott Williams & Wilkins; Simpson K, Knox G: Oxytocin as a high-alert medication: implications for perinatal patient safety, *MCN Am J Matern Child Nurs* 34(1):8–15, 2009.
FHR, Fetal heart rate; *IV,* intravenous; *MVUs,* Montevideo units.

and care measures for augmenting labor with oxytocin are similar to those used for induction of labor with oxytocin (see Medication Guide above).

Some physicians advocate *active management of labor,* that is, augmentation of labor to establish efficient labor with the aggressive use of oxytocin so that the woman gives birth within 12 hours of admission to the labor unit. Advocates of active management believe that intervening early (as soon as a nulliparous labor is not progressing at least 1 cm/hr) with use of higher (pharmacologic) oxytocin doses administered at frequent increment intervals (e.g., a starting dose of 6 milliunits/min with increases of 6 milliunits/min every 15 minutes) shortens labor (Gilbert, 2011).

Additional components of the active management of labor include:

- Strict criteria to diagnose that the woman is indeed in active labor with 100% effacement
- Amniotomy within 1 hour of admission of a woman in labor if spontaneous rupture of the membranes has not occurred
- Continuous presence of a nurse who provides one-on-one care for the woman while she is in labor

✚ EMERGENCY

Uterine Tachysystole with Oxytocin

Signs
- More than five contractions in 10 minutes *or*
- A series of single contractions lasting >2 minutes *or*
- Contractions of normal duration occurring within 1 minute of each other

Interventions (With Normal [Category I] FHR Tracing)
- Reposition or maintain woman in side-lying position (either side).
- Administer IV fluid bolus with 500 mL of lactated Ringer's solution.
- If uterine activity has not returned to normal after 10 minutes, decrease the oxytocin dose by at least half. If uterine activity has not returned to normal after another 10 minutes, discontinue the oxytocin infusion until fewer than five contractions occur in 10 minutes.

Interventions (With Indeterminate [Category II] or Abnormal [Category III] FHR Tracing)
- Discontinue oxytocin infusion immediately.
- Reposition or maintain woman in side-lying position (either side).
- Administer IV fluid bolus with 500 mL of lactated Ringer's solution.
- Consider giving oxygen at 10 L/min if the above interventions do not resolve the indeterminate or abnormal (category II or category III) FHR tracing.
- If no response, consider giving 0.25 mg terbutaline subcutaneously according to unit protocol or standing orders.
- Notify primary health care provider of actions taken and maternal and fetal response.

Resumption of Oxytocin After Resolution of Tachysystole
- If the oxytocin infusion has been discontinued for less than 20 to 30 minutes, resume at no more than one-half the rate that caused the tachysystole.
- If the oxytocin infusion has been discontinued for more than 30 to 40 minutes, resume at the initial starting dose.

Data from Simpson K: Clinicians' guide to the use of oxytocin for labor induction and augmentation, *J Midwifery Womens Health* 56(3):214–221, 2011.
FHR, Fetal heart rate.

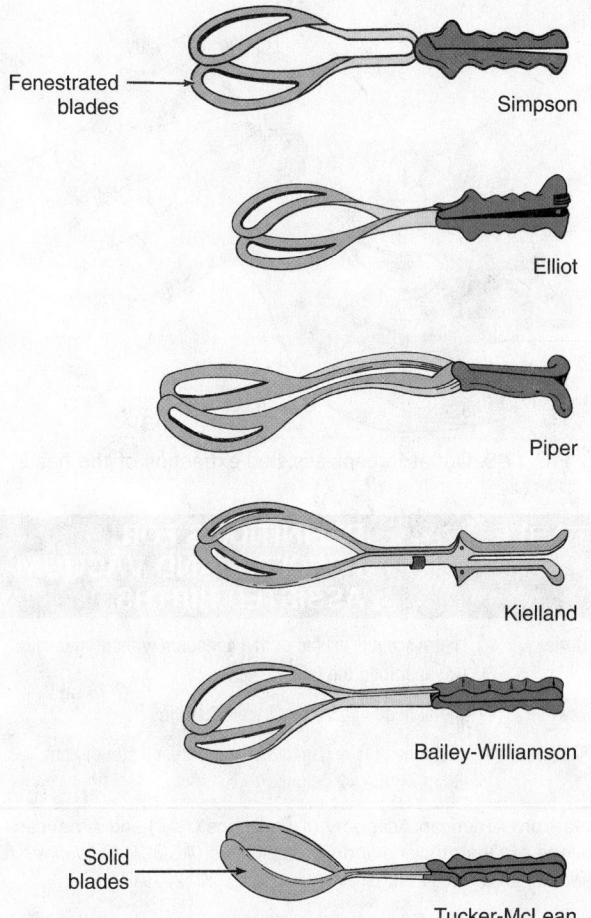

FIG 17-8 Types of forceps. Piper forceps are used to assist birth of the head in a breech birth.

The decision to use forceps or vacuum is based on the experience and personal preference of the physician performing the procedure. There are several types of operative vaginal births (American Academy of Pediatrics [AAP] and ACOG, 2012).

Forceps-Assisted Birth

A forceps-assisted birth is one in which an instrument with two curved blades is used to assist in the birth of the fetal head. The cephalic-like curve of the forceps commonly used is similar to the shape of the fetal head, with a pelvic curve to the blades conforming to the curve of the pelvic axis. The blades are joined by a pin, screw, or groove arrangement. These locks prevent the forceps from compressing the fetal skull (Fig. 17-8). There are several types of forceps-assisted births, defined primarily by the station and position of the fetal head in relationship to the maternal pelvis (Table 17-4) (AAP and ACOG, 2012).

Maternal indications for forceps-assisted birth include a prolonged second stage of labor and the need to shorten the second stage of labor for maternal reasons (e.g., maternal exhaustion or maternal cardiopulmonary or cerebrovascular disease) (Nielsen and Galan, 2012). Fetal indications include an abnormal FHR tracing or certain abnormal presentations; arrest of rotation; or extraction of the head in a breech presentation (Nielsen and Galan, 2012; Thorp, 2009).

Certain conditions are required for a forceps-assisted birth to be successful. The woman's cervix must be fully dilated to prevent

Many obstetricians in the United States emphasize using high-dose oxytocin protocols but do not implement all the other components of active management. At least one review of published studies on the effectiveness of active management of labor protocols concluded that the presence of a nurse who provides constant emotional and physical one-on-one support is the only component associated with shorter labors and lower rates of cesarean birth (Clark, Simpson, Knox, et al., 2009; Gilbert, 2011).

The original active management of labor protocols were written for nulliparous women who began laboring spontaneously. However, active management of labor protocols has been implemented by some providers in the United States on women who were not appropriate candidates (Mahlmeister, 2008).

Operative Vaginal Birth

Operative vaginal births are performed using either forceps or vacuum extractor. The use of both devices continues to decline. In 2010 fewer than 4% of all births were accomplished using forceps or vacuum assistance (Martin, Hamilton, Sutton, et al., 2012). Indications and prerequisites for the use of both instruments are similar.

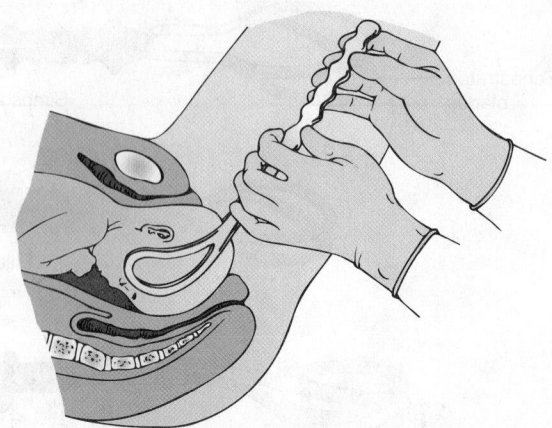

FIG 17-9 Outlet forceps-assisted extraction of the head.

TABLE 17-4	DEFINITIONS FOR FORCEPS- AND VACUUM-ASSISTED BIRTHS
Outlet	Fetal scalp is visible on the perineum without manually separating the labia
Low	Fetal head is at least at the +2 station
Midpelvis	Fetal head is engaged (no higher than 0 station) but above the +2 station

Data from American Academy of Pediatrics (AAP) and American College of Obstetricians and Gynecologists (ACOG): *Guidelines for perinatal care*, ed 7, Elk Grove Village, IL, 2012, AAP.

lacerations and hemorrhage. The bladder should be empty. The presenting part must be engaged—vertex presentation is desired. Membranes must be ruptured so the position of the fetal head can be determined precisely and the forceps can grasp the head firmly during birth (Fig. 17-9). The size of the maternal pelvis must be assessed as adequate for the estimated fetal head circumference and weight.

Management. Both blades are positioned by the physician, and the handles are locked. Traction is usually applied during contractions. The mother may or may not be instructed to push during contractions, depending on physician preference. If a decrease in the fetal heart rate occurs, the forceps are removed and reapplied.

> **⚠ NURSING ALERT**
>
> Because compression of the cord between the fetal head and the forceps will cause a decrease in FHR, the FHR is assessed, reported, and recorded before and after application of the forceps.

Nursing Considerations. When a forceps-assisted birth is deemed necessary, the nurse obtains the type of forceps requested by the physician. The nurse can explain to the mother that the forceps blades fit the same way two tablespoons fit around an egg, with the blades placed in front of the baby's ears.

After birth, the mother should be assessed for vaginal or cervical lacerations, urinary retention, and hematoma formation in the pelvic soft tissues, which may result from blood vessel damage. The infant should be assessed for bruising or abrasions at the site of the blade applications, facial palsy resulting from pressure of the

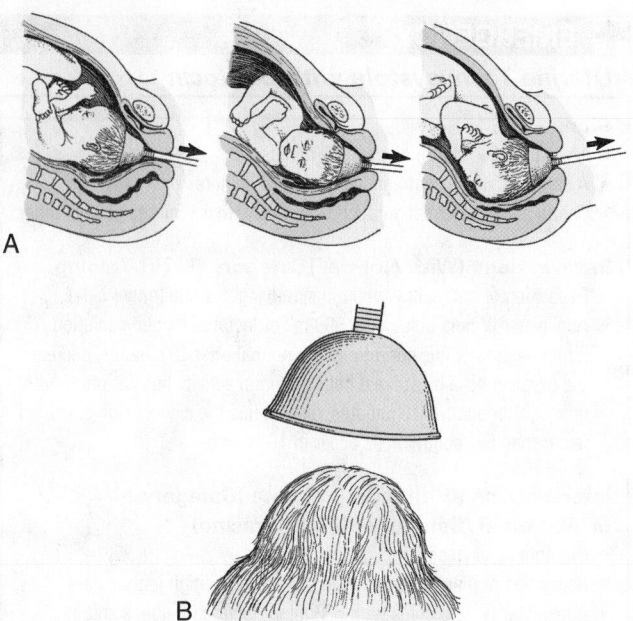

FIG 17-10 Use of vacuum extraction to rotate fetal head and assist with descent. **A,** *Arrow* indicates direction of traction on the vacuum cup. **B,** Caput succedaneum formed by the vacuum cup.

blades on the facial nerve, and subdural hematoma. Newborn and postpartum caregivers should be told that a forceps-assisted birth was performed.

Vacuum-Assisted Birth

Vacuum-assisted birth, or vacuum extraction, is a birth method involving the attachment of a vacuum cup to the fetal head, using negative pressure to assist in the birth of the head (Fig. 17-10, *A*). It is generally not used to assist birth before 34 weeks of gestation. Indications for its use are the same as those for outlet forceps. Prerequisites for use include a completely dilated cervix, ruptured membranes, engaged head, vertex presentation, and no suspicion of CPD (Cunningham, Leveno, Bloom, et al., 2010). The types of vacuum-assisted births are defined the same as for forceps-assisted births—by the station and position of the fetal head in relation to the maternal pelvis (see Table 17-4) (AAP and ACOG, 2012). Advantages of vacuum-assisted compared with forceps-assisted birth are the ease with which the vacuum can be placed and the need for less anesthesia. Also, it is far easier to learn the skills necessary to safely use the vacuum than to gain a similar level of skill with forceps (Thorp, 2009).

Management. The vacuum cup is applied to the fetal head by the physician. Basically two types of vacuum devices are in use. One is a self-contained unit, which allows the physician to both position the cup on the baby's head and generate the desired amount of negative pressure to create a vacuum. When the other type of vacuum device is used, the physician applies the cup to the baby's head, after which the nurse connects the suction tubing attached to the cup to wall suction or a separate hand pump and generates the amount of pressure requested by the physician. With both devices, a caput develops inside the cup as the pressure is initiated (see Fig. 17-10, *B*). The woman is encouraged to push as traction is applied by the physician. The vacuum cup is released and removed after birth of the head. If vacuum extraction is not successful, a forceps-assisted or cesarean birth is usually performed.

- Assess the fetal heart rate frequently during the procedure.
- Encourage the woman to push during contractions.
- If responsible for generating pressure for the vacuum, do not exceed the "green zone" indicated on the pump. Verify with the physician the amount of pressure to be generated.
- Document the number of pulls attempted, the maximum pressure used, and any pop-offs that occur.

Risks to the newborn include cephalhematoma, scalp lacerations, and subdural hematoma. Fetal complications can be reduced by strict adherence to the manufacturer's recommendations for method of application, amount of pressure to be generated, and duration of application. Maternal risks include perineal, vaginal, or cervical lacerations and soft-tissue hematomas.

Nursing Considerations. The nurse's role for the woman who has a vacuum-assisted birth is primarily one of support person and educator. The nurse can prepare the woman for birth and encourage her to remain active in the birth process by pushing during contractions. The fetal heart rate should be assessed frequently during the procedure. Documentation of the procedure in the medical record is important and is often the nurse's responsibility (Box 17-10). Neonatal caregivers should be told that the birth was vacuum assisted. After birth, the newborn must be observed for signs of trauma and infection at the application site and for cerebral irritation (e.g., poor sucking or listlessness). The newborn may also be at risk for hyperbilirubinemia and neonatal jaundice as bruising resolves. The parents may need to be reassured that the caput succedaneum usually disappears in 3 to 5 days (see Fig. 17-10, *B*) (Gilbert, 2011).

Cesarean Birth

Cesarean birth is the birth of a fetus through a transabdominal incision of the uterus. Whether cesarean birth is planned (scheduled) or unplanned, the loss of the experience of giving birth to a child in the traditional manner may have a negative effect on a woman's self-concept. An effort is therefore made to maintain the focus on the birth of the baby rather than on the operative procedure.

The purpose of cesarean birth is to preserve the life or health of the mother and her fetus. It may be the best choice for birth when evidence exists of maternal or fetal complications. Since the advent of modern surgical methods and care and the use of antibiotics, maternal and fetal morbidity and mortality have decreased. In addition, incisions are usually made into the lower uterine segment rather than in the muscular body of the uterus, thus promoting more effective healing. However, despite these advances, cesarean birth still poses threats to the health of the mother and infant.

In 2010 the cesarean birthrate in the United States was 32.8%, down from 32.9% in 2009. This was the first decrease in the overall cesarean birthrate since 1996 (Martin, Hamilton, Sutton, et al., 2012). Despite this recent small decrease, the cesarean birthrate in the United States remains very high. Part of the reason is that a number of common risk factors for cesarean birth are increasing in frequency, especially in developed countries. These factors include fetal macrosomia, advanced maternal age, obesity, gestational diabetes, and multifetal pregnancy (Thorp, 2009). Limited use of a trial of labor after a previous cesarean birth, due in part to safety and medicolegal concerns, and the advent of elective cesarean birth are other factors related to the elevated incidence. Although some women desire elective cesarean birth, fewer than 10% of all American women prefer a cesarean birth based solely on their request (Berghella and Landon, 2012). An estimate of the elective cesarean birthrate internationally is much higher compared with the United States—between 4% and 18% (Collard, Diallo, Habinsky, et al., 2008/2009).

Approaches for managing labor and birth to reduce the rate of cesarean births while increasing the rate of vaginal birth after cesarean (VBAC) are presented in Box 17-11. These approaches involve the combined efforts of health care professionals and pregnant women and their families.

Indications

Few absolute indications exist for cesarean birth. Currently, most are performed for conditions that might pose a threat to both the mother and the fetus if vaginal birth occurred, such as placenta previa or placental abruption (Berghella and Landon, 2012). Box 17-12 lists common indications for cesarean birth.

Elective Cesarean Birth

Elective cesarean birth, sometimes referred to as *cesarean on request* or *cesarean on demand,* refers to a primary cesarean birth without medical or obstetric indication. Reasons given for elective cesarean birth include fear of the pain of childbirth and the belief that the surgery will prevent future problems with pelvic support, bladder and bowel incontinence, or sexual dysfunction. Although some nulliparous women may fear the pain of labor because of no firsthand experience, multiparous women may request a cesarean birth after a previous traumatic vaginal birth. Other women desire an elective cesarean birth because of the convenience of planning a date or having control and choice about when to give birth. At this time, evidence is insufficient to recommend elective cesarean birth to prevent urinary or fecal incontinence later in life (Collard, Diallo, Habinsky, et al., 2008/2009; Roberts and Mangan, 2009; Thorp, 2009).

Potential risks of cesarean birth on request include:
- Higher rates of endometritis, blood transfusion, and venous thrombosis
- A longer hospital stay and recovery time for the woman
- An increased risk for respiratory problems for the baby
- Greater complications in subsequent pregnancies, including uterine rupture and placental implantation problems

Cesarean birth on request should not be performed unless a gestational age of 39 weeks has been accurately determined. Also, the procedure is not recommended for women who desire several additional children, because the risks for placenta previa, placenta accreta, and cesarean hysterectomy increase with each cesarean birth (Berghella and Landon, 2012).

Scheduled Cesarean Birth

Cesarean birth is scheduled or planned if:
- Labor and vaginal birth are contraindicated (e.g., complete placenta previa, active genital herpes, positive HIV status with a high viral load)
- Birth is necessary but labor is not inducible (e.g., hypertensive states that cause a poor intrauterine environment that threatens the fetus)
- This course of action has been chosen by the primary health care provider and the woman (e.g., a repeat cesarean birth)

BOX 17-11	SELECTED MEASURES TO REDUCE THE CESAREAN BIRTHRATE AND INCREASE THE RATE OF VAGINAL BIRTH AFTER CESAREAN

Educate Women Regarding:
- Advantages and safety of the home environment for early or latent labor
- Indicators for hospital admission
- Management techniques to use during labor to enhance progress
- Nonpharmacologic measures to reduce pain and discomfort and enhance relaxation
- Safety and effectiveness of TOL and VBAC

Establish Admission Criteria for Women in Labor That:
- Distinguish clinical manifestations for false labor, latent (early) labor, and active labor
- Conduct admission assessments in a separate admissions area
- Send women in false or latent (early) labor home or keep them in the admissions area
- Admit women in active labor to the labor and birth unit

Use Appropriate Assessment Techniques to:
- Determine the status of the woman and fetus
- Establish an individualized rationale for initiating labor interventions such as epidural anesthesia, induction or augmentation, amniotomy, or cesarean birth

Initiate a Doula Program That:
- Provides early, continuous one-on-one support for women in labor and for their partners

Develop a Philosophy of Labor Management That:
- Supports admission during active labor
- Uses measures that promote, support, and encourage normal spontaneous labor
- Avoids automatic interventions such as routine induction for spontaneous rupture of membranes at term or postterm pregnancy and cesarean birth for breech presentation, twin gestation, genital herpes, or failure to progress
- Relies on assessment findings reflective of the status of the woman and fetus, rather than strict adherence to set ranges for the duration of the stages and phases of labor
- Uses intermittent rather than continuous electronic fetal monitoring of low risk pregnant women
- Focuses on measures that are known to enhance the progress of labor such as one-on-one support, ambulation, upright positions, maternal position changes, oral nutrition and hydration, and nonpharmacologic pain relief
- Uses nonpharmacologic measures in a manner that reduces their labor-inhibiting effects
- Establishes criteria for elective cesarean birth and TOL
- Encourages women who have had previous cesarean birth to participate in TOL to attempt a vaginal birth

TOL, Trial of labor; *VBAC,* vaginal birth after cesarean.

BOX 17-12	INDICATIONS FOR CESAREAN BIRTH

Maternal
- Specific cardiac disease (e.g., Marfan syndrome, unstable coronary artery disease)
- Specific respiratory disease (e.g., Guillain-Barré syndrome)
- Conditions associated with increased intracranial pressure
- Mechanical obstruction of the lower uterine segment (tumors, fibroids)
- Mechanical vulvar obstruction (e.g., extensive condylomata)
- History of previous cesarean birth

Fetal
- Abnormal fetal heart rate (FHR) or pattern
- Malpresentation (e.g., breech or transverse lie)
- Active maternal herpes lesions
- Maternal human immunodeficiency virus (HIV) with a viral load of more than 1000 copies/mL
- Congenital anomalies

Maternal-Fetal
- Dysfunctional labor (e.g., cephalopelvic disproportion, "failure to progress" in labor)
- Placental abruption
- Placenta previa
- Elective cesarean birth (cesarean on maternal request)

Data from Berghella V, Landon M: Cesarean delivery. In Gabbe S, Niebyl J, Simpson J, et al, editors: *Obstetrics: normal and problem pregnancies,* ed 6, Philadelphia, 2012, Saunders; Duff P, Sweet R, Edwards R: Maternal and fetal infections. In Creasy R, Resnik R, Iams J, et al, editors: *Creasy and Resnik's maternal-fetal medicine: principles and practice,* ed 6, Philadelphia, 2009, Saunders; Thorp JM: Clinical aspects of normal and abnormal labor. In Creasy R, Resnik R, Iams J, et al, editors: *Creasy and Resnik's maternal-fetal medicine: principles and practice,* ed 6, Philadelphia, 2009, Saunders.

postoperative recovery period. They may be concerned about the added burdens of caring for the infant and perhaps other children while recovering from surgery. Others may feel glad that they have been relieved of the uncertainty about the date and time of the birth and are free of the pain of labor.

Unplanned Cesarean Birth

The psychosocial outcomes of unplanned or emergency cesarean birth are usually more pronounced and negative when compared with the outcomes associated with a scheduled or planned cesarean birth. Women and their families experience abrupt changes in their expectations for birth, postpartum care, and the care of the new baby at home. This may be an extremely traumatic experience for all.

The woman may approach the procedure tired and discouraged after an ineffective and difficult labor. Fear predominates as she worries about her own safety and well-being and that of her fetus. She may be dehydrated, with low glycogen reserves. Because preoperative procedures must be done rapidly, there is often little time for explanation of the procedures and the operation itself. Because maternal and family anxiety levels are high at this time, much of what is said may be forgotten or misunderstood. The woman may experience feelings of anger or guilt in the postpartum period. Fatigue is often noticeable in these women, and they need much supportive care.

Women who are scheduled for a cesarean birth have time to prepare for it psychologically. However, the psychologic responses of these women may differ. Those having a repeat cesarean birth may have disturbing memories of the conditions preceding the initial (primary) cesarean birth and of their experiences in the

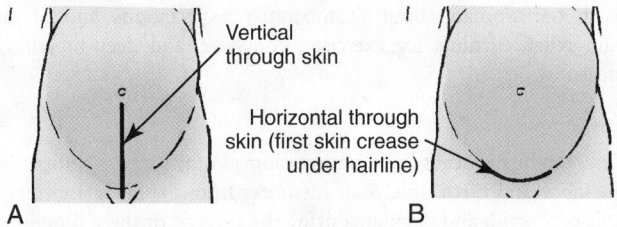

FIG 17-11 Skin incisions for cesarean birth. **A**, Vertical. **B**, Horizontal (Pfannenstiel).

Forced Cesarean Birth

A woman's refusal to undergo cesarean birth when indicated for fetal reasons is often described as a *maternal-fetal conflict*. Health care providers are ethically obliged to protect the well-being of both mother and fetus; a decision for one affects the other. If a woman refuses a cesarean birth that is recommended because of fetal jeopardy, health care providers must make every effort to find out why she is refusing and provide information that may persuade her to change her mind. If the woman continues to refuse surgery, then health care providers must decide if it is ethical to get a court order for the surgery. Every effort, however, should be made to avoid this legal step.

Surgical Techniques

The skin incision will be either vertical, extending from near the umbilicus to the mons pubis, or transverse (Pfannenstiel) in the lower abdomen (Fig. 17-11). The transverse incision, sometimes referred to as the "bikini" incision, is performed more often. The type of skin incision is generally determined by the urgency of the surgery and the presence of any prior skin incisions (Berghella and Landon, 2012). The type of skin incision does *not* necessarily indicate the type of uterine incision.

The two main types of uterine incision are the low transverse incision (Fig. 17-12, *A*) and the vertical incision, which may be either low or classic (see Fig. 17-12, *B* and *C*). Ideally, the vertical incision is contained entirely within the lower uterine segment, but extension into the contractile portion of the uterus (e.g., a classic incision) can occur (Berghella and Landon, 2012). Indications for a vertical incision include an underdeveloped lower uterine segment, a transverse lie or preterm breech presentation, certain fetal anomalies such as massive hydrocephalus, and an anterior placenta previa (Berghella and Landon, 2012). Because it is associated with a higher incidence of uterine rupture in subsequent pregnancies than is a lower-segment incision, vaginal birth after a classic uterine incision is contraindicated.

The low transverse uterine incision is performed in more than 90% of cesarean births (see Fig. 17-12, *A*). Compared with the vertical incision, the transverse incision is preferred because it does not compromise the upper uterine segment, is easier to perform and repair, and is associated with less blood loss. It also provides for the option of trial of labor and VBAC in subsequent pregnancies (Berghella and Landon, 2012).

Complications and Risks

Possible maternal complications related to cesarean birth include aspiration, hemorrhage, atelectasis, endometritis, abdominal wound dehiscence or infection, urinary tract infection, injuries to the bladder or bowel, and complications related to anesthesia (Thorp, 2009). The fetus may be born prematurely if the gestational age has not been accurately determined. Fetal asphyxia can occur if the

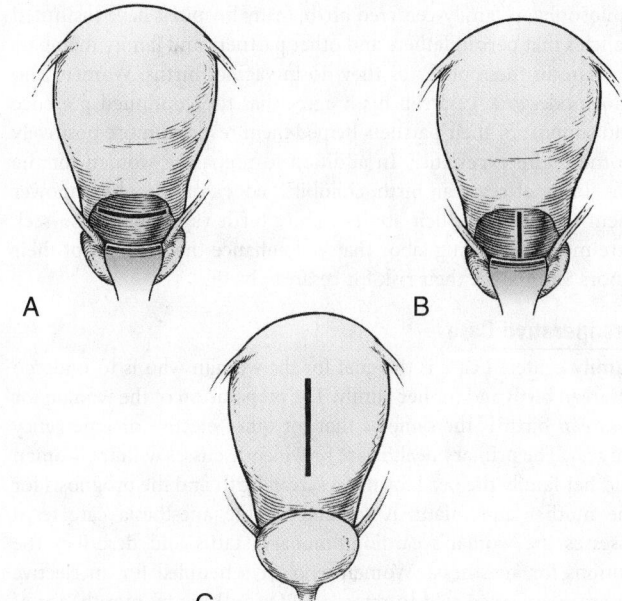

FIG 17-12 Uterine incisions for cesarean birth. **A**, Low transverse incision. **B**, Low vertical incision. **C**, Classic incision. (From Gabbe SG, Niebyl J, Simpson J, et al: *Obstetrics: normal and problem pregnancies*, ed 6, Philadelphia, 2012, Saunders.)

uterus and placenta are poorly perfused as a result of maternal hypotension caused by regional anesthesia (epidural or spinal) or maternal positioning. Fetal injuries (e.g., injuries caused by scalpel lacerations) can also occur during the surgery. The newborn is more likely to require resuscitation efforts and develop respiratory complications (Roberts and Mangan, 2009; Thorp, 2009). In addition to these risks, the woman is at economic risk because the cost of cesarean birth is higher than that of vaginal birth and a longer recovery period may require additional expenditures.

Anesthesia

Spinal, epidural, and general anesthetics are used for cesarean births. Epidural blocks are popular because women want to be awake for and aware of the birth experience. However, the choice of anesthetic depends on several factors. The mother's medical history or present condition, such as a spinal injury, hemorrhage, or coagulopathy, may rule out the use of regional anesthesia. Time is another factor, especially if there is an emergency and the life of the mother or infant is at stake. In an emergency, general anesthesia will most likely be used unless the woman already has an epidural block in effect. The woman herself is a factor. Either she may not know all the options or may have fears about having "a needle in her back" or about being awake and feeling pain. She needs to be fully informed about the risks and benefits of the different types of anesthesia so that she can participate in the decision whenever there is a choice.

Prenatal Preparation

A discussion of cesarean birth should be included in all childbirth preparation classes. No woman can be guaranteed a vaginal birth, even if she is in good health and no indication of danger to the fetus exists before the onset of labor. Therefore every woman needs to be aware of and prepared for the possibility of having a cesarean birth.

Childbirth educators should emphasize the similarities and differences between a cesarean and a vaginal birth. In support of the philosophy of family-centered birth, many hospitals have instituted policies that permit fathers and other partners and family members to share in these births as they do in vaginal births. Women who have undergone cesarean birth agree that the continued presence and support of their partners helped them respond more positively to the entire experience. In addition to preparing women for the possibility of cesarean birth, childbirth educators should empower them to believe in their ability to give birth vaginally and to seek care measures during labor that will enhance the progress of their labors and reduce their risk for cesarean birth.

Preoperative Care

Family-centered care is the goal for the woman who is to undergo cesarean birth and for her family. The preparation of the woman for cesarean birth is the same as that for other elective or emergency surgery. The primary health care provider discusses with the woman and her family the need for the cesarean birth and the prognosis for the mother and infant. A member of the anesthesia care team assesses the woman's cardiopulmonary status and describes the options for anesthesia. Women who are scheduled for an elective cesarean are often told to remain NPO (nothing by mouth) for at least 8 hours before the surgery (Roberts and Mangan, 2009). Informed consent is obtained for the procedure.

Blood tests are usually done a day or two before a planned cesarean birth or on admission to the labor and birth unit. Laboratory tests commonly ordered include a complete blood cell count and blood type and Rh status. Maternal vital signs and FHR and pattern are assessed according to hospital protocol until the operation begins. Intravenous fluids are started to maintain hydration and to provide an open line for the administration of blood or medications if needed. Other preoperative preparations include ensuring that an informed consent form has been signed, inserting a retention (Foley) catheter to keep the bladder empty, and administering prescribed preoperative medications. In addition to medications given to prevent aspiration pneumonia, women may also receive prophylactic antibiotics to prevent postoperative infection. In the rare instance that an abdominal-mons shave or a clipping of pubic hair is ordered by the primary health care provider, it is performed in the operating room just before making the incision because shaving can result in injury of the integument, thereby increasing the risk for infection. Often, TED hose and SCD boots will be placed on the woman's legs to prevent blood clot formation. Removal of contact lenses, dentures, nail polish, and jewelry may be optional, depending on hospital policies and the type of anesthesia used. If the woman wears glasses and is going to be awake, the nurse should make sure her glasses accompany her to the operating room so she can see her infant.

During the preoperative preparation, the support person is encouraged to remain with the woman as much as possible to provide continuing emotional support (if this action is culturally acceptable to the woman and support person). The nurse provides essential information about the preoperative procedures during this time. Although the nursing actions may be carried out quickly if a cesarean birth is unplanned, verbal communication, particularly explanations, is important. Silence can be frightening to the woman and her support person. The nurse's use of touch (if culturally appropriate) can communicate feelings of care and concern for the woman. The nurse can assess the woman's and her partner's perceptions about cesarean birth. As the woman expresses her feelings, the nurse may identify the potential for a disturbance in self-concept during the postpartum period that would need to be addressed. If there is time before the birth, the nurse can

teach the woman about postoperative expectations and about pain relief, turning, leg exercises, coughing, and deep-breathing measures.

Intraoperative Care

Cesarean births occur in operating rooms in the surgical suite or in the labor and birth unit. Staff members from the labor and birth unit may scrub and circulate during the surgery, or these functions may be assumed by members of the hospital's surgery staff (Fig. 17-13). If possible, the partner or another person, dressed appropriately for the operating room, accompanies the mother to the operating room and remains close to her for continued comfort and support. In unplanned cesarean birth, the nurse who cared for the

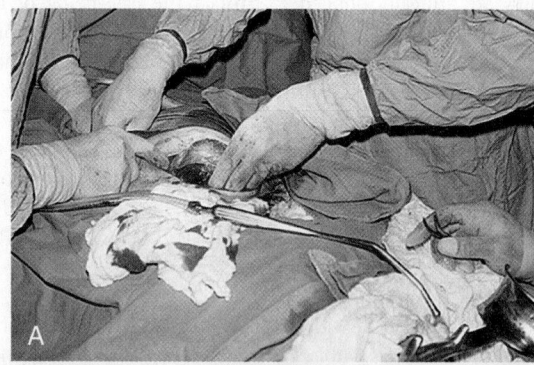

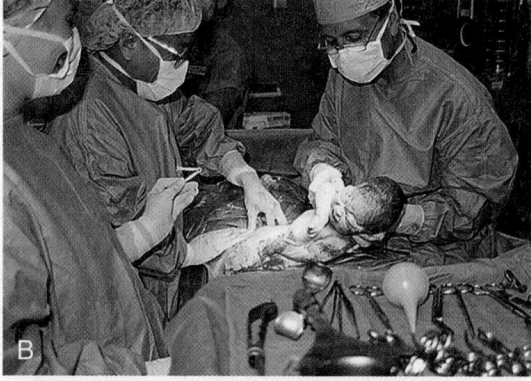

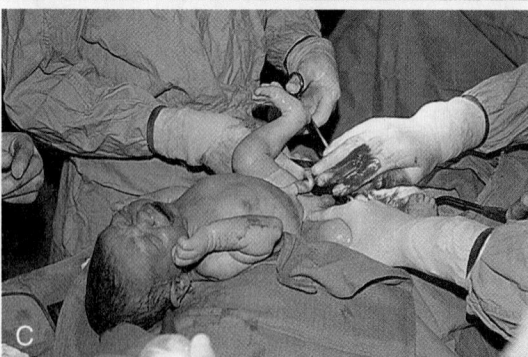

FIG 17-13 Cesarean birth. **A,** "Bikini" incision has been made, the muscle layer is separated, the abdomen is entered, and the uterus has been exposed and incised; suctioning of amniotic fluid continues as head is brought up through the incision. Note small amount of bleeding. **B,** The neonate's birth through the uterine incision is nearly complete. **C,** A quick assessment is performed; note extreme molding of head resulting from cephalopelvic disproportion. (Courtesy Marjorie Pyle, RNC, Lifecircle, Costa Mesa, CA.)

woman during labor should be part of the nursing care team in the operating room if possible.

The nurse who is circulating may assist with positioning the woman on the birth (operating) table. It is important to position her so that the uterus is displaced laterally to prevent compression of the inferior vena cava, which causes decreased placental perfusion. This is usually accomplished by placing a wedge under one hip or tilting the table to one side. The woman's legs should be strapped to the table to ensure proper positioning during the surgery. A retention (Foley) catheter is inserted into the bladder at this time if one is not already in place.

If the partner or another person is not allowed or chooses not to be present, the nurse can stay in communication with him or her and give progress reports whenever possible. If the woman is awake during the birth, the nurse, anesthesia care provider, or both can tell her what is happening and provide support. She may be anxious about the sensations she is experiencing, such as the coldness of solutions used to cleanse the abdomen and pressure or pulling during the actual birth of the infant. She also may be apprehensive because of the bright lights or the presence of unfamiliar equipment and masked and gowned personnel in the room. Explanations can help decrease the woman's anxiety.

A nurse from the labor and birth unit usually is present to provide care for the infant. A pediatrician or a nurse team skilled in neonatal resuscitation may also be present for the surgery because these infants are considered to be at risk until evidence of physiologic stability exists after the birth. A crib with resuscitation equipment is readied before surgery. Personnel who are responsible for care are expert not only in resuscitative techniques but also in detecting normal and abnormal infant responses (AAP and American Heart Association [AHA], 2011). After birth, if the infant's condition permits and the mother is awake, the baby can be placed skin-to-skin on the mother or can be given to the woman's partner or another person to hold (Fig. 17-14). The infant whose condition is compromised is transported after initial stabilization to the nursery for observation and the implementation of appropriate interventions. In some institutions, the partner or another person may accompany the infant; if not, personnel keep the family informed of the infant's progress and parent-infant contacts are initiated as soon as possible.

If family members cannot accompany the woman during surgery, they are directed to the surgical or obstetric waiting room. The physician then reports on the condition of the mother and infant to the family members after the birth is completed. Family members may be allowed to accompany the infant as he or she is transferred to the nursery, giving them an opportunity to see and admire the new baby.

LEGAL TIP: Disclosure of Patient Information

Some mothers or fathers want the privilege of informing family and friends of the sex of the infant (if it was not known before birth) or other information about the birth. Before responding to requests for such information from people waiting outside the birthing area, the nurse should check to see if the mother has given consent for such information to be released and to whom.

Immediate Postoperative Care

Once surgery is completed, the mother is transferred to a postanesthesia recovery area. After a cesarean birth, women have postoperative and postpartum needs that must be addressed. They are surgical patients as well as new mothers. Nursing assessments in this

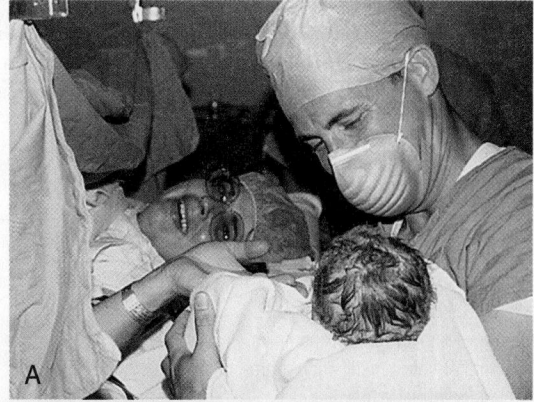

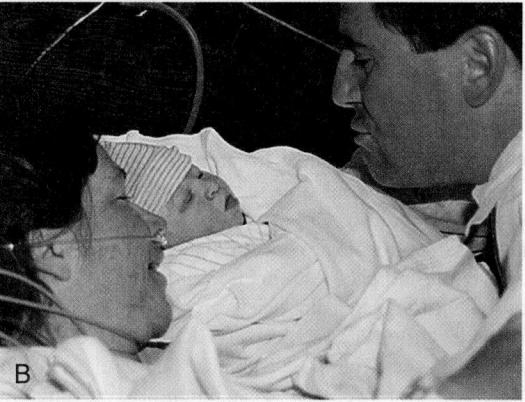

FIG 17-14 A, Parents and their newborn. The physician manually removes the placenta, suctions the remaining amniotic fluid and blood from the uterine cavity, and closes the uterine incision, peritoneum, muscle layer, fatty tissue, and finally the skin, while the new family shares some time together. **B,** Parents become better acquainted with their newborn while mother rests after surgery. (Courtesy Marjorie Pyle, RNC, Lifecircle, Costa Mesa, CA.)

immediate postbirth period follow agency protocol and include degree of recovery from the effects of anesthesia, postoperative and postbirth status, and degree of pain. A patent airway is maintained, and the woman is positioned to prevent possible aspiration. Vital signs are taken every 15 minutes for 1 to 2 hours, or until stable. The condition of the incisional dressing and the fundus and the amount of lochia are assessed, as well as the intravenous intake and the urine output through the retention (Foley) catheter. Oxytocin usually is added to at least the first liter of the intravenous infusion to ensure that the fundus remains firmly contracted, thereby reducing blood loss (Roberts and Mangan, 2009). The woman is helped to turn and do coughing, deep-breathing, and leg exercises. Medications for pain relief should be administered before postoperative pain becomes severe.

If the baby is present, the mother and her partner or another person are given some time alone with him or her to facilitate bonding and attachment. Breastfeeding can be initiated if the mother feels like trying. The woman is ready for discharge from the postanesthesia recovery area once her condition is stable and the effects of anesthesia have worn off (i.e., she is alert and oriented and able to feel and move her extremities).

Postoperative Postpartum Care

The attitude of the nurse and other health care team members can influence the woman's perception of herself after a cesarean birth.

Postpartum Pain Relief After Cesarean Birth

Incisional

- Splint incision with a pillow when moving or coughing.
- Use relaxation techniques such as music, breathing, and dim lights.

Gas

- Walk as often as you can.
- Do not eat or drink gas-forming foods, carbonated beverages, or whole milk.
- Do not use straws for drinking fluids.
- Take antiflatulence medication if prescribed.
- Lie on your left side to expel gas.
- Rock in a rocking chair.

The caregivers should stress that the woman is a new mother first and a surgical patient second. This attitude helps the woman perceive herself as having the same problems and needs as other new mothers, while requiring supportive postoperative care.

The woman's physiologic concerns may be dominated by pain at the incision site and pain resulting from intestinal gas. For the first 24 hours after surgery, pain relief can be provided by epidural opioids, patient-controlled analgesia (PCA), or intravenous or intramuscular injections. The most commonly used analgesics include opioids (e.g., hydromorphone, [Dilaudid], morphine sulfate, nalbuphine [Nubain]) and NSAIDs (e.g., ketorolac [Toradol]). If opioids are used, an antiemetic (e.g., metoclopramide [Reglan]) is often administered either as needed by the woman or around the clock as long as the opioid is used. Palpation of the fundus with the possibility of massage should be performed after an analgesic is given to decrease pain (Roberts and Mangan, 2009). By 24 hours after surgery, women are generally changed to oral analgesics. Other comfort measures such as position changes, splinting of the incision with pillows, and relaxation and breathing techniques (e.g., those learned in childbirth classes) may be implemented (see Patient Teaching box).

Women are often the best judges of what their bodies need and can tolerate, including the postoperative ingestion of foods and fluids. Some health care providers keep women NPO or allow only "sips and chips" (sips of clear fluids and teaspoons of crushed ice) until bowel sounds return. The diet is then advanced to full liquids. After women are passing flatus they can resume a regular diet (Gilbert, 2011). Because most women have an epidural or spinal anesthetic for surgery, most health care providers allow the early introduction of solid food if desired and tolerated. Intravenous fluids are usually continued until the woman is tolerating fluids orally. Ambulation and rocking in a rocking chair may relieve gas pains. Women should be taught to avoid gas-forming foods, ice chips, carbonated beverages, and using a straw to drink beverages to help limit gas formation, thereby minimizing the severity of gas pains (see Patient Teaching box above).

Nurses must be alert to a woman's physiologic needs, managing care to ensure adequate rest and pain relief. Mother-baby care (couplet care) for a cesarean birth mother may have to be modified according to her physical limitations as a surgical patient.

Daily care includes perineal care, breast care, and routine hygienic care. The woman may shower after the original incisional dressing is removed, usually on the first postoperative day (if showering is acceptable according to the woman's cultural beliefs and practices).

The indwelling (Foley) catheter is also usually removed on the first postpartum day. The woman is encouraged to be out of bed and ambulating several times each day as soon as the urinary catheter is removed. Use of TED hose or SCD boots should continue as long as the woman remains in bed. They may be removed when she begins ambulating. The nurse assesses the woman's vital signs, incision, fundus, and lochia according to hospital policies, procedures, or protocols. Breath sounds, bowel sounds, circulatory status of lower extremities, and urinary and bowel elimination patterns also are assessed. It is important to observe maternal emotional status and progress of attachment to her baby.

⚡ SAFETY ALERT

The woman should be taught to seek assistance initially when getting out of bed, especially when an intravenous line and catheter are still in place. Thereafter, when rising from a supine position, she should sit on the side of the bed first to determine if dizziness will occur, then stand at the bedside, and finally ambulate.

During the postpartum period, the nurse can provide care that meets the psychologic and teaching needs of women who have had cesarean births. She or he can explain postpartum procedures to help the woman participate in her recovery from surgery. The nurse can help the woman plan care and visits from family and friends that will allow for adequate rest periods. Providing information on and assistance with infant care can facilitate adjustment to her role as a mother. With adequate support, these women can benefit from providing baby care to facilitate attachment and enhance involvement in newborn care. The woman is supported as she breastfeeds her baby by receiving individualized assistance to comfortably hold and position the baby at her breast. Use of the side-lying or football-hold positions and supporting the newborn with pillows can enhance comfort and facilitate successful breastfeeding. The partner can be included in infant teaching sessions and in explanations about the woman's recovery (Simpson, 2008).

⚡ SAFETY ALERT

When holding her baby or breastfeeding, a woman may become drowsy and even fall asleep because of the sedation that occurs with the use of analgesics. It is important that someone be with her during these times.

The couple also should be encouraged to express their feelings about the birth experience. Some parents are angry, frustrated, or disappointed that a vaginal birth was not possible. Some women express feelings of low self-esteem or a negative self-image. Others express relief and gratitude that the baby is healthy and safely born. It may be helpful for them to have the nurse who was present during the birth visit and help fill in "gaps" about the experience.

Discharge after cesarean birth is usually by the third postoperative day. The time is often determined by criteria established by the woman's insurance carrier or the federal government (e.g., diagnosis-related groups [DRGs]). The Newborn's and Mother's Health Protection Act of 1996 provides for a length of stay of up to 96 hours after cesarean birth. These criteria may not coincide with the woman's physical or psychosocial readiness for discharge. Some states have added home care provisions for mothers who meet appropriate criteria for discharge and choose to leave sooner than the allowed length of stay. This policy recognizes that home care is

PATIENT TEACHING

Signs of Postoperative Complications After Discharge Following Cesarean Birth

Report the following signs to your health care provider:
- Temperature exceeding 38° C (100.4° F)
- Urination: painful urination, urgency, cloudy urine
- Lochia: heavier than a normal menstrual period, clots, odor
- Cesarean incision: redness, swelling, bruising, foul-smelling discharge or bleeding, wound separation
- Severe, increasing abdominal pain

BOX 17-13   **SELECTION CRITERIA FOR VAGINAL BIRTH AFTER CESAREAN**

- One or two previous low-transverse cesarean births
- Clinically adequate pelvis
- No other uterine scars or history of previous rupture
- Physicians immediately available throughout active labor capable of monitoring labor and performing an emergency cesarean birth if necessary

Data from American College of Obstetricians and Gynecologists (ACOG): *Vaginal birth after previous cesarean delivery* (ACOG Practice Bulletin No. 115), Washington, DC, 2010, Author.

---

less costly than hospital care and in most cases is more beneficial for recovery.

The nurse provides discharge teaching to prepare the woman for self-care and newborn care in a limited amount of time while still trying to ensure that she is comfortable and able to rest. Discharge teaching and planning should include information about:

- Nutrition
- Measures to relieve pain and discomfort
- Exercise and specific activity restrictions
- Time management that includes periods of uninterrupted rest and sleep
- Hygiene, breast, and incision care
- Timing for resumption of sexual activity and contraception
- Signs of complications (see Patient Teaching box)
- Infant care

The woman's family and friends should be educated regarding her needs during the recovery process, and their assistance should be coordinated before discharge. Referral to support groups (e.g., www.birthrites.org) or to community agencies may be indicated to further promote the recovery process. A postdischarge program of telephone follow-up and home visits can facilitate the woman's full recovery after cesarean birth.

Trial of Labor

A trial of labor (TOL) is the observance of a woman and her fetus for a reasonable period (e.g., 4 to 6 hours) of spontaneous active labor to assess the safety of vaginal birth for the mother and infant. It may be initiated if the mother's pelvis is of questionable size or shape or if the fetus is in an abnormal presentation or position. By far the most common reason for a TOL is if the woman wishes to have a vaginal birth after a previous cesarean birth. A woman who has had a previous cesarean birth with a low transverse uterine incision may be a candidate for a TOL. Fetal sonography, maternal pelvimetry, or both may be done before a TOL to rule out CPD. During a TOL, the woman is evaluated for active labor, including adequate contractions, engagement and descent of the presenting part, and effacement and dilation of the cervix.

The nurse assesses maternal vital signs and FHR and pattern and is alert for signs of potential complications. If complications develop, the nurse is responsible for initiating appropriate actions, including notifying the primary health care provider, and for evaluating and documenting the maternal and fetal responses to the interventions. Nurses must recognize that the woman and her partner are often anxious about her health and well-being and that of their baby. Supporting and encouraging the woman and her partner and providing information regarding progress can reduce stress and enhance the labor process and facilitate a successful outcome.

 CRITICAL THINKING CASE STUDY

Trial of Labor for Vaginal Birth After Cesarean (TOL/VBAC)

Heather, a 28-year-old G2 P1 gave birth by cesarean during her last pregnancy. During her routine prenatal visit at 32 weeks of gestation, Heather tells the nurse that she really wants to have a vaginal birth this time. Heather asks, "What do you think? Can I try for a VBAC?"

1. Evidence—Is there sufficient evidence to advise Heather about the safety and feasibility of a trial of labor (TOL) for vaginal birth after cesarean (VBAC)?
2. Assumptions—Describe an underlying assumption about each of the following issues:
   a. Risks that Heather faces if she chooses a TOL for VBAC
   b. Criteria that must be met for Heather to attempt a TOL for VBAC
   c. Labor management practices that facilitate a successful VBAC
3. What implications and priorities for nursing care can be drawn at this time?
4. Does the evidence objectively support your argument (conclusion)?

Vaginal Birth After Cesarean

Indications for primary cesarean birth, such as dysfunctional labor, breech presentation, or abnormal FHR or patterns, often are non-recurring. Therefore a woman who has had a cesarean birth with a low transverse uterine incision may subsequently become pregnant, experience no contraindications to labor and vaginal birth during the pregnancy, and choose to attempt a VBAC. Box 17-13 lists selection criteria suggested by the ACOG for identifying candidates for VBAC. Women who succeed in having a VBAC and thus avoid major abdominal surgery have less hemorrhage, fewer infections, and a shorter recovery period than do women who give birth by repeat cesarean (ACOG, 2010). The major risk associated with VBAC is uterine rupture (Berghella and Landon, 2012). Other maternal risks include operative injury, blood transfusion, hysterectomy, endometritis, and maternal death (ACOG, 2010) (see Critical Thinking Case Study).

The overall VBAC success rate is approximately 60% to 80%. The strongest predictors for a successful VBAC are a prior vaginal birth and spontaneous (rather than induced or augmented) labor (ACOG, 2010). Women whose first cesarean birth was performed because of a nonrecurring indication (e.g., breech presentation) also are likely to have a successful VBAC (Berghella and Landon, 2012). Women with the following characteristics are less likely to have a successful VBAC (ACOG, 2010):

- Recurrent indication (e.g., labor dystocia) for initial cesarean birth
- Increased maternal age
- Non-Caucasian race or ethnicity
- Gestational age >40 weeks
- Maternal obesity
- Preeclampsia
- Short interpregnancy interval
- Increased neonatal birth weight

Women are most often the primary decision makers with regard to choice of birth method. During the antepartum period, the woman should be given information about VBAC and encouraged to choose it as an alternative to repeat cesarean birth, as long as no contraindications exist. VBAC support groups (e.g., www.vbac.com) and prenatal classes can help prepare the woman psychologically for labor and vaginal birth. Women need to believe not only that their efforts during a TOL will be successful but also that they are fully capable of doing what is necessary to give birth vaginally. They must be given the opportunity to discuss their previous labor experience, including feelings of failure and loss of control, and to express concern they may have about how they will manage during their upcoming labor and birth. Not everyone is enthusiastic about TOL and VBAC. After being fully informed about the benefits and risks, more than 25% of potential candidates choose to have a repeat cesarean birth instead (Thorp, 2009).

If a woman chooses TOL, attention should be paid to her psychologic as well as physical needs during the TOL. Anxiety increases the release of catecholamines and can inhibit the release of oxytocin, thus delaying the progress of labor and possibly leading to a repeat cesarean birth. To alleviate such anxiety, the nurse can encourage the woman to use breathing and relaxation techniques and to change positions to promote labor progress. The woman's partner can be encouraged to provide comfort measures and emotional support. Collaboration among the woman in labor, her partner, the nurse, and other health care providers often results in a successful VBAC. If a TOL does not result in vaginal birth, the woman will need support and encouragement to express her feelings about having another cesarean birth. It is very important that this outcome not be labeled a failed VBAC.

Since 1996, VBAC rates have been decreasing. Both medical and nonmedical factors have contributed to this decline. In March 2010, the Eunice Kennedy Shriver National Institute of Child Health and Human Development and the NIH convened a consensus development conference to examine issues related to VBAC. The statement produced by the panel of experts affirmed that TOL is a reasonable option for many women who have had a previous cesarean birth (Berghella and Landon, 2012).

The experts found, however, that many women who were appropriate candidates for TOL and VBAC lacked access to providers and health care facilities that were able and willing to offer this option. ACOG continues to recommend that TOL and VBAC be offered only in facilities that have staff immediately available to provide emergency care. Because resources for immediate cesarean birth may not be available in all birthing facilities, the best alternative in some situations may be to refer interested women to other facilities that have the obstetric, anesthetic, pediatric, and surgical staff necessary to offer TOL and VBAC (Berghella and Landon, 2012).

OBSTETRIC EMERGENCIES

Meconium-Stained Amniotic Fluid

Meconium-stained amniotic fluid indicates that the fetus has passed meconium (first stool) before birth. Meconium-stained amniotic fluid is green. The consistency of the amniotic fluid is often described as either thin (light) or thick (heavy), depending on the amount of meconium present. Three possible reasons for the passage of meconium are:

- It is a normal physiologic function that occurs with maturity (meconium passage being infrequent before weeks 23 or 24, with an increased incidence after 38 weeks) or with a breech presentation.
- It is the result of hypoxia-induced peristalsis and sphincter relaxation.
- It may be a sequel to umbilical cord compression–induced vagal stimulation in mature fetuses.

The major risk associated with meconium-stained amniotic fluid is the development of meconium aspiration syndrome (MAS) in the newborn. MAS causes a severe form of aspiration pneumonia that occurs most often in term or postterm infants who have passed meconium in utero. MAS most likely results from a long-standing intrauterine process rather than from aspiration immediately after birth as respirations are initiated (Rozance and Rosenberg, 2012).

Management

The presence of a team skilled in neonatal resuscitation is required at the birth of any infant with meconium-stained amniotic fluid. When meconium-stained amniotic fluid is present, the AAP and the AHA Neonatal Resuscitation Program no longer recommends routine suctioning of the newborn's mouth and nose on the perineum (after the head is out but before the rest of the baby is born) followed by endotracheal suctioning after birth. Instead, management of a newborn with meconium-stained amniotic fluid is based only on assessment of the baby's condition at birth. No clinical studies warrant basing tracheal suctioning guidelines simply on meconium consistency (AAP and AHA, 2011). See the Emergency box for specific interventions.

⚡ SAFETY ALERT

Every birth should be attended by at least one person whose only responsibility is the baby and who is capable of initiating resuscitation. Either that person or someone else who is immediately available should have the skills required to perform a complete resuscitation, including endotracheal suctioning to remove meconium, if necessary.

Shoulder Dystocia

Shoulder dystocia is an uncommon obstetric emergency that increases the risk for fetal and maternal morbidity and mortality during the attempt to accomplish birth vaginally. It is a condition in which the head is born but the anterior shoulder cannot pass under the pubic arch. It is estimated that 0.6% to 1.4% of all vaginal births are complicated by shoulder dystocia (Cunningham, Leveno, Bloom, et al., 2010). The incidence of shoulder dystocia has increased in recent years, perhaps because of larger birth weights or simply because more attention is now paid to documenting the condition (Cunningham, Leveno, Bloom, et al., 2010).

Fetopelvic disproportion related to excessive fetal size (more than 4000 g) or maternal pelvic abnormalities may be a cause of shoulder dystocia, although up to half of all cases of shoulder dystocia occur with smaller fetuses (Lanni and Seeds, 2012; Thorp, 2009). Other risk factors for shoulder dystocia include maternal diabetes (risk for macrosomia) and a history of shoulder dystocia with a previous birth. In half of all cases of shoulder dystocia, however, no risk factors are identified (Thorp, 2009). Shoulder

Immediate Management of the Newborn with Meconium-Stained Amniotic Fluid

Before Birth

- Assess the amniotic fluid for the presence of meconium after rupture of membranes.
- If the amniotic fluid is meconium stained, gather equipment and supplies that might be necessary for neonatal resuscitation.
- Have at least one person capable of performing endotracheal intubation on the baby present at the birth.

Immediately After Birth

- Assess the baby's respiratory efforts, heart rate, and muscle tone.
- Suction only the baby's mouth and nose, using either a bulb syringe or a large-bore suction catheter if the baby has:
  - Strong respiratory efforts
  - Good muscle tone
  - Heart rate >100 beats/min
- Suction the trachea using an endotracheal tube connected to a meconium aspiration device and suction source to remove any meconium present before many spontaneous respirations have occurred or assisted ventilation has been initiated if the baby has:
  - Depressed respirations
  - Decreased muscle tone
  - Heart rate <100 beats/min

Data from American Academy of Pediatrics (AAP) and American Heart Association (AHA): *Textbook of neonatal resuscitation,* ed 6, Elk Grove Village, IL, 2011, AAP.

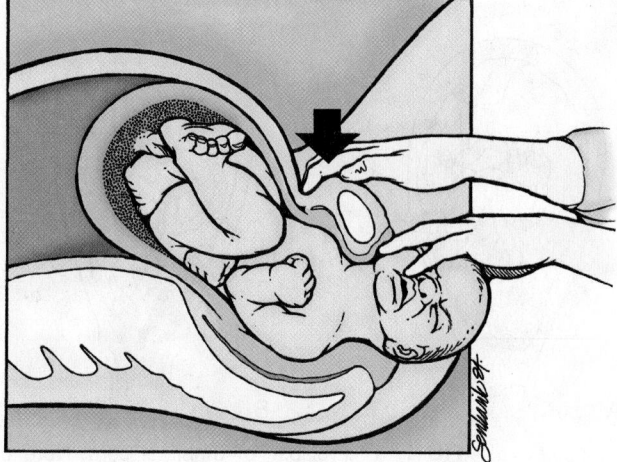

FIG 17-15 Application of suprapubic pressure. (From Gabbe S, Niebyl J, Simpson J: *Obstetrics: normal and problem pregnancies,* ed 5, Philadelphia, 2007, Churchill Livingstone.)

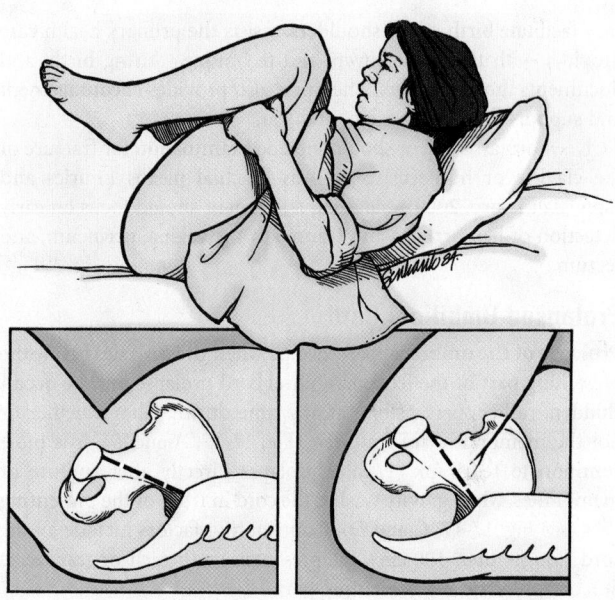

FIG 17-16 McRoberts maneuver. (From Gabbe SG, Niebyl J, Simpson J, et al: *Obstetrics: normal and problem pregnancies,* ed 6, Philadelphia, 2012, Saunders.)

dystocia cannot be accurately predicted or prevented (Cunningham, Leveno, Bloom, et al., 2010). Retraction of the fetal head against the perineum immediately after its emergence (turtle sign), however, is an early warning sign that birth of the shoulders may be difficult (Thorp, 2009).

Fetal injuries are usually caused either by asphyxia related to the delay in completing the birth or by trauma from the maneuvers used to accomplish the birth. Complications related to trauma include brachial plexus and phrenic nerve injuries and fracture of the humerus or clavicle. The most serious complication is brachial plexus injury (Erb palsy), which occurs in 10% to 20% of infants born following shoulder dystocia (Thorp, 2009). Evidence now exists that brachial plexus injuries may result from intrauterine forces during the second stage of labor rather than from the maneuvers used to accomplish birth (Lanni and Seeds, 2012). If brachial plexus injuries are recognized early and treated properly, 80% to 90% heal completely. Therefore permanent neurologic injury is rare. The major maternal complications associated with shoulder dystocia are postpartum hemorrhage and rectal injuries (Thorp, 2009).

Management

Many maneuvers and maternal position changes have been suggested and tried to free the anterior shoulder. Suprapubic pressure can be applied to the anterior shoulder (Fig. 17-15) in an attempt to push the shoulder under the symphysis pubis (Lanni and Seeds, 2012).

In the McRoberts maneuver (Fig. 17-16), the woman's legs are flexed apart with her knees on her abdomen (Lanni and Seeds, 2012). This maneuver causes the sacrum to straighten and the symphysis pubis to rotate toward the mother's head. The angle of pelvic

inclination is decreased, which frees the shoulder. Suprapubic pressure can be applied at this time. The McRoberts maneuver is the preferred method when a woman is receiving epidural anesthesia.

Having the woman move to a hands-and-knees position (the Gaskin maneuver) also has been used to resolve cases of shoulder dystocia. However, the Gaskin maneuver requires that the woman be mobile with no significant loss of motor function caused by regional anesthesia. Also, a wide and stable surface must be available (Lanni and Seeds, 2012).

Fundal pressure as a method of relieving shoulder dystocia should be avoided. Its use has been associated with neurologic complications (Gilbert, 2011).

When shoulder dystocia is diagnosed, the nurse should stay calm and immediately call for additional assistance (i.e., extra nurses, anesthesia care provider, and neonatal resuscitation team). The nurse then helps the woman assume the position or positions that

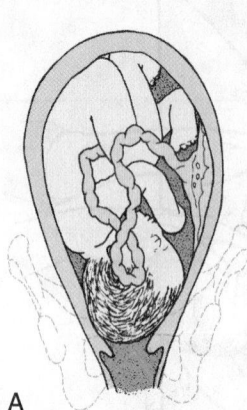 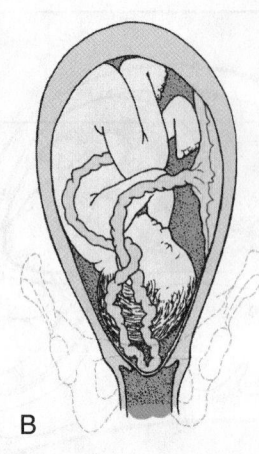 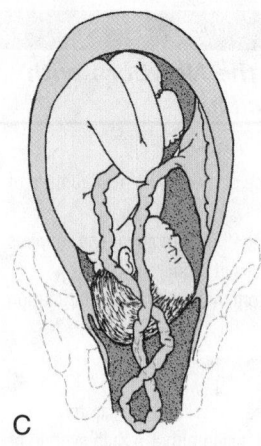 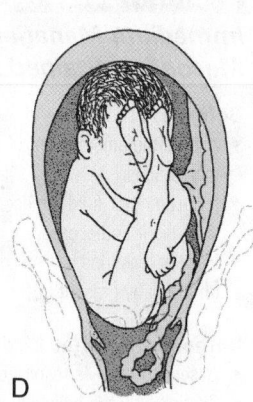

A   B   C   D

FIG 17-17 Prolapse of umbilical cord. Note pressure of presenting part on umbilical cord, which endangers fetal circulation. **A,** Occult (hidden) prolapse of cord. **B,** Complete prolapse of cord. Note that membranes are intact. **C,** Cord presenting in front of the fetal head may be seen in vagina. **D,** Frank breech presentation with prolapsed cord.

may facilitate birth of the shoulders, assists the primary health care provider with these maneuvers and techniques during birth, and documents the maneuvers. The nurse also provides encouragement and support to reduce anxiety and fear.

Newborn assessment should include examination for fracture of the clavicle or humerus as well as brachial plexus injuries and asphyxia (Thorp, 2009). Maternal assessment should focus on early detection of hemorrhage and trauma to the vagina, perineum, and rectum.

Prolapsed Umbilical Cord

Prolapse of the umbilical cord occurs when the cord lies below the presenting part of the fetus. Umbilical cord prolapse may be occult (hidden, rather than visible) at any time during labor whether or not the membranes are ruptured (Fig. 17-17, *A* and *B*). It is most common to see frank (visible) prolapse directly after rupture of membranes, when gravity washes the cord in front of the presenting part (see Fig. 17-17, *C* and *D*). Contributing factors include a long cord (longer than 100 cm), malpresentation (breech or transverse lie), or an unengaged presenting part.

If the presenting part does not fit snugly into the lower uterine segment (e.g., as in hydramnios), when the membranes rupture, a sudden gush of amniotic fluid may cause the cord to be displaced downward. Similarly, the cord may prolapse during amniotomy if the presenting part is high. A small fetus may not fit snugly into the lower uterine segment; as a result, cord prolapse is more likely to occur.

Management

Prompt recognition of a prolapsed umbilical cord is important because fetal hypoxia resulting from prolonged cord compression (i.e., occlusion of blood flow to and from the fetus for more than 5 minutes) usually results in central nervous system damage or death of the fetus. Pressure on the cord may be relieved by the examiner putting a sterile gloved hand into the vagina and holding the presenting part off the umbilical cord (Fig. 17-18, *A* and *B*). The woman may also be assisted into a position such as a modified Sims' (see Fig. 17-18, *C*), Trendelenburg, or knee-chest (see Fig. 17-18, *D*) position, in which gravity keeps the pressure of the presenting part off the cord. If the cervix is fully dilated, a forceps- or vacuum-assisted birth can be performed for the fetus in a cephalic presentation;

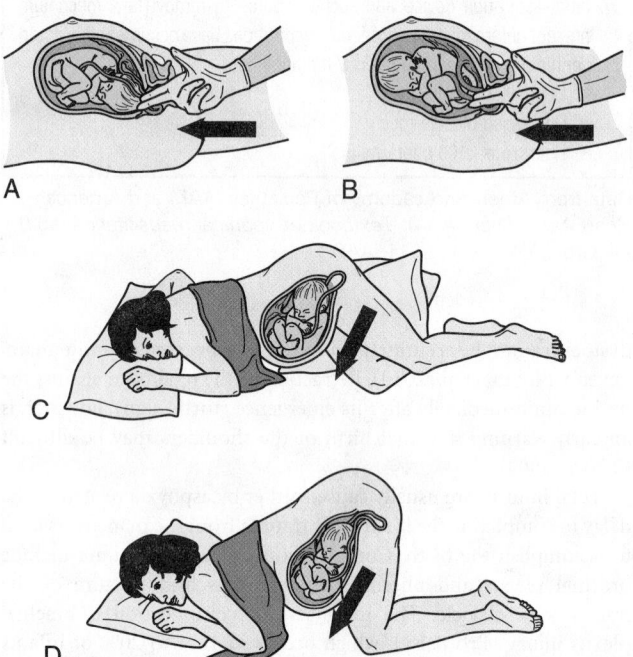

A   B

C

D

FIG 17-18 *Arrows* indicate direction of pressure against presenting part to relieve compression of prolapsed umbilical cord. Pressure exerted by examiner's fingers in **A,** vertex presentation, and **B,** breech presentation. **C,** Gravity relieves pressure when woman is in modified Sims' position with hips elevated as high as possible with pillows. **D,** Knee-chest position.

otherwise, a cesarean birth is likely to be performed. Abnormal FHR and pattern (e.g., bradycardia, absent or minimal variability, and variable or prolonged decelerations), inadequate uterine relaxation, and bleeding also can occur as a result of a prolapsed umbilical cord. Indications for immediate interventions are presented in the Emergency box. Ongoing assessment of the woman and her fetus is critical to determine the effectiveness of each action taken. The woman and her family are often aware of the seriousness of the situation; therefore the nurse must provide support by giving explanations for the interventions being implemented and their effect on the status of the fetus.

✚ EMERGENCY

Prolapsed Umbilical Cord

Signs
- Variable or prolonged deceleration during uterine contractions
- Woman reports feeling the cord after membranes rupture
- Cord is seen or felt in or protruding from the vagina

Interventions
- Call for assistance. Do not leave woman alone.
- Have someone notify the primary health care provider immediately.
- Glove the examining hand quickly and insert two fingers into the vagina to the cervix. With one finger on either side of the cord or both fingers to one side, exert upward pressure against the presenting part to relieve compression of the cord (see Fig. 17-18, *A* and *B*). Do *not* move your hand! Another person may place a rolled towel under the woman's right or left hip.
- Place woman into the extreme Trendelenburg or a modified Sims' position (see Fig. 17-18, *C*), or a knee-chest position (see Fig. 17-18, *D*).
- If cord is protruding from vagina, wrap loosely in a sterile towel saturated with warm sterile normal saline solution. Do not attempt to replace cord into cervix.
- Administer oxygen to the woman by nonrebreather mask at 8 to 10 L/min until birth is accomplished.
- Start intravenous (IV) fluids, or increase existing drip rate.
- Continue to monitor fetal heart rate (FHR) continuously, by internal fetal scalp electrode, if possible.
- Explain to woman and support person what is happening and the way it is being managed.
- Prepare for immediate vaginal birth if cervix is fully dilated, or cesarean birth if it is not.

Rupture of the Uterus

Rupture of the uterus, in which there is complete nonsurgical disruption of all uterine layers, is a rare but very serious obstetric injury that occurs in 1 in 2000 births (Francois and Foley, 2012). During labor and birth, the major risk factor for uterine rupture is a scarred uterus as a result of previous cesarean birth or other uterine surgery. Rupture usually occurs during a TOL for VBAC; symptomatic rupture is rarely observed in planned, repeat cesarean births. The likelihood of uterine rupture varies, depending on the type and location of the previous uterine incision. Uterine rupture occurs most often with a previous classic incision. Other factors that increase the risk for uterine rupture include multiple prior cesarean births, no previous vaginal births, induced or augmented labor, term gestation, multifetal gestation, fetal macrosomia, post-cesarean birth infection, and short interpregnancy interval (Berghella and Landon, 2012; Francois and Foley, 2012).

Uterine dehiscence, sometimes called *incomplete uterine rupture,* is separation of a prior scar. It may go unnoticed unless the woman undergoes a subsequent cesarean birth or other uterine surgery. The potential for maternal or fetal complications as a result of uterine dehiscence is negligible because separation of a prior scar does not result in hemorrhage (Berghella and Landon, 2012).

Signs and symptoms vary with the extent of the uterine rupture. The most common finding is an abnormal FHR tracing, particularly variable or prolonged decelerations or bradycardia. A loss of fetal station may also occur. The woman may experience constant abdominal pain, uterine tenderness, a change in uterine shape, and cessation of contractions (Berghella and Landon, 2012; Francois and

Foley, 2012). She may also exhibit signs of hypovolemic shock caused by hemorrhage (i.e., hypotension, tachypnea, pallor, and cool, clammy skin). If the placenta separates, the FHR will be absent. Fetal parts may be palpable through the abdomen.

Management

Prevention is the best treatment. Women who have had a classic uterine incision for cesarean birth are advised not to labor or attempt vaginal birth in subsequent pregnancies. Those at risk for uterine rupture are assessed closely during labor. Women whose labor is induced with oxytocin or prostaglandin (especially if their previous birth was cesarean) are monitored for signs of uterine tachysystole because this can precipitate uterine rupture. If tachysystole occurs, the oxytocin infusion is discontinued or decreased and a tocolytic medication may be given to decrease the intensity of the uterine contractions (see Emergency box on p. 467). After giving birth, the woman is assessed for excessive bleeding, especially if the fundus is firm and signs of hemorrhagic shock are present.

If rupture occurs, management depends on the severity. A small rupture may be managed with a laparotomy and birth of the infant, repair of the laceration, and blood transfusions, if needed. Hysterectomy may be necessary if the rupture is large and difficult to close or if the woman is hemodynamically unstable (Francois and Foley, 2012).

The nurse's role can include starting intravenous fluids, transfusing blood products, administering oxygen, and assisting with the preparation for immediate surgery. Supporting the woman's family and providing information about the treatment are important during this emergency. The associated fetal mortality rate is high (approximately 50% to 70%). Maternal morbidity and mortality also can be substantial (Cunningham, Leveno, Bloom, et al., 2010). Providing information about spiritual support services or suggesting that the family contact their own support system may be warranted.

Amniotic Fluid Embolus

Amniotic fluid embolus (AFE), also known as anaphylactoid syndrome of pregnancy, is a rare but devastating complication of pregnancy characterized by the sudden, acute onset of hypoxia, hypotension, cardiovascular collapse, and coagulopathy. The incidence of AFE in the United States is estimated at 1 in 8000 to 1 in 30,000 births. The true incidence is unknown because of the difficulty in confirming the diagnosis and inconsistent reporting of nonfatal cases (Jones and Clark, 2013).

AFE occurs during labor, during birth, or within 30 minutes after birth. This combination of sudden respiratory and cardiovascular collapse, along with coagulopathy, is similar to that observed in patients with anaphylactic or septic shock. In both conditions, a foreign substance is introduced into the circulation, resulting in disseminated intravascular coagulation, hypotension, and hypoxia (Martin and Foley, 2009).

In AFE, the foreign substance that initiates the condition is presumed to be present in amniotic fluid that is introduced into the maternal circulation. However, the exact factor that initiates AFE has not been identified. In the past, particles of fetal debris (e.g., vernix, hair, skin cells, or meconium) found in amniotic fluid were thought to be responsible for initiating the syndrome; however, fetal debris can be found in the pulmonary circulation of most normal laboring women. Also, fetal debris is identified in only 78% of women diagnosed with AFE. Therefore AFE is diagnosed clinically (Jones and Clark, 2013; Martin and Foley, 2009). Although AFE is rare, the mortality rate is 61% or higher (Martin and Foley, 2009). Neonatal outcome in cases of AFE is poor. If the event occurs before birth, the neonatal survival rate is approximately 80%. However, only half of these fetuses survive neurologically intact (Jones and Clark, 2013).

Maternal risk factors for AFE include advanced age, minority race, placenta previa, preeclampsia, and forceps-assisted or cesarean birth. Other factors commonly associated with the development of AFE are rapid labor and meconium staining (Cunningham, Leveno, Bloom, et al., 2010). Previously it was thought that the hypertonic uterine contractions that often accompany AFE actually caused the event. Instead, it appears that the physiologic response to AFE produces the hypertonic contractions (Jones and Clark, 2013).

Management

The immediate interventions for AFE are summarized in the Emergency box. Care must be instituted immediately. Cardiopulmonary resuscitation is often necessary. If cardiopulmonary arrest occurs, for optimal fetal survival, a perimortem cesarean birth should be accomplished within 5 minutes (Martin and Foley, 2009). The nurse's immediate responsibility is to assist with the resuscitation efforts.

If the woman survives, she is usually moved to a critical care unit. Additional interventions will likely include replacing blood and clotting factors and maintaining adequate hydration and blood pressure. The woman is usually placed on mechanical ventilation. Invasive hemodynamic monitoring may also be required (Martin and Foley, 2009).

Support of the woman's partner and family is necessary; they will be anxious and distressed. Brief explanations of what is happening are important during the emergency and can be reinforced after the immediate crisis is over. If the woman dies, emotional support and involvement of the agency's perinatal loss support team or other resource for grief counseling are needed. Later referral to community grief and loss support groups would be appropriate. The nursing staff also may need help in coping with feelings and emotions that result from a maternal death.

✚ EMERGENCY

Amniotic Fluid Embolus (Anaphylactoid Syndrome of Pregnancy)

Signs
- Respiratory Distress
  - Restlessness
  - Dyspnea
  - Cyanosis
  - Pulmonary edema
  - Respiratory arrest
- Circulatory Collapse
  - Hypotension
  - Tachycardia
  - Shock
  - Cardiac arrest
- Hemorrhage
  - Coagulation failure: bleeding from incisions, venipuncture sites, trauma (lacerations); petechiae, ecchymoses, purpura
  - Uterine atony

Interventions
- Oxygenate
  - Administer oxygen by nonrebreather facemask (8 to 10 L/min) or resuscitation bag delivering 100% oxygen.
  - Prepare for intubation and mechanical ventilation.
  - Initiate or assist with cardiopulmonary resuscitation. Tilt pregnant woman 30 degrees to side to displace uterus.
- Maintain Cardiac Output and Replace Fluid Losses
  - Position woman onto her side.
  - Administer IV fluids.
  - Administer blood products: packed cells, fresh-frozen plasma.
  - Insert indwelling catheter, and measure hourly urine output.
- Correct coagulation failure.
- Monitor fetal and maternal status.
- Prepare for emergency birth once woman's condition is stabilized.
- Provide emotional support to woman, her partner, and family.

█ KEY POINTS

- Preterm labor is uterine contractions with cervical change (e.g., effacement and dilation) that occurs between 20 and 37 completed weeks of pregnancy; preterm birth is any birth that occurs before the completion of 37 weeks of pregnancy.
- The incidence of preterm birth in the United States varies considerably by race.
- The cause of preterm labor is unknown and is assumed to be multifactorial.
- Because the onset of preterm labor can often be mistaken for normal discomforts of pregnancy, nurses should teach all pregnant women how to detect the early symptoms of preterm labor and to call their primary health care provider when symptoms occur.
- Bed rest, still a commonly prescribed intervention for preterm labor, has many deleterious side effects and has never been shown to decrease preterm birthrates; modified bed rest is recommended.
- The best reason to use tocolytic therapy is to achieve sufficient time to administer glucocorticoids in an effort to accelerate fetal

lung maturity and reduce the severity of respiratory complications in infants born preterm. In addition, time is allowed for transport of the woman before birth to a center equipped to care for preterm infants.
- If fetal or early neonatal death is expected, the parents and members of the health care team need to discuss the situation before the birth and decide on a management plan that is acceptable to everyone.
- Vigilance for signs of infection is an essential part of the care for women with preterm PROM.
- A postterm pregnancy poses a risk to both the mother and the fetus.
- Dysfunctional labor results from differences in the normal relationships among any of the five factors affecting labor and is characterized by differences in the pattern of progress in labor.
- Obese women are at risk for several complications during labor and birth, including cesarean birth. Even routine procedures require more time and effort to accomplish when the woman is obese.

- Labor should not be induced electively until the woman has reached at least 39 weeks of gestation.
- Cervical ripening using chemical or mechanical measures can increase the success of labor induction.
- Expectant parents benefit from learning about operative obstetrics (e.g., forceps- or vacuum-assisted or cesarean birth) during the prenatal period.
- The basic purpose of cesarean birth is to preserve the life and health of the mother and her fetus.
- Unless contraindicated, a vaginal birth may be possible after a previous cesarean birth.

- Labor management that emphasizes one-on-one support of the laboring woman by another woman (doula, nurse, or nurse-midwife) can reduce the rate of cesarean birth and increase the VBAC rate.
- Obstetric emergencies (e.g., meconium-stained amniotic fluid, shoulder dystocia, prolapsed cord, rupture of the uterus, and amniotic fluid embolism) occur rarely but require immediate intervention.

REFERENCES

American Academy of Pediatrics (AAP) and American College of Obstetricians and Gynecologists (ACOG): *Guidelines for perinatal care*, ed 7, Washington, DC, 2012, ACOG.

American Academy of Pediatrics (AAP) and American Heart Association (AHA): *Textbook of neonatal resuscitation*, ed 6, Elk Grove Village, IL, 2011, AAP.

American College of Obstetricians and Gynecologists (ACOG): *Induction of labor* (ACOG Practice Bulletin No. 107), Washington, DC, 2009, Author.

American College of Obstetricians and Gynecologists (ACOG): *Vaginal birth after previous cesarean delivery* (ACOG Practice Bulletin No. 115), Washington, DC, 2010, Author.

Berghella V, Landon M: Cesarean delivery. In Gabbe S, Niebyl J, Simpson J, et al, editors: *Obstetrics: normal and problem pregnancies*, ed 6, Philadelphia, 2012, Saunders.

Clark S, Simpson K, Knox G, et al: Oxytocin: new perspectives on an old drug, *Am J Obstet Gynecol* 200(1):35, e1–e6, 2009.

Collard T, Diallo H, Habinsky A, et al: Elective cesarean section: why women choose it and what nurses need to know, *Nurs Womens Health* 12(6):480–488, 2008/2009.

Craighead D: Early term birth: understanding the health risks to infants, *Nurs Womens Health* 16(2):136–144, 2012.

Cunningham F, Leveno K, Bloom S, et al: *Williams obstetrics*, ed 23, New York, 2010, McGraw-Hill.

Duff P: Maternal and perinatal infection—bacterial. In Gabbe S, Niebyl J, Simpson J, et al, editors: *Obstetrics: normal and problem pregnancies*, ed 6, Philadelphia, 2012, Saunders.

Duff P, Sweet R, Edwards R: Maternal and fetal infections. In Creasy R, Resnik R, Iams J, et al, editors: *Creasy and Resnik's maternal-fetal medicine: principles and practice*, ed 6, Philadelphia, 2009, Saunders.

Francois KE, Foley MR: Antepartum and postpartum hemorrhage. In Gabbe S, Niebyl J, Simpson J, et al, editors: *Obstetrics: normal and problem pregnancies*, ed 6, Philadelphia, 2012, Saunders.

Friedman E: Normal and dysfunctional labor. In Cohen W, Ackers D, Friedman E, editors: *Management of labor*, ed 6, Rockville, MD, 1989, Aspen.

Freda M: It's time for preconception health! *MCN Am J Matern Child Nurs* 31(6):346, 2006.

Gilbert E: *Manual of high risk pregnancy & delivery*, ed 5, St Louis, 2011, Mosby.

Hill W, Harvey C: Induction of labor. In Troiano N, Harvey C, Chez B, editors: *AWHONN's high risk & critical care obstetrics*, ed 3, Philadelphia, 2013, Wolters Kluwer/Lippincott Williams & Wilkins.

Iams J, Romero R, Creasy R: Preterm labor and birth. In Creasy R, Resnik R, Iams J, et al, editors: *Creasy and Resnik's maternal-fetal medicine: principles and practice*, ed 6, Philadelphia, 2009, Saunders.

Jones R, Clark S: Amniotic fluid embolus (anaphylactoid syndrome of pregnancy). In Troiano N, Harvey C, Chez B, editors: *AWHONN's high risk & critical care obstetrics*, ed 3, Philadelphia, 2013, Wolters Kluwer/Lippincott Williams & Wilkins.

Lanni S, Seeds J: Malpresentations and shoulder dystocia. In Gabbe S, Niebyl J, Simpson J, et al, editors: *Obstetrics: normal and problem pregnancies*, ed 6, Philadelphia, 2012, Saunders.

Macones G, Hankins G, Spong C, et al: The 2008 National Institute of Child Health and Human Development workshop report on electronic fetal monitoring: update on definitions, interpretation, and research guidelines, *J Obstet Gynecol Neonatal Nurs* 37(5):510–515, 2008.

Mahlmeister L: Best practices in perinatal care: evidence-based management of oxytocin induction and augmentation of labor, *J Perinat Neonatal Nurs* 22(4):259–263, 2008.

Malone FD, D'Alton ME: Multiple gestation: clinical characteristics and management. In Creasy R, Resnik R, Iams J, et al, editors: *Creasy and Resnik's maternal-fetal medicine: principles and practice*, ed 6, Philadelphia, 2009, Saunders.

Martin S, Foley M: Intensive care monitoring of the critically ill pregnant patient. In Creasy R, Resnik R, Iams J, et al, editors: *Creasy and Resnik's maternal-fetal medicine: principles*

and practice, ed 6, Philadelphia, 2009, Saunders.

Martin J, Hamilton B, Sutton P, et al: Births: final data for 2010, *Natl Vital Stat Rep* 61(1):1–100, 2012.

Mercer B: Assessment and induction of fetal pulmonary maturity. In Creasy R, Resnik R, Iams J, et al, editors: *Creasy and Resnik's maternal-fetal medicine: principles and practice*, ed 6, Philadelphia, 2009a, Saunders.

Mercer B: Premature rupture of the membranes. In Creasy R, Resnik R, Iams J, et al, editors: *Creasy and Resnik's maternal-fetal medicine: principles and practice*, ed 6, Philadelphia, 2009b, Saunders.

Mercer B: Premature rupture of the membranes. In Gabbe S, Niebyl J, Simpson J, et al, editors: *Obstetrics: normal and problem pregnancies*, ed 6, Philadelphia, 2012, Saunders.

Moleti C: Trends and controversies in labor induction, *MCN Am J Matern Child Nurs* 34(1):40–47, 2009.

Nielsen P, Galan H: Operative vaginal delivery. In Gabbe S, Niebyl J, Simpson J, et al, editors: *Obstetrics: normal and problem pregnancies*, ed 6, Philadelphia, 2012, Saunders.

Newman R, Unal E: Multiple gestations. In Gabbe S, Niebyl J, Simpson J, et al, editors: *Obstetrics: normal and problem pregnancies*, ed 6, Philadelphia, 2012, Saunders.

Picklesimer A, Dorman K: Maternal obesity: effects on pregnancy. In Troiano N, Harvey C, Chez B, editors: *AWHONN's high risk & critical care obstetrics*, ed 3, Philadelphia, 2013, Wolters Kluwer/Lippincott Williams & Wilkins.

Rampersad R, Macones G: Prolonged and postterm pregnancy. In Gabbe S, Niebyl J, Simpson J, et al, editors: *Obstetrics: normal and problem pregnancies*, ed 6, Philadelphia, 2012, Saunders.

Resnik J, Resnik R: Post-term pregnancy. In Creasy R, Resnik R, Iams J, et al, editors: *Creasy and Resnik's maternal-fetal medicine: principles and practice*, ed 6, Philadelphia, 2009, Saunders.

Roberts C, Mangan S: Special delivery: know the risks of cesarean section, *OR Nurse* 3(2):22–30, 2009.

Romero R, Lockwood C: Pathogenesis of spontaneous preterm labor. In Creasy R, Resnik R, Iams J, et al, editors: *Creasy and Resnik's maternal-fetal medicine: principles and practice*, ed 6, Philadelphia, 2009, Saunders.

Rozance P, Rosenberg A: The neonate. In Gabbe S, Niebyl J, Simpson J, et al, editors: *Obstetrics: normal and problem pregnancies*, ed 6, Philadelphia, 2012, Saunders.

Simhan H, Iams J, Romero R: Preterm birth. In Gabbe S, Niebyl J, Simpson J, et al, editors: *Obstetrics: normal and problem pregnancies*, ed 6, Philadelphia, 2012, Saunders.

Simpson K: Labor and birth. In Simpson K, Creehan P, editors: *AWHONN's perinatal nursing*, ed 3, Philadelphia, 2008, Lippincott Williams & Wilkins.

Simpson K: Clinicians' guide to the use of oxytocin for labor induction and augmentation, *J Midwifery Womens Health* 56(3):214–221, 2011.

Simpson K, Knox G: Oxytocin as a high-alert medication: implications for perinatal patient safety, *MCN Am J Matern Child Nurs* 34(1):8–15, 2009.

Thorp JM: Clinical aspects of normal and abnormal labor. In Creasy R, Resnik R, Iams J, et al, editors: *Creasy and Resnik's maternal-fetal medicine: principles and practice*, ed 6, Philadelphia, 2009, Saunders.

Walters M, Taylor J: Maternal obesity: consequences and prevention strategies, *Nurs Womens Health* 13(6):486–494, 2009/2010.

Wing D, Farinelli C: Abnormal labor and induction of labor. In Gabbe S, Niebyl J, Simpson J, et al, editors: *Obstetrics: normal and problem pregnancies*, ed 6, Philadelphia, 2012, Saunders.

Maternal Physiologic Changes

Kathryn R. Alden

LEARNING OBJECTIVES

On completion of this chapter, the reader will be able to:
- Describe the anatomic and physiologic changes that occur during the postpartum period.
- Discuss characteristics of uterine involution and lochial flow and describe ways to measure them.

- List expected values for vital signs and blood pressure, deviations from normal findings, and probable causes of the deviations.

The postpartum period is the interval between the birth of the newborn and the return of the reproductive organs to their normal nonpregnant state. This period is sometimes referred to as the puerperium, or **fourth trimester of pregnancy**. Although the **puerperium** has traditionally been considered to last 6 weeks, this time frame varies among women. The physiologic changes that occur during the reversal of the processes of pregnancy are distinctive, but they are normal. To provide care during the recovery period that is beneficial to the mother, her infant, and her family, the nurse must synthesize knowledge of maternal anatomy and physiology of the recovery period, the newborn's physical and behavioral characteristics, infant care activities, and the family response to the birth of the infant. This chapter focuses on anatomic and physiologic changes that occur in the mother during the postpartum period.

REPRODUCTIVE SYSTEM AND ASSOCIATED STRUCTURES

Uterus

Involution Process

The return of the uterus to a nonpregnant state after birth is called **involution**. This process begins immediately after expulsion of the placenta with contraction of the uterine smooth muscle.

At the end of the third stage of labor, the uterus is in the midline, approximately 2 cm below the level of the umbilicus, with the fundus resting on the sacral promontory. At this time, the uterus weighs approximately 1000 g (Cunningham, Leveno, Bloom, et al., 2010).

Within 12 hours, the fundus can rise to approximately 1 cm above the umbilicus (Fig. 18-1). By 24 hours after birth, the uterus is about the same size as it was at 20 weeks of gestation. Involution progresses rapidly during the next few days. The fundus descends 1 to 2 cm every 24 hours. By the sixth postpartum day, the fundus is normally located halfway between the umbilicus and the symphysis pubis. The uterus should not be palpable abdominally after 2 weeks and should have returned to its nonpregnant location by 6 weeks after birth (Blackburn, 2013).

The uterus, which at full term weighs approximately 11 times its prepregnancy weight, involutes to approximately 500 g by 1 week after birth and to 350 g by 2 weeks after birth. At 6 weeks postpartum, it weighs 60 to 80 g.

Increased estrogen and progesterone levels are responsible for stimulating the massive growth of the uterus during pregnancy. Prenatal uterine growth results from both hyperplasia (an increase in the number of muscle cells) and hypertrophy (an enlargement of the existing cells). After birth, the decrease in these hormones causes *autolysis*—the self-destruction of excess hypertrophied tissue. The additional cells laid down during pregnancy remain and account for the slight increase in uterine size after each pregnancy.

Subinvolution is the failure of the uterus to return to a nonpregnant state. The most common causes of subinvolution are retained placental fragments and infection (see Chapter 21).

Contractions

Postpartum hemostasis is achieved primarily by compression of intramyometrial blood vessels as the uterine muscle contracts rather than by platelet aggregation and clot formation. The hormone

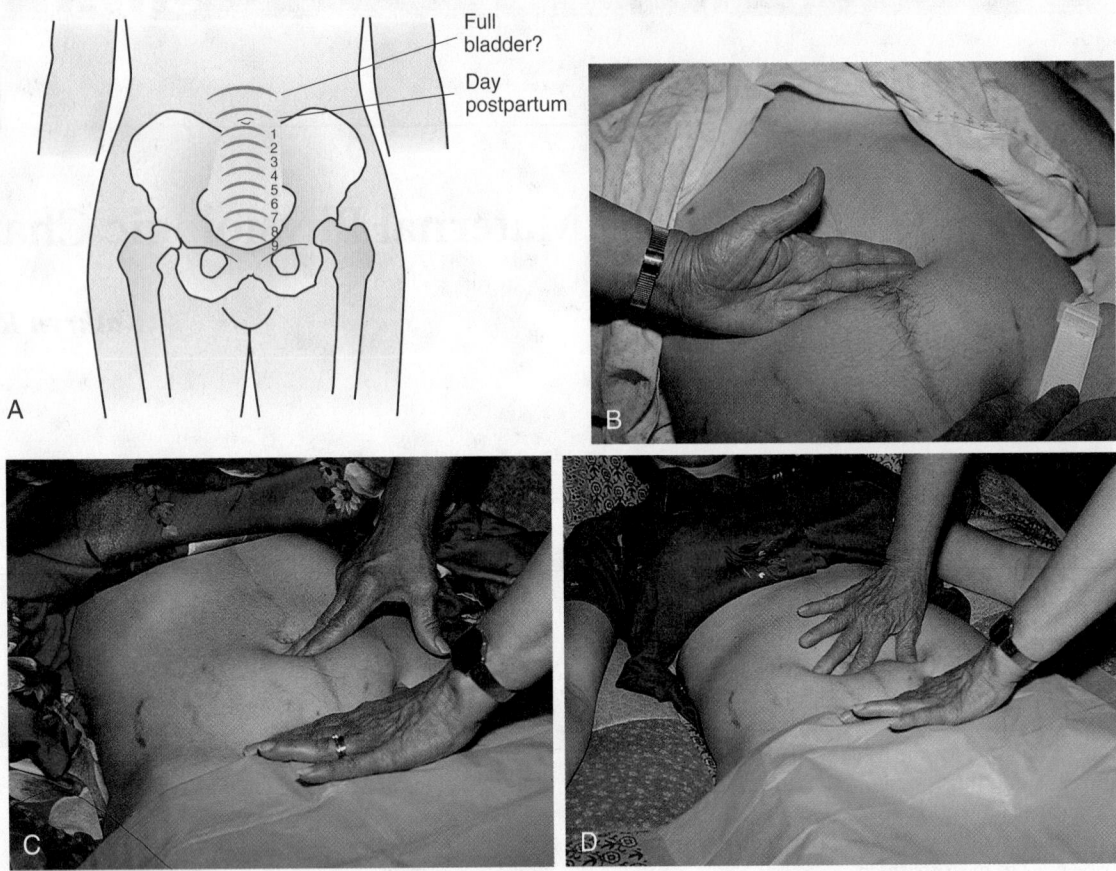

FIG 18-1 Assessment of involution of uterus after childbirth. **A,** Normal progress, days 1 through 9. **B,** Size and position of uterus 2 hours after childbirth. **C,** Two days after childbirth. **D,** Four days after childbirth. (*B* through *D*, Courtesy Marjorie Pyle, RNC, Lifecircle, Costa Mesa, CA.)

oxytocin, released from the pituitary gland, strengthens and coordinates these uterine contractions, which compress blood vessels and promote hemostasis. During the first 1 to 2 postpartum hours, uterine contractions may decrease in intensity and become uncoordinated. Because it is vital that the uterus remain firm and well contracted, exogenous oxytocin (Pitocin) is usually administered intravenously or intramuscularly immediately after expulsion of the placenta. The uterus is very sensitive to oxytocin during the first week or so after birth. Breastfeeding immediately after birth and in the early days postpartum increases the release of oxytocin, which decreases blood loss and reduces the risk for postpartum hemorrhage (Lawrence and Lawrence, 2011).

Afterpains

In first-time mothers, uterine tone is good, the fundus generally remains firm, and the woman usually perceives only mild uterine cramping. Periodic relaxation and vigorous contractions are more common in subsequent pregnancies and may cause uncomfortable cramping called **afterpains** (afterbirth pains), which typically resolve in 3 to 7 days. Afterpains are more noticeable after births in which the uterus was overdistended (e.g., macrosomic infant, multifetal gestation, polyhydramnios). Breastfeeding and exogenous oxytocic medication usually intensify these afterpains because both stimulate uterine contractions.

Placental Site

Immediately after the placenta and membranes are expelled, vascular constriction and thromboses reduce the placental site to an irregular nodular and elevated area. Upward growth of the endometrium causes sloughing of necrotic tissue and prevents the scar formation characteristic of normal wound healing. This unique healing process enables the endometrium to resume its usual cycle of changes and permit implantation and placentation in future pregnancies. Endometrial regeneration is completed by postpartum day 16, except at the placental site. Regeneration at the placental site usually is not complete until 6 weeks after birth (Blackburn, 2013).

Lochia

Postbirth uterine discharge, commonly called **lochia,** initially is bright red (lochia rubra) and may contain small clots. For the first 2 hours after birth, the amount of uterine discharge should be about that of a heavy menstrual period. After that time, the lochial flow should steadily decrease.

Lochia rubra consists mainly of blood and decidual and trophoblastic debris. The flow pales, becoming pink or brown (lochia serosa) after 3 to 4 days. Lochia serosa consists of old blood, serum, leukocytes, and tissue debris. The median duration of lochia serosa discharge is 22 to 27 days (Katz, 2012). In most women, about 10 days after childbirth the drainage becomes yellow to white (lochia alba). Lochia alba consists of leukocytes, decidua, epithelial cells, mucus, serum, and bacteria. Lochia may continue for 2 to 6 weeks after the birth but may last longer and still be normal. Thus lochia persists up to 4 to 8 weeks after birth (Cunningham, Leveno, Bloom, et al., 2010).

If the woman receives an oxytocic medication, regardless of the route of administration, the flow of lochia is often scant until the

Lochial Bleeding
- Lochia usually trickles from the vaginal opening. The steady flow is greater as the uterus contracts.
- A gush of lochia may result as the uterus is massaged. If it is dark in color, it has been pooled in the relaxed vagina, and the amount soon lessens to a trickle of bright red lochia (in the early puerperium).

Nonlochial Bleeding
- If the bloody discharge spurts from the vagina, there can be cervical or vaginal tears in addition to the normal lochia.
- If the amount of bleeding continues to be excessive and bright red, a tear can be the source.

effects of the medication wear off. The amount of lochia is usually less after a cesarean birth because the surgeon suctions the blood and fluids from the uterus or wipes the uterine lining before closing the incision. Flow of lochia usually increases with ambulation and breastfeeding. Lochia tends to pool in the vagina when the woman is lying in bed; the woman then may experience a gush of blood when she stands. This gush should not be confused with hemorrhage.

Persistence of lochia rubra early in the postpartum period suggests continued bleeding as a result of retained fragments of the placenta or membranes. Recurrence of bleeding 7 to 14 days after birth is from the healing placental site. About 10% to 15% of women will still be having normal lochia serosa discharge at their 6-week postpartum examination (Katz, 2012). However, in most women, the continued flow of lochia serosa or lochia alba by 3 to 4 weeks after birth can indicate endometritis, particularly if fever, pain, or abdominal tenderness is associated with the discharge. Lochia should smell like normal menstrual flow; an offensive odor usually indicates infection.

Not all postpartal vaginal bleeding is lochia; vaginal bleeding after birth may be caused by unrepaired vaginal or cervical lacerations. Box 18-1 distinguishes between lochial and nonlochial bleeding.

Cervix

The cervix is soft immediately after birth. The ectocervix (portion of the cervix that protrudes into the vagina) appears bruised and has some small lacerations—optimal conditions for the development of infection. Over the next 12 to 18 hours, it shortens and becomes firmer. The cervical os, which dilated to 10 cm during labor, closes gradually. Within 2 to 3 days postpartum, it has shortened, become firm, and regained its form. The cervix up to the lower uterine segment remains edematous, thin, and fragile for several days after birth. By the second or third postpartum day, the cervix is dilated 2 to 3 cm, and by 1 week after birth, it is approximately 1 cm dilated (Blackburn, 2013). The external cervical os never regains its prepregnancy appearance; it no longer has a circular shape but, instead, appears as a jagged slit often described as a "fish mouth" (see Fig. 7-2). Lactation delays the production of cervical and other estrogen-influenced mucus and mucosal characteristics.

Vagina and Perineum

Postpartum estrogen deprivation is responsible for the thinness of the vaginal mucosa and the absence of rugae. The greatly distended, smooth-walled vagina gradually decreases in size and regains tone, although it never completely returns to its prepregnancy state (Cunningham, Leveno, Bloom, et al., 2010). Rugae reappear within 3 weeks, but they are never as prominent as they are in the nulliparous woman. Most rugae are permanently flattened. The hymen remains as small tags of tissue that scar and form the myrtiform caruncles. The mucosa remains atrophic in the lactating woman, at least until menstruation resumes. Thickening of the vaginal mucosa occurs with the return of ovarian function. Estrogen deficiency is responsible for a decreased amount of vaginal lubrication. Localized dryness and coital discomfort (dyspareunia) can persist until ovarian function returns and menstruation resumes. The use of a water-soluble lubricant during sexual intercourse is usually recommended.

Immediately after birth, the introitus is erythematous and edematous, especially in the area of the episiotomy or laceration repair. It is barely distinguishable from that of a nulliparous woman if lacerations and an episiotomy have been carefully repaired, hematomas are prevented or treated early, and the woman practices good hygiene during the first 2 weeks after birth.

Most episiotomies and laceration repairs are visible only if the woman is lying on her side with her upper buttock raised or if she is placed in the lithotomy position. A good light source is essential for visualization of some repairs. Healing of an episiotomy or laceration is the same way as that of any surgical incision. Signs of infection (pain, redness, warmth, swelling, or discharge) or loss of approximation (separation of the edges of the incision) may occur. Initial healing occurs within 2 to 3 weeks, but 4 to 6 months can be required for the repair to heal completely (Blackburn, 2013). If forceps were used for the birth, the woman may have experienced vaginal or cervical lacerations; hematomas of the pelvic soft tissues can also occur with forceps-assisted birth (see Chapter 17).

Hemorrhoids (anal varicosities) are commonly seen (see Fig. 7-10). Internal hemorrhoids can evert while the woman is pushing during birth. Women often experience associated symptoms such as itching, discomfort, and bright red bleeding upon defecation. Hemorrhoids usually decrease in size within 6 weeks of childbirth.

Pelvic Muscular Support

The supporting structure of the uterus and vagina can be injured during childbirth and contributes to later gynecologic problems. Supportive tissues of the pelvic floor that are torn or stretched during childbirth can require up to 6 months to regain tone. Kegel exercises, which help strengthen perineal muscles and encourage healing, are recommended after childbirth (see Guidelines box, p. 57). Later in life, women can experience pelvic relaxation—the lengthening and weakening of the fascial supports of pelvic structures. These structures include the uterus, upper posterior vaginal wall, urethra, bladder, and rectum. Although relaxation can occur in any woman, it is commonly a direct but delayed complication of childbirth.

ABDOMEN

When the woman stands during the first days after birth, her abdomen protrudes and gives her a still-pregnant appearance. During the first 2 weeks after birth, the abdominal wall is relaxed. It takes about 6 weeks for the abdominal wall to return almost to its prepregnancy state (Fig. 18-2). The skin regains most of its previous elasticity, but some striae may persist. The return of muscle tone depends on previous tone, proper exercise, and the amount of adipose tissue. Occasionally, with or without overdistention because of a large fetus or multiple fetuses, the abdominal wall muscles separate, a condition termed *diastasis recti abdominis* (see Fig. 7-13, *B*).

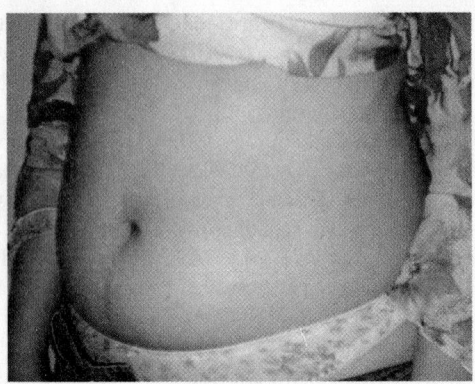

FIG 18-2 Abdominal wall 6 weeks after vaginal birth is almost back to prepregnancy appearance. Note that the linea nigra is still visible. (Courtesy Jodi Brackett, Phoenix, AZ.)

Persistence of this separation may be disturbing to the woman, but surgical correction rarely is necessary. With time, the separation becomes less apparent.

ENDOCRINE SYSTEM

Placental Hormones

Significant hormonal changes occur during the postpartal period. Expulsion of the placenta results in dramatic decreases of the hormones produced by that organ. Decreases in human chorionic somatomammotropin (also called *human placental lactogen*), estrogens, cortisol, and the placental enzyme *insulinase* reverse the diabetogenic effects of pregnancy, resulting in significantly lower blood glucose levels in the immediate puerperium. Mothers with type 1 diabetes will likely require much less insulin for several days after birth. Because these normal hormonal changes make the puerperium a transitional period for carbohydrate metabolism, it is more difficult to interpret glucose tolerance tests at this time.

Estrogen and progesterone levels drop markedly after expulsion of the placenta and reach their lowest levels 1 week after birth. Decreased estrogen levels are associated with the diuresis of excess extracellular fluid accumulated during pregnancy. In nonlactating women, estrogen levels begin to increase by 2 weeks after birth and by postpartum day 17 are higher than in women who breastfeed (Katz, 2012).

Human chorionic gonadotropin (hCG) disappears fairly quickly from maternal circulation. However, because removing hCG from the extravascular and intracellular spaces takes additional time, the hormone can be detected in the maternal system for 3 to 4 weeks after birth (Blackburn, 2013).

Pituitary Hormones and Ovarian Function

Prolactin levels in blood rise progressively throughout pregnancy. After birth, as levels of estrogen and progesterone decrease, prolactin levels increase. In women who breastfeed, prolactin levels are highest during the first month after birth and remain elevated above nonpregnant levels as long as the woman is breastfeeding. Serum prolactin levels are influenced by the frequency of breastfeeding, the duration of each feeding, and the degree to which supplementary feedings are used. Individual differences in the strength of an infant's sucking stimulus also affect prolactin levels. In nonlactating women, prolactin levels decline after birth and reach the prepregnant range by the third postpartum week (Katz, 2012).

Lactating and nonlactating women differ considerably in the timing of their first ovulation and when menstruation resumes.

Ovulation occurs as early as 27 days after birth in nonlactating women, with a mean time of about 7 to 9 weeks. About 70% of nonbreastfeeding women resume menstruating by 12 weeks after birth. The mean time to ovulation in women who breastfeed is about 6 months (Katz, 2012). The persistence of elevated serum prolactin levels in breastfeeding women appears to be responsible for suppressing ovulation. In lactating women, both the resumption of ovulation and the return of menses are determined in large part by breastfeeding patterns. For example, ovulation is delayed longer in women who breastfeed exclusively compared with women who breastfeed and offer supplemental infant formula to their infants. Because of the uncertainty about the return of ovulation and menstruation, discussion of contraceptive options early in the puerperium is necessary. The first menstrual flow after childbirth is usually heavier than normal. Within three or four cycles, the amount of menstrual flow returns to the woman's prepregnancy volume.

URINARY SYSTEM

The hormonal changes of pregnancy (i.e., high steroid levels) contribute to an increase in renal function; diminishing steroid levels after childbirth may partly explain the reduced renal function that occurs during the puerperium. Kidney function returns to normal within 1 month after birth. About 6 weeks are required for the pregnancy-induced hypotonia and dilation of the ureters and renal pelves to return to the nonpregnant state (Cunningham, Leveno, Bloom, et al., 2010). In a small percentage of women, dilation of the urinary tract can persist for 3 months or longer, increasing the chances of developing a urinary tract infection.

Urine Components

The renal glycosuria induced by pregnancy disappears by 1 week postpartum, but lactosuria may occur in lactating women. The blood urea nitrogen increases during the puerperium as autolysis of the involuting uterus occurs. Pregnancy-associated proteinuria resolves by 6 weeks after birth (Blackburn, 2013). Ketonuria may occur in women with an uncomplicated birth or after a prolonged labor with dehydration.

Postpartal Fluid Loss

Within 12 hours of birth, women begin to lose excess tissue fluid accumulated during pregnancy. Profuse diaphoresis often occurs, especially at night, for the first 2 or 3 days after childbirth. Postpartal diuresis, caused by decreased estrogen levels, removal of increased venous pressure in the lower extremities, and loss of the remaining pregnancy-induced increase in blood volume, also aids the body in ridding itself of excess fluid. Fluid loss through perspiration and increased urinary output accounts for a weight loss of approximately 2.25 kg during the puerperium.

Urethra and Bladder

Birth-induced trauma, increased bladder capacity after childbirth, and the effects of conduction anesthesia combine to cause a decreased urge to void. In addition, pelvic soreness caused by the forces of labor, vaginal lacerations, or the episiotomy reduces or alters the voiding reflex. Decreased voiding combined with postpartal diuresis can result in bladder distention.

Immediately after birth, excessive bleeding can occur if the bladder becomes distended because it pushes the uterus up and to the side and prevents it from contracting firmly. Later in the puerperium, overdistention can make the bladder more susceptible to infection and impede the resumption of normal voiding (Cunningham,

Leveno, Bloom, et al., 2010). With adequate emptying of the bladder, bladder tone is usually restored by 5 to 7 days after childbirth.

GASTROINTESTINAL SYSTEM

Appetite

The mother usually is hungry shortly after birth and can tolerate a light diet. Most new mothers are very hungry after full recovery from analgesia, anesthesia, and fatigue. Requests for extra portions of food and frequent snacks are common.

Bowel Evacuation

A spontaneous bowel evacuation may not occur for 2 to 3 days after childbirth. This delay can be explained by decreased muscle tone in the intestines during labor and the immediate puerperium, prelabor diarrhea, lack of food, or dehydration. The mother often anticipates discomfort during the bowel movement because of perineal tenderness as a result of an episiotomy, lacerations, or hemorrhoids and resists the urge to defecate. Regular bowel habits should be reestablished when bowel tone returns.

Third- and fourth-degree perineal lacerations that involve the anal sphincter are associated with an increased risk for postpartum anal incontinence. Women with this problem are more often incontinent of flatus than of stool. If anal incontinence lasts more than 6 months, studies should be conducted to determine the specific cause and appropriate treatment (Katz, 2012).

BREASTS

Promptly after birth, a decrease occurs in the concentrations of hormones (i.e., estrogen, progesterone, human chorionic gonadotropin, prolactin, cortisol, and insulin) that stimulated breast development during pregnancy. The time required for these hormones to return to prepregnancy levels is determined in part by whether the mother breastfeeds her infant.

Breastfeeding Mothers

During the first 24 hours after birth, there is little, if any, change in the breast tissue. Colostrum or early milk, a clear, yellow fluid, may be expressed from the breasts. The breasts gradually become fuller and heavier as the colostrum transitions to mature milk by about 72 to 96 hours after birth; this is often referred to as the "milk coming in." The breasts can feel warm, firm, and somewhat tender. Bluish white milk with a skim-milk appearance (true milk) can be expressed from the nipples. As milk glands and milk ducts fill with milk, breast tissue can feel somewhat nodular or lumpy. Unlike the lumps associated with fibrocystic breast changes or cancer (which can be palpated consistently in the same location), the nodularity associated with milk production tends to shift in position. Some women experience engorgement, but with frequent breastfeeding and proper care, this is a temporary condition that typically lasts only 24 to 48 hours (see Chapter 24).

Nonbreastfeeding Mothers

The breasts generally feel nodular in contrast to the granular feel of breasts in nonpregnant women. The nodularity is bilateral and diffuse. Prolactin levels drop rapidly. Colostrum is present for the first few days after childbirth. Palpation of the breast on the second or third day as milk production begins may reveal tissue tenderness in some women. On the third or fourth postpartum day, engorgement can occur. The breasts are distended (swollen), firm, tender, and warm to the touch. Breast distention is caused primarily by the temporary congestion of veins and lymphatics rather than by an accumulation of milk. Milk is present but should not be expressed. Axillary breast tissue (the tail of Spence) and any accessory breast or nipple tissue along the milk line can be involved. Engorgement resolves spontaneously, and discomfort decreases usually within 24 to 36 hours. A breast binder or well-fitted supportive bra, ice packs, fresh cabbage leaves, and/or mild analgesics may be used to relieve discomfort. Nipple stimulation is avoided. If suckling or milk expression is never begun (or is discontinued), lactation ceases within a few days to a week.

CARDIOVASCULAR SYSTEM

Blood Volume

Changes in blood volume after birth depend on several factors, such as blood loss during childbirth and the amount of extravascular water (physiologic edema) mobilized and excreted. Pregnancy-induced hypervolemia (an increase in blood volume to 40% to 45% above nonpregnancy levels [Cunningham, Leveno, Bloom, et al., 2010]) allows most women to tolerate considerable blood loss during childbirth. The average blood loss for a vaginal birth of a single fetus ranges from 300 mL to 500 mL (10% of blood volume). The typical blood loss for women who give birth by cesarean is 500 mL to 1000 mL (15% to 30% of blood volume). During the first few days after birth, the plasma volume decreases further as a result of diuresis (Blackburn, 2013).

The woman's response to blood loss during the early puerperium differs from that in a nonpregnant woman. Three postpartum physiologic changes protect the woman by increasing the circulating blood volume: (1) elimination of uteroplacental circulation reduces the size of the maternal vascular bed by 10% to 15%; (2) loss of placental endocrine function removes the stimulus for vasodilation; and (3) mobilization of extravascular water stored during pregnancy occurs. By the third postpartum day, the plasma volume has been replenished as extravascular fluid returns to the intravascular space (Katz, 2012) (see Critical Thinking Exercise).

Cardiac Output

Pulse rate, stroke volume, and cardiac output increase throughout pregnancy. Cardiac output remains increased for at least 48 hours after birth because of an increase in stroke volume. This increased stroke volume is caused by the return of blood to the maternal systemic venous circulation, a result of rapid decrease in uterine blood flow and mobilization of extravascular fluid (Monga, 2009). Stroke volume, cardiac output, end-diastolic volume, and systemic vascular resistance remain elevated over nonpregnant values for 12 weeks after birth and may not stabilize until 24 weeks after birth (Monga, 2009).

Vital Signs

Few alterations in vital signs are seen under normal circumstances. Heart rate and blood pressure return to nonpregnant levels within a few days (Katz, 2012) (Table 18-1). Respiratory function rapidly returns to nonpregnant levels after birth. After the uterus is emptied, the diaphragm descends, the normal cardiac axis is restored, and the point of maximal impulse and the electrocardiogram are normalized.

Blood Components
Hematocrit and Hemoglobin

In women with an average blood loss during birth, the hematocrit level drops moderately for 3 to 4 days, then begins to increase, and reaches nonpregnant levels by 8 weeks postpartum (Katz, 2012). A postpartum

CRITICAL THINKING EXERCISE

Maternal Postpartum Blood Loss and Fatigue

You are caring for four women on the postpartum unit, two of whom had vaginal births and two who had cesarean births. Each of the women has complained about feeling tired and has expressed concern about the amount of blood she lost during birth. Before providing patient education related to fatigue after birth and blood loss, you review the patients' records with attention to estimated blood loss, hemoglobin and hematocrit values, intake and output, and nursing notes.

1. Evidence—Is there sufficient evidence to draw conclusions about the relation between tiredness (fatigue) after birth and blood loss?
2. Assumptions—What assumptions can be made about the following factors?
   a. Comparison of amount of blood loss between women who give birth vaginally and by cesarean
   b. Postpartum norms for hematocrit and hemoglobin for women who give birth vaginally and by cesarean
   c. Causes of fatigue after birth
   d. Interventions to alleviate fatigue and replace blood lost at birth
3. What implications and priorities for nursing care can be drawn at this time?
4. Does the evidence objectively support your conclusion?

hematocrit can be lower than normal if the blood loss was increased or if the hypervolemia of pregnancy was less than normal.

White Blood Cell Count

Normal leukocytosis of pregnancy averages approximately 12,000/mm³. During the first 10 to 12 days after childbirth, values between 20,000/mm³ and 25,000/mm³ are common. Neutrophils are the most numerous white blood cells. Leukocytosis, coupled with the normal increase in erythrocyte sedimentation rate that occurs, can obscure the diagnosis of acute infections at this time.

Coagulation Factors

Clotting factors and fibrinogen are normally increased during pregnancy and remain elevated in the immediate puerperium. When combined with vessel damage and immobility, this hypercoagulable state causes an increased risk for thromboembolism, especially after a cesarean birth. Fibrinolytic activity also increases during the first few days after childbirth (Katz, 2012). Factors I, II, VIII, IX, and X decrease to nonpregnant levels within a few days. Fibrin split products, probably released from the placental site, can also be found in maternal blood.

Varicosities

Varicosities (varices) of the legs (Fig. 18-3) and around the anus (hemorrhoids) are common during pregnancy. All varices, even the less common vulvar varices, regress (empty) rapidly immediately after childbirth. Total or nearly total regression of varicosities is expected after childbirth.

RESPIRATORY SYSTEM

When birth occurs, there is an immediate decrease in intraabdominal pressure, which allows for greater excursion of the diaphragm. With decreased pressure on the diaphragm and reduced pulmonary blood flow, chest wall compliance increases. Rib cage elasticity can take months to return to a prepregnancy state. The costal angle that was increased during pregnancy may not completely return to the

TABLE 18-1   VITAL SIGNS AFTER CHILDBIRTH

NORMAL FINDINGS	DEVIATIONS FROM NORMAL FINDINGS AND PROBABLE CAUSES
Temperature During first 24 hours, temperature can increase to 38° C (100.4° F) as a result of dehydrating effects of labor. After 24 hours, the woman should be afebrile.	A diagnosis of puerperal sepsis is suggested if an increase in maternal temperature to 38° C (100.4° F) is noted after the first 24 hours after childbirth and recurs or persists for 2 days. Other possibilities are mastitis, endometritis, urinary tract infections, and other systemic infections.
Pulse Pulse, along with stroke volume and cardiac output, remains elevated for the first hour or so after childbirth. It then begins to decrease at an unknown rate to a nonpregnant rate.	A rapid pulse rate or one that is increasing can indicate hypovolemia as a result of hemorrhage.
Respirations The respiratory rate should decrease to within the woman's normal prebirth range by 6-8 weeks after childbirth.	Hypoventilation (respiratory depression) can occur after an unusually high subarachnoid (spinal) block or epidural narcotic after a cesarean birth.
Blood Pressure Blood pressure is altered slightly if at all. Orthostatic hypotension, as indicated by feelings of faintness or dizziness immediately after standing up, can develop in the first 48 hours as a result of the splanchnic engorgement that can occur after birth.	A low or decreasing blood pressure can indicate the existence of hypovolemia secondary to hemorrhage; however, it is a late sign, and other symptoms of hemorrhage usually alert the staff. An increased reading can result from excessive use of vasopressor or oxytocic medications. Because gestational hypertension can persist into or occur first in the postpartum period, routine evaluation of blood pressure is needed. If a woman complains of headache, hypertension must be ruled out as a cause before analgesics are administered.

prepregnancy level. The decline in progesterone that occurs with loss of the placenta causes $Paco_2$ levels to rise (Blackburn, 2013). The basal metabolic rate gradually returns to prepregnancy levels, usually within 1 to 2 weeks after birth.

NEUROLOGIC SYSTEM

Neurologic changes during the puerperium are those resulting from a reversal of maternal adaptations to pregnancy and those resulting from trauma during labor and birth.

Pregnancy-induced neurologic discomforts disappear after birth. Elimination of physiologic edema through the diuresis that follows

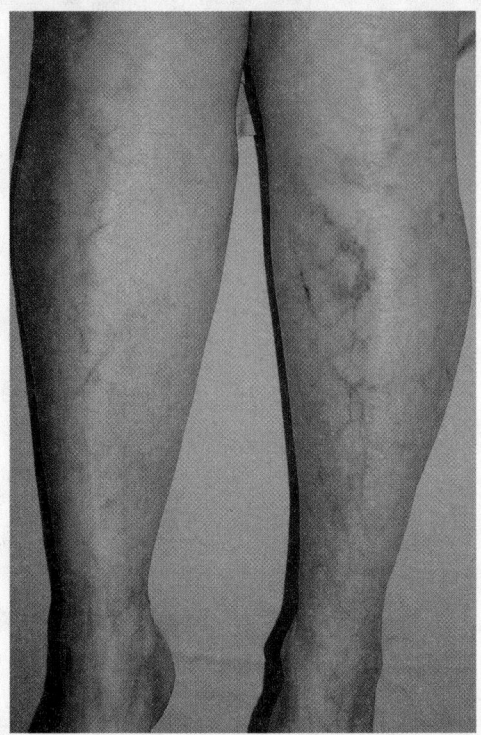

FIG 18-3 Varicosities in legs. (Courtesy Cheryl Briggs, RNC, Annapolis, MD.)

birth relieves carpal tunnel syndrome by easing compression of the median nerve. The periodic numbness and tingling of fingers usually disappear after the birth unless lifting and carrying the baby aggravate the condition.

Headache requires careful assessment. Postpartum headaches can be caused by various conditions, including postpartum-onset preeclampsia, stress, and leakage of cerebrospinal fluid into the extradural space during placement of the needle for administration of epidural or spinal anesthesia.

MUSCULOSKELETAL SYSTEM

Adaptations of the mother's musculoskeletal system that occur during pregnancy are reversed in the puerperium. These adaptations include the relaxation and subsequent hypermobility of the joints and the change in the mother's center of gravity in response to the enlarging uterus. The joints are completely stabilized by 6 to 8 weeks after birth. Although all other joints return to their normal prepregnancy state, those in the parous woman's feet do not. The new mother may notice a permanent increase in her shoe size.

INTEGUMENTARY SYSTEM

Melasma (chloasma or "mask of pregnancy") usually disappears in the postpartum period but persists in about 30% of women (Kroumpouzos, 2012). Hyperpigmentation of the areolae and linea nigra may not regress completely after childbirth. Some women will have permanent darker pigmentation of those areas. Striae gravidarum (stretch marks) on the breasts, abdomen, and thighs may fade but usually do not disappear.

Vascular abnormalities such as spider angiomas (nevi) and palmar erythema generally regress in response to the rapid decline in estrogens after the end of pregnancy. For some women, spider nevi persist indefinitely.

Hair growth slows during the postpartum period, and some hair loss is not uncommon. The abundance of fine hair seen during pregnancy usually disappears after giving birth; however, any coarse or bristly hair that appears during pregnancy usually remains. Fingernails return to their prepregnancy consistency and strength.

IMMUNE SYSTEM

In the postpartum period, the woman's immune system, which was mildly suppressed during pregnancy, gradually returns to its prepregnant state, although the exact timeline is unclear (Blackburn, 2013). This rebound of the immune system can trigger "flare-ups" of autoimmune conditions such as multiple sclerosis or lupus erythematosus (Katz, 2012).

▮ KEY POINTS

- The uterus involutes rapidly after birth and returns to the true pelvis within 2 weeks.
- The rapid decrease in estrogen and progesterone levels after expulsion of the placenta is responsible for triggering many of the anatomic and physiologic changes in the puerperium.
- Assessment of lochia and fundal height is essential to monitor the progress of normal involution and to identify potential problems.
- The return of ovulation and menses is determined in part by whether the woman breastfeeds her infant.
- Few alterations in vital signs are seen after birth under normal circumstances.
- Hypercoagulability, vessel damage, and immobility predispose the woman to thromboembolism.
- Marked diuresis, decreased bladder sensitivity, and overdistention of the bladder can lead to problems with urinary elimination.
- Pregnancy-induced hypervolemia, combined with several postpartum physiologic changes, allows the woman to tolerate considerable blood loss at birth.

REFERENCES

Blackburn ST: *Maternal, fetal, and neonatal physiology*, ed 4, St Louis, 2013, Saunders.

Cunningham F, Leveno K, Bloom S, et al: *Williams obstetrics*, ed 23, New York, 2010, McGraw-Hill.

Katz V: Postpartum care. In Gabbe SG, Niebyl JR, Simpson JL, et al, editors: *Obstetrics: normal and problem pregnancies*, ed 6, Philadelphia, 2012, Saunders.

Kroumpouzos G: Skin disease in pregnancy and puerperium. In Gabbe SG, Niebyl JR, Simpson JL, et al, editors: *Obstetrics: normal and problem pregnancies*, ed 6, Philadelphia, 2012, Saunders.

Lawrence RM, Lawrence RA: *Breastfeeding: a guide for the medical profession*, ed 7, St Louis, 2011, Mosby.

Monga M: Maternal cardiovascular, respiratory, and renal adaptation to pregnancy. In Creasy R, Resnick R, Iams J, et al, editors: *Creasy & Resnik's maternal-fetal medicine: principles and practice*, ed 6, Philadelphia, 2009, Saunders.

Nursing Care of the Family During the Postpartum Period

Kathryn R. Alden

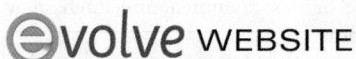 WEBSITE

http://evolve.elsevier.com/Perry/maternal

LEARNING OBJECTIVES

On completion of this chapter, the reader will be able to:
- Describe components of a systematic postpartum assessment.
- Recognize signs of potential complications in the postpartum woman.
- Identify common selection criteria for safe early postpartum discharge.
- Formulate a nursing care plan for a woman in the postpartum period.

- Explain the influence of cultural beliefs and practices on postpartum care.
- Identify psychosocial needs of the woman in the early postpartum period.
- Prepare a plan for postpartum teaching for self-management.
- Describe the nurse's role in these postpartum follow-up strategies: home visits, telephone follow-up, warm lines and help lines, support groups, and referrals to community resources.

At no other time is family-centered maternity care more important than in the postpartum period. Nursing care is provided in the context of the family unit and focuses on assessment and support of the woman's physiologic and emotional adaptation after birth. During the early postpartum period components of nursing care include assisting the mother with rest and recovery from the process of labor and birth, assessing physiologic and psychologic adaptation after birth, preventing complications, educating regarding self-management and infant care, and supporting the mother and her partner during the initial transition to parenthood. In addition, the nurse considers the needs of other family members and includes strategies in the nursing care plan to help the family adjust to the new baby.

The approach to the care of women after birth is wellness oriented. In the United States most women remain hospitalized no more than 1 or 2 days after vaginal birth and some for as few as 6 hours. Because so much important information needs to be shared with these women in a very short time, their care must be thoughtfully planned and provided. This chapter discusses nursing care of the woman and her family in the postpartum period extending into the fourth trimester—the first 3 months after birth.

TRANSFER FROM THE RECOVERY AREA

After the initial recovery period has been completed, the woman may be transferred to a postpartum room in the same or another nursing unit. In facilities with labor, delivery, recovery, postpartum (LDRP) rooms, the woman stays in the same room; the nurse who provides care during the recovery period usually continues caring for the woman. In many settings women who have received general or regional anesthesia must be cleared for transfer from the recovery area by a member of the anesthesia care team. In other settings a nurse makes the determination.

In preparing the transfer report, the recovery nurse uses information from the records of admission, labor and birth, and recovery (Fig. 19-1). Information communicated to the postpartum nurse includes identity of the health care provider; gravidity and parity; age; anesthetic used; any medications given; duration of labor and time of rupture of membranes; whether labor was induced or augmented; type of birth and repair; blood type and Rh status; group B streptococcus status; status of rubella immunity; human immunodeficiency virus (HIV), hepatitis B, and syphilis serology test results; other infections identified during pregnancy (e.g., chlamydia, gonorrhea) and whether these were treated; intravenous infusion of any fluids; physiologic status since birth; description of fundus, lochia, bladder, and perineum; sex and weight of infant; time of birth; name of pediatric care provider; chosen method of feeding; any abnormalities noted; and assessment of initial parent-infant interaction.

Most of this information is also communicated to the nurse on the mother/baby unit or the nursing staff in the newborn nursery if the infant is transferred to that unit. In addition, specific

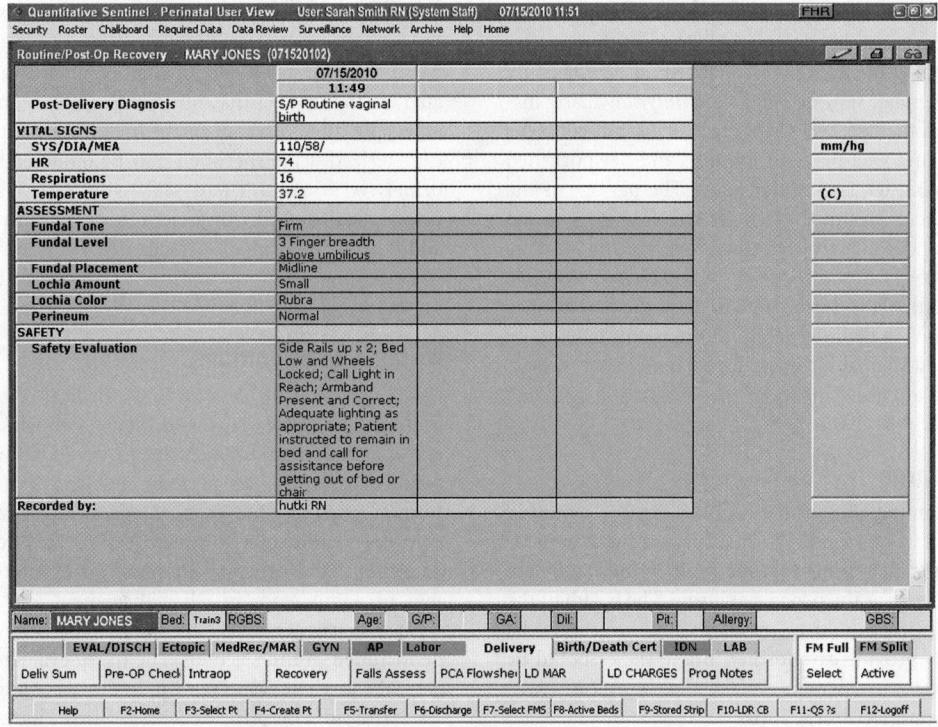

FIG 19-1 Part of a vaginal birth recovery screen in an electronic record. (Courtesy Kitty Cashion, Memphis, TN.)

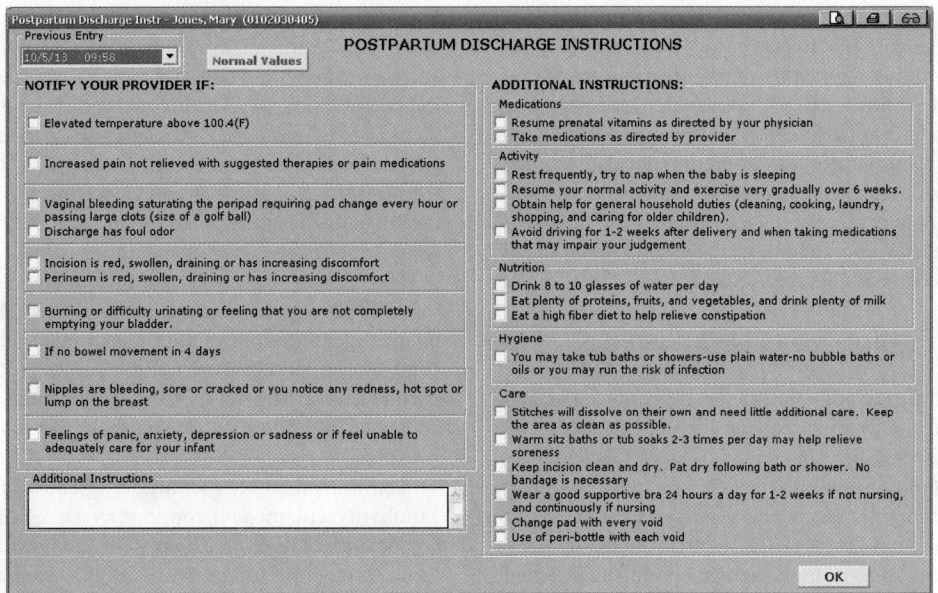

FIG 19-2 Part of a postpartum discharge teaching screen in an electronic medical record. (Courtesy Kitty Cashion, Memphis, TN.)

information should be provided regarding the infant's Apgar scores (see Chapter 23), weight, voiding, and stooling and whether fed since birth. Nursing interventions that have been completed (e.g., eye prophylaxis and vitamin K injection) and identification procedures (e.g., footprints, armbands) must be recorded.

PLANNING FOR DISCHARGE

From their initial contact with the postpartum woman, nurses prepare the new mother for the time when she will return home.

Planning for discharge begins with the first interaction between the nurse, the woman, and her family and continues until they leave the hospital or birthing facility (Fig. 19-2).

The length of stay after giving birth depends on many factors, including the physical condition of the mother and the newborn, mental and emotional status of the mother, social support at home, patient education needs for self-management and infant care, and financial constraints.

Women who give birth in birthing centers may be discharged within a few hours, after the woman's and infant's conditions are stable. Mothers and newborns who are at low risk for complications may be discharged from the hospital within 24 to 36 hours after vaginal birth. This short time frame is often called *early postpartum discharge, shortened hospital stay,* or *1-day maternity stay.* Early discharge was popular in the late 1980s and early 1990s, but concerns related to the health and well-being of mothers and newborns led to legislation promoting longer hospital stays. The passage of the Newborns' and Mothers' Health Protection Act of 1996 provided minimum federal standards for health plan coverage for mothers and their newborns (AAP Committee on Fetus and Newborn, 2010). Under this Act all health plans are required to allow the new mother and newborn to remain in the hospital for a minimum of 48 hours after an uncomplicated vaginal birth and for 96 hours after a cesarean birth, unless the attending provider in consultation with the mother decides on early discharge.

Criteria for Discharge

The AAP (2010) recommends that the hospital stay for a mother with a healthy term newborn should be of sufficient length to identify early problems and determine that the mother and family are prepared and able to care for the neonate at home. The health of the mother and her newborn should be stable; the mother should be able and confident to provide care for her infant; there should be adequate support systems in place and access to follow-up care (AAP Committee on Fetus and Newborn, 2010).

It is essential that nurses consider the individual needs of the woman and her newborn and provide care that is coordinated to meet these needs to provide timely physiologic interventions and treatment to prevent morbidity and hospital readmission. Hospital-based maternity nurses continue to play invaluable roles as caregivers, teachers, and advocates for mothers, newborns, and families in developing and implementing effective home-care strategies. Postpartum order sets and maternal-newborn teaching checklists can be used to accomplish patient care tasks and educational outcomes. With coordination, clinical care and education can be planned and provided throughout pregnancy, during the hospital stay, and in the home after discharge to promote and support the family's continued well-being (see Evidence-Based Practice box).

CARE MANAGEMENT—PHYSICAL NEEDS

The nursing plan of care includes both the postpartum woman and her infant. It is also family centered, considering the needs and concerns of the family and focusing on family unity (Waller-Wise, 2012). Although in some hospitals the nursery nurse retains primary responsibility for the infant, most perinatal settings use the couplet or mother/baby model of care (AWHONN, 2010). Nurses in these settings have been educated in both mother and infant care and function as primary nurses for both mother and infant, even if the infant is kept in the nursery. This approach is a variation of rooming-in, in which the mother and infant room together and mother and nurse share the care of the infant. The organization of the mother's care must take the newborn's feeding and care needs into consideration.

Ongoing Physical Assessment

Ongoing assessments are performed throughout hospitalization. In addition to vital signs, physical assessment of the postpartum woman focuses on evaluation of the breasts, uterine fundus, lochia, perineum, bladder and bowel function, vital signs, and legs (Table 19-1).

Routine Laboratory Tests

Several laboratory tests may be performed in the immediate postpartum period. Hemoglobin and hematocrit values are often evaluated on the first postpartum day to assess blood loss during birth, especially after cesarean birth. In some hospitals a clean-catch or catheterized urine specimen may be obtained and sent for routine urinalysis or culture and sensitivity, especially if an indwelling urinary catheter was inserted during the intrapartum period. In addition, if the woman's rubella and Rh status are unknown, tests to determine her status and need for possible treatment should be performed at this time.

Nursing Interventions

Based on the available data (e.g., medical record) and assessment findings, the nurse plans with the woman which nursing measures are appropriate and which are to be given priority. The nursing plan of care includes periodic assessments to detect deviations from normal physical changes, measures to relieve discomfort or pain, safety measures to prevent injury or infection, and teaching and counseling measures designed to promote the woman's feelings of competence in self-management and newborn care. The spouse or partner, and other family members who are present can be included in the teaching. The nurse evaluates continuously and is ready to change the plan if indicated. Almost all hospitals use standardized care plans as a base. Nurses individualize care of the postpartum woman and neonate according to their specific needs (see Nursing Care Plan). Signs of potential problems that may be identified during the assessment process are listed in Table 19-1.

Nurses assume many roles while implementing the nursing plan of care. They provide direct physical care, education about mother and baby care, counseling, and anticipatory guidance. Perhaps most important of all, they nurture the woman by providing encouragement and support as she begins to assume the many tasks of motherhood. Nurses who take the time to "mother the mother" do much to increase feelings of self-confidence in new mothers. Nurses are careful to include the woman's spouse or partner and other primary support persons in education and counseling.

The first step in providing individualized care is to confirm the woman's identity by checking her wristband. At the same time the infant's identification number is matched with the corresponding band on the mother's wrist and in some instances the father's or partner's wrist. The nurse determines how the mother wishes to be addressed and notes her preference in her record and her nursing care plan.

The woman and her family are oriented to their surroundings. Familiarity with the unit, routines, resources, and personnel reduces one potential source of anxiety—the unknown. The mother is reassured through knowing whom and how she can call for assistance and what she can expect in the way of supplies and services. If the woman's usual daily routine before admission differs from the routine of the facility, the nurse works with the woman to develop a mutually acceptable routine.

Nurses discuss infant security precautions with the mother and her family because infant abductions are an ongoing concern. Between 1983 and 2012, 130 infants were abducted from health care facilities in the United States; most (58%) of the babies were taken from the mother's room (National Center for Missing and Exploited Children, 2012). The Joint Commission (1999) calls for hospitals to have a management plan to prevent infant abductions. Such a plan might include security devices such as access control to the unit, closed-circuit television, computer monitoring systems, and

EVIDENCE-BASED PRACTICE

Perineal Trauma and Postpartum Sexual Function

Ask the Question

Which perinatal interventions for perineal trauma minimize pain and prevent sexual dysfunction?

Search for the Evidence

Search Strategies

English research-based publications on perineal trauma, birth, postpartum, sexual were included.

Databases Used

Cochrane Collaborative Database, National Guideline Clearinghouse (AHRQ), CINAHL, PubMed, and UpToDate

Critically Analyze the Evidence

- Sexual dysfunction can affect more than half of all women at 2 to 3 months after birth. One major cause is dyspareunia (painful intercourse) after perineal trauma, especially third- and fourth-degree lacerations requiring repair. Other causes can include decreased libido and lower estrogen resulting from breastfeeding, postpartum depression, and fatigue.
- Both episiotomy and second-degree lacerations with repair are associated with lower libido, orgasm, sexual satisfaction, and greater dyspareunia than in women with intact perineums (Rathfisch, Dikencik, Beji, et al., 2010). Routine episiotomy and fundal pressure during birth are not recommended.
- Warm compresses and perineal massage during first- and second-stage birth significantly decrease third- and fourth-degree tears (Aasheim, Nilsen, Lukasse, et al., 2011).
- Evidence is still mixed for whether to suture or not suture first- and second-degree lacerations. Although small studies find little difference between groups for pain and wound complications, despite slower wound healing the unsutured group still experiences greater satisfaction than the sutured group (Elharmeel, Chaudhary, Tan, et al., 2011).

Apply the Evidence: Nursing Implications

Women can be embarrassed to discuss sexual function with their partners and/or with their health care team. Nurses are ideally placed to initiate and keep the dialog going throughout childbearing. Leeman and Rogers (2012) recommend the following clinical approach for assessing and preventing postpartum sexual dysfunction:

- Discussion of anatomy, physiology, and sexual function should begin in early pregnancy and continue throughout the postpartum period, including a brief valid and reliable sexual function survey.
- Antenatal perineal massage should be taught to minimize perineal damage.
- Perineal management at birth should include limited use of instrumental delivery, especially forceps, and avoiding episiotomy, along with careful assessment and repair of anal sphincter lacerations with synthetic, absorbable sutures.

- Before hospital discharge initiate discussions with the woman and her partner regarding pain, dyspareunia, resumption of intercourse, and contraception. Women should know the hypoestogenic and sensitivity changes that they can experience as a result of breastfeeding and the need for additional vaginal lubrication.
- At postpartum visits assess urine, bowel, and sexual function; inspect perineum; and assess and discuss mood and intimacy challenges such as fatigue and timing issues. Suggest alternate positions to help increase comfort during intercourse. Evaluate satisfaction with contraceptive method.

Quality and Safety Competencies:
Evidence-Based Practice*

Knowledge

Describe Evidence-Based Practice to Include the Components of Research Evidence, Clinical Expertise, and Patient/Family Values.

Sexuality is affected by childbirth. Nurses can sensitively initiate discussion of sexual intimacy.

Skills

Base Individualized Care Plan on Patient Values, Clinical Expertise, and Evidence.

The nurse models a view of human sexuality as a healthy and normal part of one's quality of life.

Attitudes

Value the Concept of Evidence-Based Practice as Integral to Determining Best Clinical Practice.

The nurse can educate the patient and partner and dispel myths about sexuality.

References

Aasheim V, Nilsen AB, Lukasse M, et al: Perineal techniques during the second stage of labour for reducing perineal trauma. In *Cochrane Database Syst Rev* 12:CD006672.pub2. DOI: 10.1002/14651858, Chichester, UK, 2011, John Wiley & Sons.

Elharmeel SM, Chaudhary Y, Tan S, et al: Surgical repair of spontaneous perineal tears that occur during childbirth versus no intervention. In *Cochrane Database Syst Rev* 8:CD008534. DOI: 10.1002/14651858, Chichester, UK, 2011, John Wiley & Sons.

Leeman LM, Rogers RG: Sex after childbirth, *Obstet Gynecol* 119(3):647–655, 2012.

Rathfisch G, Dikencik BK, Beji NK, et al: Effects of perineal trauma on postpartum sexual function, *J Adv Nurs* 66(12):2640–2649, 2010.

Pat Mahaffee Gingrich

*Adapted from QSEN at www.qsen.org/.

electronic infant security systems in which tamper-proof tags are placed on the neonate immediately after birth and removed at the time of hospital discharge. The mother should be taught to check the identity of any person who comes to remove the baby from her room. Hospital personnel usually wear picture identification badges. On some units all staff members wear matching scrubs or special badges that are unique to the perinatal unit. As a rule the baby is never carried in a staff member's arms between the mother's room and the nursery but rather is always wheeled in a bassinet, which also contains baby care supplies. Patients and nurses must work together to ensure the safety of newborns in the hospital environment (Vincent, 2009).

TABLE 19-1 POSTPARTUM ASSESSMENT AND SIGNS OF POTENTIAL COMPLICATIONS

ASSESSMENT	NORMAL FINDINGS	SIGNS OF POTENTIAL COMPLICATIONS
Blood pressure (BP)	Consistent with BP baseline during pregnancy; can have orthostatic hypotension for 48 hours	Hypertension: anxiety, preeclampsia, essential hypertension Hypotension: hemorrhage
Temperature	36.2°-38° C (97.2° to 100.4° F)	>38° C (100.4° F) after 24 hours: infection
Pulse	50-90 beats/min	Tachycardia: pain, fever, dehydration, hemorrhage
Respirations	16-24 breaths/min	Bradypnea: effects of narcotic medications Tachypnea: anxiety; may be sign of respiratory disease
Breath sounds	Clear to auscultation	Crackles: possible fluid overload
Breasts	Days 1-2: soft	Firmness, heat, pain: engorgement
	Days 2-3: filling Days 3-5: full, soften with breastfeeding (milk is "in")	Redness of breast tissue, heat, pain, fever, body aches: mastitis
Nipples	Skin intact; no soreness reported	Redness, bruising, cracks, fissures, abrasions, blisters: usually associated with latching problems
Uterus (fundus)	Firm, midline; first 24 hours at level of umbilicus; involutes ≈1 cm/day	Soft, boggy, higher than expected level: uterine atony Lateral deviation: distended bladder
Lochia	Days 1-3: rubra (dark red) Days 4-10: serosa (brownish red or pink) After 10 days: alba (yellowish white) Amount: scant to moderate Few clots Fleshy odor	Large amount of lochia: uterine atony, vaginal or cervical laceration Foul odor: infection
Perineum	Minimal edema	Pronounced edema, bruising, hematoma
	Laceration or episiotomy: edges approximated	Redness, warmth, drainage: infection
	Pain minimal to moderate: controlled by analgesics, nonpharmacologic techniques, or both	Excessive discomfort first 1-2 days: hematoma; after day 3: infection
Rectal area	No hemorrhoids; if hemorrhoids are present, soft and pink	Discolored hemorrhoidal tissue, severe pain: thrombosed hemorrhoid
Bladder	Able to void spontaneously; no distention; able to empty completely; no dysuria	Overdistended bladder possibly causing uterine atony, excessive lochia
	Diuresis begins ≈12 hours after birth; can void 3000 mL/day	Dysuria, frequency, urgency: infection
Abdomen and bowels	Abdomen soft, active bowel sounds in all quadrants Bowel movement by day 2 or 3 after birth	No bowel movement by day 3 or 4: constipation; diarrhea
	Cesarean: incision dressing clean and dry; suture line intact	Abdominal incision—redness, edema, warmth, drainage: infection
Legs	Deep tendon reflexes (DTRs) 1+ to 2+	DTRs ≥3+: preeclampsia
	Peripheral edema possibly present Homans' sign* negative	Redness, tenderness, pain, positive Homans' sign*: venous thromboembolism (VTE)
Energy level	Able to care for self and infant; able to sleep	Lethargy, extreme fatigue, difficulty sleeping: postpartum depression
Emotional status	Excited, happy, interested or involved in infant care	Sad, tearful, disinterested in infant care: postpartum blues or depression

*Homans' sign may or may not be included in routine postpartum assessments; there is concern about its limited sensitivity and specificity in diagnosing venous thromboembolism.

⚡ SAFETY ALERT

Nurses play a critical role in educating parents about measures to prevent infant abduction. Parents should be instructed how to identify legitimate hospital personnel, to never leave the newborn in the hospital room without direct supervision, and to request a second staff member to verify the identity of any questionable person who wants to take the baby from the mother's room. Parents should be instructed to use caution when posting photos of the new baby on the Internet and publishing public notices about the birth (Vincent, 2009).

Prevention of Infection

Nurses in the postpartum setting are acutely aware of the importance of preventing infection in their patients. One important means of preventing infection is maintenance of a clean environment. Bed linens should be changed as needed. Disposable pads should be changed frequently. Women should wear shoes when walking about to avoid contaminating the linens when they return to bed. A sitz bath or heat lamp used by more than one patient must be scrubbed after each woman's use. Personnel must be conscientious about their hand hygiene to prevent cross-infection. Standard Precautions must

NURSING CARE PLAN

Postpartum Care—Vaginal Birth

NURSING DIAGNOSIS	EXPECTED OUTCOME	NURSING INTERVENTIONS	RATIONALES
Risk for Deficient Fluid Volume related to uterine atony/hemorrhage	Fundus is firm, lochia is moderate, and there is no evidence of hemorrhage.	Monitor lochia (color, amount, consistency) and count sanitary pads if lochia is heavy	To evaluate amount of bleeding
		Monitor and palpate fundus for location and tone to determine status of uterus and dictate further interventions	Because uterine atony is most common cause of postpartum hemorrhage
		Monitor intake and output, assess for bladder fullness, and encourage voiding	Because a full bladder interferes with involution of uterus
		Monitor vital signs (increased pulse and respirations, decreased blood pressure) and skin temperature and color	To detect signs of hemorrhage/shock
		Monitor postpartum hematology studies	To assess effects of blood loss
		If fundus is boggy, apply gentle massage and assess tone response.	To promote uterine contractions and increase uterine tone (Do not overstimulate because doing so can cause fundal relaxation.)
		Express uterine clots	To promote uterine contraction
		Explain to woman process of involution and teach her to assess and massage fundus and report any persistent bogginess	To involve her in self-management and increase sense of self-control
		Administer uterotonic agents per health care provider order and evaluate effectiveness	To promote continuing uterine contraction
		Administer fluids, blood, blood products, or plasma expanders as ordered	To replace lost fluid and lost blood volume
Acute Pain related to postpartum physiologic changes (hemorrhoids, episiotomy, breast engorgement, sore/damaged nipples)	Woman exhibits signs of decreased discomfort.	Assess location, type, and quality of pain	To direct intervention
		Explain to woman source and reasons for pain, its expected duration, and treatments	To decrease anxiety and increase sense of control
		Administer prescribed pain medications	To provide pain relief
		If pain is perineal (episiotomy, hemorrhoids), apply ice packs in first 24 hours	To reduce edema and vulvar irritation and reduce discomfort
		Encourage sitz baths using cool water the first 24 hours	To reduce edema and discomfort
		Use warm water for sitz baths after 24 hours	To promote circulation and reduce discomfort
		Apply witch hazel compresses	To reduce edema
		Teach woman to use prescribed perineal creams, sprays, or ointments	To depress response of peripheral nerves
		Teach woman to tighten buttocks before sitting and to sit on flat, hard surfaces	To compress buttocks and reduce pressure on perineum (Avoid donuts and soft pillows because they separate buttocks and decrease venous blood flow, increasing pain.)
		If nipples are sore or damaged, assess infant positioning and latch; assist mother to correct problems	To prevent further nipple soreness and damage
		If breasts are engorged, have woman apply ice packs and/or cabbage leaves (15-20 minutes on, 45 minutes off) between feedings	To reduce tissue swelling and promote milk flow
		Suggest that woman takes a warm shower before breastfeeding	To stimulate milk flow and relieve stasis
		If nipples are sore, have woman rub expressed milk into them after feeding and leave nipples open to air	To promote healing
		Apply hydrogel pads to sore nipples between feedings	To promote comfort
		Wear breast shell	To prevent irritation
		If pain is from breast and woman is not breastfeeding, encourage use of tight supportive bra or breast binder and application of ice packs or cold cabbage leaves	To suppress milk production and reduce tissue swelling from engorgement

Continued

◎ NURSING CARE PLAN

Postpartum Care—Vaginal Birth—cont'd

NURSING DIAGNOSIS	EXPECTED OUTCOME	NURSING INTERVENTIONS	RATIONALES
Disturbed Sleep Pattern related to excitement, discomfort, and environmental interruptions	Woman sleeps for uninterrupted periods of time and feels rested after waking.	Establish woman's routine sleep patterns and compare with current sleep pattern, exploring things that interfere with sleep	To determine scope of problem and direct interventions
		Individualize nursing routines to fit woman's natural body rhythms (i.e., wake/sleep cycles); provide a sleep-promoting environment (i.e., darkness, quiet, adequate ventilation, appropriate room temperature); prepare for sleep using woman's usual routines (i.e., back rub, soothing music, warm milk); teach use of guided imagery and relaxation techniques	To promote optimum conditions for sleep
		Avoid things or routines that can interfere with sleep (i.e., caffeine, foods that induce heartburn, fluids, strenuous mental/physical activity)	To enhance quality of sleep
		Administer sedative or pain medication as prescribed	To enhance quality of sleep
		Advise woman/partner to limit visitors and activities	To avoid further taxation and fatigue
		Teach woman to use infant nap time as a time for her also	To nap and replenish energy and decrease fatigue
Risk for Impaired Urinary Elimination related to perineal trauma and effects of anesthesia	Woman will void within 6 to 8 hours after birth and empty bladder completely.	Assess position and character of uterine fundus and bladder	To ascertain if any further interventions are indicated because of displacement of fundus or distention of bladder
		Measure intake and output	To assess adequacy of fluid intake and urine output; a full or distended bladder increases the risk for uterine atony
		Encourage voiding by assisting woman to bathroom, running water over perineum, running water in sink, and providing privacy	To encourage voiding
		Encourage oral fluid intake	To replace any fluids lost during birth and prevent dehydration
		Catheterize as necessary with indwelling or straight method	To ensure bladder emptying and prevent uterine atony

be practiced. Staff members with colds, coughs, or skin infections (e.g., a cold sore on the lips [herpes simplex virus type I]) must follow hospital protocol when in contact with postpartum patients. In many hospitals staff with open herpetic lesions, strep throat, conjunctivitis, upper respiratory infections, or diarrhea are encouraged to avoid contact with mothers and infants by staying home until the condition is no longer contagious. Visitors with signs of illness are not permitted to enter the postpartum unit.

Perineal lacerations and episiotomies can increase the risk of infection as a result of interruption in skin integrity. Proper perineal care helps prevent infection in the genitourinary area and aids the healing process. Educating the woman to wipe from front to back (urethra to anus) after voiding or defecating is a simple first step. In many hospitals a squeeze bottle filled with warm water or an antiseptic solution is used after each voiding to cleanse the perineal area. The woman should change her perineal pad from front to back each time she voids or defecates and wash her hands thoroughly before and after doing so (Box 19-1).

Prevention of Excessive Bleeding

The most frequent cause of excessive bleeding after childbirth is uterine atony (i.e., failure of the uterine muscle to contract firmly).

The two most important interventions for preventing excessive bleeding are maintaining good uterine tone and preventing bladder distention. If uterine atony occurs, the relaxed uterus distends with blood and clots, blood vessels in the placental site are not clamped off, and excessive bleeding results. Although the cause of uterine atony is not always clear, it often results from retained placental fragments.

Excessive blood loss after birth can also be caused by vaginal or vulvar hematomas or unrepaired lacerations of the vagina or cervix. These potential sources might be suspected if excessive vaginal bleeding occurs in the presence of a firmly contracted uterus.

> ### ! NURSING ALERT
>
> A perineal pad saturated in 15 minutes or less or pooling of blood under the buttocks is an indication of excessive blood loss requiring immediate assessment, intervention, and notification of the primary health care provider.

Accurate visual estimation of blood loss is an important nursing responsibility. Blood loss is usually described subjectively as scant, light, moderate, or heavy (profuse). Fig. 19-3 shows examples

BOX 19-1   INTERVENTIONS FOR EPISIOTOMY, LACERATIONS, AND HEMORRHOIDS

Explain procedure and rationale before implementation.

Cleansing

- Wash hands before and after cleansing perineum and changing pads.
- Wash perineum with mild soap and warm water at least once daily.
- Cleanse from symphysis pubis to anal area.
- Apply peripad from front to back, protecting inner surface of pad from contamination.
- Wrap soiled pad and place in covered waste container.
- Change pad with each void or defecation or at least 4 times per day.
- Assess amount and character of lochia with each pad change.

Ice Pack

- Apply a covered ice pack to perineum from front to back:
  - During first 24 hours to decrease edema formation and increase comfort.
  - After first 24 hours following birth as needed to provide anesthetic effect.

Squeeze Bottle

- Demonstrate use and assist woman; explain rationale.
- Fill bottle with tap water warmed to approximately 38° C (100.4° F) (comfortably warm on wrist).
- Instruct woman to position nozzle between her legs so squirts of water reach perineum as she sits on toilet seat. Explain that it will take whole bottle of water to cleanse perineum.
- Remind her to blot dry with toilet paper or clean wipes.
- Remind her to avoid contamination from anal area.
- Apply clean pad.

Sitz Bath
Built-In Type

- Prepare bath by thoroughly scrubbing with cleaning agent and rinsing.
- Pad with towel before filling.
- Fill one-third to one-half full with water of correct temperature 38° to 40.6° C (100.4° to 105.1° F). Some women prefer cool sitz baths. Ice is added to water to lower temperature to level comfortable for woman.
- Encourage woman to use at least twice a day for 20 minutes.
- Place call bell within easy reach.
- Teach woman to enter bath by tightening gluteal muscles and keeping them tightened and then relaxing them after she is in bath.
- Place dry towels within reach.
- Ensure privacy.
- Check woman in 15 minutes.

Disposable Type

- Clamp tubing and fill bag with warm water.
- Raise toilet seat; place bath in bowl with overflow opening directed toward back of toilet.
- Place container above toilet bowl.
- Attach tube into groove at front of bath.
- Loosen tube clamp to regulate rate of flow; fill bath to about one-half full; continue as for built-in sitz bath.

Topical Applications

- Apply anesthetic cream or spray after cleansing perineal area; use sparingly 3 to 4 times per day.
- Apply witch hazel pads (Tucks) after voiding or defecating; woman pats perineum dry from front to back and applies witch hazel pads.
- Apply hemorrhoidal cream as ordered to anal area after cleansing.

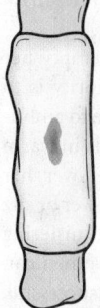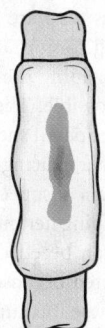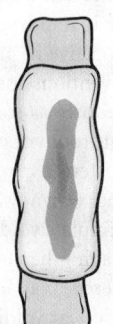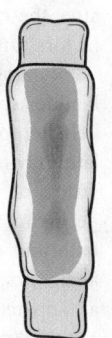

FIG 19-3 Blood loss after birth is assessed by the extent of perineal pad saturation as *(from left to right)* scant (less than 2.5 cm); light (less than 10 cm); moderate (10 cm or more); or heavy (one pad saturated within 2 hours).

of perineal pad saturation corresponding to each of these descriptions.

Although postpartal blood loss may be estimated by observing the amount of staining on a perineal pad, it is difficult to judge the amount of lochial flow based only on observation of perineal pads. More objective estimates of blood loss include measuring serial hemoglobin or hematocrit values, weighing blood clots and items saturated with blood (1 g equals 1 mL), and establishing the milliliters it takes to saturate perineal pads being used.

Any estimation of lochial flow is inaccurate and incomplete without consideration of the time factor. The woman who saturates

a perineal pad in 1 hour or less is bleeding much more heavily than the woman who saturates a pad in 8 hours.

Nurses in general tend to overestimate rather than underestimate blood loss. Different brands of perineal pads vary in their saturation volume and soaking appearance. For example, blood placed on some brands tends to soak down into the pad, whereas on other brands it tends to spread outward. Nurses should determine saturation volume and soaking appearance for the perineal pad brands used in their institution to improve accuracy of blood loss estimation.

! NURSING ALERT

The nurse always also checks for blood under the mother's buttocks. Although the amount on the perineal pad may be slight, blood may flow between the buttocks onto the linens under the mother. When this happens, excessive bleeding can go undetected.

When excessive bleeding occurs, vital signs are monitored closely. Blood pressure is not a reliable indicator of impending shock from early postpartum hemorrhage because compensatory mechanisms prevent a significant drop in blood pressure until the woman has lost 30% to 40% of her blood volume (see Chapter 21). Respirations, pulse, skin condition, urinary output, and level of consciousness are more sensitive means of identifying hypovolemic shock (see Emergency box). The frequent physical assessments performed during the fourth stage of labor are designed to provide prompt

✚ EMERGENCY

Hypovolemic Shock

Signs and Symptoms

- Persistent significant bleeding: Perineal pad is soaked within 15 minutes; initially may not be accompanied by a change in vital signs or maternal color or behavior.
- Woman states that she feels weak, light-headed, "funny," or "nauseated" or that she "sees stars."
- Woman appears anxious or exhibits air hunger.
- Skin color turns ashen or grayish.
- Skin feels cool and clammy.
- Pulse rate increases.
- Blood pressure declines.

Interventions

- Notify primary health care provider.
- If uterus is atonic, massage gently and expel clots to cause it to contract.
- Administer uterotonic medications (e.g., oxytocin, prostaglandins) as ordered to increase uterine tone.
- Give oxygen by nonrebreather face mask or nasal prongs at 8 to 10 L/min.
- Tilt the woman to her side or elevate the right hip; elevate her legs to at least a 30-degree angle.
- Provide additional or maintain existing IV infusion of lactated Ringer's solution or normal saline solution to restore circulatory volume (woman should have two patent IV lines; insert second IV infusion using 16- to 18-gauge IV catheter).
- Administer blood or blood products as ordered.
- Monitor vital signs.
- Insert an indwelling urinary catheter to monitor perfusion of kidneys.
- Administer emergency medications as ordered.
- Prepare for possible surgery or other emergency treatments or procedures.
- Record incident, medical and nursing interventions instituted, and woman's response to interventions.

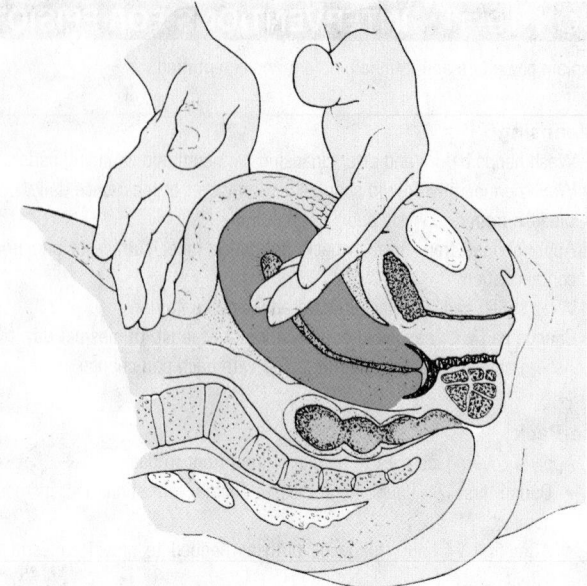

FIG 19-4 Palpating fundus of uterus during fourth stage of labor. Note that upper hand is cupped over fundus; lower hand dips in above symphysis pubis and supports uterus while it is massaged gently.

identification of excessive bleeding. Nurses maintain vigilance for excessive bleeding throughout the hospital stay as they perform periodic assessment of the uterine fundus and lochia.

Maintenance of Uterine Tone. A major intervention to restore good tone is stimulation by gently massaging the uterine fundus until firm (Fig. 19-4). Fundal massage can cause a temporary increase in the amount of vaginal bleeding seen as pooled blood leaves the uterus. Clots can be expelled. The uterus can remain boggy even after massage and expulsion of clots.

Fundal massage can be a very uncomfortable procedure. Understanding the causes and dangers of uterine atony and the purpose of fundal massage can help the woman cooperate. Teaching the woman to massage her own fundus enables her to maintain some control and decreases her anxiety.

When uterine atony and excessive bleeding occur, additional interventions likely to be used are administration of intravenous fluids and oxytocic medications (drugs that stimulate contraction of the uterine smooth muscle). (See Medication Guide in Chapter 21 for information about common oxytocic medications.)

Prevention of Bladder Distention. Uterine atony and excessive bleeding after birth can be the result of bladder distention. A full bladder causes the uterus to be displaced above the umbilicus and well to one side of the midline in the abdomen. It also prevents the uterus from contracting normally.

Women can be at risk of bladder distention resulting from urinary retention based on intrapartum factors. These risk factors include epidural anesthesia, extensive vaginal or perineal lacerations, episiotomy, instrument-assisted birth, or prolonged labor. Women who have had indwelling catheters such as with cesarean birth can experience some difficulty as they initially attempt to void after the catheter is removed. Nurses who are aware of these risk factors can be proactive in preventing complications.

Nursing interventions focus on helping the woman empty her bladder spontaneously as soon as possible. The first priority is to help her to the bathroom or onto a bedpan if she is unable to ambulate. Having her listen to running water, placing her hands in warm water, or pouring warm water from a squeeze bottle over her perineum may stimulate voiding. Helping her into the shower or sitz bath and encouraging her to void can be effective. Administering analgesics, if ordered, may be indicated because some women can anticipate pain and fear voiding. If these measures are unsuccessful, a sterile catheter can be inserted to drain the urine.

Promotion of Comfort

Most women experience some degree of discomfort during the postpartum period. Common causes of discomfort include afterbirth pains (afterpains), perineal lacerations or episiotomy, hemorrhoids, sore nipples, and breast engorgement. The woman's description of the type and severity of her pain is the best guide in choosing an appropriate intervention. To confirm the location and extent of discomfort, the nurse inspects and palpates areas of pain as appropriate for redness, swelling, discharge, and heat and observes for body tension, guarded movements, and facial tension. Blood pressure, pulse, and respirations can be elevated in response to acute pain. Diaphoresis can accompany severe pain. A lack of objective signs does not necessarily mean there is no pain because there can also be a cultural component to the expression of pain. Nursing interventions are intended to eliminate the pain sensation entirely or reduce it to a tolerable level that allows the woman to care for herself and her baby. Nurses may use both nonpharmacologic and pharmacologic interventions to promote comfort. Pain relief is enhanced by using more than one method or route.

Nonpharmacologic Interventions. A variety of nonpharmacologic measures are used to reduce postpartum discomfort. These include distraction, imagery, therapeutic touch, relaxation, acupressure, aromatherapy, hydrotherapy, massage therapy, music therapy, and transcutaneous electrical nerve stimulation (TENS).

For women who are experiencing discomfort associated with uterine contractions, applying warmth (e.g., heating pad) or lying prone may be helpful. Interaction with the infant may also provide distraction and decrease this discomfort. Because afterpains are more severe during and after breastfeeding, interventions are planned to provide the most timely and effective relief. Administering pain medication about 30 minutes before breastfeeding can help minimize afterpains that are enhanced by breastfeeding.

Simple interventions that can decrease the discomfort associated with an episiotomy or perineal lacerations include encouraging the woman to lie on her side whenever possible and use a pillow when sitting. Other interventions include application of an ice pack; topical medication (if ordered); dry heat; cleansing with a squeeze bottle; and a cleansing shower, tub bath, or sitz bath. Many of these interventions, especially ice packs, sitz baths, and topical applications (e.g., witch hazel pads), are also effective for hemorrhoids (see Box 19-1).

Sore nipples in breastfeeding mothers are most likely related to ineffective latch technique. Assessment and assistance with feeding can help alleviate the cause. To ease discomfort associated with sore nipples, the mother may apply topical preparations such as purified lanolin or hydrogel pads (see Chapter 24).

Breast engorgement can occur whether the woman is breastfeeding or formula-feeding. The discomfort associated with engorged breasts may be reduced by applying ice packs or cabbage leaves (or both) to the breasts and wearing a well-fitted support bra. Antiinflammatory medications can also help to relieve some of the discomfort. Decisions about specific interventions for engorgement are based on whether the woman chooses breastfeeding or bottle-feeding (see Chapter 24).

Pharmacologic Interventions. Pharmacologic interventions are commonly used to relieve or reduce postpartum discomfort. Most health care providers routinely order a variety of analgesics to be administered as needed, including both opioid and non-opioid (e.g., nonsteroidal antiinflammatory drugs [NSAIDs]) medications. In some hospitals NSAIDs are administered on a scheduled basis, especially if the woman had perineal repair. Topical application of antiseptic or anesthetic ointment or spray can be used for perineal pain. Patient-controlled analgesia (PCA) pumps and epidural analgesia are commonly used to provide pain relief after cesarean birth.

> ### ! NURSING ALERT
> The nurse should monitor all women receiving opioids carefully because respiratory depression and decreased intestinal motility are side effects.

Many women want to participate in decisions about analgesia. However, severe pain can interfere with active participation in choosing pain-relief measures. If an analgesic is to be given, the nurse must make a clinical judgment of the type, dosage, and frequency from the medications ordered. The woman is informed of the prescribed analgesic and its common side effects; this teaching is documented.

If acceptable pain relief has not been obtained in 1 hour and there has been no change in the initial assessment, the nurse can contact the primary care provider for additional pain-relief orders or further directions. Unrelieved pain results in fatigue, anxiety, and a worsening perception of the pain. It can also indicate the presence of a previously unidentified or untreated problem.

Breastfeeding mothers often have concerns about the effects of an analgesic on the infant. Although nearly all medications present in maternal circulation are also found in breast milk, many analgesics commonly used during the postpartum period are considered relatively safe for breastfeeding mothers. Non-opioid analgesics are preferred for pain management in postpartum breastfeeding women because they do not alter maternal or infant alertness (Lawrence and Lawrence, 2011). Timing of medications can be adjusted to minimize infant exposure. A mother may be given pain medication immediately after breastfeeding so the interval between medication administration and the next nursing period is as long as possible. The decision to administer medications of any type to a breastfeeding mother must always be made by carefully weighing the woman's need against actual or potential risks to the infant. Resources are readily accessible for nurses and health care providers to examine the safety of medications for breastfeeding mothers (e.g., LactMed [http://toxnet.nlm.nih.gov/cgi-bin/sis/htmlgen?LACT]).

Promotion of Rest

Postpartum fatigue (PPF) is more than just feeling tired; it is a complex phenomenon affected by a combination of physiologic, psychologic, and situational variables. Fatigue is common in the early postpartum period and involves both physiologic and psychologic components. Physical fatigue or exhaustion can be associated with long labors or cesarean birth; hospital routines and infant care demands such as breastfeeding also contribute to maternal fatigue. It can also be associated with anemia, infection, or thyroid dysfunction. The excitement and exhilaration experienced after the birth of the infant make resting difficult. Physical discomfort can interfere with sleep. Well-intentioned visitors can interrupt periods of rest in the hospital and at home.

Symptoms of PPF and depressive symptoms are interrelated (Doering Runquist, Morin, & Stetzer, 2009; Song, Chang, Park, et al., 2010), yet each has distinct patterns (Kuo, Yang, Kuo, et al., 2012). Depressive symptoms can affect fatigue; whereas fatigue can lead to depressive symptoms. Depression-related PPF can be differentiated from nondepression-related PPF based on whether or not depressive symptoms are reduced when fatigue is decreased (Runquist, 2007).

Fatigue is likely to worsen over the first 6 weeks after birth, often because of situational factors. After discharge from the hospital, fatigue increases as the woman provides care and feeding for the newborn in combination with other family and household responsibilities such as caring for other children, preparing meals, and doing laundry. Many women have partners, family members, or friends to provide much-needed assistance; whereas others can be without any help at all. The nurse needs to inquire about resources available to the woman after discharge and help her plan accordingly.

Interventions are planned to meet the woman's individual needs for sleep and rest while she is in the hospital. Back rubs, other comfort measures, and medication for sleep may be necessary. The side-lying position for breastfeeding minimizes fatigue in nursing mothers. Support and encouragement of mothering behaviors help reduce anxiety. Hospital and nursing routines can be adjusted to

CRITICAL THINKING CASE STUDY

Fatigue and Rest After Childbirth

Patricia gave birth to her third baby; she has two children at home, ages 3 years and 18 months. Her husband travels frequently with his job. She is breastfeeding the baby without difficulty but is concerned about how she will care for all three of her children, stating, "I remember how tired I was after my last baby. I'm not sure I can manage with three children since my husband is gone so much. Do you have any suggestions to help me?"

1. Evidence—Is there sufficient evidence to draw conclusions about whether and what support would be helpful for Patricia?
2. Assumptions—What assumptions can be made about the following factors?
   a. The relation of breastfeeding and fatigue
   b. Support in the postpartum period
   c. The role of sleep and rest in relation to fatigue and depression
   d. Spacing of pregnancies and fatigue
3. What implications and priorities for nursing care can be drawn at this time?
4. Does the evidence objectively support your conclusion?

meet the needs of individual mothers. In addition, the nurse can help the family limit visitors and provide a comfortable chair or bed for the partner or other family member who is staying with the new mother.

Because PPF can be very debilitating, follow-up after hospital discharge is important. Screening for PPF can be accomplished with a nurse-initiated telephone call at 2 weeks and at the routine 6-week postpartum visit with the health care provider. Nurses in the pediatric care provider's office or clinic should also be alert for signs of PPF. The infant will be seen within the first few days after birth—before the woman sees her obstetric care provider.

Physiologic factors contributing to PPF are amenable to intervention and may be identified even before birth. Women with sleeping problems during pregnancy, anemia, infection or inflammation, or thyroid dysfunction can be identified as having increased risk for PPF. Other physical conditions and psychologic or situational factors that might contribute to PPF can be identified during the prenatal period. The medical records of women with known risk factors can be flagged to alert hospital staff to their special needs (see Critical Thinking Case Study).

Promotion of Ambulation

Early ambulation is associated with a reduced incidence of venous thromboembolism (VTE); it also promotes the return of strength. Free movement is encouraged once anesthesia wears off unless an opioid analgesic has been administered. After the initial recovery period is over, the mother is encouraged to ambulate frequently.

In the early postpartum period women can feel light-headed or dizzy when standing. The rapid decrease in intraabdominal pressure after birth results in a dilation of blood vessels supplying the intestines (splanchnic engorgement) and causes blood to pool in the viscera. This condition contributes to the development of orthostatic hypotension and can occur when the woman who has recently given birth sits or stands, first ambulates, or takes a warm shower or sitz bath. The nurse must consider the baseline blood pressure; amount of blood loss; and type, amount, and timing of analgesic or anesthetic medications administered when helping a woman ambulate. The nurse or family member should remain nearby while the woman showers in case she becomes faint.

Women who have had epidural or spinal anesthesia may have slow return of sensory and motor function in their lower extremities, increasing the risk of falls with early ambulation. Careful assessment by the postpartum nurse can prevent falls. Factors that the nurse should consider are the time lapse since the medication was given; the woman's ability to bend both knees, place both feet flat on the bed, and lift buttocks off the bed without assistance; medications since birth; vital signs; and estimated blood loss with birth. Before allowing the woman to ambulate the nurse assesses her ability to stand unassisted beside her bed, simultaneously bending both knees slightly and then standing with knees locked. If the woman is unable to balance herself, she can be eased back into bed safely (Frank, Lane, and Hokanson, 2009).

⚡ **SAFETY ALERT**

To promote patient safety and prevent injury, it is important to have hospital personnel present at least the first time the woman gets out of bed after birth because she can feel weak, dizzy, faint, or light-headed. The woman is instructed to call for assistance before getting out of bed the first time and any time thereafter if she feels dizzy or weak. The partner or family members who are present are instructed as well.

Prevention of VTE is important. Women who must remain in bed after giving birth are at increased risk. Antiembolic stockings (TED hose) and/or a sequential compression device (SCD) boots may be ordered prophylactically, especially after cesarean birth. If a woman remains in bed longer than 8 hours (e.g., for postpartum magnesium sulfate therapy for preeclampsia), exercise to promote circulation in the legs is indicated using the following routine:

- Alternate flexion and extension of feet.
- Rotate ankles in circular motion.
- Alternate flexion and extension of legs.
- Press back of knee to bed surface; relax.

If the woman is susceptible to VTE, she is encouraged to walk about actively for true ambulation and is discouraged from sitting immobile in a chair. Women with varicosities are advised to wear support hose. If a thrombus is suspected, as evidenced by warmth, redness, or tenderness in the suspected leg, the primary health care provider should be notified immediately. Meanwhile the woman should be confined to bed with the affected limb elevated on pillows.

Promotion of Exercise

Most women who have just given birth are interested in regaining their nonpregnant figures. Postpartum exercise can begin soon after birth, although the woman should be encouraged to start with simple exercises and gradually progress to more strenuous ones. Fig. 19-5 illustrates a number of exercises appropriate for the new mother. Abdominal exercises are postponed until about 4 weeks after cesarean birth.

Kegel exercises to strengthen muscle tone are extremely important, particularly after vaginal birth. They help women regain the muscle tone that often is lost as pelvic tissues are stretched and torn during pregnancy and birth. Women who maintain muscle strength can benefit years later by maintaining urinary continence.

It is essential that women learn to perform Kegel exercises correctly (see Guidelines box on p. 57). Some women perform them incorrectly and can increase their risk of incontinence, which can occur when inadvertently bearing down on the pelvic floor muscles,

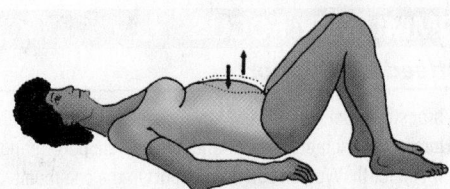

Abdominal Breathing. Lie on back with knees bent. Inhale deeply through nose. Keep ribs stationary and allow abdomen to expand upward. Exhale slowly but forcefully while contracting the abdominal muscles; hold for 3 to 5 seconds while exhaling. Relax.

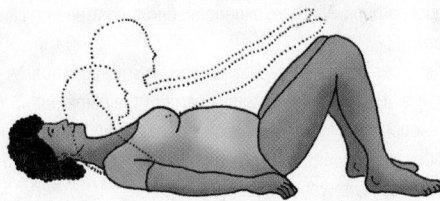

Reach for the Knees. Lie on back with knees bent. While inhaling, deeply lower chin onto chest. While exhaling, raise head and shoulders slowly and smoothly and reach for knees with arms outstretched. The body should rise only as far as the back will naturally bend while waist remains on floor or bed (about 6 to 8 inches). Slowly and smoothly lower head and shoulders back to starting position. Relax.

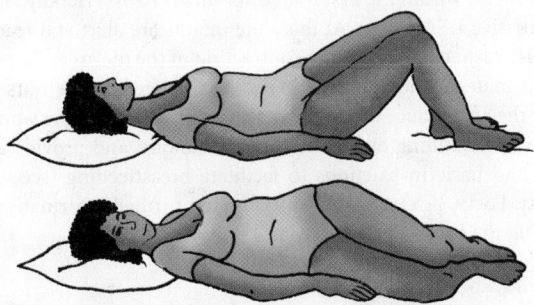

Double Knee Roll. Lie on back with knees bent. Keeping shoulders flat and feet stationary, slowly and smoothly roll knees over to the left to touch floor or bed. Maintaining a smooth motion, roll knees back over to the right until they touch floor or bed. Return to starting position and relax.

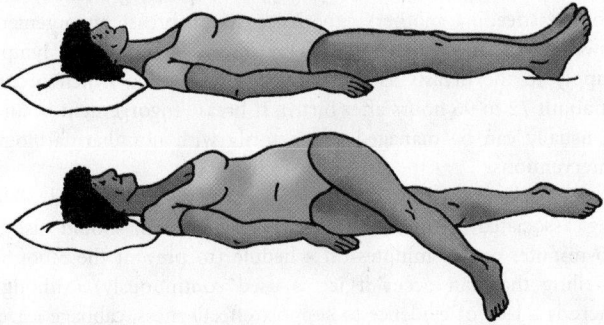

Leg Roll. Lie on back with legs straight. Keeping shoulders flat and legs straight, slowly and smoothly lift left leg and roll it over to touch the right side of floor or bed and return to starting position. Repeat, rolling right leg over to touch left side of floor or bed. Relax.

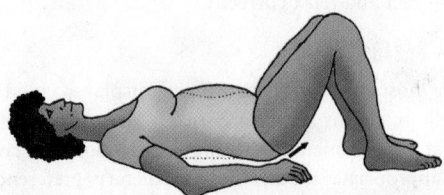

Combined Abdominal Breathing and Supine Pelvic Tilt (Pelvic Rock). Lie on back with knees bent. While inhaling deeply, roll pelvis back by flattening lower back on floor or bed. Exhale slowly but forcefully while contracting abdominal muscles and tightening buttocks. Hold for 3 to 5 seconds while exhaling. Relax.

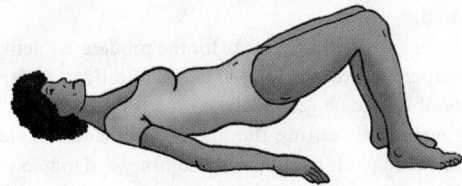

Buttocks Lift. Lie on back with arms at sides, knees bent, and feet flat. Slowly raise buttocks and arch back. Return slowly to starting position.

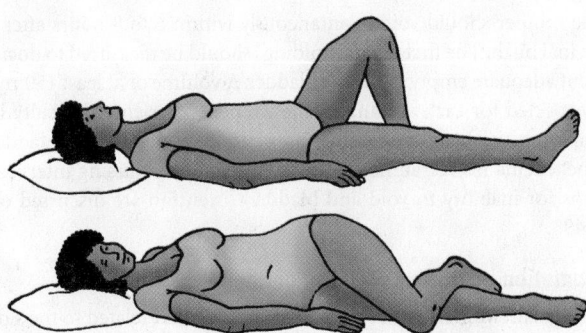

Single Knee Roll. Lie on back with right leg straight and left leg bent at the knee. Keeping shoulders flat, slowly and smoothly roll left knee over to the right to touch floor or bed and then back to starting position. Reverse position of legs. Roll right knee over to the left to touch floor or bed and return to starting position. Relax.

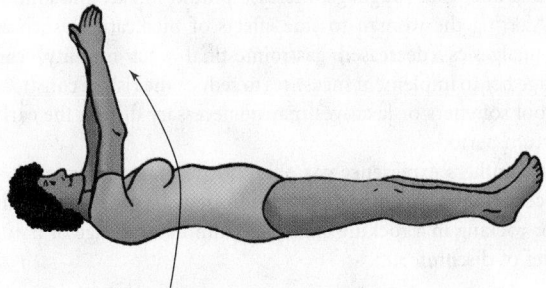

Arm Raises. Lie on back with arms extended at 90-degree angle from body. Raise arms so they are perpendicular and hands touch. Lower slowly.

FIG 19-5 Postpartum exercise should begin as soon as possible. The woman should start with simple exercises and gradually progress to more strenuous ones.

thrusting the perineum outward. The woman's technique can be assessed during the pelvic examination at her checkup by inserting two fingers intravaginally and checking whether the pelvic floor muscles contract and relax correctly.

Promotion of Nutrition

During the hospital stay most women display a good appetite and eat well; nutritious snacks are usually welcomed. Women may request that family members bring to the hospital favorite or culturally appropriate foods. Cultural dietary preferences must be respected. This interest in food presents an ideal opportunity for nutrition counseling on dietary needs after pregnancy such as for breastfeeding, preventing constipation and anemia, promoting weight loss, and promoting healing and well-being (see Chapter 9). Prenatal vitamins and iron supplements are often continued until 6 weeks after birth or until the ordered supply has been used.

The recommended caloric intake for the moderately active, non-lactating postpartum woman is 1800 to 2200 kcal/day. According to the Institute of Medicine (2005) the estimated energy requirement for a lactating woman during the first 6 months is 2700 kcal/day. Higher-than-normal caloric intake is recommended for woman who are underweight or who exercise vigorously and those who are breastfeeding more than one infant.

Promotion of Normal Bladder Function

The mother should void spontaneously within 6 to 8 hours after a vaginal birth. The first several voidings should be measured to document adequate emptying of the bladder. A volume of at least 150 mL is expected for each voiding. Some women experience difficulty in emptying the bladder, possibly as a result of diminished bladder tone, edema from trauma, or fear of discomfort. Nursing interventions for inability to void and bladder distention are discussed on p. 498.

Promotion of Normal Bowel Function

After birth, women can be at risk for constipation related to the side effects of medications (e.g., opioid analgesics, iron supplements, magnesium sulfate), dehydration, immobility, perineal lacerations or episiotomy, or hemorrhoids. Some women fear discomfort with straining to have a bowel movement. Nursing interventions to promote normal bowel elimination include educating the woman about measures to avoid constipation. These interventions include consuming adequate roughage, increasing fluid intake, and ambulating. Alerting the woman to side effects of medications such as opioid analgesics (decreased gastrointestinal tract motility) can encourage her to implement measures to reduce the risk of constipation. Stool softeners or laxatives may be necessary during the early postpartum period.

Some mothers experience gas pains; this is more common following cesarean birth. Antigas medications may be ordered. Ambulation or rocking in a rocking chair may stimulate passage of flatus and relief of discomfort.

> ### ! NURSING ALERT
> Rectal suppositories and enemas should not be administered to women with third- or fourth-degree perineal lacerations. These measures to treat constipation can be very uncomfortable and can cause hemorrhage or damage to the suture line. They can also predispose the woman to infection (AWHONN, 2006).

Promotion of Breastfeeding

The ideal time to initiate breastfeeding is within the first 1 to 2 hours after childbirth. Baby-Friendly hospitals mandate that the infant be put to breast within the first hour after birth (Baby-Friendly Hospital Initiative USA, 2010). At this time infants are alert and ready to nurse. Breastfeeding promotes contraction of the uterus and prevention of maternal hemorrhage. With the first feeding the nurse can assess the appearance of the breasts and nipples, assess the woman's basic understanding of breastfeeding technique, and provide assistance and basic instructions to facilitate breastfeeding (see Community Focus box). (See Chapter 24 for further information on assisting the breastfeeding woman.)

Lactation Suppression

Suppression of lactation is necessary when the woman has decided not to breastfeed or in the case of neonatal death. Wearing a well-fitted support bra or breast binder continuously for at least the first 72 hours after giving birth is important. Women should avoid breast stimulation, including running warm water over the breasts, newborn suckling, or expressing milk. A few nonbreastfeeding mothers experience severe breast engorgement (swelling of breast tissue caused by increased blood and lymph supply to the breasts as the body produces milk, which occurs at about 72 to 96 hours after birth). If breast engorgement occurs, it usually can be managed satisfactorily with nonpharmacologic interventions.

Ice packs to the breasts help decrease the discomfort and swelling associated with engorgement. The woman should use a 15-minutes-on, 45-minutes-off schedule (to prevent the rebound swelling that can occur if ice is used continuously). Although there is a lack of evidence to support effectiveness, cabbage leaves are often recommended to help relieve the engorgement. The woman who has chosen to formula-feed can be told to place cold cabbage leaves over her breasts inside her bra. The leaves are replaced each time they wilt. A mild analgesic or antiinflammatory medication can reduce discomfort associated with engorgement and help the mother through this uncomfortable time. Medications that were once prescribed for lactation suppression (estrogen, estrogen and testosterone, and bromocriptine) are no longer used.

Health Promotion for Planning Future Pregnancies and Children

Rubella Vaccination. For women who have not had rubella (10% to 20% of all women) or women who are serologically not immune (titer of 1:8 or enzyme immunoassay level less than 0.8), a subcutaneous injection of rubella vaccine is recommended in the immediate postpartum period to prevent the possibility of contracting rubella in future pregnancies. Seroconversion occurs in approximately 90% of women vaccinated after birth. The live attenuated rubella virus is not communicable; therefore breastfeeding mothers can be vaccinated (CDC, 2012a). However, because the virus is shed in urine and other body fluids, the vaccine should not be given if the mother or other household members are immunocompromised. Rubella vaccine is made from duck eggs; thus women who have allergies to these eggs can develop a hypersensitivity reaction to the vaccine, for which they will need adrenaline. A transient arthralgia or rash is common in vaccinated women. Because the vaccine can be teratogenic, women must be informed about this fact.

Varicella Vaccination. The CDC recommends the administration of varicella vaccine before discharge for postpartum women who have no immunity. A second dose is given 4 to 8 weeks after the first dose; this can be done at the postpartum follow-up visit. Mothers who receive the varicella vaccine can continue to breastfeed (CDC, 2012c).

LEGAL TIP: Rubella and Varicella Vaccination

Informed consent for rubella and varicella vaccination in the postpartum period includes information about possible side effects and the risk of teratogenic effects. Women must understand that they must practice contraception for 1 month after being vaccinated to avoid pregnancy (CDC, 2012c).

Tetanus-Diphtheria-Acellular Pertussis Vaccination. The tetanus-diphtheria-acellular pertussis (Tdap) vaccine is recommended for postpartum women who have not previously received the vaccine. It is given before hospital discharge or as early as possible in the postpartum period to protect women from pertussis and decrease the risk of infant exposure to pertussis. Women should be advised that other adults and children who will be around the newborn should be vaccinated with Tdap if they have not previously received the vaccine (CDC, 2012b). Women who receive the vaccine can continue to breastfeed.

Prevention of Rh Isoimmunization. Injection of Rh immune globulin (RhIg) (a solution of γ-globulin that contains Rh antibodies) within 72 hours after birth prevents sensitization in the Rh-negative woman who has had a fetomaternal transfusion of Rh-positive fetal red blood cells (RBCs) (see Medication Guide). RhIg promotes lysis of fetal Rh-positive blood cells before the mother forms her own antibodies against them.

! NURSING ALERT

After birth, Rh immune globulin is administered to all Rh-negative, antibody (Coombs' test)–negative women who give birth to Rh-positive infants. RhIg is administered to the mother intramuscularly (RhoGAM, Gamulin RH, HypRho-D, Rhophylac) or intravenously (Rhophylac). It should never be given to an infant.

The administration of 300 mcg (1 vial) of Rh immune globulin is usually sufficient to prevent maternal sensitization. If a large fetomaternal transfusion is suspected, the dosage needed should be determined by performing a Kleihauer-Betke test, which detects the

---

◆ MEDICATION GUIDE

Rh Immune Globulin, RhoGAM, Gamulin Rh, HypRho-D, Rhophylac

Action

Suppression of immune response in nonsensitized women with Rh-negative blood who receive Rh-positive blood cells because of fetomaternal hemorrhage, transfusion, or accident

Indications

Routine antepartum prevention at 28 weeks of gestation in women with Rh-negative blood; suppress antibody formation after birth, miscarriage, pregnancy termination, abdominal trauma, ectopic pregnancy, amniocentesis, version, or chorionic villi sampling

Dosage/Route

Standard dose: 1 vial (300 mcg) IM in deltoid or gluteal muscle; microdose: 1 vial (50 mcg) IM in deltoid muscle; Rho(D) immune globulin (Rhophylac) can be given IM or IV (available in prefilled syringes).

Adverse Effects

Myalgia, lethargy, localized tenderness and stiffness at injection site, mild and transient fever, malaise, headache; rarely nausea, vomiting, hypotension, tachycardia, and allergic response

Nursing Considerations

- Give standard dose to mother at 28 weeks of gestation as prophylaxis or after an incident or exposure risk that occurs after 28 weeks of gestation (e.g., amniocentesis, second-trimester miscarriage or abortion, after external version) and within 72 hours after birth if baby is Rh positive.
- Give microdose for first-trimester miscarriage or abortion, ectopic pregnancy, chorionic villi sampling.
- Verify that the woman is Rh negative and has not been sensitized; if postpartum that Coombs' test is negative; and that baby is Rh positive. Provide explanation to the woman about the procedure, including the purpose, possible side effects, and effect on future pregnancies. Have the woman sign a consent form if required by agency. Verify correct dosage and confirm lot number and woman's identity before giving injection (verify with another registered nurse or by other procedure per agency policy); document administration per agency policy. Observe patient for at least 20 minutes after administration for allergic response.
- Document lot number and expiration date in the patient record.
- The medication is made from human plasma (a consideration if woman is a Jehovah's Witness). The risk of transmitting infectious agents, including viruses, cannot be eliminated completely.

IM, Intramuscularly; *IV,* intravenously.

---

amount of fetal blood in the maternal circulation. If more than 15 mL of fetal blood is present in maternal circulation, the dosage of RhIg must be increased.

Rh immune globulin suppresses the immune response. Therefore the woman who receives both RhIg and a live virus immunization such as rubella must be tested in 3 months to see if she has developed immunity. If not, the woman will need another dose of the vaccine.

There is some disagreement about whether Rh immune globulin should be considered a blood product. Health care providers need to discuss the most current information about this issue with women whose religious beliefs conflict with having blood products administered to them (e.g., Jehovah Witnesses).

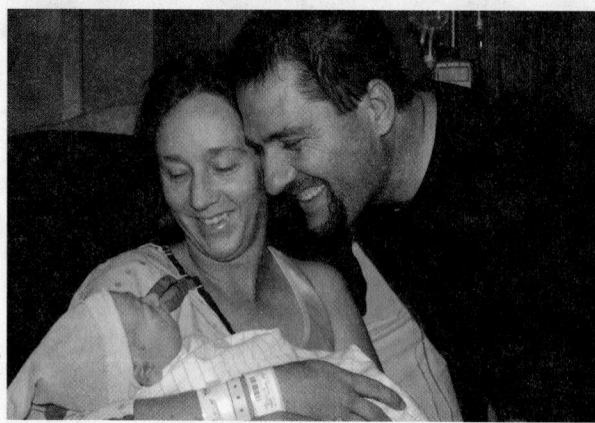

FIG 19-6 Parents getting acquainted with their new son. (Courtesy Julie and Darren Nelson, Loveland, CO.)

CARE MANAGEMENT—PSYCHOSOCIAL NEEDS

Meeting the psychosocial needs of new parents involves assessing their reactions to the birth experience, their feelings about themselves, and their interactions with the new baby (Fig. 19-6) and other family members. Specific interventions are then planned to increase the parents' knowledge and self-confidence as they assume the care and responsibility of the new baby and integrate this new member into their existing family structure in a way that meets their cultural expectations (see Chapter 20).

Taking time to assess maternal emotional needs and concerns before discharge can promote better psychologic health and adjustment to parenting. Ongoing support for postpartum women is also needed. Issues such as fatigue that often appear during the hospital stay tend to continue after discharge and can intensify. Postpartum support is especially beneficial to at-risk populations such as low-income primiparas, those at risk for family dysfunction and child abuse, and those at risk for postpartum depression (PPD).

Sometimes the psychosocial assessment indicates serious actual or potential problems that must be addressed. Box 19-2 identifies psychosocial characteristics and behaviors that may warrant ongoing evaluation after hospital discharge. Women exhibiting these needs should be referred to appropriate community resources for assessment and management.

Assessment
Effect of the Birth Experience

Many women indicate a need to examine the birth process itself and look at their own intrapartal behavior in retrospect. Their partners can express similar desires. If their birth experience was quite different from the one they planned (e.g., induction, epidural anesthesia, cesarean birth), both partners may need to mourn the loss of their expectations before they can adjust to the reality of their actual birth experience. Inviting them to review and reflect on the events and describe how they feel helps the nurse assess how well they understand what happened and how well they have been able to put their birth experience into perspective.

Maternal Self-Image

An important assessment concerns the woman's self-concept, body image, and sexuality. How this new mother feels about herself and her body during the puerperium can affect her behavior and adaptation to parenting. The woman's self-concept and body image can also affect her sexuality.

BOX 19-2 SIGNS OF POTENTIAL COMPLICATIONS: POSTPARTUM PSYCHOSOCIAL CONCERNS

The following signs can suggest potentially serious complications and should be reported to the health care provider or clinic (these may be noticed by the partner or other family members):

- Unable or unwilling to discuss labor and birth experience
- Refers to self as ugly and useless
- Excessively preoccupied with self (body image)
- Markedly depressed
- Lacks support system
- Partner and/or other family members react negatively to baby
- Refuses to interact with or care for baby (e.g., does not name baby, does not want to hold or feed baby, is upset by vomiting and wet or dirty diapers) (cultural appropriateness of actions must be considered)
- Expresses disappointment over baby's sex
- Sees baby as messy or unattractive
- Baby reminds mother of family member or friend she doesn't like
- Has difficulty sleeping
- Experiences loss of appetite

Feelings related to sexual adjustment after childbirth are often a cause of concern for new parents. Women who have recently given birth can be reluctant to resume sexual intercourse for fear of pain or worry that coitus could damage healing perineal tissue. Because many new parents are anxious for information but reluctant to bring up the subject, postpartum nurses should matter-of-factly include the topic of postpartum sexuality as a routine part of discharge teaching. Postpartum sexuality can be discussed during routine physical assessments. For example, while examining a perineal laceration or an episiotomy site, the nurse can say, "I know you're sore right now, but it probably won't be long until you (or you and your partner) are ready to make love again. Do you have any questions about resuming sex?" This approach assures the woman and her partner that resuming sexual activity is a legitimate concern for new parents and indicates the nurse's willingness to answer questions and share information.

Adaptation to Parenthood and Parent-Infant Interactions

The psychosocial assessment includes evaluating adaptation to parenthood as evidenced by the mother's and father's (partner's) reactions to and interactions with the new baby. Clues indicating successful adaptation begin to appear early in the postbirth period as parents react positively to the newborn infant and continue the process of establishing a relationship with their child.

Parents are adapting well to their new roles when they exhibit a realistic perception and acceptance of their newborn's needs and his or her limited abilities, immature social responses, and helplessness. Examples of positive parent-infant interactions include taking pleasure in the infant and the tasks done for and with him or her; understanding the infant's emotional states and providing comfort; and reading the infant's cues for new experiences and sensing his or her fatigue level (see Chapter 20).

If these indicators are missing, the nurse must investigate further in an attempt to identify what is hindering the normal adaptation process. She or he can ask several questions such as "Do you feel sad often?" or "Do you have concerns about being a good parent?" that help to determine if the woman is experiencing the

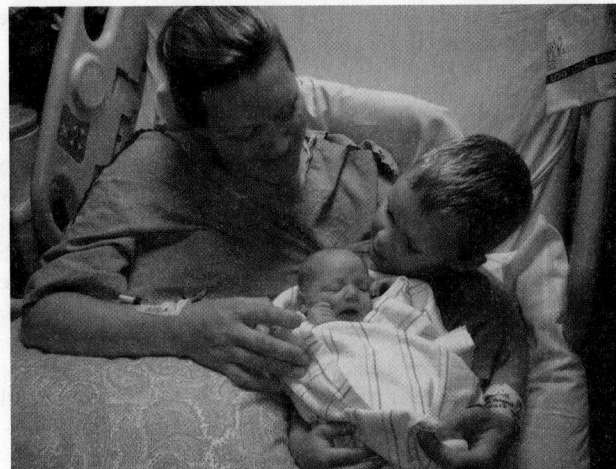

FIG 19-7 Older sibling cuddles with mother and new baby. (Courtesy Jennifer Hobgood, Creedmoor, NC.)

A Clash of Cultures

A Vietnamese woman who had been in the United States for 4 years requested rooming-in facilities after birth. Instead of participating in the care of her infant, she refused to do so, remained in bed, wore a woolen cap, and appeared distressed and angry. The staff were puzzled and upset by her behavior. One nurse decided to put into effect her newly learned concepts concerning cross-cultural nursing. She began by praising the woman's ability to speak English and, after eliciting a smile, remarked, "Every country has developed good ways to look after mothers and babies. Would you tell me about the care in Vietnam?" There was an immediate response. The woman explained that in her country women remained in bed for at least 10 days after birth and the biggest danger to their health was getting a cold. The baby was kept in the room with the mother, but either a grandmother or nurse took complete charge of the care.

With this information the nurse was able to modify her plan of care to make it culturally relevant and therefore more satisfying for the woman.

normal "baby blues" or if there is a more serious underlying condition. Screening for PPD through the use of a simple tool such as the Edinburgh Postnatal Depression Scale (EPDS) can be done before hospital discharge. Screening for PPD should also be done after discharge. The AAP recommends that pediatric care providers perform maternal screening for PPD during infant follow-up visits at 1, 2, and 4 months (AAP Committee on Psychosocial Aspects of Child and Family Health, 2010). See Chapter 21 for further discussion of PPD.

Family Structure and Functioning

A woman's adjustment to her role as mother is affected greatly by her relationships with her partner, her mother and other relatives, and any other children (Fig. 19-7). Nurses can help ease the new mother's return home by identifying possible conflicts among family members and helping the woman plan strategies for dealing with these problems before discharge. Such a conflict can arise when couples have very different ideas about parenting. Dealing with the stresses of sibling rivalry and unsolicited grandparent advice can also affect the woman's transition to motherhood. Only by asking about other nuclear and extended family members can the nurse discover potential problems in such relationships and help plan workable solutions for them.

Impact of Cultural Diversity

The final component of a complete psychosocial assessment is the woman's cultural beliefs and values. Much of a woman's behavior during the postpartum period is strongly influenced by her cultural background. Nurses are likely to come into contact with women from many different countries and cultures. All cultures have developed safe and satisfying methods of caring for new mothers and babies. The nurse can identify some cultural beliefs and practices through observation and interaction with the mother and her family. Questioning the mother and her family about their cultural practices can provide useful information to help the nurse provide optimal care. Only by understanding and respecting the values and beliefs of each woman can the nurse design a plan of care to meet individual needs (see Cultural Competence box).

Discharge Teaching

The nurse functions primarily as teacher, encourager, and supporter while implementing the psychosocial plan of care for a postpartum woman. Implementation of this care plan involves carrying out specific activities to achieve the expected outcome of care planned for each woman. Topics that should be included include promotion of parenting skills and family member adjustment to the newborn infant (see Chapter 20).

Cultural issues must also be considered when planning care. Many traditional health beliefs and practices exist among the different cultures within the North American population. Traditional health practices that are used to maintain health or avoid illnesses deal with the whole person (body, mind, and spirit) and tend to be culturally based.

Women from various cultures may view health as a balance between opposing forces (e.g., cold versus hot, yin versus yang), being in harmony with nature, or just "feeling good." Traditional practices may include the observance of certain dietary restrictions, clothing, or taboos for balancing the body; participation in certain activities such as sports and art for maintaining mental health; and use of silence, prayer, or meditation for developing spiritually. Practices such as using religious objects or eating garlic are used to protect oneself from illness and may involve avoiding people who are believed to create hexes and spells or who have an "evil eye." Restoration of health may involve a person taking folk medicines (e.g., herbs, animal substances) or using a traditional healer.

Birth occurs within this sociocultural context. Rest, seclusion, dietary restraints, and ceremonies honoring the mother are all common traditional practices that are followed for the promotion of the health and well-being of both mother and baby.

During the postpartum period there are several common traditional health practices used and beliefs held by women and their families. For example, in Southeast Asia pregnancy is considered to be a "hot" state, and childbirth results in a sudden loss of this state. Therefore balance needs to be restored by increasing the return of the hot state, which is present physically or symbolically in hot food, hot water, and warm air.

Another common belief is that the mother and baby remain in a weak and vulnerable state for a period of several weeks following birth. During this time the mother may remain in a passive role, take no baths or showers, and stay in bed to prevent cold air from entering her body. Hispanic women who have immigrated to the United States or other Western nations observe the period of 40 days (6 weeks) after birth as *la cuarentena*. During this time the woman's body is perceived to be "open" and vulnerable to drafts; la cuarentena is about "closing the body." Traditional practices associated with la cuarentena include a liquid diet of nutritious drinks, soups, and broths in the early postpartum period; binding the abdomen; avoiding cool air; and maintaining abstinence (Waugh, 2011). Without their extended families the mother may not have much help at home, making it difficult for her to observe these activity restrictions. Box 19-3 lists some common cultural beliefs about the postpartum period and family planning.

It is important that nurses consider all cultural aspects when planning care and not use their own cultural beliefs as the framework for that care. Although the beliefs and behaviors of other cultures can seem different or strange, they should be encouraged as long as the mother wants to conform to them and she and the baby have no ill effects. The nurse must determine whether a woman is using any folk medicine during the postpartum period because active ingredients in folk medicine can have adverse physiologic effects on the woman when ingested with prescribed medicines. Many young women who are first- or second-generation Americans

---

BOX 19-3   SOME CULTURAL BELIEFS ABOUT THE POSTPARTUM PERIOD AND FAMILY PLANNING

Postpartum Care

- *Chinese, Mexican, Korean,* and *Southeast Asian women* may wish to eat only warm foods and drink hot drinks to replace blood loss and restore the balance of hot and cold in their bodies. These women may also wish to stay warm and avoid bathing, exercising, and hair washing for 7 to 30 days after childbirth. Self-management may not be a priority; care by family members is preferred. The woman has respect for elders and authority. These women may wear abdominal binders. They may prefer not to give their babies colostrum.
- *Haitian women* may ask to take the placenta home to bury or burn.
- *Muslim women* follow strict religious laws on modesty and diet. A Muslim woman must keep her hair, body, arms to the wrist, and legs covered to the ankles at all times. She cannot be alone in the presence of a man other than her husband or a male relative. Observant Muslims do not eat pork or pork products and are obligated to eat meat slaughtered according to Islamic laws (halal meat). If halal meat is not available, kosher meat, seafood, or a vegetarian diet is usually acceptable.

Family Planning

- Birth control is government mandated in mainland *China*. Most *Chinese women* will have an intrauterine device inserted after the birth of their first child. Women do not want hormonal methods of contraception because they fear putting these medications in their bodies.
- *Saudi Arabian* and *Hispanic women* usually choose the rhythm method because most are Catholic.
- *(East) Indian men* are encouraged to have voluntary sterilization by vasectomy.
- *Muslim couples* may practice contraception by mutual consent as long as its use is not harmful to the woman. Acceptable contraceptive methods include foam and condoms, the diaphragm, and natural family planning.
- *Hmong women* highly value and desire large families, which limits birth control practices.
- *Mexican women* observe la cuarentena for 40 days after birth, when they observe abstinence from sexual activity.

---

follow their cultural traditions only when older family members are present or not at all.

Self-Management and Signs of Complications

Discharge planning begins at the time of admission to the unit and should be reflected in the nursing care plan developed for each woman. For example, a great deal of time during the hospital stay is usually spent in teaching about maternal self-management and care of the newborn because the goal is for all women to be capable of providing basic care for themselves and their infants at the time of discharge. In addition, every woman must be taught to recognize physical and psychologic signs and symptoms that might indicate problems and how to obtain advice and assistance quickly if these signs appear. Table 19-1 and Box 19-2, respectively, list several common indications of maternal physical and psychosocial problems in the postpartum period. (See Chapter 21 for more information on postpartum complications.) Before discharge women need basic instruction regarding a variety of self-management topics such as nutrition, exercise, family planning, the resumption of sexual intercourse, prescribed medications, and routine mother-baby follow-up care.

Because of the limited time available for teaching, nurses must target their teaching toward expressed needs of the woman. Giving the woman a list of topics and asking her to indicate her learning needs help the nurse maximize teaching efforts and can increase retention of information. Providing written materials on postpartum self-management, breastfeeding, and infant care that the woman can consult after discharge is helpful.

Just before the time of discharge the nurse reviews the woman's records to see that laboratory reports, medications, signatures, and other items are in order. Some hospitals have a checklist to use before the woman's discharge. The nurse verifies that medications, if ordered, have arrived on the unit; that any valuables kept secured during the woman's stay have been returned to her and that she has signed a receipt for them; and that the infant is ready to be discharged. The woman's and baby's identification bands are checked carefully.

⚡ **SAFETY ALERT**

No medication that can cause drowsiness should be administered to the mother before discharge if she is the one who will be holding the baby when they leave the hospital. In most instances the woman is seated in a wheelchair and given the baby to hold. Some families leave unescorted and ambulatory, depending on hospital protocol. The newborn must be secured in a car seat for the drive home (see Fig. 23-25).

In many hospitals new mothers (breastfeeding and formula feeding) are routinely presented with gift bags that contain samples of infant formula. This practice is not consistent with the Baby-Friendly Hospital USA initiative (2010).

❗ **NURSING ALERT**

Prepackaged formula should not be given to mothers who are breastfeeding. Such "gifts" are associated with earlier cessation of breastfeeding.

Sexual Activity and Contraception

Discussing sexual activity with the woman and her partner and family planning with heterosexual couples are important before they leave the hospital because many couples resume sexual activity before the traditional postpartum checkup 6 weeks after childbirth. For most women the risk of hemorrhage or infection is minimal by approximately 2 weeks after birth. Couples may be anxious about the topic but uncomfortable and unwilling to bring it up. The nurse needs to discuss the physical and psychologic effects that giving birth can have on sexual activity (see Home Care box).

Many factors can influence the timing and quality of sexual activity after birth. Postpartum perineal pain and dyspareunia (painful intercourse) are common among women with perineal lacerations or episiotomy. Discomfort is more severe and lasts longer with third- and fourth-degree lacerations. Breastfeeding mothers often experience vaginal dryness related to high levels of prolactin and low estrogen levels. Changes in family structure and altered sleep patterns can make it difficult for a couple to find time for privacy and intimacy. Postpartum depression is associated with decreased sexual desire; medication used to treat PPD can reduce sexual desire and inhibit orgasm (Leeman and Rogers, 2012).

Contraceptive options should be discussed with heterosexual women (and their partners, if present) before discharge so they can make informed decisions about fertility management before resuming sexual activity. Waiting to discuss contraception at the 6-week checkup may be too late. Ovulation can occur as soon as 1 month after birth, particularly in women who bottle-feed. Breastfeeding mothers should be informed that breastfeeding is not a reliable

means of contraception and that other methods should be used; nonhormonal methods are best because oral contraceptives can interfere with milk production. Women who are undecided about contraception at the time of discharge need information about using condoms with foam or creams until the first postpartum checkup. Contraceptive options are discussed in detail in Chapter 5.

Prescribed Medications

Women routinely continue to take their prenatal vitamins during the postpartum period. Breastfeeding mothers usually continue prenatal vitamins for the duration of breastfeeding. Supplemental iron can be prescribed for mothers with lower-than-normal hemoglobin levels. Women with extensive episiotomies or perineal lacerations (third or fourth degree) are usually prescribed stool softeners to take at home. Pain medications (opioid and non-opioid) may be prescribed, especially for women who had cesarean births. The nurse should make certain that the woman knows the route, dosage, frequency, and common side effects of all medications that she will be taking at home. Written information about the medications is usually included in the discharge instructions.

Follow-Up After Discharge

Routine Schedule of Care. Women who have experienced uncomplicated vaginal births are still commonly scheduled for the traditional 6-week postpartum examination. Women who have had a cesarean birth are often seen in the health care provider's office or clinic within 2 weeks after hospital discharge. The date and time for the follow-up appointment should be included in the discharge instructions. If an appointment is not made before the woman leaves the hospital, she should be encouraged to call the health care provider's office or clinic to schedule one.

Parents who have not already done so need to make plans for newborn follow-up at the time of discharge. Breastfeeding infants are seen routinely by the pediatric health care provider or clinic within 3 to 5 days after birth or 48 to 72 hours after hospital discharge and again at approximately 2 weeks of age (AAP, 2012). Formula-feeding infants may be seen for the first time at 2 weeks of age. If an appointment for a specific date and time was not made for the infant before leaving the hospital, the parents should be encouraged to call the office or clinic soon after their arrival home.

Home Visits. Home visits to mothers and babies within a few days of discharge can help bridge the gap between hospital care and routine visits to health care providers. Nurses can assess the mother, infant, home environment, and family interactions; answer questions and provide education and emotional support; and make referrals to community resources if necessary. Home visits have been shown to reduce the need for more expensive health care such as emergency department visits and rehospitalization; they can also reduce the incidence of PPD in women who are at risk.

The support provided by nurses and other trained community health workers can enhance parent-infant interaction and parenting skills; home visits also help to promote mutual support between the mother and her partner (De La Rosa, Perry, and Johnson, 2009). Breastfeeding outcomes can be enhanced through home visitation programs.

Home nursing care may not be available, even if needed, because no agencies are available to provide the service or no coverage is in place for payment by third-party payers. If care is available, a referral form containing information about the mother and baby should be completed at hospital discharge and sent immediately to the home care agency.

HOME CARE

Resumption of Sexual Activity

- Unless your health care provider indicates otherwise, you can safely resume sexual activity (intercourse) by the second to fourth week after birth, when bleeding has stopped and the perineum is healed. Most women resume sexual activity by 5 to 6 weeks after birth, although this varies and is often related to perineal discomfort. Perineal lacerations or episiotomy increases the chances of discomfort with intercourse. For the first 6 weeks to 6 months, vaginal lubrication can be decreased, especially among breastfeeding women. Your physiologic reactions to sexual stimulation for the first 3 months after birth may be slower and less intense. The strength of the orgasm may be reduced.
- A water-soluble gel or contraceptive cream or jelly might be recommended for lubrication. If some vaginal tenderness is present, your partner can be instructed to insert one or more clean, lubricated fingers into the vagina and rotate them to help the vagina relax and identify possible areas of discomfort. A position in which you have control of the depth of the insertion of the penis also is useful. The side-by-side or female-on-top position may be more comfortable than other positions.
- The presence of the baby influences postbirth sexual activity and enjoyment. Parents hear every sound made by the baby; conversely you may be concerned that the baby hears every sound you make. In either case any phase of the sexual response cycle may be interrupted by hearing the baby cry or move, leaving both of you frustrated and unsatisfied. In addition, the amount of psychologic energy expended by you in childcare activities may lead to fatigue. Newborns require a great deal of attention and time.
- Some women have reported feeling sexual stimulation and orgasms when breastfeeding their babies. Breastfeeding mothers often are interested in returning to sexual activity before nonbreastfeeding mothers.
- You should be instructed to perform the Kegel exercises correctly to strengthen your pubococcygeal muscle. This muscle is associated with bowel and bladder function and vaginal feeling during intercourse.

The home visit is most commonly scheduled on the woman's second day home from the hospital, but it can be scheduled on any of the first 4 days at home, depending on the individual family's situation and needs. Additional visits are planned throughout the first week as needed. The home visits may be extended beyond that time if the family's needs warrant it and if a home visit is the most appropriate option for carrying out the follow-up care required to meet the specific needs identified.

During the home visit the nurse conducts a systematic assessment of mother and newborn to determine physiologic adjustment and identify any existing complications. The assessment also focuses on the mother's emotional adjustment and her knowledge of self-management and infant care. Conducting the assessment in a private area of the home provides an opportunity for the mother to ask questions about potentially sensitive topics such as breast care, constipation, sexual activity, or family planning. Family adjustment to the newborn is assessed, and concerns are addressed during the home visit.

During the newborn assessment the nurse can demonstrate and explain normal newborn behavior and capabilities and encourage the mother and family to ask questions or express concerns that they have. The home care nurse verifies if the newborn screen for phenylketonuria and other inborn errors of metabolism has been drawn. If the baby was discharged from the hospital before 24 hours of age, a blood sample for the newborn screen can be drawn by the home care nurse, or the family needs to take the infant to the health care provider's office or clinic.

Telephone Follow-Up. In addition to or instead of a home visit, many providers are implementing one or more postpartum telephone follow-up calls to their patients for assessment, health teaching, and identification of complications to effect timely intervention and referrals. Telephone follow-up can be among the services offered by the hospital, the private health care provider or clinic, or a private agency; it can be either a separate service or combined with other strategies for extending postpartum care. Telephonic nursing assessments are frequently used after a postpartum home care visit to reassess a woman's knowledge about the signs and symptoms of adequate intake by the breastfeeding infant or, after initiating home phototherapy, to assess the caregiver's knowledge regarding equipment complications.

Warm Lines. The warm line is another type of telephone link between the new family and concerned caregivers or experienced parent volunteers. A warm line is a help line or consultation service, not a crisis intervention line. It is used appropriately for dealing with less extreme concerns that can seem urgent at the time the call is placed but are not actual emergencies. Calls to warm lines commonly relate to infant feeding, prolonged crying, or sibling rivalry. Warm-line services can extend beyond the fourth trimester. Families need to call when concerns arise and should be given telephone numbers for easy access to answers to their questions.

Support Groups. The woman adjusting to motherhood sometimes seeks a special group experience. Postpartum women who have met earlier in prenatal clinics or on the hospital unit can begin to associate for mutual support. Members of childbirth preparation classes who attend a postpartum reunion can decide to extend their relationship during the fourth trimester.

A postpartum support group enables mothers and fathers to share with and support one another as they adjust to parenting. Many new parents find it reassuring to discover that they are not alone in their feelings of confusion and uncertainty. An experienced parent can often impart concrete information to other members. Inexperienced parents can find themselves imitating the behavior of others in the group whom they perceive to be particularly capable.

Referral to Community Resources. To develop an effective referral system, it is important that the nurse have a clear understanding of the needs of the woman and family and of the organization and community resources available for meeting those needs. Locating and compiling information about available community services contribute to the development of a referral system. It is important for the nurse to develop her or his own resource file of local and national services that are frequently useful to postpartum families.

KEY POINTS

- Postpartum care is modeled on the concept of health.
- Cultural beliefs and practices affect the patient's response to the puerperium.
- The nursing care plan includes assessments to detect deviations from normal, comfort measures to relieve discomfort or pain, and safety measures to prevent injury or infection.
- Teaching and counseling measures are designed to promote the woman's feelings of competence in self-management and baby care.
- Common nursing interventions in the postpartum period include evaluating and treating the boggy uterus and the full urinary bladder; providing for nonpharmacologic and pharmacologic relief of pain and discomfort associated with the episiotomy, lacerations, afterbirth pains, or breastfeeding; and instituting measures to promote or suppress lactation.
- Meeting the psychosocial needs of new mothers involves taking into consideration the composition and functioning of the entire family.
- Early postpartum discharge will continue as a result of consumer demand, medical necessity, discharge criteria for low risk childbirth, and cost-containment measures.
- Early discharge classes, telephone follow-up, home visits, warm lines, and support groups are effective means of facilitating physiologic and psychologic adjustments in the postpartum period.

REFERENCES

American Academy of Pediatrics (AAP) Committee on Fetus and Newborn: Hospital stay for healthy term infants, *Pediatrics* 125(2):405–409, 2010.

American Academy of Pediatrics (AAP) Committee on Psychosocial Aspects of Child and Family Health: Incorporating recognition and management of perinatal and postpartum depression into pediatric practice, *Pediatrics* 126(5):1032–1039, 2010.

American Academy of Pediatrics (AAP) Section on Breastfeeding: Breastfeeding and the use of human milk, *Pediatrics* 129(3):e827–e841, 2012.

Association of Women's Health, Obstetric, and Neonatal Nurses (AWHONN): *The compendium of postpartum care*, Washington DC, 2006, AWHONN.

Association of Women's Health, Obstetric, and Neonatal Nurses (AWHONN): *Guidelines for professional registered nursing staffing for perinatal units*, Washington DC, 2010, AWHONN.

Baby-Friendly Hospital Initiative USA: The ten steps to successful breastfeeding, 2010, www.babyfriendlyusa.org/eng/10steps.html.

Centers for Disease Control and Prevention (CDC): Recommended adult immunization schedule, 2012, *MMWR Morb Mortal Wkly Rep* 61(4):1–7, 2012a.

Centers for Disease Control and Prevention (CDC): Tdap for pregnant women: information for providers, 2012b, www.cdc.gov/vaccines/vpd-vac/pertussis/tdap-pregnancy-hcp.htm#postpartum.

Centers for Disease Control and Prevention (CDC): Varicella vaccination recommendations for specific groups, 2012c, www.cdc.gov/vaccines/vpd-vac/varicella/hcp-rec-spec-groups.htm.

De La Rosa I, Perry J, Johnson V: Benefits of increased home-visitation services: exploring a case management model, *Fam Commun Health* 32(10):58–75, 2009.

Doering Runquist JJ, Morin K, Stetzer FC: Severe fatigue and depressive symptoms in lower-income urban postpartum women, *West J Nurs Res* 31(5):599–612, 2009.

Frank B, Lane C, Hokanson H: Designing a postepidural fall risk assessment score for the obstetric patient, *J Nurs Care Qual* 24(1):50–54, 2009.

Institute of Medicine: *Dietary reference intakes for energy, carbohydrate, fiber, fatty acids, cholesterol, protein, and amino acids*, Washington DC, 2005, National Academies Press.

Kuo S, Yang, Y, Kuo P, et al: Trajectories of depressive symptoms and fatigue among postpartum women, *J Obstet Gynecol Neonatal Nurs* 41(2):216–226, 2012.

Lawrence RA, Lawrence RM: *Breastfeeding: a guide for the medical profession*, ed 7, St Louis, 2011, Mosby.

Leeman LM, Rogers RG: Sex after childbirth, *Obstet Gynecol* 119(3):647–655, 2012.

National Center for Missing and Exploited Children (NCMEC): *Newborn/infant abductions*, Alexandria VA, 2012, NCMEC, www.ncmec.org/en_US/documents/InfantAbductionStats.pdf.

Runquist JJ: A depressive symptoms responsiveness model for differentiating fatigue from depression in the postpartum period, *Arch Women's Ment Health* 10(6):267–275, 2007.

Song JE, Chang SB, Park SM, et al: Empirical test of an explanatory theory of postpartum fatigue in Korea, *J Adv Nurs* 66(12):2627–2639, 2010.

The Joint Commission (TJC): Sentinel event alert: Infant abductions, preventing future occurrences, 1999, www.jointcommission.org/assets/1/18/SEA_9.pdf.

Vincent JL: Infant hospital abduction: security measures to aid in prevention, *MCN Am J Matern Child Nurs* 34(3):179–183, 2009.

Waller-Wise R: Mother-baby care: the best for patients, nurses, and hospitals, *Nurs Womens Health* 16(4):273–278, 2012.

Waugh LJ: Beliefs associated with Mexican immigrant families' practice of la cuarentena during postpartum recovery, *J Obstet Gynecol Neonatal Nurs* 40(6):732–741, 2011.

CHAPTER

20

Transition to Parenthood

Shannon E. Perry

evolve WEBSITE

http://evolve.elsevier.com/Perry/maternal

LEARNING OBJECTIVES

On completion of this chapter, the reader will be able to:
- Identify parental and infant behaviors that facilitate and those that inhibit parental attachment.
- Describe sensual responses that strengthen attachment.
- Compare maternal adjustment and paternal adjustment to parenthood.
- Describe ways in which the nurse can facilitate parent-infant adjustment.

- Examine the effects of the following on parenting responses and behavior: parental age (i.e., adolescence and older than 35 years), same-sex parenting, social support, culture, socioeconomic conditions, personal aspirations, and sensory impairment.
- Describe sibling adjustment.
- Describe grandparent adaptation.

Becoming a parent creates a period of change and instability for men and women who decide to have children. This period occurs whether parenthood is biologic or adoptive and whether the parents are married husband-wife couples, cohabiting couples, single mothers, single fathers, lesbian couples with one woman as biologic mother, or gay male couples who adopt a child. Parenting is a process of role attainment and role transition. The transition is an ongoing process as the parents and infant develop and change.

PARENTAL ATTACHMENT, BONDING, AND ACQUAINTANCE

The process by which a parent comes to love and accept a child and a child comes to love and accept a parent is known as attachment. Using the terms *attachment* and *bonding*, Klaus and Kennell (1976) originally proposed that there is a sensitive period during the first few minutes or hours after birth when mothers and fathers must have close contact with their infant to optimize the child's later development. Klaus and Kennell (1982) later revised their theory of parent-infant bonding, modifying their claim of the critical nature of immediate contact with the infant after birth. They acknowledged the adaptability of human parents, stating that more than minutes or hours were needed for parents to form an emotional relationship with their infants. The terms *attachment* and *bonding* continue to be used interchangeably.

Attachment is developed and maintained by proximity and interaction with the infant through which the parent becomes acquainted with the infant, identifies the infant as an individual, and claims the infant as a member of the family. Attachment is facilitated by positive feedback (i.e., social, verbal, and nonverbal responses, whether real or perceived, that indicate acceptance of one partner by the other). Attachment occurs through a mutually satisfying experience. A mother commented on her son's grasp reflex, "I put my finger in his hand, and he grabbed right on. It is just a reflex, I know, but it felt good anyway" (Fig. 20-1).

The concept of attachment includes mutuality; that is, the infant's behaviors and characteristics elicit a corresponding set of maternal behaviors and characteristics. The infant displays signaling behaviors such as crying, smiling, and cooing that initiate the contact and bring the caregiver to the child. These behaviors are followed by executive behaviors such as rooting, grasping, and postural adjustments that maintain the contact. Most caregivers are attracted to an alert, responsive, cuddly infant and repelled by an irritable, apparently disinterested infant. Attachment occurs more readily with the infant whose temperament, social capabilities, appearance, and sex fit the parent's expectations. If the child does not meet these expectations, the parent's disappointment can delay the attachment process. Table 20-1 presents a comprehensive list of classic infant behaviors affecting parental attachment. Table 20-2 presents a corresponding list of parental behaviors that affect infant attachment.

TABLE 20-1	INFANT BEHAVIORS AFFECTING PARENTAL ATTACHMENT	
FACILITATING BEHAVIORS	**INHIBITING BEHAVIORS**
Visually alert; eye-to-eye contact; tracking or following of parent's face	Sleepy; eyes closed most of the time; gaze aversion
Appealing facial appearance; randomness of body movements reflecting helplessness	Resemblance to person parent dislikes; hyperirritability or jerky body movements when touched
Smiles	Bland facial expression; infrequent smiles
Vocalization; crying only when hungry or wet	Crying for hours on end; colicky
Grasp reflex	Exaggerated motor reflex
Anticipatory approach behaviors for feedings; sucks well; feeds easily	Feeds poorly; regurgitates; vomits often
Enjoys being cuddled and held	Resists holding and cuddling by crying, stiffening body
Easily consolable	Inconsolable; unresponsive to parenting, caregiving tasks
Activity and regularity somewhat predictable	Unpredictable feeding and sleeping schedule
Attention span sufficient to focus on parents	Inability to attend to parent's face or offered stimulation
Differential crying, smiling, and vocalizing; recognizes and prefers parents	Shows no preference for parents over others
Approaches through locomotion	Unresponsive to parent's approaches
Clings to parent; puts arms around parent's neck	Seeks attention from any adult in room
Lifts arms to parents' in greeting	Ignores parents

Data from Gerson E: *Infant behavior in the first year of life*, New York, 1973, Raven Press.

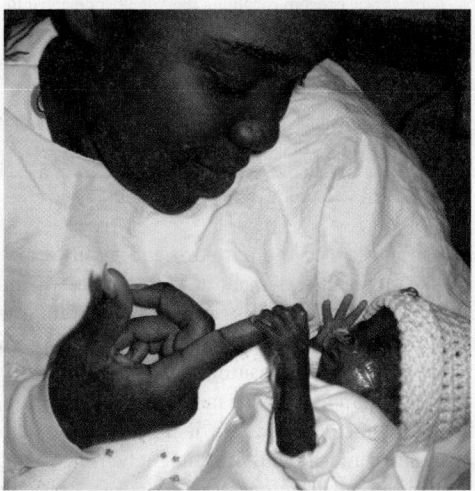

FIG 20-1 Hands. (Courtesy Cheryl Briggs, RNC, Annapolis, MD.)

TABLE 20-2	PARENTAL BEHAVIORS AFFECTING INFANT ATTACHMENT	
FACILITATING BEHAVIORS	**INHIBITING BEHAVIORS**
Looks; gazes; takes in physical characteristics of infant; assumes en face position; eye contact	Turns away from infant; ignores infant's presence
Hovers; maintains proximity; directs attention to, points to infant	Avoids infant; does not seek proximity; refuses to hold infant when given opportunity
Identifies infant as unique individual	Identifies infant with someone parent dislikes; fails to recognize any of infant's unique features
Claims infant as family member; names infant	Fails to place infant in family context or identify infant with family member; has difficulty naming
Touches; progresses from fingertip to fingers to palms to encompassing contact	Fails to move from fingertip touch to palmar contact and holding
Smiles at infant	Maintains bland countenance or frowns at infant
Talks to, coos, or sings to infant	Wakes infant when infant is sleeping; handles roughly; hurries feeding by moving nipple continuously
Expresses pride in infant	Expresses disappointment, displeasure in infant
Relates infant's behavior to familiar events	Does not incorporate infant into life
Assigns meaning to infant's actions and sensitively interprets infant's needs	Makes no effort to interpret infant's actions or needs
Views infant's behaviors and appearance in positive light	Views infant's behavior as exploiting, deliberately uncooperative; views appearance as distasteful, ugly

Data from Mercer R: Parent-infant attachment. In Sonstegard L, Kowalski K, Jennings B, editors: *Women's health* (vol 2), New York, 1983, Grune & Stratton.

An important part of attachment is acquaintance. Parents use eye contact (Fig. 20-2), touching, talking, and exploring to become acquainted with their infant during the immediate postpartum period. Adoptive parents undergo the same process when they first meet their new child. During this period, families engage in the claiming process, which is the identification of the new baby (Fig. 20-3). The child is first identified in terms of "likeness" to other family members, then in terms of "differences," and finally in terms of "uniqueness." The unique newcomer is thus incorporated into the family. Mother and father examine their infant carefully and point out characteristics that the child shares with other family members and that are indicative of a relationship between them. The claiming process is revealed by maternal comments such as "Daniel held him

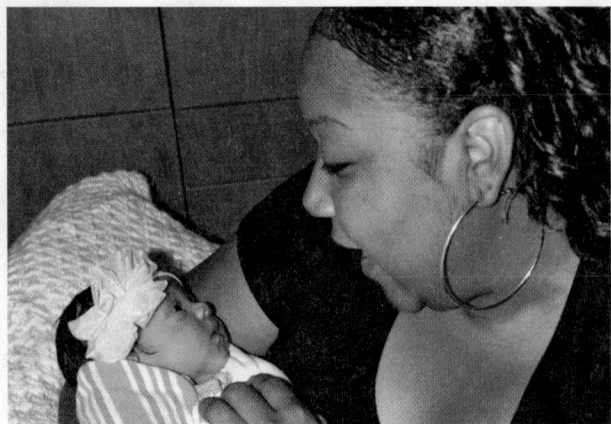

FIG 20-2 Eye-to-eye contact. (Courtesy Cheryl Briggs, RNC, Annapolis, MD.)

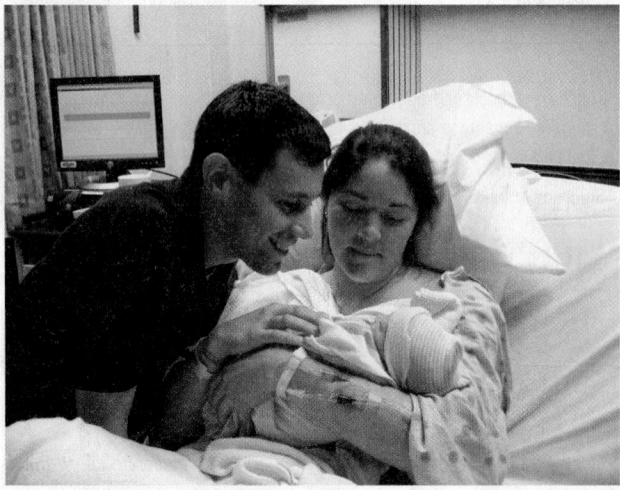

FIG 20-3 Early acquaintance between parents and infant. (Courtesy Kathryn Alden, Chapel Hill, NC.)

close and said, 'He's the image of his father,' but I found one part like me—his toes are shaped like mine."

Conversely, some mothers react negatively. They "claim" the infant in terms of the discomfort or pain the baby causes. The mother interprets the infant's normal responses as being negative toward her and reacts to her child with dislike or indifference. She does not hold the child close or touch the child to be comforting. For example, "The nurse put the baby into Marie's arms. She promptly laid him across her knees and glanced up at the television. 'Stay still until I finish watching—you've been enough trouble already.'"

Nursing interventions to facilitate parental attachment are numerous and varied (Table 20-3). They can enhance positive parent-infant contacts by heightening parental awareness of an infant's responses and ability to communicate. As the parent attempts to become competent and loving in that role, nurses can bolster the parent's self-confidence and ego. Nurses can identify actual and potential problems and collaborate with other health care professionals who will provide care for the parents after discharge. Nursing considerations for fostering maternal-infant bonding among special populations may vary (see Cultural Competence box).

Assessment of Attachment Behaviors

One of the most important areas of assessment is careful observation of specific behaviors thought to indicate the formation of

 CULTURAL COMPETENCE

Fostering Bonding in Women of Varying Ethnic and Cultural Groups

Childbearing practices and rituals of other cultures may not be congruent with standard practices associated with bonding in the Anglo-American culture. For example, Chinese families traditionally use extended family members to care for the newborn so that the mother can rest and recover, especially after a cesarean birth. Some Native American, Asian, and Hispanic women do not initiate breastfeeding until their breast milk comes in. Haitian families do not name their babies until after the confinement month. Amount of eye contact varies among cultures, too. Yup'ik Eskimo mothers almost always position their babies so that eye contact can be made.

Nurses should become knowledgeable of the childbearing beliefs and practices of diverse cultural and ethnic groups. Because individual cultural variations exist within groups, nurses need to clarify with the patient and family members or friends what cultural norms the patient follows. Incorrect judgments may be made about mother-infant bonding if nurses do not practice culturally sensitive care.

Adapted from D'Avanzo C: *Mosby's pocket guide to cultural assessment*, ed 4, St Louis, 2008, Mosby.

BOX 20-1   ASSESSING ATTACHMENT BEHAVIORS

- When the infant is brought to the parents, do they reach out for the infant and call the infant by name? (Recognize that in some cultures parents may not name the infant in the early newborn period.)
- Do the parents speak about the infant in terms of identification—whom the infant resembles, and what appears special about their infant over other infants?
- When parents are holding the infant, what kind of body contact is seen—do parents feel at ease in changing the infant's position, are fingertips or whole hands used, and does the infant have parts of the body they avoid touching or parts of the body they investigate and scrutinize?
- When the infant is awake, what kinds of stimulation do the parents provide—do they talk to the infant, to each other, or to no one, and how do they look at the infant—direct visual contact, avoidance of eye contact, or looking at other people or objects?
- How comfortable do the parents appear in terms of caring for the infant? Do they express any concern regarding their ability or disgust for certain activities, such as changing diapers?
- What type of affection do they demonstrate to the newborn, such as smiling, stroking, kissing, or rocking?
- If the infant is fussy, what kinds of comforting techniques do the parents use, such as rocking, swaddling, talking, or stroking?

emotional bonds between the newborn and family, especially the mother. Unlike physical assessment of the neonate, which has concrete guidelines to follow, assessment of parent-infant attachment relies more on skillful observation and interviewing. Rooming-in of mother and infant and liberal visiting privileges for father or partner, siblings, and grandparents provide nurses with excellent opportunities to observe interactions and identify behavior that demonstrate positive or negative attachment. Attachment behaviors can be easily observed during infant feeding sessions. Box 20-1 presents guidelines for assessment of attachment behaviors.

TABLE 20-3	EXAMPLES OF PARENT-INFANT ATTACHMENT INTERVENTIONS
INTERVENTION LABEL AND DEFINITION	**ACTIVITIES**
Attachment Promotion Facilitating the development of an affective, enduring relationship between infant and parent	Discuss with patient culture-based expressions of attachment prior to and after birth. Place newborn skin-to-skin with parent immediately after birth. Provide opportunity for parent or parents to see, hold, and examine newborn immediately after birth (i.e., delay unnecessary procedures and provide privacy). Discuss infant behavioral characteristic with parent. Assist parent of multiples in recognizing individuality of each infant. Instruct parent on attachment development, emphasizing its complexity, ongoing nature, and opportunities.
Family Integrity Promotion: Childbearing Family Facilitation of the growth of individuals or families who are adding an infant to family unit	Respect and support family's cultural value system. Assist family in developing adaptive coping mechanisms to deal with the transition to parenthood. Prepare parent(s) for expected role changes involved in becoming a parent. Prepare parent(s) for responsibilities of parenthood. Reinforce positive parenting behaviors. Identify effect of newborn on family dynamics and equilibrium.
Lactation Counseling Assisting in the establishment and maintenance of successful breastfeeding	Correct misconceptions, misinformation, and inaccuracies about breastfeeding. Provide mother the opportunity to breastfeed after birth, when possible. Instruct on infant's feeding cues (e.g., rooting, sucking, and quiet alertness). Determine frequency of normal feeding patterns, including cluster feedings and growth spurts. Discuss strategies aimed at optimizing milk supply (e.g., breast massage, frequent milk expression, complete emptying of breasts, kangaroo care, and medications). Instruct on signs and symptoms warranting reporting to a health care practitioner or lactation consultant.
Parent Education: Infant Instruction on nurturing and physical care needed during the first year of life	Determine parent(s)' knowledge and readiness and ability to learn about infant care. Provide anticipatory guidance about developmental changes during first year of life. Teach parent(s) skills to care for newborn. Demonstrate ways in which parent(s) can stimulate infant's development. Discuss infant's capabilities for interaction. Demonstrate quieting techniques.
Risk Identification: Childbearing Family Identification of individual or family likely to experience difficulties in parenting, and prioritization of strategies to prevent parenting problems	Ascertain understanding of English or other language used in community. Determine developmental stage of parent or parents. Review prenatal history for factors that predispose patient to complications. Monitor parent-infant interactions, noting behaviors thought to indicate attachment. Plan for risk-reduction activities, in collaboration with the individual or family. Refer to the appropriate community agency for follow-up if risk for parent problems or a lag in attachment has been identified.

Data from Bulechek G, Butcher H, Dochterman J, et al: *Nursing interventions classification (NIC)*, ed 6, St Louis, 2013, Mosby.

During pregnancy and often even before conception, parents develop an image of the "ideal" or "fantasy" infant. At birth, the fantasy infant becomes the real infant. How closely the dream child resembles the real child influences the bonding process. Assessing such expectations during pregnancy and at the time of the infant's birth allows identification of discrepancies in the parents' view of the fantasy child and the real child.

The labor process significantly affects the immediate attachment of mothers to their newborn infants. Factors such as a long labor, feeling tired or "drugged" after birth, problems with breastfeeding (Tharner, Luijk, Raat, et al., 2012), premature birth, and being separated from the infant at birth (Flacking, Lehtonen, Thomson, et al., 2012; Hoffenkamp, Tooten, Hall, et al., 2012) can delay the development of initial positive feelings toward the newborn. Referral to groups such as La Leche League International (www.llli.org) or Postpartum Support International (www.postpartum.net) can be useful.

PARENT-INFANT CONTACT

Early Contact

Early close contact may facilitate the attachment process between parent and child. Although a delay in contact does not necessarily mean that attachment will be inhibited, additional psychologic energy may be necessary to achieve the same effect. To date, no scientific evidence has demonstrated that immediate contact after birth is essential for the human parent-child relationship.

Early skin-to-skin contact between the mother and newborn immediately after birth and during the first hour facilitates maternal affectionate and attachment behaviors (Flacking, Lehtonen, Thomson, et al., 2012; Hung and Berg, 2011; Moore, Anderson, Bergman, et al., 2012). The newborn is placed in the prone position on the mother's bare chest; the baby and mother's chest are covered with a warm, dry blanket. This practice promotes early and effective breastfeeding and increases breastfeeding duration. It is also associated with less infant crying, improved thermoregulation (especially in low-birth-weight infants), and improved cardiorespiratory stability in late preterm infants (Moore, Anderson, Bergman, et al., 2012; Thukral, Sankar, Agarwal, et al., 2012).

Parents who cannot have early contact with their newborn (e.g., the infant was transferred to the intensive care nursery) can be reassured that such contact is not essential for optimal parent-infant interactions. Otherwise, adopted infants would not form affectionate ties with their parents. Nurses need to stress that the parent-infant relationship is a process that develops over time.

Extended Contact

Rooming-in is common in family-centered care. With this practice, the infant stays in the room with the mother. In some facilities, the newborn never leaves the mother's presence; nurses perform the initial and ongoing assessments and care in the room with the parents. In other hospitals, the infant is transferred to the postpartum or mother-baby unit from the transitional nursery (if the facility uses one) after showing satisfactory extrauterine adjustment. Nurses encourage the father or partner to participate in caring for the infant in as active a role as desired. They can also encourage siblings and grandparents to visit and become acquainted with the infant. Whether the method of family-centered care is rooming-in, mother-baby or couplet care, or a family birth unit, mothers, their partners, and family members are equal and integral parts of the developing family.

Extended contact with the infant should be available for all parents but especially for those at risk for parenting inadequacies, such as adolescents and low-income women. Postpartum nurses need to consider and encourage activities that optimize family-centered care (Welch, Hofer, Brunelli, et al., 2012). Baby Friendly status for a hospital is one means to promote family-centered care (Jaafar, Lee, and Ho, 2012; Perrine, Scanlon, Li, et al., 2012; Smith, Moore, and Peters, 2012; Vasquez and Berg, 2012).

COMMUNICATION BETWEEN PARENT AND INFANT

The parent-infant relationship is strengthened through the use of sensual responses and abilities by both partners in the interaction. The nurse should keep in mind that cultural variations are often seen in these interactive behaviors.

The Senses
Touch

Touch, or the tactile sense, is used extensively by parents as a means of becoming acquainted with the newborn. Many mothers reach out for their infants as soon as they are born and the cord is cut. Mothers lift their infants to their breasts, enfold them in their arms, and cradle them. Once the infant is close, the mother begins the exploration process with her fingertips, one of the most touch-sensitive areas of the body. Within a short time, she uses her palm

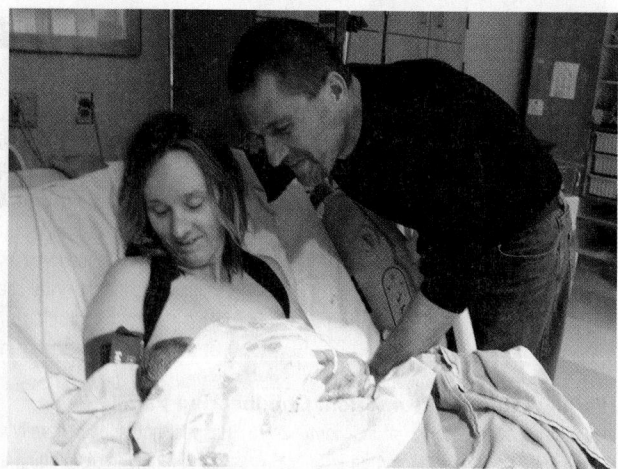

FIG 20-4 Breastfeeding in first hour after birth. (Courtesy Julie and Darren Nelson, Loveland, CO.)

to caress the baby's trunk and eventually enfolds the infant. Gentle stroking motions are used to soothe and quiet the infant; patting or gently rubbing the infant's back is a comfort after feedings. Infants also pat the mother's breast as they nurse. Both seem to enjoy sharing each other's body warmth. Parents seem to have an innate desire to touch, pick up, and hold the infant (Fig. 20-4). They comment on the softness of the baby's skin and note details of the baby's appearance. As parents become increasingly sensitive to the infant's like or dislike of different types of touch, they draw closer to the baby.

Touching behaviors of mothers vary in different cultural groups. For example, minimal touching and cuddling is a traditional Southeast Asian practice thought to protect the infant from evil spirits. Because of tradition and spiritual beliefs, women in India and Bali have practiced infant massage since ancient times (Waugh, 2011).

Eye Contact

Parents repeatedly demonstrate interest in having eye contact with the baby. Some mothers remark that once their babies have looked at them, they feel much closer to them. Parents spend much time getting their babies to open their eyes and look at them. In North American culture, eye contact appears to reinforce the development of a trusting relationship and is an important factor in human relationships at all ages. In other cultures, eye contact is perceived differently (see Cultural Competence box). For example, in Mexican culture, sustained direct eye contact is considered to be rude, immodest, and dangerous for some. This danger may arise from the *mal de ojo* (evil eye), resulting from excessive admiration. Women and children are thought to be more susceptible to the *mal de ojo* (D'Avanzo, 2008).

As newborns become functionally able to sustain eye contact with their parents, they spend time in mutual gazing, often in the en face position. In this position, the parent's face and the infant's face are approximately 8 inches apart and on the same plane (see Fig. 20-2). Nurses and nurse-midwives/physicians can facilitate eye contact immediately after birth by positioning the infant on the mother's abdomen or breasts with the mother's and the infant's faces on the same plane. Dimming the lights encourages the infant's eyes to open. To promote eye contact, instillation of prophylactic antibiotic ointment into the infant's eyes can be delayed until the infant and parents have had some time together in the first hour after birth.

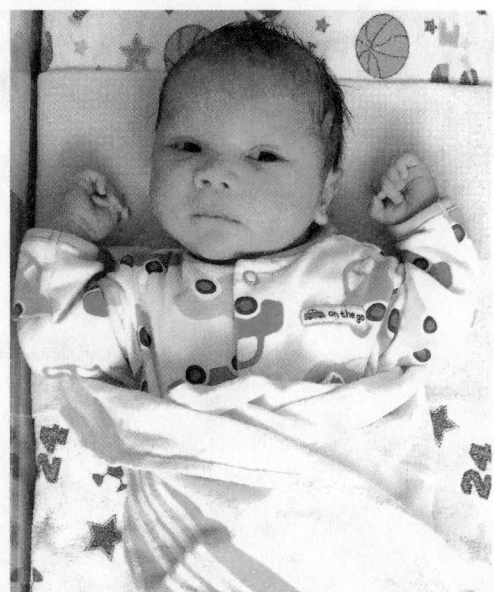

FIG 20-5 Infant in alert state. (Courtesy Cheryl Briggs, RNC, Annapolis, MD.)

Voice

The shared response of parents and infants to each other's voices is remarkable. Parents wait tensely for the first cry. Once that cry has reassured them of the baby's health, they begin comforting behaviors. As the parents speak, the infant is alerted and turns toward them. Infants respond to higher-pitched voices and can distinguish the mother's voice from others soon after birth.

Odor

Another behavior shared by parents and infants is a response to each other's odor. Mothers comment on the smell of their babies when first born and have noted that each infant has a unique odor. Infants learn rapidly to distinguish the odor of their mother's breast milk.

Entrainment

Newborns move in time with the structure of adult speech, which is termed entrainment. They wave their arms, lift their heads, and kick their legs, seemingly "dancing in tune" to a parent's voice. Culturally determined rhythms of speech are ingrained in the infant long before he or she uses spoken language to communicate. This shared rhythm also gives the parent positive feedback and establishes a positive setting for effective communication.

Biorhythmicity

The fetus is in tune with the mother's natural rhythms, biorhythmicity, such as her heartbeat. After birth, the mother's heartbeat or a recording of a heartbeat can sooth a crying infant. One task of a newborn is to establish a personal biorhythm. Parents can help in this process by giving consistent loving care and by using their infant's alert state to develop responsive behavior and increase social interactions and opportunities for learning (Fig. 20-5). The more quickly parents become competent in child care activities, the more quickly they can direct their psychologic energy toward observing the communication cues the infant gives them.

Reciprocity and Synchrony

Reciprocity is a type of body movement or behavior that provides the observer with cues. The observer or receiver interprets those cues

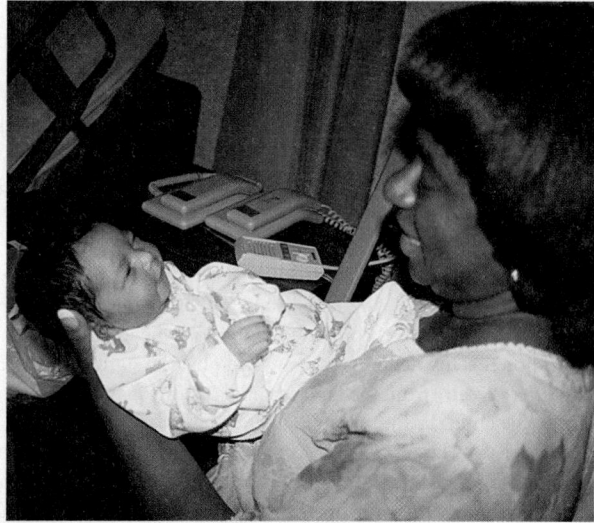

FIG 20-6 Sharing a smile; an example of synchrony. (Courtesy Marjorie Pyle, RNC, Lifecircle, Costa Mesa, CA.)

and responds to them. Reciprocity often takes several weeks to develop with a new baby. For example, when the newborn fusses and cries, the mother responds by picking up and cradling the infant; the baby becomes quiet and alert and establishes eye contact; the mother verbalizes, sings, and coos while the baby maintains eye contact. The baby then averts the eyes and yawns; the mother decreases her active response. If the parent continues to stimulate the infant, the baby may again become fussy.

Synchrony refers to the "fit" between the infant's cues and the parent's response. When parent and infant have a synchronous interaction, it is mutually rewarding (Fig. 20-6). Parents need time to learn to interpret the infant's cues correctly. For example, the infant develops a specific cry in response to different situations such as boredom, loneliness, hunger, and discomfort. The parent may need assistance in interpreting these cries, along with trial-and-error interventions, before synchrony develops.

PARENTAL ROLE AFTER BIRTH

Adaptation involves a stabilizing of tasks and a coming to terms with commitments. Parents demonstrate growing competence in child care activities and become increasingly attuned to their infant's behavior. Typically, the period from the decision to conceive through the first months of having a child is termed the transition to parenthood.

Transition to Parenthood

Historically, the transition to parenthood was viewed as a crisis. The current perspective is that parenthood is a developmental transition rather than a major life crisis. The transition to parenthood is described as a time of disorder and disequilibrium, as well as satisfaction, for mothers and their partners. Usual methods of coping often seem ineffective during this time. Some parents are so distressed that they cannot support each other. Because men typically identify their spouses as their primary or only source of support, the transition can be harder for the fathers. They often feel deprived when the mothers, who are also experiencing stress, cannot provide their usual level of support. Many parents are unprepared for the strong emotions such as the helplessness, inadequacy, and anger that arise when dealing with a crying infant.

However, parenthood allows adults to develop and display a selfless, warm, and caring side that may not be expressed in other adult roles.

For the majority of mothers and their partners, the transition to parenthood is an opportunity rather than a time of danger. Parents try new coping strategies as they work to master their new roles and reach new developmental levels. As they work through the transition, they often find personal strength and resourcefulness.

Parental Tasks and Responsibilities

Parents need to reconcile the actual child with the fantasy and dream child. This process means coming to terms with the infant's physical appearance, sex, innate temperament, and physical status. If the real child differs greatly from the fantasy child, parents may delay acceptance of the child. In some instances, they never accept the child.

Many parents know the sex of the infant before birth because of ultrasound assessments. For those who do not have this information, disappointment over the sex of the infant can take time to resolve. The parents can provide adequate physical care but find it difficult to be sincerely involved with the infant until this internal conflict has been resolved. As one mother remarked, "I really wanted a boy. I know it is silly and irrational, but when they said, 'She's a lovely little girl,' I was so disappointed and angry—yes, angry—I could hardly look at her. Oh, I looked after her okay, her feedings and baths and things, but I couldn't feel excited. To tell the truth, I felt like a monster not liking my child. Then one day she was lying there and she turned her head and looked right at me. I felt a flooding of love for her come over me, and we looked at each other a long time. It's okay now. I wouldn't change her for all the boys in the world."

The normal appearance of the neonate—size, color, molding of the head, or bowed appearance of the legs—is startling for some parents. Nurses can encourage parents to examine their babies and to ask questions about newborn characteristics.

Parents need to become adept in the care of the infant, including caregiving activities, noting the communication cues the infant gives to indicate needs and responding appropriately to those needs. Self-esteem grows with competence. Breastfeeding helps mothers feel they are contributing in a unique way to the welfare of the infant. The parent may interpret the infant's response to his or her parental care and attention as a comment on the quality of that care. Infant behaviors that parents interpret as positive responses to their care include being consoled easily, enjoying being cuddled, and making eye contact. Spitting up frequently after feedings, crying, and being unpredictable may be perceived as negative responses to parental care. Continuation of these infant responses that parents view as negative can result in alienation of parent and infant.

Some people view assistance, including advice by husbands, partners, wives, mothers, mothers-in-law, and health care professionals, as supportive. Others view advice as criticism or an indication of how inept these others judge the new parents to be. Criticism, real or imagined, of the new parents' ability to provide adequate physical care, nutrition, or social stimulation for the infant can be devastating. By providing encouragement and praise for parenting efforts, nurses can bolster the new parents' confidence.

Parents must establish a place for the newborn within the family group. Whether the infant is the firstborn or the last born, all family members must adjust their roles to accommodate the newcomer.

Becoming a Mother

Rubin (1961) identified three phases of maternal role attainment in which the mother adjusts to her parental role. These phases extend

TABLE 20-4	**PHASES OF MATERNAL POSTPARTUM ADJUSTMENT**
PHASE	**CHARACTERISTICS**
Dependent: taking-in phase	First 24 hours (range, 1 to 2 days) Focus: self and meeting of basic needs • Reliance on others to meet needs for comfort, rest, closeness, and nourishment • Excited and talkative • Desire to review birth experience
Dependent-independent: taking-hold phase	Starts second or third day; lasts 10 days to several weeks Focus: care of baby and competent mothering • Desire to take charge • Still has need for nurturing and acceptance by others • Eagerness to learn and practice— optimal period for teaching by nurses • Handling of physical discomforts and emotional changes • Possible experience with "blues"
Interdependent: letting-go phase	Focus: forward movement of family as unit with interacting members • Reassertion of relationship with partner • Resumption of sexual intimacy • Resolution of individual roles

Date from Rubin R: Basic maternal behavior, *Nurs Outlook* 9(11):683–686, 1961.

over the first several weeks and are characterized by dependent behavior, dependent-independent behavior, and interdependent behavior (Table 20-4). Rubin's research was conducted when the length of stay in the hospital was for a longer period (3 to 5 or more days). With today's early discharge, women seem to move through the phases faster.

Mercer (2004) suggested that the concept of maternal role attainment be replaced with becoming a mother to signify the transformation and growth of the mother's identity. Becoming a mother implies more than attaining a role. It includes learning new skills and increasing her confidence in herself as she meets new challenges in caring for her child or children.

Mercer (2004) identified four stages in the process of becoming a mother (Mercer and Walker, 2006, pp. 568-569):

(a) commitment, attachment to the unborn baby, and preparation for delivery and motherhood during pregnancy

(b) acquaintance/attachment to the infant, learning to care for the infant, and physical restoration during the first 2 to 6 weeks following birth

(c) moving toward a new normal

(d) achievement of a maternal identity through redefining self to incorporate motherhood (around 4 months)

The time of achievement of the stages varies, and the stages may overlap. Achievement is influenced by mother and infant variables and the social environment.

Maternal sensitivity or maternal responsiveness is an important determinant of the maternal-infant relationship. It can be defined as the quality of a mother's sensitive behaviors that are based on her awareness, perception, and responsiveness to infant cues and behaviors. Maternal sensitivity significantly influences the infant's physical, psychologic, and cognitive development. Maternal qualities inherent to this sensitivity include awareness and responsiveness to infant cues, affect, timing, flexibility, acceptance, and conflict negotiation. Maternal sensitivity is dynamic and develops over time in a reciprocal give-and-take with the infant (Shin, Park, Ryu, et al., 2008).

Not all mothers experience the transition to motherhood in the same way. For some women, becoming a mother entails multiple losses. For example, for some single women, there may be a loss of the family of origin when the family does not accept her decision to have the child. There may be loss of a relationship with the father of the baby, with friends, and with their own sense of self. Some women describe a loss of dreams including loss of job, financial security, and a future profession.

More reality-based perinatal education programs are necessary to prepare mothers better and decrease their anxiety. Live classes allow time for questions to be answered and for mothers to lend support to one another. Mothers need to know during the first months of parenthood it is common to feel overwhelmed and insecure and to experience physical and mental fatigue. They need to be assured that this situation is temporary and that 3 to 6 months may be needed to become comfortable in caregiving and in being a mother. Maternal support by professionals should not end with hospital discharge but, instead, extend over the next 4 to 6 months; long-term interventions tend to be more successful than one-time encounters. Nurses can advocate for the extension of such support services well into the postpartum period (Mercer and Walker, 2006; Shapiro, Nahm, Gottman, et al., 2011).

During pregnancy and after birth, nurses can discuss the usual postpartum concerns that mothers experience. They can provide anticipatory guidance on coping strategies, such as resting when the infant sleeps and planning with an extended family member or friend to do the housework for the first week or two after the baby is born. Once a mother is home, periodic telephone calls from a nurse who cared for her in the birth setting can provide the mother with an opportunity to vent her concerns and get support and advice from "her" nurse. Nurses should plan additional supportive counseling for first-time mothers inexperienced in child care; women whose careers had provided outside stimulation; women who lack friends or family members with whom to share delights and concerns; and adolescent mothers. When possible, postpartum home visits are included in the plan of care.

Postpartum Blues

The "pink" period surrounding the first day or two after birth, characterized by heightened joy and feelings of well-being, is often followed by a "blue" period. Up to 80% of women of all ethnic and racial groups experience the postpartum blues or "baby blues." During the blues, women are emotionally labile and often cry easily for no apparent reason. This lability seems to peak around the fifth day and subside by the tenth day. Other symptoms of postpartum blues include depression, a let-down feeling, restlessness, fatigue, insomnia, headache, anxiety, sadness, and anger. Biochemical, psychologic, social, and cultural factors have been explored as possible causes of the postpartum depressive state; however, the etiology remains unknown.

Whatever the cause, the early postpartum period appears to be one of emotional and physical vulnerability for new mothers, who are often psychologically overwhelmed by the reality of parental responsibilities. Mothers feel deprived of the supportive care they received from family members and friends during pregnancy. Some

---

PATIENT TEACHING

Coping with Postpartum Blues

- Remember that the "blues" are normal and that both the mother and the father or partner may experience them.
- Get plenty of rest; nap when the baby does if possible. Go to bed early, and let friends and family know when to visit and how they can help. (Remember, you are not "Supermom.")
- Use relaxation techniques learned in childbirth classes (or ask the nurse to teach you and your partner some techniques).
- Do something for yourself. Take advantage of the time your partner or family members care for the baby—soak in the tub (a 20-minute soak can be the equivalent of a 2-hour nap), or go for a walk.
- Plan a day out of the house—go to the mall with the baby, being sure to take a stroller or carriage, or go out to eat with friends without the baby. Many communities have churches or other agencies that provide child care programs such as Mothers' Morning Out.
- Talk to your partner about the way you feel—for example, about feeling tied down, how the birth met your expectations, and things that will help you (do not be afraid to ask for specifics).
- If you are breastfeeding, give yourself and your baby time to learn.
- Seek out and use community resources such as La Leche League or community mental health centers. One nationally recognized resource is:
Postpartum Support International
927 North Kellogg Ave.
Santa Barbara, CA 93111
(805) 967-7636
www.postpartum.net

---

mothers regret the loss of the mother–unborn child relationship and mourn its passing. Still others experience a let-down feeling when labor and birth are complete. The majority of women experience fatigue after childbirth, which is compounded by the around-the-clock demands of the new baby. Postpartum fatigue increases the risk for postpartum depressive symptoms and can have a negative effect on maternal role attainment (Hunter, Rychnovsky, and Yount, 2009; Kurth, Kennedy, Spichiger, et al., 2011; Rychnovsky and Hunter, 2009). To help mothers cope with postpartum blues, nurses can suggest various strategies (see Patient Teaching box).

A few questions on a discharge checklist can help mothers assess their level of "blues" and decide when to seek advice from their nurse, nurse-midwife, or physician. Home visits and telephone follow-up calls by a nurse are important to assess the mother's pattern of "blue" feelings and behavior over time.

Although the postpartum blues are usually mild and short lived, approximately 10% to 15% of women experience a more severe syndrome called *postpartum depression (PPD)* (see Chapter 21). Symptoms of PPD can range from mild to severe, with women having good days and bad days. Fathers can also experience PPD. Screening for PPD should be performed with both mothers and fathers. PPD can go undetected because new parents generally do not voluntarily admit to this kind of emotional distress out of embarrassment, guilt, or fear. Nurses need to include teaching about how to differentiate symptoms of the "blues" and PPD and urge parents to report depressive symptoms promptly if they occur.

Becoming a Father

The realities of the first few weeks at home with a newborn cause fathers to change their expectations, set new priorities, and redefine

TABLE 20-5	EARLY DEVELOPMENT OF THE INVOLVED FATHER ROLE
PHASE	**CHARACTERISTICS**
Expectations and intentions	Desire for emotional involvement and deep connection with infant
Confronting reality	Dealing with unrealistic expectations, frustration, disappointment, feelings of guilt, helplessness, and inadequacy
Creating the role of involved father	Altering expectations, establishing new priorities, redefining role, negotiating changes with partner, learning to care for infant, increasing interaction with infant, struggling for recognition
Reaping rewards	Infant smile, sense of meaning, completeness and immortality

Data from Goodman J: Becoming an involved father of an infant, *J Obstet Gynecol Neonatal Nurs* 34(2):190–200, 2005.

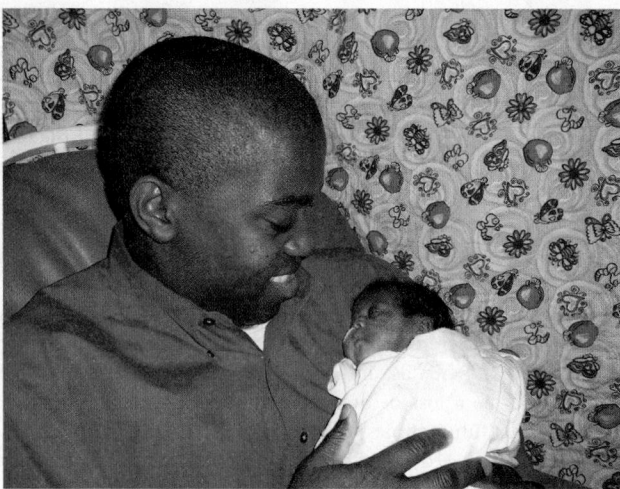

FIG 20-7 Father interacts with his newborn son. (Courtesy Cheryl Briggs, RNC, Annapolis, MD.)

their role. They develop strategies for balancing work, their own needs, and the needs of their partner and infant. Men become increasingly more comfortable with infant care. During this time, they may struggle for recognition and positive feedback from their partner, the infant, and others. They may feel excluded from support and attention by health care providers. The final phase of becoming an involved father is one of reaping rewards, the most significant being reciprocity from the infant such as a smile. This phase typically occurs around 6 weeks to 2 months. Increased sociability of the infant enhances the father-infant relationship (Table 20-5).

First-time fathers perceive the first 4 to 10 weeks of parenthood in much the same way that mothers do. It is a period characterized by uncertainty, increased responsibility, disruption of sleep, and inability to control time needed to care for the infant and reestablish the relationship with their partner (Yu, Hung, Chan, et al., 2012). Fathers express concerns about decreased attention from their partners relative to their personal relationship, the mother's lack of recognition of the father's desire to participate in decision making for the infant, and limited time available to establish a relationship with the infant (de Montigny, Lacharité, and Devault, 2012). These concerns can precipitate feelings of jealousy of the infant. The father should discuss his individual concerns and needs with the mother and become more involved with the infant. This can help alleviate feelings of jealousy.

Father-Infant Relationship

In North American culture, neonates have a powerful effect on their fathers who become intensely involved with their babies. The term used for the father's absorption, preoccupation, and interest in the infant is **engrossment**. Characteristics of engrossment include some of the sensual responses relating to touch and eye-to-eye contact that were discussed earlier and the father's keen awareness of features both unique and similar to himself that validate his claim to the infant. An outstanding response is one of strong attraction to the newborn. Fathers spend considerable time "communicating" with the infant and taking delight in the infant's response to them (Fig. 20-7). Fathers experience increased self-esteem and a sense of

being proud, bigger, more mature, and older after seeing their baby for the first time.

Fathers spend less time than mothers with infants, and their interactions with infants tend to be characterized by stimulating social play rather than caregiving. The variations in infant stimulation from both parents provide a wider social experience for the infant.

Fathers receive less interpersonal and professional support compared with mothers and can feel excluded from antenatal appointments and antenatal classes (Steen, Downe, Bamford, et al., 2012). They need information and encouragement during pregnancy and in the postnatal period related to infant care, parenting, and relationship changes. During the postpartum hospital stay, nurses can arrange to teach infant care when the father is present and provide anticipatory guidance for fathers about the transition to parenthood. Separate prenatal and parenting classes and parenting support groups for fathers can provide them with an opportunity to discuss their concerns and have some of their needs met. Postpartum telephone calls and home visits by the nurse should include time for assessment of the father's adjustment and needs (Deave, Johnson, and Ingram, 2008).

Adjustment for the Couple

The transition to parenthood brings about changes in the relationship between the mother and her partner. A strong, healthy marriage or couple relationship is the best foundation for parenthood, although even the best relationships are often shaken with the addition of a baby. During the first few weeks after birth, parents experience a plethora of emotions. Even though they may feel an overwhelming love and a sense of amazement toward their newborn, they also feel a great responsibility. Even if the mother and her partner have been to prenatal classes, read books, or sought advice from family or friends, they are usually surprised by the realities of life with a new baby and the changes in their relationship. Because men and women experience pregnancy and birth differently, the expectation is that they will also vary in their adjustment to parenthood.

Common issues that couples face as they become parents include changes in their relationship with one another, division of household and infant care responsibilities, financial concerns, balancing work and parental responsibilities, and social activities

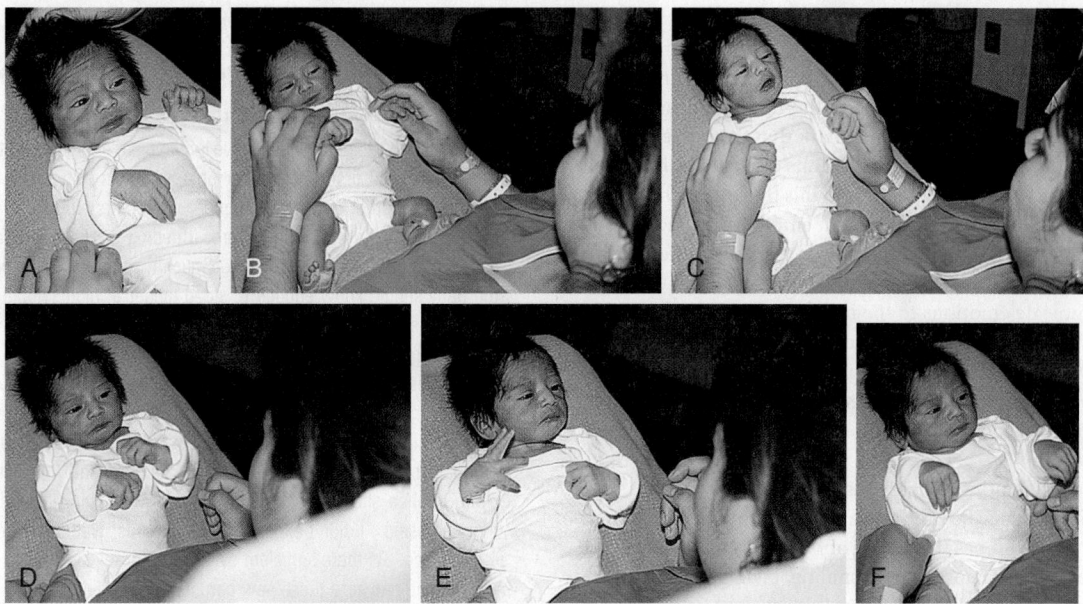

FIG 20-8 Holding newborn in en face position, mother works to alert her daughter, 6 hours old. **A,** Infant is quiet and alert. **B,** Mother begins talking to daughter. **C,** Infant responds, opens mouth like her mother. **D,** Infant gazes at her mother. **E,** Infant waves hand. **F,** Infant glances away, resting. Hand relaxes. (Courtesy Marjorie Pyle, RNC, Lifecircle, Costa Mesa, CA.)

(Menéndez, Hidalgo, Jiménez, et al., 2011). To assist new parents in their transition, nurses can encourage them during pregnancy and in the postpartum period to share personal expectations with each other and to assess their relationship periodically. Couples need to schedule time into their busy lives for one-on-one conversation and try to have regular "dates" or time apart from the infant. The mother and her partner need to express appreciation for one another as well as for their baby. Support from family, friends, and community health professionals should be identified early and used as needed during pregnancy and in the postpartum period and beyond. The couple who is willing to experiment with new approaches to their lifestyle and habits can find the transition to parenthood less difficult.

Nurses can provide opportunities for parents to discuss concerns and ask questions about resuming sexual intimacy. Sexual intimacy enhances the adult aspect of the family, and the adult pair share a closeness denied to other family members. Changes in a woman's sexuality after childbirth are related to hormonal shifts, increased breast size, uneasiness with a body that has yet to return to a prepregnant size, fatigue related to sleep deprivation, and physical exhaustion. The resumption of sexual intimacy seems to bring the parents' relationship back into focus (see Home Care box in Chapter 19).

Infant-Parent Adjustment

Newborns participate actively in shaping their parents' reaction to them. Behavioral characteristics of the infant influence parenting behaviors. The infant and the parent each have unique rhythms, behaviors, and response styles that are brought to every interaction. Infant-parent interactions can be facilitated in at least three ways: (1) modulation of rhythm, (2) modification of behavioral repertoires, and (3) mutual responsivity. Nurses can teach parents about these three aspects of infant-parent interaction through discussions, written materials, and videorecordings describing infant capabilities. A creative approach is to record the parent-infant pair during an interaction and then use the individualized recording to discuss the pair's rhythm, behavioral repertoire, and responsivity.

Rhythm. To modulate rhythm, both parent and infant must be able to interact. Therefore the infant must be in the quiet alert state, one of the most difficult of the sleep-wake states to maintain. The alert state (Fig. 20-8) occurs most often during a feeding or in face-to-face play. The parent must work hard to help the infant maintain the alert state long enough and often enough for interactions to take place. The en face position is usually assumed (Fig. 20-8, *D*). Multiparous mothers in particular are very sensitive and responsive to the infant's feeding rhythms. Mothers learn to reserve stimulation for pauses in sucking activity and not to talk or smile excessively while the infant is sucking because the infant will stop feeding to interact with her. With maturity, the infant can sustain longer interactions by modulating activity rhythms (i.e., limb movement, sucking, gaze alternation, and habituation). Meanwhile, the parent becomes more attuned to the infant's rhythms and learns to modulate the rhythms, facilitating a rhythmic turn-taking interaction.

Behavioral Repertoires. Both the infant and the parent have a repertoire of behaviors they can use to facilitate interactions. Fathers and mothers engage in these behaviors depending on the extent of contact and caregiving of the infant.

The infant's behavioral repertoire includes gazing, vocalizing, and facial expressions. The infant is able to focus and follow the human face from birth and is able to alternate the gaze voluntarily, looking away from the parent's face when understimulated or overstimulated (Fig. 20-8, *F*). Parents need to learn to be sensitive to the infant's capacity for attention and inattention and to recognize states and signs of overstimulation (see Fig. 22-13 and Family Centered Care on p. 622). Developing this sensitivity is especially important when interacting with preterm infants.

Body gestures form a part of the infant's "early language." Babies greet parents with waving hands (Fig. 20-8, *E*) or a reaching out of hands. They can raise an eyebrow or soften their expression to elicit loving attention. Game playing can stimulate them to smile or laugh.

Pouting or crying, arching of the back, and general squirming usually signal the end of an interaction.

The parents' repertoire includes various types of interactive behaviors such as constantly looking at the infant and noting the infant's response. New parents often remark that they are exhausted from looking at the baby and smiling. Adults also "infantilize" their speech to help the infant "listen." They do this by slowing the tempo, speaking loudly and rhythmically, and emphasizing key words. Phrases are repeated frequently. Infantilizing does not mean using "baby talk," which involves distortion of sounds.

To communicate emotions to the infant, parents often use facial expressions such as slow and exaggerated looks of surprise, happiness, and confusion. Games such as "peek-a-boo" and imitation of the infant's behaviors are other means of interaction. For example, if the baby smiles, so does the parent; if the baby frowns, the parent responds in kind.

Responsivity. Contingent responses (responsivity) are those that occur within a specific time and are similar in form to a stimulus behavior. The adult has the feeling of having an influence on the interaction. Infant behaviors such as smiling, cooing, and sustained eye contact, usually in en face position, are viewed as contingent responses. The infant's responses act as rewards to the initiator and encourage the adult to continue with the game when the infant responds positively. When the adult imitates the infant, the infant appears to enjoy it. A progression occurs in the types of behaviors that parents present for the baby to imitate; for example, in early interactions, the parent will grimace rather than laugh, which is in keeping with the infant's developmental level. Such behaviors sustain interactions and promote harmony in the relationship.

DIVERSITY IN TRANSITIONS TO PARENTHOOD

Various factors, including age, social networks, socioeconomic conditions, and personal aspirations for the future, influence how parents respond to the birth of a child. Cultural beliefs and practices also affect parenting behaviors. Factors that influence the risk for parenting problems include age (adolescent or older than 35 years), same-sex parenting, social support, culture, socioeconomic conditions, and personal aspirations.

Age

Maternal age has a definite effect on the outcome of pregnancy. The mother, fetus, and newborn are at highest risk when the mother is an adolescent or older than 35 years (see Critical Thinking Case Study).

The Adolescent Mother

Although becoming a parent is biologically possible for the adolescent female, her egocentricity and concrete thinking can interfere with her ability to parent effectively. Adolescent mothers are more likely to give birth to preterm and/or low-birth-weight infants (Kochanek, Kirmeyer, Martin, et al., 2012). Mortality rates are higher among infants of adolescent mothers. This can be related to inherent problems associated with preterm birth or other conditions, but it is also influenced by the mother's inexperience, lack of knowledge, and immaturity. Nevertheless, in most instances, with adequate support and developmentally appropriate teaching, adolescents can learn effective parenting skills. Strong social and functional support promote positive outcomes for adolescent mothers.

Contrary to popular beliefs related to the detrimental effects of adolescent pregnancy, research evidence suggests that the life course

❓ CRITICAL THINKING CASE STUDY

Postpartum Adjustment for the Adolescent and the Older Mother

You are a home care nurse and have had two patients referred to you. Carol is a 15-year-old first-time mother of a 5-day-old girl; she lives with her mother. The father of the baby, Robert, is 17 years old and attended childbirth classes with Carol. She is breastfeeding the baby but says that the baby sucks too slowly and takes too much time to eat. She said she thinks the baby should know enough to sleep longer at night. Robert would like to feed the baby some cereal, since he heard that will make a baby sleep longer at night.

Audrey is a 36-year-old attorney who has been practicing law for 7 years. She just gave birth to her first baby; she and her husband delayed parenting by choice until their careers were well established. She had an uneventful pregnancy, labor, and birth. During a telephone call 48 hours after discharge, when she was asked how things were going, Audrey burst into tears and said, "I didn't expect it to be like this! Nothing is going right."

1. Evidence—Is there sufficient evidence to draw conclusions about what teaching and care these new parents need?
2. Assumptions—What assumptions can be made about the following factors?
   a. The relationship of maternal age and postpartum adjustment
   b. The need for social support in the postnatal period
   c. The need for perinatal education
   d. Long-term prognosis for positive outcomes
3. What implications and priorities for nursing care can be drawn at this time?
4. Does the evidence objectively support your conclusion?

for adolescent mothers is similar to that of their socioeconomic peers (Beers and Hollo, 2009). In some families or communities, adolescent parenthood is considered a normal or positive life event. Even so, adolescent pregnancy and parenting are important public health concerns.

The transition to parenthood can be difficult for adolescent parents. Because many adolescents have their own unmet developmental needs, coping with the developmental tasks of parenthood is often difficult. Some young parents experience difficulty accepting a changing self-image and adjusting to new roles related to the responsibilities of infant care. Adolescent mothers are at increased risk for postpartum depression; this is often associated with a lack of social support and poor relations with their partner (Beers and Hollo, 2009; Molborn and Jacobs, 2011).

As adolescent parents move through the transition to parenthood, they may feel "different" from their peers, excluded from "fun" activities, and prematurely forced to enter an adult social role. The conflict between their own desires and the infant's demands, in addition to the low tolerance for frustration that is typical of adolescence, further contributes to the normal psychosocial stress of childbirth and parenting. Maintaining a relationship with the baby's father is beneficial for the teen mother and her infant, although adolescent pregnancy often heralds the departure of the young father from the relationship.

Adolescent mothers provide warm and attentive physical care; however, they use less verbal interaction than do older parents, and adolescents tend to be less responsive and to interact less positively with their infants than do older mothers. Interventions emphasizing verbal and nonverbal communication skills between mother and infant are important. Such intervention strategies must be concrete and specific because of the cognitive level of adolescents. Although some observers suggest that some adolescents may use more aggressive behaviors, a higher incidence of child abuse by adolescent mothers has not been documented. In comparison with older mothers, teenage mothers have a limited knowledge of child development. They tend to expect too much of their infants too soon and often characterize their infants as being fussy. This limited knowledge may cause teenagers to respond to their infants inappropriately.

Many young mothers pattern their maternal role on what they themselves experienced. Therefore nurses need to determine the type of support that people close to the young mother are able and prepared to give, as well as the kinds of community assistance available to supplement this support. Many teen mothers can identify a source of social support, with the predominant source being their own mothers.

Continued assessment of the new mother's parenting abilities during this postbirth period is essential. Continued support should be provided by involving the grandparents and other family members, as well as through home visits and group sessions for discussion of infant care and parenting concerns. Community-based programs for pregnant adolescents and adolescent parents improve access to health care, education, and other support services. Serious problems can be prevented through outreach programs concerned with self-management, parent-child interactions, infant development, child injuries, and failure to thrive. As the adolescent performs her mothering role within the framework of her family, she may need to address dependency versus independency issues. The adolescent's family members also need help adapting to their new roles. Some mothers and fathers of adolescents feel they are too young and unprepared to be grandparents.

The Adolescent Father

The adolescent father and mother face immediate developmental crises, which include completing the developmental tasks of adolescence, making a transition to parenthood, and sometimes adapting to marriage. These transitions are stressful. The nurse can initiate interaction with the adolescent father if he is present during prenatal visits or if he is with his partner during labor and birth. During the hospital stay, the nurse can include the adolescent father in teaching sessions about infant care and parenting. The nurse can ask him to be present during postpartum home visits and to accompany the mother and the baby to well-baby checkups at the clinic or pediatrician's office. With the adolescent mother's agreement, the nurse may contact the father directly.

Adolescent fathers need support to discuss their emotional responses to the pregnancy, birth, and fatherhood. The nurse needs to be aware of the father's feelings of guilt, powerlessness, or bravado because these feelings may have negative consequences for both the parents and the child. Counseling of adolescent fathers needs to be reality oriented and should include topics such as finances, child care, parenting skills, and the father's role in the parenting experience. Teenage fathers also need to know about reproductive physiology and birth control options, as well as sex practices that lower the risk for pregnancy and sexually transmitted infections.

The adolescent father may or may not continue to be involved in an ongoing relationship with the young mother and his baby. If he does, he can play an important role in the decisions about child care and raising the child. He may need help to develop realistic perceptions of his role as "father to a child" and is encouraged to use coping mechanisms that are not harmful to his own, his partner's, or his child's well-being. The nurse enlists support systems, parents, and professional agencies on his behalf.

Maternal Age Older Than 35 Years

Women older than 35 years have always continued their childbearing either by choice or because of a lack of or a failure of contraception during the perimenopausal years. Added to this group are women who have postponed pregnancy because of careers or other reasons, as well as women of infertile couples who finally become pregnant with the aid of technologic advances.

Support from partners aids in the adjustment of older mothers to changes involved in becoming a parent and seeing themselves as competent. Support from other family members and friends is also important for positive self-evaluation of parenting, a sense of well-being and satisfaction, and help in dealing with stress. Women who are older can experience social isolation. Older mothers may have less family and social support than younger mothers. They are less likely to live near family, and their own parents, if still living, may be unable to provide assistance or support because of age or health issues. These mothers are often caught in the "sandwich generation," taking on responsibility for care of aging parents while parenting young children. Social support may be lacking because their peers are busy with their careers and have limited time to help. Their friends are likely to have older children and have less in common with the new mother.

Changes in the sexual aspect of a relationship can create stress for new midlife parents. Mothers report that it is difficult to find time and energy for a romantic rendezvous. They attribute much of this difficulty to the reality of caring for an infant, but the decreasing libido that normally accompanies getting older also contributes.

Work and career issues are sources of conflict for older mothers. Conflicts emerge over being disinterested in work, worrying about giving enough attention to work with the distractions of a new baby, and anticipating what returning to work will entail. Child care is a major factor in causing stress about work.

Another major issue for older mothers with careers is the perception of loss of control. Mothers older than 35 years, when compared with younger mothers, are at a different stage in their careers, having attained high levels of education, career, and income. The loss of control experienced when going from the consistency of a work role to the inconsistency of the parent role comes as a surprise to many older women. Helping the older mother have realistic expectations of herself and of parenthood is essential.

New mothers who are also perimenopausal may have difficulty understanding that fatigue, loss of sleep, decreased libido, or other physiologic symptoms are the causes of the change in their sex drives. Although many women view menopause as a natural stage of life, for midlife mothers, this cessation of menstruation coincides with the state of parenthood. The changes of midlife and menopause can add more emotional and physical stress to older mothers' lives because of the time- and energy-consuming aspects of raising a young child.

Paternal Age Older Than 35 Years

Although many older fathers describe their experience of midlife parenting as wonderful, they also recognize drawbacks. Positive aspects of parenthood in older years include increased love and commitment between the two parents, a reinforcement of why one married in the first place, a feeling of being complete, experiencing of "the child" in oneself again, more financial stability than in younger years, and more freedom to focus on parenting rather than on career. Drawbacks of midlife parenting include having a young child and not being physically fit to participate in activities, being much older than other fathers, and the change that it makes in the relationship with their partner.

Parenting in Same-Sex Couples

The transition to parenting for same-sex couples can present unique challenges. Whether the couple consists of two women or two men, issues such as a lack of family acceptance and support, public ignorance, and social and legal invisibility influence their ability to adapt as new parents. The health care environment is heteronormative; for example, educational materials for new parents include information for mothers and fathers, and photos depict the traditional heterosexual couple (Röndahl, Bruhner, and Lindhe, 2009). Attitudes of health care professionals can either positively or negatively affect the care provided to same-sex couples.

Lesbian Couples

The decision for lesbian couples to conceive is intentional. Factors that influence the decision include the age, health, infertility, and career considerations of each partner. In addition, one partner may have a greater desire to experience the pregnancy and birth and to be genetically related to the infant.

Several pathways are available for two women in a same-sex or lesbian relationship who wish to become parents. The couple may decide for one of the women to conceive a child who is genetically related to her; this is usually done through donor insemination. Alternatively, the fertilized egg of one partner can be implanted into the uterus of the other partner, who carries the pregnancy. In some cases, a woman is implanted with the fertilized egg from a donor so the child is not biologically related to either partner. Another option is for a lesbian couple to adopt an infant born to a surrogate mother. They can also choose to adopt an infant through an adoption agency or by private arrangement.

Health care professionals demonstrate a variety of reactions to lesbian couples, ranging from rejection and exclusion to complete acceptance and inclusion. Some couples attempt to hide their relationship because they fear a homophobic response (Goldberg, Ryan, and Sawchyn, 2009). Judgmental attitudes, confusion, or lack of understanding can affect the quality of care provided to these families. Although the traditional roles of the mother and father in heterosexual relationships are well recognized, the role of the lesbian co-parent can be questioned, misunderstood, and ignored by society and by health care providers. Intentionally or accidentally, health care providers can exclude partners or fail to acknowledge their roles in pregnancy, birth, and parenting. Integration of the nonchildbearing partner into care includes offering opportunities afforded male partners of heterosexual women, such as cutting the cord and rooming in with the mother and baby during hospitalization.

An option not available to male partners is to actually breastfeed the infant. The nonchildbearing female partner can stimulate milk production through induced lactation using medications and regular pumping. A supplemental feeding device containing expressed breast milk or formula can be used to provide additional milk to the breastfeeding infant. Women who choose not to induce lactation yet desire to have the breastfeeding experience can put the baby to breast using a supplemental feeding device containing formula or expressed breast milk (Riordan and Wambach, 2010).

Similar to heterosexual parents, lesbian couples face challenges in adjusting to life with a new baby. After birth, the birth mother tends to be the one most responsible for child care because she is likely to be working fewer hours than her partner. Tensions can arise between the partners in relation to their roles. This can be compounded by the lack of a formal, recognized relationship between the co-parent and the infant and the issues surrounding her legal rights in relation to her partner and the infant.

Lesbian couples face strong social sanctions regarding pregnancy and parenting. Their families may not have resolved the initial dismay and guilt over learning of their daughters' homosexuality, or they may disagree with the lesbian couple's decision to conceive and be parents. Alternatively, a pregnancy or adoption can transform family relationships and open the door to acceptance by grandparents. In situations in which family support is limited or absent, the nurse can help lesbian couples locate supportive social groups, lesbian or heterosexual.

Gay Couples

Men in same-sex relationships, or gay couples, can become parents by adoption or by impregnating a surrogate by artificial insemination or sexual intercourse. Female-to-male transgender individuals in gay relationships have been known to become pregnant. Same-sex male couples face the same social sanctions regarding pregnancy and parenting that lesbian couples encounter. Both lesbian and gay couples can have children from previous heterosexual relationships.

Nurses are likely to encounter gay couples in the hospital setting if they are present for birth by a surrogate or if they are adopting a newborn and visit the hospital to spend time with the infant and learn about infant care. Nurses can help these men locate support groups that will address their needs. They need to ensure that these families receive effective health care. Data on gay parenting are limited and focus more on developmental outcomes of the children than on parenting styles or parental caregiving. Research is needed to identify the needs of gay parents and ways to support them in their parenting.

Social Support

Social support is strongly related to positive adaptation by new parents, including adolescent parents, during the transition to parenthood. Social support is multidimensional and includes the number of members in a person's social network, types of support, perceived general support, actual support received, and satisfaction with support available and received. Partner support in pregnancy has a positive influence on emotional distress in the postpartum period (Goldberg and Smith, 2011; Stapleton, Schetter, Westling, et al., 2012). The type and satisfaction of support seem to be more important than the total number of support network members.

Across cultural groups, families and friends of new parents form an important dimension of the parents' social network. Through seeking help within the social network, new mothers learn culturally valued practices and develop role competency.

Social networks provide a support system on which parents can rely for assistance, but they also can be a source of conflict. Sometimes a large network can cause problems because it results in conflicting advice that comes from numerous people. Grandparents or in-laws are most appreciated when they assist with household responsibilities and do not intrude into the parents' privacy or judge them critically.

Because of the extent of restructuring and reorganization that occur in a family with the birth of another child, the mother's moods and fatigue in the postpartum period can be helped more by situation-specific support from family and friends than by general support. General support addresses feeling loved, respected, and valued. Situation-specific support relates to practical concerns such as physical needs and child care. For example, the practical support of a grandparent bathing the infant can help lessen a second-time mother's feelings of loss by providing her time to be with her first-born child.

Culture

Cultural beliefs and practices are important determinants of parenting behaviors. Culture influences the interactions with the baby as well as the parent's or family's caregiving style. For example, the provision for a period of rest and recuperation for the mother after birth is prominent in several cultures. Asian mothers remain at home with the baby up to 30 days after birth and are not supposed to engage in household chores, including care of the baby. Often the grandmother takes over the baby's care immediately, even before discharge from the hospital (D'Avanzo, 2008). Jordanian mothers have a 40-day lying-in after birth, during which their mothers or sisters care for the baby (D'Avanzo, 2008). Japanese mothers rest for the first 2 months after childbirth. Hispanics practice an intergenerational family ritual, *la cuarentena*. For 40 days after birth, the mother is expected to recuperate and get acquainted with her infant. Traditionally, this practice involves many restrictions concerning food (spicy or cold foods, fish, pork, and citrus are avoided; tortillas and chicken soup are encouraged), exercise, and activities including sexual intercourse. Many women avoid bathing and washing their hair. Traditional Hispanic husbands do not expect to see their wives or infants until both have been cleaned and dressed after birth. *La cuarentena* incorporates individuals into the family, instills parental responsibility, and integrates the family during a critical life event (D'Avanzo, 2008).

All cultures place importance on desiring and valuing children. In Asian families, children are a source of family strength and stability, are perceived as wealth, and are objects of parental love and affection. Infants are almost always given an affectionate "cradle" name that is used during the first years of life; for example, a Filipino girl might be called "Ling-Ling" and a boy "Bong-Bong."

Differing cultural values can influence parents' interactions with health care professionals. For example, Asians are taught to be humble and obedient; to be outspoken is frowned on. They are brought up to refrain from questioning authority figures (such as a nurse), to avoid confrontation, and to respect the yin/yang balance in nature. Because of these learned values, an Asian mother might not confront the nurse about the length of time it has taken to receive the medication requested for her perineal pain. A mother may nod and say "Yes" in response to the nurse's directions for using an iced sitz bath but then will not use the sitz bath. The "yes," in this case, is a gesture of courtesy, meaning "I'm listening"; it is not an indication of agreement to comply. The mother does not use the iced sitz bath because of her traditional avoidance of bathing and cold in the puerperium. Because not all members of a cultural group adhere to traditional practices, it is necessary to validate which cultural practices are important to individual parents.

Knowledge of cultural beliefs can help the nurse make more accurate assessments and diagnoses of observed parenting behaviors. For example, nurses may become concerned when they observe cultural practices that appear to reflect poor maternal-infant bonding. Algerian mothers may not unwrap and explore their infants as part of the acquaintance process because in Algeria, babies are wrapped tightly in swaddling clothes to protect them physically and psychologically (D'Avanzo, 2008). The nurse may observe a Vietnamese woman who gives minimal care to her infant but refuses to cuddle or further interact with her baby. This apparent lack of interest in the newborn is this cultural group's attempt to ward off "evil spirits" and actually reflects an intense love and concern for the

infant (Galanti, 2008). An Asian mother might be criticized for almost immediately relinquishing the care of the infant to the grandmother and not even attempting to hold her baby when it is brought to her room. However, in Asian extended families, members show their support for a new mother's rest and recuperation by assisting with the care of the baby. Contrary to the guidance given to mothers in the United States about "nipple confusion," a mix of breastfeeding and bottle-feeding is standard practice for Japanese mothers. This tradition is related to concern for the mother's rest during the first 2 to 3 months and does not usually lead to any problems with lactation; breastfeeding is widespread and successful among Japanese women.

Cultural beliefs and values give perspective to the meaning of childbirth for a new mother and a new father. Nurses can provide an opportunity for new mothers and fathers to talk about their perceptions of the meaning of childbearing. In helping new families adjust to parenthood, nurses must provide culturally competent care by following principles that facilitate nursing practice within transcultural situations.

Socioeconomic Conditions

Socioeconomic conditions often determine access to available resources. Parents whose economic condition is made worse with the birth of each child and who cannot use an effective method of fertility management may find childbirth complicated by concern for their own health and a sense of helplessness. Mothers who are single, separated or divorced from their husbands, or without a partner, family, and friends can view the birth of a child with dread. Serious financial problems may override any desire for mothering the infant. Similarly, fathers who are overwhelmed with financial stresses may lack effective parenting skills and behaviors.

Personal Aspirations

For some women, parenthood interferes with or blocks their plans for personal freedom or advancement in their careers. Unresolved resentment can affect caregiving activities and adjustment to parenting. This situation may result in indifference and neglect of the infant or in excessive concerns; the mother may set impossibly high standards for her own behavior or the child's performance.

Nursing intervention includes providing opportunities for mothers to express their feelings freely to an objective listener, to discuss measures to permit personal growth, and to learn about the care of their infant. Referring the woman to a support group of other mothers who are in similar circumstances may also be helpful.

Nurses can be proactive in influencing changes in work policies related to maternity and paternity leaves, varying models of work sharing, and family-friendly work environments. Some corporations already structure their work sites to support new mothers (e.g., by providing on-site day care facilities and lactation rooms).

PARENTAL SENSORY IMPAIRMENT

In the early interactions between the parent and child, each uses all senses—sight, hearing, touch, taste, and smell—to initiate and sustain the attachment process. A parent who has an impairment of one or more of the senses needs to maximize use of the remaining senses. Mothers with disabilities tend to value the importance of performing parenting tasks in the perceived culturally usual way.

Visually Impaired Parent

Visual impairment alone does not seem to have a negative effect on parents' early parenting experiences. These parents, just as sighted parents, express the wonders of parenthood and encourage other visually impaired persons to become parents.

Although visually impaired parents initially feel a pressure to conform to traditional, sighted ways of parenting, they soon adapt these ways and develop methods better suited to themselves. Examples of activities that visually impaired parents do differently include preparation of the infant's nursery, clothes, and supplies. Some parents put an entire clothing outfit together and hang it in the closet rather than keeping the items separate in drawers. Some develop a labeling system for the infant's clothing and put diapering, bathing, and other care supplies where these will be easy to locate. A strength that visually impaired parents have is a heightened sensitivity to other sensory outputs. Visually impaired parents can tell when their infant is facing them because they can feel the baby's breath on their face.

One of the major difficulties that visually impaired parents experience is the skepticism, open or hidden, of health care professionals. Visually impaired people sense reluctance on the part of others to acknowledge that they have a right to be parents. Too often, nurses and physicians lack the experience to deal with the childbearing and childrearing needs of visually impaired parents, as well as parents with other disabilities (e.g., the hearing impaired, physically impaired, and mentally challenged). The nurse's best approach is to assess the parent's capabilities. From that basis, the nurse can make plans to assist the parent, often in much the same way as for a parent without impairment. Visually impaired mothers have made suggestions for providing care for women such as themselves during childbearing (Box 20-2). Such approaches can help avoid a sense of increased vulnerability on the parent's part. Childbirth education and other materials are available in Braille (www.loc.gov/nls).

Eye contact is important in North American culture. With a parent who is visually impaired, this critical factor in the parent-child attachment process is obviously missing. However, the visually impaired parent, who may never have experienced this method of strengthening relationships, does not miss it. The infant will need other sensory input from that parent. An infant looking into the eyes of a parent who is visually impaired may be unaware that the eyes are unseeing. Other people in the newborn's environment can participate in active eye-to-eye contact to supply this need. A problem may arise, however, if the visually impaired parent has an impassive facial expression. The infant, making repeated unsuccessful attempts to engage in face play with the mother, will abandon the behavior with her and intensify it with the father or other persons in the household. Nurses can provide anticipatory guidance regarding this situation and help the mother learn to nod and smile while talking and cooing to the infant.

Hearing-Impaired Parent

A parent who has a hearing impairment faces challenges in caregiving and parenting, particularly if the deafness dates from birth or early childhood. Whether one or both parents are hearing impaired, they are likely to have established an independent household. Devices that transform sound into light flashes can be fitted into the infant's room to permit immediate detection of crying. Even if the parent is not speech trained, vocalizing can serve as both a stimulus and a response to the infant's early vocalizing. Deaf parents can provide additional vocal training by use of recordings and television, so that from birth, the child is aware of the full range of the human voice. Young children acquire sign language readily, and the first sign used is as varied as the first word.

Section 504 of the Rehabilitation Act of 1973 requires that hospitals and other institutions receiving funds from the U.S. Department of Health and Human Services use various communication techniques and resources with the deaf, including having staff members or certified interpreters who are proficient in sign language. Providing written materials with demonstrations and having nurses stand where the parent can read their lips (if the parent practices lipreading) are two techniques that can be used. A creative approach is for the nursing unit to develop videos in which information on postpartum care, infant care, and parenting issues is signed by an interpreter and spoken by a nurse. A video in which a nurse signs while speaking would be ideal. With the advent of the Internet, many resources are available to the deaf parent. Box 20-3 lists suggestions for working with hearing-impaired parents.

SIBLING ADAPTATION

Because the family is an interactive, open unit, the addition of a new family member affects everyone in the family. Siblings have to assume new positions within the family hierarchy. Parents often face the task of caring for a new child while not neglecting the others and need to distribute their attention equitably. When the newborn was born prematurely or has special needs, this task can be difficult.

Reactions of siblings result from temporary separation from the mother, changes in the mother's or father's behavior, or the infant coming home. Positive behavioral changes of siblings include interest in and concern for the baby (see Fig. 20-9) and increased independence. Regression in toileting and sleep habits, aggression toward the baby, and increased seeking of attention and whining are examples of negative behaviors.

The parents' attitudes toward the arrival of the baby can set the stage for the other children's reactions (Fig. 20-9). Because the baby absorbs the time and attention of the important people in the other children's lives, jealousy (sibling rivalry) is common once the initial excitement of having a new baby in the home is over.

Parents, especially mothers, spend much time and energy promoting sibling acceptance of a new baby. Participating in sibling

---

BOX 20-2 **NURSING APPROACHES FOR WORKING WITH VISUALLY IMPAIRED PARENTS**

- Parents who are visually impaired need oral teaching by health care providers because pregnancy and childbirth information is usually not accessible to visually impaired people.
- A visually impaired parent needs an orientation to the hospital room that allows the parent to move about the room independently. For example, "Go to the left of the bed and trail the wall until you feel the first door. That is the bathroom."
- Parents who are visually impaired need explanations of routines.
- Parents who are visually impaired need to feel devices (e.g., portable sitz bath equipment, breast pump) and to hear descriptions of the devices.
- Visually impaired parents need a chance to ask questions.
- Visually impaired parents need the opportunity to hold and touch the baby after birth.
- Nurses need to demonstrate baby care by touch and to follow with, "Now show me how you would do it."
- Nurses need to give instructions such as "I'm going to give you the baby. The head is to your left side."

BOX 20-3 NURSING APPROACHES FOR WORKING WITH HEARING-IMPAIRED PARENTS

- Before initiating communication, be aware of the parents' preferences and capabilities: Do they wear a hearing aid? Do they read lips? Do they wish to have an interpreter?
- Make certain that the parent(s) sees you approaching to avoid startling the parent.
- Before speaking, be directly in front of the parent and have that person's full attention.
- When speaking, face the parent directly and be at the same level.
- Avoid standing in front of a light or a window while speaking to the parent.
- Keep your hands away from your face while speaking to minimize distractions.
- If the parent relies on lip reading, sit close enough so that the parent can easily see your lip movements.
- Speak clearly with a regular voice volume and lip movements, while maintaining eye contact.
- Speak in short, simple sentences to facilitate understanding.
- If the parent does not understand something, it is better to find a different way to say what needs to be communicated rather than repeating the same words over and over.
- Written messages aid in communication. A small white or black erasable board can be useful.
- Give educational materials to hearing-impaired parents and ask them to read the materials before doing parent teaching. They can refer to the materials after discharge.
- Use visual aids such as pictures, diagrams, or other devices when doing parent teaching.
- When doing parent teaching, it is helpful for a hearing person (partner or family member) to be present.
- Allow ample time to communicate with the hearing-impaired parent; being in a rush can evoke stress and create barriers to effective communication.

preparation classes makes a difference in the ability of parents to cope with sibling behavior (see Fig. 8-4). Older children are actively involved in preparing for the infant, and this involvement intensifies after the birth of the child. Parents have to manage their feelings of guilt that the older children are being deprived of parental time and attention and monitor the behavior of older children toward the more vulnerable infant and divert aggressive behavior. Strategies that parents have used to facilitate siblings' acceptance of a new baby are presented in the Family-Centered Care box.

FAMILY-CENTERED CARE

Strategies for Facilitating Sibling Acceptance of a New Baby

- Take your older child (or children) on a tour of your hospital room and point out similarities between this birth and his or her birth. "This is like the room I was in with you, and the baby is in the same kind of bassinet that you were in."
- Have a small gift from the baby to give to your older child each day he or she visits in the hospital.
- Give the older child a T-shirt that says "I'm a big brother" [or "sister"].
- Arrange for your children to be among the first to see the newborn. Let them hold the baby in the hospital. One mother and father arranged for their firstborn son to be present at the births of his three brothers and to be the first one to hold them.
- When the older child visits for the first time, make sure you are not holding the new baby. Your arms need to be open and available for the older child. Instruct the person accompanying the older child to call ahead or give a warning knock to give you time to lay the baby down or have someone else hold the baby.
- Plan individual time with each child. The father or partner can spend time with the older siblings while the mother is taking care of the baby and vice versa. Siblings like to have time and attention from both parents.
- Give preschool and early school-age siblings a newborn doll as "their baby." Give the sibling a photograph of the new baby to take to school to show off "his" or "her" baby. Older siblings may enjoy the responsibility of helping care for the newborn, such as learning how to give the baby a bottle or change a diaper. Remember to supervise interactions between the siblings and new baby.

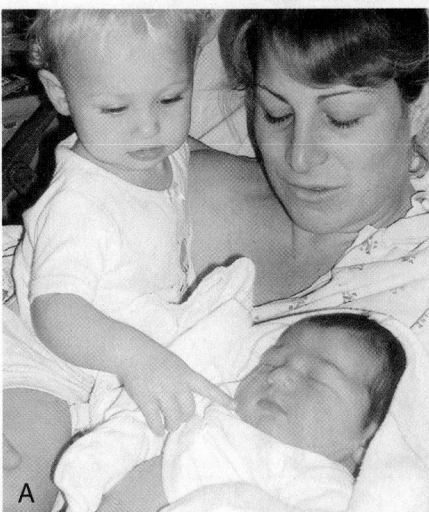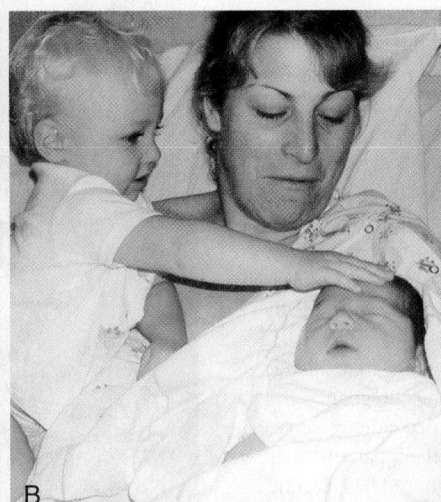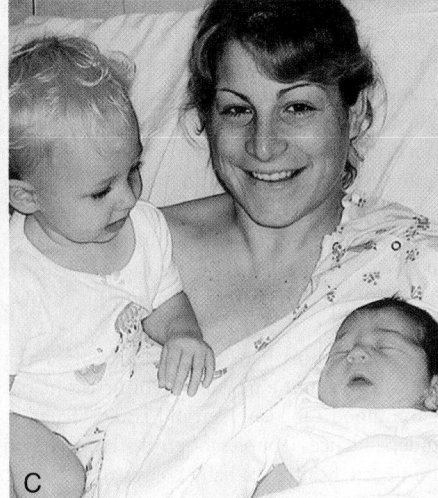

FIG 20-9 First meeting. **A,** Sister touching new sibling with fingertip. **B,** Touching with whole hand. **C,** Smiles indicate acceptance. (Courtesy Sara Kossuth, Los Angeles, CA.)

Siblings demonstrate acquaintance behaviors with the newborn. The acquaintance process depends on the information given to the child before the baby is born and on the child's cognitive development level. The initial behaviors of siblings with the newborn include looking at the infant and touching the head (see Fig. 20-9). The adjustment of older children to a newborn takes time, and parents should allow children to interact at their own pace rather than forcing them to interact. To expect a young child to accept and love a rival for the parents' affection assumes an unrealistic level of maturity. Sibling love grows as does other love, that is, by being with another person and sharing experiences. This bond between siblings involves a secure base in which one child provides support for the other, is missed when absent, and is looked to for comfort and security.

GRANDPARENT ADAPTATION

Becoming a grandparent is usually associated with great joy and happiness. Yet it is a time of transition as roles and relationships are changing and new opportunities arise. Emotions are varied and can change from day to day; feelings of joy, anticipation, and excitement are often intermingled with some degree of anxiety and uncertainty. Circumstances surrounding the pregnancy and birth influence the feelings, reactions, and responses of grandparents.

Pregnancy and birth necessitate redefining intergenerational roles and relationships within the family. A primary role of the grandparents is to support, nurture, and empower their child in his or her parenting role. Grandparents must acknowledge that things have changed since they first became parents as they deal with changes in practices and attitudes toward childbirth, childrearing, and men's and women's roles at home and in the workplace. The degree to which grandparents understand and accept current practices can influence how supportive they are to their adult children.

At the same time that they are adjusting to grandparenthood, the majority of grandparents are experiencing normative middle- and old-age life transition issues, such as retirement and a move to smaller housing, and they need support from their adult children. Some may feel regret about their limited involvement because of poor health or geographic distance.

The extent of involvement of grandparents in the care of the newborn depends on many factors, for example, the willingness of the grandparents to become involved, the proximity of the grandparents, and ethnic and cultural expectations of the grandparent's role (Fig. 20-10). If the new parents live in the United States, Asian grandparents typically are asked to come to the United States to care for the baby and the mother after birth and to care for the children once the parents return to work. In the United States, paternal grandparents, in contrast to those in other cultures, frequently consider themselves secondary to the maternal grandparents. Less seems expected of them, and they are initially less involved. Nevertheless, these grandparents are eager to help and express great pleasure in their son's fatherhood and his involvement with the baby (Fig. 20-11).

Relationships between grandparents and parents may change with the birth of a new baby. For first-time parents, pregnancy and parenthood can reawaken old issues related to dependence versus independence. Couples often do not plan on their parents' help immediately after the baby arrives. They want time "to be a family," implying a couple-baby unit, not the intergenerational family network. Contrary to their expectations, however, new parents do call on their parents for help, especially the maternal grandmother.

Many grandparents are aware of their adult children's wishes for autonomy, respect these wishes, and remain available to help when asked.

Grandparents' classes can be used to bridge the generation gap and to help the grandparents understand their adult children's parenting concepts. The classes include information on up-to-date childbearing practices; family-centered care; infant care, feeding, and safety (car seats); and exploration of roles that grandparents play in the family unit (see Community Focus box).

Increasing numbers of grandparents are providing permanent care for their grandchildren as a result of divorce, substance abuse, child abuse or neglect, abandonment, teenage pregnancy, death, human immunodeficiency virus (HIV) and acquired immunodeficiency syndrome (AIDS), unemployment, incarceration, and mental health problems. This emerging trend requires the nurse to evaluate the role of the grandparent in parenting the infant. Educational and financial considerations must be addressed and available support systems identified for these families.

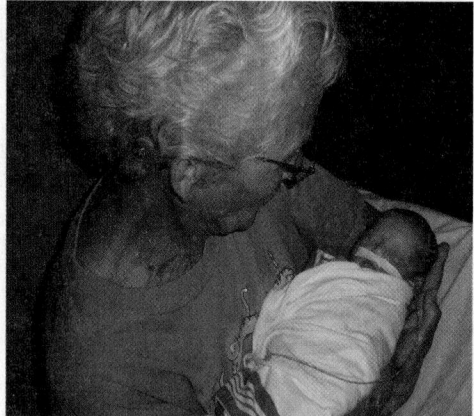

FIG 20-10 Great-grandmother and great-granddaughter get acquainted. (Courtesy Sharon Tallon, Mackinaw, IL.)

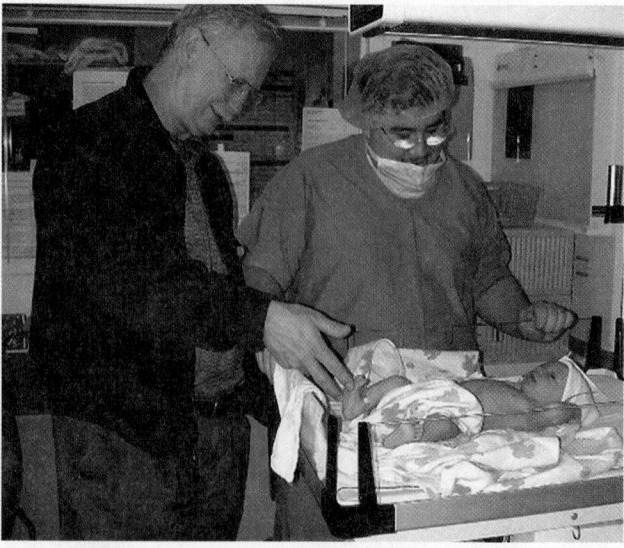

FIG 20-11 Father and grandfather becoming acquainted with new family member. (Courtesy Sharon Johnson, Petaluma, CA.)

CARE MANAGEMENT

Numerous changes occur during the first weeks of parenthood. Care management should be directed toward helping parents cope with infant care, role changes, altered lifestyle, and change in family structure resulting from the addition of a new baby. Developing skill and confidence in caring for an infant can be anxiety provoking. Anticipatory guidance can help prevent a shock of reality in the transition from hospital or birthing center to home that might negate the parents' joy or cause them undue stress.

Through education, support, and encouragement, nurses are instrumental in assisting mothers and their partners in the transition to parenthood, whether they are first-time parents or parents of several other children. Early and ongoing assessment and intervention promote positive outcomes for parents, infants, and family members (see Community Focus box and Nursing Care Plan).

🏠 COMMUNITY FOCUS

Helping Grandparents Bridge the Generation Gap

Interview a grandfather and a grandmother about their experiences with childbirth and infant care. Prepare a "letter to new parents" (written from the grandparents' perspective), which can be included in prenatal kits distributed in childbirth preparation classes and made available to all family members on the postpartum unit. Include how the birth of their adult child occurred, how things are different now, what role the grandparent can play in assisting the new parents adjust to home and child care, and what the grandparent might contribute to the family in memories.

🏠 COMMUNITY FOCUS

Identifying Parenting Resources on the Web

- Visit the website of a hospital that provides maternity services in your community. Does the hospital offer prepared childbirth, parenting, sibling, or infant/child cardiopulmonary resuscitation (CPR) classes? Are group tours of the birthing center provided for expectant parents?
- Visit the website *babycenter.com*, which provides information for parents about pregnancy, parenting, and children's health. Review the information about postpartum emotional health, causes and treatments of baby blues, and baby blues versus postpartum depression.
- Visit the website *familyandhome.org* and research the availability of support groups for parents in your community.

KEY POINTS

- The birth of a baby necessitates changes in the existing interactional structure of a family.
- Attachment is the process by which the parent and infant come to love and accept each other.
- Attachment is strengthened through the use of sensual responses or interactions by both partners in the parent-infant interaction.
- Women go through predictable stages in becoming a mother.
- Many mothers exhibit signs of postpartum blues (baby blues).
- Fathers experience emotions and adjustments during the transition to parenthood that are similar to and also distinctly different from those of mothers.
- Modulation of rhythm, modification of behavioral repertoires, and mutual responsivity facilitate infant-parent adjustment.
- Many factors influence adaptation to parenthood (e.g., age, culture, socioeconomic level, expectations of what the child will be like).
- Sibling adjustment to a new baby requires creative parental interventions.
- Grandparents can have a positive influence on the postpartum family.

REFERENCES

Beers L, Hollo R: Approaching the adolescent-headed family: a review of teen parenting, *Curr Probl Pediatr Adolesc Health Care* 39(9):216–233, 2009.

D'Avanzo C: *Mosby's pocket guide to cultural assessment*, ed 4, St Louis, 2008, Mosby.

Deave T, Johnson D, Ingram J: Transition to parenthood: the needs of parents in pregnancy and early parenthood, *BMC Pregnancy Childbirth* 8(30):1–11, 2008, www.biomedcentral.com/1471-2393/8/30.

de Montigny F, Lacharité C, Devault A: Transition to fatherhood: modeling the experience of fathers of breastfed infants, *ANS Adv Nurs Sci* 35(3):E11–E22, 2012.

Flacking R, Lehtonen L, Thomson G, et al: Closeness and separation in neonatal intensive care, *Acta Paediatr* 101(10):1032–1037, 2012.

Galanti G: *Caring for patients from different cultures*, ed 4, Philadelphia, 2008, University of Pennsylvania Press.

Goldberg AE, Smith JZ: Stigma, social context, and mental health: lesbian and gay couples across the transition to adoptive parenthood, *J Couns Psychol* 58(1):139–150, 2011.

Goldberg L, Ryan A, Sawchyn J: Feminist and queer phenomenology: a framework for perinatal nursing practice, research, and education for advancing lesbian health, *Health Care Women Int* 30(6):536–549, 2009.

Hoffenkamp HN, Tooten A, Hall RA, et al: The impact of premature childbirth on parental bonding, *Evol Psychol* 10(3):542–561, 2012.

Hung KJ, Berg O: Early skin-to-skin after cesarean to improve breastfeeding, *MCN Am J Matern Child Nurs* 36(5):318–324; quiz 325–326, 2011.

Hunter LP, Rychnovsky JD, Yount SM: A selective review of maternal sleep characteristics in the postpartum period, *J Obstet Gynecol Neonatal Nurs* 38(1):60–68, 2009.

Jaafar SH, Lee KS, Ho JJ: Separate care for new mother and infant versus rooming-in for increasing the duration of breastfeeding, *Cochrane Database Syst Rev* Sept 12(9):CD00641, 2012.

Klaus M, Kennell J: *Maternal-infant bonding*, St Louis, 1976, Mosby.

Klaus M, Kennell J: *Parent-infant bonding*, ed 2, St Louis, 1982, Mosby.

Kochanek KD, Kirmeyer SE, Martin JA, et al: Annual summary of vital statistics: 2009, *Pediatrics* 129(2):338–348, 2012.

Kurth E, Kennedy HP, Spichiger E, et al: Crying babies, tired mothers: what do we know? A systematic review, *Midwifery* 27(2):187–194, 2011.

Menéndez S, Hidalgo MV, Jiménez L, et al: Father involvement and marital relationship

◎ **NURSING CARE PLAN**

Home Care Follow-up: Transition to Parenthood

NURSING DIAGNOSIS	EXPECTED OUTCOME	INTERVENTIONS	RATIONALES
Deficient knowledge of infant care related to lack of experience or lack of support	Parents provide safe and adequate care, and infant appears healthy.	Observe infant care routines (bathing, diapering, feeding, play).	To evaluate parental ease with care and adequacy of techniques
		Observe infant's appearance (height-weight ratio, head circumference, fontanels, skin tone and turgor), and assess vital signs, overall tone, reflexes, and age-appropriate developmental skills.	To evaluate for signs indicative of inadequate care
		Explore available support systems for infant care	To determine adequacy of existing system
		Demonstrate care routines that pose difficulties, and have involved family members return demonstration	To facilitate improvements in care
		Provide ongoing follow-up and referrals as needed	To ensure that identified potential and actual care deficits are addressed and resolved
Disturbed Sleep Pattern related to infant demands and environmental interruptions	Woman sleeps for uninterrupted periods and states that she feels rested on waking	Discuss woman's routine, and specify factors that interfere with sleep	To determine scope of problem and direct interventions
		Explore ways woman and significant others can make environment more conducive to sleep (e.g., privacy, darkness, quiet, back rubs, soothing music, warm milk), and teach use of guided imagery and relaxation techniques	To promote optimal conditions for sleep
		Eliminate factors or routines that may interfere with sleep (e.g., caffeine, foods that induce heartburn, strenuous mental or physical activity)	To prevent interference with sleep.
		Advise family to limit visitors and activities	To prevent further stress and fatigue
		Have family plan specific times to care for newborn	To allow mother time to sleep
		Have mother learn to use infant nap time as time for her to nap as well	To replenish energy and decrease fatigue
		Assist family to identify persons such as family members or friends who can help with household tasks, infant care, and care of other children	To allow mother more time to rest
Impaired Home Maintenance related to addition of new family member, inadequate resources, or inadequate support systems	Home exhibits signs of safe and functional environment.	Observe home environment (e.g., available living space and sleeping arrangements; adequacy of facilities for food preparation and storage, hygiene, and toileting; overall state of repair; cleanliness; presence of safety hazards)	To determine adequacy and effective use of resources
		Observe arrangements for newborn, such as sleeping space, care equipment, and supplies (bathing, changing, feeding, transportation)	To determine adequacy of resources
		Explore who is responsible for cooking, cleaning, child care, and newborn care, and determine whether mother seems adequately rested	To determine adequacy of support systems
		Identify and arrange referrals to needed social agencies (e.g., Temporary Assistance for Needy Families [TANF]; Special Supplemental Nutrition Program for Women, Infants and Children [WIC] program; food pantries)	To address resource deficits (finances, supplies, equipment)
Interrupted Family Processes related to inclusion of new family member	Infant is successfully incorporated into family structure	Explore with family ways that birth and neonate have changed family structure and function	To evaluate functional and role adjustment
		Observe family's interaction with newborn, and note degree of bonding, evidence of sibling rivalry, and involvement in newborn care	To evaluate acceptance of newest family member
		Clarify identified misinformation and misperceptions	To promote clear communication
		Assist family in exploring options for solutions to identified problems	To promote effective problem resolution
		Support family's efforts as they move toward adjusting and incorporating new member	To reinforce new functions and roles
		If needed, make referrals to appropriate social services or community agencies	To ensure ongoing support and care

during transition to parenthood: differences between dual and single-earner families, *Span J Psychol* 14(2):639–647, 2011.

Mercer R: Becoming a mother versus maternal role attainment, *J Nurs Scholarship* 36(3):226–232, 2004.

Mercer R, Walker L: A review of nursing interventions to foster becoming a mother, *J Obst Gynecol Neonatal Nurs* 35(5):568–582, 2006.

Molborn S, Jacobs J: "We'll figure a way": teenage mothers' experiences in shifting social and economic contexts, *Qual Social* 35(1):23–46, 2011.

Moore E, Anderson G, Bergman N, et al: Early skin-to-skin contact for mothers and their healthy newborn infants, *Cochrane Database Syst Rev* 15(5):CD003519.pub3, 2012, DOI: 10.1002/14651858.

Perrine CG, Scanlon KS, Li R, et al: Baby-friendly hospital practices and meeting exclusive breastfeeding intention, *Pediatrics* 130(1):54–60, 2012.

Riordan J, Wambach K: *Breastfeeding and human lactation*, ed 4, Sudbury, MA, 2010, Jones & Bartlett.

Röndahl G, Bruhner E, Lindhe J: Heteronormative communication with lesbian families in antenatal care, childbirth and postnatal care, *J Adv Nurs* 65(11):2337–2344, 2009.

Rubin R: Basic maternal behavior, *Nurs Outlook* 9:683–686, 1961.

Rychnovsky J, Hunter LP: The relationship between sleep characteristics and fatigue in healthy postpartum women, *Womens Health Issues* 19(1):38–44, 2009.

Shapiro AF, Nahm EY, Gottman JM, et al: Bringing baby home together: examining the impact of a couple-focused intervention on the dynamics within family play, *Am J Orthopsychiatry* 81(3):337–350, 2011.

Shin H, Park Y, Ryu H, et al: Maternal sensitivity: a concept analysis, *J Adv Nurs* 64(3):304–314, 2008.

Smith PB, Moore K, Peters L: Implementing baby-friendly practices: strategies for success, *MCN Am J Matern Child Nurs* 37(4):228–233; quiz 234–235, 2012.

Stapleton LR, Schetter CD, Westling E, et al: Perceived partner support in pregnancy predicts lower maternal and infant distress, *J Fam Psychol* 26(3):453–463, 2012.

Steen M, Downe S, Bamford N, et al: Not-patient and not-visitor: a metasynthesis fathers' encounters with pregnancy, birth and maternity care, *Midwifery* 28(4):362–371, 2012.

Tharner A, Luijk MP, Raat H, et al: Breastfeeding and its relation to maternal sensitivity and infant attachment, *J Dev Behav Pediatr* 33(5):396–404, 2012.

Thukral A, Sankar MJ, Agarwal R, et al: Early skin-to-skin contact and breast-feeding behavior in term neonates: a randomized controlled trial, *Neonatology* 102(2):114–119, 2012.

Vasquez MJ, Berg OR: The baby-friendly journey in a US public hospital, *J Perinat Neonatal Nurs* 26(1):37–46, 2012.

Waugh LJ: Beliefs associated with Mexican immigrant families' practice of la cuarentena during postpartum recovery, *J Obstet Gynecol Neonatal Nurs* 40(6):732–741, 2011.

Welch MG, Hofer MA, Brunelli SA, et al; Family Nurture Intervention (FNI) Trial Group: Family nurture intervention (FNI): methods and treatment protocol of a randomized controlled trial in the NICU, *BMC Pediatr* 12:14, 2012.

Yu CY, Hung CH, Chan TF, et al: Prenatal predictors of father-infant attachment after childbirth, *J Clin Nurs* 21(11-12):1577–1583, 2012.

Postpartum Complications

Kathryn R. Alden

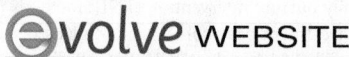 WEBSITE

http://evolve.elsevier.com/Perry/maternal

LEARNING OBJECTIVES

On completion of this chapter, the reader will be able to:

- Identify causes, signs and symptoms, possible complications, and medical and nursing management of postpartum hemorrhage.
- Describe hemorrhagic shock as a complication of postpartum hemorrhage, including medical management and nursing interventions.
- Identify causes, signs and symptoms, possible complications, and medical and nursing management of postpartum infection.
- Describe thromboembolic disorders, including incidence, etiology, signs and symptoms, and management.

- Summarize the role of the nurse in the home setting in assessing potential problems and managing care of women with postpartum complications.
- Describe structural disorders of the uterus and vagina that can result from childbearing.
- Differentiate among postpartum psychologic complications, including incidence, risk factors, signs and symptoms, severity, and management.
- Describe the nurse's role in assisting families who are grieving after maternal death.

Providing safe and effective care of the woman and family experiencing postpartum physical or psychologic complications requires a collaborative effort from all members of the health care team. This chapter focuses on the postpartum complications of hemorrhage and infection; structural disorders of the uterus, vagina, and bladder that can result from childbearing; and psychologic complications.

POSTPARTUM HEMORRHAGE

Definition and Incidence

Postpartum hemorrhage (PPH) is among the leading causes of maternal death in the United States and worldwide. It is a life-threatening event that can occur with little warning and is often unrecognized until the mother has profound symptoms. Postpartum hemorrhage occurs in approximately 3% of births (Callaghan, Kuklina, and Berg, 2010). It is preventable in more than half of the cases (Della Torre, Kilpatrick, Hibbard, et al., 2011).

PPH is defined as the loss of 500 mL or more of blood after vaginal birth and 1000 mL or more after cesarean birth. Either a 10% change in hematocrit between admission for labor and postpartum or the need for erythrocyte transfusion is used to define PPH (Francois and Foley, 2012). However, defining PPH clinically

is not a clear-cut undertaking. Diagnosis is often based on subjective observations, with blood loss often being underestimated by as much as 50% (Cunningham, Leveno, Bloom, et al., 2010).

Postpartum hemorrhage is classified as early or late with respect to the birth. Early, acute, or primary PPH occurs within 24 hours of the birth. Late or secondary PPH occurs more than 24 hours but less than 6 weeks after the birth (Francois and Foley, 2012). Today's health care environment encourages shortened hospital stays after birth, which increases the potential for acute episodes of PPH to occur outside the traditional hospital or birth center setting.

Etiology and Risk Factors

Excessive bleeding after birth can be considered with reference to the stages of labor. From birth of the fetus until separation of the placenta, the character and quantity of blood passed can suggest excessive bleeding. For example, dark blood is probably of venous origin, perhaps from varices or superficial lacerations of the birth canal. Bright blood is arterial and can indicate deep lacerations of the cervix. Spurts of blood with clots can indicate partial placental separation. Failure of blood to clot or remain clotted indicates a pathologic condition or coagulopathy such as disseminated intravascular coagulation (DIC) (see later discussion).

BOX 21-1 RISK FACTORS AND CAUSES OF POSTPARTUM HEMORRHAGE

- Uterine atony
  - Overdistended uterus—Large fetus, multiple fetuses, hydramnios, distention with clots
  - Retained placental fragments
  - Anesthesia and analgesia—Conduction anesthesia
  - Previous history of uterine atony
  - High parity
  - Prolonged labor, oxytocin-induced labor
  - Trauma during labor and birth—Forceps-assisted birth, vacuum-assisted birth, cesarean birth
- Lacerations of the birth canal
- Placenta accreta, increta, percreta
- Ruptured uterus
- Inversion of the uterus
- Coagulation disorders
- Placental abruption
- Placenta previa
- Manual removal of a retained placenta
- Magnesium sulfate administration during labor or postpartum period
- Chorioamnionitis
- Uterine subinvolution

Excessive bleeding can occur during the period from the separation of the placenta to its expulsion or removal. Commonly, such bleeding is the result of incomplete placental separation, undue manipulation of the fundus, or excessive traction on the cord. After the placenta has been expelled or removed, persistent or excessive blood loss usually is a result of uterine atony (i.e., failure to contract well or maintain contraction) or prolapse of the uterus into the vagina. Late PPH usually is the result of infection, subinvolution of the placental site, retained placental tissue, or coagulopathy (Francois and Foley, 2012). Risk factors for and causes of PPH are listed in Box 21-1.

Uterine Atony

Uterine atony is marked hypotonia (relaxation) of the uterus. Normally, placental separation and expulsion are facilitated by contraction of the uterus, which also prevents hemorrhage from the placental site. The uterine corpus is in essence a basket weave of strong, interlacing smooth-muscle bundles through which many large maternal blood vessels pass (see Fig. 3-3). If the uterus is flaccid after detachment of all or part of the placenta, brisk venous bleeding occurs and normal coagulation of the open vasculature is impaired and continues until the uterine muscle is contracted.

Uterine atony is the leading cause of early PPH. It is associated with high parity, polyhydramnios, fetal macrosomia, and multifetal gestation. In such conditions, the uterus is "overstretched" and contracts poorly after birth. Other causes of atony include traumatic birth, use of halogenated anesthetic (e.g., halothane), magnesium sulfate, rapid or prolonged labor, chorioamnionitis, use of oxytocin for labor induction or augmentation, and uterine atony in a previous pregnancy (Francois and Foley, 2012).

Retained Placenta

When the placenta has not been delivered within 30 minutes after birth despite gentle traction on the umbilical cord and uterine massage, it is described as "retained." Initial management of a retained placenta consists of manual separation and removal by the physician or nurse midwife. Supplementary anesthesia is usually not needed for women who have had regional anesthesia for birth. For other women, administration of light nitrous oxide and oxygen inhalation anesthesia or intravenous (IV) thiopental facilitates intrauterine exploration and placental separation. A tocolytic medication such as nitroglycerin IV may be given to promote uterine relaxation (Francois and Foley, 2012). After removal of a retained placenta, the woman is at continued risk for PPH and infection.

Fragments of the placenta can remain in the uterus after spontaneous separation of the placenta during the third stage of labor. In this case, the woman will have excessive bleeding and the uterus will feel boggy (soft) due to uterine atony. Ultrasonography can be used to detect placental fragments. The physician or midwife may attempt manual exploration to remove the fragments; uterine curettage (removal of uterine contents using a curette or vacuum suction) may be necessary.

In rare instances there is abnormal adherence of the placenta to the myometrium. It is unknown why this occurs, but it is thought to result from zygote implantation in an area of defective endometrium so that no zone of separation exists between the placenta and the decidua. Attempts to remove the placenta in the usual manner are unsuccessful, and laceration or perforation of the uterine wall can result, putting the woman at great risk for severe PPH and infection (Francois and Foley, 2012).

Unusual placental adherence can be partial or complete. The following degrees of attachment are recognized:

- **Placenta accreta**—Slight penetration of myometrium
- **Placenta increta**—Deep penetration of myometrium
- **Placenta percreta**—Perforation of uterus

Placenta accreta is most common, with its incidence increasing in association with the rise in cesarean birth rates (Cunningham, Leveno, Bloom, et al., 2010). Other risk factors include placenta previa, prior uterine surgery, endometrial defects, submucosal fibroids, parity, and maternal age (Francois and Foley, 2012). Placenta accreta can be diagnosed before birth using ultrasound and MRI, but often it is not recognized until there is excessive bleeding after birth. Bleeding with complete or total placenta accreta may not occur unless separation of the placenta is attempted. With more extensive involvement, bleeding becomes profuse when delivery of the placenta is attempted. Less blood is lost if the diagnosis is made antenatally and no attempt is made to manually remove the placenta. Treatment includes blood component replacement therapy. Hysterectomy can be indicated if bleeding is uncontrolled (Cunningham, Leveno, Bloom, et al., 2010).

Lacerations of the Genital Tract

Lacerations of the cervix, vagina, and perineum can cause PPH. Hemorrhage related to lacerations should be suspected if bleeding continues despite a firm, contracted uterine fundus. This bleeding can be a slow trickle, an oozing, or frank hemorrhage. Factors that influence the causes and incidence of obstetric lacerations of the lower genital tract include operative birth, precipitous birth, congenital abnormalities of the maternal soft parts, and contracted pelvis. Size, abnormal presentation, and position of the fetus; relative size of the presenting part and the birth canal; previous scarring from infection, injury, or surgery; and vulvar, perineal, and vaginal varicosities can also increase the risk for lacerations. Extreme vascularity in the labia and periclitoral areas often results in profuse bleeding if laceration occurs. Hematomas can also be present.

Lacerations of the perineum are the most common of all injuries in the lower portion of the genital tract. These are classified as first, second, third, and fourth degree (see Chapter 16). An episiotomy can extend to become either a third- or fourth-degree laceration.

Prolonged pressure of the fetal head on the vaginal mucosa ultimately interferes with the circulation and can produce ischemic or pressure necrosis. The state of the tissues in combination with the type of birth can result in deep vaginal lacerations, with consequent predisposition to vaginal hematomas.

Cervical lacerations usually occur at the lateral angles of the external os. Most are shallow, and bleeding is minimal. More extensive lacerations can extend into the vaginal vault or the lower uterine segment.

Lacerations are usually identified and sutured immediately after birth. After the bleeding has been controlled, the care of the woman with lacerations of the perineum is similar to that for women with episiotomies (i.e., analgesia as needed for pain and hot or cold applications as necessary). The need for increased roughage in the diet and increased intake of fluids is emphasized. Stool softeners may be used to assist the woman in reestablishing bowel habits without straining and putting stress on the suture lines.

> **! NURSING ALERT**
>
> To avoid injury to the suture line, a woman with third- or fourth-degree lacerations is not given rectal suppositories or enemas.

Hematomas

Pelvic hematomas (i.e., a collection of blood in the connective tissue) can be vulvar, vaginal, or retroperitoneal in origin. Vulvar hematomas are the most common. Pain is the most common symptom, and most vulvar hematomas are visible. Vaginal hematomas occur more commonly in association with a forceps-assisted birth, an episiotomy, or primigravidity (Francois and Foley, 2012).

Retroperitoneal hematomas are the least common but are life threatening. They are caused by laceration of one of the vessels attached to the hypogastric artery, usually associated with rupture of a cesarean scar during labor. During the postpartum period, if the woman reports persistent perineal or rectal pain or a feeling of pressure in the vagina, a careful examination is made. However, a retroperitoneal hematoma can cause minimal pain and the initial symptoms can be signs of shock (Francois and Foley, 2012).

Hematomas are usually surgically evacuated. Once the bleeding has been controlled, usual postpartum care is provided with paying attention to pain relief, monitoring the amount of bleeding, replacing fluids, and reviewing laboratory results (hemoglobin and hematocrit).

Inversion of the Uterus

Inversion (turning inside out) of the uterus after birth is a potentially life-threatening complication. The incidence of uterine inversion is approximately 1 in 3000 births (Cunningham, Leveno, Bloom, et al., 2010) and can recur with a subsequent birth. Uterine inversion can be incomplete, complete, or prolapsed. Incomplete inversion cannot be seen; a smooth mass can be palpated through the dilated cervix. In complete inversion, the lining of the fundus crosses through the cervical os and forms a mass in the vagina. Prolapsed inversion of the uterus is obvious—a large, red, rounded mass (perhaps with the placenta attached) protrudes 20 to 30 cm outside the introitus.

Contributing factors to uterine inversion include fundal implantation of the placenta, vigorous fundal pressure, excessive traction applied to the cord, fetal macrosomia, short umbilical cord, tocolysis, prolonged labor, uterine atony, nulliparity, and abnormally adherent placental tissue (Francois and Foley, 2012). The primary presenting signs of uterine inversion are sudden and include hemorrhage, shock, and pain. The uterus is not palpable abdominally. The uterus must be replaced into its proper position by the physician or nurse midwife.

Prevention—always the easiest, cheapest, and most effective therapy—is especially appropriate for uterine inversion. The umbilical cord should not be pulled unless the placenta has definitely separated.

Uterine inversion is an emergency situation requiring immediate interventions that include maternal fluid resuscitation, replacement of the uterus within the pelvic cavity, and correction of associated clinical conditions. Tocolytics or halogenated anesthetics may be given to relax the uterus before attempting replacement (Francois and Foley, 2012). Oxytocic agents are administered after the uterus is repositioned; broad-spectrum antibiotics are initiated. The woman's response to treatment is observed closely to prevent shock or fluid overload. If the uterus has been repositioned manually, care must be taken to avoid aggressive fundal massage.

Subinvolution of the Uterus

Late postpartum bleeding can result from **subinvolution** of the uterus (delayed return of the enlarged uterus to normal size and function). Recognized causes of subinvolution include retained placental fragments and pelvic infection. Signs and symptoms include prolonged lochial discharge, irregular or excessive bleeding, and sometimes hemorrhage. A pelvic examination usually reveals a larger-than-normal uterus that can be boggy.

Treatment of subinvolution depends on the cause. Ergonovine (Ergotrate) or methylergonovine (Methergine), 0.2 mg every 3 to 4 hours for 24 to 48 hours, is often used. Dilation and curettage (D&C) may be performed to remove retained placental fragments or to debride the placental site. If the cause of subinvolution is infection, antibiotic therapy is needed (Cunningham, Leveno, Bloom, et al., 2010).

CARE MANAGEMENT

Early recognition and treatment of PPH are critical to care management. The first step is to evaluate the contractility of the uterus. If the uterus is hypotonic, management is directed toward increasing contractility and minimizing blood loss.

If the uterus is firmly contracted and bleeding continues, the source of bleeding still must be identified and treated. Assessment may include visual or manual inspection of the perineum, the vagina, the uterus, the cervix, or the rectum and laboratory studies (e.g., hemoglobin, hematocrit, coagulation studies, platelet count). Treatment depends on the source of the bleeding.

The initial management of excessive postpartum bleeding due to uterine atony is firm massage of the uterine fundus. Expression of any clots in the uterus, elimination of bladder distention, and continuous IV infusion of 10 to 40 units of oxytocin added to 1000 mL of lactated Ringer's or normal saline solution also are primary interventions. If the uterus fails to respond to oxytocin, other uterotonic medications are administered. Misoprostol (Cytotec), a synthetic prostaglandin E_1 analog, is often used. An advantage is that it can be given by more than one route. Common dosages of misoprostol are 600 to 1000 mcg rectally or 400 mcg sublingually. A 0.2-mg dose

MEDICATION GUIDE

Uterotonic Drugs Used to Manage Postpartum Hemorrhage

DRUG	ACTION	SIDE EFFECTS	CONTRAINDICATIONS	DOSAGE AND ROUTE	NURSING CONSIDERATIONS
Oxytocin (Pitocin)	Contraction of uterus; decreases bleeding	Infrequent: water intoxication, nausea and vomiting	None for PPH	10 to 80 units/L diluted in lactated Ringer's solution or normal saline at 125 to 200 milliunits/min IV; or 10 to 20 units IM	Continue to monitor vaginal bleeding and uterine tone
Misoprostol (Cytotec)	Contraction of uterus	Headache, nausea, vomiting, diarrhea, fever, chills	None	600 to 1000 mcg rectally once or 400 mcg sublingual or PO once	Continue to monitor vaginal bleeding and uterine tone
Methylergonovine (Methergine)	Contraction of uterus	Hypertension, hypotension, nausea, vomiting, headache	Hypertension, preeclampsia, cardiac disease	0.2 mg IM every 2 to 4 hr up to five doses; may also be given intrauterine or orally	Check blood pressure before giving, and do not give if >140/90 mm Hg; continue monitoring vaginal bleeding and uterine tone
15-Methylprostaglandin $F_2\alpha$ (Prostin/15 m; Carboprost, Hemabate)	Contraction of uterus	Headache, nausea, vomiting, diarrhea, fever, chills, tachycardia, hypertension	Avoid with asthma or hypertension	0.25 mg IM or intrauterine every 15 to 90 min up to eight doses	Continue to monitor vaginal bleeding and uterine tone
Dinoprostone (Prostin E_2)	Contraction of uterus	Headache, nausea and vomiting, fever, chills, diarrhea	Use with caution with history of asthma, hypertension, or hypotension	20 mg vaginal or rectal suppository every 2 hr	Continue to monitor vaginal bleeding and uterine tone

IM, Intramuscular; *IV*, intravenous; *PPH*, postpartum hemorrhage.

of ergonovine (Ergotrate) or methylergonovine (Methergine) may be given intramuscularly to produce sustained uterine contractions; this can be repeated every 2 to 4 hours. A 0.25-mg dose of a derivative of prostaglandin $F_2\alpha$ (carboprost tromethamine [Carboprost; Hemabate]) may be given intramuscularly. It can also be given intramyometrially at cesarean birth or intraabdominally after vaginal birth. Carboprost can be repeated in recurrent doses of 0.25 mg every 15 to 90 minutes, up to 8 doses. Women with a history of asthma should not receive this medication because it can cause bronchoconstriction (Francois and Foley, 2012). Prostaglandin E_2 (Dinoprostone) 20-mg vaginal or rectal suppository can be used for postpartum hemorrhage (see the Medication Guide for a comparison of uterotonic drugs used to manage PPH). In addition to the medications used to contract the uterus, rapid administration of crystalloid solutions or blood or blood products or both will be needed to restore the woman's intravascular volume (Francois and Foley, 2012). (See Evidence-Based Practice box.)

! NURSING ALERT

Use of ergonovine or methylergonovine is contraindicated in the presence of hypertension or cardiovascular disease. Prostaglandin $F_2\alpha$ should be used cautiously in women with cardiovascular disease or asthma (Francois and Foley, 2012).

Oxygen can be given by nonrebreather facemask to enhance oxygen delivery to the cells. An indwelling urinary catheter is usually inserted to monitor urine output as a measure of intravascular volume. Laboratory studies usually include a complete blood count with platelet count, fibrinogen, fibrin split products, prothrombin time, and partial thromboplastin time. Blood type and antibody screen are done if not previously performed (Cunningham, Leveno, Bloom, et al., 2010).

If bleeding persists, bimanual compression may be performed by the obstetrician or nurse-midwife. This procedure involves inserting a fist into the vagina and pressing the knuckles against the anterior side of the uterus and then placing the other hand on the abdomen and massaging the posterior uterus with it. If the uterus still does not become firm, the physician or midwife performs manual exploration of the uterine cavity for retained placental fragments. If the preceding procedures are ineffective, surgical management is needed. Surgical management options include uterine tamponade (uterine packing or an intrauterine tamponade balloon), bilateral uterine artery ligation, ligation of utero-ovarian arteries and infundibulopelvic vessels, and selective arterial embolization. Uterine compression suturing (using, for example, B-Lynch or Hayman vertical sutures) may be performed and is sometimes combined with a tamponade balloon. If other treatment measures are ineffective, hysterectomy will likely be needed (Cunningham, Leveno, Bloom, et al., 2010; Francois and Foley, 2012).

EVIDENCE-BASED PRACTICE

Active Third-Stage Labor Management for Preventing Postpartum Hemorrhage

Ask the Question

For third-stage labor, what management techniques are most effective for prevention of postpartum hemorrhage (PPH)?

Search for the Evidence

Search Strategies

English research-based publications on uterotonics, postpartum hemorrhage (or haemorrhage), labor (or labour) bleeding, cord clamping, active management, oxytocin, prostaglandins were included.

Databases Used

Cochrane Collaborative Database, National Guideline Clearinghouse (AHRQ), CINAHL, PubMed, and UpToDate.

Critically Analyze the Evidence

PPH is still a major cause of maternal death, especially in low- and middle-income countries.

- In third-stage labor, uterine contractions expel the placenta and constrict the blood vessels of the uterine wall. To prevent PPH, health care providers actively manage third-stage labor by clamping the cord before pulsations have stopped, administering uterotonics to increase uterine contractions, and providing steady traction on the cord and counterpressure on the fundus, causing earlier expulsion of the placenta.
- Maternal effects: When compared with expectant management, the active management protocol results in less maternal blood loss and less maternal anemia (Begley, Gyte, Devane, et al., 2011). Adverse effects of active management include side effects of the uterotonics and uterine pressure: higher maternal diastolic pressure, pain requiring analgesia, nausea and vomiting. Active management is also more likely to result in readmission for bleeding, for unknown reasons.
- Effects on the newborn: Birth weight is less when the cord was clamped before cessation of pulsing, because there is less transfer of blood volume to the newborn. However, there are no differences in the number of neonatal intensive care unit (NICU) admissions nor the occurrences of neonatal jaundice (Begley, Gyte, Devane, et al., 2011).
- Uterotonics stimulate smooth muscle contraction of the uterus. Intravenous carbetocin, when compared with oxytocin, results in less need for uterine massage and use of other uterotonics, but no difference in PPH. When compared with ergometrine-oxytocin, carbetocin is associated with less blood loss and fewer side effects of nausea, vomiting, and postpartum hypertension (Su, Chong, and Samuel, 2012).
- Prostaglandins are also uterotonic. Oral or sublingual misoprostol is better than placebo for preventing blood loss and need for blood transfusion but causes dose-related shivering, increased temperature, and diarrhea and is expensive.
- Conventional injectable uterotonics such as intramuscular (IM) ergot alkaloids are the drugs of choice for preventing PPH, but prostaglandins may be useful in low-resource areas (Tuncalp, Hofmeyr, and Gülmezoglu, 2012).

Apply the Evidence: Nursing Implications

- Active management of third-stage labor is beneficial and recommended. However, it may be possible to individualize the protocol. Women should be educated before labor on their options for third-stage management and the risks and benefits of uterotonics.
- Some women request that the cord clamping be delayed until pulsations have ceased. This may benefit the newborn without significantly increasing the woman's risk for PPH.
- Nurses carefully assess the fundus and bleeding while recovering the immediate postpartum woman and are frequently the first to notice PPH.
- A protocol for PPH should be made clear to all staff. All staff should be able to identify when bleeding is too heavy and the correct steps of emptying the bladder, uterine massage, and whom to call immediately.
- Easily accessed kits of necessary medications should be available, along with training in their use.

Quality and Safety Competencies: Evidence-Based Practice*

Knowledge

Discriminate Between Valid and Invalid Reasons for Modifying Evidence-Based Clinical Practice Based on Clinical Expertise or Patient/Family Preferences.

Active management of third-stage labor may be individualized to accommodate family preferences, in collaboration with the health care provider.

Skills

Consult with Clinical Experts Before Deciding to Deviate from Evidence-Based Protocols.

Uterotonics prevent PPH but may cause adverse effects.

Attitudes

Acknowledge Own Limitations in Knowledge and Clinical Expertise Before Determining When to Deviate from Evidence-Based Best Practices.

Understanding the risks and benefits of active management are important for collaborative decision making.

References

Begley CM, Gyte GM, Devane D, et al: Active versus expectant management for women in the third stage of labour, *Cochrane Database Syst Rev* (Issue 11): DOI: 10.1002/14651858.CD007412.pub3, Chichester, UK, 2011, John Wiley & Sons.

Su L, Chong Y, Samuel M: Carbetocin for preventing postpartum haemorrhage, *Cochrane Database Syst Rev* (Issue 4): DOI: 10.1002/14651858.CD005457.pub4, Chichester, UK, 2012, John Wiley & Sons.

Tuncalp O, Hofmeyr GJ, Gülmezoglu AM: Prostaglandins for preventing postpartum haemorrhage, *Cochrane Database Syst Rev* (Issue 8):DOI: 10.1002/14651858.CD000494.pub4, Chichester, UK, 2012, John Wiley & Sons.

Pat Mahaffee Gingrich

*Adapted from QSEN at www.qsen.org/.

Herbal Remedies

Herbal remedies have been used, particularly outside the United States, with some success to control PPH after the initial management and control of bleeding. Some herbs have homeostatic actions, whereas others work as oxytocic agents to contract the uterus. However, published evidence of the safety and efficacy of herbal therapy is lacking. Evidence from well-controlled studies is needed before recommendations for practice can be made.

Nursing Interventions

The nurse must be alert to the symptoms of hemorrhage and hypovolemic shock and be prepared to act quickly to minimize blood loss

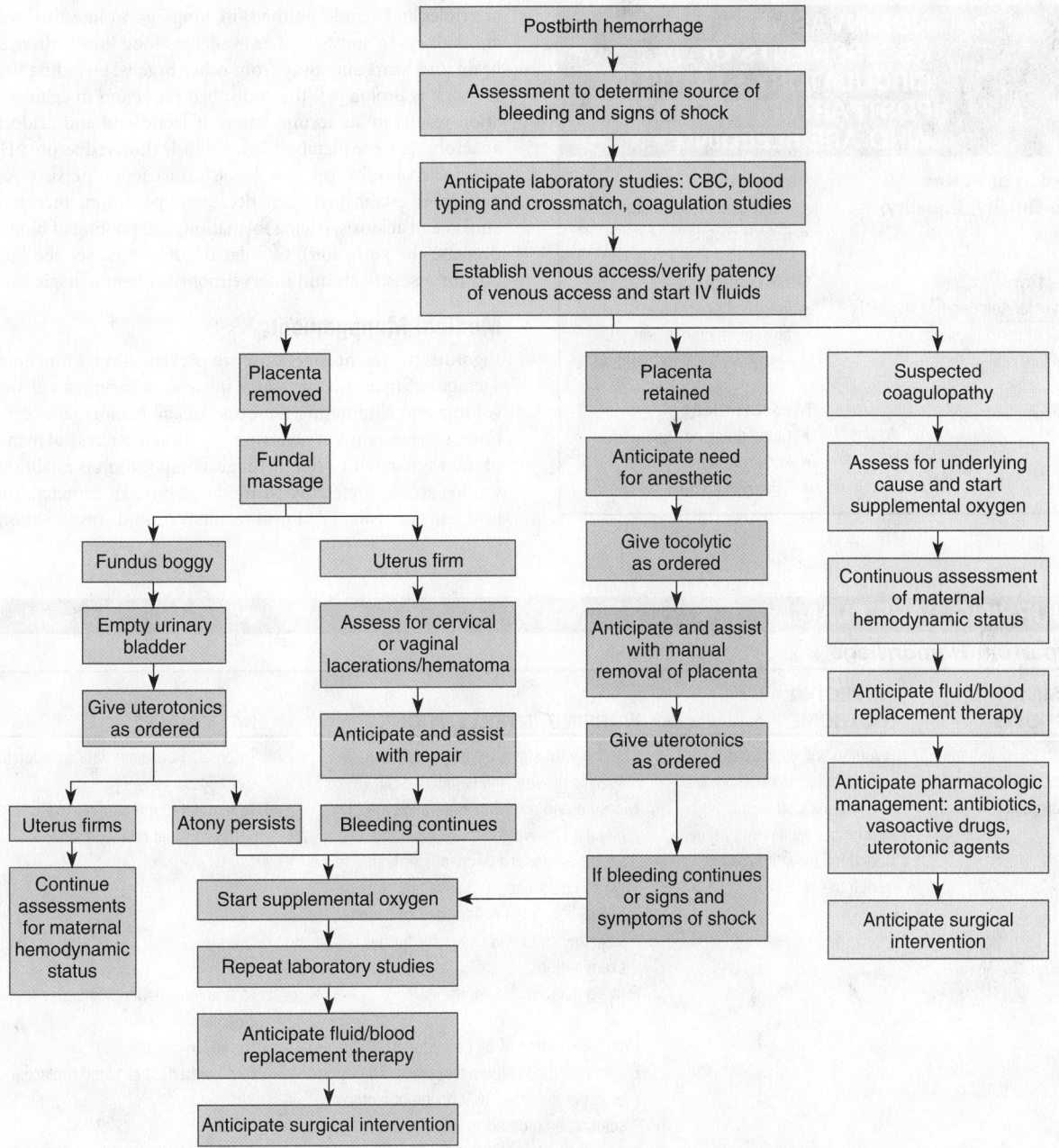

FIG 21-1 Nursing assessments for postpartum bleeding. *CBC,* Complete blood count; *IV,* intravenous; *tocolytics,* medications to relax the uterus; *uterotonics,* medications to contract the uterus.

(Fig. 21-1). Astute assessment of circulatory status can be done with noninvasive monitoring (Box 21-2). Interventions are based on the cause of PPH as previously discussed.

The woman and her family will be anxious about her condition. The nurse can intervene by calmly providing explanations about interventions being performed and the need to act quickly.

Once the woman's condition is stabilized, preparations for discharge are made. Discharge instructions for the woman who experienced PPH are similar to those for any postpartum woman. In addition, the woman should be told that she will probably feel fatigue, even exhaustion, and will need to limit her physical activities to conserve her strength. She may need instructions in increasing her dietary iron and protein intake and iron supplementation to rebuild lost red blood cell (RBC) volume. She may need assistance

with infant care and household activities until she has regained strength. Some women have problems with delayed lactation or insufficient milk production and postpartum depression (PPD). Referrals for home care follow-up or to community resources may be needed, such as to Postpartum Support International at www. chss.iup.edu/postpartum (see Nursing Care Plan).

HEMORRHAGIC (HYPOVOLEMIC) SHOCK

Hemorrhage can result in **hemorrhagic (hypovolemic) shock.** Shock is an emergency situation in which the perfusion of body organs can become severely compromised and death can occur. Physiologic compensatory mechanisms are activated in response to hemorrhage. The adrenal glands release catecholamines, causing

BOX 21-2   NONINVASIVE ASSESSMENTS OF CIRCULATORY STATUS IN POSTPARTUM PATIENTS WHO ARE BLEEDING

Palpation of Pulses (Rate, Quality, Equality)
- Arterial

Inspection
- Skin color, temperature, turgor
- Level of consciousness
- Capillary refill
- Neck veins
- Mucous membranes

Auscultation
- Heart sounds/murmurs
- Breath sounds

Observation
- Presence or absence of anxiety, apprehension, restlessness, disorientation

Measurement
- Blood pressure
- Pulse oximetry
- Urinary output

arterioles and venules in the skin, lungs, gastrointestinal tract, liver, and kidneys to constrict. The available blood flow is diverted to the brain and heart and away from other organs, including the uterus. If shock is prolonged, the continued reduction in cellular oxygenation results in an accumulation of lactic acid and acidosis (from anaerobic glucose metabolism). Acidosis (lowered serum pH) causes arteriolar vasodilation; venule vasoconstriction persists. A circular pattern is established (i.e., decreased perfusion, increased tissue anoxia and acidosis, edema formation, and pooling of blood further decrease the perfusion). Cellular death occurs. See the Emergency box for assessments and interventions for hemorrhagic shock.

Medical Management

Vigorous treatment is necessary to prevent adverse outcomes. Management of hypovolemic shock involves restoring circulating blood volume and eliminating the cause of the hemorrhage (e.g., lacerations, uterine atony, or inversion). Critical to successful management of the woman with a hemorrhagic complication is establishment of venous access, preferably with a large-bore IV catheter. The establishment of two IV lines facilitates fluid resuscitation. Fluid

NURSING CARE PLAN

Postpartum Hemorrhage

NURSING DIAGNOSIS	EXPECTED OUTCOME	NURSING INTERVENTIONS	RATIONALES
Deficient Fluid Volume related to postpartum hemorrhage	Woman will demonstrate fluid balance as evidenced by stable vital signs, prompt capillary refill time, and balanced intake and output.	Monitor vital signs, oxygen saturation, urine specific gravity, and capillary refill	To provide baseline data and detect changes
		Measure and record amount and type of bleeding by weighing and counting saturated pads; if woman is at home, teach her to count pads and save any clots or tissue; if woman is admitted to hospital, save any clots and tissue for further examination	To estimate type and amount of blood loss for fluid replacement
		Provide quiet environment	To promote rest and decrease metabolic demands
		Give explanation of all procedures	To reduce anxiety
		Begin intravenous (IV) access with 18-gauge or larger catheter for infusion of isotonic solution as ordered	To provide fluid or blood replacement
		Administer medications as ordered, such as oxytocin, misoprostol, methylergonovine, or prostaglandin $F_2\alpha$	To increase contractility of uterus
		Insert indwelling urinary catheter	To provide most accurate assessment of renal function and hypovolemia
		Prepare for surgical intervention as needed	To stop source of bleeding
Ineffective Tissue Perfusion related to hypovolemia	Woman will have stable vital signs, oxygen saturation, and arterial blood gases and adequate hematocrit and hemoglobin.	Monitor vital signs, oxygen saturation, arterial blood gases, and hematocrit and hemoglobin	To assess for hypovolemic shock and decreased tissue perfusion
		Assess capillary refill, mucous membranes, and skin temperature	To note indicators of vasoconstriction
		Give supplementary oxygen as ordered	To provide additional oxygenation to tissues
		Suction as needed, and insert oral airway	To maintain clear, open airway for oxygenation
		Monitor arterial blood gases	To provide information about acidosis or hypoxia
		Administer sodium bicarbonate if ordered	To reverse metabolic acidosis

✚ EMERGENCY

Hemorrhagic Shock

Assessments	Characteristics
• Respirations	• Rapid and shallow
• Pulse	• Rapid, weak, irregular
• Blood pressure	• Decreasing (late sign)
• Skin	• Cool, pale, clammy
• Urinary output	• Decreasing
• Level of consciousness	• Lethargy → coma
• Mental status	• Anxiety → coma
• Central venous pressure	• Decreased

Intervention

- Summon assistance and equipment.
- Start intravenous infusion per standing orders.
- Ensure patent airway; administer oxygen.
- Continue to monitor status.

resuscitation includes the administration of crystalloids (lactated Ringer's, normal saline solution), colloids (albumin), blood, and blood components. To restore circulating blood volume, a rapid IV infusion of crystalloid solution is given at a rate of 3 mL infused for every 1 mL of estimated blood loss (e.g., 3000 mL infused for 1000 mL of blood loss). Packed red blood cells (RBCs) are usually infused if the woman is still actively bleeding and no improvement in her condition is noted after the initial crystalloid infusion. Infusion of fresh frozen plasma may be needed if clotting factors and platelet counts are below normal values (Cunningham, Leveno, Bloom, et al., 2010; Francois and Foley, 2012).

Nursing Interventions

Hemorrhagic shock can occur rapidly, but the classic signs of shock may not appear until the postpartum woman has lost 30% to 40% of blood volume. The nurse must continue to reassess the woman's condition as evidenced by the degree of measurable and anticipated blood loss and mobilize appropriate resources.

Most interventions are instituted to improve or monitor tissue perfusion. Fluid resuscitation must be monitored carefully because fluid overload can occur. Intravascular fluid overload occurs most often with colloid therapy.

◎ NURSING CARE PLAN

Postpartum Hemorrhage—cont'd

NURSING DIAGNOSIS	EXPECTED OUTCOME	NURSING INTERVENTIONS	RATIONALES
Anxiety related to sudden change in health status	Woman will verbalize that anxious feelings are diminished.	Using therapeutic communication, evaluate woman's understanding of events	To provide clarification of any misconceptions
		Provide calm, competent attitude and quiet environment	To aid in decreasing anxiety
		Explain all procedures	To decrease anxiety about unknown
		Allow woman to verbalize feelings	To permit clarification of information and promote trust
		Continue to assess vital signs or other clinical indicators of hypovolemic shock	To evaluate if psychologic response of anxiety intensifies physiologic indicators
Risk for Infection related to blood loss and invasive procedures as result of postpartum hemorrhage	Woman will verbalize understanding of risk factors. Woman will demonstrate no signs of infection.	Maintain Standard Precautions and use proper hand hygiene technique when providing care	To prevent introduction of or spread of infection
		Teach woman to maintain proper hand hygiene (particularly before handling her newborn) and to maintain scrupulous perineal care with frequent change and careful disposal of perineal pads	To avoid spread of microorganisms
		Monitor vital signs	To detect signs of systemic infection
		Monitor level of fatigue and lethargy, evidence of chills, loss of appetite, nausea and vomiting, and abdominal pain	To indicate extent of infection and serve as indicators of status of infection
		Monitor lochia for foul smell	To detect sign of infection
		Assist with collection of intrauterine cultures or other specimens for laboratory analysis	To identify specific causative organism
		Monitor laboratory values (i.e., white blood cell [WBC] count, cultures)	For indicators of type and status of infection
		Ensure adequate fluid and nutritional intake	To promote healthy recovery
		Administer and monitor broad-spectrum antibiotics as ordered	To prevent or treat infection
		Administer antipyretics as ordered and necessary	To reduce elevated temperature

Transfusion reactions can follow administration of blood or blood components, including cryoprecipitates. Even in an emergency, each unit of blood or blood products should be carefully checked per hospital protocol. Complications of fluid or blood replacement therapy include hemolytic reactions, febrile reactions, allergic reactions, circulatory overloading, and air embolism.

LEGAL TIP: Standard of Care for Bleeding Emergencies
The standard of care for obstetric emergency situations such as PPH or hypovolemic shock is that provision should be made for the nurse to implement nursing actions independently. Policies, procedures, standing orders or protocols, and clinical guidelines should be established by each health care facility in which births occur and should be agreed on by health care providers involved in the care of obstetric patients.

The nurse continues to monitor the woman's pulse and blood pressure. If invasive hemodynamic monitoring is ordered, the nurse may assist with placement of a central venous pressure (CVP) or pulmonary artery (Swan-Ganz) catheter. Subsequently, the nurse monitors CVP, pulmonary artery pressure, or pulmonary artery wedge pressure as ordered (Gilbert, 2011).

Additional assessments include evaluating skin temperature, color, and turgor; and mucous membranes. Breath sounds should be auscultated before fluid volume replacement to provide a baseline for future assessment. Inspection for oozing at the sites of incisions or injections and assessment for the presence of petechiae or ecchymosis in areas not associated with surgery or trauma are critical in evaluating for disseminated intravascular coagulation (DIC) (see later discussion).

Oxygen is administered, preferably by a nonrebreather facemask, at 10 to 12 L/min to maintain oxygen saturation. Oxygen saturation should be monitored with a pulse oximeter, although measurements are not always accurate in a patient with hypovolemia or decreased perfusion. Level of consciousness is assessed frequently and provides additional indications of blood volume and oxygen saturation (Gilbert, 2011). In early stages of decreased blood flow, the woman may report "seeing stars" or feeling dizzy or nauseated. She can become restless and orthopneic. As cerebral hypoxia increases, she can become confused and react slowly to stimuli or not at all. Some women complain of headaches. An improved sensorium is an indicator of improved perfusion.

Continuous electrocardiographic monitoring may be indicated for the woman who is hypotensive or tachycardic, continues to bleed profusely, or is in shock. A Foley catheter is inserted and a urometer is attached to allow hourly assessment of urine output. The most objective and least invasive assessment of adequate organ perfusion and oxygenation is a urine output of at least 30 mL/hr (Cunningham, Leveno, Bloom, et al., 2010). Hemoglobin and hematocrit levels, platelet count, and coagulation studies are closely monitored.

COAGULOPATHIES

When bleeding is continuous and there is no identifiable source, a coagulopathy can be the cause. The woman's coagulation status must be assessed quickly and continuously. Abnormal results depend on the cause and can include increased prothrombin time, increased partial thromboplastin time, decreased platelets, decreased fibrinogen level, increased fibrin degradation products, and prolonged bleeding time. Causes of coagulopathies can include pregnancy complications such as idiopathic or immune thrombocytopenic purpura (ITP), von Willebrand disease (vWD), or DIC.

Idiopathic Thrombocytopenic Purpura

Idiopathic or immune thrombocytopenic purpura (ITP) is an autoimmune disorder in which antiplatelet antibodies decrease the life span of the platelets. Thrombocytopenia, capillary fragility, and increased bleeding time are diagnostic findings. ITP can cause severe hemorrhage after cesarean birth or cervical or vaginal lacerations. The incidence of postpartum uterine bleeding and vaginal hematomas is also increased. Neonatal thrombocytopenia can result, but serious bleeding is unusual (Rozance and Rosenberg, 2012).

Medical management focuses on control of platelet stability. If ITP was diagnosed during pregnancy, the woman likely was treated with corticosteroids or IV immune globulin. Platelet transfusions are usually given when there is significant bleeding. A splenectomy may be needed if the ITP does not respond to medical management (Cunningham, Leveno, Bloom, et al., 2010).

von Willebrand Disease

von Willebrand disease (vWD), a type of hemophilia, is probably the most common of all hereditary bleeding disorders. Although von Willebrand disease is rare, it is among the most common congenital clotting defects in U.S. women of childbearing age. It results from a deficiency or defect in a blood clotting protein called *von Willebrand factor (vWF)*. There are as many as 20 variations of vWD, most of which are inherited as autosomal dominant traits—types I and II are the most common (Cunningham, Leveno, Bloom, et al., 2010). Symptoms include recurrent bleeding episodes such as nosebleeds or after tooth extraction, bruising easily, prolonged bleeding time (the most important test), factor VIII deficiency (mild to moderate), and bleeding from mucous membranes. Although factor VIII increases during pregnancy, a risk for PPH still exists as levels of vWF begin to decrease (Cunningham, Leveno, Bloom, et al., 2010).

The woman can be at risk for bleeding for up to 4 weeks after birth. The treatment of choice is administration of desmopressin, which promotes the release of vWF and factor VIII. It can be given nasally, intravenously, or orally. Transfusion therapy with plasma products that have been treated for viruses and contain factor VIII and vWF also may be used. Concentrates of antihemophiliac factor (Humate-P or Alphanate) can be administered (Cunningham, Leveno, Bloom, et al., 2010).

Disseminated Intravascular Coagulation

Disseminated intravascular coagulation (DIC), also known as *consumptive coagulopathy*, is an imbalance between the body's clotting and fibrinolytic systems. It is a pathologic form of clotting that is diffuse and consumes large amounts of clotting factors, including platelets, fibrinogen, prothrombin, and factors V and VII. Widespread external bleeding, internal bleeding, or both can result. DIC also causes vascular occlusion of small vessels resulting from small clots forming in the microcirculation. In the obstetric population, DIC can occur as a result of acute antepartum or postpartum hemorrhage, abruptio placentae, amniotic fluid embolism, dead fetus syndrome (i.e., fetus dies but is retained in utero for at least 6 weeks), severe preeclampsia, sepsis, saline abortion, and acute fatty liver of pregnancy (Francois and Foley, 2012).

The diagnosis of DIC is made according to clinical findings and laboratory markers. Physical examination reveals unusual bleeding; spontaneous bleeding from the woman's gums or nose can occur. Petechiae can appear around a blood pressure cuff placed on the woman's arm. Excessive bleeding can occur from the site of a slight trauma (e.g., venipuncture sites, intramuscular or subcutaneous injection sites, nicks from shaving of perineum or abdomen, and injury from insertion of a urinary catheter). Hypotension is out of proportion to the observed blood loss. Other symptoms include tachycardia and diaphoresis. Laboratory tests reveal decreased levels of platelets, fibrinogen, proaccelerin, antihemophiliac factor, and prothrombin (the factors consumed during coagulation). Fibrinolysis is increased at first but is later severely depressed. Degradation of fibrin leads to the accumulation of fibrin split products in the blood; these have anticoagulant properties and prolong the prothrombin time. Bleeding time is normal, coagulation time shows no clot, clot-retraction time shows no clot, and partial thromboplastin time is increased. DIC must be distinguished from other clotting disorders before therapy is initiated.

Primary medical management in all cases of DIC involves correction of the underlying cause (e.g., removal of the dead fetus, treatment of existing infection or of preeclampsia or eclampsia, or removal of a placental abruption). Volume replacement, blood component therapy, optimization of oxygenation and perfusion status, and continued reassessment of laboratory parameters are the usual forms of treatment. Resolution of DIC usually begins with the birth of the neonate (Francois and Foley, 2012).

Nursing interventions include assessing for signs of bleeding, administering fluid or blood replacement as ordered, observing for signs of complications from the administration of blood and blood products, and protecting from injury. Because renal failure is one consequence of DIC, urinary output is closely monitored, usually by insertion of an indwelling urinary catheter. Urinary output must be maintained at more than 30 mL/hr.

The woman and her family will be anxious and concerned about her condition and prognosis. The nurse offers explanations about care and provides emotional support to them through this critical time.

VENOUS THROMBOEMBOLIC DISORDERS

Venous thromboembolism (VTE) results from the formation of a blood clot or clots inside a blood vessel and is caused by inflammation (thrombophlebitis) or partial obstruction of the vessel. Three thromboembolic conditions are of concern in the postpartum period:

- **Superficial venous thrombosis**—Involvement of the superficial saphenous venous system
- **Deep venous thrombosis (DVT)**—Occurs most often in the lower extremities; involvement varies but can extend from the foot to the iliofemoral region
- **Pulmonary embolism (PE)**—Complication of deep venous thrombosis occurring when part of a blood clot dislodges and is carried to the pulmonary artery, where it occludes the vessel and obstructs blood flow to the lungs

Incidence and Etiology

The incidence of venous thromboembolism (VTE) varies from about 1 in 1000 to 1 in 1500 pregnancies (Cunningham, Leveno, Bloom, et al., 2010; Pettker and Lockwood, 2012). VTE can occur in each trimester of pregnancy and in the postpartum period. DVT occurs most often during pregnancy, and PE is more common in the postpartum period. The incidence of VTE in the postpartum period declined in the past 30 years because early ambulation after childbirth has become standard practice. However, pulmonary embolism (PE) is a major cause of maternal death (Pettker and Lockwood, 2012). The primary causes of thromboembolic disease

are venous stasis and hypercoagulation, both of which are present in pregnancy and continue into the postpartum period. Cesarean birth nearly doubles the risk for VTE; therefore routine preoperative placement of pneumatic compression devices is recommended. Other risk factors include operative vaginal birth; history of venous thrombosis, pulmonary embolism, or varicosities; obesity; maternal age over 35; multiparity; and smoking (Pettker and Lockwood, 2012).

Clinical Manifestations

Superficial venous thrombosis is the most common form of postpartum thrombophlebitis. It is characterized by pain and tenderness in the lower extremity. Physical examination may reveal warmth; redness; and an enlarged, hardened vein over the site of the thrombosis. Deep vein thrombosis is more common during pregnancy than in the postpartum period and is characterized by unilateral leg pain, calf tenderness, and swelling. Physical examination may reveal redness and warmth, but women can have a large clot with few symptoms. A positive Homans' sign may be present, but further evaluation is needed because the calf pain can be attributed to other causes such as a strained muscle resulting from the birthing position.

Acute pulmonary embolism is usually results from dislodged deep vein thrombi. Presenting symptoms are dyspnea and tachypnea (more than 20 breaths/min). Other signs and symptoms frequently seen include tachycardia (more than 100 beats/min), apprehension, pleuritic chest pain, cough, hemoptysis, elevated temperature, and syncope (Cunningham, Leveno, Bloom, et al., 2010; Pettker and Lockwood, 2012).

Physical examination is not a sensitive diagnostic indicator for thrombosis. Venous ultrasonography with or without color Doppler is the most commonly used diagnostic test. Magnetic resonance imaging and D-dimer assays may also be used (Pettker and Lockwood, 2012). With PE, echocardiographic abnormalities may be seen in right ventricular size or function. Pregnancy limits the usefulness of arterial blood gases and oxygen saturation in diagnosis. A ventilation-perfusion scan, spiral computed tomography scan, magnetic resonance angiography, and pulmonary arteriogram may be used for diagnosis (Pettker and Lockwood, 2012).

Medical Management

Superficial venous thrombosis is treated with analgesia (nonsteroidal antiinflammatory agents), rest with elevation of the affected leg, and elastic compression stockings (Cunningham, Leveno, Bloom, et al., 2010). Heat may also be applied locally. Deep venous thrombosis is initially treated with anticoagulant therapy (usually continuous IV heparin), bedrest with the affected leg elevated, and analgesia. After the symptoms have decreased, the woman may be fitted with elastic compression stockings to wear when she is allowed to ambulate. She is taught how to put on the stockings before getting out of bed. IV heparin therapy continues for 3 to 5 days or until symptoms resolve. Oral anticoagulant therapy (warfarin [Coumadin]) is started during this time and will be continued for about 3 months. It is safe to use during lactation (see Medication Guide).

Acute pulmonary embolus is an emergent situation that requires prompt treatment. Massive pulmonary emboli can lead to pulmonary hypertension and right ventricular dysfunction; mortality is increased to 25% in these cases (Cunningham, Leveno, Bloom, et al., 2010). Immediate treatment of pulmonary embolism is anticoagulant therapy. Continuous IV heparin therapy is used for pulmonary embolism until symptoms have resolved. Intermittent subcutaneous

⬥ MEDICATION GUIDE

Warfarin Sodium (Coumadin)

Action
Blocks synthesis of clotting factors

Indications
For anticoagulation to prevent or treat blood clots

Dosage
Oral dosing depends on blood tests

Adverse Reactions
Excessive bleeding, hemorrhage, rash, gastrointestinal upset

Nursing Considerations
It is contraindicated in pregnancy (can cause fetal death or birth defects). It is usually compatible with breastfeeding (APA, 2000). Blood levels of mother should be monitored. Inform woman to avoid alcohol, avoid cranberry products and large amounts of leafy green vegetables, and watch for bruising because it can be a sign of bleeding. Avoid aspirin and nonsteroidal agents such as naproxen or ibuprofen. Coumadin may be taken with food or on empty stomach. Dose compliance is very important!

! NURSING ALERT

Medications containing aspirin are not given to women on anticoagulant therapy because aspirin inhibits synthesis of clotting factors and can lead to prolonged clotting time and increased risk for bleeding.

The woman is usually discharged home on oral anticoagulants and will need an explanation of the treatment schedule and possible side effects. If subcutaneous injections are to be given, the woman and family are taught how to administer the medication and about site rotation. They should also be given information about safe care practices to prevent bleeding and injury while she is on anticoagulant therapy (e.g., using a soft toothbrush and an electric razor). She will need information about follow-up with her health care provider to monitor clotting times and make sure that the correct dosage of anticoagulant therapy is maintained. The woman should also use a reliable form of contraception if taking warfarin because this medication is considered teratogenic (Gilbert, 2011). Oral contraceptives are contraindicated because of the increased risk for thrombosis (Cunningham, Leveno, Bloom, et al., 2010).

POSTPARTUM INFECTIONS

Postpartum infection, or *puerperal infection,* is any clinical infection of the genital tract that occurs within 28 days after miscarriage, induced abortion, or birth. The definition used in the United States continues to be the presence of a fever of 38° C (100.4° F) or more on 2 successive days of the first 10 postpartum days (not counting the first 24 hours after birth) (Katz, 2012). In the United States it occurs after approximately 2% of vaginal births and 10% to 15% of cesarean births (Katz, 2012). Other common postpartum infections include wound infections, urinary tract infections (UTIs), and respiratory tract infections. Mastitis, or breast infection, is common among breastfeeding women (see Chapter 24).

The most common infecting organisms are the numerous streptococcal and anaerobic organisms. *Staphylococcus aureus,* gonococci, coliform bacteria, and clostridia are less common but serious pathogenic organisms that can cause puerperal infection. Postpartum infections are more common in women who have concurrent medical or immunosuppressive conditions or who had a cesarean or other operative birth. Intrapartal factors such as prolonged rupture of membranes, prolonged labor, and internal maternal or fetal monitoring increase the risk for infection (Cunningham, Leveno, Bloom, et al., 2010). Factors that predispose the woman to postpartum infection are listed in Box 21-3.

Endometritis

Endometritis (infection of the lining of the uterus) is the most common postpartum infection. It usually begins as a localized infection at the placental site (Fig. 21-2) but can spread to the entire endometrium. Incidence is higher after cesarean birth. Signs of endometritis include fever (usually greater than 38° C [100.4° F]); increased pulse; chills; anorexia; nausea; fatigue and lethargy; pelvic pain; uterine tenderness; and foul-smelling, profuse lochia. Leukocytosis and a markedly increased RBC sedimentation rate are typical laboratory findings of postpartum infections. Anemia can also be present. Blood cultures or intracervical or intrauterine bacterial cultures (aerobic and anaerobic) should reveal the offending pathogens within 36 to 48 hours (Cunningham, Leveno, Bloom, et al., 2010).

Management of endometritis consists of IV broad-spectrum antibiotic therapy (cephalosporins, penicillins, or clindamycin and gentamicin) and supportive care, including hydration, rest, and pain

heparin or oral anticoagulant therapy is often continued for up to 6 months (Pettker and Lockwood, 2012).

Nursing Interventions

In the hospital, nursing care of the woman with a thrombosis consists of ongoing assessments: inspecting and palpating the affected area; palpating the peripheral pulses; checking Homans' sign; measuring and comparing leg circumferences; inspecting for signs of bleeding; monitoring for signs of pulmonary embolism, including chest pain, coughing, dyspnea, and tachypnea; and checking respiratory status for presence of crackles. Laboratory reports are monitored for prothrombin or partial thromboplastin times. The woman and her family are assessed for their level of understanding about the diagnosis and their ability to cope during the unexpected extended period of recovery.

Interventions include explanations and education about the diagnosis and the treatment. The woman will need assistance with personal care as long as she is on bed rest; the family should be encouraged to participate in the care if that is what she and they wish. While the woman is on bed rest, she should be encouraged to change positions frequently but to avoid placing her knees in a sharply flexed position that could cause pooling of blood in the lower extremities. She also should be cautioned to avoid rubbing the affected area because this action could cause the clot to dislodge. Heparin and warfarin are administered as ordered, and the physician is notified if clotting times are outside the therapeutic level. If the woman is breastfeeding, she is assured that neither heparin nor warfarin is excreted in significant quantities in breast milk. If the infant has been discharged, the family is encouraged to bring the infant for feedings as permitted by hospital policy; the mother also can express milk to be sent home.

Pain can be managed with a variety of measures. Changing positions, elevating the leg, and applying moist heat may decrease discomfort. It may be necessary to administer analgesics and anti-inflammatory medications.

BOX 21-3   PREDISPOSING FACTORS FOR POSTPARTUM INFECTION

Preconception or Antepartal Factors

- History of previous venous thrombosis, urinary tract infection, mastitis, pneumonia
- Diabetes mellitus
- Alcoholism
- Drug abuse
- Immunosuppression
- Anemia
- Malnutrition

Intrapartal Factors

- Cesarean birth
- Prolonged rupture of membranes
- Chorioamnionitis
- Prolonged labor
- Bladder catheterization
- Internal fetal/uterine pressure monitoring
- Multiple vaginal examinations after rupture of membranes
- Epidural anesthesia
- Retained placental fragments
- Postpartum hemorrhage
- Episiotomy or lacerations
- Hematomas

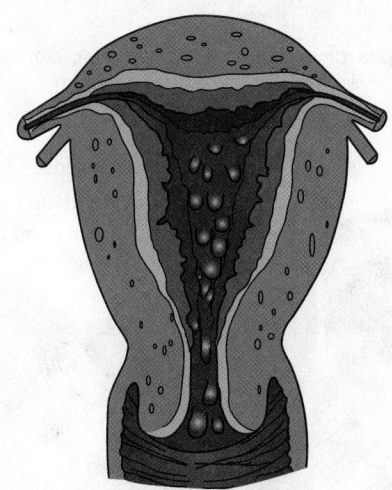

FIG 21-2 Postpartum infection—endometritis.

relief. Antibiotic therapy is usually discontinued 24 hours after the woman is asymptomatic. Assessments of lochia, vital signs, and changes in the woman's condition continue during treatment. Comfort measures depend on the symptoms and may include cool compresses, warm blankets, perineal care, and sitz baths. Teaching should include side effects of therapy, prevention of spread of infection, signs and symptoms of worsening condition, adherence to the treatment plan, and the need for follow-up care. Women may need to be encouraged or assisted to maintain mother-infant interactions and breastfeeding (if allowed during treatment).

Wound Infections

Wound infections are common postpartum infections that often develop after the woman is at home. Sites of infection include the cesarean incision and repaired laceration or episiotomy site. Predisposing factors are similar to those for endometritis (see Box 21-3). Signs of wound infection include fever, erythema, edema, warmth, tenderness, pain, seropurulent drainage, and wound separation.

Treatment of wound infections may combine antibiotic therapy with wound debridement. Wounds can be opened and drained. Nursing care includes frequent assessments of the wound and vital signs and wound care. Comfort measures include sitz baths, warm compresses, and perineal care. Teaching includes good hygiene techniques (e.g., changing perineal pads front to back, hand hygiene before and after perineal care), self-care measures, and signs of worsening conditions to report to the primary health care provider. The woman is usually discharged to home for self-care or home nursing care after treatment is initiated in the inpatient setting.

Urinary Tract Infections

UTIs occur in 2% to 4% of postpartum women. Risk factors include urinary catheterization, frequent pelvic examinations, epidural anesthesia, genital tract injury, history of UTI, and cesarean birth. Signs and symptoms include dysuria, frequency and urgency, low-grade fever, urinary retention, hematuria, and pyuria. Costovertebral angle tenderness or flank pain can indicate upper UTI. The most common infecting organism is *Escherichia coli,* although other gram-negative aerobic bacilli can cause UTIs.

Medical management for UTIs consists of antibiotic therapy, analgesia, and hydration. Postpartum women are usually treated on an outpatient basis; therefore teaching should include instructions on how to monitor temperature, bladder function, and appearance of urine. The woman should also be taught about signs of potential complications and the importance of taking all antibiotics as prescribed. Other suggestions for prevention of UTIs include proper perineal care, wiping from front to back after urinating or having a bowel movement, and increasing fluid intake.

Nursing Interventions

Women with factors that predispose them to postpartum infection (see Box 21-3) should be assessed carefully. Signs and symptoms associated with postpartum infection were discussed with each infection. Elevation of temperature, redness, and swelling are common signs. The woman may also complain of chills, fever, localized tenderness, or pain. Depending on the type of infection, laboratory tests usually performed include a complete blood count, venous blood cultures, urine cultures, and uterine tissue cultures. Review of the woman's history and the laboratory results should be included in the assessment.

The most effective and least expensive treatment of postpartum infection is prevention. Preventive measures include good prenatal nutrition to control anemia and intrapartal hemorrhage. Good maternal perineal hygiene with thorough hand hygiene is emphasized. Strict adherence to aseptic techniques by all health care personnel caring for women during labor, birth, and the postpartum period is very important.

Postpartum women are usually discharged to home by 48 hours after birth. This is often before signs of infection are evident. Nurses in birth centers and hospital settings must be able to identify women at risk for postpartum infection and provide anticipatory teaching and counseling before discharge (see Community Focus box). After discharge, telephone follow-up, hot lines, support groups, lactation counselors, home visits by nurses, and teaching materials (videos, written materials) are all interventions that can be implemented to decrease the risk for postpartum infections. Home care nurses must be able to recognize the signs and symptoms of postpartum infection and then contact the woman's primary health care provider or have the woman make the contact. These nurses must also be able to provide the appropriate nursing care for women who need follow-up home care.

STRUCTURAL DISORDERS OF THE VAGINA AND UTERUS RELATED TO CHILDBEARING

Women are at risk for problems related to the reproductive system from the age of menarche through menopause and the older years. These problems, which include structural disorders of the uterus and vagina related to pelvic relaxation and urinary incontinence (UI), are often the delayed but direct result of childbearing.

With fetopelvic disproportion, prolonged labor, or a precipitous birth, structures of the vesical and vaginal walls are stretched and can be injured. The bladder neck and urethra can be compressed between the presenting part and the pubic bones or forced downward ahead of the presenting part. Since soft-tissue damage usually occurs behind an intact vaginal epithelium, there is nothing visible to repair. However, defects can also occur in women who have never been pregnant.

Structural disorders can have far-reaching effects for the woman and her family. Beyond the obvious physiologic alterations, the woman also experiences threats to her self-concept and her ability to cope. A woman's concept of herself as a sexual being can be affected by the condition and its treatments. Her partner and family are also challenged in the way they respond to her diagnosis.

Uterine Displacement and Prolapse

Normally, the round ligaments hold the uterus in anteversion and the uterosacral ligaments pull the cervix backward and upward. Uterine displacement is a variation of this normal placement (Fig. 21-3). The most common type of displacement is posterior displacement, or retroversion, in which the uterus is tilted posteriorly and the cervix rotates anteriorly. Other variations include retroflexion and anteflexion.

By 2 months postpartum, the ligaments should return to normal length but in about one third of women, the uterus remains retroverted. This condition is rarely symptomatic, but conception can be difficult because the cervix points toward the anterior vaginal wall and away from the posterior fornix, where seminal fluid pools after coitus. If symptoms occur, they can include pelvic and low back pain, dyspareunia, and exaggeration of premenstrual symptoms.

Uterine prolapse is a more serious type of displacement. Degrees of prolapse can vary from mild to complete. In complete prolapse, the cervix and body of the uterus protrude through the vagina and the vagina is inverted (Fig. 21-4).

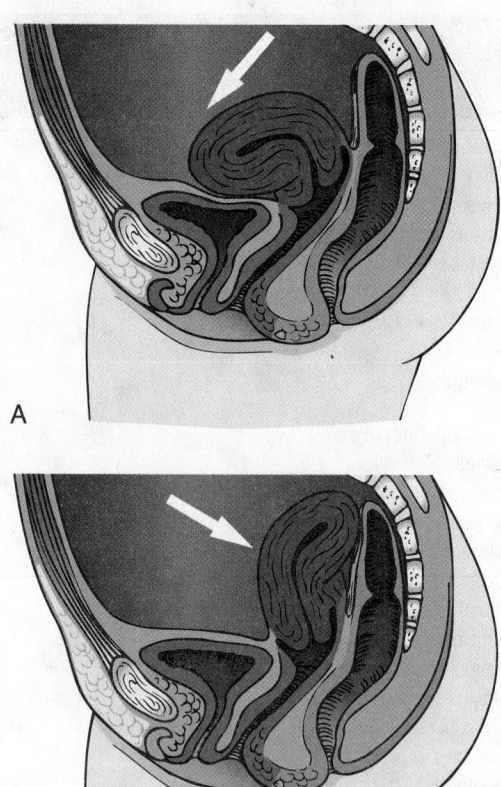

FIG 21-3 Types of uterine displacement. **A,** Anterior displacement. **B,** Retroversion (posterior displacement).

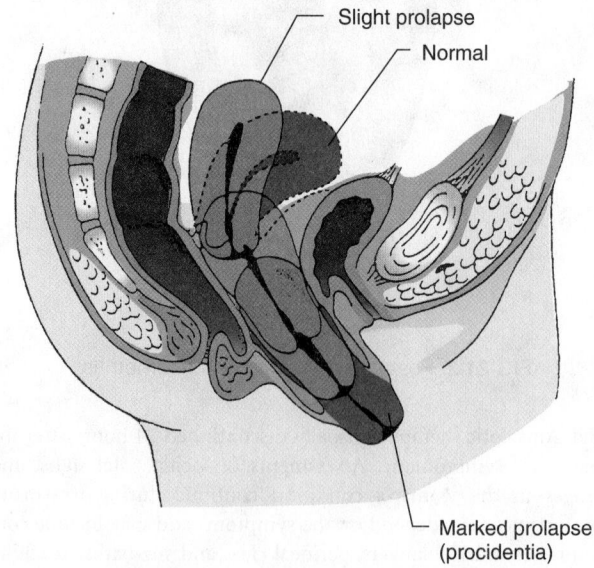

FIG 21-4 Prolapse of uterus.

Uterine displacement and prolapse can be caused by congenital or acquired weakness of the pelvic support structures (often referred to as **pelvic relaxation**). In many cases, problems can be a delayed but direct result of childbearing. Although extensive damage can be noted and repaired shortly after birth, symptoms related to pelvic relaxation most often appear during the perimenopausal period,

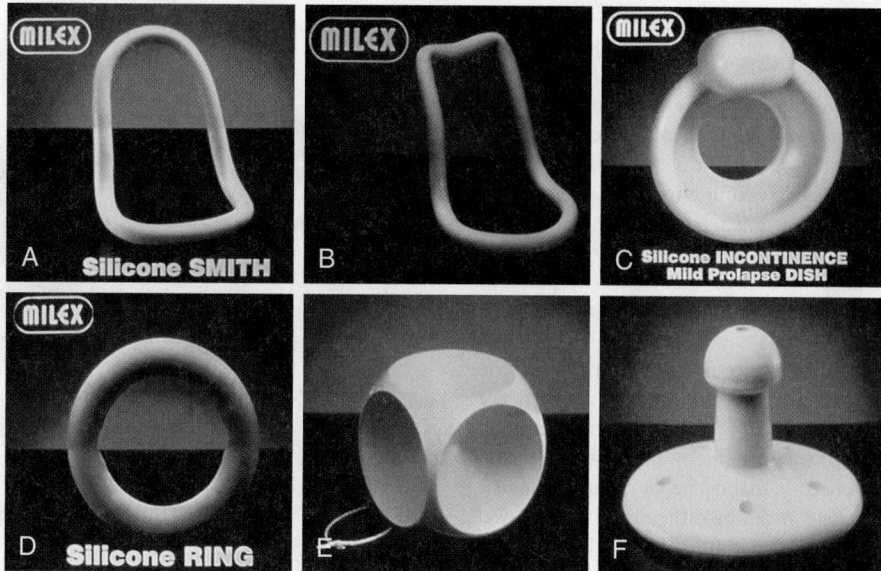

FIG 21-5 Examples of pessaries. **A,** Smith. **B,** Hodge without support. **C,** Incontinence dish with support. **D,** Ring without support. **E,** Cube. **F,** Gellhorn. (Courtesy Milex Products, Inc., a division of CooperSurgical, Trumbull, CT.)

when the effects of ovarian hormones on pelvic tissues are lost and atrophic changes begin. Pelvic trauma, stress and strain, and the aging process are contributing causes. Other causes of pelvic relaxation include reproductive surgery and pelvic radiation.

In general, symptoms of pelvic relaxation relate to the structure involved: urethra, bladder, uterus, vagina, cul-de-sac, or rectum. The most common complaints are pulling and dragging sensations, pressure, protrusions, fatigue, and low backache. Symptoms may be worse after prolonged standing or deep penile penetration during intercourse. Urinary incontinence can be present.

Medical Management

If discomfort related to uterine displacement is a problem, several interventions can be implemented to treat uterine displacement. Kegel exercises can be performed several times a day to increase muscular strength. A knee-chest position performed for a few minutes several times a day can correct a mildly retroverted uterus. A fitted *pessary* to support the uterus and hold it in the correct position may be inserted in the vagina (Fig. 21-5). Usually a pessary is used for only a short time because it can lead to pressure necrosis and vaginitis. Good hygiene is important; some women are taught to remove the pessary at night, cleanse it, and replace it in the morning. If the pessary is always left in place, regular douching with commercially prepared solutions or weak vinegar solutions (e.g., 1 tbsp to 1 qt of water) to remove increased secretions and keep the vaginal pH at 4.0 to 4.5 is suggested. After a period of treatment, most women are free of symptoms and do not require the pessary. Surgical correction is rarely indicated.

Treatment for uterine prolapse depends on the degree of prolapse. Pessaries can be useful in mild prolapse. Estrogen therapy may be used in the older woman to improve tissue tone. If these conservative treatments do not correct the problem or the degree of prolapse is significant, abdominal or vaginal hysterectomy is usually recommended.

Cystocele and Rectocele

Cystocele and rectocele often occur with uterine prolapse (although they can occur independently), causing the uterus to sag even

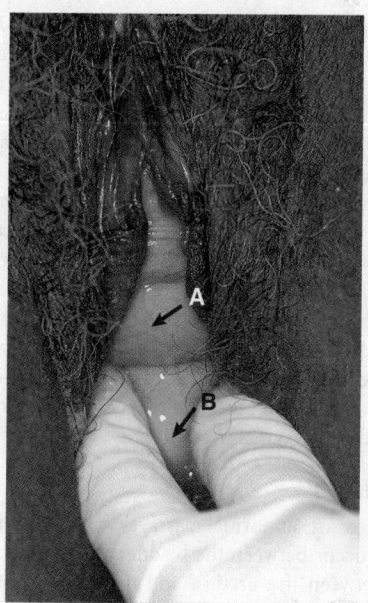

FIG 21-6 A, Cystocele. **B,** Rectocele. (From Lemmi FO, Lemmi Carlos AE: *Physical assessment findings* [multi-user CD-ROM], Philadelphia, 2000, Saunders.)

further backward and downward into the vagina. Cystocele (Fig. 21-6, *A*) is the protrusion of the bladder downward into the vagina that develops when supporting structures in the vesicovaginal septum are injured. Anterior wall relaxation develops gradually over time as a result of congenital defects of support structures, childbearing, obesity, or advanced age. When the woman stands, the weakened anterior vaginal wall cannot support the weight of the urine in the bladder; the vesicovaginal septum is forced downward, the bladder is stretched, and its capacity is increased. With time, the cystocele enlarges until it protrudes into the vagina. Complete emptying of the bladder is difficult because the cystocele sags below the bladder neck. Rectocele is the herniation of the anterior rectal wall through the relaxed or ruptured vaginal fascia and rectovaginal septum; it appears as a large bulge that may be seen through the relaxed introitus (see Fig. 21-6, *B*).

Cystoceles and rectoceles often are asymptomatic. If symptoms of cystocele are present, they can include complaints of a bearing-down sensation or that "something is in my vagina." Other symptoms include urinary frequency, retention, incontinence, and possible recurrent UTIs. On pelvic examination, the anterior wall of the vagina bulges when the woman is asked to bear down. Unless the bladder neck and urethra are damaged, urinary continence is unaffected. Women with large cystoceles complain of having to push upward on the sagging anterior vaginal wall to be able to void.

Rectoceles can be small and produce few symptoms, but some are so large that they protrude outside of the vagina when the woman stands. Symptoms are absent when the woman is lying down. A rectocele causes a disturbance in bowel function, a sensation of bearing down, or a sensation that the pelvic organs are falling out. With a very large rectocele, it can be difficult to have a bowel movement. Each time the woman strains during bowel evacuation, the feces are forced against the thinned rectovaginal wall, stretching it even more. Some women facilitate evacuation by applying digital pressure vaginally to hold up the rectal pouch.

Medical Management

Treatment for a cystocele includes use of a vaginal pessary or surgical repair. Pessaries may not be effective. An anterior repair (colporrhaphy) is the usual surgical procedure and is usually done for large symptomatic cystoceles. This involves a surgical shortening of pelvic muscles to provide better support for the bladder. An anterior repair is often combined with a vaginal hysterectomy.

Small rectoceles may not need treatment. The woman with mild symptoms may get relief from a high-fiber diet and adequate fluid intake, stool softeners, or mild laxatives. Vaginal pessaries usually are not effective. Large rectoceles that are causing significant symptoms are usually repaired surgically. A posterior repair (colporrhaphy) is the usual procedure. This surgery is performed vaginally and involves shortening the pelvic muscles to provide better support for the rectum. Anterior and posterior repairs can be performed at the same time and with vaginal hysterectomy.

Genital Fistulas

Genital fistulas are abnormal passageways between genital tract organs. Most occur between the bladder and the vagina (e.g., vesicovaginal), between the urethra and the vagina (urethrovaginal), and between the rectum or sigmoid colon and the vagina (rectovaginal) (Fig. 21-7). Genital fistulas can be a result of a congenital anomaly, gynecologic surgery, obstetric trauma, cancer, radiation therapy, gynecologic trauma, or infection (e.g., of the episiotomy site).

Signs and symptoms of vaginal fistulas depend on the site but can include the presence of urine, flatus, or feces in the vagina; odors of urine or feces in the vagina; and irritation of vaginal tissues.

Medical Management.

Management of genital fistulas depends on the location. Surgical repair is the usual treatment; however, it may not be successful.

Nursing Interventions

Nursing care of the woman with a cystocele, rectocele, or fistula requires great sensitivity because the woman's reactions are often intense. She can become withdrawn or hostile because of embarrassment about odors and soiling of her clothing that are beyond

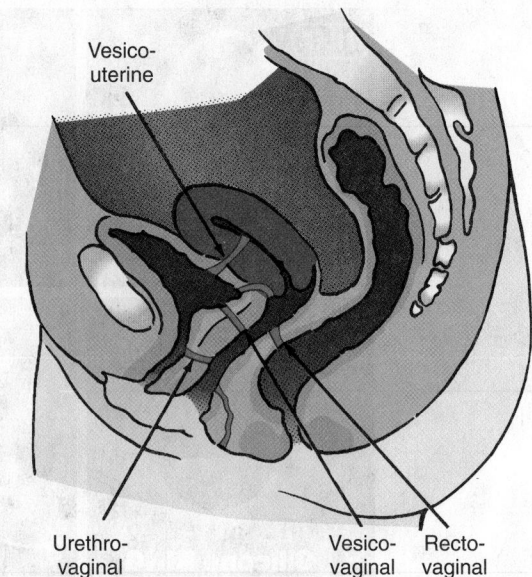

FIG 21-7 Examples of genitourinary fistulas: vesicovaginal (bladder to vagina), vesicouterine (bladder to uterus), urethrovaginal (urethra to vagina), rectovaginal (rectum to vagina). Fistulas range in size from tiny and difficult to locate to large, disfiguring the base of the bladder. (Adapted from Monahan FD, Sands J, Neighbors M, et al: *Phipps' medical-surgical nursing: health and illness perspectives,* ed 8, St Louis, 2007, Mosby.)

her control. Her sexuality is threatened; her partner may refuse sexual intimacy.

The nurse can tactfully suggest hygiene practices that reduce odor. Commercial deodorizing douches are available, or noncommercial solutions such as diluted chlorine (e.g., 1 tsp of chlorine household bleach to 1 qt of water) may be used. The chlorine solution is also useful for external perineal irrigation. Sitz baths and thorough washing of the genitalia with unscented, mild soap and warm water are helpful measures. Sparse dusting with deodorizing powders can be useful.

If a rectovaginal fistula is present, enemas given before leaving the house may provide temporary relief from oozing of fecal material until corrective surgery is performed. Irritated skin and tissues may benefit from use of a heat lamp or application of an emollient. Hygienic care is time consuming and may need to be repeated frequently throughout the day; protective pads or pants may need to be worn. All of these activities can be demoralizing to the woman and frustrating to her and her family.

Urinary Incontinence

Urinary incontinence (UI) affects young and middle-age women, with the prevalence increasing as the woman ages. The main symptom is involuntary leaking of urine, especially during coughing, laughing, or exercising. Research suggests that a significant number of women have undiagnosed urinary incontinence (Wallner, Porten, Meenan, et al., 2009).

Although nulliparous women can have UI, the incidence is higher in women who have given birth and increases with parity. Women who are overweight and those who have had a hysterectomy are also at increased risk (Sung and Hampton, 2009). Conditions that disturb urinary control include:

- Stress incontinence, caused by sudden increases in intraabdominal pressure (e.g., caused by sneezing or coughing)

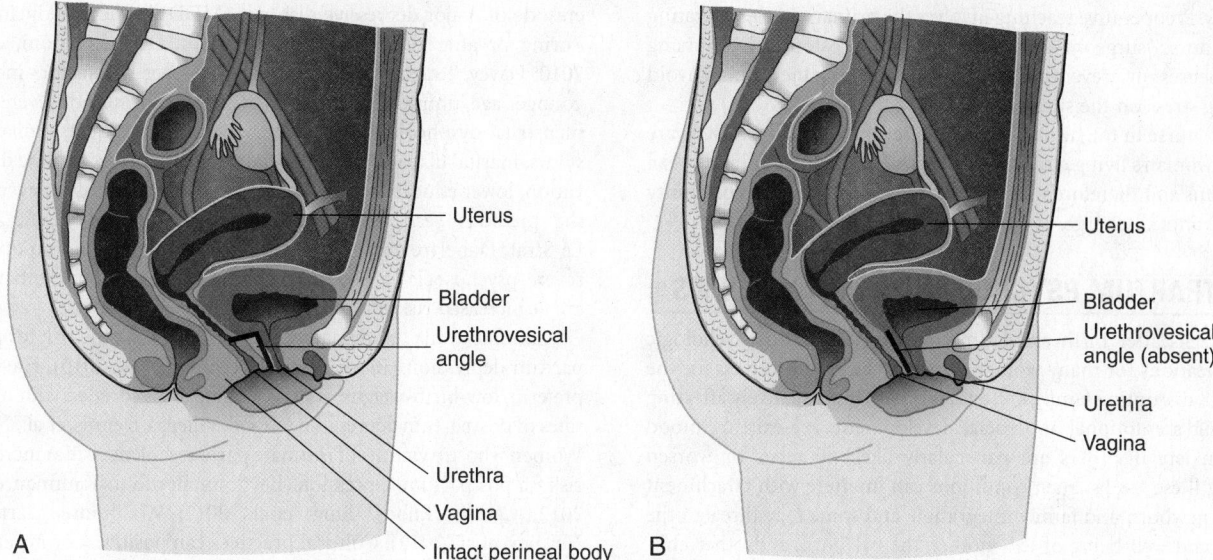

FIG 21-8 Urethrovesical angle. **A,** Normal angle. **B,** Widening (absence) of angle.

- Urge incontinence, caused by disorders of the bladder and urethra (e.g., urethritis, urethral stricture, trigonitis, and cystitis)
- Neuropathies (e.g., multiple sclerosis, diabetic neuritis, and pathologic conditions of the spinal cord)
- Congenital and acquired urinary tract abnormalities

Stress UI can follow injury to bladder neck structures. A sphincter mechanism at the bladder neck compresses the upper urethra, pulls it upward behind the symphysis, and forms an acute angle at the junction of the posterior urethral wall and the base of the bladder (Fig. 21-8). To empty the bladder, the sphincter complex relaxes and the trigone contracts to open the internal urethral orifice and pull the contracting bladder wall upward, forcing urine out. The angle between the urethra and the base of the bladder is lost or increased if the supporting pubococcygeus muscle is injured; this change, coupled with a urethrocele, causes incontinence. Urine spurts out when the woman is asked to bear down or cough while she is in the lithotomy position.

Medical Management

Mild to moderate UI can be significantly decreased or relieved in many women by bladder training and pelvic muscle (Kegel) exercises (Dumoulin and Hay-Smith, 2010). Other management strategies include pelvic flow support devices (i.e., pessaries), vaginal estrogen therapy, serotonin-norepinephrine reuptake inhibitors, electrical stimulation, insertion of an artificial urethral sphincter, and surgery (e.g., anterior repair) (Tarnay and Bhatia, 2010).

CARE MANAGEMENT

Assessment for problems related to structural disorders of the uterus and vagina focuses primarily on the genitourinary tract, the reproductive organs, bowel elimination, and psychosocial and sexual factors. A complete health history, a physical examination, and laboratory tests are done to support the appropriate medical diagnosis. The nurse must assess the woman's knowledge of the disorder, its management, and possible prognosis. Assessment for depression that can result from decreased quality of life and functional status is also important.

Possible nursing diagnoses for structural problems of the uterus and vagina include:
- Deficient Knowledge related to:
  Causes of structural disorders and treatment options
- Constipation or Diarrhea related to:
  Anatomic changes
- Acute Pain related to:
  Relaxation of pelvic support or elimination difficulties
- Ineffective Coping related to:
  Changes in body image
- Interrupted Family Processes related to:
  The woman's anatomic and functional changes
- Risk for Injury related to:
  Lack of skill in self-care procedures
  Lack of understanding of the reasons for the need to comply with therapy
- Social Isolation, Spiritual Distress, Disturbed Body Image, or Chronic Low Self-Esteem related to:
  Changes in anatomy and function
- Anxiety related to:
  Surgical procedure
  Prognosis

In general, nurses working with women with structural disorders can provide information and self-care education to prevent problems before they occur, manage or reduce symptoms and promote comfort and hygiene if symptoms are already present, and recognize when further intervention is needed. For example, women may need guidance about changes in lifestyle (e.g., losing weight) and education about pelvic muscle exercises (Sung, West, Hernandez, et al., 2009). This information can be part of all postpartum discharge teaching or provided at postpartum follow-up visits in clinics or physician or nurse-midwife offices, during postpartum home visits, or during gynecologic health examinations. Information on how to prevent or recognize problems can be a topic for workshops for women or health fairs in community settings.

Interventions for specific problems depend on the problem and the severity of the symptoms as discussed previously.

Many of the nurse's efforts with these problems are directed toward participating in a team effort to prepare the woman for surgery. Preoperative teaching involves the primary nurse, operating room nurse, surgeon, and anesthesiologist. Postoperative nursing care focuses on preventing infection and helping the woman avoid putting stress on the surgical site.

The nurse in the health-promotion setting is usually most aware of the woman's living circumstances, physical limitations, and social problems and therefore may be best suited to coordinate continuity of care after discharge.

POSTPARTUM PSYCHOLOGIC COMPLICATIONS

The weeks after birth are a time of vulnerability to psychologic complications for many women, causing significant distress for the mother, disrupting family life, and, if prolonged, negatively affecting the child's emotional and social development. Pre-existing mood and anxiety disorders are particularly likely to recur or worsen during these weeks. Such conditions can interfere with attachment to the newborn and family integration, and some may threaten the safety and well-being of the mother, the newborn, and other children. Because birth is usually thought to be a happy event, a new mother's emotional distress can puzzle and immobilize family and friends. When she most needs the caring attention of loved ones, they may either criticize or withdraw because of their anxiety. Nurses can offer anticipatory guidance, assess the mental health of new mothers, offer therapeutic interventions, and make referrals when necessary. Failure to do so can result in tragic consequences. In the rarest of cases, a disturbed mother may kill her infant, other family members, or herself.

Mood disorders are the predominant mental health disorder in the postpartum period (American Psychiatric Association [APA], 2000). Up to 80% of women experience a mild depression or "baby blues" after the birth of a child; however, functioning of the woman is usually not impaired. Baby blues are characterized by mood swings, feelings of sadness and/or anxiety, crying, difficulty sleeping, and loss of appetite. The symptoms resolve within a few days, and treatment is not needed (U.S. Department of Health and Human Services Office of Women's Health, 2009).

Postpartum Depression

Serious depression, experienced by 10% to 15% of postpartum women, can eventually incapacitate them to the point of being unable to care for themselves or their babies (Sadock, Sadock, and Ruiz, 2009). Postpartum depression affects women from all cultures, although the manifestations vary. The incidence of postpartum depression in some cultures is under-reported because of the stigma and hesitancy to seek professional help (Callister, Beckstrand, and Corbett, 2011; Goyal, Wang, Shen, et al., 2012).

The *Diagnostic and Statistical Manual of Mental Disorders (DSM-IV)* contains the official guidelines for the assessment and diagnosis of psychiatric illness (APA, 2000). However, specific criteria for *postpartum depression (PPD)* are not listed. Instead, postpartum onset can be specified for any mood disorder either without psychotic features (i.e., PPD) or with psychotic features (i.e., postpartum psychosis) if the onset occurs within 4 weeks of childbirth (APA, 2000). Clinicians and researchers often identify the postpartum period as up to 1 year after birth (O'Hara and McCabe, 2013).

The cause of PPD can be biologic, psychologic, situational, or multifactorial. Estrogen fluctuations and postpartum hypogonadism (the change from the high levels of estrogen and progesterone at the end of pregnancy to the much lower levels of both hormones that are present after birth) are important etiologic factors. Women at greatest risk for postpartum depression are those with a history of anxiety or depression and especially those who had a previous episode of major depressive disorder (MDD) in the past, including during or after pregnancy (Cunningham, Leveno, Bloom, et al., 2010; Davey, Tough, Adair, et al., 2011). Other risk factors include younger age, unintended pregnancy, personal history of severe premenstrual dysphoria, family history of mood disorder, unmarried status, marital discord, lack of social support, socioeconomic deprivation, lower education, substance abuse, and stressful life events in the previous year (Cunningham, Leveno, Bloom, et al., 2010; Le Strat, Dubertret, and Le Foll, 2011). Women facing multiple or severe psychosocial problems or chronic interpersonal difficulties are at increased risk for a major depressive episode.

Complications of pregnancy and birth increase the risk for postpartum depression (Blom, Jansen, Verhulst, et al., 2010). Having a preterm, low-birth-weight, and ill neonate are associated with higher rates of postpartum depression (Vigod, Villegas, Dennis, et al., 2010). Women who are victims of intimate partner violence are at increased risk for postpartum depression (Beydoun, Beydoun, Kaufman, et al., 2012; Cerulli, Talbor, Tang, et al., 2011; Woolhouse, Gartland, Hegarty, et al., 2012). Cultural practices can positively or negatively affect the development of PPD. Women facing multiple or severe psychosocial problems or chronic interpersonal difficulties are at increased risk for experiencing a major depressive episode. Common risk factors for postpartum depression are listed in Box 21-4.

Paternal Postpartum Depression

Often, women are not alone in their experience of postpartum depression; new fathers may have postpartum depression as well. The incidence is unclear, with reports varying from 10% to more than 50% (Paulson and Bazemore, 2010; Letourneau, Tryphonopoulos, Duffett-Leger, et al., 2012). The best predictor of paternal depression is having a partner with postpartum depression. Men may not exhibit classic symptoms of PPD but are likely to display fatigue, frustration, anger, irritability, indecisiveness, and withdrawal from social situations (Paulson and Bazemore, 2010).

Postpartum Depression Without Psychotic Features

PPD is an intense and pervasive sadness with severe and labile mood swings; it is more serious and persistent than postpartum blues. Intense fears, anger, anxiety, and despondency that persist past the baby's first few weeks are not a normal part of postpartum blues. These symptoms rarely disappear without outside help (Sadock, Sadock, and Ruiz, 2009). Most of these mothers seek help only after reaching a "crisis point."

The symptoms of postpartum major depression do not differ from those of nonpostpartum mood disorders except that the mother's ruminations of guilt and inadequacy feed her worries about being an incompetent and inadequate parent. In PPD, there can be loss of appetite or odd food cravings (often sweet desserts) and binges with abnormal appetite and weight gain. New mothers report an increased yearning for sleep, sleeping heavily but awakening instantly with any infant noise, and an inability to go back to sleep after infant feedings. Determining difficulty falling asleep is a relevant screening question to ascertain risk for PPD.

A distinguishing feature of PPD is irritability. These episodes of irritability can flare up with little provocation, and they sometimes escalate to violent outbursts or dissolve into uncontrollable sobbing. Many of these outbursts are directed against significant others (e.g., "He never helps me.") or the baby (e.g., "She cries all the time, and I feel like hitting her."). Women with postpartum major depressive episodes often have severe anxiety, panic attacks, and spontaneous crying long after the usual duration of baby blues.

Many women feel especially guilty about having depressive feelings at a time when they believe they should be happy. They can be

BOX 21-4 RISK FACTORS FOR POSTPARTUM DEPRESSION

- Prenatal anxiety or depression
- History of major depressive episode
- History of postpartum depression
- Life stress
- Lack of social support
- Unmarried
- Marital relationship problems
- Intimate partner violence
- Complicated pregnancy or birth
- Preterm or ill infant
- Postpartum blues
- Low socioeconomic status
- Unintended pregnancy

Data from Beck C: Revision of the postpartum depression predictors inventory, *J Obstet Gynecol Neonatal Nurs* 31(4):394-402, 2002; and Beck C: Predictors of postpartum depression: an update. *Nurs Res* 50(5): 275–282, 2001.

reluctant to discuss their symptoms or their negative feelings toward the infant. A prominent feature of PPD is rejection of the infant, often caused by abnormal jealousy. The mother can be obsessed by the notion that the baby will take her place in her partner's affections. Attitudes toward the infant can include disinterest, annoyance with care demands, and blaming because of her lack of maternal feeling. When observed, she can appear awkward in her responses to the baby. Obsessive thoughts about harming the infant are very frightening to her. Often she does not share these thoughts because of embarrassment; when she does, other family members become very frightened.

Medical Management. The natural course is one of gradual improvement over the 6 months after birth. However, supportive treatment alone is not efficacious for major PPD. Pharmacologic intervention is needed in most instances. Treatment options include antidepressants, antianxiety agents, mood stabilizers, and electroconvulsive therapy (ECT) (Cunningham, Leveno, Bloom, et al., 2010) (Tables 21-1 and 21-2). Alternative therapies such as herbs, dietary supplements, massage, aromatherapy, and acupuncture may be helpful. Psychotherapy focuses on the woman's fears and concerns regarding her new responsibilities and roles and monitoring for suicidal or homicidal thoughts. Support groups and marital counseling can be helpful. For some women, hospitalization is necessary.

Postpartum Depression with Psychotic Features

The most severe of the perinatal mood disorders, **postpartum psychosis,** is rare, affecting approximately 0.1% to 0.2% of postpartum women (Sadock, Sadock, and Ruiz, 2009). Once a woman has had one episode of postpartum psychosis, she has a 30% to 50% likelihood of recurrence with each subsequent birth (APA, 2000). This disorder tends to show onset within 2 weeks postpartum; however, it can present later in the course of the illness as a depression (Sadock, Sadock, and Ruiz, 2009).

Episodes of postpartum psychosis are typified by auditory or visual hallucinations, paranoid or grandiose delusions, elements of delirium or disorientation, and extreme deficits in judgment accompanied by high levels of impulsivity that can contribute to increased risks of suicide or infanticide (in 5% of psychotic women) (Sadock, Sadock, and Ruiz, 2009). Characteristically, the woman begins to complain of fatigue, insomnia, and restlessness and can have episodes of tearfulness and emotional lability. Complaints regarding

TABLE 21-1 ANTIDEPRESSANT MEDICATIONS

	PREGNANCY RISK CATEGORY*	LACTATION RISK CATEGORY*
Selective Serotonin Reuptake Inhibitors (SSRIs)		
Citalopram (Celexa)	C	L3
Escitalopram (Lexapro)	C	L3 in older infants
Fluoxetine (Prozac)	C	L2 in older infants; L3 in neonates
Fluvoxamine (Luvox)	C	L2
Paroxetine (Paxil)	D	L2
Sertraline (Zoloft)	C	L2
Serotonin/Norepinephrine Reuptake Inhibitors (SNRIs)		
Bupropion (Wellbutrin) IR & SR	B	L3
Maprotiline (Ludiomil)	B	L3
Mirtazapine (Remeron)	C	L3
Trazodone (Desyrel)	C	L2
Venlafaxine (Effexor)	C	L3
Tricyclic Antidepressants (TCAs)		
Amitriptyline (Elavil)	D	L2
Amoxapine (Asendin)	C	L2
Clomipramine (Anafranil)	C	L2
Desipramine (Norpramin)	C	L2
Doxepin (Sinequan)	C	L5
Imipramine (Tofranil)	D	L2
Nortriptyline (Pamelor)	D	L2
Monoamine Oxidase Inhibitors (MAOIs)		
Phenelzine (Nardil)	C	Unknown
Tranylcypromine (Parnate)	C	Unknown

*Sources: Hale T: *Medications and mother's milk,* ed 15, Amarillo, TX, 2012, Pharmasoft; Schatzberg A, Cole JO, DeBattista C, editors: *Manual of clinical psychopharmacology,* ed 7, Arlington, VA, 2010, American Psychiatric Publishing.
B = Animal studies have not shown fetal risk, but no controlled studies in pregnant women *or* animal studies showed adverse effect that was not confirmed in controlled studies in women in first trimester—no risk in later trimesters.
C = Animal studies show adverse effects on fetus, but no controlled studies in pregnant women *or* no studies available.
D = Positive evidence of human fetal risk.
L2 = Drug studied in limited number of breastfeeding women without an increase in adverse effects in infant *or* risk is remote.
L3 = No controlled studies in breastfeeding women *or* studies show minimal nonthreatening adverse effects.
L5 = Contraindicated because studies have shown significant and documented risk to infant.
IR, Intermediate release; *SR,* sustained release.

TABLE 21-2	ANTIANXIETY MEDICATIONS	
ANTIANXIETY MEDICATIONS	**PREGNANCY RISK CATEGORY***	**LACTATION RISK CATEGORY***
Alprazolam (Xanax)	D	L3
Buspirone (BuSpar)	C	L3
Chlordiazepoxide (Librium)	D	L3
Clonazepam (Klonopin)	C	L3
Clorazepate (Tranxene)	D	L3
Diazepam (Valium)	D	L3; L4 if used chronically
Flurazepam (Dalmane)	X	L3
Lorazepam (Ativan)	D	L3
Midazolam (Versed)	D	L3
Temazepam (Restoril)	X	L3
Triazolam (Halcion)	X	L3

*Sources: Hale T: *Medications and mother's milk,* ed 15, Amarillo, TX, 2012, Pharmasoft; Schatzberg A, Cole JO, DeBattista C, editors: *Manual of clinical psychopharmacology,* ed 7, Arlington, VA, 2010, American Psychiatric Publishing.
C = Animal studies show adverse effects on fetus, but no controlled studies in pregnant women *or* no studies available.
D = Positive evidence of human fetal risk.
X = Contraindicated because studies have shown significant and documented risk to fetus.
L3 = No controlled studies in breastfeeding women *or* studies show minimal adverse effects.
L4 = Possibly hazardous.

TABLE 21-3	MOOD STABILIZERS	
MOOD STABILIZERS	**PREGNANCY RISK CATEGORY***	**LACTATION RISK CATEGORY***
Carbamazepine (Tegretol XR)	C	L2
Clonazepam (Klonopin)	C	L3
Gabapentin (Neurontin)	C	L3
Lamotrigine (Lamictal)	C	L3
Lithium carbonate (Eskalith)	C	L4
Topiramate (Topamax)	C	L3
Valproic acid (Depakene, Depakote, Depakote ER)	D	L2

*Sources: Hale T: *Medications and mother's milk,* ed 15, Amarillo, TX, 2012, Pharmasoft; Schatzberg A, Cole JO, DeBattista C, editors: *Manual of clinical psychopharmacology,* ed 7, Arlington, VA, 2010, American Psychiatric Publishing.
C = Animal studies show adverse effects on fetus, but no controlled studies in pregnant women *or* no studies available.
D = Positive evidence of human fetal risk.
L2 = Drug studied in limited number of breastfeeding women without an increase in adverse effects in infant *or* risk is remote.
L3 = No controlled studies in breastfeeding women *or* studies show minimal nonthreatening adverse effects.
L4 = Possibly hazardous.

the inability to move, stand, or work also are common. Later, suspiciousness, confusion, incoherence, irrational statements, and obsessive concerns about the baby's health and welfare can be present. Delusions are present in 50% of women with postpartum psychosis, and hallucinations occur in approximately 25% of women with this disorder. Auditory hallucinations that command the mother to kill the infant can occur in severe cases. When delusions are present, they are often related to the infant. The mother may think the infant is possessed by the devil, has special powers, or is destined for a terrible fate (APA, 2000). Grossly disorganized behavior can be manifested as a disinterest in the infant or an inability to provide care. Some women will insist that something is wrong with the baby or accuse nurses or family members of hurting or poisoning their child.

> ! **NURSING ALERT**
>
> Nurses are advised to be alert for mothers who are agitated, overactive, confused, complaining, or suspicious.

Postpartum psychosis is most commonly associated with the diagnosis of bipolar (or manic-depressive) disorder (Sadock, Sadock, and Ruiz, 2009; Sharma, Burt, and Ritchie, 2009). This mood disorder is defined by the presence of one or more episodes of abnormally elevated energy levels, cognition, and mood and one or more depressive episodes. The elevated moods are clinically referred to as *mania*. Clinical manifestations of a manic episode include at least three of the following: grandiosity, decreased need for sleep, pressured speech, flight of ideas, distractibility, psychomotor agitation, and excessive involvement in pleasurable activities without regard for negative consequences (APA, 2000). While in a manic state, mothers need constant supervision when caring for their infant. Usually, however, they are too preoccupied to provide child care. Individuals who experience manic episodes also commonly experience depressive episodes or symptoms or mixed episodes, in which features of both mania and depression are present at the same time. These episodes are usually separated by periods of "normal" mood, but in some individuals, depression and mania may rapidly alternate. These rapid changes in mood are known as *rapid cycling*.

Medical Management. Postpartum psychosis carries a relatively good prognosis with early detection and aggressive treatment; however, if left untreated, it can progress to the second postpartum year and become more refractory to treatment (Sadock, Sadock, and Ruiz, 2009). Postpartum psychosis is a psychiatric emergency, and the mother will probably need inpatient psychiatric care. Antipsychotics and mood stabilizers such as lithium are the treatments of choice (Tables 21-3 and 21-4). Antidepressants should be used very cautiously in treating postpartum psychosis, even when depressive symptoms are present, because of the risk for precipitating rapid cycling. Because of potential risks to the breastfeeding infant, informed consent regarding the risks and benefits of exposing the newborn to a psychotropic agent and maternal mental illness must be discussed and documented (see additional discussion of lactation and psychotropic medications later in this chapter). ECT, especially when bilaterally administered, has also been shown to be highly effective in the treatment of postpartum psychosis. It is usually advantageous for the mother to have contact with her baby if she so desires, but visits must be closely supervised. Psychotherapy is indicated after the period of acute psychosis has passed.

Even though the prevalence of PPD is fairly well established, some women are unlikely to seek help from a mental health care

TABLE 21-4	ANTIPSYCHOTIC MEDICATIONS	
ANTIPSYCHOTIC MEDICATIONS	**PREGNANCY RISK CATEGORY***	**LACTATION RISK CATEGORY***
Traditional Antipsychotics		
Chlorpromazine (Thorazine)	C	L3
Fluphenazine (Prolixin)	C	L3
Haloperidol (Haldol)	C	L2
Perphenazine (Trilafon)	C	L3
Thioridazine (Mellaril)	C	L4
Thiothixene (Navane)	C	L4
Trifluoperazine (Stelazine)	Unknown	Unknown
Atypical Antipsychotics		
Aripiprazole (Abilify)	C	L3
Clozapine (Clozaril)	C	L3
Loxapine (Loxitane)	C	L4
Olanzapine (Zyprexa)	C	L2
Quetiapine (Seroquel)	C	L4
Risperidone (Risperdal)	C	L3
Ziprasidone (Geodon)	C	L4

*Sources: Hale T: *Medications and mother's milk,* ed 15, Amarillo, TX, 2012, Pharmasoft; Schatzberg A, Cole JO, DeBattista C, editors: *Manual of clinical psychopharmacology,* ed 7, Arlington, VA, 2010, American Psychiatric Publishing.
C = Animal studies show adverse effects on fetus, but no controlled studies in pregnant women *or* no studies available.
L3 = No controlled studies in breastfeeding women *or* studies show minimal nonthreatening adverse effects.
L4 = Possibly hazardous.

provider. This can be related to social stigma of mental illness, cultural beliefs, lack of knowledge, or fear of child custody implications (Yonkers, Vigod, and Ross, 2011).

CARE MANAGEMENT

Primary health care providers usually recognize severe PPD or postpartum psychosis but may miss milder forms; even if it is recognized, the woman may be treated inappropriately or subtherapeutically. Identification and treatment of maternal depression must be continued beyond the immediate postbirth period to prevent negative effects of maternal depression on the children of these mothers. To recognize symptoms of PPD as early as possible, the nurse should be an active listener and demonstrate a caring attitude. Nurses cannot depend on women to volunteer unsolicited information about their depression or ask for help. Examples of ways to initiate conversation include the following: "Now that you've had your baby, how are things going for you? Have you had to change many things in your life since having the baby?" and "How much time do you spend crying?" If the nurse assesses that the new mother is depressed, she or he must ask if the mother has thought about hurting herself or the baby. The woman may be more willing to answer honestly if the nurse says, "Many women feel depressed after having a baby, and some feel so badly that they

think about hurting themselves or the baby. Have you had these thoughts?"

> **! NURSING ALERT**
>
> Because mothers with PPD with psychotic features can harm their infants, extra precaution is needed in assessment and intervention. The nurse needs to ask specifically if the mother has had thoughts about harming her baby.

Screening for Postpartum Depression

When postpartum depression is identified early, it is highly treatable. Screening for depression during pregnancy and the postpartum period aids in prevention and early intervention for depressive symptoms. There are no national guidelines for depression screening during pregnancy and after birth. The American College of Obstetricians and Gynecologists Committee on Obstetric Practice (2010) cites a lack of sufficient evidence to warrant firm recommendations for universal screening of postpartum women, although they recognize there are benefits to screening. The U.S. Preventive Services Task Force (USPSTF, 2009) recommends screening of adults for depression, including during pregnancy and the postpartum period.

Postpartum nurses can screen for PPD before women are discharged from the hospital. While this will identify some who are at risk, it is important that follow-up screening is also done. Postpartum depression is most likely to occur around 4 weeks after birth. Follow-up assessments for risks and signs of PPD can be done by primary care providers during pediatric care visits for the infant and during postpartum follow-up visits for the mother. The American Academy of Pediatrics recommends maternal depression screening at the infant's one-, two-, and four-month visits (Earls and American Academy of Pediatrics [AAP] Committee on Psychosocial Aspects of Child and Family Health, 2010). Women with a positive screen should be referred appropriately for evaluation and treatment.

Examples of screening tools for postpartum depression include the Edinburgh Postnatal Depression Scale (EPDS), the Postpartum Depression Predictors Inventory (PDPI), and the Postpartum Depression Screening Scale (PDSS). The EPDS is a self-report assessment designed specifically to identify women experiencing PPD. It has been used and validated in studies in numerous cultures and is viewed as a valid screening tool for PPD. The assessment tool asks the woman to respond to 10 statements about the common symptoms of depression. The woman is asked to choose the response that is closest to describing how she has felt for the past week. A maximum score on the EPDS is 30; women with scores of 12 or higher may possibly have depression and need further assessment. One item on the tool addresses suicidal thoughts; responses to this item should be carefully examined (Cox, Holden, and Sagovsky, 1987).

Through focused research over at least a decade, Beck has developed and continues to refine the PDPI (PDPI-R [Revised]) (Beck, 2002) and the PDSS (Beck and Gable, 2002). The PDPI-R consists of 13 risk factors related to PPD. The PDSS is a 35-item Likert response scale that assesses for seven dimensions of depression: sleeping or eating disturbances, anxiety or insecurity, emotional lability, mental confusion, loss of self, guilt or shame, and suicidal thoughts (Beck, 2008a, 2008b). Both published tools are designed to be used by nurses and other health care professionals to elicit information from the woman during an interview to assess risk. Areas assessed include the predictors of depression as listed in Box 21-4.

In addition, a simple two-item tool has been shown to be effective in identifying women at risk for PPD. If the woman answers "Yes" to either of the two questions, the screen is considered to be positive. The questions are: "Over the past two weeks have you ever felt down, depressed, or hopeless?" and "Over the past two weeks have you felt little interest or pleasure in doing things?" (Earls and AAP Committee on Psychosocial Aspects of Child and Family Health, 2010).

If postpartum depression screening results are positive or if the woman's self-report shows signs that she might be depressed, a formal screening is needed to determine the urgency of the referral and the type of provider. Also important is the need to assess the woman's family because they may be able to offer valuable information, as well as need to express how they have been affected by the woman's emotional disorder.

Nursing Care on the Postpartum Unit

The postpartum nurse must observe the new mother carefully for any signs of tearfulness and conduct further assessments as necessary. Nurses must discuss PPD to prepare new parents for potential problems in the postpartum period and discuss ways to help prevent PPD (see Patient Teaching box and Chapter 19). The family must be able to recognize the symptoms and know where to go for help. Printed materials that explain what the woman can do to prevent depression can be used as part of discharge education (Logsdon, Tomasulo, Eckert, et al., 2012).

Women are often discharged from the hospital before the blues or depression occurs. If the postpartum nurse is concerned about the mother, a mental health consult should be requested before the mother leaves the hospital. Routine instructions regarding PPD should be given to the person who comes to take the woman home; for example, "If you notice that your wife [or partner] is upset or crying a lot, please call the postpartum care provider immediately—don't wait for the routine postpartum appointment." (See Patient Teaching box.)

Nursing Care in the Home and Community

Postpartum home visits can reduce the incidence of or complications from depression. A brief home visit or phone call at least once a week until the new mother returns for her postpartum visit may save the life of a mother and her infant; however, home visits may not be feasible or available. Supervision of the mother with emotional complications can become a prime concern. Because depression can greatly interfere with her mothering functions, family and friends may need to participate in the infant's care. This is a time for the extended family and friends to determine what they can do to help; the nurse can work with them to ensure adequate supervision and their understanding of the woman's mental illness.

When the woman has PPD, a partner often reacts with confusion, shock, denial, and anger and feels neglected and blamed. The nurse can provide nonjudgmental opportunities for the partner to verbalize feelings and concerns, help the partner identify positive coping strategies, and be a source of encouragement for the partner to continue supporting the woman. Suggestions for partners of women with PPD include helping around the house, setting limits with family and friends, going with her to appointments with the health care provider, educating himself or herself, writing down concerns and questions to take to the primary care provider or therapist, and just being with her—sitting quietly, hugging her, and demonstrating concern and compassion. Both the woman and her partner need an opportunity to express their needs, fears, thoughts, and feelings in a nonjudgmental environment.

Even if the woman is severely depressed, hospitalization can be avoided if adequate resources can be mobilized to ensure safety for both mother and infant. The nurse in home health care will need to make frequent phone calls or home visits for assessment

---

PATIENT TEACHING

Preventing Postpartum Depression

- Share knowledge about postpartum emotional problems with close family and friends.
- At least once each day or every other day, purposely relax for 15 minutes: deep breathing, meditating, taking a hot bath.
- Take care of yourself: eat a balanced diet.
- Exercise on a regular basis, at least 30 minutes a day.
- Sleep as much as possible; make a promise to yourself to try to sleep when the baby sleeps.
- Get out of the house: try to leave home for 30 minutes a day; take a walk outdoors or walk at the mall.
- Share your feelings with someone close to you; don't isolate yourself at home with the TV.
- Don't overcommit yourself or feel like you need to be a superwoman. Ask for help from family and friends.
- Don't place unrealistic expectations on yourself; you don't need to be a perfect mother.
- Be flexible with your daily activities.
- Go to a new mothers' support group: for example, take a postpartum exercise class or attend a breastfeeding support group.
- Don't be ashamed of having emotional problems after your baby is born. It happens to approximately 15% of women.

PATIENT TEACHING

Signs of Postpartum Blues, Depression, and Psychosis

Signs of baby blues (these should go away in a few days or a week):
- Sad, anxious, or overwhelmed feelings
- Crying spells
- Loss of appetite
- Difficulty sleeping

Signs of postpartum depression (can begin anytime the first year):
- Same signs as baby blues, but they last longer and are more severe
- Thoughts of harming yourself or your baby
- Not having any interest in the baby

Signs of postpartum psychosis:
- Seeing or hearing things that are not there
- Feelings of confusion
- Rapid mood swings
- Trying to hurt yourself or your baby

When to call your health care provider:
- The baby blues continue for more than 2 weeks
- Symptoms of depression get worse
- Difficulty performing tasks at home or at work
- Inability to care for yourself or your baby
- Thoughts of harming yourself or your baby

Data from U.S. Department of Health and Human Services Office of Women's Health: *Depression during and after pregnancy*, 2009, www.womenshealth.gov/publications/our-publications/fact-sheet/depression-pregnancy.pdf.

and counseling. Community resources that may be helpful are temporary child care or foster care, homemaker service, meals on wheels, parenting guidance centers, mother's-day-out programs, and telephone support groups such as Postpartum Support International (http://postpartum.net) and Depression After Delivery (www.depressionafterdelivery.com).

Referral. Women with moderate to severe cases of PPD should be referred to a mental health professional such as a psychiatric nurse practitioner or psychiatrist for evaluation and therapy. Inpatient psychiatric hospitalization may be necessary. This decision is made when the safety of the mother or children is threatened.

Providing Safety. If delusional thinking about the baby is suspected, the nurse asks, "Have you thought about hurting your baby?" When depression is suspected, the nurse asks, "Have you thought about hurting yourself?" Four criteria can be used to measure the seriousness of a suicidal plan: method, availability, specificity, and lethality. Has the woman specified a method? Is the method of choice available? How specific is the plan? If the method is concrete and detailed, with access to it right at hand, the suicide risk increases. How lethal is the method? The most lethal method is shooting, with hanging a close second. The least lethal is slashing one's wrists.

> **! NURSING ALERT**
>
> Suicidal thoughts or attempts are among the most serious symptoms of PPD and require immediate assessment and intervention.

Psychiatric Hospitalization

Women with postpartum psychosis have a psychiatric emergency and must be referred immediately to a psychiatrist who is experienced in working with women with PPD, can prescribe medication and other forms of therapy, and can assess the need for hospitalization.

> **LEGAL TIP: Commitment for Psychiatric Care**
>
> If a woman with PPD is experiencing active suicidal ideation or harmful delusions about the baby and is unwilling to seek treatment, legal intervention may be necessary to commit the woman to an inpatient setting for treatment.

If allowed within the inpatient psychiatric setting, the reintroduction of the baby to the mother can occur at the mother's own pace. A schedule is set for increasing the number of hours the mother cares for the baby over several days, culminating in the infant's staying overnight in the mother's room. This method allows the mother to experience meeting the infant's needs and giving up sleep for the baby, a situation difficult for new mothers even under ideal conditions. The mother's readiness for discharge and caring for the baby is assessed. Her interactions with her baby are carefully supervised and guided. A postpartum nurse is often asked to assist the psychiatric nursing staff in assessment of the mother-infant interactions.

Nurses should observe the mother for signs of bonding with the baby. Attachment behaviors are defined as eye-to-eye contact; physical contact that involves holding, touching, cuddling, and talking to the baby and calling the baby by name; and the initiation of appropriate care. A staff member is assigned to keep the baby in sight at all times. Indirect teaching, praise, and encouragement are designed to bolster the mother's self-esteem and self-confidence.

Psychotropic Medications

If the woman with PPD is not breastfeeding, in most cases antidepressants can be prescribed without special precautions. A variety of medications can be prescribed for these women, including tricyclic antidepressants (TCAs), selective serotonin reuptake inhibitors (SSRIs), serotonin/norepinephrine reuptake inhibitors (SNRIs), monoamine oxidase inhibitors (MAOIs), mood stabilizers, and antipsychotic medications.

MAOIs may be used for women with major depression who are not responsive to other medications and for women with panic disorder and bipolar disorder. Hypertensive crisis is the main reason that MAOIs are not prescribed more frequently than other psychotropic medications. The woman should be taught to watch for signs of hypertensive crisis—a throbbing occipital headache, stiff neck, chills, nausea, flushing, retro-orbital pain, apprehension, pallor, sweating, chest pain, and palpitations. This crisis is brought on by the woman taking any of a large variety of over-the-counter medications or eating foods that contain tyramine, which normally is broken down by the enzyme *monoamine oxidase*. The nurse must do extensive teaching about absolute avoidance of foods and medications that contain tyramine such as pseudoephedrine-containing medications, aged cheese, red wine, fava or Italian green beans, brewer's yeast, smoked fish, chicken or beef livers, and preserved meats (Hadley, Albanese, and Rochester, 2012).

The woman taking mood stabilizers (see Table 21-3) must be taught about the many side effects, and especially for those taking lithium, the need to have serum lithium levels determined every 6 months. Women with severe psychiatric syndromes such as schizophrenia, bipolar disorder, or psychotic depression will probably require antipsychotic medications (see Table 21-4). Most of these antipsychotic medications can cause sedation and orthostatic hypotension—both of which can interfere with the mother being able to care safely for her baby. They also can cause peripheral nervous system (PNS) effects such as constipation, dry mouth, blurred vision, tachycardia, urinary retention, weight gain, and agranulocytosis. Central nervous system (CNS) effects may include akathisia, dystonias, parkinsonian-like symptoms, tardive dyskinesia (irreversible), and neuroleptic malignant syndrome (potentially fatal). Medication education is especially important when caring for women who are taking antipsychotic medications. The nurse should use discretion in selecting the content to be shared because of the women's altered thought processes and the large number of side/toxic effects. The nurse may choose to do more extensive education with a close family member. The newer, atypical antipsychotic medications such as aripiprazole, olanzapine, quetiapine, risperidone, and ziprasidone are usually safer and have fewer side effects than the older, more traditional antipsychotics. Their safety in breastfeeding women, however, has not been established.

Psychotropic Medications and Lactation

Use of any psychotropic medication in a breastfeeding mother is done with consideration of risks and benefits. The risk of not treating the mother versus not breastfeeding the infant prompts providers to prescribe medications that reduce maternal symptoms without harming the infant. Concerns about many psychotropic drugs are related to the long-term use and potential effects on the infant (Lawrence and Lawrence, 2011).

Factors that affect the passage of a medication through breast milk include the size of the molecule, the solubility in lipids and water, the protein-binding capacity, the drug's pH, and the rate of diffusion. Infant factors to consider relate to the gestational and chronologic age of the infant, weight, health, and frequency and

CRITICAL THINKING CASE STUDY

Postpartum Depression

Jenna, 31, gave birth to a 7 lbs, 6 oz boy 4 weeks ago. She has been diagnosed with postpartum depression, and an SSRI (sertraline [Zoloft]) medication has been prescribed. Jenna is breastfeeding and has concerns about taking the medication.

1. Evidence—Is there sufficient evidence regarding the safety of psychotropic medications and lactation?
2. Assumptions—What assumptions can be made about the following?
   a. Lactation risk categories of SSRI medications
   b. Timing of feeding and medication administration
   c. Risks of discontinuing medications while breastfeeding
3. What is the nursing priority in this situation?
4. Does the evidence objectively support your conclusion?

SSRI, Selective serotonin reuptake inhibitor.

amount of feeding (Lawrence and Lawrence, 2011). To minimize the infant's exposure to maternal medication, the mother should avoid breastfeeding when the blood levels of the medication are peaking.

SSRIs are the most common treatment for postpartum depression; they are also prescribed for anxiety disorders. Research has shown that the majority of the SSRIs taken by breastfeeding mothers pass through the milk to the infant in small amounts and have no untoward effects on the infant (Kendall-Tackett and Hale, 2010). Paroxetine, sertraline, and nortriptyline provide less infant exposure than fluoxetine and citalopram. All breastfeeding mothers who take SSRIs should be taught to monitor their infants for signs of irritability, poor feeding, and alterations in sleep pattern (Kendall-Tackett and Hale, 2010) (see Critical Thinking Case Study).

Benzodiazepines, mood stabilizers, and antipsychotic medications are all used frequently in the treatment of postpartum psychiatric disorders despite the lack of research in this population. No long-term effects have been reported in exclusively breastfed infants whose mothers were taking benzodiazepines on a regular basis. The shorter-acting agents (alprazolam, lorazepam) are favored over those with longer half-lives (clonazepam, diazepam) (Lawrence and Lawrence, 2011).

Mood-stabilizing medications are present in the breast milk of women who take these drugs. Lithium has been the most extensively studied. Lithium has been linked to several serious adverse effects in breastfeeding infants, including hypotonia, hypothermia, cyanosis, and electrocardiogram abnormalities. Therefore its use is not recommended in breastfeeding mothers. Valproic acid and carbamazepine are considered reasonably safe for use while breastfeeding, although careful monitoring for infant hepatotoxicity is recommended. The benefits of breastfeeding and the potential risks must be carefully considered before using lithium or other mood stabilizers.

In summary, all psychotropic medications studied to date are excreted in breast milk. The best psychotropic medications for breastfeeding women are those with the greatest documentation of prior use, lower Food and Drug Administration (FDA) risk category, few or no metabolites, and fewer side effects.

When breastfeeding women have emotional complications and need psychotropic medications, referral to a mental health care provider who specializes in postpartum disorders is preferred. The woman should be informed of the risks and benefits to her and her infant of the medications to be taken. Depressed women will need the nurse to reinforce the importance of taking antidepressants as ordered. Because antidepressants usually do not exert any significant effect for approximately 2 weeks and usually do not reach full effect for 4 to 6 weeks, many women discontinue taking the medication on their own. Patient and family teaching should reinforce the schedule for taking medications until therapeutic effects are present and for as long as prescribed the health care provider.

Other Treatments for PPD

Other treatments for PPD include hormone therapy (often combined with antidepressant medication), complementary or alternative therapies (e.g., yoga, massage, relaxation techniques), ECT, and psychotherapy. ECT may be used for women with PPD who have not improved with antidepressant therapy. Psychotherapy in the form of group therapy or individual (interpersonal) therapy has been used with positive results alone and in conjunction with antidepressant therapy; however, more studies are needed to determine what types of professional support are most effective. Repetitive transcranial magnetic stimulation is a new therapy for PPD, but more studies need to be done to demonstrate the efficacy (Garcia, Flynn, Pierce, et al., 2010). Alternative therapies may be used alone but often are used with other treatments for PPD. Safety and efficacy studies of these alternative therapies are needed to ensure that care and advice are based on evidence.

NURSING ALERT

St. John's wort is often used to treat depression. It has not been proven safe for women who are breastfeeding.

Postpartum Anxiety Disorders

Anxiety disorders include generalized anxiety disorder, obsessive-compulsive disorder, panic disorder and panic attacks, specific phobias, social anxiety disorder, and post-traumatic stress disorder. Common characteristics of these disorders are irrational fear, worry, and tension; physical symptoms such as trembling, nausea and vomiting, dizziness, dyspnea, and insomnia are often seen (Cunningham, Leveno, Bloom, et al., 2010).

Women who have obsessive-compulsive disorder (OCD) often report worsening of their symptoms during pregnancy and in the postpartum period (Forray, Focseneanu, Pittman, et al., 2010). Onset of OCD can occur after birth. Compulsive checking on the sleeping baby and repetitive ritualistic washing are common. Obsessions are usually focused and specific and associated with fear of consequences (Speisman, Storch, and Abramowitz, 2011).

It is very important to distinguish between the symptoms of OCD in the postpartum patient and those of postpartum psychosis because either can involve ideation regarding harming the newborn (Speisman, Storch, and Abramowitz, 2011). Delusions and hallucinations are typical in psychosis and have implications for infant safety, but these are not found in OCD. Aggressive thoughts of women with psychoses are not distressing to them, whereas women with OCD find their obsessive thoughts are very disturbing (Speisman, Storch, and Abramowitz, 2011).

Panic attacks are discrete periods of sudden onset of intense apprehension, fearfulness, or terror (APA, 2000). During these attacks, symptoms such as shortness of breath, palpitations, chest pain, choking, smothering sensations, and fear of losing control are present. Women have reported having intrusive thoughts about terrible injury done to the infant, such as stabbing or burns, sometimes by themselves. Rarely do the women harm the baby. Nurses need only to listen to the mother to hear symptoms of panic disorder. Usually these women are so distraught that they will share with whoever will listen. Often the family has tried to tell them that what they are experiencing is normal, but they know differently. Potential nursing diagnoses for women experiencing postpartum anxiety disorders include:

- Anxiety related to:
  Postpartum adaptations and expectations
- Fear related to:
  Obsessions
  Thoughts about harming others
- Powerlessness related to:
  Feelings of losing control
- Deficient Knowledge related to:
  Postpartum mental health problems

Medical Management

There are effective treatments for anxiety disorders, and this fact should be communicated to women. Cognitive-behavioral therapy (CBT) is an attractive option because of its substantial benefits, limited duration, no drug exposure to the infant, and durability of effect. The effectiveness of treatment, widespread availability, and ease of administration make SSRIs an appealing and popular option (Cunningham, Leveno, Bloom, et al., 2010; Speisman, Storch, and Abramowitz, 2011). Medications should be prescribed with careful consideration of safety for the breastfeeding infant. Each woman should be approached on an individualized basis, assessing the severity of symptoms, obtaining the history and response to any previous treatments, understanding the woman's preferences, and educating the woman about the potential benefits and potential risk of each treatment. Treatment is usually a combination of medications, education, psychotherapy, and CBT, along with an attempt to identify any medical or physiologic contributors.

Nursing Interventions

Education is a crucial nursing intervention. New mothers should be provided with anticipatory guidance concerning the possibility of anxiety disorders during the postpartum period. Preparing for the attacks can help offset their unexpected, terrifying nature. Women can be reassured that it is common to feel a sense of impending doom and fear of insanity during panic attacks. Nurses can help women identify panic triggers that are particular to their own lives. Keeping a diary can help identify the triggers.

Family and social supports are helpful. The new mother is encouraged to put usual chores on hold and to ask for and accept help. Support groups can help these mothers to feel comfort in seeing others in similar circumstances.

A variety of other treatment options can be recommended for women with anxiety disorders. These include sensory interventions such as music therapy and aromatherapy, behavioral interventions such as breathing exercises and progressive muscle relaxation, cognitive interventions such as positive self-talk training, and exercise.

MATERNAL DEATH

Maternal death can be caused by a variety of complications, including embolism, hypertension, hemorrhage, infection, and cardiomyopathy (see Chapter 1). In many cases, the death of a mother is sudden and unexpected. Any instance of maternal death is tragic for the family as well as for the nurses and other health professionals who were involved in her care.

When a woman dies of a complication related to childbearing, the husband or partner and extended family are faced with mourning the death of a wife or partner and mother. The loss and grief are greatly compounded when there is also the death of a fetus or neonate. When the infant survives, the husband or partner is faced with parenting a baby without a surviving mother. The responsibilities of infant care can be overwhelming during this time of intense loss and grief.

Because most maternal deaths are unexpected, the grief that follows a maternal death is usually unplanned. This differs from anticipatory grief in which the loss is expected, such as with cancer. The shock and disbelief associated with unplanned grief can be engulfing and debilitating, overwhelming the normal coping abilities and creating difficulties with everyday functioning and decision making.

Nurses and other health care professionals working with families who experience maternal loss need to consider the context and implications of the maternal death on the remaining family members. Young parents may never have experienced a significant personal loss or tragedy; in many cases, their parents and grandparents are still living. Cultural beliefs and customs surrounding death can influence a family's response to maternal death (Hill, 2012). The grief response of each family member will vary; grief is an individual response, and the grieving process does not always proceed in a predictable manner.

Hospital protocols regarding maternal death are varied. When a maternal death occurs, the hospital chaplain and social worker may provide the initial contact with the family, taking them into a private room. As soon as possible, they are joined by the obstetrician, perinatologist, and nurse. This first meeting with the family is often short, providing brief explanations about the events leading up to the maternal death and attempting to answer the family's questions. The primary goal of this meeting is to show empathy and compassion for the family and to assure them of updates as soon as information becomes available (Hill, 2012). If there is a surviving infant, the family will likely want to see and hold the infant. If the neonate is in the intensive care nursery, the family can be escorted to the baby's bedside. The family will need assistance with the "next steps" in terms of making arrangements for funeral services; the nurse, chaplain, or social worker can provide the family with information and offer support during this difficult time.

Families who experience maternal loss are at risk for developing complicated bereavement and altered parenting of the surviving infant and other children in the family. A referral to social services to help the family mobilize support systems and for counseling can help combat potential problems before they develop and can be beneficial not only at the time of the loss but also in the future. Follow-up care for grieving families is essential as they progress through the stages of grief and adjust to life without the mother.

The emotional toll that a maternal death can take on the nursing and medical staff must also be addressed. Guilt, anger, fear, sadness, and depression are all common responses to a maternal death. The staff may want to participate in a debriefing session in which they can review the situation surrounding the events, their participation in caring for the mother, and their response to the death. Attending memorial or funeral services can benefit staff and family. Follow-up conferences with a social worker or grief counselor can help staff members work through their grief.

KEY POINTS

- PPH is the most common and most serious type of excessive obstetric blood loss.
- Hemorrhagic (hypovolemic) shock is an emergency situation in which the perfusion of body organs can become severely compromised and death can ensue.
- The potential hazards of therapeutic interventions can further compromise the woman with hemorrhagic disorders.
- Postpartum infection is a major cause of maternal morbidity and mortality throughout the world.
- Postpartum UTIs are common because of trauma experienced during labor.
- Structural disorders of the uterus and vagina related to pelvic relaxation are often the delayed but direct result of childbearing.

- Mood disorders account for most mental health disorders in the postpartum period.
- Suicidal thoughts or attempts are among the most serious symptoms of PPD.
- Antidepressant medications are the usual treatment for PPD; however, specific precautions are needed for breastfeeding women.
- Treatment of postpartum onset of panic disorder requires a combination of medication, education, supportive measures, and psychotherapy.
- Nurses and other health care professionals provide empathetic care and support for families who have experienced maternal loss.

REFERENCES

American College of Obstetricians and Gynecologists Committee on Obstetric Practice: Committee opinion no. 453: screening for depression during and after pregnancy, *Obstet Gynecol* 115:394–395, 2010.

American Psychiatric Association (APA): *Diagnostic and statistical manual of mental disorders*, ed 4 (revised), Washington, DC, 2000, APA Press.

Beck C: Revision of the postpartum depression predictors inventory, *J Obstet Gynecol Neonatal Nurs* 31(4):394–402, 2002.

Beck C: State of the science on postpartum depression: what nurse researchers have contributed—part 1, *MCN Am J Matern Child Nurs* 33(2):122–126, 2008a.

Beck C: State of the science on postpartum depression: what nurse researchers have contributed—part 2, *MCN Am J Matern Child Nurs* 33(3):151–156, 2008b.

Beck C, Gable R: *Postpartum depression screening scale manual*, Los Angeles, 2002, Western Psychological Services.

Beydoun HA, Beydoun MA, Kaufman JS, et al: Intimate partner violence against adult women and its association with major depressive disorder, depressive symptoms and postpartum depression: a systematic review and meta-analysis, *Soc Sci Med* 75(6):959–975, 2012.

Blom EA, Jansen PW, Verhulst FC, et al: Perinatal complications increase the risk of postpartum depression: the Generation R study, *BJOG* 117(11):1390–1398, 2010.

Callaghan WM, Kuklina EV, Berg CJ: Trends in postpartum hemorrhage: United States, 1994-2006, *Am J Obstet Gynecol* 202(4):353, e1–e6, 2010.

Callister LC, Beckstrand RL, Corbett C: Postpartum depression and help-seeking behaviors in immigrant Hispanic women, *J Obstet Gynecol Neonatal Nurs* 40(4):440–449, 2011.

Cerulli C, Talbor NL, Tang W, et al: Co-occurring intimate partner violence and mental health diagnoses in perinatal women, *J Womens Health* 20(12):1797–1803, 2011.

Cox JL, Holden JM, Sagovsky R: Detection of postnatal depression: development of the 10-item Edinburgh Postnatal Depression Scale, *Br J Psychiatry* 150:782–786, 1987.

Cunningham FG, Leveno KJ, Bloom SL, et al: *Williams obstetrics*, ed 23, New York, 2010, McGraw-Hill.

Davey HL, Tough SC, Adair CE, et al: Risk factors for sub-clinical and major postpartum depression among a community cohort of Canadian women, *Matern Child Health J* 15(7):866–875, 2011.

Della Torre M, Kilpatrick SJ, Hibbard JU, et al: Assessing preventability for obstetric hemorrhage, *Am J Perinatol* 28(10):753–760, 2011.

Dumoulin C, Hay-Smith E: Pelvic floor muscle training versus no treatment, or inactive control treatments, for urinary incontinence in women, *The Cochrane Database of Systematic Reviews* 2010. Issue 1, CD005654.

Earls MF, American Academy of Pediatrics (AAP) Committee on Psychosocial Aspects of Child and Family Health: Incorporating recognition and management of perinatal and postpartum depression into pediatric practice, *Pediatrics* 126(5):1032–1039, 2010.

Forray A, Focseneanu M, Pittman B, et al: Onset and exacerbation of obsessive-compulsive disorder in pregnancy and the postpartum period, *J Clin Psychiatr* 71(8):1061–1068, 2010.

Francois KE, Foley MR: Antepartum and postpartum hemorrhage. In Gabbe SG, Niebyl JR, Simpson JL, editors: *Obstetrics: normal and problem pregnancies*, ed 6, Philadelphia, 2012, Saunders.

Garcia KS, Flynn P, Pierce KJ, et al: Repetitive transcranial magnetic stimulation treats postpartum depression, *Brain Stimul* 3:36–41, 2010.

Gilbert E: *Manual of high risk pregnancy & delivery*, ed 5, St Louis, 2011, Mosby.

Goyal D, Wang EJ, Shen J, et al: Clinically identified postpartum depression in Asian American women, *J Obstet Gynecol Neonatal Nurs* 41(3):408–416, 2012.

Hadley DE, Albanese WP, Rochester CD: Psychiatric drug interactions explored, *Pharm Pract News*, February 2012, www.pharmacypracticenews.com/download/ppn0212_ER_WM.pdf.

Hill PE: Support and counseling after maternal death, *Semin Perinatol* 36(1):84–88, 2012.

Katz V: Postpartum care. In Gabbe SG, Niebyl JR, Simpson JL, et al, editors: *Obstetrics: normal and problem pregnancies*, ed 6, Philadelphia, 2012, Saunders.

Kendall-Tackett K, Hale TW: Review: the use of antidepressants in pregnant and breastfeeding women: a review of recent studies, *J Hum Lact* 26(2):187–195, 2010.

Lawrence RA, Lawrence RM: *Breastfeeding: a guide for the medical profession*, ed 7, St Louis, 2011, Mosby.

Le Strat Y, Dubertret C, Le Foll B: Prevalence and correlates of major depressive episode in pregnant and postpartum women in the United States, *J Affect Disord* 135(1-3):128–138, 2011.

Letourneau N, Tryphonopoulos PD, Duffett-Leger L, et al: Support intervention needs and preferences of fathers affected by postpartum depression, *J Perinat Neonatal Nurs* 26(1):69–80, 2012.

Logsdon MC, Tomasulo R, Eckert D, et al: Identification of mothers at risk for postpartum depression by hospital-based perinatal nurses, *MCN Am J Matern Child Nurs* 37(4):218–225, 2012.

O'Hara MW, McCabe JE: Postpartum depression: current status and future directions, *Annu Rev Clin Psychol* 9: 379–407, 2013.

Paulson JF, Bazemore SD: Prenatal and postpartum depression in fathers and its association with maternal depression: a meta-analysis, *JAMA* 303:1961–1969, 2010.

Pettker CM, Lockwood CJ: Thromboembolic disorders. In Gabbe SG, Niebyl JR, Simpson JL, et al, editors: *Obstetrics: normal and problem pregnancies*, ed 6, Philadelphia, 2012, Saunders.

Rozance PJ, Rosenberg AA: The neonate. In Gabbe SG, Niebyl JR, Simpson JL, et al, editors: *Obstetrics: normal and problem pregnancies*, ed 6, Philadelphia, 2012, Saunders.

Sadock B, Sadock V, Ruiz P: *Kaplan & Sadock's comprehensive textbook of psychiatry* (vol 2), ed 9, Philadelphia, 2009, Lippincott Williams & Wilkins.

Sharma V, Burt V, Ritchie H: Bipolar II postpartum depression: detection, diagnosis, and treatment, *Am J Psychiatr* 166(11):1201–1204, 2009.

Speisman BB, Storch EA, Abramowitz JS: Postpartum obsessive-compulsive disorder,

J Obstet Gynecol Neonatal Nurs 40(6):680–690, 2011.

Sung V, Hampton B: Epidemiology of pelvic floor dysfunction, *Obstet Gynecol Clin North Am* 36(3):421–443, 2009.

Sung V, West D, Hernandez A, et al: Association between urinary incontinence and depressive symptoms in overweight and obese women, *Am J Obstet Gynecol* 200(5):557, e1–e5, 2009.

Tarnay C, Bhatia N: Genitourinary dysfunction: pelvic organ prolapse, urinary incontinence, and infection. In Hacker N, Gambone J, Hobel C, editors: *Hacker and Moore's essentials of obstetrics and gynecology*, ed 5, Philadelphia, 2010, Saunders.

U.S. Department of Health and Human Services Office of Women's Health: Depression during and after pregnancy, 2009, www.womenshealth.gov/publications/ our-publications/fact-sheet/depression-pregnancy.pdf.

U.S. Preventive Services Task Force (USPSTF): *Screening for depression in adults*, Rockville,

MD, 2009, Agency for Healthcare Research and Quality, www.ahrq.gov/CLINIC/uspstf/ uspsaddepr.htm.

Vigod SN, Villegas L, Dennis CL, et al: Prevalence and risk factors for postpartum depression among women with preterm and low-birth-weight infants: a systematic review, *BJOG* 117(5):540–550, 2010.

Wallner L, Porten S, Meenan R, et al: Prevalence and severity of undiagnosed urinary incontinence in women, *Am J Med* 122(11):1037–1042, 2009.

Woolhouse H, Gartland D, Hegarty K, et al: Depressive symptoms and intimate partner violence in the 12 months after childbirth: a prospective pregnancy cohort study, *BJOG* 119(3):315–323, 2012.

Yonkers KA, Vigod S, Ross LE: Diagnosis, pathophysiology and management of mood disorders in pregnant and postpartum women, *Obstet Gynecol* 117(4):961–977, 2011.

CHAPTER

22

Physiologic and Behavioral Adaptations of the Newborn

Kathryn R. Alden

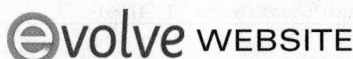 WEBSITE

http://evolve.elsevier.com/Perry/maternal

LEARNING OBJECTIVES

On completion of this chapter, the reader will be able to:
- Discuss the physiologic adaptations that the neonate must make during the period of transition from the intrauterine to the extrauterine environment.
- Describe the behavioral adaptations that are characteristic of the newborn during the transition period.
- Explain the mechanisms of thermoregulation in the neonate and the potential consequences of hypothermia and hyperthermia.

- Recognize newborn reflexes and differentiate characteristic responses from abnormal responses.
- Discuss the sensory and perceptual functioning of the neonate.
- Identify signs that the neonate is at risk related to problems with each body system.

The neonatal period includes the time from birth through day 28 of life. During this time the neonate must make many physiologic and behavioral adaptations to extrauterine life. Physiologic adjustment tasks are those that involve: (1) establishing and maintaining respirations; (2) adjusting to circulatory changes; (3) regulating temperature; (4) ingesting, retaining, and digesting nutrients; (5) eliminating waste; and (6) regulating weight. Behavioral tasks include: (1) establishing a regulated behavioral tempo independent of the mother, which involves self-regulating arousal, self-monitoring changes in state, and patterning sleep; (2) processing, storing, and organizing multiple stimuli; and (3) establishing a relationship with caregivers and the environment. The term infant usually makes these adjustments with little or no difficulty.

TRANSITION TO EXTRAUTERINE LIFE

The major adaptations associated with transition from intrauterine to extrauterine life occur during the first 6 to 8 hours after birth. The predictable series of events during transition are mediated by the sympathetic nervous system and result in changes that involve heart rate, respirations, temperature, and gastrointestinal function. This transition period represents a time of vulnerability for the neonate and warrants careful observation by nurses. To detect disorders in adaptation soon after birth, nurses must be aware of normal features of the transition period.

In their classic work on newborn adaptation to extrauterine life, Desmond, Rudolph, and Phitaksphraiwan (1966) proposed three stages of newborn transition. The stages are still considered valid today.

The first stage of the transition period lasts up to 30 minutes after birth and is called the *first period of reactivity*. The newborn's heart rate increases rapidly to 160 to 180 beats/min but gradually falls after 30 minutes or so to a baseline rate of 100 to 120 beats/min. Respirations are irregular, with a rate between 60 and 80 breaths/min. Fine crackles can be present on auscultation. Audible grunting, nasal flaring, and retractions of the chest also can be present; but these should cease within the first hour of birth. The infant is alert and may have spontaneous startles, tremors, crying, and head movement from side to side. Bowel sounds are audible, and meconium may be passed.

After the first period of reactivity the newborn either sleeps or has a marked decrease in motor activity. This *period of decreased responsiveness* lasts from 60 to 100 minutes. During this time the infant is pink, and respirations are rapid and shallow (up to 60 breaths/min) but unlabored. Bowel sounds are audible, and peristaltic waves may be noted over the rounded abdomen.

The *second period of reactivity* occurs roughly between 2 and 8 hours after birth and lasts from 10 minutes to several hours. Brief periods of tachycardia and tachypnea occur, associated with increased muscle tone, changes in skin color, and mucus production. Meconium is commonly passed at this time. Most healthy newborns experience this transition, regardless of gestational age or type of birth; extremely and very preterm infants do not because of physiologic immaturity.

PHYSIOLOGIC ADJUSTMENTS

Respiratory System

As the infant emerges from the intrauterine environment and the umbilical cord is severed, profound adaptations are necessary for survival. The most critical of these adaptations is the establishment of effective respirations. Most newborns breathe spontaneously after birth and are able to maintain adequate oxygenation. Preterm infants often encounter respiratory difficulties related to immaturity of the lungs.

Initiation of Breathing

During intrauterine life oxygenation of the fetus occurs through transplacental gas exchange. However, at birth the lungs must be established as the site of gas exchange. In utero fetal blood was shunted away from the lungs, but when birth occurs the pulmonary vasculature must be fully perfused for this purpose. Clamping the umbilical cord causes a rise in blood pressure (BP), which increases circulation and lung perfusion.

It has been recognized that there is no single trigger for newborn respiratory function. The initiation of respirations in the neonate is the result of a combination of chemical, mechanical, thermal, and sensory factors.

Chemical Factors. The activation of chemoreceptors in the carotid arteries and aorta results from the relative state of hypoxia associated with labor. With each labor contraction there is a temporary decrease in uterine blood flow and transplacental gas exchange, resulting in transient fetal hypoxia and hypercarbia. Although the fetus is able to recover between contractions, there appears to be a cumulative effect that results in progressive decline in Po_2, increased Pco_2, and lowered blood pH. Decreased levels of oxygen and increased levels of carbon dioxide seem to have a cumulative effect that is involved in initiating neonatal breathing by stimulating the respiratory center in the medulla. Another chemical factor may also play a role; it is thought that, as a result of clamping the cord, there is a drop in levels of a prostaglandin that can inhibit respirations.

Mechanical Factors. Respirations in the newborn can be stimulated by changes in intrathoracic pressure resulting from compression of the chest during vaginal birth. As the infant passes through the birth canal, the chest is compressed. With birth this pressure on the chest is released, and the negative intrathoracic pressure helps draw air into the lungs. Crying increases the distribution of air in the lungs and promotes expansion of the alveoli. The positive pressure created by crying helps to keep the alveoli open.

Thermal Factors. With birth the newborn enters the extrauterine environment, in which the temperature is significantly lower. The profound change in environmental temperature stimulates receptors in the skin, resulting in stimulation of the respiratory center in the medulla.

Sensory Factors. Sensory stimulation occurs in a variety of ways with birth. Some of these include handling the infant by the physician or midwife, suctioning the mouth and nose, and drying by the nurses. Pain associated with birth can also be a factor. The lights, sounds, and smells of the new environment can also be involved in stimulation of the respiratory center.

At term the lungs hold approximately 20 mL of fluid per kilogram. Air must be substituted for the fluid that filled the fetal respiratory tract. Traditionally it had been thought that the thoracic squeeze occurring during normal vaginal birth resulted in significant clearance of lung fluid. However, it appears that this event plays a minor role. In the days preceding labor there is reduced production of fetal lung fluid and concomitant decreased alveolar fluid volume. Shortly before the onset of labor there is a catecholamine surge that seems to promote fluid clearance from the lungs, which continues during labor (Goldsmith, 2011). The movement of lung fluid from the air spaces occurs through active transport into the interstitium, with drainage occurring through the pulmonary circulation and lymphatic system. Retention of lung fluid can interfere with the infant's ability to maintain adequate oxygenation, especially if other factors (e.g., meconium aspiration, congenital diaphragmatic hernia, esophageal atresia with fistula, choanal atresia, congenital cardiac defect, immature alveoli) that compromise respirations are present. Infants born by cesarean in which labor did not occur before birth can experience some lung fluid retention, although it typically clears without deleterious effects on the infant. These infants are also more likely to develop transient tachypnea of the newborn (TTNB) caused by the lower levels of catecholamines (Abu-Shaweesh, 2011).

The alveoli of the term infant's lungs are lined with surfactant, a protein manufactured in type II cells of the lungs. Lung expansion depends largely on chest wall contraction and adequate secretion of surfactant. Surfactant lowers surface tension, therefore reducing the pressure required to keep the alveoli open with inspiration, and prevents total alveolar collapse on exhalation, thereby maintaining alveolar stability. The decreased surface tension results in increased lung compliance, helping to establish the functional residual capacity of the lungs. With absent or decreased surfactant, more pressure must be generated for inspiration, which can soon tire or exhaust preterm or sick term infants.

Breathing movements that began in utero as intermittent become continuous after birth, although the mechanism for this is not well understood. Once respirations are established, breaths are shallow and irregular, ranging from 30 to 60 breaths/min, with periods of breathing that include pauses in respirations lasting less than 20 seconds. These episodes of periodic breathing occur most often during the active (rapid eye movement [REM]) sleep cycle and decrease in frequency and duration with age. Apneic periods longer than 20 seconds indicate a pathologic process and should be evaluated.

> **! NURSING ALERT**
>
> Newborn infants are by preference nose breathers. The reflex response to nasal obstruction is to open the mouth to maintain an airway. This response is not present in most infants until 3 weeks after birth; therefore cyanosis or asphyxia can occur with nasal blockage.

In most newborn infants auscultation of the chest reveals loud, clear breath sounds that seem very near because little chest tissue intervenes. Breath sounds should be clear and equal bilaterally. The ribs of the infant articulate with the spine at a horizontal rather than a downward slope; consequently the rib cage cannot expand with inspiration as readily as that of an adult. Because neonatal respiratory function is largely a matter of diaphragmatic contraction, abdominal breathing is characteristic of newborns. The newborn infant's chest and abdomen rise simultaneously with inspiration. Characteristics of the respiratory system of the neonate and the effects of these characteristics on respiratory function are listed in Table 22-1.

TABLE 22-1	CHARACTERISTICS OF THE RESPIRATORY SYSTEM OF THE NEONATE
CHARACTERISTIC	**EFFECT ON FUNCTION**
Immature alveoli; decreased size and number of alveoli	Risk of respiratory insufficiency and pulmonary problems
Thicker alveolar wall; decreased alveolar surface area	Less efficient gas transport and exchange
Continued development of alveoli until childhood	Possible opportunity to reduce effects of discrete lung injury
Decreased lung elastic tissue and recoil	Decreased lung compliance requiring higher pressures and more work to expand; increased risk of atelectasis
Reduced diaphragm movement and maximal force potential	Less effective respiratory movement; difficulty generating negative intrathoracic pressures; risk of atelectasis
Tendency to nose breathe; altered position of larynx and epiglottis	Enhanced ability to synchronize swallowing and breathing; risk of airway obstruction; possibly more difficult to intubate
Small compliant airway passages with higher airway resistance; immature reflexes	Risk of airway obstruction and apnea
Increased pulmonary vascular resistance with sensitive pulmonary arterioles	Risk of ductal shunting and hypoxemia with events such as hypoxia, acidosis, hypothermia, hypoglycemia, and hypercarbia
Increased oxygen consumption	Increased respiratory rate and work of breathing; risk of hypoxia
Increased intrapulmonary right-left shunting	Increased risk of atelectasis with wasted ventilation; lower P_{CO_2}
Immaturity of pulmonary surfactant system in immature infants	Increased risk of atelectasis and respiratory distress syndrome; increased work of breathing
Immature respiratory control	Irregular respirations with periodic breathing; risk of apnea; inability to rapidly alter depth of respirations

P_{CO_2}, Partial pressure of carbon dioxide.
From Blackburn S: *Maternal, fetal, and neonatal physiology: a clinical perspective*, ed 4, St Louis, 2013, Saunders.

Signs of Respiratory Distress

Signs of respiratory distress can include nasal flaring, intercostal or subcostal retractions (in-drawing of tissue between the ribs or below the rib cage), or grunting with respirations. Suprasternal or subclavicular retractions with stridor or gasping most often represent an upper airway obstruction. Seesaw or paradoxical respirations (exaggerated rise in abdomen with respiration as the chest falls) instead of abdominal respirations are abnormal and should be reported. A respiratory rate of less than 30 or greater than 60 breaths/min with the infant at rest must be evaluated. The respiratory rate of the infant can be slowed, depressed, or absent as a result of the effects of analgesics or anesthetics administered to the mother during labor and birth. Apneic episodes can be related to several events (rapid increase in body temperature, hypothermia, hypoglycemia, or sepsis) that require thorough evaluation. Tachypnea can result from inadequate clearance of lung fluid, or it can be an indication of newborn respiratory distress syndrome (RDS).

Changes in the infant's color can indicate respiratory distress. Acrocyanosis, the bluish discoloration of hands and feet, is a normal finding in the first 24 hours after birth. Transient periods of duskiness while crying are not uncommon immediately after birth; however, central cyanosis is abnormal and signifies hypoxemia. With central cyanosis the lips and mucous membranes are bluish. It can be the result of inadequate delivery of oxygen to the alveoli, poor perfusion of the lungs that inhibits gas exchange, or cardiac dysfunction. Because central cyanosis is a late sign of distress, newborns usually have significant hypoxemia when cyanosis appears (Askin, 2009).

Infants who experience mild TTNB often have signs of respiratory distress during the first 1 to 2 hours after birth as they transition to extrauterine life. Tachypnea with rates up to 100 breaths/min can be present along with intermittent grunting, nasal flaring, and mild retractions. Supplemental oxygen may be needed.

In neonates with more serious respiratory problems, symptoms of distress are more pronounced and tend to last beyond the first 2 hours after birth. Respiratory rates can exceed 120 breaths/min. Moderate-to-severe retractions, grunting, pallor, and central cyanosis can occur. The respiratory symptoms can be accompanied by hypotension, temperature instability, hypoglycemia, acidosis, and signs of cardiac problems. Common respiratory complications affecting neonates include RDS, meconium aspiration, pneumonia, and persistent pulmonary hypertension of the newborn (PPHN) (Askin, 2009) (see Chapter 25.)

Cardiovascular System

The cardiovascular system changes significantly after birth. The infant's first breaths, combined with increased alveolar capillary distention, inflate the lungs and reduce pulmonary vascular resistance to pulmonary blood flow from the pulmonary arteries. Pulmonary artery pressure drops, and pressure in the right atrium declines. Increased pulmonary blood flow from the left side of the heart increases pressure in the left atrium, which causes a functional closure of the foramen ovale. During the first few days of life crying may temporarily reverse the flow through the foramen ovale and lead to mild cyanosis.

In utero fetal P_{O_2} is 20 to 30 mm Hg. After birth, when the P_{O_2} level in the arterial blood approximates 50 mm Hg, the ductus arteriosus constricts in response to increased oxygenation. Circulating hormone prostaglandin E (PGE_2) levels also have an important role in closure of the ductus arteriosus. In term infants it functionally closes within the first hours after birth; permanent closure usually occurs within 3 to 4 weeks, and the ductus arteriosus becomes a ligament. The ductus arteriosus can open in response to low oxygen levels in association with hypoxia, asphyxia, or prematurity. With auscultation of the chest a patent ductus arteriosus can be detected as a heart murmur.

The umbilical vein and arteries constrict rapidly within the first 2 minutes after birth. It is thought that this is related to exposure of the cord to the cooler extrauterine environment and to increased oxygenation as the infant begins to breathe. With the clamping and severing of the cord, the umbilical arteries, the umbilical vein, and the ductus venosus are functionally closed; they are converted into

TABLE 22-2   CARDIOVASCULAR CHANGES AT BIRTH

PRENATAL STATUS	POSTBIRTH STATUS	ASSOCIATED FACTORS
Primary Changes		
Pulmonary circulation: High pulmonary vascular resistance, increased pressure in right ventricle and pulmonary arteries	Low pulmonary vascular resistance; decreased pressure in right atrium, ventricle, and pulmonary arteries	Expansion of collapsed fetal lung with air
Systemic circulation: Low pressures in left atrium, ventricle, and aorta	High systemic vascular resistance; increased pressure in left atrium, ventricle, and aorta	Loss of placental blood flow
Secondary Changes		
Umbilical arteries: Patent, carrying of blood from hypogastric arteries to placenta	Functionally closed at birth; obliteration by fibrous proliferation possibly taking 2 to 3 months, distal portions becoming lateral vesicoumbilical ligaments, proximal portions remaining open as superior vesicle arteries	Closure preceding that of umbilical vein, probably accomplished by smooth muscle contraction in response to thermal and mechanical stimuli and alteration in oxygen tension Mechanically severed with cord at birth
Umbilical vein: Patent, carrying of blood from placenta to ductus venosus and liver	Closed; becoming ligamentum teres hepatis after obliteration	Closure shortly after umbilical arteries; hence blood from placenta possibly entering neonate for short period after birth Mechanically severed with cord at birth
Ductus venosus: Patent, connection of umbilical vein to inferior vena cava	Closed; becoming ligamentum venosum after obliteration	Loss of blood flow from umbilical vein
Ductus arteriosus: Patent, shunting of blood from pulmonary artery to descending aorta	Functionally closed almost immediately after birth; anatomic obliteration of lumen by fibrous proliferation requiring 1 to 3 months, becoming ligamentum arteriosum	Increased oxygen content of blood in ductus arteriosus creating vasospasm of its muscular wall High systemic resistance increasing aortic pressure; low pulmonary resistance reducing pulmonary arterial pressure
Foramen ovale: Formation of a valve opening that allows blood to flow directly to left atrium (shunting of blood from right to left atrium)	Functionally closed at birth; constant apposition gradually leading to fusion and permanent closure within a few months or years in majority of persons	Increased pressure in left atrium and decreased pressure in right atrium, causing closure of valve over foramen

Data from Blackburn S: *Maternal, fetal, and neonatal physiology: a clinical perspective,* ed 4, St Louis, 2013, Saunders.

ligaments within 2 to 3 months. The hypogastric arteries also occlude and become ligaments. Table 22-2 summarizes the cardiovascular changes at birth.

Heart Rate and Sounds

The heart rate for a term newborn ranges from 120 to 160 beats/min, with brief fluctuations above and below these values usually noted during sleeping and waking states (Blackburn, 2013). The range of the heart rate in the term infant is about 85 to 100 beats/min during deep sleep and can increase to 180 beats/min or higher when the infant cries. A heart rate that is either high (more than 160 beats/min) or low (fewer than 100 beats/min) should be reevaluated within 30 minutes to 1 hour or when the activity of the infant changes. Immediately after birth the heart rate can be palpated by grasping the base of the umbilical cord.

The apical impulse (point of maximal impulse [PMI]) in the newborn is at the fourth intercostal space and to the left of the midclavicular line. The PMI is often visible and easily palpable because of the thin chest wall; this is also called *precordial activity.*

Apical pulse rates should be determined for all infants. Auscultation should be for a full minute, preferably when the infant is asleep. An irregular heart rate in newborns is not uncommon in the first few hours of life. After this time an irregular heart rate not attributed to changes in activity or respiratory pattern should be evaluated. Heart sounds during the neonatal period are of higher pitch, shorter duration, and greater intensity than during adult life. The first sound (S_1) is typically louder and duller than the second sound (S_2), which is sharp. The third and fourth heart sounds are not auscultated in newborns. Most heart murmurs heard during the neonatal period have no pathologic significance, and more than half of the murmurs disappear by 6 months. However, the presence of a murmur and accompanying signs such as poor feeding, apnea, cyanosis, or pallor are considered abnormal and should be investigated. There can be significant cardiac defects without symptoms in the early newborn period. This reinforces the importance of ongoing assessment (Sadowski, 2010).

Blood Pressure

Values for newborn BP vary with gestational age and weight. The term newborn infant's average systolic BP is 60 to 80 mm Hg, and average diastolic BP is 40 to 50 mm Hg. The mean arterial pressure (MAP) should be equivalent to the weeks of gestation. For example, an infant born at 40 weeks of gestation should have a MAP of at least 40. The BP increases by the second day of life, with minor variations noted during the first month of life. A drop in systolic BP (about 15 mm Hg) in the first hour of life is common. Crying and movement usually cause increases in the systolic BP. The measurement of BP is best accomplished with an oscillometric device while the infant is at rest. A correctly sized cuff must be used for accurate measurement of an infant's BP.

Policies on routine assessment of neonatal BP vary. In many agencies, unless a specific indication exists, BP is not measured in the newborn on a routine basis except as a baseline. In some institutions nurses obtain four extremity BPs in the presence of any cardiovascular symptoms such as tachycardia, murmur, abnormal pulses, poor perfusion, or abnormal precordial activity. If the systolic pressure is more than 10 mm Hg higher in the upper extremities than in the lower extremities, further diagnostic testing may be needed (Kenney, Hoover, Williams, et al., 2011).

Blood Volume

Blood volume in the term newborn ranges from 80 to 100 mL/kg of body weight. Immediately after birth the total blood volume averages 300 mL, but this volume can increase by as much as 100 mL, depending on the length of time to cord clamping and cutting. The infant born prematurely has a relatively greater blood volume than the term newborn. This occurs because the preterm infant has a proportionately greater plasma volume, not a greater red blood cell (RBC) mass.

Early or delayed clamping of the umbilical cord changes the circulatory dynamics of the newborn. Delayed clamping expands the blood volume from the so-called placental transfusion of blood to the newborn. Delayed cord clamping (≥2 minutes after birth) has been reported to be beneficial in improving hematocrit and iron status and decreasing anemia; such benefits can last up to 6 months (Andersson, Hellström-Westas, Andersson, et al., 2011; Arca, Botet, Palacio, et al., 2010). Polycythemia that occurs with delayed clamping is usually not harmful, although there can be an increased risk of jaundice that requires phototherapy.

Signs of Cardiovascular Problems

Close monitoring of the infant's vital signs is important for early detection of impending problems. Persistent tachycardia (more than 160 beats/min) can be associated with anemia, hypovolemia, hyperthermia, or sepsis. Persistent bradycardia (less than 100 beats/min) can be a sign of a congenital heart block or hypoxemia.

The newborn's skin color can reflect cardiovascular problems. Pallor in the immediate post birth period is often symptomatic of underlying problems such as anemia or marked peripheral vasoconstriction as a result of intrapartum asphyxia or sepsis. Any prolonged cyanosis other than in the hands or feet can indicate respiratory and/or cardiac problems. The presence of jaundice can indicate ABO or Rh factor incompatibility problems (see Chapter 25).

Congenital heart defects are the most common type of congenital malformations (see Chapter 36). Although the more serious defects such as tetralogy of Fallot are likely to have clinical manifestations such as cyanosis, dyspnea, and hypoxia, others such as small ventricular septal defects can be asymptomatic. The prenatal history can provide information regarding risk factors for congenital heart defects so the nurse knows to be more alert for symptoms. Maternal illness such as rubella, metabolic disease such as diabetes, and drug ingestion are associated with an increased risk of cardiac defects.

Hematopoietic System

The hematopoietic system of the newborn exhibits certain variations from that of the adult. Levels of RBCs and leukocytes differ, but platelets levels are relatively the same.

Red Blood Cells and Hemoglobin

Because fetal circulation is less efficient at oxygen exchange than the lungs, the fetus needs additional RBCs for transport of oxygen in utero. Therefore at birth the average levels of RBCs, hemoglobin, and hematocrit are higher than those in the adult; these levels fall slowly over the first month. At birth the RBC count ranges from 4.6 to 5.2 million/mm³ (Blackburn, 2013). The term newborn can have a hemoglobin concentration of 13.7 to 20.1 g/dL at birth, decreasing gradually to 12 to 20 g/dL during the first 2 weeks (Pagana and Pagana, 2009). Hematocrit levels at birth range from 51% to 56%, increase slightly in the first few hours or days as fluid shifts from intravascular to interstitial spaces (Blackburn, 2013), and by 8 weeks are between 39% and 59% (Pagana and Pagana, 2009). Polycythemia (central venous hematocrit greater than 65%) can occur in term and preterm infants as a result of delayed cord clamping, maternal hypertension or diabetes, or intrauterine growth restriction.

The source of the sample is a significant factor in levels of RBCs, hemoglobin, and hematocrit because capillary blood yields higher values than venous blood. The timing of blood sampling is also significant; the slight rise in RBCs after birth is followed by a substantial drop. At birth the infant's blood contains an average of 70% fetal hemoglobin; however, because of the shorter life span of the cells containing fetal hemoglobin, the percentage falls to 55% by 5 weeks and to 5% by 20 weeks. Iron stores generally are sufficient to sustain normal RBC production for 4 to 5 months in the term infant, at which time a transient physiologic anemia can occur.

Leukocytes

Leukocytosis, with a white blood cell (WBC) count of approximately 18,000/mm³ (range 9000 to 30,000/mm³), is normal at birth (Pagana and Pagana, 2009). The number of WBCs increases to 23,000 to 24,000/mm³ during the first day after birth. The initial high WBC count of the newborn decreases rapidly, and a stable level of 12,000/mm³ is normally maintained during the neonatal period. Serious infection is not tolerated well by the newborn; leukocytes are slow to recognize foreign protein and localize and fight infection early in life. Sepsis may be accompanied by a concomitant rise in neutrophils; however, some infants initially may be seen with clinical signs of sepsis without a significant elevation in WBCs. In addition, events other than infection (i.e., prolonged crying, maternal hypertension, asymptomatic hypoglycemia, hemolytic disease, meconium aspiration syndrome, labor induction with oxytocin, surgery, difficult labor, high altitude, and maternal fever) can cause neutrophilia in the newborn.

Platelets

Platelet count ranges between 150,000 and 300,000/mm³ and is essentially the same in newborns as in adults (Pagana and Pagana, 2009). The levels of factors II, VII, IX, and X found in the liver decrease during the first few days of life because the newborn cannot synthesize vitamin K. However, bleeding tendencies in the newborn are rare; and, unless the vitamin K deficiency is great, clotting is sufficient to prevent hemorrhage.

Blood Groups

The infant's blood group is determined genetically and established early in fetal life. However, during the neonatal period the strength of the agglutinogens present in the RBC membrane gradually increases. Cord blood samples may be used to identify the infant's blood type and Rh status.

Thermogenic System

Next to establishing respirations and adequate circulation, heat regulation is most critical to the newborn's survival. During the first 12 hours after birth the neonate attempts to achieve thermal balance in adjusting to the extrauterine environmental temperature. **Thermoregulation** is the maintenance of balance between heat loss and heat production. Newborns attempt to stabilize their core body temperatures within a narrow range. **Hypothermia** from excessive heat loss is a common and dangerous problem.

Anatomic and physiologic characteristics of neonates place them at risk for heat loss. Newborns have a thin layer of subcutaneous fat. The blood vessels are close to the surface of the skin. Changes in environmental temperature alter the temperature of the blood, thereby influencing temperature regulation centers in the hypothalamus. Newborns have larger body surface–to–body weight (mass) ratios than do children and adults (Blackburn, 2013).

Heat Loss

The body temperature of newborn infants depends on the heat transfer between the infant and the external environment. Factors that influence heat loss to the environment include the temperature and humidity of the air, the flow and velocity of the air, and the temperature of surfaces in contact with and around the infant. The goal of care is to maintain a neutral thermal environment for the neonate in which heat balance is maintained. The neutral thermal environment is the ideal environmental temperature that allows the neonate to maintain a normal body temperature to minimize oxygen and glucose consumption. Heat loss in the newborn occurs by four modes:

1. **Convection** is the flow of heat from the body surface to cooler ambient air. Because of heat loss by convection, the ambient temperature in the nursery is kept at approximately 24° C (75.2° F), and newborns in open bassinets are wrapped to protect them from the cold. A cap may be worn to decrease heat loss from the infant's head.
2. **Radiation** is the loss of heat from the body surface to a cooler solid surface not in direct contact but in relative proximity. To prevent this type of loss, cribs and examining tables are placed away from outside windows, and care is taken to avoid direct air drafts.
3. **Evaporation** is the loss of heat that occurs when a liquid is converted to a vapor. In the newborn heat loss by evaporation occurs as a result of vaporization of moisture from the skin. This heat loss is intensified by failing to dry the newborn directly after birth or by drying the infant too slowly after a bath. The less mature the newborn, the more severe the evaporative heat loss. Evaporative heat loss, as a component of insensible water loss, is the most significant cause of heat loss in the first few days of life.
4. **Conduction** is the loss of heat from the body surface to cooler surfaces in direct contact. When admitted to the nursery, the newborn is placed in a warmed crib to minimize heat loss. The scales used for weighing the newborn should have a protective cover to minimize conductive heat loss.

Loss of heat must be controlled to protect the infant. Control of such modes of heat loss is the basis of caregiving policies and techniques. One method for promoting thermoregulation and maternal-newborn interaction is to place the naked newborn on the mother's bare chest and cover both with a blanket (Fig. 22-1). This skin-to-skin contact reduces conductive and radiant heat loss and enhances newborn temperature control and maternal-infant interaction (Brown and Landers, 2011).

Thermogenesis

In response to cold the neonate attempts to generate heat (**thermogenesis**) by increasing muscle activity. Cold infants may cry and

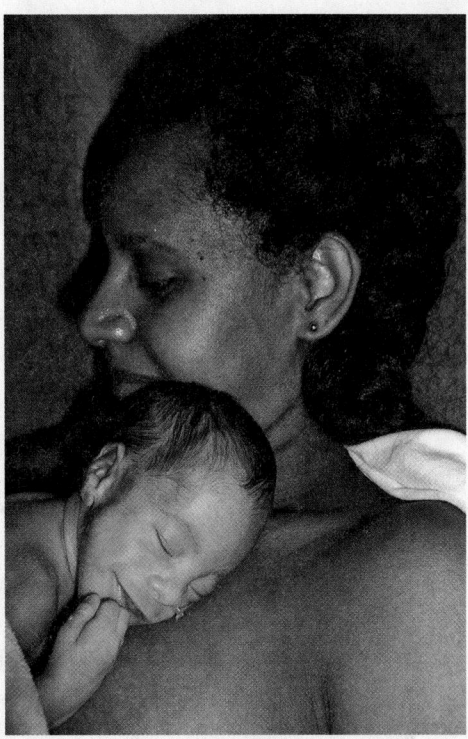

FIG 22-1 Infant in skin-to-skin contact with mother. (Courtesy Cheryl Briggs, RNC, Annapolis, MD.)

appear restless. Because of vasoconstriction the skin can feel cool to touch, and acrocyanosis can be present. There is an increase in cellular metabolic activity, primarily in the brain, heart, and liver; this also increases oxygen and glucose consumption.

In an effort to conserve heat, term newborns assume a position of flexion that helps guard against heat loss because it diminishes the amount of body surface exposed to the environment. Infants also can reduce the loss of internal heat through the body surface by constricting peripheral blood vessels.

Adults are able to produce heat through shivering; however, the shivering mechanism of heat production is rarely operable in the newborn unless there is prolonged cold exposure (Blackburn, 2013). Newborns produce heat through nonshivering thermogenesis. This is accomplished primarily by metabolism of brown fat, which is unique to the newborn; and secondarily by increased metabolic activity in the brain, heart, and liver. Brown fat is located in superficial deposits in the interscapular region and axillae and in deep deposits at the thoracic inlet, along the vertebral column, and around the kidneys. Brown fat has a richer vascular and nerve supply than ordinary fat. Heat produced by intense lipid metabolic activity in brown fat can warm the newborn by increasing heat production as much as 100%. Reserves of brown fat, usually present for several weeks after birth, are rapidly depleted with cold stress. The amount of brown fat reserve increases with the weeks of gestation. A full-term newborn has greater stores than a preterm infant.

Cold Stress

Cold stress imposes metabolic and physiologic demands on all infants, regardless of gestational age and condition. The respiratory rate increases in response to the increased need for oxygen. In the cold-stressed infant oxygen consumption and energy are diverted from maintaining normal brain and cardiac function and growth to thermogenesis for survival. If the infant cannot maintain an

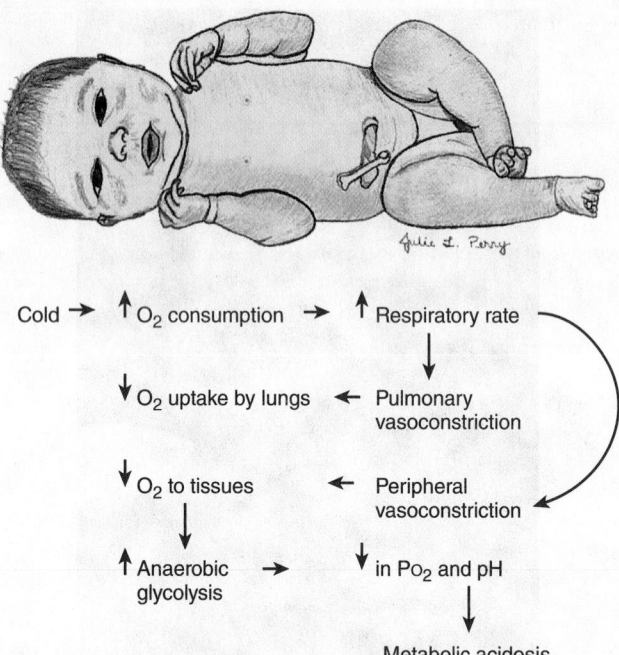

Cold → ↑ O₂ consumption → ↑ Respiratory rate

↓ O₂ uptake by lungs ← Pulmonary vasoconstriction

↓ O₂ to tissues ← Peripheral vasoconstriction

↑ Anaerobic glycolysis → ↓ in Po₂ and pH

Metabolic acidosis

FIG 22-2 Effects of cold stress. When an infant is stressed by cold, oxygen consumption increases, and pulmonary and peripheral vasoconstriction occur, thereby decreasing oxygen uptake by the lungs and oxygen to the tissues; anaerobic glycolysis increases; and there is a decrease in Po₂ and pH, leading to metabolic acidosis.

adequate oxygen tension, vasoconstriction follows and jeopardizes pulmonary perfusion. As a consequence the Po₂ is decreased, and the blood pH drops. These changes can prompt a transient respiratory distress or aggravate existing RDS. Moreover, decreased pulmonary perfusion and oxygen tension can maintain or reopen the right-to-left shunt across the ductus arteriosus.

The basal metabolic rate increases with cold stress. If cold stress is protracted, anaerobic glycolysis occurs, resulting in increased production of acids. Metabolic acidosis develops; and, if a defect in respiratory function is present, respiratory acidosis also develops (Fig. 22-2). Excessive fatty acids can displace the bilirubin from the albumin-binding sites and exacerbate hyperbilirubinemia.

Hypoglycemia is another metabolic consequence of cold stress. The process of anaerobic glycolysis uses approximately 3 to 4 times the amount of blood glucose, thereby depleting existing stores. If the infant is sufficiently stressed and low glucose stores are not replaced, hypoglycemia, which can be asymptomatic in the newborn, can develop.

Hyperthermia

Although occurring less frequently than hypothermia, hyperthermia can occur and must be corrected. A body temperature greater than 37.5° C (99.5° F) is considered to be abnormally high and is typically caused by excess heat production related to sepsis or a decrease in heat loss. Hyperthermia can result from the inappropriate use of external heat sources such as radiant warmers, phototherapy, sunlight, increased environmental temperature, and the use of excessive clothing or blankets (Brown and Landers, 2011). The clinical appearance of the infant who is hyperthermic often indicates the causative mechanism. Infants who are overheated because of environmental factors such as being swaddled in too many blankets exhibit signs of heat-losing mechanisms: skin vessels dilate, skin appears flushed,

hands and feet are warm to touch, and the infant assumes a posture of extension. The newborn who is hyperthermic because of sepsis appears stressed: vessels in the skin are constricted, color is pale, and hands and feet are cool. Hyperthermia develops more rapidly in a newborn than in an adult because of the relatively larger surface area of an infant. Sweat glands do not function well. Serious overheating of the newborn can cause cerebral damage from dehydration or even heat stroke and death (Brown and Landers, 2011).

Renal System

At term the kidneys occupy a large portion of the posterior abdominal wall. The bladder lies close to the anterior abdominal wall and is both an abdominal and a pelvic organ. In the newborn almost all palpable masses in the abdomen are renal in origin.

At birth a small quantity (approximately 40 mL) of urine is usually present in the bladder of a full-term infant. Many newborns void at the time of birth, although this is easily missed and may not be recorded. During the first few days term infants generally excrete 15 to 60 mL/kg; output gradually increases over the first month (Blackburn, 2013). The frequency of voiding varies from 2 to 6 times per day during the first and second days of life and from 5 to 25 times during the subsequent 24 hours. Approximately six to eight voidings per day of pale, straw-colored urine indicate adequate fluid intake.

> **! NURSING ALERT**
>
> Noting and recording the first voiding are important. An infant who has not voided by 24 hours should be assessed for adequacy of fluid intake, bladder distention, restlessness, and symptoms of pain. The pediatrician or neonatal nurse practitioner should be notified.

Full-term newborns have limited capacity to concentrate urine; therefore the specific gravity ranges from 1.001 to 1.020 (Pagana and Pagana, 2009). The ability to concentrate urine fully is attained by about 3 months of age. After the first voiding the infant's urine may appear cloudy (because of mucus content) and have a much higher specific gravity. This decreases as fluid intake increases. Normal urine during early infancy is usually straw colored and almost odorless. Sometimes pink-tinged uric acid crystal stains or "brick dust" appear on the diaper; these stains are normal, although they can be misinterpreted as blood. Loss of fluid through urine, feces, lungs, increased metabolic rate, and limited fluid intake results in a 5% to 10% loss of the birth weight. This usually occurs over the first 3 to 5 days of life. If the mother is breastfeeding and her milk supply has not come in yet (which occurs by the third or fourth day after birth), the neonate is somewhat protected from dehydration by its increased extracellular fluid volume. The neonate should regain the birth weight within 10 to 14 days, depending on the feeding method (breast or bottle).

Fluid and Electrolyte Balance

In the term neonate approximately 75% of body weight consists of total body water (extracellular and intracellular). A reduction in extracellular fluid occurs with diuresis during the first few days after birth. The weight loss experienced by most newborns during the first few days after birth is caused primarily by extracellular water loss (Dell, 2011).

The daily fluid requirement for neonates weighing more than 1500 g is 60 to 80 mL/kg during the first 2 days of life. From 3 to 7 days the requirement is 100 to 150 mL/kg/day; and from 8 to 30 days it is 120 to 180 mL/kg/day (Dell, 2011).

At birth the glomerular filtration rate (GFR) of a newborn is approximately 30% to 50% that of the adult. This results in a decreased ability to remove nitrogenous and other waste products from the blood. The GFR rapidly increases during the first month of life as a result of postnatal physiologic changes, including decreased renal vascular resistance, increased renal blood flow, and increased filtration pressure.

Sodium reabsorption is decreased as a result of a lowered sodium- or potassium-activated adenosine triphosphatase activity. The decreased ability to excrete excess sodium results in hypotonic urine compared with plasma, leading to a higher concentration of sodium, phosphates, chloride, and organic acids and a lower concentration of bicarbonate ions. The infant has a higher renal threshold for glucose than adults.

Bicarbonate concentration and buffering capacity are decreased. This can lead to acidosis and electrolyte imbalance.

Signs of Renal System Problems

The renal system has a wide range of functions. Dysfunction resulting from physiologic abnormalities can range from the lack of a steady stream of urine to gross anomalies such as hypospadias and exstrophy of the bladder, which can be identified easily at birth. Enlarged or cystic kidneys can be identified as masses during abdominal palpation. Some kidney anomalies also can be detected by ultrasound examination during pregnancy (see Chapter 25).

Gastrointestinal System

The full-term newborn is capable of swallowing, digesting, metabolizing and absorbing proteins and simple carbohydrates and emulsifying fats. With the exception of pancreatic amylase, the characteristic enzymes and digestive juices are present even in low-birth-weight neonates.

In the adequately hydrated infant the mucous membrane of the mouth is moist and pink; the hard and soft palates are intact. The presence of moderate-to-large amounts of mucus is common in the first few hours after birth. Small whitish areas (Epstein pearls) may be found on the gum margins and at the juncture of the hard and soft palates. The cheeks are full because of well-developed sucking pads. These, like the labial tubercles (sucking calluses) on the upper lip, disappear around the age of 12 months when the sucking period is over.

Sucking is a reflex behavior that begins in utero as early as 15 to 16 weeks. Sucking behavior is influenced by neuromuscular maturity, maternal medications received during labor and birth, and the type of initial feeding. As early as 28 weeks some infants can coordinate sucking and swallowing while breastfeeding. Bottle-feeding infants may not coordinate sucking and swallowing until 32 to 34 weeks. A special mechanism present in healthy term newborns coordinates the breathing, sucking, and swallowing reflexes necessary for oral feeding. This is well developed in most infants by 37 weeks (Gardner and Lawrence, 2011). Sucking takes place in small bursts of 3 or 4 and up to 8 to 10 sucks at a time, with a brief pause between bursts. The infant is unable to move food from the lips to the pharynx; therefore placing the nipple (breast or bottle) well inside the baby's mouth is necessary. Peristaltic activity in the esophagus is uncoordinated in the first few days of life. It quickly becomes a coordinated pattern in healthy full-term infants, and they swallow easily.

Teeth begin developing in utero, with enamel formation continuing until about 10 years of age. Tooth development is influenced by neonatal or infant illnesses and medications and by illnesses of or medications taken by the mother during pregnancy. The fluoride level in the water supply also influences tooth development. Occasionally an infant may be born with one or more teeth. These natal teeth have poorly formed roots and as they loosen place the infant at risk of aspiration. Therefore they are usually extracted.

Bacteria are not present in the infant's gastrointestinal tract at birth. Soon after birth oral and anal orifices permit entrance of bacteria and air. Generally the highest bacterial concentration is found in the lower portion of the intestine, particularly in the large intestine. Normal colonic bacteria are established within the first week after birth; and normal intestinal flora help synthesize vitamin K, folate, and biotin. Bowel sounds can usually be heard shortly after birth.

The capacity of the newborn stomach varies widely, depending on the size of the infant, from less than 30 mL on day 1 to more than 90 mL on day 3. After birth the newborn stomach becomes increasingly more compliant and relaxed to accommodate larger volumes. Several factors such as time and volume of feedings or type and temperature of food may affect the emptying time. The cardiac sphincter and nervous control of the stomach are immature; thus some regurgitation may occur. Regurgitation during the first day or two of life can be decreased by avoiding overfeeding, and burping the infant and positioning him or her with the head slightly elevated.

Digestion

The infant's ability to digest carbohydrates, fats, and proteins is regulated by the presence of certain enzymes. Most of these enzymes are functional at birth except for pancreatic amylase and lipase. Amylase is produced by the salivary glands after approximately 3 months and by the pancreas at approximately 6 months of age. This enzyme is necessary to convert starch into maltose and occurs in high amounts in colostrum. The other exception is lipase, also secreted by the pancreas; it is necessary for the digestion of fat. Therefore the normal newborn is capable of digesting simple carbohydrates and proteins but has a limited ability to digest fats. Mammary lipase in human milk aids in digestion of fats by the neonate.

Lactase levels in newborns are higher than in older infants. This enzyme is necessary for digestion of lactose, the major carbohydrate in human milk and commercial infant formula.

Stools

Meconium fills the lower intestine at birth. It is formed during fetal life from the amniotic fluid and its constituents, intestinal secretions (including bilirubin), and cells (shed from the mucosa). Meconium is greenish black and viscous and contains occult blood. The first meconium passed is usually sterile, but within hours all meconium passed contains bacteria. Most healthy term infants pass meconium within the first 12 to 24 hours of life, and almost all do so by 48 hours. The number of stools passed varies during the first week, being most numerous between the third and sixth days. Newborns fed early pass stools sooner. Progressive changes in the stooling pattern indicate a properly functioning gastrointestinal tract (Box 22-1).

Feeding Behaviors

Variations occur among infants regarding interest in food, signs of hunger, and amount ingested at one time. The amount of food that the infant takes in at any feeding depends on the size, hunger level, and alertness of the infant. When put to breast some infants feed immediately, whereas others require a longer learning period. Random hand-to-mouth movement and sucking of fingers are well

BOX 22-1 CHANGES IN STOOLING PATTERNS OF NEWBORNS

Meconium
- The infant's first stool is composed of amniotic fluid and its constituents, intestinal secretions, shed mucosal cells, and possibly blood (ingested maternal blood or minor bleeding of alimentary tract vessels).
- Passage of meconium should occur within the first 24 to 48 hours, although it can be delayed up to 7 days in very low–birth-weight infants. The passage of meconium can occur in utero and can be a sign of fetal distress.

Transitional Stools
- Usually appear by third day after initiation of feeding
- Greenish brown to yellowish brown; thin and less sticky than meconium; may contain some milk curds

Milk Stool
- Usually appears by the fourth day
- *Breastfed infants:* Stools yellow to golden, pasty in consistency; resemble a mixture of mustard and cottage cheese, with an odor similar to sour milk
- *Formula-fed infants:* Stools pale yellow to light brown, firmer consistency, with a more offensive odor

developed at birth and intensify when the infant is hungry. Caregivers should be alert and responsive to these hunger cues (Lawrence and Lawrence, 2011).

Signs of Gastrointestinal Problems

The time, color, and character of the infant's first stool should be noted. Failure to pass meconium can indicate bowel obstruction related to conditions such as an inborn error of metabolism (e.g., cystic fibrosis) or a congenital disorder (e.g., Hirschsprung's disease or an imperforate anus). An active rectal "wink" reflex (contraction of the anal sphincter muscle in response to touch) is a sign of good sphincter tone.

Fullness of the abdomen above the umbilicus can be caused by problems such as hepatomegaly, duodenal atresia, or distention. Abdominal distention at birth usually indicates a serious disorder such as a ruptured viscus (from abdominal wall defects) or tumors. Distention that occurs later can be the result of overfeeding or signal gastrointestinal disorders. A scaphoid (sunken) abdomen, with bowel sounds heard in the chest and signs of respiratory distress, indicate a diaphragmatic hernia. Fullness below the umbilicus can indicate a distended bladder.

Some infants are intolerant of certain commercial infant formulas. If an infant is allergic or unable to digest a formula, the stools can become very soft with a high water content that is signaled by a distinct water ring around the stool on the diaper. Forceful ejection of stool and a water ring around the stool are signs of diarrhea. Care must be taken to avoid misinterpreting transitional stools for diarrhea. The loss of fluid in diarrhea can rapidly lead to fluid and electrolyte imbalance. Passage of meconium from the vagina or urinary meatus is a sign of a possible fistulous tract from the rectum.

The amount and frequency of regurgitation ("spitting up") after feedings should be documented. Color change, gagging, and projectile (very forceful) vomiting occur in association with esophageal and tracheoesophageal anomalies.

Hepatic System

The liver and gallbladder are formed by the fourth week of gestation. In the newborn the liver can be palpated about 1 to 2 cm below the right costal margin because it is enlarged and occupies about 40% of the abdominal cavity. The infant's liver plays an important role in iron storage, carbohydrate metabolism, conjugation of bilirubin, and coagulation.

Iron Storage

The fetal liver, which serves as the site for production of hemoglobin after birth, begins storing iron in utero. The infant's iron store is proportional to total body hemoglobin content and length of gestation. At birth the term infant has an iron store sufficient to last 4 to 6 months. Iron stores of preterm and small-for–gestational age infants are often lower and are depleted sooner than in healthy term infants. Although both breast milk and cow's milk contain iron, the bioavailability of iron in breast milk is far superior.

The American Academy of Pediatrics (AAP) recommends that breastfed infants should receive a daily oral iron supplement (1 mg/kg) beginning at 4 months until feeding includes iron-fortified cereal or other foods fortified with iron. Formula-fed infants should receive a formula that contains supplemental iron (Baker, Greer, and the Committee on Nutrition, 2010).

Carbohydrate Metabolism

In utero the glucose concentration in the umbilical vein is approximately 80% of the maternal level. At birth the newborn is cut off from its maternal glucose supply and as a result experiences an initial decrease in serum glucose levels. Glucose levels reach a low point between 30 and 90 minutes after birth and then rise gradually. In most healthy term newborns blood glucose levels stabilize at 50 to 60 mg/dL during the first several hours after birth. Within the first week they should be approximately 60 to 80 mg/dL (Kalhan and Devaskar, 2011).

The initiation of feedings helps to stabilize the newborn's blood glucose levels. In general blood glucose levels less than 40 mg/dL are considered abnormal and warrant intervention. The hypoglycemic infant can display the classic symptoms of jitteriness, lethargy, apnea, feeding problems, or seizures; or the infant can be asymptomatic. Hypoglycemia in the initial newborn period is most often transient and easily corrected through feeding. Persistent or recurrent hypoglycemia necessitates intravenous glucose therapy and possible pharmacologic intervention.

Conjugation of Bilirubin and Newborn Jaundice

Jaundice, the visible yellowish color of the skin and sclera, is caused by elevated serum levels of unconjugated (indirect) bilirubin. The liver is responsible for the conjugation of bilirubin, which results from the breakdown of RBCs. When RBCs reach the end of their life span, their membranes rupture, and hemoglobin is released. The hemoglobin is phagocytosed by macrophages; it then splits into heme and globin. The heme is broken down by the reticuloendothelial cells, converted to bilirubin, and released in an unconjugated form. The unconjugated (indirect) bilirubin is relatively insoluble and almost entirely bound to circulating albumin, a plasma protein. Bilirubin that is not bound to albumin, or free bilirubin, can easily cross the blood-brain barrier and cause neurotoxicity.

The unconjugated bilirubin must be conjugated so it becomes soluble and excretable. In the liver the unbound bilirubin is conjugated with glucuronic acid in the presence of the enzyme glucuronyl transferase. The conjugated form of bilirubin (direct bilirubin) is soluble and excreted from liver cells as a constituent of bile. Along

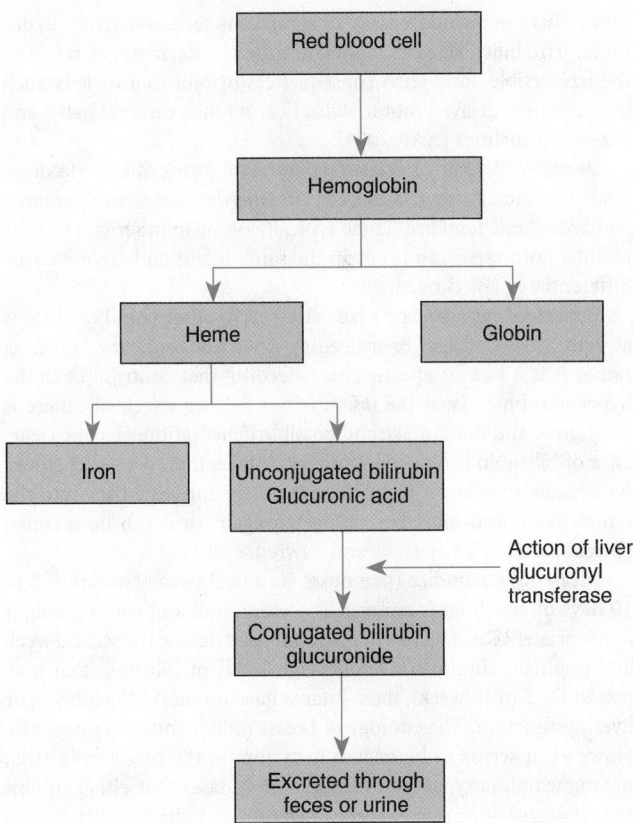

FIG 22-3 Formation and excretion of bilirubin.

with other components of bile, direct bilirubin is excreted into the biliary tract system that carries the bile into the duodenum. Bilirubin is converted to urobilinogen and stercobilinogen within the duodenum through the action of the bacterial flora. Urobilinogen is excreted in urine and feces; stercobilinogen is excreted in the feces. The effectiveness of bilirubin excretion through the feces depends on the stooling pattern of the newborn and the substances in the intestine that break down conjugated bilirubin. In the newborn intestine the enzyme β-glucuronidase is able to convert conjugated bilirubin into the unconjugated form, which is subsequently reabsorbed by the intestinal mucosa and transported to the liver; this is called *enterohepatic circulation.* Feeding is important in reducing serum bilirubin levels because it stimulates peristalsis and produces more rapid passage of meconium, thus diminishing the amount of reabsorption of unconjugated bilirubin. Feeding also introduces bacteria to aid in the reduction of bilirubin to urobilinogen. Colostrum, a natural laxative, facilitates the passage of meconium (Fig. 22-3).

When levels of unconjugated bilirubin exceed the ability of the liver to conjugate it, plasma levels of bilirubin increase, and jaundice appears. Jaundice is generally noticeable first in the head, especially in the sclera and mucous membranes, and progresses gradually to the thorax, abdomen, and extremities. The degree of jaundice is determined by serum total bilirubin measurements. Jaundice is likely to appear when bilirubin levels exceed 5 to 6 mg/dL (Blackburn, 2013).

The newborn is at risk for hyperbilirubinemia because of distinctive aspects of normal neonatal physiology. The higher RBC mass at birth and shorter life span of neonatal RBCs mean that there is the need for greater bilirubin synthesis. The ability of the liver to conjugate bilirubin is reduced during the first few days after birth; it can metabolize and excrete only about two thirds of the circulating bilirubin. In addition, there are fewer bilirubin binding sites because newborns have lower serum albumin levels. In the intestines conjugated bilirubin becomes unconjugated and recirculated through the enterohepatic circulation, which increases serum bilirubin levels (Blackburn, 2013).

Traditionally newborn jaundice has been categorized as either *physiologic* or *pathologic* (nonphysiologic), depending primarily on the time it appears and on serum bilirubin levels. Controversy surrounds the definitions of normal or physiologic ranges of total serum bilirubin. Total serum bilirubin levels in newborns are affected by variables such as length of gestation, age, weight, race, nutritional status, and mode of feeding (Blackburn, 2013). The time of onset of jaundice is a key factor in evaluating its cause and determining if treatment is needed. *Early-onset jaundice* is usually related to increased bilirubin production; *late-onset jaundice* is most often related to delayed elimination of bilirubin, with or without increased production (Kamath, Thilo, and Hernandez, 2011). Table 22-3 lists the varying causes of neonatal hyperbilirubinemia.

Among the factors that increase the risk of hyperbilirubinemia, prematurity is the most significant. Prematurity affects liver and brain metabolism and albumin binding sites, placing preterm and late preterm infants at greater risk for hyperbilirubinemia. Infants of Asian and Native American ethnicity have higher bilirubin levels. Breastfeeding infants are at greater risk of hyperbilirubinemia (see later discussion).

Although there is no consistent definition for neonatal hyperbilirubinemia, Kaplan, Wong, and Sibley (2011) define unconjugated hyperbilirubinemia as indirect bilirubin greater than 20 mg/dl. Conjugated hyperbilirubinemia is rare; it is defined as direct bilirubin levels greater than 1.5 mg/dL (Kaplan, Wong, and Sibley, 2011).

Physiologic Jaundice. Physiologic or nonpathologic jaundice occurs in approximately 60% of newborn infants born at term and 80% of preterm infants (Kaplan, Wong, and Sibley, 2011). It appears after 24 hours of age and usually resolves without treatment.

Two phases of physiologic jaundice have been identified in full-term infants. In the first phase bilirubin levels of Caucasian and African-American infants gradually increase to approximately 5 to 6 mg/dL by 72 to 96 hours of life and decrease to a plateau of 2 to 3 mg/dL by the fifth day. In Asian and Asian-American infants bilirubin levels peak between 72 and 120 hours of age and gradually fall to 2 to 3 mg/dL by the seventh to tenth days. In the second phase of physiologic jaundice bilirubin levels gradually decrease between 5 and 10 days of life, reaching normal adult levels of 2 mg/dL or less by 14 days. This pattern varies according to racial group, method of feeding (breast versus bottle), and gestational age. In preterm formula-fed infants serum bilirubin levels can peak as high as 10 to 12 mg/dL at 5 to 6 days of life and decrease slowly over a period of 2 to 4 weeks (Kaplan, Wong, and Sibley 2011).

> **⚠ NURSING ALERT**
>
> The appearance of jaundice during the first 24 hours of life or persistence beyond the ages previously delineated usually indicates a potential pathologic process that requires investigation.

Pathologic Jaundice. Although physiologic jaundice is usually considered benign, unconjugated bilirubin (indirect) can accumulate to hazardous levels and lead to a pathologic condition. Pathologic or nonphysiologic jaundice is unconjugated hyperbilirubinemia

TABLE 22-3	CAUSES OF NEONATAL UNCONJUGATED (INDIRECT) HYPERBILIRUBINEMIA
BASIS	**CAUSES**
Increased Production of Bilirubin	
Increased hemoglobin destruction	Fetomaternal blood group incompatibility (Rh, ABO)
	Congenital red blood cell abnormalities
	Congenital enzyme deficiencies (G6PD, galactosemia)
	Enclosed hemorrhage (cephalhematoma, bruising)
	Sepsis
Increased amount of hemoglobin	Polycythemia (maternal-fetal or twin-twin transfusion, SGA)
	Delayed cord clamping
Increased enterohepatic circulation	Delayed passage of meconium, meconium ileus, or plug
	Fasting or delayed initiation of feeding
	Intestinal atresia or stenosis
Altered Hepatic Clearance of Bilirubin	
Alteration in uridine diphosphate glucuronyl transferase production or activity	Immaturity
	Metabolic/endocrine disorders (e.g., Crigler-Najjar disease, hypothyroidism, disorders of amino acid metabolism)
Alteration in hepatic function and perfusion (and thus conjugating ability)	Asphyxia, hypoxia, hypothermia, hypoglycemia
	Sepsis (also causes inflammation)
	Drugs and hormones (e.g., novobiocin, pregnanediol)
Hepatic obstruction (associated with direct hyperbilirubinemia)	Congenital anomalies (biliary atresia, cystic fibrosis)
	Biliary stasis (hepatitis, sepsis)
	Excessive bilirubin load (often seen with severe hemolysis)

From Blackburn S: *Maternal, fetal, and neonatal physiology: a clinical perspective*, ed 4, St Louis, 2013, Saunders.
G6PD, Glucose-6-phosphate dehydrogenase; *SGA*, small for gestational age.

that is either pathologic in origin or severe enough to warrant further evaluation and treatment (see Chapter 23). Jaundice is usually considered pathologic or nonphysiologic if it appears within 24 hours of birth, if total serum bilirubin levels increase by more than 6 mg/dL in 24 hours, and if the serum bilirubin level exceeds 15 mg/dL at any time (Blackburn, 2013). High levels of unconjugated bilirubin are usually caused by excessive production of bilirubin through hemolysis. Hemolytic disease of the newborn caused by maternal/newborn blood group incompatibility is the most common cause of hyperbilirubinemia. It can also be caused by glucose-6-phosphate dehydrogenase (G6PD) deficiency, a genetic disorder that is more common among Asian and Native American populations. Other causes are listed in Table 22-3.

If increased levels of unconjugated bilirubin are left untreated, neurotoxicity can result as bilirubin is transferred into the brain cells. Acute bilirubin encephalopathy refers to the acute manifestations of bilirubin toxicity that occur during the first weeks after birth. This can include a range of symptoms such as lethargy, hypotonia, irritability, seizures, coma, and death. Kernicterus refers to the irreversible, long-term consequences of bilirubin toxicity such as hypotonia, delayed motor skills, hearing loss, cerebral palsy, and gaze abnormalities (AAP, 2004).

Jaundice Related to Breastfeeding. Two forms of breastfeeding-related jaundice are recognized: *breastfeeding-associated jaundice* and *breast milk jaundice*. These typically occur in otherwise healthy infants. Both types can occur in the same infant and are not easily differentiated (Blackburn, 2013).

Breastfeeding-associated jaundice (early-onset jaundice) begins at 2 to 5 days of age. Breastfeeding does not cause the jaundice; rather it is a lack of effective breastfeeding that contributes to the hyperbilirubinemia. If the infant is not feeding effectively, there is less caloric and fluid intake and possible dehydration. Hepatic clearance of bilirubin is reduced. With less intake, there are fewer stools. As a result bilirubin is reabsorbed from the intestine back into the bloodstream and must be conjugated again so it can be excreted (Blackburn, 2013; Lawrence and Lawrence, 2011).

Breast-milk jaundice (late-onset jaundice) usually occurs at 5 to 10 days of age. Infants are usually feeding well and gaining weight appropriately. Rising levels of bilirubin peak during the second week and gradually diminish. Despite high levels of bilirubin that may persist for 3 to 12 weeks, these infants have no signs of hemolysis or liver dysfunction. The etiology of breast milk jaundice is uncertain. However, it seems to be related to factors in the breast milk (e.g., pregnanediol, fatty acids, and β-glucuronidase) that either inhibit the conjugation or decrease the excretion of bilirubin (Blackburn, 2013). (See Chapter 24 for a discussion of these conditions in relation to newborn nutrition.)

Coagulation

The liver plays an important role in blood coagulation. Coagulation factors, which are synthesized in the liver, are activated by vitamin K. The lack of intestinal bacteria needed to synthesize vitamin K results in transient blood coagulation deficiency between the second and fifth days of life. The levels of coagulation factors slowly increase to reach adult levels by age 9 months. The administration of intramuscular vitamin K shortly after birth helps prevent clotting problems. Any bleeding problems noted in the newborn should be reported immediately, and tests for clotting ordered (Manco-Johnson, Rodden, and Hays, 2011).

Signs of Hepatic System Problems

Preterm infants are at risk for hepatic system problems such as hyperbilirubinemia and hypoglycemia because of their immaturity. The hematologic status of all newborns should be assessed for anemia. Because infants can develop a coagulation deficiency, a male neonate who has been circumcised must be observed closely for signs of hemorrhage. Hemorrhage also can be caused by a clotting defect, indicating a serious problem such as hemophilia.

Immune System

Beginning early in gestation the immune system of the fetus is developing the capacity to respond to foreign antigens. The development of the immune system is necessary to equip the neonate to meet the numerous environmental challenges (e.g., microorganisms) associated with life in the extrauterine world.

At birth most of the circulating antibodies in the newborn are immunoglobulin (Ig) G antibodies that were transported across the placenta from the maternal circulation. IgG is key to immunity to bacteria and viruses. This transfer of antibodies from the mother begins as early as 14 weeks of gestation and is greatest during the third trimester. By term the IgG levels in the cord blood of the infant are higher than those in maternal blood. The passive immunity afforded the infant through the placental transfer of IgG usually provides sufficient antimicrobial protection during the first 3 months of life. Production of adult concentrations of IgG is reached by 4 to 6 years of age (Kapur, Yoder, and Polin, 2011).

The fetus is capable of producing IgM by the eighth week of gestation, and low levels are present at term (less than 10% of adult levels). IgM is important for immunity to bloodborne infections and is the major immunoglobulin synthesized during the first month. By the age of 2 years, IgM reaches adult levels. The production of IgA, IgD, and IgE is much more gradual; and maximal levels are not attained until early childhood (Kapur, Yoder, and Polin, 2011).

Natural barrier mechanisms such as the acidity of the stomach and the production of pepsin and trypsin, which maintain sterility of the small intestine, are not fully developed until ages 3 to 4 weeks.

The membrane-protective IgA is missing from the respiratory and urinary tracts; and, unless the newborn is breastfed, it also is absent from the gastrointestinal tract. Breast milk provides the newborn with important immunity. The secretory IgA in human milk acts locally in the intestines to neutralize bacterial and viral pathogens. It may also lessen the risk of allergy and food intolerance through modulation of exposure to foreign milk protein antigens.

The newborn is capable of producing a protective immune response to vaccines, given as early as a few hours after birth. For example, when hepatitis B vaccine is administered at birth to the infant born to a mother with hepatitis B, there is an excellent immune response. This holds true even if the infant does not receive additional hepatitis B Ig.

The WBCs of the newborn display a delayed response to invading bacteria. The influx of phagocytic cells to areas of inflammation is somewhat slowed, although the ability of these cells to attack and destroy bacteria is equivalent to that of adults (Kapur, Yoder, and Polin, 2011).

Risk for Infection

All newborns, and preterm newborns especially, are at high risk for infection during the first several months of life. During this period infection is one of the leading causes of morbidity and mortality. The newborn cannot limit the invading pathogen to the portal of entry because of the generalized hypofunctioning of the inflammatory and immune mechanisms.

Early signs of infection must be recognized so prompt diagnosis and treatment can occur. Temperature instability or hypothermia can be symptomatic of serious infection; newborns do not typically exhibit fever, although hyperthermia can occur (temperature greater than 38° C 100.4° F]). Lethargy, irritability, poor feeding, vomiting or diarrhea, decreased reflexes, and pale or mottled skin color are some of the clinical signs that suggest infection. Respiratory symptoms such as apnea, tachypnea, grunting, or retracting can be associated with infection such as pneumonia (Lott, 2010).

Any unusual discharge from the infant's eyes, nose, mouth, or other orifice must be investigated. If a rash appears, it must be evaluated closely; many normal rashes in the newborn are not associated with any infection. Infants must be protected from infections by the use of good hand hygiene techniques.

The greatest risk factor for neonatal infection is prematurity because of immaturity of the immune system. Other risk factors include premature rupture of membranes, chorioamnionitis, maternal fever, antenatal or intrapartal asphyxia, invasive procedures, stress, and congenital anomalies (Lott, 2010).

Integumentary System

All skin structures are present at birth. The epidermis and dermis are loosely bound and extremely thin. After 35 weeks of gestation the skin is covered by vernix caseosa (a cheeselike, whitish substance) that is fused with the epidermis and serves as a protective covering. Vernix caseosa is a complex substance that contains sebaceous gland secretions. It has emollient and antimicrobial properties and prevents fluid loss through the skin; it also has antioxidant properties. Removal of the vernix is followed by desquamation of the epidermis in most infants. There is evidence that leaving residual vernix intact after birth has positive benefits for neonatal skin such as decreasing the skin pH, decreasing skin erythema, and improving skin hydration (Visscher, Utturkar, Pickens, et al., 2011).

The term infant has erythematous (red) skin for a few hours after birth, after which it fades to its normal color. The skin often appears blotchy or mottled, especially over the extremities. The hands and feet appear slightly cyanotic (acrocyanosis); this is caused by vasomotor instability and capillary stasis. Acrocyanosis is normal and appears intermittently over the first 7 to 10 days, especially with exposure to cold (Fig. 22-4).

The healthy term infant usually has a plump appearance because of large amounts of subcutaneous tissue and extracellular water content. Subcutaneous fat accumulated during the last trimester acts as insulation. Fine lanugo hair may be noted over the face, shoulders, and back. Edema of the face and ecchymosis (bruising) or petechiae may be noted as a result of face presentation, forceps-assisted birth, or vacuum extraction.

Creases are located on the palms of the hands and the soles of the feet. The simian line, a single palmar crease, is often seen in Asian infants and infants with Down syndrome. The soles of the feet should be inspected for the number of creases during the first few hours after birth; as the skin dries, more creases appear. Increasing numbers of creases correlate with a greater maturity rating. Premature newborns have few if any creases.

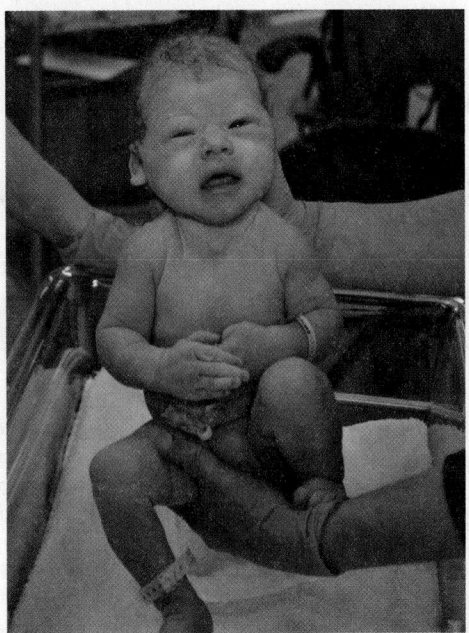

FIG 22-4 Newborn infant with acrocyanosis of upper and lower extremities. (Courtesy Barbara Wilson, West Jordan, UT.)

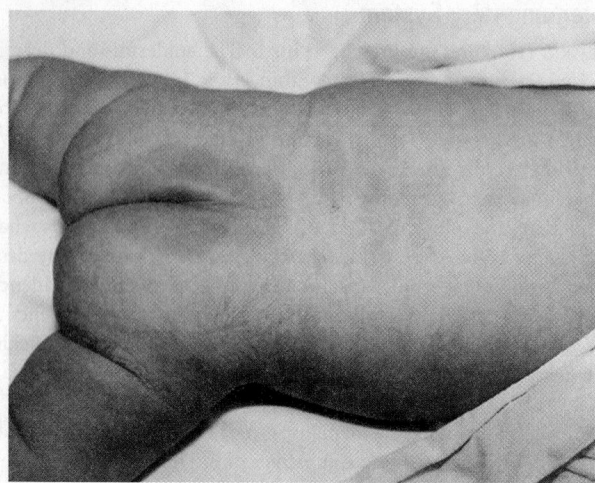

FIG 22-5 Mongolian spot.

Sweat Glands

Distended, small, white sebaceous glands noticeable on the newborn face are known as milia. Although sweat glands are present at birth, term infants usually do not sweat for the first 24 hours. By day 3 sweating begins on the face and later progresses to the palms. Infants can sweat as a function of body or environmental temperature; there can also be emotional sweating from crying or pain (Hoath and Narendran, 2011).

Desquamation

Desquamation (peeling) of the skin of the term infant does not occur until a few days after birth. Large generalized areas of skin desquamation present at birth may be an indication of postmaturity.

Mongolian Spots

Mongolian spots, bluish-black areas of pigmentation, may appear over any part of the exterior surface of the body, including the extremities. They are noted more commonly on the back and buttocks (Fig. 22-5). These pigmented areas occur most frequently in newborns whose ethnic origins are in the Mediterranean area, Latin America, Asia, or Africa. They are more common in dark-skinned individuals but may occur in 5% to 13% of Caucasians (Blackburn, 2013). They fade gradually over months or years.

> **! NURSING ALERT**
>
> The presence of any Mongolian spots on the newborn should be documented carefully in the medical record. These normal skin pigmentations can be mistaken for bruises once the infant is discharged, which can raise suspicion of physical abuse.

Nevi

Nevus simplex, also known as *salmon patches, telangiectatic nevi,* "*stork bites,*" or "*angel kisses*" are flat, pink capillary hemangiomas that are easily blanched (Fig. 22-6, *A*). They appear on the upper eyelids, nose, upper lip, lower occiput bone, and nape of the neck (Blackburn, 2013). They have no clinical significance and require no treatment. Facial lesions fade between the first and second years of life, whereas neck lesions can be visible into adulthood.

A port-wine stain, or nevus flammeus, is usually visible at birth and is composed of a plexus of newly formed capillaries in the papillary layer of the corium. It is red to purple; varies in size, shape, and

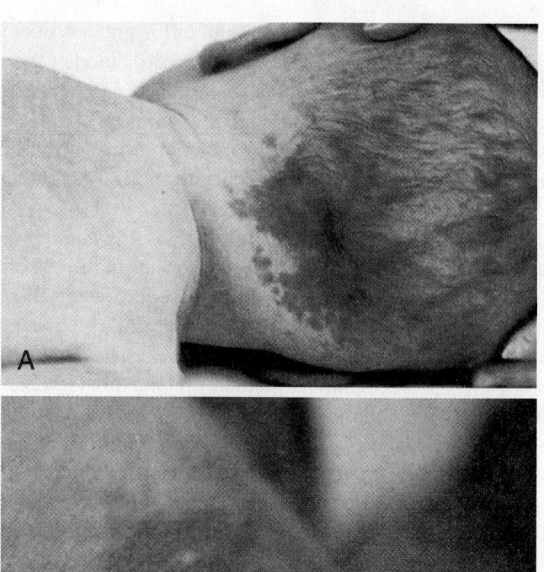

FIG 22-6 **A,** Nevus simplex or telangiectatic nevi (stork bite). **B,** Erythema toxicum. (Courtesy Mead Johnson & Co., Evansville, IN.)

location; and is not elevated. True port-wine stains do not blanch on pressure or disappear. They are found most commonly on the face and neck.

A *nevus vascularis,* or *strawberry hemangioma,* is a common type of capillary hemangioma. It consists of dilated, newly formed capillaries occupying the entire dermal and subdermal layers with associated connective tissue hypertrophy. The typical lesion is a raised, sharply demarcated, bright or dark red, rough-surfaced swelling, usually appearing on the head. These are rarely seen at birth, although 90% become visible in the neonatal period. Strawberry hemangiomas tend to grow rapidly during the first years and usually fade or shrink with time (Habif, 2009).

Erythema Toxicum

Erythema toxicum, a transient rash, is also called *erythema neonatorum, newborn rash,* or *flea bite dermatitis.* It first appears in term neonates during the first 24 to 72 hours after birth and can last up to 3 weeks of age (Blackburn, 2013). It has lesions in different stages: erythematous macules, papules, and small vesicles (see Fig. 22-6, *B*). The lesions may appear suddenly anywhere on the body. The rash is thought to be an inflammatory response. Eosinophils, which help decrease inflammation, are found in the vesicles. Although the appearance is alarming, the rash has no clinical significance and requires no treatment (see Family-Centered Care box).

Signs of Integumentary Problems

Close observation of the newborn's skin color can lead to early detection of potential problems. Any pallor, plethora (deep purplish color from increased circulating RBCs), petechiae, central cyanosis, or jaundice should be noted and described. The skin should be

Newborn Skin

A young couple with a healthy newborn girl calls the nurse because they are concerned about the small raised red dots on the baby's face and arms and that her skin is dry and flaky in certain places. The nurse assesses the newborn and concludes that the spots are not mosquito bites, as the family stated, but erythema toxicum. What further anticipatory guidance about normal newborn skin appearance could the nurse give the parents to reassure them that the newborn is healthy and "normal?"

examined for signs of birth injuries such as forceps marks and lesions related to fetal monitoring. Bruises or petechiae may be present on the head, neck, and face of an infant born with a nuchal cord (cord around the neck) or in an infant who had a face presentation at birth. Bruising can increase the risk of hyperbilirubinemia. Petechiae can be present if increased pressure was applied to an area. Petechiae scattered over the infant's body should be reported to the physician or nurse practitioner because their presence can indicate underlying problems such as low platelet count or infection. Unilateral or bilateral periauricular papillomas (skin tags) occur fairly frequently. Their occurrence is usually a family trait and of no consequence.

Reproductive System
Female

At birth the ovaries contain thousands of primitive germ cells. These represent the full complement of potential ova; no oogonia form after birth in term infants. The ovarian cortex, which is composed primarily of primordial follicles, occupies a larger portion of the ovary in the female newborn than in the adult. From birth to sexual maturity the number of ova decreases by approximately 90%.

An increase in estrogen during pregnancy followed by a drop after birth results in a mucoid vaginal discharge and even some slight bloody spotting (pseudomenstruation). External genitalia (i.e., labia majora and minora) are usually edematous with increased pigmentation. In term neonates the labia majora and minora cover the vestibule (Fig. 22-7, *A*). In preterm infants the clitoris is prominent, and the labia majora are small and widely separated. Vaginal or hymenal tags are common findings and have no clinical significance. Vernix caseosa may be present between the labia and should not be forcibly removed during bathing.

If the girl was born in the breech position, the labia may be edematous and bruised. The edema and bruising resolve in a few days; no treatment is necessary.

Male

In the uncircumcised newborn the foreskin or prepuce completely covers the glans. The foreskin adheres to the glans and is not fully retractable for 3 to 4 years. The position of the urethra should be at the tip of the penis. With **Nevus simplex,** or **epispadias** the urethral opening is located in an abnormal position, on or adjacent to the glans, although it can be placed on the penile shaft or perineum. Small, white, firm lesions called *epithelial pearls* may be seen at the tip of the prepuce.

By 28 to 36 weeks of gestation the testes can be palpated in the inguinal canal, and a few rugae appear on the scrotum. At 36 to 40 weeks of gestation the testes are palpable in the upper scrotum, and rugae appear on the anterior portion. After 40 weeks the testes can be palpated in the scrotum, and rugae cover the scrotal sac. The postterm neonate has deep rugae and a pendulous scrotum. The

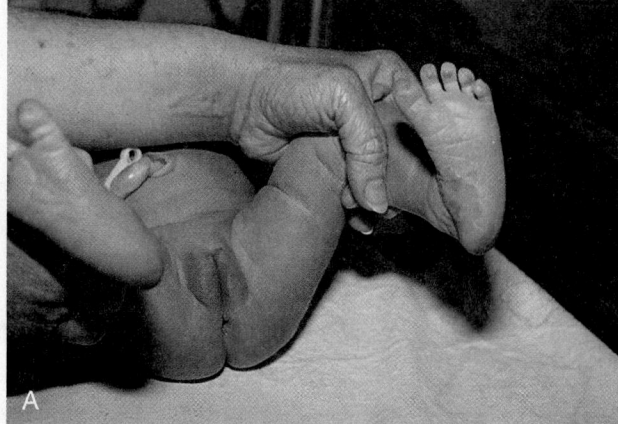

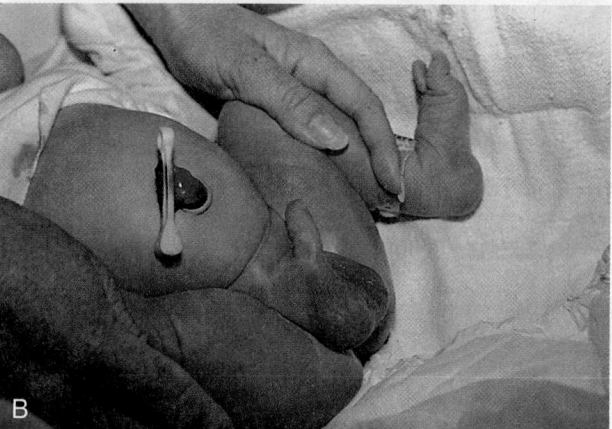

FIG 22-7 External genitalia. **A,** Genitalia in female term infant. **B,** Genitalia in uncircumcised male infant. Rugae cover scrotum, indicating term gestation. Cord has been swabbed with ethylene blue to prevent infection. (Courtesy Marjorie Pyle, RNC, Lifecircle, Costa Mesa, CA.)

incidence of undescended testes is 3.7% in term males and 21% in preterm males (Shulman, Palmert, and Wherrett, 2011). Hydroceles, caused by an accumulation of fluid around the testes, may be present. They can be easily transilluminated with a light and usually resolve without treatment.

The scrotum is usually more deeply pigmented than the rest of the skin (see Fig. 22-7, *B*), particularly in darker-skinned infants. A bluish discoloration of the scrotum suggests testicular torsion, which needs immediate attention. If the male infant is born in a breech presentation, the scrotum can be very edematous and bruised (Fig. 22-8). The swelling and discoloration subside within a few days.

Swelling of Breast Tissue

Swelling of the breast tissue in term infants of both sexes is caused by the hyperestrogenism of pregnancy. In a few infants a thin discharge (witch's milk) can be seen. This finding has no clinical significance, requires no treatment, and subsides within a few days as the maternal hormones are eliminated from the infant's body.

The nipples should be symmetric on the chest. Breast tissue and areola size increase with gestation. The areola appears slightly elevated at 34 weeks of gestation. By 36 weeks a breast bud of 1 to 2 mm is palpable; this increases to 12 mm by 42 weeks.

Signs of Reproductive System Problems

The infant must be inspected closely for ambiguous genitalia and other abnormalities. Normally in a female infant the urethral

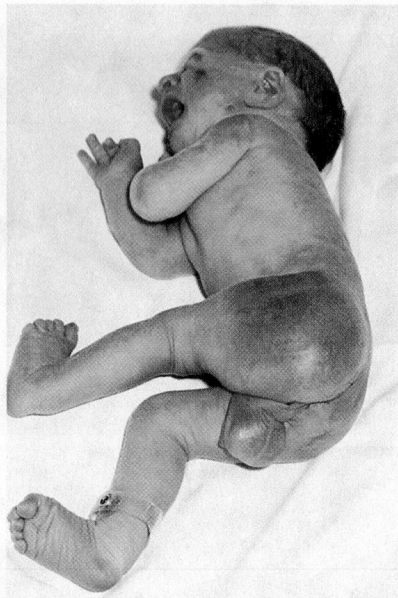

FIG 22-8 Swelling of the genitals and bruising of the buttocks after a breech birth. (From O'Doherty N: Neonatology: *Micro atlas of the newborn*, Nutley, NJ, 1986, Hoffman-LaRoche.)

opening is located behind the clitoris. Any deviation from this can incorrectly suggest that the clitoris is a small penis, which can occur in conditions such as adrenal hyperplasia. Nearly all female infants are born with hymenal tags; absence of such tags can indicate vaginal agenesis. Fecal discharge from the vagina indicates a rectovaginal fistula. Any of these findings must be reported to the physician or neonatal nurse practitioner for further evaluation.

Hypospadias or epispadias, undescended or maldescended testes, and other abnormalities of the male genitalia must be reported. Circumcision is contraindicated in the presence of hypospadias or epispadias since the foreskin is used in repair of these anomalies.

Inguinal hernias can be present and become more obvious when the infant cries. They are common, especially in African-American neonates, and usually require no treatment because they resolve with time.

Skeletal System

The infant's skeletal system undergoes rapid development during the first year of life. At birth more cartilage is present than ossified bone. Because of cephalocaudal (head-to-rump) development, the newborn looks somewhat out of proportion.

The head at term is one fourth of the total body length. The arms are slightly longer than the legs. In the newborn the legs are one third of the total body length but only 15% of the total body weight. As growth proceeds the midpoint in head-to-toe measurements gradually descends from the level of the umbilicus at birth to the level of the symphysis pubis at maturity.

The face appears small in relation to the skull. The skull appears large and heavy. Cranial size and shape can be distorted by *molding* (the shaping of the fetal head by overlapping of the cranial bones to facilitate movement through the birth canal during labor) (Fig. 22-9).

Caput Succedaneum

Caput succedaneum is a generalized, easily identifiable edematous area of the scalp, most commonly found on the occiput (Fig. 22-10, *A*). With vertex presentation the sustained pressure of the presenting vertex against the cervix results in compression of local vessels,

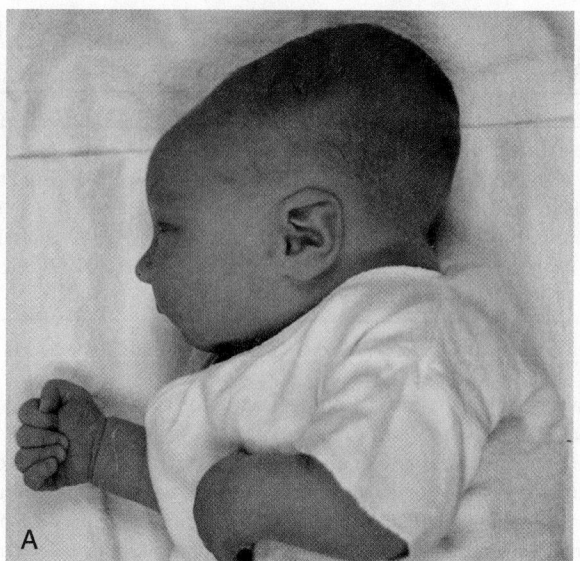

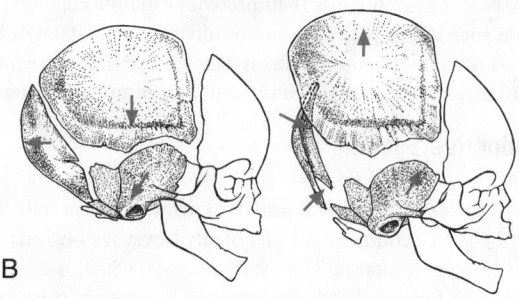

FIG 22-9 Molding. **A,** Significant molding after vaginal birth. **B,** Schematic of bones of skull when molding is present. (**A** Courtesy Kim Molloy, Knoxville, IA.)

slowing venous return. The slower venous return causes an increase in tissue fluids within the skin of the scalp, and edema develops. This edematous area, present at birth, extends across suture lines of the skull and usually disappears spontaneously within 3 to 4 days. Infants who are born with the assistance of vacuum extraction usually have a caput in the area where the cup was applied. Bruising of the scalp is often seen in the presence of caput succedaneum.

Cephalhematoma

Cephalhematoma is a collection of blood between a skull bone and its periosteum. Therefore a cephalhematoma does not cross a cranial suture line (Fig. 22-10, *B*). Often caput succedaneum and cephalhematoma occur simultaneously.

Bleeding may occur with spontaneous birth from pressure against the maternal bony pelvis. Low forceps birth and difficult forceps rotation and extraction may also cause bleeding. This soft, fluctuating, irreducible fullness does not pulsate or bulge when the infant cries. It appears several hours or the day after birth and may not become apparent until a caput succedaneum is absorbed. A cephalhematoma is usually largest on the second or third day, by which time the bleeding stops (see Family-Centered Care box). The fullness of a cephalhematoma spontaneously resolves in 3 to 6 weeks. It is not aspirated because infection may develop if the skin is punctured. As the hematoma resolves, hemolysis of RBCs occurs, and jaundice may result. Hyperbilirubinemia and jaundice may occur from a cephalhematoma after the newborn is discharged home.

Subgaleal Hemorrhage

Subgaleal hemorrhage is bleeding into the subgaleal compartment (see Fig. 22-10, C). The subgaleal compartment is a potential space that contains loosely arranged connective tissue; it is located beneath the galea aponeurosis, the tendinous sheath that connects the frontal and occipital muscles and forms the inner surface of the scalp. Subgaleal hemorrhage is commonly associated with difficult operative vaginal birth, especially vacuum extraction. With the vacuum extractor the scalp is pulled away from the bony calvarium; the vessels are torn, and blood collects in the subgaleal space. Blood loss can be severe, resulting in hypovolemic shock, disseminated intravascular coagulation (DIC), and death.

Early detection of the hemorrhage is vital; serial head circumference measurements and inspection of the back of the neck for increasing edema and a firm mass are essential. A boggy scalp, pallor, tachycardia, and increasing head circumference may also be early signs of a subgaleal hemorrhage Computed tomography or magnetic resonance imaging is useful in confirming the diagnosis. Replacement of lost blood and clotting factors is required in acute cases of hemorrhage. Another possible early sign of subgaleal hemorrhage is a forward and lateral positioning of the newborn's ears because the hematoma extends posteriorly. Monitoring the infant for changes in level of consciousness and decreases in hematocrit is also key to early recognition and management. An increase in serum bilirubin levels may be seen as a result of the degradation of blood cells within the hematoma (Mangurten and Puppala, 2011).

Spine

The bones in the vertebral column of the newborn form two primary curvatures—one in the thoracic region and one in the sacral region. Both are forward, concave curvatures. As the infant gains head control at approximately age 3 months, a secondary curvature appears in the cervical region. The newborn's spine appears straight and can be flexed easily. The newborn can lift the head and turn it from side to side when prone. The vertebrae should appear straight and flat. If a pilonidal dimple is noted, further inspection is required to determine whether a sinus is present. A pilonidal dimple, especially with a sinus and nevus pilosis (hairy nevus), is significant because it can be associated with spina bifida.

Extremities

The infant's extremities should be symmetric and of equal length. Fingers and toes should be equal in number (five fingers on each hand and five toes on each foot) and should have nails present. Digits may be missing (oligodactyly). Extra digits (polydactyly) are sometimes found on hands or feet. Fingers or toes may be fused (syndactyly).

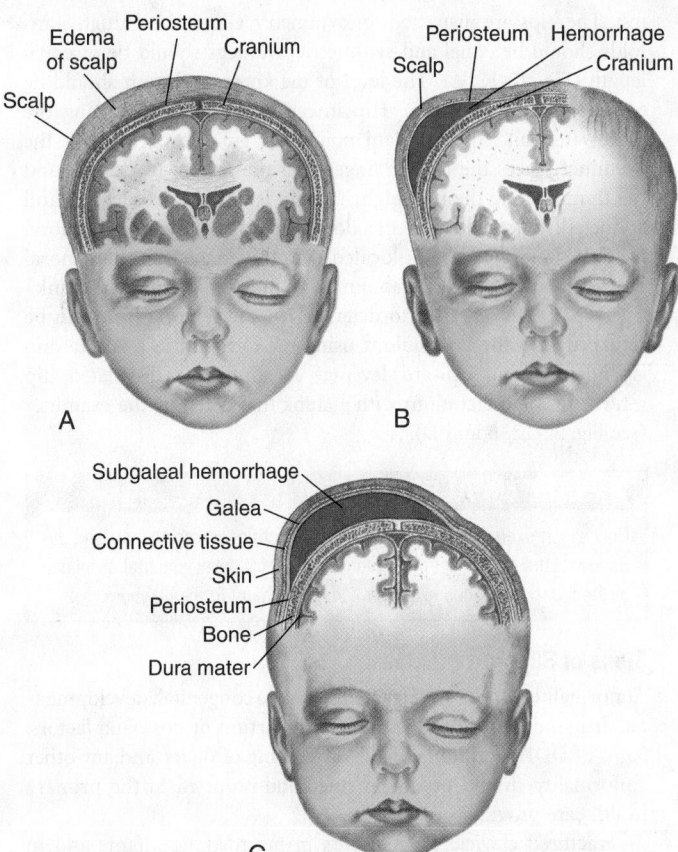

FIG 22-10 A, Caput succedaneum. **B,** Cephalhematoma. **C,** Subgaleal hemorrhage. (*A* and *B* From Seidel HM et al: *Mosby's guide to physical examination,* ed 6, St Louis, 2006, Mosby.)

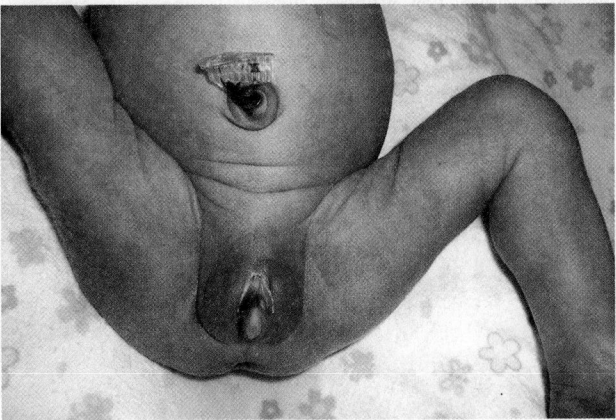

FIG 22-11 Position of infant's legs after breech birth. (Courtesy Cheryl Briggs, RNC, Annapolis, MD.)

The infant is examined for developmental dysplasia of the hip (DDH). In newborns with DDH the affected hip is unlikely to be dislocated at birth; instead it is easily dislocatable. Postnatal factors determine whether the hip dislocates, subluxates, or remains stable. DDH occurs more often in female infants, in breech presentations (Fig. 22-11), and in infants with family history of DDH (Cooperman and Thompson, 2011).

Signs of DDH are asymmetric gluteal and thigh skinfolds, uneven knee levels, a positive Ortolani test, and a positive Barlow test. The hips are inspected for symmetry. Gluteal and thigh skin-folds should be equal and symmetric, and legs should be of equal length (Fig. 22-12, *A*). The level of the knees in flexion should be equal (see Fig. 22-12, *C*). Hip integrity is assessed by using the Barlow test and the Ortolani maneuver. For the Barlow test the examiner places the middle finger over the greater trochanter and the thumb along the midthigh. The hip is flexed to 90 degrees and adducted, followed by gentle downward pushing of the femoral head. If the hip can be dislocated with this maneuver, the femoral head moves out of the acetabulum, and the examiner feels a "clunk." The hip is then checked to determine if the femoral head can be returned into the acetabulum using the Ortolani test. As the hip is abducted and upward leverage is applied, a dislocated hip returns to the acetabulum with a clunk that is felt by the examiner (see Fig. 22-12, *B* and *D*).

> ### ⚡ SAFETY ALERT
>
> Only expert examiners (physicians, nurse practitioners) should perform the Barlow test and Ortolani maneuver to assess for developmental dysplasia of the hip. An unskilled examiner can cause injury to the newborn.

Signs of Skeletal Problems

Abnormalities of the skeletal system can be congenital, developmental, drug induced, or the result of intrapartum or postnatal factors. Signs of DDH, additional digits or webbing of digits, and any other abnormality should be documented and reported to the primary health care provider.

Fractured clavicle often occurs in macrosomic infants and in those who had a difficult birth (e.g., shoulder dystocia). Unequal movement of the upper extremities or a crepitant feeling over the clavicular area can indicate fracture.

The feet of the newborn can appear to be abnormally positioned. This can indicate congenital deformity or be related to fetal positioning in utero. For example, clubfoot (talipes equinovarus), a deformity in which the foot turns inward and is fixed in a plantar-flexion position, is a congenital condition that warrants attention. If the foot is turned inward in the plantar-flexion position but can be moved into the normal position, it is likely caused by fetal positioning and should gradually resolve.

Neuromuscular System

The neuromuscular system is almost completely developed at birth. The term newborn is a responsive and reactive being with remarkable capacity for social interaction and self-organization.

Growth of the brain after birth follows a predictable pattern of rapid growth during infancy and early childhood; it becomes more gradual during the remainder of the first decade and minimal during adolescence. By the end of the first year the cerebellum ends its growth spurt, which began at approximately 30 gestational weeks.

The brain requires glucose as a source of energy and a relatively large supply of oxygen for adequate metabolism. Such requirements signal a need for careful assessment of the infant's respiratory status. The necessity for glucose requires attentiveness to neonates who are at risk for hypoglycemia (e.g., infants of mothers who have diabetes; infants who are macrosomic or small for gestational age; and newborns experiencing prolonged birth, hypoxia, or preterm birth).

Spontaneous motor activity can be seen as transient tremors of the mouth and chin, especially during crying episodes, and of the extremities, notably the arms and hands. Transient tremors are normal and can be observed in nearly every newborn. These tremors should not be present when the infant is quiet and should not persist beyond 1 month of age. Persistent tremors or tremors involving the total body can indicate pathologic conditions. Normal tremors, tremors (jitteriness) of hypoglycemia, and seizure activity must be differentiated so corrective care can be instituted as necessary.

> ### ❗ NURSING ALERT
>
> To differentiate between tremors or jitteriness and seizure activity, consider the following signs (Verklan and Lopez, 2011):
> - Tremors or jitteriness are easily elicited by motions or voice and cease with gentle restraint of the body part, whereas seizure activity continues.
> - Seizure activity is associated with ocular changes (eyes deviating or staring) and autonomic changes (apnea, tachycardia, pupil changes, increased salivation); these signs are not associated with jitteriness or tremors.

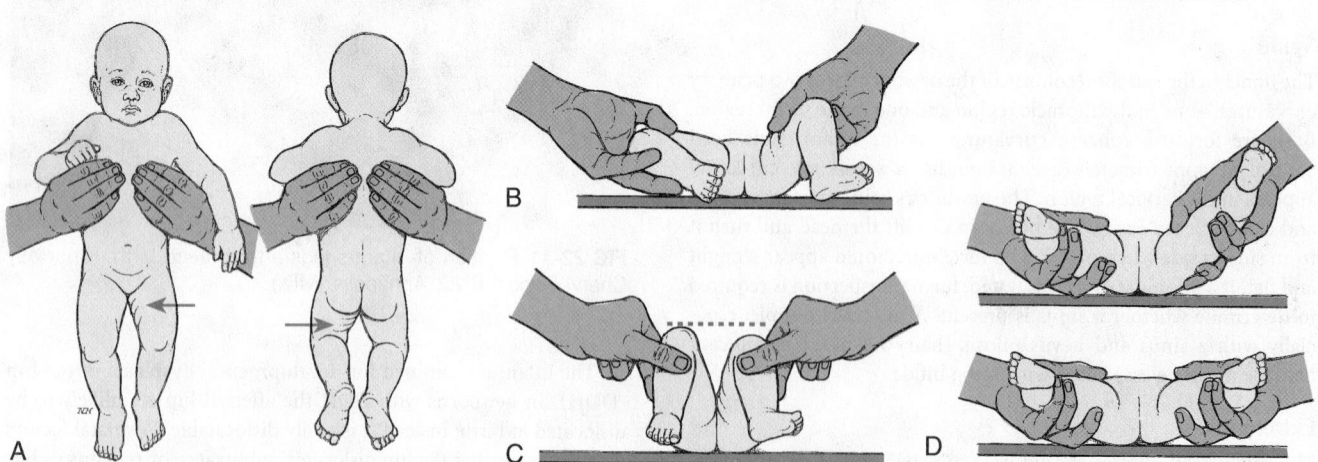

FIG 22-12 Signs of developmental dysplasia of the hip. **A,** Asymmetry of gluteal and thigh folds with shortening of the thigh (Galeazzi sign). **B,** Limited hip abduction, as seen in flexion (Ortolani test). **C,** Apparent shortening of the femur, as indicated by the level of the knees in flexion (Allis sign). **D,** Ortolani test with femoral head moving in and out of acetabulum (in infants 1 to 2 months old). (From Hockenberry MJ, Wilson D: *Wong's essentials of pediatric nursing*, ed 9, St Louis, 2013, Mosby.)

The posture of the term newborn demonstrates flexion of the arms at the elbows and the legs at the knees. Hips are abducted and partially flexed. Intermittent fisting of the hands is common.

Muscle tone and strength are directly related. The infant with normal tone and strength exhibits some resistance to passive movement such as when being pulled to sit or when the arm or leg is extended by the examiner. The hypotonic neonate shows little resistance and can feel like a "rag doll." Hypertonia is evidenced by increased resistance to passive movement.

Although neuromuscular control is very limited, it can be noted. If newborns are placed face down on a firm surface, they will turn their heads to the side. They attempt to hold their heads in line with their bodies if they are raised by their arms. Various reflexes serve to promote safety and adequate food intake.

Newborn Reflexes

The newborn has many primitive reflexes. The times at which these reflexes appear and disappear reflect the maturity and intactness of the developing nervous system. The most common reflexes found in the normal newborn are described in Table 22-4.

BEHAVIORAL CHARACTERISTICS

The healthy infant must accomplish behavioral and biologic tasks to develop normally. Behavioral characteristics form the basis of the social capabilities of the infant. Newborns progress through a hierarchy of developmental challenges as they adapt to their environment and caregivers. They must first be able to regulate their physiologic or autonomic system, including involuntary physiologic

TABLE 22-4 ASSESSMENT OF NEWBORN REFLEXES

REFLEX	ELICITING THE REFLEX	CHARACTERISTIC RESPONSE	COMMENTS
Sucking and rooting	Touch infant's lip, cheek, or corner of mouth with nipple or finger.	Infant turns head toward stimulus and opens mouth.	Response is difficult if not impossible to elicit after infant has been fed; if response is weak or absent, consider preterm birth or neurologic defect. Parental guidance: Avoid trying to turn head toward breast or nipple; allow infant to root; response disappears after 3-4* mo but can persist up to 1 yr. If response is weak or absent, can indicate prematurity or neurologic defect.
Swallowing	Feed infant; swallowing usually follows sucking and obtaining fluids.	Swallowing is usually coordinated with sucking and breathing and usually occurs without gagging, coughing, apnea, or vomiting.	If response is weak or absent, this can indicate preterm birth, effects of maternal analgesics, or illness that needs investigation. Sucking, swallowing, and breathing are often uncoordinated in preterm infant.
Grasp			
Palmar	Place finger in palm of hand.	Infant's fingers curl around examiner's fingers.	Palmar response lessens by 3-4 mo; parents enjoy this contact with infant.
Plantar	Place finger at base of toes.	Toes curl downward.	Plantar response lessens by 8 mo.

Plantar grasp reflex. (From Zitelli BJ, Davis HW: *Atlas of pediatric physical diagnosis*, ed 5, St Louis, 2007, Mosby.)

Continued

TABLE 22-4	ASSESSMENT OF NEWBORN REFLEXES—cont'd		
REFLEX	**ELICITING THE REFLEX**	**CHARACTERISTIC RESPONSE**	**COMMENTS**
Extrusion	Touch or depress tip of tongue.	Newborn forces tongue outward.	Response disappears about fourth to fifth month.
Glabellar (Myerson)	Tap over forehead, bridge of nose, or maxilla of newborn whose eyes are open.	Newborn blinks for first four or five taps.	Continued blinking with repeated taps is consistent with extrapyramidal signs.
Tonic neck or "fencing"	With infant in supine neutral position, turn head quickly to one side.	With infant facing left side, arm and leg on that side extend; opposite arm and leg flex (turn head to right, and extremities assume opposite postures).	Responses in leg are more consistent. Complete response disappears by 3-4 mo; incomplete response may be seen until third or fourth year. After 6 wk persistent response is sign of possible cerebral palsy

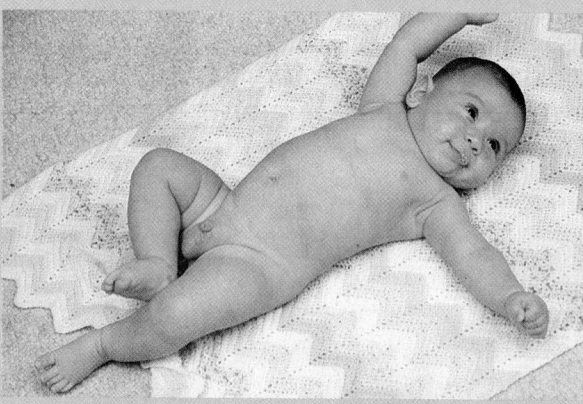

Classic pose in tonic neck reflex. (Courtesy Marjorie Pyle, RNC, Lifecircle, Costa Mesa, CA.)

Moro	Hold infant in semisitting position, allow head and trunk to fall backward to angle of at least 30 degrees (with support). Place infant supine on flat surface; perform sharp hand clap.	Symmetric abduction and extension of arms are seen; fingers fan out and form a **C** with thumb and forefinger; slight tremor may be noted; arms are adducted in embracing motion and return to relaxed flexion and movement. A cry may accompany or follow motor movement. Legs may follow similar pattern of response. Preterm infant does not complete "embrace"; instead arms fall backward because of weakness.	Response is present at birth; complete response may be seen until 8 wk; body jerk only is seen between 8 and 18 wk; response is absent by 6 mo if neurologic maturation is not delayed; response may be incomplete if infant is in deep sleep state; give parental guidance about normal response. Asymmetric response can connote injury to brachial plexus, clavicle, or humerus. Persistent response after 6 mo indicates possible neurologic abnormality.

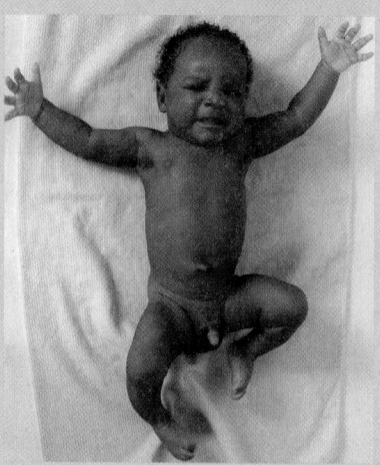

Moro reflex. (Courtesy Paul Vincent Kuntz, Texas Children's Hospital, Houston, TX.)

TABLE 22-4   ASSESSMENT OF NEWBORN REFLEXES—cont'd

REFLEX	ELICITING THE REFLEX	CHARACTERISTIC RESPONSE	COMMENTS
Stepping or "walking"	Hold infant vertically under arms or on trunk, allowing one foot to touch table surface.	Infant will simulate walking, alternating flexion and extension of feet; term infants walk on soles of their feet, and preterm infants walk on their toes.	Response is normally present for 3-4 wk.

Stepping reflex. (From Dickason EJ, Silverman BL, Kaplan JA: *Maternal-infant nursing care*, ed 3, St Louis, 1998, Mosby.)

Crawling	Place newborn on abdomen.	Newborn makes crawling movements with arms and legs.	Response should disappear about 6 wk of age.

Crawling reflex. (Courtesy Paul Vincent Kuntz, Texas Children's Hospital, Houston, TX.)

Deep tendon	Use finger instead of percussion hammer to elicit patellar, or knee jerk, reflex; newborn must be relaxed.	Reflex jerk is present; even with newborn relaxed, nonselective overall reaction may occur.	
Crossed extension	With infant in supine position, examiner extends one leg of infant and presses down knee. Stimulation of sole of foot of fixated limb should cause free leg to flex, adduct, and extend as if attempting to push away stimulating agent.	Opposite leg flexes, adducts, and then extends.	This reflex should be present during newborn period.

Crossed extension reflex. (Courtesy Marjorie Pyle, RNC, Lifecircle, Costa Mesa, CA.)

Continued

TABLE 22-4   ASSESSMENT OF NEWBORN REFLEXES—cont'd

REFLEX	ELICITING THE REFLEX	CHARACTERISTIC RESPONSE	COMMENTS
Babinski (plantar)	On sole of foot, beginning at heel, stroke upward along lateral aspect of sole; then move finger across ball of foot.	All toes hyperextend, with dorsiflexion of big toe—recorded as a positive sign.	Absence requires neurologic evaluation; should disappear after 1 yr of age. Response depends on infant's general muscle tone, maturity, and condition.

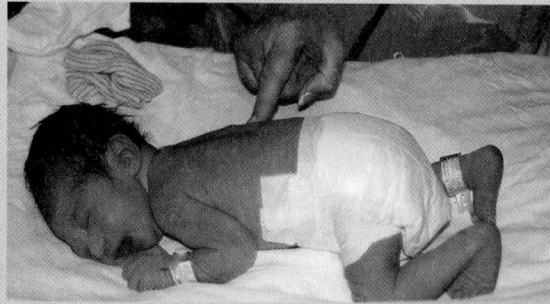

Babinski reflex. **A,** Direction of stroke. **B,** Dorsiflexion of big toe. **C,** Fanning of toes. (From Hockenberry MJ, Wilson D: *Wong's nursing care of infants and children,* ed 9, St Louis, 2013, Mosby.)

REFLEX	ELICITING THE REFLEX	CHARACTERISTIC RESPONSE	COMMENTS
Pull-to-sit (traction response); postural tone	Pull infant up by wrists from supine position with head in midline.	Head lags until infant is in upright position; then head is held in same plane with chest and shoulder momentarily before falling forward; infant attempts to right head.	Response depends on general muscle tone and maturity and condition of infant.
Truncal incurvation (Galant)	Place infant prone on flat surface; run finger down back about 4-5 cm lateral to spine, first on one side and then down other.	Trunk is flexed, and pelvis is swung toward stimulated side.	Response disappears by fourth week. Response varies but should be obtainable in all infants, including preterm ones. Absence suggests general depression of nervous system. With transverse lesions of cord, no response below level of lesion is present.

Trunk incurvation reflex. (Courtesy Marjorie Pyle, RNC, Lifecircle, Costa Mesa, CA.)

REFLEX	ELICITING THE REFLEX	CHARACTERISTIC RESPONSE	COMMENTS
Magnet	Place infant in supine position, partially flex both lower extremities, and apply light pressure with fingers to soles of feet (Fig. A). Normally, while examiner's fingers maintain contact with soles of feet, lower limbs extend.	Both lower limbs should extend against examiner's pressure (Fig. B).	Absence suggests damage to central nervous system. Weak reflex may be seen after breech presentation *without* extended legs or may indicate sciatic nerve stretch syndrome. Breech presentation *with* extended legs may evoke exaggerated response.

TABLE 22-4   ASSESSMENT OF NEWBORN REFLEXES—cont'd

REFLEX	ELICITING THE REFLEX	CHARACTERISTIC RESPONSE	COMMENTS
	Magnet reflex. (Courtesy Michael S Clement, MD, Mesa, AZ.)		
Additional newborn responses: yawn, stretch, burp, hiccup, sneeze	These are spontaneous behaviors.	Responses may be slightly depressed temporarily because of maternal analgesia or anesthesia, fetal hypoxia, or infection.	Parental guidance: Most of these behaviors are pleasurable to parents. Parents need to be assured that behaviors are normal. Sneeze is usually response to mucus in nose and not indicator of a cold (upper respiratory tract infection). No treatment is needed for hiccups; sucking may help. In preterm infant these are signs of neurodevelopmental immaturity and physiologic stress.

*All durations for persistence of reflexes are based on time elapsed after 40 weeks of gestation (i.e., if newborn was born at 36 weeks of gestation, add 1 month to all time limits given).

functions such as heart rate, respiration, and temperature. The next level is motor organization, in which infants regulate or control their motor behavior. This includes controlling random movements, improving muscle tone, and reducing excessive activity. The third level of behavior is state regulation, which refers to the ability to modulate the state of consciousness. The infant develops predictable sleep and wake states and is able to react to stress through self-regulation or through communicating with the caregiver by crying and then being consoled. Finally the infant reaches the fourth level of attention and social interaction. He or she is able to attend to visual and auditory stimulation, stay alert for long periods, and engage in social interaction (Brazelton and Nugent, 2011).

This progression in behavior is the basis for the Brazelton Neonatal Behavioral Assessment Scale (NBAS) (Brazelton and Nugent, 2011). The NBAS is an interactive examination that assesses the infant's response to 28 areas organized according to the clusters in Box 22-2. It is generally used as a research or diagnostic tool and requires special training. The NBAS helps the practitioner identify where the infant falls along the continuum of behaviors and determine the type of support needed.

The Newborn Behavioral Observations (NBO) system, based on the NBAS, is a tool that is used in clinical settings to help parents identify, understand, and respond to newborn behavior (Nugent, Keefer, Minear, et al., 2007). Karl and Keefer (2011) developed a training program using the NBO system to educate clinicians about newborn behavior, self-regulation skills, and social interaction capabilities. A major benefit of this program is that nurses and other clinicians can use the information to educate and help parents interpret newborn cues and respond appropriately, which promotes attachment (Karl and Keefer, 2011). See Chapter 20 for further discussion of attachment.

BOX 22-2   CLUSTERS OF NEONATAL BEHAVIORS IN BRAZELTON NEONATAL BEHAVIORAL ASSESSMENT SCALE

- Habituation—Ability to respond to and then inhibit responding to discrete stimulus (e.g., light, rattle, bell, pinprick) while asleep
- Orientation—Quality of alert states and ability to attend to visual and auditory stimuli while alert
- Motor performance—Quality of movement and tone
- Range of state—Measure of general arousal level or arousability of infant
- Regulation of state—How infant responds when aroused
- Autonomic stability—Signs of stress (e.g., tremors, startles, skin color) related to homeostatic (self-regulator) adjustment of the nervous system
- Reflexes—Assessment of several neonatal reflexes

From Brazelton T, Nugent J: *Neonatal behavioral assessment scale*, ed 4, London, 2011, MacKeith.

Sleep-Wake States

Healthy newborns differ in their activity levels, feeding patterns, sleeping patterns, and responsiveness. Parents' reactions to their newborns are often determined by these differences. Showing parents the unique characteristics of their infant helps them develop a more positive perception of the infant and promotes increased interaction between infant and parent. Infant responses to environmental stimuli and to their caregivers depend on the infant's state or state of consciousness.

In the early newborn period infants tend to alternate periods of sleep and wakefulness that resemble their fetal inactivity and activity patterns. Variations in the state of consciousness of infants are called

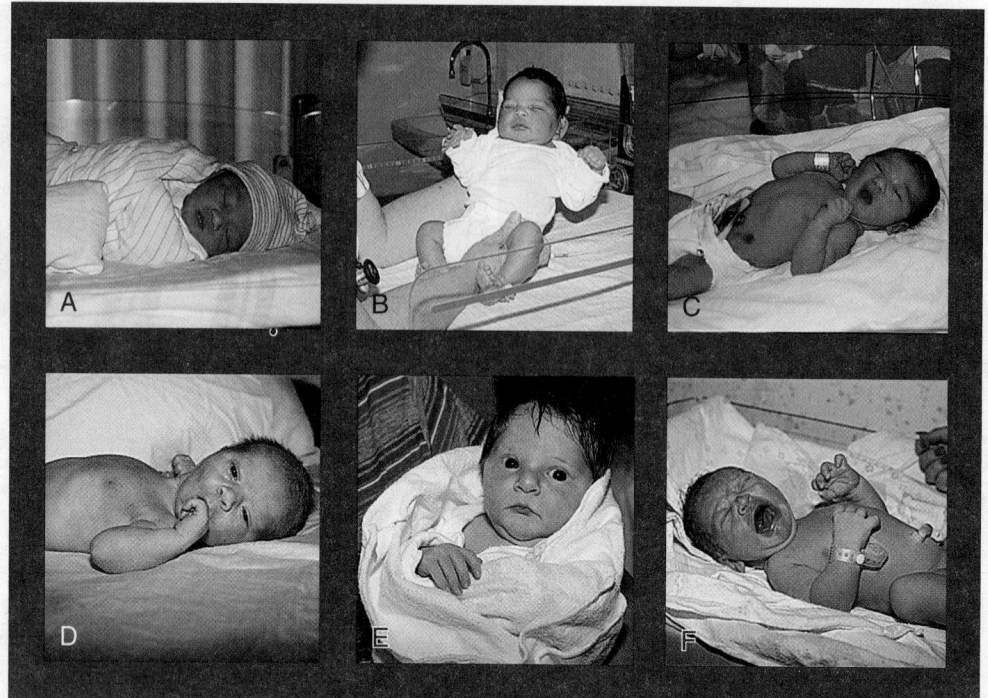

FIG 22-13 Newborn sleep-wake states. **A,** Deep sleep. **B,** Light sleep; **C,** Drowsy. **D,** Quiet alert. **E,** Active alert. **F,** Crying. (Courtesy Marjorie Pyle, RNC, Lifecircle, Costa Mesa, CA.)

sleep-wake states. The six states form a continuum from deep sleep to extreme irritability (Fig. 22-13): two sleep states (deep sleep and light sleep) and four wake states (drowsy, quiet alert, active alert, and crying) (Brazelton and Nugent, 2011). Each state has specific characteristics and state-related behaviors. The optimal state of arousal is the quiet alert state. During this state infants smile, vocalize, move in synchrony with speech, watch their parents' faces, and respond to people talking to them. They respond to internal and external environmental factors by controlling sensory input and regulating the sleep-wake states; the ability to make smooth transitions between states is called *state modulation*. The ability to regulate sleep-wake states is essential in the infant's neurobehavioral development. As infants approach term gestation, they are better able to cope with external or internal factors that affect the sleep-wake patterns.

Infants use purposeful behavior to maintain the optimal arousal state as follows: (1) actively withdrawing by increasing physical distance, (2) rejecting by pushing away with hands and feet, (3) decreasing sensitivity by falling asleep or breaking eye contact by turning the head, or (4) using signaling behaviors such as fussing and crying. These behaviors permit infants to quiet themselves and reinstate readiness to interact.

The first 6 weeks of life involve a steady decrease in the proportion of active REM sleep to total sleep. A steady increase in the proportion of quiet sleep to total sleep also occurs. Periods of wakefulness increase. For the first few weeks the wakeful periods seem dictated by hunger, but soon a need for socializing appears. The newborn sleeps on average approximately 17 hours a day, with periods of wakefulness gradually increasing. By the fourth week of life some infants stay awake from one feeding to the next.

Other Factors Influencing Newborn Behavior
Gestational Age
The gestational age of the infant and level of central nervous system (CNS) maturity affect infant behavior. In the preterm neonate with

an immature CNS the entire body responds to a pinprick of the foot, although the response may not be observed by an untrained observer. The more mature infant withdraws only the foot. CNS immaturity is reflected in reflex development, sleep-wake states, and ability (or lack thereof) to regulate or modulate a smooth transition between different states. Preterm infants have brief periods of alertness but have difficulty maintaining alertness without becoming overstimulated, which leads to autonomic instability unless intervention is implemented. Premature or sick infants show signs of fatigue or physiologic stress sooner than full-term healthy infants.

Time
The time elapsed since birth affects the behavior of infants as they attempt to become organized initially. Time elapsed since the previous feeding and time of day also can influence infants' responses.

Stimuli
Environmental events and stimuli affect the behavioral responses of infants. The newborn responds to animate and inanimate stimuli. Nurses in intensive care nurseries observe that infants respond to loud noises, bright lights, monitor alarms, and tension in the unit. If a mother is tense, nervous, or uncomfortable while feeding her infant, the infant may sense her tension and demonstrate difficulty feeding.

Medication
No conclusive evidence exists regarding the effects of maternal analgesia or anesthesia during labor on neonatal behavior. Researchers who have studied the effects of epidural medications on breastfeeding behaviors have been unable to show a cause-and-effect relationship (Hoyt, 2011).

Sensory Behaviors
From birth infants possess sensory capabilities that indicate a state of readiness for social interaction. They effectively use behavioral

responses in establishing their first dialogs. These responses, coupled with the newborns' "baby appearance" (e.g., facial proportions of forehead, eyes larger than the lower portion of the face) and their small size and helplessness, rouse feelings of wanting to hold, protect, and interact with them.

Vision

At birth the eye is structurally incomplete, and the muscles are immature. The process of accommodation is not present but improves over the first 3 months of life. The pupils react to light, the blink reflex is stimulated easily, and the corneal reflex is activated by light touch. Term newborns can see objects as far away as 50 cm (2.5 feet). The clearest visual distance is 17 to 20 cm (8 to 12 inches), which is approximately the distance between the mother's and infant's faces during breastfeeding or cuddling. Infants are sensitive to light; they frown if a bright light is flashed in their eyes and turn toward a soft, red light. If the room is darkened, they open their eyes wide and look about. By 2 months of age they can detect color; but at 5 days of age and younger they seem more attracted by black-and-white patterns.

Response to movement is noticeable. If a bright light is shown to newborns (even at 15 minutes of age), they follow it visually; some even turn their heads to do so. Because human eyes are bright shiny objects, newborns track their parents' eyes. Parents often comment on their excitement in observing this behavior. The development of eye-to-eye contact is very important for parent-infant attachment. Children of blind parents and parents who have blind children must circumvent this obstacle for the formation of a relationship.

Visual acuity is surprising. Even at 2 weeks of age infants can distinguish patterns with stripes 3 mm apart. By 6 months their vision is as acute as that of an adult. They prefer to look at patterns rather than plain surfaces, even if the latter are brightly colored. Infants prefer more complex patterns to simple ones. They prefer novelty (changes in pattern) by 2 months of age. Therefore the infant of a few weeks of age is capable of responding actively to an enriched environment.

Hearing

As soon as the amniotic fluid drains from the ears, the infant's hearing is similar to that of an adult. Loud sounds of approximately 90 decibels cause the infant to respond with a Moro reflex. The newborn responds to low-frequency sounds such as a heartbeat or lullaby by decreasing motor activity or stopping crying. High-frequency sound elicits an alerting reaction.

The sound preferred by infants is the human voice. The infant responds readily to the mother's voice. Studies indicate a selective listening to maternal voice sounds and rhythms during intrauterine life that prepares newborns for recognition and interaction with their primary caregivers—their mothers. Newborns are accustomed to hearing the regular rhythm of the mother's heartbeat in the uterus. As a result they respond by relaxing and ceasing to fuss and cry if a regular heartbeat simulator is placed in their cribs. Hearing is integral to bonding and attachment and may be more important than vision (Gardner and Goldson, 2011).

Routine hearing screening is recommended for all newborns before hospital discharge. See Chapter 23 for a discussion about screening of newborn hearing.

Smell

Newborns have a highly developed sense of smell and can detect and discriminate distinct odors. It has been shown that preterm infants as early as 28 weeks are capable of reacting to odors. They react to strong odors such as alcohol or vinegar by turning their heads away but are attracted to sweet smells. By the fifth day of life newborn infants can recognize their mother's smell. Breastfed infants are able to smell breast milk and can differentiate their mothers from other lactating women (Lawrence and Lawrence, 2011).

Taste

The newborn can distinguish among tastes, and various types of solutions elicit differing facial expressions. A tasteless solution produces no response; a sweet solution elicits eager sucking. A sour solution causes a puckering of the lips, and a bitter liquid produces a grimace.

Young infants are particularly oriented toward the use of their mouths, both for meeting their nutritional needs for rapid growth and for releasing tension through sucking. The early development of circumoral sensation, muscle activity, and taste would seem to be preparation for survival in the extrauterine environment.

Touch

The infant is responsive to touch on all parts of the body. The face (especially the mouth), the hands, and the soles of the feet seem to be the most sensitive. Reflexes can be elicited by stroking the infant. The newborn's responses to touch suggest that this sensory system is well prepared to receive and process tactile messages. Touch and motion are essential to normal growth and development. However, each infant is unique, and variations can be seen in newborns' responses to touch (see Family-Centered Care box). Birth trauma or stress and depressant drugs taken by the mother decrease the infant's sensitivity to touch or painful stimuli.

Response to Environmental Stimuli
Temperament

Classic studies have identified individual variations in the primary reaction pattern of newborns and described them as temperament. Their style of behavioral response to stimuli is guided by the temperament, affecting their sensory threshold, ability to habituate, and response to maternal behaviors. Newborns possess individual characteristics that affect selective responses to various stimuli present in the internal and external environments.

The three major patterns of behavioral style or temperament are as follows (Chess, 1969; Chess and Thomas, 1977):

1. The *easy child*, who demonstrates regularity in bodily functions, readily adapts to change, has a predominantly positive mood and moderate sensory threshold, and approaches new situations or objects with a moderate response
2. The *slow-to-warm-up child*, who has a low activity level, withdraws on first exposure to new stimuli, is slow to adapt and low in intensity of response, and is somewhat negative in mood

---

♟ FAMILY-CENTERED CARE
Newborn Behavior

A first-time single mother asks the nurse about her newborn's activity. She voices concern that the newborn cries when she changes his diaper. "He sleeps a lot and only wakes up to eat or when I change his diaper. Is that normal?" Develop a short parent-teaching lesson to present newborn behavior and care in relation to the following: sleep-wake states, newborn activities and relationship to crying behaviors in the first few days of life, and how to comfort and console the newborn.

3. The *difficult child,* who is irregular in bodily functions, intense in reactions, generally negative in mood, and resistant to change or new stimuli and often cries loudly for long periods

Habituation

Habituation is a protective mechanism that allows the infant to become accustomed to environmental stimuli. It is a psychologic and physiologic phenomenon in which the response to a constant or repetitive stimulus is decreased. In the term newborn this can be demonstrated in several ways. Shining a bright light into a newborn's eyes causes a startle or squinting the first 2 or 3 times. The third or fourth flash elicits a diminished response; and by the fifth or sixth flash the infant ceases to respond (Brazelton and Nugent, 2011). The same response pattern holds true for the sounds of a rattle or stroking the bottom of the foot.

The ability to habituate allows the healthy term newborn to select stimuli that promote continued learning about the social world, thus avoiding overload. The intrauterine environment seems to have programmed the newborn to be especially responsive to human voices, soft lights, soft sounds, and sweet tastes.

The newborn quickly learns the sounds in the home environment and is able to sleep in their midst. The selective responses of the newborn indicate cerebral organization capable of memory and making choices. The ability to habituate depends on the state of consciousness, hunger, fatigue, and temperament. These factors also affect consolability, cuddliness, irritability, and crying.

Consolability

Newborns vary in the ability to console themselves or be consoled. In the crying state most newborns initiate one of several ways to reduce their distress. Hand-to-mouth movements with or without sucking and being alert to voices, noises, or visual stimuli are common. Some infants are consoled only if they are held and rocked (Brazelton and Nugent, 2011).

Cuddliness

Cuddliness is especially important to parents because they often gauge their ability to care for the child by the child's responses to their actions. The degree to which newborns relax and mold into the contours of the person holding them varies. One extreme is the infant who always resists being held with thrashing and stiffening of the body. This is in contrast to the infant who immediately relaxes when held and molds to the body of the person. Less extreme behavior is demonstrated by infants who are passive when held and those who gradually mold after being held for a while (Brazelton and Nugent, 2011).

Irritability

Some newborns cry longer and harder than others. For some the sensory threshold seems low. They are readily upset by unusual noises, hunger, wetness, or new experiences and thus respond intensely. Others with a high sensory threshold require a great deal more stimulation and variation to reach the active, alert state.

Crying

Crying is the language an infant uses most often to communicate needs. It may signal hunger, discomfort, pain, desire for attention, or fussiness. Infants may cry in response to environmental stimuli such as cold, being overstimulated, or being held by multiple persons. Responsiveness of the caregiver to the crying creates trust as the infant learns to associate the caregiver with comfort.

The amount and tone of crying vary based on gestational age, weight, and the reason for the cry (e.g., hunger, pain). A high-pitched cry can be a sign of a neurologic disorder. Some mothers state that they learn to distinguish among the cries. The breastfeeding mother's body responds physiologically to infant crying by stimulating the milk-ejection reflex ("let-down") (Gardner and Goldson, 2011).

The duration of crying also varies greatly in each infant; newborns may cry for as little as 5 minutes or as much as 2 hours or more per day. The amount of crying peaks in the second month and then decreases. There is a diurnal rhythm of crying, with more crying occurring in the evening hours.

KEY POINTS

- By full term the newborn's various anatomic and physiologic systems have reached a level of development and functioning that permits a physical existence apart from the mother.
- The neonate's most critical adaptation to extrauterine life is to establish effective respirations.
- Heat loss in the healthy term newborn may exceed the capacity to produce heat; this can lead to metabolic and respiratory complications that threaten the newborn's well-being.
- Physiologic jaundice occurs in 60% of term infants and 80% of preterm infants.
- Jaundice is considered pathologic if it appears within the first 24 hours of life, if serum bilirubin levels increase by more than 6 mg/dL in 24 hours, or if serum bilirubin exceeds 15 mg/dL at any time.
- Some reflex behaviors are important for the newborn's survival.
- The healthy newborn has sensory abilities that indicate a state of readiness for social interaction. Sleep-wake states and other factors influence the newborn's behavior.
- Newborn behavior progresses from self-regulation of autonomic processes to social interaction.
- Each full-term newborn has a predisposed capacity to handle the multitude of stimuli in the external world.

REFERENCES

Abu-Shaweesh JM: Respiratory disorders in preterm and term infants. In Martin RJ, Fanaroff AA, Walsh MC, editors: *Fanaroff and Martin's neonatal-perinatal medicine: diseases of the fetus and infant,* ed 9, St Louis, 2011, Mosby.

American Academy of Pediatrics (AAP) Subcommittee on Hyperbilirubinemia: Clinical practice guideline: management of hyperbilirubinemia in the newborn infant 35 or more weeks of gestation, *Pediatrics* 114(1):297–316, 2004.

Andersson O, Hellström-Westas L, Andersson D, et al: Effect of delayed versus early umbilical cord clamping on neonatal outcomes and iron status at 4 months: a randomised controlled trial, *Br Med J* 343:d7157, 2011.

Arca G, Botet F, Palacio M, et al: Timing of umbilical cord clamping: new thoughts on an old discussion, *J Matern Fetal Neonatal Med* 23(11):1274–1285, 2010.

Askin D: Fetal-to-neonatal transition—what is normal and what is not? Part II: Red flags, *Neonatal Netw* 28(3):e37–e40, 2009, www.metapress.com/content/V471277271677852.

Baker RD, Greer FR, and the Committee on Nutrition: Diagnosis and prevention of iron deficiency and iron-deficiency anemia in infants and young children (0-2 years of age), *Pediatrics* 126(5):1040–1050, 2010.

Blackburn ST: *Maternal, fetal, and neonatal physiology*, ed 4, St Louis, 2013, Saunders.

Brazelton T, Nugent J: *Neonatal behavioral assessment scale*, ed 4, London, 2011, MacKeith.

Brown VD, Landers S: Heat balance. In Gardner SL, Carter BS, Enzman-Hines M, et al, editors: *Merenstein & Gardner's handbook of neonatal intensive care*, ed 7, St Louis, 2011, Mosby.

Chess S: Individuality and baby care, *Dev Med Neurol* 11(6):749–754, 1969.

Chess S, Thomas A: Temperament and the parent-child interaction, *Pediatr Ann* 6(9):574–582, 1977.

Cooperman DR, Thompson GH: Musculoskeletal disorders. In Martin RJ, Fanaroff AA, Walsh MC, editors: *Fanaroff and Martin's neonatal-perinatal medicine: diseases of the fetus and infant*, ed 9, St Louis, 2011, Mosby.

Dell KM: Fluids, electrolytes, and acid-base homeostasis. In Martin RJ, Fanaroff AA, Walsh MC, editors: *Fanaroff and Martin's neonatal-perinatal medicine: diseases of the fetus and infant*, ed 9, St Louis, 2011, Mosby.

Desmond M, Rudolph A, Phitaksphraiwan P: The transitional care nursery: a mechanism for preventive medicine in the newborn, *Pediatr Clin North Am* 13(3):651–668, 1966.

Gardner SL, Goldson E: The neonate and the environment: impact on development. In Gardner SL, Carter BS, Enzman-Hines M, et al, editors: *Merenstein & Gardner's handbook of neonatal intensive care*, ed 7, St Louis, 2011, Mosby.

Gardner SL, Lawrence RA: Breast feeding the neonate with special needs. In Gardner SL, Carter BS, Enzman-Hines M, et al, editors: *Merenstein & Gardner's handbook of neonatal intensive care*, ed 7, St Louis, 2011, Mosby.

Goldsmith JP: Delivery room resuscitation of the newborn. In Martin RJ, Fanaroff AA, Walsh MC, editors: *Fanaroff and Martin's neonatal-perinatal medicine: diseases of the fetus and infant*, ed 9, St Louis, 2011, Mosby.

Habif TP: Vascular tumors and malformations. In Habif TP, editor: *Clinical dermatology*, ed 5, Philadelphia, 2009, Mosby.

Hoath SB, Narendran V: The skin. In Martin RJ, Fanaroff AA, Walsh MC, editors: *Fanaroff and Martin's neonatal-perinatal medicine: diseases of the fetus and infant*, ed 9, St Louis, 2011, Mosby.

Hoyt MR: Anesthetic options for labor and delivery. In Martin RJ, Fanaroff AA, Walsh MC, editors: *Fanaroff and Martin's neonatal-perinatal medicine: diseases of the fetus and infant*, ed 9, St Louis, 2011, Mosby.

Kalhan SC, Devaskar SU: Metabolic and endocrine disorders. In Martin RJ, Fanaroff AA, Walsh MC, editors: *Fanaroff and Martin's neonatal-perinatal medicine: diseases of the fetus and infant*, ed 9, St Louis, 2011, Mosby.

Kamath BD, Thilo EH, Hernandez JA: Jaundice. In Gardner SL, Carter BS, Enzman-Hines M, et al, editors: *Merenstein & Gardner's handbook of neonatal intensive care*, ed 7, St Louis, 2011, Mosby.

Kaplan M, Wong RJ, Sibley E, et al: Neonatal jaundice and liver disease. In Martin RJ, Fanaroff AA, Walsh MC, editors: *Fanaroff and Martin's neonatal-perinatal medicine: diseases of the fetus and infant*, ed 9, St Louis, 2011, Mosby.

Kapur R, Yoder MC, Polin RA: Developmental immunology. In Martin RJ, Fanaroff AA, Walsh MC, editors: *Fanaroff and Martin's neonatal-perinatal medicine: diseases of the fetus and infant*, ed 9, St Louis, 2011, Mosby.

Karl DJ, Keefer CH: Use of the Behavioral Observation of the Newborn Educational Trainer for teaching newborn behavior, *J Obstet Gynecol Neonatal Nurs* 40(1):75–83, 2011.

Kenney PM, Hoover D, Williams LC, et al: Cardiovascular diseases and surgical interventions. In Gardner SL, Carter BS, Enzman-Hines M, et al, editors: *Merenstein & Gardner's handbook of neonatal intensive care*, ed 7, St Louis, 2011, Mosby.

Lawrence RA, Lawrence RM: *Breastfeeding: A guide for the medical profession*, ed 7, St Louis, 2011, Mosby.

Lott JW: Immunology and infectious disease. In Verklan MT, Walden M, editors: *Core curriculum for neonatal intensive care nursing*, ed 4, St Louis, 2010, Saunders.

Manco-Johnson M, Rodden DJ, Hays T: Newborn hematology. In Gardner SL, Carter BS, Enzman-Hines M, et al, editors: *Merenstein & Gardner's handbook of neonatal intensive care*, ed 7, St Louis, 2011, Mosby.

Mangurten HH, Puppala BL: Birth injuries. In Martin RJ, Fanaroff AA, Walsh MC, editors: *Fanaroff and Martin's neonatal-perinatal medicine: diseases of the fetus and infant*, ed 9, St Louis, 2011, Mosby.

Nugent JK, Keefer CH, Minear S, et al: *Understanding newborn behavior and early relationships: the Newborn Behavioral Observations (NBO) system handbook*, Baltimore, 2007, Brookes Publishing.

Pagana KD, Pagana TJ: *Mosby's diagnostic and laboratory test reference*, ed 9, St Louis, 2009, Mosby.

Sadowski S: Cardiovascular disorders. In Verklan MT, Walden M, editors: *Core curriculum for neonatal intensive care nursing*, ed 4, St Louis, 2010, Saunders.

Shulman RM, Palmert MR, Wherrett DK: Disorders of sex development. In Martin RJ, Fanaroff AA, Walsh MC, editors: *Fanaroff and Martin's neonatal-perinatal medicine: diseases of the fetus and infant*, ed 9, St Louis, 2011, Mosby.

Verklan MT, Lopez SM: Neurologic disorders. In Gardner SL, Carter BS, Enzman-Hines M, et al, editors: *Merenstein & Gardner's handbook of neonatal intensive care*, ed 7, St Louis, 2011, Mosby.

Visscher MO, Utturkar R, Pickens WL, et al: Neonatal skin maturation—vernix caseosa and free amino acids, *Pediatr Dermatol* 28(2):122–132, 2011.

Nursing Care of the Newborn and Family

Kathryn R. Alden

⊖volve WEBSITE

http://evolve.elsevier.com/Perry/maternal

LEARNING OBJECTIVES

On completion of this chapter, the reader will be able to:

- Explain the purpose and components of the Apgar score.
- Describe how to perform a physical assessment of a newborn.
- Describe how to perform a gestational age assessment of a newborn.
- Compare the characteristics of the preterm, late preterm, term, and postterm neonate.
- Provide nursing care to assist the newborn to transition to extrauterine life.
- Explain the elements of a safe environment.
- Discuss phototherapy and the guidelines for teaching parents about this treatment.

- Explain the purposes and methods for circumcision, the postoperative care of the circumcised infant, and parent teaching regarding circumcision.
- Review the procedures for administering an intramuscular injection, performing a heelstick, collecting urine specimens, and venipuncture.
- Evaluate pain in the newborn based on physiologic changes and behavioral observations.
- Review anticipatory guidance nurses provide to parents before discharge.

Although most infants make the necessary biopsychosocial adjustments to extrauterine existence without undue difficulty, their well-being depends on the care they receive from others. This chapter describes the assessment and care of the infant immediately after birth until discharge, as well as important anticipatory guidance related to ongoing infant care. A discussion of pain in the neonate and its management is included.

CARE MANAGEMENT: BIRTH THROUGH THE FIRST 2 HOURS

Care begins immediately after birth and focuses on assessing and stabilizing the newborn's condition. The nurse has the primary responsibility for the infant during this period because the physician or nurse midwife is involved with care of the mother. The nurse must be alert for any signs of distress and initiate appropriate interventions.

With the possibility of transmission of viruses such as hepatitis B virus (HBV) and human immunodeficiency virus (HIV) through maternal blood and blood-stained amniotic fluid, the newborn must be considered a potential contamination source until proved otherwise. As part of Standard Precautions, nurses wear gloves when handling the newborn until blood and amniotic fluid are removed by bathing.

The foundation for providing comprehensive, family-centered newborn care is awareness of the mother's preconception and prenatal history as well as intrapartal events. Recognition of risk factors (Box 23-1) enables the nurse to be more astute in observations and assessments and more likely to identify early signs of complications. This allows for earlier intervention and promotes positive outcomes.

Immediate Care After Birth

The primary goal of care in the first moments after birth is to assist the newly born infant to transition to extrauterine life by establishing effective respirations. If the infant is at term, is crying or breathing, and has good muscle tone, routine care can begin (Kattwinkel, Perlman, Aziz, et al., 2010). The infant is placed prone on the mother's abdomen or chest, and the nurse assesses the airway. Slight extension of the neck helps keep the airway patent. Drying the infant with vigorous rubbing removes moisture to prevent evaporative heat loss and provides tactile stimulation to stimulate respiratory effort. The mother and her newborn are covered with a warm blanket (Niermeyer and Clarke, 2011).

If the neonate is apneic or has gasping respirations, positive-pressure ventilation is needed. The heart rate is quickly assessed by

ink or a scanning device within 2 hours of birth (Vincent, 2009). (See later discussion of infant abduction.)

Apgar Scoring and Initial Assessment

The initial assessment of the neonate is performed immediately after birth using the Apgar score (Table 23-1) and a brief physical examination (Table 23-2). A gestational age assessment is completed within the first hours of birth in a stable newborn (Fig. 23-2). A more comprehensive physical assessment is completed within 24 hours of birth (Table 23-3).

Apgar Score

The Apgar score permits a rapid assessment of the newborn's transition to extrauterine existence based on five signs that indicate the physiologic state of the neonate: (1) heart rate, based on auscultation with a stethoscope or palpation of the umbilical cord; (2) respiratory effort, based on observed movement of the chest wall; (3) muscle tone, based on degree of flexion and movement of the extremities; (4) reflex irritability, based on response to suctioning of the nares or pharynx; and (5) generalized skin color, described as pallid, cyanotic, or pink (see Table 23-1). Evaluations are made at 1 and 5 minutes after birth and can be completed by the nurse or birth attendant. Scores of 0 to 3 indicate severe distress, scores of 4 to 6 indicate moderate difficulty, and scores of 7 to 10 indicate that the infant is having minimal or no difficulty adjusting to extrauterine life. Apgar scores do not predict future neurologic outcome but are useful for describing the newborn's transition to the extrauterine environment (Box 23-2). If resuscitation is required, it should be initiated before the 1-minute Apgar score is determined (American College of Obstetricians and Gynecologists [ACOG] Committee on Obstetric Practice, 2006, 2010).

Initial Physical Assessment

The initial examination of the newborn (see Table 23-2) can occur while the nurse is drying and wrapping the infant, or observations can be made while the infant is lying on the mother's abdomen or in her arms immediately after birth. Efforts should be directed toward minimizing interference in the initial parent-infant acquaintance process. If the infant is breathing effectively, is pink, and has no apparent life-threatening anomalies or risk factors requiring immediate attention (e.g., infant of a mother with diabetes), further examination can be delayed until after the parents have had an opportunity to interact with the infant. Routine procedures and the admission process can be carried out in the mother's room or in a separate nursery.

Physical Assessment

Although the initial assessment after birth can reveal significant anomalies, birth injuries, and cardiopulmonary problems that have immediate implications, a more detailed, thorough physical examination should follow within 12 to 18 hours after birth (see Table 23-3). The parents' presence during this and other examinations encourages discussion of their concerns and actively involves them in the health care of their infant from birth. It also affords the nurse an opportunity to observe parental interactions with the infant. The findings provide a database for implementing the nursing process with newborns and providing anticipatory guidance for the parents. Ongoing assessments are made throughout the hospital stay; another detailed physical examination is performed before discharge.

General Appearance

The neonate's maturity level can be gauged by assessment of general appearance. Features to assess in the general survey include posture,

---

BOX 23-1 ASSESSMENT OF PRECONCEPTION, PRENATAL, AND INTRAPARTUM RISK FACTORS

Preconception
- Age
- Pre-existing medical conditions: Diabetes, hypertension, cardiac disease, anemia, thyroid disorder, renal disease, obesity
- Genetic factors: Family history
- Obstetric history: Gravidity, parity, number of living children and their ages, history of stillbirth, previous infant with congenital anomalies, habitual abortion, use of assisted-reproductive technology, interpregnancy spacing
- Blood type and Rh status

Prenatal
- Prenatal care: When started
- Nutrition: Weight gain, diet, obesity, eating disorders
- Health-compromising behaviors: Smoking, alcohol use, substance abuse
- Blood group or Rh sensitization
- Medications: Prescription, over-the-counter, and complementary/alternative medications
- History of infection: Sexually-transmitted infections, TORCH infections,* group B streptococci status

Intrapartum
- Length of gestation: Preterm, late preterm, term, or postterm
- First stage of labor: Length, electronic fetal monitoring—internal or external, rupture of membranes (time, presence of meconium), signs of fetal distress (decelerations)
- Group B streptococci status: Treatment during labor
- Second stage of labor: Length, vaginal or cesarean, instrument assisted—forceps or vacuum extractor, complications (shoulder dystocia, bleeding [abruptio placentae or placenta previa]), cord prolapse, maternal analgesia and/or anesthesia

Adapted from Broussard AB and Hurst HM: Antepartum-intrapartum complications. In Verklan TM and Walden M (eds.): *AWHONN core curriculum for neonatal intensive care nursing*, ed 4, St Louis, 2010, Saunders.
*TORCH is the collective name for *t*oxoplasmosis, *o*ther infections (e.g., hepatitis), *r*ubella virus, *c*ytomegalovirus (CMV), and *h*erpes simplex virus.

---

grasping the base of the cord or by auscultating the left chest with a stethoscope. Count for 6 seconds and multiply by 10 to calculate the heart rate. It should be greater than 100 beats/min. The newborn's trunk and lips should be pink; acrocyanosis is a normal finding (see Fig. 22-4) (Niermeyer and Clarke, 2011).

If the newborn requires respiratory or circulatory support, the nurse and other members of the health care team (e.g., neonatologist, respiratory therapist) follow the American Heart Association guidelines for neonatal resuscitation (Kattwinkel, Perlman, Aziz, et al., 2010). The neonatal resuscitation algorithm directs the care (Fig. 23-1).

As soon as possible after birth, the nurse places identically numbered bands on the infant's wrist and ankle, on the mother, and on the father or significant other. An electronic infant security tag or abduction system alarm should be placed on all newborns to aid in protecting against infant abduction. The infant is footprinted with

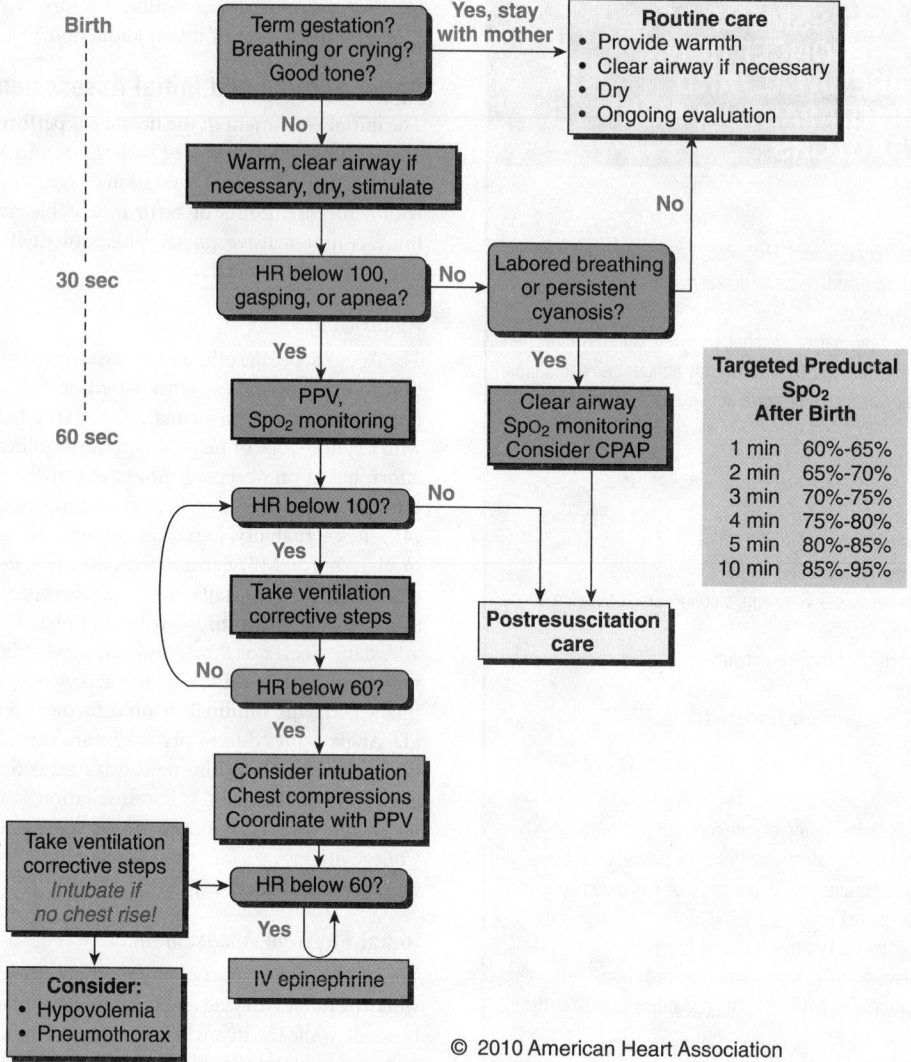

Birth

Term gestation?
Breathing or crying?
Good tone?

Yes, stay with mother →

Routine care
• Provide warmth
• Clear airway if necessary
• Dry
• Ongoing evaluation

No ↓

Warm, clear airway if
necessary, dry, stimulate

30 sec

HR below 100,
gasping, or apnea?

No →

Labored breathing
or persistent
cyanosis?

No →

Yes ↓

60 sec

PPV,
SpO₂ monitoring

Yes ↓

Clear airway
SpO₂ monitoring
Consider CPAP

**Targeted Preductal
SpO₂
After Birth**

1 min	60%-65%
2 min	65%-70%
3 min	70%-75%
4 min	75%-80%
5 min	80%-85%
10 min	85%-95%

HR below 100?

No →

Yes ↓

Take ventilation
corrective steps

**Postresuscitation
care**

No ← HR below 60?

Yes ↓

Consider intubation
Chest compressions
Coordinate with PPV

Take ventilation
corrective steps
*Intubate if
no chest rise!*

↔ HR below 60?

Yes ↓

Consider:
• Hypovolemia
• Pneumothorax

IV epinephrine

© 2010 American Heart Association

FIG 23-1 Neonatal resuscitation algorithm. *CPAP,* Continuous positive airway pressure; *HR,* heart rate; *IV,* intravenous; *PPV,* positive-pressure ventilation; *SpO₂,* blood oxygen saturation. (From Kattwinkel J, Perlman JM, Aziz K, et al: Part 15: neonatal resuscitation: 2010 American Heart Association guidelines for cardiopulmonary resuscitation and emergency cardiovascular care, *Circulation* 122(Suppl 3):S909–S919, 2010. Reprinted with permission of the American Heart Association.)

TABLE 23-1	**APGAR SCORE**		
	SCORE		
SIGN	**0**	**1**	**2**
Heart rate	Absent	Slow (<100/min)	>100/min
Respiratory effort	Absent	Slow, weak cry	Good cry
Muscle tone	Flaccid	Some flexion of extremities	Well flexed
Reflex irritability	No response	Grimace	Cry
Color	Blue, pale	Body pink, extremities blue	Completely pink

activity, any overt signs of anomalies that can cause initial distress, presence of bruising or other consequences of birth, and state of alertness. The normal resting position of the neonate is one of general flexion.

Vital Signs

The temperature, heart rate, and respiratory rate are always obtained. Blood pressure (BP) is not routinely assessed unless cardiac problems are suspected. An irregular, very slow, or very fast heart rate can indicate a need for further evaluation of circulatory status including BP measurement.

The axillary temperature is a safe, accurate measurement of temperature. Electronic thermometers have expedited this task and provide a reading within 1 minute. Temporal artery, tympanic, and oral routes for measuring temperature in the newborn are not considered accurate (Brown and Landers, 2011). Taking an infant's temperature can cause the infant to cry and struggle against the placement of the thermometer in the axilla. Before taking the

TABLE 23-2	INITIAL PHYSICAL ASSESSMENT OF THE NEWBORN
General appearance	□ Color pink □ Acrocyanosis present □ Flexed posture □ Alert □ Active
Respiratory system	□ Airway patent □ No upper airway congestion □ No retractions or nasal flaring □ Respiratory rate, 30-60 breaths/min □ Lungs clear to auscultation bilaterally □ Chest expansion symmetric
Cardiovascular system	□ Heart rate strong and regular □ No murmurs heard □ Pulses strong and equal bilaterally

Neurologic system	□ Moves extremities
	□ Normotonic
	□ Symmetric features, movement
	□ Reflexes present:
	  □ Sucking □ Rooting
	  □ Moro □ Grasp
	□ Anterior fontanel soft and flat

Gastrointestinal system	□ Abdomen soft, no distention □ Cord attached and clamped □ Anus appears patent
Eyes, nose, mouth	□ Eyes clear □ Palates intact □ Nares patent
Skin	□ No signs of birth trauma □ No lesions or abrasions
Genitourinary system	□ Normal genitalia
Other	□ No obvious anomalies

Comments:

_____

_____

_____

_____

temperature, the examiner can determine the apical heart rate and respiratory rate while the infant is quiet and at rest. The normal axillary temperature averages 37°C (98.6°F) with a range from 36.5° to 37.5°C (97.7° to 99.5°F).

⚡ SAFETY ALERT

Rectal temperatures should not be done on a newborn because of the risk for perforation.

The respiratory rate varies with the state of alertness and activity after birth. Respirations are abdominal in nature and can be counted by observing or lightly feeling the rise and fall of the abdomen. Neonatal respirations are shallow and irregular. The respirations should be counted for a full minute to obtain an accurate count because there are periods when respirations can cease for seconds (≤20) and resume again. The examiner should also

---

BOX 23-2	SIGNIFICANCE OF THE APGAR SCORE

The Apgar score was developed to provide a rapid systematic method of assessing an infant's condition at birth. When used correctly, it is useful for standardized assessment and provides a mechanism to document the neonate's transition after birth. It is designed to be used for a limited time frame. Apgar scores are affected by factors such as gestational age, maternal medications, trauma, congenital anomalies, hypovolemia, and hypoxia.

Researchers have tried to correlate Apgar scores with various outcomes in the term infant such as intelligence and neurologic development. In some instances, researchers have attempted to attribute causality to the Apgar score, that is, to suggest that the low Apgar score caused or predicted later problems. This use of the Apgar score is inappropriate.

There is a lack of evidence regarding the significance of the Apgar score in preterm infants. It should be used with this population of infants only for ongoing assessment in the delivery room.

The Apgar score is a useful index for monitoring neonatal response to resuscitation, especially in regard to a change in the score from 1 minute to 5 minutes after birth. However, assigning an Apgar score to a neonate during resuscitation is not equivalent to assigning a score to a newborn who is breathing spontaneously. It is important that health care professionals be consistent in assigning Apgar scores during a resuscitation.

Adapted from American College of Obstetricians and Gynecologists (ACOG) Committee on Obstetric Practice and American Academy of Pediatrics Committee on Fetus and Newborn: Committee opinion no. 333: the Apgar score, *Obstet Gynecol* 107:1209-1212, 2006, reaffirmed 2010.

observe for symmetry of chest movement. The average respiratory rate is 40 breaths/min but will vary between 30 and 60 breaths/min; respiratory rate can exceed 60 breaths/min if the newborn is very active or crying.

An apical pulse rate should be obtained on all newborns. Auscultation should be for a full minute, preferably when the infant is asleep or in a quiet alert state. The infant may need to be held and comforted during assessment. The normal heart rate ranges from 120 to 160 beats/min (Blackburn, 2013). It is common to detect brief irregularities in the heart rate. Heart rate varies with the newborn's behavioral state. Bradycardia is a heart rate less than 100 beats/min. However, a term infant in deep sleep may have a heart rate in the 80s or 90s; the rate should increase when the infant awakens. *Tachycardia* is defined as a sustained heart rate exceeding 160 beats/min. It is not unusual for a crying infant to have a heart rate greater than 160; the heart rate should decrease when the crying ceases (Furdon and Benjamin, 2010).

Assessment of neonatal blood pressure is based on agency policy. If BP is measured, an oscillometric monitor calibrated for neonatal pressures is preferred. An appropriate-size cuff (width-to-arm or width-to-calf ratio of 0.45 to 0.70, or approximately ½ to ¾) is essential for accuracy. Neonatal BP usually is highest immediately after birth and falls to a minimum by 3 hours after birth. It then begins to rise steadily and reaches a plateau between 4 and 6 days after birth. This measurement is usually equal to that of the immediate postbirth BP. The BP varies with the neonate's activity; accurate measurement is best obtained while the newborn is at rest. Blood pressure varies with gestational age and chronologic age. Systolic pressure in a term neonate averages 60 to 80 mm Hg; diastolic pressure averages 40 to 50 mm Hg. The mean arterial pressure should approximate the neonate's week of gestation. According to agency protocol, four extremity blood pressures may be assessed

ESTIMATION OF GESTATIONAL AGE BY MATURITY RATING

NEUROMUSCULAR MATURITY

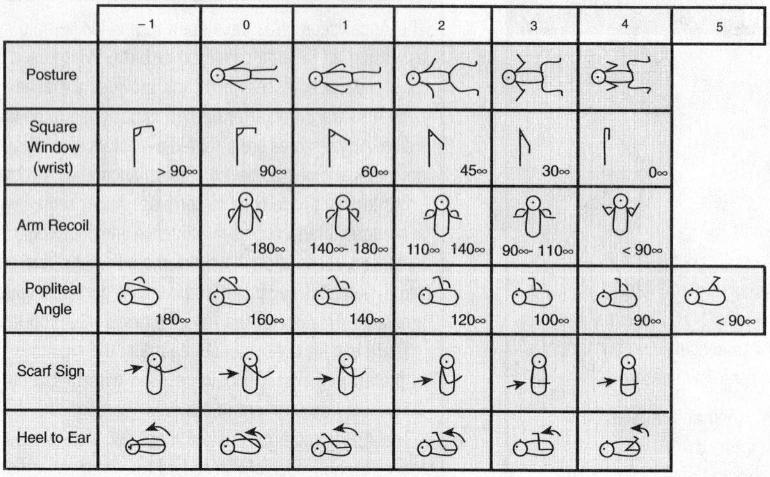

	-1	0	1	2	3	4	5
Posture							
Square Window (wrist)	> 90°	90°	60°	45°	30°	0°	
Arm Recoil		180°	140°-180°	110°-140°	90°-110°	< 90°	
Popliteal Angle	180°	160°	140°	120°	100°	90°	< 90°
Scarf Sign							
Heel to Ear							

PHYSICAL MATURITY

	-1	0	1	2	3	4
Skin	sticky friable transparent	gelatinous red, translucent	smooth pink, visible veins	superficial peeling &/or rash, few veins	cracking pale areas rare veins	parchment deep cracking no vessels
Lanugo	none	sparse	abundant	thinning	bald areas	mostly bald
Plantar Surface	heel-toe 40-50 mm: -1 <40 mm: -2	>50 mm no crease	faint red marks	anterior transverse crease only	creases ant. 2/3	creases over entire sole
Breast	imperceptible	barely perceptible	flat areola no bud	stippled areola 1-2 mm bud	raised areola 3-4 mm bud	full areola 5-10 mm bud
Eye/Ear	lids fused loosely: -1 tightly: -2	lids open pinna flat stays folded	slightly curved pinna; soft; slow recoil	well-curved pinna; soft but ready recoil	formed & firm instant recoil	thick cartilage ear stiff
Genitals (male)	scrotum flat, smooth	scrotum empty faint rugae	testes in upper canal rare rugae	testes descending few rugae	testes down good rugae	testes pendulous deep rugae
Genitals (female)	clitoris prominent labia flat	prominent clitoris small labia minora	prominent clitoris enlarging minora	majora & minora equally prominent	majora large minora small	majora cover clitoris & minora

A

MATURITY RATING

score	weeks
-10	20
-5	22
0	24
5	26
10	28
15	30
20	32
25	34
30	36
35	38
40	40
45	42
50	44

FIG 23-2 Estimation of gestational age. **A,** New Ballard Score for newborn maturity rating. Expanded scale includes extremely premature infants and has been refined to improve accuracy in more mature infants. (From Ballard JL, Khoury JC, Wedig K, et al: New Ballard Score, expanded to include extremely premature infants, *J Pediatr* 119(3):417-423, 1991.)

Continued

routinely or only when a murmur is auscultated. If the upper extremity pressures are more than 20 mm Hg greater than those in the lower extremities, the infant may have a cardiac defect such as coarctation of the aorta (Furdon and Benjamin, 2010). Peripheral pulses are also palpated as part of the assessment in any infant with a heart murmur.

> **! NURSING ALERT**
>
> To aid in identifying infants with asymptomatic congenital heart defects (CHDs), some institutions require routine pulse oximetry screening on all newborns before hospital discharge (Fig. 23-3) (see Chapter 25). Parents and care providers should be aware that this screening cannot detect all cases of CHD. A negative result does not exclude the possibility that a newborn has a congenital heart defect (Mahle, Newburger, Matherne, et al., 2009).

Baseline Measurements of Physical Growth

Baseline measurements are taken and recorded to help assess the progress and determine the growth patterns of the neonate. These measurements may be recorded on growth charts. The following measurements are made when the neonate is assessed.

Weight. The newborn is usually weighed shortly after birth. This assessment can be performed in the labor and birthing area, the mother's room, or on admission to the nursery. Care must be taken to ensure that the scales are balanced. The totally unclothed neonate is placed in the center of the scale, which is usually covered with a disposable pad or cloth to prevent heat loss via conduction and to prevent cross-infection. The nurse should place one hand over (but not touching) the neonate to be prepared to prevent the infant from falling off the scales. Weighing the infant at the same time every day is common during the hospital stay. Birth weight of a term infant typically ranges from 2500 to 4000 g (5.5 to 8.8 lb).

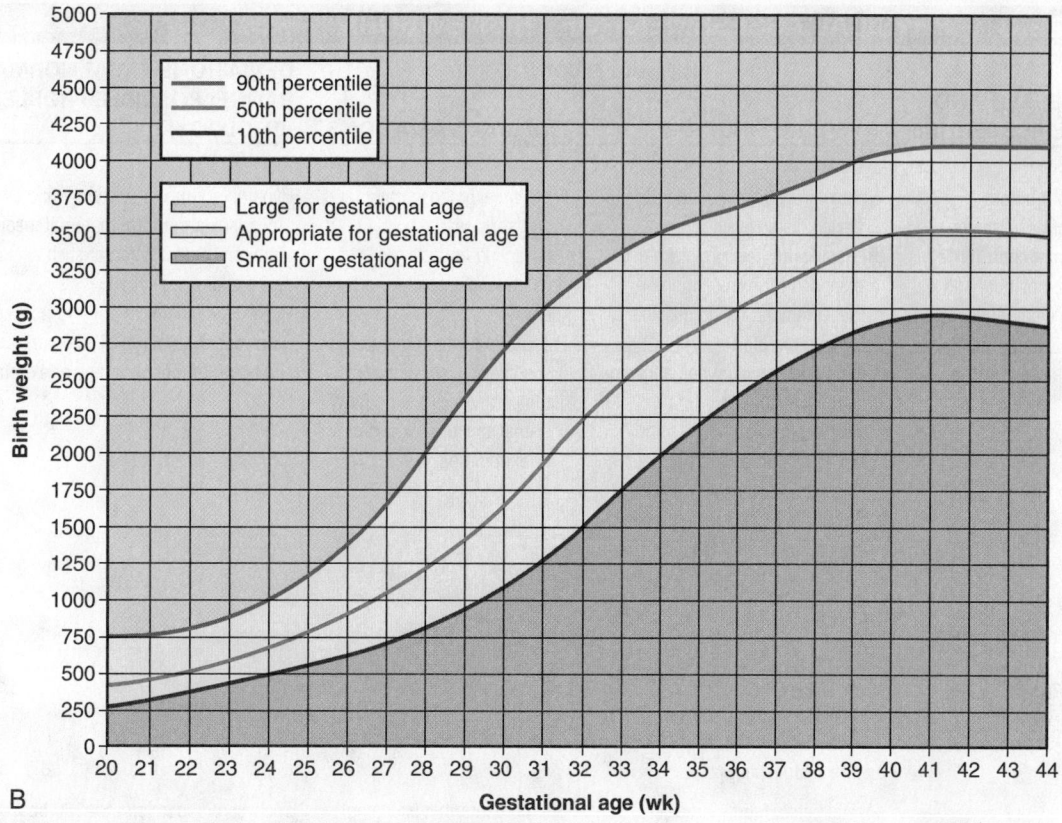

B

FIG 23-2, cont'd   B, Intrauterine growth: birth weight percentiles based on live single births at gestational ages 20 to 44 weeks. (*A*, from Ballard J, Khoury J, Wedig K, et al: New Ballard Score, expanded to include extremely premature infants, *J Pediatr* 119(3):417, 1991. *B*, Data from Alexander GR, Himes JH, Kaufman RB, et al: A United States national reference for fetal growth, *Obstet Gynecol* 87(2):163-168, 1996.)

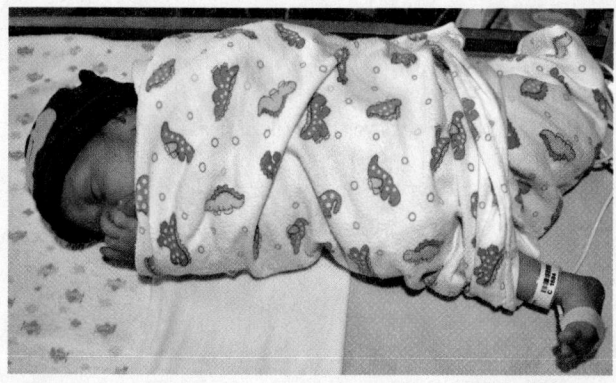

FIG 23-3 Pulse oximetry testing of a newborn. (Courtesy Cheryl Briggs, RNC, Annapolis, MD.)

Head Circumference and Body Length. The head is measured at the widest part, which is the occipitofrontal diameter. The tape measure is placed around the head just above the infant's eyebrows. The term neonate's head circumference ranges from 32 to 36.8 cm (12.6 to 14.5 in). (See Nursing Care Plan.)

The length may be difficult to obtain because of the flexed posture of the newborn. The examiner places the newborn on a flat surface and extends the leg until the knee is flat against the surface. Placing the head against a perpendicular surface and extending the leg may assist with obtaining this measurement. In the term neonate, head-to-heel length ranges from 45 to 55 cm (17.7 to 21.7 in.).

Neurologic Assessment

The physical examination includes a neurologic assessment of newborn reflexes (see Table 22-4). This assessment provides useful information about the infant's nervous system and state of neurologic maturation. Many reflex behaviors (e.g., sucking, rooting) are important for proper development. Other reflexes such as gagging and sneezing act as primitive safety mechanisms. The assessment needs to be carried out as early as possible because abnormal signs present in the early neonatal period may require further investigation before the newborn is discharged home.

Gestational Age Assessment

Assessment of gestational age is important because perinatal morbidity and mortality rates are related to gestational age and birth weight. A frequently used method of determining gestational age is the New Ballard Score, which can be used to measure gestational ages of infants as young as 20 weeks of gestation. It assesses six external physical and six neuromuscular signs. Each sign has a numeric score, and the cumulative score correlates with a maturity rating (gestational age). The examination of infants with a gestational age of 26 weeks or less should be performed at a postnatal age of less than 12 hours. For infants with a gestational age of at least 26 weeks, the examination can be performed up to 96 hours after birth. To ensure accuracy, experts recommend that the initial examination is performed within the first 48 hours of life. Neuromuscular adjustments after birth in extremely immature neonates require that

Text continued on p. 601.

TABLE 23-3 PHYSICAL ASSESSMENT OF THE NEWBORN

AREA ASSESSED AND APPRAISAL PROCEDURE	NORMAL FINDINGS		DEVIATIONS FROM NORMAL RANGE: POSSIBLE PROBLEMS (ETIOLOGY)
	AVERAGE FINDINGS	NORMAL VARIATIONS	
Posture Inspect newborn before disturbing for assessment Refer to maternal chart for fetal presentation, position, and type of birth (vaginal, surgical), given that newborn readily assumes in utero position	Vertex: arms, legs in moderate flexion; fists clenched Resistance to having extremities extended for examination or measurement, crying possible when attempted Cessation of crying when allowed to resume curled-up fetal position (lateral) Normal spontaneous movement bilaterally asynchronous (legs moving in bicycle fashion) but equal extension in all extremities	Frank breech: legs straighter and stiff, newborn assuming intrauterine position in repose for a few days Prenatal pressure on limb or shoulder possibly causing temporary facial asymmetry or resistance to extension of extremities	Hypotonia, relaxed posture while awake (preterm or hypoxia in utero, maternal medications, neuromuscular disorder such as spinal muscular atrophy) Hypertonia (chemical dependence, central nervous system [CNS] disorder) Limitation of motion in any of extremities
Vital Signs **Check heart rate and pulses:** Thorax (chest)			
Inspection	Visible pulsations in left midclavicular line, fifth intercostal space		
Palpation	Apical pulse, fourth intercostal space 120-160 beats/min when awake	80-100 beats/min (sleeping) to 180 beats/min (crying); possibly irregular for brief periods, especially after crying	Tachycardia: persistent, ≥180 beats/min (respiratory distress syndrome [RDS]; pneumonia) Bradycardia: persistent, ≤80 beats/min (congenital heart block, maternal lupus)
Auscultation Apex: mitral valve Second interspace, left of sternum: pulmonic valve Second interspace, right of sternum: aortic valve Junction of xiphoid process and sternum: tricuspid valve	Quality: *first sound* (closure of mitral and tricuspid valves) and *second sound* (closure of aortic and pulmonic valves) sharp and clear	Murmur, especially over base or at left sternal border in interspace 3 or 4 (foramen ovale anatomically closing at approximately 1 yr)	Murmur (possibly functional) Dysrhythmias: irregular rate Sounds: Distant (pneumopericardium) Poor quality Extra Heart on right side of chest (dextrocardia, often accompanied by reversal of intestines)
Peripheral pulses: femoral, brachial, popliteal, posterior tibial	Peripheral pulses equal and strong		Weak or absent peripheral pulses (decreased cardiac output, thrombus, possible coarctation of aorta if weak on left and strong on right) Bounding
Obtain temperature: Axillary: method of choice Temporal and intraauricular thermometers not effective in measuring newborn temperature	Axillary: 37° C (98.6° F) Temperature stabilized by 8-10 hr of age	36.5°-37.5° C (97.7°-100° F) Heat loss: from evaporation, conduction, convection, radiation	Subnormal (preterm birth, infection, low environmental temperature, inadequate clothing, dehydration) Increased (infection, high environmental temperature, excessive clothing, proximity to heating unit or in direct sunshine, chemical dependence, diarrhea and dehydration) Temperature not stabilized by 6-8 hr after birth (if mother received magnesium sulfate, newborn less able to conserve heat by vasoconstriction; maternal analgesics possibly reducing thermal stability in newborn)

TABLE 23-3   PHYSICAL ASSESSMENT OF THE NEWBORN—cont'd

AREA ASSESSED AND APPRAISAL PROCEDURE	NORMAL FINDINGS		DEVIATIONS FROM NORMAL RANGE: POSSIBLE PROBLEMS (ETIOLOGY)
	AVERAGE FINDINGS	NORMAL VARIATIONS	
Observe and monitor respiratory rate and effort:			

Observe respirations when infant is at rest
Observe respiratory effort
Count respirations for full minute
Auscultate breath sounds
Listen for sounds audible without stethoscope
	40/min
	Tendency to be shallow and irregular in rate, rhythm, and depth when infant is awake
	Crackles may be heard after birth
	No adventitious sounds audible on inspiration and expiration
	Breath sounds: bronchial; loud, clear
		30-60/min
		Short periodic breathing episodes and no evidence of respiratory distress or apnea (>20 sec); periodic breathing
		First period (reactivity): 50-60/min
		Second period: 50-70/min
		Stabilization (1-2 days): 30-40/min
		Crackles (fine)
			Apneic episodes: >20 sec (preterm infant: rapid warming or cooling of infant; CNS or blood glucose instability)
			Bradypnea: <25/min (maternal narcosis from analgesics or anesthetics, birth trauma)
			Tachypnea: >60/min (RDS, transient tachypnea of the newborn, congenital diaphragmatic hernia)
			Breath sounds:
			  Crackles (coarse), rhonchi, wheezing
			  Expiratory grunt (narrowing of bronchi)
			Distress evidenced by nasal flaring, grunting, retractions, labored breathing
			Stridor (upper airway occlusion)

Obtain blood pressure (BP) (usually not done in normal term infant)			

Check oscillometric monitor BP cuff: BP cuff width affects readings, use appropriate-size cuff and palpate brachial, popliteal, or posterior tibial pulse (depending on measurement site)	60-80/40-50 mm Hg (approximate ranges)
	At birth
	  Systolic: 60-80 mm Hg
	  Diastolic: 40-50 mm Hg
	At 2 weeks
	  Systolic: 68-88 mm Hg
	  Diastolic: 40-60 mm Hg
		Variation with change in activity level: awake, crying, sleeping	Difference between upper and lower extremity pressures (coarctation of aorta)
			Hypotension (sepsis, hypovolemia)
			Hypertension (coarctation of aorta, renal involvement, thrombus)

Weight			
Put cloth or paper protective liner in place and adjust scale to 0 g or pounds and ounces Weigh at same time each day Protect newborn from heat loss	Female: 3400 g (7.5 lb) Male: 3500 g (7.7 lb) Regaining of birth weight within first 2 weeks	2500-4000 g (5.5-8.8 lb) Acceptable weight loss: 10% or less in first 3-5 days Second baby weighing more than first (on average)	Weight ≤2500 g (preterm, small for gestational age, rubella syndrome) Weight ≥4000 g (large for gestational age, maternal diabetes, heredity—normal for these parents) Weight loss more than 10% to 15% (growth failure, dehydration); assess breastfeeding success

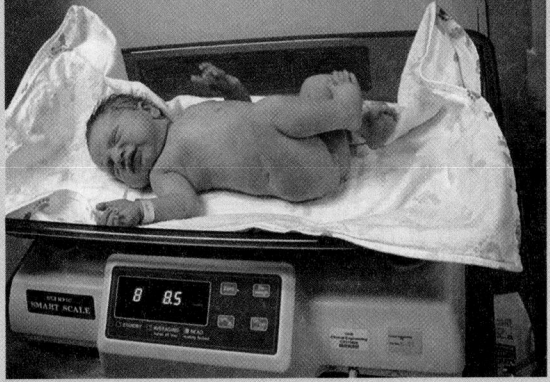

Weighing the infant. The nurse never leaves the infant alone on a scale. The scale is covered to protect against cross-infection. (Courtesy Wendy and Marwood Larson-Harris, Roanoke, VA.)

Continued

TABLE 23-3 PHYSICAL ASSESSMENT OF THE NEWBORN—cont'd

AREA ASSESSED AND APPRAISAL PROCEDURE	NORMAL FINDINGS		DEVIATIONS FROM NORMAL RANGE: POSSIBLE PROBLEMS (ETIOLOGY)
	AVERAGE FINDINGS	NORMAL VARIATIONS	
Length Measure length from top of head to heel; measuring is difficult in term infant because of presence of molding, incomplete extension of knees	50 cm (19.7 in)	45-55 cm (17.7-21.7 in)	<45 cm (17.7 in) or >55 cm (21.7 in) (chromosomal abnormality, heredity—normal for these parents); some syndromes present shorter-than-average limb length (skeletal dysplasias, achondroplasia)

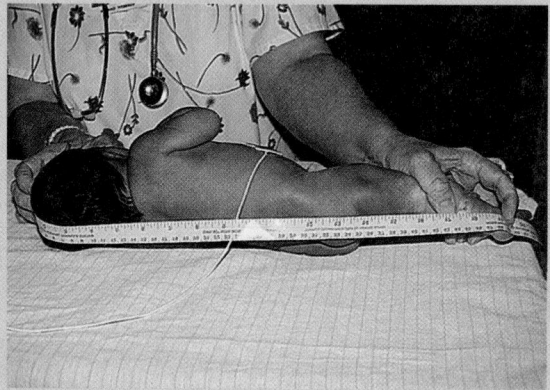

Measuring length crown to heel. To determine total length, include length of legs. If measurements are taken before the infant's initial bath, wear gloves. (Courtesy Marjorie Pyle, RNC, Lifecircle, Costa Mesa, CA.)

AREA ASSESSED AND APPRAISAL PROCEDURE	AVERAGE FINDINGS	NORMAL VARIATIONS	DEVIATIONS
Head Circumference Measure head at greatest diameter: occipitofrontal circumference May need to remeasure on second or third day after resolution of molding and caput succedaneum	33-35 cm (13-13.8 in) Circumference of head and chest approximately the same for first 1 or 2 days after birth; chest rarely measured on routine basis	32-36.8 cm (12.6-14.5 in)	Microcephaly, head ≤32 cm: (maternal rubella, toxoplasmosis, cytomegalovirus, fused cranial sutures [craniosynostosis]) Hydrocephaly: sutures widely separated, circumference ≥4 cm more than chest circumference (infection) Increased intracranial pressure (hemorrhage, space-occupying lesion)

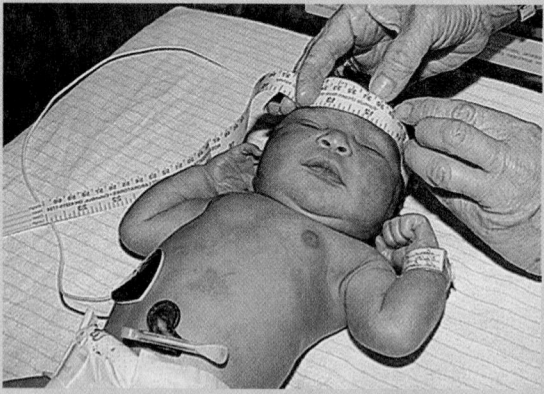

Measuring circumference of head. (Courtesy Marjorie Pyle, RNC, Lifecircle, Costa Mesa, CA.)

TABLE 23-3   PHYSICAL ASSESSMENT OF THE NEWBORN—cont'd

AREA ASSESSED AND APPRAISAL PROCEDURE	NORMAL FINDINGS		DEVIATIONS FROM NORMAL RANGE: POSSIBLE PROBLEMS (ETIOLOGY)
	AVERAGE FINDINGS	NORMAL VARIATIONS	
Chest Circumference			
Measure at nipple line	2-3 cm (0.8-1.2 in) less than head circumference; average 30-33 cm (11.8-13 in)	≤30 cm	Prematurity

Measuring circumference of chest. (Courtesy Marjorie Pyle, RNC, Lifecircle, Costa Mesa, CA.)

AREA ASSESSED AND APPRAISAL PROCEDURE	AVERAGE FINDINGS	NORMAL VARIATIONS	DEVIATIONS FROM NORMAL RANGE: POSSIBLE PROBLEMS (ETIOLOGY)
Skin			

Check color:
  Inspect and palpate
  Inspect semi-naked newborn in well-lighted, warm area without drafts; natural daylight best
  Inspect newborn when quiet and alert
	Generally pink
	Varies with ethnic origin, skin pigmentation beginning to deepen right after birth in basal layer of epidermis
	Acrocyanosis common after birth
		Mottling
		Harlequin sign
		Plethora
		Telangiectases ("stork bites" or capillary hemangiomas) (see Fig. 22-6, *A*)
		Erythema toxicum/neonatorum ("newborn rash") (see Fig. 22-6, *B*)
		Milia
		Petechiae over presenting part
		Ecchymoses from forceps in vertex births or over buttocks, genitalia, and legs in breech births
			Dark red (preterm, polycythemia)
			Gray (hypotension, poor perfusion)
			Pallor (cardiovascular problem, CNS damage, blood dyscrasia, blood loss, twin-to-twin transfusion, infection)
			Cyanosis (hypothermia, infection, hypoglycemia, cardiopulmonary diseases, neurologic or respiratory malformations)
			Generalized petechiae (clotting factor deficiency, infection)
			Generalized ecchymoses (hemorrhagic disease)

Observe for jaundice	None at birth	Physiologic jaundice in up to 60% of term infants in first week of life	Jaundice within first 24 hr (increased hemolysis, Rh isoimmunization, ABO incompatibility)
Observe for birthmarks or bruises: Inspect and palpate for location, size, distribution, characteristics, color, if obstructing airway or oral cavity		Mongolian spot (see Fig. 22-5) in infants of African-American, Asian, and Native-American origin	Hemangiomas Nevus flammeus: port-wine stain Nevus vasculosus: strawberry mark Cavernous hemangioma

Continued

TABLE 23-3 PHYSICAL ASSESSMENT OF THE NEWBORN—cont'd

AREA ASSESSED AND APPRAISAL PROCEDURE	NORMAL FINDINGS		DEVIATIONS FROM NORMAL RANGE: POSSIBLE PROBLEMS (ETIOLOGY)
	AVERAGE FINDINGS	NORMAL VARIATIONS	
Check skin condition: Inspect and palpate for intactness, smoothness, texture, edema, pressure points if ill or immobilized	Edema confined to eyelid (result of eye prophylaxis) Opacity: few large blood vessels visible indistinctly over abdomen	Possibly puffy Slightly thick; superficial cracking, peeling, especially of hands, feet No visible blood vessels, a few large vessels clearly visible over abdomen Some fingernail scratches	Edema on hands, feet; pitting over tibia; periorbital (overhydration; hydrops) Texture thin, smooth, or of medium thickness; rash or superficial peeling visible (preterm, postterm) Numerous vessels very visible over abdomen (preterm) Texture thick, parchment-like; cracking, peeling (postterm) Skin tags, webbing Papules, pustules, vesicles, ulcers, maceration (impetigo, candidiasis, herpes, diaper rash)
Weigh infant routinely	Dehydration: loss of weight best indicator	Normal weight loss after birth: up to 10% of birth weight	
Gently pinch skin between thumb and forefinger over abdomen and inner thigh to check for turgor	After pinch released, skin returns to original state immediately		Loose, wrinkled skin (prematurity, postmaturity, dehydration: fold of skin persisting after release of pinch) Tense, tight, shiny skin (edema, extreme cold, shock, infection)
Note presence of subcutaneous fat deposits (adipose pads) over cheeks, buttocks		Variation in amount of subcutaneous fat	Lack of subcutaneous fat, prominence of clavicle or ribs (preterm, malnutrition)
Check for vernix caseosa: Observe color, amount, and odor before bath or removing clothing	Whitish, cheesy, odorless	Usually more found in creases, folds	Absent or minimal (postmature infant) Abundant (preterm) Green color (possible in utero release of meconium or presence of bilirubin) Odor (possible intrauterine infection)
Assess lanugo: Inspect for this fine, downy hair, amount and distribution	Over shoulders, pinnas of ears, forehead	Variation in amount	Absent (postmature) Abundant (preterm, especially if lanugo abundant, long, and thick over back)
Head Palpate skin	(See "Skin")	Caput succedaneum, possibly showing some ecchymosis (see Fig. 22-10, *A*)	Cephalhematoma (see Fig. 22-10, *B*)
Inspect shape, size	Making up one fourth of body length Molding (see Fig. 22-9)	Slight asymmetry from intrauterine position Lack of molding (preterm, breech presentation, cesarean birth)	Severe molding (birth trauma) Indentation (fracture from trauma)
Palpate, inspect, and note size and status of fontanels (open vs. closed)	Anterior fontanel 5-cm diamond, increasing as molding resolves Posterior fontanel triangle, smaller than anterior	Variation in fontanel size with degree of molding Difficulty in feeling fontanels possible because of molding	Fontanels: Full, bulging (tumor, hemorrhage, infection) Large, flat, soft (malnutrition, hydrocephaly, delayed bone age, hypothyroidism) Depressed (dehydration)

TABLE 23-3   PHYSICAL ASSESSMENT OF THE NEWBORN—cont'd

AREA ASSESSED AND APPRAISAL PROCEDURE	NORMAL FINDINGS		DEVIATIONS FROM NORMAL RANGE: POSSIBLE PROBLEMS (ETIOLOGY)
	AVERAGE FINDINGS	NORMAL VARIATIONS	
Palpate sutures	Palpable and separated sutures	Possible overlap of sutures with molding	Sutures: Widely spaced (hydrocephaly) Premature closure (fused) (craniosynostosis)
Inspect pattern, distribution, amount of hair; feel texture	Silky, single strands lying flat; growth pattern toward face and neck	Variation in amount	Fine, wooly (preterm) Unusual swirls, patterns, or hairline; or coarse, brittle (endocrine or genetic disorders)
Eyes			
Check placement on face	Eyes and space between eyes each one-third the distance from outer-to-outer canthus	Epicanthal folds: characteristic in some ethnicities	Epicanthal folds when present with other signs (chromosomal disorders such as Down, cri-du-chat syndromes)

In pseudostrabismus, inner epicanthal folds cause the eyes to appear misaligned; however, corneal light reflexes are perfectly symmetric. Eyes are symmetric in size and shape and are well placed.

AREA ASSESSED AND APPRAISAL PROCEDURE	AVERAGE FINDINGS	NORMAL VARIATIONS	DEVIATIONS FROM NORMAL RANGE: POSSIBLE PROBLEMS (ETIOLOGY)
Check for symmetry in size, shape	Symmetric in size, shape		
Check eyelids for size, movement, blink	Blink reflex	Edema if eye prophylaxis drops or ointment instilled	
Assess for discharge	None No tears	Some discharge if silver nitrate used Occasional presence of some tears	Discharge: purulent (infection) Chemical conjunctivitis from eye medication is common—requires no treatment
Evaluate eyeballs for presence, size, shape	Both present and of equal size, both round, firm	Subconjunctival hemorrhage	Agenesis or absence of one or both eyeballs Lens opacity or absence of red reflex (congenital cataracts, possibly from rubella, retinoblastoma [cat's eye reflex]) Lesions: coloboma, absence of part of iris (congenital) Pink color of iris (albinism) Jaundiced sclera (hyperbilirubinemia)
Check pupils	Present, equal in size, reactive to light		Pupils: unequal, constricted, dilated, fixed (intracranial pressure, medications, tumor)
Evaluate eyeball movement	Random, jerky, uneven, focus possible briefly, following to midline	Transient strabismus or nystagmus until third or fourth month	Persistent strabismus Doll's eyes (increased intracranial pressure) Sunset (increased intracranial pressure)
Assess eyebrows: amount of hair, pattern	Distinct (not connected in midline)		Connection in midline (Cornelia de Lange syndrome)

Continued

TABLE 23-3 PHYSICAL ASSESSMENT OF THE NEWBORN—cont'd

AREA ASSESSED AND APPRAISAL PROCEDURE	NORMAL FINDINGS		DEVIATIONS FROM NORMAL RANGE: POSSIBLE PROBLEMS (ETIOLOGY)
	AVERAGE FINDINGS	NORMAL VARIATIONS	
Nose Observe shape, placement, patency, configuration	Midline Some mucus but no drainage Preferential nose breather Sneezing to clear nose	Slight deformity (flat or deviated to one side) from passage through birth canal	Copious drainage (rarely congenital syphilis); blockage membranous or bone with cyanosis at rest and return of pink color with crying (choanal atresia) Malformed (congenital syphilis, chromosomal disorder) Flaring of nares (respiratory distress)
Ears Observe size, placement on head, amount of cartilage, open auditory canal	Correct placement line drawn through inner and outer canthi of eyes reaching to top notch of ears (at junction with scalp) Well-formed, firm cartilage	Size: small, large, floppy Darwin's tubercle (nodule on posterior helix)	Agenesis Lack of cartilage (preterm) Low placement (chromosomal disorder, intellectual disability, kidney disorder) Preauricular tag or sinus Size: possibly overly prominent or protruding ears

Placement of ears on the head in relation to a line drawn from the inner to the outer canthus of the eye. **A,** Normal position. **B,** Abnormally angled ear. **C,** True low-set ear. (Courtesy Mead Johnson Nutritionals, Evansville, IN.)

Assess hearing	Responds to voice and other sounds	State (e.g., alert, asleep) influencing response	Lack of response to loud noise *should not* imply deafness
Perform universal newborn hearing screening to identify deficits (see Fig. 23-11)	Both ears pass		One or both ears fail
Facies Observe overall appearance and symmetry of face	Rounded and symmetric; influenced by birth type, molding, or both	Positional deformities	Usually accompanied by other features such as low-set ears, other structural disorders (hereditary, chromosomal aberration)

Mouth
Inspect and palpate
Assess buccal mucosa
   Dry or moist
   Pink
   Status intact
Assess lips for color, configuration, movement
	Symmetry of lip movement	Transient circumoral cyanosis	Gross anomalies in placement, size, shape (cleft lip or palate [or both], gums)
			Cyanosis, circumoral pallor (respiratory distress, hypothermia)
			Asymmetry in movement of lips (seventh cranial nerve paralysis)

TABLE 23-3   PHYSICAL ASSESSMENT OF THE NEWBORN—cont'd

AREA ASSESSED AND APPRAISAL PROCEDURE	NORMAL FINDINGS		DEVIATIONS FROM NORMAL RANGE: POSSIBLE PROBLEMS (ETIOLOGY)
	AVERAGE FINDINGS	NORMAL VARIATIONS	
Check gums	Pink gums	Inclusion cysts (Epstein pearls—Bohn nodules, whitish, hard nodules on gums or roof of mouth)	Teeth: predeciduous or deciduous (hereditary)
Assess tongue for color, mobility, movement, size	Tongue not protruding, freely movable, symmetric in shape, movement Sucking pads inside cheeks	Short lingual frenulum (ankyloglossia)	Macroglossia (preterm, chromosomal disorder) Thrush: white plaques on cheeks or tongue that bleed if touched (*Candida albicans*)
Assess palate (soft, hard): Arch Uvula	Soft and hard palates intact Uvula in midline	Anatomic groove in palate to accommodate nipple, disappearance by 3 to 4 yr of age Epstein pearls	Cleft hard or soft palate
Assess chin	Distinct chin		Micrognathia—recessed chin with prominent overbite (Pierre Robin or other syndrome)
Evaluate saliva for amount, character	Mouth moist, pink		Excessive salivation and choking or turning blue (esophageal atresia, tracheoesophageal fistula)
Check reflexes: Rooting Sucking Extrusion	Reflexes present	Reflex response dependent on state of wakefulness and hunger	Absent (preterm)
Neck			
Inspect and palpate for movement, flexibility, masses, bruising	Short, thick, surrounded by skin folds; no webbing		Webbing (Turner syndrome)
Check sternocleidomastoid muscles, movement and position of head	Head held in midline (sternocleidomastoid muscles equal), no masses Freedom of movement from side to side and flexion and extension, no movement of chin past shoulder	Transient positional deformity apparent when newborn is at rest: passive movement of head possible	Restricted movement, holding of head at angle (torticollis [wryneck], opisthotonos) Absence of head control (preterm birth, Down syndrome, hypotonia [spinal muscular atrophy])
Assess trachea for position and thyroid gland	Thyroid not palpable		Masses (enlarged thyroid) Distended veins (cardiopulmonary disorder) Skin tags
Chest			
Inspect and palpate shape of chest	Almost circular, barrel shaped	Tip of sternum possibly prominent	Bulging of chest, unequal movement (pneumothorax, pneumomediastinum) Malformation (funnel chest—pectus excavatum)
Observe respiratory movements	Symmetric chest movements, chest and abdominal movements synchronized during respirations	Occasional retractions, especially when crying	Retractions with or without respiratory distress (preterm, RDS) Paradoxic breathing
Evaluate clavicles	Clavicles intact		Fracture of clavicle (trauma); crepitus
Assess ribs	Rib cage symmetric, intact; moves with respirations		Poor development of rib cage and musculature (preterm)

Continued

TABLE 23-3   PHYSICAL ASSESSMENT OF THE NEWBORN—cont'd

AREA ASSESSED AND APPRAISAL PROCEDURE	NORMAL FINDINGS		DEVIATIONS FROM NORMAL RANGE: POSSIBLE PROBLEMS (ETIOLOGY)
	AVERAGE FINDINGS	NORMAL VARIATIONS	

Assess nipples for size, placement, number	Nipples prominent, well formed; symmetrically placed		Nipples
			  Supernumerary, along nipple line
			  Malpositioned or widely spaced

Check breast tissue	Breast nodule: approximately 6 mm in term infant	Breast nodule: 3-10 mm Secretion of witch's milk	Lack of breast tissue (preterm) Sounds: bowel sounds may be heard in diaphragmatic hernia (see "Abdomen")
Auscultate: Heart sounds and rate and breath sounds (see "Vital Signs")			
Abdomen			
Inspect and palpate umbilical cord	Two arteries, one vein Whitish gray Definite demarcation between cord and skin, no intestinal structures within cord Dry around base, drying Odorless Cord clamp in place for 24 to 48 hr	Reducible umbilical hernia	One artery (renal anomaly) Meconium stained (intrauterine distress) Bleeding or oozing around cord (hemorrhagic disease) Redness or drainage around cord (infection, possible persistence of urachus) Hernia: herniation of abdominal contents through cord opening (e.g., omphalocele); defect covered with thin, friable membrane, possibly extensive

Inspect size of abdomen and palpate contour	Rounded, prominent, dome shaped because abdominal musculature not fully developed
	Liver possibly palpable 1-2 cm (0.4-0.8 in) below right costal margin
	No other masses palpable
	No distention
	Few visible veins on abdominal surface
		Some diastasis recti (separation) of abdominal musculature	Gastroschisis: herniation of abdominal contents to the side or above the cord, contents not covered by membranous tissue and may include liver
			Distention at birth: ruptured viscus, genitourinary masses or malformations: hydronephrosis, teratomas, abdominal tumors
			  Mild (overfeeding, high gastrointestinal tract obstruction)
			  Marked (lower gastrointestinal tract obstruction, anorectal malformation, anal stenosis), often with bilious emesis
			  Intermittent or transient (overfeeding)
			Partial intestinal obstruction (stenosis of bowel)
			Visible peristalsis (obstruction)
			Malrotation of bowel or adhesions
			Sepsis (infection)

Auscultate bowel sounds and note number, amount, and character of stools	Sounds present within minutes after birth in healthy term infant Meconium stool passing within 24-48 hr after birth		Scaphoid, with bowel sounds in chest and severe respiratory distress (congenital diaphragmatic hernia)
Assess color		Linea nigra possibly apparent and caused by hormone influence during pregnancy	
Observe movement with respiration	Respirations primarily diaphragmatic, abdominal and chest movement synchronous		Decreased or absent abdominal movement with breathing (phrenic nerve palsy, congenital diaphragmatic hernia)

TABLE 23-3 PHYSICAL ASSESSMENT OF THE NEWBORN—cont'd

AREA ASSESSED AND APPRAISAL PROCEDURE	NORMAL FINDINGS		DEVIATIONS FROM NORMAL RANGE: POSSIBLE PROBLEMS (ETIOLOGY)
	AVERAGE FINDINGS	NORMAL VARIATIONS	
Genitalia **Female (see Fig. 22-7, A)** Inspect and palpate			
General appearance		Increased pigmentation caused by pregnancy hormones	Ambiguous genitalia—wide variation (small phallus not well distinguished from enlarged clitoris)
Clitoris	Usually edematous		Virilized female—extremely large clitoris (congenital adrenal hyperplasia)
Labia majora	Usually edematous, covering labia minora in term newborns	Edema and ecchymosis after breech birth Some vernix caseosa between labia possible	
Labia minora	Possible protrusion over labia majora		Enlarged clitoris with urinary meatus on tip, absent scrotum, micropenis, fused labia Stenosed meatus Labia majora widely separated and labia minora prominent (preterm)
Discharge	Smegma	Blood-tinged discharge from pseudomenstruation caused by pregnancy hormones	Fecal discharge (fistula)
Vagina	Open orifice Mucoid discharge Hymenal/vaginal tag		Absence of vaginal orifice
Urinary meatus	Beneath clitoris, difficult to see		Bladder exstrophy (bladder outside abdominal cavity and turned inside out)
Check urination	Voiding 2-6 times per 24 hr for first 1-2 days; voiding 6-10 times per 24 hr by day 4 or 5	Rust-stained urine (uric acid crystals)	No void within first 24 hours (renal agenesis; Potter syndrome)
Male (see Fig. 22-7, B) Inspect and palpate			
General appearance		Increased size and pigmentation caused by pregnancy hormones, (wide variation in size of genitalia)	Ambiguous genitalia Micropenis
Penis Urinary meatus appearance Prepuce (foreskin)—do not forcibly retract foreskin if uncircumcised	Foreskin covers glans (if uncircumcised), meatus at tip of penis Prepuce covering glans penis and not retractable	Prepuce removed if circumcised	Urinary meatus not on tip of glans penis (hypospadias, epispadias, foreskin may be retracted or absent) Round meatal opening
Scrotum: Rugae (wrinkles)	Large, edematous, pendulous in term infant; covered with rugae	Scrotal edema and ecchymosis if breech birth Hydrocele, small, noncommunicating	Scrotum smooth and testes undescended (preterm, cryptorchidism) Bifid scrotum Hydrocele Inguinal hernia
Testes	Palpable on each side	Bulge palpable in inguinal canal	Undescended (preterm)

Continued

TABLE 23-3   PHYSICAL ASSESSMENT OF THE NEWBORN—cont'd

AREA ASSESSED AND APPRAISAL PROCEDURE	NORMAL FINDINGS		DEVIATIONS FROM NORMAL RANGE: POSSIBLE PROBLEMS (ETIOLOGY)
	AVERAGE FINDINGS	NORMAL VARIATIONS	
Check urination	Voiding within 24 hr, stream adequate	Rust-stained urine (uric acid crystals)	No void in first 24 hr (renal agenesis; Potter syndrome)
Check reflexes:			
Cremasteric	Testes retracted, especially when newborn is chilled		
Extremities			
Make a general check: Inspect and palpate Degree of flexion Range of motion Symmetry of motion Muscle tone	Assuming of position maintained in utero Attitude of general flexion Full range of motion, spontaneous movements	Transient positional deformities	Limited motion (malformations) Poor muscle tone (preterm, maternal medications, CNS anomalies)
Check arms and hands: Inspect and palpate Color Intactness Appropriate placement	Longer than legs in newborn period Contours and movements symmetric	Slight tremors sometimes apparent Some acrocyanosis	Asymmetry of movement (fracture/crepitus, brachial nerve trauma, malformations) Asymmetry of contour (malformations, fracture) Amelia or phocomelia (teratogens) Palmar creases Simian line with short, incurved little fingers (Down syndrome)
Count number of fingers	Five on each hand Fist often clenched with thumb under fingers		Webbing of fingers: syndactyly Absence or excess of fingers Strong, rigid flexion; persistent fists; positioning of fists in front of mouth constantly (CNS disorder) Yellowed nail beds (meconium staining)
Evaluate joints: Shoulder Elbow Wrist Fingers	Full range of motion, symmetric contour		Increased tonicity, clonus, prolonged tremors (CNS disorder)
Check reflex: grasp (palmar and plantar)	Palmar: Infant's fingers flex tightly around examiner's finger when palm is stimulated Plantar: Infant's toes flex tightly around examiner's finger when base of toes on sole of foot is stimulated	Spontaneous grasp responses during sucking	Weak or absent reflexes can indicate CNS depression
Check legs and feet: Inspect and palpate Color Intactness Length in relation to arms and body and to each other	Appearance of bowing because lateral muscles more developed than medial muscles	Feet appearing to turn in but can be easily rotated externally, positional defects tending to correct while infant is crying Acrocyanosis	Amelia, phocomelia (chromosomal defect, teratogenic effect) Temperature of one leg differing from that of the other (circulatory deficiency, CNS disorder)
Number of toes	Five on each foot		Webbing, syndactyly (chromosomal defect) Absence or excess of digits (chromosomal defect, familial trait)
Femur Head of femur as legs are flexed and abducted, placement in acetabulum (see Fig. 22-12)	Intact femur		Femoral fracture (difficult breech birth) Developmental dysplasia of the hip (DDH)
Major gluteal folds	Major gluteal folds even		Gluteal folds uneven: DDH

TABLE 23-3   PHYSICAL ASSESSMENT OF THE NEWBORN—cont'd

AREA ASSESSED AND APPRAISAL PROCEDURE	NORMAL FINDINGS		DEVIATIONS FROM NORMAL RANGE: POSSIBLE PROBLEMS (ETIOLOGY)
	AVERAGE FINDINGS	NORMAL VARIATIONS	

Soles of feet	Soles well lined (or wrinkled) over two thirds of foot in term infants
	Plantar fat pad giving flat-footed effect
			Soles of feet:
			    Few creases (preterm)
			        Covered with creases (postmature)
			Congenital clubfoot

Evaluate joints:
    Hip
    Knee
    Ankle
    Toes
	Full range of motion, symmetric contour		Hypermobility of joints (Down syndrome)

Check reflexes (see Table 22-4)			Asymmetric movement (trauma, CNS disorder)

Back
Assess anatomy:
 	
    Inspect and palpate
 	
        Spine
 	
        Shoulders
        Scapulae
        Iliac crests
 	
        Base of spine—pilonidal dimple or sinus
	
	Spine straight and easily flexed
	Infant able to raise and support head momentarily when prone
	
	Shoulders, scapulae, and iliac crests lining up in same plane
		Temporary minor positional deformities, correction with passive manipulation	Limitation of movement (fusion or deformity of vertebra)
			Spina bifida cystica (meningocele, myelomeningocele)
			Pigmented nevus with tuft of hair, location anywhere along the spine often associated with spina bifida occulta
			Sinus (opening to spinal cord)

Check reflexes (spinal related): Test trunk incurvation reflex	Trunk flexed and pelvis swings to stimulated side	May not be apparent in first few days but is usually present in 5-6 days	If transverse lesion is present, no response below lesion; absence of response: central nervous system abnormality or CNS depression
Test magnet reflex	Lower limbs extend as pressure applied to feet with legs in semiflexed position	Weak or exaggerated response with breech presentation	Absence: suggestive of CNS damage or malformation

Anus
Inspect and palpate
    Placement
    Patency
    Test for sphincter response (active "wink" reflex)
Observe for the following:
    Abdominal distention
    Passage of meconium from anal opening
    Fecal drainage from perineum, penis, vagina
	One anus with good sphincter tone
	Passage of meconium within 24 hr after birth
	Anal "wink" present, anal opening patent
		Passage of meconium within 48 hr of birth	Imperforate anus without fistula
			Rectal atresia and stenosis
			Absence of anal opening; drainage of fecal material from vagina in female or urinary meatus in male (rectal fistula) or along perineal raphe (midline area between base of penis and anus)—anorectal malformation

Stools Observe frequency, color, consistency	Meconium followed by transitional and soft yellow stool		No stool (obstruction) Frequent watery stools (infection, phototherapy)

◎ NURSING CARE PLAN

The Normal Newborn

NURSING DIAGNOSIS	EXPECTED OUTCOME	NURSING INTERVENTIONS	RATIONALES
Ineffective Airway Clearance related to excess mucus production or improper positioning	Neonate's airway remains patent; breath sounds are clear, and no respiratory distress is evident.	Teach parents that gagging, coughing, and sneezing are normal neonatal responses	To assist neonate in clearing airways
		Teach parents feeding techniques that prevent overfeeding and distention of abdomen and to burp neonate frequently	To prevent regurgitation and aspiration
		Position neonate on back when sleeping	To prevent suffocation
		Suction mouth and nasopharynx with bulb syringe as needed; clean nares of crusted secretions	To clear airway and prevent aspiration and airway obstruction
		Teach parents how to use bulb syringe and how to relieve airway obstruction	To clear airway
Risk for Imbalanced Body Temperature related to larger body surface relative to mass	Neonate's temperature remains in range of 36.5° to 37.5° C (97.7° to 99.5° F).	Maintain neutral thermal environment	To identify any changes in neonate's temperature that may be related to other causes
		Monitor neonate's axillary temperature frequently	To identify any changes promptly and to prevent hypothermia and cold stress
		Bathe neonate efficiently when temperature is stable, using warm water, drying carefully, and avoiding exposing neonate to drafts	To avoid heat loss from evaporation and convection
		Report any alterations in temperature findings promptly.	To assess for signs of infection or hypoglycemia and facilitate prompt treatment
Risk for Infection related to immature immunologic defenses and environmental exposure	Neonate will be free from signs of infection.	Review maternal record for evidence of any risk factors	To ascertain whether neonate is predisposed to infection
		Monitor temperature and other vital signs	To identify early possible evidence of infection, especially temperature instability
		Have all care providers, including parents, perform proper hand hygiene before handling newborn	To protect newborn from infection
		Provide prescribed eye prophylaxis	To prevent infection
		Keep genital area clean and dry using proper cleansing techniques	To prevent skin irritation, cross-contamination, and infection
		Keep umbilical stump clean and dry	To promote drying and to minimize chance of infection
		If infant is circumcised, keep site clean and apply diaper loosely	To prevent infection and to prevent trauma
		Teach parents to keep neonate away from crowds and environmental irritants	To reduce potential sources of infection
Risk for Injury related to sole dependence on caregiver	Neonate remains free of injury.	Monitor environment for hazards such as sharp objects (e.g., long fingernails, jewelry of caregiver)	To prevent injury
		Handle neonate gently and support head, ensure use of car seat by parents, teach parents to avoid placing neonate on high surface unsupervised, and to supervise pet and sibling interactions	To prevent injury
		Assess neonate frequently for any evidence of jaundice, and teach parents to monitor for jaundice	To identify rising bilirubin levels, treat promptly, and prevent complications such as acute bilirubin encephalopathy and kernicterus

NURSING CARE PLAN

The Normal Newborn—cont'd

NURSING DIAGNOSIS	EXPECTED OUTCOME	NURSING INTERVENTIONS	RATIONALES
Readiness for Enhanced Family Coping related to anticipatory guidance regarding responses to neonate's crying	Parents will verbalize their understanding of methods of coping with neonate's crying and describe increased success in interpreting neonate's cries.	Alert parents to crying as neonate's form of communication and that cries can be differentiated to indicate hunger, wetness, pain, and loneliness	To provide reassurance that crying is not indicative of neonate's rejection of parents and that parents will learn to interpret different cries of their child
		Teach parents normal patterns of infant crying (e.g., *Period of PURPLE Crying*) and alert them to the danger of shaking a baby	To provide anticipatory guidance and to prevent injury to the infant
		Differentiate self-consoling behaviors from fussing or crying	To give parents concrete examples of interventions
		Discuss methods of consoling the crying neonate, such as changing diapers, talking softly to neonate, holding neonate's arms close to body, swaddling, picking neonate up, rocking, using pacifier, feeding, or burping	To provide anticipatory guidance and promote parental confidence

a follow-up examination is performed to further validate neuromuscular criteria (Ballard, Khoury, Wedig, et al., 1991). Box 23-3 highlights specific maneuvers used in gestational age assessment.

Classification of Newborns by Gestational Age and Birth Weight

Classification of infants at birth by both birth weight and gestational age provides a more satisfactory method for predicting mortality risks and providing guidelines for management of the neonate than estimating gestational age or birth weight alone. The infant's birth weight, length, and head circumference are plotted on standardized graphs that identify normal values for gestational age. A normal range of birth weights exists for each gestational week (see Fig. 23-2, *B*).

The infant whose weight is appropriate for gestational age (AGA) (between the 10th and 90th percentiles) can be presumed to have grown at a normal rate regardless of the length of gestation—preterm, term, or postterm. The infant who is large for gestational age (LGA) (more than the 90th percentile) can be presumed to have grown at an accelerated rate during fetal life; the small-for-gestational-age (SGA) infant (less than the 10th percentile) can be presumed to have grown at a restricted rate during intrauterine life. When gestational age is determined according to the New Ballard Score, the newborn will fall into one of the following nine possible categories for birth weight and gestational age: AGA—term, preterm, postterm; SGA—term, preterm, postterm; or LGA—term, preterm, postterm. Birth weight influences mortality: the lower the birth weight, the higher the mortality. The same is true for gestational age: the lower the gestational age, the higher the mortality (Gardner and Hernandez, 2011).

Infants may also be classified in the following ways according to gestation:

- Preterm or premature—born before completion of 37 weeks of gestation, regardless of birth weight
- Late preterm—born between 34 0/7 and 36 6/7 weeks
- Term—born between the beginning of week 37 and the end of week 42 of gestation
- Postterm (postdate)—born after completion of week 42 of gestation

- Postmature—born after completion of week 42 of gestation and showing the effects of progressive placental insufficiency

Early Term Infant

Experts have proposed another category to classify newborns. "Early term" describes infants born from 37 0/7 to 38 6/7 weeks of gestation (Fleischman, Oinuma, and Clark, 2010). A recent increase in the number of early term infants is associated with elective inductions and elective cesarean births that are scheduled before 39 weeks. Compared with full-term infants, early term infants are at greater risk for short-term and long-term health problems. Birth at 37 to 38 weeks is associated with higher incidence of breastfeeding difficulties and respiratory problems such as respiratory distress syndrome and transient tachypnea of the newborn (TTNB) (Bates, Rouse, Chapman, et al., 2010). These infants are also at increased risk for long-term problems such as learning difficulties (e.g., attention deficit hyperactivity disorder [ADHD]) (Lindstrom, Lindblad, and Hjern, 2011). Early term infants have higher neonatal, postnatal, and infant mortality rates (Reddy, Bettegowda, Dias, et al., 2011). Nurses and other health care providers need to be aware of the vulnerability of this population of neonates and monitor them closely (Craighead, 2012).

Late Preterm Infant

Seventy-one percent of preterm births in the United States are between 34⅗ and 36⅗ weeks of gestation; these late preterm infants account for 8.5% of all births (Hamilton, Martin, and Ventura, 2011). Elective vaginal and cesarean births before 39 weeks have contributed significantly to late preterm birth rates (Reddy, Ko, Raju, et al., 2009).

Late preterm infants have been called "The Great Impostors" because they are often the size and weight of term infants and are treated as healthy newborns. Despite their appearance as term infants, late preterm infants are at increased risk for respiratory distress, temperature instability, hypoglycemia, apnea, feeding difficulties, and hyperbilirubinemia (Cooper, Holditch-Davis, Verklan, et al., 2012). Nurses working with healthy term infants must be cognizant of the risk factors for late preterm infants and be

BOX 23-3   MANEUVERS USED IN ASSESSING GESTATIONAL AGE

Posture

With infant quiet and in a supine position, observe degree of flexion in arms and legs. Muscle tone and degree of flexion increase with maturity. Full flexion of the arms and legs = score 4.*

Square Window

With thumb supporting back of arm below wrist, apply gentle pressure with index and third fingers on dorsum of hand without rotating infant's wrist. Measure angle between base of thumb and forearm. Full flexion (hand lies flat on ventral surface of forearm) = score 4.*

Arm Recoil

With infant supine, fully flex both forearms on upper arms and hold for 5 seconds; pull down on hands to extend fully, and rapidly release arms. Observe rapidity and intensity of recoil to a state of flexion. A brisk return to full flexion = score 4.*

Popliteal Angle

With infant supine and pelvis flat on a firm surface, flex lower leg on thigh and then flex thigh on abdomen. While holding knee with thumb and index finger, extend lower leg with index finger of other hand. Measure degree of angle behind knee (popliteal angle). An angle of less than 90 degrees = score 5.*

Scarf Sign

With infant supine, support head in midline with one hand; use other hand to pull infant's arm across the shoulder so that infant's hand touches shoulder. Determine location of elbow in relation to midline. Elbow does not reach midline = score 4.*

Heel to Ear

With infant supine and pelvis flat on a firm surface, pull foot as far as possible (without using force) up toward ear on same side. Measure distance of foot from ear and degree of knee flexion (same as popliteal angle). Knees flexed with a popliteal angle of less than 10 degrees = score 4.*

From Hockenberry MJ, Wilson D: *Wong's nursing care of infants and children,* ed 9, St Louis, 2011, Mosby.
*See Fig. 23-2 for scale and interpretation of scores.

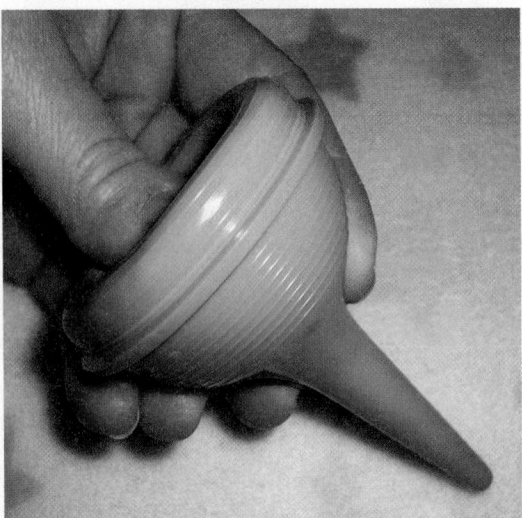

FIG 23-4 Bulb syringe. Bulb must be compressed before inserting tip into mouth. (Courtesy Cheryl Briggs, RNC, Annapolis, MD.)

GUIDELINES
Suctioning with a Bulb Syringe

- The bulb syringe should always be kept in the infant's crib.
- The mouth is suctioned first to prevent the infant from inhaling pharyngeal secretions by gasping as the nares are touched.
- The bulb is compressed (see Fig. 23-4) and the tip is inserted into one side of the mouth. The center of the infant's mouth is avoided because the gag reflex can be stimulated.
- The nasal passages are suctioned one nostril at a time.
- When the infant's cry does not sound as though it is through mucus or a bubble, suctioning can be stopped.
- The parents should be given demonstrations on how to use the bulb syringe and asked to perform a return demonstration.

continually vigilant for the development of problems related to the infant's immaturity. In an effort to identify these infants, a gestational age assessment should be performed on all newborns soon after birth (Cooper, Holditch-Davis, Verklan, et al., 2012). The late preterm infant's care is further addressed in Chapter 25.

Interventions

Changes can occur quickly in newborns immediately after birth. Assessment must be followed by the implementation of appropriate care.

Airway Maintenance

Generally, the healthy term infant born vaginally has little difficulty clearing the airway. Most secretions are moved by gravity and brought by the cough reflex to the oropharynx to be drained or swallowed or wiped away. If the infant has excess mucus in the respiratory tract, the mouth and nasal passages can be gently suctioned with a bulb syringe (see Guidelines box and Fig. 23-4). Routine chest percussion

and suctioning of healthy term or late preterm infants are avoided; evidence is insufficient to support anything other than gentle nasopharyngeal and oropharyngeal suctioning to clear secretions. The nurse should listen to the infant's respirations and lung sounds with a stethoscope to determine if crackles or inspiratory stridor is present. Fine crackles may be auscultated for several hours after birth. If the bulb syringe does not clear mucus interfering with respiratory effort, mechanical suction can be used.

If the newborn has an obstruction that is not cleared with suctioning, the neonatal or pediatric care provider should be notified. Further investigation must occur to determine if a mechanical defect (e.g., tracheoesophageal fistula, choanal atresia [see Chapter 25]) is causing the obstruction.

Deeper suctioning may be needed to remove mucus from the newborn's nasopharynx or posterior oropharynx. However, this type of suctioning should be performed only after an assessment of the risks involved.

Maintaining an Adequate Oxygen Supply

Four conditions are essential for maintaining an adequate oxygen supply:
- A clear airway
- Effective establishment of respirations

BOX 23-4   SIGNS OF POTENTIAL COMPLICATIONS: ABNORMAL NEWBORN BREATHING

- Bradypnea (≤30 respirations/min)
- Tachypnea (≥60 respirations/min)
- Abnormal breath sounds: coarse or fine crackles, wheezes, expiratory grunt
- Respiratory distress: nasal flaring, retractions, stridor, gasping, chin tug
- Seesaw or paradoxic respirations
- Skin color: cyanosis, mottling
- Pulse oximetry value: <95%

- Adequate circulation, adequate perfusion, and effective cardiac function
- Adequate thermoregulation

Newborns who encounter respiratory problems are likely to exhibit signs and symptoms that indicate some degree of distress. Preterm infants are at greatest risk for respiratory distress (Box 23-4; see also Chapter 25).

Maintaining Body Temperature

Effective neonatal care includes maintenance of a neutral thermal environment (see Chapter 22). Cold stress increases the need for oxygen and can deplete glucose stores. The infant may react to exposure to cold by increasing the respiratory rate and may become cyanotic.

The ideal method for promoting warmth and maintaining neonatal body temperature is early skin-to-skin contact (SSC) with the mother. The naked infant is placed prone directly on the mother's chest; both mother and infant are then covered with a warm blanket. Early SSC has distinct short-term and long-term benefits including temperature stabilization, reduced crying, improved breastfeeding initiation and duration, and maternal attachment (Bramson, Lee, Moore, et al., 2010; Gabriel, Martin, Escobar, et al., 2010; Moore, Anderson, Bergman, et al., 2012). Other interventions to promote warmth include drying and wrapping the newborn in warmed blankets immediately after birth, keeping the head well covered, and keeping the ambient temperature of the nursery or mother's room at 22° to 26° C (72° to 78° F) (American Academy of Pediatrics [AAP] and American College of Obstetricians and Gynecologists [ACOG], 2012).

If the infant does not remain skin-to-skin with the mother during the first 1 to 2 hours after birth, the nurse places the thoroughly dried infant under a radiant warmer or in a warm incubator until the body temperature stabilizes. The infant's skin temperature is used as the point of control in a warmer with a servo-controlled mechanism. The control panel is usually maintained between 36° and 37° C (96.8° and 98.6° F). This setting should maintain the healthy term newborn's skin temperature at approximately 36.5° to 37° C (97.7° to 98.6° F). A thermistor probe (automatic sensor) is usually placed on the upper quadrant of the abdomen immediately below the right or left costal margin (never over a bone). A reflector adhesive patch can be used over the probe to provide adequate warming. This probe is designed to detect minor temperature changes resulting from external environmental factors or neonatal factors (peripheral vasoconstriction, vasodilation, or increased metabolism) before a dramatic change in core body temperature develops. The servo-controller adjusts the temperature of the warmer to maintain the infant's skin temperature within the preset range. The sensor needs to be checked periodically

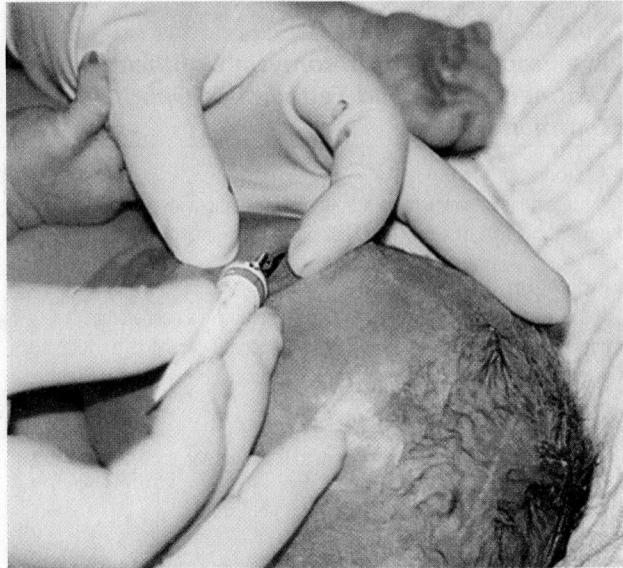

FIG 23-5 Instillation of medication into eye of newborn. Thumb and forefinger are used to open the eye; medication is placed in the lower conjunctiva from the inner to the outer canthus. (Courtesy Marjorie Pyle, Lifecircle, Costa Mesa, CA.)

to make sure it is securely attached to the infant's skin. The axillary temperature of the newborn is checked every hour (or more often as needed) until the newborn's temperature stabilizes. The length of time to stabilize and maintain body temperature varies; each newborn should therefore be allowed to achieve thermal regulation as necessary, and care should be individualized.

During all procedures, heat loss must be avoided or minimized for the newborn; therefore examinations and activities are performed with the newborn under a heat panel. The initial bath is postponed until the newborn's skin temperature is stable and can adjust to heat loss from a bath. Two to four hours may pass before this occurs.

Even a healthy term infant can become hypothermic. Inadequate drying and wrapping immediately after birth, a cold birthing room, or birth in a car on the way to the hospital can cause the newborn's temperature to fall below the normal range (hypothermia). The hypothermic infant should be warmed gradually because rapid warming can cause apneic spells and acidosis. Therefore the warming process is monitored to progress slowly over 2 to 4 hours.

Immediate Interventions

One of the nurse's responsibilities is to perform certain interventions soon after birth to provide for the safety and well-being of the newborn. Such interventions may be delayed for an hour or two to provide time for uninterrupted maternal-infant bonding.

Eye Prophylaxis. The instillation of a prophylactic agent in the eyes of all neonates (Fig. 23-5) is mandatory in the United States. This is a precautionary measure against ophthalmia neonatorum, which is an inflammation of the eyes resulting from gonorrheal or chlamydial infection contracted by the newborn during passage through the mother's birth canal. In the United States, if parents object to this treatment, they may be asked to sign an informed refusal form and their refusal is documented in the neonate's record. The agent used for prophylaxis varies according to hospital protocols but usually includes forms of erythromycin or tetracycline or silver nitrate (see Medication Guide). Canadian hospitals have not recommended the use of silver nitrate since 1986. Its use in the

💊 MEDICATION GUIDE

Eye Prophylaxis: Erythromycin Ophthalmic Ointment, 0.5%, and Tetracycline Ophthalmic Ointment, 1%

Action

These antibiotic ointments are both bacteriostatic and bactericidal. They provide prophylaxis against ophthalmia neonatorum.

Indication

These medications are applied to prevent ophthalmia neonatorum in newborns of mothers who are infected with gonorrhea and chlamydia. Eye prophylaxis for ophthalmia neonatorum is required by law in all U.S. states.

Neonatal Dosage

Apply a 1- to 2-cm ribbon of ointment to the lower conjunctival sac of each eye; can also be used in drop form.

Adverse Reactions

Can cause chemical conjunctivitis that lasts 24 to 48 hours; vision can be blurred temporarily.

Nursing Considerations

Administer within 1 to 2 hours of birth. Wear gloves. Cleanse the eyes if necessary before administration. Open the eyes by putting a thumb and finger at the corner of each lid and gently pressing on the periorbital ridges. Squeeze the tube and spread the ointment from the inner canthus of the eye to the outer canthus. Do not touch the tube to the eye. After 1 minute, excess ointment may be wiped off. Observe eyes for irritation. Explain the treatment to the parents.

💊 MEDICATION GUIDE

Vitamin K: Phytonadione (AquaMEPHYTON, Konakion)

Action

This intervention provides vitamin K because the newborn does not have the intestinal flora to produce this vitamin in the first week after birth. It also promotes formation of clotting factors (II, VII, IX, X) in the liver.

Indication

Vitamin K is used for the prevention and treatment of hemorrhagic disease in the newborn.

Neonatal Dosage

Administer a 0.5-mg to 1-mg (0.25- to 0.5-mL) dose intramuscularly (IM) within 2 hours of birth; can be repeated if the newborn shows bleeding tendencies. Vitamin K is never administered by the intravenous route for the prevention of hemorrhagic disease of the newborn except in some cases of a preterm infant who has no muscle mass. In such instances, the medication is diluted and given over 10 to 15 minutes while closely monitoring the infant with a cardiorespiratory monitor. Rapid IV administration of vitamin K can cause cardiac arrest.

Adverse Reactions

Edema, erythema, and pain at the injection site occur rarely; hemolysis, jaundice, and hyperbilirubinemia have been reported, particularly in preterm infants.

Nursing Considerations

Follow procedure for IM injection on p. 613.

United States is minimal because silver nitrate does not protect against chlamydial infection and can cause chemical conjunctivitis. Instillation of eye prophylaxis can be delayed until an hour or so (up to 2 hours in Canada) after birth so that eye contact and parent-infant attachment and bonding are facilitated.

Topical antibiotics such as tetracycline and erythromycin, silver nitrate, and a 2.5% povidone-iodine solution are not effective in the treatment of chlamydial conjunctivitis. A 14-day course of oral erythromycin or an oral sulfonamide can be given for chlamydial conjunctivitis (AAP Committee on Infectious Diseases, 2012).

Vitamin K Prophylaxis. Administering vitamin K intramuscularly is routine in the newborn period in the United States. A single intramuscular injection of 0.5 to 1 mg of vitamin K is given soon after birth to prevent hemorrhagic disease of the newborn. Administration can be delayed until after the first breastfeeding in the birthing room (AAP and ACOG, 2012). Vitamin K is synthesized by intestinal flora, which are not present at birth. The introduction of bacteria begins with the first feedings, and by the age of 7 days, healthy newborns are able to produce their own vitamin K (see Medication Guide).

⚡ SAFETY ALERT

Vitamin K is never administered by the intravenous route for the prevention of hemorrhagic disease of the newborn except in some cases of a preterm infant who has no muscle mass. In such cases, the medication should be diluted and given over 10 to 15 minutes while closely monitoring the infant with a cardiorespiratory monitor. Rapid bolus administration of vitamin K can cause cardiac arrest.

Promoting Parent-Infant Interaction. Today's childbirth practices promote the family as the focus of care. Parents generally desire to share in the birth process and to have early contact with their infants. The infant can be put to breast soon after birth. Early contact between mother and newborn can be important in developing future relationships; it also has a positive effect on the initiation and duration of breastfeeding. Early mother-infant contact produces physiologic benefits for the mother and neonate. Maternal levels of oxytocin and prolactin rise with early breastfeeding. The process of developing active immunity begins as the infant ingests antibodies from the mother's colostrum.

CARE MANAGEMENT: FROM 2 HOURS AFTER BIRTH UNTIL DISCHARGE

Depending on the model of care delivery, the mother/baby nurse or newborn nursery nurse is responsible for ongoing assessment and care of the newborn. Astute assessment skills and appropriate interventions promote positive outcomes, especially for newborns who experience any problems before going home. Newborn care is family-centered as the nurse provides education and support for the new parents throughout the hospital stay and assists them in preparing for hospital discharge.

Common Newborn Problems
Birth Injuries

Birth trauma includes any physical injury sustained by a newborn during labor and birth. Although most injuries are minor and resolve during the neonatal period without treatment, some types

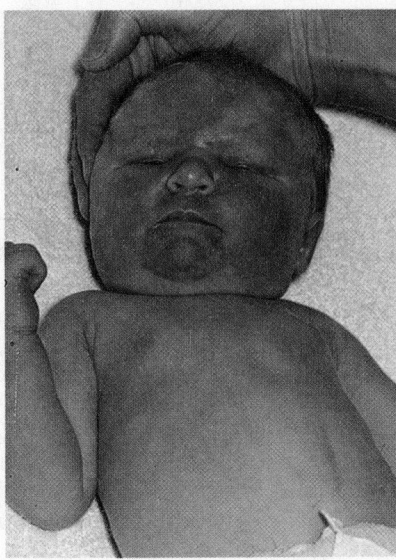

FIG 23-6 Marked bruising on the entire face of an infant born vaginally after face presentation. Less severe ecchymoses were present on the extremities. Phototherapy was required for treatment of jaundice resulting from the breakdown of accumulated blood. (From O'Doherty N: *Neonatology: micro atlas of the newborn,* Nutley, NJ, 1986, Hoffman-La Roche.)

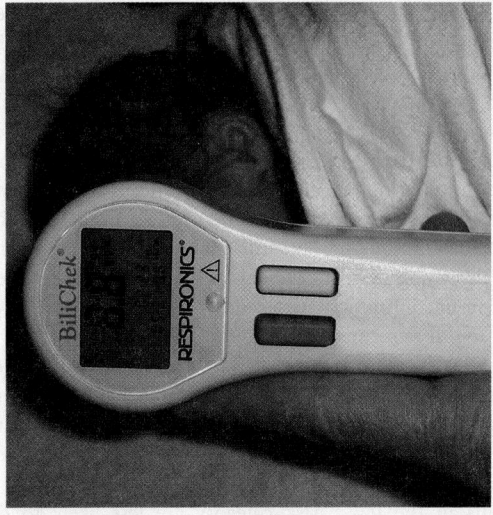

FIG 23-7 Transcutaneous monitoring of bilirubin with a transcutaneous bilirubinometry (TcB) monitor. (Courtesy Cheryl Briggs, RNC, Annapolis, MD.)

of trauma require intervention; a few are serious enough to be fatal. (See Chapter 25 for more information on birth injuries.)

Soft-Tissue Injuries. Retinal and subconjunctival hemorrhages result from rupture of capillaries caused by increased pressure during birth. These hemorrhages usually clear within 5 days after birth and present no further problems. Parents need explanation and reassurance that these injuries are harmless.

Erythema, ecchymoses, petechiae, abrasions, lacerations, or edema of the buttocks and extremities can be present. Localized discoloration can appear over the presenting part as a result of forceps- or vacuum-assisted birth. Ecchymoses and edema can appear anywhere on the body. Petechiae (pinpoint hemorrhagic areas) acquired during birth can extend over the upper trunk and face. These lesions are benign if they disappear within 2 or 3 days of birth and no new lesions appear. Ecchymoses and petechiae can be signs of a more serious disorder, such as thrombocytopenic purpura. To differentiate hemorrhagic areas from a skin rash or discolorations, try to blanch the skin with two fingers. Petechiae and ecchymoses will not blanch because extravasated blood remains within the tissues, whereas skin rashes and discolorations will blanch.

Trauma can occur during labor and birth to the presenting fetal part. Caput succedaneum and cephalhematoma are discussed in Chapter 22 (see Fig. 22-10). Forceps injury and bruising from the vacuum cup occur at the site of application of the instruments. A forceps injury commonly produces a linear mark across both sides of the face in the shape of the blades of the forceps. The affected areas are kept clean to minimize the risk for infection. These injuries usually resolve spontaneously within several days with no specific therapy. With the increased use of the vacuum extractor and the use of padded forceps blades, the incidence of these lesions can be significantly reduced.

Bruises over the face can be the result of face presentation (Fig. 23-6). In a breech presentation, bruising and swelling may be seen over the buttocks or genitalia (see Fig. 22-8). The skin over the entire head can be ecchymotic and covered with petechiae caused by a tight nuchal cord. If the hemorrhagic areas do not disappear spontaneously in 2 days or if the infant's condition changes, the primary health care provider is notified.

Accidental lacerations can be inflicted with a scalpel during a cesarean birth. These cuts may occur on any part of the body but are most often found on the scalp, buttocks, and thighs. They are usually superficial and need only to be kept clean. If skin closure is needed, an adhesive substance or strips may be applied. Rarely are sutures needed.

Physiologic Problems

Jaundice. A majority of newborn infants will experience some level of jaundice during the first few days of life, usually occurring after 24 hours. In most cases, it is *physiologic jaundice,* caused by increased levels of unconjugated bilirubin; physiologic jaundice is usually self-limiting, requires no treatment, and resolves in a few days. It must be differentiated from *pathologic jaundice,* or hyperbilirubinemia, which is associated with higher levels of unconjugated bilirubin. This type of jaundice can appear in the first 24 hours and often requires phototherapy to resolve. Jaundice can also be associated with breastfeeding (see Chapter 22).

Every newborn should be assessed for jaundice at least every 8 to 12 hours; this can be easily done when vital signs are assessed. Visual assessment of jaundice alone does not provide an accurate assessment of the level of serum bilirubin, especially in dark-skinned newborns. To differentiate cutaneous jaundice from normal skin color, the nurse applies pressure with a finger over a bony area (e.g., the nose, forehead, sternum) for several seconds to empty all the capillaries in that spot. If jaundice is present, the blanched area will appear yellow before the capillaries refill. The conjunctival sacs and buccal mucosa also are assessed, especially in darker-skinned infants. Assessing for jaundice in natural light is recommended because artificial lighting and reflection from nursery walls can distort the actual skin color.

Noninvasive monitoring of bilirubin using cutaneous reflectance measurements (transcutaneous bilirubinometry [TcB]) allows for repetitive estimations of bilirubin (Fig. 23-7). These devices work well on both dark- and light-skinned infants and demonstrate linear correlation with serum determinations of bilirubin levels in fullterm infants. TcB monitors can be used to screen for clinically significant jaundice and decrease the need for serum bilirubin measurements.

In an effort to prevent severe hyperbilirubinemia and the neurologic complications of acute bilirubin encephalopathy and kernicterus (see Chapter 22), the American Academy of Pediatrics [AAP] Subcommittee on Hyperbilirubinemia (2004) recommends routine screening of all newborns before hospital discharge using TcB or serum bilirubin measurement. If the TcB level is greater than 12 mg/dL, a serum bilirubin check is done. Total serum bilirubin levels are interpreted according to an hour-specific nomogram to determine the risk for hyperbilirubinemia (AAP Subcommittee on Hyperbilirubinemia, 2004) (Fig. 23-8). A web-based tool at www.bilitool.org facilitates calculating the risk for neonatal hyperbilirubinemia.

Infants in the lower risk category are less likely to develop hyperbilirubinemia. However, because there can be risk factors such as lower gestational age that can increase the risk for hyperbilirubinemia, the AAP warns that all infants should be considered as being at potential risk for hyperbilirubinemia, even if they were identified as being in the low risk category. This means that all newborns should be followed after hospital discharge for the development of unexpected jaundice and that parents should be given printed and verbal information about newborn jaundice (Bromiker, Bin-Nun, Schimmel, et al., 2012; Maisels, Bhutani, Bogen, et al., 2009).

> **! NURSING ALERT**
>
> Breastfeeding is essential in preventing hyperbilirubinemia. Newborns should breastfeed early (within 1 to 2 hours after birth) and often (at least 8-12 times/24 hr) (AAP Subcommittee on Hyperbilirubinemia, 2004). Colostrum acts as a laxative to promote stooling, which helps rid the body of bilirubin.

Routine assessment of risk factors for severe hyperbilirubinemia is advised. The most common risk factors include gestational age less than 38 weeks, exclusive breastfeeding (especially in association with breastfeeding difficulties and excessive weight loss), significant jaundice in a sibling, isoimmune or other hemolytic disease (e.g., glucose-6-phosphate dehydrogenase [G6PD] deficiency), cephalhematoma or significant bruising, and East Indian race (Maisels, Bhutani, Bogen, et al., 2009). Close follow-up of infants at risk for severe hyperbilirubinemia is essential; parents should be educated and encouraged to follow postdischarge recommendations (AAP Subcommittee on Hyperbilirubinemia, 2004).

If an infant is jaundiced in the first 24 hours of life, a TcB or total serum bilirubin (TSB) level should be measured and results interpreted based on the newborn's age in hours according to the hourspecific nomogram for infants born at 35 weeks of gestation or later (AAP Subcommittee on Hyperbilirubinemia, 2004). Repeat testing is based on the risk level (low, intermediate, or high), the age of the neonate, and the progression of jaundice.

Therapy for Hyperbilirubinemia. The decision to treat an infant for hyperbilirubinemia is based on serum bilirubin levels, the

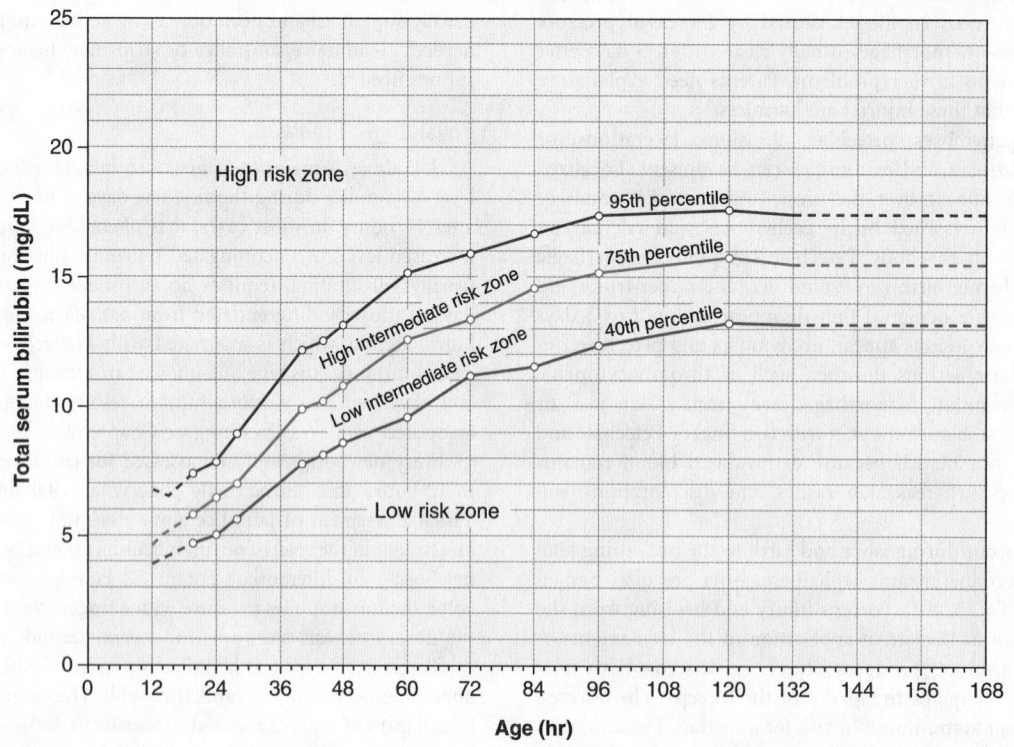

FIG 23-8 Nomogram for designation of risk in 2840 well newborns at 36 or more weeks' gestational age with birth weight of 2000 g or more or 35 or more weeks' gestational age with birth weight of 2500 g or more based on the hour-specific serum bilirubin values. (This nomogram should not be used to represent the natural history of neonatal hyperbilirubinemia.) (From Bhutani V, Johnson L, Sivieri EM: Predictive ability of a predischarge hour-specific serum bilirubin for subsequent significant hyperbilirubinemia in healthy term and near-term newborns, *Pediatrics* 103(1):6-14, 1999.)

infant's gestational age, and the presence of risk factors. The American Academy of Pediatrics provides guidelines that provide direction for health care providers in determining the need for phototherapy or exchange transfusion (AAP Committee on Hyperbilirubinemia, 2004).

The goal of treatment of hyperbilirubinemia is to help reduce the newborn's serum levels of unconjugated bilirubin. There are two ways to reduce unconjugated bilirubin levels: phototherapy and exchange blood transfusion. Exchange transfusion is used to treat those infants whose levels of serum bilirubin are rising rapidly despite the use of intensive phototherapy.

Phototherapy. The purpose of phototherapy is to reduce the level of circulating unconjugated bilirubin or to keep it from increasing. Phototherapy uses light energy to change the shape and structure of unconjugated bilirubin and convert it to molecules that can be excreted. The dose and effectiveness of phototherapy are affected by the source of light. Phototherapy units vary in the spectrum of light they deliver and in the filters that are used. The most effective therapy is achieved with special blue fluorescent tubes or a specially designed light-emitting diode (LED). Phototherapy lights do not emit significant ultraviolet radiation; the small amount that is emitted does not cause erythema. Most of the ultraviolet light is absorbed by the glass wall of the fluorescent tube and by the plastic cover of the light (AAP Subcommittee on Hyperbilirubinemia, 2004; Kamath, Thilo, and Hernandez, 2011). Phototherapy is usually effective for treatment of hyperbilirubinemia that has not reached levels associated with acute bilirubin encephalopathy or kernicterus.

The effectiveness of phototherapy is related to the distance between the light and the neonate and on the area of skin that is exposed. During phototherapy, the unclothed infant is placed under a bank of lights approximately 45 to 50 cm from the light source. Phototherapy can be used for the infant in an incubator (Fig. 23-9) or in an open crib. The distance varies according to unit protocol and type of light used. The lamp's energy output should be monitored routinely with a photometer during treatment to ensure efficacy of therapy. Phototherapy is used until the infant's serum bilirubin level decreases to within an acceptable range. The decision to discontinue therapy is based on the observation of a definite downward trend in the bilirubin values.

The infant's eyes must be protected by an opaque mask to prevent overexposure to the light. The eye shield should cover the eyes completely but not occlude the nares. Before the mask is applied, the infant's eyes should be closed gently to prevent excoriation of the corneas. The mask should be removed periodically and during infant feedings so that the eyes can be checked and cleansed with water and the parents can have visual contact with the infant (see Family-Centered Care box and Fig. 23-10).

Phototherapy can cause changes in the infant's temperature, depending partially on the bed used—bassinet, incubator, or radiant warmer. When under a phototherapy light, infants are usually clothed only with a diaper. The infant's temperature should be closely monitored. Phototherapy lights can increase the rate of insensible water loss, which contributes to fluid loss and dehydration. Therefore the infant must be adequately hydrated. Hydration maintenance in the healthy newborn is accomplished with human milk or infant formula. Feedings of glucose water or plain water have no advantage or benefit because these liquids do not promote excretion of bilirubin in the stools and can actually perpetuate enterohepatic circulation, thus delaying bilirubin excretion.

It is important to closely monitor urinary output as an indicator of hydration status while the infant is receiving phototherapy. Urine output can be decreased or unaltered; the urine can have a dark gold or brown appearance.

The number and consistency of stools are monitored. Bilirubin breakdown increases gastric motility, which results in loose stools that can cause skin excoriation and breakdown. The infant's buttocks must be cleaned after each stool to help maintain skin integrity.

If the infant is under phototherapy lights, maximizing skin exposure to the light is important. Infants need to be turned at least every 2 hours. A fine maculopapular rash can appear during phototherapy, but this condition is transient.

In addition to phototherapy lights, other systems are used for phototherapy. A bassinet system provides special blue light above and beneath the infant. Another phototherapy device is a

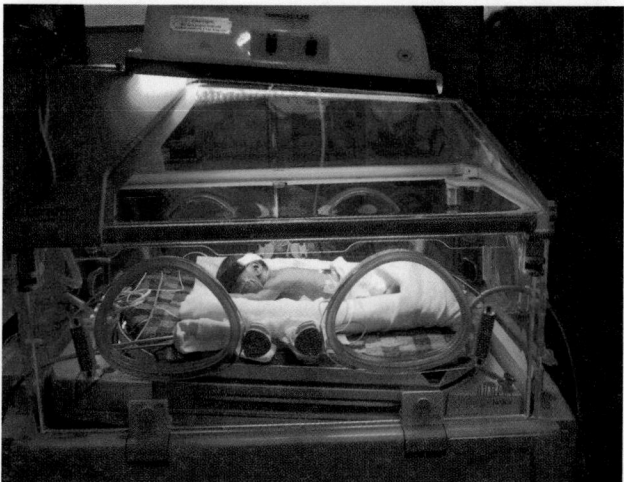

FIG 23-9 Infant under phototherapy lights while in incubator. (Courtesy Randi and Jacob Wills, Clayton, NC.)

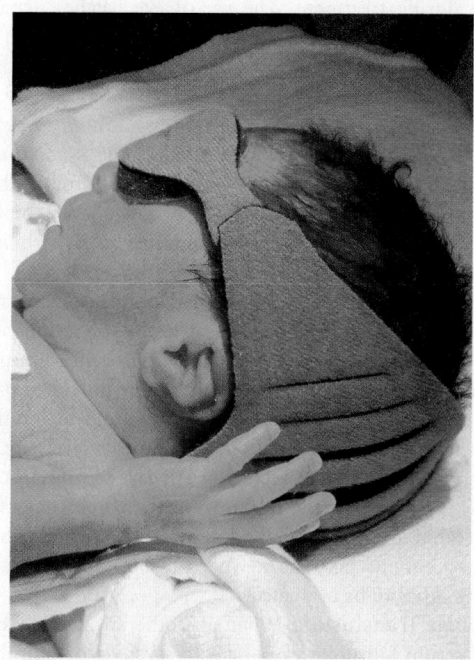

FIG 23-10 Infant with eyes covered while receiving phototherapy. (Courtesy Cheryl Briggs, RNC, Annapolis, MD.)

Phototherapy and Parent-Infant Interaction

The traditional use of phototherapy has evoked concerns regarding a number of psychobehavioral issues, including parent-infant separation, potential social isolation, decreased sensorineural stimulation, altered biologic rhythms, altered feeding patterns, and activity changes. Parental anxiety is greatly increased, particularly at the sight of the newborn blindfolded and under special lights. The interruption of breastfeeding for phototherapy is a potential deterrent to successful maternal-infant attachment and interaction. Because research has demonstrated that bilirubin catabolism occurs primarily within the first few hours of the initiation of phototherapy, there is increased support for the removal of the infant from treatment for feeding and holding. Intermittent phototherapy can be just as effective as continuous therapy when used correctly. The benefits of stopping phototherapy for short periods so parents can feed and hold the newborn should be carefully weighed by the health care team and the parents.

fiberoptic blanket that is connected to a light source. The blanket is flexible and can be placed around the infant's torso or underneath the infant in the bassinet. There are also bilirubin beds with LED lights in a pad that covers the surface of the bassinet. The LEDs do not produce heat and can be used with radiant warmers. These devices are usually less effective when used alone as compared with conventional phototherapy lights. They can be very useful in combination with overhead phototherapy lights. In certain instances, the infant's bilirubin levels increase rapidly and intensive phototherapy is required; this situation involves the use of a combination of conventional lights and fiberoptic blankets to maximize bilirubin reduction. Although fiberoptic lights do not produce heat as do conventional lights, staff should ensure that a covering pad is placed between the infant's skin and the fiberoptic device to prevent skin burns, especially in preterm infants. The newborn can remain in the mother's room in an open crib or in her arms during treatment. The use of eye patches depends on whether the devices are used alone or in combination with phototherapy lights.

Home Phototherapy. The use of home phototherapy should be reserved for healthy term infants with bilirubin levels in the "optional phototherapy" range according to the nomogram. The concern is that home phototherapy units do not provide the same level of irradiance or body surface coverage as phototherapy devices used in the hospital (AAP Committee on Hyperbilirubinemia, 2004).

Follow-up. Close follow-up is needed for infants who have been treated for hyperbilirubinemia. Repeat testing of serum bilirubin levels and follow-up visits with the pediatric health care provider are expected. Some institutions or third-party providers pay for a home visit to evaluate the infant's condition and to monitor the mother's health. When follow-up serum bilirubin levels are needed after discharge from the hospital, a health care technician or nurse may draw the blood for the specimen or the parents may take the baby to a laboratory to have blood drawn for a serum bilirubin. In some cases, parents take the newborn to an outpatient clinic or physician's office to be evaluated.

Exchange Transfusion. When phototherapy is not effective in reducing serum bilirubin levels or with severe hyperbilirubinemia such as in hemolytic disease, exchange transfusion may be needed. This procedure is done in an intensive care setting. The infant's blood is replaced with a combination of blood products such as red blood cells (RBCs) mixed with 5% albumin or fresh frozen plasma (Kaplan, Wong, Sibley, et al., 2011).

Hypoglycemia. Hypoglycemia in a term infant during the early newborn period is defined as a blood glucose concentration less than adequate to support neurologic, organ, and tissue function; however, there is a lack of consensus among experts regarding the precise level at which this concentration occurs. Similarly, there is no consensus about when to screen for hypoglycemia or the level at which treatment should be instituted (Adamkin and Committee on Fetus and Newborn, 2011). Hypoglycemia that warrants treatment is usually defined as blood glucose levels less than 40 to 45 mg/dL, although some experts recommend treatment for levels less than 50 mg/dL (Kalhan and Devaskar, 2011; McGowan, Rozance, Price-Douglas, et al., 2011).

! NURSING ALERT

Bedside glucose monitoring is performed using reagent test strips with or without a reflectance colorimeter. Because of variations in devices and operator techniques, it is recommended that any level less than 40 to 45 mg/dL should be followed up with a serum glucose level (Kalhan and Devaskar, 2011).

At birth, the maternal source of glucose is cut off with the clamping of the umbilical cord. Most healthy term newborns experience a transient decrease in glucose levels to as low as 30 mg/dL during the first 1 to 2 hours after birth, with a subsequent mobilization of free fatty acids and ketones to help maintain adequate glucose levels (Blackburn, 2013). Infants who are asphyxiated or have other physiologic stress can experience hypoglycemia as a result of a decreased glycogen supply, inadequate gluconeogenesis, or overutilization of glycogen stored during fetal life. There is concern about neurologic injury as a result of severe or prolonged hypoglycemia, especially in combination with ischemia (Kalhan and Devaskar, 2011).

There is no need to routinely assess glucose levels of healthy term infants. Breastfeeding early and often helps these neonates maintain adequate glucose levels.

Glucose levels should be measured in neonates at 34 weeks of gestation or more if risk factors or clinical manifestations of hypoglycemia are present. Infants considered to be at risk for hypoglycemia include those who are small for gestational age (SGA) or large for gestational age (LGA), infants of mothers with diabetes, and late preterm infants. The frequency of glucose testing is determined by the risk factors for each individual newborn. All at-risk infants should be fed within the first hour, with glucose testing done 30 minutes after feeding. For at least the first 24 hours after birth, late preterm and SGA neonates should be fed every 2 to 3 hours, with glucose levels measured before each feeding. LGA infants and infants of diabetic mothers should have glucose screening before feedings for at least the first 12 hours after birth; further testing is done if glucose levels are less than 45 mg/dL (Adamkin and Committee on Fetus and Newborn, 2011).

Glucose testing should be done on any infant with clinical signs of hypoglycemia. The clinical signs of hypoglycemia can be transient or recurrent and include jitteriness, lethargy, poor feeding, abnormal cry, hypotonia, temperature instability (hypothermia), respiratory distress, apnea, and seizures (Kalhan and Devaskar, 2011). It is important to remember that hypoglycemia can be present in the absence of clinical manifestations.

! NURSING ALERT

Late preterm infants are at increased risk for hypoglycemia. They have decreased glycogen stores and lack hepatic enzymes for gluconeogenesis and glycogenolysis. Their hormonal regulation and insulin secretion are immature. The increased risk of cold stress and feeding difficulties adds to the risk for hypoglycemia (Cooper, Holditch-Davis, Verklan, et al., 2012).

The at-risk asymptomatic neonate with glucose levels less than 25 mg/dL in the first 4 hours or less than 35 mg/dL from 4 to 24 hours of age should be fed. Glucose testing should be repeated 1 hour after feeding. If levels remain low despite feeding, intravenous dextrose is warranted. In such infants, the treatment should be aimed at maintaining the blood glucose levels above 45 mg/dL. For the neonate with clinical signs of hypoglycemia, regardless of cause or age, intravenous dextrose infusion is usually recommended. For any infant with hypoglycemia, follow-up glucose testing at specified intervals is needed until glucose levels are stable (Adamkin and Committee on Fetus and Newborn, 2011; McGowan, Rozance, Price-Douglas, et al., 2011).

Hypocalcemia. Hypocalcemia is defined as serum calcium levels of less than 7.8 to 8 mg/dL in term infants and slightly lower (7 mg/dL) in preterm infants. Hypocalcemia is common in critically ill neonates but also can occur in infants of mothers with diabetes or in those who had perinatal asphyxia or trauma, and in low-birth-weight and preterm infants. Infants born to mothers treated with anticonvulsants during pregnancy are also at risk (Rigo, Mohamed, and De Curtis, 2011). Early-onset hypocalcemia usually occurs within the first 24 to 48 hours after birth. Signs of hypocalcemia include jitteriness, high-pitched cry, irritability, apnea, intermittent cyanosis, abdominal distention, and laryngospasm, although some hypocalcemic infants are asymptomatic. Jitteriness is a symptom of both hypoglycemia and hypocalcemia; therefore hypocalcemia must be considered if the therapy for hypoglycemia proves ineffective.

In most instances, early-onset hypocalcemia is self-limiting and resolves within 1 to 3 days. Treatment usually includes early feeding of an appropriate source of calcium such as fortified human milk or a preterm infant formula (Jones, Hayes, Starbuck, et al., 2011).

Laboratory and Diagnostic Tests

Because newborns experience many transitional events in the first 28 days of life, laboratory samples are often collected to determine adequate physiologic adaptation and to identify disorders that can adversely affect the child's life beyond the neonatal period. Blood samples for most laboratory tests can be obtained from the neonate with a heel puncture, also known as a *heelstick*. Tests commonly performed other than blood glucose and bilirubin levels include newborn screening tests and serum drug levels. Standard laboratory values for a term newborn are given in Table 23-4.

Universal Newborn Screening

Mandated by U.S. law, newborn genetic screening is an important public health program aimed at early detection of genetic diseases that result in severe health problems if not treated early. The universal screening program is state-based and involves a variety of components including education, screening, follow-up, treatment, and a system for monitoring and evaluation. When the program began, 29 core conditions were included in the screening panel: 3 hemoglobinopathies (e.g., sickle cell disease), 20 inborn errors of metabolism (e.g., phenylketonuria [PKU], galactosemia), and 6 other disorders. Two others have since been added: severe combined

TABLE 23-4	STANDARD LABORATORY VALUES IN A TERM NEWBORN*
Hemoglobin (g/dL)	14.5 to 22.5
Hematocrit (%)	48 to 69
Red blood cells (RBCs)/mcL	4.8×10^6 to 7.1×10^6
Platelet count/mm³	150,000 to 300,000
White blood cells (WBCs)/mcL	9,000 to 30,000
Bilirubin, total	<2 mg/dL
Serum glucose	40 to 60 mg/dL
Blood gases	
Arterial	pH 7.31 to 7.49
	PCO_2 26 to 41 mm Hg
	PO_2 60 to 70 mm Hg
Venous	pH 7.31 to 7.41
	PCO_2 40 to 50 mm Hg
	PO_2 40 to 50 mm Hg

Data from Hockenberry MJ, Wilson D: *Wong's nursing care of infants and children,* ed 9, St Louis, 2011, Mosby; Pagana K, Pagana T: *Mosby's diagnostic and laboratory test reference,* ed 9, St Louis, 2009, Mosby.
PCO_2, Partial pressure of carbon dioxide; *PO_2,* partial pressure of oxygen.
**dL,* Deciliter; mcL, microliter.

immunodeficiency and critical congenital heart disease (Howell, Terry, Olney, et al., 2012). The majority of disorders included in the screening are not symptomatic at birth. Individual states select additional disorders to include in the screening. This list is available through the National Newborn Screening and Genetics Resource Center (NNSGRC) at http://genes-r-us.uthscsa.edu. Some of the major disorders for which infants are screened are described in Table 23-5.

Blood samples are obtained from newborn infants using a heel-stick; blood is collected on a special filter paper and sent to a designated state laboratory for analysis. Samples are usually collected in the hospital after 24 hours of age and before discharge; testing may be delayed for sick or preterm infants or those born outside the hospital (ACOG Committee on Genetics, 2011). The screening test should be repeated at age 1 to 2 weeks if the initial specimen was obtained when the infant was younger than 24 hours.

The American College of Medical Genetics (2009) recommends that states retain the residual dried blood filter spots. These blood samples are useful for future testing and for research purposes.

Families should be educated about universal newborn screening during the prenatal period (ACOG Committee on Genetics, 2011) (see Community Focus box). More often, discussion about the screening occurs in the hospital setting at the time of blood sample collection. Nurses can provide education for parents regarding the purpose of the screening, the procedure for blood sampling, when to expect results, and the importance of follow-up (Araia, Wilson, Chakraborty, et al., 2012).

Newborn Hearing Screening

Hearing loss is one of the genetic disorders in the universal screening program. It is the most commonly diagnosed of all the core conditions in the screening program (Howell, Terry, Olney, et al., 2012).

TABLE 23-5 SELECTED DISORDERS FROM UNIVERSAL NEWBORN SCREENING

DISORDER/EVIDENCE	SYMPTOMS	SCREENING INCIDENCE	TREATMENT
PKU (classic) Elevated phenylalanine (plasma concentrations >20 mg/dL)	Severe intellectual disability if early detection and treatment not started; eczema, seizures, behavior disorders, decreased pigmentation, distinctive musty or mouselike odor	1:16,000 More common in Caucasians and Native Americans	Lifelong dietary management with low-phenylalanine diet; possible tyrosine supplementation
Congenital hypothyroidism (primary) Low T_4, elevated TSH	Asymptomatic at birth; mental and motor delays (although neonatal detection and treatment have decreased incidence of intellectual disability); short stature; coarse, dry skin and hair; hoarse cry; constipation	1:3000 with some ethnic variation	Maintain L-thyroxine levels in upper half of normal range; periodic bone age testing to monitor growth
Galactosemia (transferase deficiency) Elevated galactose; low or absent fluorescence	Hypotonia, lethargy, vomiting, diarrhea, metabolic acidosis, *Escherichia coli* sepsis, or liver dysfunction; intellectual disability, jaundice, blindness, cataracts, long-term behavioral problems, and neurologic impairment	1:60,000	Eliminate galactose and lactose from the diet (breastfeeding is contraindicated); soy formulas in infancy; lactose-free solid foods
Maple syrup urine disease (MSUD) Elevated leucine	Poor feeding, lethargy, hypotonia, vomiting, ketoacidosis, and seizures; sweet maple syrup odor may occur in urine, cerumen, or sweat	1:185,000; higher in certain Mennonite (Older Order) populations—1:358	Branched-chain amino acid–free formula with added protein-based formula; thiamine supplement in some individuals; lifelong treatment and monitoring necessary
Homocystinuria Elevated methionine and homocysteine	Infancy: nonspecific growth failure; developmental delay; more commonly diagnosed around 3 yr Intellectual disability, seizures, behavioral disorders, early-onset thromboses, dislocated lenses, tall lanky body habitus	1:200,000 to 1:350,000; more prevalent in Ireland and New South Wales, Australia (1:60,000)	Methionine-restricted diet; vitamin B_6 supplement if responsive
Congenital adrenal hyperplasia (CAH) Elevated 24-hydroxyprogesterone; abnormal electrolytes	Hyponatremia, hyperkalemia, hypoglycemia, dehydration; weight loss; hypotension; shock in "salt wasting" type; female virilization; progressive virilization in both sexes	1:15,000 to 1:20,000; less common in African-Americans (1:42,000)	Reduce excessive corticotropins; replace glucocorticoids and mineral corticoids; corrective surgery for ambiguous genitalia (intersex assignment is controversial)
Sickle cell/hemoglobin SC (thalassemias)	Repeated infections, growth failure, pallor, hemolytic anemia; sickle cell crisis	Sickle cell anemia (SCA), 1:2647 in non–African-Americans; 1:396 in African-Americans; 1:36,000 in Hispanics	Preventive care: treatment of meningococcal and pneumococcal infections; hydroxyurea (antisickling agent); prevent human parvovirus B19 infection (limits production of reticulocytes)
Biotinidase deficiency Deficient or absent activity of biotinidase on colorimetric assay	Myoclonic seizures, hypotonia, feeding difficulties, organic aciduria, fungal infections, ataxia, skin rash, hearing loss, alopecia, optic nerve atrophy, developmental delay, coma, and death	1:60,000	5-20 mg biotin daily; less with partial deficiency

Data from DeBaun MR, Frei-Jones M, Vichinsky E: Hemoglobinopathies. In Kliegman R, Stanton B, St. Geme J, et al, editors: *Nelson textbook of pediatrics,* ed 19, Philadelphia, 2011, Saunders; Kishnani PS, Chen Y: Defects in metabolism of carbohydrates. In Kliegman R, Stanton B, St. Geme J, et al, editors: *Nelson textbook of pediatrics,* ed 19, Philadelphia, 2011, Saunders; LaFranchi S: Disorders of the thyroid gland. In Kliegman R, Stanton B, St. Geme J, et al, editors: *Nelson textbook of pediatrics,* ed 19, Philadelphia, 2011, Saunders; Rezvani I, Rosenblatt DS: Defects in metabolism of amino acid. In Kliegman R, Stanton B, St. Geme J, et al, editors: *Nelson textbook of pediatrics,* ed 19, Philadelphia, 2011, Saunders; White P: Congenital hyperplasia and related disorders. In Kliegman R, Stanton B, St. Geme J, et al, editors: *Nelson textbook of pediatrics,* ed 19, Philadelphia, 2011, Saunders.
PKU, Phenylketonuria; *SC,* sickle cell; *T_4,* thyroxine; *TSH,* thyroid-stimulating hormone.

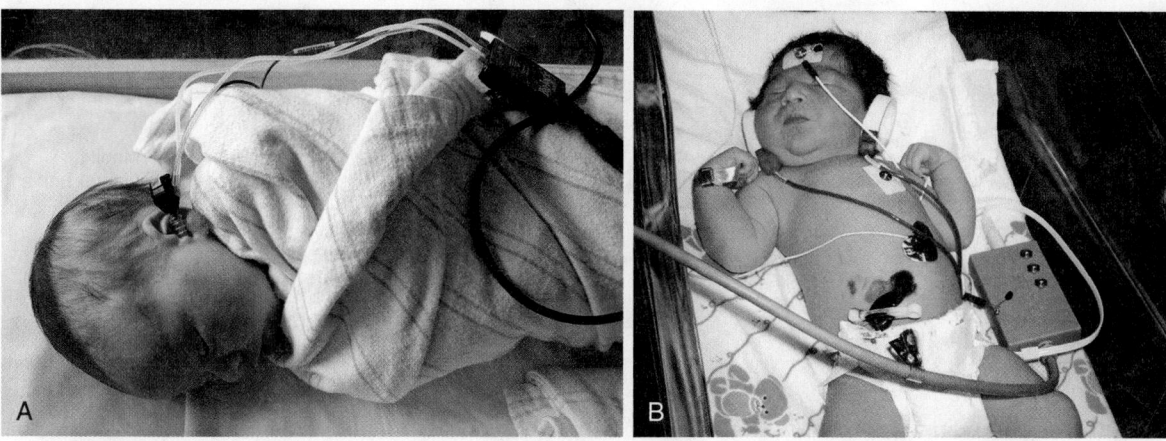

FIG 23-11 Newborn hearing screening. **A,** Evoked otoacoustic emissions (EOAE) test. **B,** Auditory brain response (ABR) test. (*A,* Courtesy Julie and Darren Nelson, Loveland, CO. *B,* Courtesy Dee Lowdermilk, Chapel Hill, NC.)

Universal Newborn Screening

- Visit the National Newborn Screening and Genetics Resource Center (NNSGRC) website (http://genes-r-us.uthscsa.edu). Review the information for parents and family about resources, disorders tested, and screening programs. What types of disorders are screened in your state? Is the screening for the condition required by law and fully implemented?
- At the NNSGRC website, visit the newborn screening program website for your state. Does your state require newborn hearing screening? Review the information for parents about diagnostic testing and community support services.

The Joint Committee on Infant Hearing (2007) recommends routine hearing screening for all newborns before hospital discharge or no later than 1 month of age. Through early hearing detection and intervention (EHDI) programs, the outcome for infants who are deaf or hard of hearing can be maximized.

Using noninvasive technology, newborn hearing screening provides information about the pathways from the external ear to the cerebral cortex. Two tests commonly are used to assess hearing function in the newborn. Initial screening is done with the evoked otoacoustic emissions (EOAE) test. The auditory brainstem response (ABR) test is used as follow-up if the initial screening is abnormal. Neither test is definitive in diagnosing hearing loss; they are used to determine whether further, more accurate hearing testing is needed through audiologic evaluation. For the EOAE test, a soft rubber earpiece that makes a soft clicking noise is placed in the baby's outer ear (Fig. 23-11, *A*). A healthy ear will "echo" the click sound back to a microphone inside the earpiece that is in the baby's ear. The ABR test is performed by attaching sensors to the baby's forehead and behind each ear. An earphone is placed in the baby's outer ear and sends a series of quiet sounds into the sleeping baby's ear (Fig. 23-11, *B*). The sensors measure the responses of the baby's acoustic nerve. The responses are recorded and stored in a computer.

Newborns who do not pass the initial screening test should have the hearing screening test repeated as part of follow-up care. If the infant still does not pass, a comprehensive audiologic evaluation should be done by 3 months of age. Regardless of the outcome of hearing testing, all infants should have regular and ongoing surveillance of developmental, hearing, and speech-language skills through regular well-child visits beginning at the age of 2 months so that any hearing loss may be promptly identified and treated (Joint Committee on Infant Hearing, 2007).

Collection of Specimens

Ongoing evaluation and screening of a newborn often requires obtaining blood by heelstick or venipuncture or the collection of a urine specimen. Laboratory tests may be ordered routinely (e.g., newborn screening) or for a specific purpose as directed by the health care provider.

Heelstick. Most blood specimens are drawn by laboratory technicians. Nurses, however, may be required to perform heelsticks to obtain blood for glucose monitoring, newborn screening, or other tests.

> ❗ **NURSING ALERT**
>
> Blood samples should be collected in a manner that minimizes pain and trauma to the infant and maximizes the accuracy of test results. If a laboratory technician is collecting the specimen, the nurse assists as needed to maximize safety and infant comfort.

Warming the heel before the sample is taken is often helpful; application of heat for 5 to 10 minutes helps dilate the vessels in the area. A cloth soaked with warm water and wrapped loosely around the foot provides effective warming (Fig. 23-12). Disposable heel warmers are available from a variety of companies but should be used with care to prevent burns. Nurses should wear gloves when collecting any specimen. The nurse cleanses the area with an appropriate skin antiseptic, restrains the infant's foot with a free hand, and then punctures the site. A spring-loaded automatic puncture device causes less pain and requires fewer punctures than a manual lance blade.

The most serious complication of an infant heelstick is necrotizing osteochondritis resulting from lancet penetration of the bone. To prevent this problem, the puncture is made at the outer aspect of the heel and penetrates no deeper than 2.4 mm. To identify the appropriate puncture site, the nurse draws an imaginary line from between the fourth and fifth toes and parallel to the lateral aspect of the foot to the heel, where the puncture is made; a second line can be drawn from the great toe to the medial aspect of the heel (see

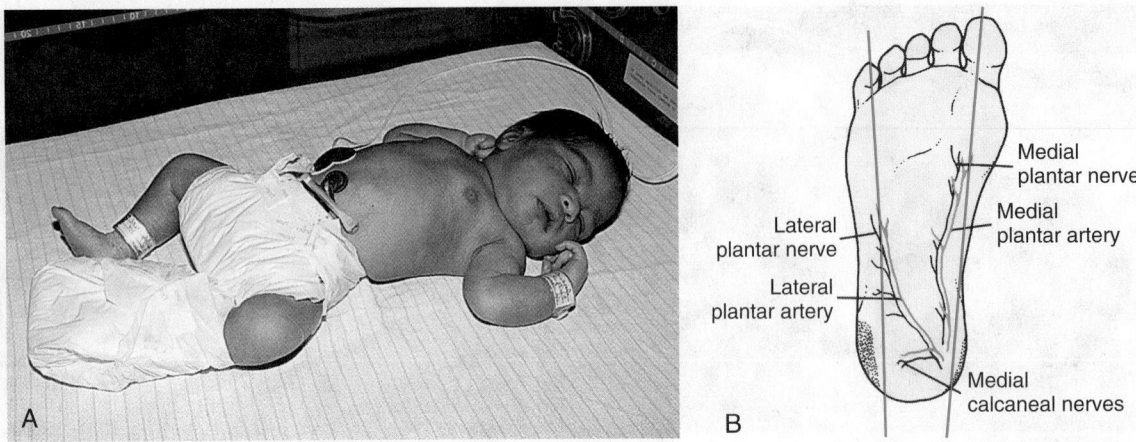

FIG 23-12 Heelstick. **A,** Newborn with foot wrapped for warmth to increase blood flow to extremity before heelstick. **B,** Heelstick sites *(shaded areas)* on infant's foot for obtaining samples of capillary blood. (*A,* Courtesy Marjorie Pyle, RNC, Lifecircle, Costa Mesa, CA.)

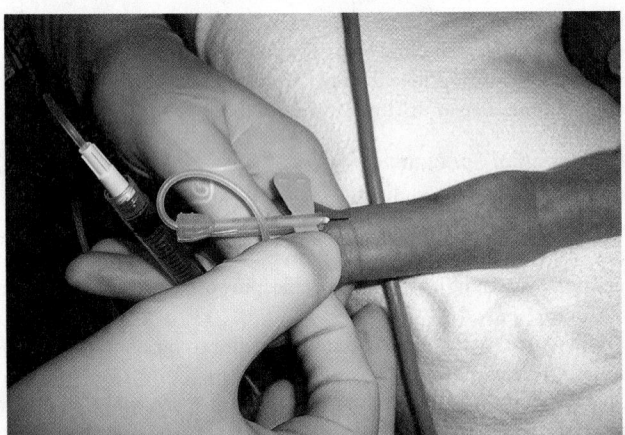

FIG 23-13 Venipuncture using a butterfly needle. (Courtesy Cheryl Briggs, RNC, Annapolis, MD.)

Fig. 23-12). Repeated trauma to the walking surface of the heel can cause fibrosis and scarring that can lead to problems with walking later in life.

After the specimen has been collected, gentle pressure is applied with a dry gauze pad. No further skin cleanser should be applied because it will cause the site to continue to bleed. The site is then covered with an adhesive bandage. The nurse ensures proper disposal of equipment used, reviews the laboratory requisition for correct identification, and checks the specimen for accurate labeling and routing.

A heelstick is traumatic for the infant and causes pain. After several heelsticks, infants have been observed to withdraw their feet when they are touched. To reassure the infant and promote feelings of safety, the neonate should be cuddled and comforted when the procedure is complete and appropriate pain management measures taken to minimize the pain.

Venipuncture. Occasionally, laboratory tests are ordered that require larger samples of blood than can be collected with a heelstick. Venous blood samples can be drawn from antecubital, saphenous, superficial wrist, and rarely, scalp veins. When venipuncture is required, positioning of the needle is extremely important. A 23- or 25-gauge butterfly needle or hypodermic needle with a syringe is used (Fig. 23-13). Patience is required during the procedure because

the blood return in small veins is slow and consequently the small needle must remain in place longer than a larger needle. A tourniquet is optional but can help increase blood flow with venipuncture. The infant is carefully restrained during the procedure to prevent injury (see Chapter 39).

If venipuncture or arterial puncture is performed for blood gas studies, crying, fear, and agitation will affect the values; therefore every effort must be made to keep the infant quiet during the procedure. Pressure must be maintained over an arterial or femoral vein puncture with a dry gauze square for 3 to 5 minutes to prevent bleeding from the site.

For an hour after any venipuncture, the nurse observes the infant frequently for evidence of bleeding or hematoma formation at the puncture site. The infant is cuddled and comforted when the procedure is completed, and appropriate pain management measures are taken. The nurse assesses and documents the infant's tolerance of the procedure.

> ! **NURSING ALERT**
>
> Only venous or capillary blood samples can be used for newborn screening and genetic studies; cord blood is not used for such samples.

Obtaining a Urine Specimen. Analysis of urine is a valuable laboratory tool for infant assessment; the way in which the specimen is collected can influence the results. The urine sample should be fresh and analyzed within 1 hour of collection. A urine collection bag is often used to obtain a specimen (see Chapter 39 for more information about the procedure for collecting a urine specimen from an infant).

Interventions
Protective Environment
The provision of a protective environment is basic to the care of the newborn. The construction, maintenance, and operation of nurseries in accredited hospitals are monitored by national professional organizations such as the American Academy of Pediatrics (AAP), The Joint Commission (TJC), the Occupational Safety and Health Administration (OSHA), and local or state governing bodies. In addition, hospital personnel develop their own policies and procedures for protecting the newborns under their care. Prescribed

standards cover areas such as environmental factors, measures to control infection, and safety factors.

Current health care trends and the focus on nonseparation of mothers and babies have prompted some hospitals to abandon having a separate newborn nursery. In the mother/baby care model of care, the infant stays in the mother's room, which reduces the need for a separate nursery.

Environmental Factors. Environmental factors include provision of adequate lighting, elimination of potential fire hazards, safety of electrical appliances, adequate ventilation, and controlled temperature (i.e., warm and free of drafts) and humidity (i.e., 40% to 60%) (AAP and ACOG, 2012).

Infection Control Factors. Measures to control infection in newborn nurseries include adequate floor space to permit the positioning of bassinets at least 3 feet apart in all directions, handwashing facilities, and areas for cleaning and storing equipment and supplies. Only specified personnel directly involved in the care of mothers and infants are allowed in these areas, thereby reducing the opportunities for the transmission of pathogenic organisms.

> **! NURSING ALERT**
>
> Proper hand hygiene is essential to preventing the spread of health care–associated infection. Personnel should wash hands with soap and water or use an alcohol-based handrub in accordance with hospital infection control policies. Hand hygiene should be performed before and after touching the infant, before an invasive procedure or medication administration, after contact with potentially contaminated objects (e.g., computer keyboards, telephone, countertop surfaces), and after removing sterile or non-sterile gloves (World Health Organization [WHO], 2009).

Health care workers must wear gloves when handling infants until blood and amniotic fluid have been removed from the skin, when drawing blood (e.g., heelstick), when caring for a fresh wound (e.g., circumcision), and during diaper changes.

Visitors such as siblings and grandparents are expected to perform hand hygiene before having contact with infants or equipment. Individuals with infectious conditions are excluded from contact with newborns or must take special precautions when working with infants. This group includes persons with upper respiratory tract infections, gastrointestinal tract infections, and infectious skin conditions.

Preventing Infant Abduction. Health care institutions must be proactive in protecting newborns from abductions. Examples of measures taken include:

- Placing matching identification bracelets on infants and their parents immediately after birth
- Using identification bands with radiofrequency transmitters (Fig. 23-14) that set off an alarm if the bracelet is removed or if a certain threshold is crossed (doorway to exit the unit or building)
- Footprinting
- Taking identification pictures immediately after birth, before the infant leaves the mother's side

Agencies must conduct periodic unit and hospital-wide drills aimed at preventing newborn abductions. Personnel caring for newborns must be clearly identified by photo identification, and parents must be educated regarding measures to prevent abduction from the mother's room (i.e., be certain they know the identity of anyone who cares for the infant and never release the infant to anyone who is not wearing the appropriate identification) (Vincent, 2009).

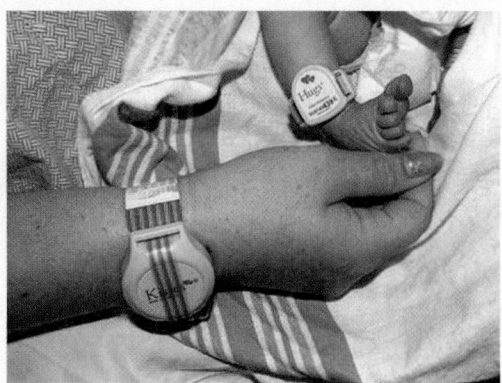

FIG 23-14 Mother and infant wear electronic bracelets as part of an infant security system. (Courtesy Shannon Perry, Phoenix, AZ.)

Therapeutic and Surgical Procedures

Intramuscular Injection. Newborns routinely receive intramuscular injections before discharge. A single dose of vitamin K is administered shortly after birth and hepatitis B (HepB) vaccine is administered before discharge. Under specific circumstances, other intramuscular injections may be ordered, such as a dose of hepatitis B immune globulin for infants born to mothers who are positive for hepatitis B.

Selection of the appropriate equipment and site for intramuscular injection is important. In most cases, a 25-gauge, ⅝-inch needle is used. Injections must be given in muscles large enough to accommodate the medication, and major nerves and blood vessels must be avoided. The muscles of newborns may not tolerate more than a 0.5 mL per intramuscular injection. The preferred injection site for newborns is the vastus lateralis (Fig. 23-15). The dorsogluteal muscle is very small, poorly developed, and dangerously close to the sciatic nerve, which occupies a proportionately larger area in infants than in older children. Therefore it is not recommended as an injection site in small children. The newborn's deltoid muscle has an inadequate amount of muscle for intramuscular administration. A key factor in preventing and minimizing local reaction to intramuscular injections is adequate deposition of the medication deep within the muscle; therefore muscle size, needle length, and amount of medication injected should be carefully considered.

The nurse wears nonsterile gloves when administering an injection. The neonate's leg should be stabilized. The nurse cleanses the injection site with an appropriate skin antiseptic and then stabilizes the infant's muscle between the thumb and forefinger. The needle is inserted into the vastus lateralis at a 90-degree angle. The medication is injected slowly. After the medication is injected, the nurse withdraws the needle quickly and places a dry gauze pad over the site, applying gentle pressure to minimize pain and bleeding.

The nurse comforts the infant after an injection and discards equipment properly. Needles are never recapped but are properly discarded in an appropriate safety container. The name of the medication, date and time, amount, route, and site of injection are documented in the newborn's record.

Immunizations. Hepatitis B (HepB) vaccination is recommended for all infants before hospital discharge. Parental consent should be obtained before administering the vaccine. Infants at highest risk for contracting hepatitis B are those born to women who have hepatitis B or whose hepatitis B status is unknown. Before administering the vaccine, it is important to note the mother's

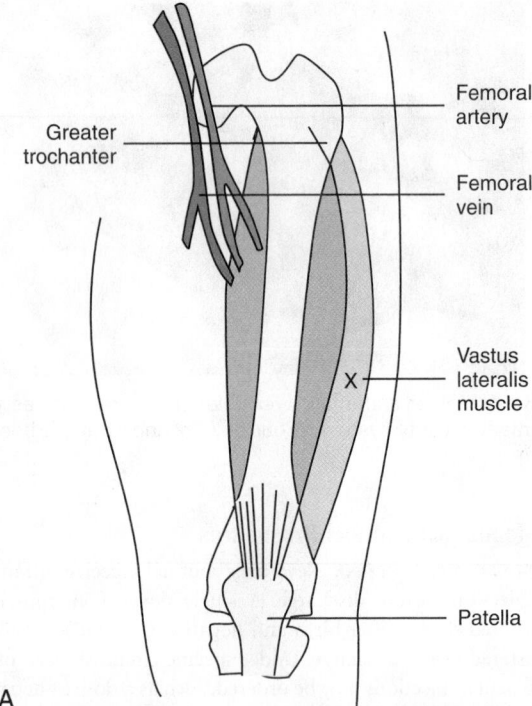

A

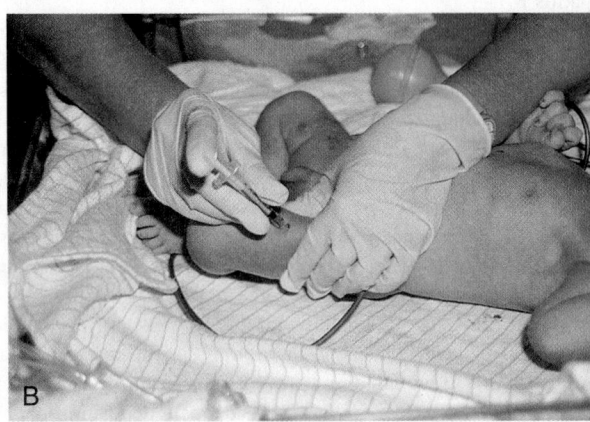

B

FIG 23-15 Intramuscular injection. **A,** Acceptable intramuscular injection site for newborn infant. *X,* injection site. **B,** Infant's leg stabilized for intramuscular injection. Nurse is wearing gloves to give injection. (*B,* Courtesy Marjorie Pyle, Lifecircle, Costa Mesa, CA.)

hepatitis B status. Infants born to hepatitis B surface antigen (HBsAg)–negative mothers should receive the vaccine before they leave the hospital. If the mother is positive for hepatitis B, the infant should receive the HepB vaccine and HepB immune globulin (HBIG) within 12 hours after birth; the injections are given in separate sites (only one injection is given in each leg). When the mother's HBsAg status is unknown, the infant who weighs 2000 g or more receives HepB vaccine within 12 hours after birth; infants who weigh 2000 g or less should receive HepB vaccine and HBIG during the first 12 hours. The mother's HBsAg status is determined as soon as possible; if the results are positive, the infant who weighs 2000 g or more needs a dose of HBIG before the age of 1 week. (See the Medication Guides.) The HepB vaccination plan is a series of three

---

MEDICATION GUIDE

Hepatitis B Vaccine (Recombivax HB, Engerix-B)

Action

Hepatitis B vaccine induces protective antihepatitis B antibodies in 95% to 99% of healthy infants who receive the recommended three doses. The duration of protection of the vaccine is unknown.

Indication

Hepatitis B vaccine is for immunization against infection caused by all known subtypes of hepatitis B virus (HBV).

Neonatal Dosage

The usual dosage is Recombivax HB 5 mg/0.5 mL or Engerix-B 10 mg/0.5 mL intramuscularly at birth, at 1 to 2 months, and at 6 months.

Adverse Reactions

Common adverse reactions are rash, fever, erythema, swelling, and pain at injection site.

Nursing Considerations

- Parental consent must be obtained before administration. Follow proper procedure for administration of intramuscular (IM) injection (see p. 613). If infant also needs hepatitis B immune globulin (HBIG), use separate sites for the two injections.
- For infants of mothers with negative hepatitis B status: administer hepatitis B (HepB) vaccine before discharge from hospital.
- For infants born to hepatitis B surface antigen (HBsAg)–positive mothers: administer HepB vaccine and HBIG within 12 hours after birth.
- For infants born to mothers whose hepatitis B status is unknown:
  - ≤2000 g: administer HepB vaccine and HBIG within 12 hours after birth
  - ≥2000 g: administer HepB vaccine as soon as possible; if mother's HepB results are positive, give HBIG by 1 week of age

---

MEDICATION GUIDE

Hepatitis B Immune Globulin

Action

Hepatitis B immune globulin (HBIG) provides a high titer of antibody to hepatitis B surface antigen (HBsAg).

Indication

The HBIG vaccine provides prophylaxis against infection in infants born of HBsAg–positive mothers.

Neonatal Dosage

Administer one 0.5-mL dose intramuscularly (IM) within 12 hours of birth.

Adverse Reactions

Hypersensitivity may occur.

Nursing Considerations

The HBIG vaccine must be given within 12 hours of birth. Follow proper procedure for administration of IM injection (see p. 613). (See guidelines for administration in Medication Guide: Hepatitis B above.) The HBIG vaccine can be given at the same time as the hepatitis B vaccine but at a different site. Document the date, time, and site of injection, as well as the lot number and expiration date of the vaccine, according to agency policy.

injections: birth, 1 to 2 months of age, and 6 to 18 months of age (Centers for Disease Control and Prevention [CDC], 2013).

The schedule for immunizations should be reviewed with the parents. Hepatitis B vaccine is currently administered to newborns before hospital discharge (depending on maternal hepatitis B status) or within 1 month of birth. See Chapter 31 for a complete discussion of infant immunizations.

Circumcision. Circumcision is the removal of all or part of the foreskin (prepuce) of the penis. Usually it is performed during the first few days of life but is sometimes done at a later time for preterm or ill neonates or for religious or cultural reasons.

Policies and Recommendations. Over the past decade, circumcision rates in the United States have steadily decreased. The Centers for Disease Control and Prevention (CDC) (Zhang, Shinde, Kilmarx, et al., 2011) reviewed data on newborn male circumcision (NMC) from three national data sources and found NMC rates ranging from 56.3% to 58.4%. One of the factors that influenced the decline is the lack of medical reimbursement for the procedure by Medicaid and some private insurers. The AAP policy on circumcision that was issued in 1999 and reaffirmed in 2005 recognized potential benefits of NMC, although the AAP did not deem them sufficient to recommend routine newborn circumcision (AAP Task Force on Circumcision, 1999, 2005). In 2012, the AAP issued a new policy statement regarding newborn male circumcision. The policy states: "Evaluation of current evidence indicates that the health benefits of newborn male circumcision outweigh the risks and that the procedure's benefits justify access to this procedure for families who choose it." (AAP Task Force on Circumcision, 2012). The health benefits of NMC cited by AAP include prevention of urinary tract infection in male infants younger than 1 year, reduced risk for penile cancer, and reduced risk for heterosexual acquisition of sexually transmitted infections, particularly HIV (AAP Task Force on Circumcision, 2012). In spite of the new evidence, AAP does not recommend the practice of routine newborn circumcision. The American College of Obstetricians and Gynecologists endorsed the new AAP policy. The World Health Organization (WHO) (2012) recognizes male circumcision as an important intervention in reducing the risk for heterosexually acquired HIV in men.

Even with the change in AAP policy on NMC, newborn male circumcision remains a controversial topic. Opponents of circumcision feel that the procedure is unnatural and unnecessary and that it violates basic human rights They cite concerns about acute pain; risks related to acute complications such as hemorrhage, infection, and penile injury (removal of excessive skin, damage to the meatus or glans); and long-term implications such as adverse effects on sexual function and pleasure. Websites such as www.intactamerica.org discourage parents from circumcising their newborn sons.

Parental Decision. Circumcision is a matter of personal parental choice. Parents usually decide to have their newborn circumcised for one or more of the following reasons: hygiene, religious conviction, tradition, culture, or social norms. Cost and insurance coverage are considerations in the parents' decision-making process. Parents need to make an informed choice regarding newborn circumcision based on the most current evidence and recommendations. Health care providers and nurses who care for childbearing families can help parents make an informed choice about newborn circumcision by providing factual, unbiased, evidence-based information. They can provide opportunities for discussion about the benefits and risks of the procedure.

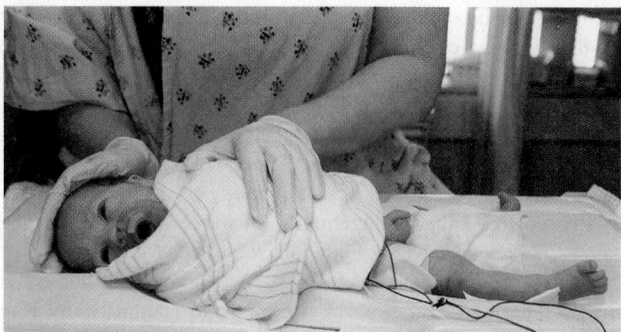

FIG 23-16 Positioning of infant in Circumstraint. (Courtesy Paul Vincent Kuntz, Texas Children's Hospital, Houston, TX.)

> **! NURSING ALERT**
>
> There are websites devoted to presenting arguments against newborn circumcision (e.g., www.intactamerica.org). The information in these sites is often not evidence-based and should be evaluated by nurses and health care professionals who work with childbearing families. Parents can be directed to websites of professional organizations that provide current, evidence-based information about newborn circumcision (e.g., www.aap.org).

Expectant parents need to begin learning about circumcision during the prenatal period, but circumcision often is not discussed with the parents before labor. In many instances, it is only when the mother is being admitted to the hospital or birth unit that she is first confronted with the decision regarding circumcision. Because the stress of the intrapartum period makes this a difficult time for parental decision making, this is not an ideal time to broach the topic of circumcision and expect a well-thought-out decision. Circumcision requires a signed consent form in addition to the safety measures that precede any surgical procedure (e.g., proper identification).

Procedure. Circumcision is not performed immediately after birth because of the danger of cold stress and decreased clotting factors but is usually done in the hospital before discharge. The circumcision of a Jewish male infant is commonly performed on the eighth day after birth at home in a ceremony called a *bris.* This timing is logical from a physiologic standpoint because clotting factors decrease somewhat immediately after birth and do not return to prebirth levels until the end of the first week.

Feedings may be withheld up to 2 to 3 hours before the circumcision to prevent vomiting and aspiration, although in some hospitals, infants are allowed to breastfeed until the time they are taken to the nursery for the procedure. To prepare the infant for the circumcision, he is positioned on a plastic restraint form (Fig. 23-16) and the penis is cleansed with soap and water or a preparatory solution such as povidone-iodine. The infant is draped to provide warmth and a sterile field, and the sterile equipment is readied for use.

In the hospital setting, newborn circumcision is usually performed using the Gomco (Yellen) or Mogen clamp or the PlastiBell device. The technique is usually based on health care provider training and preference. The procedure takes only a few minutes to perform. Use of the Gomco or Mogen clamp involves surgical removal of the foreskin. The clamp technique minimizes blood loss (Fig. 23-17). After the circumcision is completed, a small petrolatum gauze dressing or a generous amount of petrolatum or A&D

ointment may be applied to the penis for the first few days to prevent the diaper from adhering to the site. With the PlastiBell technique, the plastic bell is first fitted over the glans, a suture is tied around the rim of the bell, and excess foreskin is cut away. The plastic rim remains in place for about a week; it falls off after healing has taken place, usually within 5 to 7 days (Fig. 23-18). Petrolatum is not usually needed when the PlastiBell is used.

Procedural Pain Management. Circumcision is painful. The pain is characterized by both physiologic and behavioral changes in the infant (see discussion that follows). Four types of anesthesia and analgesia are used in newborns who undergo circumcisions: ring block, dorsal penile nerve block (DPNB), topical anesthetic such as eutectic mixture of local anesthetic (EMLA) (prilocaine-lidocaine) or LMX4 (4% lidocaine), and concentrated oral sucrose. Nonpharmacologic methods such as nonnutritive sucking and containment (swaddling) can be used to enhance pain management.

The Cochrane group exploring pain relief for neonatal circumcision (Brady-Fryer, Wiebe, and Lander, 2004) found that DPNB was the most effective intervention for decreasing the pain of circumcision. A DPNB includes subcutaneous injections of buffered lidocaine at the 2 o'clock and 10 o'clock positions at the base of the penis. A ring block is the injection of buffered lidocaine administered subcutaneously on each side of the penile shaft. The circumcision should not be performed for at least 5 minutes after these injections.

A topical anesthetic cream (eutectic mixture of local anesthetic [EMLA]) can be applied to the penis at least 1 hour before the circumcision. The area where the prepuce attaches to the glans is well coated with 1 g of the cream and then covered with a transparent occlusive dressing or finger cot. Just before the procedure, the cream is removed. Blanching or redness of the skin can occur.

After the circumcision, the infant is comforted until he is quieted. If the parents were not present during the procedure, the infant is returned to them. The infant can be fussy for several hours and can have disturbed sleep-wake states and disorganized feeding behaviors. Some infants will go into a deep sleep after circumcision until they are awakened for feeding. Oral liquid acetaminophen may be administered after the procedure and repeated every 4 hours (as ordered by the health care provider) for a maximum of five doses in 24 hours or a maximum of 75 mg/kg/day.

Care of the Newly Circumcised Infant. Postcircumcision protocols vary. In many settings, the circumcision site is assessed for bleeding every 15 to 30 minutes for the first hour and then hourly for the next 4 to 6 hours. The nurse monitors the infant's urinary output, noting the time and amount of the first voiding after the circumcision.

If bleeding occurs from the circumcision site, the nurse applies gentle pressure with a folded sterile gauze pad. A hemostatic agent such as Gelfoam® powder or sponge can be applied to help control bleeding. If bleeding is not easily controlled, a blood vessel may need to be ligated. In this event, one nurse notifies the physician and prepares the necessary equipment (i.e., circumcision tray and suture material) while another nurse maintains intermittent pressure until the physician arrives.

Nurses provide education for parents related to care of the circumcised infant, which includes observing for complications such as bleeding or infection (see Patient Teaching box). Parents need

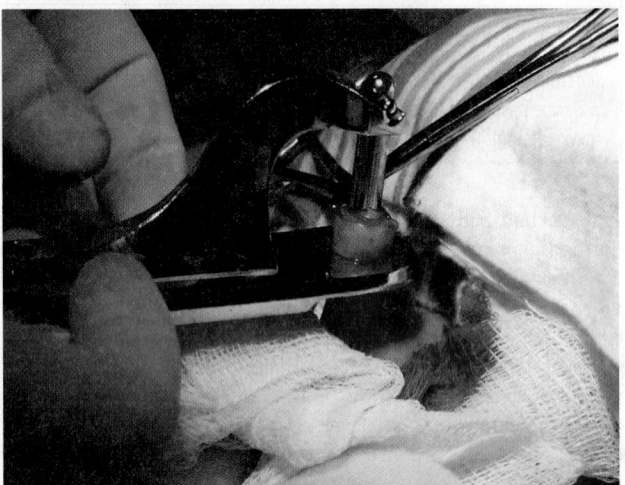

FIG 23-17 Circumcision with the Gomco (Yellen) clamp. After hemostasis occurs, the foreskin (over the metal dome) is cut away. (Courtesy Cheryl Briggs, RNC, Annapolis, MD.)

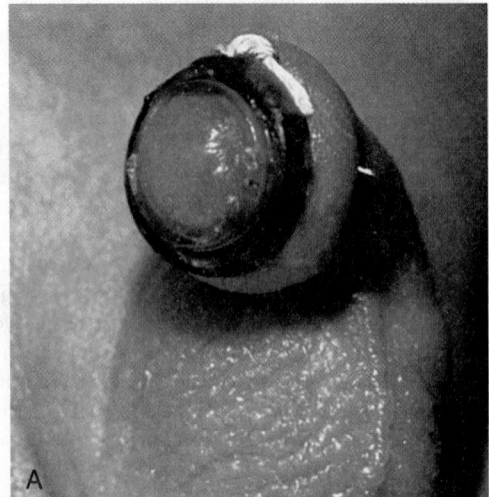 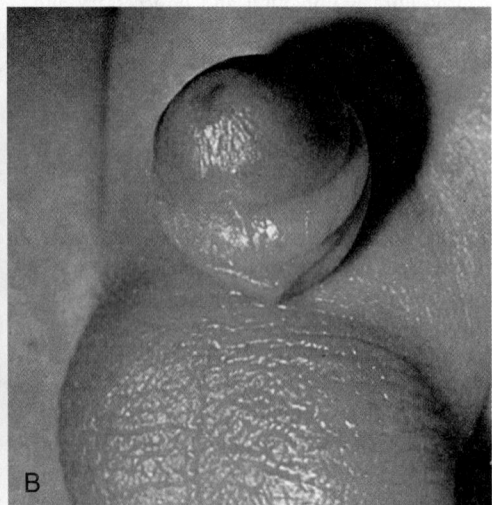

FIG 23-18 Newborn penis after circumcision using Hollister PlastiBell. **A,** Suture around rim of PlastiBell controls bleeding. **B,** Plastic rim and suture drop off in 7 to 10 days. (Permission to use and/or reproduce this copyrighted material has been granted by the owner, Hollister, Inc., Libertyville, IL.)

support and encouragement as they perform postcircumcision care. Newborns typically cry when the diaper is changed and when petrolatum gauze is removed and reapplied. This can make new parents feel anxious because they do not want to inflict pain on the infant. Nurses can inform parents that the discomfort is usually temporary and will soon subside.

Nursing actions are planned and implemented to prevent infection. Prepackaged commercial wipes are not used because they can contain alcohol, which delays healing and causes discomfort. Instead, the nurse washes the penis gently with water to remove urine and feces and, if necessary, applies fresh petrolatum around the glans after each diaper change. The glans penis, normally dark red during healing, becomes covered with a yellow exudate in about 24 hours, which is part of normal healing—not an infective process. No attempt should be made to remove the exudate, which persists for 2 to 3 days. Parents are taught to apply the diaper so that it does not press on the circumcised area. They are encouraged to change the diaper at least every 4 hours to prevent it from sticking to the penis.

PATIENT TEACHING

Care of the Circumcised Newborn at Home

Wash hands before touching the newly circumcised penis.

Check for Bleeding
- Check circumcision for bleeding with each diaper change.
- If bleeding occurs, apply gentle pressure with a folded sterile gauze square. If bleeding does not stop with pressure, notify primary health care provider.

Observe for Urination
- Check to see that the infant urinates after being circumcised.
- Infant should have a wet diaper 2 to 6 times per 24 hours the first 1 to 2 days after birth and then at least 6 to 8 times per 24 hours after 3 to 4 days.

Keep Area Clean
- Change the diaper and inspect the circumcision at least every 4 hours.
- Wash the penis gently with warm water to remove urine and feces. Apply petrolatum to the glans with each diaper change (omit petrolatum if a PlastiBell was used). Do not use baby wipes because they can contain alcohol.
- Do not wash the penis with soap until the circumcision is healed (5 to 6 days).
- Apply the diaper loosely over the penis to prevent pressure on the circumcised area.

Check for Infection
- Glans penis is dark red after circumcision and then becomes covered with yellow exudate in 24 hours, which is normal and will persist for 2 to 3 days. Do not attempt to remove it.
- Redness, swelling, discharge, or odor indicates infection. Notify the pediatric health care provider if you think the circumcision area is infected.

Provide Comfort
- Circumcision is painful. Handle the area gently.
- Provide comfort measures such as holding the baby skin-to-skin, cuddling, swaddling, or rocking.

Neonatal Pain

Neonatal Responses to Pain

There is clear evidence that neonates can feel pain, despite previous thinking that the immaturity of the nervous system prevented or blunted pain sensation and that neonates were incapable of remembering painful experiences. Pain in the neonate and pain in later life can be qualitatively different, but research has substantiated that newborns do experience pain (Blackburn, 2013).

Pain has physiologic and psychologic components. Its psychologic component and the diffuse total body response to pain exhibited by the neonate led many health care providers in the past to believe that infants, especially preterm infants, do not experience pain. The central nervous system is well developed, however, as early as 24 weeks of gestation. The peripheral and spinal structures that transmit pain information are present and functional between the first and second trimesters. The pituitary-adrenal axis is also well developed at this time, and a fight-or-flight reaction is observed in response to the catecholamines released in response to stress.

The physiologic response to pain in neonates can be life threatening. Pain response can decrease tidal volume, increase demands on the cardiovascular system, increase metabolism, and cause neuroendocrine imbalance. The hormonal-metabolic response to pain in a term infant has greater magnitude and shorter duration than that in adults. The newborn's sympathetic response to pain is less mature and therefore less predictable than an adult's.

Pain response is influenced by a variety of factors such as characteristics of the painful stimulus, gestational age, biologic factors, and behavioral state. The source, location, and timing of the pain affect the response; newborns respond differently to acute pain than to prolonged or recurrent pain. In general, infants of younger gestational ages seem to display less vigorous pain responses. There can be genetic differences in pain responses related to the amount and type of neurotransmitters and receptors available to mediate pain. The behavioral state of the neonate also affects the pain response. Those who are more awake tend to have more robust pain responses than those in sleep states (Gardner, Enzman-Hines, and Dickey, 2011).

The most common behavioral sign of pain is a vocalization or crying, ranging from a whimper to a distinctive high-pitched, shrill cry. Facial expressions include grimacing, eye squeeze, brow contraction, deepened nasolabial furrows, a taut and quivering tongue, and an open mouth (Fig. 23-19). The infant will flex and adduct the upper body and lower limbs in an attempt to withdraw from the painful stimulus. The preterm infant has a lower-than-normal threshold for initiation of this flex response. An infant who receives a muscle-paralyzing agent such as vecuronium will be unable to mount a behavioral or visible pain response.

Pain can result in significant changes in heart rate, blood pressure (increased or decreased), intracranial pressure, vagal tone, respiratory rate, and oxygen saturation. Neonates respond to painful stimuli with release of epinephrine, norepinephrine, glucagon, corticosterone, cortisol, 11-deoxycorticosterone, lactate, pyruvate, and glucose (Blackburn, 2013) (Box 23-5).

Assessment of Neonatal Pain

In assessing pain, the nurse needs to consider the health of the neonate, the type and duration of the painful stimulus, environmental factors, and the infant's state of alertness. For example, severely compromised neonates may be unable to generate a pain response although they are, in fact, experiencing pain.

Every patient should have an initial pain assessment as well as a pain management plan; this mandate includes newborns. The National Association of Neonatal Nurses (NANN) developed

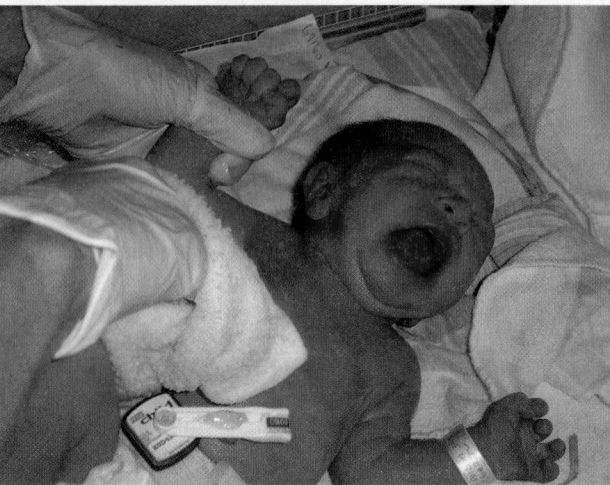

FIG 23-19 Signs of discomfort: note eye squeeze, brow bulge, nasolabial furrow, and wide-spread mouth. (Courtesy Kathryn Alden, Chapel Hill, NC.)

practice guidelines stating that all nurses who care for newborns should have education and competency validation in pain assessment. Pain should be assessed and documented on a regular basis (Walden and Gibbins, 2008).

Pain assessment tools include:
- Neonatal Infant Pain Scale (NIPS) (Lawrence, Alcock, McGrath, et al., 1993)
- Premature Infant Pain Profile (PIPP) (Stevens, Johnston, Petryshen, et al., 1996)
- Neonatal Pain Agitation and Sedation Scale (NPASS) (Hummel, Puchalski, Creech, et al., 2008)

A pain assessment tool used by nurses in some neonatal intensive care units (NICU) is CRIES (Krechel and Bildner, 1995) (Table 23-6). This tool was developed for use by nurses who work with preterm and term infants. CRIES is an acronym for the physiologic and behavioral indicators of pain used in the tool: *c*rying, *r*equiring increased oxygen, *i*ncreased vital signs, *e*xpression, and *s*leeplessness. Each indicator is scored from 0 to 2. The total possible pain score, which represents the worst pain, is 10. A pain score greater than 4 should be considered significant. This tool can be used on infants between 32 weeks of gestation and 20 weeks after birth.

Healthy term newborns are exposed to fewer sources of pain than preterm infants in a NICU where painful procedures are inherent to care management. Even in low risk newborns, nurses need to assess for signs of discomfort as part of routine assessments and especially during and after routine procedures such as heelsticks, injections, and circumcision.

Management of Neonatal Pain

The goals of the management of neonatal pain are to: (1) minimize the intensity, duration, and physiologic cost of the pain; and (2) maximize the neonate's ability to cope with and recover from the pain. Nonpharmacologic and pharmacologic strategies are used. It is important to note that despite research evidence, policies, and standards of practice focused on assessing and managing pain in newborns, acute infant pain remains undermanaged and, in some cases, unmanaged (Gardner, Enzman-Hines, and Dickey, 2011; Taddio, Appleton, Bortolussi, et al., 2010).

Nonpharmacologic Management. A variety of nonpharmacologic pain management techniques are used with neonates. Nurses and parents may combine two or more techniques as they seek to promote infant comfort and reduce pain.

BOX 23-5 MANIFESTATIONS OF ACUTE PAIN IN THE NEONATE

Physiologic Responses
- Vital signs—Observe for variations.
  - Increased heart rate
  - Increased blood pressure
  - Rapid, shallow respirations
- Oxygenation.
  - Decreased transcutaneous oxygen saturation (tcPO$_2$)
  - Decreased arterial oxygen saturation (SaO$_2$)
- Skin—Observe color and character.
  - Pallor or flushing
  - Diaphoresis
  - Palmar sweating
- Laboratory evidence of metabolic or endocrine changes.
  - Hyperglycemia
  - Lowered pH
  - Elevated corticosteroids
- Other observations.
  - Increased muscle tone
  - Dilated pupils
  - Decreased vagal nerve tone
  - Increased intracranial pressure

Behavioral Responses
- Vocalizations—Observe quality, timing, and duration.
  - Crying
  - Whimpering
  - Groaning
- Facial expression—Observe characteristics, timing, orientation of eyes and mouth.
  - Grimaces
  - Brow furrowed
  - Chin quivering
  - Eyes tightly closed
  - Mouth open and squarish
- Body movements and posture—Observe type, quality, and amount of movement or lack of movement; relationship to other factors.
  - Limb withdrawal
  - Thrashing
  - Rigidity
  - Flaccidity
  - Fist clenching
- Changes in state—Observe sleep, appetite, activity level.
  - Changes in sleep-wake cycles
  - Changes in feeding behavior
  - Changes in activity level
  - Fussiness, irritability
  - Listlessness

Modified from Blackburn S: *Maternal, fetal, and neonatal physiology: a clinical perspective,* ed 4, St Louis, 2013, Mosby; and Gardner SL, Enzman-Hines M, Dickey LA: Pain and pain relief. In Gardner SL, Carter BS, Enzman-Hines M, et al, editors: *Merenstein & Gardner's handbook of neonatal intensive care,* ed 7, St Louis, 2011, Mosby.

One of the most common measures is swaddling or snugly wrapping the infant with a blanket, although research evidence is lacking to support its effectiveness. It is thought that the security of feeling slight pressure around the body mimics the sensations of the intrauterine environment. Swaddling is most effective during the first few weeks of life (Fig. 23-20).

TABLE 23-6	CRIES NEONATAL POSTOPERATIVE PAIN SCALE*		
	0	**1**	**2**
Crying	No	High pitched	Inconsolable
Requires oxygen for saturation >95%	No	<30%	>30%
Increased vital signs	Heart rate and blood pressure equal to or less than preoperative state	Heart rate and blood pressure <20% of preoperative state	Heart rate and blood pressure >20% of preoperative state
Expression	None	Grimace	Grimace and grunt
Sleepless	No	Wakes at frequent intervals	Constantly awake

Coding Tips for Using CRIES

Crying	The characteristic cry of pain is high pitched.
	If no cry or cry that is not high pitched, score 0.
	If cry is high pitched but infant is easily consoled, score 1.
	If cry is high pitched and infant is inconsolable, score 2.
Requires oxygen for saturation >95%	Look for changes in oxygenation. Infants experiencing pain manifest decreases in oxygenation as measured by total carbon dioxide or oxygen saturation. (Consider other causes of changes in oxygenation, such as atelectasis, pneumothorax, oversedation.)
	If no oxygen is required, score 0.
	If <30% oxygen is required, score 1.
	If >30% oxygen is required, score 2.
Increased vital signs	**NOTE:** Measure blood pressure last because this may wake the infant, causing difficulty with other assessments. Use baseline preoperative parameters from a nonstressed period.
	Multiply baseline heart rate (HR) × 0.2; then add this to baseline HR to determine the HR that is 20% over baseline. Do likewise for blood pressure (BP). Use mean BP.
	If HR and BP are both unchanged or less than baseline, score 0.
	If HR or BP is increased but increase is <20% of baseline, score 1.
	If either one is increased >20% over baseline, score 2.
Expression	The facial expression most often associated with pain is a grimace.
	This may be characterized by brow lowering, eyes squeezed shut, deepening of the nasolabial furrow, open lips and mouth.
	If no grimace is present, score 0.
	If grimace alone is present, score 1.
	If grimace and noncry vocalization grunt is present, score 2.
Sleepless	This is scored based on the infant's state during the hour preceding this recorded score.
	If the child has been continuously asleep, score 0.
	If he or she has awakened at frequent intervals, score 1.
	If he or she has been awake constantly, score 2.

From Krechel SW, Bildner J: CRIES: a new neonatal postoperative pain measurement score. Initial testing of validity and reliability, *Paediatr Anaesth* 5(1):53-61, 1995.
*Neonatal pain assessment tool developed at the University of Missouri—Columbia.

❗ NURSING ALERT

Swaddling is popular among nurses and parents as a comfort measure for calming a fussy baby and for promoting sleep. However, it is important that it is done properly. Traditional swaddling involves wrapping the infant tightly in a blanket with the legs extended and close together. This position is associated with increased risk for hip dislocation (developmental dysplasia of the hip [DDH]). The correct way to swaddle an infant is with the hips in slight flexion and abducted and allowing freedom of movement of the knees (Price and Schwend, 2011).

A benefit of swaddling is that it provides warmth, but it can also cause overheating. Infants should be swaddled in a light-weight blanket and never in heavy materials.

While swaddling can help an infant remain supine for sleeping, a swaddled infant should never be placed in the prone position (on the abdomen).

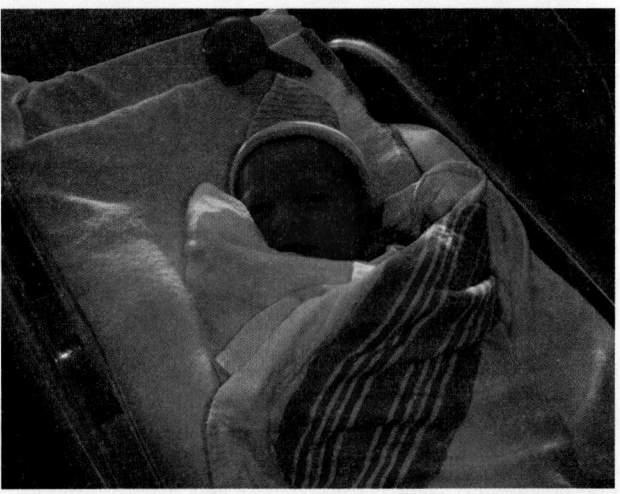

FIG 23-20 Swaddled newborn. (Courtesy Kathryn Alden, Chapel Hill, NC.)

There are other nonpharmacologic measures used by nurses and parents to promote comfort. Facilitated tucking, a hand-swaddling technique, is effective for preterm infants (Riddell, Racine, Turcotte, et al., 2011). Nonnutritive sucking (NNS) on a pacifier is a common comfort measure used with newborns. Oral sucrose in small amounts given with a syringe with or without a pacifier for sucking is safe and effective in reducing neonatal pain during single events (Cignacco, Sellam, Stoffel, et al., 2012; Kassab, Roydhouse, Fowler, et al., 2012; Riddell, Racine, Turcotte, et al., 2011; Stevens, Yamada, and Ohlsson, 2010). Oral sucrose and NNS given a few minutes before a painful procedure may help reduce the discomfort (Liaw, Zeng, Yang, et al., 2011). Skin-to-skin contact with the mother, also known as *kangaroo care,* during a painful procedure can help reduce pain (Chermont, Falcão, de Sousa Silva, et al., 2009; Riddell, Racine, Turcotte, et al., 2011). Breastfeeding helps reduce pain during heel lancing and blood collection (Leite, Linhares, Lander, et al., 2009; Weissman, Aranovitch, Blazer, et al., 2009). Other nonpharmacologic measures for reducing pain in newborns include touch, massage, rocking, holding, and environmental modification (e.g., low noise and lighting). Combining these nonpharmacologic methods results in more effective pain reduction. Distraction with visual, oral, auditory, or tactile stimulation can be helpful in term neonates or older infants (see Evidence-Based Practice box).

Pharmacologic Management. Pharmacologic agents are used to alleviate pain in neonates associated with procedures. Local anesthesia is routinely used during procedures such as circumcision and chest tube insertion. Topical anesthesia is used for circumcision, lumbar puncture, venipuncture, and heelsticks. Non-opioid analgesia (oral liquid acetaminophen) is effective for mild to moderate pain from inflammatory conditions. Morphine and fentanyl are the most widely used opioid analgesics for pharmacologic management of neonatal pain. Continuous or bolus intravenous infusion of opioids provides effective and safe pain control. Other methods for managing neonatal pain are epidural infusion, local and regional nerve blocks, and intradermal or topical anesthetics (Gardner, Enzman-Hines, and Dickey, 2011).

Promoting Parent-Infant Interaction

Nurses play an important role in promoting early social interaction between parents and their newborn infant. From birth throughout the hospital stay, nurses assess attachment behaviors (see Chapter 20) and provide support and education to parents as they become acquainted with the neonate. Nurses working in outpatient settings or home care provide follow-up assessments and care related to parent-child interactions. By teaching parents to recognize infant cues and respond appropriately, the nurse facilitates development of the parents' confidence in meeting the needs of their newborn (see Family-Centered Care box).

The sensitivity of the parent to the social responses of the infant is basic to the development of a mutually satisfying parent-child relationship. Sensitivity increases over time as parents become more aware of their infant's social capabilities. In supporting parents, nurses need to consider cultural beliefs and traditions that influence parenting behaviors and infant care practices (see Cultural Competence box).

The activities of daily care during the neonatal period are the best times for infant and family interactions. While caring for their newborn, the mother and father (or other family member) can talk to the infant, play baby games, caress and cuddle the baby, and perhaps use infant massage. Feeding is an optimal time for interaction because the infant is usually awake and alert, at least at the

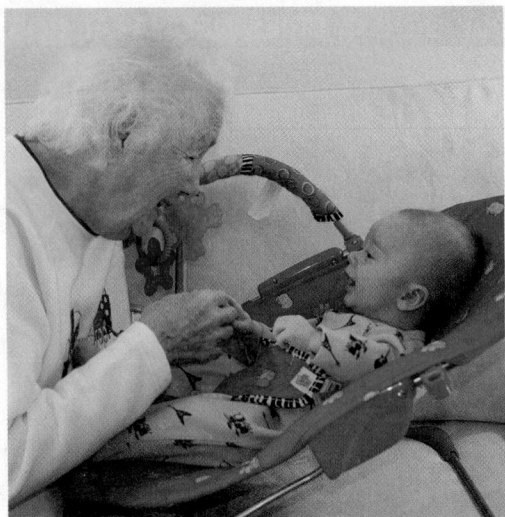

FIG 23-21 Great-grandmother and infant enjoying social interaction. (Courtesy Freida Belding, Bird City, KS.)

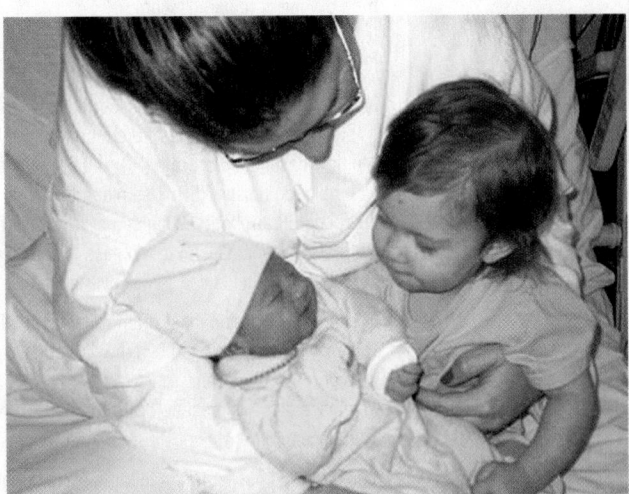

FIG 23-22 Mother supervising contact of older sibling with newborn. (Courtesy Rebekah Vogel, Fort Collins, CO.)

beginning of the feeding. Too much stimulation should be avoided after feeding and before a sleep period. In Fig. 23-21 a great-grandmother and infant are shown engaging in arousal, imitation of facial expression, and smiling. Older children's contact with a newborn is encouraged and supervised based on the developmental level of the child (Fig. 23-22). Parents often keep memento books that record the birth, the hospital stay, and their infant's progress. Other parents create blogs (e.g., www.wordpress.com) to share their development as a family.

Discharge Planning and Teaching

Infant care activities can cause anxiety for new parents. Support from nurses can be an important factor in determining whether new parents seek and accept help in the future. It is best for the nurse to avoid trying to cover all the content at one time because the parents can be overwhelmed by too much information and become more anxious. However, because hospital stays after birth are relatively short, teaching all the content that is necessary can be a challenge for the nurse. As a result, many institutions have developed home visitation programs that take the necessary teaching to the new

EVIDENCE-BASED PRACTICE

Nonpharmacologic Pain Relief for Newborns

Ask the Question

For term newborns, what complementary or alternative pain relief is effective for minor painful procedures, such as heelstick?

Search for the Evidence

Search Strategies

English research-based publications on newborn, pain, breastfeeding, heelstick, sucrose were included.

Databases Used

Cochrane Collaborative Database, National Guidelines Clearinghouse (AHRQ), CINAHL, PubMed, and UpToDate.

Critically Analyze the Evidence

- Pain scores in newborns assess physical changes to determine pain levels. Term newborns have lower pain scores during minor painful procedures when they use sucking-related interventions and are held and rocked. Preterm newborns 30 to 36 weeks benefit from kangaroo care (being carried bundled skin-to-skin upright on caregiver's chest), sucking-related interventions, and swaddling (Riddell, Racine, Turcotte, et al., 2011).
- Breastfeeding is the first choice for single painful procedures, for the multi-sensorial and synergistic comfort it brings. It also provides the parents a caregiving role (Academy of Breastfeeding Medicine [ABM] Protocol Committee, 2010).
- Skin-to-skin contact, along with 24% sucrose or 25% to 50% glucose administered via pacifier, dropper, syringe, or finger all provide significant pain relief (ABM, 2010; Kassab, Roydhouse, Fowler, et al., 2012).
- Preterm babies are at risk for more painful procedures. If breastfeeding is not possible, sucking-related interventions with sucrose decrease pain scores. However, there is concern that prolonged sucrose exposures in premature infants may lead to delays in motor skills and attention scores (ABM Protocol Committee, 2010).
- For term infants, sensory saturation uses multiple senses to diminish minor pain. A protocol of simultaneously massaging the infant's face, speaking to the infant, and instilling a sweet solution into the infant's mouth is more effective for relieving pain than the sweet solution alone (Bellieni, Tei, Coccina, et al., 2012).

Apply the Evidence: Nursing Implications

- Nonpharmacologic pain relief methods for newborns use the gate-control theory to distract the newborn's attention by using strong single or multi-sensorial stimulation. Warmth, touch, auditory and visual attention, and sucking a sweet solution decrease pain scores.
- Sensory saturation can be easily accomplished in the nursery. Parents who are taught this technique become active participants in their newborn's

procedural care. However, they need clear education that using sucrose is not an appropriate long-term strategy for use at home.

- Although skin-to-skin contact, breastfeeding, and human milk are not well researched as pain relief interventions for preterm newborns, the ABM (2010) recommends that parents be allowed to try these measures.
- Comfort measures usually work best when initiated a few minutes before the procedure to allow the newborn time to relax and reorganize (Kassab, Roydhouse, Fowler, et al., 2012).
- Procedures other than single heelsticks or needlestick should be evaluated for pharmacologic analgesia. Sucrose is not sufficient pain relief for circumcisions.

Quality and Safety Competencies:
Evidence-Based Practice*

Knowledge

Describe How the Strength and Relevance of Available Evidence Influences the Choice of Interventions in Provision of Patient-Centered Care.

Multi-sensorial stimulation that includes sucrose and sucking works best for pain relief.

Skills

Participate in Structuring the Work Environment to Facilitate Integration of New Evidence into Standards of Practice.

Parents can learn skills to manage their newborn's pain.

Attitudes

Value the Need for Continuous Improvement in Clinical Practice Based on New Knowledge.

Nurses can explain to parents the evidence for pain relief in newborns.

References

Academy of Breastfeeding Medicine (ABM) Protocol Committee: Clinical protocol #23: Non-pharmacologic management of procedure-related pain in the breastfeeding infant, *Breastfeed Med* 5(6):315–319, 2010.

Bellieni CV, Tei M, Coccina F, et al: Sensorial saturation for infants' pain, *J Matern Fetal Neonatal Med* 25(Suppl 1):79–81, 2012.

Kassab MI, Roydhouse JK, Fowler C, et al: The effectiveness of glucose in reducing needle-related procedural pain in infants, *J Pediatr Nurs* 27(1):3–17, 2012.

Riddell RP, Racine NM, Turcotte K, et al: Non-pharmacological management of infant and young child procedural pain. In *Cochrane Database Syst Rev* (Issue 10):DOI: 10.1002/14651858.CD006275.pub2, Chichester, UK, 2011, John Wiley & Sons.

Pat Mahaffee Gingrich

*Adapted from QSEN at www.qsen.org/.

parents, although the hospital nurse still provides most of the essential information for newborn care.

To set priorities for teaching, the nurse follows parental cues. Knowledge deficits or gaps should be identified before beginning to teach. Normal growth and development and the changing needs of the infant (e.g., for personal interaction and stimulation, growth milestones, exercise, injury prevention, and social contacts), as well as the topics that follow, should be included during discharge planning with parents. Safety issues should be addressed (see Home Care box).

Temperature

Parents need to understand practical information related to thermoregulation. The nurse discusses the following topics in parent teaching:

- The causes of elevation in body temperature (e.g., overwrapping, cold stress with resultant vasoconstriction, or minimal response to infection) and the body's response to extremes in environmental temperature
- Ways to promote normal body temperature, such as dressing the infant appropriately for the environmental air

FAMILY-CENTERED CARE

Helping Parents Recognize, Interpret, and Respond to Newborn Behaviors

Learning to read a baby's body language can enable parents to be more effective in preventing and solving problems around the infant's sleeping, eating, and crying and enhances parent-infant interaction. Nurses can teach new parents the following:

1. **Identify three newborn "Zones," traditionally referred to as newborn states.**
   - "Resting Zone": also known as *sleep states*
     - *Still/deep sleep:* Baby is completely still. Breathing is regular. No spontaneous activity. No movement of eyes, and eyelids stay shut. No vocalizing. Muscles are totally relaxed.
     - *Active/light sleep:* Baby may wiggle or vocalize. Eyes may flash open. Baby may make sucking movements—but still be asleep.
   - "Ready Zone": *alert state*
     - Baby's eyes are bright. Baby can focus on an object or person. Baby reacts to stimulation. Motor activity is minimal.
   - "Rebooting Zone": *fussy/crying state*
     - Baby's motor activity increases and is jerky. Baby is less responsive and moves from fussing to crying.

2. **Identify signs of stress.**
   - When babies are stressed or over-stimulated, they show changes in their body and behavior. These changes are called *SOSs* (Signs of Over-Stimulation), traditionally referred to as a baby's *stress response*.
     - *Body SOSs:* changes in color (becoming more red or pale); changes in breathing (becoming more irregular or choppy); changes in movement (becoming jerky or having more tremors)
     - *Behavioral SOSs:* "spacing out" (going from an alert state to a drowsy state); "switching off" (gaze aversion, or looking away from parent); "shutting down" (going from drowsy to a sleep state)
   - When baby shows an SOS, parents should *decrease* stimulation and *increase* support by doing one or several of the following:
     - Quiet one's voice
     - Glance away from baby
     - Encourage baby to suck a finger or mother's breast
     - Swaddle baby
     - Place baby skin to skin

3. **Help baby sleep well.**
   - Distinguish active/light sleep from still/deep sleep.
   - Parent's care:
     - *Prepare baby to sleep:* swaddling may help; feed in quiet, dark room at night and active, light environment during day.
     - *Get baby to sleep:* put baby down for sleep while he or she is still awake.
     - *Help baby stay asleep:* don't pick up during active/light sleep.
   - After breastfeeding is well established, notice when sleeping baby moves into active/light sleep. Wait and see if baby will transition from active/light sleep back to deep/still sleep—and sleep a bit longer.

4. **Help baby eat well.**
   - Recognize early signs of hunger during the first few weeks: wiggling, making sucking movements, bringing hand to mouth.
   - Notice if a fragile baby "spaces out" or "shuts down" when trying to eat. Bring this baby skin to skin and decrease stimulation before resuming feeding.
   - If a parent needs to wake a fragile or small baby to eat, do so from active/light sleep, not from still/deep sleep.

5. **Help crying baby: Consider what "TO DO."**
   - **T:** *Talk* quietly to baby in sing-song voice.
   - **O:** *Observe* to see if baby takes self-calming actions: brings his or her hand to his or her mouth, making sucking movements, or moves into the fencing reflex position.
   - **DO:** *Bring* baby's hands to his or her chest; encourage sucking; make gentle "shooshing" sounds; swaddle baby; and/or bring baby skin to skin.

6. **Play with baby so he or she can learn and grow.**
   - Demonstrate baby's ability to look at a parent's face, watch a toy move, or turn to parent's voice.
   - Watch for an SOS during play. If an SOS occurs, decrease stimulation and increase support as described earlier in box.
   - Observe baby's developing process of interaction: first, getting quiet and still; second, turning toward parent; third, turning toward and looking at parent.
   - Reinforce benefits of sensitive, face-to-face parent interaction with baby.

Data from Tedder JL: Give them the HUG: an innovative approach to helping parents understand the language of their newborn, *J Perinat Educ* 17(2):14–20, 2008; Tedder JL: *H.U.G.: help-understanding-guidance for young families,* www.hugyourbaby.org.

CULTURAL COMPETENCE

Cultural Beliefs and Practices Related to Infant Care

Nurses working with childbearing families from other cultures and ethnic groups must be aware of cultural beliefs and practices that are important to individual families. People with a strong sense of heritage may hold on to traditional health beliefs long after adopting other U.S. lifestyle practices. These health beliefs can involve practices regarding the newborn. For example, some Asians, Hispanics, Eastern Europeans, and Native Americans delay breastfeeding because they believe that colostrum is "bad." Some Hispanics and African-Americans place a belly band over the infant's umbilicus. The birth of a male child is generally preferred by Asians and Eastern Indians, and some Asians and Haitians delay naming their infants.

temperature and protecting the infant from exposure to direct sunlight
- Use of warm wraps or extra blankets in cold weather
- Technique for taking the newborn's axillary temperature, and normal values for axillary temperature
- Signs to be reported to the primary health care provider such as high or low temperatures with accompanying fussiness, lethargy, irritability, poor feeding, and excessive crying

Respirations

The nurse provides information to parents regarding the normal characteristics of newborn respirations, emergency procedures, and measures to protect the infant. It is helpful to discuss signs of the common cold and to offer suggestions related to care of the infant who experiences this type of illness. Review the following points:
- Normal variations in the rate and rhythm of respirations
- Reflexes such as sneezing to clear the airway
- Use of the bulb syringe

HOME CARE

Infant Safety

- Never leave your baby alone on a bed, couch, or table. Even newborns can move enough to eventually reach the edge and fall off.
- Never put your baby on a cushion, pillow, beanbag, or waterbed to sleep. Your baby may suffocate. Also, do not keep pillows, large floppy toys, or loose plastic sheeting in the crib.
- Always lay the baby flat in bed on his or her back for sleep. Do not place your infant on the abdomen for sleep.
- When using an infant carrier, place the carrier on the floor in a place where you can see the baby. It should never be on a high place, such as a table, sofa, or store counter.
- Infant carriers do not keep your baby safe in a car. Always place your baby in an approved car safety seat when traveling in a motor vehicle (car, truck, bus, or van). Car safety seats are recommended for travel on trains and airplanes as well. Use the car safety seat for *every* ride. Your baby should be in a rear-facing infant car safety seat from birth until age 2 years or until exceeding the car seat's limits for height and weight. The car safety seat should be in the back seat of the car (see Fig. 23-25). This precaution is especially important in vehicles with front passenger air bags because when air bags inflate, they can be fatal for infants and toddlers. If an infant must ride in the front seat, disable the air bag.
- When bathing your baby, never leave him or her alone. Newborns and infants can drown in 1 to 2 inches of water.
- Be sure that your hot water heater is set at 49° C (120° F) or less. Always check bath-water temperature with your elbow before putting your baby in the bath.
- Do not tie anything around your baby's neck. Pacifiers, for example, tied around the neck with a ribbon or string can strangle your baby.
- Check your baby's crib for safety. Slats should be no more than 2¼ inches apart. The space between the mattress and sides should be less than 2 fingerwidths. The bedposts should have no decorative knobs.
- There should be no bumper pads, blankets, stuffed toys, or other items in the baby's crib because of the risk for suffocation.
- Keep the crib or playpen away from window blind and drapery cords; your baby could strangle on them.
- Keep the crib and playpen well away from radiators, heat vents, and portable heaters. Linens in the crib or playpen can catch fire if they come into contact with these heat sources.
- Install smoke detectors on every floor of your home. Check them once a month to be sure they are working properly. Change batteries twice a year.
- Avoid exposing your baby to cigarette or cigar smoke in your home or other places. Passive exposure to tobacco smoke greatly increases the likelihood that your infant will have respiratory symptoms and illnesses.
- Be gentle with your baby. Do not pick your baby up or swing your baby by the arms or throw him or her up in the air. Never shake the baby.

- Steps to take if the infant appears to be choking
- The need to protect the infant from:
  - Exposure to people with upper respiratory tract infections and respiratory syncytial virus
  - Exposure to secondhand tobacco smoke
  - Suffocation from loose bedding, water beds, and beanbag chairs; drowning (in bath water); entrapment under excessive bedding or in soft bedding; anything tied around the infant's neck; poorly constructed playpens, bassinets, or cribs
- Sleep position—on back when put to sleep

- Avoid the use of baby powder, which is a commonly aspirated substance. If parents desire to use a powder, a cornstarch preparation can be substituted. Whenever a powder is used, it should be placed in the caregiver's hand and then applied to the skin. It is kept away from the infant's face.
- Notify the health care provider if the infant develops symptoms such as difficulty breathing or swallowing, nasal congestion, excess drainage of mucus, coughing, sneezing, decreased interest in feeding, or fever.
- If the infant has a respiratory illness such as the "common cold," the following suggestions can be helpful:
  - Feed smaller amounts more often to prevent overtiring the infant.
  - Hold the baby in an upright position to feed.
  - For sleeping, raise the infant's head and chest by raising the mattress 30 degrees. (Do *not* use a pillow.)
  - Avoid drafts; do not overdress the baby.
  - Use only medications prescribed by a physician. Do not use over-the-counter medications without physician approval.
  - Use nasal saline drops in each nostril and suction well with bulb syringe to decrease and relieve secretions.

Feeding Patterns

Nurses instruct parents about infant feeding and provide assistance based on whether they have chosen breastfeeding or formula feeding. Feeding patterns and practices for newborns are discussed in Chapter 24.

Elimination

Awareness of the normal elimination patterns of newborns helps parents recognize problems related to voiding or stooling. The following points are included in teaching about elimination:

- Color of normal urine and number of voidings to expect each day: at least two to six for the first 1 to 3 days; then a minimum of six to eight voidings per day thereafter.
- Changes to be expected in the color and consistency of the stool (i.e., meconium to transitional to soft yellow or golden yellow) and the number of bowel evacuations, plus the odor of stools for breastfed or bottle-fed infants (see Box 22-1).
- Formula-fed infants may have as few as one stool every other day after the first few weeks of life; stools are pasty to semiformed.
- Breastfed infants should have at least three stools every 24 hours for the first few weeks. The stools are looser and resemble mustard mixed with cottage cheese; the odor is less offensive than that of infants who are formula-fed.

Positioning and Holding

The AAP Task Force on Sudden Infant Death Syndrome (SIDS) (2011) recommends placing the infant in the supine position for sleep during the first year of life to prevent SIDS. Infants should lie on a firm surface, specifically on a firm crib mattress covered by a fitted sheet. Soft materials such as comforters, quilts, pillows, or sheepskins should not be placed in the crib. Room sharing, but not bed sharing, is recommended during infant sleep. Infants may be brought into the parent's bed for comforting or for breastfeeding but should be returned to the crib or bassinet before the parent goes to sleep. It is important to avoid overheating the infant.

Anatomically, the infant's shape—a barrel chest and flat, curveless spine—facilitates the infant to roll from the side to the prone position; therefore the side-lying position for sleep is not recommended.

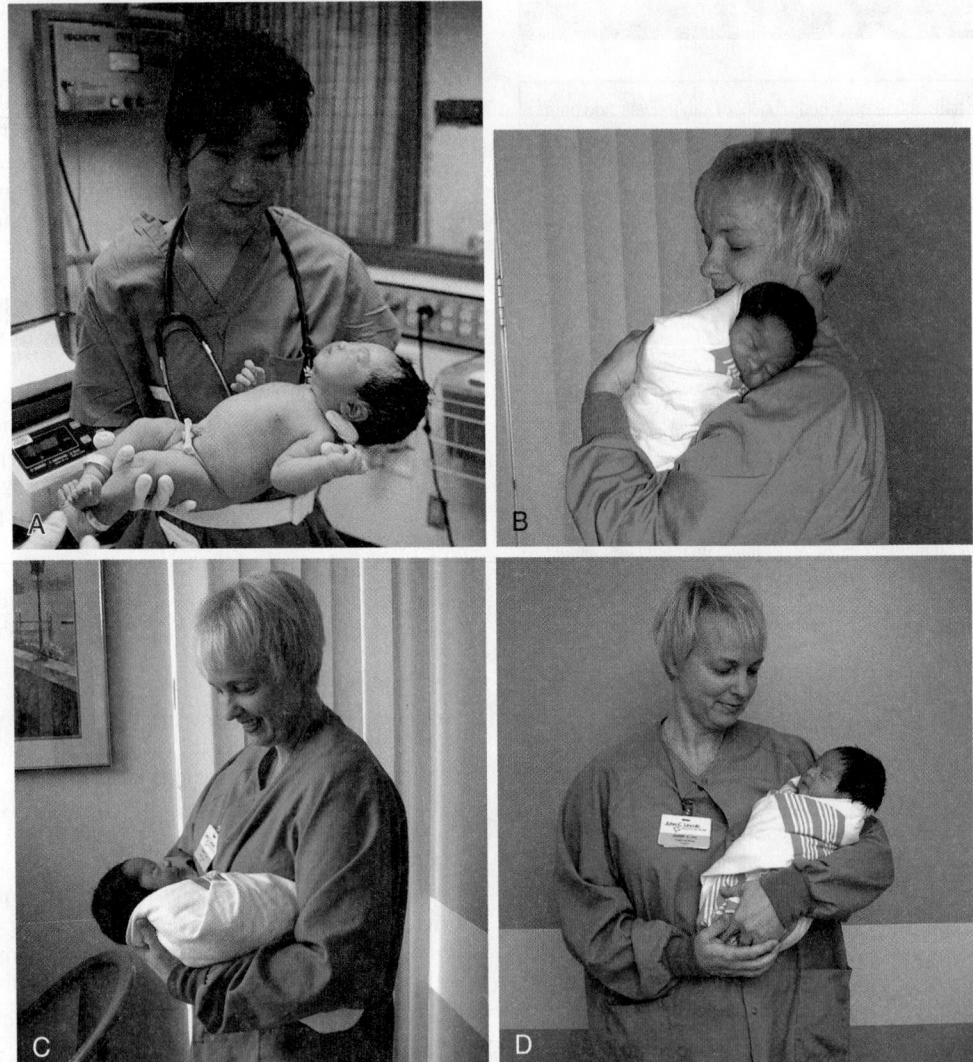

FIG 23-23 Holding the baby securely with support for head. **A,** Holding infant while moving infant from scale to bassinet. Baby is undressed to show posture. **B,** Holding baby upright in "burping" position. **C,** "Football" (under the arm) hold. **D,** Cradling hold. (**A,** Courtesy Kim Molloy, Knoxville, IA. **B, C,** and **D,** Courtesy Julie Perry Nelson, Loveland, CO.)

When the infant is awake, "tummy time" can be provided under parental supervision so the infant can begin to develop appropriate muscle tone for eventual crawling; this tummy time is also effective in the prevention of a misshaped head (positional plagiocephaly).

Care must be taken to prevent the infant from rolling off flat, unguarded surfaces. When an infant is on such a surface, the parent or nurse who must turn away from the infant even for a moment should always keep one hand placed securely on the infant. The infant is always held securely with the head supported because newborns are unable to maintain an erect head posture for more than a few moments. Fig. 23-23 illustrates various positions for holding an infant with adequate support (see Critical Thinking Case Study).

Rashes

Diaper Rash. The majority of infants develop a diaper rash at some time. This dermatitis or skin inflammation appears as redness, scaling, blisters, or papules. Various factors contribute to diaper rash including infrequent diaper changes, diarrhea, use of plastic pants to cover the diaper, a change in the infant's diet such as when solid foods are added, or when breastfeeding mothers eat certain foods.

Parents are instructed in measures to help prevent and treat diaper rash. Diapers should be checked often and changed as soon as the infant voids or stools. Plain water with mild soap is used to cleanse the diaper area; if baby wipes are used, they should be unscented and contain no alcohol. The infant's skin should be allowed to dry completely before applying another diaper. Exposing the buttocks to air can help dry up diaper rash. Because bacteria thrive in moist, dark areas, exposing the skin to dry air decreases bacterial proliferation. Zinc oxide ointments can be used to protect the infant's skin from moisture and further excoriation.

Although diaper rash can be alarming to parents and annoying to babies, most cases resolve within a few days with simple home treatments. There are instances when diaper rash is more serious and requires medical treatment.

The warm, moist atmosphere in the diaper area provides an optimal environment for *Candida albicans* growth; dermatitis appears in the perianal area, inguinal folds, and lower abdomen. The affected area is intensely erythematous with a sharply demarcated, scalloped edge, often with numerous satellite lesions that extend beyond the larger lesion. The usual source of infection is from

Late-Preterm Infant, Sudden Infant Death Syndrome, and Infant Sleep Position

Mary gave birth to a 35-week, 2250 g (4 lb 15 oz) female infant whom she named Delilah. This is her third baby; the other children are 18 and 20 years old. Mary and Delilah are being discharged home today. The nurse has given her instructions about placing Delilah on her back for sleep. Mary said that she remembers her other two children slept best when they were on their "tummies" for sleep. When Mary was in college, she worked as a unit secretary in a newborn nursery and she recalls that when babies were on their backs, they tended to "spit up" and turn blue. Recently, her sister had a baby who had to be under bilirubin lights and the nurses turned the baby on her abdomen sometimes for sleep. Mary voiced concerns to the nurse about putting Delilah down to sleep on her back at home. How should the nurse respond to Mary's concerns?

1. Evidence—Is there sufficient evidence to draw conclusions about the safety and efficacy of the supine position for sleep for the late preterm infant in reducing the incidence of sudden infant death syndrome?
2. Assumptions—What assumptions can be made about the following factors related to infant positioning?
   a. Risk for aspiration
   b. Sleep position in the nursery versus sleep position at home
   c. Sleep position for late preterm versus term infants
3. What implications and priorities for nursing care can be drawn at this time?
4. Does the evidence objectively support your conclusion?

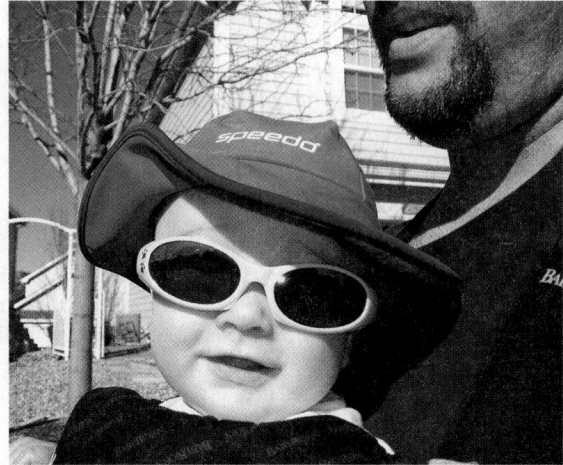

FIG 23-24 Sunglasses protect the infant's eyes. (Courtesy Julie Perry Nelson, Loveland, CO.)

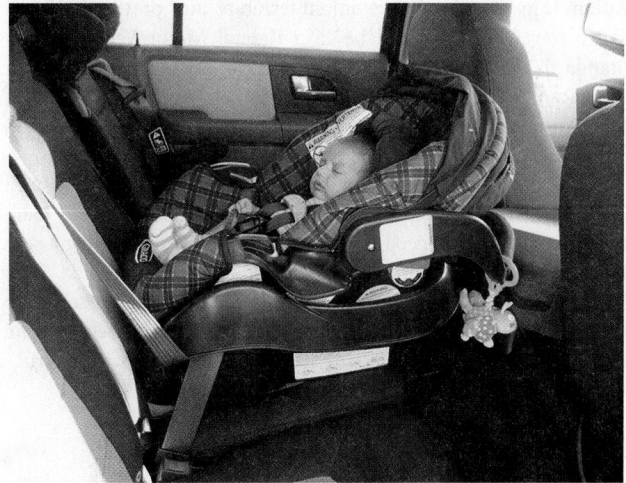

FIG 23-25 Rear-facing car seat in rear seat of car. Infant is placed in seat when going home from the hospital. (Courtesy Brian and Mayannyn Sallee, Anchorage, AK.)

handling by persons who do not practice good hand hygiene. It can also appear 2 to 3 days after an oral infection (thrush).

Therapy consists of applications of an anticandidal ointment, such as clotrimazole or miconazole, with each diaper change. Sometimes the infant is given an oral antifungal preparation such as nystatin or fluconazole to eliminate any gastrointestinal source of infection.

Other Rashes. A rash on the cheeks can result from the infant's scratching with long unclipped fingernails or from rubbing the face against the crib sheets, particularly if regurgitated stomach contents are not washed off promptly. The newborn's skin begins a natural process of peeling and sloughing after birth. Dry skin may be treated with a neutral pH lotion, but this should be used sparingly. Newborn rash, erythema toxicum, is a common finding (see Fig. 22-6, *B*) and needs no treatment.

Clothing

Parents commonly ask how warmly they should dress their infant. A simple suggestion is to dress the child for the environment as they dress themselves, adding no more than one layer more than they would be wearing as adults. Overheating should be avoided (AAP Task Force on Sudden Infant Death Syndrome, 2011). A cap or bonnet is needed to protect the scalp and minimize heat loss if the weather is cool or to protect against sunburn. Wrapping the infant snugly in a blanket maintains body temperature and promotes a feeling of security. Overdressing in warm temperatures can cause discomfort, as can underdressing in cold weather. Parents are encouraged to dress the infant at all times in flame-retardant clothing. The eyes should be shaded if it is sunny and hot. Infant sunglasses are available to protect the infant's eyes when outdoors (Fig. 23-24).

Car Seat Safety

Infants should travel only in federally approved rear-facing safety seats secured in the rear seat (Fig. 23-25).

To secure the infant in the rear-facing car safety seat, shoulder harnesses are placed in the slots at or below the level of the infant's shoulders. The harness is snug, and the retainer clip is placed at the level of the infant's armpits as opposed to on the abdomen or neck area. The car seat is secured by using the vehicle seat belts.

Infants and toddlers should use a rear-facing car seat until the age of 2 years or for as long as possible up to the weight and height limit for their particular car seat. The safest area of the car is the back seat. A car safety seat that faces the rear gives the best protection for the disproportionately weak neck and heavy head of an infant. In this position, the force of a frontal crash is spread over the head, neck, and back; the back of the car safety seat supports the spine (AAP, 2012; National Highway Traffic Safety Administration [NHTSA], 2012).

In cars equipped with front air bags, rear-facing infant seats should not be placed in the front seat. Serious injury can occur if the air bag inflates, because these types of infant seats fit close to the dashboard. If the infant must ride in the front seat, the air bag must be turned off. For cars with side air bags, parents should read the vehicle owner's manual for information about placement of car seats next to a side air bag (AAP, 2012; NHTSA, 2012).

Infants are positioned at a 45-degree angle in a car seat to prevent slumping and subsequent airway obstruction. Many seats allow for adjustment of the seat angle. For seats that are not adjustable, a tightly rolled newspaper, a solid-core Styrofoam roll, or a firm roll of fabric can be placed under the car safety seat to place the infant at a 45-degree angle (Bull, Engle, and American Academy of Pediatrics Committee on Injury, Violence, and Poison Prevention and Committee on Fetus and Newborn, 2009).

Before discharge from the birth institution, infants born at less than 37 weeks of gestation should be observed in a car seat (preferably their own) for at least 90 to 120 minutes or a period of time equal to the length of the car ride home. The infant is monitored for apnea, bradycardia, and a decrease in oxygen saturation (Fig. 23-26). If the infant exhibits any of these clinical signs, travel home should be in a Federal Motor Vehicle Safety Standard 213 (FMVSS 213)–approved car bed (Bull, Engle, and American Academy of Pediatrics Committee on Injury, Violence, and Poison Prevention and Committee on Fetus and Newborn, et al., 2009).

If the parents do not have a car safety seat, arrangements should be made to make an appropriate seat available for purchase, loan, or donation. Parents need to be cautioned about purchasing a secondhand car safety seat without knowing the seat's history. They should never use a car seat that was involved in a moderate to severe crash, is too old, has visible cracks, does not have a label with the model number and manufacture date, does not come with instructions, is missing parts, or was recalled (AAP, 2012).

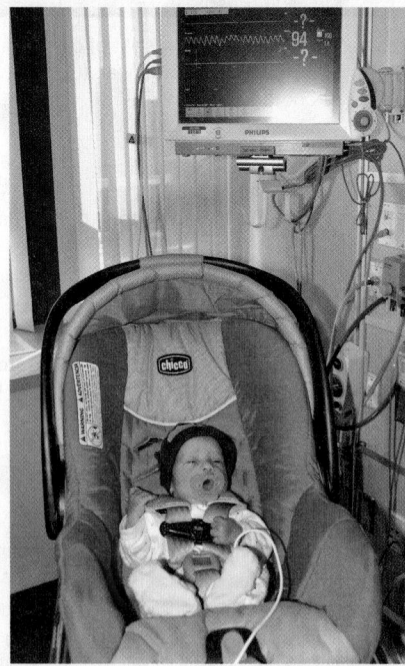

FIG 23-26 Car seat testing before discharge from the hospital: preterm infant in car seat with pulse oximetry monitoring. (Courtesy Cheryl Briggs, RNC, Annapolis, MD.)

Nonnutritive Sucking

Sucking is the infant's chief pleasure. However, sucking needs may not be satisfied by breastfeeding or bottle-feeding alone. In fact, sucking is such a strong need that infants who are deprived of sucking, such as those with a cleft lip, will suck on their tongues. Several benefits of nonnutritive sucking have been demonstrated, such as an increased weight gain in preterm infants, increased ability to maintain an organized state, and decreased crying.

There is compelling evidence that pacifiers help prevent SIDS. The AAP Task Force on Sudden Infant Death Syndrome (2011) suggests that parents consider offering a pacifier for naps and bedtime. The pacifier should be used when the infant is placed supine for sleep, and it should not be reinserted once the infant falls asleep. No infant should be forced to take a pacifier. Pacifiers are to be cleaned often and replaced regularly and should not be coated with any type of sweet solution. Pacifier use for breastfeeding infants should be delayed for 3 to 4 weeks to ensure that breastfeeding is well established.

Problems arise when parents are concerned about the sucking of fingers, thumb, or pacifier and try to restrain this natural tendency. Before giving advice, nurses should investigate the parents' feelings and base the guidance they give on the information solicited. For example, some parents see no problem with the infant sucking on a thumb or finger but find the use of a pacifier objectionable. In general, either practice need not be restrained unless thumb sucking or pacifier use persists past 4 years of age or past the time when the permanent teeth erupt. Parents are advised to consult with their pediatric health care provider or pediatric dentist about this topic.

A parent's excessive use of the pacifier to calm the infant should also be explored, however. Placing a pacifier in the infant's mouth as soon as the infant begins to cry can reinforce a pattern of distress and relief.

If parents choose to let their infant use a pacifier, they need to be aware of certain safety considerations before purchasing one. A homemade or poorly designed pacifier can be dangerous because the entire object can be aspirated if it is small or a portion can become lodged in the pharynx. Improvised pacifiers, such as those made from a padded nipple, also pose dangers because the nipple can separate from the plastic collar and be aspirated. Safe pacifiers are made of one piece that includes a shield or flange large enough to prevent entry into the mouth and a handle that can be grasped (Fig. 23-27).

Bathing and Umbilical Cord Care

Bathing. Bathing serves several purposes. It provides opportunities for (1) completely cleansing the infant, (2) observing the infant's

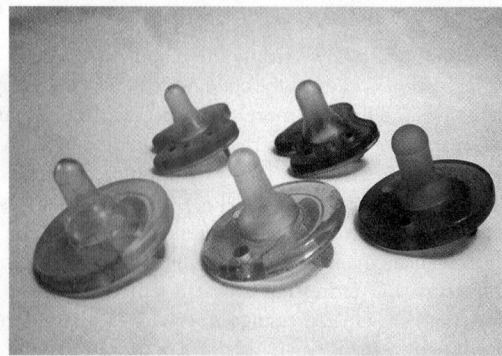

FIG 23-27 Safe pacifiers for term and preterm infants. Note one-piece construction, easily grasped handle, and large shield with ventilation holes. (Courtesy Julie Perry Nelson, Loveland, CO.)

condition, (3) promoting comfort, and (4) parent-child-family interaction.

An important consideration in skin cleansing is the preservation of the skin's acid mantle, which is formed from the uppermost horny layer of the epidermis, sweat, superficial fat, metabolic products, and external substances such as amniotic fluid and microorganisms. To protect the newborn's skin, use a cleanser with a neutral pH and preferably without preservatives (Association of Women's Health, Obstetric and Neonatal Nurses [AWHONN], 2007). Sponge baths are usually given until the infant's umbilical cord falls off and the umbilicus is healed. However, bathing the newborn by immersion has been found to allow less heat loss and provoke less crying. Immersion bathing is a safe alternative to sponge bathing, provided that the infant's condition is stable (no temperature instability, respiratory or cardiac illness) and that the infant is dried off immediately thereafter and kept warm (AWHONN, 2007). A daily bath is not necessary for achieving cleanliness and can do harm by disrupting the integrity of the newborn's skin; cleansing the perineum after a soiled diaper and daily cleansing of the face is usually sufficient. Until the initial bath is completed, personnel must wear gloves to handle the newborn.

The infant bath time provides a wonderful opportunity for parent-infant social interaction (Fig. 23-28). While bathing the baby, parents can talk to the infant, caress and cuddle the infant, and engage in arousal and imitation of facial expressions and smiling. Parents can pick a time for the bath that is easy for them and when the baby is awake, usually before a feeding.

Umbilical Cord Care. The goal of cord care is to prevent or decrease the risk for hemorrhage and infection. The umbilical cord stump is an excellent medium for bacterial growth and can easily become infected. Hospital protocol determines the technique for routine cord care. The current recommendations for cord care by the Association of Women's Health, Obstetric and Neonatal Nurses (AWHONN, 2007) include cleaning the cord with water (and cleanser if needed to remove debris) during the initial bath and subsequently cleaning with plain water if the umbilical stump is soiled with urine or stool. Evidence does not support the routine use of antiseptic or antimicrobial preparations for cord care (Lund and Durand, 2011).

The plastic cord clamp that was applied at birth is removed once the stump has started drying and is no longer bleeding

(Fig. 23-29), typically in 24 to 48 hours. The stump and base of the cord should be assessed for edema, redness, and purulent drainage with each diaper change. The area should be kept clean and dry and open to air or loosely covered with clothing. If soiled, the area is cleansed with plain water and dried with clean absorbent gauze. The diaper is folded down and away from the stump (AWHONN, 2007). The umbilical cord begins to dry, shrivel, and blacken by the second or third day of life, The stump deteriorates through the process of dry gangrene; therefore odor alone is not a positive indicator of omphalitis (infection of the umbilical stump). Cord separation time is influenced by several factors, including type of cord care, type of birth, and other perinatal events. The average cord separation time is 10 to 14 days, although it can take up to 3 weeks for this to occur. Some dried blood may be seen in the umbilicus at separation (Fig. 23-30). Parents are instructed in appropriate home cord care (per pediatric health care practitioner or institution protocol) and the expected time of cord separation.

See the Home Care box for information regarding sponge bathing, skin care, cord care, trimming nails, and dressing the infant.

Infant Follow-up Care

Follow-up care after hospital discharge usually occurs within 72 hours at the clinic or health care provider's office. This is especially important for breastfed newborns for monitoring their weight and hydration status. When infants are discharged at less than 48 hours of age, home care follow-up is an essential component of care. Home care may be provided either by a nurse as part of the routine follow-up care of infants or through a visiting nurse or community health nurse referral service.

Cardiopulmonary Resuscitation

All personnel working with infants must have current infant cardiopulmonary resuscitation (CPR) certification. Parents should receive instruction in relieving airway obstruction and CPR. Classes are often offered in hospitals and clinics during the prenatal period or to parents of newborns. Such instruction is especially important for parents whose infants were preterm or had cardiac or respiratory problems. Some grandparents take CPR classes. Babysitters should also learn CPR.

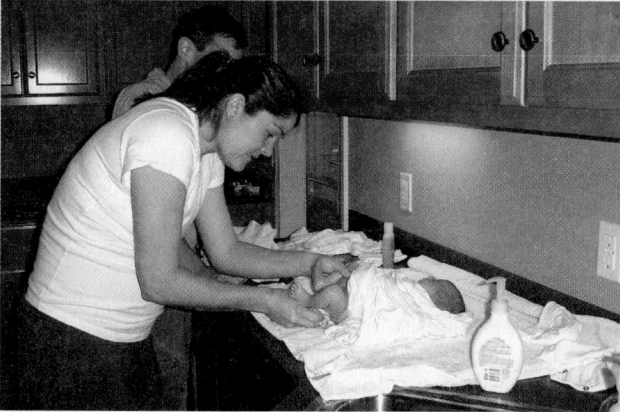

FIG 23-28 Mother giving newborn a sponge bath at home. (Courtesy Kathryn Alden, Chapel Hill, NC.)

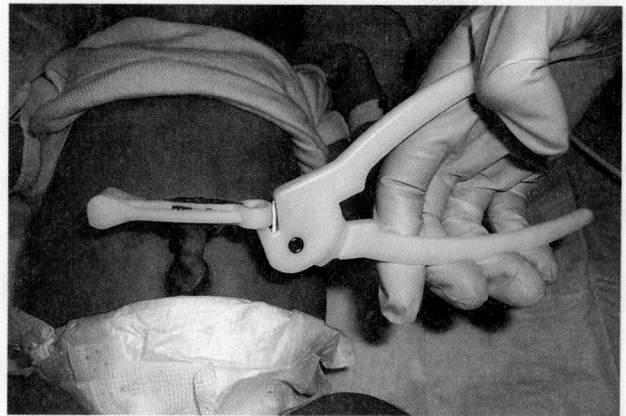

FIG 23-29 With special tool, nurse removes clamp after cord dries (approximately 24 to 48 hours after birth). (Courtesy Cheryl Briggs, RNC, Annapolis, MD.)

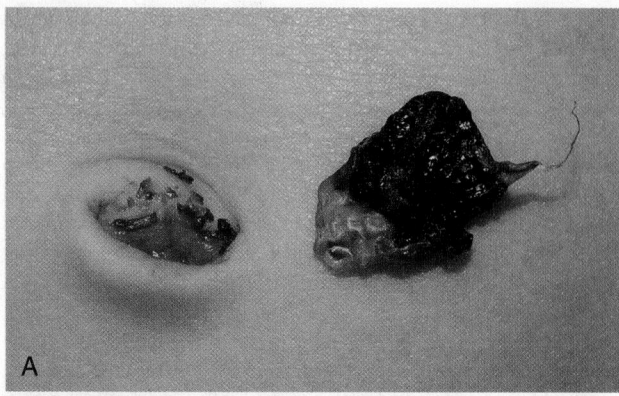

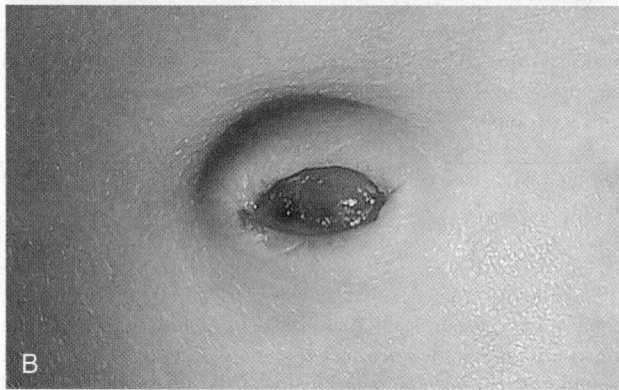

FIG 23-30 Cord separation. **A,** Cord separated with some dried blood still in the umbilicus. **B,** Umbilicus cleansed and beginning to heal. (Courtesy Cheryl Briggs, RNC, Annapolis, MD.)

Practical Suggestions for the First Weeks at Home

Numerous changes occur during the first weeks of parenthood. Care management should be directed toward helping parents cope with infant care, role changes, altered lifestyle, and change in family structure resulting from the addition of a new baby. Developing skill and confidence in caring for an infant can be especially anxiety provoking. Anticipatory guidance can help prevent a reality shock in the transition from hospital or birthing center to home that might negate the parents' joy or cause them undue stress. For example, the nurse can teach parents several strategies that help quiet a fussy baby, prevent crying, and induce quiet attention or sleep.

Parents must be helped to anticipate events during the transition from hospital to home. This is especially important for first-time parents. Even the simplest strategies can provide enormous support. Printed materials reinforcing education topics are helpful, as is a list of available community resources, both local and national, and websites that provide reliable information about child care. Classes in the prenatal period or during the postpartum stay are helpful. Instructions for the first days at home include relevant topics such as activities of daily living, dealing with visitors, and activity and rest.

Interpretation of Crying. Crying is an infant's first social communication. Some babies cry more than others, but all babies cry. They cry to communicate that they are hungry, uncomfortable, wet, ill, or bored and sometimes for no apparent reason at all. The longer parents are around their infants, the easier the task becomes of interpreting what a cry means. Many infants have a fussy period during the day, often in the late afternoon or early evening when everyone is naturally tired. Environmental tension adds to the length and intensity of crying spells. Babies also have periods of vigorous crying when no comforting can help. These periods of crying can last for long stretches until the infants seem to cry themselves to

---

HOME CARE

Bathing, Cord Care, Skin Care, and Nail Care

Timing
- Newborns do not need a bath every day. Every other day is often enough.
- Fit bath time into the family's schedule.
- Give a bath at any time convenient to you but not immediately after a feeding period because the increased handling can cause regurgitation.

Prevent Heat Loss
- The temperature of the room should be 24° C (75° F), and the bathing area should be free of drafts.
- Control heat loss during the bath to conserve the infant's energy. Bathing the infant quickly, exposing only a portion of the body at a time, and drying thoroughly are all parts of the bathing technique.

Gather Supplies and Clothing Before Starting
- Tub for water; fill only to 3 to 4 inches of water
- Towels for drying the infant and a clean washcloth
- Unscented, mild soap; with a neutral pH, and preferably with no preservatives
- Diaper
- Clothing suitable for wearing indoors: diaper, shirt; stretch suit or nightgown optional
- Cotton balls
- Receiving blanket

Bathe the Baby
- Bring the infant to the bathing area when all supplies are ready.
- Never leave the infant alone on bath table or in the bath water, not even for a second! If you have to leave, take the infant with you or place the infant back into the crib.
- Test the temperature of the water. It should feel pleasantly warm to the inner wrist—36.6° to 37.2° C (98° to 99° F).
- Do not hold the infant under running water—the water temperature can change, and the infant can be scalded or chilled rapidly. The baby can be tub-bathed after the cord drops off and the umbilicus and circumcised penis are completely healed. Some providers may say tub baths are acceptable before these events.
- If sponge bathing is to be performed, undress the baby and wrap in a towel with the head exposed. Uncover the parts of the body you are washing, taking care to keep the rest of the baby covered as much as possible to prevent heat loss.
- Begin by washing the baby's face with water; do not use soap on the face. Cleanse the eyes from the inner canthus outward using separate parts of a clean washcloth for each eye. For the first 2 to 3 days, a discharge can result from the reaction of the conjunctiva to the substance (erythromycin) used as a prophylactic measure against infection. Any discharge should be considered abnormal and reported to the pediatric health care provider.

HOME CARE

Bathing, Cord Care, Skin Care, and Nail Care—cont'd

- Cleanse the ears and nose with twists of moistened cotton or a corner of the washcloth. Do not use cotton-tipped swabs because they can cause injury. The areas behind the ears need daily cleansing.
- Wash the body with mild soap; rinse and dry to decrease heat loss. Place your hand under the baby's shoulders and lift gently to expose the neck, lift the chin, and wash the neck, taking care to cleanse between the skinfolds. Wash between the fingers and toes, and then rinse and dry thoroughly. Wash the genital area last.
- If the hair is to be washed, begin by wrapping the infant in a towel with the head exposed. Hold the infant in a football position (under the arm) with one hand, using the other hand to wash the hair. Wash the scalp with water, mild soap, and a soft brush; rinse well and dry thoroughly. Scalp desquamation, called *cradle cap,* can often be prevented by removing any scales with a fine-toothed comb or brush after washing. If the condition persists, the health care provider may prescribe a medicated shampoo to massage into the scalp. A blow dryer is never used on an infant because the temperature is too hot for a baby's skin.

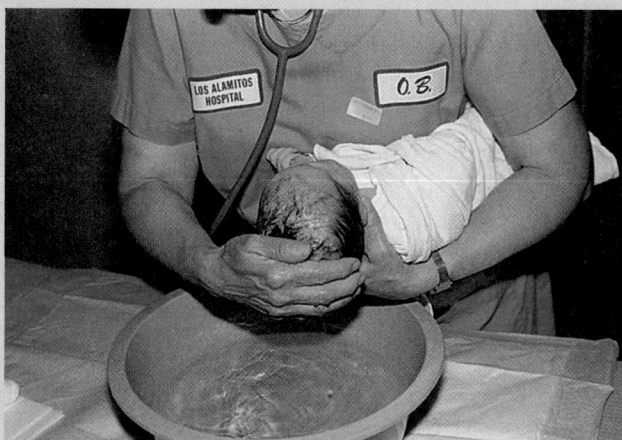

Wash hair with baby wrapped to limit heat loss. (Courtesy Marjorie Pyle, RNC, Lifecircle, Costa Mesa, CA.)

Skin Care

- The skin of a newborn is sensitive and should be cleaned only with water between baths. Soap has drying properties, and its use is limited to bathing. Creams, lotions, ointments, or powders are not recommended. If the skin seems excessively dry during the first 2 to 3 weeks after birth, an unscented, non–alcohol-based lotion may be used; checking with the pediatric health care provider for suggestions on skin care products is best. Experts advise that baby clothes be laundered separately using a mild laundry detergent (Dreft or Ivory Snow); clothes should be rinsed twice with plain water.
- The fragile skin can be injured by too vigorous cleansing. If stool or other debris has dried and caked on the skin, soak the area to remove it. Do not attempt to rub it off because abrasion can result. Gentleness, patting dry rather than rubbing, and using a mild soap without perfumes or coloring

are recommended. Chemicals in the coloring and perfume can cause rashes on sensitive skin.
- Babies are very prone to sunburn and should be kept out of direct sunlight. Use of sunscreens should be discussed with the health care provider.
- Babies often develop rashes that are normal. Neonatal acne resembles pimples and can appear at 2 to 4 weeks of age, resolving without treatment by 6 to 8 months. Heat rash is common in warm weather, which appears as a fine red rash around creases or folds where the baby sweats.

Cord Care

- Cleanse with plain water around base of the cord where it joins the skin. Notify the health care provider of any odor, discharge, or skin inflammation (redness) around the cord. The clamp is removed when the cord is dry (approximately 24 to 48 hours after birth). The diaper should not cover the cord because a wet or soiled diaper will slow or prevent drying of the cord and foster infection. When the cord drops off after 10 to 14 days, a few small drops of blood may be seen. If there is active bleeding, notify the pediatric health care provider.

Nail Care

- Do not cut fingernails and toenails immediately after birth. The nails have to grow out far enough from the skin so that the skin is not cut by mistake. If the baby scratches himself or herself, apply loosely fitted mitts over each of the baby's hands. Do so as a last resort, however, because it interferes with the baby's ability for self-consolation sucking on thumb or finger. When the nails have grown, the fingernails and toenails can be trimmed with manicure scissors or clippers; nails should be cut straight across. The ideal time to trim the nails is when the infant is sleeping. Soft emery boards may be used to file the nails. Nails should be kept short.

Genital Care

- Cleanse the genitalia of infants daily and after voiding or defecating. For girls, the genitalia are cleansed by separating the labia and gently washing from the pubic area to the anus. For uncircumcised boys, wash and rinse the penis with soap and warm water. Do not attempt to retract the foreskin. The pediatric care provider will inform you when the foreskin can safely be retracted. By age 3 years in 90% of boys, the foreskin can be retracted easily without causing pain or trauma. For others, the foreskin is not retractable until adolescence. As soon as the foreskin is partly retractable and the child is old enough, he can be taught self-care. Once healed, the circumcised penis does not require any special care other than cleansing with diaper changes.
- The infant's skin should be allowed to dry completely before applying another diaper. Exposing the buttocks to air can help dry up diaper rash. Because bacteria thrive in moist dark areas, exposing the skin to dry air decreases bacterial proliferation. Zinc oxide ointments can be used to protect the infant's skin from moisture and further excoriation.

FAMILY-CENTERED CARE

Period of PURPLE Crying®

Period of PURPLE Crying is a program to educate new parents about infant crying and the dangers of shaking a baby. Each letter in the acronym "PURPLE" represents key concepts:

P = Peak of crying. Your baby may cry more each week. The most at 2 months, then less at 3 to 5 months.

U = Unexpected. Crying can come and go and you don't know why.

R = Resists soothing. Your baby may not stop crying no matter what you try.

P = Pain-like face. A crying baby may look like they are in pain, even when they are not.

L = Long lasting. Crying can last as much as 5 hours a day, or more.

E = Evening. Your baby may cry more in the later afternoon and evening.

From Barr M: *The Period of PURPLE Crying,* from www.purplecrying.info.

sleep. The nurse informs new parents that time and infant maturation will take care of these types of cries. Many hospitals distribute a DVD on infant crying to new parents. *Period of PURPLE Crying* is an example (see Family-Centered Care box). It is intended to help parents understand that crying is normal and help them cope with infant crying. If parents have greater understanding of infant crying, they may be less likely to inflict harm such as occurs with "shaken-baby" syndrome.

Recognizing Signs of Illness. In addition to explaining the need for well-baby follow-up visits, the nurse should discuss with parents the signs of illness in newborns (see Patient Teaching box). Of particular importance is the parents' assessment of jaundice in newborns discharged early. Parents should be advised to call their pediatric care provider immediately if they notice increasing jaundice or signs of illness and to ask about over-the-counter medications, such as acetaminophen for infants, to keep at home.

PATIENT TEACHING

Signs of Illness

Notify the pediatric health care provider if any of these signs occur:

- Fever: temperature above 38°C (100.4°F) axillary; also a continual rise in temperature (**NOTE:** Tympanic (ear) thermometers are not recommended for infants younger than 3 months.)
- Hypothermia: temperature below 36.5°C (97.7°F) axillary
- Poor feeding or little interest in food: refusal to eat for two feedings in a row
- Vomiting: more than one episode of forceful vomiting or frequent vomiting (over a 6-hr period)
- Diarrhea: two consecutive green, watery stools (**NOTE:** Stools of breastfed infants are normally looser than stools of formula-fed infants. Diarrhea will leave a water ring around the stool, whereas breastfed stools will not.)
- Decreased bowel movement: in a breastfed infant, fewer than three stools per day; in a formula-fed infant, fewer than one stool every other day
- Decreased urination: fewer than six to eight wet diapers per day after 3 to 4 days of age
- Breathing difficulties: labored breathing with flared nostrils or absence of breathing for more than 15 seconds (**NOTE:** A newborn's breathing is normally irregular and between 30 to 40 breaths/min. Count the breaths for a full minute.)
- Cyanosis (bluish skin color) whether accompanying a feeding or not
- Lethargy: sleepiness, difficulty waking, or periods of sleep longer than 6 hours (most newborns sleep for short periods, usually from 1 to 4 hours, and wake to be fed)
- Inconsolable crying (attempts to quiet not effective) or continuous high-pitched cry
- Bleeding or purulent (yellowish) drainage from umbilical cord or circumcision; foul odor or redness at the site
- Drainage from the eyes

KEY POINTS

- Assessment of the newborn requires data from the prenatal, intrapartal, and postnatal periods.
- The immediate assessment of the newborn includes Apgar scoring and a general evaluation of physical status.
- Knowledge of biologic and behavioral characteristics is essential for guiding assessment and interpreting data.
- Gestational age assessment provides important information for predicting risks and guiding care management.
- Nursing care immediately after birth includes maintaining an open airway, preventing heat loss, and promoting parent-infant interaction.
- Providing a protective environment is a key responsibility of the nurse and includes such measures as careful identification

procedures, support of physiologic functions, and ways to prevent infection.

- The newborn has social and physical needs.
- Newborns require careful assessment for physiologic and behavioral manifestations of pain.
- Nonpharmacologic and pharmacologic measures are used to reduce infant pain.
- Before hospital discharge, nurses provide anticipatory guidance for parents regarding feeding and elimination patterns; positioning and holding; comfort measures; car seat safety; bathing, skin care, cord care, and nail care; and signs of illness.
- All parents should have instruction in infant CPR.

REFERENCES

Adamkin DH, Committee on Fetus and Newborn: Clinical report—postnatal glucose homeostasis in late-preterm and term infants, *Pediatrics* 127(3):575–579, 2011.

American Academy of Pediatrics (AAP): *Car seats: information for families,* Elk Grove

Village, IL, 2012, Author, www.healthychildren.org/English/safety-prevention/on-the-go/Pages/Car-Safety-Seats-Information-for-Families.aspx?nfstat.

American Academy of Pediatrics (AAP) Committee on Infectious Diseases: *Red book:*

2012 report of the Committee on Infectious Diseases, ed 29, Elk Grove Village, IL, 2012, Author.

American Academy of Pediatrics (AAP) Subcommittee on Hyperbilirubinemia: Clinical practice guideline: management of hyperbilirubinemia in the newborn infant 35 or more weeks of gestation, *Pediatrics* 114(1):297–316, 2004.

American Academy of Pediatrics (AAP) Task Force on Circumcision: Circumcision policy statement, *Pediatrics* 103(3):686–693, 1999, affirmed 2005.

American Academy of Pediatrics (AAP) Task Force on Circumcision: Circumcision policy statement, *Pediatrics* 130(3):585–586, 2012.

American Academy of Pediatrics (AAP) Task Force on Sudden Infant Death Syndrome: SIDS and other sleep-related infant deaths: expansion of recommendations for a safe infant sleeping environment, *Pediatrics* 128(5):e1341–e1367, 2011.

American Academy of Pediatrics (AAP), American College of Obstetricians and Gynecologists (ACOG): *Guidelines for perinatal care*, ed 7, Elk Grove Village, IL, 2012, Author.

American College of Medical Genetics: Position statement on importance of residual newborn screening dried blood spots, 2009, www.acmg.net/StaticContent/NewsReleases/Blood_Spot_Position_Statement2009.pdf.

American College of Obstetricians and Gynecologists (ACOG) Committee on Genetics: Committee opinion no. 481: newborn screening, *Obstet Gynecol* 117(3):762–765, 2011.

American College of Obstetricians and Gynecologists (ACOG) Committee on Obstetric Practice: Committee opinion no. 333: the Apgar score, *Obstet Gynecol* 107:1209–1212, 2006, reaffirmed 2010.

Araia MH, Wilson BJ, Chakraborty P, et al: Factors associated with knowledge of and satisfaction with newborn screening education: a survey of mothers, *Genet Med* 14(12):963–970, 2012.

Association of Women's Health, Obstetric and Neonatal Nurses: *Neonatal skin care: evidence-based clinical practice guideline*, ed 2, Washington, DC, 2007, Author.

Ballard J, Khoury J, Wedig K, et al: New Ballard Score, expanded to include extremely premature infants, *J Pediatr* 119(3):417–423, 1991.

Bates E, Rouse D, Chapman V, et al: Fetal lung maturity testing before 39 weeks and neonatal outcomes, *Obstet Gynecol* 116(6):1288–1295, 2010.

Blackburn ST: *Maternal, fetal, and neonatal physiology: a clinical perspective*, ed 4, St Louis, 2013, Saunders.

Brady-Fryer B, Wiebe N, Lander JA: Pain relief for newborn circumcision, *Cochrane Database Syst Rev* (Issue 4):CD004217, 2004.

Bramson L, Lee JW, Moore E, et al: Effect of early skin-to-skin mother-infant contact during the first 3 hours following birth on exclusive breastfeeding during the maternity hospital stay, *J Hum Lact* 26(2):130–137, 2010.

Bromiker R, Bin-Nun A, Schimmel MS, et al: Neonatal hyperbilirubinemia in the low-intermediate-risk category on the bilirubin nomogram, *Pediatrics* 130(3):e470–e475, 2012.

Brown VD, Landers S: Heat balance. In Gardner SL, Carter BS, Enzman-Hines M, et al, editors: *Merenstein & Gardner's handbook of neonatal intensive care*, ed 7, St Louis, 2011, Mosby.

Bull M, Engle WA, American Academy of Pediatrics Committee on Injury, Violence, and Poison Prevention and Committee on Fetus and Newborn: Safe transportation of preterm and low birth weight infants at hospital discharge, *Pediatrics* 123(5):1424–1429, 2009.

Centers for Disease Control and Prevention: Advisory Committee on Immunization Practices (ACIP): Recommended immunization schedule for persons aged 0 through 18 ears and adults aged 19 years and older United States 2013, *MMWR Morb Mortal Wkly Rep* 62(Suppl 1):1–21, 2013.

Chermont A, Falcão L, de Souza Silva E, et al: Skin-to-skin contact and/or oral 25% sucrose for procedural pain relief for term newborn infants, *Pediatrics* 124(6):e1102–e1107, 2009.

Cignacco EL, Sellam G, Stoffel L, et al: Oral sucrose with facilitated tucking is effective pain control for preterm infants: a randomized control trial, *Pediatrics* 129(2):299–308, 2012.

Cooper BM, Holditch-Davis D, Verklan MT, et al: Newborn clinical outcomes of the AWHONN late preterm infant research-based practice project, *J Obstet Gynecol Neonatal Nurs* 41(6):774–785, 2012.

Craighead DV: Early term birth: understanding the health risks to infants, *Nurs Womens Health* 16(2):136–145, 2012.

Fleischman AR, Oinuma M, Clark SL: Rethinking the definition of "term pregnancy", *Obstet Gynecol* 116(1):136–139, 2010.

Furdon SA, Benjamin K: Physical assessment. In Verklan MT, Walden M, editors: *Core curriculum for neonatal intensive care nursing*, ed 4, St Louis, 2010, Saunders.

Gabriel MM, Martin KL, Escobar AL, et al: Randomized controlled trial of early skin-to-skin contact: effects on the mother and the newborn, *Acta Paediatr* 99(11):1630–1634, 2010.

Gardner SL, Enzman-Hines M, Dickey LA: Pain and pain relief. In Gardner SL, Carter BS, Enzman-Hines M, et al, editors: *Merenstein & Gardner's handbook of neonatal intensive care*, ed 7, St Louis, 2011, Mosby.

Gardner SL, Hernandez JA: Initial nursery care. In Gardner SL, Carter BS, Enzman-Hines M, et al, editors: *Merenstein & Gardner's handbook of neonatal intensive care*, ed 7, St Louis, 2011, Mosby.

Hamilton BE, Martin JA, Ventura SJ: Births: preliminary data for 2010, *Natl Vital Stat Rep* 60(2):1–26, 2011, www.cdc.gov/nchs/data/nvsr/nvsr60/nvsr60_02.pdf.

Howell RR, Terry S, Olney R, et al: CDC Grand Rounds: newborn screening and improved outcomes, *MMWR Morb Mortal Wkly Rep* 61(21):390–393, 2012.

Hummel P, Puchalski M., Creech SD, et al: Clinical reliability and validity of the N-PASS: neonatal pain, agitation, and sedation scale with prolonged pain, *J Perinatol* 28(1):55–60, 2008.

Joint Committee on Infant Hearing: Year 2007 position statement: principles and guidelines for early hearing detection and intervention programs, *Pediatrics* 120(4):898–921, 2007.

Jones JE, Hayes RD, Starbuck AL, et al: Fluid and electrolyte management. In Gardner SL, Carter BS, Enzman-Hines M, et al, editors: *Merenstein & Gardner's handbook of neonatal intensive care*, ed 7, St Louis, 2011, Mosby.

Kalhan SC, Devaskar SU: Disorders of carbohydrate metabolism. In Martin RJ, Fanaroff AA, Walsh MC, editors: *Fanaroff and Martin's neonatal-perinatal medicine: diseases of the fetus and infant*, ed 9, St Louis, 2011, Mosby.

Kamath BC, Thilo EH, Hernandez JA: Jaundice. In Gardner SL, Carter BS, Enzman-Hines M, et al, editors: *Merenstein & Gardner's handbook of neonatal intensive care*, ed 7, St Louis, 2011, Mosby.

Kaplan M, Wong RJ, Sibley E, et al: Neonatal jaundice and liver disease. In Martin RJ, Fanaroff AA, Walsh MC, editors: *Fanaroff and Martin's neonatal-perinatal medicine: diseases of the fetus and infant*, ed 9, St Louis, 2011, Mosby.

Kassab MI, Roydhouse JK, Fowler C, et al: The effectiveness of glucose in reducing needle-related procedural pain in infants, *J Pediatr Nurs* 27(1):3–17, 2012.

Kattwinkel J, Perlman JM, Aziz K, et al: Part 15: neonatal resuscitation: 2010 American Heart Association guidelines for cardiopulmonary resuscitation and emergency cardiovascular care, *Circulation* 122(Suppl 3):S909–S919, 2010.

Krechel S, Bildner J: CRIES: a new neonatal postoperative pain measurement score—initial testing of validity and reliability, *Paediatr Anaesth* 5(1):53–61, 1995.

Lawrence J, Alcock D, McGrath P, et al: The development of a tool to assess neonatal pain, *Neonatal Netw* 12(6):59–66, 1993.

Leite A, Linhares M, Lander J, et al: Effects of breastfeeding on pain relief in full-term newborns, *Clin J Pain* 25(9):827–832, 2009.

Liaw J, Zeng W, Yang L, et al: Nonnutritive sucking and oral sucrose relieve neonatal pain during intramuscular injection of hepatitis vaccine, *J Pain Manag* 42(6):918–930, 2011.

Lindstrom K, Lindblad F, Hjern A: Preterm birth and attention-deficit/hyperactivity disorder, *Pediatrics* 127(5):858–865, 2011.

Lund CH, Durand DJ: Skin and skin care. In Gardner SL, Carter BS, Enzman-Hines M, et al, editors: *Merenstein & Gardner's handbook of neonatal intensive care*, ed 7, St Louis, 2011, Mosby.

Mahle WT, Newburger JW, Matherne GP, et al: Role of pulse oximetry in examining newborns for congenital heart disease: a scientific statement from the American Heart Association and the American Academy of Pediatrics, *Circulation* 120:447–458, 2009.

Maisels MJ, Bhutani VK, Bogen D, et al: Hyperbilirubinemia in the newborn infant > or = 35 weeks gestation: an update with clarifications, *Pediatrics* 124(4):1193–1198, 2009.

McGowan JE, Rozance PJ, Price-Douglas W, et al: Glucose homeostasis. In Gardner SL, Carter BS, Enzman-Hines M, et al, editors: *Merenstein & Gardner's handbook of neonatal intensive care*, ed 7, St Louis, 2011, Mosby.

Moore ER, Anderson GC, Bergman N, et al: Early skin-to-skin contact for mothers and their healthy newborn infants, *Cochrane Database Syst Rev* May 16 (Issue 5):CD003519, 2012.

National Highway Traffic Safety Administration (NHTSA) Parents Central: *From car seats to car keys: keeping kids safe*, Washington, DC, 2012, Author, www.safercar.gov/parents/ Home.htm.

Niermeyer S, Clarke SB: Delivery room care. In Gardner SL, Carter BS, Enzman-Hines M, et al, editors: *Merenstein & Gardner's handbook of neonatal intensive care*, ed 7, St Louis, 2011, Mosby.

Price CT, Schwend RM: Improper swaddling a risk factor for developmental dysplasia of hip, *AAP News* 32(9), 2011, www.aapnews.org.

Reddy UM, Bettegowda VR, Dias T, et al: Term pregnancy: a period of heterogenous risk for infant mortality, *Obstet Gynecol* 117(6):1279–1287, 2011.

Reddy UM, Ko CW, Raju TN, et al: Delivery indications at late-preterm gestations and infant mortality rates in the United States, *Pediatrics* 124(1):234–240, 2009.

Riddell RP, Racine N, Turcotte K, et al: Nonpharmacological management of procedural pain in infants and young children: an abridged Cochrane review, *Pain Res Manag* 16(5):321–330, 2011.

Rigo J, Mohamed MW, De Curtis M: Disorders of calcium, phosphorus, and magnesium metabolism. In Martin RJ, Fanaroff AA, Walsh MC, editors: *Fanaroff and Martin's neonatal-perinatal medicine: diseases of the fetus and infant*, ed 9, St Louis, 2011, Mosby.

Stevens B, Johnston C, Petryshen P, et al: Premature infant pain profile: development and initial validation, *Clin J Pain* 12(1):13–22, 1996.

Stevens B, Yamada J, Ohlsson A: Sucrose for analgesia in newborn infants undergoing painful procedures, *Cochrane Database Syst Rev* (Issue 1):CD001069, 2010.

Taddio A, Appleton M, Bortolussi R, et al: Reducing the pain of childhood vaccination: an evidence-based clinical practice guideline (summary), *CMAJ* 182(18):1989–1995, 2010.

Vincent JL: Infant hospital abduction: security measures to aid in prevention, *MCN Am J Matern Child Nurs* 34(3):179–183, 2009.

Walden M, Gibbins S: *Pain assessment & management guideline for practice*, ed 2, Glenview, IL, 2008, National Association of Neonatal Nurses.

Weissman A, Aranovitch M, Blazer S, et al: Heel-lancing in newborns: behavioral and spectral analysis assessment of pain control methods, *Pediatrics* 124(5):e921–e926, 2009.

World Health Organization (WHO): *WHO guidelines on hand hygiene in health care: a summary*, Geneva, Switzerland, 2009, WHO Press.

World Health Organization (WHO): *Voluntary medical male circumcision for HIV prevention*, 2012, www.who.int/hiv/topics/ malecircumcision/fact_sheet/en/index.html.

Zhang X, Shinde S, Kilmarx PH, et al: Trends in in-hospital newborn male circumcision— United States, 1999-2010, *MMWR Morb Mortal Wkly Rep* 60(34):1167–1168, 2011.

Newborn Nutrition and Feeding

Kathryn R. Alden

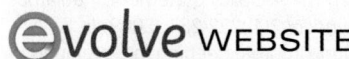 WEBSITE

http://evolve.elsevier.com/Perry/maternal

LEARNING OBJECTIVES

On completion of this chapter, the reader will be able to:

- Describe current recommendations for infant feeding.
- Explain the nurse's role in helping families choose an infant feeding method.
- Discuss benefits of breastfeeding for infants, mothers, families, and society.
- Describe nutritional needs of infants.
- Describe anatomic and physiologic aspects of breastfeeding.
- Recognize newborn feeding-readiness cues.

- Explain maternal and infant indicators of effective breastfeeding.
- Examine nursing interventions to facilitate and promote successful breastfeeding.
- Analyze common problems associated with breastfeeding and interventions to help resolve them.
- Compare powdered, concentrated, and ready-to-use forms of commercial infant formula.
- Develop a teaching plan for the formula-feeding family.

Good nutrition in infancy fosters optimal growth and development. Infant feeding is more than providing nutrition; it is an opportunity for social, psychologic, and even educational interaction between parent and infant. It can also establish a basis for developing good eating habits that last a lifetime.

Through preconception and prenatal education and counseling nurses play an instrumental role in helping parents make an informed decision about infant feeding. Scientific evidence is clear that human milk provides the best nutrition for infants, and parents should be strongly encouraged to choose breastfeeding (AAP Section on Breastfeeding, 2012). Although many consider commercial infant formula to be equivalent to breast milk, this belief is erroneous. Human milk is the gold standard for infant nutrition. It is species specific, uniquely designed to meet the needs of human infants. The composition of human milk changes to meet the nutritional needs of growing infants. It is highly complex, with antiinfective and nutritional components combined with growth factors, enzymes that aid in digestion and absorption of nutrients, and fatty acids that promote brain growth and development. Infant formulas are usually adequate in providing nutrition to maintain infant growth and development within normal limits, but they are not equivalent to human milk.

Breastfeeding is defined as the transfer of human milk from the mother to the infant; the infant receives milk directly from the mother's breast. *Exclusive breastfeeding* means that the infant receives no other liquid or solid food (AAP Section on Breastfeeding, 2012). If the infant is fed expressed breast milk from the mother or a donor milk bank, it is called *human milk feeding*.

Whether the parents choose breastfeeding, human milk feeding, or formula feeding, nurses provide support and ongoing education. Parent education and care management are necessarily based on current research findings and standards of practice. Nurses and lactation consultants (who are most often nurses) provide education, assistance, and support for mothers, infants, and families. After hospital discharge nurses and lactation consultants in primary care and community health settings provide ongoing support and assistance to promote optimal feeding practices and positive health outcomes.

This chapter focuses on meeting nutritional needs for normal growth and development from birth to 6 months, with emphasis on the neonatal period when feeding practices and patterns are established. Breastfeeding and formula feeding are addressed. Information on breastfeeding is focused on the direct transfer of milk from mother to infant.

RECOMMENDED INFANT NUTRITION

The American Academy of Pediatrics (AAP) recommends exclusive breastfeeding for the first 6 months of life and that breastfeeding be continued as complementary foods are introduced. Breastfeeding

---

TABLE 24-1   BENEFITS OF BREASTFEEDING

BENEFITS FOR THE INFANT	BENEFITS FOR THE MOTHER	BENEFITS TO FAMILIES AND SOCIETY
Reduced risk for: • Nonspecific gastrointestinal infections • Celiac disease • Childhood inflammatory bowel disease • Necrotizing enterocolitis in preterm infants • Clinical asthma, atopic dermatitis, and eczema • Lower respiratory tract infection • Otitis media • SIDS • Obesity in adolescence and adulthood • Types 1 and 2 diabetes • Acute lymphocytic and myeloid leukemia Enhanced neurodevelopmental outcomes, especially in preterm infants	Decreased postpartum bleeding and more rapid uterine involution Reduced risk for: • Ovarian cancer and breast cancer (primarily premenopausal) • Type II diabetes • Hypertension, hypercholesterolemia, and cardiovascular disease • Rheumatoid arthritis Unique bonding experience Increased maternal role attainment	• Convenient; ready to feed • No bottles or other necessary equipment • Less expensive than infant formula • Reduced annual health care costs • Less parental absence from work because of ill infant • Reduced environmental burden related to disposal of formula packaging and equipment

Data from American Academy of Pediatrics Section on Breastfeeding: Breastfeeding and the use of human milk—policy statement, *Pediatrics* 129(3):e827-e841, 2012; Stuebe A: The risks of not breastfeeding for mothers and infants, *Rev Obstet Gynecol* 2(4):222-231, 2009; Ip S, Chung M, Raman G, et al: A summary of the Agency for Healthcare Research and Quality's evidence report on breastfeeding in developed countries, *Breastfeed Med* 4(suppl 1):S17-S30, 2009.
SIDS, Sudden infant death syndrome.

should continue for 1 year and thereafter as desired by the mother and her infant (AAP Section on Breastfeeding, 2012). According to the Global Strategy for Infant and Young Child Feeding, endorsed by the World Health Organization (WHO) and United Nations Children's Fund (UNICEF), infants should be exclusively breastfed for 6 months, and breastfeeding should continue for up to 2 years and beyond (WHO and UNICEF, 2003).

Exclusive breastfeeding for the first 6 months of life is also recommended by other professional health care organizations such as the American Academy of Family Physicians (AAFP, 2012), Academy of Breastfeeding Medicine (ABM Board of Directors, 2008), the American College of Obstetricians and Gynecologists (ACOG Committee on Health Care for Underserved Women and Committee on Obstetric Practice, 2007), and the American Dietetic Association (ADA, 2009). The Association of Women's Health, Obstetric and Neonatal Nurses (AWHONN, 2007) actively supports breastfeeding as the ideal form of infant nutrition and provides guidelines for nurses in promoting breastfeeding and supporting breastfeeding families.

Breastfeeding Rates

Breastfeeding rates in the United States have risen steadily over the past decade. The Centers for Disease Control and Prevention (CDC, 2012) reported that the U.S. breastfeeding initiation rate in 2009 was 76.9%, which is the highest ever reported. The 6-month breastfeeding rate was 47.2%, and the 12-month rate was 25.5%. The rate of exclusive breastfeeding at 3 months was 36% and at 6 months, 16.3%. In spite of the increases in breastfeeding rates, the United States continues to fall short of the *Healthy People 2020* goals of 81% of infants ever breastfed, 60.6% breastfeeding at 6 months, and 34.1% at 12 months; goals for exclusive breastfeeding are 46.2% through 3 months and 25.5% through 6 months (USDHHS, 2010).

Trends remain unchanged in breastfeeding rates among minority groups in the United States. The lowest breastfeeding rates are among non-Hispanic black women (Jensen, 2012), although the overall percentage of non-Hispanic black women who breastfeed has increased in recent years. The minority group most likely to breastfeed is Hispanic women (Scanlon, Grummer-Strawn, Li et al., 2010).

Benefits of Breastfeeding

Extensive evidence exists concerning the health benefits of breastfeeding and human milk for infants, with some of the benefits extending into adulthood (Table 24-1). These benefits are optimized when infants are breastfed exclusively and when the duration of breastfeeding is increased (Mass, 2011). The evidence supporting breastfeeding as the ideal form of infant nutrition is so strong that health care professionals may need to present information about it from two perspectives: benefits of and risks of not breastfeeding (Spatz and Lessen, 2011).

Breastfeeding is associated with health benefits for mothers (see Table 24-1). The benefits are increased with the number of children who were breastfed and the total length of time of lactation.

The psychologic benefits for mothers include enhanced bonding and attachment. For many women breastfeeding is associated with a sense of empowerment in the ability to provide nutrition for the infant.

Breastfeeding is convenient. The milk is ready to feed and at the proper temperature. In most cases there is no need for bottles or other equipment.

The economic benefits of breastfeeding affect families, employers, insurers, and the entire nation. Because infant formula is expensive, breastfeeding represents a significant savings for families. It reduces health care costs and decreases employee absenteeism. It has been estimated that the United States could save $13 billion dollars per year and more than 900 infant deaths could be prevented if 90% of infants were breastfed exclusively for 6 months (Bartick and Reinhold, 2010).

Breastfeeding has environmental benefits. It reduces the waste that is deposited in landfills, including formula packaging, bottles, nipples, and other equipment. There is no need for fuel to prepare or transport human milk, which saves energy resources (USDHHS, 2011).

CHOOSING AN INFANT FEEDING METHOD

For most women there is a clear choice to either breastfeed or formula feed. In some cases women decide to combine breastfeeding and formula feeding. However, this practice may be associated with a shorter duration of breastfeeding (Holmes, Auinger, and Howard, 2011). In some instances women want their infants to receive breast milk but prefer not to feed directly from their breasts.

Choosing to Breastfeed

Women most often choose to breastfeed because they are aware of the benefits to the infant (Nelson, 2012). This reinforces the importance of prenatal education about the numerous benefits of breastfeeding.

Breastfeeding is a natural extension of pregnancy and childbirth; it is much more than simply a means of supplying nutrition for infants. Many women seek the unique bonding experience between mother and infant that is characteristic of breastfeeding.

Women tend to select the same method of infant feeding for each of their children. If the first child was breastfed, subsequent children will likely also be breastfed.

The support of the partner and family is a major factor in the mother's decision to breastfeed. Women who perceive their partners to prefer breastfeeding are more likely to breastfeed. Women are more likely to breastfeed successfully when partners and family members are positive about breastfeeding and have the skills to support it.

Cultural factors influence infant feeding decisions. For example, in the Hispanic culture breastfeeding is the norm, whereas formula feeding is more common among African-American families (see Cultural Competence box).

The decision to breastfeed exclusively is related to the mother's knowledge about the health benefits to the infant and her comfort level with breastfeeding in social settings (Stuebe and Bonuck, 2011). The likelihood that women will breastfeed exclusively may be greater if they made the decision to do so during pregnancy (Tenfelde, Finnegan, and Hill, 2011).

There appears to be a relationship between maternal weight and infant feeding decisions. Women who are overweight or obese are less likely to breastfeed than women who are underweight or of average weight (Mehta, Siega-Riz, Herring, et al., 2011).

Other factors influence decisions about infant nutrition. Social and systemic factors create obstacles or barriers to breastfeeding among women in the United States. These include a lack of broad social support for breastfeeding and the widespread marketing by infant formula companies. In addition, there is a lack of prenatal breastfeeding education for expectant parents and insufficient training/education of health care professionals about breastfeeding. In some institutions the policies and practices do not support exclusive breastfeeding (Mass, 2011). There is a lack of support for breastfeeding mothers during the first 2 to 3 weeks after birth when they are most likely to encounter difficulties.

On a more personal level, a major obstacle for women is employment and the need to return to work after birth (Mass, 2011). A lack of support from the partner and family also creates obstacles to breastfeeding for many women. In a meta-synthesis of 14 qualitative studies about infant feeding decision making, Nelson (2012) reported common barriers to breastfeeding such as lack of comfort or uneasiness with breastfeeding, pain, lifestyle incompatibility, discomfort with public breastfeeding, and a lack of formal support.

⊕ CULTURAL COMPETENCE
Breastfeeding Among African-American Women

African-American women are least likely to breastfeed than other ethnic groups in the United States. Multiple factors are involved in this phenomenon. There may be a lack of knowledge or misinformation about benefits and management of breastfeeding. Support for breastfeeding may be lacking (Lewallen and Street, 2010). They may believe that formula is nutritionally superior to breastfeeding. African-American women tend to return to work earlier and are more likely to be employed in environments that are unsupportive of breastfeeding. Stereotypes about breastfeeding and the idea that breasts are primarily sexual objects can influence the decision to choose formula feeding over breastfeeding. Cultural traditions are an important factor (Philipp and Jean-Marie, 2007). Kuae Mattox, National President of Mocha Moms, Inc., an organization that supports African-American breastfeeding mothers, writes: "…African American women have a much steeper road to climb when it comes to breastfeeding, and some believe its roots go as far back as slavery, when our ancestors were 'wet nurses', forced to breastfeed the master's children, often to the exclusion of their own. That created a negative breastfeeding cultural legacy that some believe still permeates our culture today" (Mattox, 2012, p. 2).

African-American women need information and support for breastfeeding. Many are surrounded by family and friends who advise them to formula feed (Nelson, 2012). A national, nonprofit organization called *Mocha Moms, Inc.* is reaching out to women in creative and unconventional ways. This group of stay-at-home mothers consists primarily of African-American professional women with college degrees who previously worked but have chosen to stay at home to be with their children. Mocha Moms offer support groups and provide information through Internet-based communications and peer-to-peer information sharing. Their website is www.mochamoms.org.

References
Lewallen LP, Street DJ: Initiating and sustaining breastfeeding in African American women, *J Obstet Gynecol Neonatal Nurs* 39(6):667–674, 2010.

Mattox KK: African American mothers: bringing the case for breastfeeding home, *Breastfeed Med* 7(2):1–3, 2012.

Nelson AM: A meta-synthesis related to infant feeding decision making, *MCN Am J Matern Child Nurs* 37(4):247–252, 2012.

Philipp BL, Jean-Marie S: African American women and breastfeeding: the courage to love: infant mortality commission, Washington, DC, 2007, Joint Center for Political and Economic Studies.

Choosing to Formula Feed

Parents who choose to formula feed often make this decision without complete information and understanding of the benefits of breastfeeding. Even women who are educated about the advantages of breastfeeding may still decide to formula feed. Cultural beliefs and myths and misconceptions about breastfeeding influence women's decision making. Many women see bottle-feeding as more convenient or less embarrassing than breastfeeding. Some view formula feeding as a way to ensure that the father, other family members, and day care providers can feed the baby. Some women lack confidence in their ability to produce breast milk of adequate quantity or quality. Women who have had previous unsuccessful breastfeeding experiences may choose to formula feed subsequent infants. Some women see breastfeeding as incompatible with an active social life, or they think that it will prevent them from going back to work. Modesty issues and societal barriers exist against breastfeeding in public. A major barrier for many women is the influence of family and friends (Nelson, 2012).

Women who participate in the Supplemental Nutrition Program for Women, Infants, and Children (WIC) are more likely to formula feed (Jensen, 2012; Mass, 2011). Although in recent years WIC has improved food packages for breastfeeding families, many women on WIC decide to formula feed based on the perceived monetary value of infant formula as well as convenience and social factors (Jensen, 2012).

Contraindications to Breastfeeding

Breastfeeding is contraindicated in a few circumstances. Newborns who have galactosemia should not receive human milk. Breastfeeding is contraindicated for mothers who are positive for human T-cell lymphotropic virus types I or II and those with untreated brucellosis. Women should not breastfeed if they have active tuberculosis (TB) or if they have active herpes simplex lesions on the breasts. However, neither of these conditions precludes a mother expressing milk for her infant (AAP Section on Breastfeeding, 2012). Women with active TB can breastfeed when they have been treated for at least 2 weeks and are deemed noninfectious. Varicella that occurs 5 days before or 2 days after birth and acute H1N1 infection require temporary separation of mother and infant. In both instances it is safe for infants to receive expressed milk (AAP Section on Breastfeeding, 2012).

In the United States maternal human immunodeficiency virus (HIV) infection is considered a contraindication for breastfeeding (AAP Section on Breastfeeding, 2012). However, that is not true in other countries. In developing countries where HIV is prevalent, the benefits of breastfeeding for infants outweigh the risk of contracting HIV from infected mothers (WHO, UNICEF, UNFPA, and UNAIDS, 2010).

Breastfeeding is not recommended when mothers are receiving chemotherapy or radioactive isotopes (e.g., with diagnostic procedures). Maternal use of mood-altering drugs ("street drugs") is incompatible with breastfeeding (AAP Section on Breastfeeding, 2012). Other maternal medications may also be incompatible with and require temporary or permanent cessation of breastfeeding.

Cultural Influences on Infant Feeding

Cultural beliefs and practices are significant influences on infant feeding methods. Although recognized cultural norms exist, one cannot assume that generalized observations about any cultural group hold true for all members of that group. Many regional and ethnic cultures are found within the United States. Dealing effectively with these groups requires that nurses be knowledgeable and sensitive to the cultural factors influencing infant feeding practices.

In general people who have immigrated to the United States from poorer countries often choose to formula feed their infants because they believe it is a better, more "modern" method or because they want to adapt to U.S. culture and perceive that formula feeding is the custom. Hispanic women who are more acculturated may be less likely to breastfeed and, if they do, tend to breastfeed for a shorter duration (Ahluwalia, D'Angelo, Morrow, et al., 2012).

Breastfeeding beliefs and practices vary across cultures. For example, among the Muslim culture breastfeeding for 24 months is customary. Before the first feeding rubbing a small piece of softened date on the newborn's palate is a ritual. Because of the cultural emphasis on privacy and modesty, Muslim women may choose to bottle-feed formula or expressed breast milk while in the hospital. Because of beliefs about the harmful nature or inadequacy of

colostrum, some cultures apply restrictions on breastfeeding for a period of days after birth. Such is the case for many cultures in Southern Asia, the Pacific Islands, and parts of sub-Saharan Africa. Before the mother's milk is deemed to be "in," babies are fed prelacteal food such as honey or clarified butter in the belief that these substances will help clear out meconium. Other cultures begin breastfeeding immediately and offer the breast each time the infant cries.

A common practice among Mexican women is *las dos cosas* ("both things"). This refers to combining breastfeeding and commercial infant formula. It is based on the belief that, by combining the two methods, the mother and infant receive the benefits of breastfeeding, and the infant receives the additional vitamins from infant formula (Bartick and Reyes, 2012; Rios, 2009). This practice can result in problems with milk supply and babies refusing to latch on to the breast, which can lead to early termination of breastfeeding.

Some cultures have specific beliefs and practices related to the mother's intake of foods that foster milk production. Korean mothers often eat seaweed soup and rice to enhance milk production. Hmong women believe that boiled chicken, rice, and hot water are the only appropriate nourishments during the first postpartum month. The balance between energy forces, hot and cold, or yin and yang is integral to the diet of the lactating mother. Hispanics, Vietnamese, Chinese, East Indians, and Arabs often use this belief in choosing foods. "Hot" foods are considered best for new mothers. This belief does not necessarily relate to the temperature or spiciness of foods. For example, chicken and broccoli are considered "hot," whereas many fresh fruits and vegetables are considered "cold." Families often bring desired foods into the health care setting.

NUTRIENT NEEDS

Fluids

During the first 2 days of life the fluid requirement for healthy infants (more than 1500 g) is 60 to 80 mL of water per kilogram of body weight per day. From day 3 to 7 the requirement is 100 to 150 mL/kg/day; from day 8 to day 30 it is 120 to 180 mL/kg/day (Dell, 2011). In general neither breastfed nor formula-fed infants need to be given water, not even those living in very hot climates. Breast milk contains 87% water, which easily meets fluid requirements. Feeding water to infants can decrease caloric consumption at a time when they are growing rapidly.

Infants have room for little fluctuation in fluid balance and should be monitored closely for fluid intake and water loss. They lose water through excretion of urine and insensibly through respiration. Under normal circumstances they are born with some fluid reserve, and some of the weight loss during the first few days is related to fluid loss. However, in some cases they do not have this fluid reserve, possibly because of inadequate maternal hydration during labor or birth.

Energy

Infants require adequate caloric intake to provide energy for growth, digestion, physical activity, and maintenance of organ metabolic function. Energy needs vary according to age, maturity level, thermal environment, growth rate, health status, and activity level. For the first 3 months the infant needs 110 kcal/kg/day. From 3 months to 6 months the requirement is 100 kcal/kg/day. This level decreases slightly to 95 kcal/kg/day from 6 to 9 months and increases to 100 kcal/kg/day from 9 months to 1 year (AAP Committee on Nutrition, 2009).

Human milk provides an average of 67 kcal/100 mL or 20 kcal/oz. The fat portion of the milk provides the greatest amount of energy. Infant formulas simulate the caloric content of human milk. Usually a standard formula contains 20 kcal/oz, although the composition differs among brands.

Carbohydrates

According to the Institute of Medicine (IOM, 2005), the recommended adequate intake (AI) for carbohydrates in the first 6 months of life is 60 g/day and 95 g/day for the second 6 months. Because newborns have only small hepatic glycogen stores, carbohydrates should provide at least 40% to 50% of the total calories in the diet. Moreover newborns may have a limited ability to carry out gluconeogenesis (the formation of glucose from amino acids and other substrates) and ketogenesis (the formation of ketone bodies from fat), the mechanisms that provide alternative sources of energy.

As the primary carbohydrate in human milk and commercially prepared infant formula, lactose is the most abundant carbohydrate in the diet of infants up to age 6 months. Lactose provides calories in an easily available form. Its slow breakdown and absorption also increase calcium absorption. Corn syrup solids or glucose polymers are added to infant formulas to supplement the lactose in the cow's milk and thereby provide sufficient carbohydrates.

Oligosaccharides, another form of carbohydrate found in breast milk, are critical in the development of microflora in the intestinal tract of the newborn. These prebiotics promote an acidic environment in the intestines, preventing the growth of gram-negative and other pathogenic bacteria, thus increasing the infant's resistance to gastrointestinal (GI) illness.

Fat

Fats provide a major energy source for infants, supplying as much as 50% of the calories in breast milk and formula. The recommended AI of fat for infants younger than 6 months is 31 g/day (IOM, 2005). The fat content of human milk is composed of lipids, triglycerides, and cholesterol; cholesterol is an essential element for brain growth. Human milk contains the essential fatty acids (EFAs) linoleic acid and linolenic acid and the long-chain polyunsaturated fatty acids arachidonic acid (ARA) and docosahexaenoic acid (DHA). Fatty acids are important for growth, neurologic development, and visual function. Cow's milk contains fewer of the EFAs and no polyunsaturated fatty acids. Most formula companies add DHA to their products, although there is a lack of evidence supporting the benefit (Lawrence and Lawrence, 2011b). Modified cow's milk is used in most infant formulas; but the milk fat is removed, and another fat source such as corn oil, which the infant can digest and absorb, is added in its place. If whole milk or evaporated milk without added carbohydrate is fed to infants, the resulting fecal loss of fat (and therefore loss of energy) can be excessive because the milk moves through the infant's intestines too quickly for adequate absorption to take place. This can lead to poor weight gain.

Protein

High-quality protein from breast milk, infant formula, or other complementary foods is necessary for infant growth. The protein requirement per unit of body weight is greater in the newborn than at any other time of life. For infants younger than 6 months the recommended AI for protein is 9.1 g/day (IOM, 2005).

Human milk contains the two proteins whey and casein in a ratio of approximately 70:30 compared with the ratio of 20:80 in most cow's milk–based formula (Blackburn, 2013). This whey/casein ratio in human milk makes it more easily digestible and produces the soft stools seen in breastfed infants. The primary whey protein in human milk is α-lactalbumin; this protein is high in essential amino acids needed for growth. The whey protein lactoferrin in human milk has iron-binding capabilities and bacteriostatic properties, particularly against gram-positive and gram-negative aerobes, anaerobes, and yeasts. The casein in human milk enhances the absorption of iron, thus preventing iron-dependent bacteria from proliferating in the GI tract (Lawrence and Lawrence, 2011a). The amino acid components of human milk are uniquely suited to the newborn's metabolic capabilities. For example, cystine and taurine levels are high, whereas phenylalanine and methionine levels are low.

Vitamins

With the exception of vitamin D, human milk contains all of the vitamins required for infant nutrition, with individual variations based on maternal diet and genetic differences. Vitamins are added to cow's-milk formulas to resemble levels found in breast milk. Although cow's milk contains adequate amounts of vitamins A and B complex, vitamin C (ascorbic acid), vitamin E, and vitamin D must be added.

Vitamin D facilitates intestinal absorption of calcium and phosphorus, bone mineralization, and calcium resorption from bone. According to the AAP, all infants who are breastfed or partially breastfed should receive 400 International Units of vitamin D daily, beginning the first few days of life. Nonbreastfeeding infants and older children who consume less than 1 quart per day of vitamin D–fortified milk should also receive 400 International Units of vitamin D each day (Wagner, Grier, and AAP Section on Breastfeeding and Committee on Nutrition, 2008).

Vitamin K, required for blood coagulation, is produced by intestinal bacteria. However, the gut is sterile at birth, and a few days are required for intestinal flora to become established and produce vitamin K. To prevent hemorrhagic problems in the newborn an injection of vitamin K is given at birth to all newborns, regardless of feeding method (AAP Section on Breastfeeding, 2012).

The breastfed infant's vitamin B_{12} intake depends on the mother's dietary intake and stores. Mothers who are on strict vegetarian (vegan) diets and those who consume few dairy products, eggs, or meat are at risk for vitamin B_{12} deficiency. Breastfed infants of vegan mothers should be supplemented with vitamin B_{12} from birth.

Minerals

The mineral content of commercial infant formula is designed to reflect that of breast milk. Unmodified cow's milk is much higher in mineral content than human milk, which also makes it unsuitable for infants during the first year of life. Minerals are typically highest in human milk during the first few days after birth and decrease slightly throughout lactation.

The ratio of calcium to phosphorus in human milk is 2:1, an optimal proportion for bone mineralization. Although cow's milk is high in calcium, the calcium/phosphorus ratio is low, resulting in decreased calcium absorption. Consequently young infants fed unmodified cow's milk are at risk for hypocalcemia, seizures, and tetany. The calcium/phosphorus ratio in commercial infant formula is between that of human milk and cow's milk.

Iron levels are low in all types of milk; however, iron from human milk is better absorbed than iron from cow's milk, iron-fortified formula, or infant cereals. Breastfed infants draw on iron reserves deposited in utero and benefit from the high lactose and vitamin C levels in human milk that facilitate iron absorption. Full-term infants have enough iron stores from the mother to last for the first 4 months. After 4 months of age, infants who are exclusively breastfed are at risk for iron deficiency. The AAP recommends giving exclusively breastfed infants an iron supplement (1 mg/kg/day) beginning at 4 months and continuing until the infant is consuming iron-containing complementary foods such as iron-fortified cereals. Infants who are partially breastfed should receive the same iron supplement if more than half of their daily feedings consists of human milk and they are not consuming iron-rich foods (Baker, Greer, and the AAP Committee on Nutrition, 2010). Formula-feeding infants should receive an iron-fortified commercial infant formula until 12 months of age. Infants younger than 1 year should never be fed whole milk (Baker, Greer, and the AAP Committee on Nutrition, 2010).

Fluoride levels in human milk and commercial formulas are low. This mineral, which is important in preventing dental caries, can cause spotting of the permanent teeth (fluorosis) in excess amounts. Experts recommend that no fluoride supplements be given to infants younger than 6 months. From 6 months to 3 years, fluoride supplements are based on the concentration of fluoride in the water supply (AAP Section on Breastfeeding, 2012).

BREASTFEEDING

Anatomy of the Lactating Breast

Each female breast is composed of approximately 15 to 20 segments (lobes) embedded in fat and connective tissues and well supplied with blood vessels, lymphatic vessels, and nerves (Fig. 24-1). Within each lobe is glandular tissue consisting of alveoli, the milk-producing cells, surrounded by myoepithelial cells that contract to send the milk forward to the nipple during milk ejection. Each nipple has multiple pores that transfer milk to the suckling infant. The ratio of glandular to adipose tissue in the lactating breast is approximately 2:1 compared with a 1:1 ratio in the nonlactating breast. Within each breast is a complex, intertwining network of milk ducts that transport milk from the alveoli to the nipple. The milk ducts dilate and expand at milk ejection. Previous thinking held that the milk ducts converged behind the nipple in lactiferous sinuses, which acted as reservoirs for milk. However, research based on ultrasonography of lactating breasts has shown that these sinuses do not exist and, in fact, glandular tissue can be found directly beneath the nipple (Geddes, 2007; Ramsay, Kent, Hartmann, et al., 2005) (Fig. 24-2).

The size and shape of the breast are not accurate indicators of its ability to produce milk. Although nearly every woman can

lactate, a small number have insufficient mammary gland development to breastfeed their infants exclusively. Typically these women experience few breast changes during puberty or early pregnancy. In some cases they are still able to produce some breast milk, although the quantity is not likely to be sufficient to meet the nutritional needs of the infant. These mothers can offer supplemental nutrition to support optimal infant growth. Devices are available to allow mothers to offer supplements while the baby is nursing at the breast.

Because of the effects of estrogen, progesterone, human placental lactogen, and other hormones of pregnancy, changes occur in the breasts in preparation for lactation. Breasts increase in size corresponding to growth of glandular and adipose tissue. Blood flow to the breasts nearly doubles during pregnancy. Sensitivity of the breasts increases, and veins become more prominent. The nipples become more erect, and the areolae darken. Nipples and areolae enlarge. Around week 16 of gestation the alveoli begin producing prepartum milk or colostrum. Montgomery glands on the areola enlarge. The oily substance secreted by these sebaceous glands helps provide protection against the mechanical stress of sucking and invasion by pathogens. The odor of the secretions can be a means of communication with the infant.

Lactogenesis

After the mother gives birth a precipitous fall in progesterone triggers the release of prolactin from the anterior pituitary gland. During pregnancy prolactin prepares the breasts to secrete milk and during lactation to synthesize and secrete milk. Prolactin levels are highest during the first 10 days after birth, gradually declining over time but remaining above baseline levels for the duration of lactation. Prolactin is produced in response to infant suckling and emptying of the breasts (Fig. 24-3, *A*). Milk production is a *supply-meets-demand system* (i.e., as milk is removed from the breast, more is produced). Incomplete removal of milk from the breasts can lead to decreased milk supply. Oxytocin is essential to lactation. As the nipple is stimulated by the suckling infant, the posterior pituitary is prompted by the hypothalamus to produce oxytocin. This hormone is responsible for the milk ejection reflex (MER), or *let-down reflex* (see Fig. 24-3, *B*). The myoepithelial cells surrounding the alveoli respond to oxytocin by contracting and sending the milk forward through the ducts to the nipple. The MER is triggered multiple times during a feeding session. Thoughts, sights, sounds, or odors that the mother associates with her baby (or

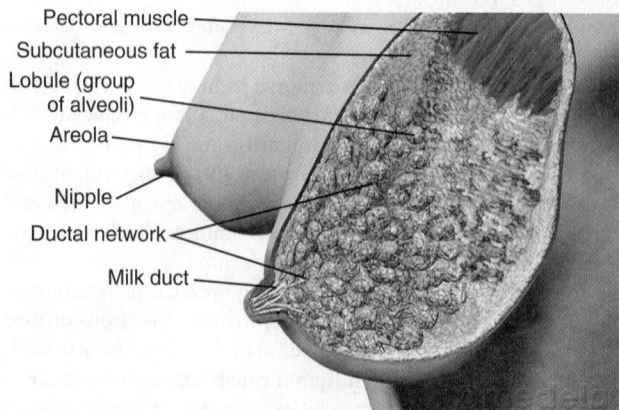

FIG 24-1 Anatomy of the lactating breast. (Copyright © 2013 Medela.)

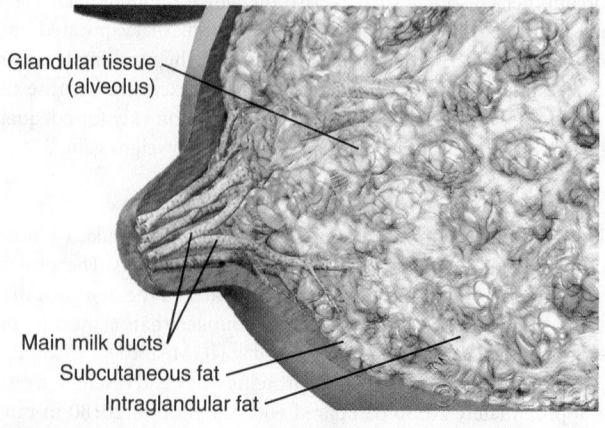

FIG 24-2 Enhanced view of milk glands and ducts. (Copyright © 2013 Medela.)

other babies) such as hearing the baby cry can trigger the MER. Many women report a tingling "pins and needles" sensation in the breasts as milk ejection occurs, although some mothers can detect milk ejection only by observing the sucking and swallowing of the infant. The MER also can occur during sexual activity because oxytocin is released during orgasm. The reflex can be inhibited by fear, stress, and alcohol consumption.

> ### ! NURSING ALERT
>
> Be cautious in referring to the MER as "let-down." Some women may interpret let-down as being associated with feelings of depression.

Oxytocin is the same hormone that stimulates uterine contractions during labor. Consequently the MER can be triggered during labor, as evidenced by leakage of colostrum. This reflex readies the breasts for immediate feeding by the infant after birth. Oxytocin has the important function of contracting the mother's uterus after birth to control postpartum bleeding and promote uterine involution. Thus mothers who breastfeed are at decreased risk for postpartum hemorrhage. Uterine contractions that occur with breastfeeding are often painful during and after feeding for the first 3 to 5 days.

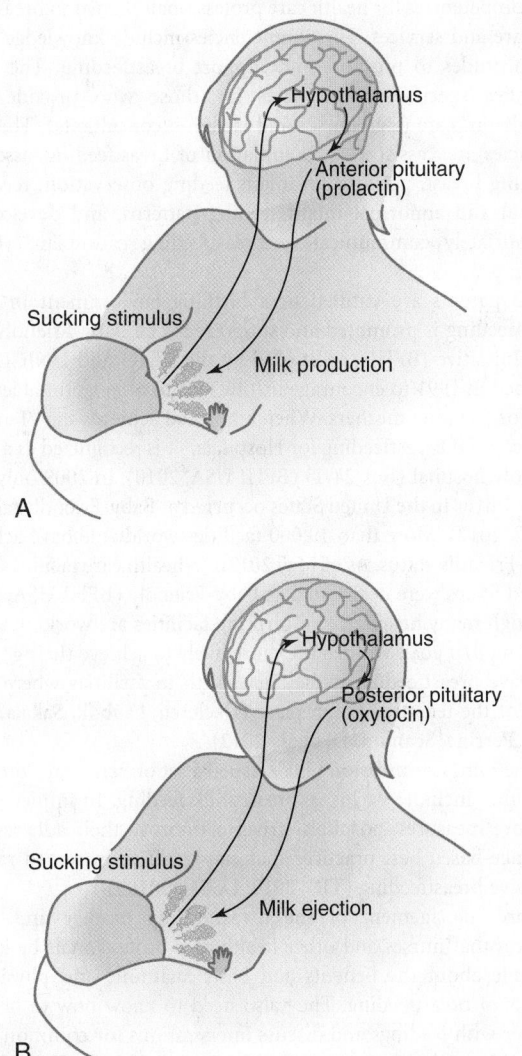

FIG 24-3 Maternal breastfeeding reflexes. **A,** Milk production. **B,** Milk ejection (let-down).

These "afterpains" are more common in multiparas and tend to resolve completely within 1 week after birth.

Prolactin and oxytocin have been called the *mothering hormones* because they affect the postpartum woman's emotions and her physical state. Many women report feeling thirsty or very relaxed during breastfeeding, probably as a result of these hormones.

The nipple-erection reflex is an important part of lactation. When the infant cries, suckles, or rubs against the breast, the nipple becomes erect, which aids in the propulsion of milk through the ducts to the nipple pores. Nipple sizes, shapes, and ability to become erect vary with individuals. Some women have flat or inverted nipples that do not become erect with stimulation; these women likely need assistance with effective latch. Their infants should not be offered bottles or pacifiers until breastfeeding is well established.

Uniqueness of Human Milk

Human milk is the ideal food for human infants. It is a dynamic substance with a composition that changes to meet the changing nutritional and immunologic needs of the growing infant. Breast milk is specific to the needs of each infant; for example, the milk produced by mothers of preterm infants differs in composition from that of mothers who give birth at term.

Human milk contains immunologically active components that provide some protection against a broad spectrum of bacterial, viral, and protozoal infections. The major immunoglobulin (Ig) in human milk is secretory IgA; IgG, IgM, IgD, and IgE are also present. Human milk also contains T and B lymphocytes, epidermal growth factor, cytokines, interleukins, bifidus factor, complement (C3 and C4), and lactoferrin, all of which have a specific role in preventing localized and systemic bacterial and viral infections (Lawrence and Lawrence, 2011a).

Human milk composition and volumes vary according to the stage of lactation. In lactogenesis stage I, beginning at approximately 16 to 18 weeks of pregnancy, the breasts are preparing for milk production by producing prepartum milk or colostrum. Stage II of lactogenesis begins with birth as progesterone levels drop sharply when the placenta is removed. For the first 2 to 3 days after birth, the baby receives colostrum, a clear, yellowish fluid that is rich in antibodies and higher in protein but lower in fat than mature milk. The high protein level of colostrum facilitates binding of bilirubin, and the laxative action of colostrum promotes early passage of meconium. Colostrum is important in the establishment of normal *Lactobacillus bifidus* flora in the infant's digestive tract. It gradually changes to transitional milk. By 3 to 5 days after birth the woman experiences a noticeable increase in milk production. This is often referred to as *the milk coming in*. Breast milk continues to change in composition for approximately 10 days, when the mature milk is established. This is stage III of lactogenesis (Lawrence and Lawrence, 2011a).

The composition of human milk changes over time as the infant grows and develops. Fat is the most variable component of human milk with changes in concentration over a feeding, over a 24-hour period, and across time. Variations in fat content exist between breasts and among individuals (Lawrence and Lawrence, 2011a). During each feeding the concentration of fat gradually increases from the lower fat foremilk to the richer hindmilk. The hindmilk contains the denser calories from fat necessary for ensuring optimal growth and contentment between feedings. Because of this changing composition of human milk during each feeding, breastfeeding the infant long enough to supply a balanced feeding is important.

Milk production gradually increases as the baby grows. Infants have fairly predictable growth spurts (at approximately 10 days, 3 weeks, 6 weeks, 3 months, and 6 months), when more frequent feedings stimulate increased milk production. These growth spurts usually last 24 to 48 hours, after which the infants resume their usual feeding pattern as the mother's milk supply increases.

CARE MANAGEMENT

Supporting Breastfeeding Mothers and Infants

The key to encouraging mothers to breastfeed is education and anticipatory guidance, beginning as early as possible during and even before pregnancy. Each encounter with an expectant mother is an opportunity to educate, dispel myths, clarify misinformation, and address concerns. Prenatal education and preparation for breastfeeding influence feeding decisions, breastfeeding success, and the amount of time that women breastfeed. Prenatal preparation ideally includes the father of the baby, partner, or another significant support person and provides information about benefits of breastfeeding and how he or she can participate in infant care and nurturing.

Connecting expectant mothers with women from similar backgrounds who are breastfeeding or have successfully breastfed is often helpful. Nursing mothers' support groups such as La Leche League or Mocha Moms provide information about breastfeeding along with opportunities for breastfeeding mothers to interact with one another and share concerns (Fig. 24-4). Peer counseling programs such as those instituted by WIC are beneficial.

For women with limited access to health care, the postpartum period may provide the first opportunity for education about breastfeeding. Even women who have indicated the desire to formula feed can benefit from information about the benefits of breastfeeding. Offering these women the chance to try breastfeeding with the assistance of a nurse or lactation consultant can influence a change in infant feeding practices.

Promoting feelings of competence and confidence in the breastfeeding mother and reinforcing the unequaled contribution she is making toward the health and well-being of her infant are the responsibility of the nurse and other health care professionals. The first 2 weeks of breastfeeding can be the most challenging as mothers are adjusting to life with a newborn, the baby is learning to latch on and feed effectively, and the mother may be experiencing nipple or breast discomfort. This is a time when support is critical. Primiparous women are most likely to experience early breastfeeding problems, which often result in less exclusive breastfeeding and shorter duration of breastfeeding (Chantry, 2011). Anticipatory guidance during the prenatal period and especially during the hospital stay after birth can provide the mother with information and increase her confidence in her ability to successfully breastfeed her infant. New mothers need access to lactation support following discharge through primary care offices or outpatient lactation services. Peer support is also helpful.

The most common reasons for breastfeeding cessation are insufficient milk supply, painful nipples, and problems getting the infant to feed (Lauwers and Swisher, 2011; Lawrence and Lawrence, 2011a). Early and ongoing assistance and support from health care professionals to prevent and address problems with breastfeeding can help promote a successful and satisfying breastfeeding experience for mothers and infants. Many health care agencies have certified lactation consultants on staff. These health care professionals, who are usually nurses, have specialized training and experience in helping breastfeeding mothers and infants.

The U.S. Breastfeeding Committee (USBC, 2010a) has identified key competencies for health care professionals related to breastfeeding care and services. The competencies include knowledge, skills, and attitudes to promote and support breastfeeding. The USBC identifies specific competencies for those who provide more "hands-on" care (e.g., nurses and lactation consultants). The competencies are: "assist in early initiation of breastfeeding, assess the lactating breast, perform an infant feeding observation, recognize normal and abnormal infant feeding patterns, and develop and appropriately communicate a breastfeeding care plan" (USBC, 2010a, p. 5).

All parents are entitled to a birthing environment in which breastfeeding is promoted and supported. The Baby-Friendly Hospital Initiative (BFHI), sponsored by the WHO and UNICEF, was founded in 1991 to encourage institutions to offer optimal levels of care for lactating mothers. When a hospital achieves the "Ten Steps to Successful Breastfeeding for Hospitals," it is recognized as a Baby-Friendly hospital (Box 24-1) (BFHI USA, 2010). In 2009 only 6.2% of live births in the United States occurred at Baby-Friendly facilities (CDC, 2012). More than 19,000 facilities worldwide have achieved Baby-Friendly status. As of May 2012 143 health care facilities in the United States were designated as Baby-Friendly (BFHI USA, 2012), although many hospitals and birthing facilities are working toward reaching that goal. Women are more likely to achieve their goals for exclusive breastfeeding if they give birth in facilities where all or most of the ten steps are in place (Declercq, Labbok, Sakala, et al., 2009; Perrine, Scanlon, Li, et al., 2012).

The Joint Commission (TJC) issued a set of Perinatal Core Measures that includes exclusive breast milk feeding. In implementing the core measures, hospitals strive to improve their adherence to evidence-based best practices that can result in increased rates of exclusive breastfeeding (TJC, 2012; USBC, 2010b).

Care management of the breastfeeding mother and infant requires that nurses and other health care professionals be knowledgeable about the benefits and basic anatomic and physiologic aspects of breastfeeding. They also need to know how to help the mother with feedings and discuss interventions for common problems. Ongoing support of the mother enhances her self-confidence and promotes a satisfying and successful breastfeeding experience. Mothers should be encouraged to ask for help with breastfeeding,

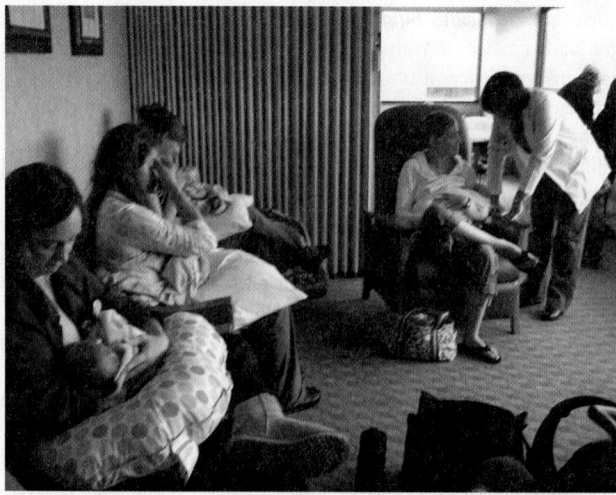

FIG 24-4 Breastfeeding mothers support group with lactation consultant. (Courtesy Shannon Perry, Phoenix, AZ.)

especially while they are in the hospital. Primiparas are likely to need the most assistance and in many facilities are routinely seen by lactation consultants. The mother needs to understand infant behaviors in relation to breastfeeding and recognize signs that the baby is ready to feed. Infants exhibit feeding-readiness cues or early signs of hunger. Instead of waiting to feed until the infant is crying in a distraught manner or withdrawing into sleep, the mother should attempt to breastfeed when the baby exhibits feeding cues (see Evidence-Based Practice box):

- Hand-to-mouth or hand-to-hand movements
- Sucking motions
- *Rooting reflex*—infant moves toward whatever touches the area around the mouth and attempts to suck
- Mouthing

Babies normally consume small amounts of milk with feedings during the first 3 days of life. As the baby adjusts to extrauterine life and the digestive tract is cleared of meconium, milk intake increases from 15 to 30 mL per feeding in the first 24 hours to 60 to 90 mL by the end of the first week.

In the postpartum period interventions focus on helping the mother and the newborn initiate successful breastfeeding. An important goal is to build maternal confidence in breastfeeding. Interventions to promote successful breastfeeding include educating and assisting mothers and their partners with basics such as latch and positioning, signs of adequate feeding, and self-care measures such as prevention of engorgement. It is important to provide the parents with a list of resources that they can contact after discharge from the hospital.

The ideal time to begin breastfeeding is within the first hour after birth (BFHI, 2010). Newborns without complications should be allowed to remain in direct skin-to-skin contact with the mother until the baby is able to breastfeed for the first time (AAP Section on Breastfeeding, 2012). This is true both for mothers who gave birth by cesarean and for those who gave birth vaginally. Early skin-to-skin contact is associated with higher rates of exclusive breastfeeding while in the hospital (Bramson, Lee, Moore, et al., 2010) and

increased duration of breastfeeding (Moore, Anderson, Bergman, et al., 2012).

Routine procedures such as vitamin K injection, eye prophylaxis, weighing, and bathing should be delayed until the neonate has completed the first feeding (AAP Section on Breastfeeding, 2012).

Positioning

For the initial feedings it can be advantageous to encourage and assist the mother to breastfeed in a semireclining position with the newborn lying prone, skin-to-skin on the mother's bare chest. Her body supports the baby. The mother is more relaxed, nipple pain is reduced or eliminated, and the mother has more freedom of movement to use her hands. The baby is able to use inborn reflexes to latch onto the breast and feed effectively. This approach to breastfeeding is based on the concept of "biological nurturing" (Colson, 2010, 2012).

The four traditional positions for breastfeeding are the football or clutch hold (under the arm), modified cradle or across-the-lap, cradle, and side-lying (Fig. 24-5). The mother should be encouraged to use the position that most easily facilitates latch while allowing maximal comfort. The football or clutch hold is often recommended for early feedings because the mother can see the baby's mouth easily as she guides the infant onto the nipple.

> ### ! NURSING ALERT
>
> To avoid confusion and misunderstanding when working with Hispanic women, avoid the term "football hold" to describe the under-the-arm or clutch position for breastfeeding—*football* refers to soccer in their culture.

Mothers who gave birth by cesarean often prefer the football or clutch hold. The modified cradle or across-the-lap hold works well for early feedings, especially with smaller babies. The side-lying position allows the mother to rest while breastfeeding. Women with perineal pain and swelling often prefer this position. Cradling is the most common breastfeeding position for infants who have learned to latch easily and feed effectively. Before discharge from the birth institution the nurse can help the mother try all of the positions so she will be confident in trying these positions at home.

During breastfeeding the mother should be as comfortable as possible. After arranging for privacy, the nurse might suggest that she empty her bladder and attend to other needs before starting a feeding session. The nurse who is assisting with breastfeeding should be at the mother's eye level. The mother holds the infant securely at the level of the breast, supported by firm pillows or folded blankets, facing toward her. The baby's mouth is directly in front of the nipple. The mother should support the baby's neck and shoulders with her hand and not push on the occiput. The baby's body is held in alignment (ears, shoulders, and hips are in a straight line) during latch and feeding.

Latch

Latch, or latch-on, is defined as placement of the infant's mouth over the nipple, areola, and breast, making a seal between the mouth and breast to create adequate suction for milk removal. In preparation for latch during early feedings the mother should manually express a few drops of colostrum or milk and spread it over the nipple. This action lubricates the nipple and entices the baby to open the mouth as the milk is tasted.

To facilitate latch the mother supports her breast in one hand with the thumb on top and four fingers underneath at the back edge of the areola. The breast is compressed slightly, as one might compress a large sandwich in preparing to take a bite, parallel to the

> ### BOX 24-1   TEN STEPS TO SUCCESSFUL BREASTFEEDING FOR HOSPITALS
>
> 1. Have a written breastfeeding policy that is communicated routinely to all health care staff.
> 2. Train all health care staff in skills necessary to implement this policy.
> 3. Inform all pregnant women about the benefits and management of breastfeeding.
> 4. Help mothers initiate breastfeeding within ½ hour of birth.
> 5. Show mothers how to breastfeed and maintain lactation, even if they should be separated from their infants.
> 6. Give newborn infants no food or drink other than breast milk unless medically indicated.
> 7. Practice rooming-in (i.e., allow mothers and infants to remain together 24 hours a day).
> 8. Encourage breastfeeding on demand.
> 9. Give no artificial teats or pacifiers (also called *dummies or soothers*) to breastfeeding infants.
> 10. Foster the establishment of breastfeeding support groups and refer mothers to them on discharge from the hospital or clinic.
>
> From WHO/UNICEF: *Baby friendly hospital initiative: revised and expanded for integrated care*, 2009, http://www.unicef.org/nutrition/index_24850.html.

EVIDENCE-BASED PRACTICE

Maternal Feeding Styles and Childhood Obesity

Ask the Question

Does caregiver responsiveness to infant feeding cues have an impact on overweight in early childhood and beyond?

Search for the Evidence

Search Strategies

English research-based publications on infant, feeding, satiety, breastfeeding, overweight, obesity were included.

Databases Used

Cochrane Collaborative Database, National Guidelines Clearinghouse (AHRQ), CINAHL, PubMed, and UpToDate

Critically Analyze the Evidence

- Childhood obesity can have its roots in the feeding patterns established in infancy. This research field for primary prevention of obesity is new, and many infant feeding studies are currently in the pipeline.
- Overfeeding can impair the infant's ability to self-regulate. Infants whose caregivers are responsive to an infant's hunger and satiety (full) cues are significantly less likely to be overweight (DiSantis, Hodges, Johnson, et al., 2011).
- Discordant responsiveness occurs when the caregiver perceives that the infant cannot recognize hunger or satiety. Restrictive feeding style is associated with maternal fear of causing obesity. Pressuring feeding style is associated with caregiver concern that the infant has poor appetite and will be underweight (Gross, Mendelsohn, Fierman, et al., 2011).
- In a Latina population a pressuring feeding style emerges as a result of belief that all infant crying or hand sucking is caused by hunger and that babies should always finish their bottles. Pressuring style is more likely in foreign-born women and women with less than a high-school education (Gross, Fierman, Mendelsohn, et al., 2010).
- Low-income, food-insecure mothers are more likely to be discordant, either restrictive or pressuring, than food-secure mothers (Gross, Mendelsohn, Fierman, et al., 2012).

Apply the Evidence: Nursing Implications

- Parental education about infant hunger and satiety cues ideally should begin in antenatal education classes and be reinforced intensively during the postpartum period. The nurse should point out the infant cues and praise the parents for appropriate responsiveness.
- Videos and printed material and warm lines should be made available to new parents. Specific suggestions about how much formula to feed initially and how voiding and stool patterns and weight gain reflect adequate nutrition can provide education guidelines.
- Assessing for familial and cultural beliefs enables the nurse to address parental and extended family concerns. The nurse can address how the

new mother might respond to well-meaning but incorrect comments from family and strangers.

- Education regarding the various newborn cries and their possible causes can reassure parents and their extended families that feeding should not be the first and only option.
- Breastfeeding is the gold standard for infant feeding because it is more difficult to overfeed.
- Nurses can advocate on a local and national level to eliminate food insecurity.

Quality and Safety Competencies:
Evidence-Based Practice*

Knowledge

Describe evidence-based practice to include the components of research evidence, clinical expertise, and patient/family values.

Parental education about correctly interpreting infant feeding cues can prevent overfeeding and childhood obesity.

Skills

Read original research and evidence reports related to area of practice.

As a new topic this field of research is developing tools to measure infant feeding cues and caregiver responsiveness and is developing interventions for clinical trials.

Attitudes

Appreciate the importance of regularly reading relevant professional journals.

As further research is published, further systematic analyses and clinical guidelines may emerge about the best interventions for healthy habits in infancy.

References

DiSantis KI, Hodges EA, Johnson SL, et al: The role of responsive feeding in overweight during infancy and toddlerhood: a systematic review, *Int J Obes (Lond)* 35(4):480–492, 2011.

Gross RS, Fierman AH, Mendelsohn AL, et al: Maternal perceptions of infant hunger, satiety, and pressuring feeding styles in an urban Latina WIC population, *Acad Pediatr* 10(1):29–35, 2010.

Gross RS, Mendelsohn AL, Fierman AH, et al: Maternal controlling feeding styles during early infancy, *Clin Pediatr (Phila)* 50(12):1125–1133, 2011.

Gross RS, Mendelsohn AL, Fierman AH, et al: Food insecurity and obesogenic maternal infant feeding styles and practices in low-income families, *Pediatrics* 130(2):254–261, 2012.

Pat Mahaffee Gingrich

*Adapted from QSEN at www.qsen.org/.

infant's lips, so an adequate amount of breast tissue is taken into the mouth with latch. Most mothers need to support the breast during feeding for at least the first days until the infant is adept at feeding.

The mother holds the baby close to the breast with the infant's mouth directly in front of the nipple. The infant who is displaying the rooting reflex with the mouth opening widely may easily latch on. If the infant is not readily opening the mouth, the mother tickles the baby's lips with her nipple, stimulating the mouth to open. When the mouth is open wide and the tongue is down, the mother quickly

"hugs" the baby to the breast, bringing him or her onto the nipple (Fig. 24-6). The amount of areola in the baby's mouth with correct latch depends on the size of the baby's mouth and the size of the areola and nipple. If breastfeeding is painful, the baby likely has not taken enough of the breast into the mouth, and the tongue is pinching the nipple.

Mothers may also use the asymmetric latch technique. When the baby's mouth opens widely, the mother moves the baby in toward her body so the chin and lower mandible make contact with the breast first followed by the top lip. When the baby is

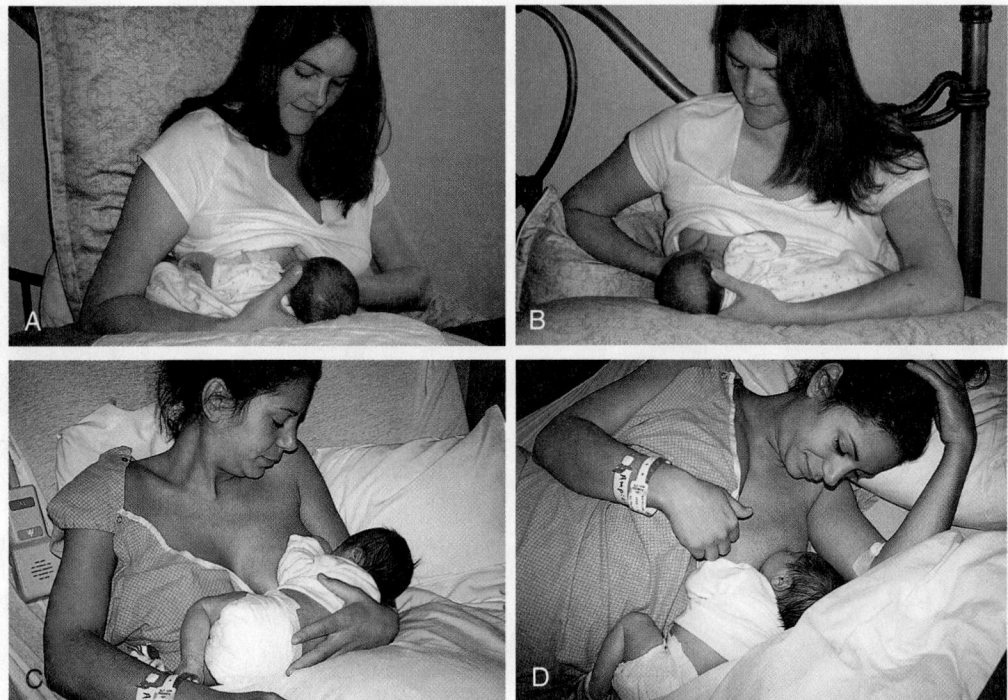

FIG 24-5 Breastfeeding positions. **A,** Football or clutch (under the arm) hold. **B,** Across the lap (modified cradle). **C,** Cradling. **D,** Lying down. (**A** and **B** Courtesy Kathryn Alden, Chapel Hill, NC. **C** and **D** Courtesy Marjorie Pyle, RNC, Lifecircle, Costa Mesa, CA.)

latched on, the nose is tilted slightly away from the mother's breast, and the chin is pressed into the underside of the breast. The infant's mouth placement is asymmetric on the areola; the lower part is covered by the baby's mouth, but the top is clearly visible above the top lip.

Once the infant is latched on and sucking, there are signs that the feeding is going well. These include: (1) the mother reports a firm tugging sensation on her nipple but feels no pinching or pain; (2) the baby sucks with cheeks rounded, not dimpled; (3) the baby's jaw glides smoothly with sucking; and (4) swallowing is usually audible. Sucking creates a vacuum in the intraoral cavity as the breast is compressed between the tongue and the palate. When the infant is latched on and sucking correctly, breastfeeding is not painful. If she feels pinching or pain after the initial sucks or does not feel a strong tugging sensation on the nipple, the latch and positioning are evaluated. Any time the signs of adequate latch and sucking are not present, the baby should be taken off the breast, and latch attempted again. To prevent nipple trauma as the baby is taken off the breast, the mother is instructed to break the suction by inserting a finger in the side of the baby's mouth between the gums and leaving it there until the nipple is completely out of the mouth (Fig. 24-7) (see Nursing Care Plan).

The nurse should observe at least one feeding every shift each day while the mother and newborn are in the hospital (AAP Section on Breastfeeding, 2012). Using a standard breastfeeding scoring tool such as the LATCH (Jenson, Wallace, and Kelsay, 1994) to document observations provides consistency in assessment criteria. With the LATCH assessment tool, each letter represents a scored item: *L*atch, *A*udible swallowing, *T*ype of nipple, *C*omfort level of the mother, and *H*old (positioning). During the feeding assessment the nurse can provide education about breastfeeding, help with feeding techniques, and offer support. If the mother's partner or other family members are present, the nurse can include them in the teaching and demonstrate how they can help the mother and provide support.

Milk Ejection or Let-Down

As the baby begins sucking on the nipple, the milk ejection, or let-down, reflex is stimulated (see Fig. 24-3, *B*). The following signs indicate that milk ejection has occurred:

- The mother may feel a tingling sensation in the nipples and breasts, although many women never feel when milk ejection (let-down) occurs.
- The baby's suck changes from quick, shallow sucks to a slower, more drawing sucking pattern.
- Audible swallowing is present as the baby sucks.
- In the early days the mother feels uterine cramping and can have increased lochia during and after feedings.
- The mother feels relaxed or drowsy during feedings.
- The opposite breast may leak.

Frequency of Feedings

Feeding patterns vary because every mother-infant dyad is unique. Breastfeeding frequency is influenced by a variety of factors, including the infant's age and weight, the infant's stomach capacity and gastric emptying time, and the storage capacity of the breast (i.e., the milk available when the breast is full).

Newborns need to breastfeed at least 8 to 12 times in a 24-hour period (AAP Section on Breastfeeding, 2012). Some infants breastfeed every 2 to 3 hours throughout a 24-hour period. Others cluster-feed, breastfeeding every hour or so for three to five feedings and then sleeping for 3 to 4 hours between clusters. During the first 24 to 48 hours after birth most babies do not awaken this often to feed. Parents need to understand that they should awaken the baby to feed at least every 3 hours during the day and at least every 4 hours at night. (Feeding frequency is determined by counting from the beginning of one feeding to the beginning of the next.) Once the infant is feeding well and gaining weight adequately, going to *demand feeding* is appropriate, in which case the infant determines the frequency of feedings. (With demand feeding the infant should still receive at least eight feedings in 24 hours.)

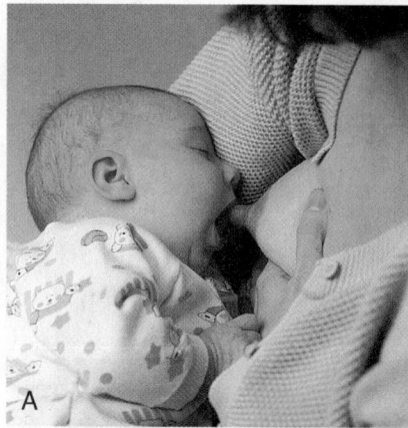

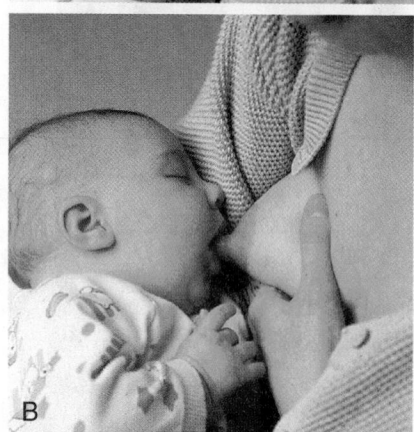

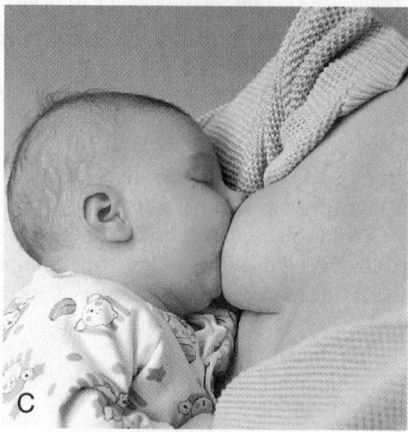

FIG 24-6 Latch. **A,** Mother tickles baby's lower lip with nipple until he or she opens wide. **B,** Once baby's mouth is opened wide, she quickly "hugs" baby to breast. **C,** Baby should have as much areola (dark area around nipple) in his or her mouth as possible, not just the nipple. (Copyright © 2013 Medela.)

! NURSING ALERT

Nurses should caution parents against attempting to place newborn infants on strict feeding schedules. Strict scheduling of feedings (forcing the baby wait for a set amount of time before feeding) can result in failure to meet the nutritional needs of infants.

Infants should be fed whenever they exhibit feeding cues. Keeping the baby close is the best way to observe and respond to these cues. Newborns should remain with mothers during the recovery period after birth and room-in during the hospital stay. At home babies should be kept nearby so parents can observe signs that the baby is

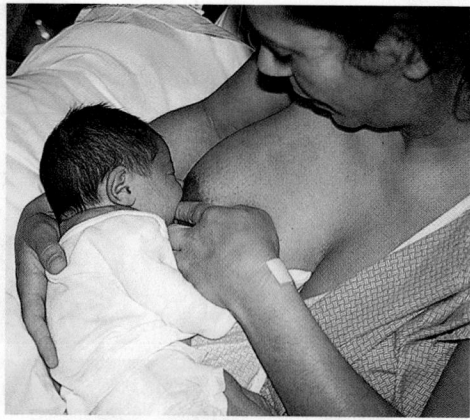

FIG 24-7 Removing infant from breast by inserting a finger to break suction. (Courtesy Marjorie Pyle, RNC, Lifecircle, Costa Mesa, CA.)

ready to feed. The mother and breastfeeding infant should sleep in proximity (in the same room but not in the same bed) to promote breastfeeding (AAP Section on Breastfeeding, 2012).

Duration of Feedings

The duration of breastfeeding sessions varies greatly because the timing of milk transfer differs for each mother-baby pair. The average time for early feedings is 30 to 40 minutes or approximately 15 to 20 minutes per breast. As infants grow they become more efficient at breastfeeding, and consequently the length of feedings decreases. The amount of time an infant spends breastfeeding is not a reliable indicator of the amount of milk the infant consumes because some of the time at the breast is spent in nonnutritive sucking.

In the early days after birth the mother may be instructed to feed on the first breast until the neonate falls asleep and try to wake the baby and offer the second breast. Some mothers prefer one-sided nursing, which means that the baby nurses only one breast at each feeding. The first breast offered should be alternated at each feeding to ensure that each breast receives equal stimulation and emptying.

Instead of instructing mothers to feed for a set number of minutes, nurses should teach them to look for signs that the baby has finished feeding (e.g., the baby's sucking and swallowing pattern has slowed, the breast is softened, the baby appears content and may fall asleep or release the nipple).

If a baby seems to be feeding effectively and the urine output is adequate but the weight gain is not satisfactory, the mother may be switching to the second breast too soon. Feeding on the first breast until it softens ensures that the baby receives the higher-fat hindmilk, which usually results in increased weight gain.

Indicators of Effective Breastfeeding

One of the most common concerns of breastfeeding mothers is how to determine if the baby is getting enough milk. In the newborn period, when breastfeeding is becoming established, parents should be taught about the signs that breastfeeding is going well. Awareness of these signs helps them recognize when problems arise so they can seek appropriate assistance (Box 24-2).

During the early days of breastfeeding, keeping a feeding diary can be helpful, recording the time and length of feedings and infant urine output and bowel movements. The data from the diary provide evidence of the effectiveness of breastfeeding and are useful to health care providers in assessing adequacy of feeding. Parents are instructed to take this feeding diary to the follow-up visit with the pediatric care provider.

⊚ NURSING CARE PLAN

Breastfeeding and Infant Nutrition

NURSING DIAGNOSIS	EXPECTED OUTCOME	NURSING INTERVENTIONS	RATIONALES
Ineffective Breastfeeding related to knowledge deficit of the mother as evidenced by ongoing incorrect latch technique	Mother will demonstrate correct latch technique. Infant will latch correctly and suck with gliding jaw movements and audible swallowing. Mother will report "tugging" but no nipple pain with infant suckling. Mother will express increased satisfaction with breastfeeding, and neonate will exhibit satisfaction of hunger and sucking needs.	Assess mother's knowledge and motivation for breastfeeding	To provide starting point for teaching
		Observe breastfeeding session at least once each shift	To provide baseline assessment for positive reinforcement and problem identification
		Describe and demonstrate ways to stimulate sucking reflex, various positions for breastfeeding, and use of pillows during session	To promote maternal and neonatal comfort and effective latch
		Monitor position of infant's mouth on areola and position of head and body	To give positive reinforcement for correct latch position or to correct poor latch position
		Teach mother ways to stimulate neonate to maintain an awake state by diapering, unwrapping, massaging, or burping	To complete breastfeeding session thoroughly and satisfactorily
		Give mother information regarding lactation diet, expression of milk by hand or pump, and storage of expressed breast milk	To provide basic information
		Provide mother with printed information on all aspects of breastfeeding	To reinforce verbal instructions and demonstrations
		Provide mother with information about follow-up care and support after discharge, including support groups, lactation consultants, and other community resources	To provide further information and group support
Ineffective Infant Feeding Pattern related to inability to coordinate sucking and swallowing	Neonate will coordinate sucking and swallowing to accomplish effective feeding pattern.	Assess for factors that can contribute to ineffective sucking and swallowing	To provide basis for plan of care
		Teach mother to observe feeding-readiness cues	To enhance effective feeding
		Modify feeding methods as needed	To maintain hydration status and nutritional requirements
		Promote calm, relaxed atmosphere	To provide pleasant breastfeeding experience for mother and neonate
		Refer to lactation consultant	To provide specialized support
Anxiety related to ineffective infant feeding pattern	Mother will report decrease in anxiety level and express satisfaction with breastfeeding.	Assess mother's feelings and anxieties about breastfeeding	To identify specific concerns
		Monitor maternal anxiety level during feeding sessions	To provide basis for care planning
		Provide education about breastfeeding	To help mother increase her knowledge about breastfeeding and improve her confidence
		Provide positive reinforcement for feeding pattern improvement	To decrease anxiety
		Monitor weight, intake, and output of neonate	To provide information regarding effective feeding
		Enlist assistance of support persons	To provide positive feedback for increasing skill
		Provide information for lactation support	To decrease anxiety after discharge
		Initiate follow-up (telephone calls, follow-up with health care provider, outpatient lactation consultant) as needed	To assess progress, detect problems, and provide support

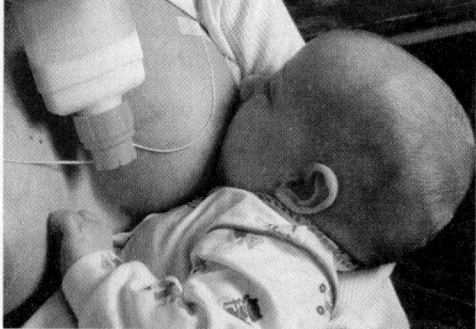

The infant's output is highly indicative of feeding adequacy. It is important that parents are aware of the expected changes in the characteristics of urine output and bowel movements during the early newborn period. As the volume of breast milk increases, urine becomes more dilute and should be light yellow; dark, concentrated urine can be associated with inadequate intake and possible dehydration. (Note: Infants with jaundice often have darker urine as bilirubin is excreted.) Infants should have at least six to eight sufficiently wet diapers (light yellow urine) every 24 hours after day 4. The first 1 to 2 days after birth newborns pass meconium stools, which are greenish black, thick, and sticky. By day 2 or 3 the stools become greener, thinner, and less sticky. If the mother's milk has come in by day 3 or 4, the stools start to appear greenish yellow and are looser. By the end of the first week breast milk stools are yellow, soft, and seedy (they resemble a mixture of mustard and cottage cheese). If an infant is still passing meconium stool by day 3 or 4, breastfeeding effectiveness and milk transfer should be assessed.

Infant should have at least three stools (quarter-size or larger) per day for the first month. Some babies stool with every feeding. The stooling pattern gradually changes; breastfed infants can continue to stool more than once per day or they may stool only every 2 or 3 days. As long as the baby continues to gain weight and appears healthy, this decrease in the number of bowel movements is normal.

Supplements, Bottles, and Pacifiers

Unless a medical indication exists, no supplements should be given to breastfeeding infants (AAP Section on Breastfeeding, 2012; ABM Protocol Committee, 2009). With sound breastfeeding knowledge and practice, supplements are rarely needed. Early supplementation by hospital staff undermines a new mother's confidence and models behavior that is counterproductive to prolonging breastfeeding.

If a supplement is deemed necessary, giving the baby expressed breast milk is best. Before supplementation it is important to perform a careful evaluation of the mother-infant dyad.

Possible indications for supplementary feeding include infant factors such as hypoglycemia, dehydration, weight loss of more than 7% associated with delayed lactogenesis, delayed passage of bowel

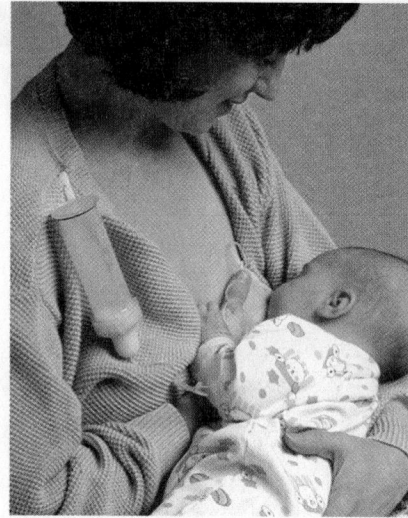

FIG 24-8 Supplemental nursing device. (Copyright © 2013 Medela.)

movements or meconium stool continued to day 5, poor milk transfer, or hyperbilirubinemia.

Maternal indications for possible supplementation include delayed lactogenesis and intolerable pain during feedings. Women who have had previous breast surgery such as augmentation or reduction may need to provide supplementary feedings for their infants (ABM Protocol Committee, 2009).

Newborns can become confused going from breast to bottle or bottle to breast when breastfeeding is first being established. Breastfeeding and bottle-feeding require different oral motor skills. It is best to avoid bottles until breastfeeding is well established, usually after 3 or 4 weeks.

If supplemental feeding is needed, nurses or lactation consultants can help parents use supplemental nursing devices. This allows the baby to be supplemented with expressed breast milk or infant formula while still breastfeeding (Fig. 24-8). Infants can also be fed with a spoon, dropper, cup, or syringe. If parents choose to use bottles, a slow-flow nipple is recommended. Although some parents combine breastfeeding and bottle-feeding, many babies never take a bottle and go directly from the breast to a cup.

Because of the correlation between pacifier use and a decreased risk of sudden infant death syndrome (SIDS), experts recommend pacifier use for healthy term infants at nap or sleep time, but only after breastfeeding is well established at about 3 or 4 weeks of age (AAP Section on Breastfeeding, 2012).

Special Considerations

Sleepy Baby. Some babies need to be awakened for feedings for the first few days after birth. If the infant is awakened from a sound sleep, attempts at feeding may be unsuccessful. Babies are more likely to feed if they are awakened from a light or active sleep state. Signs that the infant is in this sleep state are movements of the eyelids, body movements, and making sounds while sleeping. Unwrapping the baby, changing the diaper, sitting the baby upright, talking to him or her with variable pitch, gently massaging his or her chest or back, and stroking the palms or soles may bring the baby to an alert state. It is helpful to place the sleepy baby skin-to-skin with the mother; she can move the infant to the breast when feeding-readiness cues are apparent.

Fussy Baby. Babies sometimes awaken from sleep crying frantically. Although they are hungry, they cannot focus on feeding until they are calmed. Parents can swaddle the baby, hold him or her close, talk soothingly, and allow him or her to suck on a clean finger until calm enough to latch on to the breast. Placing the baby skin-to-skin with the mother can be very effective in calming a fussy infant. Fussiness during feeding can be the result of birth injury such as bruising of the head or fractured clavicle. Changing the feeding position can help alleviate this problem.

Infants who were suctioned extensively or intubated at birth can demonstrate an aversion to oral stimulation. The baby may scream and stiffen if anything approaches the mouth. Parents need to spend time holding and cuddling the baby before attempting to breastfeed.

An infant can become fussy and appear discontented when sucking if the nipple does not extend far enough into the mouth. The feeding can begin with well-organized sucks and swallows, but the infant soon begins to pull off the breast and cry. The mother should support her breast throughout the feeding so the nipple stays in the same position as the feeding proceeds and the breast softens.

Fussiness can be related to GI distress (e.g., cramping, gas pains). It can occur in response to an occasional feeding of infant formula; or it can be related to something the mother has ingested, although most women are able to eat a normal diet without causing GI distress to the breastfeeding infant. Persistent crying or refusing to breastfeed can indicate illness. Parents are instructed to notify the health care provider if either circumstance occurs.

Some mothers find that their babies are less fussy when placed in a sling or carrier. Some slings make it easy to breastfeed without removing the baby from the sling (Fig. 24-9).

Slow Weight Gain. Newborn infants typically lose 5% to 6% of body weight after birth before they begin to gain weight. Weight loss of more than 7% in a breastfeeding infant during the first 3 days of life needs to be investigated (Lauwers and Swisher, 2011). After the early milk has transitioned to mature milk, infants should gain approximately 110 to 200 g (3.9 to 7 oz) per week or 20 to 28 g (0.7 to 1 oz) per day for the first 3 months. (Breastfed infants usually do not gain weight as quickly as formula-fed infants.)

Parents are taught the warning signs of ineffective breastfeeding, including inadequate weight gain, minimal output, and feeding constantly. If any of these warning signs are present, the parent should notify the health care provider.

At times slow weight gain is related to inadequate breastfeeding. Feedings can be short or infrequent, or the infant can be latching incorrectly or sucking ineffectively or inefficiently. Other possibilities are illness or infection; malabsorption; or circumstances that increase the baby's energy needs such as congenital heart disease, cystic fibrosis, or simply being small for gestational age. Slow weight gain must be differentiated from failure to thrive; this can be a serious problem that warrants medical intervention.

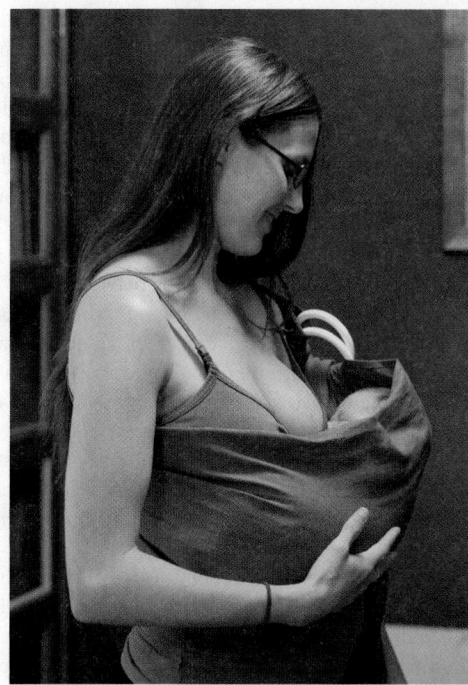

FIG 24-9 Baby breastfeeding while in sling. (Courtesy Julie Perry Nelson, Loveland, CO.)

Maternal factors can be the cause of slow weight gain. The mother can have a problem with inadequate emptying of the breasts, pain with feeding, or inappropriate timing of feedings. Inadequate glandular breast tissue or previous breast surgery can affect milk supply. Severe intrapartum or postpartum hemorrhage (Sheehan's syndrome), illness, or medications can decrease milk supply. Stress and fatigue also negatively affect milk production (Lauwers and Swisher, 2011; Lawrence and Lawrence, 2011a).

In most instances the solution to slow weight gain is to increase feeding frequency and to improve the feeding technique. Positioning and latch are evaluated, and adjustments are made. Adding a feeding or two in a 24-hour period can help. If the problem is a sleepy baby, parents are instructed in waking techniques.

Using alternate breast massage during feedings can help increase the amount of milk going to the infant. With this technique the mother massages her breast from the chest wall to the nipple whenever the baby has sucking pauses. This technique also can increase the fat content of the milk, which aids in weight gain.

When babies are calorie deprived and need supplementation, they can receive expressed breast milk or formula with a supplemental nursing device (see Fig. 24-8), spoon, cup, syringe, or bottle. In most cases supplementation is necessary only for a short time until the baby gains weight and is feeding adequately.

Jaundice. Chapter 22 discusses jaundice (hyperbilirubinemia) in the newborn in detail. Breastfeeding infants can develop *early-onset jaundice* or *breastfeeding-associated jaundice,* which is associated with insufficient feeding and infrequent stooling. Colostrum has a natural laxative effect and promotes early passage of meconium. Bilirubin is excreted from the body primarily through the intestines. Infrequent stooling allows bilirubin in the stool to be resorbed into the infant's system, thus increasing bilirubin levels (Blackburn, 2013). To prevent early-onset, breastfeeding-associated jaundice, newborns should be breastfed frequently during the first several days of life. Increased frequency of feedings is associated with decreased bilirubin levels.

To treat early-onset jaundice, breastfeeding is evaluated in terms of frequency and length of feedings, positioning, latch, and milk transfer. Factors such as a sleepy or lethargic infant or maternal breast engorgement can interfere with effective breastfeeding and should be corrected. If the infant's intake of milk needs to be increased, a supplemental feeding device can deliver additional breast milk or formula while the infant is nursing. Bilirubin levels are closely monitored (see Chapter 23).

Late-onset jaundice or *breast milk jaundice* affects a small number of breastfed infants and develops between 5 and 10 days of age. Affected infants are typically thriving, gaining weight, and stooling normally; all pathologic causes of jaundice have been ruled out. In the presence of other risk factors, hyperbilirubinemia can be severe enough to require phototherapy. In most cases of breast milk jaundice no intervention is necessary. Some health care providers recommend temporary interruption of breastfeeding for 12 to 24 hours to allow bilirubin levels to decrease, although this approach is not preferred (Blackburn, 2013; Lawrence and Lawrence, 2011a).

Any breastfeeding infant who develops jaundice should be evaluated carefully for weight loss greater than 7%, decreased milk intake, infrequent stooling (fewer than three stools per day by day 4), and decreased urine output (fewer than four to six wet diapers per day). Bilirubin levels should be assessed by serum testing or transcutaneous monitoring.

Preterm Infants. Human milk is the ideal food for preterm infants, with benefits that are unique and in addition to those received by term healthy infants. Breast milk enhances retinal maturation in the preterm infant and improves neurocognitive outcomes; it also decreases the risk of necrotizing enterocolitis. Greater physiologic stability occurs with breastfeeding compared with bottle-feeding (Lawrence and Lawrence, 2011a).

Initially preterm milk contains higher concentrations of energy, protein, sodium, chloride, potassium, iron, and magnesium than term milk. It is more similar to term milk by approximately 4 to 6 weeks. Depending on gestational age and physical condition, many preterm infants are capable of breastfeeding for at least some feedings each day. Mothers of preterm infants who are not able to breast-feed their infants should begin pumping their breasts as soon as possible after birth with a hospital-grade electric pump (Fig. 24-10). Pumping frequency depends on the mother's breastfeeding goals but may be recommended 8 to 10 times every 24 hours to establish the milk supply. These women are taught proper handling and storage of breast milk to minimize bacterial contamination and growth. Kangaroo care (skin-to-skin contact) is advised until the baby is able to breastfeed and while breastfeeding is established because it enhances milk production (Hurst and Meier, 2010; Lauwers and Swisher, 2011).

The mothers of preterm infants often receive specific emotional benefits in breastfeeding or providing breast milk for their babies. They find rewards in knowing that they can provide the healthiest nutrition for the infant and believe that breastfeeding enhances feelings of closeness to the infant.

Late Preterm Infants. Neonates born at 34 0/7 to 36 6/7 weeks of gestation are categorized as *late preterm infants*. These newborns are at risk for feeding difficulties because of their low energy stores and high energy demands (ABM, 2011a; Cooper, Holditch-Davis, Verklan et al., 2012). They tend to be sleepy, with minimal and short wakeful periods. Late preterm infants often tire easily while feeding and have a weak suck and low tone; these factors can contribute to inadequate milk intake. Early and extended skin-to-skin contact promotes breastfeeding and helps prevent hypothermia. Because these infants are more prone to positional apnea than term infants, mothers are advised to use the clutch (under the arm or football) hold for feeding, and avoid flexing the head, which can impede breathing. Often supplementation is needed; expressed breast milk is the optimal supplement, preferably at the breast using a supplemental feeding device (see Fig. 24-8) (Cleveland, 2010).

Breastfeeding Multiple Infants. Breastfeeding is especially beneficial to twins, triplets, and other higher-order multiples because of the immunologic and nutritional advantages and the opportunity for the mother to interact with each baby frequently. Most mothers are capable of producing an adequate milk supply for multiple infants. Parenting multiples can be overwhelming; mothers and their husbands or partners need extra support and help to learn how to manage feedings (Fig. 24-11).

Expressing and Storing Breast Milk

Breast milk expression is a common practice, typically performed to obtain breast milk for someone other than the mother to feed to the baby. It is most often associated with maternal employment. In some

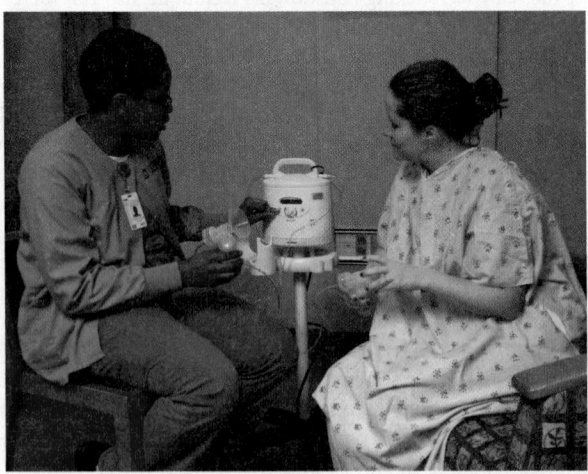

FIG 24-10 Nurse explains use of hospital-grade electric breast pump to new mother. (Courtesy Kathryn Alden, Chapel Hill, NC.)

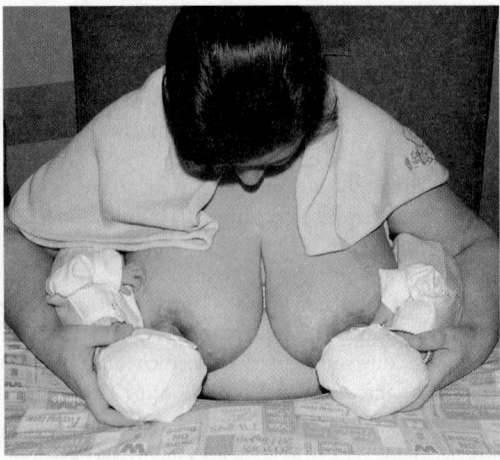

FIG 24-11 Breastfeeding twins. (Courtesy Cheryl Briggs, RNC, Annapolis, MD.)

situations expression of breast milk is necessary or desirable such as when engorgement occurs, when the mother's nipples are sore or damaged, when the mother and baby are separated as in the case of a preterm infant who remains in the hospital after the mother is discharged, or when the mother leaves the infant with a caregiver and will not be present for feeding. Some women express milk to have an emergency supply. Some women choose to pump exclusively, providing breast milk for their infants but never allowing the baby to suckle at the breast. Because pumping and hand expression are rarely as efficient as a baby in removing milk from the breast, the milk supply is never judged based solely on the volume expressed. Milk volume can be more accurately assessed using prefeeding and postfeeding infant weights, also known as *test weights* (Powers, 2010).

Hand Expression. All mothers should be instructed in hand expression. After thoroughly washing her hands, the mother places one hand on her breast at the edge of the areola. With her thumb above and fingers below, she presses in toward her chest wall and gently compresses the breast while rolling her thumb and fingers forward toward the nipple. She repeats these motions rhythmically until the milk begins to flow. The mother simply maintains steady, light pressure while the milk is flowing easily. The thumb and fingers should not pinch the breast or slip down to the nipple, and the mother should rotate her hand to reach all sections of the breast. Applying warm moist towels to the breasts and gently massaging can aid in stimulating the MER (Riordan and Hoover, 2010).

Mechanical Milk Expression (Pumping). For most women recommendations are to initiate pumping only after the milk supply is well established and the infant is latching and breastfeeding well. However, when breastfeeding is delayed after birth such as when babies are ill or preterm, mothers should begin pumping with an electric breast pump as soon as possible and continue to pump regularly until the infant is able to breastfeed effectively.

Numerous approaches to pumping can be used. Some women pump on awakening in the morning or after feedings. Others choose to pump one breast while the baby is feeding from the other; this is usually done if the baby typically feeds from only one breast at each feeding. Double pumping (pumping both breasts at the same time) saves time and can stimulate the milk supply more effectively than single pumping (Fig. 24-12).

The amount of milk obtained when pumping depends on the type of pump being used, the time of day, the time since the baby breastfed, the mother's milk supply, how practiced she is at pumping, and her comfort level (pumping is uncomfortable for some women). Breast milk can vary in color and consistency, depending on the time of day, the age of the baby, and foods the mother has eaten.

Types of Pumps. Many types of breast pumps are available, varying in price and effectiveness. Before purchasing or renting a breast pump, the mother will benefit from counseling by a nurse or lactation consultant to determine which pump best suits her needs. The flange (funnel-shaped device that fits over the nipple or areola) should fit the nipple to prevent nipple pain, trauma, and possible reduction in milk supply. Mothers are advised to use the lowest suction setting on electric pumps, increasing gradually if needed. Breast massage before and during pumping can increase the amount of milk obtained.

Manual or hand pumps are the least expensive and can be the most appropriate when portability and quietness of operation are important. These pumps are most often used by mothers who are pumping for an occasional bottle (Fig. 24-13).

Full-service electric pumps, or hospital-grade pumps (see Figs. 24-10 and 24-12), most closely duplicate the sucking action and pressure of the breastfeeding infant. When breastfeeding is delayed after birth (e.g., preterm or ill newborn) or when the mother and baby are separated for lengthy periods, these pumps are most appropriate. Because hospital-grade breast pumps are very heavy and expensive, portable versions of these pumps are available to rent for home use.

Electric self-cycling double pumps are efficient and easy to use. They are designed for working mothers. Some of these pumps come with carry bags containing coolers to store pumped milk.

Smaller electric or battery-operated pumps are typically used when pumping is performed occasionally, but some models are satisfactory for working mothers or others who pump on a regular basis.

Storage of Breast Milk. Mothers who express and feed breast milk to their infants need to be educated about safe practices for handling, storing, and feeding. Attention to hand hygiene and proper cleaning equipment can reduce the risk of bacterial contamination. This is especially important when mothers are providing milk for preterm or ill neonates (Hurst and Meier, 2010; Labiner-Wolfe and Fein, 2013). Guidelines for storing expressed breast milk for a healthy term infant are listed in the Patient Teaching box.

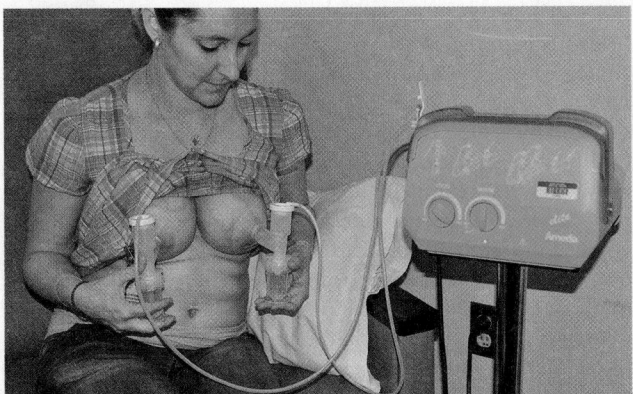

FIG 24-12 Bilateral breast pumping. (Courtesy Cheryl Briggs, RNC, Annapolis, MD.)

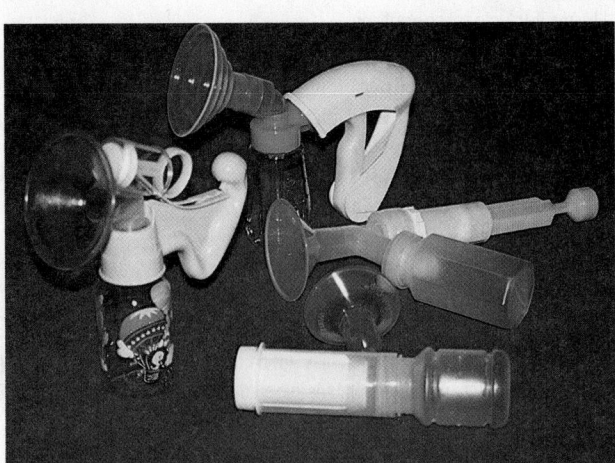

FIG 24-13 Manual breast pumps. (Courtesy Marjorie Pyle, RNC, Lifecircle, Costa Mesa, CA.)

PATIENT TEACHING

Breast Milk Storage Guidelines for Home Use for Full-Term Infants

- Before expressing or pumping breast milk, wash your hands.
- Containers for storing milk should be washed in hot, soapy water and rinsed thoroughly; they can also be washed in a dishwasher. If the water supply may not be clean, boil containers after washing. Plastic bags designed specifically for breast milk storage can be used for short-term storage (<72 hours).
- Write the date of expression on container before storing milk. A water-proof label is best.
- Store milk in serving sizes of 2 to 4 ounces to prevent waste.
- Storing breast milk in the refrigerator or freezer with other food items is acceptable.
- When storing milk in a refrigerator or freezer, place containers in the middle or back of the freezer, not on the door.
- When filling a storage container that will be frozen, fill only three quarters full, allowing space at the top of the container for expansion.
- To thaw frozen breast milk, place container in the refrigerator for gradual thawing or under warm, running water for quicker thawing. Never boil or microwave.
- Milk thawed in the refrigerator can be stored for 24 hours.
- Thawed breast milk should never be refrozen.
- Shake milk container before feeding baby and test the temperature of the milk on the inner aspect of your wrist.
- Any unused milk left in the bottle after feeding is discarded.

Human Milk Storage Guidelines for Full-Term Infants

LOCATION OF STORAGE	TEMPERATURE	RECOMMENDED SAFE DURATION FOR STORAGE
Room temperature	16-29° C (60-85° F)	3-4 hours optimal 6-8 hours acceptable*
Refrigerator	4° C (39° F) or lower	72 hours optimal 5-8 days acceptable*
Freezer	Less than −4° C (24° F)	6 months optimal 12 months acceptable

Modified from Academy of Breastfeeding Medicine Protocol Committee: ABM clinical protocol no. 8: Human milk storage information for home use for full-term infants, *Breastfeed Med* 5(3):127–130, 2010.
*Under very clean conditions.

The preferred containers for long-term storage of breast milk have hard sides such as hard plastic or glass with an airtight seal. Flexible polyethylene bags are not recommended for long-term milk storage (>72 hours) because there is a greater chance of leakage and loss of immune cells (Tully and Jones, 2010).

⚡ SAFETY ALERT

Breast milk is never thawed or heated in a microwave oven. Microwaving does not heat evenly and can cause encapsulated boiling bubbles to form in the center of the liquid, which may not be detected when drops of milk are checked for temperature. Babies have sustained severe burns to the mouth, throat, and upper GI tract as a result of microwaved milk. In addition, microwaving significantly decreases the antiinfective properties and vitamin C content. The safety of low-temperature microwaving is questionable (ABM Protocol Committee, 2010; Lawrence and Lawrence, 2011a).

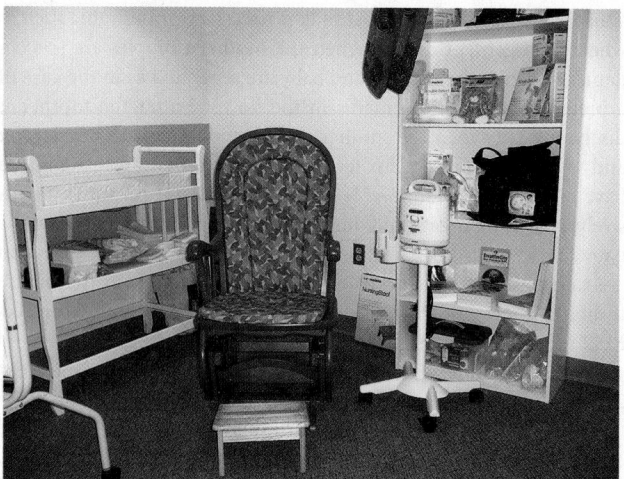

FIG 24-14 Lactation room. Note breast pump, rocking chair, nursing foot stool, changing table, books, and supplies. (Courtesy Cheryl Briggs, RNC, Annapolis, MD.)

Working and Breastfeeding

Returning to work after birth is associated with a decrease in the duration of breastfeeding. Women who return to work often face workplace challenges in breastfeeding such as lack of flexibility in work schedules, inadequate breaks to allow time for pumping, lack of privacy, lack of space for pumping, and lack of support from supervisors or co-workers. Increasing numbers of women are working from home and are likely to resume their jobs earlier than the traditional 6 week–to–3 month maternity leave. Issues that can challenge continued breastfeeding while working include fatigue, child care concerns, competing demands, and household responsibilities (Rojjanasrirat and Wambach, 2010).

Employed mothers can continue breastfeeding with appropriate guidance and support. They are encouraged to set realistic goals for employment and breastfeeding, with accurate information regarding the costs, risks, and benefits of available feeding options.

Women who are able to breastfeed their infants during the workday tend to breastfeed longer. With increasing numbers of women having the option of working from home, this situation is becoming more common. Many working mothers pump their milk while they are at work and save the milk for later feedings. Working mothers who are unable to pump or breastfeed their infants during the workday have the shortest duration of breastfeeding. Because women are a significant proportion of the workforce, many companies make provisions for breastfeeding women returning to work. Breastfeeding programs typically include on-site lactation rooms and/or education and consulting services. Lactation rooms that provide space and privacy for pumping are available at many worksites and on college campuses (Fig. 24-14). Workplace support for breastfeeding mothers has improved significantly in recent years. However, further efforts are needed to educate employers about the importance of supporting their breastfeeding employees. Employers need to realize that breastfeeding programs can provide short- and long-term cost savings with significant health benefits for mothers, infants, and families (Tuttle and Slavit, 2009). The Health Resources and Services Administration offers a free toolkit for employers: the "Business Case for Breastfeeding" outlines steps that employers can take to support breastfeeding employees (www.womenshealth.gov/breastfeeding/programs/business-case/tool-kit.cfm://aks/hrsa/gov).

Weaning

Weaning is initiated when babies are introduced to foods other than breast milk and concludes with the last breastfeeding. Gradual weaning over weeks or months is easier for mothers and infants than abrupt weaning. Abrupt weaning is likely to be distressing for mother and baby and physically uncomfortable for the mother.

Weaning is initiated by either the infant or the mother. With infant-led weaning the infant moves at his or her own pace in omitting feedings, which usually facilitates a gradual decrease in the mother's milk supply. Mother-led weaning means that the mother decides which feedings to drop. This approach is most easily undertaken by omitting the feeding of least interest to the baby or the one through which the infant is most likely to sleep. Every few days thereafter the mother drops another feeding until the infant is gradually weaned from the breast (Lauwers and Swisher, 2011).

Infants can be weaned directly from the breast to a cup. Bottles are usually offered to infants younger than 6 months. If the infant is weaned before 1 year of age, the infant should receive iron-fortified formula instead of cow's milk (AAP Section on Breastfeeding, 2012).

If abrupt weaning is necessary, breast engorgement often occurs. To relieve the discomfort the mother can take mild analgesics such as ibuprofen, wear a supportive bra, apply ice packs or cabbage leaves to the breasts, and pump small amounts if needed. When possible it is best to avoid pumping because the breasts should remain full enough to promote a decrease in the milk supply (Lauwers and Swisher, 2011).

Weaning is often a very emotional time for mothers; many believe that it is the end to a special, satisfying relationship with the infant and benefit from time to adapt to the changes. Sudden weaning can evoke feelings of guilt and disappointment. Some women go through a grieving period after weaning. Nurses and others can help the mother by discussing other ways to continue this nurturing relationship with the infant such as skin-to-skin contact while bottle-feeding or holding and cuddling the baby. Support from the father or partner and other family members is essential at this time.

Milk Banking

For infants who cannot be breastfed but who also cannot survive except on human milk, banked donor milk is critically important. Because of the antiinfective and growth-promoting properties of human milk and its superior nutrition, donor milk is used in many neonatal intensive care units for preterm or sick infants when the mother's own milk is not available. Donor milk also is used therapeutically in other situations such as for infants with short gut syndrome, infants with IgA deficiency who are not breastfed, and older children or adults with IgA deficiency (Tully and Jones, 2010).

The AAP recommends pasteurized donor milk for preterm infants if the mother's own milk is not available despite substantial lactation support (AAP Section on Breastfeeding, 2012). The value of donor milk is further emphasized by the ABM in their recommendation of pasteurized donor milk for the healthy term and preterm infant when the mother's milk is not available (ABM, 2009).

The Human Milk Banking Association of North America (HMBANA) (www.hmbana.org) has established annually reviewed guidelines for the operation of donor human milk banks. Currently there are 12 human milk banks in the United States and Canada (HMBANA, 2012). The milk banks collect, screen, process, and distribute the milk donated by lactating mothers. All donors are screened both by interview and serologically for communicable diseases. Donor milk is stored frozen until it is heat processed to kill potential pathogens; it is then refrozen for storage until it is

dispensed for use. The heat processing adds a level of protection for the recipient that is not possible with any other donor tissue or organ. Banked milk is dispensed only by prescription. A per-ounce fee is charged by the bank to pay for the processing costs, but the HMBANA guidelines prohibit payment to donors (Tully and Jones, 2010).

Care of the Mother

Nutrition. In general the breastfeeding mother should eat a healthy, well-balanced diet. Caloric intake during lactation should be sufficient to achieve the goal of balancing energy intake and expenditure. Most women are able to achieve that balance by adding 450 to 500 calories per day (AAP Section on Breastfeeding, 2012). Even with the increased caloric intake, women who are breastfeeding tend to lose weight more quickly than those who are formula feeding (Lawrence and Lawrence, 2011a).

Medications or diets that promote weight loss are not recommended for breastfeeding mothers. Rapid loss of large amounts of weight can be detrimental, given that fat-soluble contaminants to which the mother has been exposed are stored in body fat reserves and these can be released into the breast milk. Another potential consequence of weight loss is reduced milk production. For most women a weight loss of 1 to 2 kg (2.2 to 4.4 lb) per month is safe; however, if weight loss exceeds this amount, careful evaluation of infant weight and feeding pattern is recommended. The mother's diet is also evaluated.

No specific foods that the breastfeeding mother must consume or avoid have been identified. In most cases the woman can consume a normal diet, according to her personal preferences and cultural practices. Women may be told to continue taking their prenatal vitamins as long as they are breastfeeding.

It is recommended that breastfeeding mothers consume 200 to 300 mg of the ω-3 long-chain polyunsaturated fatty acids (DHA) daily. A DHA supplement and a multivitamin may be needed for women who are undernourished and those on vegan diets (AAP Section on Breastfeeding, 2012).

Mothers are encouraged to drink fluids in response to thirst (women often report feeling thirsty when they are breastfeeding). It can be helpful for the mother to know that if her urine appears light yellow (like lemonade), she is probably consuming adequate fluids. Increased consumption of water or other fluids by the mother does not increase milk supply, and overhydration can actually decrease milk production.

Rest. The breastfeeding mother should rest as much as possible, especially in the first 1 or 2 weeks after birth. Fatigue, stress, and worry can negatively affect milk production and ejection (let-down). The nurse can encourage the mother to sleep when the baby sleeps. Breastfeeding in a side-lying position promotes rest for the mother. The father, partner, grandparents, other relatives, and friends can help with household chores and caring for other children.

Breast Care. The breastfeeding mother's normal routine bathing is all that is necessary to keep her breasts clean. Soap can have a drying effect on nipples; therefore the mother should avoid washing the nipples with soap.

Breast creams should not be used routinely because they can block the natural oil secreted by the Montgomery glands on the areola.

The mother with flat or inverted nipples may benefit from wearing breast shells in her bra, although there is a lack of evidence to support the effectiveness of doing so. It is thought that these hard plastic devices exert mild pressure around the base of the nipple to encourage nipple eversion. Breast shells are also useful for sore

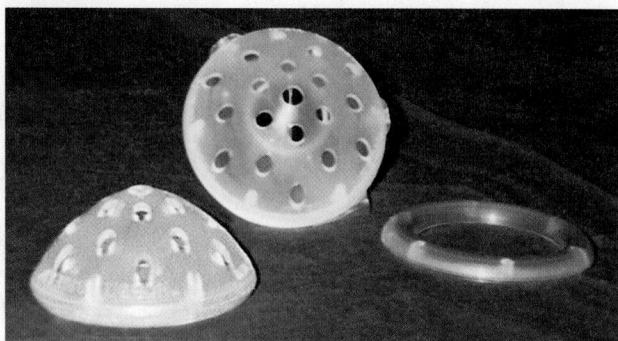

FIG 24-15 Breast shells.

nipples to keep the mother's bra or clothing from touching the nipples (Fig. 24-15).

If a mother needs breast support, she will likely be uncomfortable unless she wears a bra because otherwise the ligament that supports the breast (Cooper's ligament) will stretch and be painful. Bras should fit well and provide nonbinding support. Underwire or improperly fitting bras can cause clogged milk ducts.

If milk leakage between feedings is a problem, mothers can wear breast pads (disposable or washable) inside the bra. Plastic-lined breast pads are not recommended because they trap moisture and can contribute to sore nipples.

Breastfeeding and Contraception. Although breastfeeding confers a period of infertility, it is not considered an effective method of contraception unless the mother is strictly following guidelines for the lactational amenorrhea method of contraception (see Chapter 5). Breastfeeding delays the return of ovulation and menstruation; however, ovulation can occur before the first menstrual period after birth.

The contraceptive methods least likely to affect breastfeeding and milk production are the lactational amenorrhea method, natural family planning, barrier methods (diaphragm/cap, spermicides, condoms), and intrauterine devices. Hormonal contraceptives containing estrogen, including combined estrogen-progesterone pills or injectables, are not recommended for breastfeeding mothers because of the potential for reducing milk supply. Progestin-only contraceptives (pill, injection, or implant) are better options for breastfeeding mothers, although their use is not recommended during the first 4 weeks after birth (CDC, 2010) (see Chapter 5).

Breastfeeding During Pregnancy. Breastfeeding women can conceive and continue breastfeeding throughout the pregnancy if there are no medical contraindications (e.g., risk of preterm labor). For pregnant women who are breastfeeding, adequate nutrition is especially important to promote normal fetal growth.

Nipple tenderness associated with early pregnancy can cause discomfort when nursing the older child. The taste and composition of breast milk are altered during pregnancy, which can prompt some children to self-wean (Lawrence and Lawrence, 2011a).

When the baby is born, colostrum is produced. The practice of breastfeeding a newborn and an older child is called tandem nursing. The nurse should remind the mother always to feed the infant first to ensure that he or she is receiving adequate nutrition. The supply-meets-demand principle works in this situation, just as with breastfeeding multiples.

Breastfeeding After Breast Surgery. Previous breast surgery can affect the ability to produce breast milk and transfer it to the infant. Before undergoing breast surgery all women should discuss their lactation potential with their surgeon. Surgical procedures can damage nerves and interrupt milk ducts. Women who have had augmentation mammoplasty (breast implants) should be able to breastfeed successfully. However, if the procedure was done because of hypoplastic or asymmetric breasts, there can be concerns about adequate milk production. Reduction mammoplasty is more likely to cause problems with the ability to successfully lactate because of interference with milk ducts, removal of glandular tissue, and nerve damage. Even so, many women are still able to breastfeed completely or partially. Mothers with a history of breast surgery are instructed to monitor their infants carefully for signs of adequate feeding.

It is possible for some women with a history of breast cancer to breastfeed. However, treatment for breast cancer (surgery, radiation, chemotherapy) can result in reduced milk supply or absence of lactation in the affected breast.

Breastfeeding and Obesity. Women who are overweight or obese are more likely to experience delayed onset of lactogenesis stage II and reduced milk production compared with women of average weight. Breastfeeding duration tends to be shorter among this population of mothers (Lepe, Bacardí Gascón, Castañeda-González et al., 2011; Turcksin, Bel, Galjaard, et al., 2012; Wojcicki, 2011).

For women who have had bariatric surgery and plan to breastfeed, it is important to know when the surgery was performed. Nutrient and weight losses tend to stabilize approximately 12 to 18 months following the procedure. If the mother is consuming at least 1800 kcal/day and her weight has stabilized, her milk supply may be adequate. Breastfeeding mothers who have had a malabsorptive procedure such as a Roux-en-Y gastric by-pass should take daily dietary supplements, including a prenatal vitamin, vitamin B_{12}, and iron with vitamin C (to maximize absorption).

It is important to monitor infant weight gain. Vitamin B_{12} deficiency or decreased milk production can cause failure to thrive. In addition, vitamin B_{12} deficiency can result in infant anemia, developmental delays, and neurologic problems (Lamb, 2011).

Medications, Alcohol, Smoking, and Caffeine. Although much concern exists about the compatibility of drugs and breastfeeding, few drugs are absolutely contraindicated during lactation. Considerations in evaluating the safety of a specific medication during breastfeeding include the pharmacokinetics of the drug in the maternal system and the absorption, metabolism, distribution, storage, and excretion in the infant. The gestational and chronologic age of the infant, body weight, and breastfeeding pattern are also considered. In general any medication that is given to an infant routinely is safe for a mother who is breastfeeding. Breastfeeding mothers should be cautioned about taking any medications except those that are deemed essential. They are advised to check with their health care provider before taking any medication. Current, reliable information about the safety of medications and breastfeeding can be accessed through LactMed, a website provided by National Library of Medicine: http://toxnet.nlm.nih.gov/cgi-bin/sis/htmlgen?LACT.

Drugs that are absolutely contraindicated for breastfeeding mothers include antimetabolite and cytotoxic medications and drugs of abuse such as cocaine, heroin, amphetamines, and phencyclidine. Other medications that are generally contraindicated are amiodarone, chloramphenicol, doxepin, lithium, and radiopharmaceuticals (Hale, 2010).

It is recommended that women who have been stable on a methadone maintenance program should be allowed to breastfeed. Their infants may have decreased severity of neonatal abstinence symptoms when they are receiving breast milk (Lawrence and Lawrence, 2011a).

Certain medications can reduce maternal milk production and should be avoided. These include ergot alkaloids (bromocriptine, cabergoline, ergotamine) and pseudoephedrine (Hale, 2010).

As the use of antidepressant medications rises among childbearing women, there are increasing concerns about the effects of these medications on breastfeeding infants. A review of psychotropic medications indicates that the safest antidepressant drugs for breastfeeding mothers are sertraline, paroxetine, and fluvoxamine because there is minimal transfer into human milk. Antidepressants that are contraindicated while breastfeeding include citalopram, escitalopram, and fluoxetine because of the high levels excreted in breast milk, their long half-life, and adverse effects on the infant (Fortinguerra, Clavenna, and Bonati, 2009).

Alcohol consumption by breastfeeding mothers requires special caution. Although there is no standard recommendation about avoiding alcohol use when breastfeeding, it is important for mothers to be aware of potential risks. The AAP Section on Breastfeeding (2012) recommends that alcohol intake by breastfeeding women should be minimal. Intake of alcohol should be limited to occasional consumption of less than 0.5 g/kg of body weight (e.g., 8 oz. wine or 2 beers). Alcohol passes freely from the blood into breast milk, with peak levels occurring in 30 to 60 minutes on an empty stomach and 60 to 90 minutes when consumed with food. The MER and milk production can be adversely affected by maternal alcohol intake. If a breastfeeding mother chooses to have one or two drinks, she should not breastfeed for at least 2 hours. Contrary to popular belief, pumping and discarding milk does not accelerate removal of alcohol from the milk (Lawrence and Lawrence, 2011a).

Smoking by breastfeeding mothers should be strongly discouraged (AAP Section on Breastfeeding, 2012). It can impair milk production; it also exposes the infant to the risks of secondhand smoke. Nicotine is transferred to the infant in breast milk, whether the mother smokes or uses a nicotine patch, although the effect on the infant is uncertain. Lactating mothers who continue to smoke should be advised not to smoke within 2 hours before breastfeeding and never to smoke in the same room with the infant.

Moderate intake of caffeine by breastfeeding mothers appears to pose no risk to normal full-term infants. Minimal amounts of caffeine pass through to the infant in the breast milk. However, caffeine does accumulate in infants, especially if they are preterm (Lawrence and Lawrence, 2011a).

Herbal Preparations. Herbs and herbal preparations such as teas are often recommended for breastfeeding women, especially when there is a need to increase milk supply. Although these herbal preparations may seem to be effective for some women, the recommendations are based on anecdotal information. There is a lack of evidence related to the prevalence, effectiveness, and safety of herbs during breastfeeding. Herbals are not regulated by the Food and Drug Administration (FDA) because they are considered dietary supplements. Consequently there is a lack of quality control; unknown additives in and unknown side effects from herbal preparations can be harmful to the infant. Although some herbs may be considered safe, others contain pharmacologically active compounds that can have unfavorable effects. A thorough maternal history should include the use of any herbal remedies. Each remedy should then be evaluated for its compatibility with breastfeeding. The regional poison control center can provide information on the active properties of herbs (Lawrence and Lawrence, 2011a).

Common Concerns of the Breastfeeding Mother. The breastfeeding mother can experience some common problems. In most cases these complications are preventable if the mother receives appropriate education about breastfeeding. Early recognition and prompt resolution of these problems are important to prevent interruption of breastfeeding and promote the mother's comfort and sense of well-being. Emotional support provided by the nurse or

CRITICAL THINKING CASE STUDY

Breastfeeding: Engorgement and Nipple Soreness

The home care nurse visits Mary, a 35-year-old primipara who was discharged from the hospital 24 hours after giving birth to Matthew, a 3400 g (7.5 lb) baby boy who is now 3 days old. When Mary answers the door, she is tearful and appears very tired. Mary's mother is holding the baby, who is asleep in her arms. Mary tells the nurse that, when she awakened this morning, her breasts were very firm and "achy." She tried to latch the baby on to the breast, but the nipple was too flat, and he could not get it in his mouth; he was crying so hard that her mother gave him some formula. Mary's nipples appear irritated and cracked; she says "it hurts too much to feed him anyway." The baby has had only two wet diapers and no bowel movements in the last 24 hours. Mary says he cries much of the time and never seems to settle down to sleep for very long. Mary states, "I think it would be easier if I switch to formula."

1. Evidence—Does the nurse have enough evidence at this time to draw conclusions about the feeding difficulties experienced by this mother and infant?
2. Assumptions—What assumptions can be made about the following issues?
   a. Mary's milk supply
   b. Mary's sore nipples
   c. Matthew's urinary output and bowel elimination pattern
   d. Mary's commitment to breastfeeding
3. What implications and priorities for nursing care can be identified at this time?
4. Does the evidence objectively support your conclusion?

lactation consultant is essential to help allay the mother's frustration and anxiety and prevent early cessation of breastfeeding.

Engorgement. Engorgement is a common response of the breasts to the sudden change in hormones and the onset of significantly increased milk volume. It usually occurs 3 to 5 days after birth when the milk "comes in." As milk production rapidly increases, the volume can exceed the storage capacity of the alveoli in the breasts. If milk is not removed, the alveoli become distended, causing impairment of capillary blood flow surrounding the alveolar cells. As the blood vessels become more congested, fluid leaks into the surrounding tissue, resulting in edema. The milk ducts can be compressed by the tissue edema so milk cannot flow easily from the breasts. The breasts can become firm, tender, and hot and can appear shiny and taut. The areolae are firm, and the nipples can flatten, making it difficult for the infant in latching on to the breast (see Critical Thinking Case Study). Because back pressure on full milk glands inhibits milk production, if milk is not removed from the breasts, the milk supply can diminish.

When engorgement occurs, it is a temporary condition that is usually resolved within 24 hours. The mother is instructed to feed every 2 hours, softening at least one breast and pumping the other breast as needed to soften it. Pumping during engorgement does not cause a problematic increase in milk supply.

A variety of interventions are used to treat engorgement, although there is a lack of research evidence confirming the effectiveness of any specific intervention. Frequently used treatments for engorgement include the use of cold (ice packs, gel packs, cold compresses) after breastfeeding, chilled cabbage leaves, warmth (warm compresses, warm showers) before breastfeeding, antiinflammatory medications, breast massage, and pumping.

Because of the swelling of breast tissue surrounding the milk ducts, ice packs are often recommended in a 15- to 20-minutes on, 45-minutes off rotation between feedings. The ice packs should cover both breasts. Large bags of frozen peas make easy packs and can be refrozen between uses.

Fresh, raw cabbage leaves placed over the breasts between feedings can help relieve engorgement. It is thought that the effect of the cabbage leaves is related to the coolness of the leaves and phytoestrogens within them. They are washed, dried, chilled in the refrigerator or freezer, crushed slightly to break up the veins in the leaves, and then placed over the breasts for 15 to 20 minutes (Fig. 24-16). This treatment can be repeated for two or three sessions. Frequent application of cabbage leaves can decrease milk supply. Cabbage leaves are often very effective for formula-feeding mothers who want their milk to "dry up"; they are advised to wear the cabbage leaves constantly while engorged, replacing the leaves with fresh ones as they become wilted. Cabbage leaves should not be used if the mother is allergic to cabbage or develops a skin rash.

Antiinflammatory medications such as ibuprofen can help reduce the pain and swelling associated with engorgement. Ibuprofen also helps reduce fever and aching in the breasts that are often associated with engorgement.

Because heat increases blood flow, its application to an already congested breast is usually counterproductive. However, occasionally standing in a warm shower starts the milk leaking, or the mother may be able to manually express enough milk to soften the areola sufficiently to allow the baby to latch and breastfeed.

When engorgement occurs or as a result of excessive intravenous fluids during labor, the nipple and areola can become distended, making it difficult for the newborn to latch successfully. This can also occur in mothers who have received oxytocin for labor induction or augmentation. A technique called *reverse pressure softening* manually displaces the areolar interstitial fluid inward, softening the areola and making it easier for the infant's mouth to grasp the nipple and areola with latch (Lauwers and Swisher, 2011).

Sore Nipples. Mild nipple tenderness during the first few days of breastfeeding is common. Severe soreness or painful, abraded, cracked, or bleeding nipples are not normal and most often result from poor positioning, incorrect latch, improper suck, or infection. Severe nipple pain can be related to vasospasm or Raynaud's phenomenon (Lawrence and Lawrence, 2011a). The key to preventing sore nipples is correct breastfeeding technique. Limiting the time at the breast does not prevent sore nipples. They are often the result of the mother allowing the baby to latch onto the breast before the mouth is open wide.

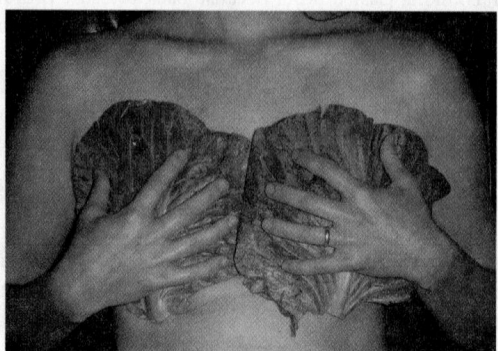

FIG 24-16 Cabbage leaves to treat engorgement. (Courtesy Kathryn Alden, Chapel Hill, NC.)

For the first few days after birth the mother can experience some mild discomfort with the infant's initial sucks. This should quickly dissipate as the milk begins to flow and acts as a lubricant. To make the initial sucks less painful the mother can express a few drops of colostrum or milk to moisten the nipple and areola before latch. If the mother continues to experience nipple pain or discomfort after the first few sucks, the nurse or lactation consultant helps her evaluate the latch and baby's position at the breast. If the nipple pain continues, the mother needs to remove the baby from the breast, breaking suction with her finger in the baby's mouth. Repositioning the mother or infant may be helpful in resolving the nipple discomfort. The mother then proceeds to attempt latch again, making sure that the baby's mouth is open wide before latching him or her on to the breast (see Fig. 24-6).

The nurse or lactation consultant can assess the infant's suck by inserting a clean, gloved finger into the mouth and stimulating the infant to suck. If the tongue is not extruding over the lower gum and the mother reports pain or pinching with sucking, the baby may have ankyloglossia, which is a short or tight frenulum (commonly known as tongue-tie). In some instances this condition is corrected surgically to free the tongue for less painful, more effective breastfeeding (Powers, 2010).

The treatment for sore nipples is first to identify the cause and then attempt to correct the problem. Early assessment and intervention are essential to increase the likelihood that the mother will continue to breastfeed. Once the problem is identified and corrected, sore nipples should heal within a few days, even though the baby continues to breastfeed regularly. When sore nipples occur, the woman is advised to start the feeding on the least sore nipple. It is important to assess the nipples for cracking or other damage to the skin integrity, which increases the risk of infection. If there is any break in the skin, the mother is advised to wipe the nipples with water after feeding to remove the baby's saliva. A thin coating of a topical antibiotic may help reduce the risk of infection and promote healing (the antibiotic cream or ointment should be removed before breastfeeding). Sore nipples should be open to air as much as possible. To promote comfort breast shells may be worn inside the bra; these devices allow air to circulate while keeping clothing off sore nipples (see Fig. 24-15).

Rapid healing of sore nipples is critical to relieve the mother's discomfort, maintain breastfeeding, and prevent mastitis. Although numerous creams, ointments, gels, and gel pads have been used to treat sore nipples, there is a lack of conclusive evidence related to the effectiveness of any particular method. However, because they have not been shown to cause harm, many health care professionals recommend their use. Some women report increased comfort for sore nipples with the application of purified lanolin or hydrogel pads (Smith and Riordan, 2010).

If nipples are extremely sore or damaged and if the mother cannot tolerate breastfeeding, she may need to use an electric breast pump for 24 to 48 hours to allow the nipples to begin healing before resuming breastfeeding. She should use a pump that effectively empties the breasts (see Figs. 24-10 and 24-12).

> **! NURSING ALERT**
>
> The mother who has a sudden onset of sore nipples or experiences sore nipples after days or weeks of comfortable breastfeeding likely has some type of nipple infection, most often bacterial or fungal (candidiasis). Other possible causes are skin problems such as psoriasis, allergic reactions, or vasospasm. Careful assessment and referral for treatment are needed (Smith and Riordan, 2010).

Insufficient Milk Supply. A major reason that women stop breastfeeding is perceived or actual insufficient milk supply (Brand, Kothari, and Stark, 2011; Lauwers and Swisher, 2011). Careful evaluation of the mother-infant dyad is needed, including assessment of infant weight gain or loss, feeding technique, and milk transfer and consideration of possible medical causes for low supply (e.g., medications, glandular insufficiency, previous breast surgery). Stress and fatigue can cause decreased milk production.

Interventions for increasing milk supply are based on causative factors. In many cases the mother is told to spend time with the baby skin-to-skin, increase feeding frequency, express milk using an electric pump, rest as much as possible, consume a healthy diet, and reduce stress. If nonpharmacologic measures to increase milk supply are not effective, galactogogues (medications or other substances that are believed to increase milk supply) may be recommended. Herbal galactagogues such as fenugreek, blessed thistle, goat's rue, and shatavari may increase milk production. However, herbal remedies should be used with caution.

Pharmaceutical galactogogues must be prescribed by the health care provider. Metoclopramide and domperidone are the most commonly prescribed medications; both are dopamine antagonists typically used to treat gastroesophageal reflux. They also increase prolactin levels, which enhances milk production. Metoclopramide has unpleasant side effects such as fatigue, irritability, and depression; there is a risk of severe allergic reaction. Domperidone is often prescribed for lactating women in Canada and other countries (Flanders, Lowe, Kramer et al., 2012), although it is not available in the United States except through some compounding pharmacies (ABM Protocol Committee, 2011b; Lauwers and Swisher, 2011). The FDA has issued a warning against the use of domperidone stating that "the importation of this drug presents a public health risk and violates the Federal Food, Drug, and Cosmetic Act (the Act)" (FDA, 2012).

Plugged Milk Ducts. A milk duct can become plugged or clogged, causing an area of the breast to become swollen and tender. This area typically does not empty or soften with feeding or pumping. A small white pearl may be visible on the tip of the nipple; this pearl is the curd of milk blocking the flow. The mother is afebrile and has no generalized symptoms.

Plugged milk ducts are most often the result of inadequate removal of milk from the breast, which can be caused by clothing that is too tight, a poorly fitting or underwire bra, or always using the same position for feeding. Application of warm compresses to the affected area and to the nipple before feeding helps promote emptying of the breast and release of the plug.

Frequent feeding is recommended, with the baby beginning the feeding on the affected side to foster more complete emptying. The mother is advised to massage the affected area while the infant nurses or while she is pumping. Varying feeding positions and feeding without wearing a bra may be useful in resolving a plugged duct (Riordan and Wambach, 2010).

Plugged milk ducts can increase susceptibility to breast infection. For recurrent plugged ducts, taking lecithin, a fat emulsifier, may be useful for the mother (Lawrence and Lawrence, 2011a).

Mastitis. Although the term mastitis means inflammation of the breast, it is most often used to refer to infection of the breast. It is characterized by the sudden onset of influenza-like symptoms, including fever, chills, body aches, and headache. The woman usually has localized breast pain and tenderness and a hot, reddened area on the breast. Mastitis most commonly occurs in the upper outer quadrant of the breast; one or both breasts can be affected. Most cases occur during the first 6 weeks of breastfeeding, but mastitis can occur at any time (Lawrence and Lawrence, 2011a).

Certain factors can predispose a woman to mastitis. Inadequate emptying of the breasts is common, which can be related to engorgement, plugged ducts, a sudden decrease in the number of feedings, abrupt weaning, or wearing underwire bras. Sore, cracked nipples can lead to mastitis by providing a portal of entry for causative organisms (*Staphylococcus, Streptococcus,* and *Escherichia coli* being most common). Stress and fatigue, maternal illness, ill family members, breast trauma, and poor maternal nutrition also are predisposing factors for mastitis (Lauwers and Swisher, 2011; Lawrence and Lawrence, 2011a). Breastfeeding mothers should be taught the signs of mastitis before they are discharged from the hospital after birth, and they need to know to call the health care provider promptly if the symptoms occur. Treatment includes antibiotics such as cephalexin or dicloxacillin for 10 to 14 days and analgesic and antipyretic medications such as ibuprofen. The mother is advised to rest as much as possible and breastfeed the baby or pump frequently, striving to empty the affected side adequately. Warm compresses to the breast before feeding or pumping can be useful. Adequate fluid intake and a balanced diet are important for the mother with mastitis (Lauwers and Swisher, 2011).

Complications of mastitis include breast abscess, chronic mastitis, and fungal infections of the breast. Most complications can be prevented by early recognition and treatment.

Follow-up After Hospital Discharge

Problems with sore nipples, engorgement, and jaundice are likely to occur after discharge from the birth institution. The nurse educates the mother about potential problems she may encounter once she is home. She should be given a list of resources for help with breastfeeding concerns. Community resources for breastfeeding mothers include lactation consultants in hospitals, primary care offices, or private practice; nurses in pediatric or obstetric offices; support groups such as La Leche League; and peer counseling programs (e.g., those offered through WIC). The Internet has many websites containing current and correct information about breastfeeding (e.g., www.breastfeeding.com) (see Community Focus box). The National Breastfeeding Helpline (1-800-994-9662) through the Office of Women's Health provides breastfeeding information and counseling by English- and Spanish-speaking counselors.

Telephone follow-up by nurses or lactation consultants in hospitals, birth centers, clinics, or offices within the first day or two after discharge can help identify problems and offer needed advice and support. Breastfeeding infants should be seen by a health care provider at 3 to 5 days of age and again at 2 to 3 weeks to assess weight

---

🏠 COMMUNITY FOCUS

Resources for Breastfeeding Mothers

- Visit the International Lactation Consultant Association (ILCA) website (www.ilca.org). What is the mission and vision of the association? Locate a board-certified lactation consultant in your community. What other resources are available for breastfeeding mothers after discharge from the hospital in your community?
- Visit the La Leche League International website (www.llli.org). What is the mission of the La Leche League? Locate a La Leche League group in your community.

gain and offer encouragement and support to the mother (AAP Section on Breastfeeding, 2012).

FORMULA FEEDING

Parent Education

The majority of infants receive at least some amount of commercial infant formula during their first year of life. Some parents choose formula feeding instead of breastfeeding; others combine the two methods. If the infant is weaned from breastfeeding before the first birthday, iron-fortified infant formula should be given (AAP Section on Breastfeeding, 2012).

It is important for nurses and other health care professionals to be intentional about providing education for parents related to formula preparation, feeding, and common problems they can encounter (Hancock and Brown, 2010). Mothers have reported that they do not get sufficient information from health care professionals about formula feeding (Lakshman, Ogilvie, and Ong, 2009). Because of the lack of clear information about the practical aspects of formula feeding, parents often rely on advice from friends and family. If that advice is incorrect and the parents use unsafe practices for formula preparation and feeding, the infant is at risk for food-borne illness and burns.

Readiness for Feeding

Ideally the first feeding of formula is given after the neonate's initial transition to extrauterine life. Feeding-readiness cues include stability of vital signs, effective breathing pattern, presence of bowel sounds, an active sucking reflex, and signs described earlier for breastfed infants.

Feeding Patterns

In the first 24 to 48 hours of life a newborn typically consumes 15 to 30 mL of formula at a feeding. Intake gradually increases during the first week of life. Most newborns are drinking 90 to 150 mL at a feeding by the end of the second week or sooner. The newborn infant should be fed at least every 3 to 4 hours, even if it is necessary to wake him or her for the feedings; however, rigid feeding schedules are not recommended. The infant showing an adequate weight gain can be allowed to sleep at night and be fed only on awakening. Most newborns need six to eight feedings in 24 hours; the number of feedings decreases as the infant matures and consumes more at each feeding. By 3 to 4 weeks after birth a fairly predictable feeding pattern has usually developed. Scheduling feedings arbitrarily at predetermined intervals may not meet a newborn's needs, but initiating feedings at convenient times often moves the feedings to times that work for the family.

Mothers usually notice increases in the infant's appetite at the age of approximately 10 days, 3 weeks, 6 weeks, 3 months, and 6 months. These appetite spurts correspond to growth spurts. Mothers should increase the amount of formula per feeding by approximately 30 mL to meet the baby's needs at these times.

Feeding Technique

Infants should be held for all feedings. During feedings parents are encouraged to sit comfortably, holding the infant close in a semi-upright position with good head support. Feedings provide opportunities to bond with the baby through touching, talking, singing, or reading to the infant. Parents should consider feedings a time of peaceful relaxation with the infant. Mothers who bottle-feed should be encouraged to spend some time with their newborns in skin-to-skin contact.

> ⚡ **SAFETY ALERT**
>
> A bottle should never be propped with a pillow or other inanimate object and left with the infant. This practice can result in choking, and it deprives the infant of important interaction during feeding. Moreover, propping the bottle has been implicated in causing nursing-bottle caries or decay of the first teeth resulting from continuous bathing of the teeth with carbohydrate-containing fluid as the infant sporadically sucks the nipple.

Newborns must learn to coordinate sucking, swallowing, and breathing as they feed. The typical fast flow of milk from bottles can create difficulty for an infant trying to learn to feed. A slow-flow nipple is often used for the first few weeks.

Traditionally parents are told to position the infant in a semi-reclining position and to hold the bottle so that fluid fills the nipple and none of the air in the bottle is allowed to enter it (Fig. 24-17, A). A more physiologic approach to bottle-feeding is called *paced bottle-feeding*. With this method of feeding the bottle is held at more of a horizontal angle; when the baby pauses between bursts of sucking, the parent withdraws the nipple, allowing it to rest on the baby's lip until he or she is ready to resume sucking (Lauwers and Swisher, 2011). This position slows the flow of milk from the bottle so the infant is more in control. Paced bottle-feeding works well for infants who are primarily breastfeeding but are occasionally fed from a bottle (see Patient Teaching box on p. 658 and Fig. 24-17, B).

If the infant falls asleep or ceases to suck, it usually indicates that he or she has consumed enough formula to feel satiated. Teach parents to look for these cues and avoid overfeeding, which can contribute to obesity.

Instruct parents to observe the infant for signs of stress during feeding, including turning the head, arching the back, choking, sputtering, changing color, moving the arms, and tensing fists (Lauwers and Swisher, 2011). When these signs occur, the parent should stop feeding and attempt to calm the infant before resuming. The signs can indicate that the infant is finished with the feeding and does not want to drink any more.

Most infants swallow air when fed from a bottle and need a chance to burp several times during a feeding. Parents are taught various positions that can be used for burping (Fig. 24-18).

Common Concerns

Parents need to know what to do if the infant spits up. They may need to decrease the amount of feeding or feed smaller amounts more frequently. Burping the infant several times during a feeding such as when the infant's sucking slows down or stops can decrease spitting. Holding the baby upright for 30 minutes after feeding and avoiding bouncing or placing him or her on the abdomen soon after the feeding is finished can also help. Spitting can be a result of overfeeding, or it can be symptomatic of gastroesophageal reflux. Parents should report vomiting one third or more of the feeding at most feeding sessions or projectile vomiting to the health care provider and should be cautioned to refrain from changing the infant's formula without consulting the health care provider.

Bottles and Nipples

Various brands and styles of bottles and nipples are available. Most babies feed well with any bottle and nipple. The bottles, nipples, rings, and caps should be washed in warm soapy water, using a bottle and nipple brush to facilitate thorough cleansing. They should be placed in boiling water for 5 minutes and allowed to air dry; this should be done at least before the first use and thereafter unless they

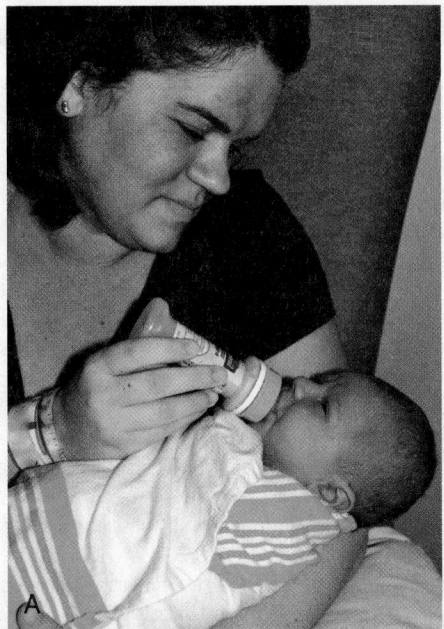

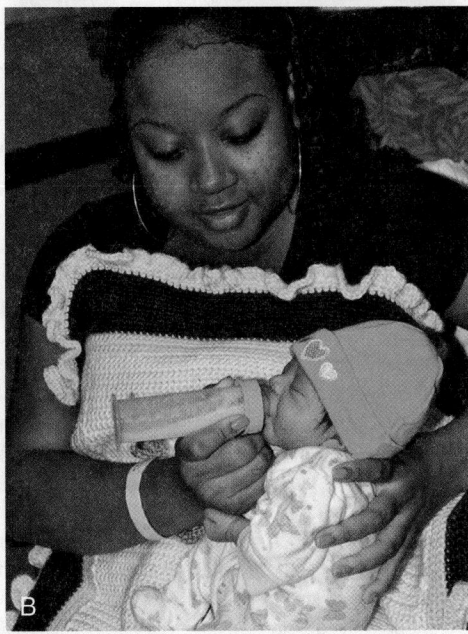

FIG 24-17 A, Bottle-feeding: traditional technique with infant semi-reclining. **B,** Paced bottle-feeding: infant is more upright. (Courtesy Cheryl Briggs, RNC, Annapolis, MD.)

are cleaned in a dishwasher (see Patient Teaching box on p. 658). Boiling of feeding equipment is recommended if the infant has oral thrush.

Infant Formulas
Commercial Formulas

Commercial infant formulas are designed to resemble human milk as closely as possible, although none has ever duplicated it. The exact composition of infant formula varies with the manufacturer, but all must meet specific standards.

Infants who are not breastfed should be given commercial iron-fortified formulas. Families with limited income may be eligible for services through the WIC program, which provides iron-fortified infant formula.

Commercially prepared formulas are cow's milk–based formulas that have been modified to closely resemble the nutritional content of human milk. The caloric content of standard infant formula is 20 kcal/oz. These formulas are altered from cow's milk by removing butterfat, decreasing the protein content, and adding vegetable oil and carbohydrate. Some have demineralized whey added to yield a whey/casein ratio of 60:40. Regardless of the commercial brand, the standard cow's milk–based formulas have essentially the same compositions of vitamins, minerals, protein, carbohydrates, and essential amino acids, with minor variations such as the source of carbohydrate; nucleotides to enhance immune function; and long-chain polyunsaturated fatty acids (DHA and ARA), which are thought to improve visual and cognitive function. Furthermore, FDA regulates the manufacture of infant formula in the United States to ensure product safety. Standard cow's milk–based formulas are sold as low-iron and iron-fortified formulas; however, only the iron-fortified formulas meet infants' requirements.

Four main categories of commercially prepared infant formulas are available: (1) cow's milk–based formulas; (2) soy-based formulas, commonly used for children who are lactose or cow's milk–protein intolerant; (3) casein- or whey-hydrolysate formulas, used primarily for children who cannot tolerate or digest cow's milk or soy-based formulas; and (4) amino acid formulas, used for infants with multiple food protein intolerances.

The AAP Committee on Nutrition indicates that few solid indications exist for the use of soy protein–based formulas instead of cow's milk–based formulas (Bhatia, Greer, and AAP Committee on Nutrition, 2008). Soy-based formulas are recommended for infants with galactosemia and congenital lactase deficiency; infants with secondary lactase deficiency may benefit as well. Infants with documented IgE allergies caused by cow's milk should be fed an extensively hydrolyzed protein formula. Soy protein–based formulas have not been proven to be effective against colic or in the prevention of allergy in healthy or high risk infants.

Alternate milk sources such as goat's milk; skim or low-fat milk; condensed milk; or raw, unpasteurized milk from any animal source should not be fed to infants because they are inadequate to support growth and can contain excess protein or an inadequate calcium/phosphorus ratio, which can cause seizures.

⚡ SAFETY ALERT

Because of concerns about potential harmful effects of bisphenol A (BPA), parents should be cautioned about using hard plastic polycarbonate baby bottles or containers. BPA is a chemical that is used to harden plastics, prevent bacterial contamination of foods, and prevent can rusting. It is in many food and liquid containers, including baby bottles. The AAP (2012) recommends avoiding clear plastic bottles or containers imprinted with the recycling number 7 and the letters PC and purchasing bottles that are certified or identified as BPA-free. Glass bottles are an alternative, but parents must be aware of the risk for injury if the bottle is dropped or broken. Because heat can cause the release of BPA from plastic, polycarbonate bottles should never be boiled, heated in the microwave, or washed in a dishwasher (AAP, 2012).

Formula Preparation

Commercial formulas are available in three forms: powder, concentrate, and ready to feed. All forms are equivalent in terms of nutritional content, but they vary considerably in cost.

- Ready-to-feed formula is the most expensive but the easiest to use. The desired amount is poured into the bottle. The

PATIENT TEACHING

Formula Preparation and Feeding

Formula Preparation

- Using warm soapy water, wash your hands, arms, and under your nails; rinse well. Clean and sanitize the surface where you will be preparing the bottles.
- Thoroughly wash bottles, nipples, rings, caps, can opener, and other preparation utensils in hot soapy water and rinse thoroughly. Squeeze water through nipples to make sure that the holes are open.
- Place bottles, nipples, rings, and caps in a pot and cover with water; boil for 5 minutes; remove items from pot with sanitized tongs and allow them to air dry. (Do this at least before using items the first time; thereafter you can continue to do this or place items in the dishwasher.)
- Note the expiration date on the formula container. It should be used before the expiration date. Any unopened expired formula should be returned to the place of purchase.
- Read the label on the container of formula and mix it exactly according to the directions.
- Mix formula with tap water deemed safe by the local health department. Allow cold water to run for 2 minutes before collecting it. Then bring it to a rolling boil and continue boiling for 1 to 2 minutes. If using bottled water, make sure that it is labeled as "sterile"; unsterile bottled water must be boiled. After boiling allow water to cool before mixing the formula but not for longer than 30 minutes.
- If using a can of ready-to-feed or concentrated formula, wash the top of the can with hot soapy water and rinse well. Shake the can before opening.
- Mixing formula
  - *Ready-to-feed:* No mixing is needed; do not add water. Pour desired amount of formula into clean bottle; add nipple and ring.
  - *Concentrate:* Pour desired amount of formula into clean bottle and add equal amount of cooled boiled water. Add nipple and ring and shake well.
  - *Powder:* When first opening the container of powder, write the date on the lid. Using the scoop from the container, add 1 scoop of powdered formula for each 2 ounces of boiled, cooled water in a clean bottle. For example, if 6 ounces of water is in the bottle, add three scoops of powder. Add nipple and ring and shake well.
- If preparing multiple bottles at the same time, place nipple right side up on each bottle and cover with a clean nipple cap. Use bottles within 48 hours.
- Opened cans of ready-to-feed or concentrated formula should be covered and refrigerated. Any unused portions must be discarded after 48 hours.
- Bottles or cans of unopened formula can be stored at room temperature.
- If the formula is refrigerated, warm it by placing the bottle in a pan of hot water. Never use a microwave to warm any food to be given to a baby. Test the temperature of the formula by letting a few drops fall on the inside of your wrist. If the formula feels comfortably warm to you, the temperature is correct.

Feeding Techniques and Tips

- Newborns should be fed at least every 3 to 4 hours and should never go longer than 4 hours without feeding until a satisfactory pattern of weight gain is established. This period can be as long as 2 weeks. If a baby cries or fusses between feedings, check to see if the diaper should be changed and if the baby needs to be picked up and cuddled. If the baby continues to cry and acts hungry, feed him or her. Babies do not get hungry on a regular schedule.
- Infants gradually increase the amount of milk they drink with each feeding. The first day or so most newborns consume 15 to 30 mL (0.5 to 1 ounce) with each feeding. This amount increases as the infant grows. If any formula remains in the bottle as the feeding ends, it must be thrown away because saliva from the baby's mouth can cause the formula to spoil.
- Keep a feeding diary, writing down the amount of formula the infant drinks with each feeding for the first week or so. Also record the wet diapers and bowel movements the baby is having. Take this diary with you when you take the baby for the first follow-up visit with the primary health care provider.
- For feeding hold the infant close in a semi-reclining position. Talk to him or her during the feeding. This time is ideal for social interaction and cuddling.
- Place the nipple in the infant's mouth on the tongue. It should touch the roof of the mouth to stimulate the baby's sucking reflex. Hold the bottle like a pencil. Keep it tipped so the nipple stays filled with milk and the baby does not suck in air.
- Taking a few sucks and then pausing briefly before continuing to suck again is normal for infants. Some infants take longer to feed than others. Be patient. Keep the baby awake; encouraging sucking may be necessary. Moving the nipple gently in the infant's mouth may stimulate sucking.
- Another technique that can be used for bottle-feeding is *paced bottle-feeding*. The infant is placed in a more upright position, and the bottle is held at a more horizontal angle. When the baby pauses between bursts of sucking, withdraw the nipple and allow it to rest on the baby's lip until he or she is ready to resume sucking. This slows the flow of milk from the bottle so the infant is more in control. Paced bottle-feeding works well for infants who are primarily breastfeeding but are occasionally fed from a bottle
- Newborns are apt to swallow air when sucking. Give the infant opportunities to burp several times during a feeding. As he or she gets older, you will know better when to stop for burping.
- After the first 2 or 3 days the stools of a formula-fed infant are yellow and soft but formed. The infant may have a stool with each feeding in the first 2 weeks, although this amount can decrease to one or two stools each day. It is not abnormal for formula-fed infants to have a stool every other day.

Safety Tips

- Infants should be held and never left alone while feeding. Never prop the bottle. The infant might inhale formula or choke on any that was spit up. Infants who fall asleep with a propped bottle of milk or juice can be prone to cavities when the first teeth come in.
- Know how to use the bulb syringe and help an infant who is choking.

---

opened can is refrigerated safely for 48 hours. This type of formula can be purchased in individual disposable bottles for the most convenient feeding.

- Concentrated formula is less expensive than ready to feed. It is diluted with equal parts of water and can be stored in the refrigerator for 48 hours after opening.

- Powdered formula is the least expensive. It is easily mixed by using one scoop for every 60 mL of water.

The commercial infant formula must include label directions for preparation and use of the formula with pictures and symbols for the benefit of individuals who cannot read. Some manufacturers translate the directions into languages such as Spanish, French,

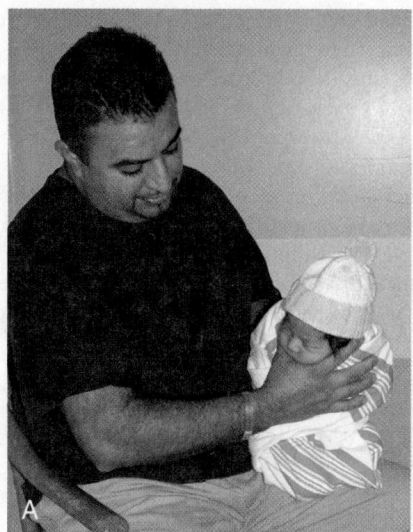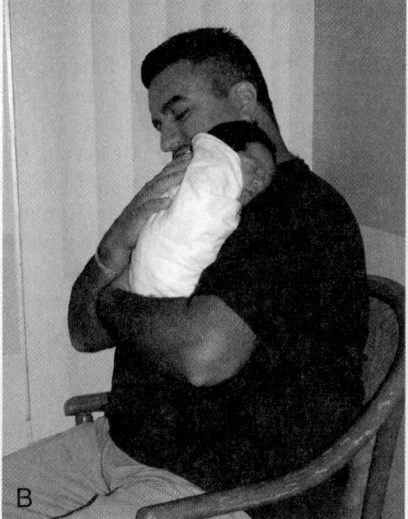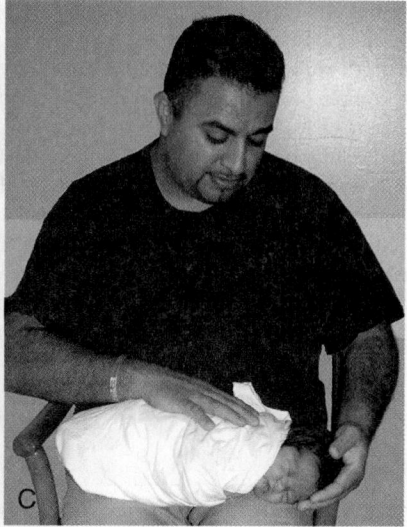

FIG 24-18 Positions for burping an infant. **A,** Sitting. **B,** On shoulder. **C,** Across lap. (Courtesy Julie Perry Nelson, Loveland, CO.)

Vietnamese, Chinese, and Arabic to prevent misunderstanding and errors in formula preparation.

The water used to mix either powdered or concentrated liquid formula need not contain any fluoride, especially in the first 6 months of life. Excess fluoride can permanently stain the teeth once they appear.

Sterilization of formula rarely is recommended when families have access to a safe public water supply. Instead formula is prepared with attention to cleanliness. When water from a private well is used, parents should be advised to contact the health department to have a chemical and bacteriologic analysis of the water performed before using the water in formula preparation. The presence of nitrates, excess fluoride, or bacteria may be harmful to the infant.

It is usually safe to mix infant formula with cold tap water that has been boiled for 1 to 2 minutes and allowed to cool. Bottled water that is labeled as "sterile" is safe for mixing formula. However, nonsterile bottled water should be boiled for 1 to 2 minutes and cooled.

If the conditions in the home appear unsanitary, the nurse should recommend the use of ready-to-feed formula or teach the mother to sterilize the formula. The two traditional methods for sterilization are terminal heating and the aseptic method. In the terminal heating method the prepared formula is placed in the bottles, which are topped with the nipples placed upside down and covered with the caps and sealed loosely with the rings. The bottles are then boiled together in a water bath for 25 minutes. In the aseptic method the bottles, rings, caps, nipples, and any other necessary equipment such as a funnel are boiled separately, after which the formula is poured into the bottles. Instructions for formula preparation and feeding are provided in the Patient Teaching box on p. 658.

Vitamin and Mineral Supplementation

Commercial iron-fortified formula has all of the nutrients that infants need for the first 6 months of life. After 6 months fluoride supplementation is recommended based on levels in the water supply. Nonbreastfeeding infants who consume less than 1 quart per day of vitamin D–fortified milk should receive 400 International Units of vitamin D each day beginning with hospital discharge (Wagner, Grier, and AAP Section on Breastfeeding and Committee on Nutrition, 2008).

Weaning

The bottle-fed infant gradually learns to use a cup, and the parents find that they are preparing fewer bottles. The bottle-feeding before bedtime is often the last one to remain. Babies have a strong need to suck, and the baby who has the bottle taken away too early or abruptly compensates with nonnutritive sucking on his or her fingers, thumb, a pacifier, or even the tongue. Therefore weaning from a bottle should be attempted gradually because the baby has learned to rely on the comfort that sucking provides.

Complementary Feeding: Introducing Solid Foods

Complementary feedings are defined as foods or liquids given to the infant in addition to breast milk or formula. The AAP Committee on Nutrition (2009) recommends introducing solid foods after 4 months of age and preferably after 6 months of age. Traditionally, the recommended first foods were single-grain cereals, followed by vegetables and fruits. However, there is a lack of evidence to support any particular order as having advantages for infants. Breastfeeding infants in particular can benefit from a source of iron such as iron-fortified cereal or meat. New foods should be introduced slowly to assess for any allergic reaction or intolerance. It is best to offer no more than three new foods per week. Fruits and vegetables should be offered to infants daily starting at 6 to 8 months. Fruit juices are not recommended before 6 months of age because it is possible that the infant who drinks juice will consume less breast milk or formula.

Consumption of low-nutrient foods such as fatty or sugary foods or restaurant foods should be limited.

In spite of the recommendations from the AAP, many parents begin complementary feedings earlier than 4 months. In a large-scale study of feeding practices, more than half of the infants had received solid foods before the age of 4 months (Grummer-Strawn, Scanlon, and Fein, 2008). The infant receives the right balance of nutrients from breast milk or formula during the first 4 to 6 months. The notion that the feeding of solids helps the infant sleep through the night is not true. Parents should not put cereal into the infant's bottle. Introduction of solid foods before the infant is 4 to 6 months of age can result in overfeeding and decreased intake of breast milk or formula.

Cultural beliefs and traditions affect complementary feeding practices. First foods given to infants vary widely. For example, first foods for Egyptian infants include bread soaked in milk and tea or yogurt sweetened with honey. Chinese and Vietnamese infants are sometimes fed prechewed rice paste, rice, or sweetened porridge (Pak-Gorstein, Haq, and Graham, 2009).

Nurses and other health care professionals educate parents regarding complementary feedings. This most often occurs during well-baby supervision visits with the pediatric health care provider. Early feeding practices have implications for long-term dietary patterns; therefore it is essential to teach parents about proper nutrition.

KEY POINTS

- Human breast milk is species-specific and is the recommended form of infant nutrition. It provides immunologic protection against many infections and diseases.
- Breast milk changes in composition with each stage of lactogenesis, during each feeding, and as the infant grows.
- During the prenatal period expectant parents should be informed of the benefits of breastfeeding for infants, mothers, families, and society.
- Infants should be breastfed within the first hour after birth and at least 8 to 12 times every 24 hours thereafter.
- Parents should be taught to recognize the signs of effective breastfeeding.
- Breast milk production is based on a supply-meets-demand principle: the more the infant nurses, the greater the milk supply.

- Infants go through predictable growth spurts.
- Sore nipples are most often caused by incorrect latch.
- Commercial infant formulas provide satisfactory nutrition for most infants.
- Infants should be held for feedings.
- Parents should be instructed about the types of infant formulas, proper preparation for feeding, and correct feeding technique.
- Solid (complementary) food should be started at about 6 months of age.
- Unmodified cow's milk is inappropriate for infants less than 1 year of age.
- Nurses must be knowledgeable about feeding methods and provide education and support for families.

REFERENCES

Academy of Breastfeeding Medicine (ABM) Board of Directors: Position on breastfeeding, *Breastfeed Med* 3(4):267–270, 2008.

Academy of Breastfeeding Medicine (ABM) Protocol Committee: ABM clinical protocol #4: Mastitis, *Breastfeed Med* 3(3):177–180, 2008.

Academy of Breastfeeding Medicine (ABM) Protocol Committee: ABM clinical protocol #3: Hospital guidelines for the use of supplementary feedings in the healthy term breastfed infant, *Breastfeed Med* 4(3):175–182, 2009.

Academy of Breastfeeding Medicine (ABM) Protocol Committee: ABM clinical protocol #8: Human milk storage information for home use for full-term infants, *Breastfeed Med* 5(3):127–130, 2010.

Academy of Breastfeeding Medicine (ABM) Protocol Committee: ABM clinical protocol #10: Breastfeeding the late preterm infant, *Breastfeed Med* 5 (3):127–130, 2011a.

Academy of Breastfeeding Medicine (ABM) Protocol Committee: ABM clinical protocol #9: Use of galactogogues in initiating or augmenting the rate of maternal milk secretion, *Breastfeed Med* 6(1):41–49, 2011b.

Ahluwalia IB, D'Angelo D, Morrow B, et al: Association between acculturation and

breastfeeding among Hispanic women: data from the Pregnancy Risk Assessment and Monitoring System, *J Hum Lact* 28(2):167–173, 2012.

American Academy of Family Physicians (AAFP): Breastfeeding policy statement, 2012, www.aafp.org/online/en/home/policy/policies/b/breastfeedingpolicy.html.

American Academy of Pediatrics (AAP): Ages and stages: baby bottles and bisphenol A (BPA), 2012, http://www.healthychildren.org/English/ages-stages/baby/feeding-nutrition/pages/Baby-Bottles-And-Bisphenol-A-BPA.

American Academy of Pediatrics (AAP) Committee on Nutrition: *Pediatric nutrition handbook*, ed 6, Elk Grove Village, IL, 2009, AAP.

American Academy of Pediatrics (AAP) Section on Breastfeeding: Breastfeeding and the use of human milk—policy statement, *Pediatrics* 129(3):e827–e841, 2012.

American College of Obstetricians and Gynecologists (ACOG) Committee on Health Care for Underserved Women and Committee on Obstetric Practice: Breastfeeding: maternal and infant aspects, *ACOG Clin Rev* 12(1):1S–16S, 2007.

American Dietetic Association (ADA): Position of the American Dietetic Association:

promoting and supporting breastfeeding, *J Am Diet Assoc* 109(11):1926–1942, 2009.

Association of Women's Health, Obstetric and Neonatal Nurses (AWHONN): *Breastfeeding and the role of the nurse in the promotion of breastfeeding*, Washington, DC, 2007, AWHONN.

Baby-Friendly USA (BFHI USA): Implementing the UNICEF/WHO baby friendly hospital initiative in the US, 2010, www.babyfriendlyusa.org.

Baby-Friendly USA (BFHI USA): Baby-Friendly hospitals and birth centers, 2012, www.babyfriendlyusa.org/eng/03.html.

Baker RD, Greer FR, and AAP Committee on Nutrition: Clinical report: diagnosis and prevention of iron-deficiency and iron-deficiency anemia in infants and young children (0-3 years of age), *Pediatrics* 126(5):1–11, 2010.

Bartick M, Reinhold A: The burden of suboptimal breastfeeding in the United States: a pediatric cost analysis, *Pediatrics* 125(5):e1048–e1056, 2010.

Bartick M, Reyes C: Las dos cosas: an analysis of attitudes of Latina women on non-exclusive breastfeeding, *Breastfeed Med* 7(1):19–24, 2012.

Bhatia J, Greer F, and American Academy of Pediatrics (AAP) Committee on Nutrition:

Use of soy protein-based formulas in infant feeding, *Pediatrics* 121(5):1062–1068, 2008.

Blackburn ST: *Maternal, fetal, and neonatal physiology*, ed 4, St Louis, 2013, Saunders.

Bramson L, Lee JW, Moore E, et al: Effect of early skin-to-skin mother-infant contact during the first 3 hours following birth on exclusive breastfeeding during the maternity hospital stay, *J Hum Lact* 26(2):130–137, 2010.

Brand E, Kothari C, Stark MA: Factors related to breastfeeding discontinuation between hospital discharge and 2 weeks' postpartum, *J Perinat Educ* 20(1):36–44, 2011.

Centers for Disease Control and Prevention (CDC): US medical eligibility criteria for contraceptive use, 2010: Adapted from the World Health Organization medical eligibility criteria for contraceptive use, ed 4, *MMWR Morb Mortal Weekly Rep* 59(RR4):1–86, 2010.

Centers for Disease Control and Prevention (CDC): Breastfeeding report card—United States, 2012, www.cdc.gov/breastfeeding/data/reportcard.htm.

Chantry CJ: Supporting the 75%: overcoming barriers after breastfeeding initiation, *Breastfeed Med* 6(5):337–339, 2011.

Cleveland K: Feeding challenges in the late preterm infant, *Neonatal Net* 29(1):37–41, 2010.

Colson S: What happens to breastfeeding when mothers lie back? *Clin Lact* 1:9–12, 2010.

Colson S: The laid-back breastfeeding revolution, *Midwifery Today* 101:9–11 and 66, 2012.

Cooper BM, Holditch-Davis D, Verklan MT, et al: Newborn clinical outcomes of the AWHONN late preterm infant research-based practice project, *J Obstet Gynecol Neonatal Nurs* 41(6):774–785, 2012.

Declercq E, Labbok MH, Sakala C, et al: Hospital practices and women's likelihood of fulfilling their intention to exclusively breastfeed, *Am J Public Health* 99(5):929–935, 2009.

Dell KM: Fluid, electrolytes, and acid-base homeostasis. In Martin RJ, Fanaroff AA, Walsh MC, editors: *Fanaroff and Martin's Neonatal-perinatal medicine: diseases of the fetus and infant*, ed 9, St Louis, 2011, Mosby.

Flanders D, Lowe A, Kramer M, et al: *A consensus statement on the use of domperidone to support lactation*, Canadian Lactation Consultant Association, 2012, www.ilca.org/i4a/pages/index.cfm?pageid=3520.

Food and Drug Administration (FDA): Import alert 61-07, 2012, www.accessdata.fda.gov/cms_ia/importalert_166.html.

Fortinguerra F, Clavenna A, Bonati M: Psychotropic drug use during breastfeeding: a review of the evidence, *Pediatrics* 124(4):e547–e556, 2009.

Geddes D: Inside the lactating breast: the latest anatomy research, *J Midwifery Women's Health* 52 (6):556–563, 2007.

Grummer-Strawn L, Scanlon K, Fein S: Infant feeding and feeding transitions during the first year of life, *Pediatrics* 122 (suppl 2):S36–S42, 2008.

Hale T: Drug therapy and breastfeeding. In Riordan J, Wambach K, editors: *Breastfeeding and human lactation*, ed 4, Sudbury Mass, 2010, Jones & Bartlett.

Hancock M, Brown J: Formula-feeding safety: what nurses need to teach parents who choose to formula-feed, *Nurs Women's Health* 14(4):303–309, 2010.

Holmes AH, Auinger P, Howard CR: Combination feeding of breast milk and formula: evidence for shorter breast-feeding duration from the National Health and Nutrition Examination Survey, *J Pediatr* 159(2):186–191, 2011.

Human Milk Banking Association of North America (HMBANA): Who do we serve? 2012 www.hmbana.org/who-do-we-serve.

Hurst NM, Meier PP: Breastfeeding the preterm infant. In Riordan J, Wambach K, editors: *Breastfeeding and human lactation*, ed 4, Sudbury, MA, 2010, Jones and Bartlett.

Institute of Medicine: *Dietary reference intakes for energy, carbohydrate, fiber, fatty acids, cholesterol, protein, and amino acids*, Washington, DC, 2005, National Academies Press.

Jensen E: Participation in the Supplemental Nutrition Program for Women, Infants, and Children (WIC) and breastfeeding: national, regional, and state level analyses, *Matern Child Health J* 16(3):624–631, 2012.

Jenson D, Wallace S, Kelsay P: LATCH: a breastfeeding charting system and documentation tool, *J Obstet Gynecol Neonatal Nurs* 23(1):27–32, 1994.

Labiner-Wolfe J, Fein SB: How US mothers store and handle their expressed breast milk, *J Hum Lact* 29(1):54–58, 2013.

Lakshman R, Ogilvie D, Ong K: Mothers' experiences of bottle-feeding: a systematic review of qualitative and quantitative studies, *Arch Dis Child* 94(8):596–601, 2009.

Lamb M: Weight-loss surgery and breastfeeding, *Clin Lact* 2(2-3):17–21, 2011.

Lauwers J, Swisher A: *Counseling the nursing mother: a lactation consultant's guide*, ed 5, Sudbury, Mass, 2011, Jones and Bartlett.

Lawrence RM, Lawrence RA: *Breastfeeding: a guide for the medical profession*, ed 7, St Louis, 2011a, Mosby.

Lawrence RM, Lawrence RA: Breastfeeding: more than just good nutrition, *Pediatr Rev* 32(7):267–280, 2011b.

Lepe M, Bacardí Gascón M, Castañeda-González LM, et al: Effect of maternal obesity on lactation: systematic review, *Nutr Hosp* 26(6):1266–1269, 2011.

Mass SB: Supporting breastfeeding in the United States: the Surgeon General's call to action, *Curr Opin Obstet Gynecol* 23(6):460–464, 2011.

Mehta UJ, Siega-Riz AM, Herring AH, et al: Maternal obesity, psychological factors, and breastfeeding duration, *Breastfeed Med* 6(6):369–376, 2011.

Moore ER, Anderson GC, Bergman N, et al: Early skin-to-skin contact for mothers and their healthy newborn infants, *Cochrane Database Syst Rev* 5:CD003519.pub3, 2012. DOI: 10.1002/1465158.

Nelson AM: A meta-synthesis related to infant feeding decision making, *MCN Am J Matern Child Nurs* 37(4):247–252, 2012.

Pak-Gorstein S, Haq A, Graham E: Cultural influences on infant feeding practices, *Pediatr Rev* 30(3):e11–e21, 2009.

Perrine CG, Scanlon KS, Li R, et al: Baby-friendly hospital practices and meeting exclusive breastfeeding intention, *Pediatrics* 130(1):1–7, 2012.

Powers NG: Low intake in the breastfed infant: maternal and infant considerations. In Riordan J, Wambach K, editors: *Breastfeeding and human lactation*, ed 4, Sudbury Mass, 2010, Jones and Bartlett.

Ramsay D, Kent J, Hartmann R, et al: Anatomy of the lactating human breast redefined with ultrasound imaging, *J Anat* 206(6):525–534, 2005.

Riordan J, Hoover K: Perinatal and intrapartum care. In Riordan J, Wambach K, editors: *Breastfeeding and human lactation*, ed 4, Sudbury, MA, 2010, Jones and Bartlett.

Riordan J, Wambach K: Breast-related problems. In Riordan J, Wambach K, editors: *Breastfeeding and human lactation*, ed 4, Sudbury, MA, 2010, Jones and Bartlett.

Rios E: Promoting breastfeeding in the Hispanic community, *Breastfeed Med* 4(suppl 1):S69–S70, 2009.

Rojjanasrirat W, Wambach K: Maternal employment and breastfeeding. In Riordan J, Wambach K, editors: *Breastfeeding and human lactation*, ed 4, Sudbury, MA, 2010, Jones and Bartlett.

Scanlon KS, Grummer-Strawn L, Li R, et al: Racial and ethnic differences in breastfeeding initiation and duration by state: national immunization survey, US, 2004-2008, *MMWR Morbid Mortal Wkly Rep* 59(11):1–21, 2010.

Smith L, Riordan J: Postpartum care. In Riordan J, Wambach K, editors: *Breastfeeding and human lactation*, ed 4, Sudbury Mass, 2010, Jones and Bartlett.

Spatz DL, Lessen R: *The risks of not breastfeeding: position statement*, Morrisville, NC, 2011, International Lactation Consultant Association.

Stuebe AM, Bonuck K: What predicts intent to breastfeed exclusively? Breastfeeding knowledge, attitudes, and beliefs in a diverse urban population, *Breastfeed Med* 6(6):413–420, 2011.

Tenfelde S, Finnegan L, Hill PD: Predictors of breastfeeding exclusivity in a WIC sample, *J Obstet Gynecol Neonatal Nurs* 40(2):179–189, 2011.

The Joint Commission (TJC): *Specifications manual for Joint Commission national quality core measures, version 2013 A1*, Washington

DC, 2012, The Joint Commission, manual.jointcommission.org/releases/TJC2013A/MIF0170.html.

Tully M, Jones F: Donor milk banking. In Riordan J, Wambach K, editors: *Breastfeeding and human lactation*, ed 4, Sudbury Mass, 2010, Jones and Bartlett.

Turcksin R, Bel S, Galjaard S, et al: Maternal obesity and breastfeeding intention, initiation, intensity and duration: a systematic review, *Matern Child Nutr* Aug 20, 2012, DOI: 10.1111/j.1740-8709.2012.00439.x, Epub ahead of print.

Tuttle C, Slavit W: Establishing the business case for breastfeeding, *Breastfeed Med* 4(suppl 1):S59–S62, 2009.

United States Breastfeeding Committee (USBC): *Core competencies in breastfeeding care and services for all health care professionals*, rev ed, Washington, DC, 2010a, USBC.

United States Breastfeeding Committee (USBC): *Implementing the Joint Commission perinatal care core measure on exclusive breast milk feeding*, rev ed, Washington, DC, 2010b, USBC.

United States Department of Health and Human Services (USDHHS): *Healthy People 2020*, Washington, DC, 2010, USDHHS, www.healthypeople.gov/hp2020/.

United States Department of Health and Human Services (USDHHS): *The Surgeon General's call to action to support breastfeeding*, Washington, DC, 2011, USDHHS, Office of the Surgeon General, *www.surgeongeneral.gov/library/calls/breastfeeding/calltoactiontosupportbreastfeeding.pdf*.

Wagner C, Grier F, AAP Section on Breastfeeding and Committee on Nutrition: Prevention of rickets and vitamin D deficiency in infants, children and adolescents, *Pediatrics* 122(5):1142–1152, 2008.

Wojcicki JM: Maternal prepregnancy body mass index and initiation and duration of breastfeeding: a review of the literature, *J Women's Health* 20(3):341–347, 2011.

World Health Organization (WHO) and United Nations Children's Fund (UNICEF): *Global strategy for infant and young child feeding*, Geneva, 2003, WHO, www.who.int/child_adolescent_health/documents/9241562218/en.

WHO, UNICEF, UNFPA, and UNAIDS: Guidelines on HIV and infant feeding, Geneva, 2010, WHO, www.whqlibdoc.who.int/publications/2010/9789241599535_eng.pdf.

The High Risk Newborn

David Wilson

LEARNING OBJECTIVES

On completion of this chapter, the reader will be able to:

- Summarize assessment and care of the newborn with soft tissue, skeletal, and neurologic injuries caused by birth trauma.
- Identify maternal conditions that place the newborn at risk for infection.
- Describe methods used to identify infection in the newborn.
- Identify the effects of maternal use of alcohol, heroin, methadone, marijuana, methamphetamine, cocaine, and tobacco on the fetus and newborn.
- Describe the assessment of a newborn exposed to harmful drugs in utero.
- Identify clinical manifestations of infection in the newborn.
- Describe the nurse's role in the diagnosis of neonatal sepsis.
- Compare characteristics of neonatal Rh and ABO incompatibility.
- Compare and contrast the physical characteristics of preterm, late preterm, term, and postterm neonates.

- Discuss respiratory distress syndrome and the approach to treatment.
- Compare methods of oxygen therapy for the high risk infant.
- Describe nursing interventions for nutritional care of the preterm infant.
- Discuss the pathophysiology of retinopathy of prematurity and bronchopulmonary dysplasia and identify the predisposing risk factors.
- Describe risk factors associated with the birth and transition of an infant of a diabetic mother.
- Plan developmentally appropriate care for the high risk infant.
- Develop a plan to address the unique needs of parents of high risk infants.
- Describe nursing care of the family in the event of a stillbirth or death of a high risk infant.
- Discuss the identification and care of infants with an inborn error of metabolism.

A high risk neonate can be defined as a newborn, regardless of gestational age or birth weight, who has a greater-than-average chance of morbidity or mortality because of conditions or circumstances associated with birth and the adjustment to extrauterine existence. The high risk period encompasses human growth and development from the time of viability (the gestational age at which survival outside the uterus is believed to be possible, or as early as 23 weeks of gestation) up to 28 days after birth; thus it includes threats to life and health that occur during the prenatal, perinatal, and postnatal periods.

High risk infants are most often classified according to birth weight, gestational age, and predominant pathophysiologic problems. The more common problems related to physiologic status are closely associated with the state of maturity of the infant and usually involve chemical disturbances (e.g., hypoglycemia, hypocalcemia) or consequences of immature organs and systems (e.g., hyperbilirubinemia, respiratory distress, hypothermia). Because high risk factors are common to several specialty areas—particularly obstetrics, pediatrics, and neonatology—specific terminology is needed to describe the developmental status of the newborn (Box 25-1).

A challenge for the nurse is the birth of an infant at risk because of conditions or circumstances that are superimposed on the normal course of events associated with birth and the adjustment to extrauterine existence. The infant may be considered high risk because of birth trauma, maternal substance abuse, infection, or congenital anomalies. Infants born preterm and postterm and those born to mothers with conditions such as diabetes are also considered high risk and warrant careful monitoring. Birth trauma includes physical injuries that a neonate sustains during labor and birth. Congenital anomalies include such conditions as gastrointestinal (GI) malformations, cleft lip and cleft palate, genitourinary defects, neural tube defects, abdominal wall defects, and cardiac defects.

At times the nurse is able to anticipate problems such as when a woman is admitted in premature labor or a congenital anomaly is

BOX 25-1 — CLASSIFICATION OF HIGH RISK INFANTS

Classification According To Size

- **Low-birth-weight (LBW) infant**—Infant whose birth weight is less than 2500 g (5 lbs 8 oz), regardless of gestational age
- **Very low–birth-weight (VLBW) infant**—Infant whose birth weight is less than 1500 g (3 lbs 5 oz)
- **Extremely low–birth-weight (ELBW) infant**—Infant whose birth weight is less than 1000 g (2 lb 3 oz)
- **Appropriate-for-gestational-age (AGA) infant**—Infant whose weight falls between the 10th and 90th percentiles on intrauterine growth curves
- **Small-for-date (SFD) or small-for-gestational-age (SGA) infant**—An infant whose rate of intrauterine growth was slowed and whose birth weight falls below the 10th percentile on intrauterine growth curves
- **Intrauterine growth restriction (IUGR)**—Found in infants whose intrauterine growth is restricted (sometimes used as a more descriptive term for SGA infants)
- **Symmetric IUGR**—Growth restriction in which the weight, length, and head circumference are all affected
- **Asymmetric IUGR**—Growth restriction in which the head circumference remains within normal parameters while the birth weight falls below the 10th percentile
- **Large-for-gestational-age (LGA) infant**—Infant whose birth weight falls above the 90th percentile on intrauterine growth charts

Classification According to Gestational Age

- **Preterm (premature) infant**—Infant born before completion of 37 weeks of gestation, regardless of birth weight
- **Full-term infant**—Infant born between the beginning of the 38 weeks and the completion of the 42 weeks of gestation, regardless of birth weight
- **Late-preterm infant**—Infant born between 34 0/7 and 36 6/7 weeks of gestation, regardless of birth weight*
- **Postterm (postmature) infant**—Infant born after 42 weeks of gestational age, regardless of birth weight

Classification According to Mortality

- **Live birth**—Birth in which neonate manifests any heartbeat, breathes, or displays voluntary movement, regardless of gestational age
- **Fetal death**—Death of fetus after 20 weeks of gestation and before birth with absence of any signs of life after birth
- **Neonatal death**—Death that occurs in the first 27 days of life; early neonatal death occurs in the first week of life; late neonatal death occurs at 7 to 27 days
- **Perinatal mortality**—Total number of fetal and early neonatal deaths per 1000 live births

*Definitions of *late-preterm infants* vary among experts, but Engle (2006) suggests this definition (which corresponds to the 239th to the 259th day from the first day of the last menstrual period).

TABLE 25-1 — TYPES OF BIRTH INJURIES

SITE OF INJURY	TYPE OF INJURY
Scalp	Caput succedaneum
	Subgaleal hemorrhage
	Cephalhematoma
Skull	Linear fracture
	Depressed fracture
	Occipital osteodiastasis
Intracranial	Epidural hematoma
	Subdural hematoma (laceration of falx, tentorium, or superficial veins)
	Subarachnoid hemorrhage
	Cerebral contusion
	Cerebellar contusion
	Intracerebellar hematoma
Spinal cord (cervical)	Vertebral artery injury
	Intraspinal hemorrhage
	Spinal cord transection or injury
Plexus	Erb palsy
	Klumpke paralysis
	Total (mixed) brachial plexus injury
	Horner syndrome
	Diaphragmatic (phrenic nerve) paralysis
	Lumbosacral plexus injury
Cranial and peripheral nerve	Radial nerve palsy
	Medial nerve palsy
	Sciatic nerve palsy
	Laryngeal nerve palsy
	Diaphragmatic paralysis
	Facial nerve palsy

From Paige PL, Moe PC: Neurologic disorders. In Merenstein GB, Gardner SL, editors: *Handbook of neonatal intensive care*, ed 6, St Louis, 2006, Mosby.

morbidity. Most birth injuries are avoidable, especially with careful assessment of risk factors and appropriate planning of the birth. The use of fetal ultrasonography allows antepartum diagnosis of certain fetal conditions that may be treated in utero or shortly after birth. Elective cesarean birth can be chosen for some pregnancies to prevent significant birth injury. A small percentage of significant birth injuries such as in especially difficult or prolonged labor or an abnormal fetal presentation are unavoidable despite skilled and competent obstetric care. Some injuries cannot be anticipated until the specific circumstances are encountered during childbirth. Emergency cesarean birth may provide a last-minute salvage, but in these circumstances the injury may be unavoidable. The same injury might be caused in several ways (e.g., a cephalhematoma could result from an obstetric technique such as forceps birth or vacuum extraction or from pressure of the fetal skull against the maternal pelvis).

Many injuries are minor and resolve readily in the neonatal period without treatment. Other trauma requires some degree of intervention; few are serious enough to be fatal. The nurse's contributions to the newborn's welfare begin with early observation of his or her transition. Promptly reporting signs that indicate deviations from normal permits early initiation of appropriate therapy. Table 25-1 provides an overview of neurologic birth injuries and the sites in which they occur.

diagnosed by ultrasound before birth. At other times the birth of a high risk infant is unanticipated. In either case the personnel and equipment necessary for immediate care of the infant must be available.

BIRTH INJURIES

Birth trauma (injury) is physical injury sustained by a neonate during labor and birth. It remains an important source of neonatal

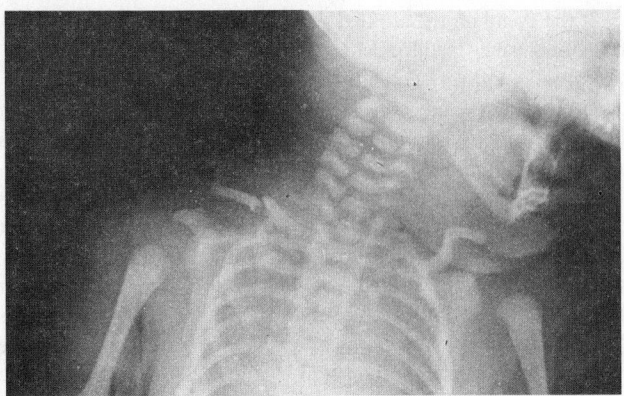

FIG 25-1 Fractured clavicle after shoulder dystocia. (From O'Doherty N: *Neonatology: micro atlas of the newborn*, Nutley, NJ, 1986, Hoffmann-La Roche.)

CARE MANAGEMENT

When the newborn is born, the nurse makes a rapid inspection and physical assessment to determine whether there are any life-threatening conditions that require immediate medical or surgical attention. A comprehensive physical assessment of the newborn is performed after the parents have had the opportunity to interact with their new baby. Because evidence of some birth injuries may not be apparent at the initial examination, assessment continues during each contact with the neonate.

Soft-tissue injuries that commonly occur at birth (i.e., caput succedaneum and cephalhematoma) are discussed in Chapter 22.

Skeletal Injuries

The newborn's immature, flexible skull can withstand a great degree of deformation (molding) before fracture results. Considerable force is required to fracture it. Two types of skull fractures typically identified in the newborn are linear and depressed fractures. The location of the fracture and involvement of underlying structures determine its significance.

If an artery lying in a groove on the undersurface of the skull is torn as a result of the fracture, increased intracranial pressure (ICP) follows. Unless a blood vessel is involved, linear fractures, which account for 70% of all fractures for this age-group, heal without special treatment. The soft skull may become indented without laceration of either the skin or the dural membrane. These depressed fractures, or Ping-Pong ball indentations, may occur during difficult births from pressure of the head on the bony pelvis. They can also occur as a result of injudicious application of forceps.

The clavicle is the bone most often fractured during birth. Generally the break is in the middle third of the bone (Fig. 25-1). Dystocia, particularly shoulder impaction, may be the predisposing problem. Limited arm motion, crepitus over the bone, and absence of the Moro reflex on the affected side are often present. Except for use of gentle rather than vigorous handling and containment of the limb against the chest, no accepted treatment for fractured clavicle of the newborn exists, and the prognosis is good. The humerus and femur are other bones that may be fractured during a difficult birth. Fractures in newborns generally heal rapidly. Immobilization is accomplished with slings, splints, swaddling, and other devices.

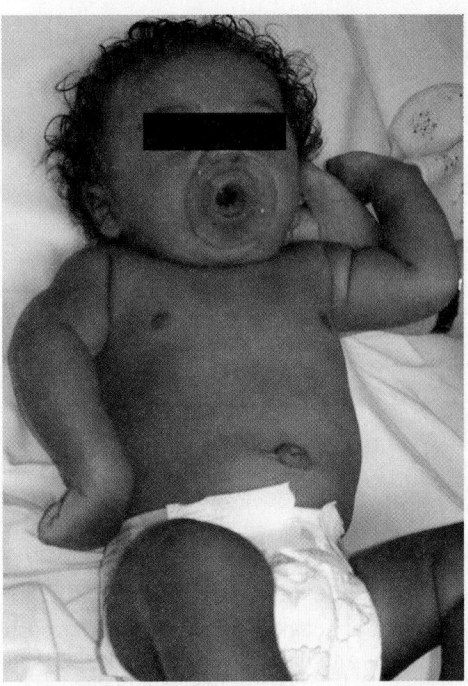

FIG 25-2 Erb-Duchenne paralysis in newborn infant. Moro reflex is absent in right upper extremity. Recovery was complete. (From Chung KC, Yang LJ-S, McGillicuddy JE: *Practical management of pediatric and adult brachial plexus palsies*, Philadelphia, 2012, Saunders.)

The parents need support in handling these infants because they often are afraid of hurting them. They are encouraged to practice handling, changing, and feeding the affected neonate under the guidance of nursery personnel. This increases their confidence and knowledge and facilitates attachment. A plan for follow-up therapy is developed with the parents so the times and arrangements for therapy are acceptable to them.

Peripheral Nervous System Injuries

Plexus injury results from forces that alter the normal position and relationship of the arm, shoulder, and neck. Erb palsy (Erb-Duchenne paralysis) is caused by damage to the upper plexus and usually results from a stretching or pulling away of the shoulder from the head such as might occur with shoulder dystocia or a difficult vertex or breech birth. The less common lower-plexus palsy, or Klumpke palsy, results from severe stretching of the upper extremity while the trunk is relatively less mobile.

The clinical manifestations of Erb palsy are related to the paralysis of the affected extremity and muscles. The arm hangs limp alongside the body. The shoulder and arm are adducted and rotated internally. The elbow is extended, and the forearm is pronated with the wrist and fingers flexed; a grasp reflex may be present because finger and wrist movement remains normal (Carlo, 2011b) (Fig. 25-2). In lower-plexus palsy the muscles of the hand are paralyzed, with consequent wrist drop and relaxed fingers. In a third and more severe form of brachial palsy, the entire arm is paralyzed and hangs limp and motionless at the side. The Moro reflex is absent on the affected side for all of the forms of brachial palsy. Total plexus is the second most common type of plexus injury.

Treatment of the affected arm is aimed at preventing contractures of the paralyzed muscles and maintaining correct placement of the humeral head within the glenoid fossa of the scapula.

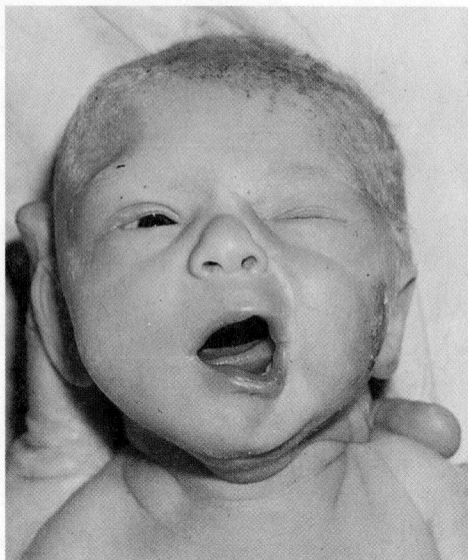

FIG 25-3 Facial paralysis 15 minutes after forceps birth. Absence of movement on affected side is especially noticeable when infant cries. (From O'Doherty N: *Neonatology: micro atlas of the newborn,* Nutley, NJ, 1986, Hoffmann-La Roche.)

Complete recovery from stretched nerves usually takes 3 to 6 months. However, avulsion of the nerves (complete disconnection of the ganglia from the spinal cord that involves both anterior and posterior roots) results in permanent damage. For injuries that do not improve by 3 months, surgical intervention may be needed to relieve pressure on the nerves or repair the nerves with grafting (Carlo, 2011b).

Nursing care of the newborn with brachial palsy is concerned primarily with proper positioning of the affected arm. The affected arm should be abducted 90 degrees with external shoulder rotation, forearm supination, and extension at the wrist with the palm facing the infant's face. Passive range-of-motion exercises of the shoulder, wrist, elbow, and fingers are initiated in the latter part of the first week. Wrist flexion contractures may be prevented with the use of a wrist splint with padding in the fist. In dressing the infant, preference is given to the affected arm. Undressing begins with the unaffected arm, and redressing begins with the affected arm to prevent unnecessary manipulation and stress on the paralyzed muscles. Instruct parents to use the football position when holding the infant and avoid picking the child up from under the axillae or pulling on the arms.

Pressure on the facial nerve (cranial nerve VII) during birth may result in injury to it. The primary clinical manifestations are loss of movement on the affected side such as an inability to completely close the eye, drooping of the corner of the mouth, and absence of wrinkling of the forehead and nasolabial fold (Fig. 25-3). Facial palsy or paralysis is most noticeable when the infant cries. The mouth is drawn to the unaffected side, the wrinkles are deeper on the normal side, and the eye on the involved side remains open. Often the condition is temporary, resolving within hours or days of birth. Permanent paralysis is rare unless the nerve fibers were torn, in which case surgical intervention may be necessary.

Nursing care of the infant with facial nerve paralysis involves helping the infant suck and the mother with feeding techniques. The infant may require gavage feeding to prevent aspiration. Breastfeeding is not contraindicated, but the mother needs additional assistance to help the infant grasp and compress the areolar area.

If the eyelid on the affected side does not close completely, artificial tears can be instilled daily to prevent drying of the conjunctiva, sclera, and cornea. The eyelid is often taped shut to prevent accidental injury. If eye care is needed at home, the parents are taught the procedure for administering eyedrops before the infant is discharged.

Phrenic nerve paralysis results in diaphragmatic paralysis as demonstrated by ultrasonography, which shows paradoxical chest movement and an elevated diaphragm. Initially radiography may not demonstrate an elevated diaphragm if the neonate is receiving positive-pressure ventilation (Volpe, 2008). The injury sometimes occurs in conjunction with brachial palsy. Respiratory distress is the most common and important sign of injury. Because injury to the phrenic nerve is usually unilateral, the lung on the affected side does not expand, and respiratory efforts are ineffectual. The infant is positioned on the affected side to facilitate maximum expansion of the uninvolved lung. Breathing is primarily thoracic; cyanosis, tachypnea, or complete respiratory failure may be seen. Pneumonia and atelectasis on the affected side may also occur.

The infant with phrenic nerve paralysis requires the same nursing care as any infant with respiratory distress. As with other birth injuries, the family's emotional needs are similar to those discussed for soft-tissue injury (see Chapter 22). Follow-up is also essential because of the extended length of recovery.

Neurologic Injuries

Neurologic injury in newborn infants is common with the increased survival of low-birth-weight and very low–birth-weight infants; in addition, the lower the gestational age, the higher the risk for certain neurologic injuries. Such infants are particularly vulnerable to ischemic injury caused by variable (both increased and decreased) cerebral blood flow subsequent to asphyxia; and preterm infants, with a fragile cerebrovascular network, are highly prone to periventricular or intraventricular hemorrhage. Fragility and increased permeability of capillaries and prolonged prothrombin time predispose preterm infants to trauma when delicate structures are subjected to the forces of labor. The more common cerebral complications and nursing care are outlined in Table 25-2.

The highest incidence of abnormal neurologic findings occurs in very low–birth-weight (VLBW) infants and those with intracranial hemorrhage. Major neurologic problems such as cerebral palsy, seizures, and hydrocephalus are usually diagnosed in the first 2 years of life. Less severe deficits such as learning disorders, attention deficit hyperactivity disorder (ADHD), and fine- and gross-motor incoordination may not be diagnosed until preschool or even school age. Cerebral palsy is one of the most common neurologic deficits in survivors of preterm birth (see Chapter 49).

Recent research has shown that therapeutic hypothermia provided by cooling either the infant's head or the whole body reduces the severity of the neurologic damage in hypoxic ischemic encephalopathy when it is applied in the early stages of injury (first 6 hours after birth) in infants with a gestational age of 35 to 36 weeks or more (Azzopardi, Strohm, Edwards, et al., 2009; Edwards, Brocklehurst, Gunn, et al., 2010; Jacobs, Hunt, Tarnow-Mordi, et al., 2007; Laptook, 2009).

NEONATAL INFECTIONS

Sepsis

Sepsis (the presence of microorganisms or their toxins in the blood or other tissues) continues to be one of the most significant causes of neonatal morbidity and mortality. Maternal immunoglobulin M

TABLE 25-2	NEUROLOGIC COMPLICATIONS		
DESCRIPTION	**CLINICAL MANIFESTATIONS**	**THERAPEUTIC MANAGEMENT**	**CARE MANAGEMENT**
Hypoxic-Ischemic Brain Injury			
Nonprogressive neurologic (brain) impairment caused by intrauterine or postnatal asphyxia resulting in hypoxemia or cerebral ischemia Hypoxic-ischemic encephalopathy—the resultant cellular damage that causes the clinical manifestations	Appears within first 6-12 hr after hypoxic episode Seizures Abnormal muscle tone (usually hypotonia) Disturbance of sucking and swallowing Apneic episodes Stupor or coma Muscular weakness in hips and shoulders (full term), lower-limb weakness (preterm)	Prevent hypoxia. Provide supportive care. Provide adequate ventilation. Maintain cerebral perfusion. Prevent cerebral edema. Treat underlying cause. Administer antiseizure drugs. Initiate therapeutic hypothermia if criteria met (see Neurologic Injuries).	See Care of the High Risk Newborn and Family (p. 696). Observe for signs that indicate cerebral hypoxia. Monitor ventilatory and intravenous therapy. Observe for and manage seizures. Support family. Provide guidelines for family management of potential mild-to-severe neurologic damage.
Germinal Matrix or Intraventricular Hemorrhage			
Hemorrhage into and around ventricles caused by ruptured vessels as a result of an event that increases cerebral blood flow to area	Sudden deterioration in condition if bleed is large Most bleeds initially asymptomatic Tense, bulging anterior fontanel Neurologic signs: • Twitching • Stupor • Apnea • Seizures Evident on cranial ultrasonography or magnetic resonance imaging	Provide supportive care. Provide ventilatory support. Maintain oxygenation. Regulate fluid, electrolytes, acid-base balance. Suppress or prevent seizures. Provide ventricular shunting or drainage.	See Care of the High Risk Newborn and Family (p. 696). Prevent increased cerebral blood pressure. Avoid events that may increase or decrease cerebral blood flow (e.g., pain, unnecessary stimulation, endotracheal suctioning, hypoxia, hyperosmolar drugs, rapid volume expansion). Elevate head of bed 20-30 degrees; keep head in midline. Support family. Monitor for posthemorrhagic hydrocephalus after diagnosis. Provide developmental care and enhancement.
Intracranial Hemorrhage			
Subdural Subarachnoid Intracerebellar	Sudden decrease in hematocrit Change in sensorium Poor feeding See Chapter 45	See Chapter 45.	Same as for germinal matrix or intraventricular hemorrhage

(IgM) does not cross the placenta. IgG levels in term infants are equal to maternal levels; however, in preterm infants the amount of IgG is directly proportional to gestational age. IgA and IgM require time to reach optimum levels after birth. Neonatal neutrophils are present in term infants but have decreased functional capabilities; response to infections is sluggish. Phagocytosis is less efficient. Serum complement levels are low in term infants and even lower in the preterm infant; serum complement (C1 through C6) is involved in immunologic reactions, some of which kill or lyse bacteria and enhance phagocytosis. The gut mucosal barrier is initially immature in both term and preterm infants; this barrier is enhanced by the ingestion of human colostrum, which contains antiinfective properties. Dysmaturity seen with intrauterine growth restriction (IUGR) and preterm and postdate birth further compromises the immune system of the neonate.

Table 25-3 outlines risk factors for neonatal sepsis. Special precautions for preventing infection and prompt recognition when it occurs are necessary for optimal newborn care. Neonatal infections may be acquired in utero, at birth or shortly thereafter, and as a health care–associated infection (HAI).

Neonatal bacterial infection is classified into two patterns according to the time of presentation. Early-onset or congenital sepsis usually manifests within 24 to 48 hours of birth, progresses more rapidly than later-onset infection, and carries a mortality rate as high as 50%. Early-onset sepsis is acquired in the perinatal period; infection can occur from direct contact with organisms from the maternal GI and genitourinary tracts. The most common infecting organisms are *Escherichia coli* and group B streptococcus (GBS) (Stoll, Hansen, Sanchez, et al., 2011). *E. coli*, which may be present in the vagina, accounts for approximately half of all cases of sepsis caused by gram-negative organisms. GBS is an extremely virulent organism in neonates, with a high (50%) death rate in affected infants. Other bacteria noted to cause early-onset infection include *Haemophilus influenzae*, *Citrobacter* and *Enterobacter* organisms, coagulase-negative staphylococci, and *Streptococcus viridans*. Other pathogens that are harbored in the vagina and may infect the infant

TABLE 25-3	**RISK FACTORS FOR NEONATAL SEPSIS**
SOURCE	**RISK FACTORS**
Maternal	Low socioeconomic status
	Poor prenatal care
	Poor nutrition
	Substance abuse
Intrapartum	Premature rupture of membranes
	Maternal fever
	Chorioamnionitis
	Prolonged labor
	Rupture of membranes >18 hr
	Premature labor
	Maternal urinary tract infection
Neonatal	Twin or multiple gestation
	Male
	Birth asphyxia
	Meconium aspiration
	Congenital anomalies of skin or mucous membranes
	Galactosemia
	Absence of spleen
	Low birth weight or preterm birth
	Malnourishment
	Prolonged hospitalization
	Invasive procedures

include gonococci, *Candida albicans,* herpes simplex virus (HSV) type 2, and chlamydia. Early-onset sepsis is associated with a history of obstetric events such as preterm birth, prolonged rupture of membranes (more than 18 hours), maternal fever during labor, and chorioamnionitis. Early-onset infection is also inversely related to infant birth weight (Polin and AAP Committee on Fetus and Newborn, 2012).

Late-onset sepsis, occurring approximately at 7 to 30 days of age, is considered primarily to be an infection acquired in the hospital or community; the offending organisms are usually staphylococci, *Klebsiella* organisms, enterococci, *E. coli,* and *Pseudomonas* or *Candida* species (Stoll, 2011). Coagulase-negative staphylococci, considered to be primarily a contaminant in older children and adults, are commonly found to be the cause of septicemia in extremely low–birth-weight (ELBW) and VLBW infants. Additional infections of concern include methicillin-resistant *Staphylococcus aureus,* vancomycin-resistant enterococci, and multidrug-resistant gram-negative pathogens. Bacterial invasion can occur through sites such as the umbilical stump; the skin; mucous membranes of the eye, nose, pharynx, and ear; and internal systems such as the respiratory, nervous, urinary, and GI systems.

Perinatally acquired infections may cause miscarriage, stillbirth, intrauterine infection, congenital malformations, and acute neonatal disease. Other viral infections such as respiratory syncytial virus (RSV), rotavirus, herpes simplex, influenza, and varicella may occur in the neonatal intensive care unit (NICU). These pathogens also may cause chronic infection, with subtle manifestations that may be recognized only after a prolonged period. It is important to recognize the manifestations of infections in the neonatal period to be able to treat the acute infection, prevent HAIs in other infants, and anticipate effects on the infant's subsequent growth and development.

Fungal infections are of greatest concern in the immunocompromised or preterm infant. Occasionally fungal infections such as thrush are found in otherwise healthy term infants.

Septicemia refers to a generalized infection in the bloodstream. Pneumonia, the most common form of neonatal infection, is one of the leading causes of perinatal death. Bacterial meningitis occurs in approximately 0.2 to 0.4 cases per 1000 live births, with a higher rate in preterm infants. Gastroenteritis is sporadic, depending on epidemic outbreaks. Local infections such as conjunctivitis and thrush occur commonly.

CARE MANAGEMENT

Review the prenatal record for risk factors associated with infection and the signs and symptoms suggestive of infection. Maternal vaginal or perineal infection may be transmitted directly to the infant during passage through the birth canal. Psychosocial history and history of sexually transmitted infections (STIs) may indicate possible human immunodeficiency virus (HIV), hepatitis B virus (HBV), herpes (type 2), or cytomegalovirus (CMV) infection.

Perinatal events should also be reviewed. Premature rupture of membranes (PROM) may be caused by maternal or intrauterine infection. Ascending infection may occur after prolonged PROM, prolonged labor, or intrauterine fetal monitoring. In some cases infection may occur with intact membranes or contribute to early rupture. A maternal history of fever during labor or the presence of foul-smelling amniotic fluid may also indicate infection. Antibiotic therapy initiated during labor should be noted. The neonate's gestational age, maturity, birth weight, and gender affect the incidence of infection. Sepsis occurs about twice as often and results in a higher mortality in male than in female infants. Assess the neonate for respiratory distress, skin abscesses, petechial rashes, and other indications of infection.

During the postnatal period note the time of onset of suspicious clinical signs. Onset within the first 48 hours of life is more often associated with prenatal or perinatal predisposing factors; onset after 2 or 3 days more often reflects an HAI.

The earliest clinical signs of neonatal sepsis are characterized by a lack of specificity. The nonspecific signs include lethargy, poor feeding, poor weight gain, and irritability. The nurse or parent may simply note that the infant is not doing as well as before. Differential diagnosis may be difficult because signs of sepsis are similar to signs of noninfectious neonatal problems such as hypoglycemia and respiratory distress. Additional clinical and laboratory information, including cultures, supplement the findings described. Table 25-4 outlines the clinical manifestations associated with neonatal sepsis.

Laboratory studies are important. Specimens for cultures include blood, cerebrospinal fluid (CSF), stool, and urine. A complete blood cell count with differential is performed to determine the presence of bacterial infection or increased or decreased white blood cell count (the latter is an ominous sign). The total neutrophil count, immature-to-total (I/T) neutrophil ratio, absolute neutrophil count, platelet count, procalcitonin, and C-reactive protein may be used to determine the presence of sepsis. It is important to note that these tests are often adjuncts for the confirmation of neonatal sepsis; a combination of these tests and clinical signs often alert the practitioner to the need for treatment. Additional diagnostic tests that may be used to identify or exclude neonatal sepsis include sedimentation rate, interleukins (IL-8, IL-2, IL-6, and IL-1β), and nucleic acid amplification testing (NAAT). Antepartum infection can now be treated successfully with a number of antiviral medications to

TABLE 25-4	CLINICAL MANIFESTATIONS OF SEPSIS*
SYSTEM	**SIGNS**
Respiratory	Apnea
	Tachypnea
	Grunting, nasal flaring
	Retractions
	Decreased oxygen saturation
	Metabolic acidosis
Cardiovascular	Decreased cardiac output
	Tachycardia
	Bradycardia
	Hypotension
	Decreased perfusion
Central nervous	Temperature instability
	Lethargy
	Hypotonia
	Irritability, seizures
Gastrointestinal	Feeding intolerance (decreased suck strength and intake; increasing residuals)
	Abdominal distention
	Vomiting, diarrhea
Integumentary	Jaundice
	Pallor
	Petechiae
	Mottling

Modified from Askin DF: Bacterial and fungal sepsis in the neonate, *J Obstet Gynecol Neonatal Nurs* 24(7):635–643, 1995.
*Laboratory findings include neutropenia, increased bands, hypoglycemia or hyperglycemia, metabolic acidosis, and thrombocytopenia.

decrease viral replication and fetal transmission of disease; neonates may also be treated with antiviral medications such as acyclovir and ganciclovir. In high risk infants with significant illness, antiviral or antibiotic treatment may begin once cultures are obtained. Once the pathogen is identified, antibiotic, antiviral, or antifungal therapy may be modified.

Vigilant assessment continues during and after treatment. Prolonged administration of antibiotics to ELBW neonates without positive cultures in the first week of life is associated with an increased incidence of necrotizing enterocolitis (NEC), mortality, and late-onset infection; therefore careful use of antibiotics and close observation of such infants are recommended (Cotten, Taylor, Stoll, et al., 2009; Kuppala, Meinzen-Derr, Morrow, et al., 2011). The newborn continues to be assessed for sequelae to septicemia, which include meningitis, disseminated intravascular coagulation (DIC), NEC, pneumonia, and septic shock. Septic shock results from the toxins released into the bloodstream. The most common signs include decreasing oxygen saturation, poor perfusion (prolonged capillary refill, cool extremities, mottling), tachycardia, respiratory distress, and hypotension.

Breastfeeding (medically stable infants) or feeding the newborn expressed breast milk from the mother is encouraged. Breast milk provides protective mechanisms. Colostrum contains IgA, which offers protection against infection in the GI tract. Human milk contains iron-binding protein that exerts a bacteriostatic effect on

E. coli. Human milk also contains macrophages and lymphocytes. The vulnerability of infants to common mucosal pathogens such as RSV may be reduced by passive transfer of maternal immunity in the colostrum and breast milk. There is evidence that early enteral feedings with human milk are beneficial in establishing a natural barrier to infection in ELBW and VLBW infants (Hanson, 2007). Human milk is also thought to provide some degree of protection from NEC.

Administering medications, taking precautions when performing treatments, and following isolation procedures are also interventions to consider in the prevention and treatment of neonatal sepsis.

Monitoring an intravenous (IV) infusion and administering antibiotics are important nursing responsibilities. It is important to administer the prescribed dose of antibiotic within 1 hour after it is prepared to avoid loss of drug stability. If the IV fluid that the infant is receiving contains electrolytes, vitamins, or other medications, the nurse should check with the hospital pharmacy before adding antibiotics. The antibiotic (or other medication) may be deactivated or may form a precipitate when combined with other medications.

Care must be taken in suctioning secretions from any newborn's oropharynx or trachea. Routine suctioning is not recommended and may further compromise the infant's immune status, cause hypoxia, and increase ICP. Efforts should also be taken to prevent ventilator-associated pneumonia in infants on mechanical ventilation (see Chapter 40). Isolation procedures are implemented as indicated according to hospital policy. Isolation protocols change rapidly, and the nurse is urged to participate in continuing education and in-service programs to remain up to date.

Prevention

Virtually all controlled clinical trials have demonstrated that effective hand washing is responsible for the prevention of HAI in nursery units. Nursing is directly or indirectly responsible for minimizing or eliminating environmental sources of infectious agents in the nursery. Measures to be taken include Standard Precautions, careful and thorough cleaning of contaminated equipment, frequent replacement of used equipment (e.g., changing IV and nasogastric [NG] tubing per hospital protocol and cleaning resuscitation and ventilation equipment, IV pumps, and incubators), and appropriate disposal of contaminated linens and diapers. Overcrowding must be avoided in nurseries. Guidelines for space, visitation, and general infection control in areas where newborns receive care have been established and published (AAP and ACOG, 2007).

Infants cared for in the NICUs are at high risk for infection. Infection rates in VLBW infants are higher in those with lower birth weights. *Hand washing is the single most effective measure to reduce HAI.* However, the rate of compliance with standards for hand hygiene is reported to be only 22% (Buus-Frank, 2004). The combined use of alcohol, hand hygiene, and gloves is effective in reducing the incidence of systemic infection. It is incumbent on caregivers to strictly adhere to recommended guidelines for hand hygiene.

Antibiotic is instilled into a newborn's eyes 1 to 2 hours after birth to prevent infection (see Fig. 23-5). The skin, its secretions, and normal flora are natural defenses that protect against invading pathogens. Warm water may be used to remove blood and meconium from the neonate's face, head, and body. A mild nonmedicated soap (in a single-use container) can be used with careful water rinsing. Vernix caseosa is not scrubbed vigorously for removal, since this further disrupts the skin barrier properties (see Guidelines box, pp. 701-702). No single method of cord care has been shown to be more effective in the promotion of drying, separating, and preventing colonization. Current recommendations for cord care by the Association of Women's Health, Obstetric and Neonatal Nurses (AWHONN) (2007) include cleaning the cord with sterile water or a neutral pH cleanser; subsequent care entails cleaning the cord with water. Nurses must follow agency protocols for cord care, but they can recommend revision of protocols based on research (see also Umbilical Cord Care, Chapter 23, p. 627). Polin, Denson, Brady, et al. (2012) provide additional strategies for the prevention of HAI in the NICU.

MATERNAL INFECTIONS

The range of pathologic conditions produced by infectious agents is large, and the difference between the maternal and fetal effects caused by any one agent is also great. Some maternal infections, especially during early gestation, can result in fetal loss or malformations because the fetus's ability to handle infectious organisms is limited and the fetal immunologic system is unable to prevent the dissemination of infectious organisms to the various tissues.

Not all prenatal infections produce teratogenic effects. Furthermore the clinical picture of disorders caused by transplacental transfer of infectious agents is not always well defined. Some viral agents can cause remarkably similar manifestations, and it is common to test for all of them when a prenatal infection is suspected. This is the so-called TORCH complex, an acronym for:

- *T*—Toxoplasmosis
- *O*—Other (e.g., HBV, parvovirus, HIV, West Nile)
- *R*—Rubella
- *C*—CMV infection
- *H*—Herpes simplex

To determine the causative agent in a symptomatic infant, tests are performed to rule out each of these infections. The *O* category may involve testing for several viral infections (e.g., HBV, varicella zoster, measles, mumps, HIV, syphilis, and human parvovirus). Bacterial infections are not included in the TORCH workup because they are usually identified by clinical manifestations and readily available laboratory tests. Gonococcal conjunctivitis (ophthalmia neonatorum) and chlamydial conjunctivitis have been reduced significantly by prophylactic measures at birth (see Critical Thinking Case Study and Chapter 22). The major maternal infections, their possible effects, and specific nursing considerations are outlined in Table 25-5.

CARE MANAGEMENT

One of the major goals in the care of infants suspected of having an infectious disease is identification of the causative organism. Standard Precautions are implemented according to institution policy. Pregnant health care personnel are cautioned to avoid contact with infants with suspected CMV and rubella infections. HSV is easily transmitted from one infant to another; therefore the risk of cross-contamination is reduced or eliminated by wearing gloves for patient contact. The *2012 Red Book: Report of the Committee on Infectious Diseases* (AAP, 2012) provides guidelines for the type and duration of precautions for most bacterial and viral exposures. Careful hand washing is the most important nursing intervention in reducing the spread of any infection.

Specimens need to be obtained for laboratory examinations, and the infant and parents need to be prepared for diagnostic

---

? CRITICAL THINKING CASE STUDY

Neonate with Chlamydia

An 8-day-old male infant is brought to the pediatric urgent care center on a Sunday morning by Maggie, an 18-year-old single mother, with a complaint of eye drainage for 2 days. Maggie is breastfeeding and states that she was diagnosed and partially treated for a couple of sexually transmitted infections in late gestation; she does not remember the name but says one started with a "C." The medications made her stomach sick, so she quit taking them after 2 days. The practitioner examines the infant, who has a purulent yellowish discharge from both eyes but otherwise appears healthy; she suspects chlamydial conjunctivitis and orders cultures of the eye drainage. The retrieved medical record from the infant's birth indicates that eye prophylaxis with erythromycin ophthalmic ointment was administered.

1. Evidence—Is there sufficient evidence to draw conclusions about the cause of the infant's eye drainage?
2. Assumptions—What assumptions can be made about the following factors:
   a. Treatment for neonatal chlamydia infection.
   b. Neonatal sequelae of inadequate chlamydia treatment in newborn.
   c. The mother's health status and possible treatment (she is not allergic to penicillin).
3. What implications and priorities for nursing care can be drawn at this time?
4. Does the evidence objectively support your conclusion?

---

procedures. When possible, long-term disabilities are prevented by early evaluation and implementation of therapy. The family is taught any special handling techniques needed for the care of their infant and signs of complications or possible sequelae. If sequelae are inevitable, the family needs assistance in determining how they can best cope with the problems such as assistance with home care, referral to appropriate agencies, or placement in an institution for care. The major goal of nursing care is prevention of these disorders with provision of adequate prenatal care for the expectant mother and precautions regarding exposure to teratogenic infections.

DRUG-EXPOSED INFANTS*

Maternal habits hazardous to the fetus and neonate include drug addiction, smoking, and alcohol abuse. Occasional withdrawal reactions have been reported in neonates of mothers who use to excess such drugs as barbiturates, alcohol, amphetamines, or antidepressants. Serious reactions are seen in neonates whose mothers abuse psychoactive drugs or are treated with methadone.

Narcotics, which have a low molecular weight, readily cross the placental membrane and enter the fetal system. Illicit substances may also be transmitted to the newborn through breast milk. When the mother is a habitual user of opiates, especially OxyContin, heroin, or methadone, the unborn child may also become chemically dependent or passively addicted to the drug, which places such infants at risk during the perinatal and early neonatal periods. Neonatal abstinence syndrome (NAS) is the term used to describe the set of behaviors exhibited by infants exposed to narcotics in utero.

---

*Unless otherwise noted, the information presented throughout this section refers to drug-exposed neonates in general, regardless of the drug to which they have been exposed.

TABLE 25-5	INFECTIONS ACQUIRED FROM THE MOTHER BEFORE, DURING, OR AFTER BIRTH*	
FETAL OR NEWBORN EFFECT	**TRANSMISSION**	**NURSING CONSIDERATIONS†**
Human Immunodeficiency Virus No significant difference between infected and uninfected infants at birth in some instances Embryopathy reported by some observers: • Depressed nasal bridge • Mild upward or downward obliquity of eyes • Long palpebral fissures with blue sclerae • Patulous lips • Ocular hypertelorism • Prominent upper vermilion border See also Chapter 43	Transplacental; during vaginal birth; potentially in breast milk	Administer combination antiretroviral prophylaxis to human immunodeficiency (HIV)–positive mother; prophylaxis to prevent perinatal transmission may begin after first trimester. Choice of regimens is determined by examining a number of factors, including mother's current treatment. Detailed recommendations can be obtained from Panel on Treatment of HIV-Infected Pregnant Women and Prevention of Perinatal Transmission (2011). During labor *ZDV is recommended for all HIV-infected pregnant women, regardless of the antepartum treatment regimen.* HIV-exposed neonates (regardless of maternal antiretroviral dosing) should receive a 6-wk course of ZDV starting as soon after birth as possible but preferably within 6 to 12 hours; nevirapine may also be given in 3 doses during the first week of life. ZDV dosing varies according to infant gestational age and route of administration (Panel on Treatment, Table 9, 2011). Cesarean birth at 38 weeks' gestation in HIV-positive mothers is recommended to reduce transmission. Avoid breastfeeding in HIV-positive mother. For chemoprophylaxis against *Pneumocystis carinii* pneumonia in HIV-exposed infants, drug of choice is trimethoprim-sulfamethoxazole (Bactrim, Septra). Documented routine HIV education and routine testing with consent for all pregnant women in United States are recommended.
Chickenpox (Varicella-Zoster Virus [VZV]) Intrauterine exposure—congenital varicella syndrome: limb dysplasia, microcephaly, cortical atrophy, chorioretinitis, cataracts, cutaneous scars, other anomalies, auditory nerve palsy, motor and cognitive delays Severe symptoms (rash, fever) and higher mortality in infant whose mother develops varicella 5 days before to 2 days after birth	First trimester (fetal varicella syndrome); perinatal period (infection)	Use varicella zoster immune globulin or IVIG to treat infants born to mothers with onset of disease within 5 days before or 2 days after birth. Healthy term infants exposed postnatally to varicella (especially if mother's rash does not appear until after 48 hours after birth) should not receive varicella zoster immune globulin (AAP, 2012). Institute isolation precautions in newborn born to mother with varicella up to 21-28 days (latter time if newborn received varicella zoster immune globulin or IVIG after birth (if hospitalized).† Prevention—Immunize all children with varicella vaccine.
Chlamydia Infection *(Chlamydia trachomatis)* Conjunctivitis, pneumonia	Last trimester or perinatal period	Standard ophthalmic prophylaxis for gonococcal ophthalmia neonatorum (topical antibiotics, silver nitrate, or povidone-iodine) is *not effective* in treatment or prevention of chlamydial ophthalmia. Treat with oral erythromycin or ethylsuccinate for 14 days; a second course of erythromycin may be required, and follow-up of exposed infant is recommended (see Critical Thinking Case Study, p. 670).

Continued

TABLE 25-5   INFECTIONS ACQUIRED FROM THE MOTHER BEFORE, DURING, OR AFTER BIRTH*—cont'd

FETAL OR NEWBORN EFFECT	TRANSMISSION	NURSING CONSIDERATIONS†
Coxsackievirus (Group B Enterovirus-Nonpolio, Parechovirus)		
Poor feeding, vomiting, diarrhea, fever; cardiac enlargement, arrhythmias, congestive heart failure; lethargy, seizures, meningoencephalitis, pneumonitis Mimics bacterial sepsis	Peripartum	Treatment is supportive. Provide IVIG in neonatal infections.
Cytomegalovirus (CMV)		
Variable manifestation from asymptomatic to severe Microcephaly, cerebral calcifications, chorioretinitis Jaundice, hepatosplenomegaly Petechial or purpuric rash (Fig. 25-4) Neurologic sequelae—seizure disorders, sensorineural hearing loss, cognitive impairment	Throughout pregnancy	Infection acquired at birth, shortly thereafter, or via human milk is not associated with clinical illness in term infants. Exposed preterm infants may have systemic infection, including interstitial pneumonia. Affected individuals excrete virus. Virus is detected in urine or tissue by electron microscopy. Pregnant women should avoid close contact with known cases. To treat infection administer antivirals such as IV ganciclovir or oral valganciclovir for 6 weeks to newborn (AAP, 2012).
Parvovirus B19 (Erythema Infectiosum)		
Fetal hydrops and death from anemia and heart failure with early exposure Anemia with later exposure No teratogenic effects established Ordinarily low risk of adverse effect to fetus	Transplacental	First-trimester infection has most serious effects. Aggressive cardiovascular and respiratory support is required in newborns with hydrops. Pregnant health care workers should not care for patients who might be highly contagious (e.g., child with sickle cell anemia, aplastic crisis). Routine exclusion of pregnant women from workplace where disease is occurring is not recommended.
Gonococcal Disease *(Neisseria gonorrhoeae)*		
Ophthalmitis Neonatal gonococcal arthritis, septicemia, meningitis	Last trimester or perinatal period	Preventive—Apply prophylactic medication to eyes at time of birth. Infant with confirmed ophthalmia, scalp abscess, or disseminated infection should be hospitalized, and cultures obtained to determine antimicrobial treatment. Consider testing infant for *Chlamydia*, HIV, and syphilis. Irrigate infant's eyes with saline until discharge is eliminated. Obtain smears for culture. To treat ophthalmia and nondisseminated infection, administer IV or IM ceftriaxone once. Disseminated disease requires cefotaxime treatment for 1 week.
Hepatitis B Virus (HBV)		
May be asymptomatic at birth; more than 90% of infants infected perinatally develop chronic Hep B infection Clinical hepatitis, jaundice, changes in liver function; possible fulminant hepatitis	Transplacental; contaminated maternal fluids or secretions during birth	Administer HBIG to all infants of HBsAG-positive mothers within 12 hr of birth; in addition, administer HepB vaccine at separate site. Prevention—Immunize all infants with HepB vaccine. Infants born to HBsAG-positive mothers and weighing <2000 g (4 lbs 7 oz) should receive 3-dose vaccine series *in addition* to birth dose (See Immunizations, Chapter 31.)
Listeriosis (Listeria monocytogenes)		
Maternal infection associated with spontaneous abortion, preterm birth, and fetal death Preterm birth, sepsis, and pneumonia seen in early-onset disease; late-onset disease usually manifests as meningitis	Transplacental by ascending infection or exposure at birth	Hand washing is essential to prevent nosocomial spread. Treat infected newborn with antibiotics—ampicillin and an aminoglycoside such as gentamicin (14- to 21-day treatment is recommended for meningitis).

TABLE 25-5   INFECTIONS ACQUIRED FROM THE MOTHER BEFORE, DURING, OR AFTER BIRTH*—cont'd

FETAL OR NEWBORN EFFECT	TRANSMISSION	NURSING CONSIDERATIONS†
Rubella, Congenital (Rubella Virus)		
Congenital rubella syndrome Eyes—retinopathy, cataracts (unilateral or bilateral), microphthalmia, retinitis, glaucoma CNS signs—microcephaly, seizures, severe cognitive impairment Congenital heart defects—patent ductus arteriosus Auditory defects—sensorineural hearing loss Dermal erythropoiesis—blueberry muffin lesions IUGR—hyperbilirubinemia, meningitis, thrombocytopenia, hepatomegaly	First trimester; early second trimester	Pregnant women should avoid contact with all affected persons, including infants with rubella syndrome. Emphasize vaccination of all unimmunized prepubertal children, susceptible adolescents, and women of childbearing age (nonpregnant). Caution women against becoming pregnant for at least 28 days after vaccination.
Syphilis, Congenital (Treponema pallidum)		
Stillbirth, prematurity, hydrops fetalis May be asymptomatic at birth and in first few weeks of life or may have multisystem manifestations: hepatosplenomegaly, lymphadenopathy, hemolytic anemia, pneumonia, and thrombocytopenia Copper-colored maculopapular cutaneous lesions (Fig. 25-5) (usually after first few weeks of life), mucous membrane patches, hair loss, nail exfoliation, snuffles (syphilitic rhinitis), profound anemia, poor feeding, pseudoparalysis of one or more limbs, dysmorphic teeth (older child)	Transplacental; can be anytime during pregnancy or at birth	This is most severe form of syphilis. Treatment consists of IV aqueous penicillin or IM procaine penicillin. Diagnostic evaluation depends on maternal serology testing, maternal therapy and response, maternal and infant serologic titers, results of nontreponemal infant tests, and infant physical examination (including ophthalmologic examinations and long-bone radiographs) and laboratory examination results (e.g., LFTs, CBC, platelets, CSF protein and cell count). Monitor closely for development of complications of disease during first year of life.
Toxoplasmosis, Congenital (Toxoplasma gondii)		
May be asymptomatic at birth (70%-90% of cases) or have maculopapular rash, lymphadenopathy, hepatosplenomegaly, jaundice, thrombocytopenia In some cases severely infected fetus may die in utero or shortly after birth Later developments— hydrocephaly, cerebral calcifications, chorioretinitis (classic triad), microcephaly, seizures, cognitive impairment, deafness, encephalitis, myocarditis, hepatosplenomegaly, anemia, jaundice, diarrhea, vomiting, purpura	Throughout pregnancy Predominant host for organism is cats May be transmitted through cat feces or poorly cooked or raw infected meats	Caution pregnant women to avoid contact with cat feces (e.g., emptying cat litter boxes). Administer sulfadiazine (with folinic acid) and pyrimethamine (Daraprim). Spiramycin may be administered to infected pregnant female to reduce transmission to fetus but has no effect if fetal infection has occurred.
Herpes Simplex Virus (HSV)		
Neonatal herpes manifests in one of three ways: (1) with SEM involvement; (2) as localized CNS disease; or (3) as disseminated disease involving multiple organs. In skin and eye disease rash appears as vesicles or pustules on erythematous base. Clusters of lesions are common. Lesions ulcerate and crust over rapidly (Fig. 25-6) Ophthalmologic clinical findings include chorioretinitis and microphthalmia; neurologic involvement such as microcephaly and encephalomalacia may also develop. Disseminated infections may involve virtually every organ system; but liver, adrenal glands, and lungs are most commonly affected. In HSV meningitis, infants develop multiple lesions of cortical hemorrhagic necrosis. It can occur alone or with SEM lesions. Presenting symptoms, which may occur in second-to-fourth weeks of life, include lethargy, poor feeding, irritability, and local or generalized seizures. Neonatal HSV has high mortality rate.	86% to 90% of cases transmitted at birth (Shet, 2011)	Absence of skin lesions in neonate exposed to maternal herpesvirus does not indicate absence of disease. Contact Precautions (in addition to Standard Precautions) should be instituted .It is recommended that swabs of mouth, nasopharynx, conjunctivae, rectum, and any skin vesicles be obtained from exposed neonate; in addition, urine, stool, blood, and CSF specimens should be obtained for culture. Therapy with IV acyclovir is initiated if culture results are positive or if there is strong suspicion of herpesvirus infection; ophthalmic treatment (e.g., 1% trifluridine or 3% vidarabine) is required for ocular involvement in addition to acyclovir. Therapy with oral acyclovir for 6 months is recommended for neonates with HSV CNS disease (AAP, 2012).

Continued

TABLE 25-5	**INFECTIONS ACQUIRED FROM THE MOTHER BEFORE, DURING, OR AFTER BIRTH*—cont'd**	
FETAL OR NEWBORN EFFECT	**TRANSMISSION**	**NURSING CONSIDERATIONS†**
Group B Streptococcus Early-onset-infection (first 24 hours of life)—pneumonia, respiratory distress, shock, apnea, and meningitis Late-onset—(3 to 4 days of age)—bacteremia or meningitis; may occur later in LBW infants	Acquired perinatally; intrapartum antibiotics decrease early-onset but not late-onset disease Risk factors include preterm birth, maternal GBS (untreated), previous birth of GBS-infected newborn, maternal chorioamnionitis	Administer ampicillin plus an aminoglycoside such as gentamicin in infant with presumptive GBS infection; in infant with positive GBS, administer penicillin G. Observe Standard Precautions, including strict hand hygiene for handling all infants

CNS, central nervous system; *CBC*, complete blood count; *CSF*, cerebrospinal fluid; *GBS*, group B streptococcus; *HBIg*, hepatitis B immunoglobulin; *HBsAG*, hepatitis B surface antigen; *IUGR*, intrauterine growth restriction; *IM*, intramuscular; *IV*, intravenous; *IVIG*, intravenous immunoglobulin; *LBW*, low-birth-weight; *LFT*, liver function test; *SEM*, skin, eye, and mouth; *ZDV*, zidovudine.

*This table is not an exhaustive representation of all perinatally transmitted infections. For further information regarding specific diseases or treatment not listed here, refer to American Academy of Pediatrics (AAP) Committee on Infectious Diseases, Pickering L, editor: *2012 Red book: report of the Committee on Infectious Diseases*, ed 29, Elk Grove Village, Ill, 2012, AAP.

†Isolation precautions depend on institutional policy.

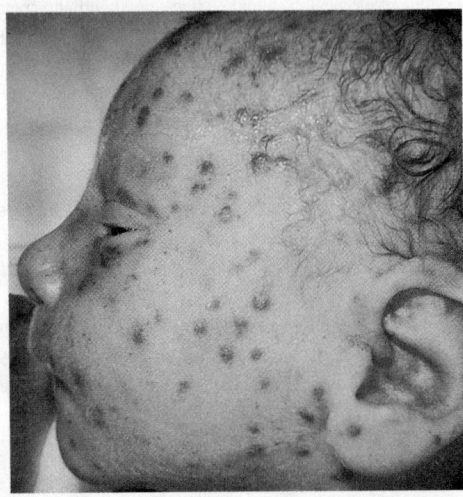

FIG 25-4 Neonatal cytomegalovirus infection. Typical rash seen in a severely affected infant. (Courtesy David A. Clarke, Philadelphia, PA.)

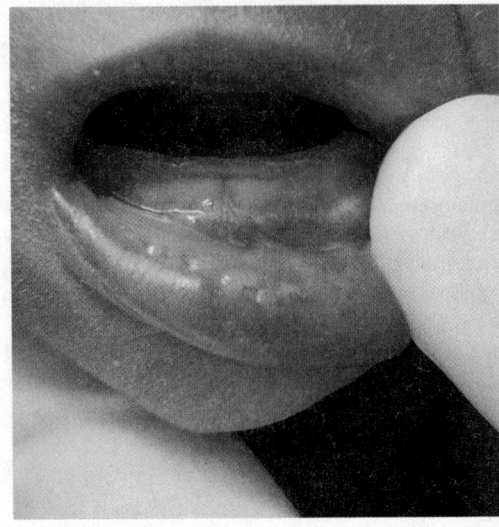

FIG 25-6 Herpes simplex virus oral lesions. (Courtesy David A. Clarke, Philadelphia, PA.)

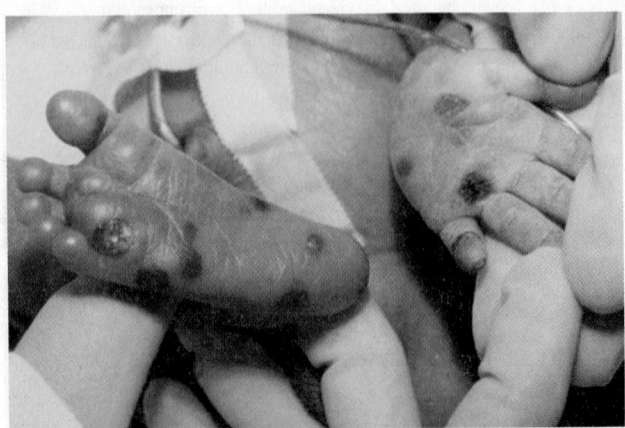

FIG 25-5 Neonatal syphilis lesions on hands and feet. (Courtesy Mahesh Kotwal, MD, Phoenix, AZ.)

The adverse effects of exposure of a fetus to drugs are varied. They include transient changes such as alterations in fetal breathing movements and irreversible effects such as fetal death, IUGR, structural malformations, behavioral problems, or cognitive impairment. Determining the specific effects of individual drugs on an individual fetus is made difficult by polydrug use, which is common; errors or omissions in reporting drug use; and variations in the strength, purity, and types of additives found in street drugs. Maternal conditions such as poverty, malnutrition, and co-morbid conditions such as STIs further compound the difficulty in identifying the presence and consequences of intrauterine drug exposure. Most infants who are exposed to drugs in utero may demonstrate no immediate untoward effects and appear normal at birth. Infants exposed only to heroin may begin to exhibit signs of drug withdrawal within 12 to 24 hours. If mothers have been taking methadone, the signs appear somewhat later (i.e., anywhere from 1 or 2 days to 2 to 3 weeks or more after birth). The clinical manifestations may fall into

BOX 25-2	SIGNS OF WITHDRAWAL IN NEONATES

Neurologic
- Irritability
- Seizures
- Hyperactivity
- High-pitched cry
- Tremors
- Exaggerated Moro reflex
- Hypertonicity of muscles

Gastrointestinal
- Poor feeding
- Diarrhea
- Dehydration
- Vomiting
- Frantic, uncoordinated sucking
- Gastric residuals

Autonomic
- Diaphoresis
- Fever
- Mottled skin
- Nasal stuffiness

Miscellaneous
- Disrupted sleep patterns
- Diaphoresis
- Tachypnea (>60 breaths/min)
- Excoriations (knees, face)
- Temperature instability

any one or all of the following categories: CNS, GI, respiratory, and autonomic nervous system signs (Burgos and Burke, 2009; Kuschel, 2007). The manifestations become most pronounced between 48 and 72 hours of age and may last from 6 days to 8 weeks, depending on the severity of the withdrawal (Box 25-2). Although these infants suck avidly on fists and display an exaggerated rooting reflex, they are poor feeders with uncoordinated and ineffectual sucking and swallowing reflexes.

Approximately 55% to 94% of infants born to narcotic-addicted mothers show signs of withdrawal (Burgos and Burke, 2009). Because of irregular and varying degrees of drug use, quality of drug, and mixed-drug usage by the mother, some infants display mild or variable manifestations. Most manifestations are the vague, nonspecific signs characteristic of all infants in general; therefore it is important to differentiate between drug withdrawal and other disorders before specific therapy is instituted. Other conditions (e.g., hypocalcemia, hypoglycemia, sepsis) often coexist with the drug withdrawal. Additional signs seen in drug-exposed newborns include loose stools; tachycardia; fever; projectile vomiting; crying; nasal stuffiness; and generalized perspiration, which is unusual in newborns.

Newborn urine, hair, or meconium sampling may be required to identify drug exposure and implement appropriate early interventional therapies aimed at minimizing the consequences of intrauterine drug exposure. Meconium sampling for fetal drug exposure is reported to provide more screening accuracy than urine screening because drug metabolites accumulate in meconium (Kuschel, 2007). Urine toxicology screening may be less accurate because it reflects only recent substance intake by the mother (Albright and Rayburn, 2009). Meconium and hair testing for drug metabolites has the advantages of being noninvasive, more accurate, and easy to collect. One study examining urine, hair, and meconium samples for drug use found that, although all of these tests were reliable to a greater or lesser degree, the single most reliable method for determining prenatal drug use was a careful history collected by an experienced interviewer (Eyler, Behnke, Wobie, et al., 2005).

The treatment of drug-exposed infants initially consists of early identification through maternal history, presenting symptoms of NAS, or toxicology screening when substance abuse is strongly suspected. Early identification and intervention are essential to prevent

further adverse effects; early discharge from the birth institution should be postponed until the maternal situation is assessed further and a treatment plan for the mother and infant is established. Drug therapies to decrease withdrawal effects include parenteral or oral administration of phenobarbital, buprenorphine, clonidine, methadone, and morphine. A combination of these drugs may be necessary to treat infants exposed to multiple drugs in utero, and careful attention should be given to possible adverse effects of the treatment drugs (Burgos and Burke, 2009).

The prognosis for drug-exposed infants depends on the type and amount of drug(s) taken by the mother and the stage(s) of fetal development in which the drug was taken. The overall mortality rate of infants born to narcotic-addicted mothers is increased; but with early recognition, proper treatment, and long-term follow-up the morbidity and mortality associated with drug exposure are decreased.

Often drug-exposed infants exhibit poor brain and body growth at birth. However, sometimes infants do not exhibit any signs that indicate exposure to harmful agents; therefore their condition may be overlooked until symptoms appear later in life. Drug-exposed infants may have chronic feeding problems; irritability; abnormal neurologic responses; abnormal parent-infant interactions; developmental and cognitive delays; learning disabilities in childhood; and behavioral problems, including ADHD.

CARE MANAGEMENT

One of the key factors in the treatment of drug-exposed neonates is early identification of substance abuse in the pregnant woman so treatment can be initiated and side effects minimized. This is especially problematic from a social and legal standpoint because the pregnant woman is often aware of the consequences of admitting to substance abuse and therefore may be less likely to readily admit to the problem for fear of social and legal repercussions. If the mother has had good prenatal care, the practitioner is aware of the problem and may have instituted therapy before birth. However, a number of mothers deliver their infants without the benefit of adequate care, and the condition is unknown to health care personnel at the time of birth.

The degree of withdrawal is closely related to the amount of drug the mother has habitually taken, the length of time she has been taking the drug, and her drug level at the time of birth. The most severe symptoms are observed in the infants of mothers who have taken large amounts of drugs over a long period. In addition, the nearer to the time of birth that the mother takes the drug, the longer it takes the child to develop withdrawal, and the more severe the manifestations. The infant may not exhibit withdrawal symptoms until 7 to 10 days after birth, by which time most newborns have been discharged from the birth center, and caregivers are less likely to recognize signs of irritability and poor feeding as withdrawal, thus predisposing the newborn to abuse or neglect and growth failure (failure to thrive). The infant may be at further risk for subsequent abuse or neglect because of home conditions that preclude adequate newborn care and follow-up.

After the presence of NAS is identified in an infant, nursing care is directed toward treating the presenting signs, decreasing stimuli that may precipitate hyperactivity and irritability (e.g., dimming the lights, decreasing noise levels), providing adequate nutrition and hydration, and promoting the mother-infant relationship. Appropriate individualized developmental care is implemented to facilitate self-consoling and self-regulating behaviors. Irritable and hyperactive infants have been found to respond to physical comforting, movement, and close contact. Wrapping infants snugly and rocking and holding them tightly limit their ability to self-stimulate. Arranging nursing activities to reduce the amount of disturbance helps decrease exogenous stimulation.

Breastfeeding is encouraged in mothers who are not using illicit substances, do not have HIV infection, and are compliant with a methadone program; breastfeeding promotes mother-infant bonding, and small quantities of methadone passed through breast milk have not proved to be harmful.

The Neonatal Abstinence Scoring System or Finnegan tool (Fig. 25-7) was developed to monitor infants in an objective manner and evaluate their response to clinical and pharmacologic interventions (Finnegan, 1985). This system is also designed to help nurses and other health care workers evaluate the severity of infants' withdrawal symptoms.

The Neonatal Intensive Care Unit Network Neurobehavioral Scale (NNNS) is a comprehensive neurologic and behavioral assessment tool that may be used to identify newborns at risk as a result of intrauterine drug exposure. The tool measures stress or abstinence, state, neurologic status, and muscle tone in the context of the newborn's medical condition at the time of examination. The NNNS may be used for medically stable newborns who are at least 30 weeks of gestation and up to 48 weeks of corrected or conceptional age (Lester, Tronick, and Brazelton, 2004).

Loose stools, poor intake, and regurgitation after feeding predispose these infants to malnutrition, dehydration, skin breakdown, and electrolyte imbalance. In addition, they burn up energy with continual activity and increased oxygen consumption at the cellular level. Frequent weighing, careful monitoring of intake and output and electrolytes, and additional caloric supplementation may be necessary. Hyperactive infants must be protected from skin abrasions on the knees, toes, and cheeks that are caused by rubbing on bed linens while in a prone position (awake). Monitoring and recording the activity level and its relationship to other activities such as feeding and preventing complication are important nursing functions.

A valuable aid to anticipating problems in the newborn is recognizing substance abuse in the mother. Unless the mother is enrolled in a methadone rehabilitation program, she seldom risks calling attention to her habit by seeking prenatal care. Consequently infants and mothers are exposed to the additional hazards of obstetric and medical complications. Moreover, the nature of substance use and addiction makes the user susceptible to disorders such as infection (HBV, HIV), and the hazards of inadequate nutrition and preterm birth. Methadone treatment does not prevent withdrawal reaction in neonates, but the clinical course may be modified. In addition, the intensive psychologic support of mothers is a factor in the treatment and reduction of perinatal mortality. Experience has indicated that these mothers are usually anxious and depressed, lack confidence, have a poor self-image, and have difficulty with interpersonal relationships. They may have a psychologic need for the pregnancy and an infant.

Initial symptoms or the recurrence of withdrawal symptoms may develop after discharge from the hospital; therefore it is important to establish rapport and maintain contact with the family so they will return for treatment if this occurs. The demands of the drug-exposed infant on the caregiver are enormous and unrewarding in terms of positive feedback. The infants are difficult to comfort, and they cry for long periods, which can be especially trying for the caregiver after the infant's discharge from the hospital. Long-term follow-up to evaluate the status of the infant and family is very important. Sudden infant death syndrome (SIDS) (see Chapter 31) and HIV infection are observed more commonly in infants born to users of methadone and heroin.

Many problems arise in relation to the disposition of infants of drug-dependent mothers. Those who advocate separation of mothers and children argue that the mothers are not capable of assuming responsibility for their infant's care, child care is frustrating to them, and their existence is too disorganized and chaotic. Others encourage the mother-infant bond and recommend a protected environment such as a therapeutic community; a halfway house; or continuous ongoing, supportive services in the home after discharge. Careful evaluation and the cooperative efforts of a variety of health professionals are required whether the choice is foster home placement or supportive follow-up care of mothers who keep their infants.

Alcohol Exposure

Alcohol ingestion during pregnancy is associated with both short- and long-term effects on the fetus and newborn. The quantity of alcohol required to produce fetal effects is unclear, but it is known that infants born to heavy drinkers have twice the risk of congenital abnormalities than those born to moderate drinkers (Carlo, 2011a). Alcohol withdrawal can occur in neonates, particularly when maternal ingestion occurs near the time of birth. Signs and symptoms include jitteriness, increased tone and reflex responses, and irritability. Seizures are also common. Fetal effects of alcohol exposure vary from subtle learning disabilities to obvious facial features and growth abnormalities. In 2004 the National Organization on Fetal Alcohol Syndrome (NOFAS) clarified terminology for fetal alcohol exposure by adopting the term fetal alcohol spectrum disorder (FASD) as an umbrella term to describe the range of clinical effects. Fetal alcohol syndrome (FAS) falls within this spectrum but is reserved for individuals who display the triad of characteristic facial features, growth restriction, and neurodevelopmental deficits with a confirmed history of maternal alcohol consumption (Banakar, Kudlur, and George, 2009). Craniofacial features include microcephaly, small eyes or short palpebral fissures, a thin upper lip, a flat midface, and an indistinct philtrum (Fig. 25-8). Neurologic problems in FAS children include some degree of IQ deficit, ADHD, diminished fine-motor skills, and poor speech. They have been shown to lack inhibition, have no stranger anxiety, and lack appropriate judgment skills.

Infants who do not display the signs of FAS but are born to mothers who are also heavy alcohol drinkers have significantly more tremors, hypertonia, restlessness, excessive mouthing movements, crying, and inconsolability than infants of substance-abusive mothers who do not consume alcohol during pregnancy. An added concern regarding substance abuse is that many of the mothers often use several drugs such as tranquilizers, sedatives, amphetamines, phencyclidine, marijuana, and other psychotropic agents. These drugs may alter the mother's perception of the newborn's cues and physical and emotional needs.

For additional details regarding diagnosis and treatment of FASD see the Centers for Disease Control and Prevention FAS website: *www.cdc.gov/ncbddd/fasd/index.html.*

Cocaine Exposure

Cocaine is a CNS stimulant and peripheral sympathomimetic. Legally it is classified as a narcotic, but it is not an opioid. The effects on fetuses are secondary to maternal effects, which include increased blood pressure (BP), decreased uterine blood flow, and increased

NEONATAL ABSTINENCE SCORING SYSTEM

System	Signs and Symptoms	Score	AM				PM				Comments
Central Nervous System Disturbances	Excessive high-pitched (or other) cry	2									Daily weight:
	Continuous high-pitched (or other) cry	3									
	Sleeps <1 hour after feeding	3									
	Sleeps <2 hours after feeding	2									
	Sleeps <3 hours after feeding	1									
	Hyperactive Moro reflex	2									
	Markedly hyperactive Moro reflex	3									
	Mild tremors disturbed	1									
	Moderate-severe tremors disturbed	2									
	Mild tremors undisturbed	3									
	Moderate-severe tremors undisturbed	4									
	Increased muscle tone	2									
	Excoriation (specific area)	1									
	Myoclonic jerks	3									
	Generalized convulsions	5									
Metabolic/Vasomotor/Respiratory Disturbances	Sweating	1									
	Fever <101° (99–100.8° F/37.2–38.2° C)	1									
	Fever >101° (38.4° C and higher)	2									
	Frequent yawning (>3 or 4 times/interval)	1									
	Mottling	1									
	Nasal stuffiness	1									
	Sneezing (>3 or 4 times/interval)	1									
	Nasal flaring	2									
	Respiratory rate >60/min	1									
	Respiratory rate >60/min with retractions	2									
Gastrointestinal Disturbances	Excessive sucking	1									
	Poor feeding	2									
	Regurgitation	2									
	Projectile vomiting	3									
	Loose stools	2									
	Watery stools	3									
	Total Score										
	Initials of Scorer										

FIG 25-7 Neonatal Abstinence Scoring (NAS) system developed by L. Finnegan. (From Nelson N: *Current therapy in neonatal-perinatal medicine*, ed 2, St Louis, 1990, Mosby.)

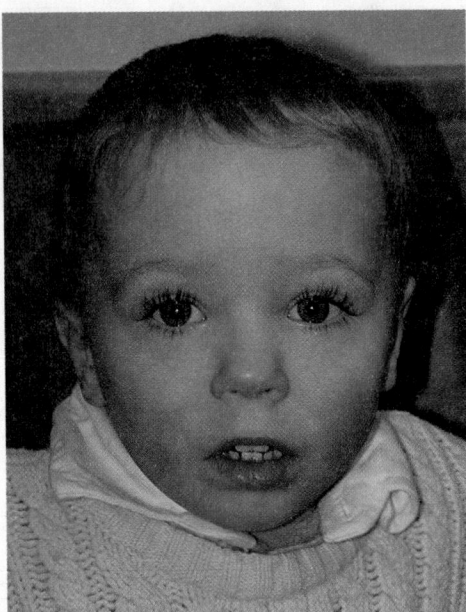

FIG 25-8 Child with fetal alcohol syndrome. (From Jorde LB, Carey JC, Bamshad MJ: *Medical genetics*, ed 4, St Louis, 2010, Mosby.)

vascular resistance. Consequently the fetus experiences decreased blood flow and oxygenation because of placental and fetal vasoconstriction. Researchers have concluded that variables such as the mother's lack of prenatal care; poor nutrition; and use of tobacco, alcohol, and other drugs during pregnancy compound the effects of cocaine exposure in the infant (Bandstra, Morrow, Mansoor, et al., 2010).

Infants may appear normal or may show neurologic problems at birth that may continue during the neonatal period. In much of the research literature these findings were transient, and evidence demonstrating permanent sequelae has varied. Either of two types of behavior may emerge as a result of the effects of cocaine on fetal development: neurobehavioral depression or excitability. The behaviors of a depressed infant include lethargy, poor suck, hypotonia, a weak cry, and difficulty in arousing. The behaviors of an excitable neonate may include a high-pitched cry, hypertonicity, rigidity, irritability, an inability to be consoled, and an intolerance to changes in routine (Bauer, Langer, Shankaran, et al., 2005; Chiriboga, Kuhn, and Wasserman, 2007).

Sequelae of prenatal cocaine exposure include preterm birth, a smaller head circumference, decreased birth length, and decreased weight. Head growth may be one of the best predictors of long-term development (Bauer, Langer, Shankaran, et al., 2005). Early studies of cocaine exposure identified an increased incidence of gastroschisis, genitourinary anomalies, and periventricular and intraventricular hemorrhage; however, meta-analyses have not confirmed these complications (Bandstra, Morrow, Mansoor, et al., 2010). Heavy cocaine exposure has been shown to result in elevated heart rate and irregular respirations after birth (Schuetze and Eiden, 2006).

Some studies found that long-term sequelae for newborns exposed to cocaine include lower language, motor, and cognitive scores and an increased risk for learning disabilities (Morrow, Culbertson, Accornero, et al., 2006); however, one study revealed no significant differences in the total or verbal intelligence quotient (IQ) scores but did note an increased risk of specific cognitive

impairments (Singer, Minnes, Short, et al., 2004). In a study that controlled for other prenatal drug exposures, a dose-related effect of cocaine was found on expressive, receptive, and total language scores at 3, 5, and 12 years of age (Bandstra, Morrow, Accornero, et al., 2011). Other investigators have found that the subtle effects of cocaine on school performance are moderated by the child's environment (Ackerman, Riggins, and Black, 2010). Studies using the Brazelton Neonatal Assessment Scale have again shown inconsistent results with subtle abnormalities in neurobehavioral clusters varying in timing of severity and according to levels of exposure (Bandstra, Morrow, Mansoor, et al., 2010).

Treatment of these infants is similar to that for other drug-exposed infants, including reduction of external stimuli, supportive treatment aimed at alleviating symptoms, and at times mild sedation.

CARE MANAGEMENT

Nursing care of cocaine-exposed infants is the same as that for other drug-exposed infants. Because they have increased flexor tone, these infants respond to swaddling (Pitts, 2010). Positioning, infant massage, and limited tactile stimulation have been shown to be effective interventions. Significant amounts of cocaine have been found in breast milk (Winecker, Goldberger, Tebbett, et al., 2001); therefore mothers should be cautioned regarding this hazard to their infants.

Referral to early intervention programs, including child health care, parental drug treatment, individualized developmental care, and parenting education, is essential in promoting optimum outcome for these children. Because they often live in impoverished environments, they are at high risk for cognitive delays, lack of child health care, and inadequate nutrition and benefit from early intervention programs.

Methamphetamine Exposure

The fetal and neonatal effects of maternal use of methamphetamines in pregnancy are not well known, and findings are often confounded by polydrug use and the effects of the newborn or child's environment. Low birth weight (LBW), preterm birth, and anomalies such as cleft lip and palate and cardiac defects have been reported in infants exposed to methamphetamines in utero (Pitts, 2010).

Methamphetamine use has increased significantly in the past 10 years in certain regions of the United States. In a report by Terplan, Smith, Kozloski, et al. (2009), 24% of pregnant women admitted to federally funded treatment centers in the United States used methamphetamines in 2006, up from 8% in 1994; 63% of pregnant women using methamphetamines reported using the drug throughout the pregnancy. A higher incidence of preterm birth and placental abruption was associated with methamphetamine use. In addition, fetal growth restriction (small for gestational age) was slightly higher in methamphetamine-exposed offspring; however, 80% of these neonates' mothers also had significant alcohol and tobacco use.

Study reports vary in the time of clinical manifestations of withdrawal from this drug; one study did not identify any signs of withdrawal in the first 3 days after birth, but long-term data were not collected (Smith, Yonekura, Wallace, et al., 2003). A study of infants exposed to methamphetamine in utero showed that such infants had significantly smaller head circumferences and birth weights than those not exposed; in addition, the exposed infants exhibited withdrawal signs of agitation, vomiting, and tachypnea, which were not observed in the unexposed infants (Chomchai, Na Manorom, Watanarungasan, et al., 2004). After birth infants may experience abnormal sleep patterns, agitation, poor feeding, and state disorganization (Pitts, 2010).

The long-term effects of methamphetamine exposure on children remain unclear; however, some studies have shown problems with mathematics and language skills. It is postulated that, similar to cocaine, methamphetamine exposure may affect areas of the brain responsible for higher-order functioning, with effects more likely to be manifest when the child reaches school age (Lester and Lagasse, 2010).

Marijuana Exposure

Marijuana has replaced cocaine as the most common illicit drug used by women ages 18 to 44 years (nonpregnant and pregnant) in the United States (Kuczkowski, 2007). Marijuana crosses the placenta; however, specific effects on the fetus have been difficult to determine. Some studies have reported an association between the chronic use of marijuana and a decrease in fetal growth and infant birth weight and length (Kuczkowski, 2007); however, this finding is confounded by cigarette smoking (Bandstra and Accornero, 2011; Schempf, 2007). More subtle effects of major exposure such as an increase in attention problems have also been identified (Marroun, Hudziak, Tiemeier, et al., 2011). Compounding the issue of the effects of marijuana, especially among women ages 18 to 30 years (Kuczkowski, 2007), is multidrug use, which combines the harmful effects of marijuana, tobacco, alcohol, opiates, and cocaine. Long-term follow-up studies on exposed infants are needed.

Selective Serotonin Reuptake Inhibitors

Studies estimate that between 15% and 25% of pregnant women experience major depression (Cantor Sackett, Weller, and Weller, 2009; Oberlander, Warburton, Misri, et al., 2006). For many of these women selective serotonin reuptake inhibitors (SSRIs) provide an important therapeutic benefit; however, these drugs may result in side effects in their newborns. Signs of withdrawal are present in up to one third of infants exposed to SSRIs in utero (Burgos and Burke, 2009). Findings include hypertonia, tremulousness, wakefulness, high-pitched crying, and feeding problems. An increased risk of persistent pulmonary hypertension has been reported in neonates exposed to SSRIs early in pregnancy (Cantor Sackett, Weller, and Weller, 2009); however, this finding has not been reported consistently (Wilson, Zelig, Harvey, et al., 2011). Some SSRIs are transferred into breast milk. Breastfeeding infants whose mothers are taking SSRIs should be monitored for sleep disturbances, irritability, and poor feeding.

CARE MANAGEMENT

The general nursing care of the newborn exposed to these drugs is directed toward identification of substance use in the mother and vigilance for signs of withdrawal in the neonate. Nurses may use the NAS tool to identify the severity of withdrawal for the implementation of specific drug treatment. Identifying specific signs and symptoms associated with drug withdrawal also assists in developing a plan of care to benefit the mother-infant pair. The nurse has an important role in helping the mother with caretaking abilities to promote self-esteem and meet the newborn's individual needs. Referral to special developmental care programs may be required to prevent serious cognitive and behavioral problems at the time of school entry.

HEMOLYTIC DISORDERS

Hyperbilirubinemia in the first 24 hours of life is most often the result of hemolytic disease of the newborn (HDN) (erythroblastosis fetalis), an abnormally rapid rate of red blood cell (RBC) destruction. Anemia caused by this destruction stimulates the production of RBCs, which in turn provides increasing numbers of cells for hemolysis. Major causes of increased erythrocyte destruction are isoimmunization (primarily Rh) and ABO incompatibility.

Blood Incompatibility

The membranes of human blood cells contain a variety of antigens, also known as agglutinogens, substances capable of producing an immune response if recognized by the body as foreign. The reciprocal relationship between antigens on RBCs and antibodies in the plasma causes agglutination (clumping). In other words antibodies in the plasma of one blood group (except the AB group, which contains no antibodies) produce agglutination when mixed with antigens of a different blood group. In the ABO blood group system, the antibodies occur naturally. In the Rh system the person must be exposed to the Rh antigen before significant antibody formation takes place and causes a sensitivity response known as isoimmunization.

Rh Incompatibility (Isoimmunization)

The Rh blood group consists of several antigens (with D being the most prevalent). For simplicity only the terms Rh positive (presence of antigen) and Rh negative (absence of antigen) are used in this discussion. The presence or absence of the naturally occurring Rh factor determines the blood type.

Ordinarily no problems are anticipated when the Rh blood types are the same in both the mother and the fetus or when the mother is Rh positive and the infant is Rh negative. Difficulty may arise when the mother is Rh negative and the infant is Rh positive. Although the maternal and fetal circulations are separate, there is evidence of a bidirectional trafficking of fetal RBCs and cell-free DNA to the maternal circulation (Moise, 2007). However, more commonly fetal RBCs enter into the maternal circulation at the time of birth. The mother's natural defense mechanism responds to these alien cells by producing anti-Rh antibodies.

Under normal circumstances this process of isoimmunization has no effect during the first pregnancy with an Rh-positive fetus because the initial sensitization to Rh antigens rarely occurs before the onset of labor. However, with the increased risk of fetal blood being transferred to the maternal circulation during placental separation, maternal antibody production is stimulated. During a subsequent pregnancy with an Rh-positive fetus, these previously formed maternal antibodies to Rh-positive blood cells may enter the fetal circulation, where they attack and destroy fetal erythrocytes (Fig. 25-9). Multiple gestations, abruptio placentae, placenta previa, manual removal of the placenta, and cesarean birth increase the incidence of transplacental hemorrhage and subsequent isoimmunization (Diehl-Jones and Fraser Askin, 2010).

Because the condition begins in utero, the fetus attempts to compensate for the progressive hemolysis and anemia by accelerating the rate of erythropoiesis. As a result, immature RBCs (erythroblasts) appear in the fetal circulation; thus the term erythroblastosis fetalis.

There is wide variability in the development of maternal sensitization to Rh-positive antigens. Sensitization may occur during the first pregnancy if the woman had previously received an Rh-positive blood transfusion. No sensitization may occur in situations in which

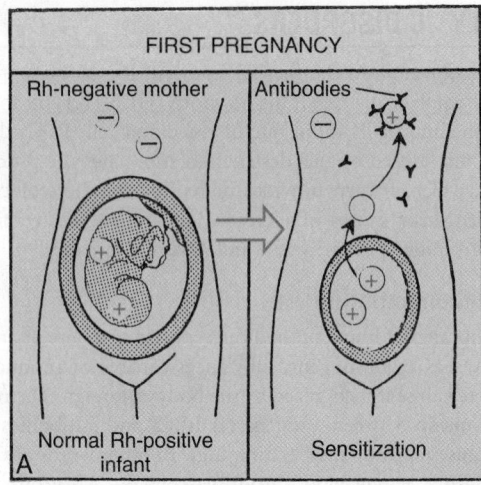

FIRST PREGNANCY

Rh-negative mother

Antibodies

Normal Rh-positive infant

A

Sensitization

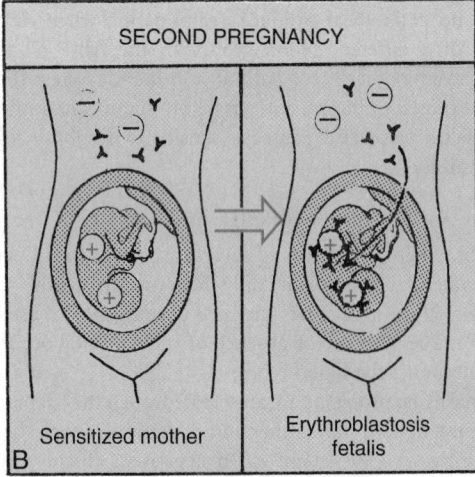

SECOND PREGNANCY

Sensitized mother

Erythroblastosis fetalis

B

FIG 25-9 Development of maternal sensitization to Rh antigens. **A,** Fetal Rh-positive erythrocytes enter the maternal system. Maternal anti-Rh antibodies are formed. **B,** Anti-Rh antibodies cross the placenta and attack fetal erythrocytes.

a strong placental barrier prevents transfer of fetal blood into the maternal circulation. In approximately 10% to 15% of sensitized mothers there is no hemolytic reaction in the newborn. In addition, some Rh-negative women, even though exposed to Rh-positive fetal blood, are immunologically unable to produce antibodies to the foreign antigen.

In the most severe form of erythroblastosis fetalis, **hydrops fetalis,** the progressive hemolysis causes fetal hypoxia; cardiac failure; generalized edema (anasarca); and fluid effusions into the pericardial, pleural, and peritoneal spaces (hydrops). The fetus may be delivered stillborn or in severe respiratory distress. Maternal RhIg administration, early intrauterine detection of fetal anemia by ultrasonography (serial Doppler assessment of the peak velocity in the fetal middle cerebral artery), and subsequent treatment by fetal blood transfusions or high-dose IVIG have dramatically improved the outcome of affected fetuses (Moise, 2008a).

ABO Incompatibility

Hemolytic disease can also occur when the major blood group antigens of the fetus are different from those of the mother. The major blood groups are A, B, AB, and O. In the North American Caucasian population 46% have type O blood, 42% have type A blood, 9% have type B blood, and 3% have type AB blood.

TABLE 25-6	POTENTIAL MATERNAL-FETAL ABO INCOMPATIBILITIES	
MATERNAL BLOOD GROUP	**INCOMPATIBLE FETAL BLOOD GROUP**	
O	A or B	
B	A or AB	
A	B or AB	

The presence or absence of antibodies and antigens determines whether agglutination will occur. Antibodies in the plasma of one blood group (except the AB group, which contains no antibodies) produce agglutination (clumping) when mixed with antigens of a different blood group. Naturally occurring antibodies in the recipient's blood cause agglutination of a donor's RBCs. The agglutinated donor cells become trapped in peripheral blood vessels, where they hemolyze, releasing large amounts of bilirubin into the circulation.

The most common blood group incompatibility in the neonate is between a mother with O blood group and an infant with A or B blood group (see Table 25-6 for possible ABO incompatibilities). Naturally occurring anti-A or anti-B antibodies already present in the maternal circulation cross the placenta and attack the fetal RBCs, causing hemolysis. Usually the hemolytic reaction is less severe than in Rh incompatibility; however, rare cases of hydrops have been reported (Black and Maheshwari, 2009). Unlike the Rh reaction, ABO incompatibility may occur in the first pregnancy. The risk of significant hemolysis in subsequent pregnancies is higher when the first pregnancy is complicated by ABO incompatibility (Sarici, Yurdakok, Serdar, et al., 2002).

Jaundice may appear shortly after birth (during the first 24 hours) in newborns affected by HDN, and serum levels of unconjugated bilirubin rise rapidly. Anemia results from the hemolysis of large numbers of erythrocytes, and hyperbilirubinemia and jaundice result from the inability of the liver to conjugate and excrete the excess bilirubin. Most newborns with HDN are not jaundiced at birth. However, hepatosplenomegaly and varying degrees of hydrops may be evident. If the infant is severely affected, signs of anemia (notably marked pallor) and hypovolemic shock are apparent. Hypoglycemia may occur as a result of pancreatic cell hyperplasia.

Early identification and diagnosis of Rh(D) sensitization are important in the management and prevention of fetal complications. A maternal antibody titer (indirect Coombs' test) should be drawn at the first prenatal visit. Genetic testing allows early identification of paternal zygosity at the Rh(D) gene locus, thus allowing earlier detection of the potential for isoimmunization and avoiding further maternal or fetal testing (Moise, 2008b). Amniocentesis can be used to test the fetal blood type of a woman whose antibody screen result is positive; the use of PCR may determine the fetal blood type and presence of maternal antibodies. The fetal hemoglobin and hematocrit can also be measured. Chorionic villus sampling has drawbacks that preclude its use, including possible spontaneous abortion of the fetus and fetomaternal hemorrhage, which would essentially make the situation worse. With either method, if the fetus is found to be Rh negative, no further treatment is required. The detection of cell-free fetal DNA in the maternal plasma of Rh(D)-negative women to detect an Rh(D)-positive fetus has been used successfully in Europe. Such testing usually negates the necessity of amniocentesis for fetal blood type (Moise and Argoti, 2012).

Ultrasonography is considered an important adjunct in the detection of isoimmunization; alterations in the placenta, umbilical cord, and amniotic fluid volume and the presence of fetal hydrops can be detected with high-resolution ultrasonography and allow early treatment before the development of erythroblastosis. Doppler ultrasonography of fetal middle cerebral artery peak velocity has been used to detect and measure fetal hemoglobin and subsequently fetal anemia (Moise and Argoti, 2012). Erythroblastosis fetalis caused by Rh incompatibility can also be monitored by evaluating rising anti-Rh antibody titers in the maternal circulation or testing the optical density of amniotic fluid (delta OD450 test) because bilirubin discolors the fluid.

The disease in the newborn is suspected on the basis of the timing and appearance of jaundice and can be confirmed postnatally by detecting antibodies attached to the circulating erythrocytes of affected infants (direct Coombs' test or direct antiglobulin test). The Coombs' test may be performed on umbilical cord blood samples from infants born to Rh-negative mothers if there is a history of incompatibility or further investigation is warranted.

The primary aim of therapeutic management of isoimmunization is prevention. Postnatal therapy is usually phototherapy for mild cases of hemolysis and exchange transfusion for more severe forms. Although phototherapy may control bilirubin levels in mild cases, the hemolytic process may continue, causing severe anemia between 7 and 21 days of life. In some institutions a metalloporphyrin is administered intramuscularly to decrease the formation of bilirubin in neonates with ABO incompatibility.

Prevention

The administration of RhIg, a human gamma globulin concentrate of anti-D, to all unsensitized Rh-negative mothers after birth or abortion of an Rh-positive infant or fetus prevents the development of maternal sensitization to the Rh factor. The injected anti-Rh antibodies are thought to destroy (by subsequent phagocytosis and agglutination) fetal RBCs passing into the maternal circulation before they can be recognized by the mother's immune system. Because the immune response is blocked, anti-D antibodies and memory cells (which produce the primary and secondary immune responses, respectively) are not formed (Bagwell, 2007; Blackburn, 2011). The inhibition of memory cell formation is especially important because memory cells provide long-term immunity by initiating a rapid immune response after the antigen is reintroduced (McCance and Huether, 2010).

To be effective, RhIg (e.g., RhoGAM) must be administered to unsensitized mothers within 72 hours (but possibly as long as 3 to 4 weeks) after the first birth or abortion and repeated after subsequent pregnancies or losses. The administration of RhIG at 26 to 28 weeks of gestation further reduces the risk of Rh isoimmunization. RhIg is not effective against existing Rh-positive antibodies in the maternal circulation.

Studies have demonstrated the effectiveness of IVIG at decreasing the severity of RBC destruction (hemolysis) in HDN and subsequent development of neonatal jaundice (Elalfy, Elbarbary, and Abaza, 2011; Mundy, 2005). IVIG administered to the neonate is believed to attack the maternal cells that destroy neonatal RBCs, slowing the progression of bilirubin production (Mundy, 2005). This therapy, often used in conjunction with phototherapy, may decrease the necessity for exchange transfusion. Maternal administration of high-dose IVIG, alone or in combination with plasmapheresis, decreases the fetal effects of Rh(D) isoimmunization (Moise, 2008b; Urbaniak, 2008).

Intrauterine Transfusion

Infants of mothers already sensitized may be treated by intrauterine transfusion, which consists of infusing blood into the umbilical vein of the fetus. The need for therapy is based on the antenatal diagnosis of fetal anemia by serial Doppler assessments of peak systolic velocity of the middle cerebral artery (Moise and Argot, 2012). With the advance of ultrasound technology, fetal transfusion may be accomplished directly via the umbilical vein, infusing type O Rh-negative packed RBCs to raise the fetal hematocrit to 40% to 50%; fetal movement and transfusion risks are minimized by administering vecuronium bromide for temporary fetal paralysis. The frequency of intrauterine transfusions may vary according to institution and fetal hydropic status, but one recommendation is for intervals of 10 days, 2 weeks, and then 3 weeks for subsequent procedures until the fetus reaches pulmonary maturity at approximately 37 to 38 weeks of gestation (Moise, 2008b; Moise and Argoti, 2012). Intraperitoneal blood transfusions are used less commonly for isoimmunization because of higher associated fetal risks; however, they may be used when intravascular access is impossible.

Exchange Transfusion

Exchange transfusion, in which the infant's blood is removed in small amounts (usually 5 to 10 mL at a time) and replaced with compatible blood (e.g., Rh-negative blood), is a standard mode of therapy for treatment of severe hyperbilirubinemia and is the treatment of choice for hyperbilirubinemia and hydrops caused by Rh incompatibility. Exchange transfusion removes the sensitized erythrocytes, lowers the serum bilirubin level to prevent bilirubin encephalopathy, corrects the anemia, and prevents cardiac failure. Indications for exchange transfusion in full-term infants may include a rapidly increasing serum bilirubin level and hemolysis despite intensive phototherapy. The criteria for exchange transfusions in preterm infants vary according to associated illness factors. The AAP Subcommittee on Hyperbilirubinemia (2004) practice parameter guidelines provide recommendations for initiating phototherapy and exchange transfusion in infants at 35 weeks of gestation or more. An infant born with hydrops fetalis or signs of cardiac failure is a candidate for immediate exchange transfusion with fresh whole blood.

For exchange transfusion fresh whole blood is typed and crossmatched to the mother's serum. The amount of donor blood used is usually double the blood volume of the infant, which is approximately 85 mL/kg body weight but is limited to no more than 500 mL. The two-volume exchange transfusion replaces approximately 85% of the neonate's blood.

An exchange transfusion is a sterile surgical procedure. A catheter is inserted into the umbilical vein and threaded into the inferior vena cava. Depending on the infant's weight, 5 to 10 mL of blood is withdrawn within 15 to 20 seconds, and the same volume of donor blood is infused over 60 to 90 seconds.

CARE MANAGEMENT

The initial nursing responsibility is recognizing jaundice in the newborn at risk. The possibility of hemolytic disease can be anticipated from the prenatal and perinatal history. Prenatal evidence of incompatibility and a positive Coombs' test result are cause for increased vigilance for early signs of jaundice in an infant. Data indicate that the hour-specific bilirubin nomogram can be used in infants born at 35 weeks or more with ABO incompatibility and a positive Coombs' test result to follow the infant's serum bilirubin to determine the need for additional follow-up after hospital discharge (Schutzman, Sekhon, and Hundalani, 2010).

If an exchange transfusion is required, the nurse prepares the infant and the family and assists the practitioner with the procedure. The infant receives nothing by mouth (NPO) during the procedure; therefore a peripheral infusion of dextrose and electrolytes is established. The nurse documents the blood volume exchanged, including the amount of blood withdrawn and infused, the time of each procedure, and the cumulative record of the total volume exchanged. Vital signs monitored electronically are evaluated frequently and correlated with the removal and infusion of blood. If signs of cardiac or respiratory problems occur, the procedure is stopped temporarily and resumed after the infant's cardiorespiratory function stabilizes. The nurse also observes for signs of blood transfusion reaction and maintains the infant's blood glucose levels and fluid balance.

Throughout the procedure attention must be given to the infant's thermoregulation. Hypothermia increases oxygen and glucose consumption, causing metabolic acidosis. Not only do these consequences hinder the infant's overall physical ability to withstand the long procedure, but they also inhibit the binding capacity of albumin and bilirubin and the hepatic enzymatic reactions, thus increasing the risk of kernicterus. Conversely hyperthermia damages the donor erythrocytes, elevating the free potassium content and predisposing the infant to cardiac arrest.

The exchange transfusion is performed with the infant in a radiant warmer. However, he or she is usually covered with sterile drapes that may prevent the radiant heat from sufficiently warming the skin. The blood may also be warmed (using specially designed blood warming devices only) before infusion.

After the procedure is completed the nurse inspects the umbilical site for evidence of bleeding. The catheter may remain in place in case repeated exchanges are required.

INFANTS OF DIABETIC MOTHERS

Before insulin therapy few women with diabetes were able to conceive; for those who did, the mortality rate for both the mother and infant was high. The morbidity and mortality of infants of diabetic mothers (IDMs) have been reduced significantly as a result of effective control of maternal diabetes and an increased understanding of fetal disorders. Because infants born to women with gestational diabetes mellitus (DM) are at risk for the same complications as IDMs, the following discussion of IDMs includes infants born to women with gestational DM.

The severity of maternal diabetes affects infant survival. It is determined by the duration of the disease before pregnancy; age of onset; extent of vascular complications; and abnormalities of the current pregnancy such as pyelonephritis, diabetic ketoacidosis, pregnancy-induced hypertension, and noncompliance. The single most important factor influencing fetal well-being is the euglycemic status of the mother. It has been found that reasonable metabolic control that begins before conception and continues during the first weeks of pregnancy can prevent malformation in an IDM. Elevated levels of hemoglobin A1c during the periconception period appear to be associated with a higher incidence of congenital malformations. In the case of gestational diabetes, macrosomia is the most common finding; serious complications are rare (Mitanchez, 2010).

Hypoglycemia may appear a short time after birth and in IDMs is associated with increased insulin activity in the blood. The serum glucose level that corresponds to clinical hypoglycemia has not been well defined. Because some infants experience metabolic complications at higher levels than previously thought, some researchers recommend that serum glucose levels be maintained above 45 mg/dL (2.5 mmol/L) in infants with abnormal clinical symptoms and as high as 50 or 60 mg/dL in other infants (Cornblath, Hawdon, Williams, et al., 2000; Deshpande and Ward Platt, 2005). The AAP recommends that symptomatic infants receive treatment if their blood glucose is less than 40 mg/dL (Adamkin and AAP Committee on Fetus and Newborn, 2011).

Hypoglycemia in IDMs is related to hypertrophy and hyperplasia of the pancreatic islet cells and thus is a transient state of hyperinsulinism. High maternal blood glucose levels during fetal life provide a continual stimulus to the fetal islet cells for insulin production (glucose easily passes the placental barrier from maternal to fetal side; however, insulin does not cross the placental barrier). Historically, maternal hyperglycemia was believed to contribute to fetal macrosomia. However, Hay (2012) suggests that maternal hyperlipidemia and increased lipid transfer to the fetus are responsible for the excessive weight gain and fat deposition seen in such infants (Hay, 2012). IDMs are more likely to have disproportionately large abdominal circumferences and shoulders, leading to an increased risk of shoulder dystocia and birth injury (Dailey and Coustan, 2010). When the neonate's glucose supply is removed abruptly at the time of birth, the continued production of insulin soon depletes the blood of circulating glucose, creating a state of hyperinsulinism and hypoglycemia within 0.5 to 4 hours, especially in infants of mothers with poorly controlled diabetes (formerly class C diabetes or beyond [class D through R]). Precipitous drops in blood glucose levels can cause serious neurologic damage or death.

IDMs have a characteristic appearance (Box 25-3 and Fig. 25-10). Infants of mothers with advanced diabetes may be small for gestational age, have IUGR, or be the appropriate size for gestational age because of the maternal vascular (placental) involvement. There is an increase in congenital anomalies in IDMs in addition to a high susceptibility to hypoglycemia, hypocalcemia, hypomagnesemia, polycythemia, hyperbilirubinemia, cardiomyopathy, and respiratory distress syndrome (RDS) (Dailey and Coustan, 2010). Central nervous system (CNS) anomalies such as anencephaly, spina bifida, and holoprosencephaly occur at rates 10 times higher than in any other population of mothers. Cardiac anomalies such as ventriculoseptal defects and coarctation of the aorta are increased fivefold in IDMs, and sacral agenesis and caudal regression occur almost exclusively in IDMs (Gabbe, Niebyl, and Simpson, 2007). Hyperinsulinemia and hyperglycemia in the diabetic mother may be factors in reducing fetal surfactant synthesis, thus contributing to the development of RDS. Although large, these infants may be delivered before term as a result of maternal complications or increased fetal size.

Congenital hyperinsulinism is a condition that causes neonatal macrosomia, and profound hypoglycemia is often present in the neonatal period. However, this condition is usually not associated

---

BOX 25-3 CLINICAL MANIFESTATIONS OF INFANTS OF DIABETIC MOTHERS

- Large for gestational age
- Very plump and full faced
- Abundant vernix caseosa
- Plethora
- Listless and lethargic
- Possibly meconium stained at birth
- Hypotonia

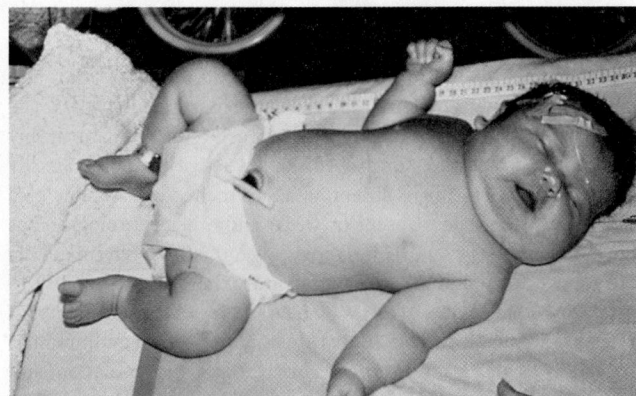

FIG 25-10 Large-for-gestational-age infant. This infant of a diabetic mother weighed 5 kg (11 lbs) at birth and exhibits the typical round facies. (From Zitelli BJ, Davis HW: *Atlas of pediatric physical diagnosis*, ed 5, Philadelphia, 2007, Mosby.)

with maternal DM, but appears to have a genetic etiology; the condition is also associated with syndromes such as Beckwith-Wiedemann syndrome (Sperling, 2011).

Some IDMs are also at increased risk for deep vein thrombosis, with renal vein thrombosis and hematuria being the most common presentation (Hay, 2012). Additional problems in IDMs include perinatal iron deficiency and neurologic impairments (seizures, lethargy, jitteriness, and changes in tone) (Hay, 2012).

The most important management of IDMs is careful monitoring of serum glucose levels and observation for accompanying complications such as RDS and cardiac anomalies. The infants are examined for the presence of any anomalies or birth injuries; and blood studies for determination of glucose, calcium, hematocrit, and bilirubin are obtained on a regular basis.

Because the hypertrophied pancreas is so sensitive to blood glucose concentrations, the administration of oral glucose may trigger a massive insulin release, resulting in rebound hypoglycemia. Therefore feedings of breast milk or formula begin within the first hour after birth, provided that the infant's cardiorespiratory condition is stable. Approximately half of these infants do well and adjust without complications. Infants born to mothers with poorly controlled diabetes may require IV dextrose infusions. Treatment with 10% dextrose and water intravenously is initiated with the goal of maintaining serum blood glucose levels between 40 and 50 mg/dL (Adamkin and AAP, Committee on Fetus and Newborn, 2011). Oral and IV intake may be titrated to maintain adequate blood glucose levels. Frequent blood glucose determinations are needed for the first 2 to 4 days of life to assess the degree of hypoglycemia present at any given time. Testing blood taken from the heel with calibrated portable reflectance meters (e.g., glucometers) is a simple and effective screening evaluation that can then be confirmed by laboratory examination.

CARE MANAGEMENT

The nursing care of IDMs involves early examination for congenital anomalies, signs of possible respiratory or cardiac problems, maintenance of adequate thermoregulation, early introduction of carbohydrate feedings as appropriate, and monitoring of serum blood glucose levels. The latter is of particular importance because many infants with hypoglycemia may remain asymptomatic. Symptomatic IDMs who are unable to feed should be started on a continuous intravenous infusion of 10% dextrose at 4 to 6 mg/min/kg unless blood glucose is below 20 mg/dL. In such cases a one-time bolus infusion of 10% dextrose (200 mg/kg) should be given over 2 to 4 minutes, followed by a constant intravenous infusion of 10% dextrose and water as noted previously (Hay, 2012). IV glucose infusion requires careful monitoring of the site and the neonate's reaction to therapy; high glucose concentrations (≥12.5%) should be infused via a central line instead of a peripheral site.

Because macrosomic infants are at risk for problems associated with a difficult birth, they are monitored for birth injuries such as brachial plexus injury and palsy, fractured clavicle, and phrenic nerve palsy. Additional monitoring of the infant for problems associated with this condition (polycythemia, hypocalcemia, poor feeding, and hyperbilirubinemia) is also a vital nursing function.

Some evidence indicates that IDMs have an increased risk of acquiring type 2 diabetes and metabolic syndrome in childhood or early adulthood (Hay, 2012); therefore nursing care should also focus on healthy lifestyle and prevention later in life with IDMs.

CONGENITAL ANOMALIES

Congenital defects are reported to occur in 2% to 3% of all live births (Bay, Steele, and Davis, 2007), but this number increases to about 6% by 5 years, when more anomalies are diagnosed. In addition, the incidence of congenital malformations in fetuses that are aborted is higher than that in infants who are born alive, thus adding to the overall incidence. Major congenital defects are the leading cause of death in infants younger than 1 year of age in the United States and account for 20% of neonatal deaths. Between 1999 and 2008 rates of cleft lip and cleft palate had the highest prevalence followed by Down syndrome, omphalocele or gastroschisis, spina bifida or myelomeningocele, and anencephaly. Prevalence of Down syndrome was highest among mothers 40 to 54 years of age, and rates of omphalocele or gastroschisis were highest among mothers younger than 20 years of age (EPA Report on the Environment, 2011). Although the incidences of other causes of neonatal mortality have decreased, the death rate associated with most congenital anomalies has essentially remained stable since 1932.

The most common major congenital anomalies that cause serious problems in the neonate are congenital heart disease, abdominal wall defects, imperforate anus, neural tube defects (NTDs), cleft lip or palate, clubfoot, and developmental dysplasia of the hip. These are thought to result from the interaction of multiple genetic and environmental factors.

Most congenital anomalies are detected at birth or shortly thereafter. Although surgical techniques and treatments have made a significant difference in the morbidity of some anomalies, these continue to be a major source of chronic illness and morbidity in the first year of life.

Ways of detecting and preventing some of these anomalies are being improved continuously, as are some surgical techniques for the care of the fetus with certain anomalies. Promoting the availability of these services to populations at risk challenges community health care systems. An interdisciplinary team approach is vital for providing holistic care: the surgical treatment, rehabilitation, and education of the child and psychosocial and financial assistance for the parents. Parental disappointment and disillusion add to the complexity of the nursing care needed for these infants.

A number of congenital anomalies are discussed in the following pediatric systems and conditions chapters:
- Cleft lip and palate, Chapter 41
- Esophageal atresia and tracheoesophageal fistula, Chapter 41
- Omphalocele and gastroschisis, Chapter 41

- Congenital cardiac defects, Chapter 42
- Congenital diaphragmatic hernia and choanal atresia, Chapter 40
- Neural tube defects and myelomeningocele, Chapter 49
- Developmental dysplasia of the hip and clubfoot, Chapter 48
- Hypospadias, Disorders of Sex Development, and Bladder Exstrophy, Chapter 44

PRETERM AND POSTERM INFANTS

Preterm Infants

Prematurity accounts for the largest number of admissions to NICUs. Immaturity of most organ systems places infants at risk for a variety of neonatal complications (e.g., hyperbilirubinemia, RDS, intellectual and motor delays). LBW and prematurity were the second leading cause of infant mortality in the United States in 2008 (Mathews and MacDorman, 2012). The actual cause of prematurity is not known in most instances. Factors such as poverty, maternal infections, previous preterm birth, multiple pregnancies, pregnancy-induced hypertension, and placental problems that interrupt the normal course of gestation before completion of fetal development are responsible for a large number of preterm births.

The outlook for preterm infants is largely but not entirely related to the state of physiologic and anatomic immaturity of the various organs and systems at the time of birth. There is a significant difference between a 24-week preterm infant and one born at 36 weeks, yet both are considered to be preterm. Therefore in the context of this discussion of prematurity, the term is relative to the gestational age of the infant. Infants at term have advanced to a state of maturity sufficient to allow a successful transition to the extrauterine environment. Preterm infants must make the same adjustments but with functional immaturity proportional to the stage of development reached at the time of birth. However, these adjustments may be limited or even hindered by the external environment to which the preterm infant is exposed. Exposure to excessive stimuli, bacteria, and viruses make the environment less conducive for preterm infants to grow and develop. The degree to which infants are prepared for extrauterine life can be predicted to some extent by birth weight and estimated gestational age.

Preterm infants have a number of distinct characteristics at various stages of development. Identification of these characteristics provides valuable clues to the gestational age and thus to the infant's physiologic capabilities. The general outward physical appearance changes as the fetus progresses to maturity. Characteristics of skin, general attitude (or posture) when supine, appearance of hair, and amount of subcutaneous fat provide cues to a newborn's physical development. Observation of spontaneous, active movements and response to stimulation and passive movement contributes to the assessment of neurologic status. The appraisal is made as soon as possible after admission to the nursery because much of the observation and management of infants depend on this information.

On inspection preterm infants are very small and appear scrawny because they have only minimal subcutaneous fat deposits (or none in some cases) and a proportionately large head in relation to the body, which reflects the cephalocaudal direction of growth. The skin is bright pink (often translucent, depending on the degree of immaturity), smooth, and shiny, with small blood vessels clearly visible underneath the thin epidermis. The fine lanugo hair is abundant over the body (depending on gestational age) but is sparse, fine, and fuzzy on the head. The ear cartilage is soft and pliable, and the soles and palms have minimal creases, resulting in a smooth appearance. The bones of the skull and the ribs feel soft, and the eyes may be closed. Male infants have few scrotal rugae, and the testes are undescended; in girls the labia and clitoris are prominent.

In contrast to full-term infants' overall attitude of flexion and continuous activity, preterm infants may be inactive and listless. The extremities maintain an attitude of extension and remain in any position in which they are placed. Reflex activity is only partially developed (i.e., sucking is absent, weak, or ineffectual; swallow, gag, and cough reflexes are absent or weak; and other neurologic signs are absent or diminished). Physiologically immature preterm infants are unable to maintain body temperature, have limited ability to excrete solutes in the urine, and have increased susceptibility to infection. A pliable thorax, immature lung tissue, and an immature regulatory center lead to **periodic breathing,** hypoventilation, and frequent periods of apnea. They are more susceptible to biochemical alterations such as hyperbilirubinemia and hypoglycemia, and they have a higher extracellular water content that renders them more vulnerable to fluid and electrolyte derangements. Preterm infants exchange fully half of their extracellular fluid volume every 24 hours compared with one seventh of the volume in adults.

The soft cranium is subject to characteristic unintentional deformation caused by positioning from one side to the other on a mattress. The head looks disproportionately longer from front to back, is flattened on both sides, and lacks the usual convexity seen at the temporal and parietal areas. This positional molding is often a concern to parents and may influence their perception of the infant's attractiveness and their responsiveness to the infant. Positioning the infant on a waterbed or gel mattress can reduce or minimize cranial molding.

Neurologic impairment (e.g., from intraventricular hemorrhage) and serious sequelae correlate with the size and gestational age of infants at birth and the severity of neonatal complications. The greater the degree of immaturity, the greater is the degree of potential disability. A greater incidence of cerebral palsy, ADHD, visual-motor deficits, and altered intellectual functioning is observed in preterm than in full-term infants. However, behavioral development can be enhanced when families are provided with support and infants are referred to appropriate services for neurologic and developmental interventions. Parental interest and involvement are important variables in the developmental progress of infants.

When the birth of a preterm infant is anticipated, the NICU is alerted, and a team approach implemented. Ideally a neonatologist, an advanced practice nurse, a staff nurse, and a respiratory therapist are present for the birth. Infants who do not require resuscitation are immediately transferred in a heated incubator to the NICU, where they are weighed and where IV lines, oxygen therapy, and other therapeutic interventions are initiated as needed. Resuscitation is conducted in the birth area until infants can be safely transported to the NICU.

Subsequent care is determined by the infant's status. The general care of preterm infants differs from that of full-term infants primarily in the areas of respiratory support, temperature regulation, nutrition, susceptibility to infection, activity intolerance, neurodevelopmental care, and other consequences of physical immaturity.

CARE MANAGEMENT

The nursing care, similar to the therapeutic management, is individualized for each infant. See appropriate discussions under Care of the High Risk Newborn and Family for additional details of care.

Late-Preterm Infants

There has been increased interest in late-preterm infants of 34 to 36⁶/₇ weeks of gestation who may receive the same treatment as term infants. Late-preterm infants often experience morbidities similar to those of preterm infants, including respiratory distress, hypoglycemia requiring treatment, temperature instability, poor feeding, jaundice, and discharge delays, as a result of illness. Therefore assessment and prompt intervention in life-threatening perinatal emergencies often make the difference between a favorable outcome and a lifetime of disability. It is estimated that late-preterm infants represent 70% of the total preterm infant population and that the mortality rate for this group is significantly higher than that of term infants (7.9 versus 2.4 per 1000 live births, respectively) (Tomashek, Shapiro-Mendoza, Davidoff, et al., 2007). Because late-preterm infants' birth weights often range from 2000 to 2500 g (4.4 to 5.5 lbs) and they appear relatively mature compared with smaller preterm infants, they may be cared for in the same manner as healthy term infants while risk factors for late-preterm infants are overlooked. Late-preterm infants are often discharged early from the birth institution and have a significantly higher rate of rehospitalization within 2 weeks of being discharged than term infants (Escobar, Clark, and Greene, 2006; National Perinatal Association, 2012). Discussions regarding high risk infants in this chapter also refer to late-preterm infants who are experiencing a delayed transition to extrauterine life. Nurses in newborn nurseries should be familiar with the characteristics of late-preterm infants and recognize the significance of serious deviations from expected observations (see Critical Thinking Case Study). When providers can anticipate the need for specialized care and plan for it, the probability of successful outcome is increased.

The AWHONN has published the *Assessment and Care of the Late Preterm Infant* (AWHONN, 2010) for the education of perinatal nurses regarding the late-preterm infant's risk factors and appropriate care and follow-up care (Table 25-7). The National Perinatal Association (2012) recently published an extensive multidisciplinary guideline for the care of late preterm infants.

Postterm Infants

Infants born of a gestation that extends beyond 42 weeks as calculated from the mother's last menstrual period (or by gestational age assessment) are considered to be postterm, or postmature, regardless of birth weight. This constitutes 3.5% to 15% of all pregnancies. The cause of delayed birth is unknown. Some infants are appropriate for gestational age but show the characteristics of progressive placental dysfunction. These infants display characteristics such as absence of lanugo, little if any vernix caseosa, abundant scalp hair, and long fingernails. The skin is often cracked, parchmentlike, and desquamating. A common finding in postterm infants is a wasted physical appearance that reflects intrauterine deprivation. Depletion of subcutaneous fat gives them a thin, elongated appearance. The little vernix caseosa that remains in the skinfolds may be stained a deep yellow or green, which is usually an indication of meconium in the amniotic fluid.

There is a significant increase in fetal and neonatal mortality in postterm infants compared with those born at term. They are especially prone to fetal distress associated with the decreasing efficiency of the placenta, macrosomia, and meconium aspiration syndrome. The greatest risk occurs during the stresses of labor and birth, particularly in infants of primigravidas, or women delivering their first child. Close surveillance with fetal assessment and induction of labor is usually recommended when infants are significantly overdue.

Complications of Preterm Birth
Respiratory Distress Syndrome

Respiratory distress is a name applied to respiratory dysfunction in neonates and is primarily a disease related to developmental delay in lung maturation. The terms respiratory distress syndrome (RDS) and hyaline membrane disease are most often applied to this severe lung disorder, which not only is responsible for more infant deaths than any other disease but also carries the highest risk in terms of long-term respiratory and neurologic complications. It is seen almost exclusively in preterm infants. The disorder is rare in drug-exposed infants and infants who have been subjected to chronic intrauterine stress (e.g., maternal preeclampsia or hypertension). Respiratory distress of a nonpulmonary origin in neonates may also be caused by sepsis, cardiac defects (structural or functional), exposure to cold, airway obstruction (atresia), intraventricular hemorrhage, hypoglycemia, metabolic acidosis, acute blood loss, and drugs. Pneumonia in the neonatal period may result in respiratory distress caused by bacterial or viral agents and may occur alone or as a complication of RDS.

Preterm infants are born before the lungs are fully prepared to serve as efficient organs for gas exchange. This appears to be a critical factor in the development of RDS. The effects of lung immaturity are compounded by the presence of more cartilage in the chest wall, leading to increased compliance of the chest wall, which collapses inward in response to less compliant (stiffer) lung tissue.

There is evidence of fetal respiratory activity before birth. The lungs make feeble respiratory movements, and fluid is excreted through the alveoli. Because the final unfolding of the alveolar septa, which increases the surface area of the lungs, occurs during the last trimester of pregnancy, preterm infants are born with numerous underdeveloped and many uninflatable alveoli. Pulmonary blood flow is limited as a result of the collapsed state of the fetal lungs, particularly poor vascular development in general, and an immature capillary network. Because of increased pulmonary vascular resistance (PVR), the major portion of fetal blood is shunted from the lungs by way of the ductus arteriosus and foramen ovale.

At birth infants must initiate breathing and keep the previously fluid-filled lungs inflated with air. At the same time the pulmonary capillary blood flow must be increased approximately 10-fold to provide for adequate lung perfusion and alter the intracardiac pressure that closes the fetal cardiac structures. Most full-term infants

---

⚡ CRITICAL THINKING CASE STUDY

Late-Preterm Infant

A 2013-g (4 lb 7 oz) male infant is born at an estimated gestational age of 35 weeks. The parents are excited about this birth because they have been trying to become pregnant for 6 years. The baby is placed on the mother's (Patti) abdomen after birth for skin contact but does not breastfeed. The nurse assessing the baby notes that he has some mild grunting, nasal flaring, and intercostal retractions; he is taken to the transitional nursery for further evaluation and treatment. Jorge, the father, speaks little English but asks when they will be able to hold their son again; Patti is crying and asks to have her baby brought back to her as soon as his condition is stable because she really wants to breastfeed him.

1. Evidence—Is there sufficient evidence to draw conclusions about what to tell Patti and Jorge about their infant son?
2. Assumptions—What assumptions can be made about the following?
   a. The mother's and father's reaction to their son's birth
   b. The infant's expected progress
   c. The possibility of Patti breastfeeding the baby
3. What implications and priorities for nursing care can be drawn at this time?
4. Does the evidence objectively support your conclusion?

TABLE 25-7	LATE PRETERM INFANT ASSESSMENT AND INTERVENTIONS	
RISK FACTORS	**ASSESSMENT**	**INTERVENTIONS***
Respiratory distress	Assess for cardinal signs of respiratory distress (nasal flaring, grunting, tachypnea, central cyanosis, retractions) and presence of apnea, especially during feedings. Assess for hypothermia, hypoglycemia.	Perform gestational age assessment. Observe for signs of respiratory distress; monitor oxygenation by pulse oximetry; provide supplemental oxygen judiciously.
Thermal instability	Monitor axillary temperature every 30 min immediately after birth until stable; thereafter every 1-4 hr, depending on gestational age and ability to maintain thermal stability.	Provide skin-to-skin care in immediate postpartum period for stable infant. Implement measures to avoid excess heat loss (adjust environmental temperature, avoid drafts). Bathe only after thermal stability has been maintained for 1 hr.
Hypoglycemia	Monitor for signs and symptoms of hypoglycemia. Assess feeding ability (latch-on, nipple feeding). Assess thermal stability and signs and symptoms of respiratory distress. Monitor bedside glucose in infants with additional risk factors (IDM, prolonged labor, respiratory distress, poor feeding).	Initiate early feedings of human milk or formula. Avoid dextrose water or water feedings. Provide IV dextrose as necessary for hypoglycemia.
Jaundice	Observe for jaundice in first 24 hr. Evaluate maternal-fetal history for additional risk factors that may cause increased hemolysis and circulating levels of unconjugated bilirubin (Rh, ABO, spherocytosis, bruising). Assess feeding method, voiding and stooling patterns.	Monitor transcutaneous bilirubin and note risk zone on hour-specific nomogram (see Fig. 23-8).
Feeding problems	Assess suck-swallow and breathing. Assess for respiratory distress, hypoglycemia, thermal stability. Assess latch-on, maternal comfort with feeding method. Determine weight loss (should be ≤10% of birth weight).	Initiate early feedings (human milk or formula). Ensure maternal knowledge of feeding method and signs of inadequate feeding (sleepiness, lethargy, color changes during feeding, apnea during feeding, decreased or absent urine output).
Neurodevelopmental problems	Assess for respiratory distress, neonatal jaundice, hypoglycemia, and thermal instability. Assess neurodevelopmental status. Assess for seizure activity.	Perform newborn screening, including hearing test. Implement individualized developmental care. Encourage parents to keep follow-up appointments with health care provider for evaluation of growth and development (including cognitive function and achievement of appropriate milestones).
Infection	Evaluate maternal-fetal history for risk factors that may contribute to neonatal septicemia. Assess for signs and symptoms of neonatal infection (see Tables 25-4 and 25-5).	Use Standard Precautions, especially hand washing between infants and after contact with surfaces that may harbor bacteria (e.g., keyboards, telephones). Maintain thermal stability. Administer hepatitis B vaccine. Encourage breastfeeding and assist mother-baby pair with breastfeeding. Encourage parents to decrease infant exposure to respiratory viruses after discharge and obtain vaccines as appropriate to prevent development of respiratory viruses (e.g., influenza).

Portions adapted from Association of Women's Health, Obstetric and Neonatal Nurses (AWHONN): *Assessment and care of the late preterm infant: Evidence-based clinical practice guideline,* Washington, DC, 2010, The Association.
IDM, Infant of diabetic mother; *IV,* intravenous.
*This is not an exhaustive list of nursing interventions; additional interventions include those discussed under the care of the high risk infant in this chapter.

successfully accomplish these adjustments, but preterm infants with respiratory distress are unable to do so. Although numerous factors are involved, immaturity of the surfactant system plays a central role.

Surfactant is a surface-active phospholipid secreted by the alveolar epithelium. Acting much like a detergent, this substance reduces the surface tension of fluids that line the alveoli and respiratory passages, resulting in uniform nexpansion and maintenance of lung expansion at low intraalveolar pressure. Immature development of

these functions produces consequences that seriously compromise respiratory efficiency. Deficient surfactant production causes unequal inflation of alveoli on inspiration and the collapse of alveoli on end expiration. Without surfactant infants are unable to keep their lungs inflated and therefore exert a great deal of effort to reexpand the alveoli with each breath. With increasing exhaustion infants are able to open fewer and fewer alveoli. This inability to maintain lung expansion produces widespread atelectasis.

BOX 25-4   CLINICAL MANIFESTATIONS OF RESPIRATORY DISTRESS SYNDROME

- Tachypnea (≥60 breaths/min) initially*
- Dyspnea
- Pronounced intercostal or substernal retractions
- Fine inspiratory crackles
- Audible expiratory grunt
- Flaring of the external nares
- Cyanosis or pallor
- Apnea
- With progression of condition, deteriorating vital signs including blood pressure, apnea, body temperature instability

*Not all infants born with respiratory distress syndrome manifest these characteristics; very low–birth-weight and extremely low–birth-weight infants may have respiratory failure and shock at birth because of physiologic immaturity.

In the absence of alveolar stability (normal functional residual capacity) and with progressive atelectasis, PVR increases; with normal lung expansion it would decrease. Consequently hypoperfusion to the lung tissue occurs, with a decrease in effective pulmonary blood flow. The increase in PVR causes partial reversion to the fetal circulation, with a right-to-left shunting of blood through the persisting fetal communications (i.e., the ductus arteriosus and foramen ovale).

Inadequate pulmonary perfusion and ventilation produce hypoxemia and hypercapnia. Pulmonary arterioles, with their thick muscular layer, are markedly reactive to diminished oxygen concentration. Thus a decrease in oxygen tension causes vasoconstriction in the pulmonary arterioles that is further enhanced by a decrease in blood pH. This vasoconstriction contributes to a marked increase in PVR. In normal ventilation with increased oxygen concentration, the ductus arteriosus constricts, and the pulmonary vessels dilate to decrease PVR.

Prolonged hypoxemia activates anaerobic glycolysis, which produces increased amounts of lactic acid. An increase in lactic acid causes metabolic acidosis; an inability of the atelectatic lungs to blow off excess carbon dioxide produces respiratory acidosis. Acidosis causes further vasoconstriction. With deficient pulmonary circulation and alveolar perfusion, partial pressure of oxygen in arterial blood continues to fall, pH falls, and the materials needed for surfactant production are not circulated to the alveoli.

The diagnosis of RDS is made on the basis of clinical manifestations (Box 25-4) and radiographic studies. Radiographic findings characteristic of RDS include (1) a diffuse granular pattern over both lung fields that closely resembles ground glass and represents alveolar atelectasis; and (2) dark streaks, or bronchograms, within the ground glass areas that represent dilated, air-filled bronchioles. It is often difficult to distinguish between RDS and pneumonia in infants with respiratory distress. The extent of respiratory function and acid-base balance is determined by blood gas analysis. Pulse oximetry, carbon dioxide monitoring, and pulmonary function studies help to differentiate pulmonary and extrapulmonary illness and are used in the management of RDS.

The treatment of RDS involves immediate establishment of adequate oxygenation and ventilation, supportive care and measures required for any preterm infant, and those instituted to prevent further complications associated with preterm birth. The supportive measures most crucial to a favorable outcome are to:

- Maintain adequate ventilation and oxygenation.
- Maintain acid-base balance.
- Maintain a neutral thermal environment.
- Maintain adequate tissue perfusion and oxygenation.
- Prevent hypotension.
- Maintain adequate hydration and electrolyte status.

Nipple and gavage feedings are contraindicated in any situation that creates a marked increase in respiratory rate because of the greater hazards of aspiration. Nutrition is provided by parenteral therapy during the acute stage of the disease, and minimal enteral feeding is provided to enhance maturation of the neonate's GI system.

The administration of exogenous surfactant to preterm neonates with RDS has become an accepted and common therapy in most neonatal centers worldwide. Numerous clinical trials involving the administration of exogenous surfactant to infants with or at high risk for RDS demonstrate improvements in blood gas values and ventilator settings, decreased incidence of pulmonary air leaks, intraventricular hemorrhage, decreased deaths from RDS, and an overall decreased infant mortality rate (AAP Committee on Fetus and Newborn, 2008; Stevens and Sinkin, 2007). The overall rates of some associated co-morbidities (bronchopulmonary dysplasia, NEC, patent ductus arteriosus) have not decreased with surfactant replacement. Currently exogenous surfactant is derived from a natural source (e.g., porcine, bovine). In 2012 a synthetic surfactant, Lucinactant, was approved for use in infants with RDS. However, clinical trials have yet to establish its effectiveness over an animal-derived surfactant (Piehl, Fernandez-Bustamante, 2012; Walsh, Daigle, Diblasi, et al., 2013).

Complications seen with surfactant administration include pulmonary hemorrhage and mucus plugging. Surfactant therapy is also being used in infants with meconium aspiration, infectious pneumonia, sepsis, persistent pulmonary hypertension, and lung hypoplasia concomitant with congenital diaphragmatic hernia (Stevens and Sinkin, 2007). Surfactant may be administered at birth as a preventive or prophylactic treatment of RDS or later in the course of RDS as a rescue treatment; however, research has demonstrated improved clinical outcomes and fewer adverse effects when surfactant is administered prophylactically to infants at risk for developing RDS (AAP Committee on Fetus and Newborn, 2008; Stevens, Harrington, Blennow, et al., 2007). Surfactant is administered via an endotracheal (ET) tube directly into the infant's trachea (Fig. 25-11). Nursing responsibilities with surfactant administration include assistance in the delivery of the product, collection and monitoring of arterial blood gases, scrupulous monitoring of oxygenation with pulse oximetry, and assessment of the infant's tolerance of the procedure. After surfactant is absorbed, respiratory compliance usually increases, which requires adjustment of ventilator settings to decrease mean airway pressure and prevent overinflation or hyperoxemia. Suctioning is usually delayed for approximately an hour (depending on the type of surfactant and unit protocol) to allow maximum effects to occur. Studies have shown the benefit of administering surfactant early (prophylactic) in infants at risk for developing RDS and then extubating and placing on nasal continuous positive airway pressure (CPAP); this decreased the overall incidence of bronchopulmonary dysplasia, need for mechanical ventilation, and fewer air leak syndromes (Stevens, Harrington, Blennow, et al., 2007). Although an aerosolized surfactant is now available and is being used in adults, further research is needed to establish protocols for the dose, preparation, and route of administration in infants (Abdel-Latif and Osborn, 2012; Walsh, Daigle, Diblasi, et al., 2013). This method would theoretically decrease the problems associated with current delivery systems (i.e., contamination of the airway, interruption of mechanical ventilation, and loss of the drug in the ET tubing from reflux).

The goals of oxygen therapy are to provide adequate oxygen to the tissues, prevent lactic acid accumulation resulting from hypoxia, and at the same time avoid the potentially negative effects of oxygen and barotrauma. Numerous methods have been devised to improve oxygenation (Table 25-8). All require that the gas be warmed and humidified before entering the respiratory tract. If the infant does not require intubation and mechanical ventilation, oxygen can be supplied by nasal cannula or via nasal prongs in conjunction with CPAP. If oxygen saturation of the blood cannot be maintained at a satisfactory level and the carbon dioxide level ($PaCO_2$) rises, infants require ventilatory assistance.

RDS is a self-limiting disease. Before the use of surfactant, infants typically experienced a period of deterioration ($\approx$48 hours) and, in the absence of complications, improved by 72 hours. Often heralded by the onset of diuresis, this improvement was attributed primarily to increased production and greater availability of surfactant. With the administration of surfactant, lung compliance begins to improve almost immediately, resulting in lower oxygen requirements and a decreased need for ventilatory support (Stevens and Sinkin, 2007).

Infants with RDS who survive the first 96 hours have a reasonable chance of recovery. However, complications of RDS include associated respiratory conditions and problems associated with prematurity, including patent ductus arteriosus and congestive heart failure, intraventricular hemorrhage, bronchopulmonary dysplasia, retinopathy of prematurity, pneumonia, air leak syndrome, sepsis, NEC, and neurologic sequelae.

CARE MANAGEMENT

Care of infants with RDS involves all of the observations and interventions previously described for high risk infants. In addition, the nurse is concerned with the complex problems related to respiratory therapy and the constant threat of hypoxemia and acidosis that complicates the care of patients in respiratory difficulty.

The respiratory therapist, an important member of the NICU team, is often responsible for maintaining respiratory equipment. Although it may be his or her responsibility to regulate the apparatus, nurses should understand the equipment and be able to recognize when it is not functioning correctly. The most essential nursing

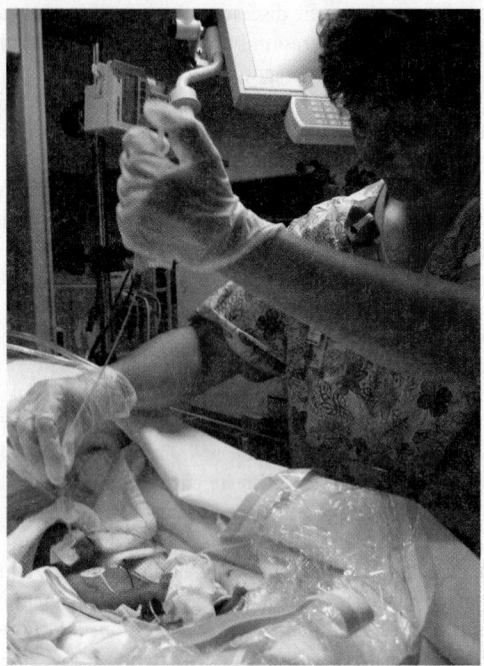

FIG 25-11 Exogenous surfactant administration via endotracheal tube. (Courtesy E. Jacobs, Texas Children's Hospital, Houston, TX.)

TABLE 25-8 COMMON METHODS FOR ASSISTED VENTILATION IN NEONATAL RESPIRATORY DISTRESS

METHOD	DESCRIPTION	HOW PROVIDED
Conventional Methods		
Continuous positive airway pressure (CPAP)	Provides constant distending pressure to airway in spontaneously breathing infant	Nasal prongs Face mask Nasal cannula
Intermittent mandatory ventilation (IMV)*	Allows infant to breathe spontaneously at own rate but provides mechanical cycled respirations and pressure at regular preset intervals	Endotracheal intubation and ventilator
Synchronized intermittent mandatory ventilation (SIMV)	Mechanically delivered breaths are synchronized to onset of spontaneous patient breaths; assist/control mode facilitates full inspiratory synchrony; involves signal detection of onset of spontaneous respiration from abdominal movement, thoracic impedance, and airway pressure or flow changes	Patient-triggered infant ventilator with signal detector and assist/control mode; endotracheal tube
Volume-guarantee ventilation	Delivers predetermined volume of gas using inspiratory pressure that varies according to infant's lung compliance (often used in conjunction with SIMV)	Volume-guarantee ventilator with flow sensor; endotracheal tube
Alternative Methods		
High-frequency oscillation (HFO)	Application of high-frequency, low-volume, sine-wave flow oscillations to airway at rates between 480 and 1200 breaths/min	Variable-speed piston pump (or loudspeaker, fluidic oscillator); endotracheal tube
High-frequency jet ventilation (HFJV)	Uses separate, parallel, low-compliant circuit and injector port to deliver small pulses or jets of fresh gas deep into airway at rates between 250 and 900 breaths/min	May be used alone or with low-rate IMV; endotracheal tube

*Also referred to *as conventional ventilation* (vs. high-frequency ventilation [HFV]).

function is to observe and assess the infant's response to therapy. Continuous monitoring and close observation are mandatory because an infant's status can change rapidly and oxygen concentration and ventilation parameters are prescribed according to the infant's blood gas measurements and pulse oximetry readings.

Changes in oxygen concentration are based on these observations. The amount of oxygen administered, expressed as the fraction of inspired air (FiO_2), is determined on an individual basis according to pulse oximetry or direct or indirect measurement of arterial oxygen concentration. Capillary samples collected from the heel are useful for pH and $PaCO_2$ determinations but not for oxygenation status. Continuous transcutaneous or pulse oximetry readings are recorded at least hourly.

Mucus may collect in the respiratory tract as a result of the infant's pulmonary condition. Secretions interfere with gas flow and predispose the infant to obstruction of the passages, including the ET tube. Suctioning should be performed only when necessary and should be based on individual infant assessment, which includes auscultation of the chest, evidence of decreased oxygenation, excess moisture in the ET tube, or increased infant irritability. During suctioning, a variety of techniques can be used to minimize complications such as increased ICP and health care-associated pneumonia, including using a closed suctioning system, placing the infant in a lateral instead of a supine position, and maintaining the ventilator circuit in a horizontal position to reduce the draining of oropharyngeal secretions into the lower respiratory tract (Polin, Denson, Brady, et al., 2012).

When nasopharyngeal passages, the trachea, or the ET tube is being suctioned, the catheter should be inserted gently but quickly; intermittent suction is applied as the catheter is withdrawn. Negative airway pressure should only be applied for no more than 10 to 15 seconds because continuous suction removes air from the lungs along with the mucus. It is recommended that the "two-person" suctioning procedure be used on infants who are acutely ill and who do not tolerate any procedure without profound decreases in oxygen saturation, BP, and heart rate. The object of suctioning an artificial airway is to maintain patency of that airway, not the bronchi. Suction applied beyond the ET tube can cause traumatic lesions of the trachea. The use of in-line suction catheters may decrease airway contamination and hypoxia. Evidence-based guidelines for ET suctioning of neonates have been published (Gardner and Shirland, 2009).

The most advantageous positions for facilitating an infant's open airway are on the side with the head supported in alignment by a small folded blanket or, when on the back, positioned to keep the neck slightly extended. With the head in the "sniffing" position, the trachea is opened at its maximum; hyperextension reduces the tracheal diameter in neonates.

Inspection of the skin is part of routine infant assessment. Position changes and the use of water pillows are helpful in guarding against skin breakdown.

Mouth care is especially important when infants are receiving NPO, and the problem is often aggravated by the drying effect of oxygen therapy. Drying and cracking can be prevented by good oral hygiene using sterile water. Irritation to the nares or mouth that occurs from appliances used to administer oxygen (e.g., nasal CPAP) may be reduced by the use of a water-soluble ointment. Routine oral hygiene care in intubated adults and older children has been shown to decrease the incidence of ventilator-associated pneumonia (see Chapter 40).

The nursing care of an infant with RDS is a demanding role; meticulous attention must be given to subtle changes in the infant's oxygenation status. The importance of attention to detail cannot be overemphasized, particularly in regard to medication administration (see Nursing Care Plan).

◎ NURSING CARE PLAN

The High Risk Infant with Respiratory Distress Syndrome

NURSING DIAGNOSIS	PATIENT OUTCOMES	NURSING INTERVENTIONS	RATIONALE
Ineffective Breathing Pattern related to pulmonary, neurologic vascular, alveolar, and muscular immaturity **Child's or Family's Defining Characteristics** *(Subjective and Objective Data)* Decreased inspiratory and expiratory pressure Decreased minute ventilation Use of accessory muscles to breathe Nasal flaring Grunting Apnea Tachypnea Altered chest excursion Respiratory rate: <20 or >60 breaths/min	High risk infant will maintain patent airway and ventilatory status adequate for oxygenation.	Position to facilitate airway expansion and prevent collection of secretions Closely monitor for deviations from desired breathing pattern—pulse oximetry, arterial blood gases, clinical signs of poor oxygenation, grunting, nasal flaring, apnea, tachypnea, retractions, and cyanosis Monitor vital signs for change in condition or status such as decreased cardiac output (poor perfusion, mottling, deteriorating respiratory status) Assist with exogenous surfactant administration and monitor patient tolerance or change in status Suction oropharynx, nasopharynx, trachea, or endotracheal tube only as necessary and based on respiratory assessment	To allow oxygen entry into bronchial tree and alveoli To facilitate proper oxygenation by implementing appropriate therapy such as supplemental oxygen, mechanical ventilation, or change of position To implement appropriate therapy such as suctioning, supplemental oxygen, or vasopressor drugs To increase alveolar expansion and enhance oxygen–carbon dioxide exchange To remove secretions that may interfere with adequate ventilation and oxygenation

Continued

◎ NURSING CARE PLAN

The High Risk Infant with Respiratory Distress Syndrome—cont'd

NURSING DIAGNOSIS	PATIENT OUTCOMES	NURSING INTERVENTIONS	RATIONALE
Ineffective Thermoregulation related to immature neurologic and metabolic temperature control	Infant will maintain stable body temperature (specify range for age).	Place ELBW or VLBW infant in polyethylene wrap or bag immediately after birth (after drying off rapidly)	To control environmental temperature and keep infant's temperature stable
Child's or Family's Defining Characteristics		Place newborn in thermally controlled incubator or radiant warmer	
(Subjective and Objective Data)		Use environmental controls for decreasing body heat loss (plastic heat shield, increased ambient temperature, servo control on warmer or incubator)	To regulate body temperature within acceptable range and minimize heat loss
Reduction in body temperature below normal range		Place knitted or cloth cap on head	To prevent heat loss from exposed scalp
Slow capillary refill			
Cool skin		Monitor axillary temperature as often as necessary or per unit protocol	To detect necessity for environmental temperature regulation and to determine infant's response to environmental thermoregulation
Increased respiratory rate			
Tachycardia			
		Check temperature of newborn in relation to environmental temperature and temperature of heating element	To detect change in thermoregulatory status, which may indicate significant disease process such as sepsis
		Monitor vital signs and skin color, perfusion, pulses, and respiratory status	To detect changes in status that require additional intervention for stabilization
		Monitor for signs of hyperthermia (flushing, tachycardia, altered level of consciousness) and hypothermia (decreased activity; respiratory distress [deterioration]; cool, mottled extremities)	To prevent untoward effects of hyperthermia (fluctuating cerebral perfusion, apnea, increased metabolism with decreased available glucose for vital functions) or hypothermia (increased glucose use, lactic acidosis, respiratory compromise)
		Monitor serum glucose levels as necessary or per unit protocol	To ensure that euglycemia is maintained
Risk for Impaired Parent-Infant Attachment	Parent(s) will form emotional bond or attachment with newborn.	Encourage parent(s) to hold and make eye contact with newborn as physical status allows	To minimize effects of physical separation from newborn
Child's or Family's Defining Characteristics		Encourage parent-newborn skin-to-skin contact in delivery room as condition of newborn allows	To facilitate parent-infant interaction that is meaningful and comforting
(Subjective and Objective Data)		Explain to parents the newborn's illness in simple terms and expectations for recovery	To enhance parental knowledge and decrease potential fear of unknown regarding infant's survival and recovery
Risk Factors			
Separation			
Preterm infant			
Physical barriers		Encourage parents to name newborn	To provide child individual identity
		Encourage parent participation in newborn care activities such as touching infant, expressing and storing maternal breast milk, and talking to infant	To facilitate parental involvement in attaining the role of parents and decrease feelings of helplessness

ELBW, Extremely low–birth-weight; *VLBW,* very low–birth-weight.

Other Respiratory Disorders

Newborn infants are vulnerable to a variety of pulmonary complications, some requiring oxygen therapy (Table 25-9). For example, the preterm infant is subject to periods of apnea; and in term, late-preterm, and postterm infants, intrauterine stress often causes fetuses to pass meconium, which may be aspirated before or during birth. Oxygen therapy, although lifesaving, is not without its hazards.

Positive pressure introduced by mechanical apparatus has created an increase in the incidence of ruptured alveoli and subsequent pneumothorax and **bronchopulmonary dysplasia (chronic lung disease).** The use of nasal CPAP (Fig. 25-13) decreases the incidence of adverse effects associated with intubation and positive-pressure ventilation in preterm infants with RDS. Retinopathy of prematurity is observed almost exclusively in preterm infants and is related

TABLE 25-9 RESPIRATORY COMPLICATIONS

DESCRIPTION	CLINICAL MANIFESTATIONS	THERAPEUTIC MANAGEMENT	CARE MANAGEMENT
Meconium Aspiration Syndrome			
Aspiration of amniotic fluid containing meconium into fetal or newborn trachea in utero or at first breath	Meconium stained at birth Tachypnea Hypoxia Acidemia Hyperventilation (early) Hypoventilation (later)	Suction hypopharynx after head is delivered (Fig. 25-12). Infants who are vigorous with strong, stable respiratory effort, good muscle tone, and heart rate >100 beats/min should not undergo tracheal suctioning but should be monitored closely. Infants who demonstrate poor respiratory effort, low heart rate, and poor tone should be intubated rapidly, suctioned appropriately, and resuscitated according to clinical status after suctioning. Monitor for respiratory distress; manage with supplemental oxygen. Prevent acidosis and hypoxemia. Exogenous surfactant, inhaled nitric oxide, or extracorporeal membrane oxygenation (ECMO) may be used	See Respiratory Distress Syndrome (p. 685).
Apnea of Prematurity			
Lapse of spontaneous breathing for ≥20 seconds, which may or may not be followed by bradycardia, oxygen desaturation, and color change	Persistent apneic spells, bradycardia, oxygen desaturation, and cyanosis	Observe for apnea. Check for thermal stability and metabolic problem such as hypoglycemia. Administer caffeine as prescribed. Administer nasal continuous positive airway pressure (CPAP).	Provide continuous electronic monitoring (respiratory and heart rates). Observe for presence of respirations. Observe color. Provide gentle tactile stimulation. Suction nose and oropharynx if still apneic. Apply artificial ventilation with bag-valve-mask using minimum of pressure needed to gently lift rib cage. Assess for and manage any precipitating factors (e.g., temperature instability, abdominal distention, ambient oxygen). Observe for signs of caffeine toxicity: tachycardia (rate ≥180 beats/min) and (later) vomiting, restlessness, irritability. Assess skin (with use of nasal CPAP) for breakdown, irritation at nasal septum.
Pneumothorax			
Presence of extraneous air in pleural space as a result of alveolar rupture	Tachypnea or apnea Systemic hypotension Sudden or persistent oxygen desaturation Grunting, nasal flaring Retractions Absent or diminished breath sounds Shift in point of maximum impulse of heart sounds Bradycardia, cyanosis	Evacuate trapped air in pleural space through needle aspiration or insertion of chest tube. In otherwise healthy term infants who do not require high oxygen concentration or mechanical ventilation, a nitrogen "washout" may be performed with 100% oxygen; this accelerates resorption of free air in pleura into blood; consider benefits and risks of hyperoxygenation.	Maintain close vigilance of infants with respiratory distress and those on assisted ventilation. Provide appropriate care of closed chest drainage apparatus. Ensure that emergency needle aspiration setup is available.

Continued

TABLE 25-9 RESPIRATORY COMPLICATIONS—cont'd

DESCRIPTION	CLINICAL MANIFESTATIONS	THERAPEUTIC MANAGEMENT	CARE MANAGEMENT
Bronchopulmonary Dysplasia			

Pathologic process related to alveolar damage from lung disease, prolonged exposure to mechanical ventilation, high peak inspiratory pressures and oxygen, and immature alveoli and respiratory tract	Dyspnea
	Barrel chest
	Inability to wean from oxygen or mechanical ventilation after course of respiratory distress syndrome (surfactant deficiency)
	Wheezing
		Prevention—Administer maternal steroids; administer exogenous surfactant postnatally.
		Provide early detection with pulmonary function tests.
		Use synchronized or volume guarantee ventilation, decreased inspiratory pressures, or nasal CPAP.
		Prevent air leaks.
		Use high-frequency ventilation.
		Prevent or control respiratory or systemic infections.
		Minimize use of high oxygen concentrations in neonatal resuscitation and with mechanical ventilation; monitor oxygen saturation and implement resuscitation according to neonate response to low oxygen administration.
		Diagnosis established:
		  Support respiratory efforts.
		  Maintain adequate oxygenation and avoid hypoxemia.
		  Administer diuretics, bronchodilators.
		  Provide supplemental oxygen in hospital or home.
		  Prevent upper respiratory infections (e.g., RSV).
		  Administer age-appropriate immunizations (e.g., pneumococcal).
			Provide individualized developmental care and enhancement.
			Monitor oxygen saturations closely in preterm infants and avoid hyperoxemia.
			Provide opportunities for additional rest during feedings.
			Observe for signs of fluid overload or pulmonary edema.
			Assist with home oxygen therapy as needed.
			Assess susceptibility to upper respiratory tract infections and need for frequent hospitalization for respiratory dysfunction.
			Provide increased caloric density (feedings) with human milk fortifier or protein supplements.

Persistent Pulmonary Hypertension of the Newborn			
Severe pulmonary hypertension and large right-to-left shunt through foramen ovale and ductus arteriosus; often associated with conditions such as meconium aspiration, congenital diaphragmatic hernia, congenital cardiac anomalies	Hypoxia Marked cyanosis Tachypnea with grunting and retractions Decreased peripheral pulses and prolonged capillary refill (poor perfusion) Shock	Provide supplemental oxygen and assisted ventilation. Administer systemic vasodilators such as sildenafil to increase pulmonary perfusion and systemic oxygenation. Maintain acid-base balance. Prevent hypoxemia and hypercarbia. Regulate intravenous fluids. Administer inhaled nitric oxide or ECMO.	See Care of the High Risk Newborn and Family (p. 696) and Respiratory Distress Syndrome (p. 685). Provide nursing care to reduce stress to infant, especially noxious stimuli that cause increased oxygen demands. Decrease physical manipulation and disturbance. Monitor oxygenation status.
Retinopathy of Prematurity			
Severe vascular constriction in immature retinal vasculature followed by hypoxemia in retina, which in turn stimulates abnormal vascular proliferation of retinal capillaries into hypoxic area; as retinal veins dilate and multiply in direction of lens, retinal detachment may occur if untreated Multifactorial etiology—preterm birth major risk factor	Progressive vascular growth of retina Eventual blindness if not treated Diagnosed by ophthalmologic examination	Prevent preterm birth. Provide early screening and detection in infants born at <28 weeks of gestation and weight <1500 g (3 lbs 5 oz). Decrease exposure to bright, direct lighting; although exposure to bright light has not been proven to contribute to retinopathy of prematurity, such exposure is undesirable from a neurobehavioral developmental perspective. Use supplemental oxygen judiciously and monitor oxygen blood levels carefully; prevent wide fluctuations in oxygen blood levels (hyperoxia and hypoxia). Arrest vascular proliferation process—cryotherapy or laser photocoagulation; surgical repair of detached retina. Recently there has been increased interest in administration of an antivascular endothelial growth factor drug bevacizumab, which arrests proliferation of vessels and prevents retinal detachment commonly seen in retinopathy of prematurity. If successful, this therapy may preclude the use of laser therapy (Mintz-Hittner and Best, 2009).	See Care of the High Risk Newborn and Family (p. 696). Provide preventive care by monitoring blood oxygen levels closely, responding promptly to saturation alarms, and preventing fluctuations in blood oxygen levels. Provide postoperative pain management if surgery is performed. Provide parental education and support. Provide nursing care using principles of individualized developmental care.

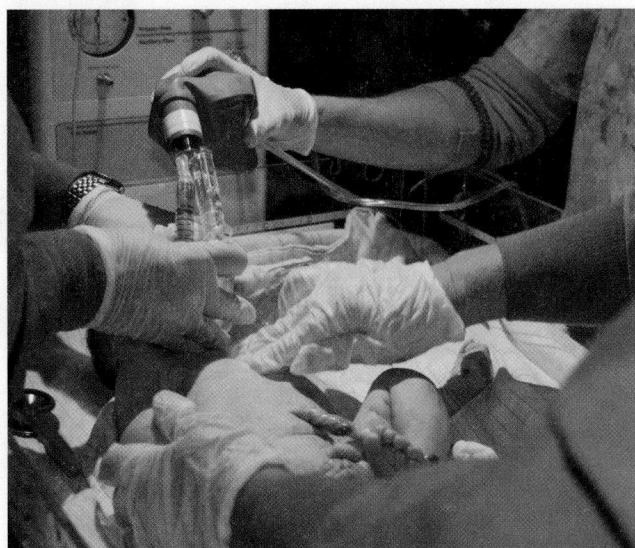

FIG 25-12 Infant being resuscitated at birth. Note presence of meconium on abdomen and umbilical cord. (Courtesy Shannon Perry, Phoenix, AZ.)

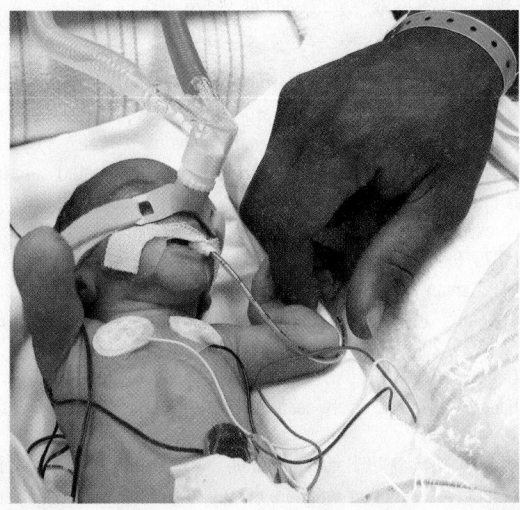

FIG 25-13 Infant on nasal continuous positive airway pressure with father's finger in hand. (Courtesy E. Jacobs, Texas Children's Hospital, Houston, TX.)

primarily to prematurity and oxygen therapy (see Table 25-9). Some evidence supports the resuscitation of asphyxiated newborns with 21% oxygen rather than 100% oxygen; preliminary studies demonstrate no significant neurologic morbidities at 18 to 24 months in newborns resuscitated with 21% oxygen (Saugstad, 2007; Saugstad, Ramji, Soll, et al., 2008). Proponents for room air resuscitation suggest that fewer complications are associated with oxidative stress and hyperoxemia when room air is administered (Vento and Saugstad, 2011). The 2010 American Heart Association Neonatal Resuscitation Guidelines recommend the initiation of neonatal resuscitation using room air (no supplemental oxygen); if the neonate does not improve within 90 seconds, the use of supplemental oxygen is recommended (see Evidence-Based Practice box). Pulse oximetry is recommended to monitor the infant's oxygenation status during resuscitation and prevent excessive use of oxygen in

both term and preterm infants (Kattwinkel, Perlman, Aziz, et al., 2010).

Inhaled nitric oxide (INO) and extracorporeal membrane oxygenation (ECMO) are additional therapies used in the treatment of respiratory distress and respiratory failure in neonates. INO is used in term and late-preterm infants with conditions such as persistent pulmonary hypertension, meconium aspiration syndrome (see Table 25-9), pneumonia, sepsis, and congenital diaphragmatic hernia to decrease or reverse pulmonary hypertension, pulmonary vasoconstriction, acidosis, and hypoxemia. Nitric oxide is a colorless, highly diffusible gas that can be administered through the ventilator circuit blended with oxygen. INO may be used in conjunction with surfactant replacement therapy, high-frequency ventilation, or ECMO. Although INO is used in preterm infants with respiratory distress and respiratory failure, its use has not proved to be significantly effective in decreasing rates of bronchopulmonary dysplasia or improving survival rates in preterm infants (Barrington and Finer, 2007; Donohue, Gilmore, Cristofalo, et al., 2011).

Sildenafil, a potent vasodilator, has demonstrated significant benefits in the treatment of persistent pulmonary hypertension in neonates (Shah and Ohlsson, 2011); the drug may be administered by NG tube or via IV route.

ECMO may be used in the management of term infants with acute severe respiratory failure for the same conditions as those mentioned for INO. This therapy involves a modified heart-lung machine, although in ECMO the heart is not stopped, and blood does not entirely bypass the lungs. Blood is shunted from a catheter in the right atrium or right internal jugular vein by gravity to a servo-regulated roller pump, pumped through a membrane lung where it is oxygenated and through a small heat exchanger, and then returned to the systemic circulation via a major artery such as the carotid artery to the aortic arch. ECMO provides oxygen to the circulation; allows the lungs to "rest"; and decreases pulmonary hypertension and hypoxemia in such conditions as persistent pulmonary hypertension of the newborn, congenital diaphragmatic hernia, sepsis, meconium aspiration, and severe pneumonia.

Necrotizing Enterocolitis

Necrotizing enterocolitis (NEC) is an acute inflammatory disease of the bowel with increased incidence in preterm infants. The precise cause of NEC is still uncertain, but it appears to occur in infants whose GI tracts have experienced vascular compromise. Intestinal ischemia of unknown etiology, immature GI host defenses, bacterial proliferation, and feeding substrate are now believed to have a multifactorial role in the etiology of NEC. Preterm birth remains the most prominent risk factor in the development of NEC (Maheshwari and Carlo, 2011).

The damage to mucosal cells lining the bowel wall may be significant. Diminished blood supply to these cells causes their death in large numbers; they stop secreting protective, lubricating mucus; and the thin, unprotected bowel wall is attacked by proteolytic enzymes. Thus the bowel wall continues to swell and break down; it is unable to synthesize protective IgM; and the mucosa is permeable to macromolecules (e.g., exotoxins), which further hampers intestinal defenses. Gas-forming bacteria invade the damaged areas to produce pneumatosis intestinalis, the presence of gas in the submucosal or subserosal surfaces of the bowel.

A consistent relationship has been observed between the development of NEC and enteric feeding of hypertonic substances (e.g., formula, hyperosmolar medications). It is unclear whether

EVIDENCE-BASED PRACTICE

Use of Room Air or Low Oxygen for Newborn Stabilization and Resuscitation in the Delivery Room

Ask the Question
PICOT Question
Is room air or low oxygen (O_2) better for newborn stabilization and resuscitation in the delivery room?

Search for Evidence
Search Strategies
Search selection included English publications on room air or low O_2 use for newborn stabilization and resuscitation in delivery room in past 3 years.

Database Used
PubMed

Critically Analyze the Evidence
- In infants weighing 1500 g (3 lbs 5 oz) or less, stabilization or resuscitation in the delivery room with fraction of inspired oxygen (FiO_2) below 100% or room air can be initiated without contributing to morbidity (Stola, Schulman, and Perlman, 2009).
- Systematic review of 21% O_2 versus 100% O_2 use for stabilization or resuscitation of newborns found a significant reduction in risk for newborn mortality and hypoxic ischemic encephalopathy when 21% O_2 was used (Saugstad, Ramji, Soll, et al., 2008).
- In neonates 24 to 28 weeks' gestational age, resuscitation with 30% O_2 vs 90% O_2 was associated with decreased oxidative stress, inflammation, need for O_2, and risk of bronchopulmonary dysplasia (Vento, Moro, Escrig, et al., 2009).
- In neonates less than or equal to 28 weeks' gestational age, use of a low FiO_2 ($\leq$30%) for resuscitation was found to be safe. The supply of O_2 should be adjusted, depending on the response of the newborn (Escrig, Arruza, Izquierdo, et al., 2008).
- In neonates less than or equal to 32 weeks' gestational age, target O_2 saturation was not achieved by 3 minutes of life when room air was used for resuscitation (Wang, Anderson, Leone, et al., 2008).
- Use of heated and humidified air in neonates less than or equal to 32 weeks' gestational age during resuscitation or stabilization in the delivery room minimized postnatal heat loss (te Pas, Lopriore, Dito, et al., 2010).
- Infants receiving 100% O_2 with positive-pressure ventilation and healthy infants transitioned in room air had similar increase in O_2 saturation, but a slower increase in O_2 saturation was observed in infants receiving 100% O_2 free flow (Rabi, Chen, Yee, et al., 2009).
- Newborns with spontaneous circulation (heart rate >60 beats/min) should be stabilized or resuscitated with room air, but asphyxiated newborns with depressed circulation (heart rate <60 beats/min) should be stabilized or resuscitated with 100% O_2 (Ten and Matsiukevich, 2009).
- In very preterm infants (<30 weeks' gestational age) stabilized or resuscitated with 100% O_2, the majority (80%) had SpO_2 $\geq$95% in the first 10 minutes. Infants stabilized or resuscitated with room air followed a course similar to that of full-term and preterm newborns when 100% O_2 was administered along with titration against SpO_2. Similar changes in heart rate were observed in both groups (Dawson, Kamlin, Wong, et al., 2009).
- Room air is as effective as 100% O_2 in stabilizing or resuscitating newborns when using short-term outcome measures (Richmond and Goldsmith, 2008).

Apply the Evidence: Nursing Implications
- There is *good evidence* with *strong recommendations* for using O_2 of various concentrations for newborn stabilization and delivery room resuscitations (Guyatt, Oxman, Vist, et al., 2008). Factors such as newborn gestational age and heart rate should be taken into consideration when determining O_2 concentration for neonatal resuscitation.

Quality and Safety Competencies:
Evidence-Based Practice*
Knowledge
Differentiate Clinical Opinion from Research and Evidence-Based Summaries
Describe the various interventions for newborn stabilization and delivery room resuscitations with room air or low O_2.

Skills
Base Individualized Care Plan on Patient Values, Clinical Expertise, and Evidence
Integrate evidence into practice by using interventions for newborn stabilization and delivery room resuscitations with room air or low O_2.

Attitudes
Value the Concept of Evidence-Based Practice as Integral to Determining Best Clinical Practice
Appreciate strengths and weakness of evidence for newborn stabilization and delivery room resuscitations with room air or low oxygen.

References
Dawson JA, Kamlin COF, Wong C, et al: Oxygen saturation and heart rate during delivery room resuscitation of infants <30 weeks' gestation with air or 100% oxygen, *Arch Dis Child Fetal Neonatal Ed* 94:F87–F91, 2009.

Escrig R, Arruza L, Izquierdo I, et al: Achievement of targeted saturation values in extremely low gestational age neonates resuscitated with low or high oxygen concentrations: a prospective, randomized trial, *Pediatrics* 121(5):875–881, 2008.

Guyatt GH, Oxman AD, Vist GE, et al: GRADE: An emerging consensus on rating quality of evidence and strength of recommendations, *BMJ* 336:924–926, 2008.

Rabi Y, Chen SY, Yee WH, et al: Relationship between oxygen saturation and the mode of oxygen delivery used in newborn resuscitation, *J Perinatol* 29:101–105, 2009.

Richmond S, Goldsmith JP: Refining the role of oxygen administration during deliver room resuscitation: what are the future goals? *Semin Fetal Neonatal Med* 13:368–374, 2008.

Saugstad OD, Ramji S, Soll RF, et al: Resuscitation of newborn infants with 21% or 100% oxygen: an updated systematic review and meta-analysis, *Neonatology* 94(3):176–182, 2008.

Stola A, Schulman J, Perlman J: Initiating delivery room stabilization/resuscitation in very low birth weight (VLBW) infants with an FiO_2 less than 100% is feasible, *J Perinatol* 29:548–552, 2009.

te Pas AB, Lopriore E, Dito I, et al: Humidified and heated air during stabilization at birth improves temperature in preterm infants, *Pediatrics* 125(6):e1427–e1432, 2010.

Ten VS, Matsiukevich D: Room air or 100% oxygen for resuscitation of infants with prenatal depression, *Curr Opin Pediatr* 21:188–193, 2009.

Vento M, Moro M, Escrig R, et al: Preterm resuscitation with low oxygen causes less oxidative stress, inflammation, and chronic lung disease, *Pediatrics* 124(3):e439–e449, 2009.

Wang CL, Anderson C, Leone TA, et al: Resuscitation of preterm neonates by using room air or 100% oxygen, *Pediatrics* 121(6):1083–1089, 2008.

Olga A. Taylor

*Adapted from QSEN at www.qsen.org.

this connection is a result of the formula imposing a stress on an ischemic bowel or serving as a substrate for bacterial growth or possibly a combination of these factors.

Radiographic studies show a sausage-shaped dilation of the intestine that progresses to marked distention and the characteristic pneumatosis intestinalis (i.e., "soapsuds," or the bubbly appearance of thickened bowel wall and ultralumina). There may be air in the portal circulation or free air observed in the abdomen, indicating perforation. Laboratory findings may include anemia, leukopenia, leukocytosis, metabolic acidosis, and electrolyte imbalance. In severe cases coagulopathy (DIC) or thrombocytopenia may be evident. Organisms are often cultured from blood, although bacteremia or septicemia may not be prominent early in the course of the disease.

Treatment of NEC begins with prevention. Oral feedings may be withheld for at least 24 to 48 hours from infants who are believed to have experienced birth asphyxia. Breast milk is the preferred enteral nutrient because it confers some passive immunity (IgA), macrophages, and lysozymes. The early clinical signs of NEC are subtle and nonspecific and may often be overlooked for other conditions; the earliest clinical signs include lethargy, abdominal distention, and high gastric residuals (Kastenberg and Sylvester, 2013).

Minimal enteral feedings (trophic feeding, GI priming) have gained acceptance with no evidence of increased incidence of NEC. In particular the use of fresh human milk has been shown to decrease the risk of NEC (Hay, 2008). Systematic reviews of the role of probiotics such as *Lactobacillus acidophilus* and *Bifidobacterium infantis* administered with enteral feedings for the prevention of NEC have demonstrated a reduced incidence of severe NEC and mortality in preterm infants (Alfaleh, Anabrees, Bassler, et al., 2011; Patel and Denning, 2013). The preferred type and optimal dosing of probiotics remain to be determined. There is evidence that the use of standardized feeding protocols that guide decisions about the initiation of feedings in preterm infants, advancement of feedings, and management of feeding intolerance may help prevent NEC (Gephart and Hanson, 2013). The role of lactoferrin (the major whey protein in human milk) in combination with lysozyme (also found in human milk) may have a significant role in the prevention of NEC and neonatal sepsis in high risk preterm infants; both act in the intestine to kill harmful bacteria and enhance intestinal immune properties (Sherman, 2013).

Medical treatment of infants with confirmed NEC consists of discontinuation of all oral feedings; institution of abdominal decompression via NG suction; administration of IV antibiotics; and correction of extravascular volume depletion, electrolyte abnormalities, acid–base imbalances, and hypoxia. Replacing oral feedings with parenteral fluids decreases the need for oxygen and circulation to the bowel. Serial abdominal radiographs (supine and left lateral decubitus) are taken in the acute phase to monitor for possible progression of the disease to intestinal perforation.

With early recognition and treatment, medical management is increasingly successful. If there is progressive deterioration under medical management or evidence of perforation, surgical resection and anastomosis are performed. Extensive involvement may necessitate surgical intervention and establishment of an ileostomy, jejunostomy, or colostomy. Sequelae in surviving infants include short-bowel syndrome (see Chapter 41), colonic stricture with obstruction, fat malabsorption, and growth failure secondary to intestinal dysfunction. A variety of surgical interventions for NEC are available and depend on the extent of bowel necrosis, associated illness factors, and infant stability. Intestinal transplantation has been successful in some former preterm infants with NEC-associated short-bowel syndrome who had already developed life-threatening total parenteral nutrition–related complications. Transplantation may be a lifesaving option for infants who previously faced high morbidity and mortality.

CARE MANAGEMENT

Nursing responsibilities begin with the prompt recognition of the early warning signs of NEC. Because the signs are similar to those observed in many other disorders of newborns, nurses must constantly be aware of the possibility of this disease in infants who are at high risk for developing it (Box 25-5).

When the disease is suspected, the nurse assists with diagnostic procedures and implements the therapeutic regimen. Vital signs, including BP, are monitored for changes that might indicate bowel perforation, septicemia, or cardiovascular shock; and measures are instituted to prevent possible transmission to other infants. It is especially important to avoid rectal temperatures because of the increased danger of perforation. To avoid pressure on the distended abdomen and facilitate continuous observation, infants are often left undiapered and positioned supine or on the side.

Observe for indications of early development of NEC by checking the appearance of the abdomen for distention (measuring abdominal girth, measuring residual gastric contents before feedings, and listening for bowel sounds) and performing all routine assessments for high risk neonates.

Conscientious attention to nutrition and hydration needs is essential; administer antibiotics as prescribed. The time at which oral feedings are reinstituted varies considerably but is usually at least 7 to 10 days after diagnosis and treatment. Feeding is usually reestablished using human milk if available.

Because NEC is an infectious disease, one of the most important nursing functions is control of infection. Strict hand washing is the primary barrier to its spread, and confirmed multiple cases are isolated. Persons with symptoms of a GI disorder should not care for these or any other infants.

Infants who require surgery require the same careful attention and observation as any infant with abdominal surgery, including ostomy care (as applicable). This condition is one of the most common reasons for performing ostomies on newborns. Throughout the medical and surgical management of infants with NEC, the nurse should be continually alert to signs of complications such as septicemia, DIC, hypoglycemia, and other metabolic derangements.

BOX 25-5   CLINICAL MANIFESTATIONS OF NECROTIZING ENTEROCOLITIS

Nonspecific Clinical Signs	Specific Signs
• Lethargy	• Distended (often shiny) abdomen
• Poor feeding	• Blood in stools or gastric contents
• Hypotension	
• Vomiting	• Gastric retention (undigested formula)
• Apnea	
• Decreased urinary output	• Localized abdominal wall erythema or induration
• Unstable body temperature	
• Jaundice	• Bilious vomitus

CARE OF THE HIGH RISK NEWBORN AND FAMILY

Assessment

A thorough systematic physical assessment is an essential component in the care of high risk infants. Subtle changes in feeding behavior, activity, color, oxygen saturation (Sao₂), or vital signs often indicate an underlying problem. LBW preterm infants, especially VLBW or ELBW infants, are ill equipped to withstand prolonged physiologic stress and may die within minutes of exhibiting abnormal symptoms if the underlying pathologic process is not corrected. Alert nurses are aware of subtle changes and react promptly to implement interventions that promote optimal functioning in high risk neonates. Changes in the infant's status are noted through ongoing observations of his or her adaptation to the extrauterine environment.

Observational assessments of high risk infants are made according to each infant's acuity; critically ill infants require close observation and assessment of respiratory function, including continuous pulse oximetry, electrolytes, and evaluation of blood gases. Accurate documentation of the infant's status is an integral component of nursing care. With the aid of continuous, sophisticated cardiopulmonary monitoring, nursing assessments and daily care may be coordinated to allow for minimal handling of the infant (especially VLBW or ELBW infants) to decrease the effects of environmental stress.

Most neonates under intensive observation are placed in a controlled thermal environment and monitored for heart rate, respiratory activity, and temperature. The monitoring devices are equipped with an alarm system that indicates when the vital signs are above or below preset limits.

BP is monitored routinely in sick neonates by either internal or external means. Direct recording with arterial catheters is often used but carries the risks inherent in any procedure in which a catheter is introduced into an artery. BP values gradually increase over the first month of life in preterm and term infants. BP norms vary by gestational age and weight, medications such as corticosteroids, and disease process. One of the primary considerations in the preterm infant is the relationship between systemic BP and the determination of adequate cerebral blood flow. In the NICU frequent laboratory examinations and their interpretation are integral parts of the ongoing assessment of infants' progress. Accurate intake and output records are kept on all acutely ill infants. An accurate output can be obtained by collecting urine in a plastic urine collection bag specifically made for preterm infants or by weighing the diapers, which is the simplest and least traumatic means of measuring urinary output. The preweighed wet diaper is weighed on a gram scale, and the gram weight of the urine is converted directly to milliliters (e.g., 25 g = 25 mL).

Blood examinations are a necessary part of the ongoing assessment and monitoring of the high risk newborn's progress. The tests most often performed are blood glucose, bilirubin, calcium, hematocrit, serum electrolytes, and blood gases. Samples may be obtained from the heel; by venipuncture; by arterial puncture; or by an indwelling catheter in an umbilical vein, an umbilical artery, or a peripheral artery.

When numerous blood samples must be drawn, it is important to maintain an accurate record of the amount of blood being removed, especially in ELBW and VLBW infants, who can ill afford to have their blood supply depleted during the acute phase of their illness. There is an increased emphasis on drawing as little blood as possible from high risk neonates to minimize the depletion of blood volume and avoid blood transfusions and associated complications. To avoid the need for repeated arterial punctures, pulse oximetry, which measures the saturation or percentage of oxygen in the hemoglobin, typically is used. Although used less frequently than pulse oximetry, transcutaneous carbon dioxide (tcPco₂) is monitored in some situations. The nurse notes changes in oxygenation (or other aspects being monitored) associated with handling and adjusts the infant's care accordingly. The frequency of vital signs is determined by the infant's acuity level (seriousness of condition) and response to handling.

Respiratory Support

The primary objective in the care of high risk infants is to establish and maintain respiration. Many infants require supplemental oxygen and assisted ventilation. All infants require appropriate positioning to maximize oxygenation and ventilation. Oxygen therapy is provided on the basis of the infant's requirements and illness (see Respiratory Distress Syndrome, p. 685).

Thermoregulation

After or concurrent with the establishment of respiration, the most crucial need of LBW infants is application of external warmth. Preventing heat loss in distressed infants is absolutely essential for survival, and maintaining a neutral thermal environment is a challenging aspect of neonatal intensive nursing care. Heat production is a complicated process that involves the cardiovascular, neurologic, and metabolic systems; and immature neonates have all of the problems related to heat production that are faced by full-term infants (see Thermogenic System, Chapter 22). However, LBW infants are placed at further disadvantage by a number of additional problems. They have an even smaller muscle mass and fewer deposits of brown fat for producing heat, lack insulating subcutaneous fat, and have poor reflex control of skin capillaries.

To delay or prevent the effects of cold stress, at-risk newborns are placed in a heated environment immediately after birth, where they remain until they are able to maintain thermal stability (i.e., the capacity to balance heat production and conservation with heat dissipation). Because overheating produces an increase in oxygen and calorie consumption, infants are also jeopardized in a hyperthermic environment. A neutral thermal environment is one that permits the infant to maintain a normal core temperature with minimum oxygen consumption and calorie expenditure (Bissinger and Annibale, 2010). Studies indicate that optimum thermoneutrality cannot be predicted for every high risk infant's needs. In healthy term infants it is recommended that axillary temperatures be maintained at 36.5° to 37.5° C (97.7° to 99.5° F); in preterm infants axillary temperatures of 36.3° and 36.9° C (97.3° and 98.4° F) are considered appropriate (Brown and Landers, 2011).

VLBW and ELBW infants, with thin skin and almost no subcutaneous fat, can control body heat loss or gain only within a limited range of environmental temperatures. In these infants heat loss from radiation, evaporation, and transepidermal water loss is 3 to 5 times greater than in larger infants, and a decrease in body temperature is associated with an increase in mortality. Further research is needed to define a neutral thermal environment for ELBW infants.

The consequences of cold stress that produce additional hazards to neonates are (1) hypoxia, (2) metabolic acidosis, and (3) hypoglycemia. Increased metabolism in response to chilling creates a compensatory increase in oxygen and calorie consumption. If available oxygen is not increased to accommodate this need, arterial oxygen tension is decreased. This is further complicated by a smaller

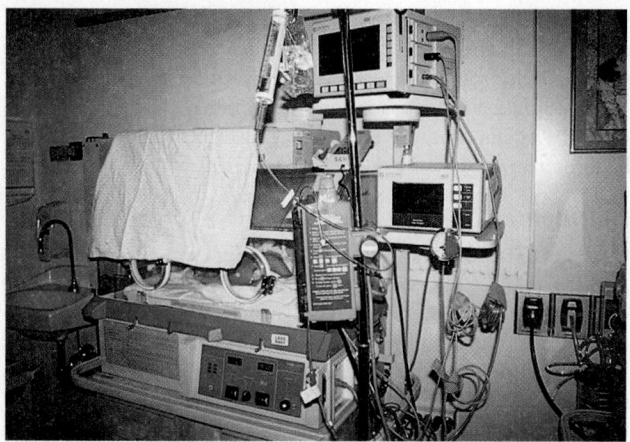

FIG 25-14 Infant in double-walled incubator with a blanket for a light shield. (Courtesy Marjorie Pyle, RNC, Lifecircle, Costa Mesa, CA.)

lung volume in relation to the metabolic rate, which creates diminished oxygen in the blood and concurrent pulmonary disorders. A small advantage is gained by the presence of fetal hemoglobin because its increased capacity to carry oxygen allows the infant to exist for longer periods in conditions of lowered oxygen tension.

The three primary methods for maintaining a neutral thermal environment are the use of an incubator (Fig. 25-14), a radiant warming panel, and an open bassinet with cotton blankets. A dressed infant under blankets can maintain a certain temperature within a wider range of environmental temperatures; however, the close observations required with a high risk infant are best accomplished if the infant remains partially unclothed. The incubator should always be prewarmed before placing an infant in it. The use of double-walled incubators significantly improves the infant's ability to maintain a desirable temperature and reduce energy expenditure related to heat regulation. Inside or outside the incubator, head coverings are effective in preventing heat loss. A fabric-insulated or wool cap is more effective than one fashioned from stockinette. The use of a heated gel mattress with radiant heat has been shown to decrease the incidence of radiation heat loss significantly and preserve an adequate neutral thermal environment for the VLBW neonate (Lewis, Sanders, and Brockopp, 2011; Soll, 2008). An effective means for maintaining the desired range of temperature in the infant is the use of a manually adjusted or automatically controlled (servo-controlled) incubator. The latter mechanism, when set at the upper and lower limits of the desired circulating air temperature range, adjusts automatically in response to signals from a thermal sensor attached to the abdominal skin. If the infant's temperature drops, the warming device is triggered to increase heat output. The servo control is usually set to a desired skin temperature between 36° and 36.5° C (96.8° and 97.7° F) (Brown and Landers, 2011).

A high-humidity atmosphere contributes to body temperature maintenance by reducing evaporative heat loss. A number of "microenvironments" may be used with VLBW and ELBW infants to minimize evaporative and insensible water losses. These include items such as food-grade plastic bags or plastic wrap, humidified reservoirs for incubators, and humidified plastic heat shields covered with plastic wrap. When such environments are used, special care must be taken to avoid bacterial contamination of the warm and humid environment by organisms such as *Pseudomonas* and *Serratia*, which have an affinity for moist environments; postnatally

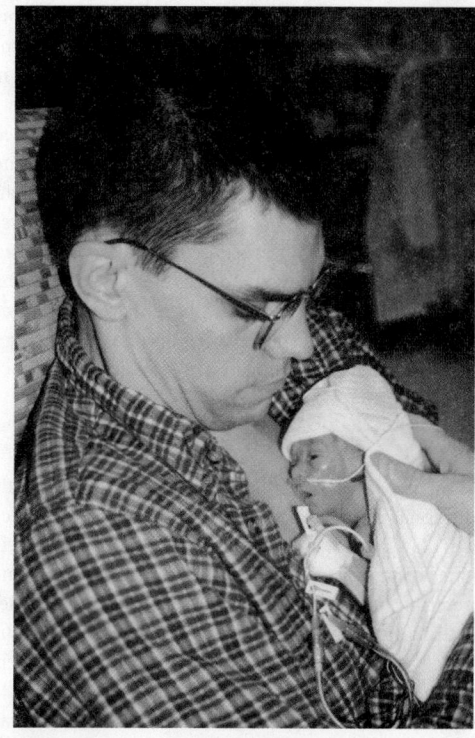

FIG 25-15 Father providing skin-to-skin care (kangaroo care). (Courtesy Judy Meyr, St Louis, MO).

acquired *pneumonia from such organisms may be fatal, particularly in VLBW infants.* A systematic review of practices to decrease hypothermia at birth in LBW infants found that plastic wraps (polyethylene) or bags kept preterm infants warmer, leading to higher temperatures on admission to neonatal units and less hypothermia (Lewis, Sanders, and Brockopp, 2011; McCall, Alderdice, Halliday, et al., 2010). This practice is now recommended in the Neonatal Resuscitation Program guidelines published by the American Heart Association (Kattwinkel, Perlman, Aziz, et al., 2010).

Skin-to-skin (kangaroo) contact (Fig. 25-15) between a stable preterm infant and parent is also a viable option for interaction because of the maintenance of appropriate body temperature by the infant. Other benefits of skin-to-skin contact are discussed later in this chapter.

Protection from Infection

Protection from infection is an integral part of all newborn care, but preterm and sick neonates are particularly susceptible. The protective environment of a regularly cleaned and changed incubator provides effective isolation from airborne infective agents. However, thorough, meticulous, and frequent hand washing is the foundation of a preventive program. This includes *all* persons who come in contact with infants and their equipment. After handling another infant or equipment, no one should ever touch an infant without first washing his or her hands.

Personnel with infectious disorders are either barred from the unit until they are no longer infectious or are required to wear suitable shields such as masks or gloves to reduce the likelihood of contamination. An annual influenza vaccination is recommended for NICU personnel. Standard Precautions as a method of infection control are instituted in all nursery areas to protect the infants and staff. The benefit of "gowning" by visitors and hospital staff to control infection is not supported by research. Sibling visitation in the NICU has not been shown to increase HAI; however, appropriate screening for upper respiratory illness in siblings is recommended.

The sources of infection rise in direct relationship to the number of persons and pieces of equipment coming in contact with the infants. Equipment used in the care of infants is cleaned on a regular basis in accordance with manufacturer recommendations or institutional protocol; this includes cleaning cribs, mattresses, incubators, radiant warmers, cardiorespiratory monitors, pulse oximeters, and vital sign–monitoring equipment after usage with one infant and before usage with another. Because organisms thrive best in water, plumbing fixtures and humidifying equipment are particularly hazardous. Disposable equipment used for water-related therapies such as nebulizers and plastic tubing is changed regularly.

Hydration

High risk infants often receive supplemental parenteral fluids to supply additional calories, electrolytes, and water. Adequate hydration is particularly important in preterm infants because their extracellular water content is higher (70% in full-term infants and up to 90% in preterm infants), their body surface is larger, and the capacity for handling fluid shifts is limited in preterm infants' underdeveloped kidneys. Therefore these infants are highly vulnerable to fluid depletion.

Parenteral fluids may be given to the high risk neonate via several routes, depending on the nature of the illness, the duration and type of fluid therapy, and unit preference. Common routes of fluid infusion include peripheral, peripherally inserted central venous (or percutaneous central venous), surgically inserted central venous, and umbilical venous catheters. The preferred sites for peripheral IV infusions in neonates are the peripheral veins on the dorsal surfaces of the hands or feet. Alternative sites are scalp veins and antecubital veins. Special precautions and frequent observations must accompany the use of peripheral lines (Beauman and Swanson, 2006). In many neonatal centers the percutaneous central venous catheter is used for parenteral therapy and medication administration because of less expense and decreased neonatal trauma.

In most facilities NICU nurses insert peripheral IV catheters and maintain the infusions. IV fluids must always be delivered by continuous infusion pumps that deliver minute volumes at a preset flow rate. The catheter is secured to the skin with a transparent dressing or minimum amount of tape (see Skin Care, p. 701), with care taken not to cause undue pressure from the catheter hub and tubing. Because all infants, especially those who are ELBW and VLBW, are highly vulnerable to any fluid shifts, infusion rates are regulated carefully and checked hourly to prevent tissue damage from extravasation, fluid overload, or dehydration. Pulmonary edema, congestive heart failure, patent ductus arteriosus, and intraventricular hemorrhage may occur with fluid overload. Dehydration may cause electrolyte disturbances with potentially serious CNS effects.

Infants who are ELBW, tachypneic, receiving phototherapy, or in a radiant warmer have increased insensible water losses that require appropriate fluid adjustments. Nurses must monitor fluid status by daily (or more frequent) weights and accurate intake and output of all fluids, including medications and blood products. Serum electrolytes are monitored per unit protocol, and urine electrolytes are obtained as warranted by the infant's condition. ELBW infants often require more frequent monitoring of these parameters because of their inordinate transepidermal fluid loss, immature renal function, and propensity to dehydration or overhydration. Intolerance of even dextrose 5% is not uncommon in ELBW infants, with

subsequent glycosuria and osmotic diuresis. Alterations in behavior, alertness, or activity level in these infants receiving IV fluids may signal an electrolyte imbalance, hypoglycemia, or hyperglycemia. Nurses should also be observant for tremors or seizures in VLBW or ELBW infants because these may be a sign of hyponatremia or hypernatremia.

Nutrition

Optimum nutrition is critical in the management of LBW and preterm infants, but there are difficulties in providing for their nutritional needs. The various mechanisms for ingestion and digestion of foods are not fully developed; the more immature the infant, the greater the problem. In addition, the nutritional requirements for this group of infants are not known with certainty. It is known that all preterm infants are at risk because of poor nutritional stores and several physical and developmental characteristics.

An infant's nutritional needs for rapid growth and daily maintenance must be met in the presence of several anatomic and physiologic disabilities. Although some sucking and swallowing activities are demonstrated before birth and in preterm infants, coordination of these mechanisms does not occur until approximately 32 to 34 weeks of gestation, and they are not fully synchronized until 36 to 37 weeks. Initial sucking is not accompanied by swallowing, and esophageal contractions are uncoordinated. Consequently infants are highly prone to aspiration and its attendant dangers. As infants mature the suck-swallow pattern develops but is slow and ineffectual, and these reflexes may also become easily exhausted.

The amount and method of feeding are determined by the infant's size and condition. Nutrition can be provided by either the parenteral or enteral route or by a combination of the two. Infants who are ELBW, VLBW, or critically ill often obtain most of their nutrients by the parenteral route because of their inability to digest and absorb enteral nutrition. Illness factors resulting in hypoxia and major organ immaturity further preclude the use of enteral feeding until the infant's condition has stabilized. NEC has previously been associated with enteral feedings in acutely ill or distressed infants (see Necrotizing Enterocolitis, p. 693). Total parenteral nutritional support of acutely ill infants may be accomplished successfully with commercially available IV solutions specifically designed to meet the infant's nutritional needs, including protein, amino acids, trace minerals, vitamins, carbohydrates (dextrose), and fat (lipid emulsion).

Studies have shown that there are benefits to the early introduction of small amounts of enteral feedings in metabolically stable preterm infants. These minimal enteral (trophic gastrointestinal priming) feedings have been shown to stimulate the infant's GI tract, preventing mucosal atrophy and subsequent enteral feeding difficulties. Enteral feedings with as little as 0.1 to 4 mL/kg of breast milk or preterm formula may be given by gavage as soon as the infant is medically stable. These enteral feedings have been shown to simulate the infant's GI tract, preventing mucosal atrophy and subsequent enteral feeding difficulties. Parenteral hydration and nutrition are continued until the infant is able to tolerate an amount of enteral feeding sufficient to sustain growth. An increased incidence of NEC in VLBW infants receiving minimal enteral nutrition has not been substantiated (Reynolds and Thureen, 2007; Terrin, Passariello, Canani, et al., 2009). Minimal enteral feedings increase mineral absorption, increase serum calcium and alkaline phosphatase activity, and substantially decrease the incidence of bilious gastric residuals and feeding intolerance in preterm infants. Minimal enteral feedings are recommended as the standard of care for feeding VLBW infants (Hay, 2008).

Although the timing of the first feeding has been a matter of controversy, most authorities now believe that early feeding (provided that the infant is medically stable) reduces the incidence of complicating factors such as hypoglycemia, dehydration, and the degree of hyperbilirubinemia. The feeding regimen used varies in different units.

Breastfeeding

Ample evidence indicates that human milk is the best source of nutrition for term and preterm infants. Studies indicate that small preterm infants are able to breastfeed if they have adequate sucking and swallowing reflexes and there are no other contraindications such as respiratory complications or concurrent illness (Dougherty and Luther, 2008). Mothers who wish to breastfeed their preterm infants are encouraged to pump their breasts until their infants are sufficiently stable to tolerate breastfeeding. Appropriate guidelines for the storage of expressed mother's milk should be followed to decrease the risk of milk contamination and destruction of its beneficial properties.

Milk produced by mothers whose infants are born before term contains higher concentrations of protein, sodium, chloride, and IgA. Growth factors, hormones, prolactin, calcitonin, thyroxine (T_4), steroids, and taurine (an essential amino acid) are also present in human milk. Secretory IgA concentration is higher in the milk from mothers of preterm infants than in the milk from mothers of full-term infants. IgA is important in the control of bacteria in the intestinal tract, where it inhibits adherence and proliferation of bacteria on epithelial surfaces. Additional protection from infection is provided by leukocytes, lactoferrin, and lysozyme, all of which are present in human milk. The milk produced by mothers for their infants changes in content over the first 30 days postnatally, at which time it is similar to full-term human milk. Despite its benefits, LBW infants (<1500 g [3 lbs 5 oz]) who are fed unfortified human milk exclusively demonstrate decreased growth rates and nutritional deficiencies even beyond the hospitalization period. These infants often have inadequacies of calcium, phosphorus, protein, sodium, vitamins, and energy. Specially designed supplements for human milk have been developed to address these deficits. Fortifiers are commercially available, usually as a liquid or powder containing protein; carbohydrate; calcium; phosphorus; magnesium; sodium; and varied amounts of zinc, copper, and vitamins. Because fortifiers do not contain sufficient iron, an exogenous source must be administered after enteral feeding.

A number of studies regarding the effects of long-chain polyunsaturated fatty acids on cognitive development, visual acuity, and physical growth in full-term and preterm infants have prompted formula companies to add docosahexaenoic acid (DHA) and arachidonic acid (AA) to their infant formulas. AA and DHA are present in human milk, and their presence has been reported to lead to an increase in cognitive development in human milk–fed infants compared with infants fed a formula without these fatty acids. However, one meta-analysis of four clinical trials demonstrated no clinically significant developmental benefits to supplementation of formula with AA and DHA in term and preterm infants at 18 months of age (Beyerlein, Hadders-Algra, Kennedy, et al., 2010).

Preterm infants may be able to breastfeed successfully earlier than previously believed (28 to 36 weeks); in addition, preterm infants who are breastfed rather than bottle-fed demonstrate fewer incidences of oxygen desaturation; absence of bradycardia; warmer skin temperature; and better coordination of breathing, sucking, and swallowing (Gardner and Lawrence, 2011). Preterm infants should be evaluated carefully for readiness to breastfeed, including assessment of behavioral state, ability to maintain body temperature outside an artificial heat source, respiratory status, and readiness to suckle at the mother's breast. Readiness to suckle may be accomplished with nonnutritive suckling at the breast during skin-to-skin (kangaroo) contact so the mother and newborn may become accustomed to one another (Gardner and Lawrence, 2011). Nasal cannula oxygen may also be provided during preterm breastfeeding on the basis of the infant's assessed requirements.

Nipple Feeding

Vigorous infants can be fed from a nipple with little difficulty, but compromised preterm infants require alternative methods. The amount to be fed is determined largely by the infant's weight gain and tolerance of previous feeding and is increased by small increments until a satisfactory caloric intake is ensured.

The rate of increase that is well tolerated varies from one infant to another, and determining this rate is often a nursing responsibility. Preterm infants require more time and patience to feed compared with full-term infants, and the oropharyngeal mechanism may be stressed by an attempt to feed too rapidly. It is important not to tire the infants or overtax their capacity to retain the feedings. When infants require a prolonged time to complete a feeding, gavage feeding may be considered for the next time.

A developmental approach to feeding considers the individual infant's readiness rather than initiating feedings based on weight and age or a predetermined time schedule. Feeding readiness is determined by each infant's medical status, energy level, ability to sustain a brief quiet alert state, gag reflex (demonstrated with a gavage tube insertion), spontaneous rooting and sucking behaviors, and hand-to-mouth behaviors (Nye, 2008) A preterm infant may experience difficulty coordinating sucking, swallowing, and breathing, with resultant apnea, bradycardia, and decreased oxygen saturation. The infant's ability to suck on a pacifier does not indicate complete readiness for nipple feeding or ability to coordinate the previously mentioned activities without some degree of stress; a gradual introduction of nippling in preterm infants is based on careful evaluation of their ability to maintain adequate cardiopulmonary functions while feeding. When infants are unable to tolerate bottle feedings, intermittent feedings by gavage are instituted until they gain enough strength and coordination to use the nipple.

The nipple used should be relatively firm and stable. Although a high-flow, pliable nipple requires less energy to use, it may provide a flow rate that is too rapid for some preterm infants to manage without a risk of aspiration. A firmer nipple facilitates a more "cupped" tongue configuration and allows for a more controlled, manageable flow rate.

The infant is positioned in the feeder's arms or placed semiupright in the lap and held with the back curved slightly to simulate the position assumed naturally by most full-term newborns. The use of gentle cheek and jaw support for preterm infants has been shown to facilitate feedings. Stroking the infant's lips, cheeks, and tongue before feeding helps promote oral sensitivity. Inward and upward support to the infant's cheeks and a slightly upward lift to the chin are provided by the fingers to assist nipple compression during feeding.

Bottle-feedings are continued if infants are able to tolerate the feedings and take the required amount. Some preterm infants respond more slowly than full-term infants; therefore the feeding interval and the amount of the feeding are individualized. Preterm infants are often slow feeders and require patience, frequent rest periods, and burping (or bubbling).

Gavage Feeding

Gavage feeding is a safe means of meeting the nutritional requirements of infants who are unable to feed orally. These infants are usually too weak to suck effectively, are unable to coordinate swallowing, and lack a gag reflex. Gavage feedings may be provided by continuous drip regulated via infusion pump or by intermittent bolus feedings. Studies have demonstrated an overall decrease in total milk fat concentration delivery when continuous gavage infusions are administered, which suggests that intermittent or bolus gavage of expressed mother's milk be administered when possible (Premji, Paes, Jacobson, et al., 2002). Intermittent gavage feeding is used as an energy-conserving technique for infants learning to nipple feed who become excessively tired, listless, or cyanotic.

A size 3.5-, 5-, 6-, or 8-Fr feeding tube is used to instill the feeding; and the methods for determining correct placement are described below (Fig. 25-16). Although the more relaxed lower esophageal sphincter makes passage of the tube easier, there may be changes in heart rate and BP in response to vagal stimulation.

When an indwelling tube is required, consideration should be given to using a product made of Silastic rather than polyvinyl chloride (PVC) because PVC becomes stiff when exposed to body fluids.

The stomach is aspirated, the contents measured, and the aspirate returned as part of the feeding. However, this practice may vary, depending on circumstances and individual unit protocol. The amount of aspirate depends on the time since the previous feeding or concurrent illness. Some advocate deducting the amount aspirated to avoid overdistending the stomach.

The milk or formula is allowed to flow by gravity, and the length of time varies. This procedure is not used as a timesaving method for the nurse. Complications of indwelling tubes include aspiration, obstructed nares, mucus plugs, purulent rhinitis, epistaxis, infection, and possible stomach perforation. Current best practice dictates a radiograph as the only certain way to determine NG tube placement in the stomach. Methods such as auscultation of an air bubble, neck-ear-xiphoid (NEX) measurements for insertion depth, or pH measurements are considered imprecise when used as the only method for determination of placement of feeding tubes in infants (de Boer, Smit, and Mainous, 2009; Ellett, Croffie, Cohen, et al., 2005; Farrington, Lang, Cullen, et al., 2009; Freeman, Saxton, and Holberton, 2012; Quandt, Schraner, Ulrich Bucher, et al., 2009; Renner, 2010). Ellett, Cohen, Perkins, et al. (2011) developed an age-related, height-based regression equation for determining adequate gastric tube insertion length for use in neonates less than 1 month old (corrected age). Others have developed guidelines for correct NG tube insertion and placement in LBW and term infants based on the infant's weight (Freeman, Saxton, and Holberton, 2012; Gallaher, Cashwell, Hall, et al., 1993). Further research is needed to determine optimal positioning of feeding tubes in high risk infants on intermittent bolus or continuous gavage feedings.

The infant may be held during gavage feedings by the caregiver or parent. If necessary, oxygen may be supplied via nasal cannula to facilitate handling. It is not recommended that the infant be removed from a primary source of oxygen for feedings because doing so decreases oxygen availability. Nonnutritive sucking (NNS) on a pacifier may help bring the infant to a quiet alert state in preparation for feeding. Proposed benefits of NNS include improved weight gain, improved milk intake, more stable heart rate and oxygen saturation, earlier age at full oral feeds, and improved behavioral state.

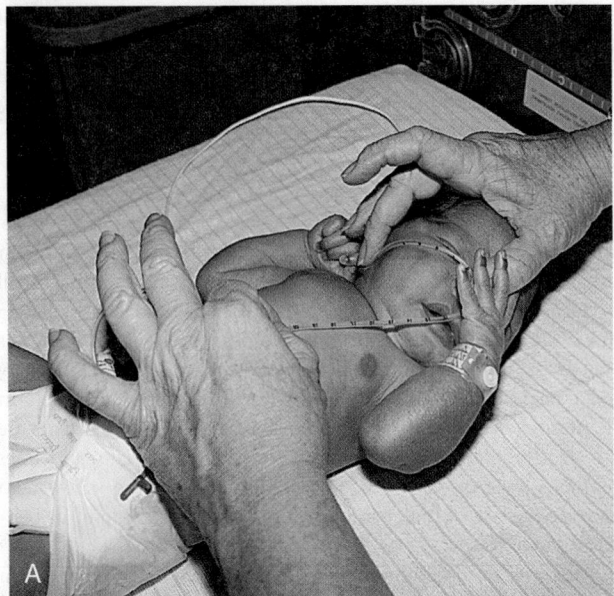

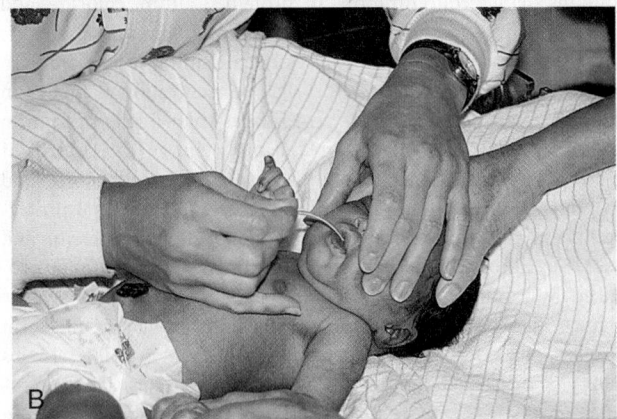

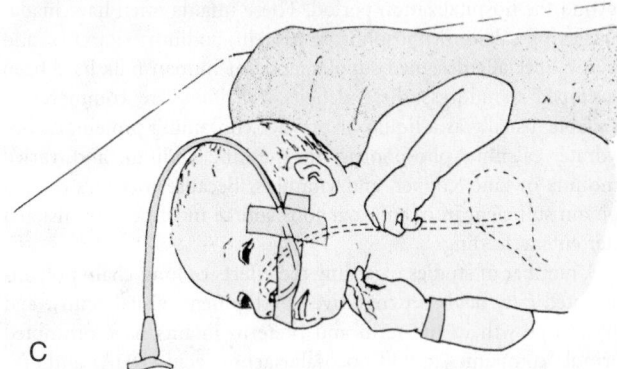

FIG 25-16 Gavage feeding. **A,** Measurement of gavage feeding tube from tip of nose to earlobe and to midpoint between end of xiphoid process and umbilicus (NEMU). Tape may be used to mark correct length on tube. **B,** Insertion of gavage tube using orogastric route. **C,** Indwelling gavage tube, nasogastric route. After feeding by orogastric or nasogastric tube, infant is propped on right side or placed prone (preterm infant) for 1 hour to facilitate emptying of stomach into small intestine. Note rolled towel for support (see the column at left for methods to determine adequate feeding tube placement). **(A** and **B,** Courtesy Marjorie Pyle, RNC, Lifecircle, Costa Mesa, CA.)

Energy Conservation

One of the major goals of care for the high risk infant is conservation of energy. Much of the care described in this section is directed toward this end (e.g., disturbing the infant as little as possible, maintaining a neutral thermal environment, gavage feeding as appropriate, promoting oxygenation, and judiciously implementing any caregiving activities that increase oxygen intake and caloric consumption). An infant who is not required to expend excess energy to breathe, eat, or alter body temperature can use this energy for growth and development. Diminishing environmental noise levels and shading the infant from bright lights also promote rest (see Developmental Outcome, p. 703).

Skin Care

The skin of preterm infants is characteristically immature relative to that of full-term infants. In most preterm infants the skin barrier properties resemble those of the term infant by 2 to 4 weeks' postnatal age, regardless of gestational age at birth. Because of its increased sensitivity and fragility, no alkaline-based soap that might destroy the acid mantle of the skin is used. The increased permeability of the skin facilitates absorption of ingredients. All skin products (e.g., alcohol, chlorhexidine, povidone-iodine) should be used with caution; the skin is rinsed with water afterward because these substances may cause severe irritation and chemical burns in VLBW and ELBW infants.

The skin is easily excoriated and denuded; therefore care must be taken to avoid damage to the delicate structure. The total skin is thinner than that of full-term infants and lacks rete pegs, appendages that anchor the epidermis to the dermis. Therefore there is less cohesion between the thinner skin layers. The use of adhesive tape or bandages may excoriate the skin or adhere to the skin surface so well that the epidermis can be separated from the dermis and pulled away with the tape, thus altering skin barrier function. Pectin barriers and hydrocolloid adhesives may be useful because these products mold well to skin contours and adhere in moist conditions. Recommendations for protecting the integrity of the skin of preterm infants include using minimal adhesive tape, backing the tape with cotton, and delaying adhesive and pectin barrier removal until adherence is reduced (Lund and Kuller, 2007). Emollients such as Eucerin or Aquaphor have been used to promote skin integrity and prevent dry, cracking, and peeling skin in infants at risk for skin breakdown. Emollients may also reduce transepidermal water loss and protect infants from HAI (Polin, Denson, Brady, et al., 2012). However, in some studies these agents have been shown to increase the risk for coagulase-negative infections in preterm infants and therefore should be used with caution. The use and effectiveness of emollients in high risk neonates is controversial, and further studies are needed (Telofski, Morello, Mack Correa, et al., 2012).

It is unsafe to use scissors to remove dressings or tape from the extremities of very small and immature infants because it is easy to snip off tiny extremities or nick loosely attached skin. Solvents used to remove tape are avoided because they tend to dry and burn the skin. Guidelines for skin care are listed in the Guidelines box.

GUIDELINES

Neonatal Skin Care

General Skin Care
Assessment
- Assess skin every day or more often as needed for redness, dryness, flaking, scaling, rashes, lesions, excoriation, and breakdown.
- Identify risk factors for skin injury: gestational age ≤30 weeks, adhesive use, nutritional compromise, high-frequency ventilation, extracorporeal membrane oxygenation, hypotension requiring vasopressors.
- Use a valid assessment tool to provide reliable and objective measurement of skin condition.
- Evaluate/report abnormal skin findings and analyze for possible causes.
- Intervene according to interpretation of findings or health care provider order.

Bathing
Initial Bath
- Assess to ensure that the infant has a stable temperature for a minimum of 2 to 4 hours before first bath.
- Use cleansing agents with neutral pH or minimal dyes or perfume in water.
- Use Standard Precautions; wear gloves.
- Do not completely remove vernix; allow it to wear off with normal care and handling.
- Bathe preterm infant younger than 32 weeks in warm water only for the first week.

Routine
- Decrease frequency of baths to every second or third day by daily cleansing of eye, oral, and diaper areas and pressure points.
- Use pH neutral cleanser or soaps no more than 2 or 3 times a week.
- Avoid rubbing skin during bathing or drying.

- Immerse stable infants fully (except head) in an appropriate-size tub.
- Use swaddled immersion bathing technique: slowly unwrap after gently lowering into water for sensitive but stable infants needing assistance with motor system reactivity.

Emollients
- Apply sparingly to dry, flaking, fissured areas as needed.
- Choose petrolatum-based products that are free of preservatives, dyes, and perfumes.
- Observe neonates ≤750 g (1 lb 10 oz) receiving emollient therapy for increased risk of coagulase-negative *Staphylococcus* infections.
- Consider dispensing emollients from hospital pharmacy, unit dose, or patient-specific container to reduce contamination.

Adhesives
- Decrease use as much as possible.
- Use semipermeable dressings to secure intravenous (IV) lines, nasogastric or orogastric tubes, silicone catheters, and central lines.
- Use hydrogel or limb electrodes.
- Consider pectin barriers beneath adhesives to protect skin.
- Secure pulse oximeter probe or electrodes with elasticized dressing material (carefully avoid restricting blood flow).
- Do not use adhesive remover, solvents, or bonding agents.
- Avoid removing adhesives for at least 24 hours after application.
- Adhesive removal can be facilitated using water, mineral oil, or petrolatum.
- Remove adhesives or skin barriers slowly, supporting the skin underneath with one hand and gently peeling away the product from the skin with the other hand.

Continued

GUIDELINES

Neonatal Skin Care—cont'd

Antiseptic Agents

- Apply before invasive procedures.
- Consider the potential for skin breakdown or irritation with disinfectant.
- No specific disinfectant is recommended over another for all neonates; remove completely with water or saline after use.
- Avoid use of isopropyl alcohol for skin preparation or removal of other disinfectants.

Transepidermal Water Loss

- Minimize transepidermal water loss (TEWL) and heat loss in small preterm infants at <30 weeks of gestation by:
  - Measuring ambient humidity during first weeks of life.
  - Applying occlusive polyethylene body bag immediately at birth and removing after infant is stabilized in the neonatal intensive care unit.
  - Considering increasing humidity to 70% to 90% by using a humidified incubator for first 7 days; decrease to 50% until 28 days of age.
  - Using supplemental conductive heat and reducing radiant heat source.
  - Applying semipermeable transparent dressings to skin surfaces on infant's chest, abdomen, and back.
  - Considering use of emollients (see Emollients above)

Skin Breakdown

Prevention

- Decrease pressure from externally applied forces using water, air, or gel mattresses; sheepskin; or cotton bedding.
- Provide adequate nutrition, including protein, fat, and zinc.
- Apply transparent adhesive dressings to protect arms, elbows, and knees from friction injury.
- Use tracheostomy and gastrostomy dressings (Hydrasorb or Lyofoam) for drainage and relief of pressure from tracheostomy or gastrostomy tube.
- Use emollient in diaper area (groin and thighs) to reduce urine irritation.

Treating Skin Breakdown

- Irrigate wound every 4 to 8 hours with warm half-strength normal saline using a 20-mL or larger syringe and 20-gauge Teflon catheter.
- Culture wound and treat if signs of infection are present (excessive redness, swelling, pain on touch, heat, or resistance to healing).
- Use transparent adhesive dressing for uninfected wounds.
- Apply hydrogel with or without antibacterial or antifungal ointments (as ordered) for infected wounds (may need to moisten before removal).
- Use hydrocolloid for deep, uninfected wounds (leave in place for 5 to 7 days) or as an ostomy barrier and to improve appliance adhesion; warm barrier in hand for several minutes to soften before applying to skin.
- Avoid use of antiseptic solutions for wound cleansing (use for intact skin only).

Treating Diaper Dermatitis

- Maintain clean, dry skin; use absorbent diapers and change often.
- If mild irritation occurs, use petrolatum barrier.
- For developing dermatitis, apply a generous quantity of zinc-oxide barrier (remove only soiled matter, leaving original barrier in place).
- For severe dermatitis identify cause and treat (frequent stooling from spina bifida, severe opiate withdrawal, or malabsorption syndrome).
- Treat *Candida albicans* with antifungal ointment or cream.
- Avoid powders and antibiotic ointments. (See Care of the Umbilicus and Circumcision in Chapter 23.)

Other Skin Care Concerns

Use of Substances on Skin

- Evaluate all substances that come in contact with infant's skin.
- Before using any topical agent, analyze components of preparation and:
  - Use sparingly and only when necessary.
  - Confine use to smallest possible area.
  - Whenever possible and appropriate, wash off with water.
  - Monitor infant carefully for signs of toxicity and systemic effects.

Use of Thermal Devices

- Avoid heat lamps because of increased potential for burns. If needed, measure actual temperature of exposed skin every 15 minutes.
- When using preheated transcutaneous electrodes:
  - Avoid use on extremely low–birth-weight infants.
  - Set at lowest possible temperature.
  - Use pulse oximetry rather than transcutaneous monitoring whenever possible.
- When prewarming heels before phlebotomy, avoid temperatures over 40° C (104.0° F).
- Provide warm ambient humidity directed away from infant; use aerosolized sterile water and maintain ambient temperature not to exceed 40° C (104.0° F).
- Document use of all heating devices.

Use of Fluid Therapy and Hemodynamic Monitoring

- Be certain that fingers or toes are visible whenever extremity is used for peripheral IV or arterial line.
- Secure catheter or needle with transparent dressing and tape to promote easy visualization of site.
- Assess site hourly for signs of ischemia, infiltration, and inadequate perfusion (check capillary refill, pulses, color).
- Avoid use of restraints (e.g., arm boards); if used, check that they are secured safely and not restricting circulation or movement (check for pressure areas).
- Use commercial IV protector (e.g., I.V. House) with minimal tape.

Data from Johnson FE, Maikler VE: Nurses' adoption of the AWHONN/NANN Neonatal Skin Care Project, *NINR* 1(1):59–67, 2001; Kuller JM: Skin breakdown: risk factors, prevention, and treatment, *Newborn Infant Nurs Rev* 1(1):33–42, 2001; Lund CH, Kuller J, Lott JW: Neonatal skin care: clinical outcomes of the AWHONN/NANN evidence-based clinical practice guideline, *J Obstet Gynecol Neonatal Nurs* 30(1):41–51, 2001; Lund CH, Kuller J, Raines DA, et al: *Neonatal skin care: evidence-based clinical practice guideline*, ed 2, Washington, DC, 2007, AWHONN; Lund C, Lane A, Raines DA: Neonatal skin care: the scientific basis for practice, *J Obstet Gynecol Neonatal Nurs* 28(3):241–254, 1999; Taquino LT: Promoting wound healing in the neonatal setting: process versus protocol, *J Perinat Neonatal Nurs* 14(1):108–118, 2000.

During skin assessment of preterm infants nurses are alert to the subtle signs that indicate zinc deficiency, a problem sometimes seen in infants who have inadequate intake or abnormal losses of zinc. Breakdown usually occurs in the areas around the mouth, buttocks, fingers, and toes. In preterm and VLBW infants it may also occur in the creases of the neck, wrists, and ankles and around wounds. Zinc deficiency is most likely to appear in preterm infants with inadequate zinc intake, an ileostomy, short-bowel syndrome, or chronic diarrhea. Suspicious lesions are reported to the practitioner so zinc supplements can be prescribed. Skin injuries have been reported during the use of phototherapy blankets. Caution is warranted in using these products in ELBW infants and infants who are at risk for skin breakdown.

Developmental Outcome

Much attention has been focused on the effects of early developmental intervention on both normal and preterm infants. Infants respond to a great variety of stimuli, and the atmosphere and activities of the NICU are overstimulating. Consequently infants in NICUs are subjected to inappropriate stimulation that can be harmful. For example, the noise level that results from monitoring equipment, alarms, and general unit activity has been correlated with the incidence of intracranial hemorrhage, especially in ELBW and VLBW infants. Personnel should reduce noise-generating activities such as closing doors (including incubator portholes), listening to loud radios, talking loudly, and handling equipment (e.g., trash containers). Byers, Waugh, and Lowman (2006) suggest monitoring sound levels in the NICU to address problem areas. Nursing care activities such as taking vital signs, changing the infant's position, weighing, and changing diapers are associated with frequent periods of hypoxia, oxygen desaturation, and elevated ICP. The more immature the infant, the less able he or she is to habituate to a single procedure such as taking an oscillometric BP without becoming overstimulated.

Twenty-four–hour surveillance of sick infants implies maximum visibility and often bright lights. Units should establish a night-day sleep pattern by darkening the room, covering cribs with blankets, or placing eye patches over the infant's eyes at night. Infants need scheduled rest periods during which the lights are dimmed, the incubators are covered with blankets, and the infants are not disturbed for handling of any kind (Altimier, 2007). Sleep periods should be undisturbed for at least 50 minutes to allow complete sleep cycles.

Infants' eyes should be shielded from bright procedure lights to prevent potential harm. Many experts suggest that the human face, especially the parent's, is the best visual stimulus and that visual stimuli be kept to a minimum early in development. Developmental care, accentuating the infant's unique ability to achieve behavioral state organization, is tailored to the developmental level and tolerance of each infant based on a comprehensive behavioral assessment. During the early stages of development (especially before 33 weeks of gestation), external stimulation produces uncoordinated, random activity such as jerky limb extension, hyperflexion, and irregular vital signs. At this stage infants need to have minimum environmental stimulation. Using the developmental model of supportive care, the nurse closely monitors physiologic and behavioral signs to promote organization and well-being of the high risk infant during handling. Softly calling the infant by name and then gently placing a hand on the body signal that care is beginning and alleviate the abrupt interruption that precedes caregiving. Infants are handled with slow, controlled movements (some infants are unstable if moved abruptly), and their random movements are controlled with

limbs held flexed close to their bodies during turning or other position changes. This containment or facilitated tucking may also be used before invasive procedures such as heelstick to alleviate distress. Blanket swaddling and nesting or containment have been shown to decrease physiologic and behavioral stress during routine care procedures such as bathing, weighing, and heelstick. A nest constructed by placing blanket rolls underneath the bed sheet helps infants maintain an attitude of flexion when prone or side lying.

Although it must be individually adjusted, skin-to-skin contact (kangaroo care) and short periods of gentle massage can help reduce stress in preterm infants. Regular passive skin-to-skin contact between parents (mother or father) and LBW infants has been shown to alleviate stress. The parent wears a loose-fitting, open-front top; and the undressed (except for diaper) infant is placed in a vertical position on the parent's bare chest, which permits direct eye contact, skin-to-skin sensations, and close proximity (see Fig. 25-15). In addition to being a safe and effective method for VLBW infant-parent acquaintance, skin-to-skin contact between the parent and infant can have a positive healing effect for the mother with a high risk pregnancy. Mothers may experience psychologic healing related to preterm birth and regain the mothering role through early skin-to-skin contact with their VLBW infants. Major neonatal benefits of skin-to-skin care include a reduced risk of mortality, fewer HAI, decreased length of hospital stay, maintenance of neonatal thermal stability and oxygen saturation, increased feeding vigor, and improved growth (Conde-Agudelo, Belizán and Diaz-Rossello, 2011; Dodd, 2005). In full-term newborns skin-to-skin contact has a strong analgesic effect during procedures such as heel lance (Cong, Ludington-Hoe, McCain, et al., 2009). LBW infants receiving skin-to-skin contact with breastfeeding mothers maintained higher oxygen saturation and were less likely to have desaturations below 90%, and their mothers were more likely to continue breastfeeding both in the hospital and for 1 month after discharge. Kangaroo care of preterm infants fosters appropriate neurobehavioral development by promoting stability of heart and respiratory function, minimizes purposeless movements, offers maternal proximity for attention, improves the infant's behavioral state, and permits self-regulating behaviors (McCain, Ludington-Hoe, Swinth, et al., 2005).

The arena of developmental care for preterm infants has expanded to include a wide variety of interventions such as infant massage, soothing soft music, recordings of parents reading stories, positioning to enhance self-regulatory abilities, enhancement of hand-to-mouth activities, uninterrupted sleep periods, decreased environmental light and noise, and even the use of stuffed animals to facilitate infant positioning. As a result of such interventions, parents may perceive the NICU environment as less threatening. Active participation in providing such an environment for their special infant also involves the parents in the provision of daily care when the newborn is critically ill and cannot be fed or held.

When infants have reached sufficient developmental organization and stability, interventions are designed and implemented to support their growing abilities. Nurses and parents become adept at learning to read infants' behavioral cues and supplying appropriate interventions (Table 25-10). Cues include both approach and avoidance behaviors. Approach behaviors that are supported and enhanced include tongue extension, hand clasp, hand-to-mouth movements, sucking, looking, and cooing. Signs of stress or fatigue that signal the infant's need for "time-out" are described in Table 25-10.

When infants are recovering and are free of support systems, medically stable, and on room air or smaller amounts of oxygen, they are assessed to document behavioral state organization and

TABLE 25-10	SIGNS OF STRESS OR FATIGUE IN NEONATES
SUBSYSTEM	**SIGNS OF STRESS**
Autonomic	Physiologic instability
Respiratory	Tachypnea, pauses, gasping, sighing
Color	Mottled, flushed, dusky, pale or gray
Visceral	Hiccups, gagging, choking, spitting up, grunting and straining as if having a bowel movement, coughing, sneezing, yawning
Autonomic	Tremors, startles, twitches
Motor	Fluctuating tone; lack of control over movement, activity, and posture
Flaccidity	Low tone in trunk; limp, floppy upper and lower extremities; limp, drooping jaw (gape face)
Hypertonicity	Arm or leg extensions, arm(s) outstretched with fingers splayed in salute gesture, fingers stiffly outstretched, trunk arching, neck hyperextended
Hyperflexion	Trunk, extremities, fisting
Activity	Squirming; frantic, diffuse activity or little or no activity or responsiveness
State	Disorganized quality to state behaviors, including available states, maintenance of state control, and transition from one state to another
Sleep	Whimpering sounds, facial twitching, irregular respirations, fussing, grimacing, restless appearance
Awake	Glazed, unfocused look; staring; worried or pained expression; hyperalert or panicked appearance; eye roving; crying; cry-face; actively averting gaze or closing eyes; irritability; prolonged awake periods; inconsolability; frenzy Abrupt or rapid state changes
Other state-related behaviors and attention interaction	Efforts to attend to and interact with environmental stimulation eliciting signs of stress and disorganized subsystem functioning
Autonomic	Physiologic instability of varying degrees with autonomic, respiratory, color, and visceral responses
Motor	Fluctuating tone, increased motor activity; progressively frantic diffuse activity if stimulation continues
State	Roving eyes; gaze averting; glazed, unfocused look or worried, panicked expression; weak cry; cry-face; irritability Closed eyes and sleeplike withdrawal Abrupt state changes Signs of stress when presented with more than one type of stimulus at a time

Data from Als H: Toward a synactive theory of development: promise for the assessment and support of infant individuality, *Infant Mental Health J* 3(4):229–243, 1982; Als H: A synactive model of neonatal behavior organization: framework for the assessment of neurobehavioral development in the premature infant and for support of infants and parents in the neonatal intensive care environment, *Phys Occup Ther Pediatr* 6:3–55, 1986; Hunter JG: The neonatal intensive care unit. In Case-Smith J, Allen AS, Pratt PN, editors: *Occupational therapy for children*, ed 4, St Louis, 2001, Mosby.

ability to self-regulate. When the infant is stable and mature enough to begin developmental intervention, activities are individualized according to each infant's cues, temperament, state, behavioral organization, and particular needs. Intervention periods are short (e.g., 2 to 3 minutes of voices, 5 minutes of quiet music). Hearing and vestibular interventions are initiated earlier than visual stimulation. One type of intervention at a time is applied to document the infant's tolerance and response. An intervention program for convalescing infants includes parents and siblings early in the infant's hospitalization; teaching parents to be responsive to the infant's individual cues is an important function of the NICU nurse. Parents, siblings, and health care providers are encouraged to adhere to the established developmental care plan to avoid disruption in sleep-wake cycles and minimize inappropriate stimuli.

Developmental care of preterm neonates is an ongoing process in the NICU and is incorporated into the daily care given to each infant. The nurse is cognizant of the preterm infant's developmental needs, temperament, and newborn state and environmental conditions that adversely affect the infant; nursing care is planned accordingly to enhance optimal physical, psychosocial, and neurologic development. This task is often difficult to accomplish when invasive treatments or interventions are required to stabilize the critically ill neonate.

Family Support and Involvement

Professional health care workers often are so absorbed in the lifesaving physical aspects of care that they ignore the emotional needs of infants and their families. The significance of early parent-child interaction and infant stimulation has been documented by reliable research. Nurses must be aware of these infant and family needs and incorporate activities that facilitate family interaction into the nursing care plan.

The birth of a preterm infant is an unexpected and stressful event for which families are emotionally unprepared. They find themselves simultaneously coping with their own needs, the needs of their infant, and the needs of their family (especially when they have other children). To compound the situation, their infant's precarious condition engenders an atmosphere of apprehension and uncertainty.

- Work through the events surrounding labor and birth.
- Acknowledge that the infant's life is endangered and begin the anticipatory grieving process.
- Confront and recognize feelings of inadequacy and guilt in not delivering a healthy child.
- Adapt to the neonatal intensive care environment.
- Resume parental relationships with the sick infant and initiate the caregiving role.
- Prepare to take the infant home.

Modified from Siegel R, Gardner SL, Dickey LA: Families in crisis: theoretical and practical considerations. In Gardner SL, Carter BS, Enzman-Hines M, et al., editors: *Merenstein and Gardner's handbook of neonatal intensive care*, ed 7, St Louis, 2011, Mosby.

They are faced with multiple crises and overwhelming feelings of responsibility, helplessness, and frustration.

All parents have some anxieties about the outcome of a pregnancy, but after a preterm birth the concern is heightened regarding both the viability and normalcy of their infant. Mothers may see their infant only briefly before the newborn is removed to the NICU or even to another hospital, leaving them with just the recollection of the infant's very small size and unusual appearance. They often feel alone or lost on the mother-baby unit, belonging neither with mothers who have lost their infants nor with those who have delivered healthy, full-term infants. The staff and physicians are often guarded in discussing the infant's condition; mothers are continually expecting to hear that their infant has died, and they are sensitive to the anxieties of other mothers and staff members. Going home without their infant only compounds their feelings of disappointment, failure, and deprivation.

When an infant is to be transported from the hospital, the parents need a description of the facility where the infant is going. They need to know the location, reputation, and nature of the facility and the care that the infant is expected to receive. The name of the infant's physician and the telephone number of the nursery should be given to them, and unfamiliar terms such as *neonatologist*, *ventilator*, *infusion*, and *incubator* should be explained. Explanations should be kept simple, and parents should be given the opportunity to ask questions. If booklets are available that describe the facility, they are given to the family.

Perhaps most important, the parents should have some contact with the infant before the transport. Being able to see, touch, and (if possible) hold their infant may help decrease parents' anxiety. Often a photograph or even a videotape of their infant can serve as tangible evidence of the newborn's existence until the parents are able to travel to the regional facility. When possible, it is often advisable to transfer the mother to the same institution as her infant.

Parents need to be informed of their infant's progress and reassured that he or she is receiving proper care. They need to understand the smallest aspects of the infant's condition and treatment. Parents need a realistic, honest, and direct assessment of the situation. Using nonmedical terminology, moving at a pace that is comfortable for parents to assimilate the information, and avoiding lengthy technical explanations facilitate communication with family members. Psychologic tasks that must be accomplished by parents during their infant's care are presented in Box 25-6.

Facilitating Parent-Infant Relationships

Because of their physiologic instability, infants are separated from their mothers immediately and surrounded by a complex, impenetrable barrier of glass windows, mechanical equipment, and special caregivers. There is some evidence indicating that the emotional separation that accompanies the physical separation of mothers and infants may interfere with the normal mother-infant attachment process discussed in Chapter 20. Maternal attachment is a cumulative process that begins before conception, strengthens by significant events during pregnancy, and matures through mother-infant contact during the neonatal period and infancy.

When an infant is sick, the necessary physical separation appears to be accompanied by an emotional estrangement by the parents, which may seriously damage the capacity for parenting their infant. This detachment is further hampered by the tenuous nature of the infant's condition. When survival is in doubt, parents may be reluctant to establish a relationship with their infant. They prepare themselves for the infant's death while continuing to hope for recovery. This anticipatory grief and hesitancy to embark on a relationship are evidenced by behaviors such as delay in giving the infant a name, reluctance in visiting the nursery (or when they do visit, focusing on equipment and treatments rather than on their infant), and hesitancy to touch or handle the infant when given the opportunity.

Family-centered care of high risk newborns includes encouraging and facilitating parental involvement rather than isolating parents from their infant and associated care. This is particularly important for mothers; to reduce the effects of physical separation, mothers are united with their newborn at the earliest opportunity.

Preparing the parents to see their infant for the first time is an important nursing responsibility. The nurse prepares them for their infant's appearance, the equipment attached to the child, and the general atmosphere of the unit. The initial encounter with the NICU is a stressful experience; and the frightening array of people, equipment, and activity is likely to be overwhelming. A book of photographs or pamphlets describing the NICU environment (infants in incubators or under radiant warmers, monitors, mechanical ventilators, and IV equipment) provides a useful and nonthreatening introduction to the NICU.

Parents are encouraged to visit their infant as soon as possible. Even if they saw the infant at the time of transport or shortly after birth, he or she may have changed considerably, especially if a number of medical and equipment requirements are associated with the hospitalization. At the bedside the nurse should explain the function of each piece of equipment and the role it plays in facilitating recovery. Explanations may often need to be patiently repeated because parents' anxiety over the infant's condition and the surroundings may prevent them from really "hearing" what is being said. When possible, some items related to therapy can be removed (e.g., phototherapy can be discontinued temporarily, and eye patches removed to permit eye-to-eye contact).

Parents appreciate the support of a nurse during the initial visit with their infant, but they may also appreciate some time alone with the infant for a short while. It is important during the early visits to emphasize the positive aspects of their infant's behavior and development so the parents can focus on their child as an individual rather than on the equipment that surrounds him or her. For example, the nurse may describe the infant's spontaneous behaviors during care such as the grasp reflex and spontaneous movement or make comments about the infant's biologic functions. Most institutions have open visiting policies so parents and siblings may visit their infant as often as they wish.

Parents vary greatly in the degree to which they are able to interact with their infant. Some may wish to touch or hold him or her during the first visit, but others may not feel comfortable enough to even enter the nursery. These reactions depend on a variety of prenatal and postnatal factors such as the parity of the mother and her preparation before birth; the infant's size, condition, and physical appearance; and the type of treatment the infant is receiving. It is essential to recognize that the individualized pacing and quality of the interactions are more important than an early onset of these interactions. Parents may not be receptive to early and extended infant contact because they need time to adjust to the impact of an infant with birth problems and must be helped to grieve before they can accept the child.

One recent study of fathers with an infant in the NICU found that common barriers to paternal involvement included the infant's small size and fragile health status, perceived infant feedback (negative), nurses' attitudes toward paternal involvement, and conflict over the demands of home, work responsibilities, and care of other children. Facilitators of paternal involvement included the support of family and friends, perceived positive infant responses, maternal encouragement, and nurses' encouraging attitudes (Feeley, Waitzer, Sherrard, et al., 2013). The study concluded that NICU nurses have a strong positive or negative influence on the father's involvement with infant care and his perception of his ability to care for the infant.

The parents' inability to focus on their infant is a clue for the nurse to help them express and deal with feelings of guilt, anxiety, helplessness, inadequacy, anger, and ambivalence. Nurses can help them recognize that they are normal responses shared by other parents. It is important to point out and reinforce the positive aspects of parents' behavior and interactions with their infant.

Most parents feel shaky and insecure about initiating interaction with their infant. Nurses can sense parents' level of readiness and offer encouragement in these initial efforts. Parents of preterm infants follow the same acquaintance process as do parents of term infants. They may quickly proceed through the process or may require several days or even weeks to complete it. They begin by touching their infant's extremities with their fingertips and poking the infant tenderly and then proceed to caresses and fondling (Fig. 25-17). Touching is the first act of communication between parents and child. Parents need to be prepared for their infant's exaggerated and generalized startle responses to touch so they do not interpret these as negative reactions to their overtures. It may be necessary to limit tactile stimuli when the infant is critically ill and labile, but the nurse can offer other options such as speaking softly or sitting at the bedside.

Parents of acutely ill preterm infants may express feelings of helplessness and lack of control. Involving the parent in some type of caregiving activity, no matter how minor it may seem to the nurse, enables the parent to "take on" a more active role. Examples of such caregiving for an acutely ill infant who cannot be held and is seemingly not responding positively include moistening the infant's lips with a small amount of sterile water on a cotton-tipped swab or pumping and storing breast milk.

Eventually parents begin to endow their infant with an identity—as part of the family. When an infant no longer appears as a foreign object and begins to take on aspects of family members such as the father's chin or the sister's nose, nurses can facilitate this incorporation. Parents are encouraged to bring in clothes, a toy, a stuffed animal, or a family snapshot for their infant; and the nurse can help them set goals for themselves and the child. Parents may become involved by reading a children's storybook or nursery rhymes in a soft, soothing voice. Some families tape record the parents' voices telling or reading stories and play the tapes when the infant is able to cope with such stimuli. The nurse must discuss feeding schedules, and parents are encouraged to visit at times when they can become involved in the care of their infant. Throughout the parent-infant acquaintance process, the nurse listens carefully to what the parents say to assess their concerns and their progress toward incorporating their infant into their lives. The manner in which parents refer to their infant and the questions they ask reveal their worries and feelings and can serve as valuable clues to future relationships with the child. The alert nurse is attuned to these subtle indications of parents' needs, which provide guidelines for nursing intervention. Often all that they need is reassurance that they will have the support of the nurse during caregiving activities and that the behaviors about which they are concerned are normal reactions and will disappear as the infant matures.

Parents need guidance in their relationships with their infant and help in their efforts to meet the child's physical and developmental needs. The nursing staff must help parents understand that their preterm infant offers few behavioral rewards and show them how to accept small rewards. The infant's reactions and behaviors are explained to parents, who take their infant's jerky, rejective behavior

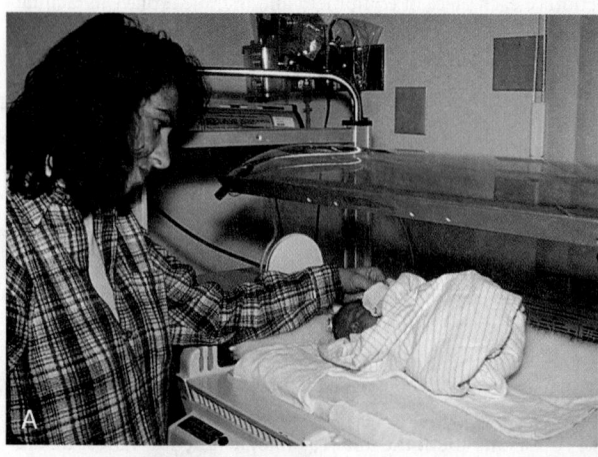
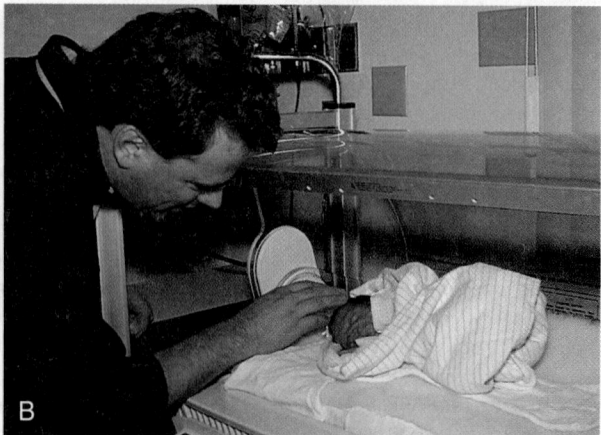

FIG 25-17 A, Mother interacts with her preterm infant by touch. **B,** Father interacts with his newborn by stroking and touching infant with fingertips. (Courtesy Michael S. Clement, MD, Mesa, AZ.).

personally. They need reassurance that these behaviors are not a reflection on their parenting skills. Parents are taught to recognize their infant's cues regarding stimulation, handling, and other interaction, especially aversive behaviors that indicate a need for rest. Nurses need to include parents in planning their infant's care and sensory stimulation materials such as a music box or recording.

Above all, nurses must encourage and reinforce parents during their caregiving activities and interactions with their infant to promote healthy parent-child relationships. It is also helpful for the parents to have contact and communication with a consistent group of nurses. This decreases the different information given to them and often instills confidence that, although they cannot be at their infant's bedside 24 hours a day, there are competent and caring nurses whom they may call to inquire about the infant's status. Periodic parent conferences involving the staff caring for the child serve to clarify misunderstandings or problems related to the infant's condition.

Discharge Planning and Home Care

Parents become apprehensive and excited as the time for discharge approaches. They have many concerns and insecurities regarding the care of their infant. They fear that the child may still be in danger, that they will be unable to recognize signs of distress or illness in their infant, and that the infant may not yet be ready for discharge. Nurses need to begin early to help parents acquire or increase their skills in the care of their infant. Appropriate instruction must be provided, and sufficient time allowed for the family to assimilate the information and learn the continuing special care requirements. Where rooming-in or other live-in arrangements are available, parents can stay for a few days and nights and assume the care of their infant under the supervision and support of the nursing staff.

There should be appropriate medical and nursing follow-up and referrals to services that can benefit the family, including developmental follow-up. Parents of preterm infants should also be given adequate information about immunizations with other discharge planning information. With the trend toward earlier discharge, many hospital-based home health care agencies become involved in the follow-up and care of NICU "graduates" in the home. For the parents of an infant being discharged with equipment such as an oxygen tank, apnea monitor, or even a ventilator, discharge planning requires multidisciplinary collaborative practice to ensure that the family has not only the appropriate resources but also the available assistance for dealing with the infant's needs. Many communities have organized support groups, including those discussed previously, those designed for parents of infants who require special care because of specific defects or disabilities, and those for parents of multiple births.

Since preterm infants remain at high risk for SIDS following discharge to the home environment, nurses should discuss safe infant sleep practices with the parents and other potential caregivers, including guidelines for safe sleep for infants with special needs (gastroesophageal reflux, mechanical ventilation, oroesophageal malformations) (see SIDS, Chapter 31).

Car-seat safety is an essential aspect of discharge planning, and infants younger than 37 weeks of gestation should have a period of observation in an appropriate car seat to monitor for possible apnea, bradycardia, and decreased SaO$_2$ (Bull, Engle, and AAP Committee on Injury, Violence, and Poison Prevention and the Committee on Fetus and Newborn, 2009) (see Community Focus box). Several models can be adapted for small infants with the placement of blanket rolls on each side of the infant to support the head and trunk. For adequate support without slumping, the seat

back–to-crotch strap distance must be 14 cm (5.5 inches) or less; a small rolled blanket may be placed between the crotch strap and the infant to reduce slouching. The distance from the lower harness strap to the seat bottom should be 25.5 cm (10 inches) or less to decrease the potential for the harness straps to cross the infant's ears. The rear-facing semiupright position provides support for the head, neck, and back, thereby reducing the stress to the neck and spinal cord in a vehicle crash. Car-seat manufacturers must specify recommended minimum and maximum weights for the occupant; therefore it is important to check the manufacturer recommendations before purchasing a car seat for a smaller infant. Additional guidelines are available from the AAP (Durbin and AAP Committee on Injury, Violence, and Poison Prevention, 2011).

An important part of discharge planning and care of preterm infants is nutrition for continued growth; thus the choice of feeding must be addressed carefully. Human milk must be fortified according to the infant's corrected age and physiologic needs. In a Cochrane review fortification of human milk with a multinutrient supplement for at least 12 weeks after hospital discharge was found to result in higher rates of growth (McCormick, Henderson, Fahey, et al., 2010). Full-term infant formulas are not considered adequate for proper growth in preterm infants.

Knowing that staff members are available for telephone or personal contact when the parents take the infant home provides a measure of security to anxious parents. Many NICU facilities maintain a policy of open communication between staff and parents both during the infant's hospitalization and after discharge. It is the responsibility of the NICU staff to make certain that parents are prepared to care for their infant both emotionally and physically. At the same time it is important that parents establish a trusting relationship with the infant's primary care provider in the community before discharge from the acute care facility.

Neonatal Loss

The precarious nature of many high risk infants makes death a real and ever-present possibility. Although infant mortality has been reduced sharply with improved technology, the mortality rate is still greatest during the neonatal period. Nurses in the NICU are usually the persons who must prepare the parents for an inevitable death, provide end-of-life care for the infant and family, and facilitate a family's grieving process after an expected or unexpected death. In the event of a stillbirth or infant death shortly after birth, the labor and birth nurse or postpartum nurse will provide the care for the infant and family. The labor and birth nurse as well as the postpartum (or mother-baby) nurse also participate in the care of the family during this time of crisis.

The loss of an infant has special meaning for the grieving parents. It represents a loss of a part of themselves (especially for mothers), a loss of the potential for immortality that offspring represent, and the loss of the dream child that has been fantasized about throughout the pregnancy. There is often a sense of emptiness and failure. In addition, when an infant has lived for such a short time, there may be few, if any, pleasant memories to serve as a basis for the identification and idealization that are part of the resolution of a loss.

To help parents understand that the death is a reality, it is important that they be encouraged to hold their infant before death and, if possible, be present at the time of death so their infant can die in their arms if they choose. Many who deny the need to hold their infant may later regret the decision.

Parents are given the opportunity to actually "parent" the infant in any manner they wish or are able to do before and after the death. This may include seeing, touching, holding, caressing, and talking

🏠 COMMUNITY FOCUS

Preterm and Late-Preterm Infant Car Seat Evaluation

The American Academy of Pediatrics (AAP) (Bull, Engle, and Committee on Injury, Violence, and Poison Prevention and the Committee on Fetus and Newborn, 2009) recommends that infants born before 37 weeks' of gestation be evaluated for apnea, bradycardia, and oxygen desaturation episodes before hospital discharge.* The AAP suggests that facilities develop policies for the implementation of a program of evaluation; however, few evidence-based practice recommendations have been published to date delineating specific requirements for such a program. Based on the available literature, suggestions for providing a car seat evaluation of infants born before 37 weeks of gestation include:

- Use the parents' car seat for the evaluation.
- Perform the evaluation 1 to 7 days before the infant's anticipated discharge.
- Secure the infant in the car seat per guidelines using blanket rolls on the side.
- Set the pulse oximeter low alarm at 88% (or per unit protocol).
- Set the heart rate low alarm limit at 80 beats/min and apnea alarm at 20 seconds (cardiorespiratory monitor).
- Leave the infant undisturbed semiupright in the car seat for a minimum of 90 to 120 minutes or for the time period parents state it takes (whichever is longer) to arrive at their home.
- Document the infant's tolerance to the car-seat evaluation.
- An episode of desaturation, bradycardia, or apnea (20 seconds or more) constitutes a failure, and evaluation by the practitioner must occur before discharge. If the infant experiences this in a semiupright position, a car bed with the infant supine should be considered, and similar testing should be undertaken in the car bed.
- Repeat the test after 24 hours after modifications have been made to the car seat, car bed, or infant's position in either restraint system.
- It is recommended that a certified car-seat technician place the infant in the car seat (or bed) if a failure occurs (see National Highway Traffic Safety Administration website† for car-seat inspection station).
- If the infant is being discharged on an apnea or cardiorespiratory monitor, this equipment should be used during the trip home.
- The technician demonstrates appropriate positioning of the infant in the restraint device to the parents and has the parents do a return demonstration.
- Document the interventions, the infant's tolerance, and the parents' return demonstration.

Modified from American Academy of Pediatrics: Safe transportation of premature and low birth weight infants, *Pediatrics* 97(5):758–760, 1996; American Academy of Pediatrics: Transporting children with special health care needs, *Pediatrics* 104(4):988–992, 1999; Bull MJ, Engle WA, and Committee on Injury, Violence, and Poison Prevention and the Committee on Fetus and Newborn: Safe transportation of preterm and low birth weight infants at hospital discharge, *Pediatrics* 123(5):1424–1429, 2009.

*Infants at risk for obstructive apnea (e.g., Pierre Robin sequence or congenital neuromuscular disorders such as spinal muscular atrophy) may also need to be evaluated in a semiupright car seat or car bed before discharge.

†www.nhtsa.gov.

to their infant privately; the parents may also wish to bathe and dress the infant. If parents are hesitant about seeing their dead infant, it is advisable to keep the body in the unit for a few hours because many parents change their minds after the initial shock of the death.

Parents may need to see and hold the infant more than once—the first time to say "hello" and the last time to say "good-bye." If parents wish to see the infant after the body has been taken to the morgue, the infant should be retrieved, wrapped in a blanket, rewarmed, and taken to the mother's room or other private place. The nurse should stay with the parents and provide them an opportunity for private time alone with their dead infant. Individual grief responses of the mother and father should be recognized and handled appropriately; gender differences and cultural and religious beliefs will affect the parents' grief responses.

A hospice approach may be implemented for families with infants for whom the decision has been made to not prolong life and who are receiving only palliative. Another approach is to send the family home with the infant and allow them to spend time together until the eventual death; hospice services may be available, and supportive care is provided in the home setting. Some families find this option less restrictive and more family oriented than being in the hospital setting. (See Chapter 36 for further discussion of hospice care.)

A photograph of the infant taken before or after death is highly desirable. Parents may wish to have a special family portrait taken with the infant and other family members; this often helps personalize and make the experience more tangible. The parents may not wish to see the photograph at the time of death, but the chance to refer to it later will help make their infant seem more real, which is a part of the normal grief process. A photograph of their infant being held by the hand or touched by an adult offers a more positive image than a morgue type of photograph. A bereavement or memory packet can be given to the grieving parents and family and may include the infant's handprints and footprints, a lock of hair, the bedside name card, the ID bracelet or armbands and, as appropriate to the family's religious beliefs, a certificate of baptism.

Naming the deceased infant is an important step in the grieving process. Some parents may hesitate to give the newborn a name that had been chosen during the pregnancy for their "special baby." However, having a tangible person for whom to grieve is an important component of the grieving process.

A nurse who is familiar to the family should be present during the discussion about the dead or dying infant. The nurse should talk with parents openly and honestly about funeral arrangements because few parents have had experience with this aspect of death. Many funeral homes now offer inexpensive arrangements for these special cases. Someone from the NICU should take the responsibility for acquiring this type of information. It is often helpful to parents for the NICU to have a list of local funeral homes, services offered, and prices. Families need to be informed of the options available, but a funeral is preferable because the ritual provides an opportunity for parents to feel the support of friends and relatives. A member of the clergy of the appropriate faith may be notified if the parents wish. Issues regarding an autopsy or organ donation (when appropriate) are approached in a multidisciplinary fashion (primary practitioner and primary nurse) with respect, sensitivity to cultural and religious beliefs, tact, and consideration of the family's wishes. Gardner and Dickey (2011) and Jansen (2003) provide additional suggestions for helping families who experience neonatal loss.

Before the parents leave the hospital, they are given the telephone number of the unit and are invited to call any time they have any further questions. Many intensive care units make a point to contact the parents several weeks after a neonatal death to assess the parents' coping mechanisms, evaluate the grieving process, and provide support as needed. Several organizations are available to offer support and understanding to families who have lost a newborn; these organization include the Compassionate Friends,* Aiding Mothers and Fathers Experiencing Neonatal Death (AMEND),† and Share Pregnancy and Infant Loss Support, Inc.‡ (See also Chapter 36 for further discussion of end-of-life care.)

Nurses who care for critically ill infants also experience grief; NICU nurses may feel helpless and sorrowful. It is important that such grief be allowed and that nurses attend the funeral or memorial service as a part of working through the grief process. Nurses may fear that showing emotion is unprofessional and that the expression of grief indicates "loss of control." These fears are unfounded. Studies have demonstrated that to continue to be effective managers and providers of care, nurses must be allowed to grieve and support each other through the process (Gardner and Dickey, 2011).

Baptism

Because many Christian parents wish to have their child baptized if death is anticipated or is a decided possibility, this may become a nursing responsibility. Whenever possible, it is most desirable that a representative of the parents' faith (e.g., a Roman Catholic priest or a Protestant minister) perform such a ritual. When death is imminent, a nurse or a physician can perform the baptism by simply pouring water on the infant's forehead (a medicine dropper is a convenient means) while repeating the words, "I baptize you in the name of the Father and of the Son and of the Holy Spirit." This includes a birth of any gestational age, particularly when the parents are Roman Catholic.

When the parents' faith is uncertain, a conditional baptism can be carried out by saying, "If you are capable of receiving baptism, I baptize you in the name of the Father and of the Son and of the Holy Spirit." The baptism is recorded in the infant's chart, and a notice is placed on the crib or incubator. Parents are informed at the first opportunity.

NEWBORN SCREENING FOR DISEASE

A number of genetic disorders can be detected in the newborn period. There is no national policy for such detection in the United States; therefore the extent of neonatal screening is determined by state laws and voluntary guidelines. Most states require screening for phenylketonuria (PKU), congenital hypothyroidism (CH), galactosemia, and hemoglobin defects such as sickle cell disease (see Chapter 43); screening for congenital hearing loss is recommended at the same time as disease screening. Because concern has been voiced regarding the inconsistency among states in screening for genetic disorders based on cost, population demographics, resource availability, and political environment, the Task Force on Newborn Screening was formed by the AAP and other federal health care agencies to address this issue (Lloyd-Puryear, Tonniges, van Dyck, et al., 2006).

The use of pulse oximetry to screen for critical congenital heart disease in healthy term infants has been endorsed by the Department of Health and Human Services and is being implemented in numerous states; this screening should be incorporated into the recommended uniform newborn screening panel (Bradshaw and Martin, 2012; Mahle, Martin, Beekman, et al., 2012). Recommendations for screening healthy term newborns include the following (Kemper, Mahle, Martin, et al., 2011):

- Screen healthy term newborns after 24 hours of life or as close to discharge from the birth hospital as possible.
- Use a motion-tolerant pulse oximeter.
- Avoid false-positive results by screening while the infant is alert.
- Obtain pulse oximeter readings from the right hand and one foot.
- Pulse oximetry ≤90% in right hand or foot is considered a positive screening, and additional evaluation is warranted (e.g., echocardiogram).
- 90% to 95% in the right hand or foot or >3% difference between the two extremities warrants a repeat test in 1 hour. If screening values remain the same as the first time, consider repeating the screen in 1 hour. If parameters remain unchanged after the second screen, repeat a third time. If unchanged consider it a positive screen.
- ≥95% in the right hand or foot and ≤3% difference between the two extremities is a negative screen (no further testing is required).

The AAP and ACOG (2007) also recommend routine prenatal and perinatal HIV counseling and testing for all pregnant women and their newborns. Benefits of early identification of HIV-infected infants are early antiretroviral therapy and aggressive nutritional supplementation; appropriate changes in their immunization schedule; monitoring and evaluation of immunologic, neurologic, and neuropsychologic functions for possible changes caused by antiretroviral therapy; initiation of interventions for special educational needs; evaluation for the need of other therapies such as IVIG for the prevention of bacterial infections; tuberculosis screening and treatment; and management of communicable disease exposures. In addition, vertical transmission of HIV from the mother to the newborn may be reduced to 2% with a cesarean birth before the rupture of membranes and onset of labor (AAP and ACOG, 2007). As a result of virologic diagnostic techniques such as HIV culture, PCR, and immune complex–dissociated p24 antigen, diagnosis of HIV infection can be made in 30% to 50% of infants at birth and in 100% of infants by 4 to 6 months of age. For information on additional diseases that may be screened in the newborn period, see Newborn Screening Fact Sheets (Kaye and AAP Committee on Genetics, 2006).

Inborn Errors of Metabolism

Inborn errors of metabolism (IEMs) constitute a large number of inherited diseases caused by the absence or deficiency of a substance essential to cellular metabolism, usually an enzyme. When the normal metabolic process is interrupted as a result of a missing enzyme, an accumulation of substances precedes the interruption, the end product of the process is absent, or the process takes an alternate metabolic pathway. The consequence is manifested as an illness. Most IEMs are characterized by abnormal protein, carbohydrate, or fat metabolism.

Newborn screening for IEMs varies from state to state; but all states test for at least seven core disorders, (i.e., phenylketonuria [PKU], CH, galactosemia, sickle cell disease, thalassemia, congenital

*PO Box 3696, Oakbrook, IL 60522-3696; 630-990-0010, 877-969-0010; http://www.compassionatefriends.org/home.aspx.
†Contact Maureen Connelly, 4324 Berrywick Terrace, St. Louis, MO 63128; 314-487-7582; or Martha Eise, Martha@amendgroup.com; http://www.amendgroup.com.
‡National Share Office, 402 Jackson Street, St. Charles, MO, 63301; 800-821-6819.

adrenal hyperplasia [CAH], and cystic fibrosis [CF].* The purpose of screening is to identify children who may have a condition that benefits from early identification and treatment to prevent cognitive impairment. The screening test is most reliable if the blood sample is taken after the infant has ingested a source of protein for 24 hours. Because of early discharge of newborns, recommendations for screening include (1) collecting the initial specimen as close as possible to discharge or no later than 7 days, (2) obtaining a subsequent sample by 2 weeks of age if the initial specimen is collected before the newborn is 24 hours old, and (3) designating a primary care provider to all newborns before discharge for adequate newborn screening follow-up (Kaye and AAP Committee on Genetics, 2006).

The nurse's responsibilities are to educate parents regarding the importance of screening and collect appropriate specimens at the recommended time (after 24 hours of age). With early newborn discharge before 24 hours, some authorities recommend a repeat screening for PKU within 2 weeks (Kaye and AAP Committee on Genetics, 2006). Accurate screening depends on high-quality blood spots on approved filter paper forms. The blood should completely saturate the filter paper spot on one side only. The paper should not be handled, placed on wet surfaces, or contaminated with any substance.

A new screening test, tandem mass spectrometry, has the potential for identifying more than 20 IEMs in addition to the standard IEMs. With tandem mass spectrometry, earlier identification may prevent further developmental delays and morbidities in affected children (Wilcken, 2010).

A major concern is that a significantly large number of infants are *not* rescreened for metabolic disorders after early discharge and are at risk for a missed or delayed diagnosis of a treatable disorder. Special consideration must be given to screening infants born at home who have no hospital contact. It is always necessary to confirm the screening results with diagnostic testing.

Congenital Hypothyroidism

CH may have a number of causes and can be either permanent or transient. Transient CH is frequently associated with maternal Graves' disease that was treated with antithyroid drugs. Most cases are sporadic (nonhereditary), but approximately 15% of all cases are transmitted as an autosomal dominant trait. The most common pathogenesis is thyroid dysgenesis, mostly with unknown causes. Worldwide the most common cause of CH resulting in hypothyroidism is iodine deficiency. However, no matter what the cause, the manifestations (Box 25-7) and management are similar. In some conditions the thyroid deficiency is severe, and manifestations develop early; in others the symptoms may be delayed for months or years. Early detection and prompt initiation of treatment are essential because their delay results in various degrees of cognitive impairment, in which the IQ loss has a direct relationship to the time that treatment is initiated. If treatment is implemented from 0 to 3 months of age, the mean IQ attained is 89 (range 64 to 107); if treatment begins at 3 to 6 months, mean IQ reaches 71 (range 36 to 96); treatment initiated after 6 months of age results in a mean IQ of 54 (range 25 to 80).

Results of screening tests in the United States indicate that CH occurs in approximately one in 4000 to one in 3000 newborns

---

BOX 25-7	CLINICAL MANIFESTATIONS OF CONGENITAL HYPOTHYROIDISM

Birth*
- Poor feeding
- Lethargy
- Prolonged jaundice (>2 weeks)
- Respiratory difficulties
- Cyanosis
- Constipation
- Bradycardia
- Hoarse cry
- Large anterior and posterior fontanels
- Postterm
- Birth weight over 4000 g (8 lbs 13 oz)

Older Child
- Short stature
- Obesity
- Varying degrees of intellectual deficits
- Abnormal tendon reflexes
- Slow, awkward movements

Ages 6 to 9 Weeks†
- Depressed nasal bridge
- Short forehead
- Puffy eyelids
- Large tongue
- Thick, dry, mottled skin
- Coarse, dry, lusterless hair
- Abdominal distention
- Umbilical hernia
- Hyporeflexia
- Bradycardia
- Hypothermia
- Hypotension
- Anemia
- Widely patent cranial sutures

*Clinical manifestations may not be obvious at birth, possibly because of maternal transfer of thyroid hormone to the fetus. Manifestations may be delayed in infants with certain types of familial hypothyroidism and in breastfed infants (may show after weaning).
†If untreated, classical features.

(Kaye and Committee on Genetics, 2006). It affects all races and ethnicities, but it is more prevalent among Hispanic and American Indian or Alaskan Native people (one in 2000 to one in 700 newborns) and less prevalent among African-Americans (one in 3200 to one in 17,000 newborns). Infants with Down syndrome have a much higher rate of either permanent or transient forms of the disorder (approximately one in 140 newborns) (Kaye and Committee on Genetics, 2006). In addition, a higher incidence of other congenital abnormalities has been observed in infants with CH. Many preterm infants have transient hypothyroidism (hypothyroxinemia) at birth as a result of hypothalamic and pituitary immaturity. Infants born before 28 weeks of gestation may require temporary thyroid hormone replacement. Some screening programs target both primary (thyroid-based) and secondary (pituitary-based) hypothyroidism.

Because CH is one of the most common preventable causes of cognitive impairment, early diagnosis and treatment of this disease are essential interventions. Neonatal screening consists of an initial filter paper blood spot T_4 measurement followed by measurement of thyroid-stimulating hormone (TSH) in specimens with low T_4 values.

Tests are mandatory in all U.S. states and territories. Although a blood sample obtained by heelstick for the spot test is best obtained between 2 and 6 days of age, specimens are usually taken within the first 24 to 48 hours or before discharge as part of a concurrent screen for other metabolic defects. Early screening can result in overdiagnosis (false positives) but is preferable to missing the diagnosis.

For screening results that show a low level of T_4 (<10%), TSH levels are obtained; if these are elevated (>40 mU/L), further tests to determine the cause of the disease should be administered (AAP and American Thyroid Association, 2006). Additional tests include serum measurement of T_4, triiodothyronine (T_3), resin uptake, free T_4, and thyroid-bound globulin. Tests of thyroid gland function (thyroid scan and uptake) usually involve oral administration of a radioactive isotope of iodine (^{131}I) and measurement of iodine uptake by the thyroid, usually within 24 hours. In CH protein-bound iodine, T_4, T_3, and free T_4 levels are low; and thyroid uptake of ^{131}I is decreased. Skeletal radiography is used to assess age.

In newborns thyroid function studies are elevated in comparison with values in older children; therefore it is important to document the timing of the tests. In preterm and sick full-term infants, thyroid function tests are usually lower than in healthy full-term infants; a repeat T_4 and TSH may be evaluated after 30 weeks (corrected age) in newborns born before that time and after resolution of the acute illness in sick full-term infants.

Treatment involves lifelong thyroid hormone replacement therapy as soon as possible after diagnosis to abolish all signs of hypothyroidism and reestablish normal physical and mental development. The drug of choice is synthetic levothyroxine sodium (Synthroid, Levothroid). Optimum dosage of L-thyroxine should be able to maintain blood TSH concentration between 0.5 and 2 mU/L during the first 3 years of life (AAP and American Thyroid Association, 2006). Regular measurement of T_4 levels is important to ensure optimum treatment. Bone age surveys are also performed to ensure optimum growth.

The most important nursing objective is early identification of the disorder. Nurses caring for neonates must be certain that screening is performed, especially in infants who are preterm, discharged early, or born at home. Approximately 10% of cases are detected only by a second screening at 2 to 6 weeks of age. Nurses in community health need to be aware of the earliest signs of the disorder. Parental remarks about an unusually "quiet and good" baby and demonstrated symptoms such as prolonged jaundice, constipation, and umbilical hernia should lead to a suspicion of hypothyroidism, which requires a referral for specific tests.

After the diagnosis is confirmed, parents need an explanation of the disorder and the necessity of lifelong treatment. The child should be referred to a pediatric endocrinologist for care. The importance of compliance with the drug regimen for the child to achieve normal growth and development must be stressed (Kaye and AAP Committee on Genetics, 2006). Because the drug is tasteless, it can be crushed and added to formula, water, or food. If a dose is missed, twice the dose should be given the next day. Unless there are maternal contraindicative factors, breastfeeding is acceptable and encouraged in infants with hypothyroidism (Lawrence and Lawrence, 2011). Parents also need to be aware of signs indicating overdose such as a rapid pulse, dyspnea, irritability, insomnia, fever, sweating, and weight loss. Ideally they should know how to count the pulse and be instructed to withhold a dose and consult their practitioner if the pulse rate is above a certain value. Signs of inadequate treatment are fatigue, sleepiness, decreased appetite, and constipation.

If the diagnosis was delayed past early infancy, the chance of permanent cognitive impairment is great. Parents need the same guidance in caring for their child as do others who have an offspring with cognitive impairment. They need an opportunity to discuss their feelings regarding late recognition of the disorder. Although treatment will not reverse the intellectual deficit, it may prevent further damage. Genetic counseling is important for the rare families in which the etiology of CH is thyroid dyshormonogenesis, which is inherited in an autosomal recessive manner.

Phenylketonuria

PKU, an inborn error of metabolism inherited as an autosomal recessive trait (the *PAH* gene is located on chromosome 12q24), is caused by a deficiency or absence of the enzyme needed to metabolize the essential amino acid phenylalanine. Classic PKU is at one end of a spectrum of conditions known as hyperphenylalaninemia. Within the spectrum of hyperphenylalaninemia are conditions with varying degrees of severity, depending on the degree of enzyme deficiency. Because rarer forms are a result of a deficiency in other enzymes and are diagnosed and treated differently, the following discussion of PKU is limited to the severe, classic form.

In PKU the hepatic enzyme phenylalanine hydroxylase, which normally controls the conversion of phenylalanine to tyrosine, is deficient. This results in the accumulation of phenylalanine in the bloodstream and urinary excretion of abnormal amounts of its metabolites, the phenyl acids. One of these phenylketones, phenylacetic acid, gives urine the characteristic musty odor associated with the disease. Another is phenylpyruvic acid, which is responsible for the term phenylketonuria.

Tyrosine, the amino acid produced by the metabolism of phenylalanine, is absent in PKU. Tyrosine is needed to form the pigment melanin and the hormones epinephrine and T_4. Decreased melanin production results in similar phenotypes of most individuals with PKU, which is blond hair, blue eyes, and fair skin that is particularly susceptible to eczema and other dermatologic problems. Children with a genetically darker skin color may be red haired or brunette.

The prevalence of PKU varies widely in the United States because different states have different definition criteria for what constitutes hyperphenylalaninemia and PKU. The reported figures for PKU in the United States are one case per 15,000 live births. The incidence of the disease varies widely by ethnic groups. In Europe the incidence is one in 10,000 births; in Asia and Africa the prevalence is quite low (Blau, van Spronsen, and Levy, 2010).

Clinical manifestations in untreated PKU include failure to thrive (growth failure); frequent vomiting; irritability; hyperactivity; and unpredictable, erratic behavior. Cognitive impairment is thought to be caused by the accumulation of phenylalanine and presumably by decreased levels of the neurotransmitters dopamine and tryptophan, which affect the normal development of the brain and CNS, resulting in defective myelinization, cystic degeneration of the gray and white matter, and disturbances in cortical lamination. Older children commonly display bizarre or schizoid behavior patterns such as fright reactions, screaming episodes, head banging, arm biting, disorientation, failure to respond to strong stimuli, and catatonia-like positions.

The objective in diagnosing and treating the disorder is to prevent cognitive impairment. Every newborn should be screened for PKU. The most commonly used test for screening newborns is the Guthrie blood test, a bacterial inhibition assay for phenylalanine in the blood. *Bacillus subtilis*, present in the culture medium, grows if the blood contains an excessive amount of phenylalanine. If performed properly, this test detects serum phenylalanine levels greater than 4 mg/dL (normal value, 1.6 mg/dL), but it will not quantify the results. Other methods for testing include quantitative fluorometric assay and tandem mass spectrometry, which give an absolute value. Only fresh heel blood, not cord blood, can be used for the test.

> **! NURSING ALERT**
>
> Avoid "layering" the blood specimen on the special Guthrie paper. Layering is placing one drop of blood on top of the other or overlapping the specimen. This practice results in a falsely high reading, or false positive, which will lead the newborn screening department to call the family and health care provider to arrange for a diagnostic blood phenylalanine test to determine whether the newborn truly has PKU. Best results are obtained by collecting the specimen with a pipette from the heelstick and spreading the blood uniformly over the blot paper.

Because of the possibility of variant forms of hyperphenylalaninemia, PKU cofactor variant screen should be performed in all children diagnosed with PKU. A major concern is that a significant number of infants are not rescreened for PKU after early discharge and are at risk for a missed or delayed diagnosis. Give special consideration to screening infants born at home who have no hospital contact and infants adopted internationally.

Treatment of PKU involves restricting phenylalanine in the diet. Because the genetic enzyme is intracellular, systemic administration of phenylalanine hydroxylase is of no value. Phenylalanine cannot be eliminated from the diet because it is an essential amino acid in tissue growth. Therefore dietary management must meet two criteria: (1) meet the child's nutritional need for optimum growth, and (2) maintain phenylalanine levels within a safe range (2 to 6 mg/dL in neonates and children up to 12 years, 2 to 10 mg/dL through adolescence, and 2 to 15 mg/dL in adults) (Kaye and AAP Committee on Genetics, 2006).

Professionals agree that infants with PKU who have blood phenylalanine levels higher than 10 mg/dL should be started on treatment to establish metabolic control as soon as possible, ideally by 7 to 10 days of age (Kaye and AAP Committee on Genetics, 2006). The daily amounts of phenylalanine are individualized for each child and require frequent changes on the basis of appetite, growth and development, and blood phenylalanine and tyrosine levels.

Because all natural food proteins contain phenylalanine and are limited, the diet must be supplemented with a specially prepared phenylalanine-free formula (e.g., Phenex-1 for infants or Phenex-2 for children and adults). The phenylalanine-free formula is an amino acid–modified formula essential in the low phenylalanine diet to provide the appropriate protein, vitamins, minerals, and calories for optimal growth and development. Because tyrosine becomes an essential amino acid, the phenylalanine-free formula supplies an adequate amount; but in some cases additional supplementation may be needed. The phenylalanine-free amino acid–modified formula for infants has all the nutrients necessary for adequate infant growth. Because of the low phenylalanine content of breast milk, total or partial breastfeeding may be possible with close monitoring of phenylalanine levels (Lawrence and Lawrence, 2011).

Most clinicians now agree that, to achieve optimal metabolic control and outcome, a restricted phenylalanine diet, including medical foods and low-protein products, most likely is medically required for virtually all individuals with classic PKU for their entire lives (Kaye and AAP Committee on Genetics, 2006). Such lifetime reduction of phenylalanine intake is necessary to prevent neuropsychologic and cognitive deficits because even mild hyperphenylalaninemia (20 mg/dL) would produce such effects. To evaluate the effectiveness of dietary treatment, frequent monitoring of blood phenylalanine and tyrosine levels is necessary.

Phenylalanine levels greater than 6 mg/dL in mothers with PKU affect the normal embryologic development of the fetus, including cognitive impairment, cardiac defects, and LBW. It is recommended that phenylalanine levels below 6 mg/dL be achieved at least 3 months before conception in women with PKU (Kaye and AAP Committee on Genetics, 2006).

The principal nursing considerations involve teaching the family regarding the dietary restrictions. Although the treatment may sound simple, the task of maintaining such a strict dietary regimen is demanding, especially for older children and adolescents. In addition, mothers of children with PKU may have to spend many hours preparing special foods such as low-phenylalanine snacks. Foods with low phenylalanine levels (e.g., vegetables; fruits; juices; some cereals, breads, and starches) must be measured to provide the prescribed amount of phenylalanine. High-protein foods such as meat and dairy products are eliminated from the diet. The sweetener aspartame (NutraSweet) should be avoided because it is composed of two amino acids, aspartic acid and phenylalanine, and if used decreases the amount of natural phenylalanine that is prescribed for the day. However, medications that use aspartame as the sweetener may be used if no other nonaspartame medications are available because the content of the artificial sweetener is minimal or can be counted in the total daily phenylalanine allowance.

Maintaining the diet during infancy presents few problems. Solid foods such as cereal, fruits, and vegetables are introduced as usual to the infant. Difficulties arise as the child gets older. Studies show a gradual decline in diet compliance with consequent increases in blood phenylalanine levels during early adolescence and young adulthood (Channon, Goodman, Zlotowitz, et al., 2007).

A decreased appetite and refusal to eat may reduce intake of the calculated phenylalanine requirement. The child's increasing independence may also inhibit absolute control of what he or she eats. Either factor can result in decreased or increased phenylalanine levels. During the school years peer pressure becomes a major force in deterring the child from eating the prescribed foods or abstaining from high-protein foods such as milkshakes and ice cream. Limitations of this diet are best illustrated by an example: a quarter-pound hamburger may provide a 2-day phenylalanine allowance for a school-age child.

The assistance of a registered dietitian is essential. Parents need a basic understanding of the disorder and practical suggestions regarding food selection and preparation. Meal planning is based on weighing the food on a gram scale; a less accurate method is the exchange list. As soon as children are old enough, usually by early preschool, they should be involved in the daily calculation, menu planning, and formula preparation. Using a computer, voice-activated calculator, cards, or colored beads can help them keep track of the daily allowance of phenylalanine foods. A system of goal setting, self-monitoring, contracts, and rewards can promote compliance in adolescents.

Preparation of the phenylalanine-free formula can present some challenges. The formula tends to be lumpy; mixing the powder with a small amount of water to make a paste and then adding the rest of the required liquid helps to alleviate this problem. A blender or mixer dissolves the powder more easily; a rechargeable hand mixer can be used when traveling. Although the taste is virtually impossible to camouflage, many new products are on the market today. Some of the complete formulas are chocolate, vanilla, strawberry, and orange flavored. Incomplete formulas that do not contain the vitamins and minerals and are plain tasting are also available; these can be added to cold foods instead of mixing them as a formula. Formula bars are convenient for active adolescents. Formula capsules are also available, but the patient would need to take 20 or more capsules per day.

Galactosemia

Galactosemia is a rare autosomal recessive disorder that results from various gene mutations leading to three distinct enzymatic deficiencies. The most common type of galactosemia (classic galactosemia) results from a deficiency of a hepatic enzyme, galactose 1-phosphate uridyltransferase (GALT), and affects approximately one of 50,000 births. The other two varieties of galactosemia involve deficiencies in the enzymes galactokinase (GALK) and galactose 4'-epimerase (GALE); these are extremely rare disorders. All three enzymes (GALT, GALK, and GALE) are involved in the conversion of galactose into glucose.

As galactose accumulates in the blood, several organs are affected. Hepatic dysfunction leads to cirrhosis, resulting in jaundice in the infant by the second week of life. The spleen subsequently becomes enlarged as a result of portal hypertension. Cataracts are usually recognizable by 1 or 2 months of age; cerebral damage, manifested by the symptoms of lethargy and hypotonia, is evident soon afterward. Infants with galactosemia appear normal at birth, but within a few days of ingesting milk (which has a high lactose content) they begin to experience vomiting and diarrhea, leading to weight loss. *E. coli* sepsis is also a common presenting clinical sign. Death during the first month of life is frequent in untreated infants. Occasionally classic galactosemia is seen with milder, chronic manifestations such as growth failure, feeding difficulty, and developmental delay. This presentation is more frequent among African-American children with galactosemia (Kaye and AAP Committee on Genetics, 2006).

Diagnosis is made on the basis of the infant's history, physical examination, galactosuria, increased levels of galactose in the blood, and decreased levels of GALT activity in erythrocytes. The infant may display characteristics of malnutrition (i.e., hypoglycemia, jaundice, hepatosplenomegaly, sepsis, cataracts, and decreased muscle tone) (Bosch, 2006). Newborn screening for this disease is required in most states. Heterozygotes can also be identified because heterozygotic individuals have significantly lower levels of the essential enzyme.

During infancy treatment consists of eliminating all milk and lactose-containing formula, including breast milk. Traditionally lactose-free formulas are used, with soy-protein formula being the feeding of choice; however, some research suggests that elemental formula (galactose-free) may be more beneficial than soy formulas (Zlatunich and Packman, 2005). However, the AAP recommends the use of soy protein–based formula for infants with galactosemia, and it is considerably less expensive than elemental formula (Bhatia, Greer, and AAP Committee on Nutrition, 2008). As the infant progresses to solids, only foods low in galactose should be consumed. Certain fruits are high in galactose, and some dietitians recommend that they be avoided. Food lists should be given to the family to ensure that appropriate foods are chosen.

If galactosemia is suspected, supportive treatment and care are implemented, including monitoring for hypoglycemia, liver failure, bleeding disorders, and *E. coli* sepsis.

Nursing interventions are similar to those for PKU except that dietary restrictions are easier to maintain because many more foods are allowed. However, reading food labels carefully for the presence of any form of lactose, especially dairy products, is mandatory. Many drugs such as some of the penicillin preparations contain lactose as filler and also must be avoided. Unfortunately lactose is an unlabeled ingredient in many pharmaceuticals. Therefore instruct parents to ask their local pharmacist about galactose content of any over-the-counter or prescription medication.

Genetic Evaluation and Counseling

Genetic counseling is a communication process concerned with the human problems associated with the occurrence, or risk of occurrence, of a genetic disorder in a family. It involves relaying information about the diagnosis, treatment options, recurrence risk, and availability of prenatal diagnosis. With the completion of the Human Genome Project, the international project to determine the total genetic information in humans, a new era of human genetics is unfolding (International Human Genome Sequencing Consortium, 2004), and it is leading to a better understanding of specifically how genetic variation contributes to health and disease. It is essential that nurses master the basic principles of heredity, understand how heredity contributes to disorders, and be aware of the types of genetic testing available.

Nurses frequently encounter children with genetic diseases and families in which there is a risk that a disorder may be transmitted to or occur in an offspring. It is their responsibility to be alert to situations in which persons could benefit from a genetic evaluation and counseling, be aware of the local genetic resources, aid families in finding services, and offer support and care for children and families affected by genetic conditions. Local genetic clinics can be located through several sites. The Genetic Alliance* is a nonprofit organization that has a database of support groups for genetic conditions. Another resource is GeneTests,† a publicly funded medical genetics information resource developed for physicians and other health care providers, is available at no cost to all interested people. A third resource is the National Society of Genetic Counselors,‡ which lists genetic counselors by states in the United States.

Maintaining contact with the family or referring them to an agency that can provide a sustained relationship, usually the public health agency in their locality, is one of the most important aspects in the care of the patient and family. In a disorder that requires conscientious diet management such as PKU or galactosemia, it is important to make certain that the family understands and follows the advice. A vital role for nurses is to advocate for the child and family as they make their way through the various specialty clinics. This is especially important for families who are more vulnerable because of cognitive, hearing, language, or financial issues and those who otherwise may have difficulty accessing health services. Nurses can reinforce the genetic information or arrange for additional genetic counseling if a family has additional questions or misunderstandings (see also Genetic Counseling, Chapter 6).

---

*Genetic Alliance, 4301 Connecticut Ave., Suite 404, Washington, D.C. 20008-2369; (202) 966-5557; www.geneticalliance.org.
†www.ncbi.nlm.nih.gov/sites/GeneTests. Sponsored by the University of Washington, 1410 NE Campus Parkway, Seattle, WA 98195; (206) 543-2100
‡NSGC Executive Office; 330 N. Wabash Avenue, Suite 2000; Chicago, IL 60611; (312) 321-6834; www.nsgc.org.

KEY POINTS

- The identification of maternal and fetal risk factors in the antepartum and intrapartum periods is vital for planning adequate care of high risk infants.
- A small percentage of significant birth injuries may occur despite skilled and competent obstetric care.
- Metabolic abnormalities of diabetes mellitus in pregnancy adversely affect embryonic and fetal development.
- Infection in the newborn may be acquired in utero, at birth, in breast milk, or from within the nursery.
- The most common maternal infections during early pregnancy that are associated with various congenital malformations include toxoplasmosis, herpes, CMV, rubella, parvovirus B19, and varicella.
- HIV transmission from mother to infant occurs transplacentally at various gestational ages, perinatally by maternal blood and secretions, and by breast milk.
- Preterm infants are at risk for problems related to the immaturity of organ systems.
- Maternal-fetal Rh and ABO incompatibility may cause significant hemolysis and jaundice in the neonatal period.

- The injection of Rho(D) immunoglobulin in Rh-negative and Coombs' test–negative women minimizes the possibility of isoimmunization.
- The nurse is often the first to observe signs of newborn drug withdrawal (NAS) and acquire information from the maternal history.
- Congenital anomalies are the leading cause of death in the first year of life.
- The curative and rehabilitative problems of a child with a congenital anomaly are often complex, requiring a multidisciplinary approach to care.
- Parents often need special instruction (e.g., cardiopulmonary resuscitation, oxygen therapy, or nutritional requirements) before they take a high risk infant home.
- The supportive care given to the parents of infants with a congenital anomaly or IEM must begin at birth or at the time of diagnosis and continue for years.

REFERENCES

Abdel-Latif ME, Osborn DA: Nebulised surfactant in preterm infants with or at risk of respiratory distress syndrome, *Cochrane Database Syst Rev* CD008310, 2012.

Ackerman JP, Riggins T, Black MM: A review of the effects of prenatal cocaine exposure among school-aged children, *Pediatrics* 125(3):554–565, 2010.

Adamkin DH, American Academy of Pediatrics, Committee on Fetus and Newborn: Postnatal glucose homeostasis in late-preterm and term infants, *Pediatrics* 127(3):575–579, 2011.

Albright BB, Rayburn WF: Substance abuse among reproductive age women, *Obstet Gynecol Clin* 36(4):891–906, 2009.

Alfaleh K, Anabrees J, Bassler D, et al: Probiotics for prevention of necrotizing enterocolitis in preterm infants, *Cochrane Database Syst Rev* 3:CD005496, 2011.

Altimier L: The neonatal intensive care unit (NICU). In Kenner C, Lott J, editors: *Comprehensive neonatal care: an interdisciplinary approach*, ed 4, St Louis, 2007, Saunders.

American Academy of Pediatrics (AAP) American Thyroid Association: Update of newborn screening and therapy for congenital hypothyroidism, *Pediatrics* 117(6):2290–2303, 2006.

American Academy of Pediatrics (AAP) Committee on Fetus and Newborn: Surfactant-replacement therapy for respiratory distress in preterm and term neonates, *Pediatrics* 121(2):419–432, 2008.

American Academy of Pediatrics (AAP) Committee on Infectious Diseases, Pickering L, editor: *2012 Red Book: Report of the Committee on Infectious Diseases*, ed 29, Elk Grove Village, Ill, 2012, Author.

American Academy of Pediatrics (AAP) Subcommittee on Hyperbilirubinemia: Management of hyperbilirubinemia in the newborn infant 35 or more weeks of gestation (clinical practice guideline), *Pediatrics* 114(1):297–316, 2004.

American Academy of Pediatrics (AAP) and American College of Obstetricians and Gynecologists (ACOG): Guidelines for perinatal care, ed 6, Elk Grove Village, Ill, 2007, The Academy.

Association of Women's Health, Obstetric and Neonatal Nurses (AWHONN): *Evidence-based clinical practice guideline: neonatal skin care*, ed 2, Washington, DC, 2007, The Association.

Association of Women's Health, Obstetric and Neonatal Nurses (AWHONN): *Assessment and care of the late preterm infant: Evidence-based clinical practice guideline*, Washington, DC, 2010, The Association.

Azzopardi DV, Strohm B, Edwards D, et al: Moderate hypothermia to treat perinatal asphyxial encephalopathy, *N Engl J Med* 361(14):1349–1358, 2009.

Bagwell GA: Hematologic system. In Kenner C, Lott J, editors: *Comprehensive neonatal care: an interdisciplinary approach*, ed 4, St Louis, 2007, Saunders.

Banakar MK, Kudlur NS, George S: Fetal alcohol spectrum disorder (FASD), *Indian J Pediatr* 76(11):1173–1175, 2009.

Bandstra ES, Accornero VH: Infants of substance abusing mothers. In Martin RJ, Fanaroff AA, Walsh MC, editors: *Fanaroff and Martin's neonatal-perinatal medicine: diseases of the fetus and infant*, ed 9, St Louis, 2011, Mosby.

Bandstra ES, Morrow CE, Mansoor E, et al: Prenatal drug exposure: infant and toddler outcomes, *J Addict Dis* 29(2):245–258, 2010.

Bandstra ES, Morrow CE, Accornero VH, et al: Estimated effects of in utero cocaine exposure on language development through early adolescence, *Neurotoxicol Teratol* 33(1):25–35, 2011.

Barrington KJ, Finer NN: Inhaled nitric oxide for preterm infants: a systematic review, *Pediatrics* 120(5):1088–1099, 2007.

Bauer CR, Langer JC, Shankaran S, et al: Acute neonatal effects of cocaine exposure during pregnancy, *Arch Pediatr Adolesc Med* 159(9):824–834, 2005.

Bay CA, Steele MW, Davis H: Genetic disorders and dysmorphic conditions. In Zitelli B, Davis H, editors: *Atlas of pediatric physical diagnosis*, ed 5, St Louis, 2007, Mosby.

Beauman SS, Swanson A: Neonatal infusion therapy: preventing complications and improving outcomes, *Newborn Infant Nurs Rev* 16(4):193–201, 2006.

Beyerlein A, Hadders-Algra M, Kennedy K, et al: Infant formula supplementation with long-chain polyunsaturated fatty acids has no effect on Bayley developmental scores at 18 months of age—IPD meta-analysis of 4 large clinical trials, *J Pediatr Gastroenterol Nutr* 50(1):79–84, 2010.

Bhatia J, Greer F, AAP Committee on Nutrition: Use of soy protein-based formulas in infant feeding, *Pediatrics* 121(5):1062–1068, 2008.

Bissinger RL, Annibale DJ: Thermoregulation in very low–birth-weight infants during the golden hour: results and implications, *Adv Neonatal Care* 10(5):230–238, 2010.

Black LV, Maheshwari A: Disorders of the fetomaternal unit: hematologic manifestations in the fetus and neonate, *Semin Perinatol* 33(1):12–19, 2009.

Blackburn ST: *Maternal, fetal, and neonatal physiology: a clinical perspective*, ed 4, Philadelphia, 2013, Saunders.

Blau N, van Spronsen FJ, Levy HL: Phenylketonuria, *Lancet* 23, 376(9750):1417–1427, 2010.

Bosch AM: Classical galactosaemia revisited, *J Inherit Metab Dis* 29(4):516–525, 2006.

Bradshaw EA, Martin GR: Screening for critical congenital heart disease: advancing detection in the newborn, *Curr Opin Pediatr* 24(5):603–608, 2012.

Brown VD, Landers S: Heat balance. In Gardner SL, Carter BS, Enzman-Hines M, et al, editors: *Merenstein and Gardner's handbook of neonatal intensive care*, ed 7, St Louis, 2011, Mosby.

Bull MJ, Engle WA, AAP Committee on Injury, Violence, and Poison Prevention, and the Committee on Fetus and Newborn: Safe transportation of preterm and low-birth-weight infants at hospital discharge, *Pediatrics* 123(5):1424–1429, 2009.

Burgos AE, Burke BL: Neonatal abstinence syndrome, *NeoReviews* 10(5):e222–e228, 2009.

Buus-Frank M: Hands that heal—hands that harm, *Adv Neonatal Care* 4(5):251–255, 2004.

Byers JF, Waugh WR, Lowman LB: Sound level exposure of high-risk infants in different environmental conditions, *Neonatal Netw* 25(1):25–32, 2006.

Cantor Sackett J, Weller RA, Weller EB: Selective serotonin reuptake inhibitor use during pregnancy and possible neonatal complications, *Curr Psychiatry Rep* 11(3):253–257, 2009.

Carlo WA: Fetal alcohol syndrome. In Kliegman RM, Stanton BF, St Geme JW, et al, editors: *Nelson textbook of pediatrics*, ed 19, Philadelphia, 2011a, Saunders.

Carlo WA: Peripheral nerve injuries. In Kliegman RM, Stanton BF, St Geme JW, et al, editors: *Nelson textbook of pediatrics*, ed 19, Philadelphia, 2011b, Saunders.

Channon S, Goodman G, Zlotowitz S, et al: Effects of dietary management of phenylketonuria on long-term cognitive outcome, *Arch Dis Child* 92(3):213–218, 2007.

Chiriboga CA, Kuhn L, Wasserman GA: Prenatal cocaine exposures and dose-related cocaine effects on infant tone and behavior, *Neurotoxicol Teratol* 29(3):323–330, 2007.

Chomchai C, Na Manorom N, Watanarungsan P, et al: Methamphetamine abuse during pregnancy and its impact on neonates born at Siriraj Hospital, Bangkok, Thailand, *Southeast Asian J Trop Med Public Health* 35(1):228–231, 2004.

Conde-Agudelo A, Belizán JM, Diaz-Rossello J: Kangaroo mother care to reduce morbidity and mortality in low birthweight infants, *Cochrane Database Syst Rev* 3:CD002771, 2011.

Cong X, Ludington-Hoe SM, McCain G, et al: Kangaroo care modifies preterm infant heart rate variability in response to heel stick pain: pilot study, *Early Hum Dev* 85(9):561–567, 2009.

Cornblath M, Hawdon JM, Williams A, et al: Controversies regarding definition of neonatal hypoglycemia: suggested operational thresholds, *Pediatrics* 105(5):1141–1145, 2000.

Cotten CM, Taylor S, Stoll B, et al: Prolonged duration of initial empirical antibiotic treatment is associated with increased rates of necrotizing enterocolitis and death for extremely low–birth-weight infants, *Pediatrics* 123(1):58–66, 2009.

Dailey TL, Coustan DR: Diabetes in pregnancy, *NeoReviews* 11(11):e619–e625, 2010.

de Boer JC, Smit BJ, Mainous RO: Nasogastric tube position and intragastric air collection in a neonatal intensive care population, *Adv Neonatal Care* 9(6):293–298, 2009.

Deshpande S, Ward Platt M: The investigation and management of neonatal hypoglycaemia, *Semin Fetal Neonatal Med* 10(4):351–361, 2005.

Diehl-Jones WL, Fraser Askin D: Hematologic disorders. In Verklan MT, Walden M, editors: *Core curriculum for neonatal intensive care nursing*, ed 4, St Louis, 2010, Saunders.

Dodd VL: Implications of kangaroo care for growth and development in preterm infants, *J Obstet Gynecol Neonatal Nurs* 34(2):218–232, 2005.

Donohue PK, Gilmore MM, Cristofalo E, et al: Inhaled nitric oxide in preterm infants: a systematic review, *Pediatrics* 127(2):e414–e422, 2011.

Dougherty D, Luther M: Birth to breast—a feeding care map for the NICU: helping the extremely low birth weight infant navigate the course, *Neonatal Netw* 27(6):371–377, 2008.

Durbin DR, AAP Committee on Injury, Violence, and Poison Prevention: Child passenger safety, *Pediatrics* 127(4):e1050–e1066, 2011.

Edwards AD, Brocklehurst P, Gunn AJ, et al: Neurological outcomes at 18 months of age after moderate hypothermia for perinatal hypoxic ischaemic encephalopathy: synthesis and meta-analysis of trial data, *BMJ* 340:c.363, 2010.

Elalfy MS, Elbarbary NS, Abaza HW: Early intravenous immunoglobulin (two-dose regimen) in the management of severe Rh hemolytic disease of newborn—a prospective randomized controlled trial, *Eur J Pediatr* 170(4):461–467, 2011.

Ellett ML, Cohen MD, Perkins SM, et al: Predicting the insertion length for gastric tube placement for neonates, *J Obstet Gynecol Neonatal Nurs* 40(4):412–421, 2011.

Ellett ML, Croffie JM, Cohen MD, et al: Gastric tube placement in young children, *Clin Nurs Res* 14(3):238–252, 2005.

Engle WA: A recommendation for the definition of "late preterm" (near term) and the birth weight-gestational age classification system, *Semin Perinatol* 30(1):2–7, 2006.

Environmental Protection Agency (EPA) Report on the Environment: *Birth defects prevalence and mortality*, Washington, DC, US EPA. 2011, cfpub.epa.gov/eroe/index.cfm?fuseaction=detail.viewInd&lv=list.listByAlpha&r=239796&subtop=381.

Escobar GJ, Clark RH, Greene JD: Short-term outcomes of infants born at 35 and 36 weeks gestation: we need to ask more questions, *Semin Perinatol* 30(1):28–33, 2006.

Eyler FD, Behnke M, Wobie K, et al: Relative ability of biologic specimens and interviews to detect prenatal cocaine use, *Neurotoxicol Teratol* 27(4):677–687, 2005.

Farrington M, Lang S, Cullen L, et al: Nasogastric tube placement verification in pediatric and neonatal patients, *Pediatr Nurs* 35(1):17–24, 2009.

Feeley N, Waitzer E, Sherrard K, et al: Fathers' perceptions of the barriers and facilitators to their involvement with their newborn hospitalized in the neonatal intensive care unit, *J Clin Nurs* 22(3-4):521–530, 2013.

Finnegan LP: Neonatal abstinence. In Nelson N, editor: *Current therapy in neonatal perinatal medicine 1985-1986*, Toronto, 1985, Decker.

Freeman D, Saxton V, Holberton J: A weight-based formula for the estimation of gastric tube insertion length in newborns, *Adv Neonatal Care* 12(3):179–182, 2012.

Gabbe SG, Niebyl JR, Simpson KL, editors: *Obstetrics: normal and problem pregnancies*, ed 5, London, 2007, Churchill Livingstone.

Gallaher KJ, Cashwell S, Hall V, et al: Orogastric tube insertion length in very low birth weight infants, *J Perinatol* 13(2):128–131, 1993.

Gardner SL, Dickey LA: Grief and perinatal loss. In Gardner SL, Carter BS, Enzman-Hines M, et al, editors: *Merenstein and Gardner's handbook of neonatal intensive care*, ed 7, St Louis, 2011, Mosby.

Gardner SL, Lawrence RA: Breast feeding the neonate with special needs. In Gardner SL, Carter BS, Enzman-Hines M, et al, editors: *Merenstein and Gardner's handbook of neonatal intensive care*, ed 7, St Louis, 2011, Mosby.

Gardner DL, Shirland L: Evidence-based guideline for suctioning the intubated neonate and infant, *Neonatal Netw* 28(5):281–302, 2009.

Gephart SM, Hanson CK: Preventing necrotizing enterocolitis with standardized feeding protocols: not only possible, but imperative, *Adv Neonatal Care* 13(1):48–54, 2013.

Hanson LA: Session 1: Feeding and infant development breast-feeding and immune function, *Proc Nutr Soc* 66(3):384–396, 2007.

Hay WW: Care of the infant of the diabetic mother, *Curr Diab Rep* 12(1):4–15, 2012.

Hay WW: Strategies for feeding the preterm infant, *Neonatology* 94(4):245–254, 2008.

International Human Genome Sequencing Consortium: Finishing the euchromatic sequence of the human genome, *Nature* 431:931–945, 2004.

Jacobs S, Hunt R, Tarnow-Mordi W, et al: Cooling for newborns with hypoxic ischaemic encephalopathy, *Cochrane Database Syst Rev* 4:CD003311, 2007.

Jansen JL: A bereavement model for the intensive care nursery, *Neonatal Netw* 22(3):17–23, 2003.

Kastenberg ZJ, Sylvester KG: The surgical management of necrotizing enterocolitis, *Clin Perinatol* 40(1):135–148, 2013.

Kattwinkel JM, Perlman JM, Aziz K, et al: Part 15: Neonatal resuscitation: 2010 American Heart Association Guidelines for Cardiopulmonary Resuscitation and Emergency Cardiovascular Care, *Circulation* 122(18 suppl):S909–S919, 2010.

Kaye CI, AAP Committee on Genetics: Newborn screening fact sheets, *Pediatrics* 118(3):e934–e963, 2006. (Note: this was reaffirmed by AAP in January 2011.)

Kemper AR, Mahle WT, Martin GR, et al: Strategies for implementing screening for critical congenital heart disease, *Pediatrics* 128(5):e1259–e1267, 2011.

Kuczkowski KM: The effects of drug abuse on pregnancy, *Curr Opin Obstet Gynecol* 19(6):578–585, 2007.

Kuppala VS, Meinzen-Derr J, Morrow AL, et al: Prolonged initial empirical antibiotic treatment is associated with adverse outcomes in premature infants, *J Pediatr* 159(5):720–725, 2011.

Kuschel C: Managing drug withdrawal in the newborn infant, *Semin Fetal Neonatal Med* 212(2):127–133, 2007.

Laptook AR: Use of therapeutic hypothermia for term infants with hypoxic-ischemic encephalopathy, *Pediatr Clin North Am* 56(3):601–616, 2009.

Lawrence RA, Lawrence RM: *Breastfeeding: a guide for the medical profession*, ed 7, St Louis, 2011, Mosby.

Lester BM, Lagasse LL: Children of addicted women, *J Addict Dis* 29(2):259–276, 2010.

Lester BM, Tronick EZ, Brazelton TB: The Neonatal Intensive Care Unit Network Neurobehavioral Scale procedures, *Pediatrics* 113(3 suppl):641–667, 2004.

Lewis DA, Sanders LP, Brockopp DY: The effect of three nursing interventions on thermoregulation in low-birth-weight infants, *Neonatal Netw* 30(3):160–164, 2011.

Lloyd-Puryear MA, Tonniges T, van Dyck PC, et al: American Academy of Pediatrics (AAP) Newborn Screening Task Force Recommendations: How far have we come? *Pediatrics* 117 suppl 3):S194–S211, 2006.

Lund CH, Kuller JM: Integumentary system. In Kenner C, Lott J, editors: *Comprehensive neonatal care: an interdisciplinary approach*, ed 4, St Louis, 2007, Elsevier.

Maheshwari A, Carlo WA: Neonatal necrotizing enterocolitis. In Kliegman RM, Stanton BF, St Geme JW, et al, editors: *Nelson textbook of pediatrics*, ed 19, Philadelphia, 2011, Saunders.

Mahle WT, Martin GR, Beekman RH, et al: Endorsement of Health and Human Services recommendation for pulse oximetry screening for critical congenital heart disease, *Pediatrics* 129(1):190–192, 2012.

Marroun HE, Hudziak JJ, Tiemeier H, et al: Intrauterine cannabis exposure leads to more aggressive behavior and attention problems in 18-month-old girls, *Drug Alcohol Depend* 118(2-3):470–474, 2011.

Mathews TJ, MacDorman MF: *Infant mortality statistics from the 2008 period linked birth/infant death data set*, *Natl Vital Stat Rep* 60(5):1–49, Atlanta, 2012, Centers for Disease Control and Prevention.

McCall EM, Alderdice FA, Halliday HL, et al: Interventions to prevent hypothermia at birth in preterm and/or low birthweight babies, *Cochrane Database Syst Rev* 3:CD004210, 2010.

McCain GC, Ludington-Hoe SM, Swinth JY, et al: Heart rate variability responses of a preterm infant to kangaroo care, *J Obstet Gynecol Neonatal Nurs* 34(6):689–694, 2005.

McCance K, Huether S: *Pathophysiology: the biological basis for disease in infants and children*, ed 6, St Louis, 2010, Mosby.

McCormick FM, Henderson G, Fahey T, et al: Multinutrient fortification of human breast milk for preterm infants following hospital discharge, *Cochrane Database Syst Rev* 7:CD004866, 2010.

Mintz-Hittner HA, Best LM: Antivascular endothelial growth factor for retinopathy of prematurity, *Curr Opin Pediatr* 21(2):182–187, 2009.

Mitanchez D: Foetal and neonatal complications in gestational diabetes: perinatal mortality, congenital malformations, macrosomia, shoulder dystocia, birth injuries, neonatal complications, *Diabetes Metab J* 36(6 Pt 2):617–627, 2010.

Moise KJ: Red cell alloimmunization. In Gabbe SG, Niebyl JR, Simpson KL, editors: *Obstetrics: normal and problem pregnancies*, ed 5, London, 2007, Churchill Livingstone.

Moise KJ: Fetal anemia due to non-Rhesus-D red-cell alloimmunization, *Semin Fetal Neonatal Med* 13(4):207–214, 2008a.

Moise KJ Jr: Management of rhesus alloimmunization in pregnancy, *Obstet Gynecol* 112(1):164–176, 2008b.

Moise KJ, Argoti PS: Management and prevention of red cell alloimmunization in pregnancy: a systematic review, *Obstet Gynecol* 120(5):1132–1139, 2012.

Morrow CE, Culbertson JL, Accornero VH, et al: Learning disabilities and intellectual functioning in school-aged children with prenatal cocaine exposure, *Dev Neuropsychol* 30(3):905–931, 2006.

Mundy CA: Intravenous immunoglobulin in the management of hemolytic disease of the newborn, *Neonatal Netw* 24(6):17–24, 2005.

National Perinatal Association: *Multidisciplinary guidelines for the care of late preterm infants*, Binghamton, NY, 2012, Author; www.nationalperinatal.org/lptguidelines/pdf/NPALatePretermGuidelines11-12.pdf.

Nye C: Transitioning premature infants from gavage to breast, *Neonatal Netw* 27(1), 2008.

Oberlander TF, Warburton W, Misri S, et al: Neonatal outcomes after prenatal exposure to selective serotonin reuptake inhibitor antidepressants and maternal depression using population-based linked health data, *Arch Gen Psychiatry* 63(8):898–906, 2006.

Panel on Treatment of HIV-Infected Pregnant Women and Prevention of Perinatal Transmission: *Recommendations for use of antiretroviral drugs in pregnant HIV-infected women for maternal health and interventions to reduce perinatal HIV transmission in the United States*, Washington, DC, 2011, National Institutes of Health, pp 1–207, aidsinfo.nih.gov/contentfiles/lvguidelines/perinatalgl.pdf.

Patel RM, Denning PW: Therapeutic use of prebiotics, probiotics, and postbiotics to prevent necrotizing enterocolitis: what is the current evidence? *Clin Perinatol* 40(1):11–25, 2013.

Piehl E, Fernandez-Bustamante A: Lucinactant for the treatment of respiratory distress syndrome in neonates, *Drugs Today (Barc)* 48(9):587–593, 2012.

Pitts K: Perinatal substance abuse. In Verklan MT, Walden M, editors: *Core curriculum for neonatal intensive care nursing*, ed 4, St Louis, 2010, Saunders.

Polin RA, AAP Committee on Fetus and Newborn: Management of neonates with suspected or proven early-onset bacterial sepsis, *Pediatrics* 129(5):1006–1015, 2012.

Polin RA, Denson S, Brady MT, et al: Strategies for prevention of health care–associated infections in the NICU, *Pediatrics* 129(4):e1085–e1093, 2012.

Premji SS, Paes B, Jacobson K, et al: Evidence-based feeding guideline for very low birthweight infants, *Adv Neonatal Care* 2(1):5–18, 2002.

Quandt D, Schraner T, Ulrich Bucher H, et al: Malposition of feeding tubes in neonates: is it an issue? *J Pediatr Gastroenterol Nutr* 48(5):608–611, 2009.

Renner M: Far from reliable: pH testing in the neonatal intensive care unit, *J Pediatr Nurs* 25(6):580–583, 2010.

Reynolds RM, Thureen PJ: Special circumstances: trophic feeds, necrotizing enterocolitis and bronchopulmonary dysplasia, *Semin Fetal Neonatal Med* 12(1):64–70, 2007.

Sarici SU, Yurdakok M, Serdar MA, et al: An early (sixth-hour) serum bilirubin measurement is useful in predicting the development of significant hyperbilirubinemia and severe ABO hemolytic disease in a selective high-risk population of newborns with ABO incompatibility, *Pediatrics* 109(4):e53, 2002.

Saugstad OD: Optimal oxygenation at birth and in the neonatal period, *Neonatology* 91(4):319–322, 2007.

Saugstad OD, Ramji S, Soll RF, et al: Resuscitation of newborn infants with 21% or 100% oxygen: an updated systematic review and meta-analysis, *Neonatology* 94(3):176–182, 2008.

Schempf AH: Illicit drug use and neonatal outcomes: a critical review, *Obstet Gynecol Surv* 62(11):749–757, 2007.

Schuetze P, Eiden RD: The association between maternal cocaine use during pregnancy and physiological regulation in 4- to 8-week-old infants: an examination of possible mediators and moderators, *J Pediatr Psychol* 31(1):15–26, 2006.

Schutzman DL, Sekhon R, Hundalani S: Hour-specific bilirubin nomogram in infants with ABO incompatibility and direct Coombs-positive results, *Arch Pediatr Adolesc Med* 164(12):1158–1164, 2010.

Shah PS, Ohlsson A: Sildenafil for pulmonary hypertension in neonates, *Cochrane Database Syst Rev* 10(8):CD005494, 2011.

Sherman MP: Lactoferrin and necrotizing enterocolitis, *Clin Perinatol* 40(1):79–91, 2013.

Shet A: Congenital and perinatal infections: throwing new light with an old TORCH, *Indian J Pediatr* 78(1):88–95, 2011.

Singer LT, Minnes S, Short E, et al: Cognitive outcomes of preschool children with prenatal cocaine exposure, *JAMA* 291(20):2448–2456, 2004.

Smith L, Yonekura ML, Wallace T, et al: Effects of prenatal methamphetamine exposure on fetal growth and drug withdrawal symptoms in infants born at term, *J Dev Behav Pediatr* 24(1):17–23, 2003.

Soll R: Heat loss prevention in neonates, *J Perinatol* 28(suppl 1):S557–S559, 2008.

Sperling MA: Hypoglycemia. In Kliegman RM, Stanton BF, St Geme JW, et al, editors: *Nelson textbook of pediatrics*, ed 19, Philadelphia, 2011, Saunders.

Stevens TP, Sinkin RA: Surfactant replacement therapy, *Chest* 131(5):1577–1582, 2007.

Stevens TP, Harrington EW, Blennow M, et al: Early surfactant administration with brief ventilation vs. selective surfactant and continued mechanical ventilation for preterm infants with or at risk for respiratory distress syndrome, *Cochrane Database Syst Rev* 4:CD003063, 2007.

Stoll BJ: Infections of the neonatal infant. In Kliegman RM, Stanton BF, St Geme JW, et al, editors: *Nelson textbook of pediatrics*, ed 19, Philadelphia, 2011, Saunders.

Stoll BJ, Hansen NI, Sanchez PJ, et al: Early-onset neonatal sepsis: the burden of group B streptococcal and *E. coli* disease continues, *Pediatrics* 127(5):817–826, 2011.

Telofski LS, Morello AP, Mack Correa MC, et al: The infant skin barrier: can we preserve, protect, and enhance the barrier? *Dermatol Res Pract* 2012:198789, 2012; DOI: 10.1155/2012/198789.

Terplan M, Smith EJ, Kozloski MJ, et al: Methamphetamine use among pregnant women, *Obstet Gynecol* 113(6):1285–1291, 2009.

Terrin G, Passariello A, Canani RB, et al: Minimal enteral feeding reduces the risk of sepsis in feed-intolerant very low–birth-weight newborns, *Acta Paediatr* 98(2):31–35, 2009.

Tomashek KM, Shapiro-Mendoza CK, Davidoff MJ, et al: Differences in mortality between late-preterm and term singleton infants in the United States, 1995-2002, *J Pediatr* 151(5):450–456, 2007.

Urbaniak SJ: Noninvasive approaches to the management of RhD hemolytic disease of the fetus and newborn, *Transfusion* 48(1):12–19, 2008.

Vento M, Saugstad OD: Oxygen therapy. In Martin RJ, Fanaroff AA, Walsh MC, editors: *Fanaroff and Martin's neonatal-perinatal medicine: diseases of the fetus and infant*, ed 9, St Louis, 2011, Mosby.

Volpe JJ: *Neurology of the newborn*, ed 5, Philadelphia, 2008, Saunders.

Walsh BK, Daigle B, Diblasi RM, et al: AARC clinical practice guideline: surfactant replacement therapy, *Respir Care* 58(2):367–375, 2013.

Wilcken B: Expanded newborn screening: reducing harm, assessing benefit, *J Inherit Metab Dis* 33(suppl 2):S205–S210, 2010.

Wilson KL, Zelig CM, Harvey JP, et al: Persistent pulmonary hypertension of the newborn is associated with mode of delivery and not with maternal use of selective serotonin reuptake inhibitors, *Am J Perinatol* 28(1):19–24, 2011.

Winecker RE, Goldberger BA, Tebbett IR, et al: Detection of cocaine and its metabolites in breast milk, *J Forensic Sci* 46(5):1221–1223, 2001.

Zlatunich CO, Packman S: Galactosaemia: early treatment with an elemental formula, *J Inherit Metab Dis* 28:163–168, 2005.

CHAPTER
26

21st Century Pediatric Nursing

Marilyn J. Hockenberry

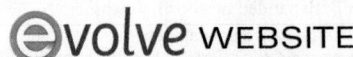
http://evolve.elsevier.com/Perry/maternal

LEARNING OBJECTIVES

On completion of this chapter, the reader will be able to:
- Define the terms *mortality* and *morbidity*.
- Identify two ways that knowledge of mortality and morbidity can improve child health.
- List three major causes of death during infancy, early childhood, later childhood, and adolescence.
- List two major causes of illness during childhood.

- Describe five broad functions of the pediatric nurse in promoting the health of children.
- Define the term *critical thinking*.
- Identify the five steps of the nursing process.
- Define the term *nursing diagnosis*.
- Define evidence-based practice.

HEALTH CARE FOR CHILDREN

The major goal for pediatric nursing is to improve the quality of health care for children and their families. In 2011, almost 74 million children 0 to 17 years of age lived in the United States, comprising 23.7% of the population (Forum on Child and Family Statistics, 2012). The health status of children in the United States has improved in a number of areas, including increased immunization rates for all children, decreased adolescent birth rate, and improved child health outcomes. Unfortunately, millions of children and their families have no health insurance, which results in a lack of access to care and health-promotion services. In addition, disparities in pediatric health care are related to race, ethnicity, socioeconomic status, and geographic factors. Patterns of child health are shaped by medical progress and societal trends (Starmer, Duby, Slaw, et al., 2010). Shifts in population demographics, family structure, income, education levels, and cultural norms directly affect the health of children (Leslie, Slaw, Edwards, et al., 2010). The *Healthy People 2020* leading health indicators (Box 26-1) provide a framework for identifying essential components for child health–promotion programs designed to prevent future health problems in our nation's children.

Health Promotion

Many leading causes of disease, disability, and death in children (i.e., prematurity, nutritional deficiencies, injuries, chronic lung disease, obesity, cardiovascular disease, depression, violence, substance abuse, and human immunodeficiency virus/acquired immunodeficiency syndrome [HIV/AIDS]) can be significantly reduced or prevented in children and adolescents by addressing six categories of behavior (World Health Organization, 2011):
1. Tobacco use
2. Behavior that results in injury and violence
3. Alcohol and substance use
4. Dietary and hygienic practices that cause disease
5. Sedentary lifestyle
6. Sexual behavior that causes unintended pregnancy and disease

Child health promotion provides opportunities to reduce differences in current health status among members of different groups and ensure equal opportunities and resources to enable all children to achieve their fullest health potential.

Nutrition

Nutrition is an essential component for healthy growth and development. Human milk is the preferred form of nutrition for all infants. Breastfeeding provides the infant with micronutrients, immunologic properties, and several enzymes that enhance digestion and absorption of these nutrients. A recent resurgence in breastfeeding has occurred because of the education of mothers and fathers regarding its benefits and increased social support.

Children establish lifelong eating habits during the first 3 years of life, and the nurse is instrumental in educating parents about the

718

process of feeding and the importance of nutrition. Most eating preferences and attitudes related to food are established by family influences and culture. During adolescence, parental influence diminishes and the adolescent makes food choices related to peer acceptability and sociability. Occasionally these choices are detrimental to adolescents with chronic illnesses like diabetes, obesity, chronic lung disease, hypertension, cardiovascular risk factors, and renal disease.

Families that struggle with lower incomes, homelessness, and migrant status generally lack the resources to provide their children with adequate food intake, nutritious foods such as fresh fruits and vegetables, and appropriate protein intake. The result is nutritional deficiencies with subsequent growth and developmental delays, depression, and behavior problems.

Dental Care

Dental caries is the single most common chronic disease of childhood (Cheng, Han, and Gansky, 2008; Heuer, 2007). Nearly one in five children between the ages of 2 and 4 years has visible cavities (Kagihara, Niederhauser, and Stark, 2009). The most common form of early dental disease is early childhood caries, which may begin before the first birthday and progress to pain and infection within the first 2 years of life (Kagihara, Niederhauser, and Stark, 2009). Preschoolers of low-income families are twice as likely to develop tooth decay and only half as likely to visit the dentist as other children. Early childhood caries is a preventable disease, and nurses play an essential role in educating children and parents about practicing dental hygiene beginning with the first tooth eruption; drinking fluoridated water, including bottled water; and instituting early dental preventive care.

Immunizations

The two public health interventions that have had the greatest impact on world health are clean drinking water and childhood vaccination programs. Immunization rates differ depending on children's race and ethnicity, family income, the state in which they live, types of vaccinations, and their age (whether adolescent or younger children). The nurse should review individual immunization records at every clinic visit, avoid missing opportunities to vaccinate, and encourage parents to keep immunizations current. Nurses are

responsible for keeping up with changes in immunization schedules, recommendations, and research related to childhood vaccines.

Childhood Health Problems

Changes in modern society, including advancing medical knowledge and technology, the proliferation of information systems, economically troubled times, and various changes and disruptive influences on the family, are leading to significant medical problems that affect the health of children (Leslie, Slaw, Edwards, et al., 2010). Recent concern has focused on groups of children who are at highest risk, such as children born prematurely or with very low birth weight (VLBW) or low birth weight (LBW), children attending child care centers, children who live in poverty or are homeless, children of immigrant families, and children with chronic medical and psychiatric illness and disabilities. In addition, these children and their families face multiple barriers to adequate health, dental, and psychiatric care. The new morbidity, also known as *pediatric social illness*, refers to the behavior, social, and educational problems that children face. Problems that can negatively impact a child's development include poverty, violence, aggression, noncompliance, school failure, and adjustment to parental separation and divorce. In addition, mental health issues cause challenges in childhood and adolescence.

Obesity and Type 2 Diabetes

Childhood obesity is the most common nutritional problem among American children, is increasing in epidemic proportions, and is associated with type 2 diabetes (Cali and Caprio, 2008; de Onis, Blössner, and Borghi, 2010; Matyka, 2008; Raj and Kumar, 2010). Obesity in children and adolescents is defined as a body mass index (BMI) at or greater than the 95th percentile for youth of the same age and gender (Schwartz and Chadha, 2008). The National Health and Nutrition Examination Survey reported that the prevalence of overweight children doubled and the prevalence of overweight adolescents tripled between 1980 and 2000 (American Dietetic Association, 2008).

Advancements in entertainment and technology such as television, computers, and video games have contributed to the growing childhood obesity problem in the United States. In the National Longitudinal Study of Adolescent Health, screen time (TV, video, computer use) interacts with genetic factors to influence BMI changes (Graff, North, Monda, et al., 2011). Lack of physical activity related to limited resources, unsafe environments, and inconvenient play and exercise facilities, combined with easy access to television and video games, increases the incidence of obesity among low-income, minority children. Overweight youth have increased risk for developing hypercholesterolemia, insulin resistance, diabetes, hypertension, and heart disease (Matyka, 2008; Schwartz and Chadha, 2008) (Fig. 26-1). The U.S. Department of Health and Human Services suggests that nurses focus on prevention strategies to reduce the incidence of overweight children from the current 20% in all ethnic groups to less than 6%.

Childhood Injuries

Injuries are the most common cause of death and disability to children in the United States (Schnitzer, 2006) (Table 26-1). Motor vehicle accidents (MVAs) continue to be the most common cause of death in children older than 1 year. Other unintentional injuries (choking, drowning, fires, and firearm accidents) take the lives of children every day. Many childhood injuries and fatalities could be prevented by implementing programs of accident prevention and health promotion.

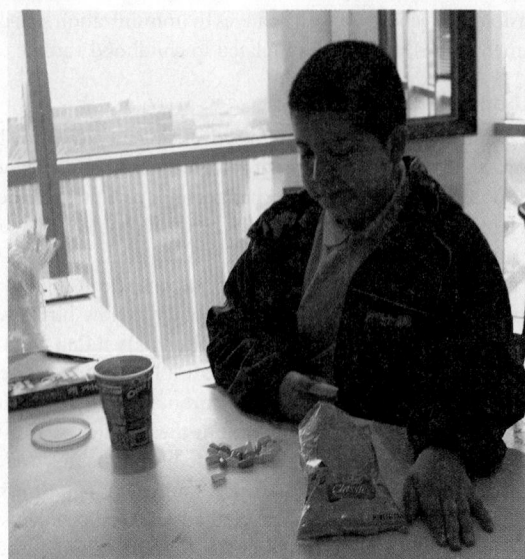

FIG 26-1 The American culture's intake of high-caloric fatty foods contributes to obesity in children.

The type of injury and the circumstances surrounding it are closely related to normal growth and development (Box 26-2). As children develop, their innate curiosity compels them to investigate the environment and to mimic the behavior of others. This is essential to acquire competency as an adult but can also predispose children to numerous hazards.

The child's developmental stage partially determines the types of injuries that are most likely to occur at a specific age and helps provide clues to preventive measures. For example, small infants are helpless in any environment. When they begin to roll over or propel themselves, they can fall from unprotected surfaces. The crawling infant, who has a natural tendency to place objects in the mouth, is at risk for aspiration or poisoning. The mobile toddler, with the instinct to explore and investigate and the ability to run and climb, may experience falls, burns, and collisions with objects. As children grow older, their absorption with play makes them oblivious to environmental hazards such as street traffic or water. The need to conform and gain acceptance compels older children and adolescents to accept challenges and dares. Although the rate of injuries is high in children younger than 9 years, most fatal injuries occur in later childhood and adolescence.

The pattern of deaths caused by unintentional injuries, especially from MVAs, drowning, and fires, is remarkably consistent in most Western societies. The leading causes of death from injuries for each age-group according to gender are presented in Table 26-1. The majority of deaths from injuries occur in boys. It is important to note that accidents continue to account for more than 3 times as many teen deaths as any other cause (Annie E. Casey Foundation, 2009). Fortunately, prevention strategies such as the use of car restraints, bicycle helmets, and smoke detectors have significantly decreased fatalities for children. Nevertheless, the overwhelming causes of death in children are MVAs, including occupant, pedestrian, bicycle, and motorcycle deaths; these account for more than half of all injury deaths (Centers for Disease Control and Prevention [CDC], 2006). Children older than 1 year of age have the highest rate of death from MVAs, primarily from a failure to properly use car restraints (Fig. 26-2).

Pedestrian accidents involving children account for significant numbers of motor vehicle–related deaths. Most of these accidents

TABLE 26-1	MORTALITY FROM LEADING TYPES OF UNINTENTIONAL INJURIES, UNITED STATES, 2008 (RATE PER 100,000 POPULATION IN EACH AGE-GROUP)			
	AGE (YR)			
TYPE OF ACCIDENT	**1**	**1-4**	**5-14**	**15-24**
Males				
All causes	716.4	31.2	15.9	108.8
Unintentional injuries (all types)	33.3	10.5	5.8	48.1
Motor vehicle	2.8 (2)	3.0 (2)	3.0 (1)	29.5 (1)
Drowning	1.1 (4)	3.4 (1)	0.9 (2)	2.3 (3)
Fires and flames	0.5 (5)	1.1 (3)	0.5 (3)	0.4 (5)
Firearms	—	—	—	—
Choking*	1.7 (3)	0.5 (5)	—	—
Falls	—	—	—	0.9 (4)
Mechanical suffocation	25.0 (1)	0.6 (4)	0.2 (4)	—
Poisoning	—	—	0.1 (5)	11.2 (2)
All other unintentional injuries	4.6	1.9	1.0	3.8
Accidents as a percent of all deaths	4.6%	33.7%	36.5%	44.2%
Females				
All causes	591.7	24.7	12.0	39.2
Unintentional injuries (all types)	28.0	6.9	3.4	16.6
Motor vehicle	2.0 (2)	2.4 (1)	2.0 (1)	11.7 (1)
Drowning	0.9 (4)	1.8 (2)	0.4 (2)	0.3 (3)
Fires and flames	0.4 (5)	0.9 (3)	0.4 (2)	0.3 (3)
Firearms	—	—	—	—
Choking*	1.1 (3)	0.3 (4)	—	—
Falls	—	—	—	0.2 (5)
Mechanical suffocation	21.4 (1)	0.3 (4)	0.1 (4)	—
Poisoning	—	—	0.1 (4)	3.4 (2)
All other unintentional injuries	2.1	1.1	0.4	0.8
Accidents as a percent of all deaths	4.7%	27.9%	28.3%	42.3%

Adapted from National Safety Council: *Injury facts*, 2012 Edition, Itaska, IL, 2012, Author. Data from National Center for Health Statistics and US Census Bureau.

occur at midblock, at intersections, in driveways, and in parking lots. Driveway injuries typically involve small children and large vehicles backing up.

Bicycle-associated injuries also cause a number childhood deaths. Children ages 5 to 9 years are at greatest risk for bicycling fatalities. The majority of bicycling deaths are from head injuries. Helmets

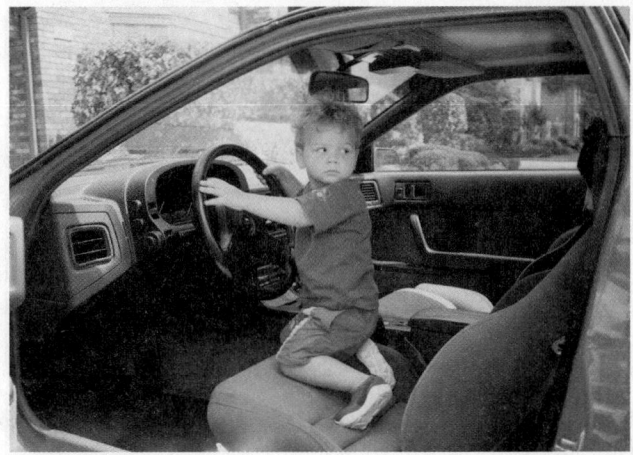

FIG 26-2 Motor vehicle injuries are the leading cause of death in children older than 1 year. The majority of fatalities involve occupants who are unrestrained.

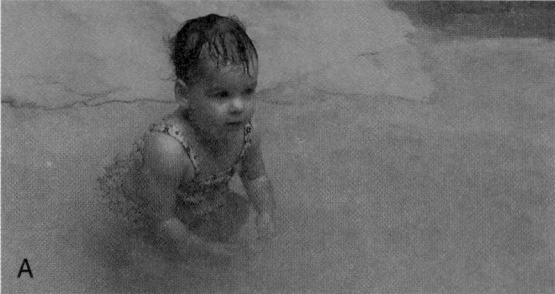
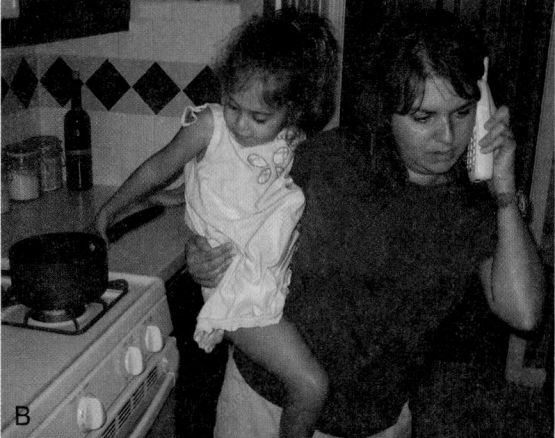

FIG 26-3 **A,** Drowning is one of the leading causes of death. Children left unattended are unsafe even in shallow water. **B,** Burn-related injuries commonly occur in the home as a result of distraction.

greatly reduce the risk for head injury, but few children wear helmets (Castle, Burke, Arbogast, et al., 2010). Community-wide bicycle helmet campaigns and mandatory-use laws have resulted in significant increases in helmet use. Still, issues such as stylishness, comfort, and social acceptability remain important factors in noncompliance. Nurses can educate children and families about pedestrian and bicycle safety. In particular, school nurses can promote helmet wearing and encourage peer leaders to act as role models.

Drowning and burns are among the top three leading causes of deaths for males and females throughout childhood (Fig. 26-3). In addition, improper use of firearms is a major cause of death among males (Fig. 26-4). During infancy, more boys die from aspiration or suffocation than do girls (Fig. 26-5). Approximately 70% of all unintentional poisonings are reported in children younger than 2 years (Bronstein, Spyker, Cantilena, et al., 2008; Franklin and Rodgers, 2008) (Fig. 26-6). By ages 4 to 5 years, unintentional poisonings are uncommon. Intentional poisoning, associated with drug and alcohol abuse and suicide attempt, is the second leading cause of death in adolescent females and third leading cause in adolescent males.

Violence

Youth violence is a high-visibility, high-priority concern in every sector of U.S. society. (U.S. Department of Health and Human Services, 2011). Strikingly higher homicide rates are found among minority populations, especially African-American children. The causes of violence against children and self-inflicted violence are not fully understood. Violence seems to permeate American households through television programs, commercials, video games, and movies, all of which tend to desensitize the child toward violence. Violence also permeates the schools with the availability of guns, illicit drugs, and gangs. The problem of child homicide is extremely

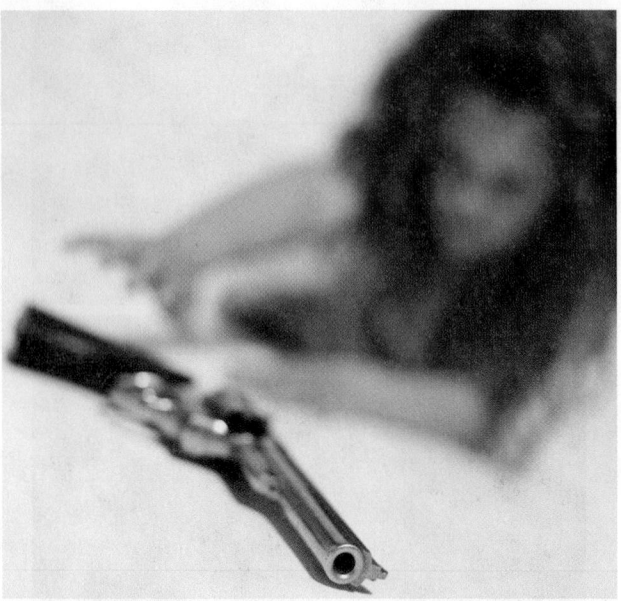

FIG 26-4 Improper storage and supervision are contributing causes of firearm-related childhood deaths. (Copyright © 2012 Photos.com, a division of Getty Images. All rights reserved.)

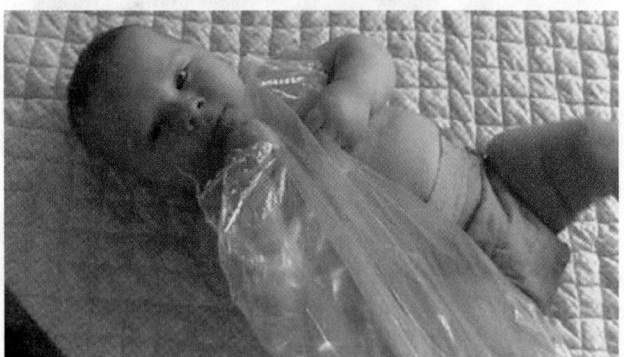

FIG 26-5 Mechanical suffocation is the leading cause of death from injury in infants.

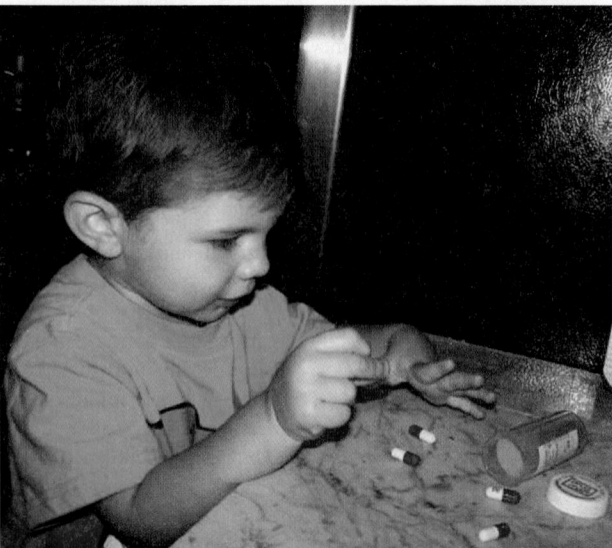

FIG 26-6 Poisoning causes a considerable number of injuries in children. Medications should never be left where children can reach them.

complex and involves numerous social, economic, and other influences. Prevention lies in better understanding of the social and psychologic factors that lead to the high rates of homicide and suicide. Nurses need to be especially aware of young people who harm animals or start fires, are depressed, are repeatedly in trouble with the criminal justice system, or are associated with groups known to be violent. Prevention requires early identification and rapid therapeutic intervention by qualified professionals.

Pediatric nurses can assess children and adolescents for risk factors related to violence. Families who own firearms must be educated about their safe use and storage. The presence of a gun in a household increases the risk for suicide by about fivefold and the risk for homicide by about threefold. Technologic changes such as childproof safety devices and loading indicators could improve the safety of firearms (see Community Focus box).

Substance Abuse

Risk-taking behaviors, particularly in males, tend to begin in the first decade of life and continue into adolescence with drinking alcohol while driving, speeding, carrying a weapon, or using illicit drugs. Adolescent trends in cigarette smoking, alcohol use, and illicit drug abuse have declined since 2002. Approximately 9.8% of youth reported cigarette smoking, 15.9% reported alcohol use, and 9.5% reported illicit drug abuse within the past month (National Survey on Drug Use and Health, 2008). The slight decline in American youth's illicit drug use is attributed to education regarding the

---

🏠 COMMUNITY FOCUS

Violence in Children

The serious problem of community violence affects the lives of many children and expands throughout the family, schools, and workplace. Nurses working with children, adolescents, and families have a critical role in reducing violence through early identification and symptom recognition of the mental-emotional stress that can result from these experiences.

Violent crimes continue to be a significant health issue for children, with homicide being the second leading cause of death in 15- to 19-year-olds (Annie E. Casey Foundation, 2009). The multifaceted origins of violence include developmental factors, gang involvement, access to firearms, drugs, the media, poverty, and family conflict. Often the silent and under-recognized victims are the children who witness acts of community violence. Studies suggest that chronic exposure to violence has a negative effect on a child's cognitive, social, psychologic, and moral development. Also, multiple exposures to episodes of violence do not inoculate children against the negative effects; continued exposure can result in lasting symptoms of stress. Children living with chronic violence may exhibit behaviors such as difficulty concentrating in school, memory impairment, aggressive play, uncaring behaviors, and constricted activities and thinking for fear of reliving the traumatic event.

National concern about the increasing prevalence of violent crimes has prompted nurses to actively participate in ensuring that children grow up in safe environments. Pediatric nurses are positioned to assess children and adolescents for signs of exposure to violence and well-known risk factors; nurses also can provide nonviolent problem-solving strategies, counseling, and referrals. These activities affect community practice and expand the nurse's role in the future health environment. Professional resources include the following:

National Domestic Violence Hotline
PO Box 161810
Austin, TX 78716
800-799-SAFE
www.ndvh.org

adverse effects of illicit drugs, parental disapproval, decreased availability of drugs, and consistent participation in church and organized activities such as scouts and sports.

Mental Health Problems

One out of 5 adolescents has a mental health problem, and 1 out of 10 has a serious emotional problem that affects daily functioning (Coury, 2006). Psychosocial problems in children seen in primary care settings in rural areas are common (Polaha, Dalton, and Allen, 2011). Children and adolescents with mental health problems are more likely to drop out of school than those with other disabilities (Polaha, Dalton, and Allen, 2011). Suicide is defined as a self-chosen death and is the third leading cause of death in children ages 10 to 19 years (Doucette, 2005). The American Association of Suicidology (2009) estimates that there are 11.5 youth suicides (15-24 years) every day. Suicide is preventable. Nurses should be alert to the symptoms of mental illness and potential suicidal ideation and be aware of potential resources for high-quality integrated mental health services.

MORTALITY AND MORBIDITY

Infant Mortality

The infant mortality rate is the number of deaths during the first year of life per 1000 live births. It may be further divided into neonatal mortality (<28 days of life) and postneonatal mortality (28 days to 11 months). In the United States, infant mortality has decreased dramatically. At the beginning of the twentieth century, the rate was approximately 200 infant deaths per 1000 live births. Based on preliminary data the infant mortality rate was 6.05 deaths per 1000 live births in 2011 (Hamilton, Hoyert, Martin, et al., 2013; Hoyert and Xu, 2012).

From a worldwide perspective, however, the United States lags behind other nations in reducing infant mortality. In 2010 the United States ranked number 30 among nations with 40,000 births or more. Hong Kong, Japan, and Finland have the three lowest rates, with the United States ranked thirtieth behind Hungary and the Slovack Republic (Hamilton, Hoyert, Martin, et al., 2013).

Birth weight is considered the major determinant of neonatal death in technologically developed countries. The lower the birth weight, the higher the mortality. The relatively high incidence of LBW (<2500 g [5.5 pounds]) in the United States is considered a key factor in its higher neonatal mortality rate when compared with other countries. Access to and the use of high-quality prenatal care is a promising preventive strategy to decrease early birth and infant mortality. Other factors that increase the risk for infant mortality include African-American race, male gender, short or long gestation, maternal age, and lower level of maternal education (Martin, Kochanek, Strobino, et al., 2005).

As Table 26-2 demonstrates, many of the leading causes of death during infancy continue to occur during the perinatal period. The first four causes—congenital anomalies, disorders relating to short gestation and unspecified LBW, sudden infant death syndrome, and newborn affected by maternal complications of pregnancy—accounted for about half (52%) of all deaths of infants younger than 1 year (Hamilton, Hoyert, Martin, et al., 2013). LBW is a major indicator of infant health and a significant predictor of infant mortality (Hamilton, Hoyert, Martin, et al., 2013). Many birth defects are associated with LBW, and reducing the incidence of LBW will help prevent congenital anomalies. Infant mortality resulting from HIV infection decreased significantly during the 1990s.

When infant death rates are categorized according to race, a disturbing difference is seen. Infant mortality for Caucasians is considerably lower than for all other races in the United States, with African-Americans having twice the rate of Caucasians. Although the infant mortality of all racial groups increased slightly between 2001 and 2002, the gap has remained constant, with the infant mortality rate expressed as a ratio of African-American to Caucasian deaths being relatively unchanged (Hamilton, Hoyert, Martin, et al., 2013). The LBW rate is also much higher for African-American infants than for any other group.

Childhood Mortality

Death rates for children older than 1 year have always been lower than those for infants. Children ages 5 to 14 years have the lowest rate of death. However, a sharp rise occurs during later adolescence, primarily from injuries, homicide, and suicide (Table 26-3). In 2011 accidental injuries accounted for 35.6% of all deaths. The second leading cause of death was homicide, accounting for 11.4% of all deaths in 2011 (Hamilton, Hoyert, Martin, et al., 2013). The trend in racial differences that occurs in infant mortality is also apparent in childhood deaths for all ages and for both sexes. Caucasians have fewer deaths for all ages, and male deaths outnumber female deaths.

After 1 year of age, the cause of death changes dramatically, with unintentional injuries (accidents) being the leading cause from the youngest ages to the adolescent years. Violent deaths have been steadily increasing among young people ages 10 through 25 years. Homicide is the third leading cause of death in the 15- to 19-year age-group (see Table 26-3). Children 12 years of age and older tend

TABLE 26-2	INFANT MORTALITY RATE AND PERCENTAGE OF TOTAL DEATHS FOR 10 LEADING CAUSES OF INFANT DEATH IN 2011 (RATE PER 1000 LIVE BIRTHS)*		
RANK	**CAUSE OF DEATH (BASED ON 10TH REVISION, INTERNATIONAL CLASSIFICATION OF DISEASES)**	**PERCENT**	**RATE**
	All races, all causes	100.00%	604.7
1	Congenital anomalies	20.8	126.1
2	Disorders relating to short gestation and unspecified low birth weight	17.2	104.1
3	Sudden infant death syndrome	7.2	43.3
4	Newborn affected by maternal complications of pregnancy	6.6	39.9
5	Accidents (unintentional injuries)	4.6	27.5
6	Newborn affected by complications of placenta, cord, and membranes	4.1	25.1
7	Bacterial sepsis of newborn	2.2	13.3
8	Respiratory distress of newborn	2.1	13.0
9	Diseases of circulatory system	2.1	12.5
10	Neonatal hemorrhage, asphyxia	1.9	11.2

Adapted from Hamilton BE, Hoyert DL, Martin JA, et al: Annual summary of vital statistics: 2010-2011, *Pediatrics* 131(3):548-558, 2013.

*Preliminary data.

TABLE 26-3	FIVE LEADING CAUSES OF DEATH IN CHILDREN IN UNITED STATES: SELECTED AGE INTERVALS, 2011* (RATE PER 100,000 POPULATION)						
	AGES 1-4 YEARS		**AGES 5-9 YEARS**		**AGES 10-14 YEARS**		**AGES 15-19 YEARS**
RANK	**CAUSE**	**RATE**	**CAUSE**	**RATE**	**CAUSE**	**RATE**	**CAUSE**	**RATE**
	All causes	26.1	All causes	12.0	All causes	14.2	All causes	48.9
1	Accidents	8.3	Accidents	3.7	Accidents	4.2	Accidents	19.6
2	Congenital anomalies	3.0	Cancer	2.2	Cancer	2.0	Suicide	8.1
3	Homicide	2.3	Congenital anomalies	0.9	Suicide	1.3	Homicide	7.7
4	Cancer	2.2	Homicide	0.6	Congenital anomalies	0.8	Cancer	3.0
5	Heart disease	1.0	Influenza and pneumonia	0.3	Homicide	0.7	Heart disease	1.4

Adapted from Hamilton BE, Hoyert DL, Martin JA, et al: Annual summary of vital statistics: 2010-2011, *Pediatrics* 131(3):548-558, 2013.
*Preliminary data.

to be killed by nonfamily members (acquaintances and gangs, typically of the same race) and most frequently by firearms. Suicide, a form of self-violence, continues to be a leading cause of death among children and adolescents 10 to 19 years of age.

Childhood Morbidity

Acute illness is defined as an illness with symptoms severe enough to limit activity or require medical attention. Respiratory illness accounts for approximately 50% of all acute conditions, 11% are caused by infections and parasitic disease, and 15% are caused by injuries. The chief illness of childhood is the common cold.

The types of diseases that children contract during childhood vary according to age. For example, upper respiratory tract infections and diarrhea decrease in frequency with age, whereas other disorders, such as acne and headaches, increase. Children who have had a particular type of problem are more likely to have that problem again. Morbidity is not distributed randomly in children. Recent concern has focused on groups of children who have increased morbidity: homeless children, children living in poverty, LBW children, children with chronic illnesses, foreign-born adopted children, and children in day-care centers. A number of factors place these groups at risk for poor health. A major cause is barriers to health care, especially for the homeless, the poverty stricken, and those with chronic health problems. Other factors include improved survival of children with chronic health problems, particularly infants of VLBW.

THE ART OF PEDIATRIC NURSING

Philosophy of Care

Nursing of infants, children, and adolescents is consistent with the definition of nursing as "the diagnosis and treatment of human responses to actual or potential health problems." This definition incorporates the four essential features of contemporary nursing practice (American Nurses Association, 2003):

1. Attention to the full range of human experiences and responses to health and illness without restriction to a problem-focused orientation
2. Integration of objective data with knowledge gained from an understanding of the patient or group's subjective experience
3. Application of scientific knowledge to the processes of diagnosis and treatment
4. Provision of a caring relationship that facilitates health and healing

Family-Centered Care

The philosophy of family-centered care recognizes the family as the constant in a child's life. Service systems and personnel must support, respect, encourage, and enhance the family's strength and competence by developing a partnership with parents (National Center for Cultural Competence, 2007). Nurses support families in their natural caregiving and decision-making roles by building on their unique strengths and acknowledging their expertise in caring for their child both within and outside the hospital setting (National Center for Cultural Competence, 2007). The nurse considers the needs of all family members in relation to the care of the child (Box 26-3). The philosophy acknowledges diversity among family structures and backgrounds; family goals, dreams, strategies, and actions; and family support, service, and information needs (Hooper, 2008).

Two basic concepts in family-centered care are enabling and empowerment. Professionals enable families by creating opportunities and means for all family members to display their current abilities and competencies and to acquire new ones to meet the needs of the child and family. Empowerment describes the interaction of professionals with families in such a way that families maintain or acquire a sense of control over their family lives and acknowledge positive changes that result from helping behaviors that foster their own strengths, abilities, and actions.

Although caring for the family is strongly emphasized throughout this text, it is highlighted in features such as Cultural Competence and Family-Centered Care boxes.

Atraumatic Care

Atraumatic care is the provision of therapeutic care in settings by personnel and through the use of interventions that eliminate or minimize the psychologic and physical distress experienced by children and their families in the health care system. Therapeutic care encompasses the prevention, diagnosis, treatment, or palliation of acute or chronic conditions. Setting refers to the place in which that care is given—the home, the hospital, or any other health care setting. Personnel includes anyone directly involved in providing therapeutic care. Interventions range from psychologic approaches, such as preparing children for procedures, to physical interventions, such as providing space for a parent to room in with a child. Psychologic distress may include anxiety, fear, anger, disappointment, sadness, shame, or guilt. Physical distress may range from sleeplessness and immobilization to disturbances from sensory stimuli such as pain, temperature extremes, loud noises, bright lights, or darkness. Thus atraumatic care is concerned with the

---

BOX 26-3   KEY ELEMENTS OF FAMILY-CENTERED CARE

- Incorporating into policy and practice the recognition that the family is the constant in a child's life while the service systems and support personnel within those systems fluctuate
- Facilitating family-professional collaboration at all levels of hospital, home, and community care:
  - Care of an individual child
  - Program development, implementation, and evaluation
  - Policy formation
- Exchanging complete and unbiased information between family members and professionals in a supportive manner at all times
- Incorporating into policy and practice the recognition and honoring of cultural diversity, strengths, and individuality within and across all families, including ethnic, racial, spiritual, social, economic, educational, and geographic diversity
- Recognizing and respecting different methods of coping and implementing comprehensive policies and programs that provide developmental, educational, emotional, environmental, and financial support to meet the diverse needs of families
- Encouraging and facilitating family-to-family support and networking
- Ensuring that home, hospital, and community service and support systems for children needing specialized health and developmental care and their families are flexible, accessible, and comprehensive in responding to diverse family-identified needs
- Appreciating families as families and children as children, recognizing that they possess a wide range of strengths, concerns, emotions, and aspirations beyond their need for specialized health and developmental services and support

From Shelton TL, Stepanek JS: Family-centered care for children needing specialized health and developmental services, Bethesda, MD, 1994, Association for the Care of Children's Health.

BOX 26-4   UNITED NATIONS' DECLARATION OF THE RIGHTS OF THE CHILD

All children need:
- To be free from discrimination
- To develop physically and mentally in freedom and dignity
- To have a name and nationality
- To have adequate nutrition, housing, recreation, and medical services
- To receive special treatment if handicapped
- To receive love, understanding, and material security
- To receive an education and develop his or her abilities
- To be the first to receive protection in disaster
- To be protected from neglect, cruelty, and exploitation
- To be brought up in a spirit of friendship among people

---

where, who, why, and how of any procedure performed on a child for the purpose of preventing or minimizing psychologic and physical stress (Wong, 1989).

The overriding goal in providing atraumatic care is, first, do no harm. Three principles provide the framework for achieving this goal: (1) prevent or minimize the child's separation from the family, (2) promote a sense of control, and (3) prevent or minimize bodily injury and pain. Examples of providing atraumatic care include fostering the parent-child relationship during hospitalization, preparing the child before any unfamiliar treatment or procedure, controlling pain, allowing the child privacy, providing play activities for expression of fear and aggression, providing choices to children, and respecting cultural differences.

Role of the Pediatric Nurse

The pediatric nurse is responsible for promoting the health and well-being of the child and family. Nursing functions vary according to regional job structures, individual education and experience, and personal career goals. Just as patients (children and their families) have unique backgrounds, each nurse brings an individual set of variables that affect the nurse-patient relationship. No matter where pediatric nurses practice, their primary concern is the welfare of the child and family.

Therapeutic Relationship

The establishment of a therapeutic relationship is the essential foundation for providing high-quality nursing care. Pediatric nurses need to have meaningful relationships with children and their families and yet remain separate enough to distinguish their own feelings and needs. In a therapeutic relationship, caring, well-defined boundaries separate the nurse from the child and family. These boundaries are positive and professional and promote the family's control over the child's health care. Both the nurse and the family are empowered and maintain open communication. In a nontherapeutic relationship, these boundaries are blurred and many of the nurse's actions may serve personal needs (e.g., a need to feel wanted and involved) rather than the family's needs.

Exploring whether relationships with patients are therapeutic or nontherapeutic helps nurses identify problem areas early in their interactions with children and families (see Guidelines box). Although questions regarding the nurse's involvement may label certain actions negative or positive, no one action makes a relationship therapeutic or nontherapeutic. For example, a nurse may spend additional time with the family but still recognize his or her own needs and maintain professional separateness. An important clue to nontherapeutic relationships is the staff's concerns about their peer's actions with the family.

Family Advocacy and Caring

Although nurses are responsible to themselves, the profession, and the institution of employment, their primary responsibility is to the consumer of nursing services: the child and family. The nurse must work with family members, identify their goals and needs, and plan interventions that best address the defined problems. As an advocate, the nurse assists the child and family in making informed choices and acting in the child's best interest. Advocacy involves ensuring that families are aware of all available health services, adequately informed of treatments and procedures, involved in the child's care, and encouraged to change or support existing health care practices. The United Nations' Declaration of the Rights of the Child (Box 26-4) provides guidelines for nursing practice to ensure that every child receives optimum care.

As nurses care for children and families, they must demonstrate caring, compassion, and empathy for others. Aspects of caring embody the concept of atraumatic care and the development of a therapeutic relationship with patients. Parents perceive caring as a sign of quality in nursing care, which is often focused on the nontechnical needs of the child and family. Parents describe "personable" care as actions by the nurse that include acknowledging the parent's presence, listening, making the parent feel comfortable in the hospital environment, involving the parent and child in the nursing care, showing interest in and concern for their welfare, showing affection and sensitivity to the parent and child,

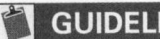

GUIDELINES

Exploring Your Relationships with Children and Families

To foster therapeutic relationships with children and families, you must first become aware of your caregiving style, including how effectively you take care of yourself. The following questions should help you understand the therapeutic quality of your professional relationships.

Negative Actions

- Are you overinvolved with children and their families?
  - Do you work overtime to care for the family?
  - Do you spend off-duty time with children's families, either in or out of the hospital?
  - Do you call frequently (either the hospital or home) to see how the family is doing?
  - Do you show favoritism toward certain patients?
  - Do you buy clothes, toys, food, or other items for the child and family?
  - Do you compete with other staff members for the affection of certain patients and families?
  - Do other staff members comment to you about your closeness to the family?
  - Do you attempt to influence families' decisions rather than facilitate their informed decision making?
- Are you underinvolved with children and families?
  - Do you restrict parent or visitor access to children, using excuses such as the unit is too busy?
  - Do you focus on the technical aspects of care and lose sight of the person who is the patient?
- Are you overinvolved with children and underinvolved with their parents?
  - Do you become critical when parents do not visit their children?
  - Do you compete with parents for their children's affection?

Positive Actions

- Do you strive to empower families?
  - Do you explore families' strengths and needs in an effort to increase family involvement?
  - Have you developed teaching skills to instruct families rather than doing everything for them?
  - Do you work with families to find ways to decrease their dependence on health care providers?
  - Can you separate families' needs from your own needs?

- Do you strive to empower yourself?
  - Are you aware of your emotional responses to different people and situations?
  - Do you seek to understand how your own family experiences influence reactions to patients and families, especially as they affect tendencies toward overinvolvement or underinvolvement?
  - Do you have a calming influence, not one that will amplify emotionality?
  - Have you developed interpersonal skills in addition to technical skills?
  - Have you learned about ethnic and religious family patterns?
  - Do you communicate directly with persons with whom you are upset or take issue?
  - Are you able to "step back" and withdraw emotionally, if not physically, when emotional overload occurs, yet remain committed?
  - Do you take care of yourself and your needs?
  - Do you periodically interview family members to determine their current issues (e.g., feelings, attitudes, responses, wishes), communicate these findings to peers, and update records?
  - Do you avoid relying on initial interview data, assumptions, or gossip regarding families?
  - Do you ask questions if families are not participating in care?
  - Do you assess families for feelings of anxiety, fear, intimidation, worry about making a mistake, a perceived lack of competence to care for their child, or fear of health care professionals overstepping their boundaries into family territory, or vice versa?
  - Do you explore these issues with family members and provide encouragement and support to enable families to help themselves?
  - Do you keep communication channels open among self, family, physicians, and other care providers?
  - Do you resolve conflicts and misunderstandings directly with those who are involved?
  - Do you clarify information for families or seek the appropriate person to do so?
- Do you recognize that from time to time a therapeutic relationship can change to a social relationship or an intimate friendship?
  - Are you able to acknowledge the fact when it occurs and understand why it happened?
  - Can you ensure that there is someone else who is more objective who can take your place in the therapeutic relationship?

---

communicating with them, and individualizing the nursing care. Parents perceive personable nursing care as being integral to establishing a positive relationship.

Disease Prevention and Health Promotion

Every nurse involved in caring for children must understand the importance of disease prevention and health promotion. A nursing care plan must include a thorough assessment of all aspects of child growth and development, including nutrition, immunizations, safety, dental care, socialization, discipline, and education. If problems are identified, the nurse intervenes directly or refers the family to other health care providers or agencies.

The best approach to prevention is education and anticipatory guidance. An appreciation of the hazards or conflicts of each developmental period enables the nurse to guide parents regarding child-rearing practices aimed at preventing potential problems. One significant example is safety. Because each age-group is at risk for special types of injuries, preventive teaching can significantly reduce injuries, lowering permanent disability and mortality rates.

Prevention also involves less obvious aspects of caring for children. The nurse is responsible for providing care that promotes mental well-being (e.g., enlisting the help of a child life specialist during a painful procedure such as an immunization).

Health Teaching

Health teaching is inseparable from family advocacy and prevention. Health teaching may be the nurse's direct goal, such as during parenting classes, or may be indirect, such as by:

- Helping parents and children understand a diagnosis or medical treatment
- Encouraging children to ask questions about their bodies
- Referring families to health-related professional or lay groups
- Supplying patients with appropriate literature
- Providing anticipatory guidance

Health teaching is one area in which nurses often need preparation and practice with competent role models, since it involves transmitting information at the child's and family's level of understanding and desire for information. As an effective educator, the nurse focuses on providing the appropriate health teaching with generous feedback and evaluation to promote learning.

Injury Prevention

Each year, injuries kill or disable more children older than 1 year than all childhood diseases combined. The nurse plays an important role in preventing injuries by using a developmental approach to safety counseling for parents of children of all ages. Realizing that safety concerns for a young infant are completely different from injury risks of adolescents, the nurse discusses appropriate injury preventions tips to parents and children as part of routine patient care.

Support and Counseling

Attention to emotional needs requires support and, sometimes, counseling. The role of child advocate or health teacher is supportive by virtue of the individualized approach. The nurse can offer support by listening, touching, and being physically present. Touching and physical presence are most helpful with children because they facilitate nonverbal communication. Counseling involves a mutual exchange of ideas and opinions that provides the basis for mutual problem solving. It involves support, teaching, techniques to foster the expression of feelings or thoughts, and approaches to help the family cope with stress. Optimally, counseling not only helps resolve a crisis or problem but also enables the family to attain a higher level of functioning, greater self-esteem, and closer relationships. Although counseling is often the role of nurses in specialized areas, counseling techniques are discussed in various sections of this text to help students and nurses cope with immediate crises and refer families for additional professional assistance.

Coordination and Collaboration

The nurse, as a member of the health care team, collaborates and coordinates nursing care with the care activities of other professionals. A nurse working in isolation rarely serves the child's best interests. The concept of holistic care can be realized through a unified, interdisciplinary approach by being aware of individual contributions and limitations and collaborating with other specialists to provide high-quality health services. Failure to recognize limitations can be nontherapeutic at best and destructive at worst. For example, the nurse who feels competent in counseling but who is really inadequate in this area may not only prevent the child from dealing with a crisis but also impede future success with a qualified professional.

Ethical Decision Making

Ethical dilemmas arise when competing moral considerations underlie various alternatives. Parents, nurses, physicians, and other health care team members may reach different but morally defensible decisions by assigning different weights to competing moral values. These competing moral values may include autonomy, the patient's right to be self-governing; nonmaleficence, the obligation to minimize or prevent harm; beneficence, the obligation to promote the patient's well-being; and justice, the concept of fairness. Nurses must determine the most beneficial or least harmful action within the framework of societal mores, professional practice standards, the law, institutional rules, the family's value system and religious traditions, and the nurse's personal values.

Nurses must prepare themselves systematically for collaborative ethical decision making. They can accomplish this through formal course work, continuing education, contemporary literature, and work to establish an environment conducive to ethical discourse. Moreover, nurses must be educated on the mechanisms for dispute resolution, case review by ethics committees, procedural safeguards, state statutes, and case law (Woods, 2005).

The nurse also uses the professional code of ethics for guidance and as a means for professional self-regulation. The Code of Ethics for Nurses by the American Nurses Association focuses on the nurse's accountability and responsibility to the patient and emphasizes the nursing role as an independent professional, one that upholds its own legal liability. Nurses may face ethical issues regarding patient care, such as the use of lifesaving measures for VLBW newborns or the terminally ill child's right to refuse treatment. They may struggle with questions regarding truthfulness, balancing their rights and responsibilities in caring for children with AIDS, whistleblowing, or allocating resources.

Research and Evidence-Based Practice

Nurses should contribute to research because they are the individuals observing human responses to health and illness. The current emphasis on measurable outcomes to determine the efficacy of interventions (often in relation to the cost) demands that nurses know whether clinical interventions result in positive outcomes for their patients. This demand has influenced the current trend toward evidence-based practice (EBP), which implies questioning why something is effective and whether a better approach exists. The concept of EBP also involves analyzing and translating published clinical research into the everyday practice of nursing. When nurses base their clinical practice on science and research and document their clinical outcomes, they will be able to validate their contributions to health, wellness, and cure, not only to their patients, third-party payers, and institutions but also to the nursing profession. Evaluation is essential to the nursing process, and research is one of the best ways to accomplish this.

EBP is the collection, interpretation, and integration of valid, important, and applicable patient-reported, nurse-observed, and research-derived information. Evidence-based nursing practice combines knowledge with clinical experience and intuition. It provides a rational approach to decision making that facilitates best practice (Scott and McSherry, 2009; van Achterberg, Schoonhoven, and Grol, 2008). EBP is an important tool that complements the nursing process by using critical thinking skills to make decisions based on existing knowledge. The traditional nursing process approach to patient care can be used to conceptualize the essential components of EBP nursing. During the assessment and diagnostic phases of the nursing process, the nurse establishes important clinical questions and completes a critical review of existing knowledge. EBP also begins with identification of the problem. The nurse asks clinical questions in a concise, organized way that allows for clear answers. Once the specific questions are identified, extensive searching for the best information to answer the question begins. The nurse evaluates clinically relevant research, analyzes findings from the history and physical examinations, and reviews the specific pathophysiology of the defined problem. The third step in the nursing process is to develop a care plan. In evidence-based nursing practice, the care plan is established on completion of a critical appraisal of what is known and not known about the defined problem. Next, in the traditional nursing process, the nurse implements the care plan. By integrating evidence with clinical expertise, the nurse focuses care on the patient's unique needs. The final step in EBP is consistent with the final phase of the nursing process: to evaluate the effectiveness of the care plan.

Searching for evidence in this modern era of technology can be overwhelming. For nurses to implement EBP, they must have access to appropriate recent resources such as online search engines and journals. In many institutions, computer terminals are available on

TABLE 26-4	THE GRADE CRITERIA TO EVALUATE THE QUALITY OF THE EVIDENCE
QUALITY	**TYPE OF EVIDENCE**
High	Consistent evidence from well-performed randomized clinical trials (RCTs) or exceptionally strong evidence from unbiased observational studies
Moderate	Evidence from RCTs with important limitations (inconsistent results, methodologic flaws, indirect evidence, or imprecise results) or unusually strong evidence from unbiased observational studies
Low	Evidence for at least one critical outcome from observational studies, from RCTs with serious flaws, or from indirect evidence
Very Low	Evidence for at least one of the critical outcomes from unsystematic clinical observations or very indirect evidence
QUALITY	**RECOMMENDATION**
Strong	Desirable effects clearly outweigh undesirable effects, or vice versa
Weak	Desirable effects closely balanced with undesirable effects

Adapted from Guyatt GH, Oxman AD, Visit GE, et al: GRADE: an emerging consensus on rating quality of evidence and strength of recommendations, *BMJ* 336:924–926, 2008.

patient care units, with the Internet and online journals easily accessible. Another important resource for the implementation of EBP is time. The nursing shortage and ongoing changes in many institutions have compounded the issue of nursing time allocation for patient care, education, and training. In some institutions, nurses are given paid time away from patient care duties to participate in activities that promote EBP. This requires an organizational environment that values EBP and its potential impact on patient care. As knowledge is generated regarding the significant impact of EBP on patient care outcomes, it is hoped that the organizational culture will change to support the staff nurse's participation in EBP. As the amount of available evidence increases, so does our need to critically evaluate the evidence.

Throughout this book, EBP boxes summarize the existing evidence that promotes excellence in clinical care. The GRADE criteria are used to evaluate the quality of research articles used to develop practice guidelines (Guyatt, Oxman, Vist, et al., 2008). Table 26-4 defines how the nurse rates the quality of the evidence using the GRADE criteria and establishes a strong versus weak recommendation. Each EBP box rates the quality of existing evidence and the strength of the recommendation for practice change.

CLINICAL REASONING AND THE PROCESS OF PROVIDING NURSING CARE TO CHILDREN AND FAMILIES

Clinical Reasoning

A systematic thought process is essential to a profession. It assists the professional in meeting the patient's needs. Clinical reasoning is a cognitive process that uses formal and informal thinking to gather and analyze patient data, evaluate the significance of the information, and consider alternative actions (Simmons, 2010). It is based on the

scientific method of inquiry, which is also the basis for the nursing process. Clinical reasoning and the nursing process are considered crucial to professional nursing in that they constitute a holistic approach to problem solving.

Clinical reasoning is a complex developmental process based on rational and deliberate thought. Clinical reasoning provides a common denominator for knowledge that exemplifies disciplined and self-directed thinking. The knowledge is acquired, assessed, and organized by thinking through the clinical situation and developing an outcome focused on optimum patient care. Clinical reasoning transforms the way in which individuals view themselves, understand the world, and make decisions. In recognition of the importance of this skill, critical thinking exercises presented in this text in *Critical Thinking Case Study* boxes demonstrate the importance of clinical reasoning. These exercises present a nursing practice situation that challenges the student to use the skills of clinical reasoning to come to the best conclusion. A series of questions lead the student to explore the evidence, assumptions underlying the problem, nursing priorities, and support for nursing interventions that allow the nurse make a rational and deliberate response. These exercises are designed to enhance nursing performance in clinical reasoning.

Nursing Process

The nursing process is a method of problem identification and problem solving that describes what the nurse actually does. The five-step nursing process model is assessment, diagnosis (problem identification), planning (with outcome development), implementation, and evaluation. The second step of the nursing process, nursing diagnosis, involves naming the child's or family's problem in standardized nursing language. In the American Nurses Association (2003) Standards of Practice, the nursing diagnosis phase of the nursing process is separated into two steps: nursing diagnosis and outcome identification.

Assessment

Assessment is a continuous process that operates at all phases of problem solving and is the foundation for decision making. Assessment involves multiple nursing skills and consists of the purposeful collection, classification, and analysis of data from a variety of sources. To provide an accurate and comprehensive assessment, the nurse must consider information about the patient's biophysical, psychologic, sociocultural, and spiritual background.

Nursing Diagnosis

The second stage of the nursing process is problem identification and nursing diagnosis. At this point, the nurse must interpret and make decisions about the data gathered. The nurse organizes or clusters these data into categories to identify significant areas and makes one of the following decisions:

- No dysfunctional health problems are evident; no interventions are indicated.
- Risk for dysfunctional health problems exists; interventions are needed for health promotion.
- Actual dysfunctional health problems are evident; interventions are needed for health promotion.

The nursing diagnosis is the naming of the cue clusters that are obtained during the assessment phase. According to NANDA International (formerly the North American Nursing Diagnosis Association), the currently accepted definition of the term nursing diagnosis is that it is a clinical judgment about individual, family, or community responses to actual and potential health problems and life processes. Nursing care plans in this text provide an

FAMILY-CENTERED CARE

Using Defining Characteristics to Select an Appropriate Nursing Diagnosis

An 18-month-old only child is admitted with respiratory distress and a presumptive diagnosis of epiglottitis. Initial nursing actions focus on the child's physiologic status. As the condition stabilizes, the nurse gathers family assessment data. The child's immunizations are current, he is clean and well nourished, and his developmental age is appropriate. The parents are both present at admission. The mother is distraught about the sudden onset of respiratory distress. She states that earlier, her child had only a "runny nose" and she thought it was just a cold. When the child suddenly began to have difficulty breathing, she felt helpless and unable to relieve her child's discomfort. She states: "Nothing I did made him any better. If I had known this could happen, I would have brought him to the hospital sooner. I feel like a bad mother." In the hospital, after explanations by the nurses, the mother understands that epiglottitis is a sudden illness that typically follows symptoms of a cold. She is cooperative and asks what she can do to make her child more comfortable. She implements all the suggestions of the health care team. The father supports both the child and mother, although he assumes a more passive, "listening" role.

Three nursing diagnoses that relate to family and parent situations may be relevant. The first step is to review the diagnoses and the defining characteristics and decide which one is most appropriate:

1. Impaired Parenting—Inability of the primary caregiver to create, maintain, or regain an environment that nurtures the child's growth and development
   Selected defining characteristics:
   - Insecure (or lack of) attachment to infant
   - Poor or inappropriate caregiving skills

2. Parental Role Conflict—Parent experience of role confusion and conflict in response to crisis
   Selected defining characteristics:
   - Parent expressing concerns about changes in parental role
   - A demonstrated disruption in care or caregiving routines
   - Parent expressing concerns or feelings of inadequacy to provide for the child's physical and emotional needs during hospitalization or in home
   - Parent verbalizing or demonstrating feelings of guilt, anger, fear, anxiety, or frustration about effect of child's illness on family process

3. Interrupted Family Processes—A change in family relationships or functioning
   Selected defining characteristics:
   - Expressions of conflict within the family
   - Changes in communication patterns among family members

Of these three diagnoses, the most relevant one is *Parental Role Conflict*. The parents demonstrate attachment behavior to their child and are attentive to his needs. They appear to have appropriate parenting skills and are able to communicate effectively with each other. Neither parent expressed any conflict within the family. The sudden onset of this child's illness has interrupted the mother's usual role and caused her to feel inadequate, anxious, and guilty. However, the mother is able to adapt to this crisis. She demonstrates an ability to cope by learning and implementing new comforting skills for her child. The defining characteristics of the other two diagnoses require maladaptive characteristics that are clearly not demonstrated by these parents.

---

understanding of the standardized language and how it relates to the individualized plan.

Not all children have actual health problems; some have a potential health problem, which is a risk state that requires nursing intervention to prevent the development of an actual problem. Potential health problems may be indicated by risk factors, or signs, that predispose a child and family to a dysfunctional health pattern and are limited to individuals at greater risk than the population as a whole. Nursing interventions are directed toward reducing risk factors. To differentiate actual from potential health problems, the word *risk* is included in the nursing diagnosis statement (e.g., Risk for Infection).

Signs and symptoms refer to a cluster of cues and defining characteristics that are derived from patient assessment and indicate actual health problems. When a defining characteristic is essential for the diagnosis to be made, it is considered critical. These critical defining characteristics help differentiate between diagnostic categories. For example, in deciding between the diagnostic categories related to family function and coping, the nurse uses defining characteristics to choose the most appropriate nursing diagnosis (see Family-Centered Care box).

Planning

After identifying the nursing diagnoses, the nurse develops a care plan and establishes outcomes or goals. The outcome is the projected or expected change in a patient's health status, clinical condition, or behavior that occurs after nursing interventions have been instituted. The ultimate goal of nursing care is to convert the nursing diagnoses into a desired health state. The care plan must be established before specific nursing interventions are developed and implemented.

Implementation

The implementation phase begins when the nurse puts the selected intervention into action and accumulates feedback data regarding its effects (or the patient's response to the intervention). The feedback returns in the form of observation and communication and provides a database on which to evaluate the outcome of the nursing intervention. It is imperative that continual assessment of the patient's status occurs throughout all phases of the nursing process, thus making the process a dynamic rather than static problem-solving method. Throughout the implementation stage, the main concerns are the patient's physical safety and psychologic comfort in terms of atraumatic care.

Evaluation

Evaluation is the last step in the decision-making process. The nurse gathers, sorts, and analyzes data to determine whether (1) the established outcome has been met, (2) the nursing interventions were appropriate, (3) the plan requires modification, or (4) other alternatives should be considered. The evaluation phase either completes the nursing process (outcome is met) or serves as the basis for selecting alternative interventions to solve the specific problem.

With the current focus on patient outcomes in health care, the patient's care is evaluated not only at discharge but thereafter as well to ensure that the outcomes are met and there is adequate care for resolving existing or potential health problems. One federal agency that has developed clinical guidelines is the Agency for Healthcare Research and Quality.*

---

*540 Gaither Road, Suite 2000, Rockville, MD 20850; 301-427-1364; info@ahrq.gov; www.ahrq.gov.

GUIDELINES
Documentation of Nursing Care

- Initial assessments and reassessments
- Nursing diagnoses and/or patient care needs
- Interventions identified to meet the patient's nursing care needs
- Nursing care provided
- Patient's response to and the outcomes of the care provided
- Abilities of patient and/or, as appropriate, significant other(s) to manage continuing care needs after discharge

Documentation

Although documentation is not one of the five steps of the nursing process, it is essential for evaluation. The nurse can assess, diagnose and identify problems, plan, and implement without documentation; however, evaluation is best performed with written evidence of progress toward outcomes. The patient's medical record should include evidence of those elements listed in the Guidelines box.

QUALITY OUTCOME MEASURES

Quality of care refers to the degree to which health services for individuals and populations increase the likelihood of desired health outcomes and are consistent with current professional knowledge (Institute of Medicine, 2000). Because nurses are the principal caregivers within health care institutions, high-quality nursing outcomes are used as an indicator of the ability to provide excellence in patient care. Nurse-sensitive indicators are chosen by using specific evaluation criteria. Specific examples of patient-centered outcome measures established by the National Quality Forum are found in Box 26-5. A comprehensive resource, the Quality and Safety Education for Nurses (QSEN), is funded by the Robert Wood Johnson Foundation.* Each EBP box in this book ends with the QSEN competences related to knowledge, skills, and attitudes for evidence-based nursing practice.

Quality outcome evaluation criteria establish a framework for measuring nursing care performance. In addition to using the National Quality Forum's measurement evaluation criteria, nurses

---

*Frances Payne Bolton School of Nursing, Case Western Reserve University, 10900 Euclid Avenue, Cleveland, OH 44106-4904; 216-368-4700; fax: 216-368-3542; e-mail: qsen.institute@gmail.com; www.qsen.org.

BOX 26-5 NATIONAL QUALITY FORUM: PATIENT-CENTERED OUTCOME MEASURES

Death among surgical inpatients with treatable serious complications (failure to rescue)—The percentage of major surgical inpatients who experience a hospital-acquired complication and die

Pressure ulcer prevalence—Percentage of inpatients who have a hospital-acquired pressure ulcer

Falls prevalence—Number of inpatient falls per inpatient days

Falls with injury—Number of inpatient falls with injuries per inpatient days

Restraint prevalence—Percentage of inpatients who have a vest or limb restraint

Urinary catheter–associated urinary tract infection for intensive care unit (ICU) patients—Rate of urinary tract infections associated with use of urinary catheters for ICU patients

Central line catheter–associated bloodstream infection rate for ICU and high-risk nursery patients—Rate of bloodstream infections associated with use of central line catheters for ICU and high-risk nursery patients

Ventilator-associated pneumonia for ICU and high-risk nursery patients—Rate of pneumonia associated with use of ventilators for ICU and high-risk nursery patients

Adapted from National Quality Forum: Nursing performance measurement and reporting: a status report, *NQF* (Issue Brief 5):July 2007, www.qualityforum.org/Publications/2007/07/Nursing_Performance_Measurement_and_Reporting_.aspx.

---

should evaluate each quality-nursing indicator to ensure it is an essential component of health care quality established by the Institute of Medicine (IOM) (2000). The IOM components include being:

- Safe
- Effective
- Patient-centered
- Timely
- Efficient
- Equitable

Throughout the chapters that focus on serious health problems, we have developed examples of quality outcome measures for specific diseases that reflect patient-centered outcomes. Quality outcome measures promote interdisciplinary teamwork and focus care on improving patient care.

KEY POINTS

- Although the infant mortality rate in the United States has declined over the past few decades, the United States lags significantly behind most other major countries, such as Canada.
- LBW, which is closely related to early gestational age, is considered the leading cause of neonatal death in the United States.
- Injuries are the leading cause of death in children older than 1 year, with the majority being MVA injuries.
- Childhood morbidity encompasses acute illness, chronic disease, and disability.
- Eighty percent of childhood illnesses are attributable to infections, with respiratory tract infections occurring 2 or 3 times more often than all other illnesses combined.

- The *new morbidity* refers to behavioral, social, and educational problems that can significantly alter a child's health.
- Developmental stage and environment are important determinants of the prevalence of injuries at a given age and thus help direct preventive measures.
- The philosophy of family-centered care recognizes that the family is the constant in a child's life and that service systems and personnel must support, respect, and enhance the family's strength and competence.
- Atraumatic care is the provision of therapeutic care in settings by personnel and by the use of interventions that eliminate or minimize the psychologic and physical distress experienced by children and their families in the health care system.

- The pediatric nurse's roles include a therapeutic relationship, family advocacy, disease prevention and health promotion, health teaching, support and counseling, coordination and collaboration, ethical decision making, and research.
- EBP is the collection, interpretation, and integration of valid, important, and applicable patient-reported, nurse-observed, and research-derived information.

- The process of nursing children and families includes accurate and comprehensive assessment, analysis, and synthesis of assessment data to arrive at a nursing diagnosis, planning of care, implementation of the plan, and evaluation of interventions.
- Because nurses are the principal caregivers within health care institutions, quality outcomes are used as a measure of the ability to provide excellence in patient care.

REFERENCES

American Association of Suicidology: Youth suicide fact sheet, 2009, www.suicidology.org.

American Dietetic Association: Position of the American Dietetic Association: nutrition guidance for healthy children ages 2 to 11 years, *J Am Dietetic Assoc* 108(6):1038–1047, 2008.

American Nurses Association: *Nursing: scope and standards of practice*, Washington, DC, 2003, Author.

Annie E Casey Foundation: *2009 Kids count data book: state profiles of child well-being*, Baltimore, 2009, Author.

Bronstein AC, Spyker DA, Cantilena LR, et al: 2007 Annual report of the American Association of Poison Control Centers' national poison data system: 25th annual report, *Clin Toxicol* 46(1):927–1057, 2008.

Cali AMG, Caprio S: Prediabetes and type 2 diabetes in youth: an emerging epidemic disease? *Curr Opin Endocrinol Diabetes Obes* 15:123–127, 2008.

Castle SL, Burke RV, Arbogast H, et al: Bicycle helmet legislation and injury patterns in trauma patients under age 18, *J Surg Res*, 2010 [Epub ahead of print].

Centers for Disease Control and Prevention (CDC): *CDC injury fact book*, Atlanta, 2006, National Center for Injury Prevention and Control.

Cheng NF, Han PZ, Gansky SA: Methods and software for estimating health disparities: the case of children's oral health, *Am J Epidemiol* 168(8):906–914, 2008.

Coury DL: Over the rainbow: advancing child health in the new millennium, *Ambul Pediatr* 6(3):134–137, 2006.

de Onis M, Blössner M, Borghi E: Global prevalence and trends of overweight and obesity among preschool children, *Am J Clin Nutr* 92(5):1257–1264, 2010.

Doucette A: Youth suicide. In Cosby AG, Greenberg RE, Southward LH, et al, editors: *About children: an authoritative resource on the state of childhood today*, Elk Grove Village, IL, 2005, American Academy of Pediatrics.

Forum on Child and Family Statistics: America's children in brief: key national indicators of well-being, 2012, www.childstats.gov/pdf/ac2012/ac_12.pdf.

Franklin RL, Rodgers GB: Unintentional child poisoning treated in the United States hospital emergency departments: national estimates of incident cases, population-based poisoning rates, and product involvement, *Pediatrics* 122(6):1244–1251, 2008.

Graff M, North KE, Monda KL, et al: The combined influence of genetic factors and sedentary activity on body mass changes from adolescence to young adulthood: the National Longitudinal Adolescent Health Study, *Diabetes Metab Res Rev* 27(1):63–69, 2011.

Guyatt GH, Oxman AD, Vist GE, et al: GRADE: an emerging consensus on rating quality of evidence and strength of recommendations, *BMJ* 336(7650):924–926, 2008.

Hamilton BE, Hoyert DL, Martin JA, et al: Annual summary of vital statistics: 2010-2011, *Pediatrics* 131(3):548–558, 2013.

Heuer S: Family-centered care, *J Spec Pediatr Nurs* 12(1):61–65, 2007.

Hooper VD: Patient-family centered care: are we there yet? *J Peri Anesthesia Nurs* 23(6):440–442, 2008.

Hoyert DL, Xu J: Deaths: preliminary data for 2011, *Natl Vital Stat Rep* 61(6):1–51, 2012.

Institute of Medicine: *Crossing the quality chasm*, Washington, DC, 2000, Author.

Kagihara LE, Niederhauser VP, Stark M: Assessment, management, and prevention of early childhood caries, *J Am Acad Nurse Pract* 21(1):1–10, 2009.

Leslie LK, Slaw KM, Edwards A, et al: Peering into the future: pediatrics in a changing world, *Pediatrics* 126(5):982–988, 2010.

Martin JA, Kochanek KD, Strobino DM, et al: Annual summary of vital statistics: 2003, *Pediatrics* 115(3):619–634, 2005.

Matyka KA: Type 2 diabetes in childhood: epidemiological and clinical aspects, *Brit Med Bull* 86:59–75, 2008.

National Center for Cultural Competence: *A guide for advancing family-centered and culturally and linguistically competent care*, Washington DC, 2007, Georgetown University Center for Child and Human Development.

National Survey on Drug Use and Health: *Trends in substance use, dependence or abuse, and treatment among adolescents: 2002–2007*, Rockville MD, 2008, Office of Applied Studies.

Polaha J, Dalton WT 3rd, Allen S: The prevalence of emotional and behavior problems in pediatric primary care serving rural children, *J Pediatr Psychol*, 2011 [Epub ahead of print].

Raj M, Kumar RK: Obesity in children & adolescents, *Indian J Med Res* 132(5):598–607, 2010.

Schnitzer PG: Prevention of unintentional childhood injuries, *Am Fam Physician* 74(11):1864–1869, 2006.

Schwartz MS, Chadha A: Type 2 diabetes mellitus in childhood: obesity and insulin resistance, *J Am Osteopath Assoc* 108:518–524, 2008.

Scott K, McSherry R: Evidence-based nursing: clarifying the concepts for nurses in practice, *J Clin Nurs* 18(8):1085–1095, 2009.

Simmons B: Clinical reasoning: concept analysis, *J Adv Nurs* 66(5):1151–1158, 2010.

Starmer AJ, Duby JC, Slaw KM, et al: Pediatrics in the year 2020 and beyond: preparing for plausible futures, *Pediatrics* 126(5):971–981, 2010.

U.S. Department of Health and Human Services: Youth violence: a report of the surgeon general, www.surgeongeneral.gov/library/youthviolence/.

van Achterberg T, Schoonhoven L, Grol R: Nursing implementation science: how evidence-based nursing requires evidence-based implementation, *J Nurs Scholarsh* 40(4):302–310, 2008.

Wong D: Principles of atraumatic care. In Feeg V, editor: *Pediatric nursing: forum on the future—looking toward the 21st century*, Pitman, NJ, 1989, Anthony J Jannetti.

Woods M: Nursing ethics education: are we really delivering the good(s)? *Nurs Ethics* 12(1):5–18, 2005.

World Health Organization: School health and youth health promotion, 2011, www.who.int/school_youth_health/en.

Family, Social, Cultural, and Religious Influences on Child Health Promotion

Marilyn J. Hockenberry

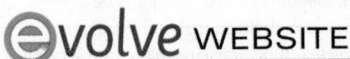 WEBSITE

http://evolve.elsevier.com/Perry/maternal

LEARNING OBJECTIVES

On completion of this chapter, the reader will be able to:
- Discuss definitions of *family*.
- Discuss the role transition experienced by new parents.
- Explain various parenting behaviors such as parenting styles, disciplinary patterns, and communication skills.
- Demonstrate an understanding of special parenting situations such as adoption, divorce, single parenting, parenting in reconstituted families, and dual-earner families.

- Define culture and cultural humility.
- Describe the subcultural influences on child development in the areas of socioeconomic class, poverty, religion, and schools.
- Identify areas of potential conflict of values and customs for a nurse interacting with a family from a different cultural or ethnic group.

DEFINITION OF FAMILY

The term *family* has been defined in many different ways according to the individual's own frame of reference, values, or discipline. There is no universal definition of family; a family is what an individual considers it to be. *Biology* describes the family as fulfilling the biologic function of perpetuation of the species. *Psychology* emphasizes the interpersonal aspects of the family and its responsibility for personality development. *Economics* views the family as a productive unit providing for material needs. *Sociology* depicts the family as a social unit interacting with the larger society, creating the context within which cultural values and identity are formed. Others define family in terms of the relationships of the persons who make up the family unit. The most common type of relationships are consanguineous (blood relationships), affinal (marital relationships), and family of origin (family unit a person is born into).

Earlier definitions of family emphasized that family members were related by legal ties or genetic relationships and lived in the same household with specific roles. Later definitions have been broadened to reflect both structural and functional changes. A family can be defined as an institution in which individuals, related through biology or enduring commitments and representing similar or different generations and genders, participate in roles involving mutual socialization, nurturance, and emotional commitment (Coehlo, Kaakinen, Hanson, et al., 2009). Nursing care of infants and children is intimately involved with care of the child *and* the family. Family structure and dynamics can have an enduring influence on a child, affecting the child's health and well-being. Consequently, nurses must be aware of the functions of the family, various types of family structures, and theories that provide a foundation for understanding the changes within a family and for directing family-oriented interventions.

Family Structure

The family structure, or family composition, consists of individuals, each with a socially recognized status and position, who interact with one another on a regular, recurring basis in socially sanctioned ways (Coehlo, Kaakinen, Hanson, et al., 2009) (Fig. 27-1). When members are gained or lost through events such as marriage, divorce, birth, death, abandonment, or incarceration, the family composition is altered and roles must be redefined or redistributed.

Traditionally, the family structure was either a nuclear or extended family. In recent years, family composition has assumed new configurations, with the single-parent family and blended family becoming prominent forms. The predominant structural pattern in any society depends on the mobility of families as

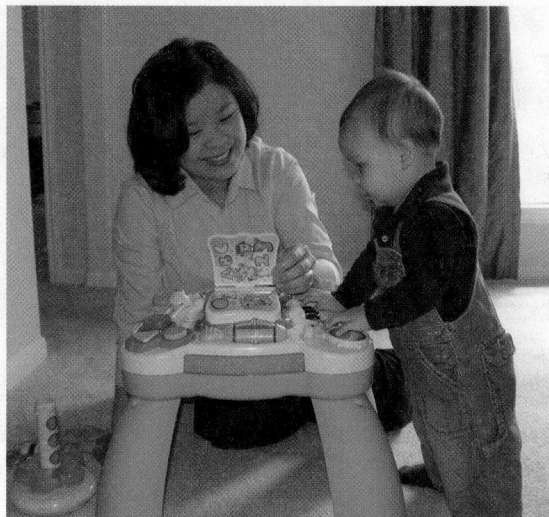

FIG 27-1 Quality time spent within the family is essential to a child's health and well-being.

they pursue economic goals and as relationships change. It is not uncommon for children to belong to several different family groups during their lifetime.

Nurses must be able to meet the needs of children from many diverse family structures and home situations. A family's particular structure affects the direction of nursing care. The U.S. Census Bureau uses four definitions for families: the traditional nuclear family, the nuclear family, the blended family or household, and the extended family or household.

Family Strengths and Functioning Style

Family function refers to the interactions of family members, especially the quality of those relationships and interactions (Bomar, 2004). Researchers are interested in family characteristics that help families function effectively. Knowledge of these factors guides the nurse throughout the nursing process and helps the nurse to predict ways that families may cope and respond to a stressful event, to provide individualized support that builds on family strengths and unique functioning style, and to assist family members in obtaining resources.

Family strengths and unique functioning styles (Box 27-1) are significant resources that nurses can use to meet family needs. Building on qualities that make a family work well and strengthening family resources make the family unit even stronger. All families have strengths as well as vulnerabilities.

Family Roles and Relationships

Each individual has a position, or status, in the family structure and plays culturally and socially defined roles in interactions within the family. Each family also has its own traditions and values and sets its own standards for interaction within and outside the group. Each determines the experiences the children should have, those they are to be shielded from, and how each of these experiences meets the needs of family members. When family ties are strong, social control is highly effective and most members conform to their roles willingly and with commitment. Conflicts arise when people do not fulfill their roles in ways that meet other family members' expectations, either because they are unaware of the expectations or because they choose not to meet them.

Parental Roles

In all family groups, the socially recognized status of father and mother exists with socially sanctioned roles that prescribe appropriate sexual behavior and childrearing responsibilities. The guides for behavior in these roles serve to control sexual conflict in society and provide for prolonged care of children. The degree to which parents are committed and the way they play their roles are influenced by a number of variables and by the parents' unique socialization experience.

Parental role definitions have changed as a result of the changing economy and increased opportunities for women (Bomar, 2004). As the woman's role has changed, the complementary role of the man has also changed. Many fathers are more active in childrearing and household tasks. As the redefinition of gender roles continues in American families, role conflicts may arise in many families because of a cultural lag of the persisting traditional role definitions.

Family Size and Configuration

Parenting practices differ between small and large families. Small families place more emphasis on the individual development of the children. Parenting is intensive rather than extensive, and there is constant pressure to measure up to family expectations. Children's development and achievement are measured against those of other children in the neighborhood and social class. In small families, children have more democratic participation than in larger families. Adolescents in small families identify more strongly with their parents and rely more on them for advice. They have well-developed, autonomous inner controls as contrasted with adolescents from larger families, who rely more on adult authority.

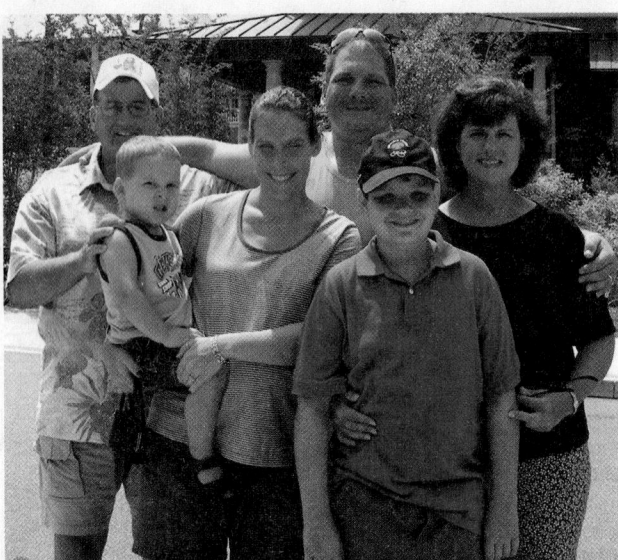

FIG 27-2 Family structure and function promote strong relationships among its members.

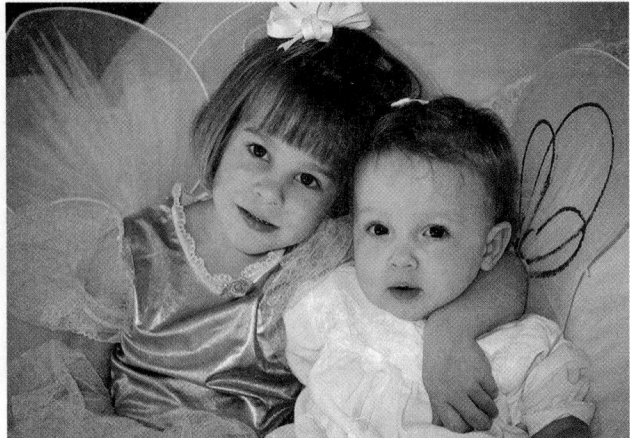

FIG 27-3 An older sister lovingly embraces her adopted sister.

Children in a large family are able to adjust to a variety of changes and crises. There is more emphasis on the group and less on the individual (Fig. 27-2). Cooperation is essential, often because of economic necessity. The large number of people sharing a limited amount of space requires a greater degree of organization, administration, and authoritarian control. A dominant family member (a parent or older child) wields control. The number of children reduces the intimate, one-to-one contact between the parent and any individual child. Consequently, children turn to each other for what they cannot get from their parents. The reduced parent-child contact encourages individual children to adopt specialized roles to gain recognition in the family.

Older siblings in large families often administer discipline. Siblings are usually attuned to what constitutes misbehavior. Sibling disapproval or ostracism is frequently a more meaningful disciplinary measure than parental interventions. In situations such as death or illness of a parent, an older sibling often assumes responsibility for the family at considerable personal sacrifice. Large families generate a sense of security in the children that is fostered by sibling support and cooperation. However, adolescents from a large family are more peer oriented than family oriented.

SPECIAL PARENTING SITUATIONS

Parenting is a demanding task under ideal circumstances, but when parents and children face situations that deviate from "the norm," the potential for family disruption is increased. Situations that are encountered frequently are divorce, single parenthood, blended families, adoption, and dual-career families. In addition, as cultural diversity increases in our communities, many immigrants are making the transition to parenthood and a new country, culture, and language simultaneously. Other situations that create unique parenting challenges are parental alcoholism, homelessness, and incarceration. Although these topics are not addressed here, the reader may wish to investigate them further.

Parenting the Adopted Child

Adoption establishes a legal relationship between a child and parents who are not related by birth but who have the same rights and obligations that exist between children and their biologic parents. In the past, the biologic mother alone made the decision to relinquish the rights to her child. In recent years, the courts have acknowledged the legal rights of the biologic father regarding this decision. Concerned child advocates have questioned whether decisions that honor the father's rights are in the best interests of the child. As the child's rights have become recognized, older children have successfully dissolved their legal bond with their biologic parents to pursue adoption by adults of their choice. Furthermore, there is a growing interest and demand within the gay and lesbian community to adopt.

Unlike biologic parents, who prepare for their child's birth with prenatal classes and the support of friends and relatives, adoptive parents have fewer sources of support and preparation for the new addition to their family. Nurses can provide the information, support, and reassurance needed to reduce parental anxiety regarding the adoptive process and refer adoptive parents to state parental support groups. Such sources can be contacted through a state or county welfare office.

The sooner infants enter their adoptive home, the better the chances of parent-infant attachment. However, the more caregivers the infant had before adoption, the greater the risk for attachment problems. The infant must break the bond with the previous caregiver and form a new bond with the adoptive parents. Difficulties in forming an attachment depend on the amount of time he or she has spent with caregivers early in life as well as the number of caregivers (e.g., the birth mother, nurse, adoption agency personnel).

Siblings, adopted or biologic, who are old enough to understand should be included in decisions regarding the commitment to adopt, with reassurance that they are not being replaced. Ways that the siblings can interact with the adopted child should be stressed (Fig. 27-3).

Issues of Origin

The task of telling children that they are adopted can be a cause of deep concern and anxiety. There are no clear-cut guidelines for parents to follow in determining when and at what age children are ready for the information. Parents are naturally reluctant to present such potentially unsettling news. However, it is important that parents not withhold the adoption from the child, since it is an essential component of the child's identity.

The timing arises naturally as parents become aware of the child's readiness. Most authorities believe that children should be informed at an age young enough so that, as they grow older, they do not remember a time when they did not know they were adopted. The time is highly individual but must be right for both the parents and the child. It may be when children ask where babies come from, at which time children can also be told the facts of their adoption. If they are told in a way that conveys the idea that they were active participants in the selection process, they will be less likely to feel that they were abandoned victims in a helpless situation. For example, parents can tell children that their personal qualities drew the parents to them. It is wise for parents who have not previously discussed adoption to tell children that they are adopted before the children enter school, to avoid having them learn it from third parties. Complete honesty between parents and children strengthens the relationship.

Parents should anticipate behavior changes after the disclosure, especially in older children. Children who are struggling with the revelation that they are adopted may benefit from individual and family counseling. Children may use the fact of their adoption as a weapon to manipulate and threaten parents. Statements such as "My real mother would not treat me like this" or "You don't love me as much because I'm adopted" hurt parents and increase their feelings of insecurity. Such statements may also cause parents to become over-permissive. Adopted children need the same undemanding love, combined with firm discipline and limit setting, as any other child.

Adolescence

Adolescence may be an especially trying time for parents of adopted children. The normal confrontations of adolescents and parents assume more painful aspects in adoptive families. Adolescents may use their adoption to defy parental authority or as a justification for aberrant behavior. As they attempt to master the task of identity formation, they may begin to have feelings of abandonment by their biologic parents. Gender differences in reacting to adoption may surface.

Adopted children fantasize about their biologic parents and may feel the need to discover their parents' identity to define themselves and their own identity. It is important for parents to keep the lines of communication open and to reassure their child that they understand the need to search for their identity. In some states, birth certificates are made legally available to adopted children when they come of age. Parents should be honest with questioning adolescents and tell them of this possibility (the parents themselves are unable to obtain the birth certificate; it is the children's responsibility if they desire it).

Cross-Racial and International Adoption

Adoption of children from racial backgrounds different from that of the family is commonplace. In addition to the problems faced by adopted children in general, children of a cross-racial adoption must deal with physical and sometimes cultural differences. It is advised that parents who adopt children with different ethnic background do everything to preserve the adopted children's racial heritage.

Although the children are full-fledged members of an adopting family and citizens of the adopted country, if they have a strikingly different appearance from other family members or exhibit distinct racial or ethnic characteristics, challenges may be encountered outside the family. Bigotry may appear among relatives and friends. Strangers may make thoughtless comments and talk about the children as though they were not members of the family. It is vital that family members declare to others that this is their child and a cherished member of the family.

In international adoptions, the medical information the parents receive may be incomplete or sketchy; weight, height, and head circumference are often the only objective information present in the child's medical record. Many internationally adopted children were born prematurely, and common health problems such as infant diarrhea and malnutrition delay growth and development. Some children have serious or multiple health problems that can be stressful for the parents.

Parenting and Divorce

Since the mid-1960s, a marked change in the stability of families has been reflected in increased rates of divorce, single parenthood, and remarriage. In 2008, the divorce rate for the United States was 3.4 per 1000 total population (Centers for Disease Control and Prevention [CDC], 2012). The divorce rate has changed little since 1987. In the decade before that, the rate increased yearly, with a peak in 1979. Although almost half of all divorcing couples are childless, it is estimated that more than 1 million children experience divorce each year.

The process of divorce begins with a period of marital conflict of varying length and intensity, followed by a separation, the actual legal divorce, and the reestablishment of different living arrangements. Because a function of parenthood is to provide for the security and emotional welfare of children, disruption of the family structure often engenders strong feelings of guilt in the divorcing parents.

During a divorce, parents' coping abilities may be compromised. The parents may be preoccupied with their own feelings, needs, and life changes and be unavailable to support their children. Newly employed parents, usually mothers, are likely to leave children with new caregivers, in strange settings, or alone after school. The parent may also spend more time away from home, searching for or establishing new relationships. Sometimes, however, the adult feels frightened and alone and begins to depend on the child as a substitute for the absent parent. This dependence places an enormous burden on the child.

Common characteristics in the custodial household after separation and divorce include disorder, coercive types of control, inflammable tempers in both parents and children, reduced parental competence, a greater sense of parental helplessness, poorly enforced discipline, and diminished regularity in household routines. Noncustodial parents are seldom prepared for the role of visitor, may assume the role of recreational and "fun" parent, and may not have a residence suitable for children's visits. They may also be concerned about maintaining the arrangement over the years to follow.

Impact of Divorce on Children

Parental divorce is an additional childhood adversity that contributes to poor mental health outcomes, especially when combined with child abuse. Parental psychopathology may be one possible mechanism to explain the relationships between child abuse, parental divorce, and psychiatric disorders and suicide attempts (Afifi, Boman, Fleisher, et al., 2009). Even when a divorce is amicable and open, children recall parental separation with the same emotions felt by victims of a natural disaster: loss, grief, and vulnerability to forces beyond their control. A recent study found that increasing one of children's most important interpersonal resources—the quality of the mother-child relationship—improved children's post-divorce adjustment (Velez, Wolchik, Tein, et al., 2011).

The impact of divorce on children depends on several factors, including the age and gender of the children, the outcome of the divorce, and the quality of the parent-child relationship and parental

BOX 27-2   FEELINGS AND BEHAVIORS OF CHILDREN RELATED TO DIVORCE

Infancy
- Effects of reduced mothering or lack of mothering
- Increased irritability
- Disturbance in eating, sleeping, and elimination
- Interference with attachment process

Early Preschool Children (Ages 2-3 Years)
- Frightened and confused
- Blame themselves for the divorce
- Fear of abandonment
- Increased irritability, whining, tantrums
- Regressive behaviors (e.g., thumb sucking, loss of elimination control)
- Separation anxiety

Later Preschool Children (Ages 3-5 Years)
- Fear of abandonment
- Blame themselves for the divorce; decreased self-esteem
- Bewilderment regarding all human relationships
- Become more aggressive in relationships with others (e.g., siblings, peers)
- Engage in fantasy to seek understanding of the divorce

Early School-Age Children (Ages 5-6 Years)
- Depression and immature behavior
- Loss of appetite and sleep disorders
- May be able to verbalize some feelings and understand some divorce-related changes
- Increased anxiety and aggression
- Feelings of abandonment by departing parent

Middle School-Age Children (Ages 6-8 Years)
- Panic reactions
- Feelings of deprivation—loss of parent, attention, money, and secure future
- Profound sadness, depression, fear, and insecurity
- Feelings of abandonment and rejection

- Fear regarding the future
- Difficulty expressing anger at parents
- Intense desire for reconciliation of parents
- Impaired capacity to play and enjoy outside activities
- Decline in school performance
- Altered peer relationships—become bossy, irritable, demanding, and manipulative
- Frequent crying, loss of appetite, sleep disorders
- Disturbed routine, forgetfulness

Later School-Age Children (Ages 9-12 Years)
- More realistic understanding of divorce
- Intense anger directed at one or both parents
- Divided loyalties
- Ability to express feelings of anger
- Ashamed of parental behavior
- Desire for revenge; may wish to punish the parent they hold responsible
- Feelings of loneliness, rejection, and abandonment
- Altered peer relationships
- Decline in school performance
- May develop somatic complaints
- May engage in aberrant behavior such as lying, stealing
- Temper tantrums
- Dictatorial attitude

Adolescents (Ages 12-18 Years)
- Able to disengage themselves from parental conflict
- Feelings of a profound sense of loss—of family, childhood
- Feelings of anxiety
- Worry about themselves, parents, siblings
- Expression of anger, sadness, shame, embarrassment
- May withdraw from family and friends
- Disturbed concept of sexuality
- May engage in acting-out behaviors

care during the years after the divorce. Family characteristics are more crucial to the child's well-being than specific child characteristics such as age or gender. High levels of ongoing family conflict are related to problems of social development, emotional stability, and cognitive skills for the child.

Feelings of children toward divorce vary with age (Box 27-2). Previously, researchers believed that divorce had a greater impact on younger children, but recent observations indicate that divorce constitutes a major disruption for children of all ages. The feelings and behaviors of children may be different for various ages and gender, but all children suffer stress second only to the stress produced by the death of a parent. Although considerable research has looked at gender differences in children's adjustments to divorce, the findings are not conclusive.

Some children feel a sense of shame and embarrassment concerning the family situation. Sometimes children see themselves as different, inferior, or unworthy of love, especially if they feel responsible for the family dissolution. Although the social stigma attached to divorce no longer produces the emotions it did in the past, such feelings may still exist in small towns or in some cultural groups and can reinforce children's negative self-image. The lasting effects of divorce depend on the children's and the parents' adjustment to the

transition from an intact family to a single-parent family and, often, to a reconstituted family.

Although most studies have concentrated on the negative effects of divorce on youngsters, some positive outcomes of divorce have been reported. A successful post-divorce family, either a single-parent or a reconstituted family, can improve the quality of life for both adults and children. If conflict is resolved, a better relationship with one or both parents may result, and some children may have less contact with a disturbed parent. Greater stability in the home setting and the removal of arguing parents can be a positive outcome for the child's long-term well-being.

Telling the Children

Parents are understandably hesitant to tell children about their decision to divorce. Most parents neglect to discuss either the divorce or its inevitable changes with their preschool child. Without preparation, even children who remain in the family home are confused by the parental separation. Frequently, children are already experiencing vague, uneasy feelings that are more difficult to cope with than being told the truth about the situation.

If possible, the initial disclosure should include both parents and siblings, followed by individual discussions with each child.

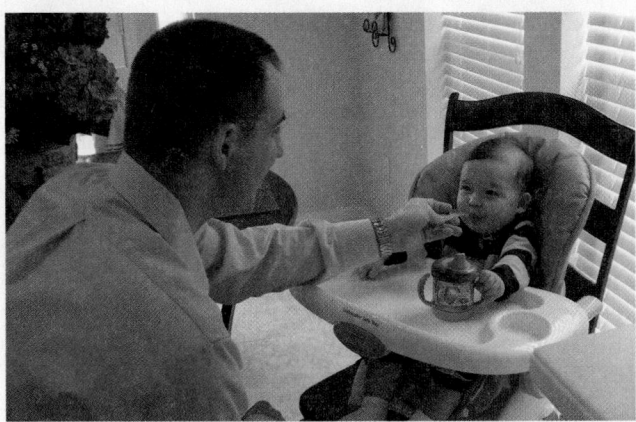

FIG 27-4 Fathers who assume care of their children may feel more comfortable and successful in their parenting role.

Sufficient time should be set aside for these discussions, and they should take place during a period of calm, not after an argument. Parents who physically hold or touch their children provide them with a feeling of warmth and reassurance. The discussions should include the reason for the divorce, if age-appropriate, and reassurance that the divorce is not the fault of the children.

Parents should not fear crying in front of the children, because their crying gives the children permission to cry also. Children need to ventilate their feelings. Children may feel guilt or a sense of failure or that they are being punished for misbehavior. They normally feel anger and resentment and should be allowed to communicate these feelings without punishment. They also have feelings of terror and abandonment. They need consistency and order in their lives. They want to know where they will live, who will take care of them, if they will be with their siblings, and if there will be enough money to live on. Children may also wonder what will happen on special days such as birthdays and holidays, whether both parents will come to school events, and whether they will still have the same friends. Children fear that if their parents stopped loving each other, they could stop loving them. Their need for love and reassurance is tremendous at this time.

Custody and Parenting Partnerships

In the past, when parents separated, the mother was given custody of the children with visitation agreements for the father. Now both parents and the courts are seeking alternatives. Current belief is that neither fathers nor mothers should be awarded custody automatically. Custody should be awarded to the parent who is best able to provide for the children's welfare. In some cases, children experience severe stress when living or spending time with a parent. Many fathers have demonstrated both their competence and their commitment to care for their children (Fig. 27-4).

Often overlooked are the changes that may occur in the children's relationships with other relatives, especially grandparents. Grandparents are increasingly involved in the care of young children (Fergusson, Maughan, and Golding, 2008). Grandparents on the noncustodial side are often kept from their grandchildren, whereas those on the custodial side may be overwhelmed by their adult child's return to the household with grandchildren.

Two other types of custody arrangements are divided custody and joint custody. Divided, or split, custody means that each parent is awarded custody of one or more of the children, thereby separating siblings. For example, sons might live with the father and daughters with the mother.

Joint custody takes one of two forms. In joint physical custody, the parents alternate the physical care and control of the children on an agreed-on basis while maintaining shared parenting responsibilities legally. This custody arrangement works well for families who live close to each other and whose occupations permit an active role in the care and rearing of the children. In joint legal custody, the children reside with one parent but both parents are the children's legal guardians and both participate in childrearing.

Coparenting offers substantial benefits for the family: children can be close to both parents, and life with each parent can be more normal (as opposed to having a disciplinarian mother and a recreational father). To be successful, parents in these arrangements must be highly committed to provide normal parenting and to separate their marital conflicts from their parenting roles. No matter what type of custody arrangement is awarded, the primary consideration is the welfare of the children.

Single Parenting

An individual may acquire single-parent status as a result of divorce, separation, death of a spouse, or birth or adoption of a child. Although divorce rates have stabilized, the number of single-parent households continues to rise. In 2009, 27.3% of children younger than 18 years lived in single-parent families and the majority of single parents were women (Kreider and Ellis, 2011). Although some women are single parents by choice, most never planned on being single parents and many feel pressure to marry or remarry.

Managing shortages of money, time, and energy is often a concern for single parents. Studies repeatedly confirm the financial difficulties of single-parent families, particularly single mothers. In 2004, only one third of mother-headed households received any child support or alimony (Annie E. Casey Foundation, 2009). In fact, the stigma of poverty may be more keenly felt than the discrimination associated with being a single parent. These families are often forced by their financial status to live in communities with inadequate housing and personal safety concerns. Single parents often feel guilty about the time spent away from their children. Divorced mothers from marriages in which the father assumed the role of breadwinner and the mother the household maintenance and parenting roles have considerable difficulty adjusting to their new role of breadwinner. Many single parents have trouble arranging for adequate child care, particularly for a sick child.

Being a teenage parent adds to the financial burden of being a single parent and can have long-term consequences for the mother and child. Poverty is a well-known predictor of adverse effects on a child's health and well-being. Approximately 78% of children born to a teenage mother who did not marry or graduate high school live in poverty. In contrast, only 9% of children born to women older than 20 years who marry and finish high school live in poverty (Annie E. Casey Foundation, 2009).

Social supports and community resources needed by single-parent families include:

- Health care services that are open on evenings and weekends
- High-quality child care
- Respite child care to relieve parental exhaustion and prevent burnout
- Parent enhancement centers for advancing education and job skills, providing recreational activities, and offering parenting education

Single parents need social contacts separate from their children for their own emotional growth and that of their children. Parents

Without Partners, Inc.* is an organization designed to meet the needs of single parents.

Single Fathers

Fathers who have custody of their children have many of the same problems as divorced mothers. They feel overburdened by the responsibility, depressed, and concerned about their ability to cope with the emotional needs of the children, especially girls. Some fathers lack homemaking skills. They may find it difficult at first to coordinate household tasks, school visits, and other activities associated with managing a household alone.

Parenting in Reconstituted Families

In the United States, many of the children living in homes where parents have divorced will experience another major change in their lives such as the addition of a stepparent or new siblings (Coehlo, Kaakinen, Hanson, et al., 2009).

The entry of a stepparent into a ready-made family requires adjustments for all family members. Some obstacles to the role adjustments and family problem solving include disruption of previous lifestyles and interaction patterns, complexity in the formation of new ones, and lack of social supports. Despite these problems, most children from divorced families want to live in a two-parent home.

Cooperative parenting relationships can allow more time for each set of parents to be alone to establish their own relationship with the children. Under ideal circumstances, power conflicts between the two households can be reduced and tension and anxiety can be lessened for all family members. In addition, the children's self-esteem can be increased and continued contact with grandparents is more likely. Flexibility, mutual support, and open communication are critical in successful relationships in stepfamilies and stepparenting situations.

Parenting in Dual-Earner Families

No change in family lifestyle has had more impact than the large numbers of women moving away from the traditional homemaker role and entering the workplace (Coehlo, Kaakinen, Hanson, et al., 2009). Working mothers have become the norm in the United States.

The trend toward increased numbers of dual-earner families is unlikely to diminish significantly. As a result, the family is subject to considerable stress as members attempt to meet often competing demands of occupational needs and those regarded as necessary for a rich family life.

Role definitions are frequently altered to arrange a more equitable division of time and labor, as well as to resolve conflict, especially conflict related to traditional cultural norms. Overload is a common source of stress in a dual-earner family, and social activities are significantly curtailed. Time demands and scheduling are major problems for all individuals who work. When the individuals are parents, the demands can be even more intense. Dual-earner couples may increase the strain on themselves to avoid creating stress for their children. Although no evidence indicates that the dual-earner lifestyle is stressful to children, the stress experienced by the parents may affect the children indirectly.

Maternal employment may have variable effects on preschool children's health (Mindlin, Jenkins, and Law, 2009). The quality of child care is a persistent concern for all working parents. Determinants of child care quality are based on health and safety requirements, responsive and warm interaction between staff and children, developmentally appropriate activities, trained staff, limited group size, age-appropriate caregivers, adequate staff-to-child ratios, and adequate indoor and outdoor space. Nurses play an important role in helping families find suitable sources of child care and prepare children for this experience.

Kinship Care

Since the 1980s, the proportion of children in out-of-home care placed with relatives has increased rapidly. More than 2.6 million U.S. children are raised by grandparents or other kin at some time in their lives (Annie E. Casey Foundation, 2012). According to U.S. Census Bureau data, kinship caregivers are more likely to be poor, single, older, less educated, and unemployed than families in which at least one parent is present.

Foster Parenting

The term foster care is defined as placement in an approved living situation away from the family of origin (Annie E. Casey Foundation, 2012). The living situation may be an approved foster home, possibly with other children, or a preadoptive home. Each state provides a standard for the role of foster parent and a process by which to become one. These "parents" contract with the state to provide a home for children for a limited duration. Most states require about 27 hours of training before being on contract and at least 12 hours of continuing education a year. Foster parents may be required to attend a foster parent support group that is often separate from a state agency. Each state has guidelines regarding the relative health of the prospective foster parents and their families, background checks regarding legal issues for the adults, personal interviews, and a safety inspection of the residence and surroundings (Chamberlain, Price, Leve, et al., 2008).

Nurses should be aware that nearly 700,000 children spend time living in foster care in a given year, many of them facing developmental concerns (Annie E. Casey Foundation, 2012). Children from lower-income, single-mother, and mother-partner families are considerably more likely to be living in foster care (Berger and Waldfogel, 2004). Children in foster care tend to have a higher-than-normal incidence of acute and chronic health problems and may experience feelings of isolation or confusion (Annie E. Casey Foundation, 2012). Foster children are often at risk because of their previous caregiving environment. Nurses should strive to implement strategies to improve the health care for this group of children. In particular, assessment and case management skills are required to involve other disciplines in meeting their needs.

SOCIAL, CULTURAL, AND RELIGIOUS INFLUENCES

Promoting the health of children requires a nurse to understand social, cultural, and religious influences on children and their families. The U.S. population is constantly evolving; patients experience negative health outcomes when social, cultural, and religious factors are not considered as influencing their health care; families may incorporate other health care systems such as Eastern medicine or traditional healing into their lives; and it is required by legislative, regulatory, and credentialing bodies (Tervalon, 2003). Educating health care providers is one way to reduce disparities in health care.

Cultural humility is a "commitment and active engagement in a lifelong process that individuals enter into for an on-going basis

---

*1650 South Dixie Hwy., Suite 402, Boca Raton, FL 33432; 800-637-7974; http://parentswithoutpartners.org.

Cultural Definitions

Culture characterizes a particular group with its values, beliefs, norms, patterns, and practices that are learned, shared, and transmitted from one generation to another (Leininger, 2001). Culture differs from both race and ethnicity. *Race* is a term with roots in anthropology, distinguishing variety in humans by physical traits. *Ethnicity* is the affiliation of a set of persons who share a unique cultural, social, and linguistic heritage. *Gender* is an individual's self-identification as man or woman, and *sex* is the biologic designation of male or female. *Social class* is a complex social construction that usually incorporates levels of education in the family, occupation, income, and access to resources. *Socialization* is the process by which society communicates its competencies, values, and expectations to children (Trawick-Smith, 2006). *Culture* is a complex whole in which each part is interrelated. It is an umbrella term that holds together many interrelated yet unique aspects of humanity, including beliefs, tradition, life ways, and heritage. It is much more than a country of origin or a demographic designation such as African-American or Caucasian.

Five Components of Cultural Competence

Cultural competence includes following five components (Munoz and Luckmann, 2005):
1. **Cultural awareness**—A cognitive process through which the nurse appreciates and is sensitive to the cultural values of the patient and family
2. **Cultural knowledge**—The foundation the nurse builds through formal and informal education that includes world views of different cultures, values, beliefs, and perceptions about health and illness
3. **Cultural skill**—The ability to include cultural data in the nursing assessment through the collection of cultural data in the health interview and observations
4. **Cultural encounter**—The process through which the nurse seeks opportunities to engage in cross-cultural interactions directly or indirectly
5. **Cultural desire**—The genuine and sincere motivation to work effectively with minority patients; can only be achieved if the individual wants to engage in the process of acquiring cultural competence

with patients, communities, colleagues, and themselves" (Tervalon and Murray-Garcia, 1998, p. 118). It requires that health care providers participate in continual process of self-reflection and self-critique that recognizes the power of the health care provider role, that views the patient and family as full members of the health care team, and that does not end after reading one chapter or attending one course but is an evolving aspect of being a health care provider. "Cultural competency is not an abdominal exam" (Kumagai and Lypson, 2009, p. 783). It is not a static endpoint to be checked off the list but an ongoing process that promotes deeper thinking and knowledge of oneself, others, and the world (Kumagai and Lypson, 2009). (See Cultural Competence box.)

It is important to understand nursing's contribution to culturally congruent care. A holistic view of care was first described by Madeleine Leininger, the recognized founder of transcultural nursing, in her culture care diversity and universality theory (Leininger, 2001; Munoz and Luckmann, 2005). The theory provides an intellectual framework and a research methodology for providing culturally congruent patient care. Nurses must remain aware that every family, child, and health care provider comes to a clinical encounter with a cultural lens through which they see and interpret the world.

Cultures and subcultures contribute to the uniqueness of child members in such a subtle way and at such an early age that children grow up to think that their beliefs, attitudes, values, and practices are the "correct" or "normal" ones. By age 5 years, children can identify persons who belong to their cultural background. During later primary years, children can identify those from different cultures (Trawick-Smith, 2006). A set of values learned in childhood is likely to characterize children's attitudes and behavior for life, influencing their long-range goals and their short-range, impulsive inclinations. Thus every ongoing society socializes each succeeding generation to its cultural heritage. (See Cultural Competence box.)

The manner and sequence of the growth and development phenomenon are universal and fundamental features of all children; however, children's varied behavioral responses to similar events are often determined by their culture. Culture plays a critical role in the parenting behaviors that facilitate children's development (Melendez, 2005). Children acquire the skills, knowledge, beliefs, and values important to their own family and culture. Cultural backgrounds can influence the pace of acquisition of cognitive and

motor skills as well as the child's social and emotional development (Trawick-Smith, 2006).

Cultures may also differ in whether status in a group is based on age or on skill. Even children's play and their types of games are culturally determined. In some cultures, children play in groups composed of members of the same gender; in others they play in mixed-gender groups. In some cultures, team games predominate; in others, most play is limited to individual games.

Standards and norms vary from culture to culture and from location to location; a practice that is accepted in one area may meet with disapproval or create tension in another. The extent to which cultures tolerate divergence from the established norm also varies among cultures and subcultural groups. Although conforming to cultural norms provides a degree of security, it is a decided deterrent to change.

⚠ **NURSING ALERT**

American cultures and subcultures can be so diverse that it is essential that nurses be aware of and knowledgeable about the predominant groups in their work community and apply this knowledge in their practice.

Social Roles

Much of children's self-concept comes from their ideas about their social roles. Roles are cultural creations; therefore the culture prescribes patterns of behavior for persons in a variety of social positions. All persons who hold similar social positions have an obligation to behave in a particular manner. A role prohibits some behaviors and allows others. Because culture outlines and clarifies roles, it is a significant influence on the development of children's self-concept (i.e., attitudes and beliefs they have about themselves).

A social group consists of a system of roles carried out in both primary and secondary groups. A **primary group** has intimate, continued, face-to-face contact; mutual support of members; and the ability to order or constrain a considerable proportion of individual members' behavior. Two such groups are the family and the peer group, both of which have a great deal of influence on the child.

Secondary groups are groups that have limited, intermittent contact and generally less concern for members' behavior. These groups offer little in terms of support or pressure toward conformity except in rigidly limited areas. Examples of secondary groups are professional associations and social organizations such as church groups.

A concept of social role also depends largely on whether a child is reared in a primary- or secondary-group community. Children are subjected to perceptibly different forms of parental training in these two types of environments. The influences, strengths, and limitations of both groups are significant.

In a primary-group community (e.g., family; peer group; some contemporary rural, religious, or ethnic communities), all members know each other, most belong to the same subgroups, and all are concerned about each member's behavior. Community members have a high degree of material and psychologic support and one traditional set of values that the entire group agrees on and supports; thus there is little conflict of values. In a stable community where the members remain within comparatively defined limits and relatives are likely to live close together, young members have ample opportunity to observe and absorb cultural practices and customs. Any member of the community feels justified in evaluating and censuring the conduct of another member.

Children reared in the relative isolation of secondary-group environmental influences tend to learn that there is only one acceptable way to respond to any given situation. The entire group agrees, and any tendency to deviate is met with collective disapproval. It is the parents' duty to see that the children learn and follow social roles and modes of behavior defined and strengthened by the views of the community.

The childrearing orientation in a secondary-group environment, such as urban communities, can differ considerably from that of a primary-group environment. The interaction between primary and secondary groups may reinforce values when both groups endorse that value or create confusion or conflict when one group rejects a value accepted by the other. An urban community is dynamic. Many of the traditional behaviors and values may not meet the needs of the changing society. Consequently, parents are often uncertain about what to teach their children. They may wish to rear their children with values consistent with their own, but the differences in experience between the generations are too great. As a result, they often grant their children autonomy in some areas of decision making early in the developmental process and other secondary groups assume a greater influence. None of the groups is highly dominant in its influence; therefore the children are exposed to an eclectic set of values and expectations, some in agreement and some in conflict. From these they must ultimately select those that they determine to be best for them and adopt them to form a consistent set of roles and behaviors to incorporate into the self-concept.

Self-Esteem and Culture

Culture influences a child's sense of self-esteem (Trawick-Smith, 2006). Some cultures are more collective in thought and action. A child from a collective culture will hold an inclusive view of himself or herself. Self-evaluation is related to the accomplishments or competencies of the entire family or community. School experiences that focus on personal achievement may promote positive self-esteem in some children but not in others who depend more on the success of a whole family or peer group. Their sense of control may not come from individual self-reliance but, rather, from a feeling of worth in their family or community (Trawick-Smith, 2006).

Families and culture also influence the criteria children use to evaluate their own abilities. In addition, cultures vary in whether they instill an internal locus of control (a belief in the ability to regulate one's own life). Effects on self-esteem are minimal if these beliefs are directed by parents and are in accordance with cultural customs (Trawick-Smith, 2006). Ethnic pride can help children maintain a positive self-image and counteract the effects of prejudice, which can have a negative impact on emotional health (Trawick-Smith, 2006).

Communities

Surveys of more than 1 million youth in the United States in grades 6 through 12 have shown that persons who experience a higher number of specific assets in their lives are more likely to make healthy choices and avoid high risk behaviors. These assets offer a framework for positive child and adolescent development. The child's or adolescent's community is made up of family, school, neighborhood, youth organization, and other members (Fig. 27-5).

Four categories of external assets that youth receive from the community are (Search Institute, 2007):

1. **Support**—Young people need to feel support, care, and love from their families, neighbors, and others. They also need organizations and institutions that offer positive, supportive environments.
2. **Empowerment**—Young people need to feel valued by their community and be able to contribute to others. They need to feel safe and secure.
3. **Boundaries and expectations**—Young people need to know what is expected of them and what activities and behaviors are within the community boundaries and what are outside of them.
4. **Constructive use of time**—Young people need opportunities for growth through constructive, enriching opportunities and through quality time at home.

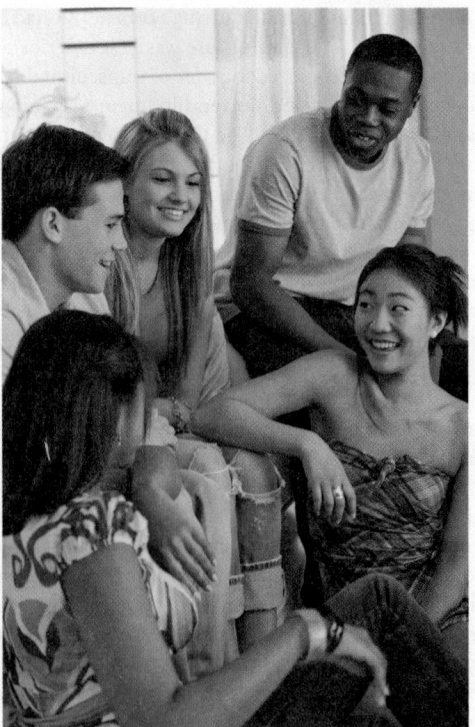

FIG 27-5 Youngsters from different cultural backgrounds interact within the larger culture. (© 2012 Photos.com, a division of Getty Images. All rights reserved.)

Internal assets must also be nurtured in the community's young members. These internal qualities guide choices and create a sense of centeredness, purpose, and focus. The four categories of internal assets are (Search Institute, 2007):

1. **Commitment to learning**—Young people need to develop a commitment to education and lifelong learning.
2. **Positive values**—Youth need to have a strong sense of values that direct their choices.
3. **Social competencies**—Young people need competencies that help them make positive choices and build relationships.
4. **Positive identity**—Young people need a sense of their own power, purpose, worth, and promise.

Peer Groups

Peer groups also have an impact on the socialization of children (Fig. 27-6). Peer relationships become increasingly important and influential as children proceed through school. In school, children have what can be regarded as a culture of their own. This is even more apparent in unsupervised playgroups because the culture in school is partly produced by adults.

During their lives, children are exposed to value systems such as those of the family, ethnic group, and social class. In peer-group interactions, they confront a variety of these sets of values. The values imposed by the peer group are especially compelling because children must accept and conform to them to be accepted as members of the group. When the peer values are not too different from those of family and teachers, the mild conflict created by these small differences serves to separate children from the adults in their lives and to strengthen the feeling of belonging to the peer group.

The kind of socialization provided by the peer group depends on the subculture that develops from its members' background, interests, and capabilities. Some groups support school achievement, others focus on athletic prowess, and still others are decidedly against educative goals. Scholastic achievement is strongly related to the peer group's value system. Many conflicts between teachers and students and between parents and students can be attributed to fear of rejection by peers. What is expected from parents regarding academic achievement and what is expected from the peer culture often conflict, especially during high school.

Although the peer group has neither the traditional authority of the parents nor the legal authority of the schools for teaching information, it manages to convey a substantial amount of information to its members, especially on taboo subjects such as sex and drugs. Children's need for the friendship of their peers brings them into an increasingly complex social system. Through peer relationships, children learn to deal with dominance and hostility and to relate with persons in positions of leadership and authority. Other functions of the peer subculture are to relieve boredom and to provide recognition that individual members do not receive from teachers and other authority figures.

The peer-group culture has secrets, mores, and codes of ethics that promote group solidarity and detachment from adults. They have traditions and folkways, including age-related games and other activities, that are transferred from "generation to generation" of schoolchildren and that have a great influence over the behavior of all group members. As children move from one level to the next, they discard the folkways of the younger group as they adopt those of the new group. For example, a school-age child rides a bicycle to school; the high school student prefers a car. As they advance, children are forward oriented only—they look forward with anticipation but may look backward with contempt.

Cultural Health Beliefs and Practices

Nurses encounter people of many different racial and ethnic origins in the process of meeting the health needs of children and families. Some of these families have become so enculturated to the majority culture that their health beliefs and practices are consistent with those of the health care system. For many families, however, traditional practices and beliefs are an integral part of their daily lives. Health care workers should be aware that other people might live by different rules and priorities, which decisively influence their health-related behavior. Guidelines for exploring a family's culture are found in Box 27-3.

A model for learning about health traditions that differ from the Western, or modern, health care system is based on three dimensions:

1. What are the physical aspects of caring for the body (e.g., are there special clothes, foods, medicines)?
2. What are the mental parts of caring for health (e.g., feelings, attitudes, rituals, actions)?
3. What are the spiritual aspects of health (who I am, spiritual customs, prayers, healers)?

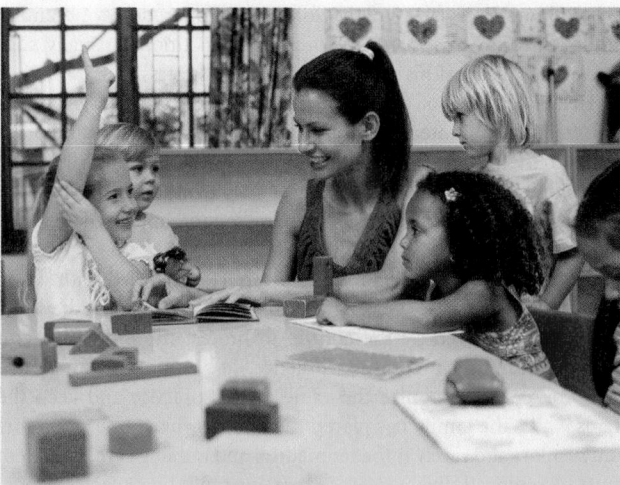

FIG 27-6 Children from a variety of cultural and ethnic backgrounds begin to socialize in the child care setting. (© 2012 Photos.com, a division of Getty Images. All rights reserved.)

BOX 27-3 EXPLORING A FAMILY'S CULTURE, ILLNESS, AND CARE

- What do you think caused your child's health problem?
- Why do you think it started when it did?
- How severe is your child's sickness? Will it have a short or long course?
- How do you think your child's sickness affects your family?
- What are the chief problems your child's sickness has caused?
- What kind of treatment do you think your child should receive?
- What are the most important results you hope to receive from your child's treatment?
- What do you fear most about your child's sickness?

Adapted from Kleinman A, Eisenberg L, Good B: Culture, illness, and care: clinical lessons from anthropologic and cross-cultural research, *Ann Intern Med* 88:251–258, 1978.

For each of these dimensions, one must consider the cultural traditions used to maintain health, protect health, and restore health (Spector, 2009).

Health Beliefs

The beliefs related to the cause of illness and the maintenance of health are integral parts of a family's cultural heritage. Often inseparable from religious beliefs, they influence the way families cope with health problems and respond to health care providers. Predominant among most cultures are beliefs related to natural forces, supernatural forces, and an imbalance between forces.

Natural Forces. The most common natural forces held responsible for ill health if the body is not adequately protected include cold air entering the body and impurities in the air. For example, a Chinese parent may overdress an infant in an effort to keep cold wind from entering the child's body. The Chinese believe that cold weather, rain, or wind is responsible for "cold" conditions. They also believe that an innate energy called *chi* enters and leaves the body through the mouth, nose, and ears and flows through the body in definite pathways, or meridians, at specific times and locations. The Chinese believe that a lack of chi and blood causes fatigue, low energy, and a variety of ailments.

Supernatural Forces. Some cultures view evil influences such as voodoo, witchcraft, or evil spirits as causes of illness, especially illnesses that cannot be explained by other means.

A health belief that is common among people from Latin American, Mediterranean, some Asian, and some African societies is the concept of the "evil eye" (Spector, 2009). It is part of the concept of health as a state of balance and illness as a state of imbalance (see following section). Strength and power are associated with the evil eye; therefore, as long as an individual's strength and weakness remain in balance, he or she is unlikely to become a victim of the evil eye. Weaknesses are not necessarily physical. For example, an excess of some emotion, such as envy, can create weakness. Infants and small children, because of immature development of their internal strength-weakness states, are especially vulnerable to the gaze of the evil eye. Consequently, the evil eye serves to rationalize an inexplicable onset of illness in children who display symptoms such as restlessness, crying, diarrhea, vomiting, and fever.

Imbalance of Forces. The concept of balance or equilibrium is widespread throughout the world. One of the most common imbalances is that which exists between "hot" and "cold." This belief derived from the ancient Greek concept of body humors (Andrews and Boyle, 2008), which states that illness is caused by an imbalance of the four humors: phlegm, blood, black bile, and yellow bile. These are balanced in healthy people and out of balance in those with illnesses. Such imbalance is thought to cause internal damage or altered function. Treatment of the illness is directed at restoring balance. The hot and cold understanding of disease is based in this concept. Diseases, areas of the body, foods, and illnesses are classified as either "hot" or "cold." Foods and beverages are designated hot or cold based on the effect they exert, not their actual temperature. In Chinese health belief, the forces are termed *yin* (cold) and *yang* (hot) (Spector, 2009).

Illness is treated by restoring normal balance through the application of appropriate "hot" or "cold" remedies. A "cold" condition such as a respiratory disease is believed to be caused by exposure to cold weather, rain, or cold wind entering the body; it is treated by administration of "hot" foods, herbs, or drugs. Menstruation is considered a "hot" condition; therefore women are cautioned against ingesting "hot" foods, which might increase menstrual flow or produce cramping. Ingesting too much of either "hot" or "cold" foods can also be interpreted as a cause of illness.

Health care workers who are aware of this belief are better able to understand why some persons refuse to eat certain foods. It is often useful to discuss the diet with the family to determine their beliefs regarding food choices. It is possible to help families devise a diet that contains the necessary balance of basic food groups prescribed by the medical subculture while conforming to the beliefs of the ethnic subculture.

The "hot-cold" food classification may have adverse effects. For example, in some cultures, newborn infants are often started on evaporated milk formulas. Whereas evaporated milk is considered a "hot" food, whole milk is viewed as a "cold" food. Infants tend to develop rashes, which are believed to be caused by "hot" foods; in such cases, parents may decide to switch to whole milk. However, parents fear that it is dangerous to change too rapidly, so they often feed the child some type of neutralizing substance, which may create additional health problems. The nurse can help avoid such a problem by determining the family's preference before discharge from the hospital and prescribing a formula that is agreeable to both the family and the practitioner.

Health Practices

Cultures have numerous similarities regarding prevention and treatment of illness. The folk healers are powerful persons in their community and can acquire information about an illness without resorting to probing questions. They "speak the language" of the family who seeks help and often combine their rituals and potions with prayer and entreaties to God. They also are able to create an atmosphere conducive to successful management. Furthermore, they exhibit a sincere interest in the family and their problem.

Some folk remedies are compatible with the medical regimen and are useful to reinforce the treatment plan. For example, aspirin (a "hot" medication) is an appropriate therapy for "cold" diseases such as arthritis. It is common to discover that a folk prescription has a scientific basis. In any case, respect practices that do not harm patients.

In cultures that believe in the concept, overcoming the effect of the evil eye usually requires specialized rituals conducted by the appropriate practitioner. For example, the Hispanic *curandero* ascertains that the condition is truly the result of the evil eye by performing an assessment ritual and then performs a curative ritual. Sometimes faith in the folk practitioner delays obtaining needed medical treatment, although the practitioner usually suggests medical care if his or her efforts are unsuccessful.

Health practices of different cultures may also present problems of assessment and interpretation. For example, certain cultural practices or remedies can be mistakenly judged as evidence of child abuse by uninformed professionals (Box 27-4). It is important to keep the lines of communication open with families and approach the situation with a sense of cultural humility.

Faith healing and religious rituals are closely allied with many folk-healing practices. Wearing of amulets, medals, and other religious relics believed by the culture to protect the individual and facilitate healing is a common practice. It is important for health care workers to recognize the value of this practice and keep the items where the family has placed them or nearby. It offers comfort and support and rarely impedes medical and nursing care. If an item must be removed during a procedure, it should be replaced, if possible, when the procedure is completed. The nurse should explain the reason for its temporary removal to the family to reassure them their wishes will be respected (see Family-Centered Care box).

BOX 27-4   CULTURAL PRACTICES POSSIBLY CONSIDERED ABUSIVE BY THE DOMINANT CULTURE

Coining—A Vietnamese practice that may produce weltlike lesions on the child's back when the edge of a coin is repeatedly rubbed lengthwise on the oiled skin to rid the body of disease.

Cupping—An Old World practice (also practiced by the Vietnamese) of placing a container (e.g., tumbler, bottle, jar) containing steam against the skin surface to "draw out the poison" or other evil element. When the heated air within the container cools, a vacuum is created that produces a bruiselike blemish on the skin directly beneath the mouth of the container.

Burning—A practice of some Southeast Asian groups whereby small areas of skin are burned to treat enuresis and temper tantrums.

Female genital mutilation (female circumcision)—Removal of or injury to any part of the female genital organ; practiced in Africa, the Middle East, Latin America, India, Asia, North America, Australia, and Western Europe.

Forced kneeling—A child discipline measure of some Caribbean groups in which a child is forced to kneel for a long time.

Topical garlic application—A practice of Yemenite Jews in which crushed garlic cloves or garlic–petroleum jelly plaster is applied to the wrists to treat infectious disease. The practice can result in blisters or garlic burns.

Traditional remedies that contain lead—*Greta* and *azarcon* (Mexico; used for digestive problems), *paylooah* (Southeast Asia; used for rash or fever), and *surma* (India; used as a cosmetic to improve eyesight).

FAMILY-CENTERED CARE

Cultural Awareness

A 15-month-old Bosnian girl in status epilepticus was carried in by her parents. They were frightened and spoke little English. I learned that the child had received a measles, mumps, and rubella (MMR) immunization the day before. As I proceeded to unwrap her from the blanket she was in, I quickly assessed the ABCs (airway, breathing, and circulation). I noticed that she was warm (probably a febrile seizure) and that a rag soaked in alcohol was tied around each thigh. Focusing on her potential airway compromise and trying to calm the parents, I proceeded to put an oxygen mask on her, undress her for a full assessment, and remove the alcohol rags. I spoke to the parents all the while in a calm, soothing voice. Once I had established an intravenous line and given her lorazepam (Ativan), the seizures stopped. So did the communication between her parents and me. I noticed that they would no longer give me eye contact, and the mother would not even speak to me after the seizures stopped. It wasn't until I was returning to the department from admitting her that I realized why they might have stopped communicating with me—I had removed the rags! Had I only thought to replace the rags or asked their permission to remove the rags, things may have been different.

Laura L. Kuensting, MSN(R), RN
Cardinal Glennon Children's Hospital
St. Louis, Missouri

Religious Beliefs and Practices

Religion and spirituality also exert a significant influence on the health of children and families and the decisions made around health and illness. Many immigrants came to the United States for religious freedom and established a religious and moral atmosphere

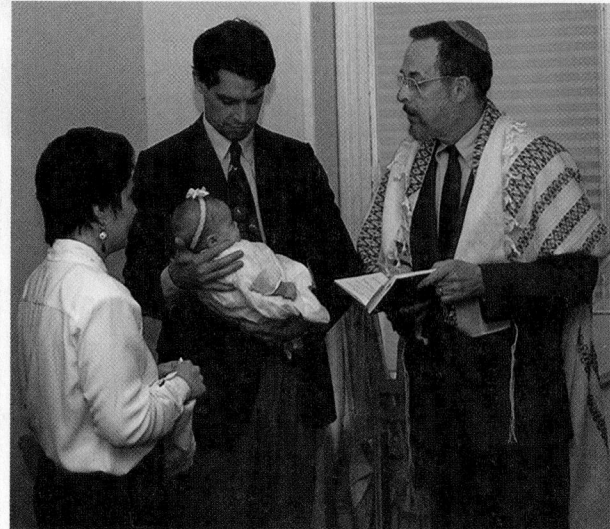

FIG 27-7 Soon after an infant is born, many families have special religious ceremonies.

that persists today. However, individual differences are part of the general culture.

The family's religious orientation dictates a code of behavior and influences the family's attitudes toward education, male and female role identity, and their ultimate destiny. It may also determine the school that the children attend, their companions, and often their mate selection. Religious beliefs are such an integral part of many cultures that it is difficult to distinguish the culture from the religion. In a few instances, such as in the Mennonite and Amish communities, religion is the basis for a common way of life that determines where the children are raised and their lifestyle. It is also important to remember that families who do not subscribe to a particular religion or who are atheist also have beliefs and convictions about family, the surrounding world, and life in general that influence children in these families.

Religious and spiritual dimensions are among the most important influences in many people's lives (Fig. 27-7). The terms *religion* and *spirituality* are often used interchangeably, but this is a mistake. Spirituality is "concerned with the deepest levels of human experiencing, the places of deepest…meaning in and for our lives" (Mercer, 2006). For children, in particular, spirituality possesses a relational consciousness; it concerns the child in relation to the source of power (God, Allah) that gives meaning to the relationship, other people, the surrounding world, and within oneself (Mercer, 2006). Religion, on the other hand, is a particular and culturally influenced representation of human spirituality. Nurses promote holistic nursing care through an integration of spiritual and psychosocial care. The care focuses on activities that support a person's system of beliefs and worship, such as praying, reading religious materials, and performing religious rituals. In addition, it means being attentive and open to the unique spiritual experiences and insight of children. Unfortunately, "such insights may be dismissed as cute or the product of an overactive imagination" (Mercer, 2006). Whereas meeting the spiritual needs of the child and family can provide strength, unmet spiritual needs can result in spiritual distress and debilitation. In practice, application of the nursing process for spiritual care (Box 27-5) can enhance the spiritual well-being of the child and family.

Religious beliefs that relate to health care and that may be a source of conflict between a family and the health care team remind

BOX 27-5	GUIDELINES FOR INTEGRATING SPIRITUAL CARE INTO PEDIATRIC NURSING PRACTICE

- Respect the child's and family's religious beliefs and practices.
- Consider the child's development when talking about spiritual concerns.
- Contact the institution's chaplaincy department for patients and families who have symptoms of spiritual distress or ask for specific religious rituals.
- Become knowledgeable about the religious worldviews of cultural groups found in the patients you care for.
- Encourage visitation with family members, members of the patient's spiritual community, and spiritual leaders.
- Allow children and families to teach you about the specifics of their religious beliefs.
- Develop awareness of your own spiritual perspective.
- Listen for understanding rather than agreement or disagreement.

Adapted from Barnes LL, Plotnikoff GA, Fox K, et al: Spirituality, religion, and pediatrics: intersecting worlds of healing, *Pediatrics* 106(Suppl 4):899–908, 2000; Brooks B: Spirituality. In Kline N, editor: *Essentials of pediatric oncology nursing: a core curriculum*, ed 2, Glenview, IL, 2004, Association of Pediatric Oncology Nurses.

us of the power of ordinary, daily life experience (e.g., childrearing and food preparation) to bring to life the concept of what is sacred (Mercer, 2006). Religion and spirituality influence how individuals view an illness, a treatment regimen, and the role and utility of the health care provider. They also influence actions of food preparation and dietary restrictions and rituals surrounding birth and death. A key role of nurses is to keep communication between the family and health care team open and ask about such influences.

Respecting these rituals is especially important during a physical examination or preparation for surgery. An important role of the nurse is to be aware of families' spiritual needs and convey an attitude of concern for this important element of the child's care. Religion, which offers families understanding and spiritual support, is a valuable asset to health care. Table 27-1 outlines characteristics of selected religions with beliefs that affect nursing care.

In some instances, the rights of the family and the responsibility of the state may be in conflict. For example, Jehovah's Witnesses refuse blood transfusions for themselves and for their children. Parents, by law, have the primary obligation to care for and make decisions about their minor children. However, the legal principle of *parens patriae* says that the state has an overriding interest in the health and welfare of its citizens. Parents' refusal of medical treatment for their child that is deemed essential can be interpreted as neglect. In addition to advocating for the child and family, the nurse's role may include assuming the role of consultant to the staff and family regarding new, alternative methods of transfusion and, if necessary, coordinating with officials to petition juvenile or family court for temporary guardianship of the child.

TABLE 27-1 RELIGIOUS BELIEFS THAT MAY AFFECT NURSING CARE

BIRTH AND DEATH	DIET AND FOOD PRACTICES	MEDICAL CARE
Buddhist		
Birth—No baptism Infant presentation **Death**—Last rite chanting is often practiced at bedside soon after death; the deceased's family or Buddhist priest should be contacted **Organ donation and transplantation**—Organ donation is a matter of individual conscience	Restrictions on some food combinations; extremes must be avoided Some sects are strictly vegetarian Discourage use of alcohol and drugs	Illness is believed to be a trial to aid development of soul; illness results from Karmic causes Surgery is permitted, but extremes must be avoided Cleanliness is of great importance Family, community, and Buddhist priest are supportive visitors
Church of Christ, Scientist (Christian Science)		
Birth—No baptism **Death**—No last rites; autopsy is not permitted except in cases of sudden death; individuals can choose burial or cremation **Organ donation and transplantation**—Church takes no specific position on transplantation as distinct from other medical or surgical procedures Individuals decide on organ donation	Abstain from alcohol and some forms of tea and coffee	Oppose human intervention with drugs or other therapies; however, accept legally required immunizations Accept physical and moral healing Family, friends, and members of spiritual community may visit
Church of Jesus Christ of Latter Day Saints (Mormon)		
Birth—No baptism Infant is blessed by church official at first opportunity after birth (in church) Baptism by immersion at 8 years **Death**—Believe that it is proper to bury the dead in the ground; cremation is discouraged **Organ donation and transplantation**—Individuals can choose whether to will organs to be used in transplants	Prohibit tea (except herbal), coffee, and alcohol Some individuals avoid chocolate and other products that contain caffeine Fasting for 24 hours each month	Devout adherents believe in divine healing Medical therapy is not prohibited Spiritual items—A "garment" (type of underwear) that is considered sacred; person may not want to remove it Family, friends, and church members are supportive visitors

TABLE 27-1   RELIGIOUS BELIEFS THAT MAY AFFECT NURSING CARE—cont'd

BIRTH AND DEATH	DIET AND FOOD PRACTICES	MEDICAL CARE
Hindu **Birth**—No baptism **Death**—Certain prescribed rites are followed after death; priest may tie thread around neck or wrist to signify blessing; family will wash the body; are particular about who touches their dead; bodies are to be cremated **Organ donation and transplantation**—No religious laws prohibiting donation; individual decision	Many dietary restrictions Eating meat is forbidden	With an amputation, loss of a limb is believed to represent sins committed in previous life Accept most modern medical practices; some belief in faith healing Spiritual item—Person may wear a thread around wrist or body; do not remove it Family, community members, and priest are supportive visitors
Islam (Muslim/Moslem) **Birth**—At birth, the first words said to the infant in his or her right ear are Allah-o-Akbar (Allah is great), and the remainder of the Call for Prayer is recited; an Aqeeqa (party) to celebrate the birth of the child is arranged by the parents; male children are circumcised **Death**—At the time of death, specific rituals (e.g., bathing, wrapping the body in cloth) must be done by same-sex Muslim; before moving and handling the body, it is preferable to contact someone from the person's mosque or the local Islamic Society to perform these rituals **Organ donation and transplantation**—Individual decides	Prohibit all pork products and alcohol Fasting is practiced during the ninth month of the Islamic year (Ramadan)	Believers are encouraged in the Qu'ran to seek treatment; it is taught that only Allah cures; however, Muslims are taught not to refuse treatment in the belief that Allah will take care of them because he also chooses at times to work through the efforts of humans Other practices—Right hand is used for eating; left hand is for hygiene Family and friends are supportive visitors
Jehovah's Witnesses **Birth**—No baptism **Death**—No official last rites are practiced when death occurs **Organ donation and transplantation**—Organ donation is forbidden	No tobacco; moderate alcohol permissible	Blood or blood products are not allowed; volume expanders are permissible if not derived from blood
Judaism (Orthodox and Conservative) **Birth**—No baptism Ritual circumcision of male infants on eighth day; performed by mohel (ritual circumciser familiar with Jewish law and aseptic technique) **Death**—According to tradition, during last moments of life, relatives and close friends remain with the deceased Amputated limbs or surgically removed tissues should be made available to family for burial Cremation not allowed **Organ donation and transplantation**—A complex issue; sometimes they are practiced	Numerous dietary kosher laws exist; followers are allowed meat only from animals that are vegetable eaters and are ritually slaughtered; predatory fowl, shellfish, and pork are prohibited Milk products served first can be followed by meat in a few minutes, but milk may not be consumed for several hours after eating meat Fasting is part of Yom Kippur observance Matzo replaces leavened bread during Passover week	May resist surgical procedures during Sabbath, which extends from sundown Friday until sundown Saturday Illness is grounds for violating dietary laws Spiritual items—Men may wear prayer shawl, yarmulke (cap) while praying Family, friends, and rabbi are supportive visitors
Roman Catholic **Birth**—Infant baptism; especially urgent if poor prognosis, when it may be performed by anyone **Death**—Sacrament of the Sick is performed if prognosis is poor while patient is alive **Organ donation and transplantation**—Transplantation of organs is viewed by Catholics as ethically and morally acceptable to the Vatican; organ donation is viewed as an act of charity	Abstaining from meat is practiced on Ash Wednesday, Good Friday, and Fridays during Lent (as a rule)	Encourage anointing of the sick Spiritual items—Rosary beads, crucifix Traditional church teaching does not approve of contraceptives or abortion

Data from Galanti G: *Caring for patients from different cultures,* ed 3, Philadelphia, 2004, University of Pennsylvania Press; Lipson JG, Dibble SL, Minarik PA: *Culture and clinical care: a pocket guide,* San Francisco, 2005, UCSF Nursing Press; Purnell LD, Paulanka BJ: *Transcultural health care: a culturally competent approach,* Philadelphia, 2003, FA Davis; Spector RE: *Cultural diversity in health and illness,* ed 6, Upper Saddle River, NJ, 2004, Pearson Prentice-Hall.

CULTURAL AND RELIGIOUS AWARENESS

Cultural and religious rituals are important practices among families from various cultures. An example is the Jewish upsherenish ceremony, which celebrates a boy's first haircut when he reaches 3 years of age. Any procedure requiring haircutting, such as placement of an intravenous line in a scalp vein, must be discussed with parents to obtain their permission.

Table 27-2 outlines some characteristics of selected cultures. Nurses must assess the cultural and religious practices of families to identify how these practices are similar to and different from those of their own cultural and religious backgrounds.

> **! NURSING ALERT**
>
> These generalizations are presented to help nurses learn the unique beliefs and practices of various groups and are not meant to be stereotypes of any group. It is critical to remember that no cultural group is homogeneous, every racial and ethnic group contains great diversity, and knowledge of a culture may not reflect an individual member's beliefs (Kleinman and Benson, 2006).

Concepts that come from medical anthropology can provide a framework for addressing health care issues. These concepts can have a direct impact on patient care. They lead the nurse away from an ethnocentric or medicocentric view of the health care encounter into the health care reality as constructed by the patient and family.

This is relevant for addressing many of the problems that plague the American health care system, including patient dissatisfaction with the health care they receive, unequal distribution of high-quality health care, and excessive costs (Kleinman and Benson, 2006).

It is also important for nurses to recognize that disease and illness are distinct entities. Clinicians diagnose and treat diseases—that is, abnormalities in the structure and function of body organs and systems. Illness and disease are not interchangeable; illness may occur even when disease is not present, and the course of a disease may vary substantially from the experience of illness.

Illness is culturally constructed; an individual's culture influences how a sickness is perceived, labeled, and explained. Culture also influences the meaning assigned to the illness, the role the individual with the sickness adopts, and the response of the family and community to the sickness.

Tension may arise when the perception of the illness and disease varies widely among the patient, family, and health care team. Failure of health care providers to recognize these disparities may be partially to blame in cases of noncompliance, delivery of inadequate care, and patient or family dissatisfaction. To begin addressing these issues, it is important for nurses to understand the various domains of health care in which individuals operate in American society, including professional (health care providers and institutions), popular (family, community, and lay literature), and folk (nonprofessional healers). Each domain possesses a method for defining and explaining the sickness and what should be done to

TABLE 27-2	BROAD CULTURAL CHARACTERISTICS RELATED TO THE HEALTH CARE OF CHILDREN AND FAMILIES		
HEALTH BELIEFS	**HEALTH PRACTICES**	**FAMILY RELATIONSHIPS**	**COMMUNICATION**
African			
Illness classified as: 　Natural—affected by forces of nature without adequate protection (e.g., cold air, pollution, food and water) 　Unnatural—God's punishment for improper behavior May see illness as the "will of God"	Self-care and folk medicine prevalent Folk therapies usually religious in origin Folk therapies often not shared with the medical provider Prayer as common means for prevention and treatment	Strong kinship bonds in extended family; members come to aid of others in crisis Less likely to view illness as a burden Place strong emphasis on work and ambition Elders cared for and respected	Alert to any evidence of discrimination Place importance on nonverbal behavior Affection shown by touching and hugging Silence may indicate lack of trust Initial eye contact to show respect; maintaining eye contact can be viewed as aggressive Best to use direct but caring approach
Chinese			
A healthy body viewed as gift from parents and ancestors and must be cared for Health seen as one of the results of balance between the forces of yin (cold) and yang (hot)—energy forces that rule the world Illness caused by an imbalance Blood believed to be source of life and is not regenerated Chi is innate energy	Goal of therapy is to restore the balance of yin and yang Acupuncturist needles applied to appropriate meridians identified in terms of yin and yang Acupressure and tai chi replacing acupuncture in some areas Moxibustion—application of heat to skin over specific meridians Wide use of medicinal herbs procured and applied in prescribed ways Meals may or may not be planned to balance hot and cold	Extended family pattern common Strong concept of loyalty of young to old Respect for elders taught at early age—acceptance without questioning or talking back Children's behavior a reflection on family Family and individual honor and "face" important Self-reliance and self-esteem highly valued; self-expression repressed	Open expression of emotions unacceptable Often smile when they do not comprehend Eye contact avoided as a sign of respect

TABLE 27-2	BROAD CULTURAL CHARACTERISTICS RELATED TO THE HEALTH CARE OF CHILDREN AND FAMILIES—cont'd		
HEALTH BELIEFS	**HEALTH PRACTICES**	**FAMILY RELATIONSHIPS**	**COMMUNICATION**
Haitian			
Illness seen as a punishment	Health a personal responsibility	Maintenance of family reputation paramount	Recent immigrants and older persons may speak only Haitian Creole
Natural cause (*maladi bone die*—disease of the Lord) caused by environmental factors, movement of blood within the body, changes between hot and cold, and bone displacement	Foods have properties of "hot" or "cold" and "light" or "heavy" and must be in harmony with one's life cycle and bodily states	Lineal authority supreme; children in a subordinate position in family hierarchy	Often smile and nod in agreement when do not understand
Supernatural (*loa*—spirits' anger)	Natural illnesses treated by home and folk remedies first	Children valued for parental security in old age and expected to contribute to family welfare at an early age	Quiet and gentle communication style and lack of assertiveness lead health care providers to falsely believe they comprehend health teaching and are compliant
Good health seen as the maintenance of equilibrium	May use religious medallions, rosary beads, or figure of saint to pray with		
Prayer and good spiritual habits important			May not ask questions if health care provider is busy or rushed
Japanese			
Shinto religious influence	Energy restored by means of acupuncture, acupressure, massage, and moxibustion along affected meridians	Close intergenerational relationships	Make significant use of nonverbal communication with subtle gestures and facial expression
Human inherently good		Generational categories:	
Evil caused by outside spirits		*Issei*—first generation to live in United States	Tend to suppress emotions
Illness caused by contact with polluting agents (e.g., blood, corpses, skin diseases)	*Kampō* medicine—use of natural herbs	*Nisei*—second generation	Will often wait silently
Health achieved through harmony and balance between self and society	Believe in removal of diseased parts	*Sansei*—third generation	
	Trend is to use both Western and Asian healing methods	*Yonsei*—fourth generation	
	Care for people with disabilities viewed as family's responsibility	Family tends to keep problems to self	
Disease caused by disharmony with society and not caring for body	Take pride in child's good health	Value self-control and self-sufficiency	
	Seek preventive care and medical care for illness	Concept of *haji* (shame) imposes strong control; unacceptable behavior of children reflects on family	
Mexican-American			
Health controlled by environment, fate, and will of God	Seek help from curandero or curandera, especially in rural areas	Strong kinship—extended families include *compadres* (godparents) established by ritual kinship	Spanish speaking or bilingual
Certain illnesses considered "hot" and "cold" states and are treated with food that complements those states	*Curandero(a)* receives position by birth, apprenticeship, or a "calling" via dream or vision	Children valued highly and desired, taken everywhere with family	May have a strong preference for native language and revert to it in times of stress
Disease based on imbalance between individual and environment	Treatments involve use of herbs, rituals, and religious artifacts	Elderly treated with respect	May shake hands or engage in introductory embrace
	Practice for severe illness—make promises, visit shrines, offer medals and candles, offer prayers		Interpret prolonged eye contact as disrespectful
	Adhere to "hot" and "cold" food prescriptions and prohibitions for prevention and treatment of illness		Relaxed concept of time—may be late to appointments
Native American			
Believe health is state of harmony with nature and universe	Distinction made between indigenous health problem requiring native healer or practice and Western disease requiring other medical care	Cultures vary in kinship structure	Use anecdotes or metaphors to discuss a situation
Respect bodies through proper management		Extended family structure—usually includes relatives from both sides of family	Long pauses indicate careful consideration
Depend on individual belief in traditional culture	Health practices include self-sufficiency and harmonious living	Elder members assume leadership roles	Nonverbal communication
Traditional health beliefs holistic and wellness oriented	Participation in religious ceremonies and prayer promotes health		Respect indicated by avoiding eye contact
			Individuals usually speak for themselves

Continued

TABLE 27-2	BROAD CULTURAL CHARACTERISTICS RELATED TO THE HEALTH CARE OF CHILDREN AND FAMILIES—cont'd		
HEALTH BELIEFS	**HEALTH PRACTICES**	**FAMILY RELATIONSHIPS**	**COMMUNICATION**
Puerto Rican			
Subscribe to the "hot-cold" theory of causation of illness Believe some illness caused by evil forces Destiny (*Si Dios quiere*—if God wants) is in control of health	Infrequent use of health care system Seek folk healers (*espiritistas*)—use of herbs, rituals Treatment classified as "hot" or "cold" Many varieties of herbal teas used to treat illness and promote healing	Family usually large and home centered—the core of existence Father has authority in family Great respect for elders Children valued—seen as a gift from God Children taught to obey and respect parents	Spanish speaking or bilingual Strong sense of family privacy—may view questions regarding family as impudent
Vietnamese			
Good health considered to be balance between yin and yang Concept of health based on harmony and balance Rituals used to prevent illness	Family uses all means possible before using outside agencies for health care Regard health as family responsibility; outside aid sought when resources run out Use herbal medicine, spiritual practices, and acupuncture May consider head sacred and feet profane; avoid touching head after feet May use cupping, coin rubbing, or pinching skin May inhale aromatic oils, take herbal teas, or wear strings tied on body	Family is revered institution Multigenerational families Family is chief social network Children highly valued Individual needs and interests subordinate to those of a family group Father is main decision maker Women taught submission to men Parents expect respect and obedience from children	May hesitate to ask questions Questioning authority is sign of disrespect; asking questions considered impolite May avoid eye contact with health care professionals as a sign of respect

Data from Galanti G: *Caring for patients from different cultures,* ed 3, Philadelphia, 2004, University of Pennsylvania Press; Lipson JG, Dibble SL, Minarik PA: *Culture and clinical care: a pocket guide,* San Francisco, 2005, UCSF Nursing Press; Purnell LD, Paulanka BJ: *Transcultural health care: a culturally competent approach,* Philadelphia, 2003, FA Davis; Spector RE: *Cultural diversity in health and illness,* ed 6, Upper Saddle River, NJ, 2004, Pearson Prentice Hall.

address it. The challenge for nurses and other health care providers is to address this disconnect with families and develop mutually agreed-on goals. Nurses are in a prime position to assume this role because understanding the human response to disease is central to their role. In addition, collaboration with the child and family is central to the role of the pediatric nurse.

Not all health care providers feel adequately prepared to care for culturally diverse populations. A study of 1700 resident physicians by Betancourt (2007) revealed that 25% to 30% of them did not feel prepared to deal with families who are mistrustful of the health care system, those with limited English proficiency, those whose health perspective differs from a Western-based model, adults who incorporate other family into the decision-making process, or those who bring their spirituality into the health care environment.

Unfortunately, the numbers may not be too different for nursing and other health care professionals. Such statistics are a wake-up call for anyone who strives for high-quality patient care.

One method of addressing this disconnect with families and beginning collaboration is by understanding the family's explanatory model of illness. The questions in Box 27-3 (Kleinman and Benson, 2006) aim to elicit an individual's beliefs about the disease or illness, the meaning attached to it, goals, and expectations of the outcome and role of the health care provider. Nurses can use these questions to discern areas of discrepancy for further dialog, negotiation, and collaboration. This discussion, when conducted with a genuine interest in the family's and child's perspective, is a significant step in building trusting relationships, promoting adherence, decreasing disparities, and increasing health care satisfaction.

KEY POINTS

- Because there is no agreement about the definition of family, a family is what an individual considers it to be.
- Three areas of special concern to adoptive families include the initial attachment process, the task of telling the children they are adopted, and identity formation during adolescence.
- Marital factors within the home significantly influence a child's development. The impact of divorce on a child depends on the child's age, the outcome, and the quality of the parent-child relationship and parental care after the divorce.

- Single parenting and stepparenting create adjustment difficulties and add stress to the already demanding parental role. Significant numbers of children will live in a single-parent or reconstituted family at some point.
- Culture is the pattern of assumptions, beliefs, and practices encompassing other products of human work and thoughts specific to members of an intergenerational group, community, or population.
- Nurses have a responsibility to understand the influences of culture, race, and ethnicity on the development of social and

emotional relationships, childrearing practices, and attitudes toward health.

- Socioeconomic influences play a major role in opportunities for health promotion and wellness.
- Religious practices greatly influence health-promotion beliefs in families.
- Because verbal and nonverbal communication are important cultural considerations, nurses need to acknowledge and respect their patients' practices for productive interaction to occur.

- Cultural beliefs related to cause of illness and maintenance of health may focus on natural forces, supernatural forces, or an imbalance of forces.
- The practice of cultural humility is continual and an important concept in the nursing process. Nurses can facilitate this process by recognizing cultural differences, integrating cultural knowledge, being aware of their own beliefs and practices, and acting in a culturally appropriate manner.
- No cultural group is homogeneous; every racial and ethnic group contains great diversity.

REFERENCES

Afifi TO, Boman J, Fleisher W, et al: The relationship between child abuse, parental divorce, and lifetime mental disorders and suicidality in a nationally representative adult sample, *Child Abuse Negl* 33(3): 139–147, 2009.

Andrews MM, Boyle JS: *Transcultural concepts in nursing care*, ed 5, Philadelphia, 2008, Lippincott.

Annie E Casey Foundation: *2009 Kids count data book: state profiles of child well-being*, Baltimore, 2009, Author.

Annie E Casey Foundation: *Kinship families*, Author, 2012, http://datacenter.kidscount. org/.

Berger L, Waldfogel J: Out-of-home placement of children and economic factors: an empirical analysis, *Rev Econo Household* 2(4):387–411, 2004.

Betancourt J: Commentary on "Current approaches to integrating elements of cultural competence in nursing education," *J Transcult Nurs* 18(Suppl 25):25S–27S, 2007.

Bomar PJ: *Promoting health in families*, ed 3, Philadelphia, 2004, Saunders.

Centers for Disease Control and Prevention (CDC): *Marriage and divorce*, Atlanta, GA, 2012, Author.

Chamberlain P, Price J, Leve LD, et al: Prevention of behavior problems for children in foster care: outcomes and mediation effects, *Prev Sci* 9(1):17–27, 2008.

Coehlo DP, Kaakinen JR, Hanson SMH, et al: *Family health care nursing*, ed 4, Philadelphia, 2009, Davis.

Fergusson E, Maughan B, Golding J: Which children receive grandparental care and what effect does it have? *Child Psychol Psychiatry* 49(2):161–169, 2008.

Kleinman A, Benson P: Anthropology in the clinic: the problem of cultural competency and how to fix it, *PLoS Med* 3(10): 1673–1676, 2006.

Kreider RM, Ellis R: *Living arrangements of children: 2009*, Curr Popul Rep, pp 70–126, Washington, DC, 2011, US Census Bureau.

Kumagai AK, Lypson ML: Beyond cultural competence: critical consciousness, social justice, and multicultural education, *Acad Med* 84(6):782–787, 2009.

Leininger MM: The theory of culture care diversity and universality. In Leininger MM, editor: *Culture care diversity and universality: a theory of nursing*, Sudbury, MA, 2001, Jones & Bartlett.

Melendez L: Parental beliefs and practices around early self-regulation: the impact of culture and immigration, *Infants Young Child* 18(2):136–146, 2005.

Mercer JA: Children as mystics, activists, sages, and holy fools: understanding the spirituality of children and its significance for clinical work, *Pastoral Psychol* 54(5):497–515, 2006.

Mindlin M, Jenkins R, Law C: Maternal employment and indicators of child health: a systematic review in pre-school children in OECD countries, *J Epidemiol Community Health* 63(5):340–350, 2009.

Munoz CC, Luckmann J: *Transcultural communication in nursing*, Clifton Park, NY, 2005, Thomson Delmar Learning.

Search Institute: Developmental assets lists, 2007, www.search-institute.org/ developmental-assets/lists.

Spector RE: *Cultural diversity in health and illness*, ed 7, Upper Saddle River, NJ, 2009, Prentice-Hall.

Tervalon M: Components of culture in health for medical students' education, *Acad Med* 78(6):570–576, 2003.

Tervalon M, Murray-Garcia J: Cultural humility versus cultural competence: a critical distinction in defining physician training outcomes in multicultural education, *J Health Care Poor Underserved* 9(2): 117–125, 1998.

Trawick-Smith J: *Early childhood development: a multicultural perspective*, ed 4, Upper Saddle River, NJ, 2006, Prentice-Hall.

Velez CE, Wolchik SA, Tein JY, et al: Protecting children from the consequences of divorce: a longitudinal study of the effects of parenting on children's coping processes, *Child Dev* 82(1):244–257, 2011.

Developmental and Genetic Influences on Child Health Promotion

Marilyn J. Hockenberry

evolve WEBSITE
http://evolve.elsevier.com/Perry/maternal

LEARNING OBJECTIVES

On completion of this chapter, the reader will be able to:
- Describe major trends in growth and development.
- Explain the alterations in the major body systems that take place during the process of growth and development.
- Discuss the development and relationships of personality, cognition, language, morality, spirituality, and self-concept.
- Describe the role of play in the growth and development of children.
- Demonstrate an understanding of the role of innate and environmental factors in the physical and emotional development of children.

GROWTH AND DEVELOPMENT

Foundations of Growth and Development

Growth and development, usually referred to as a unit, express the sum of the numerous changes that take place during the lifetime of an individual. The entire course is a dynamic process that encompasses several interrelated dimensions:
- **Growth**—Increase in number and size of cells as they divide and synthesize new proteins; results in increased size and weight of the whole or any of its parts
- **Development**—Gradual change and expansion; advancement from lower to more advanced stages of complexity; the emerging and expanding of the individual's capacities through growth, maturation, and learning
- **Maturation**—Increase in competence and adaptability; aging; usually used to describe a qualitative change; a change in the complexity of a structure that makes it possible for that structure to begin functioning; to function at a higher level
- **Differentiation**—Processes by which early cells and structures are systematically modified and altered to achieve specific and characteristic physical and chemical properties; sometimes used to describe the trend of mass to specific; development from simple to more complex activities and functions

All of these processes are interrelated, simultaneous, and ongoing; none occurs apart from the others. The processes depend on a sequence of endocrine, genetic, constitutional, environmental, and nutritional influences (Seidel, Ball, Dains, et al., 2007). The child's body becomes larger and more complex; the personality simultaneously expands in scope and complexity. Very simply, growth can be viewed as a quantitative change, and development as a qualitative change.

Stages of Development

Most authorities in the field of child development conveniently categorize child growth and behavior into approximate age stages or in terms that describe the features of a developmental age period. The age ranges of these stages admittedly are arbitrary and, because they do not take into account individual differences, cannot be applied to all children with any degree of precision. However, categorization affords a convenient means to describe the characteristics associated with the majority of children at periods when distinctive developmental changes appear and specific developmental tasks must be accomplished. (A **developmental task** is a set of skills and competencies peculiar to each developmental stage that children must accomplish or master to deal effectively with their environment.) It is also significant for nurses to know that there are characteristic health problems peculiar to each major phase of development. The

BOX 28-1   DEVELOPMENTAL AGE PERIODS

Prenatal Period—Conception to Birth

Germinal—Conception to ≈2 weeks

Embryonic—2 to 8 weeks

Fetal—8 to 40 weeks (birth)

A rapid growth rate and total dependency make this one of the most crucial periods in the developmental process. The relationship between maternal health and certain manifestations in the newborn emphasizes the importance of adequate prenatal care to the health and well-being of the infant.

Infancy Period—Birth to 12 Months

Neonatal—Birth to 27 or 28 days

Infancy—1 to ≈12 months

The infancy period is one of rapid motor, cognitive, and social development. Through mutuality with the caregiver (parent), the infant establishes a basic trust in the world and the foundation for future interpersonal relationships. The critical first month of life, although part of the infancy period, is often differentiated from the remainder because of the major physical adjustments to extrauterine existence and the psychologic adjustment of the parent.

Early Childhood—1 to 6 Years

Toddler—1 to 3 years

Preschool—3 to 6 years

This period, which extends from the time children attain upright locomotion until they enter school, is characterized by intense activity and discovery. It is a time of marked physical and personality development. Motor development advances steadily. Children at this age acquire language and wider social relationships, learn role standards, gain self-control and mastery, develop increasing awareness of dependence and independence, and begin to develop a self-concept.

Middle Childhood—6 to 11 or 12 Years

Frequently referred to as the *school age,* this period of development is one in which the child is directed away from the family group and centered around the wider world of peer relationships. There is steady advancement in physical, mental, and social development with emphasis on developing skill competencies. Social cooperation and early moral development take on more importance with relevance for later life stages. This is a critical period in the development of a self-concept.

Later Childhood—11 to 19 Years

Prepubertal—10 to 13 years

Adolescence—13 to ≈18 years

The tumultuous period of rapid maturation and change known as adolescence is considered to be a transitional period that begins at the onset of puberty and extends to the point of entry into the adult world—usually high school graduation. Biologic and personality maturation are accompanied by physical and emotional turmoil, and there is redefining of the self-concept. In the late adolescent period the young person begins to internalize all previously learned values and focus on an individual rather than a group identity.

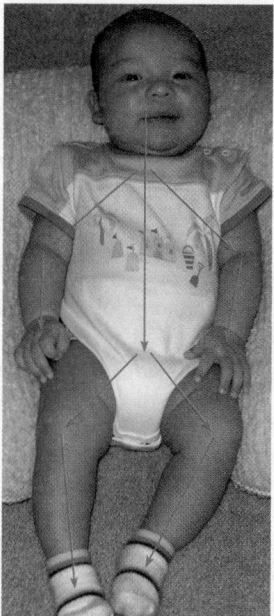

FIG 28-1 Directional trends in growth.

patterns, or trends, are universal and basic to all humans, but each person accomplishes these in a manner and time unique to that individual.

Directional Trends. Growth and development proceed in regular, related directions or gradients and reflect the physical development and maturation of neuromuscular functions (Fig. 28-1). The first pattern is the cephalocaudal, or head-to-tail, direction. The head end of the organism develops first and is large and complex; the lower end is small and simple and takes shape at a later period. The physical evidence of this trend is most apparent during the period before birth, but it also applies to postnatal behavior development. Infants achieve structural control of their heads before they have control of their trunks and extremities, hold their backs erect before they stand, use their eyes before their hands, and gain control of their hands before they have control of their feet.

Second, the proximodistal, or near-to-far, trend applies to the midline-to-peripheral concept. A conspicuous illustration is the early embryonic development of limb buds, which is followed by rudimentary fingers and toes. In infants shoulder control precedes mastery of the hands; the whole hand is used as a unit before the fingers can be manipulated; and the central nervous system develops more rapidly than the peripheral nervous system.

These trends or patterns are bilateral and appear symmetric (i.e., each side develops in the same direction and at the same rate as the other). For some of the neurologic functions this symmetry is only external because of unilateral differentiation of function at an early stage of postnatal development. For example, by the age of approximately 5 years, children have demonstrated a decided preference for the use of one hand over the other, although previously either one had been used.

The third trend, differentiation, describes development from simple operations to more complex activities and functions. From broad, global patterns of behavior, more specific, refined patterns emerge. All areas of development (physical, mental, social, and emotional) proceed in this direction. Through the process of development and differentiation, early embryonic cells with vague, undifferentiated functions progress to an immensely complex organism composed of highly specialized and diversified cells, tissues, and

sequence of descriptive age periods and subperiods that are used here and elaborated on in subsequent chapters is listed in Box 28-1.

Patterns of Growth and Development

There are definite and predictable patterns in growth and development that are continuous, orderly, and progressive. These

organs. Generalized development precedes specific or specialized development; gross, random muscle movements take place before fine-muscle control.

Sequential Trends. In all dimensions of growth and development, there is a definite, predictable sequence, with each child normally passing through every stage. Children crawl before they creep, creep before they stand, and stand before they walk. Later facets of the personality are built on the early foundation of trust. The child babbles and then forms words and finally sentences; writing emerges from scribbling.

Developmental Pace. Although development has a fixed, precise order, it does not progress at the same rate or pace. There are periods of accelerated growth and periods of decelerated growth in both total body growth and the growth of subsystems. Not all areas of development occur at the same pace. When a spurt occurs in one area such as gross motor, minimal advances may take place in language, fine motor, or social skills. After the gross motor skill has been achieved, development focus shifts to another area. The rapid growth before and after birth gradually levels off throughout early childhood. Growth is relatively slow during middle childhood, markedly increases at the beginning of adolescence, and levels off in early adulthood. Each child grows at his or her own pace. Distinct differences are observed among children as they reach developmental milestones.

Sensitive Periods. At limited times during the process of growth the organism interacts with a particular environment in a specific manner. Periods termed critical, sensitive, vulnerable, and optimal are the times in the lifetime of an organism when it is more susceptible to positive or negative influences.

The quality of interactions during these sensitive periods determines whether the effects on the organism will be beneficial or harmful. For example, physiologic maturation of the central nervous system is influenced by the adequacy and timing of contributions from the environment such as stimulation and nutrition. The first 3 months of prenatal life are sensitive periods for physical growth of fetuses.

Psychologic development also appears to have sensitive periods when an environmental event has maximal influence on the developing personality. For example, primary socialization occurs during the first year when the infant makes the initial social attachments and establishes a basic trust in the world. A warm relationship with a parent figure is fundamental to a healthy personality. The same concept might be applied to readiness for learning skills such as toilet training or reading. In these instances there appears to be an opportune time when the skill is best learned.

Individual Differences

Each child grows in his or her own unique and personal way. Great individual variation exists in the age at which developmental milestones are reached. The sequence is predictable; the exact timing is not. Rates of growth vary, and measurements are defined in terms of ranges to allow for individual differences. Some children are fast growers, others are moderate, and some are slower to reach maturity. Periods of fast growth such as the pubescent growth spurt may begin earlier or later in some children than in others. Children may grow fast or slowly during the spurt and may finish sooner or later than other children. Gender is an influential factor because girls seem to be more advanced in physiologic growth at all ages.

Biologic Growth and Physical Development

As children grow their external dimensions change. These changes are accompanied by corresponding alterations in structure and

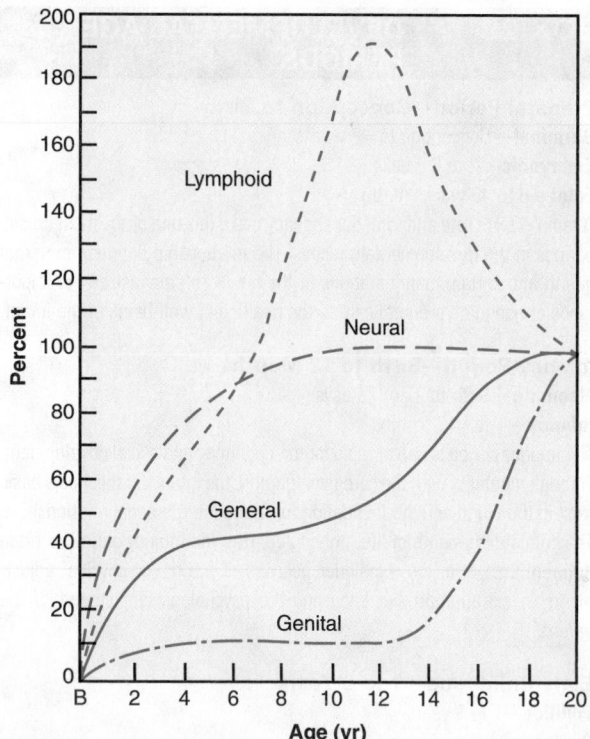

FIG 28-2 Growth rates for the body as a whole and three types of tissues. *Lymphoid:* thymus, lymph nodes, and intestinal lymph masses. *Neural:* brain, dura, spinal cord, optic apparatus, and head dimensions. *General:* body as a whole; external dimension; and respiratory, digestive, renal, circulatory, and musculoskeletal systems. (Data from Jackson JA, Patterson DG, Harris RE: *The measurement of man,* Minneapolis, 1930, University of Minnesota Press.)

function of internal organs and tissues that reflect the gradual acquisition of physiologic competence. Each part has its own rate of growth, which may be directly related to alterations in the size of the child (e.g., the heart rate). Skeletal muscle growth approximates whole body growth; brain, lymphoid, adrenal, and reproductive tissues follow distinct and individual patterns (Fig. 28-2). When growth deficiency has a secondary cause such as severe illness or acute malnutrition, recovery from the illness or the establishment of an adequate diet produces a dramatic acceleration of the growth rate that usually continues until the child's individual growth pattern is resumed.

External Proportions

Variations in the growth rate of different tissues and organ systems produce significant changes in body proportions during childhood. The cephalocaudal trend of development is most evident in total body growth as indicated by these changes. During fetal development the head is the fastest growing body part; at 2 months of gestation it constitutes 50% of total body length. During infancy growth of the trunk predominates; the legs are the most rapidly growing part during childhood; in adolescence the trunk again elongates. In newborn infants the lower limbs are one third the total body length but only 15% of the total body weight; in adults the lower limbs constitute half of the total body height and 30% or more of the total body weight. As growth proceeds the midpoint in head-to-toe measurements gradually descends from a level even with the umbilicus at birth to the level of the symphysis pubis at maturity.

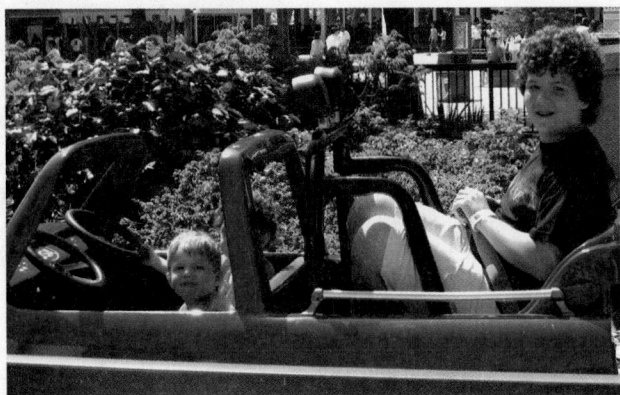

FIG 28-3 Changes in body proportions occur dramatically during childhood.

Biologic Determinants of Growth and Development

The most prominent feature of childhood and adolescence is physical growth (Fig. 28-3). Throughout development various tissues in the body undergo changes in growth, composition, and structure. In some tissues the changes are continuous (e.g., bone growth and dentition); in others significant alterations occur at specific stages (e.g., appearance of secondary sex characteristics). When these measurements are compared with standardized norms, a child's developmental progress can be determined with a high degree of confidence (Table 28-1). Growth in children with Down syndrome differs from that in other children. They have slower growth velocity between 6 months and 3 years and then again in adolescence. Puberty occurs earlier, and they achieve shorter stature. This population of patients is frequent users of the health care system, often with multiple providers, and benefit from the use of the Down syndrome growth chart to monitor their growth (Cronk, Crocker, Pueschel, et al., 1988; Myrelid, Gustafsson, Ollars, et al., 2002).

Linear growth, or height, occurs almost entirely as a result of skeletal growth and is considered a stable measurement of general growth. Growth in height is not uniform throughout life but ceases when maturation of the skeleton is complete. The maximum rate of growth in length occurs before birth, but newborns continue to grow at a rapid although slower rate.

At birth, weight varies more than height and is to a greater extent a reflection of the intrauterine environment. The average newborn weighs from 3175 to 3400 g (7 to 7.5 lbs). In general the birth weight doubles by 4 to 7 months of age and triples by the end of the first year. By the age of 2 to 2.5 years the birth weight usually quadruples. After this point the "normal" rate of weight gain, just as the growth in height, assumes a steady annual increase of approximately 2 to 2.75 kg (4.4 to 6 lbs) per year until the adolescent growth spurt.

Both bone age determinants and state of dentition are used as indicators of development. Because both are discussed elsewhere, neither is elaborated here (see next section for bone age; see also Chapter 31 for dentition).

Skeletal Growth and Maturation

The most accurate measure of general development is skeletal or bone age, the radiologic determination of osseous maturation. Skeletal age appears to correlate more closely with other measures of physiologic maturity (e.g., onset of menarche) than with chronologic age or height. Bone age is determined by comparing the mineralization of ossification centers and advancing bony form to age-related standards.

TABLE 28-1	GENERAL TRENDS IN HEIGHT AND WEIGHT GAIN DURING CHILDHOOD	
AGE-GROUP	**WEIGHT***	**HEIGHT***
Infants		
Birth-6 months	Weekly gain: 140-200 g (5-7 oz) Birth weight doubles by end of first 4-7 months†	Monthly gain: 2.5 cm (1 inch)
6-12 months	Weight gain: 85-140 g (3-5 oz) Birth weight triples by end of first year	Monthly gain: 1.25 cm (0.5 inch) Birth length increases by ≈50% by end of first year
Toddlers	Birth weight quadruples by age 2.5	Height at age 2 is ≈50% of eventual adult height Gain during second year: about 12 cm (4.7 inches) Gain during third year: about 6-8 cm (2.4-3.1 inches)
Preschoolers	Annual gain: 2-3 kg (4.5-6.5 lbs)	Birth length doubles by age 4 years Annual gain: 5-7.5 cm (2-3 inches)
School-age children	Annual gain: 2-3 kg (4.5-6.5 lbs)	Annual gain after age 7: 5 cm (2 inches) Birth length triples by about age 13 years
Pubertal Growth Spurt		
Females 10-14 years	Weight gain: 7-25 kg (15.5-55 lbs) Mean: 17.5 kg (38.5 lbs)	Height gain: 5-25 cm (2-10 inches); ≈95% of mature height achieved by onset of menarche or skeletal age of 13 years Mean: 20.5 cm (8 inches)
Males 11-16 years	Weight gain: 7-30 kg (15.5-66 lbs) Mean: 23.7 kg (52.2 lbs)	Height gain: 10-30 cm (4-12 inches); ≈95% of mature height achieved by skeletal age of 15 years Mean: 27.5 cm (11 inches)

*Annual height and weight gains for each age-group represent averaged estimates from a variety of sources.
†Jung FE, Czajka-Narins DM: Birth weight doubling and tripling times: an updated look at the effects of birth weight, sex, race, and type of feeding, *Am J Clin Nutr* 42:182–189, 1985.

Bone formation begins during the second month of fetal life when calcium salts are deposited in the intercellular substance (matrix) to form calcified cartilage first and then true bone. Bone formation exhibits some differences. In small bones the bone continues to form in the center, and cartilage continues to be laid down on the surfaces. In long bones the ossification begins in the diaphysis (the long central portion of the bone) and continues in the epiphysis (the end portions of the bone). Between the diaphysis and the epiphysis, an epiphyseal cartilage plate (or growth plate) unites with the diaphysis by columns of spongy tissue, the metaphysis. Active growth in length takes place in the epiphyseal growth plate. Interference with this growth site by trauma or infection can result in deformity.

The first centers of ossification appear in 2-month-old embryos, and at birth the number is approximately 400, about half the number at maturity. New centers appear at regular intervals during the growth period and provide the basis for assessment of bone age. Postnatally the earliest centers to appear (at 5 to 6 months of age) are those of the capitate and hamate bones in the wrist. Therefore radiographs of the hand and wrist provide the most useful areas for screening to determine skeletal age, especially before age 6 years. These centers appear earlier in girls than in boys.

Nurses must understand that the growing bones of children possess many unique characteristics. Bone fractures occurring at the growth plate may be difficult to discover and may significantly affect subsequent growth and development (Urbanski and Hanlon, 1996). Factors that may influence skeletal muscle injury rates and types in children and adolescents include (Caine, DiFiori, and Maffulli, 2006; Kaczander, 1997):

- Less protective sports equipment for children.
- Less emphasis on conditioning, especially flexibility.
- In adolescents, fractures are more common than ligamentous ruptures because of the rapid growth rate of the physeal (segment of tubular bone that is concerned mainly with growth) zone of hypertrophy.

Neurologic Maturation

In contrast to other body tissues, which grow rapidly after birth, the nervous system grows proportionately more rapidly before birth. Two periods of rapid brain cell growth occur during fetal life: a dramatic increase in the number of neurons between 15 and 20 weeks of gestation and another increase at 30 weeks, which extends to 1 year of age. The rapid growth of infancy continues during early childhood and slows to a more gradual rate during later childhood and adolescence.

Postnatal growth consists of increasing the amount of cytoplasm around the nuclei of existing cells, increasing the number and intricacy of communications with other cells, and advancing their peripheral axons to keep pace with expanding body dimensions. This allows for increasingly complex movement and behavior. Neurophysiologic changes also provide the foundation for language, learning, and behavior development. Neurologic or electroencephalographic development is sometimes used as an indicator of maturational age in the early weeks of life.

Lymphoid Tissues

Lymphoid tissues contained in the lymph nodes, thymus, spleen, tonsils, adenoids, and blood lymphocytes follow a growth pattern unlike that of other body tissues. These tissues are small in relation to total body size, but they are well developed at birth. They increase rapidly to reach adult dimensions by 6 years of age and continue to grow. At approximately 10 to 12 years of age they reach a maximum development that is approximately twice their adult size. This is followed by a rapid decline to stable adult dimensions by the end of adolescence.

Development of Organ Systems

All tissues and organ systems undergo changes during development. Some are striking; others are subtle. Many have implications for assessment and care. Because the major importance of these changes relates to their dysfunction, the developmental characteristics of various systems and organs are discussed throughout the book as

they relate to these areas. Physical characteristics and physiologic changes that vary with age are included in age-group descriptions.

Physiologic Changes

Physiologic changes that take place in all organs and systems are discussed as they relate to dysfunction. Other changes such as pulse and respiratory rates and blood pressure are an integral part of physical assessment (see Chapter 29). In addition, there are changes in basic functions, including metabolism, temperature, and patterns of sleep and rest.

Metabolism

The rate of metabolism when the body is at rest (basal metabolic rate or BMR) demonstrates a distinctive change throughout childhood. Highest in newborn infants, the BMR closely relates to the proportion of surface area to body mass, which changes as the body increases in size. In both sexes the proportion decreases progressively to maturity. The BMR is slightly higher in boys at all ages and further increases during pubescence over that in girls.

The rate of metabolism determines the caloric requirements of the child. The basal energy requirement of infants is about 108 kcal/kg of body weight and decreases to 40 to 45 kcal/kg at maturity. Water requirements throughout life remain at approximately 1.5 mL/calorie of energy expended. Children's energy needs vary considerably at different ages and with changing circumstances. The energy requirement to build tissue steadily decreases with age following the general growth curve; however, energy needs vary with the individual child and may be considerably higher. For short periods (e.g., during strenuous exercise) and more prolonged periods (e.g., illness), the needs can be very high.

Temperature

Body temperature, reflecting metabolism, decreases over the course of development (see Appendix C). Thermoregulation is one of the most important adaptation responses of infants during the transition from intrauterine to extrauterine life. In healthy neonates hypothermia can result in several negative metabolic consequences such as hypoglycemia, elevated bilirubin levels, and metabolic acidosis. Skin-to-skin care, also referred to as *kangaroo care,* is an effective way to prevent neonatal hypothermia in infants. Unclothed, diapered infants are placed on the parent's bare chest after birth, promoting thermoregulation and attachment (Galligan, 2006). After the unstable regulatory ability in the neonatal period, heat production steadily declines as the infant grows into childhood. Individual differences of 0.5° to 1° F are normal, and occasionally a child normally displays an unusually high or low temperature. Beginning at approximately 12 years of age, girls display a temperature that remains relatively stable, but the temperature in boys continues to fall for a few more years. Females maintain a temperature slightly above that of males throughout life.

Even with improved temperature regulation, infants and young children are highly susceptible to temperature fluctuations. Body temperature responds to changes in environmental temperature and is increased with active exercise, crying, and emotional stress. Infections can cause a higher and more rapid temperature increase in infants and young children than in older children. In relation to body weight, an infant produces more heat per unit than adolescents. Consequently during active play or when heavily clothed, an infant or small child is likely to become overheated.

Sleep and Rest

Sleep, a protective function in all organisms, allows for repair and recovery of tissues after activity. As in most aspects of development,

Healthy Food Choices

Current research indicates that new lower fat recipes in school lunch programs are well accepted by children (Matvienko, 2007). However, less-healthy foods are still more readily available than more-healthy foods in schools in the United States (Delva, O'Malley, and Johnston, 2007).

individual children vary widely in the amount and distribution of sleep at various ages. As they mature the total time they spend in sleep and the amount of time they spend in deep sleep changes.

Newborn infants sleep much of the time that is not occupied with feeding and other aspects of their care. As they grow older, the total time spent in sleep gradually decreases, they remain awake for longer periods, and they sleep longer at night. For example, the length of a sleep cycle increases from approximately 50 to 60 minutes in newborn infants to approximately 90 minutes in adolescents (Anders, Sadeh, and Appareddy, 2005). During the latter part of the first year, most children sleep through the night and take one or two naps during the day. By the time they are 12 to 18 months old, most children have eliminated the second nap. After age 3 years children have usually given up daytime naps except in cultures in which an afternoon nap or siesta is customary. Sleep time declines slightly from ages 4 to 10 years and increases somewhat during the pubertal growth spurt.

The quality of sleep changes as children mature. As they develop through adolescence, their need for sleep does not decline; but their opportunity for sleep may be affected by social, activity, and academic schedules. The time spent in deep, restful sleep increases from 50% in infancy to 80% in older children.

Nutrition

Nutrition is probably the single most important influence on growth. Dietary factors regulate growth at all stages of development, and their effects are exerted in numerous and complex ways. During the rapid prenatal growth period poor nutrition may influence development from the time of implantation of the ovum until birth. During infancy and childhood the demand for calories is relatively great, as evidenced by the rapid increase in both height and weight. At this time protein and caloric requirements are higher than at almost any period of postnatal development. As the growth rate slows with its concomitant decrease in metabolism, caloric and protein requirements are reduced correspondingly.

Growth is uneven during the periods of childhood between infancy and adolescence, when there are plateaus and small growth spurts. Children's appetites fluctuate in response to these variations until the turbulent growth spurt of adolescence, when adequate nutrition is extremely important but may be subjected to numerous emotional influences. Adequate nutrition is closely related to good health throughout life, and an overall improvement in nourishment is evidenced by the gradual increase in size and early maturation of children in this century (see Community Focus box).

Temperament

Temperament is defined as "the manner of thinking, behaving, or reacting characteristic of an individual" (Chess and Thomas, 1999) and refers to the way in which a person deals with life. From the time of birth children exhibit marked individual differences in the way they respond to their environment and the way others, particularly the parents, respond to them and their needs. A genetic basis has been suggested for some differences in temperament. Nine characteristics of temperament have been identified through interviews

Activity—Level of physical motion during activity such as sleeping, eating, playing, dressing, and bathing

Rhythmicity—Regularity in the timing of physiologic functions such as hunger, sleep, and elimination

Approach-withdrawal—Nature of initial responses to a new stimulus such as people, situations, places, foods, toys, and procedures. (**Approach** responses are positive and displayed by activity or expression; **withdrawal** responses are negative expressions or behaviors.)

Adaptability—Ease or difficulty with which the child adapts or adjusts to new or altered situations

Threshold of responsiveness (sensory threshold)—Amount of stimulation such as sounds or light required to evoke a response in the child

Intensity of reaction—Energy level of the child's reactions regardless of quality or direction

Mood—Amount of pleasant, happy, friendly behavior compared with unpleasant, unhappy, crying, unfriendly behavior exhibited by the child in various situations

Distractibility—Ease with which a child's attention or direction of behavior can be diverted by external stimuli

Attention span and persistence—Length of time a child pursues a given activity (**attention**) and the continuation of an activity despite obstacles (**persistence**)

with parents (Box 28-2). Temperament refers to behavioral tendencies, not to discrete behavioral acts. There are no implications of good or bad. Most children can be placed into one of three common categories based on their overall pattern of temperamental attributes:

- The easy child—Easygoing children are even tempered, are regular and predictable in their habits, and have a positive approach to new stimuli. They are open and adaptable to change and display a mild-to–moderately intense mood that is typically positive. Approximately 40% of children fall into this category.
- The difficult child—Difficult children are highly active, irritable, and irregular in their habits. Negative withdrawal responses are typical, and they require a more structured environment. These children adapt slowly to new routines, people, and situations. Mood expressions are usually intense and primarily negative. They exhibit frequent periods of crying, and frustration often produces violent tantrums. This group represents about 10% of children.
- The slow-to-warm-up child—Slow-to-warm-up children typically react negatively and with mild intensity to new stimuli and, unless pressured, adapt slowly with repeated contact. They respond with only mild but passive resistance to novelty or changes in routine. They are inactive and moody but show only moderate irregularity in functions. Fifteen percent of children demonstrate this temperament pattern.

Thirty-five percent of children either have some, but not all, of the characteristics of one of the categories or are inconsistent in their behavioral responses. Many normal children demonstrate this wide range of behavioral patterns.

Significance of Temperament

Observations indicate that children who display the difficult or slow-to-warm-up patterns of behavior are more vulnerable to the development of behavior problems in early and middle childhood. Any child can develop behavior problems if there is dissonance between his or her temperament and the environment. Demands for change and adaptation that are in conflict with the child's capacities can become excessively stressful. However, authorities emphasize that it is not the temperament patterns of children that place them at risk; rather it is the degree of fit between children and their environment, specifically their parents, that determines the degree of vulnerability. The potential for optimum development exists when environmental expectations and demands fit with the individual's style of behavior and the parents' ability to navigate this period (Chess and Thomas, 1999).

Early identification of temperament provides a useful tool for caregivers in anticipating probable areas of difficulty or risk associated with development. For example, "difficult" children may be prone to colic in infancy; active children require more vigilance to prevent injury; and school entry requires different approaches for children with different temperaments.

Research indicates that irritable and unadaptable infants can raise doubts in mothers about their competence (Beck, 1996). Additional research indicates that a child's temperament can affect parent-child interactions and influence the parents' self-esteem, marital harmony, mood, and overall satisfaction as parents (Carey, 1998). Studies on the relationship between temperament and the ability to perform a task successfully (mastery motivation) have found that infants with high mastery are more cooperative and less difficult (Morrow and Camp, 1996). Principles that can be used by nurses in direct patient care and providing anticipatory guidance are listed in Box 28-3.

DEVELOPMENT OF PERSONALITY AND MENTAL FUNCTION

Personality and cognitive skills develop in much the same manner as biologic growth—new accomplishments build on previously mastered skills. Many aspects depend on physical growth and maturation. This is not a comprehensive account of the multiple facets of personality and behavior development. Many aspects are integrated with the child's emotional and social development in a later discussion of various age-groups. Table 28-2 summarizes some of the developmental theories.

Theoretic Foundations of Personality Development
Psychosexual Development (Freud)

According to Freud all human behavior is energized by psychodynamic forces, and this psychic energy is divided among three components of personality: the id, ego, and superego (Freud, 1933). The id, the unconscious mind, is the inborn component that is driven by instincts. It obeys the pleasure principle of immediate gratification of needs, regardless of whether the object or action can actually do so. The ego, the conscious mind, serves the reality principle. It functions as the conscious or controlling self that is able to find realistic means for gratifying the instincts while blocking the irrational thinking of the id. The superego, the conscience, functions as the moral arbitrator and represents the ideal. It is the mechanism

---

BOX 28-3	ACTIVITIES TO PROMOTE MASTERY MOTIVATION

- Encourage unobtrusive assistance during play.
- Share pleasure with infant in accomplishments.
- Don't give immediate assistance during tasks.
- Don't interrupt infant during tasks.
- Let infant initiate activities.
- Limit controlling feedback during play.
- Provide audio and visually responsive toys.
- Provide early kinesthetic stimulation (picking up, rocking).

From Morrow JD, Camp BW: Mastery motivation and temperament of 7-month-old infants, *Pediatr Nurs* 22(3):211–217, 1996.

TABLE 28-2	SUMMARY OF PERSONALITY, COGNITIVE, AND MORAL DEVELOPMENT THEORIES			
PSYCHOSEXUAL (FREUD)	PSYCHOSOCIAL (ERIKSON)	COGNITIVE (PIAGET)	MORAL JUDGMENT (KOHLBERG)	SPIRITUAL (FOWLER)
I. Infancy: Birth to 1 Year				
Oral	Trust vs. mistrust	Sensorimotor (birth-2 years)		Undifferentiated
II. Toddlerhood: 1 to 3 Years				
Anal	Autonomy vs. shame and doubt	Preoperational thought, preconceptual phase (transductive reasoning [e.g., specific to specific]) (2-4 years)	Preconventional (premoral) level Punishment and obedience orientation	Intuitive-projective
III. Early Childhood: 3 to 6 Years				
Phallic	Initiative vs. guilt	Preoperational thought, intuitive phase (transductive reasoning) (4-7 years)	Preconventional (premoral) level Naive instrumental orientation	Mythical-literal
IV. Middle Childhood: 6 to 12 Years				
Latency	Industry vs. inferiority	Concrete operations (inductive reasoning and beginning logic) (7-11 years)	Conventional level Good-boy, nice-girl orientation Law-and-order orientation	Synthetic-convention
V. Adolescence: 12-18 Years				
Genital	Identity vs. role confusion	Formal operations (deductive and abstract reasoning) (11-15 years)	Postconventional or principled level Social-contract orientation	Individuating-reflexive

that prevents individuals from expressing undesirable instincts that might threaten the social order.

Freud considered the sexual instincts to be significant in the development of the personality (Freud, 1964). However, he used the term psychosexual to describe any sensual pleasure. During childhood certain regions of the body assume a prominent psychologic significance as the source of new pleasures and conflicts gradually shifts from one part of the body to another at particular stages of development:

- **Oral stage** (birth to 1 year)—During infancy the major source of pleasure seeking is centered on oral activities such as sucking, biting, chewing, and vocalizing. Children may prefer one of these over the others, and the preferred method of oral gratification can provide some indication of the personality they develop.
- **Anal stage** (1 to 3 years)—Interest during the second year of life centers in the anal region as sphincter muscles develop and children are able to withhold or expel fecal material at will. At this stage the climate surrounding toilet training can have lasting effects on children's personalities.
- **Phallic stage** (3 to 6 years)—During the phallic stage the genitalia become an interesting and sensitive area of the body. Children recognize differences between the sexes and become curious about the dissimilarities. This is the period around which the controversial issues of the Oedipus and Electra complexes, penis envy, and castration anxiety are centered.
- **Latency period** (6 to 12 years)—During the latency period children elaborate on previously acquired traits and skills. Physical and psychic energy is channeled into acquisition of knowledge and vigorous play.
- **Genital stage** (age 12 years and older)—The last significant stage begins at puberty with maturation of the reproductive system and production of sex hormones. The genital organs become the major source of sexual tensions and pleasures, but energies are also invested in forming friendships and preparing for marriage.

Psychosocial Development (Erikson)

The most widely accepted theory of personality development is that advanced by Erikson (1963). Although built on Freudian theory, it is known as psychosocial development and emphasizes a healthy personality as opposed to a pathologic approach. Erikson also uses the biologic concepts of critical periods and epigenesis, describing key conflicts or core problems that the individual strives to master during critical periods in personality development. Successful completion or mastery of each of these core conflicts is built on the satisfactory completion or mastery of the previous stage.

Each psychosocial stage has two components (i.e., the favorable and the unfavorable aspects of the core conflict), and progress to the next stage depends on resolution of this conflict. No core conflict is ever mastered completely but remains a recurrent problem throughout life. No life situation is ever secure. Each new situation presents the conflict in a new form. For example, when children who have satisfactorily achieved a sense of trust encounter a new experience (e.g., hospitalization), to master the situation they must again develop a sense of trust in those responsible for their care. Erikson's life-span approach to personality development consists of eight stages; however, only the first five relating to childhood are included here:

- **Trust versus mistrust** (birth to 1 year)—The first and most important attribute to develop for a healthy personality is basic trust. Establishing basic trust dominates the first year of life and describes all of the child's satisfying experiences at this age. Corresponding to Freud's oral stage, it is a time of "getting" and "taking in" through all the senses. It exists only in relation to something or someone; therefore consistent, loving care by a mothering person is essential for development of trust. **Mistrust** develops when trust-promoting experiences are deficient or lacking or basic needs are inconsistently or inadequately met. Although shreds of mistrust are sprinkled throughout the personality, from a basic trust in parents stems trust in the world, other people, and oneself. The result is faith and optimism.
- **Autonomy versus shame and doubt** (1 to 3 years)—Corresponding to Freud's anal stage, the problem of autonomy can be symbolized by the holding on and letting go of the sphincter muscles. The development of autonomy during the toddler period is centered on children's increasing ability to control their bodies, themselves, and their environment. They want to do things for themselves using their newly acquired motor skills of walking, climbing, and manipulating and their mental powers of selecting and decision making. Much of their learning is acquired by imitating the activities and behavior of others. Negative feelings of doubt and shame arise when children are made to feel small and self-conscious, when their choices are disastrous, when others shame them, or when they are forced to be dependent in areas in which they are capable of assuming control. The favorable outcomes are self-control and willpower.
- **Initiative versus guilt** (3 to 6 years)—The stage of initiative corresponds to Freud's phallic stage and is characterized by vigorous, intrusive behavior; enterprise; and a strong imagination. Children explore the physical world with all their senses and powers (Fig. 28-4). They develop a conscience. No longer guided only by outsiders, they have an inner voice that warns and threatens. Children sometimes undertake goals or activities that are in conflict with those of parents or others, and being made to feel that their activities or imaginings are bad produces a sense of guilt. They must learn to retain a sense of initiative without impinging on the rights and privileges of others. The lasting outcomes are direction and purpose.

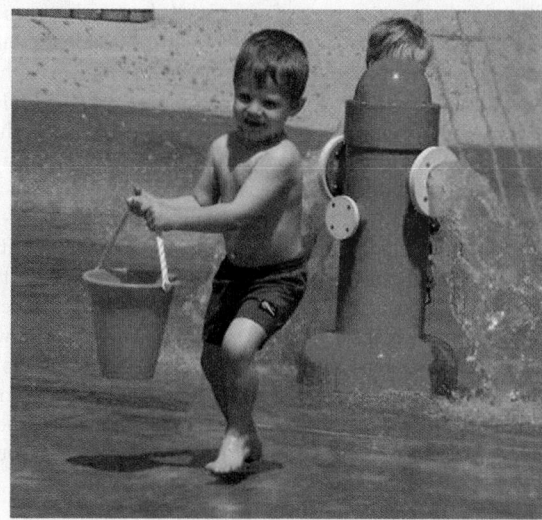

FIG 28-4 The stage of initiative is characterized by physical activity and imagination while children explore the physical world around them.

- **Industry versus inferiority** (6 to 12 years)—The stage of industry is the latency period of Freud. Having achieved the more crucial stages in personality development, children are ready to be workers and producers. They want to engage in tasks and activities that they can carry through to completion; they need and want real achievement. Children learn to compete and cooperate with others, and they learn the rules. It is a decisive period in their social relationships with others. Feelings of inadequacy and inferiority may develop if too much is expected of them or if they believe that they cannot measure up to the standards set for them by others. The ego quality developed from a sense of industry is competence.

- **Identity versus role confusion** (12 to 18 years)—Corresponding to Freud's genital period, the development of identity is characterized by rapid and marked physical changes. Previous trust in their bodies is shaken, and children become overly preoccupied with the way they appear in the eyes of others compared with their own self-concept. Adolescents struggle to fit the roles they have played and those they hope to play with the current roles and fashions adopted by their peers, to integrate their concepts and values with those of society, and to come to a decision regarding an occupation. An inability to solve the core conflict results in role confusion. The outcome of successful mastery is devotion and fidelity to others and to values and ideologies.

Theoretic Foundations of Intellectual Development

The term *cognition* refers to the process by which developing individuals become acquainted with the world and the objects it contains. Children are born with inherited potentials for intellectual growth, but they must develop that potential through interaction with the environment. By assimilating information through the senses, processing it, and acting on it, they come to understand relationships between objects and between themselves and their world. With cognitive development children acquire the ability to reason abstractly, think in a logical manner, and organize intellectual functions or performances into higher-order structures. Language, morals, and spiritual development emerge as cognitive abilities advance.

Cognitive Development (Piaget)

Cognitive development consists of age-related changes that occur in mental activities. The best-known theory regarding children's thinking, and a more comprehensive developmental theory than those already described, was developed by the Swiss psychologist Jean Piaget (1969). According to Piaget intelligence enables individuals to make adaptations to the environment that increase the probability of survival; and through their behavior individuals establish and maintain equilibrium with the environment.

Piaget (1969) proposed three stages of reasoning: (1) intuitive, (2) concrete operational, and (3) formal operational. When they enter the stage of concrete logical thought at about age 7 years, children are able to make logical inferences, classify, and deal with quantitative relationships about concrete things. Not until adolescence are they able to reason abstractly with any degree of competence. Each stage is derived from and builds on the accomplishments of the previous stage in a continuous, orderly process. The course of intellectual development is both maturational and invariant and is divided into the following stages (ages are approximate):

- **Sensorimotor** (birth to 2 years)—The sensorimotor stage of intellectual development consists of six substages (see pp. 875 to 876 and pp. 924 and 925) that are governed by sensations in which simple learning takes place. Children progress from reflex activity through simple repetitive behaviors to imitative behavior. They develop a sense of cause and effect as they direct behavior toward objects. Problem solving is primarily by trial and error. They display a high level of curiosity, experimentation, and enjoyment of novelty and begin to develop a sense of self as they are able to differentiate themselves from their environment. They become aware that objects have permanence (i.e., that an object exists even though it is no longer visible). Toward the end of the sensorimotor period, children begin to use language and representational thought.

- **Preoperational** (2 to 7 years)—The predominant characteristic of the preoperational stage of intellectual development is egocentrism, which in this sense does not mean selfishness or self-centeredness but the inability to put oneself in the place of another. Children interpret objects and events not in terms of general properties but in terms of their relationships or their use to them. They are unable to see things from any perspective other than their own; they cannot see another's point of view, nor can they see any reason to do so (see Cognitive Development, Chapter 33).

  Preoperational thinking is concrete and tangible. Children cannot reason beyond the observable, and they lack the ability to make deductions or generalizations. Thought is dominated by what they see, hear, or otherwise experience. However, they are increasingly able to use language and symbols to represent objects in their environment. Through imaginative play, questioning, and other interactions, they begin to elaborate concepts and make simple associations between ideas. In the latter stage of this period their reasoning is intuitive (e.g., the stars have to go to bed just as they do); and they are only beginning to deal with problems of weight, length, size, and time. Reasoning is also transductive (i.e., because two events occur together, they cause each other, or knowledge of one characteristic is transferred to another [e.g., all women with big bellies have babies]).

- **Concrete operations** (7 to 11 years)—At this age thought becomes increasingly logical and coherent. Children are able to classify, sort, order, and otherwise organize facts about the world to use in problem solving. They develop a new concept of permanence—conservation (see Cognitive Development [Piaget], Chapter 34) (i.e., they realize that physical factors such as volume, weight, and number remain the same even though outward appearances are changed). They are able to deal with a number of different aspects of a situation simultaneously. They do not have the capacity to deal in abstraction; they solve problems in a concrete, systematic fashion based on what they can perceive. Reasoning is inductive. Through progressive changes in thought processes and relationships with others, thought becomes less self-centered. They can consider points of view other than their own. Thinking has become socialized.

- **Formal operations** (11 to 15 years)—Formal operational thought is characterized by adaptability and flexibility. Adolescents can think in abstract terms, use abstract symbols, and draw logical conclusions from a set of observations. For example, they can solve the following question: If A is larger than B and B is larger than C, which symbol is the largest? (The answer is A.) They can make hypotheses and test them; they can consider abstract, theoretic, and philosophic matters. Although they may confuse the ideal with the practical, most contradictions in the world can be dealt with and resolved.

Language Development

Children are born with the mechanism and capacity to develop speech and language skills. However, they do not speak spontaneously. The environment must provide a means for them to acquire these skills. Speech requires intact physiologic structure and function (including respiratory, auditory, and cerebral) plus intelligence, a need to communicate, and stimulation.

The rate of speech development varies from child to child and is directly related to neurologic competence and cognitive development. Gesture precedes speech, and in this way a small child communicates satisfactorily. As speech develops gesture recedes but never disappears entirely. Research suggests that infants can learn sign language before vocal language and that it may enhance the development of vocal language (Thompson, Cotner-Bichelman, McKerchar, et al., 2007). At all stages of language development, children's comprehension vocabulary (what they understand) is greater than their expressed vocabulary (what they can say), and this development reflects a continuing process of modification that involves both the acquisition of new words and the expanding and refining of word meanings previously learned. By the time they begin to walk, children are able to attach names to objects and persons.

The first parts of speech used are nouns, sometimes verbs (e.g., "go"), and combination words (e.g., "bye-bye"). Responses are usually structurally incomplete during the toddler period, although the meaning is clear. Next they begin to use adjectives and adverbs to qualify nouns, followed by adverbs to qualify nouns and verbs. Later pronouns and gender words are added (e.g., "he" and "she"). By the time children enter school, they are able to use simple, structurally complete sentences that average five to seven words.

Moral Development (Kohlberg)

Children also acquire moral reasoning in a developmental sequence. Moral development, as described by Kohlberg (1968), is based on cognitive developmental theory and consists of the following three major levels, each of which has two stages:

- **Preconventional level**—The preconventional level of moral development parallels the preoperational level of cognitive development and intuitive thought. Culturally oriented to the labels of good/bad and right/wrong, children integrate these in terms of the physical or pleasurable consequences of their actions. At first children determine the goodness or badness of an action in terms of its consequences. They avoid punishment and obey without question those who have the power to determine and enforce the rules and labels. They have no concept of the basic moral order that supports these consequences. Later children determine that the right behavior consists of that which satisfies their own needs (and sometimes the needs of others). Although elements of fairness, give and take, and equal sharing are evident, they are interpreted in a practical, concrete manner without loyalty, gratitude, or justice.
- **Conventional level**—At the conventional stage children are concerned with conformity and loyalty. They value the maintenance of family, group, or national expectations regardless of consequences. Behavior that meets with approval and pleases or helps others is considered good. One earns approval by being "nice." Obeying the rules, doing one's duty, showing respect for authority, and maintaining the social order are the correct behaviors. This level is correlated with the stage of concrete operations in cognitive development.
- **Postconventional, autonomous, or principled level**—At the postconventional level the individual has reached the

cognitive stage of formal operations. Correct behavior tends to be defined in terms of general individual rights and standards that have been examined and agreed on by the entire society. Although procedural rules for reaching consensus become important, with emphasis on the legal point of view, there is also emphasis on the possibility for changing law in terms of societal needs and rational considerations.

The most advanced level of moral development is one in which self-chosen ethical principles guide decisions of conscience. These are abstract and ethical but universal principles of justice and human rights with respect for the dignity of people as individuals. It is believed that few people reach this stage of moral reasoning.

Spiritual Development (Fowler)

Spiritual beliefs are closely related to the moral and ethical portion of the child's self-concept and as such must be considered as part of his or her basic needs assessment. Children need to have meaning, purpose, and hope in their lives. In addition, the need for confession and forgiveness is present, even in very young children. Extending beyond religion (an organized set of beliefs and practices), spirituality affects the whole person, including the mind, body, and spirit. Fowler (1981) has identified seven stages in the development of faith, four of which are closely associated with and parallel cognitive and psychosocial development in childhood:

- **Stage 0: Undifferentiated**—This stage of development encompasses the period of infancy during which children have no concept of right or wrong, no beliefs, and no convictions to guide their behavior. However, the beginnings of a faith are established with the development of basic trust through their relationships with the primary caregiver.
- **Stage 1: Intuitive-projective**—Toddlerhood is primarily a time of imitating the behavior of others. Children imitate the religious gestures and behaviors of others without comprehending any meaning of or significance to the activities. During the preschool years they assimilate some of the values and beliefs of their parents. Parental attitudes toward moral codes and religious beliefs convey to children what they consider to be good and bad. Children still imitate behavior at this age and follow parental beliefs as part of their daily lives rather than through an understanding of their basic concepts.
- **Stage 2: Mythical-literal**—Through the school-age years spiritual development parallels cognitive development and is closely related to children's experiences and social interaction. Most children have a strong interest in religion during the school-age years. They accept the existence of a deity, and petitions to an omnipotent being are important and expected to be answered; good behavior is rewarded, and bad behavior is punished. Their developing conscience bothers them when they disobey. They have a reverence for thoughts and matters and are able to articulate their faith. They may even question the validity of their faith.
- **Stage 3: Synthetic-convention**—As children approach adolescence they become increasingly aware of spiritual disappointments. They recognize that prayers are not always answered (at least on their own terms) and may begin to abandon or modify some religious practices. They begin to reason, to question some of the established parental religious standards, and to drop or modify some religious practices.
- **Stage 4: Individuating-reflexive**—Adolescents become more skeptical and begin to compare the religious standards of their parents with those of others. They attempt to determine

which standards to adopt and incorporate into their own set of values. They also begin to compare religious standards with the scientific viewpoint. It is a time of searching rather than reaching. Adolescents are uncertain about many religious ideas but do not achieve profound insights until late adolescence or early adulthood.

Development of Self-Concept

Self-concept is how an individual describes himself or herself. The term *self-concept* includes all of the notions, beliefs, and convictions that constitute an individual's self-knowledge and influence his or her relationships with others. It is not present at birth but develops gradually as a result of unique experiences within the self, significant others, and the realities of the world. However, an individual's self-concept may or may not reflect reality.

In infancy the self-concept is primarily an awareness of one's independent existence learned in part as a result of social contacts and experiences with others. The process becomes more active during toddlerhood as children explore the limits of their capacities and the nature of their impact on others. School-age children are more aware of differences among people, are more sensitive to social pressures, and become more preoccupied with issues of self-criticism and self-evaluation. During early adolescence children focus more on physical and emotional changes taking place and on peer acceptance. Self-concept is crystallized during later adolescence as young people organize their self-concept around a set of values, goals, and competencies acquired throughout childhood.

Body Image

A vital component of self-concept, body image refers to the subjective concepts and attitudes that individuals have toward their own bodies. It consists of the physiologic (the perception of one's physical characteristics), psychologic (values and attitudes toward the body, abilities, and ideals), and social nature of one's image of self (the self in relation to others). All three of the components interrelate with one another. Body image is a complex phenomenon that evolves and changes during the process of growth and development. Any actual or perceived deviation from the "norm" (no matter how this is interpreted) is cause for concern. The extent to which a characteristic, defect, or disease affects children's body image is influenced by the attitudes and behavior of those around them.

The significant others in their lives exert the most important and meaningful impact on children's body image. Labels that are attached to them (e.g., "skinny," "pretty," or "fat") or body parts (e.g., "ugly mole," "bug eyes," or "yucky skin") are incorporated into the body image. Because they lack the understanding of deviations from the physical standard or norm, children notice prominent differences in others and unwittingly make rude or cruel remarks about such minor deviations as large or widely spaced front teeth, large or small eyes, moles, or extreme variations in height.

Infants receive input about their bodies through self-exploration and sensory stimulation from others. As they begin to manipulate their environment, they become aware of their bodies as separate from others. Toddlers learn to identify the various parts of their bodies and are able to use symbols to represent objects. Preschoolers become aware of the wholeness of their bodies and discover the genitalia. Exploration of the genitalia and the discovery of differences between the sexes become important.

School-age children begin to learn about internal body structure and function and become aware of differences in body size and configuration. They are highly influenced by the cultural norms of society and current fads. Children whose bodies deviate from the norm are often criticized or ridiculed. Adolescence is the age when children become most concerned about the physical self. The unfamiliar body changes and the new physical self must be integrated into the self-concept. Adolescents face conflicts over what they see and what they visualize as the ideal body structure. Body image formation during adolescence is a crucial element in the shaping of identity, the psychosocial crisis of adolescence.

Self-Esteem

Self-esteem is the value that an individual places on oneself and refers to an overall evaluation of oneself (Willoughby, King, and Polatajko, 1996). Whereas self-esteem is described as the affective component of the self, self-concept is the cognitive component; however, the two terms are almost indistinguishable and are often used interchangeably.

The term *self-esteem* refers to a personal, subjective judgment of one's worthiness derived from and influenced by the social groups in the immediate environment and individuals' perceptions of how they are valued by others. It changes with development. Highly egocentric toddlers are unaware of any difference between competence and social approval. On the other hand, preschool and early school-age children are increasingly aware of the discrepancy between their competencies and the abilities of more advanced children. Being accepted by adults and peers outside the family group becomes more important to them. Positive feedback enhances their self-esteem; they are vulnerable to feelings of worthlessness and anxious about failure.

As children's competencies increase and they develop meaningful relationships, their self-esteem rises. It is again at risk during early adolescence when they are defining an identity and sense of self in the context of their peer group. Unless children are continually made to feel incompetent and of little worth, a decrease in self-esteem during vulnerable times is only temporary. Children assess the following aspects of themselves in forming an overall evaluation of their self-esteem (Sieving and Zirbel-Donisch, 1990):

- **Competence**—How adequate are my cognitive, physical, and social skills?
- **Sense of control**—How well can I complete tasks needed to produce desired actions? Is someone or something specific versus luck or chance responsible for my successes and failures?
- **Moral worth**—How closely do my actions and behaviors meet moral standards that have been set?
- **Worthiness of love and acceptance**—How worthy am I of love and acceptance from parents, other significant adults, siblings, and peers?

Factors that influence the formation of a child's self-esteem include (1) the child's temperament and personality, (2) abilities and opportunities available to accomplish age-appropriate developmental tasks, (3) how significant others interact with the child, and (4) social roles assumed and the expectations of these roles (see also Psychosocial History, Chapter 29).

ROLE OF PLAY IN DEVELOPMENT

Through the universal medium of play children learn what no one can teach them. They learn about their world and how to deal with this environment of objects, time, space, structure, and people. They learn about themselves operating within that environment (i.e., what they can do, how to relate to things and situations, and how to adapt themselves to the demands society makes on them). Play is the *work* of children. In play they continually practice the

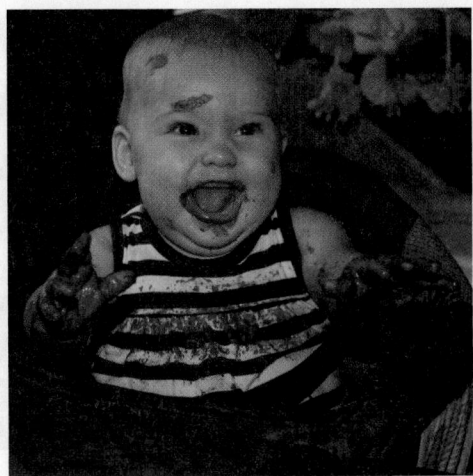

FIG 28-5 Children derive pleasure from handling raw materials. (Paints in this picture are nontoxic.)

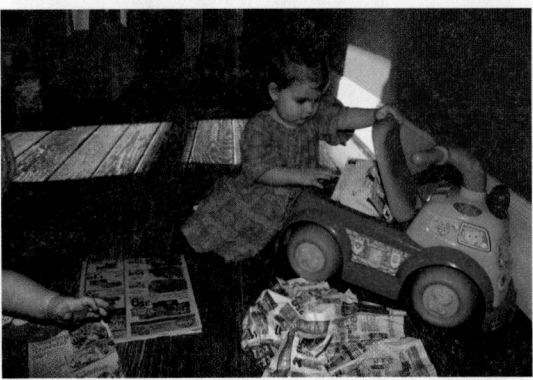

FIG 28-6 After infants develop new skills to grasp and manipulate, they begin to conquer new abilities such as putting paper in and taking it out of a toy car.

complicated, stressful processes of living, communicating, and achieving satisfactory relationships with other people.

Classification of Play

From a developmental point of view, patterns of children's play can be categorized according to content and social character. In both there is an additive effect; each builds on past accomplishments, and some element of each is maintained throughout life. At each stage in development the new predominates.

Content of Play

The content of play involves primarily the physical aspects of play, although social relationships cannot be ignored. The content of play follows the directional trend of the simple to the complex:

- **Social-affective play**—Play begins with social-affective play, wherein infants take pleasure in relationships with people. As adults talk, touch, nuzzle, and in various ways elicit responses from an infant, the infant soon learns to provoke parental emotions and responses with such behaviors as smiling, cooing, or initiating games and activities. The type and intensity of the adult behavior with children vary among cultures.
- **Sense-pleasure play**—Sense-pleasure play is a nonsocial stimulating experience that originates from without. Objects in the environment (e.g., light and color, tastes and odors, textures and consistencies) attract children's attention, stimulate their senses, and give pleasure. Pleasurable experiences are derived from handling raw materials (water, sand, food), body motion (swinging, bouncing, rocking), and other uses of senses and abilities (smelling, humming) (Fig. 28-5).
- **Skill play**—After infants have developed the ability to grasp and manipulate, they persistently demonstrate and exercise their newly acquired abilities through skill play, repeating an action over and over again. The element of sense-pleasure play is often evident in the practicing of a new ability, but all too frequently the determination to conquer the elusive skill produces pain and frustration (e.g., putting paper in and taking it out of a toy car) (Fig. 28-6).
- **Unoccupied behavior**—In unoccupied behavior children are not playful but focusing their attention momentarily on anything that strikes their interest. They daydream, fiddle with clothes or other objects, or walk aimlessly. This role differs from that of onlookers, who actively observe the activity of others.
- **Dramatic, or pretend, play**—One of the vital elements in children's process of identification is dramatic play, also known as *symbolic* or *pretend play*. It begins in late infancy (11 to 13 months) and is the predominant form of play in preschool children. After children begin to invest situations and people with meanings and attribute affective significance to the world, they can pretend and fantasize almost anything. By acting out events of daily life, they learn and practice the roles and identities modeled by the members of their family and society. Children's toys, replicas of the tools of society, provide a medium for learning about adult roles and activities that may be puzzling and frustrating to them. Interacting with the world is one way children get to know it. The simple, imitative, dramatic play of toddlers such as using the telephone, driving a car, or rocking a doll evolves into more complex, sustained dramas of preschoolers, which extend beyond common domestic matters to the wider aspects of the world and the society such as playing police officer, storekeeper, teacher, or nurse. Older children work out elaborate themes, act out stories, and compose plays.
- **Games**—Children in all cultures engage in games alone and with others. Solitary activity involving games begins as very small children participate in repetitive activities and progress to more complicated games that challenge their independent skills such as puzzles, solitaire, and computer or video games. Very young children participate in simple, imitative games such as pat-a-cake and peek-a-boo. Preschool children learn and enjoy formal games, beginning with ritualistic, self-sustaining games such as ring-around-a-rosy and London Bridge. With the exception of some simple board games, preschool children do not engage in competitive games. Preschoolers hate to lose and try to cheat, want to change rules, or demand exceptions and opportunities to change their moves. School-age children and adolescents enjoy competitive games, including cards, checkers, and chess, and physically active games such as baseball.

Social Character of Play

The play interactions of infancy are between the child and an adult. Children continue to enjoy the company of adults but are increasingly able to play alone. As age advances interaction with age-mates increases in importance and becomes an essential part of the

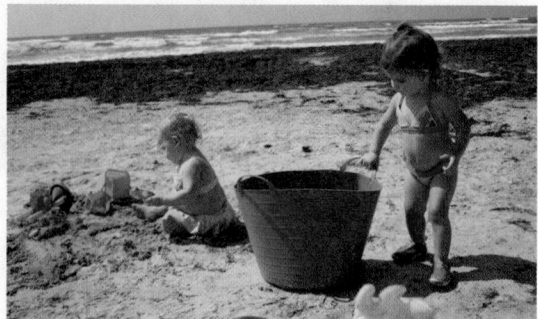

FIG 28-7 Parallel play at the beach.

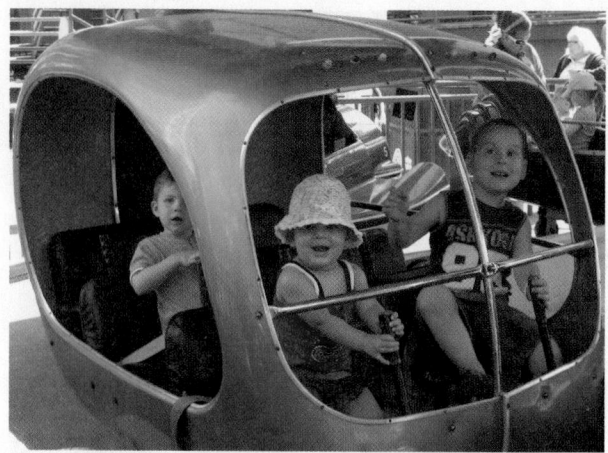

FIG 28-8 Associative play.

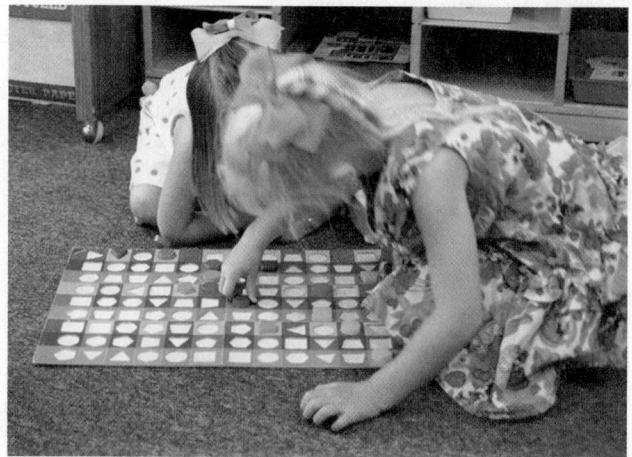

FIG 28-9 Cooperative play.

socialization process. Through interaction highly egocentric infants, unable to tolerate delay or interference, ultimately acquire concern for others and the ability to delay gratification or even to reject it at the expense of another. A pair of toddlers will engage in considerable combat because their personal needs cannot tolerate delay or compromise. By the time they reach age 5 or 6 years, children are able to arrive at compromises or make use of arbitration, usually after they have attempted but failed to gain their own way. Through continued interaction with peers and the growth of conceptual abilities and social skills, children are able to increase participation with others in the following types of play:

- **Onlooker play**—During onlooker play children watch what other children are doing but make no attempt to enter into the play activity. There is an active interest in observing the interaction of others but no movement toward participating. Watching an older sibling bounce a ball is a common example of the onlooker role.
- **Solitary play**—During solitary play children play alone with toys different from those used by other children in the same area. They enjoy the presence of other children but make no effort to get close to or speak to them. Their interest is centered on their own activity, which they pursue with no reference to the activities of the others.
- **Parallel play**—During parallel activities children play independently but among other children. They play with toys similar to those that the children around them are using but as each child sees fit, neither influencing nor being influenced by the other children. Each plays beside, but not with, other children (Fig. 28-7). There is no group association. Parallel play is the characteristic play of toddlers, but it may also occur in other groups of any age. Individuals who are involved in a creative craft with each person separately working on an individual project are engaged in parallel play.
- **Associative play**—In associative play children play together and are engaged in a similar or even identical activity, but there is no organization, division of labor, leadership assignment, or mutual goal. Children borrow and lend play materials, follow each other with wagons and tricycles, and sometimes attempt to control who may or may not play in the group. Each child acts according to his or her own wishes; there is no group goal (Fig. 28-8). For example, two children play with dolls, borrowing articles of clothing from one another and engaging in similar conversation, but neither directs the other's actions or establishes rules regarding the limits of the play session. There is a great deal of behavioral contagion: when one child initiates an activity, the entire group follows the example.

- **Cooperative play**—Cooperative play is organized, and children play in a group *with* other children (Fig. 28-9). They discuss and plan activities with the purpose of accomplishing an end (e.g., to make something, attain a competitive goal, dramatize situations of adult or group life, or play formal games). The group is loosely formed, but there is a marked sense of belonging or not belonging. The goal and its attainment require organization of activities, division of labor, and role playing. The leader-follower relationship is definitely established, and the activity is controlled by one or two members who assign roles and direct the activity of the others. The activity is organized to allow one child to supplement another's function to complete the goal.

Functions of Play
Sensorimotor Development
Sensorimotor activity is a major component of play at all ages and the predominant form of play in infancy. Active play is essential for muscle development and serves a useful purpose as a release for surplus energy. Through sensorimotor play, children explore the nature of the physical world. Infants gain impressions of themselves and their world through tactile, auditory, visual, and kinesthetic stimulation. Toddlers and preschoolers revel in body movement and exploration of objects in space. With increasing maturity sensorimotor play becomes more differentiated and involved. Whereas very young children run for the sheer joy of body movement, older

children incorporate or modify the motions into increasingly complex and coordinated activities such as races, games, roller skating, and bicycle riding.

Intellectual Development

Through exploration and manipulation children learn colors, shapes, sizes, textures, and the significance of objects. They learn the significance of numbers and how to use them; they learn to associate words with objects; and they develop an understanding of abstract concepts and spatial relationships such as *up, down, under,* and *over.* Activities such as puzzles and games help them develop problem-solving skills. Books, stories, films, and collections expand knowledge and provide enjoyment as well. Play provides a means to practice and expand language skills. Through play children continually rehearse past experiences to assimilate them into new perceptions and relationships. Play helps children comprehend the world in which they live and distinguish between fantasy and reality.

Socialization

From very early infancy children show interest and pleasure in the company of others. Their initial social contact is with the mothering person, but through play with other children they learn to establish social relationships and solve the problems associated with these relationships. They learn to give and take, which is more readily learned from critical peers than from more tolerant adults. They learn the sex role that society expects them to fulfill and approved patterns of behavior and deportment. Closely associated with socialization is development of moral values and ethics. Children learn right from wrong, the standards of the society, and to assume responsibility for their actions.

Creativity

In no other situation is there more opportunity to be creative than in play. Children can experiment and try out their ideas in play through every medium at their disposal, including raw materials, fantasy, and exploration. Creativity is stifled by pressure toward conformity; therefore striving for peer approval may inhibit creative endeavors in school-age or adolescent children. Creativity is primarily a product of solitary activity; however, creative thinking is often enhanced in group settings where listening to others' ideas stimulates further exploration of one's own ideas. After children feel the satisfaction of creating something new and different, they transfer this creative interest to situations outside the world of play.

Self-Awareness

Beginning with active explorations of their bodies and awareness of themselves as separate from their mothers, the process of developing a self-identity is facilitated through play activities. Children learn who they are and their place in the world. They become increasingly able to regulate their own behavior, learn what their abilities are, and compare their abilities with those of others. Through play children are able to test their abilities, assume and try out various roles, and learn the effects that their behavior has on others. They learn the sex role that society expects them to fulfill and approved patterns of behavior and deportment.

Therapeutic Value

Play is therapeutic at any age (Fig. 28-10). In play children can express emotions and release unacceptable impulses in a socially acceptable fashion. They are able to experiment and test fearful situations and can assume and vicariously master the roles and positions that they are unable to perform in the world of reality. Children

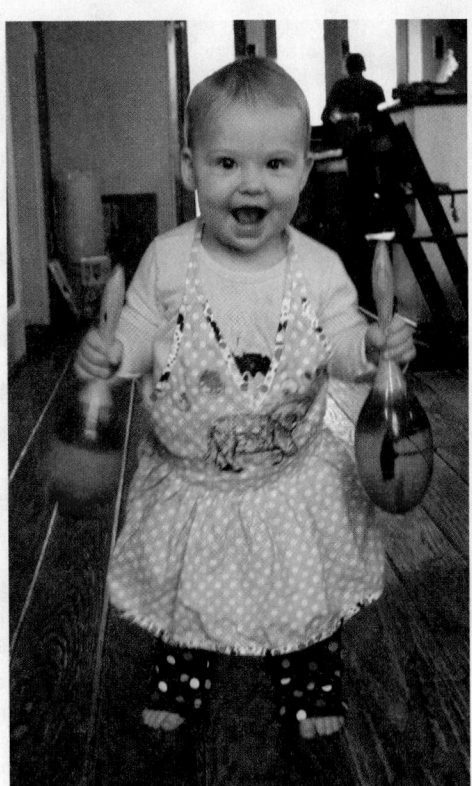

FIG 28-10 Play is therapeutic at any age and provides a means for release of tension and stress.

reveal much about themselves in play. Through play they are able to communicate to the alert observer the needs, fears, and desires that they are unable to express with their limited language skills. Throughout their play children need the acceptance of adults and their presence to help them control aggression and channel their destructive tendencies.

Morality

Although children learn at home and at school the behaviors considered right and wrong in the culture, the interaction with peers during play contributes significantly to their moral training. Nowhere is the enforcement of moral standards as rigid as in the play situation. If they are to be acceptable members of the group, children must adhere to the accepted codes of behavior of the culture (e.g., fairness, honesty, self-control, consideration for others). Children soon learn that their peers are less tolerant of violations than are adults and that, to maintain a place in the play group, they must conform to the standards of the group (Fig. 28-11).

Toys

The type of toys chosen by or provided for children can support and enhance their development in the areas just described. Although no scientific evidence shows that any toy is necessary for optimal learning, toys offer an opportunity to bring children and parents together. Research has indicated that a positive parent-child interaction can enhance early childhood brain development (AAP, 2003). Toys that are small replicas of the culture and its tools help children assimilate into their culture. Toys that require pushing, pulling, rolling, and manipulating teach them about physical properties of the items and help develop muscles and coordination. Rules and the basic elements of cooperation and organization are learned through board games.

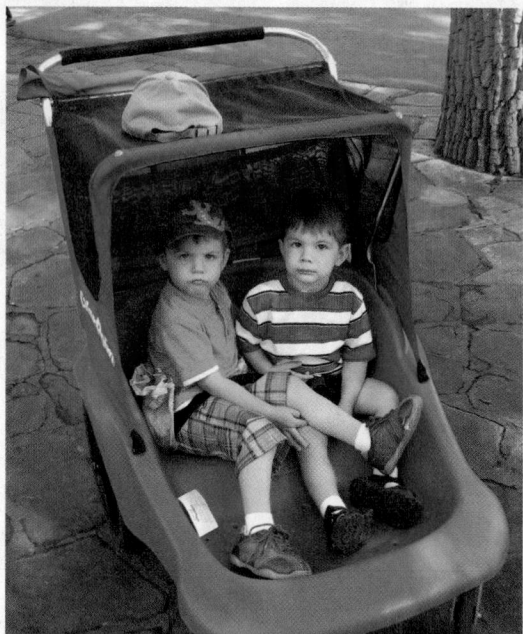

FIG 28-11 Peers become increasingly important as children develop friendships outside the family group.

Because they can be used in a variety of ways, raw materials with which children can exercise their own creativity and imaginations are sometimes superior to ready-made items. For example, building blocks can be used to construct a variety of structures, count, and learn shapes and sizes.

DEVELOPMENTAL ASSESSMENT

One of the most essential components of a complete health appraisal is assessment of developmental function. Screening procedures are designed to identify quickly and reliably children whose developmental level is below normal for their age and who therefore require further investigation. They also provide a means of recording objective measurements of present developmental function for future reference. Since the passage of Public Law 99-457, the Education of the Handicapped Act Amendments of 1986, much greater emphasis is placed on developmental assessment of children with disabilities, and nurses can play a vital role in providing this service. All the procedures discussed in this section can be administered in a variety of settings: home, school, day care center, hospital, practitioner's office, or clinic.

In the past, the most widely used developmental screening tests for young children were the series of tests known as the Denver Developmental Screening Test (DDST) and its revision, the DDST-R, which was revised, restandardized, and renamed the Denver II. The American Academy of Neurology (AAN) and the Child Neurology Society (CNS) state that research has found the Denver II to be insensitive and lacking in specificity; therefore neither the AAN nor the CNS recommends use of the Denver II for primary care developmental screening (Filipek, Accardo, Ashwal, et al., 2000). A complete list of child development assessment tools has been developed by the National Early Childhood Technical Assistance Center (NECTAC) as part of its cooperative agreement with the U.S. Office of Special Education Programs.* The pediatric health promotion

*Developmental screening and Assessment Instruments is available at http://www.nectac.org/%7Epdfs/pubs/screening.pdf

---

> **BOX 28-4** **AGES AND STAGES QUESTIONNAIRES AT A GLANCE**
>
> - Type of screening: Developmental (ASQ-3™) and social-emotional (ASQ:SE)
> - Age range: 1-66 months for ASQ-3™, 3-66 months for ASQ:SE
> - Number of questionnaires: 21 for ASQ-3™, 8 for ASQ:SE
> - Number of items: About 30 per questionnaire
> - Online components: Data management and questionnaire completion
> - Reading level of items: 4th to 6th grade
> - Who completes it: Parents
> - Time to complete: 10-15 minutes
> - Who scores it: Professionals
> - Time to score: 2-3 minutes
> - Languages: English and Spanish (for other languages, visit www.agesandstages.com)

chapters include detailed information on development and assessment that is unique to the age and stage of the child.

Ages and Stages

Ages and stages is a term used to broadly outline key periods in the human development timeline. During each stage, growth and development occur in primary developmental domains that include physical, intellectual, language, and social-emotional (Box 28-4). The Ages & Stages Questionnaires (ASQ)* are high-quality screening tools that include 19 age-specific surveys that ask parents about developmental skills common in daily life for children 1 month to 5½ years. Parents or other caregivers answer questions regarding their child's abilities (e.g., Does your child climb on an object such as a chair to reach something he wants? When your child wants something, does she tell you by pointing to it?). Children whose development appears to fall significantly below results of other children their age are flagged for further evaluation The ASQ can be used as a universal screening tool in pediatric clinics to identify children at risk for social-emotional developmental delays (Briggs, Stettler, Silver, et al., 2012).

GENETIC FACTORS THAT INFLUENCE DEVELOPMENT

Genes, Genetics, and Genomics

Nurses and other health care providers are increasingly faced with incorporating genetic and genomic information into their practice. In response to this need, the Consensus Panel on Genetic/Genomic Nursing Competencies was established in 2006. This independent panel of nurse leaders from clinical, research, and academic settings established essential minimal competencies necessary for nurses to deliver competent genetic- and genomic-focused nursing care. Subsequently the American Association of Colleges of Nursing published the revised *The Essentials of Baccalaureate Education for Professional Nursing Practice* (2008, www.aacn.nche.edu/education/pdf/BaccEssentials08.pdf) and *The Essentials of Master's Education in Nursing* (2011, www.aacn.nche.edu/education/pdf/Master's Essentials11.pdf), both of which identified genetics and genomics as strong forces influencing the role of nurses in patient care. This brief overview identifies key terms and concepts and highlights

*The ASQ can be found at www.agesandstages.com

essential genetics and genomics competencies for all nurses (2008, www.genome.gov/Pages/Careers/HealthProfessionalEducation/geneticscompetency.pdf).

Genes are segments of deoxyribonucleic acid (DNA) that specify for proteins, segments of proteins, or strands of ribonucleic acid (RNA) necessary to control physiologic functions or characteristics. These segments are often referred to as *sites* or *loci*, indicating a physical or "geographic" location on a chromosome. Variant forms of a gene commonly occur within a population. When referring to a particular form of a gene, the term *allele* is used. Specific differences within a gene are called *mutations* if they are rare within a population or are polymorphisms if they are found within more than 1% of a particular population. Mutations and polymorphisms can be inherited or acquired. Variant alleles caused by mutations or polymorphisms may lead to no measureable or observable differences, cause the person to be susceptible to clinically recognizable pathology within specific environmental contexts, cause a clinically recognized disease or disorder, or prove advantageous within a particular environmental context. Whereas genetics is the study of individual genes and the impact of their variant forms on relatively rare single gene disorders, genomics is the study of combinations of multiple genes, their interactions with one another, the environment, and other psychosocial and cultural factors (Guttmacher and Collins, 2002).

In earlier times human diseases were thought to be either clearly genetic or typically environmental. However, the observation that some genetic disorders are congenital (present at birth) but others are expressed later in life has led scientists to conclude that many, if not most, diseases are caused by a genetic predisposition that can be activated by an environmental trigger. Examples of such interactions are found in single-gene disorders such as phenylketonuria (PKU) and sickle cell disease and multifactorial conditions such as cancer and neural tube defects (NTDs). PKU is a disorder resulting from the (genetically determined) absence of an enzyme that metabolizes the amino acid phenylalanine. However, the deleterious effects in the infant are expressed only after sufficient ingestion of phenylalanine-containing substances such as milk (environmental trigger). Even in the case of a "classic" genetic condition such as sickle cell disease, its acute symptoms are precipitated by certain conditions such as lowered oxygen tension, infection, or dehydration.

Cancer is another example of genetic-environment interplay and explains the difference between inherited conditions and somatic cell genetic disorders. A normal somatic cell (any body cell other than the ova and sperm) may become a cancer cell after acquiring a series of gene changes. This process is the typical "genetic" cause of cancer. In a small subset of families a mutation in a gene normally involved in regulation of cell growth, DNA repair, or cell death (apoptosis) is transmitted through the germ cells (ova and sperm). Children who inherit the genetic mutation have it in all of their somatic cells, making them more susceptible to subsequent genetic changes in one or more cells that may transform into cancer cells. Beyond the genetic component of cancer, there is little dispute that environmental insult such as tobacco smoking, sun exposure, and radiation can be carcinogenic. Such environmental triggers are capable of spontaneously creating noninherited mutations in genes that regulate cell growth and cell response to cell abnormalities that can eventually lead to malignant transformation.

Evidence is growing that genes play an important role in human susceptibility and resistance to infection, even in cases with a clear environmental cause of the infectious disease. Evidence for this genetic element in resistance gained heightened recognition during the first decade of the acquired immunodeficiency (AIDS) epidemic.

Researchers discovered that adults with a specific deletion in both copies of their *CCR5* genes did not become infected with human immunodeficiency virus (HIV) despite repeated exposure. Later it was found that children exposed in utero to HIV typically had a significantly delayed onset of disease if at least one of their *CCR5* genes had the specific mutation (Romiti, Colognesi, Cancrini, et al., 2000).

Congenital Anomalies

Embryogenesis and fetal development are an intricate and precisely timed series of events in which all parts must be properly integrated to ensure a coordinated whole. Insults during development or abnormalities in differentiation or in the proper timing of organogenesis may result in a variety of congenital anomalies. Congenital anomalies, or birth defects, occur in 2% to 4% of all live-born children and are often classified as deformations, disruptions, dysplasias, or malformations. Deformations are often caused by extrinsic mechanical forces on normally developing tissue. Clubfoot is an example of a deformation often caused by uterine constraint. Disruptions result from the breakdown of previously normal tissue. Congenital amputations caused by amniotic bands (fibrous strands of amnion that wrap around different body parts during development) are examples of disruption anomalies. Dysplasias result from abnormal organization of cells into a particular tissue type. Congenital abnormalities of the teeth, hair, nails, or sweat glands may be manifestations of one of the more than 150 different ectodermal dysplasia syndromes (Ectodermal Dysplasia Society, 2013). Malformations are abnormal formations of organs or body parts resulting from an abnormal developmental process. Most malformations occur before 12 weeks of gestation. Cleft lip, an example of a malformation, occurs at approximately 5 weeks of gestation when the developing embryo naturally has two clefts in the area. Normally between 5 and 7 weeks cells rapidly divide and migrate to fill in these clefts. If there is an abnormality in this developmental process, the embryo is left with either a unilateral or bilateral cleft lip that may also involve the palate.

The types of anomalies that can result from genetic or prenatal environmental causes can be major structural abnormalities with serious medical, surgical, or quality-of-life consequences; or they can be minor anomalies or normal variants with no serious consequences such as a sacral dimple, an extra nipple, or a café-au-lait spot. Congenital anomalies can occur in isolation such as congenital heart defect, or multiple anomalies may be present. A recognized pattern of anomalies resulting from a single specific cause is called a syndrome (e.g., Down syndrome, fetal alcohol syndrome). A nonrandom pattern of malformations for which a cause has not been determined is called an association (e.g., VACTERL [vertebral defects, anal atresia, cardiac defect, tracheoesophageal fistula, and renal and limb defects] association). When a single anomaly leads to a cascade of additional anomalies, the pattern of defects is referred to as a sequence. Pierre Robin sequence begins with the abnormal development of the mandible, resulting in abnormal placement of the tongue during development. The normal developmental process for the palate is prevented because the tongue obstructs the migration of the palatal shelves toward the midline, and a cleft palate remains. Consequently infants born with Pierre Robin sequence have a recessed mandible and an abnormally placed tongue and are at risk for obstructive apnea. NTDs, cleft lip and palate, deafness, congenital heart defects, and cognitive impairment are examples of congenital malformations that can occur in isolation or as part of a syndrome, association, or sequence and can have different causes such as single-gene or chromosome abnormalities, prenatal exposures, or multifactorial causes.

Disorders of the Intrauterine Environment

The intrauterine environment can have a profound and permanent effect on developing fetuses with or without chromosome or single-gene abnormalities. For example, intrauterine growth restriction can occur with many genetic syndromes such as Down, Russell-Silver, Prader-Willi, and Turner syndromes (Rimoin, Connor, Pyeritz, et al., 2002); or it can be caused by nongenetic factors such as maternal alcohol ingestion. Placental abnormalities are increasingly being found to be the etiologic factor in neurodevelopmental disorders (e.g., cerebral palsy and cognitive impairment) that were previously attributed to asphyxia during delivery (Bos, Einspieler, Prechtl, et al., 2001). Teratogens, agents that cause birth defects when present in the prenatal environment, account for most adverse intrauterine effects not attributable to genetic factors. Types of teratogens include drugs (phenytoin [Dilantin], warfarin [Coumadin], isotretinoin [Accutane]), chemicals (ethyl alcohol, cocaine, lead), infectious agents (rubella, cytomegalovirus), physical agents (maternal ionizing radiation, hyperthermia), and metabolic agents (maternal PKU). Many of these teratogenic exposures and the resulting effects are completely preventable such as ingestion of alcohol resulting in fetal alcohol syndrome or fetal alcohol effects, which causes severe birth defects, including cognitive impairment.

Genetic Disorders

Genetic disorders can be caused by chromosome abnormalities as seen in Turner syndrome, Down syndrome, or velocardiofacial syndrome (VCFS); single-gene mutations as seen in sickle cell anemia, neurofibromatosis, or Duchenne muscular dystrophy; a combination of genetic and environmental factors as seen in NTDs or maturity-onset diabetes in the young; and mitochondrial DNA (mtDNA) mutations as seen in nonsyndromic deafness susceptibility caused by aminoglycoside sensitivity.

Both numeric and large structural abnormalities of autosomes (all chromosomes except the X and Y chromosomes) account for a variety of syndromes usually characterized by cognitive deficiencies. Nurses often note dysmorphic facial features, behavioral characteristics such as an unusual cry and poor feeding behavior, and other neurologic manifestations such as hypotonia or abnormal reflex responses, which may alert them to these and other chromosome abnormalities.

Somatic cells contain 44 autosomes (the 22 pairs of chromosomes that do not greatly influence sex determination at conception) and two sex chromosomes, XX in females and XY in males. For the purpose of cytogenetic studies, chromosomes are usually displayed in a karyotype, the laboratory-made arrangement of specially prepared chromosomes according to their size and centromere position. Numeric chromosome abnormalities occur whenever entire chromosomes are added or deleted. Down syndrome is an example of a condition caused by having an extra autosome, chromosome 21. Turner syndrome is the only example of a condition compatible with life that is caused by the absence of a chromosome. Children with Turner syndrome have one X chromosome. Chromosomes are subject to structural alterations resulting from breakage and rearrangement. A chromosome deletion occurs when chromosome breakage results in loss of the broken fragment at the terminal end of a chromosome or within the chromosome. Some structural chromosome abnormalities are too small to visualize reliably under a light microscope but are still clinically relevant. Fragile, or weak, sites associated with expanded triplet repeats have been identified on both the autosomes and the X chromosome. A classic example is fragile X syndrome. Contiguous gene syndromes are disorders characterized by a microdeletion or microduplication of smaller chromosome segments, which may require special analysis techniques or molecular testing to detect (Bar-Shira, Rosner, Rosner, et al., 2006).

Chromosome anomalies typically affect large numbers of genes; however, a single-gene disorder is caused by an abnormality within a gene or in the regulatory region of a gene. Single-gene disorders can affect all body systems and may have mild-to-severe expressions. They display a Mendelian pattern of dominant or recessive inheritance that was first delineated in the mid-nineteenth century by Gregor Mendel's experiments with plants.

Mendelian inheritance laws allow for risk prediction in single-gene disorders; however, phenotypic expression may be altered by incomplete penetrance or variable expressivity of the responsible allele. An allele is said to have reduced or incomplete penetrance in a population when a proportion of people who possess that allele do not express the phenotype. An allele is said to have variable expressivity when individuals possessing that allele display the features of the syndrome in various degrees from mild to severe. If a person expresses even the mildest possible phenotype, the allele is penetrant in that individual.

Role of Nurses in Genetics

All nurses need to be prepared to use genetic and genomic information and technology when providing care. Nearly 50 nursing organizations endorsed essential minimum competencies necessary for nurses to deliver competent genetic- and genomic-focused nursing care (Consensus Panel on Genetic/Genomic Nursing Competencies, 2006). The professional practice domains include applying and integrating genetic knowledge into nursing assessment; identifying and referring patients who may benefit from genetic information or services; identifying genetics resources and services to meet patients' needs; and providing care and support before, during, and after providing genetic information and services. Often a nurse is the first one to recognize the need for genetic evaluation by identifying an inherited disorder in a family history or noting physical, cognitive, or behavioral abnormalities when performing a nursing assessment (Box 28-5).

Applying and Integrating Genetic and Genomic Knowledge into Nursing Assessment

Family health history is an important tool to identify individuals and families at increased risk for disease, risk factors for disease (e.g., obesity), and inheritance patterns of diseases. Because of its importance, all nurses need to be able to elicit family history information and document the collected information in pedigree format.

When eliciting a family health history, nurses should collect information about all family members within a minimum of three generations. This process usually takes 20 to 30 minutes. When possible, it is best to include both parents in the interview to elicit information about relatives on both sides of the family. Medical records, birth and death records, family Bibles, and photograph albums are helpful resources; and people being interviewed should be instructed to bring such items if they are available. It may be necessary to consult other members of the family. The level of education and degree of understanding vary widely among informants and influence their reliability. The informants may be reticent, particularly if they view the disorder as something for which they should be ashamed or that is in some way threatening. Sometimes true relationships may be concealed such as adoption or misattributed paternity.

In addition to family history, nurses caring for children and families need to collect pregnancy, labor and delivery, perinatal,

BOX 28-5   PEDIATRIC INDICATIONS FOR GENETIC CONSULTATION

- Family history
  - Family history of hereditary diseases, birth defects, or developmental problems
  - Family history of sudden cardiac death or early-onset cancer
  - Family history of mental illness
- Medical history
  - Abnormal newborn screen
  - Abnormal genetic test result ordered by a nongenetics professional who lacks the knowledge and experience to discuss the implications of results
  - Excessive bleeding or excessive clotting
  - Progressive neurologic condition
  - Recurrent infection or immunodeficiency
- Developmental history
  - Behavioral disorders
  - Cognitive impairment or autism
  - Development and speech delays or loss of developmental milestones
- Physical assessment
  - Major congenital anomaly
  - Minor anomalies and dysmorphic features
  - Growth abnormalities
  - Skeletal abnormalities
  - Visual or hearing problems
  - Metabolic disorder (unusual odor of breath, urine, or stool)
  - Sexual development abnormalities or delayed puberty
  - Skin disorders or abnormalities
- Parental requests that child be evaluated by a genetics professional

Adapted from Pletcher BA, Toriello HV, Noblin SJ, et al: Indications for genetic referral: a guide for healthcare providers, *Genet Med* 9(6):385–389, 2007.

medical, and developmental histories. Although it is common for genetics nurses to obtain all of these histories before or during an initial genetics consultation, not all nurses are expected to obtain all of these assessment data from each patient during a pediatric visit. Electronic medical records are making it more practical to construct a comprehensive set of histories even when many health care professionals contribute only a portion of the total history.

All nurses are taught to perform physical assessments, but they are seldom taught to recognize minor anomalies and dysmorphology that may suggest a genetic disorder. Yet nurses are keen in recognizing delays in development, behavior differences, and global appearances that raise concern that a newborn, infant, child, or adolescent needs further evaluation. Although dysmorphology is beyond the scope of this chapter, readers are encouraged to review the January 2009 issue of *American Journal of Medical Genetics* (Carey, Cohen, Curry, et al., 2009). Drawings and photographs of normal and abnormal morphologic characteristics are provided for the head, face, and extremities together with accepted dysmorphology terminology. Nurses knowledgeable in dysmorphology are able to articulate specific concerns about a child's appearance rather than rely on the outdated and offensive phrase, "funny looking kid." When a major anomaly is identified, nurses should raise suspicion that the child could have additional congenital anomalies. When three or more minor anomalies are identified, nurses should suspect the possibility of an underlying syndrome. However, it is important to consider the biologic parents' physical appearance, development, and behavior when considering the relevance of the child's combination of minor anomalies.

Identifying and Referring

It is nurses' responsibility to learn basic genetic principles, be alert to situations in which families could benefit from genetic evaluation and counseling, know about special services that can help manage and support affected children, and be familiar with facilities in their areas where these services are available. In this way they are able to direct individuals and families to needed services and be active participants in the genetic evaluation and counseling process. A regularly updated resource for locating genetics clinics can be found at www.genetests.org (click on Clinic Directory tab). Contact information for specific genetics professionals can be found at the following websites: geneticists, www.acmg.net (click on Find a Geneticist); genetics nurses, www.isong.org (call or e-mail office); and genetic counselors, www.nsgc.org (click on Find a Counselor). In addition, state health departments either offer services or can help identify health professionals with specialty training in genetics.

Early identification of a genetic disorder allows anticipation of associated conditions and implementation of available preventive measures and therapy to avoid potential complications and enhance the child's health. It may also prevent the unexpected birth of another affected child in the immediate or extended family. Nurses have an important role in identifying patients and families who have or are at risk for developing or transmitting a genetic condition (see Box 28-5). When facilitating genetics consultations, nurses should share with the genetics professional the findings in the histories they collected that triggered the consultation. Nurses can also help the referral process by determining and communicating the family's initial concerns, their state of knowledge about the reason for referral, and their attitudes and beliefs concerning genetics.

Genetic evaluation for diagnostic purposes may occur at any point in the life span. In the newborn period birth defects and abnormal newborn screen results are obvious reasons for referral. Beyond the newborn period indicators for referral include metabolic disorders, developmental delays, growth delays, behavioral problems, cognitive delays, abnormal or delayed sexual development, and medical problems known to be associated with genetic diseases. For example, a preschooler with hyperactivity and autistic-like behaviors may need evaluation for fragile X syndrome, and a 17-year-old girl with primary amenorrhea and short stature should be evaluated for Turner syndrome.

With so many recent advances in genetic testing, it is not unusual for a child or adult with long-standing medical problems, including cognitive impairment, to be referred for reevaluation of his or her condition as a possible genetic disorder that might not have been diagnosable a few years earlier such as microdeletion disorders or single-gene mutations. If a genetic diagnosis is made, the patient is usually referred back to the primary care physician with recommendations for routine management.

Providing Education, Care, and Support

Maintaining contact with the family or making a referral to a health care practice or an agency that can provide a sustained relationship is critical. It is becoming more common for genetics health care professionals to provide regular follow-up and management, particularly for children with rare genetic disorders. However, some families choose not to have follow-up visits.

Regardless of whether families choose to receive continued care with a genetics center, clinic, or professional, nurses can help patients and families process and clarify the information they receive during a genetics visit. Misunderstanding of this information can have many causes, including cultural differences, the disparity of knowledge between the counselor and the family, and the heightened emotion surrounding genetic counseling. Family members have difficulty absorbing all of the information presented during a genetics evaluation and counseling session. Knowing this, genetics professionals write and send clinic summary letters to families. The nurse may need to help the family understand terminology in the letter, help them identify and articulate remaining questions or areas of clarification, and coach them through the process of accessing genetics health professionals to have remaining questions and concerns answered. Information often needs to be repeated several times before the family understands the content and its implications.

Nurses must assess for and address parents' feelings of guilt about carrying "bad genes" or having "made my child sick." Depending on the type of cytogenetic disorder, the nurse may be able to absolve the parents of guilt by explaining the random nature of segregation during both gamete formation and fertilization and that these errors in cell division unique to the pregnancy in question are not likely to happen again and are not inherited. If the condition is a Mendelian-inherited or mitochondrial disorder, it is important to assess parents' understanding of recurrence risk, help them understand the chances that a subsequent pregnancy will not be affected, and ensure they have been given information about their options for future children (preimplantation diagnosis, use of donor egg or sperm, prenatal diagnosis, or adoption). Families often try to reason that some unrelated event caused the abnormality (e.g., a fall, a urinary tract infection, or "one glass of wine") before the mother was aware that she was pregnant. These misconceptions need to be assessed and dispelled.

After, and sometimes before, a genetics visit, parents often use the Internet to find answers to their questions. During the initial genetics evaluation a diagnosis may not be possible. Instead findings in medical, developmental, and family histories lead the professional to order genetic tests and other diagnostic procedures. Diagnoses under consideration are discussed briefly with the parents. Some parents are satisfied with the brief information and do not care to find out more until the actual diagnosis is established. Others seek as much information as they can about the diagnoses under consideration. The information they find can be terrifying and overwhelming and inaccurate or misleading. Nurses can play an important role in helping parents identify reliable, accurate resources for information at whatever time they desire it. It is also important to stress that everything that is described for a genetic condition may not be relevant to their child. Before the follow-up genetics visit when test and procedure results are discussed, nurses can help parents identify and write down the questions and concerns they need addressed before leaving the clinic.

After a genetics diagnosis is made or a genetic predisposition to a delayed-onset disorder is identified, nurses need to have frequent contact with patients and families as they attempt to incorporate recommended therapies or disease-prevention strategies into their daily lives. For example, a disorder such as PKU requires conscientious diet management; therefore it is important to make certain that the family understands and follows instructions and is able to navigate the health care system to access the essential formula and low-phenylalanine food products. An infant evaluated for cleft palate and cardiac defect and subsequently found to have VCFS requires surgical intervention for the congenital malformations. Such an infant also benefits from early intervention services and eventually an individualized education plan in school because developmental delays and eventual learning problems are common.

Initial and ongoing assessment of the family's coping abilities, resources, and support systems is vital to determine their need for additional assistance and support. As with any family who has a child with chronic health care needs, nurses must teach them to become the child's advocate. Nurses can help families locate agencies and clinics specializing in a specific disorder or its consequences that can provide services (e.g., equipment, medication, and rehabilitation), educational programs, and parent support groups. Referral to local and national support groups or contact with a local family that has a child with the same condition can be helpful for new parents. Privacy and confidentiality are imperative, and both families must give permission before their contact information is given. Nurses can also be instrumental in helping parents start a support group when none is available.

Parental attachment and adjustment to the baby can be supported and facilitated by nursing interventions. Assessing the parents' understanding of the child's disorder and providing simple and truthful explanations can help them begin to understand their child's health issues. Guiding the parents in recognizing their child's cues, responses, and strengths can be helpful even for experienced parents. A caring attitude conveys the value of their child and by extension their value as parents. The nurse can help the parents identify their strengths as a family and support that is available to them.

Giving birth to and raising a child with a genetic disorder is not necessarily a lifetime burden. It is important for nurses to ask parents to describe their experience raising their child with a particular genetic condition. What has been the impact on their family? Although parents may initially experience negative outcomes such as shock, emotional distress, and grief, families can adapt and thrive. Resources for managing stress and restoring balance in the lives of families affected by a genetic condition can help. Van Riper's research (2007) has identified nursing interventions that can promote resilience and adaptation in families of children with Down syndrome. His recommendations are useful for families of children with any type of genetic disorder:

- Recognize multiple stressors, strains, and transitions in their lives (e.g., unmet family needs).
- Discuss and implement strategies for reducing family demands (e.g., setting priorities and reducing the number of outside activities family members in which are involved).
- Identify and use individual, family, and community resources (e.g., humor, family flexibility, supportive extended family, respite care, local support groups, and Internet resources).
- Expand the range and efficacy of their coping strategies (e.g., increase the use of active strategies such as reframing, mobilize their ability to acquire and accept help, and decrease the use of passive appraisal).
- Encourage the use of an affirming style of family problem-solving communication (e.g., one that conveys support and caring and exerts a calming influence).

Some families struggle after learning that their child has a genetic disorder. They may feel ashamed of a hereditary disorder and seek to blame their partner for transmitting a faulty gene or chromosome. Intrafamilial strife, hostility, and marital or couple disharmony, sometimes to the point of family disintegration, can occur. Nurses should be alert for evidence of risk factors that indicate poor adjustment (e.g., child abuse, divorce, or other maladaptive behaviors). Referral to psychosocial professionals for crisis intervention may be necessary.

KEY POINTS

- Growth is a change in quantity and occurs when cells divide and synthesize new proteins.
- Maturation, a qualitative change, is the aging process or an increase in competence and adaptability.
- Differentiation is a biologic description of the processes by which early cells and structures are modified and altered to achieve specific and characteristic physical and chemical properties.
- Development involves change from a lower to a more advanced stage of complexity.
- The five major developmental periods are prenatal, infancy, early childhood, middle childhood, and later childhood (pubescence and adolescence).
- Growth and development proceed in predictable patterns of direction, sequence, and pace.
- The directional trends in growth and development are cephalocaudal, proximodistal, and mass to specific.
- Physical development includes increase in height and weight and changes in body proportion, dentition, and some body tissues.
- The three broad classifications of child temperament are the easy child, the difficult child, and the slow-to-warm-up child.
- The developmental theories most widely used in explaining child growth and development are Freud's psychosexual stages, Erikson's stages of psychosocial development, Piaget's stages of cognitive development, Kohlberg's stages of moral development, and Fowler's stages of spiritual development.
- To develop a positive self-concept, children need recognition for their achievements and the approval of others.
- Through play children learn about their world and how to relate to objects, people, and situations.
- Play provides a means of development in the areas of sensorimotor and intellectual progress, socialization, creativity, self-awareness, and moral behavior; it serves as a means for release of tension and expression of emotions.
- Growth and development are affected by a variety of conditions and circumstances, including heredity, physiologic function, gender, disease, physical environment, nutrition, and interpersonal relationships.
- Children's vulnerability and reaction to stress depend to a large extent on their age, coping behaviors, and support systems.
- Developmental screening tools are valuable in identifying infants and children who are at risk for developmental delays.
- Genetic mutations and polymorphisms can be inherited or acquired. Mutations are rare, whereas polymorphisms occur in greater than 1% of a population.
- All nurses should be familiar with genetic or genomic information as it relates to the care of their patient.

REFERENCES

American Academy of Pediatrics (AAP) Committee on Early Childhood, Adoption, and Dependent Care: Selecting appropriate toys for young children: the pediatrician's role, *Pediatrics* 111(4):911–913, 2003.

Anders TF, Sadeh A, Appareddy V: Normal sleep in neonates and children. In Sheldon S, Ferber R, Kryger M, editors: *Principles and practice of sleep medicine in the child*, Philadelphia, 2005, Saunders.

Bar-Shira A, Rosner G, Rosner S, et al: Array-based comparative genome hybridization in clinical genetics, *Pediatr Res* 60(3):353–358, 2006.

Beck CT: A meta-analysis of the relationship between postpartum depression and infant temperament, *Nurs Res* 45(4):225–230, 1996.

Bos AF, Einspieler C, Prechtl HF, et al: Intrauterine growth retardation, general movements, and neurodevelopmental outcome: a review, *Dev Med Child Neurol* 43(1):61–68, 2001.

Briggs RD, Stettler EM, Silver EJ, et al: Social-emotional screening for infants and toddlers in primary care, *Pediatrics* 129:e377, 2012.

Caine D, DiFiori J, Maffulli N: Physeal injuries in children's and youth sports: reasons for concern? *Br J Sports Med* 40(9):749–760, 2006.

Carey JC, Cohen MM, Curry CJ, et al: Elements of morphology: standard terminology for the lips, mouth, and oral region, *Am J Med Genet A* 149A(1):77–92, 2009.

Carey WB: Teaching parents about infant temperament, *Pediatrics* 102(5 suppl E):1311–1316, 1998.

Chess S, Thomas A: *Goodness of fit: clinical applications from infancy through adult life*, London, 1999, Routledge.

Consensus Panel on Genetic/Genomic Nursing Competencies: *Essential nursing competencies and curricula guidelines for genetics and genomics*, Silver Spring, MD, 2006, American Nurses Association.

Cronk C, Crocker AC, Pueschel SM, et al: Growth charts for children with Down syndrome: 1 month to 18 years of age, *Pediatrics* 81(1):102–110, 1988.

Delva J, O'Malley PM, Johnston LD: Availability of more-healthy and less-healthy food choices in American schools: a national study of grade, racial/ethnic, and socioeconomic differences, *Am J Prev Med* 33(4 suppl):S226–S239, 2007.

Ectodermal Dysplasia Society: What is ED? 2013, http://www.ectodermaldysplasia.org/whatised.php

Erikson EH: *Childhood and society*, ed 2, New York, 1963, Norton.

Filipek PA, Accardo PJ, Ashwal S, et al: Practice parameter: screening and diagnosis of autism. Report of the Quality Standards Subcommittee of the American Academy of Neurology and the Child Neurology Society, *Neurology* 55:468–479, 2000.

Fowler J: *Stages of faith: the psychology of human development and the quest for meaning*, New York, 1981, HarperCollins.

Freud S: *New introductory lectures in psychoanalysis*, New York, 1933, Norton.

Freud S: An outline of psychoanalysis. In Strachey J, editor and translator: The standard edition of the complete psychological works of Sigmund Freud, vol 23, London, 1964, Hogarth Press.

Galligan M: Proposed guidelines for skin-to-skin treatment of neonatal hypothermia, *MCN Am J Matern Child Nurs* 31(5):298–304, 2006.

Guttmacher AE, Collins FS: Genomic medicine—a primer, *N Engl J Med* 347(19):1512–1520, 2002.

Kaczander BI: Pediatric sports medicine: a unique perspective, *Pediatr Manage* 16(2):53–60, 1997.

Kohlberg L: Moral development. In Sills DL, editor: *International encyclopedia of the social sciences*, New York, 1968, Macmillan.

Matvienko O: Impact of a nutrition education curriculum on snack choices of children ages six and seven years, *J Nutr Educ Behav* 39(5):281–285, 2007.

Morrow JD, Camp BW: Mastery motivation and temperament of 7-month-old infants, *Pediatr Nurs* 22(3):211–217, 1996.

Myrelid A, Gustafsson J, Ollars B, et al: Growth charts for Down's syndrome from birth to 18 years of age, *Arch Dis Child* 87(2):97–103, 2002.

Piaget J: *The theory of stages in cognitive development*, New York, 1969, McGraw-Hill.

Rimoin DL, Connor MJ, Pyeritz RE, et al: *Emery and Rimoin's principles and practice of medical genetics*, London, 2002, Churchill Livingstone.

Romiti ML, Colognesi C, Cancrini C, et al: Prognostic value of a CCR5 defective allele in pediatric HIV-1 infection, *Mol Med* 6(1):28–36, 2000.

Seidel HM, Ball JW, Dains JE, et al: *Mosby's guide to physical examination*, ed 6, St Louis, 2007, Mosby.

Sieving RE, Zirbel-Donisch ST: Development and enhancement of self-esteem in children, *J Pediatr Health Care* 4(6):290–296, 1990.

Thompson R, Cotner-Bichelman N, McKerchar P, et al: Enhancing early communication through infant sign training, *J Appl Behav Anal* 40(1):15–23, 2007.

Urbanski LF, Hanlon DP: Pediatric orthopedics, *Top Emerg Med* 18(2):73–90, 1996.

Van Riper M: Families of children with Down syndrome: responding to "a change in plans" with resilience, *J Pediatr Nurs* 22(2):116–128, 2007.

Willoughby C, King G, Polatajko H: A therapist's guide to children's self-esteem, *Am J Occup Ther* 50(2):124–132, 1996.

Communication, History, and Physical Assessment

Marilyn J. Hockenberry

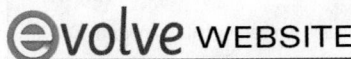

http://evolve.elsevier.com/Perry/maternal

LEARNING OBJECTIVES

On completion of this chapter, the reader will be able to:
- Identify communication strategies for interviewing parents.
- Formulate guidelines for using an interpreter.
- Identify communication strategies for communicating with children of different age-groups.
- Describe four communication techniques that are useful with children.
- State the components of a complete health history.
- List three areas that are evaluated as part of nutritional assessment.

- Prepare a child for a physical examination based on his or her developmental needs.
- Perform a comprehensive physical examination in a sequence appropriate to the child's age.
- Recognize expected normal findings for children at various ages.
- Record the physical examination according to the head-to-toe format.

GUIDELINES FOR COMMUNICATION AND INTERVIEWING

The most widely used method of communicating with parents on a professional basis is the interview process. Unlike social conversation, interviewing is a specific form of goal-directed communication. As nurses converse with children and adults, they focus on the individuals to determine the kind of persons they are, their usual mode of handling problems, whether they need help, and the way they react to counseling. Developing interviewing skills requires time and practice, but following some guiding principles can facilitate this process. An organized approach is most effective when using interviewing skills in patient teaching.

Establishing a Setting for Communication
Appropriate Introduction
Introduce yourself, and ask the name of each family member who is present. Address parents or other adults by their appropriate titles, such as "Mr." and "Mrs.," unless they specify a preferred name. Record the preferred name on the medical record. Using formal address or their preferred names, rather than using first names or "mother" or "father," conveys respect and regard for the parents or other caregivers (Seidel, Ball, Dains, et al., 2011).

At the beginning of the visit, include children in the interaction by asking them their name, age, and other information. Nurses often direct all questions to adults, even when children are old enough to speak for themselves. This only terminates one extremely valuable source of information: the patient. When including the child, follow the general rules for communicating with children given in the Guidelines box on p. 775.

Assurance of Privacy and Confidentiality
The place where the nurse conducts the interview is almost as important as the interview itself. The physical environment should allow for as much privacy as possible, with distractions, such as interruptions, noise, or other visible activity, kept to a minimum. At times it is necessary to turn off a television, radio, or cellular telephone. The environment should also have some play provision for young children to keep them occupied during the parent-nurse interview (Fig. 29-1). Parents who are constantly interrupted by their children are unable to concentrate fully and tend to give brief answers to finish the interview as quickly as possible.

Confidentiality is another essential component of the initial phase of the interview. Because the interview is usually shared with other members of the health care team or the teacher (in the case of students), be certain to inform the family of the limits regarding

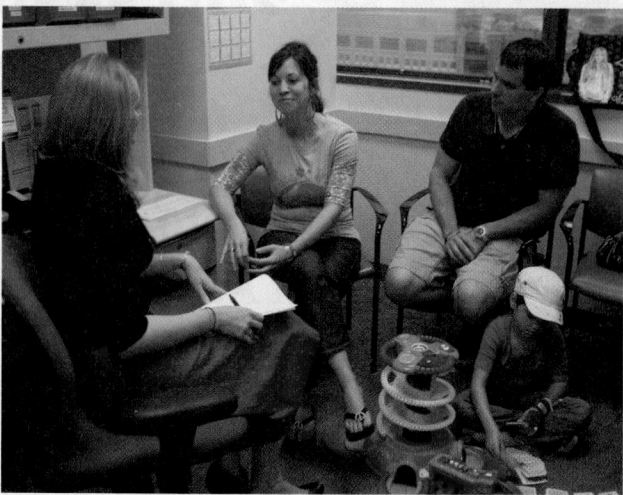

FIG 29-1 Child plays while nurse interviews parents.

BOX 29-1	TELEPHONE TRIAGE GUIDELINES

- Date and time
- Background
  - Name, age, sex
  - Chronic illness
  - Allergies, current medications, treatments, or recent immunizations
- Chief complaint
- General symptoms
  - Severity
  - Duration
  - Other symptoms
  - Pain
- Systems review
- Steps taken
  - Advised to call emergency medical services (911)
  - Advised to see practitioner
  - Advised regarding home care
  - Advised to call back if symptoms worsen or fail to improve

Resources for Telephone Triage Protocols

Beaulieu R, Jumphreys J: Evaluation of a telephone advice nurse in a nursing faculty managed pediatric community clinic, *J Pediatr Health Care* 22(3):175–181, 2008.

Marklund B, Ström M, Månsson J, et al: Computer-supported telephone nurse triage: an evaluation of medical quality and costs, *J Nurs Manage* 15:180–187, 2007.

Simonsen SM: *Telephone assessment: guidelines for practice,* ed 2, St Louis, 2001, Mosby.

confidentiality. If confidentiality is a concern in a particular situation, such as when talking to a parent suspected of child abuse or a teenager contemplating suicide, deal with this directly and inform the person that in such instances confidentiality cannot be ensured. However, the nurse judiciously protects information of a confidential nature.

Computer Privacy and Applications in Nursing

The use of computer technology to store and retrieve health information has become widespread. The health care community is increasingly concerned about the privacy and security of this health information. Any person accessing confidential health information is charged with managing safeguards for disclosure, since violations might incur civil damages.

Many institutions use computer and information applications in nursing (nursing informatics), such as electronic medical records, to record care and access information. Two important health care applications are (1) record transmission, including online access, fax, and e-mail; and (2) telemedicine. The telemedicine application is capable of two-way video conferencing, transmission of radiographs, and clinical consultation between remote sites and centralized resources.*

Telephone Triage and Counseling

Nurses are increasingly responsible for assessing children's symptoms and applying clinical judgment for further medical care (triage) via telephone report. Most often, health problems are assessed and prioritized according to urgency and nurses provide treatment via telephone services. A well-designed telephone triage program is essential for safe, prompt, and consistent quality health care (Beaulieu and Humphreys, 2008; Marklund, Ström, Månsson, et al., 2007). Telephone triage is more than "just a phone call," since a child's life is a high price to pay for poorly managed or incompetent telephone assessment skills. Typically, guidelines for telephone triage include asking screening questions; determining when to immediately refer to emergency medical services (dial 911); and determining when to refer to same-day appointments, appointments in 24 to 72 hours, appointments in 4 days or more, or home

care (Box 29-1). Successful outcomes are based on the consistency and accuracy of the information provided. Telephone triage care management has increased access to high-quality health care services and empowered parents to participate in their child's medical care. Consequently, patient satisfaction has significantly improved. Unnecessary emergency department and clinic visits have decreased, saving medical costs and time (with less absence from work) for families in need of health care.

COMMUNICATING WITH FAMILIES

Communicating with Parents

Although the parent and the child are separate and distinct individuals, the nurse's relationship with the child is frequently mediated by the parent, particularly with younger children. For the most part, nurses acquire information about the child by direct observation or through communication with the parents. Usually it can be assumed that, because of the close contact with the child, the parent gives reliable information. Assessing the child requires input from the child (verbal and nonverbal), information from the parent, and the nurse's own observations of the child and interpretation of the relationship between the child and the parent. When children are old enough to be active participants in their own health maintenance, the parent becomes a collaborator in health care.

Encouraging the Parents to Talk

Interviewing parents not only offers the opportunity to determine the child's health and developmental status but also offers information about factors that influence the child's life. Whatever the parent sees as a problem should be a concern of the nurse. These problems

---

are not always easy to identify. Nurses need to be alert for clues and signals by which a parent communicates worries and anxieties. Careful phrasing with broad, open-ended questions such as "What is Jimmy eating now?" provides more information than several single-answer questions, such as "Is Jimmy eating what the rest of the family eats?"

Sometimes the parent will take the lead without prompting. At other times it may be necessary to direct another question on the basis of an observation, such as "Connie seems unhappy today" or "How do you feel when David cries?" If the parent appears to be tired or distraught, consider asking "What do you do to relax?" or "What help do you have with the children?" A comment such as "You handle the baby very well. What kind of experience have you had with babies?" to new parents who appear comfortable with their first child gives positive reinforcement and provides an opening for questions they might have on the infant's care. Often all that is required to keep parents talking is a nod or saying "yes" or "uh-huh."

Directing the Focus

Directing the focus of the interview while allowing maximum freedom of expression is one of the most difficult goals in effective communication. One approach is the use of open-ended or broad questions, followed by guiding statements. For example, if the parent proceeds to list the other children by name, say, "Tell me their ages, too." If the parent continues to describe each child in depth, which is not the purpose of the interview, redirect the focus by stating, "Let's talk about the other children later. You were beginning to tell me about Paul's activities at school." This approach conveys interest in the other children but focuses the assessment on the patient.

Listening and Cultural Awareness

Listening is the most important component of effective communication. When the purpose of listening is to understand the person being interviewed, it is an active process that requires concentration and attention to all aspects of the conversation—verbal, nonverbal, and abstract. Major blocks to listening are environmental distraction and premature judgment.

Although it is necessary to make some preliminary judgments, listen with as much objectivity as possible by clarifying meanings and attempting to see the situation from the parent's point of view. Effective interviewers consciously control their reactions, responses, and the techniques they use (see Cultural Competence box).

Careful listening relies on the use of clues, verbal leads, or signals from the interviewee to move the interview along. Frequent references to an area of concern, repetition of certain key words, or a special emphasis on something or someone serves as a cue to the interviewer for the direction of inquiry. Concerns and anxieties are often mentioned in a casual, offhand manner. Even though they are casual, they are important and deserve careful scrutiny to identify problem areas. For example, a parent who is concerned about a child's habit of bed-wetting may casually mention that the child's bed was "wet this morning."

Using Silence

Silence as a response is often one of the most difficult interviewing techniques to learn. The interviewer requires a sense of confidence and comfort to allow the interviewee space in which to think without interruptions. Silence permits the interviewee to sort out thoughts and feelings and search for responses to questions. Silence can also be a cue for the interviewer to go more slowly, reexamine the approach, and not push too hard (Seidel, Ball, Dains, et al., 2011).

Sometimes it is necessary to break the silence and reopen communication. Do this in a way that encourages the person to continue talking about what is considered important. Breaking a silence by introducing a new topic or by prolonged talking essentially terminates the interviewee's opportunity to use the silence. Suggestions for breaking the silence include statements such as "Is there anything else you wish to say?" "I see you find it difficult to continue; how may I help?" or "I don't know what this silence means. Perhaps there is something you would like to put into words but find difficult to say."

Being Empathic

Empathy is the capacity to understand what another person is experiencing from within that person's frame of reference; it is often described as the ability to put oneself in another's shoes. The essence of empathic interaction is accurate understanding of another's feelings (Mathiasen, 2006). Empathy differs from sympathy, which is *having* feelings or emotions similar to those of another person, rather than *understanding* those feelings (Mathiasen, 2006).

Providing Anticipatory Guidance

The ideal way to handle a situation is to deal with it *before* it becomes a problem. The best preventive measure is anticipatory guidance. Traditionally, anticipatory guidance focused on providing families information on normal growth and development and nurturing childrearing practices. For example, one of the most significant areas in pediatrics is injury prevention. Beginning prenatally, parents need specific instructions on home safety. Because of the child's maturing developmental skills, parents must implement home safety changes early to minimize risks to the child.

Unprepared parents can be disturbed by many normal developmental changes, such as a toddler's diminished appetite, negativism, altered sleeping patterns, and anxiety toward strangers. The chapters on health promotion provide the nurse information for counseling parents. However, anticipatory guidance should extend beyond giving general information during brief visits to empowering families to use the information as a means of building competence in their parenting abilities (Magar, Dabova-Missova, and Gjerdingen, 2006). To achieve this level of anticipatory guidance, the nurse should:

- Base interventions on needs identified by the family, not by the professional
- View the family as competent or as having the ability to be competent
- Provide opportunities for the family to achieve competence

🌐 CULTURAL COMPETENCE

Interviewing Without Judgment

It is easy to inject one's own attitudes and feelings into an interview. Often nurses' own prejudices and assumptions, which may include racial, religious, and cultural stereotypes, influence their perceptions of a parent's behavior. What the nurse may interpret as a parent's passive hostility or lack of interest may be shyness or an expression of anxiety. For example, in Western cultures, eye contact and directness are signs of paying attention. However, in many non-Western cultures, including that of Native Americans, directness (e.g., looking someone in the eye) is considered rude. Children are taught to avert their gaze and to look down when being addressed by an adult, especially one with authority (Seidel, Ball, Dains, et al., 2011). Therefore nurses must make judgments about "listening," as well as verbal interactions, with an appreciation of cultural differences.

BOX 29-2 BLOCKS TO COMMUNICATION

Communication Barriers (Nurse)
- Socializing
- Giving unrestricted and sometimes unasked for advice
- Offering premature or inappropriate reassurance
- Giving overready encouragement
- Defending a situation or opinion
- Using stereotyped comments or clichés
- Limiting expression of emotion by asking directed, closed-ended questions
- Interrupting and finishing the person's sentence
- Talking more than the interviewee
- Forming prejudged conclusions
- Deliberately changing the focus

Signs of Information Overload (Patient)
- Long periods of silence
- Wide eyes and fixed facial expression
- Constant fidgeting or attempting to move away
- Nervous habits (e.g., tapping, playing with hair)
- Sudden interruptions (e.g., asking to go to the bathroom)
- Looking around
- Yawning, eyes drooping
- Frequently looking at a watch or clock
- Attempting to change topic of discussion

Avoiding Blocks to Communication

A number of blocks to communication can adversely affect the quality of the helping relationship. The interviewer introduces many of these blocks, such as giving unrestricted advice or forming prejudged conclusions. Another type of block occurs primarily with the interviewees and concerns information overload. When individuals receive too much information or information that is overwhelming, they often demonstrate signs of increasing anxiety or decreasing attention. Such signals should alert the interviewer to give less information or to clarify what has been said. Box 29-2 lists some of the more common blocks to communication, including signs of information overload.

The nurse can correct communication blocks by careful analysis of the interview process. One of the best methods for improving interviewing skills is audiotape or videotape feedback. With supervision and guidance, the interviewer can recognize the blocks and consciously avoid them.

Communicating with Families Through an Interpreter

Sometimes communication is impossible because two people speak different languages. In this case it is necessary to obtain information through a third party, the interpreter. When using an interpreter, the nurse follows the same interviewing guidelines. Specific guidelines for using an adult interpreter are given in the Guidelines box.

Communicating with families through an interpreter requires sensitivity to cultural, legal, and ethical considerations (see Cultural Competence box). For example, in some cultures, using a child as an interpreter is considered an insult to an adult because children are expected to show respect by not questioning their elders. In some cultures, class differences between the interpreter and the family may cause the family to feel intimidated and less inclined to offer information. Therefore it is important to choose the translator

 GUIDELINES

Using an Interpreter

- Explain to interpreter the reason for the interview and the type of questions that will be asked.
- Clarify whether a detailed or brief answer is required and whether the translated response can be general or literal.
- Introduce the interpreter to family, and allow some time before the interview for them to become acquainted.
- Communicate directly with family members when asking questions to reinforce interest in them and to observe nonverbal expressions, but do not ignore interpreter.
- Pose questions to elicit only one answer at a time, such as "Do you have pain?" rather than "Do you have any pain, tiredness, or loss of appetite?"
- Refrain from interrupting family member and interpreter while they are conversing.
- Avoid commenting to interpreter about family members, since they may understand some English.
- Be aware that some medical words, such as *allergy,* may have no similar word in another language; avoid medical jargon whenever possible.
- Be aware that cultural differences may exist regarding views on sex, marriage, or pregnancy.
- Allow time after the interview for interpreter to share something that he or she thought could not be said earlier; ask about the interpreter's impression of nonverbal clues to communication and family members' reliability or ease in revealing information.
- Arrange for family to speak with the same interpreter on subsequent visits whenever possible.

 CULTURAL COMPETENCE

Using Children as Translators

When no one else is available to translate, children within the family are often asked to assume this role. In this situation it is important to stress *literal* translation of parent responses. To ensure correct translations, it may be necessary to interrupt the parent and ask the child to translate every few sentences. When using children as interpreters, ask questions directed at specific answers and assess the interpreted translation in terms of nonverbal expressions of communication. Note that some institutions prohibit or discourage the use of children as interpreters; check institution policy for compliance.

! **NURSING ALERT**

When using translated materials, such as a health history form, be certain the informant is literate in the foreign language.

carefully and provide time for the interpreter and family to establish rapport.

Legal and ethical concerns may also arise. For example, in obtaining informed consent through an interpreter, the nurse should fully inform the family of all aspects of the particular procedure to which they are consenting. Issues of confidentiality may arise when family members related to another patient are asked to interpret for the family, thus revealing sensitive information that may be shared with other families on the unit. With increased sensitivity toward patient rights and confidentiality, many institutions now require consent forms produced in the patient's primary language.

GUIDELINES

Communicating with Children

- Allow children time to feel comfortable.
- Avoid sudden or rapid advances, broad smiles, extended eye contact, or other gestures that may be seen as threatening.
- Talk to the parent if child is initially shy.
- Communicate through transition objects such as dolls, puppets, and stuffed animals before questioning a young child directly.
- Give older children the opportunity to talk without the parents present.
- Assume a position that is at eye level with child (Fig. 29-2).
- Speak in a quiet, unhurried, and confident voice.
- Speak clearly, be specific, and use simple words and short sentences.
- State directions and suggestions positively.
- Offer a choice only when one exists.
- Be honest with children.
- Allow them to express their concerns and fears.
- Use a variety of communication techniques.

Communicating with Children

Although the greatest amount of verbal communication is usually carried out with the parent, do not exclude the child during the interview. Pay attention to infants and younger children through play or by occasionally directing questions or remarks to them. Include older children as active participants.

In communication with children of all ages, the nonverbal components of the communication process convey the most significant messages. It is difficult to disguise feelings, attitudes, and anxiety when relating to children. They are alert to surroundings and attach meaning to every gesture and move that is made; this is particularly true of very young children.

Active attempts to make friends with children before they have had an opportunity to evaluate an unfamiliar person tend to increase their anxiety. Continue to talk to the child and parent but go about activities that do not involve the child directly, thus allowing the child to observe from a safe position. If the child has a special toy or doll, "talk" to the doll first. Ask simple questions such as "Does your teddy bear have a name?" to ease the child into conversation. Other guidelines for communicating with children are in the Guidelines box. Specific guidelines for preparing children for procedures, a common nursing function, are in Chapter 39.

Communication Related to Development of Thought Processes

The normal development of language and thought offers a frame of reference for communicating with children. Thought processes progress from sensorimotor to perceptual to concrete and finally to abstract, formal operations. An understanding of the typical characteristics of these stages provides the nurse with a framework to facilitate social communication (Box 29-3).

Infancy. Because they are unable to use words, infants primarily use and understand nonverbal communication. Infants communicate their needs and feelings through nonverbal behaviors and vocalizations that can be interpreted by someone who is around them for a sufficient time. Infants smile and coo when content and cry when distressed. Crying is provoked by unpleasant stimuli from inside or outside, such as hunger, pain, body restraint, or loneliness. Adults interpret this to mean that an infant needs something and consequently try to alleviate the discomfort and reduce tension. Crying (or the desire to cry) persists as a part of everyone's communication repertoire.

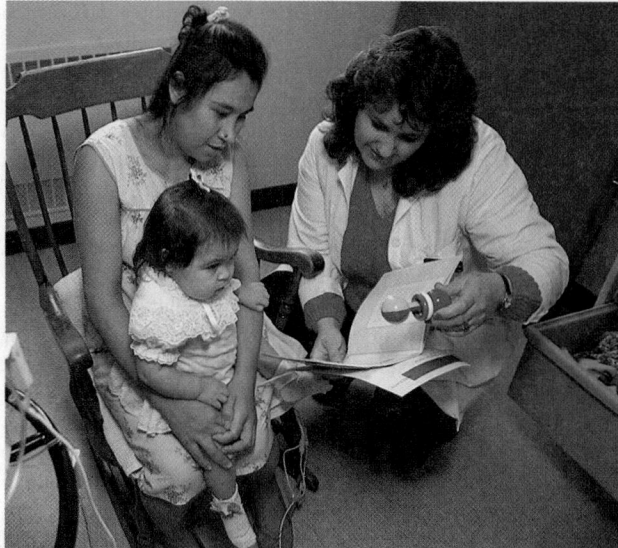

FIG 29-2 Nurse assumes position at child's level.

BOX 29-3	CHARACTERISTICS OF COMMUNICATIVE DEVELOPMENT IN YOUNG CHILDREN

Perlocutionary Stage (0 to 8-9 Months)
- Child is reflexive to stimuli.
- Child shows increasing purpose in action.

Emerging Illocutionary Stage (8-9 to 12-15 Months)
- Child communicates intentionally with signals and gestures.

Conventional Illocutionary–Emerging Locutionary Stage (12-15 to 18-24 Months)
- Child communicates intentionally with gestures, vocalizations, and verbalizations.

Adapted from Hoge DR, Parette HP: Facilitating communicative development in young children with disabilities, *Transdisc J* 5(2):113–130, 1995.

Infants respond to adults' nonverbal behaviors. They become quiet when they are cuddled, patted, or receive other forms of gentle physical contact. They receive comfort from the sound of a voice, even though they do not understand the words that are spoken. Until infants reach the age at which they experience stranger anxiety, they readily respond to any firm, gentle handling and quiet, calm speech. Loud, harsh sounds and sudden movements are frightening.

Early Childhood. Children younger than 5 years are egocentric. They see things only in relation to themselves and from their point of view. Therefore focus communication on them. Tell them what they can do or how they will feel. Experiences of others are of no interest to them. It is futile to use another child's experience in an attempt to gain the cooperation of small children. Allow them to touch and examine articles they will come in contact with. A stethoscope bell will feel cold; palpating a neck might tickle. Although they have not yet acquired sufficient language skills to express their feelings and wants, toddlers can effectively use their hands to communicate ideas without words. They push an unwanted object away, pull another person to show them something, point, and cover the mouth that is saying something they do not wish to hear.

Everything is direct and concrete to small children. They are unable to work with abstractions and interpret words literally. Analogies escape them because they are unable to separate fact from fantasy. For example, they attach literal meaning to such common phrases as "two-faced," "sticky fingers," or "coughing your head off." Children who are told they will get "a little stick in the arm" may not be able to envision an injection (Fig. 29-3). Therefore avoid using a phrase that might be misinterpreted by a small child.

School-Age Years. Younger school-age children rely less on what they see and more on what they know when faced with new problems. They want explanations and reasons for everything but require no verification beyond that. They are interested in the functional aspect of all procedures, objects, and activities. They want to know why an object exists, why it is used, how it works, and the intent and purpose of its user. They need to know what is going to take place and why it is being done to them specifically. For example, to explain a procedure such as taking blood pressure, show the child how squeezing the bulb pushes air into the cuff and makes the "silver" in the tube go up. Let the child operate the bulb. An explanation for the procedure might be as simple as "I want to see how far the silver goes up when the cuff squeezes your arm." Consequently, the child becomes an enthusiastic participant.

School-age children have a heightened concern about body integrity. Because of the special importance they place on their body, they are sensitive to anything that constitutes a threat or suggestion of injury to it. This concern extends to their possessions, so they may appear to overreact to loss or threatened loss of treasured objects. Helping children voice their concerns enables the nurse to provide reassurance and to implement activities that reduce their anxiety. For example, if a shy child dislikes being the center of attention, ignore that particular child by talking and relating to other children in the family or group. When children feel more comfortable, they will usually interject personal ideas, feelings, and interpretations of events.

Adolescence. As children move into adolescence, they fluctuate between child and adult thinking and behavior. They are riding a current that is moving them rapidly toward a maturity that may be beyond their coping ability. Therefore when tensions rise, they may seek the security of the more familiar and comfortable expectations of childhood. Anticipating these shifts in identity allows the nurse to adjust the course of interaction to meet the needs of the moment. No single approach can be relied on consistently, and encountering cooperation, hostility, anger, bravado, and a variety of other behaviors and attitudes is common. It is as much a mistake to regard the adolescent as an adult with an adult's wisdom and control as it is to assume that the teenager has the concerns and expectations of a child.

Interviewing the adolescent presents some special issues. The first may be whether to talk with the adolescent alone or with the adolescent and parents together. Of course, if the parent is not there, the only question is whether to suggest to the teenager that the parents be interviewed at another time. If the parents and teenager are together, talking with the adolescent first has the advantage of immediately identifying with the young person, thus fostering the interpersonal relationship. However, talking with the parents initially may provide insight into the family relationship. In either case, give both parties an opportunity to be included in the interview. If time is limited, such as during history taking, clarify this at the onset to avoid appearing to "take sides" by talking more with one person than with the other.

Confidentiality is of great importance when interviewing adolescents. Explain to parents and teenagers the limits of confidentiality, specifically that young persons' disclosures will not be shared unless they indicate a need for intervention, as in the case of suicidal behavior.

Another dilemma in interviewing adolescents is that two views of a problem frequently exist—the teenager's and the parents'. Clarification of the problem is a major task. However, providing both parties an opportunity to discuss their perceptions in an open and unbiased atmosphere can, by itself, be therapeutic. Demonstrating positive communication skills can help families communicate more effectively (see Guidelines box).

Communication Techniques

Nurses use a variety of verbal techniques to encourage communication. Some of these techniques are useful to pose questions or explore concerns in a less threatening manner. Others can be presented as word games, which are often well received by children.

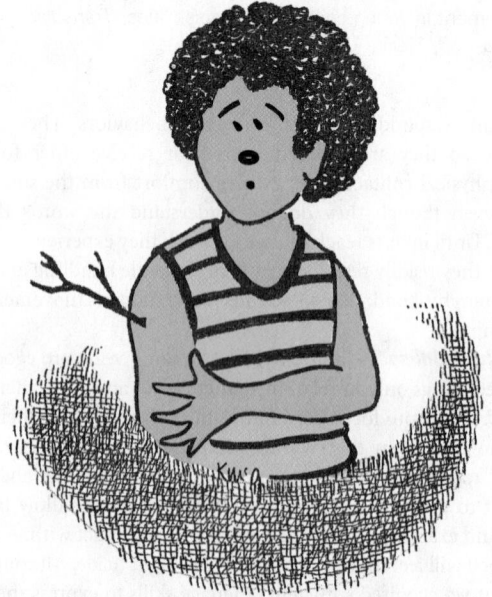

FIG 29-3 A young child may take the expression "a little stick in the arm" literally.

📋 GUIDELINES

Communicating with Adolescents

Build a Foundation	Communicate Effectively
• Spend time together.	• Give undivided attention.
• Encourage expression of ideas and feelings.	• Listen, listen, listen.
• Respect their views.	• Be courteous, calm, and open minded.
• Tolerate differences.	• Try not to overreact. If you do, take a break.
• Praise good points.	• Avoid judging or criticizing.
• Respect their privacy.	• Avoid the "third degree" of continuous questioning.
• Set a good example.	• Choose important issues when taking a stand.
	• After taking a stand:
	• Think through all options.
	• Make expectations clear.

However, for many children and adults, talking about feelings is difficult and verbal communication may be more stressful than supportive. In such instances, use several nonverbal techniques to encourage communication.

Box 29-4 describes both verbal and nonverbal techniques. Because of the importance of play in communicating with children, play is discussed more extensively in the section that follows. Any of the verbal or nonverbal techniques can give rise to strong feelings that surface unexpectedly. Be prepared to handle them or to recognize when issues go beyond your ability to deal with them. At that point, consider an appropriate referral.

Play. Play is a universal language of children. It is one of the most important forms of communication and can be an effective technique in relating to them. The nurse can often pick up on clues about physical, intellectual, and social developmental progress from the form and complexity of a child's play behaviors. Play requires minimum equipment or none at all. Many providers use therapeutic play to reduce the trauma of illness and hospitalization (see

Chapter 39) and to prepare children for therapeutic procedures (see Chapter 39).

Because their ability to perceive precedes their ability to transmit, infants respond to activities that register on their physical senses. Patting, stroking, and other skin play convey messages. Repetitive actions, such as stretching infants' arms out to the side while they are lying on their back and then folding the arms across the chest or raising and revolving the legs in a bicycling motion, will elicit pleasurable sounds. Colorful items to catch the eye or interesting sounds, such as a ticking clock, chimes, bells, or singing, can be used to attract children's attention.

Older infants respond to simple games. The old game of peek-a-boo is an excellent means of initiating communication with infants while maintaining a "safe," nonthreatening distance. After this intermittent eye contact, the nurse is no longer viewed as a stranger but as a friend. This can be followed by touch games. Clapping an infant's hands together for pat-a-cake or wiggling the toes for "this little piggy" delights an infant or small child. Talking to a

---

BOX 29-4　CREATIVE COMMUNICATION TECHNIQUES WITH CHILDREN

Verbal Techniques

"I" Messages

- Relate a feeling about a behavior in terms of "I."
- Describe effect behavior had on the person.
- Avoid use of "you."
- "You" messages are judgmental and provoke defensiveness.

   Example—"You" message: "You are being uncooperative about doing your treatments."

   Example—"I" message: "I am concerned about how the treatments are going because I want to see you get better."

Third-Person Technique

- Express a feeling in terms of a third person ("he," "she," "they"). This is less threatening than directly asking children how they feel because it gives them an opportunity to agree or disagree without being defensive.

   Example—"Sometimes when a person is sick a lot, he feels angry and sad because he cannot do what others can." Either wait silently for a response or encourage a reply with a statement such as "Did you ever feel that way?"

- This approach allows children three choices: (1) to agree and, one hopes, express how they feel; (2) to disagree; or (3) to remain silent, which means they probably have such feelings but are unable to express them at this time.

Facilitative Response

- Listen carefully and reflect back to patients the feelings and content of their statements.
- Responses are empathic and nonjudgmental and legitimize the person's feelings.
- Formula for facilitative responses: "You feel _____ because _____."

   Example—If child states, "I hate coming to the hospital and getting needles," a facilitative response is, "You feel unhappy because of all the things that are done to you."

Storytelling

- Use the language of children to probe into areas of their thinking while bypassing conscious inhibitions or fears.

- The simplest technique is asking children to relate a story about an event, such as "being in the hospital."
- Other approaches:
   - Show children a picture of a particular event, such as a child in a hospital with other people in the room, and ask them to describe the scene.
   - Cut out comic strips, remove words, and have child add statements for scenes.

Mutual Storytelling

- Reveal child's thinking and attempt to change child's perceptions or fears by retelling a somewhat different story (more therapeutic approach than storytelling).
- Begin by asking child to tell a story about something, and then tell another story that is similar to child's tale but with differences that help child in problem areas.

   Example—Child's story is about going to the hospital and never seeing his or her parents again. Nurse's story is also about a child (using different names but similar circumstances) in a hospital whose parents visit every day, but in the evening after work, until the child is better and goes home with them.

Bibliotherapy

- Use books in a therapeutic and supportive process.
- Provide children with an opportunity to explore an event that is similar to their own but sufficiently different to allow them to distance themselves from it and remain in control.
- General guidelines for using bibliotherapy are:
   1. Assess child's emotional and cognitive development in terms of readiness to understand the book's message.
   2. Be familiar with the book's content (intended message or purpose) and the age for which it is written.
   3. Read the book to the child if child is unable to read.
   4. Explore the meaning of the book with the child by having child:
      Retell the story
      Read a special section with the nurse or parent
      Draw a picture related to the story and discuss the drawing
      Talk about the characters
      Summarize the moral or meaning of the story

Continued

BOX 29-4 CREATIVE COMMUNICATION TECHNIQUES WITH CHILDREN—cont'd

Dreams

- Dreams often reveal unconscious and repressed thoughts and feelings.
- Ask child to talk about a dream or nightmare.
- Explore with child what meaning the dream could have.

"What If" Questions

- Encourage child to explore potential situations and to consider different problem-solving options.
  Example—"What if you got sick and had to go the hospital?" Children's responses reveal what they know already and what they are curious about, providing an opportunity for them to learn coping skills, especially in potentially dangerous situations.

Three Wishes

- Ask, "If you could have any three things in the world, what would they be?"
- If child answers, "That all my wishes come true," ask child for specific wishes.

Rating Game

- Use some type of rating scale (numbers, sad to happy faces) to have child rate an event or feeling.
  Example—Instead of asking youngsters how they feel, ask how their day has been "on a scale of 1 to 10, with 10 being the best."

Word Association Game

- State key words and ask children to say the first word they think of when they hear the word.
- Start with neutral words and then introduce more anxiety-producing words, such as "illness," "needles," "hospitals," and "operation."
- Select key words that relate to some relevant event in the child's life.

Sentence Completion

- Present a partial statement and have the child complete it. Some sample statements are:
  The thing I like best (least) about school is _____.
  The best (worst) age to be is _____.
  The most (least) fun thing I ever did was _____.
  The thing I like most (least) about my parents is _____.
  The one thing I would change about my family is _____.
  If I could be anything I wanted, I would be _____.
  The thing I like most (least) about myself is _____.

Pros and Cons

- Select a topic, such as "being in the hospital," and have child list "five good things and five bad things" about it.
- This is an exceptionally valuable technique when applied to relationships, such as things family members like and dislike about each other.

Nonverbal Techniques

Writing

- Writing is an alternative communication approach for older children and adults.
- Specific suggestions include:
  - Keep a journal or diary.
  - Write down feelings or thoughts that are difficult to express.
  - Write "letters" that are never mailed (a variation is making up a "pen pal" to write to).
- Keep an account of child's progress from both a physical and an emotional viewpoint.

Drawing

- Drawing is one of the most valuable forms of communication—both non-verbal (from looking at the drawing) and verbal (from child's story of the picture).
- Children's drawings tell a great deal about them because they are projections of their inner selves.
- Spontaneous drawing involves giving child a variety of art supplies and providing the opportunity to draw.
- Directed drawing involves a more specific direction, such as "draw a person" or the "three themes" approach (state three things about child and ask child to choose one and draw a picture).

Guidelines for Evaluating Drawings

- Use spontaneous drawings and evaluate more than one drawing whenever possible.
- Interpret drawings in light of other available information about child and family, including the child's age and stage of development.
- Interpret drawings as a whole rather than focusing on specific details of the drawing.
- Consider individual elements of the drawing that may be significant:
  - Sex of figure drawn first—Usually relates to child's perception of own gender role
  - Size of individual figures—Expresses importance, power, or authority
  - Order in which figures are drawn—Expresses priority in terms of importance
  - Child's position in relation to other family members—Expresses feelings of status or alliance
  - Exclusion of a member—May denote feeling of not belonging or desire to eliminate
  - Accentuated parts—Usually express concern for areas of special importance (e.g., large hands may be a sign of aggression)
  - Absence of or rudimentary arms and hands—Suggest timidity, passivity, or intellectual immaturity; tiny, unstable feet may express insecurity, and hidden hands may mean guilt feelings
  - Placement of drawing on the page and type of stroke—Free use of paper and firm, continuous strokes express security, whereas drawings restricted to a small area and lightly drawn in broken or wavering lines may be a sign of insecurity
  - Erasures, shading, or cross-hatching—Expresses ambivalence, concern, or anxiety with a particular area

Magic

- Use simple magic tricks to help establish rapport with child, encourage compliance with health interventions, and provide effective distraction during painful procedures.
- Although the "magician" talks, no verbal response from child is required.

Play

- Play is the universal language and "work" of children.
- It tells a great deal about children because they project their inner selves through the activity.
- Spontaneous play involves giving child a variety of play materials and providing the opportunity to play.
- Directed play involves a more specific direction, such as providing medical equipment or a dollhouse for focused reasons, such as exploring child's fear of injections or exploring family relationships.

foot or other part of the child's body is another effective tactic. Much of the nursing assessment can be carried out with the use of games and simple play equipment while the infant remains in the safety of the parent's arms or lap.

The nurse can capitalize on the natural curiosity of small children by playing games such as "Which hand do you take?" and "Guess what I have in my hand" or by manipulating items such as a flashlight or stethoscope. Finger games are useful. More elaborate materials, such as puppets and replicas of familiar or unfamiliar items, serve as excellent means of communicating with small children. The variety and extent are limited only by the nurse's imagination.

Through play, children reveal their perceptions of interpersonal relationships with their family, friends, or hospital personnel. Children may also reveal the wide scope of knowledge they have acquired from listening to others around them. For example, through needle play, children may reveal how carefully they have watched each procedure by precisely duplicating the technical skills. They may also reveal how well they remember those who performed procedures. In one example, a child painstakingly reenacted every detail of a tedious medical procedure, including the role of the physician who had repeatedly shouted at her to be still for the long ordeal. Her anger at him was most evident during the play session and revealed the cause for her abrupt withdrawal and passive hostility toward the medical and nursing staff after the test.

HISTORY TAKING

Performing a Health History

The format used for history taking may be (1) direct, in which the nurse asks for information via direct interview with the informant; or (2) indirect, in which the informant supplies the information by completing some type of questionnaire. The direct method is superior to the indirect approach or a combination of both. However, because time is limited, the direct approach is not always practical. If the nurse cannot use the direct approach, he or she should review parents' written responses and question them regarding any unusual answers. The categories listed in Box 29-5 encompass children's current and past health status and information about their psychosocial environment.

Identifying Information

Much of the identifying information may already be available from other recorded sources. However, if the parent and youngster seem anxious, use this opportunity to ask about such information to help them feel more comfortable.

Informant. One of the important elements of identifying information is the informant, the person(s) who furnishes the information. Record (1) who the person is (child, parent, or other), (2) an impression of reliability and willingness to communicate, and (3) any special circumstances such as the use of an interpreter or conflicting answers by more than one person.

Chief Complaint

The chief complaint is the specific reason for the child's visit to the clinic, office, or hospital. It may be the theme, with the present illness viewed as the description of the problem. Elicit the chief complaint by asking open-ended, neutral questions such as "What seems to be the matter?" "How may I help you?" or "Why did you come here today?" Avoid labeling-type questions such as "How are you sick?" or "What is the problem?" It is possible that the reason for the visit is not an illness or problem.

BOX 29-5 OUTLINE OF A PEDIATRIC HEALTH HISTORY

Identifying Information
- Name
- Address
- Telephone
- Birth date and place
- Race or ethnic group
- Sex
- Religion
- Date of interview
- Informant

Chief complaint (CC)—To establish the major specific reason for the child's and parents' seeking professional health attention

Present illness (PI)—To obtain all details related to the chief complaint

Past history (PH)—To elicit a profile of the child's previous illnesses, injuries, or operations
- Birth history (pregnancy, labor and birth, perinatal history)
- Previous illnesses, injuries, or operations
- Allergies
- Current medications
- Immunizations
- Growth and development
- Habits

Review of systems (ROS)—To elicit information concerning any potential health problem
- General
- Integument
- Head
- Eyes
- Ears
- Nose
- Mouth
- Throat
- Neck
- Chest
- Respiratory
- Cardiovascular
- Gastrointestinal
- Genitourinary
- Gynecologic
- Musculoskeletal
- Neurologic
- Endocrine

Family medical history—To identify genetic traits or diseases that have familial tendencies and to assess exposure to a communicable disease in a family member and family habits that may affect the child's health, such as smoking and chemical use

Psychosocial history—To elicit information about the child's self-concept

Sexual history—To elicit information concerning the child's sexual concerns or activities and any pertinent data regarding adults' sexual activity that influences the child

Family history—To develop an understanding of the child as an individual and as a member of a family and a community
- Family composition
- Home and community environment
- Occupation and education of family members
- Cultural and religious traditions
- Family function and relationships

Nutritional assessment—To elicit information on the adequacy of the child's nutritional intake and needs
- Dietary intake
- Clinical examination

GUIDELINES

Analyzing the Symptom: Pain

Type

Be as specific as possible. With young children, asking the parents how they know the child is in pain may help describe its type, location, and severity. For example, a parent may state, "My child must have a severe earache because she pulls at her ears, rolls her head on the floor, and screams. Nothing seems to help." Help older children describe the "hurt" by asking them if it is sharp, throbbing, dull, or stabbing. Record whatever words they use in quotes.

Location

Be specific. "Stomach pains" is too general a description. Children can better localize the pain if they are asked to "point with one finger to where it hurts" or to "point to where Mommy or Daddy would put a Band-Aid." Determine if the pain radiates by asking, "Does the pain stay there or move? Show me with your finger where the pain goes."

Severity

Severity is best determined by finding out how it affects the child's usual behavior. Pain that prevents a child from playing, interacting with others, sleeping, and eating is most often severe. Assess pain intensity using a rating scale, such as a numeric or FACES scale (see Chapter 30).

Duration

Include the duration, onset, and frequency. Describe this in terms of activity and behavior, such as "pain reported to last all night, child refused to sleep and cried intermittently."

Influencing Factors

Include anything that causes a change in the type, location, severity, or duration of the pain: (1) precipitating events (those that cause or increase the pain), (2) relieving events (those that lessen the pain, such as medications), (3) temporal events (times when the pain is relieved or increased), (4) positional events (standing, sitting, lying down), and (5) associated events (meals, stress, coughing).

Occasionally it is difficult to isolate one symptom or problem as the chief complaint because the parent may identify many. In this situation, be as specific as possible when asking questions. For example, asking informants to state which *one* problem or symptom prompted them to seek help now may help them focus on the most immediate concern.

Present Illness

The history of the present illness* is a narrative of the chief complaint from its earliest onset through its progression to the present. Its four major components are (1) the details of **onset**, (2) a complete **interval** history, (3) the **present** status, and (4) the reason for seeking help **now**. The focus of the present illness is on all factors relevant to the main problem, even if they have disappeared or changed during the onset, interval, and present.

Analyzing a Symptom. Because pain is often the most characteristic symptom denoting the onset of a physical problem, it is used as an example for analysis of a symptom. Assessment includes (1) type, (2) location, (3) severity, (4) duration, and (5) influencing factors (see Guidelines box; see also Pain Assessment, Chapter 30).

---

*The term *illness* is used in its broadest sense to denote any problem of a physical, emotional, or psychosocial nature. It is actually a history of the chief complaint.

Past History

The history contains information relating to all previous aspects of the child's health status and concentrates on several areas that are ordinarily passed over in the history of an adult, such as birth history, detailed feeding history, immunizations, and growth and development. Because this section includes a great deal of information, use a combination of open-ended and fact-finding questions. For example, begin interviewing for each section with an open-ended statement such as "Tell me about your child's birth" to provide the informants the opportunity to relate what they think is most important. Ask fact-finding questions related to specific details whenever necessary to focus the interview on certain topics.

Birth History. The birth history includes all data concerning (1) the mother's health during pregnancy, (2) the labor and birth, and (3) the infant's condition immediately after birth. Because prenatal influences have significant effects on a child's physical and emotional development, a thorough investigation of the birth history is essential. Because parents may question what relevance pregnancy and birth have on the child's present condition, particularly if the child is past infancy, explain why such questions are included. An appropriate statement may be "I will be asking you some questions about your pregnancy and ____'s [refer to child by name] birth. Your answers will give me a more complete picture of his [or her] overall health."

Because emotional factors also affect the outcome of pregnancy and the subsequent parent-child relationship, investigate (1) concurrent crises during pregnancy and (2) prenatal attitudes toward the fetus. It is best to approach the topic of parental acceptance of pregnancy through indirect questioning. Asking parents if the pregnancy was planned is a leading question because they may respond affirmatively for fear of criticism if the pregnancy was unexpected. Rather, encourage parents to state their true reactions by referring to specific facts relating to the pregnancy, such as the spacing between offspring, an extended or short interval between marriage and conception, or a pregnancy during adolescence. The parent can choose to explore such statements with further explanations or, for the moment, may not be able to reveal such feelings. If the parent remains silent, return to this topic later in the interview.

Dietary History. Because parental concerns are common and nursing interventions are important in ensuring optimum nutrition, the dietary history is discussed in detail later in this chapter in the Nutritional Assessment section.

Previous Illnesses, Injuries, and Operations. When inquiring about past illnesses, begin with a general statement such as "What other illnesses has your child had?" Because parents are most likely to recall serious health problems, ask specifically about colds; earaches; and childhood diseases such as measles, rubella (German measles), chickenpox, mumps, pertussis (whooping cough), diphtheria, tuberculosis, scarlet fever, strep throat, recurrent ear infections, gastroesophageal reflux, tonsillitis, or allergic manifestations.

In addition to illnesses, ask about injuries that required medical intervention, operations, and any other reason for hospitalization, including the dates of each incident. Focus on injuries such as accidental falls, poisoning, choking, or burns, since these may be potential areas for parental guidance.

Allergies. Ask about commonly known allergic disorders such as hay fever and asthma; unusual reactions to drugs, food, or latex products; and reactions to other contact agents such as poisonous plants, animals, household products, or fabrics. If asked appropriate questions, most people can give reliable information about drug reactions (see Guidelines box).

GUIDELINES

Taking an Allergy History

- Has your child ever taken any drugs or tablets that have disagreed with him or her or caused an allergic reaction? If yes, can you remember the name(s) of these drugs?
- Can you describe the reaction?
- Was the drug taken by mouth (as a tablet or syrup), or was it an injection?
- How soon after starting the drug did the reaction happen?
- How long ago did this happen?
- Did anyone tell you it was an allergic reaction, or did you decide for yourself?
- Has your child ever taken this drug, or a similar one, again? If yes, did your child experience the same problems?
- Have you told the doctors or nurses about your child's reaction or allergy?

! NURSING ALERT

Information about allergic reactions to drugs or other products is essential. Failure to document a serious reaction places the child at risk if the agent is given.

Current Medications. Inquire about current drug regimens, including vitamins, antipyretics (especially aspirin), antibiotics, antihistamines, decongestants, or herbs and homeopathic medications. List all medications, including name, dose, schedule, duration, and reason for administration. Often parents are unaware of the drug's actual name. Whenever possible, ask parents to bring the containers with them to the next visit, or ask for the name of the pharmacy and call for a list of all the child's recent prescription medications. However, this list will not include over-the-counter medications, which are important to know.

Immunizations. A record of all immunizations is essential. Because many parents are unaware of the exact name and date of each immunization, the most reliable source of information is a hospital, clinic, or private practitioner's record. All immunizations and "boosters" are listed, stating (1) the name of the specific disease, (2) the number of injections, (3) the dosage (sometimes lesser amounts are given if a reaction is anticipated), (4) the ages when administered, and (5) the occurrence of any reaction after the immunization.

! NURSING ALERT

Inquire about previous administration of any horse or other foreign serum. Inquire about recent administration of immune gamma globulin or blood transfusion because these necessitate a delay in giving live vaccines. And ask about anaphylactic reactions to neomycin, eggs, or any other component of a vaccine.

Growth and Development. The most important previous growth patterns to record are:

- Approximate weight at 6 months, 1 year, 2 years, and 5 years of age
- Approximate length at ages 1 and 4 years
- Dentition, including age of onset, number of teeth, and symptoms during teething

---

BOX 29-6 HABITS TO EXPLORE DURING HEALTH INTERVIEW

- Behavior patterns such as nail biting, thumb sucking, pica (habitual ingestion of nonfood substances), rituals ("security" blanket or toy), and unusual movements (head banging, rocking, overt masturbation, walking on toes)
- Activities of daily living, such as hour of sleep and arising, duration of nighttime sleep and naps, type and duration of exercise, regularity of stools and urination, age of toilet training, and daytime or nighttime bed-wetting
- Unusual disposition; response to frustration
- Use or abuse of alcohol, drugs, coffee, or tobacco

Developmental milestones include:

- Age of holding up head steadily
- Age of sitting alone without support
- Age of walking without assistance
- Age of saying first words with meaning
- Present grade in school
- Scholastic performance
- If the child has a best friend
- Interactions with other children, peers, and adults

Use specific and detailed questions when inquiring about each developmental milestone. For example, "sitting up" can mean many different activities, such as sitting propped up, sitting in someone's lap, sitting with support, sitting up alone but in a hyperflexed position for assisted balance, or sitting up unsupported with the back slightly rounded. A clue to misunderstanding of the requested activity may be an unusually early age of achievement.

Habits. Habits are an important area to explore (Box 29-6). Parents frequently express concerns during this part of the history. Encourage their input by saying, "Please tell me any concerns you have about your child's habits, activities, or development." Investigate further any concerns that parents express.

One of the most common concerns relates to sleep. Many children develop a normal sleep pattern, and all that is required during the assessment is a general overview of nighttime sleep and nap schedules. However, a number of children develop sleep problems (see Sleep Problems, Chapters 31 and 32). When sleep problems occur, the nurse needs a more detailed sleep history to guide appropriate interventions.*

Habits related to use of chemicals apply primarily to older children and adolescents. If a youngster admits to smoking, drinking, or using drugs, ask about the quantity and frequency. Questions such as "Many kids your age are experimenting with drugs and alcohol; have you ever had any drugs or alcohol?" may give more reliable data than questions such as "How much do you drink?" or "How often do you drink or take drugs?" Clarify that "drinking" includes all types of alcohol, including beer and wine. When quantities such as a "glass" of wine or a "can" of beer are given, ask about the size of the container.

If older children deny use of chemical substances, inquire about past experimentation. Asking "You mean you never tried to smoke or drink?" implies that the nurse expects some such activity, and the youngster may be more inclined to answer truthfully. Be aware of

---

*A sleep history and a sleep chart for the family to record the child's daily sleep and wake activities is available in Wilson D, Hockenberry M: *Wong's clinical manual of pediatric nursing*, ed 8, St Louis, 2011, Mosby.

the confidential nature of such questioning, the adverse effect that the parents' presence may have on the adolescent's willingness to answer, and the fact that self-reporting may not be an accurate account of chemical abuse.

Sexual History

The sexual history is an essential component of adolescents' health assessment. The history uncovers areas of concern related to sexual activity; alerts the nurse to circumstances that may indicate screening for sexually transmitted infections or testing for pregnancy; and provides information related to the need for sexual counseling, such as safer sex practices. Box 29-7 gives guidelines for anticipatory guidance topics for parents and adolescents.

One approach to initiating a conversation about sexual concerns is to begin with a history of peer interactions. Open-ended statements or questions such as "Tell me about your social life" or "Who are your closest friends?" generally lead into a discussion of dating

---

BOX 29-7 ANTICIPATORY GUIDANCE—SEXUALITY

Ages 12 to 14 Years
- Have adolescent identify supportive adult to discuss sexuality issues and concerns with.
- Discuss advantages of delaying sexual activity.
- Discuss making responsible decisions regarding normal sexual feelings.
- Discuss role of gender, peer pressure, and the media in sexual decision making.
- Discuss contraceptive options (advantages and disadvantages).
- Provide education regarding sexually transmitted infections (STIs), including human immunodeficiency virus (HIV) infection; clarify risks, and discuss condoms.
- Discuss abuse prevention: avoiding dangerous situations, role of drugs and alcohol, and use of self-defense.
- Have adolescent clarify values, needs, and ability to be assertive.
- If adolescent is sexually active, discuss limiting partners, use of condoms, and contraceptive options.
- Have confidential interview with adolescent (including a sexual history).
- Discuss the evolution of sexual identity and expression.
- Discuss breast examination or testicular examination.

Ages 15 to 18 Years
- Support delaying sexual activity.
- Discuss alternatives to intercourse.
- Discuss "When are you ready for sex?"
- Clarify values; encourage responsible decision making.
- Discuss consequences of unprotected sex: early pregnancy, STIs, including HIV infection.
- Discuss negotiating with partner and barriers to safer sex.
- If adolescent is sexually active, discuss limiting partners, use of condoms, and contraceptive options.
- Emphasize that sex should be safe and pleasurable for both partners.
- Have confidential interview with adolescent.
- Discuss concerns about sexual expression and identity.

Data from Fonseca H, Greydanus D: Sexuality in the child, teen and young adult: concepts for the clinician, *Prim Care Clin Office Pract* 34:275–292, 2007; Wright K: Anticipatory guidance: developing a healthy sexuality, *Pediatr Ann* 26(Suppl 2):S142–S144, C3, 1997.

---

and sexual issues. To probe further, include questions about the adolescent's attitudes on such topics as sex education, "going steady," "living together," and premarital sex. Phrase questions to reflect concern rather than judgment or criticism of sexual practices.

In any conversation regarding sexual history, be aware of the language that is used in either eliciting or conveying sexual information. For example, avoid asking whether the adolescent is "sexually active," since this term is broadly defined. "Are you having sex with anyone?" is probably the most direct and best understood question. Since same-sex experimentation may occur, refer to all sexual contacts in nongender terms, such as "anyone" or "partners," rather than "girlfriends" or "boyfriends."

Family Medical History

The family medical history is used primarily to discover any hereditary or familial diseases in the parents and child. In general, it is confined to first-degree relatives (parents, siblings, grandparents, and immediate aunts and uncles). Information for each family member includes age; marital status; state of health if living; cause of death if deceased; and any evidence of conditions such as early heart disease, sudden death from unknown cause, hypercholesterolemia, hypertension, cancer, diabetes mellitus, obesity, congenital anomalies, allergies, asthma, seizures, tuberculosis, sickle cell disease, cognitive impairment, hearing or visual deficits, psychiatric disorders such as depression or psychosis, and emotional problems. Confirm the accuracy of the reported disorders by inquiring about the symptoms, course, treatment, and sequelae of each diagnosis.

Geographic Location. One of the important areas to explore when assessing the family health history is geographic location, including the birthplace and travel to different areas in or outside of the country, for identification of possible exposure to endemic diseases. Although the primary interest is the child's temporary residence in various localities, also inquire about close family members' travel, especially during tours of military service or business trips. Children are especially susceptible to parasitic infestation in areas of poor sanitary conditions and to vector-borne diseases, such as those from mosquitoes or ticks in warm and humid or heavily wooded regions.

Family Structure

Assessment of the family, both its structure and function, is an important component of the history-taking process. Because the quality of the functional relationship between the child and family members is a major factor in emotional and physical health, family assessment is discussed separately and in greater detail apart from the more traditional health history.

Family assessment is the collection of data about the composition of the family and the relationships among its members. In its broadest sense, family refers to all those individuals who are considered by the family member to be significant to the nuclear unit, including relatives, friends, and social groups such as the school and church. Although family assessment is not family therapy, it can and frequently is therapeutic. Involving family members in discussing family characteristics and activities can provide insight into family dynamics and relationships.

Because of the time involved in performing an in-depth family assessment as presented here, be selective in deciding when knowledge of family function may facilitate nursing care (see Guidelines box). During brief contacts with families, a full assessment is not appropriate and screening with one or two questions from each category may reflect the health of the family system or the need for additional assessment.

The most common method of eliciting information on the family structure is to interview family members. The principal areas of concern are (1) family composition, (2) home and community environment, (3) occupation and education of family members, and (4) cultural and religious traditions (Box 29-8).

Psychosocial History

The traditional medical history includes a personal and social section that concentrates on children's personal status, such as school adjustment and any unusual habits, and the family and home environment. Because several personal aspects are covered under development and habits, only those issues related to children's ability to cope and their self-concept are presented here.

Through observation, obtain a general idea of how children handle themselves in terms of confidence in dealing with others, answering questions, and coping with new situations. Observe the parent-child relationship for the types of messages sent to children about their coping skills and self-worth. Do the parents treat the child with respect, focusing on strengths, or is the interaction one of constant reprimands, with emphasis on weaknesses and faults? Do the parents help the child learn new coping strategies or support the ones the child uses?

Parent-child interactions also convey messages about body image. Do the parents label the child and body parts, such as "bad boy," "skinny legs," or "ugly scar"? Do the parents handle the child gently, using soothing touch to calm an anxious child, or do they treat the child roughly, using slaps or restraint to make the child obey? If the child touches certain parts of the body, such as the genitalia, do the parents make comments that suggest a negative connotation?

With older children, many of the communication strategies discussed earlier in the chapter are useful in eliciting more definitive information about their coping and self-concept. Children can write down five things they like and dislike about themselves. The nurse can use sentence completion statements, such as "The thing I like best (or worst) about myself is _____"; "If I could change one thing about myself, it would be _____"; or "When I am scared, I _____."

Review of Systems

The review of systems is a specific review of each body system, following an order similar to that of the physical examination (see Guidelines box). Often the history of the present illness provides a complete review of the system involved in the chief complaint. Because asking questions about other body systems may appear irrelevant to the parents or child, precede the questioning with an explanation of why the data are necessary (similar to the explanation concerning the relevance of the birth history) and reassure the parents that the child's main problem has not been forgotten.

Begin the review of a specific system with a broad statement such as "How has your child's general health been?" or "Has your child had any problems with his eyes?" If the parent states that the child has had problems with some body function, pursue this with an encouraging statement such as "Tell me more about that." If the parent denies any problems, query for specific symptoms (e.g., "No headaches, bumping into objects, or squinting?"). If the parent reconfirms the absence of such symptoms, record positive statements in the history, such as "Mother denies headaches, bumping into objects, or squinting." In this way, anyone who reviews the health history is aware of exactly what symptoms were investigated.

Performing a Nutritional Assessment
Dietary Intake

Knowledge of the child's dietary intake is an essential component of a nutritional assessment. However, it is also one of the most difficult factors to assess. Individuals' recall of food consumption, especially amounts eaten, is frequently unreliable. The food intake history of children and adolescents is prone to reporting error, mostly in the form of under-reporting. People from different cultures may have difficulty adequately describing the types of food they eat. Despite

---

📋 GUIDELINES

Initiating a Comprehensive Family Assessment

Perform a comprehensive assessment on:
- Children receiving comprehensive well-child care
- Children experiencing major stressful life events (e.g., chronic illness, disability, parental divorce, death of a family member)
- Children requiring extensive home care
- Children with developmental delays
- Children with repeated accidental injuries and those with suspected child abuse
- Children with behavioral or physical problems that could be caused by family dysfunction

---

BOX 29-8   FAMILY ASSESSMENT INTERVIEW

General Guidelines
- Schedule the interview with the family at a time that is most convenient for all parties; include as many family members as possible; clearly state the purpose of the interview.
- Begin the interview by asking each person's name and their relationship to one another.
- Restate the purpose of the interview and the objective.
- Keep the initial conversation general to put members at ease and to learn the "big picture" of the family.
- Identify major concerns and reflect these back to the family to be certain that all parties receive the same message.
- Terminate the interview with a summary of what was discussed and a plan for additional sessions if needed.

Structural Assessment Areas
Family Composition
- Immediate members of the household (names, ages, and relationships)
- Significant extended family members
- Previous marriages, separations, death of spouses, or divorces

Home and Community Environment
- Type of dwelling, number of rooms, occupants
- Sleeping arrangements
- Number of floors, accessibility of stairs and elevators
- Adequacy of utilities
- Safety features (fire escape, smoke and carbon monoxide detectors, guardrails on windows, use of car restraint)

Continued

BOX 29-8   FAMILY ASSESSMENT INTERVIEW—cont'd

- Environmental hazards (e.g., chipped paint, poor sanitation, pollution, heavy street traffic)
- Availability and location of health care facilities, schools, play areas
- Relationship with neighbors
- Recent crises or changes in home
- Child's reaction and adjustment to recent stresses

Occupation and Education of Family Members
- Types of employment
- Work schedules
- Work satisfaction
- Exposure to environmental or industrial hazards
- Sources of income and adequacy
- Effect of illness on financial status
- Highest degree or grade level attained

Cultural and Religious Traditions
- Religious beliefs and practices
- Cultural and ethnic beliefs and practices
- Language spoken in home
- Assessment questions include:
  - Does the family identify with a particular religious or ethnic group? Are both parents from that group?
  - How is religious or ethnic background part of family life?
  - What special religious or cultural traditions are practiced in the home (e.g., food choices and preparation)?
  - Where were family members born, and how long have they lived in this country?
  - What language does the family speak most frequently?
  - Do they speak and understand English?
  - What do they believe causes health or illness?
  - What religious or ethnic beliefs influence the family's perception of illness and its treatment?
  - What methods are used to prevent or treat illness?
  - How does the family know when a health problem needs medical attention?
  - Whom does the family contact when a member is ill?
  - Does the family rely on cultural or religious healers or remedies? If so, ask them to describe the type of healer or remedy.
  - Whom does the family go to for support (clergy, medical healer, relatives)?
  - Does the family experience discrimination because of their race, beliefs, or practices? Ask them to describe.

Functional Assessment Areas
Family Interactions and Roles
- *Interactions* refer to ways family members relate to each other. Chief concern is the amount of intimacy and closeness among the members, especially spouses.
- *Roles* refer to behaviors of people as they assume a different status or position.
- Observations include:
  - Family members' responses to each other (cordial, hostile, cool, loving, patient, short-tempered)
  - Obvious roles of leadership versus submission
  - Support and attention shown to various members

- Assessment questions include:
  - What activities does the family perform together?
  - Whom do family members talk to when something is bothering them?
  - What are members' household chores?
  - Who usually oversees what is happening with the children, such as at school or health care?
  - How easy or difficult is it for the family to change or accept new responsibilities for household tasks?

Power, Decision Making, and Problem Solving
- *Power* refers to individual member's control over others in family; it is manifested through family decision making and problem solving.
- Chief concern is clarity of boundaries of power between parents and children.
- One method of assessment involves offering a hypothetical conflict or problem, such as a child failing school, and asking family how they would handle this situation.
- Assessment questions include:
  - Who usually makes the decisions in the family?
  - If one parent makes a decision, can the child appeal to the other parent to change it?
  - What input do children have in making decisions or discussing rules?
  - Who makes and enforces the rules?
  - What happens when a rule is broken?

Communication
- Communication is concerned with clarity and directness of communication patterns.
- Further assessment includes periodically asking family members if they understood what was just said and to repeat the message.
- Observations include:
  - Who speaks to whom
  - If one person speaks for another or interrupts
  - If members appear uninterested when certain individuals speak
  - If there is agreement between verbal and nonverbal messages
- Assessment questions include:
  - How often do family members wait until others are through talking before "having their say"?
  - Do parents or older siblings tend to lecture and preach?
  - Do parents tend to "talk down" to the children?

Expression of Feelings and Individuality
- Expressions are concerned with personal space and freedom to grow, with limits and structure needed for guidance.
- Observing patterns of communication offers clues to how freely feelings are expressed.
- Assessment questions include:
  - Is it OK for family members to get angry or sad?
  - Who gets angry most of the time? What do they do?
  - If someone is upset, how do other family members try to comfort this person?
  - Who comforts specific family members?
  - When someone wants to do something, such as try out for a new sport or get a job, what is the family's response (offer assistance, discouragement, or no advice)?

GUIDELINES
Review of Systems

General—Overall state of health, fatigue, recent or unexplained weight gain or loss (period of time for either), contributing factors (change of diet, illness, altered appetite), exercise tolerance, fevers (time of day), chills, night sweats (unrelated to climatic conditions), frequent infections, general ability to carry out activities of daily living

Integument—Pruritus, pigment or other color changes, acne, eruptions, rashes (location), tendency for bruising, petechiae, excessive dryness, general texture, disorders or deformities of nails, hair growth or loss, hair color change (for adolescent, use of hair dyes or other potentially toxic substances, such as hair straighteners)

Head—Headaches, dizziness, injury (specific details)

Eyes—Visual problems (behaviors indicative of blurred vision, such as bumping into objects, clumsiness, sitting close to television, holding a book close to face, writing with head near desk, squinting, rubbing the eyes, bending head in an awkward position), cross-eyes (strabismus), eye infections, edema of lids, excessive tearing, use of glasses or contact lenses, date of last optic examination

Ears—Earaches, discharge, evidence of hearing loss (ask about behaviors, such as need to repeat requests, loud speech, inattentive behavior), results of any previous auditory testing

Nose—Nosebleeds (epistaxis), constant or frequent runny or stuffy nose, nasal obstruction (difficulty breathing), alteration or loss of sense of smell

Mouth—Mouth breathing, gum bleeding, toothaches, toothbrushing, use of fluoride, difficulty with teething (symptoms), last visit to dentist (especially if temporary dentition is complete), response to dentist

Throat—Sore throats, difficulty swallowing, choking (especially when chewing food; may be from poor chewing habits), hoarseness or other voice irregularities

Neck—Pain, limitation of movement, stiffness, difficulty holding head straight (torticollis), thyroid enlargement, enlarged nodes or other masses

Chest—Breast enlargement, discharge, masses, enlarged axillary nodes (for adolescent girl, ask about breast self-examination)

Respiratory—Chronic cough, frequent colds (number per year), wheezing, shortness of breath at rest or on exertion, difficulty breathing, sputum production, infections (pneumonia, tuberculosis), date of last chest x-ray examination, skin reaction from tuberculin testing

Cardiovascular—Cyanosis or fatigue on exertion, history of heart murmur or rheumatic fever, anemia, date of last blood count, blood type, recent transfusion

Gastrointestinal (questions in regard to appetite, food tolerance, and elimination habits are asked elsewhere)—Nausea, vomiting (not associated with eating, may be indicative of brain tumor or increased intracranial pressure), jaundice or yellowing skin or sclera, belching, flatulence, recent change in bowel habits (blood in stools, change of color, diarrhea or constipation)

Genitourinary—Pain on urination, frequency, hesitancy, urgency, hematuria, nocturia, polyuria, unpleasant odor to urine, force of stream, discharge, change in size of scrotum, date of last urinalysis (for adolescent, sexually transmitted infection, type of treatment; for male adolescent, ask about testicular self-examination)

Gynecologic—Menarche, date of last menstrual period, regularity or problems with menstruation, vaginal discharge, pruritus, date and result of last Papanicolaou (Pap) test (include obstetric history, as discussed under birth history, when applicable); if sexually active, type of contraception, sexually transmitted infection and type of treatment

Musculoskeletal—Weakness, clumsiness, lack of coordination, unusual movements, back or joint stiffness, muscle pains or cramps, abnormal gait, deformity, fractures, serious sprains, activity level

Neurologic—Seizures, tremors, dizziness, loss of memory, general affect, fears, nightmares, speech problems, any unusual habits

Endocrine—Intolerance to weather changes, excessive thirst or urination, excessive sweating, salty taste to skin, signs of early puberty

---

these obstacles, a dietary evaluation is an important component of the child's assessment.

The dietary reference intakes (DRIs) are a set of four nutrient-based reference values that provide quantitative estimates of nutrient intake for use in assessing and planning dietary intake (American Academy of Pediatrics, 2009). The specific DRIs are:

- **Estimated average requirement (EAR)**—Nutrient intake estimated to meet the requirement of half the healthy individuals (50%) for a specific age and gender group.
- **Recommended dietary allowance (RDA)**—Average daily dietary intake sufficient to meet the nutrient requirement of nearly all (97% to 98%) of healthy individuals for a specific age and gender group.
- **Adequate intake (AI)**—Recommended intake level based on estimates of nutrient intake by healthy groups of individuals.
- **Tolerable upper intake level (UL)**—Highest average daily nutrient intake level likely to pose no risk for adverse health effects. As intake increases above the UL, risk for adverse effects increases.

Fig. 29-4 contains MyPlate, which describes the recommended dietary allowance. Specific questions used to conduct a nutritional assessment are given in Box 29-9. Every nutritional assessment should begin with a dietary history. The exact questions used to elicit

CULTURAL COMPETENCE
Food Practices

Because cultural practices are prevalent in food preparation, consider carefully the kinds of questions that are asked and the judgments made during counseling. For example, some cultures, such as Hispanic, African-American, and Native-American, include many vegetables, legumes, and starches in their diet that together provide sufficient essential amino acids, even though the actual amount of meat or dairy protein is low. (See Table 27-1.)

a dietary history vary with the child's age. In general, the younger the child, the more specific and detailed the history should be. The overview elicited from the dietary history can be helpful in evaluating food frequency records. The history is also concerned with financial and cultural factors that influence food selection and preparation (see Cultural Competence box).

The most common and probably easiest method of assessing daily intake is the 24-hour recall. The child or parent recalls every item eaten in the past 24 hours and the approximate amounts. The 24-hour recall is most beneficial when it represents a typical day's intake. Some of the difficulties with a daily recall are the family's inability to remember exactly what was eaten and inaccurate

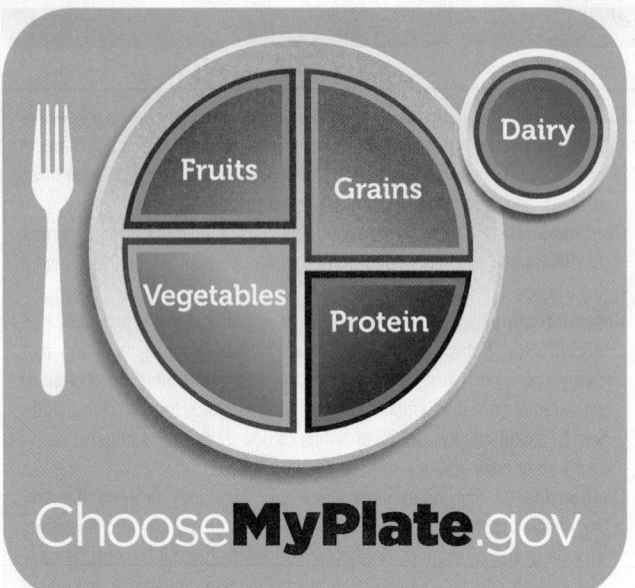

FIG 29-4 MyPlate. MyPlate advocates building a healthy plate by making half of your plate fruits and vegetables and the other half grains and protein. Avoiding oversized portions, making half your grains whole grains, and drinking fat-free or low-fat (1%) milk are additional recommendations for a healthy diet. (From U.S. Department of Agriculture: *MyPlate*, Washington, DC, June 2011, Author, www.choosemyplate.gov.)

estimation of portion size. To increase accuracy of reporting portion sizes, the use of food models and additional questions are recommended. In general, this method is most useful in providing *qualitative* information about the child's diet.

To improve the reliability of the daily recall, the family can complete a food diary by recording every food and liquid consumed for a certain number of days. A 3-day record consisting of 2 weekdays and 1 weekend day is representative for most people. Providing specific charts to record intake can improve compliance. The family should record items immediately after eating.

Clinical Examination of Nutrition

A significant amount of information regarding nutritional deficiencies comes from a clinical examination, especially from assessing the skin, hair, teeth, gums, lips, tongue, and eyes. Hair, skin, and mouth are vulnerable because of the rapid turnover of epithelial and mucosal tissue. Table 29-1 summarizes clinical signs of possible nutritional deficiency or excess. Few are diagnostic for a specific nutrient, and if suspicious signs are found, they must be confirmed with dietary and biochemical data. Generally, the clinical examination does not reveal children *at risk* for a deficiency or excess.

Anthropometry, an essential parameter of nutritional status, is the measurement of height, weight, head circumference, proportions, skinfold thickness, and arm circumference in young children. Height and head circumference reflect past nutrition, whereas weight, skinfold thickness, and arm circumference reflect present nutritional status, especially of protein and fat reserves. Skinfold

---

BOX 29-9   DIETARY REFERENCE INTAKES FOR AN INDIVIDUAL

Estimated average requirement (EAR)—Used to examine the possibility of inadequacy.

Recommended dietary allowance (RDA)—Dietary intake at or above this level usually has a low probability of inadequacy.

Adequate intake (AI)—Dietary intake at or above this level usually has a low probability of inadequacy.

Tolerable upper intake level (UL)—Dietary intake above this level usually places an individual at risk for adverse effects from excessive nutrient intake.

Dietary History

- What are the family's usual mealtimes?
- Do family members eat together or at separate times?
- Who does the family grocery shopping and meal preparation?
- How much money is spent to buy food each week?
- How are most foods prepared—baked, broiled, fried, other?
- How often does the family or your child eat out?
  - What kinds of restaurants do you go to?
  - What kinds of food does your child typically eat at restaurants?
- Does your child eat breakfast regularly?
- Where does your child eat lunch?
- What are your child's favorite foods, beverages, and snacks?
  - What are the average amounts eaten per day?
  - What foods are artificially sweetened?
  - What are your child's snacking habits?
  - When are sweet foods usually eaten?
  - What are your child's toothbrushing habits?
- What special cultural practices are followed? What ethnic foods are eaten?

- What foods and beverages does your child dislike?
- How would you describe your child's usual appetite (hearty eater, picky eater)?
- What are your child's feeding habits (breast, bottle, cup, spoon, eats by self, needs assistance, any special devices)?
- Does your child take vitamins or other supplements? Do they contain iron or fluoride?
- Does your child have any known or suspected food allergies? Is your child on a special diet?
- Has your child lost or gained weight recently?
- Are there any feeding problems (excessive fussiness, spitting up, colic, difficulty sucking or swallowing)? Are there any dental problems or appliances, such as braces, that affect eating?
- What types of exercise does your child do regularly?
- Is there a family history of cancer, diabetes, heart disease, high blood pressure, or obesity?

Additional Questions for Infants

- What was the infant's birth weight? When did it double? Triple?
- Was the infant premature?
- Are you breastfeeding or have you breastfed your infant? For how long?
- If you use a formula, what is the brand?
  - How long has the infant been taking it?
  - How many ounces does the infant drink a day?
- Are you giving the infant cow's milk (whole, low fat, skim)?
  - When did you start?
  - How many ounces does the infant drink a day?
- Do you give your infant extra fluids (water, juice)?

BOX 29-9 DIETARY REFERENCE INTAKES FOR AN INDIVIDUAL—cont'd

- If the infant takes a bottle to bed at nap time or nighttime, what is in the bottle?
- At what age did the child start on cereal, vegetables, meat or other protein sources, fruit or juice, finger food, table food?
- Do you make your own baby food or use commercial foods, such as infant cereal?
- Does the infant take a vitamin or mineral supplement? If so, what type?

- Has the infant had an allergic reaction to any food(s)? If so, list the foods and describe the reaction.
- Does the infant spit up frequently; have unusually loose stools; or have hard, dry stools? If so, how often?
- How often do you feed your infant?
- How would you describe your infant's appetite?

Adapted from Murphy SP, Poos MI: Dietary reference intakes: summary of applications in dietary assessment, *Public Health Nutr* 5(6A): 843–849, 2002.

TABLE 29-1 CLINICAL ASSESSMENT OF NUTRITIONAL STATUS

EVIDENCE OF ADEQUATE NUTRITION	EVIDENCE OF DEFICIENT OR EXCESS NUTRITION	DEFICIENCY OR EXCESS*
General Growth		
Between 5th and 95th percentiles for height, weight, and head circumference	<5th or >95th percentile for growth	Protein, calories, fats, and other essential nutrients, especially vitamin A, pyridoxine, niacin, calcium, iodine, manganese, zinc
Steady gain with expected growth spurts during infancy and adolescence	Absence of or delayed growth spurts; poor weight gain	
Sexual development appropriate for age	Delayed sexual development	Excess vitamins A, D
Skin		
Smooth, slightly dry to touch	Hardening and scaling	Vitamin A
Elastic and firm	Seborrheic dermatitis	Excess niacin
Absence of lesions	Dry, rough, petechiae	Riboflavin
Color appropriate to genetic background	Delayed wound healing	Vitamin C
	Scaly dermatitis on exposed surfaces	Riboflavin, vitamin C, zinc
	Wrinkled, flabby	Niacin
	Crusted lesions around orifices, especially nares	Protein, calories, zinc
	Pruritus	Excess vitamin A, riboflavin, niacin
	Poor turgor	Water, sodium
	Edema	Protein, thiamine
Excess sodium
	Yellow tinge (jaundice)	Vitamin B_{12}
Excess vitamin A, niacin
	Depigmentation	Protein, calories
	Pallor (anemia)	Pyridoxine, folic acid, vitamins B_{12}, C, E (in premature infants), iron
Excess vitamin C, zinc
	Paresthesia	Excess riboflavin
Hair		
Lustrous, silky, strong, elastic	Stringy, friable, dull, dry, thin	Protein, calories
	Alopecia	Protein, calories, zinc
	Depigmentation	Protein, calories, copper
	Raised areas around hair follicles	Vitamin C

Continued

TABLE 29-1   CLINICAL ASSESSMENT OF NUTRITIONAL STATUS—cont'd

EVIDENCE OF ADEQUATE NUTRITION	EVIDENCE OF DEFICIENT OR EXCESS NUTRITION	DEFICIENCY OR EXCESS*
Head		
Even molding, occipital prominence, symmetric facial features	Softening of cranial bones, prominence of frontal bones, skull flat and depressed toward middle	Vitamin D
Fused sutures after 18 months		
	Delayed fusion of sutures	Vitamin D
	Hard, tender lumps in occiput	Excess vitamin A
	Headache	Excess thiamine
Neck		
Thyroid not visible, palpable in midline	Thyroid enlarged, may be grossly visible	Iodine
Eyes		
Clear, bright	Hardening and scaling of cornea and conjunctiva	Vitamin A
Good night vision	Night blindness	Vitamin A
Conjunctiva—Pink, glossy	Burning, itching, photophobia, cataracts, corneal vascularization	Riboflavin
Ears		
Tympanic membrane—Pliable	Calcified (hearing loss)	Excess vitamin D
Nose		
Smooth, intact nasal angle	Irritation and cracks at nasal angle	Riboflavin Excess vitamin A
Mouth		
Lips—Smooth, moist, darker color than skin	Fissures and inflammation at corners	Riboflavin Excess vitamin A
Gums—Firm, coral pink, stippled	Spongy, friable, swollen, bluish red or black, bleed easily	Vitamin C
Mucous membranes—Bright pink, smooth, moist	Stomatitis	Niacin
Tongue—Rough texture, no lesions, taste sensation	Glossitis	Niacin, riboflavin, folic acid
	Diminished taste sensation	Zinc
Teeth—Uniform white color, smooth, intact	Brown mottling, pits, fissures	Excess fluoride
	Defective enamel	Vitamins A, C, D, calcium, phosphorus
	Caries	Excess carbohydrates
Chest		
In infants, shape almost circular	Depressed lower portion of rib cage	Vitamin D
In children, lateral diameter increased in proportion to anteroposterior diameter	Sharp protrusion of sternum	Vitamin D
Smooth costochondral junctions	Enlarged costochondral junctions	Vitamins C, D
Breast development—Normal for age	Delayed development	See under General Growth; especially zinc

TABLE 29-1   CLINICAL ASSESSMENT OF NUTRITIONAL STATUS—cont'd

EVIDENCE OF ADEQUATE NUTRITION	EVIDENCE OF DEFICIENT OR EXCESS NUTRITION	DEFICIENCY OR EXCESS*
Cardiovascular System		
Pulse and blood pressure (BP) within normal limits	Palpitations	Thiamine
	Rapid pulse	Potassium Excess thiamine
	Dysrhythmias	Magnesium, potassium Excess niacin, potassium
	Increased BP	Excess sodium
	Decreased BP	Thiamine Excess niacin
Abdomen		
In young children, cylindric and prominent	Distended, flabby, poor musculature	Protein, calories
	Prominent, large	Excess calories
In older children, flat	Potbelly, constipation	Vitamin D
Normal bowel habits	Diarrhea	Niacin Excess vitamin C
	Constipation	Excess calcium, potassium
Musculoskeletal System		
Muscles—Firm, well-developed, equal strength bilaterally	Flabby, weak, generalized wasting	Protein, calories
	Weakness, pain, cramps	Thiamine, sodium, chloride, potassium, phosphorus, magnesium Excess thiamine
	Muscle twitching, tremors	Magnesium
	Muscular paralysis	Excess potassium
Spine—Cervical and lumbar curves (double-S curve)	Kyphosis, lordosis, scoliosis	Vitamin D
Extremities—Symmetric; legs straight with minimum bowing	Bowing of extremities, knock-knees	Vitamin D, calcium, phosphorus
	Epiphyseal enlargement	Vitamins A, D
	Bleeding into joints and muscles, joint swelling, pain	Vitamin C
Joints—Flexible, full range of motion, no pain or stiffness	Thickening of cortex of long bones with pain and fragility, hard tender lumps in extremities	Excess vitamin A
	Osteoporosis of long bones	Calcium Excess vitamin D
Neurologic System		
Behavior—Alert, responsive, emotionally stable	Listless, irritable, lethargic, apathetic (sometimes apprehensive, anxious, drowsy, mentally slow, confused)	Thiamine, niacin, pyridoxine, vitamin C, potassium, magnesium, iron, protein, calories Excess vitamins A, D, thiamine, folic acid, calcium
Absence of tetany, convulsions	Masklike facial expression, blurred speech, involuntary laughing	Excess manganese
	Convulsions	Thiamine, pyridoxine, vitamin D, calcium, magnesium Excess phosphorus (in relation to calcium)
Intact peripheral nervous system	Peripheral nervous system toxicity (unsteady gait, numb feet and hands, fine motor clumsiness)	Excess pyridoxine
Intact reflexes	Diminished or absent tendon reflexes	Thiamine, vitamin E

*Nutrients listed are deficient unless specified as excess.

thickness is a measurement of the body's fat content, because approximately half the body's total fat stores are directly beneath the skin. The upper arm muscle circumference is correlated with measurements of total muscle mass. Because muscle serves as the body's major protein reserve, this measurement is considered an index of the body's protein stores. Ideally, growth measurements are recorded over time, and comparisons are made regarding the *velocity* of growth based on previous and present values.

Numerous biochemical tests are available for assessing nutritional status and include analysis of plasma; blood cells; urine; and tissues from liver, bone, hair, and fingernails. Many of these tests are complicated and are not performed routinely. Common laboratory procedures for nutritional status include measurement of hemoglobin, hematocrit, transferrin, albumin, creatinine, and nitrogen. Appendix B provides laboratory values for these tests and more specific nutrient measurements.

Evaluation of Nutritional Assessment

After collecting the data needed for a thorough nutritional assessment, evaluate the findings to plan appropriate counseling. From the data, assess whether the child is (1) malnourished, (2) at risk for becoming malnourished, (3) well nourished with adequate reserves, or (4) overweight or obese.

Analyze the daily food diary for the variety and amounts of foods suggested in MyPlate (see Fig. 29-4). For example, if the list includes no vegetables, inquire about this rather than assume that the child dislikes vegetables, since it is possible that none were served that day. Also, evaluate the information in terms of the family's ethnic practices and financial resources. Encouraging increased protein intake with additional meat is not always feasible for families on a limited budget and may conflict with food practices that use meat sparingly, such as in Asian meal preparation.

PHYSICAL ASSESSMENT

General Approaches Toward Examining the Child

Although the approach to and sequence of the physical examination differ according to the child's age, the following discussion outlines the traditional model for physical assessment. Because the physical examination is a vital part of preventive pediatric care, Fig. 29-5 gives a schedule for periodic health visits.

Sequence of the Examination

Ordinarily, the sequence for examining patients follows a head-to-toe direction. The main function of such a systematic approach is to provide a general guideline for assessment of each body area to

Clinical Preventive Services for Normal-Risk Children*

Age	Infancy							Early Childhood							Middle Childhood						Adolescence							
	Newborn	3-5 d	By1mo	2 mo	4 mo	6 mo	9 mo	12mo	15mo	18mo	24mo	30mo	3 y	4 y	5 y	6 y	7 y	8 y	9 y	10 y	11 y	12 y	13 y	14 y	15 y	16 y	17 y	18 y
History Initial/Interval	●	●	●	●	●	●	●	●	●	●	●	●	●	●	●	●	●	●	●	●	●	●	●	●	●	●	●	●
Measurements																												
Length/Height and Weight	●	●	●	●	●	●	●	●	●	●	●	●	●	●	●	●	●	●	●	●	●	●	●	●	●	●	●	●
Head Circumference	●	●	●	●	●	●	●	●	●	●	●																	
Weight for Length	●	●	●	●	●	●	●	●	●	●																		
Body Mass Index											●	●	●	●	●	●	●	●	●	●	●	●	●	●	●	●	●	●
Blood Pressure	★	★	★	★	★	★	★	★	★	★	★	★	●	●	●	●	●	●	●	●	●	●	●	●	●	●	●	●
Sensory Screening																												
Vision	★	★	★	★	★	★	★	★	★	★	★	★	●	●	●	●	★	●	★	●	★	●	★	★	●	★	★	●
Hearing	●	★	★	★	★	★	★	★	★	★	★	★	★	●	●	●	★	●	★	●	★	★	★	★	★	★	★	★
Developmental/ Behavioral Assessment																												
Developmental Screening							●			●		●																
Autism Screening										●	●																	
Developmental Surveillance	●	●	●	●	●	●		●	●		●		●	●	●	●	●	●	●	●	●	●	●	●	●	●	●	●
Psychosocial/ Behavioral Assessment	●	●	●	●	●	●	●	●	●	●	●	●	●	●	●	●	●	●	●	●	●	●	●	●	●	●	●	●
Alcohol and Drug Use Assessment																					★	★	★	★	★	★	★	★
Physical Examination	●	●	●	●	●	●	●	●	●	●	●	●	●	●	●	●	●	●	●	●	●	●	●	●	●	●	●	●
Procedures																												
Newborn Metabolic/ Hemoglobin Screening	◄——	●	——►																									
Immunization	●	●	●	●	●	●	●	●	●	●	●	●	●	●	●	●	●	●	●	●	●	●	●	●	●	●	●	●
Hematocrit or Hemoglobin					★			●			★	★	★	★	★	★	★	★	★	★	★	★	★	★	★	★	★	★
Lead Screening						★	★	●or★		★	●or★		★	★	★	★												
Tuberculin Test			★			★		★		★	★	★	★		★	★	★	★	★	★	★	★	★	★	★	★	★	★
Dyslipidemia Screening											★			★		★		★		★	★	★	★	★	★	★	★	●
STI Screening																					★	★	★	★	★	★	★	★
Cervical Dysplasia Screening																					★	★	★	★	★	★	★	★
Oral Health						★	★	●or★		●or★	●or★	●or★	●			●												
Anticipatory Guidance	●	●	●	●	●	●	●	●	●	●	●	●	●	●	●	●	●	●	●	●	●	●	●	●	●	●	●	●

Key: ● = To be performed; ★ = risk assessment to be performed, with appropriate action to follow, if positive; ◄——●——► = range during which a service may be provided, with the symbol indicating the preferred age.

*For current immunization schedules, see Chapter 31.

FIG 29-5 Preventive health care chart. *STI*, Sexually transmitted infection. (Adapted from American Academy of Pediatrics Committee on Practice and Ambulatory Medicine and Bright Futures Steering Committee: recommendations for preventive pediatric health care, *Pediatrics* 120[6]:1376, 2007.)

avoid omitting segments of the examination. The standard recording of data also facilitates exchange of information among different professionals. This orderly sequence is frequently altered to accommodate the child's developmental needs, although the examination is recorded following the head-to-toe model. Using developmental and chronologic age as the main criteria for assessing each body system accomplishes several goals:

- Minimizes stress and anxiety associated with assessment of various body parts
- Fosters a trusting nurse-child-parent relationship
- Allows for maximum preparation of the child
- Preserves the essential security of the parent-child relationship, especially with young children
- Maximizes the accuracy and reliability of assessment findings

Preparation of the Child

Although the physical examination consists of painless procedures, for some children the use of a tight arm cuff, probes in the ears and mouth, pressure on the abdomen, and a cold piece of metal to listen to the chest are stressful. Therefore the nurse should use the same considerations discussed in Chapter 39 for preparing children for procedures. In addition to that discussion, general guidelines related to the examining process are given in the Guidelines box.

The physical examination should be as pleasant as possible, as well as educational. The paper-doll technique is a useful approach to teaching children about the body part that is being examined (Fig. 29-6). At the conclusion of the visit, the child can bring home the paper doll as a memento.

Table 29-2 summarizes guidelines for positioning, preparing, and examining children at various ages. Because no child fits precisely into one age category, it may be necessary to vary the approach after a preliminary assessment of the child's developmental achievements and needs. Even with the best approach, many toddlers are uncooperative and inconsolable for much of the physical examination. However, some seem intrigued by the new surroundings and unusual equipment and respond more like preschoolers than toddlers. Likewise, some early preschoolers may require more of the "security measures" employed with younger children, such as continued parent-child contact, and less of the preparatory measures used with preschoolers, such as playing with the equipment before and during the actual examination (Fig. 29-7).

Growth Measurements

Measurement of physical growth in children is a key element in evaluating their health status. Physical growth parameters include weight, height (length), skinfold thickness, arm circumference, and head circumference. Values for these growth parameters are plotted on percentile charts, and the child's measurements in percentiles are compared with those of the general population.

Growth Charts

Growth charts use a series of percentile curves to demonstrate the distribution of body measurements in children. The Centers for Disease Control (CDC) recommends that the World Health Organization (WHO) growth standards be used to monitor growth for infants and children between the ages of 0 and 2 years. The CDC growth charts are used for children age 2 years and older.*

Children whose growth may be questionable include:

- Children whose height and weight percentiles are widely disparate (e.g., height in the 10th percentile and weight in the 90th percentile, especially with above-average skinfold thickness)
- Children who fail to follow the expected growth velocity in height and weight, especially during the rapid growth periods of infancy and adolescence
- Children who show a sudden increase (except during puberty), decrease, or no change in a previously steady growth pattern.

Because growth is a continuous but uneven process, the most reliable evaluation lies in comparing growth measurements over time. It is important to remember that normal growth patterns vary among children of the same age (Fig. 29-8).

Breastfed and Formula-Fed Infants. The WHO growth charts are used because they reflect growth patterns among children who were predominantly breastfed (the recommended standard for

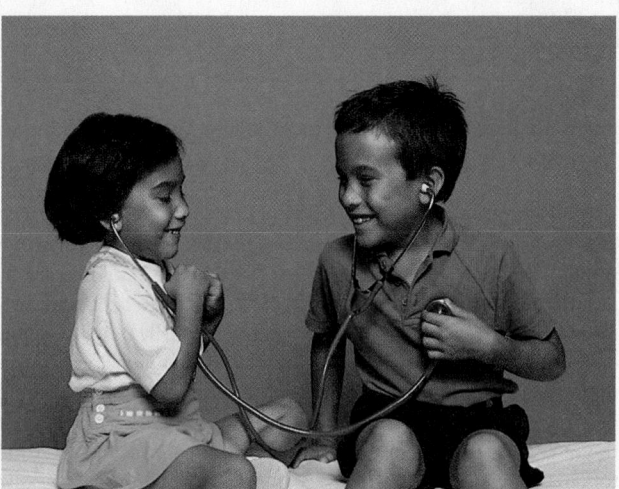

FIG 29-7 Preparing children for physical examination.

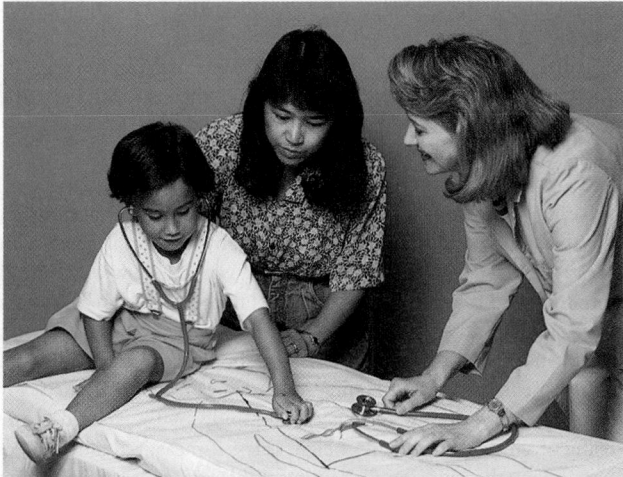

FIG 29-6 Using paper-doll technique to prepare child for physical examination.

*Growth Charts can be found on the Centers for Disease Control and Prevention website at http://www.cdc.gov/growthcharts/who_charts.htm.

GUIDELINES

Performing Pediatric Physical Examination

- Perform the examination in an appropriate, nonthreatening area:
  - Have room well lit and decorated with neutral colors.
  - Have room temperature comfortably warm.
  - Place all strange and potentially frightening equipment out of sight.
  - Have some toys, dolls, stuffed animals, and games available for child.
  - If possible, have rooms decorated and equipped for different-age children.
  - Provide privacy, especially for school-age children and adolescents.
- Provide time for play and becoming acquainted.
- Observe behaviors that signal child's readiness to cooperate:
  - Talking to the nurse
  - Making eye contact
  - Accepting the offered equipment
  - Allowing physical touching
  - Choosing to sit on examining table rather than parent's lap
- If signs of readiness are not observed, use the following techniques:
  - Talk to parent while essentially "ignoring" child; gradually focus on child or a favorite object, such as a doll.
  - Make complimentary remarks about child, such as appearance, dress, or a favorite object.
  - Tell a funny story or play a simple magic trick.
  - Have a nonthreatening "friend" available, such as a hand puppet to "talk" to child for the nurse (see Fig. 29-26, *A*).
- If child refuses to cooperate, use the following techniques:
  - Assess reason for uncooperative behavior; consider that a child who is unduly afraid may have had a traumatic experience.
  - Try to involve child and parent in process.
  - Avoid prolonged explanations about examining procedure.
  - Use a firm, direct approach regarding expected behavior.
  - Perform examination as quickly as possible.
  - Have attendant gently restrain child.
  - Minimize any disruptions or stimulation.
  - Limit number of people in room.
  - Use isolated room.
  - Use quiet, calm, confident voice.

- Begin examination in a nonthreatening manner for young children or children who are fearful:
  - Use activities that can be presented as games, such as test for cranial nerves (see Table 29-13) or parts of developmental screening tests (pp. 825-826).
  - Use approaches such as "Simon Says" to encourage child to make a face, squeeze a hand, stand on one foot, and so on.
  - Use paper-doll technique:
    1. Lay child supine on an examining table or floor that is covered with a large sheet of paper.
    2. Trace around child's body outline.
    3. Use body outline to demonstrate what will be examined, such as drawing a heart and listening with stethoscope before performing activity on child.
- If several children in the family will be examined, begin with most cooperative child to model desired behavior.
- Involve child in examination process:
  - Provide choices, such as sitting on table or in parent's lap.
  - Allow child to handle or hold equipment.
  - Encourage child to use equipment on a doll, family member, or examiner.
  - Explain each step of the procedure in simple language.
- Examine child in a comfortable and secure position:
  - Sitting in parent's lap
  - Sitting upright if in respiratory distress
- Proceed to examine the body in an organized sequence (usually head to toe) with the following exceptions:
  - Alter sequence to accommodate needs of different-age children (see Table 29-2).
  - Examine painful areas last.
  - In emergency situation, examine vital functions (airway, breathing, and circulation) and injured area first.
- Reassure child throughout the examination, especially about bodily concerns that arise during puberty.
- Discuss findings with family at the end of the examination.
- Praise child for cooperation during the examination; give a reward such as a small toy or sticker.

---

infant feeding) for at least 4 months and still breastfeeding at 12 months.

Length

The term *length* refers to measurements taken when children are supine (also referred to as recumbent length). Until children are 24 months old (or 36 months if using the chart for birth to 36 months), measure recumbent length. Because of the normally flexed position during infancy, fully extend the body by (1) holding the head in midline, (2) grasping the knees together gently, and (3) pushing down on the knees until the legs are fully extended and flat against the table. If using a measuring board, place the head firmly at the top of the board and the heels of the feet firmly against the footboard.

If such a measuring device is not available, measure length by placing the child on a paper-covered surface, marking the endpoints of the top of the head and the heels of the feet, and measuring between these two points (Fig. 29-9). For accurate measurement, hold the writing utensil at a right angle to the table

when marking the cephalic point; position the feet with the toes pointing directly to the ceiling when marking the heel point. Regardless of the method used, have someone assist in holding the child's head in midline while you extend the legs and take the measurements.

Height

The term *height* (or stature) refers to the measurement taken when a child is standing upright. Measure height by having the child, with shoes removed, stand as tall and straight as possible, with the head in midline and the line of vision parallel to the ceiling and floor. Be certain the child's back is to the wall or other vertical flat surface, with the heels, buttocks, and back of the shoulders touching the wall and the medial malleoli touching if possible (Fig. 29-10). Check for and correct bending of the knees, slumping of the shoulders, or raising of the heels. Normally, height is less if measured in the afternoon than in the morning. To minimize this variation, apply modest upward pressure under the jaw or the mastoid processes behind the ears.

TABLE 29-2   AGE-SPECIFIC APPROACHES TO PHYSICAL EXAMINATION DURING CHILDHOOD

POSITION	SEQUENCE	PREPARATION
Infant		
Before able to sit alone—Supine or prone, preferably in parent's lap; before 4-6 months, can place on examining table	If quiet, auscultate heart, lungs, abdomen. Record heart and respiratory rates. Palpate and percuss same areas. Proceed in usual head-to-toe direction. Perform traumatic procedures last (eyes, ears, mouth [while crying]). Elicit reflexes as body part is examined. Elicit Moro reflex last.	Completely undress if room temperature permits. Leave diaper on male infant. Gain cooperation with distraction, bright objects, rattles, talking. Smile at infant; use soft, gentle voice. Pacify with bottle of sugar water or feeding. Enlist parent's aid for restraining to examine ears, mouth. Avoid abrupt, jerky movements.
After able to sit alone—Sitting in parent's lap whenever possible; if on table, place with parent in full view		
Toddler		
Sitting or standing on or by parent	Inspect body area through play: "count fingers," "tickle toes." Use minimum physical contact initially. Introduce equipment slowly. Auscultate, percuss, palpate whenever quiet. Perform traumatic procedures last (same as for infant).	Have parent remove outer clothing. Remove underwear as body part is examined. Allow to inspect equipment; demonstrating use of equipment is usually ineffective. If uncooperative, perform procedures quickly. Use restraint when appropriate; request parent's assistance. Talk about examination if cooperative; use short phrases. Praise for cooperative behavior.
Prone or supine in parent's lap		
Preschool Child		
Prefer standing or sitting	If cooperative, proceed in head-to-toe direction. If uncooperative, proceed as with toddler.	Request self-undressing. Allow to wear underpants if shy. Offer equipment for inspection; briefly demonstrate use. Make up story about procedure (e.g., "I'm seeing how strong your muscles are" [blood pressure]). Use paper-doll technique. Give choices when possible. Expect cooperation; use positive statements (e.g., "Open your mouth").
Usually cooperative prone or supine		
Prefer parent's closeness		
School-Age Child		
Prefer sitting	Proceed in head-to-toe direction. May examine genitalia last in older child.	Respect need for privacy. Request self-undressing. Allow to wear underpants. Give gown to wear. Explain purpose of equipment and significance of procedure, such as otoscope to see eardrum, which is necessary for hearing. Teach about body function and care.
Cooperative in most positions		
Younger child prefers parent's presence		
Older child may prefer privacy		
Adolescent		
Same as for school-age child	Same as older school-age child. May examine genitalia last.	Allow to undress in private. Give gown. Expose only area to be examined. Respect need for privacy. Explain findings during examination: "Your muscles are firm and strong." Matter-of-factly comment about sexual development: "Your breasts are developing as they should be." Emphasize normalcy of development. Examine genitalia as any other body part; may leave to end.
Offer option of parent's presence		

For the most accurate measurement, use a wall-mounted unit (stadiometer; see Fig. 29-10). The movable measuring rod of platform scales is accurate only if it remains parallel to the floor and rests securely on the topmost part of the head. To improvise a flat surface for measuring length, attach a paper or metal tape or yardstick to the wall, position the child adjacent to the tape, and place a three-dimensional object, such as a thick book or box, on top of the head. Rest the side of the object firmly against the wall to form a right angle. Measure length or stature to the nearest 1 mm or ⅛ inch.

Weight

Weight is measured with an appropriate-size balance beam scale, which measures weight to the nearest 10 g (0.35 oz) for infants and

100 g (0.22 lb) for children. Before weighing the child, balance the scale by setting it at 0 and noting if the balance registers exactly in the middle of the mark. If the end of the balance beam rises to the top or bottom of the mark, more or less weight, respectively, is needed. Some scales are designed to self-correct, but others need to be recalibrated by the manufacturer. Scales vary in their accuracy; infant scales tend to be more accurate than adult platform scales, and newer scales tend to be more accurate than older ones, especially at the upper levels of weight measurement. When precise measurements are necessary, two nurses should take the weight independently; if there is a discrepancy, take a third reading.

Take measurements in a comfortably warm room. When the birth-to-36-month growth charts are used, children should be weighed nude. Older children are usually weighed while wearing their underpants or a light gown. However, always respect the privacy of all children. If the child must be weighed wearing some article of clothing or some type of special device, such as a prosthesis or an armboard for an intravenous device, note this when recording

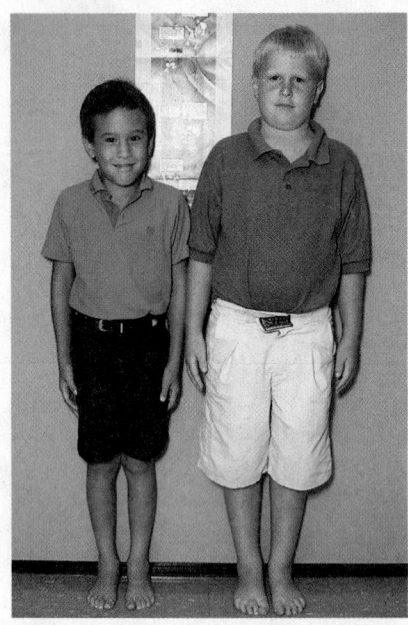

FIG 29-8 These children of identical age (8 years) are markedly different in size. Child on left, of Asian descent, is at 5th percentile for height and weight. Child on right is above 95th percentile for height and weight. However, both children demonstrate normal growth patterns.

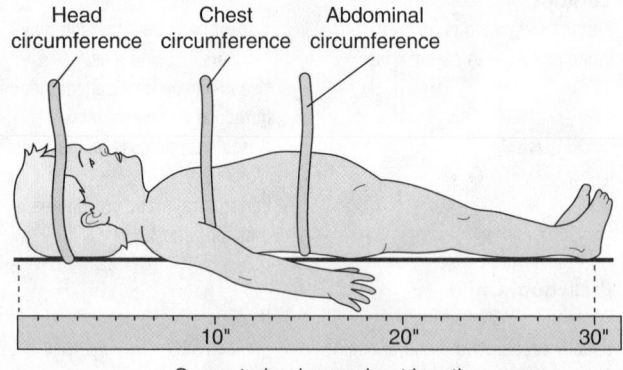

FIG 29-9 Measurement of head, chest, and abdominal circumference and crown-to-heel (recumbent) length. (From Price DL: *Pediatric nursing: an introductory text,* ed 10, St Louis, 2007, Saunders.)

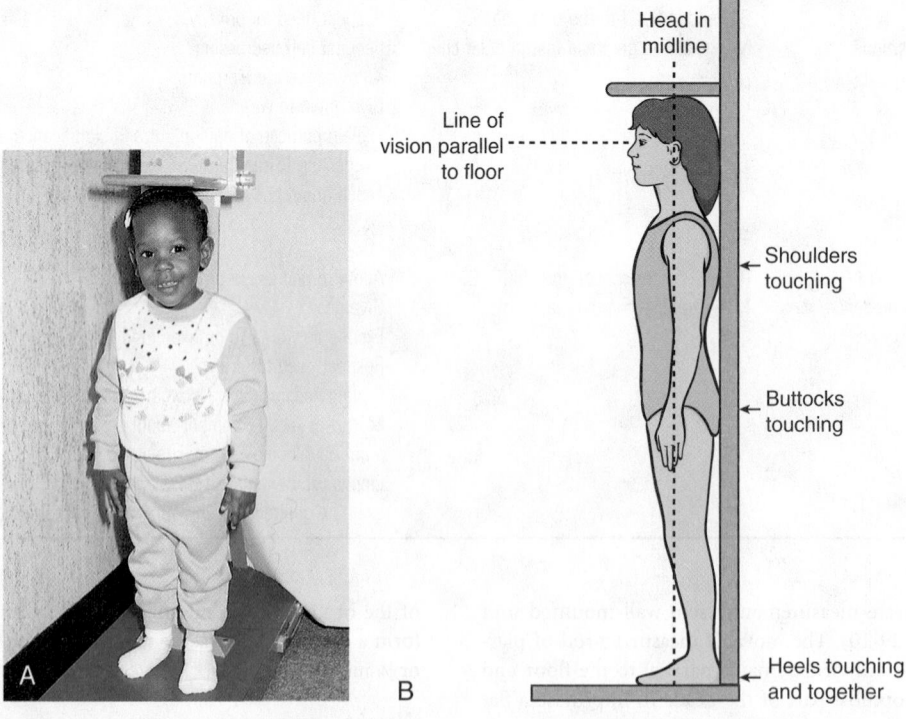

FIG 29-10 **A** and **B,** Measurement of height. (*A,* From Seidel HM, Ball JW, Dains JE, et al: *Mosby's guide to physical examination,* ed 6, St Louis, 2007, Mosby. *B,* From Wilson S: *Health assessment for nursing practice,* ed 5, St Louis, 2013, Mosby.)

the weight. Children who are measured for recumbent length are usually weighed on an infant platform scale and placed in a lying or sitting position. When weighing a child, place your hand lightly above the infant to prevent him or her from accidentally falling off the scale (Fig. 29-11, *A*) or stand close to the toddler, ready to prevent a fall (Fig. 29-11, *B*). For maximum asepsis, cover the scale with a clean sheet of paper between each child's measurement.

Skinfold Thickness and Arm Circumference

Measures of relative weight and stature cannot distinguish between adipose (fat) tissue and muscle. One convenient measure of body fat is skinfold thickness, which is increasingly recommended as a routine measurement. Measure skinfold thickness with special calipers, such as the Lange calipers. The most common sites for measuring skinfold thickness are the triceps (most practical for routine clinical use), subscapula, suprailiac, abdomen, and upper thigh. For greatest reliability, follow the exact procedure for measurement and record the average of at least two measurements of one site.

Arm circumference is an indirect measure of muscle mass. Measurement of arm circumference follows the same procedure as for skinfold thickness except the midpoint is measured with a paper or steel tape. Place the tape vertically, along the posterior aspect of the upper arm to the acromial process and to the olecranon process; half the measured length is the midpoint.

Head Circumference

Measure head circumference in children up to 36 months of age and in any child whose head size is questionable. Measure the head at its greatest circumference, usually slightly above the eyebrows and pinna of the ears and around the occipital prominence at the back of the skull (see Fig. 29-9). Because head shape can affect the location of the maximum circumference, more than one measurement at points above the eyebrows is necessary to obtain the most accurate measure. Use a paper or metal tape, since a cloth tape can stretch and give a falsely small measurement. For greatest accuracy, use devices marked with tenths of a centimeter, since the percentile charts have only 0.5-cm increments.

Plot the head size on the appropriate growth chart under head circumference. Generally, head and chest circumferences are equal at about 1 to 2 years of age. During childhood, chest circumference exceeds head size by about 5 to 7 cm (2 to 2.75 inches).

Physiologic Measurements

Physiologic measurements, key elements in evaluating physical status of vital functions, include temperature, pulse, respiration, and blood pressure. Compare each physiologic recording with normal values for that age-group. In addition, compare the values taken on preceding health visits with present recordings. For example, a falsely elevated blood pressure reading may not indicate hypertension if previous recent readings have been within normal limits. The isolated recording may indicate some stressful event in the child's life.

As in most procedures carried out with children, treat older children and adolescents much the same as adults. However, give special consideration to preschool children (see Atraumatic Care box). For best results in taking vital signs of infants, count respirations first (before the infant is disturbed), take the pulse next, and measure temperature last. If vital signs cannot be taken without disturbing the child, record the child's behavior (e.g., crying) along with the measurement.

Temperature

Temperature is the measure of heat content within an individual's body. The core temperature most closely reflects the temperature of the blood flow through the carotid arteries to the hypothalamus. Core temperature is relatively constant despite wide fluctuations in the external environment. When a child's temperature is altered, receptors in the skin, spinal cord, and brain respond in an attempt to achieve normothermia, a normal temperature state. In pediatrics, there is a lack of consensus regarding what temperature constitutes

---

ATRAUMATIC CARE

Reducing Young Children's Fears

Young children, especially preschoolers, fear intrusive procedures because of their poorly defined body boundaries. Therefore avoid invasive procedures, such as measuring rectal temperature, whenever possible. Also, avoid using the word "take" when measuring vital signs, since young children interpret words literally and may think that their temperature or other function will be taken away. Instead, say, "I want to know how warm you are."

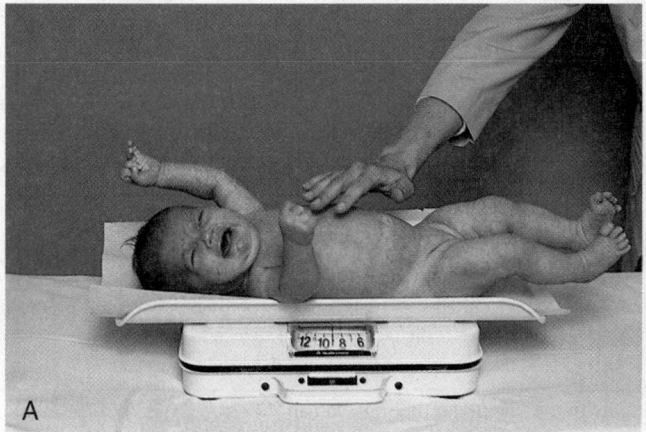
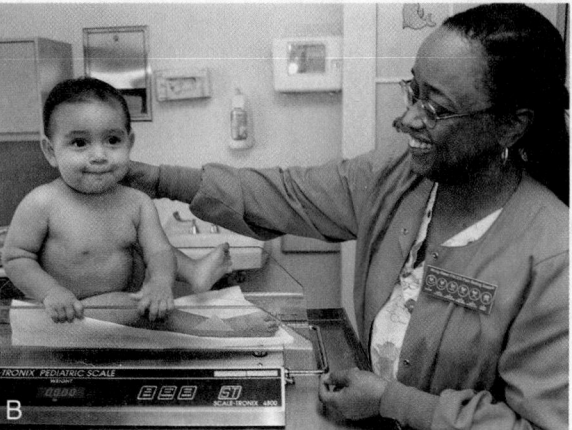

FIG 29-11 A, Infant on scale. **B,** Toddler on scale. Note presence of nurse to prevent falls. (*B,* Courtesy Paul Vincent Kuntz, Texas Children's Hospital, Houston, TX.)

normothermia for every child. For rectal temperatures in children, a value of 37° to 37.5°C (98.6° to 99.5°F) is an acceptable range, where heat loss and heat production are balanced. For neonates, a core body temperature between 36.5° and 37.6°C (97.7° and 99.7°F) is a desirable range. In the neonate, obtain temperature measurements for monitoring adequacy of thermoregulation, not fever; therefore temperature measurements in each infant should be carefully considered in the context of the *purpose* and the environment.

The nurse can measure temperature in healthy children at several body sites via oral, rectal, axillary, ear canal, tympanic membrane, temporal artery, or skin route (Box 29-10). For the ill child, other sites for temperature measurement that have been investigated include the urinary bladder, pulmonary artery, and esophageal and nasopharyngeal sites (El-Radhi and Barry, 2006; Mains, Coxall, and Lloyd, 2008) (Box 29-11). One of the most important influences on the accuracy of temperature is improper temperature-taking technique. Detailed discussion of temperature-taking methods and visual examples of proper techniques are given in Table 29-3. For a critical review of the evidence on temperature-taking methods, see the Evidence-Based Practice box.

The most frequently used temperature measurement devices in infants and children include:

- **Electronic intermittent thermometers**—Measure the patient's temperature at oral, rectal, and axillary sites and are used as primary diagnostic indicators
- **Infrared thermometers**—Measure the patient's temperature by collecting emitted thermal radiation from a particular site (e.g., ear canal)
- **Electronic continuous thermometers**—Measure the patient's temperature during the administration of general anesthesia, treatment of hypothermia or hyperthermia, and other situations that require continuous monitoring

Box 29-12 provides a detailed description of these devices.

BOX 29-10 RECOMMENDED TEMPERATURE SCREENING ROUTES IN INFANTS AND CHILDREN

Birth to 2 Years
- Axillary
- Rectal—if definitive temperature reading is needed for infants older than 1 month

2 to 5 Years
- Axillary
- Tympanic
- Oral—when child can hold thermometer under tongue
- Rectal—if definitive temperature reading is needed

Older than 5 Years
- Oral
- Axillary
- Tympanic

! NURSING ALERT

The belief that core temperature can be estimated by adding 1°C to the temperature taken in the axilla is incorrect. Do not add a degree to the finding obtained by taking a temperature by the axillary route (Craig, Lancaster, Williamson, et al., 2000).

Pulse

A satisfactory pulse can be taken radially in children older than 2 years. However, in infants and young children, the apical impulse (heard through a stethoscope held to the chest at the apex of the heart) is more reliable (see Fig. 29-33 for location of pulses). Count the pulse for 1 full minute in infants and young children because of possible irregularities in rhythm. However, when frequent apical

---

BOX 29-11 ALTERNATIVE TEMPERATURE MEASUREMENT SITES FOR THE ILL CHILD

Skin
- Probe is placed on the skin to determine heat output in response to changes in the patient's skin temperature.
- Skin temperature sensors are most often used for neonates and infants placed in radiant heat warmers or isolettes (using servo-control feature of the apparatus). In turn, the heater unit warms to a set point to maintain the infant's temperature within a specified range.
- ThermoSpot is an example of a device allowing continuous thermal monitoring in neonates.

Urinary Bladder
- A thermistor or thermocouple is placed within the indwelling bladder catheter. The catheter tip immersed in the bladder provides a continuous temperature read-out on the bedside monitor.
- This is not a true measure of core temperature but responds better than rectal and skin temperatures to core body changes.
- Because of thermistor sizes, this method is unusable with neonates and small infants.

Pulmonary Artery
- A catheter is placed into the heart to obtain a reading in the pulmonary artery.
- It is used in critical care settings or operating rooms only in patients requiring aggressive monitoring.
- Catheter is not available in sizes for neonates or small infants.

Esophageal Site
- Probe is inserted into the lower third of the esophagus at the level of the heart.
- This is used in critical care settings or operating rooms.
- Several companies have esophageal stethoscopes with temperature probe monitors for patients in the operating room that show a continuous temperature reading.

Nasopharyngeal Site
- Probe is inserted into the nasopharynx, posterior to the soft palate, and provides an estimate of hypothalamic temperature.
- This is used in critical care settings or operating rooms.

Data from Kumar PR, Nisarga R, Gowda B: Temperature monitoring in newborns using ThermoSpot, *Indian J Pediatr* 71(9):795–796, 2004; Martin SA, Kline AM: Can there be a standard for temperature measurement in the pediatric intensive care unit? *AACN Clin Issues* 15(2):254–266, 2004; Maxton FJC, Justin L, Gilles D: Estimating core temperature in infants and children after cardiac surgery: a comparison of six methods, *J Adv Nurs* 45(2):214–222, 2004.

rates are necessary, use shorter counting times (e.g., 15- or 30-second intervals). For greater accuracy, measure the apical rate while the child is asleep; record the child's behavior along with the rate. Grade pulses according to the criteria in Table 29-4. Compare radial and femoral pulses at least once during infancy to detect the presence of circulatory impairment, such as coarctation of the aorta. (See Appendix C for normal rates for pediatric age-groups.)

Respiration

Count the respiratory rate in children in the same manner as for the adult patient. However, in infants, observe abdominal movements since respirations are primarily diaphragmatic. Because the movements are irregular, count them for 1 full minute for accuracy (see also pp. 814-815). (See Appendix C for normal respiratory rates in children.)

TABLE 29-3	TEMPERATURE MEASUREMENT LOCATIONS FOR INFANTS AND CHILDREN

TEMPERATURE SITE

Oral

Place tip under tongue in right or left posterior sublingual pocket, not in front of tongue. Have child keep mouth closed, without biting on thermometer.

Pacifier thermometers measure intraoral or supralingual temperature and are available but lack support in the literature.

Several factors affect mouth temperature: eating and mastication, hot or cold beverages, open-mouth breathing, ambient temperature.

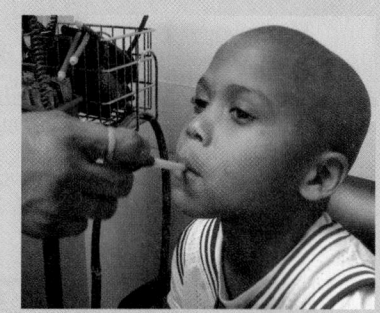

Axillary

Place tip under arm in center of axilla and keep close to skin, not clothing. Hold child's arm firmly against side. Temperature may be affected by poor peripheral perfusion (results in lower value), clothing or swaddling, use of radiant warmer, or amount of brown fat in cold-stressed neonate (results in higher value).

Advantage—Avoids intrusive procedure and eliminates risk for rectal perforation.

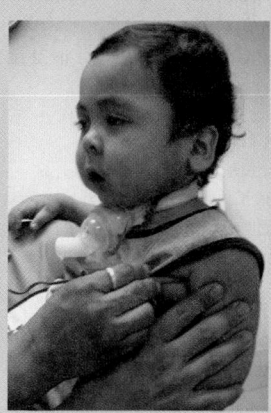

Ear-Based (Aural)

Insert small infrared probe deeply into canal to allow sensor to obtain measurement. Size of probe (most are 8 mm) may influence accuracy of result. In young children this may be a problem because of small diameter of canal. Proper placement of ear is controversial related to whether the pinna should be pulled in manner similar to that used during otoscopy (see pp. 809-810).

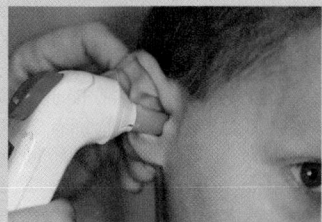

Rectal

Place well-lubricated tip at maximum 2.5 cm (1 in) into rectum for children and 1.5 cm (0.6 in) for infants; securely hold thermometer close to anus.

Child may be placed in side-lying, supine, or prone position (i.e., supine with knees flexed toward abdomen); cover penis, since procedure may stimulate urination. A small child may be placed prone across parent's lap.

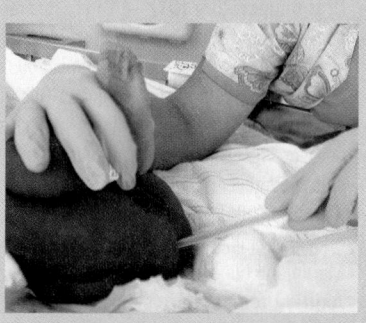

Continued

TABLE 29-3	TEMPERATURE MEASUREMENT LOCATIONS FOR INFANTS AND CHILDREN—cont'd

TEMPERATURE SITE

Temporal Artery

An infrared sensor probe scans across forehead, capturing heat from arterial blood flow. Temporal artery is only artery close enough to skin's surface to provide access for accurate temperature measurement.

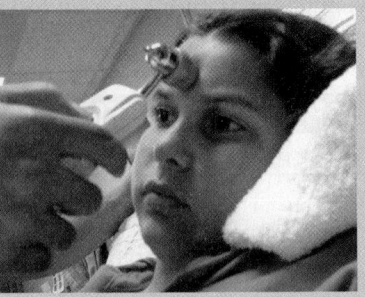

Data from Falzon A, Grech V, Caruana B, et al: How reliable is axillary temperature measurement? *Acta Paediatr* 92(3):309–313, 2003; Martin SA, Kline AM: Can there be a standard for temperature measurement in the pediatric intensive care unit? *AACN Clin Issues* 15(2):254–266, 2004. (Oral, axillary, rectal, and temporal artery images courtesy Paul Vincent Kuntz, Texas Children's Hospital, Houston, TX.)

EVIDENCE-BASED PRACTICE

Temperature Measurement in Pediatrics

Ask the Question

In infants and children, what is the most accurate method for measuring temperature in febrile children?

Search for the Evidence

Search Strategies

Clinical research studies related to this issue were identified by searching for English publications for infant and child populations; comparisons with gold standard: rectal thermometry.

Databases Used

PubMed, Cochrane Collaboration, MD Consult, Joanna Briggs Institute, National Guideline Clearinghouse (AHRQ), TRIP Database Plus, PedsCCM, BestBETs

Critically Analyze the Evidence

- **Rectal temperature**—Rectal measurement remains the clinical gold standard for the precise diagnosis of fever in infants and children compared with other methods (Fortuna, Carney, Macy, et al., 2010; Greenes and Fleisher, 2004; Holzhauer, Reith, Sawin, et al., 2009; Riddell and Eppich, 2003; University of Michigan, 2003). However, this procedure is more invasive and is contraindicated for infants younger than 1 month, children with recent rectal surgery, children with diarrhea or anorectal lesions, and children receiving chemotherapy (cancer treatment usually affects mucosa and causes neutropenia).
- **Oral temperature (OT)**—OT indicates rapid changes in core body temperature, but accuracy may be an issue when compared with the rectal site (Jensen, Jensen, Madsen, et al., 2000). OTs are considered the standard for temperature measurement (Gilbert, Barton, and Counsell, 2002) but are contraindicated in children who have an altered level of consciousness, are receiving oxygen, are mouth breathing, are experiencing mucositis, had recent oral surgery or trauma, or are younger than 5 years (Carroll, 2000; El-Radhi and Barry, 2006). Limitations of OTs include the effects of ambient room temperature and recent oral intake (Carroll, 2000; Martin and Kline, 2004).
- **Axillary temperature**—This is inconsistent and insensitive in infants and children older than 1 month (Falzon, Grech, Caruana, et al., 2003;

Jean-Mary, Dicanzio, Shaw, et al., 2002). In neonates with fever, the axillary temperature cannot be used interchangeably with rectal measurement (Hissink Muller, van Berkel, and de Beaufort, 2008).
- **Ear (aural) temperature**—This is not a precise measurement of body temperature. Meta-analysis of 101 studies comparing tympanic membrane temperatures with rectal temperatures in children concluded that the tympanic method demonstrated a wide range of variability, limiting its application in a pediatric setting (Craig, Lancaster, Taylor, et al., 2002). More recently published reviews continue to find poor sensitivity using infrared ear thermometry (Devrim, Kara, Ceyhan, et al., 2007; Dodd, Lancaster, Craig, et al., 2006). Diagnosis of fever without a focus should not be made based on tympanic thermometry, since it is not an accurate measure of core temperature (Craig, Lancaster, Taylor, et al., 2002; Devrim, Kara, Ceyhan, et al., 2007; Dodd, Lancaster, Craig, et al., 2006; Riddell and Eppich, 2003).
- **Temporal artery temperature (TAT)**—TAT is not predictable for fever in young children but can be used as a screening tool for detecting fever less than 38°C (100.4°F) in children 3 months to 4 years of age (Al-Mukhaizeem, Allen, Komar, et al., 2004; Callanan, 2003; Fortuna, Carney, Macy, et al., 2010; Greenes and Fleisher, 2001; Hebbar, Fortenberry, Rogers, et al., 2005; Holzhauer, Reith, Sawin, et al., 2009; Schuh, Komar, Stephens, et al., 2004; Siberry, Diener-West, Schappell, et al., 2002; Titus, Hulsey, Heckman, et al., 2009).

Apply the Evidence: Nursing Implications

- No single site used for temperature assessment provides unequivocal estimates of core body temperature.
- Studies show that the axillary and tympanic measures demonstrate poor agreement when these modes are compared with more accurate core temperature methods. The differences are more evident as temperature increases, regardless of age.
- TAT is not predictable for fever and should be used only as a screening tool in young children.
- When an accurate method for obtaining a correct reflection of core temperature is needed, the rectal temperature is recommended in younger children and the oral route in older children.

EVIDENCE-BASED PRACTICE

Temperature Measurement in Pediatrics—cont'd

Quality and Safety Competencies:
Evidence-Based Practice*

Knowledge

Differentiate Clinical Opinion from Research and Evidence-Based Summaries.

Demonstrate understanding of thermometry selection based on the developmental age of the child.

Skills

Base Individualized Care Plan on Patient Values, Clinical Expertise, and Evidence.

Integrate evidence into practice by using the correct type of thermometry to screen for fever compared with measures used for accurate determination of the degree of fever.

Attitudes

Value the Concept of Evidence-Based Practice (EBP) as Integral to Determining Best Clinical Practice.

Recognize strengths and weakness of evidence for the most accurate method for measuring fever in infants and children.

References

Al-Mukhaizeem F, Allen U, Komar L, et al: Comparison of temporal artery, rectal and esophageal core temperatures in children: results of a pilot study, *Paediatr Child Health* 9(7):461–465, 2004.

Callanan D: Detecting fever in young infants: reliability of perceived, pacifier, and temporal artery temperatures in infants younger than 3 months of age, *Pediatr Emerg Care* 19(4):240–243, 2003.

Carroll M: An evaluation of temperature measurement, *Nurs Stand* 14(44):39–43, 2000.

Craig JV, Lancaster GA, Taylor S, et al: Infrared ear thermometry compared with rectal thermometry in children: a systematic review, *Lancet* 360(9333):603–609, 2002.

Devrim I, Kara A, Ceyhan M, et al: Measurement accuracy of fever by tympanic and axillary thermometry, *Pediatr Emerg Care* 23(1):16–19, 2007.

Dodd SR, Lancaster GA, Craig JV, et al: In a systematic review, infrared ear thermometry for fever diagnosis in children finds poor sensitivity, *J Clin Epidemiol* 59:354–357, 2006.

El-Radhi AS, Barry W: Thermometry in paediatric practice, *Arch Dis Child* 91(4):351–356, 2006.

Falzon A, Grech V, Caruana B, et al: How reliable is axillary temperature measurement? *Acta Paediatr* 92(3):309–313, 2003.

Fortuna EL, Carney MM, Macy M, et al: Accuracy of non-contact infrared thermometry versus rectal thermometry in young children evaluated in the emergency department for fever, *J Emerg Nurs* 36(2):101–104, 2010.

Gilbert M, Barton AJ, Counsell CM: Comparison of oral and tympanic temperatures in adult surgical patients, *Appl Nurs Res* 15(1):42–47, 2002.

Greenes DS, Fleisher GR: Accuracy of a noninvasive temporal artery thermometer for use in infants, *Arch Pediatr Adolesc Med* 155(3):376–381, 2001.

Greenes DS, Fleisher GR: When body temperature changes, does rectal temperature lag? *J Pediatr* 144(6):824–826, 2004.

Hebbar K, Fortenberry JD, Rogers K, et al: Comparison of temporal artery thermometer to standard temperature measurement in pediatric intensive care unit patients, *Pediatr Crit Care Med* 6(5):557–561, 2005.

Hissink Muller PC, van Berkel LH, de Beaufort AJ: Axillary and rectal temperature measurements poorly agree in newborn infants, *Neonatology* 94(1):31–34, 2008.

Holzhauer JK, Reith V, Sawin K, et al: Evaluation of temporal artery thermometry in children 3-36 months old, *J Spec Pediatr Nurs* 14(4):239–244, 2009.

Jean-Mary MB, Dicanzio J, Shaw J, et al: Limited accuracy and reliability of infrared axillary and aural thermometers in a pediatric outpatient population, *J Pediatr* 141(5):671–676, 2002.

Jensen BN, Jensen FS, Madsen SN, et al: Accuracy of digital tympanic, oral, axillary, and rectal thermometers compared with standard rectal mercury thermometers, *Eur J Surg* 166(11):848–851, 2000.

Martin SA, Kline AM: Can there be a standard for temperature measurement in the pediatric intensive care unit? *AACN Clin Issues* 15(2):254–266, 2004.

Riddell A, Eppich W: Should tympanic temperature measurement be trusted? BestBETs, 2003, www.bestbets.org/cgi-bin/bets.pl?record=00340.

Schuh S, Komar L, Stephens D, et al: Comparison of the temporal artery and rectal thermometry in children in the emergency department, *Pediatr Emerg Care* 20(11):736–741, 2004.

Siberry GK, Diener-West M, Schappell E, et al: Comparison of temple temperatures with rectal temperatures in children under 2 years of age, *Clin Pediatr* 41(6):405–414, 2002.

Titus MO, Hulsey T, Heckman J, et al: Temporal artery thermometry utilization in pediatric emergency care, *Clin Pediatr* 48(2):190–193, 2009.

University of Michigan: Rectal temperature is still the gold standard for determining the presence or absence of fever, Evidence-Based Pediatrics website, 2003, www.med.umich.edu/pediatrics/ebm/cats/fever.htm.

*Based on Quality and Safety Education for Nurses at www.qsen.org.

Blood Pressure

Blood pressure (BP) measurement by noninvasive methods is part of a routine vital sign determination. Measure BP annually in children 3 years of age through adolescence and in children with symptoms of hypertension, children in emergency departments and intensive care units, and high risk infants (National High Blood Pressure Education Program Working Group on High Blood Pressure in Children and Adolescents, 2004).

Measurement Devices. Ambulatory BP monitoring in children and adolescents is a valuable method for assessing and managing suspected hypertension. Also measure BP using electronic devices that employ oscillometric or Doppler techniques. In oscillometry, pressure changes are transmitted through the arterial wall to the pressure cuff and the oscillations are detected by a pressure-sensitive indicator. Oscillometers have digital read-outs for systolic, diastolic, and mean arterial pressures (MAPs) and for pulse. The MAP is not the same as the mean BP (arithmetic average of systolic and diastolic pressures). Rather, it is a value somewhat lower than the arithmetic mean. BP readings using oscillometry, such as Dinamap, are generally higher (10 mm Hg higher) than measurements using auscultation (Park, Menard, and Schoolfield, 2005) (Table 29-5). Differences between Dinamap and auscultatory readings prevent the interchange of the readings by the two methods (Midgley, Wardhaugh, Macfarlane, et al., 2009).

Doppler ultrasound translates changes in ultrasound frequency caused by blood movement within the artery to audible sound by

BOX 29-12 TYPES OF THERMOMETERS USED TO MEASURE TEMPERATURE IN INFANTS AND CHILDREN

Electronic Thermometer
- Temperature is sensed with an electronic component called *thermistor* mounted at the tip of a plastic and stainless steel probe, which is connected to an electronic recorder. A disposable plastic cover is used for infection control.
- Temperature measurement appears on digital display within 60 seconds.
- Probe can be placed in mouth, axilla, or rectum.

Infrared Thermometer
- Thermal radiation is measured from axilla, ear canal, or tympanic membrane.
- Temperature measurement appears on digital display in approximately 1 second.
- Three types are available for ear-based use: tympanic, ear canal, and arterial heat balance via the ear canal (AHBE).
- Often these devices are all inappropriately referred to as *tympanic thermometers.*
- Temperatures measured in this way reflect arterial (bloodstream) temperature.

Ear-Based Temperature Sensor
- Although this is frequently used in pediatric settings (especially ambulatory clinics), debate continues on the reliability of ear-based thermometry in screening febrile children.
- Most models use "offsets" for internal calculations that transform ear temperature into supposedly equivalent oral or rectal temperatures.

Ear Sensor (LighTouch LTX)
- This measures the infrared heat energy radiating from canal opening, scans canal for highest temperature reading, and then calculates arterial temperature (correlates highly with core or internal body temperature).
- It is available in two sizes; smaller size of LighTouch Pedi-Q is for infants and toddlers.

Axillary Sensor (LighTouch LTN)
- This measures the infrared heat energy radiating from the axilla.
- It can be used on wet skin; in incubators; or under radiant heaters, warming pads, or other heat sources.

Digital Thermometer
- A probe is connected to a microprocessor chip, which translates signals into degrees and sends temperature measurement to digital display.
- It is used like an oral electronic thermometer and can be used for measuring oral, rectal, and axillary temperature.
- It is more accurate and easier to read but somewhat more expensive than plastic strip thermometer.

Liquid Crystal Skin Contact Thermometer (Chemical Dot Thermometer)
- This single-use, disposable, flexible thermometer has a specific chemical mixture in each circle that changes color to measure temperature increments of $\frac{2}{10}$ of a degree.
- There are two types:
  1. Kept in mouth (1 minute), axilla (3 minutes), or rectum (3 minutes); color change is read 10 to 15 seconds after removing thermometer.
  2. Wearable, continuous-use thermometer, which is placed under axilla; may be read within 2 to 3 minutes after placement and continuously thereafter; discard and replace every 48 hours.

TABLE 29-4 GRADING OF PULSES

GRADE	DESCRIPTION
0	Not palpable
+1	Difficult to palpate, thready, weak, easily obliterated with pressure
+2	Difficult to palpate, may be obliterated with pressure
+3	Easy to palpate, not easily obliterated with pressure (normal)
+4	Strong, bounding, not obliterated with pressure

TABLE 29-5 NORMATIVE DINAMAP BLOOD PRESSURE VALUES (SYSTOLIC/DIASTOLIC; MEAN ARTERIAL PRESSURE IN PARENTHESES)

AGE-GROUP	MEAN	90TH PERCENTILE	95TH PERCENTILE
Newborn (1-3 days)	65/41 (50)	75/49 (59)	78/52 (62)
1 month-2 years	95/58 (72)	106/68 (83)	110/71 (86)
2-5 years	101/57 (74)	112/66 (82)	115/68 (85)

From Park M, Menard S: Normative oscillometric blood pressure values in the first 5 years in an office setting, *Am J Dis Child* 143(7):860–864, 1989.

means of a transducer in the cuff. This technique is useful for systolic pressure measurement but is unreliable for diastolic pressure measurement. Oscillometric and Doppler instruments are useful in measuring BP in infants and have largely replaced the flush method, which reflects only the mean BP, and the auscultatory method.

Selection of Cuff. No matter what type of noninvasive technique is used, the most important factor in accurately measuring BP is the use of an appropriate-size cuff (cuff size refers only to the inner inflatable bladder, not the cloth covering). A technique to establish an appropriate cuff size is to choose a cuff with a bladder width that is approximately 40% of the arm circumference midway between the olecranon and the acromion. This will usually be a cuff bladder that covers 80% to 100% of the circumference of the arm (Fig. 29-12) (Beevers, Lip, and O'Brien, 2001). Cuffs that are either too narrow or too wide affect the accuracy of BP measurements. If the cuff size is too small, the reading on the device is falsely high. If the cuff size is too large, the reading is falsely low (Clark, Kieh-Lai, Sarnaik, et al., 2002).

Using limb circumference for selecting cuff width more accurately reflects direct arterial BP than using limb length, since this method takes into account variations in arm thickness and the amount of pressure required to compress the artery. For measurement on sites other than the upper arms, use the limb circumference, although the shape of the limb (e.g., conical shape of the thigh)

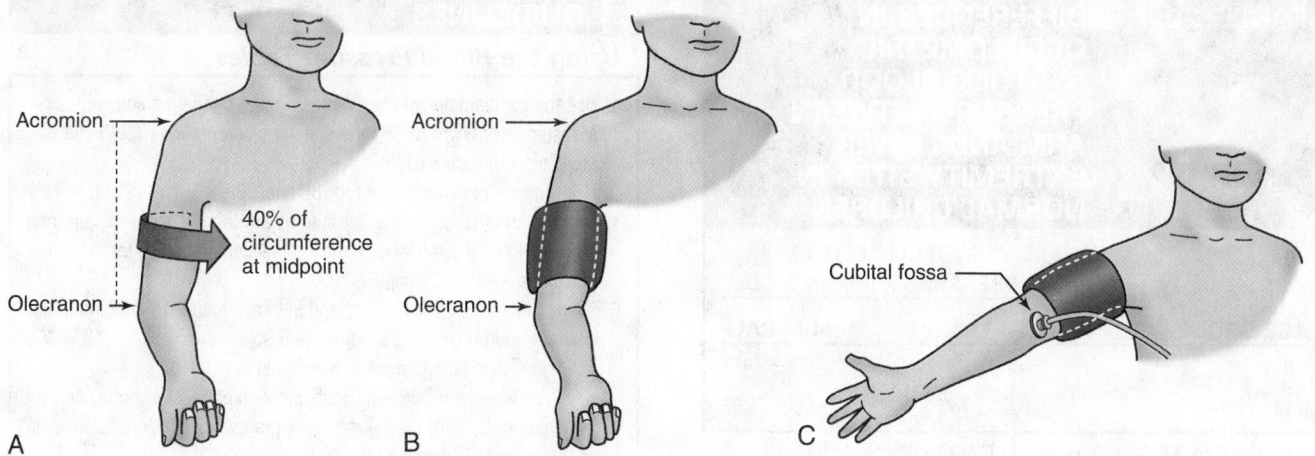

FIG 29-12 Determination of proper cuff size. **A,** Cuff bladder width should be approximately 40% of circumference of arm measured at a point midway between olecranon and acromion. **B,** Cuff bladder length should cover 80% to 100% of circumference of arm. **C,** Blood pressure should be measured with cubital fossa at heart level. Arm should be supported. Stethoscope bell is placed over brachial artery pulse, proximal and medial to cubital fossa and below bottom edge of cuff. (From National Institutes of Health, National Heart, Lung, and Blood Institute: *Update on the Task Force Report [1987] on high blood pressure in children and adolescents: a working group report from the National High Blood Pressure Education Program,* NIH Pub No 96-3790, Bethesda, MD, September 1996, Authors.)

TABLE 29-6		RECOMMENDED DIMENSIONS FOR BLOOD PRESSURE CUFF BLADDERS	
AGE	**WIDTH (CM)**	**LENGTH (CM)**	**MAXIMUM ARM CIRCUMFERENCE (CM)***
Newborn	4	8	10
Infant	6	12	15
Child	9	18	22
Small adult	10	24	26
Adult	13	30	34
Large adult	16	38	44
Thigh	20	42	52

From National High Blood Pressure Education Program Working Group on High Blood Pressure in Children and Adolescents: The fourth report on the diagnosis, evaluation, and treatment of high blood pressure in children and adolescents, http://www.nhlbi.nih.gov/health/prof/heart/hbp/hbp_ped.pdf, US Department of Health and Human Services.
*Calculated so that largest arm would still allow bladder to encircle arm by at least 80%.

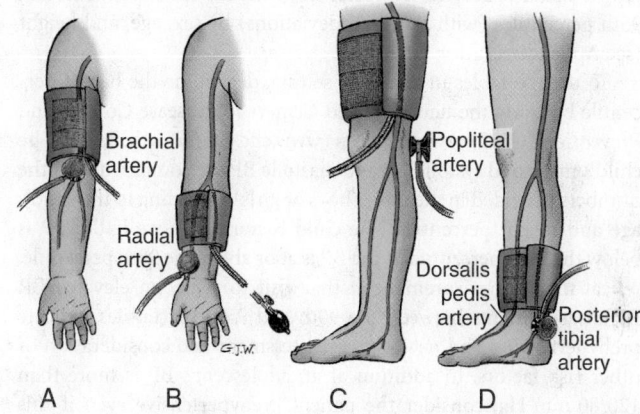

FIG 29-13 Sites for measuring blood pressure. **A,** Upper arm. **B,** Lower arm or forearm. **C,** Thigh. **D,** Calf or ankle.

> **! NURSING ALERT**
>
> When taking BP, use an appropriate-size cuff. When the correct size is not available, use an oversize cuff rather than an undersize one or use another site that more appropriately fits the cuff size. Do not choose a cuff based on the name of the cuff (e.g., an "infant" cuff may be too small for some infants).

> **! NURSING ALERT**
>
> Compare BP in the upper and lower extremities to detect abnormalities, such as coarctation of the aorta, in which the lower extremity pressure is less than the upper extremity pressure.

may prevent appropriate placement of the cuff and inaccurately reflect intraarterial BP (Table 29-6).

When using a site other than the arm, BP measurements using noninvasive techniques may differ. Generally, systolic pressure in the lower extremities (thigh or calf) is greater than pressure in the upper extremities and systolic BP in the calf is higher than that in the thigh (Fig. 29-13). Table 29-7 lists these differences that are applied to oscillometric measurements taken on the right extremities with the child supine and the cuff size based on the circumference method.

Measurement and Interpretation. Measuring and interpreting BP in infants and children require attention to correct procedure because (1) limb sizes vary and cuff selection must accommodate the circumference; (2) excessive pressure on the antecubital fossa

TABLE 29-7	DIFFERENCES IN OSCILLOMETRIC SYSTOLIC BLOOD PRESSURE BETWEEN ARM AND LOWER EXTREMITY SITES IN NORMAL CHILDREN	
	SYSTOLIC BLOOD PRESSURE × (MEAN ± SD)	
AGE-GROUP (YR)	**ARM-THIGH**	**ARM-CALF**
4-8	−7.1 ± 6.8	−9.3 ± 7.4
9-16	−2.4 ± 7.7	−5.0 ± 26.9

Data from Park M, Lee D, Johnson GA: Oscillometric blood pressures in the arm, thigh, and calf in healthy children and those with aortic coarctation, *Pediatrics* 91(4):761–765, 1993.

affects the Korotkoff sounds; (3) children easily become anxious, which can elevate BP; and (4) BP values change with age and growth. In children and adolescents, determine the normal range of BP by body size and age. BP standards that are based on sex, age, and height provide a more precise classification of BP according to body size. This approach avoids misclassifying children who are very tall or very short. The revised BP tables now include the 50th, 90th, and 95th percentiles (with standard deviations) by sex, age, and height (see Appendix C).

To use the tables in a clinical setting, determine the height percentile by using the newly revised Centers for Disease Control and Prevention (CDC) growth charts (www.cdc.gov/growthcharts). The child's measured systolic BP and diastolic BP are compared with the numbers provided in the table (boys or girls) according to the child's age and height percentile. The child is normotensive if the BP is below the 90th percentile. If the BP is at or above the 90th percentile, repeat the BP measurement at that visit to verify an elevated BP. BP measurements between the 90th and 95th percentiles indicate prehypertension and necessitate reassessment and consideration of other risk factors. In addition, if an adolescent's BP is more than 120/80 mm Hg, consider the patient prehypertensive even if this value is below the 90th percentile. This BP level typically occurs for systolic BP at 12 years old and for diastolic BP at 16 years old. If the child's BP (systolic or diastolic) is at or above the 95th percentile, the child may be hypertensive and the measurement must be repeated on at least two occasions to confirm diagnosis (National High Blood Pressure Education Program, 2004) (see Guidelines box).

Orthostatic Hypotension. Orthostatic hypotension (OH), also called *postural hypotension* or *orthostatic intolerance,* often manifests as syncope (fainting), vertigo (dizziness), or lightheadedness and is caused by decreased blood flow to the brain (cerebral hypoperfusion). Normally blood flow to the brain is maintained at a constant level by a number of compensating mechanisms that regulate systemic BP. When one assumes a sitting or standing position from a supine or recumbent position, peripheral capillary vasoconstriction occurs and blood that was pooling in the lower vasculature is returned to the heart for redistribution to the head and remainder of the body. When this mechanism fails or is slow to respond, the person may experience vertigo or syncope. One of the most common causes of OH is hypovolemia, which may be induced by medications such as diuretics, vasodilator medications, and prolonged immobility or bed rest. Other causes of OH include dehydration, diarrhea,

GUIDELINES
Using the Blood Pressure Tables

1. Use the standard height charts to determine the height percentile.
2. Measure and record the child's systolic blood pressure (SBP) and diastolic blood pressure (DBP).
3. Use the correct gender table for SBP and DBP.
4. Find the child's age on the left side of the table. Follow the age row horizontally across the table to the intersection of the line for the height percentile (vertical column).
5. There, find the 50th, 90th, 95th, and 99th percentiles for SBP in the left columns and for DBP in the right columns.
   - BP less than 90th percentile is normal.
   - BP between the 90th and 95th percentiles is prehypertension. In adolescents, BP of 120/80 mm Hg or greater is prehypertension, even if this figure is less than the 90th percentile.
   - BP over the 95th percentile may be hypertension.
6. If the BP is over the 90th percentile, the BP should be repeated twice at the same office visit, and an average SBP and DBP should be used.
7. If the BP is over the 95th percentile, BP should be staged. If BP is stage 1 (95th to 99th percentile plus 5 mm Hg), BP measurements should be repeated on two more occasions. If hypertension is confirmed, evaluation should proceed. If BP is stage 2 (>99th percentile plus 5 mm Hg), prompt referral should be made for evaluation and therapy. If the patient is symptomatic, immediate referral and treatment are indicated.

From National High Blood Pressure Education Program Working Group on High Blood Pressure in Children and Adolescents: The fourth report on the diagnosis, evaluation, and treatment of high blood pressure in children and adolescents, http://www.nhlbi.nih.gov/health/prof/heart/hbp/hbp_ped.pdf, US Department of Health and Human Services.

emesis, fluid loss from sweating and exertion, alcohol intake, dysrhythmias, diabetes mellitus, sepsis, and hemorrhage.

BP measurements taken with the child supine and then standing (at least 2 minutes in each position) may demonstrate variability and assist in the diagnosis of OH. The child with a sustained drop in systolic pressure of more than 20 mm Hg or in diastolic pressure of more than 10 mm Hg after standing for 2 minutes without an increase in heart rate of more than 15 beats/min most likely has an autonomic deficit. Nonneurogenic causes of OH have a compensatory increase in pulse of more than 15 beats/min as well as a drop in BP, as noted previously. For the child or adolescent with vertigo, lightheadedness, nausea, syncope, diaphoresis, and pallor, it is important to monitor BP and heart rate to determine the original cause. BP is an important diagnostic measurement in children and adolescents and must be a part of the routine monitoring of vital signs.

NURSING ALERT

Published norms for BP, such as those in Appendix C, are valid only if you use the same method of measurement (auscultation and cuff size determination) in clinical practice.

General Appearance

The child's general appearance is a cumulative, subjective impression of the child's physical appearance, state of nutrition, behavior, personality, interactions with parents and nurse (also siblings if present), posture, development, and speech. Although the nurse records general appearance at the beginning of the physical

TABLE 29-8	DIFFERENCES IN COLOR CHANGES OF RACIAL GROUPS	
DESCRIPTION	**APPEARANCE IN LIGHT SKIN**	**APPEARANCE IN DARK SKIN**
Cyanosis—Bluish tone through skin; reflects reduced (deoxygenated) hemoglobin	Bluish tinge, especially in palpebral conjunctiva (lower eyelid), nail beds, earlobes, lips, oral membranes, soles, and palms	Ashen gray lips and tongue
Pallor—Paleness; may be sign of anemia, chronic disease, edema, or shock	Loss of rosy glow in skin, especially face	Ashen gray appearance in black skin More yellowish brown color in brown skin
Erythema—Redness; may be result of increased blood flow from climatic conditions, local inflammation, infection, skin irritation, allergy, or other dermatoses or may be caused by increased numbers of red blood cells as compensatory response to chronic hypoxia	Redness easily seen anywhere on body	Much more difficult to assess; rely on palpation for warmth or edema
Ecchymosis—Large, diffuse areas, usually black and blue, caused by hemorrhage of blood into skin; typically result of injuries	Purplish to yellow-green areas; may be seen anywhere on skin	Very difficult to see unless in mouth or conjunctiva
Petechiae—Same as ecchymosis except for size: small, distinct, pinpoint hemorrhages ≤2 mm in size; can denote some type of blood disorder, such as leukemia	Purplish pinpoints most easily seen on buttocks, abdomen, and inner surfaces of arms or legs	Usually invisible except in oral mucosa, conjunctiva of eyelids, and conjunctiva covering eyeball
Jaundice—Yellow staining of skin usually caused by bile pigments	Yellow staining seen in sclerae of eyes, skin, fingernails, soles, palms, and oral mucosa	Most reliably assessed in sclerae, hard palate, palms, and soles

examination, it encompasses all the observations of the child during the interview and physical assessment.

Note the facies, the child's facial expression and appearance. For example, the facies may give clues to children who are in pain; have difficulty breathing; feel frightened, discontented, or unhappy; are mentally delayed; or are acutely ill.

Observe the posture, position, and types of body movement. The child with hearing or vision loss may characteristically tilt the head in an awkward position to hear or see better. The child in pain may favor a body part. The child with low self-esteem or a feeling of rejection may assume a slumped, careless, and apathetic pose. Likewise, a child with confidence, a feeling of self-worth, and a sense of security usually demonstrates a tall, straight, well-balanced posture. While observing such body language, do not interpret too freely but, rather, record objectively.

Note the child's hygiene in terms of cleanliness; unusual body odor; the condition of the hair, neck, nails, teeth, and feet; and the condition of the clothing. Such observations are excellent clues to possible instances of neglect, inadequate financial resources, housing difficulties (e.g., no running water), or lack of knowledge concerning children's needs.

Behavior includes the child's personality, activity level, reaction to stress, requests, frustration, interactions with others (primarily the parent and nurse), degree of alertness, and response to stimuli. Some mental questions that serve as reminders for observing behavior include:

- What is the child's overall personality?
- Does the child have a long attention span, or is he or she easily distracted?
- Can the child follow two or three commands in succession without the need for repetition?
- What is the youngster's response to delayed gratification or frustration?
- Does the child use eye contact during conversation?
- What is the child's reaction to the nurse and family members?
- Is the child quick or slow to grasp explanations?

Skin

Assess skin for color, texture, temperature, moisture, turgor, lesions, and rashes. Examination of the skin and its accessory organs primarily involves inspection and palpation. Touch allows the nurse to assess the texture, turgor, and temperature of the skin. The normal color in light-skinned children varies from a milky white and rose to a deeply hued pink. Dark-skinned children, such as those of Native-American, Hispanic, or African descent, have inherited various brown, red, yellow, olive green, and bluish tones in their skin. Asian persons have skin that is normally of a yellow tone. Several variations in skin color can occur, some of which warrant further investigation. The types of color change and their appearance in children with light or dark skin are summarized in Table 29-8.

Normally the skin texture of young children is smooth, slightly dry, and not oily or clammy. Evaluate skin temperature by symmetrically feeling each part of the body and comparing upper areas with lower ones. Note any difference in temperature.

Determine tissue turgor, or elasticity in the skin, by grasping the skin on the abdomen between the thumb and index finger, pulling it taut, and quickly releasing it. Elastic tissue immediately resumes its normal position without residual marks or creases. In children with poor skin turgor, the skin remains suspended or tented for a few seconds before slowly falling back on the abdomen. Skin turgor is one of the best estimates of adequate hydration and nutrition.

Accessory Structures

Inspection of the accessory structures of the skin may be performed while examining the skin, scalp, or extremities.

Inspect the hair for color, texture, quality, distribution, and elasticity. Children's scalp hair is usually lustrous, silky, strong, and elastic. Genetic factors affect the appearance of hair. For example, the hair of African-American children is usually curlier and coarser than that of Caucasian children. Hair that is stringy, dull, brittle, dry, friable, and depigmented may suggest poor nutrition. Record any bald or thinning spots. Loss of hair in infants may indicate lying in the same position and may be a cue to counsel parents concerning the child's stimulation needs.

Inspect the hair and scalp for general cleanliness. Persons in some ethnic groups condition their hair with oils or lubricants that, if not thoroughly washed from the scalp, clog the sebaceous glands, causing scalp infections. Also examine the area for lesions; scaliness; evidence of infestation, such as lice or ticks; and signs of trauma, such as ecchymosis, masses, or scars.

In children who are approaching puberty, look for growth of secondary hair as a sign of normally progressing pubertal changes. Note precocious or delayed appearance of hair growth because, although not always suggestive of hormonal dysfunction, it may be of great concern to the early- or late-maturing adolescent.

Inspect the nails for color, shape, texture, and quality. Normally the nails are pink, convex, smooth, and hard but flexible (not brittle). The edges, which are usually white, should extend over the fingers. Dark-skinned individuals may have more deeply pigmented nail beds. Short, ragged nails are typical of habitual biting. Uncut, dirty nails are a sign of poor hygiene.

The palm normally shows three flexion creases (Fig. 29-14, *A*). In some situations such as Down syndrome, the two distal horizontal creases are fused to form a single horizontal crease (the single palmar crease, or transpalmar crease) (Fig. 29-14, *B*). If grossly abnormal lines or folds are observed, sketch a picture to describe them and refer the finding to a specialist for further investigation.

Lymph Nodes

Lymph nodes are usually assessed during examination of the part of the body in which they are located. The body's lymphatic drainage system is extensive. Fig. 29-15 shows the usual sites for palpating accessible lymph nodes.

Palpate nodes using the distal portion of the fingers and gently but firmly pressing in a circular motion along the regions where nodes are normally present. During assessment of the nodes in the head and neck, tilt the child's head upward slightly but without tensing the sternocleidomastoid or trapezius muscles. This position facilitates palpation of the submental, submandibular, tonsillar, and cervical nodes. Palpate the axillary nodes with the child's arms relaxed at the sides but slightly abducted. Assess the inguinal nodes with the child in the supine position. Note size, mobility, temperature, and tenderness, as well as reports by the parents regarding any visible change of enlarged nodes. In children, small, nontender, movable nodes are usually normal. Tender, enlarged,

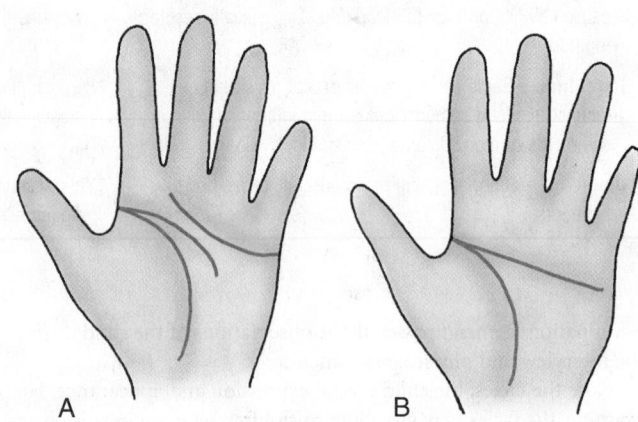

FIG 29-14 Examples of flexion creases on palm. **A,** Normal. **B,** Transpalmar crease.

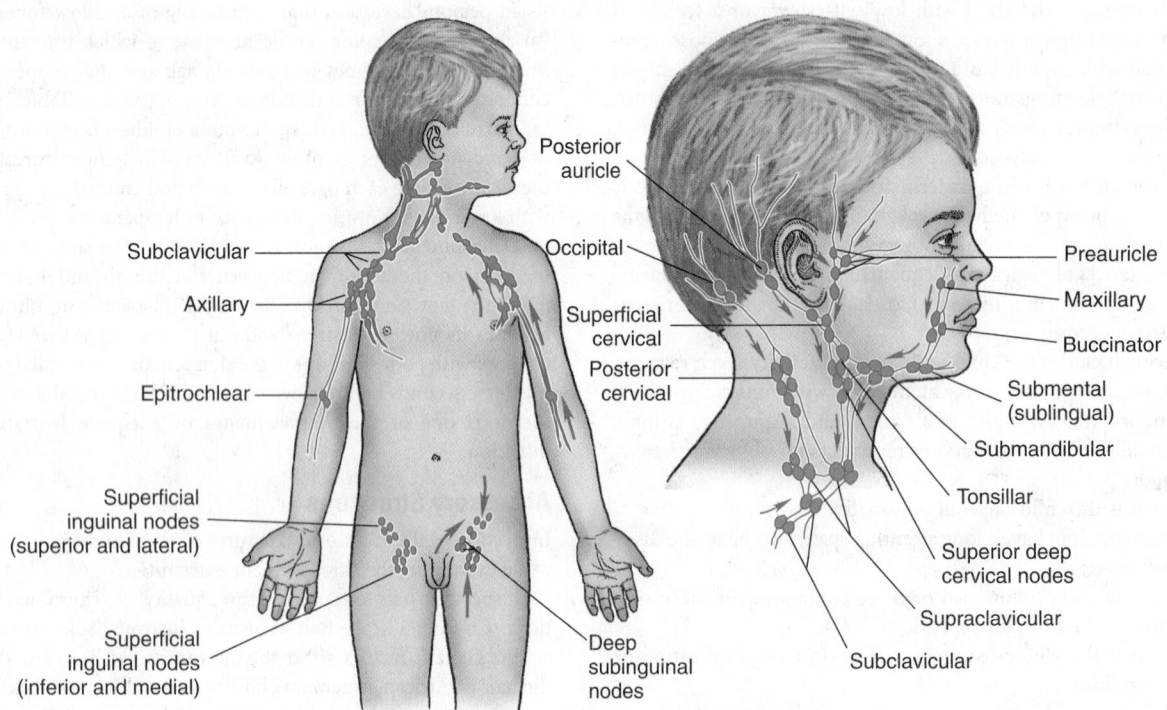

FIG 29-15 Location of superficial lymph nodes. *Arrows* indicate directional flow of lymph.

warm, erythematous lymph nodes generally indicate infection or inflammation close to their location. Report such findings for further investigation.

Head and Neck

Observe the head for general shape and symmetry. A flattening of one part of the head, such as the occiput, may indicate that the child continually lies in this position. Marked asymmetry is usually abnormal and may indicate premature closure of the sutures (craniosynostosis).

> **! NURSING ALERT**
>
> Significant head lag after 6 months of age strongly indicates cerebral injury and is referred for further evaluation.

Note head control in infants and head posture in older children. Most infants by 4 months of age should be able to hold the head erect and in midline when in a vertical position.

Evaluate range of motion by asking the older child to look in each direction (to either side, up, and down) or by manually putting the younger child through each position. Limited range of motion may indicate wryneck, or torticollis, in which the child holds the head to one side with the chin pointing toward the opposite side as a result of injury to the sternocleidomastoid muscle.

> **! NURSING ALERT**
>
> Hyperextension of the head (opisthotonos) with pain on flexion is a serious indication of meningeal irritation and is referred for immediate medical evaluation.

Palpate the skull for patent sutures, fontanels, fractures, and swellings. Normally, the posterior fontanel closes by the second month of life and the anterior fontanel fuses between 12 and 18 months. Early or late closure is noted, since either may be a sign of a pathologic condition. While examining the head, observe the face for symmetry, movement, and general appearance. Ask the child to "make a face" to assess symmetric movement and disclose any degree of paralysis. Note any unusual facial proportion, such as an unusually high or low forehead; wide- or close-set eyes; or a small, receding chin.

In addition to assessment of the head and neck for movement, inspect the neck for size and palpate its associated structures. The neck is normally short, with skinfolds between the head and shoulders during infancy; however, it lengthens during the next 3 to 4 years.

> **! NURSING ALERT**
>
> If any masses are detected in the neck, report them for further investigation. Large masses can block the airway.

Eyes

Inspection of External Structures

Inspect the lids for proper placement on the eye. When the eye is open, the upper lid should fall near the upper iris. When the eyes are closed, the lids should completely cover the cornea and sclera (Fig. 29-16).

Determine the general slant of the palpebral fissures or lids by drawing an imaginary line through the two points of the medial canthus and across the outer orbit of the eyes and aligning each eye on the line. Usually the palpebral fissures lie horizontally. However, in Asians the slant is normally upward.

Also inspect the inside lining of the lids, the palpebral conjunctivae. To examine the lower conjunctival sac, pull the lid down while the patient looks up. To evert the upper lid, hold the upper lashes and gently pull *down* and *forward* as the child looks down. Normally the conjunctiva appears pink and glossy. Vertical yellow striations along the edge are the meibomian glands, or sebaceous glands, near the hair follicle. Located in the inner or medial canthus and situated on the inner edge of the upper and lower lids is a tiny opening, the lacrimal punctum. Note any excessive tearing, discharge, or inflammation of the lacrimal apparatus.

The bulbar conjunctiva, which covers the eye up to the limbus, or junction of the cornea and sclera, should be transparent. The sclera, or white covering of the eyeball, should be clear. Tiny black marks in the sclera of heavily pigmented individuals are normal.

The cornea, or covering of the iris and pupil, should be clear and transparent. Record opacities because they can be signs of scarring or ulceration, which can interfere with vision. The best way to test for opacities is to illuminate the eyeball by shining a light at an angle (obliquely) toward the cornea.

Compare the pupils for size, shape, and movement. They should be round, clear, and equal. Test their reaction to light by quickly shining a light toward the eye and removing it. As the light approaches, the pupils should constrict; as the light fades, the pupils should dilate. Test the pupil for any response of accommodation by having the child look at a bright, shiny object at a distance and quickly moving the object toward the face. The pupils should constrict as the object is brought near the eye. Record normal findings on examination of the pupils as PERRLA, which stands for "**P**upils **E**qual, **R**ound, **R**eact to **L**ight, and **A**ccommodation."

Inspect the iris and pupil for color, size, shape, and clarity. Permanent eye color is usually established by 6 to 12 months of age. While inspecting the iris and pupil, look for the lens. Normally the lens is not visible through the pupil.

Inspection of Internal Structures

The ophthalmoscope permits visualization of the interior of the eyeball with a system of lenses and a high-intensity light. The lenses permit clear visualization of eye structures at different distances from the nurse's eye and correct visual acuity differences in the examiner and child. Use of the ophthalmoscope requires practice to know which lens setting produces the clearest image.

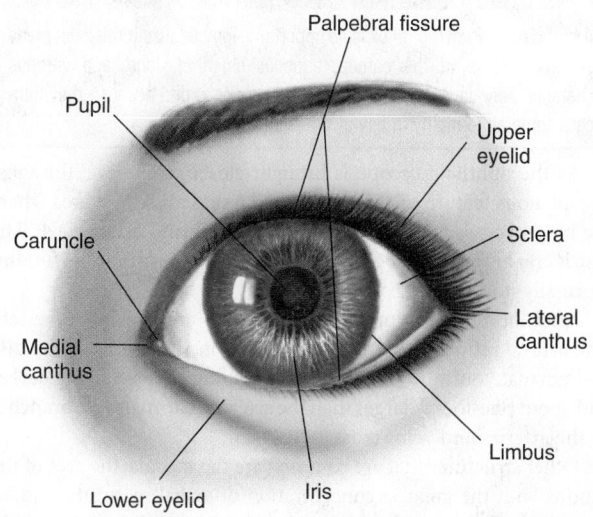

FIG 29-16 External structures of eye.

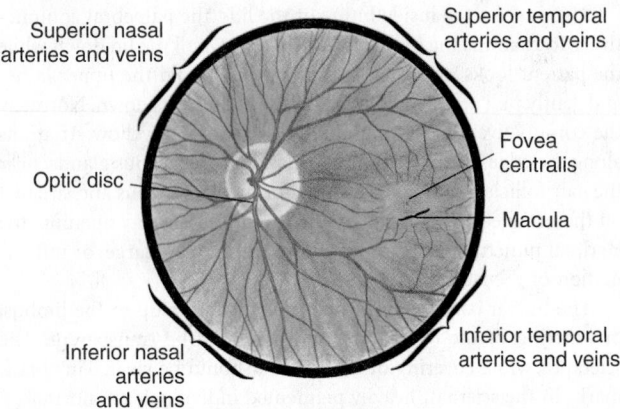

FIG 29-17 Structures of fundus. (From Seidel HM, Ball JW, Dains JE, et al: *Mosby's guide to physical examination*, ed 7, St Louis, 2011, Mosby.)

The ophthalmic and otic heads are usually interchangeable on one "body" or handle, which encloses the power source, either disposable or rechargeable batteries. The nurse should practice changing the heads, which snap on and are secured with a quarter turn, and replacing the batteries and light bulbs. Nurses who are not directly involved in physical assessment are often responsible for ensuring that the equipment functions properly.

Preparing the Child. The nurse can prepare the child for the ophthalmoscopic examination by showing the child the instrument, demonstrating the light source and how it shines in the eye, and explaining the reason for darkening the room. For infants and young children who do not respond to such explanations, it is best to use distraction to encourage them to keep their eyes open. Forcibly parting the lids results in an uncooperative, watery-eyed child and a frustrated nurse. Usually, with some practice, the nurse can elicit a red reflex almost instantly while approaching the child and may also gain a momentary inspection of the blood vessels, macula, or optic disc.

Funduscopic Examination. Fig. 29-17 shows the structures of the back of the eyeball, or the fundus. The fundus is immediately apparent as the red reflex. The intensity of the color increases in darkly pigmented individuals.

! NURSING ALERT

A brilliant, uniform red reflex is an important sign because it rules out many serious defects of the cornea, aqueous chamber, lens, and vitreous chamber. Any dark shadows or opacities are recorded because they indicate some abnormality in any of these structures.

As the ophthalmoscope is brought closer to the eye, the most conspicuous feature of the fundus is the optic disc, the area where the blood vessels and optic nerve fibers enter and exit the eye. The disc is creamy pink and lighter in color than the surrounding fundus. Normally it is round or vertically oval.

After locating the optic disc, inspect the area for blood vessels. The central retinal artery and vein appear in the depths of the disc and emanate outward with visible branching. The veins are darker and about one-fourth larger than the arteries. Normally the branches of the arteries and veins cross each other.

Other structures that are common are the macula, the area of the fundus with the greatest concentration of visual receptors, and, in the center of the macula, a minute glistening spot of reflected light called the fovea centralis; this is the area of most perfect vision.

Vision Testing

Several tests are available for assessing vision. This discussion focuses on four areas: (1) ocular alignment, (2) visual acuity, (3) peripheral vision, and (4) color vision. Vision screening should be performed by age 3 years and annually after that or more often if there are concerns (American Academy of Pediatrics, 2003a; Wall, Marsh-Tootle, Evans, et al., 2002). Chapter 37 discusses behavioral and physical signs of visual impairment.

Ocular Alignment. Normally, by the age of 3 to 4 months, children are able to fixate on one visual field with both eyes simultaneously (binocularity). One of the most important tests for binocularity is alignment of the eyes to detect nonbinocular vision, or **strabismus** (Halle, 2002). In strabismus, or cross-eye, one eye deviates from the point of fixation. If the misalignment is constant, the weak eye becomes "lazy," and the brain eventually suppresses the image produced by that eye. If strabismus is not detected and corrected by age 4 to 6 years, blindness from disuse, known as **amblyopia,** may result.

Tests commonly used to detect misalignment are the corneal light reflex and the cover tests. To perform the corneal light reflex test, or Hirschberg test, shine a flashlight or the light of the ophthalmoscope directly into the patient's eyes from a distance of about 40.5 cm (16 inches). If the eyes are orthophoric, or normal, the light falls symmetrically within each pupil (Fig. 29-18, *A*). If the light falls off center in one eye, the eyes are misaligned. Epicanthal folds, excess folds of skin that extend from the roof of the nose to the inner termination of the eyebrow and that partially or completely overlap the inner canthus of the eye, may give a false impression of misalignment (pseudostrabismus) (Fig. 29-18, *B*). Epicanthal folds are often found in Asian children.

In the cover test, one eye is covered and the movement of the *uncovered* eye is observed while the child looks at a near (33 cm [13 inches]) or distant (6 m [20 feet]) object. If the uncovered eye does not move, it is aligned. If the uncovered eye moves, a misalignment is present because, when the stronger eye is temporarily covered, the misaligned eye attempts to fixate on the object.

In the alternate cover test, occlusion shifts back and forth from one eye to the other and movement of the eye that was *covered* is observed as soon as the occluder is removed while the child focuses on a point in front of him or her (Fig. 29-19). If normal alignment is present, shifting the cover from one eye to the other will not cause the eye to move. If misalignment is present, eye movement will occur when the cover is moved. This test takes more practice than the other cover test because the occluder must be moved back and forth quickly and accurately to see the eye move. Because deviations can occur at different ranges, it is important to perform the cover tests at both close and far distances.

! NURSING ALERT

The cover test is usually easier to perform if the examiner uses his or her hand rather than a card-type occluder (see Fig. 29-19). Attractive occluders fashioned like an ice cream cone or happy-face lollipop cut from cardboard are also well received by young children.

Photoscreening is a technique used to screen for amblyopia, refractive disorders, and media opacities (American Academy of Pediatrics, 2003a). Using a camera, the nurse obtains images of the pupillary reflexes (reflections) and red reflexes (Bruckner test) (American Academy of Pediatrics, 2003a). Photoscreening offers an effective way to screen infants, preverbal children, and those with developmental delays who are difficult to screen.

Visual Acuity Testing in Children Beyond Infancy. The most common test for measuring **visual acuity** is the Snellen letter chart,

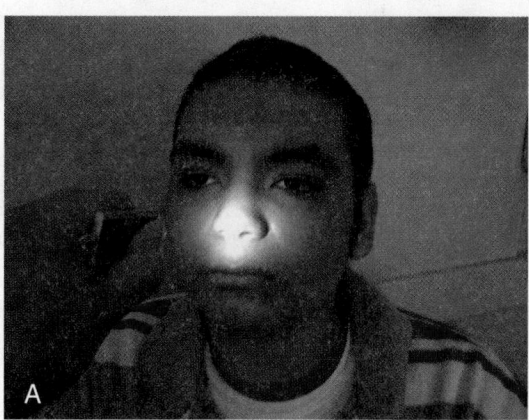
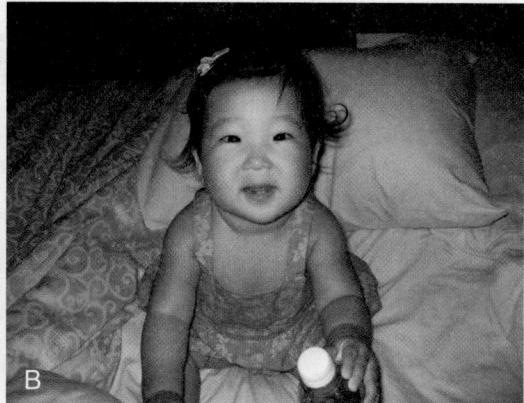

FIG 29-18 A, Corneal light reflex test demonstrating orthophoric eyes. **B,** Pseudostrabismus. Inner epicanthal folds cause eyes to appear misaligned; however, corneal light reflexes fall perfectly symmetrically.

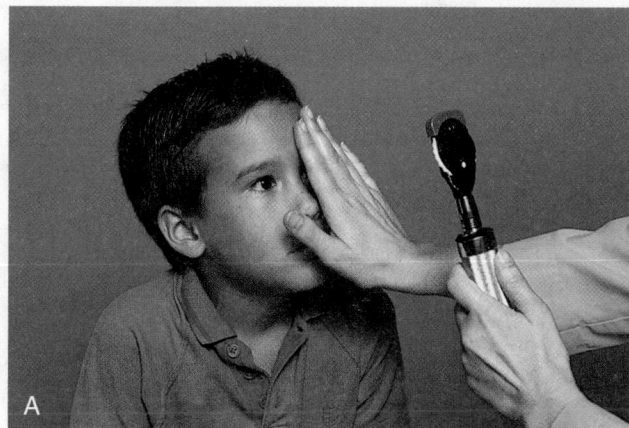
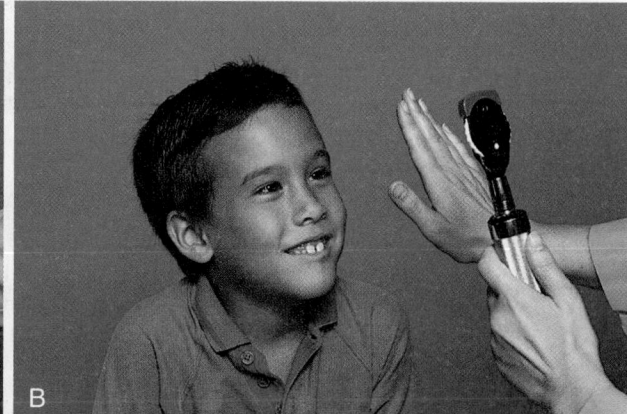

FIG 29-19 Alternate cover test to detect amblyopia in patient with strabismus. **A,** Eye is occluded, and child is fixating on light source. **B,** If eye does not move when uncovered, eyes are aligned.

which consists of lines of letters of decreasing size. The American Academy of Pediatrics (2003a) recommends that children stand 10 feet from the chart with their heels at the 10-foot line during testing. When screening for visual acuity in children, the nurse tests the child's right eye first by covering the left. Children who wear glasses should be screened with them on. Tell the child to keep both eyes open during the examination. If the child fails to read the current line, move up the chart to the next larger line. Continue up the chart until a line is found that the child can pass. Then begin moving down the chart again until the child fails to read the line. To pass each line, the child must correctly identify four of six symbols on the line. Repeat the procedure, covering the right eye. Table 29-9 provides a list of visual screening tests for children and guidelines for referral recommended by the American Academy of Pediatrics (2003a).

For children unable to read letters and numbers, the tumbling E or HOTV test is useful (Coats and Jenkins, 1997). The tumbling E test uses the capital letter E pointing in four different directions. The child is asked to point in the direction the E is facing. The HOTV test consists of a wall chart composed of the letters H, O, T, and V. The child is given a board containing a large H, O, T, and V. The examiner points to a letter on the wall chart, and the child matches the correct letter on the board held in his or her hand. The tumbling E and HOTV are excellent tests for preschool-age children.

Visual Acuity Testing in Infants and Difficult-to-Test Children. In newborns, vision is tested mainly by checking for light perception by shining a light into the eyes and noting responses such as pupillary constriction, blinking, following the light to midline, increased alertness, or refusal to open the eyes after exposure to the light. Although the simple maneuver of checking light perception and eliciting the pupillary light reflex indicates that the anterior half of the visual apparatus is intact, it does not confirm that the infant can see. In other words, this test does not assess whether the brain receives the visual message and interprets the signals.

Another test of visual acuity is the infant's ability to fix on and follow a target. Although any brightly colored or patterned object can be used, the human face is excellent. Hold the infant upright while moving your face slowly from side to side.

> **! NURSING ALERT**
>
> If visual fixation and following are not present by 3 to 4 months of age, further ophthalmologic evaluation is necessary.

Other signs that may indicate visual loss or other serious eye problems include fixed pupils, strabismus, constant nystagmus, the setting-sun sign, and slow lateral movements. Unfortunately, it is difficult to test each eye separately; the presence of such signs in one eye could indicate unilateral blindness.

TABLE 29-9   EYE EXAMINATION GUIDELINES*

FUNCTION	RECOMMENDED TESTS	REFERRAL CRITERIA	COMMENTS
Ages 3-5 Years			

Distance visual acuity	Snellen letters
	Snellen numbers
	Tumbling E
	HOTV
	Picture test:
	   Allen figures
	   LEA symbols
		1. <4 of 6 correct on 20-foot (6-m) line with either eye tested at 10 foot (3 m) monocularly (i.e., <10/20 or 20/40)
		or
		2. Two-line difference between eyes, even within passing range (i.e., 10/12.5 and 10/20 or 20/25 and 20/40)
			1. Tests are listed in decreasing order of cognitive difficulty; highest test that child is capable of performing should be used; in general, tumbling E or HOTV test should be used for children 3-5 yr of age and Snellen letters or numbers for children 6 yr and older.
			2. Testing distance of 10 feet (3 m) is recommended for all visual acuity tests.
			3. Line of figures is preferred over single figures.
			4. Nontested eye should be covered by occluder held by examiner or by adhesive occluder patch applied to eye; examiner must ensure that it is not possible to peek with nontested eye.

Ocular alignment	Cross cover test at 10 feet (3 m) Random dot E stereo test at 18 inches (40 cm) Simultaneous red reflex test (Bruckner test)	Any eye movement <4 of 6 correct Any asymmetry of pupil color, size, brightness	Child must be fixing on a target while cross cover test is performed. Use direct ophthalmoscope to view both red reflexes simultaneously in a darkened room from 2-3 feet (0.6 to 0.9 m) away; detects asymmetric refractive errors as well.
Ocular media clarity (cataracts, tumors, etc.)	Red reflex	White pupil, dark spots, absent reflex	Use direct ophthalmoscope in a darkened room. View eyes separately at 12-18 inches (30-45 cm); white reflex indicates possible retinoblastoma.
6 Years and Older			

Distance visual acuity	Snellen letters
	Snellen numbers
	Tumbling E
	HOTV
	Picture test:
	   Allen figures
	   LEA symbols
		1. <4 of 6 correct on 15-foot (4.5-m) line with either eye tested at 10 feet (3 m) monocularly (i.e., <10/15 or 20/30)
		or
		2. Two-line difference between eyes, even within the passing range (i.e., 10/10 and 10/15 or 20/20 and 20/30)
			1. Tests are listed in decreasing order of cognitive difficulty; highest test that child is capable of performing should be used; in general, tumbling E or HOTV test should be used for children 3-5 yr of age and Snellen letters or numbers for children 6 yr and older.
			2. Testing distance of 10 feet (3 m) is recommended for all visual acuity tests.
			3. Line of figures is preferred over single figures.
			4. Nontested eye should be covered by occluder held by examiner or by adhesive occluder patch applied to eye; examiner must ensure that it is not possible to peek with nontested eye.

Ocular alignment	Cross cover test at 10 feet (3 m) Random dot E stereo test at 18 inches (40 cm) Simultaneous red reflex test (Bruckner test)	Any eye movement <4 of 6 correct Any asymmetry of pupil color, size, brightness	Child must be fixing on target while cross cover test is performed. Use direct ophthalmoscope to view both red reflexes simultaneously in a darkened room from 2-3 feet (0.6 to 0.9 m) away; detects asymmetric refractive errors as well.
Ocular media clarity (cataracts, tumors, etc.)	Red reflex	White pupil, dark spots, absent reflex	Use direct ophthalmoscope in a darkened room. View eyes separately at 12-18 inches (30-45 cm); white reflex indicates possible retinoblastoma.

From American Academy of Pediatrics, Committee on Practice and Ambulatory Medicine, Section on Ophthalmology: Eye examination in infants, children, and young adults by pediatricians, *Pediatrics* 111(4):902–907, 2003.
*Assessing visual acuity (vision screening) is one of the most sensitive techniques for detection of eye abnormalities in children. The American Academy of Pediatrics Section on Ophthalmology, in cooperation with American Association for Pediatric Ophthalmology and Strabismus and American Academy of Ophthalmology, has developed these guidelines to be used by physicians, nurses, educational institutions, public health departments, and other professionals who perform vision evaluation services.

Special tests are available for testing infants and other difficult-to-test children to assess acuity or confirm blindness. For example, in visually evoked potentials, the eyes are stimulated with a bright light or pattern and electrical activity to the visual cortex is recorded through scalp electrodes. Acuity is assessed by using progressively smaller patterns.

Peripheral Vision. In children who are old enough to cooperate, estimate peripheral vision, or the visual field of each eye, by having the children fixate on a specific point directly in front of them while an object, such as a finger or a pencil, is moved from beyond the field of vision into the range of peripheral vision. As soon as children see the object, have them say "stop." At that point, measure the angle from the anteroposterior axis of the eye (straight line of vision) to the peripheral axis (point at which the object is first seen). Check each eye separately and for each quadrant of vision. Normally children see about 50 degrees upward, 70 degrees downward, 60 degrees

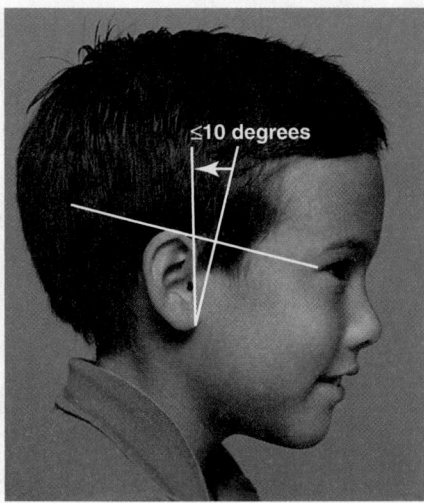

FIG 29-20 Ear alignment.

nasalward, and 90 degrees temporally. Limitations in peripheral vision may indicate blindness from damage to structures within the eye or to any of the visual pathways.

Color Vision. The tests available for color vision include the Ishihara test and the Hardy-Rand-Rittler test. Each consists of a series of cards (pseudoisochromatic) that contain a color field composed of spots of a certain "confusion" color. Against the field is a number or symbol similarly printed in dots but of a color likely to be confused with the field color by the person with a color vision deficit. As a result, the figure or letter is invisible to an affected individual but is clearly seen by a person with normal vision.

Ears

Inspection of External Structures

The entire external earlobe is called the pinna, or auricle; one is located on each side of the head. Measure the height alignment of the pinna by drawing an imaginary line from the outer orbit of the eye to the occiput, or most prominent protuberance of the skull. The top of the pinna should meet or cross this line. Low-set ears are commonly associated with renal anomalies or cognitive impairment. Measure the angle of the pinna by drawing a perpendicular line from the imaginary horizontal line and aligning the pinna next to this mark. Normally the pinna lies within a 10-degree angle of the vertical line (Fig. 29-20). If it falls outside this area, record the deviation and look for other anomalies.

Normally the pinna extends slightly outward from the skull. Except in newborn infants, ears that are flat against the head or protruding away from the scalp may indicate problems. Flattened ears in an infant may suggest a frequent side-lying position and, just as with isolated areas of hair loss, may be a clue to investigate parents' understanding of the child's stimulation needs.

Inspect the skin surface around the ear for small openings, extra tags of skin, or sinuses. If a sinus is found, note this because it may represent a fistula that drains into some area of the neck or ear. Cutaneous tags represent no pathologic process but may cause parents concern in terms of the child's appearance.

Also assess the ear for hygiene. An otoscope is not necessary for looking into the external canal to note the presence of cerumen, a waxy substance produced by the ceruminous glands in the outer portion of the canal. Cerumen is usually yellow-brown and soft. If an otoscope is used and any discharge is visible, note its color and odor. Avoid transmitting potentially infectious material to the other

ear or to another child through handwashing and using disposable specula or sterilizing reusable specula between each examination.

Inspection of Internal Structures

The head of the otoscope permits visualization of the tympanic membrane by use of a bright light, a magnifying glass, and a speculum. Some otoscopes have an attachment for a pneumonic device to insert air into the canal to determine membrane compliance (movement). The speculum, which is inserted into the external canal, comes in a variety of sizes to accommodate different canal widths. The largest speculum that fits comfortably into the ear is used to achieve the greatest area of visualization. The lens, or magnifying glass, is movable, allowing the examiner to insert an object, such as a curette, into the ear canal through the speculum while still viewing the structures through the lens.

Positioning the Child. Before beginning the otoscopic examination, position the child properly and gently restrain (have the child sit on parent's lap and hold parent's hands) if necessary. Older children usually cooperate and do not need restraint. However, prepare them for the procedure by allowing them to play with the instrument, demonstrating how it works, and stressing the importance of remaining still. A helpful suggestion is to let them observe you examining the parent's ear. Restraint is needed for younger children because the ear examination upsets them (see Atraumatic Care box).

As you insert the speculum into the meatus, move it around the outer rim to accustom the child to the feel of something entering the ear. If examining a painful ear, touch a nonpainful part of the affected ear, then examine the unaffected ear, and finally return to the painful ear. By this time the child is usually less fearful of anything causing discomfort to the ear and will cooperate more.

For their protection and safety, restrain infants and toddlers for the otoscopic examination. There are two general positions of restraint. In one, the child is seated sideways in the parent's lap with one arm hugging the parent and the other arm at the side. The ear to be examined is toward the nurse. With one arm the parent holds the child's head firmly against his or her chest and with the other arm hugs the child, thereby securing the child's free arm (Fig. 29-21, *A*). Examine the ear using the same procedure for holding the otoscope as described later.

The other position involves placing the child on the side, back, or abdomen with the arms at the side and the head turned so that the ear to be examined points toward the ceiling. Lean over the child, use the upper part of the body to restrain the arms and upper trunk movements, and use the examining hand to stabilize the head. This position is practical for young infants or for older children who need minimum restraint, but it may not be feasible for other children who protest vigorously. For safety, enlist the parent's or an assistant's help in immobilizing the head by firmly placing one hand above the ear and the other on the child's side, abdomen, or back (Fig. 29-21, *B*).

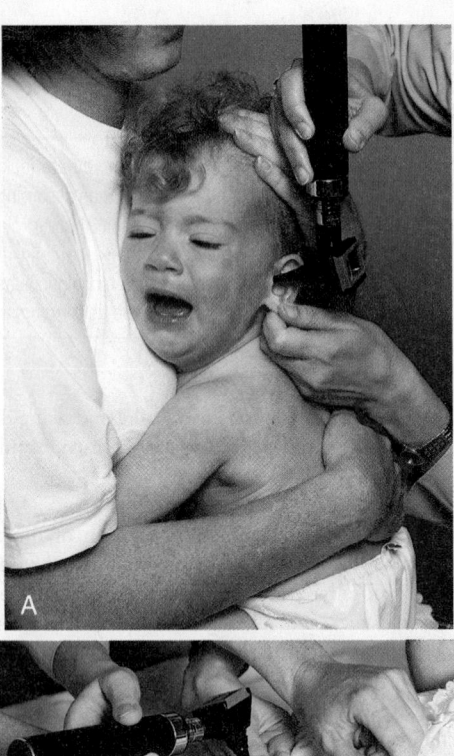

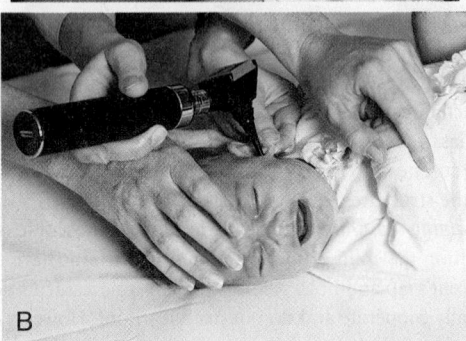

FIG 29-21 Position for restraining child **(A)** and infant **(B)** during otoscopic examination.

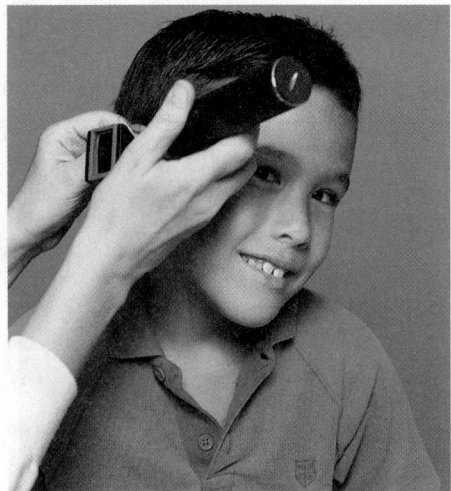

FIG 29-22 Positioning head by tilting it toward opposite shoulder for full view of tympanic membrane.

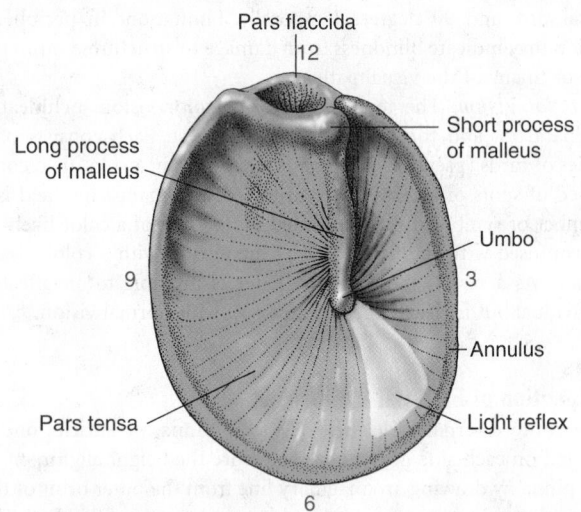

FIG 29-23 Landmarks of tympanic membrane. (From Rothrock JC: *Alexander's care of the patient in surgery,* ed 15, St Louis, 2015, Mosby.)

With cooperative children, examine the ear with the child in a side-lying, sitting, or standing position. One disadvantage to standing is that the child may "walk away" as the otoscope enters the canal. If the child is standing or sitting, tilt the head slightly toward the child's opposite shoulder to achieve a better view of the drum (Fig. 29-22).

With the thumb and forefinger of the free (usually nondominant) hand, grasp the auricle. For the two positions of restraint, hold the otoscope upside down at the junction of its head and handle with the thumb and index finger. Place the other fingers against the skull to allow the otoscope to move with the child in case of sudden movement. In examining a cooperative child, hold the handle with the otic head upright or upside down. Use the dominant hand to examine both ears or reverse hands for each ear, whichever is more comfortable.

Before using the otoscope, visualize the external ear and the tympanic membrane as being superimposed on a clock (Fig. 29-23). The numbers are important geographic landmarks. Introduce the speculum into the meatus between the 3 and 9 o'clock positions in a *downward* and *forward* position. Because the canal is curved, the speculum does not permit a panoramic view of the tympanic membrane unless the canal is straightened. In infants, the canal curves upward. Therefore pull the pinna *down* and *back* to the 6 to 9 o'clock range to straighten the canal (Fig. 29-24, *A*). With older children, usually those older than 3 years, the canal curves downward and forward. Therefore pull the pinna *up* and *back* toward a 10 o'clock

position (Fig. 29-24, *B*). If you have difficulty visualizing the membrane, try repositioning the head, introducing the speculum at a different angle, and pulling the pinna in a slightly different direction. Do not insert the speculum past the cartilaginous (outermost) portion of the canal, usually a distance of 0.60 to 1.25 cm (0.23 to 0.5 inch) in older children. Insertion of the speculum into the posterior or bony portion of the canal causes pain.

In neonates and young infants, the walls of the canal are pliable and floppy because of the underdeveloped cartilaginous and bony structures. Therefore the very small 2-mm speculum usually needs to be inserted deeper into the canal than in older children. Exercise great care not to damage the walls or drum. For this reason, only an experienced examiner should insert an otoscope into the ears of very young infants.

Otoscopic Examination. As you introduce the speculum into the external canal, inspect the walls of the canal, the color of the tympanic membrane, the light reflex, and the usual landmarks of the bony prominences of the middle ear. The walls of the external auditory canal are pink, although they are more pigmented in dark-skinned children. Minute hairs are evident in the outermost portion,

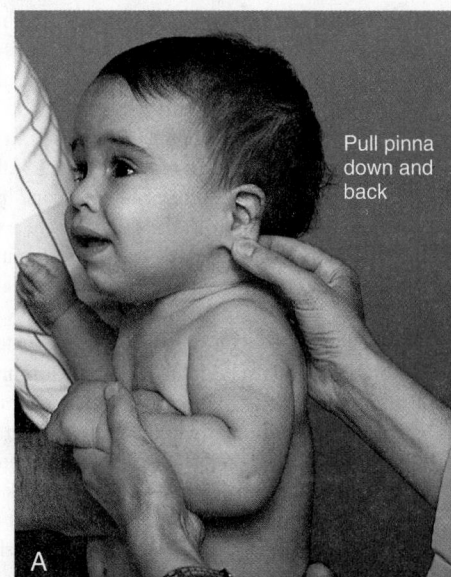
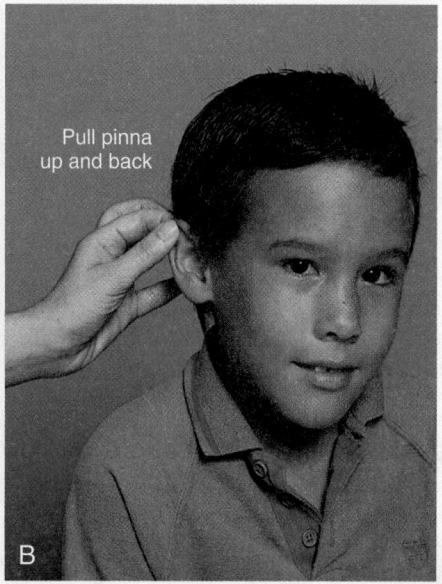

Pull pinna down and back

Pull pinna up and back

A

B

FIG 29-24 Positioning for visualizing eardrum in infant **(A)** and in child older than 3 years **(B)**.

	AUDITORY TEST AND		
AGE	**AVERAGE TIME**	**TYPE OF MEASUREMENT**	**PROCEDURE**
All ages	Evoked otoacoustic emissions, 10-min test	Physiologic test specifically measuring cochlear (outer hair cell) response to presentation of stimulus	Small probe containing sensitive microphone is placed in ear canal for stimulus delivery and response detection.
Birth-9 months	Auditory brainstem response, 15-min test	Electrophysiologic measurement of activity in auditory nerve and brainstem pathways	Placement of electrodes on child's head detects auditory stimuli presented through earphones one ear at a time.
9 months-2½ yr	Conditioned oriented responses or visual reinforced audiometry, 30-min test	Behavioral tests measuring child's responses to speech and frequency-specific stimuli presented through speakers	Both techniques condition child to associate speech or frequency-specific sound with reinforcement stimulus, such as lighted toy.

TABLE 29-10 AUDITORY TESTS FOR INFANTS AND CHILDREN

Adapted with permission from Bachmann KR, Arvedson JC: Early identification and intervention for children who are hearing impaired, *Pediatr Rev* 19:155–165, 1998.

where cerumen is produced. Note signs of irritation, foreign bodies, or infection.

Foreign bodies in the ear are not uncommon in children and range from erasers to beans. Symptoms may include pain, discharge, and affected hearing. Remove soft objects, such as paper or insects, with forceps. Remove small, hard objects, such as pebbles, with a suction tip, a hook, or irrigation. However, irrigation is contraindicated if the object is vegetative matter, such as beans or pasta, which swells when in contact with fluid.

> **! NURSING ALERT**
>
> If there is any doubt about the type of object in the ear and the appropriate method to remove it, refer the child to the appropriate practitioner.

The tympanic membrane is a translucent, light pearly pink or gray. Note marked erythema (which may indicate suppurative otitis media); a dull, nontransparent grayish color (sometimes suggestive of serous otitis media); or ashen gray areas (signs of scarring from a previous perforation). A black area usually suggests a perforation of the membrane that has not healed.

The characteristic tenseness and slope of the tympanic membrane cause the light of the otoscope to reflect at about the 5 or 7

o'clock position. The light reflex is a fairly well-defined, cone-shaped reflection, which normally points away from the face.

The bony landmarks of the drum are formed by the umbo, or tip of the malleus. It appears as a small, round, opaque, concave spot near the center of the drum. The manubrium (long process or handle) of the malleus appears to be a whitish line extending from the umbo upward to the margin of the membrane. At the upper end of the long process near the 1 o'clock position (in the right ear) is a sharp, knoblike protuberance, representing the short process of the malleus. Note the absence of the light reflex or loss or abnormal prominence of any of these landmarks.

Auditory Testing

Several types of hearing tests are available and recommended for screening in infants and children (American Academy of Pediatrics, 2003b) (Table 29-10). Universal newborn hearing screening is available in almost every state in the United States. The nurse must operate under a high index of suspicion for those children who may have conditions associated with hearing loss, whose parents are concerned about hearing loss, and who may have developed behaviors that indicate auditory impairment (Cunningham and Cox, 2003). Chapter 37 discusses types of hearing loss, causes, clinical manifestations, and appropriate treatment.

Nose

Inspection of External Structures

The nose is located in the middle of the face just below the eyes and above the lips. Compare its placement and alignment by drawing an imaginary vertical line from the center point between the eyes down to the notch of the upper lip. The nose should lie exactly vertical to this line, with each side exactly symmetric. Note its location, any deviation to one side, and asymmetry in overall size and in diameter of the nares (nostrils). The bridge of the nose is sometimes flat in Asian and African-American children. Observe the alae nasi for any sign of flaring, which indicates respiratory difficulty. Always report any flaring of the alae nasi. Fig. 29-25 illustrates the landmarks used in describing the external structures of the nose.

Inspection of Internal Structures

Inspect the anterior vestibule of the nose by pushing the tip upward, tilting the head backward, and illuminating the cavity with a flashlight or otoscope without the attached ear speculum. Note the color of the mucosal lining, which is normally redder than the oral membranes, as well as any swelling, discharge, dryness, or bleeding. There should be no discharge from the nose.

On looking deeper into the nose, inspect the turbinates, or concha, plates of bone that jut into the nasal cavity and are enveloped by mucous membrane. The turbinates greatly increase the surface area of the nasal cavity as air is inhaled. The spaces or channels between the turbinates are called the meatus and correspond to each of the three turbinates. Normally the front end of the inferior and middle turbinate and the middle meatus are seen. They should be the same color as the lining of the vestibule.

Inspect the septum, which should divide the vestibules equally. Note any deviation, especially if it causes an occlusion of one side of the nose. A perforation may be evident within the septum. If this is suspected, shine the light of the otoscope into one naris and look for admittance of light to the other. Because olfaction is an important function of the nose, testing for smell may be done at this point or as part of cranial nerve assessment (see Table 29-13).

Mouth and Throat

With a cooperative child, the nurse can accomplish almost the entire examination of the mouth and throat without the use of a tongue blade. Ask the child to open the mouth wide; to move the tongue in different directions for full visualization; and to say "ahh," which depresses the tongue for full view of the back of the mouth (tonsils, uvula, and oropharynx). For a closer look at the buccal mucosa, or lining of the cheeks, ask children to use their fingers to move the outer lip and cheek to one side (see Atraumatic Care box).

Infants and toddlers usually resist attempts to keep the mouth open. Because inspecting the mouth is upsetting, leave it for the end of the physical examination (along with examination of the ears) or do it during episodes of crying. However, the use of a tongue blade (preferably flavored) to depress the tongue may be needed. Place the tongue blade along the *side* of the tongue, not in the center back area where the gag reflex is elicited. Fig. 29-26, *B*, illustrates proper positioning of the child for the oral examination.

The major structure of the exterior of the mouth is the lips. The lips should be moist, soft, smooth, and pink, or a deeper hue than

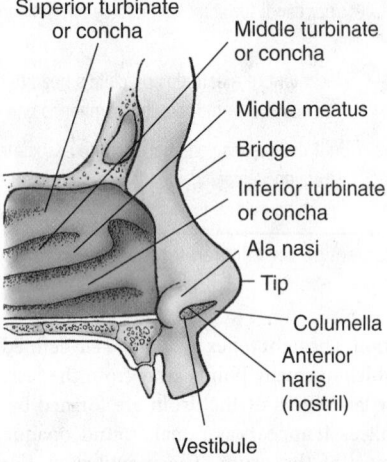

Superior turbinate
or concha

Middle turbinate
or concha

Middle meatus

Bridge

Inferior turbinate
or concha

Ala nasi

Tip

Columella

Anterior
naris
(nostril)

Vestibule

FIG 29-25 External landmarks and internal structures of nose.

ATRAUMATIC CARE

Encouraging Opening the Mouth for Examination

- Perform the examination in front of a mirror.
- Let child first examine someone else's mouth, such as the parent, the nurse, or a puppet (Fig. 29-26, *A*), and then examine child's mouth.
- Instruct child to tilt the head back slightly, breathe deeply through the mouth, and hold the breath; this action lowers the tongue to the floor of the mouth without the use of a tongue blade.
- Lightly brushing the palate with a cotton swab also may open the mouth for assessment.

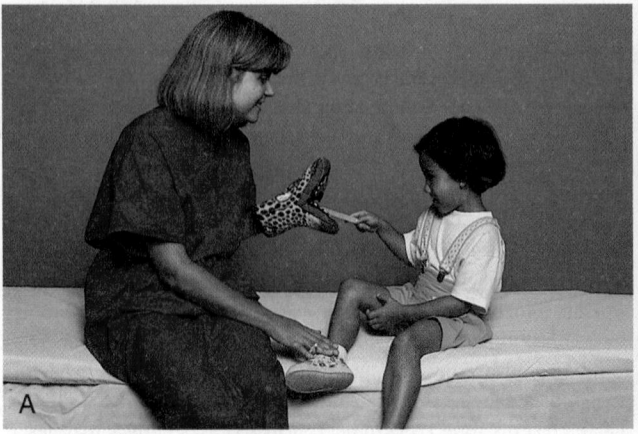

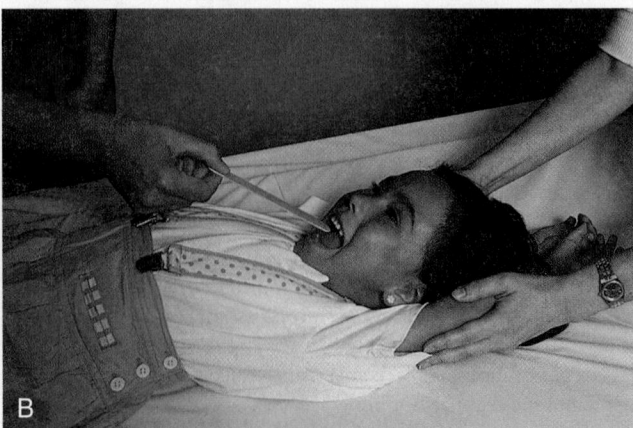

FIG 29-26 A, Encouraging child to cooperate. **B,** Positioning child for examination of mouth.

the surrounding skin. The lips should be symmetric when relaxed or tensed. Assess symmetry when the child talks or cries.

Inspection of Internal Structures

The major structures that are visible within the oral cavity and oropharynx are the mucosal lining of the lips and cheeks, gums (or gingiva), teeth, tongue, palate, uvula, tonsils, and posterior oropharynx (Fig. 29-27). Inspect all areas lined with mucous membranes (inside the lips and cheeks, gingiva, underside of the tongue, palate, and back of the pharynx) for color, any areas of white patches or ulceration, bleeding, sensitivity, and moisture. The membranes should be bright pink, smooth, glistening, uniform, and moist.

Inspect the teeth for number in each dental arch, for hygiene, and for occlusion or bite (see also Teething, Chapter 31). Discoloration of tooth enamel with obvious plaque (whitish coating on the surface of the teeth) is a sign of poor dental hygiene and indicates a need for counseling. Brown spots in the crevices of the crown of the tooth or between the teeth may be caries (cavities). Chalky white to yellow or brown areas on the enamel may indicate fluorosis (excessive fluoride ingestion). Teeth that appear greenish black may be stained temporarily from ingestion of supplemental iron.

Examine the gums (gingiva) surrounding the teeth. The color is normally coral pink, and the surface texture is stippled, similar to the appearance of an orange peel. In dark-skinned children, the gums are more deeply colored and a brownish area is often observed along the gum line.

Inspect the tongue for papillae—small projections that contain several taste buds and give the tongue its characteristic rough appearance. Note the size and mobility of the tongue. Normally the tip of the tongue should extend to the lips or beyond.

The roof of the mouth consists of the hard palate, which is located near the front of the oral cavity, and the soft palate, which is located toward the back of the pharynx and has a small midline protrusion called the uvula. Carefully inspect the palates to ensure they are intact. The arch of the palate should be dome shaped. A narrow, flat roof or a high, arched palate affects the placement of the tongue and can cause feeding and speech problems. Test movement of the uvula by eliciting a gag reflex. It should move upward to close off the nasopharynx from the oropharynx.

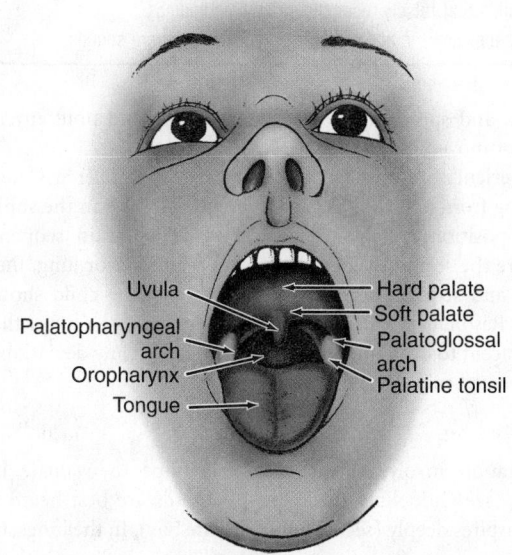

FIG 29-27 Interior structures of mouth.

Examine the oropharynx and note the size and color of the palatine tonsils. They are normally the same color as the surrounding mucosa; glandular, rather than smooth in appearance; and barely visible over the edge of the palatoglossal arches. The size of the tonsils varies considerably during childhood. However, report any swelling, redness, or white areas on the tonsils.

Chest

Inspect the chest for size, shape, symmetry, movement, breast development, and the bony landmarks formed by the ribs and sternum. The rib cage consists of 12 ribs on each side and the sternum, or breast bone, located in the midline of the trunk (Fig. 29-28). The sternum is composed of three main parts. The manubrium, the uppermost portion, can be felt at the base of the neck at the suprasternal notch. The largest segment of the sternum is the body, which forms the sternal angle (angle of Louis) as it articulates with the manubrium. At the end of the body is a small, movable process called the xiphoid. The angle of the costal margin as it attaches to the sternum is called the costal angle and is normally about 45 to 50 degrees. These bony structures are important landmarks in the location of ribs and intercostal spaces (ICSs), which are the spaces between the ribs. They are numbered according to the rib directly *above* the space. For example, the space immediately below the second rib is the second ICS.

The thoracic cavity is also divided into segments by drawing imaginary lines on the chest and back. Fig. 29-29 illustrates the anterior, lateral, and posterior divisions.

Measure the size of the chest by placing the measuring tape around the rib cage at the nipple line (see Fig. 29-9). For greatest accuracy, take two measurements—one during inspiration and the other during expiration—and record the average. Chest size is important mainly in relation to head circumference (see p. 795). Always report marked disproportions because most are caused by abnormal head growth; however, some may be a result of altered chest shape, such as barrel chest (chest is round) or pigeon chest (sternum protrudes outward).

During infancy, the chest's shape is almost circular, with the anteroposterior (front-to-back) diameter equaling the transverse, or lateral (side-to-side), diameter. As the child grows, the chest normally increases in the transverse direction, causing the anteroposterior diameter to be less than the lateral diameter. Note the angle made by the lower costal margin and the sternum, and palpate the junction of the ribs with the costal cartilage (costochondral junction) and sternum, which should be fairly smooth.

Movement of the chest wall should be symmetric bilaterally and coordinated with breathing. During inspiration the chest rises and expands, the diaphragm descends, and the costal angle increases. During expiration the chest falls and decreases in size, the diaphragm rises, and the costal angle narrows (Fig. 29-30). In children younger than 6 or 7 years, respiratory movement is principally abdominal or diaphragmatic. In older children, particularly girls, respirations are chiefly thoracic. In either case, the chest and abdomen should rise and fall together. Always report any asymmetry of movement.

While inspecting the skin surface of the chest, observe the position of the nipples and any evidence of breast development. Normally the nipples are located slightly lateral to the midclavicular line between the fourth and fifth ribs. Note symmetry of nipple placement and normal configuration of a darker-pigmented areola surrounding a flat nipple in the prepubertal child.

Pubertal breast development usually begins in girls between 10 and 14 years of age (see Chapter 35). Record early (precocious) or

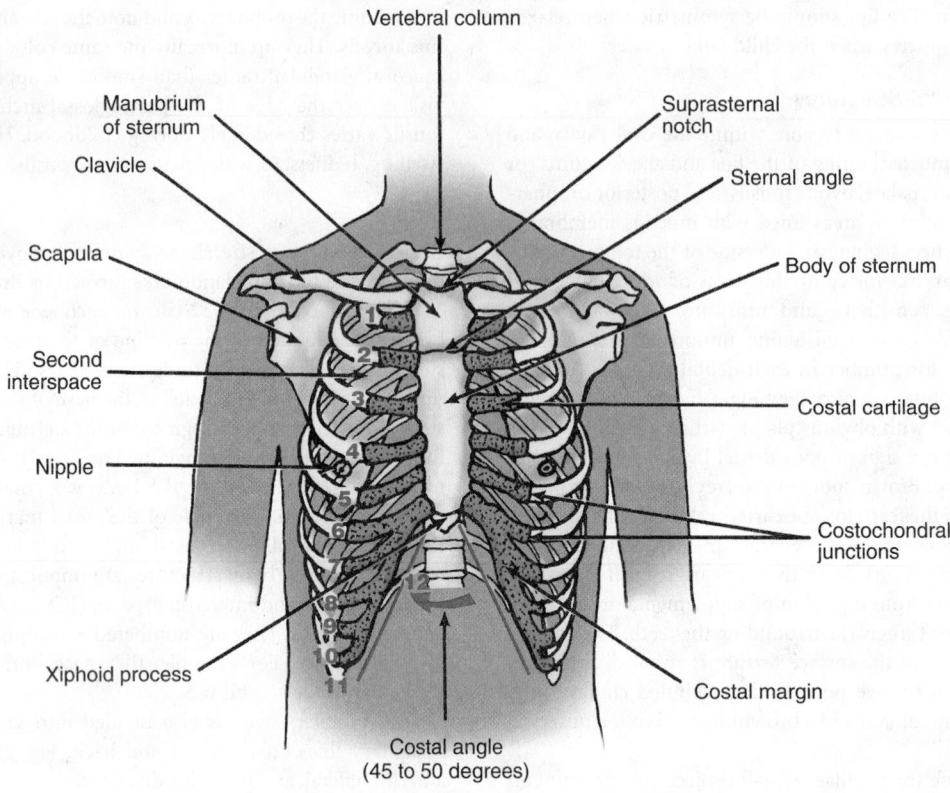

FIG 29-28 Rib cage.

delayed breast development, as well as evidence of any other second-ary sexual characteristics. In males, breast enlargement (gyneco-mastia) may be caused by hormonal or systemic disorders, but more commonly it is a result of adipose tissue from obesity or a transitory body change during early puberty. In either situation, investigate the child's feelings regarding breast enlargement.

In adolescent girls who have achieved sexual maturity, palpate the breasts for evidence of any masses or hard nodules. Use this opportunity to discuss the importance of routine breast self-examination. To decrease any fear or concern that results when a mass is felt, emphasize that most palpable masses are benign.

Lungs

The lungs are situated inside the thoracic cavity, with one lung on each side of the sternum. Each lung is divided into an apex, which is slightly pointed and rises above the first rib; a base, which is wide and concave and rides on the dome-shaped diaphragm; and a body, which is divided into lobes. The right lung has three lobes—the upper, middle, and lower. The left lung has only two lobes—the upper and lower—because of the space occupied by the heart (Fig. 29-31).

Inspection of the lungs primarily involves observation of respiratory movements. Evaluate respirations for (1) rate (number per minute), (2) rhythm (regular, irregular, or periodic), (3) depth (deep or shallow), and (4) quality (effortless, automatic, difficult, or labored). Note the character of breath sounds, such as noisy, grunting, snoring, or heavy.

Evaluate respiratory movements by placing each hand flat against the back or chest with the thumbs in midline along the lower costal margin of the lungs. The child should be sitting during this procedure and, if cooperative, should take several deep breaths. During respiration your hands will move with the chest wall. Assess the

---

📋 GUIDELINES

Effective Auscultation

- Make certain child is relaxed and not crying, talking, or laughing. Record if child is crying.
- Check that room is comfortable and quiet.
- Warm stethoscope before placing it against skin.
- Apply firm pressure on chest piece but not enough to prevent vibrations and transmission of sound.
- Avoid placing stethoscope over hair or clothing, moving it against skin, breathing on tubing, or sliding fingers over chest piece, which may cause sounds that falsely resemble pathologic findings.
- Use a symmetric and orderly approach to compare sounds.

---

amount and speed of respiratory excursion, and note any asymmetry of movement.

Experienced examiners may percuss the lungs. Percuss the anterior lung from apex to base, usually with the child in the supine or sitting position. Percuss each side of the chest in sequence to compare the sounds. When percussing the posterior lung, the procedure and sequence are the same, although the child should be sitting. Resonance is heard over all the lobes of the lungs that are not adjacent to other organs. Record and report any deviation from the expected sound.

Auscultation

Auscultation involves using the stethoscope to evaluate breath sounds (see Guidelines box). Breath sounds are best heard if the child inspires deeply (see Atraumatic Care box). In the lungs, breath sounds are classified as *vesicular, bronchovesicular,* or *bronchial* (Box 29-13).

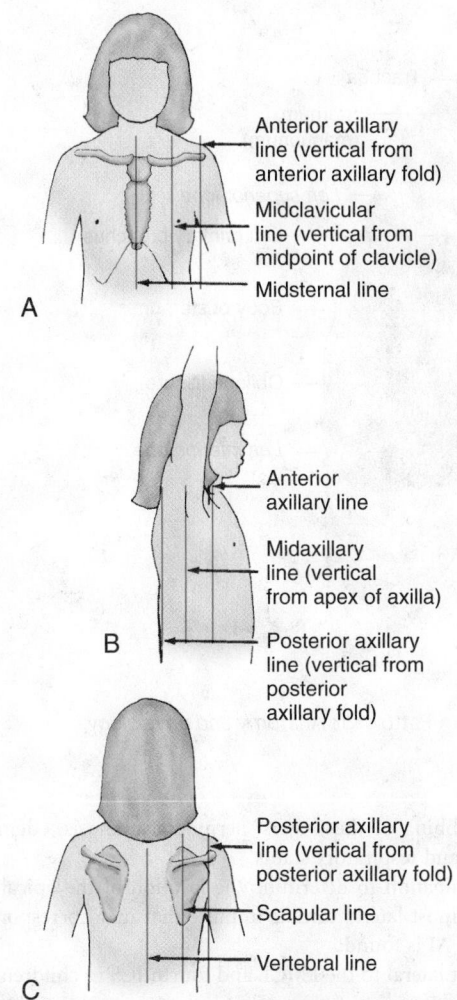

FIG 29-29 Imaginary landmarks of chest. **A,** Anterior. **B,** Right lateral. **C,** Posterior.

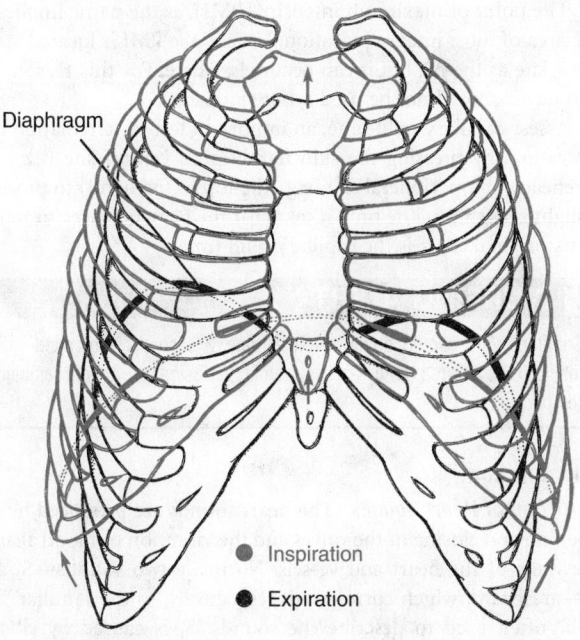

FIG 29-30 Movement of chest during respiration.

ATRAUMATIC CARE

Encouraging Deep Breaths

- Ask child to "blow out" the light on an otoscope or pocket flashlight; discreetly turn off the light on the last try so that the child feels successful.
- Place a cotton ball in child's palm; ask child to blow the ball into the air and have parent catch it.
- Place a small tissue on the top of a pencil and ask child to blow the tissue off.
- Have child blow a pinwheel, a party horn, or bubbles.

BOX 29-13 CLASSIFICATION OF NORMAL BREATH SOUNDS

Vesicular Breath Sounds
- Heard over entire surface of lungs, with exception of upper intrascapular area and area beneath manubrium.
- Inspiration is louder, longer, and higher pitched than expiration.
- Sound is soft, swishing noise.

Bronchovesicular Breath Sounds
- Heard over manubrium and in upper intrascapular regions where trachea and bronchi bifurcate.
- Inspiration is louder and higher pitched than in vesicular breathing.

Bronchial Breath Sounds
- Heard only over trachea near suprasternal notch.
- Inspiratory phase is short, and expiratory phase is long.

Absent or diminished breath sounds are always an abnormal finding warranting investigation. Fluid, air, or solid masses in the pleural space all interfere with the conduction of breath sounds. Diminished breath sounds in certain segments of the lung can alert the nurse to pulmonary areas that may benefit from chest physiotherapy. Increased breath sounds after pulmonary therapy indicate improved passage of air through the respiratory tract. Box 29-14 lists terms used to describe various respiration patterns.

Various pulmonary abnormalities produce adventitious sounds that are not normally heard over the chest. These sounds occur in addition to normal or abnormal breath sounds. They are classified into two main groups: crackles, which result from the passage of air through fluid or moisture; and wheezes, which are produced as air passes through narrowed passageways, regardless of the cause, such as exudate, inflammation, spasm, or tumor. Considerable practice with an experienced tutor is necessary to differentiate the various types of lung sounds. Often it is best to describe the type of sound heard in the lungs rather than trying to label it. Always report any abnormal sounds for further medical evaluation.

Heart

The heart is situated in the thoracic cavity between the lungs in the mediastinum and above the diaphragm (Fig. 29-32). About two thirds of the heart lies within the left side of the rib cage, with the other third on the right side as it crosses the sternum. The heart is positioned in the thorax like a trapezoid:

- **Vertically** along the right sternal border (RSB) from the second to the fifth rib
- **Horizontally** (long side) from the lower right sternum to the fifth rib at the left midclavicular line (LMCL)

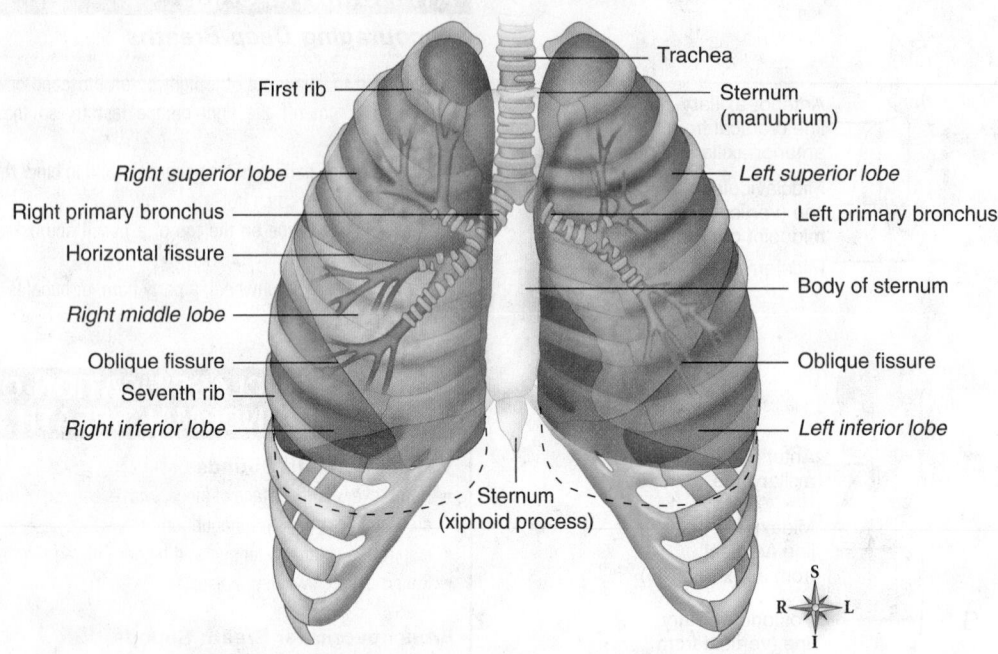

FIG 29-31 Location of lobes of lungs within thoracic cavity. (From Patton KT: *Anatomy and physiology*, ed 8, St Louis, 2013, Mosby.)

BOX 29-14 **VARIOUS PATTERNS OF RESPIRATION**

Tachypnea—Increased rate

Bradypnea—Decreased rate

Dyspnea—Distress during breathing

Apnea—Cessation of breathing

Hyperpnea—Increased depth

Hypoventilation—Decreased depth (shallow) and irregular rhythm

Hyperventilation—Increased rate and depth

Kussmaul respiration—Hyperventilation, gasping and labored respiration; usually seen in diabetic coma or other states of respiratory acidosis

Cheyne-Stokes respiration—Gradually increasing rate and depth with periods of apnea

Biot respiration—Periods of hyperpnea alternating with apnea (similar to Cheyne-Stokes except that depth remains constant)

Seesaw (paradoxic) respirations—Chest falls on inspiration and rises on expiration

Agonal—Last gasping breaths before death

- **Diagonally** from the left sternal border (LSB) at the second rib to the LMCL at the fifth rib
- **Horizontally** (short side) from the RSB and LSB at the second ICS—base of the heart

Inspection is easiest when the child is sitting in a semi-Fowler position. Look at the anterior chest wall from an angle, comparing both sides of the rib cage with each other. Normally they should be symmetric. In children with thin chest walls, a pulsation may be visible. Because comprehensive evaluation of cardiac function is not limited to the heart, also consider other findings such as the presence of all pulses (especially the femoral pulses) (Fig. 29-33), distended neck veins, clubbing of the fingers, peripheral cyanosis, edema, blood pressure, and respiratory status.

Use palpation to determine the location of the apical impulse (AI), the most lateral cardiac impulse that may correspond to the apex. The AI is found:

- Just lateral to the LMCL and fourth ICS in children younger than 7 years
- At the LMCL and fifth ICS in children older than 7 years

Although the AI gives a general idea of the size of the heart (with enlargement, the apex is lower and more lateral), its normal location is variable, making it an unreliable indicator of heart size.

The point of maximum intensity (PMI), as the name implies, is the area of most intense pulsation. Usually the PMI is located at the same site as the AI, but it can occur elsewhere. For this reason, the two terms should not be used synonymously.

Assess capillary refill time, an important test for circulation and hydration, by pressing the skin lightly on a central site (e.g., the forehead) or a peripheral site (e.g., the top of the hand) to produce a slight blanching. The time it takes for the blanched area to return to its original color is the capillary refill time.

> **! NURSING ALERT**
>
> Capillary refill should be brisk—less than 2 seconds. Prolonged refill may be associated with poor systemic perfusion or a cool ambient temperature.

Auscultation

Origin of Heart Sounds. The heart sounds are produced by the opening and closing of the valves and the vibration of blood against the walls of the heart and vessels. Normally two sounds—S_1 and S_2—are heard, which correspond, respectively, to the familiar "lub dub" often used to describe the sounds. S_1 is caused by closure of the tricuspid and mitral valves (sometimes called the

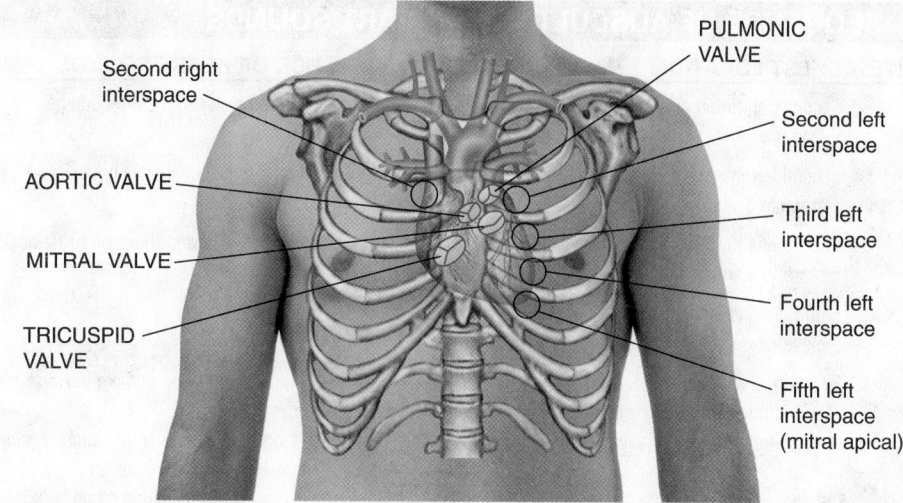

FIG 29-32 Position of heart within thorax. (From Seidel HM, Dains JE, Ball JW, et al: *Mosby's guide to physical examination*, ed 7, St Louis, 2011, Mosby.)

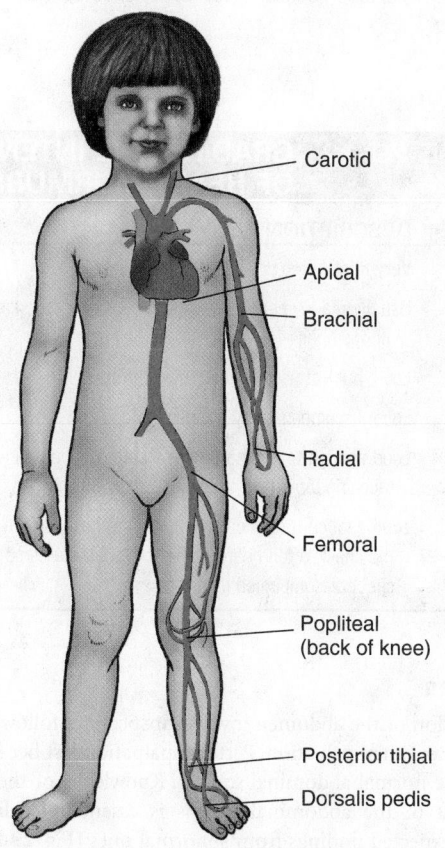

FIG 29-33 Location of pulses.

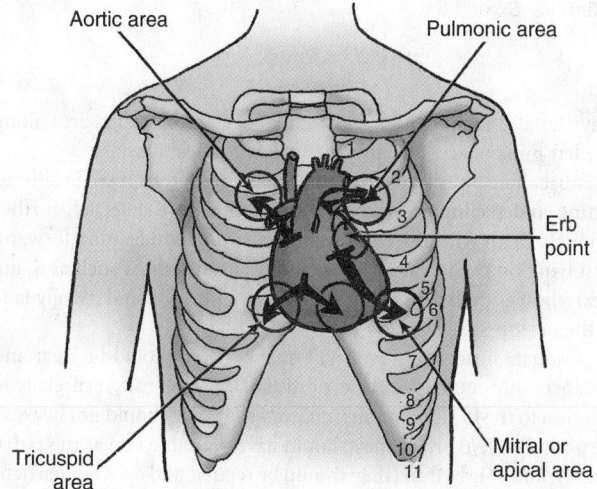

FIG 29-34 Direction of heart sounds for anatomic valve sites and areas *(circled)* for auscultation.

Two other heart sounds, S_3 and S_4, may be produced. S_3 is normally heard in some children. S_4 is rarely heard as a normal heart sound; it usually indicates the need for further cardiac evaluation.

Differentiating Normal Heart Sounds. Fig. 29-34 illustrates the approximate anatomic position of the valves within the heart chambers. Note that the anatomic location of valves does not correspond to the area where the sounds are heard best. The auscultatory sites are located in the direction of the blood flow through the valves.

Normally, S_1 is louder at the apex of the heart in the mitral and tricuspid area and S_2 is louder near the base of the heart in the pulmonic and aortic area (Table 29-11). Listen to each sound by inching down the chest. To distinguish between S_1 and S_2 heart sounds, simultaneously palpate the carotid pulse with the index and middle fingers and listen to the heart sounds; S_1 is synchronous with the carotid pulse.

Auscultate the following areas for sounds, such as murmurs, which may radiate to these sites: sternoclavicular area above the

atrioventricular valves). S_2 is the result of closure of the pulmonic and aortic valves (sometimes called semilunar valves). Normally the split of the two sounds in S_2 is distinguishable and widens during inspiration. Physiologic splitting is a significant normal finding.

> **❗ NURSING ALERT**
>
> Fixed splitting, in which the split in S_2 does not change during inspiration, is an important diagnostic sign of atrial septal defect.

TABLE 29-11	SEQUENCE OF AUSCULTATING HEART SOUNDS*	
AUSCULTATORY SITE	**CHEST LOCATION**	**CHARACTERISTICS OF HEART SOUNDS**
Aortic area	Second right intercostal space close to sternum	S_2 heard louder than S_1; aortic closure heard loudest
Pulmonic area	Second left intercostal space close to sternum	Splitting of S_2 heard best, normally widens on inspiration; pulmonic closure heard best
Erb point	Second and third left intercostal spaces close to sternum	Frequent site of innocent murmurs and those of aortic or pulmonic origin
Tricuspid area	Fifth right and left intercostal spaces close to sternum	S_1 heard as louder sound preceding S_2 (S_1 synchronous with carotid pulse)
Mitral or apical area	Fifth intercostal space, left midclavicular line (third to fourth intercostal space and lateral to left midclavicular line in infants)	S_1 heard loudest; splitting of S_1 may be audible because mitral closure is louder than tricuspid closure S_1 heard best at beginning of expiration with child in recumbent or left side-lying position; occurs immediately after S_2; sounds like word S_1 S_2 S_3: "Ken-tuc-ky" S_4 heard best during expiration with child in recumbent position (left side-lying position decreases sound); occurs immediately before S_1; sounds like word S_4 S_1 S_2: "Ten-nes-see"

*Use both diaphragm and bell chest pieces when auscultating heart sounds. Bell chest piece is necessary for low-pitched sounds of murmurs, S_3, and S_4.

clavicles and manubrium, area along the sternal border, area along the left midaxillary line, and area below the scapulae.

Auscultate the heart with the child in at least two positions: sitting and reclining. If adventitious sounds are detected, further evaluate them with the child standing, sitting and leaning forward, and lying on the left side. For example, atrial sounds such as S_4 are heard best with the person in a recumbent position and usually fade if the person sits or stands.

Evaluate heart sounds for (1) quality (they should be clear and distinct—not muffled, diffuse, or distant); (2) intensity, especially in relation to the location or auscultatory site (they should not be weak or pounding); (3) rate (they should have the same rate as the radial pulse); and (4) rhythm (they should be regular and even). A particular dysrhythmia that occurs normally in many children is sinus dysrhythmia, in which the heart rate increases with inspiration and decreases with expiration. Differentiate this rhythm from a truly abnormal dysrhythmia by having children hold their breath. In sinus dysrhythmia, cessation of breathing causes the heart rate to remain steady.

Heart Murmurs. Another important category of the heart sounds is murmurs, which are produced by vibrations within the heart chambers or in the major arteries from the back-and-forth flow of blood. (For a more detailed discussion, see Assessment of Cardiac Function, Chapter 42.) Murmurs are classified as:

- **Innocent**—No anatomic or physiologic abnormality exists.
- **Functional**—No anatomic cardiac defect exists, but a physiologic abnormality such as anemia is present.
- **Organic**—A cardiac defect with or without a physiologic abnormality exists.

The description and classification of murmurs are skills that require considerable practice and training. In general, recognize murmurs as distinct swishing sounds that occur in addition to the normal heart sounds and record the (1) location, or the area of the heart in which the murmur is heard best; (2) time of the occurrence of the murmur within the S_1-S_2 cycle; (3) intensity (evaluate in relationship to the child's position); and (4) loudness. Table 29-12 lists the usual subjective method of grading the loudness or intensity of a murmur.

TABLE 29-12	GRADING THE INTENSITY OF HEART MURMURS
GRADE	**DESCRIPTION**
I	Very faint; often not heard if child sits up
II	Usually readily heard; slightly louder than grade I; audible in all positions
III	Loud, but not accompanied by a thrill
IV	Loud, accompanied by a thrill
V	Loud enough to be heard with a stethoscope barely touching the chest; accompanied by a thrill
VI	Loud enough to be heard with the stethoscope not touching the chest; often heard with the human ear close to the chest; accompanied by a thrill

Abdomen

Examination of the abdomen involves inspection, followed by auscultation and then palpation. Perform palpation last because it may distort the normal abdominal sounds. Knowledge of the anatomic placement of the abdominal organs is essential to differentiate normal, expected findings from abnormal ones (Fig. 29-35).

For descriptive purposes, the abdominal cavity is divided into four quadrants by drawing a vertical line midway from the sternum to the symphysis pubis and a horizontal line across the abdomen through the umbilicus. The sections are named:

- Left upper quadrant
- Left lower quadrant
- Right upper quadrant
- Right lower quadrant

Inspection

Inspect the contour of the abdomen with the child erect and supine. Normally the abdomen of infants and young children is cylindric

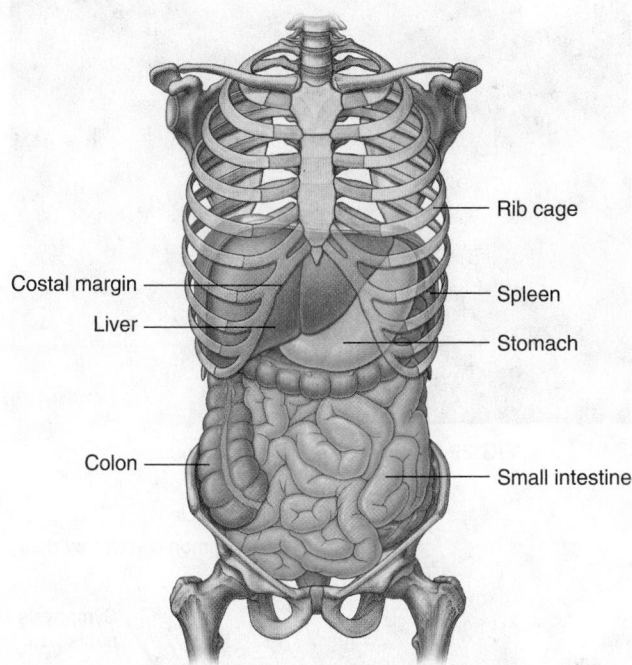

FIG 29-35 Location of structures in abdomen. (From Drake RL, Vogl W, Mitchell AWM: *Gray's anatomy for students*, New York, 2005, Churchill Livingstone.)

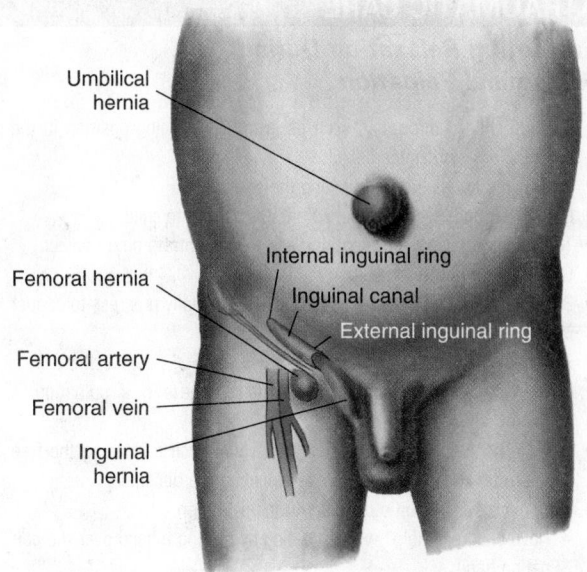

FIG 29-36 Location of hernias.

and, in the erect position, fairly prominent because of the physiologic lordosis of the spine. In the supine position, the abdomen appears flat. A midline protrusion from the xiphoid to the umbilicus or symphysis pubis is usually diastasis recti, or failure of the rectus abdominis muscles to join in utero. In a healthy child, a midline protrusion is usually a variation of normal muscular development.

> **! NURSING ALERT**
>
> A tense, boardlike abdomen is a serious sign of paralytic ileus and intestinal obstruction.

The skin covering the abdomen should be uniformly taut, without wrinkles or creases. Sometimes silvery, whitish striae ("stretch marks") are seen, especially if the skin has been stretched as in obesity. Superficial veins are usually visible in light-skinned, thin infants, but distended veins are an abnormal finding.

Observe movement of the abdomen. Normally chest and abdominal movements are synchronous. In infants and thin children, peristaltic waves may be visible through the abdominal wall; they are best observed by standing at eye level to and across from the abdomen. Always report this finding.

Examine the umbilicus for size, hygiene, and evidence of any abnormalities, such as hernias. The umbilicus should be flat or only slightly protruding. If a herniation is present, palpate the sac for abdominal contents and estimate the approximate size of the opening. Umbilical hernias are common in infants, especially in African-American children.

Hernias may exist elsewhere on the abdominal wall (Fig. 29-36). An inguinal hernia is a protrusion of peritoneum through the abdominal wall in the inguinal canal. It occurs mostly in males, is frequently bilateral, and may be visible as a mass in the scrotum. To locate a hernia, slide the little finger into the external inguinal ring at the base of the scrotum and ask the child to cough. If a hernia is

present, it will hit the tip of the finger. If the child is too young to cough, have the child blow up a balloon or laugh to raise the intraabdominal pressure sufficiently to demonstrate the presence of an inguinal hernia.

A femoral hernia, which occurs more frequently in girls, is felt or seen as a small mass on the anterior surface of the thigh just below the inguinal ligament in the femoral canal (a potential space medial to the femoral artery). Feel for a hernia by placing the index finger of your right hand on the child's right femoral pulse (left hand for left pulse) and the middle finger flat against the skin toward the midline. The ring finger lies over the femoral canal, where the herniation occurs. Palpation of hernias in the pelvic region is often part of the genital examination.

Auscultation

The most important finding to listen for is peristalsis, or bowel sounds, which sound like short metallic clicks and gurgles. Record their frequency per minute (e.g., 5 sounds/min). Stimulate bowel sounds by stroking the abdominal surface with a fingernail. Report absence of bowel sounds or hyperperistalsis, since either usually denotes an abdominal disorder.

Palpation

There are two types of palpation: superficial and deep. For superficial palpation, lightly place your hand against the skin and feel each quadrant, noting any areas of tenderness, muscle tone, and superficial lesions such as cysts. Because superficial palpation is often perceived as tickling, use several techniques to minimize this sensation and relax the child (see Atraumatic Care box). Admonishing the child to stop laughing only draws attention to the sensation and decreases cooperation.

Deep palpation is for palpating organs and large blood vessels and for detecting masses and tenderness that were not discovered during superficial palpation. Palpation usually begins in the lower quadrants and proceeds upward to avoid missing the edge of an enlarged liver or spleen. Except for palpating the liver, successful identification of other organs, such as the spleen, kidney, and part of the colon, requires considerable practice with tutored supervision. Report any questionable mass. The lower edge of the liver is

ATRAUMATIC CARE

Promoting Relaxation During Abdominal Palpation

- Position child comfortably, such as in a semireclining position in the parent's lap, with knees flexed.
- Warm your hands before touching the skin.
- Use distraction, such as telling stories or talking to child.
- Teach child to use deep breathing and to concentrate on an object.
- Give infant a bottle or pacifier.
- Begin with light, superficial palpation and gradually progress to deeper palpation.
- Palpate any tender or painful areas last.
- Have child hold the parent's hand and squeeze it if palpation is uncomfortable.
- Use the nonpalpating hand to comfort child, such as placing the free hand on the child's shoulder while palpating the abdomen.
- To minimize sensation of tickling during palpation:
  - Have children "help" with palpation by placing a hand over the palpating hand.
  - Have them place a hand on the abdomen with the fingers spread wide apart, and palpate between their fingers.

sometimes felt in infants and young children as a superficial mass 1 to 2 cm (0.4 to 0.8 inch) below the right costal margin (the distance is sometimes measured in fingerbreadths). Normally the liver descends during inspiration as the diaphragm moves downward. Do not mistake this downward displacement as a sign of liver enlargement.

⚠ NURSING ALERT

If the liver is palpable 3 cm (1.2 in) below the right costal margin or the spleen is palpable more than 2 cm (0.8 in) below the left costal margin, these organs are enlarged—a finding that is always reported for further medical investigation.

Palpate the femoral pulses by placing the tips of two or three fingers (index, middle, or ring) along the inguinal ligament about midway between the iliac crest and symphysis pubis. Feel both pulses simultaneously to make certain that they are equal and strong (Fig. 29-37).

⚠ NURSING ALERT

Absence of femoral pulses is a significant sign of coarctation of the aorta and is referred for medical evaluation.

Genitalia

Examination of genitalia conveniently follows assessment of the abdomen while the child is still supine. In adolescents, inspection of the genitalia may be left to the end of the examination. The best approach is to examine the genitalia matter-of-factly, placing no more emphasis on this part of the assessment than on any other segment. It helps to relieve children's and parents' anxiety by telling them the results of the findings; for example, the nurse might say, "Everything looks fine here."

If it is necessary to ask questions, such as about discharge or difficulty urinating, respect the child's privacy by covering the lower abdomen with the gown or underpants. To prevent embarrassing interruptions, keep the door or curtain closed and post a "do not

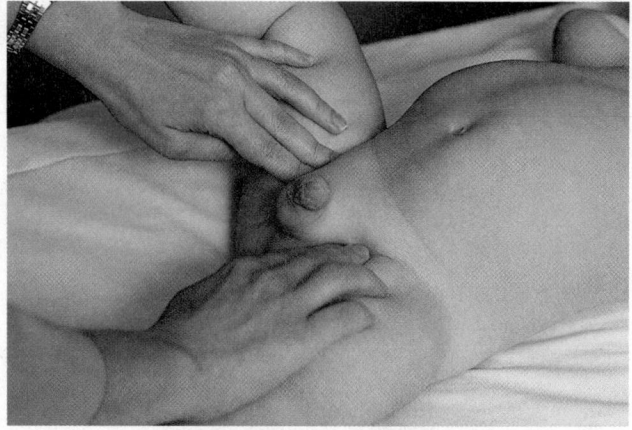

FIG 29-37 Palpating for femoral pulses.

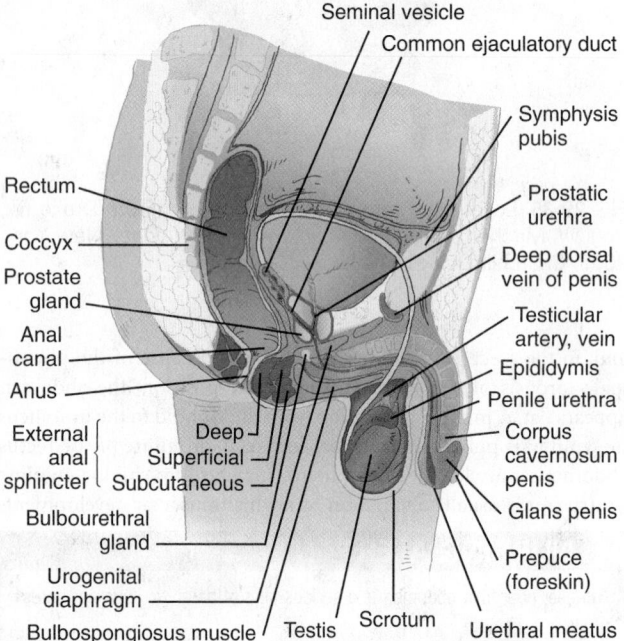

FIG 29-38 Major structures of genitalia in uncircumcised postpubertal male. (From Black JM: *Medical-surgical nursing: clinical management for positive outcomes,* ed 8, St Louis, 2008, Saunders.)

disturb" sign. Have a drape ready to cover the genitalia if someone enters the room.

In examining the genitalia, wear gloves when touching body substances. It might be helpful for the adolescent to know that wearing gloves also prevents skin-to-skin contact.

The genital examination is an excellent time for eliciting questions or concern about body function or sexual activity. Also use this opportunity to increase or reinforce the child's knowledge of reproductive anatomy by naming each body part and explaining its function. This part of the health assessment is an opportune time to teach testicular self-examination to boys.

Male Genitalia

Note the external appearance of the glans and shaft of the penis, the prepuce, the urethral meatus, and the scrotum (Fig. 29-38). The penis is generally small in infants and young boys until puberty, when it begins to increase in both length and width. In an obese child, the penis often looks abnormally small because of the folds of skin partially covering it at the base. Be familiar with normal pubertal growth of the external male genitalia to compare the findings with the expected sequence of maturation (see Chapter 35).

Examine the glans (head of the penis) and shaft (portion between the perineum and prepuce) for signs of swelling, skin lesions, inflammation, or other irregularities. Any of these signs may indicate underlying disorders, especially sexually transmitted infections.

Carefully inspect the urethral meatus for location and evidence of discharge. Normally it is centered at the tip of the glans. Also note hair distribution. Normally, before puberty, no pubic hair is present. Soft, downy hair at the base of the penis is an early sign of pubertal maturation. In older adolescents, hair distribution is diamond-shaped from the umbilicus to the anus.

Note the location and size of the scrotum. The scrota hang freely from the perineum behind the penis, and the left scrotum normally hangs lower than the right. In infants, the scrota appear large in relation to the rest of the genitalia. The skin of the scrotum is loose and highly rugated (wrinkled). During early adolescence, the skin normally becomes redder and coarser. In dark-skinned children, the scrota are usually more deeply pigmented.

Palpation of the scrotum includes identification of the testes, epididymis, and, if present, inguinal hernias. The two testes are felt as small, ovoid bodies about 1.5 to 2 cm (0.6 to 0.8 in) long—one in each scrotal sac. They do not enlarge until puberty, when they approximately double in size.

When palpating for the presence of the testes, avoid stimulating the cremasteric reflex, which is stimulated by cold, touch, emotional excitement, or exercise. This reflex pulls the testes higher into the pelvic cavity. Several measures are useful in preventing the cremasteric reflex during palpation of the scrotum. First, warm the hands. Second, if the child is old enough, examine him in a tailor or "Indian" position, which stretches the muscle, preventing its contraction (Fig. 29-39, *A*). Third, block the normal pathway of ascent of the testes by placing the thumb and index finger over the upper part of the scrotal sac along the inguinal canal (Fig. 29-39, *B*). If there is any question concerning the existence of two testes, place the index and middle fingers in a scissors fashion to separate the right and left scrota. If, after using these techniques, you have not palpated the testes, feel along the inguinal canal and perineum to locate masses that may be undescended testes. Although undescended testes may descend at any time during childhood and are checked at each visit, report any failure to palpate the testes.

Female Genitalia

The examination of female genitalia is limited to inspection and palpation of external structures. If a vaginal examination is required, the nurse should make an appropriate referral unless he or she is qualified to perform the procedure.

A convenient position for examination of the genitalia involves placing the young child supine on the examining table or in a semi-reclining position on the parent's lap with the feet supported on your knees as you sit facing the child. Divert the child's attention from the examination by instructing her to try to keep the soles of her feet pressed against each other. Separate the labia majora with the thumb and index finger and retract outward to expose the labia minora, urethral meatus, and vaginal orifice.

Examine the female genitalia for size and location of the structures of the vulva, or pudendum (Fig. 29-40). The mons pubis is a

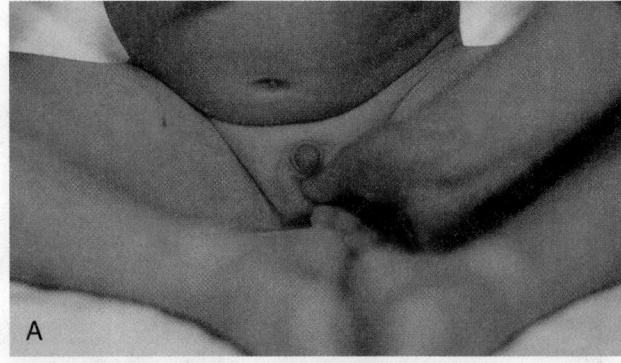
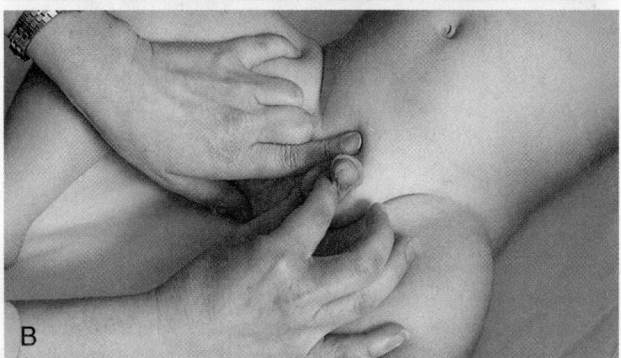

FIG 29-39 A, Preventing cremasteric reflex by having child sit in tailor position. **B,** Blocking inguinal canal during palpation of scrotum for descended testes.

pad of adipose tissue over the symphysis pubis. At puberty the mons is covered with hair, which extends along the labia. The usual pattern of female hair distribution is an inverted triangle. The appearance of soft, downy hair along the labia majora is an early sign of sexual maturation. Note the size and location of the clitoris, a small, erectile organ located at the anterior end of the labia minora. It is covered by a small flap of skin, the prepuce.

The labia majora are two thick folds of skin running posteriorly from the mons to the posterior commissure of the vagina. Internal to the labia majora are two folds of skin called the labia minora. Although the labia minora are usually prominent in the newborn, they gradually atrophy, which makes them almost invisible until their enlargement during puberty. The inner surface of the labia should be pink and moist. Note the size of the labia and any evidence of fusion, which may suggest male scrota. Normally no masses are palpable within the labia.

The urethral meatus is located posterior to the clitoris and is surrounded by the Skene glands and ducts. Although not a prominent structure, the meatus appears as a small **V**-shaped slit. Note its location, especially if it opens from the clitoris or inside the vagina. Gently palpate the glands, which are common sites of cysts and sexually transmitted lesions.

The vaginal orifice is located posterior to the urethral meatus. Its appearance varies depending on individual anatomy and sexual activity. Ordinarily, examination of the vagina is limited to inspection. In virgins, a thin crescent-shaped or circular membrane, called the hymen, may cover part of the vaginal opening. In some instances it completely occludes the orifice. After rupture, small rounded pieces of tissue called caruncles remain. Although an imperforate hymen denotes lack of penile intercourse, a perforate one does not necessarily indicate sexual activity (see also Sexual Abuse, Chapter 35).

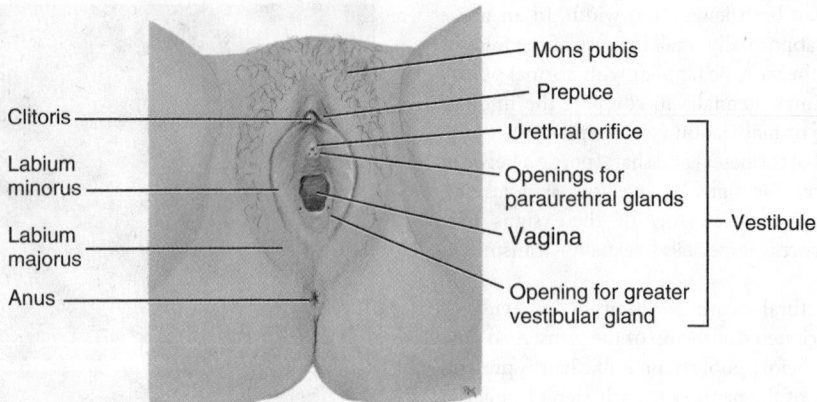

FIG 29-40 External structures of genitalia in postpubertal female. Labia are spread to reveal deeper structures. (From Applegate E: *The anatomy and physiology learning system,* ed 3, St Louis, 2006, Saunders.)

> ⚠ **NURSING ALERT**
>
> In girls who have been circumcised, the genitalia will appear different. Do not show surprise or disgust, but note the appearance and discuss the procedure with the young woman (see also Cultural Competence box, p. 59).

Surrounding the vaginal opening are Bartholin glands, which secrete a clear, mucoid fluid into the vagina for lubrication during intercourse. Palpate the ducts for cysts. Also note the discharge from the vagina, which is usually clear or white.

Anus

After examination of the genitalia, it is easy to identify the anal area, although the child should be placed on the abdomen. Note the general firmness of the buttocks and symmetry of the gluteal folds. Assess the tone of the anal sphincter by eliciting the anal reflex (anal wink). Gently scratching the anal area results in an obvious quick contraction of the external anal sphincter.

Back and Extremities
Spine

Note the general curvature of the spine. Normally the back of a newborn is rounded or C-shaped from the thoracic and pelvic curves. The development of the cervical and lumbar curves approximates development of various motor skills, such as cervical curvature with head control, and gives the older child the typical double-S curve.

Marked curvatures in posture are abnormal. Scoliosis, lateral curvature of the spine, is an important childhood problem, especially in girls. Although scoliosis may be identified by observing and palpating the spine and noting a sideways displacement, more objective tests include:

- With the child standing erect, clothed only in underpants (and bra if older girl), observe from behind, noting asymmetry of the shoulders and hips.
- With the child bending forward so that the back is parallel to the floor, observe from the side, noting asymmetry or prominence of the rib cage.

A slight limp, a crooked hemline, or complaints of a sore back are other signs and symptoms of scoliosis.

Inspect the back, especially along the spine, for any tufts of hair, dimples, or discoloration. Mobility of the vertebral column is easy to assess in most children because of their tendency to be in constant motion during the examination. However, you can test mobility by asking the child to sit up from a prone position or to do a modified sit-up exercise.

Movement of the cervical spine is an important diagnostic sign of neurologic problems, such as meningitis. Normally, movement of the head in all directions is effortless.

> ⚠ **NURSING ALERT**
>
> Hyperextension of the neck and spine, or opisthotonos, which is accompanied by pain when the head is flexed, is always referred for immediate medical evaluation.

Extremities

Inspect each extremity for symmetry of length and size; refer any deviation for orthopedic evaluation. Count the fingers and toes to be certain of the normal number. This is so often taken for granted that an extra digit (polydactyly) or fusion of digits (syndactyly) may go unnoticed.

Inspect the arms and legs for temperature and color, which should be equal in each extremity, although the feet may normally be colder than the hands.

Assess the shape of bones. There are several variations of bone shape in children. Although many of them cause parents concern, most are benign and require no treatment. Bowleg, or genu varum, is lateral bowing of the tibia. It is clinically present when the child stands with an outward bowing of the legs, giving the appearance of a bow. Usually there is an outward curvature of both femur and tibia (Fig. 29-41, *A*). Toddlers are usually bowlegged after beginning to walk until all their lower back and leg muscles are well developed. Unilateral or asymmetric bowlegs that are present beyond the age of 2 to 3 years, particularly in African-American children, may represent pathologic conditions requiring further investigation.

Knock-knee, or genu valgum, appears as the opposite of bowleg, in that the knees are close together but the feet are spread apart. It is determined clinically by using the same method as for genu varum but by measuring the distance between the malleoli, which normally should be less than 7.5 cm (3 in) (Fig. 29-41, *B*). Knock-knee is normally present in children from about 2 to 7 years of age.

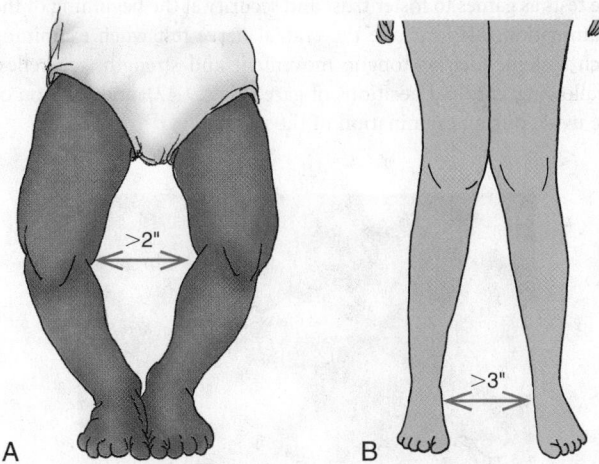

FIG 29-41 A, Bowleg. **B,** Knock-knee.

Knock-knee that is excessive, asymmetric, accompanied by short stature, or evident in a child nearing puberty requires further evaluation.

Next inspect the feet. Infants' and toddlers' feet appear flat because the foot is normally wide and the arch is covered by a fat pad. Development of the arch occurs naturally from the action of walking. Normally, at birth the feet are held in a valgus (outward) or varus (inward) position. To determine whether a foot deformity at birth is a result of intrauterine position or development, scratch the outer, then inner, side of the sole. If the foot position is self-correctable, it will assume a right angle to the leg. As the child begins to walk, the feet turn outward less than 30 degrees and inward less than 10 degrees.

Toddlers have a "toddling" or broad-based gait, which facilitates walking by lowering the center of gravity. As the child reaches preschool age, the legs are brought closer together. By school age, the walking posture is much more graceful and balanced.

The most common gait problem in young children is pigeon toe, or toeing in, which usually results from torsional deformities, such as internal tibial torsion (abnormal rotation or bowing of the tibia). Tests for tibial torsion include measuring the thigh-foot angle, which requires considerable practice for accuracy.

Elicit the plantar or grasp reflex by exerting firm but gentle pressure with the tip of the thumb against the lateral sole of the foot from the heel upward to the little toe and then across to the big toe. The normal response in children who are walking is flexion of the toes. Babinski sign, dorsiflexion of the big toe and fanning of the other toes, is normal during infancy but abnormal after about 1 year of age or when locomotion begins.

Joints

Evaluate the joints for range of motion. Normally this requires no specific testing if you have observed the child's movements during the examination. However, routinely investigate the hips in infants for congenital dislocation. Report any evidence of joint immobility or hyperflexibility. Palpate the joints for heat, tenderness, and swelling. These signs, as well as redness over the joint, warrant further investigation.

Muscles

Note symmetry and quality of muscle development, tone, and strength. Observe development by looking at the shape and contour of the body in both a relaxed and a tensed state. Estimate tone by

grasping the muscle and feeling its firmness when it is relaxed and contracted. A common site for testing tone is the biceps muscle of the arm. Children are usually willing to "make a muscle" by clenching their fist.

Estimate strength by having the child use an extremity to push or pull against resistance, as in the following examples:

- **Arm strength**—Child holds the arms outstretched in front of the body and tries to raise the arms while downward pressure is applied.
- **Hand strength**—Child shakes hands with nurse and squeezes one or two fingers of the nurse's hand.
- **Leg strength**—Child sits on a table or chair with the legs dangling and tries to raise the legs while downward pressure is applied.

Note symmetry of strength in the extremities, hands, and fingers, and report evidence of paresis, or weakness.

Neurologic Assessment

The assessment of the nervous system is the broadest and most diverse part of the examination process, since every human function, both physical and emotional, is controlled by neurologic impulses. Much of the neurologic examination has already been discussed, such as assessment of behavior, sensory testing, and motor function. The following focuses on a general appraisal of cerebellar function, deep tendon reflexes, and the cranial nerves.

Cerebellar Function

The cerebellum controls balance and coordination. Much of the assessment of cerebellar function is included in observing the child's posture, body movements, gait, and development of fine and gross motor skills. Tests such as balancing on one foot and the heel-to-toe walk assess balance. Test coordination by asking the child to reach for a toy, button clothes, tie shoes, or draw a straight line on a piece of paper (provided the child is old enough to do these activities). Coordination can also be tested by any sequence of rapid, successive movements, such as quickly touching each finger with the thumb of the same hand.

Several tests for cerebellar function can be performed as games (Box 29-15). When a Romberg test is done, stay beside the child if there is a possibility that he or she might fall. School-age children should be able to perform these tests, although in the finger-to-nose test preschoolers normally can only bring the finger within 5 to 7.5 cm (2 to 3 in) of the nose. Difficulty in performing these exercises indicates poor sense of position (especially with the eyes closed) and incoordination (especially with the eyes opened).

Reflexes

Testing reflexes is an important part of the neurologic examination. Persistence of primitive reflexes, loss of reflexes, or hyperactivity of deep tendon reflexes is usually a result of a cerebral insult.

Elicit reflexes by using the rubber head of the reflex hammer, flat of the finger, or side of the hand. If the child is easily frightened by equipment, use your hand or finger. Although testing reflexes is a simple procedure, the child may inhibit the reflex by unconsciously tensing the muscle. To avoid tensing, distract younger children with toys or talk to them. Older children can concentrate on the exercise of grasping their two hands in front of them and trying to pull them apart. This diverts their attention from the testing and causes involuntary relaxation of the muscles.

Deep tendon reflexes are stretch reflexes of a muscle. The most common deep tendon reflex is the knee jerk reflex, or patellar reflex (sometimes called the quadriceps reflex). Figs. 29-42 through 29-45 illustrate the reflexes normally elicited. Report any diminished or hyperreflexive response for further evaluation.

Cranial Nerves

Assessment of the cranial nerves is an important area of neurologic assessment (Fig. 29-46; Table 29-13). With young children, present the tests as games to foster trust and security at the beginning of the examination. Also include the cranial nerve test when examining each system, such as tongue movement and strength, gag reflex, swallowing, cardinal positions of gaze (Fig. 29-47), and position of the uvula during examination of the mouth.

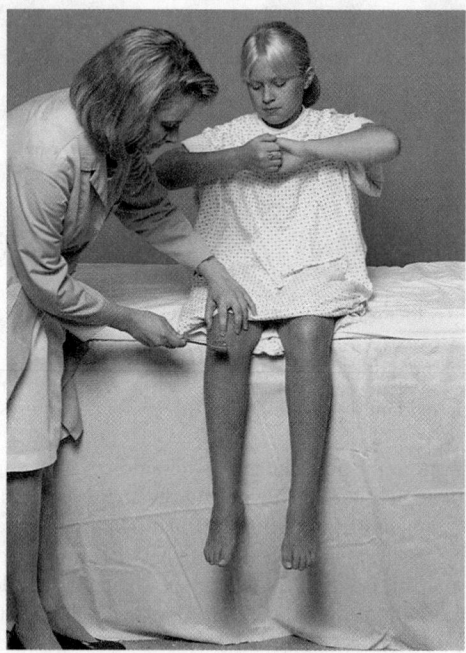

FIG 29-44 Testing for patellar, or knee jerk, reflex, using distraction. Child sits on edge of examining table (or on parent's lap) with lower legs flexed at knee and dangling freely. Patellar tendon is tapped just below kneecap. Normal response is partial extension of lower leg.

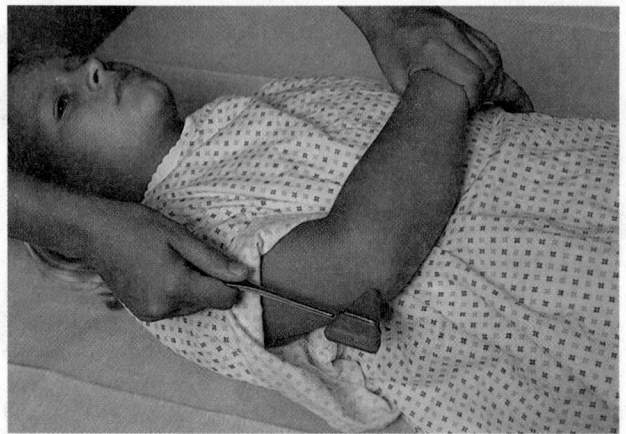

FIG 29-42 Testing for triceps reflex. Child is placed supine with forearm resting over chest, and triceps tendon is struck. Alternate procedure: child's arm is abducted, with upper arm supported and forearm allowed to hang freely. Triceps tendon is struck. Normal response is partial extension of forearm.

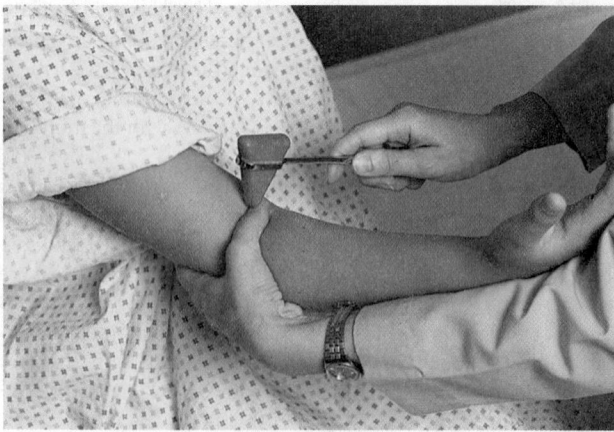

FIG 29-43 Testing for biceps reflex. Child's arm is held by placing partially flexed elbow in examiner's hand with examiner's thumb over antecubital space. Examiner's thumbnail is struck with hammer. Normal response is partial flexion of forearm.

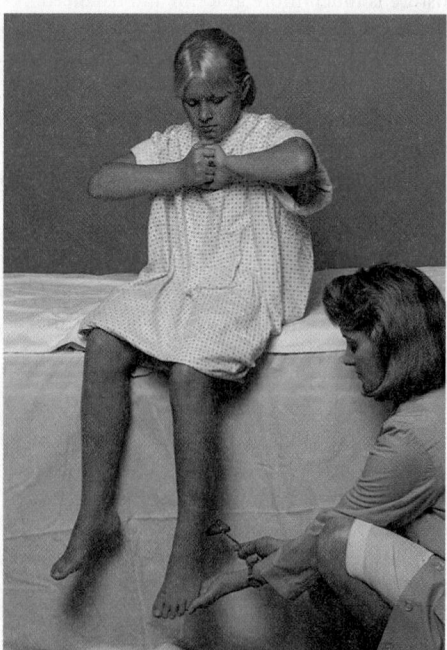

FIG 29-45 Testing for Achilles reflex. Child should be in same position as for knee jerk reflex. Foot is supported lightly in examiner's hand, and Achilles tendon is struck. Normal response is plantar flexion of foot (foot pointing downward).

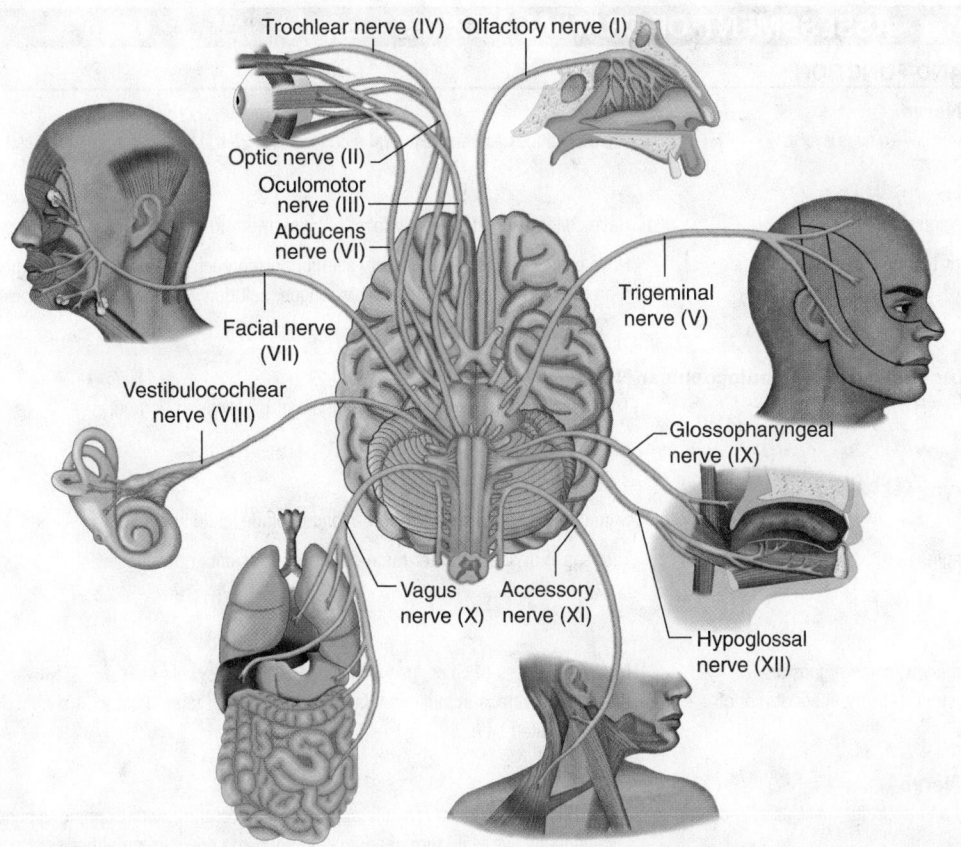

FIG 29-46 Cranial nerves. (From Patton KT, Thibodeau GA: *Anatomy & physiology*, ed 8, St Louis, 2013, Mosby.)

TABLE 29-13 ASSESSMENT OF CRANIAL NERVES

DESCRIPTION AND FUNCTION	TESTS
I—Olfactory Nerve Olfactory mucosa of nasal cavity Smell	With eyes closed, have child identify odors such as coffee, alcohol from a swab, or other smells; test each nostril separately.
II—Optic Nerve Rods and cones of retina, optic nerve Vision	Check for perception of light, visual acuity, peripheral vision, color vision, and normal optic disc.

III—Oculomotor Nerve
Extraocular muscles of eye:
  Superior rectus—moves eyeball up and in
  Inferior rectus—moves eyeball down and in
  Medial rectus—moves eyeball nasally
  Inferior oblique—moves eyeball up and out
	Have child follow an object (toy) or light in six cardinal positions of gaze (see Fig. 29-47).

Pupil constriction and accommodation	Perform *PERRLA* (**P**upils **E**qual, **R**ound, **R**eact to **L**ight, and **A**ccommodation).
Eyelid closing	Check for proper placement of lid.
IV—Trochlear Nerve Superior oblique (SO) muscle—moves eye down and out	Have child look down and in (see Fig. 29-47).
V—Trigeminal Nerve Muscles of mastication	Have child bite down hard and open jaw; test symmetry and strength.
Sensory—face, scalp, nasal, and buccal mucosa	With child's eyes closed, see if child can detect light touch in mandibular and maxillary regions. Test corneal and blink reflex by touching cornea lightly (approach from side so that child does not blink before cornea is touched).

Continued

TABLE 29-13 ASSESSMENT OF CRANIAL NERVES—cont'd

DESCRIPTION AND FUNCTION	TESTS
VI—Abducens Nerve	
Lateral rectus (LR) muscle—moves eye temporally	Have child look toward temporal side (see Fig. 29-47).
VII—Facial Nerve	
Muscles for facial expression	Have child smile, make funny face, or show teeth to see symmetry of expression.
Anterior two thirds of tongue (sensory)	Have child identify sweet or salty solution; place each taste on anterior section and sides of protruding tongue; if child retracts tongue, solution will dissolve toward posterior part of tongue.
VIII—Auditory, Acoustic, or Vestibulocochlear Nerve	
Internal ear	Test hearing; note any loss of equilibrium or presence of vertigo.
Hearing and balance	
IX—Glossopharyngeal Nerve	
Pharynx, tongue	Stimulate posterior pharynx with a tongue blade; child should gag.
Posterior third of tongue	Test sense of sour or bitter taste on posterior segment of tongue.
Sensory	
X—Vagus Nerve	
Muscles of larynx, pharynx, some organs of gastrointestinal system, sensory fibers of root of tongue, heart, and lung	Note hoarseness of voice, gag reflex, and ability to swallow. Check that uvula is in midline; when stimulated with tongue blade, it should deviate upward and to stimulated side.
XI—Accessory Nerve	
Sternocleidomastoid and trapezius muscles of shoulder	Have child shrug shoulders while applying mild pressure; with examiner's hands placed on shoulders, have child turn head against opposing pressure on either side; note symmetry and strength.
XII—Hypoglossal Nerve	
Muscles of tongue	Have child move tongue in all directions; have child protrude tongue as far as possible; note any midline deviation. Test strength by placing tongue blade on one side of tongue and having child move it away.

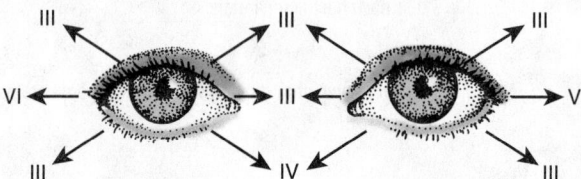

FIG 29-47 Checking extraocular movements in the six cardinal positions indicates the functioning of cranial nerves III, IV, and VI. (From Ignatavicius DD, Workman ML: *Medical-surgical nursing: patient-centered collaborative care,* ed 6, St Louis, 2009, Saunders.)

KEY POINTS

- To effectively establish a setting for communication, nurses must make an appropriate introduction and ensure privacy and confidentiality.
- When communicating with parents, nurses need to encourage parental involvement, listen carefully, use silence, and be empathic.
- Communication with children must reflect their developmental stage.
- Nonverbal communication with children may take the form of writing, drawing, and play.
- The objectives of performing a health history are to identify pertinent information, determine the chief complaint, analyze the present illness, secure the patient's health history, review biologic systems, and record a family medical history and child psychosocial and sexual history.
- Family assessment is the collection of data about family composition and relationships among its members; it also focuses on home and community environment, parents' occupation and education, and cultural and religious traditions.
- The family function interview examines interaction and roles, power, decision making, problem solving, communication, and expression of feelings and individuality.
- Nutritional assessment is performed by determination of dietary intake, clinical examination, and biochemical analysis.

- Growth measurements during the physical examination focus on length or height, weight, skinfold thickness, and arm and head circumference. Assessment of growth is measured against standard growth charts to determine a child's status in comparison with other children of the same age.
- Measurements of temperature, pulse, respiration, and BP constitute the physiologic approach to assessment.
- The child's general appearance is a cumulative, subjective impression of physical appearance, state of nutrition, behavior, personality, interactions with parents and nurse, posture, development, and speech.
- Assessment of the skin, which primarily involves inspection and palpation, focuses on color, texture, temperature, moisture, and turgor. The nurse needs to be aware of both physiologic and ethnic factors that may affect these areas.
- In assessment of the lymph nodes, the nurse examines, by palpation, the part of the body in which the glands are located.
- The head is inspected for shape, symmetry, mobility, and muscle control.
- Examination of the eyes includes placement and alignment, inspection of external and internal structures, and vision testing.
- The ear examination encompasses placement and alignment, external and internal structures, and auditory testing.
- The lungs are examined by inspection, palpation, percussion, and auscultation.
- Auscultation is the most important procedure for examining the heart.
- Abdominal assessment follows an orderly sequence of inspection, auscultation, and palpation, since palpation may distort normal abdominal sounds.
- Examination of the genitalia may provoke anxiety in the child, and the nurse must avoid any transference of anxiety.
- Neurologic assessment addresses behavior; motor, sensory, and cerebellar function; reflexes; and cranial nerves.

REFERENCES

American Academy of Pediatrics: *Pediatric nutrition handbook*, ed 6, Elk Grove Village, IL, 2009, Author.

American Academy of Pediatrics, Committee on Practice and Ambulatory Medicine, Section on Ophthalmology: Eye examination in infants, children, and young adults by pediatricians, *Pediatrics* 111(4):902–907, 2003a.

American Academy of Pediatrics, Committee on Practice and Ambulatory Medicine, Section on Otolaryngology and Bronchoesophagology: Hearing assessment in infants and children: recommendations beyond neonatal screening, *Pediatrics* 111(2):436–440, 2003b.

Beaulieu R, Humphreys J: Evaluation of a telephone advice nurse in a nursing faculty managed pediatric community clinic, *J Pediatr Health Care* 22(3):175–181, 2008.

Beevers G, Lip GYH, O'Brien E: ABC of hypertension blood pressure measurement, part I, Sphygmomanometry: factors common to all techniques, *BMJ* 322(7292):981–985, 2001.

Clark JA, Kieh-Lai MW, Sarnaik A, et al: Discrepancies between direct and indirect blood pressure measurements using various recommendations for arm cuff selection, *Pediatrics* 110(5):920–923, 2002.

Coats DK, Jenkins RH: Vision assessment of the pediatric patient: refinements, *Am Acad Ophthalmol* 1(1):1–12, 1997.

Craig JV, Lancaster GA, Williamson PR, et al: Temperature measured at the axilla compared with rectum in children and young people: systematic review, *BMJ* 320(7243):1174–1178, 2000.

Cunningham M, Cox EO: Hearing assessment in infants and children: recommendations beyond neonatal screening, *Pediatrics* 111(2):436–440, 2003.

El-Radhi AS, Barry W: Thermometry in paediatric practice, *Arch Dis Child* 91(4):351–356, 2006.

Halle C: Achieve new vision screening objectives, *Nurse Pract* 27(3):15–35, 2002.

Magar NA, Dabova-Missova S, Gjerdingen DK: Effectiveness of targeted anticipatory guidance during well-child visits: a pilot trial, *J Am Board Fam Med* 19(5):450–458, 2006.

Mains JA, Coxall K, Lloyd H: Measuring temperature, *Nurs Stand* 22(39):44–47, 2008.

Marklund B, Ström M, Månsson J, et al: Computer-supported telephone nurse triage: an evaluation of medical quality and costs, *J Nurs Manage* 15(2):180–187, 2007.

Mathiasen H: Empathy and sympathy: voices from literature, *Am J Cardiol* 97(12):1789–1790, 2006.

Midgley PC, Wardhaugh B, Macfarlane C, et al: Blood pressure in children aged 4-8 years: comparison of Omron HEM 711 and sphygmomanometer blood pressure measurements, *Arch Dis Child* 94(12):955–958, 2009.

National High Blood Pressure Education Program Working Group on High Blood Pressure in Children and Adolescents: The fourth report on the diagnosis, evaluation, and treatment of high blood pressure in children and adolescents, *Pediatrics* 114(Suppl 2, 4th Rep):555–576, 2004.

Park MK, Menard SW, Schoolfield J: Oscillometric blood pressure standards for children, *Pediatr Cardiol* 26(5):601–607, 2005.

Seidel HM, Ball JW, Dains JE, et al: *Mosby's guide to physical examination*, ed 7, St Louis, 2011, Mosby.

Wall TC, Marsh-Tootle W, Evans HH, et al: Compliance with vision-screening guidelines among a national sample of pediatricians, *Ambul Pediatr* 2(6):449–455, 2002.

Pain Assessment and Management in Children

Marilyn J. Hockenberry

evolve WEBSITE

http://evolve.elsevier.com/Perry/maternal

LEARNING OBJECTIVES

On completion of this chapter, the reader will be able to:
- Identify measures to assess pain in children.
- List various types of pain-assessment tools for use with children.
- Outline essential pain-management strategies to reduce pain in children.

- Review common types of pain experienced by children.
- Discuss evidence to support specific pain-management strategies.

PAIN ASSESSMENT

Many children and adolescents continue to suffer from inadequately treated pain of all types (Perquin, Hazebroek-Kampschreur, Hunfeld, et al., 2000). Several research studies suggest that the undertreatment of pain in children is related to inconsistent practice in pain assessment, administration of analgesics at subtherapeutic levels, prolonged intervals between medications (Jacob and Puntillo, 2000), and lack of systematic monitoring and evaluation of relief (Jacob, Miaskowski, Savedra, et al., 2003a, 2003b; Jacob and Mueller, 2008). Optimal pain management begins with thorough assessment, which guides the selection of treatments. Acute pain assessment is easier to perform than complex pain that may be chronic, recurrent, or persistent.

Assessment of Acute Pain

Acute pain in children may have several causes such as: (1) medical procedures (immunization, venipuncture for blood draw or intravenous therapy, lumbar puncture for diagnosis or treatment, bone marrow aspiration, skin debridement for severe burns; (2) surgical (appendectomy, tonsillectomy) and orthopedic (spinal fusion) procedures; (3) medical treatments (chemotherapy-induced mucositis or peripheral neuropathy); (4) injury (such as falls, burns, motor vehicle accidents, other traumatic injuries); (5) infection; and (6) exacerbation of disease-related pain (e.g., arthritis, sickle cell disease, cancer).

Pain Intensity

Traditionally assessment measures are defined as behavioral measures, physiologic measures, and measures of self-reports. These measures predominantly address the domain of pain intensity. The behavioral measures of pain (for infants and children younger than 4 years; Table 30-1) and self-reports of pain (for children 4 years and older; Table 30-2) have been developed, validated, and widely used. Self-report measures are not sufficiently valid for children below 3 years of age because many are not able to accurately self-report their pain. Distress behaviors such as vocalization, facial expression, and body movement have been associated with pain (Figs. 30-1 and 30-2; Box 30-1). These behaviors are helpful in evaluating pain in infants and children with limited communication skills. However, discriminating between pain behaviors and reactions from other sources of distress such as hunger, anxiety, or other types of discomfort is not always easy. These factors decrease the specificity and sensitivity of behavioral measures (see Table 30-1).

Behavioral assessment is useful for measuring pain in infants and preverbal children who do not have the language skills to communicate that they are in pain or in children with mental clouding and confusion that limit their ability to communicate meaningfully. Behavior provides important information that cannot be obtained from self-report. Behavioral assessment may provide a more complete picture of the total pain experience when administered in conjunction with a subjective self-report measure. However, behavioral pain scales may be more time-consuming than self-reports. These measures depend on a trained observer to watch and record children's behaviors such as vocalization, facial expression, and body movements that suggest discomfort. Behaviors are assigned numbers from 0 to 4 to represent different intensities of distress. Scores are added to determine the child's pain rating.

TABLE 30-1 SUMMARY OF SELECTED BEHAVIORAL PAIN ASSESSMENT SCALES FOR YOUNG CHILDREN

AGES OF USE	RELIABILITY AND VALIDITY	VARIABLES	SCORING RANGE
Objective Pain Score (OPS) (Hannallah, Broadman, Belman, et al., 1987)			
4 months-18 years	Concurrent validity with linear analog pain scale, Spearman's r: 0.721 with scores ≥6 and 0.419 with scores <6 Interrater agreement, coefficient alpha: 0.986 for one rater and 0.983 for the other Concurrent validity with CHEOPS, Pearson correlation coefficient: 0.88 and 0.94	Blood pressure (0-2) Crying (0-2) Moving (0-2) Agitation (0-2) Verbal evaluation or body language (0-2)	0 = no pain; 10 = worst pain
Children's Hospital of Eastern Ontario Pain Scale (CHEOPS) (McGrath, Johnson, Goodman, et al., 1985)			
1-5 years	Interrater reliability: 90%-99.5% Internal correlation: significant correlations between pairs of items Concurrent validity between CHEOPS and visual analog scale (VAS): 0.91; between individual and total scores of CHEOPS and VAS: 0.50-0.86 Construct validity with preanalgesia and postanalgesia scores: 6.3-9.9	Cry (1-3) Facial (0-2) Child verbal (0-2) Torso (1-2) Touch (1-2) Legs (1-2)	4 = no pain; 13 = worst pain
Nurses Assessment of Pain Inventory (NAPI) (Stevens, 1990)			
Newborn-16 years	Not tested by original author; later tested by Joyce, Schade, Keck, et al. (1994) Interrater agreement: weighted kappa 0.37-0.80 Discriminant validity: statistically significant differences between preanalgesia and postanalgesia scores ($p < 0.0001$) Reliability: Cronbach alpha: 0.35-0.69	Body movement (0-2) Facial (0-3) Touching (0-2)	0 = no pain; 7 = worst pain
Behavioral Pain Score (BPS) (Robieux, Kumar, Radhakrishnan, et al., 1991)			
3-36 months	Original article stated, "reliability of the VAS and BPS scores was tested by a k test"; no further testing of reliability or validity mentioned	Facial expression (0-2) Cry (0-3) Movements (0-3)	0 = no pain; 8 = worst pain
Modified Behavioral Pain Scale (MBPS) (Taddio, Nulman, Koren, et al., 1995)			
4-6 months	Concurrent validity between MBPS and VAS scores: correlation coefficient 0.68 ($p < 0.001$) and 0.74 ($p < 0.001$) Construct validity using prevaccination and postvaccination scores with EMLA vs. placebo: significantly lower scores with EMLA ($p < 0.01$) Internal consistency of items: significant correlations between items Interrater agreement ICC: 0.95, $p < 0.001$ Test-retest reliability: 0.95, $p < 0.001$	Facial expression (0-3) Cry (0-4) Movements (0, 2, 3)	0 = no pain; 10 = worst pain
Riley Infant Pain Scale (RIPS) (Schade, Joyce, Gerkensmeyer, et al., 1996)			
<36 months and for children with cerebral palsy	Interrater agreement using intraclass correlation coefficient: 0.53-0.83, $p < 0.0001$ Discriminant validity using Mann-Whitney U test with preanalgesia and postanalgesia scores: statistically significant ($p < 0.001$) Sensitivity: 0.23-0.31 Specificity: 0.86-0.90 Interrater reliability using two-way cross-tabulations and kappa statistics (r[87] = 0.94; $p < 0.001$) and kappa values above 0.50 for each category	0: Neutral face/smiling, calm, sleeping quietly, no cry, consolable, moves easily 1: Frowning/grimace, restless body movements, restless sleep, whimpering, winces with touch 2: Clenched teeth, moderate agitation, sleeps intermittently, difficult to console, cries with touch 3: Full cry expression, thrashing/flailing, sleeping prolonged periods interrupted by jerking or no sleep, screaming/high-pitched cry, inconsolable, screams when touched/moved	0 = no pain; 3 = worst pain

Continued

TABLE 30-1   SUMMARY OF SELECTED BEHAVIORAL PAIN ASSESSMENT SCALES FOR YOUNG CHILDREN—cont'd

AGES OF USE	RELIABILITY AND VALIDITY	VARIABLES	SCORING RANGE
FLACC Postoperative Pain Tool (Merkel, Voepel-Lewis, Shayevitz, et al., 1997)			
2 months-7 years	Validity using analysis of variance for repeated measures to compare FLACC scores before and after analgesia; preanalgesia FLACC scores significantly higher than postanalgesia scores at 10, 30, and 60 min ($p < 0.001$ for each time) Correlation coefficients used to compare FLACC pain scores and OPS pain scores; significant positive correlation between FLACC and OPS scores ($r = 0.80$; $p < 0.001$); positive correlation also found between FLACC scores and nurses' global ratings of pain ($r[47] = 0.41$; $p < 0.005$)	Face (0-2) Legs (0-2) Activity (0-2) Cry (0-2) Consolability (0-2)	0 = no pain; 10 = worst pain

FLACC Scale*

	0	1	2
Face	No particular expression or smile	Occasional grimace or frown, withdrawn, disinterested	Frequent- to- constant frown, clenched jaw, quivering chin
Legs	Normal position or relaxed	Uneasy, restless, tense	Kicking or legs drawn up
Activity	Lying quietly, normal position, moves easily	Squirming, shifting back and forth, tense	Arched, rigid, or jerking
Cry	No cry (awake or asleep)	Moans or whimpers, occasional complaint	Crying steadily, screams or sobs, frequent complaints
Consolability	Content, relaxed	Reassured by occasional touching, hugging, or talking to; distractible	Difficult to console or comfort

*From Merkel SI, Voepel-Lewis T, Shayevitz JR, et al: The FLACC: a behavioral scale for scoring postoperative pain in young children, *Pediatr Nurs* 23(3):293–297, 1997. Used with permission of Jannetti Publications, Inc., and the University of Michigan Health System. Can be reproduced for clinical and research use.

TABLE 30-2   PAIN-RATING SCALES FOR CHILDREN

PAIN SCALE, DESCRIPTION	INSTRUCTIONS	RECOMMENDED AGE AND COMMENTS
Wong-Baker FACES Pain-Rating Scale*		

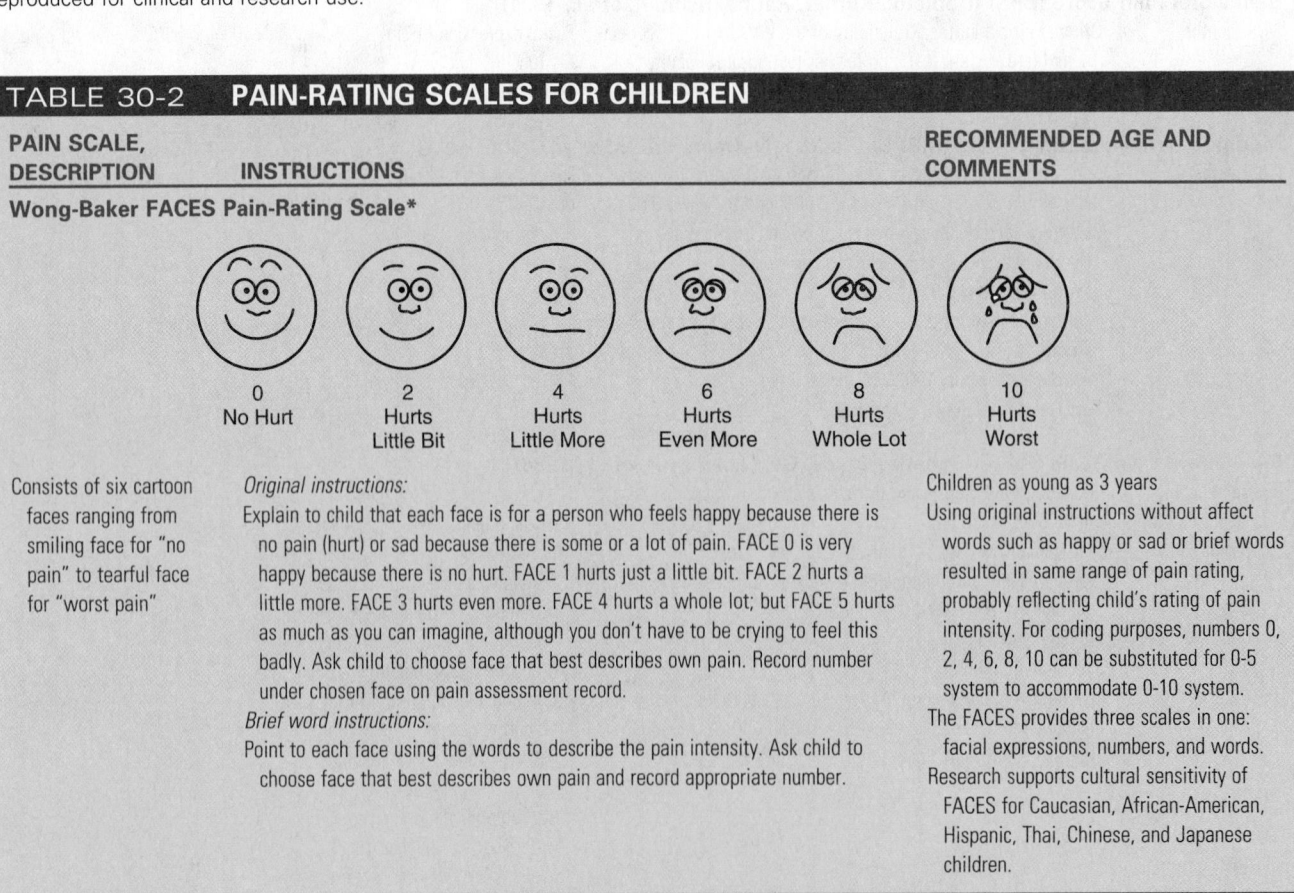

0	2	4	6	8	10
No Hurt	Hurts Little Bit	Hurts Little More	Hurts Even More	Hurts Whole Lot	Hurts Worst

| Consists of six cartoon faces ranging from smiling face for "no pain" to tearful face for "worst pain" | *Original instructions:*
 Explain to child that each face is for a person who feels happy because there is no pain (hurt) or sad because there is some or a lot of pain. FACE 0 is very happy because there is no hurt. FACE 1 hurts just a little bit. FACE 2 hurts a little more. FACE 3 hurts even more. FACE 4 hurts a whole lot; but FACE 5 hurts as much as you can imagine, although you don't have to be crying to feel this badly. Ask child to choose face that best describes own pain. Record number under chosen face on pain assessment record.
 Brief word instructions:
 Point to each face using the words to describe the pain intensity. Ask child to choose face that best describes own pain and record appropriate number. | Children as young as 3 years
 Using original instructions without affect words such as happy or sad or brief words resulted in same range of pain rating, probably reflecting child's rating of pain intensity. For coding purposes, numbers 0, 2, 4, 6, 8, 10 can be substituted for 0-5 system to accommodate 0-10 system.
 The FACES provides three scales in one: facial expressions, numbers, and words.
 Research supports cultural sensitivity of FACES for Caucasian, African-American, Hispanic, Thai, Chinese, and Japanese children. |

TABLE 30-2	**PAIN-RATING SCALES FOR CHILDREN—cont'd**	
PAIN SCALE, DESCRIPTION	**INSTRUCTIONS**	**RECOMMENDED AGE AND COMMENTS**

Oucher (Beyer, Denyes, and Villarruel, 1992)

Consists of six photographs of a Caucasian child's face representing "no hurt" to "biggest hurt you could ever have"; also includes vertical scale with numbers from 0 to 100; scales for African-American and Hispanic children have been developed (Villarruel and Denyes, 1991)	*Numeric scale:* Point to each section of scale to explain variations in pain intensity: "0 means no hurt." "This means little hurts" (pointing to lower part of scale, 1-29). "This means middle hurts" (pointing to middle part of scale, 30-69). "This means big hurts" (pointing to upper part of scale, 70-99). "100 means the biggest hurt you could ever have." Score is actual number stated by child. *Photographic scale:* Point to each photograph and explain variations in pain intensity using following language: first picture from bottom is "no hurt," second is "a little hurt," third is "a little more hurt," fourth is "even more hurt than that," fifth is "pretty much or a lot of hurt," and sixth is "biggest hurt you could ever have." Score pictures from 0 to 5, with bottom picture scored as 0. *General:* Practice using Oucher by recalling and rating previous pain experiences (e.g., falling off bike). Child points to number or photograph that describes pain intensity associated with experience. Obtain current pain score from child by asking, "How much hurt do you have right now?"	Children 3-13 years Use numeric scale if child can count of any two numbers or by tens (Jordan-Marsh, Yoder, Hall, et al., 1994). Determine whether child has cognitive ability to use photographic scale; child should be able to rate six geometric shapes from largest to smallest. Determine which ethnic version of Oucher to use. Allow child to select version of Oucher or use version that most closely matches physical characteristics of child. NOTE: Ethnically similar scale may not be preferred by child when given choice of ethnically neutral cartoon scale (Luffy and Grove, 2003).

Poker Chip Tool (Hester, Foster, Jordan-Marsh, et al., 1998)

Uses four red poker chips placed horizontally in front of child	Say to child: "I want to talk with you about the hurt you may be having right now." Align chips horizontally in front of child on bedside table, clipboard, or other firm surface. Tell child, "These are pieces of hurt." Beginning at chip nearest child's left side and ending at one nearest right side, point to chips and say, "This (first chip) is a little bit of hurt and this (fourth chip) is the most hurt you could ever have." For a young child or any child who may not fully comprehend the instructions, clarify by saying, "That means this (1) is just a little hurt, this (2) is a little more hurt, this (3) is more yet, and this (4) is the most hurt you could ever have." Do not give children an option for 0 hurt. Research with Poker Chip Tool has verified that children without pain will so indicate by responses such as, "I don't have any." Ask child, "How many pieces of hurt do you have right now?" After initial use of Poker Chip Tool, some children internalize the concept "pieces of hurt." If child gives response such as, "I have one right now," before you ask or lay out poker chips, record number of chips on Pain Flow Sheet. Clarify child's answer by statements such as, "Oh, you have a little hurt? Tell me about the hurt."	Children as young as 4 years Determine whether child has cognitive ability to use numbers by identifying larger of any two numbers.

Word-Graphic Rating Scale† (Tesler, Savedra, Holzemer, et al., 1991)

No pain	Little pain	Medium pain	Large pain	Worst possible pain

Uses descriptive words (may vary in other scales) to denote varying intensities of pain	Explain to child, "This is a line with words to describe how much pain you may have. This side of the line means no pain, and over here the line means worst possible pain." (Point with your finger where "no pain" is, and run it along the line to "worst possible pain" as you say it.) "If you have no pain, you would mark like this." (Show example.) "If you have some pain, you would mark somewhere along the line, depending on how much pain you have." (Show example.) "The more pain you have, the closer to worst pain you would mark. The worst pain possible is marked like this." (Show example.) "Show me how much pain you have right now by marking with a straight, up-and-down line anywhere along the line to show how much pain you have right now." With millimeter rule, measure from the "no pain" end to mark and record this measurement as pain score.	Children 4-17 years

Continued

TABLE 30-2   PAIN-RATING SCALES FOR CHILDREN—cont'd

PAIN SCALE, DESCRIPTION	INSTRUCTIONS	RECOMMENDED AGE AND COMMENTS

Numeric Scale

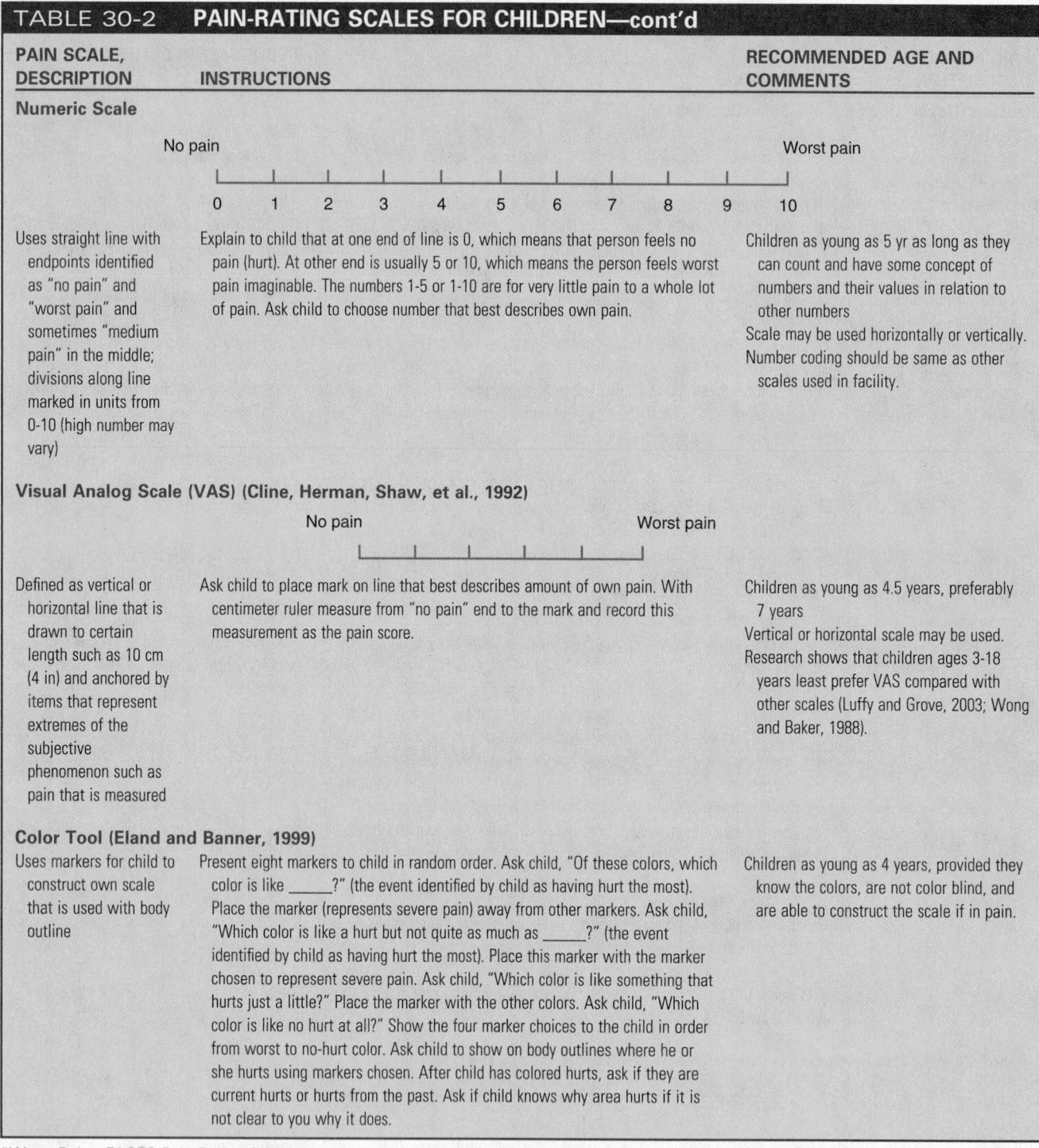

Uses straight line with endpoints identified as "no pain" and "worst pain" and sometimes "medium pain" in the middle; divisions along line marked in units from 0-10 (high number may vary)	Explain to child that at one end of line is 0, which means that person feels no pain (hurt). At other end is usually 5 or 10, which means the person feels worst pain imaginable. The numbers 1-5 or 1-10 are for very little pain to a whole lot of pain. Ask child to choose number that best describes own pain.	Children as young as 5 yr as long as they can count and have some concept of numbers and their values in relation to other numbers Scale may be used horizontally or vertically. Number coding should be same as other scales used in facility.

Visual Analog Scale (VAS) (Cline, Herman, Shaw, et al., 1992)

Defined as vertical or horizontal line that is drawn to certain length such as 10 cm (4 in) and anchored by items that represent extremes of the subjective phenomenon such as pain that is measured	Ask child to place mark on line that best describes amount of own pain. With centimeter ruler measure from "no pain" end to the mark and record this measurement as the pain score.	Children as young as 4.5 years, preferably 7 years Vertical or horizontal scale may be used. Research shows that children ages 3-18 years least prefer VAS compared with other scales (Luffy and Grove, 2003; Wong and Baker, 1988).

Color Tool (Eland and Banner, 1999)

Uses markers for child to construct own scale that is used with body outline	Present eight markers to child in random order. Ask child, "Of these colors, which color is like _____?" (the event identified by child as having hurt the most). Place the marker (represents severe pain) away from other markers. Ask child, "Which color is like a hurt but not quite as much as _____?" (the event identified by child as having hurt the most). Place this marker with the marker chosen to represent severe pain. Ask child, "Which color is like something that hurts just a little?" Place the marker with the other colors. Ask child, "Which color is like no hurt at all?" Show the four marker choices to the child in order from worst to no-hurt color. Ask child to show on body outlines where he or she hurts using markers chosen. After child has colored hurts, ask if they are current hurts or hurts from the past. Ask if child knows why area hurts if it is not clear to you why it does.	Children as young as 4 years, provided they know the colors, are not color blind, and are able to construct the scale if in pain.

*Wong-Baker FACES Pain Rating Scale reference manual describing development and research of the scale is available from City of Hope Pain/Palliative Care Resource Center, 1500 East Duarte Road, Duarte, CA 91010; (626) 359-8111, ext. 3829; fax (626) 301-8941; www.elsevierhealth.com/WOW/. Use of FACES with children is demonstrated in *Whaley and Wong's Pediatric Nursing Video Series*, "Pain Assessment and Management," narrated by Donna Wong, PhD, RN. Available from Elsevier, 3251 Riverport Lane, Maryland Heights, MO, 63043; (800) 426-4545; fax (800) 535-9935; www.elsevierhealth.com.

†Instructions for Word-Graphic Rating Scale from Acute Pain Management Guideline Panel: *Acute pain management in infants, children, and adolescents: operative and medical procedures;* quick reference guide for clinicians, ACHPR Pub No 92-0020, Rockville, MD, 1992, Agency for Health Care Research and Quality, US Department of Health and Human Services. Word-Graphic Rating Scale is part of the Adolescent Pediatric Pain Tool and is available from Pediatric Pain Study, University of California, School of Nursing, Department of Family Health Care Nursing, San Francisco, CA 94143-0606; (415) 476-4040.

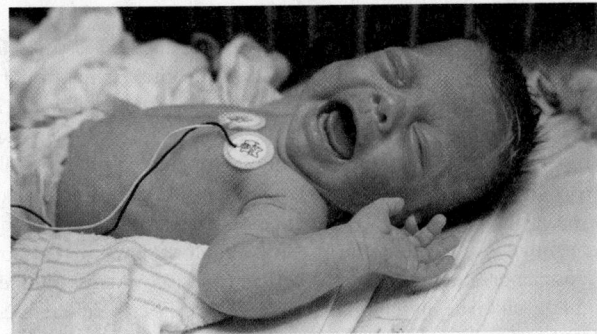

FIG 30-1 Full, robust crying of preterm infant after heelstick. (Courtesy Halbouty Premature Nursery, Texas Children's Hospital, Houston, TX; photo by Paul Vincent Kuntz.)

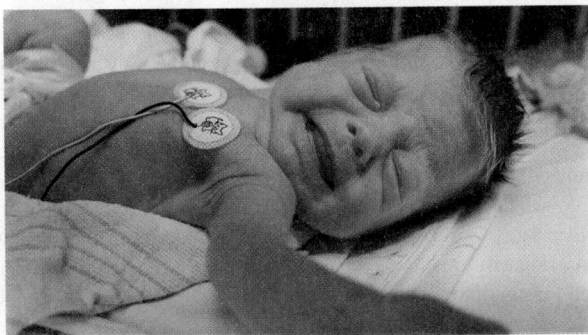

FIG 30-2 The face of pain after heelstick. Note eye squeeze, brow bulge, nasolabial furrow, and wide-spread mouth. (Courtesy Halbouty Premature Nursery, Texas Children's Hospital, Houston, TX; photo by Paul Vincent Kuntz.)

Behavioral measures are most reliable when measuring short, sharp procedural pain such as during injections or lumbar punctures and in infants. They are less reliable when measuring longer-lasting pain and in older children, when pain scores on behavioral measures do not always correlate with the children's own reports of pain intensity. Behavioral pain measures have been developed and validated on short, sharp pain or on pain in the recovery room immediately after arousal from anesthesia.

The most commonly used behavioral pain measure is the FLACC. The FLACC Pain Assessment Tool (Manworren and Hynan, 2003; Merkel, Voepel-Lewis, Shayevitz, et al., 1997) is an interval scale that includes five categories of behavior: facial expression (F), leg movement (L), activity (A), cry (C), and consolability (C). It measures pain by quantifying pain behaviors with scores ranging from 0 (no pain behaviors) to 10 (most possible pain behaviors). Other behavioral measures (see Table 30-1) include the (1) Children's Hospital of Eastern Ontario Pain Scale (CHEOPS), which was developed in collaboration with experienced recovery room nurses who were queried about which behaviors they most frequently observed to determine whether a child is in pain (McGrath, Johnson, Goodman, et al., 1985; Suraseranivongse, Montapaneewat T, Manon J, 2005); (2) Toddler-Preschooler Postoperative Pain Scale (TPPPS), which is an observational scale developed for measuring postoperative pain in children ages 1 to 5 years (Suraseranivongse, Montapaneewat T, Manon J, 2005; Tarbell, Cohen, and Marsh, 1992); (3) the Parent's Postoperative Pain Rating Scale (PPPRS), which is a scale that parents may use to rate their children's pain by noting changes in the frequency of a number of behaviors (Chambers, 2003;

BOX 30-1 DEVELOPMENTAL CHARACTERISTICS OF CHILDREN'S RESPONSES TO PAIN

Young Infant
- Generalized body response of rigidity or thrashing, possibly with local reflex withdrawal of stimulated area
- Loud crying
- Facial expression of pain (brows lowered and drawn together, eyes tightly closed, and mouth open and squarish)
- No association demonstrated between approaching stimulus and subsequent pain

Older Infant
- Localized body response with deliberate withdrawal of stimulated area
- Loud crying
- Facial expression of pain or anger
- Physical resistance, especially pushing stimulus away after it is applied

Young Child
- Loud crying, screaming
- Verbal expressions such as "Ow," "Ouch," "It hurts"
- Thrashing of arms and legs
- Attempts to push stimulus away before it is applied
- Lack of cooperation; need for physical restraint
- Requests termination of procedure
- Clings to parent, nurse, or other significant person
- Requests emotional support such as hugs or other forms of physical comfort
- May become restless and irritable with continuing pain
- Behaviors occurring in anticipation of actual painful procedure

School-Age Child
- May see all behaviors of young child, especially during actual painful procedure, but less in anticipatory period
- Stalling behavior such as, "Wait a minute" or "I'm not ready"
- Muscular rigidity such as clenched fists, white knuckles, gritted teeth, contracted limbs, body stiffness, closed eyes, wrinkled forehead

Adolescent
- Less vocal protest
- Less motor activity
- More verbal expressions such as, "It hurts" or "You're hurting me"
- Increased muscle tension and body control

Data from Craig KD, McMahon RJ, Morison JD, et al: Developmental changes in infant pain expression during immunization injections, *Soc Sci Med* 19(12):1331–1337, 1984; and Katz ER, Kellerman J, Siegel SE: Behavioral distress in children with cancer undergoing medical procedures: developmental considerations, *J Consult Clin Psychol* 48(3):356–365, 1980.

Chambers, Finley, McGrath, et al., 2003; Chambers and Craig, 1998; Finley, Chambers, and McGrath, et al., 2003); and (4) Parents' Postoperative Pain Measure (PPPM), which was developed based on cues parents reported observing in their children following surgery (e.g., changes in appetite, activity level).

In critical care settings the COMFORT scale (Ambuel, Hamlett, Marx, 1992) is recommended. The COMFORT scale is a behavioral, unobtrusive method of measuring distress in unconscious and ventilated patients. It has eight indicators: alertness, calmness/agitation, respiratory response, physical movement, blood pressure, heart rate, muscle tone, and facial tension. Each indicator is scored between 1 and 5 based on the behaviors exhibited by the patient. Patients are observed unobtrusively for 2 minutes, and the total score is derived by adding the scores of each indicator. The total scores can range between 8 and 40. A score of 17 to 26 generally indicates adequate sedation and pain control. Because of the complexity of measuring blood pressure and heart rate, this scale is used primarily for patients in a critical care setting.

For children 3 to 4 years the most frequently used measure of pain intensity is the Faces Pain Scale. There are many different "faces" scales. Faces scales provide a series of facial expressions depicting gradations of pain. They are appealing to children and easy to use because children can simply point to the face that represents how they feel. Two faces scales, the Bieri Faces Pain Scale—Revised (Hicks, von Baeyer CL, Spafford PA, et al., 2001) and the Wong-Baker FACES Pain Scale (Wong and Baker, 1988), are the most widely used. The Bieri scale is made up of six faces depicting increasing gradation of pain severity from 0 = "no pain" on the left face to 5 = "most pain possible" on the right face. In developing this scale the authors did not include a smiling face at the "no pain" end or tears at the "most pain" end and validated it so it is equivalent to a 0-to-10 metric system. The Wong-Baker FACES Pain Scale consists of six cartoon faces ranging from a smiling face for "no pain" to a tearful face for "worst pain." The child is asked to choose a face that describes his or her pain.

For children 8 years and older the numeric rating scale (NRS), specifically the 0-to-10 scale, is most widely used in clinical practice because it is easy to use and document. However, there is little research to support the reliability and validity of the NRS, except in the context of the Oucher Pain Scale (Beyer, Turner, Jones, 2005). The visual analog scale (VAS), a 10-centimeter line anchored by numbers or words *"no pain"* on the left, and *"worst pain"* on the right is another measure of pain intensity with established reliability and validity (Tesler, Savedra, and Holzemer, et al., 1991). It requires a higher degree of abstraction than the NRS, but it cannot be used in telephone follow-up.

Global Judgment of Improvement and of Satisfaction with Treatment

Although pain intensity is the dimension that is most commonly assessed, patients or patient surrogates should also be asked to rate a global judgment of satisfaction with pain treatment. The ratings mean something different from one patient or surrogate to another. Some may focus on the relief of pain; whereas others may consider side effects of the treatment. The global question should be posed with indications of what should be considered in the answer such as, "Considering pain relief, side effects, physical recovery, and emotional recovery, how satisfied were you with the treatments your child is receiving for pain?"

Adverse Events and Symptoms

After pain medications are initiated, not only should pain intensity be reassessed, but treatment-emergent adverse events should also be evaluated. Adverse events refer to newly emerging signs, symptoms, laboratory findings, or diseases that occur after medications for pain are initiated. Constipation is the most frequent symptom and is often not assessed, particularly for patients on prolonged opioid treatments. There is no particular strategy to measure either the occurrence or severity of the events. Children older than 10 years may be able to provide this information. In younger children parents or caregivers should be asked about adverse events and symptoms.

Physical Recovery

Another domain is physical recovery, which includes aspects of physical functioning that are influenced by the procedure or injury causing acute pain. For example, swallowing 50 mL of water is important after tonsillectomy. Possible assessments of the physical recovery domain include time to ambulation, time to resume swallowing, time to normal spirometry, oral intake, and time out of bed. However, measures such as tolerance of physical therapy may be inconsistent. One child may be intolerant of physical therapy because he or she did not want to go when asked, whereas another might be said to be intolerant to it only if he or she cried and refused to continue with it. These measures of physical recovery should be assessed systematically to evaluate interventions to control pain following procedures and injuries that have specific effects on physical functioning.

Emotional Response

The domain of emotional response includes all aspects of negative affect or distress secondary to pain such as anxiety, depression, fear, distress, dysphoria, or unhappiness. Behaviors indicating avoidance, withdrawal, or resistance need to be assessed. In children 8 years and older the PedIMMPACT group recommends the use of the Adolescent Pediatric Pain Tool (APPT) (Savedra, Holzemer, and Tesler, 1993), which allows children to describe the quality of the pain using a word list. The 56 words are grouped according to sensory, affective, and evaluative qualities of pain; it has been validated and can be used for children 8 years of age and over

Assessment of Chronic and Recurrent Pain

Pain that persists for 3 months or more or beyond the expected period of healing is defined as chronic pain (Merskey and Bogduk, 1994). Complex regional pain syndrome and chronic daily headache are the most common chronic pain conditions in children. Pain that is episodic and recurs is defined as *recurrent pain*. The time frame within which episodes of pain recur is at least 3 months. Recurrent pain in children includes migraine headache, episodic sickle cell pain, recurrent abdominal pain, and recurrent limb pain. van Dijk, McGrath, Pickett, et al (2006) reported that 57% of school-age children were having at least one recurrent pain (headaches, stomach pains, growing pains), and at least 6% had one or more chronic pain (disease related, back pain). Chronic and recurrent pain adversely affects the psychosocial and physical well-being of children. The domains for the assessment of chronic or recurrent pain are the same for acute pain (pain intensity global judgment of satisfaction with treatment, symptoms and adverse events, physical functioning, emotional functioning, economic factors) and two additional domains (role functioning and sleep). Because the time course of chronic and recurrent pain is different from that of acute pain, measures used to assess the impact of chronic and recurrent pain must consider timing and duration as key factors.

Pain diaries are commonly used to assess pain symptoms and response to treatment in children and adolescents with recurrent and chronic pain (Ely, Dampier, Gilday, et al., 2002; Dampier, Ely, Brodecki, et al., 2002a, 2002b; Palermo and Valenzuela, 2003; Palermo, Valenzuela, and Stork, 2004; Stinson, Stevens, Feldman, et al., 2008; Stone, Broderick, Schwartz, et al., 2003). Most pain diaries use NRSs or VASs with varying anchors such as faces scales or words. Children as young as 6 years have been included in diary studies. Conventional paper-and-pencil measures have been associated with several limitations such as poor compliance, missing data, hoarding responses, and back-and-forward filling (Palermo and Valenzuela, 2003; Stone, Broderick, Schwartz, et al., 2003). An increasing number of studies are converting paper diaries into electronic diaries for use in school-age children and adolescents with recurrent or chronic pain (Palermo, Valenzuela, and Stork, 2004; Stinson, Stevens, Feldman, et al., 2008; Stone, Broderick, Schwartz, et al., 2003). Electronic diaries were found to show higher accuracy of children's diary responses and higher compliance rates when compared to the paper format. However, electronic diaries are more expensive and may have a number of logistic issues that must be resolved.

The PedIMMPACT group recommends the same approach for measuring global judgment of satisfaction with treatment, symptoms, and adverse events. The physical functioning domain in chronic and recurrent pain is focused on activities of everyday life such as sitting or walking or more vigorous activities such as running and other sports. The recommendation is to use a measure such as the Functional Disability Inventory (Walker and Greene, 1991, No. 43) for assessing physical functioning in school-age children and adolescents. The Functional Disability Inventory assesses the child's ability to perform everyday physical activities and has established psychometric properties with different populations (Claar and Walker, 2006; Reid, Lang, and McGrath, 1997; Vervoort, Gougert, Eccleston, et al., 2006). For younger children (less than 7 years), the PedsQL developed by Varni, Seid, and Rode (1999) is recommended for assessing the physical functioning domain as it relates to pain. The PedsQL is a multidimensional scale with both parent- and child-report versions. It assesses (1) physical functioning, (2) emotional functioning, (3) social functioning, and (4) school functioning.

The emotional functioning domain most often refers to depression and anxiety because they are elevated in children with chronic and recurrent pain (Palermo, 2000). However, most of these children do not have clinical levels of anxiety or depression. The Children's Depression Inventory (Kovacs, 1981) and the Revised Child Anxiety and Depression Scale (Chorpita, Yim, and Moffitt, et al., 2000) have been used to assess anxiety and depression in children and adolescents with chronic or recurrent pain.

Chronic and recurrent pain can significantly interfere with the roles that children and adolescents perform such as being a student, friend, and family member. School attendance is used as a measure of role functioning in school-age children with chronic or recurrent pain. Absence from school is an important measure of fulfillment of the role of student. Other measures such as the PedsQL (Varni, Seid, and Rode, 1999) and PedMIDAS (Hershey, Powers, Vockell, et al., 2001; 2004) have been validated for measurement of role functioning in these children.

Sleep disruption is also common in chronic and recurrent pain. More than half of children with pain-related conditions (headache, juvenile idiopathic arthritis, or sickle cell disease) report difficulties sleeping (Walters and Williamson, 1999; Palermo and Kiska, 2005). Sleep diaries in which the child (or parent) keeps a record of the time to go to bed, fall asleep, and wake up are useful for assessment of pain interference with sleep. The sleep diary was validated with sleep actigraphy in healthy children ages 13 and 14 years (Gaina, Sekine, and Chen, 2004). In addition, the Sleep Habits Questionnaire (Owens, Spirito, McGuinn, 2000) may be useful for assessing sleep behaviors in school-age children with chronic or recurrent pain.

Multidimensional Measures

Several cognitive skills such as measurement, classification, and seriation (the ability to accurately place in ascending or descending order) become explicit between approximately 7 and 10 years of age.

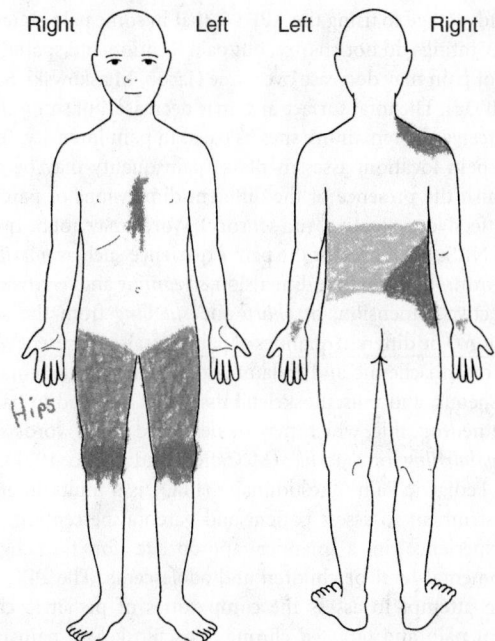

FIG 30-3 Adolescent Pediatric Pain Tool: body outlines for pain assessment. Instructions: "Color in the areas on these drawings to show where you have pain. Make the marks as big or as small as the place where the pain is." Tool has been completed by a child with sickle cell disease. (From Savedra MC, Tesler MD, Holzemer WL, Ward JA, School of Nursing, University of California–San Francisco; copyright 1989, 1992.)

Older children are able to use the 0-to-10 NRS that is currently used by adolescents and adults. However, the use of the 0-to-10 NRS is only an assessment of pain intensity, which may not change in some pain states (Jacob, Miaskowski, Savedra, et al., 2003a). Other dimensions such as pain quality, pain location, and spatial distribution of pain may change without a change in pain intensity.

Two multidimensional assessment tools that assess not only pain intensity but also pain location and pain quality have been well validated in children 8 years and older. Modeled after the McGill Pain Questionnaire (Melzack, 1975), the APPT is a multidimensional pain instrument for children and adolescents that is used to assess three dimensions of pain: location, intensity, and quality (Fig. 30-3). The APPT is a one-page, two-sided instrument with a front and back body outline on one side (Savedra, Tesler, Holzemer, et al., 1989; Savedra, Holzemer, Tesler, et al., 1993). On the back side is a 100-mm word-graphic rating scale (Tesler, Savedra, Holzemer, et al., 1991) and a pain descriptor list (Wilkie, Holzemer, Tesler, et al., 1990). Each of the three components of the APPT is scored separately. The body outline is scored by placing a clear plastic template overlay with 43 body areas on the body outline diagram. An estimate of the pervasiveness of the pain is made by counting the number of body areas marked. A ruler or micrometer preprinted on the APPT is used to score the word-graphic rating scale. The number of millimeters from the left side of the scale to the point marked by the child is measured; the numeric value provides an overall evaluation of the amount of pain the child is experiencing. The total number of words on the descriptor list is counted; scores range from 0 to 56. The clinician then counts the number of words selected in each of three categories—evaluative (0-8), sensory (0-37), and affective (0-11)—and calculates a percentage score for each one (Savedra, Holzemer, Tesler, et al., 1993).

An advantage to using the APPT is that in some pain states pain-intensity ratings do not change, but pain location and spatial distribution of pain may decrease over time (Jacob, Miaskowski, Savedra, et al., 2003a). The total surface area may decrease, but some children may perceive the remaining sites as equal in pain intensity. In addition to pain location, assessments of pain quality may be able to distinguish the presence of the different dimensions of pain (temporal, affective, evaluative, and sensory). Words may not be quantifiable on NRSs yet represent the pain experience such as *horrible* and *terrible* from the evaluative dimension, *screaming* and *terrifying* from the affective dimension, or *sharp* and *stabbing* from the sensory dimension. The different qualities of pain may also represent whether pain is of an ischemic and inflammatory nature in the cutaneous, subcutaneous, and musculoskeletal tissues, as opposed to pain that is more neuropathic, which may be described using words such as *shooting, burning,* or *shocklike* (McCaffery and Pasero, 1999).

The Pediatric Pain Questionnaire (PPQ) is a multidimensional pain instrument to assess patient and parental perceptions of the pain experience in a manner appropriate for the cognitive-developmental level of children and adolescents. The PPQ represents an attempt to assess the complexities of pediatric chronic, recurrent pain and targeted chronic musculoskeletal pain in children with juvenile rheumatoid arthritis. It consists of eight questions: (1) the pain history, (2) pain language, (3) the colors children associate with pain, (4) the emotions they experience, (5) their worst pain experiences, (6) the ways they cope with pain, (7) the positive aspects of pain, and (8) the location of their current pain. The PPQ includes three components: (1) VASs; (2) color-coded rating scales; and (3) verbal descriptors to provide information about the sensory, affective, and evaluative dimensions of chronic pain (Varni, Thompson, and Hanson, 1987). It also has information about the child's and family's pain history, symptoms, pain-relief interventions, and socioenvironmental situations that may influence pain. The child, parent, and health care provider complete the form separately.

The number of pain measures available for use in infants and young children has increased dramatically and adds a layer of complexity to the assessment of pain in children. The current trend supports a common metric for measurement of pain in children (von Baeyer and Hicks, 2000). Most instruments consist of 0 for no pain to a range of 4 to 160 for the top anchors in pain measures. A pain score of 5 may mean a lot of pain (if a 0 to 5 scale is used) or very little (if a 0 to 100 scale is used), and it may not be clearly specified which score corresponds to which scale. Other health care providers who do not specialize in pediatric pain may be confused by the available instruments and scoring methods and may not be able to determine the effectiveness of interventions by the pain score documented. An advantage to using a common metric is that a certain score may be considered as the point at which an intervention is required or a point at which relief may be considered adequate (von Baeyer and Hicks, 2000). The 0-to-10 system was reported to be preferred by health care providers and would make pain scores easier to read, interpret, and integrate into research and practice.

ASSESSMENT OF PAIN IN SPECIFIC POPULATIONS

Children with Communication and Cognitive Impairment

The assessment of pain in children with communication and cognitive impairment can be challenging. Children who have significant difficulties in communicating with others about their pain include those with significant neurologic impairments (e.g., cerebral palsy), intellectual disability, metabolic disorders, autism, severe brain injury, and communication barriers (e.g., critically ill children who are on ventilators or heavily sedated or have neuromuscular disorders, loss of hearing, or loss of vision). These children are at greater risk than other children for undertreatment of pain because they have medical problems that may cause pain and they undergo painful procedures. Their behaviors include moaning, inconsistent patterns of play and sleep, changes in facial expression, and other physical problems that may mask expression of pain and be difficult to interpret (Hadden and von Baeyer, 2002). These children often experience spasticity, contractures, and orthopedic surgical treatment that may be painful.

The mother or primary caregiver is an important source of information during assessment (Breau, MacLaren, McGrath, et al., 2003). As many as 60% of parents of children with severe cognitive impairment reported that their child experienced pain or severe discomfort that was not being managed effectively (Lenton, Stallard, Lewis, et al., 2001; Stallard, Williams, Velleman, et al., 2002). The most frequently reported pain behaviors are crying; being less active; seeking comfort; moaning; not cooperating; being irritable; being stiff, spastic, tense, or rigid; sleeping less; being difficult to satisfy or pacify; flinching or moving body part away; and being agitated or fidgety (Hadden and von Baeyer, 2002). Parents also reported that some daily living activities were painful such as assisted stretching and walking, independent standing, toileting, putting on splints, occupational therapy, range of motion, and physical therapy.

Stallard, Williams, Lenton, et al. (2001) asked the parents of cognitively impaired and noncommunicative children to assess the presence, severity, and duration of their pain during a 2-week observation period. Parents reported that 84% experienced pain on 5 or more separate days, with 32% experiencing pain on 12 or more days. Of the 74 episodes that lasted longer than 30 minutes, 33.8% occurred at night. Most pain episodes were judged to last longer than 10 minutes, with 48% of the children having episodes lasting longer than 10 minutes on 5 or more days. Although the experience of pain was common among this group of children, none was receiving treatment for relief or management of pain.

The Non-communicating Children's Pain Checklist is a pain measurement tool specifically designed for children with cognitive impairments (Breau, McGrath, Camfield, et al., 2002). The scale discriminates between periods of pain and calm and can predict behavior during subsequent episodes of pain (Fig. 30-4). The scale consists of six subscales (vocal, social, facial, activity, body and limbs, physiologic signs), which are scored based on the number of times the items are observed over a 10-minute period (0 = not at all, 1 = just a little, 2 = fairly often, 3 = very often).

Another tool, the Pain Indicator for Communicatively Impaired Children (PICIC), distinguishes between pain and nonpain in communicatively impaired children with life-threatening illness (Stallard, Williams, Velleman, et al., 2002). The PICIC has six core pain cues: (1) crying with or without tears; (2) screaming, yelling, groaning, or moaning; (3) screwed up or distressed looking face; (4) body appearing stiff or tense; (5) difficulty in comforting or consoling; and (6) flinching or moving away if touched. The items are rated using a 4-point Likert scale (1 = not at all, 2 = a little, 3 = often, 4 = all the time).

Cultural Differences

Several barriers to effective pain treatment in non-English speaking patients have been documented and include inadequate assessment

Non-communicating Children's Pain Checklist — Postoperative Version (NCCPC-PV)

NAME:_____ UNIT/FILE #:_____ DATE:_____ (dd/mm/yy)

OBSERVER:_____ START TIME:_____ AM/PM STOP TIME:_____ AM/PM

How often has this child shown these behaviors in the last 10 minutes? Please circle a number for each behavior. If an item does not apply to this child (for example, this child cannot reach with his/her hands), then indicate "not applicable" for that item.

0 = NOT AT ALL	1 = JUST A LITTLE	2 = FAIRLY OFTEN	3 = VERY OFTEN	NA = NOT APPLICABLE

I. Vocal

	0	1	2	3	NA
1. Moaning, whining, whimpering (fairly soft)	0	1	2	3	NA
2. Crying (moderately loud)	0	1	2	3	NA
3. Screaming/yelling (very loud)	0	1	2	3	NA
4. A specific sound or word for pain (e.g., a word, cry, or type of laugh)	0	1	2	3	NA

II. Social

	0	1	2	3	NA
5. Not cooperating, cranky, irritable, unhappy	0	1	2	3	NA
6. Less interaction with others, withdrawn	0	1	2	3	NA
7. Seeking comfort or physical closeness	0	1	2	3	NA
8. Being difficult to distract, not able to satisfy or pacify	0	1	2	3	NA

III. Facial

	0	1	2	3	NA
9. A furrowed brow	0	1	2	3	NA
10. A change in eyes, including squinching of eyes, eyes opened wide, eyes frowning	0	1	2	3	NA
11. Turning down of mouth, not smiling	0	1	2	3	NA
12. Lips puckering up, tight, pouting, or quivering	0	1	2	3	NA
13. Clenching or grinding teeth, chewing, or thrusting tongue out	0	1	2	3	NA

IV. Activity

	0	1	2	3	NA
14. Not moving, less active, quiet	0	1	2	3	NA
15. Jumping around, agitated, fidgety	0	1	2	3	NA

V. Body and Limbs

	0	1	2	3	NA
16. Floppy	0	1	2	3	NA
17. Stiff, spastic, tense, rigid	0	1	2	3	NA
18. Gesturing to or touching part of the body that hurts	0	1	2	3	NA
19. Protecting, favoring, or guarding part of the body that hurts	0	1	2	3	NA
20. Flinching or moving the body part away, being sensitive to touch	0	1	2	3	NA
21. Moving the body in a specific way to show pain (e.g., head back, arms down, curls up, etc.)	0	1	2	3	NA

VI. Physiologic

	0	1	2	3	NA
22. Shivering	0	1	2	3	NA
23. Change in color, pallor	0	1	2	3	NA
24. Sweating, perspiring	0	1	2	3	NA
25. Tears	0	1	2	3	NA
26. Sharp intake of breath, gasping	0	1	2	3	NA
27. Breath holding	0	1	2	3	NA

SCORE SUMMARY

Category	I	II	III	IV	V	VI	TOTAL
Score							

FIG 30-4 Non-communicating Children's Pain Checklist. (Copyright 2004, Lynn Breau, Patrick McGrath, Allen Finley, and Carol Camfield. Reprinted with permission.)

Continued

USING THE NCCPC-PV

The NCCPC-PV was designed to be used for children age 3 to 18 years who are unable to speak because of cognitive (mental/intellectual) impairments or disabilities. It can be used *whether or not* a child has physical impairments or disabilities. Descriptions of the types of children used to validate the NCCPC-PV can be found in: Breau, L.M., Finley, G.A., McGrath, P.J., & Camfield, C.S. (2002). Validation of the Non-communicating Children's Pain Checklist — Postoperative Version. *Anesthesiology, 96* (3), 528-535. The NCCPC-PV was designed to be used without training by parents and caregivers (carers), or by other adults who are not familiar with a specific child (do not know them well).

The NCCPC-PV may be freely copied for clinical use or use in research funded by not-for-profit agencies. For-profit agencies should contact Lynn Breau: Pediatric Pain Research, IWK Health Centre, 5850 University Avenue, Halifax, Nova Scotia, Canada, B3J 3G9 (lbreau@ns.sympatico.ca).

The NCCPC-PV was intended for use for pain after surgery or due to other procedures conducted in hospital. If short- or long-term pain is suspected for a child at home or in a long-term residential setting, the **Non-communicating Children's Pain Checklist — Revised** may be used. It can be obtained by contacting Lynn Breau. Information regarding the NCCPC-R can be found in: Breau, L.M., McGrath, P.J., Camfield, C.S. & Finley, G.A. (2002). Psychometric Properties of the Non-communicating Children's Pain Checklist—Revised. *Pain, 99,* 349-357.

ADMINISTRATION

To complete the NCCPC-R, base your observations on the child's behavior over **10 minutes**. *It is not necessary to watch the child continuously for this period*. However, it is recommended that the observer be in the child's presence for the majority of this time (e.g., be in the same room with the child). Although shorter observation periods may be used, the cut-off scores described below may not apply.

At the end of the observation time, indicate how frequently (how often) each item was seen or heard. This should not be based on the child's typical behavior or in relation to what he or she usually does. A guide for deciding the frequency of items is below:

> 0 = Not present at all during the observation period. (Note: If the item is not present because the child is not capable of performing that act, it should be scored as "NA").
> 1 = Seen or heard rarely (hardly at all), but is present.
> 2 = Seen or heard a number of times, but not continuous (not all the time).
> 3 = Seen or heard often, almost continuous (almost all the time); anyone would easily notice this if they saw the child for a few moments during the observation time.
> NA = Not applicable. This child is not capable of performing this action.

SCORING

1. Add up the scores for each subscale and enter below that subscale number in the Score Summary at the bottom of the sheet. Items marked "NA" are scored as "0" (zero).
2. Add up all subscale scores for Total Score.
3. Check whether the child's score is greater than the cut-off score.

CUT-OFF SCORE

Based on the scores of 24 children age 3 to 18 (Breau, Finley, McGrath, & Camfield, 2002), a **Total Score of 11 or more** indicates a child has **moderate to severe pain**. Based on unpublished data from this same sample, a *Total score of 6-10* indicates a child has **mild pain**. When parents and caregivers completed the NCCPC-PV in hospital for the study group, this was accurate 88% of the time. When other observers completed the NCCPC-PV, this was accurate 75% of the time. A Total Score of 10 or less indicates less than moderate/severe pain. This was correct in the study group for parents and caregivers 81% of the time and for other observers 63% of the time.

USE OF CUT-OFF SCORES

As with all observational tools, caution should be taken in using cut-off scores, because they may not be 100% accurate. They should not be used as the only basis for deciding whether a child should be treated for pain. In some cases children may have lower scores when pain is present. For more detailed instructions for use of the NCCPC-PV in such situations, please refer to the full manual, available from Lynn Breau: Pediatric Pain Research, IWK Health Centre, 5850 University Avenue, Halifax, Nova Scotia, Canada, B3J 3G9 (lbreau@ns.sympatico.ca).

FIG 30-4, cont'd

of pain, concern about side effects of and tolerance to analgesics, patient and family reluctance to report pain, fear that pain means worse disease, reluctance to take pain medications, and lack of adherence to prescribed analgesics (Abbe, Simon, Angiolilo, et al., 2006; Bruera, Willey, Ewert-Flannagan, et al., 2005; Flores and Vega, 1998; Flores, Abreu, Olivar, et al., 1998). Non-English speaking patients pose additional language and cultural barriers that make pain assessment and treatments more challenging.

A major challenge in the assessment and management of pain in children is the cultural appropriateness of pain assessment tools that has been validated only in Caucasian and English-speaking children. Observational scales and interview questionnaires for pain may not be as reliable for pain assessment as self-report scales in Hispanic children. In Chinese children who learned to read Chinese characters vertically downward and from right to left, the use of vertically oriented VASs resulted in less error than horizontally oriented scales. Therefore cultural background may influence the reliability of pain assessment tools developed in a single cultural context (Bernstein and Pachter, 2003).

The Oucher Pain Scale (see Table 30-2), originally developed and validated as a self-report of pain intensity for Caucasian children 3 to 12 years old, now features culturally specific photographs with pictures of children who more closely match the physical characteristics of children (Beyer and Knott, 1998). The Oucher consists of a 0-to-10 numeric scale for older children and a six-picture photographic scale for younger children. The five versions of the Oucher are: (1) White or Caucasian, (2) Black or African-American, (3) Hispanic, (4) First Nations (boy and girl), and Asian (boy and girl). They can be downloaded free of charge at www.oucher.org, and include instructions and information related to validity and reliability.

The APPT also has a Spanish version (Van Cleve, Munoz, Bossert, et al., 2001) that has been used in children and adolescents with cancer (Jacob, McCarthy, Sambuco, et al., 2008; Van Cleve, Bossert, Beecroft, et al., 2004). Jacob, McCarthy, and Sambuco et al. (2008) examined the pain experience of Spanish-speaking children with cancer who were asked about their pain during the week before a scheduled oncology clinic appointment. They found that 41% of the patients were experiencing pain. Some were experiencing moderate-to-severe pain and did not receive medications because they were not reporting their pain. The APPT has a body outline that may be useful for non-English speaking children to communicate the location and extensiveness of the pain. To minimize the risk of undertreatment of pain, non-English speaking children and adolescents may be given the body outline diagram of the APPT, and clinicians may encourage them to use the body outline diagram for communicating pain (Jacob, McCarthy, Sambuco, et al., 2008).

Children with Chronic Illness and Complex Pain

Questionnaires and pain assessment scales do not always provide the most meaningful means of assessing pain in children, particularly for those with complex pain. Some children cannot relate to a face or number that describes their pain and may not be able to isolate pain from other concurrent symptoms they are experiencing. Experiencing multiple symptoms makes the task of having to isolate the pain symptom from other symptoms difficult in children with cancer. Rating the pain does not always accurately convey to others how they really feel (Woodgate and Yanofsky, 2004).

In children with chronic illness, particularly those with complex pain, the most important aspect of the assessment is the relationship developed between the child and the family; and it is in developing this relationship that the pain team gets the sense of what the pain experience is like for the child and family. The pain experience may interfere with the child's ability to eat, sleep, and perform daily activities and routines (Miaskowski and Lee, 1999; Morin, Gibson, and Wade, 1998). It may also be complicated by pain processes that occur in the central nervous system (e.g., hyperalgesia, central sensitization, windup), by other symptoms (e.g., fatigue, nausea, vomiting, diarrhea, constipation) that accompany medical treatments, and by complications (e.g., infections, unexpected development of fistulas, typhlitis) from disease or treatments.

Other important questions to ask the family include the (1) onset of pain (i.e., was the onset sudden, unexpected, off and on, ongoing);

(2) pain duration or pattern (i.e., when did the pain start; how long does it last); (3) the effectiveness of the current treatment (i.e., which medications and doses help; what other strategies have you tried that work); (4) factors that aggravate or relieve the pain (i.e., which situations, positions, events, or activities make the pain worse, what makes the pain better); (5) other symptoms (e.g., nausea) and complications (e.g., fever, difficulty with breathing) that occur concurrently; and (6) interference with the child's sleep, mood, function, and interactions with family (McCaffery and Pasero, 1999). Asking if the pain is better or worse at certain times during the day or night can also assess variations and rhythms of pain. Other aspects warranting careful assessment that may pose barriers to effective management include family issues and relationships, fears and concerns about addictions (see Community Focus box), the clinician's and family's lack of knowledge about pain, inappropriate use of pain medications, ineffective management of adverse effects from medications, and the use of different modalities (McCaffery and Pasero, 1999).

🏠 COMMUNITY FOCUS

Fear of Opioid Addiction

One of the reasons for the unfounded but prevalent fear of addiction from opioids used to relieve pain is a misunderstanding of the differences between physical dependence, tolerance, and addiction. Health care professionals and the community often confuse addiction with the physiologic effects of opioids, when in reality these three events are unrelated.

The American Society of Addiction Medicine defines these three terms as follows:

Physical dependence on an opioid is a physiologic state in which abrupt cessation of the opioid, or administration of an opioid antagonist, results in a withdrawal syndrome. Physical dependence on opioids is an expected occurrence in all individuals in the presence of continuous use of opioids for therapeutic or nontherapeutic purposes. It does not, in and of itself, imply addiction.

Tolerance is a form of neuroadaptation to the effects of chronically administered opioids (or other medications) that is indicated by the need for increasing or more frequent doses of the medication to achieve the initial effects of the drug. A person may develop tolerance both to the analgesic effects of opioids and to some of the unwanted side effects such as respiratory depression, sedation, or nausea. Tolerance varies in occurrence, but it does not, in and of itself, imply addiction.

Addiction in the context of pain treatment with opioids is characterized by a persistent pattern of dysfunctional opioid use that may involve any or all of the following:

- Adverse consequences associated with the use of opioids
- Loss of control over the use of opioids
- Preoccupation with obtaining opioids, despite the presence of adequate analgesia

Nurses must educate older children, parents, and health professionals about the extremely low risk of real addiction (less than 1%) from the use of opioids to treat pain. Infants, young children, and comatose or terminally ill children simply cannot become addicted because they are incapable of a consistent pattern of drug-seeking behavior such as stealing, drug dealing, prostitution, and use of family income to obtain opioids for nonanalgesic reasons.

Data from American Society of Addiction Medicine: *Public policy statement on definitions related to the use of opioids for pain treatment, 2001,* www.asam.org.

PAIN MANAGEMENT

Unrelieved pain may lead to potential long-term physiologic, psychosocial, and behavioral consequences (Goldschneider and Anand, 2003; Weisman, Bernstein, and Schechter, 1998). Management of pain should be a priority for all clinicians.

Nonpharmacologic Management

Pain is often associated with fear, anxiety, and stress. A number of nonpharmacologic techniques (see Guidelines box) such as distraction, relaxation, guided imagery, and cutaneous stimulation provide coping strategies that may help reduce pain perception, make pain more tolerable, decrease anxiety, and enhance the effectiveness of analgesics or reduce the dosage required (Rusy and Weisman, 2000). In addition, these techniques decrease the perceived threat of pain, provide a sense of control, enhance comfort, and promote rest and sleep (McCaffery and Pasero, 1999). Although there is a paucity of research on the effectiveness of many of these interventions, the strategies are safe, noninvasive, and inexpensive; and most are independent nursing functions. Environmental and psychologic factors may exert a powerful influence on children's pain perceptions and may be modified by using psychosocial strategies, education, parental support, and cognitive behavioral interventions. For children undergoing repeated painful procedures, cognitive-behavioral interventions are effective for decreasing anxiety and distress (McGrath and Hillier, 2003).

If the child cannot identify a familiar coping technique, the nurse can describe several strategies and let him or her select the most appealing one. Experimentation with several strategies that are suitable to the child's age, pain intensity, and abilities is often necessary to determine the most effective approach. Parents should be involved in the selection process; they may be familiar with the child's usual coping skills and can help identify potentially successful strategies. Involving parents also encourages their participation in learning the skill with the child and acting as coach. If the parent cannot help the child, other appropriate people may include a grandparent, older sibling, nurse, or child-life specialist (McGrath and Hillier, 2003).

Children should learn to use a specific strategy before pain occurs or becomes severe. To reduce the child's effort, instructions for a strategy such as distraction or relaxation can be audiotaped and played during a period of comfort. However, even after they have learned an intervention, children often need help using it during a painful procedure. The intervention can also be used after the procedure. This gives the child a chance to recover, feel mastery, and cope more effectively (McGrath and Hillier, 2003).

Several studies have documented the effectiveness of nonpharmacologic analgesia such as containment, positioning, nonnutritive sucking (Fig. 30-5), and kangaroo holding in neonates during painful procedures. Containment is achieved through positioning and blanket rolls (Cole and Jorgensen, 1997). It provides a "nest" that enhances the infant's feelings of security and decreases stress. Comforting measures and swaddling have been demonstrated to reduce crying and heart rate after procedures such as heel punctures and injections. Infants between 27 and 34 weeks of gestational age who were swaddled after a routine heelstick procedure were able to calm crying immediately, decrease heart rate, and return to a sleep state; in comparison, infants who were not swaddled took a minimum of 10 minutes to return to baseline physiologic and behavioral levels (Fearon, Kisilevsky, Hains, et al., 1997). Proper positioning with the infant held in a midline orientation, hand-to-mouth activity, and proper flexion can promote self-soothing behaviors. "Facilitated tucking," which is holding the infant's

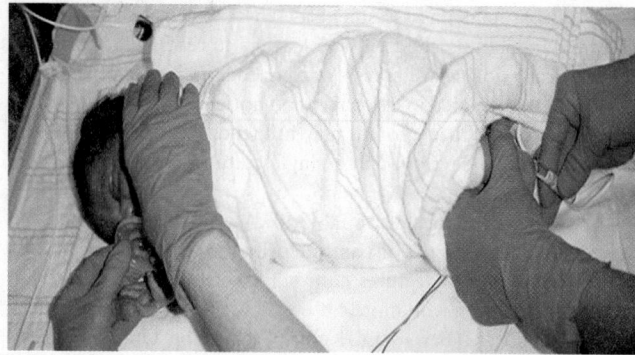

FIG 30-5 Sucking following oral sucrose can enhance analgesia before a heelstick in a preterm infant.

extremities flexed and contained close to the trunk, during heel lance procedures has been demonstrated to decrease heart rate, decrease crying time, and promote stability in the sleep-wake cycles after the lance.

Nonnutritive sucking (pacifier) attenuates behavioral, physiologic, and hormonal responses to pain from procedures such as heel punctures, venipuncture, and immunization injections. The administration of concentrated sucrose with and without nonnutritive sucking has been demonstrated to have calming and pain-relieving effects for invasive procedures in neonates (see Evidence-Based Practice box). The amount of time crying was decreased with 0.24 to 0.48 g (0.008 to 0.17 oz; 2 mL) of a 12% to 24% sucrose solution administered orally 2 minutes before a heel lance or venipuncture (Stevens, Yamada, and Ohlsson, 2005). The use of multimodal therapy, such as sucrose in combination with swaddling or nonnutritive sucking, is recommended to manage pain in neonates undergoing minor painful procedures such as heel punctures and circumcision.

Kangaroo care is a skin-to-skin holding of infants dressed only in diapers against their mother's or father's chest (Gray, Watt, and Blass, 2000; Johnston, Stevens, Pinelli, et al., 2003). Infants who spent 1-to-3 hours in kangaroo care showed increased frequency in quiet sleep, longer duration of quiet sleep, and decreased crying in the neonatal intensive care unit (NICU); and they cried less at the age of 6 months when compared with neonates who did not receive skin-to-skin contact. Significant differences were found in pain responses during heel lancing between infants who were kangaroo held and those who were not. In the study by Gray, Watt, and Blass (2000), heart rate increased by 8-to-10 beats/min in the kangaroo care group versus 36-to-38 beats/min in the control group of neonates who were swaddled in bassinets; grimacing was 64% less, and crying was 82% less. In another study infant responses to pain during heel lance procedures were compared using kangaroo holding (Fig. 30-6) with the neonate held upright at a 60-degree angle between the mother's breasts for maximal skin-to-skin contact (Johnston, Stevens, Pinelli, et al., 2003). A blanket was placed over the neonate's back, and the mother's clothes were wrapped around the neonate for 30 minutes before the lancing procedure, during, and at least 30 minutes after the heelstick. Another group remained in the isolette in a prone position, swaddled with a blanket and the heel accessible, for 30 minutes before the heel lancing procedure. Pain scores were significantly lower in kangaroo-held infants.

Many terms are used to describe approaches to health care that are outside the realm of conventional medicine as practiced in the United States. Complementary and alternative medicine (CAM), as

GUIDELINES

Nonpharmacologic Strategies for Pain Management

General Strategies

- Prepare child before potentially painful procedures but avoid "planting" the idea of pain.
  - For example, instead of saying, "This is going to (or may) hurt," say, "Sometimes this feels like pushing, sticking, or pinching, and sometimes it doesn't bother people. Tell me what it feels like to you."
  - Use "nonpain" descriptors when possible (e.g., "It feels like heat" rather than "It's a burning pain"). This allows for variation in sensory perception, avoids suggesting pain, and gives child control in describing reactions.
  - Avoid evaluative statements or descriptions (e.g., "This is a terrible procedure" or "It really will hurt a lot").
- Stay with child during a painful procedure.
  - Allow parents to stay with child if child and parent desire; encourage parent to talk softly to child and remain near child's head.
- Educate child about the pain, especially when explanation may lessen anxiety (e.g., that pain may occur after surgery and does not indicate that something is wrong); reassure child that he or she is not responsible for the pain.
- For long-term pain control give child a doll, which represents "the patient," and allow him or her to do everything to the doll that is done to the child; pain control can be emphasized through the doll by stating, "Dolly feels better after the medicine."

Specific Strategies

Distraction

- Involve child in play; use radio, tape recorder, CD player, or computer game; have child sing or use rhythmic breathing.
- Have child take a deep breath and blow it out until told to stop.
- Have child blow bubbles to "blow the hurt away."
- Have child concentrate on yelling or saying "ouch," with instructions to "yell as loud or soft as you feel it hurt; that way I know what's happening."
- Have child look through kaleidoscope (type with glitter suspended in fluid-filled tube) and encourage him or her to concentrate by asking, "Do you see the different designs?"
- Use humor such as watching cartoons, telling jokes or funny stories, or acting silly with child.
- Have child read, play games, or visit with friends.

Relaxation

- With an infant or young child:
  - Hold in a comfortable, well-supported position such as vertically against the chest and shoulder.
  - Rock in a wide, rhythmic arc in a rocking chair or sway back and forth rather than bouncing child.
  - Repeat one or two words softly such as "Mommy's here."
- With a slightly older child:
  - Ask child to take a deep breath and "go limp as a rag doll" while exhaling slowly; then ask him or her to yawn (demonstrate if needed).
  - Help child assume a comfortable position (e.g., pillow under neck and knees).
  - Begin progressive relaxation: starting with the toes, systematically instruct child to let each body part "go limp" or "feel heavy"; if child

has difficulty relaxing, instruct him or her to tense or tighten each body part and then relax it.
  - Allow child to keep eyes open, since children may respond better if eyes are open rather than closed during relaxation.

Guided Imagery

- Have child identify some highly pleasurable real or imaginary experience.
- Have child describe details of the event, including as many senses as possible (e.g., "feel the cool breezes," "see the beautiful colors," "hear the pleasant music").
- Have child write down or tape record script.
- Encourage child to concentrate only on the pleasurable event during the painful time; enhance the image by recalling specific details through reading the script or playing the tape.
- Combine with relaxation and rhythmic breathing.

Positive Self-Talk

- Teach child positive statements to say when in pain (e.g., "I'll be feeling better soon," "When I go home, I'll feel better, and we'll eat ice cream").

Thought Stopping

- Identify positive facts about the painful event (e.g., "It doesn't last long").
- Identify reassuring information (e.g., "If I think about something else, it doesn't hurt as much").
- Condense positive and reassuring facts into a set of brief statements and have child memorize them (e.g., "Short procedure, good veins, little hurt, nice nurse, go home").
- Have child repeat the memorized statements whenever thinking about or experiencing the painful event.

Behavioral Contracting

- Informal—May be used with children as young as 4 or 5 years of age:
  - Use stars, tokens, or cartoon character stickers as rewards.
  - Give child who is uncooperative or procrastinating during a procedure a limited time (measured by a visible timer) to complete the procedure.
  - Proceed as needed if child is unable to comply.
  - Reinforce cooperation with a reward if the procedure is accomplished within specified time.
- Formal—Use written contract, which includes:
  - Realistic (seems possible) goal or desired behavior.
  - Measurable behavior (e.g., agrees not to hit anyone during procedures).
  - Contract written, dated, and signed by all people involved in any of the agreements.
  - Identified rewards or consequences that are reinforcing.
  - Goals that can be evaluated.
  - Commitment and compromise requirements for both parties (e.g., while timer is used, nurse will not nag or prod child to complete procedure).

EVIDENCE-BASED PRACTICE

Reduction of Minor Procedural Pain in Infants

Ask the Question

In newborns and infants, does sucrose provide adequate analgesia during minor painful procedures? Are the effects age dependent?

Search for the Evidence
Search Strategies

Search selection criteria included English publications within the past 10 years, research-based articles (level 1 or lower) on neonates or infants undergoing venipuncture or immunizations.

Databases Used

PubMed, Cochrane Collaboration, MD Consult, Joanna Briggs Institute, National Guideline Clearinghouse (AHQR), TRIP Database Plus, PedsCCM, BestBETs

Critically Analyze the Evidence

Studies evaluated whether sucrose provides adequate analgesia for minor painful procedures.

Venipuncture vs. Heel Lance for Blood Sampling

- Venipuncture performed by skilled phlebotomists results in less pain than heelstick for blood sampling (Shah and Ohlsson, 2004).
- Decreased pain scores, cry duration, and mother's rating of infant's pain demonstrated venipuncture as the preferred method of blood collection (Shah and Ohlsson, 2004).
- Infants receiving heelstick may also require more than one stick to get enough for the sample; venipuncture reduces the risk of additional sticks (Shah and Ohlsson, 2004).

Glucose vs. EMLA cream for venipuncture in neonates

- 30% oral glucose and placebo on the skin group had significantly lower Premature Infant Pain Profile (PIPP) scores and duration of crying than the EMLA (lidocaine and prilocaine) and oral placebo group (Gradin, Lenclen, Gajdos, et al., 2002).
- Fewer patients in the glucose group were scored on the PIPP as having pain or a score above 6 (19.3% compared with 41.7%) (Gradin, Lenclen, Gajdos, et al., 2002).

Glucose compared with EMLA for venipuncture pain

- Combination of EMLA and 1 mL oral glucose (300 mg/mL) significantly reduced pain response associated with diphtheria-pertussis-tetanus immunizations in 3-month-old infants (Lindh, Wiklund, Blomquist, et al., 2003).

Sucrose for minor painful procedures (heel lance and venipuncture)

- A total of 150 full-term newborns were randomly assigned to one of six treatment groups: (1) no treatment, (2) 2 mL of sterile water placebo, (3) 2 mL of 30% glucose, (4) 2 mL of 30% sucrose, (5) 2 mL of 30% sucrose with pacifier, and (6) pacifier alone. The pacifier alone was more effective than sweet solutions; sweet solutions and the pacifier were significantly more effective than the placebo; and sucrose and glucose were equally effective in lowering pain scores (Carbajal, Chauvet, Couderc, et al., 1999).
- Behavioral state, difficulty, and duration of venipuncture were not significantly different between 2 mL of a placebo of sterile water or 25% sucrose slowly over 2 minutes into the mouth by syringe 4 minutes before

venipunctures. Heart rate, crying times, and neonatal facial coding system scores were significantly lower in the treatment group (25% sucrose) (Acharya, Annamali, Taub, et al., 2004).
- A 2-mL amount of 24% sucrose solution alone was the most effective analgesic compared with placebo (spring water), EMLA, or EMLA combined with 2 mL of sucrose. The combination of EMLA and sucrose did not enhance the analgesic effects (Abad, Diaz-Gomez, Domenech, et al., 2001).
- Sucrose in a wide variety of dosages delivered by syringe or pacifier was found to decrease crying time, heart rate, facial action, and composite pain scores during venipuncture and heel lance (Stevens, Yamada, and Ohlsson, 2005).
- Use of sucrose in a range of 0.012 to 0.12 g (0.05 to 0.5 mL) of a 24% solution 2 minutes before a single heel lance or venipuncture is safe and effective for pain relief (Stevens, Yamada, and Ohlsson, 2005).
- Concomitant use of other methods of pain relief, including use of pacifier, rocking, kangaroo care, or holding along with sucrose intervention, is recommended (Stevens, Yamada, and Ohlsson, 2005).

Apply the Evidence: Nursing Implications

There is *good evidence* with *strong recommendation* (Guyatt, Oxman, Vist, et al., 2008) for using sucrose to provide adequate analgesia during minor painful procedures. Sucrose is effective in reducing pain response in infants 6 months of age and younger undergoing minor acute painful procedures. The most effective dose has been 24% solution given at least 2 minutes before a procedure. Doses of 50% to 75% have been effective for relieving pain during immunizations in infants up to 6 months of age, suggesting that higher concentrations may be required for older infants. Effective dose volumes range from 0.05 to 2 mL, with lower volumes used for low-birth-weight infants and larger volumes used for older infants. Sucrose in combination with nonpharmacologic support during a procedure may increase the analgesic response for older infants (2 months) even with lower concentrations of sucrose. Interventions include using a pacifier, holding, swaddling, skin-to-skin contact, and rocking. Administration can be by a labeled oral syringe, dipped pacifier, or bottle, depending on the infant's ability and age. Comparisons between sucrose and glucose have been inconclusive.

Quality and Safety Competencies:
Evidence-Based Practice*
Knowledge

Differentiate clinical opinion from research and evidence-based summaries.

Describe the use of sucrose to provide analgesia during minor painful procedures.

Skills

Base the individualized care plan on patient values, clinical expertise, and evidence.

Integrate evidence into practice by using sucrose for analgesia during minor painful procedures.

Attitudes

Value the concept of evidence-based practice as integral to determining best clinical practice.

Appreciate strengths and weakness of evidence for sucrose use during minor painful procedures.

EVIDENCE-BASED PRACTICE

Reduction of Minor Procedural Pain in Infants—cont'd

References

Abad F, Diaz-Gomez NM, Domenech E, et al: Oral sucrose compares favorably with lidocaine-prilocaine cream for pain relief during venepuncture in neonates, *Acta Paediatr* 90:160–165, 2001.

Acharya AB, Annamali S, Taub NA, et al: Oral sucrose analgesia for preterm infant venepuncture, *Arch Dis Child Fetal Neonatal Educ* 89:F17–F18, 2004.

Carbajal R, Chauvet X, Couderc S, et al: Randomised trial of analgesic effects of sucrose, glucose, and pacifiers in term neonates, *BMJ* 319(7222):1393–1397, 1999.

Gradin M, Lenclen R, Gajdos V, et al: Crossover trial of analgesic efficacy of glucose and pacifier in very preterm neonates during subcutaneous injections, *Pediatrics* 110(6):1053–1057, 2002.

Guyatt GH, Oxman AD, Vist GE, et al: GRADE: an emerging consensus on rating quality of evidence and strength of recommendations, *BMJ* 336:924–926, 2008.

Lindh V, Wiklund U, Blomquist HK, et al: EMLA cream and oral glucose for immunization pain in 3-month-old infants, *Pain* 104(1-2):381–388, 2003.

Shah V, Ohlsson A: Venipuncture versus heel lance for blood sampling in term neonates, *Cochrane Database Syst Rev* (4):CD001452.pub2; DOI: 10.1002/14651858, 2004.

Stevens B, Yamada J, Ohlsson A: *Sucrose for analgesia in newborn infants undergoing painful procedures* [review], *Cochrane Neonatal Collaboration*, 2005, www.thecochranelibrary.com.

Carol Turnage Carrier; Updated by Olga A. Taylor

*Adapted from the QSEN at www.qsen.org.

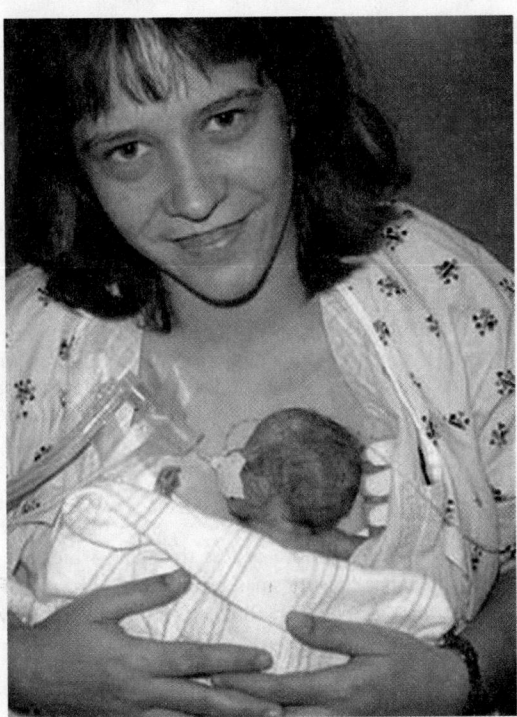

FIG 30-6 Mother using kangaroo hold with her newborn infant. Note placement of the infant directly on the mother's skin.

defined by the National Center for Complementary and Alternative Medicine, is a group of diverse medical and health care systems, practices, and products that are not currently considered part of conventional medicine (Myers, Stuber, Bonamer-Rheingans, et al., 2005). Although some scientific evidence exists regarding some CAM therapies, most key questions are yet to be answered through well-designed scientific studies (i.e., questions such as whether these therapies are safe and whether they work for the diseases or medical conditions for which they are used.

CAM therapies may be grouped into five classes: (1) biologically based (foods, special diets, herbal or plant preparations, vitamins, other supplements); (2) manipulative treatments (chiropractic, osteopathy, massage); (3) energy-based (Reiki, bioelectric or magnetic treatments, pulsed fields, alternating and direct currents); (4) mind-body techniques (mental healing, expressive treatments,

spiritual healing, hypnosis, relaxation); and (5) alternative medical systems (homeopathy, naturopathy, ayurvedic, traditional Chinese medicine that includes acupuncture and moxibustion).

Current estimates of pediatric CAM use range from 10% to 15%, derived from children sampled at health care facilities, with chronic conditions, and/or from countries other than the United States. For the U.S. population, pediatric CAM use was estimated to be 31% to 84% (Myers, Stuber, Bonamer-Rheingans, et al., 2005; Rusy and Weisman, 2000). Those who used CAM were found in each age-group, and the mean age was 10.3 years. The majority used unconventional therapy for chronic, as opposed to life-threatening, medical conditions. The therapies that are used increasingly include herbal medicine, massage, megavitamins, self-help groups, folk remedies, energy healing, and homeopathy (Myers, Stuber, Bonamer-Rheingans, et al., 2005; Rusy and Weisman, 2000).

Pharmacologic Management

For mild pain (<3 on 0-to-10 scale) or moderate pain (4 to 6 on 0-to-10 scale) acetaminophen (Tylenol, Paracetamol) and nonsteroidal antiinflammatory drugs (NSAIDs) are suitable (Table 30-3). For moderate (5 to 6) to severe pain (7 to 10 on 0-to-10 scale) opioids are needed (Table 30-4). A combination (acetaminophen with codeine) works better in some cases because nonopioids act at the peripheral nervous system and opioids act at the central nervous system. Oxycodone is available without a nonopioid in an immediate- and controlled-release preparation (OxyContin). Morphine is considered the gold standard for the management of severe pain. When morphine is not a suitable opioid, drugs such as hydromorphone (Dilaudid) and fentanyl (Sublimaze) are effective substitutes. Although fentanyl is used as an anesthetic in the operating room, it is classified as an analgesic. It can be administered safely by nurses by the intravenous (IV) (Fig. 30-7), intramuscular (IM), transmucosal, and transdermal routes (Algren, Gursoy, Johnson, et al., 1998; Golianu, Krane, Galloway, et al., 2000).

> ## ! NURSING ALERT
>
> The optimum dosage of an analgesic is one that controls pain without causing severe side effects. This usually requires titration, the gradual adjustment of drug dosage (usually by increasing the dose) until optimum pain relief without excessive sedation is achieved. Dosage recommendations are only safe initial dosages (see Tables 30-4 and 30-5), not optimum dosages.

TABLE 30-3	NONSTEROIDAL ANTIINFLAMMATORY DRUGS (NSAIDs) APPROVED FOR CHILDREN*†	
DRUG	**DOSAGE**	**COMMENTS**
Acetaminophen (Tylenol)	10-15 mg/kg/dose every 4-6 hr not to exceed 5 doses in 24 hr or 75 mg/kg/day, orally	Available in numerous preparations Nonprescription Higher dosage range may provide increased analgesia
Choline magnesium trisalicylate (Trilisate)	Children <37 kg (81.5 lbs): 50 mg/kg/day divided into 2 doses Children >37 kg (81.5 lbs): 2250 mg/day divided into 2 doses	Available in suspension, 500 mg/5 mL Prescription
Ibuprofen (children's Motrin, children's Advil)	Children >6 mo: 5-10 mg/kg/dose every 6-8 hr not to exceed 40 mg/kg/day	Available in numerous preparations Available in suspension, 100 mg/5 mL, and drops, 100 mg/2.5 mL Nonprescription
Naproxen (Naprosyn)	Children >2 yr: 10 mg/kg/day divided into 2 doses	Available in suspension, 125 mg/5 mL, and several different dosages for tablets Prescription
Tolmetin (Tolectin)	Children >2 yr: 20 g/kg/day divided into 3-4 doses	Available in 200-mg, 400-mg, and 600-mg tablets Prescription

Data from Olin BR et al: *Drug facts and comparisons,* St Louis, 2002, Facts and Comparisons.

*Newer formulations of nonsteroidal antiinflammatory drugs (NSAIDs) selectively inhibit one of the enzymes of cyclooxygenase (COX-2, which is responsible for pain transmission) but do not inhibit the other (COX-1). Inhibition of COX-1 decreases prostaglandin production, which is necessary for normal organ function. For example, prostaglandins help maintain gastric mucosal blood flow and barrier protection, regulate blood flow to the liver and kidneys, and facilitate platelet aggregation and clot formation. Theoretically the COX-2 NSAIDs provide similar analgesic and antiinflammatory benefits with fewer gastric and platelet side effects than the nonselective agents. COX-2 NSAIDs are approved for use in patients older than 18 years of age.

†All NSAIDs in this table (except acetaminophen) have significant antiinflammatory, antipyretic, and analgesic actions. Acetaminophen has a weak antiinflammatory action, and its classification as an NSAID is controversial. Patients respond differently to various NSAIDs; therefore changing from one drug to another may be necessary for maximum benefit. Acetylsalicylic acid (aspirin) is also an NSAID but is not recommended for children because of its possible association with Reye's syndrome. The NSAIDs in this table have no known association with Reye's syndrome. However, caution should be exercised in prescribing any salicylate-containing drug (e.g., Trilisate) for children with known or suspected viral infection. Side effects of ibuprofen, naproxen, and tolmetin include nausea, vomiting, diarrhea, constipation, gastric ulceration, bleeding nephritis, and fluid retention. Acetaminophen and choline magnesium trisalicylate are well tolerated in the gastrointestinal tract and do not interfere with platelet function. NSAIDs (except acetaminophen) should not be given to patients with allergic reactions to salicylates. All the NSAIDs should be used cautiously in patients with renal impairment.

Several drugs known as *coanalgesics* or adjuvant *analgesics* may be used alone or with opioids to control pain symptoms and opioid side effects. Drugs frequently used to relieve anxiety, cause sedation, and provide amnesia are diazepam (Valium) and midazolam (Versed). However, these drugs are not analgesics and should be used to enhance the effects of analgesics and not as a substitute for them. Other adjuvants include tricyclic antidepressants (e.g., amitriptyline, imipramine) and antiepileptics (e.g., gabapentin, carbamazepine, clonazepam) for neuropathic pain (Table 30-5), stool softeners and laxatives for constipation, antiemetics for nausea and vomiting, diphenhydramine for itching, steroids for inflammation and bone pain, and dextroamphetamine and caffeine for possible increased analgesia and decreased sedation (McCaffery and Pasero, 1999).

Children (except infants younger than about 3 to 6 months) metabolize drugs more rapidly than adults; younger children may require higher doses of opioids to achieve the same analgesic effect. Therefore the therapeutic effect and duration of analgesia vary. Children's dosages are usually calculated according to body weight, except in children with a weight greater than 50 kg (110 lbs), in whom the weight formula may exceed the average adult dose. In this case the adult dose is used. Conversion factors for selected opioids must be used when a change is made from IV (preferred) or IM to oral. Immediate conversion from IM or IV to the suggested equianalgesic oral dose may result in a substantial error. For example, the dose may be significantly more or less than that which the child requires. Small changes ensure small errors. Several routes of analgesic administration can be used (Box 30-2); the most effective and least traumatic route should be selected.

Transmucosal and Transdermal Analgesia

Oral transmucosal fentanyl (Oralet) provides nontraumatic preoperative and preprocedural analgesia and sedation (Golianu, Krane, Galloway, et al., 2000). Fentanyl is also available as a transdermal patch (Duragesic). Although contraindicated for acute pain management, it may be used for older children and adolescents who have cancer or sickle cell pain or patients who are opioid tolerant.

One of the most significant improvements in the ability to provide atraumatic care to children is the anesthetic cream LMX (a 4% liposomal lidocaine cream) or EMLA (eutectic mixture of local anesthetics) (Abdelkefi, Abdennebi, Mellouli, et al., 2004; Choi, Irwin, Hui, et al., 2003; Egekvist and Bjerring, 2000; Gad, Olsen, Lysgaard, et al., 2005; Rogers and Ostrow, 2004; Santiago, Abad, Fernandez, et al., 2000; Uziel, Berkovitch, Gazarian, et al., 2003). The eutectic mixture (lidocaine 2.5% and prilocaine 2.5%), the melting point of which is lower than that of the two anesthetics alone, permits effective concentrations of the drug to penetrate intact skin (Fig. 30-8).

In some situations there isn't ample time for topical preparations such as LMX or EMLA to take effect, and refrigerant sprays such as

TABLE 30-4   DOSAGE OF SELECTED OPIOIDS FOR CHILDREN

DRUG	APPROPRIATE EQUIANALGESIC	APPROXIMATE EQUIANALGESIC PARENTERAL DOSE	RECOMMENDED STARTING DOSE (CHILDREN <50 KG (110 LBS) BODY WEIGHT)*	
			ORAL	PARENTERAL*
Morphine	30 mg every 3-4 hr	10 mg every 3-4 hr	0.2-0.4 mg/kg every 3-4 hr 0.3-0.6 mg/kg time released every 12 hr	0.1-0.2 mg/kg IM every 3-4 hr 0.02-0.1 mg/kg IV bolus every 2 hr 0.015 mg/kg every 8 min PCA 0.01-0.02 mg/kg/hr IV infusion (neonates) 0.01-0.06 mg/kg/hr IV infusion (child)
Fentanyl (Sublimaze) (oral mucosal form [Actiq])†	Not available	0.1 mg IV	5-15 mcg/kg; maximum dose 400 mcg	0.5-1.5 mcg/kg IV bolus every 30 min 1-2 mcg/hr IV infusion
Codeine‡	200 mg every 3-4 hr	130 mg every 3-4 hr	1 mg/kg every 3-4 hr	Not recommended
Hydromorphone§ (Dilaudid)	7.5 mg every 3-4 hr	1.5 mg every 3-4 hr	0.04-0.1 mg/kg every 3-4 hr	0.02-0.1 mg/kg every 3-4 hr 0.005-0.2 mg/kg IV bolus every 2 hr
Hydrocodone and acetaminophen (Lorcet, Lortab, Vicodin, others)	30 mg every 3-4 hr	Not available	0.2 mg/kg every 3-4 hr	Not available
Levorphanol (Levo-Dromoran)	4 mg every 6-8 hr	2 mg every 6-8 hr	0.04 mg/kg every 6-8 hr	0.02 mg/kg every 6-8 hr
Meperidine (Demerol)‖	300 mg every 2-3 hr	100 mg every 3 hr	Not recommended	0.75 mg/kg every 2-3 hr
Methadone (Dolophine, others)¶	20 mg every 6-8 hr	10 mg every 6-8 hr	0.2 mg/kg every 6-8 hr	0.1 mg/kg every 6-8 hr
Oxycodone (Roxicodone, OxyContin; also in Percocet, Percodan, Tylox, others)	20 mg every 3-4 hr	Not available	2 mg/kg every 3-4 hr#	Not available

Data from Acute Pain Management Guideline Panel: *Acute pain management: operative or medical procedures and trauma: clinical practice guideline*, AHCPR Pub No 92-0032, Rockville, MD, 1992, Agency for Health Care Policy and Research, Public Health Service, US Department of Health and Human Services; Berde C, Ablin A, Glazer J, et al: American Academy of Pediatrics Report of the Subcommittee on Disease-Related Pain in Childhood Cancer, *Pediatrics* 86(5 pt 2):820, 1990.

IM, Intramuscularly; *IV*, intravenous; *PCA*, patient-controlled analgesia.

NOTE: Published tables vary in suggested doses that are equianalgesic to morphine. Clinical response is criterion that must be applied for each patient; titration to clinical response is necessary. Because there is incomplete cross-tolerance among these drugs, it is usually necessary to use a lower than equianalgesic dose when changing drugs and retitrate to response.

CAUTION: Recommended doses do not apply to patients with renal or hepatic insufficiency or other conditions affecting drug metabolism and kinetics.

*CAUTION: Doses listed for patients with body weight less than 50 kg (110 lbs) cannot be used as initial starting doses in infants younger than 6 months of age. For nonventilated infants younger than 6 months the initial opioid dose should be about ¼ to ⅓ of the dose recommended for older infants and children. For example, morphine could be used at a dose of 0.03 mg/kg instead of the traditional 0.1 mg/kg.

†Actiq is indicated only for management of breakthrough cancer pain in patients with malignancies who are already receiving and are tolerant to opioid therapy, but it can be used for preoperative or preprocedural sedation/analgesia.

‡CAUTION: Codeine doses above 65 mg often are not appropriate because of diminishing incremental analgesia with increasing doses but continually increasing constipation and other side effects. Dosages are from McCaffery M, Pasero C: *Pain: a clinical manual*, ed 2, St Louis, 1999, Mosby.

§For morphine, hydromorphone, and oxymorphone, rectal administration is an alternate route for patients unable to take oral medications, but equianalgesic doses may differ from oral and parenteral doses because of pharmacokinetic differences.

‖Meperidine is not recommended for continuous pain control (i.e., after surgery) because of risk of normeperidine toxicity.

¶Initial dose is 10%-25% of equianalgesic morphine dose. Parenteral Dolophine is no longer available in the United States.

#CAUTION: Doses of aspirin and acetaminophen in combination with opioid or nonsteroidal antiinflammatory drug preparations must also be adjusted to patient's body weight. Daily dose of acetaminophen should not exceed 75 mg/kg, or 4000 mg.

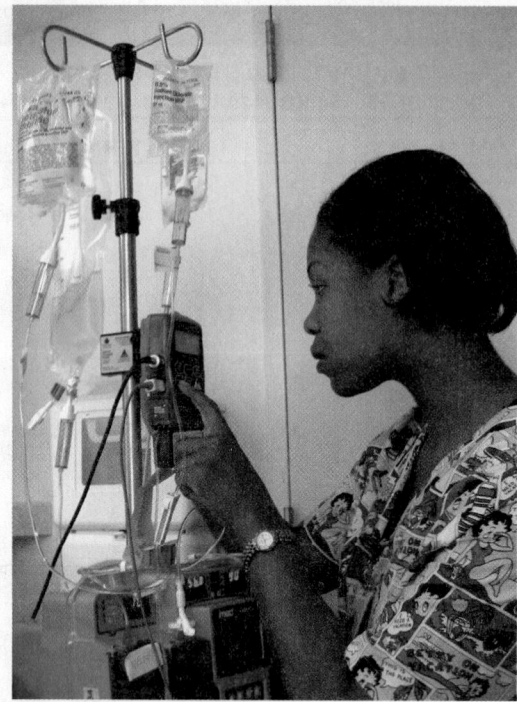

FIG 30-7 Nurse programming a patient-controlled analgesia pump to administer analgesia.

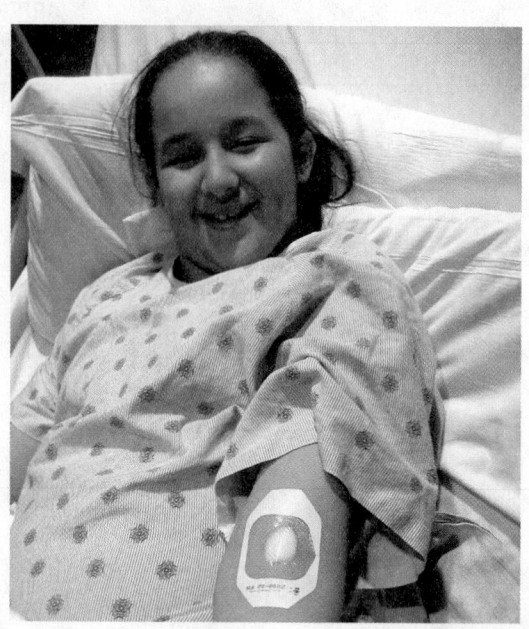

FIG 30-8 LMX is an effective analgesic before intravenous insertion or blood draw.

TABLE 30-5	MANAGEMENT OF OPIOID SIDE EFFECTS	
SIDE EFFECT	**ADJUVANT DRUGS**	**NONPHARMACOLOGIC TECHNIQUES**
Constipation	**Senna and docusate sodium** *Tablet:* 2-6 yr: Start with ½ tablet once a day; maximum: 1 tablet twice a day 6-12 yr: Start with 1 tablet once a day; maximum: 2 tablets twice a day >12 yr: Start with 2 tablets once a day; maximum: 4 tablets twice a day *Liquid:* 1 mo-1 yr: 1.25-5 mL q hs 1-5 yr: 2.5-5 mL q hs 5-15 yr: 5-10 mL q hs >15 yr: 10-25 mL q hs **Casanthranol and docusate sodium** *Liquid:* 5-15 mL q hs *Capsules:* 1 cap PO q hs **Bisacodyl:** PO or PR 3-12 yr: 5 mg/dose/day >12 yr: 10-15 mg/dose/day **Lactulose** 7.5 mL/day after breakfast Adult: 15-30 mL/day PO **Mineral oil:** 1-2 tsp/day PO **Magnesium citrate** <6 yr: 2-4 mL/kg PO once 6-12 yr: 100-150 mL PO once >12 yr: 150-300 mL PO once **Milk of Magnesia** <2 yr: 0.5 mL/kg/dose PO once 2-5 yr: 5-15 mL/day PO 6-12 yr: 15-30 mL PO once >12 yr: 30-60 mL PO once	Increase water intake Prune juice, bran cereal, vegetables

TABLE 30-5	MANAGEMENT OF OPIOID SIDE EFFECTS—cont'd	
SIDE EFFECT	**ADJUVANT DRUGS**	**NONPHARMACOLOGIC TECHNIQUES**
Sedation	**Caffeine:** single dose of 1-1.5 mg PO **Dextroamphetamine:** 2.5-5 mg PO in AM and early afternoon **Methylphenidate:** 2.5-5 mg PO in AM and early afternoon Consider opioid switch if sedation is persistent	Caffeinated drinks (e.g., Mountain Dew, cola drinks)
Nausea, vomiting	**Promethazine:** 0.5 mg/kg q 4-6 hr; maximum: 25 mg/dose **Ondansetron:** 0.1-0.15 mg/kg IV or PO q 4 hr; maximum: 8 mg/dose **Granisetron:** 10-40 mcg/kg q 2-4 hr; maximum: 1 mg/dose **Droperidol:** 0.05-0.06 mg/kg IV q 4-6 hr; can be very sedating	Imagery, relaxation Deep, slow breathing
Pruritus	**Diphenhydramine:** 1 mg/kg IV or PO q 4-6 hr prn; max: 25 mg/dose **Hydroxyzine:** 0.6 mg/kg/dose PO q 6 hr; maximum: 50 mg/dose **Naloxone:** 0.5 mcg/kg q 2 min until pruritus improves (diluted in solution of 0.1 mg of naloxone per 10 mL of saline) **Butorphanol:** 0.3-0.5 mg/kg IV (use cautiously in opioid-tolerant children; may cause withdrawal symptoms); maximum: 2 mg/dose because mixed agonist-antagonist	Oatmeal baths, good hygiene Exclude other causes of itching Change opioids
Respiratory depression: mild to moderate	Hold dose of opioid Reduce subsequent doses by 25%	Arouse gently, give oxygen, encourage to deep breathe
Respiratory depression: severe	**Naloxone** *During disease pain management:* 0.5 mcg/kg in 2-min increments until breathing improves (American Pain Society, 1999; McCaffery and Pasero, 1999) Reduce opioid dose if possible Consider opioid switch *During sedation for procedures:* 5-10 mcg/kg until breathing improves (Yaster, Krance, Kaplan, et al., 1997) Reduce opioid dose if possible Consider opioid switch	Oxygen, bag and mask if indicated
Dysphoria, confusion, hallucinations	Evaluate medications, eliminate adjuvant medications with central nervous system effects as symptoms allow Consider opioid switch if possible **Haloperidol** (Haldol): 0.05-0.15 mg/kg/day divided in 2-3 doses; maximum: 2-4 mg/day	Rule out other physiologic causes
Urinary retention	Evaluate medications, eliminate adjuvant medications with anticholinergic effects (e.g., antihistamines, tricyclic antidepressants) Occurs more frequently with spinal analgesia than with systemic opioid use **Oxybutynin** 1 yr: 1 mg tid 1-2 yr: 2 mg tid 2-3 yr: 3 mg tid 4-5 yr: 4 mg tid >5 yr: 5 mg tid	Rule out other physiologic causes In/out or indwelling urinary catheter

hs, At bedtime; *IV,* intravenously; *PO,* by mouth; *PR,* by rectum; *prn,* as needed; *q,* every; *tid,* 3 times a day.

ethyl chloride and fluoromethane can be used (Reis and Holubkov, 1997). When sprayed on the skin, these sprays vaporize, rapidly cool the area, and provide superficial anesthesia. Hospital formularies may have other products with lidocaine, prilocaine, or amethocaine topical preparations that require less time for application. A randomized controlled trial compared the efficacy and safety of amethocaine gel (which is applied for 30 minutes) and EMLA cream (which is applied for 60 minutes) before a port-a-cath puncture. Children rated the pain following the puncture using the FACES Pain Scale (coded 0 to 5). Both groups had low pain scores, less than or equal to 2, and it did not make a significant difference whether the amethocaine or the EMLA cream was used. The researchers concluded that the amethocaine was clinically equivalent to EMLA, but the amethocaine gel required less time for anesthesia (Bishai, Taddio, Bar-Oz, et al., 1999).

Monitoring Side Effects

Although both nonopioids and opioids have side effects, the major concern is with side effects from opioids (Box 30-3). Respiratory depression is the most serious complication and is most likely to occur in sedated patients. The respiratory rate may decrease gradually, or respirations may cease abruptly. Lower limits of normal are

BOX 30-2 ROUTES AND METHODS OF ANALGESIC DRUG ADMINISTRATION

Oral

- Oral route preferred because of convenience, cost, and relatively steady blood levels
- Higher dosages of oral form of opioids required for equivalent parenteral analgesia
- Peak drug effect occurs after 1 to 2 hours for most analgesics
- Delay in onset a disadvantage when rapid control of severe or fluctuating pain is desired

Sublingual, Buccal, or Transmucosal

- Tablet or liquid placed between cheek and gum (buccal) or under tongue (sublingual)
- Highly desirable because more rapid onset than oral route
- Produced less first-pass effect through liver than oral route, which normally reduces analgesia from oral opioids (unless sublingual or buccal form is swallowed, which occurs often in children)
- Few drugs commercially available in this form
- Many drugs can be compounded into sublingual troche or lozenge*
- Actiq—Oral transmucosal fentanyl citrate in hard confection base on plastic holder; indicated only for management of breakthrough cancer pain in patients with malignancies who are already receiving and are tolerant to opioid therapy, but can be used for preoperative or preprocedural sedation and analgesia

Intravenous (IV) (Bolus)

- Preferred for rapid control of severe pain
- Provides most rapid onset of effect, usually in about 5 minutes
- Advantage for acute pain, procedural pain, and breakthrough pain
- Needs to be repeated hourly for continuous pain control
- Drugs with short half-life (morphine, fentanyl, hydromorphone) preferable to avoid toxic accumulation of drug

IV (Continuous)

- Preferred over bolus and intramuscular injection for maintaining control of pain
- Provides steady blood levels
- Easy to titrate dosage

Subcutaneous (SC) (Continuous)

- Used when oral and IV routes not available
- Provides equivalent blood levels to continuous IV infusion
- Suggested initial bolus dose to equal 2-hour IV dose; total 24-hour dosage usually requires concentrated opioid solution to minimize infused volume; use smallest-gauge needle that accommodates infusion rate

Patient-Controlled Analgesia (PCA)

- Generally refers to self-administration of drugs, regardless of route
- Typically uses programmable infusion pump (IV, epidural, SC) that permits self-administration of boluses of medication at preset dose and time interval (lockout interval is time between doses)
- PCA bolus administration often combined with initial bolus and continuous (basal or background) infusion of opioid
- Optimum lockout interval not known but must be at least as long as time needed for onset of drug
    - Should effectively control pain during movement or procedures
    - Longer lockout provides larger dose

Family-Controlled Analgesia

- One family member (usually a parent) or other caregiver designated as child's primary pain manager with responsibility for pressing PCA button

- Guidelines for selecting primary pain manager for family-controlled analgesia:
    - Spends a significant amount of time with patient
    - Is willing to assume responsibility of being primary pain manager
    - Is willing to accept and respect patient's reports of pain (if able to provide) as best indicator of how much pain the patient is experiencing; knows how to use and interpret a pain-rating scale
    - Understands purpose and goals of patient's pain-management plan
    - Understands concept of maintaining steady analgesic blood level
    - Recognizes signs of pain and side effects and adverse reactions to opioid

Nurse-Activated Analgesia

- Child's primary nurse designated as primary pain manager and is only person who presses PCA button during that nurse's shift
- Guidelines for selecting primary pain manager for family-controlled analgesia also applicable to nurse-activated analgesia
- May be used in addition to basal rate to treat breakthrough pain with bolus doses; patient assessed every 30 minutes for need for bolus dose
- May be used without a basal rate as means of maintaining analgesia with around-the-clock bolus doses

Intramuscular

NOTE: Not recommended for pain control; not current standard of care
- Painful administration (hated by children)
- Some drugs can cause tissue and nerve damage
- Wide fluctuation in absorption of drug from muscle
- Faster absorption from deltoid than from gluteal sites
- Shorter duration and more expensive than oral drugs
- Time consuming for staff and unnecessary delay for child

Intranasal

- Available commercially as butorphanol (Stadol NS); approved for those older than 18 years of age
- Should not be used in patient receiving morphinelike drugs because butorphanol is partial antagonist that reduces analgesia and may cause withdrawal

Intradermal

- Used primarily for skin anesthesia (e.g., before lumbar puncture, bone marrow aspiration, arterial puncture, skin biopsy)
- Local anesthetics (e.g., lidocaine) cause stinging, burning sensation
- Duration of stinging dependent on type of "caine" used
- To avoid stinging sensation associated with lidocaine:
    - Buffer solution by adding 1 part sodium bicarbonate (1 mEq/mL) to 9 to 10 parts 1% or 2% lidocaine with or without epinephrine (see Evidence-Based Practice box on p. 855)
- Normal saline with preservative, benzyl alcohol, anesthetizes venipuncture site
- Use same dose as for buffered lidocaine (see Evidence-Based Practice box on p. 855)

Topical or Transdermal

- EMLA (eutectic mixture of local anesthetics [lidocaine and prilocaine]) cream and anesthetic disk or 4% lidocaine cream (LMX4)
    - Eliminates or reduces pain from most procedures involving skin puncture
    - Must be placed on intact skin over puncture site and covered by occlusive dressing or applied as anesthetic disc for 1 hour or more before procedure (see Evidence-Based Practice box on p. 855)

BOX 30-2   ROUTES AND METHODS OF ANALGESIC DRUG ADMINISTRATION—cont'd

- Synera, S-Caine (lidocaine/tetracaine)
  - Apply for 20-30 minutes
  - Do not apply to broken skin
- Lidocaine-adrenaline-tetracaine (LAT), tetracaine-phenylephrine (tetraphen)
  - Provides skin anesthesia about 15 minutes after application on nonintact skin
  - Gel (preferable) or liquid placed on wounds for suturing
  - Adrenaline not for use on end arterioles (fingers, toes, tip of nose, penis, earlobes) because of vasoconstriction
- Transdermal fentanyl (Duragesic)
  - Available as patch for continuous pain control
  - Safety and efficacy not established in children younger than 12 years of age
  - Not appropriate for initial relief of acute pain because of long interval to peak effect (12 to 24 hours); for rapid onset of pain relief give an immediate-release opioid
  - Orders for "rescue doses" of an immediate-release opioid recommended for breakthrough pain, a flare of severe pain that breaks through the medication being administered at regular intervals for persistent pain
  - Has duration of up to 72 hours for prolonged pain relief
  - If respiratory depression occurs, possible need for several doses of naloxone
- Vapocoolant
  - Use of prescription spray coolant such as Fluori-Methane or ethyl chloride (Pain-Ease); applied to the skin for 10 to 15 seconds immediately before needle puncture; anesthesia lasts about 15 seconds
  - Some children dislike cold; may be less uncomfortable to spray coolant on a cotton ball and then apply this to the skin
  - Application of ice to skin for 30 seconds has been found to be ineffective

Rectal
- Alternative to oral or parenteral routes
- Variable absorption rate

- Generally disliked by children
- Many drugs able to be compounded into rectal suppositories*

Regional Nerve Block
- Use of long-acting local anesthetic (bupivacaine or ropivacaine) injected into nerves to block pain at site
- Provides prolonged analgesia after surgery such as after inguinal herniorrhaphy
- May be used to provide local anesthesia for surgery such as dorsal penile nerve block for circumcision or reduction of fractures

Inhalation
- Use of anesthetics such as nitrous oxide to produce partial or complete analgesia for painful procedures
- Side effects (e.g., headache) possible from occupational exposure to high levels of nitrous oxide

Epidural or Intrathecal
- Involves catheter placed into epidural, caudal, or intrathecal space for continuous infusion or single or intermittent administration of opioid with or without a long-acting local anesthetic (e.g., bupivacaine, ropivacaine)
- Analgesia primarily from direct effect of drug on opioid receptors in spinal cord
- Respiratory depression rare but may have slow and delayed onset; can be prevented by checking level of sedation and respiratory rate and depth hourly for initial 24 hours and decreasing dose when excessive sedation is detected
- Nausea, itching, and urinary retention common dose-related side effects from the epidural opioid
- Mild hypotension, urinary retention, and temporary motor or sensory deficits common unwanted effects of epidural local anesthetic
- Catheter for urinary retention inserted during surgery to decrease trauma to child; if inserted when child is awake, anesthetize urethra with lidocaine

Data primarily from American Pain Society: *Principles of analgesic use in the treatment of acute pain and chronic cancer pain*, ed 4, Glenview, Ill, 1999, The Society; and McCaffery M, Pasero C: *Pain: a clinical manual*, ed 2, St Louis, 1999, Mosby.
*For further information about compounding drugs in troche or suppository form, contact Professional Compounding Centers of America (PCCA), 9901 S. Wilcrest Drive, Houston, TX 77009; (800) 331–2498; www.pccarx.com.

not established for children, but any significant change from a previous rate calls for increased vigilance. A slower respiratory rate does not necessarily reflect decreased arterial oxygenation; an increased depth of ventilation may compensate for the altered rate. If respiratory depression or arrest occurs, the nurse must be prepared to intervene quickly (see Guidelines box).

Although respiratory depression is the most feared side effect, constipation is a common and sometimes serious side effect of opioids. Opioids decrease peristalsis and increase anal sphincter tone. If prolonged use of opioids is expected, prevention with stool softeners and laxatives is more effective than treatment once constipation occurs. Dietary treatment such as increased fiber is usually not sufficient to promote regular bowel evacuation. However, dietary measures such as increased fluid and fruit intake and physical activity are encouraged. Another common side effect is pruritus from epidural or IV infusion. Pruritus can be treated with low doses of IV naloxone, nalbuphine, or diphenhydramine. Children may also experience nausea and vomiting; however, these subside after

2 days of opioid administration. Oral or rectal antiemetics may be necessary to minimize nausea and vomiting.

Both tolerance and physical dependence can occur with prolonged use of opioids (see Community Focus box on p. 839). Physical dependence is a normal, natural, physiologic state of "neuroadaptation." When opioids are discontinued abruptly without weaning, withdrawal symptoms occur. Symptoms of withdrawal occur at 24 hours after abrupt discontinuation and reach a peak within 72 hours. They include signs of neurologic excitability (irritability, tremors, seizures, increased motor tone, insomnia), gastrointestinal dysfunction (nausea, vomiting, diarrhea, abdominal cramps), and autonomic dysfunction (sweating, fever, chills, tachypnea, nasal congestion, rhinitis). They can be anticipated and prevented by weaning patients from opioids that were administered for more than 5 to 10 days. Adherence to a weaning protocol to prevent or minimize withdrawal symptoms from opioids is required. A weaning flow sheet (Fig. 30-9) may be used to assess the efficacy of opioid weaning in neonates (Franck and Vilardi, 1995; Franck,

BOX 30-3 SIDE EFFECTS OF OPIOIDS

General
- Constipation (possibly severe)
- Respiratory depression
- Sedation
- Nausea and vomiting
- Agitation, euphoria
- Mental clouding
- Hallucinations
- Orthostatic hypotension
- Pruritus
- Urticaria
- Sweating
- Miosis (may be sign of toxicity)
- Anaphylaxis (rare)

Signs of Tolerance
- Decreasing pain relief
- Decreasing duration of pain relief

Signs of Withdrawal Syndrome in Patients with Physical Dependence

Initial Signs of Withdrawal
- Lacrimation
- Rhinorrhea
- Yawning
- Sweating

Later Signs of Withdrawal
- Restlessness
- Irritability
- Tremors
- Anorexia
- Dilated pupils
- Gooseflesh
- Nausea, vomiting

 GUIDELINES

Managing Opioid-Induced Respiratory Depression

If Respirations Are Depressed
- Assess sedation level.
- Reduce infusion by 25% when possible.
- Stimulate patient (shake shoulder gently, call by name, ask to breathe).

If Patient Cannot Be Aroused or Is Apneic
- Administer naloxone (Narcan):
  - For children weighing less than 40 kg (88 lbs), dilute 0.1 mg naloxone in 10 mL sterile saline to make 10 mcg/mL solution and give 0.5 mcg/kg.
  - For children weighing more than 40 kg (88 lbs), dilute 0.4-mg ampule in 10 mL sterile saline and give 0.5 mL.
- Administer bolus by slow intravenous push every 2 minutes until effect is obtained.
- Closely monitor patient. Duration of antagonist action of naloxone may be shorter than that of opioid, requiring repeated doses of naloxone.
- Tolerance occurs when the dose of an opioid needs to be increased to achieve the same analgesic effect that was previously achieved at a lower dose (see Community Focus box on p. 839). Tolerance may develop after 10 to 21 days of morphine administration. Treatment of tolerance involves increasing the dose or decreasing the duration between doses. Treatment of physical dependence involves gradually reducing the dose over several days to prevent withdrawal symptoms. Following are guidelines for treating physical dependence from morphine (Max, Payne, Edwards, et al., 1999):
- Gradually reduce dose (similar to tapering of steroids).
- Give half of previous daily dose every 6 hours for first 2 days.
- Then reduce dose by 25% every 2 days. Continue this schedule until total daily dosage of 0.6 mg/kg/day of morphine (or equivalent) is reached. After 2 days on this dose discontinue opioid.
  - You may also switch to oral methadone, using one fourth of equianalgesic dose as initial weaning dose and proceeding as described previously.

NOTE: Respiratory depression caused by benzodiazepines (e.g., diazepam [Valium] or midazolam [Versed]) can be reversed with flumazenil [Romazicon]). Pediatric dosing experience suggests 0.01 mg/kg (0.1 mL/kg); if no (or inadequate) response after 1 or 2 minutes, administer same dose and repeat as needed at 60-second intervals for maximum dosage of 1 mg (10 mL) (Yaster, Krance, Kaplan, et al., 1997).

Vilardi, Durand, et al., 1998). In older infants and young children (7 months to 10 years) the Withdrawal Assessment Tool–1 may be used to assess and monitor withdrawal symptoms in pediatric critically ill children who are exposed to opioids and benzodiazepines for prolonged periods (Franck, Harris, Soetenga, et al., 2008).

Parents and older children may fear addiction when opioids are prescribed. The nurse should address these concerns with assurance that any such risk is extremely low. It may be helpful to ask the question, "If you did not have this pain, would you want to take this medicine?" The answer is invariably no, which reinforces the solely therapeutic nature of the drug. It is also important to avoid making statements to the family such as, "We don't want you to get used to this medicine," or "By now you shouldn't need this medicine," which may reinforce the fear of becoming addicted. Although both physical dependence and tolerance are physiologic states, addiction or psychologic dependence is a psychologic state and implies a "cause-effect" mode of thinking, such as, "I need the drug because it makes me feel better." Infants and children do not have the cognitive ability to make the cause-effect association and therefore cannot become addicted. The use of opioid analgesics early in life has not been demonstrated to increase the risk for addiction later in life. Nurses need to explain to parents the differences among physical dependence, tolerance, and addiction and allow them to express concerns about the use and duration of use of opioids. When infants and children are treated appropriately with opioids, they may be at risk for physical tolerance and physical dependence but not psychologic dependence or addiction (McCaffery and Pasero, 1999).

Unfortunately individuals who have severe, unrelieved pain may become intensely focused on finding relief. Sometimes behaviors such as "clock watching" make patients appear to others to be preoccupied with obtaining opioids. However, this preoccupation focuses on finding relief of pain, not on using opioids for reasons other than pain control. This phenomenon has been termed *pseudoaddiction* and must not be confused with real addiction.

Evaluation of Effectiveness of Pain Regimen

The effectiveness of analgesics can be enhanced by a supportive attitude toward the child. By reinforcing the cause and effect of the medication and analgesia, the nurse can condition the child to expect pain relief, provided the regimen is likely to be effective. A pain-relief scale or periodic ratings of pain intensity should be used for evaluation of effectiveness of pain regimens.

The response to therapy should be evaluated 15 to 30 minutes after each dose, and titration should continue to the highest achievable amount of relief (Max, Payne, Edwards, et al., 1999). In a retrospective study that examined the pain experience of children with sickle cell disease, evidence of pain relief from medications was documented for less than half (44.8%) of the patients in the emergency department (ED) (Jacob and Mueller, 2008). Even though the Joint Commission on Accreditation of Healthcare Organizations required documentation of pain assessments with vital signs, evidence of pain relief was not documented in 41.4% of the episodes. If titration methods were used in the ED or during the course of hospitalization, they were not reflected in the amount of medications received by the children (Jacob and Mueller, 2008; Jacob, Miaskowski, Savedra, et al., 2003a).

Children's Hospital Oakland Opioid Weaning Flowsheet and Guidelines for Use of the Form
Analgesia/sedation orders (drug/dose/frequency)

Date			
Drug			
Administration time			
Dose ↑ or ↓ or freq change			

Time:			
Choose one:			
Crying/agitated 25%-50% of interval	2		
Crying/agitated >50% of interval	3		
Choose one:			
Sleeps ≤25% of interval	3		
Sleeps 26%-75% of interval	2		
Sleeps >75% of interval	1		
Choose one:			
Hyperactive Moro	2		
Markedly hyperactive Moro	3		
Choose one:			
Mild tremors, disturbed	1		
Moderate/severe tremors, disturbed	2		
Increased muscle tone	2		
Temperature 37.2°-38.4°C	1		
Temperature >38.4°C	2		
Respiratory rate >60 (extubated)	2		
Suction >twice/interval (intubated)	2		
Sweating	1		
Frequent yawning (>3-4/interval)	1		
Sneezing (>3-4/interval)	1		
Nasal stuffiness	1		
Emesis	2		
Projectile vomiting	3		
Loose stools	2		
Watery stools	3		
TOTAL SCORE			
ADJUSTED SCORE			
INITIALS OF PERSON SCORING			

Directions: Score every 2-4 hours per guideline
Score greater than 8-12 may indicate withdrawal

Guidelines for use of the flow sheet

Use of form

Use the flowsheet for all infants who have received continuous or around-the-clock opioid medication for 3 days or more, or more than 3 doses per day for more than 5 days. This patient population will most often include postoperative patients, agitated intubated infants, and all post-ECMO patients.

Instructions

1. Write drug, dose, and frequency of analgesics and sedatives ordered
2. Enter date, name of drug (abbreviated MS=morphine sulfate or FENT=fentanyl), and administration time of drugs given in the appropriate boxes; indicate if dose frequency given is an increase or decrease from the ordered dose
3. Scoring must be performed every 4 hours during weaning of opioids, every 2 hours if score is 8 or greater. The score for each item indicates the presence of the sign during the previous 2-4 hours (depending on the scoring interval). Every 4-hour scoring should continue until the patient is off all opioids for 48-72 hours. Place a "0" in the column after the sign if it is not seen during the scoring period.

Central nervous system

Crying behavior: Score 2 points if patient exhibits crying or cry behavior for a duration of ≤50% of the scoring interval. Score 3 points if cumulative crying behavior totals >50% of the scoring interval.
NOTE: Crying behavior is accompanied by the facial expressions associated with crying, but without audible sounds because of endotracheal intubation.
Sleeping: Score 3 points if patient sleeps for ≤25% of the scoring interval. Score 2 points if patient sleeps for 26%-75% of the scoring interval. Score 1 point if patient sleeps for >75% of the scoring interval.
Moro (startle) reflex: Score 2 points if patient has some arm and/or leg extension when touched or when disturbed by loud noises. Score 3 points if patient has marked arm and/or leg extension that is accompanied by crying behavior, hyperalert state, or continued arm and/or leg tremors after being startled.
Tremors—disturbed: Score 1 point if patient has mild tremors when disturbed. Score 2 points if patient has moderate to severe tremors when disturbed. NOTE: Tremors are alternating movements that are rhythmic, of equal rate and amplitude, and can usually be stopped by flexion of the limb.
Increased muscle tone: Score 2 points if patient exhibits fisting or tight flexion of extremities that are difficult to extend.

Metabolic

Temperature: Score 1 point if patient's temperature is 37.2°-38.4°C. Score 2 points if patient's temperature is >38.4°C.
Respiratory rate: Score 1 point if patient's spontaneous respiratory rate is >60/minute. Score 2 points if patient's spontaneous respiratory rate is >60/minute and accompanied by retractions.
Suction: Score 2 points if patient is suctioned more than twice during a 4-hour period.
Sweating: Score 1 point if patient exhibits any type of sweating, including beads of sweat, or if skin is moist to touch.
Yawning: Score 1 point if patient yawns >3-4 times in succession or yawns 1-2 times often during a 4-hour period.
Sneezing: Score 1 point if patient sneezes >3-4 times in succession or sneezes 1-2 times during a 4-hour period.
Nasal stuffiness: Score 1 point for nasal stuffiness.

Gastrointestinal

Emesis of formula/stomach contents: Score 2 points if patient has 1 or more episodes of emesis during a 4-hour period.
Projectile vomiting: Score 3 points if patient has 1 or more episodes of projectile vomiting.
Loose stools: Score 2 points if patient has loose stools characterized by a water ring around some solid stool. The stools will often be frequent. NOTE: Do not score for "breast milk" stools: frequent, small, seedy, yellow stools.
Watery stools: Score 3 points if patient has stools that consist of only liquid. The stools will often be frequent.

Total score: Add up all the scores in the column and place the total score in this box. Clinical signs that appear continuously, such as respiratory rate >60 or regular poor feeding, should be included in the total score.
Adjusted score: The adjusted score is used when a sign is detected that is expected to occur independently of withdrawal, due to a preexisting condition (high respiratory rate in infant with bronchopulmonary dysplasia). The decision to adjust the score should be made after discussion with the health care team during rounds, and the rationale should be recorded in a problem-oriented note. Circle the signs to be excluded and deduct the points from the total score to obtain the adjusted score.
Initials of person scoring: The person scoring should write his/her initials in this space.

FIG 30-9 Weaning flow sheet to monitor opioid weaning in neonates. (Modified from Franck L, Vilardi J: Assessment and management of opioid withdrawal in ill neonates, *Neonatal Netw* 14[2]:39–48, 1995.)

Several harmful effects occur with unrelieved pain, particularly when pain is prolonged. A number of physiologic stress responses in the body are triggered during pain, and they lead to negative consequences that involve multiple systems. Unrelieved pain may prolong the stress response and adversely affect an infant's or child's recovery, whether it is from trauma, surgery, or disease. In a landmark study by Anand and Hickey (1992), 30 neonates received deep intraoperative anesthesia with high doses of the opioid sufentanil, followed after surgery with an infusion of opioids for 24 hours; and 15 neonates received lighter anesthesia with halothane and morphine followed after surgery by intermittent morphine and diazepam. The 15 neonates who received the lighter anesthesia and intermittent postoperative opioids had more severe hyperglycemia and lactic acidemia, and four postoperative deaths occurred in the group. The 30 neonates who received deep anesthesia had a lower incidence of complications (sepsis, metabolic acidosis, disseminated intravascular coagulation) and no deaths.

Poorly controlled acute pain can predispose patients to chronic pain syndromes. A guiding principle in pain management is that prevention of pain is always better than treatment (Benjamin, Swinson, and Nagel, 2000). Pain that is established and severe is often more difficult to control. When pain is unrelieved, sensory input from injured tissues reaches spinal cord neurons and may enhance subsequent responses. Long-lasting changes in cells within spinal cord pain pathways may occur after a brief painful stimulus and lead to the development of chronic pain conditions. Basbaum (1999a, 1999b) reported a series of studies that emphasize a distinct neurochemistry of acute and persistent pain and concluded that persistent pain is not merely a prolonged acute pain symptom of some other disease. Underlying physiologic mechanisms lead to the persistence of pain (Marx, 2004; Woolf and Salter, 2000).

In a study of nursing practice related to pain assessment and management in different pediatric specialty units (Jacob and Puntillo, 2000), complaints of pain were noted, but specific pain scores or notations about responses to analgesics after administration were seldom documented. Pain scores were not available before and after analgesics; therefore it was not possible to conclude whether analgesics were effective. Thus nurses need to evaluate and monitor pain in a timely fashion after administration of analgesics; titrate dosage to effect; or make recommendations for an alternate analgesic, addition of another analgesic, or a combination of analgesics, adjuvants, and nonpharmacologic strategies if pain persists.

Consequences of Untreated Pain

Despite current research on the neonate's experience of pain, infant pain often remains inadequately managed. The mismanagement of infant pain is partially the result of misconceptions regarding the effects of pain on the neonate and the lack of knowledge of immediate and long-term consequences of untreated pain. Infants respond to noxious stimuli through (1) physiologic indicators (i.e., increased heart rate and blood pressure, variability in heart rate and intracranial pressure [ICP]), (2) decreases in Sao_2 and skin blood flow, and (3) behavioral indicators (i.e., muscle rigidity, facial expression, crying, withdrawal, and sleeplessness) (Anand, Grunau, and Oberlander, 1997; Bildner and Krechel, 1996). The physiologic and behavioral changes and a variety of neurophysiologic responses to noxious stimulation are responsible for acute and long-term consequences of pain.

Anand and Hickey (1987) described responses of infants to painful stimuli. Chemical and hormonal responses were observed following noxious stimuli without the use of an anesthetic or analgesic. Such responses included increases in β-endorphin secretion (an endogenous opioid), plasma renin activity, plasma epinephrine and norepinephrine, catecholamines, growth hormone, glucagon, aldosterone, and other corticosteroids. The result of these chemical and hormonal increases includes the breakdown of fat and carbohydrate stores; prolonged hyperglycemia; and increased serum lactate, pyruvate, total ketone bodies, and nonesterified fatty acids. Such consequences can be attributed to a greater morbidity for neonates in the NICU. Several experimental studies revealed a significant decrease in these responses when adequate analgesia was used before the painful procedure. One study showed that the standardization of postoperative pain management strategies for infants in the NICU led to the following improvements: (1) decreased

---

length of time to extubation, (2) decreased length of stay, (3) better fluid management, and (4) reduced side effects of opioids. The authors also noted improved pain management documentation, decreased cost, and decreased nursing time (Furdon, Eastman, Benjamin, et al., 1998) (see Atraumatic Care box).

COMMON PAIN STATES

Pain in Primary Care

In normative problems such as teething; during immunizations and vaccinations; and in common childhood illnesses such as otitis media, pharyngitis, and viral infections, pain is the presenting symptom that can be distressing (Schechter, 2003). The inflammation or irritation of the gingiva as the tooth erupts is responsible for discomfort during teething. Teething infants show more mouthing and drooling than nonteething infants. A topical anesthetic such as benzocaine, cold or frozen teething rings, and hard crackers or bread can alleviate pain during teething.

Injections from immunizations, IM antibiotics in the ED or health care provider's office, and blood draws are common sources of pain in children (Schechter, 2003). The immunization schedule for infants and young children requires at least 19 injections in the first 6 years of childhood; children receive four or five injections at multiple visits. Potential complications to needlesticks include fibrosis, contracture, abscess, and nerve injury. Factors that affect the incidence of complication are the injection site, the injectate itself (lower pH causing more burning and stinging), needle length, and frequency of injection. Warming the injectate, using lidocaine as a diluent, and applying ice and pressure to the site immediately before the procedure may reduce the discomfort associated with IM injections. Topical analgesia such as EMLA, LMX, amethocaine, cold sprays, and iontophoresis (see Evidence-Based Practice boxes) and cognitive-behavioral techniques (distraction, bubbles, parental presence, age-appropriate explanations, kaleidoscopes, music, stories) have been used to minimize pain, stress, fear, distress, and anxiety during injections. If multiple injections are required, parents have reported that simultaneous administration is less painful and less traumatic for their children than sequential administration.

In patients with otitis media the incidence of pain is lower in those who received ibuprofen 3 times a day when compared with those children who received acetaminophen or who did not receive either ibuprofen or acetaminophen (Bertin, Pons, d'Athis, et al., 1996). Warm compresses using oatmeal or warm stones have also been found to be effective for otitis media. Local anesthetic combinations such as Auralgan (antipyrine, benzocaine, and oxyquinoline

EVIDENCE-BASED PRACTICE

Analgesic Patches: Synera to Decrease Pain During Painful Procedures

Ask the Question

Do topical analgesic patches (e.g., lidocaine-tetracaine [Synera, S-Caine]) offer additional advantages (less time, ease of use, lower cost, higher effectiveness, decreased anxiety) in relieving pain during peripheral intravenous (PIV) cannulation in children compared with lidocaine cream (LMX) and buffered lidocaine via injection?

Search for the Evidence
Search Strategies

English research-based publications on lidocaine-tetracaine patches for venipuncture without time limitation were included. Exclusions included epidural use, dermatologic procedures, and S-Caine Peel.

Databases Used

Cochrane Collaboration Database, Joanna Briggs Institute, National Guideline Clearinghouse (AHRQ), PubMed, SUMSearch, CINAHL, Scopus, Micromedex, UpToDate, BestBETs, manufacturer's websites (Endo Pharmaceuticals, ZARS Pharma)

Critically Analyze the Evidence

Studies evaluated effectiveness of Synera patch in decreasing pain during painful procedures.

- Synera is as effective as EMLA (a eutectic mix of lidocaine and prilocaine) in a much shorter time frame with fewer adverse reactions in adults (Sawyer, Febbraro, Masud, et al., 2009).
- Synera reduced PIV cannulation pain and did not alter the success rate in children 3 to 17 years old (Singer, Taira, Chisena, et al., 2008).
- Median self-reported pain using a visual analog scale or Wong-Baker FACES scale was significantly lower when the Synera patch was placed over the antecubital or hand vein vs. the placebo patch ($p = 0.04$) (Singer, Taira, Chisena, et al., 2008).
- A 20-minute application of the S-Caine patch (Synera) was effective in lessening pain in children scheduled for vascular access (Sethna, Verghese, Hannallah, et al., 2005).
- Synera pain patch significantly reduced pain compared with placebo (median Oucher scores of 0 vs. 60; $p < 0.001$); 59% of children in the pain patch group reported no pain compared with 20% in the placebo group (Sethna, Verghese, Hannallah, et al., 2005).
- Mild skin erythema (<38%) and edema (<2%) occurred with similar frequencies between the groups (Sethna, Verghese, Hannallah, et al., 2005).

Apply the Evidence: Nursing Implications

There is *good evidence* with *strong recommendation* for using Synera patches to decrease pain during painful procedures (Guyatt, Oxman, Vist, et al., 2008). Synera use during PIV cannulation in children 3 years and older decreases

pain. It should not be used in children with sensitivity to lidocaine, tetracaine, para-aminobenzoic acid (PABA), or amide- or ester-type anesthetics. Use with caution in patients with hepatic impairment and those receiving class I antiarrhythmic drugs (e.g., tocainide and mexiletine) and do not apply to broken skin. Use the patch immediately after opening the pouch; do not cut or remove any layers of the patch; and ensure that the holes on the patch are not covered by clothing. Do not keep the patch on longer than 20 to 30 minutes. As with all transdermal patches containing medication, after use fold the adhesive together and dispose of used patches in a location out of the reach of children. Do not use in a magnetic resonance imaging suite.

Quality and Safety Competencies:
Evidence-Based Practice*
Knowledge

Differentiate clinical opinion from research and evidence-based summaries.

Describe the use of Synera to decrease pain during painful procedures.

Skills

Base individualized care plan on patient values, clinical expertise, and evidence.

Integrate evidence into practice by using Synera patches to decrease pain during painful procedures.

Attitudes

Value the concept of evidence-based practice as integral to determining best clinical practice.

Appreciate strengths and weakness of evidence for use of Synera patches to decrease pain during painful procedures.

References

Guyatt GH, Oxman AD, Vist GE, et al: GRADE: an emerging consensus on rating quality of evidence and strength of recommendations, *BMJ* 336:924–926, 2008.

Sawyer J, Febbraro S, Masud S, et al: Heated lidocaine/tetracaine patch (Synera, Rapydan) compared with lidocaine/prilocaine cream (EMLA) for topical anaesthesia before vascular access, *Br J Anaesth* 102(2):210–215, 2009.

Sethna NF, Verghese ST, Hannallah RS, et al: A randomized controlled trial to evaluate S-Caine patch for reducing pain associated with vascular access in children, *Anesthesiology* 102(2):403–408, 2005.

Singer AJ, Taira BR, Chisena EN, et al: Warm lidocaine/tetracaine patch versus placebo before pediatric intravenous cannulation: a randomized controlled trial, *Ann Emerg Med* 52(1):41–47, 2008.

Terri L. Brown; Updated by Olga A. Taylor

*Adapted from the QSEN at www.qsen.org.

---

sulfate dissolved in dehydrated glycerine) have been demonstrated to provide greater relief than olive oil drops to the ear (Hoberman, Paradise, Reynolds, et al., 1997).

In children with pharyngitis, spontaneous pain resolved in 80% of children who received ibuprofen during the first 48 hours, 70% of children who received acetaminophen, and 55% of children who received neither ibuprofen nor acetaminophen (Bertin, Pons, d'Athis, et al., 1996). In patients who had culture-positive streptococcal pharyngitis, those who received IM injection of a steroid such as dexamethasone or betamethasone were able to achieve pain relief

within 6 hours compared with those who did not receive either one (Marvez-Valls, Ernst, Gray, et al., 1998). Parents have also reported using salt water gargles, lozenges, and local anesthetic sprays for alleviation of their child's pain in acute pharyngitis.

Viral infections of the mouth such as primary herpetic gingivostomatitis (herpes simplex virus 1) and herpangina ulcers (coxsackievirus A) are extremely painful; if inadequately treated the pain can inhibit oral intake in children. Viscous lidocaine can be swished and spit by children older than 3 years of age or applied with cotton-tipped applicator in children younger than 3 years. A

EVIDENCE-BASED PRACTICE

Needle-Free Injection System: J-Tip to Administer Buffered Lidocaine

Ask the Question
In pediatrics are needle-free injection systems (e.g., J-Tip) effective and safe in relieving pain during peripheral intravenous (PIV) cannulation?

Search for the Evidence
Search Strategies
English-language research-based publications on jet injectors for delivery of lidocaine during PIV cannulation without time limitation were included. Exclusions included dental products, insulin, growth factor, and medications other than lidocaine.

Databases Used
Cochrane Collaboration Database, Joanna Briggs Institute, National Guideline Clearinghouse (AHRQ), PubMed, SUMSearch, CINAHL, Scopus, UpTo-Date, BestBETs, manufacturers' or distributors' websites (National Medical Products, Bioject, and Injex)

Critically Analyze the Evidence
- J-Tip is superior in pain prevention compared with lidocaine cream (LMX) or EMLA (a eutectic mix of lidocaine and prilocaine) (Jimenez, Bradford, Seidel, et al., 2006; Spanos, Booth, Koenig, et al., 2008).
- J-Tip with 0.2 mL of 1% buffered lidocaine provided greater anesthesia than a 30-minute application of LMX in children ages 8 to 15 years undergoing 22- or 24-gauge peripheral intravenous (PIV) catheter insertion (Spanos, Booth, Koenig, et al., 2008).
- Visual analog scale (VAS) scores were significantly different immediately after PIV catheter insertion (17.3 for J-Tip vs. 44.6 for LMX; $p < 0.001$). Blinded reviewer VAS scores were not statistically significant (21.7 for J-Tip vs. 31.9 for LMX; $p = 0.23$) (Spanos, Booth, Koenig, et al., 2008).
- J-Tip did not alter the insertion site or affect the success of PIV access on the first attempt; multiple injections could be performed if necessary without causing lidocaine toxicity (Spanos, Booth, Koenig, et al., 2008).
- J-Tip with 0.25 mL of 1% buffered lidocaine provided greater anesthesia than application of 2.5 g of EMLA in a study of 116 children ages 7 to 19 years undergoing PIV catheter insertion (Jimenez, Bradford, Seidel, et al., 2006).
- Subjects' self-report median pain ratings of PIV cannulation using a 0 to 10 VAS were 0 for J-Tip and 3 for EMLA ($p = 0.0001$ for patients receiving EMLA ≥60 minutes before cannulation and $p = 0.0013$ for those receiving EMLA <60 minutes before) (Jimenez, Bradford, Seidel, et al., 2006).
- More pain scores were favorable for the J-Tip application (84% reported no pain at the time of injection) compared with EMLA application (61% reported pain at time of Tegaderm dressing removal; $p = 0.004$) (Jimenez, Bradford, Seidel, et al., 2006).
- J-Tip with 0.2 mL of 1% buffered lidocaine was no more effective than jet-delivered placebo (preservative-free normal saline) during PIV cannulation but may provide superior analgesia compared with no local anesthetic pretreatment (Auerbach, Tunik, and Mojica, 2009).
- Children 5 to 18 years of age received either J-Tip (0.2 mL of buffered 1% lidocaine) or jet-delivered placebo (0.2 mL of preservative-free normal saline) 60 seconds before PIV cannulation in an emergency department.

Subjects reported pain on injection and on PIV cannulation using a 100-mm color analog scale (Auerbach, Tunik, and Mojica, 2009).
- Mean needle insertion pain score for jet lidocaine, 28 mm, was similar to the mean score for placebo, 34 mm, and lower than the no-device group, 52 mm; most patients reported that they would request this device for future PIV access (Auerbach, Tunik, and Mojica, 2009).

Apply the Evidence: Nursing Implications
There is *good evidence* with a *strong recommendation* for using J-Tip to administer buffered lidocaine (Guyatt, Oxman, Vist, et al., 2008). J-Tip with 0.2 mL of buffered lidocaine 1% decreases pain during PIV insertion. It is recommended to wait 1 minute after administration before attempting PIV insertion. J-Tip should not be used to administer buffered lidocaine in children with a known hypersensitivity to lidocaine or other amide-type local anesthetics such as prilocaine, mepivacaine, bupivacaine, or etidocaine.

Quality and Safety Competencies: Evidence-Based Practice*
Knowledge
Differentiate clinical opinion from research and evidence-based summaries.
Describe the use of J-Tip to administer buffered lidocaine.

Skills
Base individualized care plan on patient values, clinical expertise, and evidence.
Integrate evidence into practice by using J-Tip to administer buffered lidocaine.

Attitudes
Value the concept of evidence-based practice as integral to determining best clinical practice.
Appreciate strengths and weakness of evidence for using J-Tip to administer buffered lidocaine.

References
Auerbach M, Tunik M, Mojica M: A randomized, double-blind controlled study of jet lidocaine compared to jet placebo for pain relief in children undergoing needle insertion in the emergency department, *Acad Emerg Med* 16(1):1–6, 2009.

Guyatt GH, Oxman AD, Vist GE, et al: GRADE: an emerging consensus on rating quality of evidence and strength of recommendations, *BMJ* 336:924–926, 2008.

Jimenez N, Bradford H, Seidel KD, et al: A comparison of a needle-free injection system for local anesthesia versus EMLA for intravenous catheter insertion in the pediatric patient, *Anesth Analg* 102(2):411–414, 2006.

Spanos S, Booth R, Koenig H, et al: Jet injection of 1% buffered lidocaine versus topical ELA-Max for anesthesia before peripheral intravenous catheterization in children: a randomized controlled trial, *Pediatr Emerg Care* 24(8):511–515, 2008.

Terri Brown; Updated by Olga A. Taylor

*Adapted from the QSEN at www.qsen.org.

2% viscous lidocaine solution contains 100 mg/5 mL lidocaine hydrochloride; dosages of more than 5 mg/kg every 3 hours can be potentially toxic in small children (Gonzales-Del-Rey, Wason, and Druckenbrod, 1994). Parents need careful instructions to place an accurate amount of lidocaine in the child's mouth. Benzocaine has also been used, and methemoglobinemia has been reported as a rare side effect associated with its administration in younger children. "Magic mouthwash" preparation has ingredients that adhere to the lesion and provide pain relief. It usually consists of equal parts of diphenhydramine, viscous lidocaine, and aluminum and

EVIDENCE-BASED PRACTICE

Buffered Lidocaine for Pain Reduction During Peripheral Intravenous Access in Children

Ask the Question

In children is buffered lidocaine an appropriate anesthetic for reducing pain during peripheral intravenous (PIV) access?

Search for the Evidence

Search Strategies

Search criteria included English-language publications within the past 5 years, research-based articles (level 3 or lower) on children undergoing PIV access. Two of the articles reviewed were more than 5 years old but were included based on the limited literature in this area.

Databases Used

PubMed, Cochrane Collaboration, MD Consult, Joanna Briggs Institute, National Guideline Clearinghouse (AHQR), TRIP Database, PedsCCM, BestBETs

Critically Analyze the Evidence

- Patients' comfort and satisfaction were improved when the pH of lidocaine solution was increased; it is recommended to increase pH of lidocaine solution using bicarbonate immediately before administration (Cepeda, Tzortzopoulou, Thackrey, et al., 2010).
- Buffered lidocaine vs. liposomal lidocaine cream (LMX) was evaluated before PIV access in children (4 to 17 years of age; 61% female). Both interventions decreased pain; no significant differences in pain levels between buffered lidocaine and LMX groups were noted. The LMX group stated that the pain came with the removal of the occlusive dressing from the site (Luhmann, Hurt, Shootman, et al., 2004).
- PIV access without buffered lidocaine was significantly more painful than PIV access with buffered lidocaine in children (Fein, Boardman, Stevenson, et al., 1998).
- Subcutaneous lidocaine vs. no pain-control measures was evaluated in children younger than 2 years of age before PIV access in the emergency department; no significant differences in pain levels were found (Sacchetti and Carraccio, 1996).
- PIV access without lidocaine was significantly more painful than PIV access with lidocaine regardless of catheter size (Klein, Shugerman, Leigh-Taylor, et al., 1995).

Apply the Evidence: Nursing Implications

There is *good evidence* with a *strong recommendation* (Guyatt, Oxman, Vist, et al., 2008) for using buffered lidocaine as a pain reduction measure in children before PIV access. Buffered lidocaine should be used in children older than 2 years of age. It has an immediate time of onset and a duration of about 1 hour and can be injected at multiple sites. The following dosage is recommended: 0.1 to 0.5 mL buffered 1% lidocaine to a maximum of 0.45 mL/kg/dose; can repeat dose after 2 hours. Buffered lidocaine should

not be used within 2 hours before vesicants or with abraded skin. There is a possibility of some vasoconstriction with its use, which may increase the difficulty of PIV access. An "extra stick" and ineffective buffered lidocaine administration may result in pain during both local administration and PIV access. Expertise in administering buffered lidocaine is an important factor related to its effectiveness.

Quality and Safety Competencies: Evidence-Based Practice*

Knowledge

Differentiate clinical opinion from research and evidence-based summaries.

Describe the use of buffered lidocaine for pain reduction during PIV access in children.

Skills

Base individualized care plan on patient values, clinical expertise, and evidence.

Integrate evidence into practice by using buffered lidocaine for pain reduction during PIV access in children.

Attitudes

Value the concept of evidence-based practice as integral to determining best clinical practice.

Appreciate the strengths and weakness of the evidence for using buffered lidocaine for pain reduction during PIV access in children.

References

Cepeda MS, Tzortzopoulou A, Thackrey M, et al: Adjusting the pH of lidocaine for reducing pain on injection, *Cochrane Database Syst Rev* 12:1–64, 2010.

Fein JA, Boardman CR, Stevenson S, et al: Saline with benzyl alcohol as intradermal anesthesia for intravenous line placement in children, *Pediatr Emerg Care* 14(2):119–122, 1998.

Guyatt GH, Oxman AD, Vist GE, et al: GRADE: an emerging consensus on rating quality of evidence and strength of recommendations, *BMJ* 336:924–926, 2008.

Klein EJ, Shugerman RP, Leigh-Taylor K, et al: Buffered lidocaine: analgesia for intravenous line placement in children, *Pediatrics* 95(5):709–712, 1995.

Luhmann J, Hurt S, Shootman M, et al: A comparison of buffered lidocaine versus ELA-Max before peripheral intravenous catheter insertions in children, *Pediatrics* 113(3 Pt 1):217–220, 2004.

Sacchetti AD, Carraccio C: Subcutaneous lidocaine does not affect the success rate of intravenous access in children less than 24 months of age, *Acad Emerg Med* 3(11):1016–1019, 1996.

Angela Morgan; Updated by Olga Taylor

*Adapted from the QSEN at www.qsen.org.

magnesium hydroxide (Maalox); equal parts of diphenhydramine and attapulgite suspension (Kaopectate); or a sucralfate suspension plus diphenhydramine and attapulgite suspension solutions that coat the lesions.

Painful and Invasive Procedures

Several painful and invasive procedures require the administration of anesthetics and analgesics. For circumcision pain caudal or penile blocks are used before the procedure; then parents are instructed how to apply lidocaine gels for the first 24 to 36 hours after the

circumcision. For open wounds bupivacaine may be instilled with or without epinephrine onto the dressing applied to skin to minimize pain for up to 48 hours after the procedure. For graft donor sites analgesia is maintained by using a foam dressing soaked with bupivacaine (0.25%, 2 mg/kg; 0.8 mL/kg) applied to the donor surface. A continuous infusion of 0.25% bupivacaine at 1 to 3 mL/hr via a standard 18-gauge epidural catheter is then curled on the outer or inner surface of the foam (Cousins and Power, 2003). Wound perfusion of bupivacaine is useful for iliac crest bone graft donor sites (used for alveolar bone grafting in some techniques of cleft palate repair). A standard 18-gauge epidural catheter is also used with a very low infusion rate (1 to 3 mL/hr) of bupivacaine. For minor and some intermediate procedures, the local anesthetic infiltration with bupivacaine is commonly used. Some examples of these procedures include surface wounds and tunneling procedures in the anesthetized child requiring inguinal surgery; insertion of ventriculoperitoneal shunts, central venous lines, or central venous catheter-reservoir systems; and similar procedures.

Nitrous oxide, which is taken up rapidly and eliminated by the lungs, is highly insoluble in the blood and delivered quickly to the brain to produce an analgesic effect equivalent to that of IV morphine. After approximately 2 minutes of inhalation, maximum pain relief can be achieved. The child breathes via face mask, nasal mask, or mouthpiece. It is not suitable for children younger than 3 years old and works best for children older than 5 years of age. Nitrous oxide inhalations are used frequently for a wide variety of procedures that require potent analgesia for a short time such as suture insertion or removal, dressing removal or changes (including burns), drain or catheter removal, venipuncture or cannulation, lumbar puncture, physical therapy, and biopsies (skin, muscle, renal, or bone marrow). However, the use of nitrous oxide is contraindicated in children with pneumothorax, bowel obstruction, abnormal airway, recent head injury (especially with an intracranial air pocket), chronic respiratory disease with air trapping or bullous changes in the lung, and some types of uncorrected congenital heart disease (such as pulmonary hypertension). Nitrous oxide may lead to expansion of air pockets in confined spaces (chest, cranial cavities, bowel lumens) and create an increased pressure and tension effect. Tension pneumothorax, ischemia or shift of intracranial contents, and bowel distention with risk of perforation could occur. In addition, because nitrous oxide produces a degree of sedation and potentiates the sedative effects of other central nervous system depressants, caution is required when concurrently giving opioids, benzodiazepines, antihistamines, and similar drugs. Inspired concentrations of up to 50% nitrous oxide used for less than 30 minutes do not affect airway reflexes. Only trained personnel may administer nitrous oxide and monitor the child (Cousins and Power, 2003).

Postoperative Pain

Pain associated with surgery to the chest (e.g., repair of congenital heart defects, chest trauma) or abdominal regions (e.g., appendectomy, cholecystectomy, splenectomy) may result in pulmonary complications. Pain leads to decreased muscle movement in the thorax and abdominal area and decreased tidal volume, vital capacity, functional residual capacity, and alveolar ventilation. The patient is unable to cough and clear secretions, and the risk for complications such as pneumonia and atelectasis is high. Severe postoperative pain also results in sympathetic overactivity, which leads to increases in heart rate, peripheral resistance, blood pressure, and cardiac output. The patient eventually experiences an increase in cardiac demand and myocardial oxygen consumption and a decrease in oxygen delivery to the tissues.

The basis for good postoperative pain control in children is preemptive analgesia. Preemptive analgesia involves administration of medications (e.g., local and regional anesthetics, analgesics) before the child experiences the pain or before surgery is performed so the sensory activation and changes in the pain pathways of the peripheral and central nervous system can be controlled. Preemptive analgesia has been demonstrated to lower postoperative pain, analgesic requirement, hospital stay, and complications after surgery and minimize the risks for peripheral and central

nervous system sensitization that can lead to persistent pain (Cousins and Power, 2003).

A combination of medications (multimodal or balanced analgesia) is used for postoperative pain and may include nonsteroidal antiinflammatory drugs (NSAIDs), local anesthetics, nonopioids, and opioid analgesics to achieve optimum relief and minimize side effects. Opioids administered around the clock (ATC) during the first 48 hours or via patient-controlled analgesia (PCA) are commonly prescribed after surgery. The duration of use is frequently limited to days because the cause of pain usually resolves. The combination of the IV NSAID ketorolac and morphine using a PCA device is frequently prescribed after thoracic surgery. Morphine delivered by PCA leads to a lower total dosage of opioid analgesia when compared with the administration of intermittent doses of analgesic as required. After bowel surgery a mixture of local anesthetics (bupivacaine) and a low-dose opioid (fentanyl) delivered by epidural route improves the rate of recovery and minimizes the gastrointestinal effects (e.g., bowel stasis, nausea, vomiting). Once bowel function has been restored, oral opioids such as immediate- and controlled-release preparations are preferred in older children. Controlled-release opioids facilitate ATC dosing and improve sleep. They are also associated with lower incidence of nausea, sedation, and breakthrough pain.

Burn Pain

Because burn pain has multiple components, involves repeated manipulations over the injured painful sites, and has changing pattern over time, it is difficult and challenging to control. It includes a constant background pain that is felt at the wound sites and surrounding areas and can be exacerbated (breakthrough pain) by movements such as changing position, turning in bed, walking, or even breathing. Areas of normal skin that have been harvested for skin grafts (donor sites) also elicit pain. Pain is commonly experienced with intense tingling or itching sensations when skin grafting is required. During the healing process, when the tissue and nerve regenerate, the necrotic tissue (eschar) is excised until viable tissue is reached. The healing process may last for months to years. Pain or paresthetic sensations (e.g., itching, tingling, cold sensations) may persist. In addition, discomfort may be associated with immobilization of limbs in splints or garments and multiple surgical interventions such as skin grafting and reconstructive surgery (Choiniere, 2003).

Multiple therapeutic procedures are carried out during the course of treatment. These procedures (i.e., dressing changes, wound debridement and cleansing, physical therapy sessions) occur daily or even several times a day. Providing proper analgesia without interfering with the patient's awareness during and after the procedure is the biggest challenge in the management of burn pain. Fentanyl or alfentanil has a major advantage over morphine because of the short duration. Fentanyl can prevent oversedation following the procedure. For less painful procedures premedication with oral morphine, oral ketamine, or milder opioids 15 minutes before the procedure may be sufficient. Depending on the patient's anxiety level, a benzodiazepine (e.g., lorazepam) before the procedure may be beneficial. For longer procedures morphine is the mainstay of treatment. Some patients may require moderate-to-deep sedation and analgesia. Oral oxycodone with midazolam and acetaminophen, in addition to nitrous oxide, may be needed. IV ketamine administered at subtherapeutic doses has been one of the most extensively used anesthetics for burn patients. The dysphoria and unpleasant reactions associated with ketamine administration may be minimized with premedication with a benzodiazepine. If ketamine is used with either morphine or fentanyl, the regimen could have opioid-sparing actions and reduce the opioid-related side effects.

Psychologic interventions can also be helpful in the treatment of burn pain. These interventions include hypnosis, relaxation training (breathing exercises, progressive muscle relaxation), biofeedback, stress inoculation training, cognitive-behavioral strategies (guided imagery, distraction, coping skills), and group and individual psychotherapy. They can be used alone or in combination. All of these techniques can help the patient relax and maintain a sense of control (Choiniere, 2003). A major disadvantage of these interventions is that they require time and discipline and often patients are too stressed, fatigued, disoriented, or sick to engage in them.

Recurrent Headaches

Recurrent headaches in children can have several causes, including tension, dental braces, imbalance or weakness of eye muscles causing deviation in alignment and refractive errors, sequelae to accidents, sinusitis and other cranial infection or inflammation, increased intracranial pressure, epileptic attacks, drugs, obstructive sleep apnea and, rarely, hypertension. Other causes may include arteriovenous malformations, disturbances in cerebrospinal fluid flow or absorption, intracranial hemorrhages, ocular and dental diseases, bacterial infections, and brain tumors. Severe pain is the most disturbing symptom in migraine. Tension-type headache is usually mild or moderate, often producing a pressing feeling in the temples like a "tight band around the head." Continuous, daily, or near-daily headache with no specific cause occurs in a small subgroup of children. In epilepsy headaches commonly occur immediately before, during, or after a seizure attack.

Treatment of recurrent headaches requires an understanding of the antecedents and consequences of headache pain. A headache diary can allow the child to record the time of onset, activities before the onset, any worries or concerns as far back as 24 hours before the onset, severity and duration of pain, pain medications taken, and activity pattern during headache episodes. The headache diary allows ongoing monitoring of headache activity, indicates the effects of interventions, and guides treatment planning.

There are two main approaches to management of headache using behavioral approaches: (1) teaching patients self-control skills to prevent headache (biofeedback techniques and relaxation training), and (2) modifying behavior patterns that increase the risk of headache occurrence or reinforce headache activity (cognitive-behavioral stress-management techniques). Biofeedback is a technology-based form of relaxation therapy and can be useful in assessing and reinforcing learning of relaxation skills such as progressive muscle relaxation, deep breathing, and imagery. Children as young as 7 years of age have been taught these skills and with 2 or 3 weeks of practice are able to decrease the time needed to achieve relaxation.

To modify behavior patterns that increase the risk of headache occurrence or reinforce headache activity, the nurse instructs parents to avoid giving excessive attention to their child's headache and to respond matter-of-factly to pain behavior and requests for special attention (Holden, Deichmann, and Levy, 1999). Parents are taught to assess whether school or social performance demands are being avoided because of headache. They are taught to focus attention on adaptive coping such as the use of relaxation techniques and maintenance of normal activity patterns. When using cognitive-behavioral stress-management techniques, the parents identify negative thoughts and situations that may be associated with increased risk for headache. The child is then taught to activate positive thoughts and engage in adaptive behavior appropriate to the situation.

Recurrent Abdominal Pain

Recurrent abdominal pain (RAP) or functional abdominal pain is defined as pain that occurs at least once per month for 3 consecutive months, accompanied by pain-free periods, and is severe enough that it interferes with a child's normal activities. Management of RAP is highly individualized to reflect the causes of the pain and the psychosocial needs of the child and family. A clear understanding of the child's characteristics (anxiety, physical health, temperament, coping skills, experience, learned response, depression), child's disability (school attendance, activities with family, social interactions, pain behaviors), environmental factors (family attitudes and behavioral patterns, school environment, community, friendships), and the pain stimulus (disease, injury, stress) is important in planning management strategies (Collins and Weisman, 2003).

Before any workup of the pain, the nurse informs the family that RAP is common in children and only 10% of children with RAP have an identifiable organic cause for their pain symptom. Medical workup is dictated by the child's symptoms and signs in combination with knowledge about common organic causes of RAP. If an organic cause is found, it is treated appropriately. Even if no organic cause is found, the nurse needs to communicate to the child and family a belief that the pain is real. Usually the abdominal pain goes away; however, even if problems are identified, they may not be the actual cause, and pain may persist, be replaced by another symptom, or go away on its own. The management of plan includes regular follow-up at a 3- to 4-month intervals, a list of symptoms that call for earlier contact, and biobehavioral pain-management techniques. The goal is to minimize the impact that the pain has on the child's activities and the family's life (Collins and Weisman, 2003).

Case reports have demonstrated the effectiveness of implementing a time-out procedure, token systems, and positive reinforcement based on operant theory treatment modalities. Stress-management and cognitive-behavioral strategies have also been reported to be successful. Parent training in how to avoid positive reinforcement of sick behaviors and focus on rewarding healthy behaviors is important. Over the course of several sessions parents are educated about RAP, how to distinguish between sick and well behaviors, a reward system for well behaviors, and the importance of reinforcing relaxation and stressing the teaching of coping skills to children for pain management. Treatment may consist of a varying number of sessions over 1 to 6 months and include various components such as monitoring symptoms, limited parent attention, relaxation training, increased dietary fiber, and requirements of school attendance. Response rates are 25% without abdominal pain and 56% to 75% improvements in symptoms (Collins and Weisman, 2003). The use of cognitive-behavioral therapy has been documented to reduce or eliminate pain in children with RAP and highlights the involvement of parents in supporting their child's self-management behavior. No negative side effects of symptom substitution occurred with the interventions. One study demonstrated that the combination of self-regulation and cognitive-behavioral interventions along with fiber intervention is more effective for treating RAP than using fiber alone (Weydert, Ball, and Davis, 2003).

Pain with Sickle Cell Disease

A painful episode is the most frequent cause for ED visits and hospital admissions among children with sickle cell disease. The acute painful episode in sickle cell disease is the only pain syndrome in which opioids are considered the major therapy and are started in early childhood and continued throughout adult life. A source of frustration for patients and clinicians is that the most current analgesic regimens are inadequate in controlling some of the most severe painful episodes. A multidisciplinary approach that involves both pharmacologic and nonpharmacologic modalities (cognitive-behavioral intervention, heat, massage, physical therapy) is needed but not often implemented. The goals of treatment of the acute episode may not be to take all the pain away, which is usually impossible, but to make the pain tolerable to the patient until the episode resolves and increase function and patient participation in activities of daily living (Benjamin, Dampier, Jacox, et al., 1999; Max, Payne, Edwards, et al., 1999).

Individuals coming to an ED for acute painful episodes usually have exhausted all home care options or outpatient therapy (Benjamin, Dampier, Jacox, et al., 1999; Max, Payne, Edwards, et al., 1999). The nurse should ask patients what the usual medication, dosage, and side effects were in the past; about the usual medication taken at home; and about medication taken since the onset of present pain. The patient may be on long-term opioid therapy at home and therefore may have developed some degree of tolerance. A different potent opioid or a larger dose of the same medication may be indicated. Because mixed opioid-agonist-antagonists (e.g., pentazocine, nalbuphine, butorphanol) may precipitate withdrawal syndromes, these should be avoided if patients were taking long-term opioids at home. A "passport" card with patient information about the diagnosis, previous complications, suggested pain management regimen, and name and contact information of the primary hematologist would be helpful for parents and would facilitate management of pain in the ED.

The patient is admitted for inpatient management of severe pain if adequate relief is not achieved in the ED (Benjamin, Dampier, Jacox, et al., 1999; Max, Payne, Edwards, et al., 1999). For severe pain IV administration with bolus dosing and continuous infusion using a PCA device may be necessary. Patients requiring more than 5 to 7 days of opioids should have tapering doses to avoid the physiologic symptoms of withdrawal (dysphoria, nasal congestion, diarrhea, nausea and vomiting, sweating, and seizures). Appropriate weaning of the PCA schedules starts with reduction of the continuous infusion rate before discontinuation while the patient can continue to use demand doses for analgesia. Morphine-equivalent equianalgesic conversions may be used to convert continuous infusion rates to equivalent oral analgesics. Doses of long-acting oral analgesics such as sustained-release oral morphine may also be used to replace continuous-infusion dosing. The demand doses can be reduced subsequently if analgesia remains adequate.

Some patients whose pain is managed poorly try to persuade medical staff to give them more analgesic, engage in clock watching, and request specific medications or dosages. These patients are often perceived as manipulative and demanding. Because patients with sickle cell disease have lifelong experiences with pain, they are knowledgeable about the medications and doses that are effective (Benjamin, Dampier, Jacox, et al., 1999; Max, Payne, Edwards, et al., 1999). Therefore the nurse should respect their requests for specific medications and doses and not interpret them as indications of drug-seeking behavior.

Patients who are administered doses of opioids that are inadequate to relieve their pain or whose doses are not tapered after a course of treatment may develop **iatrogenic** pseudoaddiction (Elander, Lusher, Bevan, et al., 2004), which resembles addiction. Pseudoaddiction or clock-watching behavior may be resolved by communicating with patients to ensure accurate assessment, involving them in decisions about their pain management, and administering adequate opioid doses (Elander, Lusher, Bevan, et al., 2004).

Cancer Pain

Pain is the most prevalent symptom (84.4%) and was rated as moderate to severe (86.6%) and highly distressing (52.8%) in children with cancer (Collins, Byrnes, Dunkel, et al., 2000). Pain is present before diagnosis and treatment and may resolve after initiation of anticancer therapy. However, treatment-related pain is a common occurrence. Pain may be related to an operation; mucositis; a phantom limb; infection; chemotherapy; and procedures such as bone marrow aspiration, needle puncture, and lumbar puncture (Collins, Byrnes, Dunkel, et al., 2000). Tumor-related pain frequently occurs when the child relapses or when tumors become resistant to treatment. Intractable pain may occur in patients with solid tumors that metastasize to the central or peripheral nervous system. In young adult survivors of childhood cancer, chronic pain conditions may develop, including complex regional pain syndrome of the lower extremity, phantom limb pain, avascular necrosis, mechanical pain related to bone that failed to unite after tumor resection, and postherpetic neuralgia.

Oral mucositis (ulceration of the oral cavity and throat) may occur in 40% of patients undergoing chemotherapy or radiotherapy and in 76% of patients undergoing bone marrow transplant (Berger, Henderson, Nadoolman, et al., 1995). No present therapy adequately relieves the pain of these lesions. Antihistamines, local anesthetics, and opioids provide only temporary relief, may block taste perception, or may produce additional side effects such as lethargy and constipation. Initial treatment includes single agents (saline, opioids, sodium bicarbonate, hydrogen peroxide, sucralfate suspension, clotrimazole, nystatin, viscous lidocaine, amphotericin B, dyclonine) or mouthwash mixtures using a combination of agents (lidocaine, diphenhydramine, Maalox or Mylanta, nystatin). The mucositis after bone marrow transplantation may be prolonged, continuously intense, exacerbated by mouth care and swallowing, or worse during waking hours. The patient may be unable to eat or swallow. Morphine administered as a continuous infusion or delivered by PCA device may be required until mucositis is resolved (Collins and Weisman, 2003).

Other treatment-related pain includes (1) abdominal pain after allogeneic bone marrow transplantation, which may be associated with acute graft-versus-host disease; (2) abdominal pain associated with typhlitis (infection of the cecum), which occurs when the patient is immunocompromised; (3) phantom sensations and phantom limb pain after an amputation; (4) peripheral neuropathy after administration of vincristine; and (5) medullary bone pain, which may be associated with administration of granulocyte colony–stimulating factor (Collins and Weisman, 2003).

Almost 40% of all pain episodes in children with cancer may be attributed to procedures (Ljungman, Gordh, Sorensen, et al., 1999, 2000, 2001; Ljungman, Kreuger, Andreasson, et al., 2000). Survivors of childhood cancer describe vivid memories of their experience with repeated painful procedures during treatment. These procedures include needle puncture for IM chemotherapy (L-asparaginase), IV lines, port access and blood draws, lumbar puncture, bone marrow aspiration and biopsy, removal of central venous catheters, and other invasive diagnostic procedures. Fear and anxiety related to these procedures may be minimized with parent and child preparation. The preparation starts with obtaining information from the parent about the child's coping styles, explaining the procedure, and enlisting their support, followed by an age-appropriate explanation to the child. Topical analgesics (cold sprays, EMLA, amethocaine gels), as discussed previously, have been effective in providing analgesia before needle procedures.

Lumbar puncture for administration of chemotherapy (cytarabine, methotrexate) and collection of cerebrospinal fluid may lead to a leak at the puncture site and low intracranial pressure (Collins and Weisman, 2003). Some children may experience post-dural puncture headache, which may be treated by administering nonopioid analgesics and placing the patient in the supine position for 1 hour after the procedure. The pain related to bone marrow aspiration is caused by the insertion of a large needle into the posterior iliac space and the unpleasant sensation experienced at the time of marrow aspiration. Nonpharmacologic strategies such as cognitive-behavioral therapy, guided imagery, relaxation, music therapy, hypnosis, conscious sedation, and general anesthesia have been proven effective in decreasing pain and distress during the procedure.

Morphine is the most widely used opioid for moderate-to-severe pain and may be administered via the oral (including sustained-release formulations such as MS Contin and Kadian), IV, subcutaneous, epidural, and intrathecal routes. When dose-limiting side effects of morphine develop, hydromorphone has been reported to be effective in several studies of children with cancer (Drake, Longworth, and Collins, 2004). In a study of children and adolescents with mucositis after bone marrow transplantation, which compared morphine to hydromorphone using PCA, hydromorphone was tolerated well and had a potency ratio of approximately 6:1 relative to morphine (Drake, Longworth, and Collins, 2004).

The most common clinical syndrome of neuropathic pain is painful peripheral neuropathy caused by chemotherapeutic agents, particularly vincristine and cisplatin, and rarely cytarabine (Collins and Weisman, 2003). Withdrawal of the chemotherapy may resolve the neuropathy over weeks to months, or it may persist even after withdrawal. Neuropathic pain is associated with at least one of the following: (1) pain that is described as electric or shocklike, stabbing, or burning; (2) signs of neurologic involvement (paralysis, neuralgia, pain hypersensitivity) other than those associated with the progression of the tumor; and (3) the location of the solid organ cancer consistent with neurologic damage that could give rise to neuropathic pain. Dying children with cancer who experience neuropathic pain have higher baseline requirements of morphine and require more rapid increases of morphine than dying children without neuropathic pain (Dougherty and DeBaun, 2003). Children with neuropathic pain often require massive opioid infusion (3 mg/kg/hr of IV morphine dose equivalent or approximately 100-fold greater than standard starting infusion rates). An epidural or subarachnoid infusion may be initiated if the patient experiences dose-limiting side effects of opioids or if pain was resistant to opioids.

Tricyclic antidepressants (amitriptyline, desipramine) and anticonvulsants (gabapentin, carbamazepine) have demonstrated effectiveness in neuropathic cancer pain. Randomized controlled trials showed that 60% to 70% of patients with neuropathic pain achieve relief with tricyclic antidepressants (Sindrup, Otto, Finnerup, et al., 2005). The tricyclic antidepressants have many actions that could be involved in their pain-relieving effect and have been considered the mainstay of therapy for neuropathic pain (Sindrup, Otto, Finnerup, et al., 2005).

Klepstad, Borchgrevink, Hval, et al. (2001) reported the pain experience of a 12-year-old girl with severe neuropathic pain caused by a cervical spinal tumor. Two weeks after resection of the tumor, the child experienced increased pain in her neck, which was superficial and distributed in the dermatomes below the cervical medullary lesion. Pain was provoked by touch and did not decrease in intensity despite a subcutaneous infusion of morphine at 160 mg/24 hr. The child screamed from increased pain when her parents or siblings tried to comfort her with bodily contact. Pain was relieved after administration of 7.5-to-10 mg IV ketamine. Ketamine is an N-methyl-D-aspartate (NMDA) antagonist, which has undesirable side effects (sedation, nausea, dissociative reactions, muteness, dizziness, and visual distortions) and short duration of action (Sang, 2000). After administration of ketamine the child was able to tolerate touch without pain paroxysms. A continuous IV infusion was eventually initiated for convenience, and benzodiazepines were added to avoid the psychomimetic effects associated with ketamine. More recently Finkel, Pestieau, and Quezado (2007) used subanesthetic doses of ketamine to treat 11 children and adolescents who were on high doses of opioids and had uncontrolled cancer pain. Ketamine appeared to improve pain control and have an opioid-sparing effect. Members of a pain-management consulting service directed and titrated the ketamine to address symptoms. The ketamine dosage range used (0.1 to 1 mg/kg/hr) was low-dose and is lower than that used for anesthetic purposes. Lorazepam (0.025 mg/kg every 12 hours) was administered concurrently during ketamine treatment. Heart rate, noninvasive blood pressure, respiratory rate, and oxygen saturation are monitored continuously.

Although ketamine is frequently used to ensure analgesia and sedation during painful procedures in children, its long-term use for the treatment of neuropathic pain in children has not been studied systematically and is not of clinical benefit for all patients (Klepstad, Borchgrevink, Hval, et al., 2001). In randomized studies of patients with chronic neuropathic pain, only some had a beneficial response to ketamine (Haines and Gaines, 1999; Max, Byas-Smith, Gracely, et al., 1995; Mitchell, 2001). Other NMDA antagonists (dextromethorphan, memantine) are available for clinical use, but no reports on their use in children with neuropathic pain related to cancer have been documented.

Pain and Sedation in End-of-Life Care

Many patients require doses of opioids that make them sedated but arousable as their disease progresses (cancer, human immunodeficiency virus, cystic fibrosis, neurodegenerative disease) at the end of life. Comfort can be achieved with a combination of opioids and adjuvant analgesics in most situations. Parents need reassurance that the opioids are treating pain but not causing the child's death and that the child's advancing disease is the cause of death.

A small group of patients have intolerable side effects or inadequate analgesia despite extremely aggressive use of medications to relieve pain and side effects. Continuous sedation may be a means of relieving suffering when there is no feasible or acceptable means of providing analgesia that preserves alertness. A continuing high-dose infusion of opioids along with sedation is prescribed to reduce the possibility that a child might experience unrelieved pain but be too sedated to report it. Sedation in these situations is widely regarded as providing comfort, not euthanasia. Clinicians and ethicists have a range of views regarding assisted suicide and euthanasia, but they all agree that no child or parent should choose death because of inadequate efforts to relieve pain and suffering (Berde and Collins, 2003).

KEY POINTS

- Although the ability to measure pain in children has improved dramatically in recent years, assessment of pain in children continues to be complex and challenging.
- Behavioral assessment is useful for measuring pain in infants and preverbal children who do not have the language skills to communicate that they are in pain or when mental clouding and confusion limit a child's ability to communicate.
- Physiologic measures are not able to distinguish between physical responses to pain and other forms of stress to the body.
- The number of pain measurement tools that are available for use in infants and young children has increased dramatically and adds a layer of complexity to the assessment of pain in children.
- Important components of assessment include the onset of pain; pain duration or pattern; effectiveness of the current treatment; factors that aggravate or relieve the pain; other symptoms and complications concurrently felt; and interference with the child's mood, function, and interactions with family.
- The administration of sucrose with and without nonnutritive sucking has a calming and pain-relieving effect for invasive procedures in neonates.
- One of the most significant improvements in the ability to provide atraumatic care to children is the anesthetic cream LMX or EMLA.
- Nonopioids, including acetaminophen (Tylenol, paracetamol) and NSAIDs, are suitable for mild-to-moderate pain; opioids are needed for moderate-to-severe pain.
- Several drugs known as coanalgesics or adjuvant analgesics may be used alone or with opioids to control pain symptoms and opioid side effects.
- A significant advance in the administration of IV, epidural, or subcutaneous analgesics is the use of PCA.

- Although respiratory depression is the most feared side effect of opioids, constipation is a common and sometimes serious side effect that decreases peristalsis and increases anal sphincter tone.
- Several harmful effects occur with unrelieved pain, particularly when pain is prolonged.
- Surgery and traumatic injuries (i.e., fractures, dislocations, strains, sprains, lacerations, burns) generate a *catabolic state* as a result of increased secretion of catabolic hormones and lead to alterations in blood flow, coagulation, fibrinolysis, substrate metabolism, and water and electrolyte balance and increase the demands on the cardiovascular and respiratory systems.
- Because burn pain has multiple components, involves repeated manipulations over the injured painful sites, and has changing pattern over time, it is difficult and challenging to control.
- Treatment of recurrent headaches requires an understanding of the antecedents and consequences of headache pain.
- RAP or functional abdominal pain is defined as pain that occurs at least once per month for 3 consecutive months accompanied by pain-free periods and is severe enough that it interferes with a child's normal activities.
- A painful episode is the most frequent cause for ED visits and hospital admissions among children with sickle cell disease.
- Pain is the most prevalent symptom reported by children with cancer.
- Injections from immunizations, IM antibiotics in the ED or health care provider's office, and blood draws are common sources of pain in children.
- For nonpainful procedures such as radiologic imaging studies, several medications are used to sedate, minimize anxiety, and induce amnesia.
- Several painful and invasive procedures require the administration of anesthetics and analgesics.

REFERENCES

Abbe M, Simon C, Angiolilo A, et al: A survey of language barriers from the perspective of pediatric oncologists, interpreters, and parents, *Pediatr Blood Cancer* 47(6):819–824, 2006.

Abdelkefi A, Abdennebi YB, Mellouli F, et al: Effectiveness of fixed 50% nitrous oxide oxygen mixture and EMLA cream for insertion of central venous catheters in children, *Pediatr Blood Cancer* 43(7):777–779, 2004.

Algren JT, Gursoy F, Johnson TD, et al: The effect of nitrous oxide diffusion on laryngeal mask airway cuff inflation in children, *Paediatr Anaesth* 8(1):31–36, 1998.

Ambuel B, Hamlett KW, Marx CM, et al: Assessing distress in pediatric intensive care environments: the COMFORT scale, *J Pediatr Psychol* 17(1):95–109, 1992.

American Pain Society: *Principles of analgesic use in the treatment of acute pain and chronic cancer pain*, ed 4, Glenview, Ill, 1999, The Society.

Anand KJ, Hickey P: Pain and its effects in the human neonate and fetus, *N Engl J Med* 317(21):1321–1329, 1987.

Anand KJ, Hickey PR: Halothane-morphine compared with high-dose sufentanil for anesthesia and postoperative analgesia in neonatal cardiac surgery, *N Engl J Med* 326(1):1–9, 1992.

Anand KJ, Grunau RE, Oberlander TF: Developmental character and long-term consequences of pain in infants and children, *Child Adolesc Psychiatr Clin North Am* 6(4):703–724, 1997.

Basbaum AI: Distinct neurochemical features of acute and persistent pain, *Proc Natl Acad Sci USA* 96(14):7739–7743, 1999a.

Basbaum AI: Spinal mechanisms of acute and persistent pain, *Reg Anesth Pain Med* 24(1):59–67, 1999b.

Benjamin L, Swinson G, Nagel R: Sickle cell anemia day hospital: an approach for the management of uncomplicated painful crises, *Blood* 95:1130–1137, 2000.

Benjamin LJ, Dampier CD, Jacox AK, et al: *Guideline for the management of acute and chronic pain in sickle cell disease*, Glenview, Ill, 1999, American Pain Society.

Berde C, Collins J: Cancer pain and palliative care in children. In Melzack R, Wall P,

editors: *Handbook of pain management*, St Louis, 2003, Churchill Livingstone.

Berger A, Henderson M, Nadoolman W, et al: Oral capsaicin provides temporary relief for oral mucositis pain secondary to chemotherapy/radiation therapy, *J Pain Symptom Manage* 10(3):243–248, 1995.

Bernstein B, Pachter L: Cultural considerations in children's pain. In Schechter N, Berde C, Yaster M, editors: *Pain in infants, children, and adolescents*, Philadelphia, 2003, Lippincott Williams & Wilkins.

Bertin L, Pons G, d'Athis P, et al: A randomized double blind multicentre controlled trial of ibuprofen versus acetaminophen and placebo for symptoms of acute otitis media in children, *Fundam Clin Pharmacol* 10:387–392, 1996.

Beyer JE, Knott CB: Construct validity estimation for the African-American and Hispanic versions of the Oucher scale, *J Pediatr Nurs* 13(1):20–31, 1998.

Beyer JE, Denyes MJ, Villarruel AM: The creation, validation and continuing development of the Oucher: a measure of pain intensity in children, *J Pediatr Nurs* 7(5):335–346, 1992.

Beyer JE, Turner SB, Jones L, et al: The alternate forms reliability of the Oucher pain scale, *Pain Manag Nurs* 6(1):10–17, 2005.

Bildner J, Krechel SW: Increasing staff nurse awareness of postoperative pain management in the NICU, *Neonatal Netw* 15(1):11–16, 1996.

Bishai R, Taddio A, Bar-Oz B, et al: Relative efficacy of amethocaine gel and lidocaine-prilocaine cream for port-a-cath puncture in children, *Pediatrics* 104(3):e31, 1999.

Breau LM, MacLaren J, McGrath PJ, et al: Caregivers' beliefs regarding pain in children with cognitive impairment: relation between pain sensation and reaction increases with severity of impairment, *Clin J Pain* 19(6):335–344, 2003.

Breau LM, McGrath PJ, Camfield CS, et al: Psychometric properties of the Non-communicating Children's Pain Checklist—Revised, *Pain* 99:349–357, 2002.

Bruera E, Willey JS, Ewert-Flannagan PA, et al: Pain intensity assessment by bedside nurses and palliative care consultants: a retrospective study, *Support Care Cancer* 13(4):228–231, 2005.

Chambers C: The role of family factors in pediatric pain. In McGrath PJ, Finley G, editors: *Pediatric pain: biological and social context*, Seattle, Wash, 2003, IASP Press, pp 99–130.

Chambers C, Craig K: An intrusive impact of anchors in children's faces pain scales, *Pain* 78:27–37, 1998.

Chambers CT, Finley GA, McGrath PJ, et al.: The parents' postoperative pain measure: replication and extension to 2-6-year-old children, *Pain* 105(3):437–443, 2003.

Choi WY, Irwin MG, Hui TW, et al: EMLA cream versus dorsal penile nerve block for postcircumcision analgesia in children, *Anesth Analg* 96(2):396–399, 2003.

Choiniere M: Pain of burns. In Melzack R, Wall P, editors: *Handbook of pain management*, St Louis, 2003, Churchill Livingstone.

Chorpita BF, Yim BF, Moffitt C, et al: Assessment of symptoms of DSM-IV anxiety and depression in children: a revised child anxiety and depression scale, *Behav Res Ther* 38(8):835–855, 2000.

Claar RL, Walker LS: Functional assessment of pediatric pain patients: psychometric properties of the functional disability inventory, *Pain* 121(1-2):77–84, 2006.

Cline ME, Herman J, Shaw ER, et al: Standardization of the visual analogue scale, *Nurs Res* 41(6):378–380, 1992.

Cole J, Jorgensen K: Medical, developmental, and pharmacologic intervention: the essence of collaboration, *Neonatal Netw* 16:56–58, 1997.

Collins JJ, Byrnes ME, Dunkel IJ, et al: The measurement of symptoms in children with cancer, *J Pain Symptom Manage* 19(5):363–377, 2000.

Collins J, Weisman S: Management of pain in childhood cancer. In Schechter N, Berde C, Yaster M, editors: *Pain in infants, children, and adolescents*, Philadelphia, 2003, Lippincott Williams & Wilkins.

Cousins M, Power I: Acute and postoperative pain. In Melzack R, Wall P, editors: *Handbook of pain management*, St Louis, 2003, Churchill Livingstone.

Dampier C, Ely L, Brodecki D, et al: Characteristics of pain managed at home in children and adolescents with sickle cell disease by using diary self-reports, *J Pain* 3(6):461–470, 2002a.

Dampier C, Ely L, Brodecki D, et al: Home management of pain in sickle cell disease: a daily diary study in children and adolescents, *J Pediatr Hematol Oncol* 24(8):643–647, 2002b.

Dougherty M, DeBaun MR: Rapid increase of morphine and benzodiazepine usage in the last 3 days of life in children with cancer is related to neuropathic pain, *J Pediatr* 142(4):373–376, 2003.

Drake R, Longworth J, Collins JJ: Opioid rotation in children with cancer, *J Palliat Med* 7(3):419–422, 2004.

Egekvist H, Bjerring P: Effect of EMLA cream on skin thickness and subcutaneous venous diameter: a randomized, placebo-controlled study in children, *Acta Dermatol Venereol* 80(5):340–343, 2000.

Eland JA, Banner W: Analgesia, sedation, and neuromuscular blockage in pediatric critical care. In Hazinski ME, editor: *Manual of pediatric critical care*, St Louis, 1999, Mosby.

Elander J, Lusher J, Bevan D, et al: Understanding the causes of problematic pain management in sickle cell disease: evidence that pseudoaddiction plays a more important role than genuine analgesic dependence, *J Pain Symptom Manage* 27(2):156–169, 2004.

Ely B, Dampier C, Gilday M, et al: Caregiver report of pain in infants and toddlers with sickle cell disease: reliability and validity of a daily diary, *J Pain* 3(1):50–57, 2002.

Fearon I, Kisilevsky BS, Hains SM, et al: Swaddling after heel lance: age-specific effects on behavioral recovery in preterm infants, *Develop Behav Pediatr* 18:222–232, 1997.

Finkel JC, Pestieau SR, Quezado ZM: Ketamine as an adjuvant for treatment of cancer pain in children and adolescents, *J Pain* 8(6):515–521, 2007.

Finley GA, Chambers CT, McGrath PJ, et al: Construct validity of the parents' postoperative pain measure, *Clin J Pain* 19(5):329–334, 2003.

Flores G, Vega LR: Barriers to health care access for Latino children: a review, *Fam Med* 30(3):196–205, 1998.

Flores G, Abreu M, Olivar MA, et al: Access barriers to health care for Latino children, *Arch Pediatr Adolesc Med* 152(11):1119–1125, 1998.

Franck L, Vilardi J: Assessment and management of opioid withdrawal in ill neonates, *Neonatal Netw* 14(2):39–48, 1995.

Franck LS, Vilardi J, Durand D, et al: Opioid withdrawal in neonates after continuous infusions of morphine or fentanyl during extracorporeal membrane oxygenation, *Am J Crit Care* 7(5):364–369, 1998.

Franck LS, Harris SK, Soetenga DJ, et al: The Withdrawal Assessment Tool-1 (WAT-1): an assessment instrument for monitoring opioid and benzodiazepine withdrawal symptoms in pediatric patients, *Pediatr Crit Care Med* 9(6):573–580, 2008.

Furdon SA, Eastman M, Benjamin K, et al: Outcome measures after standardized pain management strategies in postoperative patients in the neonatal intensive care unit, *J Perinat Neonatal Nurs* 12(1):58–69, 1998.

Gad LN, Olsen KS, Lysgaard AB, et al: Optimized use of EMLA cream in children—secondary publication: a randomized, prospective, controlled comparison of two application regimes, *Ugeskr Laeger* 167(4):404–407, 2005.

Gaina A, Sekine M, Chen X, et al: Validity of child sleep diary questionnaire among junior high school children, *J Epidemiol* 14(1):1–4, 2004.

Goldschneider K, Anand K: Long-term consequences of pain in neonates. In Schechter N, Berde C, Yaster M, editors: *Pain in infants, children, and adolescents*, Philadelphia, 2003, Lippincott Williams & Wilkins.

Golianu B, Krane EJ, Galloway KS, et al: Pediatric acute pain management, *Pediatr Clin North Am* 47(3):559–587, 2000.

Gonzales-Del-Rey J, Wason S, Druckenbrod R: Lidocaine overdose: another preventable case? *Pediatr Emerg Care* 10:344–346, 1994.

Gray L, Watt L, Blass E: Skin-to-skin contact is analgesic in healthy newborns, *Pediatrics* 105(1):110–111, 2000.

Hadden KL, von Baeyer CL: Pain in children with cerebral palsy: common triggers and expressive behaviors, *Pain* 99(1-2):281–288, 2002.

Haines DR, Gaines SP: N of 1 randomised controlled trials of oral ketamine in patients with chronic pain, *Pain* 83(2):283–287, 1999.

Hannallah RS, Broadman LM, Belman AB, et al: Comparison of caudal and ilioinguinal/ iliohypogastric nerve blocks for control of post-orchiopexy pain in pediatric ambulatory surgery, *Anesthesiology* 66:832–834, 1987.

Hershey AD, Powers SW, Vockell AL, et al: PedMIDAS: development of a questionnaire to assess disability of migraines in children, *Neurology* 57(11):2034–2039, 2001.

Hershey AD, Powers SW, Vockell AL, et al: Development of a patient-based grading scale for PedMIDAS, *Cephalalgia* 24(10):844–849, 2004.

Hester NO, Foster RL, Jordan-Marsh M, et al: Putting pain measurement into clinical practice. In Finley GA, McGrath PJ, editors:

Measurement of pain in infants and children, vol 10, Seattle, 1998, International Association for the Study of Pain Press.

Hicks CL, von Baeyer CL, Spafford PA, et al: The FACES pain scale—revised: toward a common metric in pediatric pain measurement, *Pain* 93(2):173–183, 2001.

Hoberman A, Paradise JL, Reynolds EA, et al: Efficacy of Auralgan for treating ear pain in children with acute otitis media, *Arch Pediatr Adolesc Med* 151:675–678, 1997.

Holden E, Deichmann M, Levy J: Empirically supported treatments in pediatric psychology: recurrent pediatric headache, *J Pediatr Psychol* 24:91–100, 1999.

Jacob E, Puntillo KA: Variability of analgesic practices for hospitalized children on different pediatric specialty units, *J Pain Symptom Manage* 20(1):59–67, 2000.

Jacob E, Mueller BU: Pain experience of children with sickle cell disease who had prolonged hospitalizations for acute painful episodes, *Pain Med* 9(1):13–21, 2008.

Jacob E, Miaskowski C, Savedra M, et al: Management of vaso-occlusive pain in children with sickle cell disease, *J Pediatr Hematol Oncol* 25(4):307–311, 2003a.

Jacob E, Miaskowski C, Savedra M, et al: Changes in intensity, location, and quality of vaso-occlusive pain in children with sickle cell disease, *Pain* 102(1-2):187–193, 2003b.

Jacob E, McCarthy KS, Sambuco G, et al: Intensity, location, and quality of pain in Spanish-speaking children with cancer, *Pediatr Nurs* 34(1):45–52, 2008.

Johnston CC, Stevens B, Pinelli J, et al: Kangaroo care is effective in diminishing pain response in preterm neonates, *Arch Pediatr Adolesc Med* 157(11):1084–1088, 2003.

Jordan-Marsh M, Yoder L, Hall D, et al: Alternate Oucher form testing gender ethnicity and age variations, *Res Nurs Health* 17:111–118, 1994.

Joyce BA, Schade JG, Keck JF, et al: Reliability and validity of preverbal pain assessment tools, *Issues Comp Pediatr Nurs* 17:121–135, 1994.

Kovacs M: Rating scales to assess depression in school-aged children, *Acta Paedopsychiatr* 46(5-6):305–315, 1981.

Klepstad P, Borchgrevink P, Hval B, et al: Long-term treatment with ketamine in a 12-year-old girl with severe neuropathic pain caused by a cervical spinal tumor, *J Pediatr Hematol Oncol* 23(9):616–619, 2001.

Lenton S, Stallard P, Lewis M, et al: Prevalence and morbidity associated with nonmalignant, life-threatening conditions in childhood, *Child Care Health Dev* 27(5):389–398, 2001.

Ljungman G, Gordh T, Sorensen S, et al: Pain in paediatric oncology: interviews with children, adolescents and their parents, *Acta Paediatr* 88(6):623–630, 1999.

Ljungman G, Gordh T, Sorensen S, et al: Pain variations during cancer treatment in children: a descriptive survey, *Pediatr Hematol Oncol* 17(3):211–221, 2000.

Ljungman G, Gordh T, Sorensen S, et al: Lumbar puncture in pediatric oncology: conscious sedation vs. general anesthesia, *Med Pediatr Oncol* 36(3):372–379, 2001.

Ljungman G, Kreuger A, Andreasson S, et al: Midazolam nasal spray reduces procedural anxiety in children, *Pediatrics* 105(1 Pt 1):73–78, 2000.

Luffy R, Grove SK: Examining the validity, reliability, and preference of three pediatric pain measurement tools in African-American children, *Pediatr Nurs* 29(1):54–60, 2003.

Manworren R, Hynan L: Clinical validation of FLACC: Preverbal Patient Pain Scale, *Pediatr Nurs* 29(2):140–146, 2003.

Marvez-Valls EG, Ernst AA, Gray J, et al: The role of betamethasone in the treatment of acute exudative pharyngitis, *Acad Emerg Med* 5:567–572, 1998.

Marx J: Pain research: prolonging the agony, *Science* 305(5682):326–329, 2004.

Max MB, Byas-Smith MG, Gracely RH, et al: Intravenous infusion of the NMDA antagonist, ketamine, in chronic posttraumatic pain with allodynia: a double-blind comparison to alfentanil and placebo, *Clin Neuropharmacol* 18(4):360–368, 1995.

Max MB, Payne R, Edwards WT, et al: *Principles of analgesic use in the treatment of acute pain and cancer pain*, Glenview, Ill, 1999, American Pain Society.

McCaffery M, Pasero C: *Pain clinical manual*, St Louis, 1999, Mosby.

McGrath P, Hillier L, editors: *Modifying the psychologic factors that intensify children's pain and prolong disability*, Philadelphia, 2003, Lippincott Williams & Wilkins.

McGrath PJ, Johnson G, Goodman JT, et al: The CHEOPS: a behavioral scale to measure postoperative pain in children. In Fields H, Dubner R, Cervero F, editors: *Advances in pain research and therapy*, New York, 1985, Raven Press.

Melzack R: The McGill pain questionnaire: major properties and scoring methods, *Pain* 1:277–299, 1975.

Merkel SI, Voepel-Lewis T, Shayevitz JR, et al: The FLACC: a behavioral scale for scoring postoperative pain in young children, *Pediatr Nurs* 23(3):293–297, 1997.

Merskey H, Bogduk N, editors: *Classification of chronic pain: descriptions of chronic pain syndromes and definitions of pain terms*, ed 2, Seattle, 1994, IASP Press.

Miaskowski C, Lee K: Pain, fatigue, and sleep disturbances in oncology outpatients receiving radiation therapy for bone metastasis: a pilot study, *J Pain Symptom Manage* 17(5):320–332, 1999.

Mitchell AC: An unusual case of chronic neuropathic pain responds to an optimum frequency of intravenous ketamine infusions, *J Pain Symptom Manage* 21(5):443–446, 2001.

Morin C, Gibson D, Wade J: Self-reported sleep and mood disturbance in chronic pain patients, *Clin J Pain* 14(4):311–314, 1998.

Myers C, Stuber ML, Bonamer-Rheingans JI, et al: Complementary therapies and childhood cancer, *Cancer Control* 12(3):172–180, 2005.

Owens JA, Spirito A, McGuinn M: The Children's Sleep Habits Questionnaire (CSHQ): psychometric properties of a survey instrument for school-aged children, *Sleep* 23(8):1043–1051, 2000.

Palermo TM: Impact of recurrent and chronic pain on child and family daily functioning: a critical review of the literature, *J Dev Behav Pediatr* 21(1):58–69, 2000.

Palermo TM, Kiska R: Subjective sleep disturbances in adolescents with chronic pain: relationship to daily functioning and quality of life, *J Pain* 6(3):201–207, 2005.

Palermo T, Valenzuela D: Use of pain diaries to assess recurrent and chronic pain in children, *Suffer Child* 3:1–14, 2003.

Palermo TM, Valenzuela D, Stork PP: A randomized trial of electronic versus paper pain diaries in children: impact on compliance, accuracy, and acceptability, *Pain* 107(3):213–219, 2004.

Perquin CW, Hazebroek-Kampschreur AA, Hunfeld JA, et al: Chronic pain among children and adolescents: physician consultation and medication use, *Clin J Pain* 16(3):229–235, 2000.

Reid GJ, Lang BA, McGrath PJ: Primary juvenile fibromyalgia: psychological adjustment, family functioning, coping, and functional disability, *Arthritis Rheum* 40(4):752–760, 1997.

Reis E, Holubkov R: Vapocoolant spray is equally effective as EMLA cream in reducing immunization pain in school-aged children, *Pediatrics* 100(6):e5, 1997.

Robieux I, Kumar R, Radhakrishnan S, et al: Assessing pain and analgesia with a lidocaine-prilocaine emulsion in infants and toddlers during venipuncture, *J Pediatr* 118(6):971–973, 1991.

Rogers TL, Ostrow CL: The use of EMLA cream to decrease venipuncture pain in children, *J Pediatr Nurs* 19(1):33–39, 2004.

Rusy L, Weisman S: Complementary therapies for acute pediatric pain management, *Pediatr Clin North Am* 47(3):589–599, 2000.

Sang CN: NMDA-receptor antagonists in neuropathic pain: experimental methods to clinical trials, *J Pain Symptom Manage* 19(1 suppl):S21–S25, 2000.

Santiago A, Abad P, Fernandez C, et al: Premedication with EMLA cream for ambulatory surgery in children, *Ambu Surg* 8(3):157, 2000.

Savedra MC, Holzemer WL, Tesler MD, et al: Assessment of postoperation pain in children and adolescents using the adolescent pediatric pain tool, *Nurs Res* 42(1):5–9, 1993.

Savedra MC, Tesler MD, Holzemer WL, et al: Pain location: validity and reliability of body outline markings by hospitalized children and adolescents, *Res Nurs Health* 12:307–314, 1989.

Schade JG, Joyce BA, Gerkensmeyer J, et al: Comparison of three preverbal scales for postoperative pain assessment in a diverse pediatric sample, *J Pain Symptom Manage* 12(6):348–359, 1996.

Schechter N: Management of common pain problems in the primary care pediatric setting. In Schechter N, Berde C, Yaster M, editors: *Pain in infants, children, and adolescents*, Philadelphia, 2003, Lippincott Williams & Wilkins.

Sindrup SH, Otto M, Finnerup NB, et al: Antidepressants in the treatment of neuropathic pain, *Basic Clin Pharmacol Toxicol* 96(6):399–409, 2005.

Stallard P, Williams L, Lenton S, et al: Pain in cognitively impaired, non-communicating children, *Arch Dis Child* 85(6):460–462, 2001.

Stallard P, Williams L, Velleman R, et al: The development and evaluation of the pain indicator for communicatively impaired children (PICIC), *Pain* 98(1-2):145–149, 2002.

Stevens B: Development and testing of a pediatric pain management sheet, *Pediatr Nurs* 16(6):543–548, 1990.

Stevens B, Yamada J, Ohlsson A: Sucrose for analgesia in newborn infants undergoing painful procedures (review), *Cochrane Neonatal Collaboration*, 2005, www.thecochranelibrary.com.

Stinson JN, Stevens BJ, Feldman BM, et al: Construct validity of a multidimensional electronic pain diary for adolescents with arthritis, *Pain* 136(3):281–292, 2008.

Stone AA, Broderick E, Schwartz JE, et al: Intensive momentary reporting of pain with an electronic diary: reactivity, compliance, and patient satisfaction, *Pain* 104(1-2):343–351, 2003.

Suraseranivongse S, Montapaneewat T, Manon J, et al: Cross-validation of a self-report scale for postoperative pain in school-aged children, *J Med Assoc Thai* 88:412–418, 2005.

Taddio A, Nulman I, Koren BS, et al: A revised measure of acute pain in infants, *J Pain Symptom Manage* 10(6):456–463, 1995.

Tarbell SE, Cohen IT, Marsh JL: The Toddler-Preschooler Postoperative Pain Scale: an observational scale for measuring postoperative pain in children aged 1-5: preliminary report, *Pain* 50(3):273–280, 1992.

Tesler MD, Savedra MC, Holzemer WL, et al: The word-graphic rating scale as a measure of children's and adolescents' pain intensity, *Res Nurs Health* 14:361–371, 1991.

Uziel Y, Berkovitch M, Gazarian M, et al: Evaluation of eutectic lidocaine/prilocaine cream (EMLA) for steroid joint injection in children with juvenile rheumatoid arthritis: a double-blind, randomized, placebo-controlled trial, *J Rheumatol* 30(3):594–596, 2003.

Van Cleve L, Bossert E, Beecroft P, et al: The pain experience of children with leukemia during the first year after diagnosis, *Nurs Res* 53(1):1–10, 2004.

Van Cleve L, Munoz C, Bossert EA, et al: Children's and adolescents' pain language in Spanish: translation of a measure, *Pain Manag Nurs* 2(3):110–118, 2001.

van Dijk A, McGrath PA, Pickett W, et al: Pain prevalence in nine- to 13-year-old schoolchildren, *Pain Res Manag* 11(4):234–240, 2006.

Varni JW, Seid M, Rode CA: The PedsQL: measurement model for the pediatric quality of life inventory, *Med Care* 37(2):126–139, 1999.

Varni JW, Thompson KL, Hanson V: The Varni/Thompson Pediatric Pain Questionnaire. Part I. Chronic musculoskeletal pain in juvenile rheumatoid arthritis, *Pain* 28:27–38, 1987.

Vervoort T, Gougert L, Eccleston C, et al: Catastrophic thinking about pain is independently associated with pain severity, disability, and somatic complaints in school children and children with chronic pain, *J Pediatr Psychol* 31(7):674–683, 2006.

Villarruel AM, Denyes MJ: Pain assessment in children: theoretical and empirical validity, *Adv Nurs Sci* 14(2):32–41, 1991.

von Baeyer C, Hicks C: Support for a common metric for pediatric pain intensity scales, *Pain Res Manage* 4(2):157–160, 2000.

Walker LS, Greene JW: The functional disability inventory: measuring a neglected dimension of child health status, *J Pediatr Psychol* 16(1):39–58, 1991.

Walters A, Williamson G: The role of activity restriction in the association between pain and depression: a study of pediatric patients with chronic pain, *Child Health Care* 28:33–50, 1999.

Weisman S, Bernstein B, Schechter N: Consequences of inadequate analgesia during painful procedures in children, *Arch Pediatr Adolesc Med* 152:147–149, 1998.

Weydert J, Ball T, Davis M: Systematic review of treatments for recurrent abdominal pain, *Pediatrics* 111(1):1–3, 2003.

Wilkie DJ, Holzemer WL, Tesler MD, et al: Measuring pain quality: validity and reliability of children's and adolescents' pain language, *Pain* 41(2):151–159, 1990.

Wong DL, Baker CM: Pain in children: comparison of assessment scales, *Pediatr Nurs* 14(1):9–17, 1988.

Woodgate R, Yanofsky R: A different perspective to approaching cancer symptoms in children, *J Pain Symptom Manage* 26(3):800–817, 2004.

Woolf CJ, Salter MW: Neuronal plasticity: increasing the gain in pain, *Science* 288(5472):1765–1769, 2000.

Yaster M, Krance EJ, Kaplan RF, et al: Pediatric pain management and sedation handbook, St Louis, 1997, Mosby.

The Infant and Family

David Wilson

⊖volve WEBSITE

http://evolve.elsevier.com/Perry/maternal

LEARNING OBJECTIVES

On completion of this chapter, the reader will be able to:

- Identify the major biologic, psychosocial, cognitive, and social developments during the first year of life.
- Relate parent-child attachment, separation anxiety, and stranger fear to developmental achievements during infancy.
- Provide anticipatory guidance to parents regarding common parental concerns during infancy.
- Provide anticipatory guidance to parents regarding recommendations for feeding infants.
- Outline immunization requirements during infancy, early childhood, and adolescence.
- List general contraindications, precautions, and administration routes for immunizations.

- Provide anticipatory guidance to parents regarding injury prevention based on the infant's developmental achievements.
- Provide principles of anticipatory guidance in the care of the family with an infant who is experiencing colic.
- Plan nursing care that meets the physical and emotional needs of the child and family with growth failure.
- Provide nursing care that meets the immediate and long-term needs of the family who lost a child from sudden infant death syndrome.
- Provide anticipatory guidance for the prevention of sudden infant death syndrome.
- Identify the needs of the family whose child is home-monitored for apnea.

PROMOTING OPTIMAL GROWTH AND DEVELOPMENT

Biologic Development

At no other time in life are physical changes and developmental achievements as dramatic as during infancy. All major body systems undergo progressive maturation, and there is concurrent development of skills that increasingly allow infants to respond to and cope with the environment. Acquisition of these fine and gross motor skills occurs in an orderly head-to-toe and center-to-periphery (cephalocaudal and proximodistal) sequence.

Proportional Changes

Growth is very rapid during the first year, especially the initial 6 months. Infants gain 150 to 200 g (5 to 7 oz) weekly until approximately age 5 to 6 months, when the birth weight has at least doubled. An average weight for a 6-month-old child is 7.26 kg (16 lb). Weight gain slows during the second 6 months. By 1 year of age, the infant's birth weight has tripled, for an average weight of 9.75 kg (21.5 lb). *Height* increases by 2.5 cm (1 in) a month during the first 6 months and also slows during the second 6 months. Increases in length occur in sudden spurts, rather than in a slow, gradual pattern. Average height is 65 cm (25.5 inches) at 6 months and 74 cm (29 inches) at 12 months. By 1 year, the birth length has increased by almost 50%. This increase occurs mainly in the trunk, rather than in the legs, and contributes to the infant's characteristic physique.

Head growth is also rapid. During the first 6 months, head circumference increases approximately 1.5 cm (0.6 inch) a month, but the rate of increase falls to only 0.5 cm (0.2 inch) monthly during the second 6 months. The average size is 43 cm (17 inches) at 6 months and 46 cm (18 inches) at 12 months. By 1 year, head size has increased by almost 33%. Closure of the cranial sutures occurs, with the posterior fontanel closing by 6 to 8 weeks of age and the anterior fontanel closing by 12 to 18 months of age (the average age being 14 months).

Expanding head size reflects the growth and differentiation of the *nervous system*. By the end of the first year, the brain has increased in weight about 2.5 times. Maturation of the brain is exhibited in the dramatic developmental achievements of infancy (Table 31-1). Primitive reflexes are replaced by voluntary, purposeful movement, and new reflexes that influence motor development appear.

Text continued on p. 869

TABLE 31-1   GROWTH AND DEVELOPMENT DURING INFANCY

AGE (MO)	PHYSICAL	GROSS MOTOR	FINE MOTOR	SENSORY	VOCALIZATION	SOCIALIZATION/ COGNITION
1	Weight gain of 150-200 g (5-7 oz) weekly for first 6 mo Height gain of 2.5 cm (1 inch) monthly for first 6 mo Head circumference increases by 1.5 cm (⁶/₁₀ inch) monthly for first 6 mo Primitive reflexes present and strong Doll's eye reflexes and dance reflex fading Obligatory nose breathing (most infants)	Assumes flexed position with pelvis high but knees not under abdomen when prone (at birth, knees flexed under abdomen)* Can turn head from side to side when prone; lifts head momentarily from bed (see Fig. 31-3, *A*)* Has marked head lag, especially when pulled from lying to sitting position (see Fig. 31-2, *A*) Holds head momentarily parallel and in midline when suspended in prone position Assumes asymmetric tonic neck reflex position when supine When held in standing position, body is limp at knees and hips In sitting position, back is uniformly rounded, absence of head control	Hands predominantly closed Grasp reflex strong Hand clenches on contact with rattle	Able to fixate on moving object in range of 45 degrees when held at a distance of 20-25 cm (8-10 inches) Visual acuity approaches 20/100† Follows light to midline Quiets when hears a voice	Cries to express displeasure Makes small, throaty sounds Makes comfort sounds during feeding	Is in sensorimotor phase—stage I, use of reflexes (birth–1 mo), and stage II, primary circular reactions (1-4 mo) Watches parent's face intently as parent talks to infant
2	Posterior fontanel closed Crawling reflex disappears	Assumes less flexed position when prone—hips flat, legs extended, arms flexed, head to side* Less head lag when pulled to sitting position (see Fig. 31-2, *B*) Can maintain head in same plane as rest of body when held in ventral suspension When prone, can lift head almost 45 degrees off table When moved to sitting position, head is held up but bends forward (see Fig. 31-5, *B*) Assumes asymmetric tonic neck reflex position intermittently	Hands often open Grasp reflex fading	Binocular fixation and convergence to near objects beginning When supine, follows dangling toy from side to point beyond midline Visually searches to locate sounds Turns head to side when sound is made at level of ear	Vocalizes, distinct from crying* Crying becomes differentiated Coos Vocalizes to familiar voice	Demonstrates social smile in response to various stimuli*

Continued

TABLE 31-1   GROWTH AND DEVELOPMENT DURING INFANCY—cont'd

AGE (MO)	PHYSICAL	GROSS MOTOR	FINE MOTOR	SENSORY	VOCALIZATION	SOCIALIZATION/ COGNITION
3	Primitive reflexes fading	Able to hold head more erect when sitting, but still bobs forward Has only slight head lag when pulled to sitting position Assumes symmetric body positioning Able to raise head and shoulders from prone position to a 45- to 90-degree angle from table; bears weight on forearms When held in standing position, able to bear slight fraction of weight on legs Regards own hand	Actively holds rattle but will not reach for it* Grasp reflex absent Hands kept loosely open Clutches own hand; pulls at blankets and clothes	Follows object to periphery (180 degrees)* Locates sound by turning head to side and looking in same direction* Begins to have ability to coordinate stimuli from various sense organs	Squeals aloud to show pleasure* Coos, babbles, chuckles Vocalizes when smiling "Talks" a great deal when spoken to Less crying during periods of wakefulness	Displays considerable interest in surroundings Ceases crying when parent enters room Can recognize familiar faces and objects, such as feeding bottle Shows awareness of strange situations
4	Drooling begins Moro, tonic neck, and rooting reflexes have disappeared*	Has almost no head lag when pulled to sitting position (see Fig. 31-2, C)* Balances head well in sitting position (see Fig. 31-5, C)* Back less rounded, curved only in lumbar area Able to sit erect if propped up Able to raise head and chest off surface to angle of 90 degrees (see Fig. 31-3, B) Assumes predominant symmetric position Rolls from back to side*	Inspects and plays with hands; pulls clothing or blanket over face in play* Tries to reach objects with hand but overshoots Grasps object with both hands Plays with rattle placed in hand, shakes it, but cannot pick it up if dropped Can carry objects to mouth	Able to accommodate to near objects Binocular vision fairly well established Can focus on a 1.25 cm (½-inch) block Beginning eye-hand coordination	Makes consonant sounds n, k, g, p, b Laughs aloud* Vocalization changes according to mood	Is in stage III, secondary circular reactions Demands attention by fussing; becomes bored if left alone Enjoys social interaction with people Anticipates feeding when sees bottle or mother if breastfeeding Shows excitement with whole body, squeals, breathes heavily Shows interest in strange stimuli Begins to show memory
5	Beginning signs of tooth eruption as bumps on gums are palpable Birth weight doubles	No head lag when pulled to sitting position When sitting, able to hold head erect and steady Able to sit for longer periods when back is well supported Back straight When prone, assumes symmetric positioning with arms extended Can turn over from abdomen to back* When supine, puts feet to mouth	Able to grasp objects voluntarily* Uses palmar grasp, bidextrous approach Plays with toes Takes objects directly to mouth Holds one cube while regarding a second one	Visually pursues a dropped object Is able to sustain visual inspection of an object Can localize sounds made below ear	Squeals Makes cooing vowel sounds interspersed with consonant sounds (e.g., ah-goo)	Smiles at mirror image Pats bottle or breast with both hands More enthusiastically playful, but may have rapid mood swings Is able to discriminate strangers from family Vocalizes displeasure when object is taken away Discovers parts of body

TABLE 31-1 GROWTH AND DEVELOPMENT DURING INFANCY—cont'd

AGE (MO)	PHYSICAL	GROSS MOTOR	FINE MOTOR	SENSORY	VOCALIZATION	SOCIALIZATION/ COGNITION
6	Growth rate may begin to decline Weight gain of 90-150 g (3-5 oz) weekly for next 6 mo Height gain of 1.25 cm (0.5 inch) monthly for next 6 mo Teething may begin with eruption of two lower central incisors* Chewing and biting occur*	When prone, can lift chest and upper abdomen off surface, bearing weight on hands (see Fig. 31-3, C) When about to be pulled to a sitting position, lifts head Sits in high chair with back straight Rolls from back to abdomen When held in standing position, bears almost all of weight Hand regard absent	Resecures a dropped object Drops one cube when another is given Grasps and manipulates small objects Holds bottle Grasps feet and pulls to mouth	Adjusts posture to see an object Prefers more complex visual stimuli Can localize sounds made above ear Will turn head to the side, then look up or down	Begins to imitate sounds* Babbling resembles one-syllable utterances—*ma, mu, da, di, hi* Vocalizes to toys, mirror image Takes pleasure in hearing own sounds (self-reinforcement)	Recognizes parents; begins to fear strangers Holds arms out to be picked up Has definite likes and dislikes Begins to imitate (cough, protrusion of tongue) Excites on hearing footsteps Laughs when head is hidden in a towel Briefly searches for a dropped object (object permanence beginning)* Frequent mood swings—from crying to laughing with little or no provocation
7	Sits alone without support	When supine, spontaneously lifts head off surface Sits, leaning forward on hands (see Fig. 31-5, D)* When prone, bears weight on one hand Sits erect momentarily Bears full weight on feet (see Fig. 31-6, A) When held in standing position, bounces actively	Transfers objects from one hand to the other (see Fig. 31-5, E)* Has unidextrous approach and grasp Holds two cubes more than momentarily Bangs cube on table Rakes at a small object	Can fixate on very small objects* Responds to own name Localizes sound by turning head in a curving arch Beginning awareness of depth and space Has taste preferences	Produces vowel sounds and chained syllables—*baba, dada, kaka* Vocalizes four distinct vowel sounds "Talks" when others are talking	Increasing fear of strangers; shows signs of fretfulness when parent disappears* Imitates simple acts and noises Tries to attract attention by coughing or snorting Plays peekaboo Demonstrates dislike of food by keeping lips closed Exhibits oral aggressiveness in biting and mouthing Demonstrates expectation in response to repetition of stimuli
8	Begins to show regular patterns in bladder and bowel elimination Parachute reflex appears (see Fig. 31-4) Eruption of upper central incisors	Sits steadily unsupported (see Fig. 31-5, E)* Readily bears weight on legs when supported; may stand holding onto furniture Adjusts posture to reach an object	Has beginning pincer grasp using index, fourth, and fifth fingers against lower part of thumb Releases objects at will Rings bell purposely Retains two cubes while regarding third cube Secures an object by pulling on a string Reaches persistently for toys out of reach		Makes consonant sounds *t, d, w* Listens selectively to familiar words Utterances signal emphasis and emotion Combines syllables, such as *dada*, but does not ascribe meaning to them	Increasing anxiety over loss of parent, particularly mother, and fear of strangers Responds to word "no" Dislikes dressing, undressing, and diaper change

Continued

TABLE 31-1 GROWTH AND DEVELOPMENT DURING INFANCY—cont'd

AGE (MO)	PHYSICAL	GROSS MOTOR	FINE MOTOR	SENSORY	VOCALIZATION	SOCIALIZATION/ COGNITION
9	Eruption of upper lateral incisor may begin	Creeps on hands and knees Sits steadily on floor for prolonged time (10 min) Recovers balance when leaning forward but cannot do so when leaning sideways Pulls self to standing position and stands holding onto furniture (see Fig. 31-6, B and C)*	Uses thumb and index fingers in crude pincer grasp (see Fig. 31-1)* Preference for use of dominant hand now evident Grasps third cube Compares two cubes by bringing them together	Localizes sounds by turning head diagonally and directly toward sound Depth perception increasing	Responds to simple verbal commands Comprehends "no-no"	Parent (mother) is increasingly important for own sake Shows increasing interest in pleasing parent Begins to show fears of going to bed and being left alone Puts arms in front of face to avoid having it washed
10	Labyrinth-righting reflex is strongest—when infant is in prone or supine position, is able to raise head	Can change from prone to sitting position Stands while holding onto furniture, sits by falling down Recovers balance easily while sitting While standing, lifts one foot to take a step (see Fig. 31-6, D)	Crude release of an object beginning Grasps bell by handle		Says "dada," "mama" with meaning* Comprehends "bye-bye" May say one word (e.g., "hi," "bye," "no")	Inhibits behavior to verbal command of "no-no" or own name Imitates facial expressions; waves bye-bye Extends toy to another person but will not release it Develops object permanence* Repeats actions that attract attention and cause laughter Pulls clothes of another to attract attention Plays interactive game such as pat-a-cake Reacts to adult anger; cries when scolded Demonstrates independence in dressing, feeding, locomotive skills, and testing of parents Looks at and follows pictures in a book
11	Eruption of lower lateral incisor may begin	When sitting, pivots to reach toward back to pick up an object Cruises or walks holding onto furniture or with both hands held*	Explores objects more thoroughly (e.g., clapper inside bell) Has neat pincer grasp Drops object deliberately for it to be picked up Puts one object after another into a container (sequential play) Able to manipulate an object to remove it from tight-fitting enclosure		Imitates definite speech sounds	Experiences joy and satisfaction when a task is mastered Reacts to restrictions with frustration Rolls ball to another on request Anticipates body gestures when a familiar nursery rhyme or story is being told (e.g., holds toes and feet in response to "This little piggy went to market") Plays game up-down, "so big," or peekaboo Shakes head for "no"

TABLE 31-1	GROWTH AND DEVELOPMENT DURING INFANCY—cont'd					
AGE (MO)	PHYSICAL	GROSS MOTOR	FINE MOTOR	SENSORY	VOCALIZATION	SOCIALIZATION/ COGNITION
12	Birth weight tripled*	Walks with one hand held*	Releases cube in cup	Discriminates simple geometric forms (e.g., circle)	Says three to five words besides "dada," "mama"*	Shows emotions such as jealousy, affection (may give hug or kiss on request), anger, fear
	Birth length increased by 50%*	Cruises well	Attempts to build two-block tower but fails	Amblyopia may develop with lack of binocularity	Comprehends meaning of several words (comprehension always precedes verbalization)	Enjoys familiar surroundings and explores away from parent
	Head and chest circumference equal (head circumference 46 cm [18 inches])	May attempt to stand alone momentarily; may attempt first step alone*	Tries to insert a pellet into a narrow-necked bottle but fails	Can follow rapidly moving object	Recognizes objects by name	Is fearful in strange situation; clings to parent
	Has total of six to eight deciduous teeth	Can sit down from standing position without help	Can turn pages in a book, many at a time	Controls and adjusts response to sound; listens for sound to recur	Imitates animal sounds	May develop habit of "security blanket" or favorite toy
	Anterior fontanel almost closed				Understands simple verbal commands (e.g., "Give it to me," "Show me your eyes")	Has increasing determination to practice locomotor skills
	Landau reflex fading					Searches for an object even if it has not been hidden, but searches only where object was last seen*
	Babinski reflex disappears					
	Lumbar curve develops; lordosis evident during walking					

*Milestones that represent essential integrative aspects of development that lay the foundation for the achievement of more advanced skills.
†Degree of visual acuity varies according to vision measurement procedure used.

Because of the complexity of the developmental process during the first 12 months, Table 31-1 is presented to help organize and clarify the data already discussed. Although all milestones are important, some represent essential integrative aspects of development that lay the foundation for achievement of more advanced skills. These essential milestones are designated by an asterisk in the table. The table represents the average monthly age at which various skills are attained. It must be remembered that although the sequence is the same, the rate will vary among children.

The *chest* assumes a more adult contour, with the lateral diameter becoming larger than the anteroposterior diameter. The chest circumference approximately equals the head circumference by the end of the first year. The heart grows less rapidly than the rest of the body. Its weight is usually doubled by 1 year of age; in comparison, body weight triples during the same period. The size of the heart is still large in relation to the chest cavity; its width is approximately 55% of the chest width.

Maturation of Systems

Other organ systems also change and grow during infancy. The *respiratory* rate slows somewhat (see Appendix C) and is relatively stable. Respiratory movements continue to be abdominal. Several factors predispose the infant to more severe and acute respiratory problems. The close proximity of the trachea to the bronchi and its branching structures rapidly transmits infectious agents from one anatomic location to another. The short, straight eustachian tube closely communicates with the ear, allowing infection to ascend from the pharynx to the middle ear. In addition, the inability of the immune system to produce sufficient immunoglobulin A (IgA) in

the mucosal lining provides less protection against infection in infancy than during later childhood.

The *heart rate* slows (see Appendix C), and the rhythm is often *sinus dysrhythmia* (i.e., rate increases with inspiration and decreases with expiration). Blood pressure also changes during infancy (see Appendix C). Systolic pressure rises during the first 2 months as a result of the increasing ability of the left ventricle to pump blood into the systemic circulation. Diastolic pressure decreases during the first 3 months and then gradually rises to values close to those at birth. Fluctuations in blood pressure occur during varying states of activity and emotion.

Significant *hematopoietic changes* occur during the first year (see Appendix B). Fetal hemoglobin (HgbF) is present in large quantities for the first 5 months, with adult hemoglobin steadily increasing through the first half of infancy. Fetal hemoglobin has a shorter life span than adult hemoglobin; therefore there is an increased turnover of these cells and a gradual decrease in hemoglobin. This process results in a *physiologic anemia* around 3 to 6 months of age. High levels of HgbF depress the production of erythropoietin, a hormone released by the kidney that stimulates red blood cell production. Hemoglobin levels decrease to a certain point at which tissue oxygenation needs stimulate erythropoietin, and erythropoiesis resumes, forming new red blood cells.

Maternally derived iron stores are present for the first 5 to 6 months and gradually diminish, which also accounts for lowered hemoglobin levels toward the end of the first 6 months. The occurrence of physiologic anemia is not affected by an adequate supply of iron. However, when erythropoiesis is stimulated, iron supplies are necessary for the formation of hemoglobin.

The *digestive processes* are immature at birth. Although term newborn infants have some limitations in digestive function, human milk has properties that partially compensate for decreased digestive enzymatic activity, thus enabling breastfed infants to receive optimal nutrition during the first several months of life. Saliva is secreted in small amounts, but the majority of the digestive processes do not begin functioning until age 3 months, when drooling is common because of the poorly coordinated swallowing reflex. The enzyme *amylase* (also called *ptyalin*) is present in small amounts but usually has little effect on the foodstuffs because of the small amount of time the food stays in the mouth. Gastric digestion in the stomach consists primarily of the action of hydrochloric acid and rennin, an enzyme that acts specifically on the casein in milk to cause the formation of curds (i.e., coagulated semisolid particles of milk). The curds cause the milk to be retained in the stomach long enough for digestion to occur.

Digestion also takes place in the duodenum, where pancreatic enzymes and bile begin to break down protein and fat. Secretion of the pancreatic enzyme *amylase,* which is needed for digestion of complex carbohydrates, is deficient until about the fourth to sixth month of life. *Lipase* is also limited, and infants do not achieve adult levels of fat absorption until 4 to 5 months of age. *Trypsin* is secreted in sufficient quantities to catabolize protein into polypeptides and some amino acids.

The immaturity of the digestive processes is evident in the appearance of stools. During infancy, solid foods (e.g., peas, carrots, corn, and raisins) are passed incompletely broken down in the feces. An excess quantity of fiber easily disposes the child to loose, bulky stools. During infancy, the stomach enlarges to accommodate a greater volume of food. By the end of the first year, the infant is able to tolerate three meals a day and an evening bottle and may have one or two bowel movements daily. With any type of gastric irritation, however, the infant is vulnerable to diarrhea, vomiting, and dehydration (see Chapter 41).

The *liver* is the most immature of all the gastrointestinal organs throughout infancy. The ability to conjugate bilirubin and secrete bile is achieved after the first couple of weeks of life. However, the capacities for gluconeogenesis, formation of plasma protein and ketones, storage of vitamins, and deaminization of amino acids remain relatively immature for the first year of life.

Maturation of the suckling, sucking, and swallowing reflexes and the eruption of teeth (see Teething, p. 881) parallel the changes in the gastrointestinal tract and prepare the infant for the introduction of solid foods.

The immunologic system undergoes numerous changes during the first year. Full-term newborns receive significant amounts of maternal immunoglobulin G (IgG), which, for approximately 3 months, confers immunity against antigens to which their mothers were exposed. During this time, infants begin to synthesize IgG; approximately 40% of adult levels are reached by 1 year of age. Significant amounts of immunoglobulin M (IgM) are produced at birth, and adult levels are reached by 9 months of age. Secretory IgA is not present at birth but is found in saliva and tears by 2 to 5 weeks.

Prebiotic oligosaccharides found in breast milk produce probiotic bacteria such bifidobacteria and lactobacilli, which in turn stimulate synthesis and secretion of secretory IgA (sIgA). Secretory IgA is present in large amounts in colostrum; IgA confers protection to the mucous membranes of the gastrointestinal tract (Blackburn, 2013; Lawrence and Lawrence, 2011) against many bacteria, such as *Escherichia coli*, and viruses, such as rubella, poliovirus, and the enteroviruses. The development of the mucosa-associated lymphoid tissue occurs during infancy; in part, this system is believed to prevent colonization and passage of bacteria across the infant's mucosal barrier (Lawrence and Lawrence, 2011). The function and quantity of T-lymphocytes, lymphokines, interferon-γ, interleukins, tumor necrosis factor-α, and complement are reduced in early infancy, thus preventing optimal response to certain bacteria and viruses. The production of IgA and immunoglobulins D and E (IgD and IgE) is much more gradual, and maximum levels are not attained until early childhood. Probiotics may have a significant role in helping the gastrointestinal tract establish a "good" bacterial colonization in the gut to prevent many illnesses, including antibiotic-induced diarrhea and possibly *Helicobacter pylori* gastritis (Thomas, Greer, American Academy of Pediatrics [AAP], et al., 2010).

There is evidence that vernix caseosa, a white oily substance that coats the term infant's body and is often found in abundance in creases of the axilla and groin, has innate immunologic properties that serve to protect the newborn from infection (Narendran and Hoath, 2006). Vernix also appears to have a role in maintaining the integrity of the stratum corneum and facilitating acid mantle development (Hoath, Pickens, and Visscher, 2006). The epidermis of the full-term infant undergoes maturation during the first month of life; the newborn's skin acts as a barrier to infection, assists in thermal regulation, and prevents transepidermal water loss in term infants.

During infancy, *thermoregulation* becomes more efficient; the ability of the skin to contract and of muscles to shiver in response to cold increases. The peripheral capillaries respond to changes in ambient temperature to regulate heat loss. The capillaries constrict in response to cold, conserving core body temperature and decreasing potential evaporative heat loss from the skin surface. The capillaries dilate in response to heat, decreasing internal body temperature through evaporation, conduction, and convection. Shivering (*thermogenesis*) causes the muscles and muscle fibers to contract, generating metabolic heat that is distributed throughout the body. Increased adipose tissue during the first 6 months insulates the body against heat loss.

A shift in the *total body fluid* occurs. At birth, 75% of the term infant's body weight is water, with a large percentage being extracellular fluid (ECF). As the percentage of body water decreases, so does the amount of ECF—from 40% at term to 20% in adulthood. The high proportion of ECF, which is composed of blood plasma, interstitial fluid, and lymph, predisposes the infant to a more rapid loss of total body fluid and, consequently, dehydration. The loss of 5% to 10% of the term newborn's initial birth weight in the first 5 days of life is attributed to ECF compartment contraction, enhanced renal tubular function, and rapidly increasing glomerular filtration rate.

The immaturity of the *renal structures* also predisposes the infant to dehydration. Complete maturity of the kidney occurs during the latter half of the second year, when the cuboidal epithelium of the glomeruli becomes flattened. Before this time, the glomeruli's filtration capacity is reduced. Urine is voided frequently and has a low specific gravity (i.e., 1.000 to 1.010). At term, most infants produce and excrete approximately 15 to 60 mL/kg/24 hr, and an output of less than 0.5 mL/kg/hr after 48 hours of age is considered to be oliguria (Blackburn, 2013).

Auditory acuity is at adult levels during infancy. Visual acuity begins to improve, and binocular fixation is established. Binocularity, or the fixation of two ocular images into one cerebral picture (fusion), begins to develop by 6 weeks of age and should be well established by age 4 months. Depth perception (stereopsis) begins

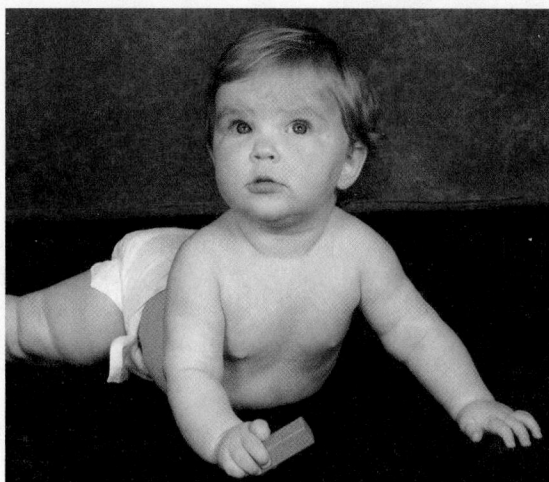

FIG 31-1 Crude pincer grasp at 8 to 10 months. (Photo by Paul Vincent Kuntz, Texas Children's Hospital, Houston, TX.)

to develop by age 7 to 9 months but may not be fully mature until 2 to 3 years of age, thus increasing the infant's and younger toddler's risk for falling.

Fine Motor Development

Fine motor behavior includes the use of the hands and fingers in the prehension (grasp) of an object. Grasping occurs during the first 2 to 3 months as a reflex and gradually becomes voluntary. At 1 month of age, the hands are predominantly closed, and by 3 months, they are mostly open. By this time, infants demonstrate a desire to grasp an object but they "grasp" it more with the eyes than with the hands. If a rattle is placed in the hand, the infant will actively hold onto it. By 4 months of age, the infant regards both a small pellet and the hands and then looks from the object to the hands and back again. By 5 months, the infant is able to voluntarily grasp an object.

Gradually the palmar grasp (using the whole hand) is replaced with a pincer grasp (using the thumb and index finger). The infant uses a crude pincer grasp by 8 to 9 months of age and has progressed to a neat pincer grasp by 11 months (Fig. 31-1).

By 6 months of age, infants have increased manipulative skill: they hold their bottle, grasp their feet and pull them to their mouth, and feed themselves a cracker. By 7 months, they transfer objects from one hand to the other, use one hand for grasping, and hold a cube in each hand simultaneously. They enjoy banging objects and will explore the movable parts of a toy.

By 10 months of age, the pincer grasp is sufficiently established to enable infants to pick up a raisin and other finger foods. They can deliberately let go of an object and will offer it to someone. By 11 months, they put objects into a container and like to remove them. By age 1 year, infants try to build a tower of two blocks but fail.

Gross Motor Development

Head Control. The full-term newborn can momentarily hold the head in midline and parallel when the body is suspended ventrally and can lift and turn the head from side to side when prone. This is not the case when the infant is lying prone on a pillow or soft surface; infants do not have the head control to lift their head out of the depression of the object and therefore risk possible suffocation in the prone position early in infancy (see Sudden Infant Death

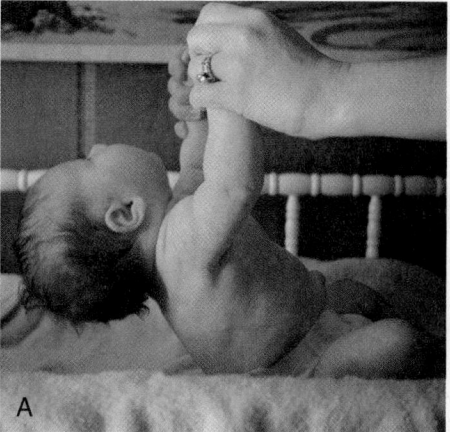

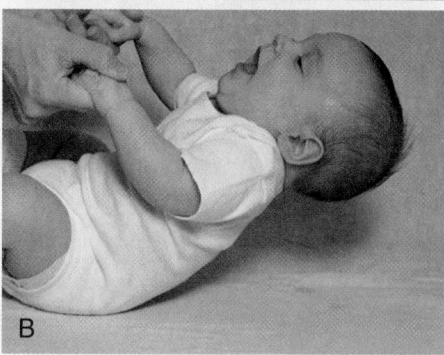

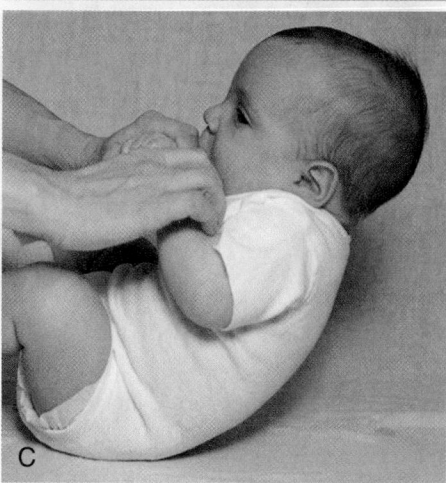

FIG 31-2 Head control while pulled to sitting position. **A,** Complete head lag at 1 month. **B,** Partial head lag at 2 months. **C,** Almost no head lag at 4 months.

Syndrome, p. 910). Marked head lag is evident when the infant is pulled from a lying to a sitting position. By 3 months of age, infants can hold their head well beyond the plane of the body. By 4 months of age, infants can lift the head and front portion of the chest approximately 90 degrees above the table, bearing their weight on the forearms. Only slight head lag is evident when the infant is pulled from a lying to a sitting position, and by 4 to 6 months, head control is well established (Figs. 31-2 and 31-3).

> ### ! NURSING ALERT
>
> An infant who displays head lag at 6 months of age should have a developmental and neurologic evaluation.

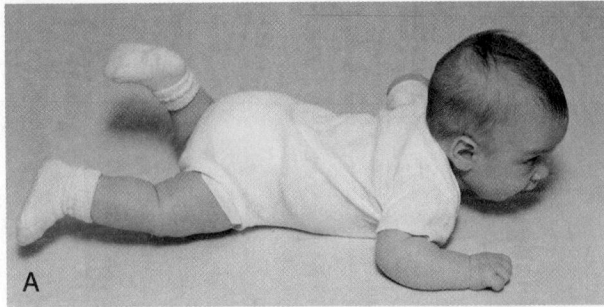

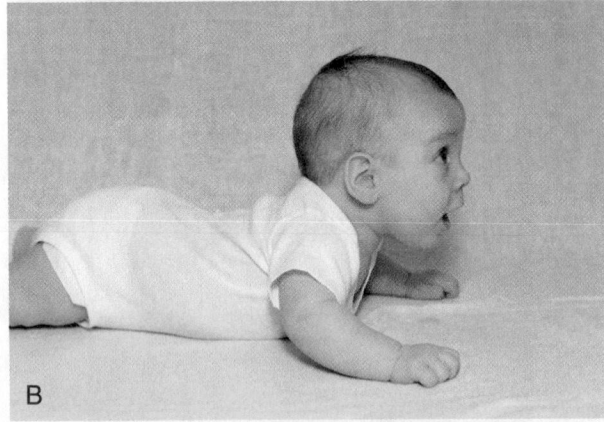

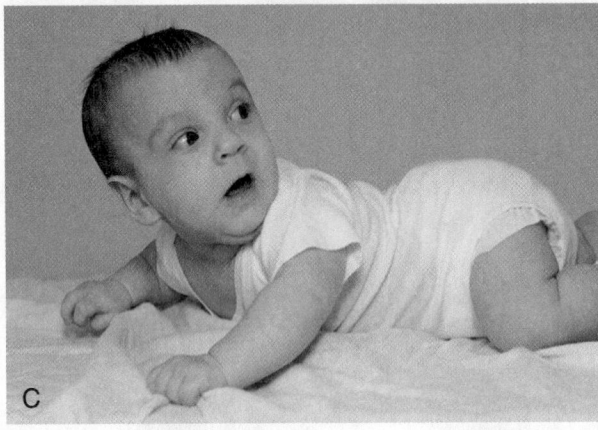

FIG 31-3 Head control while prone. **A,** Infant momentarily lifts head at 1 month. **B,** Infant lifts head and chest 90 degrees and bears weight on forearms at 4 months. **C,** Infant lifts head, chest, and upper abdomen and can bear weight on hands at 6 months. Note how this position facilitates turning from abdomen to back.

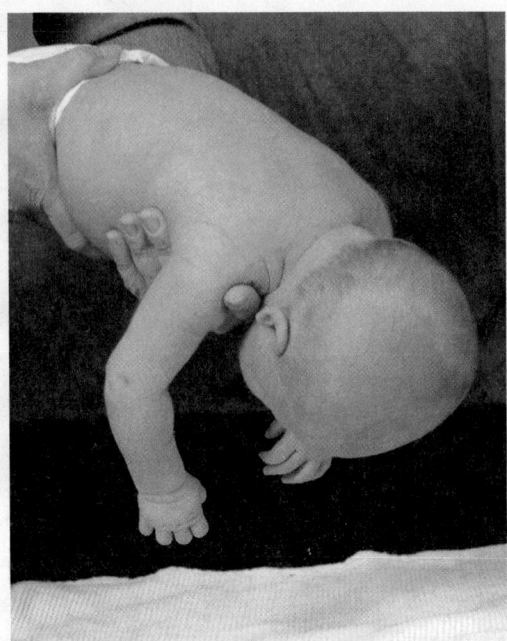

FIG 31-4 Parachute reflex. Infant extends arms to protect from falling. (Photo by Paul Vincent Kuntz, Texas Children's Hospital, Houston, TX.)

> **! NURSING ALERT**
>
> In the first several months, before the infant can roll over, the head should be positioned on alternating sides to prevent positional plagiocephaly (when asleep or awake in the supine position).

Rolling Over. Newborns may roll over accidentally because of their rounded back. The ability to willfully turn from the abdomen to the back occurs at 5 months, and the ability to turn from the back to the abdomen occurs at 6 months. Infants put to sleep on their sides may easily roll over to a prone (face-down) position, thus placing them at higher risk for sudden infant death syndrome (SIDS). It is therefore important to place infants in a supine position for sleep. While the infant is awake, a prone position (tummy time) is acceptable to enhance achievement of milestones such as head control, crawling, creeping, and turning over. It is noteworthy that the parachute reflex (Fig. 31-4), a protective response to falling, appears at 7 months.

Sitting. The ability to sit follows progressive head control and straightening of the back (Fig. 31-5). For the first 2 to 3 months, the back is uniformly rounded. The convex cervical curve forms at approximately 3 to 4 months of age, when head control is established. The convex lumbar curve appears when the child begins to sit, at about age 4 months. As the spinal column straightens, the infant can be propped in a sitting position. By age 7 months, infants can sit alone, leaning forward on their hands for support. By age 8 months, they can sit well while unsupported and begin to explore their surroundings in this position rather than in a lying position. By 10 months, they can maneuver from a prone to a sitting position.

Locomotion. Locomotion involves acquiring the ability to bear weight, propel forward on all four extremities, stand upright with support, and, finally, walk alone (Fig. 31-6). Following a cephalocaudal pattern, infants 4 to 6 months old have increasing coordination in their arms. Initial locomotion results in infants propelling themselves backward by pushing with the arms. By 6 to 7 months of age, they are able to bear all their weight on their legs with assistance. *Crawling* (propelling forward with belly on floor) progresses to *creeping* (on hands and knees with belly off floor) by 9 months. At this time, they stand while holding onto furniture and can pull themselves to the standing position but they are unable to maneuver back down except by falling, usually on their bottom. By 11 months, they walk while holding onto furniture or with both hands held, and by age 1 year, they may be able to walk with one hand held. A number of infants attempt their first independent steps by their first birthday. Although there is considerable variation among infants for the achievement of these milestones, they provide guidelines for early intervention.

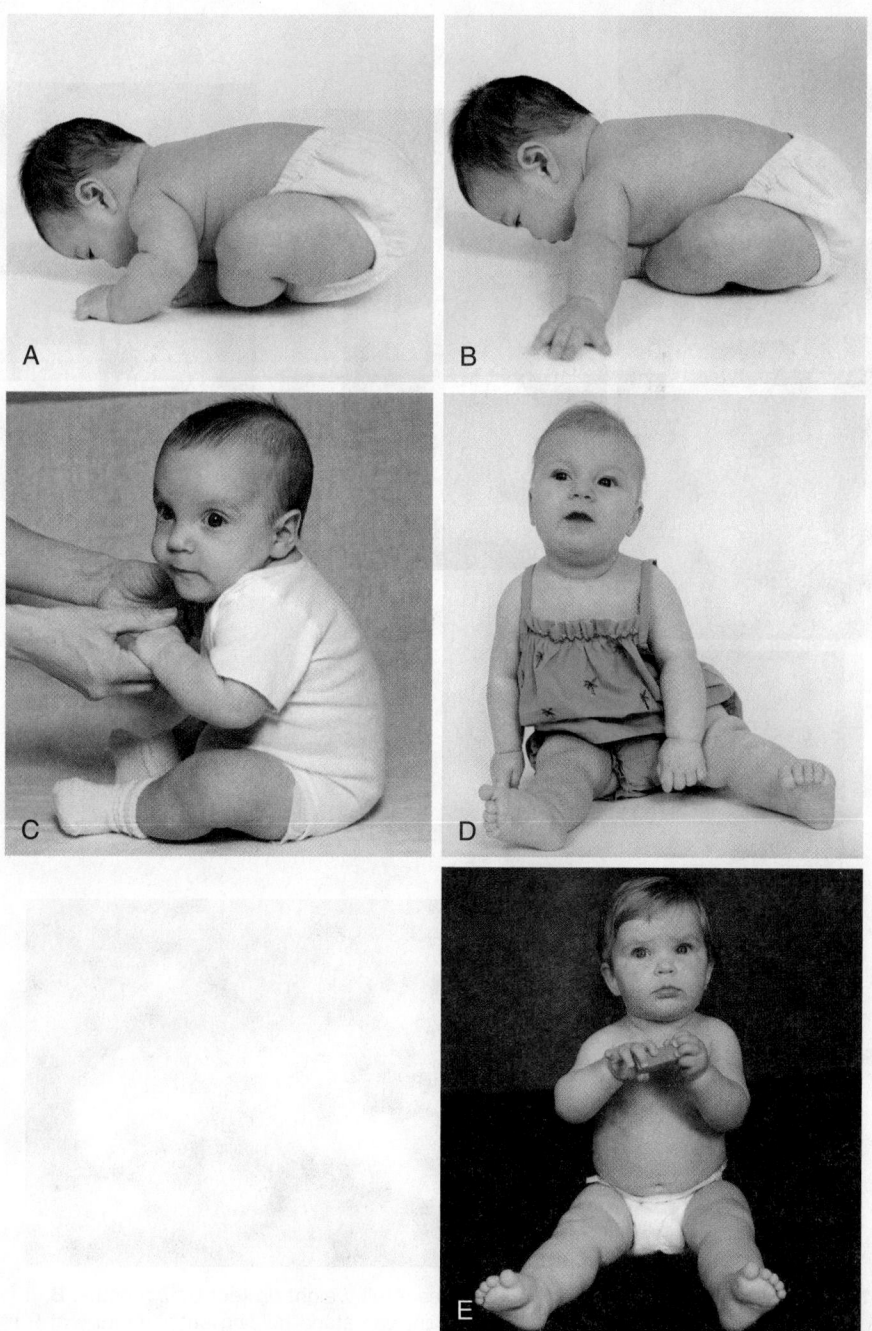

FIG 31-5 Development of sitting. **A,** Back is completely rounded and infant has no ability to sit upright at 1 month. **B,** At 2 months, infant exhibits more control; back is still rounded, but infant can sit up momentarily with some head control. **C,** Back is rounded only in lumbar area and infant is able to sit erect with good head control at 4 months. **D,** Infant can sit alone, leaning on hands for support, at 7 months. **E,** Infant sits without support at 8 months. Note the transferring of objects that occurs beginning at 7 months. (Photos by Paul Vincent Kuntz, Texas Children's Hospital, Houston, TX.)

! NURSING ALERT

An infant who does not pull to a standing position by 11 to 12 months of age should be further evaluated for possible developmental dysplasia of the hip (see Chapter 48).

Psychosocial Development

Developing a Sense of Trust (Erikson)

Erikson's (1963) phase I (birth to 1 year) is concerned with *acquiring a sense of trust* while *overcoming a sense of mistrust*. The trust that develops is a trust of self, of others, and of the world. Infants "trust" that their feeding, comfort, stimulation, and caring needs will be met. The crucial element for the achievement of this task is the quality of both the parent-child (or caregiver-child) relationship and

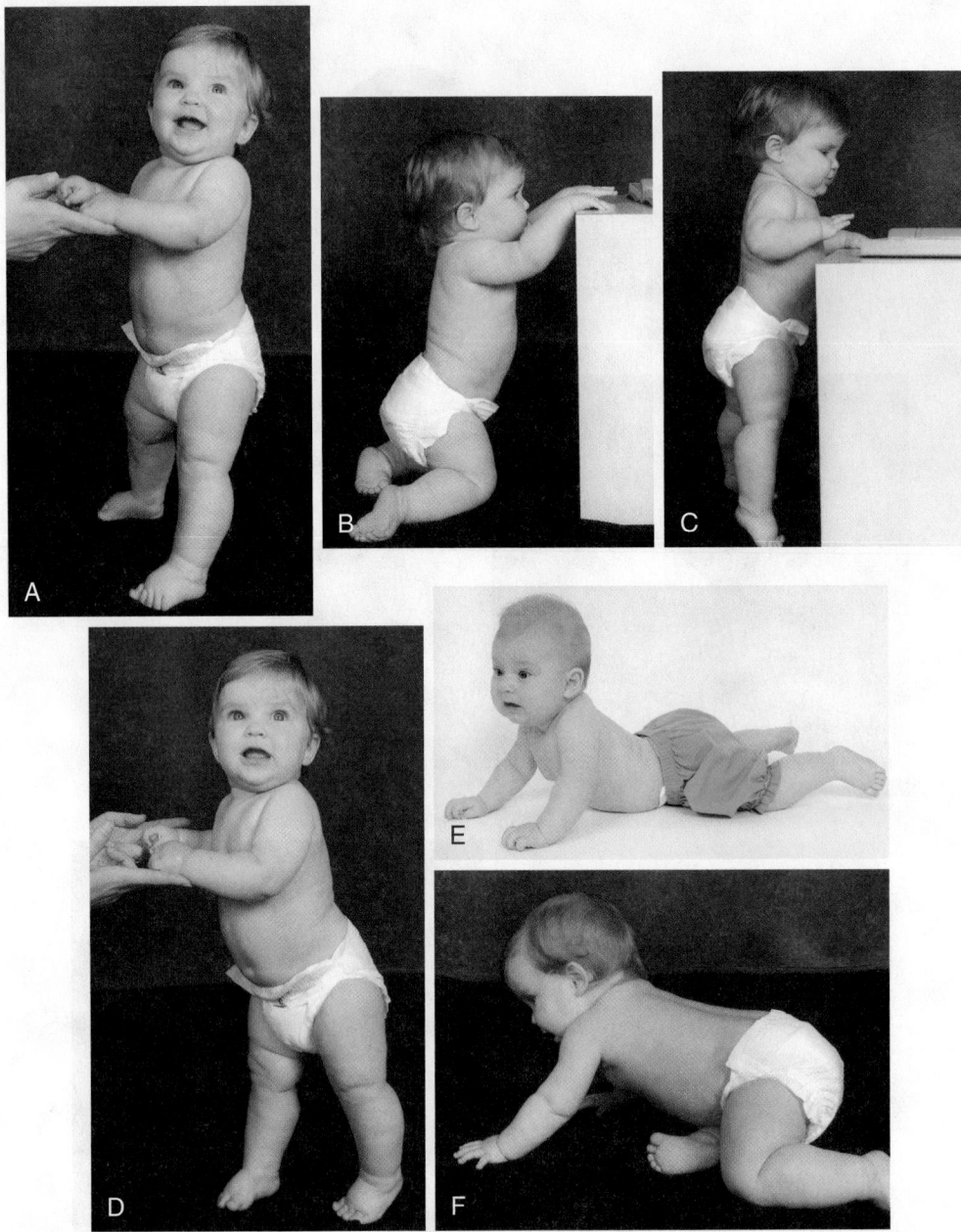

FIG 31-6 Development of locomotion. **A,** Infant bears full weight on feet by 7 months. **B,** Infant can maneuver from sitting to kneeling position. **C,** Infant can stand holding onto furniture at 9 months. **D,** While standing, infant takes deliberate step at 10 months. **E,** Infant crawls with abdomen on floor and pulls self forward, and then, **F,** creeps on hands and knees at 9 months. (Photos by Paul Vincent Kuntz, Texas Children's Hospital, Houston, TX.)

the care the infant receives. The provision of food, warmth, and shelter by itself is inadequate for the development of a strong sense of self. The infant and parent must jointly learn to satisfactorily meet their needs in order for mutual regulation of frustration to occur. When this synchrony fails to develop, mistrust is the eventual outcome.

Failure to learn *delayed gratification* leads to mistrust. Mistrust can result from either too much or too little frustration. If parents always meet their children's needs before the children signal their readiness, infants will never learn to test their ability to control the environment. If the delay is prolonged, infants experience constant frustration and eventually mistrust others in their efforts to satisfy them. Therefore consistency of care is essential.

The trust acquired in infancy provides the foundation for all succeeding phases. Trust allows infants a feeling of physical comfort and security, which assists them in experiencing unfamiliar situations with a minimum of fear. Erikson has divided the first year of life into two oral/social stages. During the first 3 to 4 months, food intake is the most important social activity in which the infant engages. The newborn can tolerate little frustration or delay of gratification. Primary narcissism (total concern for oneself) is at its height. However, as bodily processes such as vision, motor movements, and vocalization become better controlled, infants use more advanced behaviors to interact with others. For example, rather than cry, infants may put their arms up to signify a desire to be held.

The next social modality involves a mode of reaching out to others through *grasping*. Grasping is initially reflexive, but even as a reflex, it has a powerful social meaning for the parents. The reciprocal response to the infant's grasping is the parents' holding on and touching. There is pleasurable tactile stimulation for both the child and the parents.

Tactile stimulation is extremely important in the total process of acquiring trust. The degree of mothering skill, the quantity of food, or the length of sucking does not determine the quality of the experience. Rather, it is the overall quality of the interpersonal relationship that influences the infant's formulation of trust.

During the second stage, the more active and aggressive modality of *biting* occurs. Infants learn that they can hold onto what is their own and can more fully control their environment. During this stage, infants may be confronted with one of their first conflicts. If they are breastfeeding, they quickly learn that biting causes the mother to become upset and withdraw the breast. Yet biting also brings internal relief from teething discomfort and a sense of power or control.

This conflict may be solved in a variety of ways. The mother may wean the infant from the breast and begin bottle-feeding, or the infant may learn to bite substitute "nipples," such as a pacifier, and retain pleasurable breastfeeding. The successful resolution of this conflict strengthens the mother-child relationship because it occurs at a time when infants are recognizing the mother as the most significant person in their life.

Cognitive Development
Sensorimotor Phase (Piaget)

The theory most commonly used to explain *cognition*, or the ability to know, is that of Piaget (1952). The period from birth to 24 months is termed the *sensorimotor phase* and is composed of six stages; however, because this discussion is concerned with ages birth to 12 months, only the first four stages are discussed. The last two stages occur during the toddler period of 12 to 24 months and are discussed in Chapter 32.

During the sensorimotor phase, infants progress from reflex behaviors to simple repetitive acts to imitative activity. Three crucial events take place during this phase. The first event involves *separation*, in which infants learn to separate themselves from other objects in the environment. They realize that others besides themselves control the environment and that certain readjustments must take place for mutual satisfaction to occur. This coincides with Erikson's concept of the formation of trust.

The second major accomplishment is achieving the concept of object permanence, or the realization that objects that leave the visual field still exist. A typical example of the development of object permanence is when infants are able to pursue objects they observe being hidden under a pillow or behind a chair (Fig. 31-7). This skill develops at approximately 9 to 10 months of age, which corresponds to the time of increased locomotion skills.

The last major intellectual achievement of this period is the ability to use *symbols*, or *mental representation*. The use of symbols allows the infant to think of an object or situation without actually experiencing it. The recognition of symbols is the beginning of the understanding of time and space.

Piaget's first stage, from birth to 1 month, is identified by the infant's *use of reflexes*. At birth, the infant's individuality and temperament are expressed through the physiologic reflexes of sucking, rooting, grasping, and crying. The repetitious nature of the reflexes is the beginning of associations between an act and a sequential response. When infants cry because they are hungry, a nipple is put

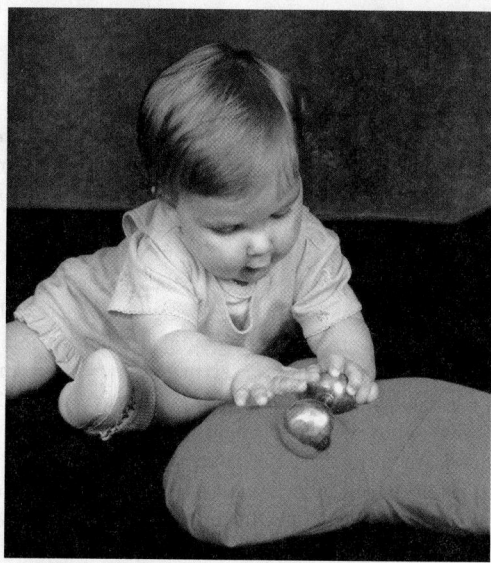

FIG 31-7 Nine-month-old infant actively searches for object hidden behind pillow. (Photo by Paul Vincent Kuntz, Texas Children's Hospital, Houston, TX.)

in the mouth and they suck, feel satisfaction, and sleep. They are assimilating this experience while perceiving auditory, tactile, and visual cues. This experience of perceiving certain patterns, or "ordering," provides a foundation for the subsequent stages.

The second stage, *primary circular reactions*, marks the beginning of the replacement of reflexive behavior with voluntary acts. During the period from 1 to 4 months, activities such as sucking or grasping become deliberate acts that elicit certain responses. The beginning of accommodation is evident. Infants incorporate and adapt their reactions to the environment and recognize the stimulus that produced a response. Previously they would cry until the nipple was brought to the mouth. Now they associate the nipple with the sound of the parent's voice. They accommodate this new piece of information and adapt by ceasing to cry when they hear the voice—before receiving the nipple. What is taking place is a realization of causality and a recognition of an orderly sequence of events. The environment is taken in with all of the senses and with whatever motor ability is present.

The *secondary circular reactions* stage is a continuation of primary circular reactions and lasts until 8 months of age. In this stage, the primary circular reactions are repeated and prolonged for the response that results. Grasping and holding now become shaking, banging, and pulling. Shaking is performed to hear a noise, not solely for the pleasure of shaking. The quality and quantity of an act become evident. More or less shaking produces different responses. Understanding of causality, time, deliberate intention, and separateness from the environment begins to develop.

Three new processes of human behavior occur. *Imitation* requires the differentiation of selected acts from several events. By the second half of the first year, infants can imitate sounds and simple gestures. *Play* becomes evident as they take pleasure in performing an act after they have mastered it. Many of the infant's waking hours are absorbed in sensorimotor play. *Affect* (the outward manifestation of emotion and feeling) is seen as infants begin to develop a sense of permanency. During the first 6 months, infants believe that an object exists only for as long as they can visually perceive it. In other words, out of sight, out of mind. Affect in relation to external objects is evident when the object continues to be present or remembered even though it is beyond the range of perception. Object permanence is a critical component of parent-child attachment and is seen in the development of separation anxiety at 6 to 8 months of age (see p. 877).

During the fourth sensorimotor stage, *coordination of secondary schemas and their application to new situations,* infants use previous behavioral achievements primarily as the foundation for adding new intellectual skills to their expanding repertoire. This stage is largely transitional. Increasing motor skills allow for greater exploration of the environment. They begin to discover that hiding an object does not mean that it is gone but that removing an obstacle will reveal the object. This marks the beginning of intellectual reasoning. Furthermore, they can experience an event by observing it and they begin to associate symbols with events (e.g., "bye-bye" with "Mommy goes to work"), but the classification is purely their own. In this stage, they learn from the object itself; this is in contrast to the second stage, in which infants learn from the type of interaction between objects or individuals. Intentionality is further developed in that infants now actively attempt to remove a barrier to the desired (or undesired) action (see Fig. 31-7). If something is in their way, they attempt to climb over it or push it away. Previously, an obstacle would cause them to give up any further attempt to achieve the desired goal.

Development of Body Image

The development of body image parallels sensorimotor development. Infants' kinesthetic and tactile experiences are the first perceptions of their body, and the mouth is the principal area of pleasurable sensations. Other parts of the body are primarily objects of pleasure—the hands and fingers to suck and the feet to play with. As physical needs are met, they feel comfort and satisfaction with their body. Messages conveyed by the caregivers reinforce these feelings. For example, when infants smile, they receive emotional satisfaction from others who smile back.

Achieving the concept of object permanence is basic to the development of self-image. By the end of the first year, infants recognize that they are distinct from their parents. At the same time, they have increasing interest in their image, especially in the mirror (Fig. 31-8). As motor skills develop, they learn that parts of the body are useful; for example, the hands bring objects to the mouth and the legs help them move to different locations. All of these achievements transmit messages to them about themselves. Therefore it is important to transmit positive messages to infants about their bodies.

Social Development

Infants' social development is initially influenced by their reflexive behavior, such as the grasp, and eventually depends primarily on the interaction between them and the principal caregivers. **Attachment** to the parent is increasingly evident during the second half of the first year. In addition, tremendous strides are made in communication and personal-social behavior. Whereas crying and reflexive behavior are methods to meet one's needs in the neonatal period, the social smile is an early step in social communication. This has a profound effect on family members and is a tremendous stimulus for evoking continued responses from others. By 4 months, infants laugh aloud.

Play is a major socializing agent and provides stimulation needed to learn from and interact with the environment. By age 6 months, infants are personable. They play games such as peekaboo when their head is hidden in a towel, they signal their desire to be picked up by extending their arms, and they show displeasure when a toy is removed or their face is washed.

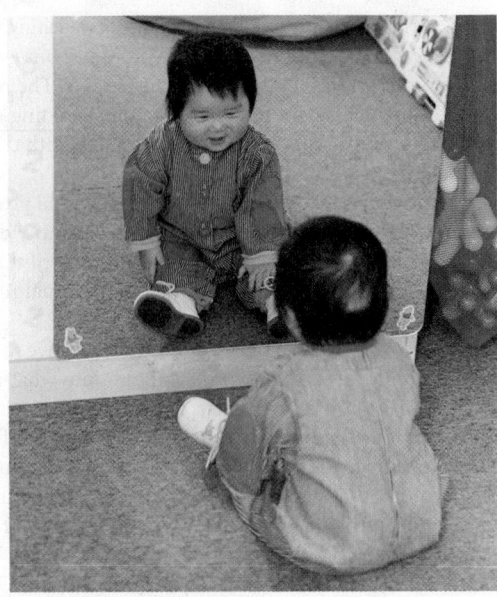

FIG 31-8 Nine-month-old infant enjoying own image in mirror.

Attachment

The importance of human physical contact to infants cannot be overemphasized. Parenting is not an instinctual ability but, instead, a learned, acquired process. The attachment of parent and child, which begins before birth, assumes even more importance at birth and continues during the first year. In the following discussion of attachment, the term *mother* is used in the broad context of the consistent caregiver with whom the child relates more than anyone else. However, in society's changing social climate and gender-role stereotypes, this person may very well be the father or a grandparent. Studies on paternal-infant attachment demonstrate that stages similar to those in maternal attachment occur and that fathers are often more involved in child care when mothers are employed (although many mothers continue to do the majority of infant care). Additional research has shown that inexperienced, first-time fathers are as capable as experienced fathers of developing a close attachment with their infants. Studies of fathers of high risk infants demonstrate that fathers experience feelings of love and affection toward their offspring during the newborn period; fathers in one study verbalized more positive feelings of love and affection toward the newborn when they were able to have close physical contact such as holding the child (Sullivan, 1999). The father has also been reported to have a significant role in supporting the mother in the perinatal period; fathers of high risk infants reported concern about their mates' well-being in addition to the status of the ill infant (Lundqvist and Jakobsson, 2003). Research demonstrates that fathers develop feelings of attachment with their offspring and that their relationship with the infant is an important factor in the mother's emotional well-being. With many single-parent families in existence, a grandmother (or other significant caregiver) may become the primary caregiver. It is important for nurses to recognize that infant-parent attachments may be present or absent in situations wherein caregiver roles are less well defined by those involved.

When the infant is not provided a safe haven and consistent and loving care, an *insecure attachment* develops; such infants do not feel they can trust the world in which they live. This insecure attachment may result in psychosocial difficulties as the child grows and may persist even into adulthood. Insecure attachment may also exist in homes where there is domestic violence and maternal postnatal depression.

Attachment progresses during infancy, with the child assuming an increasingly significant role. Two components of cognitive development are required for attachment: (1) the ability to discriminate the mother from other individuals, and (2) the achievement of object permanence. Both of these processes prepare the infant for an equally important aspect of attachment: separation from the parent. Separation-individuation should occur as a harmonious, parallel process with emotional attachment.

During the formation of attachment to the parent, the infant progresses through four distinct but overlapping stages. For the first few weeks, infants respond indiscriminately to anyone. Beginning at approximately 8 to 12 weeks of age, they cry, smile, and vocalize more to the mother than to anyone else but continue to respond to others, whether familiar or not. At approximately 6 months of age, infants show a distinct preference for the mother. They follow her more, cry when she leaves, enjoy playing with her more, and feel most secure in her arms. About 1 month after showing attachment to the mother, many infants begin attaching to other members of the family, most often the father.

Infants acquire other developmental behaviors that influence the attachment process. These include:

- Differential crying, smiling, and vocalization (more to the mother than to anyone else)
- Visual-motor orientation (looking more at the mother, even if she is not close)
- Crying when the mother leaves the room
- Approaching through locomotion (crawling, creeping, or walking)
- Clinging (especially in the presence of a stranger)
- Exploring away from the mother while using her as a secure base

Reactive attachment disorder (RAD) is a psychologic and developmental problem that stems from maladaptive or absent attachment between the infant and parent and may persist into childhood and even adulthood (Zeanah and Gleason, 2010). Infants at risk for RAD include those who have been victims of physical or sexual abuse or neglect; infants exposed to parental alcoholism, mental illness, and substance abuse; and infants who have experienced the absence of a consistent primary caregiver as a result of foster care, institutionalization, parental abandonment, or parental incarceration. RAD is a form of extreme insecure attachment. Historically, two different patterns of RAD were described: the emotionally withdrawn–inhibited pattern and an indiscriminate-disinhibited pattern (Zeanah and Fox, 2004). Recently Zeanah and Gleason (2010) have proposed classifying these two subtypes into separate disorders: disinhibited social engagement disorder of childhood and reactive attachment disorder of infancy or early childhood. These researchers postulate that children who experience grossly inadequate child care will develop severe attachment disorder. Signs of RAD are usually seen before the age of 5 years in infants who had insecure attachments to the mother or other primary caregiver. The child may manifest behaviors such as not being cuddly with parents, failing to make eye contact with significant others, having poor impulse control, and being destructive to self and others. Maltreated and orphaned children may be diagnosed with this complex disorder. Without early intervention, some of these children fail to develop a conscience and suffer from an antisocial personality disorder that may lead to criminal acts. Children with autism or other pervasive developmental disorders have

behaviors that are categorically different from those with RAD (Zeanah and Gleason, 2010).

Separation Anxiety. Between ages 4 and 8 months, the infant progresses through the first stage of separation-individuation and begins to have some awareness of self and mother as separate beings. At the same time, object permanence is developing and the infant is aware that the parent can be absent. Therefore separation anxiety develops and is manifested through a predictable sequence of behaviors.

During the early second half of the first year, infants protest when placed in their crib, and a short time later they object when the mother leaves the room. Infants may not notice the mother's absence if they are absorbed in an activity. However, when they realize her absence, they protest. From this point on, they become very alert to her activities and whereabouts. By 11 to 12 months, they are able to anticipate her imminent departure by watching her behaviors and they begin to protest before she leaves. At this point, many parents learn to postpone alerting the child to their departure until just before leaving.

Stranger Fear. As infants demonstrate attachment to one person, they correspondingly exhibit less friendliness to others. Between ages 6 and 8 months, fear of strangers and stranger anxiety become prominent and are related to infants' ability to discriminate between familiar and unfamiliar people. Behaviors such as clinging to the parent, crying, and turning away from the stranger are common (Fig. 31-9).

Language Development

The infant's first means of verbal communication is crying. Crying as a biologic sign conveys a message of urgency and signals displeasure, such as hunger. However, crying is also a social event that affects the development of the parent-infant relationship—either by its absence, which usually has a positive effect on parents, or its presence, which may involve a negative response or persuade parents to minister to the child's physical or emotional needs.

In the first few weeks of life, crying has a reflexive quality and is mostly related to physiologic needs. Infants cry for 1 to 1.5 hours a day up to 3 weeks of age and then build up to 2 and even 4 hours by 6 weeks. Crying tends to decrease by 12 weeks of age. It is thought

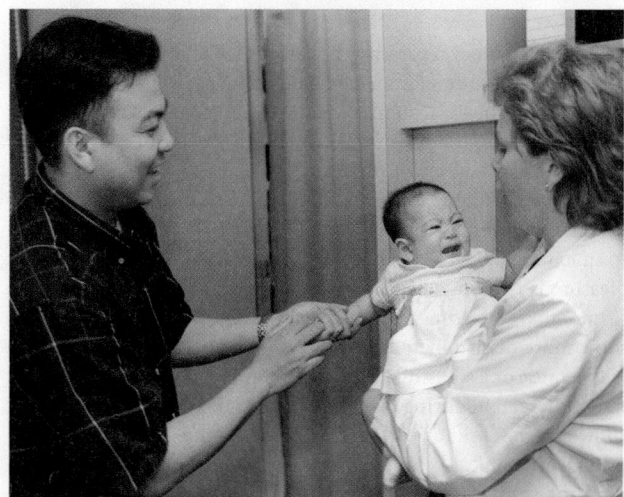

FIG 31-9 Behaviors related to fear of strangers include clinging to the parent and turning away from the stranger. (Photo by Paul Vincent Kuntz, Texas Children's Hospital, Houston, TX.)

FAMILY-CENTERED CARE

Child's Developing Language Skills

During the acquisition of new language skills the child temporarily may stop using other recently learned sounds or words. This is often distressing for parents, who have waited in anticipation for the words "dada" or "mama," because these sounds are commonly replaced by other vocalizations and may not be repeated for several weeks. Nurses can reassure parents that the child will again say these special words, and with increased meaning.

that the increase in crying for no apparent reason during the first few months may be related to the discharge of energy and the maturational changes in the central nervous system. During the end of the first year, infants cry for attention; from fear (especially stranger fear); and from frustration, usually in response to their developing but inadequate motor skills.

! NURSING ALERT

Be alert to parents' reports about maternal postpartum depression and infant crying, since these concerns may indicate a stressed mother-infant relationship.

Vocalizations heard during crying eventually become syllables and words (e.g., the "mama" heard during vigorous crying). Infants vocalize as early as 5 to 6 weeks of age by making small throaty sounds. By 2 months, they make single vowel sounds such as *ah, eh,* and *uh.* By 3 to 4 months, the consonants *n, k, g, p,* and *b* are added and the infants coo, gurgle, and laugh aloud. By 8 months, they imitate sounds; add the consonants *t, d,* and *w;* and combine syllables (e.g., "dada") but they do not ascribe meaning to the word until 10 to 11 months of age (see Family-Centered Care box). By 9 to 10 months, they comprehend the meaning of the word "no" and obey simple commands. By age 1 year, they can say three to five words with meaning.

Play

Play during infancy represents the various social modalities observed during cognitive development. Infants' activity is primarily narcissistic and revolves around their own body. As discussed under Development of Body Image (p. 876), body parts are primarily objects of play and pleasure.

During the first year, play becomes more sophisticated and interdependent. From birth to 3 months, infants' responses to the environment are global and largely undifferentiated. Play is dependent; pleasure is demonstrated by a quieting attitude (1 month), a smile (2 months), or a squeal (3 months). From 3 to 6 months, infants show more discriminate interest in stimuli and begin to play alone with a rattle or a soft stuffed toy or with someone else. There is much more interaction during play. By 4 months of age, they laugh aloud, show a preference for certain toys, and become excited when food or a favorite object is brought to them. They recognize an image in a mirror, smile at it, and vocalize to it.

By 6 months to 1 year, play involves sensorimotor skills. Actual games such as peekaboo and pat-a-cake are played. Verbal repetition and imitation of simple gestures occur in response to

demonstration. Play is much more selective, not only in terms of specific toys but also in terms of "playmates." Although play is solitary or one-sided, infants choose with whom they will interact. At 6 to 8 months, they usually refuse to play with strangers. Parents are definite favorites, and infants know how to attract their attention. At 6 months, they extend the arms to be picked up; at 7 months, cough or squeal to make their presence known; at 10 months, pull the parent's clothing; and at 12 months, call them by name. This represents a tremendous advance from the newborn, who signaled biologic needs by crying to express displeasure.

Stimulation is as important for psychosocial growth as food is for physical growth. Knowledge of developmental milestones allows nurses to guide parents regarding proper play for infants. It is not sufficient to place a mobile over a crib and toys in a play yard for a child's optimal social, emotional, and intellectual development. Likewise, the television or recorded videos, for the most part, do not provide infants with appropriate sensory stimulation, do not increase language skills, and should therefore be restricted in children younger than 2 years (AAP Council on Communications and Media, 2011). Play must provide interpersonal contact and recreational and educational stimulation. Infants need to be *played with,* not merely *allowed to play.* Although the type of play infants engage in is called *solitary,* this is a figurative, not literal, term to denote one-sided play. The type of toys given to the child is much less important than the quality of personal interaction that occurs.

Temperament

The infant's temperament or behavioral style influences the type of interaction that occurs between the child and parents, especially the mother, and other family members (see general discussion of temperament in Chapter 28). In assessments of a child's temperament, it is the parents' perception of the child and the degree of fit between their expectations and the child's actual temperament that are important. The more dissonance, or lack of harmony, between the child's temperament and the parent's ability to accept and deal with the behavior, the more risk for subsequent parent-child conflicts.

Although most behavioral researchers agree that there is a strong biologic component to temperament, researchers also suggest that temperament may be modified by the environment, particularly the family (Wilson, White, Cobb, et al., 2000). Family interaction with the infant is perceived as a circular process wherein each family member affects each other and the family as a unit. With these concepts in mind, the nurse has an important role in helping the family understand the infant's temperament as it relates to family dynamics and the eventual well-being of the child and family unit (Wilson, White, Cobb, et al., 2000).

Some researchers speculate that infant temperament may contribute to maternal depression. Indeed, when reciprocity is lacking between the infant and the mother or when the infant's behavior does not meet maternal expectations, there is increased risk for discord. Beck's (2001) meta-analysis found that infant temperament was a mild risk factor for postpartum depression, whereas self-esteem, marital status, socioeconomic status, and unplanned or unwanted pregnancy were much more significant in predicting maternal depression. Fragmented maternal sleep rather than infant temperament was positively correlated to maternal depression in another study (Goyal, Gay, and Lee, 2009). Others (McGrath, Records, and Rice, 2008) found that depressed mothers (vs. nondepressed mothers) rated their infant's temperament at 2 and 6 months of age as more difficult. The researchers stress that depressed mothers need to be identified and assisted in making the transition to motherhood and in developing synchronicity with their newborn infants. Researchers have correlated fussy infant temperament with the introduction of early complementary feedings (at 3 months of age) (Wasser, Bentley, Borja, et al., 2011) and feeding infants foods that may contribute to obesity (Vollrath, Tonstad, Rothbart, et al., 2011).

The Revised Infant Temperament Questionnaire (RITQ) (Carey and McDevitt, 1978) can be used as a screening tool with parents. The questionnaire focuses on nine temperament variables, but the 95 questions relate specifically to activities such as sleeping, feeding, playing, diapering, and dressing. The scores from the RITQ help identify the child's temperamental style. Use of the RITQ is well accepted by parents and should be accompanied by an adequate explanation of the results. In discussing the results, the nurse should avoid descriptors such as *difficult* and describe such infants in terms such as *intense* or *less predictable*. The Early Infancy Temperament Questionnaire is a 76-item parent questionnaire that was adapted from the RITQ to specifically evaluate temperament characteristics of infants 1 to 4 months old, whereas the RITQ is best suited for infants 4 months old and older (Medoff-Cooper, Carey, and McDevitt, 1993).

With knowledge of the infant's temperament, nurses are better able to (1) provide parents with background information that will help them see their child in a better perspective, (2) offer a more organized picture of their child's behavior and possibly reveal distortions in their perceptions of the behavior, and (3) guide parents regarding appropriate childrearing techniques. Appropriate counseling based on awareness of the child's temperament can greatly enhance the quality of interaction between parents and infant. Even just letting parents know that "difficult" traits are innate can relieve feelings of guilt and incompetence.

Knowledge of the developmental sequence allows the nurse to assess normal growth and minor or abnormal deviations. It also helps parents gain realistic expectations of their child's ability and provides guidelines for suitable play and stimulation. Parents who lack knowledge of child growth and development may set inappropriate behavioral expectations for their child. Emphasizing the child's developmental rather than chronologic age strengthens the parent-child relationship by fostering trust and lessening frustration. Therefore thorough understanding and appreciation of children's growth and development are essential.

Coping with Concerns Related to Normal Growth and Development
Separation and Stranger Fear

A number of fears can appear during infancy. However, the fear that causes parents the most concern is fear related to strangers and separation. Although erroneously interpreted by some as a sign of undesirable, antisocial behavior, stranger fear and separation anxiety are important components of a strong, healthy, parent-child attachment. Nevertheless, this period can present difficulties for the parent and child. Parents may experience guilt at having to leave the infant because he or she violently protests being separated from the parents. To accustom the infant to new people, parents are encouraged to have close friends or relatives visit often. This provides other persons with whom the child is comfortable and who can give parents time for themselves.

Infants also need opportunities to safely experience strangers. Usually toward the end of the first year, infants begin to venture away from the parent and demonstrate curiosity about strangers. If

allowed to explore at their own rate, many infants eventually "warm up." If parents hold the child away from their face, the infant can observe while maintaining close physical contact.

The best approach for the stranger (who may be the nurse) is to talk softly; meet the child at eye level (to appear smaller); maintain a safe distance from the infant; and avoid sudden, intrusive gestures, such as holding the arms out and smiling broadly.

Parents also may wonder whether they should encourage the child's clinging, dependent behavior, especially if there is pressure from others who view this as "spoiling." Parents need to be reassured that such behavior is healthy, desirable, and necessary for the child's optimal emotional development. If parents can reassure the infant of their presence, the infant will learn to realize that they are still there even if not physically present. Talking to infants when leaving the room, allowing them to hear one's voice on the telephone, and using transitional objects (e.g., a favorite blanket or toy) reassure them of the parent's continued presence.

Alternative Child Care Arrangements

For many parents, especially working mothers, locating safe and competent child care facilities for the infant is an increasingly difficult problem—one that is compounded by the number of mothers working outside the home. Over the past 40 years, there has been a marked shift in child care arrangements; whereas the majority of children are cared for in group centers or other settings, an increasing number of children are being cared for in home settings.

The basic types of care are (1) in-home care, either in the parents' or caregivers' home (family day care) and (2) center-based care, usually in a day care center. *In-home care* may consist of a full-time baby-sitter who lives in the home, a full-time baby-sitter who comes to the home, cooperative arrangements such as exchange baby-sitting, and family day care. A licensed *small family child day care home* typically provides care and protection for up to six children for part of a day and does not include informal arrangements such as exchange baby-sitting or caregivers in the child's own home. The six children include the family day care provider's own children younger than 5 years living in the home. *Large family child day care homes* may provide care for eight to twelve children. Unfortunately, many family child day care homes operate without a license and may care for large numbers of infants without adequate staff and facilities.

Child center-based care usually refers to a licensed day care facility that provides care for six or more children for 6 or more hours a day. *Work-based group care* is another option that is becoming increasingly popular as employers recognize the benefit of providing high-quality and convenient child care to their employees. *Sick-child care* may also be available for times when the child is ill. Such programs are often located in community hospitals or in work settings.

Nurses may fulfill a unique role in guiding parents in locating suitable facilities that have a well-qualified staff. State licensing agencies can help parents identify day care centers that accept children of specific age-groups and that are convenient to home and work. Their records are available to the public and provide reports from the health, safety, and fire departments; periodic evaluations from the licensing agency; complaints filed against the center; and qualifications of the center's employees. State-licensed programs are supposed to abide by established standards, which represent the minimum requirements and safeguards; however, enforcement of the standards is sometimes inadequate. Early childhood programs may also belong to a voluntary accreditation system, the National

Association for the Education of Young Children, which serves as a model for optimal care.*

The same attention should be applied to locating competent baby-sitters. References from other parents are essential, and there is no substitute for observing the interaction between the individual and the child. Although very young infants need little if any preparation for the introduction of a new caregiver, older infants may benefit from a gradual placement to reduce stranger anxiety. At all times the parent should have the right to visit the child, and regular conferences should be established to review the child's progress. Some child care centers provide a service whereby the parent may log on to the Internet from work and view the child's activity at the center for reassurance that the child is well.

Important areas for parents to evaluate are the center's daily program, teacher qualifications, nurturing qualities of caregivers, child-to-staff ratio, discipline policy, environmental safety precautions, provision of meals, sanitary conditions, adequate indoor and outdoor space per child, and fee schedule. Although fees vary considerably, a program that charges a minimum fee may also be providing minimum services. Parents should arrange to meet the director and some of the employees, especially those who would be caring for the child. Resources to familiarize parents with characteristics of quality child care and checklists to systematically evaluate the center and compare it with other facilities can help parents make successful choices.

One of the areas that is increasingly important in selecting child care is the center's health practices; however, parents often do not check the center for health and safety features. Evidence shows that children, especially those younger than 3 years in day care centers, have more illnesses—especially diarrhea, otitis media, respiratory tract infections (especially if the caregiver smokes), hepatitis A, meningitis, and cytomegalovirus—than children cared for in their home. The strongest predictor of risk for illness is the number of unrelated children in the room. Proactive infection control measures and education of staff have been effective in reducing the incidence of upper respiratory tract infections, diarrhea, and rotavirus. It has been reported that families who have children in out-of-home child care lose an estimated 13 days of work per year as a result of infections (Brady, 2005). Parents should inquire about the center's policy regarding the attendance and care of sick children. Parents with children in day care or even in-home care need to discuss safe sleep positions and environments for infants in order to prevent SIDS (Matthews and Moore, 2013).

Limit Setting and Discipline

As infants' motor skills advance and mobility increases, parents face the need to set safe limits to protect the child and establish a positive and supportive parent-child relationship (see Nurse's Role in Injury Prevention, p. 903). Although there are numerous disciplinary techniques, some are more appropriate for this age than others. An effective approach used in disciplining a child is the use of "time-out." The important principle to consider is that the place for

time-out needs to be commensurate with the child's abilities. For example, the play yard is better for most infants than a chair. Although parents may be concerned with instituting discipline during infancy, it is important to stress that the earlier effective disciplinary methods are employed, the easier it is to continue these approaches.

Parents must recognize the child's cognitive and behavioral limitations; adequate protection from hazards must be implemented because infants and toddlers do not understand a cause-effect relationship between dangerous objects and physical harm. Children will innately test limits and explore during the exploratory phase of growth; instead of discouraging exploration, parents should provide safe alternatives, put away dangerous household items, and provide consistent discipline and nurturing.

Effective teaching for injury prevention optimally begins in infancy by helping parents understand the nature of their child's normal development. It must be reiterated continually that infants cry because a need is not being met, not to intentionally irritate an adult. The fussy or irritable infant is a potential victim of shaken baby syndrome (or other bodily harm), since adults and caregivers may not understand the nature of the infant's crying.*

Thumb-Sucking and Use of a Pacifier

Sucking is the infant's chief pleasure and may not be satisfied by breastfeeding or bottle-feeding. It is such a strong need that infants who are deprived of sucking, such as those with a cleft lip repair, will suck on their tongues. Some newborns are born with sucking blisters on their hands from in utero sucking activity.

Problems arise when parents are overly concerned about the sucking of the fingers, thumb, or pacifier and attempt to restrain this natural tendency. Before giving advice, nurses should investigate the parents' feelings and base guidance on this information.

Pacifier use, particularly in the early days after birth and in the birth hospital, has gained considerable attention in the scientific literature. Biancuzzo (2003) suggests that it cannot be stated with absolute certainty that pacifier use is bad in every situation but warns of a potential harm in the use of pacifiers based on available evidence. Furthermore, she cautions health care workers to be informed regarding potential harm in pacifier use and to inform parents of the potential. Lawrence and Lawrence (2011), as well as other experts in breastfeeding, recommend that health care workers not introduce pacifiers to breastfed infants unless the parent requests it. Pacifier use is not recommended as part of the Baby-Friendly Hospital Initiative. O'Connor, Tanabe, Siadaty, et al. (2009) reviewed 29 studies and concluded that pacifier use did not adversely affect breastfeeding duration or exclusivity. They further concluded that pacifier use and shortened breastfeeding in many studies likely represented a number of other complex factors such as breastfeeding difficulties or intent to wean.

Pacifier use has been associated with an increased risk for otitis media in several studies (Niemelä, Pihakari, Pokka, et al., 2000; Rovers, Numans, Langenbach, et al., 2008). The American Academy of Pediatrics (AAP) and American Academy of Family Physicians recommend use of pacifier during the first 6 months because of the benefit in regard to pain management and prevention of sudden infant death syndrome (SIDS) but recommend the child be weaned from the pacifier during the second 6 months of life

---

*Information about accreditation criteria and procedures of the National Academy for Early Childhood Program Accreditation/NAEYC is available from the National Association for the Education of Young Children, 1313 L St. NW, Suite 500, Washington, DC 20005; 800-424-2460 or 202-232-8777; www.naeyc.org. These criteria are excellent guidelines for evaluating child care facilities. Other resources are (1) *Choosing Quality Childcare: What's Best for Your Family?* and a number of other child care articles and pamphlets from American Academy of Pediatrics, 141 Northwest Point Blvd., Elk Grove Village, IL 60007; 847-434-4000; http://aap.org; and (2) Child Care Aware, 800-424-2246; www.childcareaware.org.

*One resource for parents and health care professionals is the National Center on Shaken Baby Syndrome, and the Period of Purple Crying Program®; 1433 North Highway 89, Suite 110, Farmington, UT, 84025; 801-447-9360; www.dontshake.org.

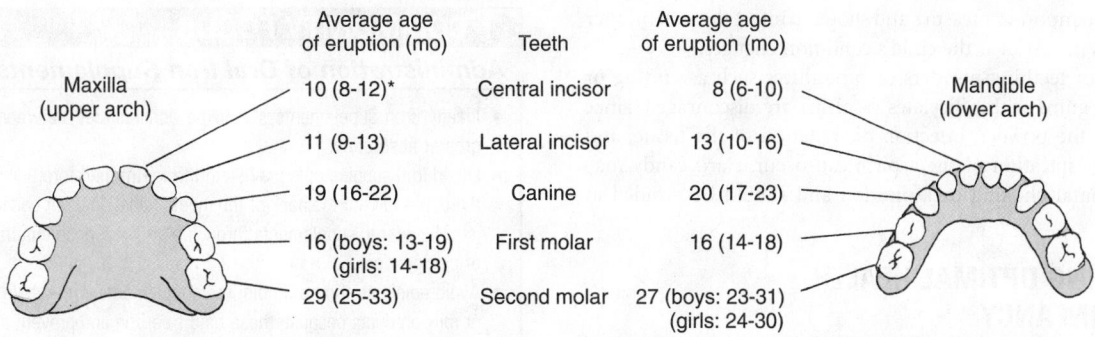

FIG 31-10 Sequence of eruption of primary teeth. *Range represents ±1 standard deviation, or 67% of subjects studied. (Data from American Dental Association, http://www.mouthhealthy.org/en/az-topics/e/eruption-charts.aspx.)

(Sexton and Natale, 2009). Pacifier use during painful procedures in neonates has been shown to produce an analgesic effect when combined with a concentrated sucrose solution (Carbajal, 2005) (see Chapter 30).

A review of studies by the Joanna Briggs Institute (2005) found an association between pacifier use in infancy and a reduction in breastfeeding and exclusive breastfeeding. However, the authors concluded that pacifier use did not cause a reduction in breastfeeding; rather, it was a "marker for socioeconomic, demographic, psychosocial and cultural factors that determine pacifier use and breastfeeding." In addition, the researchers examined studies related to pacifier use and prevention of SIDS; infants put to sleep with a pacifier had a *reduced* risk for SIDS. Because of the limited number of studies correlating pacifier use and increased risk for infections or dental malocclusion, the authors were unable to make any recommendations for or against pacifier use in relation to these practices (Joanna Briggs Institute, 2005).

A recent Cochrane review found that pacifier use in full-term healthy infants, started from birth or after lactation was established, did not significantly affect the prevalence or duration of exclusive and partial breastfeeding up to 4 months of age (Jaafar, Jahanafar, Angolkar, et al., 2011).

The AAP Task Force on Sudden Infant Death Syndrome (2005), recommends limited pacifier use in infants, citing the strong evidence for pacifier use and its protective effect in SIDS reduction. The exact mechanism involved in the protection for SIDS is not known. Still, pacifier use should not replace actual feeding or suckling; prohibiting pacifier use will not ensure an increase in the length of breastfeeding; and there should be an emphasis on allowing the infant to control the pace, frequency, and termination of feeding rather than allowing the pacifier (or anything else) to become the focus of the interaction.

To decrease dependence on nonnutritive sucking in young infants, sucking pleasure can be increased by prolonging feeding time. Also, the parent's excessive use of the pacifier to calm the child should be explored. It is not unusual for parents to place a pacifier in the infant's mouth as soon as crying begins, thus reinforcing a pattern of distress-relief.

If the child uses a pacifier, stress safety considerations in purchasing one. During infancy and early childhood there is no need to restrain nonnutritive sucking of the fingers. Malocclusion may occur if thumb-sucking persists past approximately 4 years of age, or when the permanent teeth erupt. Some parents may perceive pacifiers as less damaging because they are discarded by 2 to 3 years of age, whereas thumb-sucking may persist well into school-age years. Both pacifier use and thumb-sucking may also have significant cultural variations. Thumb-sucking reaches its peak at age 18 to 20 months and is most prevalent when the child is hungry, tired, or feeling insecure. Persistent thumb-sucking in a listless, apathetic child always warrants investigation. It may be a sign of an emotional problem between parent and child or of boredom, isolation, and lack of stimulation.

At the time of this writing, there is no evidence that pacifier use and nonnutritive sucking in *preterm infants* have any effect on the initiation and length of breastfeeding. Nonnutritive sucking should not be withheld from preterm infants, especially when used in conjunction with concentrated sucrose for pain management.

Teething

One of the more difficult periods in the infant's (and parents') life is the eruption of the deciduous (primary) teeth, often referred to as *teething*. The age of tooth eruption shows considerable variation among children, but the order of their appearance is fairly regular and predictable (Fig. 31-10). The first primary teeth to erupt are the lower central incisors, which appear at approximately 6 to 10 months of age (average 8 months). These are followed closely by the upper central incisors. The following is a quick guide to assessment of deciduous teeth during the first 2 years:

Age of the child in months − 6 = Number of teeth.

For example, 8 months of age − 6 = 2 teeth at this time.

Teething is a physiologic process; some discomfort is common as the crown of the tooth breaks through the periodontal membrane. Some children show minimal evidence of teething, such as drooling, gum rubbing, increased finger sucking, or biting on hard objects. Others are very irritable, have difficulty sleeping, and refuse to eat solid foods. Generally, signs of illness such as fever, vomiting, or diarrhea are not symptoms of teething but of illness and may warrant further investigation. Because teething pain is a result of inflammation, cold is soothing. Giving the child a cold teething ring helps relieve the inflammation (do not freeze liquid-filled teething rings). Several nonprescription topical anesthetic ointments are available, such as Baby Ora-Jel, although parents and health care workers should be aware of the risks of using topical anesthetic products (absorption rates vary in infants) (Markman, 2009). The active ingredient in most of them is benzocaine, which may rarely cause methemoglobinemia. If such products are used, parents are advised to apply them correctly. In the event of persistent irritability that affects sleeping and feeding, systemic analgesics such as acetaminophen or ibuprofen can be given (if age appropriate) for no more than 3 days (Anderson, 2004); however, parents should know that this is a temporary measure and should contact the practitioner if symptoms persist or if the child's condition changes.

The use of teething powders or procedures such as cutting or rubbing the gums with salicylates (aspirin) are discouraged, since ingestion of the powder, infection or irritation of the tissue, and ingestion or aspiration of the aspirin can occur. Hard candy may cause accidental choking or aspiration and should be avoided at this age.

PROMOTING OPTIMAL HEALTH DURING INFANCY

Nutrition

Ideally, discussion of optimal nutrition should begin prenatally with a discussion regarding maternal intake of adequate nutrition in the form of a balanced diet and adequate amounts of protein, vitamins, and minerals, all of which have an impact on the growing fetus. Nurses should encourage and provide information for parents to discuss the options of breastfeeding or bottle-feeding the infant well in advance of the birth date. The choice for either is highly individual and is discussed in Chapter 24. This section is concerned primarily with infant nutrition during the months when growth needs and developmental milestones ready the child for the introduction of solid foods.

Despite adequate availability of optimal nutrient sources, health care experts are concerned that infants are not fed appropriately. Infants may be given solid foods when their digestive system is not ready to completely absorb such foods. In addition, drinks that are inappropriate for growing infants may be given in place of enriched infant milk and may only provide "empty" calories and contribute to childhood and adult cardiovascular disease or obesity and place the infant at risk for iron deficiency anemia, vitamin D deficiency, and rickets. A survey of infant feeding practices found that about 40% of infants had consumed infant cereal, fruit, or vegetables by 4 months of age, despite recommendations that such foods not be introduced until 4 to 6 months (Grummer-Strawn, Scanlon, and Fein, 2008). In the same study, 50% of infants were consuming cake, fried potatoes, candy, and cookies by age 12 months. There is some preliminary evidence that accelerated weight gain in the first 6 months of life may be correlated with obesity later in life (Taveras, Rifas-Shiman, Belfort, et al., 2009). Infant health practices, including nutrition, may have a far-reaching, long-term impact on the child's life. Growth and development could be negatively affected, as could the risk for acquiring certain chronic health conditions. Nurses must be proactive in teaching parents what constitutes appropriate infant nutrition and nutritional habits, which provide the child with an optimal opportunity to grow and develop into a healthy child and adult.

The First 6 Months

Human milk is the most desirable complete diet for the infant during the first 6 months. The healthy term infant receiving breast milk from a well-nourished mother usually requires no specific vitamin and mineral supplements, with a few exceptions. Daily supplements of vitamin D and vitamin B_{12} may be indicated if the mother's intake of these vitamins is inadequate. The AAP (2008) recommends that all infants (including those exclusively breastfed) receive a daily supplement of 400 international units (IU) of vitamin D beginning in the first few days of life to prevent rickets and vitamin D deficiency. Vitamin D supplementation should occur until the infant is consuming at least 1 L/day (or 1 quart/day) of vitamin D–fortified formula (AAP, 2008). Non-breastfed infants

COMMUNITY FOCUS

Administration of Oral Iron Supplements

- Ideally, iron supplements should be administered between meals for greater absorption.
- Liquid iron supplements may stain the teeth; therefore administer with a dropper toward the back of the mouth (side). In older children, administer liquid iron supplements through a straw or rinse mouth thoroughly after ingestion.
- Avoid administration of liquid iron supplements with whole cow's milk or milk products because these bind free iron and prevent absorption.
- Educate parents that iron supplements will turn stools black or tarry green.
- Iron supplements may cause transient constipation. Caution parents not to switch to a low-iron–containing formula or whole milk, which are poor sources of iron and may lead to iron deficiency anemia (see Iron Deficiency Anemia, Chapter 43).
- In older children, follow liquid iron supplement with a citrus fruit or juice drink (no more than 3-4 oz).
- Avoid administration of iron supplements with foods or drinks that bind iron and prevent absorption (see p. 935).

who are taking less than 1 L/day of vitamin D–fortified formula should also receive a daily vitamin D supplement of 400 IU (see Safety Alert). If the infant is being exclusively breastfed after 4 months (when fetal iron stores are depleted), iron supplementation (1 mg/kg/day) is recommended until appropriate iron-containing complementary foods such as iron-fortified cereal are introduced (Baker, Greer, and AAP Committee on Nutrition, 2010) (see Community Focus box). Infants, whether breastfed or bottle-fed, do not require additional fluids, especially water or juice, during the first 4 months of life. Excessive intake of water in infants may result in water intoxication and hyponatremia.

SAFETY ALERT

There are reports of accidental overdoses of liquid vitamin D in infants because of packaging errors; the syringe for liquid administration may not be labeled clearly for 400 IU. Nurses should educate parents to read the syringe and to avoid administering more than 400 IU of vitamin D (FDA Consumer Health Information, 2010).

Employed mothers can continue breastfeeding with guidance and encouragement.* Mothers are encouraged to set realistic goals for employment and breastfeeding, with accurate information regarding the costs, risks, and benefits of available feeding options. Barriers encountered by working breastfeeding mothers include lack of employer or co-worker support, unavailable or inadequate facilities for pumping and storing milk, lack of time to express milk while at work, and real or perceived low milk supply (Johnston and Esposito, 2007; Rojjanasrirat, 2004; Shealey, Li, Benton-Davis, et al., 2005). Important themes that emerged in the study by Rojjanasrirat (2004) of working breastfeeding mothers included support (emotional, informational, and instrumental), attitude, and psychologic distress. Johnston and Esposito (2007) found flexible scheduling and increased paid maternity leave time (at least 12 weeks vs. 10 weeks) to be key to encouraging mothers to continue breastfeeding.

---

*See also *The CDC Guide to Breastfeeding Interventions* (Shealy, Li, Benton-Davis, et al., 2005), which includes information for working and breastfeeding, www.cdc.gov/breastfeeding/pdf/breastfeeding_interventions.pdf.

Many mothers may find that a program of breast pumping when away from home and bottle-feeding the infant the expressed milk with or without formula supplementation is successful. Expressed breast milk may be stored in the refrigerator (4°C [39°F]) without danger of bacterial contamination for up to 5 days (Lawrence and Lawrence, 2011). Although feeding the infant at home may occur on a demand basis, pumping milk away from home may be needed every 3 to 4 hours to maintain adequate supply. Breast milk may be expressed by hand or pump (manual or electric) and stored in an appropriate air-tight glass or plastic container. Expressed breast milk may be frozen (−18°C [0°F] or lower) for up to 6 months (depending on the type of freezer used), but care should be taken to prevent freezer burn (see Lawrence and Lawrence, 2011, for further guidelines on storing and freezing human milk).

In addition to efficient breast pumping, mothers also need child care by a trusted individual or agency and support and assistance from significant others. As with all breastfeeding mothers, these women must have proper nutrition and rest for adequate lactation. Maternal fatigue is considered the biggest threat to successful breastfeeding in employed mothers.

> ## ! NURSING ALERT
>
> Warming expressed milk in a microwave decreases the availability of antiinfective properties and vitamin C and causes a separation of milk layers, which affects fat content (Lawrence and Lawrence, 2011). To prevent oral burns from uneven warming of the milk, breast milk should never be thawed or rewarmed in a microwave oven. To thaw the frozen milk, either place container under a lukewarm water bath (<40.5°C [105°F]) or place in refrigerator overnight.

An acceptable alternative to breastfeeding is commercial iron-fortified formula. Like human milk, it supplies all nutrients needed by the infant for the first 6 months. Unmodified whole cow's milk, low-fat cow's milk, skim milk, other animal milks, and imitation milk drinks are not acceptable as a major source of nutrition for infants because of their limited digestibility, increased risk for contamination, and lack of components needed for appropriate growth. Whole milk can cause iron deficiency anemia in infants, possibly as a result of occult gastrointestinal blood loss. Pasteurized whole cow's milk is deficient in iron, zinc, and vitamin C and has a high renal solute load, which makes it undesirable for infants younger than 12 months (AAP, 2009).

> ## ! NURSING ALERT
>
> Neither infant formula nor breast milk should be warmed in a microwave oven because this may cause oral burns as a result of uneven heating in the container; the bottle or container may remain cool while hot spots develop in the formula (Food and Drug Administration [FDA], 2012; Morin, 2009a).

> ## ! NURSING ALERT
>
> Dietary fat in infants younger than 6 months should not be restricted unless on specific medical advice. Substituting skim or low-fat milk is unacceptable, since the essential fatty acids are inadequate and the solute concentration of protein and electrolytes, such as sodium, is too high.

The amount of formula per feeding and the number of feedings per day vary among infants. Infants being fed on demand usually determine their own feeding schedule, but some infants may need

> ## ⊕ CULTURAL COMPETENCE
>
> ### Multicultural Feeding Practices
>
> Cultural beliefs and values often influence infant feeding practices. Health care professionals may benefit from understanding the multicultural feeding practices that parents choose for their infant. Traditional feeding practices include offering a variety of liquids or foods, such as sugared wine, water, or honey during the first few days of life and thereafter.

a more planned schedule based on average feeding patterns to ensure sufficient nutrients. In general, the number of feedings decreases from six at 1 month of age to four or five at 6 months. Regardless of the number of feedings, the total amount of formula ingested will usually level off at about 32 ounces (946 mL) per day.

Honey should be avoided in the first 12 months because of the risk for botulism (see Chapter 49); a pacifier should not be coated with honey to encourage the infant to take it. Socializing the infant to food flavors of the family's culture is common in addition to continuing breastfeeding for 2 to 4 years (see Cultural Competence box).

Bottled water for mixing powdered or concentrated formula is a relatively safe alternative to tap water if available tap water has a high content of contaminants such as lead. Do not assume, however, that bottled water is sterile unless specifically stated on the container. Fluoridated bottled water is not necessary for mixing powdered formula unless the local water source is low in fluoride, in which case fluoride supplementation is recommended after age 6 months (see Dental Health, p. 885).

The addition of solid foods before 4 to 6 months of age is not recommended. During the early months, solid foods are not compatible with the ability of the gastrointestinal tract and infant's nutritional needs. Feeding solids to young infants exposes them to food antigens that may produce food protein allergy. There is ample evidence that early introduction of foods other than maternal milk in the first 6 months of life predisposes children to an increased risk for food allergy development; foods known to be allergenic (e.g., peanuts, eggs, fish, seafood) should be introduced later than 12 months according to the child's risk for atopy (AAP, 2009).

Developmentally, infants are not ready for solid food. The extrusion (protrusion) reflex is strong and often causes them to push food out of the mouth. Infants instinctively suck when given food. Because of their limited motor abilities, infants are unable to deliberately push food away or avoid feeding. Therefore early introduction of solids is a type of forced feeding that may lead to excessive weight gain and increased predisposition to allergies and iron deficiency anemia. Parents should be cautioned concerning the use of juices and nonnutritive drinks such as fruit-flavored drinks or carbonated beverages (soda or pop) during this period. Many juices and nonnutritive drinks, although readily available to consumers, do not provide sufficient and appropriate caloric intake for infants younger than 12 months; such drinks may replace the nutrients in breast milk or formula and lead to growth or health problems. Fruit juices are not required in the first 6 months; there are no studies demonstrating benefits of giving fruit juice to infants.

The World Health Organization growth charts released in 2006 are now recommended as reference growth charts in children 0 to 59 months of age (Grummer-Strawn, Reinold, Krebs, et al., 2010) (cdc.gov/growthcharts/who_charts.htm).

The Second 6 Months

During the second half of the first year, human milk or formula should optimally continue to be the primary source of nutrition.

Fluoride supplementation should begin, depending on the infant's intake of fluoride (in formula mixed with tap water or bottled water [containing fluoride] as appropriate) (see Dental Health, p. 885). If breastfeeding is discontinued, a commercial iron-fortified formula should be substituted. Follow-up or transition formulas marketed for older infants offer no special advantages over other infant formulas and provide excessive protein (AAP, 2009).

The major change in feeding habits is the addition of solid foods to the infant's diet. Physiologically and developmentally, the infant 4 to 6 months of age is in a transition period. By this time, the gastrointestinal tract has matured sufficiently to handle more complex nutrients and is less sensitive to potentially allergenic foods. Tooth eruption is beginning and facilitates biting and chewing. The extrusion reflex has disappeared, and swallowing is more coordinated to allow the infant to accept solids easily. Head control is well developed, which permits infants to sit with support and purposely turn the head away to communicate lack of interest in food. Voluntary grasping and improved eye-hand coordination gradually allow infants to pick up finger foods and feed themselves. Their increasing sense of independence is evident in their desire to hold the bottle and try to "help" during feeding.

Selection and Preparation of Solid Foods

The choice of solid foods to introduce first is variable but should meet the reasons for feeding solids, such as supplying nutrients not found in formula or breast milk. Iron-fortified infant cereal is generally introduced first because of its high iron content (7 mg/3 tbsp of prepared dry cereal). Commercially prepared ready-to-serve dry cereals for infants include rice, barley, oatmeal, and high-protein cereals; rice is usually suggested as an initial food because of its easy digestibility and low allergenic potential. Cereals such as cream of farina should not be used, since infant commercial cereals are a better source of iron. Some of the commercial baby cereals are combined with fruit. There is little nutritional benefit from these preparations, and they are more expensive. New foods should be added one at a time; therefore parents should avoid cereal combinations when beginning a new grain.

Infant cereal (iron fortified) may be mixed with expressed breast milk or water until whole milk is given. After 6 months of age, small amounts of 100% fruit juices can be mixed with the dry cereal; the vitamin C content of the juice enhances the absorption of iron in the cereal. Because of their benefit as a source of iron, infant cereals should be continued until the child is 18 months of age.

Fruit juice can be offered from a cup for its rich source of vitamin C and as a substitute for milk for one feeding a day. Large quantities of certain juices (e.g., apple, pear, prune, sweet cherry, peach, grape) should be avoided because they may cause abdominal pain, diarrhea, or bloating in some children. Avoid fruit-flavored drinks, which may be marketed as juices but contain high concentrations of complex sugars. White grape juice (no more than 5 oz/day) may be better absorbed and safe for infants this age without causing gastrointestinal distress. The AAP (2009) recommends that fruit juice intake not exceed 4 to 6 ounces per day and that juices not be given to infants younger than 4 to 6 months. Because vitamin C is naturally destroyed by heat, juice is not warmed. Juice containers are always kept covered and refrigerated to prevent further vitamin loss.

The addition of other foods is arbitrary. A common sequence is to introduce strained fruits followed by vegetables and, finally, meats; however, some clinicians prefer to add vegetables before fruit. If foods are introduced early, citrus fruits, meats, and eggs are delayed until after 6 months of age because of their potential to result in allergy. At 6 months, foods such as a cracker or zwieback can be offered as finger and teething foods. By 8 to 9 months, junior foods and nutritious finger foods such as firmly cooked vegetable, raw pieces of fruit, or cheese can be given. By 1 year, well-cooked table foods are served.

The introduction of solid foods into the infant's diet at this age is primarily for taste and chewing experience, not for growth. The majority of the infant's caloric needs are derived from the primary milk source (human or formula); therefore solids should not be perceived as a substitute for milk until the child is older than 12 months. Portion sizes may vary according to the infant's taste. In general, 1 tablespoon per year of age (i.e., ½ to ¾ tablespoon for most infants younger than 12 months) is adequate for most infants. In most cases, 2 tablespoons may be served, but because of the infant's focus on the texture and feel of the food, smaller amounts will be consumed. Another reason for smaller portions is the concern over feeding habits in early childhood and obesity; early feeding of smaller portions may help prevent the "clean your plate" or "eat all your food or you can't get down from the table" concepts, which are known to contribute to overeating in later life. The addition of solid foods to the exclusively breastfed infant's diet does not significantly increase overall caloric intake or weight gain.

Commercially prepared baby foods are the most common type of food served to infants in the United States. They are convenient but sometimes contain added salt or sugar and can be relatively expensive. An alternative is to prepare baby foods at home, which is a simple and inexpensive process. Fruits and vegetables can be steamed in a small amount of water and pureed in a blender or food processor. Many of them, such as ripe banana, can be mashed fine with a fork. Fruits such as apples or pears require little or no water in the cooking process. Vegetables such as carrots, potatoes, or string beans require additional water in the cooking and blending process.

In general, low-calorie milk and foods should be avoided in infants and toddlers unless a strict medically prescribed diet is required. The infant's growth during this phase is crucial to future health status. Although saturated fat restriction is desirable after 2 years of age, the AAP (2009) cautions against excessive restriction of dietary fat in infancy. One suggestion is to limit the *amount* (serving size) of dietary fat in foods provided rather than eliminate them altogether, especially during infancy. However, it is important to recognize that certain types of dietary fat are unacceptable for infants; fried potatoes, candy, ice cream, cake, soda pop and other sweetened drinks, and other such items are not appropriate for infants and may contribute to childhood cardiovascular disease and obesity.

Parents are cautioned to avoid reliance on food supplements marketed as iron- or vitamin-fortified as primary sources of minerals. Instead, encourage parents to offer the child a variety of fruits, vegetables, and whole grains, including those known to naturally be rich in iron (Fox, Reidy, Novak, et al., 2006).

Introduction of Solid Foods

When the spoon is first introduced, infants often push it away and appear dissatisfied. Patience and skill are required to overcome this initial response. A small-bowled, straight, long-handled spoon, similar to a demitasse spoon, allows a small portion of food to be placed toward the back of the tongue. Food that is placed on the front of the tongue and pushed out is simply scooped up and refed. As infants become accustomed to the spoon, they more eagerly accept the food and eventually will open the mouth in anticipation (or keep it closed in dislike). Because the first introduction of food is a new experience, spoon feeding should be attempted after

PATIENT TEACHING

Introducing Solid Foods to Infants

- Introduce solids when infant is hungry.
- Begin spoon-feeding by pushing food to back of tongue because of infant's natural tendency to thrust the tongue forward.
- Use a small spoon with a straight handle; begin with 1 or 2 teaspoons of food; gradually increase to a couple of tablespoons per feeding.
- Introduce one food at a time, usually at intervals of 4 to 7 days, to allow for identification of food allergies.
- As the amount of solid food increases, decrease the quantity of milk to prevent overfeeding.
- Do not introduce foods by mixing them with formula in the bottle.

ingestion of some breast milk or formula to associate this activity with a pleasurable and satisfying experience. Trying to introduce a food *after* the entire milk feeding is usually useless because the infant is satiated and has no inclination to try something new.

After several spoon feedings, food can be introduced at the beginning of a meal. It is best to introduce many foods during the first year, when the infant is more likely to eat them because of a hearty appetite resulting from a rapid growth rate. During the toddler years, eating becomes less of an adventure and strong food preferences become evident.

One food item is introduced at intervals of 4 to 7 days to allow for identification of food allergies. New foods are fed in small amounts, from 1 teaspoon to a few tablespoons. As the amount of solid food increases, the quantity of milk is decreased to less than 1 L daily to prevent overfeeding.

Because feeding is a learning process as well as a means of nutrition, new foods are given alone to allow the child to learn new tastes and textures. Food should not be mixed in the bottle and fed through a nipple with a large hole; this deprives the child of the pleasure of learning new tastes and of developing a discriminating palate. It can also cause problems with poor chewing of food later in life because of lack of experience. Guidelines for the introduction of new foods are given in the Patient Teaching box.

The infant's first, second, and often twentieth try at self-feeding or cup feeding is a sloppy experience. Finger foods such as soft fruits or vegetables are just as good as playthings as food; they can be squeezed, smeared, squashed, and thoroughly painted on oneself, others, and the surrounding environment. However, all of this is part of learning, and mastery follows many accidents.

Parents are encouraged to interpret the infant's signals of discomfort and intervene in ways other than through feeding. Crying, fussiness, and sucking do not necessarily indicate hunger. Rocking, stroking, holding, and offering a toy or a pacifier may be more appropriate than automatically responding with food.

Weaning

Defined as the process of giving up one method of feeding for another, *weaning* usually refers to relinquishing the breast or bottle for a cup. In Western societies this is generally regarded as a major task for infants and is often seen as a potentially traumatic experience. It is psychologically significant because the infant is required to give up a major source of oral pleasure and gratification. Other cultural groups define weaning in relation to significant life events (e.g., teething) or reaching a specific age. No one time for weaning is best for every child, but generally, most infants show signs of

readiness during the second half of the first year. It is recommended that weaning be accomplished with the infant's needs as a guide (Lawrence and Lawrence, 2011).

Infants have learned that good things come from a spoon. Their increasing desire for freedom of movement may lessen their desire to be held close for feedings. They are acquiring more control over their actions and can easily manipulate a cup to their lips (even if it is held upside down!). Imitation becomes a powerful motivator by age 8 or 9 months, and they enjoy using a cup or glass like others do. Weaning should be gradual, replacing one bottle-feeding or breastfeeding at a time. The nighttime feeding is usually the last feeding to be discontinued. It is advisable never to begin allowing a child to take a bottle of milk to bed; this is a major cause of early childhood caries in deciduous teeth. If breastfeeding is terminated before 5 or 6 months of age, weaning should be to a bottle to provide for the infant's continued sucking needs. If breastfeeding is discontinued later, weaning can be directly to a cup, especially by age 12 to 14 months. Any sweet liquid, such as fruit juice, should be given in a cup.

Sleep and Activity

Sleep patterns vary among infants, with active infants typically sleeping less than placid children. Generally, by 3 to 4 months of age, most infants have developed a nocturnal pattern of sleep that lasts 9 to 11 hours. The total daily sleep is approximately 15 hours. In a study of Swiss children, Iglowstein, Jenni, Molinari, et al. (2003) found that the average number of hours of sleep in 6-month-olds was 14.2 hours. Consolidation of nocturnal sleep hours occurred during the first 12 months with decreasing daytime sleep and increasing nighttime sleep (approximately 11.7 hours) by 1 year of age. The number of naps per day varies, but infants may take one or two naps by the end of the first year. Breastfed infants usually sleep for shorter periods, with more frequent waking, especially during the night, compared with bottle-fed infants (Quillin and Glenn, 2004); average total sleep for 4-week-old infants in this study was 14 hours. Because of the trend toward breastfeeding, sleep norms such as those previously described, which were based primarily on bottle-fed infants, may not be relevant.

Most infants are naturally active and need no encouragement to be mobile. Problems can arise when devices such as play yards, strollers, commercial swings, and mobile walkers are used excessively. These items restrict movement and prevent infants from exploring and developing gross motor skills. Contrary to popular belief, mobile walkers do not enhance coordination and are dangerous if tipped over or placed near stairs (see also Sleep Problems in Chapter 32).

Dental Health

Good infant dental hygiene begins with appropriate maternal dental health before and during the pregnancy and counseling during early infancy regarding dietary intake for the promotion of optimal oral hygiene. Parents are counseled early regarding feeding practices that increase the risk for poor dental health. Some of these, as previously mentioned, include propping the milk bottle, giving the milk bottle in the bed, or giving fruit juices in a bottle, especially before 6 months of age. These contribute to enamel erosion and early childhood caries (previously called *baby bottle tooth decay*). Parents should also be made aware that dental caries is contagious and can be prevented with optimal oral hygiene starting in infancy (Peterson-Sweeney and Stevens, 2010).

Once the primary teeth erupt, cleaning should begin. The teeth and gums are initially cleaned by wiping with a damp cloth;

toothbrushing is too harsh for the tender gingiva. The caregiver can stabilize the infant by cradling the child with one arm and using the free hand to cleanse the teeth. Oral hygiene can be made pleasant by singing or talking to the infant. It is recommended that the infant have a brief oral health examination by 6 months of age from a qualified pediatric health care practitioner; infants at high risk for caries are identified, and oral health counseling is implemented. It is also recommended that the infant have an established dental home by 1 year of age (American Academy of Pediatric Dentistry, 2012). It is generally recommended that a small, soft-bristled toothbrush be used as more teeth erupt and the infant adjusts to the routine of cleaning. Water is preferred to toothpaste, which the infant will swallow (and if the toothpaste is fluoridated, the infant may ingest excessive amounts of fluoride). The American Academy of Pediatric Dentistry (2012) recommends a "smear" of toothpaste for children younger than 2 years and a pea-size amount for those 2 to 5 years old.

Fluoride, an essential mineral for building caries-resistant teeth, is needed beginning at 6 months of age if the infant does not receive water with adequate fluoride content. The AAP (2009) recommends that children 6 months to 3 years of age take 0.25 mg fluoride daily if water fluoride content is less than 0.3 ppm. The fluoride dosage has been decreased from earlier recommendations because of an increased occurrence of dental fluorosis from excessive fluoride ingestion. If bottled water is used to reconstitute powdered or concentrated formula, it should either be fluoride-free or contain low levels of fluoride.

Dietary considerations are also important because habits begun during infancy tend to continue into later years. Avoid foods with concentrated sugar (sucrose) in the infant's diet. Parents should be counseled regarding the detrimental effects of frequent and prolonged bottle-feeding or breastfeeding during sleep, when the milk or other fluid, such as juice, bathes the teeth, causing early childhood caries.

Immunizations

One of the most dramatic advances in pediatrics has been the decline of infectious diseases during the twentieth century because of the widespread use of immunization for preventable diseases. However, childhood vaccines have been widely criticized in recent years, and fear related to vaccine components has prompted some families to avoid childhood vaccines. In addition, many of the diseases for which children are vaccinated are rarely seen on a large-scale basis, leading some parents to believe that such vaccines are no longer necessary in the twenty-first century. The Internet provides a variety of information suggesting parents avoid childhood vaccines; a number of "vaccine myths" exist, which are based on erroneous information. The nurse is in an optimal position to provide parents with accurate information regarding childhood illnesses and available vaccines; the parent must then make an informed decision regarding the child's vaccinations. Nurses should address parents' concerns about childhood vaccines and avoid judgmental attitudes regarding the parents' decision to not vaccinate children.

Although many of the immunizations can be given to individuals of any age, the recommended primary schedule begins during infancy and, with the exception of boosters, is completed during early childhood. Therefore the discussion of childhood immunizations for diphtheria, tetanus, pertussis; polio; measles, mumps, rubella; *Haemophilus influenzae* type b; hepatitis A virus (HAV), hepatitis B virus (HBV); pneumococcus; influenza; meningococcus; and chickenpox is included in this chapter. Selected vaccines

generally reserved for children considered at high risk for the disease are discussed here and as appropriate throughout the text. (See also Communicable Diseases, Chapter 33, for a discussion of several of the diseases for which vaccines are available.)

Schedule for Immunizations

In the United States, two organizations—the Advisory Committee on Immunization Practices of the Centers for Disease Control and Prevention (CDC) and the Committee on Infectious Diseases of the American Academy of Pediatrics (AAP)—govern the recommendations for immunization policies and procedures. In Canada, recommendations are from the National Advisory Committee on Immunization under the authority of the Minister of Health and Public Health Agency of Canada. The policies of each committee are *recommendations,* not rules, and they change as a result of advances in the field of immunology. Pediatric nurses must stay informed of the latest advances and changes in policy.

In the United States, the recommended age for beginning primary immunizations of infants is within 2 weeks of birth or, in special circumstances, at birth (Figs. 31-11 and 31-12). Infants born preterm should receive the full dose of each vaccine at the appropriate chronologic age. Recommended schedules for children not immunized during infancy are available at the Centers for Disease Control and Prevention (CDC) website *www.cdc.gov/vaccines/recs/schedules/child-schedule.htm.* Immunization schedules for Canadian children are available from the Public Health Agency of Canada (*http://www.phac-aspc.gc.ca/im/is-cv/index-eng.php*).

Children who began primary immunizations at the recommended age but fail to receive all of the doses do not need to begin the series again but, instead, receive only the missed doses. For situations in which there is doubt that the child will return for immunization according to the optimal schedule, the following vaccines can be administered simultaneously:

- HepA (HAV)
- HepB (HBV)
- DTaP (diphtheria, tetanus, acellular pertussis)
- IPV (inactivated poliovirus)
- MMR (measles, mumps, rubella)
- Varicella
- Hib (*Haemophilus influenzae* type b)

Parenteral vaccines are given in separate syringes in different injection sites (AAP Committee on Infectious Diseases, 2012).

Recommendations for Routine Immunizations*

Hepatitis A Virus. Hepatitis A has been recognized as a significant child health problem, particularly in communities with unusually high infection rates. HAV is spread by the fecal-oral route and from person-to-person contact, by ingestion of contaminated food or water, and rarely by blood transfusion. The illness has an abrupt onset, with fever, malaise, anorexia, nausea, abdominal discomfort, dark urine, and jaundice being the most common clinical signs of infection. In children younger than 6 years, who represent approximately one third of all cases of hepatitis A, the disease may be asymptomatic, and jaundice is rarely evident.

---

*Because of constant changes in the pharmaceutical industry, trade names of single and combination vaccines in this section may differ from those currently available. The reader is encouraged to access the vaccine page of the Center for Biologics Evaluation and Research (CBER) of the Food and Drug Administration for the latest licensed vaccine trade names: http://www.fda.gov/BiologicsBloodVaccines/default.htm.

These recommendations must be read with the footnotes that follow. For those who fall behind or start late, provide catch-up vaccination at the earliest opportunity as indicated by the green bars in Figure 1. To determine minimum intervals between doses, see the catch-up schedule (Figure 2). School entry and adolescent vaccine age groups are in bold.

Vaccines	Birth	1 mo	2 mos	4 mos	6 mos	9 mos	12 mos	15 mos	18 mos	19–23 mos	2-3 yrs	**4-6 yrs**	7-10 yrs	**11-12 yrs**	13–15 yrs	16–18 yrs
Hepatitis B¹ (HepB)	◄1st dose►	◄─── 2nd dose ───►			◄──────────────── 3rd dose ────────────────►											
Rotavirus² (RV) RV-1 (2-dose series); RV-5 (3-dose series)			◄1st dose►	◄2nd dose►	See footnote 2											
Diphtheria, tetanus, & acellular pertussis³ (DTaP: <7 yrs)			◄1st dose►	◄2nd dose►	◄3rd dose►		◄──────── 4th dose ────────►					◄5th dose►				
Tetanus, diphtheria, & acellular pertussis⁴ (Tdap: ≥7 yrs)														(Tdap)		
Haemophilus influenzae type b⁵ (Hib)			◄1st dose►	◄2nd dose►	See footnote 5		◄─ 3rd or 4th dose, see footnote 5 ─►									
Pneumococcal conjugate⁶ᵃ'ᶜ (PCV13)			◄1st dose►	◄2nd dose►	◄3rd dose►		◄──────── 4th dose ────────►									
Pneumococcal polysaccharide⁶ᵇ'ᶜ (PPSV23)																
Inactivated Poliovirus⁷ (IPV) (<18 years)			◄1st dose►	◄2nd dose►	◄──────────────── 3rd dose ────────────────►							◄4th dose►				
Influenza⁸ (IIV; LAIV) 2 doses for some : see footnote 8							Annual vaccination (IIV only)					Annual vaccination (IIV or LAIV)				
Measles, mumps, rubella⁹ (MMR)							◄──── 1st dose ────►					◄2nd dose►				
Varicella¹⁰ (VAR)							◄──── 1st dose ────►					◄2nd dose►				
Hepatitis A¹¹ (HepA)							◄──── 2 dose series, see footnote 11 ────►									
Human papillomavirus¹² (HPV2: females only; HPV4: males and females)														(3-dose series)		
Meningococcal¹³ (Hib-MenCY ≥ 6 weeks; MCV4-D≥9 mos; MCV4-CRM ≥ 2 yrs.)					◄──────────────── see footnote 13 ────────────────►									◄1st dose►		booster

▓ Range of recommended ages for all children	▓ Range of recommended ages for catch-up immunization	▓ Range of recommended ages for certain high-risk groups	▓ Range of recommended ages during which catch-up is encouraged and for certain high-risk groups	☐ Not routinely recommended

This schedule includes recommendations in effect as of January 1, 2013. Any dose not administered at the recommended age should be administered at a subsequent visit, when indicated and feasible. The use of a combination vaccine generally is preferred over separate injections of its equivalent component vaccines. Vaccination providers should consult the relevant Advisory Committee on Immunization Practices (ACIP) statement for detailed recommendations, available online at http://www.cdc.gov/vaccines/pubs/acip-list.htm. Clinically significant adverse events that follow vaccination should be reported to the Vaccine Adverse Event Reporting System (VAERS) online (http://www.vaers.hhs.gov) or by telephone (800-822-7967). Suspected cases of vaccine-preventable diseases should be reported to the state or local health department. Additional information, including precautions and contraindications for vaccination, is available from CDC online (http://www.cdc.gov/vaccines) or by telephone (800-CDC-INFO [800-232-4636]).

This schedule is approved by the Advisory Committee on Immunization Practices (http://www.cdc.gov/vaccines/acip/index.html), the American Academy of Pediatrics (http://www.aap.org), the American Academy of Family Physicians (http://www.aafp.org), and the American College of Obstetricians and Gynecologists (http://www.acog.org).

NOTE: The above recommendations must be read along with the footnotes of this schedule.

Footnotes — Recommended immunization schedule for persons aged 0 through 18 years—United States, 2013

For further guidance on the use of the vaccines mentioned below, see: http://www.cdc.gov/vaccines/pubs/acip-list.htm.

1. **Hepatitis B (HepB) vaccine. (Minimum age: birth)**
   Routine vaccination:
   At birth
   - Administer monovalent HepB vaccine to all newborns before hospital discharge.
   - For infants born to hepatitis B surface antigen (HBsAg)–positive mothers, administer HepB vaccine and 0.5 mL of hepatitis B immune globulin (HBIG) within 12 hours of birth. These infants should be tested for HBsAg and antibody to HBsAg (anti-HBs) 1 to 2 months after completion of the HepB series, at age 9 through 18 months (preferably at the next well-child visit).
   - If mother's HBsAg status is unknown, within 12 hours of birth administer HepB vaccine to all infants regardless of birth weight. For infants weighing <2,000 grams, administer HBIG in addition to HepB within 12 hours of birth. Determine mother's HBsAg status as soon as possible and, if she is HBsAg-positive, also administer HBIG for infants weighing ≥2,000 grams (no later than age 1 week).
   Doses following the birth dose
   - The second dose should be administered at age 1 or 2 months. Monovalent HepB vaccine should be used for doses administered before age 6 weeks.
   - Infants who did not receive a birth dose should receive 3 doses of a HepB-containing vaccine on a schedule of 0, 1 to 2 months, and 6 months starting as soon as feasible. See Figure 2.
   - The minimum interval between dose 1 and dose 2 is 4 weeks and between dose 2 and 3 is 8 weeks. The final (third or fourth) dose in the HepB vaccine series should be administered no earlier than age 24 weeks, and at least 16 weeks after the first dose.
   - Administration of a total of 4 doses of HepB vaccine is recommended when a combination vaccine containing HepB is administered after the birth dose.
   Catch-up vaccination:
   - Unvaccinated persons should complete a 3-dose series.
   - A 2-dose series (doses separated by at least 4 months) of adult formulation Recombivax HB is licensed for use in children aged 11 through 15 years.
   - For other catch-up issues, see Figure 2.

2. **Rotavirus (RV) vaccines. (Minimum age: 6 weeks for both RV-1 [Rotarix] and RV-5 [RotaTeq]).**
   Routine vaccination:
   - Administer a series of RV vaccine to all infants as follows:
     1. If RV-1 is used, administer a 2-dose series at 2 and 4 months of age.
     2. If RV-5 is used, administer a 3-dose series at ages 2, 4, and 6 months.
     3. If any dose in series was RV-5 or vaccine product is unknown for any dose in the series, a total of 3 doses of RV vaccine should be administered.
   Catch-up vaccination:
   - The maximum age for the first dose in the series is 14 weeks, 6 days.
   - Vaccination should not be initiated for infants aged 15 weeks 0 days or older.
   - The maximum age for the final dose in the series is 8 months, 0 days.
   - If RV-1 (Rotarix) is administered for the first and second doses, a third dose is not indicated.
   - For other catch-up issues, see Figure 2.

3. **Diphtheria and tetanus toxoids and acellular pertussis (DTaP) vaccine. (Minimum age: 6 weeks)**
   Routine vaccination:
   - Administer a 5-dose series of DTaP vaccine at ages 2, 4, 6, 15–18 months, and 4 through 6 years. The fourth dose may be administered as early as age 12 months, provided at least 6 months have elapsed since the third dose.
   Catch-up vaccination:
   - The fifth (booster) dose of DTaP vaccine is not necessary if the fourth dose was administered at age 4 years or older.
   - For other catch-up issues, see Figure 2.

4. **Tetanus and diphtheria toxoids and acellular pertussis (Tdap) vaccine. (Minimum age: 10 years for Boostrix, 11 years for Adacel).**
   Routine vaccination:
   - Administer 1 dose of Tdap vaccine to all adolescents aged 11 through 12 years.
   - Tdap can be administered regardless of the interval since the last tetanus and diphtheria toxoid-containing vaccine.
   - Administer one dose of Tdap vaccine to pregnant adolescents during each pregnancy (preferred during 27 through 36 weeks gestation) regardless of number of years from prior Td or Tdap vaccination.
   Catch-up vaccination:
   - Persons aged 7 through 10 years who are not fully immunized with the childhood DTaP vaccine series, should receive Tdap vaccine as the first dose in the catch-up series; if additional doses are needed, use Td vaccine. For these children, an adolescent Tdap vaccine should not be given.
   - Persons aged 11 through 18 years who have not received Tdap vaccine should receive a dose followed by tetanus and diphtheria toxoids (Td) booster doses every 10 years thereafter.
   - An inadvertent dose of DTaP vaccine administered to children aged 7 through 10 years can count as part of the catch-up series. This dose can count as the adolescent Tdap dose, or the child can later receive a Tdap booster dose at age 11–12 years.
   - For other catch-up issues, see Figure 2.

5. ***Haemophilus influenzae* type b (Hib) conjugate vaccine. (Minimum age: 6 weeks)**
   Routine vaccination:
   - Administer a Hib vaccine primary series and a booster dose to all infants. The primary series doses should be administered at 2, 4, and 6 months of age; however, if PRP-OMP (PedvaxHib or Comvax) is administered at 2 and 4 months of age, a dose at age 6 months is not indicated. One booster dose should be administered at age 12 through15 months.
   - Hiberix (PRP-T) should only be used for the booster (final) dose in children aged 12 months through 4 years, who have received at least 1 dose of Hib.

FIG 31-11 Recommended immunization schedule for persons ages 0 through 18 years. (From Centers for Disease Control and Prevention: *Recommended immunization schedules for persons aged 0 through 18 years—United States,* 2013.)

Continued

For further guidance on the use of the vaccines mentioned below, see: http://www.cdc.gov/vaccines/pubs/acip-list.htm.

Catch-up vaccination:

- If dose 1 was administered at ages 12-14 months, administer booster (as final dose) at least 8 weeks after dose 1.
- If the first 2 doses were PRP-OMP (PedvaxHIB or Comvax), and were administered at age 11 months or younger, the third (and final) dose should be administered at age 12 through 15 months and at least 8 weeks after the second dose.
- If the first dose was administered at age 7 through 11 months, administer the second dose at least 4 weeks later and a final dose at age 12 through 15 months, regardless of Hib vaccine (PRP-T or PRP-OMP) used for first dose.
- For unvaccinated children aged 15 months or older, administer only 1 dose.
- For other catch-up issues, see Figure 2.

Vaccination of persons with high-risk conditions:

- Hib vaccine is not routinely recommended for patients older than 5 years of age. However one dose of Hib vaccine should be administered to unvaccinated or partially vaccinated persons aged 5 years or older who have leukemia, malignant neoplasms, anatomic or functional asplenia (including sickle cell disease), human immunodeficiency virus (HIV) infection, or other immunocompromising conditions.

6a. **Pneumococcal conjugate vaccine (PCV). (Minimum age: 6 weeks)**

Routine vaccination:

- Administer a series of PCV13 vaccine at ages 2, 4, 6 months with a booster at age 12 through 15 months.
- For children aged 14 through 59 months who have received an age-appropriate series of 7-valent PCV (PCV7), administer a single supplemental dose of 13-valent PCV (PCV13).

Catch-up vaccination:

- Administer 1 dose of PCV13 to all healthy children aged 24 through 59 months who are not completely vaccinated for their age.
- For other catch-up issues, see Figure 2.

Vaccination of persons with high-risk conditions:

- For children aged 24 through 71 months with certain underlying medical conditions (see footnote 6c), administer 1 dose of PCV13 if 3 doses of PCV were received previously, or administer 2 doses of PCV13 at least 8 weeks apart if fewer than 3 doses of PCV were received previously.
- A single dose of PCV13 may be administered to previously unvaccinated children aged 6 through 18 years who have anatomic or functional asplenia (including sickle cell disease), HIV infection or an immunocompromising condition, cochlear implant or cerebrospinal fluid leak. See MMWR 2010;59 (No. RR-11), available at http://www.cdc.gov/mmwr/pdf/rr/rr5911.pdf.
- Administer PPSV23 at least 8 weeks after the last dose of PCV to children aged 2 years or older with certain underlying medical conditions (see footnotes 6b and 6c).

6b. **Pneumococcal polysaccharide vaccine (PPSV23). (Minimum age: 2 years)**

Vaccination of persons with high-risk conditions:

- Administer PPSV23 at least 8 weeks after the last dose of PCV to children aged 2 years or older with certain underlying medical conditions (see footnote 6c). A single revaccination with PPSV should be administered after 5 years to children with anatomic or functional asplenia (including sickle cell disease) or an immunocompromising condition.

6c. **Medical conditions for which PPSV23 is indicated in children aged 2 years and older and for which use of PCV13 is indicated in children aged 24 through 71 months:**

- Immunocompetent children with chronic heart disease (particularly cyanotic congenital heart disease and cardiac failure); chronic lung disease (including asthma if treated with high-dose oral corticosteroid therapy), diabetes mellitus; cerebrospinal fluid leaks; or cochlear implant.
- Children with anatomic or functional asplenia (including sickle cell disease and other hemoglobinopathies, congenital or acquired asplenia, or splenic dysfunction);
- Children with immunocompromising conditions: HIV infection, chronic renal failure and nephrotic syndrome, diseases associated with treatment with immunosuppressive drugs or radiation therapy, including malignant neoplasms, leukemias, lymphomas and Hodgkin disease; or solid organ transplantation, congenital immunodeficiency.

7. **Inactivated poliovirus vaccine (IPV). (Minimum age: 6 weeks)**

Routine vaccination:

- Administer a series of IPV at ages 2, 4, 6–18 months, with a booster at age 4–6 years. The final dose in the series should be administered on or after the fourth birthday and at least 6 months after the previous dose.

Catch-up vaccination:

- In the first 6 months of life, minimum age and minimum intervals are only recommended if the person is at risk for imminent exposure to circulating poliovirus (i.e., travel to a polio-endemic region or during an outbreak).
- If 4 or more doses are administered before age 4 years, an additional dose should be administered at age 4 through 6 years.
- A fourth dose is not necessary if the third dose was administered at age 4 years or older and at least 6 months after the previous dose.
- If both OPV and IPV were administered as part of a series, a total of 4 doses should be administered, regardless of the child's current age.
- IPV is not routinely recommended for U.S. residents aged 18 years or older.
- For other catch-up issues, see Figure 2.

8. **Influenza vaccines. (Minimum age: 6 months for inactivated influenza vaccine [IIV]; 2 years for live, attenuated influenza vaccine [LAIV])**

Routine vaccination:

- Administer influenza vaccine annually to all children beginning at age 6 months. For most healthy, nonpregnant persons aged 2 through 49 years, either LAIV or IIV may be used. However, LAIV should NOT be administered to some persons, including 1) those with asthma, 2) children 2 through 4 years who had wheezing in the past 12 months, or 3) those who have any other underlying medical conditions that predispose them to influenza complications. For all other contraindications to use of LAIV see MMWR 2010; 59 (No. RR-8), available at http://www.cdc.gov/mmwr/pdf/rr/rr5908.pdf.
- Administer 1 dose to persons aged 9 years and older.

For children aged 6 months through 8 years:

- For the 2012–13 season, administer 2 doses (separated by at least 4 weeks) to children who are receiving influenza vaccine for the first time. For additional guidance, follow dosing guidelines in the 2012 ACIP influenza vaccine recommendations, MMWR 2012; 61: 613–618, available at http://www.cdc.gov/mmwr/pdf/wk/mm6132.pdf.
- For the 2013–14 season, follow dosing guidelines in the 2013 ACIP influenza vaccine recommendations.

9. **Measles, mumps, and rubella (MMR) vaccine. (Minimum age: 12 months for routine vaccination)**

Routine vaccination:

- Administer the first dose of MMR vaccine at age 12 through 15 months, and the second dose at age 4 through 6 years. The second dose may be administered before age 4 years, provided at least 4 weeks have elapsed since the first dose.
- Administer 1 dose of MMR vaccine to infants aged 6 through 11 months before departure from the United States for international travel. These children should be revaccinated with 2 doses of MMR vaccine, the

- For vaccination of persons with primary and secondary immunodeficiencies, see Table 13, "Vaccination of persons with primary and secondary immunodeficiencies," in General Recommendations on Immunization (ACIP), available at http://www.cdc.gov/mmwr/preview/mmwrhtml/rr6002a1.htm; and American Academy of Pediatrics. Immunization in Special Clinical Circumstances. In: Pickering LK, Baker CJ, Kimberlin DW, Long SS eds. Red book: 2012 report of the Committee on Infectious Diseases. 29th ed. Elk Grove Village, IL: American Academy of Pediatrics.

first at age 12 through 15 months (12 months if the child remains in an area where disease risk is high), and the second dose at least 4 weeks later.

- Administer 2 doses of MMR vaccine to children aged 12 months and older, before departure from the United States for international travel. The first dose should be administered on or after age 12 months and the second dose at least 4 weeks later.

Catch-up vaccination:

- Ensure that all school-aged children and adolescents have had 2 doses of MMR vaccine; the minimum interval between the 2 doses is 4 weeks.

10. **Varicella (VAR) vaccine. (Minimum age: 12 months)**

Routine vaccination:

- Administer the first dose of VAR vaccine at age 12 through 15 months, and the second dose at age 4 through 6 years. The second dose may be administered before age 4 years, provided at least 3 months have elapsed since the first dose. If the second dose was administered at least 4 weeks after the first dose, it can be accepted as valid.

Catch-up vaccination:

- Ensure that all persons aged 7 through 18 years without evidence of immunity (see MMWR 2007;56 [No. RR-4], available at http://www.cdc.gov/mmwr/pdf/rr/rr5604.pdf) have 2 doses of varicella vaccine. For children aged 7 through 12 years the recommended minimum interval between doses is 3 months (if the second dose was administered at least 4 weeks after the first dose, it can be accepted as valid); for persons aged 13 years and older, the minimum interval between doses is 4 weeks.

11. **Hepatitis A vaccine (HepA). (Minimum age: 12 months)**

Routine vaccination:

- Initiate the 2-dose HepA vaccine series for children aged 12 through 23 months; separate the 2 doses by 6 to 18 months.
- Children who have received 1 dose of HepA vaccine before age 24 months, should receive a second dose 6 to 18 months after the first dose.
- For any person aged 2 years and older who has not already received the HepA vaccine series, 2 doses of HepA vaccine separated by 6 to 18 months may be administered if immunity against hepatitis A virus infection is desired.

Catch-up vaccination:

- The minimum interval between the two doses is 6 months.

Special populations:

- Administer 2 doses of Hep A vaccine at least 6 months apart to previously unvaccinated persons who live in areas where vaccination programs target older children, or who are at increased risk for infection.

12. **Human papillomavirus (HPV) vaccines. (HPV4 [Gardasil] and HPV2 [Cervarix]). (Minimum age: 9 years)**

Routine vaccination:

- Administer a 3-dose series of HPV vaccine on a schedule of 0, 1-2, and 6 months to all adolescents aged 11-12 years. Either HPV4 or HPV2 may be used for females, and only HPV4 may be used for males.
- The vaccine series can be started beginning at age 9 years.
- Administer the second dose 1 to 2 months after the **first** dose and the third dose 6 months after the **first** dose (at least 24 weeks after the first dose).

Catch-up vaccination:

- Administer the vaccine series to females (either HPV2 or HPV4) and males (HPV4) at age 13 through 18 years if not previously vaccinated.
- Use recommended routine dosing intervals (see above) for vaccine series catch-up.

13. **Meningococcal conjugate vaccines (MCV). (Minimum age: 6 weeks for Hib-MenCY, 9 months for Menactra [MCV4-D], 2 years for Menveo [MCV4-CRM]).**

Routine vaccination:

- Administer MCV4 vaccine at age 11–12 years, with a booster dose at age 16 years.
- Adolescents aged 11 through 18 years with human immunodeficiency virus (HIV) infection should receive a 2-dose primary series of MCV4, with at least 8 weeks between doses. See MMWR 2011; 60:1018–1019 available at: http://www.cdc.gov/mmwr/pdf/wk/mm6030.pdf.
- For children aged 2 months through 10 years with high-risk conditions, see below.

Catch-up vaccination:

- Administer MCV4 vaccine at age 13 through 18 years if not previously vaccinated.
- If the first dose is administered at age 13 through 15 years, a booster dose should be administered at age 16 through 18 years with a minimum interval of at least 8 weeks between doses.
- If the first dose is administered at age 16 years or older, a booster dose is not needed.
- For other catch-up issues, see Figure 2.

Vaccination of persons with high-risk conditions:

- For children younger than 19 months of age with anatomic or functional asplenia (including sickle cell disease), administer an infant series of Hib-MenCY at 2, 4, 6, and 12-15 months.
- For children aged 2 through 18 months with persistent complement component deficiency, administer either an infant series of Hib-MenCY at 2, 4, 6, and 12 through 15 months or a 2-dose primary series of MCV4-D starting at 9 months, with at least 8 weeks between doses. For children aged 19 through 23 months with persistent complement component deficiency who have not received a complete series of Hib-MenCY or MCV4-D, administer 2 primary doses of MCV4-D at least 8 weeks apart.
- For children aged 24 months and older with persistent complement component deficiency or anatomic or functional asplenia (including sickle cell disease), who have not received a complete series of Hib-MenCY or MCV4-D, administer 2 primary doses of either MCV4-D or MCV4-CRM. If MCV4-D (Menactra) is administered to a child with asplenia (including sickle cell disease), do not administer MCV4-D until 2 years of age and at least 4 weeks after the completion of all PCV13 doses. See MMWR 2011;60:1391–2, available at http://www.cdc.gov/mmwr/pdf/wk/mm6040.pdf.
- For children aged 9 months and older who are residents of or travelers to countries in the African meningitis belt or to the Hajj, administer an age appropriate formulation and series of MCV4 for protection against serogroups A and W-135. Prior receipt of Hib-MenCY is not sufficient for children traveling to the meningitis belt or the Hajj. See MMWR 2011;60:1391–2, available at http://www.cdc.gov/mmwr/pdf/wk/mm6040.pdf.
- For children who are present during outbreaks caused by a vaccine serogroup, administer or complete an age and formulation-appropriate series of Hib-MenCY or MCV4.
- For booster doses among persons with high-risk conditions refer to http://www.cdc.gov/vaccines/pubs/acip-list.htm#mening.

Additional information

- For contraindications and precautions to use of a vaccine and for additional information regarding that vaccine, vaccination providers should consult the relevant ACIP statement available online at http://www.cdc.gov/vaccines/pubs/acip-list.htm.
- For the purposes of calculating intervals between doses, 4 weeks = 28 days. Intervals of 4 months or greater are determined by calendar months.
- Information on travel vaccine requirements and recommendations is available at http://wwwnc.cdc.gov/travel/page/vaccinations.htm.

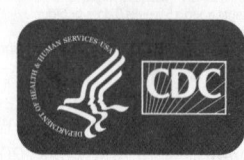

U.S. Department of Health and Human Services
Centers for Disease Control and Prevention

FIG 31-11, cont'd

The figure below provides catch-up schedules and minimum intervals between doses for children whose vaccinations have been delayed. A vaccine series does not need to be restarted, regardless of the time that has elapsed between doses. Use the section appropriate for the child's age. Always use this table in conjunction with Figure 1 and the footnotes that follow.

Vaccine	Minimum Age for Dose 1	Minimum Interval Between Doses			
		Dose 1 to dose 2	Dose 2 to dose 3	Dose 3 to dose 4	Dose 4 to dose 5
Persons aged 4 months through 6 years					
Hepatitis B[1]	Birth	4 weeks	8 weeks and at least 16 weeks after first dose; minimum age for the final dose is 24 weeks		
Rotavirus[2]	6 weeks	4 weeks	4 weeks[2]		
Diphtheria, tetanus, pertussis[3]	6 weeks	4 weeks	4 weeks	6 months	6 months[3]
Haemophilus influenzae type b[5]	6 weeks	4 weeks if first dose administered at younger than age 12 months 8 weeks (as final dose) if first dose administered at age 12–14 months No further doses needed if first dose administered at age 15 months or older	4 weeks[5] if current age is younger than 12 months 8 weeks (as final dose)[5] if current age is 12 months or older and first dose administered at younger than age 12 months and second dose administered at younger than 15 months No further doses needed if previous dose administered at age 15 months or older	8 weeks (as final dose) This dose only necessary for children aged 12 through 59 months who received 3 doses before age 12 months	
Pneumococcal[6]	6 weeks	4 weeks if first dose administered at younger than age 12 months 8 weeks (as final dose for healthy children) if first dose administered at age 12 months or older or current age 24 through 59 months No further doses needed for healthy children if first dose administered at age 24 months or older	4 weeks if current age is younger than 12 months 8 weeks (as final dose for healthy children) if current age is 12 months or older No further doses needed for healthy children if previous dose administered at age 24 months or older	8 weeks (as final dose) This dose only necessary for children aged 12 through 59 months who received 3 doses before age 12 months or for children at high risk who received 3 doses at any age	
Inactivated poliovirus[7]	6 weeks	4 weeks	4 weeks	6 months[7] minimum age 4 years for final dose	
Meningococcal[13]	6 weeks	8 weeks[13]	see footnote 13	see footnote 13	
Measles, mumps, rubella[9]	12 months	4 weeks			
Varicella[10]	12 months	3 months			
Hepatitis A[11]	12 months	6 months			
Persons aged 7 through 18 years					
Tetanus, diphtheria; tetanus, diphtheria, pertussis[4]	7 years[4]	4 weeks	4 weeks if first dose administered at younger than age 12 months 6 months if first dose administered at 12 months or older	6 months if first dose administered at younger than age 12 months	
Human papillomavirus[12]	9 years	Routine dosing intervals are recommended[12]			
Hepatitis A[11]	12 months	6 months			
Hepatitis B[1]	Birth	4 weeks	8 weeks (and at least 16 weeks after first dose)		
Inactivated poliovirus[7]	6 weeks	4 weeks	4 weeks[7]	6 months[7]	
Meningococcal[13]	6 weeks	8 weeks[13]			
Measles, mumps, rubella[9]	12 months	4 weeks			
Varicella[10]	12 months	3 months if person is younger than age 13 years 4 weeks if person is aged 13 years or older			

NOTE: The above recommendations must be read along with the footnotes of this schedule.

FIG 31-12 Catch-up immunization schedule for persons ages 4 months through 18 years who start late or are more than 1 month behind. (From Centers for Disease Control and Prevention: *Catch-up immunization schedule for persons aged 4 months through 18 years—United States*, 2013.)

HepA vaccine is now recommended for all children beginning at age 1 year (i.e., 12 months to 23 months). The second dose in the two-dose series may be administered no sooner than 6 months after the first dose. For further information, see Fig. 31-11.

Hepatitis B Virus. Hepatitis B is a significant pediatric disease because HBV infections that occur during childhood and adolescence can lead to fatal consequences from cirrhosis or liver cancer during adulthood. Up to 90% of infants infected perinatally and 25% to 50% of children infected before age 5 years become HBV carriers. In addition, the incidence of HBV infection increases rapidly during adolescence. It is recommended that newborns receive the HepB vaccine before hospital discharge if the mother is hepatitis B surface antigen (HBsAg) negative. Monovalent HepB vaccine should be given as the birth dose, whereas a combination vaccine containing HepB may be given for subsequent doses in the series (see also Fig. 31-11). Both full-term and preterm infants born to mothers whose HBsAg status is positive or unknown should receive the HepB vaccine and hepatitis B immune globulin (HBIG) within 12 hours of birth at two different injection sites. Because the immune response to the HepB vaccine is not optimal in newborns weighing less than 2000 g (4 lb 7 oz), the first HepB vaccine dose should be given to such infants at 1 month, as long as the mother's HBsAg status is negative (AAP Committee on Infectious Diseases, 2012). In the event that the preterm infant is given a dose at birth, the current recommendation is that the infant be given the full series (three additional doses) at 1, 2, and 6 months of age. The AAP

Committee on Infectious Diseases (2012) also encourages immunization of all children by age 11 years.

In the late 1990s, the HepB vaccine contained small amounts of mercury (thimerosal) as a preservative, which generated concern regarding possible mercury poisoning in infants and led to a subsequent decrease in HepB immunization rates in newborns. However, a preservative-free HepB vaccine (Recombivax HB, pediatric-adolescent formulation) is available, and the Centers for Disease Control and Prevention (CDC) (2011a) strongly recommends that HepB immunization occur in newborns before discharge from the birth hospital. Studies have not found any association between thimerosal in vaccines and neurologic developmental disorders such as autism spectrum disorder (Miller and Reynolds, 2009; Price, Thompson, Goodson, et al., 2010) (see Critical Thinking Case Study).

The vaccine is given intramuscularly in the vastus lateralis in newborns or in the deltoid for older infants and children. One study found that needle length affected the immune response of obese adolescents receiving the HBV vaccine; according to this study, obese adolescents immunized with a 1.5-inch (38-mm) needle achieved significantly higher antibody titers to hepatitis B than those immunized with a standard 1-inch needle (Middleman, Anding, and Tung, 2010). Regardless of age, avoid the dorsogluteal site because it has been associated with low antibody seroconversion rates, indicating a reduced immune response. No data exist regarding the seroconversion when the ventrogluteal site is used. The vaccine can be safely administered simultaneously at a separate site with DTaP, MMR, and Hib vaccines.

Diphtheria. Although cases of diphtheria are rare in the United States, the disease can result in significant morbidity. Respiratory manifestations include respiratory nasopharyngitis or obstructive laryngotracheitis with upper airway obstruction. The cutaneous manifestations of the disease include vaginal, otic, conjunctival, or cutaneous lesions, which are seen primarily in urban homeless persons and in the tropics. Administer a single dose of equine antitoxin (currently not available in the United States) intravenously to the child with clinical symptoms because of the often fulminant progression of the disease (AAP Committee on Infectious Diseases, 2012). Diphtheria vaccine is commonly administered:

1. In combination with tetanus and pertussis vaccines (DTaP) or DTaP and Hib vaccines for children younger than 7 years
2. In combination with a conjugate *H. influenzae* type B vaccine (see Fig. 31-11)
3. In a combined vaccine with tetanus (DT) for children younger than 7 years who have some contraindication to receiving pertussis vaccine
4. In combination with tetanus and acellular pertussis (Tdap) for children 11 years and older
   OR
5. As a single antigen when combined antigen preparations are not indicated

Although the diphtheria vaccine does not produce absolute immunity, protective antitoxin persists for 10 years or more when given according to the recommended schedule, and boosters are given every 10 years for life (see discussion below for adolescent diphtheria and acellular pertussis and tetanus toxoid recommendation). Several vaccines contain diphtheria toxoid (Hib, meningococcal, pneumococcal), but this does not confer immunity to the disease.

Tetanus. Three forms of tetanus vaccine—tetanus toxoid, tetanus immunoglobulin (TIG) (human), and tetanus antitoxin (equine antitoxin)—are available; however, tetanus antitoxin is no longer available in the United States. Tetanus toxoid is used for routine primary immunization, usually in one of the combinations listed for diphtheria, and provides protective antitoxin levels for approximately 10 years.

Tetanus and diphtheria toxoids along with acellular pertussis vaccine (Tdap, adolescent formulation) are now recommended for children ages 11 to 12 years who have completed the recommended DTaP/DTP vaccine series but have not received the tetanus (Td) booster dose. Children ages 7 through 10 years who are not fully vaccinated for pertussis (did not receive 5 doses of DTaP or 4 doses of DTaP with the fourth dose being administered on or after the fourth birthday) should receive a dose of Tdap (CDC, 2011b). Boostrix (Tdap) is currently licensed for children 10 to 18 years of age, whereas Adacel (Tdap) is licensed for individuals 11 to 64 years of age. For more information see Fig. 31-11.

For wound management, passive immunity is available with TIG. Persons with a history of two previous doses of tetanus toxoid can receive a booster dose of the toxoid. Separate syringes and different sites are used when tetanus toxoid and TIG are given concurrently.

For children older than 7 years who require wound prophylaxis, tetanus immunization may be accomplished by administering Td (adult-type diphtheria and tetanus toxoids). If TIG is not available, the equine antitoxin (not available in the United States) may be administered after appropriate testing for sensitivity. The antitoxin is administered in a separate syringe and at a separate intramuscular site if given concurrently with tetanus toxoid. For further

---

? CRITICAL THINKING CASE STUDY

Childhood Immunizations and Autism

Monica, a 26-year-old mother of 2 children, ages 8 months and 2 years, brings them to the clinic for a well-child check. When asked if the children are up to date on their immunization schedule, Monica replies that she and her partner have decided not to have the children immunized. She states that a neighbor has a 9-year-old with autism and her Internet research and talks with various neighbors have convinced them that autism may possibly be caused by all of the immunizations children are receiving. Monica also points out that her children do not go to day care and that she plans to home school them; therefore she believes the risk for communicable disease contraction is low. "Besides, none of our neighborhood kids have ever had any of those diseases like measles or chickenpox because their parents get them immunized," she states. Upon physical examination, the two children appear to be in excellent health and their previous health history and family health history do not reveal any major health risk factors.

1. Evidence—Is there sufficient evidence to draw any conclusions about Monica's concerns about childhood immunizations?
2. Assumptions—Describe any underlying assumptions about the following:
   a. Childhood immunizations and autism
   b. Monica's reasons for not immunizing her children
   c. The concept of herd immunity
3. What approach would be the best to address Monica's concerns about not immunizing her children?
4. Is there objective evidence to support your conclusions?

information on wound prophylaxis, see the *2012 Red Book* (AAP Committee on Infectious Diseases, 2012).

Pertussis. Pertussis vaccine is recommended for all children 6 weeks through 6 years of age (up to the seventh birthday) who have no neurologic contraindications to its use. Concerns over outbreaks of the disease in the past decade have prompted discussion about vaccinating infants and adults. Many cases of pertussis have occurred in children younger than 6 months or persons older than 7 years, both groups falling in the category for which pertussis immunization previously was not recommended (CDC, 2005b). The tetanus and diphtheria toxoids and acellular pertussis vaccine (Tdap) is now recommended at ages 11 to 12 years for children who have completed the DTaP/DTP childhood series. The Tdap is also recommended for adolescents 13 to 18 years old who have not received a tetanus booster (Td) or Tdap dose and have completed the childhood DTaP/DTP series. In June 2013 the Advisory Committee on Immunization Practices (ACIP) recommended against universal revaccination with Tdap for adolescents and adults who have previously been vaccinated for pertussis; this recommendation was based on data indicating a low burden of pertussis illness in this age-group and an increased cost of universal revaccination (Long, 2013). Children ages 7 through 10 years who are not fully vaccinated for pertussis (did not receive 5 doses of DTaP or 4 doses of DTaP with the fourth dose being administered on or after the fourth birthday), should receive a dose of Tdap (CDC, 2011b) (see discussion in the Tetanus section).

Currently, two forms of pertussis vaccine are available in the United States. The whole-cell pertussis vaccine is prepared from inactivated cells of *Bordetella pertussis* and contains multiple antigens. In contrast, the acellular pertussis vaccine contains one or more immunogens derived from the *B. pertussis* organism. The highly purified acellular vaccine is associated with fewer local and systemic reactions than those occurring with the whole-cell vaccine in children of similar age. The acellular pertussis vaccine is recommended for the first three immunizations and is usually given at 2, 4, 6 months, 15 to 18 months, and 4 to 6 years of age with diphtheria and tetanus (DTaP). Several forms of acellular pertussis vaccine are currently licensed for use in infants: Daptacel, Pediarix, Kinrix (DTaP and IPV), and Infanrix (diphtheria, tetanus toxoid, and acellular pertussis conjugate). Pentacel is licensed for use in infants 4 weeks old and older; in addition to acellular pertussis, diphtheria, and tetanus, this vaccine also contains inactivated poliovirus (IPV) and Hib conjugate. Either the acellular or whole-cell vaccine may be given for the fourth and fifth doses, but the acellular is preferred. It is also recommended that the first three DTaP vaccinations be from the same manufacturer. The fourth dose may be from a different manufacturer. The child who has received one or more whole-cell vaccines may complete the series of five with the acellular vaccine.

Health care workers who may be susceptible to pertussis as a result of waning immunity and who have potential exposure to children or adults with pertussis should receive a single dose of Tdap (if not previously vaccinated with same) and take the necessary protective precautions against droplet contamination (wear procedural or surgical masks and practice hand washing). The diagnosis of pertussis may be missed or delayed in unvaccinated infants, who often are seen with respiratory distress and apnea without the typical cough. Additional guidelines for prevention and treatment of pertussis among health care workers and close contacts are available from the Centers for Disease Control and Prevention (CDC) website: www.cdc.gov/vaccines/.

The ACIP and American College of Obstetricians and Gynecologists recently recommended that pregnant women who are not protected against pertussis receive the Tdap vaccine anytime after 20 weeks of gestation or after birth before discharge from the hospital; breastfeeding is not a contraindication to Tdap vaccination (CDC, 2012).

Polio. An all-IPV (inactivated poliovirus) vaccine schedule for routine childhood polio vaccination is now recommended for children in the United States. All children should receive a dose of IPV at 2 months, 4 months, 6 to 18 months, and 4 to 6 years of age, for a total of four doses (AAP Committee on Infectious Diseases, 2012).

The change from the exclusive use of oral polio vaccine (OPV) to the exclusive use of the IPV vaccine is related to the rare risk for vaccine-associated polio paralysis (VAPP) from OPV. The exclusive use of the IPV vaccine eliminates the risk for VAPP but is associated with an increased number of injections and increased cost. Since IPV vaccine usage was instituted in the United States in 2000, no new cases of VAPP have occurred. PEDIARIX is a combination vaccine containing DTaP, hepatitis B, and IPV; this may be used as the primary immunization beginning at 2 months of age (AAP Committee on Infectious Diseases, 2012). KINRIX contains DTaP and IPV, and it may be used as the 5th dose in the DTaP series and the 4th dose in the IPV series in children ages 4 to 6 years whose previous vaccine doses have been with INFANRIX and/or PEDIARIX for the first three doses and INFANRIX for the 4th dose. As just noted, Pentacel is also licensed for use in infants 4 weeks old and older and contains DTaP, Hib, and inactivated poliovirus. PEDIARIX has been licensed for use in children as young as 6 weeks and contains DTaP, Hep B, and inactivated poliovirus.

Measles. The measles (rubeola) vaccine is given at 12 to 15 months of age. During the course of measles outbreaks, the vaccine can be given any time after 6 months of age, followed by a second inoculation after age 12 months. The second measles immunization is recommended at 4 to 6 years of age (at school entry) but may be given earlier provided that 4 weeks have elapsed since the administration of the previous dose. Revaccination should occur by 11 to 12 years of age if the measles vaccine was not administered at school entry (4 to 6 years). Any child who is vaccinated before 12 months of age should receive two additional doses beginning at 12 to 15 months and separated by at least 4 weeks (AAP Committee on Infectious Diseases, 2012). Revaccination should include all individuals born after 1956 who have not received two doses of measles vaccine after 12 months of age. Individuals born before this date are thought to be immune from exposure to natural measles virus. Because of the continuing occurrence of measles in older children and young adults, identify potentially susceptible adolescents and young adults and immunize them if two doses of measles vaccine have not been administered previously or the person had a confirmed case of the illness. The National Institute of Allergy and Infectious Diseases (NIAID), in collaboration with 34 other professional organizations, published new evidence-based guidelines for the diagnosis and management of food allergy; the NIAID recommends that children receive the MMR or MMRV (measles, mumps, rubella, and varicella) vaccine despite a history of severe egg allergy reaction (Boyce, Assa'ad, Burks, et al., 2010).

The MMRV vaccine (ProQuad) is an attenuated live virus vaccine and may be given to children 12 months to 12 years of age concurrent with other vaccines. Concerns for increased risk for febrile seizures in children 12 months to 23 months of age after administration of MMRV vaccine initially prompted the ACIP (CDC, 2008) to remove its recommendation for MMRV being the preferred vaccine (vs. separate injections of MMR and varicella vaccines). However, after further review, the ACIP amended that recommendation and now recommends either administering MMR and varicella vaccines (two separate vaccines) or the MMRV vaccine as the first vaccination in children ages 12 to 47 months. For children 48 months and older, the first dose with MMRV is recommended to decrease the number of injections. For the same reason, MMRV is also recommended for the second dose at any age (15 months through 12 years).

The risks and benefits of administering the MMRV vaccine should be fully explained to the parent or caregiver; the risk for a febrile seizure at 5 to 12 days in children 12 to 23 months old remains relatively low and should be weighed with the benefit of one less intramuscular injection (AAP, 2012).

Mumps. Mumps virus vaccine is recommended for children at 12 to 15 months of age and is typically given in combination with measles and rubella. It should not be administered to infants younger than 12 months because persisting maternal antibodies can interfere with the immune response.

Because of recent outbreaks of the disease, especially in children 10 to 19 years of age, mumps immunization is recommended for all individuals born after 1957 who may be susceptible to mumps (i.e., those who have no history of having had the disease or vaccine and who have no laboratory evidence of immunity).

Rubella. Rubella is a relatively mild infection in children, but in a pregnant woman the actual infection presents serious risks to the developing fetus. Therefore the aim of rubella immunization is actually protection of the unborn child rather than the recipient of the immunization.

Rubella immunization is recommended for all children at 12 to 15 months of age and is administered in a combined form with measles and mumps vaccine. Increased emphasis should also be placed on vaccinating all unimmunized prepubertal children and susceptible adolescents and adult women in the childbearing age-group. Because the live attenuated virus may cross the placenta and theoretically present a risk to the developing fetus, rubella vaccine is currently not given to any pregnant woman. Although this is standard practice, current evidence from women who received the vaccine while pregnant and delivered unaffected offspring indicates that the risk to the fetus is negligible. In addition, there is no reported danger of administering rubella vaccine to a child if the mother is pregnant. Postpubertal females without evidence of rubella immunity should be immunized unless they are pregnant; they should be counseled not to become pregnant for 28 days after receiving the rubella-containing vaccine (AAP, 2012).

Pneumococcal Infections. Streptococcal pneumococci are responsible for a number of bacterial infections in children younger than 2 years, which may cause serious morbidity and mortality. Among these are generalized infections such as septicemia and meningitis or localized infections such as otitis media, sinusitis, and pneumonia. These illnesses are particularly problematic in children who attend day care facilities (the incidence in day care children is 2 or 3 times higher than in children not attending out-of-home day care) and in those who are immunocompromised. In 2010, a 13-valent pneumococcal conjugate vaccine (PCV 13 [Prevnar 13]) was licensed for use and is currently recommended as the standard pneumococcal vaccine for children ages 6 weeks to 24 months. Children who have started the PCV series with PCV 7 may complete the vaccine series with PCV 13 (CDC, 2010).

The PCV 13 vaccine is administered at 2, 4, and 6 months, with a fourth dose at 12 to 15 months of age. A single supplemental dose of PCV 13 is recommended for children 14 through 59 months who have received an age-appropriate series of PCV 7, and a single supplemental dose of PCV 13 is also recommended for children ages 60 through 71 months who received a series of PCV 7. PCV 13 is also recommended for all children younger than 24 months and for older children (24 to 71 months) with sickle cell disease; functional or anatomic asplenia; nephrotic syndrome or chronic renal failure; conditions associated with immunosuppression, such as solid organ transplantation, drug therapy, or cytoreduction therapy (including long-term systemic corticosteroid therapy); diabetes mellitus; cochlear implants; congenital immunodeficiency; human immunodeficiency virus (HIV) infection; cerebrospinal fluid leaks; chronic cardiovascular disease (e.g., congestive heart failure or cardiomyopathy); chronic pulmonary disease (e.g., emphysema or cystic fibrosis, but not asthma); chronic liver disease (e.g., cirrhosis); or exposure to living environments or social settings in which the risk for invasive pneumococcal disease or its complications is very high (e.g., Alaskan Native, African-American, and certain Native-American populations) The PCV 13 vaccine may be administered in conjunction with all other immunizations in a separate syringe and at a separate intramuscular site. For further information, see Fig. 31-11.

The PPV (pneumococcal polysaccharide [23-valent] vaccine) is not recommended for children younger than 24 months who do not have one of the high risk conditions described previously. One dose of PPV is recommended in children older than 23 months who have one of the high risk conditions after primary immunization with PCV 13 (see Fig. 31-11).

Haemophilus influenzae Type B. Hib conjugate vaccines protect against a number of serious infections caused by Hib, especially bacterial meningitis, epiglottitis, bacterial pneumonia, septic arthritis, and sepsis (Hib is not associated with the viruses that cause influenza, or "flu"). Hib vaccines that are currently available include PedvaxHIB, Pentacel, and Comvax, which are combination vaccines; Hiberix; and ActHIB. Pentacel is described in the previous section on Pertussis. MenHibrix has been licensed for administration to children ages 6 weeks to 18 months and provides protection against meningococcal (groups A, C, Y, and W-135) as well as *Haemophilus influenzae* type b (Hib) infections. MenHibrix is administered in a four-dose series at 2, 4, 6, and 12 to 15 months of age. These conjugate vaccines connect Hib to a nontoxic form of another organism, such as meningococcal protein, tetanus toxoid, or diphtheria protein. There is no antibody response to these nontoxic proteins, but they significantly improve the antibody response to Hib, especially in infants. The use of combination vaccines provides equivalent immunogenicity and decreases the number of injections an infant receives. However, it is important that they be given to the appropriate-age child. Hiberix is a conjugate vaccine licensed for use as the booster (final) dose of the Hib vaccine series for children ages 15 months to 4 years (CDC, 2009). In 2013 the AAP Committee on Infectious Diseases clarified that only one dose of Hib vaccine should be given to children 15 months of age or older who have not been previously vaccinated (AAP Committee on Infectious Diseases, 2013).

When possible, the Hib conjugate vaccine used at the first vaccination should be used for all subsequent vaccinations in the primary series. All Hib vaccines are administered by intramuscular injection using a separate syringe and at a site separate from any concurrent vaccinations. For more information, see Fig. 31-11.

Varicella. Administration of the cell-free live-attenuated varicella vaccine is recommended for any susceptible child (one who lacks proof of varicella vaccination or has a reliable history of varicella infection). A single dose of 0.5 mL should be given by subcutaneous injection. The first dose of varicella vaccine is recommended for children ages 12 to 15 months, and to ensure adequate protection, a second varicella vaccine is recommended for children at 4 to 6 years of age. The second varicella vaccine may be administered before 4 years of age as long as a period of 3 months occurs between the first and second dose. Children 13 years of age or older who are susceptible should receive two doses administered at least 4 weeks apart. Children in the same age-group (13 to 18 years) who have received only one previous varicella vaccine should receive a second varicella vaccine. The two-dose regimen was adopted to protect children who did not have adequate protection with one dose, not because of waning immunity to the vaccine (AAP Committee on Infectious Diseases, 2012). The combination vaccine MMRV (ProQuad) is licensed for use in children ages 12 months to 12 years (see discussion in the Measles section).

According to the AAP Committee on Infectious Diseases (2012), children who have received two doses of the varicella vaccine are one-third less likely to have breakthrough illness in the first 10 years of immunization in comparison with those who have received one dose. Children who do contract varicella after immunization reportedly have milder cases with fewer vesicles, lower degree of fever, and faster recovery. Antibodies persist for at least 8 years.

Keep the vaccine frozen in the lyophilic form (stable particles that readily go into solution) and use it within 30 minutes of being reconstituted to ensure viral potency.

Varicella vaccine may be administered simultaneously with MMR. However, separate syringes and injection sites should be used. If they are not administered simultaneously, the interval between administration of varicella vaccine and MMR should be at least 1 month. Varicella vaccine may also be given simultaneously with DTaP, IPV, HepB, or Hib vaccine (AAP Committee on Infectious Diseases, 2012). The vaccine is administered subcutaneously. For more information, see Fig. 31-11.

Influenza. The influenza vaccine is recommended annually for children ages 6 months to 18 years. Influenza vaccine (inactivated influenza vaccine [IIV*]) may be given to any healthy children 6 months old and older. The vaccine is administered in early fall before the flu season begins and is repeated yearly for ongoing protection. The intramuscular vaccine is administered as two separate doses 4 weeks apart in first-time recipients younger than 9 years. The dose is 0.25 mL for children ages 6 to 35 months and 0.5 mL for children 3 years and older. An intradermal form of IIV has been licensed for persons 18 to 64 years of age. The vaccine may be given simultaneously with other vaccines but in a separate syringe and at a separate site. The vaccine is administered yearly because different strains of influenza are used each year in the manufacture of the vaccine. The NIAID 2010 guidelines (Boyce, Assa'ad, Burks, et al., 2010) state that there is insufficient evidence to recommend administering either one of the available influenza vaccines to patients with a history of severe reactions to egg proteins; however the guidelines also point out that egg protein allergy is relatively common in individuals who would benefit from the influenza vaccine (e.g., children with asthma). The AAP Committee on Infectious Diseases (2012) recommends an assessment of the egg allergenic reaction, mild versus severe, before making a decision about the vaccine administration to children who have a history of egg allergy. Several options for administering the influenza vaccine are described in the literature, and individuals should discuss the risks and benefits with a knowledgeable health care practitioner.

The live attenuated influenza vaccine (LAIV) is an acceptable alternative to the intramuscular vaccine in specific age-groups. The vaccine is given nasally as two doses at least 28 days apart in healthy persons ages 2 to 49 years. The LAIV form is not recommended for children 2 to 4 years of age with wheezing in the previous 12 months or diagnosed asthma (AAP Committee on Infectious Diseases, 2012). Although it is an alternative to the injection, it costs more and may not be covered by insurance companies. Either IIV or LAIV may be given to healthy, nonpregnant persons ages 2 to 49 years (AAP Committee on Infectious Diseases, 2012). Yearly influenza vaccine should be administered to health care workers and to children ages 6 to 59 months with medical conditions (including asthma, cardiac disease, HIV, diabetes, and sickle cell disease) that place them at risk for influenza-related complications.

The H1N1 virus (swine flu) is a subtype of influenza type A. Previous outbreaks of H1N1 influenza occurred in 1918, and the mortality rates were significant both in the United States and worldwide. The 2009 pandemic of H1N1 caused significant morbidity and mortality worldwide, but particularly in Mexico and the United States. Antigenic shift occurs when influenza A viruses undergo significant changes that result in new infection subtypes; such is the case in the pandemic of 2009.

Meningococcal Infections. Invasive meningococcal disease continues to be the cause of high morbidity in children in the United States. Infants younger than 1 year are particularly susceptible, yet the highest fatalities occur in adolescents (approximately 20%). There is also evidence that the risk for meningococcal infections is high in college freshmen living in dormitories. Meningococcal infections are also responsible for significant morbidities, including limb or digit amputation, skin scarring, hearing loss, and neurologic disabilities.

Neisseria meningitidis is the leading cause of bacterial meningitis in the United States. It is not recommended that children 9 months to 10 years old routinely receive the meningococcal conjugate vaccines because the infection rate is low in this age-group. Children at increased risk for meningococcal infection should receive a two-dose series of a meningococcal conjugate vaccine (MCV4) given at least 2 months apart. These include children with terminal complement component deficiency, anatomic or functional asplenia, or HIV. In such cases, these children should receive two doses of either MenACWY-D (Menactra) or MenACWY-CRM (Menveo), both of

---

*The trivalent inactivated influenza vaccine (TIV) was changed to Inactivated Influenza Vaccine (IIV) because of the anticipated quadrivalent influenza vaccine in the 2013-2014 season (AAP Committee on Infectious Diseases, 2013).

which are MCV4 vaccines (AAP Committee on Infectious Diseases, 2012). A meningococcal and Hib vaccine, MenHibrix (Hib-MenCY-TT), has been licensed for administration to children ages 6 weeks to 18 months and provides protection against meningococcal infections (groups A, C, Y, and W-135) and *Haemophilus influenzae* type b (Hib) infections. MenHibrix is administered in a four-dose series at 2, 4, 6, and 12 to 15 months of age and is recommended for infants at increased risk for meningococcal disease rather than as a routinely recommended vaccine (CDC, 2013). Children ages 2 to 18 years who travel to or reside in countries where *N. meningitidis* is hyperendemic or epidemic or who are at risk during a community outbreak should receive one dose of MCV4 (either Menveo or Menactra). Menactra is licensed for administration in children as young as 9 months, whereas Menveo is licensed only for children 2 years of age and older.

Children and adolescents 11 to 12 years of age should receive a single immunization of MCV4 (either Menactra or Menveo) and a booster of the same at age 16 to 18 years. Others at high risk who should receive MCV4 include college freshmen living in dormitories and military recruits. For more information see Fig. 31-11.

Persons who are at high risk for the disease and previously received MPSV4 (meningococcal polysaccharide vaccine) 3 or more years previously should be reimmunized with MCV4. MCV4 (Menveo or Menactra) is administered as an intramuscular injection (0.5 mL) and may be administered in conjunction with other vaccines in a separate syringe and at a separate site. Immunization with MCV4 is contraindicated in persons with hypersensitivity to any components of the vaccine, including diphtheria toxoid, and to rubber latex (part of vial stopper).

Recommendations for Selected Immunizations

Two additional vaccines are recommended for children and adolescents at high risk for particular diseases. Two rotavirus vaccines, RotaTeq and Rotarix, have received a license from the U.S. Food and Drug Administration for distribution in the United States. Rotavirus is one of the leading causes of severe diarrhea in infants and young children. RotaTeq is licensed for administration to infants at 6 to 12 weeks of age, with two additional doses administered at 4- to 10-week intervals but not after 32 weeks of age; the dose is 2 mL, and the product must be protected from light until administration (AAP Committee on Infectious Diseases, 2012). Rotarix (1 mL) may be administered beginning at 6 weeks of age with a second dose at least 4 weeks after the first dose but before 24 weeks of age. Both vaccines are administered orally.

Two human papillomavirus (HPV) vaccines have been licensed for use in adolescents; a quadrivalent HPV4 vaccine, Gardasil, has been approved and is recommended for female children and adolescents to prevent HPV-related cervical cancer. The vaccine is administered intramuscularly in three separate doses; the first dose in the series may be given at 11 to 12 years of age (minimum age, 9 years), and the second dose is administered 2 months after the first, with the third dose being given 6 months after the first dose. The HPV4 vaccine may also be administered to boys and men ages 9 to 26 years in a three-dose series to reduce the likelihood of genital warts (AAP Committee on Infectious Diseases, 2012). The bivalent vaccine (HPV2), Cervarix, is licensed for use in girls and women ages 10 to 25 years for the prevention of HPV-related cervical cancer; this vaccine is given in a three-dose series.

Immunizations that may be used in older children and adolescents in the future and that are being evaluated include vaccines for preventing diseases such as herpes simplex virus, human cytomegalovirus, and Epstein-Barr virus. Others, such as the rabies vaccine, are discussed elsewhere in this text.

Reactions

Vaccines for routine immunizations are among the safest and most reliable drugs available. However, minor side effects do occur after many of the immunizations, and, rarely, a serious reaction may result from the vaccine.

With inactivated antigens, such as DTaP, side effects are most likely to occur within a few hours or days of administration and are usually limited to local tenderness, erythema, and swelling at the injection site; low-grade fever; and behavioral changes (drowsiness, fretfulness, eating less, prolonged or unusual cry). Rarely, more severe reactions may occur, especially with pertussis. Reactions to DTaP tend to be more severe if they occurred with a previous immunization; fever, swelling, irritability, and pain are more common after the fourth DTaP vaccination in the series. Acetaminophen may help reduce this discomfort and should be given in an age-appropriate dose and time interval.

Hib vaccine is one of the safest vaccines available but may be associated with low-grade fever and mild local reactions at the site of injection, which resolve rapidly. Fever (temperature >38.5°C [101.3°F]) may rarely occur.

A number of inactive components are incorporated in vaccines to enhance their effectiveness and safety. Some of these components include preservatives, stabilizers, adjuvants, antibiotics, and purified culture medium proteins to enhance effectiveness. A child may react to the preservative in the vaccine rather than the vaccine component; an example of this is the HepB vaccine, which is prepared from yeast cultures. Yeast hypersensitivity might preclude one from receiving that particular vaccine. Trace amounts of neomycin are used to decrease bacterial growth within certain vaccine preparations, and persons with documented anaphylactic reactions to neomycin should avoid those vaccines. Most vaccine preparations now contain vial stoppers with a synthetic rubber to prevent latex allergy reactions; however, health care personnel administering vaccines should make sure that the package insert specifies there is no latex in the stopper. In the event that an individual has had a severe reaction to a vaccine and subsequent immunizations are required, an allergist should be consulted to determine the best course of action. The influenza vaccine contains small amounts of egg protein; thus children who have severe allergy to egg should seek the advice of an allergist regarding this vaccine. Most children with egg allergy are reported to be likely to develop a tolerance to small amounts over time (Settipane, Siri, and Bellanti, 2009).

Some vaccines contain a preservative, thimerosal, which contains ethylmercury. Concerns regarding possible mercury poisoning in the 1990s prompted many to put off vaccination of infants and small children for fear of childhood developmental problems such as autism. A number of manufacturers have since stopped producing vaccines containing thimerosal. No local hypersensitivity reactions to thimerosal have been recorded, and studies on thimerosal and the potential link to autism or any other pervasive developmental disorder failed to establish a causal relationship between the two (Hviid, Stellfeld, Wohlfahrt, et al., 2003; Parker, Schwartz, Todd, et al., 2004; Price, Thompson, Goodson, et al., 2010; Schultz, 2010). The Institute of Medicine (2004), following an in-depth 3-year study, concluded that there was no link between autism and the MMR vaccine or vaccines containing the preservative *thimerosal*.

A commonly observed reaction includes localized erythema and induration, which may occur when the vaccine is not administered deeply enough into the muscle. This reaction can be prevented by

ATRAUMATIC CARE

Immunizations

Needle length is an important factor and must be considered for each individual child; fewer reactions to immunizations are observed when the vaccine is given deep into the muscle rather than into subcutaneous tissue. Contrary to previous belief, deep intramuscular tissue has a better blood supply and fewer pain receptors than adipose tissue, thus providing an optimal site for immunizations with fewer side effects (Zuckerman, 2000).

To minimize local reactions from vaccines:

- Recommended needle length for newborn to 2 months is 16 mm (⅝ inch).
- Select a needle of adequate length (25 mm [1 in] in infants) to deposit the antigen deep in the muscle mass.
- Toddlers and older children require a needle length of 16 to 25 mm (⅝ to 1 inch) for deltoid, or 25 to 32 mm (1 to 1¼ in) for vastus lateralis (Schechter, Zempsky, Cohen, et al., 2007).
- Adolescents require a needle length of 25 to 51 mm (1 to 2 in) in deltoid or vastus lateralis (Schechter, Zempsky, Cohen, et al., 2007) depending on size of muscle mass.
- Inject into the vastus lateralis or ventrogluteal muscle; the deltoid may be used in children 18 months of age or older.

Use one or more of the following techniques to minimize pain:

- Apply the topical anesthetic *EMLA* (lidocaine-prilocaine) to the injection site and cover with an occlusive dressing for at least 1 hour before the injection.
- Apply the topical anesthetic *LMX4* (4% lidocaine) to the injection site 30 minutes before the injection; there is no evidence that an occlusive dressing is required except to prevent ingestion or accidental application to the eyes in infants (Wong, 2003).
- Apply a vapocoolant spray (e.g., ethyl chloride or Fluori-Methane) directly to the skin or to a cotton ball, which is placed on the skin for 15 seconds immediately before the injection (Reis and Holubkov, 1997).

- There is evidence that a concentrated oral sucrose solution (24%) and nonnutritive sucking (NNS) (pacifier) decrease the pain related to minor invasive procedures in neonates (Stevens, Johnston, Franck, et al., 1999; Stevens, Yamada, and Ohlsson, 2001). Most studies have focused on heel lance, venipuncture, and circumcision (neonatal period), but one institution has incorporated a neonatal oral sucrose pain protocol for painful procedures, including intramuscular injections (Thompson, 2005). Hatfield (2008) found that 2- and 4-month-old infants who received a 0.6 mL/kg dose of 24% sucrose and NNS 2 minutes before immunization administration had decreased pain behavioral responses compared with a control group of infants who received only sterile water and NNS 2 minutes before the injection. Liaw, Zeng, Yang, et al., (2011) found that NNS and oral sucrose provided analgesia to newborns receiving the hepatitis B vaccine. Therefore it is recommended that a concentrated oral sucrose solution (1 to 2 mL) be administered orally 2 minutes before the injection, during the injection, and up to 3 minutes after the procedure to decrease neonatal pain with immunizations.
- In preschool children, use distraction, such as telling the child to "take a deep breath and blow and blow and blow until I tell you to stop."
- A combination of pharmacologic and nonpharmacologic interventions including breastfeeding, oral sucrose, and NNS has been found to decrease the pain sensation in infants receiving their childhood immunizations (Shah, Taddio, Rieder, et al., 2009).

NOTE: Changing the needle on the syringe after drawing up the vaccine and before injecting it has not been shown to decrease local reactions. In children 4 to 6 years of age, the administration of sequential injections or simultaneous injections of vaccines did not alter their perceptions of distress, but parents preferred the simultaneous method (Horn and McCarthy, 1999).

---

ensuring that needle length is appropriate for the child's muscle size. Although many vaccine preparations are commercially available in prepackaged form, the enclosed needle may not be of adequate length to penetrate the muscle in certain children (see Atraumatic Care box above and Administration, p. 896).

Unlike the inactivated antigens, live attenuated virus vaccines such as MMR multiply for days or weeks, and unfavorable reactions and vaccine-associated disorders can occur for 30 to 60 days. These reactions are usually mild, although reactions to rubella tend to be more troublesome in older children and adults.

Contraindications and Precautions

Nurses need to be aware of the reasons for withholding immunizations—both for the child's safety in terms of avoiding reactions and for the child's maximum benefit from receiving the vaccine. Unfounded fears and lack of knowledge regarding contraindications can needlessly prevent a child from having protection from life-threatening diseases. Issues that have surfaced regarding vaccines include the misconception that administering combination vaccines may overload the child's immune system; the combined vaccines have undergone rigorous study in relation to side effects and immunogenicity rates following administration. Others may express concern that vaccines are not a part of the individual's natural immunity and that administering too many vaccines may decrease the child's immunity to such diseases. Parents may also voice concerns that vaccines may cause diseases such as asthma,

multiple sclerosis, or diabetes mellitus (Kimmel, Burns, Wolfe, et al., 2007). Another concern of parents is the number of vaccines or "shots" given to infants at any given time and the pain and discomfort this may cause.

A *contraindication* is considered as a condition in an individual that increases the risk for a serious adverse reaction (e.g., not administering a live virus vaccine to a severely compromised child). A *precaution* is a condition in a recipient that might increase the risk for a serious adverse reaction or that might compromise the ability of the vaccine to produce immunity (CDC, 2011c).

The general contraindication for all immunizations is a severe febrile illness. This precaution avoids adding the risk for adverse side effects from the vaccine to an already ill child or mistakenly identifying a symptom of the disease as having been caused by the vaccine. The presence of minor illnesses such as the common cold is not a contraindication. Live virus vaccines are generally not administered to anyone with an altered immune system, since multiplication of the virus may be enhanced, causing a severe vaccine-induced illness.

In general, live virus vaccines such as varicella and MMR should not be administered to persons who are severely immunocompromised (National Center for Immunization and Respiratory Diseases, 2011). Another contraindication to live virus vaccines (e.g., MMR and varicella) is the presence of recently acquired passive immunity through blood transfusions, immunoglobulin, or maternal antibodies. Administration of MMR and varicella vaccines should be postponed for a minimum of 3 months after passive immunization with immunoglobulins and blood transfusions (except washed red blood cells (RBCs), which do not interfere with the immune response). Suggested intervals between administration of immunoglobulin preparations and MMR and varicella vaccines depend on the type of immune product and dosage. If the vaccine and immunoglobulin are given simultaneously because of imminent exposure to disease, the two preparations are injected at sites far from each other. Vaccination should be repeated after the suggested intervals unless there is serologic evidence of antibody production.

A family history of seizures or any other adverse events following vaccination, penicillin allergy, allergies to duck meat or duck feathers, and a family history of SIDS are not considered contraindications to receiving childhood vaccines (AAP Committee on Infectious Diseases, 2012).

A final contraindication is a known allergic response to a previously administered vaccine or a substance in the vaccine. MMR vaccines contain minute amounts of neomycin; measles and mumps vaccines, which are grown on chick embryo tissue cultures, are not believed to contain significant amounts of egg cross-reacting proteins. Therefore only a history of anaphylactic reaction to neomycin, gelatin, or the vaccine itself is considered a contraindication to their use.

Pregnancy is a contraindication to MMR vaccines, although the risk for fetal damage is primarily theoretical. Breastfeeding is not a contraindication for any vaccine. The only vaccine virus that has been isolated in human milk is rubella, and there is no indication this is harmful to infants. Rubella infection in an infant as a result of exposure to the rubella virus in human milk would likely be well tolerated since the vaccine is attenuated (AAP Committee on Infectious Diseasaes, 2012). See also Family-Centered Care box.

Administration

The principal precautions in administering immunizations include proper storage of the vaccine to protect its potency and institution of recommended procedures for injection. The nurse must be familiar with the manufacturer's directions for storage and reconstitution of the vaccine. For example, if the vaccine is to be refrigerated, it should be stored on a center shelf, not in the door, where frequent temperature increases from opening the refrigerator can alter the vaccine's potency. For protection against light, the vial can be wrapped in aluminum foil. Periodic checks are established to ensure that no vaccine is used after its expiration date.

The DTaP vaccines contain the adjuvant *alum* to retain the antigen at the injection site and prolong the stimulatory effect. Because subcutaneous or intracutaneous injection of the adjuvant can cause local irritation, inflammation, or abscess formation, attention to excellent intramuscular injection technique must be used (see Atraumatic Care box, p. 895). Ipp, Parkin, Lear, et al. (2009) evaluated the administration order of the vaccines diphtheria-tetanus–acellular pertussis–*Haemophilus influenzae* type b (DTaP-Hib) and pneumococcal conjugate vaccine (PCV) and pain perception in 120 infants 2 to 6 months of age. The infants who were given the primary DTaP-Hib vaccine before the PCV vaccine had significantly lower pain scores as measured by the Modified Behavioral Pain Scale than those who received the PCV vaccine first. Both groups of infants were given both vaccines. Additional pain measures included crying as measured by video recording and parent perception of child pain using the Visual Analog Scale. The researchers recommend giving the primary DTaP-Hib vaccine before the PCV to reduce pain in infants receiving routine immunizations.

One of the most important features of injecting vaccines is adequate penetration of the muscle for deposition of the drug

FAMILY-CENTERED CARE

Communicating with Parents About Immunizations

- Provide accurate and user-friendly information on vaccines (the necessity for each one, the disease each prevents, potential adverse effects).
- Realize that the parent is expressing concern for the child's health.
- Acknowledge the parent's concerns in a genuine, empathetic manner.
- Tailor the discussion to the needs of the parent.
- Avoid judgmental or threatening language.
- Be knowledgeable about the benefits of individual vaccines, the common adverse effects, and how to minimize those effects.
- Give the parent the vaccine information statement (VIS) beforehand and be prepared to answer any questions that may arise.
- Help the parent make an informed decision regarding the administration of each vaccine.
- Be flexible and provide parents options regarding the administration of multiple vaccines, especially in infants, who must receive multiple injections at 2, 4, and 6 months (i.e., allow parents to space the vaccinations at different visits to decrease the total number of injections at each visit; make provisions for office visits for immunization purposes only [does not incur a practitioner fee except for administration of vaccine], provided the child is healthy).
- Involve the parent in minimizing the potential adverse effects of the vaccine (e.g., administering an appropriate dose of acetaminophen 45 minutes before administering the vaccine [as warranted]; applying EMLA [lidocaine-prilocaine] or LMX4 [4% lidocaine] to the injection sites before administration; following up to check on the child if untoward reactions have occurred in the past or parent is especially anxious about the child's well-being).
- Respect the parent's ultimate wishes.

Data from Coyer SM: Understanding parental concerns about immunizations, *J Pediatr Health Care* 16(4):193–196, 2002; Fredrickson DD, Davis TC, Bocchini JA: Explaining the risks and benefits of vaccines to parents, *Pediatr Ann* 30(7):400–406, 2001; Rosenthal P: Overcoming skepticism toward vaccines: a look at the real benefits and risks, *Consult Pediatr* 4(Suppl):S3–S7, 2004.

intramuscularly and not subcutaneously (depending on the manufacturer's recommendation for administration). The use of appropriate needle length is an essential component of administering vaccines. In two studies, the use of longer needles significantly decreased the incidence of localized edema and tenderness when vaccines were administered to a group of infants (Diggle and Deeks, 2000; Diggle, Deeks, and Pollard, 2006) (see Evidence-Based Practice box). Similar findings have been recorded for children 4 to 6 years of age receiving the 5th DTaP vaccine (Jackson, Yu, Nelson, et al., 2011). In some studies the site of administration influenced pain perception and localized reactions. Cook and Murtagh (2006) found that administration of the pertussis vaccine in the ventrogluteal muscle in children ages 2 months to 18 months was safe and had few localized reactions compared with anterolateral thigh administration. Junqueira, Tavares, Martins, et al. (2010) found that administration of the hepatitis B vaccine in the ventrogluteal muscle (vs. anterolateral thigh) of 580 infants resulted in a lower incidence of fever and localized reactions (see Intramuscular Administration, Chapter 39).

The total series requires several injections, and every attempt is made to rotate the sites and administer the injections as painlessly as possible (see Intramuscular Administration, Chapter 39). When two or more injections are given at separate sites, the order of

EVIDENCE-BASED PRACTICE

Appropriate Site, Technique, Needle Size, and Dose for Intramuscular Injections in Infants, Toddlers, and Small Children

Ask the Question
In infants, toddlers, and small children, what is the best site, technique, needle size and gauge, and dosage for intramuscular (IM) injections?

Search the Evidence
Search Strategies
Literature from 1990 to 2009 was reviewed to obtain clinical research studies related to this issue.

Databases Used
CINAHL, PubMed

Critically Analyze the Evidence
Searches reviewed were small studies. There were no randomized trials, double-blind trials, or large clinical studies addressing the subject of IM injections in children.

Infants and Toddlers
- A 16-mm needle was sufficient to penetrate the anterolateral thigh muscle if the needle is inserted at a 90° angle without pinching the muscle in children ages 2, 4, 6, and 18 months (Cook and Murtagh, 2002).
- A 25-mm needle is necessary to penetrate the thigh muscle when a 45° injection technique was employed. Longer needle length is needed to fully deposit the medication into the muscle in children ages 2, 4, 6, and 18 months (Cook and Murtagh, 2002).
- When diphtheria-tetanus-pertussis (DTP) immunizations were administered to infants ≤7 months of age, 84.6% of injections were administered at the correct site (anterior thigh). Incorrect sites of administration included 5.1% dorsogluteal and 2.6% deltoid muscles (Daly, Johnston, and Chung, 1992).
- Vaccines containing adjuvant such as alum (e.g., DTaP, hepatitis A and hepatitis B, diphtheria-tetanus [DT or Td]) should be given deep into the muscle to prevent local reactions (American Academy of Pediatrics [AAP], 2012; Centers for Disease Control and Prevention [CDC], 2002; Petousis-Harris, 2008; Taddio, Ilersich, Ipp, et al., 2009).
- Injecting adjuvant-containing vaccines into subcutaneous tissue increases the incidence of local reactions (Taddio, Ilersich, Ipp, et al., 2009; Zuckerman, 2000).
- 4-month-old infants experienced fewer local side effects (redness, tenderness, and swelling) when immunizations were administered into the anterior aspect of the thigh with a 25-mm (1-inch) needle versus shorter 16-mm (⅝-inch) needle (Diggle and Deeks, 2000).
- Localized vaccine reactions were significantly reduced when long needles (25 mm) were used for infant immunizations (Diggle, Deeks, and Pollard, 2006; Petousis-Harris, 2008).
- A 16-mm needle may be adequate for injections in small infants, and a 22- to 25-mm (⅞- to 1-inch) needle can be used in infants 2 months and older (AAP, 2012).
- A 22- to 32-mm (⅞- to 1¼-inch) needle is recommended for injections in toddlers if deltoid muscle size is adequate (CDC, 2002).
- A minimum of a 25-mm long needle is recommended for anterolateral thigh injection in toddlers (CDC, 2002).
- Dorsogluteal muscle should be avoided in infants and toddlers, and in smaller preschoolers with smaller muscle mass, because of the possibility of damaging the sciatic nerve (AAP, 2012).

- In children >1 year old, deltoid muscle is recommended for IM injections. When multiple vaccines are given, two may be given in the thigh (anterior and lateral) because of its larger size (Diggle, 2003).
- Injections in the anterolateral thigh should be given at least 2.5 cm (1 inch) apart so local reactions are less likely to overlap (AAP, 2012).
- No research or supportive data were found regarding the amount of medication to be given at the different sites in infants and toddlers.

Children and Adolescents
- A 22- to 25-gauge needle for all IM childhood immunizations is recommended (AAP, 2012; CDC, 2002).
- Deltoid muscle may be used for immunizations in toddlers, older children, and adolescents (AAP, 2012; CDC, 2002).
- 16-mm needle for children <60 kg and 25-mm needle for children 60-70 kg are appropriate for IM injections in the deltoid injection site (Koster, Stellato, Kohn, et al., 2009).
- Ventrogluteal site is relatively free of important nerves and vascular structures and is the site of choice for pediatric IM injections in children of all ages; no complications at this site were reported (Beecroft and Kongelbeck, 1994).
- Longer needle (25 mm) was preferred for injection when bunching the skin and injecting; shorter needle (16 mm) was perceived as causing fewer localized reactions when the injection was administered with the skin being held taut (Groswasser, Kahn, Bouche, et al., 1997).
- Needle length found to be the most significant variable for local reactions in children after injection: 25-mm needle was associated with fewer localized reactions versus 16-mm needle (Davenport, 2004).
- In children older than 1 year, deltoid muscle is recommended for IM injections. When multiple vaccines are given, two may be given in the thigh (anterior and lateral) because of its larger size (Diggle, 2003).
- Injections in the anterolateral thigh should be given at least 2.5 cm (1 inch) apart so local reactions are less likely to overlap (AAP, 2012).
- IM injections in the buttocks with longer needles and 90° angle are associated with less reactogenicity (Petousis-Harris, 2008).

Apply the Evidence: Nursing Implications
There is **low quality evidence** with **strong recommendation** to continue administering IM injections to children in the anterolateral thigh (up to 12 months old), deltoid (12 months and older), and ventrogluteal site (Guyatt, Oxman, Vist, et al., 2008). Needle length is an important factor in decreasing local reactions; the length should be adequate to deposit the medication into the muscle for IM injections. Recommendations are for a 25-mm (1-inch) needle in infants, a 25- to 32-mm (1- to 1¼-inch) needle for toddlers, and a 38- to 51-mm (1½- to 2-inch) needle for older children; preterm and small emaciated infants may require a shorter needle (16 to 25 mm [⅝ to 1 inch]) based on weight and muscle mass size.

Quality and Safety Competencies:
Evidence-Based Practice*
Knowledge
Differentiate clinical opinion from research and evidence-based summaries
Describe various methods for identifying appropriate site, technique, needle size, and dose for intramuscular injections in infants, toddlers, and small children.

Continued

Appropriate Site, Technique, Needle Size, and Dose for Intramuscular Injections in Infants, Toddlers, and Small Children—cont'd

Skills

Base individualized care plan on patient values, clinical expertise, and evidence.

Integrate evidence into practice by using the techniques for intramuscular injections in clinical care.

Attitudes

Value the concept of evidence-based practice (EBP) as integral to determining best clinical practice.

Appreciate strengths and weakness of evidence for identifying appropriate site, technique, needle size, and dose for intramuscular injections in infants, toddlers, and small children.

References

American Academy of Pediatrics (AAP) Committee on Infectious Diseases, Pickering L, editor: *Red Book: report of the Committee on Infectious Diseases*, ed 29, Elk Grove Village, IL, 2012, Author.

Beecroft PC, Kongelbeck SR: How safe are intramuscular injections? *AACN Clin Issues* 5(2):207–215, 1994.

Centers for Disease Control and Prevention (CDC): General recommendations on immunization, *MMWR Recomm Rep* 51(RR-2):12–14, 2002.

Cook IF, Murtagh J: Needle length required for intramuscular vaccination of infants and toddlers: an ultrasonographic study, *Austral Fam Phys* 31(3):295–297, 2002.

Daly JM, Johnston W, Chung Y: Injection sites utilized for DPT immunizations in infants, *J Comm Health Nurs* 9(2):87–94, 1992.

Davenport JM: A systematic review to ascertain whether the standard needle is more effective than a longer or wider needle in reducing the incidence of local reaction in children receiving primary immunization, *J Adv Nurs* 46(1):66–77, 2004.

Diggle L: The administration of child vaccines, part 11, Childhood vaccinations, *Practice Nurse* 25(12):63–69, 2003.

Diggle L, Deeks J: Effect of needle length on incidence of local reactions to routine immunisation in infants aged 4 months: randomised controlled trial, *BMJ* 321(7266):931–933, 2000.

Diggle L, Deeks JJ, Pollard AJ: Effect of needle size on immunogenicity and reactogenicity of vaccines in infants: randomized controlled trial, *BMJ* 333(7568):571, 2006.

Groswasser J, Kahn A, Bouche B, et al: Needle length and injection technique for efficient intramuscular vaccine delivery in infants and children evaluated through an ultrasonographic determination of subcutaneous and muscle layer thickness, *Pediatrics* 100(3 Part 1):400–403, 1997.

Guyatt GH, Oxman AD, Vist GE, et al: GRADE: an emerging consensus on rating quality of evidence and strength of recommendations, *BMJ* 336(7650):924–926, 2008.

Koster M, Stellato N, Kohn N, et al: Needle length for immunizations of early adolescents as determined by ultrasound, *Pediatrics*, 124:667–672, 2009.

Petousis-Harris H: Vaccine injection technique and reactogenicity: evidence for practice, *Vaccine* 26:6299–6304, 2008.

Taddio A, Ilersich AL, Ipp M, et al: Physical interventions and injection techniques for reducing injection pain during routine childhood immunizations: systematic review of randomized controlled trials and quasi-randomized controlled trials, *Clin Ther* 31:S48–S76, 2009.

Zuckerman J: The importance of injecting vaccines into muscle, *BMJ* 321(7271):1237–1238, 2000.

Updated by Olga Taylor

*Adapted from the QSEN.

injections is arbitrary. Because allergic reactions can occur after injection of vaccines, appropriate precautions are taken (see Anaphylaxis, Chapter 42).

Nurses administer vaccines and thus have the responsibility for adequately informing parents of the nature, prevalence, and risks of the disease; the type of immunization product to be used; the expected benefits and the risk for side effects of the vaccine; and the need for accurate immunization records. Referring to immunizations as "baby shots" and limiting the discussion to vague statements about the vaccines are unacceptable practices.

Another important nursing responsibility is accurate documentation. Each child should have an immunization record for parents to keep, especially for families who move frequently. Although immunization rates have increased significantly, health care professionals should use every opportunity to encourage complete immunization of all children (see Family-Centered Care box on p. 896). Blank immunization records may be downloaded from a number of websites, including the Immunization Action Coalition,* which has vaccine information and records in a number of languages.

The following information is documented on the medical record: day, month, and year of administration; manufacturer and lot number of vaccine; and the name, address, and title of the person administering the vaccine. Additional data to record are the site and route of administration and evidence that the parent or legal guardian gave informed consent before the immunization was administered. Any adverse reactions after the administration of any vaccine are reported to the Vaccine Adverse Event Reporting System.*

An additional source of vaccine information that must be given to parents (by law; National Childhood Vaccine Injury Act of 1986) before the administration of vaccines is the vaccine information statement (VIS) for the particular vaccine being administered. Health care practitioners are required to fully inform families of the risks and benefits of the vaccines. VISs are designed to provide updated information to the adult vaccinee or parents or legal guardians of children being vaccinated regarding the risks and benefits of each vaccine. Questions regarding the information in the VISs should be answered by the practitioner. VISs are available for the following vaccines: anthrax, tetanus, diphtheria, pertussis, MMR, MMRV, IPV, varicella, Hib, influenza, meningococcal, pneumococcal, rabies, shingles, smallpox, yellow fever, Japanese encephalitis, rotavirus, human papillomavirus, typhoid, HPV, HepA, and HepB. An updated VIS should be provided, and

*www.immunize.org.

*For information call (800) 822-7967 or visit www.fda.gov/cber/vaers/vaers.htm.

documentation in the patient's chart should state that the VIS was given and include the publication date of the VIS; this represents informed consent once the parent or caregiver gives permission to administer the vaccines. VISs are available from state or local health departments or from the Immunization Action Coalition* and Centers for Disease Control and Prevention (CDC) in various languages.†

In response to the concerns of manufacturers, practitioners, and parents of children with serious vaccine-associated injuries, the National Childhood Vaccine Injury Act of 1986 and the Vaccine Compensation Amendments of 1987 were passed. These laws are designed to provide fair compensation for children who are inadvertently injured and provide greater protection from liability for vaccine manufacturers and providers. For further information, contact the National Vaccine Injury Compensation Program: 800 338-2382; www.hrsa.gov/vaccinecompensation/.

Safety Promotion and Injury Prevention

Injuries are a major cause of death during infancy, especially for children 6 to 12 months old. According to a Canadian survey (Flavin, Dostaler, Simpson, et al., 2006), the top leading causes of injury to infants were falls, ingestion injuries, and burns. The three leading causes of accidental death injury in infants were suffocation, motor vehicle–related injuries, and drowning (CDC, 2007). Mack, Gilchrist, and Ballesteros (2008) report that fall-related injuries in the home were the most common reason for emergency department visits in infants ages 0 to 12 months; according to these authors, one infant is injured every 1½ minutes. In a similar study of infants treated for accidents, the bed was commonly listed as being involved, whereas car seat at 2 months of age and stairs at 12 months were reported to be the cause of the accidental injury (Mack, Gilchrist, and Ballesteros, 2008). According to a recent Cochrane study, one third of all injuries occur in the home, yet there is insufficient evidence to demonstrate that modification of the home environment has an impact on the rate of injuries (Turner, Arthur, Lyons, et al., 2011). Constant vigilance, awareness, and supervision are essential as the child gains increased locomotor and manipulative skills that are coupled with an insatiable curiosity about the environment. Box 31-1 lists the major developmental achievements of each period during infancy and the appropriate injury prevention plan. Table 31-2 lists common types of injuries and associated objects that predispose to such injuries. Suggestions for promoting safety in the home environment are given for specific types of injuries. The acronym *S-A-F-E P-A-D* shown in Table 31-2 may be used to identify common types of injuries to infants and older children.

Motor Vehicle Safety

Automobile injuries are the leading cause of accidental death in children between the ages of 1 and 9 years (Bernard, Paulozzi, and Wallace, 2007). A significant number of nonfatal vehicle-related injuries in children between 1 and 4 years of age occur as a result of back-over while children are playing in a driveway (CDC, 2005a). In addition, a significant number of infants are injured or die from improper restraint within the vehicle, most often from riding on the lap of another occupant. Desapriya, Joshi, Subwarzi, et al. (2008) found that falls accounted for a significant proportion of injuries (98%) in infants from birth to 4 months of age as a result of inappropriate use of a car restraint system. Reports indicate that child

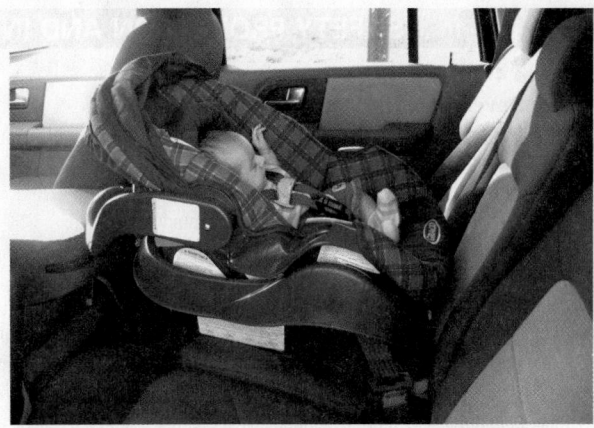

FIG 31-13   Rear-facing infant seat in rear seat of car. The infant is placed in the seat when going home from the hospital. (Courtesy Brian and Mayannyn Sallee, Anchorage, AK.)

restraint use decreases with increasing age of children and increasing number of occupants. Lack of proper child restraint continues to be a major factor in fatal accidents involving children. All infants must be secured in a federally approved restraint rather than held or placed on the seat of the car. There is no safe alternative.

Infant restraints are designed either as an infant-only model or as a convertible infant-toddler model. Either restraint is a semireclined seat that faces the rear of the car. A rear-facing car seat provides the best protection for the disproportionately heavy head and weak neck of an infant (Fig. 31-13). This position minimizes the stress on the neck by spreading the forces of a frontal crash over the entire back, neck, and head; the spine is supported by the back of the car seat. If the seat were faced forward, the head would whip forward because of the force of the crash, creating enormous stress on the neck. It is now recommended that all infants and toddlers ride in rear-facing car safety seats until they reach the age of 2 years or the height recommended by the car seat manufacturer (AAP, 2011).* Some infant-only rear-facing infant car safety seats can accommodate children weighing up to a maximum of 35 pounds. Studies indicate that toddlers up to 24 months of age are safer riding in convertible seats in the rear-facing position (Bull and Durbin, 2008; Henary, Sherwood, Crandall, et al., 2007).

The restraint is anchored to the vehicle with the vehicle's seat belt, and the restraint has a harness system for securing the infant. Some harness systems require a clip to keep the shoulder straps correctly positioned. Newer vehicles (manufactured after 1999) have tether straps that attach to anchors in the car seat to better secure the seat and minimize forward movement of the forward-facing convertible seats in the event of an accident. The LATCH (lower anchor and tether for children) system provides car seat anchors between the front cushion and backrest so that the seat belt does not have to be used. However, the National Highway Traffic Safety Administration (NHTSA) recommends (as of February 2014) that the seat belt be used to anchor the car seat instead of the LATCH system if the combined weight of the child and car seat exceeds 65 pounds. Some automobiles have tether straps for

---

*Car seat information is available from the AAP at www.aap.org/healthtopics/carseatsafety.cfm; and from the Insurance Institute for Highway Safety, 1005 N. Glebe Road, Suite 800, Arlington, VA 22201; 703-247-1500; fax: 703-247-1588; www.iihs.org. The National Highway Traffic Safety Administration, www.nhtsa.gov, also provides child passenger safety and air bag safety information for parents.

BOX 31-1 SAFETY PROMOTION AND INJURY PREVENTION DURING INFANCY

Birth to 4 Months
Major Developmental Accomplishments
- Exhibits involuntary reflexes (e.g., crawling reflex may propel infant forward or backward; startle reflex may cause the body to jerk)
- May roll over
- Has increasing eye-hand coordination and voluntary grasp reflex

Injury Prevention
Aspiration
- Aspiration is not as great a danger to this age-group, but parents should begin practicing safeguarding early (see under Age 4 to 7 Months).
- Never shake baby powder directly on infant; place powder in hand and then on infant's skin; store container closed and out of infant's reach.
- Hold infant for feeding; do not prop bottle.
- Know emergency procedures for choking.
- Use pacifier with one-piece construction and loop handle.

Burns
- Install smoke detectors in home.
- Do not microwave infant formula or breast milk because this can cause burns because of uneven warming.
- Check bathwater temperature.
- Do not pour hot liquids when infant is close by, such as sitting on lap.
- Beware of cigarette ashes that may fall on infant.
- Do not leave infant in sun for more than a few minutes; keep skin covered.
- Wash flame-retardant clothes according to label directions.
- Use cool-mist vaporizers.
- Do not leave child in parked car.
- Check surface heat of car restraint before placing child in seat.

Suffocation and Drowning
- Keep all plastic bags stored out of infant's reach; discard large plastic garment bags after tying in a knot.
- Do not cover mattress with plastic.
- Use firm mattress and loose blankets, with no pillows.
- Make certain crib design follows federal regulations and mattress fits snugly—crib slats 2.375 inches (6 cm) apart.*
- Position crib away from other furniture and away from heat radiators.
- Do not tie pacifier on a string around infant's neck.
- Remove bibs at bedtime.
- Never leave infant alone in bath.
- Do not leave infant younger than 12 months alone on adult or youth mattress or "beanbag" type seats.
- Install carbon monoxide monitor.

Motor Vehicles
- Transport infant in federally approved, rear-facing car seat, preferably in back seat.†
- Do not place infant on seat (of car) or in lap.
- Do not place child in a carriage or stroller behind a parked car.
- Do not place infant or child in front passenger seat with an air bag.
- Do not leave infant unattended in car, especially in environmental temperatures above 70° F.

Falls
- Crib rails are fixed and firmly latched. As of 2011, only beds with fixed rails are recommended, but some older models may be in use (suggest purchasing a rail-latching mechanism for older models).

- Never leave infant alone on a raised, unguarded surface.
- When in doubt as to where to place child, use floor.
- Restrain child in infant seat, and never leave child unattended while the seat is resting on a raised surface.
- Avoid using a high chair until child can sit well with support.

Poisoning
- Poisoning is not as great a danger to this age-group, but parents should begin practicing safeguards early (see under Age 4 to 7 Months).

Bodily Damage
- Keep sharp or jagged objects such as knives and broken glass out of child's reach.
- Keep diaper pins closed and away from infant.

Age 4 to 7 Months
Major Developmental Accomplishments
- Rolls over
- Sits momentarily
- Grasps and manipulates small objects
- Resecures a dropped object
- Has well-developed eye-hand coordination
- Can focus on and locate very small objects
- Has prominent mouthing (oral fixation)
- Can push up on hands and knees
- Crawls backward

Injury Prevention
Aspiration
- Keep buttons, beads, syringe caps, and other small objects out of infant's reach.
- Keep floor free of any small objects.
- Do not feed infant hard candy, nuts, food with pits or seeds, or whole or circular pieces of hot dog.
- Exercise caution when giving teething biscuits, since large chunks may be broken off and aspirated.
- Do not feed infant while he or she is lying down.
- Inspect toys for removable parts.
- Keep baby powder, if used, out of reach.
- Avoid storing large quantities of cleaning fluid, paints, pesticides, and other toxic substances.
- Discard used containers of poisonous substances.
- Do not store toxic substances in food or drink containers.
- Discard used button-size batteries; store new batteries in safe area.
- Know telephone number of local poison control center ([800] 222-1222) (usually listed in front of telephone directory).

Suffocation
- Keep all latex balloons out of reach.
- Remove all crib toys that are strung across crib or play yard when child begins to push up on hands or knees or is 5 months old.

Burns
- Keep water faucets out of reach.
- Place hot objects (cigarettes, candles, incense) on high surface out of child's reach.
- Limit exposure to sun; apply sunscreen.

BOX 31-1 SAFETY PROMOTION AND INJURY PREVENTION DURING INFANCY—cont'd

Falls
- Restrain in a high chair.
- Crib rails are fixed and firmly latched. As of 2011, only beds with fixed rails are recommended.

Motor Vehicles
- See under Birth to 4 Months.

Poisoning
- Make certain that paint for furniture or toys does not contain lead.
- Place toxic substances on a high shelf or in locked cabinet.
- Hang plants or place on high surface rather than on floor.
- Know telephone number of local poison control center ([800] 222-1222) (usually listed in front of telephone directory).

Bodily Damage
- Give toys that are smooth and rounded, preferably made of wood or plastic.
- Avoid long, pointed objects as toys.
- Avoid toys that are excessively loud.
- Keep sharp objects out of infant's reach.

Age 8 to 12 Months
Major Developmental Accomplishments
- Crawls or creeps
- Stands, holding onto furniture
- Stands alone
- Cruises around furniture
- Walks
- Climbs
- Pulls on objects
- Throws objects
- Is able to pick up small objects; has pincer grasp
- Explores by putting objects in mouth
- Dislikes being restrained
- Explores away from parent
- Increasingly understands simple commands and phrases

Injury Prevention
Aspiration
- Keep small objects off floor, off furniture, and out of reach of children.
- Take care in feeding solid table food to give very small pieces.
- Do not use beanbag toys or allow child to play with dried beans.
- See also under Age 4 to 7 Months.

Bodily Damage
- See under Age 4 to 7 Months.
- Avoid placing televisions or other large objects on top of furniture, which may be overturned when infant pulls self to standing position.

Falls
- Avoid walkers, especially near stairs.*
- Ensure that furniture is sturdy enough for child to pull self to standing position and cruise.
- Fence stairways at top and bottom if child has access to either end.*
- Dress infant in safe shoes and clothing (soles that do not "catch" on floor, tied shoelaces, pant legs that do not touch floor).

Suffocation and Drowning
- Keep doors of ovens, dishwashers, refrigerators, coolers, and front-loading clothes washers and dryers closed at all times.
- If storing an unused large appliance, such as a refrigerator, remove the door.
- Supervise contact with inflated balloons; immediately discard popped balloons, and keep uninflated balloons out of reach.
- Fence swimming pools and other bodies of standing water such as decorative fountains; lock gate to swimming pools so only adult can access.
- Always supervise when near any source of water, such as cleaning buckets, drainage areas, ponds, toilets.
- Keep bathroom doors closed.
- Eliminate unnecessary pools of water.
- Keep one hand on child at all times when in bathtub.

Poisoning
- Administer medications as a drug, not as a candy.
- Do not administer medications unless prescribed by a practitioner.
- Return medications and poisons to safe storage area immediately after use; replace caps properly if a child-protector cap is used.
- Have poison control center number ([800] 222-1222) on telephone and refrigerator.

Burns
- Place guards in front of or around any heating appliance, fireplace, or furnace.
- Keep electrical wires hidden or out of reach.
- Place plastic guards over electrical outlets; place furniture in front of outlets.
- Keep hanging tablecloths out of reach (child may pull down hot liquids or heavy or sharp objects).

*Information on many items such as cribs or walkers is available from U.S. Consumer Product Safety Commission, (800) 638-2772; www.cpsc.gov/.
†See footnote on p. 899.

rear-facing infant-only seats as well. Although many infant restraints can be recliners, they are used in the car only in the position specified by the manufacturer.

Severe injuries and deaths in children have occurred from air bags deploying on impact in the front passenger seat. The back seat is the safest area of the car for children. For restraints to be effective, they must be used properly. Dressing the infant in an outfit with sleeves and legs allows the harness to hold the child securely in the seat. A small blanket or towel rolled tightly can be placed on either side of the head to minimize movement and keep the infant's hips against the back of the seat. Padding between the infant's legs and

crotch is added to prevent slouching. Thick, soft padding is not placed under the infant or behind the back because during the impact, the padding will compress, leaving the harness straps loose. Preterm infants being discharged home from the hospital should be placed in an appropriate car seat restraint as it would be placed in the car, and the infant's heart rate and oxygen saturation are monitored for a minimum of 1 hour and maximum of 3 hours (depending on the length of the trip to the home) to detect any potential problems with airway occlusion. (See Community Focus, p. 708, for preterm infant restraint; for further discussion of car seat restraints, see Chapter 25.)

TABLE 31-2   COMMON INFANT INJURIES, ASSOCIATED RISK FACTORS, AND SAFETY PROMOTION

SAFE PAD	RISK FACTORS	SUGGESTED SAFETY INTERVENTIONS
S—Suffocation, Sleep position	Latex balloons	Avoid latex balloons except with close adult supervision.
	Plastic bags	Tie unused plastic bags in a knot and dispose of in a safe container.
	Bed surface (noninfant) such as sofa or adult bed	Avoid placing infants to sleep on sofas, soft bedding, or adult bed.
	Pillows	Avoid use of pillows for sleep.
	Soft cushions and blankets	Clear bedding of soft cushions and blankets.
	Prone sleeping	Place infant to sleep on back at all times.
A—Asphyxia, animal bites	Food items: cylindric items such as hot dogs, hard candy, peanuts, almonds	Cut hot dogs lengthwise; avoid hard candy in infants and toddlers. Infants should completely chew up each food item in mouth; do not feed more until item is swallowed.
	Toys: small toys such as Legos	As a general rule of thumb, if the toy fits into a toilet paper cardboard roll, it can be swallowed by a small child.
	Small objects: batteries, buttons, beads, dried beans, syringe caps, safety pins	Keep out of reach of infants, who are naturally inquisitive.
	Pacifiers	Pacifiers should be one piece.
	Baby (talc) powder	Avoid shaking powder over infant; if used, place on adult's hand and then place on infant's skin.
	Domestic dogs, cats	Supervise child around domestic animals; teach not to approach dog that is eating, has puppies, or is not feeling well. Animals that are "tame" can be unpredictable. Small children are the right size for most domesticated animals to come face to face. Closely supervise child around visiting pets. (See Pet and Wild Animal Bites, Chapter 47.)
F—Falls	Stairs	Infants like to climb; place childproof gate at top and bottom of stairs.
	Diaper changing table	Infants do not have depth perception and cannot perceive a dangerous height from one that is safe. Never leave infants unattended on a flat surface, even if not rolling over.
	Crib, bed-crib sides can fall when infant leans on them	In 2011, a mandate was made to stop selling drop-side infant cribs.*
	Infant carriers	Never leave infant unattended in a carrier on top of a surface such as a shopping cart, clothes dryer, washer, kitchen cabinet; place carrier on floor.
	Car seat restraints	Secure infant in car seat restraint and never leave unattended if unrestrained.
	High chair	Restrain infant in high chair; avoid using high chair except for feeding and only if adult supervision is adequate; even restrained infants can squirm out of some restraints and fall.
	Infant walkers	Use only stationary walkers. There is no evidence that walkers help infants "walk" any sooner. Wheeled walkers can easily be propelled off stairs and other platforms such as porches or decks, causing significant injury.
	Windows, screens	Avoid placing furniture next to a window. Infants learn to climb and can fall out of open windows, even with screens.
	Television, stereos, sound systems	These must be secured to the stand; infants can pull the stand over, causing the TV or sound system to land on their heads, causing significant injury.
E—Electrical burns or burns	Electrical outlets	Place safety cap over electrical outlets; infants may be burned by placing conductive object into outlet.
	Hot hair combs, curlers	Keep out of reach of infant and keep turned off when not in use.
	Water	Infants may turn on tap or faucet in bathtub and burn self. Lower the water heater to a safe temperature of 49° C (120° F). Before placing infant in tub, check temperature of water and completely turn off faucet so child cannot alter temperature of water. NEVER leave infant unattended in tub or sink of water.
	Fireplace	Place a childproof screen in front of fireplace.
	Stove, hot liquids	Keep top front burners off and keep pot handles turned toward back to avoid infant pulling hot pot onto self and causing burn injuries.
	Cigarettes	Avoid smoking and holding infant on lap while smoking cigar or cigarette.

TABLE 31-2	COMMON INFANT INJURIES, ASSOCIATED RISK FACTORS, AND SAFETY PROMOTION—cont'd	
SAFE PAD	**RISK FACTORS**	**SUGGESTED SAFETY INTERVENTIONS**
P—Poisoning, ingestions	Medication, ointments, cream, lotions	Medications left in purses or handbags or on a table top can often be ingested by the curious infant. Keep Poison Control Center number readily available ([800]-222-1222).
	Plants: household plants may be a source of accidental poisoning	Keep plants out of child's reach.
	Cleaning solutions	Store in locked cabinet or in top cabinet where there are no drawers or shelves for infant to climb on. Avoid storing cleaning and caustic solutions in containers such as a soda bottle or jar—infants and toddlers cannot differentiate a soda from a caustic drain cleaner.
	Inhalation or oral or nasal ingestion of poisonous or harmful chemicals such as methamphetamine, gasoline, turpentine	Keep gasoline and turpentine stored in a locked cabinet or closet out of child's reach. Avoid storing in containers that are also used to keep drinks or food.
A—Automobile safety	Car or truck and hot weather	An automobile-related hazard for infants is overheating (hyperthermia) and subsequent death when left in a vehicle in hot weather (>26.4° C [80° F]). Infants dissipate heat poorly, and an increase in body temperature may cause death in a few hours. Caution parents against leaving infants in a vehicle alone for *any reason*.
	Air bags	Avoid placing infant in a car restraint behind an air bag. Deactivate the air bag (available in certain models) or place the infant in the back seat in a proper car seat restraint.
	Car seat restraint	See discussion on p. 899.
D—Drowning	Bath tub	NEVER leave infant unattended in tub or sink of water.
	Swimming pools, bird baths, decorative ponds of water, splash pads	Place fence around pools with gate lock that is out of child's reach. Supervise infants in water at ALL times; an infant may drown in as little as 2 inches of water. Swimming lessons are encouraged but are not foolproof for drowning if infant or child hits head on hard object and becomes unconscious as falling into the water.
	5-gal buckets	Keep 5-gal buckets empty of water or elevated out of child's reach.

*A number of parent education pamphlets—such as Crib Safety Tips and Is Your Used Crib Safe?—are available in English and Spanish from the U.S. Consumer Product Safety Commission, 4330 East West Highway, Bethesda, MD 20814; (800) 638-2772; www.cpsc.gov/.

! NURSING ALERT

Rear-facing infant safety seats must not be placed in the front seats of cars equipped with an air bag on the passenger side. If an infant safety seat is placed in the passenger seat with an air bag, the child could be seriously injured if the air bag is released, since rear-facing infant seats extend closer to the dashboard.

Another automobile-related hazard for infants is *overheating* (hyperthermia) and subsequent death when left in a vehicle in hot weather (over 26.4° C [80° F]). Infants dissipate heat poorly, and an increase in body temperature may cause death in a few hours. Parents are cautioned against leaving infants in a vehicle alone for *any reason*. A small sign or placard has been designed to hang in the rear-view mirror to remind the parent that there is a child in the back seat. Busy parents may forget the child in the back when preoccupied with errands, children's school and extracurricular activities, and busy work schedules.

Nurse's Role in Injury Prevention

The task of injury prevention begins to be appreciated only when the potential environmental dangers to which infants are vulnerable are considered. Injury prevention and parent education should be handled on a growth and developmental basis. It is simply impossible to completely protect infants and small children from all potential dangers without placing them in a sterile, impractical environment. However, a large percentage of childhood deaths continue to occur as a result of *preventable* injuries (Martin, Kochanek, Strobino, et al., 2005; Schnitzer, 2006). Nurses must be aware of the possible causes of injury in each age-group to provide anticipatory, preventive teaching. For example, the nurse should discuss guidelines for injury prevention during infancy (see Box 31-1) before the child reaches the susceptible age-group. Preventive teaching ideally begins during pregnancy.

One third of all injuries to children occur in the home, and therefore the importance of safety cannot be overemphasized. The Patient Teaching box summarizes a home safety checklist that can be presented to parents to increase their awareness of danger areas in the home and assist them in implementing safety devices and practices *before* their absence can inflict injury on infants. Hands-on displays such as cabinet latches or toilet seat locks can familiarize parents with inexpensive, commercial devices that can be used in the home to prevent injuries.

Injury prevention requires protection of the child and education of the caregiver. Nurses in ambulatory care settings, health maintenance centers, and visiting nurse agencies are in a most favorable position for injury education. This does not exclude nurses in inpatient facilities, who could use visiting times as an excellent opportunity for discussing this topic. Although early discharge after birth may be restrictive for parent teaching, this is an excellent opportunity to introduce the family to infant safety and safety for other

PATIENT TEACHING

Child Home Safety Checklist

Safety: Fire, Electrical, Burns
- Guards in front of or around any heating appliance, fireplace, or furnace (including floor furnace)*
- Electrical wires hidden or out of reach*
- No frayed or broken wires; no overloaded sockets
- Plastic guards or caps over electrical outlets; furniture in front of outlets*
- Hanging tablecloths out of reach, away from open fires*
- Smoke detectors tested and operating properly
- Kitchen matches stored out of child's reach*
- Large, deep ashtrays throughout house (if used)
- Small stoves, heaters, and other hot objects (cigarettes, candles, coffee pots, slow cookers) placed where they cannot be tipped over or reached by children
- Hot water heater set at 49° C (120° F) or lower
- Pot handles turned toward back of stove, center of table
- No loose clothing worn near stove
- No cooking or eating hot foods or liquids with child standing nearby or sitting in lap
- All small appliances, such as iron, turned off, disconnected, and placed out of reach when not in use
- Cool, not hot, mist vaporizer if used
- Fire extinguisher available on each floor and checked periodically
- Electrical fuse box and gas shutoff accessible
- Family escape plan in case of a fire practiced periodically; fire escape ladder available on upper-level floors
- Telephone number of fire or rescue squad and address of home with nearest cross street posted near phone

Safety: Suffocation and Aspiration
- Small objects stored out of reach*
- Toys inspected for small removable parts or long strings*
- Hanging crib toys and mobiles placed out of reach
- Plastic bags stored away from young child's reach; large plastic garment bags discarded after tying in knots*
- Mattress or pillow not covered with plastic or in manner accessible to child*
- Crib design according to federal regulations (crib slats less than 2.375 inches [6 cm] apart) with snug-fitting mattress*†
- Crib positioned away from other furniture or windows*
- Portable play yard gates up at all times while in use*
- Accordion-style gates not used*
- Bathroom doors kept closed and toilet lids down*
- Faucets turned off firmly*
- Pool fenced with locked gate
- Proper safety equipment at poolside
- Electronic garage door openers stored safely and garage door adjusted to rise when door strikes object
- Doors of ovens, trunks, dishwashers, refrigerators, and front-loading clothes washers and dryers kept closed*
- Unused appliance, such as a refrigerator, securely closed with lock or doors removed*

- Food served in small, non-cylindric pieces*
- Toy chests without lids or with lids that securely lock in open position*
- Buckets and wading pools kept empty when not in use*
- Clothesline above head level
- At least one member of household trained in basic life support (cardiopulmonary resuscitation), including first aid for choking

Safety: Poisoning
- Toxic substances, including batteries, placed on a high shelf, preferably in locked cabinet
- Toxic plants hung or placed out of reach*
- Excess quantities of cleaning fluid, paints, pesticides, drugs, and other toxic substances not stored in home
- Used containers of poisonous substances discarded where child cannot obtain access
- Telephone number of local poison control center ([800] 222-1222) and home address with nearest cross street posted near phone
- Medicines clearly labeled in childproof containers and stored out of reach
- Household cleaners, disinfectants, and insecticides kept in their original containers, separate from food and out of reach
- Smoking in areas away from children

Safety: Falls
- Nonskid mats, strips, or surfaces in tubs and showers
- Exits, halls, and passageways in rooms kept clear of toys, furniture, boxes, or other items that could be obstructive
- Stairs and halls well lighted, with switches at both top and bottom
- Sturdy handrails for all steps and stairways
- Nothing stored on stairways
- Treads, risers, and carpeting in good repair
- Glass doors and walls marked with decals
- Safety glass used in doors, windows, and on walls
- Gates on top and bottom of staircases and elevated areas, such as porch, fire escape*
- Guardrails on upstairs windows with locks that limit height of window opening and access to areas such as fire escape*
- Crib side rails raised to full height; mattress lowered as child grows*
- Restraints used in high chairs, walkers, or other baby furniture; preferably walkers not used*
- Scatter rugs secured in place or used with nonskid backing
- Walks, patios, and driveways in good repair

Safety: Bodily Injury
- Knives, power tools, and unloaded firearms stored safely or placed in locked cabinet
- Garden tools returned to storage racks after use
- Pets properly restrained and immunized for rabies
- Swings, slides, and other outdoor play equipment kept in safe condition
- Yard free of broken glass, nail-studded boards, other litter
- Cement birdbaths placed where young child cannot tip them over*
- Furniture anchored so child cannot pull down on top of self when climbing or pulling to stand

*Safety measures are specific for homes with young children. All safety measures should be implemented in homes where children reside and visit frequently, such as those of grandparents or baby-sitters.

†Federal regulations are available from U.S. Consumer Product Safety Commission, (800) 638–2772; www.cpsc.gov.

children as well. Parents should be encouraged to take an infant cardiopulmonary resuscitation (CPR) class to deal effectively with potential problems. This tool further empowers the parents to raise their new infant in the best environment possible.

One approach to teaching injury prevention is to relate why children in various age-groups are prone to specific types of injuries. Stressing prevention is just as important as emphasizing the *why* of the injury. However, injury prevention must also be practical. Asking parents for their ideas leads to realistic suggestions that can be followed. For instance, bathroom cleaning agents, cosmetics, and personal care items can be placed on a top shelf in the linen closet and towels or sheets can be stored on the lower shelves and floor.

If an injury has occurred, the nurse should not be too quick to admonish the parent. Injuries do not always indicate neglect. It is a difficult task to watch children carefully without overprotecting or unnecessarily confining them. Allowing children to explore while maintaining consistent, age-appropriate limits is sound advice.

Parents need to remember that infants and young children cannot anticipate danger or understand when it is or is not present. Also, infants have no cognitive concept of cause and effect and therefore cannot relate meaning to experiences or potential dangers. A dead electrical wire may present no actual harm, but if the child is allowed to play with it, a poor behavior is enforced and will be practiced when the child encounters a live wire. Although it is always wise to explain why something is dangerous, it must be remembered that small children need to be physically removed from the situation.

It is not easy to teach safety, supervise closely, and refrain from saying "no" a hundred times a day. Parents become acutely aware of this dilemma as soon as the infant learns to crawl. Preventing injuries to children is usually the first reason for limit setting and discipline, but limits are also set to prevent damage to valuable household objects. When small children are in the home, dangerous objects must be removed or guarded and valuable articles placed out of reach.

When children are taught the meaning of "no," they should also be taught what "yes" means. Children should be praised for playing with suitable toys, their efforts at behaving or listening should be reinforced, and innovative and creative recreational toys should be provided for them. Infants love to tear paper and avidly pursue books, magazines, or newspapers left on the floor. Instead of always scolding them for destroying a valued book, parents should provide child-safe books (e.g., those constructed of fabric) for them to play with. If they enjoy pots and pans, a cabinet can be arranged with safe utensils for them to explore.

One additional factor must be stressed concerning injury prevention and education. Children are imitators; they copy what they see and hear. *Practicing safety teaches safety,* which applies to parents and their children and to nurses and their patients. Saying one thing but doing another confuses children and can lead to difficulties as the child grows older.

Anticipatory Guidance—Care of Families

Childrearing is no easy task; it presents challenges to both new and "seasoned" parents. Society's changing roles and mores, combined with a highly mobile population, leave little stability for traditional role models and time-honored methods of raising children. As a result, parents look to health care professionals for guidance. Nurses are in an advantageous position to render assistance and offer suggestions. Every phase of a child's life has its particular traumas—toilet training for toddlers, unexplained fears for preschoolers, and identity crises for adolescents. For parents of an infant, some

PATIENT TEACHING

Guidance During Infant's First Year

First 6 Months
- Teach car safety with use of federally approved restraint, facing rearward, in the middle of the back seat—not in a front seat with an air bag.
- Understand each parent's adjustment to the newborn, especially mother's emotional needs after birth.
- Teach care of infant and help parents understand his or her individual needs and temperament and that the infant expresses wants through crying.
- Reassure parents that infant cannot be spoiled by too much attention during the first 4 to 6 months.
- Encourage parents to establish a schedule that meets needs of child and themselves.
- Help parents understand infant's need for stimulation in environment.
- Support parents' pleasure in seeing child's growing friendliness and social response, especially smiling.
- Plan anticipatory guidance for safety.
- Stress need for routine childhood immunizations.
- Prepare for introduction of solid foods.

Second 6 Months
- Prepare parents for child's "stranger anxiety."
- Encourage parents to allow child to cling to them and avoid long separation from either.
- Guide parents concerning discipline because of infant's increasing mobility.
- Encourage use of negative voice and eye contact rather than physical punishment as a means of discipline.
- Encourage showing most attention when infant is behaving well, rather than when infant is crying.
- Teach injury prevention because of child's advancing motor skills and curiosity.
- Encourage parents to leave child with suitable caregiver to allow some free time.
- Discuss readiness for weaning (as desired).
- Explore parents' feelings regarding infant's sleep patterns.

challenges center around dependency, discipline, increased mobility, and safety. Major areas for parental guidance during the first year are listed in the Patient Teaching box.

SPECIAL HEALTH PROBLEMS

Colic (Paroxysmal Abdominal Pain)

Colic is reported to occur in 15% to 40% of all infants (Morin, 2009b), yet it has no particular affinity in regard to the sex, race, or socioeconomic status (Ellett, 2003). An organic cause may be identified in fewer than 5% of infants seen by physicians because of excessive crying (Roberts, Ostapchuk, and O'Brien, 2004). The condition is generally described as abdominal pain or cramping that is manifested by loud crying and drawing the legs up to the abdomen. Other definitions include variables such as duration of cry greater than 3 hours a day occurring more than 3 days per week and for more than 3 weeks and parental dissatisfaction with the child's behavior. Some studies report an increase in symptoms (fussiness and crying) in the late afternoon or evening (Morin, 2009b); however, in some infants, the onset of symptoms occurs at another time. Colic is more common in infants younger than 3 months than in older infants, and infants with difficult temperaments are more likely to be colicky.

Despite the obvious behavioral indications of pain, the infant with colic gains weight and usually thrives. There is no evidence of a residual effect of colic on older children except perhaps a strained parent-child relationship in some cases. In other words, infants who are colicky grow up to be normal children and adults. Colic is self-limiting and in most cases resolves as infants mature, generally around 12 to 16 weeks of age (Lobo, Kotzer, Keefe, et al., 2004; O'Connor, 2009).

Among the theories investigated as potential causes are too rapid feeding, overeating, swallowing excessive air, improper feeding technique (especially in positioning and burping), and emotional stress or tension between the parent and child. Although all of these may occur, there is no evidence that one factor is consistently present. Infants with cow's milk allergy (CMA) symptoms have a high rate of colic (44%), and eliminating cow's milk products from the infant's diet can reduce the symptoms. However, there is considerable controversy about the role of allergy and colic because there does not appear to be an increased incidence of atopy in infants with colic (Sicherer, 2003).

Keefe, Lobo, Froese-Fretz, et al. (2006) propose that colic has origins in the infant's inability to self-regulate the sleep-wake cycles based on central nervous system (CNS) immaturity rather than gastrointestinal (GI) system dysfunction. These researchers implemented a home-based intervention program aimed at promoting infant state regulation (sleep-wake cycles), promoting synchrony between parent and child, providing parental support, and decreasing infant irritability. The results of the study found that infants in the treatment group cried 1.7 hours less per day than infants in the control group. In addition, families in both the treatment and control group reported benefitting from a nurse visiting in the home and listening to parents' concerns about the infant's and the family's well-being.

Parental smoking, strained parent-infant interaction, lactase deficiency, difficult infant temperament, difficulty regulating emotions, overstimulation, CNS immaturity, and neurochemical dysregulation in the brain have also been proposed as potential causes of colic (Ellett, 2003; Neu and Robinson, 2003). A positive association between consumption of fruit juices (carbohydrate malabsorption) and colic has been demonstrated in some cases (Duro, Rising, Cedillo, et al., 2002). Some experts have suggested that gastroesophageal reflux is a cause of colic, but studies have not supported this theory (St. James-Roberts, 2008). The consensus of many experts who study colic is that it is multifactorial and that no single treatment for every colicky infant will be effective in alleviating the symptoms. Some researchers have found an association between colic in infancy and later childhood physical conditions such as abdominal pain and allergic disorders; however, causality was not confirmed in this group of children (Savino, Castagno, Bretto, et al., 2005).

Therapeutic Management

Management of colic should begin with an investigation of possible organic causes, such as CMA, intussusception, or other GI problem. If a sensitivity to cow's milk is strongly suspected, a trial substitution of another formula such as an extensively hydrolyzed (Nutramigen, Alimentum, Pregestimil), whey hydrolysate, or amino acid (Neocate, EleCare) formula is warranted. Soy formulas are usually avoided because of the possibility of sensitivity to soy protein as well (AAP, 2009). Oral administration of *Lactobacillus reuteri* to colicky exclusively breastfed infants decreased crying symptoms to less than 3

hours per day within 21 days of initiation in a randomized, double-blind, placebo-controlled trial of 50 colicky infants (Savino, Cordisco, Tarasco, et al., 2010). Savino, Palumeri, Castagno, et al. (2006) found that infants fed a partially hydrolyzed whey protein formula supplemented with oligosaccharides had decreased crying time after 7 days when compared with infants fed a standard formula and simethicone.

When no specific inciting agent can be found, the supportive measures discussed under Care Management are used.

The use of drugs, including sedatives, antispasmodics, antihistamines, and antiflatulents, is sometimes recommended. The most commonly used sedatives are phenobarbital, hydroxyzine hydrochloride (Atarax), and chloral hydrate. Simethicone (Mylicon) may also help allay the symptoms of colic. However, in most controlled studies, none of these drugs completely reduced the symptoms of colic. Behavioral interventions have not proved effective at reducing the symptoms of colic but have helped parents deal with their crying infants in a more positive manner. The addition of lactase to infant formula has produced mixed results as far as abatement of overall symptoms.

An extensive review of a wide variety of interventions for colic indicates no specific safe remedies are available to alleviate symptoms of colic in every infant. Dietary changes, such as eliminating cow's milk protein from the lactating mother's diet, and behavioral interventions were shown to be effective in helping parents reduce stimulation and respond to the infant's crying, yet these interventions are perceived only as moderately effective (Joanna Briggs Institute, 2008). Administering sucrose was effective at reducing crying in colicky infants for a short period (3-30 minutes) (Joanna Briggs Institute, 2008). A recent position statement by the Canadian Paediatric Society, Nutrition and Gastroenterology Committee (Critch, 2011) concluded that dietary modifications are beneficial in some cases but not all; the use of lactate, probiotics, prebiotics, or soy formula independently to decrease symptoms of colic had insufficient evidence to support their use. The use of complementary medicines for infantile colic, namely fennel extract, herbal tea, and sugar solutions, reportedly lack sufficient evidence to recommend their use (Perry, Hunt, and Ernst, 2011).

Another study found that a combination of interventions—massage, herbal tea, sucrose solution, and hydrolyzed formula—decreased crying in reported colicky infants; the administration of the hydrolyzed formula achieved best results, whereas massage was least effective at reducing crying (Arikan, Alp, Gozum, et al., 2008).

CARE MANAGEMENT

The initial step in managing colic is to take a thorough, detailed history of the usual daily events. Areas that should be stressed include (1) the infant's diet; (2) the diet of the breastfeeding mother; (3) the time of day when crying occurs; (4) the relationship of crying to feeding time; (5) the presence of specific family members during crying and habits of family members, such as smoking; (6) activity of the mother or usual caregiver before, during, and after crying; (7) characteristics of the cry (duration, intensity); (8) measures used to relieve crying and their effectiveness; and (9) the infant's stooling, voiding, and sleeping patterns. Of special emphasis is a careful assessment of the feeding process via demonstration by the parent.

If cow's milk sensitivity is suspected, breastfeeding mothers should follow a milk-free diet for a minimum of 3 to 5 days in an attempt to reduce the infant's symptoms. Caution mothers that some nondairy creamers may contain calcium caseinate, a cow's

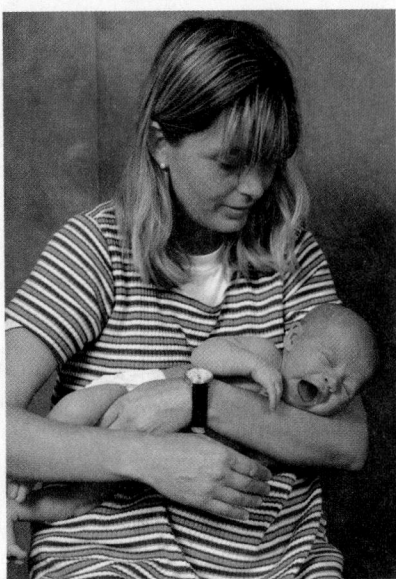

FIG 31-14 The "colic carry" may be comforting to an infant with colic. (Photo by Paul Vincent Kuntz, Texas Children's Hospital, Houston, TX.)

milk protein. If a milk-free diet is helpful, lactating mothers may need calcium supplements to meet the body's requirement. Bottle-fed infants may improve with the same dietary modifications as for infants with CMA. Additional approaches for managing colic are listed in the Patient Teaching box (see also Fig. 31-14).

One important nursing intervention (before or after an organic cause has been eliminated) is reassuring both parents that they are not doing anything wrong and that the infant is not experiencing any physical or emotional harm. Parents, especially mothers, become easily frustrated with their infant's crying and perceive this as a sign that something is horribly wrong. In addition, colicky infants may be at increased risk for being shaken or otherwise abused by their caregivers and experiencing traumatic brain injury. A survey of fathers of colicky infants revealed that professional assistance was limited. The fathers described the experience of having a colicky infant as similar to falling into an abyss from which they had to climb with the assistance of family and friends, thus reinforcing the importance of empathetic nurses (Ellett, Appleton, and Sloan, 2009). An empathetic, gentle, and reassuring attitude, in addition to suggestions for treatment, will help allay parents' anxieties, which are usually exacerbated by loss of sleep and preoccupation over the infant's welfare. Colic disappears spontaneously, usually by 3 to 4 months of age, although guarantees should never be given since it may continue for much longer. Other support persons and extended family members may be enlisted to support the parents during this difficult time.

Failure to Thrive (Growth Failure)

Failure to thrive (FTT), or growth failure, is a sign of inadequate growth resulting from an inability to obtain or use calories required for growth. FTT has no universal definition, although one of the more common criteria is a weight (and sometimes height) that falls below the 5th percentile for the child's age. Another definition of FTT includes a weight for age (height) z value of less than -2.0 (a z value is a standard deviation value that represents anthropometric data normalizing for sex and age with greater precision than growth percentile curves [Markowitz, Watkins, and Duggan, 2008]). A third

way to define FTT is a weight curve that crosses more than 2 percentile lines on a standardized growth chart after previous achievement of a stable growth pattern. Weight for length is reported to be a better indicator of acute undernutrition (Cole and Lanham, 2011). Growth measurements alone are not used to diagnose children with FTT. Rather, the finding of a pattern of persistent deviation from established growth parameters is cause for concern. In addition to lack of consensus on the precise definition of FTT, some advocate for a change in terminology; thus terms such as *growth failure*, *growth faltering*, and *pediatric undernutrition* are used in the literature for FTT (Locklin, 2005). The term *FTT* will be used in the following discussion. According to Cole and Lanham (2011), approximately 5% to 10% of children in primary care in the United States have FTT, with the majority presenting before the age of 18 months.

Some experts suggest that the previously used classifications of *organic FTT* and *nonorganic FTT* are too simplistic because most cases of growth failure have mixed causes; they suggest that FTT be classified according to pathophysiology in the categories in Box 31-2.

The cause of FTT is often multifactorial and involves a combination of infant organic disease, dysfunctional parenting behaviors, subtle neurologic or behavioral problems, and disturbed parent-child interactions (Block, Krebs, and AAP Committee on Child Abuse and Neglect and Committee on Nutrition, 2005). However, the primary etiology is inadequate caloric intake, regardless of the cause.

BOX 31-2   **PATHOPHYSIOLOGIC CAUSES OF FAILURE TO THRIVE**

Inadequate caloric intake—Incorrect formula preparation, neglect, food fads, excessive juice consumption, poverty, breastfeeding problems, behavioral problems affecting eating, or central nervous system problems affecting intake

Inadequate absorption—Cystic fibrosis, celiac disease, vitamin or mineral deficiencies, HIV infection, biliary atresia, or hepatic disease

Increased metabolism—Hyperthyroidism, congenital heart disease, or chronic immunodeficiency

Defective utilization—Genetic anomaly such as trisomy 21 or 18, chronic infection, or metabolic storage diseases

Adapted from Krugman SD, Dubowitz H: Failure to thrive, *Am Fam Physician* 68(5):879–886, 2003.

Infants who are born preterm and with very low birth weight (VLBW) or extremely low birth weight (ELBW), as well as those with intrauterine growth restriction (IUGR), are often referred for FTT within the first 2 years of life because they typically do not grow physically at the same rate as term cohorts even after discharge from the acute care facility. Catch-up growth has been shown to be much more difficult to achieve in ELBW and VLBW infants. As children, former VLBW and ELBW infants are more likely to have small stature and demonstrate lower cognitive and academic achievement scores than term cohorts (Casey, Whiteside-Mansell, Barrett, et al., 2006). Children with congenital heart disease are also more likely to develop FTT in infancy as a result of inadequate caloric intake, malabsorption, increased energy expenditure that superseded caloric intake, and pulmonary hypertension (Cook and Higgins, 2010).

Other factors that can lead to inadequate caloric intake in infancy include poverty, health or childrearing beliefs such as fad diets, child neglect, inadequate nutritional knowledge, family stress, feeding resistance, and insufficient breast milk intake. In infants younger than 8 weeks, breastfeeding problems as a result of inadequate latch or uncoordinated sucking and swallowing may occur (Cole and Lanham, 2011). One account reports a 6-month-old term infant with FTT as a result of severe ankyloglossia (tongue tie) (Forlenza, Paradise Black, McNamara, et al., 2010).

Diagnostic Evaluation

Diagnosis is initially made from evidence of FTT. If FTT is recent, the weight but not the height is below accepted standards (usually the 5th percentile); if FTT is longstanding, both weight and height are low, indicating chronic malnutrition. The use of weight velocities (according to the World Health Organization growth charts at http://www.who.int/childgrowth/standards/en/ may be a better indicator of short-term growth failure while considering age-dependent changes in growth (Cole and Lanham, 2011). Perhaps as important as anthropometric measurements are a complete health and dietary history (including perinatal history), physical examination for evidence of organic causes, developmental assessment, and family assessment. A dietary intake history, either a 24-hour food intake or a history of food consumed over a 3- to 5-day period, is also essential. In addition, explore the child's activity level, parental height, perceived food allergies, and dietary restrictions. An assessment of household organization and mealtime behaviors and rituals is important in the collection of pertinent data. It is often helpful to obtain the growth patterns of the affected child's parents and siblings; these can be compared with norm-referenced standards to evaluate the child's growth (Markowitz, Watkins, and Duggan, 2008). An assessment of the home environment and child-parent interaction may be helpful as well. Other tests (lead toxicity, anemia, stool-reducing substances, occult blood, ova and parasites, alkaline phosphatase, and zinc levels) are selected only as indicated to rule out organic problems. In most cases, laboratory studies are of little diagnostic value (AAP, 2009; Cole and Lanham, 2011). To prevent the overuse of diagnostic procedures, consider FTT early in the differential diagnosis. To avoid the social stigma of FTT during the early investigative phase, some health care workers use the term *growth delay* (or *failure*) until the actual cause is established.

Therapeutic Management

The primary management of FTT is aimed at reversing the cause of the growth failure. If malnutrition is severe, the initial treatment is directed at reversing the malnutrition while avoiding the refeeding syndrome. The goal is to provide sufficient calories to support "catch-up" growth—a rate of growth greater than the expected rate for age.

In addition to adding caloric density to feedings, the child may require multivitamin supplements and dietary supplementation with high-calorie foods and drinks. Any coexisting medical problems are treated.

In most cases of FTT, an interdisciplinary team of physician, nurse, dietitian, child life specialist, occupational therapist, pediatric feeding specialist, and social worker or mental health professional is needed to deal with the multiple problems. Make efforts to relieve any additional stresses on the family by offering referrals to welfare agencies or supplemental food programs. In some cases, family therapy may be required. Temporary placement in a foster home may relieve the family's stress, protect the child, and allow the child some stability if insurmountable obstacles are preventing appropriate family function. Behavior modification aimed at mealtime rituals (or lack thereof) and family social time may be required. Hospitalization admission is indicated for (1) evidence (anthropometric) of severe acute malnutrition, (2) child abuse or neglect, (3) significant dehydration, (4) caregiver substance abuse or psychosis, (5) outpatient management that does not result in weight gain, and (6) serious intercurrent infection (AAP, 2009; Block, Krebs, and AAP Committee on Child Abuse and Neglect and Committee on Nutrition, 2005).

Prognosis. The prognosis for children with FTT is related to the cause. If the parents have simply not understood the infant's needs, teaching may remedy the child's limited caloric intake and permanently reverse the growth failure. Inadequate or infrequent feeding periods by the infant's primary caregiver, in conjunction with family disorganization, are often observed to be the cause of FTT.

Few long-term studies provide data on the prognosis for children with FTT; however, some studies indicate that children who had FTT as infants had shorter heights, lower weights, and lower scores on measures of psychomotor development than peers (Black, Dubowitz, Krishnakumar, et al., 2007; Rudolf and Logan, 2005). Low-birth-weight preterm infants are also at high risk for faltering growth and cognitive delays as a result of poor growth (Cole and Lanham, 2011). Factors related to poor prognosis are severe feeding resistance, lack of awareness in and cooperation from the parent(s), low family income, low maternal educational level, adolescent mother, preterm birth, IUGR, and early age of onset of FTT. Because later cognitive and motor function are affected by malnourishment

- Growth failure (see p. 907 for definitions)
- Developmental delays—social, motor, adaptive, language
- Undernutrition
- Apathy
- Withdrawn behavior
- Feeding or eating disorders, such as vomiting, feeding resistance, anorexia, pica, rumination
- No fear of strangers (at age when stranger anxiety is normal)
- Avoidance of eye contact
- Wide-eyed gaze and continual scan of the environment ("radar gaze")
- Stiff and unyielding or flaccid and unresponsive
- Minimal smiling

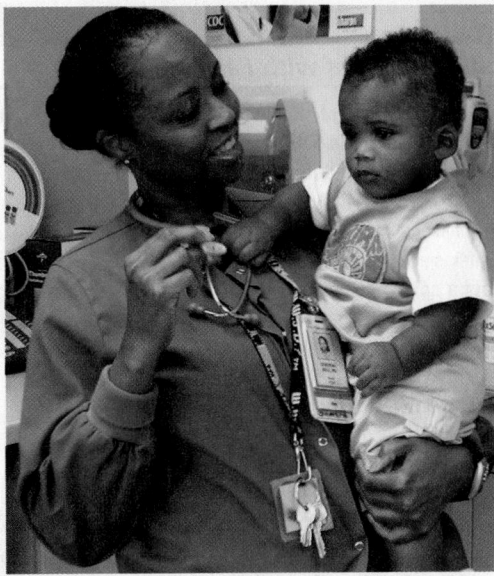

FIG 31-15 Consistent nursing contact is important in developing trust in infants with failure to thrive.

in infancy, many of these children are below normal in intellectual development, have poorer language development and less well-developed reading skills, attain lower social maturity, and have a higher incidence of behavioral disturbances (Markowitz, Watkins, and Duggan, 2008). Such findings indicate that a long-term plan and follow-up care are needed for the optimal development of these children.

CARE MANAGEMENT

Nurses play a critical role as part of the interdisciplinary team in the diagnosis of FTT through their assessment of the child, parents, and family interactions. Knowledge of the characteristics of children with FTT and their families is essential in helping identify these children and hastening the confirmation of a diagnosis (Box 31-3). Accurate assessment of initial weight and height and daily weight, as well as recording of all food intake, is imperative. The nurse documents the child's feeding behavior and the parent-child interaction during feeding, other caregiving activities, and play.

Besides showing signs of malnutrition and delayed social development, children with FTT may exhibit altered behavioral interactions. They may display intense interest in inanimate objects, such as toys, but much less interest in social interactions. They are often watchful of people at a distance but become increasingly distressed as others come closer. They may dislike being touched or held and avoid face-to-face contact. However, when held, they protest briefly on being put down and are apathetic when left alone.

Children with FTT may have a history of difficult feeding, vomiting, sleep disturbance, and excessive irritability. Patterns such as crying during feedings; vomiting; hoarding food in the mouth; ruminating after feeding; refusing to switch from liquids to solids; and displaying aversion behavior, such as turning from food or spitting food, become attention-seeking mechanisms to prolong the attention received at mealtime. In some cases, the child may use feeding as a control mechanism in a poorly organized or chaotic family situation; parents may allow the child to dictate the norms for behavior and feeding because of inexperience with parenting or poor parenting role models. Thus refusing to eat or eating only sweets and snacks with nonnutritive value may be the child's norm based on food availability and family tradition. In such cases, family therapy is essential to reverse the trend and assist the parents and child in understanding each others' roles.

Some parents are at increased risk for attachment problems because of (1) isolation and social crisis; (2) inadequate support systems, such as teenage and single mothers; and (3) poor parenting

role models as a child. Other factors that should be considered are lack of education; physical and mental health problems such as physical and sexual abuse, depression, or drug dependence; immaturity, especially in adolescent parents; and lack of commitment to parenting, such as giving priority to entertainment or employment. Often these parents and their families are under stress and in multiple chronic emotional, social, and financial crises.

Because part of the difficulty between parent and child is dissatisfaction and frustration, the child should have a primary core of nurses (Fig. 31-15). The nurses caring for the child can learn to perceive the child's cues and reverse the cycle of dissatisfaction, especially in the area of feeding.

Because many of these children are responding to stimuli that have led to the negative feeding patterns, an important primary intervention is to structure the feeding environment to encourage healthful eating. Initially, staff members and a feeding specialist may need to feed these children to thoroughly assess the difficulties encountered during the feeding process and to devise strategies that eliminate or minimize such problems. General guidelines for the feeding process are outlined in the Guidelines box.

Four primary goals in the nutritional management of children with FTT are to (1) correct nutritional deficiencies and achieve ideal weight for height, (2) provided adequate calories for catch-up growth, (3) restore optimal body composition, and (4) educate the parents or primary caregivers regarding the child's nutritional requirements and appropriate feeding methods (Corrales and Utter, 2005; Maggioni and Lifshitz, 1995). For infants, 24 kcal/oz formulas may be provided to increase caloric intake; older children (1 to 6 years) may benefit from a 30-kcal/oz formula (AAP, 2009). Other carbohydrate additives include fortified rice cereal and vegetable oil. Because vitamin and mineral deficiencies may occur, multivitamin supplementation, including zinc and iron, is recommended. For toddlers, a high-calorie milk drink such as PediaSure may be used to increase caloric intake. Carefully monitor for signs of intolerance to the formula.

Because maladaptive feeding practices often contribute to growth failure, give parents specific step-by-step directions for formula preparation, as well as a written schedule of feeding times. Restrict

GUIDELINES

Feeding the Child with Failure to Thrive

Provide a primary core of staff to feed the child. The same nurses are able to learn the child's cues and respond consistently.

Provide a quiet, unstimulating atmosphere. A number of children with failure to thrive (FTT) are very distractible and their attention is diverted with minimal stimuli. Older children do well at a feeding table; bottle-fed infants and children should always be held.

Maintain a calm, even temperament throughout the meal. Negative outbursts may be commonplace in this child's habit formation. Limits on eating behavior definitely need to be provided, but they should be stated in a firm, calm tone. If the nurse is hurried or anxious, the feeding process will not be optimized.

Talk to the child by giving directions about eating. "Take a bite, Lisa" is appropriate and directive. The more distractible the child, the more directive the nurse should be to refocus attention on feeding. Positive comments about feeding are actively given.

Be persistent. This is perhaps one of the most important guidelines. Parents often give up when the child begins negative feeding behavior. Calm perseverance through 10 to 15 minutes of food refusal will eventually diminish negative behavior. Although forced feeding is avoided, "strictly encouraged" feeding is essential.

Maintain a face-to-face posture with the child when possible. Encourage eye contact and remain with the child throughout the meal.

Introduce new foods slowly. Often these children have been exclusively bottle-fed. If acceptance of solids is a problem, begin with pureed food and, after it is accepted, advance to junior and regular solid foods.

Follow the child's rhythm of feeding. The child will set a rhythm when the previous conditions are met.

Develop a structured routine. Disruption in other activities of daily living has great impact on feeding responses, so bathing, sleeping, dressing, playing, and feeding are structured. The nurse should feed the child in the same way and place as often as possible. The length of the feeding should also be established (usually 30 minutes).

---

juice intake in children with FTT until adequate weight gain has been achieved with appropriate milk sources; thereafter give no more than 4 oz/day of juice.

Behavior modification techniques may be used with older infants and toddlers to interrupt poor feeding patterns. Feeding times may actually involve "struggles of will" in cases of maladaptive feedings that result in FTT. These behaviors are different from the occasional toddler behavior of food refusal, which is primarily developmental, not pathologic. The association of appropriate food with good or bad behaviors and consequent rewards may be part of the complex problem. In severe cases of malnourishment, tube feedings or intravenous therapy may be required.

In addition to attending to the child's physical needs, the interdisciplinary team must plan care for appropriate developmental stimulation. After an approximate developmental age is established, a planned program of play is begun. Ideally, a child life specialist is involved to implement and supervise the stimulation program. Every effort is made to teach the parent how to play and interact with the child.

Nursing care of children with FTT involves a "family systems" approach. In other words, for the entire family to become healthy, each member must be helped to change. Care of the parents is aimed at helping them improve their self-esteem by acquiring positive, successful parenting skills. Initially, this necessitates providing an

environment in which they feel welcomed and accepted. Depending on the cause of FTT, many children are treated on an outpatient basis.

Sudden Infant Death Syndrome

Sudden infant death syndrome (SIDS) is defined as the sudden death of an infant younger than 1 year that remains unexplained after a complete postmortem examination, including an investigation of the death scene and a review of the case history. Since 1992, the incidence of SIDS in the United States has decreased by 53% to an all-time low of 0.57 per 1000 live births in 2002 (AAP Task Force on Sudden Infant Death Syndrome, 2005). The dramatic decrease is attributed to the Back to Sleep campaign.* SIDS is the third leading cause of infant deaths (birth to 12 months) and the leading cause of postneonatal deaths (between 1 and 12 months). SIDS claimed the lives of 2145 infants in the United States in 2006; preliminary data from 2011 indicate there were 1711 deaths from SIDS (Hoyert and Xu, 2012). For the years 2010 to 2011 infant mortality rates decreased by 16.1% for SIDS, whereas other causes of infant mortality remained static (Hoyert and Xu, 2012). Despite dramatic decreases in SIDS rates, rates for African-American, Native-American, and American-Alaskan infants remains disproportionately higher than for the rest of the population. In 2007, SIDS rates were 2.4 times higher for Native-American mothers and 1.9 times higher for African-American mothers compared with non-Hispanic Caucasian mothers (Mathews and MacDorman, 2011; Mathews and MacDorman, 2012). It is also important to note that overall infant death rates for 2006 and 2007 were significantly higher for African-American infants (13.59 per 1000 live births) than for Hispanic (5.59 per 1000 live births) and Caucasian (5.70 per 1000 live births) infants. Likewise, the percentage of infants born preterm (<37 weeks) was significantly higher (18.5%) in African-American women than Caucasian women (11.7%) (MacDorman and Mathews, 2011). Preterm births rank second as cause of infant death; this trend has been constant since the mid-1990s when the rates of SIDS deaths significantly decreased in the United States.

The SIDS rate remained fairly static between 1999 and 2001. This has been attributed to improved death scene investigation and determination of non-SIDS causes of postneonatal mortality. In addition, there is speculation that deaths attributed to SIDS during the period of 1992 to 2001 may have been a result of other causes (AAP Task Force on Sudden Infant Death Syndrome, 2005). Table 31-3 summarizes the major epidemiologic characteristics of SIDS.

There has been considerable debate over the term *SIDS*, yet the definition noted above remains for the time being. Other terms have been developed to explain sudden deaths in infants. *Sudden unexpected early neonatal death* (SUEND) and *sudden unexpected infant death* (SUID) share similar features but differ in regard to the timing of death: whereas SUID is considered a death in the postneonatal period, SUEND occurs in the first week of life. The AAP Task Force on Sudden Infant Death Syndrome (2011) policy statement considers SIDS to be a component of SUID.

Etiology

There are numerous theories regarding the etiology of SIDS; however, the cause remains unknown. One hypothesis is that SIDS is related to a brainstem abnormality in the neurologic regulation

---

*Back to Sleep materials may be ordered by contacting the National Institute of Child Health and Human Development Information Resource Center, Back to Sleep, PO Box 3006, Rockville, MD 20847; 800-505-CRIB (2742); fax: 866-760-5947; www.nichd.nih.gov/sids.

TABLE 31-3   EPIDEMIOLOGY OF SUDDEN INFANT DEATH SYNDROME

FACTOR	OCCURRENCE
Incidence	55.4 per 100,000 live births (2008)*
Peak age	2–3 mo; 95% occur by 6 mo; preterm infants die from sudden infant death syndrome (SIDS) at mean age of 6 wk later than mean age of death from SIDS for term infants
Sex	Higher percentage of boys affected
Time of death	During sleep
Time of year	Increased incidence in winter
Racial	Greater incidence in African Americans and Native Americans. (See Sudden Infant Death Syndrome, p. 910.)
Socioeconomic	Increased occurrence in lower socioeconomic class
Birth	Higher incidence in: • Preterm infants, especially infants of extremely and very low birth weight • Multiple births[†] • Neonates with low Apgar scores • Infants with central nervous system disturbances and respiratory disorders such as bronchopulmonary dysplasia • Increasing birth order (subsequent siblings as opposed to firstborn child)
Health status	Infants with a recent history of illness; lower incidence in immunized infants
Sleep habits	Highest risk associated with prone position; use of soft bedding; overheating (thermal stress); cosleeping with adult, especially on sofa or noninfant bed; higher incidence in cosleeping with adult smoker Infants cosleeping with adult at higher risk if younger than 11 weeks
Feeding habits	Lower incidence in breastfed infants
Pacifier	Lower incidence in infants put to sleep with pacifier
Siblings	May have greater incidence in siblings of SIDS victims
Maternal	Young age; cigarette smoking, especially during pregnancy; poor prenatal care; substance abuse (heroin, methadone, cocaine). A few studies have shown an increased risk in infants exposed to second-hand environmental tobacco smoke.

Data from American Academy of Pediatrics Task Force on Infant Sleep Position and Sudden Infant Death Syndrome: Changing concepts of sudden infant death syndrome: implications for infant sleeping environment and sleep position, *Pediatrics* 105(3):650–656, 2000; American Academy of Pediatrics Task Force on Sudden Infant Death Syndrome: The changing concept of sudden infant death syndrome: diagnostic coding shifts, controversies regarding the sleeping environment, and new variables to consider in reducing risk, *Pediatrics* 116(5):1245–1255, 2005; American Academy of Pediatrics Task Force on Sudden Infant Death Syndrome: SIDS and other sleep-related infant deaths: expansion of recommendations for a safe infant sleeping environment, *Pediatrics* 128(5):1030–1038, 2011.
*Heron M: Deaths: Leading causes for 2008, *Natl Vital Stat Rep* 60(6):1–94, 2012.
[†]Although a rare event, simultaneous death of twins from SIDS can occur.

of cardiorespiratory control. This maldevelopment affects arousal and physiologic responses to a life-threatening challenge during sleep (AAP Task Force on Sudden Infant Death Syndrome, 2005). Abnormalities include prolonged sleep apnea, increased frequency of brief inspiratory pauses, excessive periodic breathing, and impaired arousal responsiveness to increased carbon dioxide or decreased oxygen. However, *sleep apnea is not the cause of SIDS.* The vast majority of infants with apnea do not die, and only a minority of SIDS victims have documented apparent life-threatening events (ALTEs) (see Apparent Life-Threatening Event, p. 915). Numerous studies indicate that no association exists between SIDS and any childhood vaccine.

A genetic predisposition to SIDS has been postulated as a cause. In one study, a genetic mutation on chromosome 6q 22.1-22.31 was positively linked to a syndrome of SIDS and dysgenesis of the testis (Puffenberger, Hu-Lince, Parod, et al., 2004). Three triple-risk hypotheses have been proposed to explain the etiology of SIDS. Proposed factors include an underlying infant vulnerability factor (e.g., brain abnormality), a critical incident in the fetal developmental period or in early neonatal life, and an environmental stressor such as prone sleep positioning (Filiano and Kinney, 1994; Guntheroth and Spiers, 2002; Matthews and Moore, 2013). However, the

triple-risk theories have not been fully accepted by all experts as a cause for SIDS, and further data are needed to identify a single cause or combination of causes for SIDS deaths (Guntheroth and Spiers, 2002).

Risk Factors for SIDS

Maternal smoking during pregnancy has emerged in numerous epidemiologic studies as a major factor in SIDS, and tobacco smoke in the infant's environment after birth has also been shown to have a possible relationship to the incidence of SIDS (AAP Task Force on Sudden Infant Death Syndrome, 2005, 2011). Data show that exposure to tobacco smoke increased an infant's risk for SIDS 1.9 times over infants not exposed; 59% of SIDS deaths in smoke-exposed infants were attributed to maternal smoking (Anderson, Johnson, and Batal, 2005). It has been postulated that 12% of all SIDS deaths could be prevented with prenatal maternal smoking cessation (Pollack, 2001). Increased nicotine concentrations in lung tissue were found in children who died from SIDS compared with a group of control children (McMartin, Platt, Hackman, et al., 2002).

Cosleeping, or an infant sharing a bed with an adult or older child on a noninfant bed, has been reported to have a positive association with SIDS. One survey found a high association between infant deaths, nonstandard beds (sofa, day bed), and bed sharing; a large percentage of infants were found dead on their backs when bed sharing, suggesting suffocation (Unger, Kemp, Wilkins, et al., 2003). A study from Scotland indicates that the risk for SIDS when bed sharing is significantly increased for infants younger than 11 weeks (Tappin, Ecob, and Brooke, 2005). Vennemann, Bajanowski, Brinkmann, et al. (2009) identified infant sleeping in the house of a friend or relative and sleeping in the family living room as significant risk factors for SIDS. Other studies correlated higher incidences of SIDS and infant cosleeping with maternal smoking, cosleeping with multiple family members, sleeping on a couch, use of a pillow in the infant's bed, maternal overweight, soft bedding, and unintentional asphyxiation resulting from adult intoxication (overlaying) (AAP Task Force on Infant Sleep Position and Sudden Infant Death Syndrome, 2000; AAP Task Force on Sudden Infant Death Syndrome, 2005, 2011; Blair, Sidebotham, Evason-Coombe, et al., 2009; Carroll-Pankhurst and Mortimer, 2001; Hauck, Herman, Donovan, et al., 2003; Li, Zhang, Zielke, et al., 2009; McGarvey, McDonnell, Chong, et al., 2003; Person, Lavezzi, and Wolf, 2002).

Studies from countries other than the United States link sleep habits with an increased risk for SIDS. Prone sleeping may cause oropharyngeal obstruction or affect thermal balance or arousal state. One study found that healthy full-term infants had significantly impaired arousal from active and quiet sleep states when sleeping prone (Horne, Ferens, Watts, et al., 2001). Rebreathing of carbon dioxide by infants in the prone position is also a possible cause of SIDS. Infants sleeping prone and on soft bedding may not be able to move their heads to the side, thus increasing the risk for suffocation and lethal rebreathing. Evidence from other countries and the United States shows an increased incidence of SIDS in infants placed in a side-lying position; thus *the side-lying position is no longer recommended* for infants sleeping at home, day care, or hospitals (unless medically indicated). Most preterm infants being discharged from the hospital should be placed in a supine sleeping position unless special factors predispose them to airway obstruction.

One postulated cause of SIDS has been a prolonged Q-T interval; however, there has been no strong evidence to support this as a cause of SIDS or universal testing of newborns for prolonged Q-T interval (AAP Task Force on Sudden Infant Death Syndrome, 2005).

Soft bedding such as waterbeds, sheepskins, beanbags, pillows, and quilts should be avoided for infant sleeping surfaces. Bedding items such as stuffed animals and toys should be removed from the crib while the infant is asleep. Head covering by a blanket has also been found to be a risk factor for SIDS, thus supporting the recommendation to avoid extra bed linens and other items (Mitchell, Thompson, Becroft, et al., 2008). Crib bumper pads have not been shown to reduce infant injury and should therefore be avoided (AAP Task Force on Sudden Infant Death Syndrome, 2011).

In a recent retrospective study of SIDS deaths, Ostfield, Esposito, Perl, et al. (2010) found that at least one modifiable risk factor such as those previously listed was present in 96% of the deaths; a total of 78% of the deaths had anywhere from two to seven risk factors.

Protective Factors for SIDS

One study indicated that breastfeeding during the first 16 weeks of life decreased the likelihood of SIDS (Alm, Wennergren, Norvenius, et al., 2002). A subsequent meta-analysis confirmed that exclusive breastfeeding for any period of time decreased the overall risk for SIDS (Hauck, Thompson, Tanabe, et al., 2011). Some studies have found pacifier use in infants to be a protective factor

against the occurrence of SIDS; the data for pacifier use in infants in the first year of life are said to be more compelling than data linking pacifier use to the development of dental complications and the inhibition of breastfeeding (AAP Task Force on Sudden Infant Death Syndrome, 2005, 2011). Therefore the AAP recommends using a pacifier at naptime and bedtime, using a pacifier only if the infant is breastfeeding successfully, not using a sweetened coating on the pacifier, and avoiding forcing the infant to use the pacifier.

The AAP Task Force on Sudden Infant Death Syndrome (2005, 2011) recommends that all infants be placed to sleep in the supine (on the back) position. The AAP Task Force on Sudden Infant Death Syndrome (2011) emphasizes that medically stable preterm infants and infants diagnosed with gastroesophageal reflux (GER) be placed in a supine sleep position unless there is a specific upper airway disorder wherein the risk for death from the condition is greater than the risk for SIDS. The supine sleep position has not demonstrated an increased risk for choking and aspiration in infants, including those with GER (AAP Task Force on Sudden Infant Death Syndrome, 2011).

Since the Back to Sleep campaign in 1992 advocating nonprone sleeping for infants, an increased incidence of positional plagiocephaly has been observed (see p. 914). It is recommended that an infant's head position be alternated during sleep time to prevent plagiocephaly. Infants may be placed prone during awake periods to prevent positional plagiocephaly and to encourage development of upper shoulder girdle strength (AAP Task Force on Sudden Infant Death Syndrome, 2005, 2011). Updated childhood immunization status has also been shown to be protective against SIDS.

Although the cause of SIDS is unknown, autopsies reveal consistent pathologic findings, such as pulmonary edema and intrathoracic hemorrhages, that confirm the diagnosis. Consequently, autopsies should be performed on all infants suspected of dying of SIDS, and findings should be shared with the parents as soon as possible after the death. Postmortem findings in SIDS and accidental suffocation or intentional suffocation such as in Munchausen syndrome by proxy (see Child Maltreatment, Chapter 33) are practically the same. Individuals with less experience and training in performing autopsies, such as coroners instead of medical examiners, may not correctly identify some deaths as SIDS. Therefore mortality statistics can vary in different regions.

Infant Risk Factors

Certain groups of infants are at increased risk for SIDS:
- Low birth weight
- Low Apgar scores
- Recent viral illness
- Siblings of two or more SIDS victims
- Male sex
- Infants of Native-American or African-American ethnicity

No diagnostic tests exist to predict which infants, including those in the above groups, will survive, and home apnea monitoring is no guarantee of survival. Whether subsequent siblings of one SIDS infant are at increased risk for SIDS is unclear. Even if the risk is increased, families have a 99% chance that their subsequent child will *not* die of SIDS. A review of sibling deaths attributed to SIDS in England failed to ascertain a precise risk for recurrence; previous studies suggested a recurrence risk range of 1.7 to 10.1, yet the researchers concluded the studies had too many methodologic flaws to draw any firm conclusions (Bacon, Hall, Stephenson, et al., 2008). Others report that recurrence risks for a SIDS death in a family with a previous infant SIDS death range from 2% to 6% (AAP Task Force on Sudden Infant Death Syndrome, 2005). ***Home apnea monitoring is not recommended*** for this group of children, but it is often used by health care practitioners and may even be requested by parents (AAP Task Force on Sudden Infant Death Syndrome, 2005, 2011). There is no evidence that home apnea monitoring prevents SIDS (Strehle, Gray, Gopisetti, et al., 2012). Monitoring is best initiated on an individual basis.

CARE MANAGEMENT

Nurses have a vital role in preventing SIDS by educating families about the risk of prone sleeping position in infants from birth to 6 months of age, the use of appropriate bedding surfaces, the association with maternal smoking, and the dangers of cosleeping on non-infant surfaces with adults or other children. Also, nurses have an important role in modeling behaviors for parents to foster practices that decrease the risk for SIDS, including placing infants in a supine sleeping position in the hospital. Data indicate that a small percentage of nurses still place healthy infants in a side-lying position in the hospital (Bullock, Mickey, Green, et al., 2004; Thompson, 2005). Statistics for infants being placed in a prone sleeping position in the United States decreased from 70% in 1992 to 13% in 2004 (AAP Task Force on Sudden Infant Death Syndrome, 2005). One study of neonatal intensive care unit (NICU) nurses indicated that 52% routinely provided discharge instructions that promote supine sleep positions at home; common nonsupine positions recommended by the nurses included either supine or side or exclusive side-lying sleep position (Aris, Stevens, Lemura, et al., 2006). A survey of levels II and III NICU nurses found that nurses still positioned infants in a side-lying position for fear of aspiration (29%), for comfort reasons (28%), and for infant safety (20%) (Grazel, Phalen, and Palomano, 2010). Nurses ***must*** be proactive in further decreasing the incidence of SIDS; after-birth discharge planning, newborn discharges, follow-up home visits, well-baby clinic visits, and immunization visits provide excellent opportunities to educate parents in these matters.

Many health care workers are concerned that infants placed on the back to sleep will aspirate emesis or mucus, yet studies fail to show an increase in infant deaths, spitting up during sleep, aspiration, asphyxia, or respiratory failure as a result of supine sleep positioning (AAP Task Force on Sudden Infant Death Syndrome, 2011; Malloy, 2002; Tablizo, Jacinto, Parsley, et al., 2007).

Research findings have important implications for practices that may reduce the risk for SIDS, such as avoiding smoking during pregnancy and near the infant; using the supine sleeping position; avoiding soft, moldable mattresses, blankets, and pillows; avoiding bed sharing; breastfeeding; and avoiding overheating during sleep. Nurses must continue to take every opportunity to advocate for infants by providing information for parents and caregivers about the modifiable risk factors for SIDS that can be implemented to prevent its occurrence across all sectors of the population.

Loss of a child from SIDS presents several crises with which the parents must cope. In addition to grief and mourning the death of their child, the parents must face a tragedy that was sudden, unexpected, and unexplained. The psychologic intervention for the family must deal with these additional variables. This discussion focuses primarily on the objectives of care for families experiencing SIDS rather than on the process of grief and mourning, which is explored in Chapter 36.

Care of the Family of a SIDS Infant. The first persons to arrive at the scene may be the police and emergency medical service personnel. They should handle the situation by asking few questions; giving no indication of wrongdoing, abuse, or neglect; making sensitive judgments concerning any resuscitation efforts for the child; and comforting the family members as much as possible. A compassionate, sensitive approach to the family during the first few minutes can help spare them some of the overwhelming guilt and anguish that commonly follow this type of death.

The medical examiner or coroner may go to the home or place of death and make the death pronouncement; until then, the sleep environment should remain as it was when the infant was initially found (Koehler, 2008). If the infant is not pronounced dead at the scene, he or she may be transported to the emergency department to be pronounced by a physician. Usually there is no attempt at resuscitation in the emergency department. While they are in the emergency department, the parents should be asked only factual questions, such as when they found the infant, how he or she looked, and whom they called for help. The nurse should avoid any remarks that may suggest responsibility, such as "Why didn't you go in earlier?" "Didn't you hear the infant cry out?" "Was the head buried in a blanket?" or "Were the siblings jealous of this child?" It is the coroner's responsibility to document these findings at the scene rather than have parents recount the experience in the emergency department (Koehler, 2008). Parents may also express feelings of guilt about administering cardiopulmonary resuscitation (CPR) correctly or the timing of CPR in relation to finding the infant.

At this time, the physician should initiate the discussion of an autopsy, often with the nurse being present to support the family. The physician or medical examiner, depending on the circumstances, should emphasize that a diagnosis cannot be confirmed until the postmortem examination is completed. Nurses may balk at the idea of requesting an autopsy because of the parents' emotional state; however, an autopsy may clear up possible misconceptions regarding the death. Instructions about the autopsy and funeral arrangements may need to be repeated or put in writing. If the mother was breastfeeding, she needs information about abrupt discontinuation of lactation. The nurse or physician should contact the primary care practitioner for the infant and the mother to avoid any miscommunications or telephone calls at a later date inquiring about the child's health status.

A review of 60 studies shows that parents experiencing perinatal death perceive health care workers' responses as having a significant impact on the parents' grieving process; parents perceived the behavior of many health care workers as thoughtless or insensitive. The findings suggest that nurses and physicians would benefit from more bereavement training (Gold, 2007).

An important aspect of compassionate care for these parents is allowing them to say good-bye to their child. These are the parents' last moments with their child, and they should be as quiet, meaningful, peaceful, and undisturbed as possible. Encourage parents to hold their infant before leaving the emergency department. Because the parents leave the hospital without their infant, it is helpful to accompany them to the car or arrange for someone else to take them home. A debriefing session may help health care workers who dealt with the family and deceased infant to cope with emotions that are often engendered when a SIDS victim is brought into the acute care facility. Comprehensive guidelines have been published for health care professionals involved in SIDS investigations to assist the family and at the same time to determine that the infant's death was not the result of other factors such as child maltreatment (AAP Committee on Child Abuse and Neglect, 2001).

When the parents return home, a competent, qualified professional should visit them as soon after the death as possible. They should receive printed material that contains excellent information about SIDS (available from the national organizations*).

During the initial visit, help the parents gain an intellectual understanding of the condition. The nursing objectives are to assess what the parents have been told about SIDS; what they think happened; and how they explained this to the other siblings, family members, and friends. One question that the nurse will never be able to answer and therefore should not attempt to is, "Why did this happen to our baby?" or "Who is responsible for this tragedy?" These and other questions may linger in the parents' minds for months or even years.

When the unexpected death of a child occurs, it is common for one parent to blame the other for the child's death. Parents may also experience guilt over the child's death; if they had checked earlier, the child might still be alive. It is important that the nurse assist parents in working through these feelings to prevent marital disruption in addition to the loss of the loved child.

Some parents are able to discuss their feelings openly, and the nurse should be supportive of this coping skill. However, others may be reluctant to express their grief, and the nurse can encourage the expression of emotions by asking about crying and feeling sad, angry, or guilty. This is an attempt to provoke a display of emotion, not just an admission of a feeling. During this session, help the parents explore their usual coping mechanisms and, if these are ineffectual, to investigate new approaches. For example, one parent may refrain from discussing the death for fear of upsetting the other parent, but each may need to hear how the other feels.

Ideally, the number of visits and plans for subsequent intervention need to be flexible. Parents facing the question of having a subsequent child will need support. Both the birth of a subsequent child and the survival of that child, especially past the age of death of the previous child, are important transitional stages for parents.

Positional Plagiocephaly

Since the Back to Sleep campaign began in 1992 advocating non-prone sleeping for infants to prevent sudden infant death syndrome (SIDS), an increase in the incidence of positional plagiocephaly has been observed (AAP Task Force on Sudden Infant Death Syndrome, 2005; Littlefield, Saba, and Kelly, 2004). The prevalence of positional plagiocephaly at 4 months is reported to range from slightly less than 20% to as much as 48% (Robinson and Proctor, 2009). The term *plagiocephaly* connotes an oblique or asymmetric head; *positional plagiocephaly, deformational plagiocephaly*, or *nonsynostotic plagiocephaly* implies an acquired condition that occurs as a result of cranial molding during infancy (Hummel and Fortado, 2005). Because infants' sutures are not closed, the skull is pliable and, when infants are placed on their backs to sleep, the posterior occiput flattens over time (Fig. 31-16, *A*). A typical bald spot develops, which is usually transient. As a result of prolonged pressure on one side of the skull, that side becomes misshapen; mild facial asymmetry may develop. The sternocleidomastoid muscle may tighten on the preferential side, and torticollis may also develop. Congenital or acquired torticollis may cause plagiocephaly; other causes of deformational plagiocephaly include certain craniofacial syndromes. This

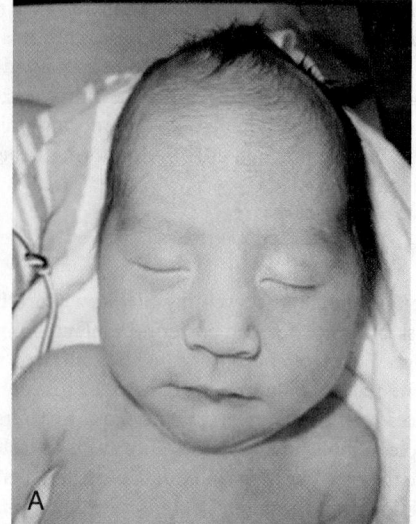

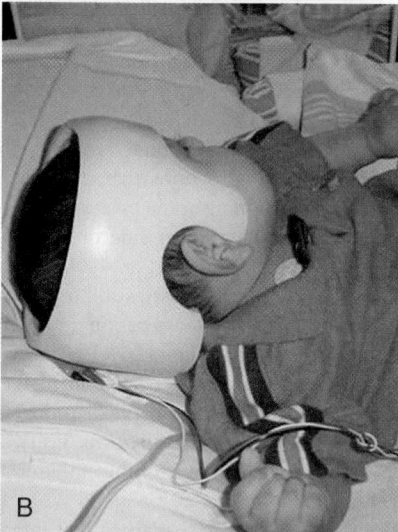

FIG 31-16 A, Plagiocephaly. **B,** Helmet used to correct plagiocephaly. (Courtesy Dr. Gerardo Cabrera-Meza, Department of Neonatology, Baylor College of Medicine, Houston, TX.)

discussion centers only on positional plagiocephaly caused by supine sleeping position.

Diagnostic Evaluation

The diagnosis of positional plagiocephaly may be made on physical examination of the infant's head; the infant's head is viewed frontally and from above. The typical infant's head shape will resemble a parallelogram, with unilateral flattening of the occiput, frontal and parietal bossing, a prominent cheekbone, and an anterior ear displacement. An evaluation of neck movement and range of motion is also made to determine the presence of torticollis. In most cases, skull films and further radiologic studies (computed tomographic scan) are used only to rule out craniosynostosis or other cranial deformity that may affect brain growth.

Therapeutic Management

Prevention of positional plagiocephaly may begin shortly after birth by placing the infant to sleep supine and alternating the infant's head position nightly, avoiding prolonged placement in car safety seats and swings, and using prone positioning or "tummy time" for

*American SIDS Institute, 528 Ravens Way, Naples, FL 34110, (239) 431-5425, www.sids.org; First Candle, 1314 Bedford Ave., Suite 210, Baltimore, MD 21208, (800) 221-7437, www.firstcandle.org; National Sudden and Unexpected Infant/Child Death and Pregnancy Loss Resource Center, Georgetown University, Box 571272, Washington, DC 20057-1272, (866) 866-7437, 202-687-7466, www.sidscenter.org.

approximately 30 to 60 minutes per day when the infant is awake (Laughlin, Luerssen, Dias, et al., 2011).

Treatment of torticollis and plagiocephaly initially involves exercises to loosen the tight muscle and switching head position sides during feeding, carrying, and sleep. If the plagiocephaly is not resolved within 4 to 8 weeks of physical therapy, a customized helmet may be worn to decrease the pressure on the affected side of the skull (Fig. 31-16, B). If no improvement occurs with physical therapy or a molded helmet over a period of 2 to 3 months, the infant may be referred to a pediatric neurosurgeon or craniofacial surgeon; the referral should optimally occur by 4 to 6 months of age (Laughlin, Luerssen, Dias, et al., 2011).

The helmet is worn 23 hours a day for a prescribed period (usually 3 months). Repositioning and physical therapy are said to be more effective when used before the infant can roll over or move his or her head alone (i.e., before approximately 3 to 4 months of age) (Robinson and Proctor, 2009). Reports of developmental delay in infants with positional plagiocephaly (nonsynostotic) vary in regard to outcomes, but current studies do not conclusively prove that such infants are at higher risk for developmental delays (Robinson and Proctor, 2009).

CARE MANAGEMENT

Minor skull flattening is not considered significant, but parents should learn to prevent plagiocephaly by altering the infant's head position during sleep. Infants should be placed prone on a firm surface during awake time (tummy time) for at least 15 to 20 minutes, which prevents plagiocephaly and facilitates development of upper shoulder girdle strength; the latter helps in the progressive development of movements such as rolling over and starting to rise up on all fours, which are precursors to crawling and eventually walking. A total of thirty to sixty minutes of supervised tummy time per day in infants younger than 6 months is recommended (Laughlin, Luerssen, Dias, et al., 2011; Robinson and Proctor, 2009).

Despite the perceived increase in the incidence of positional plagiocephaly, the supine sleeping position is still recommended because it has led to a significant decrease in loss of infant lives from SIDS (AAP Task Force on Sudden Infant Death Syndrome, 2011). Additional measures to prevent positional plagiocephaly include avoiding excessive time spent in car restraint seats, infant seats, and bouncers. Alternating the infant's head position for sleep times can also prevent unilateral molding. When a nurse or parent notices plagiocephaly, a consultation with the primary health care practitioner is recommended to evaluate the head shape and ascertain the need for early intervention.

Nurses are in a unique position in well-child care settings to encourage parents to follow guidelines for preventing plagiocephaly, demonstrate alternating head placement for sleeping, demonstrate sternocleidomastoid muscle exercises (as appropriate to the condition), and encourage tummy time for infants during awake periods. Most important, nurses should continue to encourage parents to place the infant in a supine sleep position despite the development of plagiocephaly. Nurses can also assist parents in the proper use of a skull-molding helmet and reassure them of the high rate of success with the helmet. Allowing parents to verbalize concerns and feelings related to the health status of the child as well as provision of current best practice is an important nursing function. Parents should not become so alarmed by plagiocephaly that they abandon supine sleeping position for the infant but should consult with the health care practitioner for further advice.

Apparent Life-Threatening Event

An apparent life-threatening event (ALTE), formerly referred to as *aborted SIDS death* or *near-miss SIDS*, generally refers to an event that is sudden and frightening to the observer in which the infant exhibits a combination of apnea, change in color (pallor, cyanosis, redness), change in muscle tone (usually hypotonia), and choking, gagging, or coughing and that usually involves a significant intervention and even CPR by the caregiver who witnesses the event (National Institutes of Health, 1987). The definition of *ALTE* may include apnea, but ALTE may occur without apnea (Silvestri, 2012; Silvestri and Weese-Mayer, 2003). It is erroneous to characterize ALTE as a near-miss SIDS incident (Adams, Good, and Defranco, 2009). Infants with ALTE are at increased risk for SIDS; the risk for SIDS may be 3 to 5 times greater in infants who experienced an ALTE (Hunt and Hauck, 2011).

Results from the Collaborative Home Infant Monitoring Evaluation (CHIME) study found that apnea and bradycardia occurred at conventional and extreme alarm thresholds in all groups of infants studied—siblings of SIDS infants, infants with ALTEs, symptomatic (of apnea and bradycardia) and asymptomatic preterm infants weighing less than 1750 g (3 lb 13 oz) at birth, and healthy term infants. Approximately 30% of infants with ALTE were born at less than 37 weeks of gestation. The researchers concluded that many infants experience apnea and bradycardia in each of these groups yet do not die (Jobe, 2001; Ramanathan, Corwin, Hunt, et al., 2001). Furthermore, it was reported that apnea does not appear to be an immediate precursor to SIDS and that cardiorespiratory monitoring is not an effective tool for identifying infants at greater risk for SIDS (AAP Committee on Fetus and Newborn, 2003). CHIME data indicate that infants with ALTE did not have some of the typical characteristics associated with SIDS infants; these include fewer infants with low birth weight and who are small for gestational age at birth, fewer teenage pregnancies, and a younger infant age at the time of ALTE. The researchers concluded that despite some similar characteristics between ALTE and SIDS, the differences warrant a separate focus on ALTE events (Esani, Hodgman, Ehsani, et al., 2008).

Diagnostic Evaluation

An essential component of the diagnostic process includes a detailed description of the event, including who witnessed the event; where the infant was during the event; and what, if any, activities were involved (e.g., during or after a feeding, riding in a car seat restraint, presence of siblings or any minor children, what clothing the infant was wearing). In addition, a prenatal and postnatal history must be obtained. A short period of observation in the emergency department may be appropriate to observe the infant's respiratory pattern and response to feeding. A careful evaluation of late preterm and preterm infants in the car restraints currently in use is essential; upper airway occlusion and subsequent apnea and cyanosis may occur if the infant is not positioned properly. Reported diagnoses in infants with ALTE include a neurologic event such as a seizure (30% of cases seen); GI problem, including gastroesophageal reflux (50%); respiratory conditions (20%); and metabolic conditions, cardiac anomaly, or child abuse (each <5%). In some cases, multiple diagnoses may be made (Hall and Zalman, 2005).

In the event that an underlying diagnosis such as those mentioned previously is not established, home monitoring may be recommended. The most commonly used monitoring is continuous recording of cardiorespiratory patterns (cardiopneumogram or pneumocardiogram). Four-channel pneumocardiograms (or multichannel pneumogram) monitor heart rate, respirations (chest impedance), nasal airflow, and oxygen saturation. A more sophisticated test, polysomnography (sleep study), also records brain waves, eye and body movements, esophageal manometry, and end-tidal carbon dioxide measurements. However, none of these tests can predict risk. Some children with normal results may still have subsequent apneic episodes.

Therapeutic Management

The treatment of an infant with an ALTE depends on the underlying condition (see p. 915). Treatment of recurrent apnea (without an underlying organic problem) usually involves continuous home monitoring of cardiorespiratory rhythms and, in some cases, the use of methylxanthines (respiratory stimulant drugs, such as caffeine). The decision to discontinue the monitoring is based on the infant's clinical condition. A general guideline for discontinuation is when infants with ALTEs have gone 2 or 3 months without significant numbers of episodes requiring intervention. Silvestri (2012) notes that the challenge in treating an infant with an ALTE is to determine if the infant is at further risk for a recurrent event and significant morbidity and death.

Newer home apnea monitors allow download of information that assists the health care practitioner in deciding when to discontinue home monitoring. It is imperative to remember, however, that the *home apnea monitor will not predict or prevent SIDS* (Strehle, Gray, Gopisetti, et al., 2012). Furthermore, impedance-based monitors detect chest wall movement and will not detect obstructive apnea unless the episode involves significant bradycardia. Monitors with respiratory impedance plethysmography (RIP) are capable of detecting obstruction as well as central apnea (Silvestri, 2012).

CARE MANAGEMENT

The diagnosis of an ALTE causes great anxiety and concern in parents, and the institution of home monitoring presents additional physical and emotional burdens. Parents of infants on home apnea monitors report experiencing emotional distress, especially depression and hostility, during the first few weeks after hospital discharge. For parents of a SIDS victim who have a new infant on home apnea monitoring, the anxiety is compounded by the uncertainty of the future of the living child and grief for the lost child. Home apnea monitoring may offer some predictability and control over the current child's survival through the period of uncertainty.

If home monitoring is required, the nurse can be a major source of support to the family in terms of education about the equipment; education regarding observation of the infant's status; and instructions regarding immediate intervention during apneic episodes, including CPR. Several reports indicate that the first week to month after discharge is the most stressful for parents, particularly when the rate of false alarms is high (Bennett, 2002). To help the family cope with the numerous procedures they must learn, adequate preparation before discharge and written instructions are essential. In the first few weeks after discharge, parents may benefit by having a practitioner readily available to answer questions regarding false alarms and for other technical assistance.

Several types of home monitors are available and are set up by either a home monitor equipment company or home health staff. Nurses, especially those involved in the care at home, must become familiar with the equipment, including its advantages and disadvantages. Safety is a major concern because monitors can cause electrical burns and electrocution. The following precautions are recommended:

- Remove leads from infant when not attached to the monitor.
- Unplug the power cord from the electrical outlet when the cord is not plugged into the monitor.

- Use safety covers on electrical outlets to discourage children from inserting objects into sockets.

Additional home use instructions should focus on troubleshooting the monitor alarms. *Encourage parents to first look at the infant if an alarm goes off to ensure the infant is breathing and then to determine the cause of the alarm.* Parents also need information about traveling or running necessary errands with an infant on an apnea monitor, what to do in case of power failure, and whom to contact if the monitor alarm goes off continuously but the infant appears well. Siblings should also be supervised when near the infant and taught that the monitor is not a toy. Other safety practices include informing local utility and rescue squads (fire and/or emergency services) of the home monitoring in case of an emergency, especially if the family lives in a remote rural area. Telephone numbers for these services should be posted in the home or set up as speed dial on certain phones in the event that a universal 911 system is not available. Post instructions for infant CPR in a central location of the house and encourage parents to tell visitors and other family members about the location of such instructions. If a cellular phone is the main house phone, make sure it stays in a central location for all family members to access in an emergency.

> ### ❗ NURSING ALERT
>
> If the infant is apneic, gently stimulate the trunk by patting or rubbing it. Call loudly for help even if alone. If the infant is prone, turn to the back and flick the heels of the feet. If there is still no response, immediately begin CPR. After approximately 2 minutes of CPR, activate the emergency medical service—"Call 911!" and then resume CPR until emergency responders arrive or the infant starts breathing. Never vigorously shake the child. No more than 10 seconds are spent on stimulation before implementing CPR.

Caregivers need detailed information regarding proper attachment of the electrodes to the infant's chest with impedance monitors that detect chest movement. The electrodes are placed in the midaxillary line at a space one or two fingerbreadths below the nipple. For home use, electrodes attached to a belt that is placed around the child's trunk are preferred (Fig. 31-17). The belt is positioned so that

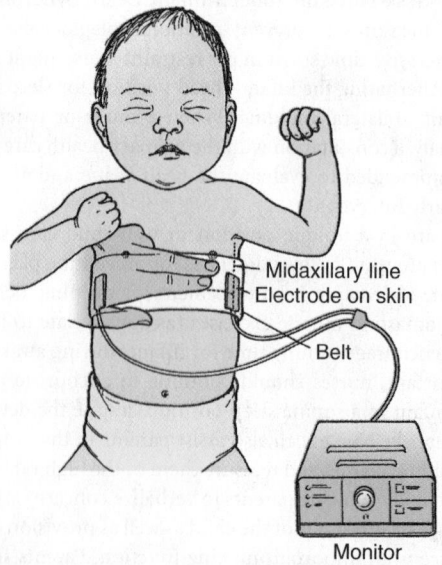

FIG 31-17 Placement of electrodes or belt for apnea monitoring. In small infants, one fingerbreadth below the nipple line may be used to determine correct placement of the monitor belt.

the electrodes contact the skin in the same area. Monitors may have memory chips that allow for event recording, which can be an effective tool in evaluating the use of the monitor, events immediately before and after the ALTE, and reported frequency of alarms.

Monitors are effective only if they are used. They do not prevent death but alert the caregiver to the ALTE in time to intervene. The need to use the monitor and to respond appropriately to alarms must be stressed. Noncompliance can result in the infant's death.

Family Support. Many of the stresses observed during the home monitoring period are characteristic of families with chronically ill children. The child with an apnea or cardiorespiratory monitor may have additional health care needs such as a gastrostomy, tracheostomy, and myriad medications or treatments that exacerbate the parents' stress. Parents report increased stress, including concern for the child's survival, fear of incompetence in assuming home responsibility, inadequate respite care, lack of time for other children and spouse, social isolation from friends and extended family, constant work, and fatigue. The monitored child is at risk for vulnerable child syndrome, which may lead to lack of parental separation and preferential treatment, causing further family disruption. To deal with these potential effects, nurses need to use the same interventions as those discussed for children with chronic illness and be aware of the need for referral when difficulties are suspected.

To lessen the continuous responsibility of monitoring, other family members, such as grandparents and other immediate family members should be taught how to manipulate the equipment, read and interpret the signals, and administer CPR. They are encouraged to stay with the infant for regular periods to allow the parents respite. Support groups of other families who have successfully completed monitoring can also be of benefit. Because reliable babysitters are difficult to locate, support group members and nursing students may be potential sources of qualified caregivers.

KEY POINTS

- Biologic development of the child encompasses proportional changes; sensory changes, including binocularity, depth perception, and visual preference; maturation of biologic systems; fine motor development; and gross motor development.
- Erikson's theory of psychosocial development (birth to 1 year) is concerned with acquiring a sense of trust while overcoming a sense of mistrust.
- Piaget's theory of cognitive development, as it applies to the infant, focuses on the sensorimotor phase, which includes the use of reflexes, primary circular reactions, secondary circular reactions, and coordination of secondary schemata and their application to new situations.
- Development of body image begins in infancy; by 1 year of age, infants recognize that they are distinct from their parents.
- Social development of the infant is guided by attachment, language development, personal-social behavior, and participation in play.
- Temperament influences the type of interaction that occurs between the child and parents and siblings.
- Parents are faced with many concerns, including selecting an appropriate day care, limit setting and discipline, thumb-sucking and pacifier use, and teething.
- Breast milk provides optimal nutrition for the infant during the first 6 months, followed by gradual introduction of solid food during the second 6 months. Commercial iron-fortified infant formula is a safe alternative to human milk. Whole milk is not recommended until after 12 months.
- Cleaning the teeth regularly in early childhood and appropriate dietary intake promote good dental health.
- Recommended routine immunizations in childhood include those for HBV, HAV, diphtheria, tetanus, pertussis, polio, measles, mumps, rubella, pneumococcus, meningococcus, chickenpox, influenza, and Hib.

- Recommended immunizations for selected groups of children and adolescents include the rotavirus and HPV vaccines.
- Because injuries are a major cause of death during infancy, parents should be alerted to aspiration of foreign objects, suffocation, falls, poisoning, burns, motor vehicle injuries, and bodily damage, as well as preventive actions needed to make the environment safe for infants.
- Treatment of colic may involve change in feeding practices, correction of a stressful environment, behavior modification, and support of the parent.
- FTT may occur in children who have a chronic illness, or it may occur in a family environment wherein healthy infant feeding practices are poorly managed or understood. The etiology of FTT is often multifactorial and not always associated with a pattern of disturbed maternal-infant relationship.
- SIDS is the third leading cause of infant death in the United States.
- Factors that place the infant at high risk for SIDS include prone sleeping position, soft bedding, sleeping in a noninfant bed with an adult or older child, and maternal prenatal smoking.
- Positional plagiocephaly can be easily prevented by allowing the awake infant to have periods of tummy time and by alternating the infant's head position during sleep.
- The primary nursing responsibility in care associated with sudden infant death is educating the family of newborns about the risks for SIDS, modeling appropriate behaviors in the hospital such as placing the infant in a supine sleep position, and providing emotional support of the family who have experienced a SIDS loss.
- Infants with an ALTE are carefully evaluated for clues to the underlying cause.
- Home apnea or cardiorespiratory monitors do not prevent SIDS.

REFERENCES

Adams SM, Good MW, Defranco GM: Sudden infant death syndrome, *Am Fam Physician* 79(10):870–874, 2009.

Alm B, Wennergren G, Norvenius SG, et al: Breast-feeding and the sudden infant death syndrome in Scandinavia, 1992-1995, *Arch Dis Child* 86(6):400–402, 2002.

American Academy of Pediatric Dentistry: Guideline on infant oral health care. In *AAPD Reference Manual 2010-2011* 33(6):12, 114, 2012, www.aapd.org/media/Policies_Guidelines/G_InfantOralHealthCare.pdf.

American Academy of Pediatrics (AAP): Prevention of rickets and vitamin D deficiency in infants, children, and adolescents, *Pediatrics* 122(5):1142–1148, 2008.

American Academy of Pediatrics (AAP): *Pediatric nutrition handbook,* ed 6, Elk Grove Village, IL, 2009, Author.

American Academy of Pediatrics (AAP): Policy statement—child passenger safety, *Pediatrics* 127(4):788–793, 2011.

American Academy of Pediatrics (AAP) Committee on Child Abuse and Neglect: Distinguishing sudden infant death syndrome from child abuse fatalities, *Pediatrics* 107(2):437–441, 2001.

American Academy of Pediatrics (AAP) Committee on Fetus and Newborn: Apnea, sudden infant death syndrome, and home monitoring, *Pediatrics* 111(4):914–917, 2003.

American Academy of Pediatrics (AAP) Committee on Infectious Diseases, Pickering L, editor: *2012 Red Book: report of the Committee on Infectious Diseases*, ed 29, Elk Grove Village, IL, 2012, Author.

American Academy of Pediatrics (AAP) Committee on Infectious Diseases: Recommended childhood and adolescent immunization schedule—United States, 2013, *Pediatrics* 131(2):397–398, 2013.

American Academy of Pediatrics (AAP) Council on Communications and Media: Media use by children younger than 2 years, *Pediatrics* 128(5):1040–1045, 2011.

American Academy of Pediatrics Task Force on Infant Sleep Position and Sudden Infant Death Syndrome: Changing concepts of sudden infant death syndrome: implications for infant sleeping environment and sleep position, *Pediatrics* 105(3):650–656, 2000.

American Academy of Pediatrics (AAP) Task Force on Sudden Infant Death Syndrome: The changing concept of sudden infant death syndrome: diagnostic coding shifts, controversies regarding the sleeping environment, and new variables to consider in reducing risk, *Pediatrics* 116(5):1245–1255, 2005.

American Academy of Pediatrics (AAP) Task Force on Sudden Infant Death Syndrome: SIDS and other sleep-related infant deaths: expansion of recommendations for a safe infant sleeping environment, *Pediatrics* 128(5):1030–1038, 2011.

Anderson JE: "Nothing but the tooth": dispelling myths about teething, *Contemp Pediatr* 21(7):75–83, 2004.

Anderson ME, Johnson DC, Batal HA: Sudden infant death syndrome and prenatal maternal smoking: rising attributed risk in the Back to Sleep era, *BMC Med* 3(1):4, 2005.

Arikan D, Alp H, Gozum S, et al: Effectiveness of massage, sucrose solution, herbal tea or hydrolyzed formula in the treatment of infantile colic, *J Clin Nurs* 17(13):1754–1761, 2008.

Aris C, Stevens TP, Lemura C, et al: NICU nurses' knowledge and discharge teaching related to infant sleep position and risk of SIDS, *Adv Neonatal Care* 6(5):281–294, 2006.

Bacon CJ, Hall DB, Stephenson TJ, et al: How common is repeat sudden infant death syndrome? *Arch Dis Child* 93(4):323–326, 2008.

Baker RD, Greer FR, American Academy of Pediatrics (AAP) Committee on Nutrition: Clinical report—diagnosis and prevention of iron deficiency and iron-deficiency anemia in infants and young children (0-3 years of age), *Pediatrics* 126(5):1040–1050, 2010.

Beck CT: Predictors of postpartum depression: an update, *Nurs Res* 50(5):275–285, 2001.

Bennett AD: Home apnea monitoring for infants: a discussion of primary care issues, *Adv Nurs Pract* 10(3):48–53, 2002.

Bernard SJ, Paulozzi LJ, Wallace DL; Centers for Disease Control and Prevention (CDC): Fatal injuries among children by race and ethnicity—United States, 1999-2002, *MMWR Surveill Summ* 56(SS-5):1–16, 2007.

Biancuzzo M: *Breastfeeding the newborn: clinical strategies for nurses*, ed 2, St Louis, 2003, Mosby.

Black MM, Dubowitz H, Krishnakumar A, et al: Early intervention and recovery among children with failure to thrive: follow-up at age 8, *Pediatrics* 120(1):59–69, 2007.

Blackburn ST: *Maternal, fetal, & neonatal physiology: a clinical perspective*, ed 4, St Louis, 2013, Saunders.

Blair PS, Sidebotham P, Evason-Coombe C, et al: Hazardous cosleeping environments and risk factors amenable to change: case-control study of SIDS in southwest England, *BMJ* 339:b3446, 2009.

Block RW, Krebs NF, American Academy of Pediatrics (AAP) Committee on Child Abuse and Neglect and Committee on Nutrition: Failure to thrive as a manifestation of child neglect, *Pediatrics* 116(5):1234–1237, 2005.

Boyce JA, Assa'ad A, Burks AW, et al: Guideline for the diagnosis and management of food allergy in the United States: summary of the NIAID-sponsored expert panel report, *J Allergy Clin Immunol* 126(6):1005–1118, 2010.

Brady MT: Infectious disease in pediatric out-of-home child care, *Am J Infect Control* 33(5):276–285, 2005.

Bull MJ, Durbin DR: Rear-facing car safety seats: getting the message right, *Pediatrics* 121(3):619–620, 2008.

Bullock LFC, Mickey K, Green J, et al: Are nurses acting as role models for the prevention of SIDS? *MCN Am J Matern Child Nurs* 29(3):172–177, 2004.

Carbajal R: Nonpharmacologic management of pain in infants, *Arch Pediatr* 12(1):110–116, 2005 (article in French).

Carey WB, McDevitt SC: Revision of the infant temperament questionnaire, *Pediatrics* 61(5):735–739, 1978.

Carroll-Pankhurst C, Mortimer EA: Sudden infant death syndrome, bedsharing, parental weight, and age of death, *Pediatrics* 107(3):530–536, 2001.

Casey PH, Whiteside-Mansell L, Barrett K, et al: Impact of prenatal and/or postnatal growth problems in low birth weight preterm infants on school-age outcomes: an 8-year longitudinal evaluation, *Pediatrics* 118(3):1078–1086, 2006.

Centers for Disease Control and Prevention (CDC): Nonfatal motor-vehicle-related backover injuries among children—United States, 2001-2003, *MMWR Morb Mortal Weekly Rep* 54(06):144–146, 2005a.

Centers for Disease Control and Prevention (CDC): Outbreaks of pertussis associated with hospitals—Kentucky, Pennsylvania, and Oregon, 2003, *MMWR Morb Mortal Weekly Rep* 54(03):67–71, 2005b.

Centers for Disease Control and Prevention: Fatal injuries among children by race and ethnicity—United States, 1999–2002, *MMWR Morb Mortal Wkly Rep Surveill Summ* 56(SS05):1–16, 2007.

Centers for Disease Control and Prevention (CDC): Update: recommendations from the Advisory Committee on Immunization Practices (ACIP) regarding administration of combination MMRV vaccine, *MMWR Morb Mortal Weekly Rep* 57(10):258–260, 2008.

Centers for Disease Control and Prevention (CDC): Licensure of a *Haemophilus influenzae* type b (Hib) vaccine (Hiberix) and updated recommendations for use of Hib vaccine, *MMWR Morb Mortal Weekly Rep* 58(36):1008–1009, 2009.

Centers for Disease Control and Prevention (CDC): Prevention of pneumococcal disease among infants and children—use of 13-valent pneumococcal conjugate vaccine and 23-valent pneumococcal polysaccharide vaccine: recommendations of the Advisory Committee on Immunization Practices (ACIP), *MMWR Recomm Rep* 59(RR-11):1–18, 2010.

Centers for Disease Control and Prevention (CDC): Recommended immunization schedules for persons aged 0 through 18 years—United States, 2011, *MMWR Morb Mortal Weekly Rep* 60(5):1–4, 2011a.

Centers for Disease Control and Prevention (CDC): Updated recommendations for use of tetanus toxoid, reduced diphtheria toxoid and acellular pertussis (Tdap) vaccine from the Advisory Committee on Immunization Practices, 2010, *MMWR Morb Mortal Weekly Rep* 60(01):13–15, 2011b.

Centers for Disease Control and Prevention (CDC): Updated recommendations for use of meningococcal conjugate vaccines—Advisory Committee on Immunization Practices (ACIP), 2010, *MMWR Morb Mortal Weekly Rep* 60(03):72–76, 2011c.

Centers for Disease Control and Prevention (CDC): Recommended adult immunization schedule—United States, 2012, *MMWR Morb Mortal Weekly Rep* 61(4):1–5, 2012, www.cdc.gov/vaccines/schedules/hcp/adult.html.

Centers for Disease Control and Prevention (CDC): Infant meningococcal vaccination: Advisory Committee on Immunization Practices (ACIP) recommendation and rationales, *MMWR Weekly Rep* 62(3):52–54, 2013.

Cole SZ, Lanham JS: Failure to thrive: an update, *Am Fam Physician* 83(7):829–834, 2011.

Cook EH, Higgins SS: Congenital heart disease. In Allen PJ, Vessey JA, Schapiro NA, editors: *Primary care of the child with a chronic condition*, ed 5, St Louis, 2010, Mosby.

Cook IF, Murtagh J: Ventrogluteal area: a suitable site for intramuscular vaccination in infants and toddlers, *Vaccine* 24(13):2403–2408, 2006.

Corrales KM, Utter SL: Growth failure. In Samour PQ, King K, editors: *Handbook of pediatric nutrition*, ed 3, Sudbury, MA, 2005, Jones & Bartlett.

Critch JN: Infantile colic: is there a role for dietary interventions? *Paediatr Child Health* 16(1):47–49, 2011, www.cps.ca/english/statements/N/InfantileColic.htm.

Desapriya EB, Joshi P, Subwarzi S, et al: Infant injuries from child restraint safety seat misuse at British Columbia Children's Hospital, *Pediatr Int* 50(5):674–678, 2008.

Diggle L, Deeks J: Effect of needle length on incidence of local reactions to routine immunizations in infants aged 4 months: randomized controlled trial, *BMJ* 321(7266):931–993, 2000.

Diggle L, Deeks JJ, Pollard AJ: Effect of needle size and immunogenicity and reactogenicity of vaccines in infants: a randomized controlled trial, *BMJ* 333(7568):571, 2006.

Duro D, Rising R, Cedillo M, et al: Association between infantile colic and carbohydrate malabsorption from fruit juices in infancy, *Pediatrics* 109(5):797–805, 2002.

Ellett MLC: What is known about colic? *Gastroenterol Nurs* 26(2):60–65, 2003.

Ellett ML, Appleton MM, Sloan RS: Out of the abyss of colic: a view through the father's eyes, *MCN Am J Matern Child Nurs* 34(3):164–171, 2009.

Erikson EH: *Childhood and society*, ed 2, New York, 1963, Norton.

Esani N, Hodgman JE, Ehsani N, et al: Apparent life-threatening events and sudden infant death syndrome: comparison of risk factors, *J Pediatr* 152(3):A2, 2008.

FDA Consumer Health Information: *Infant overdose risk with liquid vitamin D*, Washington, DC, 2010, U.S. Food and Drug Administration, www.fda.gov/downloads/ForConsumers/ConsumerUpdates/UCM215586.pdf.

Filiano JJ, Kinney HC: A perspective on neuropathologic findings in victims of the sudden infant death syndrome: the triple-risk model, *Biol Neonate* 65(3-4):194–197, 1994.

Flavin MP, Dostaler SM, Simpson K, et al: Stages of development and injury patterns in the early years: a population-based analysis, *BMC Public Health* 6(July 18):187–197, 2006.

Food and Drug Administration (FDA): *FDA 101: infant formula, consumer updates*, Washington, DC, 2012. Author, www.fda.gov/ForConsumers/ConsumersUpdates/ucm048694.htm.

Forlenza GP, Paradise Black NM, McNamara EG, et al: Ankyloglossia, exclusive breastfeeding, and failure to thrive, *Pediatrics* 125(6):e1500–e1504, 2010.

Fox MK, Reidy K, Novak T, et al: Sources of energy and nutrients in the diets of infants and toddlers, *J Am Diet Assoc* 106(Suppl 1):S28–S42, 2006.

Gold KJ: Navigating care after a baby dies: a systematic review of parent experiences with health providers, *J Perinatol* 27(4):230–237, 2007.

Goyal D, Gay C, Lee K: Fragmented maternal sleep is more strongly correlated with depressive symptoms than infant temperament at three months postpartum, *Arch Womens Ment Health* 12(4):229–237, 2009.

Grazel R, Phalen AG, Palomano RC: Implementation of the American Academy of Pediatrics recommendations to reduce sudden infant death syndrome risk in neonatal intensive care units: an evaluation of nursing knowledge and practice, *Adv Neonatal Care* 10(6):332–342, 2010.

Grummer-Strawn LM, Reinold C, Krebs NF, et al: Use of World Health Organization and CDC growth charts for children aged 0-59 months in the United States, *MMWR Recomm Rep* 59(RR-9):1–15, 2010.

Grummer-Strawn LM, Scanlon KS, Fein SB: Infant feeding and feeding transitions during the first year of life, *Pediatrics* 122(Suppl 2):S36–S42, 2008.

Guntheroth WG, Spiers PS: The triple risk hypotheses in sudden infant death syndrome, *Pediatrics* 110(5):e64, 2002.

Hall KL, Zalman B: Evaluation and management of apparent life threatening events in children, *Am Fam Physician* 71(12):2301–2308, 2005.

Hatfield LA: Sucrose decreases infant neurobehavioral pain response to immunizations: a randomized controlled trial, *J Nurs Scholarship* 40(3):219–225, 2008.

Hauck FR, Herman SM, Donavan M, et al: Sleep environment and the risk of sudden infant death syndrome in an urban population: the Chicago Infant Mortality Study, *Pediatrics* 111(5 Part 2):1207–1214, 2003.

Hauck FR, Thompson JM, Tanabe KO, et al: Breastfeeding and reduced risk of sudden infant death syndrome: a meta-analysis, *Pediatrics* 128(1):103–110, 2011.

Henary B, Sherwood CP, Crandall JR, et al: Car safety seats for children: rear facing for best protection, *Inj Prev* 13(6):398–402, 2007.

Hoath SB, Pickens WL, Visscher MO: The biology of vernix caseosa, *Int J Cosmet Sci* 28(5):319–333, 2006.

Horn MI, McCarthy AM: Children's responses to sequential versus simultaneous immunization injections, *J Pediatr Health Care* 13(1):18–23, 1999.

Horne RS, Ferens D, Watts AM, et al: The prone sleeping position impairs arousability in term infants, *J Pediatr* 138(6):793–795, 2001.

Hoyert DL, Xu JQ: Deaths: preliminary data for 2011, *Nat Vital Stat Rep* 61(6):1–53, Hyattsville, MD, 2012, National Center for Health Statistics.

Hummel P, Fortado D: Impacting infant head shapes, *Adv Neonatal Care* 5(6):329–342, 2005.

Hunt CE, Hauck FR: Sudden infant death syndrome. In Kliegman RM, Stanton BF, St. Geme JW, et al, editors: *Nelson textbook of pediatrics*, ed 19, Philadelphia, 2011, Saunders.

Hviid A, Stellfeld M, Wohlfahrt J, et al: Association between thimerosal-containing vaccine and autism, *JAMA* 290(13):1763–1766, 2003.

Iglowstein I, Jenni OG, Molinari L, et al: Sleep duration from infancy to adolescence: reference values and generational trends, *Pediatrics* 111(2):302–307, 2003.

Institute of Medicine: *Immunization safety review: vaccines and autism*, Washington, DC, 2004, National Academies Press.

Ipp M, Parkin PC, Lear N, et al: Order of vaccine injection and infant pain response, *Arch Pediatr Adolesc Med* 163(5):469–472, 2009.

Jaafar SH, Jahanafar S, Angolkar M, et al: Pacifier use versus no pacifier use in breastfeeding term infants for increasing duration of breastfeeding, *Cochrane Database Syst Rev* (3):CD007202, 2011.

Jackson LA, Yu O, Nelson JC, et al: Injection site and risk of medically attended local reactions to acellular pertussis vaccine, *Pediatrics* 127(3):e681–e687, 2011.

Joanna Briggs Institute: Early childhood pacifier use in relation to breastfeeding, SIDS, infection, and dental occlusion, *Best Practice Information Sheet* 9(3):1–6, 2005.

Joanna Briggs Institute: Best practice: the effectiveness of interventions for infant colic, *Best Practice Information Sheet* 12(6):1–4, 2008, www.joannabriggs.edu.au/pdf/BPIScolic.pdf.

Jobe AH: What do home monitors contribute to the SIDS problem? (editorial), *JAMA* 285(17):2244–2245, 2001.

Johnston ML, Esposito N: Barriers and facilitators for breastfeeding among working women in the United States, *J Obstetr Gynecol Neonat Nurs* 36(1):9–20, 2007.

Junqueira ALN, Tavares VR, Martins RMB, et al: Safety and immunogenicity of hepatitis B vaccine administered into ventrogluteal vs. anterolateral thigh sites in infants: a randomized controlled trial, *Int J Nurs Stud* 47(9):1074–1079, 2010.

Keefe MR, Lobo ML, Froese-Fretz A, et al: Effectiveness of an intervention for colic, *Clin Pediatr* 45(2):123–133, 2006.

Kimmel SR, Burns IT, Wolfe RM, et al: Addressing immunization barriers, benefits, and risks, *J Fam Pract* 56(2):S61–S69, 2007.

Koehler SA: Sudden infant death syndrome deaths: the role of forensic nurses, *J Forensic Nurs* 4(3):141–142, 2008.

Laughlin J, Luerssen TG, Dias MS, et al: Prevention and management of positional skull deformities in infants, *Pediatrics* 128(6):1236–1241, 2011.

Lawrence RA, Lawrence RM: *Breastfeeding: a guide for the medical profession*, ed 7, St Louis, 2011, Mosby.

Li L, Zhang Y, Zielke RH, et al: Observations on increased accidental asphyxia deaths in infancy while cosleeping in the state of Maryland, *Am J Forensic Med Pathol* 30(4):318–321, 2009.

Liaw JJ, Zeng WP, Yang L, et al: Nonnutritive sucking and oral sucrose relieve neonatal pain during intramuscular injection of hepatitis vaccine, *J Pain Symptom Manage* 42(6):918–930, 2011.

Littlefield TR, Saba NM, Kelly KM: On the current incidence of deformational plagiocephaly: an estimation based on prospective registration at a single center, *Semin Pediatr Neurol* 11(4):301–304, 2004.

Lobo ML, Kotzer AM, Keefe MR, et al: Current beliefs and management strategies for treating infant colic, *J Pediatr Health Care* 18(3):115–122, 2004.

Locklin M: The redefinition of failure to thrive from a case study perspective, *Pediatr Nurs* 31(6):474–479, 495, 2005.

Long SS: ACIP: routine booster dose of Tdap not recommended, *AAP News* 34(8):10, 2013.

Lundqvist P, Jakobsson L: Swedish men's experiences of becoming fathers to their preterm infants, *Neonat Netw* 22(6):25–31, 2003.

MacDorman MF, Mathews TJ, Centers for Disease Control and Prevention (CDC): Infant deaths—United States, 2000-2007, *MMWR Surveill Summ* 60(Suppl):49–51, 2011.

Mack KA, Gilchrist J, Ballesteros MF: Injuries among infants treated in the emergency departments in the United States, 2001-2004, *Pediatrics* 121(5):930–937, 2008.

Maggioni A, Lifshitz F: Nutritional management of failure to thrive, *Pediatr Clin North Am* 42(4):791–810, 1995.

Malloy MH: Trends in postneonatal aspiration deaths and reclassification of sudden infant death syndrome: impact of the "Back to Sleep" program, *Pediatrics* 109(4):661–665, 2002.

Markman L: Teething: facts and fiction, *Pediatr Rev* 30(8):e59–e64, 2009.

Markowitz R, Watkins JB, Duggan C: Failure to thrive: malnutrition in the pediatric outpatient setting. In Markowitz R, Watkins JB, Duggan C, editors: *Nutrition in pediatrics*, ed 4, Hamilton, Ontario, 2008, BC Decker.

Martin JA, Kochanek KD, Strobino DM, et al: Annual summary of vital statistics—2003, *Pediatrics* 115(3):619–634, 2005.

Mathews TJ, MacDorman MF: Infant mortality statistics from the 2007 period linked birth/infant death data set, *Natl Vital Stat Rep* 59(6):8–30, 2011.

Mathews TJ, MacDorman MF: Infant mortality statistics from the 2008 period linked birth/infant death data set, *Nat Vital Stat Rep* 60(5):1–27, Hyattsville, MD, 2012, National Center for Health Statistics.

Matthews R, Moore A: Babies are still dying of SIDS, *AJN* 113(2):59–64, 2013.

McGarvey C, McDonnell M, Chong A, et al: Factors relating to the infant's last sleep environment in sudden infant death syndrome in the Republic of Ireland, *Arch Dis Child* 88(12):1058–1064, 2003.

McGrath JM, Records K, Rice M: Maternal depression and infant temperament characteristics, *Infant Behav Dev* 31(1):71–80, 2008.

McMartin KI, Platt MS, Hackman R, et al: Lung tissue concentrations of nicotine in sudden infant death syndrome (SIDS), *J Pediatr* 140(2):205–209, 2002.

Medoff-Cooper B, Carey WB, McDevitt SC: The early infancy temperament questionnaire, *J Dev Behav Pediatr* 14(4):230–235, 1993.

Middleman AB, Anding R, Tung C: Effect of needle length when immunizing obese adolescents with hepatitis B vaccine, *Pediatrics* 125(3):e508–e512, 2010.

Miller L, Reynolds J: Autism and vaccination—the current evidence, *J Spec Pediatr Nurs* 14(3):166–172, 2009.

Mitchell EA, Thompson JM, Becroft DM, et al: Head covering and the risk for SIDS: findings from the New Zealand and German SIDS case-control studies, *Pediatrics* 121(6):e1478–e1483, 2008.

Morin K: Preparing infant formula: increasing caregiver knowledge, *MCN Am J Matern Child Nurs* 34(6):387, 2009a.

Morin K: The challenge of colic in infants, *MCN Am J Matern Child Nurs* 34(3):192, 2009b.

Narendran V, Hoath SB: The skin. In Martin RJ, Fanaroff AA, Walsh MC, editors: *Fanaroff and Martin's neonatal-perinatal medicine*, ed 8, St Louis, 2006, Mosby.

National Center for Immunization and Respiratory Diseases: General recommendations on immunization: recommendations of the Advisory Committee on Immunization Practices (ACIP), *MMWR Recomm Rep* 60(2):1–64, 2011.

National Institutes of Health: Consensus Development Conference on Infantile Apnea and Home Monitoring, Sept 29 to Oct 1, 1986, *Pediatrics* 79(2):292–299, 1987.

Neu M, Robinson JA: Infants with colic: their childhood characteristics, *J Pediatr Nurs* 18(1):12–20, 2003.

Niemelä M, Pihakari O, Pokka T, et al: Pacifier as a risk factor for acute otitis media: a randomized, controlled trial of parental counseling, *Pediatrics* 106(3):483–488, 2000.

O'Connor NR: Infant formula, *Am Fam Physician* 79(7):565–570, 2009.

O'Connor NR, Tanabe KO, Siadaty MS, et al: Pacifiers and breastfeeding: a systematic review, *Arch Pediatr Adolesc Med* 163(4):378–382, 2009.

Ostfield BM, Esposito L, Perl H, et al: Concurrent risks of sudden infant death syndrome, *Pediatrics* 125(3):447–453, 2010.

Parker SK, Schwartz B, Todd J, et al: Thimerosal-containing vaccines and autistic spectrum disorder: a critical review of published original data, *Pediatrics* 114(3):793–804, 2004.

Perry R, Hunt K, Ernst E: Nutritional supplements and other complementary medicines for infantile colic: a systematic review, *Pediatrics* 127(4):720–733, 2011.

Person TL, Lavezzi WA, Wolf BC: Cosleeping and sudden unexpected death in infancy, *Arch Pathol Lab Med* 126(3):343–345, 2002.

Peterson-Sweeney K, Stevens J: Optimizing the health of infants and children: their oral health counts! *J Pediatr Nurs* 25(4):244–249, 2010.

Piaget J: *The origins of intelligence in children*, New York, 1952, International Universities Press.

Pollack HA: Sudden infant death syndrome, maternal smoking during pregnancy and effectiveness of smoking cessation intervention, *Am J Public Health* 91(3):432–436, 2001.

Price CS, Thompson WW, Goodson B, et al: Prenatal and infant exposure to thimerosal from vaccines and immunoglobulins and risk of autism, *Pediatrics* 126(4):656–664, 2010.

Puffenberger EG, Hu-Lince D, Parod JM, et al: Mapping of sudden infant death with dysgenesis of the testes syndrome (SIDDT) by a SNP genome scan and identification of TSPYL loss of function, *Proc Natl Acad Sci USA* 101(32):11689–11694, 2004.

Quillin SI, Glenn LL: Interaction between feeding method and co-sleeping on maternal-newborn sleep, *J Obstet Gynecol Neonatal Nurs* 33(5):580–588, 2004.

Ramanathan R, Corwin MJ, Hunt CE, et al: Cardiorespiratory events recorded on home monitors: comparison of healthy infants with those at increased risk for SIDS, *JAMA* 285(17):2199–2243, 2001.

Reis EC, Holubkov R: Vapocoolant spray is equally effective as EMLA cream in reducing immunization pain in school-aged children, *Pediatrics* 100(6):1025, 1997.

Roberts DM, Ostapchuk M, O'Brien J: Infantile colic, *Am Fam Physician* 70(4):735–740, 2004.

Robinson S, Proctor M: Diagnosis and management of deformational plagiocephaly: a review, *J Neurosurg Pediatr* 3(4):284–295, 2009.

Rojjanasrirat W: Working women's breastfeeding experiences, *MCN Am J Matern Child Nurs* 29(4):222–227, 2004.

Rovers MM, Numans ME, Langenbach E, et al: Is pacifier use a risk factor for otitis media? A dynamic cohort study, *Fam Pract* 25(4):233–236, 2008.

Rudolf MCJ, Logan S: What is the long term outcome for children who fail to thrive? A systematic review, *Arch Dis Child* 90(9):925–931, 2005.

Savino F, Castagno E, Bretto R, et al: A prospective 10-year study on children who had severe infantile colic, *Acta Paediatr Suppl* 94(449):129–132, 2005.

Savino F, Cordisco L, Tarasco V, et al: Lactobacillus reuteri DSM 17938 in infantile colic: a randomized, double-blind, placebo-controlled trial, *Pediatrics* 126(3):e526–e533, 2010.

Savino F, Palumeri E, Castagno E, et al: Reduction of crying episodes owing to infantile colic: a randomized controlled study on the efficacy of a new infant formula, *Eur J Clin Nutr* 60(11):1304–1310, 2006.

Schechter NL, Zempsky WT, Cohen LL, et al: Pain reduction during pediatric immunizations: evidence-based review and recommendations, *Pediatrics* 119(5):e1184–e1198, 2007.

Schnitzer PG: Prevention of unintentional childhood injuries, *Am Fam Physician* 74(11):1864–1869, 2006.

Schultz ST: Does thimerosal or other mercury exposure increase the risk for autism? *Acta Neurobiol Exp (Wars)* 70(2):187–195, 2010.

Settipane RA, Siri D, Bellanti JA: Egg allergy and influenza vaccination, *Allergy Asthma Proc* 30(6):660–665, 2009.

Sexton S, Natale R: Risks and benefits of pacifiers, *Am Fam Physician* 79(8):681–685, 2009.

Shah V, Taddio A, Rieder MJ, et al: Effectiveness and tolerability of pharmacologic and combined interventions for reducing injection pain during routine childhood immunizations: systematic review and meta-analyses, *Clin Ther* 31(Suppl 2):S104–S151, 2009.

Shealy KR, Li R, Benton-Davis S, et al: *The CDC guide to breastfeeding interventions*, Atlanta, 2005, U.S. Department of Health and Human Services, Centers for Disease Control and Prevention.

Sicherer SH: Clinical aspects of gastrointestinal food allergy in children, *Pediatrics* 111(6 Part 3):1609–1616, 2003.

Silvestri J: Indications for home monitoring (or not), *Clin Perinatol* 36(1):87–99, 2012.

Silvestri JM, Weese-Mayer D: Disorders of respiratory control: apnea and SIDS. In Rudolph CD, Rudolph AM, Hostetter MK, editors: *Rudolph's pediatrics*, ed 21, New York, 2003, McGraw-Hill.

Stevens B, Johnston C, Franck L, et al: The efficacy of developmentally sensitive interventions and sucrose for relieving procedural pain in very low birth weight neonates, *Nurs Res* 48(1):35–43, 1999.

Stevens B, Yamada J, Ohlsson A: Sucrose for analgesia in newborn infants undergoing painful procedures, *Cochrane Database Syst Rev* (4):CD001069, 2001.

St. James-Roberts I: Infant crying and sleeping: helping parents to prevent and manage problems, *Primary Care* 35(3):547–567, 2008.

Strehle EM, Gray WK, Gopisetti S, et al: Can home monitoring reduce mortality in infants at increased risk of sudden infant death syndrome? A systematic review, *Acta Paediatr* 101(1):8–13, 2012.

Sullivan JR: Development of father-infant attachment in fathers of preterm infants, *Neonatal Netw* 18(7):33–39, 1999.

Tablizo MA, Jacinto P, Parsley D, et al: Supine sleeping position does not cause clinical aspiration in neonates in hospital newborn nurseries, *Arch Pediatr Adolesc Med* 161(5):507–510, 2007.

Tappin D, Ecob R, Brooke H: Bedsharing, roomsharing, and sudden infant death syndrome in Scotland: a case-control study, *J Pediatr* 147(1):32–37, 2005.

Taveras EM, Rifas-Shiman SL, Belfort MB, et al: Weight status in the first 6 months of life and obesity at 3 years of age, *Pediatrics* 123(4):1177–1183, 2009.

Thomas DW, Greer FR, American Academy of Pediatrics (AAP) Committee on Nutrition and Section on Gastroenterology, Hepatology, and Nutrition: Probiotics and prebiotics in pediatrics, *Pediatrics* 126(6):1217–1231, 2010.

Thompson DG: Safe sleep practices for hospitalized infants, *Pediatr Nurs* 31(5):400–403, 409, 2005.

Turner S, Arthur G, Lyons RA, et al: Modification of the home environment for the reduction of injuries, *Cochrane Database Syst Rev* (2):CD003600, 2011.

Unger B, Kemp, JS, Wilkins D, et al: Racial disparity and modifiable risk factors among infants dying suddenly and unexpectedly, *Pediatrics* 111(2):E127–E131, 2003.

Vennemann MM, Bajanowski T, Brinkmann B, et al: Sleep environment risk factors for sudden infant death syndrome: the German Sudden Infant Death Syndrome Study, *Pediatrics* 123(4):1162–1170, 2009.

Vollrath ME, Tonstad S, Rothbart MK, et al: Infant temperament is associated with potentially obesogenic diet at 18 months, *Int J Pediatr Obes* 6(2-2):e408–e414, 2011.

Wasser H, Bentley M, Borja J, et al: Infants perceived as "fussy" are more likely to receive complementary foods before 4 months, *Pediatrics* 127(2):229–237, 2011.

Wilson ME, White MA, Cobb B, et al: Family dynamics, parental-fetal attachment and infant temperament, *J Adv Nurs* 31(1):204–210, 2000.

Wong DL: Topical local anesthetics: two products for pain relief during minor procedures, *Am J Nurs* 103(6):42–45, 2003.

Zeanah CH, Fox NA: Temperament and attachment disorders, *J Clin Child Adolesc Psychol* 33(1):82–87, 2004.

Zeanah CH, Gleason MM: *Reactive attachment disorder: a review for DSM-V*, Washington, DC, 2010, American Psychiatric Association, pp 1-53, www.dsm5.org/Proposed%20 Revision%20Attachments/APA%20 DSM-5%20Reactive%20Attachment%20 Disorder%20Review.pdf.

Zuckerman J: The importance of injecting vaccines into muscle, *BMJ* 321(7271):1237–1238, 2000.

The Toddler and Family

David Wilson

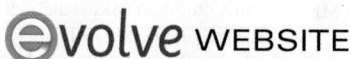 WEBSITE

http://evolve.elsevier.com/Perry/maternal

LEARNING OBJECTIVES

On completion of this chapter, the reader will be able to:
- Identify the major biologic, psychosocial, cognitive, and social developments during the toddler years.
- Relate separation anxiety and negativism to developmental tasks.
- Recognize readiness for toilet training and offer parents guidelines.

- Prepare parents of toddlers for the birth of a sibling.
- Provide parents with guidelines for handling temper tantrums.
- Provide parents with feeding recommendations for the toddler.
- Outline a preventive dental hygiene plan for toddlers.
- Provide anticipatory guidance to parents regarding injury prevention based on the toddler's developmental achievements.

PROMOTING OPTIMAL GROWTH AND DEVELOPMENT

The term *terrible twos* has often been used to describe the toddler years, the period from 12 to 36 months of age. Although the term may be used often to describe the toddler's *behavior,* it is not meant to typify or label the child. It is a time of intense exploration of the environment as children attempt to find out how things work and how to control others through temper tantrums, negativism, and obstinacy. Although this can be a challenging time for parents and child as each learns to know the other better, it is an extremely important period for developmental achievement and intellectual growth. Toddlers are very lovable at times; however, because of their search for autonomy, they may test parents' and caregivers' patience.

Biologic Development
Proportional Changes
Growth slows considerably during toddlerhood. The average *weight* gain is 1.8 to 2.7 kg (4 to 6 lbs). The birth weight is quadrupled by 2½ years of age. The rate of increase in height also slows. The usual increment is an addition of 7.5 cm (3 inches) per year and occurs mainly in elongation of the legs rather than the trunk. The average *height* of a 2-year-old is 86.6 cm (34 inches). In general adult height is about twice the 2-year-old child's height. Accurate measurement of height and weight during the toddler years should reveal a steady growth curve that is *steplike* in nature rather than linear (straight),

which is characteristic of the growth spurts during the early childhood years.

The rate of increase in *head circumference* slows somewhat by the end of infancy, and head circumference is usually equal to chest circumference by 1 to 2 years of age. The usual total increase in head circumference during the second year is 2.5 cm (1 inch). Then the rate of increase slows until at age 5 years the increase is less than 1.25 cm (0.5 inch) per year. The anterior fontanel closes between 12 and 18 months of age.

Chest circumference continues to increase in size and exceeds head circumference during the toddler years. Its shape also changes as the transverse, or lateral, diameter exceeds the anteroposterior diameter. After the second year the chest circumference exceeds the abdominal measurement; this, in addition to the growth of the lower extremities, gives the child a taller, leaner appearance. However, the toddler still appears relatively squat and "pot-bellied" because of the less well-developed abdominal musculature and short legs. The legs remain slightly bowed or curved during the second year from the weight of the relatively large trunk.

Sensory Changes
Visual acuity of 20/40 is considered acceptable during the toddler years. Full binocular vision is well developed, and any evidence of persistent strabismus requires professional attention as early as possible to prevent amblyopia. Depth perception continues to develop but, because of the child's lack of motor coordination, falls from heights are a persistent danger.

The senses of *hearing, smell, taste,* and *touch* become increasingly well developed, coordinated with one another, and associated with other experiences. All of the senses are used to explore the environment. Toddlers visually inspect an object by turning it over; they may taste it, smell it, and touch it several times before they are satisfied with their investigation. They shake it to see if it makes noise and vigorously test its durability.

Another example of the integrated function of the senses is the toddler's development of specific *taste preferences.* The toddler is much less likely than an infant to try a new food because of its appearance, texture, or smell, not just its taste.

Maturation of Systems

Most of the physiologic systems are relatively mature by the end of toddlerhood. Volume of the *respiratory tract* and growth of associated structures continue to increase during early childhood, lessening some of the factors that predisposed the child to frequent and serious infections during infancy. The internal structures of the ear and throat continue to be short and straight, and the lymphoid tissue of the tonsils and adenoids continues to be large. As a result otitis media, tonsillitis, and upper respiratory tract infections are common. The respiratory and heart rates slow, and the blood pressure increases (see Appendix C). Respirations continue to be abdominal.

Under conditions of moderate variation in temperature the toddler rarely has the difficulties of the young infant in maintaining *body temperature.* The mature functioning of the renal system serves to conserve fluid under times of stress, decreasing the risk of dehydration.

The *digestive processes* are fairly complete by the beginning of toddlerhood. The acidity of the gastric contents continues to increase and has a protective function because it is capable of destroying many types of bacteria. Stomach capacity increases to allow for the usual schedule of three meals a day.

One of the more prominent changes of the gastrointestinal system is the voluntary control of elimination. With complete myelination of the spinal cord, control of the anal and urethral sphincters is gradually achieved. The *physiologic* ability to control the sphincters probably occurs somewhere between ages 18 and 24 months. Bladder capacity also increases considerably, and by 14 to 18 months of age the child is able to retain urine for up to 2 hours or longer.

The *defense mechanisms* of the skin and blood, particularly phagocytosis, are much more efficient in toddlers than in infants. The production of antibodies is well established. However, many young children have a sudden increase in colds and minor infections when they enter preschool or other group situations such as day care because of their exposure to pathogens and the lack of understanding of general hygiene measures such as hand washing.

Gross and Fine Motor Development

The major *gross motor skill* during the toddler years is the development of locomotion. By 12 to 13 months of age toddlers walk alone using a wide stance for extra balance, and by 18 months they try to run but fall easily (Fig. 32-1). Between 2 and 3 years of age refinement of the upright, biped position is evident in improved coordination and equilibrium. At age 2 years toddlers can walk up and down stairs; by age 2½ years they can jump using both feet, stand on one foot for a second or two, and manage a few steps on tiptoe. By the end of the second year they can stand on one foot, walk on tiptoe, and climb stairs with alternate footing.

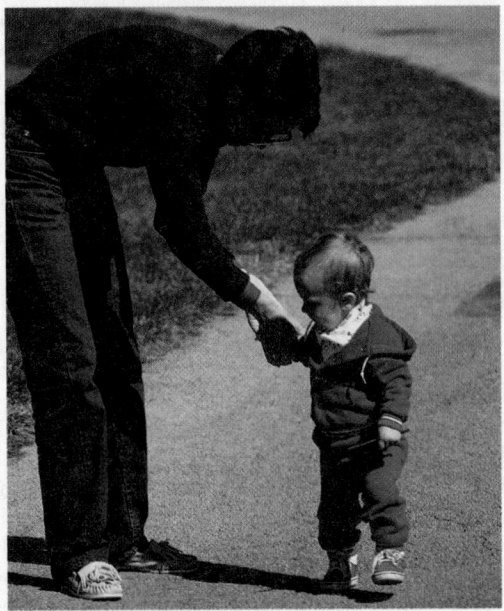

FIG 32-1 Typical toddling gait.

Fine motor development is demonstrated in increasingly skillful manual dexterity. For example, by age 12 months toddlers are able to grasp a very small object but are unable to release it at will. At 15 months they can drop a pellet into a narrow-necked bottle. Casting or throwing objects and retrieving them become almost obsessive activities at about 15 months. By 18 months of age toddlers can throw a ball overhand without losing their balance.

Mastery of gross and fine motor skills is evident in all phases of the child's activity such as play, dressing, language comprehension, response to discipline, social interaction, and propensity for injuries. Activities occur less in isolation and more in conjunction with other physical and mental abilities to produce a purposeful result. For example, the toddler walks to reach a new location, releases a toy to pick it up or to choose a new one, and scribbles to look at the image produced. The possibilities of the exploration, investigation, and manipulation of the environment—and its hazards—are endless.

Psychosocial Development

Toddlers are faced with the mastery of several important tasks. If the need for basic trust has been satisfied, they are ready to give up dependence for control, independence, and autonomy. Some of the specific tasks to be dealt with include:

- Differentiation of self from others, particularly the mother.
- Toleration of separation from parent.
- Ability to delay gratification.
- Control over bodily functions.
- Acquisition of socially acceptable behavior.
- Verbal means of communication.
- Ability to interact with others in a less egocentric manner.

Mastery of these goals is only begun during late infancy and the toddler years, and tasks such as developing interpersonal relationships with others may not be completed until adolescence. However, crucial foundations for successful completion of such developmental tasks are established during these early formative years.

Developing a Sense of Autonomy (Erikson)

According to Erikson (1963), the developmental task of toddlerhood is acquiring a sense of *autonomy* while overcoming a sense of *doubt* and *shame.* As infants gain trust in the predictability and reliability of their parents, environment, and interaction with others, they begin to discover that their behavior is their own and that it has a predictable, reliable effect on others. However, although they realize their will and control over others, they are confronted with the conflict of exerting autonomy and relinquishing the much-enjoyed dependence on others. Exerting their will has definite negative consequences, whereas retaining dependent, submissive behavior is generally rewarded with affection and approval. At the same time continued dependency creates a sense of doubt regarding their potential capacity to control their actions. This doubt is compounded by a sense of shame for feeling this urge to revolt against others' will and a fear that they will exceed their own capacity for manipulating the environment.

Just as the infant has the social modalities of grasping and biting, the toddler has the newly gained modality of holding on and letting go. To hold on and let go is evident with the use of the hands, mouth, eyes, and eventually the sphincters when toilet training is begun. These social modalities are expressed constantly in the child's play activities such as casting or throwing objects; taking objects out of boxes, drawers, or cabinets; holding on tighter when someone says, "No, don't touch"; and spitting out food as taste preferences become strong.

Several characteristics, especially negativism and ritualism, are typical of toddlers in their quest for autonomy. As they attempt to express their will, they often act with negativism, the persistent negative response to requests. The words "no" or "me do" can be the sole vocabulary. Emotions are expressed strongly, usually in rapid mood swings. One minute toddlers can be engrossed in an activity, and the next minute they might be extremely frustrated because they are unable to manipulate a toy or open a door. If scolded for doing something wrong, they can have a temper tantrum and almost instantaneously pull at the parent's legs to be picked up and comforted. Understanding and coping with these swift changes in behavior is often difficult for parents. Many find the negativism exasperating and, instead of dealing constructively with it, give in to it, which further threatens children in their search for learning acceptable methods of interacting with others (see Temper Tantrums, p. 932; see Negativism, p. 933).

In contrast to negativism, which often disrupts the environment, ritualism, the need to maintain sameness and reliability, provides a sense of comfort. Toddlers can venture out with security when they know that familiar people, places, and routines still exist. One can easily understand why change such as hospitalization represents such a threat to these children. Without the comfortable rituals there is little opportunity to exert autonomy. Consequently dependency and regression occur (see Regression, p. 933).

Erikson focuses on the development of the *ego,* which may be thought of as reason or common sense, during this phase of psychosocial development. There is a struggle as the child deals with the impulses of the *id* and attempts to tolerate frustration and learn socially acceptable ways of interacting with the environment. The *ego* is evident as the child is able to tolerate delayed gratification.

There is also a rudimentary beginning of the *superego,* or conscience, which is the incorporation of the morals of society and the process of acculturation. With the development of the ego children further differentiate themselves from others and expand their sense of trust within themselves. However, as they begin to develop awareness of their own will and capacity to achieve, they also become aware of their ability to fail. This ever-present awareness of potential failure creates doubt and shame. Successful mastery of the task of autonomy necessitates opportunities for self-mastery while withstanding the frustration of necessary limit setting and delayed gratification. Opportunities for self-mastery are present in appropriate play activities, toilet training, the crisis of sibling rivalry, and successful interactions with significant others.

Cognitive Development
Sensorimotor and Preoperational Phase (Piaget)

The period from 12 to 24 months of age is a continuation of the final two stages of the sensorimotor phase. During this time the cognitive processes develop rapidly and at times seem similar to those of mature thinking. However, reasoning skills are still primitive and need to be understood to deal with the typical behaviors of a child of this age effectively.

Tertiary Circular Reactions

In the fifth stage of the sensorimotor phase (13 to 18 months of age), the child uses active experimentation to achieve previously unattainable goals. Newly acquired physical skills are increasingly important for the function they serve rather than for the acts themselves. The child incorporates the old learning of secondary circular reactions with new skills and applies the combined knowledge to new situations, with emphasis on the results of the experimentation. In this way there is the beginning of rational judgment and intellectual reasoning. During this stage there is further differentiation of one's self from objects. This is evident in the child's increasing ability to venture away from the parent and tolerate longer periods of separation.

Awareness of a causal relationship between two events is apparent. After flipping a light switch, toddlers are aware that a reciprocal response occurs. However, they are not able to transfer that knowledge to new situations. Therefore, every time they see what appears to be a light switch, they must reinvestigate its function. Such behavior demonstrates the beginning of *categorizing data into distinct classes and subclasses.* Examples of this type of behavior are innumerable as toddlers continuously explore the same object each time it appears in a new place.

Because classification of objects is still rudimentary, the *appearance* of an object denotes its function. For example, if the child's toys are stored in a paper bag or large container, that toy receptacle is no different from the garbage pail or laundry basket. If allowed to turn over the toy receptacle, the child will just as quickly do the same to other similar containers because in the child's mind there is no difference. Expecting the child to judge which receptacles are permissible to explore and which are not is inappropriate for this age-group. Instead the forbidden object such as the garbage pail should be placed out of reach. This has significance in relation to protecting the toddler from injury; the toddler is not able to differentiate between safe objects with which he or she can play and objects which are unsafe under similar circumstances. For example, if the child is allowed to throw a toy ball, he or she does not necessarily understand why a toy block that may harm someone cannot be thrown.

The discovery of objects as objects leads to the awareness of their spatial relationships. Children are able to recognize different shapes and their relationship to one another. For example, they can fit slightly smaller boxes into one another (nesting) and can place a round object into a hole, even if the board is turned around, upside down, or reversed. Children are also aware of space and the relationship of their body to dimensions such as height. They stretch, stand on a low stair or stool, and pull a string to reach an object.

Object permanence has also advanced. Although they still cannot find an object that has been invisibly displaced or moved from under one pillow to another without actually seeing the change, toddlers are increasingly aware of the existence of objects behind closed doors, in drawers, on countertops, and under tables. Parents are usually acutely aware of this developmental achievement and find high places and locked cabinets to be the only places inaccessible to toddlers.

Invention of New Means Through Mental Combinations

From ages 19 to 24 months the child is in the final sensorimotor stage. During this stage he or she completes the more primitive, autistic-like thought processes of infancy and is prepared for the more complex mental operations that occur during the phase of preoperational thought. One of the most dramatic achievements of this stage is in the area of object permanence. Children now actively search for an object in several potential hiding places. In addition, they can infer a cause when only experiencing the effect. They can infer that an object was hidden in any number of places even if they only saw the original hiding place.

Imitation displays deeper meaning and understanding. There is greater symbolization to imitation. The child is acutely aware of others' actions and attempts to copy them in gestures and words. Domestic mimicry (imitating household activities) and gender-role behavior become increasingly common during this stage, especially during the second year. Identification with the parent of the same gender becomes apparent by the second year and represents the child's intellectual ability to identify different models of behavior and imitate them appropriately (Fig. 32-2).

The concept of time is still embryonic; but children have some sense of timing in terms of anticipation, memory, and a limited ability to wait. They may listen to the command, "Just a minute," and behave appropriately. However, their sense of time is exaggerated; 1 minute can seem like an hour. Toddlers' limited attention spans also indicate their sense of immediacy and concern for the present.

Preoperational Phase

At approximately 2 years of age the child enters the preconceptual phase of cognitive development, which lasts until about age 4 years. The preconceptual phase is a subdivision of the preoperational phase, which spans ages 2 to 7 years. It is primarily one of transition that bridges the purely self-satisfying behavior of infancy and the rudimentary socialized behavior of latency. *Preoperational thought* implies that children cannot think in terms of *operations* (i.e., the ability to manipulate objects in relation to one another in a logical fashion). Rather toddlers think primarily on the basis of their perception of an event. Problem solving is based on what they see or hear directly rather than on what they recall about objects and events. Several characteristics are unique to preoperational thought (Box 32-1).

Within the second year the child increasingly uses language symbolically and is concerned with the "why" and "how" of things. For example, a pencil is "something to write with," and food is "something to eat." However, such mental symbolization is closely associated with prelogical reasoning. For instance, a needle is "something that hurts." Such painful experiences take on new significance because memory is associated with the specific event, and fears are likely to develop such as resistance to people who wear a uniform or rooms that look like the practitioner's office. Because of the vulnerability of these early years, it is essential to prepare children for any new experience, whether it is a new baby-sitter or a visit to the practitioner or dentist.

Spiritual Development

Spiritual development in children is often discussed in terms of the child's developmental level because the evolution of spirituality often parallels cognitive development (Elkins and Cavendish, 2004). The child's family and environment strongly influence his or her perception of the world around him or her, and this often includes spirituality. Furthermore, family values, beliefs, customs, and expressions of these influence the child's perception of his or her spiritual self (Elkins and Cavendish, 2004). Neuman (2011) proposes that Fowler's stages of faith (Fowler, 1981) be used to better understand children and spirituality; she provides an excellent overview of the stages of faith in childhood. The relationship among spirituality, illness in childhood, and nursing has been studied in the context of suffering, terminal illness such as cancer, and end-of-life care. In the past decade there has been an increased interest in and focus on spiritual care in adults and children as further understanding of the influence of one's spirituality on health, illness, and well-being has progressed.

Toddlers learn about God through the words and actions of those closest to them. They have only a vague idea of God and religious teachings because of their immature cognitive processes; however, if God is spoken about with reverence, young children associate God with something special. During this period the assignment of powerful religious symbols and images is strongly influenced by the manner in which it is presented; therein lies the potential for the development of guilt and fear or conversely love and companionship with religious symbols (Roehlkepartain, King, Wagener, et al., 2006). Toddlers are said to be in the intuitive-projective phase of Fowler's faith construct (Fowler, 1981) wherein thinking is largely based on fantasy and rather fluid in relation to reality and fantasy. God may be described as being around like air by the toddler because of the fluidity in dividing fantasy and reality (Neuman, 2011).

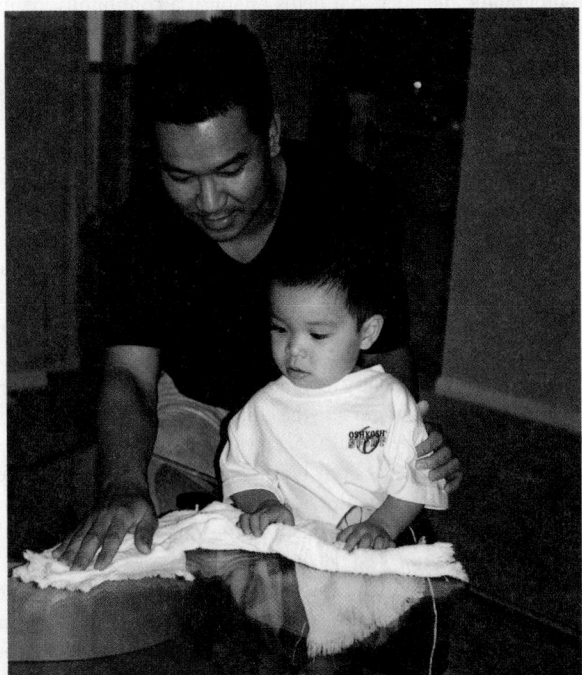

FIG 32-2 Domestic mimicry and sex-role behavior are common during toddlerhood.

BOX 32-1 CHARACTERISTICS OF PREOPERATIONAL THOUGHT

Egocentrism—Inability to envision situations from perspectives other than one's own

Example—If a person is positioned between the toddler and another child, the toddler, who is facing the person, will explain that both children can see the middle person's face. The young child is unable to realize that the other person views the middle person from a different perspective, the back.

Implication—Avoid moralizing about "why" something is wrong if it requires an understanding of someone else's feelings or opinion. Telling a child to stop hitting because hitting hurts the other person is often ineffective because to the aggressor it feels good to hit someone else. Instead emphasize that hitting is not allowed.

Transductive reasoning—Reasoning from the particular to the particular

Example—Child refuses to eat a food because something previously eaten did not taste good.

Implication—Accept child's reasoning; offer refused food at different time.

Global organization—Reasoning that changing any one part of the whole changes the entire whole

Example—Child refuses to sleep in room because location of bed is changed.

Implication—Accept child's reasoning; use same bed position or introduce change slowly.

Centration—Focusing on one aspect rather than considering all possible alternatives

Example—Child refuses to eat a food because of its color, even though its taste and smell are acceptable.

Implication—Accept child's reasoning.

Animism—Attributing lifelike qualities to inanimate objects

Example—Child scolds stairs for making child fall down.

Implication—Join child in the "scolding." Keep frightening objects out of view.

Irreversibility—Inability to undo or reverse actions initiated physically

Example—When told to stop doing something such as talking, child is unable to think of positive activity.

Implication—State requests or instructions *positively* (e.g., "Be quiet.")

Magical thinking—Believing that thoughts are all-powerful and can cause events

Examples—Child wishes someone died; then if the person dies, child feels at fault because of the "bad" thought that made the death happen.

- Calling children "bad" because they did something wrong makes them feel as if they are bad.

Implications—Clarify that thoughts do not make things happen and that child is not responsible.

- Use "I" rather than "you" messages to communicate thoughts, feelings, expectations, or beliefs without imposing blame or criticism. Emphasize that the act is bad, not the child.

Inability to conserve—Inability to understand the idea that a mass can be changed in size, shape, volume, or length without losing or adding to the original mass (instead children judge what they see by the immediate perceptual clues given to them)

Example—If two lines of equal length are presented in such a way that one appears longer than the other, child will state that one line is longer even if he or she measures both lines with a ruler or yardstick and finds that each has the same length.

Implications—Change the most obvious perceptual clue to reorient child's view of what is seen. For example, give medicine in a small medicine cup rather than a large cup because child will imagine that the large vessel contains more liquid. If child refuses the medicine in the small cup, pour it into a large cup, because the liquid will appear to be less in a tall, wide container.

- Give a large, flat cookie rather than a thick, small one or do the reverse with meat or cheese; child will usually eat larger size of favorite food and smaller size of less favorite food.

Toddlers begin to assimilate behaviors associated with the divine (folding hands in prayer). Routines such as saying prayers before meals or at bedtime can be important and comforting. Because toddlers tend to find solace in ritualistic behavior and routines, they incorporate routines associated with religious practices into their behavioral patterns without understanding all of the implications of the rituals until later. Near the end of toddlerhood, when children use preoperational thought, there is some advancement of their understanding of God. Religious teachings such as reward or fear of punishment (heaven or hell) and moral development (see Chapter 28), may influence their behavior (Fosarelli, 2003).

Development of Body Image

As in infancy the development of body image closely parallels cognitive development. Developing psychologic understanding provides greater self-awareness, and young children learn to answer the question, "Who am I?" During the second year children recognize themselves in a mirror and make verbal references to themselves ("Me big"). With increasing motor ability toddlers recognize the usefulness of body parts and gradually learn their names. They also learn that certain parts of the body have various meanings (e.g., during toilet training the genitalia become significant, and cleanliness is emphasized). By 2 years of age they recognize gender differences and refer to self by name and then by pronoun. Gender identity is developed by age 3 years. By this time the child also begins to remember events with reference to their personal significance, forming an autobiographic memory that helps establish a continuous identity throughout the events of life.

Once they begin preoperational thought, toddlers can use symbols to represent objects, but their thinking may lead to inaccuracies. For example, if someone who is pregnant is called "fat," they describe all "fat" women as having babies. There is a beginning recognition of words used to describe physical appearance such as "pretty," "handsome," or "big boy." Such expressions eventually influence how children view their own bodies.

Although little research has been done on body-image development in young children, it is evident that body integrity is poorly understood and intrusive experiences are threatening. For example, toddlers forcefully resist procedures such as examining the ear or mouth and taking an axillary temperature. The procedure itself (e.g., taking vital signs) is not hurting the child, but it represents an intrusion into the child's personal space, which elicits a strong protest. Toddlers also have unclear body boundaries and may associate nonviable parts such as feces with essential body parts. This can be seen in a toddler who is upset by flushing the toilet and watching the stool disappear.

Nurses can help parents foster a positive body image in their child by encouraging them to avoid negative labels such as "skinny arms" or "chubby legs," self-perceptions that can last a lifetime. Body parts, especially those related to elimination and reproduction, should be called by their correct names. Respect for the body should be practiced.

Development of Gender Identity

Just as toddlers explore their environment, they also explore their bodies and find that touching certain body parts is pleasurable. Genital fondling (masturbation) can occur and involves manual stimulation and posturing movements (especially in young girls) such as tightening the thighs or applying mechanical pressure to the pubic or suprapubic area. Other demonstrations of pleasurable activities include rocking, swinging, and hugging people and toys. Parental reactions to toddlers' sexual behavior influence the children's own attitudes and should be accepting rather than critical. If such acts are performed in public, parents should not condone or bring attention to the behavior but should teach the child that it is more acceptable to perform the behavior in private.

Children in this age-group are learning vocabulary associated with anatomy, elimination, and reproduction. Certain associations between words and functions become significant and can influence future sexual attitudes. For example, if parents refer to the genitalia as dirty, especially in the context of elimination, this association between "genitalia" and "dirty" may be transferred to sexual functions later in life. Sex-role differences become obvious to children and are evident in much of toddlers' imitative play. Although current research indicates that prenatal exposure to testosterone strongly influences the individual's gender identity, researchers also indicate that there are sensitive periods (e.g., puberty) that may influence the development of gender identity (Berenbaum and Beltz, 2011; Hines, 2011; Savic, Garcia-Falqueras, and Swaab, 2010). A sense of maleness or femaleness, or gender identity, is formed by age 3 years, and the child's feelings about being male or female begin to form (Fonseca and Greydanus, 2007). Early attitudes are formed about affectionate behaviors between adults from observing parental and other adult sexual or sensual activities. (See also Sex Education, Chapter 33.) The quality of relationships with parents is important to the child's capacity for sexual and emotional relationships later in life.

Social Development

A major task of the toddler period is differentiation of self from significant others, usually the mother. The differentiation process consists of two phases: *separation* (i.e., the child's emergence from a symbiotic fusion with the mother) and *individuation* (i.e., achievements that mark the child's expressions of his or her individual characteristics in the environment). Although the process begins during the latter half of infancy, the major achievements occur during the toddler years.

Toddlers have an increased understanding and awareness of object permanence and some ability to withstand delayed gratification and tolerate moderate frustration. As a result toddlers react differently to strangers than do infants. The appearance of unfamiliar people does not represent such a significant threat to their attachment to mother. They have learned from experience that parents still exist when physically absent. Repetition of events such as going to bed without the parents but waking to find them there again (in the household) reinforces the reliability of such brief separations. Consequently toddlers are able to venture away from their parents for brief periods.

According to Harpaz-Rotem and Bergman (2006), the separation-individuation phase encompasses the phenomenon of rapprochement; as the toddler separates from the mother and begins to make sense of experiences in the environment, he or she is drawn back to the mother for assistance in verbally articulating the meaning of the experiences. Developmentally the term *rapprochement* means the child moves away and returns for reassurance. If the mother's response to the toddler is inappropriate, the toddler may experience insecurity and confusion.

Transitional objects such as a favorite blanket or toy provide security for children, especially when they are separated from parents, dealing with a new stress, or just fatigued (Fig. 32-3). Security objects often become so important to toddlers that they refuse to have them taken away. Such behavior is normal; there is no need to discourage this tendency. During separations such as day care, hospitalization, or even overnight stays with relatives, transitional objects should be provided to minimize any feelings of fear or loneliness.

Learning to tolerate and master brief periods of separation is an important developmental task of children in this age-group. In addition, it is a necessary component of parenting because brief periods of separation allow parents to regain their energy and patience and minimize any tendency to direct their irritations and frustrations at the children.

Language

The most striking characteristic of language development during early childhood is the increasing level of comprehension. Although the number of words acquired (i.e., from about four at 1 year of age to approximately 300 at age 2 years is notable, *the ability to comprehend and understand speech is much greater than the number of words the child can say.* Bilingual children can also achieve their early linguistic milestones in each of the languages at the same time and produce a substantial number of semantically corresponding words in each of their two languages from the very first words or signs.

At age 1 year children use one-word sentences or holophrases. The word "up" can mean "pick me up" or "look up there." For children the one word conveys the meaning of a sentence, but to others it may mean many things or nothing. At this age about 25% of the vocalizations are intelligible. By the age of 2 years children use

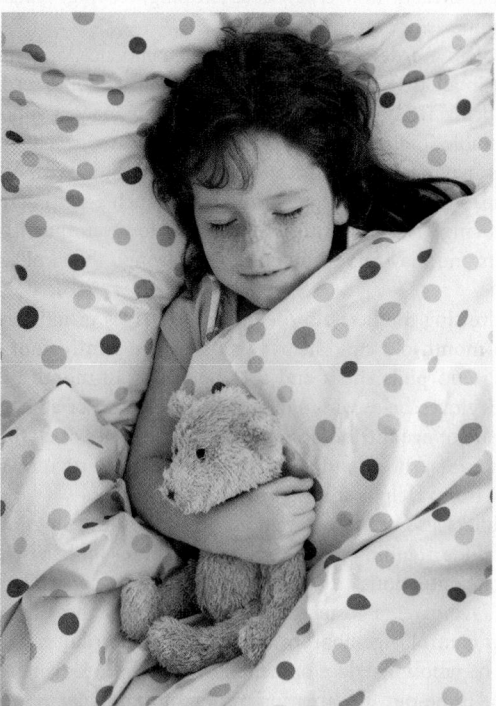

FIG 32-3 Transitional objects such as a fuzzy stuffed animal are sources of security to a toddler. (Copyright © 2011 Photos.com, a division of Getty Images. All rights reserved.)

multiword sentences by stringing together two or three words such as the phrases "mama go bye-bye" or "all gone," and approximately 65% of their speech is understandable. By 3 years the children put words together into simple sentences, begin to master grammatical rules, acquire five or six new words daily, know their age and gender, and can count three objects correctly. Looking at books during this period provides an ideal setting for further language development (Feigelman, 2011). Authorities have evaluated the impact of television viewing on toddler language development and found that those who started watching television at younger than 12 months of age and who watched longer than 2 hours per day had significant language delays (Chonchaiva and Pruksananonda, 2008). Adult-child conversations with infants and toddlers have been shown to positively affect language development; the researchers recommend reading, storytelling, and interactive adult-child communication (Zimmerman, Gilkerson, Richards, et al., 2009). The American Academy of Pediatrics (AAP) Council on Communications and Media (2011) reaffirms that televised or recorded media usage in children younger than 2 years of age decreases language skills and the time parents interact with the child. Furthermore, educational programs have not been shown to increase cognitive skills in young children (AAP Council on Communications and Media, 2011).

Gestures precede or accompany each of the language milestones up to 30 months of age (putting phone to ear, pointing). After sufficient language development, gestures phase out, and the pace of word learning increases (Bates and Dick, 2002).

Personal-Social Behavior

Perhaps one of the most dramatic aspects of development in the toddler is personal-social interaction. Parents often wonder why their manageable, docile, lovable infant has turned into a determined, strong-willed, volatile little tyrant. In addition, the tyrant of the terrible twos can swiftly and unpredictably revert back to the adorable, cuddly child. All of this is part of growing up and is evident in such areas as dressing, feeding, playing, and establishing self-control.

Toddlers are developing skills of independence, and these are evident in all areas of behavior. By 15 months children feed themselves, drink well from a covered cup, and manage a spoon with considerable spilling. By 24 months they use a spoon well and by 36 months may be using a fork. Between ages 2 and 3 years they eat with the family and like to help with chores such as setting the table or removing dishes from the dishwasher. However, they lack table manners and may find it difficult to sit through the family's entire meal.

In dressing toddlers also demonstrate strides in independence. The 15-month-old child helps by putting the arm or foot out for dressing and pulls shoes and socks off. The 18-month-old child removes gloves, helps with pullover shirts, and may be able to unzip. By 2 years of age the toddler removes most articles of clothing and puts on socks, shoes, and pants without regard to right or left and back or front. Help is still needed to fasten clothes.

Toddlers also begin to develop concern for the feelings of others and an understanding of how adult expectations for behavior apply to specific situations (e.g., causing a sibling to cry while playing rough). As parents foster their understanding, they are able to develop control. Age-appropriate discipline contributes to healthy social and emotional development. Positive reinforcement, redirecting, and time-out are appropriate for most toddlers. Social and emotional problems can develop in the youngest children. Early screening and intervention promote more positive developmental outcomes as the young child grows and develops.

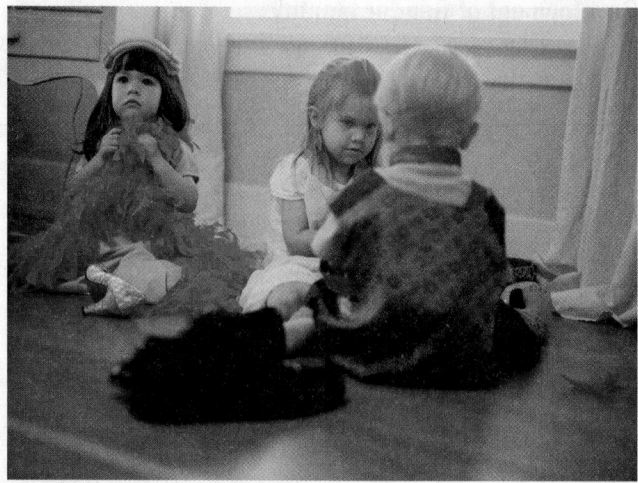

FIG 32-4 Young children enjoy dressing up. (Copyright © 2011 Photos.com, a division of Getty Images. All rights reserved.)

Play

Play magnifies toddlers' physical and psychosocial development. Interaction with people becomes increasingly important. The solitary play of infancy progresses to parallel play (i.e., toddler play alongside, not with, other children). Although sensorimotor play is still prominent, there is much less emphasis on the exclusive use of one sensory modality. Toddlers inspect toys, talk to toys, test toys' strength and durability, and invent several uses for toys. Imitation is one of the most distinguishing characteristics of play and enriches children's opportunity to engage in fantasy. With less emphasis on gender-stereotyped toys, play objects such as dolls, carriages, dollhouses, balls, dishes, cooking utensils, child-size furniture, trucks, and dress-up clothes are suitable for both genders (Fig. 32-4); however, boys may be more interested than girls in activities related to trucks, trailers, action figures, and building blocks, and girls may prefer doll-related activities.

Increased locomotive skills make push-pull toys, straddle trucks or cycles, a small gym and slide, balls of various sizes, and riding toys appropriate for energetic toddlers. Finger paints; thick crayons; chalk; blackboard; paper; and puzzles with large, simple pieces use toddlers' developing fine motor skills. Interlocking blocks in various sizes and shapes provide hours of fun and during later years are useful objects for creative and imaginative play. The most educational toy is the one that fosters the interaction of an adult with a child in supportive, unconditional play. Toys should not be substitutes for the attention of devoted caregivers, but they can enhance these interactions (Glassy, Romano, and AAP Committee on Early Childhood, 2003). Parents and other providers are encouraged to allow children to play with a variety of simple toys that foster creative thinking (e.g., blocks, dolls, and clay) rather than passive toys that the child observes (battery-operated or mechanical). Active play time should also be encouraged over the use of computer or video games, which are more passive (Ginsburg and AAP Committee on Communications, 2007).

Certain aspects of play are related to emerging linguistic abilities. Talking is a form of play for toddlers, who enjoy musical toys such as age-appropriate compact disk (CD) players, "talking" dolls and animals, and toy telephones. Children's television programs are appropriate for some children over 2 years of age who learn to associate words with visual images. However, total media time should be limited to 1 hour or less of quality programming per day. Parents are encouraged to allow the child to engage in unstructured playtime, which is considered much more beneficial than any electronic media exposure (AAP Council on Communications and Media, 2011). Toddlers also enjoy "reading" stories from a picture book and imitating the sounds of animals.

Tactile play is also important for exploring toddlers. Water toys, a sandbox with a pail and shovel, finger paints, soap bubbles, and clay provide excellent opportunities for creative and manipulative recreation. Adults sometimes forget the fascination of feeling textures such as slippery cream, mud, or pudding; catching air bubbles; squeezing and reshaping clay; or smearing paints. These types of unstructured activities are as important as educational play to allow children the freedom of expression.

Selection of appropriate toys must involve safety factors, especially in relation to size and sturdiness. The oral activity of toddlers puts them at risk for aspirating small objects and ingesting toxic substances. Parents need to be especially vigilant of toys played with in other children's homes and those of older siblings. Toys are a potential source of serious bodily damage to toddlers, who may have the physical strength to manipulate them but not the knowledge to appreciate their danger (Stephenson, 2005). Government agencies do not inspect and police all toys on the market. Therefore adults who purchase play equipment, supervise purchases, or allow children to use play equipment need to evaluate its safety, including toys that are gifts or those that are purchased by the children themselves. Adults should also be alert to notices of toys determined to be defective and recalled by the manufacturers. Parents and health care workers can obtain information on a variety of recalled products and report potentially dangerous toys and child products to the U.S. Consumer Product Safety Commission* or, in Canada, the Canadian Toy Testing Council.† Printable tips on toy safety are also available from Safe Kids Worldwide (www.safekids.org).

Table 32-1 summarizes the major features of growth and development for the age-groups of 15, 18, 24, and 30 months.

---

*800-638-2772; http://www.cpsc.gov (assistance is also available in Spanish).
†1973 Baseline Road, Ottawa, Ontario K2C 0C7 Canada; 613-228-3155; fax: 613-228-3242; www.toy-testing.org.

TABLE 32-1   GROWTH AND DEVELOPMENT DURING TODDLER YEARS

AGE (mo)	PHYSICAL	GROSS MOTOR	FINE MOTOR	SENSORY	LANGUAGE	SOCIALIZATION
15	Steady growth in height and weight Head circumference 48 cm (19 inches) Weight 11 kg (24 lbs) Height 78.7 cm (31 inches)	Walks without help (usually since age 13 mo) Creeps up stairs Kneels without support Cannot walk around corners or stop suddenly without losing balance Cannot throw ball without falling Runs clumsily; falls often	Constantly casting objects to floor Builds tower of two cubes Holds two cubes in one hand Releases pellet into narrow-necked bottle Scribbles spontaneously Uses cup well but rotates spoon before it reaches mouth	Able to identify geometric forms; places round object into appropriate hole Binocular vision well developed Displays intense and prolonged interest in pictures	Uses expressive jargon Says four to six words, including names "Asks" for objects by pointing Understands simple commands May use head-shaking gesture to denote "no" Uses "no" even while agreeing to the request Uses common repetitive gestures such as putting cup to mouth when empty	Tolerates some separation from parent Less likely to fear strangers Beginning to imitate parents such as cleaning house (sweeping, dusting), folding clothes May discard bottle Kisses and hugs parents; may kiss pictures in a book
18	Picky eater from decreased growth needs Anterior fontanel closed Physiologically able to control sphincters	Assumes standing position without support Walks up stairs with one hand held Pulls and pushes toys Jumps in place with both feet Seats self on chair Throws ball overhand without falling	Builds tower of three or four cubes Release, prehension, and reach well developed Turns pages in book two or three at a time In drawing makes stroke imitatively Manages spoon without rotation		Says 10 or more words Points to common object such as shoe or ball and to two or three body parts Forms word combinations Forms gesture-word combinations Forms gesture-gesture combinations	Expresses emotions; has temper tantrums Great imitator (domestic mimicry) Takes off gloves, socks, and shoes and unzips Temper tantrums may be more evident Beginning awareness of ownership ("my toy") May develop dependence on transitional objects such as "security blanket"

Continued

TABLE 32-1	GROWTH AND DEVELOPMENT DURING TODDLER YEARS—cont'd				
AGE (mo)	PHYSICAL	GROSS MOTOR	FINE MOTOR	SENSORY	LANGUAGE	SOCIALIZATION
24	Head circumference 49-50 cm (19.3-20 inches) Chest circumference exceeds head circumference Lateral diameter of chest exceeds anteroposterior diameter Usual weight gain of 1.8-2.7 kg (4-6 lbs) Usual gain in height of 10-12.5 cm (4-5 inches) Adult height approximately double height at 2 years of age May have achieved readiness for beginning daytime control of bowel and bladder Primary dentition of 16 teeth	Goes up and down stairs alone with two feet on each step Runs fairly well, with wide stance Picks up object without falling Kicks ball forward without overbalancing	Builds tower of six or seven cubes Aligns two or more cubes like a train Turns pages of book one at a time In drawing imitates vertical and circular strokes Turns doorknob; unscrews lid	Accommodation well developed In geometric discrimination able to insert square block into oblong space	Has vocabulary of approximately 300 words Uses two- or three-word phrases Uses pronouns "I," "me," "you" Understands directional commands Gives first name; refers to self by name Verbalizes need for toileting, food, or drink Talks incessantly	Stage of parallel play Has sustained attention span Temper tantrums decreasing Pulls people to show them something Increased independence from parent Dresses self in simple clothing Develops visual recognition and verbal self-reference ("Me big")
30	Birth weight quadrupled Primary dentition (20 teeth) completed (30-33 months) May have daytime bowel and bladder control	Jumps with both feet Jumps from chair or step Stands on one foot momentarily Takes a few steps on tiptoe	Builds tower of eight cubes Adds chimney to train of cubes Good hand-finger coordination; holds crayon with fingers rather than fist Moves fingers independently In drawing imitates vertical and horizontal strokes; makes two or more strokes for cross		Gives first and last name Refers to self by appropriate pronoun Uses plurals Names one color	Separates more easily from parent In play helps put things away; can carry breakable objects; pushes with good steering Begins to notice gender differences; knows own gender May attend to toilet needs without help except for wiping Emotions expand to include pride, shame, guilt, embarrassment

Coping with Concerns Related to Normal Growth and Development

Toilet Training

One of the major tasks of toddlerhood is toilet training. Anticipatory guidance and clinical intervention for families surrounding toilet training should begin during routine well-child visits before the child's developmental readiness to toilet train. Preparation and education reveal and allay misconceptions; lead to the development of appropriate expectations; and provide information, guidance, and support to parents for managing this potentially frustrating process.

Voluntary control of the anal and urethral sphincters is achieved sometime after the child is walking, probably between ages 18 and 24 months. However, complex psychophysiologic factors are required for readiness. The child must be able to recognize the urge to let go and hold on and communicate this sensation to the parent. In addition, some motivation is probably involved in the desire to please the parent by holding on rather than pleasing oneself by letting go. Cultural beliefs may also affect the age at which children demonstrate readiness (Feigelman, 2011).

Schmitt (2004) notes that comparative studies over the past 5 decades indicate that children in the 1990s in the United States were toilet trained at a later age (18 months in the 1960s versus 36 months in the 1990s); one possible contributing factor is the availability and convenience of disposable diapers. Another study found that the child's average age at initiation of toilet training was 20.6 months (Horn, Brenner, Rao, et al., 2006).

GUIDELINES

Assessing Toilet Training Readiness

Physical Readiness

• Voluntary control of anal and urethral sphincters, usually by 18 to 24 months of age
• Ability to stay dry for 2 hours; decreased number of wet diapers; waking dry from nap
• Regular bowel movements
• Gross motor skills of sitting, walking, and squatting
• Fine motor skills to remove clothing

Mental Readiness

• Recognizing urge to defecate or urinate
• Verbal or nonverbal communicative skills to indicate when wet or has urge to defecate or urinate
• Cognitive skills to imitate appropriate behavior and follow directions

Psychologic Readiness

• Expressing willingness to please parent
• Ability to sit on toilet for 5 to 10 minutes without fussing or getting off
• Curiosity about adults' or older sibling's toilet habits
• Impatience with soiled or wet diapers; desire to be changed immediately

Parental Readiness

• Recognizing child's level of readiness
• Willingness to invest time required for toilet training
• Absence of family stress or change such as a divorce, moving, new sibling, or imminent vacation

---

Five markers signal a child's readiness to toilet train: bladder readiness, bowel readiness, cognitive readiness, motor readiness, and psychologic readiness (Schmitt, 2004). According to some experts, physiologic and psychologic readiness is not complete until ages 22 to 30 months (Schum, Kolb, McAuliffe, et al., 2002); however, Schmitt (2004) emphasizes that parents should begin preparing their children for toilet training earlier than 30 months. By this time children have mastered most essential gross motor skills, can communicate intelligibly, are in less conflict with their parents in terms of self-assertion and negativism, and are aware of the ability to control the body and please their parents. Both the AAP and the Canadian Paediatric Society recommend starting toilet training by 18 months of age and suggest that the child must be interested in the process (Kiddoo, 2012). There is no universal right age to begin toilet training or an absolute deadline to complete it. An important role for the nurse is to help parents identify the readiness signs in their children (see Guidelines box).* On average girls are developmentally ready to begin toilet training 2 to 2½ months before boys (Schum, Kolb, McAuliffe, et al., 2002).

Nighttime bladder control normally takes several months to years after daytime training begins. This is because the sleep cycle needs to mature so the child can awake in time to urinate. Feigelman (2011) indicates that bed-wetting is normal in girls up to age 4 years and boys up to age 5 years. Few children have night-wetting episodes after daytime dryness is totally achieved; however, children who do

*A helpful book is *Guide to Toilet Training*, available from the AAP, 847-434-4000; www.aap.org/bookstore. Additional resources are listed in the Schmitt (2004) reference.

not have nighttime dryness by the age of 6 years are likely to require intervention (Mercer, 2003).

Bowel training is usually accomplished before bladder training because of its greater regularity and predictability. The sensation for defecation is stronger than that for urination and easier for children to recognize. A well-balanced diet that includes dietary fiber helps keep stool soft and supports the development and maintenance of regular bowel movements.

A number of techniques are helpful when initiating training, and cultural differences should be considered. In the United States some of the options recommended by practitioners include the Brazelton child-oriented approach, the AAP guidelines (which are similar to Brazelton method), Dr. Spock's training method, and the intensive "toilet-training-in-a-day" (operant conditioning) approach by Azrin and Foxx (Choby and George, 2008). An extensive study and review by the Agency for Healthcare Research and Quality in 2006 (Klassen, Kiddoo, Lang, et al., 2006) concluded that the child-oriented method and the Azrin and Foxx method were effective at toilet training healthy children (Choby and George, 2008). Another method emerging in the literature involves early assisted toilet training of infants around 2 to 3 weeks of age, but there are no studies assessing this method (Kiddoo, 2012). The following discussion of toilet training methods includes suggestions from the child-oriented approach.

Parents should begin the readiness phase of toilet training by teaching the child about how the body functions in relation to voiding and having a stool. Schmitt (2004) suggests that parents talk about how adults and animals perform such functions on a routine basis. Another suggestion is to make toilet training as easy and simple as possible. Important considerations are the selection of the child's clothing and the potty chair or use of the toilet. A freestanding potty chair allows children a feeling of security (Fig. 32-5, *A*). Planting the feet firmly on the floor also facilitates defecation. Another option is a portable seat attached to the regular toilet, which may ease the transition from potty chair to regular toilet. Placing a small bench under the feet helps stabilize the child's position. It is probably best to keep the potty in the bathroom and let the child observe the excreta being flushed down the toilet to associate these activities with usual practices. If a potty chair is not available, having the child sit facing the toilet tank provides added support (Fig. 32-5, *B*). Practice sessions should be limited to 5 to 8 minutes; a parent should stay with the child, practicing sanitary habits after every session. Children should be praised for cooperative behavior and successful evacuation. Dressing children in easily removed clothing; using training pants, "pull-on" diapers, or underwear; and encouraging imitation by watching others are other helpful suggestions.

When the child begins to experience regular daytime dryness, parents may experiment with underwear during the day. Daytime accidents are common, particularly during periods of intense activity. Young children become so engrossed in play activity that, if they are not reminded, they will wait until it is too late to reach the bathroom. Therefore frequent reminders and trips to the toilet are necessary. Parents often forget to plan ahead when their toddlers are being toilet trained; before trips outside the house it is important to remind children to at least try to urinate to decrease the chance of needing to use the toilet while the car is stuck in traffic.

As the child masters each step of toileting (discussion, undressing, going, wiping, dressing, flushing, and hand washing), he or she gains a sense of accomplishment that parents should reinforce. If the parent-child relationship becomes strained, both may need a break to focus on enjoyable activities together. Regression may coincide

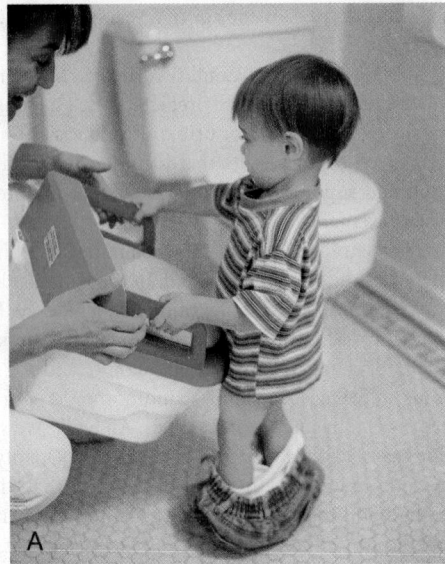

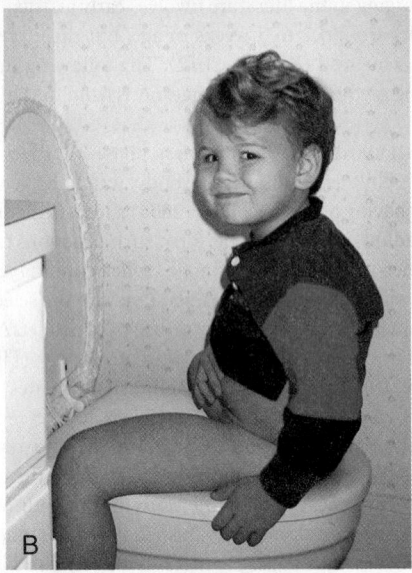

FIG 32-5 A, Children may begin toilet training sitting on a small potty chair. **B,** Sitting in reverse fashion on a regular toilet provides additional support to a young child. (**A,** Copyright © 2011 Photos.com, a division of Getty Images. All rights reserved.)

with a stressful family situation or the child being pushed too hard and too fast. It is a normal part of toilet training and does not mean failure but should be viewed as a temporary setback to a more comfortable place for the child.

Day care providers also play a role in the support and education of parents regarding toilet training practices. It is important for parents to inform all caregivers of their individual family values and the child's specific needs when planning for training away from home. Ensuring consistency in care of toddlers and healthy practices in a sanitary environment allow for safe and effective toilet practices in all settings.

Sibling Rivalry

The natural jealousy and resentment of children to a new child in the family is referred to as *sibling rivalry.* The arrival of a new infant represents a crisis for even the best-prepared toddlers. It is not the infant that toddlers resent but the changes that this additional sibling produces, especially the separation from mother during the

birth. The parents now share their love and attention with someone else, the usual routine is disrupted, and toddlers may lose their crib or room, all at a time when they thought they were in control of their world. Sibling rivalry tends to be most pronounced in the firstborn, who experiences *dethronement* (i.e., loss of sole parental attention). It also seems to be most difficult for young children, particularly in terms of mother-child interaction.

Preparation of children for the birth of a sibling is individual, but age dictates some important considerations. Time for toddlers is a vague concept. Tomorrow could be yesterday or next week, and a month from now could be never. Preparing children too soon for the birth may lessen their interest by the time the event occurs. A good time to start talking about the new baby is when the toddler becomes aware of the pregnancy and the changes taking place in the home in anticipation of the new member.

Toddlers need to have a realistic idea of what the newborn will be like. Telling them that a new playmate will come home soon sets up unrealistic expectations. Rather parents should stress the activities that will take place when the baby arrives home such as diapering, bottle-feeding or breastfeeding, bathing, and dressing. At the same time parents should emphasize which routines will stay the same such as reading stories or going to the park. The disruption of the toddler's routine is significant but can be restored with some effort by the parents. It may be helpful for the father to spend more quality time with the toddler in the evening in anticipation of the mother's time being occupied with the new baby. If toddlers have had no contact with an infant, it is a good idea to introduce them to one if feasible.

A new sibling in the home is stressful; thus any additional stresses for the toddler should be avoided or minimized. For example, moving the toddler to a regular bed or a different room should be done well in advance of the infant's arrival.

Pregnancy is an abstraction for toddlers. They need concrete illustrations of how the baby is growing inside the mother. It is an excellent opportunity for introducing aspects of reproduction and sexuality. Seeing simple pictures of the uterus and fetus and feeling the fetus move help the child feel involved in the experience (see Fig. 8-3). Children also benefit from classes for siblings that may be part of prenatal sessions (see Fig. 8-4).

When the newborn arrives, toddlers keenly feel the changed focus of attention. Visitors may initiate problems when they inadvertently shower the infant with attention and presents while neglecting the older child. Parents can minimize this by alerting visitors to the toddler's needs and including the child in the visits as much as possible. The toddler can also help with the care of the newborn by getting diapers and doing other small tasks (Fig. 32-6).

How children exhibit jealousy is complex. Some overtly hit the infant, push the child off the mother's lap, or pull the bottle or breast from the infant's mouth. For this reason infants must be protected by parental supervision of the interaction between the siblings. More often the expressions of hostility and resentment are more subtle and covert. Toddlers may verbally express a wish that the infant "go back inside mommy"; or they revert to more infantile forms of behavior such as demanding a bottle, soiling their underpants, clinging for attention, using baby talk, or aggressively acting out toward others.

Temper Tantrums

Toddlers may assert their independence by violently objecting to discipline. They may lie down on the floor, kick their feet, and scream as loud as possible. Some have learned the effectiveness of holding their breath until the parent relents. Although holding one's

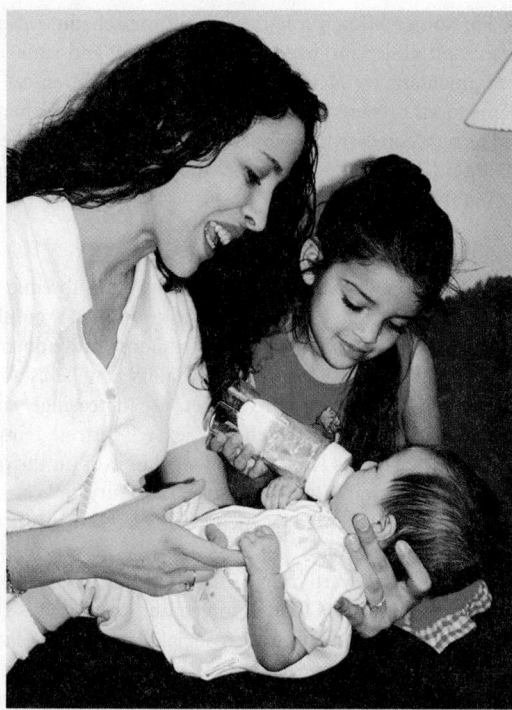

FIG 32-6 To minimize sibling rivalry, parents should include the toddler during caregiving activities.

breath may cause fainting from lack of oxygen, the accumulation of carbon dioxide stimulates the respiratory control center, resulting in no physical harm. Rarely breath-holding spells can involve symmetric tonic-clonic movements, which can be frightening to parents; the child recovers quickly when the spell is over, and there is no residual damage (Stein, 2003). Tantrums are an indication of the child's inability to control emotions; toddlers are particularly prone to tantrums because their strong drive for mastery and autonomy is frustrated by adult figures or lack of motor and cognitive skills (Needlman, Howard, and Zuckerman, 1995).

The best approach toward tapering temper tantrums requires consistency and developmentally appropriate expectations and rewards. Ensuring consistency among all caregivers in expectations, prioritizing which rules are important, and developing consequences that are reasonable for the child's level of development help manage the behavior. For example, a popular time for a tantrum is before bed; mealtime is also a common time for temper tantrums to occur (Luangrath and Hiscock, 2011). Active toddlers often have trouble slowing down and, when placed in bed, resist staying there. Parents can reinforce consistency and expectations by stating, "After this story it is bedtime." Starting at 18 months time-outs work well for managing temper tantrums. One key to handling the child's behavior is to demonstrate consistency in dealing with both the behavior and the situation that seemingly precipitated the tantrum; inconsistency reinforces the negative behavior because the child cannot cognitively comprehend the ambiguous messages being received from the parents. Another favorite time for temper tantrums is in the store, especially at the end of the day when the child is tired. Avoid the "set up" for a negative outcome by recognizing the child's limitations and work around the situation for a positive outcome.

During tantrums ignore the behavior, provided it is not injurious to the child such as violently banging the head on the floor. Continue to be present to provide a feeling of control and security to the child once the tantrum has subsided. (See also Limit Setting and Discipline, Chapter 27.) When the child starts demonstrating appropriate behavior, provide positive feedback about that behavior. During periods of no tantrums practice developmentally appropriate positive reinforcement.

Other suggestions for handling tantrums include (Needlman, Howard, and Zuckerman, 1995):

- Offering the child options instead of an "all or none" position.
- Picking one's battles carefully and ignoring small skirmishes over unimportant issues.
- Giving comfort once the child is able to control emotions but not giving in to the original request.
- Praising the child for positive behavior when he or she is not having a tantrum.

Temper tantrums are common during the toddler years and essentially represent normal developmental behaviors. However, they can be signs of serious problems. Nurses should be alert to situations that require further evaluation.

Negativism

One of the more difficult aspects of rearing children in this age-group is their persistent "no" response to every request. The negativism is not an expression of being stubborn or insolent but a necessary assertion of self-control. Children test limits to gain understanding of the world and to learn to modify their behavior to fit the expectations of society. Negativism begins to subside as most children prepare to enter kindergarten.

One method of dealing with the negativism is to reduce the opportunities for a "no" answer. Asking the child, "Do you want to go to sleep now?" is an example of a question that will almost certainly be answered with an emphatic "no." Instead, tell the child that it is time to go to sleep and proceed accordingly. In their attempt to exert control, children like to make choices. When confronted with appropriate choices such as, "You may have a peanut butter and jelly sandwich or chicken noodle soup for lunch," they are more likely to choose one rather than automatically say no. However, if their response is negative, parents should make the choice for the child.

Nurses working with children and parents can help parents understand this concept by role modeling. For example, when the nurse approaches the toddler to take vital signs, instead of asking, "Can I listen to your heart?" the nurse can say, "I'm going to listen to your heart." Because of normal developmental behavior, toddlers vigorously resist first attempts at taking vital signs because it is an intrusion on their bodies. Second, they are most likely going to answer "no," not because they necessarily fear the procedure itself but because of the tendency to answer all questions with a negative response. If the nurse asks the question, and the toddler says, "No," but the nurse proceeds anyway, the toddler starts to mistrust the nurse's actions because they contradict his or her words.

Regression

The retreat from one's present pattern of functioning to past levels of behavior is referred to as *regression*. It usually occurs in instances of discomfort or stress when one attempts to conserve psychic energy by reverting to patterns of behavior that were successful in earlier stages of development. Regression is common in toddlers because almost any additional stress hinders their ability to master present developmental tasks. Any threat to their autonomy such as illness, hospitalization, separation from parents, or adjustment to a new sibling represents a need to revert to earlier forms of behavior such as increased dependency; refusal to use the potty chair; temper tantrums; demand for the bottle, stroller, or crib; and loss of newly learned motor, language, social, and cognitive skills.

At first such regression appears acceptable and comfortable for children, but the loss of newly acquired achievements is actually frightening and threatening because they are aware of their helplessness. Parents become concerned about regressive behavior and often, in their efforts to deal with it, force the child to cope with an additional source of stress (i.e., the pressure to live up to expected standards). Brazelton (1999) suggests that these predictable times of regression, or *touchpoints,* are an opportunity to prepare parents for the next step in their child's development.

When regression does occur, the best approach is to ignore it while praising existing patterns of appropriate behavior. Regression is a child's way of saying, "I can't cope with this present stress and perfect this skill as well, but I will if given patience and understanding." For this reason it is advisable not to attempt new areas of learning when an additional crisis is present or expected such as beginning toilet training shortly before a sibling is born or attempting new areas of learning during a brief period of hospitalization.

PROMOTING OPTIMAL HEALTH DURING TODDLERHOOD

Nutrition

During the period from 12 to 18 months of age the growth rate slows, decreasing the child's need for calories, protein, and fluid. However, the protein (13 g/day) and energy requirements are still relatively high to meet the demands for muscle tissue growth and high activity level. The need for minerals such as iron, calcium, and phosphorus may be difficult to meet, considering the characteristic food habits of children in this age-group. Parents may be tempted to rely on vitamin supplementation rather than a well-balanced diet to meet these requirements. Toddlers usually require three meals and two snacks per day; however, the portions consumed are generally much smaller compared with those of older children.

The 2008 Feeding Infants and Toddlers Study (FITS) (Butte, Fox, Briefel, et al., 2010) found that in general toddlers met or exceeded the requirements for daily energy and protein requirements. The FITS recommended that toddlers be fed a more balanced diet of vegetables, fruits, and whole grains.

At approximately 18 months of age most toddlers manifest this decreased nutritional need with a decreased appetite, a phenomenon known as physiologic anorexia. They become picky, fussy eaters with strong taste preferences. They may eat large amounts one day and almost nothing the next. They are increasingly aware of the nonnutritive function of food (i.e., the pleasure of eating, the social aspect of mealtime, and the control of refusing food). They are influenced by factors other than taste when choosing food. If a family member refuses to eat something, toddlers are likely to imitate that response. If the plate is overfilled, they are likely to push it away, overwhelmed by its size. If food does not appear or smell appetizing, they will probably not agree to try it. In essence mealtime is more closely associated with psychologic rather than nutritional components.

The ritualism of this age also dictates certain principles in feeding practices. Toddlers like to have the same dish, cup, or spoon every time they eat. They may reject a favorite food simply because it is served in a different dish. If one food touches another, they often refuse to eat it. Mixed foods such as stews or casseroles are rarely favorites. Because toddlers have unpredictable table manners, it is best to use plastic dishes and cups for both economic and safety

reasons. For some children a regular mealtime schedule also contributes to their desire and need for predictability and ritualism.

Developmentally by 12 months of age most children eat many of the same foods prepared for the rest of the family. Some may have mastered using a cup with occasional spilling, although most cannot use a spoon adeptly until 18 months of age or later and generally prefer using their fingers.

Nutritional Counseling

The emphasis on preventing childhood obesity and subsequent cardiovascular disease in the United States has prompted a number of changes in dietary recommendations for children and adults alike. It is now recognized that lifetime eating habits may be established in early childhood; and health care workers are increasingly emphasizing the role of food selection choices, exercise, stress reduction, and other lifestyle choices (tobacco and alcohol use) on the quality of adult life and survival. Conditions such as obesity and cardiovascular disease can be prevented by encouraging healthy eating habits in toddlers and their families.

If food is used as a reward or sign of approval, a child may overeat for nonnutritive reasons. If food is forced and mealtime is consistently unpleasant, the usual pleasure associated with eating may not develop. Mealtimes should be enjoyable rather than times for discipline or family arguments. The social aspect of mealtime may be distracting for young children; therefore an earlier feeding hour may be appropriate. Young children are unable to sit through a long meal and become restless and disruptive. This is particularly common when children are brought to the table just after active play. Calling them in from play 15 minutes before mealtime allows them ample opportunity to get ready for eating while settling down their active minds and bodies.

The method of serving food also takes on more importance during this period. Toddlers need to have a sense of control and achievement in their abilities. Giving them large, adult-size portions can overwhelm them. In general, what is eaten is much more significant than how much is consumed. Toddlers usually restrict their food preference to four or five main foods and rarely try new foods; in some cases a toddler may insist on one food such as mashed potatoes for lunch and dinner. Small amounts of meat and vegetables supply greater food value than a large consumption of bread or potato. Serving sizes need to be appropriate for age. Young children tend to like less spicy, bland food, although this is a culturally determined preference. Substitutions can be provided for foods that they do not enjoy, although parents need not cater to all of their desires. Frequent nutritious snacks can replace a meal. Grazing (i.e., nibbling and snacking) is a good way to ensure proper nutrition, provided that appropriate foods are offered.

To determine serving size for young children, use the following guidelines:

- A general guide to the serving size of food is 1 tbsp of solid food per year of age, or one fourth to one third of the adult portion size.
- Use the tablespoon guide for easily measured foods such as vegetables or rice.
- Use the fraction guide for bread or milk.

Mastication skills continue to mature, putting children at risk for choking; therefore large round foods (e.g., hot dogs, grapes, peas, carrots, popcorn, fruit gel snacks) should be avoided until the child is able to chew them effectively. Active play while eating should be discouraged to prevent choking. Appetite and food preferences are sporadic. Often the interest in food parallels a growth spurt; thus periods of good eating are interspersed with phases of poor eating.

If exposed to the same food every day, a young toddler does not learn how to manage the complex sensory information needed to eat new, more difficult foods (e.g., vegetables with a different texture versus pureed, slippery fruits). To help prevent "food jags" it is recommended that parents present food in various physical forms. The child may need to progress to eating new foods in a stepwise fashion such as visually tolerating the food, interacting with it, smelling it, touching it, tasting it, and then eating it.

This period of picky eating can be trying for both parents and child. Many authorities consider it to be a developmental phase and stress that most toddlers will consume the necessary amount of food required for growth (Cathey and Gaylord, 2004). It has also been suggested that parents plan a nutritionally balanced week instead of day because of the way toddlers restrict food intake in their effort to exert control over their environment (Morin, 2007).

Dietary Guidelines

Dietary guidelines are necessary to promote adequate energy and nutrient intake to support physical, emotional, psychologic, and cognitive development. A number of new dietary guidelines have been developed to address the issues of childhood obesity, sedentary lifestyles, and increase in cardiovascular disease mortality in the United States.

The Institute of Medicine (IOM) (2005) has developed guidelines for nutritional intake that encompass the Recommended Daily Allowances (RDAs) yet extend their scope to include additional parameters related to nutritional intake. The Dietary Reference Intakes (DRIs)* are composed of four categories: estimated average requirements (EARs) for age and gender categories, tolerable upper-limit (UL) nutrient intakes that are associated with a low risk of adverse effects, adequate intakes (AIs) of nutrients, and new standard RDAs. The guidelines present information about lifestyle factors that may affect nutrient function such as caffeine intake and exercise and about how the nutrient may be related to chronic disease. An important factor in the development of the DRIs that affects children, particularly infants from birth to age 6 months, is that the AIs are based on the nutrient intake of full-term, healthy, breastfed infants (by well-nourished mothers), which now represents the gold standard for infant nutrition in this age-group. In 2010 new DRIs for vitamin D and calcium were released by the IOM.

The 2010 Dietary Guidelines for Americans may also be used to encourage healthy dietary intakes and regular exercise designed to decrease obesity, cardiovascular risk factors, and subsequent cardiovascular disease, which is now known to occur in both young children and adults. They recommend a caloric intake for a moderately active boy, ages 2 to 3 years, of 1000 to 1400 calories per day. The emphasis in the Dietary Guidelines is in decreasing overall fat and sodium intakes and increasing the amount of daily exercise to reduce the incidence of obesity and cardiovascular disease. The 2010 Dietary Guidelines† are for children ages 2 years and older. They encourage a variety of fruits, vegetables, whole grains, and low-fat and nonfat dairy products in addition to fish, beans, and lean meat.

Additional resources for dietary counseling include MyPlate,‡ recently developed by the U.S. Department of Agriculture to replace MyPyramid. This colorful plate shows the five main food groups (i.e., fruits, grains, vegetable, protein, and dairy) with the intended purpose to involve children and their families in making appropriate food choices for meals and decrease the incidence of overweight and obesity in the United States. MyPlate provides an online interactive feature that allows the individual to select (click on) an individual food group and see choices for foods in that group. Approximate serving sizes are suggested, and vegetarian substitutions are also provided.

Nutrition during toddlerhood involves a transition as a young toddler is weaned off milk- or formula-based diets. Milk intake, the chief source of calcium and phosphorus, should average two or three servings (24 to 30 oz) a day. Consuming more than a quart of milk daily considerably limits the intake of solid foods, resulting in a deficiency of dietary iron and other nutrients. After 2 years of age children can be given low-fat milk to reduce daily total fat to less than 30% of calories, saturated fatty acids to less than 10% of calories, and cholesterol to less than 300 mg. Other measures to reduce dietary fat include using lean meats, fat-modified products (e.g., low-fat cheese), and low-fat cooking. Because less fat in children's diets can also mean fewer calories and nutrients, caregivers must know what kinds of food to choose. However, *trans* fatty acids and saturated fats should be avoided.

Iron-fortified cereals and iron-rich foods are recommended for all children older than 6 months of age. Parents should be encouraged to provide an iron-rich diet that includes heme and nonheme iron sources (red meats, poultry, fish, green leafy vegetables, dried fruit, beans) and limits whole-milk consumption. Iron supplementation may be necessary in some cases (see Community Focus, p. 882).

Calcium and vitamin D are essential for healthy bone development. An AI of calcium for children 1 to 3 years of age is 500 mg/day. Whole milk, cheese, yogurt, legumes (beans), and vegetables (broccoli, collard greens, kale) are good sources for calcium. Popular calcium-fortified foods include waffles, cereals and cereal bars, orange juice, and some white breads. Adequate vitamin D intake is essential to prevent rickets; it is now recommended that children and adolescents have an intake of at least 400 IU of vitamin D daily (AAP, 2008). Multivitamin preparations containing 400 IU of vitamin D (by tablet or liquid) are adequate if food intake is poor or exposure to sunlight is minimal; vitamin D–only preparations containing 400 IU are also available commercially (Wagner, Greer, and AAP Section on Breastfeeding and Committee on Nutrition, 2008). Sources of vitamin D include fish, fish oils, and egg yolks. Fortified cereals, dairy products, and meat are also good sources of zinc and vitamin E.

It is also recommended that toddlers have 1 cup of fruit each day. Vitamin C enhances iron absorption. Toddlers should consume approximately 4 to 6 oz of juice per day. It tastes good to toddlers and is readily available. A 6-oz glass of fruit juice equals one fruit serving; however, juices lack the fiber of whole fruit and should not be a substitution for whole fruit. High intake of juice can contribute to diarrhea, overnutrition or undernutrition, and the development of caries; thus only 4 to 6 oz of 100% fruit juice per day is recommended for toddlers (AAP Committee on Nutrition, 2009). Fruit-flavored drinks advertised as juices may not actually contain 100% juice and should be avoided.

Vegetarian Diets

Vegetarian diets have become increasingly popular in the United States because people are concerned about hypertension; cholesterol; obesity; cardiovascular disease; cancer of the stomach, intestine, and colon; and the influence of the animal rights movement. The American Dietetic Association and Dietitians of Canada (2003) issued a statement endorsing vegetarian diets for adults and

---

*www.iom.edu/Activities/Nutrition/SummaryDRIs/DRI-Tables.aspx.
†www.cnpp.usda.gov/DietaryGuidelines.htm.
‡www.choosemyplate.gov/.

children; the statement further notes that well-planned vegetarian diets are adequate for all stages of the life cycle and promote normal growth. Children and adolescents on vegetarian diets have the potential for lifelong healthy diets and have been shown to have lower intakes of cholesterol, saturated fat, and total fat and higher intakes of fruits, fiber, and vegetables than nonvegetarians (American Dietetic Association and Dietitians of Canada, 2003). In 2009 the American Dietetic Association published another position paper supporting vegetarian diets in pregnancy, infancy, and childhood, indicating that vegetarian diets in childhood do not result in lower stature. However, the ADA does emphasize that vegetarian diets may vary considerably and that assessment of dietary adequacy is essential to ensure children are receiving adequate nutrients (Craig, Mangels, and American Dietetic Association, 2009).

The major types of vegetarianism are:

- Lacto-ovo vegetarians, who exclude meat from their diet but consume dairy products and rarely fish
- Lactovegetarians, who exclude meat and eggs but drink milk
- Pure vegetarians (vegans), who eliminate all foods of animal origin, including milk and eggs
- Macrobiotics, who are even more restrictive than pure vegetarians, allowing only a few types of fruits, vegetables, and legumes
- Semi-vegetarians, who consume a lacto-ovo vegetarian diet with some fish and poultry. This is an increasingly popular form of vegetarianism and poses little or no nutritional risk to infants unless dietary fat and cholesterol intake is severely restricted.

Many individuals who are concerned about healthy diets subscribe to vegetarian diets that may not be typified by the previous categories. Therefore during nutritional assessment it is necessary to clearly list exactly what the diet includes and excludes.*

The major deficiencies that may occur in the stricter vegan diets are inadequate protein for growth; inadequate calories for energy and growth; poor digestibility of many of the bulky natural, unprocessed foods, especially for infants; and deficiencies of vitamin B_6, niacin, riboflavin, vitamin D, iron, calcium, and zinc. Vitamin D is essential if exposure to sunlight is inadequate ($\cong$5 to 15 min/day on the hands, arms, and face of light-skinned persons; slightly more in darker-pigmented individuals) or in people who are dark skinned or who live in northern latitudes or cloudy or smoky areas. Many of these deficiencies can be avoided with a multivitamin and mineral supplement in children who are not consuming 100% of the RDA of vitamins and minerals (Dunham and Kollar, 2006).

Evaluate for iron-deficiency anemia and rickets in children on strict vegetarian and macrobiotic diets; this may occur as a result of consuming plant foods such as unrefined cereals, which impair the absorption of iron, calcium, and zinc. The American Dietetic Association and Dietitians of Canada (2003) and AAP Committee on Nutrition (2009) recommend iron supplementation of 1 mg/kg/day in infants exclusively breastfed after 4 to 6 months of age by vegetarian mothers and no dietary fat restrictions in vegetarian children younger than age 2 years. Other factors that affect iron absorption are listed in Box 32-2.

Achieving a nutritionally adequate vegetarian diet is not difficult (except with the strictest diets), but it requires careful planning and knowledge of nutrient sources (AAP Committee on Nutrition,

---

*Additional information regarding vegetarian diets may be found at the Vegetarian Resource Group; 410-366-8343; www.vrg.org. Another helpful resource for adolescents and parents is the KidsHealth website: kidshealth.org/parent/nutrition_center/dietary_needs/vegetarianism.html.

| BOX 32-2 | FACTORS THAT AFFECT IRON ABSORPTION |

Increase

- Acidity (low pH)—Administer iron between meals (gastric hydrochloric acid).
- Ascorbic acid (vitamin C)—Administer iron with juice, fruit, or multivitamin preparation.
- Vitamin A
- Tissue (cellular) need
- Meat, fish, poultry
- Cooking in cast iron pots

Decrease

- Alkalinity (high pH)—Avoid any antacid preparation.
- Phosphates—Milk is unfavorable vehicle for iron administration.
- Phytates—Found in cereals
- Oxalates—Found in many fruits and vegetables (plums, currants, green beans, spinach, sweet potatoes, tomatoes)
- Tannins—Found in tea, coffee
- Tissue (cellular) saturation
- Malabsorptive disorders
- Disturbances that cause diarrhea or steatorrhea
- Infection
- Calcium (possibly dose-dependent, therefore some recommend taking calcium supplements at bedtime and limiting dietary calcium intake to 300 mg or less at each meal [Hallberg, 1998]; long-term calcium supplementation has no effect on iron absorption [Lönnerdal, 2010])

2009). For children the lacto-ovo vegetarian diet is nutritionally adequate; however, the vegan diet requires supplementation with vitamins D and B_{12} for children ages 2 to 12 years.

To ensure sufficient protein in the diet, foods with incomplete proteins (i.e., those that do not have all the essential amino acids) must be eaten at the same meal with other foods that supply the missing amino acids. The three basic combinations of foods consumed by vegetarians that generally provide the appropriate amounts of essential amino acids follow:

1. Grains (cereal, rice, pasta) and legumes (beans, peas, lentils, peanuts)
2. Grains and milk products (milk, cheese, yogurt)
3. Seeds (sesame, sunflower) and legumes

Complementary and Alternative Medicine

There are four complementary and alternative medicine (CAM) domains according to the National Center for Complementary and Alternative Medicine (NCCAM); this discussion centers only on one of those biologically based practices that include herbs, vitamins, and foods. The NCCAM (2010) classifies probiotics as a type of natural product and CAM. Many CAM products are sold over the counter as dietary supplements, but the use of some dietary supplements such as calcium for bone health or a multivitamin supplement are not considered to be CAM (NCCAM, 2010). The NCCAM (2010) reports that natural products are the most commonly used CAM products in children and most often these products are used for chronic conditions such as neck and back pain and for head and chest colds. Other surveys confirm that CAM is often used for children's chronic remedies for which traditional therapy is not effective (Huillet, Erdie-Lalena, Norvell, et al., 2011).

The misuse of vitamins as a part of CAM has the potential for placing some children at risk for health problems. Sawni,

Ragothaman, Thomas, et al. (2007) noted that of people reportedly using CAM, the most common CAM remedies used in children seen in the emergency department were home or folk remedies (59%), herbs (41%), prayer for healing (14%), and massage therapy (10%). A survey in a Women, Infants, and Children (WIC) clinic found that child herbal use was common, especially among Hispanic children attending the clinic. Some of the herbs used by the children in the survey (St. John's wort, dong quai, and kava) have questionable safety (Lohse, Stotts, and Priebe, 2006). A recent study of CAM use in children on a military base found that 23% of parents reported using CAM in their children, with herbal therapy being the most common type of CAM reported; 50% of the parents who used CAM for their children reported the use of vitamins and minerals in amounts that exceeded the RDA (Huillet, Erdie-Lalena, Norvell, et al., 2011).

There is concern that terms often used to market supplements such as megavitamins may mislead parents regarding the actual benefits (or harm) of such therapies. The intention herein is not to discredit the use of CAM such as vitamin supplements; rather it is to ensure safety and efficacy in children who may experience inadvertent harm. The use of various herbal therapies, or intake of herbs, is also becoming more popular; many of these have been a part of medicine since early days and are beneficial in some cases. Many mind-body CAM therapies (e.g., guided imagery, distraction) have proved beneficial for children undergoing cancer treatment, but the small sample sizes of the groups being studied may preclude generalization to a larger population group until further studies are undertaken (Landier and Tse, 2010).

Herbs known to have adverse effects in children include ephedra, comfrey, and pennyroyal; some herbs may not be harmful taken alone but may counteract or potentiate prescription medications when taken together. Parents should be fully informed of the use of herbs to ensure that there is more benefit than potential harm in the ingredients being used. Health care workers also need to be knowledgeable of the benefits or potential harm in herbs to counsel parents and address their concerns appropriately. Little research has been performed in children on many over-the-counter (OTC) herbal medicines, yet some herbs are known to cause harm (Gardiner and Kemper, 2011; Lanski, Greenwald, Perkins, et al., 2003; Loman, 2003). Parents should be cautioned not to exceed the ULs of vitamin intake according to the new DRIs (see p. 935).*

Sleep and Activity

Total sleep decreases only slightly during the second year and averages about 11 to 12 hours a day. Most children take one nap a day but may relinquish this habit by the end of the second or third year. Children reach an adult pattern of sleep by 3 to 4 years of age.

Sleep problems are common, especially going to bed and falling asleep, and are a response to fears and awareness of separation. Toddlers are more prone to having bedtime resistance (refusal to go to bed) and frequent night waking; during later toddlerhood this group of children may become more resistant about going to bed and express fears about monsters (Meltzer and Mindell, 2006). Sleep problems, especially going to bed and falling asleep, are common and probably related to fears of separation. Fears can be provoked by a child's daily stressors such as pressure to toilet train, moves, sibling birth, experiences of loss, or separation from parents.

Establishing a regular bedtime and routine before bedtime is helpful, and providing transitional objects such as a favorite stuffed animal or blanket can ease the child's insecurity at bedtime (see Fig. 32-3). Children may need a light snack before bedtime; a heavy meal immediately before bedtime may interfere with sleep. Other suggestions to help small children sleep better include keeping the television out of the child's room, making the hour before bedtime a quiet time of reading stories, and avoiding stimulating activities such as computer games and roughhousing (Owens, 2011). Toddlers no longer sleeping in a crib may come out of their rooms after being put to bed. Limit prolonged bedtime rituals by defining a length of time and set of activities (one more story, one more drink of water). Toddlers who are too immature to respond to the measures identified may need their doorways gated.

A toddler's activity level is high, and there is rarely a problem with too little physical exercise, provided inappropriate restrictions are not instituted. However, recently there has been concern that decreased time spent in actual physical play and more time involved with computers and television watching have increased the tendency toward being overweight. This is especially true in large urban centers during the winter months where there may not be adequate "safe" play and physical exercise space. With increasing numbers of young children being cared for outside the home, attention to the kinds of activity provided is important. For example, children with high activity levels may benefit from an environment that encourages vigorous play, whether outside or in a large indoor play area.

Sleep Problems

A number of sleep problems are identified in small children. The two major categories are the dyssomnias: the child has trouble either falling or staying asleep at night or has difficulty staying awake during the day. The second category, parasomnias, is characterized as confusional arousals, sleepwalking, sleep terrors, nightmares, and rhythmic movement disorders; these typically occur in children 3 to 8 years old (Ward, Rankin, and Lee, 2007) and decline in incidence as the child matures (Davis, Parker, and Montgomery, 2004). This discussion focuses on minor sleep issues in toddlers such as refusal to go to sleep and frequent waking during the night (Table 32-2). Other sleep disturbances such as obstructive sleep-disordered breathing and sleep terrors are discussed elsewhere in this text.

Concerns regarding sleep are common during infancy. Sometimes these concerns are as basic as parents' questioning whether the infant needs additional sleep. In this case it is best to investigate the reason for their concern, stressing the individual needs of each child. Infants who are active during wakeful periods and growing normally are sleeping a sufficient amount of time.

When a sleeping problem is presented, a careful assessment is essential. Charting sleep habits both before and after interventions is also an important strategy. Questions regarding the frequency and duration of waking, the usual bedtime routine, the number of nighttime feedings, the perceived problem (e.g., how much disruption the behavior generates), and the attempted interventions are important in planning effective approaches designed for the specific sleep problem.

One suggestion given for any type of sleep problem, "Let the child cry until he or she falls asleep," is very difficult to implement and is inappropriate for certain conditions. After the parents relent and console the child, they have only reinforced the crying. This approach is called the *extinction method* and is still used by some; parental consistency is essential for this approach (Moore, Meltzer, and Mindell, 2008).

---

*Helpful websites for health care and consumer information concerning herbs are NCCAM, www.nccam.nih.gov; American Botanical Council, abc. herbalgram.org; and Herb Research Foundation, http://www.herbs.org.

TABLE 32-2	SELECTED SLEEP DISTURBANCES DURING INFANCY AND EARLY CHILDHOOD
CONDITION AND DESCRIPTION	**MANAGEMENT**
Nighttime Feeding Child has prolonged need for middle-of-night bottle or breastfeeding. Child goes to sleep at breast or with bottle. Awakenings are frequent (may be hourly). Child returns to sleep after feeding; other comfort measures (e.g., rocking or holding) are usually ineffective.	Increase daytime feeding intervals to 4 hours or more (may need to be done gradually). Offer last feeding as late as possible at night; may need to gradually reduce amount of formula or length of breastfeeding. Offer no bottles in bed. Put to bed awake. When child is crying, check at progressively longer intervals each night; reassure child but do not hold, rock, take to parent's bed, or give bottle or pacifier.
Developmental Nighttime Crying Child age 6-12 months with undisturbed nighttime sleep now awakens abruptly; may be accompanied by nightmares.	Reassure parents that this phase is temporary. Enter room immediately to check on child but keep reassurances brief. Avoid feeding, rocking, taking to parent's bed, or any other routine that may initiate trained nighttime crying.
Refusal to Go to Sleep Child resists bedtime and comes out of room repeatedly. Nighttime sleep may be continuous, but frequent awakenings and refusal to return to sleep may occur and become a problem if parent allows child to deviate from usual sleep pattern.	Evaluate if hour of sleep is too early (child may resist sleep if not tired). Help parents establish consistent before-bedtime routine and enforce consistent limits regarding child's bedtime behavior. If child persists in leaving bedroom, close door for progressively longer periods. Use reward system with child to provide motivation.
Trained Nighttime Crying (Inappropriate Sleep Associations) Child typically falls asleep in place other than own bed (e.g., rocking chair or parent's bed) and is brought to own bed while asleep; on awakening, cries until usual routine is instituted (e.g., rocking).	Put child in own bed when awake. If possible, arrange sleeping area separate from other family members. When child is crying, check at progressively longer intervals each night; reassure child but do not resume usual routine.
Nighttime Fears Child resists going to bed or wakes during night because of fears. Child seeks parent's physical presence and falls asleep easily with parent nearby unless fear is overwhelming.	Evaluate if hour of sleep is too early (child may fantasize when nothing to do but think in dark room). Calmly reassure frightened child; keeping night light on may be helpful. Use reward system with child to provide motivation to deal with fears. Avoid patterns that can lead to additional problems (e.g., sleeping with child or taking child to parent's room). If child's fear is overwhelming, consider desensitization (e.g., progressively spending longer periods of time alone; consult professional help for protracted fears). Distinguish between nightmares and sleep terrors (confused partial arousals).

Modified from Ferber R: Behavioral "insomnia" in the child, *Psychiatr Clin North Am* 10(4):641–653, 1987.

Another approach to night crying is known as graduated extinction. This involves letting the child cry for progressively longer times between brief parental interventions that consist only of reassurance—not rocking, holding, or using a bottle or pacifier. For example, the parents may check on the child every 5 minutes (of crying) during the first night and progressively extend this interval by 5 minutes on successive nights.

Families that cannot tolerate unexpected crying spells while everyone else is asleep can try the two-step approach. Graduated extinction is used during naps and at bedtime until the parents retire for the night. If the child cries during the night, the parents use comforting measures. However, after the child is partially trained, step 2 is initiated (i.e., the use of graduated extinction at all times).

Another approach includes the positive routine and faded bedtime. In this approach the parents schedule some quiet activities close to bedtime to calm the child for approximately 20 minutes and then place him or her to sleep. Gradually the bedtime is moved 10 to 15 minutes earlier until a suitable time is set. This approach requires parental consistency and cooperation (Moore, Meltzer, and Mindell, 2008). It is appropriate for toddlers who thrive on rituals and routines. Additional methods for dealing with specific sleep problems may be found in the Moore, Meltzer, and Mindell (2008) reference.

Children who learn to fall asleep on their own at bedtime have longer sustained sleep periods than those who fall asleep with a parent present (Davis, Parker, and Montgomery, 2004). In addition, comforting children outside their own bed at night when they awaken was associated with poor sleep consolidation. Feeding 5-month-old infants after awakening at night has been associated with fewer consecutive sleep hours (Touchette, Petit, Paquet, et al., 2005). The authors of this study recommend parental presence at bedtime until the child is drowsy and then placing the child in his or her own bed for a night's sleep.

The best way to prevent sleep problems is to encourage parents to establish bedtime rituals that do not foster problematic patterns. One of the most constructive is placing infants awake in their own crib. When infants are accustomed to falling asleep somewhere else such as in their parent's arms and then being transferred to their crib, they awaken in unfamiliar surroundings and are unable to fall asleep until the routine is repeated. In addition, the bed should be used for sleeping only—not as a play yard. It is advisable not to hang playthings over or on the bed so the child associates the bed with sleep and not with activity. Although the interventions described previously and in Table 32-2 are usually successful, it is much easier to prevent the problem with appropriate counseling during the early months of the infant's life.

Dental Health

Regular Dental Examinations

The American Academy of Pediatric Dentistry (2011a) recommends that every child have an oral health examination by a practitioner by 6 months of age; if the child is in a high-risk category for caries, it is recommended that an initial visit to a dentist or pedodontist (pediatric dentist) occur by age 6 months or within 6 months of the eruption of the first tooth. Every child should have an established dental home by the age of 12 months (American Academy of Pediatric Dentistry, 2011a). Initial visits to the dentist should be non-traumatizing. Because toddlers react negatively to new and potentially frightening experiences, the initial visit can center around meeting the dentist, seeing the equipment, and sitting in the chair. If the child is cooperative, the dentist may just look at the teeth but reserve a more thorough examination for another visit. Modeling, in which the child observes procedures performed on the parent or a cooperative sibling, can also be effective but may not work on all toddlers.

Plaque Removal

Oral hygiene measures should be implemented according to the suggested schedule noted in the previous paragraph to remove plaque (i.e., soft bacterial deposits that adhere to the teeth and cause dental caries [decay or cavities] and periodontal [gum] disease). Poor oral hygiene and dietary habits are associated with the development of caries in children.

The most effective methods for plaque removal are brushing and flossing. Several brushing techniques exist, although there is no universal agreement regarding the best method. One that is suitable for cleaning the primary teeth is the scrub method. The tips of the bristles are placed firmly at a 45-degree angle against the teeth and gums and moved back and forth in a vibratory motion. The ends of the bristles should be wiggling but not moving forcefully back and forth, which can damage the gums and enamel. All the surfaces of the teeth are cleaned in this manner except the lingual (inner) surfaces of the anterior teeth. To clean these surfaces the toothbrush is placed vertical to the teeth and moved up and down. Only a few teeth are brushed at one time, using six to eight strokes for each section. A systematic approach is used so all surfaces are thoroughly cleaned (Fig. 32-7).

For young children the most effective cleaning is done by parents (Fig. 32-8). Several positions can be used that facilitate access to the mouth and help stabilize the head for comfort:

- Stand with the child's back toward the adult. (When done in front of a bathroom mirror, both the child and adult can see what is being done in the mirror.)

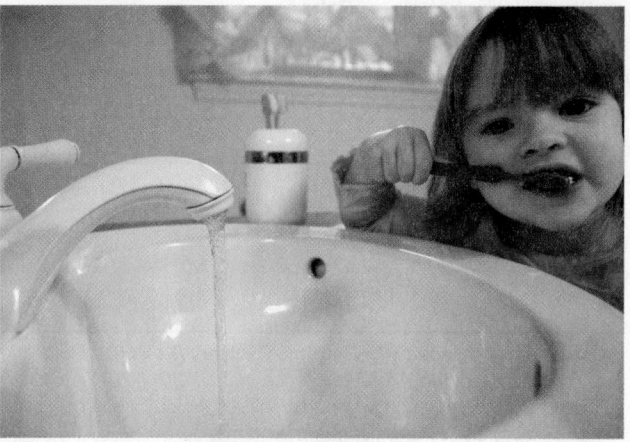

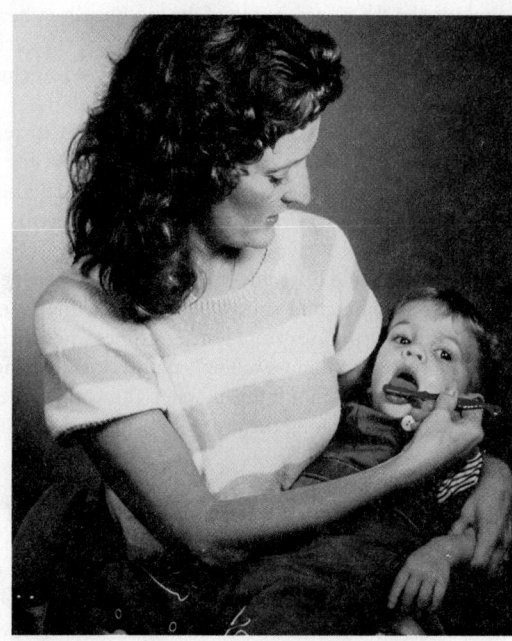

FIG 32-8 The most effective teeth cleaning is done by parents.

- Sit on a couch or bed with the child's head resting in the adult's lap.
- Sit on the floor or a stool with the child's head resting between the adult's thighs.

Use one hand to cup the chin and one to brush the teeth. For easier access to back teeth, hold the mouth partially open. After brushing with an appropriate amount of fluoridated paste or gel, avoid rinsing the mouth to maximize the beneficial effects of the fluoride (American Academy of Pediatric Dentistry, 2011b).

For effective cleaning a small toothbrush with soft, rounded, multitufted nylon bristles that are short and uniform in length is recommended. Nylon bristles dry more rapidly after use and retain their shape better than natural bristles. Toothbrushes are replaced as soon as the bristles are frayed or bent. With young children brushing may be accomplished more easily using only water because many children dislike the foam from toothpaste, and the foam interferes with visibility. Introduce toothpaste around 2 years of age and allow

TABLE 32-3	**FLUORIDE SUPPLEMENTATION***	
	WATER FLUORIDE CONTENT (PPM)	
AGE	**0.3**	**0.3–0.6**
Birth–6 months	0	0
6 months–3 years	0.25	0
3-6 years	0.50	0.25
6-16 years	1.00	0.50

From American Academy of Pediatric Dentistry 9 (AAPD): Guideline on fluoride therapy. In *AAPD reference manual 2011-2012*, 2012, retrieved from www.aapd.org/media/policies_guidelines.asp.
*Fluoride daily doses are given in milligrams.
ppm, Parts per million.

children to select the flavor they like to encourage the brushing habit. Use a pea-size amount of toothpaste for children 2 to 5 years of age (apply across the narrow width of the toothbrush rather than along its length to decrease the chance of applying an excessive amount); only a "smear" of toothpaste should be used in children younger than 2 years of age if paste is used.

After the teeth have been cleaned, they are flossed to remove plaque and debris from between the teeth and below the gum margin, where brushing is ineffective. Because young children do not have the dexterity to manipulate dental floss, parents must perform the procedure.

Ideally the teeth should be cleaned after each meal and especially before bedtime, and the child should be given nothing to eat or drink after the night brushing except water. At times when brushing is impractical, the "swish-and-swallow" method of cleaning the mouth is taught; with a mouthful of water the child rinses the mouth and swallows, repeating the procedure 3 or 4 times.*

Fluoride

Fluoride supplementation should be considered for any child older than the age of 6 months whose drinking water is deficient in fluoride. Supplementation based on fluoride concentration of water supply less than 0.3 ppm (parts per million) is 0.25 mg for a child 6 months to 3 years of age and 0.5 mg for a child 3 to 6 years of age (American Academy of Pediatric Dentistry, 2011b).

Fluoride, a mineral, is found in water, foods, or drinks in which fluoridated water was used as part of the processing system. Because the water fluoridation process and manufacturing of fluoride toothpaste are almost impossible to standardize in the United States, the dosage of fluoride supplements has been lowered to reduce the incidence of fluorosis (Table 32-3). Increased fluoride ingestion leads to enamel protein retention, hypomineralization of the enamel and dentin, and disturbance of crystal formation. The effects caused by this change range from barely discernible white fiberlike lines or spots to gray-brown stains or pitted areas. Parents should be cautioned against regular use of fluoridated water or beverages such as bottled water containing fluoride if the community water supply already has an adequate amount of fluoride.

Topical fluoride treatments (e.g., fluoride varnish) performed in the dental home are also effective in decreasing caries (American Academy of Pediatric Dentistry, 2011b).

*More detailed information can be obtained from the American Academy of Pediatric Dentistry, *www.aapd.org*.

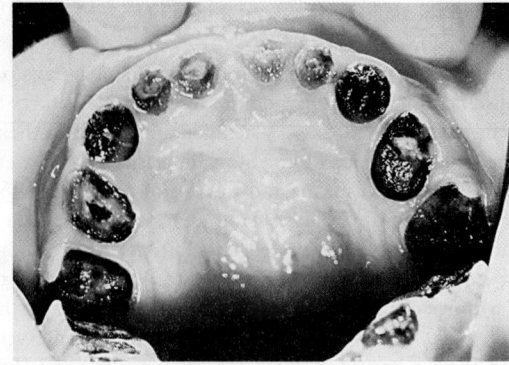

FIG 32-9 Nursing caries. Note extensive carious involvement of maxillary primary incisors. (Courtesy Bruce Carter, DDS, Texas Children's Hospital, Houston, TX.)

Dietary Factors

Diet is critical to developing good teeth because the carious process depends primarily on fermentable sugars, especially sucrose, and other carbohydrates. Refined table sugar, honey, molasses, corn syrup, and dried fruits such as raisins are highly cariogenic. Complex carbohydrates such as breads, potatoes, and pasta also contribute to caries because they lower the plaque pH. Beverages that are commonly consumed by children and adolescents and snacks are also highly cariogenic and may contribute to the incidence of overweight and obesity (American Academy of Pediatric Dentistry, 2011c).

Ideally highly cariogenic foods, especially those containing complex sugars, should be eliminated. However, because this is impractical some suggestions can be helpful. First, *the frequency with which sugar is consumed is more important than the total amount eaten.* Therefore, when sweets are eaten, they are less damaging if consumed immediately after a meal rather than as a snack between meals. When they are served as the dessert, the teeth can be cleaned afterward, decreasing the amount of time the sugar is in the mouth.

Second, the form of sugar (sucrose) is important. The more cariogenic foods are those that are sticky or hard because they remain in the mouth longer. Consequently sucking on lollipops is more cariogenic than eating a chocolate bar. Sometimes the source of the sugar is "hidden," as in numerous prescription and nonprescription drugs and many popular cereals, including the "all-natural" variety. Reading food labels is essential in eliminating sources of sucrose.

Some snacks do not contribute to tooth decay. Aged cheeses such as cheddar may alter the pH and retard bacterial growth. Sugarless gum chewed after eating may actually protect against cavities by stimulating saliva that neutralizes acid.

A special form of tooth decay in children between 18 months and 3 years of age is early childhood caries (ECC) (historically called *nursing caries* or *baby bottle tooth decay*) (Fig. 32-9). This often occurs when a child is routinely given a bottle of milk or juice at naptime or bedtime or uses the bottle as a pacifier while awake. Frequent nocturnal breastfeeding for prolonged periods also leads to extensive destruction of the teeth. The practice of coating pacifiers in honey can also contribute to caries and may be a potential source of botulism poisoning. As the sweet liquid pools in the mouth, the teeth are bathed for several hours in this cariogenic environment. Prolonged bottle-feeding well into toddler years in some cultures may contribute to significant ECC (Brotanek, Schroer, Valentyn, et al., 2009). In one group prolonging bottle-feeding into toddlerhood was perceived as "buying time" to decrease the child's crying (Freeman and Stevens, 2008). The maxillary (upper) incisors and molars are affected most because the mandibular (lower) incisors are protected by the lower lip, tongue, and saliva. Severely decayed teeth may require the application of stainless steel bands to preserve the spacing until the permanent teeth erupt.

Early childhood caries is now considered to be an infectious disease of childhood. There is evidence that *Streptococcus mutans* is a highly cariogenic bacteria (American Academy of Pediatric Dentistry, 2011d). One of the early origins of *S. mutans* is the mother's saliva; infants of mothers with high counts of the bacteria have a greater incidence of ECC. Therefore it is important to discuss oral hygiene with pregnant women because of its impact on their children's tooth development.

Prevention involves eliminating the bedtime bottle completely, feeding the last bottle before bedtime, substituting a bottle of water for milk or juice, not using the bottle as a pacifier, and never coating pacifiers in sweet substances. Juice in bottles, especially commercially available ready-to-use bottles, is discouraged; these beverages are especially damaging because the sugar is more readily converted to acid. Juice should always be offered in a cup to avoid prolonging the bottle-feeding habit. Toddlers should be encouraged to drink from a cup at the first birthday and weaned from a bottle by 14 months of age. Nurses are in an excellent position to counsel parents regarding the dangers of this habit and other aspects of dental care.*

Safety Promotion and Injury Prevention

According to recent data from the Centers for Disease Control and Prevention (CDC) (Borse, Gilchrist, Delinger, et al., 2008), children ages 1 to 4 years had the second highest rate of deaths from accidental injuries in the United States during the period from 2000 to 2006; the group with the highest number of deaths (56%) from accidental injuries were children ages 15 to 19 years. Boys were involved almost twice as often as girls in deaths attributed to unintentional injury. Among children ages 1 to 4 years of age, the leading causes for death were transportation related (including motor vehicle occupant, pedestrian, and pedal cyclist), drowning, and fires or burns. Deaths from accidental poisoning were higher among infants and adolescents than among toddlers. Nonfatal injuries in children ages 1 to 4 years of age occurred as a result of falls (leading cause), followed by being struck by or against something and bites or stings (including dog bites and bee or other insect attacks). Nonfatal drowning injury rates and nonfatal poisoning were higher among children ages 1 to 4 years than any other age-group.

A major factor in the critical increase of injuries during early childhood is the unrestricted freedom achieved through locomotion combined with an unawareness of danger within the environment. Toddlers delight in the repetitive use of gross motor skills, and with increasing age these skills are refined. This age-group is also very curious about how things work, and exploration of previously unknown or unseen objects and places is common. Toddlers also have not fully developed or do not understand the cause-and-effect principles that older children have and often are unable to gauge danger; poorly developed depth perception may also

contribute to falls and tumbles as does the general bodily structure of toddlers.

Nonaccidental trauma is a term used to denote child physical abuse, whether the etiology is suspected or confirmed, yet without the stigma of the term *child abuse*. Toddlers are at particular risk for nonaccidental trauma because of their tendency to be mobile and curious yet clumsy and uncoordinated; the toddlers' inability to control emotions at times and the tendency toward negativism further place the child at high risk for nonaccidental trauma.

Specific categories of injuries and appropriate prevention are best understood by associating them with the major growth and developmental achievements of this age (Table 32-4). The discussions of injuries in Chapters 31 and 33 are also relevant to safety concerns at this age.

Motor Vehicle Safety

Motor vehicle injuries cause more accidental deaths in all pediatric age-groups after 1 year of age than any other type of injury or disease and are responsible for almost half of all accidental deaths among children ages 1 to 4 years. Many of the deaths are caused by injuries within the car when restraints have not been used or have been used improperly. Unrestrained children riding in the front seat of the vehicle are at highest risk for injury. Approved restraints properly installed and applied can prevent many fatalities and injuries. Motor vehicle back-over injuries and deaths, along with deaths or serious injury resulting from heat stroke when left in a car, account for a large number of motor vehicle–related injuries in children (CDC, 2005; McLaren, Null, and Quinn, 2005).

Car Restraints. Nurses are responsible for educating parents regarding the importance of car restraints and their proper use. Five types of restraints are available: (1) infant-only devices, (2) convertible models for both infants and toddlers, (3) boosters, (4) safety belts, and (5) devices for children with disabilities (see Chapter 36). Chapter 31 discusses the infant-type restraints; convertible restraints and boosters are included here. Convertible restraints are suitable for infants and toddlers in the rearward-facing position (Fig. 32-10). It is now recommended that all infants and toddlers ride in rear-facing car safety seats until they reach the age of 2 years or height recommended by the car seat manufacturer (Durbin and AAP Committee on Injury, Violence, Poison Prevention, 2011). Many rear-facing car safety seats can accommodate children weighing up to a maximum of 35 pounds (according to manufacturer specifications).* Studies indicate that toddlers up to 24 months of age are safer riding in convertible seats in the rear-facing position (Bull and Durbin, 2008; Henary, Sherwood, Crandall, et al., 2007). In Sweden children ride in a rear-facing car safety seat until the age of 4 years, at which time they transition to a booster seat (Durbin and Committee on Injury, Violence, and Poison Prevention, 2011).

Children 2 years old and older (or those younger than 2 years) who have outgrown the rear-facing height or weight limit for their car safety seat should use a forward-facing car safety seat with a harness up to the maximum height or weigh recommended by the manufacturer (Durbin and Committee on Injury, Violence, and Poison Prevention, 2011).

Convertible restraints use different types of harness systems: a five-point harness that consists of a strap over each shoulder, one on each side of the pelvis, and one between the legs (all five come together at a common buckle) and a padded overhead shield that uses shoulder straps attached to a shield that is held in place by a crotch strap. The overhead shield convertible seats are no longer

---

*Sources of information about nursing caries and other aspects of child dental health include the National Institute of Dental and Craniofacial Research, National Institutes of Health, Bethesda, MD 20892-2190, 301-496-4261, www.nidcr.nih.gov; American Academy of Pediatric Dentistry, 211 E. Chicago Ave., Suite 1700, Chicago, IL 60611, 312-337-2169 , www.aapd.org; American Dental Association, 211 E. Chicago Ave., Chicago, IL 60611, 312-440-2500, www.ada.org/; and Canadian Dental Association, 1815 Alta Vista Drive, Ottawa, Ontario K1G 3Y6, 613-523-1770, www.cda-adc.ca.

*www.carseat.org.

TABLE 32-4 INJURY PREVENTION DURING EARLY CHILDHOOD

DEVELOPMENTAL ABILITIES RELATED TO RISK OF INJURY	INJURY PREVENTION
Motor Vehicles	
Walks, runs, and climbs	Use federally approved car restraint.
Able to open doors and gates	Supervise child while playing outside.
Can ride tricycle and other toy vehicles	Do not allow child to play on curb or behind parked car.
Can throw ball and other objects	Do not permit child to play in pile of leaves, snow, or large cardboard container in trafficked area.
	Supervise tricycle riding.
	Lock fences and doors if not directly supervising children.
	Teach child to obey pedestrian safety rules:
	• Obey traffic regulations; cross only at crosswalks and only when traffic signal indicates that it is safe.
	• Stand back a step from curb until it is time to cross.
	• Look left, right, and left again and check for turning cars before crossing street.
	• Use sidewalks; when there is no sidewalk, walk on left, facing traffic.
	• Wear light colors at night and attach fluorescent material to clothing.
Drowning	
Able to explore if left unsupervised	Supervise closely when near any source of water regardless of depth, including buckets.
Has great curiosity	Keep bathroom doors closed and lid down on toilet (or install latch).
Helpless in water; unaware of its danger— may consider "play" in any body of water same as in bath; depth of water has no significance	Have fence around swimming pool and lock gate.
	Teach swimming and water safety (however, this is not a substitute for safety).
	Supervise small children when swimming by "touch" (adult can reach out and touch child at all times).
Burns	
Able to reach heights by climbing, stretching, and standing on toes	Turn pot handles toward back of stove.
Pulls objects	Place electrical appliances such as coffee maker and popcorn machine toward back of counter.
Explores any holes or opening	Place guardrails in front of radiators, fireplaces, or other heating elements.
Can open drawers and closets	Store matches and cigarette lighters in locked or inaccessible area; discard carefully.
Unaware of potential sources of heat or fire	Place burning candles, incense, hot foods, and cigarettes out of reach.
Plays with mechanical objects	Do not let tablecloth hang within child's reach.
	Do not let electric cord from iron, curling iron, or other appliance hang within child's reach.
	Cover electrical outlets with protective plastic caps.
	Keep electrical wires hidden or out of reach.
	Do not allow child to play with electrical appliance, wires, or lighters.
	Stress danger of open flames; teach what "hot" means.
	Always check bath-water temperature; adjust water heater temperature to 49° C (120° F) or lower; do not allow children to play with faucets.
	Apply sunscreen when child is exposed to sunlight.
Accidental Poisoning	
Explores by putting objects in mouth	Place all potentially toxic agents out of reach or in locked cabinet.
Can open drawers, closets, boxes, and most containers	Caution against eating nonedible items such as plants.
Climbs	Replace medications or poisons immediately in proper storage and out of child's reach; replace child-guard caps properly.
Cannot read labels	Administer medications as drug, not as candy.
Does not know safe dose or amount	Do not store surplus toxic agents.
	Promptly discard empty poison containers; never reuse to store food item or other poison.
	Teach child not to play in trash containers.
	Never remove labels from containers of toxic substances.
	Do not store toxic liquids in containers not specifically intended for their storage (e.g., empty soda bottle that child may drink from, unaware of difference in contents).
	Know number of nearest poison control center (800-222-1222).

TABLE 32-4 INJURY PREVENTION DURING EARLY CHILDHOOD—cont'd

DEVELOPMENTAL ABILITIES RELATED TO RISK OF INJURY	INJURY PREVENTION
Falls	
Able to open doors and some windows	Use window guardrail; fasten securely.
Goes up and down stairs	Place gates at top and bottom of stairs.
Depth perception unrefined	Keep doors locked or use child-proof doorknob covers at entry to stairs, high porch, or other elevated area, including laundry chute.
Climbs on higher surfaces	Remove unsecured or scatter rugs.
	Apply nonskid decals in bathtub or shower.
	Keep crib rails fully raised and mattress at lowest level.
	Place carpeting under crib and in bathroom.
	Keep large toys and bumper pads out of crib or play yard (child can use these as "stairs" to climb out); move child to youth bed when he or she is able to climb out of crib.
	Avoid using wheeled walkers, especially near stairs and floor furnace.
	Dress in safe clothing (soles that do not "catch" on floor, tied shoelaces, pant legs that do not touch floor).
	Keep child restrained in vehicles; never leave unattended in shopping cart.
	Supervise at playgrounds; select play areas with soft ground cover and safe equipment.
Choking and Suffocation	
Puts things in mouth	Avoid large, round chunks of meat such as whole hot dogs (slice lengthwise into short pieces).
May swallow hard or nonedible pieces of food	Avoid fruit with pits, fish with bones, dried beans, hard candy, chewing gum, nuts, popcorn, grapes, marshmallows.
	Choose large, sturdy toys without sharp edges or small removable parts.
	Discard old refrigerators, ovens, and other appliances after removing door.
	Select safe toy boxes or chests without heavy, hinged lids.
	Keep Venetian blind (or shade) cords out of child's reach. Use split cords.
	Remove drawstrings from clothing.
Bodily Damage	
Still clumsy in many skills	Avoid giving sharp or pointed objects such as knives, scissors, or toothpicks, especially when walking or running.
Easily distracted from tasks	Do not allow lollipops or similar objects in mouth when walking or running.
Unaware of potential danger from strangers or other people	Teach safety precautions (e.g., to carry knife or scissors with pointed end away from face).
	Store all dangerous tools, garden equipment, and firearms in locked cabinet.
	Be alert to danger of supervised animals and household pets.
	Use safety glass and decals on large glassed areas such as sliding glass doors.
	Teach child name, address, and phone number and to ask for help from appropriate people (cashier, security guard, policeman) if lost; have identification on child (sewn in clothes, inside shoe).
	Teach stranger safety:
	• Avoid personalized clothing in public places.
	• Never go with a stranger.
	• Tell parents if anyone makes child feel uncomfortable in any way.
	Always listen to child's concerns regarding others' behavior.
	Teach child to say "no" when confronted with uncomfortable situations.

manufactured but if in one's possession may be used until the manufacturer's weight limit is reached. With both the infant and toddler restraints it is important not to add extra blankets, head cushions, or padding between the child and the restraint straps that did not come as original equipment because these "add-ons" create spaces of air between the child and the restraint and decrease support for the back, head, and neck. Cars with free-sliding latch plates on the lap or shoulder belt require the use of a metal locking clip to keep the belt in a tight-holding position. The locking clip is threaded onto the belt above the latch plate (Fig. 32-11, *A*). If parents have newer cars with automatic lap and shoulder belts, they need to have additional lap belts installed to properly secure the restraint. A 3-in-1 convertible seat is also available and can be used rear-facing, forward-facing, and as a belt-positioning seat for toddlers. This seat is larger than other convertible seats, so it is

important to verify that the seat fits in the car in the rear-facing position (AAP, 2013).

Booster seats are not restraint systems like the convertible devices because they depend on the vehicle belts to hold the child and booster seat in place. Three booster models have been approved by the National Highway Traffic Safety Administration (NHTSA): the high-back belt-positioning seat (Fig. 32-11, *B*), which provides head and neck support for the child riding in a vehicle seat without a head rest; the no-back belt-positioning seat, which should be used only if the vehicle seat has a head rest; and a combination seat, which converts from a forward-facing toddler seat to a booster seat. This last model is equipped with a harness for use by toddlers; the harness may be removed, and a belt used when the child outgrows the harness. The belt-positioning booster seats are used for children who are less than 145 cm (4 feet, 9 inches) tall and weigh

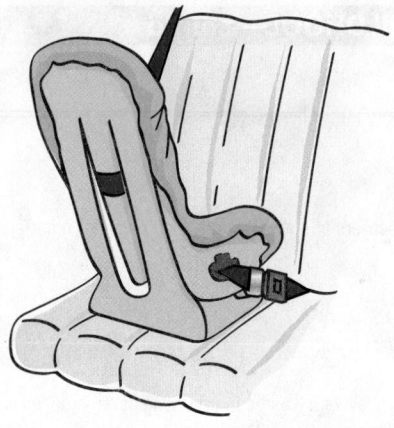

FIG 32-10 Rear-facing convertible car seat.

👪 FAMILY-CENTERED CARE

Using Car Safety Seats

- Read manufacturer directions and follow them exactly.
- Anchor safety seat securely to automobile seat and apply harness snugly to child.
- Do not start the car until everyone is properly restrained.
- *Always* use the restraint, even for short trips.
- If child begins to climb out or undo the harness, firmly say, "No." It may be necessary to stop the car to reinforce the expected behavior. Use rewards to encourage cooperative behavior.
- Encourage child to help attach buckles, straps, and shields but always double-check fastenings.
- Decrease boredom on long trips. Keep soft toys in the car for quiet play; talk to child; point out objects and teach child about them. Stop periodically. If child wishes to sleep, make certain that he or she stays in the restraint.
- Insist that others who transport children also follow these safety rules.

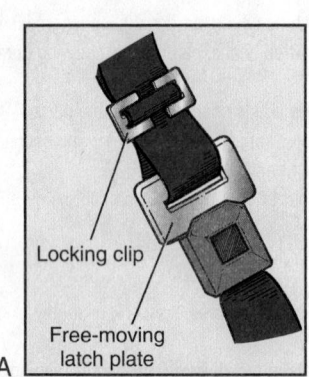

Locking clip

Free-moving latch plate

A

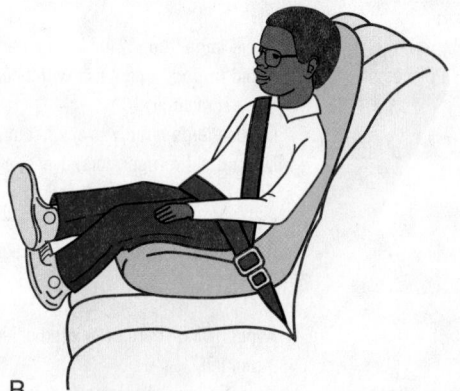

B

FIG 32-11 A, Locking clip used with free-sliding lap or shoulder belt to keep the belt in a tight-holding position. **B,** Automobile booster seat. Note placement of the shoulder strap (away from the neck and face).

15.9 kg to 36.3 kg (35 to 80 lbs, depending on the type of booster seat). In general school-age children should ride in a belt-positioning booster seat until approximately 7 to 8 years of age. However, note that, because children's sizes vary considerably, manufacturer recommendations should be followed regarding height and weight limitations. A booster seat should be used until the child is able to sit against the back of the seat with feet hanging down and legs bent at the knees. The belt-positioning booster model raises a child higher in the seat, moving the shoulder part of the belt off the neck and the lap portion off the abdomen onto the pelvis. Children who outgrow the convertible restraint may still be able to ride safely in a booster seat until the midpoint of the head is higher than the vehicle seat back.

Children should use specially designed car restraints until they are 145 cm (4 feet, 9 inches) in height or 8 to 12 years old (AAP, 2013). Shoulder-lap safety belts should be worn low on the hips, snug, and not on the abdominal area. Children should be taught to sit up straight to allow for proper fit. The shoulder belt is used only if it does not cross the child's neck or face.

Shoulder-only automatic belts are designed to protect adults. Children should use the manual shoulder belts in the rear seat. Air bags do not take the place of child safety seats or seat belts and can be lethal to young children. The safest area of the car for children is the back seat.

For any restraint to be effective, it must be used consistently and properly. Examples of misuse include misrouting the vehicle seat belt through the restraint; failing to use the vehicle seat belt to secure the restraint; failing to use a tether strap; failing to use the restraint harness system; and incorrectly positioning the child, especially by facing infants forward instead of rearward. To address these issues nurses must stress correct use of car restraints and rules that ensure compliance (see Family-Centered Care box). Children riding in car safety seats are generally much better behaved than children left unrestrained, which can be a major benefit to parents and should be emphasized as an additional advantage of restraints. Additional information about child safety restraints is available from various sources.*

The LATCH (lower anchors and tethers for children) universal child safety seat system was implemented as a requirement starting in 2002 for all new automobiles and child safety seats. This system provides uniform anchorage consisting of two lower anchorages and one upper anchorage in the rear seat of the vehicle (Fig. 32-12). When used appropriately the top anchor (tether) strap prevents the

---

*AAP, 141 Northwest Point Blvd., Elk Grove Village, IL 60007, 847-434-4000, www.aap.org; and local division of traffic safety or NHTSA, 1200 New Jersey Ave. SE, West Building, Washington, DC 20590, 888-327-4236, www.nhtsa.dot.gov.

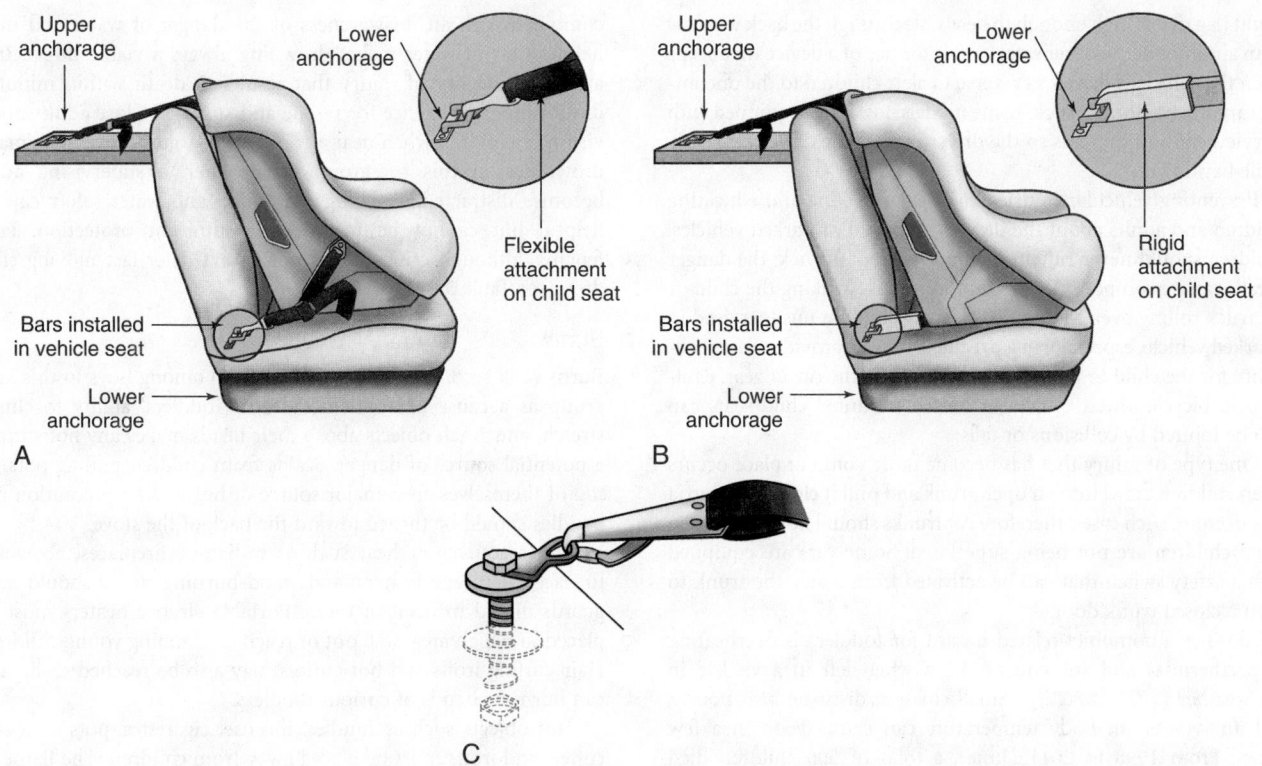

FIG 32-12 Lower anchors and tethers for children (LATCH). **A,** Flexible two-point attachment with top tether. **B,** Rigid two-point attachment with top tether. **C,** Top tether. (Courtesy U.S. Department of Transportation, National Highway Traffic Safety Administration.)

child from pitching forward in a crash. If the tether strap is not used, up to 90% of the protection of the restraint is lost. Instructions for proper installation of the tether strap and permanent bracket are included with the car restraint. New child safety seats have a hook, buckle, strap, or other connector that attaches to the anchorage. Concerns about the increased weight of children in the United States has led some to question the safety of the LATCH system with child restraints (car seats) and the child whose combined weight is more than 29.5 kg (65 lbs). The NHTSA recently changed the rule about the use of the LATCH system if the child's weight and that of the car seat weighs more than 65 lbs; in 2014 parents will be instructed to use the shoulder-lap belt restraint to restrain the child in the car seat instead of relying on the LATCH system for maximum protection if the combined weight of the child and car seat is more than 29.5 kg (65 lbs).

Children with disabilities may require a restraint system that secures them appropriately in the event of a crash. Examples of such devices include car-bed restraints for infants who cannot tolerate a semireclining position and specially adapted molded-plastic chairs for children who have spica casts. The E-Z-On vest is a special safety harness for larger children with poor trunk control. A HIPPO (Spica Cast) Car Seat is available for transporting children with spica casts; these are sold only in the United States. Additional safety restraints and a list of distributors are available at the SafetyBeltSafe U.S. website.* See also Chapter 25 for a discussion of preterm infants being discharged home and car-seat evaluation.

Optimally children should not ride in the front seat of any car with an activated air bag; if they do, the seat should be pushed as far back as possible to prevent serious harm or critical injury from front seat air bags. Many of the newer-model vehicles have side impact air bags for collision protection; these air bags are reported to be safe as long as the child is in a proper restraint system. The NHTSA (2010) recommends that children not lean on chest-only or head-chest combination side air bags. Some of the newer-model child car seats include side bumpers at head and neck height to protect children in side-impact collisions. Built-in seats are available in some cars and vans. They eliminate installation problems; however, weight and height limits vary. Reinforce that owners must verify with vehicle manufacturers details about built-in seats.

Motor Vehicle–Related Injuries. Injuries may also occur during sudden stops when objects are left unrestrained. On sudden impact a loose ball becomes a projectile missile. Therefore all items should be secured or stored in the trunk or behind a barrier such as netting in vans and wagons.

Children older than 3 years of age are often involved in pedestrian traffic injuries. Because of their gross motor skills of walking, running, and climbing and their fine motor skills of opening doors and fence gates, they are likely to be in hazardous areas when unsupervised. Unaware of danger and unable to approximate the speed of cars, they are hit by moving vehicles. Running after a ball, riding a tricycle, and playing behind a parked car are common activities that may result in a vehicular tragedy.

Toddlers playing in driveways or farmyards are at risk of back-over injury from vehicles in reverse gear. A precaution when children are playing in driveways is attaching to the tricycle a pole with a

*www.carseat.org.

bright flag that is high enough to be visible through the back window of an automobile. Another safeguard is the use of a device that beeps when the vehicle is driven in reverse to alert children to the oncoming car, van, tractor, or truck. Some models now come equipped with rearview motion cameras so the driver can see the driveway clearly while backing out.

Preventing vehicular injuries involves protecting and educating children and adults about the danger of moved or parked vehicles. Children should never ride in the open back of a truck; the danger of falls can be compounded by another vehicle striking the child or the truck rolling over. In addition, leaving children unsupervised in a parked vehicle, especially in a private driveway, provides an opportunity for the child to release the brake or put the car in gear. Children in bicycle-towed trailers or bicycle-mounted child seats can also be injured by collisions or falls.

One type of injury that has become more commonplace occurs when children crawl into an open trunk and pull it closed. Asphyxia may occur in such cases; therefore car trunks should not be left open when children are not being supervised. Some cars are equipped with a safety switch that can be activated from inside the trunk to open a closed trunk door.

Another automobile-related hazard for toddlers is overheating (hyperthermia) and subsequent death when left in a vehicle in hot weather (>27°C [80°F]). Small children dissipate heat poorly, and an increase in body temperature can cause death in a few hours. From 1998 to 2011 (June), a total of 506 children died from hyperthermia when left alone in parked cars; in 2010 the total number of child deaths was 49, and it is estimated that an average of 38 children die each year from overheating in cars (Null, 2011). It is estimated that, with the ambient temperature at 22° to 35.5°C (72° to 96°F), the vehicle interior temperature rises by 10.5° to 11°C (19° to 20°F) for each 10 minutes, even with a window cracked (Null, 2011). In a study of 171 child fatalities from overheating in a car, 50% of adults who left a child in a car either forgot or were unaware that the child was still in the car. A significant number of those children (32) were left by family members who intended to take the child to day care but forgot the child in the car at the workplace; 22 children were left in the car by a day care worker or driver (Guard and Gallagher, 2005). Parents are cautioned against leaving infants alone in a vehicle for *any reason*.

Preventing vehicular injuries involves protecting and educating children about the danger of moving and parked vehicles. Although preschool children are too young to be trusted to always obey, parents should emphasize looking for moving vehicles before crossing the street, recognizing the stop and go colors of traffic lights, and following traffic officers' signals. Physical barriers limiting children from playing near vehicles help prevent these injuries. Most important, what is preached must be practiced. Children learn through imitation, and consistency reinforces learning.

Drowning

The highest rate of drowning in the years 2000 to 2006 was in children ages 0 to 4 years; children ages 12 to 36 months are at highest risk for drowning during the same time period (Weiss and AAP Committee on Injury, Violence, and Poison Prevention, 2010). Drowning deaths in infants occur most commonly in the bathtub and large buckets. With well-developed skills of locomotion, toddlers are able to reach potentially dangerous areas such as bathtubs, toilets, buckets, swimming pools, hot tubs, and ponds or lakes. Toddlers' intense drive for exploration and investigation

combined with an unawareness of the danger of water and their helplessness in water makes drowning always a viable threat. It is also one category of injury that results in death within minutes, diminishing the chance for rescue and survival. Close adult supervision of children when near any source of water is essential; many drownings in this age-group occur when a supervising adult becomes distracted. Teaching swimming and water safety can be helpful but cannot be regarded as sufficient protection. Pool fencing, although critical, does not always deter fast-moving children (see Table 32-4).

Burns

Burns rank second among girls and third among boys in this age-group as a cause of accidental death. Toddlers' ability to climb, stretch, and reach objects above their heads makes any hot surface a potential source of danger. Scalds from children pulling pots on top of themselves are a major source of burns. As a precaution pot handles should be turned toward the back of the stove.

Other sources of heat such as radiators, fireplaces, accessible furnaces, kerosene heaters, and wood-burning stoves should have guards placed in front of them. Portable electric heaters must be placed in a high area, well out of reach of climbing young children. Hair curling irons and hot curlers may also be reached easily and can burn the hands of curious toddlers.

Hot objects such as candles, incense, cigarettes, pots of tea or coffee, and irons must be placed away from children. The flame of a candle and the smoke of a cigarette invite investigation. Flame burns represent one of the most fatal types of burns and commonly occur when children play with matches and accidentally set themselves (and the home) on fire. To prevent flame burns, matches and lighters must be stored safely away from children, and parents need to teach children the dangers of playing with such objects. In addition, all homes, apartments, and any other type of dwelling where people sleep should have smoke detectors installed to alert the occupants of a fire. A safety plan for immediate escape is also essential.

Electrical burns represent an immediate danger to children. Young toddlers may explore outlets with conductive articles and wires by mouthing them. Because water is an excellent conductor, the chance for a severe circumoral electrical burn is great. Electrical outlets should have protective guards (or sliding guards) plugged into them when not in use (Fig. 32-13) or be made inaccessible by having furniture placed in front of them when feasible.

Scald burns are the most common type of thermal injury in children. A scalding burn is often caused by high-temperature tap water, with which children come in contact as a result of turning on the hot-water faucet, falling into a bathtub of hot water, pulling hot pots onto themselves, or suffering deliberate abuse. Limiting household water temperatures to less than 49°C (120°F) is highly recommended. At this temperature it takes 10 minutes of exposure to the water to cause a full-thickness burn. Conversely water temperatures of 54°C (130°F), the usual setting of most water heaters, expose household members to the risk of full-thickness burns within 30 seconds. Nurses can help prevent such burns by advising parents of this common household danger and recommending that they readjust their water heaters to a safe temperature.

Sunburns are a year-round concern in certain regions. Children spend a large amount of time outdoors. Their increased mobility makes it difficult to prevent sun exposure. Sunburn can be prevented by applying a sunscreen with a sun protection factor (SPF) of 15 or

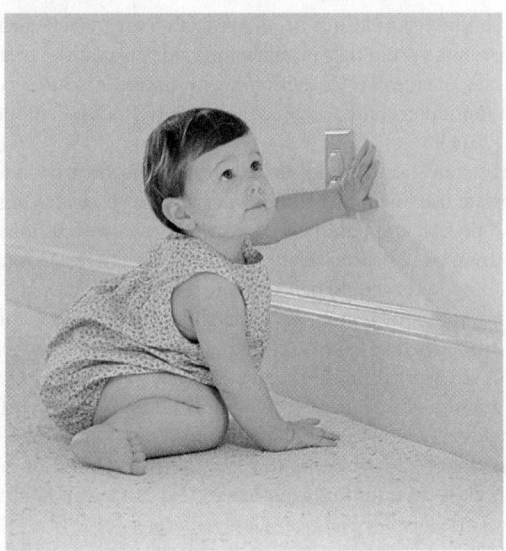

FIG 32-13 Special plastic caps in electrical sockets prevent young fingers from exploring dangerous areas. (Copyright © 2011 Photos.com, a division of Getty Images. All rights reserved.)

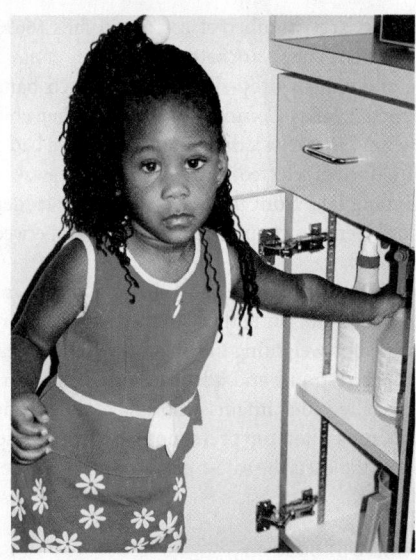

FIG 32-14 Children are most likely to ingest substances that are on their level such as cleaning agents stored under sinks, rat poison, plants, or diaper pail deodorants.

greater, dressing in protective clothing (wide-brimmed hat, protective cotton clothing with a tight weave), and avoiding sun exposure between 10 AM and 2 PM.

Accidental Poisoning

Toddlers are at the highest risk for accidental poisoning because of their innate curiosity and ability to open "childproof" containers. Mouthing activity continues to be prevalent after 1 year of age, and exploring objects by tasting them is part of children's curious investigation. Toddlers' curiosity and inability to understand logical consequences further place them at risk for ingesting harmful substances. Many household products, medications, and plants can be poisonous if swallowed, if they come in contact with the skin or eyes, or if they are inhaled. Although in many instances poisoning does not result in death, it may cause significant morbidity such as esophageal stricture from lye ingestion. Toddlers are able to climb most heights, open most drawers or closets, and unscrew most lids. By trial and error younger children also manage to undo tops of bottles, plastic containers, aerosol cans, and jars, including those with child-resistant lids. Newer forms of drugs such as transdermal patches and cough-suppressant lozenges have created additional dangers because they are not packaged with safety caps and the lozenges look like candy.

The major reason for poisoning is improper storage (Fig. 32-14). The guidelines suggested in Chapter 31 apply to children in this age-group as well. However, unlike infants, who are confined to certain heights and unable to unlatch inventive locks, young children manage to find access to many high-level, tight-security places. For this age-group only a locked cabinet is safe.

Recent attention has focused on the use of OTC medications used for cough and colds as a common cause of accidental poisonous ingestion in toddlers. Ingestion of acetaminophen is also a common cause of morbidity because it is found in many combination OTC products; caregivers may unknowingly administer a dose of acetaminophen in addition to an OTC drug containing the product without knowing the danger.

Emergency and preventive measures for accidental poisoning are discussed in Chapters 31 and 41. Parents should have ready access to the telephone number for the poison control center (National Poison Control, 800-222-1222) and be prepared to act on the advice of the center.

Falls

Falls are still a hazard to children in this age-group, although by the later part of early childhood gross and fine motor skills are well developed, decreasing the incidence of falls down stairs and from chairs. However, playground injuries are common. Children need to be taught safety at play areas such as no horseplay on high slides or jungle gyms, *sitting* on swings, and staying away from moving swings. Passive prevention includes placement of grass, sand, or wood chips under play equipment. Swing seats should be made of plastic, canvas, or rubber and have smooth or rounded edges. Slides should have inclines of no more than 30 degrees, evenly spaced rungs for climbing, and protective "tunnels."

The climbing and running of the typical toddler are complicated by the child's total disregard and lack of appreciation for danger. Gates must be placed at both ends of stairs. Accessible windows must have window guards, not screens, to prevent falls to the ground below. Falling from open windows is a major cause of accidental death in urban, lower socioeconomic groups. Doors leading to stairwells or porches must be locked because preschoolers can open them easily. A convenient type of lock is a sliding bar or hook that can be attached to the door and frame at a level higher than the child can reach; such locks also have safety clasps or devices that prevent children from being able to open them. Falls from balconies, porches, decks, and bleachers are all possible for active toddlers.

Cribs and vehicles are other sources of falls. To avoid injury crib rails should be fully raised, the mattress should be kept at the lowest position, and toys or bumper pads that may be used as steps to climb out should be removed. Rails need to be sized appropriately because most children younger than 6 years of age can slip through a 6-inch opening; however, no children older than 1 year can usually pass through a 4-inch opening. Ideally the floor under the crib should be carpeted or have a throw rug. Cribs, bassinets, and play yards were associated with a large number of accidental falls (66% of all fall injuries to children) (Yeh, Rochette, McKenzie, et al., 2011). The manufacture and sale of drop-side cribs has been banned by the Consumer Product Safety Commission (2010). When children reach a height of 89 cm (35 inches), they should sleep in a bed rather than a crib. If a bunk bed is selected, parents should be aware of possible dangers, including falls from the top bed and the ladder and head entrapment between the mattress and guardrail or between the supporting mattress slats.

Children can fall from high chairs, shopping carts, carriages, car seats, and strollers if not properly restrained or because of a change in balance created by weighting the object down with heavy objects. Therefore proper restraint and adequate supervision are essential. Children, especially older infants who are mobile, should not be placed in an infant seat on top of a shopping cart because the infant seat may fall off the cart; the safest place for an infant seat is inside the bed of the cart.

Aspiration and Suffocation

Foreign body aspiration is most common during the second year of life. Usually by 1 year of age children chew well, but they may have difficulty with large pieces of food (e.g., meat and whole hot dogs) and hard foods (e.g., nuts). Young children cannot discard pits from fruit or bones from fish. It takes practice to learn how to chew gum without swallowing it. Gel snacks that are sealed in plastic wrappers can also be difficult to manage, and the plastic wrapper can be aspirated. Therefore parents must implement the same precautions as discussed for infants regarding food selection (see Chapter 31).

Play objects for toddlers must still be chosen with an awareness of danger from small parts. Large, sturdy toys without sharp edges or removable parts are safest. Small plastic toys such as Legos can cause choking or be aspirated; such plastic items often do not appear on radiographic films. Balloons, coins, paper clips, pins, bells, button batteries, pull-tabs on cans, thumbtacks, nails, screws, jewelry (especially pierced earrings), and all types of pins are common household objects that can cause significant harm if swallowed or aspirated. Because of the danger of aspiration, parents should be taught emergency procedures for choking.

Suffocation from causes seen during infancy is less frequent; but old refrigerators, ovens, and other large appliances are an ever-present threat. Toddlers can climb inside these appliances and, if they close the door behind them, can be trapped. Removing all doors before discarding or storing old appliances prevents such tragic deaths. Toddlers may also suffocate when unsafe toy box lids accidentally close on their heads or necks.

Because some of the older heating systems and hot-water heaters may emit carbon monoxide, which is undetectable by human smell, each house should have a carbon monoxide detector in addition to a smoke detector.

Bodily Injury

Toddlers are still clumsy in many of their skills and can seriously harm themselves when walking while holding a sharp or pointed object or having food or objects such as spoons in their mouths. Preventing such occurrences is the best approach. With preschoolers teaching safety is most important. The child should be taught that, when walking with a pointed object such as a knife or scissors, the pointed end is held away from the face. Dangerous garden or workshop equipment and all firearms should be stored in locked cabinets. Power lawn mowers and weed eaters are especially dangerous because they can throw rocks and other solid items (projectiles), and

young children should not be allowed in an area where such tools are in use; nor should they be taken for a ride on a mower or allowed to operate the device. Television tip-overs are a source of head trauma in toddlers and preschool age-group (Rutkoski, Sippey, and Gaines, 2011).

Safety education should include respect for firearms and their appropriate use, including nonpowder guns such as air guns, rifles (BB and pellet), and paintball guns, which can cause serious penetrating injuries. Firearm safety devices such as trigger locks and personalized locks should be used to prevent unintentional firing of guns and subsequent injuries or fatalities. In addition, the child should be warned of and protected against potential danger from animals (see Animal Bites, Chapter 47).

An additional safeguard for young children is the use of safety glass in doors, windows, and tabletops and the application of decals on glass doors and windows to reduce the likelihood of running through glass. In addition, children should not be allowed to run, jump, wrestle, or play ball near glass structures.

A discussion of bodily injury must also include alerting the parent to threats to the child's well-being from adults or other children who might take advantage of the toddler who cannot protect himself or herself. Because toddlers are often not able to verbalize their emotions and feelings or may not understand inappropriate touching behavior by a family member or friend, it is important for parents to protect children by not leaving them in situations where there is a potential for bodily harm. The "stranger danger" concept is still important to teach, yet statistics show that personal harm more often comes from relatives or family friends who are not considered strangers. Therefore it is important to discuss appropriate and inappropriate touching (what feels comfortable and what does not) in a manner that will not frighten or overwhelm the child. Child abductions can be prevented with close adult supervision; additional safeguards include screening for risk factors for missing children such as divorce, family discord, and substance abuse. Encourage parents to have a current, high-quality picture of the child. The goal is not to induce fear about such events but to make nurses and parents aware so they can take steps to keep each child safe from bodily harm.

Household safety should be practiced and includes the usual precautions recommended for any age-group (see Patient Teaching box: Child Home Safety Checklist, p. 904).

Anticipatory Guidance—Care of Families

Understanding toddlers is fundamental to successful child rearing. Nurses, particularly those in ambulatory or child health centers, are in a favorable position to help parents facilitate the tasks and meet the needs of children in this age-group. Prevention yields better results than treatment. Anticipatory guidance is paramount if one wishes to prevent future problems (see Family-Centered Care box).

Advice is sometimes not the sole answer. Actual assistance such as being available for home visiting or telephone consulting should be part of the nurse's flexible repertoire of interventions. Whether parents are experiencing the dilemmas of rearing a first or a subsequent child, they benefit from sharing their feelings, frustrations, and satisfactions. They need adult companionship, freedom from childrearing responsibilities, and periodic separations from their children. Part of a nurse's responsibility is to provide opportunities for parents to express their feelings and to meet their physical, mental, and spiritual needs.

FAMILY-CENTERED CARE

Guidance During Toddler Years

Ages 12 to 18 Months

- Prepare parents for expected behavioral changes of toddler, especially negativism and ritualism.
- Assess present feeding habits and encourage gradual weaning from bottle and increased intake of solid foods.
- Stress expected feeding changes of picky eating habits, food fads, and strong taste preferences; need for scheduled routine at mealtimes; inability to sit through an entire meal; and lack of table manners.
- Prepare parents for potential dangers of the home, particularly motor vehicle injuries, poisoning, and falling injuries; give appropriate suggestions for safety proofing the home.
- Discuss need for firm but gentle discipline and ways to deal with negativism and temper tantrums; stress positive benefits of appropriate discipline.
- Emphasize importance for both child and parents of brief, periodic separations.
- Discuss new toys that use developing gross and fine motor, language, cognitive, and social skills.
- Emphasize need for dental supervision, types of basic dental hygiene at home, and food habits that predispose to caries; stress importance of supplemental fluoride (according to age [older than 6 months] and fluoride content of local water supply).

Ages 18 to 24 Months

- Stress importance of peer companionship in play.
- Explore need for preparation for additional sibling (as appropriate); stress importance of preparing child for new experiences.
- Assess sleep patterns at night, particularly the habit of a bedtime bottle, which is a major cause of dental caries, and behaviors that delay hour of sleep.
- Discuss present discipline methods, their effectiveness, and parents' feelings about child's negativism; stress that negativism is an important

aspect of developing self-assertion and independence and is not a sign of spoiling.

- Discuss signs of readiness for toilet training; emphasize importance of waiting for physical and psychologic readiness.
- Discuss development of fears such as fear of darkness or loud noises and habits such as security blanket or thumb sucking; stress normalcy of these transient behaviors.
- Prepare parents for signs of regression in time of stress.
- Assess child's ability to separate easily from parents for brief periods under familiar circumstances.
- Allow parents opportunity to express their feelings of weariness, frustration, and exasperation; be aware that it is often difficult to love toddlers when they are not asleep!
- Point out some of the expected changes of the next year such as longer attention span, somewhat less negativism, and increased concern for pleasing others.

Ages 24 to 36 Months

- Discuss importance of imitation and domestic mimicry and need to include child in activities.
- Discuss approaches toward toilet training, particularly realistic expectations and attitude toward accidents.
- Stress uniqueness of toddlers' thought processes, especially through their use of language, poor understanding of time, view of causal relationships in terms of proximity of events, and inability to see events from another's perspective.
- Stress that discipline still must be structured and concrete and that relying solely on verbal reasoning and explanation leads to injuries, confusion, and misunderstanding.
- Discuss investigation of preschool or day care center toward completion of second year.

KEY POINTS

- The toddler stage, extending from 12 to 36 months, is a period of intense exploration of the environment.
- Biologic development during the toddler years is characterized by the acquisition of fine and gross motor skills that allow children to master a wide range of activities.
- Although most of the physiologic systems are mature by the end of toddlerhood, development of certain areas of the brain is still occurring, allowing for greater intellectual capacity.
- Locomotion is the major gross motor skill acquired during toddlerhood, followed by increased eye-hand coordination.
- Specific tasks in the psychosocial development of a toddler include differentiating self from others, tolerating separation from parent, coping with delayed gratification, controlling bodily functions, acquiring socially acceptable behavior, communicating verbally, and interacting with others in a less egocentric manner.
- According to Erikson the major developmental task of toddlerhood is acquiring a sense of autonomy while overcoming a sense of doubt and shame.
- In Piaget's sensorimotor and preconceptual phases of development, the toddler experiments by incorporating the old learning of secondary circular reactions with new skills and applies this

knowledge to new situations. There is the beginning of rational judgment, an understanding of causal relationships, and discovery of objects as objects.

- Preconceptual thought is characterized by egocentrism, centration, global organization of thought processes, animism, and irreversibility.
- Language is the major cognitive achievement in toddlerhood.
- The most striking characteristic of language development during early childhood is the increasing level of comprehension.
- Development of body image occurs with increasing motor ability, at which point toddlers recognize the importance and capacity of body parts.
- The two phases of differentiation of self from significant others are separation and individuation.
- Parental concerns during the toddler years include toilet training; coping with sibling rivalry; limit setting and discipline; and dealing with temper tantrums, negativism, and regression.
- Effective discipline techniques for toddlers include reward, ignoring or extinction, and time-out.
- Nutrition is important during the toddler stage because eating habits established in this period have lasting effects in subsequent years.

- Regular dental examinations, fluoride supplementation, removal of plaque, and provision of a low-cariogenic diet promote optimum dental health.
- Common sleep problems that develop during early childhood (and that are easily prevented) are associated with night crying and refusal to go to sleep.

- Because of increased locomotion, toddlers are at high risk for sustaining injuries. Fatal injuries are primarily a result of motor vehicle accidents, drownings, and burns.
- Motor vehicle injuries are responsible for almost half of all accidental deaths among children ages 1 to 4 years.

REFERENCES

American Academy of Pediatric Dentistry (AAPD): Guideline on infant oral health care, *AAPD reference manual 2010-2011* 33(6):12, 114, 2011a, www.aapd.org/media/Policies_Guidelines/G_InfantOralHealthCare.pdf.

American Academy of Pediatric Dentistry (AAPD): Policy on early childhood caries (ECC): classifications, consequences, and preventive strategies, *AAPD reference manual 2010-2011* 32(6):41–43, 2011b.

American Academy of Pediatric Dentistry (AAPD): Policy on use of fluoride, *AAPD reference manual 2010-2011* 32(6):34–35, 2011c.

American Academy of Pediatric Dentistry (AAPD): Policy on dietary recommendations for infants, children and adolescents, *AAPD reference manual 2010-2011* 32(6):48–49, 2011d.

American Academy of Pediatrics (AAP): Prevention of rickets and vitamin D deficiency in infants, children, and adolescents, *Pediatrics* 122(5):1142–1148, 2008.

American Academy of Pediatrics (AAP) Committee on Nutrition: *Pediatric nutrition handbook*, ed 6, Elk Grove Village, Ill, 2009, Author.

American Academy of Pediatrics (AAP) Council on Communications and Media: Media use by children younger than 2 years, *Pediatrics* 128(5):1040–1045, 2011.

American Academy of Pediatrics (AAP): Car seats: Information for families for 2013, 2013, http://www.healthychildren.org/English/safety-prevention/on-the-go/pages/Car-Safety-Seats-Information-for-Families.aspx.

American Dietetic Association (ADA): Dietitians of Canada: Position of the American Dietetic Association and Dietitians of Canada: vegetarian diets, *J Am Diet Assoc* 103(6):748–765, 2003.

Bates E, Dick F: Language, gesture, and the developing brain, *Dev Psychobiol* 40:293–310, 2002.

Berenbaum SA, Beltz AM: Sexual differentiation of human behavior: effects of prenatal and pubertal organizational hormones, *Front Neuroendocrinol* 32(2):183–200, 2011.

Borse NN, Gilchrist J, Delinger AM, et al: *CDC Childhood Injury Report: patterns of unintentional injuries among 0-19 year olds in the United States, 2000-2006*, Atlanta, 2008, Centers for Disease Control and Prevention.

Brazelton TB: How to help parents of young children: the touchpoints model, *J Perinatol* 19(6 Pt 2):S6–S7, 1999.

Brotanek JM, Schroer D, Valentyn L, et al: Reasons for prolonged bottle-feeding and iron deficiency among Mexican-American toddlers: an ethnographic study, *Acad Pediatr* 9(1):17–25, 2009.

Bull MJ, Durbin DR: Rear-facing car safety seats: getting the message right, *Pediatrics* 121(3):619–620, 2008.

Butte NF, Fox MK, Briefel RR, et al: Nutrient intakes of US infants, toddlers, and preschoolers meet or exceed dietary reference intakes, *J Am Diet Assoc* 110(12 suppl 3):S27–S37, 2010.

Cathey M, Gaylord N: Picky eating: a toddler's continuing approach to mealtime, *Pediatr Nurs* 30(2):101–107, 2004.

Centers for Disease Control and Prevention (CDC): Nonfatal motor-vehicle-related backover injuries among children—United States, 2001-2003, *MMWR Morb Mortal Wkly Rep* 54(06):144–146, 2005.

Choby BA, George SA: Toilet training, *Am Family Physician* 78(9):1059–1064, 2008.

Chonchaiva W, Pruksananonda C: Television viewing associates with delayed language development, *Acta Paediatr* 97(7):977–982, 2008.

Consumer Product Safety Commission: Full-size baby cribs and non–full-size baby cribs: safety standards, *Fed Reg* 75(248):81766–81788, 2010.

Craig WJ, Mangels AR, and American Dietetic Association: Position of the American Dietetic Association: vegetarian diets, *J Am Diet Assoc* 109(7):1266–1282, 2009.

Davis KF, Parker K, Montgomery GL: Sleep in infants and young children. Part 2. Common sleep problems, *J Pediatr Health Care* 18(3):130–137, 2004.

Dunham L, Kollar L: Vegetarian eating for children and adolescents, *J Pediatr Health Care* 20(1):27–34, 2006.

Durbin DR, American Academy of Pediatrics (AAP) Committee on Injury, Violence, and Poison Prevention: Technical report—child passenger safety, *Pediatrics* 127(4):e1050–e1066, 2011.

Elkins M, Cavendish R: Developing a plan for pediatric spiritual care, *Holistic Nurs Pract* 18(4):179–184, 2004.

Erikson EH: *Childhood and society*, ed 2, New York, 1963, Norton.

Feigelman S: The second year. In Kliegman RM, Stanton BF, St. Geme JW, et al, editors: *Nelson textbook of pediatrics*, ed 19, Philadelphia, 2011, Saunders.

Fonseca H, Greydanus DE: Sexuality in the child, teen, and young adult: concepts for the clinician, *Prim Care Clin Office Pract* 34 (2):275–292, 2007.

Fosarelli P: Children and the development of faith: implications for pediatric practice, *Contemp Pediatr* 20(1):85–98, 2003.

Fowler JW: *Stages of faith: the psychology of human development and the quest for meaning*, San Francisco, 1981, Harper & Row.

Freeman R, Stevens A: Nursing caries and buying time: an emerging theory of prolonged bottle-feeding, *Community Dent Oral Epidemiol* 36(5):425–433, 2008.

Gardiner P, Kemper KJ: Herbs, complementary therapies, and integrative medicine. In Kliegman RM, Stanton BF, St. Geme JW, et al, editors: *Nelson textbook of pediatrics*, ed 19, Philadelphia, 2011, Saunders.

Ginsburg KR, American Academy of Pediatrics (AAP) Committee on Communications: The importance of play in promoting healthy child development and maintaining strong parent-child bonds, *Pediatrics* 119(1):182–191, 2007.

Glassy D, Romano J, and American Academy of Pediatrics (AAP) Committee on Early Childhood, Adoption, and Dependent Care: Selecting appropriate toys for young children: the pediatrician's role, *Pediatrics* 111(4):911–913, 2003.

Guard A, Gallagher SS: Heat-related deaths in young children in parked cars: an analysis of 171 fatalities in the United States, 1995-2002, *Inj Prev* 11(1):33–37, 2005.

Hallberg L: Does calcium interfere with iron absorption? (editorial), *Am J Clin Nutr* 68(1):3–4, 1998.

Harpaz-Rotem I, Bergman A: On an evolving theory of attachment: rapprochement theory of a developing mind, *Psychoanal Study Child* 61:170–189, 2006.

Henary B Sherwood CP, Crandall JR, et al: Car safety for children: rear facing for best protection, *Inj Prev* 13(6):398–402, 2007.

Hines M: Gender development and the human brain, *Annu Rev Neurosci* 34:69–88, 2011.

Horn IB, Brenner R, Rao M, et al: Beliefs about the appropriate age for initiating toilet training: are there racial and socioeconomic differences? *J Pediatr* 149(2):165–168, 2006.

Huillet A, Erdie-Lalena C, Norvell D, et al: Complementary and alternative medicine used by children in military pediatric clinics, *J Altern Complement Med* 17(6):531–537, 2011.

Institute of Medicine (IOM): *Dietary reference intakes for energy, carbohydrate, fiber, fat, fatty acids, cholesterol, protein, and amino acids*, Washington, DC, 2005, The Institute, National Academies Press.

Kiddoo DA: Toilet training children: when to start and how to train, *CMAJ* 184(5): 511–512, 2012.

Klassen TP, Kiddoo D, Lang ME, et al: The effectiveness of different methods of toilet training for bowel and bladder control, *Evid Rep Technol Assess (Full Rep)* Dec(147):1–57, 2006.

Landier W, Tse AM: Use of complementary and alternative medical interventions for the management of procedural-related pain, anxiety, and distress in pediatric oncology: an integrative review, *J Pediatr Nurs* 25(6):566–579, 2010.

Lanski SL, Greenwald M, Perkins A, et al: Herbal therapy in a pediatric emergency department population: expect the unexpected, *Pediatrics* 111(5 Pt 1):981–985, 2003.

Lohse B, Stotts JL, Priebe JR: Survey of herbal use by Kansas and Wisconsin WIC participants reveals moderate, appropriate use and identifies herbal education needs, *J Am Diet Assoc* 106(2):227–237, 2006.

Loman DG: The use of complementary and alternative health care practices among children, *J Pediatr Health Care* 17(2):58–63, 2003.

Lönnerdal B: Calcium and iron absorption—mechanisms and public health relevance, *Int J Vitamin Nutr Res* 80(4-5):293–299, 2010.

Luangrath A, Hiscock H: Problem behavior in children: an approach for general practice, *Aust Fam Physician* 40(9): 678–681, 2011.

McLaren C, Null J, Quinn J: Heat stress from enclosed vehicles: moderate ambient temperatures cause significant temperature rise in enclosed vehicles, *Pediatrics* 116(1):e109–e112, 2005.

Meltzer LJ, Mindell JA: Sleep and sleep disorders in children and adolescents, *Psychiatr Clin North Am* 29(4):1059–1076, 2006.

Mercer R: Treating nocturnal enuresis, *Adv Nurs Pract* 11(2):26–31, 2003.

Moore M, Meltzer LJ, Mindell JA: Bedtime problems and night waking in children, *Prim Care Clin Office Pract* 35(3):569–581, 2008.

Morin K: Infant nutrition: toddlers: start off on the right foot, *MCN Am J Matern Child Nurs* 32(2):122, 2007.

National Center for Complementary and Alternative Medicine (NCCAM): *What is complementary and alternative medicine?* Bethesda, MD, 2010, National Institutes of Health, National Center for Complementary and Alternative Medicine, www.anccam.nih.gov/health/whatiscam.

National Highway Traffic Safety Administration (NHTSA): *A parent's guide to booster seats (pamphlet)*, Washington, DC, 2010, The Administration, nhtsa.gov.org.

Needlman R, Howard B, Zuckerman B: Helping parents get beyond the terrible 2's, *Patient Care* 29(1):52–61, 1995.

Neuman ME: Addressing children's beliefs through Fowler's stages of faith, *J Pediatr Nurs* 26(1):44–50, 2011.

Null J: *Hyperthermia deaths of children in vehicles*, 2011, San Francisco State University, Department of Geosciences, www.ggweather.com/heat.

Owens JA: Sleep medicine. In Kliegman RM, Stanton BF, St. Geme JW, et al, editors: *Nelson textbook of pediatrics*, ed 19, Philadelphia, 2011, Saunders.

Roehlkepartain EC, King PE, Wagener LM, et al, editors: *The handbook of spiritual development in childhood and adolescence*, Thousand Oaks, CA, 2006, Sage.

Rutkoski JD, Sippey M, Gaines BA: Traumatic television tip-overs in the pediatric population, *J Surg Res* 166(2):199–204, 2011.

Savic I, Garcia-Falqueras A, Swaab DF: Sexual differentiation of the human brain in relation to gender identity and sexual orientation, *Prog Brain Res* 186:41–62, 2010.

Sawni A, Ragothaman R, Thomas RL, et al: The use of complementary/alternative therapies among children attending an urban pediatric emergency department, *Clin Pediatr* 46(1):36–41, 2007.

Schmitt BD: Toilet training: getting it right the first time, *Contemp Pediatr* 21(3):105–108, 111–112, 115–116, 2004.

Schum TR, Kolb TM, McAuliffe TL, et al: Sequential acquisition of toilet-training skills: a descriptive study of gender and age differences in normal children, *Pediatrics* 109(3):e48, 2002.

Stein MT: Difficult behavior: temper tantrums to conduct disorders. In Rudolph CD, Rudolph AM, Hostetter MK, editors: *Rudolph's pediatrics*, ed 21, New York, 2003, McGraw-Hill.

Stephenson M: Danger in the toy box, *J Pediatr Health Care* 19(3):187–189, 2005.

Touchette E, Petit D, Paquet J, et al: Factors associated with fragmented sleep at night across early childhood, *Arch Pediatr Adolesc Med* 159(3):242–249, 2005.

Wagner CL, Greer FR, American Academy of Pediatrics (AAP) Section on Breastfeeding and Committee on Nutrition: Prevention of rickets and vitamin D deficiency in infants, children, and adolescents, *Pediatrics* 122(5):1142–1148, 2008.

Ward TM, Rankin S, Lee KA: Caring for children with sleep problems, *J Pediatr Nurs* 22(4):283–296, 2007.

Weiss J, Committee on Injury, Violence, and Poison Prevention: technical report—prevention of drowning, *Pediatrics* 126(1):e253–e262, 2010.

Yeh ES, Rochette LM, McKenzie LB, et al: Injuries associated with cribs, playpens, and bassinets among young children in the US—1990-2008, *Pediatrics* 127(3):479–486, 2011.

Zimmerman FJ, Gilkerson J, Richards JA, et al: Teaching by listening: the importance of adult-child conversations to language development, *Pediatrics* 124(1):342–349, 2009.

The Preschooler and Family

David Wilson

℮volve WEBSITE

http://evolve.elsevier.com/Perry/maternal

LEARNING OBJECTIVES

On completion of this chapter, the reader will be able to:
- Identify the major biologic, psychosocial, cognitive, moral, spiritual, and social developments that occur during the preschool years.
- List the benefits of imaginary playmates.
- Prepare preschoolers for preschool or day care experience.
- Provide parents with guidelines for sex education.
- Provide parents with guidelines for dealing with a child's fears, stresses, aggression, and sleep problems.

- Recognize the causes of stuttering during the preschool years.
- Offer parents suggestions for preventing speech problems.
- Recognize feeding patterns of preschoolers.
- Provide anticipatory guidance to parents regarding injury prevention based on the preschooler's developmental achievements.

PROMOTING OPTIMAL GROWTH AND DEVELOPMENT

The combined biologic, psychosocial, cognitive, spiritual, and social achievements during the *preschool period* (3 to 5 years of age) prepare preschoolers for their most significant change in lifestyle: entrance into school. Their control of bodily functions, experience of brief and prolonged periods of separation, ability to interact cooperatively with other children and adults, use of language for mental symbolization, and increased attention span and memory prepare them for the next major period: the school years. Successful achievement of previous levels of growth and development is essential for preschoolers to refine many of the tasks that were mastered during the toddler years.

Biologic Development

The rate of physical growth slows and stabilizes during the preschool years. The average *weight* is 14.5 kg (32 lbs) at 3 years, 16.7 kg (36.8 lbs) at 4 years, and 18.7 kg (41.5 lbs) at 5 years. The average weight gain per year remains approximately 2 to 3 kg (4.5 to 6.5 lbs). Growth in *height* also remains steady, with an annual increase of 6.5 to 9 cm (2.5 to 3.5 inches), and generally occurs by elongation of the legs rather than the trunk. The average height is 95 cm (37.5 inches) at 3 years, 103 cm (40.5 inches) at 4 years, and 110 cm (43.5 inches) at 5 years.

Physical proportions no longer resemble those of the squat, pot-bellied toddler. The preschooler is slender but sturdy, graceful, agile, and posturally erect. There is little difference in physical characteristics according to gender, except as dictated by such factors as dress and hairstyle.

Most organ systems can adjust to moderate stress and change. During this period most children are toilet trained. For the most part motor development consists of increases in strength and refinement of previously learned skills such as walking, running, and jumping. However, muscle development and bone growth are still far from mature. Excessive activity and overexertion can injure delicate tissues. Good posture, appropriate exercise, and adequate nutrition and rest are essential for optimal development of the musculoskeletal system.

Gross and Fine Motor Skills

Walking, running, climbing, and jumping are well established by age 36 months. Refinement in eye-hand and muscle coordination is evident in several areas. At age 3 the preschooler rides a tricycle,

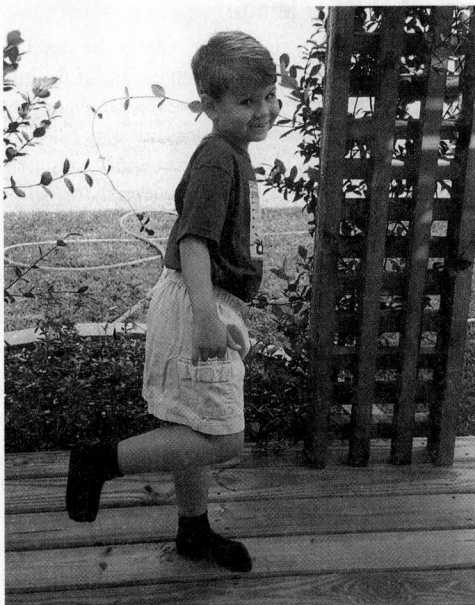

FIG 33-1 A 4-year-old child has sufficient balance to stand or hop on one foot.

walks on tiptoe, balances on one foot for a few seconds, and broad jumps. By age 4 the child skips and hops proficiently on one foot (Fig. 33-1) and catches a ball reliably. By age 5 he or she skips on alternate feet, jumps rope, and begins to skate and swim.

Fine motor development is evident in the child's increasingly skillful manipulation such as in drawing and dressing. These skills provide readiness for learning and independence for entry into school.

Psychosocial Development
Developing a Sense of Initiative (Erikson)

After preschoolers have mastered the tasks of the toddler period, they are ready to face the developmental endeavors of the preschool period. Erikson (1963) maintained that the chief psychosocial task of this period is acquiring a sense of *initiative*. Children are in a stage of energetic learning. They play, work, and live to the fullest and feel a real sense of accomplishment and satisfaction in their activities. Conflict arises when they overstep the limits of their ability and inquiry and experience a sense of *guilt* for not having behaved appropriately. Feelings of guilt, anxiety, and fear may also result from thoughts that differ from expected behavior.

A particularly stressful thought is wishing one's parent dead. As a sense of rivalry or competition develops between the child and same-sex parent, the child may think of ways to get rid of the interfering parent. In most situations this rivalry is resolved when the child strongly identifies with the same-sex parent and peers during the school years. However, if that parent dies before the identification process is completed, the preschooler may be overwhelmed with guilt for having wished and therefore "caused" the death. Clarifying for children that wishes cannot and do not make events occur is essential in helping them overcome their guilt and anxiety.

Development of the *superego*, or *conscience*, begins toward the end of the toddler years and is a major task for preschoolers (see Cultural Competence box). Learning right from wrong and good from bad is the beginning of morality (see section on Moral Development).

🌐 CULTURAL COMPETENCE
Learning Sociocultural Mores

Developing a conscience implies learning the sociocultural mores of the family's heritage. Depending on the type of attitudes conveyed, children learn not only appropriate behaviors but also tolerant, biased, or prejudicial values concerning their ethnic, religious, and social background and those of other groups. Much of this influence may remain dormant until they associate with children or adults of a different ethnic background. Then, depending on the particular group, they may be accepted or ostracized for their attitudes.

Cognitive Development

One of the tasks related to the preschool period is readiness for school and scholastic learning. Many of the thought processes of this period are crucial for achieving such readiness, and it is intentional that the child begins school between ages 5 and 6 rather than at an earlier age.

Preoperational Phase (Piaget)

Piaget's cognitive theory does not include a period specifically for children who are 3 to 5 years old. The *preoperational phase* covers the age span from 2 to 7 years and is divided into two stages: the *preconceptual phase*, ages 2 to 4, and the phase of *intuitive thought*, ages 4 to 7. One of the main transitions during these two phases is the shift from totally egocentric thought to social awareness and the ability to consider other viewpoints. However, egocentricity is still evident.

Language continues to develop during the preschool period. Speech remains primarily a vehicle of egocentric communication. Preschoolers assume that everyone thinks as they do and that a brief explanation of their thinking makes the entire thought understood by others. Because of this self-referenced, egocentric verbal communication, it is often necessary to explore and understand the young child's thinking through other, nonverbal approaches. For children in this age-group, the most enlightening and effective method is *play*, which becomes the child's way of understanding, adjusting to, and working out life's experiences.

Preschoolers increasingly use language without comprehending the meaning of words, particularly concepts of right and left, causality, and time. Children may use the concepts correctly but only in the circumstances in which they have learned them. For example, they may know how to put on shoes by remembering that the buckle is always on the outside of the foot. However, if different shoes have no buckles, they cannot reason which shoe fits which foot. In other words, they do not understand the concept of *right and left.*

Superficially, *causality* resembles logical thought. Preschoolers explain a concept as they heard it described by others, but their understanding is limited. An example is the concept of time. Because *time* is still incompletely understood, the child interprets it according to his or her own frame of reference, such as "A long time means until Christmas." Consequently time is best explained in relationship to an event such as, "Your mother will visit you after you finish your lunch." Avoiding words such as *yesterday, tomorrow, next week,* or *Tuesday* to express when an event is expected to occur and instead associating time with expected daily events help children learn about temporal relationships while increasing their trust in others' predictions.

Preschoolers' thinking is often described as *magical thinking.* Because of their egocentrism and transductive reasoning, they believe that thoughts are all-powerful. Such thinking places them in the vulnerable position of feeling guilty and responsible for bad thoughts, which may coincide with the occurrence of a wished event. Their inability to logically reason the cause and effect of an illness or injury makes it especially difficult for them to understand such events.

> **! NURSING ALERT**
>
> Counseling children whose parents are going through a divorce or separation should involve a discussion with the child about her or his role. Because of magical thinking the child may believe that she or he wished the other parent away. The child should be reassured that this is not the case.

Preschoolers believe in the power of words and accept their meaning literally. An example of this type of thinking is calling children "bad" because they did something wrong. In the preschooler's mind calling them bad means that he or she is a bad person; thus it is better to say that the actions were bad (e.g., "That was a bad thing to do").

Moral Development

Preconventional or Premoral Level (Kohlberg)

Young children's development of moral judgment is at the most basic level. They have little, if any, concern about why something is wrong. They behave because of the freedom or restriction that is placed on actions. In the *punishment and obedience orientation,* children (from about 2 to 4 years) judge whether an action is good or bad depending on whether it results in reward or punishment. If children are punished for it, the action is bad. If they are not punished, the action is good regardless of the meaning of the act. For example, if parents allow hitting, the child perceives that hitting is good because it is not associated with punishment.

From approximately 4 to 7 years of age children are in the stage of *naive instrumental orientation,* in which actions are directed toward satisfying their needs and less frequently the needs of others. They have a concrete sense of justice and fairness during this period of development.

Spiritual Development

Children generally learn about faith and religion from significant others in their environment, usually from parents and their religious beliefs and practices. However, young children's understanding of spirituality is influenced by their cognitive level. Preschoolers have a concrete concept of a God with physical characteristics, often similar to an imaginary friend. They understand simple Bible stories, memorize short prayers, and imitate the religious practices of their parents without fully understanding the significance of these rituals. Preschoolers benefit from concrete representations of religious practices such as picture Bible books and small statues such as those of the Nativity scene.

Development of the conscience is strongly linked to spiritual development. At this age children are learning right from wrong and behaving correctly to avoid punishment. Wrongdoing provokes feelings of guilt, and preschoolers often misinterpret illness as a punishment for real or imagined transgressions. Observing religious traditions and participating in a religious community can help children cope during stressful periods such as illness and hospitalization (Speraw, 2006).

In many religious faiths cultural practices and religion are closely intertwined (McEvoy, 2003) and are an important part of the child's and family's life.

Development of Body Image

The preschool years play a significant role in the development of body image. With increasing comprehension of language, preschoolers recognize that individuals have desirable and undesirable appearances. They recognize differences in skin color and racial identity and are vulnerable to learning prejudices and biases. They are aware of the meaning of words such as *pretty* or *ugly,* and they reflect the opinions of others regarding their own appearance. By 5 years of age children compare their size with that of their peers and can become conscious of being large or short, especially if others refer to them as "so big" or "so little" for their age. Research indicates that girls as young as preschool age already show concern about appearance and weight (Skouteris, McCabe, Swinburn, et al., 2010). Because these are formative years for both boys and girls, parents should make efforts to instill *positive* principles regarding body image, give their children encouraging feedback regarding their appearance, and emphasize the importance of accepting individuals no matter how their appearances differ. Children at this age should be educated regarding the benefits of physical activity and nutrition on health rather than focusing on weight.

Despite the advances in body-image development, preschoolers have poorly defined body boundaries and little knowledge of their internal anatomy. Intrusive experiences are frightening, especially those that disrupt the integrity of the skin such as injections and surgery. They fear that, if their skin is "broken," all of their blood and "insides" can leak out. Therefore bandages are critical to "keep everything from coming out."

Development of Sexuality

Sexual development during these years is an important phase in the formation of a person's overall sexual identity and beliefs. Preschoolers are forming strong attachments to the opposite-sex parent while identifying with the same-sex parent. *Sex-typing,* or the process by which an individual develops the behavior, personality, attitudes, and beliefs appropriate for his or her culture and sex, occurs through several mechanisms during this period. Probably the most powerful mechanisms are childrearing practices and imitation. Gender identification is a result of complex prenatal and postnatal psychologic factors and biologic or genetic factors. Most children are aware of their gender and the expected sets of related behaviors by 1.5 to 2.5 years of age.

As sexual identity develops beyond gender recognition, modesty may become a concern. Sex-role imitation and "dressing up" like Mommy or Daddy are important activities. Attitudes and responses of others to role-playing can condition the child to accept the views of others. For example, comments such as "Boys shouldn't play with dolls" can influence a boy's self-concept of masculinity.

Sexual exploration may be more pronounced now than ever before, particularly in terms of exploring and manipulating the genitalia. Questions about sexual reproduction may come to the forefront in the preschooler's search for understanding (see Chapters 34 and 35).

Social Development

During the preschool period the *separation-individuation process* is completed. Preschoolers have overcome much of the anxiety associated with strangers and the fear of separation of earlier years. They relate to unfamiliar people easily and tolerate brief separations from parents with little or no protest. However, they still need parental security, reassurance, guidance, and approval, especially when entering preschool or elementary school. Prolonged separation such as that imposed by illness and hospitalization is difficult, but

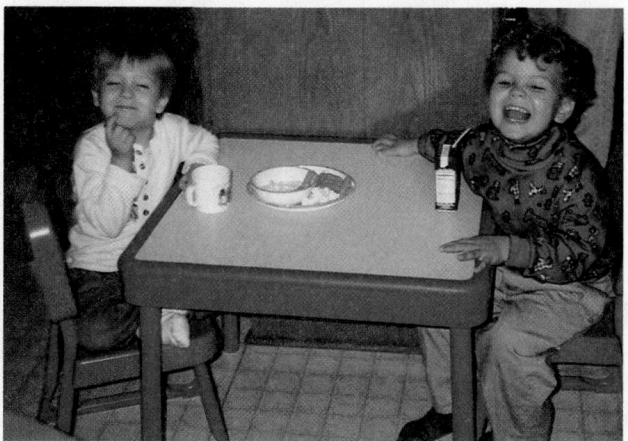

FIG 33-2 Preschool children enjoy friends and often use nonverbal messages to communicate.

preschoolers respond to anticipatory preparation and concrete explanation. Maintaining an established routine is still important in early preschoolers regardless of home, school, or hospital environment. They can cope with changes in daily routine much better than toddlers, although they may develop more imaginary fears. Preschoolers gain security and comfort from familiar objects such as toys, dolls, or photographs of family members. They are able to work through many of their unresolved fears, fantasies, and anxieties through play, especially if guided with appropriate play objects (e.g., dolls, puppets) that represent family members, health care professionals, and other children.

Language

During the preschool years language becomes more sophisticated and complex and the major mode of communication and social interaction (Fig. 33-2). Through language preschool children learn to express feelings of frustration or anger without acting them out. Both cognitive ability and environment—particularly consistent role models—influence vocabulary, speech, and comprehension. Vocabulary increases dramatically, from 300 words at age 2 years to more than 2100 words at the end of 5 years. Sentence structure, grammatic usage, and intelligibility also advance to a more adult level. Language development during these early years predicts school readiness (Harrison and McLeod, 2010) and sets the stage for later success in school (Reilly, Wake, Ukoumunne, et al., 2010).

Children between the ages of 3 and 4 years form sentences of about three or four words and include only the most essential words to convey a meaning. Such speech is often termed telegraphic for its brevity. Three-year-old children ask many questions and use plurals, correct pronouns, and the past tense of verbs. They name familiar objects such as animals, parts of the body, relatives, and friends. They can give and follow simple commands. They talk incessantly regardless of whether anyone is listening or answering them. They enjoy musical or talking toys or dolls and imitate new words proficiently. Preschoolers also benefit from "reading" picture books with a parent or adult figure; this provides immediate feedback to the child and helps develop vocabulary as he or she hears the pronunciation of words from an adult (Feigelman, 2011). There is evidence that reading and speaking to a child in early life programs words into the child's memory bank for use at a later time.

From ages 4 to 5 years preschoolers use longer sentences of four or five words and more parts of speech to convey a message (e.g., prepositions, adjectives, and a variety of verbs). They can follow

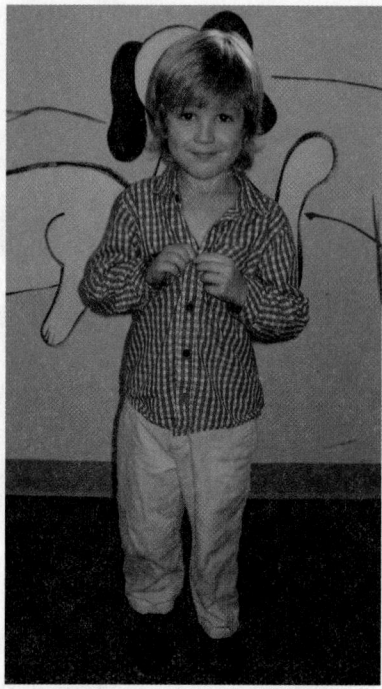

FIG 33-3 Most preschoolers are able to dress themselves but need help with more difficult items of clothing.

simple directional commands such as, "Put the ball on the chair," but can carry out only one request at a time. They answer questions such as, "What do you do when you're hungry?" by describing the appropriate action. The pattern of asking questions is at its peak, and children usually repeat a question until they receive an answer. Preschoolers also are incapable of understanding figurative speech and are very literal in their understanding of the meaning of words (Feigelman, 2011). For example, saying that an IV cannula to be inserted for hydration is a straw is interpreted by the preschooler as literally a drinking straw because that is his or her common frame of reference for that object.

By 6 years of age children can use all parts of speech correctly except for deviations from the rule. They can define simple things by describing their use, shape, or general category of classification rather than simply describing their outward appearance. For example, they define a ball as "round," "something you bounce," or "a toy," rather than only describing its color. They can give some opposites such as, "If Mommy is a woman, Daddy is a man." They can also describe an object according to its composition such as, "A spoon is made of metal."

Personal-Social Behavior

The pervasive ritualism and negativism of toddlerhood gradually diminish during the preschool years. Although self-assertion is still a major theme, preschoolers demonstrate their sense of autonomy differently. They are able to verbalize their request for independence and perform independently because of their much-refined physical and cognitive development. By 4 or 5 years of age they need little if any assistance with dressing, eating, or toileting (Fig. 33-3). They can be trusted to obey warnings of danger, although 3- or 4-year-old children may exceed their boundaries at times.

They are also much more sociable and willing to please. They have internalized many of the standards and values of the family and culture. However, by the end of early childhood they begin to question parental values and compare them with those of their peer

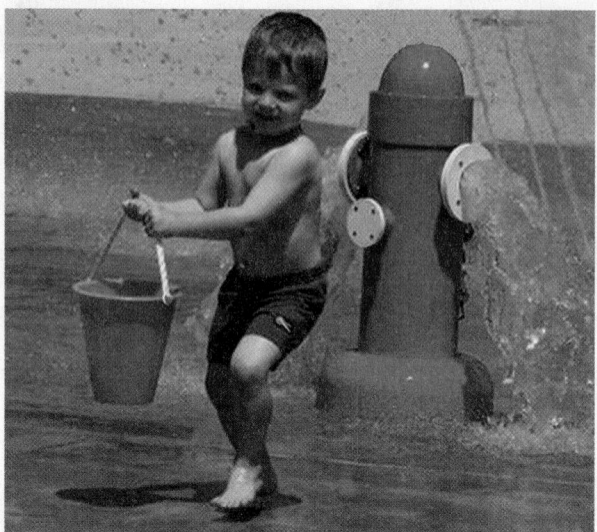

FIG 33-4 Preschoolers enjoy play activities that promote motor skills such as jumping and running. Water play is an exciting activity for preschooler.

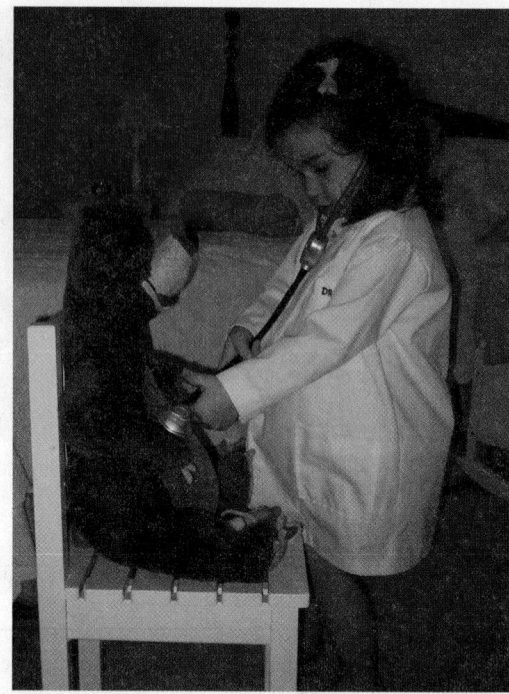

FIG 33-5 Imaginative and imitative play is typical of preschoolers.

group and other authority figures. As a result they may be less willing to abide by the family's code of conduct. Preschoolers become increasingly aware of their position and role within the family. Although this is a more secure age for experiencing the addition of another sibling, relinquishing the position of first or youngest is still difficult and requires appropriate preparation (see Sibling Rivalry, Chapter 32).

Play

Various types of play are typical of this period, but preschoolers especially enjoy associative play (i.e., group play in similar or identical activities but without rigid organization or rules). Play should provide for physical, social, and mental development.

Play activities for physical growth and refinement of motor skills include jumping, running, and climbing. Tricycles, wagons, gym and sports equipment, sandboxes, wading pools, and activities at water parks can help develop muscles and coordination (Fig. 33-4). Activities such as swimming and skating teach safety and muscle development and coordination. Children involved in the work of play do not require expensive toys and gadgets to keep them entertained but often enjoy playing with common household items such as a broom handle or even items that adults consider junk (boxes, sticks, rocks, and dirt). The imaginative mind of the preschooler enjoys playing for play's sake.

Manipulative, constructive, creative, and educational toys provide for quiet activities, fine motor development, and self-expression. Easy construction sets, large blocks of various sizes and shapes, a counting frame, alphabet or number flash cards, paints, crayons, simple carpentry tools, musical toys, illustrated books, simple sewing or handicraft sets, large puzzles, and clay are suitable toys. Electronic games and computer programs are especially valuable in helping children learn basic skills such as letters and simple words.

Probably the most characteristic and pervasive preschool activity is imitative, imaginative, and dramatic play. Dress-up clothes, dolls, housekeeping toys, dollhouses, play store toys, telephones, farm animals and equipment, village sets, trains, trucks, cars, planes, hand puppets, and medical kits provide hours of self-expression (Fig. 33-5). Probably at no other time is the reproduction of adult

behavior so faithful and absorbing as in 4- and 5-year-old children. Toward the end of the preschool period children are less satisfied with make-believe or pretend objects and enjoy doing the actual activity such as cooking and carpentry.

Television and other media also have their place in children's play, although each should be only one part of children's total repertoire of social and recreational activities. Parents and other caregivers should supervise the selection of programs, watch and discuss programs with their children, schedule limited time for television viewing, and set a good example of television viewing (American Academy of Pediatrics [AAP], 2007). Children enjoy and learn from educational programs; however, television viewing may limit time spent in other meaningful activities such as reading, physical activity, and socialization (AAP, 2007). Prolonged television viewing by young children has been linked to an increase in psychologic distress and decreased time spent in active playing, which increases the risk for obesity among certain children (Hamer, Stamatakis, and Mishra, 2009). Fast-paced television cartoons have been linked to a temporary decrease in executive functioning in 4-year-olds (self-regulation and working memory) (Lilard and Peterson, 2011).

Although the potential negative effects of television viewing have been well documented in literature, research has also shown that prosocial behavior and later academic achievement can result from viewing educational media during the preschool years; however, positive effects depend on the media content, the age of the viewer, the length of viewing time, and the presence of a co-viewing parent (Kirkorian, Wartella, and Anderson, 2008). When parents view media with their children, the activity can become interactive, with parents and children discussing program content. Considering the significant increase in media accessibility through various portable electronic devices and cell phones, parents need to be aware of the potential positive and negative effects of media exposure.

Play is so much a part of young children's lives that reality and fantasy become blurred. Make-believe is reality during play and only becomes fantasy when the toys are put away or the dress-up clothes are removed. It is no wonder that imaginary playmates are so much a part of this age period. The appearance of imaginary companions usually occurs between 2½ and 3 years of age, and for the most part such playmates are relinquished when the child enters school. Differences in birth order and gender have been noted in studies of imaginary companion play. Firstborn children have a higher incidence of imaginary companions as do young girls; young boys more often tend to impersonate characters (Trionfi and Reese, 2009).

Imaginary companions serve many purposes: they become friends in times of loneliness, accomplish what the child is still attempting, and experience what the child wants to forget or remember. It is not unusual for the "friend" to have myriad vices and be blamed for wrongdoing. Sometimes the child hopes to escape punishment by saying, "My friend George broke the glass." At other times the child may fantasize that the companion misbehaved and play the role of the parent. This becomes a way of assuming control and authority in a safe situation.

Parents often worry about the imaginary playmates, not realizing how normal and useful they are. They need to be reassured that the child's fantasy is a sign of health that helps differentiate make-believe and reality. Parents can acknowledge the presence of the imaginary companion by calling him or her by name and even agreeing to simple requests such as setting an extra place at the table, but they should not allow the child to use the playmate to avoid punishment or responsibility. For example, if the child blames the companion for messing up a room, parents need to state clearly that the child is the only one they see; therefore the child is responsible for cleaning up.

Children also benefit from play that occurs between them and a parent. Mutual play fosters development from birth through the school years and provides enriched opportunities for learning. Through mutual play parents can provide tactile and kinesthetic experiences, maximize verbal and language abilities, and offer praise and encouragement for exploration of the world. In addition, mutual play encourages positive interactions between the parent and child, strengthening their relationship.

Table 33-1 summarizes the major developmental achievements for children 3, 4, and 5 years of age.

Coping with Concerns Related to Normal Growth and Development

Preschool and Kindergarten Experience

Some children are home schooled, but many attend some type of early childhood program, usually preschool or a day care center. Group care has become commonplace with the large number of parents currently employed outside the home (see Alternate Child Care Arrangements, Chapter 31). The effects of early education and stimulation on children have increasingly gained recognition. (For a discussion of the effects of day care on young children, see Working Mothers, Chapter 27.) Because social development widens to include age mates and other significant adults, preschool provides an excellent vehicle for expanding children's experiences with others. It is also excellent preparation for entrance into elementary school.

In preschool or day care centers children are exposed to opportunities for learning group cooperation; adjusting to sociocultural differences; and coping with frustration, dissatisfaction, and anger. If activities are tailored to provide mastery and achievement, children increasingly have feelings of success, self-confidence, and personal competence. Whether structured learning is imposed is less important than the social climate, type of guidance, and attitude toward the children that is fostered by the teacher or leader. With a teacher who is aware of preschoolers' developmental abilities and

needs, children learn from the activity that is provided. Most programs incorporate a daily schedule of quiet play, active outdoor activity, group activities such as games and projects, creative or free play, and snack and rest periods. Preschool is particularly beneficial for children who lack a peer-group experience such as only children and for children from impoverished homes.

One of the issues that parents face is their children's readiness for preschool or kindergarten. There are no absolute indicators for school readiness; but children's social maturity, especially attention span, is as important as their academic readiness. Using a developmental screening tool that addresses cognitive (especially language), social, and physical milestones can identify children who may benefit from diagnostic testing and early-intervention programs before starting school. Parents play an integral role in their children's school readiness. They should promote a positive attitude toward learning, read to their children, encourage their children to participate in a variety of activities to explore their talents and interests, and choose appropriate child care or preschool programs (Hagan, Shaw, and Duncan, 2008).

Nurses and other health care workers can guide parents in selecting enriched social and educational early-intervention programs, schools, and child care centers. Careful selection of early-childhood education is intrinsic to future learning and development. Licensed and regulated programs are mandated to abide by established standards, which represent minimum requirements and safeguards. Regulation is important to protect children from harm and promote the conditions essential for a child's healthy development and learning. The National Association for the Education of Young Children (NAEYC) serves as the model for optimal care of small children.*

Areas for parents to evaluate include the daily program of the facility, teacher qualifications, staff-to-student ratio, discipline policy, environmental safety precautions, provision of meals, sanitary conditions, adequate indoor and outdoor space per child, safety and injury prevention, and fee schedule. A plan for emergency response in case of fire or other hazard [flooding, tornado] should also be well established (with evacuation drills) by the program. References from other parents help in evaluating a facility, but personal observation of the facility is recommended. Encourage parents to meet the director and some of the employees at a few facilities to make an informed choice.

Evaluation of the health practices of the facility is extremely important. Children in day care centers have more illnesses than those not in day care centers, especially gastrointestinal tract infections; respiratory tract infections; and hepatitis A, varicella-zoster virus, and cytomegalovirus infections (Nesti and Goldbaum, 2007). Nurses play an important role in infection control. Not only can they advise parents regarding the evaluation of the sanitary practices of a facility, but they can also take an active part in educating staff in measures to minimize transmission of infection (Fig. 33-6). Proactive infection control measures and education of staff have been effective in reducing the incidence of upper respiratory tract infections, diarrhea, and rotavirus (Kotch, Isbell, Weber, et al., 2007). Day care staff should also have updated routine immunizations according to the adult immunization recommendations, including the annual influenza vaccine, to protect the children in the center (AAP

---

*Information about accreditation criteria and procedures of the NAEYC Academy for Early Childhood Program Accreditation is available from the National Association for the Education of Young Children, 1313 L St. NW, Suite 500, Washington, DC 20005, 800-424-2460 or 202-232-8777, fax: 202-328-1846, www.naeyc.org. These criteria are excellent guidelines for evaluating preschools and day care centers.

TABLE 33-1 GROWTH AND DEVELOPMENT DURING PRESCHOOL YEARS

PHYSICAL	GROSS MOTOR	FINE MOTOR	LANGUAGE	SOCIALIZATION	COGNITION	FAMILY RELATIONSHIPS
Age 3 Yr						
Usual weight gain of 1.8-2.7 kg (4-6 lbs)	Rides tricycle	Builds tower of 9-10 cubes	Has vocabulary of about 900 words	Dresses self almost completely if helped with back buttons and told which shoe is right or left	Is in preconceptual phase	Attempts to please parents and conform to their expectations
Average weight of 14.5 kg (32 lbs)	Jumps off bottom step	Builds bridge with three cubes	Uses primarily telegraphic speech	Pulls on shoes	Is egocentric in thought and behavior	Is less jealous of younger sibling
Usual gain in height of 7.5 cm (3 inches) per year	Stands on one foot for a few seconds	Adeptly places small pellets in narrow-necked bottle	Uses complete sentences of three or four words	Has increased attention span	Has beginning understanding of time; uses many time-oriented expressions, talks about past and future as much as about present, pretends to tell time	Is aware of family relationships and sex-role functions
Average height of 95 cm (37.5 inches)	Goes up stairs using alternate feet; may still come down using both feet on step	In drawing, copies a circle, imitates a cross, names what has been drawn; cannot draw stick figure but may make circle with facial features	Talks incessantly regardless of whether anyone is paying attention	Feeds self completely	Has improved concept of space, as demonstrated by understanding of prepositions and ability to follow directional command	Boys tend to identify more with father or other male figure
May have achieved nighttime control of bowel and bladder	Broad jumps		Repeats sentence of six syllables	Can prepare simple meals such as cold cereal and milk	Has beginning ability to view concepts from another perspective	Has increased ability to separate easily and comfortably from parents for short periods
	May try to dance, but balance may not be adequate		Asks many questions	Can help to set table; can dry dishes without breaking any		
				May have fears, especially of dark and going to bed		
				Knows own gender and gender of others		
				Play is parallel and associative; begins to learn simple games but often follows own rules; begins to share		
Age 4 Yr						
Pulse and respiration rates decrease slightly	Skips and hops on one foot	Uses scissors successfully to cut out picture following outline	Has vocabulary of 1500 words or more	Very independent	Is in phase of intuitive thought	Rebels if parents expect too much such as impeccable table manners
Growth rate is similar to that of previous year	Catches ball reliably	Can lace shoes but may not be able to tie bow	Uses sentences of four or five words	Tends to be selfish and impatient	Causality is still related to proximity of events	Takes aggression and frustration out on parents or siblings
Average weight of 16.7 kg (36.8 lbs)	Throws ball overhead	In drawing, copies a square, traces a cross and diamond, adds three parts to stick figure	Questioning is at peak	Aggressive physically and verbally	Understands time better, especially in terms of sequence of daily events	Do's and don'ts become important
Average height of 103 cm (40.5 inches)	Walks down stairs using alternate footing		Tells exaggerated stories	Takes pride in accomplishments	Unable to conserve matter	May have rivalry with older or younger siblings; may resent older sibling's privileges and younger sibling's invasion of privacy and possessions
Birth length has doubled			Knows simple songs	Has mood swings	Judges everything according to one dimension such as height, width, or order	May "run away" from home
Maximum potential for development of amblyopia			May be mildly profane if associates with older children	Shows off dramatically, enjoys entertaining others	Immediate perceptual clues dominate judgment	Identifies strongly with parent of opposite sex
			Obeys four prepositional phrases such as under, on top of, beside, in back of, or in front of	Tells family tales to others with no restraint	Is beginning to develop less egocentrism and more social awareness	Is able to run simple errands outside the home
			Names one or more colors	Still has many fears	May count correctly but has poor mathematic concept of numbers	
			Comprehends analogies such as, "If ice is cold, fire is _____."	Play is associative	Obeys because parents have set limits, not because of understanding of right or wrong	
				Imaginary playmates are common		
				Uses dramatic, imaginative, and imitative devices		
				Sexual exploration and curiosity demonstrated through play such as being "doctor" or "nurse" (see text)		

TABLE 33-1 GROWTH AND DEVELOPMENT DURING PRESCHOOL YEARS—cont'd

PHYSICAL	GROSS MOTOR	FINE MOTOR	LANGUAGE	SOCIALIZATION	COGNITION	FAMILY RELATIONSHIPS
Age 5 Yr Pulse and respiration rates decrease slightly Average weight of 18.7 kg (41.2 lbs) Average height of 110 cm (43.5 inches) Eruption of permanent dentition may begin Handedness is established (about 90% are right-handed)	Skips and hops on alternate feet Throws and catches ball well Jumps rope Skates with good balance Walks backward with heel to toe Jumps from height of 12 inches and lands on toes Balances on alternate feet with eyes closed	May begin to tie shoelaces but still needs some help Uses scissors, simple tools, or pencil very well In drawing copies a diamond and triangle; adds seven to nine parts to stick figure; prints a few letters, numbers, or words such as first name	Has vocabulary of about 2100 words Uses sentences of six to eight words, with all parts of speech Names coins (e.g., nickel, dime) Names four or more colors Describes drawing or pictures with much comment and elaboration Knows days of week, months, and other time-associated words Knows composition of objects, such as "A shoe is made of _____" Can follow three commands in succession	Less rebellious and quarrelsome than at age 4 yr More settled and eager to get down to business Not as open and accessible in thoughts and behavior as in earlier years Independent but trustworthy, not foolhardy; more responsible Has fewer fears; relies on outer authority to control world Eager to do things right and to please; tries to "live by the rules" Has better manners Cares for self totally, occasionally needing supervision in dress or hygiene Not ready for concentrated close work or small print because of slight farsightedness and still unrefined eye-hand coordination Play is associative; tries to follow rules but may cheat to avoid losing	Begins to question what parents think by comparing them with age-mates and other adults May notice prejudice and bias in outside world Is more able to view other's perspective but tolerates rather than understands differences May begin to show understanding of conservation of numbers through counting objects regardless of arrangement Uses time-oriented words with increased understanding Cautious about accepting or believing information	Gets along well with parents May seek out parent more often than at age 4 yr for reassurance and security, especially when entering school Begins to question parents' thinking and principles Strongly identifies with parent of same sex, especially boys with their fathers Enjoys activities such as sports, cooking, and shopping with parent of same sex

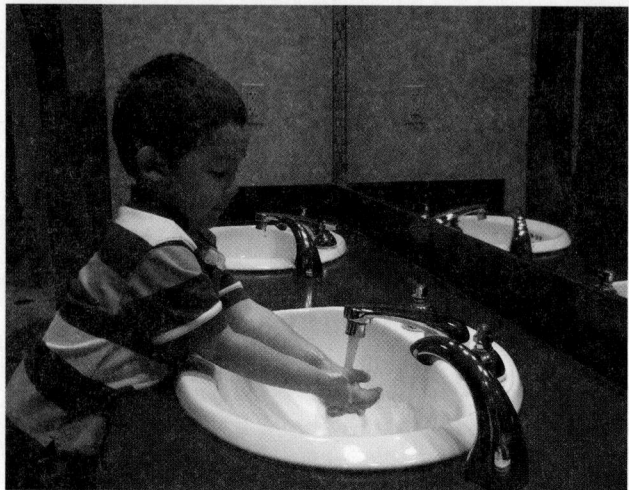

FIG 33-6 Thorough hand washing is the single most effective method of preventing infection.

Committee on Infectious Diseases, 2012). Parents should inquire about the policy of the center regarding the attendance and care of sick children.

The American Academy of Pediatrics' *2012 Red Book: Report of the Committee of Infectious Diseases* (2012) contains additional infection control guidelines regarding day care hand washing; cleaning sleep equipment, toys, and food; care of pets; and conditions or illnesses for which children should be kept out of day care to prevent the spread of illness.

Children need preparation for the preschool or kindergarten experience. For young children it represents a change from their usual home environment and prolonged separation from their parents. Before children begin school, parents should present the idea as exciting and pleasurable. Talking to children about activities such as painting, building with blocks, or enjoying swings and other outdoor equipment allows children to fantasize about the forthcoming event in a positive manner. When the first day of school arrives, parents should behave confidently. Such behavior requires them to have resolved their own feelings regarding the experience.

Parents should introduce their child to the teacher and the facility. In some instances it is helpful for parents to remain with the child for at least part of the first day until the child is comfortable and at ease. Other specific actions that can help reduce separation anxiety include providing the school with detailed information about the child's home environment such as familiar routines, favorite activities, food preferences, names of siblings or pets, and personal habits. Such information helps the child feel familiar in the strange surroundings. When schools automatically request this information, the parent has a valuable clue to evaluating the quality of the program because the request represents the staff's awareness of each child's needs. Transitional objects such as a favorite toy may also help the child bridge the gap from home to school.

Sex Education

Preschoolers have assimilated a tremendous amount of information during their short lifetimes. Although their thinking may not be mature, they search constantly for explanations and reasons that are logical and reasonable to them. The word "why" seems to supplant the word "no," which was common in toddlerhood. It is only natural that, as they learn about "me," they will also want to know "why me" and "how me." Questions such as, "Where do babies come from?"

are as casual as, "What makes it rain?" or "Who is that?" It is the *way* in which questions about procreation are answered that conditions children, even the youngest, to separate these questions from others about their world.

Two rules govern answering sensitive questions about topics such as sex. The first is to *find out what children know and think.* By investigating the theories that children have produced as a reasonable explanation, parents can give correct information and help them understand why their explanation is inaccurate. Another reason for ascertaining what the child thinks before offering any information is that the "unasked for" answer may be given. For example, 4-year-old Sally asked her father, "Where did I come from?" Both parents quickly took this inquiry as a clue for offering sex education. After the explanation Sally exclaimed, "I don't know about all that! All I know is that Mary came from New York, and I want to know where I was born."

The second rule for giving information is to *be honest.* It is true that the preschooler will forget or misunderstand much of the correct information, but the correct information can be restated until the child absorbs and comprehends the facts. Even though the correct anatomic words may be hard to pronounce or even more difficult to remember, they become foundational content for explaining other concepts at a later time.

Honesty does not imply imparting to children every fact of life or allowing excessive permissiveness in sexual curiosity. When children ask one question, they are looking for one answer. When they are ready, they will ask about the other "unfinished" parts of the story. Sooner or later they will wonder how the "sperm meets the egg" and "how the baby gets out," but during this period it is best to wait until they ask.

Regardless of whether or not children are given sex education, they will engage in games of sexual curiosity and exploration. At about 3 years of age children are aware of the anatomic differences between the sexes and concerned with how the other "works." This is not really "sexual" curiosity because many children are still unaware of the reproductive function of the genitalia. Their curiosity is for the eliminative function of the anatomy. Little boys wonder how girls can urinate without a penis, so they watch girls go to the bathroom. Because they cannot see anything but the stream of urine coming out, they want to observe further. "Doctor play" is often a game invented for just such investigation. Little girls are no less curious about boys' anatomy. It is intriguing to closely inspect this "thing" that girls do not have.

One question that parents often have is how to handle such sexual curiosity. A positive approach is to neither condone nor condemn it but to express that if children have questions, they should ask the parents; the parents should then encourage them to engage in some other activity. In this way children can be helped to understand that there are ways to satisfy their sexual curiosity other than through investigative games. This in no way condemns the act but stresses alternate methods to seek solutions and answers. Allowing children unrestricted permissiveness only intensifies their anxiety and concern, since exploring and searching usually yield little evidence to satisfy their curiosity.

Many excellent books on sex education are available for preschool children at public libraries. The Sexuality Information and Education Council of the United States (SIECUS)* and the AAP†

*SIECUS, 1706 R St., NW, Washington, DC 20009, 202-265-2405, fax: 202-462-2340, www.siecus.org.
†AAP, 141 Northwest Point Blvd, Elk Grove Village, IL 60007, 847-434-4000, fax: 847-434-8000, www.aap.org.

have bibliographies of suggested reading material. Parents should read the book themselves *before* giving or reading them to their children.

Another concern for some parents is *masturbation*, or self-stimulation of the genitalia. This occurs at any age for a variety of reasons and, if not excessive, is normal and healthy. It is most common at 4 years of age and during adolescence. For preschoolers it is a part of sexual curiosity and exploration. If parents are concerned about their children masturbating, it is essential for nurses to investigate the circumstances associated with the activity because it may be an expression of anxiety, boredom, or unresolved conflicts. Children who openly and publicly masturbate are inviting a reaction such as discipline, punishment, or criticism. They may be overwhelmed by their sexual feelings and are asking others to help channel them into more constructive outlets. Like other forms of sex play, masturbation is a private act, and parents should emphasize this to children when teaching them socially acceptable behavior.

Fears

A great number and variety of real and imagined fears are present during the preschool years, including fear of the dark, being left alone (especially at bedtime), animals (particularly large dogs), ghosts, sexual matters (castration), and objects or persons associated with pain. The exact cause of children's fears is often unknown. Parents often become perplexed about handling the fears because no amount of logical persuasion, coercion, or ridicule sends away the ghosts, boogeymen, monsters, and devils. Inappropriate television viewing by preschoolers may increase fears and anxieties because of the inability to separate reality-based experiences from fantasy portrayed on television.

The concept of animism (i.e., ascribing lifelike qualities to inanimate objects) helps explain why children fear objects. For example, a child may refuse to use the toilet after watching a television commercial in which the toilet bowl is portrayed as turning into a monster.

Preschoolers also experience fear of annihilation. Because of poorly defined body boundaries and improved cognitive abilities, young children develop concerns related to loss of body parts. They fear losing body parts with certain medical procedures such as an intravenous insertion or cast application on a limb and may see these procedures as real threats to their existence. Preschoolers are often fearful when approaching the health care environment (office or hospital) and are especially fearful of pain. Because of their inability to sometimes discern reality from the imagined, a painful procedure such as a vaccination may be perceived as the end of existence (death) *to* the child; the preschooler is often unable to see beyond that experience. It is helpful to discuss the child's fears but maintain honesty and openness when working with preschoolers in the health care setting.

The best way to help children overcome their fears is by actively involving them in finding practical methods to deal with the frightening experience. This may be as simple as keeping a night-light on in the child's bedroom for assurance that no monsters lurk in the dark. Exposing children to the feared object in a safe situation also provides a type of conditioning, or *desensitization*. For instance, children who are afraid of dogs should never be forced to approach or touch one, but they may be introduced gradually to the experience by watching other children play with the animal. This type of modeling, with others demonstrating fearlessness, can be effective if the child is allowed to progress at his or her own rate.

Usually by 5 or 6 years of age children relinquish many of their fears. Explaining the developmental sequence of fears and their gradual disappearance may help parents feel more secure in handling preschoolers' fears. Sometimes fears do not subside with simple measures or developmental maturation. When children experience severe fears that disrupt family life, professional help is required.

Stress

Although for parents the preschool years generally are less troublesome than toddlerhood, this period of life presents children with many unique stresses. Some such as fears are innate and stem from preschoolers' unique understanding of the world. Others such as beginning school are imposed. Although minimal amounts of stress are beneficial during the early years to help children develop effective coping skills, excessive stress is harmful. Young children are especially vulnerable because of their limited capacity to cope. Expression of frustration, fear, or anxiety is hampered by inadequate expressive language.

To help parents deal with stress in their child's life, they must be aware of its signs (see Stress in Childhood, Chapter 28) and be helped to identify the source. Any number of stressors may be present such as the birth of a sibling, marital discord, divorce and separation, relocation, or illness.

The best approach to dealing with stress is prevention (i.e., monitoring the amount of stress in children's lives so levels do not exceed their coping ability and informing them of anticipated changes on a short-term basis) and education. In many instances structuring children's schedules to allow rest and preparing them for change such as entering school are sufficient measures.

Aggression

The term *aggression* refers to behavior that attempts to hurt a person or destroy property. Aggression differs from anger, which is a temporary emotional state, but anger may be expressed through aggression. Hyperaggressive behavior in preschoolers is characterized by unprovoked physical attacks on other children and adults, destruction of others' property, frequent intense temper tantrums, extreme impulsivity, disrespect, and noncompliance. Aggression is influenced by a complex set of biologic, sociocultural, and familial variables. Factors that tend to increase aggressive behavior are gender, frustration, modeling, and reinforcement.

Evidence indicates that types of aggression differ between genders. Boys exhibit more physical aggression than girls during preschool years (Benzies, Keown, and Magill-Evans, 2009); however, preschool girls exhibit more relational aggression than preschool boys (Ostrov and Bishop, 2008). Frustration, or the continual thwarting of self-satisfaction by disapproval, humiliation, punishment, or insults, can lead children to act out against others as a means of release. Especially if they fear their parents, these children displace their anger on others, particularly peers and other authority figures. This type of aggression often applies to children who are well-behaved at home but have a discipline problem at school or are bullies among their playmates.

Modeling, or imitating the behavior of significant others, is a powerful influencing force in preschoolers. Children who see their parents as physically abusive are observing behavior that they come to know as acceptable and therefore may exhibit with others (Benzies, Keown, and Magill-Evans, 2009). Another aspect of modeling is the "double standard" for acceptable conduct. For example, in some families aggression is synonymous with masculinity, and boys are encouraged to defend themselves. Television is also a significant source for modeling at this impressionable age. Research indicates that there is a direct correlation between media exposure, both violent and educational media, and preschoolers exhibiting physical and relational aggression (Ostrov, Gentile, and Crick, 2006). Therefore parents should be encouraged to supervise television viewing. The AAP (2007) offers a list of recommendations for healthy television viewing.

Reinforcement can also shape aggressive behavior. Sometimes the reward for aggression is negative (e.g., punishment) yet reinforcing because it brings attention. For example, children who are ignored by a parent until they hit a sibling or the parent learn that this act garners attention.

When children exhibit extreme behaviors such as aggression, parents may be concerned about the need for professional help. Generally the difference between "normal" and "problematic" behavior is not the behavior itself but its quantity (number of occurrences), severity (interference with social or cognitive functioning), distribution (different manifestations), onset (when behavior started), and duration (at least 4 weeks).*

Speech Problems

The most critical period for speech development occurs between 2 and 4 years of age. During this period children are using their rapidly growing vocabulary faster than they can produce the words. Failure to master sensorimotor integrations results in stuttering or stammering as children try to say the word about which they are already thinking. This dysfluency in speech pattern is common during language development in children 2 to 5 years of age (National Institute on Deafness and Other Communication Disorders, 2010). Stuttering affects boys more frequently than girls, has been shown to have a genetic link, and usually resolves during childhood (Prasse and Kikano, 2008). The National Institute on Deafness and Other Communication Disorders (2010) encourages parents and caregivers of children who stutter to speak slowly and relaxed, refrain from criticizing the child's speech, resist completing the child's sentences, and take time to listen attentively.

The best therapy for speech problems is prevention and early detection. Common causes of speech problems include hearing loss or impairment, oropharyngeal structural anomalies, developmental disorders such as autism, brain injuries and other neuromotor impairments, lack of a verbally stimulating environment, and change in language exposure as in international adoption (Sharp and Hillenbrand, 2008). Referral for further evaluation and treatment may be necessary to prevent a problem from interfering with learning. Anticipatory preparation of parents for expected developmental norms may allay caregiver concerns.

Children pressured into producing sounds ahead of their developmental level may develop dyslalia (articulation problems) or revert to using infantile speech. Prevention involves educating parents regarding the usual achievement of speech production during childhood. The Denver Articulation Screening Exam is an excellent tool for assessing articulation skills of a child and explaining to parents the expected progression of sounds.

PROMOTING OPTIMAL HEALTH DURING THE PRESCHOOL YEARS

Nutrition

Healthy nutrition during childhood should include eating a variety of foods and consuming sufficient energy to promote growth and development while avoiding the development of obesity (AAP Committee on Nutrition, 2009). The 2010 Dietary Guidelines for Americans (U.S. Department of Agriculture, 2010) recommend an average intake of 1400 to 1600 calories per day for a moderately active child 4 to 8 years of age; these guidelines emphasize the reduction of sugar-sweetened beverages and excess intake of juices for young children and an overall increase in the amount of whole grains, vegetables, and fruits.* A daily intake of 16 oz/day of milk for preschoolers is recommended; this can be whole milk, 2%, or 1% milk. The Dietary Guidelines indicate that there is moderate evidence that consumption of milk and other dairy products does not contribute significantly to weight gain in young children. Fluid requirements may also decrease slightly to approximately 100 mL/kg/day but depend on the child's activity level, climatic conditions, and state of health. Protein requirements increase with age, and the recommended intake for preschoolers is 13 to 19 g/day (0.45 to 0.67 oz/day) (Otten, Hellwig, and Meyers, 2006).

The AAP Committee on Nutrition (2009) recommends the following guidelines for children older than 2 years of age: saturated fatty acid consumption should be less than 10% of total caloric intake; total fat over several days should be 20% to 30% of total caloric intake; and cholesterol consumption should be less than 300 mg/day. Fiber intake for children 3 years of age should be 19 mg/day and 25 mg/day for children 4 to 8 years of age (AAP, 2009). Research supports the efficacy of following these recommendations, and negative health effects have not been reported (American Heart Association, Gidding, Dennison, et al., 2006). These efforts are important in preventing childhood obesity, cardiovascular disease, diabetes, and metabolic syndrome. There is now sufficient evidence that the incidence of coronary heart disease, obesity, and chronic health problems such as diabetes mellitus can be influenced by early eating patterns (Barlow and Expert Committee, 2007). Evidence suggests that children who participate in family meal times in the home (three or more meals together) have a decreased risk for obesity and unhealthy eating patterns that may contribute to overweight and subsequent cardiovascular disease (Dattilo, Birch, Krebs, et al., 2012).

In addition to limiting fat consumption, it is also important to ensure that diets contain adequate nutrients such as calcium. The recommendation for daily calcium intake for children 1 to 3 years of age is 500 mg; for children 4 to 8 years of age is it 800 mg (Otten, Hellwig, and Meyers, 2006). Milk and dairy products are excellent sources of calcium and vitamin D (fortified). Low-fat milk may be substituted; thus the quantity of milk may remain the same while limiting fat intake overall.

Excessive consumption of fruit juices and other sweetened beverages has been associated with adverse health effects such as dental caries, gastrointestinal conditions such as chronic diarrhea, and diets poor in nutritive value (Allen and Myers, 2006). The AAP recommends limiting the intake of 100% fruit juice to 4 to 6 oz/day for children 1 to 6 years of age (AAP, 2009). Parents should be educated regarding nonnutritious fruit drinks, which usually contain less than 10% fruit juice yet are often advertised as healthy and nutritious; sugar content is dramatically increased and often precludes an adequate intake of milk by the child. When counseling parents regarding moderation in fruit juice consumption, providers should offer suggestions for more appropriate sources of nutrients such as ascorbic acid, folate, and potassium. In young children intake of

---

*Information on child development and behavior can be obtained through the AAP Section on Developmental and Behavioral Pediatrics, www.aap.org/sections/dbpeds.

---

*For a more comprehensive understanding, readers are urged to review Promoting Optimal Health During Toddlerhood, Chapter 32.

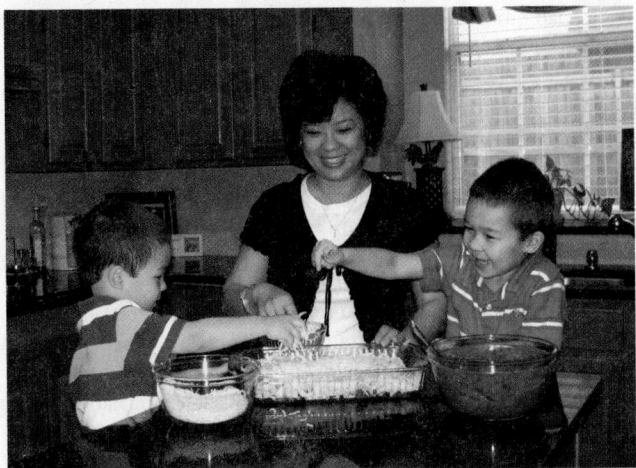

FIG 33-7 Preschool-age children enjoy helping adults and are more likely to try new foods if they can help in the preparation.

carbonated beverages that are acidic or contain high amounts of sugar is also known to contribute to dental caries; large amounts of nonnutritive calories in such beverages may also displace or preclude intake of nutrients necessary for growth.

An additional resource for dietary counseling includes MyPlate,* recently developed by the U.S. Department of Agriculture to replace MyPyramid. This colorful plate shows the five main food groups—fruits, grains, vegetable, protein, and dairy—with the intended purpose to involve children and their families in making appropriate food choices for meals and decrease the incidence of overweight and obesity in the United States. MyPlate provides an online interactive feature that allows the individual to select an individual food group and see choices for foods in that group. Approximate serving sizes are suggested, and vegetarian substitutions are also provided. This system is comprehensive and provides information for developing a healthy lifestyle at an early age. Parents can use this information to help their children make healthy lifestyle choices and prevent adverse health conditions secondary to poor nutrition. The importance of role-modeling by parents cannot be overemphasized in regard to food intake and dietary habits; if parents will not eat a particular food or if their dietary habits are poor, children are likely to develop the same habits.

Some preschoolers still have food habits that are typical of toddlers such as food fads and strong taste preferences. When they reach 4 years of age, they seem to enter another period of finicky eating, which is generally characteristic of the more rebellious behavior of children in this age-group. As with toddlers, small portions of each item being served should be offered. The practice of having children remain at the table until the "plate is clean" should be avoided because this may contribute to overeating and the development of poor eating habits that contribute to poor health later in life. By 5 years of age children are more agreeable to trying new foods, especially if they are encouraged by an adult who allows them to help with food preparation or experiment with a new taste or different dish (Fig. 33-7). Mealtimes can become battlegrounds if parents expect perfect table manners.† Usually 5-year-old children are ready

for the "social" side of eating, but 3- or 4-year-old children still have difficulty sitting quietly through long family meals.

The amount and variety of foods consumed by young children vary greatly from day to day. Consequently parents sometimes worry about the quantity and quality of food that preschoolers consume. In general the quality is much more important than the quantity, a fact that should be stressed during nutrition counseling. Eating habits are well established by 5 years of age, with the major contributing factor being the family, especially the parents.

> ### ! NURSING ALERT
>
> Obesity has increased over the past several decades in young children. Efforts to provide a healthy diet and encourage physical activity should begin early to help children achieve optimal health.

One way to lessen parental concern is to advise parents to keep a weekly record of everything the child eats. In particular the parents can measure the amount of food such as setting aside a half cup of vegetables and serving the child from this premeasured amount to provide a more accurate estimate of food intake at each meal. When parents look at the food chart at the end of the week, they are usually amazed by how much the child has consumed. In general preschoolers consume only slightly more than toddlers, or about half an adult's portion.

In addition to unhealthy eating habits, experts recognize that a sedentary lifestyle contributes to cardiovascular disease and obesity. Therefore the 2010 Dietary Guidelines also encourage 60 minutes of physical activity per day for children 6 years of age and older (U.S. Department of Agriculture, 2010). One program recommends that preschoolers be encouraged to be involved in at least 2 hours of cumulative activity per 8-hour day in day care, including unstructured free playtime (Larson, Ward, Neelon, et al., 2011).

Sleep and Activity

Sleep patterns vary widely, but the average preschooler sleeps about 12 hours a night and infrequently takes daytime naps. Waking during the night is common throughout early childhood and may be related to social and environmental factors rather than developmental or physiologic causes (Moore, Meltzer, and Mindell, 2008). Motor activity levels continue to be high and allow preschoolers to explore their environment, begin learning physical games and sports, and interact with others. Sedentary activities such as television and video or computer games are increasingly appealing and can become unhealthy substitutes for active play.

Preschoolers' increased gross motor abilities and coordination allow them to engage in many physical activities, if only at a novice level. Whether young children should begin formalized training in an activity at this early age is controversial. Training programs must consider the child's physical and psychologic immaturity, and readiness to participate in organized sports should be determined individually. The decision to participate should be based on the child's, not the parent's, motivation and enjoyment. The AAP Committee on Sports Medicine and Fitness and the AAP Committee on School Health (2006) encourages free play and a variety of physical activities; however, the AAP also supports organized play when it is developmentally appropriate and occurs in a nonthreatening, fun, and safe environment.

Sleep Problems

The preschool years are a prime time for sleep disturbances. Such disturbances are typically related to increasing autonomy, negative sleep associations, nighttime fears, inconsistent bedtime routines,

---

*http://www.choosemyplate.gov/.

†Excellent resources for parents related to mealtimes with toddlers and preschoolers include Jana LA, Shu J: *Food fights: winning the nutritional challenges of parenthood armed with insight, humor, and a bottle of ketchup,* Elk Grove Village, Ill, 2008, AAP; and Satter E: *How to get your kid to eat . . . but not too much,* Boulder, CO, 1987, Bull Publishing.

and lack of limit setting (Moore, Meltzer, and Mindell, 2008). Sleep disturbances may also be caused by nightmares and sleep terrors. Consequences of inadequate sleep include daytime tiredness, irritability and other negative behaviors, hyperactivity, difficulty concentrating, impaired learning ability, poor control of emotions and impulses, and strain on family relationships (Mindell, Kuhn, Lewin, et al., 2006).

Recommendations for handling sleep disturbances are offered only *after* a thorough assessment of the problem. Cultural traditions may dictate sleep practices that are contrary to certain well-accepted professional recommendations; therefore parents may not perceive a particular sleep practice to be a problem.

Interventions differ greatly; for example, nightmares (frightening dreams that are followed by full arousal) and sleep terrors (partial arousal from deep, nondreaming sleep) require different approaches (see Table 32-2).

For children who delay going to bed, a recommended approach involves counseling parents about the importance of a consistent bedtime ritual and emphasizing the normalcy of this type of behavior in young children. Parents should ignore attention-seeking behavior and not take the child into the parents' bed or allow him or her to stay up past a reasonable hour. Other measures that may be helpful include keeping a light on in the room, providing transitional objects such as a favorite toy, or leaving a drink of water by the bed. Parental consistency is paramount to all treatment approaches.

Helping children slow down *before* bedtime also reduces the resistance to going to bed. One strategy is to establish limited rituals that signal readiness for bed such as a bath or story. Parents can reinforce the pattern by stating, "After this story it's bedtime," and consistently carrying out the routine. If anticipated extra stimulation such as having visitors arrive at bedtime disrupts this routine, it is advisable to settle children in bed beforehand. Television viewing before bedtime may cause bedtime resistance and delay sleep.

Dental Health

By the beginning of the preschool period the eruption of the deciduous (primary) teeth is complete. Dental care is essential to preserve these temporary teeth and teach good dental habits (see Chapter 32). Although preschoolers' fine motor control is improved, they still require assistance and supervision with brushing, and flossing should be performed by parents. Professional care and prophylaxis, especially fluoride supplements (if needed), should be continued. The frequency of professional dental care should be based on a child's individual risk assessment, including family history, socioeconomic status, dental development, presence or absence of dental disease, special health care needs, and dietary habits (Kagihara, Niederhauser, and Stark, 2009). For children cared for away from home, parents should be encouraged to monitor the dental care provided by others, including minimizing cariogenic foods in the diet. Trauma to teeth during this period is common, and prompt evaluation by a dentist is warranted if oral trauma occurs. Preservation of the space previously occupied by an avulsed tooth is necessary for proper eruption of the secondary tooth.

Safety Promotion and Injury Prevention

Because of improved gross and fine motor skills, coordination, and balance, preschoolers are less prone to falls than toddlers. They tend to be less reckless; listen more to parental rules; and are aware of potential dangers such as hot objects, sharp instruments, and dangerous heights. Putting objects in the mouth as part of exploration has all but ceased, although accidental poisoning is still a danger.

Pedestrian motor vehicle injuries increase because of activities such as playing in the parking lot, driveway, or street; riding tricycles, bicycles, and other play vehicles; running after balls; or forgetting safety regulations when crossing streets.

In general the guidelines suggested for injury prevention in Table 32-4 apply to children in this age-group as well. However, emphasis is now on *education* concerning safety and potential hazards *in addition* to appropriate protection. This is an excellent time to start enforcing the use of safety items such as bicycle helmets to prevent head trauma; children are less likely to warm to the idea later in life because of peer pressure. Because preschoolers are great imitators, it is essential that parents set a good example by "practicing what they preach." Children quickly observe discrepancies in what they are told to do and what they see others do. Establishing habits at this time such as wearing protective equipment can create long-term safety behaviors.

Anticipatory Guidance—Care of Families

The preschool years present fewer childrearing difficulties than do earlier years, and this stage of development is facilitated by appropriate anticipatory guidance in the areas already discussed (see Family-Centered Care box). There is a shift in childrearing practices from protection to education, but protection is still often needed. Injury prevention previously focused on safeguarding the immediate environment with less emphasis on reasoning; now the protective guardrails or electrical outlet caps may be replaced by verbal explanations of why danger exists and how to avoid it.

During this period an emotional transition between parent and child occurs. Although children are still attached to their parents and accept all their values and beliefs, they are nearing the period of life when they will question previous teachings and prefer the companionship of peers. Entry into school marks a separation for parents and for children. Parents may need help in adjusting to this change, particularly if one parent has focused his or her daily activities primarily on home responsibilities. All family members must adjust to changes, which is part of the process of growth and development.

INFECTIOUS CONDITIONS: COMMUNICABLE DISEASES

The incidence of childhood communicable diseases has declined significantly since the advent of immunizations. Serious complications resulting from such infections have been reduced further with the use of antibiotics and antitoxins. However, infectious diseases do occur, and nurses must be familiar with the infectious agent to recognize the disease and institute appropriate preventive and supportive interventions (Table 33-2).

CARE MANAGEMENT

Table 33-2 describes the more common communicable diseases of childhood, their therapeutic management, and specific nursing care. The following is a general discussion of nursing care management for communicable diseases.

Identification of the infectious agent is of primary importance to prevent exposure of susceptible individuals. Nurses in ambulatory care settings, child care centers, and schools are often the first people to see signs of a communicable disease such as a rash or sore throat. The nurse must operate under a high index of suspicion for common childhood diseases to identify potentially infectious cases and recognize diseases that require medical intervention. An example is the

FAMILY-CENTERED CARE

Guidance During Preschool Years

Age 3 Years

- Prepare parents for child's increasing interest in widening relationships.
- Encourage enrollment in preschool.
- Emphasize importance of setting limits.
- Prepare parents to expect exaggerated tension-reduction behaviors such as need for a "security blanket."
- Encourage parents to offer child choices.
- Prepare parents to expect marked changes at 3½ years, when child becomes insecure and exhibits emotional extremes.
- Prepare parents for normal dysfluency in speech and advise them to avoid focusing on the pattern.
- Prepare parents to expect extra demands on their attention as a reflection of child's emotional insecurity and fear of loss of love.
- Warn parents that the equilibrium of a 3-year-old will change to the aggressive, out-of-bounds behavior of a 4-year-old.
- Inform parents to anticipate a more stable appetite with more food selections.
- Stress need for protection and education of child to prevent injury (see Safety Promotion and Injury Prevention, Chapter 32).

Age 4 Years

- Prepare parents for more aggressive behavior, including motor activity and offensive language.
- Prepare parents to expect resistance to parental authority.
- Explore parental feelings regarding child's behavior.
- Suggest some type of respite for primary caregivers such as placing child in preschool for part of the day.
- Prepare parents for child's increasing sexual curiosity.
- Emphasize importance of realistic limit setting on behavior and appropriate disciplinary techniques.
- Prepare parents for the highly imaginative 4-year-old who indulges in "tall tales" (to be differentiated from lies) and develops imaginary playmates.
- Prepare parents to expect nightmares or an increase in them.
- Help parents understand the nature of the child's fears and how to deal with them effectively and in a constructive manner.
- Provide reassurance that period of calmness begins at 5 years of age.

Age 5 Years

- Inform parents to expect tranquil period at 5 years of age.
- Help parents prepare children for entrance into school environment.
- Make certain that childhood immunizations are up to date before child enters school.
- Suggest that unemployed parental caregivers consider own activities when children begin school.

common complaint of sore throat. Although most often a symptom of a minor viral infection, it can signal an infection such as group A streptococcal pharyngitis. Each of these bacterial conditions requires appropriate medical treatment to prevent serious sequelae.

When a communicable disease is suspected, it is important to assess:

- Recent exposure to a known case.
- Prodromal symptoms (symptoms that occur between early manifestations of the disease and its overt clinical syndrome) or evidence of constitutional symptoms such as a fever or rash (see Table 33-2).

- Immunization history.
- History of having the disease.

Immunizations are available for many diseases, and infection usually confers lifelong immunity; therefore the possibility of many infectious agents can be eliminated based on these criteria.

Prevent Spread

Prevention consists of two components: prevention of the disease and control of its spread to others. Primary prevention rests almost exclusively on immunization. (Chapter 31 discusses the nurse's role in childhood immunization.)

Control measures to prevent spread of disease should include techniques to reduce risk of cross-transmission of infectious organisms between patients and protect health care workers from organisms harbored by patients. If a child is hospitalized, facility policies for infection control should be followed (see Chapter 39). The most important procedure is *hand washing*. People directly caring for children and handling contaminated articles must wash their hands and practice effective Standard Precautions in care of their patients.

Instruct children to practice good hand-washing technique before eating and after toileting. For diseases spread by droplets, instruct the parents in measures to reduce airborne transmission. Children who are old enough should use a tissue to cover their faces when coughing or sneezing; otherwise the parent should cover the child's mouth with a tissue and then discard it. Stress to the family the usual hygiene measures of not sharing eating and drinking utensils.

Prevent Complications

Although most children recover without difficulty, certain groups are at risk for serious, even fatal, complications from communicable diseases, especially the viral diseases chickenpox and erythema infectiosum (EI) (fifth disease) caused by human parvovirus B19.

Children with immunodeficiency (i.e., those receiving steroid or other immunosuppressive therapy, those with a generalized malignancy such as leukemia or lymphoma, and those with an immunologic disorder) are at risk for viremia from replication of the varicella-zoster virus (VZV)* in the blood. VZV is so named because it causes two distinct diseases: varicella (chickenpox) and zoster (herpes zoster or shingles). Varicella occurs primarily in children younger than 15 years of age. However, it leaves the threat of herpes zoster, an intensely painful varicella that is localized to a single dermatome (body area innervated by a particular segment of the spinal cord). In children the dermatomes most likely affected by herpes zoster are the cervical and sacral dermatomes (Leung, Robson, and Leong, 2006). Immunocompromised patients and healthy infants younger than 1 year of age (who also have reduced immunity) are at a higher risk for reactivation of VZV-causing herpes zoster, probably as a result of a deficiency in cellular immunity (AAP Committee on Infectious Diseases, 2012). One population-based study found that the incidence of herpes zoster infection in children was rare; rates were higher among children vaccinated after 5 years of age (versus those vaccinated at 12 to 18 months of age), children with severe asthma, or those with developmental disorders (Tseng, Smith, Marcy, et al., 2009). Complications of herpes zoster virus in children include secondary bacterial infection, depigmentation, and scarring. Postherpetic neuralgia in children is uncommon (Leung, Robson,

Text continued on p. 973

---

*Educational materials may be obtained from the National Shingles Foundation, 603 West 115th St, Suite 371, New York, NY 10025, 212-222-3390, www.vzvfoundation.org.

TABLE 33-2 COMMUNICABLE DISEASES OF CHILDHOOD

DISEASE	CLINICAL MANIFESTATIONS	THERAPEUTIC MANAGEMENT AND COMPLICATIONS	NURSING CARE MANAGEMENT
Chickenpox (Varicella) (Fig. 33-8) **Agents**—Varicella-zoster virus (VZV) **Source**—Primary secretions of respiratory tract of infected people; to a lesser degree skin lesions (scabs not infectious) **Transmission**—Direct contact, droplet (airborne) spread, and contaminated objects **Incubation period**—2-3 wk, usually 14-16 days **Period of communicability**—Probably 1-2 days before eruption of lesions (prodromal period) until all lesions have crusted	**Prodromal stage**—Slight fever, malaise, and anorexia for first 24 hr; rash highly pruritic; begins as macule, rapidly progresses to papule and then vesicle (surrounded by erythematous base, becomes umbilicated and cloudy, breaks easily and forms crusts); all three stages (papule, vesicle, crust) present in varying degrees at one time **Distribution**—Centripetal, spreading to face and proximal extremities but sparse on distal limbs and less on areas not exposed to heat (i.e., from clothing or sun) **Constitutional signs and symptoms**—Elevated temperature from lymphadenopathy, irritability from pruritus Breakthrough varicella seen in previously vaccinated; primarily maculopapular, with 50 lesions or fewer that often appear to be insect bites; heals faster than varicella and fever lasts fewer days; one-third less contagious to other people	**Supportive**—Diphenhydramine hydrochloride or antihistamines to relieve itching; skin care to prevent secondary bacterial infection **Specific**—Antiviral agent acyclovir or valacyclovir for children at high risk (see text); varicella-zoster immunoglobulin or immunoglobulin intravenous (IGIV) after exposure in high risk children only (see text) **Complications**—Secondary bacterial infections (group A streptococcus; abscesses, cellulitis, necrotizing fasciitis, pneumonia, sepsis) Encephalitis Varicella pneumonia (rare in healthy children) Hemorrhagic varicella (tiny hemorrhages in vesicles and numerous petechiae in skin) Chronic or transient thrombocytopenia	Maintain Standard, Airborne, and Contact Precautions if hospitalized until all lesions are crusted; for immunized child with mild breakthrough varicella, isolate until no new lesions are seen. Keep child in home away from susceptible individuals until vesicles have dried (usually 1 wk after onset of disease) and isolate high risk children from infected children. Provide skin care; give bath and change clothes and linens daily; administer topical calamine lotion; keep child's fingernails short and clean; apply mittens if child scratches. Goal is to prevent secondary infection and make child comfortable. Administer antipyretics and mild antihistamine for pruritus. Keep child cool (may decrease number of lesions). Minimize pruritus; keep child distracted; use oatmeal or baking soda baths to minimize pruritus. Remove loose crusts that rub and irritate skin. *Avoid use of aspirin* (possible association with Reye syndrome). Administer acetaminophen for fever.

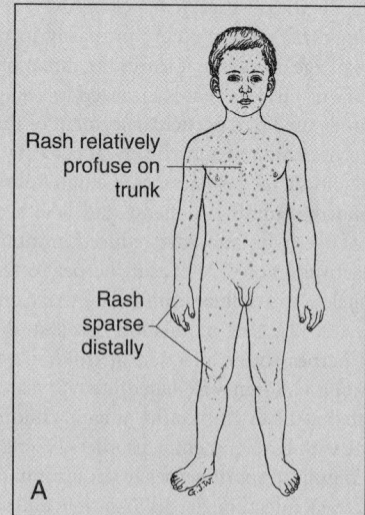
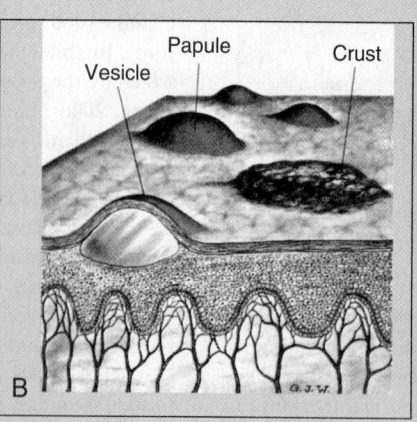
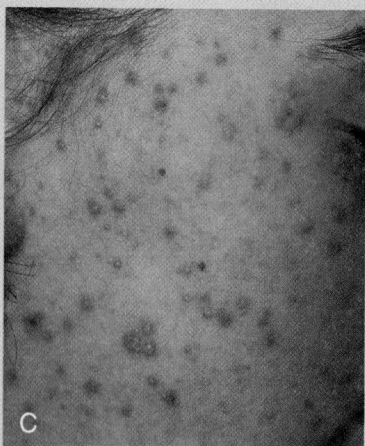

FIG 33-8 Chickenpox (varicella). **A,** Progression of disease. **B,** Simultaneous stages of lesions. **C,** Clinical view. (*C* From Habif TP: *Clinical dermatology: a color guide to diagnosis and therapy*, ed 5, St Louis, 2010, Mosby.)

TABLE 33-2	COMMUNICABLE DISEASES OF CHILDHOOD—cont'd		
DISEASE	**CLINICAL MANIFESTATIONS**	**THERAPEUTIC MANAGEMENT AND COMPLICATIONS**	**NURSING CARE MANAGEMENT**
Diphtheria **Agent**—*Corynebacterium diphtheriae* **Source**—Discharges from mucous membranes of nose and nasopharynx, skin, and other lesions of infected person **Transmission**—Direct contact with infected person, a carrier, or contaminated articles **Incubation period**—Usually 2-7 days, possibly longer **Period of communicability**—Varies; until virulent bacilli are no longer present (identified by three negative cultures); usually 2 wk but as long as 4 wk	Vary according to anatomic location of pseudomembrane **Nasal**—Resembles common cold, serosanguineous mucopurulent nasal discharge without constitutional symptoms; may be frank epistaxis **Tonsillar/pharyngeal**—Malaise; anorexia; sore throat; low-grade fever; pulse increased above expected within 24 hr; smooth, adherent, white or gray membrane; lymphadenitis possibly pronounced ("bull's neck"); in severe cases toxemia, septic shock, and death within 6-10 days **Laryngeal**—Fever, hoarseness, cough, with or without previous signs listed; potential airway obstruction, apprehensive, dyspneic retractions, cyanosis	Equine antitoxin (usually intravenously); preceded by skin or conjunctival test to rule out sensitivity to horse serum (antitoxin available only through CDC in United States) Antibiotics (penicillin G procaine, penicillin G, or erythromycin) in addition to equine antitoxin Tracheostomy for airway obstruction Treatment of infected contacts and carriers **Complications**—Toxic cardiomyopathy (second to third week) Toxic neuropathy	Follow Standard and Droplet Precautions until two cultures are negative for *C. diphtheriae*; Contact Precautions with cutaneous manifestations. Administer antibiotics in timely manner. Participate in sensitivity testing; have epinephrine available. Observe respiration for signs of obstruction.
Erythema Infectiosum (Fifth Disease) (Fig. 33-9) **Agent**—Human parvovirus B19 **Source**—Infected persons, mainly school-age children **Transmission**—Respiratory secretions, blood, blood products **Incubation period**—4-14 days; may be as long as 21 days **Period of communicability**—Uncertain but before onset of symptoms in children with aplastic crisis	Rash appearing in three stages: **I**—Erythema on face, chiefly on cheeks, "slapped face" appearance; circumoral pallor; disappears by 1-4 days **II**—About 1 day after rash appears on face maculopapular red spots appear, symmetrically distributed on upper and lower extremities; rash progresses from proximal (trunk) to distal surfaces and may last a week or more **III**—Rash subsiding but reappearing if skin is irritated or traumatized (sun, heat, cold, friction) In children with aplastic crisis rash usually absent; and prodromal illness includes fever, myalgia, lethargy, nausea, vomiting, and abdominal pain Possible concurrent vasoocclusive crisis in child with sickle cell disease	**Symptomatic and supportive**—Antipyretics, analgesics, antiinflammatory drugs Possible blood transfusion for transient aplastic anemia **Complications**—Self-limited arthritis and arthralgia (arthritis may become chronic); more common in adult women May result in serious complications (anemia, hydrops) or fetal death if mother infected during pregnancy (primarily second trimester) Aplastic crisis in children with hemolytic disease or immunodeficiency Myocarditis (rare)	Isolation of child is not necessary, except that hospitalized child (immunosuppressed or with aplastic crises) suspected of human parvovirus infection is placed on Droplet Precautions and Standard Precautions. Pregnant women need not be excluded from workplace where human parvovirus infection is present; they should not care for patients with aplastic crises; explain low risk of fetal death to those in contact with affected children; help with routine fetal ultrasound for detection of fetal hydrops. Neonate with intrauterine hydrops does not need to be isolated.

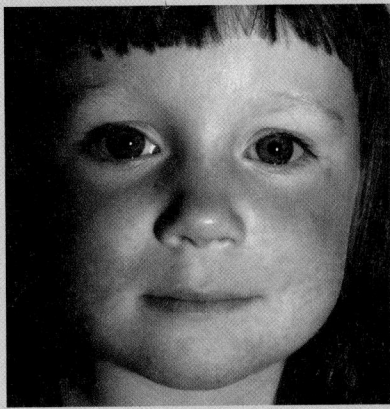

FIG 33-9 Erythema infectiosum. (From Habif TP: *Clinical dermatology: a color guide to diagnosis and therapy,* ed 5, St Louis, 2010, Mosby.)

Continued

TABLE 33-2   COMMUNICABLE DISEASES OF CHILDHOOD—cont'd

DISEASE	CLINICAL MANIFESTATIONS	THERAPEUTIC MANAGEMENT AND COMPLICATIONS	NURSING CARE MANAGEMENT
Exanthem Subitum (Roseola Infantum; Sixth Disease) (Fig. 33-10)			
Agent—Human herpesvirus type 6 (HHV-6; rarely HHV-7) **Source**—Possibly acquired from saliva of healthy adult; entry via nasal, buccal, or conjunctival mucosa **Transmission**—Year-round; no reported contact with infected individual in most cases (virtually limited to children under 3 yr, but peak age is between 6 and 15 mo of life) **Incubation period**—Usually 9-10 days for HHV-6; unknown for HHV-7 **Period of communicability**—Unknown	Persistent high fever for 3-4 days in child who appears well Precipitous drop in fever to normal with appearance of rash **Rash**—Discrete rose-pink macules or maculopapules appearing first on trunk, then spreading to neck, face, and extremities; nonpruritic, fades on pressure, lasts 1-2 days **Associated signs and symptoms**—Cervical/postauricular lymphadenopathy, inflamed pharynx, cough, coryza	Nonspecific Antipyretics to control fever **Complications**—Recurrent febrile seizures (possibly from latent infection of central nervous system that is reactivated by fever) Encephalitis, myocarditis, hepatitis, acute cerebellitis (all rare)	Teach parents measures for lowering temperature (antipyretic drugs); ensure adequate parental understanding of specific antipyretic dosage to prevent accidental overdose. If child is prone to febrile seizures, discuss appropriate precautions and possibility of recurrent febrile seizures. Ensure adequate oral fluid intake.

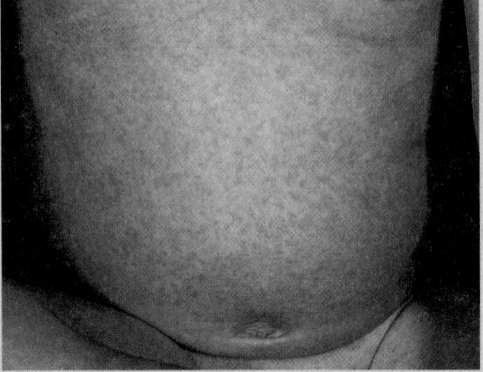

FIG 33-10 Roseola infantum. (From Habif TP: *Clinical dermatology: a color guide to diagnosis and therapy*, ed 5, St Louis, 2010, Mosby.)

DISEASE	CLINICAL MANIFESTATIONS	THERAPEUTIC MANAGEMENT AND COMPLICATIONS	NURSING CARE MANAGEMENT
Measles (Rubeola) (Fig. 33-11)			
Agent—Virus **Source**—Respiratory tract secretions, blood, and urine of infected person **Transmission**—Usually by direct contact with droplets of infected person; primarily in winter **Incubation period**—8-12 days **Period of communicability**—From 4 days before to 4 days after rash appears but mainly during prodromal (catarrhal) stage	**Prodromal (catarrhal) stage**—Fever and malaise, followed in 24 hr by coryza, cough, conjunctivitis, Koplik's spots (small, irregular red spots with a minute, bluish-white center first seen on buccal mucosa opposite molars 2 days before rash); symptoms gradually increasing in severity until second day after rash appears, when they begin to subside **Rash**—Appears 3-4 days after onset of prodromal stage; begins as erythematous maculopapular eruption on face and gradually spreads downward; more severe in earlier sites (appears confluent) and less intense in later sites (appears discrete); after 3-4 days assumes brownish appearance, and fine desquamation occurs over area of extensive involvement **Constitutional signs and symptoms**—Anorexia, abdominal pain, malaise, generalized lymphadenopathy	Vitamin A supplementation for children with acute illness (WHO recommendation): 200,000 IU for children 12 months and older, 100,000 IU for children 6 through 11 months of age, 50,000 IU for infants younger than 6 months (AAP Committee on Infectious Diseases, 2012) **Supportive**—Bed rest during febrile period; antipyretics Antibiotics to prevent secondary bacterial infection in high risk children **Complications**—Otitis media Pneumonia (bacterial) Obstructive laryngitis and laryngotracheitis Encephalitis (rare but has high mortality)	Isolate until fourth day of rash; if hospitalized, institute Droplet and Airborne Precautions. Encourage rest during prodromal stage; provide quiet activity. **Fever**—Instruct parents to administer antipyretics; avoid chilling; if child is prone to seizures, institute appropriate precautions. **Eye care**—Dim lights if photophobia present; clean eyelids with warm saline solution to remove secretions or crusts; keep child from rubbing eyes. **Coryza, cough**—Use cool-mist vaporizer; protect skin around nares with layer of petrolatum; encourage fluids and soft, bland foods. **Skin care**—Keep skin clean.

TABLE 33-2   **COMMUNICABLE DISEASES OF CHILDHOOD—cont'd**

DISEASE	CLINICAL MANIFESTATIONS	THERAPEUTIC MANAGEMENT AND COMPLICATIONS	NURSING CARE MANAGEMENT
Mumps **Agent**—Paramyxovirus **Source**—Saliva of infected persons **Transmission**—Direct contact with or droplet spread from an infected person **Incubation period**—16-18 days **Period of communicability**—Most communicable immediately before and after swelling begins	**Prodromal stage**—Fever, headache, malaise, and anorexia for 24 hr, followed by "earache" that is aggravated by chewing **Parotitis**—Parotid gland(s) (either unilateral or bilateral) enlarges and reaches maximum size in 1-3 days; accompanied by pain and tenderness; other exocrine glands (submandibular) possibly swollen	**Symptomatic and supportive**—Analgesics for pain and antipyretics for fever Intravenous fluid may be necessary for child refusing to drink or vomiting because of meningoencephalitis **Complications**—Sensorineural hearing loss (rare) Postinfectious encephalitis Myocarditis Arthritis Hepatitis Orchitis Oophoritis Pancreatitis Sterility is extremely rare in adult males Meningitis Thyroiditis (rare)	Isolate during period of communicability; institute Droplet and Contact Precautions during hospitalization. Encourage rest and decreased activity during prodromal phase until swelling subsides. Give analgesics for pain; if child is unable to swallow pills or tablets, use elixir form. Encourage fluids and soft, bland foods; avoid foods requiring chewing. Apply hot or cold compresses to neck or groin, whichever are more comforting.

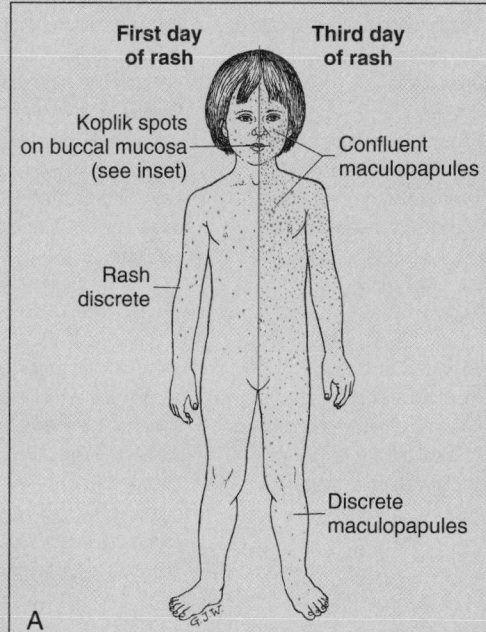

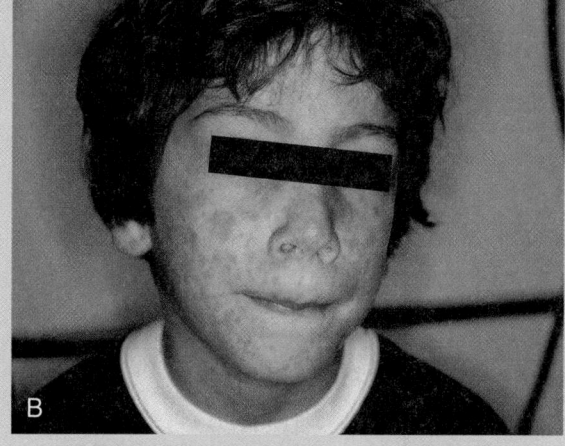

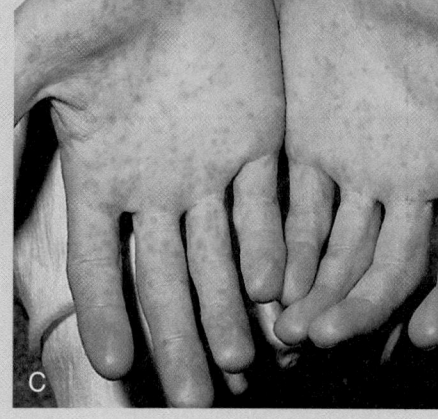

FIG 33-11 Measles (rubeola). **A,** Progression of disease. **B,** Exanthem first appears at hairline and spreads from head to toe over 3 days. **C,** Measles ultimately involves palms and soles. (*B* from Paller SA, Mancini AJ: *Hurwitz clinical pediatric dermatology,* ed 4, St Louis, 2011, Saunders; *C* from Habif TP: *Clinical dermatology: a color guide to diagnosis and therapy,* ed 5, St Louis, 2010, Mosby.)

Continued

TABLE 33-2	COMMUNICABLE DISEASES OF CHILDHOOD—cont'd		
DISEASE	**CLINICAL MANIFESTATIONS**	**THERAPEUTIC MANAGEMENT AND COMPLICATIONS**	**NURSING CARE MANAGEMENT**
Pertussis (Whooping Cough) **Agent**—*Bordetella pertussis* **Source**—Discharge from respiratory tract of infected person **Transmission**—Direct contact or droplet spread from infected person; indirect contact with freshly contaminated articles **Incubation period**—7-10 days, range 5-21 days **Period of communicability**—Greatest during catarrhal stage and the first 2 weeks after cough onset	**Catarrhal stage**—Begins with symptoms of upper respiratory tract infection (cold) such as coryza, sneezing, lacrimation, cough, and low-grade fever; symptoms continue for 1-2 wk when dry, hacking cough becomes more severe **Paroxysmal stage**—Cough most often occurs at night and consists of short, rapid coughs followed by sudden inspiration associated with a high-pitched crowing sound or "whoop"; during paroxysms cheeks become flushed or cyanotic, eyes bulge, and tongue protrudes; paroxysm may continue until thick mucus plug is dislodged; vomiting frequently follows attack; stage generally lasts 4-6 wk, followed by convalescent stage Infants under 6 mo of age may not have characteristic whoop cough but have difficulty maintaining adequate oxygenation with amount of secretions, frequent vomiting of mucus and formula or breast milk (see also Immunization, Chapter 31 for discussion of pertussis in adolescents)	Antimicrobial therapy (e.g., erythromycin, clarithromycin, azithromycin) **Supportive treatment**— Hospitalization sometimes required for infants, children who are dehydrated, or those who have difficulty maintaining adequate oxygenation Supplemental oxygen Adequate fluid intake Intensive care and mechanical ventilation may be necessary for infant <6 mo **Complications**—Pneumonia (usual cause of death) **Adolescents and adults**—complications include syncope, pneumonia, sleep disturbances, fractured ribs, incontinence; complications increase with age Atelectasis Otitis media Seizures Hemorrhage (scleral, conjunctival, epistaxis; pulmonary hemorrhage in neonate) Weight loss and dehydration Hernias (umbilical and inguinal) Prolapsed rectum	Isolate during catarrhal stage; if hospitalized, institute Droplet Precautions and Standard Precautions. Obtain nasopharyngeal culture for diagnosis. Encourage oral fluids; offer small amount of fluids frequently. Ensure adequate oxygenation during paroxysms; position infant on side to decrease chance of aspiration with vomiting. Provide high humidity (humidifier); suction as needed to prevent choking on secretions. Observe for signs of airway obstruction (infants), such as increased restlessness, apprehension, retractions, cyanosis. Encourage compliance with antibiotic therapy for household contacts. Encourage adolescents to obtain pertussis booster (Tdap) (see also Chapter 31, Immunizations). Use Standard Precautions and Droplet Precautions in health care workers exposed to children with persistent cough and high suspicion of pertussis.
Polioviruses **Agent**—Enteroviruses, three types: type 1, most frequent cause of paralysis (paralytic form), both epidemic and endemic; type 2, least frequently associated with paralysis (nonparalytic form); type 3, second most frequently associated with paralysis **Source**—Feces, urine, CNS, and oropharyngeal secretions of infected persons, especially young children	May be manifested in three different forms: **Abortive or inapparent**—Fever, uneasiness, sore throat, headache, anorexia, vomiting, abdominal pain; lasts few hours to few days **Nonparalytic**—Same manifestations as abortive but more severe, with pain and stiffness in neck, back, and legs	Treatment supportive Mechanical or assisted ventilation in case of respiratory paralysis Physical therapy for muscles following acute stage of nonparalytic form	Nursing care for paralytic form similar to child with muscular dystrophy, spinal muscular atrophy, and prolonged immobilization (see Chapter 49). Participate in physical therapy procedures (use of moist hot packs and range-of-motion exercises).

Continued

TABLE 33-2   COMMUNICABLE DISEASES OF CHILDHOOD—cont'd

DISEASE	CLINICAL MANIFESTATIONS	THERAPEUTIC MANAGEMENT AND COMPLICATIONS	NURSING CARE MANAGEMENT
Transmission—Direct contact with persons with apparent or inapparent active infection; spread is via fecal-oral and pharyngeal-oropharyngeal routes Vaccine-acquired paralytic polio may occur as result of live oral polio vaccination (no longer available in the United States) **Incubation period**—nonparalytic form, 6-7 days; paralytic form, usually 7-21 days **Period of communicability**—Not exactly known; virus present in throat and feces shortly after infection and persists for about 1 wk in throat and 4-6 wk in feces **1993**—Last known imported polio case in United States; child was transported to the United States for medical care **1979**—Last cases of indigenously acquired polio in the United States	**Paralytic**—Initial course similar to nonparalytic type, followed by recovery and then signs of central nervous system paralysis	**Complications**—Permanent paralysis Respiratory arrest Kidney stones from demineralization of bone during prolonged immobility	Position child to maintain body alignment and prevent contractures or skin breakdown; use footboard or appropriate orthoses to prevent footdrop; use pressure mattress for prolonged immobility. Encourage child to perform activities of daily living to capability, early ambulation with adjuncts; administer analgesics for maximum comfort during physical activity. Provide high-protein diet and bowel management for prolonged immobility. Observe for respiratory paralysis (difficulty in talking, ineffective cough, inability to hold breath, shallow and rapid respirations); report such signs and symptoms to practitioner.
Rubella (German Measles) (Fig. 33-12) **Agent**—Rubella virus **Source**—Primarily nasopharyngeal secretions of person with apparent or inapparent infection; virus also present in blood, stool, and urine **Incubation period**—14-21 days **Period of communicability**—2-3 days before to about 7 days after appearance of rash Congenital rubella syndrome–may result in mild-to-severe ophthalmologic, cardiac, auditory, and neurologic complications; chance of congenital defects highest (50% to 85%) if mother acquires illness (rubella) in first two trimesters of pregnancy	**Constitutional signs and symptoms**—Occasionally low-grade fever, headache, malaise, and lymphadenopathy **Prodromal stage**—Absent in children, present in adults and adolescents; consists of low-grade fever, headache, malaise, anorexia, mild conjunctivitis, coryza, sore throat, cough, and lymphadenopathy; lasts 1-5 days, subsides 1 day after appearance of rash **Rash**—First appears on face and rapidly spreads downward to neck, arms, trunk, and legs; by end of first day body is covered with discrete, pinkish-red, maculopapular exanthema; disappears in same order as it began and is usually gone by third day	No treatment necessary other than antipyretics for low-grade fever and analgesics for discomfort **Complications**—Rare (arthritis, encephalitis, or purpura); most benign of all childhood communicable diseases; greatest danger is teratogenic effect on fetus; miscarriage and fetal death may occur	Reassure parents of benign nature of illness in affected child. Use comfort measures as necessary. Avoid contact with pregnant woman. Monitor rubella titers in pregnant adolescent. Standard Precautions for hospitalized child; Droplet Precautions for 7 days after onset of rash. Contact isolation for infant with suspected or confirmed congenital rubella or until two cultures are negative for rubella.

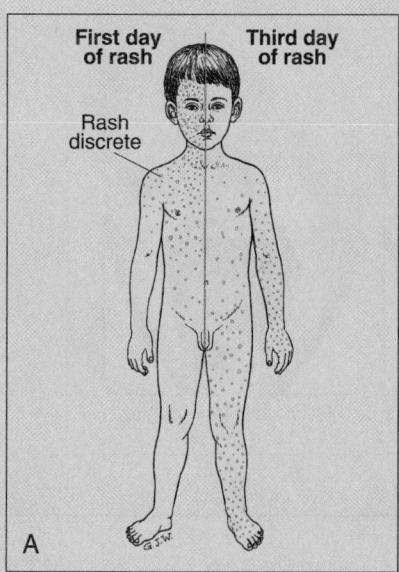

First day of rash   Third day of rash

Rash discrete

A

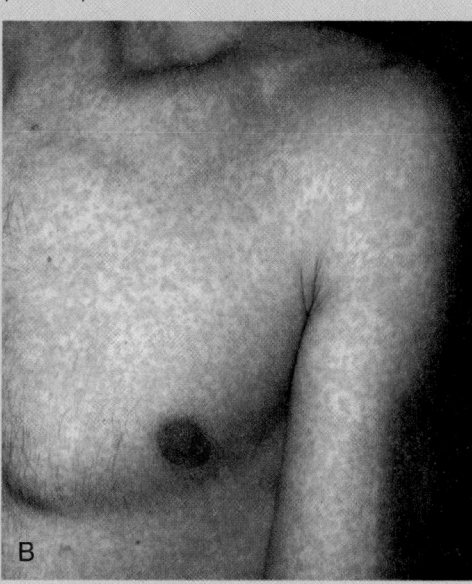

B

FIG 33-12 Rubella (German measles). **A,** Progression of rash. **B,** Clinical view. (*B* from Habif TP: *Clinical dermatology: a color guide to diagnosis and therapy,* ed 5, St Louis, 2010, Mosby.)

Continued

TABLE 33-2   COMMUNICABLE DISEASES OF CHILDHOOD—cont'd

DISEASE	CLINICAL MANIFESTATIONS	THERAPEUTIC MANAGEMENT AND COMPLICATIONS	NURSING CARE MANAGEMENT
Scarlet Fever* (Fig. 33-13) **Agent**—Group A β-hemolytic streptococci (GAS) **Source**—Usually from nasopharyngeal secretions of infected persons and carriers **Transmission**—Direct contact with infected person or droplet spread; indirectly by contact with contaminated articles or ingestion of contaminated milk or other food **Incubation period**—2-5 days, with range of 1-7 days **Period of communicability**—During incubation period and clinical illness, approximately 10 days; during first 2 wk of carrier phase, although may persist for months Severe cases now rare	**Prodromal stage**—Abrupt high fever, pulse increased out of proportion to fever, vomiting, headache, chills, malaise, abdominal pain, halitosis **Enanthema**—Tonsils enlarged, edematous, reddened, and covered with patches of exudates; in severe cases appearance resembles membrane seen in diphtheria; pharynx edematous and beefy red; during first 1-2 days tongue coated and papillae become red and swollen (white strawberry tongue); by fourth or fifth day white coat sloughs off, leaving prominent papillae (red strawberry tongue); palate covered with erythematous punctate lesions **Exanthema**—Rash appears within 12 hr after prodromal signs; red pinhead-size punctate lesions rapidly become generalized but are absent on face, which becomes flushed with striking circumoral pallor; rash more intense in folds of joints; by end of first week desquamation begins (fine, sandpaper-like on torso; sheetlike sloughing on palms and soles), which may be complete by 3 wk or longer	**Treatment of choice**—Full course of penicillin (or erythromycin in penicillin-sensitive children), or oral cephalosporin **Supportive measures**—Rest during febrile phase, analgesics for sore throat; antipruritics for rash if bothersome **Complications**—Peritonsillar and retropharyngeal abscess Sinusitis Otitis media Acute glomerulonephritis Acute rheumatic fever Polyarthritis (uncommon) Toxic shock syndrome Osteomyelitis	Institute Standard and Droplet Precautions until 24 hr after initiation of treatment. Ensure compliance with oral antibiotic therapy; intramuscular benzathine penicillin G [Bicillin] may be given if parents' reliability in giving oral drugs is questionable. Encourage rest during febrile phase; provide quiet activity during convalescent period. Relieve discomfort of sore throat with analgesics, gargles, lozenges, and antiseptic throat sprays. Encourage oral fluids during febrile phase; avoid irritating liquids (certain citrus juices) or rough foods (chips); when child is able to eat, begin with soft diet. Advise parents to consult practitioner if fever persists after beginning therapy. Discuss procedures for preventing spread of infection; discard toothbrush; avoid sharing drinking and eating utensils. Monitor for sequelae of GAS-acute rheumatic fever and acute glomerulonephritis.

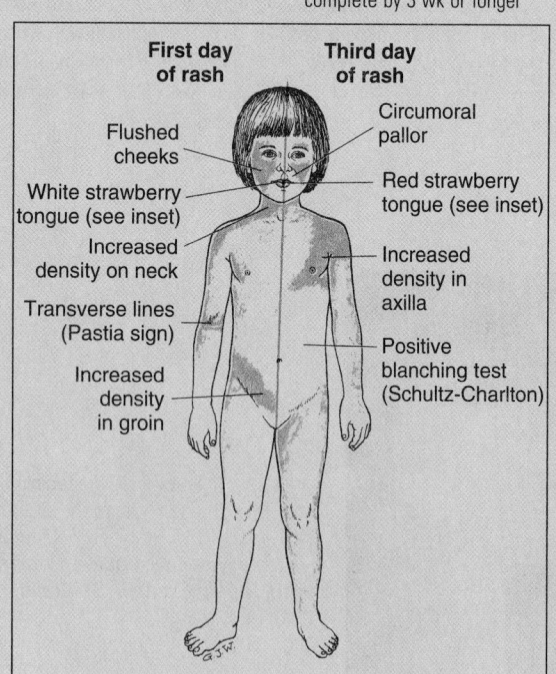

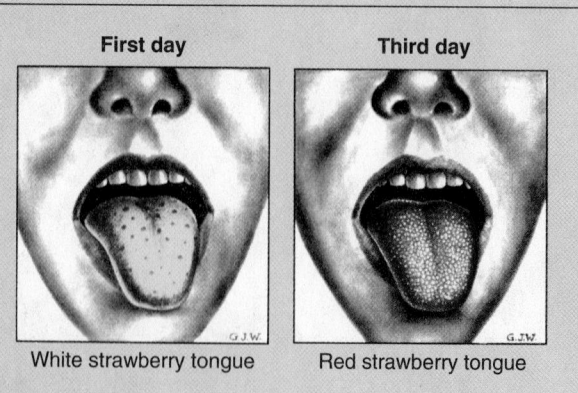

White strawberry tongue   Red strawberry tongue

FIG 33-13 Scarlet fever.

*Commonly called *streptococcal pharyngitis;* with the exception of the characteristic rash, scarlet fever and streptococcal pharyngitis have the same epidemiology, features, symptoms, signs, sequelae, and treatment (AAP Committee on Infectious Diseases, 2012). Also note that GAS is a common cause of many infections in children, including impetigo, cellulitis, and necrotizing fasciitis.

and Leong, 2006). Fetal infection after maternal varicella, especially if infection occurs before the 20th week of gestation, may be fatal or result in congenital varicella syndrome. Varicella infection occurring in infants exposed to maternal varicella from a period 5 days before birth to 2 days after birth have an increased likelihood of becoming infected and should be treated with varicella-zoster immunoglobulin intravenous (IGIV) (AAP Committee on Infectious Diseases, 2012).

The use of varicella-zoster IGIV is recommended for children who are immunocompromised, who have no previous history of varicella, and who are likely to contract the disease and have complications as a result (AAP Committee on Infectious Diseases, 2012). The antiviral agents acyclovir or valacyclovir may be used to treat varicella infections in susceptible immunocompromised persons. It is effective in decreasing the number of lesions; shortening the duration of fever; and decreasing itching, lethargy, and anorexia.

Children with hemolytic disease such as sickle cell disease are at risk for aplastic anemia from EI. Human parvovirus B19 infects and lyses red blood cell (RBC) precursors, thus interrupting the production of RBCs. Therefore the virus may precipitate a severe aplastic crisis in patients who need increased RBC production to maintain normal RBC volumes. Thrombocytopenia and neutropenia may also occur as a result of human parvovirus B19 infection. Fetuses have a relatively high rate of RBC production and immature immune systems; they may develop severe anemia and hydrops as a result of maternal human parvovirus infection. Fetal death rates as a result of human parvovirus B19 have been estimated to be between 2% and 6% (AAP Committee on Infectious Diseases, 2012).

In the past decade the incidence of pertussis has increased, particularly in infants younger than 6 months old and children 10 to 14 years of age. Early clinical manifestations of pertussis in infants may include gagging, coughing, emesis, and apnea; the typical "whoop" associated with the disease is absent (Teng and Wang, 2011; Wood and McIntyre, 2008). In older children the disease may manifest as a common cold (see Table 33-2). It is now recommended that children 11 to 18 years old receive a booster pertussis vaccine (tetanus and acellular pertussis [Tdap]) to prevent the disease (see Immunizations, Chapter 31). Because pertussis is contagious, especially among close household members, identify it early and initiate treatment for the child and those who have been exposed. Azithromycin (for infants younger than 1 month old) and clarithromycin or azithromycin should be administered to infants and children with pertussis. Although the risk of contracting hypertrophic pyloric stenosis is increased in infants younger than 1 month old taking azithromycin, it remains the drug of choice for the treatment of pertussis in this age-group (AAP Committee on Infectious Diseases, 2012).

Prevention of complications from diseases such as diphtheria, pertussis, and scarlet fever requires compliance with antibiotic therapy. With oral preparations stress the need to complete the entire course of therapy.

Evidence suggests that vitamin A supplementation reduces both morbidity and mortality in measles and that all children with severe measles should receive vitamin A supplements. A single oral or parenteral dose of 200,000 IU for children at least 1 year old is recommended (use half that dose for children 6 to 12 months of age). The higher dose may be associated with vomiting and headache for a few hours. The dose should be repeated the next day and at 4 weeks for children with ophthalmologic evidence of vitamin A deficiency (AAP Committee on Infectious Diseases, 2012) (see also Table 33-2).

> **! NURSING ALERT**
>
> Although the risk of vitamin A toxicity from these doses (they are 100 to 200 times the recommended dietary allowance) is relatively low, nurses should instruct parents on safe storage of the drug. Ideally, vitamin A should be dispensed in the age-appropriate unit dose to prevent excessive administration and possible toxicity.

Provide Comfort

Many communicable diseases cause skin manifestations that are bothersome to children. The chief discomfort from most rashes is itching, and measures such as cool baths (usually without soap) and lotions (e.g., calamine) are helpful.

> **! NURSING ALERT**
>
> When lotions with active ingredients such as diphenhydramine in Caladryl are used, they should be applied sparingly, especially over open lesions, where excessive absorption can lead to drug toxicity. These lotions should be used with caution in children who are simultaneously receiving an oral antihistamine. Cooling the lotion in the refrigerator beforehand often makes it more soothing on the skin than at room temperature.

To avoid overheating, which increases itching, children should wear lightweight, loose, nonirritating clothing and keep out of the sun. If the child persists in scratching, keep the nails short and smooth or use mittens and clothes with long sleeves or legs. For severe itching antipruritic medication such as diphenhydramine (Benadryl) or hydroxyzine (Atarax) may be required, especially when the child has trouble sleeping because of itching. Loratadine, cetirizine, and fexofenadine do not cause drowsiness and may be preferred for urticaria during the day.

An elevated temperature is common, and both antipyretic medicine (acetaminophen or ibuprofen) and environmental manipulation are implemented (see Controlling Elevated Temperatures, Chapter 39). Acetaminophen is effective in lowering the fever but does not significantly reduce the symptoms of itching, anorexia, abdominal pain, fussiness, or vomiting.

A sore throat, another frequent symptom, is managed with lozenges, saline rinses (if the child is old enough to cooperate), and analgesics. Because most children are anorectic during an illness, bland foods and increased liquids are usually preferred. During the early stages of the disease children voluntarily curtail their activity; and, although bed rest is beneficial, it should not be imposed unless specifically indicated. During periods of irritability quiet activity (e.g., reading, music, television, video games, puzzles, coloring) helps distract children from the discomfort.

Support Child and Family

Most communicable diseases are benign, but they may produce considerable concern and anxiety for parents. Often the occurrence of a disease such as chickenpox is the first time the child is acutely uncomfortable. Parents need assistance to cope with manifestations of the illness such as intense itching. The family and child need reassurance that generally recovery is rapid. However, visible signs of the dermatosis may be present for some time after the child is well enough to resume usual activities.

CHILD MALTREATMENT

The broad term *child maltreatment* includes intentional physical abuse or neglect; emotional abuse or neglect; and sexual abuse of children, usually by adults. It is one of the most significant social problems affecting children. In 2010 child protective service (CPS) agencies in the United States confirmed that an estimated 794,000 children were victims of child maltreatment. Of the confirmed cases approximately 17.6% suffered physical abuse, 9.2 % sexual abuse, 2.4% medical neglect, and 8.1 % psychologic maltreatment or emotional abuse. In 2010 there were an estimated 1560 child fatalities as a result of child abuse and neglect (U.S. Department of Health and Human Services, 2012). Children under 1 year of age had the highest rate of victimization (20.6 per 1000 children in the population of the same age), whereas children 1 to 3 years of age had rates of 11.9, 11.4, and 11.0 per 1000 children, respectively (U.S. Department of Health and Human Services, 2012). However, reported statistics only partially represent the actual incidence of child maltreatment because many cases are believed to be unreported.*

Child Neglect

Child neglect is the most common form of maltreatment. More than half of all reported cases are associated with deprivation of necessities, and 34% of deaths from maltreatment are in this group (U.S. Department of Health and Human Services, 2012). Neglect is generally defined as the failure of a parent or other person legally responsible for the child's welfare to provide for her or his basic needs and an adequate level of care.

Important contributing factors for child neglect are lack of knowledge of the child's needs, lack of resources, and caregiver substance abuse. For example, neglectful parents often demonstrate poor parenting skills. They may be unaware that an infant needs to be fed every 3 to 4 hours, may not know what to feed the child, and may have insufficient funds to buy food. The most serious lack of knowledge is failure to recognize emotional nurturing as an essential need of children (see also Failure to Thrive, Chapter 31).

Types of Neglect

Neglect takes many forms and can be classified broadly as physical or emotional maltreatment. Physical neglect involves the deprivation of necessities such as food, clothing, shelter, supervision, medical care, and education. Emotional neglect generally refers to failure to meet the child's needs for affection, attention, and emotional nurturance.

Neglect may also include lack of intervention for or fostering of maladaptive behavior such as delinquency or substance abuse. Emotional abuse or psychologic maltreatment, an even more difficult aspect of maltreatment to define, refers to the deliberate attempt to destroy or significantly impair a child's self-esteem or competence. Emotional abuse may take the form of rejecting, isolating, terrorizing, ignoring, corrupting, verbally assaulting, or overpressuring the child.

Physical Abuse

The deliberate infliction of physical injury on a child, usually by the child's caregiver, is termed *physical abuse.* Nonaccidental trauma is the term used to describe the injury resulting from the abuse. Legal definitions of physical abuse are found in state and federal statutes. The Child Abuse Prevention and Treatment Act of 1996 defines abuse as "any recent act or failure to act that results in imminent risk of serious harm, death, serious physical or emotional harm of a child (<18 years) by a parent or caregiver who is responsible for

the child's welfare." Each state defines abuse according to its reporting laws. Minor physical injury is responsible for more reported cases of maltreatment than major physical injury, but major physical abuse causes more deaths. Despite the importance of the problem, a universally accepted definition of what constitutes minor and major physical abuse does not exist. Rather each state in the United States defines abuse according to its individual reporting laws.

Shaken Baby Syndrome/Traumatic Brain Injury

Shaken baby syndrome (SBS) is a serious form of child abuse caused by violent shaking of infants and is one form of abusive head trauma. Physicians commonly use more general terms, including *abusive head trauma, nonaccidental head injury, traumatic brain injury (TBI),* or *neuroinflicted brain injury;* these terms do not assume the mechanism of injury but rather describe the injury itself (AAP Committee on Child Abuse and Neglect, 2009; Chiesa and Duhaime, 2009; Squier, 2011). This violent shaking would be easily recognized by others as dangerous (AAP Committee on Child Abuse and Neglect, 2009) and is most often a result of the caregiver's frustration with crying. Every year in the United States an estimated 1200 to 1400 children are shaken, and 25% to 30% of these victims die as a result of their injuries. The rest have lifelong complications (Barr, 2012; Keenan, Runyan, Marshall, et al., 2004; National Center on Shaken Baby Syndrome, n.d.).* The peak incidence of SBS/TBI is in the third month of life; the majority of victims are male, and the perpetrators are most often related males in the victim's household (Barr, 2012).

It is important to understand what happens in SBS. Infants have a large head-to-body ratio, weak neck muscles, and a large amount of water in the brain. Violent shaking causes the brain to rotate within the skull, resulting in shearing forces that tear blood vessels and neurons. The characteristic injuries that occur are intracranial bleeding (subdural hematoma) and in approximately 85% of cases retinal hemorrhages, which are classic results of repetitive acceleration-deceleration head trauma (Levin, 2009). Injuries may also include fractures of the ribs and long bones; however, most often there are no signs of external injury. SBS is often not an isolated event. Victims can be seen with a variety of symptoms, from generalized flulike symptoms to unresponsiveness with impending death (Mraz, 2009). Many of the presenting symptoms such as vomiting, irritability, poor feeding, and listlessness are often mistaken for common infant and childhood ailments. In more severe forms presenting symptoms may include seizures, posturing, alterations in level of consciousness, apnea, bradycardia, or death. The long-term outcomes of SBS include seizure disorders; visual impairments, including blindness; developmental delays; hearing loss; cerebral palsy; and mild-to-profound mental, cognitive, or motor impairments (Walls, 2006). Nurses can take an active role in preventing SBS by teaching all caregivers about crying and techniques to cope with inconsolable crying (Altman, Canter, Patrick, et al., 2011; Carbaugh, 2004). Two studies report significant reductions in the incidence of SBS when programs aimed at educating parents about the nature of the infant's crying and associated infant behavior and preventing shaking as a form of dealing with the infant's crying behavior are presented to mothers and families in the immediate postpartum period (Barr, 2012). Barr (2012) notes that preventive programs are effective in the prevention of SBS. Nurses in the mother-baby unit should talk with parents about infant behavior, including crying and sleep patterns. Other caregivers should also be educated regarding infant crying behavior and consoling methods

---

*Additional information is available from the Children's Bureau, Administration for Children and Families, 370 L'Enfant Promenade SW, Washington, DC 20447, 800-422-4453, www.acf.hhs.gov.

---

*National Center on Shaken Baby Syndrome: www.dontshake.com.

aimed at preventing violent shaking (Barr, 2012). An educational tool for parents is the Period of PURPLE Crying* program, which presents material for parents about infant crying and resources to cope with infant crying.

> ## ! NURSING ALERT
>
> Nurses should emphasize to parents and caregivers the danger of shaking infants. Education must include coping mechanisms for caring for infants with inconsolable crying.

CARE MANAGEMENT

Nursing care of the infant with SBS/TBI should immediately focus on recognizing the condition and attention given to the ABCs (airway, breathing, circulation), spinal cord immobilization, and prevention of hypoxemia by monitoring oxygen saturation. Because some infants demonstrate no outward signs and symptoms in the acute phase, the nurse should be alert for subtle signs such as alternating levels of consciousness, poor feeding, and decreased activity level. If SBS is suspected, the infant may be sent for a CT scan for diagnostic purposes. Additional nursing care should focus on preventing hypotension (monitor perfusion and BP), and fluids may be needed to maintain adequate vascular volume. ICP is monitored, and increased intracranial pressure (target of 15 mm Hg in infant; 18 mm Hg in child, and 20 mm Hg in adolescent) is prevented by avoiding suctioning unless absolutely necessary. Mannitol or 3% normal Saline IV is administered, the head of the bed is elevated 30 degrees, and sedative medication or neuromuscular blockade is given as warranted. Hypoglycemia should be avoided to maintain adequate brain function.

Depending on the infant's status, short-term and long-term care often includes administering enteral feedings if the child is unable to feed and H2 blockers to prevent stress ulcers and monitoring for signs of cerebral edema and seizure activity (see also Chapter 45, Head Injury). The care of the mother and other family members should not be forgotten. Often there is much blaming and increased emotional tension; law enforcement will likely be involved in an investigation, and this engenders additional family stress. The nurse supports the family by adopting a nonjudgmental attitude and focusing on the immediate medical needs of the child. A multidisciplinary team of health care workers may assist in caring for the needs of the family and in protecting the child and family from further physical and emotional harm.

Munchausen Syndrome by Proxy

Munchausen syndrome by proxy (MSBP), also known as *medical child abuse* or *factitious disorder by proxy,* is a rare but serious form of child abuse in which caregivers deliberately exaggerate or fabricate histories and symptoms or induce symptoms. It is a form of child maltreatment that may include physical, emotional, and psychologic abuse for the gratification of the caregiver. In most cases the perpetrator is the biologic mother with some degree of health care knowledge and training. Health care providers can become easily misled and unknowingly enable the perpetrator (Leider, Irving, Mauricio, et al., 2005). Because of the history of symptoms provided by the caregiver, the child endures painful and unnecessary medical testing and procedures. Common symptoms presented are seizures, nausea and vomiting, diarrhea, and altered mental status; they are usually witnessed only by the perpetrator.

Considerations when determining whether a child is a victim of MSBP include:

- Is the child's condition consistent with the reported history?
- Does diagnostic evidence support the reported history?
- Has anyone other than the caregiver witnessed the symptoms?
- Is treatment being provided primarily because of the caregiver's demands?

The resolution of symptoms after separation from the perpetrator confirms the diagnosis.

Factors Predisposing to Physical Abuse

The causes of child abuse are multifaceted. Child maltreatment occurs across all socioeconomic, religious, cultural, racial, and ethnic groups (Goldman, Salus, Wolcott, et al., 2003). Three risk factors are commonly identified in child abuse: parental characteristics, characteristics of the child, and environmental characteristics. However, no single factor or group of factors is predictive of abuse. Rather the interaction of these factors is thought to increase the risk of abuse occurring in a particular family.

Parental Characteristics. Some identified characteristics occur more frequently in parents who abuse their children and therefore are considered risk factors. Younger parents more often abuse their children. Single-parent families are at higher risk for abuse; in single-parent families that include an unrelated partner, the partner is sometimes the abuser, although a biologic parent is most commonly the perpetrator (U.S. Department of Health and Human Services, 2012).

Abusive families are often socially isolated and have few supportive relationships. They often have additional stressors such as low-income circumstances with little education. Parents with substance-abuse problems pose a greater risk for abuse and neglect because of a variety of factors. The additional stressors of substance abuse with the demands of normal care of children create situations in which abuse and neglect can occur because these parents have impaired judgment and may react with violence while under the influence of drugs or alcohol (Wells, 2009). With little or no available support system and concurrent stressors imposed by the child or environment, these parents are vulnerable to additional crises of any nature and may strike out at the child as a method of releasing their frustration and anxiety.

Other factors identified in abusive parents include low self-esteem and little knowledge of appropriate parenting skills. Parenting skills are learned behaviors, and parents who grew up with poor parental role models may have difficulty parenting their own children. Approximately one third of parents who were maltreated as children will subject their children to similar maltreatment (Gara, Allen, Herzog, et al., 2000).

Characteristics of the Child. The onus for child abuse is always on the abuser. However, children who are abused do have some common characteristics. Children from birth to 1 year of age are at highest risk for being abused (U.S. Department of Health and Human Services, 2012). Infants and small children require constant attention and must have all their needs met by others. This can result in parental or caregiver fatigue that results in striking out at the child with physical force, shaking the child, or ignoring his or her needs.

The physical and emotional demands placed on the parents or caregiver of an unwanted, brain-damaged, hyperactive, or physically disabled child may overwhelm them, resulting in abuse. Children with disabilities may not understand that abusive behaviors are not appropriate; thus they may not tell others or defend

---

*www.purplecrying.info/sections/index.php?sct=1&.

themselves. Premature infants may be at risk for maltreatment because of failure of parent-child bonding during early infancy, increased physical care needs, or irritability. One child may be singled out in an abusive family. Removing that child from the home often places the other siblings at risk for abuse. Therefore no child is safe if left in the abusive environment unless the parents can be helped to learn new parenting skills, meet the children's needs, and release their frustration through alternatives other than attacking their children.

Environmental Characteristics. The environment is a significant part of the potentially abusive situation. A typical environment is one of chronic stress, including problems of divorce, poverty, unemployment, poor housing, frequent relocation, alcoholism, and drug addiction. Increased exposure between children and parents such as that which occurs in crowded living conditions also increases the likelihood of abuse.

Although most reporting of abuse has been from lower socioeconomic populations as stated previously, child abuse is not a problem of any one societal group. Stresses imposed by poverty predispose lower socioeconomic families to abusive situations, and abuse in these groups is more likely to be reported. However, concealed crises may also be present in upper-class families. Families who have substitute caregivers such as day care providers and babysitters may also be at risk for child abuse, especially if the family has not fully evaluated the caregiver. Nurses need to be aware of all these factors to identify the less obvious examples of child abuse and neglect.

Sexual Abuse

Sexual abuse is one of the most devastating types of child maltreatment, and estimates indicate that it has increased significantly during the past decade (U.S. Department of Health and Human Services, 2012). Some of the apparent increase is because of increased awareness (Putnam, 2003).

As with all forms of child maltreatment, no universal definition for sexual abuse exists. Definitions cover a range of acts, including involvement of children in sexual acts they do not understand, to which they cannot give consent, or that violate social taboos (Finkel and DeJong, 2001). The Child Abuse and Prevention Act defines sexual abuse as "the use, persuasion, or coercion of any child to engage in sexually explicit conduct (or any simulation of such conduct) or producing any visual depiction of such conduct, or rape, molestation, prostitution, or incest with children."

Sexual abuse includes the following types of sexual maltreatment (see also Rape, Chapter 35):

Incest—Any physical sexual activity between family members; blood relationship is not required (abusers can include stepparents, unrelated siblings, grandparents, uncles, and aunts); does not include sexual relations between legally sanctioned partners such as spouses

Molestation—Vague term that includes "indecent liberties" such as touching, fondling, kissing, single or mutual masturbation, or oral-genital contact

Exhibitionism—Indecent exposure, usually exposure of the genitalia by an adult man to children or women

Child pornography—Arranging and photographing, in any media, sexual acts involving children, alone or with adults or animals, regardless of consent by the child's legal guardian; also may denote distribution of such material in any form with or without profit

Child prostitution—Involving children in sex acts for profit and usually with changing partners

Pedophilia—Literally means "love of child" and does not denote a type of sexual activity but rather the preference of an adult for prepubertal children as the means of achieving sexual excitement

Human trafficking often involves some form of coerced sexual activity and thus sexual abuse that may also often involve physical and mental abuse. Many victims of human trafficking are females under the age of 18 years who are forced to perform sexual acts for the monetary profit of the perpetrators. One form of sex trafficking called sex tourism involves adult men traveling to developing nations to have sex with young children (Sabella, 2011). Nurses may encounter victims of sex trafficking and subsequent sexual and physical abuse who are seeking medical care in outpatient and emergent health care settings for a plethora of health problems (STIs, bruises, wound infections, PTSD, suicidal ideation, and addiction). However, nurses may not be aware of the victim's plight unless he or she delves further into the person's history and background (Sabella, 2011).

Characteristics of Abusers and Victims

Anyone, including siblings and mothers, can be sexual abusers; but a typical abuser is a man whom the victim knows. Offenders come from all levels of society. Adults comprise 80% of sexual abuse offenders; the remaining 20% is composed of adolescents and preadolescents (Johnson, 2003). Many offenders hold full-time jobs, are active in community affairs, and may not have prior criminal records (Finkel and DeJong, 2001). Offenders often are employed (or volunteers) in positions such as teaching or coaching that bring them into contact with young girls and boys. Child sexual abuse may be generational unless discovered and stopped (Johnson, 2003). Offenders may commit many assaults before being caught.

Incestuous relationships between father or stepfather and daughter are generally prolonged, and the victims are usually reluctant to report the situation because of fear of retaliation and fear that they will not be believed. Typically incestuous relationships begin later than other forms of child abuse. The eldest daughter is usually abused, but in her absence another sister may be substituted. Sibling incest may also occur. Sexual abuse by relatives with a strong emotional bond with the victim such as a parent is often the most devastating to the child.

Boys are also victims of both intrafamilial and extrafamilial abuse. Compared with female victims, male victims are much less likely to report abuse, and they may suffer much greater emotional harm from incestuous relationships. Boys are likely to be subjected to anal penetration and oral-genital contact. They often have subtle physical findings and are abused by a father, stepfather, or mother's boyfriend.

Significant risk factors for child sexual abuse include parental unavailability, lack of emotional closeness and flexibility, social isolation, emotional deprivation, and communication difficulties. Most sexual abuse is committed by men and people known to the child, with family members constituting as many as two thirds of the perpetrators.

Initiation and Perpetuation of Sexual Abuse

The cycle of sexual abuse often starts insidiously unless it involves an isolated attack such as rape. Often offenders spend time with the victims to gain their trust before initiating any sexual contact. Most victims are then pressured into being an accessory to the sexual activity through various means (Box 33-1) and may be unaware that sexual activity is part of the offer. Children may not reveal the truth for fear that their parents would not believe them if they told, especially if the offender is a trusted member of the family. Some fear

BOX 33-1   METHODS USED TO PRESSURE CHILDREN INTO SEXUAL ACTIVITY

- The child is offered gifts or privileges.
- The adult misrepresents moral standards by telling the child that it is "okay to do."
- Isolated and emotionally and socially impoverished children are enticed by adults who meet their needs for warmth and human contact.
- The offender asks the child for help in finding a favorite pet or object with which the child can easily identify.
- The successful sex offender pressures the victim into secrecy regarding the activity by describing it as a "secret between us" that other people may take away if they find out.
- The offender plays on the child's fears, including fear of punishment by the offender, fear of repercussions if the child tells, and fear of abandonment or rejection by the family.

BOX 33-2   WARNING SIGNS OF ABUSE

- Physical evidence of abuse or neglect, including previous injuries
- Conflicting stories about the "accident" or injury from the parents or others
- Cause of injury blamed on sibling or other party
- An injury inconsistent with the history such as a concussion and broken arm from falling off a bed
- History inconsistent with child's developmental level such as a 6-month-old turning on the hot water
- A complaint other than the one associated with signs of abuse (e.g., a chief complaint of a cold when there is evidence of first- and second-degree burns)
- Inappropriate response of caregiver such as an exaggerated or absent emotional response, refusal to sign for additional tests or agree to necessary treatment, excessive delay in seeking treatment, or absence of parents for questioning
- Inappropriate response of child such as little or no response to pain, fear of being touched, excessive or lack of separation anxiety, indiscriminate friendliness to strangers
- Child's report of physical or sexual abuse
- Previous reports of abuse in the family
- Repeated visits to emergency facilities with injuries
- Parent or caregiver report of being gone and finding the child unresponsive, indicating absence during the supposed event that resulted in harm

that they will be blamed for the situation; and many young children with limited vocabulary have difficulty describing the activity when they do have the courage or opportunity to reveal the abuse.

Incest most frequently occurs between fathers and daughters, but it may also be between grandfather and granddaughter or brother and sister. Brother-sister incest has been found to be just as damaging as father-daughter abuse (Cyr, Wright, McDuff, et al., 2002). Victims may take years to disclose this abuse. However, not all incestuous relationships follow this pattern of silence. Reports of father-daughter incest during child custody conflicts have become more common and have raised serious concerns regarding the possibility of false accusation. Rather than tolerating or denying the child's sexual abuse, the other parent (usually the mother) is typically the chief accuser.

Nursing Care of the Maltreated Child

A critical responsibility of health professionals is identifying abusive situations as early as possible. Nurses who increase their knowledge of the different types of abuse and neglect and underlying causes enhance their ability to identify, intervene, and prevent children from maltreatment and neglect (Giardino and Giardino, 2003). The characteristics that may predispose members of some families to commit abuse can serve as a framework for assessing vulnerability but are never predictive of actual abuse. A careful, detailed history and interview combined with a thorough physical examination are the diagnostic tools needed to identify abuse. Nurses have a special role because they may be the first person to see the child and parent and are the consistent caregivers if the child is hospitalized (see Guidelines box).

In interviewing the child and family the nurse must be careful to avoid biasing the child's retelling of the events. Some experts suggest that health professionals limit the interview to the child's physical and mental health concerns and leave topics of the family's social, legal, or other problems to law enforcement or the CPS (Kellogg, 2005; McClain, Giardet, Lahoti, et al., 2000). If this is not possible, make an effort to coordinate the interview process so all pertinent health care professionals can be present for the interview.

Recognition of abuse or neglect necessitates a familiarity with both physical and behavioral signs that suggest maltreatment (Box 33-2). No one indicator can be used to diagnose maltreatment. It is a pattern or combination of indicators that should arouse suspicion and lead to further investigation. It is important to note that some

GUIDELINES

Talking with Children Who Reveal Abuse

- Provide a private time and place to talk.
- Do not promise not to tell; tell them that you are required by law to report the abuse.
- Do not express shock or criticize their family.
- Use their vocabulary to discuss body parts.
- Avoid using any leading statements that can distort their report.
- Reassure them that they have done the right thing by telling.
- Tell them that the abuse is not their fault, that they are not bad or to blame.
- Determine their immediate need for safety.
- Let the child know what will happen when you report.

situations such as bleeding disorders, osteogenesis imperfecta, or sudden infant death syndrome may be misinterpreted as abuse. In addition, some cultural practices such as cupping or coin rubbing (see Health Practices, Chapter 27), may mimic physical abuse. Unintentional injuries such as burns from metal buckles on car seats, bruising from seat belts, or spiral fractures from a twist and fall injury may also be wrongly diagnosed as abuse. Normal variants such as mongolian spots and congenital anomalies of genitalia can be mistaken for abuse.

Caregiver-Child Interaction

The nurse can use the initial contact with the family to assess the interaction between the caregiver and the child. Observations of the caregivers should include emotional support for the child, attentiveness to his or her needs, and concern for his or her injury. Although caregivers and children may vary in responses to a stressful event, note an unusual caregiver-child relationship and factor this into the overall evaluation of the child.

Certain behavioral responses of the parents to their child and to the interviewer should alert the nurse to the possibility of maltreatment. Abusive parents may have difficulty showing concern for their child. They may be unable or unwilling to comfort the child. Abusers may blame the child for the injuries or belittle her or him for being clumsy or stupid. When interacting with health care workers, the parent may become hostile or uncooperative. During the child's hospitalization they may not participate in her or his care and may show little concern for her or his progress, eventual discharge, or need for follow-up care.

Abused children's responses to their parents or the injury may also support the suspicion of abuse. Although no one pattern is typical, extremes of behavior may be observed. Children may be unresponsive to the parent or excessively clinging and intolerant of separation. They may be overly attached to the abusive parent, possibly in the hope of preventing any upset that may precipitate anger and another attack. During care of the injury children may be passive and accepting of the discomfort or uncooperative and fearful of any physical contact. They may avoid eye contact. Some children maintain a wary watchfulness of all strangers; some shy away from strangers as if frightened; others are unusually affectionate and outgoing.

History and Interview

Child Physical Abuse. It is often difficult to distinguish child maltreatment from accidental injuries. Caregivers whose history of events may be deceptive or incomplete and children who are nonverbal may make the assessment more complex. A purposeful, skilled history and appropriate interview questions help the nurse ensure the right course of action. Knowledge of mechanism of injury and child development is essential. Cases of abuse are often detected when the child or caregiver history of events does not match with physical findings. Children who are verbal can often give a history of the injury. Separating the child from the caregiver may provide a more reliable history. It is important to ask nonleading, open-ended questions. The history should include a narrative of the injury from both caregiver and child (if verbal). Date, time, and location where the injury took place along with who was present at the time of the injury are essential questions. Family history for bleeding and bone disorders is important. Box 33-3 outlines areas of history that are of concern for potential abuse.

Neglect and Emotional Abuse. Each child may manifest different responses to neglect, depending on the situation and the child's developmental age. The goal of the interview is to determine whether the child is in a safe environment and whether the caregiver has the skills and resources to care for the child. It is often difficult to determine whether the circumstances constitute poor parenting skills or true neglect. Warning signals for behaviors for which to look are found in Box 33-2.

Sexual Abuse. An essential component to identifying sexual abuse is the interview. Several dynamics may impede the child's revelation of sexual abuse. Child sexual abuse is often perpetrated by someone known to the child, including family members. In some cases the child may have been sworn to secrecy. He or she may have been told that no one will believe the story or that the family would be harmed if he or she told someone about the abuse. Small children may imitate behaviors they have had perpetrated on themselves or have seen others do. The nurse must be able to recognize normal, age-related sexual curiosity and self-stimulating behaviors. Typically children do not act out specific details of the sexual act or perform intrusive acts on others unless they have sexual knowledge beyond their normal age-related development (Johnson, 2003).

Children's reports of sexual abuse may vary from contradictory stories to unwavering versions of the experience. Stories that sound contradictory may reflect the child's experiences in several instances of abuse. In addition, children who repeatedly tell identical facts may have been prompted to do so.

Increasing evidence suggests that the types of interrogation to which children are exposed after reports of sexual abuse shape their thinking. To avoid biasing the interaction, nurses must be skillful interviewers when questioning children who may be victims of abuse. Medical records should include verbatim statements made by the child and interviewer that reflect appropriate nonleading questions and statements (Hornor, 2001; Kellogg, 2005; McClain, Girardet, Lahoti, et al., 2000). The child may not be emotionally ready to discuss the abuse. Establishing rapport with the child is essential to gaining his or her trust. Interviews should not be rushed. Engaging the child in play activities while encouraging conversation may help her or him to discuss the abuse. It may take several interviews or psychologic counseling for the child to be forthcoming about the abuse. Information regarding the last sexual contact is important because it determines the need for a forensic evaluation. Children who have been sexually abused within the past 72 to 96 hours should be considered for forensic testing.

Unfortunately there is no typical profile of the victim, and the nurse must have a high index of suspicion to identify these children. Physical signs vary and may include any of those listed for sexual abuse. The victim may exhibit various behavioral manifestations, but none of these behaviors is diagnostic. When abused children exhibit these behaviors, the signs may be incorrectly attributed to the normal stresses of childhood, especially in older school-age children or adolescents. Even signs considered most predictive of sexual abuse such as certain genital findings, sexually inappropriate behavior for age, enactment of adult sexual activity, and intense focus on sexual activity (e.g., masturbation) do not always indicate that sexual abuse has occurred. Conversely abused children may not demonstrate more knowledge of sexual activity than nonabused children. However, one difference in the abused child's explanation of sexual activity may be unusual affective responses. For example, abused children may have an increased incidence of sleep disorders, temper tantrums, and depression.

> ### ! NURSING ALERT
>
> When children report potentially sexually abusive experiences, their reports need to be taken seriously but also cautiously to avoid alarming the child or falsely accusing someone.

Physical Assessment

Child Physical Abuse. The goal of the physical assessment for child physical abuse is identification of all injuries. A systems approach ensures that the whole body is evaluated. In instances of severe abuse and injuries the assessment should begin with a rapid assessment of airway, breathing, circulation, and neurologic systems. A systematic head-to-toe examination follows. Attention to areas often overlooked such as the scalp, behind the ears, and the frenulum is essential. The child's exterior genital area and posterior surface should be examined completely.

Record the location and a detailed description of all injuries. Note the color, size, and location of all bruising. Burn documentation should include the location, pattern, demarcation lines, and presence of eschar or blisters. Diagrams of the injuries using a body

BOX 33-3 CLINICAL MANIFESTATIONS OF POTENTIAL CHILD MALTREATMENT

Physical Neglect
Suggestive Physical Findings
- Failure to thrive (growth failure)
- Signs of undernutrition such as thin extremities, abdominal distention, lack of subcutaneous fat
- Poor personal hygiene
- Unclean or inappropriate dress
- Evidence of poor health care such as delayed immunizations, untreated infections, frequent colds
- Frequent injuries from lack of supervision

Suggestive Behaviors
- Dull and inactive affect; excessively passive or sleepy
- Self-stimulatory behaviors such as finger sucking or rocking
- Begging or stealing food
- Absenteeism from school
- Substance abuse
- Vandalism or shoplifting

Emotional Abuse and Neglect
Suggestive Physical Findings
- Failure to thrive (growth failure)
- Eating or feeding disorder
- Enuresis
- Sleep disorder

Suggestive Behaviors
- Self-stimulatory behaviors such as biting, rocking, sucking
- During infancy lack of social smile and stranger anxiety
- Withdrawal from environment and people
- Unusual fearfulness
- Antisocial behavior such as destructiveness, stealing, cruelty to animals or people
- Extremes of behavior such as overcompliant and passive or aggressive and demanding
- Lags in emotional and intellectual development, especially language
- Suicide attempts or attempts to harm self

Physical Abuse
Suggestive Physical Findings
- Bruises and welts
  - On face, lips, mouth, back, buttocks, thighs, or areas of torso
  - Regular patterns descriptive of object used such as belt buckle, hand, wire hanger, chain, wooden spoon, squeeze or pinch marks
  - May be present in various stages of healing
- Burns
  - On soles of feet, palms of hands, back, or buttocks
  - Patterns descriptive of object used such as round cigar or cigarette burns; sharply demarcated areas from immersion in scalding water; rope burns on wrists or ankles from being bound; burns in the shape of an iron, radiator, or electric stove burner
  - Absence of "splash" marks and presence of symmetric burns
  - Stun gun injury: lesions circular, fairly uniform (up to 0.5 cm), and paired about 5 cm (1¾ in) apart
- Fractures and dislocations
  - Skull, nose, or facial structures
  - Injury denoting type of abuse such as spiral fracture or dislocation from twisting an extremity or whiplash from shaking child
  - Multiple new or old fractures in various stages of healing

- Lacerations and abrasions
  - On backs of arms, legs, torso, face, or external genitalia
  - Unusual symptoms such as abdominal swelling, pain, and vomiting from punching
  - Descriptive marks such as from human bites or pulling out of hair
- Chemical
  - Unexplained repeated poisoning, especially drug overdose
  - Unexplained sudden illness such as hypoglycemia from insulin administration

Suggestive Behaviors
- Wary of physical contact with adults
- Apparent fear of parents or going home
- Lying very still while surveying environment
- Inappropriate reaction to injury such as failure to cry from pain
- Lack of reaction to frightening events
- Apprehension when hearing other children cry
- Indiscriminate friendliness and displays of affection
- Superficial relationships
- Acting-out behavior such as aggression to seek attention
- Withdrawal behavior

Sexual Abuse
Suggestive Physical Findings
- Bruises, bleeding, lacerations, or irritation of external genitalia, anus, mouth, or throat
- Torn, stained, or bloody underclothing
- Pain on urination or pain, swelling, and itching of genital area
- Penile discharge
- Sexually transmitted infection, nonspecific vaginitis, or venereal warts
- Difficulty in walking or sitting
- Unusual odor in genital area
- Recurrent urinary tract infections
- Presence of sperm
- Pregnancy in young adolescent

Suggestive Behaviors
- Sudden emergence of sexually related problems, including excessive or public masturbation, age-inappropriate sexual play, promiscuity, or overtly seductive behavior
- Withdrawn behavior, excessive daydreaming
- Preoccupation with fantasies, especially in play
- Poor relationships with peers
- Sudden changes such as anxiety, loss or gain of weight, clinging behavior
- In incestuous relationships excessive anger at mother for not protecting daughter
- Regressive behavior such as bed-wetting or thumb-sucking
- Sudden onset of phobias or fears, particularly fears of dark, men, strangers, or particular settings or situations (e.g., undue fear of leaving house or staying at day care center or baby-sitter's house)
- Running away from home
- Substance abuse, particularly of alcohol or mood-elevating drugs
- Profound and rapid personality changes, especially extreme depression, hostility, and aggression (often accompanied by social withdrawal)
- Rapidly declining school performance
- Suicidal attempts or ideation

diagram form are helpful. If possible obtain photographs of the injuries with a measurement tool.

Not all forms of physical abuse have obvious signs. Intraabdominal organ injury from blunt trauma to the abdomen can occur without signs of external abdominal bruising. Nurses should consider intraabdominal injury in infants and children who have any other signs of abuse.

All evidence collected must adhere to strict guidelines for legal purposes; the chain of custody must be appropriately maintained with local law enforcement personnel. Documentation on the chain of custody form should include the names of people collecting and receiving evidence (e.g., photographs and deoxyribonucleic acid [DNA] samples), types of evidence collected and received, and date of receipt (Kaczor, Pierce, Makoroff, et al., 2006; Kellogg, 2005).

> **! NURSING ALERT**
>
> Incompatibility between the history and the injury is probably the most important criterion on which to base the decision to report suspected abuse.

Neglect and Emotional Abuse. Neglect from deprivation of necessities is easier to identify than emotional neglect or psychologic maltreatment because physical signs are usually evident. Assessment of the child's height, weight, nutritional status, hygiene, and age-appropriate interactions is important for the overall picture of potential neglect. Emotional maltreatment may be readily suspected, but it is difficult to substantiate. Physical signs are often nonspecific; and nurses must rely on behavioral indicators, which range from depression to acting-out behavior, to help identify a possibly abusive situation. Any persistent and unexplained change in the child's behavior is an important clue to possible emotional abuse.

Sexual Abuse. Identifying instances of sexual abuse is particularly difficult because often few if any obvious physical indications of the activity exist. Physical signs vary and may include any of those listed in Box 33-3 for sexual abuse. The goal of the physical examination is to document genital findings. In most cases the genital examination findings are normal, which does not mean that sexual abuse did not occur. Fondling or genital-to-genital contact without penetration may leave no physical findings. Forensic evidence obtained directly from a prepubertal victim's body diminishes greatly after 24 hours, with the best chance for evidence collection coming from bed linens or the child's underwear (Christian, Lavelle, DeJong, et al., 2000). The female genital examination should include a description of the vulva, hymen, and surrounding tissue. Abnormal findings of concern are injuries to the posterior vulva or the lower half of the hymenal ring or abrasions, bruising, or bleeding of the genital or anal tissue. It is often helpful to use a magnifying instrument (colposcope) to detect subtle injuries. There are many variants of normal findings for female genital anatomy; thus it is recommended that the examination be done by a practitioner experienced with these types of cases. Contrary to popular myth, the size of the hymenal opening does not predict the likelihood of sexual abuse (Christian and Rubin, 2002). For male victims swelling, abrasions, or bruising of the genital tissue raises concerns. Examine the anal area for symmetry, tone, fissures, or scars. Genital tissue heals very quickly and most often without scars. Therefore, unless the child is seen within a few days of injury, the genital tissue may appear normal. In addition, the vaginal and anal mucosa is elastic; therefore penetration without disruption of tissue is possible. This defies another myth that there is always evidence of female virginity. Consider the collection of specimens for determining the presence of sexually transmitted infections, which may have been contracted during the sexual contact.

CARE MANAGEMENT

Protect Child from Further Abuse. Initially identification of instances of suspected abuse or neglect is essential. The nurse may come in contact with abused children in an emergency department, practitioner's office, home, day care center, or school.

> **! NURSING ALERT**
>
> The priority is to remove the child from the abusive situation to prevent further injury.

All states and provinces in North America have laws for mandatory reporting of child maltreatment. Suspected child abuse is reported to the local authorities.* Referrals usually come to the state child welfare department and are assigned to a caseworker in an agency such as CPS. After a referral has been made, a caseworker is assigned to investigate the report. Based on the findings, the child is left in the home or removed temporarily.

A court proceeding may be necessary before the child can be placed outside the home or when parental rights are to be terminated. When the courts are involved, they usually require firsthand testimony by the referring parties. Nurses may be subpoenaed to appear in court, or their notes may be introduced as evidence in court hearings. Accurate and factual documentation is essential. Behaviors are described, not interpreted, and are recorded daily to establish a progress record (see Guidelines box). Conversations among the nurse, child, and parent are recorded verbatim as much as possible.

Support Child. Children suspected of being abused are often hospitalized for medical management of their injuries and to allow further assessment of their safety needs. The needs of these children are the same as those of any hospitalized child. The child should be treated as a child with the usual physical needs, developmental tasks, and play interests—not as a victim of abuse. The goal of the nurse-child relationship is to provide a role model for the parents in helping them relate positively and constructively to their child and to foster a therapeutic environment for the child in his or her reprieve from the abusing situation.

Support Family. The nurse also encourages the child's relationship with nonoffending parents. The nurse does not become a substitute parent but rather acts as a role model for parents in helping them relate positively and constructively to their child. When parental ignorance of childrearing practices has played a part in the abuse, the nurse can educate the parent regarding children's physical and emotional needs. Because of the parents' own childrearing, they may not be aware of nonviolent methods of discipline such as time-outs. They may also need help in dealing with their frustration so they do not vent anger on the child. Because these parents may be sensitive to criticism or resistant to authority

---

*Telephone numbers are usually listed under "Child Abuse" in the business white pages of the local directory or you can call the emergency child abuse hotline: 800-422-4453 (800-4-A-CHILD).

GUIDELINES

Recording Assessment Data in Suspected Abuse

History of Injury

- Date, time, and place of occurrence
- Sequence of events with recorded times
- Presence of witnesses, especially person caring for child at time of incident
- Time lapse between occurrence of injury and initiation of treatment
- Interview with child when appropriate, including verbal quotations and information from drawing or other play activities
- Interview with parent, witnesses, or other significant persons, including verbal quotations
- Description of parent-child interactions (verbal interactions, eye contact, touching, parental concern)
- Name, age, and condition of other children in home (if possible)

Physical Examination

- Location, size, shape, and color of bruises; approximate location, size, and shape on drawing of body outline
- Distinguishing characteristics such as a bruise in the shape of a hand; round burn (possibly caused by cigarette)
- Symmetry or asymmetry of injury; presence of other injuries
- Degree of pain; any bone tenderness
- Evidence of past injuries; general state of health and hygiene
- Developmental level of child; perform screening test (see Developmental Assessment, Chapter 28)

figures, teaching is implemented through demonstration and example rather than through lecturing. Praise any competent parenting abilities they demonstrate to promote their sense of parental adequacy.

Advise family members to encourage the child to resume normal activities and observe her or him for signs of distress. (See Posttraumatic Stress Disorder, Chapter 34.) Children express their feelings primarily through behavior. Parents should be alert for changes in behavior that indicate distress resulting from the incident such as remaining in the house, refusal to go to school, changes in sleeping patterns, and frequency of dreams and nightmares.

Referral to appropriate social service agencies is also essential. Many abusive parents live in poverty, and the daily stresses imposed by their circumstances are overwhelming. Seek resources for financial aid, improved housing, and child care. Self-help groups also provide important services. One such group is Parents Anonymous,* a group for parents who have abused or fear that they may abuse their child but only in terms of physical abuse, not sexual abuse.

Plan for Discharge. Discharge planning should begin as soon as the legal disposition for placement has been decided, which may be temporary foster home placement; return to the parents; or permanent termination of parental rights, which is the most drastic solution, but necessary in situations of life-threatening abuse. Whenever children are sent to a foster home or juvenile institution, they must be allowed an opportunity to express their feelings. No matter how severe the abuse, they usually mourn the loss of their parents. They need help to understand why they must not return home and that

this new home is in no way a punishment. Whenever possible, foster parents are encouraged to visit in the hospital, and the nurse should take an active role in helping the new parents understand the child and his or her health care needs because studies have shown that the health care needs of children in foster care often go unmet (Mekonnen, Noonan, and Rubin, 2009).

Prevent Abuse. Prevention of child maltreatment has been an extremely difficult goal. However, nurses have played an important role in such programs. The Nurse-Family Partnership is one such program that has demonstrated evidence-based interventions resulting in the prevention of child maltreatment (Donelan-McCall, Eckenrode, and Olds, 2009).

Nurses in a variety of settings can implement similar activities. For example, nurses in prenatal clinics can prepare expectant families for adjustment to parenthood. Nursery and postpartum nurses can foster the attachment process by encouraging parents to hold and look at their infant and by teaching coping mechanisms for prolonged crying. Nurses in neonatal intensive care units can minimize the effects of separation by encouraging parents to visit and can help parents become comfortable caring for their child. Nurses in ambulatory settings can teach parents appropriate methods of bathing, feeding, toileting, disciplining, and preventing injuries while stressing the normal needs and developmental characteristics of children. Nurses must be sensitive to parental needs for attention, reassurance, and reinforcement and should refer parents to community services and self-help groups.

Unlike preventive efforts for neglect and physical abuse, which have been aimed at the potential offender, prevention of child sexual abuse has centered on education of children to protect themselves. Materials are available for parents that describe sexual abuse and its prevention.* Helpful games such as, "What if the babysitter wants to wrestle and hug but tells you to keep it a secret?" can be used to explore dangerous situations in advance and help children learn the importance of saying "no." They need reassurance that, no matter what the other person says or does, the parents want to know about it and will not punish them. Even if children participate in the activity before telling their parents, they must be reassured that it was not their fault. It is equally important to teach children safety in terms of potential risk situations. Several suggestions for parents regarding protecting and educating children against possible molestation are presented in the Family-Centered Care box. The nurse is frequently in a position to discuss the topic of abuse with parents and provide guidelines. In addition, parents need to be made aware that "nice" people, including friends and relatives, can be offenders; they should carefully observe how others act toward the child. A sudden change in the child's behavior and a response such as, "I don't like Uncle anymore" are clues to investigate the relationship. In the event of any doubt, prevent further solitary encounters between this person and the child. It is sometimes to the child's great misfortune that parents do not take certain comments seriously such as, "He hugs me too tight" or "I don't want to go with him." Casual parental statements such as, "He just loves you" or "You do whatever adults tell you to do" can place children in jeopardy. Health professionals must alert parents to such dangers and guide them toward an appreciation of the problem, providing concrete guidelines toward child education and protection.

*675 W. Foothill Blvd., Suite 220, Claremont, CA 91711, 909-621-6184, www.parentsanonymous.org.

*Sources of information are Prevent Child Abuse America, 228 S. Wabash Ave., 10th Floor, Chicago, IL 60604, 312-663-3520 or 800-Children, www.preventchildabuse.org; and American Humane, 63 Inverness Drive East, Englewood, CO 80112, 800-227-4645 (outside Colorado) or 303-792-9900, www.americanhumane.org.

FAMILY-CENTERED CARE

Preventing or Dealing with Sexual Abuse of Children

Sexual assault of children is much more common than most people realize. It may be preventable if children have proper preparation. *To provide protection and preparation:*

- Pay careful attention to who is around children. (Unwanted touch may come from someone liked and trusted.)
- Back up a child's right to say "no."
- Encourage communication by taking seriously what children *say.*
- Take a second look at signals of potential danger.
- Refuse to leave children in the company of those not trusted.
- Include information about sexual assault when teaching about safety.
- Provide specific definitions and examples of sexual assault.
- Remind children that even "nice" people sometimes do mean things.
- Urge children to tell about *anybody* who causes them to be uncomfortable.
- Prepare children to deal with bribes, threats, and possible physical force.
- Virtually eliminate secrets between children and parents.

- Teach children how to say "no," ask for help, and control who touches them and how.
- Model self-protective and limit-setting behavior for children.

Should it ever become necessary to help a child recover from a sexual assault:

- Listen carefully to understand children.
- Support the child for telling through praise, belief, sympathy, and lack of blame.
- Know local resources and choose help carefully.
- Provide opportunities to talk about the assault.
- Provide opportunities for entire family to go through recovery process.

Sexual assault affects everyone. To help deal with this social problem:

- Provide care and support to those who have been victimized.
- Recognize that offenders do not change without intervention.
- Organize neighborhood programs to support each other's efforts to protect children.
- Encourage schools to provide information about sexual assault as a problem of health and safety.
- Organize community groups to support educational-treatment and law-enforcement programs.

KEY POINTS

- The preschool years consist of the period from 3 to 5 years of age, a time that is considered critical for emotional and psychologic development.
- Biologic development in the preschool period is characterized by mature body systems and refinement in gross and fine motor behavior, as evidenced by activities such as running, riding a tricycle, and drawing.
- According to Erikson, acquiring a sense of initiative is the chief psychosocial task of the preschooler. Development of the superego occurs during this period as conscience begins to emerge.
- According to Piaget the preschool age is characterized by intuitive (or prelogical) thinking and a move toward logical thought processes through advanced, complex learning; language; and understanding of causality.
- The seeds of moral development are planted during the preschool period. According to Kohlberg, preschool children are in the stage of naive instrumental orientation, in which they are concerned with satisfying their own needs and less frequently the needs of others.
- Preschoolers often have difficulty discerning reality from fiction and believe that their thoughts are all powerful.
- Animism and magical thinking are hallmarks of preschool thinking.
- Eating habits are usually well established during the preschool years; therefore eating healthy and minimizing the intake of saturated fats and empty carbohydrate calories is an important part of educating for healthy living.
- Social development includes further separation-individuation; more sophisticated language; greater independence; and more complex, imaginative forms of play.

- Areas of special concern to parents during the preschool period are the preschool and kindergarten experience, sex education, fears, stress, and speech problems.
- In selecting an early-learning program, parents should inquire about daily activities, teacher qualifications, accreditation, student-staff ratio, safety, meals, fees, and health practices.
- Two rules that govern how parents answer questions about sex and other sensitive issues are to find out what the child knows and be honest.
- Fears constitute a great part of the preschool period; fear of objects or potential annihilation and parent-induced fears are common.
- Preschool aggression may result from frustration, modeling behavior, and reinforcement.
- Hesitancy or dysfluency in speech patterns is a normal characteristic of language development. Speech problems can occur when parents express excessive concern over this pattern.
- Health promotion continues to be directed toward proper nutrition, adequate sleep, proper dental care, and injury prevention.
- Child maltreatment may take the form of physical abuse or neglect, emotional abuse or neglect, or sexual abuse.
- Parental, child, and environmental characteristics are criteria that may predispose children to maltreatment.
- Identification of abuse entails securing evidence of maltreatment, taking a history pertaining to the incident, and assessing parental and child behaviors.
- The reported incidence of sexual abuse has increased in the past decade; common forms are incest, molestation, rape, exhibitionism, child pornography, child prostitution, and pedophilia.

REFERENCES

Allen RE, Myers AL: Nutrition in toddlers, *Am Fam Physician* 74(9):1527–1532, 2006.

Altman RL, Canter J, Patrick PA et al: Parent education by maternity nurses and prevention of abusive head trauma, *Pediatrics* 128(5):e1164–e1172, 2011.

American Academy of Pediatrics: TV and your family, 2007, www.aap.org/publiced/ BR_TV.htm.

American Academy of Pediatrics (AAP) Committee on Child Abuse and Neglect: Abusive head trauma in infants and children, *Pediatrics* 123(5):1409–1411, 2009.

American Academy of Pediatrics Committee (AAP) on Infectious Diseases, Pickering L, editor: *2012 Red Book: Report of the Committee on Infectious Diseases*, ed 29, Elk Grove Village, Ill, 2012, The Academy.

American Academy of Pediatrics (AAP) Committee on Nutrition: *Pediatric nutrition handbook*, ed 6, Elk Grove Village, Ill, 2009, The Academy.

American Academy of Pediatrics Committee (AAP) on Public Education: Children, adolescents, and television, *Pediatrics* 107(2):423–426, 2001.

American Academy of Pediatrics (AAP) Committee on Sports Medicine and Fitness and Committee on School Health: Active healthy living: prevention of childhood obesity through increased physical activity, *Pediatrics* 117(5): 1832–1842, 2006.

American Heart Association, Gidding SS, Dennison BA, et al: Dietary recommendations for children and adolescents: a guide for practitioners, *Pediatrics* 117(2):544–559, 2006.

Barlow SE, Expert Committee: Expert Committee recommendations regarding the prevention, assessment, and treatment of child and adolescent overweight and obesity: summary report, *Pediatrics* 120(suppl 4): S164–S192, 2007.

Barr RG: Preventing abusive head trauma resulting from a failure of normal interaction between infants and their caregivers, *Proc Natl Acad Sci USA* 109 (Suppl 2):17294–17301, 2012.

Benzies K, Keown L, Magill-Evans J: Immediate and sustained effects of parenting on physical aggression in Canadian children aged 6 years and younger, *Can J Psychiatry* 54(1):55–64, 2009.

Carbaugh SF: The long road home: understanding shaken baby syndrome, *Adv Neonat Care* 4:105–117, 2004.

Chiesa A, Duhaime A: Abusive head trauma, *Pediatr Clin North Am* 56(2):317–331, 2009.

Christian CW, Rubin DM: Sexual abuse. In Giardino AP, Giardino ER, editors: *Recognition of child abuse for the mandated reporter*, St Louis, 2002, GW Medical Publishing.

Christian C, Lavelle JM, DeJong AR , et al: Forensic evidence findings in prepubertal victims of sexual assault, *Pediatrics* 106:100–104, 2000.

Cyr M, Wright J, McDuff P, et al: Intrafamilial sexual abuse: brother-sister incest does not differ from father-daughter incest and stepfather-stepdaughter incest, *Child Abuse Neglect* 26(9):957–973, 2002.

Dattillo AM, Birch L, Krebs NF, et al: Need for early intervention in the prevention of pediatric overweight: a review and upcoming directions, *J Obesity* 2012:1–18, 2012.

Donelan-McCall N, Eckenrode J, Olds D: Home visiting for the prevention of child maltreatment: lessons learned during the past 20 years, *Pediatr Clin North Am* 56(2):389–403, 2009.

Erikson E: *Childhood and society*, New York, 1963, WW Norton.

Feigelman S: The preschool years. In Kliegman RM, Stanton BF, St. Geme JW, et al, editors: *Nelson textbook of pediatrics*, ed 19, Philadelphia, 2011, Saunders.

Finkel MA, DeJong AR: Medical findings in child sexual abuse. In Reece RM, Ludwig S, editors: *Child abuse medical diagnosis and management*, Philadelphia, 2001, Lippincott Williams & Wilkins.

Gara MA, Allen LA, Herzog EP, et al: The abused child as parent: the structure and content of physically abused mothers' perceptions of their babies, *Child Abuse Neglect* 24(5): 627–639, 2000.

Giardino ER, Giardino AP, editors: *Nursing approach to the evaluation of child maltreatment*, St Louis, 2003, GW Medical Publishing.

Goldman J, Salus MK , Wolcott D, et al: What factors contribute to child abuse and neglect? In Goldman J, et al, editors: *A coordinated response to child abuse and neglect: the foundation for practice*, Washington, DC, 2003, Child Welfare Information, www.childwelfare.gov/pubs/ usermanuals/foundation/foundatione.cfm.

Hagan JF, Shaw JS, Duncan PM, editors: *Bright futures: guidelines for health supervision of infants, children, and adolescents*, ed 3, Elk Grove Village, Ill, 2008, American Academy of Pediatrics.

Hamer M, Stamatakis E, Mishra G: Psychological distress, television viewing, and physical activity in children aged 4 to 12 years, *Pediatrics* 123(5):1263–1268, 2009.

Harrison LJ, McLeod S: Risk and protective factors associated with speech and language impairment in a nationally representative sample of 4- to 5-year-old children, *J Speech Lang Hear Res* 53(2):508–529, 2010.

Hornor G: Repeated sexual abuse allegations: a problem for primary care providers, *J Pediatr Health Care* 15(2):71–76, 2001.

Johnson M: Child sexual abuse. In Thomas DO, Bernardo LM, Herman B, editors: *Core curriculum for pediatric emergency nursing*, Sudbury, Mass, 2003, Jones & Bartlett.

Kaczor K, Pierce MC, Makoroff K, et al: Bruising and physical child abuse, *Clin Pediatr Emerg Med* 7(3):153–160, 2006.

Kagihara LE, Niederhauser VP, Stark M: Assessment, management, and prevention of early childhood caries, *J Am Acad Nurse Pract* 21(1):1–10, 2009.

Keenan HT, Runyan DK, Marshall SW, et al: A population-based comparison of clinical and outcome characteristics of young children with serious inflicted and noninflicted traumatic brain injury, *Pediatrics* 114(3):633–639, 2004.

Kellogg N: The evaluation of sexual abuse in children, *Pediatrics* 116(2):506–512, 2005.

Kirkorian HL, Wartella EA, Anderson DR: Media and young children's learning, *Future Child* 18(1):39–61, 2008.

Kotch JB, Isbell P, Weber DJ, et al: Hand-washing and diapering equipment reduces disease among children in out-of-home child care centers, *Pediatrics* 120(1):e29–e36, 2007.

Larson N, Ward D, Neelon SB, et al: *Preventing obesity among preschool children: how can child-care settings promote healthy eating and physical activity? Research synthesis*, Princeton, NJ, 2011, Robert Wood Johnson Foundation, http://www. healthyeatingresearch.org/images/RS_ ChildCare_For_posting_on_web_FINAL_ 10-27-11.pdf.

Leider HS, Irving SY, Mauricio R, et al: Munchausen syndrome by proxy: a case report, *AACN Clin Issues* 16(2):178–184, 2005.

Leung AK, Robson WL, Leong AG: Herpes zoster in childhood, *J Pediatr Health Care* 20(5):1783–1785, 2006.

Levin A: Retinal hemorrhages: advances in understanding, *Pediatr Clin North Am* 56(2): 333–344, 2009.

Lilard AS, Peterson J: The immediate impact of different types of television on young children's executive function, *Pediatrics* 128(4):644–649, 2011.

McClain N, Giardet R, Lahoti S, et al: Evaluation of sexual abuse in the pediatric patient, *J Pediatr Health Care* 14(3):93–102, 2000.

McEvoy M: Culture and spirituality as an integrated concept in pediatric care, *MCN Am J Matern Child Nurs* 28(1):39–43, 2003.

Mekonnen R, Noonan K, Rubin D: Achieving better healthcare outcomes for children in foster care, *Pediatr Clin North Am* 56(2): 405–415, 2009.

Mindell JA, Kuhn B, Lewin DS, et al: Behavioral treatment of bedtime problems and night wakings in infants and young children, *Sleep* 29(10):1263–1276, 2006.

Moore M, Meltzer LJ, Mindell JA: Bedtime problems and night waking in children, *Prim Care Clin Office Pract* 35(3):569–581, 2008.

Mraz MA: The physical manifestations of shaken baby syndrome, *J Forensic Nurs* 5(1):26–30, 2009.

National Center on Shaken Baby Syndrome: About the Center, n.d., www.dontshake.org/sbs.php?topNavID=2&subNavID=10.

National Institute on Deafness and Other Communication Disorders, National Institutes of Health: Stuttering, 2010, www.nidcd.nih.gov/health/voice/stutter.htm.

Nesti MMM, Goldbaum M: Infectious diseases and daycare and preschool education, *J Pediatr (Rio J)* 83(4):299–312, 2007.

Ostrov JM, Bishop CM: Preschoolers' aggression and parent-child conflict: a multi-informant and multimethod study, *J Experiment Child Psychol* 99(4):309–322, 2008.

Ostrov JM, Gentile DA, Crick NR: Media exposure, aggression and prosocial behavior during early childhood: a longitudinal study, *Soc Dev* 15(4):612–627, 2006.

Otten JJ, Hellwig JP, Meyers LD, editors: *Dietary reference intakes: the essential guide to nutrient requirements*, Washington, DC, 2006, National Academies Press.

Prasse JE, Kikano GE: Stuttering: an overview, *Am Fam Physician* 77(9):1271–1276, 2008.

Putnam FW: Ten year update review: child sexual abuse, *J Am Acad Child Adolesc Psychiatry* 42(3):269–278, 2003.

Reilly S, Wake M, Ukoumunne OC, et al: Predicting language outcomes at 4 years of age: findings from Early Language in Victoria Study, *Pediatrics* 126(6):1530–1537, 2010.

Sabella D: The role of the nurse in combating human trafficking, *AJN* 111(2):28–37, 2011.

Sharp HM, Hillenbrand K: Speech and language development and disorders in children, *Pediatr Clin North Am* 55(5):1159–1173, 2008.

Skouteris H, McCabe M, Swinburn B, et al: Healthy eating and obesity prevention for preschoolers: a randomized controlled trial, *BMC Public Health* 10:220, 2010.

Speraw S: Spiritual experiences of parents and caregivers who have children with disabilities or special needs, *Issues Mental Health Nurs* 27(2):213–230, 2006.

Squier W: The "shaken baby "syndrome: pathology and mechanisms, *Acta Neuropathol* 122(5):519–542, 2011.

Teng MS, Wang NW: Whooping cough: management and diagnosis of pertussis, *Pediatric Emergency Medicine Reports*, Health Reference Center Academic, March 1, 2011, www.find.galegroup.com.ezproxyhost.library.tmc.edu/gtx/start.do?prodId=HRCA&userGroupName=txshracd2509.

Tseng HF, Smith N, Marcy SM, et al: Incidence of herpes zoster among children vaccinated with varicella vaccine in a prepaid health care plan in the United States, 2002-2008, *Pediatr Infect Dis J* 28(12):1069–1072, 2009.

Trionfi G, Reese E: Good story: children with imaginary companions create richer narratives, *Child Dev* 4(80):1301–1313, 2009.

US Department of Agriculture: *Dietary Guidelines for Americans*, Washington, DC, 2010, US Government Printing Office, 2011, www.cnppusda.gov/dgas2010-policydocument.htm.

US Department of Health and Human Services, Administration on Children, Youth, and Families: *Child maltreatment, 2010*, Washington, DC, 2012, Government Printing Office, www.acf.hhs.gov/programs/cb/pubs/cm10/cm10.pdf.

Walls C: Shaken baby syndrome education: a role for nurse practitioners working with families of small children, *J Pediatr Health Care* 20(5):304–310, 2006.

Wells K: Substance abuse and child maltreatment, *Pediatr Clin North Am* 56(2):354–362, 2009.

Wood N, McIntyre P: Pertussis: review of epidemiology, diagnosis, management and prevention, *Paediatr Respir Rev* 9(3):201–212, 2008.

The School-Age Child and Family

Marilyn J. Hockenberry

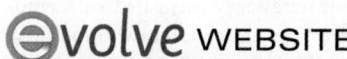 WEBSITE

http://evolve.elsevier.com/Perry/maternal

LEARNING OBJECTIVES

On completion of this chapter, the reader will be able to:

- Describe the physical, cognitive, and moral changes that take place during the middle childhood years.
- Describe ways to help a child develop a sense of accomplishment.
- Demonstrate an understanding of the changing interpersonal relationships of school-age children.
- Discuss the role of the peer group in the socialization of the school-age child.

- Discuss the role of schools in the development and socialization of the school-age child.
- Outline an appropriate health teaching plan for the school-age child.
- Plan a sex education session for a group of school-age children.
- Identify the causes and discuss the preventive aspects of injury in middle childhood.

PROMOTING OPTIMAL GROWTH AND DEVELOPMENT

The segment of the life span that extends from age 6 years to approximately age 12 years has a variety of labels, each of which describes an important characteristic of the period. These middle years are most often referred to as school-age or the school years. This period begins with entrance into the school environment, which has a significant impact on development and relationships.

Physiologically, the middle years begin with the shedding of the first deciduous tooth and end at puberty with the acquisition of the final permanent teeth (with the exception of the wisdom teeth). Before 5 or 6 years of age, children have progressed from helpless infants to sturdy, complicated individuals with an ability to communicate, conceptualize in a limited way, and become involved in complex social and motor behaviors. Physical growth is also rapid during the preschool-age years. In contrast, the period of middle childhood, between the rapid growth of early childhood and the prepubescent growth spurt, is a time of gradual growth and development with more even progress in both physical and emotional aspects.

Biologic Development

During middle childhood, growth in height and weight assumes a slower but steady pace as compared with the earlier years. Between ages 6 and 12 years, children grow an average of 5 cm (2 inches) per year to gain 30 to 60 cm (1-2 feet) in height and almost double their weight, increasing 2 to 3 kg (4.5-6.5 pounds) per year. The average 6-year-old child is about 116 cm (45.7 inches) tall and weighs about 21 kg (46 pounds); the average 12-year-old child is about 150 cm (59 inches) tall and weighs approximately 40 kg (88 pounds). During this period, girls and boys differ little in size, although boys tend to be slightly taller and somewhat heavier than girls. Toward the end of the school-age years, both boys and girls begin to increase in size although most girls begin to surpass boys in both height and weight, to the acute discomfort of both girls and boys.

Proportional Changes

School-age children are more graceful than they were as preschoolers, and they are steadier on their feet. Their body proportions take on a slimmer look, with longer legs, varying body proportion, and a lower center of gravity. Posture improves over that of the preschool period to facilitate locomotion and efficiency in using the arms and

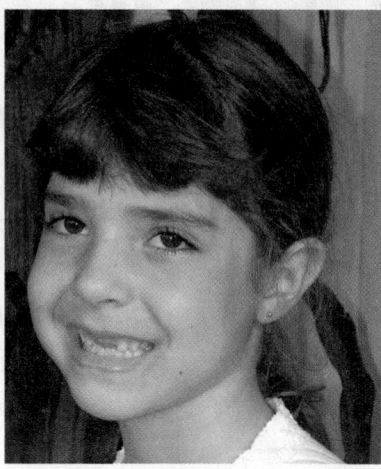

FIG 34-1 Middle childhood is the stage of development when deciduous teeth are shed.

trunk. These proportions make climbing, bicycle riding, and other activities easier. Fat gradually diminishes, and its distribution patterns change, contributing to the thinner appearance of children during the middle years.

Accompanying the skeletal lengthening and fat diminution is an increase in the percentage of body weight represented by muscle tissue. By the end of this age period, both boys and girls double their strength and physical capabilities and their steady and relatively consistent development of coordination increases their poise and skill. However, this increased strength can be misleading. Although strength increases, muscles are still functionally immature when compared with those of adolescents and they are more readily damaged by muscular injury caused by overuse.

The most pronounced changes that indicate increasing maturity in children are a decrease in head circumference in relation to standing height, a decrease in waist circumference in relation to height, and an increase in leg length in relation to height. These observations often provide a clue to a child's degree of physical maturity and have proved useful in predicting readiness for meeting the demands of school. There appears to be a correlation between physical indications of maturity and success in school.

Specific physiologic and anatomic characteristics are typical of children in middle childhood. Facial proportions change as the face grows faster in relation to the remainder of the cranium. The skull and brain grow very slowly during this period and increase little in size. Because all of the primary (deciduous) teeth are lost during this age span, middle childhood is sometimes known as the age of the loose tooth (Fig. 34-1). The early years of middle childhood, when the new secondary (permanent) teeth appear too large for the face, are known as the ugly duckling stage.

Maturation of Systems

Maturity of the gastrointestinal system is reflected in fewer stomach upsets; better maintenance of blood glucose levels; and an increased stomach capacity, which permits retention of food for longer periods. School-age children do not need to be fed as promptly or as frequently as preschool-age children. Caloric needs are less than they were in the preschool years.

Physical maturation is evident in other body tissues and organs. Bladder capacity, although differing widely among individual children, is generally greater in girls than in boys. The heart grows more slowly during the middle years and is smaller in relation to the rest of the body than at any other period of life. Heart and respiratory

rates steadily decrease, and blood pressure increases from ages 6 to 12 years (see Appendix C).

The immune system becomes more competent in its ability to localize infections and to produce an antibody-antigen response. However, children have several infections in the first 1 to 2 years of school because of increased exposure to other children.

Bones continue to ossify throughout childhood but yield to pressure and muscle pulls more readily than with mature bones. Children need ample opportunity to move around, but they should observe caution in carrying heavy loads. For example, they should shift books or tote bags from one arm to the other. Backpacks distribute weight more evenly than tote bags.

Wider differences between children are observed at the end of middle childhood than at the beginning. These differences become increasingly apparent and, if they are extreme or unique, may create emotional problems. The associated characteristics of height and weight relationships, rapid or slow growth, and other important features of development should be explained to children and their families. Physical maturity is not necessarily correlated with emotional and social maturity. Seven-year-old children who look like 10-year-old children will, in fact, think and act like 7-year-old children. To expect behaviors appropriate for the older age is unrealistic and can be detrimental to their development of competence and self-esteem. Conversely, to treat 10-year-old children who look young physically as though they were younger is an equal disservice to them.

Prepubescence

Preadolescence is the period of approximately 2 years that begins at the end of middle childhood and ends with the thirteenth birthday. Because puberty signals the beginning of the development of secondary sex characteristics, prepubescence typically occurs during preadolescence.

Toward the end of middle childhood, the discrepancies in growth and maturation between boys and girls become apparent. On the average, there is a difference of approximately 2 years between girls and boys in the age of onset of pubescence. This is a period of rapid growth in height and weight, especially for girls.

There is no universal age at which children assume the characteristics of prepubescence. The first physiologic signs appear at about 9 years of age (particularly in girls) and are usually clearly evident in 11- to 12-year-old children. Although preadolescent children do not want to be different, variability in physical growth and physiologic changes among children of the same sex and between the two sexes is often striking at this time. This variability, especially in relation to the onset of secondary sexual characteristics, is of great concern to preadolescents. Either early or late appearance of these characteristics is a source of embarrassment and uneasiness to both sexes.

Preadolescence is a period of considerable overlapping of developmental characteristics of both middle childhood and early adolescence. However, several unique characteristics set this period apart from others. Generally, puberty begins at 10 years in girls and 12 years in boys, but it can be normal for either sex after the age of 8 years. Boys experience little visible sexual maturation during preadolescence.

Psychosocial Development
Developing a Sense of Industry (Erikson)

Freud described middle childhood as the latency period, a time of tranquility between the Oedipal phase of early childhood and the eroticism of adolescence. During this time, children experience

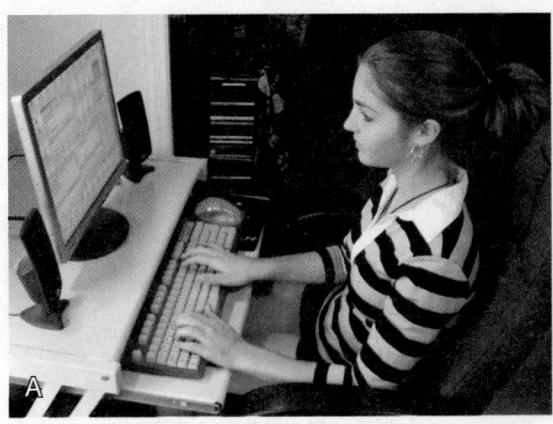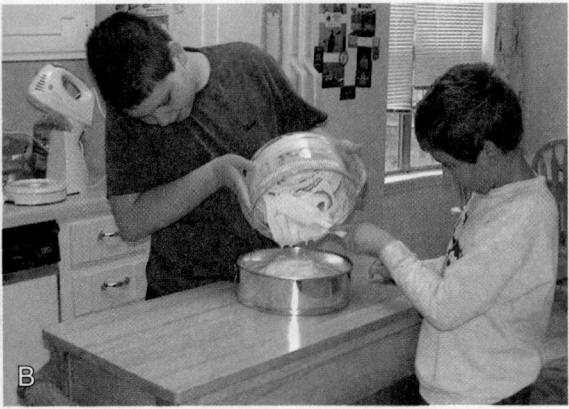

FIG 34-2 School-age children are motivated to complete tasks. **A,** Working alone. **B,** Working with others.

relationships with same-sex peers following the indifference of earlier years and preceding the heterosexual fascination that occurs for most boys and girls in puberty.

Successful mastery of Erikson's first three stages of psychosocial development is important in terms of development of a healthy personality. Successful completion of these stages requires a loving environment within a stable family unit. These experiences prepare the child to engage in experiences and relationships beyond the intimate family group.

A sense of industry or a stage of accomplishment is achieved somewhere between age 6 years and adolescence. School-age children are eager to develop skills and participate in meaningful and socially useful work. They acquire a sense of personal and interpersonal competence; receive the systematic instruction prescribed by their individual cultures; and develop the skills needed to become useful, contributing members of their social communities.

Interests expand in the middle years, and with a growing sense of independence, children want to engage in tasks that can be carried through to completion (Fig. 34-2). They gain satisfaction from independent behavior in exploring and manipulating their environment and from interaction with peers. Often the acquisition of skills provides a way to achieve success in social activities. Reinforcement in the form of grades, material rewards, additional privileges, and recognition provides encouragement and stimulation.

A sense of accomplishment also involves the ability to cooperate, to compete with others, and to cope effectively with people. Middle childhood is the time when children learn the value of doing things with others and the benefits derived from division of labor in the accomplishment of goals. Peer approval is a strong motivating power.

The danger inherent in this period of development is the occurrence of situations that might result in a sense of inferiority. Children with physical and mental limitations may be at a disadvantage in the acquisition of certain skills. When the reward structure is based on evidence of mastery, children who are incapable of developing these skills risk feeling inadequate and inferior. Even children without chronic disabilities may experience feelings of inadequacy in some areas. No child is able to do everything well, and children must learn that they will not be able to master every skill they attempt. All children, even children who usually have positive attitudes toward work and their own abilities, will feel some degree of inferiority when they encounter specific skills that they cannot master.

Children need and want real achievement. Children achieve a sense of industry when they have access to tasks that need to be done and they are able to complete the tasks well despite individual differences in their innate capacities and emotional development.

Cognitive Development (Piaget)

When children enter the school years, they begin to acquire the ability to relate a series of events to mental representations that can be expressed both verbally and symbolically. This is the stage Piaget describes as concrete operations, when children are able to use thought processes to experience events and actions. The rigid, egocentric view of the preschool years is replaced by mental processes that allow children to see things from another's point of view.

During this stage, children develop an understanding of relationships between things and ideas. They progress from making judgments based on what they see (perceptual thinking) to making judgments based on what they reason (conceptual thinking). They are able to master symbols and to use their memories of past experiences to evaluate and interpret the present.

One cognitive task of school-age children is mastering the concept of conservation (Fig. 34-3). At an early age (≈5-7 years), children grasp the concept of reversibility of numbers as a basis for simple mathematics problems (e.g., $2 + 4 = 6$ and $6 - 4 = 2$). They learn that simply altering their arrangement in space does not change certain properties of the environment, and they are able to resist perceptual cues that suggest alterations in the physical state of an object. For example, they recognize that changing the shape of a substance such as a lump of clay does not alter its total mass. They no longer perceive a tall, thin glass of water as containing a greater volume than a short, wide glass; they can distinguish between the weight of items regardless of their size. They recognize that size is not necessarily related to weight or volume. There is a developmental sequence in children's capacity to conserve matter. Conservation of mass usually is accomplished first, weight some time later, and volume last.

School-age children also develop classification skills. They can group and sort objects according to the attributes they share, place things in a sensible and logical order, and hold a concept in mind while making decisions based on that concept. Another characteristic of middle childhood is that children derive enjoyment from classifying and ordering their environment. They become occupied with collections of objects, such as stickers, shells, dolls, cars, cards, and stuffed animals. They may even begin to order friends and relationships (e.g., best friend, second-best friend).

They develop the ability to understand relational terms and concepts, such as bigger and smaller; darker and paler; heavier and lighter; to the right of and to the left of; and more than and less than.

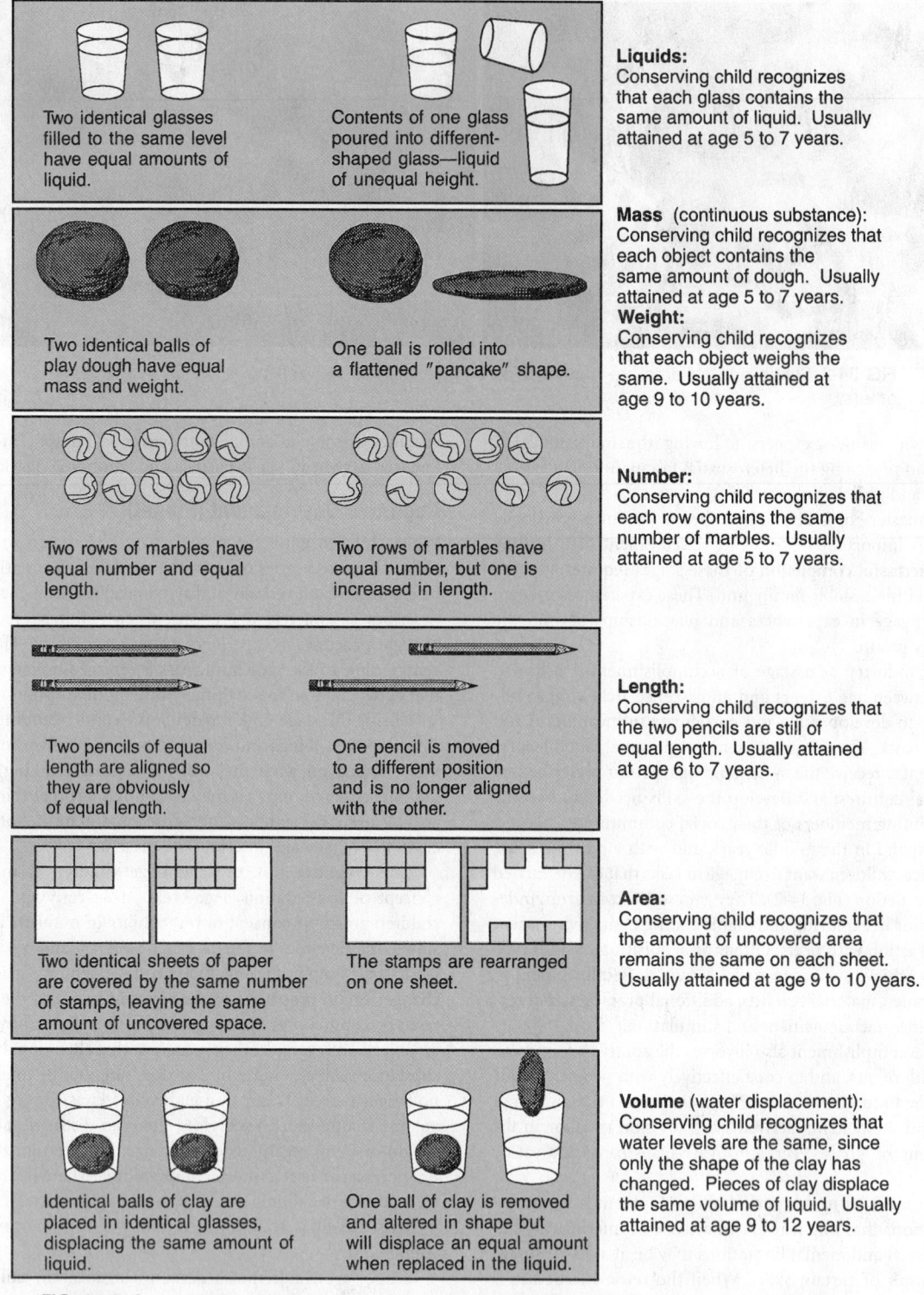

Liquids:
Conserving child recognizes that each glass contains the same amount of liquid. Usually attained at age 5 to 7 years.

Two identical glasses filled to the same level have equal amounts of liquid.

Contents of one glass poured into different-shaped glass—liquid of unequal height.

Mass (continuous substance):
Conserving child recognizes that each object contains the same amount of dough. Usually attained at age 5 to 7 years.
Weight:
Conserving child recognizes that each object weighs the same. Usually attained at age 9 to 10 years.

Two identical balls of play dough have equal mass and weight.

One ball is rolled into a flattened "pancake" shape.

Number:
Conserving child recognizes that each row contains the same number of marbles. Usually attained at age 5 to 7 years.

Two rows of marbles have equal number and equal length.

Two rows of marbles have equal number, but one is increased in length.

Length:
Conserving child recognizes that the two pencils are still of equal length. Usually attained at age 6 to 7 years.

Two pencils of equal length are aligned so they are obviously of equal length.

One pencil is moved to a different position and is no longer aligned with the other.

Area:
Conserving child recognizes that the amount of uncovered area remains the same on each sheet. Usually attained at age 9 to 10 years.

Two identical sheets of paper are covered by the same number of stamps, leaving the same amount of uncovered space.

The stamps are rearranged on one sheet.

Volume (water displacement):
Conserving child recognizes that water levels are the same, since only the shape of the clay has changed. Pieces of clay displace the same volume of liquid. Usually attained at age 9 to 12 years.

Identical balls of clay are placed in identical glasses, displacing the same amount of liquid.

One ball of clay is removed and altered in shape but will displace an equal amount when replaced in the liquid.

FIG 34-3 Common examples that demonstrate the child's ability to conserve (ages are only approximate).

They view family relationships in terms of reciprocal roles (e.g., to be a brother, one must have a sibling).

School-age children learn the alphabet and the world of symbols called *words*, which can be arranged in terms of structure and their relationship to the alphabet. They learn to tell time, to see the relationship of events in time (history) and places in space (geography), and to combine time and space relationships (geology and astronomy).

The ability to read is acquired during the school years and becomes the most significant and valuable tool for independent inquiry. Children's capacity to explore, imagine, and expand their knowledge is enhanced by reading.

Moral Development (Kohlberg)

As children move from egocentrism to more logical patterns of thought, they also move through stages in the development of conscience and moral standards. Young children do not believe that standards of behavior come from within themselves but, instead, that rules are established and set down by others. During the preschool years, children adopt and internalize the moral values of their parents. They learn standards for acceptable behavior, act according to these standards, and feel guilty when they violate them. Although children 6 or 7 years of age know the rules and behaviors expected of them, they do not understand the reasons behind them. Rewards and punishments guide their judgment; a "bad act" is one that breaks a rule or causes harm. Young children believe that what other people tell them to do is right and that what they themselves think is wrong. Consequently, children 6 or 7 years old may interpret accidents or misfortunes as punishment for "bad" acts.

Older school-age children are able to judge an act by the intentions that prompted it rather than just its consequences. Rules and judgments become less absolute and authoritarian and begin to be founded on the needs and desires of others. For older children, a rule violation is likely to be viewed in relation to the total context in which it appears. The situation, as well as the morality of the rule itself, influences reactions. Although younger children judge an act only according to whether it is right or wrong, older children take into account different points of view. They are able to understand and accept the concept of treating others as they would like to be treated.

Spiritual Development

Children at this age think in concrete terms but are avid learners and have a great desire to learn about their God. They picture God as human and use adjectives such as "loving" and "helping" to describe their deity. They are fascinated by the concepts of hell and heaven, with a developing conscience and concern about rules. They may fear going to hell for misbehavior. School-age children want and expect to be punished for misbehavior and, when given the option, tend to choose a punishment that "fits the crime." However, they may view illness or injury as a punishment for a real or imagined misdeed. The beliefs and ideals of family and religious persons are more influential than those of their peers in matters of faith.

School-age children begin to learn the difference between the natural and the supernatural but have difficulty understanding symbols. Consequently, religious concepts must be presented to them in concrete terms. Prayer or other religious rituals comfort them, and if these activities are a part of their daily lives, they can help them cope with threatening situations. Their petitions to their God in prayers tend to be for tangible rewards. Although younger children expect their prayers to be answered, as they get older, they begin to recognize that this does not always occur and they become less concerned when their prayers are not answered. They are able to discuss their feelings about their faith and how it relates to their lives (see Cultural Competence box).

Social Development

One of the most important socializing agents in the school-age years is the peer group. In addition to parents and schools, the peer group conveys a substantial amount of information to its members. Peer groups have a culture of their own with secrets, traditions, and codes of ethics that promote feelings of solidarity and detachment from adults. Through peer relationships, children learn how to deal with dominance and hostility, how to relate to persons in positions of

---

🌐 CULTURAL COMPETENCE

Religious Orientation

Many schools and communities have a Judeo-Christian orientation toward prayer, holidays, and values. This may result in conflict and discomfort for children of other religious or ethnic groups. Sensitivity must be exercised so as not to offend and confuse children from other religious backgrounds, such as the Buddhist, Hindu, and Muslim faiths, and those with no religious backgrounds.

---

leadership and authority, and how to explore ideas and the physical environment.

Peer-group identification is an important factor in gaining independence from parents. The aid and support of the group provide children with enough security to risk the moderate parental rejection brought about by small victories in the development of independence.

A child's concept of the appropriate gender role is also influenced by relationships with peers. During the early school years, few gender differences exist in the play experiences of children. Both girls and boys share games and other activities. However, in the later school years, the differences in the play of boys and girls becomes more marked.

Social Relationships and Cooperation

Daily relationships with peers provide important social interactions for school-age children. For the first time, children join group activities with unrestrained enthusiasm and steady participation. Previous interactions were limited to short periods under considerable adult supervision. With increased skills and wider opportunities, children become involved with one or more peer groups in which they can gain status as respected members.

Valuable lessons are learned from daily interaction with age mates. First, children learn to appreciate the numerous and varied points of view that are represented in the peer group. As children interact with peers who see the world in ways that are somewhat different from their own, they become aware of the limits of their own point of view. Because age mates are peers and are not forced to accept each other's ideas as they are expected to accept those of adults, other children have a significant influence on decreasing the egocentric outlook of the child. Consequently, children learn to argue, persuade, bargain, cooperate, and compromise to maintain friendships.

Second, children become increasingly sensitive to the social norms and pressures of the peer group. The peer group establishes standards for acceptance and rejection, and children are often willing to modify their behavior to be accepted by the group. The need for peer approval becomes a powerful influence toward conformity. Children learn to dress, talk, and behave in a manner acceptable to the group. A variety of roles, such as class joker or class hero, may be assumed by individual children to gain approval from the group.

Third, the interaction among peers leads to the formation of intimate friendships between same-sex peers. The school-age period is the time when children have "best friends" with whom they share secrets, private jokes, and adventures; they come to one another's aid in times of trouble. In the course of these friendships, children also fight, threaten each other, break up, and reunite. These relationships, in which the child experiences love and closeness with a peer, may be important as a foundation for relationships in adulthood (Fig. 34-4).

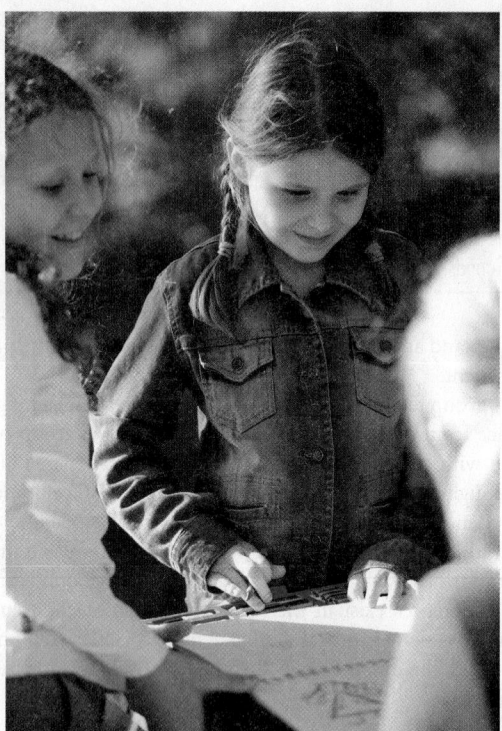

FIG 34-4 School-age children enjoy engaging in activities with a "best friend." (© 2011 Photos.com, a division of Getty Images. All rights reserved.)

Clubs and Peer Groups. One of the outstanding characteristics of middle childhood is the formation of formalized groups, or clubs. A prominent feature of these groups is the rigid rules imposed on the members. There is exclusiveness in the selection of persons who have the privilege of joining. Acceptance in the group is often determined on a pass-fail basis according to social or behavioral criteria. Conformity is the core of the group structure. There are often secret codes, shared interests, and special modes of dress, and each child must abide by a standard of behavior established by the members. Conforming to the rules provides children with feelings of security and relieves them of the responsibility of making decisions. By merging their identities with those of their peers, children are able to move from the family group to an outside group as a step toward seeking further independence. Peer groups and clubs allow children to substitute conformity to a peer group for conformity to a family at a time when children are still too insecure to function independently.

During the early school years, groups are usually small and loosely organized, with changing membership and no formal structure. The clubs and groups usually do not display elements of cooperation and order that are seen in groups of older children. In general, girls' groups are less formalized than boys' are, and although there may be a mixture of both sexes in the early school years, the groups of later school years are composed predominantly of children of the same sex. Common interests are the basis around which the group is structured.

Peer-group identification and association are essential to a child's socialization. Poor relationships with peers and a lack of group identification can contribute to bullying. Bullying is any recurring activity that intends to cause harm, distress, or control toward another in which there is a perceived imbalance of power between the aggressor(s) and the victim (Lamb, Pepler, and Craig, 2009).

Although bullying can occur in any setting, it most often occurs at school during unstructured times such as recess (Arseneault, Bowes, and Shakoor, 2010). Children who are targeted for bullying often have internalizing characteristics such as withdrawal, anxiety, depression, low self-esteem, and reduced assertiveness that may make them an easy target for bullying (Arseneault, Bowes, and Shakoor, 2010). Bullies are generally defiant toward adults, antisocial, and likely to break school rules. They have dominant personalities, may come from homes where parental involvement and nurturing are lacking, and may experience or witness violence or abuse at home (Bowes, Arseneault, Maughan, et al., 2009). Boys who bully tend to use physical force, referred to as *direct bullying*, but girls usually use indirect bullying methods, such as exclusion, gossip, or rumors (Arseneault, Bowes, and Shakoor, 2010). Cyberbullying is a new form of bullying and involves the use of cellular telephones, digital cameras, or social networking Internet sites to cause distress on an individual (American Academy of Pediatrics [AAP] Committee on Injury, Violence, and Poison Prevention, 2009).

The long-term consequences of bullying are significant. Chronic bullies seem to continue their behaviors into adulthood, negatively influencing their ability to develop and maintain relationships. Victims of bullying often experience psychologic distress such as worry, sadness, anxiety, depression, and nightmares and can have increased self-harm behaviors, social isolation, suicidal ideation, and violent behaviors (Arseneault, Bowes, and Shakoor, 2010). School personnel play an important role in implementing antibullying interventions in schools; however, research has recognized that involving the whole family in antibullying programs greatly increases success (Arseneault, Bowes, and Shakoor, 2010).

There are also dangers in peer-group attachments that are too strong. Peer pressures force some children to take risks or engage in behaviors that are against their better judgment. A child's membership in a gang is associated with marked increases in serious delinquent behavior (Fisher, Montgomery, and Gardner, 2008). Peer-group activities that result in unlawful or criminal gang violence are increasing in the United States. An integration of family-centered and school-based programs is needed to reduce the influences for children to become affiliated with gangs.

Relationships with Families

Although the peer group is influential and necessary for normal child development, parents are the primary influence in shaping their children's personalities, setting standards for behavior, and establishing value systems. Family values usually take precedence over peer value systems. Although children may appear to reject parental values while testing the new values of the peer group, ultimately they retain and incorporate into their own value systems the parental values they have found to be of worth.

In the middle school years, children want to spend more time in the company of peers and they often prefer peer-group activities to family activities. This can be disturbing to parents. Children become intolerant and critical of their parents, especially when their parents' ways deviate from those of the group. They discover that parents can be wrong, and they begin to question the knowledge and authority of their parents, who were previously considered to be all-knowing and all-powerful.

Although increased independence is the goal of middle childhood, children are not prepared to abandon all parental control. They need and want restrictions placed on their behavior, and they are not prepared to cope with all of the problems of their expanding environment. They feel more secure knowing there is an authority figure to implement controls and restrictions. Children may complain loudly about restrictions and try to break down parental barriers, but they are uneasy if they succeed in doing so. They respect adults who prevent them from acting on every urge. Children view this behavior as an expression of love and concern for their welfare.

Children also need their parents to be adults, not friends. Sometimes parents, hurt by their children's rejection, attempt to maintain their love and gratitude by assuming the role of "pals." Children need the stable, secure strength provided by mature adults to whom they can turn during troubled relationships with peers or stressful changes in their world. With a secure base in a loving family, children are able to develop the self-confidence and maturity needed to break loose from the group and stand independently.

Play

Play takes on new dimensions that reflect a new stage of development in the school years. Play involves increased physical skill, intellectual ability, and fantasy. In addition, children develop a sense of belonging to a team or club by forming groups and cliques.

Rules and Rituals. The need for conformity in middle childhood is strongly manifested in the activities and games of school-age children. In the preschool years, children's games were either invented for them or played in the company of a friend or an adult. Now children begin to see the need for rules, and their games have fixed and unvarying rules that may be bizarre and extraordinarily rigid. Part of the enjoyment of the game is knowing the rules, because knowing means belonging. Conformity and ritual permeate their play and are also evident in their behavior and language. Childhood is full of chants and taunts, such as: "Eeny, meeny, miney, mo," "Last one is a rotten egg," and "Step on a crack, break your mother's back." Children derive a sense of pleasure and power from such sayings, which have been handed down with few changes through generations.

Team Play. A more complex form of play that evolves from the need for peer interaction is team games and sports. A referee, umpire, or person of authority may be required so that the rules can be followed more accurately. Team play teaches children to modify or exchange personal goals for goals of the group; it also teaches them that division of labor is an effective strategy for attaining a goal. Children learn about competition and the importance of winning—an attribute highly valued in the United States.

Team play can also contribute to children's social, intellectual, and skill growth. Children work hard to develop the skills needed to become team members, to improve their contribution to the group, and to anticipate the consequences of their behavior for the group. Team play helps stimulate cognitive growth because children are called on to learn many complex rules, make judgments about those rules, plan strategies, and assess the strengths and weaknesses of members of their own team and members of the opposing team.

Quiet Games and Activities. Although play at this age is highly active, school-age children also enjoy quiet and solitary activities. The middle years are the time for collections, which constitute another ritual. Young school-age children's collections are an odd assortment of unrelated objects in messy, disorganized piles. Collections of later school years are more orderly, selective, and organized in scrapbooks, on shelves, or in boxes.

School-age children become fascinated with complex board, card, or computer games that they can play alone, with a best friend, or with a group. As in all games, adherence to the rules is fanatic. Disagreements over rules can cause much discussion and argument but are easily resolved by reading the rules of the game.

The newly acquired skill of reading becomes increasingly satisfying as school-age children expand their knowledge of the world

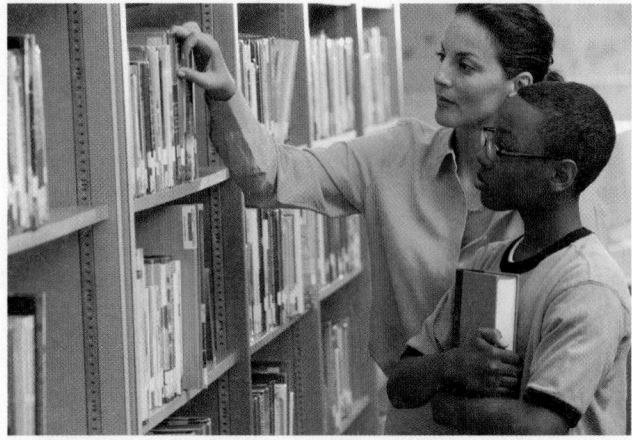

FIG 34-5 Selecting a book with the assistance of an adult. (© 2011 Photos.com, a division of Getty Images. All rights reserved.)

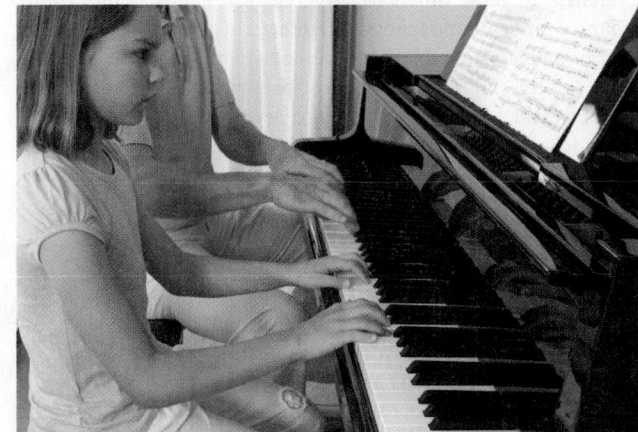

FIG 34-6 School-age children take pride in learning new skills. (© 2011 Photos.com, a division of Getty Images. All rights reserved.)

through books (Fig. 34-5). School-age children never tire of stories and, as with preschool children, love to have stories read aloud. They also enjoy sewing, cooking, carpentry, gardening, and creative activities such as painting. Many creative skills such as music and art, as well as athletic skills such as swimming, karate, dancing, and skating, are learned during these years and continue to be enjoyed into adolescence and adulthood (Fig. 34-6).

Development of a Self-Concept

The term *self-concept* refers to a conscious awareness of self-perceptions, such as one's physical characteristics, abilities, values, self-ideals and expectancy, and idea of self in relation to others. It also includes one's body image, sexuality, and self-esteem. Although primary caregivers continue to exert influence on children's self-evaluation, the opinions of peers and teachers provide valuable input during middle childhood. With the emphasis on skill building and broadened social relationships, children are continually engaged in the process of self-evaluation.

Significant adults can often manage to unobtrusively manipulate the environment so that children experience success. Each small success increases a child's self-image. The more positive children feel about themselves, the more confident they will be in trying for success in the future. All children profit from feeling that they are in some way special to a significant adult. A positive self-concept makes children feel likeable, worthwhile, and capable of significant contributions. These feelings lead to self-respect, self-confidence, and happiness. Negative feelings lead to self-doubt.

Development of a Body Image

School-age children have a relatively accurate and positive perception of their physical selves, but in general, they like their physical selves less as they grow older. The head appears to be the most important part of the school-age child's perceived image of self, with hair and eye color the characteristics used most frequently to describe the physical self.

Body image is influenced, but not solely determined, by significant others. The number of significant others who influence children's perception of themselves increases with age. Children are acutely aware of their own bodies, the bodies of their peers, and those of adults. They are also aware of deviations from the norm. Physical impairments, such as hearing or visual defects, ears that "stick out," or birthmarks, assume great importance. Increasing awareness of these differences, especially when accompanied by unkind comments and taunts from others, may cause a child to feel inferior and less desirable. This is especially true if the defect interferes with the child's ability to participate in games and activities.

Table 34-1 summarizes the major developmental achievements of the school-age years.

Coping with Concerns Related to Normal Growth and Development

School Experience

School serves as the agent for transmitting the values of society to each succeeding generation of children. School is also the setting for relationships with peers. After the family, schools are the second most important socializing agent in the lives of children.

Entrance into school causes a sharp break in the structure of the child's world. For many children, it is their first experience in conforming to a group pattern imposed by an adult who is not a parent and who has responsibility for too many children to be constantly aware of each child as an individual. Children want to go to school and usually adapt to the new conditions with little difficulty. Successful adjustment is related to the child's physical and emotional maturity and the parent's readiness to accept the separation associated with school entrance. Unfortunately, some parents express their unconscious attempts to delay the child's maturity by clinging behavior, particularly with their youngest child.

By the time they enter school, most children have a fairly realistic concept of what school involves. They receive information regarding the role of a student from parents, siblings, playmates, and the media. In addition, most children have had some experience with day care, preschool, or kindergarten. Middle-class children have fewer adjustments to make and less to learn about expected behavior because schools tend to reflect dominant middle-class customs and values. If the child has attended a preschool program, the focus of the preschool program also affects the child's adjustment. Some preschool programs provide custodial care only, but others emphasize emotional, social, and intellectual development.

Classmates have a significant impact on the socialization of children. School is the first time that most children become members of a large group of individuals their own age. Peer relationships become increasingly important and influential as children proceed through school. The specific influence exerted by the peer group depends on the background, interests, and abilities of the individual child.

Teachers. Children respond best to teachers who possess the characteristics of a warm, loving parent. Teachers in the early grades perform many of the activities formerly assumed by the parent, such as recognizing the child's personal needs (e.g., the need to go to the bathroom, need for help with clothing) and helping to develop their social behavior (e.g., manners).

Teachers, like parents, are concerned about the child's psychologic and emotional welfare. Although the functions of teachers and parents differ, both place constraints on behavior and both are in a position to enforce standards of conduct. However, the teacher's primary responsibility involves stimulating and guiding children's intellectual development, as opposed to providing for their physical welfare beyond the school setting.

TABLE 34-1 GROWTH AND DEVELOPMENT DURING THE SCHOOL-AGE YEARS

PHYSICAL AND MOTOR	MENTAL	ADAPTIVE	PERSONAL-SOCIAL
Age 6 Years			
Height and weight gain continues slowly	Develops concept of numbers	At table, uses knife to spread butter or jam on bread	Can share and cooperate better
Weight, 16-26.3 kg (35.5-58 pounds)	Can count 13 pennies	At play, cuts, folds, pastes paper; sews crudely if needle is threaded	Has great need for children of own age
Height, 106.7-122 cm (42-48 inches)	Knows whether it is morning or afternoon		Will cheat to win
Central mandibular incisors erupt	Defines common objects such as fork and chair in terms of their use	Takes bath without supervision; performs bedtime activities alone	Often engages in rough play
Loses first tooth	Obeys three commands in succession	Reads from memory; enjoys oral spelling game	Often jealous of younger brother or sister
Gradual increase in dexterity	Knows right and left hands	Likes table games, checkers, simple card games	Does what adults are seen doing
Active age; constant activity	Says which is pretty and which is ugly of a series of drawings of faces	Giggles a lot	May have occasional temper tantrums
Often returns to finger feeding	Describes the objects in a picture rather than simply enumerating them	Sometimes steals money or attractive items	Is a boaster
More aware of hand as a tool	Attends first grade	Has difficulty owning up to misdeeds	Is more independent, probably an influence of school
Likes to draw, print, color		Tries out own abilities	Has own way of doing things
Vision reaches maturity			Increases socialization

TABLE 34-1 GROWTH AND DEVELOPMENT DURING THE SCHOOL-AGE YEARS—cont'd

PHYSICAL AND MOTOR	MENTAL	ADAPTIVE	PERSONAL-SOCIAL
Age 7 Years			
Begins to grow at least 5 cm (2 inches) in height per year	Notices that certain items are missing from pictures	Uses table knife for cutting meat; may need help with tough or difficult pieces	Is becoming a real member of the family group
Weight, 17.7-30 kg (39-66.5 pounds)	Can copy a diamond	Brushes and combs hair acceptably without help	Takes part in group play
Height, 112-130 cm (44-51 inches)	Repeats three numbers backward	Likes to help and have a choice	Boys prefer playing with boys; girls prefer playing with girls
Maxillary central incisors and lateral mandibular incisors erupt	Develops concept of time; reads ordinary clock or watch correctly to nearest quarter hour; uses clock for practical purposes	Is less resistant and stubborn	Spends a lot of time alone; does not require a lot of companionship
More cautious in approaches to new performances	Attends second grade		
Repeats performances to master them	More mechanical in reading; often does not stop at the end of a sentence; skips words such as "it," "the," and "he"		
Jaw begins to expand to accommodate permanent teeth			
Ages 8 to 9 Years			
Continues to gain 5 cm (2 inches) in height per year	Gives similarities and differences between two things from memory	Makes use of common tools such as hammer, saw, screwdriver	Is easy to get along with at home
Weight, 19.5-39.5 kg (43-87 pounds)	Counts backward from 20 to 1; understands concept of reversibility	Uses household and sewing utensils	Likes the reward system
Height, 117-142 cm (46-56 inches)	Repeats days of the week and months in order; knows the date	Helps with routine household tasks such as dusting, sweeping	Dramatizes
Lateral incisors (maxillary) and mandibular cuspids erupt	Describes common objects in detail, not merely their use	Assumes responsibility for share of household chores	Is more sociable
Movement fluid; often graceful and poised	Makes change out of a quarter	Looks after all of own needs at table	Is better behaved
Always on the go; jumps, chases, skips	Attends third and fourth grades	Buys useful articles; exercises some choice in making purchases	Is interested in boy-girl relationships but will not admit it
Increased smoothness and speed in fine motor control; uses cursive writing	Reads more; may plan to wake up early just to read	Runs useful errands	Goes about home and community freely, alone or with friends
Dresses self completely	Reads classic books but also enjoys comics	Likes pictorial magazines	Likes to compete and play games
Likely to overdo; hard to quiet down after recess	More aware of time; can be relied on to get to school on time	Likes school; wants to answer all the questions	Shows preference in friends and groups
More limber; bones grow faster than ligaments	Can grasp concepts of parts and whole (fractions)	Is afraid of failing a grade; is ashamed of bad grades	Plays mostly with groups of own sex but is beginning to mix
	Understands concepts of space, cause and effect, nesting (puzzles), conservation (permanence of mass and volume)	Is more critical of self	Develops modesty
	Classifies objects by more than one quality; has collections	Takes music and sport lessons	Compares self with others
	Produces simple paintings or drawings		Enjoys organizations, clubs, and group sports
Ages 10 to 12 Years			
Weight, 24.5-58 kg (54-128 pounds)	Writes brief stories	Makes useful tools or does easy repair work	Loves friends; talks about them constantly
Height, 127-162.5 cm (50-64 inches)	Attends fifth to seventh grades	Cooks or sews in small way	Chooses friends more selectively; may have a "best friend"
Posture is more similar to an adult's; will overcome lordosis	Writes occasional short letters to friends or relatives on own initiative	Raises pets	Enjoys conversation
Remainder of teeth will erupt and tend toward full development (except wisdom teeth)	Uses telephone for practical purposes	Washes and dries own hair; is responsible for a thorough job of cleaning hair but may need reminding to do so	Develops beginning interest in opposite sex
Girls—Pubescent changes may begin to appear; body lines soften and round out	Responds to magazine, radio, or other advertising	Is sometimes left alone at home for an hour or so	Is more diplomatic
Boys—Slow growth in height and rapid weight gain; may become obese in this period	Reads for practical information or own enjoyment—stories or library books of adventure or romance, animal stories	Is successful in looking after own needs or those of other children left in his or her care	Likes family; family really has meaning
			Likes mother and wants to please her in many ways
			Demonstrates affection
			Likes father, who is admired and may be idolized
			Respects parents

Teachers serve as models that children try to emulate. Children seek their teachers' approval and avoid their disapproval. The teacher is a significant person in the life of the early school-age child, and hero worship of a teacher may extend into late childhood and pre-adolescence. Teachers who make supportive statements that reassure or commend children, use accepting and clarifying statements that help children refine ideas and feelings, and provide assistance that aids children with their own problem solving contribute to the development of a positive self-concept in the school-age child.

Parents. Parents share responsibility for helping children achieve their maximal potential. Parents can supplement the school program in numerous ways (see Family-Centered Care box). Cultivating responsibility is the goal of parental assistance. Being responsible for schoolwork helps children learn to keep promises, meet deadlines, and succeed at their jobs as adults. Responsible children may occasionally ask for help (e.g., with a spelling list), but usually they prefer to think through their work by themselves. Excessive pressure or lack of encouragement from parents may inhibit the development of these desirable traits.

Latchkey Children

The term latchkey children is used to describe children who are left to care for themselves before or after school without the supervision of an adult. The large numbers of single-parent families and working mothers, together with the lack of available child care, have created a stress-provoking situation for many school-age children. Some of these children may have a chronic illness as well.

Inadequate adult supervision after school leaves children at greater risk for injury and delinquent behavior. In some instances, outside activities are curtailed and relationships with peers may be significantly diminished. Latchkey children may feel more lonely, isolated, and fearful than children who have someone to care for them. To cope with their fears and anxieties while alone, these children may devise strategies such as hiding, playing the television at a loud volume, or using pets for comfort.

Many communities and persons concerned about the welfare of latchkey children are trying to help these children and their parents deal with this potentially serious problem. Some communities and employers have implemented after-school programs or telephone "hotlines" that provide check-in and reassurance for children. Nurses should be aware of these community services and encourage parents to teach self-help skills to these children.

Limit Setting and Discipline

Many factors influence the amount and manner of discipline and limit setting imposed on school-age children. Some of these factors are the parents' psychosocial maturity, the parents' childhood and childrearing experiences, the children's temperament, the context of the children's misconduct, and the children's response to rewards and punishments. When children develop an ability to see a situation from another's point of view, they are also able to understand the effects of their reactions on others and themselves.

Discipline should take place in a positive, supportive environment with the use of strategies to instruct and guide desired behaviors and eliminate undesired behaviors (Knox, 2010). Reasoning is an effective technique for middle school–age children. With advancing cognitive skills, they are able to benefit from more complex disciplinary strategies. For example, withholding privileges, requiring compensation, imposing penalties, and contracting can be used with great success. Problem solving is the best approach to limit setting, and children themselves can be included in the process of determining appropriate disciplinary measures.

FAMILY-CENTERED CARE
Helping Children in School

General Guidelines

- Be supportive—provide companionship; share ideas and thoughts.
- Be positive—every child should experience some success each day.
- Share an interest in reading—use the library; discuss books they are reading.
- Support and encourage activity rather than passivity.
- Encourage originality—help children make their own projects from discarded articles or other available materials.
- Foster the development of hobbies and collections.
- Encourage children to wonder and reflect during free time.
- Encourage family experiences and trips to places of interest.
- Encourage questions—help children discover sources for information or places to explore and investigate.
- Stimulate creative thinking and problem solving—help children try out new solutions to problems without fear of making mistakes.
- Use rewards rather than punishment.

Specific Guidelines

- Meet the teacher at the beginning of school, and plan to visit the school to see what is taught and expected.
- Send the child to school every day. Teachers are concerned when parents make other plans for their children; it conveys the impression that school is unimportant.
- Demonstrate an interest in what the child is learning.
- Demonstrate an interest in content and growth more than in grades.
- Make it clear to the child that schoolwork is between the child and the teacher; the teacher and child should set goals for better school performance to allow the child to feel responsible for school successes and failures.
- Take advantage of situations that support and reinforce school learning.
- Share information with teachers that will help them understand the child better.
- Communicate with the teacher if there appears to be a problem; avoid waiting for a scheduled conference.
- Provide a quiet, well-lit area for study that is safe from interruption; do not allow television or radio.
- Avoid dictating a study time, but do enforce rules, such as no television until homework is done; accept the child's word that work is complete.
- Help with homework should focus on explaining the question, not giving the answer.
- Teach the child to break large tasks (e.g., a report) into smaller, manageable tasks spread over the allotted time rather than attempting the entire project the night before it is to be completed.
- Limit home tutoring to special circumstances, such as when the teacher requests parental assistance after a child's prolonged absence.
- Request special help for children with learning problems.
- Support the school staff by showing respect for both the school system and the teacher, at least in the child's presence.

Dishonest Behavior

During middle childhood, children may engage in what is considered to be antisocial behavior. Previously well-behaved children may engage in lying, stealing, and cheating. Such behaviors are disturbing and challenging to parents.

Lying can occur for a number of reasons. By the time children enter school, they still "tell stories," often exaggerating a story or situation as a means of impressing their family or friends. However, during middle childhood, children become able to distinguish between fact and fantasy. If children do not develop this characteristic, parents need to teach them what is real and what is make-believe.

Young children may lie to escape punishment or to get out of some difficulty even when their misbehavior is evident. Older children may lie to meet expectations set by others to which they have been unable to measure up. However, most children know that lying and cheating are wrong, and they are concerned when it is observed in their friends. They are quick to tell on others when they detect cheating.

Parents need to be reassured that all children lie occasionally and that sometimes children may have difficulty separating fantasy from reality. Parents should be helped to understand the importance of being truthful in their relationships with children.

Cheating is most common in young children 5 to 6 years of age. They find it difficult to lose at a game or contest, so they may cheat to win. They have not yet realized that this behavior is wrong, and they do it almost automatically. This behavior usually disappears as they mature. However, because children model observed behaviors, parents need to be aware of their own behavior. When parents set examples of honesty, children are more likely to conform to these standards.

As with other ethically related behavior, stealing is not unexpected in younger children. Between 5 and 8 years of age, children's sense of property rights is limited and they tend to take things simply because they are attracted to them or to take money for what it will buy. They are equally likely to give away something valuable that belongs to them. When young children are caught and punished, they are penitent—they "didn't mean to" and "promise to never do it again"—but they are likely to repeat the performance the following day. Often they not only steal but also lie about their behavior or attempt to justify it with excuses. It is seldom helpful to trap children into admission by asking directly if they committed the offense. Children do not take responsibility for these behaviors until the end of middle childhood. Stealing can be an indication that something is seriously wrong or lacking in the child's life. For example, children may steal to make up for love or another satisfaction that they feel is lacking. In most situations, it is wise not to attempt to attach a hidden or deep meaning to the stealing. An admonition, together with an appropriate and reasonable punishment, such as having the older child pay back the money or return the stolen items, takes care of most cases. Most children can be taught to respect the property rights of others with little difficulty despite numerous temptations and opportunities. If children's personal rights are respected, they are likely to respect the rights of others. Some children simply need more time to learn the rules regarding private property.

Stress and Fear

Children today experience significant amounts of stress, which can cause long-term adjustment and health problems. Stress in childhood comes from a variety of sources such as conflict within the family, interpersonal relationships, and poverty. The school environment and participation in multiple organized activities can be additional sources of stress. The demands from coaches and parents, in addition to school requirements and pressure from teachers to do well on proficiency testing, can cause unrealistic expectations on school-age children (Schredl, Biernelt, Roos, et al., 2008). In addition, with the increased exposure to sexuality and provocative clothing and behaviors, children of this age-group may feel pressured to have a girlfriend or boyfriend, which their maturity level cannot handle and which causes additional stress (McLeod and Knight, 2010).

The increasing violence in society has infiltrated into the school setting. In the present information age in which tragedy is broadcast daily in the media, children come to school knowing more about the latest world events than any previous generation of children. Many children know other children who have been killed or children who have brought weapons to school. School-age children can be victims of bullying, verbal insults, unwanted sexual remarks, damaged or stolen property, and physical abuse in the school environment (Fredland, 2008).

To help children cope with stress, parents, teachers, and health care providers need to frequently reassure children that they are safe, have honest and open communication, encourage children to express their feelings, and provide time for unstructured play (Washington, 2009). Adults must recognize signs that indicate a child is undergoing stress, identify the source of the stress promptly, and refer those children who need specialized treatment.

> **! NURSING ALERT**
>
> The nurse who observes the following signs of stress in a child should explore the situation further:
> - Stomach pains or headache
> - Changes in sleep patterns or nightmares
> - Bed-wetting
> - Changes in eating habits
> - Aggressive or stubborn behavior
> - Withdrawal or reluctance to participate
> - Regression to earlier behaviors (e.g., thumb-sucking)
> - Trouble concentrating or changes in academic performance

Children 7 to 12 years of age are capable of identifying their own physiologic responses to stress. Common physiologic signs of stress include tight muscles, hot or red in the face, jittery, fast heartbeat, breathing difficulties, headache, neck pain, and abdominal pain (Washington, 2009). Children should be taught to recognize these signs as indicators of stress and to use techniques to manage their stress. Children can learn relaxation techniques such as deep-breathing exercises, progressive relaxation of muscle groups, and positive imagery to immediately reduce stress (Kostenius and Ohrling, 2009). Encouraging them to "blow off steam" through physical activity reduces tension and anxiety. Children can be encouraged to observe effective coping strategies in others and adopt them for their own use (Kostenius and Ohrling, 2009). When an effective strategy has been developed for one situation, parents can show the child how to transfer the coping strategy or technique to other situations.

In addition to stress, school-age children experience a wide variety of fears, including fear of the dark, excessive worry about past behavior, self-consciousness, social withdrawal, and an excessive need for reassurance. These fears are considered normal for children this age. During the middle-school years, children become less fearful of body safety than they were as preschoolers but they still fear being hurt, being kidnapped, or having to undergo surgery. They also fear death and are fascinated by all the aspects of death and dying. The fears of noises, darkness, storms, and dogs lessen, but new fears related predominantly to school and family bother children during this time.

PROMOTING OPTIMAL HEALTH DURING THE SCHOOL YEARS

Nutrition

Although caloric needs are diminished in relation to body size during middle childhood, resources are being laid down at this time for the increased growth needs of adolescence. Parents and children need to be aware of the value of a balanced diet to promote growth because children usually eat what their family members eat. The quality of the child's diet depends on the family's pattern of eating.

Likes and dislikes established at an early age continue in middle childhood, although preferences for single foods subside and children develop a taste for a variety of foods. However, the easy availability of fast-food restaurants, the influence of the mass media, and the temptation of "junk food" make it easy for children to fill up on empty calories. Foods that do not promote growth, such as sugars, starches, and excess fats, are common in school-age children's diets. The easy availability of high-calorie foods, combined with the tendency toward more sedentary activities, has also contributed to an epidemic of childhood obesity.

Parents are unable to monitor what their children eat when they are away from home. A parent may pack a lunch for school but is unaware of how much is eaten, traded, sold, or thrown away. Nutrition education can and should be integrated in the curriculum throughout the school years. Important aspects of nutrition education include the U.S. Food and Drug Administration's MyPlate; elements of a wholesome diet; and how food products are grown, processed, and prepared. However, school cafeterias may not always provide healthy, nutritious meals. School nurses can take an active role in nutrition education by working with teachers to plan and implement units on nutrition instruction and by working with parents and children to give nutritional guidance.

Sleep and Rest

The amount of sleep and rest required during middle childhood is highly individualized. The amount of sleep depends on the child's age, activity level, and state of health. The growth rate slows in the school-age years, and less energy is expended in growth than during preceding years.

School-age children usually do not require naps, but they do need to sleep approximately 11 hours at age 5 years and 9 hours at age 12 years each night (Smaldone, Honig, and Byrne, 2007). Although fewer bedtime problems occur during these years, occasional difficulties are still associated with the bedtime ritual. Usually children 6 or 7 years old exhibit few bedtime problems, and encouraging quiet activity before bedtime, such as coloring or reading, facilitates the task of going to bed. However, most children in middle childhood must be reminded frequently to go to bed; 8- to 9-year-old children and 11-year-old children are particularly resistant. Often these children are unaware that they are tired; if they are allowed to remain up later than usual, they are fatigued the following day. Sometimes bedtime resistance can be resolved by allowing a later bedtime as the child gets older. Twelve-year-old children usually offer no resistance at bedtime; some even retire early to read a book or listen to music.

Exercise and Activity

The improved capabilities and adaptability of school-age children permit greater speed and effort in motor activities. Larger, stronger muscles permit longer and increasingly strenuous play without exhaustion. School-age children acquire the coordination, timing, and concentration that are required to participate in adult-type activities, but they may lack the strength, stamina, and control of adolescents and adults. They can engage in a greater amount of physical activity during the school years. However, parents, teachers, and coaches must remember that although children this age are large and appear strong, they may not be ready for strenuous competitive athletics.

All growing children need regular exercise and opportunities for satisfying experiences consistent with individual likes and dislikes. Appropriate activities during the school-age years include running, jumping rope, swimming, roller skating, ice skating, dancing, and bicycle riding. Positive reinforcement achieved by experiencing increasingly smooth, rhythmic, and efficient use of the body conditions the child toward regular physical activity. Exercise is essential for muscle development and tone, refinement of balance and coordination, increased strength and endurance, and stimulation of body functions and metabolic processes. Children need ample space to run, jump, skip, and climb in addition to safe indoor and outdoor facilities and equipment. Most children have abundant energy and need little encouragement to engage in physical activity. Children with disabling conditions or those who hesitate to become involved in active play (e.g., obese children) require special assessment and help so that activities appeal to them and are compatible with their limitations while also meeting their developmental needs.

Sports

Considerable controversy surrounds the trend toward early participation in competitive athletics and the amount and type of competitive sports that are appropriate for children in the elementary grades. The current view is that virtually every child is suited for some sport, and authorities do not discourage participation if children are matched to the type of sport appropriate to their abilities and to their physical and emotional constitution. School-age children enjoy competition (Fig. 34-7). However, teachers and coaches must understand the physical limitations of children this age and teach them the proper techniques and safety measures needed to avoid injuries. A safe and appropriate sport can be identified for even the most unskilled and uncompetitive child, including children with chronic illnesses and intellectual disability. Common activities for school-age children include baseball, soccer, gymnastics, and swimming. Equipment must be maintained in safe condition, and protective apparatus should be worn to prevent serious injury.

During the school-age years, girls have the same basic body structure as boys and have a similar response to systematic exercise training. However, at puberty, boys become larger and have more muscle mass, and at this stage, it is usually recommended that girls compete only against other girls. Before puberty, there is no essential difference in strength and size between girls and boys, making these precautions unnecessary.

Preadolescence is a time to teach fundamental motor skills; develop fitness in a practical, safe, and gradual manner; and promote healthy attitudes and values. Activities should include both practice sessions and unstructured play; the actual game or event should be managed in a manner that stresses mastery of the sport and enhancement of self-image rather than winning or pleasing others. All children should have an opportunity to participate, and special ceremonies should recognize all participants, not just individuals who excel in sports or athletics.

Acquisition of Skills

School-age children demonstrate increasing fine motor abilities and complex artistic skills. Handedness is well established by the beginning of the school years, and children make great strides in

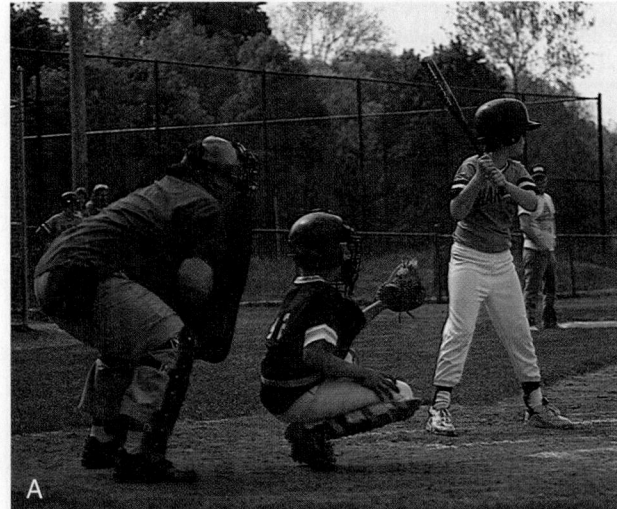

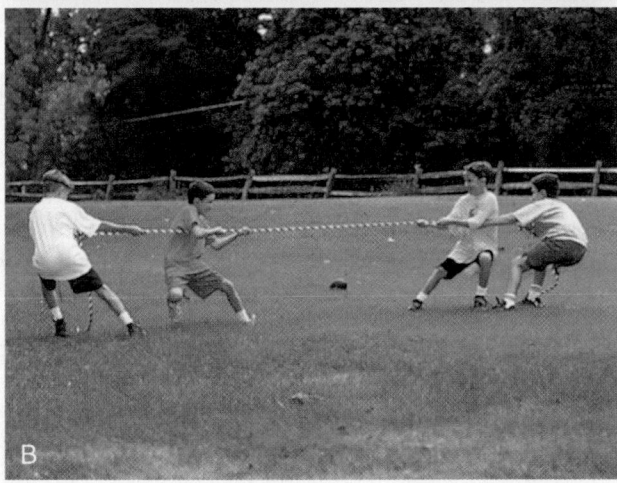

FIG 34-7 The activities engaged in by school-age children vary according to interest and opportunity. **A,** Little League competitors. **B,** Playing tug-of-war.

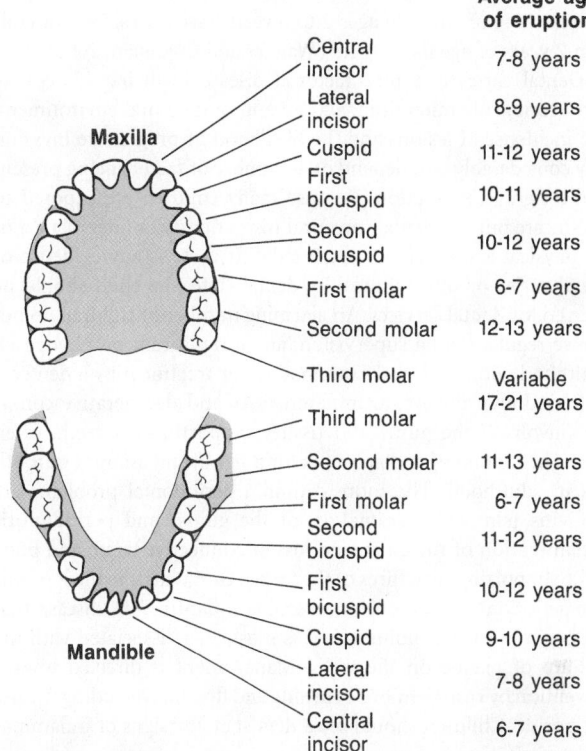

	Average age of eruption
Central incisor	7-8 years
Lateral incisor	8-9 years
Cuspid	11-12 years
First bicuspid	10-11 years
Second bicuspid	10-12 years
First molar	6-7 years
Second molar	12-13 years
Third molar	Variable 17-21 years
Third molar	
Second molar	11-13 years
First molar	6-7 years
Second bicuspid	11-12 years
First bicuspid	10-12 years
Cuspid	9-10 years
Lateral incisor	7-8 years
Central incisor	6-7 years

FIG 34-8 Sequence of eruption of the secondary teeth. (Data from Dean JA, Avery DR, McDonald RE: *McDonald and Avery dentistry for the child and adolescent*, ed 9, St Louis, 2011, Mosby.)

writing and drawing during this period. It is a time of energetic and vibrant creative productivity. With the tools of language and reading, children create poems, stories, and plays. With more advanced fine motor skills, they are able to master an unlimited variety of handicrafts, such as ceramics, needlework, woodworking, and beadwork. They avidly pursue these skills in solitude, with a friend, or through organized groups such as boys' or girls' clubs or special interest groups that use crafts or other activities as a means to occupy, entertain, and educate children.

School-age children are capable of assuming responsibility for their own needs, although their distaste for soap and water and "dress" clothes is legendary. School-age children can and want to assume their share of household tasks, which usually are related to the male and female roles that have been defined by their culture. Many children also assume responsibility for tasks outside the home, such as baby-sitting, mowing lawns, or paper routes.

Dental Health

The first permanent (secondary) teeth erupt at about 6 years of age, beginning with the 6-year molar, which erupts posterior to the deciduous molars. Other permanent teeth appear in approximately the same order as eruption of the primary teeth (see Teething, Chapter 31) and follow shedding of the deciduous teeth (Fig. 34-8).

With the appearance of the second permanent (12-year) molar, most permanent teeth are present. Permanent dentition is more advanced in girls than in boys.

Because the permanent teeth erupt during the school-age years, dental hygiene and regular attention to dental caries are important parts of health supervision during this period (see Dental Health, Chapter 33). Correct brushing techniques should be taught or reinforced, and the role that fermentable carbohydrates play in production of dental caries should be emphasized. It is important to be alert to possible malocclusion problems that may result from irregular eruption of permanent teeth and that may impair function. Regular dental supervision and continued fluoride supplementation are integral parts of the health maintenance program.

The most effective means of preventing dental caries is proper oral hygiene. Children should be taught to perform their own dental care with the supervision and guidance of the parents. Parents should learn the correct brushing technique with their children, and they should monitor their child's efforts until the child can assume full responsibility.

Dental Problems

Limited or inadequate dental care results in the most common dental problems: dental caries, malocclusion, and periodontal disease. Trauma, especially tooth avulsion, is another important dental problem. All of these conditions benefit from early intervention to prevent tooth loss.

Dental caries (cavities) is the principal oral problem in children and adolescents. Reducing the incidence and consequences of dental caries is extremely important in childhood. If untreated, dental caries can result in total destruction of the involved teeth. The prevalence rate of caries increases steadily across the life span; whereas 28% of children ages 2 to 5 years have caries, 59% of children 7 years of age have caries (Wagner and Oskouian, 2008).

Dental caries is a multifactorial disease involving susceptible teeth, cariogenic microflora, and an appropriate oral environment. The incidence of lesions and the likelihood of progressive invasion vary considerably and depend on a number of factors being present in the right combination. Because many children are exposed to health care but not dental care, oral inspection is an integral part of the physical assessment of every child. If there is any evidence of dental caries or other unhealthy dental state, the child should be referred for dental services. An alarming number of children do not receive regular dental supervision, and a significant number reach adulthood without dental examinations or treatment by a dentist.

Periodontal disease, an inflammatory and degenerative condition involving the gums and tissues supporting the teeth, often begins in childhood and accounts for a significant amount of tooth loss in adulthood. The more common periodontal problems are gingivitis (simple inflammation of the gums) and periodontitis (inflammation of the gums and loss of connective tissue and bone in the supporting structures of the teeth). Gingivitis, the most prevalent periodontal disease, is a reversible inflammatory disease that can begin in early childhood and is most often associated with the buildup of plaque on the teeth. Management is directed toward prevention by conscientious brushing and flossing, including the use of fluoride. Children should see a dentist at any signs of inflammation or irritation.

Malocclusion occurs when teeth of the upper and lower dental arches do not approximate in the proper relationships. As a result, the physiologic function of chewing is less effective and the cosmetic effect is displeasing. Teeth that are uneven, crowded, or overlapping are unable to meet their counterparts in the opposite jaw in the appropriate relationships and may be predisposed to disease in later years.

Orthodontic treatment is most successful when it is started in the late school-age or early teenage years after the last primary teeth have been shed and before growth ceases. However, referral should be made as soon as malocclusion is evident because some deformities can be corrected at an earlier age.

Dental injury may occur in childhood and includes fractures of varying degrees of severity, chipping, dislocation, or avulsion. All tooth injuries require prompt treatment by a competent dentist to prevent permanent displacement or loss. Delayed examination and diagnosis of tooth damage can result in infection or pulp involvement. Because it can affect the remaining teeth, replacement of the lost tooth is needed to maintain normal alignment and position of the other teeth.

A tooth that is avulsed (exarticulated, or "knocked out") should be replanted by the child, parent, or nurse and stabilized as soon as possible so the blood supply to the tooth can be reestablished and the tooth kept alive (see Emergency box). A tooth that is replanted promptly has a good survival rate. Avulsed primary teeth are usually not reimplanted.

As with all injuries to the mouth, an avulsed tooth causes a large amount of bleeding, which is frightening to children and their families; therefore the nurse or anyone faced with dental trauma should be prepared to provide support and reassurance during the dental trauma.

Sex Education

Many children experience some form of sex play during or before preadolescence as a response to normal curiosity, not as a result of

---

✚ EMERGENCY

Avulsed Permanent Tooth

- Recover tooth.
- Hold tooth by crown; avoid touching root area.
- If tooth is dirty, rinse it gently under running water or saline; be certain to insert stopper in sink or basin (to avoid tooth loss).

To Reimplant the Tooth
- Insert tooth into socket; be certain that the lip side (or convex surface) is facing front.
- Have child maintain tooth in place by slowly biting down on a piece of gauze.
- Transport child to dentist immediately.
- Avoid sudden stops or sharp turns to prevent dislodging tooth.

If Reluctant to Reimplant the Tooth
- Place avulsed tooth in suitable medium for transport:
  - Cold milk
  - Saliva—under child's or parent's tongue
- If child is holding tooth in the mouth, avoid sudden stops to prevent swallowing tooth.
- DO NOT FORGET TO TAKE THE TOOTH.

---

love or sexual urges. Children are experimentalists by nature, and sex play is incidental and transitory. Any adverse emotional consequences or guilt feelings depend on how the behavior is managed by the parents if it is discovered or whether children view their actions as wrong in the eyes of significant persons, particularly the parents.

The child's attitude toward sex is acquired indirectly at an early age. Initial curiosity about differences in body structure between boys and girls and between children and adults arises in the preschool years. Middle childhood is an ideal time for formal sex education, and many authorities believe that the topic is best presented from a life span approach. Information about sexual maturation and the process of reproduction minimizes children's uncertainty, embarrassment, and feelings of isolation that often accompany puberty.

An important component of ongoing sex education is effective communication with parents. If parents either repress the child's sexual curiosity or avoid dealing with it, the sexual information that the child receives may be acquired almost entirely from peers. When peers are the primary source of sexual information, it is transmitted and exchanged in secret conversation and contains a large amount of misinformation.

Nurse's Role in Sex Education

No matter where nurses practice, they can provide information on human sexuality to both parents and children. To discuss the topic adequately, nurses must have an understanding of the physiologic aspects of sexuality; knowledge of the cultural and societal values; and an awareness of their own attitudes, feelings, and biases about sexuality.

When presenting sexual information to school-age children, nurses should treat sex as a normal part of growth and development. Questions should be answered honestly, matter of factly, and to the same extent as questions about other topics. Answers should be at the child's level of understanding. There may be times when boys and girls should be taught content separately.

Children need help to differentiate sex and sexuality. Exercises on clarifying values, identifying role models, engaging in problem-solving skills, and practicing responsibility are important to prepare children for early adolescence and puberty. In addition, children need explanations of sexual information that is provided via the media or jokes. Information concerning pregnancy, contraceptives, and sexually transmitted diseases, including those caused by human immunodeficiency virus and human papillomavirus, should be presented in simple, accurate terms.

Preadolescents need precise and concrete information that will answer questions such as, "What if I start my period in the middle of class?" or "How can I keep people from telling I have an erection?" It is important to tell children what they want to know and what they can expect to happen as they become mature sexually.

During encounters with parents, nurses can be open and available for questions and discussion. They can set an example by the language they use in discussing body parts and their function and by the way in which they deal with problems that have emotional overtones, such as exploratory sex play and masturbation. Parents need help to understand normal behaviors and to view sexual curiosity in their children as a part of the developmental process. Assessing the parents' level of knowledge and understanding of sexuality provides cues to their need for supplemental information that will prepare them for the increasingly complex explanations they will need to provide as their children grow older.

School Health

Child health maintenance is ultimately the responsibility of the parents; however, the public schools and health departments in the United States have contributed to the improvement of child health by providing a healthful school environment, health services, and health education that emphasize sound health practices. Most of these functions constitute major components of community health services and involve large amounts of public funds and large numbers of health care professionals, including nurses.

A school health program is involved in ongoing health maintenance through assessment, screening, and referral activities. Routine health services provided by most schools include health appraisal, emergency care, safety education, communicable disease control, counseling, and follow-up care. Health education of school-age children is directed toward providing knowledge of health and influencing habits, attitudes, and conduct in relation to health and injury prevention.

Traditionally, school nurses were viewed as the individuals who detected diseases in the school, applied bandages, and cared for students who were ill or injured. Although these functions remain important parts of the school nurse's job, the role has expanded considerably. Today, school nurses manage and coordinate all the care required by regular students and students with special health care needs. In many settings, school health services have enlarged into family health centers that meet the needs of not only school-age children but also their families and the community. In these settings, school nurse practitioners provide health care that includes assessment of physical, psychomedical, psychoeducational, behavioral, and learning problems, as well as comprehensive well-child care (AAP, 2008).

The passage of the Education for All Handicapped Children Act and its amendments (Public Laws 94-142 and 99-457) mandated the integration of children with chronic illnesses and disabilities into the least restrictive environments, including regular classrooms whenever possible. School nurses are responsible for the medical and nursing needs of these children while they are in the school setting. School nurses develop, implement, and evaluate individualized health care plans for these children. Not all schools have a school nurse, and the use of unlicensed assistive personnel (UAP) is needed in some cases. After appropriate training and supervision, UAP can provide standardized routine health care to students. Delegation and supervision of UAP require skillful nursing assessment, effective communication, and professional judgment (AAP Council on School Health, 2009).

Injury Prevention

Because school-age children have developed more refined muscular coordination and control and can apply their cognitive capacities to their behavior, the number of injuries in middle childhood is diminished compared with the number in early childhood. The most common cause of severe injury and death in school-age children is motor vehicle accidents—either as a pedestrian or passenger (Centers for Disease Control and Prevention [CDC], 2010). It is important that nurses continue to emphasize three automobile safety measures that have been found to reduce the severity of injuries: effective car restraint systems, door-lock mechanisms, and appropriate passenger seating locations in the motor vehicle (Table 34-2). The rear vehicle seat is the safest place for children younger than 13 years, and booster seats should be used until 8 years of age (CDC, 2010).

School-age children's desire for riding bicycles increases the risk for injury on streets. Other serious injuries include accidents on skateboards, roller skates, in-line skates, scooters, and other sports equipment. All-terrain vehicles (ATVs) are popular with children

TABLE 34-2	INJURY PREVENTION DURING THE SCHOOL-AGE YEARS
DEVELOPMENTAL ABILITIES RELATED TO RISK FOR INJURY	**INJURY PREVENTION**
Motor Vehicle Accidents	
Is increasingly involved in activities away from home	Educate child regarding proper use of seat belts while a passenger in a vehicle.
Is excited by speed and motion	Maintain discipline while a passenger in a vehicle (e.g., keep arms inside, do not lean against doors, do not interfere with driver).
Is easily distracted by environment	Remind parents and children that no one should ride in the bed of a pickup truck.
Can be reasoned with	Emphasize safe pedestrian behavior.
	Insist on child wearing safety apparel (e.g., helmet) when applicable, such as riding bicycle, motorcycle, moped, or all-terrain vehicle (see Family-Centered Care box, p. 1001).

Continued

TABLE 34-2 INJURY PREVENTION DURING THE SCHOOL-AGE YEARS—cont'd

DEVELOPMENTAL ABILITIES RELATED TO RISK FOR INJURY	INJURY PREVENTION
Drowning Is apt to overdo May work hard to perfect a skill Has cautious, but not fearful, gross motor actions Likes swimming	Teach child to swim. Teach basic rules of water safety. Select safe and supervised places to swim. Check sufficient water depth for diving. Swim with a companion. Use an approved flotation device. Advocate for legislation requiring fencing around pools. Learn cardiopulmonary resuscitation.
Burns Has increasing independence Is adventurous Enjoys trying new things	Make certain home has smoke detectors. Set water heaters to 48.9° C (120° F) to avoid scald burns. Instruct child in behavior in areas involving contact with potential burn hazards (e.g., gasoline, matches, bonfires or barbecues, lighter fluid, firecrackers, cigarette lighters, cooking utensils, chemistry sets). Instruct child to avoid climbing or flying kite around high-tension wires. Instruct child in proper behavior in the event of fire (e.g., fire drills at home and school). Teach child safe cooking (use low heat; avoid any frying; be careful of steam burns, scalds, or exploding foods, especially from microwaving).
Poisoning Adheres to group rules May be easily influenced by peers Has strong allegiance to friends	Educate child regarding hazards of taking nonprescription drugs and chemicals, including aspirin and alcohol. Teach child to say "no" if offered illegal or dangerous drugs or alcohol. Keep potentially dangerous products in properly labeled receptacles, preferably out of reach.

Bodily Damage
Has increased physical skills
Needs strenuous physical activity
Is interested in acquiring new skills and perfecting attained skills
Is daring and adventurous, especially with peers
Frequently plays in hazardous places
Confidence often exceeds physical capacity
Desires group loyalty and has strong need for friends' approval
Delights in physical activity
Takes risks
Is likely to overdo
Growth in height exceeds muscular growth and coordination
	Help provide facilities for supervised activities.
	Encourage playing in safe places.
	Keep firearms safely locked up except under adult supervision.
	Teach proper care of, use of, and respect for devices with potential danger (e.g., power tools, firecrackers).
	Teach children not to tease or surprise dogs, invade their territory, take dogs' toys, or interfere with dogs' feeding.
	Stress eye, ear, or mouth protection when using potentially hazardous objects or devices or when engaging in potentially hazardous sports.
	Teach safety regarding use of corrective devices (glasses); if child wears contact lenses, monitor duration of wear to prevent corneal damage.
	Stress careful selection, use, and maintenance of sports and recreation equipment, such as skateboards and in-line skates (see Family-Centered Care box, p. 1001).
	Emphasize proper conditioning, safe practices, and use of safety equipment for sports or recreational activities.
	Caution against engaging in hazardous sports, such as those involving trampolines.
	Use safety glass and decals on large glassed areas, such as sliding glass doors.
	Use window guards to prevent falls.
	Teach name, address, and phone number and emphasize that child should ask for help from appropriate people (e.g., cashier, security guard, police) if lost; have identification on child (e.g., sewn in clothes, inside shoe).
	Teach stranger safety:
	  Avoid clothing displaying the child's name or family name in public places. Caution child to never go with a stranger.
	  Have child tell parents if anyone makes child feel uncomfortable in any way.
	Always listen to child's concerns regarding others' behavior.
	Teach child to say "no" when confronted by uncomfortable situations.

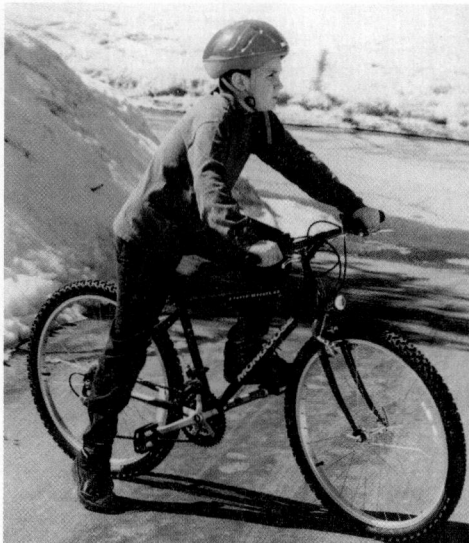

FIG 34-9 The right size bike is important; the child should be able to sit on the bike and place the balls of both feet on the ground. The foot should comfortably reach and manipulate the pedal in the down position. Wearing a protective helmet is mandatory. The helmet should be positioned so it sits low on the forehead and parallel to the ground when the head is held upright. It should not rock back and forth or shift from side to side. The strap should fasten securely under the chin.

but are unstable, difficult to handle, and responsible for a large number of childhood injuries. Several national organizations have developed policy and position statements to discourage the use of ATVs in any child younger than 16 years (American Pediatric Surgical Association, 2009).

Most injuries occur in or near the home or school. The most effective means of prevention is education of the child and family regarding the hazards of risk taking and the improper use of equipment. Safety helmets, protective eye and mouth shields, and protective padding are strongly recommended for children engaging in active sports even though they may not be required equipment. Falls from bicycles are the cause of a significant number of head injuries in school-age children, and the most important aspect of bicycle safety is to encourage children to wear protective helmets (Fig. 34-9) (Okun and Adam, 2008). Family-Centered Care boxes provide guidelines for bicycle, skateboard, and in-line skate safety and guidance during the school years.

Physically active school-age children are also highly susceptible to cuts and abrasions, and the incidence of childhood fractures, strains, and sprains is high. Trampoline injuries are highest in children ages 5 through 14 years and account for numerous fractures, sprains, and head injuries. Trampolines in the home environment, routine physical education classes, or outdoor playgrounds are not recommended for children of any age (Eberl, Schalamon, Singer, et al., 2009).

SCHOOL-AGE DISORDERS WITH BEHAVIORAL COMPONENTS

Attention Deficit Hyperactivity Disorder and Learning Disability

Attention deficit hyperactivity disorder (ADHD) refers to developmentally inappropriate degrees of inattention, impulsiveness, and

---

🏃 FAMILY-CENTERED CARE

Bicycle Safety

- Always wear a properly fitted bicycle helmet that is approved by the U.S. Consumer Product Safety Commission (CPSC); encourage parents to look for the CPSC approval sticker on the inside liner of the helmet.
- Replace a helmet every 5 years or sooner if manufacturer recommends it. **Never use a damaged or outgrown helmet.**
- Ride bicycles with traffic and away from parked cars.
- Ride single file.
- Walk bicycles through busy intersections only at crosswalks.
- Give hand signals well in advance of turning or stopping.
- Keep as close to the curb as practical.
- Watch for drain grates, potholes, soft shoulders, loose dirt, and gravel.
- Keep both hands on handlebars except with signaling.
- Never ride double on a bicycle.
- Do not carry packages that interfere with vision or control; do not drag objects behind a bike.
- Watch for and yield to pedestrians.
- Watch for cars backing up or pulling out of driveways; be especially careful at intersections.
- Look left, right, and then left before turning into traffic or roadway.
- Never hitch a ride on a truck or other vehicle.
- Learn rules of the road and respect for traffic officers.
- Obey all local ordinances.
- Wear shoes that fit securely while riding.
- Wear light colors at night and attach fluorescent material to clothing and bicycle.
- Equip the bicycle with proper lights and reflectors.
- Be certain the bicycle is the correct size for rider (see Fig. 34-9).
- Have the bicycle inspected to ensure good mechanical condition.
- Children riding as passengers must wear appropriate-size helmets and sit in specially designed protective seats.

Adapted from American Academy of Pediatrics Committee on Injury and Poison Prevention: Bicycle helmets, *Pediatrics* 122(2):450, 2008.

🏃 FAMILY-CENTERED CARE

Skateboard, In-Line Skate, and Scooter Safety

- Children younger than 5 years should not use skateboards or in-line skates because they are not developmentally prepared to protect themselves from injury. Children ages 6 to 10 years should use these only with close adult supervision.
- Children younger than 8 years should ride scooters only with close adult supervision.
- Children who ride skateboards, in-line skates, or scooters should wear helmets and other protective equipment, especially on their knees, wrists, and elbows, to prevent injury.
- Skateboards, in-line skates, and scooters should never be used near traffic or in streets. Their use should be prohibited at night. Activities that bring skateboards together (e.g., "catching a ride") are especially dangerous.
- Some types of use, such as riding homemade ramps on hard surfaces, may be particularly hazardous.

Data from Brudvik C: Injuries caused by small wheel devices, *Prev Sci* 7:313-320, 2006.

FAMILY-CENTERED CARE

Guidance During School Years

Age 6 Years
- Prepare parents to expect strong food preferences and frequent refusal of specific food items.
- Prepare parents to expect an increasingly ravenous appetite.
- Prepare parents for emotionality as child experiences erratic mood changes.
- Help parents anticipate continued susceptibility to illness.
- Teach injury prevention and safety, especially bicycle safety.
- Encourage parents to respect child's need for privacy and to provide a separate bedroom for child, if possible.
- Prepare parents for child's increasing interests outside the home.
- Help parents understand the need to encourage child's interactions with peers.

Ages 7 to 10 Years
- Prepare parents to expect improvement in health with fewer illnesses, but warn them that allergies may increase or become apparent.
- Prepare parents to expect an increase in minor injuries.
- Emphasize caution in selecting and maintaining sports equipment, and reemphasize safety.
- Prepare parents to expect increased involvement with peers and interest in activities outside the home.
- Emphasize the need to encourage independence while maintaining limit setting and discipline.
- Prepare mothers to expect more demands at 8 years.
- Prepare fathers to expect increasing admiration at 10 years; encourage father-child activities.
- Prepare parents for prepubescent changes in girls.

Ages 11 to 12 Years
- Help parents prepare child for body changes of pubescence.
- Prepare parents to expect a growth spurt in girls.
- Make certain child's sex education is adequate with accurate information.
- Prepare parents to expect energetic but stormy behavior at 11 years, becoming more even-tempered at 12 years.
- Encourage parents to support child's desire to "grow up" but to allow regressive behavior when needed.
- Prepare parents to expect an increase in child's masturbation.
- Instruct parents that the amount of rest the child needs may increase.
- Help parents educate child regarding experimentation with potentially harmful activities.

Health Guidance
- Help parents understand the importance of regular health and dental care for the child.
- Encourage parents to teach and model sound health practices, including diet, rest, activity, and exercise.
- Stress the need to encourage children to engage in appropriate physical activities.
- Emphasize providing a safe physical and emotional environment.
- Encourage parents to teach and model safety practices.

BOX 34-1 CHARACTERISTICS OF ATTENTION DEFICIT HYPERACTIVITY DISORDER

Inattention
Appears careless in schoolwork and activities at home, easily distracted by external stimuli, forgetful in daily activities, avoids or dislikes engaging in tasks that require sustained mental effort

Hyperactivity
Fidgety, squirms in seat, restless, has difficulty in playing quietly or engaging in quiet-time games or activities, talks excessively

Impulsivity
Has poor impulse control, has difficulty waiting for turn or waiting in line, interrupts others' conversations

Modified from American Psychiatric Association: *Diagnostic and statistical manual of mental disorders,* ed 4, text rev (DSM-IV TR), Washington, DC, 2000, Author.

disability (LD) refers to a heterogeneous group of disorders manifested by significant difficulties in the acquisition and use of listening, speaking, reading, writing, reasoning, or mathematic skills.

Learning disabilities and ADHD affect every aspect of a child's life but are most obvious in the classroom. Early identification of affected children is important because the characteristics of these disorders significantly interfere with the normal course of emotional and psychologic development. Many children develop maladaptive behavior patterns that impede psychosocial adjustment while they try to cope with cognitive dysfunction. Their behavior evokes negative responses from others, and repeated exposure to negative feedback adversely affects their self-concept. The characteristics of ADHD affect the child's written and adaptive skills, social status, and self-esteem (Cunningham and Jensen, 2011; Myers, Eisenhauer, and Ryan, 2003).

Diagnostic Evaluation

The behaviors exhibited by children with ADHD are not unusual. The difference lies in the quality of motor activity and the developmentally inappropriate inattention, impulsivity, and hyperactivity displayed by children with ADHD. The manifestations may be numerous or few and mild or severe, and they vary with the child's developmental level. Any given child will not have every manifestation characteristic of the syndrome, and the degree of severity is highly variable. Mild manifestations of symptoms may not be apparent in some educational and family environments, but severe symptoms will be recognizable in most environments. Every child with ADHD is different from all other children with ADHD. The clinical manifestations of ADHD are outlined in Box 34-1.

Most behavioral manifestations of ADHD are apparent at an early age, but the LDs may not become evident until the child enters school. The disorder is unpredictable; it may remit spontaneously at any age, and the number of years that a child will require treatment is unknown.

A major clinical manifestation is distractibility. The stimuli may come from external sources or internal sources. Children often demonstrate immaturity relative to chronologic age. Selective attention is often seen, in which the child has difficulty attending to "nonpreferred" tasks such as completing chores or finishing homework. The child may not consider the consequences of behavior, may take excessive physical risks (often beginning early in life), and may demonstrate inappropriate social skills.

hyperactivity. To be diagnosed as ADHD, the symptoms must have been present between 4 and 18 years of age and must be present in more than one major setting (AAP, Clinical Practice Guideline, 2011). In addition, the persistence of developmentally inappropriate and marked inattention must not be a symptom of another disorder (American Psychiatric Association [APA], 2000). A learning

Children with ADHD demonstrate one of three subtypes (APA, 2000):

1. Combined type—Six (or more) symptoms of inattention and six (or more) symptoms of hyperactivity-impulsivity that persist for at least 6 months. Most children and adolescents with ADHD have the combined type.
2. Predominantly inattentive type—Six (or more) symptoms of inattention (but fewer than six symptoms of hyperactivity-impulsivity) that persist for at least 6 months.
3. Predominantly hyperactive-impulsive type—Six (or more) symptoms of hyperactivity-impulsivity (but fewer than six symptoms of inattention) that persist for at least 6 months. Inattention may often still be a significant clinical feature in such cases.

A diagnosis of ADHD is established based on characteristics in the APA's (2000) *Diagnostic and Statistical Manual of Mental Disorders (DSM-IV-TR)* and a thorough evaluation of the child. It is important to emphasize the need for a complete and thorough multidisciplinary evaluation that incorporates the efforts of the pediatrician (often a developmental pediatrician or pediatric neurologist), psychologist, pediatric nurse, classroom teacher, reading and math specialist, special education teacher, possibly a speech therapist, and the child's parents. The clinicians and professionals must first determine whether the child's behavior is age appropriate or truly problematic.

A history (both medical and developmental) and a description of the child's behavior should be obtained from as many observers of the child as possible (especially the parents and teachers), along with the health care professionals involved. Descriptions of the child's behavior in home and school situations should be included. In obtaining descriptive material, the interviewer must question the observers carefully because some persons, especially parents, may be so concerned with gross behaviors that they overlook less distressing but equally important symptoms. For example, parents may report a "colicky" infant, a child who began to run soon after walking, a toddler who was compelled to touch everything in sight, and a child who resisted sleep until exhausted. A pregnancy and birth history may provide clues to a situation that might have produced an episode of hypoxia.

A physical examination, including vision and hearing screening and a detailed neurologic evaluation, will help rule out any severe neurologic disorders. Psychologic testing, especially projective tests, is valuable in identifying visual-perceptual difficulties, problems with spatial organization, and other phenomena that suggest cortical or diencephalic involvement; it also helps to identify the child's intelligence and achievement levels.

Behavioral checklists and adaptive scales are also helpful in measuring social adaptive functioning in children with ADHD. Psychiatric disorders, medical problems, and traumatic experiences are ruled out, including lead poisoning, seizures, partial hearing loss, psychosis, and the witnessing of sexual activity or violence.

Therapeutic Management

Management of the child with ADHD usually involves multiple approaches that include family education and counseling, medication, proper classroom placement, environmental manipulation, and behavioral therapy or psychotherapy. Interventions for children with LD are primarily educational.

Pharmacologic Therapy. The most commonly used medications for AHDH are the psychostimulants methylphenidate hydrochloride (Ritalin) and dextroamphetamine sulfate (Dexedrine). The majority of patients with ADHD are treated with the psychostimulant methylphenidate (AAP, Clinical Practice Guideline, 2011). Psychostimulants cause an increase in dopamine and norepinephrine levels, which leads to stimulation of the inhibitory system of the central nervous system (CNS). Children are given a small dosage initially, and the dosage is gradually increased until the desired response is achieved. Children who receive stimulants should be monitored carefully for the development of tics during initial treatment, and stimulants should be avoided in children who have a history of ticlike behaviors, a family history of Tourette syndrome (TS), or ADHD combined with TS.

The stimulant dextroamphetamine may be used in children younger than 6 years of age to treat ADHD, but evidence of its safety and efficacy in young children and adolescents has been questioned. Lisdexamfetamine (Vyvanse) reportedly has less substance abuse potential that dextroamphetamine; it is metabolized to dextroamphetamine only after ingestion and thus may be more suitable for children and adolescents who may abuse dextroamphetamine (AAP, Clinical Practice Guideline, 2011). Other medications include the mixed amphetamine salts (Adderall), which are available in extended release form. In some cases a nonstimulant may be added to the medication regimen along with a stimulant to achieve optimal therapeutic effects. Many of the stimulant drugs are available in short-acting and long-acting form to better meet the child's need for therapeutic management. An additional consideration in the administration of medications is the child's ability to swallow pills; some come in capsule form and can be sprinkled on applesauce (Ryan-Krause, 2011).

Other nonstimulant medications recommended by the AAP Clinical Practice Guideline (2011) include the selective norepinephrine reuptake inhibitor atomoxetine (Strattera), and the selective alpha adrenergic agonists guanfacine (Tenex, Intuniv) and clonidine. Guanfacine and clonidine are available in extended-release form but are reported to have limited evidence of efficacy and safety in preschool children with ADHD (AAP, Clinical Practice Guideline, 2011).

It is important to remember that, except for atomoxetine, these medications are not prescribed based on the child's weight but rather on resolution of the symptoms; therefore it is important to follow the child closely and evaluate for therapeutic effects and potential side effects. With all of these medications, regularly scheduled reevaluation of the child is essential to determine medication effectiveness, detect and evaluate any side effects, monitor development and health status (especially growth and blood pressure), and assess family interaction (see Critical Thinking Case Study). Children taking stimulant drugs for ADHD should undergo an extensive physical examination and history, including a family history of cardiac disease or cardiac problems. Currently, electrocardiography screening is recommended only for children taking stimulant drugs for ADHD who have a close member with a history of cardiac arrhythmia or structural heart defect (Perrin, Friedman, Knilans, et al., 2008). Medication therapy alone is not adequate to manage the child's symptoms, and other treatment modalities such as behavioral therapy should also be used for successful treatment.

Behavioral Therapy. Behavioral therapy focuses on the prevention of undesired behavior. The nurse should help families identify new appropriate contingencies and reward systems to meet the child's developing needs. They may also receive instruction in effective parenting skills, such as delivering positive reinforcement, rewarding small increments of desired behaviors, and providing age-appropriate consequences (e.g., time-out, response cost). The use of organizational charts for completing self-care activities and the use of a word processor instead of manually writing assignments

CRITICAL THINKING CASE STUDY
Attention Deficit Hyperactivity Disorder

Johnnie, age 8 years, is a third grader who was recently diagnosed with ADHD. He has been taking methylphenidate (Ritalin) for about 1 month. In the short time that Johnnie has been taking this medication, his math teacher has noticed an improvement in his performance in math class. He is receiving a grade of B instead of his previous grades of D on most math quizzes. The math teacher has also noted that Johnnie is socializing more with his classmates and now has a "best friend" in math class. Johnnie usually receives his methylphenidate from the school nurse before lunch. Yesterday Johnnie's mother told the school nurse that he has not eaten his lunch for the past week and is not hungry.

What important issues regarding Johnnie's medication should the nurse consider in her discussions with Johnnie's mother?

Questions

1. Evidence—Is there sufficient evidence to draw conclusions about Johnnie's medication from his behavior?
2. Assumptions—Describe some underlying assumptions about the following:
   a. Pharmacologic action of methylphenidate in ADHD
   b. Side effects of methylphenidate
   c. Management of side effects
3. What implications for nursing care can be drawn at this time?
4. Does the evidence objectively support your conclusion?

ADHD, Attention deficit hyperactivity disorder.

are emphasized. Through collaborative teamwork, parents learn techniques to help the child become more successful at home and in school.

Counseling or therapy can be helpful for children who demonstrate signs of anxiety or depression. Therapy can help children develop healthier self-esteem and practice problem-solving strategies. Adolescents may benefit from group work that focuses on social skill development. Parents of children with ADHD can face a lot of stress, and therapy may be indicated for parents and other family members.

Multimodal Treatment. The results of several studies suggest that multimodal treatment that involves the use of pharmacotherapy and behavioral intervention as well as close follow-up and feedback from school personnel is more effective than intensive behavioral treatment alone (Selekman, 2010).

Environmental Manipulation. Encourage families to learn how to modify the environment to allow the child to be more successful. Consistency is especially important for children with ADHD. Consistency between families and teachers in terms of reinforcing the same goals is essential. Fostering improved organizational skills requires a more highly structured environment than most children need. Children should be encouraged to make more appropriate choices and to take responsibility for their actions.

Other helpful interventions include teaching parents how to make organizational charts (e.g., listing all activities that must be performed before leaving for school) and how to decrease distractions in the environment while the child is completing homework (e.g., turning off the television, having a consistent study area equipped with needed supplies), as well as helping parents understand ways to model positive behaviors and problem solving. The focus is on strategies to help the child succeed and cope with deficits while emphasizing strengths.

Appropriate Classroom Placement. Children with ADHD need an orderly, predictable, and consistent classroom environment with clear and consistent rules. Homework and classroom assignments may need to be reduced, and more time may need to be allotted for tests to allow the child to complete the task. Verbal instructions should be accompanied by visual references such as written instructions on the blackboard. Schedules may need to be arranged so that academic subjects are taught in the morning when the child is experiencing the effects of the morning dose of medication. Low-interest and high-interest classroom activities should be intermingled to maintain the child's attention and interest. Regular and frequent breaks in activity are helpful because sitting in one place for an extended time may be difficult. Computers are helpful for children who have difficulty with writing (**dysgraphia**) and fine motor skills; in such children, handwriting will *not* improve. They need to find alternatives to physical competition that requires coordination of movement.

If the child has an LD, special training activities may be accomplished in self-contained classes limited to six to eight children, in special resource rooms with equipment and teaching teams, by mobile consultants who move from room to room to provide assistance to teachers and children, and in special first-grade programs in which high-risk children receive special attention to prevent or reduce the need for services as they progress. The purpose of programs for children with LDs is to assist them toward more successful achievement, personal adjustment, and retention in the regular classroom. Selekman (2010) lists additional behavioral, educational, and environmental strategies for children and adolescents with ADHD.

Growth and Development. Children with ADHD who are taking stimulant medications need to be assessed for the achievement of appropriate growth and development milestones at least every 6 months (Pliszka and AACAP Work Group on Quality Issues, 2007; Selekman, 2010). The side effects of these drugs often include appetite suppression, nausea, and vomiting; suppression of growth acceleration and sleep disturbances have also been recorded in children taking stimulant drugs (Selekman, 2010).

Prognosis. With appropriate intervention, ADHD is relatively stable through early adolescence for most children. Some children experience decreased symptoms during late adolescence and adulthood, but a significant number of these children carry their symptoms into adulthood. The goal for children with LDs is to help them identify their areas of weakness and learn to compensate for them.

CARE MANAGEMENT

Nurses, especially school nurses, are active participants in all aspects of the management of children with ADHD and LDs. Nurses in the community work with families and school personnel on a long-term basis to help plan and implement therapeutic regimens and to evaluate the effectiveness of therapy. They coordinate services and serve as a liaison between health and education professionals directly involved in the child's therapy program. School nurses understand the child's special needs and work with teachers (see Family-Centered Care box). Nurses in any setting (community, school, hospital, practitioner's office) provide support and guidance to children and families during the difficult period of the child's growing up with a disabling condition.

Management begins with an explanation to the parents and the child about the diagnosis, including the nature of the problem and the practitioner's concept of the underlying CNS basis for the

FAMILY-CENTERED CARE

A Child's Perception of Taking Ritalin at School

I feel embarrassed by having to leave class early to go take my medication. The other kids always ask where I'm going and why. It would be better if we could leave class at the same time as everyone else, go take the medication, and then just be a little late to the next class. Students don't ask why people are late for class, only why they leave early. It also bothers me when kids tell other kids, "Go take a pill" and other mean things just because someone is acting up.

  What could nurses and teachers do to help? Most kids do not understand why other kids have to take medication. I think it would help if a nurse or teacher talked with the other kids and explained why some children take the medication and how ADHD affects people. That way there would be more understanding among all the kids.

—**Marissa White, age 16 years**

ADHD, Attention deficit hyperactivity disorder.

disorder. Most parents are confused and feel some measure of guilt. To some parents, a diagnosis of ADHD is confirmation of the fear that their child has some irreversible, serious disease; to others, it is a relief. All parents need the opportunity to vent their feelings and suspicions. A common complaint of parents is that health care professionals do not listen to what they have to say about their children. The health care professional should focus on building self-esteem by encouraging the family to focus on developing the child's strengths (e.g., sports, hobbies, and talents) rather than just the weaknesses (Jellinek, 2008).

Parents need to be informed of the possible side effects of medications. The psychostimulants have similar side effects that include weight loss, abdominal pain, headaches, decreased appetite, sleeplessness, increased crying and irritability, nervous stimulation, and cardiovascular stimulation. The use of caffeine decreases the efficacy of these drugs, and insulin requirements may also be altered. If decreased appetite is a concern, helpful interventions include giving the psychostimulants with or after meals rather than before, encouraging consumption of nutritious snacks in the evening when the effects of the medication are decreasing, and serving frequent small meals with healthy "on-the-go" snacks. Sleeplessness is reduced by administering the medication early in the day.

Children and adolescents with ADHD are at increased risk for accidents and unintentional injuries because of their impulsivity and decreased judgment of dangerous activities. Therefore measures should be taken to protect such children from personal injury (Selekman, 2010).

Children taking tricyclic antidepressants display a dramatic increase in the incidence of dental caries. The marked anticholinergic action of the drugs increases saliva viscosity and produces a dry mouth. Emphasis on rigorous dental hygiene, conscientious home fluoride treatments, regular visits to the dentist, limited intake of refined carbohydrates, and use of artificial saliva is an important nursing function. The child should drink plenty of fluids and be well hydrated.

Parents often express concern that their children will become addicted to the psychostimulants or antidepressant drugs. Both types of drugs have the potential for abuse, and all children taking these drugs should be monitored closely for psychologic dependence, tolerance, depression, and other adverse behavior changes or idiosyncratic effects. Most children with ADHD are not interested in abusing their drugs because the effect of the drugs in these children is opposite that produced in normal individuals. However, caution parents to keep these drugs safely stored away from young children who may inadvertently ingest them and adolescents who may abuse them.

Parents need information about the prognosis and an understanding of the treatment plan. The greater their understanding of the disorder and its effects, the more likely they will be to carry out the recommended program of therapy. It is important that they understand that the therapy is not necessarily a panacea and that it will extend over a long period. This has particular significance for changes they need to make in environmental management. Reading material to help the child and family can be obtained from a variety of sources.

Posttraumatic Stress Disorder

Posttraumatic stress disorder (PTSD) refers to the development of characteristic symptoms after exposure to an extremely traumatic experience or catastrophic event. The traumatic experience is typically life threatening to oneself or a significant other and may involve grotesque mutilation or death, serious injury, or physical coercion (e.g., an assault, a natural disaster, sexual abuse, witnessing violence). It is important to note that PTSD is not limited to children who have lived in "war-torn" countries. Events such as automobile, school, or recreational accidents and bullying have also been identified as causes of PTSD. The characteristic symptoms are persistent re-experiencing of the traumatic event, avoidance of stimuli associated with the event or trauma, numbing of general responsiveness, and increased arousal.

Acute PTSD is diagnosed if symptoms are present after the first month but before the third month after the initial traumatic event. Acute stress disorder may also occur with acute PTSD. Chronic PTSD is diagnosed if the symptoms persist beyond 3 months (Cohen and AACAP Work Group on Quality Issues, 2010).

The response to the event takes place in three stages. The initial response involves intense arousal, which usually lasts for a few minutes to 1 or 2 hours. The stress hormones are at the maximum as the individual prepares for "fight or flight." A prolonged arousal phase may indicate psychosis.

The second phase, which lasts approximately 2 weeks, is one in which defense mechanisms are mobilized. It is a period of calm in which the event appears to have produced no impression. The child feels numb, and stress hormone secretion is absent. Defense mechanisms are less adaptive to specific situations and may not be what the situation demands. Denial that anything is wrong is a commonly observed defense mechanism.

The third phase is one of coping and consciously directed inquiry, which normally extends over 2 to 3 months. The victims want to know what happened and appear to be getting worse when actually they are getting better. Numerous psychologic symptoms such as depression, repetitive phenomena, phobic symptoms, anxiety, and conversion reactions may be present. Children often display repetitive actions. They play out the situation over and over again in an attempt to come to terms with their fear. Flashbacks are common. This phase can be self-perpetuating, and a prolonged reaction can develop into an obsession with the traumatic event. Some traumatic effects remain indefinitely.

Trauma-focused psychotherapy is considered first-line therapy, and selective serotonin reuptake inhibitor (SSRI) drugs may be considered on an individual basis. Rebirthing therapies or restrictive treatments that bind or withhold water or food are not recommended (Cohen and AACAP Work Group on Quality Issues, 2010).

A practice parameter for the assessment and management of PTSD in children and adolescents is published elsewhere (Cohen and AACAP Work Group on Quality Issues, 2010).

CARE MANAGEMENT

Children need to deal with all traumatic events. Their reactions depend heavily on their social environment and the way in which their caregiving adults react to the event. In the second phase of PTSD, the appropriateness of the defense mechanism must be assessed, and children must be assisted in the application of their defense. Children who do not engage in some catharsis or who have a prolonged defense phase need referral for special psychologic help.

Coping is a learned response, and children in the third phase of PTSD can be helped to deal with their fear. Children usually are willing to accept reasoning. Those who are assisted in their catharsis and are allowed expression will survive without serious lasting effects. They should be encouraged to play out the stress and to discuss their feelings about the event. If they are unable to do this, they may become obsessed with the traumatic event and require professional help. Conversion reactions are common obsessive behaviors in children with PTSD.

Children need professional help if any of the phases of PTSD are prolonged. Boys tend to have a prolonged defense phase more often than girls. Occasionally the event will be unrecognized, and the affected child will engage in what is considered to be unusual behavior. Children exhibiting any sudden change in behavior need to be assessed for a traumatic event. When the change in behavior is traced to a traumatic event, treatment can be implemented.

Nurses in settings such as the emergency department, pediatric intensive care unit, and neonatal intensive care unit should also recognize that parents of children who experience a traumatic acute trauma, life-threatening illness, or chronic illness may also experience symptoms of PTSD. PTSD may occur more often in mothers than in fathers, but some evidence indicates that fathers may have delayed symptoms (Mowery, 2011). Appropriate nursing interventions include allowing parents to discuss their feelings about the incident or threat (to themselves or their children), encouraging support from other parents in similar situations, avoiding interjecting one's own experience or feelings, and evaluating the child's reaction to the parents' symptoms (Mowery, 2011).

School Phobia

Children (other than beginning students) who resist going to school or who demonstrate extreme reluctance to attend school for a sustained period as a result of severe anxiety or fear of school-related experiences are said to have school phobia. The terms *school refusal* and *school avoidance* are also used to describe this behavior. School phobia occurs in children of all ages but is more common in children 10 years of age and older. School avoidance behaviors occur in both boys and girls and in children from all socioeconomic levels.

Anxiety that often verges on panic is a constant manifestation, and children can develop symptoms as a protective mechanism to keep them from facing the situation that distresses them. Physical symptoms are prominent and may affect any part of the body and include anorexia, nausea, vomiting, diarrhea, dizziness, headache, leg pains, and abdominal pains. Children may even develop a low-grade fever. A striking feature of school phobia is the prompt subsiding of symptoms when it is evident that the child can remain at home. Another significant observation is an absence of symptoms on weekends and holidays unless they are related to other places such as Sunday school or parties. Occasional mild reluctance to attend school is common among schoolchildren, but if the fear continues for longer than a few days, it must be considered a serious problem.

The onset of school phobia is usually sudden and precipitated by a school-related incident. By taking a careful history, nurses find out whether a poor attendance record is caused by trivial reasons.

CARE MANAGEMENT

Treatment for school phobia depends on the cause. The primary goal is to return the child to school. The longer a child is permitted to stay out of school, the more difficult it is for him or her to reenter. Parents must be convinced gently but firmly that an immediate return to school is essential and that it is their responsibility to insist on school attendance.

A school reentry protocol may be necessary for the child with severe symptoms. In reentry programs, the child role-plays routines that are involved in getting ready for school and occur at school. Relaxation techniques are also used. The child usually goes to school initially for a half day and then progresses to a full day. Often the school nurse is asked to provide support to the parents and the teacher during the reentry process. If the problem persists, professional help is recommended.

Bullying

Bullying is a form of aggression in which a person asserts power over another who is considered weaker through social, emotional, and physical means. The consequences of bullying include depression, long-term psychopathology, suicidality, psychosomatic symptoms, and psychoses. Bullying involves aggression in which the behavior is intended to harm or embarrass the victim; it occurs repeatedly over time, and there is an imbalance of power, with the bully exerting dominance over the victim (Liu and Graves, 2011). The behavior may be carried out by one person or several people who isolate the victim for purposes of harming and embarrassing through an imbalance of power. Bullying may be perceived by some as a normal social developmental step in childhood, and in some cases the bully may perceive the behavior as being fun rather than harmful. Some may view bullying with a "boys will be boys" attitude and ignore the behavior. Research has shown that bullying occurs more often in boys, but girls may also be involved in what is called *relational bullying*—a more subtle and indirect form of bullying. Bullying is more common in middle school than in high school (Liu and Graves, 2011).

Because most bullying occurs in and around the school, there has been more emphasis on recognizing and dealing with the behaviors in schools.* Interventions should include recognizing the behavior in both the bully and the victim, protecting the victim, and stopping the behavior altogether. To be effective, behavioral changes from the bully and social changes in the school environment with the assistance of parents and adults in the school should occur. The school nurse and community nurse are likely to come in contact with victims and bullies alike; the practitioner may also be involved in caring for the physical and emotional health of the victim. School and community-lead programs to heighten awareness of the consequences of bullying are reported to have been ineffective in stopping bullying; however, further studies are needed (Liu and Graves, 2011).

---

*Resources on bullying include the following: www.eyesonbullying.org; and stopbullyingnow.hrsa.gov/kids/.

Conversion Reaction

A conversion reaction (also known as hysteria, hysterical conversion reaction, and childhood hysteria) is a sudden-onset psychophysiologic disorder that can usually be traced to a precipitating environmental event. The disorder is observed with equal frequency in both sexes in childhood, but affected girls outnumber affected boys during adolescence. Manifestations of conversion reaction involve primarily the voluntary musculature and special senses and include abdominal pain, fainting, pseudoseizures, paralysis, headaches, and visual field restriction. Once considered rare in childhood, this disorder occurs more frequently than has generally been acknowledged. The most commonly observed symptom is seizure activity that can be differentiated from symptoms of neurogenic origin by formal tests, the most useful of which are normal electroencephalogram findings.

Many children with conversion reaction experienced a major family crisis before the onset of symptoms, such as the loss of a parent or other significant person through death, divorce, or moving. Children with conversion reaction characteristically come from families with communication problems or have a parent with depression or hypochondriasis.

Educating the child and family about the cause of emotional stresses or feelings and alternative approaches to coping with stress may alleviate the child's symptoms. If deep personality problems are evident, psychiatric consultation is indicated. Nursing care is similar to that for the child with recurrent abdominal pain.

Childhood Depression

Depression in childhood is often difficult to detect because children may be unable to express their feelings and tend to act out their problems and concerns. Some states of depression are temporary, such as acute depression precipitated by a traumatic event. The event might include a period of hospitalization, the loss of a parent through death or separation, or the loss of a significant relationship with something (a pet), a person (a friend, significant other, or family member), or a place (move from a familiar home, neighborhood, or city). Children with depression may demonstrate a variety of behaviors. Most responses in children are not sustained and can be modified with social and family support.

More serious and less common are the depressive responses to more chronic stress and loss. These are often observed in children with chronic illness or disability. There is no apparent precipitating event, but there is often a history of frequent disruptions in important relationships. A history of depressive illness in one or both parents during the child's lifetime is also common. Manifestations in the child are similar to those observed in acute reactions, but they occur more frequently and extend over a longer period.

▌CARE MANAGEMENT

Depressed children are managed by a health care team that is specially trained in the care of children with mental disorders. Treatment is highly individualized and undertaken in the least restrictive environment. Suicidal children are admitted to the hospital for protection if the family is unable to provide constant monitoring. Pharmacotherapy may involve TCAs or SSRIs such as fluoxetine, trazodone (Desyrel), sertraline, and paroxetine (Paxil), as well as bupropion (Wellbutrin) and venlafaxine (Effexor). There have been reports that antidepressant medications may cause increased suicidal thinking and behaviors in pediatric patients. This prompted the U.S. Food and Drug Administration (FDA) to require black box drug labeling detailing the potential suicide-related risks for pediatric patient. This warning was updated, and it was noted that the risk of suicide was highest among adolescents and young adults ages 18 to 24 years. Some data suggest that the suicide rate among adolescents taking therapeutic doses of SSRIs was lower than among those who were not being treated with antidepressant medication (Gibbons, Hur, Bhaumik, et al., 2006). However, the issue remains controversial because study results are mixed, and further studies are needed (Walter and DeMaso, 2011). Patients taking SSRIs should be followed closely (once a week) for the first 4 weeks of therapy before a dose increase is made. After 4 weeks it is recommended that follow-up occur biweekly and that children and adolescents with a risk for suicidality be referred for specialized treatment (Walter and DeMaso, 2011).

Nurses should be aware that depression is a problem that can be easily overlooked in children and can interrupt normal growth and development. Recognizing depression and suicidal tendencies in depressed adolescents and making appropriate referrals are important nursing functions. Identification of a depressed child requires a careful history (health, growth and development, social and family health), interviews with the child, and observations by the nurse, parents, and teachers. If antidepressants are prescribed, the child and family need to know that antidepressants must be at a therapeutic level for 2 to 4 weeks to achieve a beneficial effect. The child and family also need to monitor the child for side effects of the specific drug prescribed and any interactions with other drugs.

Childhood Schizophrenia

Childhood schizophrenia is a term that refers to severe deviations in ego functioning and is generally reserved for psychotic disorders that appear in children younger than 15 years of age. Childhood schizophrenia is a rare illness among children in the general population; among children with mental illness, only about 2 in every 1000 have childhood schizophrenia.

Childhood schizophrenia is characterized by symptoms that last for at least 6 months and seriously interfere with the child's functioning in school, at home, or in other social situations. The basic disturbance is a lack of contact with reality and the subsequent development of a world of the child's own. Other areas of development that may be impaired include cognition, perception, emotion, language, and physical motor control. The most common manifestations involve language disturbances, impaired interpersonal relationships, and inappropriate affect (outward expression of emotion). Treatment involves management of the symptoms, prevention of relapse, and social and occupational rehabilitation. Antipsychotic drugs that may be used include haloperidol, clozapine, chlorpromazine, olanzapine, quetiapine fumarate, and risperidone. Family interventions and family therapy often result in improvements in psychotic symptoms, thought disorders, and social functioning among children with schizophrenia.

▌CARE MANAGEMENT

Nursing care of children with psychotic disorders is a highly specialized area. Nurses should be alert to the possibility that schizophrenia can occur in children and refer children to a psychiatrist for evaluation if they consistently demonstrate abnormal behavior. In addition, nurses need to teach family members of children taking antipsychotic medications to observe for possible side effects. Common side effects include dizziness, drowsiness, tachycardia, hypotension, and extrapyramidal effects such as abnormal movements and seizures.

KEY POINTS

- Middle childhood, also known as the *school years,* is the period of life that extends from 6 to 12 years of age.
- Although growth is slower in middle childhood than in previous years, there is a steady gain in height and weight, with maturation of body systems; primary teeth are lost and replaced by permanent teeth.
- A major task during the middle school years is developing a sense of industry or accomplishment (Erikson).
- Piaget's period of concrete operations refers to the school-age period when children are able to use their thought processes to experience events and actions and make judgments based on reasoning.
- The child develops a conscience and is able to understand and adhere to rules and standards set by others.
- Entertaining different points of view, becoming sensitive to social norms, and forming peer friendships are important features of social development during the school years.
- Cooperative play, team activities, and the acquisition of skills are prime elements of play during the school years; rules and rituals assume greater importance.

- Parental concerns during middle childhood include lying, cheating, stealing, and school achievement.
- The availability of junk foods, irregular family meals, and schedules of working parents often interfere with optimal nutrition.
- Dental care is important during this time; potential dental problems include caries, periodontal disease, malocclusion, and dental injury.
- Increased socialization and media exposure make the school years an ideal time for sex education.
- School health programs ideally include health appraisal, emergency care, safety education, communicable disease control, counseling, guidance, and health education with adjustment to individual student needs.
- Injury prevention is directed toward safety education, provision of safe play areas and equipment, and well-supervised sports activities.

REFERENCES

American Academy of Pediatrics, Clinical Practice Guideline: ADHD: Clinical practice guideline for the diagnosis, evaluation, and treatment of attention-deficit/hyperactivity disorder in children and adolescents, *Pediatrics* 128(5):1007–1022, 2011.

American Academy of Pediatrics (AAP) Committee on Injury, Violence, and Poison Prevention: Policy statement: role of the pediatrician in youth violence prevention, *Pediatrics* 124(1):393–402, 2009.

American Academy of Pediatrics (AAP) Council on School Health: Role of the school nurse in providing school health services, *Pediatrics* 121(5):1052–1056, 2008.

American Academy of Pediatrics (AAP) Council on School Health: Policy statement: guidance for the administration of medication in school, *Pediatrics* 124(4):1244–1251, 2009.

American Pediatric Surgical Association Trauma Committee: Position statement on the use of all-terrain vehicles by children and youth, *J Pediatr Surg* 44:1638–1639, 2009.

American Psychiatric Association: *Diagnostic and statistical manual of mental disorders,* ed 4 (text rev) (DSM-IV TR), Washington, DC, 2000, Author.

Arseneault L, Bowes L, Shakoor S: Bullying victimization in youths and mental health problems: 'much ado about nothing?' *Psychol Med* 40:717–729, 2010.

Bowes L, Arseneault L, Maughan B, et al: School, neighborhood, and family factors are associated with children's bullying involvement: a nationally representative longitudinal study, *J Am Child Adolesc Psychiatry* 48(5):545–553, 2009.

Centers for Disease Control and Prevention (CDC) National Center for Injury Prevention and Control: *Child passenger safety,* 2010, Author, www.cdc.gov/ncipc/factsheets/childpas.htm.

Centers for Disease Control and Prevention (CDC): Vital signs: teen pregnancy—United States, 1991-2009, *MMWR Morb Mortal Wkly Rep* 60(13):414–420, 2011.

Cohen JA, AACAP Work Group on Quality Issues: Practice parameter for the assessment and treatment of children and adolescents with posttraumatic stress disorder, *J Am Acad Child Adolesc Psychiatry* 49(4):414–430, 2010.

Cunningham NR, Jensen P: Attention-deficit/hyperactivity disorder. In Kliegman RM, Stanton BF, St. Geme JW, et al, editors: *Nelson textbook of pediatrics,* ed 19, Philadelphia, 2011, Saunders.

Eberl R, Schalamon J, Singer G, et al: Trampoline-related injuries in childhood, *Eur J Pediatr* 168:1171–1174, 2009.

Fisher H, Montgomery P, Gardner F: Opportunities provision for preventing youth gang involvement for children and young people (7-16), *Cochrane Database Syst Rev* (2):CD007002, 2008.

Fredland N: Nurturing hostile environments: the problem of school violence, *Fam Community Health* 31(Suppl 18):S32–S41, 2008.

Jellinek M: ADHD treatments: going beyond the meds, *Contemp Pediatr* 25(5):39–48, 2008.

Knox M: On hitting children: a review of corporal punishment in the United States, *J Pediatr Health Care* 24(2):103–107, 2010.

Kostenius C, Ohrling K: Being relaxed and powerful: children's lived experiences of coping with stress, *Child Soc* 23:203–213, 2009.

Lamb J, Pepler D, Craig W: Approach to bullying and victimization, *Can Fam Physician* 55:356–390, 2009.

Liu J, Graves N: Childhood bullying: a review of constructs, concepts, and nursing implications, *Public Health Nurs* 28(6):556–568, 2011.

McLeod J, Knight S: The association of socioemotional problems with early sexual initiation, *Perspect Sex Reprod Health* 42(2):93–101, 2010.

Mowery BD: Post-traumatic stress disorder (PTSD) in parents: is this a significant problem? *Pediatr Nurs* 37(2):89–92, 2011.

Myers SM, Eisenhauer NJ, Ryan ME: ADHD: it is real, and it can be treated, *Clin Advisor* 6(3):15–25, 2003.

Okun A, Adam H: Safety on bicycles, skateboards, scooters, and skates, *Pediatr Rev* 29(10):366–367, 2008.

Perrin JM, Friedman RA, Knilans TK, et al: Cardiovascular monitoring and stimulant drugs for attention-deficit/hyperactivity disorder, *Pediatrics* 122(2):451–453, 2008.

Pliszka S, AACAP Work Group on Quality Issues: Practice parameter for the assessment and treatment of children, adolescents, and adults with attention-deficit/hyperactivity disorder, *J Am Acad Child Adolesc Psychiatry* 46(7):894–921, 2007.

Ryan-Krause P: Attention deficit hyperactivity disorder: Part III, *J Pediatr Health Care* 25(1):50–56, 2011.

Schredl M, Biernelt J, Roos K, et al: Nightmares and stress in children, *Sleep Hypnosis* 10(1):19–25, 2008.

Selekman J: Attention-deficit/hyperactivity disorder. In Jackson P, Vessey JA, Schapiro NA, editors: *Primary care of children with chronic conditions*, ed 5, St Louis, 2010, Mosby.

Smaldone A, Honig J, Byrne M: Sleepless in America: inadequate sleep and relationships to health and well-being of our nation's children, *Pediatrics* 119(Suppl 1):S29–S37, 2007.

Wagner R, Oskouian R: The ECC epidemic, *Contemp Pediatr* 25(9):60–79, 2008.

Walter HJ, DeMaso DR: Major depression. In Kliegman RM, Stanton BF, St. Geme JW, et al, editors: *Nelson textbook of pediatrics*, ed 19, Philadelphia, 2011, Saunders.

Washington T: Psychological stress and anxiety in middle to late childhood and early adolescence: manifestations and management, *J Pediatr Nurs* 24(4):302–313, 2009.

The Adolescent and Family

David Wilson

evolve WEBSITE

http://evolve.elsevier.com/Perry/maternal

LEARNING OBJECTIVES

On completion of this chapter, the reader will be able to:
- Describe the physical changes that occur at puberty.
- Discuss the reactions of the adolescent to physical changes that take place at puberty.
- Demonstrate an understanding of the processes by which the adolescent develops a sense of identity.
- Discuss the significance of the changing interpersonal relationships and the role of the peer group during adolescence.
- Outline a health teaching plan for adolescents.

- Identify the causes and discuss the preventive aspects of injuries during adolescence.
- Demonstrate an understanding of common disorders of the male and female reproductive systems.
- Demonstrate an understanding of health problems related to adolescent sexuality.
- Outline a care plan for the child or adolescent with an eating disorder.
- Discuss the manifestations and nursing management of selected emotional and/or behavioral problems.

PROMOTING OPTIMAL GROWTH AND DEVELOPMENT

Adolescence is a period of transition between childhood and adulthood—a time of rapid physical, cognitive, social, and emotional maturing as the boy prepares for manhood and the girl prepares for womanhood. The precise boundaries of adolescence are difficult to define, but this period is customarily viewed as beginning with the gradual appearance of secondary sex characteristics at about 11 or 12 years of age and ending with cessation of body growth at 18 to 20 years.

Several terms are used to refer to this stage of growth and development. *Puberty* refers to the maturational, hormonal, and growth process that occurs when the reproductive organs begin to function and the secondary sex characteristics develop. This process is sometimes divided into three stages: *prepubescence,* the period of about 2 years immediately before puberty when the child is developing preliminary physical changes that herald sexual maturity; *puberty,* the point at which sexual maturity is achieved, marked by the first menstrual flow in girls but by less obvious indications in boys; and *postpubescence,* a 1- to 2-year period following puberty during which skeletal growth is completed and reproductive functions become fairly well established. *Adolescence,* which literally means "to grow into maturity," is generally regarded as the psychologic, social, and maturational process initiated by the pubertal changes. It involves three distinct subphases: *early adolescence* (ages 11 to 14), *middle adolescence* (ages 15 to 17), and *late adolescence* (ages 18 to 20). The term *teenage years* is used synonymously with *adolescence* to describe ages 13 through 19.

Biologic Development

The physical changes of puberty are primarily the result of hormonal activity under the influence of the central nervous system, although all aspects of physiologic functioning are mutually interacting. The obvious physical changes are noted in increased physical growth and in the appearance and development of secondary sex characteristics; less obvious are physiologic alterations and neurogonadal maturity, accompanied by the ability to procreate. Physical distinction between the sexes is made on the basis of distinguishing characteristics. Primary sex characteristics are the external and internal organs that carry out the reproductive functions (e.g., ovaries, uterus, breasts, penis). *Secondary sex characteristics* are the changes that occur throughout the body as a result of hormonal changes (e.g., voice alterations, development of facial and pubertal hair, fat deposits) but that play no direct part in reproduction.

Hormonal Changes of Puberty

The events of puberty are caused by hormonal influences and controlled by the anterior pituitary (adenohypophysis) in response to a stimulus from the hypothalamus. Stimulation of the gonads has a dual function: (1) production and release of gametes—production of sperm in the male and maturation and release of ova in the female; and (2) secretion of sex-appropriate hormones—estrogen and progesterone from the ovaries (female) and testosterone from the testes (male).

The ovaries, testes, and adrenals secrete sex hormones. These hormones are produced in varying amounts by both sexes throughout the life span. The adrenal cortex is responsible for the small amounts secreted before the pubescent years, but the sex hormone production that accompanies maturation of the gonads is responsible for the biologic changes observed during puberty.

Estrogen, the feminizing hormone, is found in low quantities during childhood. This hormone is secreted in slowly increasing amounts until about age 11 years. In males, this gradual increase continues through maturation. In females, the onset of estrogen production in the ovary causes a pronounced increase that continues until about 3 years after the onset of menstruation, at which time it reaches a maximum level that continues throughout the reproductive life of the female.

Androgens, the masculinizing hormones, are also secreted in small and gradually increasing amounts up to about 7 to 9 years of age, at which time there is a more rapid increase in both sexes, especially boys, until about age 15 years. These hormones appear to be responsible for most of the rapid growth changes of early adolescence. With the onset of testicular function, the level of androgens (principally *testosterone*) in males increases over that in females and continues to increase until a maximum level is attained at maturity.

Sexual Maturation

The visible evidence of sexual maturation is achieved in an orderly sequence, and the state of maturity can be estimated on the basis of the appearance of these external manifestations. The age at which these changes are observed and the time required to progress from one stage to another may vary among children. The time from the appearance of breast buds to full maturity may be 1½ to 6 years for adolescent girls. It may take 2 to 5 years for male genitalia to reach adult size. The stages of development of secondary sex characteristics and genital development have been defined as a guide for estimating sexual maturity and are referred to as the *Tanner stages* (Box 35-1). The usual sequence of appearance of maturational changes is presented in Box 35-2.

Sexual Maturation in Girls. In most girls, the initial indication of puberty is the appearance of breast buds, an event known as *thelarche,* which occurs between 8 and 13 years of age (Fig. 35-1). This is followed in approximately 2 to 6 months by growth of pubic hair on the mons pubis, known as *adrenarche* (Fig. 35-2). In a minority of normally developing girls, however, pubic hair may precede breast development. The average age of thelarche for Caucasian girls is 10 years, with a range of 8 to 12¾ years; for African-American girls, the average age of thelarche is earlier, around 9 years, with a range of 7 to 11 years (Herman-Giddens, 2006). The average age of thelarche for Hispanic girls falls somewhere between the other two groups.

The initial appearance of menstruation, or menarche, occurs about 2 years after the appearance of the first pubescent changes, approximately 9 months after attainment of peak height velocity, and 3 months after attainment of peak weight velocity. There is evidence that girls are developing secondary sex characteristics at a younger age with differences noted between Caucasian and African-American girls. The explanation for this is not yet clear but appears to be influenced by being overweight as well as environmental influences. The normal age range of menarche is usually 10½ to 15 years, with the average age being 12 years, 4 months for North American girls (Wu, Mendola, and Buck, 2002). Ovulation and regular menstrual periods usually occur 6 to 14 months after menarche. Girls may be considered to have pubertal delay if breast development has not occurred by age 13 years or if menarche has not occurred within 4 years of the onset of breast development.

Sexual Maturation in Boys. The first pubescent changes in boys are testicular enlargement accompanied by thinning, reddening, and increased looseness of the scrotum (Fig. 35-3). These events usually occur between 9½ and 14 years of age. Early puberty is also characterized by the initial appearance of pubic hair. Penile enlargement begins, and testicular enlargement and pubic hair growth continue throughout midpuberty. During this period, there is also increasing muscularity, early voice changes, and development of early facial hair. Temporary breast enlargement and tenderness, *gynecomastia,* are common during midpuberty, occurring in up to one third of boys. The spurts in height and weight occur concurrently toward the end of midpuberty. For most boys, breast enlargement disappears within 2 years. By late puberty, there is a definite

---

BOX 35-1 TANNER STAGES

The Tanner stages were developed by Dr. J.M. Tanner and colleagues. Tanner stages describe the stages of pubertal growth and are numbered from stage 1 (immature) to stage 5 (mature) for both males and females. In girls and young women, the Tanner stages describe pubertal development based on breast size and the shape and distribution of pubic hair. In boys and young men, the Tanner stages describe pubertal development based on the size and shape of the penis and scrotum and the shape and distribution of pubic hair.

Data from Tanner JM: *Growth of adolescents,* Oxford, 1962, Blackwell Scientific Publications.

BOX 35-2 USUAL SEQUENCE OF MATURATIONAL CHANGES

Girls
- Breast changes
- Rapid increase in height and weight
- Growth of pubic hair
- Appearance of axillary hair
- Menstruation (usually begins 2 years after first signs noted above)
- Abrupt deceleration of linear growth

Boys
- Enlargement of testicles
- Growth of pubic hair, axillary hair, hair on upper lip, hair on face and elsewhere on body (facial hair usually appears about 2 years after appearance of pubic hair)
- Rapid increase in height
- Changes in the larynx and consequently the voice (usually take place along with growth of penis)
- Nocturnal emissions
- Abrupt deceleration of linear growth

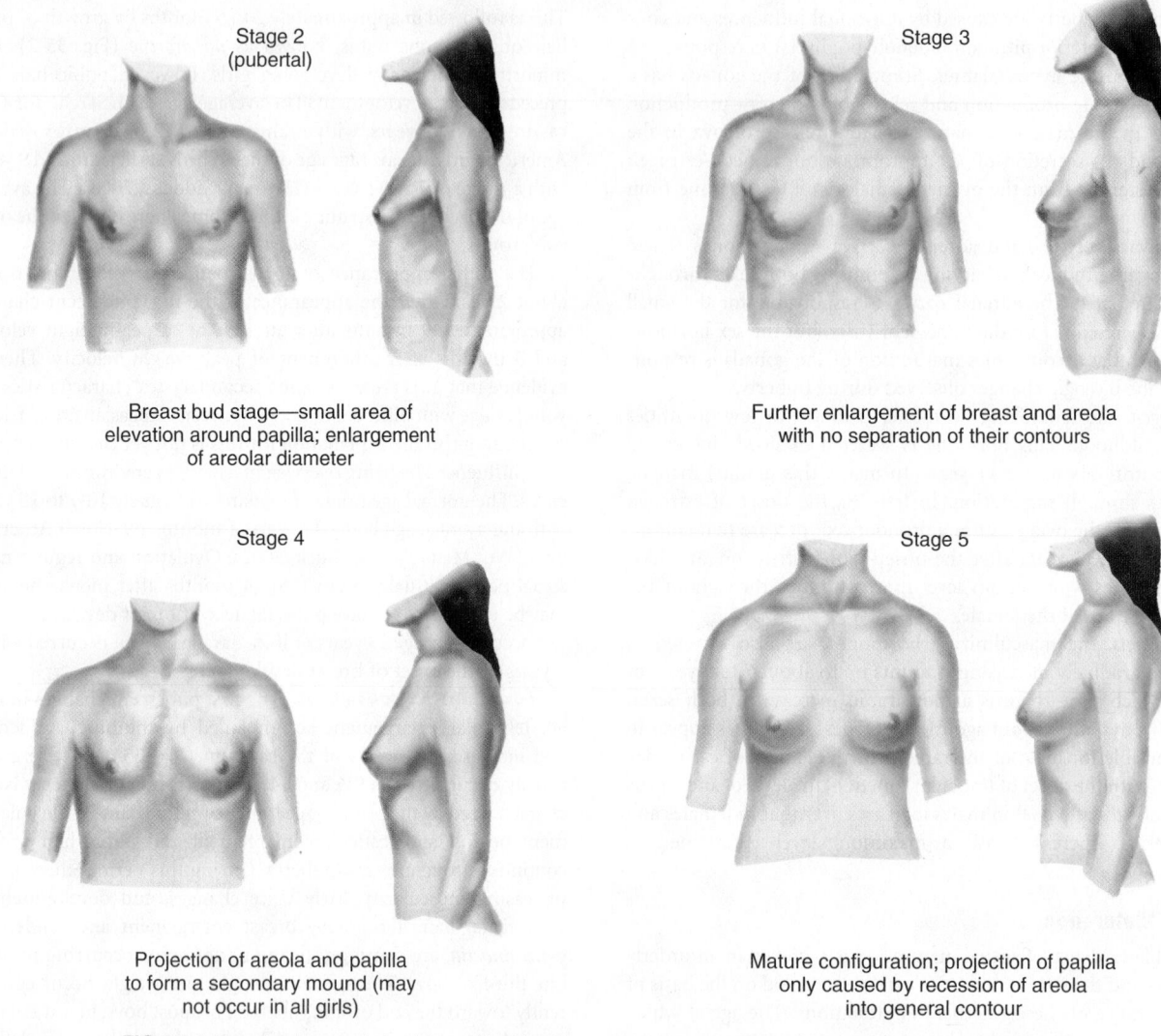

Stage 2
(pubertal)

Breast bud stage—small area of
elevation around papilla; enlargement
of areolar diameter

Stage 3

Further enlargement of breast and areola
with no separation of their contours

Stage 4

Projection of areola and papilla
to form a secondary mound (may
not occur in all girls)

Stage 5

Mature configuration; projection of papilla
only caused by recession of areola
into general contour

FIG 35-1 Development of the breast in girls—average age span: 8 to 13 years. Stage 1 (prepubertal, elevation of papilla only) is not shown. (Adapted from Daniel WA, Paulshock BZ: A physician's guide to sexual maturity, *Patient Care* 13:122–124, 1979; Marshall WA, Tanner JM: Variations in pattern of pubertal changes in girls, *Arch Dis Child* 44:291, 1969.)

increase in the length and width of the penis, testicular enlargement continues, and first ejaculation occurs. Axillary hair develops, and facial hair extends to cover the anterior neck. Final voice changes occur secondary to the growth of the larynx. Concerns about *pubertal delay* should be considered for boys who exhibit no enlargement of the testes or scrotal changes by 13½ to 14 years of age or if genital growth is not complete 4 years after the testicles begin to enlarge.

Physical Growth

A constant phenomenon associated with sexual maturation is a dramatic increase in growth. The final 20% to 25% of height is achieved during puberty, and most of this growth occurs during a 24- to 36-month period—the adolescent growth spurt. This accelerated growth occurs in all children but, as in other areas of development, is highly variable in age of onset, duration, and extent. The growth spurt begins earlier in girls, usually between ages 9½ and 14½ years; on average, it begins between ages 10½ and 16 years in boys. During this period, the average boy gains 10 to

30 cm (4-12 inches) in height and 7 to 30 kg (15.5-66 pounds) in weight. The average girl, in whom the growth spurt is slower and less extensive, gains 5 to 20 cm (2-8 inches) in height and 7 to 25 kg (15.5-55 pounds) in weight. Growth in height typically ceases 2 to 2½ years after menarche in girls and at age 18 to 20 years in boys.

This increase in size is acquired in a characteristic sequence. Growth in length of the extremities and neck precedes growth in other areas, and because these parts are the first to reach adult length, the hands and feet appear larger than normal during adolescence. Increases in hip and chest breadth take place in a few months, followed several months later by an increase in shoulder width. These changes are followed by increases in length of the trunk and depth of the chest. This sequence of changes is responsible for the characteristic long-legged, gawky appearance of early adolescent children.

Sex Differences in General Growth Patterns. Sex differences in general growth and distribution patterns are apparent in skeletal growth, muscle mass, adipose tissue, and skin. Skeletal

Stage 1
(prepubertal)

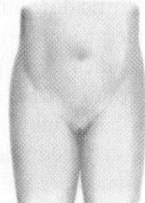

No pubic hair; essentially the same as
during childhood; no distinction between
hair on pubis and over the abdomen

Stage 2

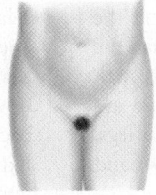

Sparse growth of long, straight, downy, and
slightly pigmented hair extending along labia;
between stages 2 and 3 begins to appear on pubis

Stage 3

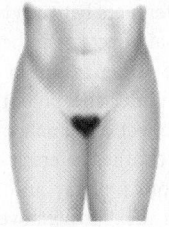

Hair darker, coarser, and curly and
spread sparsely over entire pubis in
the typical female triangle

Stage 4

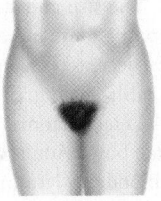

Pubic hair denser, curled, and adult in distribution
but less abundant and restricted to the pubic area

Stage 5

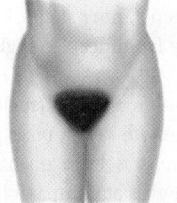

Hair adult in quantity, type, and pattern
with spread to inner aspect of thighs

FIG 35-2 Growth in pubic hair in girls—average age span for stages 2 through 5: 11 to 14 years.
(Adapted from Daniel WA, Paulshock BZ: A physician's guide to sexual maturity, *Patient Care* 13:122–
124, 1979; Marshall WA, Tanner JM: Variations in pattern of pubertal changes in girls, *Arch Dis Child*
44:291, 1969.)

Stage 1
(prepubertal)

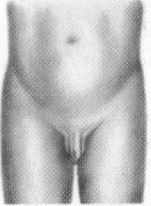

No pubic hair; essentially the same as
during childhood; no distinction between
hair on pubis and over the abdomen

Stage 2 (pubertal)

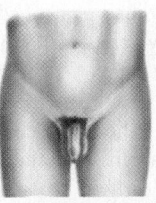

Initial enlargement of scrotum and testes;
reddening and textural changes of scrotal skin;
sparse growth of long, straight, downy, and
slightly pigmented hair at base of penis

Stage 3

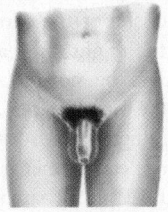

Initial enlargement of penis, mainly in
length; testes and scrotum further enlarged;
hair darker, coarser, and curly and spread
sparsely over entire pubis

Stage 4

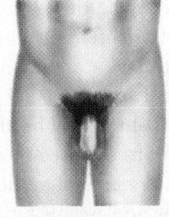

Increased size of penis with growth in diameter and
development of glans; glans larger and broader; scrotum
darker; pubic hair more abundant with curling but
restricted to pubic area

Stage 5

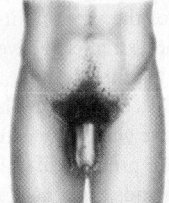

Testes, scrotum, and penis adult in size and shape;
hair adult in quantity and type with spread to inner
surface of thighs

FIG 35-3 Developmental stages of secondary sex characteristics and genital development in boys—
average age span: 12½ to 16 years. (Adapted from Daniel WA, Paulshock BZ: A physician's guide to
sexual maturity, *Patient Care* 13:122–124, 1979; Marshall WA, Tanner JM: Variations in pattern of
pubertal changes in girls, *Arch Dis Child* 44:291, 1969.)

growth differences between boys and girls are apparently a function of hormonal effects at puberty and are evident primarily in limb length. The earlier cessation of growth in girls is caused by epiphyseal unity under the potent effect of estrogen secretion, and the hormonal effect on female bone growth is much stronger than the similar effect of testosterone in boys. In boys, the prolonged growth period before puberty and the less rapid epiphyseal closure are reflected in their greater overall height and longer arms and legs. Other skeletal differences are increased shoulder width in boys and broader hip development in girls.

Hypertrophy of the laryngeal mucosa and enlargement of the larynx and vocal cords occur in both boys and girls to produce voice changes. Girls' voices become slightly deeper and considerably fuller, but the effect in boys is striking. The change in the voice of adolescent boys occurs between Tanner stages 3 and 4, with the voice often shifting uncontrollably from deep to high tones in the middle of a sentence.

Growth of lean body mass, principally muscle, which tends to occur after the bone growth spurt, takes place steadily during adolescence. Lean body mass is both quantitatively and qualitatively greater in boys than in girls at comparable stages of pubertal development. Muscle development, under the influence of androgenic hormones, increases steadily. Muscles become remarkably well developed in boys, whereas in girls, muscle mass increase is proportionate to general tissue growth.

Nonlean body mass, primarily fat, is also increased but follows a less orderly pattern. There may be a transient increase in subcutaneous fat just before the skeletal growth spurt, especially in boys. This is followed 1 to 2 years later by a modest to marked decrease, which is again more notable in boys. Later, variable amounts of fat are deposited to fill out and contour the mature physique in patterns characteristic of the adolescent's gender, particularly in the regions over the thighs, hips, and buttocks and around the breast tissue. It should be noted, however, that pediatric obesity has increased in the United States, and it is believed that obesity can change the timing of puberty. Girls with thelarche as the first sign of puberty have earlier menarche and greater body fat and body mass index (BMI) at menarche than girls with adrenarche as the first pubertal sign. Kaplowitz (2008) points out that there is evidence of a causal relationship between obesity and onset of early puberty in girls rather than earlier puberty causing an increase in body fat; no correlations between body fat and earlier puberty in boys have been reported.

Hormonal influences during puberty cause acceleration in growth and maturation of the skin and its structural appendages. Sebaceous glands become extremely active at this time, especially those on the genitalia and in the "flush areas" of the body (i.e., face, neck, shoulders, upper back, and chest). This increased activity and the structural nature of the glands are extremely important in the pathogenesis of a common problem of puberty: acne (see Chapter 47). The eccrine sweat glands, present almost everywhere on the human skin, become fully functional and respond to emotional and thermal stimulation. Heavy sweating appears to be more pronounced in boys than in girls. The apocrine sweat glands, nonfunctional in childhood, reach secretory capacity during puberty. Unlike the eccrine sweat glands, the apocrine glands are limited in distribution and grow in conjunction with hair follicles in the axillae, around the areola of the breast, around the umbilicus, on the external auditory canal, and in the genital and anal regions. Apocrine glands secrete a thick substance as a result of emotional stimulation that, when acted on by surface bacteria, becomes highly odoriferous.

Body hair assumes very characteristic distribution patterns and changes texture during puberty. Under the influence of gonadal and adrenal androgens, hair coarsens, darkens, and lengthens at sites related to secondary sex characteristics. Pubic and axillary hair appear in both sexes, although pubic hair is more extensive in males than in females. Beard, mustache, and body hair on the chest, upward along the linea alba, and sometimes on other areas (e.g., back and shoulders) appears in males and is androgen dependent. Extremity hair appears in varying amounts in both males and females but is also more prolific in the male.

Physiologic Changes

A number of physiologic functions are altered in response to some of the pubertal changes. The size and strength of the heart, blood volume, and systolic blood pressure increase, whereas the pulse rate and basal heat production decrease (see Appendix C). Blood volume, which has increased steadily during childhood, reaches a higher value in boys than in girls, a fact that may be related to the increased muscle mass in pubertal boys. Adult values are reached for all formed elements of the blood. Respiratory rate and basal metabolic rate, decreasing steadily throughout childhood, reach the adult rate in adolescence. Respiratory volume and vital capacity are increased and to a far greater extent in males than in females. During this period, physiologic responses to exercise change drastically: performance improves, especially in boys, and the body is able to make the physiologic adjustments needed for normal functioning after exercise is completed. These capabilities are a result of the increased size and strength of muscles and the increased level of cardiac, respiratory, and metabolic functioning.

Psychosocial Development
Developing a Sense of Identity (Erikson)

Traditional psychosocial theory holds that the developmental crisis of adolescence leads to the formation of a sense of identity (Erikson, 1963). Throughout childhood, individuals have been going through the process of identification as they concentrate on various parts of the body at specific times. During infancy, children identify themselves as being separate from the mother; during early childhood, they establish a gender-role identification with the appropriate-sex parent; and in later childhood, they establish who they are in relation to others. In adolescence, they come to see themselves as distinct individuals, somehow unique and separate from every other individual.

Adolescence begins with the onset of puberty and extends to relative physical and emotional stability at or near graduation from high school. During this time, the adolescent is faced with the crisis of *group identity versus alienation*. In the period that follows, the individual strives to attain autonomy from the family and develop a sense of *personal identity* as opposed to *role diffusion*. A sense of group identity appears to be essential to the development of a sense of personal identity. Young adolescents must resolve questions concerning relationships with a peer group before they are able to resolve questions about who they are in relation to family and society.

Group Identity. During the early stage of adolescence, pressure to belong to a group is intensified. Adolescents find it essential to have a group to which they feel they can belong and that provides them with status. Belonging to a crowd helps adolescents establish the differences between themselves and their parents. They dress as the group dresses and wear makeup and hairstyles according to group criteria, all of which are different from those of the parental generation. Language, music, and dancing reflect a culture that is exclusive to the adolescent. When adults begin to emulate these fashions and interests, the style changes immediately. The evidence of adolescent conformity to the peer group and nonconformity to the adult group provides teenagers with a frame of reference in which they can display their own self-assertion while they reject the identity of their parents' generation. To be different is to be unaccepted and alienated from the group.

Individual Identity. The quest for personal identity is part of the ongoing identification process. As adolescents establish identity within a group, they also attempt to incorporate multiple body changes into a concept of the self. Body awareness is part of self-awareness. In their search for identity, adolescents consider the relationships that have developed between themselves and others in the past, as well as the directions they hope to take in the future.

Significant others hold expectations for the adolescent's behavior. Often these expectations or demands are persistent enough to result in certain decisions that might be made differently or not at all if the individual could be solely responsible for identity formation. It is all too easy to slip into the roles that are expected by these external influences without incorporating personal goals or questioning these decisions. Thus individuals may become what parents or others wish them to be, based on these premature decisions. Adolescents might form a negative identity when society or their culture provides them with a self-image that is contrary to the values of the community. Labels such as "loser," "punk," "troublemaker," or "failure" are applied to certain adolescents, who then accept and live up to these labels with behaviors that validate and strengthen them.

The process of evolving a personal identity is time-consuming and fraught with periods of confusion, depression, and discouragement. Determining an identity and a place in the world is a critical and perilous feature of adolescence (see Critical Thinking Case Study). However, as the pieces gradually shift and settle into place, a positive identity eventually emerges. Role diffusion results when the individual is unable to formulate a satisfactory identity from the multiplicity of aspirations, roles, and identifications.

Sex-Role Identity. Adolescence is the time for consolidation of a sex-role identity. During early adolescence, the peer group begins to communicate expectations regarding heterosexual relationships, and as development progresses, adolescents encounter expectations for mature sex-role behavior from both peers and adults. Expectations vary from culture to culture, among geographic areas, and among socioeconomic groups.

Emotionality. Adolescents vacillate in their emotional states between considerable maturity and childlike behavior. One minute they are exuberant and enthusiastic; the next minute they are depressed and withdrawn. Unpredictable but essentially normal mood swings are common during this time. As the tension is relieved, emotion is brought under control and individuals retreat to review what has happened, to attempt to master their anger, and to increase their ability to control their emotions and gain from the new experience. Because of these mood swings, adolescents are frequently labeled as unstable, inconsistent, and unpredictable. Little things can cause an emotional upheaval and, depending on the teenager's interpretation, can mean a great deal.

Teenagers are better able to control their emotions in later adolescence. They can approach problems more calmly and rationally, and although they are still subject to periods of sadness, their feelings are less vulnerable and they begin to demonstrate more mature emotions. Whereas early adolescents react immediately and emotionally, older adolescents can control their emotions until socially acceptable times and places for expression present themselves. They are still subject to heightened emotion, and when it is expressed, their behavior reflects feelings of insecurity, tension, and indecision.

Cognitive Development (Piaget)

Cognitive thinking culminates with the capacity for *abstract thinking*. This stage, the period of *formal operations*, is Piaget's fourth and last stage. Adolescents are no longer restricted to the real and actual, which was typical of the period of concrete thought; now they are also concerned with the possible. They now think beyond the present. Without having to center attention on the immediate situation, they can imagine a sequence of events that might occur, such as college and occupational possibilities; how things might change in the future, such as relationships with parents; and the consequences of their actions, such as dropping out of high school. At this time, their thoughts can be influenced by logical principles rather than just their own perceptions and experiences. They become increasingly capable of scientific reasoning and formal logic.

Adolescents are capable of mentally manipulating more than two categories of variables at the same time. For example, they can consider the relationship between speed, distance, and time in planning a trip. They can detect logical consistency or inconsistency in a set of statements and evaluate a system or set of values in a more analytic manner. For instance, they question the parent who insists on honesty in the teenager but at the same time cheats on an income tax report or expense account.

In adolescence, young people begin to think about both their own thinking and the thinking of others. They wonder what opinion others have of them, and they are able to imagine the thoughts of others. With this capacity comes the ability to differentiate between others' thoughts and their own and to interpret the thoughts of others more accurately. They are able to understand that few concepts are absolute or independent of other influencing factors. As they become aware that other cultures and communities have different norms and standards from their own, it becomes easier for them to accept members of these other cultures, and the decision to behave in their own culture in an accepted manner becomes a more conscious commitment.

? CRITICAL THINKING CASE STUDY

Discussing the Future

Jeremy, age 17, will be graduating from high school in the spring. His mother, a single parent, tells you that she is concerned because graduation is quickly approaching and Jeremy has made no plans for what he will do with his life after graduation. Whenever Jeremy mentions the topic, his mother tells him "This is what you must do" and begins to outline the steps he must take. Jeremy just walks away. She asks, "What should I do?" What advice should you give Jeremy's mother?

1. Evidence—Is there sufficient evidence to draw any conclusions about what advice the nurse should give Jeremy's mother?
2. Assumptions—Describe an underlying assumption about each of the following issues:
   a. Adolescents and the search for personal identity
   b. The influence of others on the adolescent's search for personal identity
   c. Ways to communicate with adolescents
3. What implications and priorities for nursing care can be drawn at this time?
4. Does the evidence objectively support your argument (conclusion)?

Moral Development (Kohlberg)

Although younger children merely accept the decisions or point of view of adults, adolescents, to gain autonomy from adults, must substitute their own set of morals and values. When old principles are challenged but new independent values have not yet emerged to take their place, young people search for a moral code that preserves their personal integrity and guides their behavior, especially in the face of strong pressure to violate the old beliefs. Their decisions involving moral dilemmas must be based on an *internalized set of moral principles* that provides them with the resources to evaluate the demands of the situation and to plan actions that are consistent with their ideals.

Late adolescence is characterized by serious questioning of existing moral values and their relevance to society and the individual. Adolescents can easily take the role of another. They understand duty and obligation based on reciprocal rights of others, as well as the concept of justice that is founded on making amends for misdeeds and repairing or replacing what has been spoiled by wrongdoing. However, they seriously question established moral codes, often as a result of observing that some adults verbally ascribe to a code but do not adhere to it.

Spiritual Development

As adolescents move toward independence from parents and other authorities, some begin to question the values and ideals of their families. Others adhere to these values as a stable element in their lives as they struggle with the conflicts of this turbulent period. Adolescents need to work out these conflicts for themselves, but they also need support from authority figures or peers for their resolution.

Adolescents are capable of understanding abstract concepts and of interpreting analogies and symbols. They are able to empathize, philosophize, and think logically. Most teens search for ideals and speculate about illogical statements and conflicting ideologies. Their tendency toward introspection and emotional intensity often makes it difficult for others to know what they are thinking. They tend to keep their thoughts private, fearing that no one will understand these feelings that they perceive to be unique and special. However, they may reveal deep spiritual concerns. They need support and encouragement in their struggle for understanding and the freedom to question without censure.

Generally, the stated importance of participation in organized religion declines somewhat during the adolescent years. More high school students than post–secondary school young people attend religious services regularly, and, not surprisingly, the younger the adolescents, the more likely they are to view religion as being important to them. Among older adolescents, the importance of organized religion declines more among college students than among those not in college. Late adolescence appears to be a time when individuals reexamine and reevaluate many of the beliefs and values of their childhood. Consistent with developmental changes in value autonomy, the religious beliefs of young people are likely to become more personalized and less bound to the traditional religious practices they may have been exposed to when they were younger. As adolescents mature and form an identity, they may either reject their family's traditional beliefs or they may decide to conform to those beliefs (Neuman, 2011).

Neuman (2011) suggests that adolescents, who are searching for an identity and personal growth, may perceive God as one who accepts them and confirms their self-identity. Religious beliefs in adolescence are also strongly influenced by interpersonal relationships with peers as well as adults in their environment.

Greater levels of religiosity and spirituality are associated with fewer high risk behaviors and more health-promoting behaviors, especially for youth living in environments lacking positive influences (Regnerus and Glen, 2003). Nurses play an important role for teens by providing an opportunity to discuss issues regarding spirituality.

Social Development

To achieve full maturity, adolescents must free themselves from family domination and define an identity independent of parental authority. However, this process is fraught with ambivalence on the part of both teenagers and their parents. Adolescents want to grow up and be free of parental restraints, but they are fearful as they try to comprehend the responsibilities that are linked with independence. Feelings of immortality and exemption from the consequences of risk-taking behavior, although viewed as negative, can serve an important developmental function at this time. These feelings give adolescents the courage to separate from their parents and become independent. Part of this emancipation involves developing social relationships outside the family that help adolescents identify their role in society. Adolescence is a time of intense sociability and often a time of equally intense loneliness. Acceptance by peers, a few close friends, and the secure love of a supportive family are requisites for interpersonal maturation.

Relationships with Parents

During adolescence, the parent-child relationship changes from one of protection-dependency to one of *mutual affection and equality*. The process of achieving independence often involves turmoil and ambiguity as both parent and adolescent learn to play new roles and work toward this end while, at the same time, resolving the often painful series of rifts essential to establishing the ultimate relationship.

Most behavior observed in the adolescent is related to the struggle for independence and the external restrictions and checks and balances that are placed on this spontaneous maturation process. On the one hand, adolescents are accepted as maturing preadults. They are allowed privileges heretofore denied, and they are provided with increasing responsibilities. On the other hand, because of their unpredictability and insecurity in evaluating situations and making sound judgments, they must conform to regulations and restrictions set by adults. This state of affairs is particularly exemplified by the struggle between parents and adolescents concerning curfews and the use of social media.

As teenagers assert their rights for grown-up privileges, they frequently create tensions within the home. They resist parental control, and conflicts can arise from almost any situation or any subject. Favorite topics of dispute include whether or not the adolescent has his or her own cell phone, Internet and cell phone use, manners, dress, chores and duties, homework, disrespectful behavior, friendships, dating and relationships, money, automobiles, alcohol and other substance abuse, and time schedules. Present in these areas of conflict is the overriding argument that "everyone else has one" or is allowed the desired item or privilege and the ever-present assertions that "You don't understand me or trust me" and "You always treat me like a child." Spoken or unspoken, parents' reactions consist of "Is this all the thanks I get for what I have done for you?"

Adolescents' earliest attempts to achieve emancipation from parental controls are manifested in a period of rejection of the parents. They absent themselves from home and family activities and spend increasing time with the peer group. They confide less in

FAMILY-CENTERED CARE

Communication with Adolescents: The Art of Listening

Conflicts between parents and their adolescents are often a result of a natural characteristic of parenthood: the desire to protect one's offspring from harm or from simply doing something "stupid" or embarrassing or something they may later regret. Teenagers sometimes "bounce" their thoughts and ideas off adults. At times they really want some feedback; at other times they simply want to elicit a reaction.

I found it easy to listen openly, thoughtfully, and without interrupting when my teenagers' friends discussed troublesome topics. However, one day, when one of my own teenagers had a similar conversation with me, the parent part kicked in. I felt responsible and spoke my piece on the spot. This brought communication to a halt and resulted in defensiveness. It was a long time before my child tried to talk to me about anything controversial again. The next time one of my teenagers started a similar conversation, I decided to try to trick myself.

Throughout the entire conversation, I told myself over and over again to act as if this were not my teenager but, rather, someone else's child. I found this actually worked quite well, and I was able to listen without interrupting. I continued to use the system, sometimes with more success than at other times.

—Mother of Four

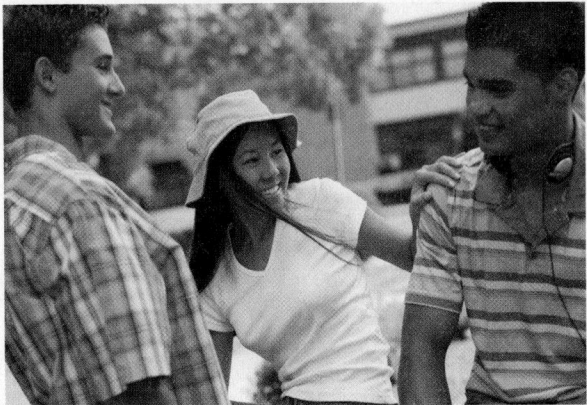

FIG 35-4 Teenagers like to gather in small groups. (Copyright © 2011 Photos.com, a division of Getty Images. All rights reserved.)

their parents, but parents continue to play an important role in their personal and health-related decision making.

With advancing adolescence, teenagers become more competent and with this competence comes a need for more autonomy. Although they may be psychologically prepared for independence, they are often thwarted in their efforts by lack of money or other parental barriers. Conflict arises in relation to the teenagers' outside activities and the elements of privacy and trust. Parental monitoring remains important throughout adolescence and may have a direct influence on adolescent sexual and substance-use behavior. Parents should be guided toward an authoritative style of parenting in which authority is used to *guide* the adolescent while allowing developmentally appropriate levels of freedom and providing clear, consistent messages regarding expectations. Consistency in guidance and establishing ground rules is extremely important for adolescents even though they may fiercely reject the parents' wishes. Authoritative style of parenting has been shown to have both immediate and long-term protective effects toward adolescent risk reduction (DeVore and Ginsburg, 2005). However, to gain the trust of adolescents, parents must respect their adolescent's privacy and show an honest and sincere interest in what the adolescent believes and feels (see Family-Centered Care box).

Relationships with Peers

Although parents remain the primary influence in their lives, for the majority of teenagers, peers assume a more significant role in adolescence than they did during childhood. The peer group serves as a strong support to teenagers, individually and collectively, providing them with a sense of belonging and a feeling of strength and power. The peer group forms the transitional world between dependence and autonomy.

Peer Group. Adolescents are usually social, gregarious, and group minded. Thus the peer group has an intense influence on adolescents' self-evaluation and behavior. To gain acceptance by a group, younger teenagers tend to conform completely in such things

as mode of dress, hairstyle, taste in music, and vocabulary. Teenagers use the peer group as a standard measure of what is normal.

The school is psychologically important to adolescents as a focus of social life. Teenagers usually distribute themselves into a relatively predictable social hierarchy. They know to which groups they and others belong. A sense of school connectedness has been found to predict decreased risk-taking behaviors in adolescents (Bond, Butler, Thomas, et al., 2007). School connectedness is correlated with caring teachers and the absence of prejudice or discrimination from peers. A sense of school connectedness is less dependent on class size, attendance, academic preparation, and parental involvement (Maes and Lievens, 2003).

Within the larger groups are smaller, distinct, and rather exclusive crowds or cliques of selected close friends who are emotionally attached to each other. The selection is based on common tastes, interests, and background. Although cliques may become formalized, most remain informal and small. However, each has an identifying feature that proclaims its difference from others and its solidarity within itself, in much the same manner as the adolescent generation as a whole sets itself apart from the adult generation. Cliques are usually made up of one gender, and girls tend to be more cliquish than boys and to have a greater need for close friendships (Fig. 35-4). Within the intimacy of the group, adolescents gain support in learning about themselves, consideration for the feelings of others, and increased ego development and self-reliance.

To *belong* is of utmost importance; thus adolescents behave in a way that will ensure their establishment in a group. Adolescents are highly susceptible to social approval, acceptance, and demands. To be ignored or criticized by peers creates feelings of inferiority, inadequacy, and incompetence.

Best Friends. Personal friendships of the one-on-one variety usually develop between same-sex adolescents. This relationship is closer and more stable than it is in middle childhood, and it is important in the quest for identity. A best friend is the best audience on whom to try out possible roles and identities that an adolescent wants to test. Best friends may try a role together, each supporting the other. Each cares about what the other thinks and feels. Because a sense of intimacy grows within a permanent relationship, the stability of this same-sex friendship is an important link in the progress toward an intimate relationship in young adulthood.

Interests and Activities

Adolescents spend a large amount of time engaging in leisure-time activities. As teenagers progress through the developmental stages of

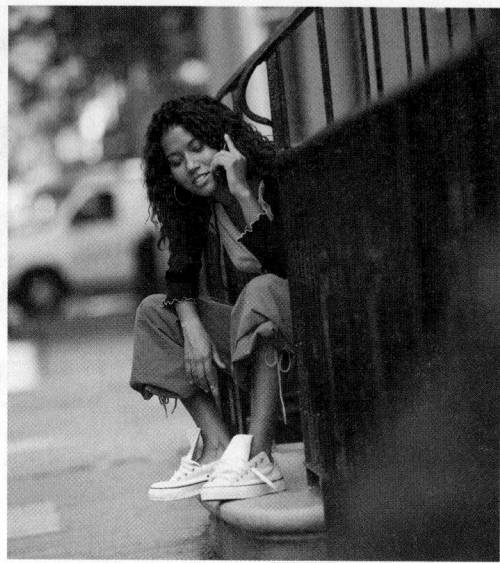

FIG 35-5 The cell phone allows adolescents to talk for hours with peers. (Copyright © 2011 Photos.com, a division of Getty Images. All rights reserved.)

adolescence, these leisure-time activities move from being family centered to being peer centered. In addition to providing teenagers with fun and enjoyment, leisure-time activities assist in the development of social, physical, and cognitive skills. Leisure-time activities also allow teenagers the opportunity to learn to set priorities and structure their time (Fig. 35-5).

The role of social media and advanced technology are nowhere more prominent than in the lives of today's adolescents. The widespread availability of the Internet and access to social networking websites such as FaceBook, chatrooms, free e-mail, blogs, and Twitter have created "virtual" communities and ways for young people to interact with others; web cameras even allow those interactions to include real-time video communication. Cellular telephones offer more mobile opportunities to talk on the phone, send text messages or instant messaging, send photos, or use video phone capabilities.

Internet chatrooms and social networking sites have created a more public arena for trying out identities and developing interpersonal skills with a wider network of people, occasionally with anonymity. This can create opportunities for young people who have a limited access to friends (because of rural location, shyness, or rare chronic conditions) to interact with people like themselves. However, most adolescents appear to be using the online social environment to interact with the same peers they spend their day with at school.

Text messaging and instant messaging via cell phones has become a common activity and can sometimes be disruptive during school. In addition, both the online and text environment can create opportunities for cyberbullying, in which teens engage in insults, harassment, and publicly humiliating statements online or on cell phones. There is increased danger of adolescents coming in contact and sharing personal information with sexual predators who pose as adolescents in an attempt to make personal contact with underage victims or engage them in sexting (sending sexually explicit or suggestive pictures or messages online) (Dowdell, Burgess, and Flores, 2011). Adolescent sexting, rather than being an innocent anonymous activity, has been linked to risky sexual behaviors in a few studies (Rice, Rhoades, Winetrobe, et al., 2012; Temple, Paul, van den Berg, et al., 2012).

Today, many adolescents must learn to juggle their time between school, activities, and job responsibilities. Adolescent work experiences provide many benefits, including time management, teamwork skills, and increased income. However, many jobs available to teenagers do not provide opportunities to apply the skills they learn in school, and jobs often have high demands for quick work with low rewards. Few apprentice opportunities are available for teenagers in the United States. It is generally recommended that adolescents limit their work to no more than 20 hours per week during the school year.

Adolescent Sexuality

Sexual activity is common by the late teen years, but only 13% of teens have ever had vaginal intercourse by age 15 years. The average age of sexual initiation is about age 17 years. The top three reasons teenagers report for waiting to have sex include religious or moral beliefs, desire to postpone motherhood, and "haven't found the right person yet" (Abma, Martinez, and Copen, 2010).

Adolescence represents a critical time in the development of sexuality. Hormonal, physical, cognitive, and social changes that occur during adolescence all have an impact on sexual development. Of all the developmental changes that affect adolescent sexuality, none is more obvious than the impact of puberty. Adolescents must come to terms with hormonal influences, physiologic manifestations such as menstruation and ejaculation, and physical changes such as breast and genital development. All of these changes have a profound impact on the way teenagers perceive their bodies (i.e., body image). In addition to transitions in body image, increasing levels of pubertal hormones contribute to increased levels of sexual motivation among both boys and girls.

Changes in sexual motivations and feelings, happening at the same time as shifts in cognitive skills, contribute to painful conjectures ("Is what I'm feeling normal?"), self-conscious concern ("Am I good-looking enough?"), and hypothetical thinking ("What if she wants to have sex?"). The emergence of formal operational thinking also increases adolescents' decision-making capabilities concerning sexual issues. As they mature, teenagers become better able to think through potential risks and benefits of sexual behaviors before they engage in any behavior. Older adolescents may also be able to conceptualize more long-term consequences of present behaviors. One of the important tasks of adolescence is to incorporate sexuality successfully into close, intimate relationships. This task is made possible by the advanced cognitive abilities that emerge over the course of adolescence.

Part of adolescent identity formation involves the development of sexual identity. As they begin to integrate changes involved with puberty, young adolescents also develop emotional and social identities separate from their families'. For young adolescents, the process of sexual identity development usually involves forming close friendships with same-sex peers, with whom they may experiment sexually, often to satisfy curiosity. Sexual activity among young teenagers varies by gender. Masturbation provides an opportunity for sexual self-exploration; participation in this behavior is influenced by learned cultural attitudes and sex-role expectations.

Many teenagers begin to make a shift from relationships with same-sex peers to intimate relationships with members of the opposite sex during middle adolescence (Fig. 35-6). Opposite-sex relationships typically begin with peer activities involving both boys and girls. Pairing off as couples becomes more common as middle adolescence progresses. The type and degree of seriousness of partner relationships vary. Initial relationships are usually noncommittal, extremely mobile, and seldom characterized by any deep romantic

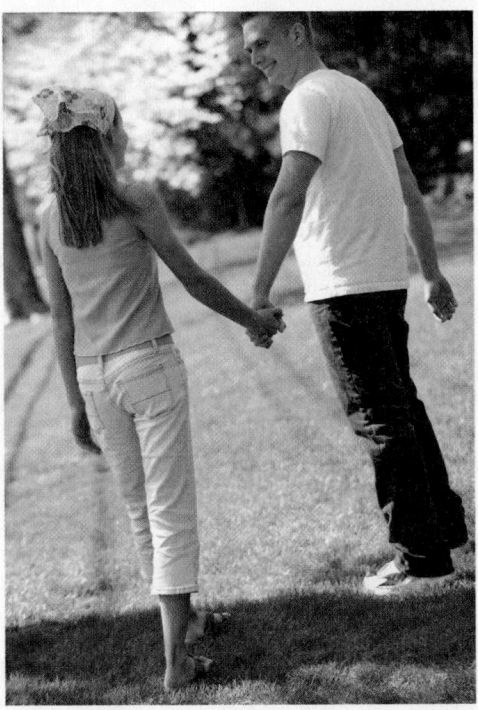

FIG 35-6 Relationships with peers of the opposite sex are an important part of adolescence. (Copyright © 2011 Photos.com, a division of Getty Images. All rights reserved.)

attachments. Sexual activity becomes more common during middle adolescence. The relationship between love and sexual expression is brought into focus during middle adolescence. Most young people oppose exploitation, pressure, or force in sex as well as sex solely for the sake of physical enjoyment without a personal relationship. Adolescents find it hard to believe that sex can exist without love; therefore they view each relationship as real love.

An integrated sexual identity often emerges during late adolescence as individuals incorporate sexual experiences, feelings, and knowledge. For most, this identity is consistent with their own physical and mental capacities and with societal limits and expectations. Most older adolescents identify themselves as being predominantly heterosexual; about 3% of males and 8% of females identify themselves as bisexual or homosexual (Mosher, Chandra, and Jones, 2005). Whatever their sexual orientation, most older teenagers possess the capacity to have intimate relationships that satisfy the emotional and sexual needs of both partners.

Sexual orientation is an important aspect of sexual identity. Sexual orientation is defined as a pattern of sexual arousal or romantic attraction toward persons of the opposite gender (heterosexual), of the same gender (homosexual, often called *gay* or *lesbian*), or of both genders (bisexual). Sexual orientation encompasses several dimensions, including attraction, fantasy, actual sexual behavior, and self-labeling or group affiliation. In individuals, the direction and intensity of each dimension are not necessarily consistent with any of the others. For example, individuals may be attracted most strongly to their same gender, fantasize about both genders, have sexual activity only with the opposite gender, and identify as gay or lesbian. Other individuals may engage in same-gender sexual behavior and fantasize about both genders but identify as heterosexual. As with all aspects of sexual identity, the dimensions of sexual orientation are influenced by cultural meaning and expectation, by gender, by peer groups, and by other environmental contexts.

Adolescence is the period during which individuals commonly begin to identify their sexual orientation as part of their developing sexual identity. However, this identification process can be profoundly influenced by cultural beliefs and values, by societal and family pressures, or by a lack of similar peers. The majority of adolescents eventually report an orientation toward exclusively heterosexual relationships. For adolescents whose orientation encompasses any same-sex dimensions, the identity process during adolescence can be complicated, especially when community norms disapprove of orientations other than heterosexual. Adolescents who have witnessed harassment or violence directed at gay, lesbian, and bisexual people, for example, may be reluctant to self-identify even when their attractions and behaviors are exclusively same-sex or bisexual.

The development of sexual orientation as part of sexual identity includes several developmental milestones during late childhood and throughout adolescence. These milestones do not necessarily occur in the same order for everyone, nor are they completed in the same amount of time. They include:

1. The realization of romantic or erotic attraction to people of one (or both) genders
2. Erotic daydreaming about one or both genders
3. Romantic partners or dates without sexual activity
4. Sexual activity with people of the preferred gender or genders (also, for some teens, sexual activity with a nonpreferred gender, out of curiosity or through social pressure)
5. Self-identification of the orientation that best fits one's current circumstances and understanding
6. Publicly self-identifying that orientation, usually to intimate friends and family first and then the wider social group
7. An intimate, committed sexual relationship with a person of the gender appropriate to one's orientation

There is no evidence that gay, lesbian, or bisexual adults are more or less likely to create long-term, stable relationships than are heterosexual couples. It should be noted that bisexual adolescents and adults do not generally engage in sexual relationships with both genders concurrently; self-identification as bisexual usually refers to the ability to be attracted to either gender but does not imply that such a person requires partners of both genders or that one must be equally attracted to and have sexual experience with both genders to be bisexual.

Although the order of these milestones varies greatly among adolescents, adolescents who identify as gay, lesbian, or bisexual tend to publicly self-identify later than heterosexual peers. Without positive gay, lesbian, or bisexual role models or a supportive peer group, sexual-minority teens can feel isolated and they may not share their orientation with anyone for fear of rejection or violence (see Critical Thinking Case Study). A comparison of bisexual youth and heterosexual youth found that bisexual adolescents, especially girls, reported lower levels of connection to family and school than did heterosexual adolescents. Nurses should be alert to these lower levels of protective relationships for bisexual youth because it may lead to poor health outcomes (Saewyc, Homma, Skay, et al., 2009).

Development of Self-Concept and Body Image

The sudden growth that takes place in early adolescence creates feelings of confusion for adolescents. They have lost the security of a familiar body and feel uncomfortable with their altered body. Consequently, they may try to either hide their body or advertise it or they may alternate between the two extremes. Teenagers are acutely aware of their appearance as they begin to acquire images of

? CRITICAL THINKING CASE STUDY

Discussing Sexual Orientation with Adolescents

John, a 17-year-old adolescent, comes into the school-based clinic and tells the nurse practitioner that he thinks he is homosexual. What is the most appropriate response for the nurse practitioner?

1. Evidence—Is there sufficient evidence to draw any conclusions about John's sexual orientation at this time?
2. Assumptions—Describe an underlying assumption about each of the following issues:
   a. Sexual orientation in adolescents
   b. Society's reaction to homosexuality
   c. Health care professionals and sexuality
3. What implications and priorities for nursing care can be drawn at this time?
4. Does the evidence objectively support your argument (conclusion)?

themselves as adults, but they see discrepancies between their ideal and actual skills and abilities.

Adolescents are continually comparing themselves with their peers and making judgments about their own normality based on these observations. Pubertal children feel most comfortable when they are just like their friends and age-mates. Perceived defects or deviations from the group average are threatening to their idealized image. Any blemish is likely to be magnified out of proportion, and any delay of the visible evidence of maturity is cause for worry. Unfortunately, this is also the time when the hormonal effect of the sebaceous glands produces acne, which creates problems for some adolescents. To the adolescent, even the most insignificant pimple may be viewed as a gross disfigurement. The diagnosis of chronic disease or a permanent physical disability has special significance during adolescence and creates additional stresses for both adolescents with the condition and health care providers.

Experts have determined that the body image established during adolescence is the one that individuals retain throughout life. Much of adolescents' search for identity takes place before a mirror as they try to read from the reflected features just who they are and what they look like to other people. Adolescents practice facial expressions and postures, try out hair arrangements, worry about a pimple, and in other ways attempt to assess the best means to achieve a maximum effect—to reveal the "true self."

The self-concept becomes more differentiated as adolescents acquire a more complex picture of themselves, one that takes situational factors into account. The self-concept gradually becomes more individualized and more distinct from the concepts of others. Although younger teenagers describe themselves in terms of similarities with peers, as adolescence advances, young people describe themselves in terms of their special characteristics.

Responses to Puberty

The response to the physical changes of pubertal growth and development is manifested differently depending on the stage of development. During early adolescence, young adolescents become preoccupied with the rapid changes in their body and are interested in the anatomy, physiology, and function of their sexual organs. Boys must also confront the sexual feelings and tensions that accompany puberty, and the appearance of nocturnal emissions may be puzzling, troublesome, or embarrassing. Unless the boy has been prepared in advance, he may find it difficult to discuss his feelings with his parents and may turn to his friends for information and

guidance. Many girls also find the rapid changes in their body to be sources of concern. Some girls perceive the increase in weight and associated fat deposition as evidence of obesity and may indulge in fad diets. Although many girls look forward to menstruation and take this event in stride, others may find the first menstrual period a distressing and frightening event. All teenagers, regardless of gender, are concerned with the question "Am I normal?" To answer this question, they compare their body with those of their peers and with images in the media. This leads to a great deal of uncertainty about their appearance and attractiveness.

If an adolescent does not enter puberty at the same time as his or her peers, considerable inner conflict may occur. Early-maturing girls and boys have higher rates of sexual risk-taking behaviors, delinquency, and substance abuse than their on-time peers (Costello, Sung, Worthman, et al., 2007; Lynne, Graber, Nichols, et al., 2007). Early puberty onset in females who are offspring of adolescent mothers may also be a significant factor in teenage pregnancies (De Genna, Larkby, and Cornelius, 2011). Nurses who work with adolescents must provide teaching and health care interventions that are appropriate for the adolescent's chronologic and cognitive development rather than the stage of physical maturation.

As growth and development proceed through middle adolescence, the rapid body changes diminish and the adolescent has time to try to make the body more attractive. Adolescents strive to achieve the perfect body within their own cultural norms. The "right" clothes and hairstyle become very important. By late adolescence, the heightened concern with body image has ended and is replaced by a general comfort with the body.

The changes that occur during the early, middle, and late phases of adolescence are summarized in Table 35-1.

PROMOTING OPTIMAL HEALTH DURING ADOLESCENCE

The major causes of morbidity and mortality in adolescence are not diseases but, instead, health-damaging behaviors. New sources of morbidity in adolescence include injury, depression, violence, sexually transmitted infections (STIs), and pregnancy; obesity may begin in childhood or adolescence, but the health consequences are more evident in early and middle adulthood. Health promotion for this age-group consists mainly of teaching and guidance to avoid risk-taking activities and health-damaging behaviors. Adolescence provides an opportunity for teenagers to incorporate healthy lifestyle behaviors that will benefit them not only during the teenage years but also throughout the life span.

Effective health education for adolescents should incorporate a developmentally appropriate, multifaceted approach. Motivational interviewing has been shown to improve adherence to health care advice by using a collaborative approach (Gance-Cleveland, 2007). In this process, the adolescent is encouraged to introspectively explore ambivalence and develop solutions for effecting change. Education alone is not enough to change behavior. Effective programs for adolescents must include opportunities to improve communication skills and enhance their social network to make more positive connections (Tuttle, Campbell-Heider, and David, 2006).

As adolescents progress through adolescence, they are able to assume additional responsibility for their own health, including maintaining health practices, taking prescribed medications, keeping appointments, and performing procedures when necessary. Health care professionals who work with adolescents should consider the adolescent's increasing independence and responsibility while

TABLE 35-1   GROWTH AND DEVELOPMENT DURING ADOLESCENCE

EARLY ADOLESCENCE (11-14 YR)	MIDDLE ADOLESCENCE (15-17 YR)	LATE ADOLESCENCE (18-20 YR)
Growth		
Rapidly accelerating growth	Growth decelerating in girls	Physically mature
Reaches peak velocity	Stature reaches 95% of adult height	Structure and reproductive growth almost complete
Secondary sex characteristics appear	Secondary sex characteristics well advanced	
Cognition		
Explores newfound ability for limited abstract thought	Developing capacity for abstract thinking	Established abstract thought
Clumsy groping for new values and energies	Enjoys intellectual powers, often in idealistic terms	Can perceive and act on long-range options
Comparison of "normality" with peers of same sex	Concern with philosophic, political, and social problems	Able to view problems comprehensively
		Intellectual and functional identity established
Identity		
Preoccupied with rapid body changes	Modifies body image	Body image and gender-role definition nearly secured
Trying out of various roles	Very self-centered; increased narcissism	Mature sexual identity
Measurement of attractiveness by acceptance or rejection of peers	Tendency toward inner experience and self-discovery	Phase of consolidation of identity
Conformity to group norms	Has a rich fantasy life	Stability of self-esteem
	Idealistic	Comfortable with physical growth
	Able to perceive future implications of current behavior and decisions; variable application	Social roles defined and articulated
Relationships with Parents		
Defining independence-dependence boundaries	Major conflicts over independence and control	Emotional and physical separation from parents completed
Strong desire to remain dependent on parents while trying to detach	Low point in parent-child relationship	Independence from family with less conflict
No major conflicts over parental control	Greatest push for emancipation; disengagement	Emancipation nearly secured
	Final and irreversible emotional detachment from parents; mourning	
Relationships with Peers		
Seeks peer affiliations to counter instability generated by rapid change	Strong need for identity to affirm self-image	Peer group recedes in importance in favor of individual friendship
Upsurge of close, idealized friendships with members of the same sex	Behavioral standards set by peer group	Testing of romantic relationships against possibility of permanent alliance
Struggle for mastery takes place within peer group	Acceptance by peers extremely important—fear of rejection	Relationships characterized by giving and sharing
	Exploration of ability to attract opposite sex	
Sexuality		
Self-exploration and evaluation	Multiple plural relationships	Forms stable relationships and attachment to another
Limited dating, usually group	Internal identification of heterosexuality, homosexual, or bisexual attractions	Growing capacity for mutuality and reciprocity
Limited intimacy	Exploration of "self appeal"	Dating as a romantic pair
	Feeling of "being in love"	May publicly identify as gay, lesbian, or bisexual
	Tentative establishment of relationships	Intimacy involves commitment rather than exploration and romanticism
Psychologic Health		
Wide mood swings	Tendency toward inner experiences; more introspective	More constancy of emotion
Intense daydreaming	Tendency to withdraw when upset or feelings are hurt	Anger more apt to be concealed
Anger outwardly expressed with moodiness, temper outbursts, and verbal insults and name-calling	Vacillation of emotions in time and range	
	Feelings of inadequacy common; difficulty in asking for help	

GUIDELINES

Interviewing Adolescents

- Ensure confidentiality and privacy; interview adolescent without parents present.
- Show concern for adolescent's perspective: "First, I'd like to talk about your main concerns" and "I'd like to know what you think is happening."
- Offer a nonthreatening explanation for the questions you ask: "I'm going to ask a number of questions to help me better understand your health."
- Maintain objectivity; avoid assumptions, judgments, and lectures.
- Ask open-ended questions when possible; move to more directive questions if necessary.
- Begin with less sensitive issues and proceed to more sensitive ones.
- Use language that both the adolescent and you understand. Clarify terms, such as "having sex."
- Restate or summarize: reflect back to adolescents what they have said, along with feelings that may be associated with their descriptions.
- Ask the adolescent if he or she minds if the practitioner shares general (or specific) information gathered in the health examination and interview with the parent. Reiterate that the teen's confidentiality will be maintained if he or she refuses to give permission (unless life-threatening information is shared).

CRITICAL THINKING CASE STUDY

Respecting Privacy

Jamie, a 17-year-old girl, arrives at the adolescent clinic with her mother, Mrs. S, for a routine history and physical examination with the nurse practitioner. As the nurse practitioner walks with Jamie to an examination room, Mrs. S whispers to the nurse practitioner, "I need to speak with you in private." How should the nurse practitioner respond to Mrs. S's request?

1. Evidence—Is there sufficient evidence to formulate a response to Jamie's mother?
2. Assumptions—Describe an underlying assumption about each of the following topics:
   a. The role of the adolescent in health care
   b. The role of the parents in the health of their adolescent
   c. Adolescents and confidentiality
3. What implications for nursing care should be established at this time?
4. Does the evidence objectively support your argument (conclusion)?

maintaining privacy and ensuring confidentiality (see Guidelines box and Critical Thinking Case Study). Parents should also respect their teenager's independence and move toward the role of consultant about health issues while also maintaining some level of parental involvement throughout adolescence.

Several professional organizations have published guidelines aimed at improving and maintaining health care for adolescents and young adults. The American Academy of Pediatrics (AAP), American Academy of Family Physicians, American Medical Association, and U.S. Preventive Services Task Force have similar guidelines for health supervision of adolescents. These guidelines emphasize the need to provide health services to adolescents that meet their physical and emotional needs. They place great import on provision of health care by health care providers who are trained in meeting the adolescents' needs. Bright Futures (Duncan and Pirretti, 2009) emphasizes the following issues be addressed with adolescents at each health visit:

- Physical growth and development (physical and dental health, body image, healthy nutrition, physical activity)
- Social and academic competence (relationships with peers and family, school performance, interpersonal relationships)
- Emotional well-being (mental health, sexuality)
- Risk reduction (tobacco, alcohol, other drugs, pregnancy, STIs)
- Violence and injury prevention

Some practical suggestions for addressing the adolescent's individual health care needs are found in the following mnemonic*:

H—Home environment, belonging, decision making
E—Education/Employment
E—Eating/nutrition
A—Activities, physical activities
D—Drugs (including smoking and alcohol use)
S—Sexuality
S—Suicide/depression
S—Safety

The following discussion of adolescent health will focus on some of the topics from this mnemonic as well as the Bright Futures topics listed above; other adolescent health issues are discussed later in this chapter.

Immunizations

An immunization update is an important part of adolescent preventive care. Obtaining a record of the teenager's prior immunizations is important. The Tdap (tetanus, diphtheria, acellular pertussis) vaccine is recommended for adolescents 11 to 18 years old who have not received a tetanus booster (Td) or Tdap dose and have completed the childhood DTaP/DTP series. When the Tdap is used as a booster dose, it may be administered earlier than the previous 5-year interval to provide adequate pertussis immunity (regardless of interval from the last Td dose) (Centers for Disease Control and Prevention [CDC], 2011). Meningococcal vaccine (MenACWY-D [Menactra] or MenACWY-CRM [Menveo]) should be given to adolescents 11 to 12 years of age with a booster dose before 16 years of age. If not previously vaccinated, they should receive 1 dose between 13 and 18 years of age (CDC, 2013a) (see also Immunizations, Chapter 31).

The quadrivalent human papillomavirus (HPV) vaccine or the bivalent HPV vaccine is recommended for the prevention of cervical precancers and cancers for girls beginning at a minimum age of 9 years. The quadrivalent HPV vaccine is recommended for males ages 9 through 18 years to reduce their likelihood of genital warts (CDC, 2013b). Each one of the HPV vaccines is administered in a three-dose series; it is important to follow the recommended dose intervals for optimal effectiveness.

All adolescents who have not previously received three doses of hepatitis B vaccine should be vaccinated against hepatitis B virus. The hepatitis A vaccine should be given to adolescents who live in areas where vaccination programs target older children or who are at increased risk for infection or for whom immunity against hepatitis A is desired (CDC, 2013b). Annual influenza vaccination with either the live attenuated influenza vaccine or inactivated influenza vaccine is recommended for all children and adolescents. All adolescents should also be assessed for previous history of varicella infection or vaccination. Vaccination with the varicella vaccine is

---

*From Duncan P, Pirretti AE: Bright futures for the busy clinical practice, American Academy of Pediatrics, *Adolescent Health Update* 22(1):1–10, 2009; Goldenring JM, Rosen DS: Getting into adolescent heads: an essential update, *Contemp Pediatr* 21:64–90, 2004.

recommended for those with no previous history; for those with no previous infection or history, the varicella vaccine may be given in two doses 4 or more weeks apart to adolescents 13 years of age or older (CDC, 2013b). Adolescents should receive a tuberculin skin test if they have been exposed to active tuberculosis (TB), have lived in a homeless shelter, have been incarcerated, have lived in or come from an area with a high prevalence of TB, or currently work in a health care setting.

Nutrition

The rapid and extensive increase in height, weight, muscle mass, and sexual maturity of adolescence is accompanied by increased nutritional requirements. Because nutritional needs are closely related to the increase in body mass, the peak requirements occur in the years of maximum growth, during which the body mass almost doubles. The caloric and protein requirements during this time are higher than at almost any other time of life. As a result of this increased anabolic need, the adolescent is highly sensitive to caloric restrictions.

Current guidelines for caloric intake are provided by a number of sources. The Dietary Reference Intakes (DRIs) provide age-specific guidelines for nutrients (see Chapters 29 and 32). The 2010 Dietary Guidelines for Americans* recommend specific caloric intakes for adolescents based on their levels of activity (sedentary, moderately active, and active) as well as a recommendation to decrease the amount of fat to approximately 25% to 36% of total daily intake. A recent change in guidelines is reflected in the new MyPlate,† which takes the place of MyPyramid as a scheme for eating a balanced diet of the five main food groups—fruits, grains, protein, vegetables, and dairy products. Recent guidelines by the National Heart, Lung, and Blood Institute (NHLBI) include dietary recommendations to reduce the risk for cardiovascular disease. Included in these guidelines for adolescents is a total daily fat intake of 25% to 30% of estimated energy requirements, with emphasis on a reduction of saturated fat and avoidance of *trans* (unsaturated) fat. The guidelines also address the need for an increased intake of dietary fiber (26 grams/day [females 14 to 18 years old] and 38 grams/day [males 14 to 18 years old]), consumption of three meals per day, avoidance of tobacco, and routine screening for hyperlipidemia and hypertension in children and adolescents. Estimated energy requirements for adolescents of both sexes are provided based on three levels of activity: sedentary, moderately active, and active (National Heart, Lung, and Blood Institute, 2011). Caloric intake can be tailored to meet adolescents' increased growth needs as well as activity level such as involvement in sports. Additional guidelines recommend the reduction in added sugars; adolescents consume most of their added sugars in sweetened beverages such as soda and energy and sports drinks (Van Horn, Johnson, Flickinger, et al., 2010). Studies have shown that decreasing the daily intake of sugar-sweetened beverages resulted in significant BMI reductions in children and adolescents (Clabaugh and Neuberger, 2011; Levy, Friend, and Wang, 2011).

Adolescents usually have sufficient intake of protein to meet their needs except for those who limit their food intake because of economic problems or in an attempt to lose weight. There is a substantial increase in the need for the minerals *calcium, iron,* and *zinc* during periods of rapid growth: calcium for skeletal growth, iron for expansion of muscle mass and blood volume, and zinc for the generation of both skeletal and bone tissue. The estimated average requirement (EAR) for calcium in adolescents 14 to 18 years of age is 1100 mg (Institute of Medicine, 2010). Girls with heavy or frequent menses may be especially susceptible to iron deficiency resulting from blood loss. Calcium intake from food sources is essential during adolescence to assist in the prevention of osteoporosis. Eventual bone mass is a balance between the amount of bone laid down during adolescence and the amount later lost with aging. Overall, osteoporosis is a result of polygenic and multiple environmental factors such as nutrition, economics, and exercise (Ongphiphadhanakul, 2007). Dietary intervention should promote the regular consumption of breakfast and a balanced intake of a variety of foods.

Eating Habits and Behavior

Eating and attitudes toward food are primarily family centered during early and middle childhood, and food habits are largely related to cultural and individual family preferences and patterns. With adolescence and the move toward independence, family influences on the child diminish. Children's interests, attitudes, and routines are altered as an increasing number of meals are eaten away from home. These changes are largely a result of the high value that teenagers place on peer acceptability and sociability. Their peers easily influence their eating habits.

Pressure for time and commitments to activities adversely affect teenagers' eating habits. Omitting breakfast or eating a breakfast that is nutritionally poor in quality is frequently a problem. Snacks, usually selected on the basis of accessibility rather than nutritional merit, become increasingly a part of the habitual eating pattern during adolescence (Fig. 35-7). Excess intake of calories, sugar, fat, cholesterol, and sodium is common among adolescents and is found in all income and racial or ethnic groups and both sexes. Inadequate intake of certain vitamins (folic acid, vitamin B_6, vitamin A) and minerals (iron, calcium, zinc) is also evident, particularly among

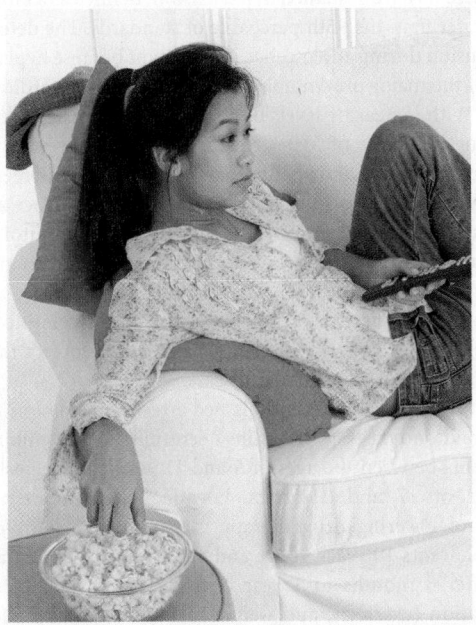

FIG 35-7 Snacking on empty calories is common among adolescents, especially during inactivity. (Copyright © 2011 Photos.com, a division of Getty Images. All rights reserved.)

---

*Dietary Guidelines for Americans, Institute of Medicine, www.health.gov/dietaryguidelines.
†MyPlate, www.choosemyplate.gov.

girls and teenagers of low socioeconomic status. In combination with other factors, these dietary patterns could result in increased risk for obesity and chronic diseases such as heart disease, osteoporosis, and some types of cancer later in life. Maximum bone mass is also acquired during adolescence; therefore the calcium deposited during these years determines the risk for osteoporosis. Milk is usually passed over in favor of soft drinks.

Overeating or undereating during adolescence presents special problems. When they experience the normal increase in weight and fat deposition of the growth spurt, teenage girls often resort to dieting. The desire for a slim figure and a fear of becoming "fat" prompt teenage girls to embark on nutritionally inadequate reducing regimens that drain their energy and deprive their growing bodies of essential nutrients. They resort to diets on their own or with peers in an effort to conform. Many adopt current fad diets and are victims of food misinformation. Boys are less inclined to undereat. They are more concerned about gaining size and strength. However, they tend to eat foods high in calories but low in other essential nutrients.

Obesity is increasing among both children and adolescents in the United States. Poor dietary habits and increasingly sedentary lifestyles have caused this obesity epidemic. Currently 16.9% of children ages 2 to 19 years are obese. The vast majority (90%) of obese adolescents remain obese into their 30s: 94% of women overall and 88% of men (Gordon-Larsen, The, and Adair, 2010).

Health problems traditionally thought of as adult comorbidities of obesity, including type 2 diabetes mellitus, obstructive sleep apnea, and nonalcoholic steatohepatitis, are occurring in adolescents. Lifestyle changes necessary for adolescents to lose weight require the involvement of family members who provide support and encourage active participation.

Hypertension and Hyperlipidemia

As adolescents experience sexual maturation, along with increases in height and weight, blood pressure increases from the onset of adolescence and continues to rise until the end of pubertal growth. This trend is especially apparent among males. Approximately 1% of adolescents have sustained hypertension, defined as a blood pressure greater than the 95th percentile of standards. The detection of hypertension during adolescence is important because hypertension is one of the major preventable risk factors for adult cardiovascular disease. With increasing levels of obesity, there have been reports of increasing incidence of hypertension among adolescents (Hansen, Gunn, and Kaelber, 2007; LaRosa and Meyers, 2010). Screening for hypertension and associated risk factors should take place annually beginning at age 3 years. Specific guidelines for monitoring and treatment of hypertension in adolescents are found in the 2011 NHLBI summary report (see also Chapter 42).

Along with hypertension, smoking, and obesity, elevated serum cholesterol and triglyceride levels are major risk factors for the development of adult cardiovascular disease.

The NHLBI (2011) recently issued a recommendation for universal lipid (nonfasting or fasting) screening of all children and adolescents between the ages of 9 and 11 years and again between the ages of 17 and 21 years. Low-density lipoprotein (LDL) cholesterol–lowering drug therapy is recommended for children and adolescents 10 years of age and older whose LDL remains elevated after 6 months to 1 year on a restricted fat diet, lifestyle modification (exercise), and weight management (NHLBI, 2011). Additional information and practice guidelines for monitoring cholesterol levels and initiation of cholesterol–lowering medication as well as specific dietary modifications are found in the 2011

NHLBI summary report at www.nhlbi.nih.gov/guidelines/cvd_ped/summary.htm#chap5.

CARE MANAGEMENT

Adolescents should receive at a minimum an annual assessment of weight, height, and BMI for age plotted on a standard growth chart. Healthy dietary habits should be discussed with all adolescents. The frequency of eating at fast-food and other restaurants, consumption of sweetened beverages, and consumption of excessive portion sizes should be identified. In addition to food intake, the nurse should assess the level of physical activity, sedentary behaviors, and sleep patterns. Readiness to change; environmental supports and barriers; and family history of diabetes, heart disease, and early stroke must be considered when planning nutritional education and guidance. Nurses in the school setting can assist in advocating for comprehensive nutritional services for preschool through grade 12 students.

Sleep and Rest

Teenagers vary in their need for sleep and rest. Rapid physical growth, the tendency toward overexertion, and the overall increased activity of this age contribute to fatigue in adolescents. During growth spurts, the need for sleep is increased. Their propensity for staying up late makes it difficult to arise in the morning, and they may sleep late at every opportunity. Adequate sleep and rest at this time are important to a total health regimen.

Exercise and Activity

Although today's youth are less fit than children 20 years ago, adolescents probably spend more time and energy practicing and participating in sports activities than members of any other age-group. Many adolescents participate in sports within school settings (Fig. 35-8). School-based, health-oriented physical education may provide both immediate effects of the activity and sustained effects

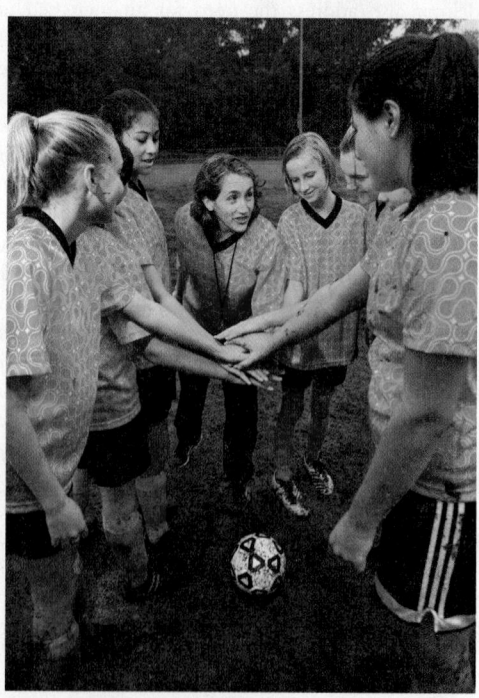

FIG 35-8 Adolescents should be encouraged to participate in activities that contribute to lifelong physical fitness. (Copyright © 2011 Photos.com, a division of Getty Images. All rights reserved.)

through encouragement of lifelong activity patterns. High schools continue to cut physical education classes, with only half of high school students attending physical education classes in 2011. Fewer than half of students (31.5%) attended these classes daily, and the majority of classes included only 20 minutes of exercise (CDC, 2012b). To improve health outcomes, school-age children and adolescents should engage in 60 minutes or more of moderate to vigorous physical activity daily (U.S. Department of Health and Human Services, 2008b).

The practice of sports, games, and even dancing contributes significantly to growth and development, the education process, and better health. These activities provide exercise for growing muscles, interactions with peers, and a socially acceptable means of enjoying stimulation and conflict. In addition, competitive activities help teenagers in the process of self-appraisal and the development of self-respect and concern for others. Because physical fitness appears to be a major influence on one's lifelong health status, children should be encouraged to participate in activities that contribute to lifelong physical fitness. Nurses can encourage participation as a way to promote health and build self-esteem. However, adolescents should not be encouraged to engage in physical activities that are beyond their physical or emotional capacity (see Sports Participation and Injury, Chapter 48).

Dental Health

Dental health should not be neglected during adolescence, although the rate of caries formation is not as great as in childhood. Dental care is an aspect of preventive care that is not received by substantial proportions of children in the United States. It is recommended that an evaluation for caries takes place at a minimum of every year and optimally at 6-month intervals. Pit and fissure sealants are a safe and effective technique for dental caries prevention. Early adolescence is usually when corrective orthodontic appliances are worn, and these are frequently a source of embarrassment and concern to teens. Reassurance regarding the temporary nature of the annoyance and anticipation of an improved appearance help adolescents tolerate the inconvenience. It is also important to reinforce the orthodontist's directions regarding use and care of the appliances and to emphasize careful attention to toothbrushing during this time (see also Chapters 32 and 33). During late adolescence, the third molars (wisdom teeth) should be evaluated to determine appropriate management (American Academy of Pediatric Dentistry, 2012).

Personal Care

Body-conscious teenagers are highly amenable to discussion and counseling about personal care and hygiene. Body changes associated with puberty bring special needs for cleanliness. The hyperactive sebaceous glands and newly functioning apocrine glands make frequent bathing or showering a necessity, and underarm deodorants assume an important place in personal care. Adolescents discover that hair requires more frequent shampooing, and girls often have questions about hair removal, use of cosmetics, and menstrual hygiene. Peer-group discussions center on the advantages of particular products or methods. Adolescents are continually bombarded with messages from the media regarding the best way to enhance their popularity and attractiveness. Nurses are in a position to help them evaluate the relative merits of commercial products.

Vision

Regular vision testing is an important part of health care and supervision during adolescence. During adolescence, visual refractive difficulties reach a peak that is not exceeded until the fifth decade of life. The increased demands of schoolwork make adequate vision essential for academic success. Consequently, teenagers are more likely to be referred for visual evaluation. The need for corrective lenses can create psychologic problems for teenagers if they believe that glasses spoil their appearance or do not fit their body image. Contact lenses may be a preferred solution; a variety of lenses are now available at fairly reasonable prices. For some, the impact of a visual defect, no matter how slight, may be stressful.

Hearing

Considerable concern has focused on current teenage practices that damage hearing. Cochlear damage from relatively continuous exposure to the loud sound levels of rock music has been documented. The popularity of personal music players with lightweight earphones that are inserted into the ear canal is of particular concern to health care professionals. When these units are used for extended periods, permanent hearing loss can occur. Although appeals for more judicious use are not always successful, teenagers should be informed of the risk. (See Chapter 37 for a discussion of noise-related hearing loss.)

Posture

Many adolescents demonstrate altered posture. Rapid skeletal growth is often associated with slower muscular growth, and as a result, some teenagers may appear awkward or slump and fail to stand or sit upright. However, some postural defects of adolescence require early medical intervention. Scoliosis is a defect of the spine that occurs frequently in adolescence and is more common in girls than in boys (see Idiopathic Scoliosis, Chapter 48). The majority of cases are idiopathic, and the defect manifests as a painless curvature of the spine. Fortunately, most of these spinal curvatures will not require treatment. However, because there is no way to predict which curvatures will progress, all curvatures of the spine should be referred for further evaluation.

Body Art

Body art (piercing and tattooing) is an aspect of adolescent identity formation. The skin has become the latest source of parent-adolescent conflict. Adolescents often seek body art as an expression of their personal identity and style. Tattoos may mark significant life events such as new relationships, births, and deaths. Piercing the ear, nose, nipple, eyebrow, labia, navel, penis, or tongue may sometimes create a health problem. It is a nursing responsibility to caution girls and boys against having piercing performed by friends, parents, or themselves. Although in most cases piercings have few, if any, serious side effects, there is always a risk for complications such as infection, cyst or keloid formation, bleeding, dermatitis, or metal allergy. Using the same unsterilized needle to pierce body parts of multiple teenagers presents the same risk for human immunodeficiency virus (HIV), hepatitis C virus, and hepatitis B virus transmission as occurs with other needle-sharing activities. A recent report highlighted the danger of contaminated tattoo ink, which occurred in association with an outbreak of non-tuberculous *Mycobacterium chelonae* skin infections (Kennedy, Bedard, Younge, et al., 2012).

A qualified operator using proper sterile technique should perform the procedure. This is especially important if an adolescent has a history of diabetes, allergies, or skin disorders. Adolescents should be informed about the approximate time for healing after body piercing and the care of the pierced area during and after healing. Some body sites need extra precautions. For example, cartilage (ear, nose) has a poor blood supply and heals slowly and scars easily; nipple piercing puts adolescents at risk for breast abscesses. Finally, migration of the piercing is common with naval and other flat skin surface piercing. Piercing guns should not be used for piercing anything other than the earlobe because guns place the piercing too deeply.

The presence of body art in the form of tattoos and branding is common among adolescents and young adults. Professionals as well as amateur artists administer tattoos. The risk to adolescents receiving tattoos is low. The greatest risk is for the tattoo artist, who comes in contact with the client's blood. Adolescents who are amateur tattoo artists benefit from discussions about Standard Precautions and the hepatitis B vaccination. Many states either have no regulations or do not enforce existing regulations of piercing and tattooing facilities. The local health department is a source of information about local regulatory requirements. The Centers for Disease Control and Prevention (CDC) has an excellent website that outlines safety concerns for persons performing and receiving body art (http://www.cdc.gov/niosh/topics/body_art/).

Tanning

The quest for an attractive appearance leads many teenagers to excessive sunbathing and artificial means for tanning. However, this practice has serious long-term risks, and adolescents should be educated regarding the detrimental effects of sunlight on the skin (see Sunburn, Chapter 47). Long-term effects include premature aging of the skin; increased risk for skin cancer; and, in susceptible individuals, phototoxic reactions.

The increasing popularity of artificial tanning has prompted concern from health care professionals regarding the use of sunlamps and tanning machines. The long-term effects of tanning machines are similar to those of the sun; dermatologists do not recommend tanning by this means. Those who insist on using tanning equipment should be warned that goggles must be worn in tanning booths to prevent serious corneal burning. Education on the use of sunscreens, including hypoallergenic products, with a sun protective factor (SPF) of at least 15 and a nonalcohol base without lanolin, parabens, or fragrance, is important. Broad-spectrum sunscreens that protect against both ultraviolet A and ultraviolet B (UV-A and UV-B) are the most effective. Self-tanning creams safely simulate the appearance of a tan; however, teens using these products should be cautioned that sun protection is still required. Targeting health education messages to adolescents and incorporating educational components relating to sun protection behaviors in school health curricula and in health care visits will increase adolescents' knowledge and awareness.

Stress Reduction

The multiple changes occurring in adolescence can result in great stress (Fig. 35-9 and Box 35-3). Adolescents are faced with pressures from peers that often involve taking serious health risks, including pressures for sexual experimentation; use of drugs, alcohol, and cigarettes; and potentially dangerous physical activities.

Early-maturing girls and late-maturing children are especially sensitive to the stresses of being different from their peers. Many feel intense anxiety over their identity. Both early- and late-maturing children feel out of place among their classmates, but slow-maturing children appear to experience the most pronounced inner turmoil and may be hesitant to voice their concerns. Slow-maturing adolescents need support and reassurance that they are not abnormal and need only be patient until the time comes when they, too, will mature physically.

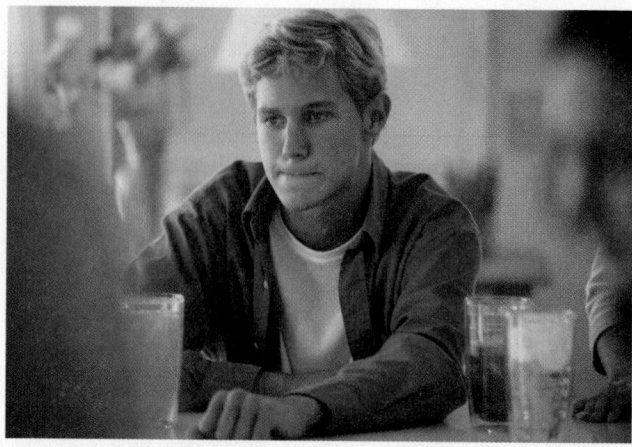

FIG 35-9 Adolescents use being alone as a method of coping with stress. Health care professionals need to assess whether this indicates clinical depression. (Copyright © 2011 Photos.com, a division of Getty Images. All rights reserved.)

BOX 35-3	AREAS OF STRESS IN ADOLESCENCE
• Body image • Sexuality conflicts • Scholastic pressures • Competitive pressures • Relationships with parents • Relationships with siblings	• Relationships with peers • Dating • Finances • Decisions about present and future roles • Career planning • Ideologic conflicts

Sexuality Education and Guidance

The average American teenager spends more than 7 hours every day in front of some type of medium. This potentially exposes them to unrealistic sexual messages and images, usually without adult supervision or interaction. Research has demonstrated that adolescents whose parents limit their television viewing are less likely to engage in earlier sex (American Academy of Pediatrics [AAP] Council on Communications and Media, 2010). In addition, social media use is a routine part of contemporary adolescents' daily lives, and there are many positive benefits including enhancing communication, social connection, and computer skills. However, some evidence indicates that there are often online expressions of sexual experimentation, including sending and receiving sexually explicit messages, photographs, or images via cell phones and computers (O'Keeffe and Clarke-Pearson, 2011). All media sources provide adolescents potential exposure to information that may be inaccurate, riddled with cultural and moral judgments, and not very helpful.

The responsibility for providing sexuality education has been assumed by parents; schools; churches; community agencies such as Planned Parenthood Federation of America, Inc.;* and health care professionals, especially nurses. Many adolescents perceive nurses, especially school nurses, as individuals who possess important information and who are willing to discuss sex with them. To be able to discuss the topic adequately, nurses must have not only an understanding of the physiologic aspects of sexuality and a knowledge of cultural and societal values but also an awareness of their own attitudes, feelings, and biases about sexuality.

*434 West 33rd St., New York, NY 10001; 800-230-PLAN (7526); www.plannedparenthood.org.

Comprehensive information about sexuality education is offered by the Sexuality Information and Education Council of the United States (SIECUS)* and the Sex Information and Education Council of Canada.† The SIECUS maintains that every sexuality education program should present the topic from six aspects, including biologic, social, health, personal adjustments and attitudes, interpersonal associations, and the establishment of values.

Whether nurses counsel young people on an individual basis, in mixed groups, or in groups segregated by gender makes little difference. Ideally, boys and girls should be able to discuss sexuality objectively with one another and in groups, but this is not always possible. The differences in the rate of maturation between boys and girls and among different members of the same sex often make it desirable to discuss certain aspects of sexuality in segregated groups for early adolescents. As a rule, the need for separate discussion groups diminishes as young people mature.

Sexuality education should consist of instruction concerning normal body functions and should be presented in a straightforward manner using correct terminology. When discussing sex and sexual activities, nurses should use simple but correct language—not street language, highly scientific terminology, or evasive jargon. After they understand the meaning of biologic terms such as uterus, testicles, and vagina, most teenagers prefer to use them in their discussions.

Many girls arrive at menarche with ambivalent attitudes, myths, and illogical beliefs. Even girls adequately prepared for menstruation do not always understand its relationship to the total process of reproduction. Many are under the incorrect impression that the "safe" time for sexual intercourse is midway between menstrual periods.

Teenagers' curiosity and desire for information extend beyond the need for anatomic and physiologic knowledge. They need to know more than the mechanics of conception, pregnancy, and birth. Adolescents, girls in particular, want answers to questions such as: "What is it like?" "Does it hurt?" "What happens when …?" and "Is it all right if you …?" Boys are often concerned about the fallacy that a relationship exists between penis size and sexual function. They need reassurance that masturbation is a normal and common practice, that some degree of homosexuality in early adolescence is not unusual, and that oral-genital relations can be normal substitutes for intercourse.

Teenagers need to discuss intercourse, alternative methods of sexual satisfaction, and how to resist peer pressure. With the increased incidence of sexually transmitted infections, especially HIV infection, the topic of "safe sex," especially abstinence or the use of condoms, is essential. Role playing can help teenagers learn effective approaches to dealing with difficult situations. Sex and sexuality cannot be taught without discussions of mature decision making, sexual responsibility, and values clarification. Adolescents may receive inaccurate and ambiguous messages regarding sexual behavior; for example, an adolescent may be told that abstinence from vaginal intercourse will prevent transmission of a sexually transmitted infection. Accurate and unbiased information regarding sexual practices should be provided in a setting wherein the adolescent feels comfortable asking questions without being degraded or made to feel uncomfortable for seeking information.

Adolescents need role models and life experiences with delayed gratification. Most important, they need problem-solving experience and decision-making skills so they can anticipate the positive and negative outcomes of their decisions. With this type of assistance, teenagers can become sexually responsible young adults (see also Contraception, Chapter 5).

Safety Promotion and Injury Prevention

Physical injuries are the greatest single cause of death in the adolescent age-group and claim more lives than all other causes combined. The most vulnerable ages are the years 15 to 24 years, when accidental injuries account for a significant percentage of fatalities. Motor-vehicle traffic-related deaths decreased 41% during the years 2000 to 2009 among adolescents ages 15 to 19 years, yet these accidents account for the leading cause of unintentional injury among persons from birth to 19 years of age (CDC, 2012a).

During adolescence, peak physical, sensory, and psychomotor function give teenagers a feeling of strength and confidence that they have never experienced before, and the physiologic changes of puberty give impetus to many basic instinctual forces. One manifestation of this is an increase in energy that simply must be discharged through action, often at the expense of logical thinking and other control mechanisms. Their propensity for risk-taking behavior plus feelings of indestructibility makes adolescents especially prone to injuries. Some of the developmental characteristics of teenagers and injury prevention suggestions are outlined in Box 35-4.

Motor Vehicle–Related Injuries

Adolescents' newly acquired ability to drive and the normal developmental need for independence and freedom make automobiles an attractive part of their lives. Motor vehicle crashes are the single greatest source of unintentional injury and death in young people in the United States. Many factors contribute to the higher rate of crashes among young drivers, including lacking driving experience and maturity, following too closely, driving too fast, having other teen passengers in the car, texting or answering a cell phone while driving, and driving under the influence of alcohol. Young drivers' elevated crash risk is highest between ages 16 and 17 years but persists through age 19 or 20 years. These data lend support to efforts in the United States to delay full licensure beyond age 16 years. There is also evidence that graduated licensing systems that phase in unsupervised driving in higher risk situations such as nighttime driving and having passengers in the car are effective in decreasing the motor vehicle crash risk for adolescents (McCartt, Mayhew, Braitman, et al., 2009).

There has been recent attention on distracted teenage driving and cell phone talking or texting while driving. Studies have shown that drivers using handheld devices are considerably more distracted and spend less time looking at the road or paying attention to driving conditions (Hosking, Young, and Regan, 2009; Owens, McLaughlin, and Sudweeks, 2011). According to the 2011 Youth Risk Behavior Surveillance, 32.8% of adolescents nationwide reportedly texted or e-mailed while driving a car or other vehicle at least 1 day during a 30-day period before the survey (CDC, 2012b).

Nurses should educate teenagers and their parents about the risk of driving while drinking alcohol or of riding in an automobile with a drunk driver. Many families arrange a no-questions-asked ride home to prevent an adolescent from riding with a drunk driver. Families should also require adolescents to log several hours of supervised practice driving before taking the car out alone. Educational efforts should also discuss that the major risk for death in a motor vehicle accident is failure to use a safety restraint.

Other Vehicle Injuries. The increasing use of motorcycles, all-terrain vehicles, jet skis, and snowmobiles has caused an increase in

*90 John St., Suite 402, New York, NY 10038; 212-819-9770; www.siecus.org.
†850 Coxwell Ave., Toronto, Ontario M4C 5R1; 416-466-5304; www.sieccan.org.

BOX 35-4 **INJURY PREVENTION DURING ADOLESCENCE**

Developmental Abilities Related to Risk for Injury
- Need for independence and freedom
- Testing independence
- Age permitted to drive a motor vehicle (varies)
- Inclination for risk-taking behaviors
- Feeling of indestructibility
- Need for discharging energy, often at expense of logical thinking and other control mechanisms
- Strong need for peer approval
- Desire to attempt hazardous feats
- Peak incidence for practice and participation in sports
- Access to more complex tools, objects, and locations
- Can assume responsibility for own actions

Injury Prevention
Pedestrian
- Emphasize and encourage safe pedestrian behavior:
  - At night, walk with a friend.
  - If someone is following you, go to nearest place with people.
  - Do not walk in secluded areas; take well-traveled walkways.

Motor or Nonmotor Vehicles
- Passenger—Promote appropriate behavior while riding in a motor vehicle.
- Driver—Provide competent driver education; encourage judicious use of vehicle; discourage drag racing on regular streets, "playing chicken"; discourage text messaging; maintain vehicle in proper condition (brakes, tires, etc.).
- Teach and promote safety and maintenance of two-wheeled vehicles.
- Encourage wearing of safety apparel such as helmet, long trousers.
- Reinforce the dangers of drugs, including alcohol, when operating a motor vehicle.

Falls
- Teach and encourage general safety measures in all activities.

Drowning
- Teach nonswimmer to swim.
- Teach basic rules of water safety:
  - Judicious selection of place to swim
  - Sufficient water depth for diving
  - Swimming with companion
  - Wear life vest with water sports (e.g., boating, skiing)
  - Avoid swimming, boating, or other water sports after or during alcohol consumption

Burns
- Reinforce proper behavior in areas involving contact with burn hazards (gasoline, electric wires, fires).
- Advise regarding excessive exposure to natural or artificial sunlight (ultraviolet burn).
- Discourage smoking.
- Encourage use of sunscreen.

Poisoning
- Educate in hazards of drug use, including alcohol.

Bodily Damage
- Promote acquisition of proper instruction in sports and use of sports equipment.
- Instruct in safe use of and respect for firearms and other devices with potential danger (e.g., power tools, fireworks).
- Provide and encourage use of protective equipment when using potentially hazardous devices (e.g., motorcycles, power tools) or when engaging in sports activities such as skate boarding.
- Promote access to and/or provision of safe sports and recreational facilities.
- Be alert for signs of depression (potential suicide).
- Instruct regarding proper use of corrective devices (e.g., glasses, contact lenses, hearing aids).
- Encourage and foster judicious application of safety principles and prevention.

---

injuries among young people who are below the legal age for driving automobiles. Many adolescents ride bicycles without helmets and without lights at night, and the overwhelming majority of deaths from bicycle injuries (primarily head injuries) involve teenagers. In-line skating and skateboarding without protective gear also contribute to a significant number of traumatic brain injuries in U.S. adolescents and young people.

Firearms

Firearms are the major cause of intentional fatal injuries in the United States. Adolescence is the peak age for being either a victim or an offender in an injury involving a firearm. Gun carrying among adolescents is on the rise and is not limited to the stereotypic inner-city youth. Family members and acquaintances are a common source of guns for young people. Gun availability in the home is strongly linked to unintentional death and injury to children (Glatt, 2005). In addition, the presence of a gun in the home increases the risk for adolescent suicide and homicide. All families should be assessed for the presence of a gun in the home and informed of this risk. They must take preventive action to ensure that the guns are never loaded, that guns are locked up in a safe place, and that ammunition is stored and locked up separately in a location accessible only to appropriate adults.

Sports Injuries

Because the degree of physical maturation, size, coordination, and endurance varies greatly among adolescents of the same age, sports competition among young people who differ greatly in strength and agility is unfair and hazardous. Matching candidates for sports should be done relative to physical maturity, height, weight, and physical fitness and skills, particularly in sports involving rigorous body contact. Age is a less important consideration.

Every sport has some potential for injury, whether one participates in serious competition or engages in the activity for pure enjoyment. Overuse injuries are common in adolescents and result in more time missed from the activity than fractures. The increase in strength and vigor in adolescence may tempt adolescents to overextend themselves. Injuries sustained in sports or recreational activities can involve any part of the body and range from relatively minor cuts, bruises, and abrasions to totally incapacitating central nervous system injuries or death. Recently attention has focused on traumatic brain injuries resulting from concussions incurred in contact sports.

CARE MANAGEMENT

Safety promotion and injury prevention is an ongoing part of nursing responsibility throughout the teenage years. Anticipatory guidance to parents and children regarding the expected problems and hazards related to growth and development does not end as adolescents approach maturity. They need education in basic safety precautions, instruction in skills required in the performance of activities such as sports, instruction in handling motor vehicles, and information about using proper protective equipment and properly maintaining equipment. During adolescence, however, health and safety education and guidance are more effective when the young people are involved directly. Parents and health care professionals can emphasize the importance of safety during performance of activities and the proper conditioning and preparation for sports.

Prevention can occur on a variety of levels. Safety advocacy, public policy changes, and legislation can curtail injuries. Examples of such approaches are laws that mandate wearing seat belts, prohibiting handheld cell phone usage while the car is in motion, using helmets while driving moving vehicles other than automobiles, keeping the legal drinking age at 21 years, and instituting curfews for teen drivers. In addition to improvements in the environment, health education for teenagers and significant adults is essential. Helping adolescents understand their need for engaging in risky behavior, exploring possible negative outcomes, and weighing possible alternatives are critical components of injury prevention.

Anticipatory Guidance—Care of Families

Both adolescents and their parents are often confused and perplexed about the changes and behavior of this stage of development. Parents need support and guidance to help them through this period. They need to understand the changes taking place and to accept the expected behaviors that accompany the process of detachment. Parents may need help to "let go" and to promote the changed relationship from one of dependence to one of mutuality (see Patient Teaching box).

SPECIAL HEALTH PROBLEMS

DISORDERS OF THE FEMALE REPRODUCTIVE SYSTEM

Disorders related to the female reproductive system such as amenorrhea and dysmenorrhea are discussed in Chapter 4. Sexually transmitted infections are also discussed in Chapter 4.

DISORDERS OF THE MALE REPRODUCTIVE SYSTEM

Many obvious anomalies, such as hypospadias, hydrocele, phimosis, and cryptorchidism, are identified with corrective measures instituted during early childhood. The most frequent problems related to the reproductive organs in later childhood are:

- Infections, such as urethritis (see Urinary Tract Infection, Chapter 44)
- Hematuria
- Penile problems, such as nonretractable foreskin in uncircumcised males, drug-induced priapism, carcinoma, and trauma
- Scrotal conditions, such as varicocele (elongation, dilation, and tortuosity of the veins superior to the testicle)
- Testicular torsion (a condition in which the testicle hangs free from its vascular structures, which can result in partial or complete venous occlusion with rotation)

Tumors of the testes are not common (≈8000 cases per year in the United States [Feldman, Bosl, Sheinfeld, et al., 2008]), but when

---

PATIENT TEACHING

Guidance During Adolescence

Encourage Parents to:
- Accept adolescent as a unique individual
- Respect adolescent's ideas, likes and dislikes, and wishes
- Be involved with school functions and attend adolescent's performances, whether it be a sporting event or a school play
- Listen and try to be open to teenager's views, even when they disagree with parental views
- Avoid criticism about no-win topics
- Provide opportunity for choosing options and accept natural consequences of these choices
- Allow young person to learn by doing, even when choices and methods differ from those of adults
- Provide adolescent with clear, reasonable limits
- Clarify house rules and consequences for breaking them
- Let society's rules and consequences teach responsibility outside the home
- Allow increasing independence within limitations of safety and well-being
- Be available but avoid pressing teenager too far
- Respect adolescent's privacy
- Try to share adolescent's feelings of joy or sorrow
- Respond to feelings, as well as words
- Be available to answer questions, give information, and provide companionship
- Try to make communication clear
- Avoid comparisons with siblings
- Assist adolescent in selecting appropriate career goals and preparing for adult role
- Welcome adolescent's friends into the home and treat them with respect
- Provide unconditional love
- Be willing to apologize when mistaken

Be Aware That Adolescents:
- Are subject to turbulent, unpredictable behavior
- Are struggling for independence
- Are trying to establish their own identity separate from parents and family
- Are extremely sensitive to feelings and behavior that affect them
- May receive a different message from what was sent
- Consider friends extremely important
- Have a strong need to belong to a peer group of friends and not necessarily to family (except in certain circumstances)

---

manifested in adolescence, they are generally malignant and demand immediate evaluation. Testicular cancer is the most common solid tumor in adolescent boys and men 15 to 34 years of age. The usual presenting symptom for testicular cancer is a heavy, hard mass (either smooth or nodular) that is palpated on the testis; approximately 40% of men present with a painful mass. If a firm swelling is noted, the adolescent should be evaluated by ultrasonography and immediately referred for direct biopsy if the mass is found to be solid.

Treatment involves surgical removal of the affected testicle (orchiectomy) and adjacent lymph nodes (if affected) and possibly chemotherapy and radiation following surgery. Fertility may be regained after chemotherapy and surgery; however, sperm banking before the initiation of chemotherapy is recommended. Assisted

Testicular Self-Examination

At a recent faculty meeting, Paul, the pediatric nurse practitioner who runs the school-based health clinic, presented his plan for a class on testicular self-examination (TSE) to be delivered to the sophomore boys. Several teachers questioned the value of providing such a class when there is limited time to deliver content relating to "routine academic subjects." What important issues regarding testicular cancer and TSE should Paul use to justify providing this class to the sophomore boys?

1. Evidence—Is there sufficient evidence to justify teaching sophomore boys about TSE?
2. Assumptions—Describe the underlying assumption about each of the following:
   a. Detection of testicular cancers in adolescence
   b. Usual presenting symptom of testicular cancer
   c. Knowledge of genital anatomy among adolescent boys
   d. Ways to teach adolescent boys about their anatomy
3. What priorities and implications for nursing care can be drawn at this time?
4. Does the evidence objectively support your argument (conclusion)?

reproduction is also an option, and successful paternity is reported to be between 50% and 85% (Feldman, Bosl, Sheinfeld, et al., 2008). Recurrence of testicular cancer in the contralateral testis may occur; therefore follow up is essential.

CARE MANAGEMENT

Adolescent boys are also self-conscious about their changing bodies and need preparation for a genital examination. The most successful approach is to assume a matter-of-fact attitude toward the examination, explain precisely what will take place, and maintain a continuous commentary about what is being done and the findings at each phase of the examination.

The routine health assessment of every adolescent boy should include teaching about testicular cancer and how to perform a testicular self-examination (TSE) every month. This rare malignancy is curable if detected early. Nurses are in an ideal position to teach TSE in a manner that is respectful of the adolescent boy's anxieties and that promotes early treatment (see Critical Thinking Case Study).

In the TSE, each testicle is examined individually, preferably after a warm bath or shower when scrotal skin is more relaxed, using the thumbs and fingers of both hands and applying a small amount of firm, gentle pressure. The normal testicle is a firm organ with a smooth, egg-shaped contour; the epididymis is palpated as a raised swelling on the superior aspect of the testicle and should not be taken for an abnormality.

Gynecomastia

Male breasts, although not strictly part of the male reproductive system, respond to hormonal changes. Some degree of bilateral or unilateral breast enlargement occurs frequently in boys during puberty. It is estimated that approximately half of adolescent boys have transient gynecomastia, usually lasting less than 1 year, which subsides spontaneously with achievement of male development. A careful assessment of the pubertal stage at the onset of gynecomastia; medication history, including anabolic steroids; and the exclusion of renal, liver, thyroid, and endocrine disorders or dysfunction allow the examiner to reassure the adolescent that the changes are pubertal gynecomastia and that no further assessment is indicated. Gynecomastia may also be drug induced; calcium channel blockers, cancer chemotherapeutic agents, histamine$_2$-receptor blockers, and oral ketoconazoles have all been shown to cause the condition.

If the condition persists or is extensive enough to cause embarrassment or excessive stress in the young boy, plastic surgery may be indicated for cosmetic and psychologic considerations. Administration of testosterone has no effect on breast development or regression and may aggravate the condition.

CARE MANAGEMENT

Treatment of gynecomastia usually consists of assurance to the adolescent and his parents that this is a benign and temporary situation. A physical examination with palpation is necessary to differentiate gynecomastia from increased adiposity caused by being overweight. Adolescents who are distressed about physical integrity and masculinity may benefit from the knowledge that this condition occurs in more than 50% of all adolescent boys.

NUTRITIONAL AND EATING DISORDERS

Obesity

Few problems in childhood and adolescence are so obvious to others, are so difficult to treat, and have such long-term effects on health as obesity. Several different definitions have been proposed for obesity and overweight. Obesity has been defined as an increase in body weight resulting from an excessive accumulation of body fat relative to lean body mass. Overweight refers to the state of weighing more than average for height and body build. Currently, the body mass index (BMI) measurement is recommended as the most accurate method for screening children and adolescents for obesity. The BMI measurement is strongly associated with subcutaneous and total body fat and with skinfold thickness measurements. It is also highly specific for children with the greatest amount of body fat. Pediatric growth charts that include BMI for age and sex are available from the CDC.* Children with a BMI between the 85th and 95th percentiles are considered overweight, and obesity is defined by a BMI greater than or equal to the 95th percentile (Gahagan, 2011).

Regardless of the definition used, the number of overweight children in the United States is increasing and has reportedly reached epidemic status (Spruijt-Metz, 2011). Approximately 12.5 million children are overweight or obese (Ogden, Carroll, and Flegal, 2008). Numerous studies dating back to the early 1960s have documented childhood overweight through comprehensive evaluations of dietary intake, physical activity, and anthropometric measures (CDC using the various National Health and Nutrition Examination Surveys [NHANES], I, II, III, and IV) (Ogden, Carroll, and Flegal, 2008; Ogden, Kuczmarski, Flegal, et al., 2002; Ogden, Troiano, Briefel, et al., 1997). In children ages 6 to 11 years, the prevalence of childhood overweight remained fairly constant in between 1963 and 1974 at approximately 4% and 5.5%, respectively. However, more recent NHANES surveys have seen these numbers steadily climb to reach 17% in 2- to 19-year-old children. Between 1999/2000 and 2009/2010, a significant increase in obesity was observed in males 2 to 19 years of age but not in females of the same age (Ogden, Carroll, Kit, et al., 2012). African-American and Hispanic children are disproportionately represented by a higher

---

*www.cdc.gov/growthcharts.

prevalence of overweight and obesity (23.1% and 21.0%, respectively) compared with non-Hispanic white children (15.9%) (Ogden, Carroll, and Flegal, 2008). A study of 9464 Native-American schoolchildren ages 5 to 18 years found that 39% were overweight, and a further review of tribes across the United States found that 30% to 46% of Native Americans were at risk for overweight (Hardy, Harrell, and Bell, 2004).

Because adult obesity is associated with increased mortality and morbidity from a variety of complications, both physical and psychologic, adolescent obesity is a serious condition. Research indicates that overweight children and adolescents are at risk for continuing to be obese as adults, thereby experiencing the health and social consequences of obesity much earlier than children and adolescents of normal weight. Parental obesity increases the risk for overweight by twofold to threefold (Baker, Barlow, Cochran, et al., 2005). The probability that overweight school-age children will become obese adults is estimated at 50%, and the likelihood that overweight adolescents will become obese adults is estimated at 70% to 80% (National Institute for Health Care Management Foundation, 2003).

Obesity in childhood and adolescence has been related to elevated blood cholesterol, high blood pressure, respiratory disorders, orthopedic conditions, cholelithiasis, some types of adult-onset cancer, nonalcoholic fatty liver disease (NAFLD), and type 2 diabetes mellitus. The incidence of metabolic syndrome was 50% in a study group of overweight and obese adolescents (Weiss, Dziura, Burgert, et al., 2004). Common emotional consequences of obesity include poor body image, low self-esteem, social isolation, and feelings of depression and rejection (Sjöberg, Nilsson, and Leppert, 2005).

Etiology and Pathophysiology

Obesity results from a caloric intake that consistently exceeds caloric requirements and expenditure and may involve a variety of interrelated influences, including metabolic, hypothalamic, hereditary, social, cultural, and psychologic factors (Fig. 35-10). Because the etiology of obesity is multifactorial, the treatment requires multilevel interventions.

A balance between energy intake and energy expenditure is a critical factor in regulating body weight. Factors that raise energy intake or decrease energy expenditure by even small amounts can have a long-term impact on the development of overweight and obesity. For example, a positive balance of one serving of a sweetened juice or soft drink (≈120 kcal) per day would produce a 50-kg (110-pound) increase in body mass over a 10-year period (Hill, Wyatt, Reed, et al., 2003).

Familial influence is an epidemiologic consideration in regard to children's weight. Twin studies suggest that approximately 35% to 50% of the tendency toward obesity is inherited (Beaty, 2007). Twin studies have also suggested that this tendency is a combination of genetic and environmental factors. Mothers seem to play a greater role in the gestational weight of their children (Jaquet, Swaminathan, Alexander, et al., 2005). When both parents are obese, there is a 60% to 80% increase in the likelihood of the child becoming obese (Koeppen-Schomerus, Wardle, and Plomin, 2001; Wardle, Carnell, Haworth, et al., 2008). The specific influences of genes and environment within developing children are not well defined. The increasing rates of obesity within genetically stable populations suggest that environmental and some perinatal factors (e.g., bottle feeding) are contributors to the current increases in childhood obesity (National Institute for Health Care Management Foundation, 2003).

Birth weight does not seem to be a long-term contributing factor in detection and prediction of childhood obesity (Kain, Corvalán,

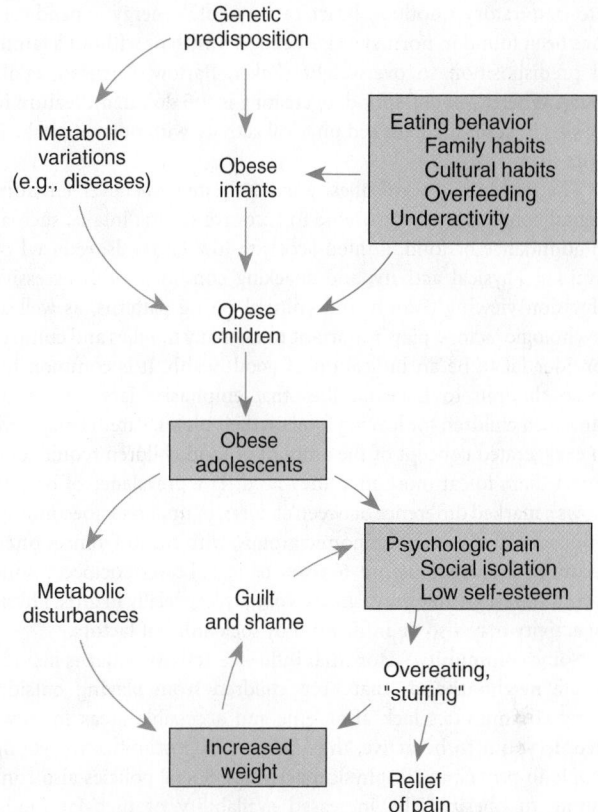

FIG 35-10 Complex relationships in obesity.

Lera, et al., 2009; McCarthy, Hughes, Tilling, et al., 2007); obese children do not have higher birth weights than nonobese children. There is, however, a high correlation between childhood adiposity and parental adiposity (Boney, Verma, Tucker, et al., 2005; Bouchard, 2009; Li, Kaur, Choi, et al., 2005). One study found that the best determinant of adult obesity was the child's weight at 5 years of age or an increased weight gain from 1 to 5 years of age (McCarthy, Hughes, Tilling, et al., 2007).

Fewer than 5% of the cases of childhood obesity can be attributed to an underlying disease. Such diseases include hypothyroidism; adrenal hypercorticoidism; hyperinsulinism; and dysfunction or damage to the central nervous system (CNS) as a result of tumor, injury, infection, or vascular accident. Obesity is a frequent complication of muscular dystrophy, paraplegia, Down syndrome, spina bifida, and other chronic illnesses that limit mobility.

A major focus of obesity research has been on appetite regulation. The expression of appetite is chemically coded in the hypothalamus by distinctive circuitry. Orexigenic substances produce signals that promote eating behaviors, and anorexigenic substances promote the cessation of eating behaviors. Feedback loops between signals have been identified where one signal peptide is able to alter the secretion of another signal peptide. No one signal has been identified as the gatekeeper of appetite. It is apparent that an entire network of signals, including their frequency and amplitude, is responsible for triggering eating behaviors.

There is little evidence to support a relationship between obesity and "low metabolism." Small differences may exist in regulation of dietary intake or metabolic rate between obese and nonobese children that could lead to an energy imbalance and inappropriate weight gain, but these small differences are difficult to accurately quantify. No differences in basal metabolic rate, sleeping metabolic rate, respiratory quotient, heart rate, or total energy expenditure have been found in normal weight children with or without a familial predisposition to overweight (Baker, Barlow, Cochran, et al., 2005). Whereas in childhood, overeating is the dominant feature in obesity, in adult life, reduced physical activity with normal intake is more likely.

The tendency toward obesity is manifested whenever environmental conditions are favorable to excessive caloric intake, such as an abundance of food, limited access to low-fat foods, reduced or minimal physical activity, and snacking combined with excessive television viewing. Family and cultural eating patterns, as well as psychologic factors, play important roles; many families and cultures consider fat to be an indication of good health. It is common for obese children to have families that emphasize large meals or admonish children for leaving food on their plates. Parents may have an exaggerated concept of the amount of food children require and expect them to eat more than they need. The prevalence of obesity shows a marked difference between children in upper-socioeconomic groups and lower-socioeconomic groups, with the differences often becoming apparent before 6 years of age. Lower socioeconomic groups have a greater prevalence of obesity, especially in girls. Physical activity may also be influenced by sociocultural factors.

Some community factors that influence activity patterns include unsafe neighborhoods that keep children from playing outside. Many communities lack affordable and accessible areas for low-income youth to be active, thus limiting opportunities for young people to participate in physical activities. Social policies also contribute to obesity. The increased availability of high-fat foods, pricing strategies that promote unhealthy food choices, and over-zealous food advertising that targets children and adolescents with high-fat and high-sugar foods are some examples.

Institutional factors also influence patterns of obesity and decreased physical activity. Many school policies allow students to leave school for lunch. Vending machines in school often are filled with high-fat and high-calorie foods and soft drinks. Although well-balanced, nutritious school lunches may be available to students, they often opt for less nutritious choices such as high-fat snacks.

Physical inactivity has also been identified as an important contributing factor in the development and maintenance of childhood overweight. There is little doubt that physical activity has decreased in elementary and secondary schools in the United States in past years. Although there have been positive attempts to incorporate more physical activity into schools within the past several years, most of children's physical activity must occur within the family or outside of school. Decreased physical activity within the family is a powerful influence on children because children imitate their parents and other adults. Parental obesity and low levels of physical activity are correlated with decreased physical activity in children.

The growing attraction and availability of many sedentary activities, including television, handheld video games, computers, and the Internet, have also greatly influenced the amount of time that children spend participating in sedentary behaviors. When combining television viewing with video games, it is estimated that children may spend as much as 6 hours per day on various media, which takes time away from meaningful activities such as exercise and reading (Roberts and Foehr, 2008). The AAP (2011) recently issued a policy statement encouraging parents to limit media viewing in children to 2 hours or less per day. The AAP asserts that media time, especially advertisements of food products, has a direct correlation with the increased incidence of childhood obesity in the United States.

Psychologic factors also affect eating patterns. In infancy, children experience relief from discomfort through feeding and learn to associate eating with a sense of well-being, security, and the comforting presence of a nurturing person. Eating is soon associated with the feeling of being loved. In addition, the pleasurable oral sensation of sucking provides a connection between emotions and early eating behavior. Many parents use food as a positive reward for desired behaviors. This practice may become a habit, and the child may continue to use food as a reward, a comfort, and a means of dealing with depression or hostility. Many individuals eat when they are not hungry or in response to boredom, loneliness, sadness, depression, or tiredness. Difficulty in determining feelings of satiety can lead to weight problems and may compound the factor of eating in response to emotional rather than physical hunger cues.

Eating behaviors are closely related to memory. Memory and appetite are chemically encoded, with each individual having his or her own circuitry relating to eating behaviors. Similar to memory, the circuitry can be modified over time (Feldman, Friedman, and Sleisenger, 2002).

Diagnostic Evaluation

A careful history is obtained regarding the development of obesity, and a physical examination is performed to differentiate simple obesity from increased fat that results from organic causes. A family history of obesity, diabetes, coronary heart disease, and dyslipidemia should be obtained for all children who are overweight or at risk for overweight. Specific information from the patient and family about the effects of obesity on daily functioning—for example, problems with nighttime breathing and sleep, daytime sleepiness, joint pain, inability to keep up with family activities and peers at school—is helpful. The physical examination should focus on identifying comorbid conditions and identifiable causes of obesity. For some, psychologic assessment by interviews and standardized personality tests may provide insight into the personality and emotional problems that contribute to obesity and that might interfere with therapy.

It is useful to estimate the degree of obesity to determine the component of body weight that can be modified. All of the following methods have been used to assess obesity: BMI, body weight, weight-height ratios, weight-age ratios, hydrostatic (underwater) weight, skinfold measurements, bioelectrical analysis, computed tomography, magnetic resonance imaging, and neutron activation. Each of these methods has advantages and disadvantages. Hydrostatic, or underwater, weighing provides the most accurate measurement of lean body weight.

Body mass index is currently considered the best method to assess weight in children and adolescents. The calculation is based on the individual's height and weight. In adults, BMI definitions are fixed measures without regard for sex and age. The BMI in children and adolescents varies to accommodate age- and sex-specific changes in growth. The formula for BMI calculation is:

$$\text{Weight in pounds} \div (\text{Height in inches})^2 \times 703$$
$$\text{OR}$$
$$\text{Weight in kilograms} \div (\text{Height in meters})^2$$

BMI measures in children and adolescents are plotted on growth charts that enable health care professionals to determine BMI for age for the patient (see Appendix A).

The initial assessment of obese children and adolescents should include screening to evaluate for comorbidities. The history is an important guide to determine the workup. A complete physical examination is important. Some areas to focus on include (1) skin for stretch markings and discolorations (e.g., acanthosis nigricans), (2) joints for swelling and evidence of pain, and (3) airway for evidence of obstruction and enlarged tonsils. Basic laboratory studies include a fasting lipid panel; fasting insulin level; fasting glucose hepatic enzymes, including γ-glutamyltransferase (GGT); and in some institutions, hemoglobin A1$_c$. Other studies, such as a sleep study, metabolic studies, and radiographic evaluations, may be added based on the history and physical examination. These assessments may determine whether the patient needs a referral to specialty services for more focused evaluation and treatment, such as endocrinology (insulin resistance, diabetes), hepatology (elevated liver enzymes, NAFLD), orthopedics (Blount disease), or pulmonary medicine (sleep-disordered breathing, noninvasive continuous positive airway pressure).

Therapeutic Management

The best approach to the management of obesity is a preventive one. Early recognition and control measures are essential before the child or adolescent reaches an obese state. Health care providers must educate families about the medical complications of obesity, and families are encouraged to be involved in the treatment plan.

The treatment of obesity is difficult. Many approaches do not achieve long-term success. The average individual loses only about 5% to 10% of his or her weight with available therapies. Losing weight can have a significant positive effect on many comorbidities, but unfortunately, the lost weight is frequently regained in a year or two.

Diet modification is an essential part of weight-reduction programs. Dietary counseling is directed toward improving the nutritional quality of the diet rather than toward dietary restriction. Children and adolescents should avoid fad diets. Most dietitians and nutrition experts recommend a diet with no *trans* fats, low-saturated fat, moderate total fat (≤30%) and a half plate of fruits and vegetables daily, consistent with the MyPlate* food guide for children. Also, promoting high-fiber foods and avoiding highly refined starches and sugars decrease caloric intake. The Dietary Guidelines for Americans† may be used as a guide for caloric intake for adolescents concerned about weight control; these guidelines also emphasize daily exercise in weight management for children and adolescents. Many programs recommend using a food diary as a helpful tool to increase awareness of food choices and eating behaviors. The goal is to encourage the individual to make healthy choices in food selection and discourage eating food by habit or to appease boredom. Box 35-5 contains helpful suggestions.

In patients with severe obesity, strict diets have been used, such as the protein-sparing modified fast—a hypocaloric, ketogenic diet that is designed to provide enough protein to minimize loss of lean body mass during weight loss. Such diets need to be closely monitored and should be used only with multidisciplinary teams that include a physician, nutritionist, and behavioral therapist. Generally, the diet consists of 1.5 to 2.5 g of protein per kilogram. The intake of carbohydrates is low enough to induce ketosis. The benefits of the diet are relatively rapid weight loss and anorexia induced by ketosis. Potential complications include protein losses, hypokalemia, hypoglycemia, inadequate calcium intake, and orthostatic hypotension. Potassium and calcium supplements and adequate calorie-free beverages can minimize these complications (Baker, Barlow, Cochran, et al., 2005). It is difficult to sustain such diets over the long term,

---

> ### BOX 35-5   RECOMMENDED BEHAVIORS FOR PREVENTING OBESITY
>
> In counseling adolescents whose body mass index is between the 5th and 84th percentiles, physicians and health care providers should recommend the following steps to prevent obesity:
> - Limit or avoid consumption of sugar-sweetened beverages.
> - Consume recommended quantities of fiber, fruits, and vegetables.
> - Limit television and other screen time to no more than 2 hours per day.
> - Remove television and computer screens from primary sleeping areas.
> - Eat breakfast daily.
> - Limit eating at fast food restaurants.
> - Have frequent family meals in which parents and youth eat together.
> - Limit portion sizes.

Adapted from Davis DM, Gance-Cleveland B, Hassink S, et al: Recommendations for prevention of childhood obesity, *Pediatrics* 120(Suppl):S229–S253, 2007.

---

and the long-term outcomes of using these diets have not been established.

Researchers continue searching for medications that will successfully treat obesity. The Food and Drug Administration (FDA) has approved sibutramine, an appetite suppressant, for use in adolescents 16 years old and older for the treatment of obesity (U.S. Preventive Services Task Force, 2010). Orlistat, a lipase inhibitor, has been approved for adolescents 12 to 18 years of age who have BMIs more than 2 units above the 95th percentile for age and sex; however, side effects of the drug include fatty or oily stools and possible malabsorption of fat-soluble vitamins (Kanekar and Sharma, 2010). There are currently no drugs approved for use in overweight or obese children younger than the age of 12 years. Other drugs have been used to promote weight loss in children with certain conditions, such as metformin in obese adolescents with insulin resistance and hyperinsulinism, octreotide for hypothalamic obesity caused by intracranial tumors, growth hormone in children with Prader-Willi syndrome, and leptin for congenital leptin deficiency.

Combining behavioral modifications with pharmacologic therapy in children 12 years and older have produced mixed results referent to total weight loss maintained over a significant period of time (U.S. Preventive Services Task Force, 2010). Reports suggest modest benefits with moderate to high behavioral interventions (measured in number of contact hours) in decreasing mean BMI of children and adolescents involved in such programs over a period of 6 to 12 months (Whitlock, O'Connor, Williams, et al., 2010). Programs including family-based behavioral modification, dietary modification, and exercise have been shown to be successful in reducing obesity in some children (AAP, 2006).

Bariatric surgery may be the only practical alternative for increasing numbers of severely overweight adolescents who have failed organized attempts to lose or maintain weight loss through conventional nonoperative approaches and who have serious life-threatening conditions. Until recently, there were few studies in adolescents that suggested surgical weight loss improved the early mortality of patients with severe obesity. In recent years, there has been an increase in bariatric surgery among teens, especially involving the laparoscopic adjustable gastric band procedure (although the FDA has not approved its use in adolescents). The laparoscopic Roux-en-Y gastric bypass is commonly performed for weight loss in adolescents. Data suggest that bariatric surgery in adolescents

---

*www.choosemyplate.gov/index.html.
†www.health.gov/dietaryguidelines.

results in sustained weight loss, a decrease in BMI, and a decrease in the incidence of comorbidities such as type II diabetes (Barnett, 2011). Best practice recommendations for childhood and adolescent weight loss surgery are published elsewhere (Pratt, Lenders, Dionne, et al., 2009). Physicians must define clear, realistic, and restrictive guidelines to apply with younger patients when surgery is considered. Candidates for surgery should be referred to centers that offer a multidisciplinary team experienced in the management of childhood and adolescent obesity. The surgery should be performed by surgeons who have participated in subspecialty training in bariatric medical and surgical care as detailed by the American College of Surgeons and the American Society for Metabolic and Bariatric Surgery.

CARE MANAGEMENT

Nurses play a key role in the adherence and maintenance phases of many weight-reduction programs. Nurses assess, manage, and evaluate the progress of many overweight adolescents. They also play an important role in recognizing potential weight problems and assisting parents and adolescents in preventing obesity.

The presence of obesity may not be obvious from appearance alone. Regular assessment of height and weight and computation of the BMI facilitate early recognition. Published guidelines are available for childhood obesity prevention and treatment (Barlow and Expert Committee, 2007). Children with BMIs greater than or equal to the 95th percentile for age and sex should receive in-depth medical assessment. Children with BMIs in the 85th to 95th percentile range should be evaluated for secondary complications (e.g., diabetes, hypertension, and hyperlipidemia) and family history. Evaluation includes a height and weight history of the adolescent and family members, eating habits, appetite and hunger patterns, and physical activities. A psychosocial history is also helpful in understanding the impact of obesity on the child's life.

Before initiating a treatment plan, it is important to be certain that the family is ready for change. Lack of readiness may result in failure, frustration, and reluctance to address the problem in the future. The nurse should explore with adolescents the reasons behind the desire to lose weight because motivation to lose weight is the key to success. Adolescents need to take a personal responsibility for their dietary habits and physical activity. Young persons who are forced by their parents to seek help are seldom motivated, become rebellious, and are unwilling to control their dietary intake.

Nutritional Counseling. Preventing an increase in body fat during growth is a realistic approach. This is often accomplished by adjusting four aspects of eating: (1) reducing the quantity eaten by purchasing, preparing, and serving smaller portions; (2) altering the quality consumed by substituting low-calorie, low-fat foods for high-calorie foods (especially for snacks); (3) eating regular meals and snacks, particularly breakfast; and (4) altering situations by severing associations between eating and other stimuli, such as eating while watching television.

The most successful diets are those that use ordinary foods in controlled portions rather than diets that require the avoidance of specific foods.

Teach adolescents and parents how to incorporate favorite foods into their diet and to select satisfying substitutes. Dieting teens should eat what the rest of the family eats but less of it. When parents buy and prepare smaller amounts, they eliminate tempting second helpings and leftovers. To maintain a healthy diet, it is necessary to

encourage the consumption of high-nutrient foods such as fruits, vegetables, whole grains, and low-fat dairy protein products. Keep calories and fat to a healthy level without being significantly restricted. To be successful, a dietary program should be nutritionally sound with sufficient satiety value, produce the desired weight loss, and be accompanied by nutrition education and continued support. Children and adolescents should not initiate a reduction diet without health assessment and counseling. Davis, Gance-Cleveland, Hassink, et al. (2007) describe steps to approaching behavior change with youth (Box 35-6).

Behavioral Therapy. Altering eating behavior and eliminating inappropriate eating habits are essential to weight reduction, especially in maintaining long-term weight control. Most behavioral modification programs include the following concepts:

- A description of the behavior to be controlled, such as eating habits
- Attempts to modify and control the stimuli that govern eating
- Development of eating techniques designed to control speed of eating
- Positive reinforcement for these modifications through a suitable reward system that does not include food

Box 35-5 includes specific strategies to modify eating habits.

Group Involvement. Commercial groups (e.g., Weight Watchers) and diet workshops composed primarily of adults may be helpful to some teenagers; however, a peer group is often more effective. Teenage groups include summer camps designed for obese young people and conducted by health care professionals, school groups organized and led by a school nurse, and groups associated with special clinics.

These groups are concerned not only with weight loss but also with the development of a positive self-image and the encouragement of physical activity. Nutrition education, diet planning, and the improvement of social skills are essential components of these groups. Improvement is determined by positive changes in all aspects of behavior.

Family Involvement. There is a definite connection among family environment, interaction, and obesity. The nurse needs to educate parents in the purposes of the therapeutic measures and their role in management. The family needs nutrition education and counseling regarding the reinforcement plan, alterations in the food environment, and ways to maintain proper attitudes. They can support their child in efforts to change eating behaviors, food intake, and physical activity.

Research indicates that family meals may also play a role in decreasing obesity and high risk behaviors among adolescents by promoting healthy eating habits; however, more quality research is needed to clarify the protective role of such interactions in regard to adolescent obesity (Fulkerson, Neumark-Sztainer, Hannan, et al., 2008; Fulkerson, Story, Mellin, et al., 2006; Larson, Neumark-Sztainer, Hannan, et al., 2007).

Parents can also affect the child's eating habits by decreasing media time viewed by the entire family and by discussing food advertisements that promote unhealthy food and eating habits.

Physical Activity. The current recommendation for physical activity for children and adolescents is to participate in a combined total of 60 minutes of physical activity daily; this can be moderate to vigorous intensive exercise or activity (U.S. Department of Health and Human Services, 2008b). Regular physical activity is incorporated into all weight-reduction programs. Any form of increased physical activity is beneficial, provided that the activities are age-appropriate and enjoyable. Recommendations for physical activity

BOX 35-6	PEDIATRIC OBESITY PREVENTION PROTOCOL FOR PRIMARY CARE

Step 1: Assess
- Explain and conduct assessments of:
  - Weight, height, and body mass index percentile
  - Dietary intake (fruit, vegetables, sweetened beverages, and fast food)
  - Activity (screen time, moderate to vigorous activity)
  - Eating behaviors (breakfast, portion sizes, family meals)
- Provide and elicit feedback on body mass index and behaviors found to be inside and outside the optimal range.

Step 2: Set Agenda
- Explore interest in changing behaviors not in the optimal range.
- Agree on target behaviors with the patient and caregiver.

Step 3: Assess Motivation and Confidence
- With regard to interest in changing weight status or behaviors, assess:
  - Willingness
  - Perceived importance
  - Confidence in having success
- Probe the patient regarding ratings of willingness, perceived importance, and confidence to explore the advantages and disadvantages of changing.

Step 4: Summarize and Probe Possible Changes
- Summarize the advantages and disadvantages of change.
- Query possible next steps.
- Offer ideas for getting started in making a change as needed.
- Summarize the change plan.
- Provide positive feedback.

Step 5: Schedule Follow-Up Visit
- If a change plan is made, agree on a follow-up appointment within a specified number of weeks or months.
- If no change plan is made, agree to revisit the topic within a specific number of weeks or months.

Adapted from Davis DM, Gance-Cleveland B, Hassink S, et al: Recommendations for prevention of childhood obesity, *Pediatrics* 120(Suppl):S229–S253, 2007.

need to consider the current health status and developmental level of the child or adolescent. The best choice for exercise is any form that is enjoyable and likely to be sustainable. Aerobic and endurance exercises help oxidize body fats. Light exercises such as walking may provide an opportunity for the family to increase time together and increase caloric expenditure. Walking for 30 minutes each day and decreasing caloric intake by 500 calories per day may significantly reduce the risk for chronic disease. Weight training can increase the basal metabolic rate and replace fat mass with muscle mass. However, weight training is not generally recommended for prepubertal children until they have reached physical and skeletal maturity. In prepubertal children, increasing outdoor playtime is likely to be beneficial. Many children find exercise videos and treadmills boring and may not continue these activities. There are a great variety of physical activities to choose from that are likely to appeal to different people. Team sports and individual sports such as dance, bike riding, swimming, and karate are some examples. Limiting sedentary

activities such as television viewing (while eating snacks!) is the most effective way to encourage physical activity.

Prevention. Weight loss programs do not enjoy the success of therapeutic interventions for other disorders. Gradual accumulation of adipose tissue during childhood establishes a pattern of eating that is difficult to reverse in adolescence. Prevention of obesity should begin in early childhood with the development of healthy eating habits, regular exercise patterns, and a positive relationship between parents and children. Prevention of adolescent obesity is best accomplished by early identification of obesity in the preschool, school-age, and preadolescent periods. Health care professionals should encourage frequent health care visits for children who are overweight or obese and incorporate a dietary history and counseling into each well-infant, well-child, and well-adolescent visit.

Anorexia Nervosa and Bulimia Nervosa

Anorexia nervosa (AN) is an eating disorder characterized by a refusal to maintain a minimally normal body weight and by severe weight loss in the absence of obvious physical causes. Approximately 5% of adolescent girls in the United States have AN, and 5% to 10% of all cases occur in boys and men (AAP Committee on Adolescence, 2010). The average age of onset is 13 years, but the disorder can occur as early as 10 years of age and as late as 25 years of age. Individuals with AN are described as perfectionists, academically high achievers, conforming, and conscientious. Typically, they have high energy levels even with marked emaciation. Patients with AN may eventually develop bulimia.

Bulimia (from the Greek meaning "ox hunger") refers to an eating disorder similar to AN. Bulimia nervosa (BN) is observed more commonly in older adolescent girls and young women; boys and men with bulimia are less common. BN patients may be of average or slightly above average weight. BN is characterized by repeated episodes of binge eating followed by inappropriate compensatory behaviors, such as self-induced vomiting; misuse of laxatives, diuretics, or other medications; fasting; or excessive exercise (AAP Committee on Adolescence, 2010). The binge behavior consists of secretive, frenzied consumption of large amounts of high-calorie (or "forbidden") foods during a brief time (usually <2 hours). The binge is counteracted by a variety of weight control methods (purging). These binge-purge cycles are followed by self-deprecating thoughts, a depressed mood, and an awareness that the eating pattern is abnormal. Nonpurging bulimic individuals may use other inappropriate compensatory behaviors such as fasting or excessive exercising but do not regularly engage in self-induced vomiting or the abuse of laxatives, enemas, or diuretics (American Psychiatric Association [APA], 2000).

Although persons with BN have many issues in common with those who have other eating disorders, impulse control and satiety regulation are important problems in BN. Many individuals with BN begin with only occasional binges and purges "just for fun," enjoying the control over their weight while eating amounts of food that would normally produce obesity. As the condition progresses, the frequency of binges increases, the amount of food consumed increases, and they gradually lose control over the binge-purge cycle. The frequency of binging can be anywhere from once per week to 7 or 8 times per day. Because persons with BN usually binge on high-calorie foods, especially sweets, ice cream, and pastries, insulin production is stimulated to cope with the added carbohydrates. When the food is vomited, the unused insulin stimulates hunger and the desire to eat.

A third eating disorder, identified as eating disorder not otherwise specified (EDNOS), has components of both AN and BN with varying degrees of symptomatology that are not always characteristic of the established diagnostic criteria for AN and BN (American Dietetic Association, 2006). Binge eating disorder (BED) is a type of EDNOS. Persons with BED may diet in an attempt to control their weight but without the extreme weight control compensatory practices of vomiting, laxative use, diuretics, and excessive exercise (American Dietetic Association, 2006; Forman, 2011).

A fourth type of eating disorder, avoidant/restrictive food intake disorder (ARFID), has been proposed and is scheduled to appear in the American Psychiatric Association's (APA's) *DSM-V* classification of eating disorders of children. In this disorder, there is an apparent lack of interest in eating or food with significant weight loss, nutritional deficiency, and dependence on enteral feeding; there is also significant psychosocial functioning with this disorder, and it is not associated with AN or BN (APA, 2010).

Etiology and Pathophysiology

The etiology of these disorders remains unclear. There is a distinct psychologic component, and the diagnosis is based primarily on psychologic and behavioral criteria. Dieting appears to be common to the initiation of both AN and BN. The disorders appear to be caused by a combination of genetic, neurochemical, psychodevelopmental, and sociocultural factors. The dominant aspects of AN are a relentless pursuit of thinness and a fear of fatness, usually preceded by a period of mood disturbances and behavior changes.

Weight loss may be triggered by a typical adolescent crisis such as the onset of menstruation or a traumatic interpersonal incident that precipitates serious, out-of-control dieting. Situations of severe family stress (e.g., parental separation or divorce) or circumstances in which the adolescent perceives a lack of personal control (e.g., teasing at school, changing schools, or going to college) may precipitate a desire for control and the decision not to eat. Frequently, there is an exaggerated misinterpretation of the normal fat deposition characteristic of early adolescence or anxiety because of comments that the adolescent is putting on weight.

Many experts have associated the development of an eating disorder with family characteristics such as an adolescent perception of high parental expectations for achievement and appearance, difficulty managing conflict and poor communication styles, enmeshment and occasionally estrangement among family members, devaluation of the mother or the maternal role, and marital tension. Families struggling with an eating disorder have been characterized as often having difficulties responding positively to the changing physical and emotional needs of the adolescent. Family stress of any kind may become a significant factor in the development of an eating disorder (Forman, 2011).

Society's emphasis and the media's focus on tall, thin individuals may also play a role. Studies evaluating the possible association of eating disorders and sexual abuse have been conflicting. Childhood sexual abuse may be a factor in some cases of AN.

Patients with eating disorders commonly have psychiatric problems, including affective disorder, anxiety disorder, obsessive-compulsive disorder (OCD), and personality disorder. Adult women with eating disorders were found to have higher rates of obsessive-compulsive behavior traits in their childhoods. Patients with eating disorders have also been found to have higher reported rates of substance abuse, with alcohol problems being more common in those with BN than AN (Forman, 2011). It is important to note that many of the clinical findings are directly related to the state of starvation and improve with weight gain.

Many sports and artistic endeavors that emphasize leanness (e.g., ballet and running) and sports in which the scoring is partly subjective (e.g., gymnastics) have been associated with a higher incidence of eating disorders such as AN. The term **female athlete triad,** characterized by disordered eating behavior, amenorrhea, and osteoporosis, has been applied to young women with restrictive eating disorders and amenorrhea (Landry, 2011).

A genetic role has been postulated for eating disorders; a significant number of young women with a first-degree relative having an eating disorder were at a significantly higher rate of having an eating disorder (Forman, 2011). However, some consider these eating disorders to not be a direct result of family inheritance but, rather, a secondary effect of the manifestations of conditions such as anxiety, depression, and OCD " that may be modulated through the internal milieu of puberty" (Landry, 2011).

Diagnostic Evaluation

Diagnosis of AN is made on the basis of clinical manifestations (Box 35-7) and conformity to the criteria established by the APA (2000). Diagnosis of BN is confirmed, according to the APA's *DSM* (2000), by at least two binge eating episodes per week for the preceding 3 months. Characteristics of BN and AN are listed in Table 35-2.

A complete history and physical examination are important to rule out other causes of weight loss. The medical assessment of an eating disorder focuses on the complications of altered nutritional status and purging. A careful history assesses weight changes, dietary patterns, and the frequency and severity of purging and excessive exercise. The patient's weight and height should be measured and evaluated for appropriateness according to standard weight for height, age, and sex determined according to the percentile of his or her expected body weight or BMI.

The diagnosis of eating disorder (ED) is made clinically, but additional laboratory diagnostic tests may be obtained to identify malnutrition or other associated complications. Additional diagnostic measures may include a complete blood count to evaluate for anemia and other hematologic abnormalities; erythrocyte sedimentation rate or C-reactive protein to detect evidence of inflammation; electrolytes as well as calcium, magnesium, phosphorus, blood urea nitrogen, and creatinine; urinalysis, including specific gravity; and bone density studies for osteopenia, which is commonly observed in patients with AN. In patients with prolonged amenorrhea, human chorionic gonadotropin is assessed to determine the presence of pregnancy. Other tests for patients with amenorrhea include thyroid function tests and measurement of serum prolactin and follicle-stimulating hormone to help rule out prolactinoma (hormone-secreting pituitary tumor), hyperthyroidism, hypothyroidism, or ovarian failure. In addition, a comprehensive cardiac evaluation is often recommended in those with AN. Further

---

BOX 35-7   CLINICAL MANIFESTATIONS OF ANOREXIA NERVOSA

- Severe and profound weight loss
- Secondary amenorrhea (if menarche attained)
- Primary amenorrhea (if menarche not attained)
- Sinus bradycardia
- Lowered body temperature
- Hypotension
- Intolerance to cold
- Dry skin and brittle nails
- Appearance of lanugo hair
- Thinning hair
- Abdominal pain
- Bloating
- Constipation
- Fatigue
- Lightheadedness
- Evidence of muscle wasting (cachectic appearance)
- Bone pain with exercise

TABLE 35-2   CHARACTERISTICS OF INDIVIDUALS WITH EATING DISORDERS

FACTORS	ANOREXIA NERVOSA	BULIMIA
Food	Turns away from food to cope	Turns to food to cope
Personality	Introverted Avoids intimacy Negates feminine role	Extroverted Seeks intimacy Aspires to feminine role
Behavior	"Model" child Obsessive-compulsive	Often acts out Impulsive
School	High achiever	Variable school performance
Control	Maintains rigid control	Loses control
Body image	Body image distortion	Less frequent body image distortion
Health	Denies illness	Recognizes illness Health fluctuates
Weight	Body weight <85% of expected norm	Within 2.3-7 kg (5-15 lb) of normal body weight or may be overweight
Sexuality	Usually not sexually active	Often sexually active

diagnostic tests may be required based on the history and findings from these diagnostic tests.

Screening Tools. All patients in high risk categories for eating disorders should be screened during routine office visits. The medical history is most important for diagnosing eating disorders because the physical examination findings may be normal, especially early in the illness. A number of screening questionnaires are available to assist with the interview. For example, with the SCOFF questionnaire, 1 point is scored for every "yes." A score of 2 or more indicates a likely case of AN or BN. The questions related to the mnemonic SCOFF are (1) Do you make yourself *sick* because you feel uncomfortably full? (2) Do you worry that you have lost *control* over how much you eat? (3) Have you recently lost more than 6.4 kg (14 pounds or *one* stone) in a 3-month period? (4) Do you believe yourself to be *fat* when others say that you are too thin? and (5) Would you say that *food* dominates your life? (Morgan, Reid, and Lacey, 1999).

Therapeutic Management

The treatment and management of AN involve three major goals: (1) reinstitution of normal nutrition or reversal of the severe state of malnutrition, (2) resolution of disturbed patterns of family interaction, and (3) individual psychotherapy to correct deficits and distortions in psychologic functioning. The treatment of eating disorders requires the cooperative efforts of an interdisciplinary team composed of a primary care practitioner, nurse, dietitian, and mental health care provider with pediatric and adolescent health care experience. Because of the psychogenic nature of the disorder,

the treatment may be long. Recent studies suggest that family-based therapy is more effective than individual cognitive behavioral therapy in reducing the maladaptive eating behaviors in adolescents with AN (Lock, 2010).

Most adolescents are treated on an outpatient basis, but those with problems requiring immediate medical attention, such as severe malnutrition or electrolyte or psychiatric disturbances (severe depression or suicidal ideation), require hospitalization. Persons with BN may benefit from cognitive behavioral therapy, other psychotherapy, antidepressant medications, or a combination of antidepressant medication and psychotherapy (Kreipe, 2011).

Nutrition Therapy. The most important goal is to treat any life-threatening malnutrition and to restore dietary stability and weight gain. This may require the administration of tube feedings or intravenous fluids if the malnutrition is severe. In most cases, it is best to reintroduce food and snacks slowly in a stepwise manner. A reasonable goal is to reach an eventual intake of 2000 to 3000 kcal per day and a weight gain of 0.22 to 0.45 kg (0.5-1 pound) per week (American Dietetic Association, 2006). When restoring nutrition, health care professionals must avoid the **refeeding syndrome,** which consists of cardiovascular, neurologic, and hematologic complications that occur when nutritional replacement is given too rapidly. This syndrome can be avoided with slow refeeding and the addition of phosphorus when total body phosphorus is depleted. Treatment goal weights are individualized and based on age, height, stage of puberty, premorbid weight, and previous growth charts. In young women who have reached menarche, resumption of menses is an objective measure of return to biologic health.

Dietary interventions are combined with behavioral therapy to improve the underlying psychologic misconceptions about weight loss. Another aspect of treatment is to relieve the anxiety related to eating and the depression that accompanies the disorder. The administration of antianxiety or antidepressant medications is beneficial. However, when these drugs are used, patients should be carefully monitored for cardiovascular side effects.

Cognitive Behavioral Therapy. Behavioral interventions are often necessary to encourage patients to accomplish the desired caloric intake and weight gain. Weight restoration as an outpatient is accomplished with behavioral contracts negotiated between the therapists and patient. The goal is to increase the patient's feelings of control and responsibility toward achieving recovery. The contract can stipulate at what weight tube feedings will be implemented. Individual psychotherapy is aimed at helping the young person resolve the adolescent identity crisis, particularly as it relates to a distorted body image. If the disorder is related to a dysfunctional family situation, therapy is most successful when it is started soon after the onset of illness and directed toward disengagement and redirection of malfunctioning processes in the family.

Pharmacotherapy. Pharmacotherapy in the treatment of AN has been disappointing so far. None of the randomized controlled trials (RCTs) have shown improvement in weight gain in adults treated with pharmacotherapy, and no studies have been conducted in children and adolescents (Golden and Attia, 2011). The few studies that have been done have primarily evaluated medications' efficacy in the treatment of comorbid disorders such as OCD and depression. Anxiolytic medications may be helpful before meals to relieve some patients' anxiety.

Tricyclic antidepressants (TCAs) and fluoxetine belong to a group of medications known as *selective serotonin reuptake inhibitors (SSRIs),* which have been more successful when used with BN. There is also some evidence that TCAs such as desipramine, imipramine, and amitriptyline; monoamine oxidase inhibitors; and buspirone

? CRITICAL THINKING CASE STUDY

Anorexia Nervosa

Jane is a 13-year-old girl whose grades have been excellent and whom the teachers describe as a "model student." Recently, Jane's teacher told the nurse practitioner that Jane's parents were in the middle of a "messy divorce." In addition, several of Jane's friends told the nurse practitioner that they are concerned about Jane because she runs every day at lunchtime and seldom eats lunch with them. Jane told her friends that she gained weight over the winter months and that she is running because she wants to qualify for the track team this spring. At the time of her routine health interview and sports physical examination, the nurse practitioner notes that Jane's oral temperature is 36° C (96.8° F) and that she weighs 34 kg (75 pounds). Jane has lost 9 kg (20 pounds) since her last sports physical. Jane tells the nurse practitioner that she has not had her menstrual period for 3 months.

1. Evidence—Is there sufficient evidence to draw any conclusions about Jane's behavior?
2. Assumptions—Describe some underlying assumptions about the following:
   a. Personality characteristics of individuals with anorexia nervosa (AN)
   b. Factors influencing the development of AN
   c. Clinical manifestations of AN
   d. Treatment of AN
3. What priorities for nursing care should be established for Jane at this time?
4. Does the evidence objectively support your argument (conclusion)?

are more effective compared with a placebo in decreasing binging and vomiting in patients with BN. Some of the latter medications, however, may have side effects that may preclude their utility in such patients (Golden and Attia, 2011). Topiramate, an antiepileptic agent, and the selective serotonin antagonist *ondansetron* have demonstrated some benefit in treating patients with BN. As with AN, pharmacotherapy should be an adjunct to behavioral therapy.

CARE MANAGEMENT

Nurses need to adopt and maintain a kind and supportive yet firm manner in managing the care of the adolescent with eating disorders without creating a passive-dependent attitude. The individual requires sustained support and reassurance to cope with ambivalent feelings related to body concept and the desire to be seen as cooperative, reliable, and worthy of receiving kindness. Encouraging the adolescent with education and activities that strengthen self-esteem facilitates the resocialization process and promotes social acceptance among peers. The nursing process in the care of adolescents with an eating disorder such as overweight or obesity is outlined in the Nursing Care Plan.

It is important for nurses to be aware of the physical side effects of AN. Patients frequently limit their fluid intake. Urinary tract problems are common, and ketones and protein may be detected in the urine as a result of breakdown of fat and protein. Vital sign instability can be severe and can include orthostatic hypotension; the pulse becomes irregular, and the rate decreases markedly. Electrolyte imbalances can be life threatening, and bradycardia and hypothermia can result in cardiac arrest (see Critical Thinking Case Study).

The team responsible for the management of young people with AN arranges a carefully structured environment. First, there must be consistency. The team decides on an approach and adheres to it.

The plan is structured with reality testing regarding caloric intake and body image perception as an essential component. The team members provide a unified front to avoid any possibility of manipulation or inconsistency. Second, all team members are involved; responsibility for the program cannot be left to one person. The role and boundaries of each member are clearly spelled out. Third, continuity of team members is important; it is helpful to have the same team members all the time.

Fourth, communication among team members is essential. Communication with the patient regarding what is expected is also important. Sometimes the limit setting may seem unreasonable; if the adolescent does not understand the rationale for the limits, he or she may sabotage the entire program. It is also important to communicate with the family. Fifth, the plan must provide for support of the adolescent, the family, and team members. The adolescent's efforts should be supported, and positive feedback should be provided for accomplishments made in normalizing eating habits. Meetings are held to discuss the feelings and concerns of the patient, immediate caregivers, and team members.

A behavioral contract, an agreement that the adolescent makes with others to change a maladaptive behavior, has proved to be effective in some cases. The written contract is constructed by the therapeutic team and approved and signed by the adolescent. Unless the adolescent agrees to its terms, the contract can become the source of a power struggle. However, it can be an effective tool that places the responsibility for weight gain or other behavioral change on the adolescent.

Family-based therapy is often used in the treatment of adolescent eating disorders, specifically in the treatment of AN. In particular, the Maudsley approach aims to help parents rediscover their own resources and take an active role in their children's recovery. Encourage families to explore how it has become problematic to follow the normal developmental course of their family life cycle by looking at how the eating disorder and the interactional patterns in the family have become entangled.

Nursing care of the adolescent with BN is similar to care of the patient with AN. Acute care involves careful monitoring of fluid and electrolyte alterations and observation for signs of cardiac complications. Nutritional consultation and follow-up care are essential. The nurse should encourage the adolescent and family members to structure the environment to reduce the binging behavior. Getting rid of binge foods; restricting eating to one room of the house; not engaging in other activities while eating; and substituting exercise, crafts, visualization, and relaxation techniques for binging are helpful interventions.

Nurses, patients, and families can find assistance and information from several organizations. The National Association of Anorexia Nervosa and Associated Eating Disorders* provides counseling, referral, and self-help programs for young people with AN. The National Eating Disorders Association† provides information and support services for both patients and families.

HEALTH PROBLEMS WITH A BEHAVIORAL COMPONENT

Substance Abuse

Although experimentation with drugs during childhood and adolescence is widespread, most children and teens do not become high

---

*Helpline 630-577-1330, available 9 AM to 5 PM Central Time, Monday through Friday; e-mail: anadhelp@anad.org; www.anad.org.
†603 Stewart St., Suite 803, Seattle, WA 98101; 800-931-2237; www.edap.org.

◎ NURSING CARE PLAN

The Adolescent with an Eating Disorder

NURSING DIAGNOSIS	EXPECTED OUTCOME	INTERVENTIONS	RATIONALES
Imbalanced Nutrition: Less Than Body Requirements related to altered self-image, inadequate nutrient intake, and chronic vomiting **Child's/Family's Defining Characteristics (Subjective and Objective Data)** Body weight 20% or more under ideal	Nutrient intake is sufficient to maintain optimal cellular and metabolic function.	If adolescent's life is in immediate danger as result of malnutrition, implement plan for restoring physiologic homeostasis: electrolyte and fluid replacement, enteral feedings as required, monitoring of vital signs, and restoration of fluid and electrolyte balance	To prevent death or multiorgan failure To restore fluid balance and prevent life-threatening electrolyte imbalance
		Develop mutually agreeable targeted daily caloric intake goal (specify goal)	To give adolescent sense of control over nutrient intake and establish realistic plan for weight gain
		Observe eating behaviors	To detect detrimental habits such as purging or binging after meals
		Monitor nutritional intake and behavior thereafter for 1 hour	To detect physiologic changes that may be life threatening
		Monitor vital signs as warranted by patient status; obtain baseline vitals on admission	To detect life-threatening conditions such as dehydration or hyponatremia
		Monitor fluid and electrolyte status	To detect early warning signs of dehydration or fluid and electrolyte imbalance
		Set mutually agreeable target intake of fluids per day	To prevent further weight loss
		Establish mutually agreeable targeted goal for daily exercise that is congruent with nutrient intake and weight gain	To prevent self-harm
		Monitor activities for detrimental behaviors such as administering enemas, purging, binging (bulimic), and excessive exercise	To clarify expectations and provide limits for control of behaviors that are not acceptable
		Set limits and clearly define expectations in relation to therapeutic plan to increase nutrient intake	To establish mutually agreed-on plan for nutrient intake and weight gain
		Develop behavioral contract for nutrient intake and cessation of behaviors related to eating that are detrimental	To promote verbalization of concerns and fears
Disturbed Body Image related to altered self-perception **Child's/Family's Defining Characteristics (Subjective and Objective Data)** Negative feelings about body	Adolescent displays evidence of developing and maintaining positive self-image.	Encourage adolescent to verbalize feelings and concerns regarding view of self in relation to peers and family members	To enhance self-esteem and alter misconception of self in relation to others
		Provide opportunity for adolescent to engage in activities that have potential to build self-esteem	To promote self-esteem
		Encourage self-care in relation to dietary management and weight control	To set limits for behavior
		Encourage discussion of maladaptive behaviors surrounding food and fluid intake: binging, purging, laxative use, excess exercise	To provide consistency in therapy and allow mutual discussion
		Provide therapeutic discussion (over time) of personal attributes perceived as positive	To enhance reality-based self-perception
		Involve adolescent in activities designed to promote positive image of self-worth and accomplishment	To promote sense of accomplishment and enhance self-image
		Involve family members and adolescent in group family counseling to discuss expectations and members' roles within family	To promote expression of perceptions about self within family and identify any distorted patterns of interaction that require clarification or modification

risk users. *Monitoring the Future* has been providing long-term research about the rates of substance use among adolescents, young adults, and adults since 1975. The 2010 survey found that marijuana use and acceptance of marijuana use have been on the rise since 2007. Alcohol use has been on the decline since the early 1980s and reached historically low levels in 2010. Cigarette use was on a steady decline since the mid-1990s but showed some increase in 2010, which followed a leveling off of the perceived risk of cigarette use. The use of illicit drugs other than marijuana has shown minimal change. However, 15% of 12th graders in 2010 reported the use of prescription drugs without medical supervision (Johnston, O'Malley, Bachman, et al., 2011).

Drug abuse, misuse, and addiction are culturally defined and are voluntary behaviors. Drug tolerance and physical dependence are involuntary physiologic responses to the pharmacologic characteristics of drugs, such as opioids and alcohol. Consequently, an individual can be addicted to a narcotic with or without being physically dependent. A person can also be physically dependent on a narcotic without being addicted (e.g., patients who use opioids to control pain).

The CRAFFT questionnaire is a brief screening tool which can be used in the primary care setting to identify adolescent substance abuse; the mnemonic stands for C-car; R-relax; A-alone; F-forget; F-friends; T-trouble. The six questions relate to the use of drugs in the settings described by the mnemonic. Two or more positive answers to the items in the tool indicate the need for further referral for possible substance abuse (Knight, Sherritt, Shrier, et al., 2002).

Motivation

Most drug use begins with experimentation. The drug may be used only once, may be used occasionally, or may become part of a drug-centered lifestyle. Children and adolescents initiate drug use out of curiosity. Adolescents who use drugs may fall into one of two broad categories—experimenters and compulsive users—or they may fall into a third category somewhere on the continuum between these extremes, referred to as *recreational users*, principally of drugs such as marijuana, cocaine, alcohol, and prescription drugs. For many, the goal is peer acceptance; these users fit more closely with the experimenting, intermittent users. For others, the goal is intoxication or the sustained intense effects from using a particular drug; these users resemble the compulsive users. These users may engage in periodic heavy use, or binges. The groups of greatest concern to health care workers are those whose patterns of use involve high doses or mixed drugs with the danger of overdose and compulsive users with the threat of dependence, withdrawal syndromes, and altered lifestyle.

Types of Drugs Abused

Any drug can be abused, and most are potentially harmful to adolescents still going through formative life experiences. Although rarely considered drugs by society, the chemically active substances frequently abused are the xanthines and theobromines contained in chocolate, tea, coffee, and colas. Ethyl alcohol and nicotine are other drugs that are legal and socially sanctioned. Any of these substances can produce mild to moderate euphoric or stimulant effects and can lead to physical and psychologic dependence.

Drugs with mind-altering abilities that are available on the "street" and are of medical and legal concern are the hallucinogenic, narcotic, hypnotic, and stimulant drugs. In addition, health care professionals are concerned about the use of alcohol and volatile substances that are inhaled to achieve altered sensation (e.g., gasoline, antifreeze, plastic model airplane cement, typewriter correction fluid, organic solvents). The abuse of prescription and synthetic drugs such as oxycodone, alprazolam (Xanax), dextromethorphan, and amphetamine-dextroamphetamine (Adderall) has been reported to have reached epidemic proportions among adolescents and young people (Bryner, Wang, Hui, et al., 2006; Maxwell, 2011). Studies show that adolescents prefer pain relievers to stimulants, sedatives, or tranquilizers; females tend to prefer pain relievers to stimulants, and abuse of these substances was also strongly correlated with other illicit substances (Young, Glover, and Havens, 2012). Others report that adolescents believe that prescription medications, although not taken under practitioner orders, are safer than illicit substances. Cough and cold preparations such as NyQuil, Coricidin, and Robitussin were reported in 2006 to be favorite substances abused to get high among persons ages 12 to 25 years (U.S. Department of Health and Human Services, 2008a). Many of the prescription drugs are available at a decreased cost compared with the more exotic drugs of abuse and are often found in the medicine or kitchen cabinet at home. Websites also promote the "safe use" of some psychoactive drugs and supply information on new "designer" drugs that are not detectable on a standard urine drug screening test.

Tobacco. Cigarette smoking has been on a slow decline since the peak in 1999 despite multiple efforts, including increased costs, changes in community attitudes about smoking among adults, media campaigns with counter-advertising, and tobacco-free environments (CDC, 2010a). Use of all tobacco products among youth did not change between 2006 and 2009 (CDC, 2010b).

Although the number of adult and adolescent smokers has declined in recent years, cigarette smoking is still considered the chief avoidable cause of death. The hazards of smoking at any age are undisputed; however, a preventive approach to teenage smoking is especially important. Because of its addictive nature, smoking begun in childhood and adolescence can result in a lifetime habit, with increased morbidity and early mortality.

The effects of secondhand smoke exposure are also well known and include increased incidence of low birth weight and subsequent illness, increased incidence of sudden infant death syndrome (maternal smoking during and after pregnancy), increased incidence of acute lower respiratory tract infections, and exacerbation of asthma symptoms (wheezing, cough, phlegm, breathlessness) in children with asthma (U.S. Department of Health and Human Services, 2006).

Etiology. Teenagers begin smoking for a variety of reasons, including imitation of adult behavior; peer pressure; a desire to imitate behaviors and lifestyles portrayed in movies and advertisements; and a desire to control weight, especially among young women. Teenagers who do not smoke usually have family members and friends who do not smoke or who oppose smoking. Most teens who refrain from smoking have a desire to succeed in academics or athletics (particularly high-performance sports, such as basketball, swimming, and track) and plans to go to college (see Community Focus box). Although smoking among college students has increased in recent years, rates of smoking are highest among adolescents who do not complete high school.

Smokeless Tobacco. The term *smokeless tobacco* refers to tobacco products that are placed in the mouth but not ignited (e.g., snuff and chewing tobacco). This substitute for cigarettes continues to pose a hazard to adolescents, although use had steadily declined by about 50% since the peak prevalence in 1995; the 2010 data showed a slight increase. Children and adolescents continue to recognize the risk of smokeless tobacco and have expressed high rates of disapproval (Johnston, O'Malley, Bachman, et al., 2011). These

🏠 COMMUNITY FOCUS

Early Sexual Maturation, Alcohol, and Cigarettes

Smoking cigarettes and drinking alcohol among adolescents are complex behaviors that are not explained by any one factor. Some theorists and investigators believe there is a relationship between biologic maturation and risk-taking behaviors. For example, young girls who are sexually mature at an earlier age than their peers are often attracted to older girls and boys who may engage in risk-taking behaviors. If older teens smoke, drink, and drive while under the influence of alcohol with no adverse consequences (e.g., no motor vehicle accidents), young girls may believe that they, too, will be safe while smoking, drinking, or riding in an automobile with friends who are drinking.

Although parents and nurses cannot influence the time of biologic maturation, they can identify young girls who are at risk for the initiation of risk-taking behaviors because of early puberty. Parents need to understand that an early-maturing daughter might be uncomfortable with her body, and they should take advantage of opportunities to build her self-esteem. Parental sensitivity to the importance of peer-group acceptance and parental support of a teenage daughter who feels left out or different are crucial. School nurses can provide anticipatory guidance to these girls and help them role-play coping strategies for situations that involve offers to smoke and drink. In addition, school nurses can provide information about physical development during puberty and emphasize that not all teenagers mature at the same time or rate.

Teachers, coaches, and community and church leaders can provide opportunities for these girls to "fit in" with their same-age peers through activities that stress mutual goals. For example, an early-maturing girl is typically taller than her age-mates and can be an asset in sports such as basketball and track-and-field events.

products have also been proved to be carcinogenic, and regular use can cause dental problems, foul-smelling breath, and tooth erosion or loss.

CARE MANAGEMENT

Prevention of regular smoking in teenagers is the most effective way to reduce the overall incidence of smoking. A variety of methods have been used. Posters, charts, displays, statistics, and the use of examples of actual damaged lungs to communicate the hazards of smoking all have their supporters and doubters. Some schools also use films and demonstrations in science classes.

For the most part, smoking prevention programs that focus on the negative, long-term effects of smoking on health have been ineffective. Youth-to-youth programs and those emphasizing the immediate effects are more effective but primarily in improving teenagers' attitudes toward not smoking. Because smoking and smoking-related behaviors are social symbols, antismoking campaigns must address the norms of potential smokers. Anything that ridicules or threatens the social norms of the peer group can be unproductive or counterproductive. Investigators have found that teaching resistance to peer pressure to smoke is effective in early adolescence. Although the effects of these programs may decrease with time, the effects can be enhanced in older adolescents by presenting information in class instead of simply handing out written material to the students.

Two areas of focus for antismoking programs are peer-led programs and use of media in smoking prevention (e.g., CDs,

videotapes, and films). Peer-led programs emphasizing the social consequences of smoking have proved most successful. If a significant number of influential peers can "sell" their classmates on the idea that the habit is not popular, the followers will imitate their behavior. Such programs emphasize short-term rather than long-term consequences (e.g., the effects of smoking on personal appearance, such as unattractive stains on teeth and hands and unpleasant odor of breath and clothing).

The use of pharmacologic agents for smoking cessation include nicotine replacement therapy, bupropion, and varenicline. Varenicline taken orally for 12 weeks was shown to be safe and effective in assisting persons who wish to stop smoking (Cahill, Stead, and Lancaster, 2011), but side effects such as nausea and abdominal distention may make the drug less palatable for some. None of these three drugs has been specifically approved for use in children and adolescents for smoking cessation.

The impact of school-based antismoking programs can be strengthened by expanding these programs to include parents, mass media, youth groups, and community organizations. For example, mass media efforts that involve antismoking radio campaigns have been identified as the most cost-effective mass media intervention.

Smoking bans in schools also accomplish several goals: (1) they discourage students from starting to smoke; (2) they reinforce knowledge of the health hazards of cigarette smoking and exposure to environmental tobacco smoke; and (3) they promote a smoke-free environment as the norm (see Community Focus box).

Alcohol. Acute or chronic abuse of alcohol (ethanol) is responsible for many acts of violence, suicide, accidental injury, and death. Alcohol drinking is likely to begin in the middle-school years and increases with age. By 18 years of age, 80% to 90% of adolescents have tried alcohol. Ethanol is a depressant that reduces inhibitions against aggressive and sexual acting out. Severe physical and psychologic symptoms accompany abrupt withdrawal, and long-term use leads to slow tissue destruction, especially of the brain and liver cells. The most noticeable effects of alcohol occur within the CNS and include changes in cognitive and autonomic functions such as judgment, memory, learning ability, and other intellectual capacities. Young people with alcoholism often drink alone and cannot control their use of alcohol. They often rely on the substance as a defense against depression, anxiety, fear, or anger. Not all of these characteristics are observed in adolescents who are abusing alcohol, but if several signs are evident, the child or adolescent should be considered at risk. Referral to a health care professional and detoxification therapy may be necessary. Information about alcohol and answers to questions are available through the Alcohol Hotline.* Other groups that provide support and counseling for families are Al-Anon, Ala-Teen, Ala-Tot, and Alcoholics Anonymous (an organization that has listings in all local directories).

Cocaine. Although cocaine is not pharmacologically considered a narcotic, it is legally categorized as such. Cocaine is available in two forms: water-soluble cocaine hydrochloride, which is administered by "snorting" or intravenous injection; and nonsoluble alkaloid (freebase) cocaine, which is used primarily for smoking. Crack, or "rock," is a purer, more menacing form of the drug. It can be produced cheaply and smoked in either water pipes or mentholated cigarettes.

Cocaine creates a sense of euphoria, or an indefinable high. Withdrawal does not produce the dramatic symptoms observed in

---

*Toll free 866-925-4030.

COMMUNITY FOCUS

Nonsmoking Strategies

Nurses who work in schools, hospitals, and community agencies can take advantage of all opportunities to provide education about the dangers of smoking, to discourage smoking initiation by children and adolescents, to encourage smoking cessation, and to promote smoke-free environments. In particular, school nurses must be alert to the vulnerability of young preteens when they enter junior high or middle school. These nurses are in an ideal position to assess stress, personal conflict, weight concerns, peer pressures, and other factors that place preteens at risk for smoking initiation. Nurses should serve as counselors to student, teacher, and parent groups and as advocates for antismoking legislative efforts. The following additional strategies are recommended:*

- Provide only brief information about long-term health consequences (e.g., cardiovascular and cancer risks).
- Discuss immediate physiologic consequences (e.g., changes in heart rate, blood pressure, respiratory symptoms, and blood carbon monoxide concentrations).
- Mention alternatives to smoking that also establish a self-image that appears independent, mature, or sophisticated (e.g., weight lifting; jogging; dancing; joining a boys' or girls' club; engaging in volunteer work for a hospital, political, religious, or community group).
- Mention the negative effects in detail (e.g., earlier wrinkling of skin; yellow stains on teeth and fingers; tobacco odor on breath, hair, and clothing).
- Mention the increasing ostracism of smokers by nonsmokers, both legal and informal, in the workplace and in public places.
- Mention the increasing evidence that secondhand smoke is injurious to the health of nonsmokers who are regularly exposed, especially small children.
- Acknowledge that many adults, who were enticed to start smoking as teenagers because of its social benefits, now wish they could stop smoking.
- Give cooperative adolescents effective arguments to deal with peer pressure (e.g., by not smoking, a teenager demonstrates independence and nonconformity, traits normally prized by youth).
- Request posters or pamphlets from local agencies (e.g., American Cancer Society, American Heart Association, and American Lung Association) to display in prominent places at school.

*The Centers for Disease Control and Prevention has information on the effects of tobacco, smoking cessation, and tobacco control programs; 1600 Clifton Road, Atlanta, GA 30333; 800-232-4636; e-mail: tobaccoinfo@cdc.gov; www.cdc.gov/tobacco.

withdrawal from other substances. The effects are those commonly seen in depression, including lack of energy and motivation, irritability, appetite changes, psychomotor delay, and irregular sleep patterns. More serious symptoms include cardiovascular manifestations and seizures. Physical withdrawal should not be confused with the so-called *crash* after a cocaine high, which consists of a long period of sleep. Answers to questions about the risks of using cocaine are available at the National Cocaine Hotline,* which also provides referrals to support groups and treatment centers.

*800-COCAINE (800-262-2463).

Narcotics. Narcotic drugs include opiates, such as heroin and morphine, and opioids (opiate-like drugs), such as hydromorphone (Dilaudid), hydrocodone, fentanyl, meperidine (Demerol), and codeine. These drugs produce a state of euphoria by removing painful feelings and creating a pleasurable experience and a sense of success accompanied by clouding of the consciousness and a dreamlike state. Physical signs of narcotic abuse include constricted pupils; respiratory depression; and, often, cyanosis. Needle marks may be visible on the arms or legs in chronic users. Physical withdrawal from opiates is extremely unpleasant unless controlled with supervised tapering doses of the opioid or substitution of methadone.

As important as the physical effects are the indirect consequences related to the illegal status of narcotic use and the problems associated with securing the drug (e.g., the time-consuming searches to obtain the drug and the often illegal methods used to meet the high cost of purchasing it). Health problems also result from self-neglect of physical needs (nutrition, cleanliness, dental care); overdose; contamination; and infection, including HIV and hepatitis B and hepatitis C infection.

Central Nervous System Depressants. Central nervous system depressants include a variety of hypnotic drugs that produce physical dependence and withdrawal symptoms on abrupt discontinuation. They create a feeling of relaxation and sleepiness but impair general functioning. Drugs in this category include barbiturates, nonbarbiturates, and alcohol. Barbiturates combined with alcohol produce a profound depressant effect. Flunitrazepam (Rohypnol), known as the "date rape drug," is a hypnotic drug abused by adolescents. Many women and men report being raped after unknowingly being given Rohypnol in a drink. Rohypnol is 10 times more powerful than diazepam (Valium). It produces prolonged sedation, a feeling of well-being, and short-term memory loss.

Central Nervous System Stimulants. Amphetamines and cocaine do not produce strong physical dependence and can be withdrawn without much danger. However, psychologic dependence is strong, and acute intoxication can lead to violent aggressive behavior or psychotic episodes characterized by paranoia, uncontrollable agitation, and restlessness. When combined with barbiturates, the euphoric effects are particularly addictive.

Methamphetamine can be snorted, injected, swallowed, or smoked and produces a burst of energy in its users, along with intense, alternating attacks of boldness and paranoia. It provokes excitement far more intense than that caused by cocaine. The drug, with the street names *crank, meth,* and *crystal,* is inexpensive and has a longer period of action than cocaine. Instead of a short (few minutes) high, as achieved with cocaine, a user can remain "up" for hours on a similar dose of crank.

Health care professionals are concerned about the use of various volatile substances, or inhalants such as gasoline, model airplane cement, and organic solvents; these substances are inhaled by the user to achieve an altered sensation, and the most recent surveillance has indicated a modest increase in use after nearly a decade of decline. Adolescents breathe or place these substances into paper or plastic bags or soda cans from which they rebreathe the fumes to produce a feeling of euphoria and altered consciousness. These substances contain chemical solvents and are extremely hazardous. Dusters contain Freon, a substance that can cause fatal cardiac dysrhythmias. Inhalants are the only substance that has a higher incidence of use among young adolescents. This is probably related to the fact that the products are readily available and may be the only substances available for young teens. Many young children are unaware of the dangers of "sniffing" or "huffing." In addition to rapid loss of consciousness and respiratory arrest, these substances may cause visual scanning problems, language deficiencies, motor instability, memory deficits, and attention and concentration problems.

Mind-Altering Drugs. Hallucinogens (psychedelics, psychotomimetics, psychotropics, or illusionogenics) are drugs that produce vivid hallucinations and euphoria. These drugs do not produce physical dependence, and they can be abruptly withdrawn without ill effect. However, the acute and long-term effects are variable, and in some individuals, the dissociative behavior may be prolonged. Cannabis (marijuana, hashish) and lysergic acid diethylamide (LSD) are also included in this category of drugs.

CARE MANAGEMENT

Nurses who have contact with children and adolescents are in an excellent position to provide information about substance abuse and to serve as patient advocates. Nurses most often encounter young substance abusers when they are (1) experiencing overdose or withdrawal symptoms, (2) manifesting bizarre behavior or confusion secondary to drug ingestion, (3) worried that they are or will become addicted, or (4) worried about a friend or family member who is addicted.

In particular, nurses who care for hospitalized adolescents need to know if these youths use drugs compulsively. Drug withdrawal can seriously complicate other illnesses. Nurses should be alert for any physical or behavioral clues that indicate the onset of withdrawal or the effects of drugs. School nurses and nurses who work in the community play an essential role in identifying children, adolescents, and families with substance abuse problems. The school nurse may be the first to identify a child or adolescent who has ingested a particular drug by the child's erratic behavior in class or on the school grounds (see Critical Thinking Case Study). Early identification of those at risk for substance abuse problems is an essential aspect of prevention. Pediatric health care professionals also prevent substance abuse by creating trusting relationships so that children and adolescents feel comfortable asking questions about drugs, and health care professionals can alert them to websites and other aspects of society that encourage experimentation with drugs.

Acute Care. Adolescents experiencing toxic drug effects or withdrawal symptoms are usually seen initially in the emergency department. Experienced emergency department personnel are familiar with the management of acute drug toxicity and the signs, symptoms, and behavioral characteristics associated with a variety of substances. When the drug is questionable or unknown, knowledge of these factors facilitates management and treatment. Often, observation or description of the child's or adolescent's behavior is more valuable than reports by patients or their friends.

The treatment for drug toxicity or withdrawal varies according to the drug and the method used. Every effort is made to determine the type, time of ingestion, amount of drug taken, mode of administration, and factors related to the onset of presenting symptoms. It is helpful to know the individual's pattern of use. For example, if two types of drugs are involved, they may require different treatments. Historically, gastric lavage has been used when the drug has been ingested recently and the cough reflex is intact, but it is of little value when the drug has been administered by the intravenous ("mainlined") or intranasal ("sniffed") route.

CRITICAL THINKING CASE STUDY
Prescription Medication Abuse in Adolescence

An eighth grade teacher calls the school nurse, Sally, to her classroom and reports that a girl is behaving "strangely"; the girl slept most of the period before lunch and has not participated in class discussions. Sally, RN, takes the girl to her office and performs an initial assessment. Upon assessment, the girl demonstrates short-term memory lapse and has slightly slurred speech and her pupillary reaction to light is delayed; her blood pressure is 112/68 mm Hg, respirations are 14 breaths/min and regular, and heart rate is 102 beats/min. She denies taking any pills or liquid initially but then states she had a migraine on arrival to school and a friend gave her two blue pills to help with the headache. She refuses to say who gave her the pills and does not know what they were but thought they were Tylenol. She states that she does not know where her mother or father are but thinks they are at work.

1. Evidence—Is there sufficient evidence for Sally to implement a plan of care for this adolescent?
2. What should Sally's next course of action involve? What is her professional responsibility in this case?
3. Assumptions—Describe the underlying assumptions about the following:
   a. The school nurse's physical assessment findings
   b. The misuse of prescription medications by adolescents
4. What nursing priorities and implications for care can be made at this time? What type of care should this eighth grader receive?

Single-dose activated charcoal has been used for acute poisoning, but there is considerable controversy regarding the benefits and effects over time (Chyka, Seger, Krenzelok, et al., 2005; Elder, 2010; Isbister and Kumar, 2011). Some experts recommend supportive care as the mainstay of overdose treatment in pediatrics (Hanhan, 2008). The administration of a drug antidote such as naloxone and the early (within 1-2 hours of ingestion) administration of activated charcoal may be used for opioid overdose. Because the actual content of most street drugs is highly questionable, other pharmaceutic agents are administered with caution except perhaps the narcotic antagonists in cases of suspected opiate overdoses. It is also necessary to assess for possible trauma sustained while the patient was under the influence of the drug.

Long-Term Management. A major factor in the treatment and rehabilitation of young drug users is careful assessment in the nonacute stage to determine the function that the drug plays in the adolescent's life. The motivation phase is directed toward exploring the factors that influence drug use. It also involves establishing a feeling of self-worth and a commitment to self-help in the teen.

Rehabilitation begins when adolescents decide that they can and are willing to change. Rehabilitation involves fostering healthy interdependent relationships with caring and supportive adults and exploring alternate mechanisms for problem solving while simultaneously reducing or eliminating drug use. Persons working with troubled youth must be prepared for recidivism, or the tendency to relapse, and maintain a plan for reentry into the treatment process.

Family Support. Most treatment programs for substance abusers are based on adult 12-step models such as Alcoholics Anonymous. Research is needed to determine whether these adult models are effective for adolescents. Tough Love* is one program that is based on the conviction that parents have the right and responsibility to be the policymakers in the family, to set limits on the behavior of their children, and to take control of the household from out-of-control adolescents. The premise is that allowing teenagers to experience the negative consequences of their behavior will bring them closer to accepting help or changing their behavior. Another group that provides support and counseling for families experiencing substance abuse and seeking strategies to cope with their children is Parents Anonymous.† Another source of information is the Substance Abuse and Mental Health Services Administration's National Clearinghouse for Alcohol and Drug Information.‡ The National Institute on Drug Abuse (NIDA) also contains an abundance of information for adolescents on the effects of abused substances, prevention, and treatment (www.drugabuse.gov/students-young-adults).

Prevention. Nurses play an important role in education efforts, as well as in individual observation, assessment, and therapy related to substance abuse. In recent years, a variety of educational programs have been applied with promising results. The most effective prevention strategies are those that are part of a broader, more general effort to promote overall health and success. Health-compromising behaviors are often interconnected and have common antecedents. Prevention efforts that focus on changing only one behavior (e.g., alcohol, other drug use) are less likely to be successful. Successful programs are those that have promoted parenting skills, social skills among distractible children, academic achievement, and skills to resist peer pressure.

Peer pressure is a powerful tool and can be used effectively in substance abuse prevention. A group that has had some success in reducing injury from drunk driving is Students Against Destructive Decisions (SADD).§ Techniques used by this group include peer counseling, parental guidelines for teenage parties, and community awareness. Nurses should encourage the formation of SADD chapters in the high schools in their communities.

Suicide

Suicide is defined as the deliberate act of self-injury with the intent that the injury results in death. Most experts distinguish among suicidal ideation, suicide attempt (or parasuicide), and suicide.

Suicidal ideation involves a preoccupation with thoughts about committing suicide and may be a precursor to suicide. Although it is common for adolescents to experience occasional suicidal thoughts, expressions of preoccupation with suicide should be taken seriously and an assessment should be conducted for appropriate referral. A suicide attempt is intended to cause injury or death. The term parasuicide is used to refer to behaviors ranging from gestures to serious attempts to kill oneself. *Parasuicide* is a preferred term because it makes no reference to intent and because a person's motive may be too difficult or complex to determine. However, all parasuicidal activity should be taken seriously.

> ⚠ **NURSING ALERT**
>
> A history of a previous suicide attempt is a serious indicator for possible suicide completion in the future. Studies of adolescent suicides have found that as many as half of the adolescents had made previous attempts.

Results from the 2011 Youth Risk Behavior Surveillance indicated that 7.8% of students nationwide had attempted suicide at least once during the 12 months preceding the survey; the range of suicide attempts by adolescents across the states varied from 3.6% to 11.3% (CDC, 2012b). The overall incidence of youth suicide has decreased since 1992, yet the CDC and other experts note that the incidence is still too high. Approximately 12.8% of the students in this survey reported that they had made a specific plan to attempt suicide in the 12 months preceding the survey. Suicide is currently the third leading cause of death during the teenage years, surpassed only by death from motor vehicle crashes and homicides (see Chapter 27).

Etiology

Individual, family, and social or environmental factors have all been implicated in suicide. The single most important individual factor is the presence of an active psychiatric disorder (depression, bipolar disorder, psychosis, substance abuse, or conduct disorder). Alcohol use in particular has been associated with more than 50% of suicides (Shain and AAP Committee on Adolescence, 2007). For some teens, suicide becomes the final pathway for release from their psychiatric and social problems. Child and adolescent suicide victims are reported to have higher rates not only of depression but also of conduct disorders; bipolar disorders; substance abuse; interpersonal problems with parents; and a family history of depression, substance abuse, and suicidal behavior.

Gay, lesbian, and bisexual adolescents are at particularly high risk for suicide attempts, especially if raised in an environment where they are denied support systems (Saewyc, Skay, Hynds, et al., 2007) (see Community Focus box). Family factors influencing suicide include parental loss; family disruption; a family history of suicide, depression, substance abuse, or emotional disturbance; child abuse or neglect; unavailable parents; poor communication and isolation within the family; family conflict; and unrealistically high parental expectations or parental indifference with low expectations. Families who respect individuality, are cohesive and caring, balance discipline with a supportive and understanding relationship, have good systems of communication, and have at least one attentive and caring parent available to the child protect adolescents from suicidal outcomes. Social or environmental factors include incarceration, isolation, acute loss of a boyfriend or girlfriend, lack of future options, and availability of firearms in the home.

Methods

Firearms are by far the most commonly used instruments in completed suicides among males and females (Shain and AAP Committee on Adolescence, 2007). For adolescent males, the second and third most common means of suicide are hanging and overdose, respectively; for females, the second and third most common means are overdose and strangulation, respectively.

The most common method of suicide *attempt* is overdose or ingestion of a potentially toxic substance, such as drugs. The second most common method of suicide attempt is self-inflicted laceration.

---

*www.toughlove.com.
†675 W. Foothill Blvd., Suite 220, Claremont, CA 91711; 909-621-6184; www.parentsanonymous.org.
‡1 Choke Cherry Road, Rockville, MD 20857; 877-SAMHSA-7; http://ncadi.samhsa.gov.
§255 Main St., Marlborough, MA 01752; 877-SADD-INC; www.sadd.org.

COMMUNITY FOCUS

Suicide, Sexual Identity, and Sexual Orientation

A significant number of teenage suicides occur among homosexual youths. Gay or lesbian adolescents who live in families or communities that do not accept homosexuality are likely to suffer low self-esteem, self-loathing, depression, and hopelessness as a result. Such internalization, without treatment and support, can lead to substance abuse and, eventually, suicide. Youths most at risk are those who struggle with gender identity issues such as gay identity formation at a young age, intrapersonal conflict regarding sexuality, and nondisclosure of orientation to others.

Supportive parents, friends, or relationships serve as protective factors against suicide. However, many gay, lesbian, and bisexual adolescents do not feel supported, understood, or accepted by their friends, parents, and families. Nurses who interact with adolescents must be aware of the association between suicide and adolescent homosexuality and gender nonconformity. School nurses may be the first individuals to discuss issues of sexual identity and orientation with adolescents or their families. In their professional capacity, nurses can serve as support persons for these adolescents. Nurses can also provide guidance and resources to families so that they understand how best to nurture and support their child.

Nurses must also capitalize on opportunities or experiences that promote the healthy development of self-esteem in youths who choose nontraditional or alternative sexual orientation. Educational programs to raise the level of consciousness about the risk factors for and warning signs of suicide are one example. Another possibility could be programs conducted in or outside of school that are designed to foster peer relationships and competency in social skills among high risk adolescents and young adults, such as support groups and social organizations for these young people.

! NURSING ALERT

Given what is known about youth suicide, nurses should ask parents, especially those with at-risk teenagers, if firearms are available in the house and, if so, recommend their removal. Parents must ensure that their children—especially those who are depressed, have poor problem-solving skills, or use drugs or alcohol—do not have access to firearms. Parents must also be educated on the warning signs of suicide (Box 35-8).

Motivation

Suicidal ideation is common in adolescents. It represents numerous fantasies, such as relief from suffering, a means of gaining comfort and sympathy, or a means of revenge against those who have hurt them. Adolescents have the erroneous perception that the act of suicide will evoke remorse and pity and that they will be able to return and witness the grief. Angry children or adolescents who are unable to directly punish those who have injured or insulted them may take revenge on those who love them through self-destruction ("They'll be sorry when they find me dead"; "They'll be sorry they were mean to me").

For adolescents who are severely depressed, suicide seems to be the only release from their despair. These adolescents rarely provide evidence of their intent and frequently conceal their suicidal thoughts. Many adolescents, however, tell their peers of their suicidal thoughts or plans but avoid telling adults. Social isolation is a significant factor in distinguishing adolescents who will kill themselves from those who will not. It is also more characteristic of those who complete suicide than of those who make attempts or threats.

BOX 35-8 WARNING SIGNS OF SUICIDE

- Preoccupation with themes of death—focuses on morbid thoughts
- Wants to give away cherished possessions
- Talks of own death, desire to die
- Loss of energy, loss of interest, listlessness
- Exhaustion without obvious cause
- Changes in sleep patterns—too much or too little
- Increased irritability, argumentativeness, or stubbornness
- Physical complaints—recurrent stomachaches, headaches
- Repeated visits to physician, nurse practitioner, or emergency department for treatment of injuries
- Reckless behavior
- Antisocial behavior—engages in drinking, uses drugs, fights, commits acts of vandalism, runs away from home, becomes sexually promiscuous
- Sudden change in school performance—lowered grades, cutting classes, dropping out of activities
- Resists or refuses to go to school
- Remains distant, sad, remote—flat affect, frozen facial expression
- Describes self as worthless
- Sudden cheerfulness after deep depression
- Social withdrawal from friends, activities, interests that were previously enjoyed
- Impaired concentration
- Dramatic change in appetite

The frequency of contagion or copycat suicides (i.e., an increase in youth suicide that occurs after the suicide of one teenager is publicized) is disturbing and may indicate that teenagers perceive suicide as glamorous. In addition, young people may not realize the finality of suicide because they have become desensitized from constantly viewing violence and death on television.

Diagnostic Evaluation

Depression is common among adolescents who attempt suicide. Depression is characterized by both subjective symptoms and objective signs that reflect the adolescent's sadness and despair. Adolescents describe feelings of sadness, despair, helplessness, hopelessness, boredom, loss of interest, and isolation. They may also feel self-reproach, self-deprecation, and guilt. Subjective symptoms of depression or specific changes in behavior place an adolescent at risk for suicide (Box 35-9).

Therapeutic Management

Threats of suicide should always be taken seriously. There has been a tendency to dismiss suicide attempts as impulsive acts resulting from temporary crises or depression. If a suicide attempt fails to draw attention to their problems or makes them worse, the child or adolescent may conclude that suicide is the only answer. Children and adolescents need to know that someone cares and must be provided with swift and efficient crisis intervention. Although ordinary practitioners can manage an acute depressive reaction without difficulty, the adolescent who has made a serious attempt or has a specific plan for suicide should receive immediate attention and competent psychiatric care.

Youths who are actively suicidal need inpatient care, monitoring, and treatment. Medications for depression and bipolar disorder often take several weeks to reach therapeutic levels. The time until

BOX 35-9 CHARACTERISTICS OF CHILDREN OR ADOLESCENTS WITH DEPRESSION

Behavior

- Predominantly sad facial expression with absence or diminished range of affective response (most of the day)
- Solitary play or work; tendency to be alone; lack of interest in play with friends
- Withdrawal from previously enjoyed activities and relationships
- Lowered grades in school; lack of interest in doing homework or achieving in school; refuses to wake up for school
- Diminished motor activity; tiredness
- Tearfulness or crying
- Inability to concentrate
- Dependent and clinging or aggressive and disruptive
- Recurrent suicidal thoughts or talk

Internal States

- Utterance of statements reflecting lowered self-esteem, sense of hopelessness, or guilt
- Suicidal ideations

Physiology

- Constipation
- Loss of energy; fatigue
- Nonspecific complaints of not feeling well
- Change in appetite resulting in weight loss or gain
- Alterations in sleeping pattern, sleeplessness, or hypersomnia

medications and therapy begin to take effect can be trying for the adolescent and the family. It is important to encourage families to support their teen in adherence to the regimen prescribed. The SSRIs are often prescribed for depression, but teens who are taking such medications need careful, frequent monitoring.

> **! NURSING ALERT**
>
> Adolescents who express suicidal feelings and have a specific plan should be monitored at all times. They should not have access to firearms, prescription or over-the-counter drugs, belts, scarves, shoestrings, sharp objects, matches, or lighters. If they are intoxicated, they must be restrained or placed in a protective environment until a psychiatrist or psychologist can assess them.

CARE MANAGEMENT

Nurses play a pivotal role in reducing adolescent suicide. Nurses have the opportunity to provide anticipatory guidance to parents and adolescents. They can teach parents to be supportive and to develop positive communication patterns that help teens feel connected with and loved by their families. To foster healthy development, parents can be encouraged to provide teens with creative outlets and to assist young people in accepting strong emotions—pain, anger, and frustration—as a normal part of the human experience.

Care of suicidal adolescents includes early recognition, management, and prevention. The most important aspect of management is the recognition of warning signs that indicate that an adolescent

is troubled and might attempt suicide. The nurse must take any suicidal remarks seriously and not leave the young person alone until the degree of suicidality is assessed. A mnemonic for the assessment process is *SLAP*: specificity, lethality, accessibility, and proximity. The first step (specificity) is to ask adolescents whether they feel suicidal or as though they would like to take their own lives. If so, have they chosen a means of suicide and do they have a specific plan? The second stage of assessment (lethality) involves determining the lethality of the methods available to them. Do they plan to use a gun or knife? Have they chosen highly lethal medications, hanging, or carbon monoxide poisoning? The third stage (accessibility) involves determining the availability of the means of suicide, and the fourth stage (proximity) involves assessing whether they have determined a time to commit suicide and when.

Health care professionals must be alert to the signs of depression, and anyone who exhibits such behavior should be referred for thorough psychologic assessment. Depression is manifested differently in children and adolescents than in adults. In teens, it may be masked by impulsive aggressive behaviors. Defiance, disobedience, behavior problems, and psychosomatic disturbances can indicate underlying depression, suicidal ideation, and impending suicide attempts.

> **! NURSING ALERT**
>
> No threat of suicide should be ignored or challenged. Threats are a symptom that must be taken seriously. Too often, suicidal threats or minor attempts are confused with bids for attention. It is also a mistake to be lulled into a false sense of security when an adolescent's depression is apparently relieved. The improvement in attitude may mean that the adolescent has made the decision and found the means to carry out the threat.

Peers and other confidants are valuable observers and excellent sources of information about potential suicide attempts. They may not be able to diagnose depression, but they are able to sense when a friend has undergone a marked personality change. It is important to emphasize that the peer who detects any changes in a friend is a potential rescuer and should not remain silent about the observations. Friendship does not imply collusion. A peer who believes that a friend may be suicidal should alert someone who can help (e.g., a parent, teacher, guidance counselor, school nurse).

Routine health assessments of adolescents should include questions that assess the presence of suicidal ideation or intent. The following questions can be asked (Greydanus and Pratt, 1995):

1. Do you consider yourself more a happy person, an unhappy person, or somewhere in the middle?
2. Have you ever been so unhappy or upset that you felt like being dead?
3. Have you ever thought about hurting yourself?
4. Have you ever developed a plan to hurt yourself or kill yourself?
5. Have you ever attempted to kill yourself?

If adolescents answer "yes" to questions 2, 3, or 4, they should be asked if they feel that way now to assess for current suicidality. If teens say they have attempted suicide in the past, assess the number of times and ask them to describe what they were feeling, which method they used, what happened, if they would make a similar attempt, and how they would handle their despair now. Any previous suicide attempt indicates an increased risk for a future attempt. The risk for a suicide attempt in the near future increases as the frequency of suicidal ideation increases.

If children or adolescents express suicidal intent, nurses make a contract, asking them to sign an agreement that they will not attempt suicide during an agreed-on period and that they will call the 24-hour crisis line immediately if they feel that they cannot keep to their contract. The amount of time an adolescent feels comfortable contracting is usually an indication of his or her risk and stability.

Because a suicide attempt is frequently an outgrowth of family distress, it is essential to intervene with the family. It is important to assess family interactions and to recognize disturbed relationships. The most effective approach is recognition of susceptible adolescents during the early stages of family distress so that family counseling can be started. Prevention must be directed toward improving childrearing practices through support and education of parents and changing societal conditions that generate defeat, despair, and maladaptive behavior.

Although confidentiality is an essential part of adolescent counseling, in the case of self-destructive behaviors, confidentiality cannot be honored. Suicidal behavior is reported to the family and other professionals, and adolescents are informed that this will be done. Such action conveys an important message to the youth: that the professionals understand and care.

Many schools have instituted suicide prevention programs. These programs include services such as drop-in counseling and a peer counseling telephone line. Information can also be obtained from the American Association of Suicidology.*

---

*5221 Wisconsin Ave. NW, Washington, DC 20015; 202-237-2280; www.suicidology.org.

KEY POINTS

- The pubescent growth spurt that begins around age 10 years in girls and age 12 years in boys signals the beginning of adolescence.
- Biologic development during puberty is characterized by increased activity of the pituitary gland, which results in sexual maturity and the appearance of secondary sex characteristics.
- According to Erikson, the major developmental crisis of adolescence is establishing a sense of identity.
- Spiritual development is characterized by the questioning of family values and ideals, a move to more philosophic thinking, and emphasis on personal religion.
- Adolescent relationships with parents may be strained; the influence of the peer group increases, and intimate relationships assume importance.
- Teenagers demonstrate a wide variety of interests, and their increased physical and cognitive skills allow them to engage in increasingly difficult and complex activities.
- Adolescents' emotions fluctuate.
- Nutritional needs may not be met by teenagers' eating habits, such as snacking and irregular mealtimes.
- Motor vehicle injuries are the primary cause of death from injury in the adolescent years.
- The rapid changes, growth, and stress accompanying the transition to adulthood may predispose adolescents to faulty problem solving.

- Cognitive development in adolescence includes abstract thought, thinking beyond the present, logical reasoning, and a sense of idealism.
- Development of body image is closely tied to body changes and social interactions.
- According to Kohlberg's theory of moral development, adolescents begin to question existing moral values and learn to make choices.
- Eating disorders observed in middle and late childhood are obesity, AN, BN, and EDNOS.
- Tobacco smoking is a widespread problem among teenagers. Reasons for smoking include social pressure, mass media influence, and a need to develop a self-concept.
- The substances abused by children and adolescents are alcohol, marijuana, narcotics, central nervous system depressants, central nervous system stimulants, hydrocarbons and fluorocarbons, and mind-altering drugs.
- Suicide, the deliberate act of self-injury with the intent to kill, may occur because of difficulties coping with stress, disturbed family environment, substance abuse or dependency, or mental health disorder.
- No threat of suicide by an adolescent should be ignored.
- Signs of depression in children and adolescents are often subtle and require astute observation by parents and health care professionals.

REFERENCES

Abma JC, Martinez GM, Copen CE: Teenagers in the United States: sexual activity, contraceptive use, and childbearing, National Survey of Family Growth 2006-2008, National Center for Health Statistics, *Vital Health Stat* 23(30):1–47, 2010.

American Academy of Pediatric Dentistry: Guideline on periodicity of examination, preventive dental services, anticipatory guidance/counseling and oral treatment for infants, children, and adolescents, *AAPD*

Reference Manual 2011-2012 33(6):103–108, 2012.

American Academy of Pediatrics (AAP): Active healthy living: prevention of childhood obesity through increased physical activity, *Pediatrics* 117(5):1834–1842, 2006.

American Academy of Pediatrics (AAP): Policy statement—children, adolescents, obesity, and the media, *Pediatrics* 128(1):201–208, 2011.

American Academy of Pediatrics (AAP) Committee on Adolescence: Identification and management of eating disorders in children and adolescents, *Pediatrics* 126(6):1240–1253, 2010.

American Academy of Pediatrics (AAP) Council on Communications and Media: Policy statement: sexuality, contraception and the media, *Pediatrics* 126(3):576–582, 2010.

American Dietetic Association: Position of the American Dietetic Association: nutrition intervention in the treatment of anorexia nervosa, bulimia nervosa, and other eating disorders, *J Am Diet Assoc* 106(12):2073–2082, 2006.

American Psychiatric Association (APA): *Diagnostic and statistical manual of mental disorders*, ed 4 (DSM-IV TR), Washington, DC, 2000, Author.

American Psychiatric Association (APA): *DSM-V development: proposed revisions*, Arlington, VA, 2010, Author, www.dsm5.org/ProposedRevisions/Pages/proposedrevision.aspx?rid=110.

Baker S, Barlow S, Cochran W, et al: Overweight children and adolescents: a clinical report of the North American Society for Pediatric Gastroenterology, Hepatology and Nutrition, *J Pediatr Gastroenterol Nutr* 40:533–543, 2005.

Barlow SE, Expert Committee: Expert Committee recommendations regarding the prevention, assessment, and treatment of child and adolescent overweight and obesity: summary report, *Pediatrics* 120(Suppl 4): S164–S192, 2007.

Barnett SJ: Contemporary surgical management of the obese adolescent, *Curr Opin Pediatr* 23(3):351–355, 2011.

Beaty TH: Invited commentary: two studies of genetic control of birth weight where large data sets were available, *Am J Epidemiol* 165:753–755, 2007.

Bond L, Butler H, Thomas L, et al: Social and school connectedness in early secondary school as predictors of late teenage substance use, mental health, and academic outcomes, *J Adolesc Health* 40(4):357.e9–e18, 2007.

Boney C, Verma A, Tucker R, et al: Metabolic syndrome in childhood: association with birth weight, maternal obesity, and gestational diabetes mellitus, *Pediatrics* 115:290–296, 2005.

Bouchard C: Childhood obesity: are genetic differences involved? *Am J Clin Nutr* 89(5):1494S–1501S, 2009.

Bryner JK, Wang UK, Hui JW, et al: Dextromethorphan abuse in adolescents: an increasing trend: 1999-2004, *Arch Pediatr Adolesc Med* 160(12):1217–1222, 2006.

Cahill R, Stead LF, Lancaster T: Nicotine receptor partial agonists for smoking cessation, *Cochrane Database Syst Rev 2011*, 2:CD006103, 2011.

Centers for Disease Control and Prevention (CDC): Cigarette use among high school students—United States, 1991-2009, *MMWR Morb Mortal Wkly Rep* 59(26):797–801, 2010a.

Centers for Disease Control and Prevention (CDC): Tobacco use among middle and high school students—United States, 2000-2009, *MMWR Morb Mortal Wkly Rep* 59(33):1063–1068, 2010b.

Centers for Disease Control and Prevention (CDC): Updated recommendations for use of tetanus toxoid, reduced diphtheria toxoid and acellular pertussis (Tdap) vaccine from the Advisory Committee on Immunization Practices, 2010, *MMWR Morb Mortal Wkly Rep* 60(01):13–15, 2011.

Centers for Disease Control and Prevention (CDC): Vital signs: unintentional injury deaths among persons aged 0-19 years—United States, 2000-2009, *MMWR Morb Mortal Wkly Rep* 61(15):270–276, 2012a.

Centers for Disease Control and Prevention (CDC): Youth risk behavior surveillance—United States, 2011, *MMWR Morb Mortal Wkly Rep Surv Summ* 61(4):1–162, 2012b.

Centers for Disease Control and Prevention: Prevention and control of meningococcal disease: Recommendations of the Advisory Committee on Immunization Practices (ACIP), *MMWR Recomm Rep* 62(2):1–28, 2013a.

Centers for Disease Control and Prevention (CDC): Advisory Committee on Immunization Practices (ACIP) recommended immunization schedules for persons aged 0 through 18 years—United States, 2013, *MMWR Morb Mortal Wkly Rep Suppl* 62(01):2–8, 2013b.

Chyka PA, Seger D, Krenzelok EP, et al: Position paper: single-dose activated charcoal, *Clin Toxicol (Phila)* 43(2):61–87, 2005.

Clabaugh K, Neuberger GB: Research evidence for reducing sugar sweetened beverages in children, *Issues Compr Pediatr Nurs* 34(3):119–130, 2011.

Costello EJ, Sung, M, Worthman C, et al: Pubertal maturation and the development of alcohol use and abuse, *Drug Alcohol Depend* 88(Suppl 1):S50–S59, 2007.

Davis DM, Gance-Cleveland B, Hassink S, et al: Recommendations for prevention of childhood obesity, *Pediatrics* 120(Suppl):S229–S253, 2007.

De Genna NM, Larkby C, Cornelius MD: Pubertal timing and early sexual intercourse in the offspring of teenage mothers, *J Youth Adolesc* 40(10):1315–1328, 2011.

DeVore ER, Ginsburg KR: The protective effects of good parenting on adolescents, *Curr Opin Pediatr* 17(4):460–465, 2005.

Dowdell EB, Burgess AW, Flores JR: Online social networking patterns among adolescents, young adults, and sexual offenders, *Am J Nurs* 111(7):28–36, 2011.

Duncan P, Pirretti AE: Bright futures for the busy clinical practice, American Academy of Pediatrics, *Adolescent Health Update* 22(1):1–10, 2009.

Elder GM: Activated charcoal: to give or not?, *Int Emerg Nurs* 18(3):154–157, 2010.

Erikson EH: *Childhood and society*, ed 2, New York, 1963, WW Norton.

Feldman DR, Bosl GJ, Sheinfeld J, et al: Medical treatment of advanced testicular cancer, *JAMA* 299(6):672–684, 2008.

Feldman M, Friedman LS, Sleisenger MH, editors: Obesity: a historical perspective and disease prevalence estimates. In Feldman M, Friedman LS, Sleisenger MH, editors: *Sleisenger and Fordtran's gastrointestinal and liver disease*, ed 7, Philadelphia, 2002, Saunders.

Forman SF: Eating disorders: epidemiology, pathogenesis, and clinical features, *UpToDate*, 2011, www.uptodate.com/contents/eating-disorders-epidemiology-pathogenesis-and-overview-of-clinical-features.

Fulkerson JA, Neumark-Sztainer D, Hannan P, et al: Family meal frequency and weight status among adolescents: cross-sectional and 5-year longitudinal associations, *Obesity* 16(11):2529–2534, 2008.

Fulkerson JA, Story M, Mellin A, et al: Family dinner meal frequency and adolescent development: relationships with developmental assets and high-risk behaviors, *J Adolesc Health* 39(3):337–345, 2006.

Gahagan S: Overweight and obesity. In Kliegman RM, Stanton BF, St. Geme JW, et al, editors: *Nelson textbook of pediatrics*, ed 19, Philadelphia, 2011, Saunders.

Gance-Cleveland B: Motivational interviewing: improving patient education, *J Pediatr Health* 21(2):81–88, 2007.

Glatt K: Child-to-child unintentional injury and death from firearms in the United States: what can be done? *J Pediatr Nurs* 10(6):448–452, 2005.

Golden NH, Attia E: Psychopharmacology of eating disorders in children and adolescents, *Pediatr Clin North Am* 58(1):121–138, 2011.

Gordon-Larsen P, The NS, Adair LS: Longitudinal trends in obesity in the United States from adolescence to the third decade of life, *Obesity* 18(9):1801–1804, 2010.

Greydanus DE, Pratt HD: Emotional and behavioral disorders of adolescence (Part 2), *Adolesc Health Update* 8(1):1–8, 1995.

Hanhan UA: The poisoned child in the pediatric intensive care unit, *Pediatr Clin North Am* 55(3): 669–686, 2008.

Hansen ML, Gunn PW, Kaelber DC: Underdiagnosis of hypertension in children and adolescents, *JAMA* 298(8):874–879, 2007.

Hardy LR, Harrell JS, Bell RA: Overweight in children: definitions, measurements, confounding factors, and health consequences, *J Pediatr Nurs* 19(6):376–383, 2004.

Herman-Giddens ME: Recent data on pubertal milestones in United States children: the secular trend toward earlier development, *Int J Androl* 29(1):241–246, 2006.

Hill JO, Wyatt HR, Reed GW, et al: Obesity and the environment: where do we go from here? *Science* 299(5608):853–855, 2003.

Hosking SG, Young KL, Regan MA: The effects of text messaging on young drivers, *Hum Factors* 51(4):582–592, 2009.

Isbister GK, Kumar VV: Indications for single-dose activated charcoal administration in acute overdose, *Curr Opin Crit Care* 17(4):351–357, 2011.

Institute of Medicine: *Report at a glance: dietary reference intakes for calcium and vitamin D*, Author, 2010, www.iom.edu/Reports/2010/Dietary-Reference-Intakes-for-Calcium-and-Vitamin-D/Report-Brief.aspx.

Jaquet D, Swaminathan S, Alexander GR, et al: Significant paternal contribution to the risk of small for gestational age, *BJOG* 112:1539, 2005.

Johnston LD, O'Malley PM, Bachman JG, et al: *Monitoring the future—national results on adolescent drug use: overview of key findings, 2010*, Ann Arbor, 2011, Institute for Social Research, The University of Michigan.

Kain J, Corvalán C, Lera L, et al: Accelerated growth in early life and obesity in preschool Chilean children, *Obesity* 17(8):1603–1608, 2009.

Kanekar A, Sharma M: Pharmacological approaches for management of child and adolescent obesity, *J Clin Med Res* 2(3):105–111, 2010.

Kaplowitz PB: Link between body fat and the timing of puberty, *Pediatrics* 121(Suppl 3):S208–S217, 2008.

Kennedy BS, Bedard B, Younge M, et al: Outbreak of *Mycobacterium chelonae* infection associated with tattoo ink, *N Engl J Med* 367(11):1020–1024, 2012.

Knight JR, Sherritt L, Shrier LA, et al: Validity of the CRAFFT substance abuse screening test among adolescent clinic patients, *Arch Pediatr Adolesc Med* 156(6):607–614, 2002.

Koeppen-Schomerus G, Wardle J, Plomin R: A genetic analysis of weight and overweight in 4-year-old twin pairs, *Int J Obes Relat Metab Dis* 25(6):838–844, 2001.

Kreipe RE: Eating disorders. In Kliegman RM, Stanton BF, St. Geme JW, et al, editors: *Nelson textbook of pediatrics*, ed 19, Philadelphia, 2011, Saunders.

Landry GL: Female athletes: menstrual problems and the risk of osteopenia. In Kliegman RM, Stanton BF, St. Geme JW, et al, editors: *Nelson textbook of pediatrics*, ed 19, Philadelphia, 2011, Saunders.

LaRosa C, Meyers K: Epidemiology of hypertension in children and adolescents, *J Med Liban* 58(3):132–136, 2010.

Larson NI, Neumark-Sztainer D, Hannan PJ, et al: Family meals during adolescence are associated with higher diet quality and healthful meal patterns during young adulthood, *J Am Diet Assoc* 107(9):1502–1510, 2007.

Levy DT, Friend KB, Wang YC: A review of the literature on policies directed at the youth consumption of sugar sweetened beverages, *Adv Nutr* 2(2):S182–S200, 2011.

Li C, Kaur H, Choi WS, et al: Additive interactions of maternal prepregnancy BMI and breast-feeding on childhood overweight, *Obesity Res* 13:362–371, 2005.

Lock J: Treatment of adolescent eating disorders: progress and challenges, *Minerva Psichiatr* 51(3):207–216, 2010.

Lynne SD, Graber JA, Nichols TR, et al: Links between pubertal timing, peer influences and externalizing behaviors among urban students followed through middle school, *J Adolesc Health* 40(2):181.e7–e13, 2007.

Maes L, Lievens J: Can the school make a difference? A multilevel analysis of adolescent risk and health behaviour, *Soc Sci Med* 56(3):517–529, 2003.

Maxwell JC: The prescription drug epidemic in the United States: a perfect storm, *Drug Alcohol Rev* 30(3):264–270, 2011.

McCarthy A, Hughes R, Tilling K, et al: Birth weight; postnatal, infant, and childhood growth; and obesity in young adulthood: evidence from the Barry Caerphilly Growth Study, *Am J Clin Nutr* 86(4):907–913, 2007.

McCartt AT, Mayhew DR, Braitman KA, et al: Effects of age and experience on young driver crashes: review of recent literature, *Traffic Inj Prev* 10:209–219, 2009.

Morgan JF, Reid F, Lacey JH: The SCOFF questionnaire: assessment of a new screening tool for eating disorders, *BMJ* 319(7223):1467–1468, 1999.

Mosher WD, Chandra A, Jones J: Sexual behavior and selected health measures: men and women 15-44 years of age, United States, 2002, *Adv Data*, 15(362):1–55, 2005.

National Heart, Lung, and Blood Institute (NHLBI): *Expert panel on integrated guidelines for cardiovascular health and risk reduction in children and adolescents: summary report*, Bethesda, MD, 2011, U.S. Department of Health and Human Services, NHLBI, www.nhlbi.nih.gov/guidelines/cvd_ped/summary.htm#chap5.

National Institute for Health Care Management Foundation: *Childhood obesity—advancing effective prevention and treatment: an overview for health professionals*, prepared for National Institute for Health Care Management Foundation Forum, Washington, DC, April 9, 2003.

Neuman ME: Addressing children's beliefs through Fowler's stages of faith, *J Pediatr Nurs* 26(1):44–50, 2011.

Ogden CL, Carroll MD, Flegal KM: High body mass index for age among U.S. children and adolescents, 2003-2006, *JAMA* 299(20):2401–2405, 2008.

Ogden CL, Carroll MD, Kit BK, et al: Prevalence of obesity and trends in body mass index among US children and adolescents, 1999-2010, *JAMA* 307(5):483–490, 2012.

Ogden CL, Kuczmarski RJ, Flegal KM, et al: Centers for Disease Control and Prevention 2000 growth charts for the United States: improvements to the 1977 National Center for Health Statistics version, *Pediatrics* 109(1):141–142, 2002.

Ogden CL, Troiano RP, Briefel RR, et al: Prevalence of overweight among preschool children in the United States, 1971 through 1994, *Pediatrics* 99(4):e1, 1997.

O'Keeffe SG, Clarke-Pearson KC: Clinical report: the impact of social media on children, adolescents and families, *Pediatrics* 127(4):800–804, 2011.

Ongphiphadhanakul B: Osteoporosis: the role of genetics and the environment, *Forum Nutr* 60:158–167, 2007.

Owens JM, McLaughlin SB, Sudweeks J: Driver performance while text messaging using handheld and in-vehicle systems, *Accid Anal Prev* 43(3):939–947, 2011.

Pratt JSA, Lenders CM, Dionne EA, et al: Best practice updates for pediatric/adolescent weight loss surgery, *Obesity* 17(5):901–910, 2009.

Regnerus MD, Glen HE: Religion and vulnerability among low risk adolescents, *Soc Sci Res* 32(4):633–658, 2003.

Rice E, Rhoades H, Winetrobe H, et al: Sexually explicit cell phone messaging associated with sexual risk among adolescents, *Pediatrics* 130(4):667–673, 2012.

Roberts DF, Foehr UG: Children and electronic media, *Future Child* 8(1):235–253, 2008.

Saewyc EM, Homma Y, Skay CL, et al: Protective factors in the lives of bisexual adolescents in North America, *Am J Pub Health* 99(1):110–117, 2009.

Saewyc EM, Skay CL, Hynds P, et al: Suicidal ideation and attempts among adolescents in North American school-based surveys: are bisexual youth at increasing risk? *J LGBT Health Res* 3:25–36, 2007.

Shain B, AAP Committee on Adolescence: Suicide and suicide attempts in adolescents, *Pediatrics* 120(3):669–676, 2007.

Sjöberg RL, Nilsson KW, Leppert J: Obesity, shame, and depression in school-aged children: a population-based study, *Pediatrics* 116(3):e389–e393, 2005.

Spruijt-Metz D: Etiology, treatment and prevention of obesity in childhood and adolescence: a decade in review, *J Res Adolesc* 21(1):129–152, 2011.

Temple JR, Paul JA, van den Berg P, et al: Teen sexting and its association with sexual behaviors, *Arch Pediatr Adolesc Med* 166(9):828–833, 2012.

Tuttle J, Campbell-Heider N, David TM: Positive adolescent life skills training for high-risk teens: results of a group intervention study, *J Pediatr Health* 20(3):184–191, 2006.

U.S. Department of Health and Human Services: *The health consequences of involuntary exposure to tobacco smoke: a report of the surgeon general*, Washington, DC, 2006, Author.

U.S. Department of Health and Human Services: National Survey on Drug Use and Health: misuse of over-the-counter cough and cold medications among persons aged 12 to 25, SAMHSA, Rockville, MD, 2008a, www.oas.samhsa.gov/2k8/cough/cough.htm.

U.S. Department of Health and Human Services: *2008 physical activity guidelines for Americans*, 2008b, www.health.gov/PAGuidelines/guidelines.

U.S. Preventive Services Task Force: Screening for obesity in children and adolescents: U.S.

Preventive Services Task Force recommendation statement, *Pediatrics* 125(2):361–367, 2010.

Van Horn L, Johnson RK, Flickinger BD, et al: Translation and implementation of added sugars consumption recommendations: a conference report from the American Heart Association Added Sugars Conference 2010, *Circulation* 122(23):2470–2490, 2010.

Wardle J, Carnell S, Haworth CMA, et al: Evidence for a strong genetic influence on childhood adiposity despite the force of the obesogenic environment, *Am J Clin Nutr* 87(2):398–404, 2008.

Weiss R, Dziura J, Burgert TS, et al: Obesity and the metabolic syndrome in children and

adolescents, *N Engl J Med* 350(23):2362–2374, 2004.

Whitlock EP, O'Connor EA, Williams SB, et al: Effectiveness of weight management interventions in children: a targeted systematic review for the USPSTF, *Pediatrics* 125(2):e396–e418, 2010.

Wu T, Mendola P, Buck GM: Ethnic differences in the presence of secondary sex characteristics and menarche among U.S. girls: the Third National Health and Nutrition Examination Survey, 1988-1994, *Pediatrics* 10(4):752–757, 2002.

Young AM, Glover N, Havens JR: Nonmedical use of prescription medications among adolescents in the United States: a systematic review, *J Adolesc Health* 51(1):6–17, 2012.

Chronic Illness, Disability, and End-of-Life Care

Marilyn J. Hockenberry

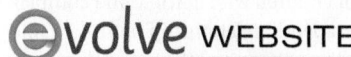

http://evolve.elsevier.com/Perry/maternal

LEARNING OBJECTIVES

On completion of this chapter, the reader will be able to:
- Identify the scope of and changing trends in care of children with special needs.
- Identify the major reactions of and effects on the family of a child with a special need.
- Define the stages of adjustment to the diagnosis of a chronic condition.

- Recognize the impact of the illness or condition on the developmental stages of childhood.
- Outline nursing interventions that promote the family's optimal adjustment to the child's chronic disorder.
- Outline nursing interventions that support the family at the time of death.
- Define the usual symptoms of normal grief.

PERSPECTIVES ON THE CARE OF CHILDREN AND FAMILIES LIVING WITH OR DYING FROM CHRONIC OR COMPLEX DISEASES

Scope of the Problem

Advances in medical and nursing care such as the increasing viability of extremely preterm infants, the portability of life-sustaining technology (e.g., total parental nutrition, ventilatory support), and life-extending treatments for children with conditions that previously would have led to an early death (e.g., malignancies, genetic conditions) (Burke and Alverson, 2010) have led to an exponential rise in the prevalence of children with complex and chronic diseases. These children have complex conditions involving several organ systems and require multiple specialists, technologic supports, and community services to help them function to their healthiest potential. The complexity, high level of skill required to meet their daily health care needs, and continuous nature and potential volatility of the condition sets this group apart from the broader population of children with special health care needs (Harrigan, Ratliffe, Patrinos, et al., 2002; Rehm and Bradley, 2005). A range of terms such as *medically complex, technology dependent,* and *multiply handicapped* have been used to describe this vulnerable population of children (Carnevale, Rehm, Kirk, et al., 2008; Cohen, Friedman, Nicholas, et al., 2008; Harrigan, Ratliffe, Patrinos, et al., 2002; Miles, Holditch-Davis, Burchinal, et al., 1999; O'Brien and Wegner, 2002; Watson, Townsley, and Abbott, 2002).

Frequent and prolonged hospitalizations; complex and multisystem health and developmental needs; and reliance on technology and care that cross hospital, clinic, and home settings are the key characteristics that all of these terms seek to signify about the children they are used to represent (Harrigan, Ratliffe, Patrinos, et al., 2002).

The nature and severity of childhood chronic and complex conditions is widely heterogeneous. However, it is the health and developmental consequences of these diagnoses such as ongoing functional impairment; neurodevelopmental disability; dependence on medical technology; and the need for ongoing skilled, supportive care from health care providers and family members that render these children and families particularly vulnerable. The impact of chronic and complex illness in children is wide ranging. Although many authors have described the rise in prevalence that has come about because of advances in medical care (Cohen, Friedman, Nicholas, et al., 2008; Council on Children with Disabilities, 2005; Haffner and Schurman, 2001; Mentro, 2003), accurate estimates of the numbers of affected families are not known (Carnevale, Rehm, Kirk, et al., 2008). These conditions present most families with additional tasks, responsibilities, and concerns (Ray, 2002). A child's activity level and developmental opportunities can be affected. Days can be lost from school. Children with complex chronic conditions may be at increased risk for behavior or emotional problems. Parents may lose days from work, experience financial strain, and be challenged both emotionally and physically as they cope with care of the child.

Siblings are also affected by having a "different" brother or sister and may simultaneously feel guilt and anger or jealousy toward their ill sibling. Clinicians need to know that siblings of children with chronic illnesses are at risk for negative psychologic effects (Sharpe and Rossiter, 2002). Parents need encouragement and assistance in understanding the reactions of siblings to having a chronically ill family member (e.g., behavioral regression, anxiety, withdrawal, apathy). In addition, secondary losses such as the ability to participate in extracurricular activities or social events occur because of routines imposed by the affected child's chronic condition.

Trends in Care

Developmental Focus

Focusing on the child's developmental level rather than chronologic age or diagnosis emphasizes the child's abilities and strengths rather than disabilities. Attention is directed to normalizing experiences, adapting the environment, and promoting coping skills. Nurses often are in vital positions to redirect attention from the pathologic model with its focus on weaknesses and problems to the developmental model to meet the unique needs of the child and family.

A developmental focus also considers family development. The life cycle of the family unit reflects both the changing ages and needs of family members and changing external demands. A family member's serious illness can cause significant stress or crisis at any stage of the family life cycle. Just as with individual development, family development may be interrupted or even regress to an earlier level of functioning. Nurses can use the concept of family development to plan meaningful interventions and evaluate care.

Family-Centered Care

Children's physical and emotional health and their cognitive and social functioning are strongly influenced by how well their families function (Schor, 2003). The importance of family-centered care—a philosophy that considers the family as the constant in the child's life—is especially evident in the care of children with special needs (see also Family-Centered Care, Chapter 26). As parents learn about the child's health care needs, they often become experts in delivering care. Health care providers, including nurses, are adjuncts to the child's care and need to form partnerships with parents. Effective communication and negotiation between parents and nurses are essential to forming trusting and effective partnerships and finding the best ways to meet the needs of the child and family (Corlett and Twycross, 2006). Collaborative relationships are characterized by communication, dialog, active listening, awareness, and acceptance of others' differences (Schor, 2003).

Family–Health Care Provider Communication. The disclosure of a serious chronic or complex condition in a child is one of the most stressful aspects of communication between families and health care professionals. Often parents have suspected for some time that something is wrong with their child and believe that their concerns were minimized or ignored by health care professionals (Smaldone and Ritholz, 2011; Thomlinson, 2002; Whitehead and Gosling, 2003). After a diagnosis is made, numerous studies have shown that parents are not always satisfied with the way in which information is given. Factors that influence parent dissatisfaction with communication include disrespectful attitudes, breaking bad news in an insensitive manner, withholding information, and changing a treatment course without preparing the child and family (Hsiao, Evan, and Zeltzer, 2007). Conversely parents report satisfaction when they perceive health

care providers to be available, demonstrate competence, and engage the child and parent in care decision making (Hsiao, Evan, and Zeltzer, 2007). Similar factors are important in communication of changes in the child's condition throughout the course of the illness.

Providing information to families with a chronically ill child should be a process of repeated discussions to allow the family to process the information and their reactions to that information and to ask for clarification and further information. Nurses play an important role in ensuring that families' needs are met during discussions related to the child's diagnosis, condition, and treatment. This requires assessing the amount of information with which the family is comfortable, how much they understand of the information already given to them, and how they are coping with the information both cognitively and emotionally. Nurses should ensure that the appropriate health care professionals address any concerns or further questions that families may have.

Establishing Therapeutic Relationships. Another important aspect of family-centered care of children with chronic and complex conditions is establishing a therapeutic relationship with the child and family, which has been shown to predict improved health-related outcomes (Denboba, McPherson, Kenney, et al., 2006). Families, most often the mother, take on enormous responsibility in providing technical care and symptom management of their child's condition outside the health care institution (O'Brien and Wegner, 2002; Raina, O'Donnell, Rosenbaum, et al., 2005; Swallow and Jacoby, 2001). To build successful therapeutic relationships with families, it is necessary for nurses to recognize parents' expertise with regard to their child's condition and needs. Care conferences, especially multidisciplinary meetings that include the family and key health professionals, provide an opportunity for sharing ideas and expressing feelings or concerns. Health care environments for children with serious illnesses are fraught with obstacles that serve as barriers to successful therapeutic relationships with families. For example, the complex, multidisciplinary care required is often characterized by fragmented, noncohesive approaches to care. Continuity of care can be a challenge in acute care hospitals today, and this makes it difficult to establish relationships and understand communication styles.

Individual discussions, especially with the case manager, primary nurse, clinical nurse specialist, or nurse practitioner, help establish a consistent and flexible care plan that can prevent conflicts or deal with these conflicts before they disrupt care. In family-centered care the goal is to maintain the integrity of the leadership role and support the family during times of crisis or stress.

The Role of Culture in Family-Centered Care. Issues of culture, ethnicity, and race affect access to services, use, and follow-through with referrals and recommendations (Coker, Rodriguez, and Flores, 2010; van Dyck, Kogan, McPherson, et al., 2004; Wise, Wampler, Chavkin, et al., 2002; Wood, Smith, Romero, et al., 2002; Zuvekas and Taliaferro, 2003). For some ethnic and minority populations, cultural understandings of illness, the structure of family life, social roles for individuals with disabilities, and other factors related to the perception of children may differ from those of mainstream American culture. These factors may affect family needs and choices regarding the care of their child with special needs.

Although culture cannot completely explain how an individual will think and act, understanding cultural perspectives can help the nurse anticipate and understand why families may make certain decisions. Cultural attributes such as values and beliefs regarding illness or chronic condition and its causation, social roles for people who are ill or disabled, family structure, the role of children, child-rearing practices, self-versus-group orientation, spirituality, and time orientation also affect a family's response to illness or chronic condition in a child (Carnevale, Alexander, Davis, et al., 2006; Carter, 2002; Marshall, Olsen, Mandleco, et al., 2003; Rehm, 1999; Sterling and Peterson, 2003).

When parents are informed of their child's chronic illness, interpreters familiar with both culture and language should be used. Children, family members, and friends of the family should not be used as translators because their presence may prevent parents from openly discussing the issues. When working with people of cultural backgrounds different from their own, nurses must listen carefully with an initial goal of understanding and articulating the family's perspective. The ability to interpret the mainstream medical culture to the family is also important. Furthermore, every effort is made to incorporate traditional cultural beliefs of a family into treatment plans. It is important to keep in mind that "cultural norms" may not always apply to every family from a shared background. Nurses who assess the unique needs of each family, listen, and keep themselves open to novel ways of meeting the individual needs of the child and family will likely be successful in establishing a therapeutic relationship. Developing a care plan in conjunction with the family, considering their preferences and priorities, is an important first step in formulating a plan that best meets the family's needs, no matter what their cultural background (Ahmann, 1994; Coker, Rodriguez, and Flores, 2010; Ochieng, 2003).

Shared Decision Making

Shared decision making among the child, family, and health care team can result from open, honest, culturally sensitive communication and the establishment of a therapeutic relationship among the family and health care providers. In a shared decision-making model, the health care professionals provide honest, clear information regarding diagnosis, prognosis, treatment options, and risk-benefit assessment. The patient and family then share information with the health care team regarding important family values, acceptable levels of discomfort or inconvenience, and the ability to comply with treatments being recommended (Charles, Gafni, and Whelan, 1997; Kon, 2010). This process allows them to discuss all options in terms of the risks and benefits to the child and family, the prognosis or expected course of the illness, and the impact on the family's resources (Box 36-1). Together the parents and health care team can make decisions that are best for the family and child at the time the decision is made (Kon, 2010).

BOX 36-1 FACILITATING SHARED DECISION MAKING

- Continually assess the impact of the child's illness and treatment on the family.
- Provide honest, accurate information regarding the trajectory of the disease, anticipated complications, and prognostic information.
- Discuss what the family desires for the child's quality of life.
- Avoid personal opinion or judgment of the family's questions and decisions.
- Be aware of nurses' personal and cultural assumptions and the ways these assumptions impact communication, decision making, and judgment.

Normalization

Normalization refers to the efforts that family members make to create a normal family life, their perceptions of the consequences of these efforts, and the meanings they attribute to their management efforts (Knafl, Darney, Gallo, et al., 2010). For chronically ill children such efforts may include attending school, pursuing hobbies and recreational interests, and achieving employment and a level of independence. For their families it may entail adapting the family routine to accommodate the ill or disabled child's health and physical needs (McDougal, 2002).

Children with chronic and complex conditions and their families face numerous challenges in achieving normalization. Families move between the "normal" of living with the experience of chronic childhood illness and the "normal" of the healthy outside world; they often redefine "normal" based on their particular experiences, needs, and circumstances (Deatrick, Knafl, Murphy-Moore, 1999; Gantt, 2002; Nelson, 2002). Normalization may be an important mediator of illness-related stressors (e.g., treatment demands, uncertainty) on family outcomes.

Nurses can help families normalize their lives by assessing their everyday life, social support systems, coping strategies, family cohesiveness, and family and community resources. Interventions could include encouraging families to reduce stress through delegation of care and family tasks, identifying ways to incorporate care into current routines, structuring the home environment to encourage the child's engagement in age-appropriate activities, and ensuring that families have access to appropriate community support services (Jokinen, 2004; Shepard and Mahon, 2000). Being supportive of the child's illness and treatment and actively including the family in all aspects of care improves their self-esteem and promotes further development (Shepard and Mahon, 2000).

Home care represents the return to a system and set of priorities in which family values are as important in the care of a child with a chronic health problem as they are in the care of other children. Home care seeks to achieve goals that are consistent with the developmental model (Stein, 1985):

- Normalize the life of the child, including those with technologically complex care, in a family and community context and setting.
- Minimize the disruptive impact of the child's condition on the family.
- Foster the child's maximum growth and development.

With appropriate training and support, families provide complex procedures and treatments in the home. Parents are challenged to retain a homelike setting among monitors, ventilators, and other sophisticated equipment. Throughout this text home care is discussed as appropriate for specific conditions. The process of transition from hospital to home is elaborated on in Chapters 20 and 21.

Paralleling normalization and home care is the process of mainstreaming, or integrating children with disabilities into regular classrooms. Just as the home is the natural environment for children, so school must also be included as an essential component of children's overall physical, intellectual, and social development. Children who attend school have the advantages of learning and socializing with a wide group of peers. There is an increased focus on individualization as plans are made to meet the academic needs of these children along with those of the rest of the students.

A variety of supplemental programs have been designed in the school system to accommodate special needs, both at school age and younger, through early intervention, which consists of any sustained and systematic effort to assist children from birth to age 3 years who have disabilities and are developmentally vulnerable. This change and increasing opportunities for normalization for children with disabilities in large part have resulted from the passage of (1) the Education for All Handicapped Children Act of 1975 (Public Law 94-142) and its 1990 amendments (Public Law 101-476), which changed the name of the act to the Individuals with Disabilities Education Act (IDEA); (2) the Education of the Handicapped Act Amendments of 1986 (Public Law 99-457), which directs states to develop and implement statewide comprehensive, coordinated, multidisciplinary interagency programs of early intervention services for infants and toddlers with disabilities and support services for their families; and (3) the Americans with Disabilities Act of 1990. Nurses can provide parents with information about these laws and in some cases may participate in the development of individualized educational programs (IEPs) or individualized family service plans (IFSPs) for children with disabilities.

Managed Care

Managed care programs have become the major form of health care provision in the United States (Jackson, 2000). This model of care has brought both opportunities and challenges with respect to the care of children with chronic and complex conditions. Although managed care may promote continuity and coordination of care for children and families with private insurance, it has had an unfavorable impact on relatively resource-limited families caring for children with complex chronic illnesses (Huffman, Brat, Chamberlain, et al., 2010). Children rely on adults for access to health care and follow-up with treatment regimens, making it necessary to manage the child's care in the context of the family (McPherson, Weissman, Strickland, et al., 2004; van Dyck, Kogan, McPherson, et al., 2004).

THE FAMILY OF THE CHILD WITH A CHRONIC OR COMPLEX CONDITION

A major goal in working with the family of a child with chronic or complex illness is to support the family's coping and promote their optimal functioning throughout the child's life. Long-term, comprehensive, family-centered approaches extend beyond supporting the child and family during the critical periods of diagnosis and hospitalization. Rather, comprehensive care involves forming parent-professional partnerships that can support a family's adaptation across the trajectory of the illness to the many changes that may be necessary in day-to-day life, determining expectations of and for the child, and providing a long-term perspective (Box 36-2).

BOX 36-2 ADAPTIVE TASKS OF PARENTS HAVING CHILDREN WITH CHRONIC CONDITIONS

1. Accept child's condition.
2. Manage child's condition on a day-to-day basis.
3. Meet child's normal developmental needs.
4. Meet developmental needs of other family members.
5. Cope with ongoing stress and periodic crises.
6. Help family members manage their feelings.
7. Educate others about child's condition.
8. Establish support system.

From Canam C: Common adaptive tasks facing parents of children with chronic conditions, *J Adv Nurs* 18:46–53, 1993.

The impact of a child's medical or developmental condition is often experienced over time, initially as a crisis at the time of diagnosis, which may occur at birth, after a long period of diagnostic testing, or immediately after a tragic injury. The impact may also be felt before the diagnosis is made, when parents are aware that something is wrong with their child but before medical confirmation (Thomlinson, 2002; Whitehead and Gosling, 2003).

The diagnosis and initial discharge home are critical times for parents (Coffey, 2006). Several factors can make it particularly difficult, including a long duration of uncertainty in the diagnostic process, negative perceptions of chronic illness, insufficient information, and lack of mutual trust between parents and their child's health care team (Garwick, Patterson, Bennett, et al., 1995; Monterosso, Kristjanson, Aoun, et al., 2007; Nuutila and Salanterä, 2006). Parental feelings of shock, helplessness, isolation, fear, and depression are common (Coffey, 2006; Nuutila and Salanterä, 2006). Throughout the first year parents struggle to accept the child's diagnosis, care, and uncertainty of the future (Coffey, 2006). Providing explicit and uncomplicated information to parents in an empathic way (Nuutila and Salanterä, 2006); assessing the family's daily routine, living conditions, background knowledge, skills and abilities, and coping behaviors; and evaluating the family's understanding of the information can encourage optimal support at the time of diagnosis and initial discharge home. It is also necessary to reassess parents' needs for information and support on a routine basis (Nuutila and Salanterä, 2006).

Other critical times include the exacerbation of the child's physical symptoms, which increases parental care. These crises often involve medical intervention and rehospitalization. Frequently the child does not return to his or her precrisis level of functioning, and parents and family must adapt to new care needs and schedules. Instability may also follow transition points on the illness trajectory. For example, changes in caregivers and significant chronologic age milestones can increase parental stress, and advocating for the child during these times is essential. Supporting parents, respecting their stress and emotions, and acknowledging their role as team members in the care of their child are important aspects of nursing care (Coffey, 2006; Nuutila and Salanterä, 2006).

Impact of the Child's Chronic Illness

Each member of a family who has a child with a chronic or complex illness is affected by the experience (Sullivan-Bolyai, Sadler, Knafl, et al., 2003). The effects on the parents and their responses may be so intense that they directly influence the other members' reactions and the child's own coping.

Parents

In addition to the stress of grieving for the loss of a perfect child, parents are affected by whether or not they receive positive feedback from interactions with their child. Many parents feel satisfaction and fulfillment from the parenting role. For others parenting may be a series of unrewarding experiences that contribute to feelings of inadequacy and failure (Box 36-3). These responses may be most evident in parents who are responsible for the child's care. For example, parents may become preoccupied with their ability to carry out certain procedures, overlooking the child's personal comfort and satisfaction or failing to offer praise for anything less than perfect cooperation or performance. They may pursue a frustrating activity until they achieve "success"—long after the child has become irritable and uncooperative. As a result parents can become caught in a pattern of interaction that is mutually unrewarding and minimally productive. This situation may become exacerbated by disagreements or lack of support from other family members and judgment from caregivers and others in the community. For these parents several strategies may be helpful, including education regarding what can reasonably be expected of their child, assistance in identifying the child's strengths, praise for a parental job well done, and respite care so parents can renew their energies.

Parental Roles. Parenting a child with a complex chronic condition requires much more than raising a typical child. In addition to attending to the routine aspects of parenting, parents of chronically ill children take on the added responsibility of performing complex technical care and symptom management, advocating for their child, and seeking and coordinating health and social services for their ill or disabled child (Kirk, Glendinning, and Callery, 2005). These added responsibilities must then be balanced with the needs of other family members, extended family and friends, and personal health and obligations to minimize consequences to the overall functioning of the family (Coffey, 2006; Ray, 2002). Enormous demands may be placed on parental time, energy, and financial resources.

Often one parent or partner remains at home to manage existing family responsibilities while the other remains with the ill child. The partner who is not included in the caregiving activities may feel neglected because all of the attention is directed toward the child and resentful that he or she is not sufficiently informed to be competent in the care. Without active participation in the child's care, the parent has little appreciation of the time and energy involved in performing these activities. When this partner does attempt to participate, the other parent may criticize the less skillful efforts. As a result, communication and support for one another may be adversely affected.

The nurse can help parents avoid role conflicts by providing anticipatory guidance early in the process. Teaching should address stressors often identified as having an impact on the marriage, including (1) the burden of care at home assumed by primarily one parent, (2) the financial burden, (3) the fear of the child dying, (4) pressure from relatives, (5) the hereditary nature of the disease (if applicable), and (6) fear of pregnancy. Other causes of tension may center on the inconveniences associated with care such as long waits for an appointment, lack of parking near care facilities, or lack of overnight accommodations. Certainly these last stressors are within health professionals' domain to minimize, if not eliminate.

BOX 36-3 ANTICIPATED PARENTAL STRESS POINTS

Diagnosis of the condition—Parents require considerable education while dealing with an emotional response.

Developmental milestones—Times that children normally achieve walking, talking, and self-care are delayed or impossible for the child.

Start of schooling—Particularly stressful are situations in which appropriate schooling will not be in a regular class placement.

Reaching the ultimate attainment—Parents must handle situations such as realizing that ambulation will be impossible or that the child will not learn to read.

Adolescence—Issues such as sexuality and independence become prominent.

Future placement—Decisions about placement must be made when the child becomes an adult or when the parents can no longer care for the child.

Death of the child

Mother-Father Differences. Mothers and fathers in the same family often adjust and cope differently as parents of a child with a complex condition. Some mothers experience a peaks-and-valleys periodic crisis pattern, whereas most fathers tend to experience a steady, gradual recovery. Some research suggests that mothers of children with certain conditions may be more susceptible to psychologic distress and fatigue than fathers (Tong, Kandala, Haig, et al., 2002). Mothers are most often the primary caregiver and are more likely than fathers to give up their jobs to care for their children, often resulting in social isolation (Coffey, 2006). Mothers often have greater needs for social support and positive appraisal of the situation, whereas fathers are more likely to use self-controlling behaviors to cope (Goldbeck, 2001; Mastroyannopoulou, Stallard, Lewis, et al., 1997).

Fathers of children with disabilities struggle with issues that may be distinct from those of the mothers (Swallow, Macfadyen, Santacroce, et al., 2012). Fathers may think that their role of protector is challenged because they do not know how to help and cannot protect their family from the seemingly overwhelming recurring problems. With today's increased emphasis on fathers' involvement in the lives of their children, this loss is felt more profoundly than in the past. The extensive stresses in the family can leave fathers feeling depressed, weak, guilty, powerless, isolated, embarrassed, and angry. However, fearful that they will lose control or be viewed as weak or ineffectual, they often hide their feelings and display an outward confidence that may lead others to believe that everything is fine. They worry about what the future holds for their children, their ability to manage the increasing financial burden, and the daily disruptions of the entire family (Davies, Gudmundsdottir, Worden, et al., 2004; Swallow, Macfadyen, Santacroce, et al., 2012). Some fathers use work as an escape to dull the pain. In addition to withdrawal, common coping strategies are problem oriented and include praying, getting information, looking at options, and weighing choices (Mastroyannopoulou, Stallard, Lewis, et al., 1997).

Single-Parent Families. Single-parent families are of special concern. The absence of a parent may result from divorce or death, or the parents may never have married. As the only parent of a child who may require extensive, sophisticated, and lifelong care, the single parent may feel an enormous burden. Available financial and emotional resources may already be stretched to the limit. A special effort should be made to help the single parent find financial and support services that can ease the burden of care. Nurses can also help the single parent identify helping roles that may be acceptable to relatives and friends.

Siblings

Results of studies on how siblings are affected by having a brother or sister with a complex condition are unclear (Anderson and Davis, 2011; Barlow and Ellard, 2006). Generally evidence shows a negative effect on siblings of children with chronic illnesses compared with siblings of healthy children (Gold, Treadwell, Weissman, et al., 2011). Siblings of children with chronic illnesses report psychosocial problems more often than their peers (Gold, Treadwell, Weissman, et al., 2011; Rossiter and Sharpe, 2001). A number of factors increase the risk of negative effects for siblings of ill children. Responsibility for caregiving, differential treatment by parents, and limitations in family resources and recreational time are often the experiences of siblings of ill or disabled children (Lobato and Kao, 2002) (Box 36-4).

An important factor in sibling adjustment and coping is information and knowledge regarding their brother's or sister's illness or complex condition. What siblings piece together or overhear is often

---

BOX 36-4 **SUPPORTING SIBLINGS OF CHILDREN WITH SPECIAL NEEDS**

Promote Healthy Sibling Relationships

- Value each child individually and avoid comparisons. Remind each child of his or her positive qualities and contribution to other family members.
- Help siblings see the differences and similarities between themselves and the child with special needs. Create a climate in which children can achieve successes without feeling guilty.
- Teach siblings ways to interact with the child.
- Seek to be fair in terms of discipline, attention, and resources; require the affected child to do as much for himself or herself as possible.
- Let siblings settle their own differences; intervene only to prevent siblings from hurting one another.
- Legitimize reasonable anger. Even children with special needs behave badly sometimes.
- Respect a sibling's reluctance to be with or to include the child with special needs in activities.

Help Siblings Cope

- Listen to siblings to let them know that their thoughts and suggestions are valued.
- Praise siblings when they have been patient, have sacrificed, or have been particularly helpful. Do not expect them to always act in this manner.
- Acknowledge the personal strengths that siblings have and their ability to cope with stress successfully.
- Provide age-appropriate information about the child's condition and update it when appropriate.

- Let teachers know what is happening so they can be understanding and helpful.
- Recognize special stress times for siblings and plan to minimize negative effects.
- Schedule special time with siblings; have a friend or family member substitute when parent is unavailable.
- Encourage siblings to join or help establish a sibling support group.
- Use the services of professionals when needed. If parent thinks that such a service is necessary, it should be provided in as vigorous a manner as a service for the child with special needs.

Involve Siblings

- Seek out ways to realistically include siblings in the care and treatment of the child with special needs.
- Limit caregiving responsibilities and give recognition when siblings perform them.
- Develop a library of children's books on special needs.
- Invite siblings to attend meetings to develop plans for the child with special needs (e.g., individualized educational program, individualized family service plan).
- Discuss future plans with them.
- Solicit their ideas on treatment and service needs.
- Have them visit professionals who work with the child.
- Help them develop competencies to teach the child new skills.
- Provide opportunities for siblings to advocate for the child.
- Allow siblings to set their own pace for learning and involvement.

Data from Powell T, Ogle P: *Brothers and sisters—a special part of exceptional families,* Baltimore, 1985, Paul H Brooks; Spokane Washington Deaconess Medical Center, Pediatric Oncology Unit: Tips for dealing with siblings, *Candlelighters Childhood Cancer Found Q Newslett* 11(3,4):7, 1987; and Carlson J, Leviton A, Mueller M: Services to siblings: an important component of family-centered practice, *ACCH Advocate* 1(1):53–56, 1993.

---

much worse than the truth. Often they imagine gruesome things regarding the experiences related to the illness, treatment, and hospitalization (Shepard and Mahon, 2000). Latino siblings have reported less accurate information about their siblings' condition than non-Latino siblings (Lobato, Kao, and Plante, 2005). Parents are usually in the best position to impart information, although they are often overwhelmed with the medical crisis at hand (Fleitas, 2000). Nurses can encourage parents to talk with the siblings about how they perceive their sick brother or sister and to be accepting of the siblings' feelings. Nurses can be ideal educators and counselors of siblings during the course of their brother's or sister's illness (Shepard and Mahon, 2000).

Coping with Ongoing Stress and Periodic Crises

Professionals can help families cope with stress by providing anticipatory guidance, providing emotional support, helping the family assess and identify specific stressors, helping them develop coping mechanisms and problem-solving strategies, and working collaboratively with parents so they become empowered in the process (Anderson and Davis, 2011).

Concurrent Stresses Within the Family

The ability to deal with the overwhelming stress of a chronic illness is challenged further when additional stresses are present. Stressors may be situational or developmental. They may be related to marital difficulties, sibling needs, homelessness, or social isolation. Some families may simultaneously be struggling with a family member's alcohol or other drug problem. Even relatively minor stressors such

as arranging care for siblings, managing the home, and traveling to distant treatment centers can challenge a family's ability to cope successfully.

Most families, regardless of their income or insurance coverage, have financial concerns. The costs of caring for a child with a complex illness can be overwhelming. Nurses and social workers can help a family review various options for financial assistance, including insurance, managed care, or health maintenance organization policies; Medicaid; Supplemental Security Income; Women, Infants, and Children (WIC) program; the state Program for Children with Special Health Needs; disease-related associations; and local philanthropic organizations.

Coping Mechanisms

Coping mechanisms are behaviors aimed at reducing the tension caused by a crisis. Approach behaviors are coping mechanisms that result in movement toward adjustment and resolution of the crisis. Avoidance behaviors result in movement away from adjustment and represent maladaptation to the crisis. Several approach and avoidance behaviors used in coping with a chronic illness are listed in the Guidelines box on p. 1057. None of the indexes can be used singly to assess the possible success or failure in resolving the crisis. Each behavior must be viewed in the context of all of the variables affecting the family. For example, observing several avoidance behaviors in an emotionally healthy family may denote significantly less risk to the successful resolution of the crisis than an equal number of avoidance behaviors in an individual who has few available supports.

Parental Empowerment

Empowerment can be seen as a process of recognizing, promoting, and enhancing competence. For parents of children with chronic conditions, empowerment may occur gradually as strength and capabilities are drawn on to master the child's care, manage family life, and plan for the future. Advocating for the child and developing parent-professional partnerships are part of taking charge (Ray, 2002).

Helping Family Members Manage Their Feelings

Although some previous research has postulated stages of adaptation to a chronic illness, there is a great deal of individual variation in responses to the diagnosis, adjustments made, and time frames for coming to terms with a diagnosis. It is important that professionals recognize and respect a wide range of reactions and coping mechanisms. In fact, members of the family of a child with a complex chronic condition may experience a number of difficult emotions, including fear, guilt, anger, resentment, and anxiety. Learning to manage these emotions promotes adaptive coping (see Guidelines box). Support from professionals, other family members, and friends can help family members manage their feelings. The following discussion examines some common phases of adjustment and emotional reactions.

Shock and Denial

The initial diagnosis of a chronic illness or complex condition is often met with intense emotion and is characterized by shock, disbelief, and sometimes denial, especially if the disorder is not obvious, as in chronic illness. Denial as a defense mechanism is a necessary cushion to prevent disintegration and is a normal response to grieving for any type of loss. Probably all family members experience various degrees of adaptive denial as they learn of the impact that the diagnosis has on their lives.

Shock and denial can last from days to months, sometimes even longer. Examples of denial that may be exhibited at the time of diagnosis include the following:

- Health care provider shopping
- Attributing the symptoms of the actual illness to a minor condition
- Refusing to believe the diagnostic tests
- Delaying consent for treatment
- Acting happy and optimistic despite the revealed diagnosis
- Refusing to tell or talk to anyone about the condition
- Insisting that no one is telling the truth regardless of others' attempts to do so
- Denying the reason for admission
- Asking no questions about the diagnosis, treatment, or prognosis.

Generally these mechanisms should be respected as short-term responses that allow individuals to distance themselves from the tremendous emotional impact and to collect and mobilize their energies toward goal-directed, problem-solving behaviors.

In children the importance of denial has repeatedly been demonstrated as a factor in their positive coping with the diagnosis. Denial allows the child to maintain hope in the face of overwhelming odds and function adaptively and productively. Similar to hope, denial may be an adaptive mechanism for dealing with loss that persists until a family or patient is ready or needs other responses.

Denial is probably the least understood and most poorly handled reaction. Health professionals typically label denial as maladaptive and act inappropriately by attempting to strip it away by repeated

---

GUIDELINES

Assessing Coping Behaviors

Approach Behaviors

- Asks for information regarding diagnosis and child's present condition
- Seeks help and support from others
- Anticipates future problems; actively seeks guidance and answers
- Endows the chronic illness or complex condition with meaning
- Shares burden of disorder with others
- Plans realistically for the future
- Acknowledges and accepts child's awareness of diagnosis and prognosis
- Expresses feelings such as sorrow, depression, and anger and realizes reason for the emotional reaction
- Realistically perceives child's condition; adjusts to changes
- Recognizes own growth through passage of time such as earlier denial and nonacceptance of diagnosis
- Verbalizes possible loss of child

Avoidance Behaviors

- Fails to recognize seriousness of child's condition despite physical evidence
- Refuses to agree to treatment
- Intellectualizes about the illness but in areas unrelated to child's condition
- Is angry and hostile to members of the staff regardless of their attitude or behavior
- Avoids staff, family members, or child
- Entertains unrealistic future plans for child with little emphasis on the present
- Is unable to adjust to or accept a change in progression of disease
- Continually looks for new cures with no perspective toward possible benefit
- Refuses to acknowledge child's understanding of disease and prognosis
- Uses magical thinking and fantasy; may seek "occult" help
- Places complete faith in religion to point of relinquishing own responsibility
- Withdraws from outside world; refuses help
- Punishes self because of guilt and blame
- Makes no change in lifestyle to meet needs of other family members
- Resorts to excessive use of alcohol or drugs to avoid problems
- Verbalizes suicidal intents
- Is unable to discuss possible loss of child or previous experiences with death

---

and sometimes blunt explanations of the prognosis. However, denial becomes maladaptive only when it prevents recognition of treatment or rehabilitative goals necessary for the child's optimal survival or development.

Adjustment

For most families adjustment gradually follows shock and is usually characterized by an open admission that the condition exists. This stage may be accompanied by several responses, which are normal parts of the adaptation process. Probably the most universal of these feelings are guilt and self-accusation. Guilt is often greatest when the cause of the disorder is directly traceable to the parent, as in genetic diseases or accidental injury. However, it can occur even without any scientific or realistic basis for parental responsibility. Frequently the guilt stems from a false assumption that the child's condition is a result of personal failure or wrongdoing such as not doing something correctly during pregnancy or the birth. Guilt may also be associated with cultural or religious beliefs. Some parents are convinced that they are being punished for some previous misdeed. Others may see the illness as a trial sent by God to test their religious strength and faith. With correct information, support, and time, most parents master guilt and self-accusation. The ability to master resentful and self-accusatory feelings of having "caused" the child's disorder is a crucial factor in determining the parents' acceptance of their child.

Children, too, may interpret their serious illness as retribution for past misbehavior. The nurse should be particularly sensitive to the child who passively accepts all painful procedures. This child may believe that such acts are inflicted as deserved punishment. It is vital that parents and health care professionals reassure children that their illnesses are not their fault.

Other common and normal reactions to a diagnosis are bitterness and anger. Anger directed inward may be evident as self-reproaching or punitive behavior such as neglecting one's health and verbally degrading oneself. Anger directed outward may be manifested in either open arguments or withdrawal from communication and may be evident in the person's relationship with any number of individuals (e.g., the spouse, the child, and siblings). Passive anger toward the ill child may be evident in decreased visiting, refusal to believe how sick the child is, or an inability to provide comfort. Among the most common targets for parental anger are members of the staff. Parents may complain about the nursing care, the insufficient time health care providers spend with them, or the lack of skill of those who draw blood or start intravenous infusions.

Children are apt to respond with anger as well, and this includes the affected child and the well siblings. Children are aware of the loss engendered by their illness or complex condition and may react angrily to the restrictions imposed or the feelings of being different. Siblings may also feel anger and resentment toward the ill child and parents for the loss of routine and parental attention. It is difficult for older children and almost impossible for younger children to comprehend the plight of the affected child. Their perception is of a brother or sister who has the undivided attention of their parents, is showered with cards and gifts, and is the focus of everyone's concern.

During the period of adjustment four types of parental reactions to the child influence the child's eventual response to the disorder:

1. *Overprotection,* in which the parents fear letting the child achieve any new skill, avoid all discipline, and cater to every desire to prevent frustration
2. *Rejection,* in which the parents detach themselves emotionally from the child but usually provide adequate physical care or constantly nag and scold the child
3. *Denial,* in which the parents act as if the disorder does not exist or attempt to have the child overcompensate for it
4. *Gradual acceptance,* in which the parents place necessary and realistic restrictions on the child, encourage self-care activities, and promote reasonable physical and social abilities

Reintegration and Acknowledgment

For many families the adjustment process culminates in the development of realistic expectations for the child and reintegration of family life with the illness or complex condition in a manageable perspective. Because a large portion of this phase is one of grief for a loss, total resolution is not possible until the child dies or leaves home as an independent adult. Therefore one can regard adjustment

as "increased comfort" with everyday living rather than a complete resolution.

This adjustment phase also involves social reintegration in which the family broadens its activities to include relationships outside of the home with the child as an acceptable and participating member of the group. This last criterion often differentiates the reaction of gradual acceptance during the adjustment period from total acceptance or perhaps is more descriptive of the acknowledgment process.

Many parents of children with chronic illnesses experience chronic sorrow (i.e., feelings of sorrow and loss that recur in waves over time). As the child's condition progresses, they experience repeated losses that represent further declines and new caregiving demands. Consequently families must be assessed on an ongoing basis and offered appropriate support and resources as their needs change over time (Bettle and Latimer, 2009; Gordon, 2009). This represents a critical period of time as the approach and support provided by the nursing and medical team during this period of time can directly impact the experience of complicated grief after the death of the child. Complicated grief (Meert, Shear, Newth, 2011), characterized as persistent distress and chronic stress response, may last 6 months or longer after the death of a child and has a significant impact on quality of life of the family left behind. It has been proposed as a new diagnostic entity to be included in the fifth edition of the *Diagnostic and Statistical Manual of Mental Disorders* (Meert, Shear, Newth, 2011).

Establishing a Support System

The diagnosis of a child with a complex chronic condition is a major situational crisis that affects the entire family system. However, families can experience positive outcomes as they successfully deal with the many challenges that accompany a child with chronic illness (Hungerbuehler, Vollrath, and Landolt, 2011).

One nursing goal is to assess which families are at greater or lesser risk for succumbing to the effects of the crisis. Several variables (i.e., available support system, perception of the event, coping mechanisms, reactions to the child, available resources, and concurrent stresses within the family) influence the resolution of a crisis. Although most families cope well, the needs of families at risk are great. If they receive emotional support and guidance early, there is an increased likelihood that they will also cope successfully.

Although it is easy to assume that families of children with the most severe illnesses or disabilities would have the poorest adjustment, the severity of the condition reflects only one part of the overall picture. The level of adjustment is significantly influenced by the functional burden on the individual family (Stein, 1985). This concept considers the issues related to caring for and living with the child in relation to the family's resources and ability to cope (Box 36-5). If a family of a child with a high level of technology dependence who demands complex care has many resources and coping skills, they may adjust more successfully to the child's situation than the family of a child with a less serious condition and few resources to counterbalance.

Intrafamilial resources, social support from friends and relatives, parent-to-parent support, parent-professional partnerships, and community resources interweave to provide a flexible web of support for families of children with chronic conditions.

THE CHILD WITH A CHRONIC OR COMPLEX CONDITION

The child's reaction to chronic illness depends to a great extent on his or her developmental level, temperament, and available coping

Data from Stein REK: Home care: a challenging opportunity, *Child Health Care* 14(2):90–95, 1985.

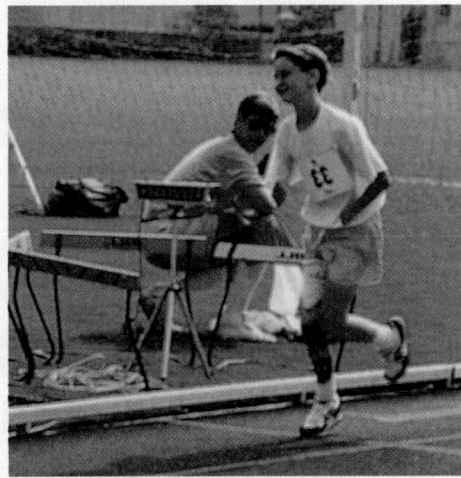

FIG 36-1 Children with any type of impairment should have the opportunity to develop their skills. (Courtesy Poyo/Hinton Photography.)

mechanisms; on the reactions of family members or significant others; and to a lesser extent on the condition itself. A child's conceptual understanding of his or her own illness is based not only on age and developmental level but also on the duration and type of experience accumulated with the disease. Knowledge of these variables is essential in providing the kind of information and support needed by these children to cope with an often overwhelming situation.

Developmental Aspects

The impact of a complex chronic illness is influenced by the age at onset. Chronic illness affects children of all ages, but the developmental aspects of each age-group dictate particular stresses and risks for the child. The nurse must also recognize that children need to redefine their condition and its implications as they develop and grow. For example, appearance, skills, and abilities are highly valued by peers (Fig. 36-1); a teenager who is limited in any of these qualities is subject to rejection. This is especially marked when an illness interferes with sexual attractiveness.

Children's developmental concepts of illness are discussed in Chapter 38. An understanding of these developmental factors

facilitates planning care to support the child and minimize the risks. Developmental aspects of chronic illness on children are described in Table 36-1.

Coping Mechanisms

Children with chronic conditions tend to use five distinct patterns of coping (Box 36-6). Children with more positive and accepting attitudes about their chronic illness use a more adaptive coping style characterized by optimism, competence, and compliance. They show fewer behavior problems at home and school. The two maladaptive coping patterns—"Feels different and withdraws" and "Is irritable, is moody, and acts out"—are associated with poorer adaptation; children using these strategies have poorer self-concepts, more negative attitudes about their conditions, and more behavior problems at home and school.

Well-adapted children gradually learn to accept their physical limitations and find achievement in a variety of compensatory motor and intellectual pursuits. They function well at home, at school, and with peers. They have an understanding of their disorder that allows them to accept their limitations, assume responsibility for their care, and assist in treatment and rehabilitation regimens. They express appropriate emotions such as sadness, anxiety, and anger at times of exacerbations but confidence and guarded optimism during periods of clinical stability (Fig. 36-2). They are able to identify with other similarly affected individuals, promoting positive self-images and displaying pride and self-confidence in their ability to master a productive, successful life despite their illnesses.

Hopefulness

Children, particularly adolescents, are sensitive to the presence or absence of hope. Hopefulness is an internal quality that mobilizes humans into goal-directed action that may be satisfying and life sustaining. A sense of hopefulness can produce increased participation in health-seeking behaviors and an improved sense of well-being (Ritchie, 2001).

Health Education and Self-Care

Health education is an intervention that promotes coping. Children need information about their condition, the therapeutic plan, and how the disease or therapy might affect their particular situation. Children nearing puberty also need to understand the maturation process and how their chronic illness may alter this event. For example, a youngster with Crohn's disease should understand that this disorder is associated with growth failure and delayed puberty; a child with diabetes needs to know that hormonal changes and increased growth needs alter food and insulin requirements at this time; and a sexually active girl with sickle cell anemia or systemic lupus erythematosus needs to be aware of the risks of pregnancy. The information should not be given all at once but timed appropriately to meet the changing needs of the youngsters, and it should be described and repeated as often as the situation demands.

NURSING CARE OF THE FAMILY AND CHILD WITH A CHRONIC OR COMPLEX CONDITION

Perform an Assessment

Because the nurse may meet a family during any phase of the adjustment process, several assessment areas are important. The family's ability to cope with previous stresses influences the current situation, and answers to questions about their usual coping skills are

TABLE 36-1 DEVELOPMENTAL EFFECTS OF CHRONIC ILLNESS OR DISABILITY ON CHILDREN

DEVELOPMENTAL TASKS	POTENTIAL EFFECTS OF CHRONIC ILLNESS OR DISABILITY	SUPPORTIVE INTERVENTIONS
Infancy		
Develop sense of trust	Multiple caregivers and frequent separations, especially if hospitalized	Encourage consistent caregivers in hospital or other care settings.
	Deprived of consistent nurturing	Encourage parental presence, "rooming in" during hospitalization, and participation in care.
Bond, or attach, to parent	Delayed because of separation; parental grief for loss of "dream" child; parental inability to accept condition, especially visible defect	Emphasize healthy, perfect qualities of infant. Help parents learn special care needs of infant for them to feel competent.
Learn through sensorimotor experiences	More exposure to painful experiences than pleasurable ones	Expose infant to pleasurable experiences through all senses (touch, hearing, sight, taste, movement).
	Limited contact with environment from restricted movement or confinement	Encourage age-appropriate developmental skills (e.g., holding bottle, finger feeding, crawling).
Begin to develop sense of separateness from parent	Increased dependency on parent for care	Encourage all family members to participate in care to prevent overinvolvement of one member.
	Overinvolvement of parent in care	Encourage periodic respite from demands of care responsibilities.
Toddlerhood		
Develop autonomy	Increased dependency on parent	Encourage independence in as many areas as possible (e.g., toileting, dressing, feeding).
Master locomotor and language skills	Limited opportunity to test own abilities and limits	Provide gross motor skill activity and modification of toys or equipment such as modified swing or rocking horse.
Learn through sensorimotor experience; beginning preoperational thought	Increased exposure to painful experiences	Give choices to allow simple feeling of control (e.g., choice of which book to look at, which kind of sandwich to eat).
		Institute age-appropriate discipline and limit setting.
		Recognize that negative and ritualistic behaviors are normal.
		Provide sensory experiences (e.g., water play, sandbox play, finger painting).
Preschool Age		
Develop initiative and purpose Master self-care skills	Limited opportunities for success in accomplishing simple tasks or mastering self-care skills	Encourage mastery of self-help skills. Provide devices that make tasks easier (e.g., self-dressing).
Begin to develop peer relationships	Limited opportunities for socialization with peers; may appear "like a baby" to age mates	Encourage socialization (e.g., inviting friends to play, day care experience, trips to park).
	Protection within tolerant and secure family, causing child to fear criticism and withdraw	Provide age-appropriate play, especially associative play opportunities.
		Emphasize child's abilities; dress appropriately to enhance desirable appearance.
Develop sense of body image and sexual identification	Awareness of body centering on pain, anxiety, and failure	Encourage relationships with same-sex and opposite-sex peers and adults.
	Sex-role identification focused primarily on mothering skills	
Learn through preoperational thought (magical thinking)	Guilt (thinking he or she caused the illness or disability or is being punished for wrongdoing)	Help child deal with criticisms; realize that too much protection prevents him or her from realities of world.
		Clarify that cause of child's illness or disability is not his or her fault or a punishment.

TABLE 36-1	DEVELOPMENTAL EFFECTS OF CHRONIC ILLNESS OR DISABILITY ON CHILDREN—cont'd	
DEVELOPMENTAL TASKS	POTENTIAL EFFECTS OF CHRONIC ILLNESS OR DISABILITY	SUPPORTIVE INTERVENTIONS
School Age		
Develop sense of accomplishment	Limited opportunities to achieve and compete (e.g., many school absences, inability to join regular athletic activities)	Encourage school attendance; schedule medical visits at times other than school; encourage child to make up missed work.
Form peer relationships	Limited opportunities for socialization	Educate teachers and classmates about child's condition, abilities, and special needs. Encourage sports activities (e.g., Special Olympics). Encourage socialization (e.g., Girl Scouts, Campfire, Boy Scouts, 4-H Club; having a best friend or club membership).
Learn through concrete operations	Incomplete comprehension of imposed physical limitations or treatment of disorder	Provide child with information about his or her condition. Encourage creative activities (e.g., VSA arts).
Adolescence		
Develop personal and sexual identity	Increased sense of feeling different from peers and reduced ability to compete with peers in appearance, abilities, special skills	Help child realize that many difficulties that teenager is experiencing are part of normal adolescence (rebelliousness, risk taking, lack of cooperation, hostility toward authority).
Achieve independence from family	Increased dependency on family; limited job or career opportunities	Provide instruction on interpersonal and coping skills. Encourage increased responsibility for care and management of disease or condition (e.g., assuming responsibility for making and keeping appointment [ideally alone], sharing assessment and planning stages of health care delivery, contacting resources). Discuss planning for future and how condition can affect choices.
Form heterosexual relationships	Limited opportunities for heterosexual friendships; less opportunity to discuss sexual concerns with peers Increased concern with issues such as why did he or she got the disorder and whether he or she can marry and have a family	Encourage socialization with peers, including peers with and without special needs. Encourage activities appropriate for age (e.g., attending mixed-sex parties, sports activities, driving a car). Be alert to cues that signal readiness for information regarding implications of condition on sexuality and reproduction. Emphasize good appearance and wearing stylish clothes, use of makeup. Understand that adolescent has same sexual needs and concerns as any other teenager.
Learn through abstract thinking	Decreased opportunity for earlier stages of cognition impeding achievement of level of abstract thinking	Provide instruction on decision making, assertiveness, and other skills necessary to manage personal plans.

enlightening. Knowledge of concurrent stresses such as financial, marital or nonmarital, and career or unemployment helps identify families who may have fewer resources to cope with the child's needs.

Finally awareness of the family members' reactions to the child and the illness or condition is important. Sample questions that the nurse and family can use to evaluate the support system, perception of the illness, coping mechanisms, resources, and concurrent stresses are listed in Table 36-2. Because factors affecting the family's response may change at any point during the illness, assessment must be a continuous process.

Special challenges exist in assessing the child's feelings about having a chronic condition. Chapter 29 presents several approaches to encourage children to discuss their feelings about their conditions. The nurse should use a variety of communication techniques such as drawing and play as assessment tools rather than relying solely on parental reports. Often children are neglected partners in their care, and their unique needs are not identified (Dixon-Woods, Young, and Henry, 1999; Young, Dixon-Woods, Windridge, et al., 2003).

The needs of working parents and siblings also should be assessed, a goal that requires flexibility in scheduling appointments to include these important family members. When working parents know that their input is valuable, they often change their work schedule to meet with a health professional. Because siblings can be

BOX 36-6   COPING PATTERNS USED BY CHILDREN WITH SPECIAL NEEDS

Develops competence and optimism—Accentuates the positive aspects of the situation and concentrates more on what he or she has or can do than on what is missing or on what he or she cannot do; is as independent as possible

Feels different and withdraws—Sees self as being different from other children because of the chronic health condition; views being different as negative; sees self as less worthy than others; focuses on things that he or she cannot do and sometimes overrestricts activities needlessly

Is irritable, is moody, and acts out—Uses proactive and self-initiated coping behaviors, although usually counterproductive in that the behaviors are not ego enhancing or socially responsible and do not result in desired outcomes; acts out irritability, which may or may not be associated with symptoms of condition

Complies with treatment—Takes necessary medications, treatments; adheres to activity restrictions; also uses behaviors that indicate developing independence (e.g., assumes responsibility for taking medication)

Seeks support—Talks with adults, children, health care providers, and nurses; develops plans to handle problems as they occur; uses downward comparison (i.e., realizes that others have it worse)

Modified from Austin J, Patterson J, Huberty T: Development of the Coping Health Inventory for children, *J Pediatr Nurs* 6(3):166–174, 1991.

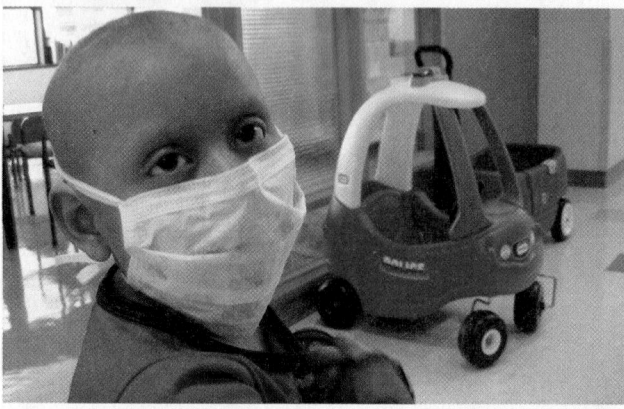

FIG 36-2 Periods of sadness and anger are appropriate in the child's adjustment to a chronic illness or disability, especially during exacerbations of the disorder.

TABLE 36-2   ASSESSMENT OF FACTORS AFFECTING FAMILY ADJUSTMENT

FACTORS AFFECTING ADJUSTMENT	ASSESSMENT QUESTIONS
Available Support System	
Status of marital relationship	To whom do you talk when you have something on your mind? (If answer is not the spouse, ask for the reason.)
Alternate support systems	When something is worrying you, what do you do? What helps you most when you are upset?
Ability to communicate	Does talking seem to help when you feel upset?
Perception of the Illness or Disability	
Previous knowledge of disorder	Have you ever heard the word (name of diagnosis) before? Tell me about it (if answer is yes).
Imagined cause of disorder	What are your thoughts about the causes of the disorder?
Effects of illness or disability on family	How has your child's illness or disability affected you and your family? How has your lifestyle changed?
Coping Mechanisms	
Reactions to previous crises	Tell me one time you've had another crisis (problem, bad time) in your family. How did you solve that problem?
Reactions to child	Do you find yourself being a little more cautious with this child than with your other children?
Childrearing practices	Do you feel as comfortable disciplining this child as your other children?
Influence of religion	Has your religion or faith been of help to you? Tell me how (if answer is yes).
Attitudes	How is this child different from the siblings or other children of similar age? Describe your child's personality. Is it easy, difficult, or in between? When you think of your child's future, what thoughts come to mind?
Available Resources	
	Which parts of your child's care are causing the most difficulty for you or your family? Which services are available to help? Which services do you need that currently are not available?
Concurrent Stresses	
	What other problems are you facing now? (Be specific; ask about financial, marital, sibling, and extended family or friends concerns.)

of any age, the use of appropriate communication strategies for assessment must be considered. Nonverbal techniques such as those discussed in Chapter 29 should be considered for these children.

Provide Support at the Time of Diagnosis

The diagnosis is a critical time for parents and can influence how they perceive their health care providers throughout care. Although they may not hear or remember all that is said to them, they frequently sense a certain attitude of acceptance, rejection, hope, or despair that may influence their ability to absorb the shock and begin adapting to the family's altered future.

Parents may be encouraged to be together when they are informed of their child's condition, thus avoiding the problem of one parent having to interpret complex findings and deal with the

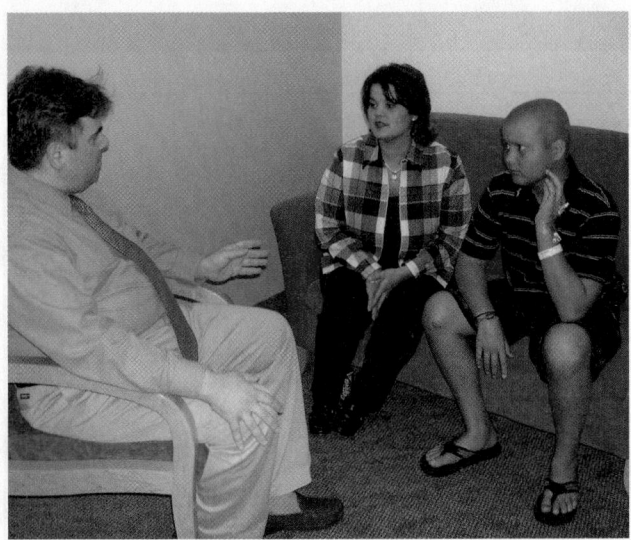

FIG 36-3 Information sessions should take place in a private, comfortable setting free of distractions and interruptions.

initial emotional reaction of the other. The informing session should take place in a private, comfortable setting free of distractions and interruptions in an atmosphere in which the parents feel free to express their emotions (Fig. 36-3). Their emotional needs are acknowledged by showing acceptance of such expressions as crying, sadness, anger, and disappointment. Emotional support is offered by having tissues available if a family member cries and demonstrating through facial and body language that indeed this is a difficult and painful period. Although touching is a powerful expression of empathy, it must be used wisely. For example, it can prematurely terminate free expression of feelings, especially when combined with statements such as, "Everything will be all right." Nurses should also be aware of cultural issues regarding touching (see Chapter 27).

Parents should receive the kind of information they desire. This can be assessed by asking questions such as, "Do you prefer to hear detailed information?" Parents or other family members may have different preferences regarding the amount of information they wish to hear. Most parents want a clear, simple explanation of the diagnosis; a prediction of possible future for the child; advice on what to do next; an opportunity to ask questions; a warm, sympathetic listener; and, most important, time. Understanding of explanations is elicited with such questions as: "Do you see what I mean?" or "Is this clear to you?" Technical terms are used with simple definitions. If the parents are unaware of the term, they are given written literature or at least a written summary of the diagnosis.

Finally the informing conference does not end with the presentation of devastating news. Instead the child's strengths, appealing behaviors, and potential for development are stressed, as are available rehabilitation efforts or treatments. Parents can be encouraged to view their experiences as a series of challenges that they are capable of handling, particularly with available professional feedback. The parents are assured that the nurse will be available to answer questions and provide further assistance as needed.

The preceding discussion relates primarily to the initial informing interview. However, because of the need for long-term follow-up, it is only one in a series of continuing discussions. In all interactions the family's input is solicited and incorporated into the care plan. Some situations require consideration of special problems (see Guidelines box).

Support the Family's Coping Methods

For the family to meet the stresses of optimally adjusting to the child's condition, each member must be supported individually so the family system is strong. Although the family can indefinitely support a member who is in need of assistance, its greatest strength lies in every member supporting one another. The nurse should bear in mind that the family member in greatest need is not necessarily the affected child but may be a parent or sibling who is dealing with stresses that require intervention.

Parents

The nurse can provide support by being attentive to families' responses to their children. Mothers and fathers need to experience success, joy, and pride in their children to give the support they need. Children, too, require support for their interactions, adjustments, and efforts. They must be reinforced for attempts to get to know their care providers and communicate their needs to them.

It is important for nurses to examine their attitudes to determine their ability to engage in parent-professional partnerships. An essential characteristic is the belief that parents are equal to professionals and are experts regarding their child (see Guidelines box on p. 1065).

Communication among all family members is encouraged. Parent group sessions can help parents verbalize thoughts and feelings to one another but often do not take into account siblings' or the child's viewpoint. Therefore the nurse may need to set up a family session such as during a home or clinic visit. Although the ideal situation is to have all the members present at one time, often this is not possible. Inviting members to participate at various visits is an appropriate alternative.

Parents can be encouraged to discuss their feelings toward the child, the impact of this event on their marriage, and associated stresses such as financial burdens. For most families, regardless of their income or insurance coverage, financial concerns exist. The costs of caring for a child with special needs can be overwhelming. In addition, the family wage earner may have to sacrifice job opportunities to remain close to a medical facility or avoid losing insurance benefits.*

The nurse regards fathers as able, effective parents who are competent and capable of coping with the challenges they face. Every effort is made to include the father in visits such as to the nursery, clinic, special school, and stimulation programs. He is included in the assessment process, with specific emphasis on having him describe the child's strengths and difficulties. It is not unusual to find two parents who have differing views of the child's abilities, especially in the area of developmental disabilities.

Numerous volunteer and community resources are available that provide assistance, rehabilitation, equipment, and funding for a variety of health problems.† National and local disease-oriented organizations may provide needed assistance and support to

---

*Information regarding financial issues is available from the Federation for Children with Special Needs, 529 Main Street, Suite 1102, Boston, MA 02129, 617-236-7210, www.fcsn.org.

†General sources of information are the Clearinghouse on Disability Information, 550 12th St SW, Room 5133, Washington, DC 20202-2550, 202-245-7307, www.ed.gov; National Dissemination Center for Children with Disabilities, 1825 Connecticut Ave NW, Washington, DC 20009, 202-884-8411 or 800-695-0285, www.nichcy.org. A comprehensive list of books and pamphlets for parents and teachers is available from the Easter Seals, 230 South Wacker Drive, Suite 2400, Chicago, IL 60606, 312-726-6200, www.easterseals.com. In Canada: Council of Canadians with Disabilities, 926-294 Portage Ave, Winnipeg, Manitoba, Canada R3C 0B9; 204-947-0303, www.ccdonline.ca.

GUIDELINES

Situations Requiring Special Consideration

Congenital Anomaly

- Tension in the delivery room conveys the sense that something is seriously wrong. Communication is often delayed while the physician is involved with the mother's care. The manner in which the infant is presented may well set the tone for the early parent-child relationship.
- Clarify role with physician in regard to revealing information to enable immediate parental support.
- Explain to parents briefly in simple language what the defect is and something concerning the immediate prognosis before showing them the infant, at which point they may be more ready to "hear" what is said.
- Be aware of nonverbal communication. Parents watch facial expressions of others for signs of revulsion or rejection.
- Present infant as something precious.
- Emphasize well-formed aspects of infant's body.
- Allow time and opportunity for parents to express their initial response.
- Encourage parents to ask questions and provide honest, straightforward answers without undue optimism or pessimism.

Cognitive Impairment

- Unless cognitive impairment is associated with other physical problems, it is often easy for parents to miss clues to its presence or make defensive excuses regarding the diagnosis.
- Plan situations that help parents become aware of the problem.
- Encourage parents to discuss their observations of child but withhold diagnostic opinions.
- Focus on what the child can do and appropriate interventions to promote progress (e.g., infant stimulation programs) to involve parents in their child's care while helping them gain an awareness of his or her condition.

Physical Disability

- If loss of motor or sensory ability occurs during childhood, the diagnosis is readily apparent. The challenge lies in helping the child and parents over the period of shock and grief and toward the phase of acceptance and reintegration.
- Institute early rehabilitation (e.g., using a prosthetic limb, learning to read braille, learning to read lips).
- Be aware that physical rehabilitation usually precedes psychologic adjustment.
- When the cause of the disability is accidental, avoid implying that parents or child was responsible for the injury but allow them the opportunity to discuss feelings of blame.
- Encourage expression of feelings (see Communication Techniques, Chapter 29).

Chronic Illness

- Realization of the true impact may take months or years. Conflict over parent's versus child's concerns may result in serious problems. When condition is inherited, parents may blame themselves, or child may blame his or her parents.
- Help each family member gain an appreciation of the others' concerns.
- Discuss hereditary aspect of condition with parents at time of diagnosis to lessen guilt and accusatory feelings.
- Encourage child to express feelings by using third-person technique (e.g., "Sometimes when a person has an illness that was passed on by the parents, that person feels angry or bitter toward them").

Multiple Disabilities

- The child or parent may require additional time for the shock phase and may be able to attend to only one diagnosis before hearing significant information regarding other disorders.
- Acknowledge parents' understanding and acceptance of all diagnoses, especially when an obvious and more hidden disability coexists.
- Appreciate the devastating consequences of more than one disability for a child, especially if they interfere with expressive-receptive abilities.

Terminal Illness

- Parents require much support to deal with their own feelings and guidance in how to tell the child the diagnosis. They may want to conceal the diagnosis from the child. They may believe that the child is too young to know, will not be able to cope with the information, or will lose hope and the will to live.
- Approach the subject of disclosure in a positive way by asking, "How will you tell your child about the diagnosis?"
- Help parents understand the disadvantages of not telling children (e.g., deprives them of the opportunity to discuss their feelings openly and ask questions, incurs the risk of their learning the truth from outside and sometimes less tactful sources, may lessen children's trust and confidence in their parents after they learn the truth).
- Guide parents to see the potential problems involved in fostering a conspiracy.
- Offer parents guidelines for how and what to tell children about their disease or the possibility of death. Explanations should be tailored to child's cognitive ability, be based on knowledge child already has, and be honest. Honesty must be tempered with concern for child's feelings.
- Assure parents that telling a child the name of the illness and the reason for treatment instills hope, provides support from others, and serves as a foundation for explaining and understanding subsequent events.
- Acknowledge that being honest is not always easy because the truth may prompt children to ask other distressing questions such as, "Am I going to die?" However, even this difficult question must be answered.

families that qualify. Many of these are discussed elsewhere in this text under the specific diagnosis. State and federal departments of health, mental health, social service, and labor may be able to help locate appropriate regional resources. For example, state programs for Children with Special Health Needs (formerly Crippled Children's Services) provide financial assistance for children with many disabling conditions. Local and national sources of respite care and medical day care may be useful to families. Nurses should become acquainted with those in their communities and with vocational programs for special groups.

Parent-to-Parent Support. Just being with another parent who has shared similar experiences is helpful. It may not need to be a parent of a child with the same diagnosis because parents in the process of adjusting to a child with special needs—or finding respite services, educational or rehabilitative services, special equipment vendors, and financial counseling—tread a common path. If the agency does not have a parent staff position, the nurse can contact parent groups who will often send a representative. Another strategy is to ask another parent to talk to the parents. The nurse should seek out a parent who is a good listener, has a nonjudgmental approach

GUIDELINES

Developing Successful Parent-Professional Partnerships

- Promote primary nursing; in nonhospital settings, designate a case manager.
- Acknowledge parents' overall competence and their unique expertise with their child.
- Respect parents' time as having value equal to that of other members of child's health care team.
- Explain or define any medical, technical, or discipline-specific terms.
- Tell families, "I am not sure" or "I don't know" when appropriate.
- Facilitate family's effectiveness in team meetings (e.g., provide parents with same information as other participants).

GUIDELINES

Promoting Normalization

Preparation—Prepare child in advance for changes that may occur from the chronic or complex condition.
Example—Tell the child in advance the possible side effects of drug therapy.

Participation—Include child in as many decisions as possible, especially those relating to his or her care regimen.
Example—The child is responsible for taking medications or scheduling home treatments.

Sharing—Allow both family members and child's peers to be a part of the care regimen whenever possible.
Examples—Give the child his or her medication when the other siblings receive their vitamins.
The parent cooks the same menu for the whole family.
If the child is invited to another's home, the parent advises the family of the child's dietary restrictions.

Control—Identify areas in which child can be in control so feelings of uncertainty, passivity, and helplessness are decreased.
Example—The child identifies activities that are appropriate to his or her energy level and chooses to rest when fatigued.

Expectation—Apply the same family rules to the child with a complex chronic illness as to the well siblings or peers.
Example—The child is disciplined, is expected to fulfill household responsibilities, and attends school in accordance with abilities.

to differences in families, and possesses good advocacy and problem-solving skills.

The parent self-help group is another way to promote parent-to-parent support.* Group members feel less alone and have the opportunity to observe both coping and mastery role modeling from other members. Parents' groups are rich resources for information. Even if parents are unable to attend meetings, they can still benefit from group newsletters and other literature that often accompany membership. The nurse can foster parent participation in self-help groups by serving as a referral agent, a group advisory board member, a resource person, a group member, or an assistant in founding a group. Sometimes all that is required in starting a group is to identify one or two parents as leaders; share with them the names, telephone numbers, and addresses of other families who have expressed both an interest and a willingness to release their phone number and address; and guide them in how to initiate a first meeting.

Advocate for Empowerment. Nurses can advocate for methods that foster opportunities for parent empowerment. For example, they can suggest reimbursement for travel and child care plus stipends to enable parents' voices to be heard at meetings and conferences. They can encourage parent membership on committees and advisory boards. They can keep parents informed of pending legislation on child health issues or take action when parents inform them.

The Child

Through ongoing contacts with the child, the nurse (1) observes his or her responses to the disorder, ability to function, and adaptive behaviors within the environment and with significant others; (2) explores the child's own understanding of his or her illness or condition; and (3) provides support while the child learns to cope with his or her feelings. Children are encouraged to express their concerns rather than allow others to express them for them because open discussions may reduce anxiety.

One of the most important interventions is alleviating the child's feeling of being different and normalizing his or her life as much as possible (see Guidelines box). Whenever possible, the nurse helps the family assess the child's daily routine for indications of a need for normalizing practices. For example, the child who remains in a bedroom all day requires a restructured daily routine to provide

activities in different parts of the house such as eating in the kitchen or dining room with the family. Such children may also be deprived of social, recreational, and academic activities that can be better accommodated by applying normalization practices. For example, home and out-of-home health-related treatments should be planned at times that least interfere with normal daily activities.

Children who are concerned that their condition detracts from their physical attractiveness need attention focused on the normal aspects of appearance and capabilities. Health professionals help strengthen and consolidate the self-image by emphasizing the normal while allowing children to express anger, isolation, fear of rejection, feelings of sadness, and loneliness. The children need positive reinforcement for compliance and any evidence of improvement. Anything that might improve attractiveness and contribute to a positive self-image is used such as makeup for a teenager with a scar, clothing that disguises a prosthesis, or a hairstyle or wig to cover a deformity or lost hair.

Siblings

The presence of a child with special needs in a family may result in parents paying less attention to the other children. Siblings may respond by developing negative attitudes toward the child or expressing anger in different forms. The nurse can help by using anticipatory guidance, questioning the parents about what they believe is the best way to have siblings respond to the child, and guiding them through ways to meet their other children's needs for attention. This questioning should take place before serious negative effects occur.

Siblings may also experience embarrassment associated with having a brother or sister with a chronic or complex condition. Parents are then faced with the difficulty of responding to this embarrassment in an understanding and appropriate manner without punishing the siblings for how they feel. They are

---

*Information about self-help groups is available from the American Self-Help Group Clearinghouse, www.selfhelpgroups.org.

encouraged to talk with the siblings about how they view their affected sibling. For example, siblings of a child with developmental disabilities may express fears about their ability to bear normal children. Adolescents in particular may not be able to discuss these vital issues with their parents and may prefer to consult with the nurse. Many siblings benefit from sharing their concerns with other young people who are experiencing a similar situation. Support groups for siblings can help decrease isolation, promote expression of feelings, and provide examples of effective coping skills.

Many parents express concern about when and how to inform the other children in the family about a sibling's illness or disability. The answer depends on each child's level of sophistication and understanding. However, it is usually best to inform the siblings before a neighbor or other nonfamily member does so. Uninformed siblings may fantasize or develop apprehensions that are out of proportion to the child's actual condition. Furthermore, if parents choose to be silent or deceptive about the issue, they are setting a negative precedent for the siblings to follow rather than encouraging them to cope with the experience in a healthy and nurturing way.

The nurse is sensitive to the reactions of siblings and whenever possible intervenes to promote more positive adjustment. For example, siblings often mention that they are expected to take on additional responsibilities to help the parents care for the child. It is not unusual for them to express a positive reaction to assuming the extra duties but a negative response to feeling unappreciated for doing so. Such feelings can often be minimized by encouraging siblings to discuss this with the parents and suggesting to parents ways of showing gratitude such as an increase in allowance; special privileges; and, most significantly, verbal praise.

Educate About the Disorder and General Health Care

Educating the family about the disorder is actually an extension of revealing the diagnosis. Education involves not only supplying technical information but also discussing how the condition will affect the child. Parents may be able to digest only so much information at a time. It may be helpful to provide essential information and then follow by asking, "What else would you like to know about your child's condition?" Responding to parents' questions and concerns ensures that their information needs are met.

Activities of Daily Living

Parents also need guidance in how the condition may interfere with or alter activities of daily living such as eating, dressing, sleeping, and toileting. One area frequently affected is nutrition. Common problems are undernutrition resulting from food being inappropriately restricted or loss of appetite, vomiting, or motor deficits that interfere with feeding; overnutrition may also occur, usually because of a caloric intake in excess of energy expenditure or boredom and lack of stimulation in other areas. Although the child requires the same basic nutrients as other children, the daily requirements may differ. Special nutritional considerations are discussed as appropriate throughout this text.

Safe Transportation

Modifications may also be needed regarding car safety. Children with conditions such as low birth weight or orthopedic, neuromuscular, or respiratory impairments often cannot safely use conventional car restraints. For example, children with hip spica casts cannot sit properly in child safety seats (see Developmental Dysplasia of the Hip, Chapter 48). Modifications can be made to some commercial models, and for older children a special vest is available that secures the child to the back seat in a lying-down position.*

If a child requires a wheelchair, the family should consult the wheelchair manufacturer for specific instructions regarding safe car transportation. Considerations for wheelchairs used with vehicle transportation must address securing both the wheelchair and the occupant in the wheelchair. Wheelchairs should be secured facing forward with tie downs at four points. The tie-down system should be dynamically crash tested, as should the occupant securement system that secures the child in the wheelchair. For example, use of trays is not recommended for transportation. With children who must travel with additional medical equipment, this equipment (e.g., oxygen, monitors, or ventilators) should be anchored to the floor or underneath the vehicle seat or wheelchair. Soft padding should be added around the equipment to reduce movement. A second adult should be present to monitor the condition of a medically fragile child while traveling.

Primary Health Care

Children with special needs require all the usual health care recommended for any child. Attention to injury prevention, immunizations, dental health, and regular physical examinations is essential. Nurses can play an important role in reminding parents of these aspects of care that are so often neglected when the concern is focused on the child's chronic condition. Specific discussions of nutrition, sleep and activity, dental health, and injury prevention are presented in the chapters on health promotion for specific age-groups. Immunizations are discussed in Chapter 31.

Parents also need to be aware of the importance of communicating the child's condition in the event of a medical emergency. Young children are unable to give information about their disorders; and, although older children may be reliable sources, after an accident they may be physically unable to speak. Therefore all children with any type of chronic condition that may affect medical care should wear some type of identification such as a MedicAlert bracelet† or carry a card in their wallet that lists the medical condition and a phone number for emergency medical records and other personal information.

Promote Normal Development

Aside from knowledge of the condition and its effect on the child's abilities, the family must be guided toward fostering appropriate development in their child. Although each stage may take longer to achieve, parents are guided toward helping the child fully realize his or her potential in preparation for the next developmental stage. Table 36-1 outlines developmental aspects of complex conditions and supportive interventions. With appropriate planning and knowledge of strategies to improve the child's functional abilities, most children can live fulfilling and productive lives.

One important aspect of promoting normal development is to encourage the child's self-care abilities in both activities of daily living and the medical regimen. An assessment of the child's age and physical, emotional, and mental capacities together with the support and structure provided by the family should be considered in determining the appropriate level of self-care in the medical regimen.

---

*Information on car safety restraints for children with special needs is available from the Automotive Safety Program, 1120 South Drive, Fesler Hall Room 207, Indianapolis, IN 46202, 800-543-6227 or 317-274-2997, www.preventinjury.org.
†MedicAlert Foundation International, 2323 Colorado Ave, Turlock, CA 95382, 888-633-4298, www.medicalert.org.

BOX 36-7   CHARACTERISTICS OF PARENTAL OVERPROTECTION

- Sacrifices self and rest of family for child
- Continually helps child even when child is capable
- Is inconsistent with regard to discipline or uses no discipline; frequently applies different rules to siblings
- Is dictatorial and arbitrary, making decisions without considering child's wishes such as keeping child from attending school
- Hovers and offers suggestions; calls attention to every activity; overdoes praise
- Protects child from every possible discomfort
- Restricts play, often because of fear that child will be injured
- Denies child opportunities for growing up and assuming responsibility such as learning to give own medications or perform treatments
- Does not understand child's capabilities and sets goals too high or too low
- Monopolizes child's time such as sleeping with child, permitting few friends, or refusing participation in social or educational activities

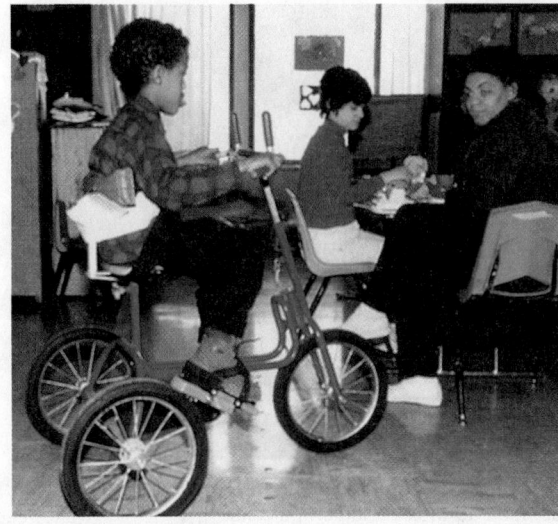

FIG 36-4 A modified tricycle with block pedals, self-adhesive straps for support, and a modified seat and handle bars can help a child with disabilities gain mobility.

Even toddlers can be involved in their own care by holding supplies for the parent during a procedure. Over time children should be encouraged toward greater autonomy in the self-care arena.

Early Childhood

During infancy the child is achieving basic trust through a satisfying, intimate, consistent relationship with his or her parents. However, affected children's early existence may be stressful, chaotic, and unsatisfying. Consequently they may need more parental support and expressions of affection to achieve trust. Likewise the parents require assistance in finding ways to meet the infant's needs such as how to hold a rigid or flaccid infant, how to feed a child with tongue thrust or episodes of dyspnea, and how to stimulate a child who seems incapable of achieving any skills. If hospitalizations are frequent or prolonged, every effort is made to preserve the parent-child relationship (see also Chapter 38). Hospital policies should promote visitation by and involvement of families.

During early childhood the goal is to achieve separation from parents, autonomy, and initiative. However, the natural parental response to having a sick child is overprotection (Box 36-7). Parents need help in realizing the importance of the child's brief separations from them and others involved in his or her care and of providing social experiences outside the home whenever possible. Respite care, which provides temporary relief for family members, can be essential in allowing caregivers time away from the daily burdens.

Young children also need the opportunity to develop independence. Frequently the child is able to learn self-help skills such as holding a bottle, finger feeding, and removing simple articles of clothing; but the parent continues to perform the act. The nurse can guide parents to the usual milestones expected from the child. When a child is unable to perform a skill independently, functional aids should be used. With innovation many adaptations can be implemented in children's environments to increase their mobility and independence and allow them to play like other children their age. For example, with slight modifications a child with physical limitations may be able to ride a tricycle (Fig. 36-4).

Another critical component for normal child development is discipline. Discipline and guidance serve several purposes (e.g., providing children with boundaries on which to test their behavior and

teaching them socially acceptable behavior). Resentment and hostility can arise among siblings if different standards are applied to each child. The nurse's responsibility is to help parents learn successful methods of managing a child's behaviors before they become problems.

School Age

For school-age children the major tasks are entry into school and achieving a sense of industry. Although the importance of school in the life of all children is well known, school absences are significantly higher among children with chronic illnesses than among their healthy peers. The more school absences the child experiences, the more difficult it is to resume attendance, and school phobia may result. The child should return to school as soon as possible after diagnosis or treatments.

Preparation for entry into or resumption of school is best accomplished through a team approach with the parents, child, teacher, school nurse, and primary nurse in the hospital. Ideally this planning should begin before hospital discharge, provided that the child is well enough to resume usual activities. A structured plan should be developed, with attention to aspects of care that must be continued during school hours such as administration of medication or other treatments.

Children also need preparation before entering or resuming school. Having a tutor in the hospital or home as soon as children are physically able helps them realize that school will continue and gives them time to consider this prospect (Fig. 36-5). They need to investigate possible answers to the many questions others will ask. One method of anticipatory preparation is to role-play, with the child as the "returned pupil" and the nurse or parent as "other schoolmates." If the child returns to school with some obvious physical change such as hair loss, amputation, or a visible scar, the nurse might also ask questions about these alterations to prompt preparatory responses from the child.

Classroom peers also need preparation; a joint plan of the teacher, nurse, and child is best. At a minimum classmates should be given a description of the child's condition, prepared for any visible changes in the child, and allowed an opportunity to ask questions. The child should have the option of attending this session. As the child's condition changes, particularly if the illness is potentially

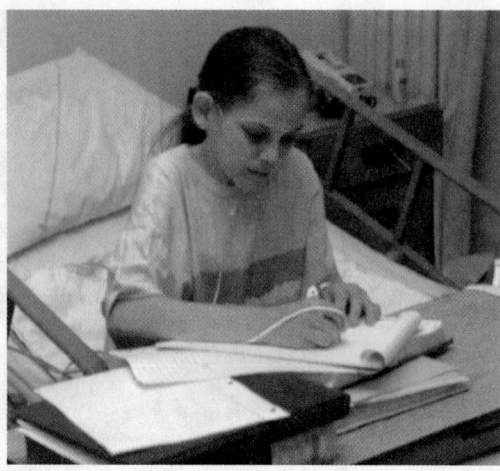

FIG 36-5 Children with disabilities should continue their schooling as soon as their condition permits.

fatal, school personnel, including the students, need periodic appraisal of his or her status and preparation for what to expect.

Children with special needs are encouraged to maintain or reestablish relationships with peers and participate according to their capabilities in any age-appropriate activities. Alternative activities may be substituted for those that are impossible or place a strain on the child's condition. Programs such as the Special Olympics* offer children an opportunity to compete with their peers and achieve athletic skill. Summer camps† allow children to associate with peers and develop a wide variety of skills. Children with special needs can derive enormous benefits from expressive activities such as art, music, poetry, dance, and drama. With adaptive equipment and imagination children can participate in a variety of activities. Organizations such as VSA Arts allow children to celebrate and share their accomplishments.‡ They need the opportunity to interact with healthy peers and engage in activities with groups or clubs composed of similarly affected age-mates. Such organizations as ostomy clubs, diabetes clubs, and cerebral palsy groups share information and provide support related to the special problems the members face.

Adolescence

Adolescence can be a particularly difficult period for the teenager and family. All of the needs discussed previously apply to this age-group as well. However, developing independence or autonomy is a major task for the adolescent as planning for the future becomes a prominent concern. Although the emphasis in the past has been on achieving independence from physical assistance, recent developments in the fields of special education, adolescent development, and family systems suggest redefining autonomy in terms of individuals' capacities to take responsibility for their own behavior, make decisions regarding their own lives, and maintain supportive social relationships. Given this understanding, even individuals with severe impairments can be viewed as autonomous if they perceive their own needs and take responsibility for meeting them, either directly or by engaging the assistance of others. As adolescents become more autonomous, the nurse can help them articulate their needs, participate in developing their own care plans, and discover and express how others can be of greatest assistance.

Physical symptoms are high on teenagers' list of health-related concerns. Because adolescence is a time of enormous physical and emotional changes, it is important for the nurse to distinguish between body changes that are related to the child's complex condition and those that are a result of normal body development. It can be a great comfort for teenagers with disabling conditions to know that many of the changes they experience are normal developmental outcomes.

A sense of feeling different from peers can lead to loneliness, isolation, and depression. Participation in groups of teenagers with chronic conditions or disabilities can alleviate feelings of isolation and smooth the transition to a meaningful relationship with one person in adulthood.

Establish Realistic Future Goals

One of the most difficult adjustments is setting realistic future goals for the child that are based on the child's own goals and values. Sometimes the impact of this decision does not surface until the child finishes school or the parents approach retirement, when a crisis can arise because of disruption of all of the family roles and relationships that maintained stability.

Planning for the future should be a gradual process. All along the parents should cultivate realistic vocations for the child. For example, if children have physical disabilities, they are directed to intellectual, artistic, or musical pursuits. Children with developmental disabilities are taught manual skills. In this way the child's development proceeds in the direction of self-support through gainful employment.

With prolonged survival young people with chronic illnesses must deal with new decisions and problems such as marriage, employment, and insurance coverage. With appropriate guidance individuals with disabilities can attain gainful employment, marriage, and a family. For those whose conditions are genetic, counseling is needed regarding future offspring. Prospective spouses often benefit from an opportunity to discuss their feelings regarding marriage to an individual with continued health needs and possibly a limited life span. Health insurance coverage is a critical issue for chronically ill children because of their enormous health care costs over time. The Affordable Care Act allows young adults to remain on their parents' insurance until 26 years of age and prevents private insurance carriers from denying them coverage. Life insurance is another dilemma, especially when children have serious conditions such as congenital heart anomalies.

PERSPECTIVES ON THE CARE OF CHILDREN AT THE END OF LIFE

Although most childhood illnesses and many injuries and other trauma respond favorably to treatment, some do not. When a child and family face a prolonged and life-limiting illness, health

---

*1133 19th St NW, Washington, DC 20036, 202-628-3630, www.specialolympics.org. Several pamphlets on sports and recreation for children with disabilities are available from Easter Seals (see footnote, p. 1063) and American Alliance for Health, Physical Education, Recreation and Dance, 1900 Association Drive, Reston, VA 20191, 703-476-3400 or 800-213-7193, www.aahperd.org.

†A directory of private and paying camps for children with a variety of chronic illnesses and general physical disabilities is available from the American Camp Association, 5000 State Road 67 North, Martinsville, IN 46151-7902, 765-342-8456 or 800-428-2267, www.acacamps.org.

‡VSA Arts has affiliate chapters in all 50 states and in selected sites internationally; annual festivals are held throughout the world. Information is available from The John F Kennedy Center for the Performing Arts, VSA Arts, 2700 F Street, NW Washington, DC 20566, 202-467-4600 or 800-444-1324, www.vsarts.org.

professionals must confront the challenge of providing the best possible care to meet the physical, psychologic, spiritual, and emotional needs of the child and family during the uncertain course of the illness and at the time of death. When death is sudden and unexpected, nurses are challenged to respond to grief and shock in families and provide comfort and support in the absence of a prior relationship.

Many factors affect the causes of death that nurses are likely to encounter in children, including developmental factors, medical advances and technology, and changing social patterns. In infants the leading causes of death are congenital anomalies, respiratory distress syndrome, disorders related to short gestation and low birth weight, and sudden infant death syndrome (Arias, MacDorman, Strobino, et al., 2003) (see Chapter 26). The leading causes of death in children 5 to 9 years of age include injuries (accidents), malignant neoplasms, congenital anomalies, assault (homicide), and heart disease. In children 10 to 14 years of age suicide is the third leading cause of death after injuries (accidents) and malignant neoplasms. In youths 15 to 19 years of age assault (homicide), suicide, malignant neoplasms, and heart disease follow accidents as the most prevalent causes of death (Anderson and Smith, 2005).

A child who is diagnosed with a life-threatening illness or suffering serious, life-threatening trauma needs medical diagnosis and intervention and nursing assessment and care—sometimes for a short time and sometimes over a lengthy period. When cure is no longer possible and life-prolonging measures result in pain and distress to the child, parents need information about care options that are available to help them decide how they want the remaining time with their child to be managed by the health care team. It is important that families be reassured that, although their child cannot be cured, active care will continue to be provided to maintain his or her comfort. Support is provided to assist the child and family during the dying process. As a result nurses may care for children and families who are making the difficult transition from curative or restorative treatments to palliative care.

Principles of Palliative Care

Palliative care involves a multidisciplinary approach to the care of children living with or dying from chronic, complex or potentially life-limiting conditions with a primary focus on symptom control, supportive care, and quality of life rather than on cure or life prolongation in the absence of the possibility of a cure (Field and Behrman, 2004). The World Health Organization (WHO) (1996) defines palliative care as the "active total care of patients whose disease is not responsive to curative treatment. Control of pain; other symptoms; and psychologic, social, and spiritual problems is paramount. The goal of palliative care is the achievement of the best possible quality of life for patients and their families." This goal is certainly compatible with care for patients who are pursuing curative or life-prolonging therapy. Therefore there should be a distinction between palliative and end-of-life care: end-of-life care is a part of palliative care, but the goals of palliative care extend to all aspects of a patient's quality of life and can be established early in the trajectory of a patient's disease. The WHO (1998) amended the definition of palliative care for children to include:

- Palliative care for children is the active total care of the child's body, mind, and spirit and involves giving support to the family.
- It begins when illness is diagnosed and continues regardless of whether or not a child receives treatment directed at the disease.

- Health providers must evaluate and alleviate the child's physical, psychologic, and social distress.
- Effective palliative care requires a broad multidisciplinary approach that includes the family and makes use of available community resources; it can be implemented successfully even if resources are limited.
- It can be provided in tertiary care facilities, in community health centers, and even in children's homes.

Palliative care interventions do not serve to hasten death; rather they provide pain and symptom management, attention to issues faced by the child and family with regard to death and dying, and promotion of optimal functioning and quality of life during the time the child has remaining. The implementation of neonatal and pediatric palliative care consulting services within hospitals has led to enhanced quality of life and end-of-life care for children and their families and support for their care providers (Jennings, 2005; Pierucci, Kirby, and Leuthner, 2001). Several principles are hallmarks of palliative care.

The child and family are considered the unit of care. The death of a child is an extremely stressful event for a family because it is out of the natural order of things. Children represent health and hope, and their death calls into question the understanding of life. A multidisciplinary team of health care professionals consisting of social workers, chaplains, nurses, personal care aides, and health care providers skilled in caring for dying patients assist the family by focusing care on the complex interactions among physical, emotional, social, and spiritual issues.

Palliative care seeks to create a therapeutic environment as homelike as possible, if not in the child's own home. Through education and support of family members, an atmosphere of open communication is provided regarding the child's dying process and its impact on all members of the family (see Evidence-Based Practice box).

Decision Making at the End of Life

Discussions concerning the possibility that a child's illness or condition is not curable and that death is an inevitable outcome cause everyone involved a great deal of stress. Physicians, other members of the health care team, and families must consider all information regarding the child's situation and make decisions to which all parties agree and that will have a profound impact on the child and family.

Ethical Considerations in End-of-Life Decision Making

A number of ethical concerns arise when parents and health care professionals are deciding on the best course of care for the dying child. Many parents and health care providers are concerned that not offering treatment that would cause potential pain and suffering but might extend life would be considered euthanasia or assisted suicide. To eliminate such concerns it is necessary to understand the various terms. Euthanasia involves an action carried out by a person other than the patient to end the life of the patient suffering from a terminal condition. The intent of this action is based on the belief that the act is "putting the person out of his or her misery"; this action has also been called mercy killing. Assisted suicide occurs when someone provides the patient with the means to end his or her life and the patient uses that means to do so. The important distinction between these two actions involves who is actually acting to end the person's life.

The American Nurses Association *Code of Ethics for Nurses* (2001) does not support the active intent on the part of a nurse to end a person's life. However, it does permit the nurse to provide

EVIDENCE-BASED PRACTICE

Pediatric Pain and Symptom Management at the End of Life

Ask the Question

In children, what is the pain and symptom experience at the end of life?

Search for Evidence

Search Strategies

Published studies from 2000 to 2005 using the subject terms *child, palliative care, pain,* and *symptoms* were identified and examined. Retrospective descriptive studies dominated the findings describing infants' and children's end-of-life experiences through the use of medical record reviews and provider and parental surveys.

Databases Used

PubMed, CINAHL

Critically Analyze the Evidence

Children experienced an average of 11 symptoms during their last week of life (Drake, Frost, and Collins, 2003). Pain, dyspnea, and fatigue were the most frequently documented symptoms experienced by most children at the end of life (Bradshaw, Hinds, Lensing, et al., 2005; Carter, Howenstein, Gilmer, et al., 2004; Drake, Frost, and Collins, 2003; Hongo, Chieko, Okada, et al., 2003). Children and their parents report high distress with pain and symptoms at the end of life. Parents reported pain and suffering as one of the most important factors in deciding to withhold or withdraw life support from their child in the pediatric intensive care unit (Meert, Thurston, and Sarnaik, 2000).

Documentation was scarce related to symptom management. Morphine was the most commonly prescribed pain medication (Drake, Frost, and Collins, 2003; Hongo, Chieko, Okada, et al., 2003). Parents reported their children as experiencing high levels of pain near the end of life (Contro, Larson, Scofield, et al., 2002). Physicians were more likely than nurses or parents to report that a child's pain and symptoms were well managed at the end of life, but the majority of both provider groups believed that the child's physical management was difficult (Andresen, Seecharan, and Toce, 2004; Wolfe, Grier, Klar, et al., 2000).

Barriers to the adequate provision of pediatric palliative care include developmental issues specific to infants and children; symptoms, their causes, how they are related, and effective treatment strategies; lack of education; and reimbursement issues (Harris, 2004). Physicians report reliance on trial and error as they learn to care for children at the end of life and the need for specialty consultations with palliative care service providers (Hilden, Emanuel, Fairclough, et al., 2001).

Apply the Evidence: Nursing Implications

There is *moderate quality evidence with strong recommendations* for better pain management at the end of life (Guyatt, Oxman, Vist, et al., 2008). Although the philosophy of palliative care encompasses pain and symptom management for infants and children who may not outlive their disease, making that care available to ease suffering and provide comfort to those who will die continues to lag. Studies show that children experience significant pain and other distressing symptoms at the end of life that are not well managed. Discrepancies in perceptions of infants' and children's pain and suffering continue to exist between providers and parents. Barriers to

providing pediatric palliative care exist. Improvements are needed in the management of pain and symptoms at the end of life for infants and children.

Quality and Safety Competencies:
Evidence-Based Practice*

Knowledge

Differentiate clinical opinion from research and evidence-based summaries.

Describe common symptoms experienced at the end of life.

Skills

Base individualized care plan on patient values, clinical expertise, and evidence.

Integrate evidence into practice by carefully assessing pain and other symptoms in children at the end of life.

Attitudes

Value the concept of evidence-based practice as integral to determining best clinical practice.

Appreciate strengths and weakness of evidence for symptom assessment and management at the end of life.

References

Andresen EM, Seecharan GA, Toce SS: Provider perceptions of child deaths, *Arch Pediatr Adolesc Med* 158:430–435, 2004.

Bradshaw G, Hinds PS, Lensing S, et al: Cancer-related deaths in children and adolescents, *J Palliat Med* 8(1):86–95, 2005.

Carter BS, Howenstein BS, Gilmer MJ, et al: Circumstances surrounding the deaths of hospitalized children: opportunities for pediatric palliative care, *Pediatrics* 114(3):361–366, 2004.

Contro N, Larson J, Scofield S, et al: Family perspectives on the quality of pediatric palliative care, *Arch Pediatr Adolesc Med* 156:1–29, 2002.

Drake R, Frost J, Collins JJ: The symptoms of dying children, *J Pain Symptom Manage* 26(1):594–603, 2003.

Guyatt GH, Oxman AD, Vist GE, et al: GRADE: an emerging consensus on rating quality of evidence and strength of recommendations, *BMJ* 336:924–926, 2008.

Harris B: Palliative care in children with cancer: which child and when? *J Natl Cancer Institute Mono* 32:144–149, 2004.

Hilden JM, Emanuel EJ, Fairclough DL, et al: Attitudes and practices among pediatric oncologists regarding end-of-life care: results of the 1998 American Society of Clinical Oncology Survey, *J Clin Oncol* 19(1):205–212, 2001.

Hongo T, Chieko W, Okada S, et al: Analysis of the circumstances at the end of life in children with cancer: symptoms, suffering and acceptance, *Pediatr Int* 45:60–64, 2003.

Meert KL, Thurston CS, Sarnaik AP: End-of-life decision-making and satisfaction with care: parental perspectives, *Pediatr Crit Care Med* 1(2):179–185, 2000.

Wolfe J, Grier HE, Klar N, et al: Symptoms and suffering at the end of life in children with cancer, *N Engl J Med* 342(5):326–333, 2000.

*Adapted from the QSEN at www.qsen.org/.

interventions to relieve symptoms in the dying patient even when the interventions involve substantial risks of hastening death. When the prognosis for a patient is poor and death is the expected outcome, it is ethically acceptable to withhold or withdraw treatments that may cause pain and suffering and provide interventions that promote comfort and quality of life. Therefore providing palliative care for patients is the ethically correct choice in such a circumstance.

Physician–Health Care Team Decision Making

Decisions by health care providers regarding care are often made on the basis of the progression of the disease or amount of trauma, the availability of treatment options that would provide cure from disease or restoration of health, the impact of such treatments on the child, and the child's overall prognosis (Davis and Eng, 1998). Often the main determinants prompting health care providers to discuss end-of-life issues and options for children with critical illnesses include the child's age, premorbid cognitive condition and functional status, pain or discomfort, probability of survival, and quality of life (Masri, Farrell, Lacroix, et al., 2000). When the health care provider discusses this information openly with families, a shared decision-making process can occur regarding do not resuscitate (DNR) orders and care that is focused on the comfort of the child and family during the dying process.

Unfortunately many families are not given the option of terminating treatment and pursuing care that is focused on comfort and quality of life when cure is unlikely, and staff may be reluctant to raise the question of DNR orders. This occurs for a number of reasons, including the belief that not being able to "save" a child is a "failure." In addition, the physician and other members of the health care team may lack knowledge of and experience with the principles of palliative care (Field and Behrman, 2004; Sahler, Frager, Levetown, et al., 2000; Sumner, 2003).

Parental Decision Making

Rarely are families prepared to cope with the numerous decisions that must be made when a child is dying. When the death is unexpected, as in the case of an accident or trauma, the confusion of emergency services and possibly an intensive care setting presents challenges to parents as they are asked to make difficult choices. If the child has either experienced a life-threatening illness such as cancer or lived with a chronic illness that has now reached its terminal phase, parents are often unprepared for the reality of their child's impending death (see Family-Centered Care box). Numerous studies have found that families facing the impending death of a child depend on information provided to them by the health care team, particularly an honest appraisal of the child's prognosis, to make difficult decisions regarding care options for their children (Hinds, Oakes, Furman, et al., 2001; James and Johnson, 1997; Wolfe, Friebert, and Hilden, 2002).

As the group of health professionals that is most involved with families, nurses are in an excellent position to ensure that families are presented with the options available to them. The nurse's first responsibility is to explore the family's wishes. This is best done in concert with the physician but at times may need to be initiated by the nurse. Statements such as, "Tell me about your thoughts for the type of care you want your child to receive when he is dying." or "Have you considered the types of interventions you would like us to use when your child is near death?" can begin discussion of this sensitive but critical aspect of terminal care.

👪 FAMILY-CENTERED CARE

Family of the Dying Child

No matter whether you have a PhD or many children, when your child dies it is a new experience, and nothing can prepare you for it. Like so many things in life, experience is the best teacher.

Three of our children have died, and by the time the third was dying, we handled many things differently. We learned a lot about dignity and the rights of the child and family. For example, at first we didn't know that we had a right to have our child die at home. We also didn't understand pain medications and that, if children are taking these medicines and are still in agony, they have not overdosed on the medication.

We learned a lot about case management. With our first two children, lots of different people were making decisions and disagreeing about what was best and what should be done. No one had primary authority. With our third child, one doctor took a primary role. Any questions and problems were handled by one person. I could call him 24 hours a day. It made a lot of difference, and I felt our concerns and needs were better heard and respected.

The nurses caring for our third child at home enabled me to step back and just be his mommy. When I could do this, I realized that we were fighting so hard for his life that we weren't really letting him die. His nurses had worked with him for a long time and really loved him. It was hard for them when we decided to let him die. In his last several days we wanted a lot of family time with our son, and I think the nurses felt left out. Something about their reaction to our increased time with him in the last few days made us feel guilty. If we had all been able to communicate a little more openly, I would have understood that they needed more time with him at the end, too. Everyone's needs could have been met.

Jeni Stepanek
Mother
Upper Marlboro, MD

The Dying Child

Children need honest and accurate information about their illness, treatments, and prognosis; this information needs to be given in clear, simple language. In most situations this best occurs as a gradual process over time characterized by increasingly open dialog among parents, professionals, and the child (Young, Dixon-Woods, Windridge, et al., 2003). Providing an atmosphere of open communication early in the course of an illness facilitates answering difficult questions as the child's condition worsens. Providing appropriate literature about the disease and the experience of illness and possible death is also helpful. Exactly how and when to involve children in decisions regarding care during their dying process and death is an individual matter. The child's age or developmental level is an important consideration in the process (Table 36-3). In general parents should be asked how they would like their child to be told of his or her prognosis, and they should be included in his or her care. Some parents may request that their child not be told that he or she is dying even if the child asks. This often places health care providers in a difficult situation. Children, even at a young age, are perceptive. Even if they are not told outright that they are dying, they realize that something is seriously wrong and that it involves them. Often helping parents understand that honesty and shared decision making between them and their child are important to the child's and family's emotional health encourages parents to allow discussion of dying with their child. Parents may require professional support and guidance in this process from a nurse, social worker, or child life specialist who has a good relationship with the child and family.

If given the opportunity, children will tell others how much they want to know. Asking questions such as, "If the disease came back, would you want to know?" "Do you want others to tell you everything even if the news isn't good?" or "If someone were not getting better [or more directly, "were dying"], do you think he would want to know?" helps children set the limits of how much truth they can cope with and accept. Children need time to process many feelings and much information so they can assimilate and ideally accept the inevitable fact of mortality.

Care of dying adolescents requires the nurse to become knowledgeable about any possible delays or alterations in normal growth and development. Legal and ethical issues also come to the forefront with respect to the age at which an adolescent should have autonomy in decision making with regard to care and treatment. Effective communication among the patient, family, and health care team is an important part of optimal care for dying adolescents (Freyer, 2004).

Treatment Options for Terminally Ill Children

Based on the child and family's decision regarding their wishes for terminal care, they have several options from which to choose.

Hospital. Families may choose to remain in the hospital to receive care if the child's illness or condition is unstable and home care is not an option or the family is uncomfortable with providing care at home. If a family chooses to remain at the hospital for terminal care, the setting should be made as homelike as possible. Families are encouraged to bring familiar items from the child's

TABLE 36-3	CHILDREN'S UNDERSTANDING OF AND REACTIONS TO DEATH	
CONCEPTS OF DEATH	**REACTIONS TO DEATH**	**NURSING CARE MANAGEMENT**
Infants and Toddlers		
Death has least significance to children younger than 6 months of age. After parent-child attachment and trust are established, the loss, even if temporary, of the significant person is profound. Prolonged separation during the first several years is thought to be more significant in terms of future physical, social, and emotional growth than at any subsequent age. Toddlers are egocentric and can only think about events in terms of their own frame of reference—living. Their egocentricity and vague separation of fact and fantasy make it impossible for them to comprehend absence of life. Instead of understanding death, this age-group is affected more by any change in lifestyle.	With the death of someone else, they may continue to act as though the person is alive. As children grow older, they are increasingly able and willing to let go of the dead person. Ritualism is important; a change in lifestyle could be anxiety producing. This age-group reacts more to the pain and discomfort of a serious illness than to the probable fatal prognosis. They also react to parental anxiety and sadness.	Help parents deal with their feelings, allowing them greater emotional reserves to meet the needs of their children. Encourage parents to remain as near to child as possible yet be sensitive to parents' needs. Maintain as normal an environment as possible to retain ritualism. If a parent has died, encourage having consistent caregiver for child. Promote primary nursing.
Preschool Children		
Preschoolers believe that their thoughts are sufficient to cause death; the consequence is the burden of guilt, shame, and punishment. Their egocentricity implies a tremendous sense of self-power and omnipotence. They usually have some understanding of the meaning of death. Death is seen as a departure, a kind of sleep. They may recognize the fact of physical death but do not separate it from living abilities. Death is seen as temporary and gradual; life and death can change places with one another. They have no understanding of the universality and inevitability of death.	If they become seriously ill, they conceive of the illness as a punishment for their thoughts or actions. They may feel guilty and responsible for the death of a sibling. Greatest fear concerning death is separation from parents. They may engage in activities that seem strange or abnormal to adults. Because they have fewer defense mechanisms to deal with loss, young children may react to a less significant loss with more outward grief than to the loss of a very significant person. The loss is so deep, painful, and threatening that the child must deny it for a time to survive its overwhelming impact. Behavior reactions such as giggling, joking, attracting attention, or regressing to earlier developmental skills indicate children's need to distance themselves from tremendous loss.	Help parents deal with their feelings, allowing them greater emotional reserves to meet the needs of their children. Help parents understand behavioral reactions of their children. Encourage parents to remain near the child as much as possible to minimize the child's great fear of separation from parents. If a parent has died, encourage having a consistent caregiver for the child. Promote primary nursing.

TABLE 36-3	CHILDREN'S UNDERSTANDING OF AND REACTIONS TO DEATH—cont'd	
CONCEPTS OF DEATH	**REACTIONS TO DEATH**	**NURSING CARE MANAGEMENT**
School-Age Children		
Children still associate misdeeds or bad thoughts with causing death and feel intense guilt and responsibility for the event.	Because of their increased ability to comprehend, they may have more fears, for example:	Help parents deal with their feelings, allowing them greater emotional reserves to meet the needs of their children.

Because of their higher cognitive abilities, they respond well to logical explanations and comprehend the figurative meaning of words.	The reason for the illness
	  Communicability of the disease to themselves or others
	  Consequences of the disease
		Encourage parents to remain near child as much as possible yet be sensitive to parents' needs.

They have a deeper understanding of death in a concrete sense.	The process of dying and death itself Their fear of the unknown is greater than their fear of the known.	Because of children's fear of the unknown, anticipatory preparation is important.
They particularly fear the mutilation and punishment they associate with death.	The realization of impending death is a tremendous threat to their sense of security and ego strength.	Because the developmental task of this age is industry, interventions of helping children maintain control over their bodies and
They personify death as the devil, a monster, or the bogeyman.	They are likely to exhibit fear through verbal uncooperativeness rather than actual physical aggression.	increasing their understanding allow them to achieve independence, self-worth, and self-esteem and avoid a sense of inferiority.
They may have naturalistic or physiologic explanations of death.	They are interested in postdeath services. They may be inquisitive about what happens to the body.	Encourage children to talk about their feelings and provide aggressive outlets.
By age 9 or 10 years, children have an adult concept of death, realizing that it is inevitable, universal, and irreversible.		Encourage parents to honestly answer questions about dying rather than avoiding the subject or fabricating euphemisms. Encourage parents to share their moments of sorrow with their children. Provide preparation for postdeath services.
Adolescents		
Adolescents have a mature understanding of death.	Adolescents straddle transition from childhood to adulthood.	Help parents deal with their feelings, allowing them greater emotional reserves to meet the needs of their children.
They are still influenced by remnants of magical thinking and are subject to guilt and shame.	They have the most difficulty in coping with death. They are least likely to accept cessation of life, particularly if it is their own.	Avoid alliances with either parent or child. Structure hospital admission to allow for maximum self-control and independence.
They are likely to see deviations from accepted behavior as reasons for their illness.	Concern is for the present much more than for the past or the future. They may consider themselves alienated from their peers and unable to communicate with their parents for emotional support, feeling alone in their struggle.	Answer adolescents' questions honestly, treating them as mature individuals and respecting their needs for privacy, solitude, and personal expressions of emotions. Help parents understand their child's reactions to death and dying, especially that concern
	Adolescents' orientation to the present compels them to worry about physical changes even more than the prognosis. Because of their idealistic view of the world, they may criticize funeral rites as barbaric, money making, and unnecessary.	for present crises, such as loss of hair, may be much greater than for future ones, including possible death.

room at home. In addition, there should be a consistent and coordinated care plan for the child's and family's comfort.

Home Care. Some families prefer to take their child home and receive services from a home care agency. Generally these services entail periodic nursing visits to administer a treatment or provide medications, equipment, or supplies. The child's care continues to be directed by the primary health care provider. Home care is often the option chosen by health care providers and families because of the traditional view that a child must be considered to have a life expectancy of less than 6 months to be referred to hospice care. Fortunately a number of hospice organizations are expanding their services to children based on the presence of a life-limiting disease process for which cure is not possible rather than on the sole criteria of a limited-time projected prognosis.

Hospice Care. Parents should be offered the option of caring for their child at home during the final phases of an illness with the assistance of a hospice organization. Hospice is a community health care organization that specializes in the care of dying patients by combining the hospice philosophy with the principles of palliative care. Hospice philosophy regards dying as a natural process and care of dying patients as including management of the physical, psychosocial, and spiritual needs of the patient and family. Care is provided by a multidisciplinary group of professionals in the patient's home or an inpatient facility that uses the hospice philosophy. Hospice care for children was introduced in the 1970s, and a number of community hospice organizations now accept children into their care (Davies, Davis, and Sibert, 2003; Faulkner and Armstrong-Dailey, 1997; Forrester, 2003; Winkler and Mardegian,

2001). Collaboration between the child's primary treatment team and the hospice care team is essential to the success of hospice care. Families may continue to see their primary care physicians as they choose.*

Hospice care is based on a number of important concepts that significantly set it apart from hospital care:

- Family members are usually the principal caregivers and are supported by a team of professional and volunteer staff.
- The priority of care is comfort. The child's physical, psychosocial, and spiritual needs are considered. Pain and symptom control are primary concerns, and no extraordinary efforts are used to attempt a cure or prolong life.
- The family's needs are considered to be as important as those of the patient.
- Hospice is concerned with the family's postdeath adjustment, and care may continue for a year or more.

The goal of hospice care is for children to live life to the fullest without pain, with choices and dignity, in the familiar environment of their home, and with the support of their family. Hospice care is covered under state Medicaid programs and by most insurance plans. The service provides home visits from nurses, social workers, chaplains, and in some cases physicians. Medications, medical equipment, and any necessary medical supplies are all provided by the hospice organization providing care.

With children the home has been the more common environment for implementing the hospice concept; it benefits the family in a variety of ways. Children who are dying are allowed to remain with those they love and with whom they feel secure. Many children who were thought to be in imminent danger of death have gone home and lived longer than expected. Siblings can feel more involved in the care and often have more positive perceptions of the death. Parental adaptation is often more favorable, demonstrated by their perceptions of how the experience at home affected their marriage, social reorientation, religious beliefs, and views on the meaning of life and death.

If the home is chosen for hospice care, the child may or may not die in the home. Reasons for final admission to a hospital vary but may be related to the parents' or siblings' wish to have the child die outside the home; exhaustion on the part of the caregivers; and physical problems such as sudden, acute pain or respiratory distress.

NURSING CARE OF THE CHILD AND FAMILY AT THE END OF LIFE

Regardless of where the child is cared for during the terminal stage of illness, both the child and family usually experience fear of (1) pain and suffering, (2) dying alone (child) or not being present when the child dies (parent), and (3) actual death. Nurses can help families by lessening their fears through attention to the care needs of the child and family (see Nursing Care Plan).

Fear of Pain and Suffering

The presence of unrelieved pain in a terminally ill child can have detrimental effects on the quality of life experienced by the child and family. Parents feel that having their child in pain is unendurable and results in feelings of helplessness and a sense that they must be present and vigilant to get the necessary pain medications. Persistent pain also has an impact on the family as a whole. Nurses can alleviate the fear of pain and suffering by providing interventions aimed at treating the pain and symptoms associated with the terminal process in children.

Pain and Symptom Management

Pain control for children in the terminal stages of illness or injury must be given the highest priority. Despite ongoing efforts to educate physicians and nurses on pain-management strategies in children, studies have reported that children continue to be undermedicated for their pain (Wolfe, Grier, Klar, et al., 2000). Nearly all children experience some amount of pain in the terminal phase of their illness. The current standard for treating children's pain follows the WHO analgesic stepladder (1996), which promotes tailoring the pain interventions to the child's level of reported pain. Children's pain should be assessed frequently, and medications adjusted as necessary. Pain medications should be given on a regular schedule, and extra doses for breakthrough pain should be available to maintain comfort. Opioid drugs such as morphine should be given for severe pain, and the dose should be increased as necessary to maintain optimal pain relief. Techniques such as distraction, relaxation techniques, and guided imagery should be combined with drug therapy to provide the child and family strategies to control pain (see Chapter 30 for further discussion of pain-management strategies) (Lambert, 1999).

In addition to pain, children experience a variety of symptoms during their terminal course as a result of their disease process or as a side effect of medicines used to manage pain or other symptoms. These symptoms include fatigue, nausea and vomiting, constipation, anorexia, dyspnea, congestion, seizures, anxiety, depression, restlessness, agitation, and confusion (Hellsten, Hockenberry, Lamb, et al., 2000; Wolfe, Friebert, and Hilden, 2002). Each of these symptoms should be managed aggressively with appropriate medications or treatments and interventions such as repositioning, relaxation, massage, and other measures to maintain the child's comfort and quality of life.

Occasionally children require very high doses of opioids to control pain. This may occur for several reasons. Children on long-term opioid pain management can become tolerant of the drug, meaning that it is necessary to give more drugs to maintain the same level of pain relief. This should not be confused with addiction, which is a psychologic dependence on the side effects of opioids. Addiction is not a factor in managing terminal pain in children. Other obvious reasons for requiring increased doses of opioids include progression of disease and other physiologic experiences of pain. It is important to understand that there is no maximum dose that can be given to control pain. However, nurses often express concern that administering doses of opioids that exceed that which they are familiar will hasten the child's death. The principle of double effect (Box 36-8) addresses such concerns. It provides an ethical standard that supports the use of interventions intended to relieve pain and suffering, even though there is a foreseeable possibility that death may be hastened (Rousseau, 2001). In cases in which the child is terminally ill and in severe pain, using large doses of opioids and sedatives to manage pain is justified when no other treatment options are available that would relieve the pain but make the risk of death less likely (Hawryluck and Harvey, 2000). See Chapter 30 for an extensive discussion of pain assessment and management.

---

*For more information, contact National Hospice and Palliative Care Organization, 1731 King Street, Alexandria, VA 22314; 703-837-1500, fax: 703-837-1233, www.nho.org; and Children's Hospice International, 1101 King S., Suite 360, Alexandria, VA 22314, 703-684-0330 or 800-24-CHILD, www.chionline.org.

⊚ NURSING CARE PLAN

The Child Who Is Terminally Ill or Dying

NURSING DIAGNOSIS	EXPECTED OUTCOMES	NURSING INTERVENTIONS	RATIONALE
Anxiety related to fear or worry about dying **Child's or Family's Defining Characteristics (Subjective and Objective Data)** Unstable emotions Aggressive behavior Withdrawn behavior Depression	Child and family will receive appropriate emotional support during terminal phase of child's illness. Child will express fears and anxiety related to dying. Family will support child's ability to express fears and anxiety. Child and family will be informed of symptoms to expect as child nears end of life. Child and family will be informed of procedures and therapies necessary to promote comfort. Child and family will be able to cope with dying process.	Encourage family to remain near child as much as possible. Encourage child to talk about feelings; help family as they encourage child to express feelings. Provide safe, acceptable outlets for aggression and for grieving. Answer questions as honestly as possible while maintaining positive, hopeful approach. Explain progression of physical symptoms as child nears end of life. Explain all procedures and therapies, especially physical effects child will experience. Help child distinguish between consequences of treatment and manifestations of the disease. Structure hospital or home environment to allow for maximum self-control and independence within limitations imposed by child's developmental level and physical condition. The following NIC concepts apply to these interventions: 　Active Listening 　Coping Enhancement 　Simple Relaxation 　Touch	To provide support through presence of loved one To provide sense of closeness and understanding among family members To establish that anger and sadness are normal reactions To promote trust as major strength for therapeutic relationships To promote trust and decrease anxiety To decrease fear of unknown, which may be more of concern than actual procedure or therapy To focus on interventions that can minimize discomfort To minimize fear and loss of control
Chronic Pain related to disease process **Characteristics (Subjective and Objective Data)** Crying Withdrawal Aggression Fear of touch Fear of movement	Child will exhibit minimal or no evidence of physical discomfort. Family will be able to participate in child's care without causing discomfort. Family will be able to provide comfort measures for child.	Assess child's level of comfort. Provide pain management around the clock. Assess child for symptoms associated with pain or its treatment. Provide stool softener, laxative, or diphenhydramine as needed. Provide nonpharmacologic interventions that child prefers. Administer anticholinergic drugs as needed. Encourage family to provide comfort measures that child prefers. Provide soothing surroundings for child. Avoid excessive noise and light. Ensure pleasant smell, touch, temperature. Place all commodities within easy reach of child. Use gentle touch when required to perform physical procedures. Avoid pressure on painful areas. Avoid pressure on bony prominences and painful sites. Use pillows and other supports to prop child in comfortable position. Place absorbent pads under hips if child is incontinent. Limit care to essential needs.	To ensure that child is treated for changes in pain To prevent recurrence or escalation of pain To ensure that child is treated for symptoms accompanying pain or its management To prevent or treat symptoms related to pain or its management To aid pharmacologic management of pain, helping to prevent recurrence or escalation of pain and accompanying symptoms To reduce secretions and lessen "death rattle," which can be distressing to family To provide comfort To minimize irritation and maximize comfort To minimize discomfort from movement To minimize pain when possible To make it easier for child to breathe To prevent skin breakdown To minimize fatigue

Continued

⊚ **NURSING CARE PLAN**

The Child Who Is Terminally Ill or Dying—cont'd

NURSING DIAGNOSIS	EXPECTED OUTCOMES	NURSING INTERVENTIONS	RATIONALE
Anticipatory Grieving related to impending loss of child	Family will express fears, concerns, and any special desires for terminal care.	Discuss with family and child the grieving process and differences in grieving among men, women, and children.	To facilitate understanding of what family members are feeling and experiencing
Child's or Family's Defining Characteristics	Family will demonstrate an understanding of their children's needs.	Provide opportunities for family members to express emotions independently or together as desired.	To provide an outlet for their emotions
(Subjective and Objective Data)	Family members will be actively involved in their child's care.	Facilitate child's or sibling's expression of emotions through art or play activities.	To facilitate expression of their emotions
Parents' feelings and physical responses of loss and depression	Family members will seek resources needed to help them during grieving process.	Help parents and siblings deal with their feelings about child's death.	To provide support
Parents' feelings of loss of control and uncertainty		Encourage parents to remain as near to child as possible.	To allow parents to feel they are doing something for their child
Child's or sibling's feelings and physical responses of loss and depression		Provide family with information regarding child's status.	To promote understanding and communication
Child's or sibling's feelings of loss of control and uncertainty		Provide family with information on common behavioral reactions.	To promote understanding of their children's behaviors
		Encourage family's assistance with child's care.	To assist with coping and minimize loss of control
		Provide information to family on how to maintain own health care needs.	To give families approval to take care of themselves
		Provide as much privacy as possible without isolating family from nurse's care.	To provide dignity for grieving process
		Help family assess their needs for referral services.	To facilitate support for families
		Encourage parents to honestly answer children's questions about dying.	To decrease children's fear and anxiety
		Provide resources for family to facilitate discussions with children about dying.	To provide support and facilitate parents' discussion
		Encourage parents to share their moments of sorrow with their children.	To promote grief expression of children
		Assist family and child with memory-making opportunities.	To facilitate emotions and sharing between family and child
		Assist child as needed to complete any unfinished business.	To facilitate support of child
		Discuss with parents appropriate involvement of siblings.	To prevent siblings from feeling excluded
		Identify family's religious and cultural beliefs related to death.	To provide support and spiritual care
		Provide preparation for postdeath services.	To provide support and guidance
		Discuss with parents the frequent need of children to be given permission to die.	To provide support and guidance
		Discuss with family their preferences for care if death is imminent.	To allow families to be in control
		Facilitate appropriate spiritual care in accordance with family's beliefs or affiliations.	To provide support
		Provide support for families who choose home care for their child.	To allow families to choose where the child is to die and provide guidance for this to occur

Parents' and Siblings' Need for Education and Support

Parents are the primary caregivers when the child is at home, and nurses providing care to the child and family need to teach the family about the medications being given to the child, how to administer them, and the use of nonpharmacologic techniques. Parents are kept informed of all medications and treatments given to a child in the hospital, and they are encouraged to participate in the child's care to the extent that they desire. This empowers parents and provides a sense of control over the child's comfort and well-being, reducing their fear that their child will be in pain or suffering as he or she is dying. In addition, better bereavement outcomes (e.g., adaptive coping; family cohesion; less anxiety, stress, and

- An action that has one good (intended) and one bad (unintended but foreseeable) effect is permissible if the following conditions are met:
- The action itself must be good or indifferent. Only the good consequences of the action must be sincerely intended.
- The good effect must not be produced by the bad effect.
- There must be a compelling or proportionate reason for permitting the foreseeable bad effect to occur.

depression) have been reported by parents who were actively involved in the care of their child (Goodenough, Drew, Higgins, et al., 2004; Lauer, Mulhern, Schell, et al., 1989). The grief work of fathers in particular seems to be facilitated when their child dies in the home setting. This finding may be related to the increased opportunity of working fathers to provide care to and spend time with their child at home versus in the hospital setting.

Siblings may feel isolated and displaced during the time that their brother or sister is dying. Parents devote the majority of their time to the care and comfort of the dying child, causing siblings to feel left out of the parent–sick child relationship. Siblings may become resentful of their sick sibling and begin to feel guilty or ashamed about such feelings (Murray, 1999). Nurses can assist the family by helping the parents identify ways to involve siblings in the caring process, perhaps by bringing some supplies or favorite toy, game, or food item. Parents should also be encouraged to schedule time to spend with the other children during which their focus is on them. Helping parents identify a trusted friend or family member who can sit with the ill child for a short period allows them to attend to their own needs or those of their other children.

Fear of Dying Alone or of Not Being Present When the Child Dies

When a child is being cared for at home, the burden of care on parents and family members can be great. Often, as the child's condition declines, family members begin the "death vigil." Rarely is a child left alone for any length of time. This can be exhausting for family members, and nurses can assist the family by helping them arrange shifts so friends or family members can be present with the child and allow others to rest. If the family has limited resources, community organizations such as hospice or churches often have volunteers who are willing to visit and sit with children. It is important that whoever is sitting with the child be aware of when the parent(s) would like to be notified to return to his or her bedside (Fig. 36-6).

When a child is dying in the hospital, the parents should be given full access to him or her at all times. If the parents need to leave they should be provided with a pager or other means of immediate communication and alerted if staff members note any change in the child that may indicate imminent death. Nurses should advocate for parents' presence in intensive care and emergency departments and attend to the parents' needs for food, drinks, comfortable chairs, blankets, and pillows.

Fear of Actual Death
Home Deaths

Most children receiving hospice care die at home, often in their own room with family, pets, and loved possessions around them. The physical process of dying can be distressing to parents because often

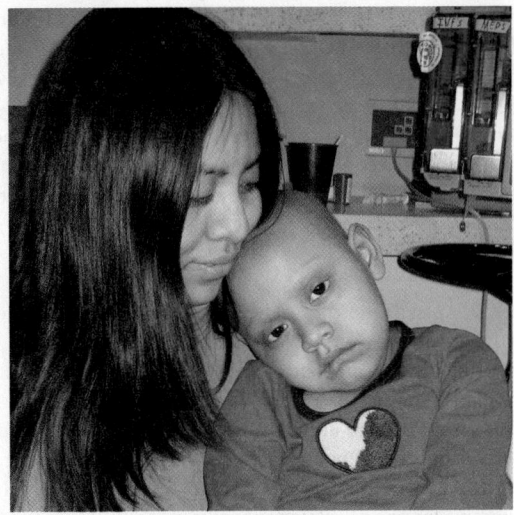

FIG 36-6 For a dying child there is no greater comfort than the security and closeness of a parent.

- Loss of sensation and movement in lower extremities, progressing toward upper body
- Sensation of heat, although body feels cool
- Loss of senses:
  - Tactile sensation decreasing
  - Sensitivity to light
  - Hearing the last sense to fail
- Confusion, loss of consciousness, slurred speech
- Muscle weakness
- Loss of bowel and bladder control
- Decreased appetite and thirst
- Difficulty swallowing
- Change in respiratory pattern:
  - Cheyne-Stokes respirations (waxing and waning of depth of breathing with regular periods of apnea)
  - "Death rattle" (noisy chest sounds from accumulation of pulmonary and pharyngeal secretions)
  - Weak, slow pulse; decreased blood pressure

the child slowly becomes less alert in the days before the actual death. The nurse can help the family by providing them with information about what changes will occur as the child progresses through the dying process (Box 36-9). During this time nursing visits often become more frequent and longer in duration to provide the family with additional support as the death nears. The most distressing change for parents to observe is the change in the respiratory pattern. In the final hours of life the dying patient's respirations may become labored, with deep breaths and long periods of apnea referred to as *Cheyne-Stokes respirations*. Families are reassured that this is not distressing to the child and that it is a normal part of the dying process. However, the use of opioids can slow the respirations to make the child breathe more easily; and scopolamine, usually applied as a topical patch, can help reduce noisy respirations known as the "death rattle." Noisy respirations are more likely to occur if the child is overhydrated.

All families have the option of admitting their child to the hospital if they feel unable to deal with the death. The child who dies at home must be pronounced dead; hospice programs typically have provisions so this proceeds smoothly. In some circumstances the police may be notified, with an explanation of the circumstances to prevent unnecessary concern regarding abuse. Providing the police with the number of the responsible practitioner is usually all that is necessary to confirm the cause of death.

Hospital Deaths

Children dying in the hospital of terminal illnesses who are receiving supportive care interventions experience a similar process. Again increased nursing presence and attendance to the child's and family's needs provide comfort and support for many families.

Death resulting from accident or trauma or acute illness in settings such as the emergency department or intensive care unit often requires the active withdrawal of some form of life-supporting intervention such as a ventilator or bypass machine. These situations often raise difficult ethical issues (Sine, Sumner, Gracy, et al., 2001), and parents are often less prepared for the actual moment of death. Nurses can help these parents by providing detailed information about what will happen as supportive equipment is withdrawn, ensuring that appropriate pain medications are administered to prevent pain during the dying process and allowing the parents time before the start of the withdrawal to be with and speak to their child. It is important that the nurse attempt to control the environment around the family at this time by providing privacy, asking if they would like to play music, softening lights and monitor noises, and arranging for any religious or cultural rituals that the family may want performed.

After the child's death the family should be allowed to remain with the body and hold or rock the child if they desire. After the nurse has removed all tubes and equipment from the body, the parents should be given the option of helping with the preparation of the body such as bathing and dressing. It is important for the nurse to determine whether the family has any specific needs because many cultures have adopted specific methods for coping with and mourning death, and impeding these practices may interfere with the grieving process (Clements, Vigil, Manno, et al., 2003).

At some point the nurse discusses whether the family has made preparations for the burial service and whether the staff can help in any way. Parents often have concerns about the funeral such as siblings' involvement in the death rituals. Although no absolute answers exist regarding the question of siblings attending the funeral or burial services, the consensus is that the surviving children benefit from being involved in these events. However, children need preparation for postdeath services. They should be told what to expect, particularly how the deceased person will look if the coffin is open; allowed their private time to say good-bye; and permitted to stay as long as they wish. Ideally the parents should prepare the siblings. If the parents' grief prevents this communication, a significant family member or friend should substitute (see Family-Centered Care box).

Organ or Tissue Donation and Autopsy

For some families organ or tissue donation may be a meaningful act (i.e., one that benefits another human being despite the loss of their child). Unfortunately initiating a discussion about tissue donation is often stressful for staff, and there may be confusion regarding whose responsibility this is. In centers in which transplants are performed, a full-time transplant coordinator is usually available to inform the family about organ donation and take care of details. If

---

FAMILY-CENTERED CARE

Children Need to Say Good-Bye

As a nurse and grief counselor, I conduct grief workshops with children who have experienced the death of someone special. Children often communicate their feelings of being excluded through drawings. They may draw a picture of the dying person in a hospital bed that is raised too high for them to see the person's face clearly. Sometimes children reveal that they did not get to say good-bye because a family member told them, for example, "You don't want to see your grandma this way. She is too sick for you to visit." If the special person died at home, the children had to stay in their room when the funeral home staff took away the body.

I have learned never to underestimate the importance of allowing children to be involved with the dying person and the significance of a child's loss. Once, when I asked a 6-year-old girl to draw a picture with the theme "This is what I was doing when my _____ died," she drew a picture and completed the sentence with "when my home died." Her grandmother had been like her mother; to the child, her home was gone. We need to give children the choice of being included in the family's activities of saying good-bye.

Barbara Bilderback, MS, MA, RN
Bereavement Supervisor, Saint Francis Hospice
Tulsa, OK

---

such services are not available, the staff needs to determine which members should discuss this topic with the family. Ideally the person who knows the family best, knows when the death is expected, or has the opportunity to spend time with the family when the death is unexpected takes the role. Often nurses are in an optimal position to suggest tissue donation after consultation with the attending physician. When possible the topic should be raised before death occurs. The request should be made in a private and quiet area of the hospital and should be simple and direct, with questions such as, "Are you a donor family?" or "Have you ever considered organ donation?"

Many states have legislated a mandatory request for organ or tissue donation when a child dies, especially if the patient is brain dead. Written consent from the family is required before donation can proceed. When requests for organ donation are made, health care practitioners must address common misunderstandings that families have about brain death and organ donation (Franz, DeJong, Wolfe, et al., 1997). Training health care professionals about sensitive approaches to requests for organ donation has been shown to increase families' willingness to consent to organ donation (American Academy of Pediatrics, 2002; Evanisko, Beasley, Brigham, et al., 1998). The option to donate organs should always be separate from the communication of impending or actual death.

Nurses need to be aware of common questions about organ donation to help families make an informed decision. Healthy children who die unexpectedly are excellent candidates for organ donation. Children with cancer, chronic disease, or infection and those who have suffered prolonged cardiac arrest may not be suitable candidates, although this is determined individually. The nurse should ask whether organ donation was discussed with the child or whether the child ever expressed such a wish. Any number of body tissues or organs can be donated (skin, corneas, bone, kidney, heart, liver, pancreas), and their removal does not mutilate or desecrate the body or cause any suffering. The family may have an open casket, and there is no delay in the funeral. There is no cost to the donor family, but organ donation does not eliminate funeral or cremation responsibilities. Most religions permit organ donation as long as the recipient benefits from the transplant, although Orthodox Judaism forbids it.

In cases of unexplained death, violent death, or suspected suicide, autopsy is required by law. In other instances it may be optional, and parents should be informed of this choice. The procedure and the forms that require signing should be explained. The family should know that the child can be in an open casket after an autopsy.

Grief and Mourning

Grief is a process, not an event, of experiencing physiologic, psychologic, behavioral, social, and spiritual reactions to the loss of a child. It is highly individualized, encompassing a broad range of manifestations from person to person. It is a natural and expected reaction to loss. It is neither orderly nor predictable. Grieving in any form is necessary for healing to occur. When death is the expected or a possible outcome of a disorder, the child and family members may experience anticipatory grief. Anticipatory grief may be manifested in varying behaviors and intensities and may include denial, anger, depression, and other psychologic and physical symptoms.

Anticipatory guidance may help grieving family members. Health care professionals should emphasize that grief reactions such as hearing the dead person's voice, feeling distant from others, or seeking reassurance that they did everything possible for the lost person are normal, necessary, and expected. They in no way signify poor coping, insanity, or an approaching mental breakdown. On the contrary such behaviors signify that the survivor is working through the acute grief. They are a necessary part of grief work. Anticipatory guidance regarding the mourning process may help families recognize the normalcy of their experiences.

It is important to recognize that some family members may experience complicated grief. Complicated grief reactions (>1 year after the loss) include such symptoms as intense intrusive thoughts, pangs of severe emotion, distressing yearnings, feelings of excessive loneliness and emptiness, unusual sleep disturbance, and maladaptive levels of loss of interest in personal activities (Meert, Shear, Newth, et al., 2011). Bereaved persons experiencing such prolonged and complicated grief should be referred to an expert in grief and bereavement counseling.

Another important aspect of grief is the individual nature of the grief experience. Each member of the family experiences the grief of the child's death in his or her own way based on the particular relationship with that child. This can create potential conflict for families because each family member has expectations that the other family members should feel and grieve as they do. Nurses caring for families experiencing grief should be aware of the different grieving styles and help the family learn to recognize and support the uniqueness of one another's grief.

Parental Grief

Parental grief after the death of a child has been found to be the most intense, complex, long-lasting, and fluctuating grief experience compared with that of other bereaved individuals. Although parents experience the primary loss of their child, many secondary losses are felt such as the loss of part of one's self, hopes and dreams for the child's future, the family unit, prior social and emotional community supports, and often spousal support. It is common for parents of the same child to experience different grief reactions.

Studies with bereaved parents have shown that grieving does not end with the severing of the bond with the deceased child but rather involves a continuing bond between the parent and that child (Klass, 2001). Parental resolution of grief is a process of integrating the dead child into daily life in which the pain of losing a child is never completely gone but lessens. There are occasions of brief relapse but not to the degree experienced when the loss initially occurred. Thus parental grief work is never completed and is a timeless process of accommodating the new reality of being without a child as it changes over time (Davies, 2004). A child's death can also challenge the marital relationship in several ways. Maternal and paternal reactions often differ (Birenbaum, Stewart, and Phillips, 1996; Moriarty, Carroll, and Cotroneo, 1996; Vance, Najman, Thearle, et al., 1995). Different grieving styles between the couple may hinder communication and support for one another. Differing needs and expectations can place a strain on the marriage.

Sibling Grief

Each child grieves in his or her own way and on his or her own timeline. Children, even adolescents, grieve differently than adults. Adults and children differ more widely in their reactions to death than in their reactions to any other phenomenon. Children of all ages grieve the loss of a loved one, and their understanding and reactions to death depend on their age and developmental level. Children grieve for a longer duration, revisiting their grief as they grow and develop new understandings of death. However, they do not grieve 100% of the time. They grieve in spurts and can be emotional and sad in one instance and then, just as quickly, off and playing. Children express their grief through play and behavior. They can be exquisitely attuned to their parents' grief and try to protect them by not asking questions or trying not to upset them. This can set the stage for the sibling to try to become the "perfect child." Children exhibit many of the grief reactions of adults, including physical sensations and illnesses, anger, guilt, sadness, loneliness, withdrawal, acting out, sleep disturbances, isolation, and search for meaning. Again nurses should be attentive for signs that siblings are struggling with their grief and provide guidance to parents when possible.

At times family members may need assistance in their grieving (see Guidelines box). Communication with the bereaved family is essential, but often nurses do not know what to say and feel helpless in offering words of comfort. The most supportive approach is to avoid judging the family's reactions or offering advice or rationalizations and to focus on feelings. Perhaps the most valuable supportive measure the nurse can perform for families is to listen. Families understand that no words will relieve their pain; all they want is acceptance, understanding, and respect for their grief.

It is important for families to understand that mourning takes a long time. Acute grief may last only weeks or months, but resolving the loss is measured in years. Holidays and anniversaries can be particularly difficult, and people who previously had been supportive may now expect the family to have "adjusted." Consequently prolonged mourning is often silent and lonely.

Many families never receive the support and guidance that could help them resolve the loss. A plan for regular follow-up with bereaved families can be beneficial. At minimum one follow-up phone call or meeting with the family should be arranged. Families can also be referred to self-help groups. When such groups are not available, nurses can be instrumental in bringing families together or facilitating parent and sibling groups. Formal bereavement programs or bereavement counseling can be helpful as well.

GUIDELINES

Supporting Grieving Families*

General

- Stay with the family; sit quietly if they prefer not to talk; cry with them if desired.
- Accept the family's grief reactions; avoid judgmental statements (e.g., "You should be feeling better by now").
- Avoid offering rationalizations for the child's death (e.g., "Your child isn't suffering anymore").
- Avoid artificial consolation (e.g., "I know how you feel," or "You're still young enough to have another baby").
- Deal openly with feelings such as guilt, anger, and loss of self-esteem.
- Focus on feelings by using a feeling word in the statement (e.g., "You're still feeling all the pain of losing a child").
- Refer the family to an appropriate self-help group or for professional help if needed.

At the Time of Death

- Reassure the family that everything possible is being done for the child if they want lifesaving interventions.
- Do everything possible to ensure the child's comfort, especially relieving pain.
- Provide the child and family with the opportunity to review special experiences or memories in their lives.
- Express personal feelings of loss or frustrations (e.g., "We'll miss him so much," "We tried everything; we feel so sorry that we couldn't save her").

- Provide information that the family requests and be honest.
- Respect the emotional needs of family members such as siblings, who may need brief respites from the dying child.
- Make every effort to arrange for family members, especially the parents, to be with the child at the moment of death if they want to be present.
- Allow the family to stay with the dead child for as long as they wish and to rock, hold, or bathe the child.
- Provide practical help when possible such as collecting the child's belongings.
- Arrange for spiritual support based on the family's religious beliefs; pray with the family if no one else can stay with them.

Postdeath

- Attend the funeral or visitation if there was a special closeness with the family.
- Initiate and maintain contact (e.g., sending cards, telephoning, inviting them back to the unit, making a home visit).
- Refer to the dead child by name; discuss shared memories with the family.
- Discourage the use of drugs and alcohol as a method of escaping grief.
- Encourage all family members to communicate their feelings rather than remain silent to avoid upsetting another member.
- Emphasize that grieving is a painful process that often takes years to resolve.

*Family refers to all significant persons involved in the child's life such as the parents, siblings, grandparents, and other close relatives or friends.

Nurses' Reactions to Caring for Dying Children

The death of a patient is one of the most stressful aspects of critical care and oncology nursing (see Family-Centered Care box).* Nurses experience reactions to a fatal illness that are very similar to the responses of family members, including denial, anger, depression, guilt, and ambivalent feelings.

Strategies that can help nurses maintain the ability to work effectively in these settings include maintaining good general health, developing well-rounded interests, using distancing techniques such as taking time off when needed, developing and using professional and personal support systems, cultivating the capacity for empathy, focusing on the positive aspects of the caregiver role, and basing nursing interventions on sound theory

*Other sources of publications on life-threatening illness and death are the Compassionate Friends, 900 Jonie Blvd, Suite 78, Oak Brook, IL 60523, 630-990-0010 or 877-969-0010, www.compassionatefriends.org; Centering Corporation, 7230 Maple St, Omaha, Neb 68134, 866-218-0101, www.centering.org; Children's Hospice International, 1104 King St, Suite 360, Alexandria, VA 22314, 800-24-CHILD or 703-684-0330, e-mail: info@chionline.org, www.chionline.org; and National Cancer Institute, Cancer Information Service, 6116 Executive Boulevard, Bethesda, MD 20892-8322, 800-422-6237, www.cancer.gov.

FAMILY-CENTERED CARE

A Dying Child: A Nurse's Perspective

Claire was unresponsive with slow, gasping breathing. Her mother asked me what I thought was happening. I replied honestly, "Your baby is dying because of her brain tumor." The mother put her arms around me and cried. We arranged for Claire to be baptized.

Honesty. As painful as the loss of a child is, my job is to assist the family through this experience. Although I usually wait until a private moment such as driving home, I found tears streaming down my face as family and friends gathered for Claire's baptism. I went into the kitchen to compose myself, only to find several of my colleagues crying as well. Saying goodbye to a dying child will always be a difficult but shared experience.

Jeanne O'Connor Egan, RN, MSN
Pediatric Clinical Specialist, Children's Hospital Washington, DC

and empiric observations. Attending shared-remembrance rituals helps some nurses resolve grief (Davis and Eng, 1998). Similarly, attending the funeral services can be a supportive act for both the family and the nurse and in no way detracts from the professionalism of care.

KEY POINTS

- Trends in the treatment of children with chronic illnesses and disabilities have focused on developmental age, the child's strengths and uniqueness, family-centered care, normalization, early discharge, home care, mainstreaming, and early intervention.

- In response to the child with chronic conditions, parents may be affected by feelings of inadequacy and failure; excessive demands on time, energy, and financial resources; and strain on the marital relationship.

- Families' reactions to chronic conditions are manifested in the following stages: shock and denial, adjustment, reintegration, and acknowledgment.
- The child's reaction to chronic conditions depends on his or her developmental level and coping mechanisms, others' reactions, and the illness itself.
- Assessment of the family's adjustment to a child's chronic illness, disability, or death includes the availability of a support system, their perception of the event, their coping mechanisms, concurrent stressors, and their response to the child.
- To help parents cope with their child's chronic and complex conditions, nurses must offer attentiveness, humanistic support, solicitation of suggestions for care, facilitation of communication, verbalization of feelings, and referral to volunteer and community agencies.
- Supporting the child involves encouraging self-expression, alleviating feelings of being different, and strengthening the child's self-image.
- Children's concept of death is determined by their cognitive ability and experience with life-threatening illness.
- Young children see death as temporary and reversible and mainly fear separation.
- School-age children view death as irreversible but not necessarily inevitable and may fear mutilation.

- Children beyond 9 to 10 years of age realize that death is irreversible, universal, and inevitable but may resist the thought of their own death.
- Siblings have special needs, including the need for information, reassurance about their own health status, assurance that they are not responsible for the illness or death, and support for their own grieving process.
- Special needs of the family facing the unexpected death of a child include support while awaiting news of the child's status; a sensitive pronouncement of death; acknowledgment of feelings of denial, guilt, and anger; an opportunity to view the body; and referrals for support.
- Special decisions at the time of dying and death may involve hospital or hospice care, visualization of the body, tissue donation and autopsy, and siblings' attendance at the funeral.
- Acute grief is a syndrome with intense and distressing psychologic and somatic symptoms that appear at the time of death.
- In dealing with stress related to the dying patient, the nurse can cope successfully through self-awareness, consciousness raising, knowledge and practice, an available support system, and maintenance of general good health and by focusing on the positive rewards of involvement with dying children and their families.

REFERENCES

Ahmann E: "Chunky stew": appreciating cultural diversity while providing health care for children, *Pediatr Nurs* 20(3):320–324, 1994.

American Academy of Pediatrics Committee on Hospital Care and Section on Surgery: Pediatric organ donation and transplantation, *Pediatrics* 109(5):982–984, 2002.

American Nurses Association: *Code of ethics for nurses with interpretive statements*, Washington, DC, 2001, ANA Publishing.

Anderson T, Davis C: Evidence-based practice with families of chronically ill children: a critical literature review, *J Evid Based Soc Work* 8(4):416–425, 2011.

Anderson RN, Smith BL: Deaths: leading causes, *Natl Vital Stat Rep* 53(17):1–89, 2005.

Arias E, MacDorman MF, Strobino DM, et al: Annual summary of vital statistics—2002, *Pediatrics* 112(6):1215–1230, 2003.

Barlow JH, Ellard DR: The psychosocial well-being of children with chronic disease, their parents and siblings: an overview of the research evidence base, *Child Care Health Dev* 32(1):19–31, 2006.

Bettle AM, Latimer MA: Maternal coping and adaptation: a case study examination of chronic sorrow in caring for an adolescent with a progressive neurodegenerative disease, *Can J Neurosci Nurs* 31(4):15–21, 2009.

Birenbaum LK, Stewart BJ, Phillips DS: Health status of bereaved parents, *Nurs Res* 45(2):105–109, 1996.

Burke RT, Alverson B: Impact of children with medically complex conditions, *Pediatrics* 126(4):789–790, 2010.

Carnevale FA, Alexander E, Davis M, et al: Daily living with distress and enrichment: the moral experience of families with ventilator-assisted children at home, *Pediatrics* 117(1):e48–e60, 2006.

Carnevale FA, Rehm RS, Kirk S, et al: What we know (and don't know) about raising children with complex continuing care needs, *J Child Health Care* 12:4–6, 2008.

Carter B: Chronic pain in childhood and the medical encounter: professional ventriloquism and hidden voices, *Qual Health Res* 12:28–41, 2002.

Charles C, Gafni A, Whelan T: Shared decision making in the medical encounter: what does it mean? *Soc Sci Med* 44:681–692, 1997.

Clements PT, Vigil GJ, Manno MS, et al: Cultural perspectives of death, grief, and bereavement, *J Psychosoc Nurs Ment Health Serv* 41(7):18–26, 2003.

Coffey JS: Parenting a child with chronic illness: a metasynthesis, *Pediatr Nurs* 32(1):51–59, 2006.

Cohen E, Friedman J, Nicholas DB, et al: A home for medically complex children: the role of hospital programs. *J Health Care Quality* 30(3):7–15, 2008.

Coker TR, Rodriguez MA, Flores G: Family-centered care for US children with special health care needs: who gets it and why? *Pediatrics* 125(6):1159–1167, 2010.

Corlett J, Twycross A: Negotiation of parental roles within family-centered care: a review of the research, *J Clin Nurs* 15(10):1308–1316, 2006.

Council on Children with Disabilities: Care coordination in the medical home:

integrating health and related systems of care for children with special health care needs, *Pediatrics* 116(5):1238–1244, 2005.

Davies B, Gudmundsdottir M, Worden B, et al: "Living in the dragon's shadow": fathers' experiences of a child's life-limiting illness, *Death Studies* 28(2):111–135, 2004.

Davies R: New understandings of parental grief: literature review, *J Adv Nurs* 46(5):506–513, 2004.

Davies R, Davis B, Sibert J: Parents' stories of sensitive and insensitive care by paediatricians in the time leading up to and including diagnostic disclosure of a life-limiting condition in their child, *Child Care Health Dev* 29(1):77–82, 2003.

Davis B, Eng B: Special issues in bereavement and staff support. In Doyle D, Hanks GWC, MacDonald N, editors: *Oxford textbook of palliative medicine*, ed 2, Oxford, 1998, Oxford University Press.

Deatrick JA, Knafl KA, Murphy-Moore C: Clarifying the concept of normalization, *Image J Nurs Sch* 31:209–214, 1999.

Denboba D, McPherson MG, Kenney MK, et al: Achieving family and provider partnerships for children with special health care needs, *Pediatrics* 118(4):1607–1615, 2006.

Dixon-Woods M, Young B, Henry D: Partnerships with children, *BMJ* 319:778–780, 1999.

Evanisko MJ, Beasley CL, Brigham LE, et al: Readiness of critical care physicians and nurses to handle requests for organ donation, *Am J Crit Care* 7(1):4–12, 1998.

Faulkner KW, Armstrong-Dailey A: Care of the dying child. In Pizzo PA, Poplack DG, editors: *Principles and practice of pediatric oncology*, Philadelphia, 1997, Lippincott-Raven.

Field MJ, Behrman RE, editors: *When children die: improving palliative and end-of-life care for children and their families*, Washington, DC, 2004, National Academies Press.

Fleitas J: When Jack fell down … Jill came tumbling after: siblings in the web of illness and disability, *MCN Am J Matern Child Nurs* 25:267–273, 2000.

Forrester L: One to one care in children's hospice, *Nurs Times* 99(16):44–45, 2003.

Franz HG, DeJong W, Wolfe SM, et al: Explaining brain death: a critical feature of the donation process, *J Transplant Coord* 7(1):14–21, 1997.

Freyer DR: Care of the dying adolescent: special considerations, *Pediatrics* 113(2):381–388, 2004.

Gantt L: As normal a life as possible: mothers and their daughters with congenital heart disease, *Health Care Women Int* 23(5):481–491, 2002.

Garwick AW, Patterson J, Bennett FC, et al: Breaking the news: how families first learn about their child's chronic condition, *Arch Pediatr Adolesc Med* 149(9):991–997, 1995.

Gold JI, Treadwell M, Weissman L, et al: The mediating effects of family functioning on psychosocial outcomes in healthy siblings of children with sickle cell disease, *Pediatr Blood Cancer* 57(6):1055–1061, 2011.

Goldbeck L: Parental coping with the diagnosis of childhood cancer: gender effects, dissimilarity within couples, and quality of life, *Psychooncology* 10:325–335, 2001.

Goodenough B, Drew D, Higgins S, et al: Bereavement outcomes for parents who lose a child to cancer: are place of death and sex of parent associated with differences in psychological functioning? *Psychooncology* 13(11):779–791, 2004.

Gordon J: An evidence-based approach for supporting parents experiencing chronic sorrow, *Pediatr Nurs* 35(2):115–119, 2009.

Haffner JC, Schurman SJ: The technology dependent child, *Pediatr Clin North Am* 48:751–764, 2001.

Harrigan RC, Ratliffe C, Patrinos ME, et al: Medically fragile pediatric patients: an integrative review of the literature and recommendations for future research, *Issues Compr Pediatr Nurs* 25:1–20, 2002.

Hawryluck LA, Harvey WR: Analgesia, virtue, and the principle of double effect, *J Palliat Care* 16(suppl):S24–S30, 2000.

Hellsten MB, Hockenberry M, Lamb D, et al: *End-of-life care for children*, Austin, Tex, 2000, Texas Cancer Council.

Hinds PS, Oakes L, Furman W, et al: End-of-life decision making by adolescents, parents, and healthcare providers in pediatric oncology: research to evidence-based practice guidelines, *Cancer Nurs* 24:122–134, 2001.

Hsiao JL, Evan EE, Zeltzer LK: Parent and child perspectives on physician communication in

pediatric palliative care, *Palliat Support Care* 5(4):355–365, 2007.

Huffman LC, Brat GA, Chamberlain LJ, et al: Impact of managed care on publicly insured children with special health care needs, *Acad Pediatr* 10(1):48–55, 2010.

Hungerbuehler I, Vollrath ME, Landolt MA: Posttraumatic growth in mothers and fathers of children with severe illnesses, *J Health Psychol* 16(8):1259–1267, 2011.

Jackson PL: The primary care provider and children with chronic conditions. In Jackson PL, Vessey PA, editors: *Primary care of the child with a chronic condition*, ed 3, St Louis, 2000, Mosby.

James L, Johnson B: The needs of parents of pediatric oncology patients during the palliative care phase, *J Pediatr Oncol Nurs* 14(2):83–95, 1997.

Jennings PD: Providing pediatric palliative care through a pediatric supportive care team, *Pediatr Nurs* 31(3):195–200, 2005.

Jokinen P: The family life-path theory: a tool for nurses working in partnership with families, *J Child Health Care* 8(2):124–133, 2004.

Kirk S, Glendinning C, Callery PJ: Parent or nurse? The experience of being the parent of a technology-dependent child, *Adv Nurs* 51(5):456–464, 2005.

Klass D: The inner representation of the dead child in the psychic and social narratives of bereaved parents. In Neimeyer RA, editor: *Meaning reconstruction and the experience of loss*, Washington, DC, 2001, American Psychological Association.

Knafl KA, Darney BG, Gallo AM, et al: Parental perceptions of the outcome and meaning of normalization, *Res Nurs Health* 33(2):87–98, 2010.

Kon AA: The shared decision-making continuum, *JAMA* 304(8):903–904, 2010.

Lambert S: Distraction, imagery, and hypnosis techniques for management of children's pain, *J Child Fam Nurs* 2(1):5–15, 1999.

Lauer ME, Mulhern RK, Schell MJ, et al: Long-term follow-up of parental adjustment following a child's death at home or hospital, *Cancer* 63(5):988–994, 1989.

Lobato DJ, Kao BT: Integrated sibling-parent group intervention to improve sibling knowledge and adjustment to chronic illness and disability, *J Pediatr Psychol* 27:711–716, 2002.

Lobato DJ, Kao BT, Plante W: Latino sibling knowledge and adjustment to chronic illness, *J Fam Psychol* 19(4):625–632, 2005.

Marshall ES, Olsen SF, Mandleco BL, et al: "This is a spiritual experience": perspectives of Latter-Day Saint families living with a child with disabilities, *Qual Health Res* 13:57–76, 2003.

Masri C, Farrell CA, Lacroix J, et al: Decision making and end-of-life care in critically ill children, *J Palliative Care* 16(suppl):S45–S52, 2000.

Mastroyannopoulou K, Stallard P, Lewis M, et al: The impact of childhood non-malignant life threatening illness on parents: gender

differences and predictors of parental adjustment, *J Child Psychol Psychiatry* 38(7):823–829, 1997.

McDougal J: Promoting normalization in families with preschool children with type 1 diabetes, *J Spec Pediatr Nurs* 7(3):113–120, 2002.

McPherson M, Weissman G, Strickland BB, et al: Implementing community-based systems of services for child and youths with special health care needs: how well are we doing? *Pediatrics* 113(5):1538–1544, 2004.

Meert KL, Shear K, Newth CJ, et al: Eunice Kennedy Shriver National Institute of Child Health and Human Development Collaborative Pediatric Critical Care Research Network. Follow-up study of complicated grief among parents eighteen months after a child's death in the pediatric intensive care unit, *J Palliat Med* 14(2):207–214, 2011.

Mentro A: Health care policy for medically fragile pediatric patients, *J Pediatr Nurs* 18(4):22, 2003.

Miles M, Holditch-Davis D, Burchinal M, et al: Distress and growth outcomes in mothers of medically fragile infants, *Nurs Res* 48:129–140, 1999.

Monterosso L, Kristjanson LJ, Aoun S, et al: Supportive and palliative care needs of families of children with life-threatening illnesses in Western Australia: evidence to guide the development of a palliative care service, *Palliat Med* 1(8):689–696, 2007.

Moriarty H, Carroll R, Cotroneo M: Differences in bereavement reactions within couples following the death of a child, *Res Nurs Health* 19:461–469, 1996.

Murray JS: Siblings of children with cancer: a review of the literature, *J Pediatr Oncol Nurs* 16(1):25–34, 1999.

Nelson AM: A metasynthesis: mothering other-than-normal children, *Qual Health Res* 12:515–530, 2002.

Nuutila L, Salanterä S: Children with a long-term illness: parents' experiences of care, *J Pediatr Nurs* 21(2):153–160, 2006.

O'Brien ME, Wegner CB: Rearing the child who is technology dependent: perceptions of parents and home care nurses, *J Spec Pediatr Nurs* 7:7–15, 2002.

Ochieng BM: Minority ethnic families and family-centered care, *J Child Health Care* 7(2):123–132, 2003.

Pierucci RL, Kirby RS, Leuthner SR: End-of-life for neonates and infants: the experience and effects of a palliative care consultation service, *Pediatrics* 108(3):653–660, 2001.

Raina P, O'Donnell M, Rosenbaum P, et al: The health and well-being of caregivers of children with cerebral palsy, *Pediatrics* 115(6):e626–e636, 2005.

Ray LD: Parenting and childhood chronicity: making visible the invisible work, *J Pediatr Nurs* 17(6):424–438, 2002.

Rehm RS: Religious faith in Mexican-American families dealing with chronic childhood illness, *Image J Nurs Sch* 31:33–38, 1999.

Rehm RS, Bradley JF. The search for social safety and satisfaction in families raising children with complex chronic conditions, *J Fam Nurs* 11(1):59–78, 2005.

Ritchie MA: Self-esteem and hopefulness in adolescents with cancer, *J Pediatr Nurs* 16:35–42, 2001.

Rossiter L, Sharpe D: The siblings of individuals with mental retardation: a quantitative integration of the literature, *J Child Fam Studies* 10(1):65–84, 2001.

Rousseau P: Ethical and legal issues in palliative care, *Prim Care* 28:391–400, 2001.

Sahler O, Frager G, Levetown M, et al: Medical education about end-of-life care in the pediatric setting: principles, challenges, and opportunities, *Pediatrics* 105:575–584, 2000.

Schor EL: Family pediatrics: report of the Task Force on the Family, *Pediatrics* 111:1541–1571, 2003.

Sharpe D, Rossiter L: Siblings of children with a chronic illness: a meta-analysis, *J Pediatr Psychol* 27:699–710, 2002.

Shepard MP, Mahon MM: Chronic conditions and the family. In Jackson PL, Vessey JA, editors: *Primary care of the child with a chronic condition*, ed 3, St Louis, 2000, Mosby.

Sine D, Sumner L, Gracy D, et al: Pediatric extubation: "pulling the tube," *J Palliat Med* 4:519–524, 2001.

Smaldone A, Ritholz MD: Perceptions of parenting children with type 1 diabetes diagnosed in early childhood, *J Pediatr Health Care* 25(2):87–95, 2011.

Stein REK: Home care: a challenging opportunity, *Child Health Care* 14(2):90–95, 1985.

Sterling YM, Peterson JW: Characteristics of African American women caregivers of children with asthma, *MCN Am J Matern Child* 28:32–38, 2003.

Sullivan-Bolyai S, Sadler L, Knafl KA, et al: Great expectations: a position description for parents as caregivers, part I, *Pediatr Nurs* 29(6):52–56, 2003.

Sumner LH: Lighting the way: improving the way children die in America, *Caring* 22:14–18, 2003.

Swallow VM, Jacoby A: Mothers' evolving relationships with doctors and nurses during the chronic childhood illness trajectory, *J Adv Nurs* 36:755–764, 2001.

Swallow V, Macfadyen A, Santacroce SJ, et al: Fathers' contributions to the management of their child's long-term medical condition: a narrative review of the literature, *Health Expect* 15(2):157–175, 2012.

Thomlinson EH: The lived experience of families of children who are failing to thrive, *J Adv Nurs* 39:537–545, 2002.

Tong H, Kandala G, Haig AJ, et al: Physical functioning in female caregivers of children with physical disabilities compared with female caregivers of children with a chronic medical condition, *Arch Pediatr Adolesc Med* 156:1138–1142, 2002.

Vance JC, Najman JM, Thearle MJ, et al: Psychological changes in parents eight months after the loss of an infant from stillbirth, neonatal death, or sudden infant death syndrome—a longitudinal study, *Pediatrics* 96(5):933–938, 1995.

van Dyck PC, Kogan MD, McPherson MG, et al: Prevalence and characteristics of children with special health care needs, *Arch Pediatr Adolesc Med* 158(9):884–890, 2004.

Watson D, Townsley R, Abbott D: Exploring multi-agency working in services to disabled children with complex health care needs and their families, *J Clin Nurs* 11:367–375, 2002.

Whitehead LC, Gosling V: Parent's perceptions of interactions with health professionals in the pathway to gaining a diagnosis of tuberous sclerosis (TS) and beyond, *Res Dev Disabil* 24:109–119, 2003.

Winkler WD, Mardegian CA: Completing the continuum of care: the growth of a pediatric hospice program, *Caring* 20:22–25, 2001.

Wise PH, Wampler NS, Chavkin W, et al: Chronic illness among poor children enrolled in the temporary assistance for needy families program, *Am J Public Health* 92:1458–1461, 2002.

Wolfe J, Friebert S, Hilden J: Caring for children with advanced cancer integrating palliative care, *Pediatr Clin North Am* 49(5):1043–1062, 2002.

Wolfe J, Grier HE, Klar N, et al: Symptoms and suffering at the end of life in children with cancer, *N Engl J Med* 342(5):326–333, 2000.

Wood PR, Smith LA, Romero D, et al: Relationships between welfare status, health insurance status, and health and medical care among children with asthma, *Am J Public Health* 92:1446–1452, 2002.

World Health Organization: *Cancer pain relief and palliative care*, Geneva, 1996, Author.

World Health Organization: Definition of palliative care for children, 1998, www.who.int/cancer/palliative/definition/en.

Young B, Dixon-Woods M, Windridge KC, et al: Managing communication with young people who have a potentially life-threatening chronic illness: qualitative study of patients and parents, *BMJ* 326(7384):305, 2003.

Zuvekas SH, Taliaferro GS: Pathways to access: health, insurance, the health care delivery system and racial/ethnic disparities, 1996-1999, *Health Affairs* 22(2):139–153, 2003.

Impact of Cognitive or Sensory Impairment on the Child and Family

Marilyn J. Hockenberry

evolve WEBSITE

http://evolve.elsevier.com/Perry/maternal

LEARNING OBJECTIVES

On completion of this chapter, the reader will be able to:
- Define the classifications of intellectual disability.
- Define developmental delay.
- Outline nursing interventions for the child with cognitive impairment that promote optimal development, including during hospitalization.
- Identify the major biologic and cognitive characteristics of children with Down syndrome.
- Outline nursing interventions for children with Down syndrome.
- Identify the major characteristics associated with fragile X syndrome.

- List the general classifications of hearing impairment and the effect on speech.
- Outline nursing interventions for children with hearing impairment, including during hospitalization.
- List the common types of visual impairments in children.
- Outline nursing interventions for children with visual impairment, including during hospitalization.
- Outline nursing interventions for children with retinoblastoma.
- Outline nursing interventions for children with an autism spectrum disorder.

COGNITIVE IMPAIRMENT

General Concepts

Cognitive impairment (CI) is a general term that encompasses any type of mental difficulty or deficiency. In this chapter the term is used synonymously with intellectual disability and replaces the term mental retardation (MR), defined by the American Association on Intellectual and Developmental Disabilities (AAIDD, 2010). Although the needs and concerns of the family are a primary focus throughout the chapter, readers are encouraged to review Chapter 36, which details the family's adjustment to disabilities in general.

The definition of intellectual disability in children consists of three components: intellectual functioning, functional strengths and weaknesses, and age younger than 18 years at time of diagnosis. Intellectual functioning is measured by the intelligence quotient (IQ) of 70 to 75 or below. The child with an intellectual disability must demonstrate functional impairment in at least 2 of 10 different adaptive skill areas: communication, self-care, home living, social skills, leisure, health and safety, self-direction, functional academics, community use, and work (American Psychiatric Association, 2013) or have deficits in one or more adaptive domains (AAIDD, 2010). The classification system by the AAIDD allows for identification of

the individual's specific needs in four established dimensions of care (Box 37-1). Careful evaluation to identify the needs of individuals with CI is focused on promoting habilitation for each person. It is anticipated that the functional capabilities of children with CI will improve over time when support is provided.

Diagnosis and Classification

The diagnosis of CI is usually made after a period of suspicion, by professionals or the family, that the child's developmental progress is delayed. In some cases it is confirmed at birth because of recognition of distinct syndromes such as Down syndrome and fetal alcohol syndrome. At the other extreme the diagnosis is made when problems such as speech delays arouse concern. In all cases a high index of suspicion for developmental delay and behavioral signs (Box 37-2) is necessary for early diagnosis; routine developmental screening can help in early identification (see Chapter 29). Delays are typically seen in gross and fine motor and speech development, although the latter is most predictive. Developmental delay can be described as any significant lag in a child's physical, cognitive, behavioral, emotional, or social development when compared against developmental norms. CI is a permanent impairment encompassing cognitive ability and adaptive behavior that are

DIMENSIONS OF CARE FOR INTELLECTUALLY DISABLED PATIENTS

- *Dimension I*—Intellectual functioning and adaptive skills
- *Dimension II*—Psychologic and emotional considerations
- *Dimension III*—Physical, health, and etiology considerations
- *Dimension IV*—Environmental considerations

EARLY BEHAVIORAL SIGNS SUGGESTIVE OF COGNITIVE IMPAIRMENT

- Dysmorphic features (e.g., Down syndrome, fragile X syndrome)
- Irritability or unresponsiveness to contact
- Abnormal eye contact
- Gross motor delay
- Decreased alertness to voice or movement
- Language difficulties or delay
- Feeding difficulties

Modified from Shapiro B, Batshaw M: Mental retardation (intellectual disability). In Kliegman RM, Behrman RE, Jenson HB, editors: *Nelson textbook of pediatrics*, ed 18, Philadelphia, 2007, Saunders; Wilks T, Gerber J, Erdie-Lalena C: Developmental milestones: cognitive development, *Pediatr Rev* 31(9):364–367, 2010.

functioning significantly below average (see Box 37-2). In the absence of clear-cut evidence of CI, it is more appropriate to use a diagnosis of developmental delay.

Results of standardized tests are used in making the diagnosis of intellectual disability based on cognitive deficits. Tests for assessing adaptive behaviors include the Vineland Social Maturity Scale and the American Association of Mental Retardation (AAMR) Adaptive Behavior Scale. Informal appraisal of adaptive behavior may be made by those fully acquainted with the child (e.g., teachers, parents, other care providers). Frequently these observations lead parents to seek evaluation of the child's development.

A more useful approach for clinical application is classification based on educational potential or symptom severity. For educational purposes the mildly impaired group (educable MR) constitutes about 85% of all people with CI, and the group with moderate levels of CI (trainable MR) accounts for about 10% of the intellectually disabled population (American Psychiatric Association, 2000; Katz and Lazcano-Ponce, 2008; Walker and Johnson, 2006) (Table 37-1). Although nurses may be familiar with the approximate range of IQ for classifying severity, they should refrain from using numbers as the criterion for assessing or evaluating the child's abilities because numbers are of little value in counseling parents or training these children.

Etiology

The causes of severe CI are primarily genetic, biochemical, and infectious. Although the etiology is unknown in most cases,

TABLE 37-1   CLASSIFICATION OF COGNITIVE IMPAIRMENT

LEVEL (IQ)*	PRESCHOOL (BIRTH–5 YEARS)—MATURATION AND DEVELOPMENT	SCHOOL AGE (6-21 YEARS)— TRAINING AND EDUCATION	ADULT (≥21 YEARS)— SOCIAL AND VOCATIONAL ADEQUACY
Mild—50-55 to ≈70-75	Often not noticed as delayed by casual observer but is slower to walk, feed self, and talk than most children; follows same sequence in development as normal children	Can acquire practical skills and useful reading and arithmetic to a third- to sixth-grade level with special education; can be guided toward social conformity; achieves mental age of 8-12 years	Can usually achieve social and vocational skills adequate to self-maintenance; may need occasional guidance and support when under unusual social or economic stress; can adjust to marriage but not childrearing
Moderate—35-40 to 50-55	Noticeable delays in motor development, especially in speech; responds to training in various self-help activities	Can learn simple communication, elementary health and safety habits, and simple manual skills; does not progress in functional reading or arithmetic; achieves mental age of 3-7 years	Can perform simple tasks under sheltered conditions; participates in simple recreation; travels alone in familiar places; usually incapable of self-maintenance
Severe—20-25 to 35-40	Marked delay in motor development; little or no communication skills; may respond to training in elementary self-care (e.g., self-feeding)	Usually walks, barring specific disability; has some understanding of speech and some response; can profit from systematic habit training; achieves mental age of toddler	Can conform to daily routines and repetitive activities; needs continuing direction and supervision in protective environment
Profound—below 20-25	Gross delay; minimum capacity for functioning in sensorimotor areas; needs total care	Obvious delays in all areas of development; shows basic emotional responses; may respond to skillful training in use of legs, hands, and jaws; needs close supervision; achieves mental age of young infant	May walk; needs complete custodial care; has primitive speech; usually benefits from regular physical activity

*Data from American Psychiatric Association: *Diagnostic and statistical manual of mental disorders (DSM-5)*, ed 5, Washington, DC, 2013, The Association; and Rittey CD: Learning difficulties: what the neurologist needs to know, *J Neurol Neurosurg Psychiatry* 74(suppl 1): 30–36, 2005.
IQ, intelligence quotient.

familial, social, environmental, and organic causes may predominate. Among individuals with CI, a sizable proportion of the cases are linked to Down syndrome, fragile X syndrome, or fetal alcohol syndrome. General categories of events that may lead to CI include the following (Katz and Lazcano-Ponce, 2008; Walker and Johnson, 2006):

- Infection and intoxication such as congenital rubella, syphilis, maternal drug consumption (e.g., fetal alcohol syndrome), chronic lead ingestion, or kernicterus
- Trauma or physical agent (i.e., injury to the brain experienced during the prenatal, perinatal, or postnatal period)
- Inadequate nutrition and metabolic disorders such as phenylketonuria or congenital hypothyroidism
- Gross postnatal brain disease such as neurofibromatosis and tuberous sclerosis
- Unknown prenatal influence, including cerebral and cranial malformations such as microcephaly and hydrocephalus
- Chromosome abnormalities resulting from radiation, viruses, chemicals, parental age, and genetic mutations such as Down syndrome and fragile X syndrome
- Gestational disorders, including prematurity, low birth weight, and postmaturity
- Psychiatric disorders that have their onset during the child's developmental period up to age 18 years such as autism spectrum disorders (ASDs)
- Environmental influences, including evidence of a deprived environment associated with a history of intellectual disability among parents and siblings

Nursing Care of Children with Impaired Cognitive Function

Nurses play a major role in identifying children with CI. In the newborn and early infancy periods few signs are present, with the exception of Down syndrome (see p. 1090). However, after this age delayed developmental milestones are the major clues to CI. In addition, nurses must have a high index of suspicion for early behavior patterns that may suggest CI (see Box 37-2). Parental concerns such as delayed development compared with siblings need to be taken seriously. All children should receive regular developmental assessment, and the nurse is often the person responsible for performing such assessments (see Chapter 29). When delays are found, the nurse must use sensitivity and discretion in revealing this finding to parents.

Educate Child and Family

To teach children with CI, it is necessary to investigate their learning abilities and deficits. This is important for the nurse who may be involved in a home care program or caring for the child in a health care setting. The nurse who understands how these children learn can teach them basic skills or prepare them for various health-related procedures effectively.

Children with CI have a marked deficit in their ability to discriminate between two or more stimuli because of difficulty in recognizing the relevance of specific cues. However, these children can learn to discriminate if the cues are presented in an exaggerated, concrete form and if all extraneous stimuli are eliminated. For example, the use of colors to emphasize visual cues or the use of singing or rhymes to stress auditory cues can help them learn. Their deficit in discrimination also implies that concrete ideas are learned much more effectively than abstract ideas. Therefore demonstration is preferable to verbal explanation, and learning should be directed

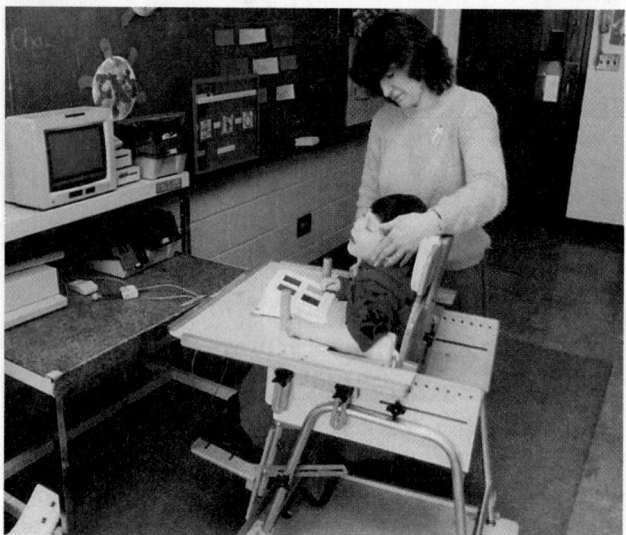

FIG 37-1 A push panel allows a child with cognitive impairment to turn a computer on and off.

toward mastering a skill rather than understanding the scientific principles underlying a procedure.

Another cognitive deficit is in short-term memory. Children of average intelligence can remember several words, numbers, or directions at one time; children with CI are less able to do so. Therefore they need simple, one-step directions. Learning through a step-by-step process requires a task analysis in which each task is separated into its necessary components and each step is taught completely before proceeding to the next activity.

One critical area of learning that has had a tremendous impact on education for cognitively impaired individuals is motivation. Programs based on the motivational principles of behavior modification, using positive reinforcement for specific tasks or behaviors, have demonstrated marked improvement in children's ability to learn. Advances in technology have greatly aided in providing reinforcement, especially in children with severe disabilities and who may have physical disabilities that limit their range of capabilities. For example, with the use of specially designed switches, children are given control of some event in the environment such as turning on the television (Fig. 37-1). The television picture becomes the reinforcement for activating the switch. Repetitive use of these switches provides an early, simplistic association with a technical device that may progress to increasingly complex aids.

Early-intervention program is a systematic program of therapy, exercises, and activities designed to address developmental delays in disabled children to help achieve their full potential (American Academy of Pediatrics [AAP] Committee on Genetics, 2001; National Down Syndrome Society, 2011a; Weijerman and de Winter, 2010). Considerable evidence indicates that these programs are valuable for cognitively impaired children. Nurses working with these families need to be aware of the types of programs in their community. Under the Individuals with Disabilities Education Act (IDEA) of 1990 (Public Law 101-476), states are encouraged to provide full early-intervention services and are required to provide educational opportunities for all children with disabilities from birth to 21 years of age. Services may be provided under state Programs for Children with Special Health Needs or Head Start or by private organizations such as National Down Syndrome

Society,* Easter Seals,† or the Arc of the United States.‡ Parents should inquire about these programs by contacting the appropriate agencies. The child's education should begin as soon as possible. As children grow older, their education should be directed toward vocational training that prepares them for as independent a lifestyle as possible within their scope of abilities.

Teach Child Self-Care Skills

When a child with CI is born, parents need help in promoting normal developmental skills that are almost automatically learned by other children. These include self-care skills such as feeding, toileting, dressing, and grooming. Teaching these skills requires a basic knowledge of the developmental sequence in learning the skills demonstrated by children of average intelligence. For example, children with subaverage intelligence would not be expected to dress themselves as early as unaffected youngsters.

Teaching self-care skills also necessitates a working knowledge of the individual steps needed to master a skill. For example, before beginning a self-feeding program, the nurse performs a task analysis. After a task analysis the child is observed in a particular situation such as eating to determine what skills the child possesses and his or her developmental readiness to learn the task. Family members are included in this process because their "readiness" is as important as the child's. Numerous self-help aids are available to facilitate independence and can help eliminate some of the difficulties of learning such as using a plate with suction cups to prevent accidental spills.§

Promote Child's Optimal Development

Optimal development involves more than achieving independence. It requires appropriate guidance for establishing acceptable social behavior and personal feelings of self-esteem, worth, and security. These attributes are not simply learned through a stimulation program. Rather they must arise from the genuine love and caring that exist among family members. However, families need guidance in providing an environment that fosters optimal development. Often the nurse can provide this help.

Another important area for promoting optimal development and self-esteem is ensuring the child's physical well-being. Any congenital defects such as cardiac, gastrointestinal, or orthopedic anomalies should be repaired. Plastic surgery may be considered when the child's appearance can be improved substantially. Dental health is significant, and orthodontic and restorative procedures can improve facial appearance immensely.

Encourage Play and Exercise

Children who are cognitively impaired have the same needs for recreation and exercise as other children. However, because of the children's slower development, parents may be less aware of these needs. Therefore the nurse guides parents toward selection of suitable play and exercise activities (Fig. 37-2). Because play has been

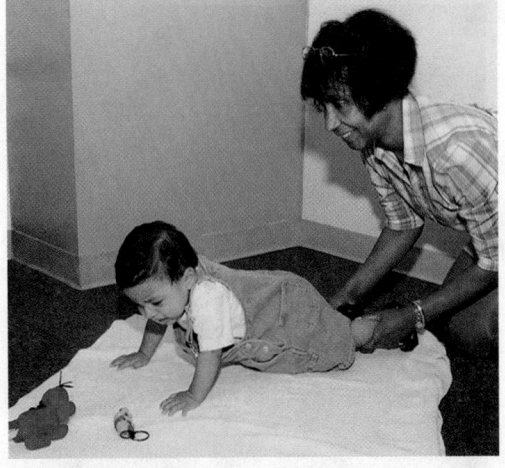

FIG 37-2 Placing an attractive object outside the child's reach encourages crawling movements. (Courtesy James DeLeon, Texas Children's Hospital, Houston, TX.)

discussed for children in each age-group in earlier chapters, only the exceptions are presented here.

The type of play is based on the child's developmental age, although the need for sensorimotor play may be prolonged for several years. Parents should use every opportunity to expose the child to as many different sounds, sights, and sensations as possible. Appropriate play includes musical mobiles, stuffed toys, water play, floating toys, a rocking chair or horse, a swing, bells, and rattles. The child should be taken on outings such as trips to the grocery store or shopping center; other people should be encouraged to visit in the home; and the child should be related to directly such as by cuddling, holding, rocking, talking to him or her in the en face (face-to-face) position, and giving "rides" on the parents' shoulders.

Toys are selected for their recreational and educational value. For example, a large inflatable beach ball is a good water toy; it encourages interactive play and can be used to learn motor skills such as balance, rocking, kicking, and throwing. A doll with removable clothes and different types of closures can help the child learn dressing skills. Musical toys that mimic animal sounds or respond with social phrases are excellent ways of encouraging speech. Toys should be simple in design so the child can learn to manipulate them without help. For children with severe cognitive and physical impairment, electronic switches can be used to allow them to operate toys (Fig. 37-3).

Suitable activities for physical activity are based on the child's size, coordination, physical fitness and maturity, motivation, and health (Fig. 37-4). Some children may have physical problems that prevent participation in certain sports such as atlantoaxial instability in children with Down syndrome (see p. 1090). These children often have greater success in individual and dual sports than in team sports and enjoy themselves most with children of the same developmental level. The Special Olympics* provides these children with a unique competitive opportunity.

Safety is a major consideration in selecting recreational and exercise activities. For example, toys that may be appropriate

---

*Information on early intervention programs in each state is available from the National Down Syndrome Society, 666 Broadway 8th Floor, New York, NY 10012-2317, 800-221-4602, fax: 212-979-2873, email: info@ndss.org, www.ndss.org.

†233 South Wacker Dr., Suite 2400, Chicago, Ill 60606-4802, 800-221-6827, TTY: 312-726-4258, fax: 312-726-1494, www.easterseals.com.

‡1825 K Street NW, Suite 1200, Washington DC, 20006, 301-565-3842 or 800-433-5255, fax: 301-565-5342, www.thearc.org.

§A resource for a variety of self-help equipment is Sammons Preston, 1000 Remington Blvd, Suite 210, Bolingbrook, IL 60440-5071, 800-323-5547, fax: 800-547-4333, www.sammonspreston.com. In Canada: 800-665-9200.

*1133 19th St. NW, Washington, DC 20036, 800-700-8585 or 202-628-3630, fax: 202-824-0200, www.specialolympics.org. (Website includes listing of state offices.) In Canada: Special Olympics Canada, 21 St Clair Avenue East, Suite 600, Toronto, Ontario M4T 1L9, 888-888-0608 or 888-888-0608 or 416-927-9050, fax: 416-927-8475, www.specialolympics.ca.

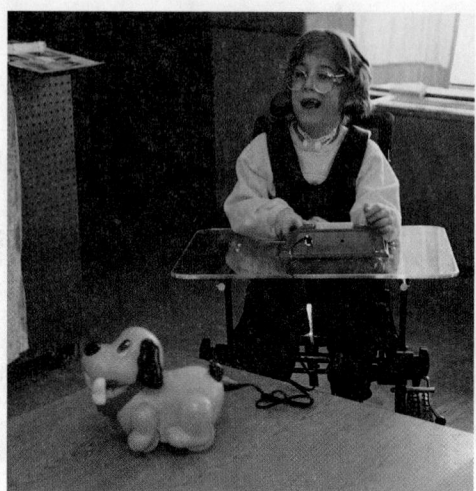

FIG 37-3 A manual switch allows a child with cognitive impairment to play with a battery-operated toy.

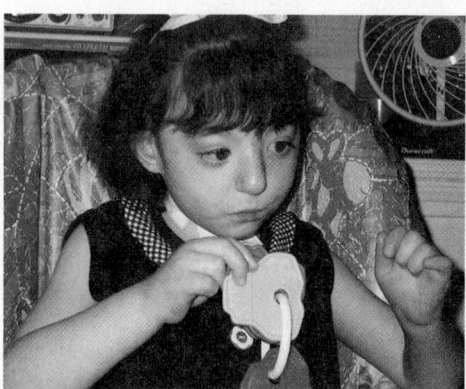

FIG 37-4 A favorite toy provides stimulation for a young child.

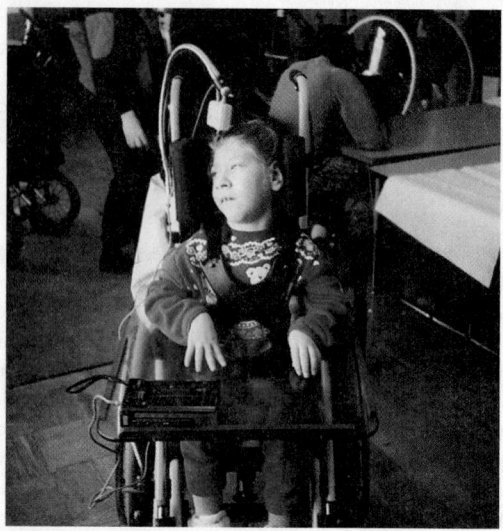

FIG 37-5 A child with cognitive and physical impairments can activate electronic and communication equipment by moving a device near her head.

developmentally may present dangers to a child who is strong enough to break them or use them incorrectly.

Provide Means of Communication

Verbal skills typically are delayed more than other physical skills. Speech requires hearing and interpretation (receptive skills) and facial muscle coordination (expressive skills). Because both types of skills may be impaired, these children need frequent audiometric testing and should be fitted with hearing aids if indicated. In addition, they may need help to learn to control their facial muscles. For example, some children may need tongue exercises to correct the tongue thrust or gentle reminders to keep the lips closed.

Nonverbal communication may be appropriate for some of these children, and various devices are available. For the child without associated physical disabilities a talking picture board is helpful. For children with physical limitations several adaptations or types of communication devices are available to facilitate selection of the appropriate picture or word (Fig. 37-5). Some children may be taught sign language or Blissymbols (i.e., a highly stylized system of graphic symbols representing words, ideas, and concepts). Although the symbols require education to learn their meaning, no reading skill is needed. The symbols are usually arranged on a board, and the person points or uses some type of selector to convey a message.

Establish Discipline

Discipline must begin early. Limit-setting measures need to be simple, consistently applied, and appropriate for the child's mental age. Control measures are based primarily on teaching a specific behavior rather than on understanding the reasons behind it. Stressing moral lessons is of little value to a child who lacks the cognitive skills to learn from self-criticism or from a lesson based on previous wrong-doing. Behavior modification, especially reinforcement of desired actions, and time-out are appropriate forms of behavior control.

Encourage Socialization

Acquiring social skills is a complex task, as is learning self-care procedures. Active rehearsals with role-playing and practice sessions and positive reinforcement for desired behavior have been the most successful approaches. Parents should be encouraged early to teach their child socially acceptable behavior: waving goodbye, saying "hello" and "thank you," responding to his or her name, greeting visitors, and sitting modestly. The teaching of socially acceptable sexual behavior is especially important to minimize sexual exploitation. Parents also need to expose the child to strangers so he or she can practice manners because there is no automatic transfer of learning from one situation to another.

Dressing and grooming are also important aspects of socialization. A child who is dressed in age-appropriate clothing and well groomed is much more likely to be accepted and develop positive self-esteem. Clothes should be clean, up-to-date, and well fitted. Many attractive outfits can be adapted with self-adhering fasteners and elastic openings to facilitate self-dressing.

As soon as possible parents should enroll the child in appropriate preschool programs. Not only do these programs provide education and training, but they also offer an opportunity for social experiences among the children. As children grow older, they should have peer experiences similar to those of other children, including group outings, sports, and organized activities such as scouts and Special Olympics. Nurses can assess the child's abilities and encourage others (e.g., parents, teachers) to promote developmentally appropriate peer interaction (Johnson and Walker, 2006; National Down Syndrome Society, 2011a; Shapiro and Batshaw, 2007).

Provide Information on Sexuality

Adolescence may be a particularly difficult time for the family, especially in terms of the child's sexual behavior, possibility of pregnancy, future plans to marry, and ability to be independent. Frequently little anticipatory guidance has been offered parents to prepare the child for physical and sexual maturation. The nurse can help in this area by providing parents with information about sex education that is geared to the child's developmental level. For example, adolescent girls need a *simple* explanation of menstruation and instructions on personal hygiene during the menstrual cycle.

These adolescents also need practical sexual information regarding anatomy, physical development, and conception.* Because of their easy persuasion and lack of judgment, they need a well-defined, concrete code of conduct. The subtleties of social sexual behavior are less beneficial than specific instructions for handling certain situations. For example, an adolescent should be told firmly never to go alone anywhere with any person that he or she does not know well. To protect him or her from abusive sexual activities, parents must observe their teenager's activities and associates closely. The question of contraceptive protection for these adolescents is often a parental concern.

Parents of these adolescents are often concerned about the advisability of marriage between two individuals with intellectual disabilities. There is no conclusive answer; each situation must be judged individually. In some instances marriage is possible, but parenthood may not be desirable because of the complexity of childrearing and the potential problem of perpetuating mental deficiency. The nurse should discuss this topic with parents and with the prospective couple, stressing suitable living accommodations and contraceptive methods to prevent pregnancy. If children are conceived, these parents require specialized help to learn to meet the needs of their offspring (Johnson and Walker, 2006).

Help Family Adjust to Future Care

Not all families are able to cope with home care of their affected child, especially one who is severely or profoundly impaired or has multiple disabilities. Older parents may not be able to assume care responsibilities after they reach retirement or older age. For these parents the decision regarding residential placement is a difficult one, and the availability of such facilities varies widely. The nurse working with a family should help them investigate and evaluate various programs and adjust to the decision for placement.

Care for Child During Hospitalization

Caring for the child during hospitalization can be a special challenge. Frequently nurses are unfamiliar with children who are cognitively impaired, and they may cope with their feelings of insecurity and fear by ignoring or isolating the child. Not only is this approach nonsupportive, but it may also be destructive for the child's sense of self-esteem and optimal development, and it may hamper the parents' ability to cope with the stress of the experience. One method that successfully avoids this nontherapeutic approach is the use of the mutual-participation model in planning the child's care. Parents are encouraged to stay with their child but should not be made to feel as if the responsibility is theirs alone.

When the child is admitted, a detailed history is taken (see Chapter 29), especially in terms of all self-care activity. During the interview the child's developmental age is assessed. It is best to avoid asking directly about IQ levels because this may make the parents uncomfortable and often tells little about the child's actual abilities. Questions are approached positively. For example, rather than asking, "Is your child toilet trained yet?" the nurse may state, "Tell me about your child's toileting habits." The assessment should also focus on any special devices the child uses, effective measures of limit setting, unusual or favorite routines, and any behaviors that may require intervention. If the parent states that the child engages in self-injurious activities (e.g., head banging, self-biting), the nurse should inquire about events that precipitate them and techniques (e.g., distraction, medication) that the parents use to manage them (Johnson and Walker, 2006; Oliver and Richards, 2010).

The nurse also assesses the child's functional level of eating and playing; ability to express needs verbally; progress in toilet training; and relationship with objects, toys, and other children. The child is encouraged to be as independent as possible in the hospital.

Realizing that the child may be lonely in the hospital, the nurse makes certain that toys and other activities are provided. The child is placed in a room with other children of approximately the same developmental age, preferably a room with only two beds to avoid overstimulation. The nurse discusses with the other parents the child's abilities and introduces the parents and children to one another. By the nurse's example of treating the child with dignity and respect, others who may fear what they do not understand are encouraged to accept the child.

Procedures are explained to the child through methods of communication that are at the appropriate cognitive level. Generally explanations should be simple, short, and concrete, emphasizing what the child will experience *physically*. Demonstration either through actual practice or with visual aids is always preferable to verbal explanation. The nurse repeats instructions often and evaluates the child's understanding by asking questions such as, "What will it feel like?" "Show me how you must lie," or "Where will the dressing be?" Parents are included in preprocedural teaching for their own learning and to help the nurse learn effective methods of communicating with the child.

During hospitalization the nurse should also focus on growth-promoting experiences for the child. For example, hospitalization may be an excellent opportunity to emphasize to parents abilities that the child does have but has not had the opportunity to practice such as self-dressing. It may also be an opportunity for social experiences with peers, group play, or new educational and recreational activities. For example, one child who had the habit of screaming and kicking demonstrated a definite decrease in these behaviors after he learned to pound pegs and use a punching bag. Through social services the parents may become aware of specialized programs for the child. Hospitalization may also offer parents a respite from everyday care responsibilities and an opportunity to discuss their feelings with a concerned professional.

Assist in Measures to Prevent Cognitive Impairment

Besides having a responsibility to families with a child with CI, nurses also need to be involved in programs aimed at preventing CI. Many of the familial, social, and environmental factors known to cause mild impairment are preventable. Counseling and education can reduce or eliminate such factors (e.g., poor nutrition, cigarette smoking, chemical abuse), which increase the risk of prematurity and intrauterine growth restriction. Interventions are directed toward improving maternal health by educating women regarding the dangers of chemicals, including prenatal alcohol exposure, which affects organogenesis; craniofacial development; and

---

*Sources of information on sexuality and conception are the Arc of the United States (see footnote, p. 1087) and Planned Parenthood Federation of America, 434 W. 33rd St., New York, NY 10001, 212-541-7800 or 800-230-7526, fax: 212-245-1845, www.plannedparenthood.org.

cognitive ability (Defendi, 2010; Wilton and Plane, 2006). Other preventive strategies that play an important role include adequate prenatal care; optimal medical care of high-risk newborns; rubella immunization; genetic counseling and prenatal screening, especially in terms of Down or fragile X syndrome; use of folic acid supplements to prevent neural tube defects during pregnancy and the childbearing years; newborn screening for treatable inborn errors of metabolism such as congenital hypothyroidism, phenylketonuria, and galactosemia; and early appropriate therapies and rehabilitation services for children with developmental disabilities.

Down Syndrome

Down syndrome is the most common chromosome abnormality of a generalized syndrome, occurring in one in 691 to 1000 live births (National Down Syndrome Society, 2011b; Weijerman and de Winter, 2010). It occurs in people of all races and economic levels.

Etiology

The cause of Down syndrome is not known, but evidence from cytogenetic and epidemiologic studies supports the concept of multiple causality. Approximately 95% of all cases of Down syndrome are attributable to an extra chromosome 21 (group G); thus the name nonfamilial trisomy 21 (National Down Syndrome Society, 2011b; Walker and Johnson, 2006). Although children with trisomy 21 are born to parents of all ages, there is a statistically greater risk in older women, particularly those older than 35 years of age. For example, in women 35 years of age the chance of conceiving a child with Down syndrome is about 1 in 350 live births, but in women age 40 it is approximately 1 in 100. However, the majority (≈80%) of infants with Down syndrome are born to women younger than 35 years of age because younger women have higher fertility rates (National Down Syndrome Society, 2011b). Approximately 3% to 4% of the cases may be caused by translocation of chromosomes 15 and 21 or 22. This type of genetic aberration is usually hereditary and is not associated with advanced parental age. of affected people, 1% to 2% demonstrate mosaicism, which refers to a mixture of normal and abnormal cell types. The degree of cognitive and physical impairment is related to the percentage of cells with the abnormal chromosome makeup.

Diagnostic Evaluation

Down syndrome can usually be diagnosed by the clinical manifestations alone (Box 37-3 and Fig. 37-6), but a chromosome analysis should be done to confirm the genetic abnormality.

Several physical problems are associated with Down syndrome. Many of these children have congenital heart malformations, the most common being septal defects. Respiratory tract infections are prevalent and, when combined with cardiac anomalies, are the chief causes of death, particularly during the first year of life. Hypotonicity of chest and abdominal muscles and dysfunction of the immune system probably predispose the child to the development of respiratory tract infection. Other physical problems include thyroid dysfunction, especially congenital hypothyroidism, and an increased incidence of leukemia.

Therapeutic Management

Although no cure exists for Down syndrome, a number of therapies such as surgery to correct serious congenital anomalies (e.g., heart defects, strabismus) are advocated. These children also benefit from evaluative echocardiography soon after birth and regular medical care. Evaluation of sight and hearing is essential; and treatment of otitis media is required to prevent auditory loss, which can influence

---

BOX 37-3   CLINICAL MANIFESTATIONS OF DOWN SYNDROME

Head and Eyes
- Separated sagittal suture*
- Brachycephaly
- Rounded and small skull
- Flat occiput
- Enlarged anterior fontanel
- Oblique palpebral fissures (upward, outward slant)*
- Inner epicanthal folds
- Speckling of iris (Brushfield spots)

Nose and Ears
- Small nose*
- Depressed nasal bridge (saddle nose)*
- Small ears and narrow canals
- Short pinna (vertical ear length)
- Overlapping upper helices
- Conductive hearing loss

Mouth and Neck
- High, arched, narrow palate*
- Protruding tongue
- Hypoplastic mandible
- Delayed teeth eruption and microdontia
- Alignment teeth abnormalities common
- Periodontal disease
- Neck skin excess and laxity*
- Short and broad neck

Chest and Heart
- Shortened rib cage
- Twelfth-rib anomalies
- Pectus excavatum or carinatum
- Congenital heart defects common (e.g., atrial septal defect, ventricular septal defect)

Abdomen and Genitalia
- Protruding, lax, and flabby abdominal muscles
- Diastasis recti abdominis
- Umbilical hernia
- Small penis
- Cryptorchidism
- Bulbous vulva

Hands and Feet
- Broad, short hands and stubby fingers
- Incurved little finger (clinodactyly)
- Transverse palmar crease
- Wide space between big and second toes*
- Plantar crease between big and second toes*
- Broad, short feet and stubby toes

Musculoskeletal and Skin
- Short stature
- Hyperflexibility and muscle weakness*
- Hypotonia
- Atlantoaxial instability
- Dry, cracked, and frequent fissuring
- Cutis marmorata (mottling)

Other
- Reduced birth weight
- Learning difficulty (average intelligence quotient of 50)
- Hypothyroidism common
- Impaired immune function
- Increased risk of leukemia
- Early-onset dementia (in one third)

*Most common findings in modified chart (Pueschel, 1999).

---

cognitive function. Periodic testing of thyroid function is recommended, especially if growth is severely delayed. Children participating in sports that may involve stress on the head and neck such as gymnastics, diving, butterfly stroke in swimming, high jump, and soccer should be evaluated radiologically for atlantoaxial instability. Symptoms of the disorder include neck pain, weakness, and torticollis. Affected children are at risk for spinal cord compression.

! NURSING ALERT

Report immediately any child with the following signs of spinal cord compression:
- Persistent neck pain
- Loss of established motor skills and bladder or bowel control
- Changes in sensation

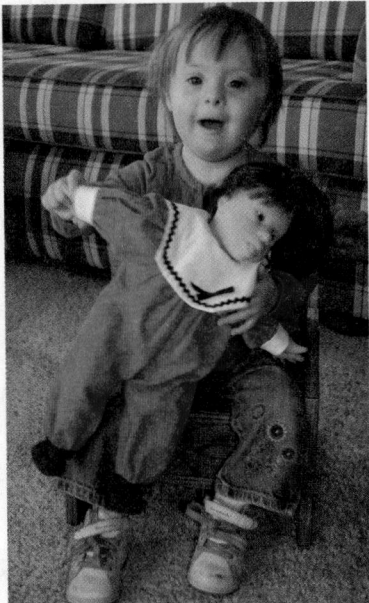

FIG 37-6 Down syndrome in an infant. Note the infant's small, square head with upward slant to the eyes; flat nasal bridge; protruding tongue; mottled skin; and hypotonia. (Courtesy Shannon E. Perry, San Francisco, CA.)

Prognosis. Life expectancy for those with Down syndrome has improved in recent years but remains lower than for the general population. More than 80% survive to age 60 years and beyond (National Down Syndrome Society, 2011b; Weijerman and de Winter, 2010). As the prognosis continues to improve for these individuals, it will be important to provide for their long-term health care and social and leisure needs.

CARE MANAGEMENT

Support Family at Time of Diagnosis. Because of the unique physical characteristics, infants with Down syndrome are usually diagnosed at birth, and parents should be informed of the diagnosis at this time. Parents usually prefer that both of them be present during the informing interview so they can support one another emotionally. They appreciate receiving reading material about the syndrome* and being referred to others such as parent groups or professional counseling for help or advice.

After parents are aware of the diagnosis, they are confronted with the crisis of losing their perfect or dream child and grieving for and accepting their reality child. Consequently the parents' responses to the child may greatly influence decisions regarding future care. Some families willingly take the child home, whereas others consider immediate residential placement. The nurse must carefully answer questions regarding developmental potential. Institutionalization is no longer an option. For families unable or ill prepared to choose taking the newborn home, specialized foster care and adoption are other options (see Critical Thinking Case Study).

---

*Sources of information include the Arc of the United States (see footnote, p. 1087); the AAIDD, 501 3rd Street NW, Suite 200, Washington, DC 20001, 800-424-3688, fax: 202-387-2193, www.aamr.org; the National Down Syndrome Society (see footnote, p. 1087); and the National Down Syndrome Congress, 30 Mansell Court, Suite 108, Roswell, GA 30076, 800-232-6372 or 770-604-9500, www.ndsccenter.org.

? CRITICAL THINKING CASE STUDY

Diagnosis of Down Syndrome

The parents of Melissa, a newborn diagnosed as having Down syndrome, ask the nurse, "What are we supposed to do with her?" They further state that they already have three other children at home.
1. Evidence—Is there sufficient evidence to draw conclusions about the parents' concerns regarding their newborn daughter?
2. Assumptions—Describe an underlying assumption about each of the following:
   a. Newborn diagnosed with Down syndrome
   b. Parental care of a newborn with Down syndrome
   c. Newborn with Down syndrome and older siblings
3. What priorities for the nursing response should be established?
4. Does the evidence support your nursing intervention?

Assist Family in Preventing Physical Problems. Many of the physical characteristics of infants with Down syndrome present nursing problems. The hypotonicity of muscles and hyperextensibility of joints complicate positioning. The limp, flaccid extremities resemble the posture of a rag doll; as a result, holding the infant is difficult and cumbersome. Sometimes parents perceive this lack of molding to their bodies as evidence of inadequate parenting. The extended body position promotes heat loss because more surface area is exposed to the environment. Parents are encouraged to swaddle or wrap the infant tightly in a blanket before picking him or her up to provide security and warmth. The nurse also discusses with parents their feelings concerning attachment to the child, emphasizing that the child's lack of clinging or molding is a physical characteristic, not a sign of detachment or rejection.

Decreased muscle tone compromises respiratory expansion. In addition, the underdeveloped nasal bone causes a chronic problem of inadequate drainage of mucus. The constant stuffy nose forces the child to breathe by mouth, which dries the oropharyngeal membranes, increasing the susceptibility to upper respiratory tract infections. Measures to lessen these problems include clearing the nose with a bulb-type syringe, rinsing the mouth with water after feedings, increasing fluid intake, and using a cool-mist vaporizer to keep the mucous membranes moist and the secretions liquefied. Other helpful measures include changing the child's position frequently, performing postural drainage with percussion if necessary, practicing good hand washing, and properly disposing of soiled articles such as tissues. If antibiotics are ordered, the nurse stresses the importance of completing the full course of therapy for successful eradication of the infection and prevention of growth of resistant organisms.

Inadequate drainage resulting in pooling of mucus in the nose also interferes with feeding. Because the child breathes by mouth, sucking for any length of time is difficult. When eating solids, the child may gag on the food because of mucus in the oropharynx. Parents are advised to clear the nose before each feeding; give small, frequent feedings; and allow opportunities for rest during mealtime.

The protruding tongue also interferes with feeding, especially of solid foods. Parents need to know that the tongue thrust is not an indication of refusal to feed but a physiologic response. They are advised to use a small but long, straight-handled spoon to push the food toward the back and side of the mouth. If food is thrust out, it should be fed again.

Dietary intake needs supervision. Decreased muscle tone affects gastric motility, predisposing the child to constipation. Dietary measures such as increased fiber and fluid promote evacuation. The child's eating habits may need careful scrutiny to prevent obesity. Height and weight measurements should be obtained on a serial basis, especially during infancy. Because these children grow more slowly than the general pediatric population, special growth charts developed for them should be used (AAP, Committee on Genetics, 2001; National Down Syndrome Society, 2011c).

During infancy the child's skin is pliable and soft. However, it gradually becomes rough and dry and is prone to cracking and infection. Skin care involves the use of minimum soap and application of lubricants. Lip balm is applied to the lips, especially when the child is outdoors, to prevent excessive chapping.

Assist in Prenatal Diagnosis and Genetic Counseling. Prenatal diagnosis of Down syndrome is possible through chorionic villus sampling and amniocentesis because chromosome analysis of fetal cells can detect the presence of trisomy or translocation. However, analysis will not identify sporadic cases in young women when there is no indication for prenatal testing. Testing for low maternal serum α-fetoprotein, high chorionic gonadotropin, low unconjugated estriol levels, maternal serum fetal cell markers, and measurement of the first-trimester nuchal transparency ultrasound marker may identify an affected fetus in women, who can then undergo amniocentesis (Bahado-Singh and Argoti, 2010; Benn and Chapman, 2009; National Down Syndrome Society, 2011b).

Prenatal testing and genetic counseling should be offered to women of advanced maternal age and those who have a family history of the disorder. If prenatal testing indicates that the fetus is affected, the nurse must allow the parents to express their feelings concerning elective abortion and support their decision to terminate or proceed with the pregnancy.

Fragile X Syndrome

Fragile X syndrome is the most common inherited cause of CI and the second most common genetic cause of CI after Down syndrome. It has been described in all ethnic groups and races. The incidence of affected boys is one in 3600; the incidence of affected girls is one in 4000 to 6000; the incidence of carrier girls is one in 100 to 260; and the incidence of carrier boys is one in 250 to 800 worldwide (Hagerman, 2008; National Fragile X Foundation, 2010).

The syndrome is caused by an abnormal gene on the lower end of the long arm of the X chromosome. Chromosome analysis may demonstrate a fragile site (a region that fails to condense during mitosis and is characterized by a nonstaining gap or narrowing) in the cells of affected males and females and in carrier females. This fragile site is caused by a gene mutation that results in excessive repeats of nucleotide in a specific deoxyribonucleic acid (DNA) segment of the X chromosome. The number of repeats in a normal individual is between 6 and 50. An individual with 50 to 200 base-pair repeats is said to have a permutation and therefore is a carrier. When passed from a parent to a child, these base-pair repeats can expand from 200 or more, which is termed a full mutation. This expansion occurs only when a carrier mother passes the mutation to her offspring; it does not occur when a carrier father passes the mutation to his daughters.

The inheritance pattern has been termed X-linked dominant with reduced penetrance. This is in distinct contrast to the classic X-linked recessive pattern in which all carrier females are normal, all affected males have symptoms of the disorder, and no males are carriers. Consequently genetic counseling of affected

BOX 37-4   CLINICAL MANIFESTATIONS OF FRAGILE X SYNDROME

Physical Features
- Increased head circumference
- Long, wide, or protruding ears
- Long, narrow face with prominent jaw
- Strabismus
- Mitral valve prolapse, aortic root dilation
- Hypotonia
- Enlarged testicles (postpubertally)

Behavioral Features
- Mild-to-severe cognitive impairment
- Speech delay; may be rapid speech with stuttering and word repetition
- Short attention span, hyperactivity
- Hypersensitivity to taste, sounds, touch
- Intolerance to change in routine
- Autistic-like behaviors such as social anxiety and gaze aversion

families is more complex than that for families with a classic X-linked disorder such as hemophilia. Prenatal diagnosis of the fragile X gene mutation is now possible with direct DNA testing in a family with an established history using amniocentesis or chorionic villus sampling (National Fragile X Foundation, 2010). Both affected sexes are capable of transmitting the fragile X disorder.

Clinical Manifestations

The classic trend of physical findings in adult men with fragile X syndrome consists of a long face with a prominent jaw (prognathism); large, protruding ears; and large testes (macroorchidism). However, in prepubertal children these features may be less obvious, and behavioral manifestations may initially suggest the diagnosis (Box 37-4). In carrier females the clinical manifestations vary greatly.

Therapeutic Management

Fragile X syndrome has no cure. Medical treatment may include the use of serotonin agents such as carbamazepine (Tegretol) or fluoxetine (Prozac) to control violent temper outbursts and central nervous system stimulants or clonidine (Catapres) to improve attention span and decrease hyperactivity. Protein replacement and gene therapy are treatment options that are being investigated (Kuehn, 2011).

All affected children require referral to early-intervention program (speech and language therapy, occupational therapy, and special education assistance) and multidisciplinary assessment, including cardiology, neurology, and orthopedic anomalies.

Prognosis. Individuals with fragile X syndrome are expected to live a normal life span. Their CI may be improved by behavioral and educational interventions that usually begin in preschool age children.

CARE MANAGEMENT

Because CI is a fairly consistent finding in individuals with fragile X syndrome, the care given to these families is the same as for any child with CI. Because the disorder is hereditary, genetic counseling is necessary to inform parents and siblings of the risks of transmission. In addition, any male or female with unexplained or nonspecific mental impairment should be referred for genetic testing and, if needed, counseling. Families with a member affected by the disorder should be referred to the National Fragile X Foundation.*

SENSORY IMPAIRMENT

Hearing Impairment

Hearing impairment is one of the most common disabilities in the United States. An estimated one to six per 1000 well infants have hearing loss of varying degrees (AAP Task Force on Newborn and Infant Hearing, 1999; Gifford, Holmes, and Bernstein, 2009). For infants admitted to neonatal intensive care units, the incidence rises sharply to approximately 2 to 4 per 100 neonates (AAP Task Force on Newborn and Infant Hearing, 1999). In the United States there are about 1 million children with hearing impairment ranging in age from birth to 21 years, and almost one third of these children have other disabilities such as visual or cognitive deficits.

Definition and Classification

Hearing impairment is a general term indicating disability that may range in severity from slight to profound hearing loss. *Slight-to-moderately severe hearing loss* describes a person who has residual hearing sufficient to enable successful processing of linguistic information through audition, generally with the use of a hearing aid. *Severe-to-profound hearing loss* describes a person whose hearing disability precludes successful processing of linguistic information through audition with or without a hearing aid. Hearing-impaired persons who are speech impaired tend not to have a physical speech defect other than that caused by the inability to hear.

Hearing defects may be classified according to etiology, pathology, or symptom severity. Each is important in terms of treatment, possible prevention, and rehabilitation.

Etiology

Hearing loss may be caused by a number of prenatal and postnatal conditions. These include a family history of childhood hearing impairment, anatomic malformations of the head or neck, low birth weight, severe perinatal asphyxia, perinatal infection (cytomegalovirus, rubella, herpes, syphilis, toxoplasmosis, bacterial meningitis), chronic ear infection, cerebral palsy, Down syndrome, prolonged neonatal oxygen supplementation or administration of ototoxic drugs (Botelho, Bouzada, de Resende, et al., 2010; Haddad, 2007; Robertson, Howarth, Bork, et al., 2009; Weijerman and de Winter, 2010).

In addition, high-risk neonates who survive formerly fatal prenatal or perinatal conditions may be susceptible to hearing loss from the disorder or its treatment. For example, sensorineural hearing loss may be a result of continuous humming noises or high noise levels associated with incubators, oxygen hoods, or intensive care units, especially when combined with the use of potentially ototoxic antibiotics.

Environmental noise is a special concern. Sounds loud enough to damage sensitive hair cells of the inner ear can produce irreversible hearing loss. Very loud, brief noise such as gunfire can cause immediate, severe, and permanent loss of hearing. Longer exposure to less intense but still hazardous sounds such as loud persistent music via headphones, sound systems, concerts, or industrial noises may also produce hearing loss (Daniel, 2007; Henderson, Testa, and Hartnick, 2011). Loud noises combined with toxic substances such as smoking or secondhand smoke produce a synergistic effect on hearing that causes hearing loss (Fabry, Davila, Arheart, et al., 2011; Mohammadi, Mazhari, Mehrparvar, et al., 2009).

Pathology

Disorders of hearing are divided according to the location of the defect. Conductive or middle-ear hearing loss results from interference of transmission of sound to the middle ear. It is the most common of all types of hearing loss and most frequently a result of recurrent serous otitis media. Conductive hearing impairment mainly involves interference with loudness of sound.

Sensorineural hearing loss involves damage to the inner ear structures or the auditory nerve. The most common causes are congenital defects of inner ear structures or consequences of acquired conditions such as kernicterus, infection, administration of ototoxic drugs, or exposure to excessive noise. Sensorineural hearing loss results in distortion of sound and problems in discrimination. Although the child hears some of everything going on around him or her, the sounds are distorted, severely affecting discrimination and comprehension.

Mixed conductive-sensorineural hearing loss results from interference with transmission of sound in the middle ear and along neural pathways. It frequently results from recurrent otitis media and its complications.

Central auditory imperception includes all hearing losses that are not linked to defects in the conductive or sensorineural structures. They are usually divided into organic or functional losses. In the organic type of central auditory imperception, the defect involves the reception of auditory stimuli along the central pathways and the expression of the message into meaningful communication. Examples are aphasia, the inability to express ideas in any form, either written or verbal; agnosia, the inability to interpret sound correctly; and dysacusis, difficulty in processing details or discriminating among sounds. In the functional type of hearing loss no organic lesion exists to explain a central auditory loss. Examples of functional hearing loss are conversion hysteria (an unconscious withdrawal from hearing to block remembrance of a traumatic event), infantile autism, and childhood schizophrenia.

Symptom Severity. Hearing impairment is expressed in terms of a decibel (dB), a unit of loudness; hearing is measured at various frequencies such as 500, 1000, and 2000 cycles/sec (i.e., the critical listening speech range). Hearing impairment can be classified according to hearing threshold level (the measurement of an individual's hearing threshold by means of an audiometer) and the degree of symptom severity as it affects speech (Table 37-2). These classifications offer only general guidelines regarding the effect of the impairment on any individual child because children differ greatly in their ability to use residual hearing.

Therapeutic Management

Conductive Hearing Loss. Treatment of hearing loss depends on the cause and type of hearing impairment. Many conductive hearing defects respond to medical or surgical treatment such as antibiotic therapy for acute otitis media or insertion of tympanostomy tubes for chronic otitis media. When the conductive loss is permanent, hearing can be improved with the use of a hearing aid to amplify sound.

The nurse should be familiar with the types, basic care, and handling of hearing aids, especially when the child is hospitalized.*

---

*1615 Bonanza St, Suite 202, Walnut Creek, CA 94596, 800-688-8765 or 925-938-9300, fax: 925-938-9315, www.fragilex.org.

*Information about hearing aids is available from the International Hearing Society, 16880 Middlebelt Road, Suite 4, Livonia, MI 48154, 800-521-5247 or 734-522-7200, fax: 734-522-0200, ihsinfo.org.

TABLE 37-2	CLASSIFICATION OF HEARING IMPAIRMENT BASED ON SYMPTOM SEVERITY	
HEARING LEVEL (DB)	**EFFECT**
Slight—16-25	Has difficulty hearing faint or distant speech Usually is unaware of hearing difficulty Likely to achieve in school but may have problems No speech defects
Mild to moderate—26-55	May have speech difficulties Understands face-to-face conversational speech at 0.9-1.5 m (3-5 ft)
Moderately severe—56-70	Unable to understand conversational speech unless loud Considerable difficulty with group or classroom discussion Requires special speech training
Severe—71-90	May hear a loud voice if nearby May be able to identify loud environmental noises Can distinguish vowels but not most consonants Requires speech training
Profound—91	May hear only loud sounds Requires extensive speech training

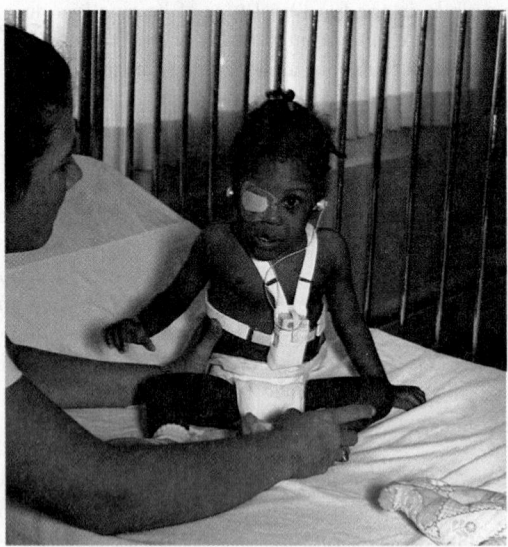

FIG 37-7 On-the-body hearing aids are convenient for young children such as this child with severe bilateral hearing loss. Note eye patching for strabismus.

Types of aids include those worn in or behind the ear, models incorporated into an eyeglass frame, and types worn on the body with a wire connection to the ear (Fig. 37-7). One of the most common problems with a hearing aid is acoustic feedback, an annoying whistling sound usually caused by improper fit of the ear mold. Sometimes the whistling may be at a frequency that the child cannot hear but that is annoying to others. In this case, if children are old enough, they are told of the noise and asked to readjust the aid.

As children grow older they may be self-conscious about the device. Effort may be made to make the aid inconspicuous such as styling the hair to cover behind-the-ear or in-the-ear models and encourage the use of attractive frames for glasses with connected hearing aids. Give children responsibility for the care of the device as soon as they are able because fostering independence is a primary goal of rehabilitation.

> **! NURSING ALERT**
>
> Stress to parents the importance of storing batteries for hearing aids in a safe location out of reach of children and teaching children not to remove the battery from the hearing aid (or supervising young children when they do so). Battery ingestion requires immediate emergency management.

Sensorineural Hearing Loss. Treatment for sensorineural hearing loss is much less satisfactory. Because the defect is not one of intensity of sound, hearing aids are of less value in this type of defect. The use of cochlear implants* (a surgically implanted prosthetic device) provides a sensation of hearing for individuals who have severe or profound hearing loss (Gifford, Holmes, and Bernstein, 2009; Zeng and Liu, 2006). Children with sensorineural hearing loss have lost or damaged some or all of their hair cells or auditory nerve fibers. Often these children cannot benefit from conventional hearing aids because they only amplify sound that cannot be processed by a damaged inner ear. A cochlear implant bypasses the hair cells to directly stimulate surviving auditory nerve fibers so they can send signals to the brain. These signals can be interpreted by the brain to produce sound and sensations (Baldassari, Schmidt, Schubert, et al., 2009; Gifford, Holmes, and Bernstein, 2009).

Multichanneled implants are now available. This more sophisticated device stimulates the auditory nerve at a number of locations with differently processed signals. It allows a person to use the pitch information present in speech signals, leading to better understanding of speech. The trend is toward early use of cochlear implants, usually by 18 months of age, to give the child maximum opportunity to develop listening, language, and speaking skills.

CARE MANAGEMENT

Assessment of children for hearing impairment is a critical nursing responsibility. Identification of hearing loss within the first 3 to 6 months of life is essential to improve the language and educational outcomes for children with hearing impairments (Gifford, Holmes, and Bernstein, 2009; Tierney and Brown, 2008). The Joint Committee on Infant Hearing (2000) issued guidelines on auditory screening of newborns and infants to detect early hearing loss and implement intervention programs. Auditory testing is presented in Chapter 29.

Infancy. At birth the nurse can observe the neonate's response to auditory stimuli, as evidenced by the startle reflex, head turning, eye blinking, and cessation of body movement. The infant may vary in the intensity of the response, depending on the state of alertness.

---

*Hearing Enrichment Language Program of the Hough Ear Institute, 3434 N.W. 56th St., Oklahoma City, Ok 73112, 405-945-7186, fax: 405-947-6266, www.integris-health.com/INTEGRIS/en-US/Specialties/EarInstitute/HELP.

BOX 37-5   CLINICAL MANIFESTATIONS OF HEARING IMPAIRMENT

Infants
- Lack of startle or blink reflex to a loud sound
- Failure to be awakened by loud environmental noises
- Failure to localize a source of sound by 6 months of age
- Absence of babble or voice inflections by age 7 months
- Lack of response to the spoken word; failure to follow verbal directions
- Response to loud noises as opposed to the voice

Children
- Using gestures rather than verbalization to express desires, especially after age 15 months
- Failure to develop intelligible speech by age 24 months
- Monotone and unintelligible speech; lessened laughter
- Vocal play, head banging, or foot stomping for vibratory sensation
- Yelling or screeching to express pleasure, needs, or annoyance
- Asking to have statements repeated or answering them incorrectly
- Greater response to facial expression and gestures than to verbal explanation
- Avoiding social interaction; preferring to play alone
- Inquiring, sometimes confused facial expression
- Suspicious alertness alternating with cooperation
- Frequently stubbornness because of lack of comprehension
- Irritability at not making themselves understood
- Shy, timid, and withdrawn behavior
- Frequently appearing "dreamy" or "in a world of their own" or exhibiting inattentiveness

GUIDELINES
Facilitating Lipreading

- Attract child's attention before speaking; use light touch to signal speaker's presence.
- Stand close to child.
- Face child directly or move to a 45-degree angle.
- Stand still; do not walk back and forth or turn away to point or look elsewhere.
- Establish eye contact and show interest.
- Speak at eye level and with good lighting on speaker's face.
- Be certain that nothing interferes with speech patterns such as chewing food or gum.
- Speak clearly and at a slow and even rate.
- Use facial expression to help convey messages.
- Keep sentences short.
- Rephrase message if child does not understand the words.

However, a consistent absence of a reaction should lead to suspicion of hearing loss. Box 37-5 summarizes other clinical manifestations of hearing impairment in infants.

Childhood. Children who are profoundly hearing impaired are much more likely to be diagnosed during infancy than less severely affected ones. If the defect is not detected during early childhood, it likely becomes evident during entry into school, when the child has difficulty learning. Unfortunately some of these children are mistakenly placed in special classes for students with learning disabilities or CI. Therefore it is essential that the nurse suspect a hearing impairment in any child who demonstrates the behaviors listed in Box 37-5.

! NURSING ALERT

When parents express concern about their child's hearing and speech development, refer the child for a hearing evaluation. Absence of well-formed syllables *(da, na, yaya)* by 11 months of age should result in immediate referral.

Of primary importance is the effect of hearing impairment on speech development.* A child with a mild conductive hearing loss may speak fairly clearly but in a loud, monotone voice. A child with

a sensorineural defect usually has difficulty in articulation. For example, an inability to hear higher frequencies may result in the word *spoon* being pronounced "poon." Children with articulation problems need to have their hearing tested.

Lipreading. Even though the child may become an expert at lipreading, only about 40% of the spoken word is understood, less if the speaker has an accent, mustache, or beard. Exaggerating pronunciation or speaking in an altered rhythm further reduces comprehension. Parents can help the child understand the spoken word by using the suggestions in the Guidelines box. The child learns to supplement the spoken word with sensitivity to visual cues, primarily body language and facial expression (e.g., tightening the lips, muscle tension, eye contact).

Cued Speech. This method of communication is an adjunct to straight lipreading. It uses hand signals to help the child with a hearing impairment distinguish between words that look alike when formed by the lips (e.g., mat, bat). It is most often used by children with hearing impairments who are using speech rather than those who are nonverbal.

Sign Language. Sign language such as American Sign Language (ASL) or British Sign Language (BSL) is a visual gestural language that uses hand signals that roughly correspond to specific words and concepts in the English language. Family members are encouraged to learn signing because using or watching hands requires much less concentration than lipreading or talking. In addition, a symbol method enables some children to learn more faster.

Speech Language Therapy. The most formidable task in the education of a child who is profoundly hearing impaired is learning to speak. Speech is learned through a multisensory approach using visual, tactile, kinesthetic, and auditory stimulation. Parents are encouraged to participate fully in the learning process.

Additional Aids. Everyday activities present problems for older children with hearing impairment. For example, they may not be able to hear the telephone, doorbell, or alarm clock. Several commercial devices are available to help them adjust to these dilemmas. Flashing lights can be attached to a telephone or doorbell to signal its ringing. Trained hearing-ear dogs can provide great assistance because they alert the person to sounds such as someone approaching, a moving car, a signal to wake up, or a child's cry. Special teletypewriters or telecommunications devices for the deaf (TTY or TDD) help people with impaired hearing communicate

---

*Other sources of information on several aspects of hearing loss are the Alexander Graham Bell Association for the Deaf and Hard of Hearing, 3417 Volta Place NW, Washington, DC 20007; voice: 202-337-5220; TTY: 202-337-5221; fax: 202-337-8314; listeningandspokenlanguage.org; and Canadian Hearing Society, voice: 877-347-3427; TTY: 877-347-3429; www.chs.ca.

with one another over the telephone; the typed message is conveyed via the telephone lines and displayed on a small screen.*

Any audiovisual medium presents dilemmas for these children, who can see the picture but cannot hear the message. However, with closed captioning a special decoding device is attached to the television, and the audio portion of a program is translated into subtitles that appear on the screen.†

Socialization. As children learn to compensate for their lack of hearing, they become extremely perceptive to visual and vibratory changes. They often know when another person wants to talk to them because the person walks close by but does not pass. They learn to be alert to other people approaching them by seeing their shadows or feeling the vibrations of their footsteps. They are acutely aware of facial expressions and may comprehend unspoken messages more quickly than the spoken word.

Socialization is extremely important to children's development. If they attend a special school for the hearing impaired, they are able to socialize with peers in that setting. Classmates become a potential source of close friendships because they communicate more easily among themselves. Encourage parents to promote these relationships whenever possible.

Children with a hearing impairment may need special help with school or social activities. For children wearing hearing aids, background noise should be kept to a minimum. Because many of these children are able to attend regular classes, the teacher may need help to adapt methods of teaching for the child's benefit. The school nurse is often in an optimal position to emphasize methods of facilitated communication such as lipreading (see Guidelines box on p. 1095). Because group projects and audiovisual teaching aids may hinder the child's learning, these educational methods should be evaluated carefully.

In a group setting it is helpful for the other members to sit in a semicircle in front of the child. Because one of the difficulties in following a group discussion is that the child is unaware of who will speak next, someone should point out each speaker. Speakers can also be given numbers, or their names can be written down as each person talks. If one person writes down the main topic of the discussion, the child is able to follow lipreading more closely. Such suggestions can increase the child's ability to participate in sports, organizations such as scouts, and group projects.

Supporting the Child and Family. After the diagnosis of hearing impairment is made, parents need extensive support to adjust to the shock of learning about their child's disability and an opportunity to realize the extent of the hearing loss. If the hearing loss occurs during childhood, the child also requires sensitive, supportive care during the long and often difficult adjustment to this sensory loss. Early rehabilitation is one of the best strategies for fostering adjustment. However, progress in learning communication may not always coincide with emotional adjustment. Depression or anger is common, and such feelings are a normal part of the grieving process. (See also Chapter 38 for an extensive discussion of the emotional support of the child and family.)

---

*Other sources of information on several aspects of hearing loss and on the International Parents' Organization are the Alexander Graham Bell Association for the Deaf and Hard of Hearing, 3417 Volta Place NW, Washington, DC 20007, voice: 202-337-5220, TTY: 202-337-5221, fax: 202-337-8314, listeningandspokenlanguage.org; and Canadian Hearing Society, 271 Spadina Road, Toronto, Ontario, Canada M5R 2V3, voice: 877-347-3427 or 416-928-2500, TTY: 416-964-0023, fax: 416-928-2506, www.chs.ca.
†Additional information is available from the National Captioning Institute, 3725 Concord Pkwy., Suite 100, Chantilly, VA 20151, voice/TTY: 703-917-7600, fax: 703-917-9853, www.ncicap.org.

 CRITICAL THINKING CASE STUDY

Hearing Impairment

Four-year-old Jason has a severe congenital hearing impairment. Jason has been admitted to the outpatient surgery PACU after a herniorrhaphy and regional block. As he emerges from anesthesia, he becomes more and more agitated.

1. Evidence—Is there sufficient evidence to draw conclusions about Jason's increasing agitation after surgery?
2. Assumptions—Describe an underlying assumption about each of the following:
   a. Severe congenital hearing impairment in a preschool child
   b. Preschooler with severe congenital hearing impairment awakening in the PACU after surgery
   c. Preschooler with severe congenital hearing impairment awakening from herniorrhaphy and after regional block
3. What priorities for nursing care should be established for Jason?
4. Does the evidence support your nursing intervention?

PACU, Postanesthesia care unit.

Caring for the Child During Hospitalization. The needs of the hospitalized child with impaired hearing are the same as those of any other child, but the disability presents special challenges to the nurse (see Critical Thinking Case Study). For example, verbal explanations must be supplemented by tactile and visual aids such as books or actual demonstration and practice. Children's understanding of the explanation needs to be reassessed constantly. If their verbal skills are poorly developed, they can answer questions through drawing, writing, or gesturing. For example, if the nurse is attempting to clarify where a spinal tap is done, the child is asked to point to where the procedure will be done on the body. Because these children often need more time to grasp the full meaning of an explanation, the nurse needs to be patient, allowing ample time for understanding.

When communicating with the child, the nurse should use the same principles as those outlined for facilitating lipreading. Ideally nurses without foreign accents should be assigned to the child. The child's hearing aid is checked to ensure that it is working properly. If it is necessary to awaken the child at night, the nurse should gently shake him or her or turn on the hearing aid before arousing him or her. The nurse should always make certain that the child can see him or her before any procedures, even routine ones such as changing a diaper or regulating an infusion. It is important to remember that the child may not be aware of one's presence until alerted through visual or tactile cues.

Ideally parents are encouraged to room with the child. However, it must be conveyed to them that this is not to serve as a convenience to the nurse but as a benefit to the child. Although the parents' aid can be enlisted in familiarizing the child with the hospital and explaining procedures, the nurse also talks directly to the youngster, encouraging expression of feelings about the experience. If the child's speech is difficult to understand, the nurse makes an effort to become familiar with his or her pronunciation of words. Parents often can be helpful by explaining the child's usual speech habits. Nonverbal communication devices that use pictures or words to which the child can point are also available. Such boards can also be made by drawing pictures or writing the words of common needs on cardboard such as *parent, food, water,* or *toilet.*

The nurse has a special role as child advocate and is in a strategic position to alert other health team members and patients to the child's special needs regarding communication. For example, the nurse should accompany other practitioners on visits to the child's room to ensure that they speak to the child and that he or she understands what is said. Caregivers sometimes forget that the child has the abilities to perceive and learn despite a hearing loss; consequently they communicate only with the parents. As a result, the child's needs and feelings remain unrecognized and unmet.

Because children with impaired hearing may have difficulty forming social relationships with other children, the child is introduced to roommates and encouraged to engage in play activities. The hospital setting can provide growth-promoting opportunities for social relationships. With the assistance of a child life specialist, the child can learn new recreational activities, experiment with group games, and engage in therapeutic play. The use of puppets, dollhouses, role-playing with dress-up clothes, building with a hammer and nails, finger painting, and water play can help the child express feelings that previously were suppressed.

Assisting in Measures to Prevent Hearing Impairment. A primary nursing role is prevention of hearing loss. Because the most common cause of impaired hearing is chronic otitis media, it is essential that appropriate measures be instituted to treat existing infections and prevent recurrences (see Chapter 40). Children with a history of ear or respiratory infections or any other condition known to increase the risk of hearing impairment should receive periodic auditory testing.

To prevent the causes of hearing loss that begin prenatally and perinatally, pregnant women need counseling regarding the necessity of early prenatal care, including genetic counseling for known familial disorders; avoidance of all ototoxic drugs, especially during the first trimester; tests to rule out syphilis, rubella, or blood incompatibility; medical management of maternal diabetes; strict control of alcohol intake; adequate dietary intake; and avoidance of smoke exposure. The necessity of routine immunization during childhood to eliminate the possibility of acquired sensorineural hearing loss from rubella, mumps, or measles (encephalitis) is stressed.

Excessive noise pollution is a well-established cause of sensorineural hearing loss. The nurse should assess the possibility of environmental noise pollution routinely and advise children and parents of the potential danger. When individuals engage in activities associated with high-intensity noise such as flying model airplanes, target shooting, or snowmobiling, they should wear ear protection such as earmuffs or earplugs. Even common household equipment such as lawn mowers, vacuum cleaners, and cordless telephones can be harmful.

> **! NURSING ALERT**
>
> Suspect hazardous noise if the listener experiences (1) difficulty in communication while hearing the sound, (2) ringing in the ears (tinnitus) after exposure to the sound, or (3) muffled hearing after leaving the sound.

Visual Impairment

Visual impairment is a common problem during childhood. In the United States the prevalence of serious visual impairment in the pediatric population is estimated at 30 to 64 children per 100,000 population. Vision impairment such as refractive error, strabismus, and amblyopia occur in 5% to 10% of all preschoolers, who are usually identified through vision screening programs (Rahi, Cumberland, Perkham, et al., 2010; Tingley, 2007; U.S. Preventive Services

Task Force, 2011). The nurse's role is one of assessment, detection, prevention, referral, and in some instances rehabilitation.

Definition and Classification

Visual impairment is a general term that encompasses both partial sight and legal blindness. Partial sight or partial visual impairment is defined as a visual acuity between 20/70 and 20/200. The child can generally use normal-size print because near vision is almost always better than distance vision. Legal blindness or severe permanent visual impairment is defined as a visual acuity of 20/200 or lower or a visual field of 20 degrees or less in the better eye. It is important to keep in mind that legal blindness is not a medical diagnosis but a legal definition. Educational and governmental agencies in the United States use the legal definition of blindness to determine tax status, eligibility for entrance into special schools, eligibility for financial aid, and other benefits.

Etiology

Visual impairment can be caused by a number of genetic and prenatal or postnatal conditions. These include perinatal infections (herpes, Chlamydia, gonococci, rubella, syphilis, toxoplasmosis); retinopathy of prematurity; trauma; postnatal infections (meningitis); and disorders such as sickle cell disease, juvenile rheumatoid arthritis, Tay-Sachs disease, albinism, and retinoblastoma. In many instances such as with refractive errors the cause of the defect is unknown.

Refractive errors are the most common types of visual disorders in children. The term refraction means bending and refers to the bending of light rays as they pass through the lens of the eye. Normally light rays enter the lens and fall directly on the retina. However, in refractive disorders the light rays either fall in front of the retina (myopia) or beyond it (hyperopia). Other eye problems such as strabismus may or may not include refractive errors, but they are important because, if untreated, they result in severe permanent visual impairment from amblyopia. These, along with other less frequent visual disorders, are summarized in Box 37-6. In addition to these disorders, other visual problems can be a result of trauma or infection.

Trauma. Trauma is a common cause of visual impairment in children. Injuries to the eyeball and adnexa (supporting or accessory structures such as eyelids, conjunctiva, or lacrimal glands) can be classified as penetrating or nonpenetrating. Penetrating wounds are most often a result of sharp instruments such as sticks, knives, or scissors or propulsive objects such as firecrackers, guns, arrows, or slingshots. Nonpenetrating injuries may be a result of foreign objects in the eyes, lacerations, a blow from a blunt object such as a ball (baseball, softball, basketball, racquet sports) or fist, or thermal or chemical burns.

Treatment is aimed at preventing further ocular damage and is primarily the responsibility of the ophthalmologist. It involves adequate examination of the injured eye (with the child sedated or anesthetized in severe injuries); appropriate immediate intervention such as removal of the foreign body or suturing of the laceration; and prevention of complications such as administration of antibiotics or steroids and complete bed rest to allow the eye to heal and blood to resorb (see Emergency box). The prognosis varies according to the type of injury. It is usually guarded in all cases of penetrating wounds because of the high risk of serious complications.

Infections. Infections of the adnexa and structures of the eyeball or globe may occur in children. The most common eye infection is conjunctivitis. Treatment is usually with ophthalmic antibiotics. Severe infections may require systemic antibiotic therapy. Steroids are used cautiously because they exacerbate viral infections such

BOX 37-6 **TYPES OF VISUAL IMPAIRMENT**

Refractive Errors

Myopia

- *Nearsightedness*—Ability to see objects clearly at close range but not at a distance

Pathophysiology

- Results from eyeball that is too long, causing images to fall in front of the retina

Clinical Manifestations

- Headaches
- Dizziness
- Excessive eye rubbing
- Head tilt or forward head thrusts
- Difficulty reading or doing other close work
- Clumsiness; walking into objects
- Blinking more than usual or irritability when doing close work
- Inability to see objects clearly
- Poor school performance, especially in subjects that require demonstration such as arithmetic

Treatment

- Corrected with biconcave lenses that focus rays on retina
- May be corrected with laser surgery

Hyperopia

Farsightedness—Ability to see objects at a distance

Pathophysiology

- Results from eyeball that is too short, causing image to focus beyond retina

Clinical Manifestations

- Because of accommodative ability, child can usually see objects at all ranges
- Most children normally hyperopic until about 7 years of age

Treatment

- When required, corrected with convex lenses that focus rays on retina
- May be corrected with laser surgery

Astigmatism

- Unequal curvatures in refractive apparatus

Pathophysiology

- Results from unequal curvatures in cornea or lens that cause light rays to bend in different directions

Clinical Manifestations

- Depend on severity of refractive error in each eye
- Possible clinical manifestations of myopia

Treatment

- Corrected with special lenses that compensate for refractive errors
- May be corrected with laser surgery

Anisometropia

- Different refractive strength in each eye

Pathophysiology

- May develop amblyopia because weaker eye is used less

Clinical Manifestations

- Depend on severity of refractive error in each eye
- Possible clinical manifestations of myopia

Treatment

- Treated with corrective lenses, preferably contact lenses, to improve vision in each eye so they work as a unit
- May be corrected with laser surgery

Amblyopia

- Lazy eye—Reduced visual acuity in one eye

Pathophysiology

- Results when one eye does not receive sufficient stimulation
- Each retina receives different images, resulting in diplopia (double vision)
- Brain accommodates by suppressing less intense image
- Visual cortex eventually does not respond to visual stimulation, with resultant loss of vision in that eye

Clinical Manifestations

- Poor vision in affected eye

Treatment

- Preventable if treatment of primary visual defect such as anisometropia or strabismus begins before 6 years of age

Strabismus

- *"Squint"* or malalignment of eyes
- *Esotropia*—Inward deviation of eye
- *Exotropia*—Outward deviation of eye

Pathophysiology

- May result from muscle imbalance or paralysis, poor vision, or congenital defect
- Because visual axes are not parallel, brain receives two images, and amblyopia can result

Clinical Manifestations

- Squints eyelids together or frowns
- Difficulty in focusing from one distance to another
- Inaccurate judgment in picking up objects
- Unable to see print or moving objects clearly
- Closing one eye to see
- Tilting head to one side
- If combined with refractive errors, may see any of the manifestations listed for refractive errors
  - Diplopia
  - Photophobia
  - Dizziness
  - Headaches

Treatment

- Depends on cause of strabismus
- May involve occlusion therapy (patching stronger eye) or surgery to increase visual stimulation to weaker eye
- Early diagnosis essential to prevent vision loss

BOX 37-6   TYPES OF VISUAL IMPAIRMENT—cont'd

Cataracts
- Opacity of crystalline lens

Pathophysiology
- Prevents light rays from entering eye and refracting on retina

Clinical Manifestations
- Gradual decrease in ability to see objects clearly
- Possible loss of peripheral vision
- Nystagmus (with severe permanent visual impairment)
- Gray opacities of lens
- Strabismus
- Absence of red reflex

Treatment
- Requires surgery to remove cloudy lens and replace lens (with intraocular lens implant, removable contact lens, prescription glasses)
- Must be treated early to prevent severe permanent visual impairment from amblyopia

Glaucoma
- Increased intraocular pressure

Pathophysiology
- Congenital type results from defective development of some component related to flow of aqueous humor
- Increased pressure on optic nerve causes eventual atrophy and severe permanent visual impairment

Clinical Manifestations
- Loss of peripheral vision—mostly seen in acquired types
- Possible bumping into objects
- Perception of halos around objects
- Possible complaint of pain or discomfort (pain, nausea, or vomiting if sudden rise in pressure)
- Eye redness
- Excessive tearing (epiphora)
- Photophobia
- Spasmodic winking (blepharospasm)
- Corneal haziness
- Enlargement of eyeball (buphthalmos)

Treatment
- Requires surgical treatment (goniotomy) to open outflow tracts
- May require more than one procedure

✚ EMERGENCY

Eye Injuries

Foreign Object
- Examine eye for presence of a foreign body (evert upper eyelid to examine upper eye).
- Remove a freely movable object with pointed corner of gauze pad lightly moistened with water.
- Do not irrigate eye or attempt to remove a penetrating object (see Penetrating Injury).
- Caution child against rubbing eye.

Chemical Burns
- Irrigate eye copiously with tap water for 20 minutes.
- Evert upper eyelid to flush thoroughly.
- Hold child's head with eye under a tap of running lukewarm water.
- Take child to emergency department.
- Have child rest with eyes closed.
- Keep room darkened.

Ultraviolet Burns
- If skin is burned, patch both eyes (make certain that eyelids are completely closed); secure dressing with Kling bandages wrapped around head rather than with tape.
- Have child rest with eyes closed.
- Refer to an ophthalmologist.

Hematoma ("Black Eye")
- Use a flashlight to check for gross hyphema (hemorrhage into anterior chamber; visible fluid meniscus across iris; more easily seen in light-colored than in brown eyes).
- Apply ice for first 24 hours to reduce swelling if no hyphema is present.
- Refer to an ophthalmologist immediately if hyphema is present.
- Have child rest with eyes closed.

Penetrating Injuries
- Take child to emergency department.
- Never remove an object that has penetrated eye.
- Follow strict aseptic technique in examining eye.
- Observe for:
  - Aqueous or vitreous leaks (fluid leaking from point of penetration).
  - Hyphema.
  - Shape and equality of pupils, reaction to light, prolapsed iris (not perfectly circular).
- Apply a Fox shield if available (not a regular eye patch) and apply patch over unaffected eye to prevent bilateral movement.
- Maintain bed rest with child in a 30-degree Fowler position.
- Caution child against rubbing eye.
- Refer to an ophthalmologist.

as herpes simplex, increasing the risk of damage to the involved structures.

CARE MANAGEMENT

Assessment of children for visual impairment is a critical nursing responsibility. Discovery of a visual impairment as early as possible is essential to prevent social, physical, and psychologic damage to the child. Assessment involves (1) identifying children who by virtue of their history are at risk, (2) observing for behaviors that indicate a vision loss, and (3) screening all children for visual acuity and signs of other ocular disorders such as strabismus. This discussion focuses on clinical manifestations of various types of visual problems (see Box 37-6). Vision testing is discussed in Chapter 29.

Infancy. At birth the nurse should observe the neonate's response to visual stimuli such as following a light or object and cessation of body movement. The infant may vary in the intensity of the response, depending on the state of alertness.

Of special importance in detecting visual impairment during infancy are the parents' concerns regarding visual responsiveness in their child. Their concerns such as lack of eye contact from the infant must be taken seriously. During infancy the child should be tested for strabismus. Lack of binocularity after 4 months of age is considered abnormal and must be treated to prevent amblyopia.

> **! NURSING ALERT**
>
> Suspect visual impairment in an infant who does not react to light and in a child of any age if the parents express concern.

Childhood. Because the most common visual impairment during childhood is refractive errors, testing for visual acuity is essential. The school nurse usually assumes major responsibility for vision testing in schoolchildren. Besides refractive errors, the nurse should be aware of signs and symptoms that indicate other ocular problems. If a referral is made to the family requesting further eye testing, the nurse is responsible for follow-up concerning the recommendation.

The shock of learning that their child has severe permanent visual impairment precipitates an immense crisis for families. The family is encouraged to investigate appropriate stimulation and educational programs for their child as soon as possible. Sources of information include state commissions for the visually impaired, local schools for children with visual impairments, the American Foundation for the Blind,* the National Federation of the Blind,† the National Association for Parents of Children with Visual Impairments,‡ the National Association for Visually Handicapped,§ the American Council of the Blind,‖ and CNIB.¶

Promoting Parent-Child Attachment. A crucial time in the life of visual impaired infants is when they and their parents are getting acquainted with one another. Pleasurable patterns of interaction between the infant and parents may be lacking if there is not enough reciprocity. For example, if the parent gazes fondly at the infant's face and seeks eye contact but the infant fails to respond because he or she cannot see the parent, a troubled cycle of responses may occur. The nurse can help parents learn to look for other cues that indicate that the infant is responding to them such as whether the eyelids blink, whether the activity level accelerates or slows, whether respiratory patterns change such as faster or slower breathing when the parents come near, and whether the infant makes throaty sounds when they speak to him or her. In time parents learn that the infant has unique ways of relating to them. They are encouraged to show affection using nonvisual methods such as talking or reading, cuddling, and walking the child.

Promoting Child's Optimal Development. Promoting the child's optimal development requires rehabilitation in a number of important areas, including learning self-help skills and appropriate communication techniques to become independent. Although nurses may not be directly involved in such programs, they can provide direction and guidance to families regarding the availability of programs and the need to promote these activities in their child.

Development and Independence. Motor development depends on sight almost as much as verbal communication depends on hearing. From earliest infancy parents are encouraged to expose the infant to as many visual-motor experiences as possible such as sitting supported in an infant seat or swing and being given opportunities for holding up the head, sitting unsupported, reaching for objects, and crawling.

Despite visual impairment the child can become independent in all aspects of self-care. The same principles used for promoting independence in sighted children apply, with additional emphasis on nonvisual cues. For example, the child may need help in dressing such as special arrangement of clothing for style coordination and braille tags to distinguish colors and prints.

The severe permanent visually impaired child also must learn to become independent in navigational skills. The two main techniques are the tapping method (use of a cane to survey the environment for direction and avoid obstacles) and guides such as a sighted human guide or a dog guide such as a seeing-eye dog. Children who are partially sighted may benefit from ocular aids such as a monocular telescope.

Play and Socialization. Children with severe permanent visual impairments do not learn to play automatically. Because they cannot imitate others or actively explore the environment as sighted children do, they depend much more on others to stimulate and teach them how to play. Parents need help in selecting appropriate play materials, especially those that encourage fine and gross motor development and stimulate the senses of hearing, touch, and smell. Toys with educational value such as dolls with various clothing closures are especially useful.

Children with severe permanent visual impairments have the same needs for socialization as sighted children. Because they have little difficulty learning verbal skills, they are able to communicate with age mates and participate in suitable activities. The nurse should discuss with parents opportunities for socialization outside the home, especially regular preschools. The trend is to include these children with sighted children to help them adjust to the outside world for eventual independence.

To compensate for inadequate stimulation, these children may develop self-stimulatory activities such as body rocking, finger flicking, or arm twirling. Discourage such habits because they delay the child's social acceptance. Behavior modification is often successful in reducing or eliminating self-stimulatory activities.

Education. The main obstacle to learning is the child's total dependence on nonvisual cues. Although the child can learn via verbal lecturing, he or she is unable to read the written word or write without special education. Therefore the child must rely on braille, a system that uses raised dots to represent letters and numbers. He or she can then read braille with the fingers and write messages using a braille writer. However, unless others read braille, this system is not useful for communicating with others. A more portable system for written communication is the use of a braille slate and stylus or a microcassette tape recorder. A recorder is especially helpful for leaving messages for others and taking notes during classroom

---

*Two Penn Plaza, Suite 1102, New York, NY 10021, 800-232-5463 or 212-502-7600, fax: 212-502-7777, www.afb.org.

†200 E. Wells St., Baltimore, MD 21230, 410-659-9314, fax: 410-685-5653, www.nfb.org.

‡PO Box 317, Watertown, Ma 02471, 800-562-6265, fax: 617-972-7444, www.napvi.org.

§22 W. 21st St., 6th Floor, New York, NY 10010, 212-889-3141, fax: 212-727-2931, www.navh.org.

‖2200 Wilson Blvd., Suite 650, Arlington, VA 22201, 800-424-8666, 202-467-5081, fax 202-465-5085, www.acb.org.

¶1929 Bayview Ave., Toronto, Ontario, Canada M4G 3E8, Canada, 800-563-2642, fax: 416-480-7700, www.cnib.ca.

lectures. For mathematic calculations, portable calculators with voice synthesizers are available.*

Records and tapes are significant sources of reading material other than braille books, which are large and cumbersome. The Library of Congress† has talking books, braille books, and a special records program, which are available at many local and state libraries and directly from the Library of Congress. The talking book machine and tape player are provided at no cost to families, and there is no postage fee for returning the materials. Learning Ally‡ also provides texts and tapes of books, which are helpful for secondary and college students who are blind. A means of writing is learning to use a home computer with a voice synthesizer that can be adapted to speak each letter or word typed.

Children with partial sight benefit from specialized visual aids that produce a magnified retinal image. The basic devices are accommodation (e.g., bringing the object closer), special plus lenses, handheld and stand magnifiers, telescopes, video projection systems, and large print. Special equipment is available to enlarge print. Information about services for the partially sighted is available from the National Association for Visually Handicapped and American Foundation for the Blind. Children with diminished vision often prefer to do close work without their glasses and compensate by bringing the object very near to their eyes. This should be allowed. The exception is children with vision in only one eye, who should always wear glasses for protection.

Caring for the Child During Hospitalization. Because nurses are more likely to care for children who are hospitalized for procedures that involve temporary loss of vision than for children who have severe permanent visual impairments, the following discussion concentrates primarily on the needs of such children. The nursing care objectives in either situation are to (1) reassure the child and family throughout every phase of treatment, (2) orient the child to the surroundings, (3) provide a safe environment, and (4) encourage independence. Whenever possible, the same nurse should care for the child to ensure consistency in the approach.

When sighted children temporarily lose their vision, almost every aspect of the environment becomes bewildering and frightening. They are forced to rely on nonvisual senses for help in adjusting to the visual impairment without the benefit of any special training. Nurses have a major role in minimizing the effects of temporary loss of vision. They need to talk to the child about everything that is occurring, emphasizing aspects of procedures that are felt or heard. They should approach the child by always identifying themselves as soon as they enter the room. Because unfamiliar sounds are especially frightening, these are explained. Parents are encouraged to room with their child and participate in the care. Familiar objects such as a teddy bear or doll should be brought from home to help lessen the strangeness of the hospital. As soon as the child is able to

be out of bed, he or she is oriented to the immediate surroundings. If the child is able to see on admission, this opportunity is taken to point out significant aspects of the room. He or she is encouraged to practice ambulating with the eyes closed to become accustomed to this experience.

The room is arranged with safety in mind. For example, a stool or chair is placed next to the bed to help the child climb in and out of bed. The furniture is always placed in the same position to prevent collisions. Cleaning personnel are reminded of the need to keep the room in order. If the child has difficulty navigating by feeling the walls, a rope can be attached from the bed to the point of destination such as the bathroom. Attention to details such as well-fitting slippers and robes that do not drag on the floor is important in preventing tripping. Unlike children who have permanent visual impairments, children with temporary visual impairments are not familiar with navigating with a cane.

The child is encouraged to be independent in self-care activities, especially if the visual loss may be prolonged or potentially permanent. For example, during bathing the nurse sets up all of the equipment and encourages the child to participate. At mealtimes the nurse explains where each food item is on the tray, opens any special containers, prepares cereal or toast, and encourages the child to self-feed. Favorite finger foods such as sandwiches, hamburgers, hot dogs, or pizza may be good selections. The child is praised for efforts at being cooperative and independent. Any improvements made in self-care, no matter how small, are stressed.

Appropriate recreational activities are provided; if a child life specialist is available, such planning is done jointly. Because children with temporary visual impairment have a wide variety of play experiences on which to draw, they are encouraged to select activities. For example, if they like to read, they may enjoy having someone read to them. If they prefer manual activity, they may appreciate playing with clay or building blocks or feeling different textures and naming them. If they need an outlet for aggression, activities such as pounding or banging on a drum can be helpful. Simple board and card games can be played with a "seeing partner" or an opponent who helps with the game. They should have familiar toys from home with which to play because familiar items are more easily manipulated than new ones. If parents want to bring presents, they should be objects that stimulate hearing and touch such as a radio, music box, or stuffed animal.

Occasionally children who are visually impaired come to the hospital for procedures to restore their vision. Although this is an extremely happy time, it also requires intervention to help them adjust to sight. They need an opportunity to take in all that they see. They should not be bombarded with visual stimuli. They may need to concentrate on people's faces or their own to become accustomed to this experience. They often need to talk about what they see and to compare the visual images with their mental ones. The children may also go through a period of depression, which must be respected and supported. The nurse or parents should encourage the child to discuss how it feels to see, especially in terms of seeing themselves.

Newly sighted children also need time to adjust and engage in activities that were impossible before. For example, they may prefer to use braille to read rather than learning a new "visual approach" because of familiarity with the touch system. Eventually, as they learn to recognize letters and numbers, they will integrate these new skills into reading and writing. However, parents and teachers must be careful not to push them before they are ready. This applies to social relationships, physical activities, and learning situations.

---

*A catalog of numerous products for people with vision problems is available from American Foundation for the Blind (see previous footnote) and from Lighthouse International, 111 E. 59th St., New York, NY 10022-1202, 212-821-9200 or 800-829-0500;TTY, 212-821-9713, fax: 212-821-9707, www.lighthouse.org.

†National Library Service for the Blind and Physically Handicapped, Library of Congress, 1291 Taylor St., NW, Washington DC 20011, 202-707-5100, 888-657-7323, TTD: 202-707-0744, fax: 202-707-0712, www.loc.gov/nls. (A state listing of libraries for readers with severe permanent visual impairments and physical disabilities and other reference circulars is available from this office.)

‡20 Roszel Road, Princeton, NJ 08540, 800-221-4792 or 866-RFBD-585, www.rfbd.org.

Assisting in Measures to Prevent Visual Impairment. An essential nursing goal is to prevent visual impairment. This involves many of the same interventions discussed for hearing impairments:

- Prenatal screening for pregnant women at risk such as those with rubella or syphilis infection and family histories of genetic disorders associated with visual loss
- Adequate prenatal and perinatal care to prevent prematurity
- Periodic screening of all children, especially newborns through preschoolers, for congenital and acquired visual impairments caused by refractive errors, strabismus, and other disorders
- Rubella immunization of all children
- Safety counseling regarding the common causes of ocular trauma, including safe practices when working with, playing with, and carrying objects such as scissors, knives, and balls

> **! NURSING ALERT**
>
> A helmet with a face mask should be required for children playing football, hockey, and baseball.

After detection of eye problems, the nurse has a responsibility to prevent further ocular damage by ensuring that corrective treatment is used. For children with strabismus, this often necessitates occlusion patching of the stronger eye. Compliance with the procedure is greatest during the early preschool years. It is more difficult to encourage school-age children to wear the occlusive patch because the poor visual acuity of the uncovered weaker eye interferes with school work and the patch sets them apart from their peers. In school they benefit from being positioned favorably (closer to the white board or other visual media) and allowed extra time to read or complete an assignment. If treatment of the eye disorder requires instillation of ophthalmic medication, the family is taught the correct procedure (see Chapter 39).

The nurse helps children with refractive errors adjust to wearing glasses. Young children who often pull off glasses benefit from temporal pieces that wrap around the ears or an elastic strap attached to the frames and around the back of the head to hold the glasses on securely. After children appreciate the value of clear vision, they are more likely to wear the corrective lenses.

Glasses should not interfere with any activity. Special protective guards are available during contact sports to prevent accidental injury; and all corrective lenses should be made from safety glass, which is shatterproof. Often corrective lenses improve visual acuity so dramatically that children are able to compete more effectively in sports. This in itself is a tremendous inducement to continue wearing glasses.

Contact lenses are a popular alternative, especially for adolescents. Several types are available such as hard lenses, including gas-permeable ones, and soft lenses, which may be designed for daily or extended wear. Contact lenses offer several advantages over glasses such as greater visual acuity, total corrected field of vision, convenience (especially with the extended-wear type), and optimal cosmetic benefit. Unfortunately they are usually more expensive and require much more care than glasses, including considerable practice to learn techniques for insertion and removal. If they are prescribed, the nurse can help to teach parents or older children how to care for them.

Because trauma is the leading cause of visual impairment, the nurse has the major responsibility of preventing further eye injury

until specific treatment is instituted. The major principles to follow when caring for an eye injury are outlined in the Emergency box on p. 1099. Because patients with a serious eye injury fear visual impairment, the nurse should stay with the child and family to provide support and reassurance.

Hearing-Visual Impairment

The most traumatic sensory impairment is loss of both vision and hearing, which may have profound effects on the child's development. They interfere with the normal sequence of physical, intellectual, and psychosocial growth. Although such children often achieve the usual motor milestones, their rate of development is slower. They learn communication only with specialized training. Finger spelling is one desirable method often taught. Words are spelled letter by letter into the child's hand, and the child spells into the other person's hand. Some children with hearing-visual impairment, especially those with residual hearing or sight, can learn to speak. Whenever possible, speech is encouraged because it allows communication with other individuals.

The future prospects for children with hearing-visual impairment are at best unpredictable. Congenital hearing-visual impairment may be accompanied by other physical or neurologic problems, which further diminish the child's learning potential. The most favorable prognosis is for children who have acquired hearing-visual impairment with few, if any, associated disabilities. Their learning capacity is greatly potentiated by their developmental progress before the sensory impairments. Although total independence, including gainful vocational training, is the goal, some children with hearing-visual impairment are unable to develop to this level. They may require lifelong parental or residential care. The nurse working with such families helps them deal with future goals for the child, including possible alternatives to home care during the parents' advancing years.

Retinoblastoma

Retinoblastoma, which arises from the retina, is the most common congenital malignant intraocular tumor of childhood. Approximately 11 cases per million occur annually, primarily in children younger than 5 years of age. Retinoblastoma is caused by a mutation in a gene and may occur sporadically or be inherited (Hurwitz, Shields, Shields, et al., 2011; Parulekar, 2010). It develops when the mutated gene is unable to produce the natural signals to stop the growth of retinal cells. Of all cases, the majority are nonhereditary and unilateral, with the remainder divided between hereditary and unilateral and hereditary and bilateral. Hereditary retinoblastomas are transmitted with few exceptions as an autosomal dominant trait with high but incomplete penetrance (Hurwitz, Shields, Shields, et al., 2011; Parulekar, 2010).

Diagnostic Evaluation

Retinoblastoma has few grossly obvious signs (Box 37-7). Typically the most common sign is observed by the parent as a whitish "glow" in the pupil, known as the white reflex or leukocoria. Leukocoria

> **BOX 37-7** **CLINICAL MANIFESTATIONS OF RETINOBLASTOMA**
>
> - White eye reflex (most common sign)
> - Strabismus (second most common sign)
> - Red, painful eye, often with glaucoma
> - Severe permanent visual impairment (late sign)

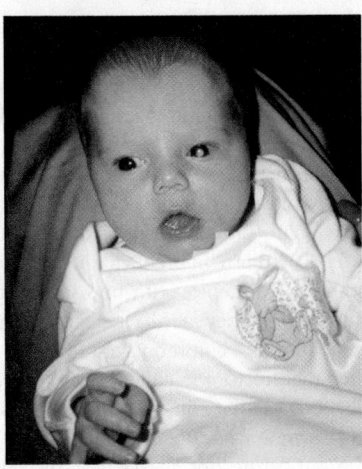

FIG 37-8 White reflex. Whitish appearance of lens is produced as light falls on tumor mass in left eye.

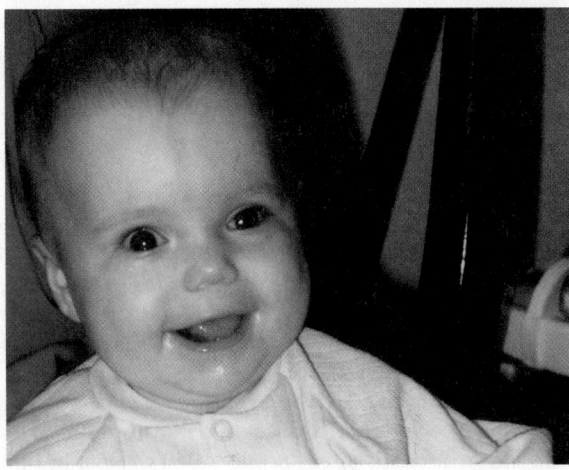

FIG 37-9 The same infant with a left prosthetic eye.

represents visualization of the tumor as the light momentarily falls on the mass (Fig. 37-8). The second most common sign of retinoblastoma is acquired strabismus (Hurwitz, Shields, Shields, et al., 2011; Phan and Stout, 2010).

The first step in diagnosis is carefully listening to and recognizing the significance of reports from family members regarding suspected abnormalities within the eye. Eye abnormalities, including white reflex, strabismus, decreased vision, and persistent painful erythematous eyes, are referred to an ophthalmologist. Definitive diagnosis is usually based on ophthalmoscopic examination with the patient under general anesthesia. Imaging studies, including ultrasonography and computed tomography of the orbit, are done to determine the extent of the disease.

Therapeutic Management

Treatment of retinoblastoma is complex. Enucleation may be used to treat advanced disease with optic nerve invasion in which there is no hope for salvage of vision. Irradiation can be used when there is vitreous seeding; and chemotherapy has been used more recently to decrease the size of the tumor, which would then allow treatment with local therapies such as plaque brachytherapy (surgical implantation of an iodine-125 applicator on the sclera until the maximum radiation dose has been delivered to the tumor), photocoagulation (use of a laser beam to destroy retinal blood vessels that supply nutrition to the tumor), and cryotherapy (freezing of the tumor, which destroys the microcirculation to the tumor and the cells themselves through microcrystal formation). Vincristine, carboplatin, and etoposide are the agents most commonly used.

The use of chemotherapy in advanced disease is controversial and has not shown improved survival. Drugs that may be used in the treatment of metastatic disease include vincristine, cyclophosphamide, doxorubicin, cisplatin, carboplatin, and etoposide. In the case of central nervous system disease, intrathecal chemotherapy may be administered (Hurwitz, Shields, Shields, et al., 2011; Lanzkowsky, 2005).

Prognosis

The overall prognosis for retinoblastoma is favorable; with early appropriate treatment the survival rate is nearly 95% for both unilateral and bilateral tumors. Retinoblastoma is one of the tumors that may spontaneously regress. Of major concern in long-term survivors is the development of decreased visual acuity; facial disfiguration; and secondary tumors, especially osteogenic sarcoma, other sarcomas, and melanoma. Children with bilateral disease (hereditary form) are more likely to develop secondary cancers than are children with unilateral disease. It is thought that these individuals are predisposed to developing cancer and that radiation increases their risk.

CARE MANAGEMENT

One of the most important nursing goals is to have a high index of suspicion for this rare malignancy. If parents report noticing a strange light in the eye or expression, these concerns must be taken seriously. Families with a history of retinoblastoma require follow-up, and the nurse can be instrumental in reminding parents of appointments and the importance of genetic counseling

Because the tumor is usually diagnosed in infants or very young children, most of the preparation for diagnostic tests and treatment involves parents. After indirect ophthalmoscopy the child may not see clearly, or the eyes may be sensitive to light because of pupillary dilation. The parents are made aware of these normal reactions before the procedure.

The treatment plan may include focal intraocular therapy with or without chemotherapy; external-beam radiation; and, if necessary, enucleation. Enucleation is the treatment of choice if there is extensive disease threatening metastasis or no chance for useful vision. The enucleation procedure and the positive benefits of a prosthesis are explained to the parents. Showing them pictures of another child with an artificial eye may help them adjust to the thought of disfigurement (Fig. 37-9).

After surgery the parents are prepared for the child's facial appearance. An eye patch is in place, and the child's face may be edematous or ecchymotic. Parents often fear seeing the surgical site because they imagine a cavity in the skull. A surgically implanted sphere maintains the shape of the eyeball, and the implant is covered with conjunctiva. When the eyelids are open, the exposed area resembles the mucosal lining of the mouth. After the child is fitted for a prosthesis, usually within 3 weeks, the facial appearance returns to normal. Initial instructions for care of the prosthesis are given by the ocularist who manufactures and fits the device.

Care of the socket is minimal and easily accomplished. The wound itself is clean and has little or no drainage. If an antibiotic ointment is prescribed, it is applied in a thin line on the surface of the tissues of the socket. To cleanse the site, an irrigating solution may be ordered and is instilled daily or more frequently *before* application of the antibiotic ointment. The dressing, consisting of an eye pad taped over the surgical site, is changed daily. After the socket has healed completely, a dressing is no longer necessary, although it is a preventive measure against infection.

Autism Spectrum Disorders

Autism spectrum disorders (ASDs) are complex neurodevelopmental disorders of unknown etiology composed of qualitative alterations in social interaction and verbal impairment with repetitive, restricted, and stereotype behavioral patterns (American Psychiatric Association, 2013; Amin, Smith, and Wang, 2011; Grynszpan, Nadel, Constant, et al., 2011).

ASD impairments range from mild to severe (Johnson, 2008). ASD is manifested during early childhood, primarily from 18 to 36 months of age. It occurs in one in 100 to 150 children in United States; is about 4 times more common in boys than in girls (although girls are more severely affected); and is not related to socioeconomic level, race, or parenting style (Centers for Disease Control and Prevention, 2009; Johnson, 2008; Shah, Dalton, and Boris, 2007).

Etiology

The cause of ASD is unknown. Researchers are investigating a number of theories, including a link between hereditary, genetics, and medical problems. Immune and environmental factors (e.g., viral infections) may interact with the genetic susceptibility to increase the incidence of ASD (Bloom-DiCicco, Lord, Zwaigenbaum, et al., 2006). Individuals with ASD may have abnormal electroencephalograms, epileptic seizures, delayed development of hand dominance, persistence of primitive reflexes, metabolic abnormalities (elevated blood serotonin), cerebellar vermal hypoplasia (part of the brain involved in regulating motion and some aspects of memory), and infantile abnormal head enlargement (Dawson, 2007; Rutter, 2011).

The strong evidence for a genetic basis in twins is consistent with an autosomal recessive pattern of inheritance. Twin studies demonstrate a high concordance (60% to 96%) for monozygotic (identical) twins and less than 5% concordance for dizygotic (nonidentical) twins. In addition, between 5% and 16% of boys with ASD are positive for the fragile X chromosome (Clifford, Dissanayake, Bui, et al., 2007).

There is a relatively high risk of recurrence of ASD in families with one affected child (Rutter, 2011; Schaefer and Lutz, 2006; Yoder, Stone, and Walden, 2009). Several genes have been suggested as possible causative factors in ASD (Dawson, 2007; Kolevzon, Gross, and Reichenberg, 2007).

The scientific evidence to date supports that there is no link between measles, mumps, and rubella (MMR) and thimerosal-containing vaccines and ASDs (Price, Thompson, Goodson, et al., 2010; Schultz, 2010) (see Evidence-Based Practice box). ASD has been reported in association with a number of conditions such as fragile X syndrome, tuberous sclerosis, metabolic disorders, fetal rubella syndrome, *Haemophilus influenzae* meningitis, and structural brain anomalies (Dawson, 2007). Recent reports have retrospectively tied ASD to prenatal and perinatal events such as maternal and paternal ages over 40 years (for fathers, one in 116 births; for mothers, one in 123 births), uterine bleeding during pregnancy, low Apgar score, fetal distress, and neonatal hyperbilirubinemia (Amin, Smith, and Wang, 2011; Croen, Najjar, Fireman, et al., 2007; Kolevzon, Gross, and Reichenberg, 2007; Rutter, 2011). However, these same researchers urge caution in interpreting these findings.

Clinical Manifestations and Diagnostic Evaluation

Children with ASD demonstrate several peculiar and often seemingly bizarre characteristics, primarily in social interactions, communication, and behavior. One hallmark characteristic is the inability to maintain eye contact with another person. Parents of autistic children have noted that their infants had difficulties with eye contact, avoidance of body contact, and language delay at a very early age (Belschner, 2007; Golnik and Maccabee-Ryaboy, 2010; Kirchner, Hatri, Heekeren, et al., 2011). Children with ASD also display limited functional play and may interact with toys in an unusual or odd manner (Belschner, 2007). They may have significant gastrointestinal symptoms. Constipation is a common symptom and can be associated with acquired megarectum in children with ASD (Buie, Campbell, Fuchs, et al., 2010). Other clinical manifestations typically seen in children with autism are described in Box 37-8.

Children with autism do not always have the same manifestations, from mild forms requiring minimal supervision to severe forms in which self-abusive behavior is common. The majority (50% to 70%) of children with autism have some degree of CI, with scores typically in the moderate-to-severe range. More girls than boys tend to have very low intelligence scores. Despite their relatively moderate-to-severe disability, some children with autism (known as savants) excel in particular areas such as art, music, memory, mathematics, or perceptual skills such as puzzle building.

Speech and language delays are also common in children with ASD. Any child who does not display such language skills as babbling or gesturing by 12 months, single words by 16 months, and two-word phrases by 24 months is recommended for immediate hearing and language evaluation. A sudden deterioration in extant expressive speech is also a red-flag event for further evaluation.

Early recognition, referral, diagnosis, and intensive early intervention tend to improve outcomes for children with ASD (Dawson, Rogers, Munson, et al., 2009; Golnik and Maccabee-Ryaboy, 2010; Zwaigenbaum, 2010). Unfortunately diagnosis is often not made until 2 to 3 years after symptoms are first recognized, which is based on the diagnostic criteria of *Diagnostic and Statistical Manual of Mental Disorders (DSM-5-TR)* (see Box 37-8).

> **! NURSING ALERT**
>
> Claims of beneficial results from the use of secretin, a peptide hormone that stimulates pancreatic secretion, have not been substantiated by scientific study (Shah, Dalton, and Boris, 2007; Welch, Ludwig, Opler, et al., 2006).*

Prognosis

ASD is usually a severely disabling condition. However, some children improve with acquisition of language skills and communication with others (Golnik and Maccabee-Ryaboy, 2010; Zwaigenbaum, 2010). Some ultimately achieve independence, but most require lifelong adult supervision. Aggravation of psychiatric symptoms occurs in about half of the children during adolescence, with girls having a tendency for continued deterioration.

Early recognition of behaviors associated with ASD is critical to implement appropriate interventions and family involvement. The prognosis is most favorable for children with higher intelligence, functional speech, and less behavioral impairment (Shah, Dalton, and Boris, 2007; Solomon, Buaminger, and Rogers, 2011).

---

*Additional information on secretin may be found by contacting the Autism Society, 4340 East-West Hwy., Suite 350, Bethesda, MD 20814-3067, 800-3AUTISM or 301-657-0881, www.autism-society.org.

EVIDENCE-BASED PRACTICE

Thimerosal-Containing Vaccines and Autism Spectrum Disorders

Ask the Question

Is the incidence of ASDs increased in children receiving vaccines containing thimerosal?

Search for Evidence

Search Strategies

Search selection criteria included English language, publication within the past 8 years, research-based articles, and infant and child populations.

Databases Used

PubMed, Cochrane Collaboration, MD Consult, Vaccine Adverse Events Reporting System (VAERS) database, American Academy of Pediatrics, Autism Research Institute

Critically Analyze the Evidence

- Evidence does not support an association between autism and mercury exposure from the pharmaceutical preservative thimerosal use in vaccinations until 2001.
- A Cochrane systematic review of 31 studies evaluating trivalent MMR in healthy individuals up to 15 years of age found no evidence that MMR is associated with autism (Demicheli, Jefferson, Rivetti, et al., 2005). Two other reviews reached similar conclusions. An additional two reviews found no evidence to support an association between autism disorders and thimerosal-containing vaccines (Parker, Schwartz, Todd, et al., 2004; Schultz, 2010).
- Two large studies in Europe found no evidence that childhood vaccination with thimerosal-containing vaccines was associated with the development of ASDs. One longitudinal study evaluated more than 14,000 children in the United Kingdom. The mercury exposure from thimerosal-containing vaccines was recorded and calculated at ages 3, 4, and 6 months and compared with cognitive and behavioral-developmental assessments performed from 6 to 91 months of age (Heron, Golding, and the ALSPAC study team, 2004). The second study, a cohort of 467,450 children in Denmark, compared the incidence of ASDs in children vaccinated with thimerosal-containing vaccines with that of ASDs in children vaccinated with a thimerosal-free formulation of the same vaccine.
- Smaller case-control studies have also found no relationships between childhood vaccination with thimerosal-containing vaccines and the development of ASDs (Baird, Pickles, Simonoff, et al., 2007; Hviid, Stellfeld, Wohlfahrt, et al., 2003; Price, Thompson, Goodson, et al., 2010).
- In 2004 the Institute of Medicine (2004) completed an update to the review of the evidence and concluded that the epidemiologic evidence supports the rejection of a causal relationship between thimerosal exposure from childhood vaccines and the onset of autism. Based on guidelines established by the U.S. Food and Drug Administration (2010) and other government monitoring agencies, no children will be exposed to excessive mercury from childhood vaccines.

Apply the Evidence: Nursing Implications

There is *good evidence with strong recommendations* (Guyatt, Oxman, Vist, et al., 2008) published that there is no link between vaccines containing thimerosal and autism or other neurodevelopmental disorders.

Quality and Safety Competencies:
Evidence-Based Practice*

Knowledge

Compare research summaries that provide evidence of the lack of association between vaccines containing thimerosal and autism or other neurodevelopmental disorders.

Skills

Integrate evidence into practice by sharing results with parents regarding the benefits of vaccinating their children and the evidence regarding lack of association between immunizations and autism disorders.

Attitudes

Appreciate strengths and weakness of the evidence that confirms the lack of a link between vaccines containing thimerosal and autism or other neurodevelopmental disorders.

References

Baird A, Pickles A, Simonoff E, et al: Measles vaccination and antibody response in autism spectrum disorders, *Arch Dis Child* 93:832–837, 2007.

Demicheli V, Jefferson T, Rivetti A, et al: Vaccines for measles, mumps and rubella in children, *Cochrane Database Syst Rev* (4):CD004407, 2005.

Guyatt GH, Oxman AD, Vist GE, et al: GRADE: an emerging consensus on rating quality of evidence and strength of recommendations, *BMJ* 336:924–926, 2008.

Heron J, Golding J, ALSPAC study team: Thimerosal exposure in infants and developmental disorders: a prospective cohort study in the United Kingdom does not support a causal association, *Pediatrics* 114(3):577–583, 2004.

Hviid A, Stellfeld M, Wohlfahrt J, et al: Association between thimerosal-containing vaccine and autism, *JAMA* 290(13):1763–1766, 2003.

Institute of Medicine: Immunization safety review: vaccines and autism, Washington, DC, 2004, National Academies Press.

Parker SK, Schwartz B, Todd J, et al: Thimerosal-containing vaccines and autistic spectrum disorder: a critical review of published original data, *Pediatrics* 114(3):793–804, 2004.

Price CS, Thompson WW, Goodson B, et al: Prenatal and infant exposure to thimerosal from vaccines and immunoglobulins and risk of autism, *Pediatrics* 126:656–664, 2010.

Schultz ST: Does thimerosal or other mercury exposure increase the risk for autism? *Acta Neurobiol Exp* 70:187–195, 2010.

US Food and Drug Administration: *Vaccines, blood and biologics: thimerosal in vaccines,* 2010, www.fda.gov/BiologicsBloodVaccines/SafetyAvailability/vaccineSafety/UCM096228.

Rosalind Bryant

*Based on QSEN at www.qsen.org.

ASD, Autism spectrum disorder; *MMR,* measles, mumps, and rubella.

CARE MANAGEMENT

Therapeutic intervention for children with ASD is a specialized area involving professionals with advanced training. Although there is no cure for ASD, numerous therapies have been used. The most promising results have been through highly structured and intensive behavior modification programs. In general the objective in treatment is to promote positive reinforcement, increase social awareness of others, teach verbal communication skills, and decrease unacceptable behavior. Providing a structured routine for the child to follow is a key in the management of ASD.

BOX 37-8	DIAGNOSTIC CRITERIA FOR AUTISM SPECTRUM DISORDERS

A. A total of six (or more) items from 1, 2, and 3, with at least two from 1 and one each from 2 and 3:

1. Qualitative impairment in social interaction as manifested by at least two of the following:

   (a) Marked impairment in the use of multiple nonverbal behaviors such as eye-to-eye gaze, facial expression, body postures, and gestures to regulate social interaction

   (b) Failure to develop peer relationships appropriate to developmental level

   (c) Lack of spontaneous seeking to share enjoyment, interests, or achievements with other people (e.g., by a lack of showing, bringing, pointing out objects of interest)

   (d) Lack of social or emotional reciprocity

2. Qualitative impairments in communication as manifested by at least one of the following:

   (a) Delay in or total lack of the development of spoken language (not accompanied by an attempt to compensate through alternative modes of communication such as gestures or mime)

   (b) In individuals with adequate speech, marked impairment in the ability to initiate or sustain a conversation with others

   (c) Stereotyped and repetitive use of language or idiosyncratic language

   (d) Lack of varied, spontaneous make-believe play or social imitative play appropriate to developmental level

3. Restricted repetitive and stereotyped patterns of behavior, interests, and activities as manifested by at least one of the following:

   (a) Encompassing preoccupation with one or more stereotyped and restricted patterns of interest that is abnormal either in intensity or focus

   (b) Apparently inflexible adherence to specific, nonfunctional routines or rituals

   (c) Stereotyped and repetitive motor mannerisms (e.g., hand or finger flapping or twisting, complex whole-body movements)

   (d) Persistent preoccupation with parts of objects

B. Delays or abnormal functioning in at least one of the following areas, with onset before age 3 years: (1) social interaction, (2) language as used in social communication, or (3) symbolic or imaginative play.

C. The disturbance is not better accounted for by Rett disorder or childhood disintegrative disorder.

From American Psychiatric Association: *Diagnostic and statistical manual of mental disorders*, ed 4, rev trans (DSM-IV TR), Washington, DC, 2000, Author.
Reprinted with permission from the Diagnostic and Statistical Manual of Mental Disorders, Fourth Edition, Text Revision (Copyright © 2000). American Psychiatric Association.

When these children are hospitalized, the parents are essential to planning care and ideally should stay with the child as much as possible. Nurses should recognize that not all children with ASD are the same and require individual assessment and treatment. Decreasing stimulation by using a private room, avoiding extraneous auditory and visual distractions, and encouraging the parents to bring in possessions to which the child is attached may lessen the disruptiveness of hospitalization. Because physical contact often upsets these children, minimum holding and eye contact may be necessary to avoid behavioral outbursts. Care must be taken when performing procedures on, administering medicine to, and feeding these children because they may be either fussy eaters who willfully starve themselves or gag to prevent eating or indiscriminate hoarders, swallowing any available edible or inedible items such as a thermometer. Eating habits of ASD children may be particularly problematic for families and may involve food refusal accompanied by mineral deficiencies, mouthing objects, eating nonedibles, and smelling and throwing food (Belschner, 2007; Caronna, Augustyn, and Zuckerman, 2007; Herndon, DiGuiseppi, Johnson et al., 2009).

Children with ASD need to be introduced to new situations slowly, with visits with staff caregivers kept short whenever possible. Because these children have difficulty organizing their behavior and redirecting their energy, they need to be told directly what to do. Communication should be at the child's developmental level, brief, and concrete.

Family Support

As with so many other chronic conditions, ASD involves the entire family and often becomes "a family disease." Nurses can help alleviate the guilt and shame often associated with this disorder by stressing what is known from a biologic standpoint and providing family support. It is imperative to help parents understand that they are not the cause of the child's condition.

Parents need expert counseling early in the course of the disorder and should be referred to the Autism Society website.* The society provides information about education, treatment programs and techniques, and facilities such as camps and group homes. Other helpful resources for parents of children with ASD are the local and state departments of mental health and developmental disabilities; these organizations provide important programs and in-school programs throughout the United States for children with ASD.

As much as possible the family is encouraged to care for the child in the home. With the help of family support programs in many states, families are often able to provide home care and assist with the educational services the child needs. As the child approaches adulthood and the parents become older, the family may require assistance in locating a long-term placement facility.

*See footnote on p. 1104.

KEY POINTS

- The AAIDD defines *intellectual disability* as significantly subaverage general intellectual functioning existing concurrently with deficits in adaptive behavior and manifested during the developmental period.

- Causes of severe CI are primarily genetic, biochemical, and infectious. Mild CI is associated primarily with familial, social, and environmental causes; severe CI is more likely to be associated with specific syndromes.

- Education of children with CI emphasizes sensory and verbal discrimination, improvement of short-term memory, motivation, and technologic support.

- Optimal development may be promoted through family guidance regarding play, communication, discipline, socialization, and sexuality.

- Prevention of CI focuses on support for preterm neonates and other high-risk newborns, rubella immunization, genetic counseling, and maternal education regarding the risks of chemical use (e.g., alcohol ingestion) and the importance of adequate nutrition.

- Down syndrome, a chromosome abnormality, is characterized by mild-to-moderate range of CI (most often), physical characteristics, slowed language development, congenital anomalies, sensory problems, and diminished growth and sexual development.

- Fragile X syndrome is characterized by CI and phenotypic findings in affected boys. It is considered the most common hereditary cause and the second leading chromosomal cause of CI after Down syndrome.

- Hearing disorders may be classified according to the location of the defect: conductive, sensorineural, mixed conductive-sensorineural, and central auditory imperception.

- Rehabilitation for hearing loss involves parent education and support, hearing aids, lipreading, sign language, speech therapy, and promotion of socialization.

- Prevention of hearing loss includes treatment of infection, universal newborn screening and child auditory testing, immunization, pregnancy and genetic counseling, and reduction of noise pollution.

- Common visual impairments in childhood include refractive errors, amblyopia, strabismus, cataracts, glaucoma, trauma, and infections.

- Prevention of visual impairment focuses on prenatal screening, prenatal and perinatal care, periodic vision screening, immunization, and safety counseling.

- Nursing goals in visual rehabilitation include helping the family and child adjust to the child's visual impairment, promoting parent-child attachment, fostering optimal development and independence, providing for play and socialization, and being aware of educational facilities.

- For a child undergoing ocular surgery, nursing care is aimed at reassuring the child and family throughout treatment, orienting the child to the surroundings, providing a safe environment, and encouraging independence.

- Retinoblastoma is a rare congenital malignant tumor; its most common clinical manifestations are white pupil reflex and strabismus.

- ASDs are a complex neurodevelopmental disorder of brain function accompanied by a broad range and severity of intellectual and behavioral deficits.

REFERENCES

American Academy of Pediatrics Committee on Genetics: Health supervision for children with Down syndrome, *Pediatrics* 107(2):442–449, 2001.

American Academy of Pediatrics Task Force on Newborn and Infant Hearing: Newborn and infant hearing loss: detection and intervention, *Pediatrics* 103(2):527–530, 1999.

American Association on Intellectual and Developmental Disabilities (AAIDD), Intellectual Disability: *Definition, classification, and systems of supports*, ed 11, Washington, DC, 2010.

American Psychiatric Association (APA): *Diagnostic and statistical manual of mental disorders (DSM-5)*, ed 5, Washington, DC, 2013, The Association.

Amin SB, Smith T, Wang H: Is neonatal jaundice associated with autism spectrum disorders: a systematic review, *J Autism Dev Disord* 29:1169–1176, 2011.

Bahado-Singh RO, Argoti P: An overview of first-trimester screening for chromosomal abnormalities, *Clin Lab Med* 30:545–555, 2010.

Baldassari CM, Schmidt C, Schubert CM, et al: Receptive language outcomes in children after cochlear implantation, *Otolaryngol Head Neck Surg* 140:114–119, 2009.

Belschner RA: Stop, assess and motivate: the SAM approach to autism spectrum disorder, *Am J Nurse Pract* 11(4):43–50, 2007.

Benn PA, Chapman AR: Practical and ethical considerations of noninvasive prenatal diagnosis, *JAMA* 301(2), 2009.

Bloom-DiCicco E, Lord C, Zwaigenbaum L, et al: The development neurobiology of autism spectrum disorder, *J Neurosci* 26(26):6897–6906, 2006.

Botelho FA, Bouzada MCF, de Resende LM, et al: Prevalence of hearing impairment in children at risk, *Braz J Otorhinolaryngol* 76(6):739–744, 2010.

Buie T, Campbell DB, Fuchs GJ, et al: Evaluation, diagnosis, and treatment of gastrointestinal disorders in individuals with ASDs: a consensus report, *Pediatrics* 125(suppl 1):S1–S18, 2010.

Caronna EB, Augustyn M, Zuckerman B: Revisiting parental concerns in the age of autism spectrum disorders, *Arch Pediatr Adolesc Med* 161:406–407, 2007.

Centers for Disease Control and Prevention (CDC): Prevalence of autism spectrum disorders: autism and developmental disorders monitoring network—United States, 2006, *MMWR Surveill Summ* 58(SS10):1–20, 2009.

Clifford S, Dissanayake C, Bui QM, et al: Autism spectrum phenotype in males and females with fragile X full mutation and permutation, *J Autism Dev Disord* 37:738–747, 2007.

Croen LA, Najjar DV, Fireman B, et al: Maternal and paternal age and the risk of autism spectrum disorders, *Arch Pediatr Adolesc Med* 161:334–340, 2007.

Daniel E: Noise and hearing loss: a review, *J School Health* 77(5):225–231, 2007.

Dawson G: Despite major challenges, autism research continues to offer hope, *Arch Pediatr Adolesc Med* 161:411–412, 2007.

Dawson G, Rogers S, Munson J, et al: Randomized, controlled trial of an intervention for toddlers with autism: the early start Denver model, *Pediatrics* 125:e17–e23, 2009.

Defendi GL: Fetal alcohol spectrum disorder: how to recognize the various manifestations, *Consult Ped* 9(10):343–351, 2010.

Fabry DA, Davila EP, Arheart KL, et al: Secondhand smoke exposure and the risk of hearing loss, *Tobacco Control* 20:82–85, 2011.

Gifford KA, Holmes MG, Bernstein HH: Hearing loss in children, *Pediatr Rev* 30(6):207–216, 2009.

Golnik A, Maccabee-Ryaboy, N: Autism: clinical pearls for primary care, *Contemp Pediatr* 42–60, 2010.

Grynszpan O, Nadel J, Constant J, et al: A new virtual environment paradigm for high-functioning autism intended to help attentional disengagement in a social context, *J Phys Ther Educ* 25(1):42–47, 2011.

Haddad J: Hearing loss. In Kliegman RM, Behrman RE, Jenson HB, et al, editors: *Nelson textbook of pediatrics*, ed 18, Philadelphia, 2007, Saunders.

Hagerman RJ: The fragile X prevalence paradox, *J Med Genet* 45:498–499, 2008.

Henderson E, Testa MA, Hartnick C: Prevalence of noise-induced hearing-threshold shifts and hearing loss among US youths, *Pediatrics* 127(1):e39–e46, 2011.

Herndon AC, DiGuiseppi C, Johnson SL, et al: Does nutritional intake differ between children and autism spectrum disorders and children with typical development? *J Autism Dev Disord* 39:212–222, 2009.

Hurwitz RL, Shields CL, Shields JA, et al: Retinoblastoma. In Pizzo PA, Poplack DG, editors: *Principals and practice of pediatric oncology*, ed 6, Philadelphia, 2011, Lippincott.

Johnson CP: Recognition of autism before age 2 years, *Pediatr Rev* 29(3):86–96, 2008.

Johnson CP, Walker WO: Mental retardation: management and prognosis, *Pediatr Rev* 27(7):249–256, 2006.

Joint Committee on Infant Hearing: Year 2000 position statement: principles and guidelines for early hearing detection and intervention programs, *Pediatrics* 106(4):798–817, 2000.

Katz G, Lazcano-Ponce E: Intellectual disability: Definition, etiological factors, classification, diagnosis, treatment and prognosis, *Salud Publica de Mexico*, 50(suppl 2):S132–S141, 2008.

Kirchner JC, Hatri A, Heekeren HR, et al: Autistic symptomatology, face processing abilities, and eye fixation patterns, *J Autism Dev Disord* 41:158–167, 2011.

Kolevzon A, Gross R, Reichenberg A: Prenatal and perinatal risk factors for autism: a review and integration of findings, *Arch Pediatr Adolesc Med* 161:326–333, 2007.

Kuehn BM: Scientists find promising therapies for fragile X and Down syndromes, *JAMA* 305(4):344–346, 2011.

Lanzkowsky P: *Manual of pediatric hematology and oncology*, ed 4, San Diego, 2005, Academic Press.

Mohammadi S, Mazhari MM, Mehrparvar AH, et al: Cigarette smoking and occupational noise-induced hearing loss, *Eur J Public Health* 20(4):452–455, 2009.

National Down Syndrome Society: Education, development, and community life, 2011a, www.ndss.org.

National Down Syndrome Society: About Down syndrome, 2011b, www.ndss.org.

National Down Syndrome Society: Healthcare, 2011c, www.ndss.org.

National Fragile X Foundation: Prevalence of fragile X syndrome, 2010, www.fragilex.org/html/prevalence.htm.

Oliver C, Richards C: Self-injurious behavior in people with intellectual disability, *Curr Opin Psychiatr* 23:412–416, 2010.

Parulekar MV: Retinoblastoma-current treatment and future direction, *Early Hum Dev* 86:619–625, 2010.

Phan IT, Stout T: Retinoblastoma presenting as strabismus and leukocoria, *J Pediatr* 157:858, 2010.

Price CS, Thompson WW, Goodson B, et al: Prenatal and infant exposure to thimerosal from vaccines and immunoglobulins and risk of autism, *Pediatrics* 126:656–664, 2010.

Pueschel SM: The child with Down syndrome. In Levine MD, Carey WB, Crocker AC, editors: *Developmental-behavioral pediatrics*, ed 3, Philadelphia, 1999, Saunders.

Rahi JS, Cumberland PM, Peckham CS, et al: Improving detection of blindness in childhood: the British childhood vision impairment study, *Pediatrics* 126:e895–e903, 2010.

Robertson CMT, Howarth TM, Bork DLR, et al: Permanent bilateral sensory and neural hearing loss of children after neonatal intensive care because of extreme prematurity: a thirty-year study, *Pediatrics* 123(5):e797–e807, 2009.

Rutter ML: Progress in understanding autism: 2007-2010, *J Autism Dev Disord* 41:395–404, 2011.

Schaefer GB, Lutz RE: Diagnostic yield in the clinical genetic evaluation of autism spectrum disorders, *Genet Med* 8(9):549–556, 2006.

Schultz ST: Does thimerosal or other mercury exposure increase the risk for autism? *Acta Neurobiol Exp* 70:187–195, 2010.

Shah PE, Dalton R, Boris NW: Pervasive developmental disorders and childhood psychosis. In Kliegman RM, Behrman RE, Jenson HB, et al, editors: *Nelson textbook of pediatrics*, ed 18, Philadelphia, 2007, Saunders.

Shapiro BK, Batshaw ML: Mental retardation (intellectual disability). In Kliegman RM,

Behrman RE, Jenson HB, et al, editors: *Nelson textbook of pediatrics*, ed 18, Philadelphia, 2007, Saunders.

Solomon M, Buaminger N, Rogers SJ: Abstract reasoning and friendship in high-functioning preadolescents with autism spectrum disorders, *J Autism Dev Disord* 41:32–43, 2011.

Tierney CD, Brown PJ: Development of children who have hearing impairment, *Pediatr Rev* 29(12):e72–e73, 2008.

Tingley DH: Vision screening essentials: screening today for eye disorders in the pediatric patient, *Pediatr Rev* 28(2):54–61, 2007.

US Preventive Services Task Force: Vision screening for children 1 to 5 years of age, *Pediatrics* 127:340–346, 2011.

Walker WO, Johnson CP: Mental retardation: overview and diagnosis, *Pediatr Rev* 27(6):204–212, 2006.

Weijerman ME, de Winter JP: Clinical practice: the care of children with Down syndrome, *Eur J Pediatr* 169:1445–1452, 2010.

Welch MG, Ludwig RJ, Opler M, et al: Secretin's role in the cerebellum: a larger biological context and implications for developmental disorders, *Cerebellum* 5:2–6, 2006.

Wilton G, Plane MB: The family empowerment network: a service model to address the needs of children and families affected by fetal alcohol spectrum disorders, *Pediatr Nurs* 32(4):299–305, 2006.

Yoder P, Stone WL, Walden T: Predicting social impairment and ASD diagnostic in younger siblings of children with autism spectrum disorder, *J Autism Dev Disord* 39:1381–1391, 2009.

Zeng FG, Liu S: Speech perception in individuals with auditory neuropathy, *J Speech Lang Hearing Res* 49:367–380, 2006.

Zwaigenbaum L: Advances in the early detection of autism, *Curr Opin Neurol* 23:97–102, 2010.

Family-Centered Care of the Child During Illness and Hospitalization

Marilyn J. Hockenberry

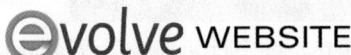

WEBSITE

http://evolve.elsevier.com/Perry/maternal

LEARNING OBJECTIVES

On completion of this chapter, the reader will be able to:
- Identify the stressors of illness and hospitalization for children during each developmental stage.
- List essential priorities of nursing care on a child's admission to the hospital.
- Review nursing interventions that prevent or minimize the stress of separation during hospitalization.
- Discuss nursing interventions that minimize the stress of loss of control during hospitalization.
- Describe nursing interventions that minimize the fear of bodily injury during hospitalization.
- Outline nursing interventions that support parents, siblings, and family during a child's illness and hospitalization.
- Describe nursing interventions needed when children are admitted to special units such as the emergency department.

STRESSORS OF HOSPITALIZATION AND CHILDREN'S REACTIONS

Often illness and hospitalization are the first crises children must face. Especially during the early years, children are particularly vulnerable to these stressors because (1) stress represents a change from the usual state of health and environmental routine, and (2) children have a limited number of coping mechanisms to resolve stressors. Major stressors of hospitalization include separation, loss of control, bodily injury, and pain. Children's reactions to these crises are influenced by their developmental age; their previous experience with illness, separation, or hospitalization; their innate and acquired coping skills; the seriousness of the diagnosis; and the support system available. Children also expressed fears caused by the unfamiliar environment or lack of information; child-staff relations; and the physical, social, and symbolic environment (Samela, Salanterä, and Aronen, 2009).

Separation Anxiety

The major stress from middle infancy throughout the preschool years, especially for children ages 6 to 30 months, is separation anxiety, also called anaclitic depression. The principal behavioral responses to this stressor during early childhood are summarized in Box 38-1. During the stage of protest, children react aggressively to the separation from the parent. They cry and scream for their parents, refuse the attention of anyone else, and are inconsolable in their grief (Fig. 38-1). In contrast, through the stage of despair, the crying stops, and depression is evident. The child is much less active, is uninterested in play or food, and withdraws from others (Fig. 38-2).

The third stage is detachment, also called denial. Superficially it appears that the child has finally adjusted to the loss. He or she becomes more interested in the surroundings, plays with others, and seems to form new relationships. However, this behavior is the result of resignation and is not a sign of contentment. The child detaches from the parent in an effort to escape the emotional pain of desiring the parent's presence and copes by forming shallow relationships with others, becoming increasingly self-centered, and attaching primary importance to material objects. This is the most serious stage because reversal of the potential adverse effects is less likely to occur after detachment is established. However, in most situations the temporary separations imposed by hospitalization do not cause such prolonged parental absences that the child enters into detachment. In addition, considerable evidence suggests that, even with stressors such as separation, children are remarkably adaptable, and permanent ill effects are rare.

Although progression to the stage of detachment is uncommon, the initial stages are observed frequently, even with brief separations from either parent. Unless health team members understand the meaning of each stage of behavior, they may erroneously label the

BOX 38-1   MANIFESTATIONS OF SEPARATION ANXIETY IN YOUNG CHILDREN

Stage of Protest

- Behaviors observed during later infancy include the following:
  - Cries
  - Screams
  - Searches for parent with eyes
  - Clings to parent
  - Avoids and rejects contact with strangers
- Additional behaviors observed during toddlerhood include the following:
  - Verbally attacks strangers (e.g., "Go away")
  - Physically attacks strangers (e.g., kicks, bites, hits, pinches)
  - Attempts to escape to find parent
  - Attempts to physically force parent to stay
- Behaviors may last from hours to days.
- Protest such as crying may be continuous, ceasing only with physical exhaustion.
- Approach of stranger may precipitate increased protest.

Stage of Despair

- Observed behaviors include the following:
  - Is inactive
  - Withdraws from others
  - Is depressed, sad
  - Lacks interest in environment
  - Is uncommunicative
  - Regresses to earlier behavior (e.g., thumb sucking, bed-wetting, use of pacifier, use of bottle)
- Behaviors may last for variable length of time.
- Child's physical condition may deteriorate from refusal to eat, drink, or move.

Stage of Detachment

- Observed behaviors include the following:
  - Shows increased interest in surroundings
  - Interacts with strangers or familiar caregivers
  - Forms new but superficial relationships
  - Appears happy
- Detachment usually occurs after prolonged separation from parent; it is rarely seen in hospitalized children.
- Behaviors represent a superficial adjustment to loss.

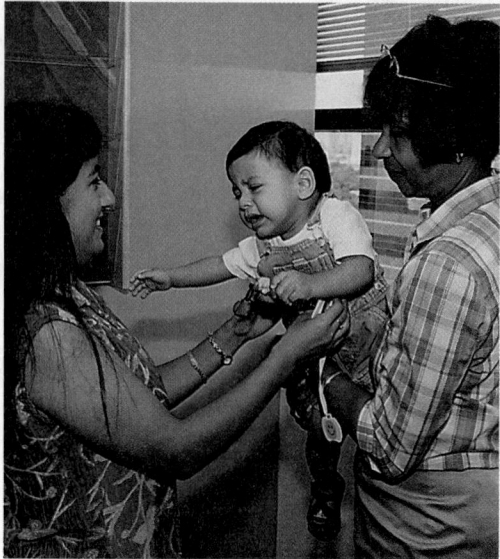

FIG 38-1 In the protest phase of separation anxiety, children cry loudly and are inconsolable in their grief for the parent. (Courtesy James DeLeon, Texas Children's Hospital, Houston, TX.)

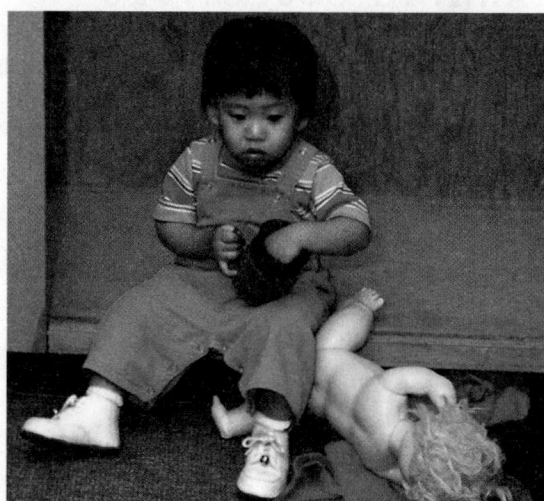

FIG 38-2 During the despair phase of separation anxiety, children are sad, lonely, and uninterested in food and play.

behaviors as positive or negative. For example, they may see the loud crying of the protest phase as "bad" behavior. Because the protests increase when a stranger approaches the child, they may interpret that reaction as meaning they should stay away. During the quiet, withdrawn phase of despair, health team members may think that the child is finally "settling in" to the new surroundings, and they may see the detachment behaviors as proof of a "positive adjustment." The faster this stage is reached, the more likely it is that the child will be regarded as the "ideal patient."

Because children seem to react "negatively" to visits by their parents, uninformed observers feel justified in restricting parental visiting privileges. For example, during the protest stage children outwardly do not appear happy to see their parents (Fig. 38-3). In fact, they may even cry louder. If they are depressed, they may reject their parents or begin to protest again. Often they cling to their parents in an effort to ensure their continued presence.

Consequently such reactions may be regarded as "disturbing" the child's adjustment to the new surroundings. If the separation has progressed to the phase of detachment, children respond no differently to their parents than they would to any other person.

Such reactions are distressing to parents, who are unaware of their meaning. If parents are regarded as intruders, they see their absence as "beneficial" to the child's adjustment and recovery. They may respond to the child's behavior by staying for only short periods, visiting less frequently, or deceiving the child when it is time to leave. The result is a destructive cycle of misunderstanding and unmet needs.

Early Childhood

Separation anxiety is the greatest stress imposed by hospitalization during early childhood. If separation is avoided, young children have a tremendous capacity to withstand any other stress. During this age

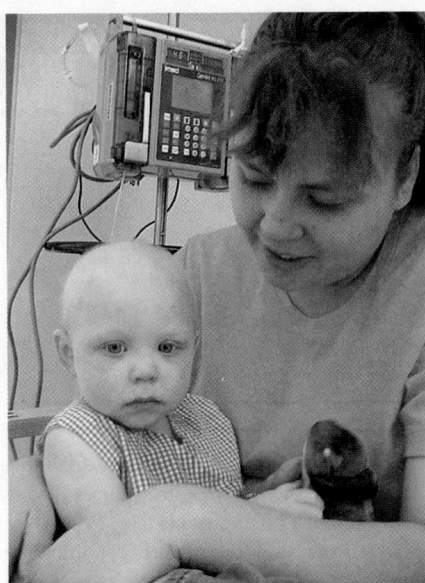

FIG 38-3 Young children may appear withdrawn and sad even in the presence of a parent. (Courtesy E. Jacob, Texas Children's Hospital, Houston, TX.)

period the typical reactions just described are seen. However, children in the toddler stage demonstrate more goal-directed behaviors. For example, they may plead with the parents to stay and physically try to keep the parents with them or try to find parents who have left. They may demonstrate displeasure on the parents' return or departure by having temper tantrums; refusing to comply with the usual routines of mealtime, bedtime, or toileting; or regressing to more primitive levels of development. However, temper tantrums, bed-wetting, or other behaviors may also be expressions of anger, a physiologic response to stress, or symptoms of illness.

Because preschoolers are more secure interpersonally than toddlers, they can tolerate brief periods of separation from their parents and are more inclined to develop substitute trust in other significant adults. However, the stress of illness usually renders preschoolers less able to cope with separation; as a result they manifest many of the stage behaviors of separation anxiety, although in general the protest behaviors are more subtle and passive than those seen in younger children. Preschoolers may demonstrate separation anxiety by refusing to eat, experiencing difficulty in sleeping, crying quietly for their parents, continually asking when the parents will visit, or withdrawing from others. They may express anger indirectly by breaking their toys, hitting other children, or refusing to cooperate during usual self-care activities. Nurses need to be sensitive to these less obvious signs of separation anxiety to intervene appropriately.

Later Childhood and Adolescence

Previous research, usually based on adult recollections, indicated that the family does not play as important a role for school-age children as it does during the toddler and preschool years. However, in a recent study that asked children about their fears when hospitalized, children listed their greatest fears regarding hospitalization as being separated from family and friends, being in an unfamiliar environment, receiving investigations or treatments, and losing self-determination or choices (Coyne, 2006). In a qualitative study of children ages 5 to 9 years, children described hospitalization in stories that focused on being alone and feeling scared, angry, or sad.

These children also described the need for protection and companionship while hospitalized (Wilson, Megel, Enenbach, et al., 2010).

Although school-age children are better able to cope with separation in general, the stress and often accompanying regression imposed by illness or hospitalization may increase their need for parental security and guidance. This is particularly true for young school-age children who have only recently left the safety of the home and are struggling with the crisis of school adjustment. Middle and late school-age children may react more to the separation from their usual activities and peers than to the absence of their parents. These children have a high level of physical and mental activity that frequently finds no suitable outlets in the hospital environment; and, even when they dislike school, they admit to missing its routine and worry that they will not be able to compete or "fit in" with their classmates when they return. Feelings of loneliness, boredom, isolation, and depression are common. Such reactions may occur more as a result of separation than of concern over the illness, treatment, or hospital setting.

School-age children may need and desire parental guidance or support from other adult figures but may be unable or unwilling to ask for it. Because the goal of attaining independence is so important to them, they are reluctant to seek help directly, fearing that they will appear weak, childish, or dependent. Cultural expectations to "act like a man" or "be brave and strong" weigh heavily on these children, especially boys, who tend to react to stress with stoicism, withdrawal, or passive acceptance. Often the need to express hostile, angry, or other negative feelings finds outlets in alternate ways such as irritability and aggression toward parents, withdrawal from hospital personnel, inability to relate to peers, rejection of siblings, or subsequent behavioral problems in school.

For adolescents separation from home and parents may produce varied emotions, ranging from difficulty coping to welcoming the event. However, loss of peer-group contact may pose a severe emotional threat because of loss of group status, inability to exert group control or leadership, and loss of group acceptance. Deviations within peer groups are poorly tolerated; and, although group members may express concern for the adolescent's illness or need for hospitalization, they continue their group activities, quickly filling the gap of the absent member. During the temporary separation from their usual group, ill adolescents may benefit from group associations with other hospitalized teens.

Effects of Hospitalization on the Child

Children may react to the stresses of hospitalization before admission, during hospitalization, and after discharge. A child's concept of illness is even more important than age and intellectual maturity in predicting the level of anxiety before hospitalization (Clatworthy, Simon, and Tiedeman, 1999). This may or may not be affected by the duration of the condition or prior hospitalizations; therefore nurses should avoid overestimating the illness concepts of children with prior medical experience (Box 38-2).

Individual Risk Factors

A number of risk factors make certain children more vulnerable than others to the stresses of hospitalization (Box 38-3). Rural children may exhibit significantly greater degrees of psychologic upset than urban children, possibly because urban children have opportunities to become familiar with a local hospital. Because separation is such an important issue surrounding hospitalization for young children, children who are active and strong willed tend to fare better when hospitalized than youngsters who are passive. Consequently nurses should be alert to children who passively accept all changes

BOX 38-2 POSTHOSPITAL BEHAVIORS IN CHILDREN

Young Children

- They show initial aloofness toward parents; this may last from a few minutes (most common) to a few days.
- This is frequently followed by dependency behaviors:
  - Tendency to cling to parents
  - Demands for parents' attention
  - Vigorous opposition to any separation (e.g., staying at preschool or with a babysitter)
- Other negative behaviors include the following:
  - New fears (e.g., nightmares)
  - Resistance to going to bed, night waking
  - Withdrawal and shyness
  - Hyperactivity
  - Temper tantrums
  - Food peculiarities
  - Attachment to blanket or toy
  - Regression in newly learned skills (e.g., self-toileting)

Older Children

- Negative behaviors include the following:
  - Emotional coldness followed by intense, demanding dependence on parents
  - Anger toward parents
  - Jealousy toward others (e.g., siblings)

BOX 38-3 RISK FACTORS THAT INCREASE CHILDREN'S VULNERABILITY TO THE STRESSES OF HOSPITALIZATION

- "Difficult" temperament
- Lack of fit between child and parent
- Age (especially between 6 months and 5 years)
- Male gender
- Below-average intelligence
- Multiple and continuing stresses (e.g., frequent hospitalizations)

BOX 38-4 FACTORS AFFECTING PARENTS' REACTIONS TO THEIR CHILD'S ILLNESS

- Seriousness of the threat to the child
- Previous experience with illness or hospitalization
- Medical procedures involved in diagnosis and treatment
- Available support systems
- Personal ego strengths
- Previous coping abilities
- Additional stresses on the family system
- Cultural and religious beliefs
- Communication patterns among family members

newborns and children with severe injuries or disabilities who have survived because of major technologic advances yet have been left with chronic or disabling conditions that require frequent and lengthy hospital stays. The nature of their conditions increases the likelihood that they will experience more invasive and traumatic procedures while they are hospitalized. These factors make them more vulnerable to the emotional consequences of hospitalization and result in their needs being significantly different from those of the short-term patients of the past (see Chapter 36 for further discussion on children with special needs). Most of these children are infants and toddlers, the age-group most vulnerable to the effects of hospitalization.

Concern in recent years has focused on the increasing length of hospitalization because of complex medical and nursing care, elusive diagnoses, and complicated psychosocial issues. Without special attention devoted to meeting children's psychosocial and developmental needs in the hospital environment, the detrimental consequences of prolonged hospitalization may be severe.

Beneficial Effects of Hospitalization

Although hospitalization can be and usually is stressful for children, it can also be beneficial. The most obvious benefit is the recovery from illness, but hospitalization also can present an opportunity for children to master stress and feel competent in their coping abilities. The hospital environment can provide children with new socialization experiences that can broaden their interpersonal relationships. The psychologic benefits need to be considered and maximized during hospitalization. Appropriate nursing strategies to achieve this goal are presented on pp. 1121-1122.

STRESSORS AND REACTIONS OF THE FAMILY OF THE CHILD WHO IS HOSPITALIZED

Parental Reactions

The crisis of childhood illness and hospitalization affects every member of the family. Parents' reactions to illness in their child depend on a variety of factors. Although one cannot predict which factors are most likely to influence their response, a number of variables have been identified (Box 38-4).

Recent research has identified common themes among parents whose children were hospitalized, including feeling an overall sense of helplessness, questioning the skills of staff, accepting the reality of hospitalization, needing to have information explained in simple language, dealing with fear, coping with uncertainty, and seeking reassurance from caregivers. This reassurance involves staff being compassionate, expressing concern for the child, and attending to detail in the child's care (Stranton, 2004).

and requests; these children may need more support than "oppositional" children.

The stressors of hospitalization may cause young children to experience short- and long-term negative outcomes. Adverse outcomes may be related to the length and number of admissions, multiple invasive procedures, and the parents' anxiety. Common responses include regression, separation anxiety, apathy, fears, and sleeping disturbances, especially for children younger than 7 years of age (Melnyk, 2000). Supportive practices such as family-centered care and frequent family visiting may lessen the detrimental effects of such admissions. Nurses should attempt to identify children at risk for poor coping strategies (Small, 2002).

Changes in the Pediatric Population

The pediatric population in hospitals has changed dramatically over the past two decades. With a growing trend toward shortened hospital stays and outpatient surgery, a greater percentage of the children hospitalized today have more serious needs complex problems than those hospitalized in the past. Many of these children are fragile

Sibling Reactions

Siblings' reactions to a sister's or brother's illness or hospitalization are discussed in Chapter 36 and differ little when a child becomes temporarily ill. Siblings experience loneliness, fear, worry, anger, resentment, jealousy, and guilt. Illness may also result in children's loss of status within their family or social group. Various factors have been identified that influence the effects of the child's hospitalization on siblings. Although these factors are similar to those seen when a child has a chronic illness, Craft (1993) reported that the following factors regarding siblings are related specifically to the hospital experience and increase the effects on the sibling:

- Being younger and experiencing many changes
- Being cared for outside the home by care providers who are not relatives
- Receiving little information about their ill brother or sister
- Perceiving that their parents treat them differently compared with before their sibling's hospitalization

Parents are often unaware of the number of effects that siblings experience during the sick child's hospitalization and the benefit of simple interventions to minimize these effects such as explicit explanations about the illness and provisions for the siblings to remain at home. Sibling visitation is usually beneficial to the patient, sibling, and parent but should be evaluated on an individual basis. Siblings should be prepared for the visit with developmentally appropriate information and be given the opportunity to ask questions.

NURSING CARE OF THE CHILD WHO IS HOSPITALIZED

Preparation for Hospitalization

Children and families require individualized care to minimize the potential negative effects of hospitalization. One method that can decrease negative feelings and fear in children is preparation for hospitalization. The rationale for preparing children for the hospital experience and related procedures is based on the principle that a fear of the unknown (fantasy) exceeds fear of the known. When children do not have paralyzing fear with which to cope, they are able to direct their energies toward dealing with the other unavoidable stresses of hospitalization.

Although preparation for hospitalization is a common practice, there is no universal standard or program for all settings. The preparation process may be elaborate with tours, puppet shows, and play-time with miniature hospital equipment; it may involve the use of books, videos, or films; or it may be limited to a brief description of the major aspects of any hospital stay. No consensus exists on the timing of preparation. Some authorities recommend preparing children 4 to 7 years of age about 1 week in advance so they can assimilate the information and ask questions. For older children the time may be longer. However, for young children who may begin to fantasize about what they observed, 1 or 2 days before admission is sufficient time for anticipatory preparation. The length of the session should be tailored to the child's attention span (i.e., the younger the child, the shorter the program). The optimal approach is one that is individualized for each child and family.

Regardless of the specific type of program, all children, even those who have been hospitalized before, benefit from an introduction to the environment and routine of the unit. Sometimes it is not possible to prepare children and families for hospitalization such as in the event of sudden, acute illness. However, care should be taken to orient them to hospital routines, establish expectations, and allow for questions.

> **! NURSING ALERT**
>
> In many hospitals child life specialists (i.e., health care professionals with extensive knowledge of child growth and development and the special psychosocial needs of children who are hospitalized and their families) help prepare children for hospitalization, surgery, and procedures. Although the structure of a program may vary, depending on the size of the pediatric facility, the patient population, and the availability of ancillary services, the two primary program objectives for child life are consistent: (1) to reduce the stress and anxiety related to the hospitalization or health care–related experiences, and (2) to promote normal growth and development in the health care setting and at home (Thompson, 2009).

A collaborative effort among the nurse, child life specialist, and other members of the child's health care team helps ensure the best possible hospital experience for the child and family.

Admission Assessment

The nursing admission history refers to a systematic collection of data about the child and family that allows the nurse to plan individualized care. The nursing admission history presented in Box 38-5 is organized according to the Functional Health Patterns outlined by Gordon (2002) (see Nursing Diagnosis, Chapter 26). This assessment framework is a guideline for formulating nursing diagnoses. One of the main purposes of the history is to assess the child's usual health habits at home to promote a more normal environment in the hospital. Therefore questions related to activities of daily living in the nutritional-metabolic, elimination, sleep-rest, and activity-exercise patterns are a major part of the assessment. The questions found under the health perception–health management pattern are directed toward evaluation of the child's preparation for hospitalization and are key factors in determining whether additional preparation is needed. The questions included in the self-perception–self-concept and role-relationship patterns offer insight into the child's potential reaction to hospitalization, especially in terms of separation.

The nurse should also inquire about the use of any medications at home, including complementary medicine practices (Box 38-6). In a study of children with cancer, 42% had used alternative or complementary therapies simultaneously with or after conventional treatments (Fernandez, Pyesmany, and Stutzer, 1999). It is important that the use of any herbal or complementary therapy be noted in a preoperative assessment because of possible anesthesia or surgical complications related to herbal products (Flanagan, 2001) (see Critical Thinking Case Study).

In addition to completing the nursing admission history, nurses should also perform a physical assessment (see Chapter 29) before planning care. At the very least the nurse's physical assessment of the child should include observation of the body for any bruises, rashes, signs of neglect, deformities, or physical limitations. The nurse should also listen to the heart and lungs to assess overall physical status. For example, it is impossible to evaluate improvement in respiratory function in a child admitted with pulmonary disease unless there are baseline data with which to compare subsequent findings.

Preparing the Child for Admission

The preparation that children require on the day of admission depends on the kind of prehospital counseling that they have received. If they have been prepared in a formalized program, they usually know what to expect in terms of initial medical procedures,

BOX 38-5 NURSING ADMISSION HISTORY ACCORDING TO FUNCTIONAL HEALTH PATTERNS*

Health Perception–Health Management Pattern
- Why has your child been admitted?
- How has your child's general health been?
- What does your child know about this hospitalization?
  - Ask the child why he or she came to the hospital.
  - If the answer is: "For an operation or for tests," ask the child to tell you about what will happen before, during, and after the operation or tests.
- Has your child ever been in the hospital before?
- How was that hospital experience?
- What things were important to you and your child during that hospitalization? How can we be most helpful now?
- What medications does your child take at home?
  - Why are they given?
  - When are they given?
  - How are they given (if a liquid, with a spoon; if a tablet, swallowed with water; or other)?
  - Does your child have any trouble taking medication? If so, what helps?
  - Is your child allergic to any medications?
- Which, if any, forms of complementary medicine practices are being used?

Nutrition–Metabolic Pattern
- What is the family's usual mealtime?
- Do family members eat together or at separate times?
- What are your child's favorite foods, beverages, and snacks?
  - Average amounts consumed or usual size of portions
  - Special cultural practices such as family eats only ethnic food
- Which foods and beverages does your child dislike?
- What are your child's feeding habits (bottle, cup, spoon, eats by self, needs assistance, any special devices)?
- How does your child like the food served (warmed, cold, one item at a time)?
- How would you describe your child's usual appetite (hearty eater, picky eater)?
- Has being sick affected your child's appetite? In what ways?
- Are there any known or suspected food allergies?
- Is your child on a special diet?
- Are there any feeding problems (excessive fussiness, spitting up, colic); any dental or gum problems that affect feeding?
  - What do you do for these problems?

Elimination Pattern
- What are your child's toileting habits (diaper, toilet trained—day only or day and night, use of word to communicate urination or defecation, potty chair, regular toilet, other routines)?
- What is your child's usual pattern of elimination (bowel movements)?
- Do you have any concerns about elimination (bed-wetting, constipation, diarrhea)?
  - What do you do for these problems?
- Have you ever noticed that your child sweats a lot?

Sleep-Rest Pattern
- What is your child's usual hour of sleep and awakening?
- What is your child's schedule for naps; length of naps?
- Is there a special routine before sleeping (bottle, drink of water, bedtime story, night-light, favorite blanket or toy, prayers)?
- Is there a special routine during sleep time such as waking to go to the bathroom?
- In which type of bed does your child sleep?

- Does your child have a separate room or share a room; if shares, with whom?
- Does your child sleep with someone or alone (e.g., sibling, parent, other person)?
- What is your child's favorite sleeping position?
- Are there any sleeping problems (falling asleep, waking during night, nightmares, sleep walking)?
- Are there any problems in awakening and getting ready in the morning?
  - What do you do for these problems?

Activity-Exercise Pattern
- What is your child's schedule during the day (preschool, day care center, regular school, extracurricular activities)?
- What are your child's favorite activities or toys (both active and quiet interests)?
- What is your child's usual television-viewing schedule at home?
- What are your child's favorite programs?
- Are there any television restrictions?
- Does your child have any illness or disabilities that limit activity? If so, how?
- What are your child's usual habits and schedule for bathing (bath in tub or shower, sponge bath, shampoo)?
- What are your child's dental habits (brushing, flossing, fluoride supplements or rinses, favorite toothpaste); schedule of daily dental care?
- Does your child need help with dressing or grooming such as hair combing?
- Are there any problems with these patterns (dislike of or refusal to bathe, shampoo hair, or brush teeth)?
  - What do you do for these problems?
- Are there special devices that your child requires help in managing (eyeglasses, contact lenses, hearing aid, orthodontic appliances, artificial elimination appliances, orthopedic devices)?
- NOTE: Use the following code to assess functional self-care level for feeding, bathing and hygiene, dressing and grooming, toileting:
  0—Full self-care
  I—Requires use of equipment or device
  II—Requires assistance or supervision from another person
  III—Requires assistance or supervision from another person and equipment or device
  IV—Is totally dependent and does not participate

Cognitive-Perceptual Pattern
- Does your child have any hearing difficulty?
  - Does your child use a hearing aid?
  - Have "tubes" been placed in your child's ears?
- Does your child have any vision problems?
  - Does your child wear glasses or contact lenses?
- Does your child have any learning difficulties?
- What is the child's grade in school?
- For information on pain see Chapter 30.

Self-Perception–Self-Concept Pattern
- How would you describe your child (e.g., takes time to adjust, settles in easily, shy, friendly, quiet, talkative, serious, playful, stubborn, easygoing)?
- What makes your child angry, annoyed, anxious, or sad? What helps?
- How does your child act when annoyed or upset?
- What have your child's experiences been with temporary separation from you (parent) and his or her reactions to it?

BOX 38-5   NURSING ADMISSION HISTORY ACCORDING TO FUNCTIONAL HEALTH PATTERNS*—cont'd

- Does your child have any fears (places, objects, animals, people, situations)?
  - How do you handle them?
- Do you think your child's illness has changed the way he or she thinks about himself or herself (e.g., more shy, embarrassed about appearance, less competitive with friends, stays at home more)?

Role-Relationship Pattern

- Does your child have a favorite nickname?
- What are the names of other family members or others who live in the home (relatives, friends, pets)?
- Who usually takes care of your child during the day and night (especially if other than parent such as babysitter, relative)?
- What are the parents' occupations and work schedules?
- Are there any special family considerations (adoption, foster child, step-parent, divorce, single parent)?
- Have any major changes in the family occurred lately (death, divorce, separation, birth of a sibling, loss of a job, financial strain, mother beginning a career, other)? Describe child's reaction.
- Who are your child's play companions or social groups (peers, younger or older children, adults, or prefers to be alone)?
- Do things generally go well for your child in school or with friends?
- Does your child have "security" objects at home (pacifier, bottle, blanket, stuffed animal or doll)? Did you bring any of these to the hospital?
- How do you handle discipline problems at home? Are these methods always effective?
- Does your child have any condition that interferes with communication? If so, what are your suggestions for communicating with your child?
- Will your child's hospitalization affect the family's financial support or care of other family members (e.g., other children)?
- What concerns do you have about your child's illness and hospitalization?
- Who will be staying with your child while hospitalized?
- How can we contact you or another close family member outside of the hospital?

Sexuality-Reproductive Pattern
(Answer questions that apply to your child's age-group.)
  - Has your child begun puberty (developing physical sexual characteristics, menstruation)? Have you or your child had any concerns?
  - Does your daughter know how to do breast self-examination?
  - Does your son know how to do testicular self-examination?

- How have you approached topics of sexuality with your child?
- Do you think you might need some help with some topics?
- Has your child's illness affected the way he or she feels about being a boy or a girl? If so, how?
- Do you have any concerns with behaviors in your child such as masturbation, asking many questions or talking about sex, not respecting others' privacy, or wanting too much privacy?
- Initiate a conversation about an adolescent's sexual concerns with open-ended to more direct questions, using the terms "friends" or "partners" rather than "girlfriend" or "boyfriend":
  - Tell me about your social life.
  - Who are your closest friends? (If one friend is identified, could ask more about that relationship such as how much time they spend together, how serious they are about each other, if the relationship is going the way the teenager hoped.)
  - Might ask about dating and sexual issues such as the teenager's views on sexuality education, "going steady," "living together," or premarital sex.
  - Which friends would you like to have visit in the hospital?

Coping–Stress Tolerance Pattern
(Answer questions that apply to your child's age-group.)
  - What does your child do when tired or upset?
    - If upset, does your child want a special person or object?
    - If so, explain.
  - If your child has temper tantrums, what causes them, and how do you handle them?
  - To whom does your child talk when worried about something?
  - How does your child usually handle problems or disappointments?
  - Have there been any big changes or problems in your family recently? If so, how have you handled them?
  - Has your child ever had a problem with drugs or alcohol or tried to commit suicide?
  - Do you think your child is "accident prone?" If so, explain.

Value-Belief Pattern
- What is your religion?
- How is religion or faith important in your child's life?
- Which religious practices would you like continued in the hospital (e.g., prayers before meals or bedtime; visit by minister, priest, or rabbi; prayer group)?

*The focus of the admission history is the child's psychosocial environment. Most of the questions are worded in terms of parental responses. Depending on the child's age, they should be addressed directly to the child when appropriate.

inpatient facilities, and nursing staff. However, prehospital counseling does not preclude the need for support during procedures such as obtaining blood specimens, x-ray film tests, or physical examination. For example, undressing young children before they feel comfortable in their new surroundings can be upsetting. Causing needless anxiety and fear during admission may adversely affect the nurse's establishment of trust with these children. Therefore nursing assistance during the admission procedure is vital regardless of how well prepared any child is for the experience of hospitalization. In addition, spending this time with the child gives the nurse an opportunity to evaluate his or her understanding of subsequent procedures (Fig. 38-4). Ideally a primary nurse is assigned whenever possible to allow for individualized care and provide a substitute support person for the child.

When a child is admitted, nurses follow several fairly universal admission procedures (Box 38-7). The minimum considerations for room assignment are age, sex, and nature of the illness. No absolute rules govern room selection, but in general placing children of the same age-group and with similar types of illness in the same room is both psychologically and medically advantageous. However, there are many exceptions. For example, a child in traction may be therapeutic for another child confined to bed because of a serious illness. A child who is independent despite physical disabilities may help another child with similar or different limitations, and the parents of the child with disabilities may achieve deeper insight and acceptance of their child's disorder.

Age-grouping is especially important for adolescents. Many hospitals make an effort to place teenagers on their own unit or in a

---

BOX 38-6   COMPLEMENTARY MEDICINE PRACTICES AND EXAMPLES

Nutrition, diet, and lifestyle or behavioral health changes—Macrobiotics, megavitamins, diets, lifestyle modification, health risk reduction and health education, wellness

Mind-body control therapies—Biofeedback, relaxation, prayer therapy, guided imagery, hypnotherapy, music or sound therapy, massage, aromatherapy, education therapy

Traditional and ethnomedicine therapies—Acupuncture, ayurvedic medicine, herbal medicine, homeopathic medicine, Native American medicine, natural products, traditional Asian medicine

Structural manipulation and energetic therapies—Acupressure, chiropractic medicine, massage, reflexology, rolfing, therapeutic touch, Qi Gong

Pharmacologic and biologic therapies—Antioxidants, cell treatment, chelation therapy, metabolic therapy, oxidizing agents

Bioelectromagnetic therapies—Diagnostic and therapeutic application of electromagnetic fields (e.g., transcranial electrostimulation, neuromagnetic stimulation, electroacupuncture)

? CRITICAL THINKING CASE STUDY

Complementary and Alternative Medicine

Maria, a 13-year-old Hispanic girl, has had severe nosebleeds. She is admitted to the hospital for a complete workup in an attempt to determine the cause. Her parents and grandparents have gathered around her bed. When you enter her room to begin admitting procedures, you notice an unusual scent. Maria's mother is rubbing the contents from an unfamiliar bottle of liquid on Maria. Meanwhile the grandmother is rubbing Maria's head. She is startled at your entry and drops something on the floor near your feet. You bend over to pick it up and discover that it is a penny.

1. Evidence—Is there sufficient evidence to draw any conclusions?
2. Assumptions—What are some underlying assumptions that may be drawn from the data about the following:
   a. Complementary or alternative medical remedies
   b. The role of ethnic or folk remedies in modern health care practice
   c. The nurse's role in cases in which alternative medicine is practiced (versus traditional medicine)
3. What implications and priorities for nursing care can be drawn at this time?
4. Does the evidence objectively support your argument (conclusion)?

---

separate designated section of the pediatric or general unit whenever possible.

Nursing Interventions

Preventing or Minimizing Separation

A primary nursing goal is to prevent separation, particularly in children younger than 5 years of age. Many hospitals have developed a system of family-centered care. This philosophy of care recognizes the integral role of the family in a child's life and acknowledges the family as an essential part of the child's care and illness experience. The family is considered to be partners in the care of the child (Smith and Conant Rees, 2000) (see Chapter 26). Family-centered care also supports the family by establishing priorities based on the needs and values of the family unit (Lewandowski and Tesler, 2003).

BOX 38-7   GUIDELINES FOR ADMISSION

Preadmission

- Assign a room based on developmental age, seriousness of diagnosis, communicability of illness, and projected length of stay.
- Prepare roommate(s) for the arrival of a new patient; when children are too young to benefit from this consideration, prepare parents.
- Prepare room for child and family with admission forms and equipment nearby to eliminate need to leave child.

Admission

- Introduce primary nurse to child and family.
- Orient child and family to inpatient facilities, especially to assigned room and unit; emphasize positive areas of pediatric unit.
  - *Room*—Explain call light, bed controls, television, bathroom, telephone, and so on.
  - *Unit*—Direct to playroom, desk, dining area, or other areas.
- Introduce family to roommate and his or her parents.
- Apply identification band to child's wrist, ankle, or both (if not already done).
- Explain hospital regulations and schedules (e.g., visiting hours, mealtimes, bedtime, limitations [give written information if available]).
- Perform nursing admission history (see Box 38-5).
- Take vital signs, blood pressure, height, and weight.
- Obtain specimens as needed and order needed laboratory work.
- Support child and assist practitioner with physical examination (for purposes of nursing assessment).

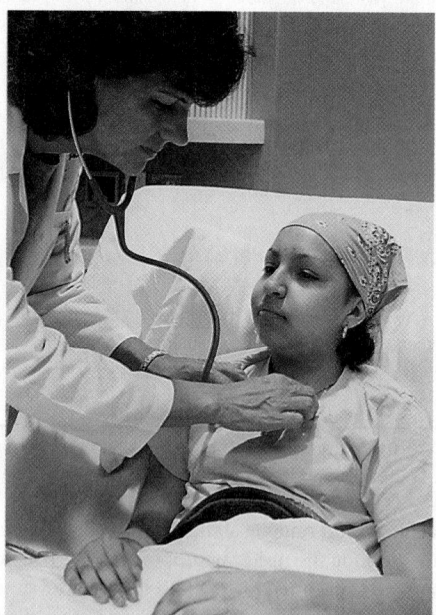

FIG 38-4 The initial admission procedures give the nurse an opportunity to get to know the child and assess his or her understanding of the hospital experience.

At the very least most hospitals welcome parents at any time. Many provide facilities such as a chair or bed for at least one person per child, unit kitchen privileges, and other amenities that create a welcoming atmosphere for parents. However, not all hospitals provide such amenities, and parents' own schedules may prevent rooming-in. In such instances strategies to minimize the effects of separation must be implemented.

Nurses must have an appreciation of the child's separation behaviors. As discussed earlier, the phases of protest and despair are normal. The child is allowed to cry. Even if the child rejects strangers, the nurse provides support through physical presence. Presence is defined as spending time being physically close to the child while using a quiet tone of voice, appropriate choice of words, eye contact, and touch in ways that establish rapport and communicate empathy. If detachment behaviors are evident, the nurse maintains the child's contact with the parents by talking about them frequently; encouraging the child to remember them; and stressing the significance of their visits, telephone calls, or letters. The use of cellular phones can increase the contact between the hospitalized child and parents or other significant family members and friends. However, wireless technology devices may not be compatible with medical equipment, and use may be restricted in certain areas within the hospital.

Parental Absence During Infant Hospitalization

Familiar surroundings also increase the child's adjustment to separation. If the parents cannot stay with the child, they should leave favorite articles from home such as a blanket, toy, bottle, feeding utensil, or article of clothing with him or her. Because young children associate such inanimate objects with significant people, they gain comfort and reassurance from these possessions. They make the association that, if the parents left this, they will surely return. Placing an identification band on the toy lessens the chances of it being misplaced and provides a symbol that the toy is experiencing the same needs as the child. Other reminders of home include photographs and recordings of family members reading a story, singing a song, saying prayers before bedtime, relating events at home, or taking a "talking walk" through the home. These reminders can be played at lonely times such as on awakening or before sleeping. Some units allow pets to visit, which can have therapeutic benefits for a child. Older children also appreciate familiar articles from home, particularly photographs, a radio, a favorite toy or game, and their own pajamas. Often the importance of treasured objects to school-age children is overlooked or criticized. However, many school-age children have a special object to which they formed an attachment in early childhood. Therefore such treasured or transitional objects can help even older children feel more comfortable in a strange environment.

The strange sights, smells, and sounds in the hospital that are commonplace for the nurse can be frightening and confusing for children. It is important for the nurse to try to evaluate stimuli in the environment from the child's point of view (considering also what the child may see or hear happening to other patients) and make every effort to protect the child from frightening and unfamiliar sights, sounds, and equipment. The nurse should offer explanations or prepare the child for experiences that are unavoidable. Combining familiar or comforting sights with the unfamiliar can relieve much of the harshness of medical equipment.

Helping children maintain their usual contacts also minimizes the effects of separation imposed by hospitalization. This includes continuing school lessons during the illness and confinement, visiting with friends either directly or through letter writing or telephone calls, age-appropriate social media, and participating in stimulating projects whenever possible (Fig. 38-5). For extended hospitalizations youngsters enjoy personalizing the hospital room to make it "home" by decorating the walls with posters and cards, rearranging the furniture, and displaying a collection or hobby.

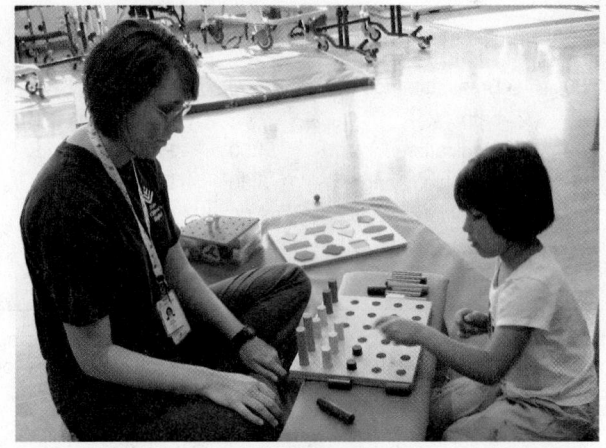

FIG 38-5 For extended hospitalizations, children enjoy doing projects to occupy time.

Minimizing Loss of Control

Feelings of loss of control result from separation, physical restriction, changed routines, enforced dependency, and magical thinking. Although some of these cannot be prevented, most can be minimized through individualized planning of nursing care.

Promoting Freedom of Movement. Younger children react most strenuously to any type of physical restriction or immobilization. Although temporary immobilization may be necessary for some interventions such as maintaining an intravenous line, most physical restriction can be prevented if the nurse gains the child's cooperation.

For young children, particularly infants and toddlers, preserving parent-child contact is the best means of decreasing the need for or stress of restraint. For example, almost the entire physical examination can be done in a parent's lap with the parent hugging the child for procedures such as an otoscopic examination. For painful procedures the nurse should assess the parents' preferences for helping, observing, or waiting outside the room.

Environmental factors may also restrict movement. Keeping children in cribs or play yards may not represent immobilization in a concrete sense, but it certainly limits sensory stimulation. Increasing mobility by transporting children in carriages, wheelchairs, carts, or wagons provides them with a sense of freedom.

In some cases physical restraint or isolation is necessary because of the child's medical diagnosis. In these cases the environment can be altered to increase sensory freedom (e.g., moving the bed toward the window; opening window shades; providing musical, visual, or tactile activities).

Maintaining the Child's Routine. Altered daily schedules and loss of rituals are particularly stressful for toddlers and early preschoolers and may increase the stress of separation. The nursing admission history provides a baseline for planning care around the child's usual home activities. A frequently neglected aspect of altered routines is the change in the child's daily activities. A typical child's day, especially during the school years, is structured with specific times for eating, dressing, going to school, playing, and sleeping. However, this time structure vanishes when the child is hospitalized. Although nurses have a set schedule, the child is frequently unaware of it, and the new schedules that are imposed may be rigid. For example, some units have uniform nap times and bedtimes for all children, but others allow children to stay up late at night. Many children obtain significantly less sleep in the hospital than at home;

Eric's Daily Schedule	
7:30 AM – Breakfast, morning bath	3:00 PM – Tutor (M, W, F) – Study time (T, Th)
9:00 – Medications, dressing change	4:00 – Physical therapy 5:30 – Dinner
11:00 – Physical therapy	9:00 – Medications, dressing change
12:00 PM – Lunch	9:15 – Bedtime

FIG 38-6 Time structuring is an effective strategy for normalizing the hospital environment and increasing the child's sense of control.

the primary causes are a delay in sleep onset and early termination of sleep because of hospital routines. Not only are hours of sleep disrupted, but waking hours are spent in passive activities. For example, few institutions impose any limits on the amount of time the child spends watching television. This may lead to children's being less "tired" at bedtime and delay the onset of sleep.

One technique that can minimize the disruption in the child's routine is establishing a daily schedule. This approach is most suitable for noncritically ill school-age and adolescent children who have mastered the concept of time. It involves scheduling the child's day to include all the activities that are important to the child and nurse such as treatment procedures, schoolwork, exercise, television, playroom, and hobbies. Together the nurse, parent, and child then plan a daily schedule with times and activities written down (Fig. 38-6). This is left in the child's room, and a clock or watch is available for his or her use. Whenever possible a calendar is also constructed with special events such as favorite television programs, visits by friends or relatives, events in the playroom, and holidays or birthdays marked. If specific changes in treatment are expected (e.g., "beginning physical therapy in 2 days"), these are added.

> **⚠ NURSING ALERT**
>
> Ask the young child to select or draw pictures or symbols to represent daily or weekly fun activities (e.g., favorite television programs, family visits, and playroom times). Draw a clock face with the hands of the clock depicting the time that each event will occur next to the child's representation. Have the child compare the clock on the schedule with a clock or watch in the room. When the two match, the child knows that it is time for a favorite activity.

Encouraging Independence. The dependent role of the hospitalized patient imposes tremendous feelings of loss on older children. Principal interventions should focus on respect for individuality and the opportunity for decision making. Although these sound simple, their efficacy lies with nurses who are flexible and tolerant. It is also important for the nurse to empower the patient while not feeling threatened by a sense of lessened control.

Enabling children's control involves helping them maintain independence and promoting the concept of self-care. Self-care refers to the practice of activities that individuals personally initiate and perform on their own behalf in maintaining life, health, and well-being (Orem, 2001). Although self-care is limited by the child's age and physical condition, most children beyond infancy can perform some activities with little or no help. Whenever possible, these activities are encouraged in the hospital. Other approaches include jointly

BOX 38-8	**BILL OF RIGHTS FOR CHILDREN AND TEENS**

In this hospital you and your family have the right to:
- Respect and personal dignity.
- Care that supports you and your family.
- Information you can understand.
- Quality health care.
- Emotional support.
- Care that respects your need to grow, play, and learn.
- Make choices and decisions.

From Association for the Care of Children's Health: *A pediatric bill of rights*, Bethesda, MD, 1991, Author.

planning care, time structuring, wearing street clothes, making choices in food selections and bedtime, continuing school activities, and rooming with an appropriate age mate.

Promoting Understanding. Loss of control can occur from feelings of having too little influence on one's destiny or sensing overwhelming control or power over fate. Although preschoolers' cognitive abilities predispose them most to magical thinking and delusions of power, all children are vulnerable to misinterpreting causes for stresses such as illness and hospitalization.

Most children feel more in control when they know what to expect because the element of fear is reduced. Anticipatory preparation and provision of information help to lessen stress and increase understanding (see Preparation for Diagnostic and Therapeutic Procedures, Chapter 39).

Informing children of their rights while hospitalized fosters greater understanding and may relieve some of the feelings of powerlessness that they typically experience. An increasing number of hospitals and organizations have developed a patient "bill of rights" that is prominently displayed throughout the hospital or presented to children and their families on admission (Box 38-8).

Preventing or Minimizing Fear of Bodily Injury

Beyond early infancy all children fear bodily injury from mutilation, bodily intrusion, body image change, disability, or death. In general preparation of children for painful procedures decreases their fears and increases cooperation. Modifying procedural techniques for children in each age-group also minimizes fear of bodily injury. For example, because toddlers and young preschoolers are traumatized by insertion of a rectal thermometer, axillary temperatures or temperatures taken with electronic or tympanic membrane devices can be substituted effectively. Whenever procedures are performed on young children, the most supportive intervention is to do the procedure as quickly as possible while maintaining parent-child contact.

Because of toddlers' and preschool children's poorly defined body boundaries, the use of bandages may be particularly helpful. For example, telling children that the bleeding will stop after the needle is removed does little to relieve their fears, but applying a small Band-Aid usually reassures them. The size of bandages is also significant to children in this age-group; the larger the bandage, the more importance is attached to the wound. Watching their surgical dressings become successively smaller is one way that young children can measure healing and improvement. Prematurely removing a dressing may cause these children considerable concern for their well-being. Specific pain management strategies are discussed in Chapter 30.

For children who fear mutilation of body parts, it is essential that the nurse repeatedly stress the reason for a procedure and evaluate the child's understanding. For example, explaining cast removal to preschoolers may seem simple enough, but children's comprehension of the details may vary considerably from the explanation. Asking the child to draw a picture of what they foresee happening presents substantial evidence of how they perceive events.

Children may fear bodily injury from a great variety of sources. Imaging machines, strange equipment used for examination, unfamiliar rooms, and awkward positions can be perceived as potentially hazardous. In addition, thoughts and actions can be imagined sources of bodily damage. Therefore it is important to investigate imagined reasons, particularly of a sexual nature, for illness. Because children may fear revealing such thoughts, using techniques such as drawing or doll play may elicit previously undisclosed misconceptions.

Older children fear bodily injury of both internal and external origins. For example, school-age children are aware of the significance of the heart and may fear the actual operation as much as the pain, the stitches, and the possible scar. Adolescents may express concern about the actual procedure but be much more anxious over the resulting scar.

Children can grasp information only if it is presented on or close to their level of cognitive development. This necessitates an awareness of the words used to describe events or processes. For example, young children told that they are going to have a CAT (i.e., computed tomography [CT]) scan may wonder, "Will there be cats? Or something that scratches?" It is clearer to describe the procedure in simple terms and explain what the letters of the common name stand for. Therefore to prevent or alleviate fears nurses must be keenly aware of the medical terminology and vocabulary that they use every day.

When children are upset about their illness, their perception can be changed by (1) providing a somewhat different and less negative account of the disease, or (2) offering an explanation that is characteristic of the next stage of cognitive development. An example of the first strategy is reassuring a preschooler who fears that after a tonsillectomy another sore throat means a second operation. Explaining that after tonsils are "fixed" they do not need fixing again can help relieve the fear. An example of the latter strategy is to explain that germs made the tonsils sick but, even though germs can cause another sore throat, they cannot cause the tonsils to ever be sick again. This higher-level explanation is based on the school-age child's concept of germs as a cause of disease.

Providing Developmentally Appropriate Activities

A primary goal of nursing care for the child who is hospitalized is to minimize threats to the child's development. Many strategies (e.g., minimizing separation) have been discussed and may be all that the short-term patient requires. However, children who experience prolonged or repeated hospitalization are at greater risk for developmental delays or regression. The nurse who provides opportunities for the child to participate in developmentally appropriate activities further normalizes his or her environment and helps reduce interference with the child's ongoing development.

Interference with normal development may have long-term implications for developing infants and toddlers. The nurse plays a primary role in identifying children at risk and helping to plan, implement, and evaluate developmental intervention.

School is an integral part of the school-age child's and adolescent's development. Accreditation standards for hospitals serving children consider access to appropriate educational services to be a key factor in the accreditation decision process when a child's treatment requires a significant absence from school (The Joint Commission, 2011). The nurse can encourage children to resume schoolwork as quickly as their condition permits, help them schedule and protect a selected time for studies, and help the family coordinate hospital educational services with their children's schools. Children should have the opportunity to continue art and music classes and their academic subjects.

To meet the unique developmental needs of adolescents, special units may be developed that provide privacy, increased socialization, and appropriate activities for these young people. Typically these units can be set apart from the general pediatric facility so the teenagers do not share space with younger children, who are often perceived as a threat to their maturity.

In caring for adolescent patients it is essential to provide flexible routines and activities such as more group activity, wearing of street clothes, and access to the items so critical to adolescents (i.e., wireless technology devices, MP3 players, DVD players, computers, e-mail, electronic video game systems, and high-definition televisions). Because adolescents' food habits are rarely limited to the three traditional meals a day, a ready supply of snacks should be available. However, the most important benefit of these units is increased socialization with peers. In addition, staff members usually enjoy working with this age-group and are able to establish the trust that is so essential for communication.

> **! NURSING ALERT**
>
> When adolescents must share a common activity room with younger patients, referring to the area as the "activity" room rather than the "playroom" may entice them to visit the room and participate in activities.

Although regression is expected and normal for all age-groups, nurses are responsible for fostering the child's growth and development. Hospitalization can become a significant opportunity for learning and advancing. Extended hospitalizations for long-term chronic illness or situations of failure to thrive, abuse, or neglect represent instances in which regression must be seen as an adjustment period to be followed by plans for promoting appropriate developmental skills.

Providing Opportunities for Play and Expressive Activities

Play is one of the most important aspects of a child's life and one of the most effective tools for managing stress. Because illness and hospitalization constitute crises in a child's life and often involve overwhelming stresses, children need to act out their fears and anxieties as a means of coping with these stresses. Play is essential to children's mental, emotional, and social well-being; it doesn't stop when children are ill or in the hospital. On the contrary, play in the hospital serves many functions (Box 38-9). Of all hospital facilities, no room probably alleviates the stressors of hospitalization more than the playroom (or activity room). In the playroom children temporarily distance themselves from their illness, hospitalization, and the associated stressors. This room should be a safe haven for children, free from medical or nursing procedures (including medication administration), strange faces, and probing questions. The playroom becomes a sanctuary in an otherwise frightening environment.

Engaging in play activities gives children a sense of control. In the hospital environment most decisions are made for the child; play and other expressive activities offer the child much-needed opportunities to make choices for themselves. Even if a child chooses not to participate in a particular activity, the nurse has offered him or

BOX 38-9	FUNCTIONS OF PLAY IN THE HOSPITAL

- Provides diversion and brings about relaxation
- Helps the child feel more secure in a strange environment
- Lessens the stress of separation and the feeling of homesickness
- Provides a means for release of tension and expression of feelings
- Encourages interaction and development of positive attitudes toward others
- Provides an expressive outlet for creative ideas and interests
- Provides a means for accomplishing therapeutic goals (see Use of Play in Procedures, Chapter 39)
- Places child in active role and provides opportunity to make choices and be in control

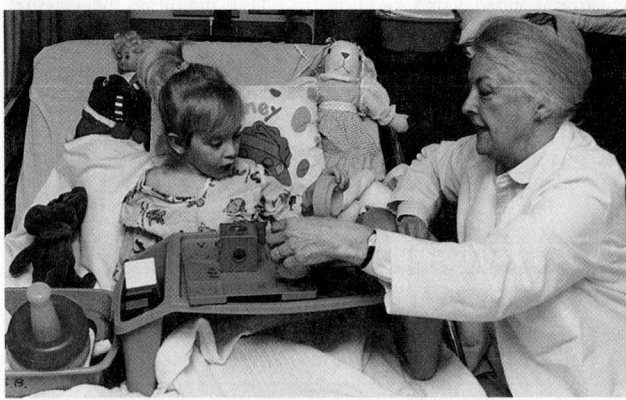

FIG 38-7 Play materials for children in the hospital need to be appropriate for their age, interests, and limitations.

her a choice, perhaps one of only a few real choices the child has had that day.

Hospitalized children typically have lower energy levels than healthy children of the same age. Therefore children may not appear engaged and enthusiastic about an activity even though they are enjoying the experience. Activities may need to be adjusted or limited based on the child's age, endurance, and any special needs.

Diversional Activities. Almost any form of play can be used for diversion and recreation, but the activity should be selected on the basis of the child's age, interests, and limitations (Fig. 38-7). Children do not necessarily need special direction for using play materials. All they require are the raw materials with which to work and adult approval and supervision to help keep their natural enthusiasm or expression of feelings from getting out of control. Small children enjoy a variety of small, colorful toys with which they can play in bed or in their room or more elaborate play equipment such as playhouses, sandboxes, rhythm instruments, or large boxes and blocks that may be a part of the hospital playroom.

Games that can be played alone or with another child or an adult are popular with older children, as are puzzles; reading material; quiet, individual activities such as sewing, stringing beads, and weaving; and Lego blocks and other building materials. Assembling models is an excellent pastime, but one should make certain that all pieces and necessary materials are included in the package so the child is not disappointed and frustrated.

Well-selected books are of infinite value to children. Children never tire of stories; having someone read aloud gives them endless hours of pleasure and is of special value to children who have limited

energy to expend in play. A radio, DVD player, electronic games, and television, included among most hospital room equipment, are useful tools for entertaining children. Computers with access to the Internet can provide diversion, educational opportunities, and online support groups.

When supervising play for ill or convalescent children, it is best to select activities that are simpler than would normally be chosen for the child's specific developmental level. These children usually do not have the energy to cope with more challenging activities. Other limitations also influence the type of activities. Special consideration must be given to children who are confined in terms of movement, have a restricted extremity, or are isolated. Toys for isolated children must be disposable or need to be disinfected after every use.

Toys. Parents of hospitalized children often ask nurses about the types of toys that would be best to bring for their child. Although they want to buy new toys for the hospitalized child to offer cheer and comfort, it is often better to wait to bring new things, especially in the case of younger children. Small children need the comfort and reassurance of familiar things such as the stuffed animal the child hugs for comfort and takes to bed at night. These familiar items are a link with home and the world outside the hospital. All toys brought into the hospital should be assessed for safety.

Large numbers of toys often confuse and frustrate small children. A few small, well-chosen toys are usually preferred to one large, expensive one. Children who are hospitalized for an extended time benefit from changes. Rather than a confusing accumulation of toys, older toys should be replaced periodically as interest wanes.

A highly successful diversion for a child who is hospitalized for a length of time and whose parents are unable to visit frequently is having the parents bring a box with several small, inexpensive, brightly wrapped items with a different day of the week printed on the outside of each package. The child will eagerly anticipate the time for opening each one. If the parents know when their next visit will be, they can provide the number of packages that corresponds to the time between visits. In this way the child knows that the diminishing packages also represent the anticipated visit from the parent.

Expressive Activities. Play and other expressive activities provide one of the best opportunities for encouraging emotional expression, including the safe release of anger and hostility. Nondirective play that allows children freedom for expression can be tremendously therapeutic. However, therapeutic play should not be confused with play therapy, a psychologic technique reserved for use by trained and qualified therapists as an interpretative method with emotionally disturbed children. On the other hand, therapeutic play is an effective, nondirective modality for helping children deal with their concerns and fears; at the same time it often helps the nurse gain insights into children's needs and feelings.

Tension release can be facilitated through almost any activity; with younger ambulatory children, large-muscle activity such as use of tricycles and wagons is especially beneficial. Much aggression can be safely directed into pounding and throwing games or activities. Beanbags are often thrown at a target or open receptacle with surprising vigor and hostility. A pounding board is used with enthusiasm by young children; clay and play dough are beneficial for use at any age.

Creative Expression. Although all children derive physical, social, emotional, and cognitive benefits from engaging in art and other creative activities, children's need for such activities is intensified when they are hospitalized. Drawing and painting are excellent media for expression. Children are more at ease expressing their

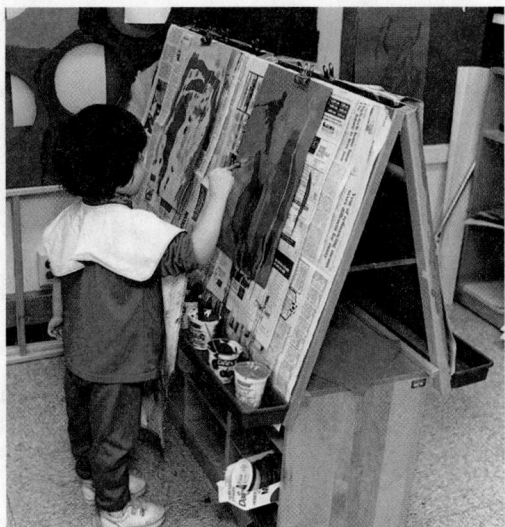

FIG 38-8 Drawing and painting are excellent media for expression.

thoughts and feelings through art because humans think first in images and later learn to translate these images into words. Children need only to be supplied with the raw materials such as crayons and paper, large brushes, an ample supply of newsprint supported on easels, or materials for finger painting (Fig. 38-8). They can work individually or together on a group project such as a mural painted on a long piece of paper.

Although interpretation of children's drawings requires special training, observing changes in a series of the child's drawings over time can be helpful in assessing psychosocial adjustment and coping. The nurse can use children's drawings, stories, poetry, and other products of creative expression as a springboard for discussion of thoughts, fears, and understanding of concepts or events (see Communication Techniques, Chapter 29). For example, a child's drawing before surgery may reveal unvoiced concerns about mutilation, body changes, and loss of self-control.

Nurses can incorporate opportunities for musical expression into routine nursing care. For example, simple musical instruments such as bracelets with bells can be placed on infants' legs for them to shake to accompany mealtime music or dressing changes. Dance and movement suggestions may encourage a child to ambulate.

Dramatic Play. Dramatic play is a well-recognized technique for emotional release, allowing children to reenact frightening or puzzling hospital experiences. Through use of puppets, replicas of hospital equipment, or actual hospital equipment, children can act out the situations that are a part of their hospital experience. Dramatic play enables children to learn about procedures and events that concern them and assume the roles of the adults in the hospital environment.

Puppets are universally effective for communicating with children. Most children see them as peers and readily communicate with them. Children will tell the puppet feelings that they hesitate to express to adults. Puppets can share children's own experiences and help them find solutions to their problems. Puppets dressed to represent figures in the child's environment (e.g., a health care provider, nurse, child patient, therapist, and members of the child's own family) are especially useful. Small, appropriately attired dolls are equally effective in encouraging the child to play out situations, although puppets are usually best for direct conversation.

Play must consider medical needs, but at times a procedure can be postponed briefly to allow the child to complete a special activity (see Critical Thinking Case Study). Play must consider any limitations imposed by the child's condition. For example, small children may eat paste and other creative media; therefore a child who is allergic to wheat should not be given finger paint made from wallpaper paste or modeling dough made with flour. A child on a restricted salt intake should not play with modeling dough because salt is one of its major constituents. At home the play program can be planned around the therapy regimen. However, play can be satisfactorily incorporated into the child's care if the nurse and others involved allow some flexibility and use creativity in planning for it.

Maximizing Potential Benefits of Hospitalization

Although hospitalization generally represents a stressful time for children and families, it also represents an opportunity for facilitating positive change within the child and among family members. For some families the stress of a child's illness, hospitalization, or both can lead to strengthening of family coping behaviors and the emergence of new coping strategies.

Fostering Parent-Child Relationships. The crisis of illness or hospitalization can mobilize parents into more acute awareness of their child's needs. For example, hospitalization provides opportunities for parents to learn more about their children's growth and development. When parents are helped to understand children's usual reactions to stress such as regression or aggression, not only are they better able to support the child through the hospital experience, but they also may extend their insights into childrearing practices after discharge.

Difficulties in parent-child relationships that existed before hospitalization (i.e., characterized by feeding problems, negative behavior, and sleep disturbances) may decrease during hospitalization. The temporary cessation of such problems sometimes alerts parents to the role that they may be playing in propagating the negative behavior. With help from health professionals, parents can restructure ways of relating to their children to foster more positive behavior.

Hospitalization may also represent a temporary reprieve or refuge from a disturbed home. Typically abused or neglected children's dramatic physical and social improvement during hospitalization is proof of the benefits and potential growth that can occur during hospitalization. These children temporarily are able to seek support, reassurance, and security from new relationships, particularly with nurses and hospitalized peers.

Providing Educational Opportunities. Illness and hospitalization represent excellent opportunities for children and other family members to learn more about their bodies, one another, and the health professions. For example, during a hospital admission for a diabetic crisis the child may learn about the disease; the parents may learn about the child's needs for independence, normalcy, and appropriate limits; and each of them may find a new support system in the hospital staff.

Illness or hospitalization can also help older children choose a career. Frequently children have impressions of physicians or nurses that are disproportionately positive or negative. Actual experience with different health professionals can influence their attitude about them and even a decision regarding a career in health care.

Promoting Self-Mastery. The experience of facing a crisis such as illness or hospitalization, coping successfully with it, and maturing as a result of it constitutes an opportunity for self-mastery. Younger children have the chance to test fantasy-versus-reality fears. They realize that they were not abandoned, mutilated, or punished. In fact, they were loved, cared for, and treated with respect for their individual concerns. It is not unusual for children who have undergone hospitalization or surgery to tell others that "it was nothing" or to display proudly their scars or bandages. For older children hospitalization may represent an opportunity for decision making, independence, and self-reliance. They are proud of having survived the experience and may feel a genuine self-respect for their achievements. Nurses can facilitate such feelings of self-mastery by emphasizing aspects of personal competence in the child and not focusing on uncooperative or negative behavior.

Providing Socialization. Hospitalization may offer children a special opportunity for social acceptance. Lonely, asocial, and even delinquent children find a sympathetic environment in the hospital. Children who have a physical disability or are in some other way "different" from their age mates may find an accepting social peer group (Fig. 38-9). Although this does not always occur spontaneously, nurses can structure the environment to foster a supportive child group. For example, selection of a compatible roommate can help children gain a new friend and learn more about themselves. Forming relationships with significant members of the care team such as the health care provider, nurse, child life specialist, or social worker can greatly enhance children's adjustment in many areas of life.

Parents may also encounter a new social group in other parents who have similar problems. The waiting room or hallway "self-help" groups are inherent to every institution. Parents meet while in the hospital or clinic and discuss their children's illnesses and treatments. Nurses can capitalize on this informal gathering by encouraging parents to discuss collectively their concerns and feelings. They can also refer parents to organized parent groups or use the help and support of parents of recovered hospitalized patients. It is important that nurses emphasize to families that each child responds differently to disease, treatments, and care. Any questions raised during group discussions should be clarified with a nurse or health care provider.

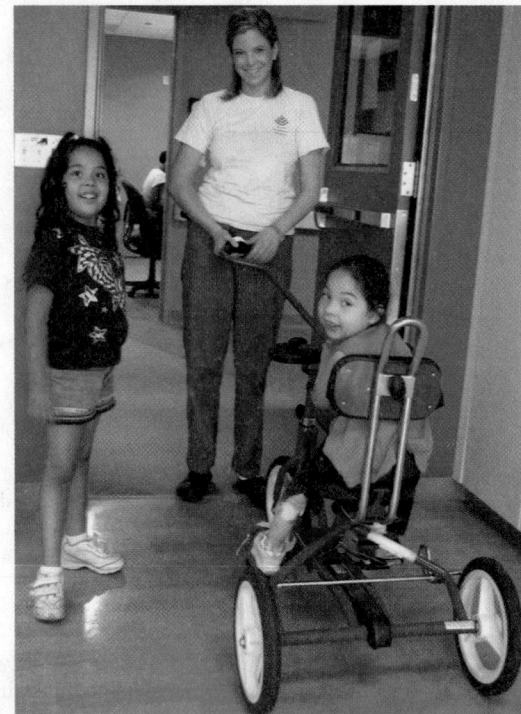

FIG 38-9 Placing children of the same age-group with similar illnesses near one another on the unit is both psychologically and medically supportive. (Courtesy E. Jacob, Texas Children's Hospital, Houston, TX.)

NURSING CARE OF THE FAMILY

Although it is not possible to predict exactly which factors are most likely to have an effect on a family's reactions, important variables are (1) the seriousness of the child's illness, (2) the family's previous experience with hospitalization, and (3) the medical procedures involved in the diagnosis and treatment. Important information is also obtained in the nursing admission history (see Box 38-5).

Supporting Family Members

Support involves the willingness to stay and listen to parents' verbal and nonverbal messages. Sometimes the nurse does not give this support directly. For example, he or she may offer to stay with the child to allow the parents time alone or may discuss with other family members the parents' need for extra relief. Often relatives and friends want to help but do not know how. Suggesting ways such as babysitting, preparing meals, doing laundry, or transporting the siblings to school can prompt others to help reduce the responsibilities that burden parents.

Support may also be provided through the clergy. Parents with deep religious beliefs may appreciate the counsel of a clergy member; but, because of their stress, they may not have sufficient energy to initiate the contact. Nurses can be supportive by arranging for clergy to visit, upholding parents' religious beliefs, and respecting the individual meaning and significance of those beliefs (Feudtner, Haney, and Dimmers, 2003).

Support involves accepting cultural, socioeconomic, and ethnic values. For example, health and illness are defined differently by various ethnic groups. For some a disorder that has few outward manifestations of illness such as diabetes, hypertension, or cardiac problems is not a sickness. Consequently following a prescribed

FAMILY-CENTERED CARE

Supporting Siblings During Hospitalization

- Trade off staying at the hospital with spouse or have a surrogate who knows the siblings well stay in the home.
- Offer information about the child's condition to both young and older siblings; respect the sibling who avoids information as a means of coping with the situation.
- Arrange for children to visit their brother or sister in the hospital if possible.
- Encourage phone visits and mail between brothers and sisters; provide children with phone numbers, writing supplies, and stamps.
- Help each sibling identify an extended family member or friend to be his or her support person and provide extra attention during parental absence.
- Make or buy inexpensive toys or trinkets for siblings, one gift for each day the child will be hospitalized.
  - Wrap each gift separately and place them in a basket, box, or other container at the child's bedside.
  - Instruct siblings to open one gift at bedtime and to remember that he or she is in their parent's thoughts.
- If the child's condition is stable and distance is not prohibitive, plan a special time at home with the siblings or have spouse or another relative or friend bring the children to meet parent(s) at a restaurant or other location near the hospital.
  - Have extended family members or friends schedule a visit to the child in the hospital during parental absence.
  - Arrange a pass for the child to leave the hospital to join the family if his or her condition permits.

Modified from Craft M, Craft J: Perceived changes in siblings of hospitalized children: a comparison of sibling and parent reports, *Child Health Care* 18(1):42-48, 1989; Rollins J: *Brothers and sisters: a discussion guide for families*, Landover, MD, 1992, Epilepsy Foundation of America.

treatment may be seen as unnecessary. Nurses who appreciate the influences of culture are more likely to intervene therapeutically. (See also Cultural Influences, Chapter 27.)

Parents need help in accepting their own feelings toward the ill child. If given the opportunity, they often disclose their feelings of loss of control, anger, and guilt. They often resist admitting to such feelings because they expect others to disapprove of behavior that is less than perfect. Unfortunately health personnel, including nurses, sometimes do exercise little tolerance for deviation from the norm. This only increases the psychologic impact of a child's illness on family members. Helping parents identify the specific reason for such feelings and emphasizing that each is a normal, expected, and healthy response to stress may reduce the parents' emotional burden.

Family-centered care also addresses the needs of siblings. Support may involve preparing siblings for hospital visits, assessing their adjustment, and providing appropriate interventions or referrals when needed. The Family-Centered Care box suggests ways that parents can support siblings during hospitalization.

Providing Information

One of the most important nursing interventions is providing information about (1) the disease, its treatment, prognosis, and home care; (2) the child's emotional and physical reactions to illness and hospitalization; and (3) the probable emotional reactions of family members to the crisis.

For many families the child's illness is the first contact they have with the hospital experience. Often parents are not prepared for the child's behavioral reactions to hospitalization such as separation behaviors, regression, aggression, and hostility. Providing the parents with information about these normal and expected behavioral responses can lessen the parents' anxiety during the hospital admission. The family is equally unfamiliar with hospital rules, which often compounds their confusion and anxiety. Therefore they need clear explanations about what to expect and what is expected of them.

Parents also need to be aware of the effects of illness on the family and strategies that prevent negative changes. Specifically parents should keep the family well informed and communicate with everyone as much as possible. They should treat all the children equally and as normally as before the illness occurred. Discipline, which initially may be lessened for the ill child, should be continued to provide a measure of security and predictability. When ill children know that their parents expect certain standards of conduct from them, they feel certain that they will recover. Conversely, when all limits are removed, they fear that something catastrophic will happen.

Helping parents understand the meaning of posthospitalization behaviors in the sick child is necessary for them to tolerate and support such behaviors. In addition, parents should be forewarned of the common reactions after discharge (see Box 38-2). Parents who do not expect such reactions may misinterpret them as evidence of the child's "being spoiled" and demand perfect behavior at a time when the child is still reacting to the stress of illness and hospitalization. If the behaviors, especially the demand for attention, are dealt with in a supportive manner, most children are able to relinquish them and assume prior levels of functioning.

Nurses should also prepare parents for the reactions of siblings, particularly anger, jealousy, and resentment. Older siblings may deny such reactions because they provoke feelings of guilt. However, everyone needs outlets for emotions, and the repressed feelings may surface as problems in school or with age mates, as psychosomatic illnesses, or in delinquent behavior.

Probably one of the most neglected areas of communication involves giving information to siblings. Frequently age becomes the only factor that leads to an awareness of this problem because older children may begin to ask questions or request explanations. However, even in this situation the information may be seriously inadequate. Children in every age-group deserve some explanation of the sibling's illness or hospitalization. In addition, nurses can minimize a sibling's fear of also getting sick or having caused the illness.

Encouraging Parent Participation

Preventing or minimizing separation is a key nursing goal with the child who is hospitalized, but maintaining parent-child contact is also beneficial for the family. One of the best approaches is encouraging parents to stay with their child and participate in the care whenever possible. Although some health facilities provide special accommodations for parents, the concept of rooming-in can be instituted anywhere. The first requirement is the staff's positive attitude toward parents. A negative attitude toward parent participation can create barriers to collaborative working relationships.

When hospital staff genuinely appreciate the importance of continued parent-child attachment, they foster an environment that encourages parents to stay. When parents are included in the care planning and understand that they are a contributing factor to the child's recovery, they are more inclined to remain with their child and have more emotional reserves to support themselves and the child through the crisis. An empowerment model of helping allows the nurse to focus on parents' strengths and seek ways to promote growth and family functioning so the parents become empowered in caring for their child. Strategies such as bedside reporting that allow parents to be involved in the discussion of the child's current status are moving health care settings closer to family-centered care (Anderson and Mangino, 2006). Liaison nursing roles in tertiary care settings are also focused on improving communication between parents and health care providers (Caffin, Linton, and Pellegrini, 2007).

Because the mother tends to be the usual family caregiver, she usually spends more time in the hospital than the father. However, not all parents feel equally comfortable assuming responsibility for their child's care. Some may be under such great emotional stress that they need a temporary reprieve from total participation in caregiving activities. Others may feel insecure in participating in specialized areas of care such as bathing the child after surgery. On the other hand, some mothers may feel a great need to control their child's care. This seems particularly true of young mothers who have recently established their role as a parent, mothers of children too young to verbalize their needs, and ethnic minority mothers when the hospital setting is predominantly staffed by nonminority personnel. Individual assessment of each parent's preferred involvement is necessary to prevent the effects of separation while supporting parents in their needs as well.

With lifestyles and gender roles changing, fathers may assume all or some of the usual "mothering" roles in the household. In these cases it may be the father-child relationship that needs to be preserved. Fathers need to be included in the care plan and respected for their parental role. For some fathers the child's hospitalization may represent an opportunity to alter their usual caregiving role and increase their involvement. In single-parent families the caregiver may not be a parent but an extended family member such as a grandparent or aunt.

One of the potential problems with continuous parent involvement is neglect of the parent's need for sleep, nutrition, and relaxation. Often the sleeping accommodations are limited to a chair, and sleep is disrupted by nursing procedures. Encouraging the parents to leave for brief periods, arranging for sleeping quarters on the unit but outside the child's room, and planning a schedule of alternating visits with another family member can minimize the stresses for the parent.

All too often nurses respond to parent participation by abandoning their patient responsibilities. They need to restructure their roles to complement and augment the caregiving functions of parents (Hopia, Tomlinson, Paavilainen, et al., 2005). Even in units structured to provide care by parents, parents frequently feel anxiety in their caregiving responsibilities; those more involved in direct care may feel more anxiety than those less involved. Therefore 24-hour responsibility may be too much for some parents. Assistance and relief by nursing personnel should always be available to these families, and nurses may need to work diligently to establish the strong bond of trust that some parents need to take advantage of these opportunities.

Preparing for Discharge and Home Care

Most hospitalizations necessitate some type of discharge preparation. Often this involves education of the family for continued care and follow-up in the home. Depending on the diagnosis, this may be relatively simple or highly complex. Preparing the family for home care demands a high degree of competence in planning and implementing discharge instructions.

Nurses are often key individuals in initiating and carrying out the discharge process. They collaborate with others in the planning and implementation phases to ensure appropriate care after hospitalization. Throughout the hospitalization the nurse should be aware of the need for discharge planning and the assessment factors that affect the family's ability to provide home care. A thorough assessment of the family and home environment should be performed to ensure that the family's emotional and physical resources are sufficient to manage the tasks of home care. (For a discussion of family and home assessment strategies, see Chapter 29.) In addition to adequate family resources, an investigation of community services, including respite care, is needed to ensure that appropriate support agencies such as emergency facilities, home health agencies, and equipment vendors are available. Financial resources are also a consideration. To coordinate the immense task of assessment and plan implementation, a care coordinator or manager should be appointed early in the discharge process.

The preparation for hospital discharge and home care begins during the admission assessment. Short- and long-term goals are established to meet the child's physical and psychosocial needs. For children with complex care needs, discharge planning focuses on obtaining appropriate equipment and health care personnel for the home. It is also concerned with treatments that parents or children are expected to continue at home. In planning appropriate teaching, nurses need to assess (1) the actual and perceived complexity of the skill, (2) the parents' or child's ability to learn the skill, and (3) the parents' or child's previous or present experience with such procedures.

The teaching plan incorporates levels of learning such as observing, participating with assistance, and finally acting without help or guidance. The skill is divided into discrete steps, and each step is taught to the family member until it is learned. Return demonstration of the skill is requested before new skills are introduced. A record of teaching and performance provides an efficient checklist for evaluation. All families need to receive detailed *written* instructions about home care with telephone numbers for assistance before they leave the hospital. Communication between the nurse performing discharge planning and home health care is essential for ensuring a smooth transition for the child and family.

After the family is competent in performing the skill, they are given responsibility for the care. When possible the family should have a transition or trial period to assume care with minimal health care supervision. This may be arranged on the unit, during a home pass, or in a facility such as a motel near the hospital. Such transitions provide a safe practice period for the family with assistance readily available when needed and are especially valuable when the family lives far from the hospital.

In many instances parents need only simple instructions and understanding of follow-up care. However, the often overwhelming care assumed by some families coupled with other stressors they may be experiencing necessitates continued professional support after discharge. A follow-up home visit or telephone call gives the nurse an opportunity to individualize care and provide information in perhaps a less stressful learning environment than the hospital. Appropriate referrals and resources may include visiting nurse or home health agencies, private nurse services, the school system, a physical therapist, a mental health counselor, a social worker, and any number of community agencies. Sharing the important issues surrounding the child's and family's needs is essential. Referral summaries should be concise, specific, and factual. When numerous support services are required, periodic collaboration among the professionals involved and the family is an excellent strategy to ensure efficient use and comprehensive delivery of services.

CARE OF THE CHILD AND FAMILY IN SPECIAL HOSPITAL SITUATIONS

In addition to a general pediatric unit, children may be admitted to special facilities such as an ambulatory or outpatient setting, an isolation room, or intensive care.

Ambulatory or Outpatient Setting

The ambulatory or outpatient setting provides needed medical services for the child while eliminating the necessity of overnight admission. The benefits of ambulatory care are (1) minimized stressors of hospitalization, especially separation from the family; (2) reduced chances of infection; and (3) increased cost savings. Admission to the ambulatory or outpatient hospital setting usually is for surgical or diagnostic procedures such as insertion of tympanostomy tubes, hernia repair, adenoidectomy, tonsillectomy, cystoscopy, or bronchoscopy.

In the ambulatory or outpatient setting adequate preparation is particularly challenging. Ideally the child and parents should receive preadmission preparation, including a tour of the facility and a review of the day's events. Parents need information in advance to help prepare the child and themselves for surgery and enable them to care for the child at home after the procedure. They also appreciate suggestions for items to bring to the hospital such as blankets or stuffed animals. When preadmission preparation is not possible, time should be allowed on the day of the procedure for children to become acquainted with their surroundings and for nurses to assess, plan, and implement appropriate teaching.

Explicit discharge instructions are important after outpatient surgery (see Family-Centered Care box). Parents need guidelines on when to call their practitioner regarding a change in the child's condition. A follow-up telephone call system allows for nurses to check on the child's progress within 48 to 72 hours after discharge. It also provides an opportunity for the nurse to review discharge information and answer questions.

> **! NURSING ALERT**
>
> Help the family prepare for the transportation home by offering these suggestions:
> - Have a blanket and pillow in the car. (Always use the car safety restraint system.)
> - Take a basin or plastic bag in case of vomiting.
> - Use a cup with a cap and straw for the child to drink fluids (except in cases of oral facial surgery in which a straw may be contraindicated).
> - Give any prescribed pain medication before leaving facility.
>
> Provide parents verbal and written information regarding potential side effects of pain medication for which they should be vigilant after discharge.

Isolation

Admission to an isolation room increases all of the stressors typically associated with hospitalization. There is further separation from familiar persons; additional loss of control; and added environmental changes such as sensory deprivation and the strange appearance of visitors. Orientation to time and place is affected. These stressors

---

> **👪 FAMILY-CENTERED CARE**
>
> ### *Discharge from Ambulatory Settings*
>
> 1. Before beginning, explain that all instructions will also be presented in writing for the family to reference later.
> 2. Provide an overview of the typical trajectory (expected pattern) of recovery.
> 3. Discuss expected progression of the child's activity level during the postdischarge period (e.g., "Mary will probably sleep for the rest of the day and feel kind of tired most of tomorrow but will be back to her usual activities the next day.").
> 4. Explain which activities the child is allowed and what is not permitted (e.g., bed rest, bathing).
> 5. Discuss dietary restrictions, being very specific and giving examples of "clear fluids" or what is meant by a "full liquid diet."
> 6. Discuss nausea and vomiting, if applicable, explaining how much is "normal" and what to do if more occurs (e.g., "Juan may be sick to his stomach and vomit. This is normal. However, if he vomits more than 3 times, please call us at this number right away.").
> 7. Discuss fever and appropriate comfort measures, explaining how much fever is considered "normal" and specifically what to do if the child goes beyond the range.
> 8. Explain the amount, location, and kind of pain or discomfort the child may experience.
>   - Give any prescribed medication before leaving the facility.
>   - Send a pain scale home with the family.
>   - Explain how much pain and discomfort is "normal" and what to do if the child surpasses that level or if pain-management interventions are unsuccessful.
>   - Discuss pain management, including dosage for pain medications and details on how to administer them.
>   - Describe appropriate nonpharmacologic comfort measures such as holding, rocking, or swaddling.
> 9. Provide information about each medication that the child will be taking at home.
>   - Review the details, including dose and route.
>   - Demonstrate how to administer medications if necessary (e.g., how to take outer packaging off suppositories, how to insert).
>   - Discuss guidelines for requesting other medications.
>   - Request that all prescriptions be filled and given to the family before discharge.
> 10. Make certain that the family has all of the equipment and supplies (e.g., gauze and tape for dressing changes) that they will need at home.
> 11. Discuss complications that may occur and the steps to take if they do.
> 12. Ensure that appropriate measures are in place for safe transport home.
>   - Remind family to use a seat belt or car seat for the child.
>   - Determine if there will be one person whose sole responsibility is helping ensure the child's safety and comfort during transport.
>   - Discuss measures the driver may need to take if this is impossible (e.g., be certain a basin is within the child's reach in case vomiting occurs; take a route that permits slower traffic and has places along the roadside to stop if necessary).
>   - Determine the availability of a blanket, pillow, and cup with a lid and straw for the child's use in the car.
> 13. Provide emergency phone numbers for the family to call with any concerns.
> 14. Explain that the family will be contacted (give an approximate time) to follow up on the child but that they should not hesitate to call if concerns arise before then.
> 15. Ask the family and child, if appropriate, if they have any questions and problem solve with family members to meet their unique needs.

are compounded by children's limited understanding of isolation. Preschool children have difficulty understanding the rationale for isolation because they cannot comprehend the cause-and-effect relationship between germs and illness. They are likely to view isolation as punishment. Older children understand the causality better but still require information to decrease fantasizing or misinterpretation.

When a child is placed in isolation, preparation is essential for him or her to feel in control. With young children the best approach is a simple explanation such as, "You need to be in this room to help you get better. This is a special place to make all the germs go away. The germs made you sick, and you could not help that."

All children, but especially younger ones, need preparation in terms of what they will see, hear, and feel in isolation. Therefore they are shown the mask, gloves, and gown and encouraged to "dress up" in them. Playing with the strange apparel lessens the fear of seeing "ghostlike" people walk into the room. Before entering the room, nurses and other health personnel should introduce themselves and let the child see their faces before donning masks. In this way the child associates them with significant experiences and gains a sense of familiarity in an otherwise strange and lonely environment.

When the child's condition improves, appropriate play activities are provided to minimize boredom, stimulate the senses, provide a real or perceived sense of movement, orient the child to time and place, provide social interaction, and reduce depersonalization. For example, the environment can be manipulated to increase sensory freedom by moving the bed toward the door or window. Opening window shades; providing musical, visual, or tactile toys; and increasing interpersonal contact can substitute mental mobility for the limitations of physical movement. Rather than dwelling on the negative aspects of isolation, the child can be encouraged to view this experience as challenging and positive. For example, the nurse can help the child look at isolation as a method of keeping others out and letting only special people in. Children often think of intriguing signs for their doors such as, "Enter at your own risk." These signs also encourage people "on the outside" to talk with the child about the ominous greeting.

Emergency Admission

One of the most traumatic hospital experiences for the child and parents is an emergency admission. The sudden onset of an illness or the occurrence of an injury leaves little time for preparation and explanation. Sometimes the emergency admission is compounded by admission to an intensive care unit (ICU) or the need for immediate surgery. However, even in instances requiring only outpatient treatment, the child is exposed to a strange, frightening environment and experiences that may elicit fear or cause pain.

There is a wide discrepancy between what constitutes a medically defined emergency and a patient-defined emergency. A growing concern is the use of major emergency departments for routine primary care health visits. To offset overcrowding in emergency departments, many facilities have minor emergency units or pediatric minor emergency units for after-hours' health care. Telephone triage for minor illnesses for patients is also emerging as a health care delivery mode to differentiate illnesses such as a common cold from true life-threatening conditions that require immediate practitioner attention and intervention. Other factors contributing to the overuse of emergency departments (as opposed to the primary practitioner's office) include the increasing number of uninsured persons and households in which both parents work full time and cannot afford to take off during the daytime to take the sick child to a practitioner.

In pediatric populations most visits to an emergency department are for respiratory infections, with skin conditions, gastrointestinal disorders, and trauma such as poisoning accounting for the remainder of cases. The most common reason parents give for bringing the child to the emergency department is concern about the illness worsening. However, practitioners may not think that the progressive symptoms necessitate immediate or emergency care. One of the nurse's primary goals is to assess the parents' perception of the event and their reasons for considering it serious or life threatening.

Lengthy preparatory admission procedures are often inappropriate for emergency situations. In such instances nurses must focus their nursing interventions on the essential components of admission counseling (Box 38-10) and complete the process as soon as the child's condition has stabilized.

Unless an emergency is life threatening, children need to participate in their care to maintain a sense of control. Because emergency departments are frequently hectic, there is a tendency to rush through procedures to save time. However, the extra few minutes needed to allow children to participate may save many more minutes of useless resistance and lack of cooperation during subsequent procedures. Other supportive measures include ensuring privacy, accepting various emotional responses to fear or pain, preserving parent-child contact, explaining all events before or as they occur, and personally remaining calm. Pain management strategies are discussed in Chapter 30.

At times, because of the child's physical condition, little or no preparatory counseling for emergency hospitalization can be done. In such situations counseling subsequent to the event has therapeutic value. Counseling should focus on evaluating children's thoughts regarding admission and related procedures. It is similar to precounseling techniques; however, instead of supplying information, the nurse listens to the explanations offered by the child. Projective techniques such as drawing, doll play, or storytelling are especially effective. The nurse then bases additional information on what has already been understood.

Intensive Care Unit

Admission to an ICU can be traumatic for both the child and parents (Fig. 38-10). The nature and severity of the illness and the

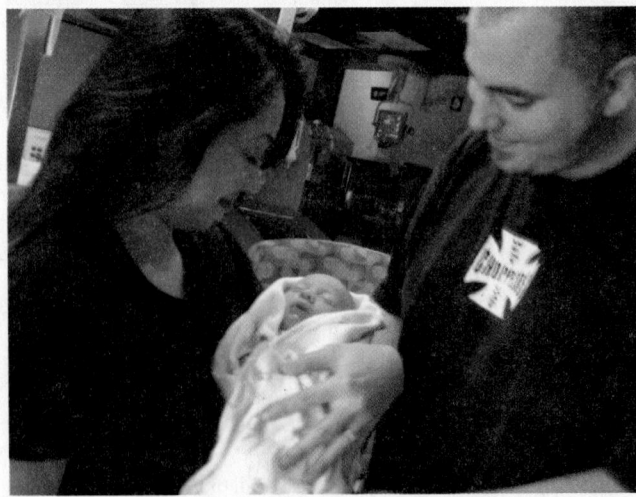

FIG 38-10 Parental presence during hospitalization provides emotional support for the child and increases the parent's sense of empowerment in the caregiver role. (Courtesy E. Jacob, Texas Children's Hospital, Houston, TX.)

circumstances surrounding the admission are major factors, especially for parents. Parents experience significantly more stress when the admission is unexpected rather than expected. Although several studies have described what parents perceive to be most stressful, the most effective strategy may simply be to ask parents what is stressful and implement interventions that will enhance their ability to cope (Board and Ryan-Wenger, 2003). Assessment should be repeated periodically to account for changes in perceptions over time. The use of daily patient goal sheets has been successful in improving communication among health care providers caring for children in the ICU (Agarwal, Frankel, Tourner, et al., 2008; Phipps and Thomas, 2007). By clearly defining daily patient care goals, health care providers believed that care was improved.

The family's emotional needs are paramount when a child is admitted to an ICU. A major stressor for parents of a child in the ICU is the child's appearance (Latour, van Goudoever, and Hazelzet, 2008). Although the same interventions discussed earlier for the stressors of separation and loss of control apply here, additional interventions may also benefit the family and child. In a qualitative study of 19 parents of 10 children in an ICU, parents reported that they simply wanted nurses to nurture the child in the same way the family would (Harbaugh, Tomlinson, and Kirschbaum, 2004). Nurse behaviors that exemplified caring and affection were perceived as helpful in decreasing stress. Behaviors perceived as not helpful included separating the child from the parents and communicating poorly with parents. Therefore even critical care must be centered on the family. It is important that visiting hours be liberal and flexible enough to accommodate parental needs and involvement.

Critically ill children become the focus of the parents' lives, and parents' most pressing need is for information. They want to know if their child will live and, if so, whether the child will be the same as before. They need to know why various interventions are being done for the child, that the child is being treated for pain or is

---

BOX 38-10 GUIDELINES FOR SPECIAL HOSPITAL ADMISSION*

Emergency Admission

- Lengthy preparatory admission procedures are often impossible and inappropriate for emergency situations.
- Focus assessment on airway, breathing, and circulation; weigh child whenever possible for calculation of drug dosages.
- Unless an emergency is life threatening, children need to participate in their care to maintain a sense of control.
- Focus on essential components of admission counseling, including the following:
  - Appropriate introduction to the family
  - Use of child's name, not terms such as "honey" or "dear"
  - Determination of child's age and some judgment about developmental age (If the child is of school age, asking about the grade level offers some evidence of intellectual ability.)
  - Information about child's general state of health, any problems that may interfere with medical treatment (e.g., allergies), and previous experience with hospital facilities
  - Information about the chief complaint from both the parents and the child

Admission to Intensive Care Unit

- Prepare child and parents for elective intensive care unit (ICU) admission such as for postoperative care after cardiac surgery.
- Prepare child and parents for unanticipated ICU admission by focusing primarily on the sensory aspects of the experience and usual family concerns (e.g., people in charge of child's care, schedule for visiting, area where family can stay).
- Prepare parents regarding child's appearance and behavior when they first visit child in ICU.
- Accompany family to bedside to provide emotional support and answer questions.
- Prepare siblings for their visit; plan length of time for sibling visitation; monitor siblings' reactions during visit to prevent them from becoming overwhelmed.
- Encourage parents to stay with their child:
  - If visiting hours are limited, allow flexibility in schedule to accommodate parental needs.
  - Give family members a written schedule of visiting times.
  - If visiting hours are liberal, be aware of family members' needs and suggest periodic respites.
  - Assure family they can call the unit at any time.

- Prepare parents for expected role changes and identify ways for them to participate in child's care without overwhelming them with responsibilities:
  - Help with bath or feeding.
  - Touch and talk to child.
  - Help with procedures.
- Provide information about child's condition in understandable language:
  - Repeat information often.
  - Seek clarification of understanding.
  - During bedside conferences interpret information for family members and child or, if appropriate, conduct report outside room.
- Prepare child for procedures even if it involves explanation while procedure is performed.
- Assess and manage pain; recognize that a child who cannot talk such as an infant or child in a coma or on mechanical ventilation can be in pain.
- Establish a routine that maintains some similarity to daily events in child's life whenever possible:
  - Organize care during normal waking hours.
  - Keep regular bedtime schedules, including quiet times when television or radio is lowered or turned off.
  - Provide uninterrupted sleep cycles (60 minutes for infants; 90 minutes for older children).
  - Close and open drapes and dim lights to allow for day and night.
  - Place curtain around bed for privacy.
  - Orient child to day and time; have clocks or calendars in easy view for older children.
- Schedule a time when child is left undisturbed (e.g., during naps, visit with family, playtime, or favorite program).
- Provide opportunities for play.
- Reduce stimulation in environment:
  - Refrain from loud talking or laughing.
  - Keep equipment noise to a minimum:
    - Turn alarms as low as safely possible.
    - Perform treatments requiring equipment at one time.
    - Turn off bedside equipment that is not in use such as suction and oxygen.
  - Avoid loud, abrupt noises.

*See also Box 38-7.

comfortable, and that the child may be able to hear them even though not awake. When parents first visit the child in the ICU, they need preparation regarding his or her appearance. Ideally the nurse should accompany the parents to the bedside to provide emotional support and answer any questions.

Despite the stresses normally associated with ICU admission, a special security develops from being monitored carefully and receiving individualized care. Therefore planning for transition to the regular unit is essential and should include the following:

- Assignment of a primary nurse on the regular unit
- Continued visits by the ICU staff to assess the child's and parents' adjustment and act as a temporary liaison with the nursing staff
- Explanation of the differences between the two units and the rationale for the change to less intense monitoring of the child's physical condition
- Selection of an appropriate room such as one that is close to the nursing station and a compatible roommate

KEY POINTS

- Children are particularly vulnerable to the stressors of illness and hospitalization because stress represents a change from the usual state of health and routine and because they possess limited coping mechanisms.
- The three stages of separation anxiety are protest, despair, and detachment.
- Feelings of loss of control are caused by unfamiliar environmental stimuli, physical restriction, altered routine, and dependency.
- Fear of bodily pain may be manifested in the following ways: infants—facial expressions and body movements; toddlers—intense emotional upset and physical resistance; preschoolers—aggression, verbal expression, and dependency; school-age children—precise verbalization of pain, passive requests for support or help, and procrastination technique; and adolescents—self-control and limited movement.
- Because of their separation from significant people, children who are hospitalized may lack the opportunity to form new attachments in the strange environment of the hospital and exhibit negative behaviors after discharge.
- Nursing care of children in the hospital is aimed at preventing or minimizing separation, decreasing loss of control, minimizing fear of bodily injury, using play or expressive activities to lessen stress, and maximizing the potential benefits of hospitalization.

- The nurse can maximize potential benefits of hospitalization by fostering parent-child relations, providing educational opportunities, promoting self-mastery, and encouraging socialization.
- Family reactions are influenced by the seriousness of the illness, experience with illness or hospitalization and diagnostic or therapeutic procedures, available support systems, personal ego strengths, coping abilities, presence of additional stressors, cultural and religious beliefs, and family communication patterns.
- Fear of contracting illness, their younger age, a close relationship with the ill sibling, substitute child care, minimal explanation of the illness, and perceived changes in parenting all increase the deleterious effects of a brother's or sister's illness and hospitalization on siblings.
- Nursing care of the family involves listening to parents' verbal and nonverbal messages; providing clergy support; accepting cultural, socioeconomic, and ethnic values; giving information to families and siblings; and preparing for discharge and home care.
- Admission to an outpatient setting, emergency department, isolation room, or ICU requires additional intervention strategies to meet the child's and family's needs.

REFERENCES

Agarwal S, Frankel L, Tourner S, et al: Improving communication in a pediatric intensive care unit using daily patient goal sheets, *J Crit Care* 23(2):227–235, 2008.

Anderson CD, Mangino RR: Nurse shift report: who says you can't talk in front of the patient? *Nurs Adm Q* 30(2):112–122, 2006.

Board R, Ryan-Wenger N: Stressors and symptoms of mothers with children in the PICU, *J Pediatr Nurs* 18(3):195–201, 2003.

Caffin CL, Linton S, Pellegrini J: Introduction of a liaison nurse role in a tertiary paediatric ICU, *Intensive Crit Care Nurs* 23(4):226–233, 2007.

Clatworthy S, Simon K, Tiedeman ME: Child drawing: hospital—an instrument designed to measure the emotional status of

hospitalized school-aged children, *J Pediatr Nurs* 14(1):2–9, 1999.

Coyne I: Children's experiences of hospitalization, *J Child Health Care* 10(4):326–336, 2006.

Craft MJ: Siblings of hospitalized children: assessment and intervention, *J Pediatr Nurs* 8(5):289–297, 1993.

Fernandez C, Pyesmany A, Stutzer C: Alternative therapies in childhood cancer, *N Engl J Med* 340(7):569–570, 1999.

Feudtner HJ, Haney J, Dimmers MA: Spiritual care needs of hospitalized children and their families: a national survey of pastoral care providers' perceptions, *Pediatrics* 111(1):e67–e72, 2003.

Flanagan K: Preoperative assessment: safety considerations for patients taking herbal products, *J Perianesth Nurs* 16(1):19–26, 2001.

Gordon M: *Manual of nursing diagnosis*, ed 10, St Louis, 2002, Mosby.

Harbaugh BL, Tomlinson PS, Kirschbaum M: Parents' perceptions of nurses' caregiving behaviors in the pediatric intensive care unit, *Issues Compr Pediatr Nurs* 27(3):163–178, 2004.

Hopia H, Tomlinson PS, Paavilainen E, et al: Child in hospital: family experiences and expectations of how nurses can promote family health, *J Clin Nurs* 14(2):212–222, 2005.

Latour JM, van Goudoever JB, Hazelzet JA: Parent satisfaction in the pediatric ICU, *Pediatr Clin North Am* 55(3):779–790, 2008.

Lewandowski LA, Tesler MD: *Family centered care: putting it into action*, Washington, DC, 2003, American Nurses Association.

Melnyk BM: Intervention studies involving parents of hospitalized young children: an analysis of the past and future recommendations, *J Pediatr Nurs* 15(1):4–13, 2000.

Orem D: *Nursing: concepts of practice*, ed 5, New York, 2001, Mosby.

Phipps LM, Thomas NJ: Hepatitis C: The use of a daily goals sheet to improve communication in the paediatric intensive care unit, *Intensive Crit Care Nurs* 23(5):264–271, 2007.

Samela M, Salanterä S, Aronen E: Child-reported hospital fears in 4 to 6-year-old children, *Pediatr Nurs* 35(5):269–276, 303, 2009.

Small L: Early predictors of poor coping outcomes in children following intensive care hospitalization and stressful medical encounters, *Pediatr Nurs* 28(4):393–401, 2002.

Smith T, Conant Rees HL: Making family-centered care a reality, *Semin Nurs Manage* 8(3):136–142, 2000.

Stranton KM: Parents' experiences of their child's care during hospitalization, *J Cult Divers* 11(1):4–11, 2004.

The Joint Commission: *Comprehensive accreditation manual for hospitals (CAMH)*, Oakbrook Terrace, Ill, 2011, Author.

Thompson R: *The handbook of child life: a guide for pediatric psychosocial care*, Springfield, Ill, 2009, Charles C Thomas.

Wilson ME, Megel ME, Enenbach L, et al: The voices of children: stories about hospitalization, *J Pediatr Health Care* 24(2):95–102, 2010.

Pediatric Variations of Nursing Interventions

Marilyn J. Hockenberry

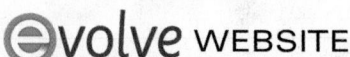 WEBSITE

http://evolve.elsevier.com/Perry/maternal

LEARNING OBJECTIVES

On completion of this chapter, the reader will be able to:
- Identify instances in which informed consent is required and in which minors may be considered emancipated.
- Formulate general guidelines for preparing children for procedures, including surgery.
- Implement play in therapeutic procedures.
- List general strategies for enhancing compliance in children and families.
- Outline general hygiene and care procedures for hospitalized children.
- Implement feeding techniques that encourage food and fluid intake.

- Describe methods of reducing the temperature in a child with fever or hyperthermia.
- Describe systems that can be used for infection control.
- Describe safe methods of administering oral, parenteral, rectal, optic, otic, and nasal medications to children.
- Identify nursing responsibilities in maintaining fluid balance.
- Demonstrate correct procedures for postural drainage and tracheostomy care.
- Describe the procedures involved in providing nutrition via gavage, gastrostomy, and parenteral routes.
- Describe the procedures involved in administering an enema and ostomy care to children.

GENERAL CONCEPTS RELATED TO PEDIATRIC PROCEDURES

Informed Consent

Before undergoing any invasive procedure, the patient or the patient's legal surrogate must receive sufficient information on which to make an informed health care decision. Informed consent should include the expected care or treatment; potential risks, benefits, and alternatives; and what might happen if the patient chooses not to consent. To obtain valid informed consent, health care providers must meet the following three conditions:

1. The person must be capable of giving consent; he or she must be over the age of majority (usually age 18 years) and considered competent (i.e., possessing the mental capacity to make choices and understand their consequences).
2. The person must receive the information needed to make an intelligent decision.
3. The person must act voluntarily when exercising freedom of choice without force, fraud, deceit, duress, or other forms of constraint or coercion.

The patient has the right to accept or refuse any health care. If a patient is treated without consent, the hospital or health care provider may be charged with assault and held liable for damages.

Requirements for Obtaining Informed Consent

Written informed consent of the parent or legal guardian is usually required for medical or surgical treatment of a minor, including many diagnostic procedures. One universal consent is not sufficient. Separate informed permissions must be obtained for each surgical or diagnostic procedure, including the following:
- Major surgery
- Minor surgery (e.g., cutdown, biopsy, dental extraction, suturing a laceration [especially one that may have a cosmetic effect], removal of a cyst, closed reduction of a fracture)
- Diagnostic tests with an element of risk (e.g., bronchoscopy, angiography, lumbar puncture [LP], cardiac catheterization, bone marrow aspiration)
- Medical treatments with an element of risk (e.g., blood transfusion, thoracentesis or paracentesis, radiotherapy)

Other situations that require patient or parental consent include the following:

- Photographs for medical, educational, or public use
- Removal of the child from the health care institution against medical advice
- Postmortem examination, except in unexplained deaths such as sudden infant death, violent death, or suspected suicide
- Release of medical information

Decision making involving the care of older children and adolescents should include the patient's assent (if feasible) and the parent's consent. Assent means that the child or adolescent has been informed about the proposed treatment, procedure, or research and is willing to allow a health care provider to perform it. Assent should include the following:

- Helping the patient achieve a developmentally appropriate awareness of the nature of his or her condition
- Telling the patient what he or she can expect
- Making a clinical assessment of the patient's understanding
- Soliciting an expression of the patient's willingness to accept the proposed procedure

Health care providers should use multiple methods to provide information, including age-appropriate methods (e.g., videos, peer discussion, diagrams, and written materials). The nurse should provide an assent form for the child to sign, and the child should keep a copy. By including the child in the decision-making process and gaining his or her acceptance, staff members demonstrate respect for the child. Assent is not a legal requirement but an ethical one to protect the rights of children.

Eligibility for Giving Informed Consent

Informed Consent of Parents or Legal Guardians. Parents have full responsibility for the care and rearing of their minor children, including legal control over them. As long as children are minors, their parents or legal guardians are required to give informed consent before medical treatment is rendered or any procedure is performed. If the parents are married to one another, consent from only one parent is required for nonurgent pediatric care. If the parents are divorced, consent usually rests with the parent who has legal custody (Berger and AAP Committee on Medical Liability, 2003). Parents also have a right to withdraw consent later.

Evidence of Consent. Regulations on obtaining informed consent vary from state to state, and policies differ at each health care facility. It is the health care provider's legal responsibility to explain the procedure, risks, benefits, and alternatives. The nurse witnesses the patient's, parent's, or legal guardian's signature on the consent form and may reinforce what the patient has been told. A signed consent form is the legal document that signifies that the process of informed consent has occurred. If parents are unavailable to sign consent forms, verbal consent may be obtained via the telephone in the presence of two witnesses. Both witnesses record that informed consent was given and by whom. Their signatures indicate that they witnessed the verbal consent.

Informed Consent of Mature and Emancipated Minors. State laws differ with regard to the age of majority (i.e., the age at which a person is considered to have all the legal rights and responsibilities of an adult). In most states 18 years is the age of majority. Competent adults can give informed consent on their own behalf. An emancipated minor is one who is legally under the age of majority but is recognized as having the legal capacity of an adult under circumstances prescribed by state law such as pregnancy, marriage, high school graduation, independent living, or military service.

Treatment Without Parental Consent. Exceptions to requiring parental consent before treating minor children occur in situations in which children need urgent medical or surgical treatment and a parent is not readily available or refuses to give consent. For example, a child may be brought to an emergency department accompanied by a grandparent, child care provider, teacher, or others. In the absence of parents or legal guardians, people in charge of the child may be given permission by the parents to give informed consent by proxy. In emergencies, including danger to life or the possibility of permanent injury, appropriate care should not be withheld or delayed because of problems obtaining consent (AAP, 2003; Berger and AAP Committee on Medical Liability, 2003). The nurse should document any efforts made to obtain consent.

Refusal to give consent can occur when the treatment such as blood transfusions conflicts with the parents' religious beliefs. All states recognize such exceptions and have statutory procedures to permit treatment if the life or health of such a minor is in jeopardy or if delayed treatment would create a risk to the minor's health. Evaluation for child abuse or neglect can occur without parental consent and without notification to the state before evaluation in most states.

Adolescents, Consent, and Confidentiality. The Health Insurance Portability and Accountability Act of 1996 (HIPAA) was passed to help protect and safeguard the security and confidentiality of health information. Because adolescents are not yet adults, parents have the right to make most decisions on their behalf and receive information. However, adolescents are more likely to seek care in a setting in which they believe their privacy will be maintained. All 50 states have enacted legislation that entitles them to consent to treatment for one or more "medically emancipated" conditions such as sexually transmitted infections, mental health services, alcohol and drug dependency, pregnancy, and contraceptive advice without the parents' knowledge (AAP, 2003; Anderson, Schaechter, and Brosco, 2005; Tillett, 2005). Consent to abortion is controversial, and statues vary widely by state. State law preempts HIPAA, regardless of whether that law prohibits, mandates, or allows discretion about a disclosure.

Preparation for Diagnostic and Therapeutic Procedures

Technologic advances and changes in health care have resulted in more pediatric procedures being performed in a variety of settings. Many procedures are both stressful and painful experiences. For most procedures the focus of care is psychologic preparation of the child and family. However, some procedures require the administration of sedatives and analgesics.

Psychologic Preparation

Preparing children for procedures decreases their anxiety, promotes their cooperation, supports their coping skills and may teach them new ones, and facilitates a feeling of mastery in experiencing a potentially stressful event. Many institutions have developed preadmission teaching programs designed to educate the pediatric patient and family by offering hands-on experience with hospital equipment, the procedure performed, and departments they will visit. Preparatory methods may be formal such as group preparation for hospitalization. Most preparation strategies are informal, focus on providing information about the experience, and are directed at stressful or painful procedures. The most effective preparation includes providing sensory-procedural information and helping the child develop coping skills such as imagery, distraction, or relaxation.

The Guidelines boxes describe general guidelines for preparing children for procedures along with age-specific guidelines that consider their developmental needs and cognitive abilities. In addition to these suggestions, nurses should consider the child's temperament, existing coping strategies, and previous experiences in individualizing the preparatory process. Children who are distractible and highly active or those who are "slow to warm up" may need individualized sessions (i.e., shorter for active children and more slowly paced for shy children). Youngsters who tend to cope well may need more emphasis on using their present skills, whereas those who appear to cope less adequately can benefit from more time devoted to simple coping strategies such as relaxing, breathing, counting, squeezing a hand, or singing. Children with previous health-related experiences still need preparation for repeat or new procedures; however, the nurse must assess what they know, correct their misconceptions, supply new information, and introduce new coping skills as indicated by their previous reactions. Especially for painful procedures, the most effective preparation includes providing sensory-procedural information and helping the child develop coping skills such as imagery or relaxation (see Guidelines boxes).

Children differ in their "information-seeking dimension." Some actively ask for information about the intended procedure, but others characteristically avoid it. Parents can often guide nurses in deciding how much information is enough for the child because they know whether he or she is typically inquisitive or satisfied with short answers. Asking older children their preferences about the amount of explanation is also important.

The exact timing of the preparation for a procedure varies with the child's age and the type of procedure. No exact guidelines govern timing; but in general the younger the child, the closer the explanation should be to the actual procedure to prevent undue fantasizing and worrying. With complex procedures more time may be needed for assimilation of information, especially with older children. For example, the explanation for an injection can immediately precede the procedure for all ages; but preparation for surgery may begin the day before for young children and a few days before for older children, although the nurse should elicit older children's preferences.

Establish Trust and Provide Support. The nurse who has spent time with and established a positive relationship with a child usually finds it easier to gain cooperation. If the relationship is based on trust, the child associates the nurse with caregiving activities that give comfort and pleasure most of the time rather than discomfort and stress. If the nurse does not know the child, it is best for he or she to be introduced by another staff person whom the child trusts. The first visit with the child should not include any painful procedure and ideally should focus on the child first and then on an explanation of the procedure.

Parental Presence and Support. Children need support during procedures, and for young children the greatest source of support is the parents. They represent security, protection, safety, and comfort. Several studies have reported a positive impact on parental distress and satisfaction and no difference in technical complications when parents remain with children (Piira, Sugiura, Champion, et al., 2005). Controversy exists regarding the role parents should assume during the procedure, especially if discomfort is involved. Several professional associations support the option of family presence during invasive procedures (American Association of Critical Care Nurses, 2006; Emergency Nurses Association, 2005). The nurse should assess the parents' preferences for assisting, observing, or waiting outside the room and the child's preference for parental presence. Respect the child's and parents' choices. Give parents who wish to stay appropriate explanation about the procedure and coach them about where to sit or stand and what to say or do to help the child through it. Support parents who do not want to be present in

---

GUIDELINES

Preparing Children for Procedures

- Determine details of exact procedure to be performed.
- Review parents' and child's present understanding.
- Base teaching on developmental age and existing knowledge.
- Incorporate parents in teaching if they desire, especially if they plan to participate in care.
- Inform parents of their supportive role during procedure such as standing near child's head or in child's line of vision and talking softly to child and the typical responses to be expected from children undergoing the procedure.
- Allow for ample discussion to prevent information overload and ensure adequate feedback.
- Use concrete, not abstract, terms and visual aids to describe procedure. For example, use a simple line drawing of a boy or girl and mark the body part that will be involved in the procedure. Use nonthreatening but realistic models.*
- Emphasize that no other body part will be involved.
- If the body part is associated with a specific function, stress the change or noninvolvement of that ability (e.g., after tonsillectomy, child can still speak).
- Use words and sentence length appropriate to child's level of understanding (a rule of thumb for the number of words in a child's sentence is equal to his or her age in years plus 1).
- Avoid words and phrases with dual meanings (see Table 39-1, p. 1135) unless child understands such words.
- Clarify all unfamiliar words (e.g., "Anesthesia is a *special* sleep").
- Emphasize sensory aspects of procedure—what child will feel, see, hear, smell, and touch and what he or she can do during procedure (e.g., lie still, count out loud, squeeze a hand, hug a doll).
- Allow child to practice procedures that require cooperation (e.g., turning, deep breathing, using an incentive spirometry).
- Introduce anxiety-inducing information last (e.g., starting an intravenous line).
- Be honest with child about unpleasant aspects of a procedure but avoid creating undue concern. When discussing that a procedure may be uncomfortable, state that it feels differently to different people.
- Emphasize end of procedure and any pleasurable events afterward (e.g., going home, seeing parents).
- Stress positive benefits of procedure (e.g., "After your tonsils are fixed, you won't have as many sore throats").
- Provide a positive ending, praising efforts at cooperation and coping.

*Soft-sculptured dolls and customized adapters and overlays for preparing children and families about procedures and as teaching models for technical care are available from Legacy Products, Inc., 120 West Main Street, PO Box 267, Cambridge City, IN 47327, 800-238-7951, e-mail: info@legacyproductsinc.com, www.legacyproductsinc.com.

their decision and encourage them to remain close by so they can be available to support the child immediately after the procedure. Parents should also know that someone will be with their child to provide support. Ideally this person should inform the parents after the procedure about how the child did.

Provide an Explanation. Age-appropriate explanations are one of the most widely used interventions for reducing anxiety in children undergoing procedures. Before performing a procedure, explain what is to be done and what is expected of the child. The explanation should be short, simple, and appropriate to the child's

GUIDELINES

Age-Specific Preparation of Children for Procedures Based on Developmental Characteristics

Infant—Developing Trust and Sensorimotor Thought
Attachment to Parent
- Involve parent in procedure if desired.*
- Keep parent in infant's line of vision.
- If parent is unable to be with infant, place familiar object with him or her (e.g., stuffed toy).

Stranger Anxiety
- Have usual caregivers perform or assist with procedure.*
- Make advances slowly and in nonthreatening manner.
- Limit number of strangers entering room during procedure.*

Sensorimotor Phase of Learning
- During procedure use sensory soothing measures (e.g., stroking skin, talking softly, giving pacifier).
- Use analgesics (e.g., topical anesthetic, intravenous opioid) to control discomfort.*
- Cuddle and hug infant after stressful procedure; encourage parent to comfort infant.

Increased Muscle Control
- Expect older infants to resist.
- Restrain adequately.
- Keep harmful objects out of reach.

Memory for Past Experiences
- Realize that older infants may associate objects, places, or people with prior painful experiences and will cry and resist at the sight of them.
- Keep frightening objects out of view.*
- Perform painful procedures in a separate room, not in crib (or bed).*
- Use nonintrusive procedures whenever possible (e.g., axillary or tympanic temperatures, oral medications).*

Imitation of Gestures
- Model desired behavior (e.g., opening mouth).

Toddler—Developing Autonomy and Sensorimotor to Preoperational Thought
Use same approaches as for infant plus the following.

Egocentric Thought
- Explain procedure in relation to what child will see, hear, taste, smell, and feel.
- Emphasize aspects of procedure that require cooperation (e.g., lying still).
- Tell child that it is okay to cry, yell, or use other means to express discomfort verbally.
- Designate one health care provider to speak during procedure. Hearing more than one can be confusing to child.*

Negative Behavior
- Expect treatments to be resisted; child may try to run away.
- Use firm, direct approach.
- Ignore temper tantrums.
- Use distraction techniques (e.g., singing a song *with* child).
- Restrain adequately.

Animism
- Keep frightening objects out of view (young children believe that objects have lifelike qualities and can harm them).

Limited Language Skills
- Communicate using gestures or demonstrations.
- Use a few simple terms familiar to child.
- Give child one direction at a time (e.g., "Lie down" and then "Hold my hand").
- Use small replicas of equipment; allow child to handle equipment.
- Use play; demonstrate on doll but avoid child's favorite doll because child may think doll is really "feeling" procedure.
- Prepare parents separately to avoid child's misinterpreting words.

Limited Concept of Time
- Prepare child shortly or immediately before procedure.
- Keep teaching sessions short (≈5-10 minutes).
- Have preparations completed before involving child in procedure.
- Have extra equipment nearby (e.g., alcohol swabs, new needle, adhesive bandages) to avoid delays.
- Tell child when procedure is completed.

Striving for Independence
- Allow choices whenever possible but realize that child may still be resistant and negative.
- Allow child to participate in care and help whenever possible (e.g., drink medicine from a cup, hold a dressing).

Preschooler—Developing Initiative and Preoperational Thought
Egocentric
- Explain procedure in simple terms and in relation to how it affects child (as with toddler, stress sensory aspects).
- Demonstrate use of equipment.
- Allow child to play with miniature or actual equipment.
- Encourage "playing out" experience on a doll both before and after procedure to clarify misconceptions.
- Use neutral words to describe the procedure (see Table 39-1, p. 1135).

Increased Language Skills
- Use verbal explanation but avoid overestimating child's comprehension of words.
- Encourage child to verbalize ideas and feelings.

Limited Concept of Time and Frustration Tolerance
- Implement same approaches as for toddler but may plan longer teaching session (10-15 minutes); may divide information into more than one session.

Illness and Hospitalization Viewed As Punishment
- Clarify why each procedure is performed; child will find it difficult to understand how medicine can make him or her feel better and can taste bad at the same time.
- Ask child thoughts regarding why a procedure is performed.
- State directly that procedures are never a form of punishment.

*Applies to any age.   *Continued*

GUIDELINES

Age-Specific Preparation of Children for Procedures Based on Developmental Characteristics—cont'd

Animism
- Keep equipment out of sight except when shown to or used on child.

Fears of Bodily Harm, Intrusion, and Castration
- Point out on drawing, doll, or child where procedure is performed.
- Emphasize that no other body part will be involved.
- Use nonintrusive procedures whenever possible (e.g., axillary temperatures, oral medication).
- Apply adhesive bandage over puncture site.
- Encourage parental presence.
- Realize that procedures involving genitalia provoke anxiety.
- Allow child to wear underpants with gown.
- Explain unfamiliar situations, especially noises or lights.

Striving for Initiative
- Involve child in care whenever possible (e.g., hold equipment, remove dressing).
- Give choices whenever possible but avoid excessive delays.
- Praise child for helping and attempting to cooperate; never shame child for lack of cooperation.

School-Age Child—Developing Industry and Concrete Thought
Increased Language Skills; Interest in Acquiring Knowledge
- Explain procedures using correct scientific and medical terminology.
- Explain procedure using simple diagrams and photographs.
- Discuss why procedure is necessary; concepts of illness and bodily functions are often vague.
- Explain function and operation of equipment in concrete terms.
- Allow child to manipulate equipment; use doll or another person as model to practice using equipment whenever possible (doll play may be considered childish by older school-age child).
- Allow time before and after procedure for questions and discussion.

Improved Concept of Time
- Plan for longer teaching sessions (≈20 minutes).
- Prepare up to 1 day in advance of procedure to allow for processing information.

Increased Self-Control
- Gain child's cooperation.
- Tell child what is expected.
- Suggest several ways of maintaining control from which the child may select (e.g., deep breathing, relaxation, counting).

Striving for Industry
- Allow responsibility for simple tasks (e.g., collecting specimens).
- Include child in decision making (e.g., time of day to perform procedure, preferred site).
- Encourage active participation (e.g., removing dressings, handling equipment, opening packages).

Developing Relationships with Peers
- Prepare two or more children for same procedure or encourage one to help prepare another.
- Provide privacy from peers during procedure to maintain self-esteem.

Adolescent—Developing Identity and Abstract Thought
Increasing Abstract Thought and Reasoning
- Discuss why procedure is necessary or beneficial.
- Explain long-term consequences of procedures; include information about body systems working together.
- Realize that adolescent may fear death, disability, or other potential risks.
- Encourage questioning regarding fears, options, and alternatives.

Consciousness of Appearance
- Provide privacy; describe how body will be covered and what will be exposed.
- Discuss how procedure may affect appearance (e.g., scar) and what can be done to minimize it.
- Emphasize any physical benefits of procedure.

Concern More with Present Than with Future
- Realize that immediate effects of procedure are more significant than future benefits.

Striving for Independence
- Involve adolescent in decision making and planning (e.g., time, place, clothing, individuals present during procedure, whether they will watch procedure).
- Impose as few restrictions as possible.
- Explore which coping strategies have worked in the past; children may need descriptions to identify various techniques.
- Accept regression to more childish methods of coping.
- Realize that adolescent may have difficulty accepting new authority figures and resist complying with procedures.

Developing Peer Relationships and Group Identity
- Same as for school-age child but assumes even greater significance.
- Allow adolescents to talk with other adolescents who have had same procedure.

level of comprehension. Long explanations may increase anxiety in a young child. When explaining the procedure to parents with the child present, the nurse uses language appropriate to the child because unfamiliar words can be misunderstood (Table 39-1). If the parents need additional preparation, it is done in an area away from the child. Teaching sessions are planned at times most conducive to the child's learning (e.g., after a rest period) and for the usual span of attention.

Special equipment is not necessary for preparing a child; but for young children who cannot yet think conceptually, using objects to supplement verbal explanation is important. Allowing children to handle actual items that will be used in their care such as a stethoscope, sphygmomanometer, or oxygen mask helps them develop familiarity with these items and reduces the fear often associated with their use. Miniature versions of hospital items such as gurneys and x-ray and intravenous (IV) equipment can be used to explain what the children can expect and permit them to safely experience situations that are unfamiliar and potentially frightening. Use photographs of children in different areas of the hospital (e.g., radiology department, operating room) to give children a more realistic idea

TABLE 39-1	SELECTING NONTHREATENING WORDS OR PHRASES
WORDS AND PHRASES TO AVOID	**SUGGESTED SUBSTITUTIONS**
Shot, bee sting, stick	Medicine under the skin
Organ	Special place in body
Test	To see how (specify body part) is working
Incision, cut	Special opening
Edema	Puffiness
Stretcher, gurney	Rolling bed, bed on wheels
Stool	Child's usual term
Dye	Special medicine
Pain	Hurt, discomfort, "owie," "boo-boo," sore, achy, scratchy
Deaden	Numb, make sleepy
Fix	Make better
Take (as in "take your temperature")	See how warm you are
Take (as in "take your blood pressure")	Check your pressure; hug your arm
Put to sleep, anesthesia	Special sleep so you won't feel anything
Catheter	Tube
Monitor	Television screen
Electrodes	Stickers, ticklers
Specimen	Sample

of equipment they may encounter. Written and illustrated materials are also valuable aids to preparation.*

Physical Preparation

One area of special concern is the administration of appropriate sedation and analgesia before stressful procedures. Chapter 30 describes sedative medications used for procedures.

Performance of the Procedure

Supportive care continues during the procedure and can be a major factor in a child's ability to cooperate. Ideally the same nurse who explains the procedure should perform or assist with the procedure. Before beginning, all equipment is assembled, and the room is readied to prevent unnecessary delays and interruptions that increase the child's anxiety. To avoid a delay during a procedure, have extra supplies handy. For example, have tape, bandages, alcohol

---

*Preparatory materials, such as *Going to the Doctor*, are available from The Fred Rogers Company, 4802 Fifth Ave., Pittsburgh, PA 15213; 412-687-2990, www.fci.org. *Hospital Friends* is available from Centering Corporation, 7230 Maple St., Omaha, NE 68134, 866-218-0101, www.centering.org. Other resources include *Berenstein Bears Go to the Doctor* and *Berenstein Bears Visit the Dentist* (New York, Random House).

swabs, and an extra needle when performing an injection or venipuncture. Minimizing the number of people present during the procedure also can decrease the child's anxiety.

To promote long-term coping and adjustment, give special consideration to the patient's age, coping skills, and procedure to be performed in determining where a procedure will occur. Treatment rooms should be used for procedures requiring sedation such as bone marrow aspirates and LPs in younger children. Traumatic procedures should never be performed in "safe" areas such as the playroom. If the procedure is lengthy, avoid conversation that could be misinterpreted by the child. As the procedure is nearing completion, the nurse should inform the child that it is almost over in language the child understands.

Expect Success. Nurses who approach children with confidence and convey the impression that they expect to be successful are less likely to encounter difficulty. It is best to approach a child as though cooperation is expected. Children sense anxiety and uncertainty in an adult and respond by striking out or actively resisting. Although it is not possible to eliminate such behavior in every child, a firm approach with a positive attitude tends to convey a feeling of security to most children.

Involve the Child. Involving children helps to gain their cooperation. Permitting choices gives them some measure of control. However, a choice is given only in situations in which one is available. Asking children, "Do you want to take your medicine now?" leads them to believe that they have an option and provides them the opportunity to legitimately refuse or delay the medication. This places the nurse in an awkward, if not impossible, position. It is much better to state firmly, "It's time to drink your medicine now." Children usually like to make choices, but the choice must be one that they do indeed have (e.g., "It's time for your medicine. Do you want to drink it plain or with a little water?").

Many children respond to tactics that appeal to their maturity or courage. This also gives them a sense of participation and achievement. For example, preschool children are proud that they can hold the dressing during the procedure or remove the tape. The same is true for school-age children, who often cooperate with minimal resistance.

Provide Distraction. Distraction is a powerful coping strategy during painful procedures (Uman, Chambers, McGrath, et al., 2006). It is accomplished by focusing the child's attention on something other than the procedure. Singing favorite songs, listening to music with a headset, counting aloud, or blowing bubbles to "blow the hurt away" are effective techniques. (For other nonpharmacologic interventions, see Chapter 30.)

Allow Expression of Feelings. The child should be allowed to express feelings of anger, anxiety, fear, frustration, or any other emotion. It is natural for children to strike out in frustration or try to avoid stress-provoking situations. The child needs to know that it is all right to cry. Behavior is children's primary means of communication, and coping and should be permitted unless it inflicts harm on them or those caring for them.

Postprocedural Support

After the procedure the child continues to need reassurance that he or she performed well and is accepted and loved. If the parents did not participate, the child is united with them as soon as possible so they can provide comfort.

Encourage Expression of Feelings. Planned activity after the procedure is helpful in encouraging constructive expression of feelings. For verbal children reviewing the details of the procedure can clarify misconceptions and garner feedback for improving the

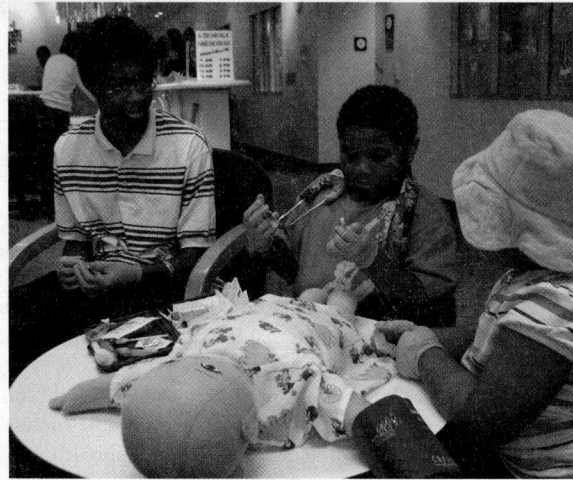

FIG 39-1 Playing with medical objects provides children with the opportunity to play out fears and concerns with supervision by a nurse or child life specialist.

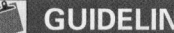

GUIDELINES
Family Preparation for Procedures

Family education for specific procedures is included throughout this unit. General concepts applicable to most family education sessions include the following:

- Name of procedure
- Purpose of procedure
- Length of time anticipated to complete procedure
- Anticipated effects
- Signs of adverse effects
- Assessment of family's level of understanding
- Demonstration and having family return it (if appropriate)

nurse's preparatory strategies. Play is an excellent activity for all children. Infants and young children should have the opportunity for gross motor movement. Older children are able to vent their anger and frustration in acceptable pounding or throwing activities. Play-Doh is a remarkably versatile medium for pounding and shaping. Dramatic play provides an outlet for anger and places the child in a position of control in contrast to the position of helplessness in the real situation. Puppets also allow the child to communicate feelings in a nonthreatening way. One of the most effective interventions is therapeutic play, which includes well-supervised activities such as permitting the child to give an injection to a doll or stuffed toy to reduce the stress of injections (Fig. 39-1).

Positive Reinforcement. Children need to hear from adults that they did the best they could in the situation, no matter how they behaved. It is important for them to know that their worth is not being judged on the basis of their behavior in a stressful situation. Reward systems such as earning stars, stickers, or a badge of courage are appealing to children.

Returning to the child a short while after the procedure helps the nurse strengthen a supportive relationship. Relating with the child in a relaxed and nonstressful period allows him or her to see the nurse not only as someone associated with stressful situations but also as someone with whom to share pleasurable experiences.

Use of Play in Procedures

The use of play is an integral part of relationships with children. As such its value in specific situations is discussed throughout this book such as in Chapter 26 in relation to hospitalization. Many institutions have elaborate and well-organized play areas and programs under the direction of child life specialists. Other institutions have limited facilities. No matter what the institution provides for children, nurses can include play activities as part of nursing care. Play can be used to teach, express feelings, or achieve a therapeutic goal. Consequently it should be included in preparing children for and encouraging their cooperation during procedures. Play sessions after procedures can be structured such as directed toward needle play or general, with a wide variety of equipment available with which children can play.

Routine procedures such as measuring blood pressure and oral administration of medication may be of concern to children.

Box 39-1 describes suggestions for incorporating play into nursing procedures and activities for the hospitalized child that facilitate learning and adjustment to a new situation.

Preparing the Family

The process of patient education involves giving the family information about the child's condition, the regimen that must be followed and why, and other health teaching as indicated. The goal of this education is to enable the family to modify behaviors and adhere to the regimen that has been mutually established.

If equipment will be needed at home (e.g., suction machines, syringes), begin making the necessary arrangements in advance so discharge can proceed smoothly. Whenever possible, make arrangements for the family to use the same equipment in the home that they are using in the hospital. This allows them to become familiar with the items. In addition, the staff can help troubleshoot the equipment in a controlled environment. Plan the teaching sessions well in advance of the time the family will be responsible for performing the care. The more complex the procedure, the more time is needed for training.

Review the instructions with family members (see Guidelines box). Encourage note taking if they desire. Allow ample practice time under supervision. At least one family member, but preferably two members, should demonstrate the procedure before they are expected to care for the child at home. Provide the family with the telephone numbers of resource individuals who are available to help them in the event of a problem.

Surgical Procedures
Preoperative Care

Children experiencing surgical procedures require both psychologic and physical preparation. An important concern is restriction of food and fluids before surgery to avoid aspiration during anesthesia. Infants require special attention to fluid needs. They should not be without oral fluids for an extended period before surgery to avoid glycogen depletion and dehydration. Table 39-2 contains current preoperative fasting guidelines.

In general, psychologic preparation is similar to that discussed earlier for any procedure and incorporates many of the same techniques used in preparing a child for hospitalization such as films, books, brochures, play, and tours (see Chapter 38). Stress points before and after surgery include the admission process, blood tests, injection of preoperative medication (if prescribed), transport to the operating room, the mask on the face during induction, and the stay in the postanesthesia care unit (PACU). Wearing a hospital gown without the security of underpants or pajama bottoms can also be

BOX 39-1 PLAY ACTIVITIES FOR SPECIFIC PROCEDURES

Fluid Intake

- Make ice pops using child's favorite juice.
- Cut gelatin into fun shapes.
- Make a game out of taking a sip when turning page of a book or in games such as Simon Says.
- Use small medicine cups; decorate the cups.
- Color water with food coloring or powdered drink mix.
- Have a tea party; pour at a small table.
- Let child fill a syringe and squirt it into mouth or use it to fill small decorated cups.
- Cut straws in half and place in a small container (much easier for child to suck liquid).
- Use a "crazy" straw.
- Make a "progress poster"; give rewards for drinking a predetermined quantity.

Deep Breathing

- Blow bubbles with a bubble blower.
- Blow bubbles with a straw (no soap).
- Blow on a pinwheel, feather, whistle, harmonica, balloon, or party blower.
- Practice band instruments.
- Have a blowing contest using balloons,* boats, cotton balls, feathers, marbles, Ping-Pong balls, pieces of paper; blow such objects on a table top over a goal line, over water, through an obstacle course, up in the air, against an opponent, or up and down a string.
- Suck paper or cloth from one container to another using a straw.
- Dramatize stories such as, "I'll huff and puff and blow your house down" from the "Three Little Pigs."
- Do straw-blowing painting.
- Take a deep breath and "blow out the candles" on a birthday cake.
- Use a little paint brush to "paint" nails with water and blow nails dry.

Range of Motion and Use of Extremities

- Throw beanbags at a fixed or movable target or wadded-up paper into a wastebasket.
- Touch or kick Mylar balloons held or hung in different positions (if child is in traction, hang balloon from a trapeze).
- Play "tickle toes"; have the child wiggle them on request.
- Play Twister game or Simon Says.
- Play pretend and guessing games (e.g., imitate a bird, butterfly, or horse).
- Have tricycle or wheelchair races in safe area.
- Play kickball or throw ball with a soft foam ball in a safe area.
- Position bed so child must turn to view television or doorway.
- Climb wall with fingers like a "spider."
- Pretend to teach aerobic dancing or exercises; encourage parents to participate.
- Encourage swimming if feasible.

- Play video games or pinball (fine-motor movement).
- Play hide and seek: hide toy somewhere in bed (or room if ambulatory) and have child find it using specified hand or foot.
- Provide clay to mold with fingers.
- Paint or draw on large sheets of paper placed on floor or wall.
- Encourage combing own hair; play "beauty shop" with "customer" in different positions.

Soaks

- Play with small toys or objects (cups, syringes, soap dishes) in water.
- Wash dolls or toys.
- Pick up marbles or pennies* from bottom of bath container.
- Make designs with coins on bottom of container.
- Pretend a boat is a submarine by keeping it immersed.
- Read to child during soaks; sing with child; or play game such as cards, checkers, or other board game (if both hands are immersed, move board pieces for child).
- Sitz bath: give child something to listen to (music, stories) or look at (View-Master, book).
- Punch holes in bottom of plastic cup, fill with water, and let it "rain" on child.

Injections

- Let child handle syringe, vial, and alcohol swab and give an injection to doll or stuffed animal.
- Use syringes to decorate cookies with frosting, squirt paint, or target shoot into a container.
- Draw a "magic circle" on area before injection; draw smiling face in circle after injection but avoid drawing on puncture site.
- Allow child to have a "collection" of syringes (without needles); make "wild" creative objects with syringes.
- If multiple injections or venipunctures are planned, make a "progress poster"; give rewards for predetermined number of injections.
- Have child count to 10 or 15 during injection.

Ambulation

- Give child something to push:
  - Toddler: push-pull toy
  - School-age child: wagon or a doll in a stroller or wheelchair
  - Adolescent: decorated intravenous stand
- Have a parade; make objects such as hats and drums.

Extending Environment (e.g., for Patients in Traction)

- Make bed into a pirate ship or airplane with decorations.
- Put up mirrors so patient can see around room.
- Move bed frequently to playroom, hallway, or outside.

*Small objects such as marbles, coins, gloves, and balloons are unsafe for young children because of possible aspiration. Latex products also carry the risk of an allergic reaction.

traumatic. Therefore these articles of clothing should be allowed to be worn into the operating room and removed after induction of anesthesia. Children are at higher risk of ineffective response to anesthesia because of higher anxiety associated with stranger anxiety (infants), separation anxiety (toddlers and preschoolers), and fear of injury or death (adolescents) (Romino, Keatley, Secrest, et al., 2005).

Psychologic intervention consisting of systematic preparation, rehearsal of the forthcoming events, and supportive care at each of these points has shown to be more effective than a single-session preparation or consistent supportive care without systematic preparation and rehearsal (Kain, Caldwell-Andrews, Mayes, et al., 2007). A family-centered preoperative preparation program may consist of a tour of the perioperative areas with short explanations of the events 5 to 7 days before surgery, a video to take home and review a couple of times with additional explanations and demonstrations of perioperative processes, a mask to take home with which to practice, pamphlets to guide parents on supporting children during

TABLE 39-2	FASTING RECOMMENDATIONS TO REDUCE THE RISK OF PULMONARY ASPIRATION*
INGESTED MATERIAL	**MINIMUM FASTING PERIOD (hr)†**
Clear liquids‡	>2
Breast milk	4
Infant formula	6
Nonhuman milk§	6
Light meal¶	6

From American Society of Anesthesiologists: Practice guidelines for preoperative fasting and the use of pharmacologic agents to reduce the risk of pulmonary aspiration: application to healthy patients undergoing elective procedures, *Anesthesiology* 90(3):896-905, 1999.

*These recommendations apply to healthy patients who are undergoing elective procedures. They are not intended for women in labor. Following the guidelines does not guarantee that complete gastric emptying has occurred.

†Fasting periods noted in chart apply to all ages.

‡Examples of clear liquids include water, fruit juices without pulp, carbonated beverages, clear tea, and black coffee.

§Because nonhuman milk is similar to solids in gastric emptying time, the amount ingested must be considered when determining appropriate fasting period.

¶A light meal typically consists of toast and clear liquids. Meals that include fried or fatty foods or meat may prolong gastric emptying time. Both the amount and type of foods ingested must be considered when determining an appropriate fasting period.

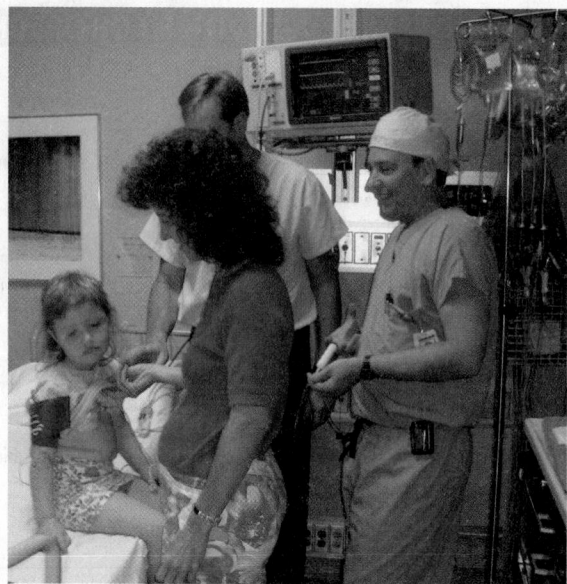

FIG 39-2 Parental presence during induction of anesthesia can minimize the child's and parents' anxiety during the preoperative period.

induction, phone calls to coach parents on preparing children 1 or 2 days before surgery, and toys and supplies in the holding area. Therapeutic play is an effective strategy in preparing children, and increased familiarity with medical procedures decreases anxiety (Li, Lopez, and Lee, 2007).

Parental Presence. Some institutions support parental presence during induction of anesthesia (Fig. 39-2). Appropriate education is essential to help parents understand the stages of anesthesia, what to expect, and how to support their child. When parents choose not to or are not allowed to attend the induction, leaving a favorite possession with the child and uniting the child and parents as soon as possible after surgery (preferably in the PACU) are important interventions. During surgery the family should have a designated place to wait and be kept informed of the child's progress. They also should know where and when they can visit the child after surgery.

According to research conducted by Kain, Caldwell-Andrews, Mayes, et al. (2007), benefits of well-prepared children and parents along with parental presence during induction of anesthesia include reduced anxiety for children and parents, lower doses of postoperative analgesia, lower incidence of severe emergence delirium symptoms, and shorter discharge time for short procedures. Other studies have not universally supported these benefits. Concern exists regarding the appropriateness of this practice for all parents. Some parents may become upset by the rapid succession of induction events, by observing their child becoming limp, and by leaving the child in the care of strangers. Even though some parents may become anxious, most control their anxiety, do not disrupt the induction, and support the child (Munro and D'Errico, 2000). Parents who are anxious before surgery tend to become even more anxious after the induction; the reverse is true of parents with little anxiety.

Preoperative Sedation. Historically the most upsetting event for children has been the preoperative injection. An increasing number of anesthesiologists use preoperative sedative premedication, usually midazolam (Versed), and parental presence for children undergoing surgery (Kain, Caldwell-Andrews, Krivutza, et al., 2004).

The goals for using preoperative medications include (1) anxiety reduction, (2) amnesia, (3) sedation, (4) antiemetic effect, and (5) reduction of secretions (Manworren and Fledderman, 2000). Chapter 30 includes a discussion of pain management strategies for children undergoing surgery. When drugs are administered, they should be delivered atraumatically via oral or IV routes. Numerous preanesthetic drug regimens are used with children, and no consensus exists on the optimal method. However, if children have no preoperative pain, are well prepared psychologically for surgery, and have their parents nearby, preoperative medication may be unnecessary.

Postoperative Care

Various psychologic and physical interventions and observations help prevent or minimize possible unpleasant effects from anesthesia and the surgical procedure. Although the incidence of serious postoperative complications in healthy children undergoing surgery is less than 1% (Maxwell and Yaster, 2000), continuous monitoring of the child's cardiopulmonary status is essential during the immediate postoperative period. Postanesthesia complications such as airway obstruction, postextubation croup, laryngospasm, and bronchospasm make maintaining a patent airway and maximum ventilation critical.

Monitoring the patient's oxygen saturation and providing supplemental oxygen as needed, maintaining body temperature, and promoting fluid and electrolyte balance are important aspects of immediate postoperative care. Vital signs are monitored continuously, and each vital sign is evaluated in terms of side effects from anesthesia, shock, or respiratory compromise (Table 39-3).

TABLE 39-3	POTENTIAL CAUSES OF POSTOPERATIVE VITAL SIGN ALTERATIONS IN CHILDREN	
ALTERATION	**POTENTIAL CAUSE**	**COMMENTS**
Heart Rate		
Increase	Decreased perfusion (shock)	Heart rate may increase to maintain cardiac output.
	Elevated temperature	
	Pain	
	Respiratory distress (early)	
	Medications (atropine, morphine, epinephrine)	
	Hypoxia	
Decrease	Vagal stimulation	Bradycardia is of more concern in young child than tachycardia.
	Increased intracranial pressure	
	Respiratory distress (late)	
	Medications (neostigmine [Prostigmin])	
Respiratory Rate		
Increase	Respiratory distress	Body responds to respiratory distress primarily by increasing rate.
	Fluid volume excess	
	Hypothermia	
	Elevated temperature	
	Pain	
Decrease	Anesthetics, opioids	Decreased respiratory rate from opioids may be compensated for by increased depth of respiration.
	Pain	
Blood Pressure		
Increase	Excess intravascular volume	This is serious in premature infants because it increases risk of intraventricular hemorrhage.
	Increased intracranial pressure	
	Carbon dioxide retention	
	Pain	
	Medication (ketamine, epinephrine)	
Decrease	Vasodilating anesthetic agents (halothane, isoflurane, enflurane)	Decreased blood pressure is late sign of shock because of elasticity and constriction of vessels to maintain cardiac output.
	Opioids (e.g., morphine)	
Temperature		
Increase	Shock (late sign)	Fever associated with infection usually occurs later than fever of noninfectious origin. Absence of fever does not rule out infection, especially in infants.
	Infection	
	Environmental causes (warm room, excess coverings)	
	Malignant hyperthermia	Malignant hyperthermia requires immediate treatment.
Decrease	Vasodilating anesthetic agents (halothane, isoflurane, enflurane)	Neonates are especially susceptible to hypothermia, with serious or fatal consequences.
	Muscle relaxants	
	Environmental causes (cool room)	
	Infusion of cool fluids or blood	

From Smith DP: *Comprehensive child and family nursing skills*, St Louis, 1991, Mosby.

A change in vital signs that demands immediate attention in the perioperative period is caused by malignant hyperthermia (MH), a potentially fatal pharmacogenetic disorder involving a defective calcium channel in the sarcoplasmic reticulum membrane. In susceptible children inhaled anesthetics and the muscle relaxant succinylcholine trigger the disorder, producing hypermetabolism. Symptoms of MH include hypercarbia (increasing end-tidal carbon dioxide), elevated temperature, tachycardia, tachypnea, acidosis, muscle rigidity, and rhabdomyolysis (Rosenberg, Davis, and James, 2007). A family or previous history of sudden high fever associated with a surgical procedure and myotonia increase the risk for MH. Children who have successfully undergone prior surgery without adverse effects may still be considered susceptible.

Treatment of MH includes immediate discontinuation of the triggering agent, hyperventilation with 100% oxygen, and IV dantrolene sodium. If the child is hyperthermic, initiate cooling measures such as ice packs to the groin, axillae, and neck and iced nasogastric (NG) lavage. The surgery may be discontinued; or, if it is emergent, it may be continued with a different anesthetic agent. The patient should be transferred to an intensive care unit for at least 36 hours and is closely monitored for stabilization of vital signs, metabolic state, and possible recurrence of symptoms.

Managing pain is a major nursing responsibility after surgery. The nurse should assess pain frequently and administer analgesics to provide comfort and facilitate cooperation with postoperative care such as ambulation and deep breathing. Opioids are the most commonly used analgesics. Routinely scheduled IV analgesics, patient-controlled analgesia, and epidural infusions, rather than as-needed orders, provide excellent analgesia in postoperative pediatric patients.

Because respiratory tract infections are a potential complication of anesthesia, make every effort to aerate the lungs and remove secretions. Auscultate the lungs regularly to identify abnormal sounds or any areas of diminished or absent breath sounds. To prevent pneumonia encourage respiratory movement with incentive spirometers or other motivating activities (see Box 39-1). If these measures are presented as games, the child is more likely to comply. The child's position is changed every 2 hours, and deep breathing is encouraged.

During the recovery period spend some time with the child to assess his or her perceptions of surgery. Play, drawing, and storytelling are excellent methods of discovering the child's thoughts. With such information the nurse can support or correct the child's perceptions and boost his or her self-esteem for having endured a stressful procedure.

Many pediatric patients are discharged shortly after surgery. Preparation for discharge begins with the preadmission preparation visit. The nurse should discuss instructions for postoperative care and review them throughout the perioperative visit. After discharge the nursing staff often makes phone calls to check the patient's status. Patient education and compliance with discharge instructions can also be assessed during these phone calls (Barnes, 2000) (see Guidelines box).

GENERAL HYGIENE AND CARE

Maintaining Healthy Skin

Maintaining an IV line, removing a dressing, positioning a child in bed, changing a diaper, using electrodes, or using restraints have the potential to contribute to skin injury. General guidelines for skin care are listed in the Guidelines box on p. 1141.

Assessment of the skin is easiest to accomplish during the bath. Examine for early signs of injury. Risk factors include impaired mobility, protein malnutrition, edema, incontinence, sensory loss, anemia, infection, failure to turn the patient, and intubation. Critically ill children are at a higher risk of pressure ulcers and skin breakdown because they often have several risk factors combined. The incidence in these children has been reported as high as 27% (Curley, Quigley, and Lin, 2003). Identification of risk factors helps to determine children who need a more thorough skin assessment. Several risk assessment scales are available for use in pediatrics such as the Braden Q Scale (Curley, Razmus, Roberts, et al., 2003) and the Glamorgan Scale (Willock, Baharestani, and Anthony, 2009). Assessment should occur within 24 hours of admission to identify pressure ulcers and wounds that occurred before admission. Pressure ulcers in children typically occur on the occiput, ears, sacrum, and scapula (Amlung, Miller, and Bosley, 2001); the heels and sacrum are common sites in adults.

When capillary blood flow is interrupted by pressure, the blood flows back into the tissue when the pressure is relieved. As the body attempts to reoxygenate the area, a bright red flush appears. This reactive hyperemia, or flush, is the earliest sign of tissue compromise and pressure-related ischemia. If pressure is prolonged, reactive hyperemia is not sufficient to revitalize ischemic tissue. Pressure ulcers in hospitalized children are uncommon, with reported rates of 1% to 13% (Noonan, Quigley, and Curley, 2006). Risk factors associated with pressure ulcers in pediatric intensive care unit patients include edema, length of stay, increasing positive

GUIDELINES

Postoperative Care

- Ensure that preparations are made to receive child:
  - Bed or crib is ready.
  - Intravenous pumps and poles, suction apparatus, and oxygen flow meter are at bedside.
- Obtain baseline information:
  - Take vital signs, including blood pressure; keep blood pressure cuff in place and deflated to lessen disturbance to child.
  - Take and record vital signs more frequently if any value fluctuates.
- Inspect operative area.
- Check dressing if present.
  - Outline any bleeding area on dressing or cast with pen.
  - Reinforce, but do not remove, loose dressing.
  - Observe areas below surgical site for blood that may have drained toward bed.
  - Assess for bleeding and other symptoms in areas not covered with a dressing such as throat after tonsillectomy.
- Assess skin color and characteristics.
- Assess level of consciousness and activity.
- Notify health care provider of any irregularities in child's condition.
- Assess for evidence of pain. (See Pain Assessment, Chapter 30.)
- Review surgeon's orders after completing initial assessment and check that any preoperative orders such as seizure or cardiac medications have been reordered and can be given by available routes (oral preparations may be contraindicated).
- Monitor vital signs as ordered and more often if indicated.
- Check dressings for bleeding or other abnormalities.
- Check bowel sounds.
- Observe for signs of shock, abdominal distention, and bleeding.
- Assess for bladder distention.
- Observe for signs of dehydration.
- Detect presence of infection:
  - Take vital signs every 2 to 4 hours as ordered.
  - Collect or request needed specimens.
  - Inspect wound for signs of infection—redness, swelling, heat, pain, and purulent drainage.

end-expiratory pressure, lack of turning, use of a specialty bed in the turning mode, and weight loss (McCord, McElvain, Sachdeva, et al., 2004). Medical devices such as pulse oximeter probes, bilevel and continuous positive airway pressure masks, oxygen cannulas, orthotics, and casts can also cause pressure ulcers.

Pressure ulcers are staged to classify the amount of tissue damage that has occurred.* Necrotic tissue must be removed so the tissue depth can be assessed accurately. Accurate documentation of redness or obvious skin breakdown is essential. Color, size (diameter and depth), location, presence of sinus tracts, odor, exudate, and response to treatment are observed and recorded at least daily.

Pressure ulcers can develop when the pressure on the skin and underlying tissues is greater than the capillary closing pressure, causing capillary occlusion. If the pressure remains unrelieved, vessels can collapse, resulting in tissue anoxia and cellular death. Pressure ulcers most often occur over bony prominences. These lesions are usually very deep (stage IV), extending into subcutaneous tissue or even more deeply into muscle, tendon, or bone.

---

*Staging of pressure ulcers and guidelines for prevention and management of pressure ulcers are available from the National Pressure Ulcer Advisory Panel, npuap.org.

Skin Care

- Keep skin free of excess moisture (e.g., urine or fecal incontinence, wound drainage, excessive perspiration).
- Cleanse skin with mild nonalkaline soap or soap-free cleaning agents for routine bathing.
- Provide daily cleansing of eyes, oral and diaper or perineal areas, and any areas of skin breakdown.
- Apply non–alcohol-based moisturizing agents after cleansing to retain moisture and rehydrate skin.
- Use minimum amount of tape and adhesives. On very sensitive skin use a protective, pectin-based or hydrocolloid skin barrier between skin and tape or adhesives.
- Place pectin-based or hydrocolloid skin barriers directly over excoriated skin. Leave barrier undisturbed until it begins to peel off or for 5 to 7 days. With wet, oozing excoriations, place a small amount of stoma powder on site, remove excess powder, and apply skin barrier. Hold barrier in place for several minutes to allow it to soften and mold to skin surface.
- Alternate electrode and probe placement sites and thoroughly assess underlying skin typically every 8 to 24 hours.
- Eliminate pressure secondary to medical devices such as tracheostomy tubes, wheelchairs, braces, and gastrostomy tubes.
- Be certain that fingers or toes are visible whenever extremity is used for intravenous (IV) or arterial line.
- Use a drawsheet to move child in bed or onto a stretcher; do not drag child from under arms.
- Position in neutral alignment; pillows, cushions, or wedges may be needed to prevent hip abduction and pressure to bony prominences such as heels, elbows, and sacral and occipital areas. When child is positioned laterally, pillows or cushions between knees, under head, and under upper arm helps promote neutral body alignment. Avoid donut cushions because they can cause tissue ischemia. Elevate head of bed 30 degrees or less to reduce pressure unless contraindicated.
- Do not massage reddened bony prominences because this can cause deep tissue damage; provide pressure relief to those areas instead.
- Routinely assess the child's nutritional status. A child who is NPO (nothing by mouth) for several days and is receiving only IV fluids is nutritionally at risk, which can also affect the ability of the skin to maintain its integrity. Consider parenteral nutrition.

A pressure-reduction device reduces pressure but does not prevent it from causing capillary closure; therefore turning and repositioning are always included when using these devices. Most of these items are overlays that are placed on top of the regular mattress. A pressure-relief device maintains pressure below that which would cause capillary closure. These devices are usually high-technology beds that are used for patients who have multiple problems and cannot be turned effectively.

Friction and shear contribute to pressure ulcers. Friction occurs when the surface of the skin rubs against another surface such as bedsheets. The skin may have the appearance of an abrasion. Skin damage is usually limited to the epidermal and upper layers. It most often occurs over the elbows, heels, or occiput. Prevention of friction injury includes the use of customized splinting over infants' heels; gel pillows under the heads of infants and toddlers; moisturizing agents; transparent dressings over susceptible areas; and soft, smooth bed linens and clothing (Baharestani and Ratliff, 2007). By itself friction does not cause tissue necrosis; however, when it acts with gravity, it results in shear injury.

Shear is the result of the force of gravity pushing down on the body and friction of the body against a surface such as the bed or chair. For example, when a patient is in the semi-Fowler position and begins to slide to the foot of the bed, the skin over the sacral area remains in the same place because of the resistance of the bed surface. The blood vessels in the area are stretched and may cause small-vessel thrombosis and tissue death (Bryant and Doughty, 2000). Prevention of shear injury includes using lift sheets when repositioning a patient, elevating the bed no more than 30 degrees for short periods, and using the knee gatch to interrupt the pull of gravity on the body toward the foot of the bed.

Epidermal stripping results when the epidermis is removed unintentionally when tape is removed. These lesions are usually shallow and irregularly shaped. Babies are at increased risk for epidermal injury. Prevention includes using no tape when possible, securing dressings with laced binders (Montgomery straps) or stretchy netting (Spandage or stockinette). Using porous or low-tack tapes (e.g., Medipore, paper, hydrogel), using alcohol-free skin sealants (No Sting Barrier Film), or picture framing wounds with hydrocolloid or wafer barriers (e.g., DuoDERM, Coloplast, Stomahesive) and then taping on top of the barrier also reduces epidermal stripping.

Tape is placed so there is no tension, traction, or wrinkles on the skin. To remove tape, slowly peel it away while stabilizing the underlying skin. Adhesive remover may be used to break the adhesive bond but may be drying to the skin. Avoid adhesive removers in preterm neonates because absorption rates vary and toxicity may occur. Remove the adhesive with water to prevent absorption and irritation. Wetting the tape with water or alcohol-based foam hand cleansers may facilitate removal.

Chemical factors can also lead to skin damage. Fecal incontinence, especially when mixed with urine; wound drainage; or gastric drainage around gastrostomy tubes can erode the epidermis. The skin can quickly progress from redness to denudement if exposure continues. Moisture barriers, gentle cleansing as soon after exposure as possible, and skin barriers can be used to prevent damage caused by chemical factors. In addition, foam dressings that wick moisture away from the skin are helpful around gastrostomy tubes and tracheostomy sites.

Bathing

Most infants and children can be bathed in a basin at the bedside or on the bed in a standard bathtub or shower. For infants and young children confined to bed, use the towel method. Immerse two towels in a dilute soap solution and wring them damp. With the child lying supine on a dry towel, place one damp towel on top of the child and use it to gently clean the body. Discard the towel, dry the child, and turn him or her prone. Repeat the procedure using the second damp towel.

School-age children and adolescents may shower or bathe. Nurses need to use judgment regarding the amount of supervision the child requires. Some can assume this responsibility unaided, but others need someone in constant attendance. Children with cognitive impairments, physical limitations such as severe anemia or leg deformities, or suicidal or psychotic problems (who may commit bodily harm) require close supervision.

Areas that require special attention are the ears, between skinfolds, the neck, the back, and the genital area. The genital area should be cleansed carefully and dried, with particular care given to skinfolds. In uncircumcised boys, usually those older than 3 years of age, the foreskin should be retracted gently, the exposed surfaces cleansed, and the foreskin then replaced. If the condition of the glans indicates inadequate cleaning such as accumulated smegma, inflammation, phimosis, or foreskin adhesions, teaching proper hygiene is indicated. In the Vietnamese and Cambodian cultures the foreskin traditionally is not retracted until adulthood. Older children have a tendency to avoid cleaning the genitalia; therefore they may need a gentle reminder.

Oral Hygiene

Mouth care is an integral part of daily hygiene and should be continued in the hospital. For some young children this is their first introduction to the use of a toothbrush. Infants and debilitated children require the nurse or a family member to perform mouth care. Although young children can manage a toothbrush and are encouraged to use it, most need assistance to perform satisfactorily. Although older children are capable of brushing and flossing without assistance, they sometimes need to be reminded.

Hair Care

Children should have their hair brushed and combed at least once daily. The hair is styled for comfort and in a manner pleasing to the child and parents. It should not be cut without parental permission, although clipping hair to provide access to a scalp vein for IV insertion may be necessary.

If children are hospitalized for more than a few days, the hair may need to be shampooed. Infants' hair may be washed during the daily bath or less frequently. For most children washing the hair and scalp once or twice weekly is sufficient unless there is an indication for more frequent washing such as after a high fever and profuse sweating. Adolescents normally have increased oily sebaceous secretions that require frequent hair care and more frequent shampoos.

Almost any child can be transported to an accessible sink for shampooing. Those who are unable to be transported can receive a shampoo in their beds with adequate protection, specially adapted equipment or positioning, or dry shampoo caps. When necessary a shampoo basin may be used or the child may be positioned near the edge of the bed, towels placed under the shoulders, a large plastic garbage bag draped at the edge of the bed with one open end under the shoulders, and the hair placed inside the opening. The other end is opened and placed in a collection container. Water can be transported in a basin.

Feeding the Sick Child

Loss of appetite is a symptom common to most childhood illnesses. Because an acute illness is usually short, the nutritional state is seldom compromised. Urging food on the sick child may precipitate nausea and vomiting. In most cases children can usually determine their own need for food.

Refusing to eat may also be one way children can exert power and control in an otherwise helpless situation. For young children loss of appetite may be related to depression caused by separation from their parents. Parents' concern with eating can intensify the problem. Forcing a child to eat meets with rebellion and reinforces the behavior as a control mechanism. Encourage parents to relax any pressure during an acute illness. Although it is best to provide high-quality, nutritious foods, the child may desire foods and liquids that contain mostly empty or nonnutritional calories. Some well-tolerated foods include gelatin, diluted clear soups, carbonated drinks, flavored ice pops, dry toast, and crackers. Even though these substances are not nutritious, they can provide necessary fluid and calories.

Dehydration is always a hazard when children have a fever or anorexia, especially when accompanied by vomiting or diarrhea.

GUIDELINES

Feeding a Sick Child

- Take a dietary history (see Chapter 29) and use information to make eating time as similar to eating at home as possible.
- Encourage parents or other family members to feed child or be present at mealtimes.
- Make mealtimes pleasant; avoid any procedures immediately before or after eating; make certain that child is rested and pain free.
- Serve small, frequent meals rather than three large meals or serve three meals and nutritious between-meal snacks.
- Provide finger foods for young children.
- Involve children in food selection and preparation whenever possible.
- Serve small portions and serve each course separately such as soup first followed by meat, potatoes, and vegetables and ending with dessert. With young children camouflage size of food by cutting meat thicker so less appears on plate or folding a cheese slice in half. Offer second helpings.
- Ensure a variety of foods, textures, and colors.
- Provide food selections that are favorites of most children such as peanut butter and jelly sandwiches, hot dogs, hamburgers, macaroni and cheese, pizza, spaghetti, tacos, fried chicken, corn, and fruit yogurt.
- Avoid foods that are highly seasoned, have strong odors, or are all mixed together unless typical of cultural practices.
- Provide fluid selections that are favorites of most children such as fruit punch, cola, ginger ale, sweetened tea, flavored ice pops, sherbet, ice cream, milk, milkshakes, pudding, gelatin, clear broth, or creamed soups.
- Offer nutritious snacks such as frozen yogurt or pudding, ice cream, oatmeal or peanut butter cookies, hot cocoa, cheese slices, pieces of raw vegetable or fruit, and dried fruit or cereal.
- Make food attractive and different; for example:
  - Serve a "picnic lunch" in a paper bag.
  - Pack food in a Chinese take-out container; decorate container.
  - Put a "face" or a "flower" on a hamburger or sandwich with pieces of vegetable.
  - Use a cookie cutter to shape a sandwich.
  - Serve pudding, yogurt, or juice frozen as an ice pop.
  - Make Slurpies or snow cones by pouring flavored syrup on crushed ice.
  - Add food coloring to water or milk.
  - Serve fluids through brightly colored or unusually shaped straws.
  - Make "bowtie" sandwiches by cutting them in triangles and placing two points together.
  - Slice sandwiches into "fingers."
  - Grate mounds of cheese.
  - Cut apples horizontally to make circles.
  - Put a banana on a hot dog bun and spread with peanut butter.
  - Break uncooked spaghetti into toothpick lengths and skewer cheese, cold meat, vegetables, or fruit chunks.
- Praise children for what they do eat.
- Do not punish children for not eating by removing their dessert or putting them to bed.

Fluids should not be forced, and the child is not awakened to take fluids. Forcing fluids may create the same difficulties as urging the child to eat unwanted food. Gentle persuasion with preferred beverages will usually meet with success. Using play techniques can also be effective (see Guidelines box).

When the child is feeling better, appetite usually begins to improve. It is best to take advantage of any hungry period by serving high-quality foods and snacks. If the child still refuses to eat, offer nutritious fluids such as prepared breakfast drinks. Parents can help by bringing in food items from home, especially if the family's cultural eating habits differ from the hospital food. A clinical dietitian may be consulted for alternative food choices.

When children are placed on special diets such as clear liquids after surgery or during episodes of diarrhea, it is essential to assess their intake and readiness to advance to more complex foods.

Regardless of the type of diet, charting the amount consumed is an important nursing responsibility. Descriptions need to be detailed and accurate such as "4 oz of orange juice, one pancake, and 8 oz of milk." Comments such as "ate well" or "ate poorly" are inadequate. Charting the percentage of the meal eaten is also inadequate unless food is measured before serving.

If the parents are involved in the child's care, encourage them to keep a list of everything he or she eats. Using a premeasured cup for fluids ensures a more accurate estimate of intake. A comparison of the intake at each meal can isolate food deficiencies such as insufficient intake of meat or vegetables. Behaviors associated with mealtime also identify possible factors influencing appetite. For example, the observation, "Child eats well when with other children but plays with food if left alone in room," helps the nurse plan mealtime activities that stimulate the child's appetite.

Although sick children's appetites may be poor and not characteristic of their home eating habits, the hospital stay provides numerous opportunities for nurses to assess the family's knowledge of good nutrition and to implement teaching as needed to improve nutritional intake.

Controlling Elevated Temperatures

An elevated temperature, most frequently from fever but occasionally caused by hyperthermia, is one of the most common symptoms of illness in children. This manifestation is a great concern to parents. To facilitate an understanding of fever, the following terms are defined:

- *Set point*—The temperature around which body temperature is regulated by a thermostat-like mechanism in the hypothalamus
- *Fever (hyperpyrexia)*—An elevation in set point such that body temperature is regulated at a higher level; may be arbitrarily defined as temperature above 38° C (100.4° F)
- *Hyperthermia*—Body temperature exceeding the set point, which usually results from the body or external conditions creating more heat than the body can eliminate such as in heat stroke, aspirin toxicity, seizures, or hyperthyroidism

Body temperature is regulated by a thermostat-like mechanism in the hypothalamus. This mechanism receives input from centrally and peripherally located receptors. When temperature changes occur, these receptors relay the information to the thermostat, which either increases or decreases heat production to maintain a constant set point temperature. However, during an infection pyrogenic substances cause an increase in the normal set point of the body, a process that is mediated by prostaglandins. Consequently the hypothalamus increases heat production until the core temperature reaches the new set point.

During the fever (febrile) state shivering and vasoconstriction generate and conserve heat during the chill phase of fever, raising central temperatures to the level of the new set point. The temperature reaches a plateau when it stabilizes in the higher range. When the temperature is greater than the set point or when the pyrogen is no longer present, a crisis, or defervescence, of the temperature occurs.

Most fevers in children are of brief duration with limited consequences and are viral in origin. When fever is caused by bacteria, endotoxins are produced that activate the inflammatory process and produce fever (Rote, Huether, and McCance, 2000). Fever has physiologic benefits, including increased white blood cell activity, interferon production and effectiveness, and antibody production and enhancement of some antibiotic effects (Considine and Brennan, 2007). Contrary to popular belief, neither the rise in temperature nor its response to antipyretics indicates the severity or etiology of the infection, which casts doubt on the value of using fever as a diagnostic or prognostic indicator.

Therapeutic Management

Treatment of elevated temperature depends on whether it is attributable to a fever or hyperthermia. Because the set point is normal in hyperthermia but increased in fever, different approaches must be used to lower body temperature successfully.

Fever. The principal reason for treating fever is the relief of discomfort. Relief measures include pharmacologic and environmental intervention. The most effective intervention is the use of antipyretics to lower the set point.

Antipyretics include acetaminophen, aspirin, and nonsteroidal antiinflammatory drugs (NSAIDs). Acetaminophen is the preferred drug. Aspirin should not be given to children because of its association in children with influenza virus or chickenpox and Reye syndrome. One nonprescription NSAID, ibuprofen, is approved for fever reduction in children as young as 6 months of age. The dosage is based on the initial temperature level: 5 mg/kg of body weight for temperatures less than 39.2° C (102.6° F) or 10 mg/kg for temperatures greater than 39.2° C. The recommended dosage for pain is 10 mg/kg every 6 to 8 hours, and the recommended maximum daily dose for pain and fever is 40 mg/kg. The duration of fever reduction is generally 6 to 8 hours and is longer with the higher dose.

The recommended doses of acetaminophen should never be exceeded. Acetaminophen should be given every 4 hours but no more than 5 times in 24 hours. Because body temperature normally decreases at night, three or four doses in 24 hours will control most fevers. The temperature is usually retaken 30 minutes after the antipyretic is given to assess its effect but should not be measured repeatedly. The child's level of discomfort is the best indication for continued treatment.

The nurse can use environmental measures to reduce fever if they are tolerated by the child and if they do not induce shivering. Shivering is the way that the body has of maintaining the elevated set point by producing heat. Compensatory shivering greatly increases metabolic requirements above those already caused by the fever.

Traditional cooling measures such as wearing minimum clothing; exposing the skin to air; reducing room temperature; increasing air circulation; and applying cool, moist compresses to the skin (e.g., the forehead) are effective if used approximately 1 hour after an antipyretic is given so the set point is lowered. Cooling procedures such as sponging or tepid baths are ineffective in treating febrile children (these measures are effective for hyperthermia) either when used alone or in combination with antipyretics, and they cause considerable discomfort (Axelrod, 2000).

Seizures associated with a fever occur in 3% to 4% of all children, usually in those between 6 months and 6 years of age. Approximately 30% of children have subsequent febrile seizures; a younger age at onset and a family history of febrile seizures are associated with increased incidence of recurring episodes. There is little evidence to support the use of antipyretic drugs or anticonvulsants to prevent a second febrile seizure; nursing intervention should focus on ways to provide care and comfort during a febrile illness. Simple febrile seizures lasting less than 10 minutes do not cause brain damage or other debilitating effects (Jones and Jacobsen, 2007; Sadleir and Scheffer, 2007). (See Febrile Seizures, Chapter 45.)

Hyperthermia. Unlike in fever, antipyretics are of no value in hyperthermia because the set point is already normal. Consequently cooling measures are used. Cool applications to the skin help reduce the core temperature. Cooled blood from the skin surface is conducted to inner organs and tissues; and warm blood is circulated to the surface, where it is cooled and recirculated. The surface blood vessels dilate as the body attempts to dissipate heat to the environment and facilitate this cooling process.

Commercial cooling devices such as cooling blankets or mattresses are available to reduce body temperature. Place the patient on the bed and cover with a sheet or lightweight blanket. Frequent temperature monitoring is essential to prevent excessive cooling of the body.

Traditionally cool compresses decrease high temperature. For tepid tub baths it is usually best to start with warm water and gradually add cool water until the desired water temperature of 37° C (98.6° F) is reached to acclimate the child to the lower water temperature. Generally the temperature of the water only has to be 1° C (or 2° F) less than the child's temperature to be effective. The child is placed directly in the tub of tepid water for 15 to 20 minutes while water is gently squeezed from a washcloth over the back and chest or gently sprayed over the body from a sprayer. In the bed or crib cool washcloths or towels are used, exposing only one area of the body at a time. Continue sponging for approximately 20 minutes.

After the tub or sponge bath the child is dried and dressed in lightweight pajamas, a nightgown, or a diaper and placed in a dry bed. He or she is dried by gently rubbing the skin surface with a towel to stimulate circulation. The temperature is retaken 30 minutes after the tub or sponge bath. The tub or sponge bath should not be continued or restarted until the skin surface is warm or if the child feels chilled. Chilling causes vasoconstriction, which defeats the purpose of the cool applications. In this condition little blood is carried to the skin surface; the blood remains primarily in the viscera to become heated.

Whether a temperature elevation in the critically ill child is caused by fever or hyperthermia, it should be treated aggressively. The metabolic rate increases 10% for every 1° C increase in temperature and 3 to 5 times during shivering, thus increasing oxygen, fluid, and caloric requirements. If the child's cardiovascular or neurologic system is already compromised, these increased needs are especially hazardous. In all children with an elevated temperature, attention to adequate hydration is essential. Most children's needs can be met through additional oral fluids.

Family Teaching and Home Care

Fever is one of the most common problems for which parents seek health care. High levels of parental anxiety (fever phobia) surrounding potential complications of fever such as seizures and dehydration are prevalent and can result in overusing antipyretics (Purssell, 2008). Parents need to know that sponging is indicated for elevated temperatures from hyperthermia rather than fever and that ice water and alcohol are inappropriate, potentially dangerous solutions (Axelrod, 2000). They should know how to take the child's temperature, how to read the thermometer accurately, and when to seek professional care (see Family-Centered Care box). Some of the newer temperature-measuring devices such as plastic strip or digital thermometers may be better suited for home use. (See Temperature, Chapter 29.) If the use of acetaminophen or ibuprofen is indicated,

---

FAMILY-CENTERED CARE
The Child with Fever

Call Office Immediately If:
- Your child is younger than 2 months old.
- The fever is over 40.6° C (105° F).
- Your child looks or acts very sick, including a stiff neck, persistent vomiting, purplish spots on the skin, confusion, trouble breathing after you have cleaned his or her nose, or inability to be comforted.

Call Within 24 Hours If:
- The fever is between 40° and 40.6° C (104° and 105° F), especially if your child is younger than 2 years old.
- Your child has had a fever for more than 24 hours without an obvious cause or location of infection.
- Your child has had a fever for more than 3 days.
- Your child has burning or pain with urination.
- Your child has a history of febrile seizures.
- The fever went away for more than 24 hours and then returned.
- You have other concerns or questions.

Modified from Schmitt BD: *Instructions for pediatric patients*, ed 2, Philadelphia, 1999, Saunders.

---

the parents need instructions in administering the drug. Emphasize accuracy in both the amount of drug given and the time intervals at which the drug is administered. Along with reduced activity, encourage small, frequent sips of clear liquids. Dress the child in light clothing; use a light blanket for children who are cold or shivering (Walsh and Edwards, 2006).

SAFETY

Safety is an essential component of any patient's care, but children have special characteristics that require an even greater concern for safety. Because small children in the hospital are separated from their usual environment and do not possess the capacity for abstract thinking and reasoning, it is the responsibility of everyone who comes in contact with them to maintain protective measures throughout their hospital stay. Nurses need to understand the age level at which each child is operating and plan for safety accordingly.

Identification (ID) bands are particularly important for children. Infants and unconscious patients are unable to tell or respond to their names. Toddlers may answer to any name or to a nickname only. Older children may exchange places, give an erroneous name, or choose not to respond to their own names as a joke, unaware of the hazards of such practices.

Environmental Factors

All of the environmental safety measures for the protection of adults apply to children, including good illumination, floors that are clear of fluid and objects that might contribute to falls, and nonskid surfaces in showers and tubs. All staff members should be familiar with the area-specific fire plan. Elevators and stairways should be made safe.

All windows should be secured. Window blind and curtain cords should be out of reach with split cords to prevent strangulation. Pacifiers should not be tied around the neck or attached to an infant by string.

Electrical equipment should be in proper working order and used only by personnel familiar with its use. It should not be in contact with moisture or situated near tubs. Electrical outlets should have covers to prevent burns in small children, whose exploratory activities may extend to inserting objects into the small openings.

Staff members should practice proper care and disposal of small objects such as syringe caps, needle covers, and temperature probes. Staff also must check bathwater carefully before placing the child in it and never leave children alone in a bathtub. Infants are helpless in water, and small children (and some older ones) may turn on the hot water faucet and be burned severely.

Furniture is safest when it is scaled to the child's proportions, sturdy, and well balanced to prevent it being tipped over easily. A special hazard for children is the danger of entrapment under an electronically controlled bed when it is activated to descend. Infants and small children must be securely strapped into infant seats, feeding chairs, and strollers. Baby walkers should not be used because they provide access to hazards, resulting in burns, falls, and poisonings. Infants; young children; and children who are weak, paralyzed, agitated, confused, sedated, or cognitively impaired are never left unattended on treatment tables, on scales, or in treatment areas. Even premature infants are capable of surprising mobility; therefore portholes in incubators must be securely fastened when not in use.

Crib sides up should always be raised and fastened securely. Use cribs that meet federal safety standards (www.cpsc.gov/info/cribs/index.html). Anyone attending an infant or small child on a stretcher or table should never turn away without maintaining hand contact with the child (i.e., keeping one hand on the child's back or abdomen to prevent rolling, crawling, or jumping from the open crib (Fig. 39-3).

The safest sleeping position to prevent sudden infant death syndrome is wholly supine (AAP, Task Force on Sudden Infant Death Syndrome, 2005). No pillows should be placed in a young infant's crib while the infant is sleeping.

Toys

Toys play a vital role in the everyday lives of children, and they are no less important in the hospital setting. Nurses are responsible for assessing the safety of toys brought to the hospital by well-meaning parents and friends. They should be appropriate to the child's age, condition, and treatment. For example, if the child is receiving oxygen, electrical or friction toys or equipment are not safe because sparks can cause oxygen to ignite. Inspect toys to ensure that they are nonallergenic, washable, and unbreakable and that they have no small, removable parts that can be aspirated or swallowed or otherwise inflict injury on a child. All objects within reach of children younger than 3 years of age should pass the choke tube test. A toilet

paper roll is a handy guide. If a toy or object fits into the cylinder (items <1¼ inches [3.175 cm] across or balls <1¾ inches [4.45 cm] in diameter), it is a potential choking danger to the child. Latex balloons pose a serious threat to children of all ages. If the balloon breaks, a child may put a piece of the latex in his or her mouth. If it is aspirated or swallowed, the latex piece is difficult to remove, resulting in choking. Latex balloons should never be permitted in the hospital setting.

Preventing Falls

Falls prevention begins with identification of children most at risk for falls. Pediatric hospitals use various methods to identify a child's risk for falls (Child Health Corporation of America, 2009). After a risk assessment is performed, multiple interventions are needed to minimize pediatric patients' risk of falling, including education of patient, family, and staff.

To identify children at risk of falling, perform a fall risk assessment on patients on admission and throughout hospitalization. Risk factors for hospitalized children include the following:

- Medication effects—Postanesthesia or sedation; analgesics or narcotics, especially in those who have never had narcotics in the past and in whom effects are unknown
- Altered mental status—Secondary to seizures, brain tumors, or medications
- Altered or limited mobility—Reduced skill at ambulation secondary to developmental age, disease process, tubes, drains, casts, splints, or other appliances; new to ambulation with assistive devices such as walkers or crutches
- Postoperative children—Risk of hypotension or syncope secondary to large blood loss, a heart condition, or extended bed rest
- History of falls
- Infants or toddlers in cribs with side rails down or on the daybed with family members
- Once children at risk for falls have been identified, alert other staff members by posting signs on the door and at the bedside, applying a special colored armband labeled "Fall Precautions," labeling the chart with a sticker, or documenting information on the chart.

Prevention of falls requires alterations in the environment, including the following:

- Keep the bed in the lowest position with the breaks locked and the side rails up.
- Place the call bell within reach.
- Ensure that all necessary and desired items are within reach (e.g., water, glasses, tissues, snacks).
- Offer toileting on a regular basis, especially if the patient is taking diuretics or laxatives.
- Keep lights on at all times, including dim lights while sleeping.
- Lock wheelchairs before transferring patients.
- Ensure that the patient has an appropriate-size gown and nonskid footwear. Do not allow gowns or ties to drag on the floor during ambulation.
- Keep the floor clean and free of clutter. Post a "wet floor" sign if the floor is wet.
- Ensure that the patient has glasses on if he or she normally wears them.

Preventing falls also relies on age-appropriate education of patients. Help the child ambulate even though he or she may have ambulated well before hospitalization. Patients who have been lying in bed need to get up slowly, sitting on the side of the bed before standing.

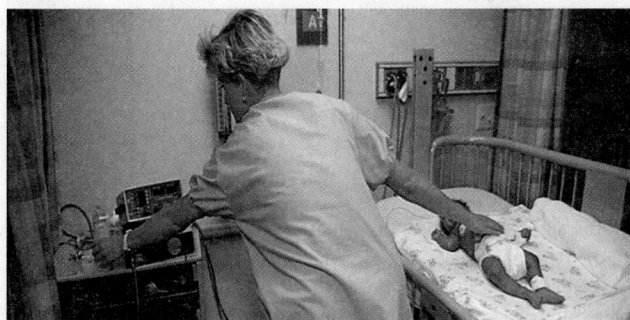

FIG 39-3 The nurse maintains hand contact when her back is turned.

The nurse also needs to educate family members:

- Call the nursing staff for assistance and do not allow patients to get up independently.
- Keep the side rails of the crib or bed up whenever patient is in it.
- Do not leave infants on the daybed; put them in the crib with the side rails up.
- When all family members need to leave the bedside, notify the staff and ensure that the patient is in the bed or crib with the side rails up and call bell within reach (if appropriate).

Infection Control

According to the Centers for Disease Control and Prevention (CDC), approximately 2 million patients each year develop nosocomial (hospital-acquired) infections. These infections occur when there is interaction among patients, health care personnel, equipment, and bacteria (Quality, Equipment Hold Keys to Infection Control, 2006). Nosocomial infections are preventable if caregivers practice meticulous cleaning and disposal techniques.

Standard Precautions synthesize the major features of universal (blood and body fluid) precautions (designed to reduce the risk of transmission of bloodborne pathogens) and body substance isolation (designed to reduce the risk of transmission of pathogens from moist body substances). Standard Precautions involve the use of barrier protection such as gloves, goggles, gown, or mask to prevent contamination from (1) blood; (2) all body fluids, secretions, and excretions except sweat, regardless of whether they contain visible blood; (3) nonintact skin; and (4) mucous membranes. They are designed for the care of all patients to reduce the risk of transmission of microorganisms from both recognized and unrecognized sources of infection.

Transmission-based precautions are designed for patients with documented or suspected infection or colonization (presence of microorganisms in or on patient but without clinical signs and symptoms of infection) with highly transmissible or epidemiologically important pathogens for which additional precautions beyond Standard Precautions are needed to interrupt transmission in hospitals. There are three types of transmission-based precautions: Airborne Precautions, Droplet Precautions, and Contact Precautions. They may be combined for diseases that have multiple routes of transmission (Box 39-2). They are to be used in addition to Standard Precautions.

Airborne Precautions reduce the risk of airborne transmission of infectious agents. Airborne transmission occurs by dissemination of either airborne droplet nuclei (small-particle residue [<5 mm] of evaporated droplets that may remain suspended in the air for long periods) or dust particles containing the infectious agent. Microorganisms carried in this manner can be dispersed widely by air currents and may become inhaled by or deposited on a susceptible host within the same room or over a longer distance from the source patient, depending on environmental factors. Special air handling and ventilation are required to prevent airborne transmission. Airborne Precautions apply to patients with known or suspected infection with pathogens transmitted by the airborne route such as measles, varicella, and tuberculosis.

Droplet Precautions reduce the risk of droplet transmission of infectious agents. Droplet transmission involves contact of the conjunctivae or the mucous membranes of the nose or mouth of a susceptible person with large-particle droplets (>5 mm) containing microorganisms generated from a person who has a clinical disease or who is a carrier of the microorganism. Droplets are generated from the source person primarily during coughing, sneezing, or

---

BOX 39-2 TYPES OF PRECAUTIONS AND PATIENTS REQUIRING THEM

Standard Precautions for Preventing Transmission of Pathogens

Use Standard Precautions for the care of all patients.

Airborne Precautions

In addition to Standard Precautions, use Airborne Precautions for patients known or suspected to have serious illnesses transmitted by airborne droplet nuclei. Examples of such illnesses include measles, varicella (including disseminated zoster), and tuberculosis.

Droplet Precautions

In addition to Standard Precautions, use Droplet Precautions for patients known or suspected to have serious illnesses transmitted by large-particle droplets. Examples of such illnesses include the following:

- Invasive *Haemophilus influenzae* type b disease, including meningitis, pneumonia, epiglottitis, and sepsis
- Invasive *Neisseria meningitidis* disease, including meningitis, pneumonia, and sepsis
- Other serious bacterial respiratory tract infections spread by droplet transmission, including diphtheria (pharyngeal), mycoplasmal pneumonia, pertussis, pneumonic plague, streptococcal pharyngitis, pneumonia, and scarlet fever in infants and young children
- Serious viral infections spread by droplet transmission, including adenovirus, influenza, mumps, parvovirus B19, and rubella

Contact Precautions

In addition to Standard Precautions, use Contact Precautions for patients known or suspected to have serious illnesses easily transmitted by direct patient contact or contact with items in the patient's environment. Examples of such illnesses include the following:

- Gastrointestinal, respiratory, skin, or wound infections or colonization with multidrug-resistant bacteria judged by the infection control program based on current state, regional, or national recommendations to be of special clinical and epidemiologic significance
- Enteric infections with a low infectious dose or prolonged environmental survival, including *Clostridium difficile;* for diapered or incontinent patients: enterohemorrhagic *Escherichia coli* O157:H7, *Shigella* organisms, hepatitis A, or rotavirus
- Respiratory syncytial virus, parainfluenza virus, or enteroviral infections in infants and young children.
- Skin infections that are highly contagious or that may occur on dry skin, including diphtheria (cutaneous), herpes simplex virus (neonatal or mucocutaneous), impetigo, major (noncontained) abscesses, cellulitis or decubitus, pediculosis, scabies, staphylococcal furunculosis in infants and young children, zoster (disseminated or in the immunocompromised host)
- Viral or hemorrhagic conjunctivitis
- Viral hemorrhagic infections (Ebola, Lassa, or Marburg)

Modified from Garner JS: Guidelines for isolation precautions in hospitals, *Infect Control Hosp Epidemiol* 17(1):66, 1996.

---

talking and during procedures such as suctioning and bronchoscopy. Transmission requires close contact between source and recipient persons because droplets do not remain suspended in the air and generally travel only short distances, usually 3 feet or less, through the air. Because droplets do not remain suspended in the air, special air handling and ventilation are not required to prevent droplet transmission. Droplet Precautions apply to any patient with known or suspected infection with pathogens that can be transmitted by infectious droplets (see Box 39-2).

Contact Precautions reduce the risk of transmission of microorganisms by direct or indirect contact. Direct-contact transmission involves skin-to-skin contact and physical transfer of microorganisms to a susceptible host from an infected or colonized person such as occurs when turning or bathing patients. Direct-contact transmission also can occur between two patients (e.g., by hand contact). Indirect contact transmission involves contact of a susceptible host with a contaminated intermediate object, usually inanimate, in the patient's environment. Contact Precautions apply to specified patients known or suspected to be infected or colonized with microorganisms that can be transmitted by direct or indirect contact.

> **! NURSING ALERT**
>
> The most common piece of medical equipment, the stethoscope, can be a potent source of harmful microorganisms and nosocomial infections.

Nurses caring for young children are frequently in contact with body substances, especially urine, feces, and vomitus. They need to exercise judgment concerning situations when gloves, gowns, or masks are necessary. For example, nurses should wear gloves and possibly gowns for changing diapers when there are loose or explosive stools. Otherwise the plastic lining of disposable diapers provides a sufficient barrier between the hands and body substances.

Antimicrobial-resistant organisms are causing increasing numbers of nosocomial infections. In hospitals patients are the most significant sources of methicillin-resistant *Staphylococcus aureus,* and the main mode of transmission is patient to patient via the hands of a health care provider (Eaton, 2005; Quality, Equipment Hold Keys to Infection Control, 2006). Hand washing is the most critical infection control practice.

During feedings wear a gown if the child is likely to vomit or spit up, which often occurs during burping. When wearing gloves, wash the hands thoroughly after removing them because gloves fail to provide complete protection. The absence of visible leaks does not indicate that the gloves are intact.

Another essential practice of infection control is that all needles (uncapped and unbroken) are disposed of in a rigid, puncture-resistant container located near the site of use. Consequently these containers are installed in patients' rooms. Because children are naturally curious, extra attention is needed in selecting a suitable type of container and a location that prevents access to the discarded needles (Fig. 39-4). The use of needleless systems allows secure syringe or IV tubing attachment to vascular access devices without the risk of needlestick injury to the child or nurse.

Transporting Infants and Children

Infants and children need to be transported within the unit and to areas outside the pediatric unit. Infants and small children can be carried for short distances within the unit, but for more extended trips the child should be securely transported in a suitable conveyance.

Small infants can be held or carried in the horizontal position with the back supported and the thigh grasped firmly by the carrying arm (Fig. 39-5, *A*). In the football hold the infant is carried on the nurse's arm with the head supported by the hand and the body held securely between the nurse's body and elbow (Fig. 39-5, *B*). Both of these holds leave the nurse's other arm free for activity. The

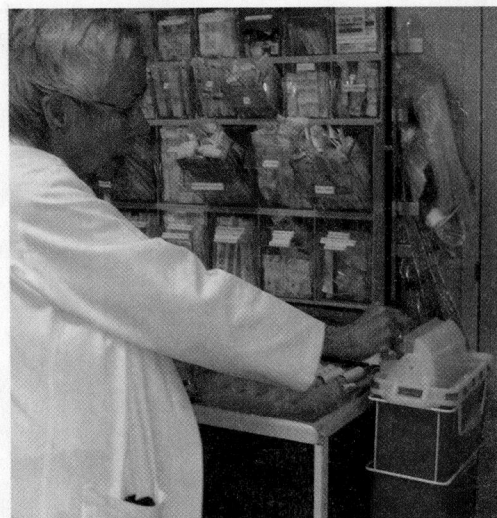

FIG 39-4 To prevent needlestick injuries, used needles (and other sharp instruments) are not capped or broken and are disposed of in rigid, puncture-resistant container located near site of use. Note placement of container to prevent children's access to contents.

infant also can be held in the upright position with the buttocks on the nurse's forearm and the front of the body resting against the nurse's chest. The infant's head and shoulders are supported by the nurse's other arm in case the infant moves suddenly (Fig. 39-5, *C*). Older infants are able to hold their heads erect but are still subject to sudden movements.

Special care is needed in transporting critically ill patients in the hospital. Critically ill children should always be transported on a stretcher or bed (rather than carried) by at least two staff members with monitoring continued during transport. A blood pressure monitor (or standard blood pressure cuff), pulse oximeter, and cardiac monitor/defibrillator should accompany every patient (Warren, Fromm, Orr, et al., 2004). Airway equipment and emergency medications should accompany the patient.

Restraining Methods and Therapeutic Holding

The Joint Commission (Joint Commission on Accreditation of Healthcare Organizations, 2001) defines restraint as "any method, physical or mechanical, which restricts a person's movement, physical activity, or normal access to his or her body." Before initiating restraints the nurse completes a comprehensive assessment of the patient to determine whether the need for a restraint outweighs the risk of not using one. Restraints can result in loss of dignity, violation of patient rights, psychologic harm, physical harm, and even death.

Consider alternative methods first and document them in the patient's record. Some examples of alternative measures include bringing a child to the nurses' station for continuous observation, providing diversional activities such as music, encouraging the participation of the parents, or therapeutic holding. Therapeutic holding is the use of a secure, comfortable, temporary holding position that provides close physical contact with the parent or caregiver for 30 minutes or less. The use of restraints can often be avoided with adequate preparation of the child, parental or staff supervision of the child, or adequate protection of a vulnerable site such as an infusion device.

The nurse needs to assess the child's development, mental status, potential to hurt others or self, and safety. He or she is responsible

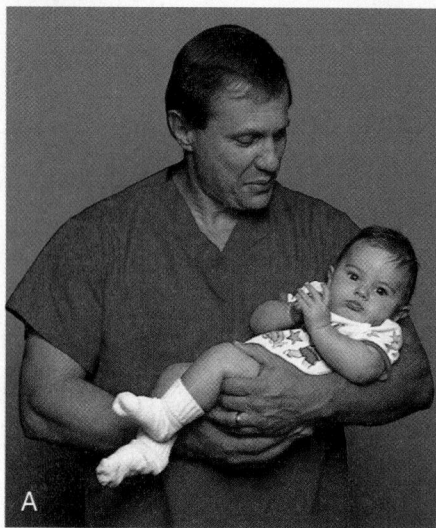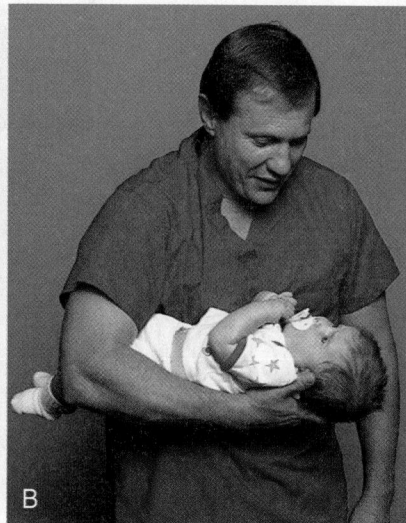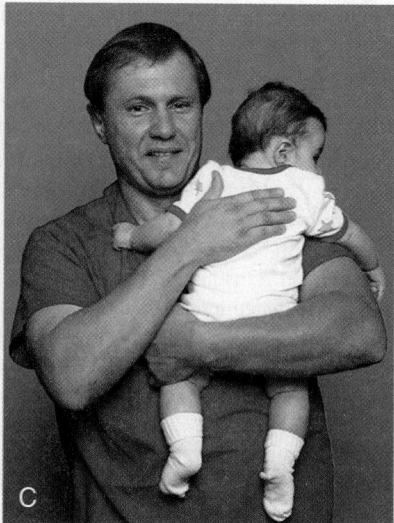

FIG 39-5 Transporting infants. **A,** Infant's thigh firmly grasped in nurse's hand. **B,** Football hold. **C,** Back supported.

for selecting the least restrictive type of restraint. Using less restrictive restraints is often possible by gaining the cooperation of the child and parents. Examples of less restrictive restraints are provided in Table 39-4.

The two types of restraints used with children are classified as medical-surgical and behavioral restraints. When a standard or protocol states that immobilization is required 100% of the time as part of the procedure or postprocedural care process, the restraint device is considered a part of routine care. For example, the postoperative use of elbow restraints after a cleft lip repair, if written in the protocol or standard of care and used for 100% of patients, would not fall under The Joint Commission or Centers for Medicare and Medicaid Services mandates concerning restraints.

Medical-surgical restraints are used for children with an artificial airway or airway adjunct for delivery of oxygen, indwelling catheters, tubes, drains, lines, pacemaker wires, or suture sites. The medical-surgical restraint is used to ensure that safe care is given to the patient. The potential risks of the restraint are offset by the potential benefit of providing safer care. Medical-surgical restraints may be instituted for any of the following reasons:

- Risk for interruption of therapy used to maintain oxygenation or airway patency
- Risk of harm if indwelling catheter, tube, drain, line, pacemaker wire, or suturing is removed, dislodged, or ruptured
- Patient confusion, agitation, unconsciousness, or developmental inability to understand direct requests or instructions

Medical-surgical restraints can be initiated by an individual order or protocol; the use of protocol must be authorized by an individual order. The order for continued use of restraints must be renewed each day. Patients are monitored at least every 2 hours.

Behavioral restraints are limited to situations in which there is a significant risk of patients physically harming themselves or others because of behavior and when nonphysical interventions are not effective. Before initiating a behavioral restraint, the nurse should assess the patient's mental, behavioral, and physical status to determine the cause for the child's potentially harmful behavior. If behavioral restraints are indicated, a collaborative approach involving the patient (if appropriate), the family, and the health care team should be used. An order must be obtained as soon as possible but no longer than 1 hour after the initiation of behavioral restraints. Behavioral

TABLE 39-4	RESTRAINING CHILDREN: LESS RESTRICTIVE TO MORE RESTRICTIVE TECHNIQUES				
TECHNIQUE OR DEVICE	**LESS RESTRICTIVE TO MORE RESTRICTIVE**				
Extremities					
Sleeves	X				
Hand mitts, mittens	X				
Stockinette		X			
Elbows (no-no's)			X		
Arm board				X	
One or two limbs					X
Three or four limbs					X
Chest and Body					
Belts, safety belts	X				
Posey vest, safety jacket			X		
Mummy restraint					X
Papoose board					X
Environment					
Side rails		X			
Crib tops		X			
Seclusion					X
Other					
Chemical			X		

Adapted from Selekman J, Snyder B: Uses of and alternatives to restraints in pediatric settings, *AACN Clin Issues* 7(4):603–610, 1996.

restraints for children must be reordered every 1 to 2 hours based on age. A licensed independent practitioner must conduct an in-person evaluation within 1 hour and again every 4 hours until restraints are discontinued. Children in behavioral restraints must be observed continuously and assessed every 15 minutes. Assessment components include signs of injury associated with applying restraint, nutrition and hydration, circulation and range-of-motion of extremities, vital signs, hygiene and elimination, physical and psychologic status and comfort, and readiness for discontinuation of restraint. The nurse must use clinical judgment in setting a schedule for when each of these parameters needs to be evaluated because every parameter must be assessed during each 15-minute physical assessment.

Restraints with ties must be secured to the bed or crib frame, not the side rails. Suggestions for increasing safety and comfort while the child is in a restraint include leaving one finger breadth between skin and the device and tying knots that allow for quick release. The nurse can also increase safety by ensuring that the restraint does not tighten as the child moves and decreasing wrinkles or bulges in it. Placing jacket restraints over an article of clothing; placing limb restraints below waist level, below knee level, or distal to the IV; and tucking in dangling straps also increase safety and comfort.

Mummy Restraint or Swaddle

When an infant or small child requires short-term restraint for examination or treatment that involves the head and neck (e.g., venipuncture, throat examination, gavage feeding), a papoose board with straps or a mummy wrap effectively controls the child's movements. A blanket or sheet is opened on the bed or crib with one corner folded to the center. The infant is placed on the blanket with the shoulders at the fold and feet toward the opposite corner. With the infant's right arm straight down against the body, the right side of the blanket is pulled firmly across the infant's right shoulder and chest and secured beneath the left side of the body. The left arm is placed straight against the infant's side, and the left side of the blanket is brought across the shoulder and chest and locked beneath the body on the right side. The lower corner is folded and brought over the body and tucked or fastened securely with safety pins. Safety pins can be used to fasten the blanket in place at any step in the process. To modify the mummy restraint for chest examination, bring the folded edge of the blanket over each arm and under the back and then fold the loose edge over and secure it at a point below the chest to allow visualization and access to the chest (Fig. 39-6, *A*).

Jacket Restraint

A jacket restraint is sometimes used to keep the child safe in various chairs. The jacket is put on the child with the ties in back so he or she is unable to manipulate them. The jacket restraint is also useful as a means of maintaining the child in a desired horizontal position. The long tapes secured to the understructure of the crib keep the child inside the crib.

Arm and Leg Restraints

Occasionally the nurse needs to restrain one or more extremities or limit their motion. Several commercial restraining devices are available, including disposable wrist and ankle restraints (Fig. 39-6, *B*). Restraints must be appropriate to the child's size and padded to prevent undue pressure, constriction, or tissue injury; and the extremity must be observed frequently for signs of irritation or impaired circulation. The ends of the restraints are never tied to the

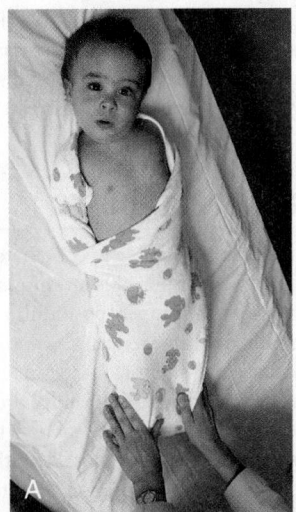

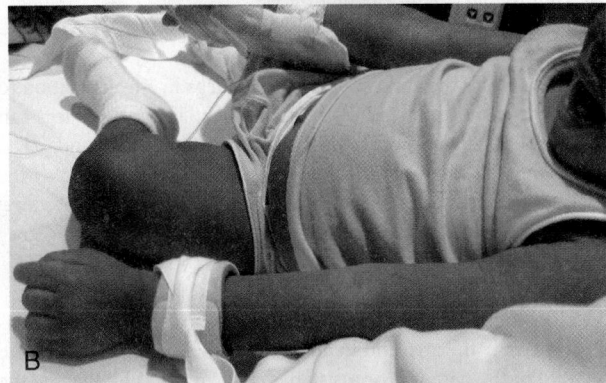

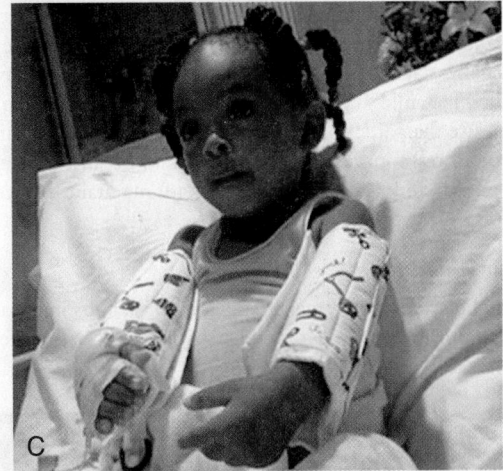

FIG 39-6 Restraint examples from most restrictive to least restrictive. **A,** Mummy restraint. **B,** Wrist restraints. **C,** Elbow restraints.

side rails because lowering the rail disturbs the extremity, frequently with a jerk that may hurt or injure the child.

Elbow Restraint

Sometimes it is important to prevent the child from reaching the head or face (e.g., after lip surgery, when a scalp vein infusion is in place, or to prevent scratching in skin disorders). Elbow restraints fashioned from a variety of materials function well (Fig. 39-6, *C*). Commercial elbow restraints are available. An improvised form of elbow restraint consists of a piece of muslin long enough to reach comfortably from just below the axilla to the wrist with a number of vertical pockets into which tongue depressors are inserted. The restraint is wrapped around the arm and secured with tapes or pins. It may be necessary to pin the top of the restraint to the undershirt sleeve to prevent the restraint from slipping.

POSITIONING FOR PROCEDURES

Infants and small children are unable to cooperate for many procedures. Therefore the nurse is responsible for minimizing their movement and discomfort with proper positioning. Older children usually need only minimal, if any, restraint. Careful explanation and preparation beforehand and support and simple guidance during the procedure are usually sufficient. For painful procedures the child should receive adequate analgesia and sedation to minimize pain and the need for excessive restraint. For local anesthesia use buffered lidocaine to reduce the stinging sensation or a topical anesthetic. (See Pain Management, Chapter 30.)

Femoral Venipuncture

The nurse places the child supine with the legs in a frog position to provide extensive exposure of the groin area. The infant's legs can be controlled effectively by the nurse's forearms and hands (Fig. 39-7). Only the side used for the venipuncture is uncovered so the practitioner is protected if the child urinates during the procedure. Pressure is applied to the site to prevent oozing from it.

Extremity Venipuncture or Injection

The most common sites of venipuncture are the veins of the extremities, especially the arm and hand. A convenient position is to place the child in the parent's (or assistant's) lap with the child facing the parent and in the straddle position. Next place the child's arm for venipuncture on a firm surface such as a treatment table. The nurse can partially stabilize the child's outstretched arm and have the parent hug the child's upper body, preventing movement; the nurse can then use the parent's arm to immobilize the venipuncture site. This type of restraint also comforts the child because of the close body contact and allows each person to maintain eye contact (Fig. 39-8).

Lumbar Puncture

Pediatric LP sets contain smaller spinal needles, but sometimes the practitioner will specify a different size or type of needle. The technique for LP in infants and children is similar to that in adults, although modifications are suggested in neonates, who have less distress in a side-lying position with modified neck extension than in flexion or a sitting position.

Children are usually easiest to control in the side-lying position, with the head flexed and the knees drawn up toward the chest. Even cooperative children need to be held gently to prevent possible trauma from unexpected, involuntary movement. They can be reassured that, although they are trusted, holding will serve as a reminder to maintain the desired position. It also provides a measure of support and reassurance to them.

A flexed sitting or side-lying position may be used, depending on the child's ability to cooperate and whether sedation will be used. In the sitting position with the hips flexed the interspinous space is maximized (Abo, Chen, Johnston, et al., 2010). The child is placed with the buttocks at the edge of the table. The nurse's hands immobilize the infant's arms and legs. Neck flexion is not necessary (Fig. 39-9).

> **! NURSING ALERT**
>
> The sitting position may interfere with chest expansion and diaphragm excursion; and in infants the soft, pliable trachea may collapse. Therefore observe the child for difficulty breathing.

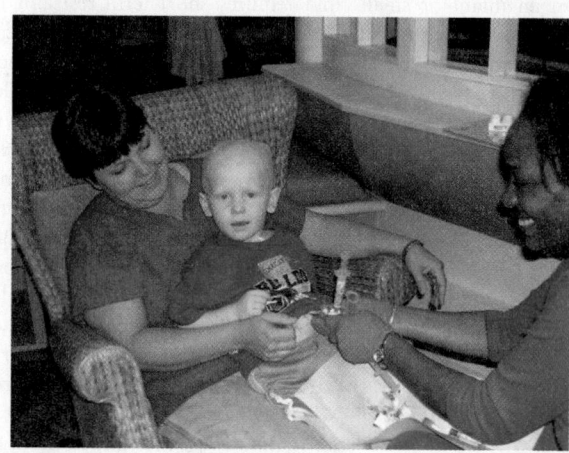

FIG 39-8 Therapeutic holding of child for extremity venipuncture with parental assistance.

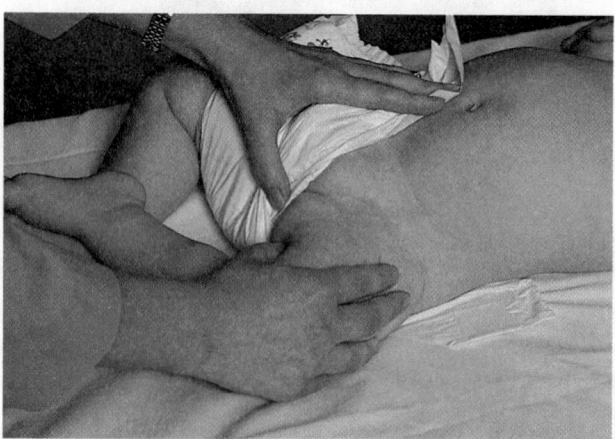

FIG 39-7 Positioning infant for femoral venipuncture.

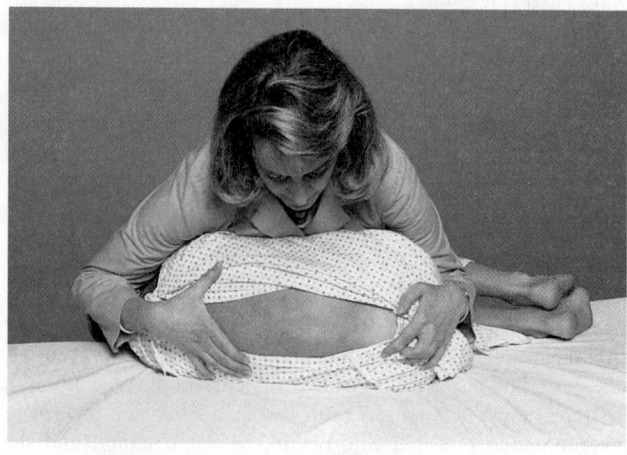

FIG 39-9 Side-lying position for lumbar puncture.

Specimens and spinal fluid pressure are obtained, measured, and sent for analysis in the same manner as for adult patients. Take vital signs as ordered and observe the child for any changes in level of consciousness, motor activity, and other neurologic signs. Post-LP headache may occur and is related to postural changes; this is less severe when the child lies flat. Headache is seen much less frequently in young children than in adolescents.

Bone Marrow Aspiration or Biopsy

The position for a bone marrow aspiration or biopsy depends on the chosen site. In children the posterior or anterior iliac crest is used most frequently, but in infants the tibia may be selected because it is easy to access the site and hold the child.

If the posterior iliac crest is used, the child is positioned prone. Sometimes a small pillow or folded blanket is placed under the hips to facilitate obtaining the bone marrow specimen. Children should receive adequate analgesia or anesthesia to relieve pain. If the child might awaken, he or she may need to be held, preferably by two people (i.e., one person to immobilize the upper body and a second person to immobilize the lower extremities).

COLLECTION OF SPECIMENS

Many of the specimens needed for diagnostic examination of children are collected in much the same way as they are for adults. Older children are able to cooperate if given proper instruction regarding what is expected of them. However, infants and small children are unable to follow directions or control body functions sufficiently to help in collecting some specimens.

Fundamental Procedure Steps Common to All Procedures

The following steps are very important for every procedure and should be considered fundamental aspects of care. Although these steps are important, they are not listed in each of the specimen collection procedures.

1. Assemble the necessary equipment.
2. Identify the child using two patient identifiers (e.g., patient name and medical record or birth date; neither can be a room number). Compare the same two identifiers with the specimen container and order.
3. Perform hand hygiene, maintain aseptic technique, and follow Standard Precautions.
4. Explain the procedure to parents and child according to the developmental level of the child; reassure the child that the procedure is not a punishment.
5. Provide atraumatic care and position the child securely.
6. Prepare area with antiseptic agent.
7. Place specimens in appropriate containers and apply a patient identification label to the specimen container in the presence of the child and family.
8. Discard puncture device in puncture-resistant container near the site of use.
9. Wash the procedural preparation agent off if povidone-iodine is used, if skin is sensitive, and for infants.
10. Remove gloves and perform hand hygiene after the procedure. Have children wash their hands if they have helped.
11. Praise the child for helping.
12. Document pertinent aspects of the procedure such as number of attempts, site and amount of blood or urine withdrawn, and type of test performed.

Urine Specimens

Older children and adolescents can use a bedpan or urinal or be trusted to follow directions for collection in the bathroom. However, they may have special needs. School-age children are cooperative but curious. They are concerned about the reasons behind things and are likely to ask questions regarding the disposition of their specimen and what one expects to discover from it. Self-conscious adolescents may be reluctant to carry a specimen through a hallway or waiting room and appreciate a paper bag for disguising the container. The presence of menses may be an embarrassment or a concern to teenage girls; therefore it is a good idea to ask them about this and make adjustments as necessary. The specimen can be delayed, or a notation made on the laboratory slip to explain the presence of red blood cells.

Preschoolers and toddlers are usually unable to void on request. It is often best to offer them water or other liquids that they enjoy and wait about 30 minutes until they are ready to void voluntarily.

Children better understand what is expected if the nurse uses familiar terms such as "pee-pee," "wee-wee," or "tinkle." Some have difficulty voiding in an unfamiliar receptacle. Potty chairs or a potty hat placed on the toilet is usually satisfactory. Toddlers who have recently acquired bladder control may be especially reluctant because they undoubtedly have been admonished for "going" in places other than those approved by parents. Enlisting the parents' help usually leads to success. For infants and toddlers who are not toilet trained, special urine collection bags with self-adhering material around the opening at the point of attachment are used. To prepare the infant, the genitalia, perineum, and surrounding skin are washed and dried thoroughly because the adhesive does not stick to a moist, powdered, or oily skin surface. The collection bag is easiest to apply if attached first to the perineum, progressing to the symphysis pubis (Fig. 39-10). With girls the perineum is stretched taut during application to ensure a leakproof fit. With boys the penis and sometimes the scrotum are placed inside the bag. The adhesive portion of the bag must be applied to the skin firmly all around the genital area to avoid leakage. The bag is checked frequently and removed as soon as the specimen is available because the moist bag may become loosened on an active child. For some types of urine testing such as specific gravity, ketones, glucose, and protein, the nurse can aspirate urine directly from the diaper. If the urine is not tested within 30 minutes, the specimen is refrigerated or placed in a sterile container with a preservative. Superabsorbent disposable diapers may absorb all urine and may also produce a false crystalluria. Specific gravity measurements are accurate for up to 4 hours provided that the disposable diapers are kept folded. Urine samples collected by the cotton-ball method were accurate for pH and specific gravity and were atraumatic to the skin of newborns (Burke, 1995).

> ### ! NURSING ALERT
>
> When using a urine collection bag, cut a small slit in the diaper and pull the bag through to allow room for urine to collect and to facilitate checking on the contents. To obtain small amounts of urine use a syringe without a needle to aspirate urine directly from the diaper. If diapers with absorbent gelling material that trap urine are used, place a small gauze dressing, some cotton balls, or a urine collection device inside the diaper to collect urine and aspirate it with a syringe.

Clean-Catch Specimens

Clean-catch specimen traditionally refers to a urine sample obtained for culture after the urethral meatus is cleaned and the first few

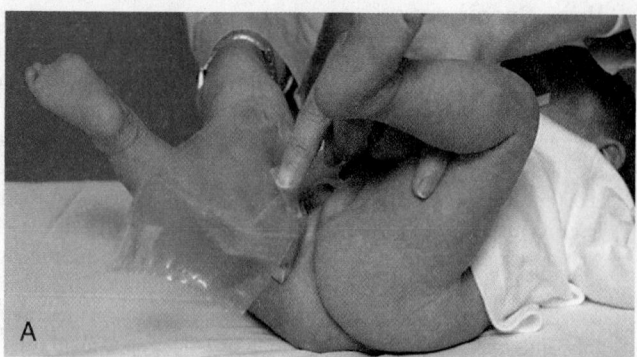
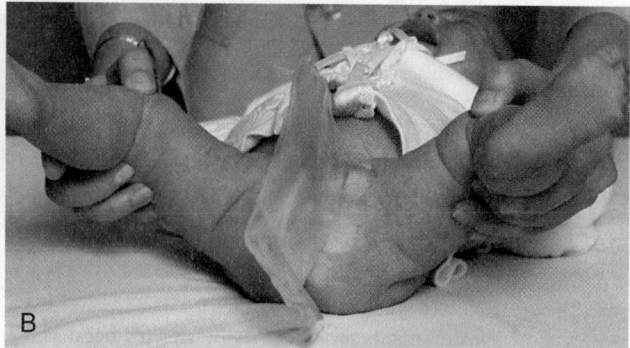

FIG 39-10 Application of urine collection bag. **A,** On female infants adhesive portion is applied to exposed and dried perineum first. **B,** Bag adheres firmly around the perineal area to prevent urine leakage.

milliliters of urine are voided (midstream specimen). In girls the perineum is wiped with an antiseptic pad from front to back. In boys the tip of the penis is cleansed.

Twenty-Four-Hour Collection

Collection bags are required in infants and small children for a 24-hour collection. Older children require special instruction about notifying someone when they need to void or have a bowel movement so urine can be collected separately and is not discarded. Some older school-age children and adolescents can take responsibility for collection of their own 24-hour specimens, keep output records, and transfer each voiding to the 24-hour collection container.

The collection period always starts and ends with an empty bladder. At the time the collection begins, instruct the child to void and discard the specimen. All urine voided in the subsequent 24 hours is saved in a container with a preservative or placed on ice. Twenty-four hours from the time that the precollection specimen was discarded, the child is again instructed to void, the specimen is added to the container, and the entire collection is taken to the laboratory.

Infants and small children who are bagged for 24-hour urine collection require a special collection bag. Frequent removal and replacement of adhesive collection devices can produce skin irritation. A thin coating of sealant such as Skin-Prep applied to the skin helps to protect it and aids adhesion (unless its use is contraindicated such as in premature infants or children with irritated skin). Plastic collection bags with collection tubes attached are ideal when the container must be left in place for a time. These can be connected to a collecting device or emptied periodically by aspiration with a syringe. When such devices are not available, a regular bag with a feeding tube inserted through a puncture hole at the top of the bag serves as a satisfactory substitute. However, take care to empty the bag as soon as the infant urinates to prevent leakage and loss of contents. An indwelling catheter may also be placed for the collection period.

Bladder Catheterization and Other Techniques

Bladder catheterization or suprapubic aspiration is used when a specimen is urgently needed or a child is unable to void or otherwise provide an adequate specimen. In infants younger than 3 months of age who are febrile, urine specimens should be collected by bladder catheterization (McGillivray, Mok, Mulrooney, et al., 2008). The AAP recommends that urine collected by the bag can be used to determine whether it is necessary to obtain a catheterized urine specimen for culture (Wald, 2005).

TABLE 39-5	**STRAIGHT CATHETER OR FOLEY CATHETER***	
	SIZE (LENGTH OF INSERTION [CM]) FOR GIRLS	**SIZE (LENGTH OF INSERTION [CM]) FOR BOYS**
Term neonate	5-6 (5)	5-6 (6)
Infant-3 yr	5-8 (5)	5-8 (6)
4-8 yr	8 (5-6)	8 (6-9)
8 yr-prepubertal	10-12 (6-8)	8-10 (10-15)
Pubertal	12-14 (6-8)	12-14 (13-18)

*Foley catheters are approximately 1 Fr size larger because of the circumference of the balloon. Example: 10-Fr Foley catheter = ≈12-Fr calibration.

Preparation for catheterization includes instruction on pelvic muscle relaxation whenever possible. The toddler, preschooler, or younger child should blow on a pinwheel and press the hips against the bed or procedure table during catheterization to relax the pelvic and periurethral muscles. The nurse describes the location and function of the pelvic muscles briefly to the older child or adolescent. The patient then contracts and relaxes the pelvic muscles, and the relaxation procedure is repeated during catheter insertion. If the patient vigorously contracts the pelvic muscles when the catheter reaches the striated sphincter (proximal urethra in boys and midurethra in girls), catheter insertion is stopped temporarily. The catheter is neither removed nor advanced; instead the child is helped to press the hips against the bed or examining table and relax the pelvic muscles. The catheter is then gently advanced into the bladder (Gray, 1996).

Catheterization is a sterile procedure, and Standard Precautions for body substance protection should be followed. If the catheter is to remain in place, a Foley catheter is used. Table 39-5 lists guidelines for choosing the appropriate-size catheter and length of insertion. The supplies needed for this procedure include sterile gloves, sterile lubricant anesthetic, the appropriate-size catheter, povidone-iodine (Betadine) swabs or an alternative cleansing agent and 4 × 4–inch gauze squares, a sterile drape, and a syringe with sterile water if a Foley catheter is used. Test the balloon of the Foley catheter by injecting sterile water before catheter insertion.

Adolescent boys and children with a history of urethral surgery may be catheterized with a coudé-tipped catheter. Children with myelodysplasia and those who have been identified as being sensitive or allergic to latex are catheterized with catheters manufactured from an alternative material. When an indwelling catheter is indicated for urinary drainage, a lubricious-coated or silicone catheter is selected because these materials produce less irritation of the urethral mucosa compared with Silastic or latex catheters when left in place for more than 72 hours.

A 2% lidocaine lubricant with applicator is assembled according to manufacturer instructions, and several drops of the lubricant are placed at the meatus. The child is advised that the lubricant is used to reduce any discomfort associated with inserting the catheter and that introduction of the catheter into the urethra will produce a sensation of pressure and a desire to urinate (Gray, 1996).

In male patients grasp the penis with the nondominant hand and retract the foreskin. In uncircumcised newborns and infants the foreskin may be adhered to the shaft; use care when retracting. If the penis is pendulous, place a sterile drape under the penis. Using the sterile hand, swab the glans and meatus 3 times with povidone-iodine. Gently introduce the tip of the lidocaine jelly applicator into the urethra 1 to 2 cm (0.4 to 0.8 inch) so the lubricant flows only into the urethra; insert 5 to 10 mL 2% lidocaine lubricant into the urethra and hold it in place for 2 to 3 minutes by gently squeezing the distal penis. Lubricate the catheter and insert it into the urethra while gently stretching the penis and lifting it to a 90-degree angle to the body. Resistance may occur when the catheter meets the urethral sphincter. Ask the patient to inhale deeply and advance the catheter. Do not force a catheter that does not easily enter the meatus, particularly if the child has had corrective surgery. For indwelling catheters, after urine is obtained, advance the catheter to the hub, inflate the balloon with sterile water, pull it back gently to test inflation, and connect it to the closed drainage system. Cleanse the glans and meatus and replace retracted foreskin. If blood is seen at any time during the procedure, discontinue the procedure and notify the practitioner.

In female patients place a sterile drape under the buttocks. Use the nondominant hand to gently separate and pull up the labia minora to visualize the meatus. Swab the meatus from front to back 3 times using a different povidone-iodine swab each time. Place 1 to 2 mL 2% lidocaine lubricant on the periurethral mucosa and insert the lubricant 1 to 2 mL into the urethral meatus. Delay catheterization for 2 to 3 minutes to maximize absorption of the anesthetic into the periurethral and intraurethral mucosa. Add lubricant to the catheter and gently insert it into the urethra until urine returns; then advance the catheter an additional 2.5 to 5 cm (1 to 2 inches). When using an indwelling Foley catheter, inflate the balloon with sterile water and gently pull back; then connect to a closed drainage system. Cleanse the meatus and labia (see Cultural Competence box). Because the use of lidocaine jelly can increase the volume of intraurethral lubricant, urine return may not be as rapid as when minimal lubrication is used.

CULTURAL COMPETENCE

Bladder Catheterization

Parents may be upset when their child is catheterized. Aside from the trauma the child experiences, some parents may fear that the procedure affects the daughter's virginity. To correct this misconception, the family may benefit from a detailed explanation of the genitourinary anatomy, preferably with a model that shows the separate vaginal and urethral openings. The nurse can also indicate that catheterization has no effect on virginity.

⚡ SAFETY ALERT

Do not advance the catheter too far into the bladder. Knotting of catheters and tubes within the bladder has been reported in several case studies. Feeding tubes should not be used for urinary catheterization because they are more flexible, longer, and prone to knotting compared with commercially designed urinary catheters (Foster, Ritchey, and Bloom, 1992; Gonzalez and Palmer, 1997; Kilbane, 2009; Levison and Wojtulewicz, 2004; Lodha, Ly, Brindle, et al., 2005; Turner, 2004).

Suprapubic aspiration is mainly used when the bladder cannot be accessed through the urethra (e.g., with some congenital urologic birth defects) or to reduce the risk of contamination that may be present when passing a catheter. With the advent of small catheters (5- and 6-Fr straight catheters), the need for suprapubic aspiration has decreased. Access to the bladder via the urethra has a much higher success rate than suprapubic aspiration, in which success depends on the practitioner's skill at assessing the location of the bladder and the amount of urine in the bladder.

Suprapubic aspiration involves aspirating bladder contents by inserting a 20- or 21-gauge needle in the midline approximately 1 cm (0.4 inch) above the symphysis pubis and directed vertically downward. The nurse prepares the skin as for any needle insertion, and the bladder should contain an adequate volume of urine. This can be assumed if the infant has not voided for at least 1 hour or the bladder can be palpated above the symphysis pubis. This technique is useful for obtaining sterile specimens from young infants because the bladder is an abdominal organ and easily accessed. Suprapubic aspiration is painful; therefore pain management during the procedure is important (see Atraumatic Care box).

Stool Specimens

Stool specimens are frequently collected from children to identify parasites and other organisms that cause diarrhea, assess gastrointestinal function, and check for occult (hidden) blood. Ideally stool should be collected without contamination with urine, but in children wearing diapers this is difficult unless a urine bag is applied. Children who are toilet trained should urinate first, flush the toilet, and then defecate into the toilet or a bedpan (preferably one that is placed on the toilet to avoid embarrassment) or a commercial potty hat.

Stool specimens should be large enough to obtain an ample sampling, not merely a fecal fragment. Specimens are placed in an

ATRAUMATIC CARE

Bladder Catheterization or Suprapubic Aspiration

- Use distraction to help the child relax (e.g., blowing bubbles, deep breathing, singing a song).
- Use lidocaine jelly to anesthetize the area before insertion of the catheter. EMLA cream (a eutectic mix of lidocaine and prilocaine) or LMX cream (lidocaine) may lessen an infant's discomfort as the needle passes through the skin for suprapubic aspiration, but care should be taken that the site is thoroughly cleaned and prepped before the procedure.
- Children often become agitated at being restrained for either procedure. Use comfort measures through touch and voice, both during and after the procedure, to help reduce the child's distress.

appropriate container, which is covered and labeled. If several specimens are needed, mark the containers with the date and time and keep them in a specimen refrigerator. Exercise care in handling the specimen because of the risk of contamination.

Blood Specimens

Whether the specimen is collected by the nurse or others, the nurse is responsible for making certain that specimens such as serial examinations and fasting specimens are collected on time and that the proper equipment is available. Collecting, transporting, and storing specimens can have a major impact on laboratory results.

Venous blood samples can be obtained by venipuncture or by aspiration from a peripheral or central access device. Withdrawing blood specimens through peripheral lock devices in small peripheral veins has varying degrees of success. Although it avoids an additional venipuncture for the child, attempting to aspirate blood from the peripheral lock may shorten the life of the device. However, the nurse can use central lines to withdraw blood samples (see Atraumatic Care box). When using an IV infusion site for specimen collection, consider the type of fluid being infused. For example, a specimen collected for glucose determination would be inaccurate if removed from a catheter through which glucose-containing solution was being administered.

The needed specimens are collected quickly, and pressure is applied to the puncture site with dry gauze until bleeding stops. The arm should be extended, not flexed, while pressure is applied for a few minutes after venipuncture in the antecubital fossa to reduce bruising. The nurse then covers the site with an adhesive bandage. In young children adhesive bandages pose an aspiration hazard; thus avoid using them or remove the adhesive bandage as soon as the bleeding stops. Applying warm compresses to ecchymotic areas increases circulation, helps remove extravasated blood, and decreases pain.

Arterial blood samples are sometimes needed for blood gas measurement, although noninvasive techniques such as transcutaneous oxygen monitoring and pulse oximetry are used frequently. Arterial samples may be obtained by arterial puncture using the radial, brachial, or femoral arteries or from indwelling arterial catheters. Assess adequate circulation before arterial puncture by observing capillary refill or performing the Allen test, a procedure that assesses the circulation of the radial, ulnar, or brachial arteries. Because unclotted blood is required, use only heparinized collection tubes or syringes. In addition, no air bubbles should enter the tube because they can alter blood gas concentration. Crying, fear, and agitation affect blood gas values; therefore make every effort to comfort the child. Pack the blood samples in

ATRAUMATIC CARE

Guidelines for Skin and Vessel Punctures

To Reduce the Pain Associated with Heel, Finger, Venous, or Arterial Punctures

- Apply EMLA (a eutectic mix of lidocaine and prilocaine) topically over the site if time permits (>60 minutes). LMX cream (lidocaine) also may be used and requires a shorter application time (30 minutes). To remove the transparent dressing atraumatically, grasp opposite sides of the film and pull the sides away from one another to stretch and loosen the film. After the film begins to loosen, grasp the other two sides and pull. Use iontophoresis (Numby Stuff) over the site if time permits (8 to 20 minutes, depending on the amount of current), a vapocoolant spray, or buffered lidocaine (injected intradermally near the vein with a 30-gauge needle) to numb the skin.
- Use nonpharmacologic methods of pain and anxiety control (e.g., ask the child to take a deep breath when the needle is inserted and again when the needle is withdrawn, to exhale a large breath or blow bubbles to "blow hurt away," or to count slowly and then faster and louder if pain is felt).
- Keep all equipment out of sight until used.
- Enlist parents' presence or assistance if they wish.
- Restrain child *only as needed* to perform the procedure safely; use therapeutic holding (see p. 1150).
- Allow the skin preparation to dry completely before penetrating the skin.
- Use the smallest gauge needle (e.g., 25 gauge) that permits free flow of blood; a 27-gauge needle can be used for obtaining 1 to 1.5 mL of blood and for prominent veins (needle length is only 1.25 cm [0.5 inch]).
- If possible, avoid putting an IV line in the dominant hand or the hand the child uses to suck the thumb.
- Use an automatic lancet device for precise puncture depth of the finger or heel; press the device lightly against the skin; avoid steadying the finger against a hard surface.
- Have a "two-try" only policy to reduce excessive insertion attempts (i.e., two operators each have two insertion attempts). If insertion is not successful after four punctures, consider alternative venous access such as a PICC; have a policy for identifying children with difficult access and

appropriate interventions (e.g., most experienced operator for the first attempt, use transilluminator or ultrasonography for insertion guidance).

For Multiple Blood Samples

- Use an intermittent infusion device (saline lock) to collect additional samples from an existing IV line; consider PICC lines early, not as a last resort.
- Coordinate care to allow several tests to be performed on one blood sample using micromethods of testing.
- Anticipate tests (e.g., drug levels, chemistry, immunoglobulin levels) and ask the laboratory to save blood for additional testing.

For Heel Lancing in Newborns

- Heel lancing has shown to be more painful than venipuncture (Shah and Ohlsson, 2007); consider venipuncture when the amount of blood from the heel would require much squeezing (e.g., genetic screening tests).
- The effectiveness of EMLA is controversial, although application of 0.5 g for 30 minutes 4 times a day in preterm infants was found to be safe (Essink-Tebbes, Wuis, Liem, et al., 1999).
- Place diapered newborn against mother's bare chest in skin-to-skin contact 10 to 15 minutes before and during heel lance (Gray, Watt, and Blass, 2000).
- During the procedure administer sucrose and encourage the newborn to suck a pacifier. When commercially manufactured 24% sucrose solution is unavailable, add 1 tsp of table sugar to 4 tsp of sterile water. Use this solution to coat the pacifier or administer 2 mL to the tongue 2 minutes before the procedure. (See Evidence-Based Practice Box, Reduction of Minor Procedural Pain in Infants, p. 842.)
- One study found that breastfeeding during a neonatal heel lance was more effective than sucrose in reducing pain (Codipietro, Ceccarelli, and Ponzone, 2008).

IV, Intravenous; *PICC,* peripherally inserted central catheter.

ice to reduce blood cell metabolism and take it to the laboratory immediately.

Take capillary blood samples from children by fingerstick. A common method for taking peripheral blood samples from infants younger than 6 months of age is by a heelstick. Before the blood sample is taken, warm the heel for 3 minutes and cleanse the area with alcohol. Holding the infant's foot firmly with the free hand, the nurse then punctures the heel with an automatic lancet device. An automatic device delivers a more precise puncture depth and is less painful than using a lance (Vertanen, Fellman, Brommels, et al., 2001). A surgical blade of any kind is contraindicated. An example of a safe device is the BD Quickheel Safety Lancet. The Tenderfoot Preemie device* was compared with the Monolet lancet and was found to be safer than the lancet and required fewer heel punctures, less collection time, and lower recollection rates (Kellam, Sacks, Wailer, et al., 2001). Shepherd, Glenesk, Niven, and others (2005) reported that the Tenderfoot device was more effective and safer than a lancet for newborn screening tests. Although obtaining capillary blood gases is a common practice, these measures may not reflect arterial values accurately.

The most serious complications of infant heel puncture are necrotizing osteochondritis from lancet penetration of the underlying calcaneus bone, infection, and abscess of the heel. To avoid osteochondritis the puncture should be no deeper than 2 mm and should be made at the outer aspect of the heel. The boundaries of the calcaneus can be marked by an imaginary line extending posteriorly from a point between the fourth and fifth toes and running parallel with the lateral aspect of the heel and another line extending posteriorly from the middle of the great toe and running parallel with the medial aspect of the heel (Fig. 39-11). Repeated trauma to the walking surface of the heel can cause fibrosis and scarring that may interfere with locomotion.

No matter how or by whom the specimen is collected, children, even some older ones, fear the loss of their blood. This is particularly true for children whose condition requires frequent blood specimens. They mistakenly believe that blood removed from their body is a threat to their lives. Explaining to them that their body continuously produces blood provides them a measure of reassurance. When the blood is drawn, a comment such as, "Just look how red it is. You're really making a lot of nice red blood," confirms this information and affords them an opportunity to express their concern.

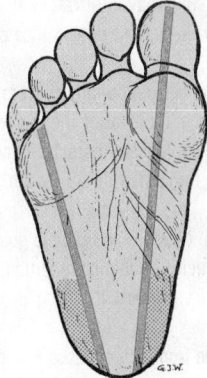

FIG 39-11 Puncture site (colored stippled area) on sole of infant's foot.

*The Tenderfoot Preemie device is manufactured by ITC, Edison, NJ, www.itcmed.com/products/tenderfoot-heel-incision-device.

An adhesive bandage gives them added assurance that the vital fluids will not leak out through the puncture site.

Children also dislike the discomfort associated with venous, arterial, and capillary punctures. They have identified these procedures as the ones most frequently causing pain during hospitalization and an arterial puncture as being one of the most painful of all procedures experienced. Toddlers are most distressed by venipuncture followed by school-age children and then adolescents. Consequently nurses need to institute pain-reduction techniques to lessen the discomfort of these procedures. (See Pain Management, Chapter 30.)

Respiratory Secretion Specimens

Collection of sputum or nasal discharge is sometimes required for the diagnosis of respiratory infections, especially tuberculosis and respiratory syncytial virus (RSV). Older children and adolescents are able to cough as directed and supply sputum specimens when given proper directions. The nurse must make it clear to them that a coughed specimen, not mucus cleared from the throat, is needed. It is helpful to demonstrate a deep cough. Infants and small children are unable to follow directions to cough and will swallow any sputum produced; therefore gastric washings (lavage) may be used to collect a sputum specimen. Sometimes a satisfactory specimen can be obtained using a suction device such as a mucus trap if the catheter is inserted into the trachea and the cough reflex elicited. A catheter inserted into the back of the throat is not sufficient. For children with a tracheostomy, a specimen is easily aspirated from the trachea or major bronchi by attaching a collecting device to the suction apparatus.

Nasal washings are usually obtained to diagnose an infection of RSV. The child is placed supine, and 1 to 3 mL of sterile normal saline is instilled with a sterile syringe (without needle) into one nostril. The contents are aspirated using a small, sterile bulb syringe and placed in a sterile container. Another method uses a syringe with 5 cm (2 inches) of 18- to 20-gauge tubing. The saline is instilled quickly and then aspirated to recover the nasal specimen. To prevent any additional discomfort, all of the equipment should be ready before beginning the procedure.

Other respiratory secretion collection methods include nasopharyngeal swabs to diagnose *Bordetella* pertussis and throat cultures. The nurse swabs both the tonsils and the posterior pharynx when obtaining a throat culture. The swab stick is inserted into the culture tube. Some culture kits require squeezing an ampule to release the culture medium.

ADMINISTRATION OF MEDICATION

Determination of Drug Dosage

Nurses must have an understanding of the safe dosages of medications they administer to children and the expected actions, possible side effects, and signs of toxicity. Unlike with adult medications, there are few standardized pediatric dosage ranges; and with a few exceptions drugs are prepared and packaged in average adult-dosage strengths.

Factors related to growth and maturation significantly alter an individual's capacity to metabolize and excrete drugs. Immaturity or defects in any of the important processes of absorption, distribution, biotransformation, or excretion can significantly alter the effects of a drug. Newborn and premature infants with immature enzyme systems in the liver (where most drugs are broken down and detoxified), lower plasma concentrations of protein for binding with drugs, and immaturely functioning kidneys (where most drugs are excreted) are particularly vulnerable to the harmful effects of drugs. Beyond the newborn period many drugs are metabolized more rapidly by the liver, necessitating larger doses or more frequent administration. This is particularly important in pain control, when the dosage of analgesics may need to be increased or the interval between doses decreased.

Various formulas involving age, weight, and body surface area (BSA) as the basis for calculations have been devised to determine children's drug dosages. Because the administration of medication is a nursing responsibility, nurses need to have not only knowledge of drug action and patient responses but also resources for estimating safe dosages for children. Children's dosages are most often expressed in units of measure per body weight (mg/kg). Some medications such as chemotherapy are more precisely dosed using BSA. The ratio of BSA to weight varies inversely with length; therefore an infant who is shorter and weighs less than an older child or adult has relatively more BSA than would be expected from the weight. BSA is based on the West nomogram and is easily determined using conversion programs widely available on the Internet.

Checking Dosage

Administering the correct dosage of a drug is a shared responsibility between the practitioner who orders the drug and the nurse who carries out that order. Children react with unexpected severity to some drugs, and ill children may be especially sensitive to drugs. When a dose is ordered that is outside the usual range or when there is some question regarding the preparation or the route of administration, the nurse should check with the prescribing practitioner before proceeding with the administration because the nurse is legally liable for any drug administered.

Even when it has been determined that the dosage is correct for a particular child, many drugs are potentially hazardous or lethal. Most facilities have regulations requiring specified drugs to be double checked by another nurse before giving them to the child. Among drugs that require such safeguards are antiarrhythmics, anticoagulants, chemotherapeutic agents, and insulin. Others frequently included are epinephrine, opioids, and sedatives. Even if this precaution is not mandatory, nurses are wise to take such precautions. Errors in decimal point placement may occur and result in a 10-fold or greater dosage error.

Identifying the Child

Before the administration of any medication, the child must be identified correctly using two identifiers (e.g., name and medical record number or birth date). With an infant, young child, or nonverbal child, the parent or guardian (if present) can verify the child's identity. After verbal verification of the child's identity (by the parent, guardian, or child), the ID band should be verified using two identifiers. Bedside computers to scan the ID bracelet for electronic record updating may also be used.

Preparing the Parents

Nearly all parents have given some type of medication to their child and can describe the approaches they have found successful. In some cases it is less traumatic for the child if a parent gives the medication, provided that the nurse prepares the medication and supervises its administration. Children being given daily medications at home are accustomed to the parent's functioning in this capacity and are less likely to fuss than if a stranger administers the medication. Individual decisions need to be made regarding parental presence and participation such as holding the child during injections.

Preparing the Child

Every child requires psychologic preparation for parenteral administration of medication and supportive care during the procedure (see p. 1137). Even if children have received several injections, they rarely become accustomed to the discomfort and have as much right as any other child to understanding and patience from those giving the injection.

Oral Administration

The oral route is preferred for administering medications to children because of the ease of administration. Most medications are dissolved or suspended in liquid preparations. Although some children are able to swallow or chew solid medications at an early age, solid preparations are not recommended for young children because of the danger of aspiration.

Most pediatric medications come in palatable and colorful preparations for added ease of administration. Some have a slightly unpleasant aftertaste, but most children swallow these liquids with little, if any, resistance. Complaints of dislike from the child can be accepted, and the taste camouflaged whenever possible. Most pediatric units have preparations available for this purpose (see Atraumatic Care box).

Preparation

The devices available to measure medicines are not always sufficiently accurate for measuring the small amounts needed in pediatric nursing practice. Molded plastic cups offer reasonable accuracy in measuring moderate doses of liquids; on the other hand, paper cups are likely to have irregularly shaped or crumpled bottoms and retain considerable amounts of thick medication. Measures less than 1 tsp are impossible to determine accurately with a medicine cup.

ATRAUMATIC CARE

Encouraging a Child's Acceptance of Oral Medication

- Give the child a flavored ice pop or small ice cube to suck to numb the tongue before giving the drug.
- Mix the drug with a small amount (≈1 tsp) of sweet-tasting substance such as honey (except in infants because of the risk of botulism), flavored syrups, jam, fruit purees, sherbet, or ice cream; avoid essential food items because the child may later refuse to eat them.
- Give a "chaser" of water, juice, soft drink, or ice pop or frozen juice bar after the drug.
- If nausea is a problem, give a carbonated beverage poured over finely crushed ice before or immediately after the medication.
- When medication has an unpleasant taste, have the child pinch the nose and drink the medicine through a straw. Much of what we taste is associated with smell.
- Flavorings such as apple, banana, and bubble gum (e.g., FLAVORx) can be added at many pharmacies at nominal additional cost. An alternative is to have the pharmacist prepare the drug in a flavored, chewable troche or lozenge.*
- Infants will suck medicine from a needleless syringe or dropper in small increments (0.25 to 0.5 mL) at a time. Use a nipple or special pacifier with a reservoir for the drug.

*For information about compounding drugs, contact Technical Staff, Professional Compounding Centers of America, 9901 S. Wilcrest Drive, Houston, TX 77099, 800-331-2498, www.pccarx.com.

The teaspoon is an inaccurate measuring device and is subject to error. Teaspoons vary greatly in capacity, and different persons using the same spoon pour different amounts. Therefore measure a drug ordered in teaspoons in milliliters; the established standard is 5 mL/tsp. A convenient hollow-handled medicine spoon is available to measure and administer the drug accurately. Household measuring spoons can also be used when other devices are not available. A device called the *Medibottle* has shown to be more effective in delivering oral medication to infants than an oral syringe (Kraus, Stohlmeyer, Hannon, et al., 2001).

Another unreliable device for measuring liquids is the dropper, which varies to a greater extent than the teaspoon or measuring cup. The volume of a drop varies according to the viscosity (thickness) of the liquid measured. Viscous fluids produce much larger drops than thin liquids. Many medications are supplied with caps or droppers designed for measuring each specific preparation. These are accurate when used to measure that specific medication but are not reliable for measuring other liquids. Emptying dropper contents into a medicine cup invites additional error. Because some of the liquid clings to the sides of the cup, a significant amount of the drug can be lost.

The most accurate means for measuring small amounts of medication is the plastic disposable syringe, especially the tuberculin syringe for volumes less than 1 mL. Not only does the syringe provide a reliable measure, but it also serves as a convenient means for transporting and administering the medication. The medication can be placed directly into the child's mouth from the syringe.

Young children and some older children have difficulty swallowing tablets or pills. Because a number of drugs are not available in pediatric preparations, tablets need to be crushed before being given to these children. Commercial devices* are available, or simple methods can be used for crushing tablets. Not all drugs can be crushed (e.g., medication with an enteric or protective coating or formulated for slow release).

The nurse can teach children who must take solid oral medication for an extended period to swallow tablets or capsules. Training sessions include using verbal instruction, demonstration, reinforcement for swallowing progressively larger candy or capsules, no attention for inappropriate behavior, and gradual withdrawal of guidance after children can swallow their medication.

Because pediatric doses often require dividing adult preparations of medication, the nurse may be faced with the dilemma of accurate dosage. Only tablets that are scored can be halved or quartered accurately. If the medication is soluble, the tablet or contents of a capsule can be mixed in a small premeasured amount of liquid, and the appropriate portion given. For example, if half a dose is required, the tablet is dissolved in 5 mL of water, and 2.5 mL is given.

Administration

Although administering liquids to infants is relatively easy, the nurse must take care to prevent aspiration. While holding the infant in a semireclining position, place the medication in the mouth from a spoon, plastic cup, dropper, or syringe (without a needle). It is best to place the dropper or syringe along the side of the infant's tongue and administer the liquid slowly in small amounts, waiting for the child to swallow between deposits.

Medicine cups can be used effectively for older infants who are able to drink from a cup. Because of the natural outward tongue

thrust in infancy, medications may need to be retrieved from the lips or chin and refed. Allowing the infant to suck the medication that has been placed in an empty nipple or inserting the syringe or dropper into the side of the mouth parallel to the nipple while the infant nurses is another convenient method for giving liquid medications to infants. Medication is not added to the infant's formula feeding because the child may subsequently refuse the formula. Dispose of any plastic covers that may be on the ends of syringes because these covers are choking hazards.

Young children who refuse to cooperate or resist consistently despite explanation and encouragement may require mild physical coercion. If so, it is carried out quickly and carefully. Make every effort to determine why the child resists and explain the reasons for the coercion in such a way that the child knows that it is being carried out for his or her well-being and is not a form of punishment. There is always a risk in using even mild forceful techniques. A crying child can aspirate a medication, particularly when lying on the back. If the nurse holds the child in the lap with the child's right arm behind the nurse, the left hand firmly grasped by the nurse's left hand, and the head securely cradled between the nurse's arm and body, the medication can be poured into the mouth slowly (Fig. 39-12).

Intramuscular Administration
Selecting the Syringe and Needle

The volume of medication prescribed for small children and the small amount of tissue available for injection necessitate selection of a syringe that can measure small amounts of solution. For volumes less than 1 mL the tuberculin syringe calibrated in 0.01-mL increments is appropriate. Minute doses may require the use of a 0.5-mL, low-dose syringe. These syringes, along with specially constructed needles, minimize the possibility of inadvertently administering incorrect amounts of a drug because of dead space, which allows fluid to remain in the syringe and needle after the plunger is

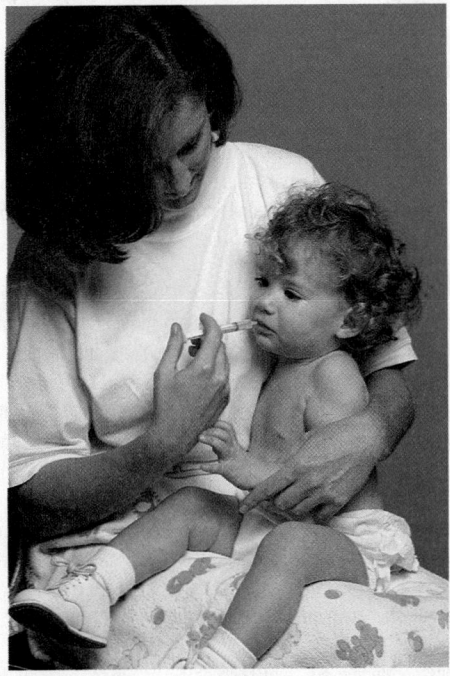

FIG 39-12 Nurse partially restrains child for easy and comfortable administration of oral medication.

---

*Several styles of pill crushers are available from Trademark Medical, 449 Sovereign Court, St. Louis, MO 63011, 800-325-9044, www.trademarkmedical.com.

pushed completely forward. A minimum of 0.2 mL of solution remains in a standard needle hub; therefore, when very small amounts of two drugs are combined in the syringe such as mixtures of insulin, the ratio of the two drugs can be altered significantly. Measures that minimize the effect of dead space are (1) when two drugs are combined in the syringe, always draw them up in the same order to maintain a consistent ratio between the drugs; (2) use the same brand of syringe (dead space may vary between brands); and (3) use one-piece syringe units (needle permanently attached to the syringe).

Dead space is also an important factor to consider when injecting medication because flushing the syringe with an air bubble adds an additional amount of medication to the prescribed dose. This can be hazardous when very small amounts of a drug are given. Consequently, flushing is not recommended, especially when less than 1 mL of medication is given. Syringes are calibrated to deliver a prescribed drug dose, and the amount of medication left in the hub and needle is not part of the syringe barrel calibrations. Certain drugs such as iron dextran and diphtheria and tetanus toxoid may cause irritation when tracked into the subcutaneous tissue. The **Z**-track method is recommended for use in infants and children rather than an air bubble. Changing the needle after withdrawing the fluid from the vial is another technique to minimize tracking.

The needle length must be sufficient to penetrate the subcutaneous tissue and deposit the medication into the body of the muscle. The needle gauge should be as small as possible to deliver the fluid safely. Smaller-diameter (25- to 30-gauge) needles cause the least discomfort, but larger gauges are needed for viscous medication and prevention of accidental bending of longer needles (see Evidence-Based Practice box).

Determining the Site

Factors to consider when selecting a site for an intramuscular (IM) injection on an infant or child include the following:

- The amount and character of the medication to be injected
- The amount and general condition of the muscle mass
- The frequency or number of injections to be given during the course of treatment
- The type of medication being given
- Factors that may impede access to or cause contamination of the site
- The child's ability to assume the required position safely

Older children and adolescents usually pose few problems in selecting a suitable site for IM injections; but infants, with their small and underdeveloped muscles, have fewer available sites. It is sometimes difficult to assess the amount of fluid that can be injected into a single site safely. Usually 1 mL is the maximum volume that should

---

EVIDENCE-BASED PRACTICE

Appropriate Site, Technique, Needle Size, and Dose for Intramuscular Injections in Infants, Toddlers, and Small Children

Ask the Question

In infants, toddlers, and small children, which site, technique, needle size and gauge, and dosage are best for intramuscular (IM) injections?

Search the Evidence

Search Strategies

Literature from 1990 to 2011 was reviewed to obtain clinical research studies related to this issue.

Databases Used

CINAHL, PubMed

Critically Analyze the Evidence

Searches reviewed were small studies. There were no randomized trials, double-blind trials, or large clinical studies addressing the subject of IM injections in children.

Infants and Toddlers

- A 16-mm needle is sufficient to penetrate the anterolateral thigh muscle if the needle is inserted at a 90-degree angle without pinching the muscle in children ages 2, 4, 6, and 18 months (Cook and Murtagh, 2002).
- A 25-mm needle is necessary to penetrate the thigh muscle when a 45-degree injection technique was used. Longer needle length is needed to fully deposit the medication into the muscle in children ages 2, 4, 6, and 18 months (Cook and Murtagh, 2002).
- For diphtheria–tetanus–pertussis (DTP) immunizations administered to infants 7 months of age and younger, 84.6% of injections were administered at the correct site (anterior thigh); 5.1% dorsogluteal and 2.6% deltoid muscles were administered at the incorrect sites (Daly, Johnston, and Chung, 1992).
- Vaccines containing adjuvant such as aluminum (e.g., DTaP, hepatitis A and B, diphtheria-tetanus [DT or Td]) should be given deep into the muscle

to prevent local reactions (AAP Committee on Infectious Diseases and Pickering, 2009; CDC, 2002; Petousis-Harris, 2008; Taddio, Ilersich, Ipp, et al., 2009).

- Injecting adjuvant-containing vaccines into subcutaneous tissue increases the incidence of local reactions (Taddio, Ilersich, Ipp, et al., 2009; Zuckerman, 2000).
- Infants 4 months old experienced fewer local side effects (redness, tenderness, and swelling) when immunizations were administered into the anterior aspect of the thigh with a 25-mm (1-inch) needle vs. shorter 16-mm ($\frac{5}{8}$-inch) needle (Diggle and Deeks, 2000).
- Localized vaccine reactions were significantly reduced when long needles (25 mm) were used for infant immunizations (Diggle, Deeks, and Pollard 2006, Petousis-Harris, 2008).
- A 16-mm needle may be adequate for injections in small infants, and a 22- to 25-mm ($\frac{7}{8}$- to 1-inch) needle can be used in infants 2 months and older (AAP Committee on Infectious Diseases and Pickering, 2009).
- A 22- to 32-mm ($\frac{7}{8}$- to $1\frac{1}{4}$-inch) needle is recommended for injections in toddlers if deltoid muscle size is adequate (CDC, 2002).
- A minimum of a 25-mm-long needle is recommended for anterolateral thigh injection in toddlers (CDC, 2002).
- Dorsogluteal muscle should be avoided in infants, toddlers, and smaller preschoolers with smaller muscle mass because of the possibility of damaging the sciatic nerve (AAP Committee on Infectious Diseases and Pickering, 2009).
- In children older than age 1 year, deltoid muscle is recommended for IM injections. When multiple vaccines are given, two may be given in the thigh (anterior and lateral) because of its larger size (Diggle, 2003).
- Injections in the anterolateral thigh should be given at least 2.5 cm (1 inch) apart so local reactions are less likely to overlap (AAP Committee on Infectious Diseases and Pickering, 2009).

EVIDENCE-BASED PRACTICE

Appropriate Site, Technique, Needle Size, and Dose for Intramuscular Injections in Infants, Toddlers, and Small Children—cont'd

- No research or supportive data were found regarding the amount of medication to be given at the different sites in infants and toddlers.
- Small and preterm infants may only tolerate up to 0.5 mL in each muscle to prevent local complications, and 1 mL of medication is recommended for infants less than 12 months; no data can be found to refute or support such a recommendation.

Children and Adolescents

- A 22- to 25-gauge needle for all IM childhood immunizations is recommended (AAP Committee on Infectious Diseases and Pickering, 2009; CDC, 2002).
- Deltoid muscle may be used for immunizations in toddlers, older children, and adolescents (AAP Committee on Infectious Diseases and Pickering, 2009; CDC, 2002).
- 16-mm for children <60 kg and 25-mm needle for children 60-70 kg are appropriate for IM injections in the deltoid injection site (Koster, Stellato, Kohn, et al., 2009).
- Ventrogluteal site is relatively free of important nerves and vascular structures and is the site of choice for pediatric IM injections in children of all ages; no complications at this site were reported (Beecroft and Kongelbeck, 1994).
- Longer needles (25 mm) were preferred for injection when bunching the skin and injecting; shorter needles (16 mm) were perceived as causing fewer localized reactions when the injection was administered with the skin held taut (Groswasser, Kahn, Bouche, et al., 1997).
- Needle length was found to be the most significant variable for local reactions in children after injection: 25-mm needle was associated with fewer localized reactions vs. 16-mm needle (Davenport, 2004).
- In children older than age 1 year deltoid muscle is recommended for IM injections. When multiple vaccines are given, two may be given in the thigh (anterior and lateral) because of its larger size (Diggle, 2003).
- Injections in the anterolateral thigh should be given at least 2.5 cm (1 inch) apart so local reactions are less likely to overlap (AAP Committee on Infectious Diseases and Pickering, 2009).
- IM injections in the buttocks with longer needles using a 90-degree angle are associated with less reactogenicity (Petousis-Harris, 2008).

Apply the Evidence: Nursing Implications

There is *low-quality evidence with strong recommendation* (Guyatt, Oxman, Vist, et al., 2008) to continue administering IM injections to children in the anterolateral thigh (up to 12 months old), deltoid (12 months and older), and ventrogluteal site.. Needle length is an important factor in decreasing local reactions; the length should be adequate to deposit the medication into the muscle for IM injections. Recommendations are for a 25-mm (1-inch) needle in infants, a 25- to 32-mm (1- to 1¼-inch) needle for toddlers, and a 38- to 51-mm (1½- to 2-inch) needle for older children; preterm and small emaciated infants may require a shorter needle (16 to 25 mm [⅝ to 1 inch]) based on weight and muscle mass size.

Quality and Safety Competencies: Evidence-Based Practice*

Knowledge

Differentiate clinical opinion from research and evidence-based summaries

Describe various methods for identifying the appropriate site, technique, needle size, and dose for IM injections in infants, toddlers, and small children.

Skills

Base individualized care plan on patient values, clinical expertise, and evidence

Integrate evidence into practice by using the techniques for IM injections in clinical care.

Attitudes

Value the concept of evidence-based practice as integral to determining best clinical practice

Appreciate the strengths and weakness of evidence for identifying appropriate site, technique, needle size, and dose for IM injections in infants, toddlers, and small children.

References

American Academy of Pediatrics (AAP) Committee on Infectious Diseases, Pickering L, editor: *Red book: report of the Committee on Infectious Diseases*, ed 28, Elk Grove Village, Ill, 2009, Author.

Beecroft PC, Kongelbeck SR: How safe are intramuscular injections? *AACN Clin Issues* 5(2):207–215, 1994.

Centers for Disease Control and Prevention (CDC): General recommendations on immunization, *MMWR Morb Mortal Wkly Rep* 51(RR-2):12–14, 2002.

Cook IF, Murtagh J: Needle length required for intramuscular vaccination of infants and toddlers: an ultrasonographic study, *Austral Fam Phys* 31(3):295–297, 2002.

Daly JM, Johnston W, Chung Y: Injection sites utilized for DPT immunizations in infants, *J Comm Health Nurs* 9(2):87–94, 1992.

Davenport JM: A systematic review to ascertain whether the standard needle is more effective than a longer or wider needle in reducing the incidence of local reaction in children receiving primary immunization, *J Adv Nurs* 46(1):66–77, 2004.

Diggle L: The administration of child vaccines. Part 11, Childhood vaccinations, *Practice Nurse* 25(12):63–69, 2003.

Diggle L, Deeks J: Effect of needle length on incidence of local reactions to routine immunisation in infants aged 4 months: randomised controlled trial, *BMJ* 321(7266):931–933, 2000.

Diggle L, Deeks JJ, Pollard AJ: Effect of needle size on immunogenicity and reactogenicity of vaccines in infants: randomized controlled trial, *BMJ* 333(7568):571, 2006.

Groswasser J, Kahn A, Bouche B, et al: Needle length and injection technique for efficient intramuscular vaccine delivery in infants and children evaluated through an ultrasonographic determination of subcutaneous and muscle layer thickness, *Pediatrics* 100(3 Pt 1):400–403, 1997.

Guyatt GH, Oxman AD, Vist GE, et al: GRADE: an emerging consensus on rating quality of evidence and strength of recommendations, *BMJ* 336(7650):924–926, 2008.

Koster M, Stellato N, Kohn N, et al: Needle length for immunizations of early adolescents as determined by ultrasound, *Pediatrics* 124:667–672, 2009.

Petousis-Harris H: Vaccine injection technique and reactogenicity—evidence for practice, *Vaccine* 26:6299–6304, 2008.

Taddio A, Ilersich AL, Ipp M, et al: Physical interventions and injection techniques for reducing injection pain during routine childhood immunizations: systematic review of randomized controlled trials and quasi-randomized controlled trials, *Clin Ther* 31(suppl):S48–S76, 2009.

Zuckerman J: The importance of injecting vaccines into muscle, *BMJ* 321(7271):1237–1238, 2000.

Updated by Olga A. Taylor

*Adapted from the QSEN at www.qsen.org.

TABLE 39-6   INTRAMUSCULAR INJECTION SITES IN CHILDREN

SITE	DISCUSSION

Vastus Lateralis

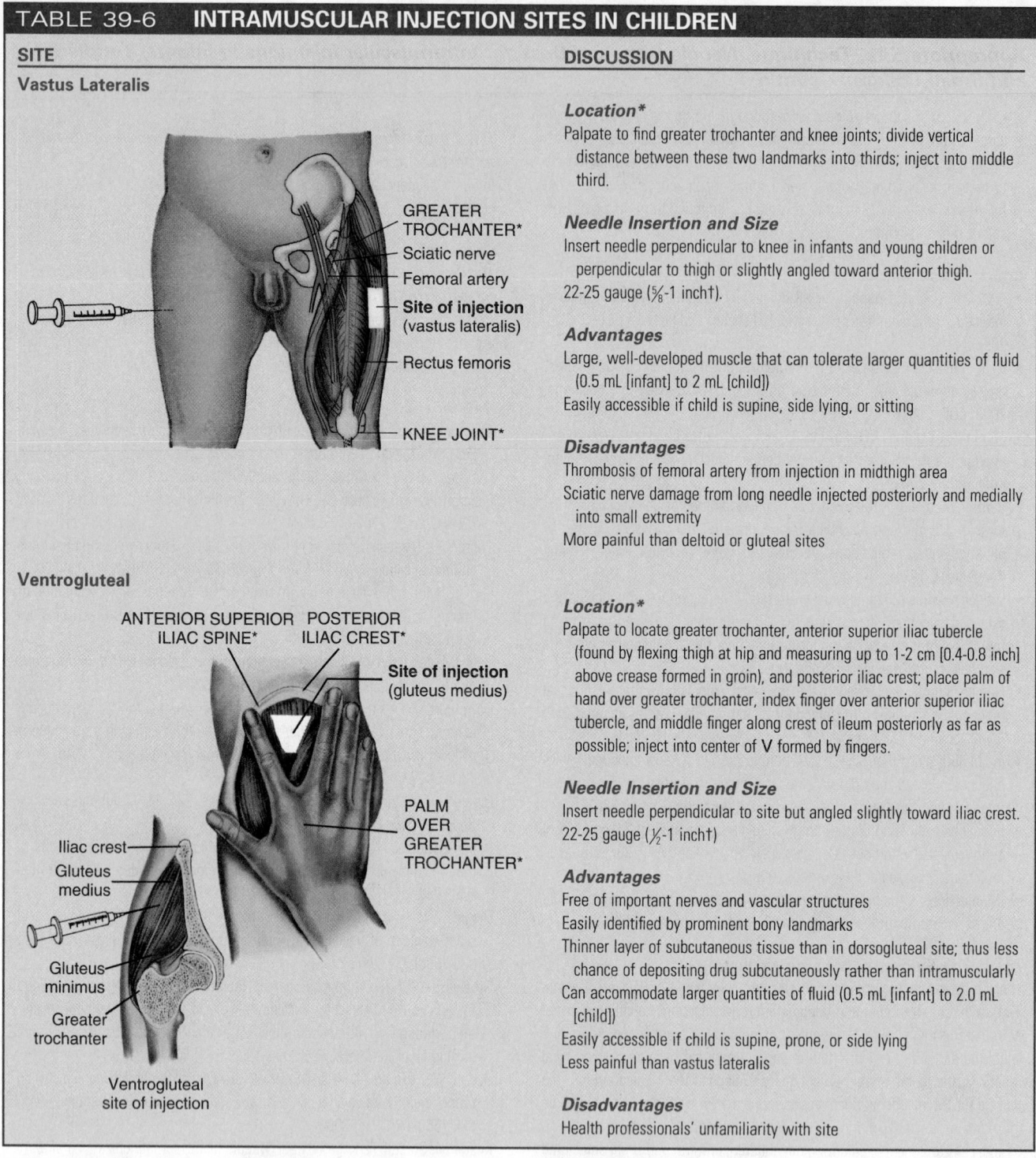

GREATER TROCHANTER*
Sciatic nerve
Femoral artery
Site of injection (vastus lateralis)
Rectus femoris
KNEE JOINT*

Ventrogluteal

ANTERIOR SUPERIOR ILIAC SPINE*   POSTERIOR ILIAC CREST*
Site of injection (gluteus medius)
PALM OVER GREATER TROCHANTER*
Iliac crest
Gluteus medius
Gluteus minimus
Greater trochanter
Ventrogluteal site of injection

Vastus Lateralis

Location*
Palpate to find greater trochanter and knee joints; divide vertical distance between these two landmarks into thirds; inject into middle third.

Needle Insertion and Size
Insert needle perpendicular to knee in infants and young children or perpendicular to thigh or slightly angled toward anterior thigh. 22-25 gauge (⅝-1 inch†).

Advantages
Large, well-developed muscle that can tolerate larger quantities of fluid (0.5 mL [infant] to 2 mL [child])
Easily accessible if child is supine, side lying, or sitting

Disadvantages
Thrombosis of femoral artery from injection in midthigh area
Sciatic nerve damage from long needle injected posteriorly and medially into small extremity
More painful than deltoid or gluteal sites

Ventrogluteal

Location*
Palpate to locate greater trochanter, anterior superior iliac tubercle (found by flexing thigh at hip and measuring up to 1-2 cm [0.4-0.8 inch] above crease formed in groin), and posterior iliac crest; place palm of hand over greater trochanter, index finger over anterior superior iliac tubercle, and middle finger along crest of ileum posteriorly as far as possible; inject into center of V formed by fingers.

Needle Insertion and Size
Insert needle perpendicular to site but angled slightly toward iliac crest. 22-25 gauge (½-1 inch†)

Advantages
Free of important nerves and vascular structures
Easily identified by prominent bony landmarks
Thinner layer of subcutaneous tissue than in dorsogluteal site; thus less chance of depositing drug subcutaneously rather than intramuscularly
Can accommodate larger quantities of fluid (0.5 mL [infant] to 2.0 mL [child])
Easily accessible if child is supine, prone, or side lying
Less painful than vastus lateralis

Disadvantages
Health professionals' unfamiliarity with site

be administered in a single site to small children and older infants. The muscles of small infants may not tolerate more than 0.5 mL. As the child approaches adult size, the nurse can use volumes approaching those given to adults. However, the larger the amount of solution, the larger the muscle at the injection site must be.

Injections must be placed in muscles large enough to accommodate the medication while avoiding major nerves and blood vessels. The IM immunization site recommended by the Centers for Disease Control and Prevention (CDC), World Health Organization, and AAP for infants is the anterolateral thigh or vastus lateralis (Table 39-6). However, in two studies immunizations at the

ventrogluteal site have been found to have fewer local reactions and fever (Cook and Murtagh, 2003; Junqueira, Tavares, Martins, et al., 2010). Cook and Murtagh (2003) also found fewer systemic reactions (irritability and persistent crying or screaming) and greater parental acceptance for the ventrogluteal site. It is relatively free of major nerves and blood vessels, is a relatively large muscle with less subcutaneous tissue than the dorsal site, has well-defined landmarks for safe site location, and is easily accessible in several positions. Distraction and prevention of unexpected movement may be more easily achieved by placing the child supine on a parent's lap for ventrogluteal site use (Cook and Murtagh, 2006).

TABLE 39-6	INTRAMUSCULAR INJECTION SITES IN CHILDREN—cont'd
SITE	**DISCUSSION**

Deltoid

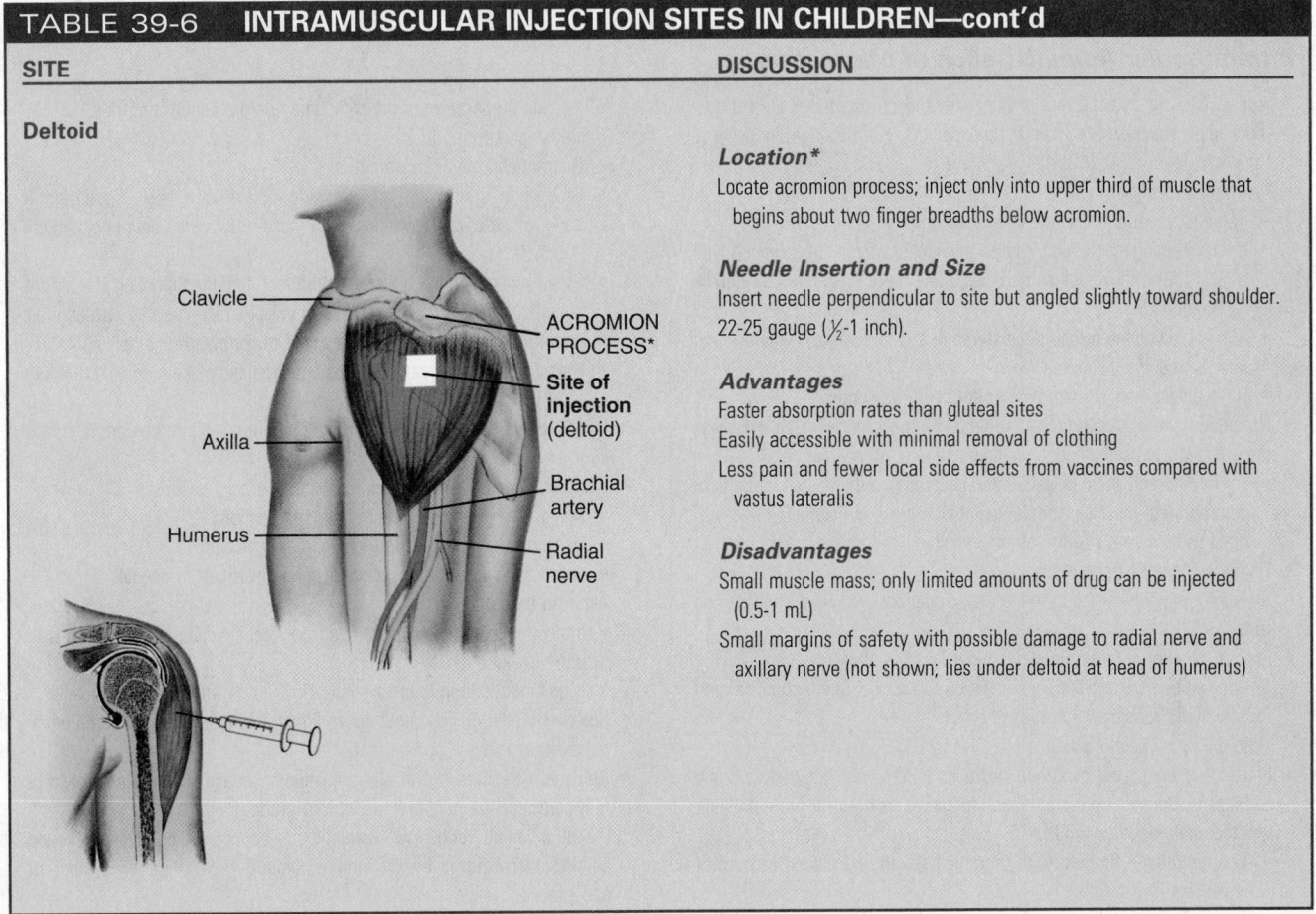

Location*

Locate acromion process; inject only into upper third of muscle that begins about two finger breadths below acromion.

Needle Insertion and Size

Insert needle perpendicular to site but angled slightly toward shoulder. 22-25 gauge (½-1 inch).

Advantages

Faster absorption rates than gluteal sites

Easily accessible with minimal removal of clothing

Less pain and fewer local side effects from vaccines compared with vastus lateralis

Disadvantages

Small muscle mass; only limited amounts of drug can be injected (0.5-1 mL)

Small margins of safety with possible damage to radial nerve and axillary nerve (not shown; lies under deltoid at head of humerus)

Labels on illustration: Clavicle, ACROMION PROCESS, Site of injection (deltoid), Axilla, Brachial artery, Humerus, Radial nerve*

*Locations are indicated by asterisks on illustrations.

†Research has shown that a 1-inch needle is needed for adequate muscle penetration in infants 4 months old and possibly in infants as young as 2 months old. (From Cook IF, Murtagh J: Needle length required for intramuscular vaccination of infants and toddlers: an ultrasonographic study, *Austral Fam Phys* 31(3):295-297, 2002.)

The deltoid muscle, a small muscle near the axillary and radial nerves, can be used for small volumes of fluid in children as young as 18 months of age. Its advantages are less pain and fewer side effects from the injectate (as observed with immunizations) compared with the vastus lateralis. Table 39-6 summarizes the three major injection sites and illustrates the location of the preferred IM injection sites for children.

Administration

Although injections that are executed with care seldom cause trauma to children, there have been reports of serious disability related to IM injections in children. Repeated use of a single site has been associated with fibrosis of the muscle with subsequent muscle contracture. Injections close to large nerves such as the sciatic nerve have been responsible for permanent disability, especially when potentially neurotoxic drugs are administered. One of the difficulties in administering the opaque preparations such as penicillin G (Bicillin) is that aspirated blood cannot be detected at the bottom of the syringe, thus increasing the risk of injecting into a blood vessel. When such drugs are injected, use great care in locating the correct site. When aspirating, the nurse should look for blood at the top of the syringe near the plunger because blood may be drawn up through the column of penicillin. One study of IM injection techniques revealed that the straighter the path of needle insertion (e.g.,

90-degree angle), the less displacement and shear to tissue, causing less discomfort (Katsma and Smith, 1997).

A reported potential hazard with medication in glass ampules is the presence of glass particles in the ampule after the container is broken. When the medication is withdrawn into the syringe, the glass particles are also withdrawn and subsequently injected into the patient. As a precaution medication from glass ampules is only drawn through a needle with a filter.

Most children are unpredictable, and few are totally cooperative when receiving an injection. Even children who appear to be relaxed and constrained can lose control under the stress of the procedure. It is advisable to have someone available to help hold the child if needed. Because children often jerk or pull away unexpectedly, the nurse should carry an extra needle to exchange for the contaminated one so the delay is minimal. The child, even a small one, is told that he or she is receiving an injection (preferably using a phrase such as "putting the medicine under the skin"); the procedure then is carried out as quickly and skillfully as possible to avoid prolonging the stressful experience. Invasive procedures such as injections are especially anxiety provoking in young children, who may associate any assault to the "behind" with punishment. Because injections are painful, the nurse should use excellent injection techniques and effective pain reduction measures to reduce discomfort (see Guidelines box).

GUIDELINES

Intramuscular Administration of Medication

- Apply EMLA (a eutectic mix of lidocaine and prilocaine) or LMX cream (lidocaine) topically over site if time permits. (See Pain Management, Chapter 30.)
- Prepare medication.
  - Select appropriate-size needle and syringe.
  - If withdrawing medication from an ampule, use a needle equipped with a filter that removes glass particles; then use a new, nonfilter needle for injection.
  - Maximum volume to be administered in a single site is 1 mL for older infants and small children.
  - Have medication at room temperature before injection.
- Determine site of injection (see Table 39-6); make certain that muscle is large enough to accommodate volume and type of medication.
  - For infants and small or debilitated children use the vastus lateralis or ventrogluteal muscles; the dorsogluteal muscle is insufficiently developed to be a safe site for infants and small children.
- Obtain sufficient help in restraining child.
- Explain briefly what is to be done and, if appropriate, what child can do to help.
- Expose injection area for unobstructed view of landmarks.
- Select a site where skin is free of irritation and danger of infection; palpate for and avoid sensitive or hardened areas.
- With multiple injections rotate sites.
- Place child in a lying or sitting position; child is not allowed to stand because landmarks are more difficult to assess, restraint is more difficult, and the child may faint and fall.
  - *Ventrogluteal*—On side with upper leg flexed and placed in front of lower leg
  - *Vastus lateralis*—Supine, lying on side, or sitting
- Use a new, sharp needle (not one that has pierced rubber stopper on vial) with smallest diameter that permits free flow of the medication.
- Grasp muscle firmly between thumb and fingers to isolate and stabilize it for deposition of drug in its deepest part; in obese children spread skin with thumb and index finger to displace subcutaneous tissue and grasp muscle deeply on each side.

- Allow skin preparation to dry completely before penetrating skin.
- Decrease perception of pain.
  - Distract child with conversation.
  - Give child something on which to concentrate (e.g., squeezing a hand or side rail, pinching own nose, humming, counting, yelling "Ouch!").
  - Spray vapocoolant (e.g., ethyl chloride or fluoromethane) on site before injection, place a cold compress or wrapped ice cube on site about 1 minute before injection, or apply cold to contralateral site.
  - Have child hold a small adhesive bandage and place it on puncture site after intramuscular injection is given.
- Insert needle quickly using a dartlike motion at a 90-degree angle unless contraindicated.
- Avoid tracking any medication through superficial tissues:
  - Replace needle after withdrawing medication.
  - Use Z-track or air-bubble technique as indicated.
  - Avoid any depression of plunger during insertion of needle.
- Aspirate for blood.
  - If blood is found, remove syringe from site, change needle, and reinsert into new location.
  - If no blood is found, inject medication slowly into a relaxed muscle.
- Remove needle quickly; hold gauze firmly against skin near needle when removing it to avoid pulling on tissue.
- Apply firm pressure to site after injection; massage site to hasten absorption unless contraindicated, as with irritating drugs.
- Place a small adhesive bandage on puncture site; with young children decorate it by drawing a smiling face or other symbol of acceptance.
- Hold and cuddle young child and encourage parents to comfort him or her; praise older child.
- Allow expression of feelings.
- Discard syringe and uncapped, uncut needle in puncture-resistant container located near site of use.
- Record time of injection, drug, dose, and injection site.

Small infants offer little resistance to injections. Although they squirm and may be difficult to hold in position, they can usually be restrained without assistance. A larger infant's body can be securely restrained between the nurse's arm and body. To inject into the body of a muscle, the nurse firmly grasps the muscle mass between the thumb and fingers to isolate and stabilize the site (Fig. 39-13). However, in obese children it is preferable to first spread the skin with the thumb and index finger to displace subcutaneous tissue and then grasp the muscle deeply on each side.

If medication is given around the clock, the nurse must wake the child. Although it may seem easier to surprise the sleeping child and do it quickly, this can cause him or her to fear going back to sleep. When awakened first, children will know that nothing will be done to them unless they are forewarned. The Guidelines box above summarizes administration techniques that maximize safety and minimize the discomfort often associated with injections.

A needleless injection system (e.g., Biojector) delivers IM or subcutaneous injections without the use of a needle and eliminates the risk of accidental needle puncture. This needle-free injection system uses a carbon dioxide cartridge to power the delivery of medication through the skin. Although it is not painless, it may reduce pain and the anxiety of seeing the needle.

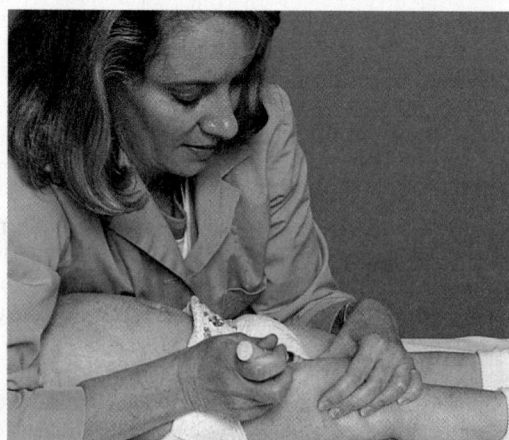

FIG 39-13 Holding small child for intramuscular injection. Note how nurse isolates and stabilizes muscle.

Subcutaneous and Intradermal Administration

Subcutaneous and intradermal injections are administered to children frequently, but the technique differs little from the method used with adults. Examples of subcutaneous injections include insulin, hormone replacement, allergy desensitization, and some vaccines. Tuberculin testing, local anesthesia, and allergy testing are examples of frequently administered intradermal injections.

Techniques to minimize the pain associated with these injections include changing the needle if it pierced a rubber stopper on a vial, using 26- to 30-gauge needles (only to inject the solution), and injecting small volumes (≤0.5 mL). The angle of the needle for the subcutaneous injection is typically 90 degrees. In children with little subcutaneous tissue, some practitioners insert the needle at a 45-degree angle. However, the benefit of using the 45-degree angle rather than the 90-degree angle remains controversial.

Although subcutaneous injections can be given anywhere there is subcutaneous tissue, common sites include the center third of the lateral aspect of the upper arm, the abdomen, and the center third of the anterior thigh. Some practitioners believe that it is not necessary to aspirate before injecting subcutaneously (e.g., this is an accepted practice in the administration of insulin). Automatic injector devices do not aspirate before injecting.

When giving an intradermal injection into the volar surface of the forearm, the nurse should avoid the medial side of the arm where the skin is more sensitive.

Intravenous Administration

The IV route for administering medications is frequently used in pediatric therapy. For some drugs it is the only effective route. This method is used for giving drugs to children who:

- Have poor absorption as a result of diarrhea, vomiting, or dehydration.
- Need a high serum concentration of a drug.
- Have resistant infections that require parenteral medication over an extended time.
- Need continuous pain relief.
- Require emergency treatment.

The nurse needs to consider several factors in relation to IV medication. When a drug is administered intravenously, the effect is almost instantaneous, and further control is limited. Most drugs for IV administration require a specified minimum dilution, rate of flow, or both; and many drugs are highly irritating or toxic to tissues outside the vascular system. In addition to the precautions and nursing observations commonly related to IV therapy, factors to consider when preparing and administering drugs to infants and children by the IV route include the following:

- Amount of drug to be administered
- Minimum dilution of drug and whether child is fluid restricted
- Type of solution in which drug can be diluted
- Length of time over which drug can be safely administered
- Rate limitations of child, vascular system, and infusion equipment
- Time that this or another drug is to be administered
- Compatibility of all drugs that child is receiving intravenously
- Compatibility with infusion fluids

Before any IV infusion check the site of insertion for patency. Never administer medications with blood products. Only one antibiotic should be administered at a time. Extra fluids needed to administer IV medications can be problematic for infants and fluid-restricted children. Syringe pumps are often used to deliver IV medication

TABLE 39-7	INTRAVENOUS CATHETER FLUSHES FOR LINES WITHOUT CONTINUOUS FLUID INFUSIONS
TYPE OF LINE	**TYPE OF FLUSH**
Peripheral lines (Hep-Lock or saline locks)	NS* after medications or every 8 hr for dormant lines; instill 2½ times tubing volume 24-g catheters: NS* or heparin 2 units/mL 2 mL
Midline	Heparin 10 units/mL; 3 ml in a 10-mL syringe† after medications or every 8 hours if dormant Newborns: heparin 1-2 units/mL to run continuously at ordered rate
External central line (nonimplanted, nontunneled, tunneled, or PICC)	Heparin 10 units/mL; 3 mL in a 10-mL syringe† after medications or once daily if dormant Newborns: heparin 2 units/mL; 2-3 ml after medications or to check line patency or heparin 1-2 units/mL to run continuously at ordered rate
Totally implanted central line (TIVAS, implanted port)	Heparin 10 units/mL; 5 mL after medications or once daily if dormant and accessed; if not accessed, heparin 100 units/mL; 5 mL every month
Arterial and central venous pressure continuous monitored lines	Heparin 2 units/mL in 55-mL syringe to run continuously at 1 mL/hr

NS, Normal saline; *PICC*, peripherally inserted central catheter; *TIVAS*, totally implantable venous access device.
*Use 5% dextrose in water when medication is incompatible with saline.
†Smaller syringes may be used when flush is delivered by a pump.

because they minimize fluid requirements and more precisely deliver small volumes of medication compared with large-volume infusion pumps. Regardless of the technique, the nurse must know the minimum dilutions for safe administration of IV medications to infants and children.

Peripheral Intermittent Infusion Device

The peripheral lock, also known as an intermittent infusion device or saline or heparin lock, is an alternative to a keep-open infusion when extended access to a vein is required without the need for continuous fluid. It is most frequently used for intermittent infusion of medication into a peripheral venous route. A short, flexible catheter is used as the lock device, and a site is selected where there will be minimal movement such as the forearm. The catheter is inserted and secured in the same manner as for any IV infusion device, but the hub is occluded with a stopper or injection cap.

The type of device used may vary, and the care and use of the peripheral lock are carried out according to the protocol of the institution or unit. However, the general concept is the same. The catheter remains in place and is flushed with saline after infusion of the medication. See the Evidence-Based Practice box and Table 39-7 on flushing with normal saline or heparin.

EVIDENCE-BASED PRACTICE

Normal Saline or Heparinized Saline Flush Solution in Pediatric Intravenous Lines

Ask the Question

Is there a significant difference in the longevity of IV intermittent infusion locks in children when NS is used as a flush instead a HS solution?

Search for the Evidence

Search Strategies

Selection criteria included evidence during the years 1992 to 2011 with the following terms: saline vs. heparin intermittent flush, children's heparin lock flush, heparin lock patency, peripheral venous catheter in children.

Databases Used

CINAHL, PubMed

Critically Analyze the Evidence

- In trials of HS administration vs. NS, placebo, or no treatment in neonates, no strong evidence regarding the effectiveness and safety of heparin in prolonging catheter life was found (Shah, Ng, and Sinha, 2005)
- No significant statistical difference was found between HS and NS flushes for maintaining catheter patency in children (Hanrahan, Kleiber, and Berends, 2000; Hanrahan, Kleiber, and Fagan, 1994; Heilskov, Kleiber, Johnson, et al., 1998; Kotter, 1996; Mok, Kwong, and Chan, 2007; Schultz, Drew, and Hewitt, 2002).
- Increased incidence of pain or erythema was associated with HS flushing of infusion devices (Hanrahan, Kleiber, and Fagan, 1994; McMullen, Fioravanti, Pollack, et al., 1993; Nelson and Graves, 1998; Robertson, 1994).
- Increased patency or longer dwell times were found with HS solutions vs. NS in 24-gauge catheters (Beecroft, Bossert, Chung, et al., 1997; Danek and Noris, 1992; Gyr, Burroughs, Smith, et al., 1995; Hanrahan, Kleiber, and Berends, 2000; Mudge, Forcier, and Slattery, 1998; Tripathi, Kaushik, and Singh, 2008).
- Younger children and preterm neonates with lower gestational ages were associated with shorter patency of IV catheters (McMullen, Fioravanti, Pollack, et al., 1993; Paisley, Stamper, Brown, et al., 1997; Robertson, 1994; Tripathi, Kaushik, and Singh, 2008).
- Infusion devices flushed with NS lasted longer than those flushed with HS (Goldberg, Sankaran, Givelichian, et al., 1999; Le Duc, 1997; Nelson and Graves, 1998).
- When measured and reported, the length of time between flushing peripheral devices affected the dwell time (Crews, Gnann, Rice, et al., 1997; Gyr, Burroughs, Smith, et al., 1995).
- Preterm neonates are at higher risk for development of clotting problems as a result of heparin; none of the studies cited anticoagulation-associated complications with HS (Klenner, Fusch, Rakow, et al., 2003).
- 0.9% sodium chloride injection is safe for maintaining patency of peripheral locks in adults and children older than age 12 years (American Society of Hospital Pharmacists, 2006).
- Either preservative-free heparin or preservative-free 0.9% sodium chloride may be used to flush a peripheral IV line; however, catheter patency may be maintained by flushing with saline when converting from continuous to intermittent use (Infusion Nurses Society, 2006).
- After each catheter use peripheral catheters should be locked with preservative-free 0.9% sodium chloride (Infusion Nurses Society, 2011).
- No recommendation is made for use of preservative-free 0.9% sodium chloride vs. heparin for locking peripheral catheters (Infusion Nurses Society, 2011).

Apply the Evidence: Nursing Implications

There is *low-quality evidence with a weak recommendation* (Guyatt, Oxman, Vist, et al., 2008) for using NS vs. HS flush solution in pediatric IV lines. Further research is still needed with larger samples of children, especially preterm neonates, using small-gauge catheters (24 gauge) and other gauge catheters flushed with NS and HS as intermittent infusion devices only (no continuous infusions). Variables to be considered include catheter dwell time; medications administered; period between regular flushing and flushing associated with medication administration; pain, erythema, and other localized complications; concentration and amount of HS used; flush method (positive-pressure technique vs. no specific technique); reason for IV device removal; and complications associated with either solution. NS is a safe alternative to HS flush in infants and children with intermittent IV locks larger than 24 gauge; smaller neonates may benefit from HS flush (longer dwell time), but the evidence is inconclusive for all weight ranges and gestational ages.

Quality and Safety Competencies:
Evidence-Based Practice*
Knowledge

Differentiate clinical opinion from research and evidence-based summaries

Describe methods for using NS or HS flush solution in pediatric IV lines.

Skills

Base individualized care plan on patient values, clinical expertise, and evidence

Integrate evidence into practice on NS or HS flush solution in pediatric IV lines.

Attitudes

Value the concept of evidence-based practice as integral to determining best clinical practice

Appreciate the strengths and weakness of evidence for NS or HS flush solution in pediatric IV lines.

References

American Society of Hospital Pharmacists Commission on Therapeutics: ASHP therapeutic position statement on the institutional use of 0.9% sodium chloride injection to maintain patency of peripheral indwelling intermittent infusion devices, *Am J Health Syst Pharm* 63(13):1273–1275, 2006.

Beecroft PC, Bossert E, Chung K, et al: Intravenous lock patency in children: dilute heparin versus saline, *J Pediatr Pharm Practice* 2(4):211–223, 1997.

Crews BE, Gnann KK, Rice MH, et al: Effects of varying intervals between heparin flushes on pediatric catheter longevity, *Pediatr Nurs* 23(1):87–91, 1997.

Danek GD, Noris EM: Pediatric IV catheters: efficacy of saline flush, *Pediatr Nurs* 18(2):111–113, 1992.

Goldberg M, Sankaran R, Givelichian L, et al: Maintaining patency of peripheral intermittent infusion devices with heparinized saline and saline: a randomized double blind controlled trial in neonatal intensive care and a review of literature, *Neonat Intensive Care* 12(1):18–22, 1999.

EVIDENCE-BASED PRACTICE

Normal Saline or Heparinized Saline Flush Solution in Pediatric Intravenous Lines—cont'd

Guyatt GH, Oxman AD, Vist GE, et al: GRADE: An emerging consensus on rating quality of evidence and strength of recommendations, *BMJ* 336(7650):924–926, 2008.

Gyr P, Burroughs T, Smith K, et al: Double-blind comparison of heparin and saline flush solutions in maintenance of peripheral infusion devices, *Pediatr Nurs* 21(4):383–389, 1995.

Hanrahan KS, Kleiber C, Berends S: Saline for peripheral intravenous locks in neonates: evaluating a change in practice, *Neonat Netw* 19(2):19–24, 2000.

Hanrahan KS, Kleiber C, Fagan C: Evaluation of saline for IV locks in children, *Pediatr Nurs* 20(6):549–552, 1994.

Heilskov J, Kleiber C, Johnson K, et al: A randomized trial of heparin and saline for maintaining intravenous locks in neonates, *J Soc Pediatr Nurs* 3(3):111–116, 1998.

Infusion Nurses Society: *Policies and procedures for infusion nursing*, ed 3, Norwood, Mass, 2006, Author.

Infusion Nurses Society: Infusion nursing standards of practice, *J Infus Nurs* 34(1S):S63–S64, 2011.

Klenner AF, Fusch C, Rakow A, et al: Benefit and risk of heparin for maintaining peripheral venous catheters in neonates: a placebo-controlled trial, *J Pediatr* 143(6):741–745, 2003.

Kotter RW: Heparin vs. saline for intermittent intravenous device maintenance in neonates, *Neonat Netw* 15(6):43–47, 1996.

Le Duc K: Efficacy of normal saline solution versus heparin solution for maintaining patency of peripheral intravenous catheters in children, *J Emerg Nurs* 23(4):306–309, 1997.

McMullen A, Fioravanti ID, Pollack D, et al: Heparinized saline or normal saline as a flush solution in intermittent intravenous lines in infants and children, *MCN Am J Matern Child Nurs* 18(2):78–85, 1993.

Mok E, Kwong TK, Chan ME: A randomized controlled trial for maintaining peripheral intravenous lock in children, *Int J Nurs Pract* 13(1):33–45, 2007.

Mudge B, Forcier D, Slattery MJ: Patency of 24-gauge peripheral intermittent infusion devices: a comparison of heparin and saline flush solutions, *Pediatr Nurs* 24(2):142–149, 1998.

Nelson TJ, Graves SM: 0.9% Sodium chloride injection with and without heparin for maintaining peripheral indwelling intermittent infusion devices in infants, *Am J Heath Syst Pharm* 55:570–573, 1998.

Paisley MK, Stamper M, Brown T, et al: The use of heparin and normal saline flushes in neonatal intravenous catheters, *J Pediatr Nurs* 23(5):521–527, 1997.

Robertson J: Intermittent intravenous therapy: a comparison of two flushing solutions, *Contemp Nurs* 3(4):174–179, 1994.

Schultz AA, Drew D, Hewitt H: Comparison of normal saline and heparinized saline for patency of IV locks in neonates, *Appl Nurs Res* 15(1):28–34, 2002.

Shah PS, Ng E, Sinha AK: Heparin for prolonging peripheral intravenous catheter use in neonates, *Cochrane Database Syst Rev* (4):CD002774, 2005.

Tripathi S, Kaushik V, Singh V: Peripheral IVs: factors affecting complications and patency—a randomized controlled trial, *J Infus Nurs* 31(3):182–188, 2008.

Updated by Olga A. Taylor

*Adapted from the QSEN at www.qsen.org.
HS, Heparinized saline; *IV*, intravenous; *NS*, normal saline.

Children may be discharged with a peripheral lock in place to continue receiving medications without hospitalization; this is usually reserved for children who require medications on a short-term basis and are referred to a home-based infusion company. Those with chronic illnesses who require repeated blood sampling or medications, long-term chemotherapy, or frequent hyperalimentation or antibiotic therapy are best managed with a central venous catheter.

Central Venous Access Device

Central venous access devices (CVADs) have several different characteristics. Factors that can influence the type of CVAD include the reason for placement of the catheter (diagnosis), length of therapy, risk to the patient in placement of the catheter, and availability of resources to help the family maintain the catheter.

Short-term or nontunneled catheters are used in acute care, emergency, and intensive care units. These catheters are made of polyurethane and placed in large veins such as the subclavian, femoral, or jugular. Insertion is by surgical incision or large percutaneous threading. A chest x-ray film should be taken to verify placement of the catheter tip before administration of fluids or medications.

Peripherally inserted central catheters (PICCs) can be used for short-term to moderate-length therapy. These catheters consist of silicone or polymer material and are placed by specially trained nurses, physicians, or interventional radiologists (Gamulka, Mendoza, and Connolly, 2005). The most common insertion site is above the antecubital area using the median, cephalic, or basilic vein. The catheter is threaded either with or without a guidewire into the superior vena cava. PICCs can be trimmed before insertion; and the decision can be made to insert the catheter midline, which is considered between the insertion site and the axilla. If the catheter is threaded midline, total parenteral nutrition (TPN) or any other drug known to irritate a peripheral vein (e.g., chemotherapy drugs) should not be administered. The high concentration of glucose in TPN makes it irritating to the vessel; it should be infused through a central catheter.

The decision to insert a PICC needs to be made before several attempts at IV insertion are made. When the antecubital veins have been punctured repeatedly, they are not considered candidates for this type of catheter. Because it is the least costly and has less chance of complications than other CVADs, it is an excellent choice for many pediatric patients.

! NURSING ALERT

Most PICC lines are not sutured into place; thus care is needed when changing the dressing.

Long-term CVADs include tunneled catheters and implanted infusion ports (Table 39-8 and Fig. 39-14). They may have single, double, or triple lumens. Several lumens (multilumen) catheters allow more than one therapy to be administered at the same time. Reasons to use multilumen catheters include repeated blood sampling, TPN, administration of blood products or infusion of large quantities or concentrations of fluids, administration of incompatible drugs or fluids at the same time (through different lumens), and central venous pressure monitoring.

TABLE 39-8   COMPARISON OF LONG-TERM CENTRAL VENOUS ACCESS DEVICES

DESCRIPTION	BENEFITS	CARE CONSIDERATIONS
Tunneled Catheter (e.g., Hickman or Broviac Catheter)		
Silicone, radiopaque, flexible catheter with open ends or VitaCuffs (biosynthetic material impregnated with silver ions) on catheter(s) enhances tissue ingrowth May have more than one lumen	Reduced risk of bacterial migration after tissue adheres to cuff One or two Dacron cuff Easy to use for self-administered infusions Removal requires pulling catheter from site (nonsurgical procedure)	Requires daily heparin flushes Must be clamped or have clamp nearby at all times Must keep exit site dry Heavy activity restricted until tissue adheres to cuff Water sports may be restricted (risk of infection) Risk of infection still present Protrudes outside body; susceptible to damage from sharp instruments and may be pulled out; may affect body image More difficult to repair Patient or family must learn catheter care
Groshong Catheter		
Clear, flexible, silicone, radiopaque catheter with closed tip and two-way valve at proximal end Dacron cuff or VitaCuff on catheter enhances tissue ingrowth May have more than one lumen	Reduced time and cost for maintenance care; no heparin flushes needed Reduced catheter damage; no clamping needed because of two-way valve Increased patient safety because of minimal potential for blood backflow or air embolism Reduced risk of bacterial migration after tissue adheres to cuff Easily repaired Easy to use for self-administered intravenous infusions	Requires weekly irrigation with normal saline Must keep exit site dry Heavy activity restricted until tissue adheres to cuff Water sports may be restricted (risk of infection) Risk of infection still present Protrudes outside body; susceptible to damage from sharp instruments and may be pulled out; can affect body image Patient or family must learn catheter care
Implanted Ports (e.g., Port-A-Cath, Infus-A-Port, Mediport, Norport, Groshong Port)		
Totally implantable metal or plastic device that consists of self-sealing injection port with top or side access with preconnected or attachable silicone catheter that is placed in large blood vessel	Reduced risk of infection Placed completely under skin and therefore much less likely to be pulled out or damaged No maintenance care and reduced cost for family Heparinized monthly and after each infusion to maintain patency (only Groshong port requires saline) No limitations on regular physical activity, including swimming Dressing needed only when port accessed with Huber needle that is not removed No or only slight change in body appearance (slight bulge on chest)	Must pierce skin for access; pain with insertion of needle; can use local anesthetic (EMLA, LMX) or intradermal buffered lidocaine before accessing port Special noncoring needle (Huber) with straight or angled design must be used to inject into port Skin preparation needed before injection Difficult to manipulate for self-administered infusions Catheter may dislodge from port, especially if child "plays" with port site (twiddler syndrome) Vigorous contact sports generally not allowed Removal requires surgical procedure

EMLA, Eutectic mix of lidocaine and prilocaine; *LMX,* lidocaine.

With any of the central venous catheters, medication is easily instilled through the injection cap. Maintenance of the catheter includes dressing changes, flushing to maintain patency, and prevention of occlusion or dislodgment.

With the implanted device the port must be palpated for placement and stabilized; the overlying skin cleansed; and only special noncoring Huber needles used to pierce the diaphragm of the port on the top or side, depending on the style. To avoid repeated skin punctures a special infusion set with a Huber needle and extension tubing with a Luer connection can be used (see Fig. 39-14). With this attached the injection procedure is the same as for an intermittent infusion device or a central venous catheter. To prevent infection, meticulous aseptic technique must be used any time the devices are entered, including instillation of heparin or saline to prevent clotting. There should be a protocol stating that the Huber needle needs to be changed at established intervals, usually 5 to 7 days.

The children and parents are taught the procedure for care of the CVAD before discharge from the hospital, including preparation

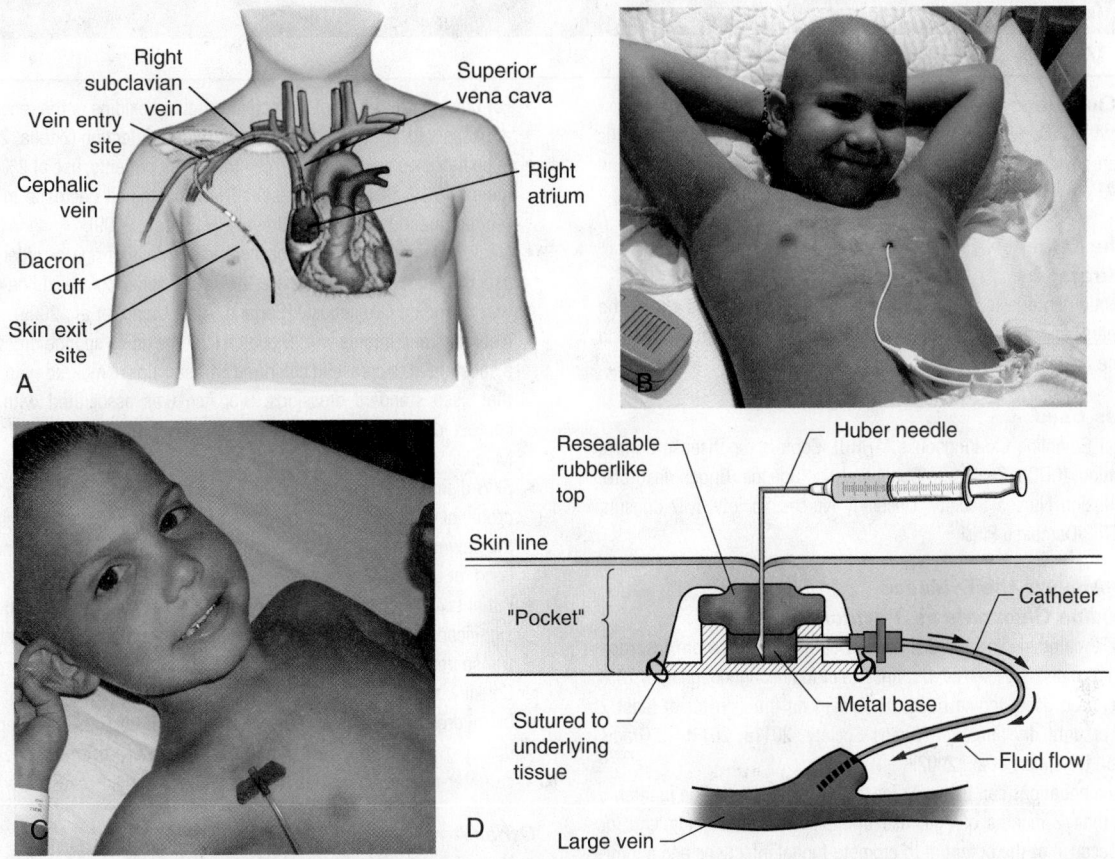

FIG 39-14 Venous access devices. **A,** External central venous catheter insertion and exit site. **B,** Child with external central venous catheter (dressing removed for photo). **C,** Child with implanted port with Huber needle in place (dressing removed for photo). **D,** Side view of implanted port.

and injection of the prescribed medication, the flush, and dressing changes. A protective device may be recommended for some active children to prevent their accidentally dislodging the needle. Many children take responsibility for preparing and administering medications. Both verbal and written step-by-step instructions are provided for the learners. See the Evidence-Based Practice box for CVAD site care.

Infection and catheter occlusion are two of the most common complications of central venous catheters. They require treatment with antibiotics for infection and a fibrinolytic agent such as alteplase for thrombus formation (Blaney, Shen, Kerner, et al., 2006; Fisher, Deffenbaugh, Poole, et al., 2004; Kerner, Garcia-Careaga, Fisher, et al., 2006; Shen, Li, Murdock, et al., 2003). Uncapping can be prevented by taping the cap securely to the catheter and the clamped line to the dressing. Leaks can be prevented by using a smooth-edged clamp only. The parents are cautioned to keep scissors away from the child to prevent accidental cutting of the catheter. If the catheter leaks, the parents are instructed to tape it above the leak and then clamp it at the taped site. The child should be taken to the practitioner as soon as possible to prevent infection or clotting after a catheter leak.

! NURSING ALERT

If a central venous catheter is removed accidentally, apply pressure to the entry site to the vein, not the exit site on the skin.

Nasogastric, Orogastric, and Gastrostomy Administration

When a child has an indwelling feeding tube or a gastrostomy, oral medications are usually given via that route. An advantage of this method is the ability to administer oral medications around the clock without disturbing the child. A disadvantage is the risk of occluding, or clogging, the tube, especially when giving viscous solutions through small-bore feeding tubes. The most important preventive measure is adequate flushing after the medication is instilled (see Guidelines box on p. 1170).

Rectal Administration

The rectal route for administration is less reliable but is sometimes used when the oral route is difficult or contraindicated. It is also used when oral preparations are unsuitable to control vomiting. Some of the drugs available in suppository form are acetaminophen, aspirin, sedatives, analgesics (morphine), and antiemetics. The difficulty in using the rectal route is that, unless the rectum is empty at the time of insertion, the absorption of the drug may be delayed, diminished, or prevented by the presence of feces. Sometimes the drug is evacuated later, securely surrounded by stool.

Remove the wrapping on the suppository and lubricate the suppository with warm water (water-soluble jelly may affect medication absorption). Rectal suppositories are traditionally inserted with the apex (pointed end) foremost. Reverse contractions or the pressure gradient of the anal canal may help the suppository slip higher into the canal. Using a glove or finger cot, quickly but gently insert the

EVIDENCE-BASED PRACTICE
Central Venous Catheter Site Care

Ask the Question

In children with CVCs, is chlorhexidine gluconate a more effective antiseptic solution than povidone-iodine in preventing CVC-related site infections and bacteremia?

Search the Evidence
Search Strategies

Search selection criteria included English language publications within the past 10 years and research-based articles on catheter site care and chlorhexidine.

Databases Used

The National Guideline Clearinghouse (AHRQ), Centers for Disease Control and Prevention (CDC), Cochrane Collaboration, Joanna Briggs Institute, PubMed, Infusion Nurses Society, Oncology Nurses Society, MD Consult, BestBETs, TRIP Database Plus

Critically Analyze the Evidence
Chlorhexidine Gluconate vs. Povidone-Iodine

- Use of 2% chlorhexidine for disinfecting catheter site before insertion (allowing it to dry) is preferred; but tincture of iodine, an iodophor, or 70% alcohol can be used. Iodine needs to remain on the skin for at least 2 minutes or until dry (Infusion Nurses Society, 2011a, 2011b; O'Grady, Alexander, Dellinger, et al., 2002).
- No recommendations can be made for the use of chlorhexidine in infants younger than 2 months of age, use of topical antibiotic ointments or creams because of the potential to promote fungal infections and antimicrobial resistance, or use of impregnated catheters and chlorhexidine sponge dressings to reduce the incidence of infection (Infusion Nurses Society, 2011a, 2011b; O'Grady, Alexander, Dellinger, et al., 2002).
- Avoid use of sponges in infants younger than 7 days old and 26 weeks' gestation. Replace the catheter-site dressing when it becomes damp, loosened, or soiled or when inspection of the site is necessary (O'Grady, Alexander, Dellinger, et al., 2002).
- Replace dressings used on short-term CVC sites every 2 days for gauze dressings and at least every 7 days for transparent dressings except in pediatric patients in whom the risk for dislodging the catheter outweighs the benefit of changing the dressing (Infusion Nurses Society, 2011a; O'Grady, Alexander, Dellinger, et al., 2002)
- Use of alcohol, chlorhexidine gluconate, povidone-iodine, and tincture of iodine (allow to dry) is recommended. If using povidone-iodine, do not apply alcohol as a second antiseptic (Infusion Nurses Society, 2006, 2011a, 2011b; Marlowe, Mistry, Coffin, and others, 2010).
- Dress the vascular access site with sterile gauze and cover it with sterile transparent dressings. Gauze dressings should be changed every 48 hours (Camp-Sorrell, 2004; Infusion Nurses Society, 2006, 2011a, 2011b).
- Semipermeable transparent dressings should be changed at least every 5 to 7 days; the interval depends on the dressing material, age and condition of the patient, infection rate reported by the organization, environmental conditions, and manufacturer labeled uses and directions (Infusion Nurses Society, 2006, 2011a, 2011b)
- Chlorhexidine for preinsertion and postinsertion site catheter care was found superior to alcohol and povidone-iodine (Camp-Sorrell, 2004; Carson 2004; Chaiyakunapruk, Veenstra, Lipsky, et al., 2002).
- Routine application of antibiotic ointment is not recommended because of the risk of fungal infections and antimicrobial resistance.

- For bone marrow transplant recipients, chlorhexidine is the recommended antisepsis for prevention of catheter-related infection (Zitella, 2003).
- In pediatric hemopoietic stem cell transplant patients, use of 2% chlorhexidine in 70% isopropanol resulted in a sustained decrease in catheter-related infections (Soothill, Bravery, Ho, et al., 2009).
- Neonates weighing 1500 g or more and 7 days of age or older tolerated use of chlorhexidine-gluconate; however, some chlorhexidine-gluconate was absorbed cutaneously (Garland, Alex, Uhing, et al., 2009).
- Neonates and infants with Biopatch (chlorhexidine sponge dressings) had a substantial decrease in colonized catheter tips compared with the group that used standard dressings. Biopatch was associated with localized contact dermatitis in infants of very low birth weight (Garland, Alex, Mueller, et al., 2001).
- Skin disinfection before CVC insertion and daily dressing changes with propanol-chlorhexidine followed by povidone-iodine was associated with the lowest rate of microbial catheter colonization (Langgartner, Linde, Lehn, et al., 2004).
- Patients with chlorhexidine-impregnated CVC dressing (Biopatch) had a significantly reduced risk of CVC colonization compared with patients with transparent dressing alone (Levy, Katz, Solter, et al., 2005; Onder, Chandar, Coakley, et al., 2009).
- In children older than 2 years of age, use of chlorhexidine-impregnated dressing should be considered as an extra prevention measure for catheter-related bloodstream infection (Infusion Nurses Society, 2011a).

Other Antiseptics

- Use of ethanol locks in children on parental nutrition (median age, 18.3 months) significantly decreased the rate of CVC infections (9.9 per 1000 to 2.1 per 1000 catheter days) (Jones, Hull, Richardson, et al., 2010).
- In pediatric patients with hemophilia (3, 11, and 13 years of age), ethanol lock therapy cleared catheter-related infection (Rajpurkar, Boldt-Macdonald, Mclenon, et al., 2009).
- In pediatric cancer patients, taurolidine/citrate (TauroLock) reduced catheter-related blood infections (Simon, Ammann, Wiszniewsky, et al., 2008).

Apply the Evidence: Nursing Implications

There is *moderate-quality evidence with a strong recommendation* (Guyatt, Oxman, Vist, et al., 2008) for CVC care. Two percent chlorhexidine should be used for catheter site antisepsis. Two percent chlorhexidine should be used with caution in premature and low-birth-weight infants. Chlorhexidine-impregnated sponges (Biopatch) should be used around the catheter site except in low-birth-weight infants in the first 2 weeks of life.

Quality and Safety Competencies:
Evidence-Based Practice*
Knowledge
Differentiate clinical opinion from research and evidence-based summaries
Describe methods for CVC care.

Skills
Base individualized care plan on patient values, clinical expertise, and evidence
Integrate evidence into practice by using appropriate CVC care.

EVIDENCE-BASED PRACTICE

Central Venous Catheter Site Care—cont'd

Attitudes

Value the concept of evidence-based practice as integral to determining best clinical practice

Appreciate the strengths and weakness of evidence for CVC care.

References

Camp-Sorrell D, editor: *Access device guidelines: recommendations for nursing practice and education*, ed 2, Pittsburgh, 2004, Oncology Nursing Society.

Carson S: Chlorhexidine versus povidone-iodine for central venous catheter site care in children, *J Pediatr Nurs* 19(1):74–80, 2004.

Chaiyakunapruk N, Veenstra D, Lipsky B, et al: Chlorhexidine compared with povidone-iodine solution for vascular catheter-site care: a meta-analysis, *Ann Intern Med* 136(11):792–801, 2002.

Garland J, Alex C, Mueller C, et al: A randomized trial comparing povidone-iodine to a chlorhexidine-impregnated dressing for prevention of central venous catheter infections in neonates, *Pediatrics* 107(6):1431–1436, 2001.

Garland JS, Alex CP, Uhing MR, et al: Pilot trial to compare tolerance of chlorhexidine gluconate to povidone-iodine antisepsis for central venous catheter placement in neonates, *J Perinatol* 29:808–813, 2009.

Guyatt GH, Oxman AD, Vist GE, et al: GRADE: an emerging consensus on rating quality of evidence and strength of recommendations, *BMJ* 336(7650):924–926, 2008.

Infusion Nurses Society: *Policies and procedures for infusion nursing*, ed 3, Norwood, Mass, 2006, Author.

Infusion Nurses Society: Infusion nursing standards of practice, *J Infus Nurs* 34(1S):S63–S64, 2011a.

Infusion Nurses Society: *Policies and procedures for infusion nursing*, ed 4, South Norwood, Mass, 2011b, Author.

Jones BA, Hull MA, Richardson DS, et al: Efficacy of ethanol locks in reducing central venous catheter infections in pediatric patients with intestinal failure, *J Pediatr Surg* 45:1287–1293, 2010.

Langgartner J, Linde H, Lehn N, et al: Combined skin disinfection with chlorhexidine/propanol and aqueous povidone-iodine reduces bacterial colonisation of central venous catheters, *Intensive Care Med* 30(6):1081–1088, 2004.

Levy I, Katz J, Solter E, et al: Chlorhexidine-impregnated dressing for prevention of colonization of central venous catheters in infants and children: a randomized controlled study, *Pediatr Infect Dis* 24(8):676–679, 2005.

Marlowe L, Mistry RD, Coffin S, et al: Blood culture contamination rates after skin antisepsis with chlorhexidine gluconate versus povidone-iodine in a pediatric emergency department, *Infect Control Hosp Epidemiol* 31(2):171–176, 2010.

O'Grady N, Alexander M, Dellinger EP, et al: Guidelines for the prevention of intravascular catheter-related infections, *MMWR Morb Mortal Wkly Rep* 51(RR–10):1–29, 2002.

Onder AM, Chandar J, Coakley S, et al: Controlling exit site infections: does it decrease the incidence of catheter-related bacteremia in children on chronic hemodialysis? *Hemodial Int* 13:11–18, 2009.

Rajpurkar M, Boldt-Macdonald K, Mclenon R, et al: Ethanol lock therapy for the treatment of catheter-related infections in haemophilia patients, *Haemophilia* 15:1267–1271, 2009.

Simon A, Ammann RA, Wiszniewsky G, et al: Taurolidine-citrate lock solution (TauroLock) significantly reduces CVAD-associated gram-positive infections in pediatric cancer patients, *BMC Infect Dis* 8:102–109, 2008.

Soothill JS, Bravery K, Ho A: A fall in bloodstream infections followed a change to 2% chlorhexidine in 70% isopropanol for catheter connection antisepsis: a pediatric single center before/after study on a hemopoietic stem cell transplant ward, *Am J Infect Control* 37:626–630, 2009.

Zitella L: Central venous catheter site care for blood and marrow transplant recipients, *Clin J Oncol Nurs* 7(3):289–298, 2003.

Brandi Horvath; updated by Olga A. Taylor

CVC, Central venous catheter.
*Adapted from the QSEN at www.qsen.org.

suppository into the rectum beyond both of the rectal sphincters. Then hold the buttocks together firmly to relieve pressure on the anal sphincter until the urge to expel the suppository has passed, which occurs within 5 to 10 minutes. Sometimes the amount of drug ordered is less than the dose available. The irregular shape of most suppositories makes the process of dividing them into a desired dose difficult if not dangerous. If it must be halved, it should be cut lengthwise. However, there is no guarantee that the drug is evenly dispersed throughout the petrolatum base.

If medication is administered via a retention enema, the same procedure is used. Drugs given by enema are diluted in the smallest amount of solution possible to minimize the likelihood of being evacuated.

Optic, Otic, and Nasal Administration

There are few differences in administering eye, ear, and nose medication to children and adults. The major difficulty is gaining children's cooperation. Older children need only an explanation and direction. Although the administration of optic, otic, and nasal medication is not painful, these drugs can cause unpleasant sensations, which can be eliminated with various techniques.

To instill eye medication place the child supine or sitting with the head extended and ask him or her to look up. Use one hand to pull the lower eyelid downward; the hand that holds the dropper rests on the head so it may move synchronously with the child's head, thus reducing the possibility of trauma to a struggling child or dropping medication on the face (Fig. 39-15). When the lower eyelid is pulled down, a small conjunctival sac is formed; apply the solution or ointment to this area rather than directly on the eyeball. Another effective technique is to pull the lower eyelid down and out to form a cup effect, into which the medication is dropped. Gently close the eyelids to prevent expression of the medication. Wipe excess medication from the inner canthus outward to prevent contamination to the contralateral eye.

> **! NURSING ALERT**
>
> To reduce unpleasant sensations when administering medications:
> *Eye*—Apply finger pressure to the lacrimal punctum at the inner aspect of the eyelid for 1 minute to prevent drainage of medication to the nasopharynx and the unpleasant "tasting" of the drug.
> *Ear*—Allow medications stored in the refrigerator to warm to room temperature before instillation.
> *Nose*—Position the child with the head hyperextended to prevent strangling sensations caused by medication trickling into the throat rather than up into the nasal passages.

GUIDELINES

Nasogastric, Orogastric, or Gastrostomy Medication Administration in Children

- Use elixir or suspension (rather than tablet) preparations of medication whenever possible.
- Dilute viscous medication or syrup with a small amount of water if possible.
- If administering tablets, crush tablet to a fine powder and dissolve drug in small amount of warm water.
- Never crush enteric-coated or sustained-release tablets or capsules.
- Avoid oily medications because they tend to cling to side of tube.
- Do not mix medication with enteral formula unless fluid is restricted. If adding a drug:
  - Check with pharmacist for compatibility.
  - Shake formula well and observe for any physical reaction (e.g., separation, precipitation).
  - Label formula container with name of medication, dosage, date, and time infusion started.
- Check for correct placement of nasogastric or orogastric tube (see Evidence-Based Practice box, pp. 1185-1186).
- Attach syringe (with adaptable tip but without plunger) to tube.
- Pour medication into syringe.
- Unclamp tube and allow medication to flow by gravity.
- Adjust height of container to achieve desired flow rate (e.g., increase height for faster flow).
- As soon as syringe is empty, pour in water to flush tubing.
  - Amount of water depends on length and gauge of tubing.
  - Determine amount before administering any medication by using a syringe to fill completely an unused nasogastric or orogastric tube with water. Amount of flush solution is usually 1.5 times this volume.
  - With certain drug preparations (e.g., suspensions), more fluid may be needed.
- If administering more than one drug at the same time, flush tube between each medication with clear water.
- Clamp tube after flushing unless it is left open.

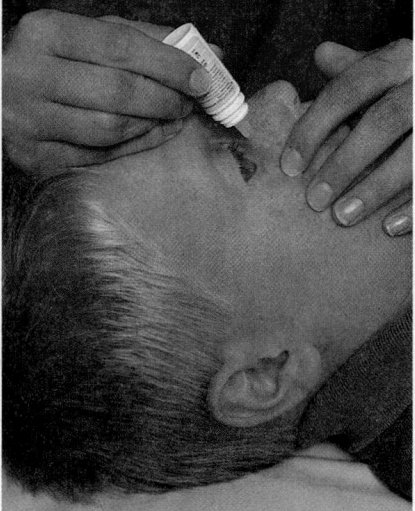

FIG 39-15 Administering eyedrops.

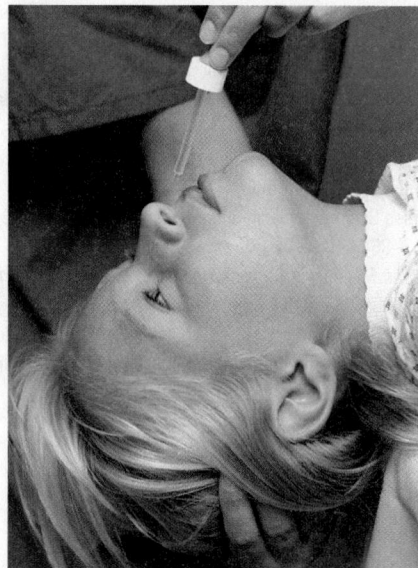

FIG 39-16 Proper position for instilling nose drops.

Instilling eyedrops in infants can be difficult because they often clench the eyelids tightly closed. One approach is to place the drops in the nasal corner where the eyelids meet. The medication pools in this area; and, when the child opens the eyelids, the medication flows onto the conjunctiva. For young children playing a game can be helpful such as instructing the child to keep the eyes closed to the count of three and then open them, at which time the drops are quickly instilled. Ointment can be applied by gently pulling down the lower eyelid and placing the ointment in the lower conjunctival sac.

💊 **MEDICATION ALERT**

If both eye ointment and drops are ordered, give drops first, wait 3 minutes, and then apply the ointment to allow each drug to work. When possible, administer eye ointments before bedtime or naptime because the child's vision will be blurred temporarily.

Ear drops are instilled with the child in the prone or supine position and the head turned to the appropriate side. For children younger than 3 years of age, the external auditory canal is straightened by gently pulling the pinna downward and straight back. The pinna is pulled upward and back in children older than 3 years of age. To place the drops deep into the ear canal without contaminating the tip of the dropper, place a disposable ear speculum in the canal and administer the drops through the speculum. Position the bottle so the drops fall against the side of the ear canal. After instillation the child should remain lying on the unaffected side for a few minutes. Gentle massage of the area immediately anterior to the ear facilitates the entry of drops into the ear canal. The use of cotton pledgets prevents medication from flowing out of the external canal. However, they should be loose enough to allow any discharge to exit from the ear. Premoistening the cotton with a few drops of medication prevents the wicking action from absorbing the medication instilled in the ear.

Nose drops are instilled in the same manner as in the adult patient. Remove mucus from the nose with a clean tissue or washcloth. Unpleasant sensations associated with medicated nose drops are minimized when care is taken to position the child with the head extended well over the edge of the bed or pillow (Fig. 39-16). Depending on size, infants can be positioned in the football hold (see Fig. 39-5, *B*), in the nurse's arm with the head extended and stabilized between the nurse's body and elbow and the arms and hands immobilized with the nurse's hands, or with the head extended over the edge of the bed or a pillow. After instillation of the drops, the child should remain in position for 1 minute to allow the drops to come in contact with the nasal surfaces. Insert nasal spray dispensers into the naris vertically and then angle them to avoid trauma to the septum and direct medication toward the inferior turbinate.

Aerosol Therapy

Aerosol therapy can be effective in depositing medication directly into the airway. The value of aerosolized water, or "mist therapy," is controversial. This route of administration can be useful in avoiding the systemic side effects of certain drugs and reducing the amount of drug necessary to achieve the desired effect. Bronchodilators, steroids, mucolytics, and antibiotics suspended in particulate form can be inhaled so the medication reaches the small airways. Aerosol therapy is particularly challenging in children who are too young to cooperate with controlling the rate and depth of breathing. Administration of this therapy requires skill, patience, and creativity.

> ### ! MEDICATION ALERT
>
> Medications can be aerosolized or nebulized with air or oxygen-enriched gas. The metered-dose inhaler (MDI) is a self-contained, handheld device that allows for intermittent delivery of a specified amount of medication. Many bronchodilators are available in this form and are used successfully by children with asthma. For children younger than the age of 5 or 6 years, a spacer device attached to the MDI can help with coordination of breathing and aerosol delivery. It also allows the aerosolized particles to remain in suspension longer. Handheld nebulizers discharge a medicated mist into a small plastic mask, which the child holds over the nose and mouth. To avoid particle deposition in the nose and pharynx, the child is instructed to take slow, deep breaths through an open mouth during the treatment. For home use an air compressor is necessary to force air through the liquid medication to form the aerosol. Compact, portable units can be obtained from health equipment companies.

Breath sounds and work of breathing should be assessed before and after treatments. Young children who become upset by having a mask held close to the face may become fatigued with fighting the procedure and actually appear worse during and immediately after the therapy. It may be necessary to spend a few minutes calming the child and allowing the vital signs to return to baseline to accurately assess changes in breath sounds and work of breathing.

Family Teaching and Home Care

The nurse usually assumes responsibility for preparing families to administer medications at home. The family should understand why the child is receiving the medication; the effects that might be expected; and the amount, frequency, and length of time the drug is to be administered. Instruction should be carried out in an unhurried, relaxed manner, preferably in an area away from a busy ward or office.

Instruct the caregiver carefully regarding the correct dosage. Some people have difficulty understanding medical terminology; the nurse should not assume that the message is clear just because they nod or otherwise indicate that they understand. For example, it is important to ascertain their interpretation of a teaspoon and be certain that they have acceptable devices for measuring the drug. If the drug is packaged with a dropper, syringe, or plastic cup, the nurse should show or mark the point on the device that indicates the prescribed dose and demonstrate how the dose is drawn up into a dropper or syringe, measured, and the bubbles eliminated. If the nurse has any doubts about the parent's ability to administer the correct dose, the parent should give a return demonstration. This is essential when a drug such as insulin or digoxin has potentially serious consequences from incorrect dosage or when more complex administration such as parenteral injections is required. When teaching a parent to give an injection, the nurse must allot adequate time for instruction and practice.

Home modifications are often necessary because the availability of equipment or assistance can differ from the hospital setting. For example, the parent may need guidance in devising methods that allow one person to hold the child and safely give the drug.

> ### ! NURSING ALERT
>
> To administer oral, nasal, or optic medication when only one person is available to hold the child, use the following procedure:
> - Place child supine on a flat surface (bed, couch, floor).
> - Sit facing child so his or her head is between operator's thighs and child's arms are under operator's legs.
> - Place lower legs over child's legs to restrain lower body if necessary.
> - To administer oral medication, place a small pillow under child's head to reduce risk of aspiration.
> - To administer nasal medication, place a small pillow under child's shoulders to aid flow of liquid through nasal passages.

The nurse should clarify with parents the time that the drug is to be administered. For instance, when a drug is prescribed in association with meals, the number of meals that the family is accustomed to eating influences the amount of drug the child receives. Does the family have meals twice a day or 5 times a day? When a drug is to be given several times during the day, together the nurse and parents can work out a schedule that accommodates the family's routine. This is particularly significant if a drug must be given at equal intervals throughout a 24-hour period. For example, telling parents that the child needs 1 tsp of medicine 4 times a day is subject to misinterpretation because the parents may routinely schedule the doses at incorrect times. Instead a preplanned schedule based on 6-hour intervals should be set up with the number of days required for the therapeutic dosage listed. Modification should also be made to accommodate sleep schedules. Written instructions should accompany all drug prescriptions.

> ### ! NURSING ALERT
>
> If parents have difficulty reading or understanding English, use colors to convey instructions. For example, mark each drug with a color and place the appropriate color on a calendar chart or on a drawing of a clock to identify when the drug needs to be given. If a liquid medication and syringe are used, also mark the syringe at the place the plunger needs to be with color-coded tape.

MAINTAINING FLUID BALANCE

Measuring Intake and Output

Accurate measurements of fluid intake and output (I&O) are essential to the assessment of fluid balance. Measurements from all sources—including gastrointestinal and parenteral I&O from urine, stools, vomitus, fistulas, NG suction, sweat, and drainage from wounds—must be taken and considered. Although the practitioner usually indicates when I&O measurements are to be recorded, it is a nursing responsibility to keep an accurate I&O record on certain children, including those:

- Receiving IV therapy.
- Who underwent major surgery.
- Receiving diuretic or corticosteroid therapy.
- With severe thermal burns or injuries.
- With renal disease or damage.
- With congestive heart failure.
- With dehydration.
- With diabetes mellitus.
- With oliguria.
- In respiratory distress.
- With chronic lung disease.

Infants and small children who are unable to use a bedpan and those who have bowel movements with every voiding require the application of a collecting device. If collecting bags are not used, wet diapers or pads are carefully weighed to ascertain the amount of fluid lost, including liquid stool, vomitus, and other losses. The volume of fluid in milliliters is equivalent to the weight of the fluid measured in grams. The specific gravity as a measure of osmolality helps to assess the degree of hydration.

For infants with diapers weigh all dry diapers to be used and note in an indelible marker the dry weight of the diaper; when there is fluid (urine or liquid stool) in the diaper, the amount of output can be approximated by subtracting the weight of the dry diaper from the weighed amount of the wet diaper.

Disadvantages of the weighed-diaper method of fluid measurement include (1) an inability to differentiate one type of loss from another because of admixture, (2) loss of urine or liquid stool from leakage or evaporation (especially if the infant is under a radiant warmer), and (3) additional fluid in the diaper (superabsorbent disposable type) from absorption of atmospheric moisture (in high-humidity incubators).

Special Needs When the Child Is NPO

Infants or children who are unable or not permitted to take fluids by mouth (NPO) have special needs. To ensure that they do not receive fluids, a sign can be placed in some obvious place such as over their beds or on their shirts to alert others to the NPO status. To prevent the temptation to drink, fluids should not be left at the bedside.

Oral hygiene, a part of routine hygienic care, is especially important when fluids are restricted or withheld. For young children who cannot brush their teeth or rinse their mouth without swallowing fluid, the mouth and teeth can be cleaned and kept moist by swabbing with saline-moistened gauze.

The child who is fluid restricted presents an equal challenge. Limiting fluids is often more difficult for the child than being NPO, especially when IV fluids are also eliminated. To make certain that the child does not drink the entire amount allowed early in the day, the daily allotment is calculated to provide fluids at periodic intervals throughout his or her waking hours. Serving the fluids in small containers gives the illusion of larger servings. No extra liquid is left at the bedside.

Parenteral Fluid Therapy
Site and Equipment

The site selected for PIV infusion depends on accessibility and convenience. Although it is possible to use any accessible in older

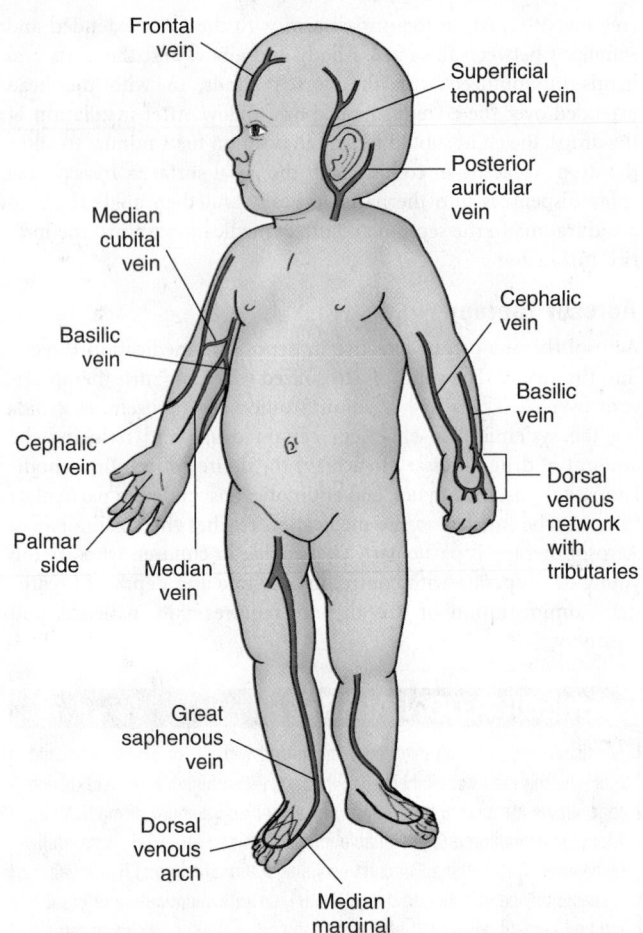

FIG 39-17 Preferred sites for venous access in infants.

children, the child's developmental, cognitive, and mobility needs must be considered when selecting a site. Ideally in older children the superficial veins of the forearm should be used, leaving the hands free. An older child can help select the site and thereby maintain some measure of control. For veins in the extremities it is best to start with the most distal site and avoid the child's favored hand to reduce the disability related to the procedure. Restrict the child's movements as little as possible; avoid a site over a joint in an extremity such as the antecubital space. In small infants a superficial vein of the hand, wrist, forearm, foot, or ankle is usually most convenient and most easily stabilized (Fig. 39-17). Foot veins should be avoided in children learning to walk and those already walking. Superficial veins of the scalp have no valves, insertion is easy, and they can be used in infants up to about 9 months of age; but they should be used only when other site attempts have failed. A transilluminator (Fig. 39-18) can aid in finding and evaluating veins for access.

Selection of a scalp vein may require clipping the area around the site to better visualize the vein and provide a smoother surface on which to tape the catheter hub and tubing. Clipping a portion of the infant's hair is upsetting to parents; therefore they should be told what to expect and reassured that the hair will grow in again rapidly (save the hair because parents often wish to keep it). Remove as little as possible directly over the insertion site and taping surface. A rubber band slipped onto the head from brow to occiput usually suffices as a tourniquet; although, if the vessel is visible, a tourniquet may not be necessary.

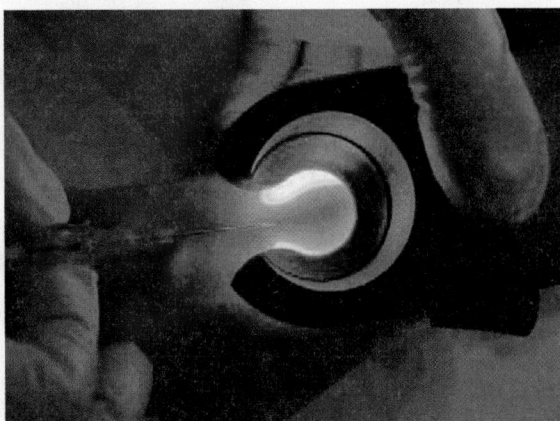

FIG 39-18 Transilluminator: low-heat light-emitting diode (LED) light placed on skin to illuminate veins; an opening allows cannulation of vein. (Courtesy Professor Mark Waltzman, Children's Hospital, Boston, MA.)

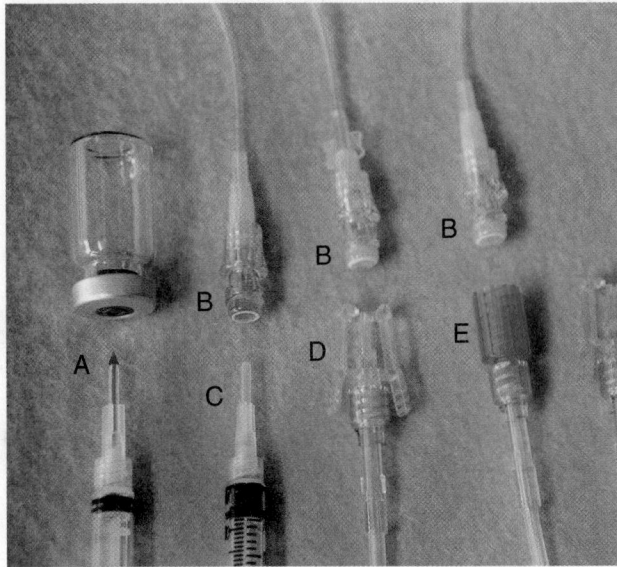

FIG 39-19 Interlink intravenous access systems. **A,** Blue spike syringe. **B,** Preslit injection port (needleless). **C,** Blunt plastic cannula syringe. **D,** Lever lock cannula. **E,** Threaded lock cannula.

Situations may occur in which rapid establishment of systemic access is vital; and venous access may be hampered by peripheral circulatory collapse, hypovolemic shock (secondary to vomiting or diarrhea, burns, or trauma), cardiopulmonary arrest, or other conditions (de Caen, Reis, and Bhutta, 2008; Hazinski, Zaritsky, Nadkarni, et al., 2002). Intraosseous infusion provides a rapid, safe, and lifesaving alternate route for administration of fluids and medications until intravascular access can be attained, especially in children who are 6 years of age and younger.

A large-bore needle such as a bone marrow aspiration needle (e.g., Jamshidi) or an intraosseous needle (e.g., Cook), is inserted into the medullary cavity of a long bone, most often the proximal tibia. This procedure is usually reserved for children who are unconscious or for those who are receiving analgesia because the procedure is painful. Local anesthesia should be used for semiconscious patients. Observe the dependent tissue closely for swelling because extravasation may be hidden under the leg and compartment syndrome may result.

For most IV infusions in children a 22- to 24-gauge catheter may be used if therapy is expected to last less than 5 days. The smallest-gauge and shortest-length catheter that will accommodate the prescribed therapy should be chosen. The length of the catheter may be directly related to infection or embolus formation (i.e., the shorter the catheter, the fewer the complications). The gauge of the catheter should maintain adequate flow of the infusate into the cannulated vein while allowing adequate blood flow around the catheter walls to promote proper hemodilution of the infusate.

Determining the best catheter for the patient early in the therapy provides the best chance of avoiding catheter-related complications. As the length of therapy increases, decisions regarding the type of infusion device (short peripheral, midline, PICC, or central venous catheter) should be explored. Guidelines such as flow charts and algorithms are available to help in these decisions.

Safety Catheters and Needleless Systems

Over-the-needle IV catheters with hollow-bore needles carry a high risk for transmission of bloodborne pathogens from needlestick injuries. Safety catheters prevent accidental needlesticks with the use of over-the-needle IV catheters (Whitby, McLaws, and Slater, 2008).

Needleless IV systems are designed to prevent needlestick injuries during administration of IV push medications and IV piggyback medications. Some needleless devices can be used with any tubing, but others require use of the entire IV delivery system for compatibility. Needleless IV systems rely on prepierced septa that are accessed by blunted plastic cannulas or systems that use valves that open and close a fluid path when activated by insertion of a syringe.

Blunt plastic cannulas and preslit injection port sites (Fig. 39-19) eliminate the need for steel needles and conventional injection port sites but remain accessible via hypodermic needles, a drawback except in emergent situations. Systems that do not permit needled access enhance safety by preventing health care workers from attempting to use needles. A syringe with a blue spike is available to access a single-dose vial (Fig. 39-19, *A*). The preslit injection port sites are identified by a white ring surrounding the port; this ring alerts users that the system is needleless (Fig. 39-19, *B*). Syringes are available with the blunt plastic cannula for accessing these sites (Fig. 39-19, *C*). A lever lock (Fig. 39-19, *D*) or threaded lock cannula (Fig. 39-19, *E*) attaches to an IV line, IV Y site, or peripheral intermittent infusion device. A preslit universal vial adapter (not pictured) provides access to standard multiple-dose vials, and syringe cannulas are then used to access the adapter. Valve technology allows syringes and IV tubing to connect directly in-line without the use of an adapter.

> ### ! NURSING ALERT
>
> Misconnections of tubing have occurred, resulting in patient deaths. Many needleless IV systems allow other types of tubing such as blood pressure and oxygen tubing to connect and instill air directly into the IV line. Before tubing is connected or reconnected to a patient, trace it completely from the patient to the point of origin for verification.

Infusion Pumps

A variety of infusion pumps are available and used in nearly all pediatric infusions to accurately administer medication and minimize the possibility of overloading the circulation. It is important

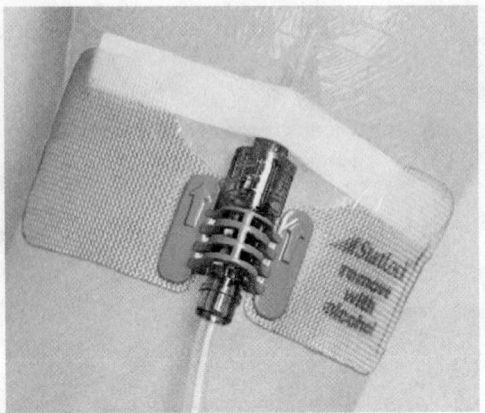

FIG 39-20 StatLock securement devices enhance peripheral intravenous line dwell time and decrease phlebitis.

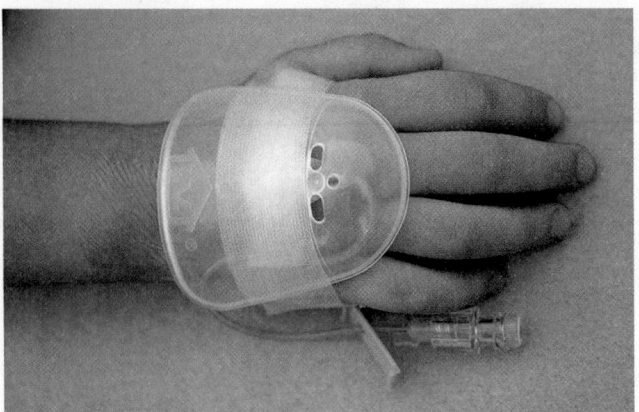

FIG 39-21 I.V. House used to protect intravenous site.

to calculate the amount to be infused in a given length of time, set the infusion rate, and monitor the apparatus frequently (at least every 1 to 2 hours) to make certain that the desired rate is maintained, the integrity of the system remains intact, the site remains intact (free of redness, edema, infiltration, or irritation), and the infusion does not stop. Continuous infusion pumps, although convenient and efficient, are not without risks. Overreliance on the accuracy of the machine can cause either too much or too little fluid to be infused; therefore its use does not eliminate careful periodic assessment by the nurse. Excess pressure can build up if the machine is set at a rate faster than the vein is able to accommodate (or continues to pump when the needle is out of the lumen).

Securing a Peripheral Intravenous Line

To maintain the integrity of the IV line, adequate protection of the site is required. The catheter hub is secured firmly at the puncture site with a transparent dressing and commercial securement device (e.g., StatLock) (Fig. 39-20) or clear nonallergenic tape. Transparent dressings are ideal because the insertion site is easily observed. Minimal tape should be used at the puncture site and on about 1 to 2 inches (2.54 to 5.08 cm) of skin beyond the site to avoid obscuring the insertion site for early detection of infiltration.

A protective cover is applied directly over the catheter insertion site to protect the infusion site. Easy access to the IV site for frequent (hourly) assessments must be considered (Infusion Nurses Society, 2006). Improvised plastic cups that are cut in half with the ridged edges covered with tape should not be used because they have injured patients. A commercial site protector, I.V. House, is available in different sizes (Fig. 39-21). Its ventilation holes prevent moisture from accumulating under the dome. This device is designed to protect the IV site and allows for visibility of the site. It also minimizes use of padded boards, splints, or other restraints and tape and maintains skin integrity. The connector tubing or extension tubing can be looped to make it small enough to fit under the protective cover to prevent accidental snagging of the catheter. It is important to secure the IV tubing safely to prevent infants and children from becoming entangled in it and from accidentally pulling the catheter or needle out. Securing the tubing in this manner also eliminates movement of the catheter hub at the insertion site (mechanical manipulation). A colorful and interesting sticker can be applied to the protecting device to add a positive note to the procedure.

Finger and toe areas are left unoccluded by dressings or tape to allow for assessment of circulation. The thumb is never immobilized because of the danger of contractures with limited movement later on. An extremity should never be encircled with tape. The use of roll gauze, self-adhering stretch bandages (Coban), and Ace bandages can cause the same constriction and hide signs of infiltration.

> ### ! NURSING ALERT
>
> Opaque covering should be avoided; however, if any type of opaque covering is used to secure the IV line, the insertion site and extremity distal to the site should be visible to detect an infiltration. If these sites are not visible, they must be checked frequently to detect problems early.

Traditionally padded boards and splints have been used to partially immobilize the IV site. Padded boards and splints and restraints were appropriate when metal needles were inserted into the vein to prevent the sharp end from puncturing the vessel, especially at a joint. With the more recent use of soft, pliable catheters, arm or leg boards may not be necessary and have several disadvantages. They obscure the IV site, can constrict the extremity, may excoriate the underlying tissue and promote infection, can cause a contracture of a joint, restrict useful movement of the extremity, and are uncomfortable. Unfortunately no research has been conducted to demonstrate their proposed benefit of increasing dwell time (patency of the IV line). Adequate securement should eliminate the need for padded boards in most circumstances. Older children who are alert and cooperative can usually be trusted to protect the IV site (see Evidence-Based Practice box).

Removing a Peripheral Intravenous Line

When it is time to discontinue an IV infusion, many children are distressed by the thought of catheter removal. Therefore they need a careful explanation of the process and suggestions for helping. Encouraging children to remove or help remove the tape from the site provides them with a measure of control and often fosters their cooperation. The procedure consists of turning off any pump apparatus, occluding the IV tubing, removing the tape, pulling the catheter out of the vessel in the opposite direction of insertion, and exerting firm pressure at the site. A dry dressing (adhesive bandage strip) is placed over the puncture site. The use of adhesive-removal pads can decrease the pain of tape removal, but the skin should be washed after use to avoid irritation. To remove transparent dressings (e.g., OpSite, Tegaderm), pull the opposing edges parallel to the skin

EVIDENCE-BASED PRACTICE

Peripheral Intravenous Care

Ask the Question

What site preparation and stabilization measures for PIV catheters are optimum for preventing complications and extending dwell time in children?

Search for Evidence

Search Strategies

Search selection criteria included English language and research-based publications within the past 20 years on PIV catheter site care.

Databases Used

National Guidelines Clearinghouse (AHQR), Cochrane Collaboration, Joanna Briggs Institute, PubMed, TRIP Database Plus, MD Consult, PedsCCM, BestBETs

Critically Analyze the Evidence

Site Preparation

- The skin should be disinfected with an appropriate antiseptic before PIV catheter insertion; allow it to dry before catheter insertion (Infusion Nurses Society, 2011a, 2011b; O'Grady, Alexander, Dellinger, et al., 2002; Registered Nurses' Association of Ontario, 2008).
- A 2% chlorhexidine-based preparation is preferred; but tincture of iodine, an iodophor, or 70% alcohol can be used. There is no recommendation for the use of chlorhexidine in infants younger than 2 months old (Infusion Nurses Society, 2011a; O'Grady, Alexander, Dellinger, et al., 2002).
- Cleansing the skin with a preparation that combines alcohol with either chlorhexidine gluconate or povidone-iodine before PIV catheter insertion is recommended (Infusion Nurses Society, 2006, 2011a, 2011b).
- All disinfectants have risks for neonates. Chlorhexidine gluconate with alcohol should not be used in neonates; aqueous chlorhexidine or povidone-iodine should be used in premature infants. Remove cleansers from infants using sterile water or normal saline to prevent absorption of the disinfectant (AWHONN, 2007).

Stabilization or Securement Devices

- PIV catheters must be stabilized for easy monitoring and evaluation of the access site; to promote delivery of therapy; and to prevent damage, dislodgement, or migration of the catheter (Infusion Nurses Society, 2011a; Registered Nurses' Association of Ontario, 2008).
- To avoid catheter movement and damage, the catheter and hub should be secured firmly with Steri-Strips and clear occlusive dressing; tape should not be placed directly to the catheter (Infusion Nurses Society, 2011a; Paulson and Miller, 2008).
- The catheter site should be assessed every 7 to 8 hours to ensure that the catheter has not migrated (Infusion Nurses Society, 2011a; Paulson and Miller, 2008).
- The traditional transparent dressing (Tegaderm) and tape group had a 65% complication rate (dislodgments, infiltration, and phlebitis) vs. a 20% complication rate in the transparent dressings and a catheter securement device (StatLock) group, indicating a 45% reduction in overall PIV therapy complications in the StatLock group (Wood, 1997).
- When comparing tape, StatLock, and Hub-Guard for a 96-hour PIV protocol change, it was found that PIV catheters with StatLock produced a statistically significant improved survival rate (52%) compared with tape (8%) or HubGuard (9%) (Smith, 2006).

Dwell Time

- In pediatric patients PIV catheters may remain in place until a complication occurs or the therapy is complete (O'Grady, Alexander, Dellinger, et al., 2002).
- In pediatric patients with PIV catheters the overall risk of PIV catheter complications was extremely low and would not be reduced substantially by routine catheter replacement (Shimandle, Johnson, Baker, et al., 1999).
- Evidence is insufficient regarding the effect of heparin use for extending PIV catheter use in neonates (Shah, Ng, and Sinha, 2005).
- An increase in complications and obstructions of PIV catheters was related to younger patient age, insertion into the wrist and scalp, and use of a 24-gauge catheter (Tripathi, Kaushik, and Singh, 2008).

Apply the Evidence: Nursing Implications

There is *low-quality evidence with strong recommendation* (Guyatt, Oxman, Vist, et al., 2008) for site preparation and stabilization measures for PIV catheters in children. For children older than 2 months of age chlorhexidine is the preferred skin cleanser. For younger infants non–alcohol-based cleansers are preferred and should be removed with sterile water or sterile normal saline to prevent absorption. The most distal vein on the extremity that allows the child optimum movement (avoid over the joint) should be selected. Veins on the scalp may be used in infants. Subsequent PIV catheters should be proximal to the previous IV site. If the child is mobile, consider using a securement or protection device (e.g., StatLock, HubGuard, Ray-Marshall Shield, IV House, IV Shield, IV Pro). Discontinue the PIV catheter if complications occur or when it is no longer needed.

Quality and Safety Competencies: Evidence-Based Practice*

Knowledge

Differentiate clinical opinion from research and evidence-based summaries

Describe methods for site preparation and stabilization measures of PIV catheters for preventing complications and extending dwell time in children.

Skills

Base individualized care plan on patient values, clinical expertise, and evidence

Integrate evidence into practice by using techniques for site preparation and stabilization measures for PIV catheters in children.

Attitudes

Value the concept of evidence-based practice as integral to determining best clinical practice

Appreciate the strengths and weakness of evidence for site preparation and stabilization measures for PIV catheters in children.

References

Association of Women's Health, Obstetric and Neonatal Nurses (AWHONN): *Neonatal skin care: evidence-based clinical practice guideline*, ed 2, Washington, DC, 2007, Author.

Guyatt GH, Oxman AD, Vist GE, et al: GRADE: An emerging consensus on rating quality of evidence and strength of recommendations, *BMJ* 336(7650):924–926, 2008.

Continued

EVIDENCE-BASED PRACTICE

Peripheral Intravenous Care—cont'd

Infusion Nurses Society: *Policies and procedures for infusion nursing*, ed 3, Norwood, Mass, 2006, Author.

Infusion Nurses Society: Infusion Nursing Standards of Practice, *J Infus Nurse* 34(1S), 2011a.

Infusion Nurses Society: *Policies and procedures for infusion nursing*, ed 4, South Norwood, Mass, 2011b, Author.

O'Grady N, Alexander M, Dellinger E, et al: Guidelines for the prevention of intravascular catheter–related infections, *MMWR Morb Mortal Wkly Rep* 51(RR-10):1–29, 2002.

Paulson PR, Miller KM: Neonatal peripherally inserted central catheters: recommendations for prevention of insertion and postinsertion complications, *Neonatal Netw* 27:245–257, 2008.

Registered Nurses' Association of Ontario: *Care and maintenance to reduce vascular access complications, guideline supplement*, Toronto, 2008, Author.

Shah PS, Ng E, Sinha AK: Heparin for prolonging peripheral intravenous catheter use in neonates, *Cochrane Database Syst Rev* (4):CD002774, 2005.

Shimandle R, Johnson D, Baker M, et al: Safety of peripheral intravenous catheters in children, *Infect Control Hosp Epidemiol* 20:736–740, 1999.

Smith B: Peripheral intravenous catheter dwell times: a comparison of three securement methods for implementation of a 96-hour scheduled change protocol, *J Infus Nurs* 29(1):14–17, 2006.

Tripathi S, Kaushik V, Singh V: Peripheral IVs: factors affecting complications and patency—a randomized controlled trial, *J Infus Nurs* 31:182–188, 2008.

Wood D: A comparative study of two securement techniques for short peripheral intravenous catheters, *J Intraven Nurs* 20(6):280–285, 1997.

Joy Hesselgrave; updated by Olga A. Taylor

IV, Intravenous; *PIV*, peripheral intravenous.
*Adapted from the QSEN at www.qsen.org.

---

to loosen the bond. Inspect the catheter tip to ensure that the catheter is intact and that no portion remains in the vein.

> **! NURSING ALERT**
>
> Consider the child's age, development, and neurologic status and his or her predictability (i.e., how the child responds to painful treatments) when determining the need for assistance to maintain safety. Manual removal of tape is the preferred method. Only if absolutely necessary should a small cut be made in the tape, using bandage scissors, to facilitate its removal. Before cutting the tape:
> - Ensure that all digits are visible.
> - Remove any barrier that hinders visibility, such as a protective covering.
> - Protect the child's skin and digits by sliding own finger(s) between the tape and the child's skin so the scissors do not touch the patient.
> - Cut on the tape on the medial aspect (thumb side) of the extremity.

Complications

The same precautions regarding maintenance of asepsis, prevention of infection, and observation for infiltration are carried out with patients of any age. However, infiltration is more difficult to detect in infants and small children than in adults. The increased amount of subcutaneous fat and the amount of tape used to secure the catheter often obscure the early signs of infiltration. When the fluid appears to be infusing too slowly or ceases, the usual assessment for obstruction within the apparatus (i.e., kinks, screw clamps, shutoff valve, and positioning interference [e.g., a bent elbow]) often locates the difficulty. When these actions fail to detect the problem, it may be necessary to carefully remove some of the dressing to obtain a clear view of the venipuncture site. Dependent areas such as the palm and undersides of the extremity or the occiput and behind the ears are examined.

Whenever possible the IV infusion should be placed in an extremity to which the ID band (or bracelet) is not attached. Serious circulatory impairment can result from infiltrated solution distal to the band, which acts as a tourniquet preventing adequate venous return. To check for return blood flow through the catheter, the tubing is removed from the infusion pump, and the bag is lowered below the level of the infusion site. Resistance during flushing or

aspiration for blood return also indicates that the IV infusion may have infiltrated surrounding tissue. A good blood return or lack thereof is not always an indicator of infiltration in small infants. Flushing the catheter and observing for edema, redness, or streaking along the vein are appropriate for assessment of the IV.

IV therapy in pediatrics tends to be difficult to maintain because of mechanical factors such as vascular trauma resulting from the catheter, the insertion site, vessel size, vessel fragility, pump pressure, the patient's activity level, operator skill and insertion technique, forceful administration of boluses of fluid, and infusion of irritants or vesicants through a small vessel. These factors cause infiltration and extravasation injuries. Infiltration is defined as inadvertent administration of a nonvesicant solution or medication into surrounding tissue. Extravasation is defined as inadvertent administration of vesicant solution or medication into surrounding tissue (Infusion Nurses Society, 2006). A vesicant or sclerosing agent causes varying degrees of cellular damage when even minute amounts escape into surrounding tissue. Guidelines are available for determining the severity of tissue injury by staging characteristics such as the amount of redness, blanching, the amount of swelling, pain, the quality of pulses below infiltration, capillary refill, and warmth or coolness of the area (Infusion Nurses Society, 2006).*

Treatment of infiltration or extravasation varies according to the type of vesicant. Guidelines are available outlining the sequence of interventions and specific treatment of infiltration or extravasation with antidotes.

> **! NURSING ALERT**
>
> When infiltration or extravasation is observed (signs include erythema, pain, edema, blanching, streaking on the skin along the vein, and darkened area at the insertion site), immediately stop the infusion, elevate the extremity, notify the practitioner, and initiate the ordered treatment as soon as possible. Remove the IV line when it is no longer needed (e.g., after infusing an antidote).

---

*Guidelines for determining tissue injury severity are available from the Infusion Nurses Society, 315 Norwood Park South, Norwood, MA 02062, 781-440-9408, www.ins1.org.

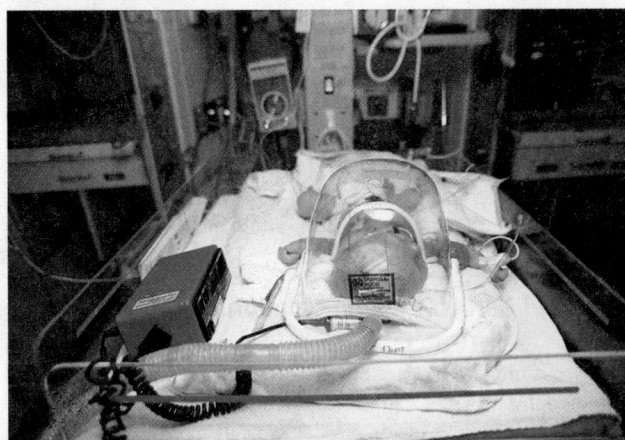

FIG 39-22 Oxygen administered to infant by means of a plastic hood. Note oxygen analyzer (blue machine).

Phlebitis, or inflammation of the vessel wall, may also develop in children who require IV therapy. Lamagna and MacPhee (2004) describe three types of phlebitis: mechanical (caused by rapid infusion rate, manipulation of the IV), chemical (caused by medications), and bacterial (caused by staphylococcal organisms). The initial sign of phlebitis is erythema (redness) at the insertion site. Pain may or may not be present.

PIV catheters are the most commonly used intravascular device. Heavy cutaneous colonization of the insertion site is the single most important predictor of catheter-related infection with all types of short-term, percutaneously inserted catheters. Phlebitis, largely a mechanical rather than infectious process, remains the most important complication associated with the use of peripheral venous catheters.*

> **! NURSING ALERT**
>
> The most effective ways to prevent infection of an IV site are to cleanse hands between each patient, wear gloves when inserting a catheter, and inspect the insertion site and physical condition of the dressing closely. Proper education of the patient and family regarding signs and symptoms of an infected site can help prevent infections from going unnoticed.

PROCEDURES FOR MAINTAINING RESPIRATORY FUNCTION

Inhalation Therapy

Oxygen Therapy

Oxygen is administered for hypoxemia and may be delivered by mask, nasal cannula, face tent, hood, face mask, or ventilator. The mode of delivery is selected on the basis of the concentration needed and the child's ability to cooperate in its use. Oxygen therapy is frequently administered in the hospital, although increasing numbers of children are receiving oxygen in the home. Oxygen is dry and therefore must be humidified.

Oxygen delivered to infants is well tolerated by using a plastic hood (Fig. 39-22). At least 4 to 5 L/min of flow is necessary to

---

*Guidelines for prevention of health care–associated infections are available from the CDC, 1600 Clifton Road, Atlanta, GA 30333, 800-232-4636 or 404-639-1515, www.cdc.gov/hai.

maintain oxygen concentrations and remove the exhaled carbon dioxide. The humidified oxygen should not be blown directly into the infant's face. Older cooperative infants and children can use a nasal cannula or prongs, which can supply a concentration of oxygen of about 50%.

Oxygen masks are available in pediatric sizes but may not be tolerated well in children because a snug fit is required to ensure adequate oxygen delivery. A face tent or bucket is often tolerated better because this soft piece of plastic sits beneath the child's chin and allows oxygen to be directed to the mouth and nose without enclosure (Curley and Moloney-Harmon, 2001). Oxygen tents (croup tents) are rarely used today in developed countries. Oxygen concentration is difficult to control, and the child's clothing can become saturated with water from the humidification and cause hypothermia.

> **⬭ MEDICATION ALERT**
>
> Prolonged exposure to high oxygen tensions can damage some body tissues and functions. The organs most vulnerable to the adverse effects of excessive oxygenation are the retinas of extremely preterm infants and the lungs of people at any age.

> **! NURSING ALERT**
>
> Inspect all toys for safety and suitability (e.g., vinyl or plastic, not stuffed items that absorb moisture and are difficult to keep dry). The high-level oxygen environment makes any source of sparks (e.g., mechanical or electrical toys) a potential fire hazard.

Oxygen-induced carbon dioxide narcosis is a physiologic hazard of oxygen therapy that may occur in people with chronic pulmonary disease such as cystic fibrosis. In these patients the respiratory center has adapted to the continuously higher arterial carbon dioxide tension ($PaCO_2$) levels; therefore hypoxia becomes the more powerful stimulus for respiration. When the arterial oxygen tension (PaO_2) level is elevated during oxygen administration, the hypoxic drive is removed, causing progressive hypoventilation and increased $PaCO_2$ levels, and the child rapidly becomes unconscious. Carbon dioxide narcosis can also be induced by the administration of sedation in these patients.

Monitoring Oxygen Therapy

Pulse oximetry is a continuous, noninvasive method of determining oxygen saturation (SaO_2) to guide oxygen therapy. A sensor composed of a light-emitting diode (LED) and a photodetector is placed in opposition around a foot, hand, finger, toe, or earlobe, with the LED placed on top of the nail when digits are used (Fig. 39-23). The diode emits red and infrared lights that pass through the skin to the photodetector. The photodetector measures the amount of each type of light absorbed by functional hemoglobins. Hemoglobin saturated with oxygen (oxyhemoglobin) absorbs more infrared light than does hemoglobin not saturated with oxygen (deoxyhemoglobin). Pulsatile blood flow is the primary physiologic factor that influences accuracy of the pulse oximeter. In infants reposition the probe at least every 3 to 4 hours to prevent pressure necrosis; poor perfusion and very sensitive skin may necessitate more frequent repositioning.

Another noninvasive method is transcutaneous monitoring (TCM), which provides continuous monitoring of transcutaneous partial pressure of oxygen in arterial blood ($tcPaO_2$) and with some

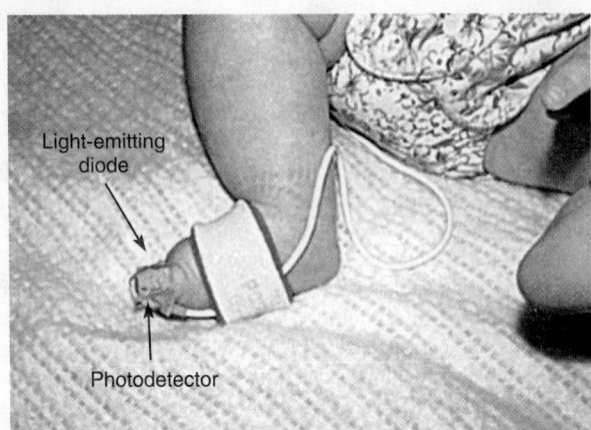

FIG 39-23 Oximeter sensor on great toe. Note that sensor is positioned with a light-emitting diode (LED) opposite photodetector. Cord is secured to foot to minimize movement of sensor.

devices of carbon dioxide in arterial blood (tcPaCO$_2$). An electrode is attached to the warmed skin to facilitate arterialization of cutaneous capillaries. The site of the electrode must be changed every 3 to 4 hours to avoid burning the skin, and the machine must be calibrated with every site change. TCM is used frequently in neonatal intensive care units, but it may not reflect PaO$_2$ in infants with impaired local circulation or older infants whose skin is thicker.

Oximetry is insensitive to hyperoxia because hemoglobin approaches 100% saturation for all PaO$_2$ readings greater than approximately 100 mm Hg, which is a dangerous situation for preterm infants at risk for developing retinopathy of prematurity (see Chapter 25). Therefore preterm infants being monitored with oximetry should have their upper limits identified such as 90% to 95%, and a protocol should be established for decreasing oxygen when saturations are high.

Oximetry offers several advantages over TCM. It (1) does not require heating the skin, thus reducing the risk of burns; (2) eliminates a delay period for transducer equilibration; and (3) maintains an accurate measurement regardless of the patient's age or skin characteristics or the presence of lung disease.

> **! NURSING ALERT**
>
> It is important to make certain that sensor connectors and oximeters are compatible. Wiring that is incompatible can generate considerable heat at the tip of the sensor, causing second- and third-degree burns under the sensors. Pressure necrosis can also occur from sensors attached too tightly. Therefore inspect the skin under the sensor frequently.

Applying the sensor correctly is essential for accurate SaO$_2$ measurements. Because the sensor must identify every pulse beat to calculate the SaO$_2$, movement can interfere with sensing. Some devices synchronize the SaO$_2$ reading with the heartbeat, thereby reducing the interference caused by motion. Sensors are not placed on extremities used for blood pressure monitoring or with indwelling arterial catheters because pulsatile blood flow may be affected.

Ambient light from ceiling lights and phototherapy and high-intensity heat and light from radiant warmers can interfere with readings. Therefore the sensor should be covered to block these light sources. IV dyes; green, purple, or black nail polish; nonopaque synthetic nails; and possibly ink used for footprinting can also cause inaccurate SaO$_2$ measurements. The dyes should be removed; or, in the case of porcelain nails, a different area used for the sensor. Skin color, thickness, and edema do not affect the readings.

Blood gas measurements are sensitive indicators of change in respiratory status in acutely ill patients. They provide valuable information regarding lung function, lung adequacy, and tissue perfusion. The pH, PaCO$_2$, HCO$_3$, and PaO$_2$ levels can provide information about whether the child is compensating and guide critical treatment decisions.

End-Tidal Carbon Dioxide Monitoring

End-tidal CO$_2$ (ETCO$_2$) monitoring measures exhaled carbon dioxide noninvasively. Capnometry provides a numeric display, and capnography provides a graph over time. Continuous capnometry is available in many bedside physiologic and stand-alone monitors. ETCO$_2$ differs from pulse oximetry in that it is more sensitive to the mechanics of ventilation rather than oxygenation. Hypoxic episodes can be prevented through the early detection of hypoventilation, apnea, or airway obstruction.

Children who are experiencing an asthma exacerbation, receiving procedural sedation, or mechanically ventilated may have ETCO$_2$ monitoring. Special sampling cannulas are used for nonintubated patients, and a small device is placed between the endotracheal (ET) tube and the ventilator tubing in intubated patients. Although ETCO$_2$ monitoring is not a substitute for arterial blood gases, it does provide ventilation information continuously and noninvasively. Normal ETCO$_2$ values are 30 to 43 mm Hg, which is slightly lower than normal arterial PCO$_2$ of 35 to 45 mm Hg. During CPR, ETCO$_2$ values consistently below 15 mm Hg indicate ineffective compressions or excessive ventilation. Changes in waveform and numeric display follow changes in ventilation by a very few seconds and precede changes in respiratory rate, skin color, and pulse oximetry values.

For years disposable colormetric ETCO$_2$ detectors have been used to assess ET tube placement. A color change with each exhaled breath when there is adequate systemic perfusion indicates that the tube is in the lungs. These devices do not provide numbers or graphic representation and the same early detection of hypoventilation as the continuous quantitative monitors.

Additional uses of ETCO$_2$ monitoring have limited supporting research. Although waveform analysis does not yet have standardized nomenclature, some clinicians use the angles of the waveform coupled with the quantitative value of ETCO$_2$ to classify the severity of asthma exacerbations. The severity of diabetic ketoacidosis (Fearon and Steele, 2002) and acidosis from gastroenteritis (Nagler, Wright, and Krauss, 2006) has also been researched in children and is used in some facilities.

When there is a change in the ETCO$_2$ value or waveform, assess the patient quickly for adequate airway, breathing, and circulation. Sedated patients may be hypoventilating and need stimulation. Intubated patients may need suctioning, have self-extubated or dislodged the tube, or have equipment failure or disconnection. Patients with asthma may have a worsening condition. Problems with the ETCO$_2$ monitoring system can include a kink in the sample line or disconnection. In general check the patient first and then the equipment.

Bronchial (Postural) Drainage

Bronchial drainage is indicated whenever excessive fluid or mucus in the bronchi is not being removed by normal ciliary activity and cough. Positioning the child to take maximum advantage of gravity facilitates removal of secretions. Postural drainage can be effective in children with chronic lung disease characterized by thick mucus such as cystic fibrosis.

Postural drainage is carried out 3 or 4 times daily and is more effective when it follows other respiratory therapy such as bronchodilator or nebulization medication. Bronchial drainage is generally performed before meals (or 1 to 1½ hours after meals) to minimize the chance of vomiting and is repeated at bedtime. The duration of treatment depends on the child's condition and tolerance; it usually lasts 20 to 30 minutes. Several positions facilitate drainage from all major lung segments.

Chest Physical Therapy

Chest physical therapy (CPT) usually refers to the use of postural drainage in combination with adjunctive techniques that are thought to enhance the clearance of mucus from the airway. These techniques include manual percussion, vibration, and squeezing of the chest; cough; forceful expiration; and breathing exercises. Special mechanical devices are also currently used to perform CPT (e.g., vest-type percussors). Postural drainage in combination with forced expiration has been shown to be beneficial.

Common techniques used in association with postural drainage include manual percussion of the chest wall and percussion with mechanical devices such as a high-frequency handheld chest compression device. A "popping," hollow sound, not a slapping sound, should be the result. The procedure should be done over the rib cage only and should be painless. Percussion can be performed with a soft circular mask (adapted to maintain air trapping) or a percussion cup marketed especially for the purpose of aiding in loosening secretions. CPT is contraindicated when patients have pulmonary hemorrhage, pulmonary embolism, end-stage renal disease, increased intracranial pressure, osteogenesis imperfecta, or minimal cardiac reserves.

Intubation

Rapid-sequence intubation (RSI) is commonly performed in pediatric (and some neonatal) patients to induce an unconscious, neuromuscular blocked condition to avoid the use of positive-pressure ventilation and the risk of possible aspiration (Bottor, 2009). Atropine, fentanyl, and vecuronium or rocuronium are drugs commonly used during RSI. In neonates ET tube intubation is often a stressful event, and hypoxia and pain are commonly associated with it; RSI in neonates may serve to prevent such adverse events (Bottor, 2009).

Indications for intubation include the following:

- Respiratory failure or arrest, agonal or gasping respirations, apnea
- Upper airway obstruction
- Significant increase in work of breathing, use of accessory muscles
- Potential for developing partial or complete airway obstruction—respiratory effort with no breath sounds, facial trauma, and inhalation injuries
- Potential for or actual loss of airway protection, increased risk for aspiration
- Anticipated need for mechanical ventilation related to chest trauma, shock, increased intracranial pressure
- Hypoxemia despite supplemental oxygen
- Inadequate ventilation

In preparation for intubation the child should be preoxygenated with 100% oxygen using an appropriate-size bag and mask. Only uncuffed ET tubes should be used in children younger than 8 years of age (Curley and Moloney-Harmon, 2001). Air or gas delivered directly to the trachea must be humidified. During intubation the cardiac rhythm, heart rate, and oxygen saturation should be monitored continuously with audible tones. ET tube placement should be verified by at least one clinical sign and at least one confirmatory technology:

- Visualization of bilateral chest expansion
- Auscultation over the epigastrium (breath sounds should not be heard) and the lung fields bilaterally in the axillary region (breath sounds should be equal and adequate)
- Water vapor in the tube (helpful; not definitive)
- Color change on end-tidal carbon dioxide detector during exhalation after at least 3 to 6 breaths or waveform/value verification with continuous capnography
- Chest radiography

Apply a protective skin barrier and secure the ET tube with tape or a securement device. An NG tube typically is inserted after intubation.

Mechanical Ventilation

ET intubation can be accomplished by the nasal (nasotracheal), oral (orotracheal), or direct tracheal (tracheostomy) routes. Although it is more difficult to place, nasotracheal intubation is preferred to orotracheal intubation because it facilitates oral hygiene and provides more stable fixation, which reduces the complication of tracheal erosion and the danger of accidental extubation.

Basic ongoing assessment of the mechanically ventilated patient includes observing the chest rise and fall for symmetry, bilateral breath sounds equal or unchanged from last assessment, level of consciousness, capillary refill and skin color, and vital signs. A heart rate that is too fast or too slow is a possible indication of hypoxemia, air leak, or low cardiac output. Pulse oximetry and end-tidal carbon dioxide monitoring is also routine along with periodic arterial blood gas analysis. If sudden deterioration of an intubated patient occurs, consider the following etiologies.

DOPE*

Displacement—Tube not in the trachea or has moved into a bronchus (right mainstream most common)

Obstruction—Secretions or kinking of the tube

Pneumothorax—Chest trauma, barotraumas, or noncompliant lung disease

Equipment failure—Check the oxygen source, Ambu bag, and ventilator

Verify placement again during each transport and when patients are moved to different beds

To maintain skin integrity in the mechanically ventilated patient, reposition the patient at least every 2 hours as the patient's condition tolerates. Apply a hydrocolloid barrier to protect the facial cheeks. Place gel pillows under pressure points such as occiput, heels, elbows, and shoulders. Allow no tubes, lines, wires, or wrinkles in bedding under the patient. Provide meticulous skin care.

Provide analgesia and sedation as needed. Use a system for communication that includes sign boards, pointing, and opening and closing eyes. To maintain safety use soft restraints if necessary to maintain a critical airway.

Ventilator-associated pneumonia is a complication that can be prevented through the use of aggressive hand hygiene, oral care, and elevation of the head of the bed between 30 and 45 degrees (unless contraindicated). Enteral nutrition is often provided to decrease the risk of bacterial translocation. Routinely assess the patient's intestinal motility (e.g., by auscultating for bowel sounds and measuring

---

*American Heart Association, 2010.

residual gastric volume or abdominal girth) and adjust the rate and volume of enteral feeding to avoid regurgitation. In high risk patients (decreased gag reflex, delayed gastric emptying, gastroesophageal reflux, severe bronchospasm), postpyloric (duodenal or jejunal) feeding tubes are often used. To prevent the aspiration of pooled secretions, suction the hypopharynx before suctioning the ET tube, before repositioning the ET tube, and before repositioning the patient. Prevent ventilator circuits' condensate from entering ET tube or in-line medication nebulizers.

Assess readiness to extubate daily. Indications that a child is ready to be extubated include an improvement in underlying condition, hemodynamic stability, and mechanical support no longer being necessary. Assess level of consciousness and ability to maintain a patent airway by mobilizing pulmonary secretions through effective coughing. Maintain NPO status 4 hours before extubation. After extubation monitor for respiratory distress, which may develop within minutes or hours. Signs of postintubation respiratory distress include stridor, hoarseness, increased work of breathing, unstable vital signs, and desaturations.

Tracheostomy

A tracheostomy is a surgical opening in the trachea; the procedure may be done on an emergency basis or elective, and it may be combined with mechanical ventilation. Pediatric tracheostomy tubes are usually made of plastic or Silastic (Fig. 39-24). The most common types are the Hollinger, Jackson, Aberdeen, and Shiley tubes. These tubes are constructed with a more acute angle than adult tubes; and they soften at body temperature, conforming to the contours of the trachea. Because these materials resist the formation of crusted respiratory secretions, they are made without an inner cannula.

Children who have undergone a tracheostomy must be monitored closely for complications such as hemorrhage, edema, aspiration, accidental decannulation, tube obstruction, and the entrance of free air into the pleural cavity. The focuses of nursing care are maintaining a patent airway, facilitating the removal of pulmonary secretions, providing humidified air or oxygen, cleansing the stoma, monitoring the child's ability to swallow, and teaching while simultaneously preventing complications.

Because the child may be unable to signal for help, direct observation and use of respiratory and cardiac monitors are essential. Respiratory assessments include breath sounds and work of breathing, vital signs, tightness of the tracheostomy ties, and the type and amount of secretions. Large amounts of bloody secretions are uncommon and should be considered a sign of hemorrhage. The practitioner should be notified immediately if this occurs.

The child is positioned with the head of the bed raised or in the position most comfortable to the child with the call light easily available. Suction catheters, suction source, gloves, sterile saline, sterile gauze for wiping away secretions, scissors, an extra tracheostomy tube of the same size with ties already attached, another tracheostomy tube one size smaller, and the obturator are kept at the bedside. A source of humidification is provided because the normal humidification and filtering functions of the airway have been bypassed. IV fluids ensure adequate hydration until the child is able to swallow sufficient amounts of fluids.

Suctioning

The airway must remain patent and may require frequent suctioning during the first few hours after a tracheostomy to remove mucus plugs and excessive secretions. Proper vacuum pressure and suction catheter size are important to prevent atelectasis and decrease hypoxia from the suctioning procedure. Vacuum pressure should range from 60 to 100 mm Hg for infants and children and from 40 to 60 mm Hg for preterm infants. Unless secretions are thick and tenacious, the lower range of negative pressure is recommended. Tracheal suction catheters are available in a variety of sizes. The catheter selected should have a diameter that is half the diameter of the tracheostomy tube. If it is too large, it can block the airway. The catheter is constructed with a side port so that it is introduced without suction and removed while simultaneous intermittent suction is applied by covering the port with the thumb (Fig. 39-25). It is inserted just to the end of the tracheostomy tube. The practice of instilling sterile saline in the tracheostomy tube before suctioning is not supported by research and is no longer recommended (see Evidence-Based Practice box).

The child is allowed to rest for 30 to 60 seconds after each aspiration to allow oxygen saturation to return to normal; then the process is repeated until the trachea is clear. Suctioning should be limited to

---

! NURSING ALERT

Suctioning should require no more than 5 seconds. Counting one one-thousand, two one-thousand, three one-thousand, and so on while suctioning is a simple means for monitoring the time. Without a safeguard the airway may be obstructed for too long. Hyperventilating the child with 100% oxygen before and after suctioning (using a bag-valve-mask or increasing the fraction of inspired oxygen concentration [FiO$_2$] ventilator setting) may be performed to prevent hypoxia. Closed tracheal suctioning systems that allow for uninterrupted oxygen delivery may also be used.

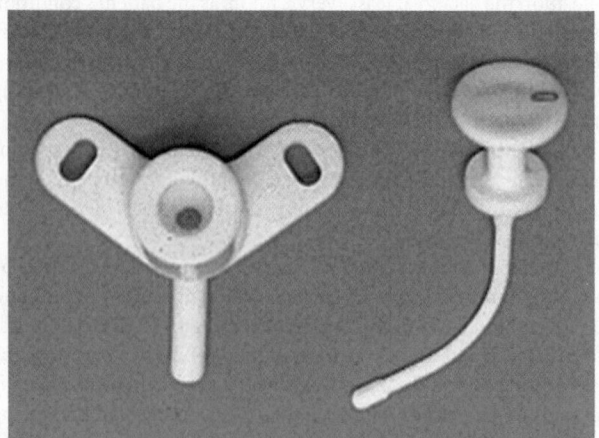

FIG 39-24 Silastic pediatric tracheostomy tube and obturator.

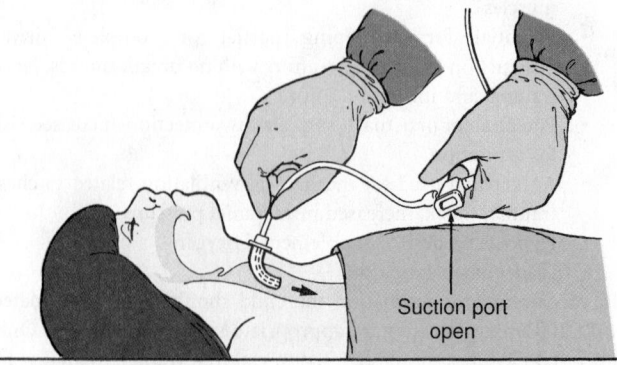

Suction port open

FIG 39-25 Tracheostomy suction catheter insertion. Note that catheter is inserted just to the end of the tracheostomy tube.

EVIDENCE-BASED PRACTICE

Normal Saline Instillation Before Endotracheal or Tracheostomy Suctioning—Helpful or Harmful?

Ask the Question
In intubated children and those with tracheostomy, is NS instillation before suctioning helpful or harmful?

Search for Evidence
Search Strategies
Searched all literature from 1980 to 2011.

Databases Used
PubMed, Cochrane Collaboration, MD Consult, BestBETs, PedsCCM, AHRQ

Critically Analyze the Evidence
- Adult studies have found decreased oxygen saturation, increased frequency of nosocomial pneumonia, and increased intracranial pressure after instillation of NS before suctioning (Ackerman, 1993; Ackerman and Gugerty, 1990; Bostick and Wendelgass, 1987; Hagler and Traver, 1994; Kinlock, 1999; O'Neal, Grap, Thompson, et al., 2001; Reynolds, Hoffman, Schlichtig, et al., 1990).
- No significant differences in oxygenation, heart rate, or blood pressure were found before or after suctioning in a group of 27 intubated neonates (Shorten, Byrne, and Jones, 1991).
- No adverse effects on lung mechanics were found after NS instillation and suctioning in neonates (Beeram and Dhanireddy, 1992).
- Children ages 10 weeks to 14 years experienced significantly greater oxygen desaturation after suctioning if NS was instilled (Ridling, Martin, and Bratton, 2003).
- With tracheostomies NS should not be instilled before suctioning (American Thoracic Society, 2005).
- Evidence does not support routine instillation of NS in neonates; however, abundant evidence indicates the adverse effects of NS instillation (Gardner and Shirland, 2009).
- Evidence indicating the detriment of the use of saline for suctioning is lacking in the pediatric population. However, saline should not be used routinely for suctioning infants and children (Morrow and Argent, 2008).
- ET suctioning performed with saline solution was associated with an increase in episodes of bradycardia, desaturations, and need for increase in the fraction of inspired oxygen (Trevisanuto, Doglioni, and Zanardo, 2009).
- Potential harms that may be associated with use of NS installation include increased coughing, oxygen desaturation, bronchospasms, tachycardia, pain, anxiety, dyspnea, increased intracranial pressure, and loosened bacterial biofilm that may colonize the ET tube (American Association for Respiratory Care, 2010).
- Use of low-sodium solution for airway suctioning in neonates significantly decreased VAP and rates of chronic lung disease (Christensen, Henry, Baer, et al., 2010).

Apply the Evidence: Nursing Implications
There is *moderate-quality evidence with a strong recommendation* (Guyatt, Oxman, Vist, et al., 2008) that adverse effects of NS instillation before suctioning in children are similar to those found for adults. This technique causes a significant reduction in oxygen saturation that can last up to 2 minutes after suctioning. The evidence does not support the use of NS instillation before ET suctioning in children.

Quality and Safety Competencies:
Evidence-Based Practice*
Knowledge
Differentiate clinical opinion from research and evidence-based summaries
Describe methods for using NS instillation before ET or tracheostomy suctioning.

Skills
Base individualized care plan on patient values, clinical expertise, and evidence
Integrate evidence into practice on NS instillation before ET or tracheostomy suctioning.

Attitudes
Value the concept of evidence-based practice as integral to determining best clinical practice
Appreciate the strengths and weakness of evidence for NS instillation before ET or tracheostomy suctioning.

References
Ackerman MH: The effect of saline lavage prior to suctioning, *Am J Crit Care* 2(4):326–330, 1993.

Ackerman MH, Gugerty B: The effect of normal saline bolus instillation in artificial airways, *J Soc Otorhinolaryngol Head Neck Nurs* 8:14–17, 1990.

American Association for Respiratory Care: AARC Clinical Practice Guidelines: endotracheal suctioning of mechanically ventilated patients with artificial airways, *Respir Care* 55(6):758–764, 2010.

American Thoracic Society: *Care of the child with a chronic tracheostomy*, 2005, www.thoracic.org/sections/publications/statements/pages/respiratory-disease-pediatric/childtrach1-12.html.

Beeram MR, Dhanireddy R: Effects of saline instillation during tracheal suction on lung mechanics in newborn infants, *J Perinatol* 12(2):120–123, 1992.

Bostick J, Wendelgass ST: Normal saline instillation as part of the suctioning procedure: effects of PaO₂ and amount of secretions, *Heart Lung* 16(5):532–537, 1987.

Christensen RD, Henry E, Baer VL, et al: A low-sodium solution for airway care: results of a multicenter trial, *Respir Care* 5(12):1680–1685, 2010.

Gardner DL, Shirland L: Evidence-based guideline for suctioning the intubated neonate and infant, *Neonat Netw* 28(5):281–302, 2009.

Guyatt GH, Oxman AD, Vist GE, et al: GRADE: an emerging consensus on rating quality of evidence and strength of recommendations, *BMJ* 336(7650):924–926, 2008.

Hagler DA, Traver GA: Endotracheal saline and suction catheters: sources of lower airway contamination, *Am J Crit Care* 3(6):444–447, 1994.

Kinlock D: Instillation of normal saline during endotracheal suctioning: effects on mixed venous oxygen saturation, *Am J Crit Care* 8(4):231–240, 1999.

Morrow BM, Argent AC: A comprehensive review of pediatric endotracheal suctioning: effects, indications, and clinical practice, *Pediatr Crit Care Med* 9(5):465–477, 2008.

O'Neal PV, Grap MJ, Thompson C, et al: Level of dyspnoea experienced in mechanically ventilated adults with and without saline instillation prior to endotracheal suctioning, *Intensive Crit Care Nurs* 17(6):356–363, 2001.

Reynolds P, Hoffman LA, Schlichtig R, et al: Effects of normal saline instillation on secretion volume, dynamic compliance, and oxygen saturation [abstract], *Am Rev Respir Dis* 141:A574, 1990.

Ridling DA, Martin LD, Bratton SL: Endotracheal suctioning with or without instillation of isotonic sodium chloride in critically ill children, *Am J Crit Care* 12(3):212–219, 2003.

Shorten DR, Byrne PJ, Jones RL: Infant responses to saline instillations and endotracheal suctioning, *J Obstet Gynecol Neonatal Nurs* 20(6):464–469, 1991.

Trevisanuto D, Doglioni N, Zanardo V: The management of endotracheal tubes and nasal cannulae: the role of nurses, *Early Hum Dev* 85:S85–S87, 2009.

Updated by Olga A. Taylor

ET, Endotracheal; *NS*, normal saline; *VAP*, ventilator-associated pneumonia.
*Adapted from the QSEN at www.qsen.org.

about three aspirations in one period. Oximetry is used to monitor suctioning and prevent hypoxia.

In the acute care setting aseptic technique is used during care of the tracheostomy. Secondary infection is a major concern because the air entering the lower airway bypasses the natural defenses of the upper airway. Gloves are worn during the aspiration procedure, although a sterile glove is needed only on the hand touching the catheter. A new tube, gloves, and sterile saline solution are used each time.

Routine Care

The tracheostomy stoma requires daily care. Assessments of the stoma area include observations for signs of infection and breakdown of the skin. The skin is kept clean and dry, and crusted secretions around the stoma may be gently removed with half-strength hydrogen peroxide. Hydrogen peroxide should not be used with sterling silver tracheostomy tubes because it tends to pit and stain the silver surface. The nurse should be aware of wet tracheostomy dressings, which can predispose the peristomal area to skin breakdown. Several products are available to prevent or treat excoriation. The Allevyn tracheostomy dressing is a hydrophilic sponge with a polyurethane back that is highly absorptive. Other possible barriers to help maintain skin integrity include the use of hydrocolloid wafers (e.g., DuoDERM CGF, Hollister Restore) under the tracheostomy flanges and extra-thin hydrocolloid wafers under the chin.

The tracheostomy tube is held in place with tracheostomy ties made of a durable, nonfraying material. The ties are changed daily and when soiled. Ties fastened with self-adhering Velcro closures are commonly used. If Velcro ties are not available, cotton ties are looped through the flanges and tied snugly in a triple knot at the side of the neck before the soiled ties are cut and removed. The ties should be tight enough to allow just a fingertip to be inserted between the ties and the neck (Fig. 39-26). It is easier to ensure a snug fit if the child's head is flexed rather than extended while the ties are being secured.

Routine tracheostomy tube changes are usually carried out weekly after a tract has been formed to minimize the formation of granulation tissue. The first change is usually performed by the

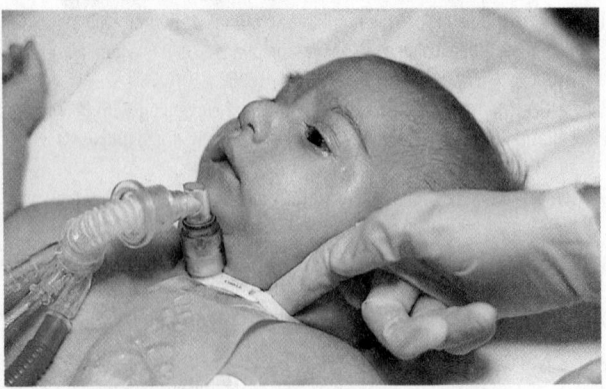

FIG 39-26 Tracheostomy ties are snug but allow one finger to be inserted.

surgeon; subsequent changes are performed by the nurse, and, if the child is discharged home with the tracheostomy, by either a parent or a visiting nurse. Ideally two caregivers participate in the procedure to help position the child.

Changing the tracheostomy tube is accomplished using sterile technique. Tube changes should occur before meals or 2 hours after the last meal. Continuous feedings should be turned off at least an hour before a tube change. The new sterile tube is prepared by inserting the obturator and attaching new ties. The child may be suctioned if necessary before the procedure and then restrained and positioned with the neck slightly extended. One caregiver removes the old ties and removes the tube from the stoma. The new tube is inserted gently into the stoma (using a downward and forward motion that follows the curve of the trachea), the obturator is removed, and the ties are secured. The adequacy of ventilation must be assessed after a tube change because the tube can be inserted into the soft tissue surrounding the trachea; therefore, breath sounds and respiratory effort are monitored carefully.

Supplemental oxygen is always delivered with a humidification system to prevent drying of the respiratory mucosa. Humidification of room air for an established tracheostomy can be intermittent if secretions remain thin enough to be coughed or suctioned from the tracheostomy. Direct humidification via a tracheostomy mask can be provided during naps and at night so the child is able to be up and around unencumbered during much of the day. Room humidifiers are also used successfully.

If the inner cannula is used, it should be removed with each suctioning, cleaned with sterile saline and pipe cleaners to remove crusted material, dried thoroughly, and reinserted.

Emergency Care: Tube Occlusion and Accidental Decannulation

Occlusion of the tracheostomy tube is life threatening, and infants and children are at greater risk than adults because of the smaller diameter of the tube. Maintaining patency of the tube is accomplished with suctioning and routine tube changes to prevent the formation of crusts that can occlude it.

Accidental decannulation also requires immediate tube replacement. Some children have a fairly rigid trachea; thus the airway remains partially open when the tube is removed. However, others have malformed or flexible tracheal cartilage, which causes the airway to collapse when the tube is removed or dislodged. Because many infants and children with upper airway problems have little airway reserve, if replacement of the dislodged tube is impossible, a smaller-size tube should be inserted. If the stoma cannot be cannulated with another tracheostomy tube, oral intubation should be performed.

Chest Tube Procedures

A chest tube is placed to remove fluid or air from the pleural or pericardial space. Chest tube drainage systems collect air and fluid while inhibiting backflow into the pleural or pericardial space. Indications for chest tube placement include pneumothorax, hemothorax, chylothorax, empyema, pleural or pericardial effusion, and prevention of accumulation of fluid in the pleural and pericardial space after cardiothoracic surgery. Nursing responsibilities include assisting with chest tube placement, managing chest tubes, and assisting with chest tube removal.

Before chest tube insertion assess hematologic and coagulation studies for any risk of bleeding during the procedure. Notify the health care provider of abnormal findings. Prepare the drainage system with sterile water as described in the package insert (some systems may not require this step). Administer pain and sedation medications as ordered. Monitor airway, breathing, circulation, and pulse oximetry throughout the procedure.

After the tube has been inserted and connected to the chest drainage system, secure the tubing so it does not become disconnected. If suction is required, use connection tubing to join the drainage system to a wall suction adapter and adjust suction on the drainage system as ordered (usually −10 to −20 cm H_2O). There should be gentle, continuous bubbling in the suction control chamber. Place occlusive dressing over the chest tube insertion site per hospital policy. Note the date, time, and your initials on the dressing. If gauze is used, use presplit gauze; "homemade" split gauze may leave loose threads in the wound. Ensure that the drainage system is positioned below the patient's chest and secured to the floor or bed. Keep the drainage tubing free of dependent loops. Obtain a chest radiograph to confirm placement of the chest tube. Ensure that daily chest radiographs are scheduled to monitor placement of the chest tube and resolution of the pneumothorax or effusion.

Disposable chest drainage systems typically consist of three chambers next to one another in one drainage unit (Fig. 39-27). The fluid collection chamber collects drainage from the patient's pleural or pericardial space. The water-seal chamber is connected directly to the fluid collection chamber and acts as a one-way valve, protecting patients from air returning to the pleural or pericardial space. The suction chamber may be a dry suction or calibrated water chamber. It is connected to external vacuum suction set to the amount of suction ordered and controls the amount of suction that patients experience.

Assess for blood clots and fibrin strands in tubes with sanguineous or serosanguineous drainage and ensure that there are no obstructions to drainage in the tube. Maintain chest tube clearance per hospital policy. Milking or stripping of chest tubes is not recommended for chest tube clearance because of the high negative intrathoracic pressure that is created. However, some special circumstances such as maintaining chest tube patency while a patient is bleeding warrant chest tube clearance with these methods. Notify the health care provider immediately if chest tube obstruction is suspected. Generally chest tubes should not be clamped. However, it may be necessary to clamp a chest tube when exchanging the collection chamber or determine the site of an air leak (see Guidelines box).

ALTERNATIVE FEEDING TECHNIQUES

Some children are unable to take nourishment by mouth because of anomalies of the throat, esophagus, or bowel; impaired swallowing capacity; severe debilitation; respiratory distress; or unconsciousness. These children are frequently fed by way of a tube inserted orally or nasally into the stomach (orogastric [OG] or NG gavage) or duodenum-jejunum (enteral gavage) or by a tube inserted directly into the stomach (gastrostomy) or jejunum (jejunostomy). Such feedings may be intermittent or by continuous drip. Feeding resistance, a problem that may result from any long-term feeding method that bypasses the mouth, is discussed in

Chapter 25. During gavage or gastrostomy feedings infants are given a pacifier. Nonnutritive sucking has several advantages such as increased weight gain and decreased crying. However, only pacifiers with a safe design can be used to prevent the possibility of aspiration. Using improvised pacifiers made from bottle nipples is not a safe practice.

When a child is concurrently receiving continuous-drip gastric or enteral feedings and parenteral (IV) therapy, the potential exists for inadvertent administration of the enteral formula through the

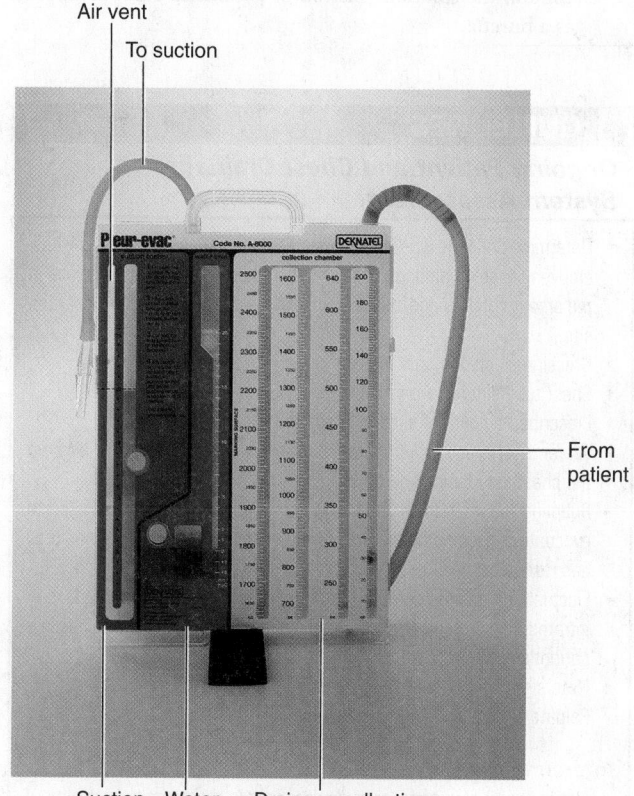

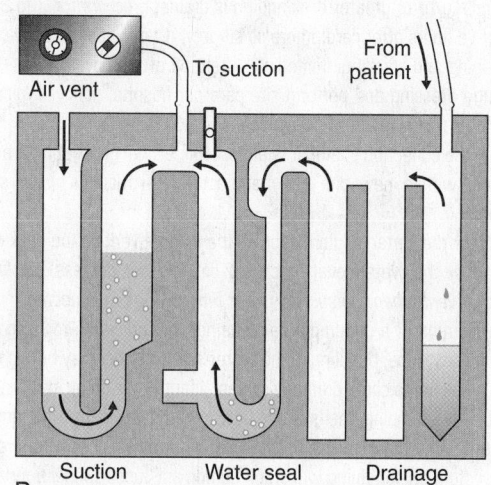

FIG 39-27 **A,** Pleur-Evac drainage system, a commercial three-bottle chest drainage device. **B,** Schematic of drainage device. (From Ignatavicius, DD, Workman, LM: *Medical-surgical nursing: patient-centered collaborative care*, ed 6, Philadelphia, 2010, Saunders.)

circulatory system. The possibility for error increases when the parenteral solution is a fat emulsion (i.e., a milky-appearing substance). Safeguards to prevent this potentially serious error include:

- Using a separate, specifically designed enteral feeding pump mounted on a separate pole for continuous-feeding solutions.
- Labeling all tubing of continuous enteral feeding with brightly colored tape or labels.
- Using specifically designed continuous-feeding bags to contain the solutions instead of parenteral equipment such as a burette.

📋 GUIDELINES

Ongoing Patient and Chest Drainage System Assessment

- Determine drainage type (sanguinous, serosanguineous, serous, chylous, empyemic), color, amount, consistency. If there is a marked decrease in the amount of drainage, assess for drainage around chest tube insertion site.
- Dressing clean, dry, and intact.
- Chest tube sutures are intact.
- Prescribed amount of suction is applied.
- Water level is at 2 cm. If water column is too high, the flow of air from the chest may be impeded.
- Bubbling in water-seal chamber is normal if chest tube was placed to evacuate a pneumothorax. Bubbling will stop when the pneumothorax has resolved.
- Fluctuations may be seen in the water column because of changes in intrathoracic pressure. Substantial fluctuations may reflect changes in a patient's respiratory status.
- Note signs and symptoms of infection or skin breakdown.
- Palpate for presence of subcutaneous air.

Interventions

- Notify health care provider of any changes in the quantity or quality of drainage.
- If 3 mL/kg/hr or greater of sanguinous drainage occurs for 2 to 3 consecutive hours after cardiothoracic surgery, it may indicate active hemorrhaging and warrants immediate attention of the physician.
- Change dressing and perform site care per hospital policy. Typically a minimal, occlusive dressing is applied.
- When the collection chamber is almost full, exchange existing drainage system with a new one per manufacturer instructions using sterile technique.
- To lower the water column, depress the manual vent on the back of the unit until the water level reaches 2 cm. *Do not depress the filtered manual vent when the suction is not functioning or connected.*
- If evacuation of a pneumothorax was not the indication for placement of the chest tube, bubbling in the water-seal chamber may be the result of a break in the chest drainage system. Identify the break in the system by briefly clamping the system between the drainage unit and the patient. When the clamp is placed between the unit and the break in the system, the bubbling will stop. Tighten any loose connections. If the air leak is suspected to be at the patient's chest wall, notify the health care provider.
- Encourage patient ambulation. Secure chest tube drainage system to prevent chest tube dislodgment from patient or disconnection from drainage system.

- Whenever access or connections are made, tracing the tubing all the way from the patient to the bag to ensure that the correct tubing source is selected.

Gavage Feeding

Infants and children can be fed simply and safely by a tube passed into the stomach through either the nares or the mouth. The tube can be left in place or inserted and removed with each feeding. In older children it is usually less traumatic to tape the tube securely in place between feedings. When this alternative is used, the tube should be removed and replaced with a new tube according to hospital policy, specific orders, and the type of tube used. Meticulous hand washing is practiced during the procedure to prevent bacterial contamination of the feeding, especially during continuous-drip feedings.

Preparation

The equipment needed for gavage feeding includes the following:

- A suitable tube selected according to the child's size, the viscosity of the solution being fed, and anticipated duration of treatment
- A receptacle for the fluid; for small amounts a 10- to 30-mL syringe barrel or Asepto syringe is satisfactory; for larger amounts a 60-mL syringe with a catheter tip is more convenient
- A 10-mL barrel syringe to aspirate stomach contents after the tube has been placed
- Water or water-soluble lubricant to lubricate the tube; sterile water is used for infants
- Paper or nonallergenic tape to mark the tube and to attach the tube to the infant's or child's cheek (and nose if placed through the nares)
- pH paper to determine the correct placement in the stomach
- The solution for feeding

Not all feeding tubes are the same. Polyethylene and polyvinylchloride types lose their flexibility and need to be replaced frequently, usually every 3 or 4 days. Polyurethane and silicone tubes remain flexible; thus they can remain in place up to 30 days. Advantages of small-bore tubes include a reduced incidence of pharyngitis, otitis media, aspiration, and discomfort. Disadvantages include difficulty during insertion (may require a stylet or metal guidewire), collapse of the tube during aspiration of gastric contents to test for correct placement, dislodgment during forceful coughing, migration out of position, knotting, occlusion, and unsuitability for thick feedings.

Procedure

Infants are easier to control if they are first wrapped in a mummy restraint (see Fig. 39-6, *A*). Even tiny infants with random movements can grasp and dislodge the tube. Preterm infants do not ordinarily require restraint; but, if they do, a small blanket folded across the chest and secured beneath the shoulders is usually sufficient. Be careful so breathing is not compromised.

Whenever possible the infant should be held and provided with a means for nonnutritive sucking during the procedure to associate the comfort of physical contact with the feeding. When this is not possible, gavage feeding is carried out with the infant or child on the back or toward the right side and the head and chest elevated. Feeding the child in a sitting position helps maintain placement of the tube in the lowest position, thus increasing the likelihood of correct placement in the stomach.

Although the most accurate method for testing tube placement is radiography, this practice is not always possible before each feeding. Research indicates that bedside assessment of gastrointestinal aspirate color and pH is useful in predicting feeding tube placement (see Evidence-Based Practice box below). If doubt exists regarding correct placement, consult the practitioner. The Guidelines box on p. 1187 describes the procedure for gavage feeding.

Studies evaluating NG and OG tube length in infants and children found that age-specific methods for predicting the distance based on height is a more accurate estimate of internal distance to the stomach (Beckstrand, Ellett, and McDaniel, 2007; Klasner, Luke, and Scalzo, 2002). The morphologic measure most commonly used by clinicians (i.e., nose-ear-xiphoid distance) is often too short to locate the entire tube pore span in the stomach. However, the nose-ear-midxiphoid umbilicus span approached the accuracy of the

age-specific prediction equations and is easier to use in a clinical setting. The best option is to adapt the nose-ear-midxiphoid umbilicus measurement for NG or OG tube length (Fig. 39-28, *A*) (see Guidelines box on p. 1187).

Ellett and Beckstrand (1999) found significant tube placement errors (43.5%) in a study of 39 hospitalized children. Children who were comatose or semicomatose, were inactive, had swallowing difficulty, or had Argyle tubes experienced increased tube placement errors. Findings supported the effectiveness of radiographs in documenting tube placement.

In a survey of 113 level II and III nurseries, 98% of the nurseries measured from the nose or mouth to the earlobe and then to the xiphoid process to calculate the length of the feeding tube for

EVIDENCE-BASED PRACTICE

Confirming Nasogastric Tube Placement in Pediatric Patients

Ask the Question
In children how should correct placement of NG tubes be assessed during hospitalization?

Search for Evidence
Search Strategies
Search selection criteria included English, research-based articles, and children and adolescents requiring NG tube placement. Search areas included aspirate, auscultation and radiology methods, NG tube length prediction methods, age-related height based methods, and accurate NG tube placement. Searches excluded newborns and preterm infants.

Databases Used
PubMed, Cochrane Collaboration, MD Consult, Joanna Briggs Institute, AHRQ-National Guideline Clearinghouse, TRIP database Plus, PedsCCM, BestBETS

Critically Analyze the Evidence
Studies compared various methods used to evaluate correct placement of the NG tube.

Accurate NG Tube Length Measurement
- Children 8 years, 4 months of age or younger: use age-related height-based equation for NG length predictions.
- Children older than 8 years, 4 months of age, short stature, or when you cannot obtain accurate height: use nose-ear-midxiphoid-umbilicus (NEMU) (Beckstrand, 1990; Beckstrand, Cirgin-Ellett, and McDaniel, 2007; Ellett, Beckstrand, Welch, et al., 1992; Strobel, Byrne, Ament, et al., 1979).

Nonradiologic Verification Methods
- A pH of 6.0 or less supports that the tip of the tube is in the gastric location (Ellett and Beckstrand, 1999; Ellett, Croffie, Cohen, et al., 2005; Huffman, Pieper, Jarczyk, et al., 2004; Metheny and Stewart, 2002; Metheny, Reed, Wiersema, et al., 1993; Metheny, Stewart, Smith, et al., 1999; Metheny, Stewart, Smith, et al., 1997; Neumann, Meyer, Dutton, et al., 1995; Nyqvist, Sorell, and Ewald, 2005; Phang, Marsh, Barlows, et al., 2004; Westhus, 2004).
- A pH greater than 5.0 does not predict correct distal tip location reliably. This may indicate respiratory or esophageal placement or the presence of medications to suppress acid secretion. Gastric aspirate pH means are statistically significantly lower compared with means from intestinal and respiratory pH aspirates (Ellett, Croffie, Cohen, et al., 2005; Metheny and Stewart, 2002; Metheny, Stewart, Smith, et al., 1999; Metheny, Stewart, Smith, et al., 1997; Phang, Marsh, Barlows, et al., 2004; Westhus, 2004).

Visual Inspection of Aspirate
- Visual inspection is less accurate than pH to confirm placement. Aspirate colors are specific to the intended placement location. Gastric contents are clear, off-white, or tan or may be brown-tinged if blood is present. Respiratory secretions may look the same. Intestinal contents are often bile stained, light to dark yellow, or greenish-brown (Metheny, Reed, Berglund, et al., 1994; Metheny and Stewart, 2002; Metheny, Stewart, Smith, et al., 1999; Phang, Marsh, Barlows, et al., 2004; Westhus, 2004).

Enzyme Testing
- Aspirate testing of enzyme levels for bilirubin, pepsin, and trypsin is highly accurate but limited to laboratory assessment (Ellett, Croffie, Cohen, and Perkins, 2005; Metheny and Stewart, 2002; Metheny, Stewart, Smith, et al., 1999; Westhus, 2004).

CO_2 Monitoring
- CO_2 monitoring is a reliable method to determine incorrect tube placement in the respiratory tract; it requires a capnograph monitor (Ellett, Croffie, Cohen, and Perkins, 2005; Metheny and Stewart, 2002; Metheny, Stewart, Smith, et al., 1999).

Gastric Auscultation
- Auscultation as a verification tool is reliable only 60% to 80% of the time and should not be used without additional methods (Ellett and Beckstrand, 1999; Metheny, McSweeney, Wehrle, et al., 1990; Neumann, Meyer, Dutton, and Smith, 1995).
- Using aspirate and nonaspirate NG tube placement verification methods in combination increases the likelihood for accurate NG tube placement to 97% to 99%, similar to the radiologic chest radiography gold standard of 99% (Ellett and Beckstrand, 1999; Ellett, Croffie, Cohen, and Perkins, 2005; Metheny and Stewart, 2002; Metheny, Reed, Berglund, et al., 1994; Metheny, Reed, Wiersema, et al., 1993; Metheny, Stewart, Smith, et al., 1999; Neumann, Meyer, Dutton, et al., 1995; Phang, Marsh, Barlows, et al., 2004; Westhus, 2004).

Apply the Evidence: Nursing Implications
There is *good evidence with strong recommendations* (Guyatt, Oxman, Vist, et al., 2008) that a combination of verification methods to confirm NG tube placement reduces the required number of x-ray films in children (Cincinnati Children's Hospital Medical Center, 2011). These methods include pH testing and visual inspection of the pH aspirate. There is also good evidence that improving the accuracy of predicting NG tube length before insertion enhances the precision of successful NG tube placement. Auscultation is used in combination with other NG tube verification methods.

Continued

EVIDENCE-BASED PRACTICE

Confirming Nasogastric Tube Placement in Pediatric Patients—cont'd

Quality and Safety Competencies:
Evidence-Based Practice*
Knowledge
Differentiate clinical opinion from research and evidence-based summaries
Describe the various verification methods to confirm NG tube placement.

Skills
Base individualized care plan on patient values, clinical expertise, and evidence
Integrate evidence into practice by using the techniques for NG tube placement verification in clinical care.

Attitudes
Value the concept of evidence-based practice as integral to determining best clinical practice
Appreciate the strengths and weakness of evidence for confirming NG tube placement.

References
Beckstrand J: The distance to the stomach for feeding tube placement in children predicted from regression on height, *Res Nurs Health* 13:411–420, 1990.
Beckstrand J, Cirgin-Ellett M, McDaniel A: Predicting internal distance to the stomach for positioning nasogastric and orogastric feeding tubes in children, *J Adv Nurs* 59:274–289, 2007.
Cincinnati Children's Hospital Medical Center: *Best evidence statement (BEST): Confirmation of nasogastric tube placement in pediatric patients*, Cincinnati, 2011, Author.
Ellett M, Beckstrand J: Examination of gavage tube placement in children, *J Soc Pediatr Nurs* 4:52–60, 1999.
Ellett M, Beckstrand J, Welch J, et al: Predicting the distance for gavage tube placement in children, *Pediatr Nurs* 18:119–121, 1992.
Ellett ML, Croffie JM, Cohen MD, et al: Gastric tube placement in young children, *Clin Nurs Res* 14:238–252, 2005.

Guyatt GH, Oxman AD, Vist GE, et al: GRADE: an emerging consensus on rating quality of evidence and strength of recommendations, *BMJ* 336:924–926, 2008.
Huffman S, Pieper P, Jarczyk KS, et al: Methods to confirm feeding tube placement: application of research in practice, *Pediatr Nurs* 30:10–13, 2004.
Metheny NA, Stewart BJ: Testing feeding tube placement during continuous tube feedings, *Appl Nurs Res* 15:254–258, 2002.
Metheny N, McSweeney M, Wehrle MA, et al: Effectiveness of the auscultatory method in predicting feeding tube location, *Nurs Res* 39:262–267, 1990.
Metheny N, Reed L, Berglund B, et al: Visual characteristics of aspirates from feeding tubes as a method for predicting tube location, *Nurs Res* 43:282–287, 1994.
Metheny N, Reed L, Wiersema L, et al: Effectiveness of pH measurements in predicting feeding tube placement: an update, *Nurs Res* 42:324–331, 1993.
Metheny NA, Stewart BJ, Smith L, et al: pH and concentrations of pepsin and trypsin in feeding tube aspirates as predictors of tube placement, *JPEN J Parenter Enteral Nutr* 21:279–285, 1997.
Metheny NA, Stewart BJ, Smith L, et al: pH and concentration of bilirubin in feeding tube aspirates as predictors of tube placement, *Nurs Res* 48:189–197, 1999.
Neumann MJ, Meyer CT, Dutton JL, et al: Hold that x-ray: aspirate pH and auscultation prove tube placement, *J Clin Gastroenterol* 20:293–295, 1995.
Nyqvist KH, Sorell A, Ewald U: Litmus tests for verification of feeding tube location in infants: evaluation of their clinical use, *J Clin Nurs* 14:486–495, 2005.
Phang JS, Marsh WA, Barlows TG, et al: Determining feeding tube location by gastric and intestinal pH values, *Nutr Clin Pract* 19:640–644, 2004.
Strobel CT, Byrne WJ, Ament ME, et al: Correlation of esophageal lengths in children with height: application to the Tuttle test without prior esophageal manometry, *J Pediatr* 94:81–84, 1979.
Westhus N: Methods to test feeding tube placement in children, *MCN Am J Matern Child Nurs* 29:282–291, 2004.

Marilyn Hockenberry; updated by Olga Taylor

*Adapted from the QSEN at www.qsen.org.
NG, Nasogastric.

placement in preterm infants. For very low–birth-weight infants, daily weight can be used to predict insertion length. Until more definitive data are available, no method that results in a shorter distance than these methods should be used.

Gastrostomy Feeding

Feeding by way of gastrostomy, or G tube, is often used for children in whom passage of a tube through the mouth, pharynx, esophagus, and cardiac sphincter of the stomach is contraindicated or impossible. It is also used to avoid the constant irritation of an NG tube in children who require tube feeding over an extended period. A gastrostomy tube may be placed with the child under general anesthesia or percutaneously using an endoscope with the patient sedated and under local anesthesia (percutaneous endoscopic gastrostomy [PEG]). The tube is inserted through the abdominal wall into the stomach about midway along the greater curvature and secured by a purse-string suture. The stomach is anchored to the peritoneum at the operative site. The tube used can be a Foley, wing-tip, or mushroom catheter. Immediately after surgery the catheter may be left open and attached to gravity drainage for 24 hours or more.

Direct postoperative care of the wound site toward prevention of infection and irritation. Cleanse the area at least daily or as often as needed to keep the area free of drainage. After healing, meticulous care is needed to keep the area surrounding the tube clean and dry to prevent excoriation and infection. Daily applications of antibiotic ointment or other preparations may be prescribed to aid in healing and prevent irritation. Exercise care to prevent excessive pull on the catheter that might cause widening of the opening and subsequent leakage of highly irritating gastric juices. Secure the tube to the abdomen, leaving a small loop of tubing at the exit site to prevent tension on the site (see Evidence-Based Practice box on p. 1188).

Granulation tissue may grow around a gastrostomy site (Fig. 39-29). This moist, beefy red tissue is not a sign of infection. However, if it continues to grow, the excess moisture can irritate the surrounding skin.

For children receiving long-term gastrostomy feeding, a skin-level device (e.g., MIC-KEY, Bard Button) offers several advantages.

GUIDELINES

Nasogastric Tube Feedings in Children

- Place child supine with head slightly hyperflexed or in a sniffing position (nose pointed toward ceiling).
- Measure the tube for approximate length of insertion and mark the point with a small piece of tape.
- Insert a tube that has been lubricated with sterile water or water-soluble lubricant through either the mouth or one of the nares to the predetermined mark. Because most young infants are obligatory nose breathers, insertion through the mouth causes less distress and helps stimulate sucking. In older infants and children the tube is passed through the nose and alternated between nostrils. An indwelling tube is almost always placed through the nose.
  - When using the nose, slip the tube along the base of the nose and direct it straight back toward the occiput.
  - When entering through the mouth, direct the tube toward the back of the throat (see Fig. 39-28, *B*).
  - If the child is able to swallow on command, synchronize passing the tube with swallowing.
- Confirm placement (see Evidence-Based Practice box, pp. 1185-1186).
- Stabilize the tube by holding or taping it to the cheek, not to the forehead, because of possible damage to the nostril. To maintain correct placement, measure and record the amount of tubing extending from the nose or mouth to the distal port when the tube is first positioned. Recheck this measurement before each feeding.
- Warm the formula to room temperature. Do not microwave! Pour formula into the barrel of the syringe attached to the feeding tube. To start the flow, give a gentle push with the plunger but then remove the plunger and allow the fluid to flow into the stomach by gravity. The rate of flow should not exceed 5 mL every 5 to 10 minutes in premature and very small infants and 10 mL/min in older infants and children to prevent nausea and regurgitation. The rate is determined by the diameter of the tubing and the height of the reservoir containing the feeding and is regulated by adjusting the height of the syringe. A usual feeding may take 15 to 30 minutes to complete.
- Flush the tube with sterile water (1 or 2 mL for small tubes to 5 to 15 mL or more for large ones) or see discussion of flushing for administering medication through nasogastric tubes in the Guidelines box on p. 1170 to clear it of formula.
- Cap or clamp indwelling tubes to prevent loss of feeding.
  - If the tube is to be removed, first pinch it firmly to prevent escape of fluid as the tube is withdrawn. Withdraw the tube quickly.
- Position the child with the head elevated 30 to 45 degrees or on the right side for 30 to 60 minutes in the same manner as after any infant feeding to minimize the possibility of regurgitation and aspiration. If the child's condition permits, bubble the youngster after the feeding.
- Record the feeding, including the type and amount of residual, the type and amount of formula, and how it was tolerated.
  - For most infant feedings any amount of residual fluid aspirated from the stomach is refed to prevent electrolyte imbalance, and the amount is subtracted from the prescribed amount of feeding. For example, if the infant is to receive 30 mL and 10 mL is aspirated from the stomach before the feeding, the 10 mL of aspirated stomach contents is refed along with 20 mL of feeding. Another method can be used in children. If residual fluid is more than one fourth of the last feeding, return the aspirate and recheck in 30 to 60 minutes. When residual fluid is less than one fourth of the last feeding, give the scheduled feeding. If large amounts of aspirated fluid persist and the child is due for another feeding, notify the practitioner.

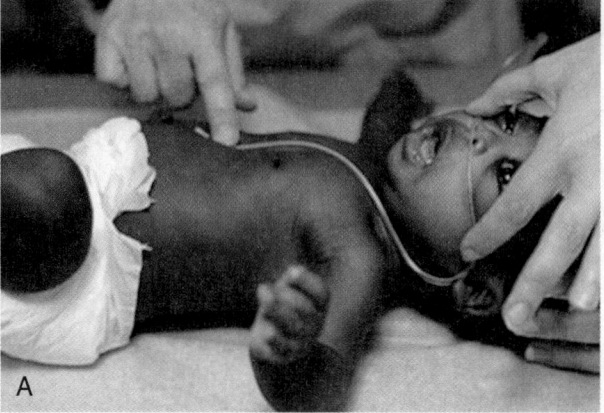

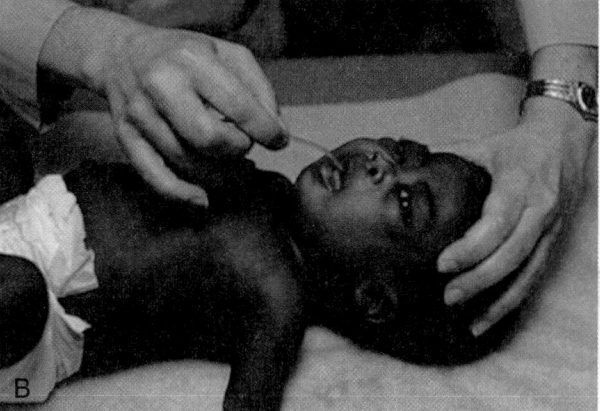

FIG 39-28 Gavage feeding. **A,** Measuring tube for orogastric feeding from tip of nose to earlobe and to midpoint between end of xiphoid process and umbilicus. **B,** Inserting tube.

The small, flexible silicone device protrudes slightly from the abdomen, is cosmetically pleasing, affords increased comfort and mobility to the child, is easy to care for, and is fully immersible in water. The one-way valve at the proximal end minimizes reflux and eliminates the need for clamping. However, the skin-level device requires a well-established gastrostomy site and is more expensive than the conventional tube. In addition, the valve may become clogged. When functioning, the valve prevents air from escaping; therefore the child may require frequent bubbling. With some devices, during feedings the child must remain fairly still because the tubing easily disconnects from the opening if the child moves. With other devices extension tubing can be attached securely to the opening (Fig. 39-30). The feeding is instilled at the other end of the tubing in a manner similar to that for a regular gastrostomy. The extension tubing may also have a separate medication port. Both the feeding and medication ports have plugs attached. Some skin-level devices require a special tube to be able to decompress the stomach (to check residual or decompress air).

Feeding of water, formula, or pureed foods is carried out in the same manner and rate as for gavage feeding. A mechanical pump may be used to regulate the volume and rate of feeding. After feedings the infant or child is positioned on the right side or in the Fowler position, and the tube may be clamped or left open and suspended between feedings, depending on the child's condition. A clamped tube allows more mobility but is only appropriate if the child can tolerate intermittent feedings without vomiting or prolonged backup of feeding into the tube. Sometimes a Y tube is used to allow for simultaneous decompression during feeding. If a Foley

EVIDENCE-BASED PRACTICE

Skin Care: Prevention and Management of Gastrostomy Button and Gastrostomy Tube Breakdown

Ask the Question

In children with skin breakdown around the gastrostomy device (tube or skin-level button), which interventions are recommended for management of skin issues?

Search for the Evidence
Search Strategies

Search selection criteria included English language publications on children and adults published on gastrostomy, care practice guidelines, and manufacturer product information.

Databases Used

Cochrane Collaboration Database, Joanna Briggs Institute, Proquest, PubMed, Scopus, National Guideline Clearinghouse (AHRQ), SUMSearch, CINAHL, Wound Ostomy and Continence Nurses Society, American Pediatric Surgical Nurses Association, patient and family listservs

Critically Analyze the Evidence
Skin Care of the Gastrostomy Tube

- The American Pediatric Surgical Nurses Association (2006) recommends cleaning the skin around the gastrostomy twice daily and as needed with warm soap and water and keeping the area dry. It is important to remove crusted areas around the G tube. Diluted half-strength hydrogen peroxide may be used to clean for the first 2 weeks.
- The Wound Ostomy and Continence Nurses Society clinical guidelines (2008) identify the use of hydrogen peroxide as one of the possible causes of hypergranulation tissue. The guidelines recommend routine assessment of the site and keeping the skin around the G tube dry to prevent complications.
- McClave and Neff (2006) suggest cleaning the skin around the G tube with mild antibacterial soap and water. The use of hydrogen peroxide is discouraged because it is corrosive to the skin and leads to excessive drying of the tissue. Prompt treatment of skin irritation is vital in preventing further skin breakdown.
- Borkowski (2004, 2005) discourages the use of hydrogen peroxide because it can cause skin irritation and may be cytotoxic, disrupting wound healing. The author recommends gently cleaning the skin with water and patting dry because aggressive cleaning around the G tube may also interfere with the healing process.
- Product information by the manufacturer of MIC-KEY (Kimberly-Clark, 2006) advises cleaning the skin around the G button with soap and water using a soft cotton tip applicator or washcloth. The document recommends inspecting the skin daily and reporting any complications to a health care provider.

Skin Barriers

- The Wound Ostomy and Continence Nurses Society clinical guidelines (2008) recommend the use of barrier ointments such as zinc oxide and nonalcohol skin barrier film to control leakage. If skin irritation is present, the guidelines recommend adding absorptive powders and skin barrier wafers to help manage leakage and promote healing.
- Borkowski (2004, 2005) uses protective barriers such as zinc oxide and petrolatum to provide skin protection. For maceration around the stoma, the use of a solid skin barrier (pectin-based wafer Stomahesive) to provide an environment for protection and healing of the skin is recommended.

Stabilization

- The Wound Ostomy and Continence Nurses Society (2008) recommends that the stabilizer be placed on the skin without excessive tension and pulling. If a long tube is not stabilized, it can increase the risk for infection, cause hyperplasia, and lead to skin breakdown.
- In three patients with peristomal irritation caused by G tube mobility, Borkowski (2004) successfully managed two patients by applying a stabilization method to the G tube. In the third patient, despite the author's recommendation, the family refused to stabilize the G tube and preferred to treat the irritation with protective barrier ointments only. This finding illustrates the need to individualize care. There was no follow-up reported in the article regarding the success of the family's methods.
- McClave and Neff (2006) reported on their experience with percutaneous endoscopic gastrostomy (PEG) tubes. PEG tubes have increased risk for mobility and migration, which leads to ulceration and enlargement of the stoma. This can be prevented by stabilizing the tube.
- Crawley-Coha (2004) strongly recommends the use of stabilizing techniques to promote healing after surgery and prevent dislodgment. In active children the use of additional products such as elastic wraps and flexible dressings to immobilize the gastrostomy device is recommended.

Hypergranulation

- In a longitudinal study of 40 children with G tubes, granulation tissue occurred 2 times more often in children with long tube devices than in those who had skin-level devices (Thorne, Radford, Onyskiw, et al., 1998).
- In a prospective study of eight patients, granulation tissue was the complication that prompted the most hospital and physician visits. Granulation tissue affected five patients (63%). Although families and caregivers were educated about the potential complications, this did not eliminate unscheduled health care contacts (Crosby and Duerksen, 2007).
- Borkowski (2004, 2005) recommends the use of triamcinolone (0.5%-0.1%) cream as a less painful alternative to the traditional silver nitrate sticks. Polyurethane foam may be used to absorb moisture and keep the skin dry to prevent further breakdown. One 2 × 2 gauze may be placed to create a snug fit for an ill-fitting low-profile device and help keep the skin dry. Stabilization of the tube is a priority to prevent the development of hypergranulation.
- In the experience of Crawley-Coha (2004) hypergranulation tissue can occur, regardless of the type of G tube placed and method of stabilization used. Treatment options include the application of silver nitrate, sharp debridement, and topical steroids. This author used triamcinolone cream (0.5%) 3 times a day with great success for the previous 6 years. In some patients polyurethane foam dressing is also used to manage hypergranulation tissue.
- The Wound Ostomy and Continence Nurses Society clinical guidelines (2008) recommend managing hypergranulation by stabilizing the tube, keeping the peristomal area dry by applying polyurethane foam, and using triamcinolone (0.5%) 3 times a day. Silver nitrate may also be used for hypergranulation.

Individualizing Care

- Borkowski (2004) acknowledges that, when children with G tube develop complications despite family education on alternative management options, families may have chosen to continue to use familiar techniques.

EVIDENCE-BASED PRACTICE

Skin Care: Prevention and Management of Gastrostomy Button and Gastrostomy Tube Breakdown—cont'd

The care plan for managing complications should consider the child's developmental age, activity level, and parental preferences.

- Crawley-Coha (2004) recommends providing parents with individualized written instructions before discharge. Ongoing support should be provided by the child's medical team. To help with transition to the home, information on support groups for patients with G tubes may be offered (e.g., Oley Foundation, www.oley.org).

Apply the Evidence: Nursing Implications

There is *very low evidence with strong recommendations* for the following (Guyatt, Oxman, Vist, et al., 2008):

1. Use mild soap and water to clean the peristomal area.
2. If skin irritation or breakdown is noted, use appropriate skin barriers:
   - Zinc oxide–based ointment, petrolatum-based ointment, or nonalcohol skin barrier for prevention or treatment of breakdown
   - Solid pectin-based wafer for maceration
3. Stabilize long G tube using one of the three methods: commercial stabilization device, polyurethane foam, or the H tape method.
4. Request an order for triamcinolone cream for short-term treatment of hypergranulation.
5. Individualize skin care management.

Quality and Safety Competencies:
Evidence-Based Practice*
Knowledge
Differentiate clinical opinion from research and evidence-based summaries

Recommend interventions for management of skin breakdown around the gastrostomy device (tube or skin-level button).

Skills
Base individualized care plan on patient values, clinical expertise, and evidence

Integrate evidence into practice by using recommended interventions for management of skin breakdown around the gastrostomy device (tube or skin-level button).

Attitudes
Value the concept of evidence-based practice as integral to determining best clinical practice

Appreciate the strengths and weakness of evidence for using interventions for management of skin breakdown around the gastrostomy device (tube or skin-level button).

References

American Pediatric Surgical Nurses Association: *Gastrostomy*, 2006, data.memberclicks.com/site/aps/GASTROSTOMY.doc.

Borkowski S: Similar gastrostomy peristomal skin irritations in three pediatric patients, *J Wound Ostomy Contin Nurs* 31(4):201–206, 2004.

Borkowski S: G tube care: managing hypergranulation tissue, *Nursing* 35(8):24, 2005.

Crawley-Coha T: A practical guide for the management of pediatric gastrostomy tubes based on 14-year experience, *J Wound Ostomy Contin Nurs* 31(4):193–200, 2004.

Crosby J, Duerksen D: A prospective study of tube- and feeding-related complications in patients receiving long-term home enteral nutrition, *J Parenter Enter Nutr* 31(4):274–277, 2007.

Guyatt GH, Oxman AD, Vist GE, et al: GRADE: an emerging consensus on rating quality of evidence and strength of recommendations, *BMJ* 336:924–926, 2008.

Kimberly-Clark: *MIC-KEY: low profile gastrostomy feeding tube—your guide to proper care*, 2006, kchealthcare.com/docs/R8201B%20MIC-KEY%20Care%20guide%20English.pdf.

McClave S, Neff R: Care and long-term maintenance of percutaneous endoscopic gastrostomy tubes (electronic version), *J Parenter Enter Nutr* 30(1):S27–S38, 2006.

Thorne S, Radford J, Onyskiw J, et al: A comparative longitudinal study of gastrostomy devices in children (electronic version), *West J Nurs Res* 20(2):145–165, 1998.

Wound Ostomy and Continence Nurses Society: *Management of gastrostomy tube complications for the pediatric and adult patient*, 2008, www.wocn.org/WOCN_Library.

Caterina Nicole Landry, Andrea J. Harrison, Mary Hershey Pascual, and Barbara Montagnino

*Adapted from the QSEN at www.qsen.org.

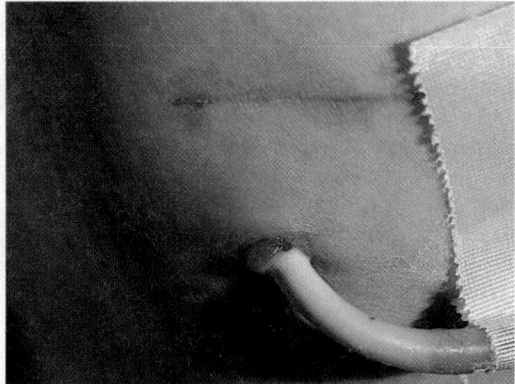

FIG 39-29 Appearance of healthy granulation tissue around stoma.

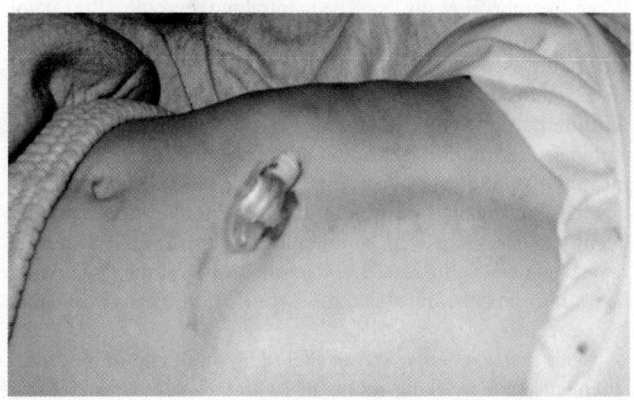

FIG 39-30 Child with skin-level gastrostomy device (MIC-KEY), which provides for secure attachment of extension tubing to gastrostomy opening.

catheter is used as the gastrostomy tube, apply very slight tension. The tube is securely taped to maintain the balloon at the gastrostomy opening and prevent leakage of gastric contents and the progression of the tube toward the pyloric sphincter, where it may occlude the stomach outlet. As a precaution the length of the tube is measured after surgery and measured again each shift to be certain that it has not slipped. The nurse can make a mark above the skin level to further ensure its placement. When the gastrostomy tube is no longer needed, it is removed; the skin opening usually closes spontaneously by contracture.

Nasoduodenal and Nasojejunal Tubes

Children at high risk for regurgitation or aspiration such as those with gastroparesis, mechanical ventilation, or brain injuries may require placement of a postpyloric feeding tube. A trained practitioner inserts the nasoduodenal or nasojejunal tube because of the risk of misplacement and potential for perforation in tubes requiring a stylet. Accurate placement is verified by radiography. Small-bore tubes may easily clog. Flush the tube when feeding is interrupted, before and after medication administration, and routinely every 4 hours or as directed by institutional policy. Tube replacement should be considered monthly to ensure optimal tube patency. Continuous feedings are delivered by a mechanical pump to regulate their volume and rate. Bolus feeds are contraindicated. Tube displacement is suspected in children showing signs of feeding intolerance such as vomiting. In these cases stop the feedings and notify the practitioner.

Total Parenteral Nutrition

TPN provides for the total nutritional needs of infants and children whose lives are threatened because feeding by way of the gastrointestinal tract is impossible, inadequate, or hazardous.

TPN therapy involves IV infusion of highly concentrated solutions of protein, glucose, and other nutrients. The solution is infused through conventional tubing with a special filter attached to remove particulate matter or microorganisms that may have contaminated the solution. The highly concentrated solutions require infusion into a vessel with sufficient volume and turbulence to allow for rapid dilution. The wide-diameter vessels selected are the superior vena cava and innominate or intrathoracic subclavian veins approached by way of the external or internal jugular veins. The highly irritating nature of concentrated glucose precludes the use of the small peripheral veins in most instances. However, diluted glucose-protein hydrolysates that are appropriate for infusing into peripheral veins are being used with increasing frequency. When peripheral veins are used, intralipid becomes the major calorie source. For long-term alimentation central venous catheters are usually used.

The infusion is maintained at a constant rate by means of an infusion pump to ensure the proper concentrations of glucose and amino acids. Accurate calculation of the rate is required to deliver a measured amount in a given length of time. Because alterations in flow rate are relatively common, the drip should be checked frequently to ensure an even, continuous infusion. The TPN infusion rate should not be increased or decreased without the practitioner being informed because alterations can cause hyperglycemia or hypoglycemia.

General assessments such as vital signs, input and output measurements, and checking results of laboratory tests facilitate early detection of infection or fluid and electrolyte imbalance. Additional amounts of potassium sand sodium chloride are often required in hyperalimentation; therefore observation for signs of

TABLE 39-9	ADMINISTRATION OF ENEMAS TO CHILDREN	
AGE	**AMOUNT (mL)**	**INSERTION DISTANCE**
Infant	120-240	2.5 cm (1 inch)
2-4 yr	240-360	5 cm (2 inch)
4-10 yr	360-480	7.5 cm (3 inch)
11 yr	480-720	10 cm (4 inch)

potassium or sodium deficit or excess is part of nursing care. This is rarely a problem except in children with reduced renal function or metabolic defects. Hyperglycemia may occur during the first day or two as the child adapts to the high-glucose load of the hyperalimentation solution. Although hyperglycemia occurs infrequently, insulin may be required to help the body adjust. When this occurs, nursing responsibilities include blood glucose testing. To prevent hypoglycemia when the hyperalimentation is disconnected, the rate of the infusion and the amount of insulin are decreased gradually.

Family Teaching and Home Care

When alternative feedings are needed for an extended period, the family needs to learn how to feed the child with an NG, gastrostomy, or TPN feeding regimen. The same principles apply as discussed earlier in this chapter for compliance, especially in terms of education, and in Chapter 21 for discharge planning and home care. Plan ample time for the family to learn and perform the procedures under supervision before they assume full responsibility for the child's care. Refer the family to community agencies that provide support and practical assistance. The Oley Foundation* is a non-profit research and education organization that assists persons receiving enteral nutrition and home TPN.

PROCEDURES RELATED TO ELIMINATION

Enema

The procedure for giving an enema to an infant or child does not differ essentially from that for an adult except for the type and amount of fluid administered and the distance for inserting the tube into the rectum (Table 39-9). Depending on the volume, use a syringe with rubber tubing, an enema bottle, or an enema bag.

An isotonic solution is used in children. Plain water is not used because, being hypotonic, it can cause rapid fluid shift and fluid overload. The Fleet enema (pediatric or adult sized) is not advised for children because of the harsh action of its ingredients (sodium biphosphate and sodium phosphate). Commercial enemas can be dangerous to patients with megacolon and dehydrated or azotemic children. The osmotic effect of the Fleet enema may produce diarrhea, which can lead to metabolic acidosis. Other potential complications are extreme hyperphosphatemia, hypernatremia, and hypocalcemia, which may lead to neuromuscular irritability and coma (Walton, Thomas, Aly, et al., 2000).

Because infants and young children are unable to retain the solution after it is administered, the buttocks must be held together for

---

*214 Hun Memorial, MC-28, Albany Medical Center, Albany, NY 12208, 800-776-OLEY, www.oley.org.

a short time to retain the fluid. The enema is administered and expelled while the child is lying with the buttocks over the bedpan and with the head and back supported by pillows. Older children are ordinarily able to hold the solution if they understand what to do and if they are not expected to hold it for too long. The nurse should have the bedpan handy or for ambulatory children ensure that the bathroom is available before beginning the procedure. An enema is an intrusive procedure and thus threatening to preschool children; therefore a careful explanation is especially important to ease possible fear.

A preoperative bowel preparation solution given orally or through an NG tube is being used increasingly instead of an enema. The polyethylene glycol–electrolyte lavage solution (GoLYTELY) mechanically flushes the bowel without significant absorption, thereby avoiding potential fluid and electrolyte imbalances. NuLYTELY, a modification of GoLYTELY, has the same therapeutic advantages as GoLYTELY and was developed to improve on the taste. Another effective oral cathartic is magnesium citrate solution.

Ostomies

Children may require stomas for various health problems. The most frequent causes in infants are necrotizing enterocolitis, imperforate anus, and less often Hirschsprung disease. In older children the most frequent causes are inflammatory bowel disease, especially Crohn disease (regional enteritis), and ureterostomies for distal ureter or bladder defects.

Care and management of ostomies in older children differ little from the care of ostomies in adult patients. The major emphasis in pediatric care is preparing the child for the procedure and teaching care of the ostomy to the child and family. The basic principles of preparation are the same as for any procedure (see p. 1131). Simple, straightforward language is most effective, together with the use of illustrations and a replica model (e.g., drawing a picture of a child with a stoma on the abdomen and explaining it as "another opening where bowel movements [or any other term the child uses] will come out"). At another time the nurse can draw a pouch over the opening to demonstrate how the contents are collected. Using a doll to demonstrate the process is an excellent teaching strategy, and special books are available.

Children with ileostomies are fitted immediately after surgery with an appliance to protect the skin from the proteolytic enzymes in the liquid stool. Infants may not be fitted with a pouch in the immediate postoperative period. When stomal drainage is minimal, as is often the case in small or preterm infants, a gauze dressing suffices. Give parents a choice of caring for the colostomy with or without an appliance. Pediatric appliances are available in a variety of sizes to ensure an adequate fit.*

Ostomy equipment consists of a one- or two-piece system with a hypoallergenic skin barrier to maintain peristomal skin integrity. The pouch should be large enough to contain a moderate amount of stool and flatus but not so large as to overwhelm the infant or child. A backing helps minimize the risk of skin breakdown from moisture trapped between the skin and pouch. Avoid small clips and rubber bands to prevent choking in young children.

Protection of the peristomal skin is a major aspect of stoma care. Well-fitting appliances are important to prevent leakage of contents. Before applying the appliance, prepare the skin with a skin sealant that is allowed to dry. Then apply stoma paste around the base of the stoma or to the back of the wafer. The sealant and paste work together to prevent peristomal skin breakdown.

In infants with a colostomy left unpouched, skin care is similar to that of any diapered child. However, protect the peristomal skin with a barrier substance (e.g., zinc oxide ointment [Sensi-Care] or a mixture of zinc oxide ointment and stoma powder [Stomahesive]). A diaper larger than the one usually worn may be needed to extend upward over the stoma and absorb drainage. If the skin becomes inflamed, denuded, or infected, the care is similar to the interventions used for diaper dermatitis. A zinc-based product helps protect healthy skin, heal excoriated skin, and minimize pain associated with skin breakdown. The skin protectant adheres to denuded, weeping skin. The nurse can apply zinc-based products over topical antifungal and antibacterial agents if infection is present. No-sting barrier film is a skin sealant that has no alcohol base and can be used on open skin without stinging.

Preventing young children from pulling off the pouch is also an important consideration. One-piece outfits keep exploring hands from reaching the pouch, and the loose waist avoids any pressure on the appliance. Keeping the child occupied with toys during the pouch change is also helpful. As children mature, encourage their participation in ostomy care. Even preschoolers can help by holding supplies, pulling paper backings from the appliance, and helping clean the stoma area. Toilet training for bladder control needs to begin at the appropriate time as for any other child.

Older children and adolescents should eventually have total responsibility for ostomy care just as they would for usual bowel function. During adolescence concerns for body image and the impact of the ostomy on intimacy and sexuality emerge. The nurse should stress to teenagers that the presence of a stoma need not interfere with their activities. These youngsters can choose which ostomy equipment is best suited to their needs. Attractively designed and decorated pouch covers are well liked by teenagers.

Children with familial adenomatous polyposis may require a colectomy with ileoanal reservoir to prevent or treat carcinoma of the colon. Peristomal skin care for these children is particularly challenging because of increased liquid stools, increased digestive enzymes that may cause skin breakdown, and the stoma being at skin level rather than raised. Additional care with this condition includes close monitoring of fluid and electrolyte status and increased incidence of bowel obstruction.

An enterostomal therapy nurse specialist is an important member of the health care team and will have additional suggestions and assistance with skin care information and ostomy pouching options. The nurse can obtain further information by contacting the Wound, Ostomy and Continence Nurses Society.*

Family Teaching and Home Care

Because these children are almost always discharged with a functioning colostomy, preparation of the family should begin as early as possible in the hospital. The nurse instructs the family in the application of the device (if used), care of the skin, and appropriate action in case skin problems develop. Early evidence of skin breakdown or stomal complication, such as ribbonlike stools, excessive diarrhea, bleeding, prolapse, or failure to pass flatus or stool is brought to the attention of the health care provider, nurse, or stoma specialist. The same principles are applied as discussed earlier in this chapter for compliance, especially in terms of education, and in Chapter 38 for discharge planning and home care.

---

*Parents may find helpful information from ConvaTec, www.convatec.com.

*888-224-9626, www.wocn.org.

KEY POINTS

- Informed consent is valid when the person is capable of giving consent (is over the age of majority and competent), is supplied with information needed to make an intelligent decision, and acts voluntarily when exercising freedom of choice.
- Informed consent is needed for major surgery, minor surgery, and diagnostic tests and medical treatments with an element of risk.
- The major principles in psychologic preparation of the child for surgery are to establish trust, provide support, and give an explanation in easy-to-understand terms.
- Preparation for procedures should be based on developmental characteristics of the child and family, emphasizing the importance of the parents' role.
- Most parents and children want to be together during stressful procedures and should be offered this opportunity, with guidance on how the parent can comfort the child.
- The use of play activities to provide teaching about necessary nursing and medical interventions is an effective tool for use with children.
- In the performance of a procedure, the nurse should expect success, involve the child when possible in the procedure, provide distraction, and allow for expression of feelings.
- Proper positioning of infants and small children for procedures is essential to minimize movement and discomfort.
- In giving postprocedural support, the nurse should encourage children to express their feelings and praise them for completion of the procedure.
- Stressful times before and after surgery that produce anxiety in children are admission, blood tests, injection of preoperative medication (if used), transportation to the operating room, and return from the PACU.
- Assessment of compliance entails measuring factors that affect compliance through clinical judgment, self-reporting, direct observation, monitoring of appointments and therapeutic response, pill counts, and chemical assay.
- Compliance strategies may be classified as organizational, educational, and behavioral.
- Knowledge of the ill child's eating habits and favorite foods can help maintain adequate nutrition.
- Skin care is essential to prevent skin breakdown.

- Control of fever may be accomplished by administration of antipyretics; hyperthermia is controlled by environmental means (minimum clothing, increased air circulation, hypothermia mattress, or cool compresses).
- Infection control is based on two systems. Standard Precautions provide protection when the infected person is undiagnosed. Transmission-based precautions add extra interventions for patients diagnosed with or suspected of having an infection.
- Ensuring safety in the hospital setting is a major concern and can be achieved through environmental measures, infection control measures, limit setting, and safe transportation.
- Restraints are used cautiously and require a medical order. Therapeutic hugging can avoid the use of restraints.
- Factors that affect drug dosage determination are growth and maturation, difficulty in evaluating drug response, and BSA.
- Family teaching regarding medication administration includes telling parents why the child is receiving the drug; its possible effects; and the amount, frequency, and length of time the drug is to be administered.
- The preferred sites for IM injection in children are the vastus lateralis and ventrogluteal areas.
- Intermittent venous access is accomplished by a peripheral intermittent infusion device, a PICC, a central venous catheter, or an implanted port.
- Several safety catheters and needleless device systems are available to reduce the risk of needlestick injuries in patients and caregivers.
- Nursing assessment of fluid and electrolyte disturbances entails observation of general appearance, vital signs, and measurement of I&O.
- Oxygen can be administered by hood, mask, nasal cannula, prongs, or face tent.
- Tracheostomy suctioning involves premeasured insertion of the catheter, application of suction for 5 seconds when withdrawing the catheter, and supplemental oxygen before and after suctioning.
- Alternative forms of feeding include gavage feeding, gastrostomy feeding, and TPN.
- In the care of children with ostomies, nurses play an important role in family support and instruction in care of the stoma site.

REFERENCES

Abo A, Chen L, Johnston P, et al: Positioning for lumbar puncture in children evaluated by bedside ultrasound, *Pediatrics* 125:e1149–e1153, 2010.

American Academy of Pediatrics (AAP): Consent for emergency medical services for children and adolescents, *Pediatrics* 111(3):703–706, 2003.

American Academy of Pediatrics (AAP) Committee on Pediatric Emergency Medicine, American College of Emergency Physicians, Pediatric Emergency Medicine Committee, et al: Patient- and family-centered care and the role of the emergency physician providing care to a child in the emergency department, *Pediatrics* 118(5):2242–2244, 2006.

American Academy of Pediatrics (AAP) Task Force on Sudden Infant Death Syndrome: The changing concept of sudden infant death syndrome: diagnostic coding shifts, controversies regarding the sleeping environment, and new variables to consider in reducing risk, *Pediatrics* 116(5):1245–1255, 2005.

American Association of Critical Care Nurses: Practice alert: family presence during CPR and invasive procedures, 2006, www.aacn.org.

American Heart Association: 2010 American Heart Association guidelines for CPR and ECC, *Circulation* 122(suppl 2), 2010.

Amlung SR, Miller WL, Bosley LM: The 1999 national pressure ulcer prevalence survey: a benchmarking approach, *Adv Skin Wound Care* 14:297–301, 2001.

Anderson SL, Schaechter J, Brosco JP: Adolescent patients and their confidentiality: staying within legal bounds, *Contemp Pediatr* 22(7):54, 2005.

Axelrod P: External cooling in the management of fever, *Clin Infect Dis* 31(suppl 5):S224–S229, 2000.

Baharestani MM, Ratliff CR: Pressure ulcers in neonates and children: an NPUAP white paper, *Adv Skin Wound Care* 20(4):208–220, 2007.

Barnes S: Not a social event: the follow-up phone call, *J Perianesth Nurs* 14(4):223–255, 2000.

Beckstrand J, Ellett MLC, McDaniel A: Predicting internal distance to the stomach for positioning NG and OG feeding tubes in children, *J Adv Nurs* 59(3):274–289, 2007.

Berger JE, American Academy of Pediatrics (AAP) Committee on Medical Liability: Consent by proxy for nonurgent pediatric care, *Pediatrics* 112(5):1186–1195, 2003.

Blaney M, Shen V, Kerner JA, et al: Alteplase for the treatment of central venous catheter occlusion in children: results of a prospective, open-label, single-arm study (the Cathflo Activase Pediatric Study), *J Vasc Interv Radiol* 17(11 Pt 1):1745–1751, 2006.

Bottor LT: Rapid sequence intubation in the neonate, *Adv Neonat Care* 9(3):111–117, 2009.

Bryant RA, Doughty D, editors: *Acute and chronic wounds: nursing management*, ed 2, St Louis, 2000, Mosby.

Burke N: Alternative methods for newborn urine sample collection, *Pediatr Nurs* 21(6):546–549, 1995.

Child Health Corporation of America: Pediatric falls: state of the science, *Pediatr Nurs* 35(4):227–231, 2009.

Codipietro L, Ceccarelli M, Ponzone A: Breastfeeding or oral sucrose solution in term neonates receiving heel lance: a randomized, controlled trial, *Pediatrics* 122(3):e716–e721, 2008.

Considine J, Brennan D: Effect of an evidence-based education programme on ED discharge advice for febrile children, *J Clin Nurs* 16:1687–1694, 2007.

Cook IF, Murtagh J: Comparative reactogenicity and parental acceptability of pertussis vaccines administered into the ventrogluteal area and anterolateral thigh in children aged 2, 4, 6, and 18 months, *Vaccine* 4(21):3330–3334, 2003.

Cook IF, Murtagh J: Ventrogluteal area—a suitable site for intramuscular vaccination of infants and toddlers, *Vaccine* 24(13):2403–2408, 2006.

Curley MAQ, Moloney-Harmon PA: *Critical care nursing of infants and children*, ed 2, Philadelphia, 2001, Saunders.

Curley MAQ, Quigley SM, Lin M: Pressure ulcers in pediatric intensive care: incidence and associated factors, *Pediatr Crit Care Med* 4:284–290, 2003.

Curley MAQ, Razmus IS, Roberts KE, et al: Predicting pressure ulcer risk in pediatric patients: the Braden Q scale, *Nurs Res* 52:22–33, 2003.

de Caen AR, Reis A, Bhutta A: Vascular access and drug therapy in pediatric resuscitation, *Pediatr Clin North Am* 55(4):909–927, 2008.

Eaton L: Hand washing is more important than cleaner wards in controlling MRSA, *BMJ* 330(7497):922, 2005.

Ellett ML, Beckstrand J: Examination of gavage tube placement in children, *J Soc Pediatr Nurs* 4(2):51–60, 1999.

Emergency Nurses Association: Family presence at the bedside during invasive procedures and resuscitation, 2005, www.ena.org.

Essink-Tebbes CM, Wuis EW, Liem KD, et al: Safety of lidocaine-prilocaine cream application four times a day in premature neonates: a pilot study, *Eur J Pediatr* 158(5):421–423, 1999.

Fearon DM, Steele DW: End-tidal carbon dioxide predicts the presence and severity of acidosis in children with diabetes, *Acad Emerg Med* 9(12):1373–1379, 2002.

Fisher AA, Deffenbaugh C, Poole RL, et al: The use of alteplase for restoring patency to occluded central venous access devices in infants and children, *J Infus Nurs* 27(3):171–174, 2004.

Foster H, Ritchey M, Bloom D: Adventitious knots in urethral catheters: report of 5 cases, *J Urol* 148(5):1496–1498, 1992.

Gamulka B, Mendoza C, Connolly B: Evaluation of a unique, nurse-inserted, peripherally inserted central catheter program, *Pediatrics* 6(115):1602–1606, 2005.

Gonzalez CM, Palmer LS: Double-knotted feeding tube in a child's bladder, *Urology* 49(5):772, 1997.

Gray L, Watt L, Blass EM: Skin-to-skin contact is analgesic in healthy newborns, *Pediatrics* 105(1):110–111, 2000, www.pediatrics.org/cgi/content/full/105/1/E14.

Gray M: Atraumatic urethral catheterization of children, *Pediatr Nurs* 22(4):306–310, 1996.

Hazinski MF, Zaritsky AL, Nadkarni VM, et al: *PALS provider manual*, Dallas, 2002, American Heart Association.

Infusion Nurses Society: *Policies and procedures for infusion nursing*, ed 3, Norwood, Mass, 2006, Author.

Joint Commission on Accreditation of Healthcare Organizations (JCAHO): *Comprehensive accreditation manual for hospitals: restraint and seclusion standards, TX7.1-TX7.5.5*, Oakbrook Terrace, Ill, 2001, Author.

Jones T, Jacobsen SJ: Childhood febrile seizures: overview and implications, *Int J Med Sci* 4(2):110–114, 2007.

Junqueira AL, Tavares VR, Martins RM, et al: Safety and immunogenicity of hepatitis B vaccine administered into ventrogluteal vs. anterolateral thigh sites in infants: a randomized controlled trial, *Int J Nurs Stud* 47(9):1074–1079, 2010.

Kain ZN, Caldwell-Andrews AA, Krivutza DM, et al: Trends in the practice of parental presence during induction of anesthesia and the use of preoperative sedative premedication in the United States, 1995–2002: results of a follow-up national survey, *Anesth Analg* 98(5):1252–1259, 2004.

Kain ZN, Caldwell-Andrews AA, Mayes LC, et al: Family-centered preparation for surgery improves perioperative outcomes in children, *Anesthesiology* 106(1):65–74, 2007.

Katsma D, Smith G: Analysis of needle path during intramuscular injection, *Nurs Res* 46(5):288–292, 1997.

Kellam B, Sacks LM, Wailer JL, et al: Tenderfoot Preemie vs a manual lancet: a clinical evaluation, *Neonatal Netw* 20(7):31–36, 2001.

Kerner JA, Garcia-Careaga MG, Fisher AA, et al: Treatment of catheter occlusion in pediatric patients, *J Parenter Enteral Nutr* 30(suppl 1):S73–S81, 2006.

Kilbane BJ: Images in emergency medicine: knotting of a urinary catheter, *Ann Emerg Med* 53(5):e3–e4, 2009.

Klasner AE, Luke DA, Scalzo AJ: Pediatric orogastric and nasogastric tubes: a new formula evaluated, *Ann Emerg Med* 39(3):268–272, 2002.

Kraus D, Stohlmeyer LA, Hannon DR, et al: Effectiveness and infant acceptance of the Rx Medibottle versus the oral syringe, *Pharmacotherapy* 21(4):416–423, 2001.

Lamagna P, MacPhee M: Phlebitis and infiltration: troubleshooting pediatric peripheral IVs, *Nurse Week (Heartland ed)* 5(4):20, 26, 28, 2004.

Levison J, Wojtulewicz J: Adventitious knot formation complicating catheterization of the infant bladder, *J Paediatr Child Health* 40(8):493–494, 2004.

Li HCW, Lopez V, Lee TLI: Psychoeducational preparation of children for surgery: the importance of parental involvement, *Patient Educ Counsel* 65:34–41, 2007.

Lodha A, Ly L, Brindle M, et al: Intraurethral knot in a very-low-birth-weight infant: Radiological recognition, surgical management and prevention, *Pediatr Radiol* 35(7):713–716, 2005.

Manworren R, Fledderman M: Preparation of the child and family for surgery. In Wise BV, McKenna C, Garvin G, et al, editors: *Nursing care of the general pediatric surgical patient*, Gaithersburg, MD, 2000, Aspen.

Maxwell LG, Yaster M: Perioperative management issues in pediatric patients, *Anesthesiol Clin North Am* 18(3):601–632, 2000.

McCord S, McElvain V, Sachdeva R, et al: Risk factors associated with pressure ulcers in the pediatric intensive care unit, *J Wound Ostomy Continence Nurs* 31(4):179–183, 2004.

McGillivray D, Mok E, Mulrooney E, et al: A head-to-head comparison: "clean-void" bag versus catheter urinalysis in the diagnosis of urinary tract infection in young children, *J Pediatr* 147(4):451–456, 2008.

Munro H, D'Errico FC: Parental involvement in perioperative anesthetic management, *J Perianesth Nurs* 15(6):397–400, 2000.

Nagler J, Wright R, Krauss B: End-tidal carbon dioxide as a measure of acidosis among children with gastroenteritis, *Pediatrics* 118(1):260–267, 2006.

Noonan C, Quigley S, Curley MAQ: Skin integrity in hospitalized infants and children: a prevalence survey, *J Pediatr Nurs* 21(6):445–453, 2006.

Piira T, Sugiura T, Champion GD, et al: The role of parental presence in the context of children's medical procedures: a systematic review, *Child Care Health Dev* 31(2):233–243, 2005.

Purssell E: Parental fever phobia and its evolutionary correlates, *J Clin Nurs* 18:210–218, 2008.

Quality, equipment hold keys to infection control, *ED Manage* 18(2):19–21, 2006.

Romino SL, Keatley VM, Secrest J, et al: Parental presence during anesthesia induction in children, *AORN J* 81(4):780–792, 2005.

Rosenberg H, Davis M, James D: Malignant hyperthermia, *Orphanet J Rare Dis* 2:21, 2007.

Rote N, Huether S, McCance K: Infections and alterations in immunity and inflammation. In Huether S, McCance K, editors: *Understanding pathophysiology*, ed 2, St Louis, 2000, Mosby.

Sadleir LG, Scheffer IE: Febrile seizures, *BMJ* 334:307–311, 2007.

Shah V, Ohlsson A: Venepuncture versus heel lance for blood sampling in term neonates, *Cochrane Database Syst Rev* (4):CD001452, 2007.

Shen V, Li X, Murdock M, et al: Recombinant tissue plasminogen activator (alteplase) for restoration of function to occluded central venous catheters in pediatric patients, *J Pediatr Hematol Oncol* 25(1):38–45, 2003.

Shepherd AJ, Glenesk A, Niven CA, et al: A Scottish study of heel-prick blood sampling in newborn babies, *Midwifery* 22(2):158–168, 2005.

Tillett J: Adolescents and informed consent: ethical and legal issues, *J Perinat Neonat Nurs* 19(2):112–121, 2005.

Turner TW: Intravesical catheter knotting: an uncommon complication of urinary catheterization, *Pediatr Emerg Care* 20(2):115–117, 2004.

Uman LS, Chambers CT, McGrath PJ, et al: Psychological interventions for needle-related procedural pain and distress in children and adolescents, *Cochrane Database Syst Rev* (4):CD005179, 2006.

Vertanen H, Fellman V, Brommels M, et al: An automatic incision device for obtaining blood samples from the heels of the preterm infants causes less damage than a conventional manual lancet, *Arch Dis Child Fetal Neonatal Educ* 84:F53–F55, 2001.

Wald ER: To bag or not to bag, *J Pediatr* 174(4):418–419, 2005.

Walsh A, Edwards H: Management of childhood fever by parents: literature review, *J Adv Nurs* 54(2):217–222, 2006.

Walton DM, Thomas DC, Aly HZ, et al: Morbid hypocalcemia associated with phosphate enema in a 6-week-old infant, *Pediatrics* 106:e37, 2000.

Warren J, Fromm RE Jr, Orr RA, et al: Guidelines for the inter- and intrahospital transport of critically ill patients, *Crit Care Med* 32(1):256–262, 2004.

Whitby M, McLaws ML, Slater K: Needlestick injuries in a major teaching hospital: the worthwhile effect of hospital-wide replacement of conventional hollow-bore needles, *Am J Infect Control* 36(3):180–186, 2008.

Willock J, Baharestani M, Anthony D: The development of the Glamorgan paediatric pressure ulcer risk assessment scale, *J Wound Care* 18(1):17–21, 2009.

Respiratory Dysfunction

David Wilson

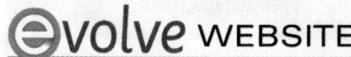 WEBSITE

http://evolve.elsevier.com/Perry/maternal

LEARNING OBJECTIVES

On completion of this chapter, the reader will be able to:
- Identify the factors leading to respiratory tract infection in the infant and young child.
- Contrast the effects of various respiratory infections observed in infants and children.
- Describe the postoperative nursing care of the child with an adenotonsillectomy.
- Outline a nursing care plan for a child with croup.
- Outline a nursing care plan for a child with acute otitis media.
- Demonstrate an understanding of the ways in which inhalation of noninfectious irritants produce pulmonary dysfunction.

- Describe the ways in which the various therapeutic measures relieve the symptoms of asthma.
- Outline a plan for teaching home care for the child with asthma.
- Describe the physiologic effects of cystic fibrosis on the gastrointestinal, endocrine, reproductive, and pulmonary systems.
- Outline a plan of care for the child with cystic fibrosis.
- List the major signs of respiratory distress in infants and children.
- Describe the nursing care for a child with respiratory failure.

RESPIRATORY INFECTION

General Aspects of Respiratory Infections

Infections of the respiratory tract are described according to the anatomic area of involvement. The *upper respiratory tract,* or *upper airway,* consists of the oronasopharynx, pharynx, larynx, and upper part of the trachea. The *lower respiratory tract* consists of the lower trachea, mainstem bronchi, segmental bronchi, subsegmental bronchioles, terminal bronchioles, and alveoli. In this discussion, the trachea is considered with lower tract disorders and infections of the epiglottis and larynx are categorized as croup syndromes. However, respiratory infections seldom fall into discrete anatomic areas. Infections often spread from one structure to another because of the contiguous nature of the mucous membrane lining the entire tract. Consequently, respiratory tract infections involve several areas rather than a single structure, although the effect on one area may predominate in any given illness.

Etiology and Characteristics

Respiratory infections account for the majority of acute illnesses in children. The etiology and course of these infections are influenced by the age of the child, the season, living conditions, and preexisting medical problems.

Infectious Agents. The respiratory tract is subject to a wide variety of infective organisms. Most infections are caused by viruses, particularly respiratory syncytial virus (RSV), nonpolio enteroviruses A, B, C, and D (formerly coxsackieviruses A and B), adenoviruses, parainfluenza viruses, and human meta-pneumoviruses. Other agents involved in primary or secondary invasion include group A β-hemolytic streptococci (GABHS), staphylococci, *Haemophilus influenzae, Chlamydia trachomatis, Mycoplasma* organisms, and pneumococci.

Age. Healthy full-term infants younger than 3 months are presumed to have a lower infection rate than older infants because of the protective function of maternal antibodies; however, infants may be susceptible to specific respiratory tract infections, namely pertussis, during this period. The infection rate increases from 3 to 6 months of age—the time between the disappearance of maternal antibodies and the infant's own antibody production. The viral infection rate remains high during the toddler and preschool years. By 5 years of age, viral respiratory tract infections are less frequent but the incidence of *Mycoplasma pneumoniae* and GABHS infections increases. The amount of lymphoid tissue increases throughout middle childhood, and repeated exposure to organisms confers increasing immunity as children grow older.

Some viral or bacterial agents produce a mild illness in older children but severe lower respiratory tract illness or croup in infants.

For example, pertussis causes a relatively harmless tracheobronchitis in childhood but is a serious disease in infancy.

Size. Anatomic differences influence the response to respiratory tract infections. The diameter of the airways is smaller in young children and subject to considerable narrowing from edematous mucous membranes and increased production of secretions. The distance between structures within the respiratory tract is also shorter in the young child, and organisms may move rapidly down the respiratory tract, causing more extensive involvement. The relatively short and open eustachian tube in infants and young children allows pathogens easy access to the middle ear.

Resistance. The ability to resist invading organisms depends on several factors. Deficiencies of the immune system place the child at risk for infection. Other conditions that decrease resistance are malnutrition, anemia, fatigue, and chilling of the body. Conditions that weaken defenses of the respiratory tract and predispose children to infection also include allergies (e.g., allergic rhinitis), preterm birth, bronchopulmonary dysplasia (BPD), asthma, history of RSV infection, cardiac anomalies that cause pulmonary congestion, and cystic fibrosis (CF). Day care attendance and exposure to secondhand smoke increase the likelihood of infection.

Seasonal Variations. The most common respiratory pathogens appear in epidemics during the winter and spring months. Mycoplasmal infections occur more often in autumn and early winter. Infection-related asthma occurs more frequently during cold weather, whereas winter and spring are typically the "RSV seasons."

Clinical Manifestations

Infants and young children, especially those between 6 months and 3 years of age, react more severely to acute respiratory tract infection than do older children. Young children display a number of generalized signs and symptoms and local manifestations (Box 40-1).

BOX 40-1 SIGNS AND SYMPTOMS ASSOCIATED WITH RESPIRATORY INFECTIONS IN INFANTS AND SMALL CHILDREN

Fever
- May be absent in newborn infants
- Greatest at ages 6 months to 3 years
- Temperature may reach 39.5° to 40.5° C (103° to 105° F) even with mild infections
- Often appears as first sign of infection
- May be listless and irritable or somewhat euphoric and more active than normal temporarily
- Tendency to develop high temperatures with infection in certain families
- May precipitate febrile seizures (see Chapter 45)
- Febrile seizures uncommon after 3 or 4 years of age

Meningismus
- Meningeal signs without infection of the meninges
- Occurs with abrupt onset of fever
- Accompanied by the following:
  - Headache
  - Pain and stiffness in the back and neck
  - Presence of Kernig and Brudzinski signs
- Subsides as the temperature decreases

Anorexia
- Common with most childhood illnesses
- Frequently the initial evidence of illness
- Persists to a greater or lesser degree throughout febrile stage of illness; often extends into convalescence

Vomiting
- Small children vomit readily with illness
- Clue to onset of infection
- May precede other signs by several hours
- Usually short-lived but may persist during the illness
- Frequent cause of dehydration if fluid intake is impaired

Diarrhea
- Usually mild, transient diarrhea but may become severe
- Often accompanies viral respiratory infections
- Frequent cause of dehydration

Abdominal Pain
- Common complaint
- Sometimes indistinguishable from pain of appendicitis

- Mesenteric lymphadenitis may be cause
- Muscle spasms from vomiting may be a factor, especially in nervous, tense child

Nasal Blockage
- Small nasal passages of infants easily blocked by mucosal swelling and exudation
- Can interfere with respiration and feeding in infants
- May contribute to the development of otitis media and sinusitis

Nasal Discharge
- Frequent occurrence
- May be thin and watery (rhinorrhea) or thick and purulent
- Depends on the type or stage of infection
- Associated with itching
- May irritate upper lip and skin surrounding the nose

Cough
- Common feature
- May be evident only during acute phase
- May persist several months after a disease

Respiratory Sounds
- Sounds associated with respiratory disease:
  - Cough
  - Hoarseness
  - Grunting
  - Stridor
  - Wheezing
- Auscultation:
  - Wheezing
  - Crackles
  - Absence of air movement

Sore Throat
- Frequent complaint of older children
- Young children (unable to describe symptoms) may not complain even when highly inflamed
- Child will often refuse to take oral fluids or solids

CARE MANAGEMENT

Assessment of the respiratory system follows the guidelines described in Chapter 29 (for assessment of the ears, nose, mouth and throat, chest, and lungs). The assessment should include respiratory rate, depth, and rhythm; heart rate; oxygenation; hydration status; body temperature; activity level; and level of comfort. Special attention should also be given to the components and observations listed in Box 40-2. A noninvasive pulse oximeter (oxygen saturation) measurement should be performed on *all* children as part of the routine physical assessment. The nursing process in the care of the child with acute respiratory tract infection is outlined in the Nursing Care Plan.

Ease Respiratory Efforts. Many acute respiratory tract infections are mild and cause few symptoms. Although children may feel uncomfortable and have a "stuffy" nose and some mucosal swelling, respiratory distress occurs infrequently. Interventions delivered at home are usually sufficient to relieve minor discomfort and ease respiratory efforts. However, in some cases, the infant or child may require close observation by health care professionals for adequate oxygenation and fluid and electrolyte status.

Warm or cool mist is a common therapeutic measure for symptomatic relief of respiratory discomfort. The moisture soothes inflamed membranes and is beneficial when there is hoarseness or laryngeal involvement. The use of steam vaporizers in the home is often discouraged because of the hazards related to their use and limited evidence to support their efficacy.

A time-honored method of producing steam is the shower. Running a shower of hot water into the empty bathtub or open shower stall with the bathroom door closed produces a quick source of steam. Keeping a child in this environment for approximately 10 to 15 minutes humidifies inspired air and can help relieve symptoms. A small child can be held on the lap of a parent or other adult. Older children can sit in the bathroom under the supervision of an adult.

Promote Rest. Children who have an acute febrile illness usually have limited activity. One of the cardinal signs that the child is feeling better is the increase in activity; this may, however, be temporary if a high fever returns after a few hours of increased activity. Children should be encouraged to rest or play quietly to avoid exacerbating symptoms.

Promote Comfort. Older children are usually able to manage nasal secretions with little difficulty. For very young infants, who normally breathe through their noses, an infant nasal aspirator or a bulb syringe is helpful in removing nasal secretions, especially before being put to bed to sleep and before feeding. This practice, preceded by instillation of saline nose drops as needed, may clear nasal passages and promote feeding. Saline nose drops can be prepared at home by dissolving 1 tsp of salt in 1 pint of warm water.

For older infants and children who can tolerate decongestants, vasoconstrictive nose drops may be administered 15 to 20 minutes before feeding and at bedtime. Two drops are instilled, and because this shrinks only the anterior mucous membranes, two more drops are instilled 5 to 10 minutes later. Phenylephrine 0.25% (for infants and children older than 6 months), ephedrine 1% (for children older than 6 years), or oxymetazoline 0.05% (for children older than 6 years) is sometimes prescribed. Older cooperative children often prefer nasal sprays. They are taught to compress the plastic container at the moment of inspiration while occluding the other nostril. Bottles of nose drops should be used for only one child and one illness because they are easily contaminated with bacteria and

viruses. To avoid rebound congestion, nose drops or sprays should not be administered for more than 3 days. To prevent cross-contamination with nose drops, draw the nose spray solution into a clean tuberculin syringe. Inject the nose spray solution into the child's nostrils using the blunt syringe.

Hot or cold applications sometimes provide relief for children with painful cervical adenitis. An ice bag or heating pad applied

---

BOX 40-2 COMPONENTS FOR ASSESSING RESPIRATORY FUNCTION

Respirations

The pattern of respirations is observed for rate, depth, ease, and rhythm of breathing:

- Rate—Rapid *(tachypnea)*, normal, or slow for the particular child
- Depth—Normal depth, too shallow *(hypopnea)*, too deep *(hyperpnea)*; usually estimated from the amplitude of thoracic and abdominal excursion
- Ease—Effortless, labored *(dyspnea)*, difficult breathing except in upright position *(orthopnea)*; associated with intercostal or substernal retractions (inspiratory "sinking in" of soft tissues in relation to the cartilaginous and bony thorax); flaring nares; head bobbing (head of sleeping child with suboccipital area supported on caregiver's forearm bobs forward in synchrony with each inspiration); grunting; or wheezing
- Labored breathing—Continuous, intermittent, becoming steadily worse, sudden onset, at rest or on exertion, associated with wheezing or grunting, associated with pain
- Rhythm—Variation in rate and depth of respirations

Other Observations

In addition to respirations, particular attention is addressed to the following:

- Evidence of infection—Check for elevated temperature; enlarged cervical lymph nodes; inflamed mucous membranes; and purulent discharges from the nose, ears, or lungs (sputum).
- Cough—Observe characteristics of cough (if present); under what circumstances cough is heard (e.g., night only, on arising); nature of cough (paroxysmal with or without wheeze; "croupy" or "brassy"); frequency of cough; associated with swallowing or other activity; character of cough (moist and dry); productivity.
- Wheeze—Note if expiratory or inspiratory, high-pitched or musical, prolonged, slowly progressive or sudden, associated with labored breathing.
- Cyanosis—Note distribution (peripheral, perioral, facial, trunk, and face), degree, duration, associated with activity or feeding (infant).
- Abdominal pain—May be a complaint in preschooler and school-age children; probably represents referred pain from chest; may be a complaint in children with pneumonia.
- Chest pain—May be a complaint of older children; note location and circumstances: localized or generalized, referred to base of neck or abdomen, dull or sharp, deep or superficial, associated with rapid, shallow respirations or grunting.
- Sputum—Older children may provide sputum sample by coughing, whereas young children may need use of bulb suction to provide a sample; note volume, color, viscosity, and odor.
- Bad breath—May be associated with some lung infections.
- Stridor—A high-pitched wheezing sound; may be present on inspiration, exhalation, or both and is a sign of upper airway edema or obstruction by mass or object.

◎ NURSING CARE PLAN

The Child with Acute Respiratory Tract Infection

NURSING DIAGNOSIS	EXPECTED OUTCOME	NURSING INTERVENTIONS	RATIONALES
Ineffective Breathing Pattern related to inflammatory process	Child's respirations will be nonlabored.	Position child for maximum ventilatory efficiency and airway patency	To allow increased chest expansion
Child's Defining Characteristics		Position child to facilitate drainage of secretions	To maintain patent airway and prevent airway obstruction
(Subjective and Objective Data)			
Use of accessory muscles to breathe		Provide humidified oxygen as prescribed	To improve oxygenation
Dyspnea		Monitor oxygenation status, including vital signs, for changes in condition	To determine need for additional interventions
Shortness of breath		Suction airway (nose, trachea) as necessary	To remove secretions and maintain airway patency
Nasal flaring			
Altered chest excursion		Administer prescribed antibiotics (if bacterial)	To treat infection source
Assumption of three-point position (tripod)		Administer bronchodilator medications as prescribed	To promote bronchodilation and improve ventilation
Respiratory rate outside normal parameter for child's age (increased or decreased rate)		Administer antiinflammatory medications as prescribed	To decrease airway inflammation and inflammatory response
		Assist with coughing	To remove secretions and clear airway
Ineffective Airway Clearance related to inflammation, mechanical obstruction, increased secretions	Child's airways will remain patent.	Position child to facilitate drainage of secretions	To prevent airway obstruction
		Perform chest percussion and postural drainage only as prescribed	To loosen and remove secretions
Child's Defining Characteristics		Suction airway as necessary	To remove secretions
(Subjective and Objective Data)		Provide humidified oxygen as prescribed	To moisten secretions and prevent airway drying
Dyspnea			
Difficulty vocalizing		Assist with coughing (as developmentally or age appropriate)	To remove secretions
Orthopnea		Avoid throat examination if epiglottitis is suspected	To prevent airway compromise
Adventitious breath sounds (crackles, wheezing, rhonchi)		Assure child (as appropriate) all measures will be taken to ensure adequate airway is maintained	To allay anxiety
Cough ineffective or absent		Implement comfort measures such as allowing parental presence, parental holding, favorite blanket or stuffed animal at side; explain all procedures beforehand	To reduce anxiety and decrease effects of medical therapy, including hospitalization if required
Restlessness			
Changes in respiratory rate and rhythm			
Risk for Injury related to presence (only as indicated) of infective organisms	Child will remain free from complications of infection.	Maintain aseptic environment using sterile suction equipment and technique	To prevent spread of infectious organisms in child and family
		Implement and practice Standard Precautions	
Child's or Family's Defining Characteristics		Implement Contact and Airborne Precautions as necessary	
(Subjective and Objective Data)		Obtain (secretion, tissue, or blood) specimen as indicated and prescribed	To identify infective organism
Tissue hypoxia			
Abnormal blood profile		Encourage child and family contacts to practice frequent hand hygiene and avoid hand-to-eye and hand-to-mouth contact	To prevent spread of infection
People or health care provider (HAI [health care–associated infection])			
		Teach child (as age appropriate) and family how to decrease spread of organisms through coughing and other secretions (e.g., by covering mouth when coughing; disposing of secretions to avoid cross-contamination)	To prevent spread of infection
Mode of transport			
Developmental age			
		Administer antibiotic or antiviral medications as prescribed	To treat infection source
		Administer fever reduction medication(s) as prescribed	To promote comfort if fever is present
		Monitor and assess for signs and symptoms of secondary complications: hypoxia, skin breakdown, poor nutrient and fluid intake, increased work of breathing, deteriorating cardiorespiratory status	To implement therapy for prevention of secondary complications
		Encourage small amounts of oral clear liquids as condition allows	To promote hydration

◎ NURSING CARE PLAN

The Child with Acute Respiratory Tract Infection—cont'd

NURSING DIAGNOSIS	EXPECTED OUTCOME	NURSING INTERVENTIONS	RATIONALES
Interrupted Family Processes related to child's illness, hospitalization, and medical or therapeutic regimen	Family will demonstrate ability to cope with child's illness.	Encourage family to remain with child	To decrease effects of separation
		Promote family-centered care	To promote family integrity
Child's or Family's Defining Characteristics		Explain procedures and therapeutic regimen to family	To provide accurate information regarding therapy and child's condition
(Subjective and Objective Data)		Keep family informed of child's status	To promote family sense of control and involvement in care
Communication patterns		Encourage family involvement in child's care	
Participation in decision making		Provide support and referral for continued support as necessary	
Availability for emotional support			
Expressions of conflict within family			
Patterns and rituals			

to the neck may decrease the discomfort, but safety precautions must be observed to prevent burns. The ice bag or heating device must be covered, and the heating pad should not be set at high settings.

Prevent Spread of Infection. Careful hand washing is important when caring for children with respiratory tract infections. Older children should use a tissue or their arm to cover their nose and mouth when they cough or sneeze, dispose of the tissues properly, and wash their hands. Remembering to cover the nose or mouth is often difficult for small children. Used tissues should be immediately thrown into the wastebasket and not allowed to accumulate in a pile. Children with respiratory tract infections should not share drinking cups, eating utensils, washcloths, or towels. Well individuals generally should not touch their eyes or nose with unwashed hands. Parents should try to remove affected children from contact with other children. Parents should also keep affected children out of school or day care settings to prevent the spread of infection. This may be a problem when living arrangements are crowded and the family has several children. An effort should be made to teach well children to stay away from ill children, to wash their hands frequently, and to avoid eating and drinking from the same utensils or cups.

Reduce Temperature. If the child has a significantly elevated body temperature, controlling the fever is important. Parents should know how to take a child's temperature and read a thermometer accurately. Nurses should not assume that all parents can read a thermometer and should provide education when needed.

If the health care practitioner prescribes acetaminophen or ibuprofen (for infants and children 6 months and older), parents will need instruction on how to administer it. Most parents can read the label and calculate the desired dosage, but parents of infants and toddlers require detailed instruction and dosing parameters. It is important to emphasize accuracy in determining both the amount of drug to be given and the time intervals for administration.

Cool liquids are encouraged to reduce the temperature and minimize the chances of dehydration (see Controlling Elevated Temperatures, Chapter 39).

! NURSING ALERT

Caution parents about the use of over-the-counter combination "cold" remedies, since these often include acetaminophen. Careful calculation of both the acetaminophen given separately and the acetaminophen in combination medications is necessary to avoid an overdose.

Promote Hydration. Dehydration is a potential complication when children have respiratory tract infections and are febrile or anorectic, especially when vomiting or diarrhea is present. Infants are especially prone to fluid and electrolyte deficits when they have a respiratory illness because a rapid respiratory rate that accompanies such illnesses precludes adequate oral fluid intake. In addition, the presence of fever increases the total body fluid turnover in infants. If the infant has nasal secretions, this further prevents adequate respiratory effort by blocking the narrow nasal passages when the infant reclines to bottle feed or breastfeed and ceases the compensatory mouth breathing effort, thus causing the child to limit intake of fluids. Adequate fluid intake is encouraged by offering small amounts of favorite fluids (clear liquids if vomiting) at frequent intervals. Oral rehydration solutions, such as Infalyte or Pedialyte, should be considered for infants, and water or a low-carbohydrate (≤5 g per 8 oz) flavored drink should be considered for older children. Fluids with caffeine (tea, coffee) should be avoided because these may act as diuretics and promote fluid loss. Sports drinks and energy drinks are not recommended for oral rehydration (American Academy of Pediatrics [AAP], 2011); some sports drinks may be diluted for older children. When encouraging oral fluids to prevent dehydration, sports drinks with "replacement electrolytes" offer no benefit over water and should be used cautiously in small children. Breastfeeding infants should continue to be breastfed because human milk confers some degree of protection from infection (see Chapter 23). Fluids should not be forced, and children should not be awakened to take fluids. Forcing fluids creates the same problem as urging unwanted food. Gentle persuasion with preferred beverages or sugar-free popsicles is usually more successful. Younger children may like to drink smaller amounts from a plastic medicine cup.

To assess their child's level of hydration (see Chapter 41), parents are advised to observe the frequency of voiding and to notify the nurse or health care practitioner if there is insufficient voiding. Counting the number of wet diapers in a 24-hour period is a satisfactory method to assess output in infants and toddlers. In the hospital, diapers are weighed to assess output, which should be at least 1 mL/kg/hr up to 30 kg in child's weight. Then it should be at least 30 mL per hour in patients weighing more than 30 kg. The practitioner should be notified if the urine output is low.

Provide Nutrition. Loss of appetite is characteristic of children with acute infections. In most cases, children can be permitted to determine their own need for food. Many children show no decrease in appetite, and others respond well to foods such as gelatin, soup, and puddings (see Feeding the Sick Child, Chapter 39). Urging foods on anorexic children may precipitate nausea and vomiting and cause an aversion to feeding that may extend into the convalescent period and beyond.

Young children with respiratory tract infections are irritable and difficult to comfort; therefore the family needs support, encouragement, and practical suggestions concerning comfort measures and administration of medication. In addition to antipyretics and nose drops, the child may require antibiotic therapy. Parents of children receiving oral antibiotics must understand the importance of regular administration and continuing the drug for the prescribed length of time, regardless of whether the child appears ill. Parents should be cautioned against giving their child any medications that are not approved by the health care practitioner and to avoid giving antibiotics left over from a previous illness or prescribed for another child. Administering unprescribed antibiotics can produce serious side effects and adverse reactions (see Chapter 39 for administration of medications and teaching parents). See also the Nursing Care Plan on p. 1198.

UPPER RESPIRATORY TRACT INFECTIONS

Nasopharyngitis

Acute nasopharyngitis, or the equivalent of the "common cold," is caused by the rhinovirus, RSV, adenoviruses, enteroviruses, influenza virus, and parainfluenza virus. Symptoms are more severe in infants and children than in adults. Fever is common in young children, and older children have low-grade fevers, which appear early in the course of the illness. Other clinical manifestations are listed in Box 40-3. Symptoms may last up to 10 days.

Therapeutic Management

Children with nasopharyngitis are managed at home. There is no specific treatment, and effective vaccines are not available. Antipyretics may be indicated for mild fever and discomfort (see Chapter 39 for management of fever). Rest is recommended. The provision of a humidified environment and increasing oral fluids may be beneficial to some children with a cold.

Cough suppressants containing dextromethorphan should be used with caution (cough is a protective way of clearing secretions) but may be prescribed for a dry, hacking cough, especially at night. However, some preparations contain 22% alcohol and can cause adverse effects such as confusion, hyperexcitability, dizziness, nausea, and sedation. Parents should monitor the child carefully for potential adverse effects. Recent concerns regarding serious side effects of cough and cold preparations in young children, particularly infants, and lack of convincing evidence that such medications are effective in reducing symptoms have prompted recommendations by health care experts to carefully evaluate the benefits and risks of recommending such

preparations for children younger than 6 years (Bell and Tunkel, 2010; Ryan, Brewer, and Small, 2008; Vassilev, Kabadi, and Villa, 2010). Over-the-counter cold preparation such as pseudoephedrine and some antihistamines are not appropriate for the treatment of the common cold in infants and toddlers; these may cause serious side effects in such children and have been associated with death in infants (Rimsza and Newberry, 2008; Ryan, Brewer, and Small, 2008).

Antihistamines are largely ineffective in treatment of nasopharyngitis (Kinyon Munch, 2010). These drugs have a weak atropine-like effect that dries secretions, but they can cause drowsiness or, paradoxically, have a stimulatory effect on children. Second-generation antihistamines such as loratadine or cetirizine are non-sedating but also have not been shown to be effective in relieving the symptoms of the common cold in small children and are not recommended by the American College of Chest Physicians (Pratter, 2006). There is no support for the usefulness of expectorants, and antibiotics are usually not indicated because most infections are viral.

Supportive treatment with antipyretics, nasal saline irrigation, and adequate fluid hydration is still the safest and most often recommended therapy for infants and small children with the common cold (Kinyon Munch, 2010).

Prevention

Nasopharyngitis is so widespread in the general population that it is impossible to prevent. Children are more susceptible because they

---

BOX 40-3   CLINICAL MANIFESTATIONS OF NASOPHARYNGITIS AND PHARYNGITIS

Nasopharyngitis
Younger Child
- Fever
- Irritability, restlessness
- Sneezing
- Vomiting or diarrhea

Older Child
- Dryness and irritation of nose and throat
- Sneezing, chilling sensation
- Muscular aches
- Cough, sometimes

Physical Signs
- Edema and vasodilation of mucosa

Pharyngitis
Younger Child
- Fever
- General malaise
- Anorexia
- Moderate sore throat
- Headache

Older Child
- Fever (may reach 40° C [104° F])
- Headache
- Anorexia
- Dysphagia
- Abdominal pain
- Vomiting

Physical Signs
Younger Child
- Mild to moderate hyperemia

Older Child
- Mild to fiery red, edematous pharynx
- Hyperemia of tonsils and pharynx; may extend to soft palate and uvula
- Often abundant follicular exudate that spreads and coalesces to form pseudomembrane on tonsils
- Cervical glands enlarged and tender

have not yet developed resistance to many viruses. Young infants and those with decreased resistance and pulmonary illness are subject to serious complications, so attempts should be made to protect them from exposure.

CARE MANAGEMENT

A cold is often the parents' first introduction to an illness in their infant. Most discomfort of nasopharyngitis is related to the nasal obstruction, especially in small infants. Elevating the head of the bed or crib mattress assists with drainage of secretions. Suctioning and vaporization may also provide relief. Saline nose drops and gentle suction with a bulb syringe before feeding and sleep time may be useful.

Maintaining adequate fluid intake is essential. Although a child's appetite for solid foods is usually diminished for several days, it is important to offer appropriate fluids to prevent dehydration.

Because nasopharyngitis is spread from secretions, the best means for prevention is avoiding contact with affected persons. This goal is difficult to accomplish in family settings, classrooms, and day care centers. Family members with a cold should try to "keep it to themselves" by carefully disposing of tissues; not sharing towels, glasses, or eating utensils; covering the mouth and nose with tissues when coughing or sneezing; and washing the hands thoroughly after nose blowing or sneezing. The most frequent carriers of infection are the human hands, which deposit viruses on doorknobs, faucets, and other everyday objects. Children should be taught to wash their hands thoroughly and avoid touching their eyes, nose, and mouth.

Support and reassurance are important elements of care for families of young children with recurrent upper respiratory infections (URIs). Because URIs are frequent in children younger than 3 years, families may feel they are on an endless roller coaster of illness. They need reassurance that frequent colds are a normal part of childhood and that by 5 years of age, their children will have developed immunity to many viruses. When children spend time in day care centers, their infection rate is higher than if they are cared for in the home because of increased exposure. Parents should know the signs of respiratory complications and should notify a health care professional if complications occur or the child does not improve within 2 to 3 days (Box 40-4).

Acute Streptococcal Pharyngitis

Children who experience GABHS infection of the upper airway (strep throat) are at risk for rheumatic fever (RF), an inflammatory disease of the heart, joints, and central nervous system (CNS) (see Chapter 42), and acute glomerulonephritis (AGN), an acute kidney infection (see Chapter 44). Permanent damage can result from these sequelae, especially RF. GABHS may also cause skin manifestations, including impetigo and pyoderma.

Clinical Manifestations

Group A β-hemolytic streptococci infection is generally a relatively brief illness that varies in severity from subclinical (no symptoms) to severe toxicity. The onset is often abrupt and characterized by pharyngitis, headache, fever, and abdominal pain. The tonsils and pharynx may be inflamed and covered with exudate (Fig. 40-1), which usually appears by the second day of illness. However, streptococcal infections should be suspected in children older than 2 years who have pharyngitis without exudate or nasal symptoms. The tongue may appear edematous and red (strawberry tongue), and the child may have a fine sandpaper rash on the trunk, axillae, elbows, and groin seen in scarlet fever (caused by a strain of group A streptococcus). The uvula is edematous and red. Anterior cervical lymphadenopathy (in ≈30% to 50% of cases) usually occurs early, and the nodes are often tender. Pain can be relatively mild to severe enough to make swallowing difficult. Clinical manifestations usually subside in 3 to 5 days unless complicated by sinusitis or parapharyngeal, peritonsillar, or retropharyngeal abscess. Nonsuppurative complications may appear after the onset of GABHS—AGN in about 10 days and RF in an average of 18 days.

Children who are GABHS carriers may have a positive throat culture but often experience a coincidental viral illness. Although antibiotic administration is not indicated for most GABHS carriers, some conditions require antibiotic therapy; these are published in the AAP's *Red Book* (American Academy of Pediatrics [AAP] Committee on Infectious Diseases, 2012).

Diagnostic Evaluation

Although 80% to 90% of all cases of acute pharyngitis are viral, a throat culture or rapid streptococcal identification test should be performed to rule out GABHS. Most streptococcal infections are short-term illnesses, and antibody responses (e.g., antistreptolysin-O titer) appear later than symptoms and are useful only for retrospective diagnosis.

Rapid identification of GABHS with diagnostic test kits (rapid antigen detection test) is possible in the office or clinic setting. Because of the high specificity of these rapid tests, a positive test

---

BOX 40-4	EARLY EVIDENCE OF RESPIRATORY COMPLICATIONS

Parents are instructed to notify the health care professional if any of the following are noted:

- Evidence of earache (see p. 1205)
- Respirations faster than 50 to 60 breaths/min
- Fever over 38.3° C (101° F)
- Listlessness
- Increasing irritability with or without fever
- Persistent cough for 2 days or more
- Wheezing
- Crying
- Refusal to eat
- Restlessness and poor sleep patterns

Adapted from National Association of Pediatric Nurse Associates and Practitioners (NAPNAP): *Baby's first cold*, New York, 1989, Winthrop Consumer Products. Copies available from NAPNAP, 1101 Kings Hwy. N., No. 206, Cherry Hill, NJ 08034; phone: 609-667-1773; website: www.napnap.org.

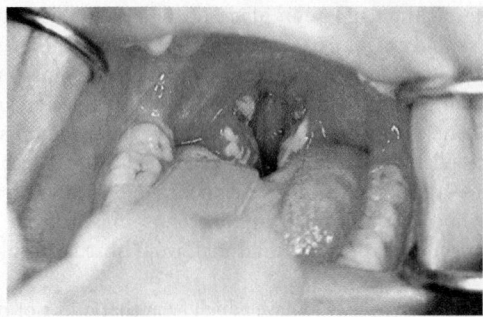

FIG 40-1 Tonsillitis and pharyngitis. (Courtesy Dr. Edward L. Applebaum, Head, Department of Otolaryngology, University of Illinois Medical Center, Chicago.)

result generally does not require throat culture confirmation. However, the sensitivities of these kits vary considerably and a confirmatory throat culture is recommended in patients who have a negative test result (AAP Committee on Infectious Diseases, 2012).

Therapeutic Management

If streptococcal sore throat infection is present, oral penicillin is prescribed in a dose sufficient to control the acute local manifestations and to maintain an adequate level for at least 10 days to eliminate any organisms that might remain to initiate RF symptoms. Penicillin does not prevent the development of AGN in susceptible children; however, it may prevent the spread of a nephrogenic strain of GABHS to others in the family. Penicillin usually produces a prompt response within 24 hours. Patients who have a history of RF or who remain symptomatic after a full course of antibiotics may require a follow-up throat swab.

Intramuscular (IM) benzathine penicillin G is an appropriate therapy, but it is painful and is not the first choice for children. Oral erythromycin is indicated for children who are allergic to penicillin. Other antibiotics used to treat GABHS are azithromycin, clarithromycin, oral cephalosporins, amoxicillin, and amoxicillin with clavulanic acid (AAP Committee on Infectious Diseases, 2012; Wessels, 2011).

CARE MANAGEMENT

The nurse often obtains a throat swab for culture or rapid antigen testing and instructs the parents about administering oral antibiotics and analgesics as prescribed. Cold or warm compresses to the neck may provide relief. In children who can cooperate, warm saline gargles may offer relief of throat discomfort. Acetaminophen and ibuprofen may be effective in decreasing the throat pain; liquid preparations or chewable forms may be preferable because of the pain associated with swallowing. Pain may interfere with oral intake, and children should not be forced to eat, but fluid intake is essential. Cool liquids or ice chips may be more acceptable than solids.

Special emphasis is placed on correct administration of oral medication and completion of the course of antibiotic therapy (see Administration of Medication, and Compliance, Chapter 39). If an injection is required, it must be administered deep into a large muscle mass (e.g., vastus lateralis or ventrogluteal muscle). To prevent pain, application of a topical anesthetic cream such as EMLA (an eutectic mixture of lidocaine and prilocaine) over the injection site $2\frac{1}{2}$ hours before the injection or LMX4 (4% lidocaine) over the site 30 minutes before the injection is helpful (see Administration of Medication: Intramuscular Administration, Chapter 39). The injection site may be tender for 1 to 2 days.

Children are considered infectious to others at the onset of symptoms and up to 24 hours after initiation of antibiotic therapy, but they should not return to school or day care until they have been taking antibiotics for a full 24-hour period. Nurses should remind the children to discard their toothbrushes and replace them with new ones after they have been taking antibiotics for 24 hours. Orthodontic appliances should be washed thoroughly because they may harbor the organisms. Parents are cautioned to prevent other household members, especially if immunocompromised, from having close contact with the sick child and avoid sharing drinking or eating items.

If the child continues to have a high fever that does not respond to antipyretics, has an extremely sore throat, refuses liquids, and appears toxic 24 to 48 hours after starting antibiotics, further evaluation by the health care practitioner is recommended.

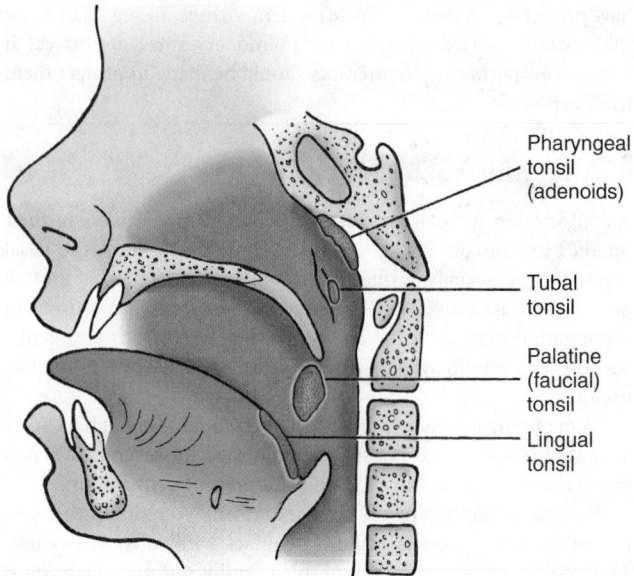

FIG 40-2 Location of various tonsillar masses.

Tonsillitis

The tonsils are masses of lymphoid tissue located in the pharyngeal cavity. They filter and protect the respiratory and alimentary tracts from invasion by pathogenic organisms and play a role in antibody formation. Although tonsil size varies, children generally have much larger tonsils than do adolescents or adults. This difference is thought to be a protective mechanism because young children are especially susceptible to URIs.

Pathophysiology

Several pairs of tonsils are part of a mass of lymphoid tissue encircling the nasal and oral pharynx, known as the Waldeyer tonsillar ring (Fig. 40-2). The palatine, or faucial, tonsils are located on either side of the oropharynx behind and below the pillars of the fauces (opening from the mouth). A surface of the palatine tonsils is usually visible during oral examination. The palatine tonsils are those removed during tonsillectomy. The pharyngeal tonsils, also known as the adenoids, are located above the palatine tonsils on the posterior wall of the nasopharynx. Their proximity to the nares and eustachian tubes causes difficulties in instances of inflammation. The lingual tonsils are located at the base of the tongue. The tubal tonsils, found near the posterior nasopharyngeal opening of the eustachian tubes, are not part of the Waldeyer tonsillar ring.

Etiology

Tonsillitis often occurs with pharyngitis. Because of the abundant lymphoid tissue and the frequency of URIs, tonsillitis is a common cause of illness in young children. The causative agent may be viral or bacterial.

Clinical Manifestations

The manifestations of tonsillitis are caused by inflammation. As the palatine tonsils enlarge from edema, they may meet in the midline (kissing tonsils), obstructing the passage of air or food. The child has difficulty swallowing and breathing. When enlargement of the adenoids occurs, the space behind the posterior nares becomes blocked, making it difficult or impossible for air to pass from the nose to the throat. As a result, the child breathes through the mouth.

Therapeutic Management

Because tonsillitis is self-limiting, treatment of viral pharyngitis is symptomatic. Throat cultures positive for GABHS infection warrant antibiotic treatment. It is important to differentiate between viral and streptococcal infection in febrile exudative tonsillitis. Because most infections are of viral origin, early rapid tests can eliminate unnecessary antibiotic administration.

Tonsillectomy is the surgical removal of the palatine tonsils. Absolute indications for a tonsillectomy are recurrent peritonsillar abscess, airway obstruction, tonsillitis resulting in febrile seizures, and tonsils requiring tissue pathology (American Academy of Otolaryngology—Head and Neck Surgery, 2011). Relative indications include three or more tonsil infections per year, persistent foul taste or breath caused by chronic tonsillitis, unilateral tonsil hypertrophy presumed to be malignant, and chronic tonsillitis in a streptococcus carrier who fails to respond to antibiotics (American Academy of Otolaryngology—Head and Neck Surgery, 2011).

Adenoidectomy (the surgical removal of the adenoids) is recommended for children who have hypertrophied adenoids that obstruct nasal breathing; additional indications for adenoidectomy include recurrent adenoiditis and sinusitis, chronic otitis media (OM) with effusion (especially if associated with hearing loss), airway obstruction and subsequent sleep-disordered breathing, persistent mouth-breathing, nasal speech, and recurrent nasopharyngitis (Benninger and Walner, 2007a). For some children, the effectiveness of tonsillectomy or adenoidectomy is modest and may not justify the risk of surgery. In practice, many physicians rely on individualized decision making and do not subscribe to an absolute set of eligibility criteria for these surgical procedures. Contraindications to either tonsillectomy or adenoidectomy are (1) cleft palate because the tonsils help minimize escape of air during speech; (2) acute infections at the time of surgery because locally inflamed tissues increase the risk for bleeding; (3) uncontrolled systemic diseases or blood dyscrasias; and (4) poor anesthetic risk.

CARE MANAGEMENT

Nursing care of tonsillitis involves providing comfort and minimizing activities or interventions that precipitate bleeding. Patients with sleep-disordered breathing require close monitoring of airway and breathing postoperatively. A soft to liquid diet is preferred. A cool-mist vaporizer keeps the mucous membranes moist during periods of mouth breathing. Warm salt-water gargles, throat lozenges, and analgesic–antipyretic drugs such as acetaminophen are used to promote comfort. Opioids are often needed to reduce pain so the child can drink. Combination non-opioid and opioid elixirs such as acetaminophen with codeine or with hydrocodone (Lortab) relieve pain and should be given routinely every 4 hours.

If surgery is required, the child requires the same psychologic preparation and physical care as for any other surgical procedure. Most tonsillectomy and adenoidectomy (T&A) surgeries now take place in outpatient settings; however, the priorities of preoperative and postoperative care remain the same. The following discussion focuses on postoperative nursing care for tonsillectomy and adenoidectomy, although both procedures may not be performed.

Until fully awake, the child is placed on his or her abdomen or side to facilitate drainage of secretions. Routine suctioning is avoided, but when performed, it is done carefully to avoid trauma to the oropharynx. When alert, the child may prefer sitting up. The child is discouraged from coughing frequently, clearing the throat, blowing the nose, and any other activity that may aggravate the operative site.

Some secretions are common, particularly dried blood from surgery. All secretions and vomitus are inspected for evidence of fresh bleeding (some blood-tinged mucus is expected). Dark brown (old) blood is usually present in the emesis, in the nose, and between the teeth. If parents do not expect this, they often become frightened at a time when they need to be calm and reassuring.

The throat is sore after surgery. An ice collar may provide relief, but many children find it bothersome and refuse to use it. Most children experience moderate pain after a T&A and need pain medication regularly for at least the first few days. Analgesics may be given rectally or intravenously to avoid the oral route. Because the pain is continuous, analgesics should be administered at regular intervals, even at night (see Pain Management, Chapter 30). An antiemetic such as ondansetron (Zofran) may be administered postoperatively if nausea or vomiting is present.

Food and fluids are restricted until the child is fully alert and there are no signs of hemorrhage. Cool water, crushed ice, flavored ice pops, or diluted fruit juice may be given, but fluids with a red or brown color are avoided to distinguish fresh or old blood in emesis from the ingested liquid. Citrus juice may cause discomfort and is usually poorly tolerated. Soft foods, particularly gelatin, cooked fruits, sherbet, soup, and mashed potatoes, are started on the first or second postoperative day or as the child tolerates feeding. The pain from surgery often inhibits fluid intake, reinforcing the need for adequate pain control. Milk, ice cream, and pudding are usually not offered because milk products coat the mouth and throat and may cause the child to clear the throat, which can initiate bleeding.

Postoperative hemorrhage is uncommon but can occur in up to 5% of patients up to 14 days after surgery. The nurse observes the throat directly for evidence of bleeding—using a good source of light and, if necessary, carefully inserting a tongue depressor. Other signs of hemorrhage are tachycardia, pallor, frequent clearing of the throat or swallowing by a younger child, and vomiting of bright red blood. Restlessness, an indication of hemorrhage, may be difficult to differentiate from general discomfort after surgery. Decreasing blood pressure is a late sign of shock.

Surgery may be required to ligate a bleeding vessel. Airway obstruction may also occur as a result of edema or accumulated secretions and is indicated by signs of respiratory distress, such as stridor, drooling, restlessness, agitation, increasing respiratory rate, and progressive cyanosis. Suction equipment and oxygen should be available after tonsillectomy.

! NURSING ALERT

The most obvious early sign of bleeding is the child's continuous swallowing of the trickling blood. While the child is sleeping, note the frequency of swallowing. If continuous bleeding is suspected, notify the surgeon immediately.

Discharge instructions include (1) avoiding irritating and highly seasoned foods, (2) avoiding gargles or vigorous toothbrushing, (3) avoiding coughing or clearing of the throat or putting objects in the mouth (e.g., a straw), (4) using analgesics or an ice collar for pain, and (5) limiting activity to decrease the potential for bleeding. Chewing gum may prevent throat and ear pain in older children. Objectionable mouth odor and slight ear pain with a low-grade fever are common for 5 to 10 days postoperatively. However, persistent severe earache, fever, or cough requires medical evaluation. Most children are ready to resume normal activity within 1 to

2 weeks after the operation. The child's voice may sound different postoperatively, especially if the tonsils were large.

Children who have received codeine after tonsillectomy or adenoidectomy or who are prescribed codeine should be observed closely for adverse effects (disorientation, confusion, unusual sleepiness, difficult to awaken, labored breathing) (FDA, 2013).

Influenza

Influenza, or the "flu," is caused by three orthomyxoviruses, which are antigenically distinct: types A and B, which cause epidemic disease; and type C, which is unimportant from an epidemiologic standpoint. Influenza is spread from one individual to another by direct contact (large-droplet infection) or by articles recently contaminated by nasopharyngeal secretions. There is no predilection for a specific age-group, but attack rates are highest in young children who have had no previous contact with a strain. Influenza is frequently most severe in infants. During epidemics, infection among school-age children is believed to be a major source of transmission in a community. The disease is more common during the winter months and has a 1- to 3-day incubation period. Affected persons are most infectious for 24 hours before and after the onset of symptoms. The virus has a peculiar affinity for epithelial cells of the respiratory tract mucosa, where it destroys ciliated epithelium with metaplastic hyperplasia of the tracheal and bronchial epithelium with associated edema. The alveoli may also become distended with a hyaline-like material. The viruses can be isolated from nasopharyngeal secretions early after the onset of infection, and serologic tests identify the type by complement fixation or the subgroups by hemagglutination inhibition.

H1N1 (swine flu) is a subtype of influenza type A. In 2009, a pandemic of H1N1 caused significant morbidity and mortality, particularly in Mexico and the United States; it was declared at an end in August 2010. A *pandemic* is defined by the World Health Organization (WHO) (2011) as the spread of a new disease to which the population has little or no immunity and that spreads rapidly from human to human. The signs and symptoms of H1N1 are the same as those mentioned below for influenza. H1N1 vaccine was combined with the seasonal influenza vaccine in the 2012 to 2013 season.

Clinical Manifestations

The manifestations of influenza may be subclinical, mild, moderate, or severe. Most patients have a dry throat and nasal mucosa, a dry cough, and a tendency toward hoarseness. A flushed face, photophobia, myalgia, hyperesthesia, and sometimes exhaustion and lack of energy accompany a sudden onset of fever and chills. Subglottal croup is common, especially in infants. The symptoms of influenza last for 4 to 5 days. Complications include severe viral pneumonia (often hemorrhagic); encephalitis; and secondary bacterial infections such as OM, sinusitis, or pneumonia.

Therapeutic Management

Uncomplicated influenza in children usually requires only symptomatic treatment, including acetaminophen or ibuprofen for fever and sufficient fluids to maintain hydration. Amantadine hydrochloride (Symmetrel) has been effective in reducing symptoms associated with type A disease if administered within 24 to 48 hours after their onset; the symptoms associated with influenza are reportedly shortened by 24 hours, but the drug does not "cure" the disease. It is ineffective against type B or C influenza or other viral diseases. It should not be given to children younger than 1 year but is recommended for unvaccinated high risk children.

Rimantadine has been approved for the treatment of flu symptoms in children and adults, but it is effective only for type A virus; this drug is taken orally in tablet or syrup twice daily for 7 days. It cannot be used for children younger than 1 year.

Zanamivir can be used for treatment of influenza in patients 7 years of age and older and for prophylaxis of influenza in patients 5 years of age and older. Both medications must also be started within 48 hours of symptom onset. Zanamivir is an inhaled medication effective for type A and type B influenza. The drug is taken twice daily for 5 days and is administered by a specially designed oral inhaler (Diskhaler).

A fourth drug, oseltamivir (Tamiflu), is a neuraminidase inhibitor that may be administered orally for 5 days to any child—from newborns to adolescents—and to adults to decrease the flu symptoms; as with other antiviral drugs, this drug must be taken within 2 days of the onset of symptoms. It is reported to be effective for types A and B influenza (AAP Committee on Infectious Diseases, 2012). Bronchospasm and a decline in lung function can occur when zanamivir is used in patients with underlying airway disease such as asthma or chronic obstructive pulmonary disease (COPD). At the time of this writing, oseltamivir and zanamivir are the only antiviral medications recommended for treatment during the 2012 to 2013 flu season because of widespread resistance to amantidine and rimantadine (AAP Committee on Infectious Diseases, 2012).

Prevention

The influenza vaccine is now recommended annually for children 6 months to 18 years of age. Influenza vaccine (inactivated influenza vaccine [IIV]) may be given to healthy children 6 months old and older. The inactivated influenza viral (IIV) vaccines are safe and effective provided the antigens in the vaccine correlate with the circulating influenza viruses (see Immunizations, Chapter 31) but are contraindicated in patients who developed Guillain-Barré syndrome within 6 weeks of receiving the vaccine in the past. The live-attenuated influenza vaccine (LAIV) is a nasal spray flu vaccine approved by the U.S. Food and Drug Administration (FDA) that is licensed for administration in persons ages 2 to 49 years. However, this preparation contains a live virus and should not be used in individuals who are immunocompromised, have reactive airway disease, are receiving immunosuppressive therapy, have a febrile illness, are receiving aspirin therapy, have a chronic respiratory condition, have received a live vaccine in the previous 28 days, are or could be pregnant, or have a history of Guillain-Barré syndrome. Patients who have had anaphylactic reactions to egg protein should receive a risk assessment evaluation by a physician with expertise in the management of allergic conditions (Centers for Disease Control and Prevention, [CDC], 2012). The Centers for Disease Control and Prevention (CDC) (2012) recommends that persons who have only experienced hives after an influenza vaccine receive the IIV. Note that children ages 6 months through 8 years now require 2 doses of influenza vaccine when it is their first season of receiving an influenza vaccine, to optimize immune response (CDC, 2012).

CARE MANAGEMENT

Nursing care for influenza is the same as for any child with a URI, including implementing measures to relieve symptoms. The greatest danger to affected children is development of a secondary infection. Prolonged fever or the appearance of fever during early convalescence is a sign of secondary bacterial infection and should be reported to the health care practitioner for antibiotic therapy.

BOX 40-5	STANDARD TERMINOLOGY FOR OTITIS MEDIA

Otitis media (OM)—An inflammation of the middle ear without reference to etiology or pathogenesis

Acute otitis media (AOM)—An inflammation of the middle ear with a rapid onset of the signs and symptoms of acute infection (i.e., fever and otalgia [ear pain])

Otitis media with effusion (OME)—Inflammation and fluid in the middle ear without symptoms of acute infection

Middle ear effusion (MEE)—Fluid in the middle ear without reference to etiology, pathogenesis, pathology, or duration

BOX 40-6	CLINICAL MANIFESTATIONS OF OTITIS MEDIA

Acute Otitis Media
- Follows an upper respiratory infection
- Otalgia (ear pain)
- Fever
- Purulent discharge (otorrhea) may or may not be present

Infant or Very Young Child
- Crying
- Fussy, restless, irritable
- Tendency to rub, hold, or pull affected ear
- Rolls head from side to side
- Difficulty comforting child
- Refuses to nurse or take bottle
- Loss of appetite

Older Child
- Crying or verbalizing feelings of discomfort
- Irritability
- Lethargy
- Loss of appetite

Chronic Otitis Media
- Hearing loss
- Difficulty communicating
- Possible feeling of fullness, tinnitus, or vertigo

Children with influenza (or other similar viruses) should not receive aspirin because of its possible link with Reye syndrome.

Otitis Media

Otitis media is one of the most prevalent diseases of early childhood. Its incidence is highest in the winter months. Many cases of bacterial OM are preceded by a viral respiratory infection. The two viruses most likely to precipitate OM are RSV and influenza. Most episodes of acute otitis media (AOM) occur in the first 24 months of life, but the incidence decreases with age except for a small increase at age 5 or 6 years when children enter school. OM occurs infrequently in children older than 7 years. Preschool-age boys are affected more frequently than preschool-age girls. Children who have siblings or parents with a history of chronic OM have a higher incidence of OM. Children living in households with many members (especially smokers) are more likely to have OM than those living with fewer persons. Passive smoking increases the risk for persistent middle ear effusion by enhancing attachment of the pathogens that cause otitis to the respiratory epithelium in the middle ear space, by prolonging the inflammatory response, and by impeding drainage through the eustachian tube (AAP, 2004a). Family socioeconomic status and extent of exposure to other children are the two most important identifiable risk factors for the occurrence of OM (AAP, 2004a).

OM has been defined in a variety of ways. The standard terminology used to define OM is outlined in Box 40-5, and AOM treatment guidelines have been published (Lieberthal, Carroll, and Chonmaitree, 2013).

Etiology

Streptococcus pneumoniae, H influenzae, and *Moraxella catarrhalis* are the three most common bacteria causing AOM. The etiology of noninfectious OM is unknown, but OM may occur because of blocked eustachian tubes, which results in negative ear pressure. Fluid is pulled from the mucosal lining, which accumulates and becomes colonized by infectious organisms. Predisposing factors include URIs, allergies, Down syndrome, cleft palate, day care attendance, exposure to secondhand smoke, and bottle propping during feeding. Breastfed infants have a lower incidence of OM than formula-fed infants. Breastfeeding may protect infants against respiratory viruses and allergy because it contains secretory immunoglobulin A, which limits the exposure of the eustachian tube and middle ear mucosa to microbial pathogens and foreign proteins. Exclusive breastfeeding for at least 4 to 6 months shows a protective effect for prevention of OM and recurrent AOM (Lieberthal, Carroll, and Chonmaitree, 2013). Reflux of milk up the eustachian tubes is less likely in breastfed infants because of the semivertical positioning during breastfeeding compared with bottle feeding.

Pathophysiology

Otitis media is primarily a result of malfunctioning eustachian tubes. Eustachian tubes have three functions relative to the middle ear: (1) protection of the middle ear from nasopharyngeal secretions; (2) drainage of secretions produced in the middle ear into the nasopharynx; and (3) ventilation of the middle ear to equalize air pressure within the middle ear and atmospheric pressure in the external ear canal and to replenish oxygen that has been absorbed.

Mechanical or functional obstruction of the eustachian tube causes accumulation of secretions in the middle ear. Intrinsic obstruction can be caused by infection or allergy; extrinsic obstruction is usually a result of enlarged adenoids or nasopharyngeal tumors. When the passage is not totally obstructed, contamination of the middle ear can take place by reflux, aspiration, or insufflation during crying, sneezing, nose blowing, and swallowing when the nose is obstructed.

Diagnostic Evaluation

Careful assessment of tympanic membrane mobility with a pneumatic otoscope is essential to differentiate AOM from OM with effusion (OME) (Lieberthal, Carroll, and Chonmaitree, 2013). A diagnosis of AOM is made if visual inspection of the tympanic membrane reveals a purulent discolored effusion and a bulging or full, opacified, or reddened immobile membrane, as well as an acute onset of ear pain for less than 48 hours (Lieberthal, Carroll, and Chonmaitree, 2013). An immobile tympanic membrane or an orange, discolored membrane indicates OME. Clinical symptoms of otitis are also helpful in making the diagnosis (Box 40-6). In AOM, symptoms such as acute onset of ear pain, fever, and a bulging yellow or red tympanic membrane are usually present. In OME, these symptoms may be absent and other nonspecific symptoms such as rhinitis, cough, or diarrhea are often present. OME may precede

AOM or predispose to its development, but OME does not represent an acute infectious process that requires antibiotic therapy (Lieberthal, Carroll, and Chonmaitree, 2013).

Therapeutic Management

Treatment for AOM is one of the most common reasons for antibiotic use in the ambulatory setting. Recently, however, concerns about drug-resistant *S. pneumoniae* and other drug resistances have led infectious disease authorities to recommend careful and judicious use of antibiotics for the treatment of this illness. Current recommendations regarding antibiotic administration to children with AOM are as follows (Lieberthal, Carroll, Chonmaitree, et al., 2013):

- Prescribe antibiotics for children 6 months of age and older who have severe signs or symptoms of AOM (moderate or severe otalgia for at least 48 hours or temperature 102.2° F [39° C]).
- Prescribe antibiotics for bilateral AOM in children younger than 24 months of age who do not have severe signs or symptoms (moderate or severe otalgia for at least 48 hours or temperature 102.2° F [39° C])
- Either prescribe antibiotics *or* offer observation with close follow-up (based on joint decision making with parent or caregiver) for unilateral AOM in children 6 months to 23 months of age who do not have severe signs or symptoms (moderate or severe otalgia for at least 48 hours or temperature 102.2° F [39° C]); if child does not improve within 48 to 72 hours, begin antibiotic therapy
- Either prescribe antibiotics *or* offer observation with close follow-up (based on joint decision making with parent or caregiver) for unilateral or bilateral AOM in children 24 months of age or older who do not have severe signs and symptoms (moderate or severe otalgia for at least 48 hours or temperature 102.2° F [39° C])

The latest AAP recommendations also place emphasis on the assessment and management of pain in children with AOM. For fever or discomfort associated with OM, analgesic-antipyretic drugs such as acetaminophen or ibuprofen may be given. The health care practitioner may prescribe topical pain relief drops such as benzocaine or lidocaine. A narcotic analgesic with codeine may be required for children with severe pain; however, side effects are common and the child should be closely monitored for GI upset, constipation, respiratory depression, and altered mental status (Lieberthal, Carroll, Chonmaitree, et al., 2013).

When antibiotics are warranted, oral amoxicillin in high doses (80-90 mg/kg/day divided twice daily) is the treatment of choice for initial episodes of AOM in children who have not received amoxicillin within the past month (Lieberthal, Carroll, and Chonmaitree, 2013). The recommendation for the duration of antibiotic therapy in severe AOM is 10 days. A 5- to 7-day course may be sufficient in children 6 years of age and older with uncomplicated AOM or a moderate or mild infection, whereas children 2 to 5 years of age with mild or moderate AOM may benefit from a 7-day course of antibiotics (Lieberthal, Carroll, Chonmaitree, et al., 2013).

Second-line antibiotics used to treat OM include amoxicillin-clavulanate; azithromycin; and cephalosporins such as cefdinir, cefuroxime, and cefpodoxime. Alternative dosing schedules and conditions are discussed in the 2013 AAP clinical practice guidelines. IM ceftriaxone is used if the causative organism is a highly resistant pneumococcus or if the parents are noncompliant with the therapy. An important consideration with the use of single-dose IM injections is the pain involved in this therapy. One strategy to minimize pain at the injection site is to reconstitute the cephalosporin with 1% lidocaine. A topical analgesic cream such as EMLA or LMX4 can also be applied to the site beforehand to reduce pain. The use of steroids, decongestants, and antihistamines to treat AOM is not recommended.

Myringotomy, a surgical incision of the eardrum, may be necessary to alleviate the severe pain of AOM. A myringotomy is also performed to provide drainage of infected middle ear fluid in the presence of complications (mastoiditis, labyrinthitis, or facial paralysis) or to allow purulent middle ear fluid to drain into the ear canal for culture. A minimally invasive laser-assisted myringotomy procedure may be performed in outpatient settings. These procedures should be performed only by ear, nose, and throat (ENT) specialists.

Tympanostomy tube placement and adenoidectomy are surgical procedures that may be done to treat recurrent chronic AOM (defined as three bouts in 6 months, six in 12 months, or six by 6 years of age). Tympanostomy tubes are pressure-equalizer (PE) tubes or grommets that facilitate continued drainage of fluid and allow ventilation of the middle ear. They are inserted to treat severe eustachian tube dysfunction, OM with effusion, or complications of OM (mastoiditis, facial nerve paralysis, brain abscess, labyrinthitis). Adenoidectomy is not recommended for treatment of AOM and is performed only in children with recurrent AOM or chronic OME with postnasal obstruction, adenoiditis, or chronic sinusitis.

In some children, residual middle ear effusions remain after episodes of AOM. Some children have fluid that persists in the middle ear for weeks or months. Antibiotics are not required for initial treatment of OME but may be indicated for children with persistent effusion for more than 3 months (AAP, 2004a). Placement of tympanostomy tubes is recommended after a total of 4 to 6 months of bilateral effusion with a bilateral hearing deficit (AAP, 2004b). This therapy allows for mechanical drainage of the fluid, which promotes healing of the membrane and prevents scar formation and loss of elasticity. Myringotomy with or without insertion of PE tubes should not be performed for initial management of OME but may be recommended for children who have recurrent episodes of OME with a long cumulative duration (AAP, 2004b).

Otitis media with effusion is frequently associated with mild to moderate impairment of hearing; therefore a hearing test should also be performed if OME persists for 3 months or more or if there is evidence of language or learning delays. Follow-up examinations of children with chronic OME should be maintained on a 3- to 6-month basis until the OME is resolved, a significant hearing loss is identified, or structural defect of the tympanic membrane or middle ear is identified (AAP, 2004a). Children with hearing loss should be referred to an otolaryngologist and should receive a speech and language evaluation as necessary.

Prevention

Routine immunization with the pneumococcal conjugate vaccine PCV7 (Prevnar 7) has reduced the incidence of AOM in many infants and children (Rodgers and Klugman, 2011). In 2010, the FDA approved a new conjugate vaccine, Prevnar 13, which replaces Prevnar 7. The vaccine is administered as a four-dose series beginning at 2 months of age; infants and children who have started the series with Prevnar 7 may complete the series with Prevnar 13 (CDC, 2010). The latest AAP clinical guidelines also recommend an annual influenza vaccination as a prevention for AOM (Lieberthal, Carroll, Chonmaitree, et al., 2013).

Parents are encouraged to reduce risk factors for AOM by breastfeeding infants for at least the first 6 months of life, avoid propping the formula bottle, decrease or discontinue pacifier use after 6 months, and prevent exposure to tobacco smoke (Lieberthal, Carroll, Chonmaitree, et al., 2013; AAP, 2004a). Xylitol or birch sugar, either in chewing gum or lozenge form, may be beneficial in preventing recurrent AOM in children over 2 years of age when used 3 to 5 times a day (Lieberthal, Carroll, Chonmaitree, et al., 2013).

CARE MANAGEMENT

Nursing objectives for children with AOM include (1) relieving pain, (2) facilitating drainage when possible, (3) preventing complications or recurrence, (4) educating the family in care of the child, and (5) providing emotional support to the child and family.

Analgesic drugs such as acetaminophen (all ages) and ibuprofen (6 months of age and older) are used to treat mild pain. For more severe pain, the AAP (Lieberthal, Carroll, Chonmaitree, et al., 2013) guidelines recommend a stronger analgesic such as codeine.

If the ear is draining, the external canal may be cleaned with sterile cotton swabs or pledgets coupled with topical antibiotic treatment. If ear wicks or lightly rolled sterile gauze packs are placed in the ear after surgical treatment, they should be loose enough to allow accumulated drainage to flow out of the ear; otherwise, infection may be transferred to the mastoid process. The wicks need to stay dry during shampoos or baths. Occasionally, drainage is so profuse that the auricle and the skin surrounding the ear become excoriated from the exudate. This is usually prevented by frequent cleansing and application of various moisture barriers (e.g., Proshield Plus), zinc oxide–based products, or petrolatum jelly (e.g., Vaseline).

Tympanostomy tubes may allow water to enter the middle ear, but recommendations for earplugs are inconsistent. Research evidence indicates that swimming without earplugs poses a slight increased risk for infection (Goldstein, Mandel, Kurs-Lasky, et al., 2005). However, lake and river water are potentially contaminated and wearing earplugs while swimming in a lake prevents total flooding of the external canal. Bathwater and shampoo water should be kept out of the ear, if possible, because soap reduces the surface tension of water and facilitates entry through the tube. Parents should be aware of the appearance of a grommet (usually a tiny, white, plastic spool-shaped tube) so that they can recognize it if it falls out. They are reassured that this is normal and requires no immediate intervention, although they should notify the health care practitioner.

Prevention of recurrence requires adequate education regarding antibiotic therapy. The symptoms of pain and fever usually subside within 24 to 48 hours, but nurses must emphasize that all of the prescribed medication should be taken. Parents should be aware that potential complications of OM, such as hearing loss, can be prevented with adequate treatment and follow-up care.

Parents also need anticipatory guidance regarding methods to reduce the risks of OM, especially in children younger than 2 years. Reducing the chances of OM is possible with simple measures, such as sitting or holding an infant upright for feedings, maintaining routine childhood immunizations, and exclusively breastfeeding until at least 6 months of age. Propping bottles is discouraged to avoid pooling of milk while the child is in the supine position and to encourage human contact during feeding. Eliminating tobacco smoke and known allergens is also recommended. Early detection of middle ear effusion is essential to prevent complications. Infants and preschool children should be screened for effusion, and all schoolchildren, especially those with learning disabilities, should be tested for hearing deficits related to a middle ear effusion.

BOX 40-7 CLINICAL MANIFESTATIONS OF INFECTIOUS MONONUCLEOSIS

Early Signs
- Headache
- Malaise
- Fatigue
- Chills
- Low-grade fever
- Loss of appetite
- Puffy eyes

Acute Disease

Cardinal Features
- Fever
- Sore throat
- Cervical adenopathy

Common Features
- Splenomegaly (may persist for several months)
- Palatine petechiae
- Macular eruption (especially on trunk)
- Exudative pharyngitis or tonsillitis

Infectious Mononucleosis

Infectious mononucleosis is an acute, self-limiting infectious disease that is common among adolescents. Symptoms include fever, exudative pharyngitis, lymphadenopathy, hepatosplenomegaly, and an increase in atypical lymphocytes. The course is usually mild but occasionally can be severe or, rarely, accompanied by serious complications.

Etiology and Pathophysiology

The herpes-like Epstein-Barr virus (EBV) is the principal cause of infectious mononucleosis. It appears in both sporadic and epidemic forms, but the sporadic cases are more common. The mechanism of spread has not been proven, but it is believed to be transmitted in saliva by direct intimate contact, although it survives in saliva for many hours outside of the body. The incubation period after exposure is approximately 30 to 50 days (AAP Committee on Infectious Diseases, 2012).

Diagnostic Tests

The onset of symptoms may be acute or insidious and may appear anywhere from 10 days to 6 weeks after exposure. The presenting symptoms vary greatly in type, severity, and duration (Box 40-7). The clinical manifestations of infectious mononucleosis are usually less severe (often subclinical or unapparent) and the convalescent phase is shorter in younger children than in older children and young adults. Heterophil antibody tests (Paul-Bunnell or Monospot) determine the extent to which the patient's serum will agglutinate sheep red blood cells; the response in these tests is primarily to immunoglobulin M, which is present in the first 2 weeks of the illness in adolescents. The spot test (Monospot) is a slide test of venous blood that has high specificity. It is rapid, sensitive, inexpensive, and easy to perform and has the advantage over the Paul-Bunnell test in that it can detect significant agglutinins at lower levels, thus allowing earlier diagnosis. Blood is usually obtained for the test by finger puncture or venous sampling and is placed on special paper. If the blood agglutinates, forming fragments or clumps, the test result is positive for the infection.

Therapeutic Management

No specific treatment exists for infectious mononucleosis. A mild analgesic is often sufficient to relieve the headache, fever, and malaise. Rest is encouraged for fatigue but is not imposed for any specific period. Affected persons are instructed to regulate activities according to their own tolerance unless complicating factors are present. Contact sports are discouraged in the presence of splenomegaly.

Antibiotics are contraindicated unless β-hemolytic streptococci are present (amoxicillin or ampicillin can cause a rash in patients with EBV infection). If sore throat is severe, effective therapies include gargles; hot drinks; anesthetic troches; or analgesics, including opioids. Corticosteroids have been used to treat respiratory distress from significant tonsillar inflammation, myocarditis, hemolytic anemia, thrombocytopenia, and neurologic complications; however, routine use of steroids is not recommended (AAP Committee on Infectious Diseases, 2012).

Prognosis. The course of this disease is usually self-limiting and uncomplicated. Acute symptoms often disappear within 7 to 10 days, and persistent fatigue subsides within 2 to 4 weeks. Some adolescents may need to restrict their activities for 2 to 3 months, but the disease rarely extends for longer periods. The adolescent is encouraged to maintain limited exercise to prevent deconditioning.

CARE MANAGEMENT

Nursing responsibilities for infectious mononucleosis are directed toward providing comfort measures to relieve symptoms and helping affected adolescents and their families determine appropriate activities for the stage of the disease. The adolescent is advised to limit exposure to persons outside the family, especially during the acute phase of illness. It may be more comfortable to limit intake to liquids during the acute phase; milkshakes are a good alternative to solid foods on a temporary basis. Throat pain may be severe enough to require an analgesic such as acetaminophen, ibuprofen, or even codeine. Careful nursing assessment of swallowing ability is essential to detect serious airway edema and airway compromise.

> **! NURSING ALERT**
>
> Advise the family to seek medical evaluation of the child or adolescent if:
> * Breathing becomes difficult.
> * Severe abdominal pain develops.
> * Sore throat pain is so severe that the child is unable drink liquids.
> * Respiratory stridor is observed.

CROUP SYNDROMES

Croup is a general term applied to a symptom complex characterized by hoarseness, a resonant cough described as "barking" or "brassy" (croupy), varying degrees of inspiratory stridor, and varying degrees of respiratory distress resulting from swelling or obstruction in the region of the larynx. Acute infections of the larynx are important in infants and small children because of their increased incidence in these age-groups and because the small diameter of the airway in infants and children places them at risk for significant narrowing with inflammation.

Croup syndromes can affect the larynx, trachea, and bronchi. However, laryngeal involvement often dominates the clinical picture because of the severe effects on the voice and breathing. Croup syndromes are described according to the primary anatomic area affected (i.e., epiglottitis [or supraglottitis], laryngitis, laryngotracheobronchitis [LTB], and tracheitis). In general, LTB occurs in very young children and epiglottitis is more common in older children. A comparison of croup syndromes is provided in Table 40-1.

With widespread immunization programs aimed at preventing *H. influenzae* type b, the cause of most cases of croup in the United States is attributed to viruses, namely parainfluenza virus, human metapneumovirus, influenza types A and B, adenovirus, and measles.

TABLE 40-1 COMPARISON OF CROUP SYNDROMES

	ACUTE EPIGLOTTITIS	ACUTE LARYNGOTRACHEOBRONCHITIS (LTB)	ACUTE SPASMODIC LARYNGITIS	ACUTE TRACHEITIS
Age-group affected	2-5 years but varies	Infant or child younger than 5 years	1-3 years	1 month–6 years (mean 5 to 7 years)
Etiologic agent	Bacterial	Viral	Viral with allergic component	Viral or bacterial with allergic component
Onset	Rapidly progressive	Slowly progressive	Sudden; at night	Moderately progressive
Major symptoms	Dysphagia Stridor aggravated when supine Drooling High fever Toxic appearance Rapid pulse and respirations	URI Stridor Brassy cough Hoarseness Dyspnea Restlessness Irritability Low-grade fever Nontoxic appearance	URI Croupy cough Stridor Hoarseness Dyspnea Restlessness Symptoms awakening child but disappearing during day Tendency to recur	URI Croupy cough Purulent secretions High fever No response to LTB therapy
Treatment	Airway protection Corticosteroids Fluids Antibiotics Reassurance	Racemic epinephrine Corticosteroids Fluids Reassurance	Cool mist Reassurance	Antibiotics Fluids

URI, Upper respiratory infection.

Acute Epiglottitis

A presumptive diagnosis of acute epiglottitis, or acute supraglottitis, is a medical emergency. It is a serious obstructive inflammatory process that occurs predominantly in children ages 2 to 5 years but can occur from infancy to adulthood. The obstruction is supraglottic as opposed to the subglottic obstruction of laryngitis. The responsible organism is usually *H. influenzae*. LTB and epiglottitis do not occur together.

Clinical Manifestations

The onset of epiglottitis is abrupt, and it can rapidly progress to severe respiratory distress. The child usually goes to bed asymptomatic to awaken later, complaining of sore throat and pain on swallowing. The child has a fever; appears sicker than clinical findings suggest; and insists on sitting upright and leaning forward with the chin thrust out, mouth open, and tongue protruding (**tripod position**). Drooling of saliva is common because of the difficulty or pain on swallowing and excessive secretions.

 NURSING ALERT

> Three clinical observations that are predictive of epiglottitis are absence of spontaneous cough, presence of drooling, and agitation.

The child is irritable; extremely restless; and has an anxious, apprehensive, and frightened expression. The voice is thick and muffled, with a froglike croaking sound on inspiration, but the child is not hoarse. Suprasternal and substernal retractions may be evident. The child seldom struggles to breathe, and slow, quiet breathing provides better air exchange. The throat is red and inflamed, and a distinctive large, cherry red, edematous epiglottis is visible on careful throat inspection.

! NURSING ALERT

> Throat inspection should be attempted only when immediate endotracheal intubation can be performed if needed.

Therapeutic Management

The course of epiglottitis may be fulminant, with respiratory obstruction appearing suddenly. Progressive obstruction leads to hypoxia, hypercapnia, and acidosis followed by decreased muscular tone; reduced level of consciousness; and, when obstruction becomes more or less complete, a rather sudden death.

The child who is suspected of having epiglottitis should be examined in a setting where emergency airway equipment is readily available. Examination of the throat with a tongue depressor is contraindicated until experienced personnel and equipment are available to proceed with immediate intubation or tracheostomy in the event that the examination precipitates further or complete obstruction.

Nasotracheal intubation or tracheostomy is usually considered for the child with epiglottitis with severe respiratory distress. It is recommended that the intubation or tracheostomy and any invasive procedure, such as starting an intravenous (IV) infusion, be performed in an area where emergency airway maintenance can be easily and quickly accomplished. Humidified oxygen is administered as necessary either via mask in older children or flow-by in younger children to avoid further agitation. Whether or not there is an artificial airway, the child requires intensive observation by experienced

personnel. The epiglottal swelling usually decreases after 24 hours of antibiotic therapy (ceftriaxone sodium or alternate cephalosporin), and the epiglottis is near normal by the third day. Intubated children are generally extubated at this time. The use of corticosteroids for reducing edema may be beneficial during the early treatment phase.

Children with suspected bacterial epiglottitis are given antibiotics intravenously followed by oral administration to complete a 7- to 10-day course. Family contacts with children younger than 4 years and any contacts younger than 4 years are treated with rifampin for 4 days (AAP Committee on Infectious Diseases, 2012).

■ CARE MANAGEMENT

Epiglottitis is a serious and frightening disease for the child and family. It is important to act quickly but calmly and to provide support without increasing anxiety. The child is allowed to remain in the position that provides the most comfort and security, and the parents are reassured that everything possible is being done to obtain relief for their child.

 NURSING ALERT

> When epiglottitis is suspected, the nurse should not attempt to visualize the epiglottis directly with a tongue depressor or take a throat culture but should refer the child for medical evaluation immediately (see Critical Thinking Case Study).

Acute care of the child is the same as that described later for the child with LTB. Continuous monitoring of respiratory status, including pulse oximetry (and blood gases if the patient is intubated), is an important part of nursing observations, and the IV infusion is maintained as described in Chapter 39.

Acute Laryngotracheobronchitis

Laryngotracheobronchitis is the most common croup syndrome. It affects primarily children younger than 5 years, and the causative organisms are viral agents, particularly the parainfluenza virus types 2 and 3, human metapneumovirus, RSV, influenza A, and influenza B. Other causative agents include *M. pneumoniae*, pneumococcus, and staphylococcus. The disease is usually preceded by a

 CRITICAL THINKING CASE STUDY

Croup Syndrome

Kim, a 4-year-old, is admitted to the emergency department with a sore throat, pain on swallowing, drooling, and a fever of 39° C (102.2° F). She looks ill, is agitated, and prefers to sit up leaning on her arms. What nursing interventions should the nurse implement in this situation?

1. Evidence—Is there sufficient evidence to draw any conclusions about Kim's condition at this time?
2. Assumptions—Describe some underlying assumptions about each of the following:
   a. Epiglottitis in children
   b. Symptoms of epiglottitis
   c. Precautions to be taken when a child has suspected epiglottitis
   d. Immediate nursing interventions when caring for a child with epiglottitis
3. What priorities for nursing care can be drawn at this time?
4. Does the evidence objectively support your argument (conclusion)?

URI, which gradually descends to adjacent structures. It is characterized by a gradual onset of low-grade fever, and the parents often report that the child went to bed and later awoke with a barky, brassy cough. Inflammation of the mucosa lining the larynx and trachea causes a narrowing of the airway. When the airway is significantly narrowed, the child inspires air past the obstruction and into the lungs, producing the characteristic inspiratory stridor and suprasternal retractions. Other classic manifestations include cough and hoarseness. Respiratory distress in infants and toddlers may be manifested by nasal flaring, intercostal retractions, tachypnea, and continuous stridor. The typical child with LTB develops the classic barking or seal-like cough and acute stridor after several days of rhinitis. When the child is unable to inhale a sufficient volume of air, symptoms of hypoxia become evident. Obstruction that is severe enough to prevent adequate ventilation and exhalation of carbon dioxide can cause respiratory acidosis and eventually respiratory failure.

Therapeutic Management

The major objective in medical management is maintaining the airway and providing adequate respiratory exchange. Children with mild croup (no stridor at rest) can be managed at home. Parents are taught the signs of respiratory distress and instructed to summon professional help early if needed. Children with labored respirations and stridor or other respiratory symptoms should receive medical attention.

The application of humidity with cool mist provides relief for most children. A cool-air vaporizer can be used at home. In the hospital, a nebulized mist for older infants and toddlers may be used to provide increased humidity and supplemental oxygen. However, controversy surrounds the use of mist therapy to treat croup. Studies have failed to demonstrate any significant improvement in subglottic edema with mist therapy (Moore and Little, 2007). A ride in the car with the windows down may help relieve symptoms.

Nebulized epinephrine (racemic epinephrine) is often used in children with severe disease, stridor at rest, retractions, or difficulty breathing. The α-adrenergic effects cause mucosal vasoconstriction and subsequently decrease subglottic edema. The onset of action is rapid, and the peak effect is observed in 2 hours. Children may be discharged home following racemic epinephrine after a 2- to 3-hour period of observation for return of acute symptoms.

Oral steroids (dexamethasone) have proven effective in the treatment of croup (often as a single dose) and are considered standard treatment for this condition (Zoorob, Sidani, and Murray, 2011); IM dexamethasone may be given to children who are unable to tolerate oral dosing. Nebulized budesonide may be administered in conjunction with IM dexamethasone.

In severe cases of LTB, the administration of heliox may be used to reduce the work of breathing and relieve airway obstruction. It reduces airway turbulence but is not recommended as a standard treatment of croup.

CARE MANAGEMENT

The most important nursing function in the care of children with LTB is continuous, vigilant observation and accurate assessment of respiratory status. Pulse oximetry is commonly used for monitoring oxygenation status. Changes in therapy are frequently based on the nurses' observations and assessments, the child's response to therapy, and tolerance of procedures. The trend away from early intubation of children with LTB emphasizes the importance of nursing observations and the ability to recognize

impending respiratory failure so that intubation can be implemented without delay.

> **! NURSING ALERT**
>
> Early signs of impending airway obstruction include increased pulse and respiratory rate; substernal, suprasternal, and intercostal retractions; flaring nares; and increased restlessness.

Infants or small children find that being treated with cool mist, coughing, having laryngeal spasms, and needing IV therapy are additional sources of distress. In many acute care facilities, the infant is allowed to be held by the parent; if cool mist is used in the treatment, it can be administered through a tube held in front of the patient while the child is held on the parent's lap.

Children with mild croup are allowed to drink the beverages they like as long as their respiratory status is stable, and parents are encouraged to try whatever comforting measures work best (e.g., holding their child, rocking, singing). If the child is unable to take oral fluids, IV fluids may be required, and steroids may need to be given intravenously.

The rapid progression of croup, the alarming sound of the cough and stridor, and the child's apprehensive behavior and ill appearance combine to create a frightening experience for the parents and family. The family should be allowed to remain with their child as much as possible.

Parents need frequent reassurance provided in a calm, quiet manner and education regarding what they can do to make their child more comfortable. Home care includes monitoring for worsening symptoms, continued humidity, adequate hydration, and nourishment.

Acute Spasmodic Laryngitis

Acute spasmodic laryngitis (spasmodic croup) is distinct from laryngitis and LTB and is characterized by recurrent paroxysmal attacks of laryngeal obstruction that occur chiefly at night. Signs of inflammation are absent or mild, and it is followed by an uneventful recovery. The child feels well the next day. Some children appear to be predisposed to the condition; allergies or hypersensitivities may be implicated in some cases. Management is the same as for infectious croup.

Bacterial Tracheitis

Bacterial tracheitis, an infection of the mucosa of the upper trachea, is a distinct entity with features of both croup and epiglottitis. The disease occurs typically at a mean age between 5 and 7 years and may cause severe airway obstruction (Roosevelt, 2011). It is believed to be a complication of LTB, and although *Staphylococcus aureus* is the most frequent organism responsible, *M. catarrhalis, S. pneumonia*, and *H. influenzae* have also been implicated.

Many of the manifestations of bacterial tracheitis are similar to those of LTB but are unresponsive to LTB therapy. The child has a history of previous URI with croupy cough, stridor unaffected by position, toxicity, absence of drooling, absence of dysphagia, and high fever. Thick, purulent tracheal secretions are common, and respiratory difficulties are secondary to these copious secretions and mucosal edema at the level of the cricoid cartilage. The child's white cell count will be elevated. Children with this condition may develop a life-threatening upper airway obstruction, respiratory failure, acute respiratory distress syndrome (ARDS), and multiple organ dysfunction (Hopkins, Lahiri, Salerno, et al., 2006).

THERAPEUTIC MANAGEMENT AND CARE MANAGEMENT

Bacterial tracheitis requires vigorous management with oxygen therapy, antipyretics, and antibiotics. Many younger children require endotracheal intubation and mechanical ventilation; patients are closely monitored for impending respiratory failure if not intubated. Early recognition to prevent life-threatening airway obstruction is essential.

INFECTIONS OF THE LOWER AIRWAYS

The reactive portion of the lower respiratory tract includes the bronchi and bronchioles in children. Cartilaginous support of the large airways is not fully developed until adolescence. Consequently, the smooth muscle in these structures represents a major factor in the constriction of the airway, particularly in the bronchioles—the portion that extends from the bronchi to the alveoli. Table 40-2 compares some of the major features of bronchial and bronchiolar infections.

Bronchitis

Bronchitis (sometimes referred to as tracheobronchitis) is an inflammation of the large airways (trachea and bronchi), which is frequently associated with URIs. Viral agents are the primary cause of the disease, although *M. pneumoniae* is a common cause in children older than 6 years. A dry, hacking, nonproductive cough that worsens at night and becomes productive in 2 to 3 days characterizes this condition.

Bronchitis is a mild, self-limiting disease that requires only symptomatic treatment, including analgesics, antipyretics, and humidity. Cough suppressants may be useful to allow rest but can interfere with clearance of secretions. Most patients recover uneventfully in 5 to 10 days. It can be associated with other underlying conditions such as CF and bronchiectasis and can become chronic in nature (cough >3 months). Adolescents with bronchitis should be screened for tobacco or marijuana use.

Respiratory Syncytial Virus and Bronchiolitis

Bronchiolitis is a common, acute viral infection with maximum effect at the bronchiolar level. The infection occurs primarily in winter and early spring. By age 3 years, most children have been infected at least once. RSV infection is the most frequent cause of hospitalization in children younger than 1 year. In addition, severe RSV infections in the first year of life represent a significant risk factor for the development of asthma up to age 13 years (Chávez-Bueno, Mejías, Jafri, et al., 2005). However, a strong causal relationship between RSV and the subsequent development of asthma has not been conclusively demonstrated (Wu and Hartert, 2011). Significant RSV infection may also occur in children older than 1 year who have a chronic or serious disabling illness. Although most cases of bronchiolitis are caused by RSV, adenoviruses and parainfluenza viruses are also implicated; recently, human metapneumovirus and human bocavirus have also been associated with bronchiolitis in children. It can also rarely be caused by *M. pneumoniae*. Occasionally, infants with RSV may have a concurrent viral or bacterial infection (e.g., otitis media, pertussis) (Watts and Goodman, 2011).

TABLE 40-2	COMPARISON OF CONDITIONS AFFECTING THE BRONCHI		
	ASTHMA*	**BRONCHITIS**	**BRONCHIOLITIS**
Description	Exaggerated response of bronchi to a trigger such as URI, animal dander, cold air, exercise Bronchospasm, exudation, and edema of bronchi, airway obstruction Inflammatory response	Usually occurs in association with URI Seldom an isolated entity	Most common infectious disease of lower airways Maximum obstructive impact at bronchiolar level
Age-group affected	Infancy to adolescence	First 4 years of life	Usually children 2 to 12 mo of age; rare after age 2 yr
Etiologic agents	Most often viruses such as RSV in infants but may be any of a variety of URI pathogens	Usually viral Other agents (e.g., bacteria, fungi, allergic disorders, airborne irritants) can trigger symptoms	Peak incidence, ≈age 6 mo Viruses, predominantly RSV; also adenoviruses, parainfluenza viruses, human metapneumovirus, and *Mycoplasma pneumoniae*
Predominant characteristics	Wheezing, cough	Persistent dry, hacking cough (worse at night) becoming productive in 2-3 days	Labored respirations, poor feeding, cough, tachypnea, retractions, nasal flaring, emphysema, increased nasal mucus, wheezing, may have fever
Treatment	Inhaled corticosteroids, bronchodilators, leukotriene modifiers, allergen and "triggers" control, long-term antiinflammatory medications	Cough suppressants if needed	Supplemental oxygen if saturations ≤90%; bronchodilators (optional) Suctioning nasopharynx Ensure adequate fluid intake Maintain adequate oxygenation

RSV, Respiratory syncytial virus; *URI*, upper respiratory infection.
*See Asthma, p. 1223.

Respiratory syncytial virus is transmitted from exposure to contaminated secretions. RSV can live on fomites for several hours and on hands for 30 minutes (AAP Committee on Infectious Diseases, 2012). The incubation period is 2 to 8 days.

Pathophysiology

Respiratory syncytial virus affects the epithelial cells of the respiratory tract. The ciliated cells swell, protrude into the lumen, and lose their cilia. RSV produces a fusion of cell membranes, forming a giant cell. The bronchiolar mucosa swells, and lumina are subsequently filled with mucus and exudate. The walls of the bronchi and bronchioles are infiltrated with inflammatory cells, and peribronchiolar interstitial pneumonitis is usually present. The varying degrees of intraluminal obstruction lead to hyperinflation, obstructive emphysema resulting from partial obstruction, and patchy areas of atelectasis. Dilation of bronchial passages on inspiration allows sufficient space for intake of air, but narrowing of the passages on expiration prevents air from leaving the lungs. Thus air is trapped distal to the obstruction and causes progressive overinflation (emphysema).

Clinical Manifestations

The illness usually begins with a URI after an incubation of about 5 to 8 days. Symptoms such as rhinorrhea and low-grade fever often appear first. OM and conjunctivitis may also be present. In time, a cough may develop. If the disease progresses, it becomes a lower respiratory tract infection and manifests typical symptoms (Box 40-8). Infants may have several days of URI symptoms or no symptoms except slight lethargy, poor feeding, or irritability.

When the lower airway is involved, classic manifestations include signs of altered air exchange, such as wheezing, retractions, crackles, dyspnea, tachypnea, and diminished breath sounds. Apnea may be the first recognized indicator of RSV infection in very young infants (younger than 1 month). Risk factors for the development of RSV infection include male gender, birth within 6 months of the start of RSV season, multiple birth, non-breastfed infants, young mothers and young mothers who smoke during pregnancy or thereafter, family history of atopy, low socioeconomic status and education, and living in crowded conditions; older family members may transmit the infection although they remain primarily asymptomatic or may only have a cold (Watts and Goodman, 2011). Preterm birth, chronic lung disease, congenital heart disease, neuromuscular disease, and immunodeficiency place children at higher risk for the development of severe RSV infection (AAP, 2006; Checchia, 2008).

BOX 40-8	**SIGNS AND SYMPTOMS OF RESPIRATORY SYNCYTIAL VIRUS**

Initial
- Rhinorrhea
- Pharyngitis
- Coughing/sneezing
- Wheezing
- Possible ear or eye drainage
- Intermittent fever

With Progression of Illness
- Increased coughing and wheezing
- Tachypnea and retractions
- Cyanosis

Severe Illness
- Tachypnea greater than 70 breaths/min
- Listlessness
- Apneic spells
- Poor air exchange; decreased breath sounds

Diagnostic Evaluation

Identification has been simplified by the development of tests done on nasopharyngeal secretions, using either a rapid immunofluorescent antibody–direct fluorescent antibody (DFA) staining or an enzyme-linked immunosorbent assay (ELISA) for RSV antigen detection (see Respiratory Secretion and Throat Specimens, Chapter 39). Hyperinflation of the lungs is generally seen on the chest radiograph.

Therapeutic Management

Children with bronchiolitis are treated symptomatically with humidified oxygen, adequate fluid intake, airway maintenance, and medications. Most children with bronchiolitis can be managed at home. Hospitalization is usually recommended for children with respiratory distress and those who cannot maintain adequate hydration. Other reasons for hospitalization include complicating conditions, such as underlying lung or heart disease or associated debilitated states, or a home environment where adequate management is questionable. An infant who is tachypneic or apneic, has marked retractions, appears listless, has a history of poor fluid intake, or is dehydrated should be closely observed for respiratory failure.

Humidified oxygen is administered in concentrations sufficient to maintain adequate oxygenation (Spo_2) at or above 90% as measured by pulse oximetry. Humidified mist may be administered. Routine chest percussion and postural drainage (formerly CPT) are not recommended (Roque Figuls, Gine-Garriga, Granados Rugeles, et al., 2012); infants with abundant nasal secretions benefit from periodic suctioning. Fluids by mouth may be contraindicated because of tachypnea, weakness, and fatigue; therefore IV fluids may be used until the acute stage of the disease has passed. Nasogastric fluids may be required if the infant is unable to tolerate oral fluids and a peripheral IV is difficult to establish.

Clinical assessments, noninvasive oxygen monitoring, and blood gas values may guide therapy. Medical therapy for bronchiolitis is primarily supportive and aimed at decreasing airway hyperresonance and inflammation and promoting adequate fluid intake. Bronchodilators may provide short-term benefits, yet overall significant improvement in the child's condition is not always appreciable. A single dose of bronchodilator therapy is often prescribed to assess for a clinical response. If it improves symptoms, it may be prescribed on an ongoing basis. If no response is evident, no further doses are given. Racemic epinephrine has been shown to produce modest improvement in ventilation status. Nebulized hypertonic saline (3%) treatments may decrease hospital length of stay and improve mucociliary clearance (Wright and Piedimonte, 2011).

Corticosteroids (inhaled or systemic) and antihistamines have not been shown to be effective in controlled studies and are not recommended for routine use. Antibiotics are not part of the treatment of RSV infection unless there is a coexisting bacterial infection such as OM (AAP, 2006). Additional recommendations in the AAP (2006) practice guideline are to encourage breastfeeding; avoid passive tobacco smoke exposure; and promote preventive measures, including hand washing.

Ribavirin, an antiviral agent (synthetic nucleoside analog), is the only specific therapy approved for hospitalized children; however, use of this drug is controversial because of concerns about the high cost, aerosol route of administration, potential toxic effects among exposed health care personnel (teratogenicity), and conflicting results of efficacy trials (AAP, 2006; Chávez-Bueno, Mejías, Jafri, et al., 2005; Ventre and Randolph, 2007).

Prevention of Respiratory Syncytial Virus Infection

The only product available in the United States for prevention of RSV infection is palivizumab (Synagis), a monoclonal antibody, which is given monthly in an IM injection to prevent hospitalization associated with RSV. According to the American Academy of Pediatrics (AAP) (Meissner and Bocchini, 2009), candidates for palivizumab include infants born before 32 weeks' gestation, infants with chronic lung disease, infants born at 32 to less than 35 weeks' gestation who attend day care or have a sibling younger than 5 years, children younger than 2 years with hemodynamically significant congenital heart disease, and children with severe immunodeficiencies (e.g., severe combined immunodeficiency or acquired immunodeficiency syndrome [AIDS]). Prophylaxis for RSV should be initiated at the onset of the RSV season and terminated at the end of the season (November to March or April). Additional age and condition recommendations are outlined in the AAP practice guideline (2006).

 MEDICATION ALERT

The lyophilized powder form of palivizumab should be administered within 6 hours of being reconstituted with sterile water because it is preservative free. A new liquid form of the drug may be available for future use.

CARE MANAGEMENT

Children admitted to the hospital with suspected RSV infection are usually assigned separate rooms or grouped with other RSV-infected children. Contact and Standard Precautions are used, including hand washing, not touching the nasal mucosa or conjunctiva, and using gloves and gowns when entering the patient's room. The 2007 CDC isolation guidelines emphasize that, although RSV may be transmitted via the droplet route, direct contact with infected respiratory secretions is the most common method of transmission; the CDC recommends Standard and Contact Precautions with RSV (Siegel, Rhinehart, Jackson, et al., 2007). The AAP Committee on Infectious Diseases (2012) also recommends these precautions but suggests that Droplet Precautions be used if persons are closer than 3 feet; Droplet Precautions are not recommended by the AAP in the routine care of persons with RSV. Other isolation procedures of potential benefit are those aimed at limiting the number of hospital personnel, visitors, and uninfected children in contact with the child. Another measure is to make patient assignments so that nurses assigned to children with RSV infection are not caring for other patients who are considered high risk.

Infants with RSV infection often have copious nasal secretions, making breathing and breastfeeding or bottle feeding difficult. This engenders concerns that the child will lose weight or stop breastfeeding altogether. Encourage breastfeeding mothers to continue feeding the infant or, if feedings are contraindicated because of the acuity of the illness, mothers should pump their milk and store it appropriately for later use (see Chapter 24). Parents are taught how to instill normal saline drops into the nares and suction the mucus with a bulb syringe or portable suction machine before feedings and before bedtime so the child may eat and rest better; unfortunately, no medications appropriate for infants can help with these symptoms. To address the issue of decreased fluid intake, parents may offer small amounts of fluids frequently to maintain adequate hydration. Infants may cough or vomit as the secretions settle in the stomach and make them prone to emesis of such secretions.

Additional nursing care is aimed at monitoring oxygenation with pulse oximetry, ensuring any bronchodilator therapy is optimized

by using a small mask for delivery, and providing information for the parent and family regarding the infant's status. For the most part, infants recover quickly from the disease and resume normal daily activities, including fluid intake. Such infants are at risk for further episodes of wheezing that may or may not involve another RSV infection; parents, however, may be concerned that the infant has another serious case of RSV infection.

Pneumonias

Pneumonia, inflammation of the pulmonary parenchyma, is common in childhood but occurs more frequently in early childhood. Clinically, pneumonia may occur either as a primary disease or as a complication of another illness. The causative agent is either inhaled into the lungs directly or comes from the bloodstream.

The most useful classification of pneumonia is based on the etiologic agent (e.g., viral, bacterial, mycoplasmal, or aspiration of foreign substances) (see Aspiration Pneumonia, p. 1220). Many organisms can cause pneumonia, and these vary according to the child's age (Ranganathan and Sonnappa, 2009):

- **Neonates**—Group B streptococci, gram-negative enteric bacteria, cytomegalovirus, *Ureaplasma urealyticum, Listeria monocytogenes, C. trachomatis*
- **Infants**—RSV, parainfluenza virus, influenza virus, adenovirus, metapneumovirus, *S. pneumoniae, H. influenzae, M. pneumoniae, Mycobacterium tuberculosis*
- **Preschool-age children**—RSV, parainfluenza virus, influenza virus, adenovirus, metapneumovirus, *S. pneumoniae, H. influenzae, M. pneumoniae, M. tuberculosis*
- **School-age children**—*M. pneumoniae, Chlamydophila pneumoniae, M. tuberculosis*, respiratory viruses

Histomycosis, coccidioidomycosis, and other fungi also cause pneumonia. Pneumonitis is a localized acute inflammation of the lung without the toxemia associated with lobar pneumonia.

The clinical manifestations of pneumonia vary depending on the etiologic agent, the child's age, the child's systemic reaction to the infection, the extent of the lesions, and the degree of bronchial and bronchiolar obstruction. The causative agent is identified from the clinical history, the child's age, the general health history, the physical examination, radiography, and the laboratory examination.

Viral Pneumonia

Viral pneumonias, which occur more frequently than bacterial pneumonias, are seen in children of all ages and are often associated with viral URIs. Viruses that cause pneumonia include RSV in infants and parainfluenza, influenza, human bocavirus (HBoV), human metapneumovirus, enterovirus, and adenovirus in older children. Differentiation among viruses is usually made by clinical features such as the child's age, medical history, season of the year, and radiographic and laboratory examination (Box 40-9).

Viral infections of the respiratory tract render the affected child more susceptible to secondary bacterial infection, especially when there is denuded bronchial mucosa. Treatment is symptomatic and includes measures to promote oxygenation and comfort, such as oxygen administration with cool mist, antipyretics for fever management, monitoring fluid intake, and family support. Antimicrobial therapy is usually reserved for children in whom a bacterial infection is demonstrated by appropriate cultures.

Primary Atypical Pneumonia

Atypical pneumonia refers to pneumonia that is caused by pathogens other than the traditionally most common and readily cultured bacteria (e.g., *S. pneumoniae*). In the category of atypical

BOX 40-9 **GENERAL SIGNS OF PNEUMONIA**

- Fever—Usually quite high (≥39.5° C [103° F])
- Respiratory
  - Cough—Nonproductive to productive with whitish sputum
  - Tachypnea
  - Breath sounds—Rhonchi or fine crackles
  - Dullness with percussion
  - Chest pain; abdominal pain with lower lobe involvement
  - Retractions
  - Nasal flaring
  - Pallor to cyanosis (depends on severity)
- Chest x-ray film—Diffuse or patchy infiltration with peribronchial distribution
- Behavior—Irritable, restless, lethargic
- Gastrointestinal—Anorexia, vomiting, diarrhea, abdominal pain

BOX 40-10 **PNEUMOTHORAX**

Pneumothorax occurs when there is an accumulation of air in the pleural space; this air increases intrapleural pressure, making it more difficult to expand the affected lung and thus the clinical manifestations of dyspnea, chest pain and often back pain, labored respirations, tachycardia, and decreased oxygen saturation. In neonates and infants on mechanical ventilation, the first clinical signs of a pneumothorax are oxygen desaturation and hypotension. The three major types of pneumothorax are tension, spontaneous, and traumatic. The definitive diagnosis of pneumothorax is a chest radiograph. The emergent treatment involves needle aspiration of the air within the pleural space; subsequently a chest tube to closed drainage is usually inserted to prevent the reaccumulation of air. *Pleural effusion* occurs when there is an excessive accumulation of fluid in the pleural space. The diagnosis is made by chest radiography, and the treatment involves evacuation of the fluid by needle aspiration followed by insertion of a chest tube to closed drainage.

pneumonias, *M. pneumoniae* and *C. pneumonia* are the most common causes of community-acquired pneumonia in children 5 years of age or older (Sandora and Sectish, 2011). It occurs in the fall and winter months and is more prevalent in crowded living conditions. Most affected persons recover from acute illness at home in 7 to 10 days with symptomatic treatment followed by 1 week of convalescence. The incubation period is 2 to 3 weeks, but the cough may last several weeks.

Chlamydial pneumonia, caused by *C. trachomatis,* can occur in infants and generally appears between 3 and 19 weeks of age. The infant contracts this from the infected genital tract of the mother at birth.

Erythromycin (for those younger than 9 years), azithromycin, and clarithromycin are the primary agents used for treating atypical pneumonia.

Bacterial Pneumonia

S. pneumoniae is the most common bacterial pathogen responsible for community-acquired pneumonia in both children and adults (Rafei and Lichenstein, 2006). Other bacteria that cause pneumonia in children are pneumococcus, group A streptococcus, *S. aureus, M. catarrhalis,* and *C. pneumoniae.*

Beyond the neonatal period, bacterial pneumonias display distinct clinical patterns that facilitate their differentiation from other forms of pneumonia. The onset of illness is abrupt and generally follows a viral infection that disturbs the natural defense mechanisms of the upper respiratory tract.

The child with bacterial pneumonia usually appears ill. Symptoms include fever, malaise, rapid and shallow respirations, cough, and chest pain. The pain of pneumonia may be referred to the abdomen in young children and confused with appendicitis. Chills and meningeal symptoms (meningism) without meningitis are common.

Most older children with pneumonia can be treated at home if the condition is recognized and treatment is initiated early. Antibiotic therapy, rest, liberal oral intake of fluid, and administration of an antipyretic for fever are the principal therapeutic measures. Chest percussion and postural drainage may be indicated; however, this is controversial. Follow-up examination is recommended for small infants and toddlers. Hospitalization is indicated when pleural effusion or empyema accompanies the disease, when respiratory distress occurs, in situations in which compliance with therapy is estimated to be poor, in infants younger than 1 month, and when there are

chronic illnesses such as congenital heart disease or BPD (Rafei and Lichenstein, 2006). IV fluids may be necessary to ensure adequate hydration, and oxygen is required if the child is in respiratory distress; some children may require initial therapy with parenteral antibiotics because of the severity of illness.

Complications. At present, the classic features and clinical course of pneumonia are seen infrequently because of early and vigorous antibiotic and supportive therapy. However, some children, especially infants, with staphylococcal or GABHS pneumonia develop empyema, pyopneumothorax, or tension pneumothorax. AOM and pleural effusion are common in children with pneumococcal pneumonia (Box 40-10) (see Evidence-Based Practice box).

Continuous closed chest drainage may be instituted when purulent fluid is aspirated. If a large amount of purulent drainage is obtained, an appropriate antibiotic may be instilled into the chest cavity, and chest drainage is discontinued for approximately 1 hour after the instillation. Closed drainage via a chest tube is continued until drainage fluid is minimal, which rarely requires more than 5 to 7 days. Sometimes repeated pleural taps are sufficient to remove fluid; however, if the purulent drainage accumulates rapidly and is highly viscous, continuous drainage is preferred. Thoracotomy with open debridement of the infected lung tissue may be required; if empyema and pneumothorax tend to recur, a partial thoracoscopic lobectomy may be performed. Alternatively, video-assisted thoracoscopy (VATS) and intrapleural fibrinolytic therapy may preclude the use of open debridement and thoracotomy (Sandora and Sectish, 2011).

Prevention

In February 2010, a 13-valent pneumococcal conjugate vaccine (PCV13) was approved for use in children ages 6 weeks to 71 months to protect against 13 pneumococcal serotypes. The Advisory Committee on Immunization Practices (ACIP) recommends routine vaccination with PCV13 of all children ages 2 to 59 months, children ages 60 to 71 months with underlying medical conditions that increase their risk for pneumococcal disease or complications, and children who previously received 1 or more doses of PCV7 (CDC, 2010). (See Immunizations, Chapter 31.)

CARE MANAGEMENT

Nursing care of the child with pneumonia is primarily supportive and symptomatic but necessitates thorough respiratory assessment

EVIDENCE-BASED PRACTICE

Nursing Interventions for Prevention of Ventilator-Associated Pneumonia in Children

Ask the Question

What nursing interventions prevent VAP in children?

Search for Evidence

Search Strategies

Search selection included English publications on nursing interventions for prevention of VAP in children and adolescents.

Databases Used

PubMed, AHRQ

Critically Analyze the Evidence

- Implementation of VAP bundle resulted in a decreased VAP rate from 5.6 infections per 1000 ventilator days at baseline to 0.3 per 1000 ventilator days (Bigham, Amato, Bondurrant, et al., 2009).
- Common VAP prevention interventions include (Bigham, Amato, Bondurrant, et al., 2009; Garland, 2010; Morrow, Argent, Jeena, et al., 2009; Norris, Barnes, and Roberts, 2009):
  - Change ventilator circuits and in-line suction catheters only when soiled.
  - Every 2 to 4 hours, drain condensate from ventilator circuit (use heated wire circuits to reduce rainout).
  - Rinse oral suction devices after use and store in a nonsealed plastic bag at the bedside.
  - Hand hygiene should be used before and after contact with ventilator circuit.
  - Wear PPE before providing care to patients when soiling from respiratory secretions is anticipated.
  - Every 2 to 4 hours, follow unit mouth care policy.
  - Unless contraindicated, elevate head of bed to 30 to 45 degrees.
  - Before repositioning patient, always drain ventilator circuit.
  - For patients older than 12 years, when possible, use ET tube with dorsal lumen above ET tube cuff to help suction secretions above the cuff.
  - Evaluate daily for possible extubation.
  - Avoid reintubation.
  - Provide deep vein thrombosis and peptic ulcer disease prophylaxis.
- Infants in supine position (infant lying on back with ET tube held upright in the vertical position) had increased colony counts or new organisms in tracheal aspirate than infants in lateral position (infant lying on side with ET tube at same level as the trachea) (Aly, Badawy, El-Kholy, et al., 2008).
- Staff education on VAP and improvements to practice changes can have a substantial impact on reducing VAP (Garland, 2010; Richardson, Hines, Dixon, et al., 2010; Turton, 2008).
- A 7-day versus 3-day ventilator circuit change was not associated with increased VAP rates (Samransamruajkit, Jirapaiboonsuk, Siritantiwat, et al., 2010).
- Use of low-sodium solution for airway care was associated with a decrease in VAP as well as chronic lung disease (Christensen, Henry, Baer, et al., 2010).
- In bronchoalveolar lavage fluid, PAI-1 levels can aid in early diagnosis of VAP (Srinivasan, Song, Wiener-Kronish, et al., 2011).
- Reduced mortality rates were observed in patients with VAP when silver-coated ET tube was used versus uncoated ET tube (Afessa, Shorr, Anzueto, et al., 2010).

Apply the Evidence: Nursing Implications

There is **good evidence** with **strong recommendations** for use of interventions to prevent VAP in children (Guyatt, Oxman, Vist, et al., 2008). Some of the prevention methods included in VAP bundles are hand hygiene, oral hygiene, use of PPE, and elevation of head of bed 30 to 45 degrees. Staff education and engagement in VAP prevention initiatives are important.

Quality and Safety Competencies:

Evidence-Based Practice*

Knowledge

Differentiate clinical opinion from research and evidence-based summaries

Describe the various interventions for prevention of VAP in children.

Skills

Base individualized care plan on patient values, clinical expertise, and evidence

Integrate evidence into practice by using interventions for prevention of VAP in children.

Attitudes

Value the concept of evidence-based practice (EBP) as integral to determining best clinical practice

Appreciate strengths and weakness of evidence for preventions of VAP in children.

References

Afessa B, Shorr AF, Anzueto AR, et al: Association between a silver-coated endotracheal tube and reduced mortality in patients with ventilator-associated pneumonia, *Chest* 137(5):1015–1021, 2010.

Aly H, Badawy M, El-Kholy A, et al: Randomized, controlled trial on tracheal colonization of ventilated infants: can gravity prevent ventilator-associated pneumonia? *Pediatrics* 122:770–774, 2008.

Bigham MT, Amato R, Bondurrant P, et al: Ventilator-associated pneumonia in the pediatric intensive care unit: characterizing the problem and implementing a sustainable solution, *J Pediatr* 154:582–587, 2009.

Christensen RD, Henry E, Baer VL, et al: A low-sodium solution for airway care: results of a multicenter trial, *Respir Care* 55(12):1680–1685, 2010.

Garland JS: Strategies to prevent ventilator-associated pneumonia in neonates, *Clin Perinatol* 37:629–643, 2010.

Guyatt GH, Oxman AD, Vist GE, et al: GRADE: an emerging consensus on rating quality of evidence and strength of recommendations, *BMJ* 336:924–926, 2008.

Morrow BM, Argent AC, Jeena PM, et al: Guideline for the diagnosis, prevention and treatment of paediatric ventilator-associated pneumonia, *S Afr Med J* 99(4):255–267, 2009.

Norris SC, Barnes AK, Roberts TD: When ventilator-associated pneumonias haunt your NICU: one unit's story, *Neonatal Netw* 28(1):59–66, 2009.

Richardson M, Hines S, Dixon G, et al: Establishing nurse-led ventilator-associated pneumonia surveillance in paediatric intensive care, *J Hosp Infect* 75(3):220–224, 2010.

Samransamruajkit R, Jirapaiboonsuk S, Siritantiwat S, et al: Effect of frequency of ventilator circuit changes (3 vs 7 days) on the rate of ventilator-associated pneumonia in PICU, *J Crit Care* 25(1):56–61, 2010.

Srinivasan R, Song Y, Wiener-Kronish J, et al: Plasminogen activation inhibitor concentrations in bronchoalveolar lavage fluid distinguishes ventilator-associated pneumonia from colonization in mechanically ventilated pediatric patients, *Pediatr Crit Care Med* 12(1):21–27, 2011.

Turton P: Ventilator-associated pneumonia in paediatric intensive care: a literature review, *Nurs Crit Care* 13(5):241–248, 2008.

Olga A. Taylor

*Adapted from the QSEN at www.qsen.org.

ET, Endotracheal; *PAI,* plasminogen activation inhibitor; *PPE,* personal protection equipment; *VAP,* ventilator-associated pneumonia.

and administration of supplemental oxygen (as required), fluids, and antibiotics. The child's respiratory rate, rhythm, and depth, oxygenation, general disposition, and level of activity are frequently assessed. To prevent dehydration, fluids are frequently administered intravenously during the acute phase.

Nursing care of the child with a chest tube requires close attention to respiratory status, as noted previously; the chest tube and drainage device used are monitored for proper function (i.e., drainage is not impeded, vacuum setting is correct, tubing is free of kinks, dressing covering chest tube insertion site is intact, water seal is maintained [if used], and chest tube remains in place). Movement in bed and ambulation with a chest tube are encouraged according to the child's respiratory status, but children require frequent doses of an analgesic. Supplemental oxygen may be required in the acute phase of the illness and may be administered by nasal cannula, face mask, or flow-by. Children are usually more comfortable in a semi-erect position (Fig. 40-3) but should be allowed to determine the position of comfort. Lying on the affected side if the pneumonia is unilateral ("good lung up") splints the chest on that side and reduces the pleural rubbing that often causes discomfort. Fever is controlled by the cool environment and administration of antipyretic drugs. Children, especially infants, with ineffectual cough or difficulty handling secretions may require suctioning to maintain a patent airway. A simple bulb suction syringe is usually sufficient for clearing the nares and nasopharynx of infants, but mechanical suction should be readily available if needed. A noninvasive suction device (BBG nasal aspirator) may be used to suction the infant's nares without the danger of causing nasal trauma; the device may be connected to mechanical suction for best results. Older children can usually handle secretions without assistance. Chest percussion, postural drainage, and nebulized bronchodilator treatments may be prescribed depending on the child's condition. Chest percussion and postural drainage currently lack empirical support for improving the child's condition or decreasing the length of stay in children with community-acquired pneumonia. For the child being cared for at home, the nurse educates the parent regarding observation for worsening symptoms, antibiotic and antipyretic administration, and encouragement of oral fluid intake. If the child is ill, solid foods may be rejected; fluid intake is encouraged until the child feels well enough to eat solids. Return to school or day care is usually permitted according to the type of pneumonia, severity of illness, and health care practitioner recommendation. It should

be emphasized that the infection may be transmitted to other children with close contact.

The hospitalized child may be apprehensive, and the treatments and tests are frightening and stress producing. It is important to involve the entire family in the care as appropriate and to encourage questions and facilitate effective communication. Reducing anxiety and apprehension reduces psychologic distress in the child, and when the child is more relaxed, the respiratory efforts are lessened. Easing respiratory efforts makes the child less apprehensive, and encouraging the presence of the caregiver provides the child with a source of comfort and support.

OTHER RESPIRATORY TRACT INFECTIONS

Pertussis (Whooping Cough)

Pertussis, or whooping cough, is an acute respiratory tract infection caused by *Bordetella pertussis*, which in the past occurred primarily in children younger than 4 years who were not immunized. It is highly contagious and is particularly threatening in young infants, who have a higher morbidity and mortality rate. It can result in encephalopathy, seizures, and pneumonia. Infants younger than 6 months may not come to the health care practitioner with the typical cough; in this age-group, apnea is a common presenting manifestation (AAP Committee on Infectious Diseases, 2012). Likewise, older children are known to manifest the disease with a persistent cough and the absence of the characteristic whoop (see Table 33-2 for signs, symptoms, and management of pertussis). The incidence is highest in the spring and summer months, and a single attack confers lifetime immunity. The resurgence of pertussis in the United States, particularly among children 10 years old and older, has prompted concerns of the long-term effects of the pertussis vaccine. Consequently, two acellular pertussis booster vaccines have been approved for children: Boostrix (for persons ages 10 years and older) and Adacel (for persons ages 11 to 64 years). (See also Immunizations, Chapter 31.) Most children with pertussis can be managed at home; care is supportive in nature, including encouraging adequate hydration and administering antipyretics. When coughing spasms occur in small children, they can be frightening for the parent and family. Admission to the hospital occurs if respiratory symptoms are severe or if apnea occurs. Treatment with antibiotics (erythromycin, clarithromycin, or azithromycin) in the catarrhal stage may result in a milder form of the infection, but treatment also prevents spread to others (AAP Committee on Infectious Diseases, 2012). Family contacts may also be treated. Pertussis symptoms usually last for 6 to 10 weeks but may persist for longer.

Tuberculosis

Tuberculosis (TB) is the second leading cause of death from an infectious disease. Ten million to 15 million persons in the United States are infected with TB. Case rates of TB for all ages are higher in urban, low-income areas and among non-white racial and ethnic groups. In recent years, foreign-born children have accounted for more than one fourth of newly diagnosed cases of TB in children 14 years of age or younger in the United States (AAP Committee on Infectious Diseases, 2012). The following groups have the greatest rates of latent TB infection: immigrants, international adoptees, refugees from or travelers to high-prevalence regions (Asia, Africa, Latin America, and countries of the former Soviet Union), homeless individuals, and inmates of correctional facilities (AAP Committee on Infectious Diseases, 2012). In addition, adolescents and adults being treated with tumor necrosis factor (TNF)-alpha antagonists

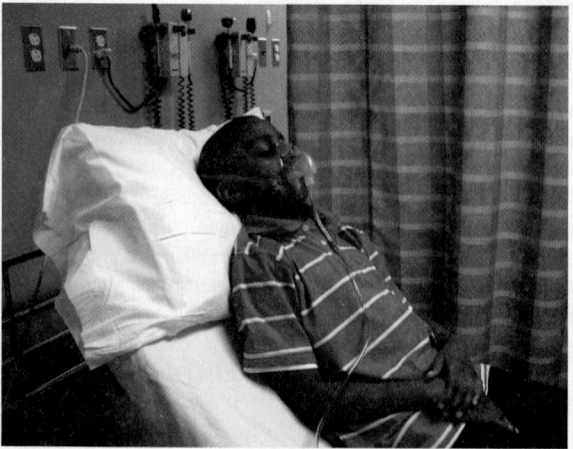

FIG 40-3 Child placed in semi-erect position is often more comfortable, and this position enhances diaphragmatic expansion.

for conditions such as inflammatory bowel disease or arthritis have been identified as having contracted TB; therefore it is recommended that screening for TB occurs in such persons before the use of TNF-alpha antagonists (AAP Committee on Infectious Diseases, 2012).

Tuberculosis is caused by *M. tuberculosis*, an acid-fast bacillus. Children are susceptible to the human *(M. tuberculosis)* and the bovine *(Mycobacterium bovis)* organisms. In parts of the world where TB in cattle is not controlled or milk is not pasteurized, the bovine type is a common source of infection.

Certain factors influence the degree to which the organism produces an altered state in the host. These factors include heredity (resistance to the infection may be genetically transmitted), gender (higher rates in adolescent girls), age (lower resistance in infants; higher incidence during adolescence), stress (emotional or physical), nutritional status, and intercurrent infection (especially human immunodeficiency virus [HIV], measles, and pertussis). Children with HIV infection have an increased incidence of TB disease, and all children with TB should be tested for HIV.

The source of TB infection in children is usually an infected member of the household or a frequent visitor to the home such as a babysitter or domestic worker. The airway is the usual portal of entry for the organism. In the lungs, a proliferation of epithelial cells surrounds and encapsulates the multiplying bacilli in an attempt to wall it off, thus forming the typical tubercle. Extension of the primary lesion at the original site causes progressive tissue destruction as it spreads within the lung, discharges material from foci to other areas of the lungs (e.g., bronchi, pleura), or produces pneumonia. Erosion of blood vessels by the primary lesion can cause widespread dissemination of the tubercle bacillus to near and distant sites (miliary TB). Extrapulmonary (miliary) TB may be manifested as malaise, fever, weight loss, superior lymphadenitis, meningitis, hepatomegaly, splenomegaly, and osteoarthritis (AAP Committee on Infectious Diseases, 2012). With the exception of meningitis, the treatment for extrapulmonary TB may be the same drug regimen as for pulmonary TB. Infants and children younger than 3 years are more likely to develop miliary TB.

Diagnostic Evaluation

Diagnosis of TB is based on information derived from physical examination, history, tuberculin skin testing, radiographic examinations, and cultures of the organism. The clinical manifestations of the disease are extremely variable (Box 40-11).

The tuberculin skin test (TST) is the most important indicator of whether a child has been infected with the tubercle bacillus. The standard dose of purified protein derivative (PPD) is 5 tuberculin units, which is administered using a 27-gauge needle and a 1-mL syringe intradermally into the volar aspect of the forearm. Creation of a visible wheal is crucial to accurate testing. The AAP (AAP Committee on Infectious Diseases, 2012) recommends that administration of the TST and interpretation of the results be performed and read only by specially educated health care professionals. Universal testing of all children for TB is no longer recommended. A targeted testing method is employed wherein only children and adolescents at high risk for contracting the disease, in addition to patients at risk for progression to TB disease, are screened. A risk factor questionnaire (Box 40-12) has been developed to facilitate screening pediatric populations at high risk.

The IGRA (interferon gamma release assay) does not cross-react with the bacille Calmette-Guérin (BCG) and is the preferred test for the diagnosis of latent tuberculosis infection (LTBI) in an asymptomatic BCG-immunized child over the age of 4 years. The IGRA cannot distinguish between latent infection and TB disease, and a negative or indeterminate result does not exclude TB infection. The cost of the blood IGRA is considerably more than the TST, and it is reported to be more involved technically; therefore the TST remains the more favored option for testing as a public health intervention (Perez-Velez, 2012). The usefulness and ability of IGRA to detect TB infection in children younger than 2 years is limited. The recommendations for use of IGRA include the following (AAP Committee on Infectious Diseases, 2012):

- Children ≥5 years who have received the BCG vaccine
- Children ≥5 who are unlikely to return for further testing
- Nontuberculous mycobacterium disease is suspected and the TST is positive
- When additional evidence is necessary to increase compliance

A positive reaction indicates that the individual has been infected and has developed sensitivity to the tubercle bacillus. The test is usually positive 2 to 10 weeks after initial infection with the organism. It does not, however, confirm the presence of active disease. Once an individual reacts positively, he or she will always react positively. A previously negative reaction that becomes positive indicates that the person has been infected since the previous test. Prompt radiographic evaluation of all children with a positive TST reaction is recommended.

BOX 40-11	**CLINICAL MANIFESTATIONS OF TUBERCULOSIS**

May be asymptomatic or produce a broad range of symptoms:
- Fever
- Malaise
- Anorexia
- Weight loss (or failure to grow in child)
- Cough (may or may not be present; progresses slowly over weeks to months)
- Aching pain and tightness in the chest
- Hemoptysis (rare)

With progression:
- Increased respiratory rate
- Poor expansion of lung on the affected side
- Diminished breath sounds and crackles
- Dullness on percussion
- Persistent fever
- Pallor, anemia, weakness, and weight loss

BOX 40-12	**VALIDATED QUESTIONS FOR DETERMINING RISK OF LTBI IN CHILDREN IN THE UNITED STATES**

- Has a family member or contact had tuberculosis disease?
- Has a family member had a positive tuberculin skin test result?
- Was your child born in a high risk country (countries other than the United States, Canada, Australia, New Zealand, or Western or Northern European countries)?
- Has your child traveled (had contact with resident populations) to a high risk country for more than 1 week?

From American Academy of Pediatrics (AAP) Committee on Infectious Diseases, Pickering L, editor: *Red book: 2012 report of the Committee on Infectious Diseases,* ed 29, Elk Grove Village, IL, 2012, Author.

LTBI, Latent tuberculosis infection.

The term *latent tuberculosis infection (LTBI)* is used to indicate infection in a person who has a positive TST, no physical findings of disease, and normal chest radiograph findings. The majority of children are asymptomatic when a positive skin test result is found, and most of them do not go on to develop the disease. The term tuberculosis disease or clinically active TB is used when a child has clinical symptoms or radiographic manifestations caused by the *M. tuberculosis* organism. A diagnosis of TB disease represents recent transmission of the *M. tuberculosis* organism and is an urgent event for public health. Prompt evaluation, treatment, and identification and treatment of contacts are key components to managing TB.

In 2010, the WHO recommended that previously treated patients should have access to drug-susceptibility testing and culture at the beginning of treatment to identify possible multidrug–TB resistance. The WHO also updated recommendations for individuals with HIV and TB; these include starting antiretroviral therapy within 8 weeks after the initiation of antituberculosis treatment and the use of a clinical algorithm to screen for TB in persons with HIV, those at high risk for HIV, or those living in congregate settings (Perez-Velez, 2012).

Therapeutic Management

Medical management of TB disease in children consists of adequate nutrition, pharmacotherapy, prevention of unnecessary exposure to other infections that further compromise the body's defenses, and sometimes surgical procedures. Family members and other contacts should also be assessed for symptoms by public health practitioners and treated accordingly.

The recommended drug regimen for LTBI in children and adolescents includes a daily dose of isoniazid (INH) for 9 months or, if daily treatment is not possible, 2 times per week with directly observed therapy (DOT). *DOT* means that a health care worker or other responsible, mutually agreed-on individual is present when medications are administered to the patient. An alternative schedule for children ages 12 years and older is to administer INH and rifapentine, once a week under strict DOT for 12 weeks (AAP Committee on Infectious Diseases, 2012).

For the child with clinically active TB disease, the goal is to achieve sterilization of the tuberculous lesion. Recommended drug therapy for treating TB disease includes combinations of INH, rifampin, pyrazinamide (PZA), and ethambutol. The AAP (AAP Committee on Infectious Diseases, 2012) recommends a 6-month regimen consisting of INH, rifampin, ethambutol, and PZA given daily for the first 2 months followed by INH and rifampin given 2 or 3 times a week by DOT for the remaining 4 months. DOT decreases the rates of relapse, treatment failures, and drug resistance and is recommended for treatment of children and adolescents with TB in the United States.

If the child is suspected of having multidrug-resistant TB, optimal therapy should consist of 4 antituberculous drugs to which the child's disease is susceptible administered daily (DOT) for 12 to 24 months from the time of culture conversion (AAP Committee on Infectious Diseases, 2012). Optimal therapy for TB in children with HIV infection has not been established, and consultation with a specialist is advised.

Surgical procedures may be required to remove the source of infection in tissues that are inaccessible to pharmacotherapy or that are destroyed by the disease. Orthopedic procedures may be performed for correction of bone deformities, and bronchoscopy may be done for removal of a tuberculous granulomatous polyp.

Prognosis. Most children recover from primary TB infection and are often unaware of its presence. However, very young children have a higher incidence of disseminated disease. TB is a serious disease during the first 2 years of life, during adolescence, and in children who are HIV positive. Except in cases of tuberculous meningitis, death seldom occurs in treated children. Antibiotic therapy has decreased the death rate and the hematogenous spread from primary lesions.

Prevention

The only definite means to prevent TB is to avoid contact with the tubercle bacillus. Maintaining an optimal state of health with adequate nutrition and avoiding fatigue and debilitating infections promote natural resistance but do not prevent infection. Pasteurization and routine testing of milk and elimination of diseased cattle have reduced the incidence of bovine TB.

Limited immunity can be produced by administration of bacille Calmette-Guérin (BCG), a live vaccine containing bovine bacilli with reduced virulence (attenuated). In most instances, positive tuberculin reactions develop after inoculation with BCG. The distribution of BCG is controlled by local or state health departments, and the vaccine is not used extensively, even in areas with a high prevalence of disease. BCG vaccination is not generally recommended for use in the United States. However, it may be recommended for long-term protection of infants and children with negative TST results who are not infected with HIV and who (1) are at high risk for continuing exposure to persons with infectious pulmonary TB or (2) are continuously exposed to persons with TB who have bacilli resistance to both INH and rifampin when the child cannot be removed from the environment or given antituberculosis drug therapy (AAP Committee on Infectious Diseases, 2012).

CARE MANAGEMENT

Children with TB receive their nursing care in ambulatory settings, outpatient departments, schools, and public health settings. Most children are not contagious and require only Standard Precautions. Children with no cough and negative sputum smears can be hospitalized in a regular patient room. However, Airborne Precautions and a negative-pressure room are required for children who are contagious and hospitalized with active TB disease. Infection control for hospital personnel in contagious cases should include the use of a personally fitted air-purifying N95 or N100 respirator (PAPR) for all patient contacts. (See AAP Committee on Infectious Diseases, 2012, for additional information on isolation of children with suspected or confirmed TB.)

Asymptomatic children with TB can attend school or day care facilities if they are receiving pharmacotherapy. They can return to regular activities as soon as effective therapy has been instituted, adherence to therapy has been documented, and clinical symptoms have diminished. Children receiving pharmacotherapy for TB can receive measles and other age-appropriate live virus vaccines unless they are receiving high-dose corticosteroids, are severely ill, or have specific contraindications to immunization.

Skin tests must be carried out correctly to obtain accurate results. The tuberculin is injected intradermally with the bevel of the needle pointing upward. A wheal 6 to 10 mm in diameter should form between the layers of the skin when the solution is injected properly. If the wheal is not formed, the procedure is repeated. The volar or dorsal surface of the forearm is the usual injection site. The reaction to the skin test is determined in 48 to 72 hours; reactions occurring after 72 hours should be measured and considered the result. The size of the transverse diameter of induration, not the erythema, is measured. The diameter transverse to the long axis of the forearm is the only one standardized for measurement purposes (AAP Committee on Infectious Diseases, 2012).

Sputum specimens are difficult or impossible to obtain from infants and young children because they swallow any mucus coughed from the lower respiratory tract. The best means for obtaining material for smears or culture is by gastric washing (i.e., aspiration of lavaged contents from the fasting stomach with a nasogastric tube). The procedure is carried out and the specimen obtained early in the morning before the customary breakfast time. In some cases, an induced sputum specimen may be obtained by administering aerosolized normal saline for 10 to 15 minutes followed by chest percussion and postural drainage and suctioning of the nasopharynx for sputum collection.

Because the success of therapy depends on compliance with the drug regimen, parents are instructed about the importance and rationale for DOT. Case finding in the community and follow-up of known contacts—individuals from whom the affected child may have acquired the disease and persons who may have been exposed to the child with the disease—are essential control measures.

PULMONARY DYSFUNCTION CAUSED BY NONINFECTIOUS IRRITANTS

Foreign Body Aspiration

Small children characteristically explore matter with their mouth and are prone to aspirate foreign bodies (FBs). Small children also place objects such as beads, paper clips, small magnets, or food items in the nose, which can easily be aspirated into the trachea. FB aspiration can occur at any age but is most common in children 1 to 3 years of age. Severity is determined by the location, type of object aspirated, and extent of obstruction. For example, dry vegetable matter (e.g., a seed, nut, or piece of carrot or popcorn) that does not dissolve and that may swell when wet creates a particularly difficult problem. The high fat content of potato chips and peanuts may cause the added risk for lipoid pneumonia. "Fun foods" are the worst offenders in terms of potential for choking. Offending foods in the order of frequency of choking are hot dogs, round candies, peanuts or other nuts, grapes, cookies or biscuits, other meats, caramels, carrots, peas, apples, celery, popcorn, sunflower seeds, orange seeds, cherry pits, watermelon seeds, gum, and peanut butter. Other items include burst latex balloons, plastic or glass beads, marbles, pen or marker caps, button or disc batteries, and coins. Objects such as small lithium or cadmium batteries may cause esophageal or tracheal corrosion.

Diagnostic Evaluation

The diagnosis of FB aspiration is suspected on the basis of the history and physical signs. Initially, a FB in the air passages produces choking, gagging, wheezing, or coughing. Laryngotracheal obstruction most commonly causes dyspnea, cough, stridor, and hoarseness because of decreased air entry. Up to half of all children with FB ingestion may be asymptomatic. Cyanosis may occur if the obstruction becomes worse. Bronchial obstruction usually produces cough (frequently paroxysmal), wheezing, asymmetric breath sounds, decreased airway entry, and dyspnea. When an object is lodged in the larynx, the child is unable to speak or breathe. If the obstruction progresses, the child's face may become livid, and if the obstruction

is total, the child can become unconscious and die of asphyxiation. If obstruction is partial, hours, days, or even weeks may pass without symptoms after the initial period. Secondary symptoms are related to the anatomic area in which the object is lodged and are usually caused by a persistent respiratory tract infection distal to the obstruction. FB aspiration should also be suspected in the presence of acute or chronic pulmonary lesions. Often, by the time secondary symptoms appear, the parents have forgotten the initial episode of coughing and gagging. Nasal FBs often manifest by unilateral purulent drainage that does not improve with time.

Radiographic examination reveals opaque FBs but is of limited use in localizing nonradiographic matter. Bronchoscopy is required for a definitive diagnosis of objects in the larynx and trachea. Fluoroscopic examination is valuable in detecting FBs in the bronchi. The mainstay of diagnosis and management of FBs is endoscopy. If there is doubt about the presence of an FB, endoscopy can be diagnostic and therapeutic.

Therapeutic Management

Foreign body aspiration may result in life-threatening airway obstruction, especially in infants because of the small diameters of their airways. Current recommendations for the emergency treatment of the choking child include the use of abdominal thrusts for children older than 1 year and back blows and chest thrusts for children younger than 1 year.

A FB is rarely coughed up spontaneously. Usually it must be removed instrumentally by endoscopy. Endoscopy and bronchoscopy require sedation with an agent such as IV propofol or midazolam. The procedure is carried out as quickly as possible because the progressive local inflammatory process triggered by the foreign material hampers removal. A chemical pneumonia soon develops, and vegetable matter begins to macerate within a few days, making it even more difficult to remove. After removal of the FB, the child is usually observed for any complications such as laryngeal edema and then discharged home within a matter of hours if vital signs are stable and recovery is satisfactory.

Prevention

Nurses are in a position to teach prevention in a variety of settings. They can educate parents singly or in groups about hazards of aspiration in relation to the developmental level of their children and encourage them to teach their children safety. Parents should be cautioned about behaviors that their children might imitate (e.g., holding foreign objects, such as pins, nails, and toothpicks, in their lips or mouth). (Prevention based on the child's age is discussed in Chapters 31 and 32.)

CARE MANAGEMENT

A major role of nurses caring for a child who has aspirated an FB is to recognize the signs of FB aspiration, observe for worsening of respiratory symptoms, and implement immediate measures to relieve an emergency obstruction. Choking on food or other material should not be fatal. Back blows and chest thrusts in infants and abdominal thrusts in children are simple procedures that can be used by both health care professionals and laypersons to save lives. To aid a child who is choking, nurses must recognize the signs of distress. A blind sweep of the child's mouth should never be performed because it may lodge the agent farther into the airway. Not every child who gags or coughs while eating is truly choking.

Aspiration Pneumonia

Aspiration pneumonia occurs when food, secretions, inert materials, volatile compounds, or liquids enter the lung and cause inflammation and a chemical pneumonitis. Aspiration of fluid or foods is a particular hazard in the child who has difficulty with swallowing or is unable to swallow because of paralysis, weakness, debility, congenital anomalies, or absent cough reflex or in the child who is force-fed, especially while crying or breathing rapidly. Clinical signs of the aspiration of oral secretions may not be distinguishable from those of other forms of acute bacterial pneumonia. For example, if vegetable matter has been aspirated, manifestations may not appear for several weeks after the event. Classic symptoms include an increasing cough or fever with foul-smelling sputum, deteriorating oxygenation, evidence of infiltrates on chest radiographs, and other signs of lower airway involvement. These deviations may persist for weeks, however, while the child starts to feel better. Rarely, aspiration causes immediate death from asphyxia; more often, the irritated mucous membrane becomes a site for secondary bacterial infection. In addition to fluids, food, vomitus, and nasopharyngeal secretions, other substances that may cause pneumonia are hydrocarbons, lipids, powder, and contrast dye or barium. The severity of the lung injury depends on the pH of the aspirated material.

CARE MANAGEMENT

Care of the child with aspiration pneumonia is the same as that described for the child with pneumonia from other causes. However, the major focus of nursing care is on prevention of aspiration. Proper feeding techniques should be carried out, and preventive measures should be used to prevent aspiration of any material that might enter the nasopharynx. The presence of a nasogastric feeding tube or a history of gastroesophageal reflux disease places the child at risk for aspiration. Nasogastric tubes used for feedings should be checked before the initiation of bolus feedings; continuous nasogastric tube feedings should also be evaluated periodically for proper tube placement. Children who are at risk for swallowing difficulties as a result of illness, physical debilitation, anesthesia, or sedation are kept on nothing by mouth (NPO) status until they can properly swallow fluids effectively. The child may receive nutrition by alternate means such as an enteral feeding tube. The child who is at risk for vomiting and incapable of protecting the airway should be positioned in a side-lying recovery position. Educating parents on its prevention is important.

Pulmonary Edema

Pulmonary edema (PE) is the movement of fluid into the alveoli and interstitium of the lungs caused by extravasation of fluid from the pulmonary vasculature (Mazor and Green, 2011). There are two main types of PE—cardiogenic and noncardiogenic.

Cardiogenic (hydrostatic, hemodynamic) PE is caused by an increase in pulmonary capillary pressure because of an increase in pulmonary venous pressure. It can be caused by excessive IV fluid administration, left ventricular failure, heart valve disorder (aortic regurgitation, aortic stenosis, mitral regurgitation), myocardial ischemia, myocarditis, sepsis, acute tachydysrhythmia, or coronary arteriosclerosis (Sovari and Ooi, 2008).

Noncardiogenic PE is caused by various conditions that result in increased pulmonary capillary permeability. Some subtypes of noncardiogenic PE include permeability PE (caused by ARDS or acute lung injury [ALI]), high altitude PE (caused by rapid ascension to heights above 12,000 feet), or neurogenic PE (after CNS insult such as seizures, head injury, or cerebral hemorrhage). Some less common forms of PE are reperfusion PE (after removal of thromboemboli from the lung or a lung transplant), reexpansion PE (caused by rapid reexpansion of a collapsed lung), or PE that results from opiate overdose (methadone or heroin), salicylate toxicity (chronic), aspiration (FB inhalation), inhalation injuries, near drowning, pulmonary embolism, viral infections, or pulmonary venoocclusive disease. Other causes include traumatic injury, organ dysfunction caused by sepsis, multiorgan failure, alcoholism or substance abuse, pregnancy (eclampsia), chronic renal impairment, malnutrition, hypertension, or a blood transfusion (transfusion-related ALI).

Pathophysiology

Fluid flows from the pulmonary vasculature into the alveolar interstitial space and then returns to the systemic circulation in a normal lung. Movement of this fluid is controlled by the net difference between hydrostatic and osmotic pressures and the permeability of the capillary membrane (Sovari and Ooi, 2008). Increased pulmonary hydrostatic pressure or increased permeability of the vascular membrane results in movement of fluid into the alveoli and interstitium of the lung. The pulmonary lymph system normally drains away any fluid from the alveoli, but when the amount of fluid present in the alveoli exceeds lymph drainage, PE occurs.

Symptoms include extreme shortness of breath, cyanosis, tachypnea, diminished breath sounds, anxiety, agitation, confusion, diaphoresis, orthopnea, respiratory crackles, expiratory wheezing (in young infants), heart murmur, third heart sound (S3) gallop, cool extremities, jugular venous distention, nocturnal dyspnea, cough, pink frothy sputum (if severe), tachycardia, hypertension, or hypotension (if caused by left ventricle dysfunction).

Therapeutic Management

Management of PE depends on the cause but can include oxygen therapy, peak end-expiratory pressure (PEEP) via continuous positive airway pressure (CPAP), and intubation with ventilatory support if respiratory failure occurs. If ventricular failure is the cause, medications such as diuretics, digoxin, positive inotropes, and vasodilators (nitroglycerin) may be started and the child may be placed on a fluid and sodium restriction. Morphine may be prescribed to relieve dyspnea. The primary goal of management is to determine why PE occurred and treat the underlying condition.

CARE MANAGEMENT

Nursing care of the child with PE is similar to that for any other acute respiratory condition. Pulse oximetry is monitored, and vital signs are observed closely for any deterioration. The nurse should note changes in oxygen saturation (Sao_2), end-tidal carbon dioxide (CO_2), and arterial blood gas (ABG) values. An ongoing assessment of the child's cardiopulmonary status is needed by checking lung sounds and observing respiratory rate, rhythm, depth, and effort. Oxygen, medications, and other respiratory treatments are administered as prescribed. Close monitoring of intake and output, electrolytes, and comfort is important. The child should be monitored for restlessness, anxiety, and air hunger. Placing the child in a high Fowler position may help with lung expansion. Because this position places pressure on bony prominences in the sacrum and hips, pressure areas must be relieved at intervals. Most of the care of PE occurs in the intensive care unit, which is anxiety provoking for the child and family. They should be given the opportunity to express their fears and anxieties and to ask questions. (For other nursing care activities, see the following section on ARDS and ALI.)

Acute Respiratory Distress Syndrome and Acute Lung Injury

ARDS and ALI are potentially life-threatening inflammatory lung conditions that may occur in both children and adults. The syndromes may be caused by direct injury to the lungs or by systemic insults that lead indirectly to lung injury, categorized by acute onset of bilateral infiltrates consistent with PE, but there is no indication of elevated left atrial pressure. They result in hypoxemia and respiratory failure. Sepsis, trauma, viral pneumonia, aspiration, fat emboli, drug overdose, reperfusion injury after lung transplantation, smoke inhalation, and near-drowning, among others, have been associated with ALI and ARDS. Both conditions are characterized by respiratory distress and hypoxemia that occur within 72 hours of a serious injury or surgery in a person with previously normal lungs. Acute pulmonary inflammation with alveolar capillary membrane destruction results in significant hypoxemia. Mechanical ventilation is often required.

Diagnostic criteria were established by the American European Consensus Conference (Bernard, Artigas, Brigham, et al., 1994) and include radiographic evidence of bilateral alveolar infiltrates, the absence of left-sided heart failure, and hypoxemia. Hypoxemia is expressed in terms of the ratio of partial pressure of oxygen (Pao_2) to the fraction of inspired oxygen (Fio_2) (P/F ratio). ALI is differentiated from the more severe syndrome of ARDS by the severity of hypoxemia. In ALI, the P/F ratio is less than or equal to 300; in ARDS, the P/F ratio is less than or equal to 200. ARDS is the more severe in the spectrum of illnesses in relation to the degree of hypoxemia.

Pathologically, the hallmark of ARDS is increased permeability of the alveolar-capillary membrane that results in PE. During the acute phase of ARDS, inflammatory mediators damage the alveolocapillary membrane, with an increasing pulmonary capillary permeability with resulting interstitial edema. Later stages are characterized by pneumocyte and fibrin infiltration of the alveoli, with the start of either the healing process or fibrosis. When fibrosis occurs, the child may demonstrate respiratory distress and the need for mechanical ventilation. In ARDS, the lungs become stiff as a result of surfactant inactivation; gas diffusion is impaired; and eventually, bronchiolar mucosal swelling and congestive atelectasis occur. The net effect is decreased functional residual capacity, pulmonary hypertension (see Chapter 42), and increased intrapulmonary right-to-left shunting of pulmonary blood flow. Surfactant secretion is reduced, and the atelectasis and fluid-filled alveoli provide an excellent medium for bacterial growth. Hypoxemia or increased work of breathing may require ventilatory support.

The child with ARDS may first demonstrate only symptoms caused by an injury or infection, but as the condition deteriorates, hyperventilation, tachypnea, increasing respiratory effort, cyanosis, and decreasing oxygen saturation occur. At times, the developing hypoxemia is not responsive to oxygen administration.

Treatment involves supportive measures to maintain adequate oxygenation and pulmonary perfusion, treatment of infection (or the precipitating cause), and maintenance of adequate cardiac output. After the underlying cause has been identified, specific treatment (e.g., antibiotics for infection) is initiated. Many patients require mechanical ventilatory support. This is usually achieved invasively (i.e., after endotracheal intubation), but occasionally noninvasive ventilation is used in milder cases. Patients requiring invasive mechanical ventilation usually require sedation, at least initially, to allow for ventilatory synchrony. Fluid administration to maintain adequate intravascular volume and end-organ perfusion must be balanced against the desire to decrease lung fluid to improve oxygenation. The provision of adequate nutrition, maintenance of patient comfort, and prevention of complications such as gastrointestinal ulceration are essential. Psychologic support of the patient and family is also important.

It has been demonstrated that inappropriate use of mechanical ventilatory support may worsen the lung injury by causing volutrauma, barotrauma, atelectrauma, and biotrauma to the injured lungs. Protective ventilatory strategies using low tidal volumes (6 mL/kg ideal body weight) have been demonstrated to improve outcomes in adults and theoretically are also appropriate in children. PEEP is applied to decrease atelectasis and maintain an "open" lung. Permissive hypercapnia may also be used. Other strategies used in the support of patients with ARDS include use of the prone position, inhaled nitric oxide, inhaled prostaglandins, high-frequency oscillatory ventilation, and extracorporeal membrane oxygenation (ECMO), although evidence to support these therapies is scant.

Prognosis

The prognosis for patients with ARDS is improving. Nonetheless, the mortality rate remains high, and in children, it ranges from 18% to 49% (Albuali, Singh, Fraser, et al., 2007; Randolph, 2009). The precipitating disorder influences the outcome; the worst prognosis is associated with uncontrolled sepsis, bone marrow transplantation, cancer, and multisystem involvement with hepatic failure. Children who recover may have persistent cough and exertional dyspnea.

CARE MANAGEMENT

The child with ARDS is cared for in the intensive care unit during the acute stages of illness. Nursing care involves close monitoring of oxygenation and respiratory status as well as assessment of cardiac output, perfusion, fluid and electrolyte balance, and renal function (urinary output). Acid-base status and pulse oximetry are important evaluation tools. Diuretics may be administered to reduce pulmonary fluid, and vasodilators may be administered to decrease pulmonary vascular pressure. Nutritional support is often required because of the prolonged acute phase of the illness. Nursing management also includes monitoring the effects of the numerous parenteral fluids and drugs used to stabilize the child and monitoring for changes in the child's hemodynamic status. Most children with ARDS require invasive monitoring via a central venous catheter. The nursing care of the child with ARDS also involves close observance of skin condition, prevention of skin breakdown by pressure area relief, and passive range of motion for prevention of muscle atrophy and contractures. Respiratory distress is a frightening situation for both the child and the parents, and attention to their psychologic needs is a major element in the care of these children. The child is often sedated during the acute phase of the illness, and weaning from sedation requires close monitoring for anxiety reduction and comfort.

Smoke Inhalation Injury

A number of noxious substances that may be inhaled are toxic to humans. They are primarily products of incomplete combustion and cause more deaths from fires than flame injuries. The severity of the injury depends on the nature of the substances generated by the material burned, whether the victim is confined in a closed space, and the duration of contact with the smoke. Three distinct syndromes of pulmonary complications may occur in children with inhalation injury: (1) early carbon monoxide (CO) poisoning, airway obstruction, and PE; (2) ARDS occurring at 24 to 48 hours or later in some cases; and (3) late complications of bronchopneumonia and pulmonary emboli (Antoon and Donovan, 2011). Smoke inhalation results in three types of injury: heat, chemical, and systemic.

Heat injury involves thermal injury to the upper airway. Air has low specific heat; therefore the injury goes no farther than the upper airway. Reflex closure of the glottis prevents injury to the lower airway.

Chemical injury involves gases that may be generated during the combustion of materials such as clothing, furniture, and floor coverings. Acids, alkalis, and their precursors in smoke can produce chemical burns. These substances can be carried deep into the respiratory tract, including the lower respiratory tract, in the form of insoluble gases. Soluble gases tend to dissolve in the upper respiratory tract.

Synthetic materials are especially toxic, producing gases such as oxides of sulfur and nitrogen, acetaldehyde, formaldehyde, hydrocyanic acid, and chlorine. Heated plastics are the source of extremely toxic vapors, including (1) chlorine and hydrochloric acid from polyvinylchloride, and (2) hydrocarbons, aldehydes, ketones, and acids from polyethylene. Irritant gases such as nitrous oxide and carbon dioxide combine with water in the lungs to form corrosive acids; aldehydes cause denaturation of proteins, cellular damage, and edema of pulmonary tissues. Chemical burns to the airways are similar to burns on the skin, except they are painless because the tracheobronchial tree is relatively insensitive to pain.

Inhalation of small amounts of noxious irritants produces alveolar and bronchiolar damage that can lead to obstructive bronchiolitis. Severe exposure causes further injury, including alveolocapillary damage with hemorrhage, necrotizing bronchiolitis, inhibited secretion of surfactant, and formation of hyaline membranes—manifestations of ARDS.

Systemic injury occurs from gases that are nontoxic to the airways (e.g., CO, hydrogen cyanide). However, these gases cause injury and death by interfering with or inhibiting cellular respiration. CO is responsible for more than half of all fatal inhalation poisonings in the United States. CO is a colorless, odorless gas with an affinity for hemoglobin 230 times greater than that of oxygen. When it enters the bloodstream, CO combines readily with hemoglobin to form carboxyhemoglobin (COHb). Because it is released less readily, tissue hypoxia reaches dangerous levels before oxygen is available to meet tissue needs.

Accidental CO poisoning is usually a result of exposure to fumes of heaters or smoke from structural fires, although poorly ventilated recreational vehicles with improperly operated or maintained gas lamps or stoves and cooking in underventilated areas with charcoal grills are also frequent causes. CO is produced by incomplete combustion of carbon or carbonaceous material such as wood or charcoal.

The signs and symptoms of CO poisoning are secondary to tissue hypoxia and vary with the level of COHb. Mild manifestations include headache, visual disturbances, irritability, and nausea; more severe intoxication causes confusion, hallucinations, ataxia, and coma. The bright, cherry red lips and skin often described are less often observed; pallor and cyanosis are seen more frequently.

Therapeutic Management

Treatment of children with smoke inhalation injury is largely symptomatic. The most widely accepted treatment is placing the child on humidified 100% oxygen as quickly as possible and monitoring for signs of respiratory distress and impending failure. Baseline ABGs and COHb levels are obtained. Pao_2 may be within normal limits unless there is marked respiratory depression. If CO poisoning is confirmed, 100% oxygen is continued until COHb levels fall to the nontoxic range of about 10%. If CO poisoning is severe, the patient may benefit from hyperbaric oxygen therapy. Hyperbaric oxygen therapy may be useful in the treatment of neurologic complications related to CO poisoning. Pulmonary care may be facilitated by bronchodilators, inhaled corticosteroids, humidification, and chest percussion and postural drainage to enhance the removal of necrotic material, minimize bronchoconstriction, and avoid atelectasis. Bronchoscopy may be needed to clear heavy secretions.

Respiratory distress may occur early in the course of smoke inhalation as a result of hypoxia, or patients who are breathing well on admission may suddenly develop respiratory distress. Therefore intubation equipment should be readily available. Transient edema of the airways can occur at any level in the tracheobronchial tree. Assessment and localization of the obstruction should be accomplished before severe swelling of the head, neck, or oropharynx occurs. Intubation is often necessary when (1) severe burns in the area of the nose, mouth, and face increase the likelihood of developing oropharyngeal edema and obstruction; (2) vocal cord edema causes obstruction; (3) the patient has difficulty handling secretions; and (4) progressive respiratory distress requires artificial ventilation. Controversy surrounds tracheostomy, but many prefer this procedure when the obstruction is proximal to the larynx and reserve nasotracheal intubation for lower tract involvement.

CARE MANAGEMENT

Nursing care of the child with inhalation injury is the same as that for any child with respiratory distress. Vital signs and other respiratory assessments (oxygenation, work of breathing, acid-base status) are performed frequently, and the pulmonary status is carefully observed and maintained. Chest physical therapy is often part of the therapy, as well as mechanical ventilation if needed. Fluid requirements for children experiencing inhalation injury are greater than for those with surface burns alone; however, one concern is the development of PE. Therefore accurate monitoring of fluid intake and output is essential.

In addition to observation and management of the physical aspects of inhalation injury, the nurse also deals with the psychologic needs of a frightened child and distraught parents. As with any accidental injury, the parents may feel overwhelming guilt even

---

> **! NURSING ALERT**
>
> The oxygen saturation (Sao_2) obtained by pulse oximetry will be normal because the device measures only oxygenated and deoxygenated hemoglobin; it does not measure dysfunctional hemoglobin, such as COHb.

when the injury occurred through no fault of their own. Parents need support, reassurance, and information regarding the child's condition, treatment, and progress.

The nurse can provide anticipatory guidance and educate families on prevention of inhalation injuries and the importance of CO detectors in the home.

Environmental Tobacco Smoke Exposure

Numerous investigations indicate that parental or family smoking is an important cause of morbidity in children. Children exposed to (secondhand) passive or environmental tobacco smoke have an increased number of respiratory illnesses, increased respiratory symptoms (i.e., cough, sputum, and wheezing), and reduced performance on pulmonary function tests (PFTs). AOM and OME are also increased in children who have smoking parents. Indoor exposure to tobacco smoke has been linked to asthma in children. Among children with asthma, there is an association between parental cigarette smoking and asthma exacerbations, trips to the emergency department (ED), medication use, and impaired recovery after hospitalization for acute asthma. Maternal cigarette smoking is associated with increased respiratory symptoms and illnesses in children; decreased fetal growth; increased births of low-birth-weight, preterm, and stillborn infants; and a greater incidence of sudden infant death syndrome (SIDS). Antenatal maternal smoking has emerged as a significant risk factor for SIDS (AAP Task Force on Sudden Infant Death Syndrome, 2005; Zhang and Wang, 2012). The risk for diagnosis of early-onset asthma in the first 3 years of life is associated with in utero exposure to maternal smoking; grandmaternal smoking was also associated with an increased risk for early-onset asthma in the grandchild even if the mother did not smoke during pregnancy (Li, Langholz, Salam, et al., 2005). Exposure to tobacco smoke during childhood may also contribute to the development of chronic lung disease in the adult.

CARE MANAGEMENT

Nurses must provide information about the hazards of environmental smoke exposure in all of their interactions with children and their family members. This information is especially important for children with respiratory and allergic illnesses. In families in which smokers refuse to quit, appropriate guidance is provided for reducing smoke in the child's environment (see Family-Centered Care box). Nurses should set an example for children and families and become advocates for "no smoking" ordinances in public places, prohibition of advertising tobacco products in the media, and inclusion of health warnings of sidestream smoke on tobacco products.* Nurses have an important role in providing parents with affordable smoking cessation education resources, including the appropriate use of smoking cessation pharmacologic aids (Sheahan and Free, 2005). Nurses also have a role in educating adolescents about avoiding using tobacco products or smoking marijuana.

LONG-TERM RESPIRATORY DYSFUNCTION

Asthma

Asthma is a chronic inflammatory disorder of the airways characterized by recurring symptoms, airway obstruction, and bronchial hyperresponsiveness (National Asthma Education and Prevention

---

FAMILY-CENTERED CARE

Decreasing Childhood Exposure to Environmental Tobacco Smoke*

- Maintain a smoke-free home.
- Avoid exposing an infant to environmental smoke.
- Use an air-purifying filter in the home where smoking is unavoidable.
- Encourage exclusive breastfeeding for the first 6 months.
- If smoking cessation is in progress by breastfeeding mother, suggest she change upper clothing after smoking and before breastfeeding infant.
- Do not smoke around children.
- Change clothing after smoking and before holding an infant in close proximity.
- Restrict smoking to an isolated area of the house where the children do not play or sleep.
- Do not smoke in motor vehicles with children.
- Do not smoke in rooms children use.
- Do not allow visitors to smoke in the home.

*For further information on the effects of secondhand smoke on child health, go to www.cdc.gov/tobacco/secondhand_smoke/index.htm.

Program [NAEPP], 2007). In susceptible children, inflammation causes recurrent episodes of wheezing, breathlessness, chest tightness, and cough, especially at night or in the early morning. The airflow limitation or obstruction is reversible either spontaneously or with treatment. Inflammation causes an increase in bronchial hyperresponsiveness to a variety of stimuli (NAEPP, 2007). Recognition of the key role of inflammation has made the use of antiinflammatory agents, especially inhaled corticosteroids, a major component in the treatment of asthma.

Asthma is classified into four categories based on the symptom indicators of disease severity. These categories are *intermittent, mild persistent, moderate persistent,* and *severe persistent.* Symptoms increase in frequency or intensity until the last category of severe persistent asthma (Box 40-13). These categories provide a stepwise approach to the pharmacologic management, environmental control, and educational interventions needed for each category (NAEPP, 2007). The stepwise approach is meant to assist in the clinical decision-making approach to effective individualized management of the child's symptoms. These categories emphasize the multifaceted aspect of the disease for consideration of effects on present quality of life and functional capacity and the future risk for adverse events (NAEPP, 2007).

Asthma prevalence, morbidity, and mortality are increasing in the United States, especially among African Americans (Akinbami, Moorman, Garbe, et al., 2009). These increases may result from worsening air pollution, poor access to medical care, or underdiagnosis and undertreatment. Asthma is the most common chronic disease of childhood, the primary cause of school absences, and the third leading cause of hospitalizations in children younger than 15 years. Although the onset of asthma may occur at any age, 80% to 90% of children have their first symptoms before 4 or 5 years of age. Boys are affected more frequently than girls until adolescence, when the trend reverses.

Etiology

Studies of children with asthma indicate that allergies influence both the persistence and the severity of the disease. In fact, **atopy,** or the

---

*For further information on the effects of secondhand smoke on child health, go to www.cdc.gov/Features/WorldCancerDay.

BOX 40-13 ASTHMA SEVERITY CLASSIFICATION IN CHILDREN: AGES 0 TO 11 YEARS*

Step 5 or 6: Severe Persistent Asthma
- Continual symptoms throughout the day
- Frequent nighttime symptoms (>1 time/wk ages 0-4 years and 7 nights/wk, ages 5 years and older)
- PEF: <60%
- FEV_1: <75% of predicted value
- Interference with normal activity: extremely limited
- Use of short-acting β-agonist for symptom control: several times a day

Step 3 or 4: Moderate Persistent Asthma
- Daily symptoms
- Nighttime symptoms: 3 to 4 times a month (ages 0-4 years), >1/wk but not nightly (ages 5-11 years)
- PEF: 60% to 80% of predicted value (ages 5 years and older)
- FEV_1: 75% to 80% (ages 5 years and older)
- PEF variability: >30%
- Interference with normal activity: some limitation
- Use of short-acting β-agonist for symptom control: daily

Step 2: Mild Persistent Asthma
- Symptoms >2 times/wk but <1 time/day
- Nighttime symptoms: 1 to 2 times a month (ages 0-4 years), 3 to 4 times a month (ages 5-11 years)
- PEF or FEV_1: ≥80% of predicted value
- PEF variability: 20% to 30%
- Interference with normal activity: minor limitation
- Use of short-acting β-agonist for symptom control: >2 days/wk but not daily

Step 1: Intermittent Asthma
- Symptoms ≤2 days/wk
- Nighttime symptoms (awakenings): ≤2 nights per month
- PEF or FEV_1: ≤80% of predicted value
- PEF variability: <20%
- Interference with normal activity: none
- Use of short-acting β-agonist for symptom control: <2 days/wk

From National Asthma Education and Prevention Program (NAEPP): *Guidelines for the diagnosis and management of asthma: summary report 2007*, from www.nhlbi.nih.gov/guidelines/asthma/index.htm. *FEV₁*, Forced expiratory volume in 1 second; *PEF*, peak expiratory flow.
*The presence of one clinical feature of severity is sufficient to place a patient in that category. An individual should be assigned to the most severe grade in which any feature occurs. The characteristics in this box are general and may overlap because asthma is highly variable. An individual's classification may change over time. Risk factors for each category are not presented in this box. See the original table shown in the 2007 NAEPP reference for additional classification data. Asthma treatment should not be based on this box.

BOX 40-14 TRIGGERS TENDING TO PRECIPITATE OR AGGRAVATE ASTHMATIC EXACERBATIONS

- Allergens
  - Outdoor—Trees, shrubs, weeds, grasses, molds, pollens, air pollution, spores
  - Indoor—Dust or dust mites, mold, cockroach antigen
- Irritants—Tobacco smoke, wood smoke, odors, sprays
- Exposure to occupational chemicals
- Exercise
- Cold air
- Changes in weather or temperature
- Environmental change—Moving to new home, starting new school, etc.
- Colds and infections
- Animals—Cats, dogs, rodents, horses
- Medications—Aspirin, nonsteroidal antiinflammatory drugs (NSAIDs), antibiotics, β-blockers
- Strong emotions—Fear, anger, laughing, crying
- Conditions—Gastroesophageal reflux, tracheoesophageal fistula
- Food additives—Sulfite preservatives
- Foods—Nuts, milk/dairy products
- Endocrine factors—Menses, pregnancy, thyroid disease

(Box 40-14). Evidence shows that viral respiratory infections, including RSV infection, may also have a significant role in the development and expression of asthma (NAEPP, 2007).

Pathophysiology

There is general agreement that inflammation contributes to heightened airway reactivity in asthma. The mechanisms contributing to airway inflammation are multiple and involve a number of different pathways. It is unlikely that asthma is caused by either a single cell or a single inflammatory mediator; rather, it appears that asthma results from complex interactions among inflammatory cells, mediators, and the cells and tissues present in the airways (NAEPP, 2007). However, recognition of the importance of inflammation has made the use of antiinflammatory agents a key component of asthma therapy.

Another important component of asthma is bronchospasm and obstruction. The mechanisms responsible for the obstructive symptoms in asthma include (1) inflammatory response to stimuli; (2) airway edema and accumulation and secretion of mucus; (3) spasm of the smooth muscle of the bronchi and bronchioles, which decreases the caliber of the bronchioles; and (4) airway remodeling, which causes permanent cellular changes (NAEPP, 2007) (Fig. 40-4).

Airflow is determined by the size of the airway lumen, degree of bronchial wall edema, mucus production, smooth muscle contraction, and muscle hypertrophy. Bronchial constriction is a normal reaction to foreign stimuli; however, with asthma, it is abnormally severe, producing impaired respiratory function. Because the bronchi normally dilate and elongate during inspiration and contract and shorten on expiration, the respiratory difficulty is more pronounced during the expiratory phase of respiration.

Increased resistance in the airway causes forced expiration through the narrowed lumen. The volume of air trapped in the lungs increases as airways are functionally closed at a point between the alveoli and the lobar bronchi. This trapping of gas

genetic predisposition for the development of an immunoglobulin E (IgE)–mediated response to common aeroallergens, is the strongest identifiable predisposing factor for developing asthma (NAEPP, 2007). However, 20% to 40% of children with asthma have no evidence of allergic disease. In addition to allergens, other substances and conditions can serve as triggers that may exacerbate asthma

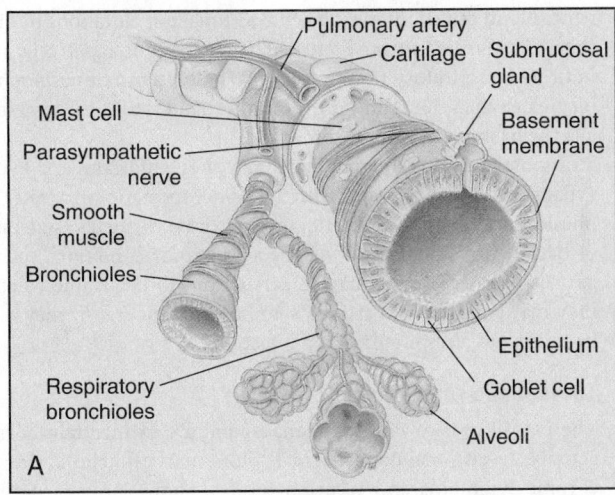
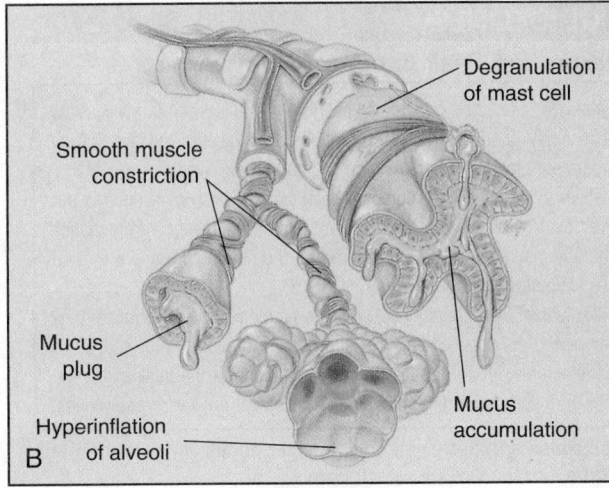

FIG 40-4 Airway obstruction caused by asthma. **A,** A normal lung. **B,** Bronchial asthma: thick mucus, mucosal edema, and smooth muscle spasm causing obstruction of small airways; breathing becomes labored, and expiration is difficult. (Adapted from Des Jardins T, Burton GG: *Clinical manifestations and assessment of respiratory disease,* ed 3, St Louis, 1995, Mosby.)

forces the individual to breathe at higher and higher lung volumes. Consequently, the person with asthma fights to inspire sufficient air. This expenditure of effort for breathing causes fatigue, decreased respiratory effectiveness, and increased oxygen consumption. The inspiration occurring at higher lung volumes hyperinflates the alveoli and reduces the effectiveness of the cough. As the severity of obstruction increases, there is a reduced alveolar ventilation with carbon dioxide retention; hypoxemia; respiratory acidosis; and, eventually, respiratory failure.

Chronic inflammation may also cause permanent damage (airway remodeling) to airway structures, which cannot be prevented by and is not responsive to current treatments (NAEPP, 2007).

Diagnostic Evaluation

The classic manifestations of asthma are dyspnea, wheezing, and coughing. An attack may develop gradually or appear abruptly and may be preceded by a URI. The age of the child is often a significant factor because the first attack frequently occurs before the age of 5 years, with some children manifesting clinical signs and symptoms in infancy. In infancy, an attack usually follows a respiratory infection. Some children may experience a prodromal itching at the front of the neck or over the upper part of the back just before an attack, especially if the attack is related to allergies (Box 40-15).

! NURSING ALERT

Shortness of breath with air movement in the chest restricted to the point of absent breath sounds (silent chest) accompanied by a sudden rise in respiratory rate is an ominous sign indicating ventilatory failure and imminent respiratory arrest.

The diagnosis is determined primarily on the basis of clinical manifestations, history, physical examination, and, to a lesser extent, laboratory tests. Generally, chronic cough in the absence of infection or diffuse wheezing during the expiratory phase of respiration is sufficient to establish a diagnosis.

Pulmonary function tests provide an objective method of evaluating the presence and degree of lung disease, as well as the response

BOX 40-15 CLINICAL MANIFESTATIONS OF ASTHMA

Cough
- Hacking, paroxysmal, irritative, and nonproductive
- Becomes rattling and productive of frothy, clear, gelatinous sputum

Respiratory-Related Signs
- Shortness of breath
- Prolonged expiratory phase
- Audible wheeze
- May have a malar flush and red ears
- Lips deep dark red color
- Possible progression to cyanosis of nail beds or circumoral cyanosis
- Restlessness
- Apprehension
- Sweating may be prominent as the attack progresses
- Posture—Older children may sit upright with shoulders in a hunched-over position, hands on the bed or chair, and arms braced (tripod position)
- Speech—May speak in short, panting, broken phrases

Chest
- Hyperresonance on percussion
- Coarse, loud breath sounds
- Wheezes throughout the lung fields
- Prolonged expiration
- Crackles
- Generalized inspiratory and expiratory wheezing; increasingly high pitched

With Repeated Episodes
- Barrel chest
- Elevated shoulders
- Use of accessory muscles of respiration
- Facial appearance: flattened malar bones, circles beneath the eyes, narrow nose, prominent upper teeth

GUIDELINES

Interpreting Peak Expiratory Flow Rates*

- Green (80% to 100% of personal best) signals *all clear*. Asthma is under reasonably good control. No symptoms are present, and the routine treatment plan for maintaining control can be followed.
- Yellow (50% to 79% of personal best) signals *caution*. Asthma is not well controlled. An acute exacerbation may be present. Maintenance therapy may need to be increased. Call the health care practitioner if the child stays in this zone.
- Red (below 50% of personal best) signals a *medical alert*. Severe airway narrowing may be occurring. A short-acting bronchodilator should be administered. Notify the health care practitioner if the peak expiratory flow rate does not return immediately and stay in yellow or green zones.

*These zones are guidelines only. Specific zones and management should be individualized for each child.

to therapy. Spirometry can generally be performed reliably on children by the age of 5 or 6 years. The NAEPP (2007) recommends that spirometry testing be done at the time of initial assessment of asthma, after treatment is initiated and symptoms have stabilized, and at least every 1 to 2 years to assess the maintenance of airway function.

Another measurement to consider is the peak expiratory flow rate (PEFR), which measures the maximum flow of air that can be forcefully exhaled in 1 second. PEFR is measured in liters per minute using a peak expiratory flow meter (PEFM). Three zones of measurement are typically used to interpret PEFR. The zone system is patterned after a traffic light to make the categories easy to understand and remember (see Guidelines box). Each child needs to establish his or her personal best value. A personal best value should be established during a 2- to 3-week period when the child's asthma is stable. During this period, the child records the PEFR at least twice a day. After the personal best value has been established, the child's current PEFR on any occasion can be compared with the personal best value. Although it can be a helpful tool in assessing a child's asthma control, it is important to note that its results depend on the child's ability to use the PEFM and willingness to participate. In some cases, a low PEFR may not truly mean that the child's asthma is poorly controlled. Each individual child's PEFR varies according to age, height, gender, and race.

Bronchoprovocation testing—direct exposure of the mucous membranes to a suspected antigen in increasing concentrations— helps identify inhaled allergens. Exposure to methacholine (methacholine challenge), histamine, or cold or dry air may be performed to assess airway responsiveness or reactivity. Exercise challenges may be used to identify children with exercise-induced bronchospasm. These tests are highly specific and sensitive and should be done under close observation in a qualified laboratory or clinic.

Skin prick testing (SPT) and serologic testing (with quantification of sIgE) for allergen-specific immunoglobulin E (sIgE) may be used to identify environmental allergens that trigger asthma (Sicherer, Wood, and AAP Section on Allergy and Immunology, 2012). It is recommended that all patients with year-round asthma symptoms be tested with skin tests or laboratory blood analysis to determine sensitization to perennial allergens (e.g., house dust mites, cats, dogs, cockroaches, molds, and fungus) (NAEPP, 2007).

In addition to these tests, other tests may be performed, including laboratory tests (complete blood count [CBC] with differential) and chest radiographs. The CBC may show a slight elevation in the white blood cell count during acute asthma, but elevations to more than 12,000/mm^3 or an increased percentage of band cells may indicate a respiratory tract infection. The presence of eosinophilia of greater than 500/mm^3, on the other hand, tends to suggest an allergic or inflammatory disorder.

Frontal and lateral radiographs may show infiltrates and hyperexpansion of the airways, with the anteroposterior diameter on physical examination indicating an increased diameter (suggestive of barrel chest). Additional diagnostic tests for conditions such as gastroesophageal reflux may be carried out to determine whether they may contribute to asthma symptoms. Radiography may assist in ruling out a respiratory tract infection.

Therapeutic Management

The overall goals of asthma management are to maintain normal activity levels, maintain normal pulmonary function, prevent chronic symptoms and recurrent exacerbations, provide optimal drug therapy with minimal or no adverse effects, and assist the child in living as normal and happy a life as possible. This includes facilitating the child's social adjustments in the family, school, and community and normal participation in recreational activities and sports. To accomplish these goals, several treatment principles need to be followed (NAEPP, 2007):

- A continuous care approach with regular visits to the health care provider is necessary to control symptoms and prevent exacerbations.
- Prevention of exacerbations includes avoiding triggers, avoiding allergens, and using medications as needed.
- Therapy includes efforts to reduce underlying inflammation and to relieve or prevent symptomatic airway narrowing.
- Therapy includes patient education, environmental control, pharmacologic management, and the use of objective measures to monitor the severity of disease and guide the course of therapy.

Allergen Control. Nonpharmacologic therapy is aimed at the prevention and reduction of exposure to airborne allergens and irritants. House dust mites and other components of house dust are frequent agents identified in children who are allergic to inhalants. The cockroach, another common household inhabitant, is an important allergen in many locations. Exterminating live cockroaches, carefully cleaning kitchen floors and cabinets, putting food away after eating, and taking trash out in the evening are essential measures to control cockroaches. The mouse allergen is the most recent allergen to be identified in the homes of inner-city children with asthma. The role of cat and dog dander in allergen-induced asthma has also been studied. Although some studies suggest sensitized persons should carefully evaluate having such pets in the household, the overall data are inconsistent on the effect of cat or dog exposure and subsequent asthma development (Chen, Tischer, Schnappinger, et al., 2010). Additional sources of pollutants include ozone, particulate matter produced by tobacco smoke, woodburning stoves, pesticides, lead, mold spores, nitrogen dioxide, and sulfur dioxide; these are believed to contribute to asthma morbidity in children and should be avoided or minimized. Living in homes close to busy roads, damp homes with mold, and exposure to tobacco smoke are significant contributing factors in the development of asthma in infants and small children (Heinrich, 2011). Recommendations for controlling allergens are found in the Patient Teaching box.

Skin testing identifies specific allergens so steps can be taken to eliminate or avoid them. Often, simply removing the offending environmental allergens or irritants (e.g., removing carpeting from the

PATIENT TEACHING

"Allergy-Proofing" the Home and Community

- Keep humidity between 30% and 50%; use dehumidifier or air conditioner if available; keep air conditioners clean and free of mold; do not use vaporizers or humidifiers.
- Encase pillows in zippered allergen-impermeable covers or wash pillows in hot water every week.
- Encase mattress and box springs in zippered allergen-impermeable cover.
- Use foam rubber mattress and pillows or Dacron pillows and synthetic blankets.
- Wash bed linens every 7 to 10 days in hot water (at least 54.4° C).
- Encase polyester comforters in allergen-impermeable covers or wash in hot water (at least 54.4° C) every week; if possible, do not use comforters and use cotton blankets.
- Store nothing under the bed; keep clothing in a closet with the door shut.
- Use washable window shades; avoid heavy curtains; if curtains are used, launder them frequently.
- Remove all carpeting if possible; if not possible, vacuum carpet once or twice a week while the child wears a mask; have child remain out of the room while vacuuming occurs and for 30 minutes after vacuuming.
- If possible, use a central vacuum cleaner with a collecting bag outside of the home or use cleaner filters (e.g., high-efficiency particulate air [HEPA] filters).

- Have air and heating ducts cleaned annually; change or clean air filters every 3 months; cover heating vents with filter material (e.g., cheesecloth) to prevent circulation of dust, especially when heat is turned on after summer.
- Use wipeable furniture (wood, plastic, vinyl, or leather) in place of upholstered furniture; avoid rattan or wicker furniture.
- Keep child indoors while lawn is being mowed, bushes/trees are being trimmed, or pollen count is high.
- Keep windows and doors closed during pollen season; use air conditioner if possible or go to places that are air conditioned, such as libraries and shopping malls, when the weather is hot.
- Wet-mop bare floors weekly; wet-dust and clean child's room weekly; child should not be present during cleaning activities.
- Limit or avoid child's exposure to tobacco and wood smoke; do not allow cigarette smoking in the house or car; select day care centers, play areas, and shopping malls that are smoke-free.
- Avoid cellar (basement) as a play area if it is damp, and use a dehumidifier in damp basement.
- Use pesticide sprays, roach bait traps, and boric acid powder to kill cockroaches; if living in an apartment or adjacent housing, encourage neighbors to work together to get rid of cockroaches and mice.
- Decrease child's exposure to air pollution from vehicle exhaust, outdoor grills, and environmental tobacco. Limit outside play on ozone alert days.

home of a child sensitive to mold and dust particles) will decrease the frequency of asthma episodes. Dehumidifiers or air conditioners may control nonspecific factors that trigger an episode, such as extremes of temperature.

Drug Therapy. Pharmacologic therapy is used to prevent and control asthma symptoms, reduce the frequency and severity of asthma exacerbations, and reverse airflow obstruction. A stepwise approach is recommended based on the severity of the child's asthma. Because inflammation is considered an early and persistent feature of asthma, therapy is directed toward long-term suppression of inflammation.

Asthma medications are categorized into two general classes: *long-term control medications* (preventive medications) to achieve and maintain control of inflammation; and *quick-relief medications* (rescue medications) to treat symptoms and exacerbations (NAEPP, 2007).

Quick-relief and long-term medications are often used in combination. Inhaled corticosteroids, cromolyn sodium and nedocromil, long-acting β_2-agonists, methylxanthines, and leukotriene modifiers are used as long-term control medications. Short-acting β_2-agonists, anticholinergics, and systemic corticosteroids are used as quick-relief or rescue medications.

Many asthma medications are given by inhalation with a nebulizer or a metered-dose inhaler (MDI). The MDI should always be attached to a spacer, especially when an inhaled corticosteroid is administered, to prevent yeast infections in the mouth. The spacer and holder can be equipped with a mask or a mouthpiece (Fig. 40-5). Pharmaceutical companies are currently mandated to produce inhalers that do not contain chlorofluorocarbons (CFCs) as the propellant because CFCs have been linked to damage and depletion of the earth's ozone level. Several currently available CFC-free MDI devices use dry powder (and are called *dry powder inhalers*); these include the Diskus inhaler and the Turbuhaler. These devices are

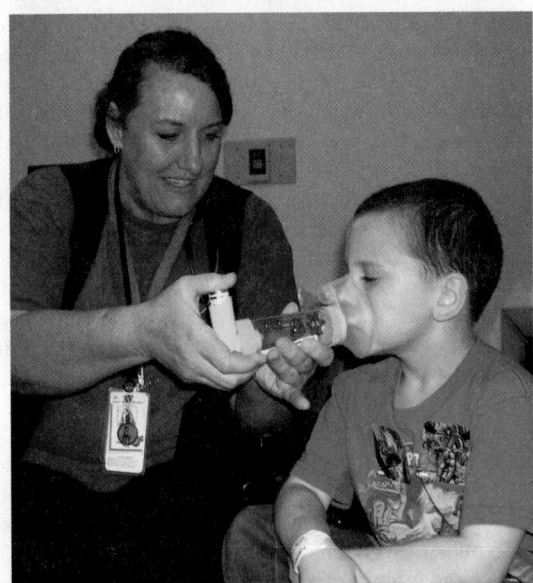

FIG 40-5 Child using metered-dose inhaler with spacer and face mask.

breath activated, and the child needs to inhale as quickly and deeply as possible to use them effectively. The Diskhaler and Aerosolizer are similar, but with the Aerosolizer, the medication must be loaded into the inhaler before use. Children who have difficulty using MDIs or other inhalers can receive their asthma medications via a nebulizer, which administers the medication via compressed air or oxygen. Children are instructed to breathe normally with the mouth open to provide a direct route to the trachea.

Corticosteroids are antiinflammatory drugs used to treat reversible airflow obstruction, control symptoms, and reduce bronchial hyperresponsiveness in chronic asthma. Inhaled corticosteroids are used as first-line therapy in children older than 5 years. Clinical studies of corticosteroids have indicated significant improvement of all asthma parameters, including decreases in symptoms, emergency visits, and medication requirements (NAEPP, 2007).

Corticosteroids may be administered parenterally, orally, or by inhalation. Oral medications are metabolized slowly, with an onset of action up to 3 hours after administration and peak effectiveness occurring within 6 to 12 hours. Oral systemic steroids may be given for short periods (e.g., 3- or 10-day "bursts") to gain prompt control of inadequately controlled persistent asthma or to manage severe persistent asthma. These drugs should be given in the lowest effective dose. These medications have few side effects (cough, dysphonia, and oral thrush), and strong evidence indicates that they improve the long-term outcomes for children of all ages with mild or moderate persistent asthma. Some studies have monitored children for 6 years after starting inhaled corticosteroids, and they indicate that when used at recommended doses, they do not have long-term significant effects on growth, bone mineral density, ocular toxicity, or suppression of the adrenal-pituitary axis (NAEPP, 2007). However, primary care providers should frequently monitor the growth of children and adolescents taking corticosteroids to assess the systemic effects of these drugs and make appropriate reductions in dosages or changes to other types of asthma therapy when necessary. Inhaled corticosteroids include budesonide and fluticasone.

β-Adrenergic agonists (short acting) (primarily albuterol, levalbuterol [Xopenex], and terbutaline) are used for treatment of acute exacerbations and for the prevention of exercise-induced bronchospasm. These drugs bind with the β-receptors on the smooth muscle of airways, where they activate adenylate cyclase and convert adenosine monophosphate (AMP) to cyclic AMP (cAMP). It is believed that the increased cAMP enhances binding of intracellular calcium to the cell membrane, reducing the availability of calcium and thus allowing smooth muscle to relax. Other effects of the drug help stabilize mast cells to prevent release of mediators. Most β-adrenergics used in asthma therapy affect predominantly the $β_2$-receptors, which help eliminate bronchospasm. $β_1$-receptor effects, such as increased heart rate and gastrointestinal disturbances, have been minimized. Albuterol is given orally (liquid or pill) or via a nebulizer or inhaler. Levalbuterol is given via nebulizer only. Terbutaline is given orally, via nebulizer, subcutaneously, or intravenously. The inhaled drugs have a more rapid onset of action than oral forms. Inhalation also reduces troublesome systemic side effects, including irritability, tremor, nervousness, and insomnia.

Salmeterol (Serevent) is a *long-acting $β_2$-agonist* (bronchodilator) that is used twice a day (no more frequently than every 12 hours). This drug is added to antiinflammatory therapy and used for long-term prevention of symptoms, especially nighttime symptoms, and exercise-induced bronchospasm. Salmeterol is not used in children younger than 12 years, and it is not used to treat acute symptoms or exacerbations. The 2007 NAEPP guidelines recommend the addition of a long-acting $β_2$-agonist (e.g., salmeterol) to a low- or medium-dosage inhaled corticosteroid to improve lung function and asthma symptoms and decrease the need for a short-acting $β_2$-agonist. Currently, the FDA is requiring studies be conducted by drug manufacturers to evaluate the safety of long-acting $β_2$-agonists (LABAs) when combined with inhaled corticosteroids versus inhaled corticosteroids alone. LABAs can increase the risk for severely worsening asthma symptoms, potentially leading to hospitalizations and death (Food and Drug Administration [FDA], 2011).

Theophylline is a methylxanthine drug used for decades to relieve symptoms and prevent asthma attacks; however, it is now used primarily in the ED when the child is not responding to maximal therapy. Therapeutic levels should be obtained with this drug because it has a narrow therapeutic window.

Cromolyn sodium is a medication used in maintenance therapy for asthma. It stabilizes mast cell membranes; inhibits activation and release of mediators from eosinophil and epithelial cells; and inhibits the acute airway narrowing after exposure to exercise, cold dry air, and sulfur dioxide. It does not result in immediate relief of symptoms and has minimal side effects (occasional coughing on inhalation of the powder formulation). It may be given via nebulizer or MDI. *Nedocromil sodium* inhibits the bronchoconstrictor response to inhaled antigens and inhibits the activity of and release of inflammatory cell types such as histamine, leukotrienes, and prostaglandins. The drug has few side effects and is used for maintenance therapy in asthma; it is not effective for reversal of acute exacerbations and is not used in children younger than 5 years.

Leukotrienes are mediators of inflammation that cause increases in airway hyperresponsiveness. Leukotriene modifiers (e.g., zafirlukast [Accolate] and montelukast sodium [Singulair]) block inflammatory and bronchospasm effects. These drugs are not used to treat acute episodes but are given orally in combination with β-agonists and steroids to provide long-term control and prevent symptoms in mild persistent asthma. Montelukast is approved for children 12 months old and older, and zafirlukast is approved for children 7 years old and older.

Anticholinergics (atropine and ipratropium [Atrovent]) may also be used for relief of acute bronchospasm. However, these drugs have adverse side effects that include drying of respiratory secretions, blurred vision, and cardiac and CNS stimulation. The primary anticholinergic drug used is ipratropium, which does not cross the blood-brain barrier and therefore elicits no CNS effects. Ipratropium, when used in combination with albuterol, has been shown to be effective during acute severe asthma in significantly improving lung function and reducing hospitalizations in children coming to the ED.

A fairly new asthma drug, omalizumab (Xolair), is a *monoclonal antibody* that blocks the binding of IgE to mast cells. Blocking this interaction eventually inhibits the inflammation that is associated with asthma. It is used in patients with moderate to persistent asthma who have confirmed perennial aeroallergen sensitivity and have had poor control of symptoms on inhaled steroids. Many patients with asthma are atopic and possess specific IgE antibodies to allergens responsible for airway inflammation. Xolair has been approved for use in children 12 years old and older. The drug is administered once or twice a month by subcutaneous injection. Efficacy of omalizumab is not immediate. In early 2007, the FDA added a "black box warning" to the drug, which highlights the risk for anaphylaxis; however, recent studies indicate the risk for anaphylaxis is reported to occur infrequently. More than half of all anaphylactic reactions occurred in the first 2 hours after administration (FDA, 2009; Thomson and Chaudhuri, 2012). In summary, omalizumab is considered effective for children and adults 12 years of age and older whose asthma symptoms are poorly controlled with inhaled corticosteroids (Thomson and Chaudhuri, 2012).

Some children with severe asthma and a history of severe life-threatening episodes may need a primary care practitioner prescription for an EpiPen (subcutaneous injectable epinephrine).

Exercise. Exercise-induced bronchospasm (EIB) is an acute, reversible, usually self-terminating airway obstruction that develops during or after vigorous activity, reaches its peak 5 to 10 minutes after stopping the activity, and usually stops in another 20 to 30 minutes. Patients with EIB have cough, shortness of breath, chest pain or tightness, wheezing, and endurance problems during exercise, but an exercise challenge test in a laboratory is necessary to make the diagnosis.

The problem is rare in activities that require short bursts of energy (e.g., baseball, sprints, gymnastics, skiing) and more common in those that involve endurance exercise (e.g., soccer, basketball, distance running). Swimming is well tolerated by children with EIB because they are breathing air fully saturated with moisture and because of the type of breathing required in swimming.

Children with asthma are often excluded from exercise by parents, teachers, and health care practitioners, as well as by the children themselves because they are reluctant to provoke an attack. However, this practice can seriously hamper peer interaction and physical health. Exercise is advantageous for children with asthma, and most children can participate in activities at school and in sports with minimal difficulty, provided their asthma is under control. Appropriate prophylactic treatment with β-adrenergic agents or cromolyn sodium before exercise usually permits full participation in strenuous exertion.

Breathing Exercises. Breathing exercises and physical training help produce physical and mental relaxation, improve posture, strengthen respiratory musculature, and develop more efficient patterns of breathing. For motivated children, breathing exercises and controlled breathing are of value in preventing overinflation and improving efficiency of the cough. However, these exercises are not recommended during acute, uncomplicated exacerbation of asthma.

Hyposensitization. The role of hyposensitization in childhood asthma has become controversial. In the past, immunotherapy was used for seasonal allergies and when single substances were identified as the offending allergen. It is not recommended for allergens that can be eliminated, such as foods, drugs, and animal dander.

The NAEPP guidelines (2007) recommend immunotherapy for asthma patients in the following situations:

- When there is evidence of a relationship between asthma symptoms and unavoidable exposure to an allergen to which the patient is sensitive
- When symptoms occur all year or at least during a major portion of the year
- When symptom control is difficult with drug therapy because multiple medications are required, the patient is not responsive to available drugs, or the patient refuses to take the medications

Injection therapy is usually limited to clinically significant allergens. The initial dose of the offending allergen(s), based on the size of the skin reaction, is injected subcutaneously. The amount is increased at weekly intervals until a maximum tolerance is reached, after which a maintenance dose is given at 4-week intervals. This may be extended to 5- or 6-week intervals during the off-season for seasonal allergens. Successful treatment is continued for a minimum of 3 years and then stopped. If no symptoms appear, acquired immunity is assumed; if symptoms recur, treatment is reinstituted. Hyposensitization injections should be administered only with emergency equipment and medications readily available in the event of an anaphylactic reaction.

Status Asthmaticus. Status asthmaticus is a medical emergency that can result in respiratory failure and death if untreated. Children who continue to display respiratory distress despite vigorous therapeutic measures, especially the use of sympathomimetics (e.g., albuterol, epinephrine), are considered to be in status asthmaticus. The condition may develop gradually or rapidly, often coincident with complicating conditions, such as pneumonia or a respiratory

! NURSING ALERT

A child with asthma who sweats profusely, remains sitting upright, and refuses to lie down is in severe respiratory distress. Also, a child who suddenly becomes agitated or an agitated child who suddenly becomes quiet may have serious hypoxia and requires immediate intervention.

virus, that can influence the duration and treatment of the exacerbation.

Therapy for status asthmaticus is aimed at improving ventilation, decreasing airway resistance and relieving bronchospasm, correcting dehydration and acidosis, allaying child and parent anxiety related to the severity of the event, and treating any concurrent infection. Humidified oxygen is recommended and should be given to maintain an oxygen saturation greater than 90%. Inhaled aerosolized short-acting β$_2$-agonists are recommended for all patients. Three treatments of β$_2$-agonists spaced 20 to 30 minutes apart are usually given as initial therapy, and continuous administration of β$_2$-agonists may be initiated. A systemic corticosteroid (oral, IV, or IM) may also be given to decrease the effects of inflammation. An anticholinergic agent such as ipratropium bromide may be added to the aerosolized solution of the β$_2$-agonist. Anticholinergics have been shown to result in additional bronchodilation in patients with severe airflow obstruction. An IV infusion is often initiated to provide a means for hydration and to administer medications. Correction of dehydration, acidosis, hypoxia, and electrolyte disturbance is guided by frequent determination of arterial pH, blood gases, and serum electrolytes.

Additional therapies in acute asthma attacks include the use of IV magnesium sulfate, a potent muscle relaxant that acts to decrease inflammation and improves pulmonary function and peak flow rate among pediatric patients treated in the ED with moderate to severe asthma. Heliox may be administered to decrease airway resistance and thereby decrease the work of breathing; heliox can be delivered via a nonrebreathing face mask from premixed tanks, which may be blended in a stand-alone unit or within a ventilator. Heliox may be used in acute exacerbations as an adjunct to β$_2$-agonist and IV corticosteroid therapy to improve pulmonary function until the two latter medications have time to take full effect in decreasing bronchospasm; whereas the effects of heliox are usually seen within 20 minutes of administration, other drugs may take longer to exert the desired effect. Ketamine, a dissociative anesthetic, is believed to cause smooth muscle relaxation and decrease airway resistance caused by severe bronchospasm in acute asthma; it may be administered as an adjunct to other therapies mentioned previously.

Antibiotics should not be used to treat acute asthma attacks except when a bacterial infection resulting from another condition such as pneumonia or sinusitis is present (NAEPP, 2007). A child suspected of having status asthmaticus is usually seen in the ED and is often admitted to a pediatric intensive care unit for close observation and continuous cardiorespiratory monitoring. A key component in the prevention of morbidity is helping the child, parents, teachers, coaches, and other adults recognize features of deteriorating respiratory status, use the correct rescue drugs effectively, and immediately place the child with deteriorating respiratory status into the care of health care professionals instead of waiting to see if the asthma improves on its own. For the child going into early status asthmaticus, immediate medical care is required to prevent irreversible respiratory failure and possible death (see Nursing Care Plan).

Prognosis. Although deaths from asthma have been relatively uncommon since the 1980s, the rate of death from asthma increased steadily in the United States until it peaked in the mid-1990s. Asthma-related deaths decreased between 1996 and 2005 by approximately 3.9% per year (Akinbami, Moorman, Garbe, et al., 2009). Data for the year 2008 indicate a significant increase in asthma symptoms, ED visits, and hospitalization among boys from birth to 4 years of age. African-American children have hospitalization and death rates 3 times higher than those of white and Hispanic children (Liu, Covar, Spahn, et al., 2011). Most asthma deaths in children occur in the home, school, or community before lifesaving medical care can be administered.

Some children's asthma symptoms may improve at puberty, but up to two thirds of children with asthma continue to have symptoms through puberty and into adulthood. The prognosis for control or disappearance of symptoms varies in children from those who have

---

◎ NURSING CARE PLAN

The Child with Acute Asthma Exacerbation

NURSING DIAGNOSIS	EXPECTED OUTCOMES	NURSING INTERVENTIONS	RATIONALES
Ineffective Airway Clearance related to inflammation and constriction (spasm) of bronchial tree	Child will exhibit effective ventilatory capacity (specify). Child will breathe easily without dyspnea.	Allow child to assume position of comfort (tripod or other)	To promote maximum ventilatory function
Child's Defining Characteristics		Administer oxygen by face mask to maintain oxygen saturation >90%	To enhance oxygenation of tissues
(Subjective and Objective Data)		Provide reassurance that symptoms will be managed and air hunger will subside	To decrease anxiety related to hypoxia
Dyspnea		Administer rescue medications (as prescribed) (NAEPP, 2007):	To open constricted airways and allow air exchange
Diminished breath sounds (air movement)		Inhaled β_2-agonist by metered-dose inhaler or aerosolized nebulization (up to three treatments in first 60 minutes) *or*	To maintain adequate tissue oxygenation
Adventitious breath sounds (wheezing)		Inhaled high-dose β_2-agonist (albuterol) and anticholinergic (ipratropium bromide [as age appropriate]) in nebulized form with oxygen (as necessary to keep saturation >90%)	
Difficulty vocalizing			
Changes in respiratory rate and rhythm			
Related Factors		Administer oral corticosteroid	To decrease inflammation
Allergen exposure		Assess child's response to rescue medications	To determine need for more aggressive interventions
Allergic airway		Administer the above rescue medications ordered as appropriate until optimum response is obtained	To control asthma symptoms and improve oxygenation
Respiratory tract infection		Observe for exacerbation of asthma symptoms	To prevent recurrence of acute episode
		Encourage small amounts of clear oral fluids as condition allows	To maintain hydration
		For severe, unresponsive exacerbation, initiate peripheral intravenous line	To maintain hydration and administer medications
		Titrate or wean oxygen concentration according to patient's response to rescue medications (based on work of breathing and oxygen saturation)	To prevent hyperoxemia
		Collaboratively evaluate cause of asthma exacerbation and treat if infection	To prevent recurrence
		Provide discharge instructions for continued control of asthma symptoms	To educate for management of symptoms and prevention of exacerbations
		Review home medication use	
		Review written action plan for asthma symptom control	To provide sense of control
		Review signs and symptoms requiring immediate medical attention	To enhance self-esteem
		Control or eradicate allergens, irritants, and other precipitating factors	
		Follow up with health care practitioner	

rare and infrequent attacks to those who are constantly wheezing or are subject to status asthmaticus. In general, when symptoms are severe and numerous, when symptoms have been present for a long time, and when there is a family history of allergy, there is a greater likelihood of a poor prognosis. Risk factors that may predict the persistence of symptoms into childhood (from infancy) include atopy, male gender, exposure to environmental tobacco, and maternal history of asthma. Many children who outgrow their exacerbations continue to have airway hyperresponsiveness and cough as adults. Furthermore, airway hyperresponsiveness in adults appears to be associated with decreased lung function.

The adolescent age-group appears to be the most vulnerable, with the greatest increase occurring in children 10 to 14 years of age. No reliable data exist to explain this increase. Factors that have been postulated include exposure of atopic persons to more allergens (particularly in large urban centers), change in severity of the disease, abuse of drug therapy (toxicity), failure of families and practitioners to recognize the severity of asthma, and psychologic factors such as denial and refusal to accept the disease. On the other hand, studies have shown that children living in rural areas and farming communities have a decreased incidence of asthma and allergy (Liu, Covar, Spahn, et al., 2011).

Risk factors for asthma deaths include early onset, frequent attacks, difficult-to-manage disease, adolescence, history of respiratory failure, psychologic problems (refusal to take medications), dependency on or misuse of asthma drugs (high use), presence of physical stigmata (barrel chest, intercostal retractions), and abnormal PFT results.

CARE MANAGEMENT

The nursing care of the child with asthma begins with a review of the child's health history; the home, school, and play environment; parent and child attitudes about the child's condition; and a comprehensive physical assessment with focus on the respiratory system. Nursing care of children with asthma involves both acute and long-term care. Nurses who are involved with children in the home, hospital, school, outpatient clinic, or health care practitioner's office play an important role in helping children and their families learn to live with the condition. The disease can be managed so that it does not require hospitalization or interfere with family life, physical activity, or school attendance. The nursing process in the care of the child with asthma is outlined in the Nursing Care Plan.

Physical assessment of asthma involves the same observations and techniques described in Chapter 29. In addition, the nurse notes and evaluates physical characteristics of a chronic respiratory condition, including chest configuration (e.g., barrel chest), posturing, and type of breathing. A history of the current and previous episodes and precipitating factors or events is important.

Nurses may perform a variety of functions in asthma care. These may include asthma education in the primary care setting and in schools and other community settings, care of the child with asthma in the acute care setting, ambulatory care, emergency department, and intensive care. Nurses also obtain information on how asthma affects the child's everyday activities and self-concept, the child's and family's adherence to the prescribed therapy, and their personal treatment goals. Every effort is made to build a partnership between the child and family and the health care team, and effective communication is an essential part of this partnership. In particular, the child's and family's satisfaction with asthma control and with the quality of care should be assessed. The nurse should also assess the child's and family's perception of the severity of the disease and their level of social support.

One of the major emphases of nursing care is outpatient management by the family. Parents are taught how to prevent exacerbations, to recognize and respond to symptoms of bronchospasm, to maintain health and prevent complications, and to promote normal activities. The nurse should determine any cultural or ethnic beliefs or practices that influence self-management and that may necessitate modifications in educational approaches to meet the family's needs. Inconsistent home care, either on the part of the child or the parents, often leads to unnecessary ED visits for management (Volpe, Smith, and Sultan, 2011). Parents and older children often need education reinforced about the maintenance aspect of asthma management; children benefit from drug therapy even when asthma manifestations are not evident.

Provide Acute Asthma Care. Children who are admitted to the hospital with acute asthma are ill, anxious, and uncomfortable. The importance of continual observation and assessment cannot be overemphasized.

When β_2-agonists, supplemental oxygen, and corticosteroids are given, the child is monitored closely and continuously for relief of respiratory distress and signs of side effects or toxicity. Pulse oximetry is monitored along with rate and depth of breathing, auscultation of air movement, adventitious sounds, and any signs of respiratory distress (e.g., nasal flaring, tachypnea, retractions). The child on supplemental oxygen requires intermittent or continuous oxygenation monitoring depending on severity of respiratory compromise and initial oxygenation status. The child in status asthmaticus should be placed on continuous cardiorespiratory (including blood pressure) and pulse oximetry monitoring. Oral fluid intake may be limited during the acute phase; IV fluid replacement may be required to provide adequate tissue hydration.

Older children may be more comfortable standing (Fig. 40-6), sitting upright, or leaning slightly forward (Fig. 40-7). Shortness of breath makes talking difficult.

The calm, efficient presence of a nurse helps reassure children that they are safe and will be cared for during this stressful period. It is important to assure children that they will not be left alone and that their parents are allowed to remain with them. Parents need

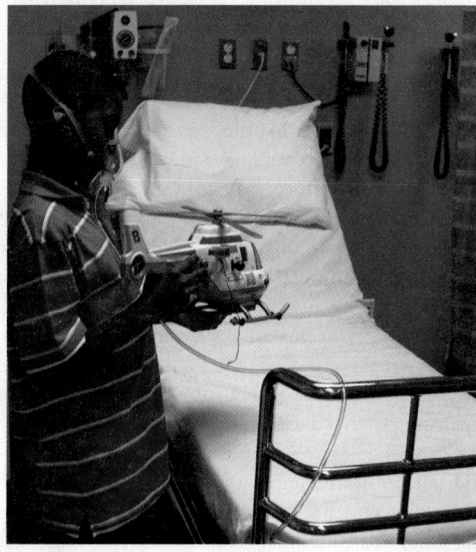

FIG 40-6 Child with asthma is allowed play activity as tolerated.

⊚ NURSING CARE PLAN

The Child with Asthma

NURSING DIAGNOSIS	EXPECTED OUTCOMES	NURSING INTERVENTIONS	RATIONALES
Risk for Suffocation related to interaction between individual and triggering factors (allergens, respiratory tract infection, exercise, irritants, emotions, temperature changes)	Child will have adequate airway exchange. Family and child will assume responsibility for asthma symptom management.	Assist child and family in recognizing factors such as allergens, irritants, temperature changes, and upper respiratory infections that trigger asthma symptoms	To avoid asthma exacerbations
Child's Defining Characteristics (Subjective and Objective Data)		Assist child (according to developmental age) and family in recognizing early signs of an asthmatic episode (use PEFM)	To control symptoms with medication
Wheezing		Educate child and family in use of inhaled corticosteroids and bronchodilator	To control symptoms and minimize shortness of breath
Dry cough		Educate child and family regarding proper use of rescue medications in case of illness exacerbation	To prevent illness exacerbations and hospitalization; to prevent side effects from improper use of certain asthma drugs
Labored respirations			
Dyspnea			
Intercostal retractions			
Complaints of tightness in chest, shortness of breath		Educate child and family regarding proper use of MDI with spacer, aerosolized nebulizer, and PEFM (know child's personal best)	To help child and family effectively manage asthma symptoms independently
Bronchial inflammation and airway constriction			
Interrupted Family Processes related to child with chronic illness	Family will cope with effects of disease. Family will provide child appropriate protective environment.	Provide family and child (as age appropriate) explanations about the disease and management	To provide adequate information To provide realistic expectations
Child's and Family's Defining Characteristics (Subjective and Objective Data)		Cooperate with family to develop written action plan for asthma management	To provide family and child sense of control
Anxiety		Discuss facilitators and barriers to effective asthma management	To assist family members in understanding their role as being vital in management of asthma
Disruptive family interactions with child and members			
Family conflicts		Encourage family and child (as age appropriate) to discuss impact of illness on family's lifestyle	To provide opportunity to verbalize frustrations and challenges of having child with chronic illness
Inadequate child support			
Child's health status ignored		Evaluate family resources for asthma management in relation to the following:	To enhance family's ability to cope with child's chronic illness
Family ignoring other members' needs for those of child with asthma		Access to health care Medication availability in home and school (or day care as appropriate) Allergen exposure control and eradication	

MDI, Metered-dose inhaler; *PEFM,* peak expiratory flow meter.

reassurance and want to be informed of their child's condition and therapies. They may believe that they have in some way contributed to the child's condition or could have prevented the episode. Reassurance regarding their efforts expended on the child's behalf and their parenting capabilities can help alleviate their stress. Efforts to reduce parental apprehension will also reduce the child's distress. Anxiety is easily communicated to the child from parents and members of the staff.

Avoid Allergens. One goal of asthma management is avoidance of an exacerbation. Parents need to know how to avoid allergens that precipitate asthma episodes. The nurse assists the parent in modifying the environment to reduce contact with the offending allergen(s). Parents are cautioned to avoid exposing a sensitive child to excessive cold, wind, and other extremes of weather; smoke (open fire or tobacco); sprays; scents; and other irritants. Foods known to provoke symptoms should be eliminated from the diet.

Approximately 2% to 6% of children with asthma are sensitive to aspirin; therefore nurses should caution parents to use other analgesic–antipyretic drugs for discomfort or fever and to read package labeling. Although aspirin is not routinely given to children in the United States, salicylate compounds are in other common medicines such as Pepto-Bismol. Children with aspirin-induced asthma may also be sensitive to nonsteroidal antiinflammatory drugs and tartrazine (yellow dye number 5, a common food coloring).

❗ NURSING ALERT

Parents are encouraged to avoid administering aspirin to any child unless specifically recommended by and under the supervision of a health care practitioner. Acetaminophen is safe for children and is the analgesic of choice.

Relieve Bronchospasm. Teach parents and older children to recognize early signs and symptoms of an impending attack so it

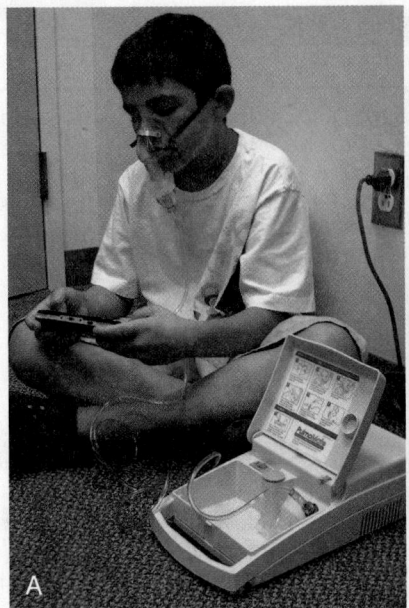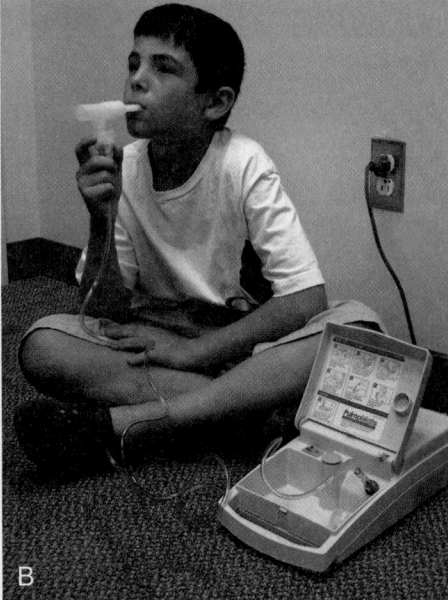

FIG 40-7 Children with asthma may take a nebulized aerosol treatment with a mask **(A)** or mouthpiece **(B)**. (Courtesy Texas Children's Hospital, Houston.)

can be controlled before symptoms become distressing. Most children can recognize prodromal symptoms well before an attack (≈6 hours) and implement preventive therapy. Objective signs that parents may observe include rhinorrhea, cough, low-grade fever, irritability, itching (especially in front of the neck and chest), apathy, anxiety, sleep disturbance, abdominal discomfort, and loss of appetite. A variety of easy-to-use, inexpensive PEFMs are available for use in the home and at school to assess changes in pulmonary function (see Patient Teaching box). In general, children 5 years of age and older are able to use a PEFM successfully. However, young children need to be supervised while they are learning to use their PEFM, and their technique should be checked frequently to ensure it is correct. Children should use the same peak flow meter over time because different brands can give significantly different values. The use of a PEFM provides objective monitoring regarding the severity of asthma and can decrease asthma episodes, health care visits, and missed school days (Burkhart, Rayens, Revelette, et al., 2007).

The family should obtain a PEFM and learn to use this device to monitor the child's asthma if the child is 5 years of age and older. A written *asthma action plan* that includes the three peak flow meter zones and the child's asthma medications may be obtained from the child's primary care provider. A home asthma action plan may reduce the risk for asthma death by 70% (Liu, Covar, Spahn, et al., 2011). Medications used for asthma exacerbations are also included in the asthma plan. This action plan should be used to make decisions about asthma management at home and at school. The nurse may assist the child and family in understanding the written action plan, emphasizing that the child and family determine the success of the plan, not the health care professionals. Teach parents how to read labels on prepared foods and snacks to determine the presence of allergens.

Children who use a nebulizer, MDI, Diskus, or Turbuhaler to deliver drugs need to learn how to use the device correctly. The MDI device delivers medication directly to the airways; therefore the child needs to learn to breathe slowly and deeply for better distribution to narrowed airways (see Patient Teaching box on. p. 1234).

A spacer or AeroChamber device should be used with MDI inhalers. These devices allow the parent or child to deliver the medication from the MDI and slowly inhale it. Spacers also help prevent yeast infections in the mouth when corticosteroids are inhaled via an MDI (see Fig. 40-5).

The child and parents also need to be cautioned about the adverse effects of prescribed drugs and the dangers of overuse of β_2-agonists. They should know that it is important to use these drugs when needed but not indiscriminately or as a substitute for avoiding the symptom-provoking allergen.

PATIENT TEACHING

Use of a Metered-Dose Inhaler*

Steps for Checking How Much Medicine Is in the Canister

1. If the canister is new, it is full.
2. If the canister has been used repeatedly, it might be empty. (Check product label to see how many inhalations should be in each canister.)
3. The most accurate way to determine how many doses remain in a MDI is to count and record each actuation as it is used.
4. Many dry powder inhalers have a dose-counting device or dose indicator on the canister to let you know when the canister is empty.
5. Do not place inhalers with hydrofluoroalkanes in water to determine whether doses remain; it will destroy them.

Steps for Using the Inhaler with Mouthpiece

1. Remove the cap and hold inhaler upright.
2. Shake the inhaler.
3. Attach spacer, as appropriate.
4. Tilt the head back slightly and breathe out slowly.
5. With the inhaler in an upright position, insert the mouthpiece:
   a. About 3 to 4 cm (1-1½ inches) from the mouth *or*
   b. Into the mouth, forming an airtight seal between the lips and the mouthpiece
6. At the end of a normal expiration, depress the top of the inhaler canister firmly to release the medication (into the mouth) and breathe in slowly (about 3 to 5 seconds). Relax the pressure on the top of the canister.
7. Hold the breath for at least 5 to 10 seconds to allow the aerosol medication to reach deeply into the lungs.
8. Remove the inhaler and breathe out slowly through the nose.

9. Wait 1 minute between puffs (if an additional puff is needed) when using a bronchodilator.

Steps for Using the Inhaler with an AeroChamber (see Fig. 40-5)

1. Remove the cap and hold inhaler upright.
2. Shake the inhaler.
3. Attach the AeroChamber.
4. With the inhaler in an upright position, insert the mouthpiece into the back of the AeroChamber.
5. Apply the AeroChamber mask to child's face and make sure there is a good seal.
6. Have child breathe slow, regular breaths. Depress the top of the inhaler canister firmly to release the medication (into the AeroChamber) as the child breathes slowly in and out. Relax the pressure on the top of the canister.
7. Hold the AeroChamber in place over the child's face until six breaths have been taken. Give one puff at a time.
8. Remove the inhaler and AeroChamber.
9. Wait 1 minute between puffs (if an additional puff is needed) when using a bronchodilator.

Common Problems for Children Using Inhalers

- Child refuses or resists treatment.
- Inhalation is too rapid.
- Child is unable to coordinate the spray with inhalation.
- Breath is not held long enough after inhalation.

*Inhaled dry powder such as budesonide (Pulmicort) requires a different inhalation technique. To use a dry powder inhaler, the base of the device is turned until a click is heard. It is important to close the mouth tightly around the mouthpiece of the inhaler and inhale rapidly. *MDI,* Metered-dose inhaler.

The child should be protected from a respiratory tract infection that can trigger an attack or aggravate the asthmatic state, especially in young children whose airways are mechanically smaller and more reactive. Annual influenza vaccinations are recommended for all children. Pneumococcal vaccines should also be maintained. Equipment used for the child, such as nebulizers, must be kept absolutely clean to decrease the chances of contamination with bacteria and fungi.

Breathing exercises and controlled breathing are taught and encouraged for motivated children, and the nurse should provide information concerning activities that promote diaphragmatic breathing, side expansion, and improved mobility of the chest wall. Play techniques that can be used for younger children to extend their expiratory time and increase expiratory pressure include blowing cotton balls or a Ping-Pong ball on a table, blowing a pinwheel, blowing bubbles, or preventing a tissue from falling by blowing it against the wall.

Self-care and asthma self-management programs are important in helping the child and family cope with asthma. They are based on the following principles:

- Asthma is a common disease that can be controlled with appropriate drug therapy, environmental control, education, and management skills.
- It is much easier to prevent than to treat an asthma episode, and adherence to a therapeutic program is necessary to prevent exacerbations
- Children with asthma can live full and active lives.

Self-contained programs and brochures for patient education are available from the Asthma and Allergy Foundation of America* and the American Lung Association.† The National Heart, Lung, and Blood Institute‡ provides educational materials for asthma education in the school setting and also copies of the *Guidelines for the Diagnosis and Management of Asthma* for the health care practitioner (NAEPP, 2007). Another publication designed for health care practitioners, *Pediatric Asthma: Promoting Best Practice,* can be obtained from the American Academy of Allergy Asthma & Immunology.§

Support Child or Adolescent and Family. The nurse working with children with asthma can provide support in a number of ways. Many children voice frustration because their exacerbations interfere with their daily activities and social lives. Children need education on their condition and reassurance from the health care team that they can learn to control and cope with their asthma and live a normal life.

Children in disruptive family situations (divorce, separation, violence, custodial battles) may disregard their daily asthma medication

---

*8201 Corporate Drive, Suite 1000, Landover, MD 20785; 800-7-Asthma; www.aafa.org.
†1301 Pennsylvania Ave., NW, Suite 800, Washington, DC 20004; 800-548-8252; national headquarters: 202-785-3385; www.lungusa.org.
‡NHLBI Health Information Center, PO Box 30105, Bethesda, MD 20824-0105; 301-592-8573; fax: 240-629-3246; www.nhlbi.nih.gov.
§555 E. Wells St., Suite 1100, Milwaukee, WI 53202; 414-272-6071; http://aaaai.org.

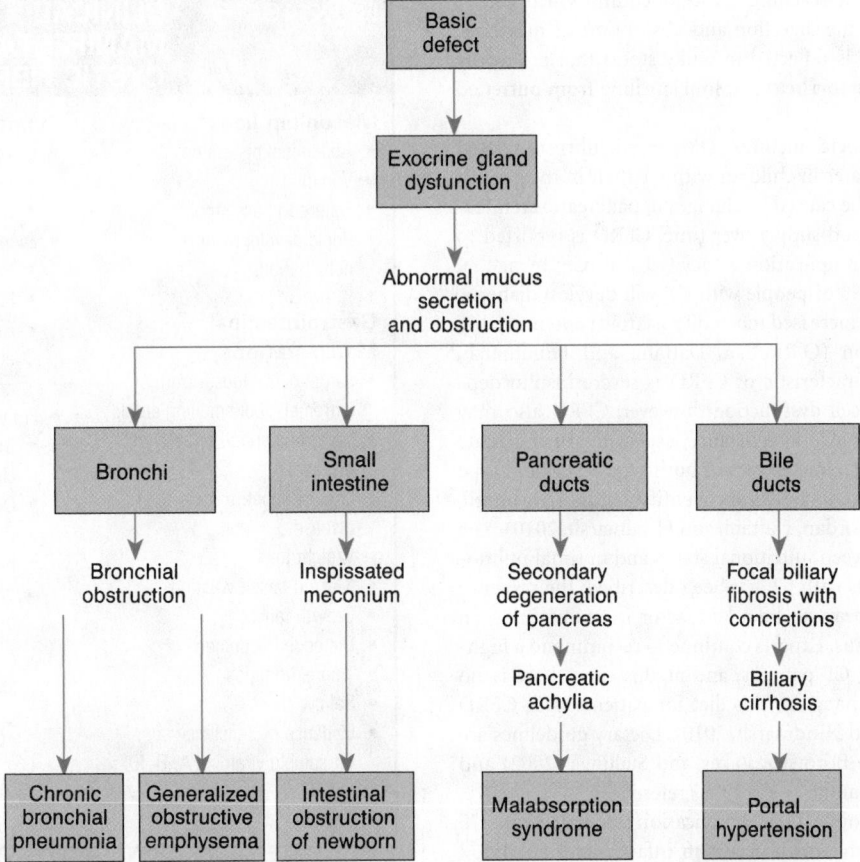

FIG 40-8 Various effects of exocrine gland dysfunction in cystic fibrosis.

regimen or may be at higher risk as a result of neglect by adults who are in charge of their care. Adolescents struggling with a sense of identity and body image often regard asthma as a condition that will "go away," especially if there is a time lapse between symptoms, and may abandon the therapeutic regimen. Referral for counseling and guidance is appropriate when the child's or adolescent's life is potentially in harm's way and the therapeutic regimen for asthma is abandoned because of personal or family crises.

The task of living day to day with affected children involves the entire family. There are periodic crises and the ever-present threat of a crisis, requiring parental vigilance; sleepless nights; frequent trips to the health care provider, ED, or hospital; and often overwhelming medical expenses. Throughout these stresses, parents are encouraged to promote as normal a life as possible for their children.

Cystic Fibrosis

Cystic fibrosis (CF) is inherited as an autosomal recessive trait; the affected child inherits the defective gene from both parents, with an overall risk of one in four if both parents carry the gene. The mutated gene responsible for CF is located on the long arm of chromosome 7. This gene codes a protein of 1480 amino acids called the **cystic fibrosis transmembrane regulator (CFTR)**. The CFTR protein is related to a family of membrane-bound glycoproteins. The glycoproteins constitute a cAMP-activated chloride channel and regulate other chloride and sodium channels at the surfaces of the epithelial cells.

Pathophysiology

Cystic fibrosis is characterized by several clinical features, which are increased viscosity of mucous gland secretions, a striking elevation of sweat electrolytes, an increase in several organic and enzymatic constituents of saliva, and abnormalities in autonomic nervous system function. Although both sodium and chloride are affected, the defect appears to be primarily a result of abnormal chloride movement; the CFTR appears to function as a chloride channel. Children with CF demonstrate an increase in sodium and chloride in both saliva and sweat. This characteristic is the basis for the sweat chloride diagnostic test. The sweat electrolyte abnormality is present from birth, continues throughout life, and is unrelated to the severity of the disease or the extent to which other organs are involved.

The primary factor, and the one that is responsible for many of the clinical manifestations of the disease, is mechanical obstruction caused by the increased viscosity of mucous gland secretions (Fig. 40-8). Instead of forming a thin, freely flowing secretion, the mucous glands produce a thick mucoprotein that accumulates and dilates them. Small passages in organs such as the pancreas and bronchioles become obstructed as secretions precipitate or coagulate to form concretions in glands and ducts. The earliest postnatal manifestation of CF is often meconium ileus in the newborn, in which the small intestine is blocked with thick, puttylike, tenacious, mucilaginous meconium.

In the pancreas, the thick secretions block the ducts, eventually causing pancreatic fibrosis. This blockage prevents essential pancreatic enzymes from reaching the duodenum, which causes marked impairment in the digestion and absorption of nutrients. The disturbed function is reflected in bulky stools that are frothy from undigested fat (steatorrhea) and foul smelling from putrefied protein (azotorrhea).

The incidence of diabetes mellitus (DM) (cystic fibrosis–related diabetes [CFRD]) is greater in children with CF than in the general population, which may be caused by changes in pancreatic architecture and diminished blood supply over time. CFRD is reported to be the most common complication associated with CF; by age 30 years, approximately 50% of people with CF will develop diabetes, which is associated with increased morbidity (sixfold) and mortality and poor lung function (O'Riordan, Dattani, and Hindmarsh, 2010). The primary characteristic of CFRD is severe insulin deficiency as a result of β-cell dysfunction; however, CFRD also may demonstrate fluctuating insulin resistance, especially during acute illness. Thus CFRD has characteristics of both type 1 DM and type 2 DM but is considered to be its own entity (Moran, Brunzell, Cohen, et al., 2010; O'Riordan, Dattani, and Hindmarsh, 2010). The positive correlation between nutritional status and optimal pulmonary function in patients with CF has been described; the presence of adequate insulin appears to be a key factor in maintaining an adequate nutritional status. Experts continue to recommend a high-fat, high-calorie diet in CF patients, and at this time there is no evidence to support a change in this diet for patients with CFRD (O'Riordan, Dattani, and Hindmarsh, 2010). Dietary guidelines are described further in the Borowitz, Baker, and Stallings (2002) and the Michel, Maqbool, Hanna, et al. (2009) references.

An uncommon gastrointestinal complication associated with CF is prolapse of the rectum, which occurs in infancy and childhood and is related to large, bulky stools; malabsorption; and increased intra-abdominal pressure secondary to paroxysmal cough. This is seen less frequently in children who receive pancreatic enzymes. Affected children of all ages are subject to intestinal obstruction from inspissated or impacted feces. Gumlike masses can obstruct the bowel and produce a partial or complete obstruction, a condition that is referred to as distal intestinal obstruction syndrome.

Pulmonary complications are present in almost all children with CF, but the onset and extent of involvement are variable. Symptoms are produced by stagnation of mucus in the airways, with eventual bacterial colonization leading to destruction of lung tissue. The abnormally viscous and tenacious secretions are difficult to expectorate and gradually obstruct the bronchi and bronchioles, causing scattered areas of bronchiectasis, atelectasis, and hyperinflation. The stagnant mucus also offers a favorable environment for bacterial growth. The most common pathogens are *Pseudomonas aeruginosa, Burkholderia cepacia, S. aureus, H. influenzae, Escherichia coli,* and *Klebsiella pneumoniae.*

The reproductive systems of both males and females with CF are affected. Females with CF have normal fallopian tubes and ovaries. Fertility can be inhibited by highly viscous cervical secretions, which act as a plug, blocking sperm entry. Women with CF who become pregnant have an increased incidence of premature labor and birth and infant low birth weight. Favorable nutritional status and pulmonary function are positively correlated with favorable pregnancy outcomes. Most men (95%) with CF are sterile, which may be caused by blockage of the vas deferens with abnormal secretions or by failure of normal development of the wolffian duct structures (vas deferens, epididymis, and seminal vesicles), resulting in decreased or absent sperm production.

Growth and development are often affected in children with moderate to severe forms of CF. Physical growth may be restricted

---

BOX 40-16   CLINICAL MANIFESTATIONS OF CYSTIC FIBROSIS

Meconium Ileus*
- Abdominal distention
- Vomiting
- Failure to pass stools
- Rapid development of dehydration

Gastrointestinal Manifestations
- Large, bulky, loose, frothy, extremely foul-smelling stools
- Voracious appetite (early in disease)
- Loss of appetite (later in disease)
- Weight loss
- Marked tissue wasting
- Growth failure
- Distended abdomen
- Thin extremities
- Sallow skin
- Evidence of deficiency of fat-soluble vitamins A, D, E, and K
- Anemia

Pulmonary Manifestations
- Initial signs:
  - Wheezing respirations
  - Dry, nonproductive cough
- Eventually:
  - Increased dyspnea
  - Paroxysmal cough
  - Evidence of obstructive emphysema and patchy areas of atelectasis
- Progressive involvement:
  - Overinflated, barrel-shaped chest
  - Cyanosis
  - Clubbing of fingers and toes
  - Repeated episodes of bronchitis and bronchopneumonia

*In about 10% of cases.

---

as a result of decreased absorption of nutrients, including vitamins and fat; increased oxygen demands for pulmonary function; and delayed bone growth. The often seen pattern is one of growth failure (failure to thrive) with increased weight loss despite an increased appetite and gradual deterioration of the respiratory system. Clinical manifestations of CF are listed in Box 40-16.

Diagnostic Evaluation

Traditionally, the diagnosis of CF was based on a positive sweat chloride test result, absence of pancreatic enzymes, radiography, COPD, and family history. Newer diagnostic methods make it possible to diagnose CF early in infancy so therapies can be implemented to increase the child's overall survival and quality of life. In addition to the sweat chloride test and factors just listed, diagnosis may be confirmed by any one of the following: newborn screening, DNA identification of mutant genes, and abnormal nasal potential difference measurement.

Universal newborn screening for CF is now required by law or rule in all of the continental United States, Hawaii, and Alaska (National Newborn Screening and Genetics Resource Center, 2013). The newborn screening test consists of an immunoreactive trypsinogen (IRT) analysis performed on a dried spot of blood, which may be followed by direct analysis of DNA for the presence of the ΔF508 mutation or other mutations on the same dried blood spot. Benefits of early screening and detection include earlier nutritional intervention for identified infants; disadvantages include the parental anxiety false-positive results may generate. Children who were identified and treated early in infancy with aggressive nutritional support had improved height and weight well into adolescence.

Although the technology is available to conduct carrier screening for the general population, this issue remains controversial, and widespread implementation of carrier screening programs is not recommended. An in utero diagnosis of CF is also possible based on detection of two CF mutations in the fetus.

The consistent finding of abnormally high sodium and chloride concentrations in the sweat is a unique characteristic of CF. Parents may report that their infant tastes "salty" when they kiss him or her. The quantitative sweat chloride test (pilocarpine iontophoresis) involves stimulating the production of sweat with a special device (involves stimulation with 3-mA electric current), collecting the sweat on filter paper, and measuring the sweat electrolytes. The quantitative analysis requires a sufficient volume of sweat (>75 mg). Two separate samples are collected to ensure the reliability of the test for any individual. Normally, sweat chloride content is less than 40 mEq/L, with a mean of 18 mEq/L. A chloride concentration greater than 60 mEq/L is diagnostic of CF; in infants younger than 3 months, a sweat chloride concentration greater than 40 mEq/L is highly suggestive of CF. In some situations, DNA testing may be substituted for the sweat test. The presence of a mutation known to cause CF on each CFTR gene predicts with a high degree of certainty that the individual has CF; however, multiple CFTR mutations may also be present and detected with DNA assay. More than 1800 different mutations have been found on the CF gene.

Chest radiography reveals characteristic patchy atelectasis and obstructive emphysema. PFTs are sensitive indexes of lung function, providing evidence of abnormal small airway function in CF. Other diagnostic tools that may aid in diagnosis include stool fat or enzyme analysis. Stool analysis requires a 72-hour sample with accurate recording of food intake during that time. Radiographs, including a contrast (dye) enema, are used for diagnosis of meconium ileus.

Therapeutic Management

Improved survival among patients with CF during the past 2 decades is attributable largely to antibiotic therapy and improved nutritional and respiratory management. Goals of CF therapeutic management are to (1) prevent or minimize pulmonary complications, (2) ensure adequate nutrition for growth, (3) encourage appropriate physical activity, and (4) promote a reasonable quality of life for the child and the family. A multidisciplinary approach to treatment is needed to accomplish these goals.

Management of Pulmonary Problems. Management of pulmonary problems is directed toward prevention and treatment of pulmonary infection by improving ventilation, removing mucopurulent secretions, and administering antimicrobial agents. Many children develop respiratory symptoms by 3 years of age. The large amounts and viscosity of respiratory secretions in children with CF contribute to the likelihood of respiratory tract infections. Recurrent pulmonary infections in children with CF result in greater damage to the airways; small airways are destroyed, causing bronchiectasis.

The most common pathogens responsible for pulmonary infections are *P. aeruginosa, B. cepacia, S. aureus, H. influenzae, E. coli,* and *K. pneumoniae. P. aeruginosa* and *B. cepacia* are particularly pathogenic for children with CF, and infections with these organisms are difficult to clear from the system. In addition, children with CF who are chronically colonized with these organisms have poorer survival rates than children who are not colonized. Colonization and infection with methicillin-resistant *S. aureus* (MRSA) has recently emerged as a critical factor in lung infection and pulmonary function in patients with CF. Patients with MRSA require longer hospitalization and multiple antibiotic regimens (Ren, Morgan, Konstan, et al., 2007). Fungal colonization with *Candida*

or *Aspergillus* organisms in the respiratory tract is also common in patients with CF.

Until recently, CPT has been the cornerstone of airway clearance; however, other airway clearance therapies (ACTs) have replaced this modality; these treatments often require more active involvement by the patient (Newton, 2009). The ACTs include the following: percussion and postural drainage, positive expiratory pressure (PEP), active-cycle-of-breathing technique, autogenic drainage, oscillatory PEP, high-frequency chest compressions (HFCC), and exercise. Studies have demonstrated that no particular ACT has any advantage over the other in relation to outcomes of sputum production; however, it is recommended that individualized assessment occur to determine the best ACT for each patient (Flume, Robinson, O'Sullivan, et al., 2009). It is not within the scope of this chapter to discuss the many different ACTs.

Airway clearance therapies such as percussion and postural drainage are usually performed on average twice daily (on rising and in the evening) and more frequently if needed, especially during pulmonary infection. The Flutter mucus clearance device is a small handheld plastic pipe with a stainless-steel ball on the inside that facilitates removal of mucus. It has the advantage of increasing sputum expectoration and being used without an assistant. Handheld percussors may be used to loosen secretions. Another method to clear mucus is high-frequency chest compression in which the child temporarily wears a mechanical vest device that provides high-frequency chest wall oscillation. Some children and adolescents with an implantable port may experience localized pain with the vest.

Patients with CF have been found to regress when conventional percussion and postural drainage is discontinued. Forced expiration, or "huffing," with the glottis partially closed helps move secretions from the small airways so that subsequent coughing can move secretions forcefully from the large airways. Several studies indicate that this maneuver enhances the pulmonary function of patients with CF. Autogenic drainage involves a variety of breathing techniques, which older children can use to force mucus in lower lobes up into the airways so it can be successfully expelled. Another mucus-clearing technique involves use of a positive expiratory pressure mask; this technique involves breathing into a mask attached to a one-way valve, which creates resistance—as the patient exhales, the airway is kept open by the pressure and mucus is forced into the upper airway for expulsion.

Bronchodilator medication delivered in an aerosol opens bronchi for easier expectoration and is administered before percussion and postural drainage when the patient exhibits evidence of reactive airway disease or wheezing. Another aerosolized medication is recombinant human deoxyribonuclease (DNase, known generically as *dornase alfa* [Pulmozyme]), which decreases the viscosity of mucus. It is well tolerated and has no major adverse effects; minor reactions are voice alterations and laryngitis. This medication, given daily via nebulization generally before or with percussion and postural drainage, has resulted in improvements in spirometry, PFTs, dyspnea scores, and perceptions of well-being and has reduced the viscosity of sputum.

Nebulized hypertonic saline (6%-7%) has been shown to be effective in improving airway hydration and increases mucus clearance in patients with CF; this treatment, however, causes bronchospasm and may not be recommended for patients with severe disease (Redding, 2009).

Physical exercise is an important adjunct to daily ACT. Exercise stimulates mucus excretion and provides a sense of well-being and increased self-esteem. Any aerobic exercise that the patient enjoys should be encouraged. The ultimate aim of exercise is to increase lung vital capacity, remove secretions, increase pulmonary blood flow, and maintain healthy lung tissue for effective ventilation.

Pulmonary infections are treated as soon as they are recognized. In patients with CF, characteristic signs of pulmonary infection—fever, tachypnea, and chest pain—may be absent; therefore a careful history and physical examination are essential. The presence of anorexia, weight loss, and decreased activity alerts the practitioner to pulmonary infection and the need for an antibiotic regimen. Aerosolized antibiotics such as tobramycin, ticarcillin, and gentamicin are beneficial for patients with frequent pulmonary exacerbations (Redding, 2009).

Intravenous antibiotics may be administered at home as an alternative to hospitalization. The use of peripherally inserted central catheters (PICCs) for the administration of antibiotics in children with CF is a viable option with limited complications and fewer needle punctures to obtain blood specimens and to maintain often lengthy treatment with parenteral antibiotics. Alternatively, an implanted port offers the advantage of access for blood draws and antibiotic infusion. When pulmonary function does not improve with outpatient management, hospitalization may be recommended for continued antibiotic therapy and vigorous postural drainage. Some health care practitioners hospitalize patients for IV antibiotic therapy and percussion and postural drainage periodically (a "tune up) to keep them well; others may be treated on an outpatient basis. Oxygen administration is used for children with acute episodes but must be used cautiously because many children with CF have chronic carbon dioxide retention, and the unsupervised use of oxygen can be harmful. With repeated infection and inflammation, bronchial cysts and emphysema may develop. These cysts may rupture, resulting in a pneumothorax.

> **! NURSING ALERT**
>
> Signs of a pneumothorax are usually nonspecific and include tachypnea, tachycardia, dyspnea, pallor, and cyanosis. A subtle drop in oxygen saturation (measured by pulse oximetry) may be an early sign of pneumothorax.

Children with a specific CF mutation (G551D) may benefit by taking ivacaftor (Kalydeco). This CF transmembrane conductance regulator (CFTR) modulator allows salt and fluid to move through the airways and prevent the buildup of thick mucus in the airways, with concomitant improvement of pulmonary function. This drug was recently approved by the FDA for children over 6 years of age (Pettit, 2012).

Blood streaking of the sputum is usually associated with increased pulmonary infection and often requires no specific treatment. Hemoptysis greater than 250 mL/24 hr for an older child (less for a younger child) indicates a potentially life-threatening event and needs to be treated immediately. Sometimes bleeding can be controlled with bed rest, IV antibiotics, replacement of acute blood loss, IV conjugated estrogens (Premarin) or vasopressin (Pitressin), and correction of any coagulation defects with vitamin K or fresh-frozen plasma. If hemoptysis persists, the site of bleeding should be localized via bronchoscopy and cauterized or embolized.

Treatment of nasal polyps includes intranasal corticosteroids, oral antihistamines, and decongestants. If these measures are ineffective, surgical interventions such as cauterization may be necessary.

Because pulmonary damage in patients with CF is believed to be caused by the inflammatory process that occurs with frequent infections, the use of corticosteroids has been studied; however, treatment with corticosteroids for prolonged periods has been associated with linear growth restriction, glucose tolerance abnormalities, and cataract formation. Antiinflammatory medications such as ibuprofen are becoming more important in the treatment of CF, but careful monitoring for adverse effects (gastrointestinal bleeding) is essential.

Management of Gastrointestinal Problems. The principal treatment for pancreatic insufficiency is replacement of pancreatic enzymes, which are administered with meals and snacks to ensure that digestive enzymes are mixed with food in the duodenum. Enteric-coated products prevent the neutralization of enzymes by gastric acids, thus allowing activation to occur in the alkaline environment of the small bowel. The amount of enzymes depends on the severity of the insufficiency, the child's response to enzyme replacement, and the health care practitioner's philosophy. Usually one to five capsules (or 2500 lipase units per kg) are administered with a meal, and a smaller amount is taken with snacks. Capsules can be swallowed whole or taken apart and the contents sprinkled on a small amount of food to be taken at the beginning of the meal. The amount of enzyme is adjusted to achieve normal growth and a decrease in the number of stools to one or two per day. Pancreatic enzymes should be taken within 30 minutes of eating. The enteric-coated beads should not be chewed or crushed because destroying the enteric coating can lead to inactivation of the enzymes and excoriation of oral mucosa. The powder form should be used cautiously because inhalation of the powder may precipitate acute bronchospasm and, if mixed with food, predigests the food, making it unpalatable.

Children with CF require a well-balanced, high-protein, high-caloric diet (because of their impaired intestinal absorption). In fact, they often require up to 150% of the recommended daily allowances to meet their needs for growth. Breastfeeding with enzyme supplementation should be continued whenever possible for parents who prefer this method and, when necessary, supplemented with a higher-calorie-per-ounce formula. For formula-fed infants, commercial cow's milk–based formulas are usually adequate, although frequently a partial hydrolysate formula with medium-chain triglycerides (e.g., Pregestimil, Alimentum) may be recommended. Enzymes are mixed into cereal or fruit, such as applesauce. Because the uptake of fat-soluble vitamins is decreased, water-miscible forms of these vitamins (A, D, E, and K) are given along with multivitamins and the enzymes. When high-fat foods are eaten, the child is encouraged to add extra enzymes. Growth failure despite adequate nutritional support may indicate deterioration of pulmonary status. Patients with CF may experience frequent anorexia as a result of the copious amounts of mucus produced and expectorated, persistent cough, effect of medications, fatigue, and sleep disruption. They may be placed on nighttime supplemental gastrostomy or nasogastric tube feedings or, rarely, parenteral alimentation in an effort to build up nutritional reserves if there has been a history of inability to maintain weight.

Meconium ileus and meconium ileus equivalent, or total or partial intestinal obstruction, can occur at any age. Constipation is often the result of a combination of malabsorption (either from inadequate pancreatic enzyme dosage or a failure to take the enzymes), decreased intestinal motility, and abnormally viscous intestinal secretions. These problems usually do not require surgical intervention and may be treated with GoLYTELY or Colyte (osmotic solutions given orally or by nasogastric tubes), other laxatives, stool softeners, or rectal administration of meglumine diatrizoate (Gastrografin).

Rectal prolapse occurs only in a small number of individuals; fewer are affected as result of early diagnosis and administration of pancreatic enzymes (Egan, 2011). The first episode of rectal prolapse is frightening to both the parents and child. Its reduction usually requires immediate guidance and intervention, which is managed by simply guiding the rectum back into place with a gloved, lubricated finger. Further management usually involves attempting to decrease the bulk of daily stools through enzyme replacement.

Children with CF often experience transient or chronic gastroesophageal reflux, which should be treated with the appropriate histamine-receptor antagonist and gastrointestinal motility drug, dietary modifications, and an upright position after feedings and meals (Hazle, 2010).

Management of Endocrine Problems. The management of CFRD is critical in the therapeutic treatment of the child with CF. CFRD presents a combination of insulin resistance and insulin deficiency, with unstable glucose homeostasis in the presence of acute lung infection and treatment. Children with CFRD require close monitoring of blood glucose, administration of oral glucose-lowering agents or insulin injections, and diet and exercise management; children with CF may be at increased risk for glucose management problems as a result of decreased nutrient absorption, anorexia, and severity of pulmonary illness. The prevalence of CFRD increases with age, and there is increased morbidity and mortality among children with CFRD compared with those without. Microvascular complications such as retinopathy and nephropathy may occur in children and adolescents with CFRD (O'Riordan, Dattani, and Hindmarsh, 2010). However, ketoacidosis is reported to be rare in individuals with CFRD (Egan, 2011). Children with CFRD should perform self–blood glucose monitoring (SBGM) 3 times daily and should be on an insulin regimen. Target glucose levels should be the same as for any other patient with diabetes. There is no evidence that oral glycemic agents are effective. During acute CF exacerbations, the nondiabetic child should be monitored closely for hyperglycemia; glycosylated hemoglobin is reportedly a poor predictor of CFRD, so an oral glucose tolerance test is the preferred screening tool (Moran, Brunzell, Cohen, et al., 2010).

Bone health is of concern in children and adults with CF. The pancreatic insufficiency of CF and chronic steroid use present potential risks for less-than-optimum bone growth in such children. Assessment of bone health by history and bone mass density evaluation should be considered in assessing the child's (8 years old and older) health status to detect and prevent osteoporosis and osteopenia.

Prognosis. The median predicted survival age for the patient with CF in 2009 was 37.4 years, and approximately 45% of patients are 18 years old and older (Cystic Fibrosis Foundation, 2011). Lung, heart, pancreas, and liver transplantation have increased survival rates among some patients with CF. Heart-lung and double-lung transplants have been successfully performed in children with advanced pulmonary vascular disease and hypoxia. The obstacles surrounding this technique are availability of donated organs; complications from surgery; pulmonary infections; and recurrence of obstructive bronchiolitis, which decreases transplanted lung function.

Despite considerable progress and a recent surge in new treatment modalities, CF remains a progressive and incurable disease. The pulmonary involvement ultimately determines the patient's outcome because pancreatic enzyme deficiency is less of a problem if adequate nutrition is ensured. With advances in technology, parents and adolescents are challenged to set future goals that may include college, careers, social relationships, and marriage. Concurrently, they are faced with increasing morbidity and higher rates of CF complications as they grow older.

CARE MANAGEMENT

Assessment of the child with CF involves both pulmonary and gastrointestinal observations. Pulmonary assessment is the same as that described for asthma, with special attention to lung sounds, observation of cough, and evidence of decreased activity or fatigue. Gastrointestinal assessment primarily involves observing the frequency and nature of the stools and abdominal distention. The observer is also alert to evidence of growth failure (e.g., weight loss, muscle wasting, pallor, anorexia, decreased activity [from baseline norm]). Family members are interviewed to determine the child's or adolescent's eating and eliminating habits and to confirm a history of frequent respiratory tract infections or bowel obstruction in infancy.

The nurse assesses the newborn for feeding and stooling patterns, which may indicate a potential problem such as meconium ileus. The nurse also participates in diagnostic testing such as the initial newborn screening, IRT, DNA analysis, or sweat chloride test.

Parents are often anxious and puzzled about the diagnostic tests and the possible implications of the test results. They need careful explanations of the disease, how it might affect their family, and what they can do to provide the best possible care for their child. It is crucial to involve the parents in the follow-up for early diagnostic testing; the neonate may require several follow-up visits in the first few weeks of life if initial test results are not conclusive.

The uncertainty, fear, and initial shock associated with the diagnosis are overwhelming to parents. They must face the impact of the chronic, life-threatening nature of the disease and the prospect of intensive treatment, for which they must assume a major part of the responsibility and for which they are ill prepared. They often fear that they will be unable to provide the care the child needs.

Hospital Care. Most patients with CF require hospitalization only for treatment of pulmonary infection, uncontrolled diabetes, or a coexisting medical problem that cannot be treated on an outpatient basis. Therefore, when patients with CF are hospitalized, Standard Precautions with meticulous hand washing should be implemented to decrease the health care–associated infection (HAI) spread of organisms to the CF patient and among other hospitalized CF patients (especially when MRSA is prevalent). Contact Precautions may be required for specific infections.

When the child with CF is hospitalized for diagnosis or treatment of pulmonary complications, aerosol therapy, percussion, and postural drainage are instituted or continued. Respiratory therapists often initiate, supervise, and provide these treatments; however, it is the nurse's responsibility to monitor the patient's tolerance to the procedure and evaluate the effectiveness of the procedure in relation to treatment goals. The nurse may at times administer aerosol therapy, perform chest percussion and postural drainage, assist with ACTs such as the mechanical vest, and teach breathing exercises. Chest percussion and postural drainage should not be performed before or immediately after meals. Planning percussion and postural drainage so it does not coincide with meals is difficult in the hospital situation but is essential to the effectiveness of this treatment.

Nursing assessments, including observation of respiratory pattern, work of breathing, and lung auscultation, are vital assessments. Noninvasive pulse oximetry provides valuable data about the patient's oxygenation status. Supplemental oxygen therapy is administered to the child with mild or moderate respiratory distress, and the child requires frequent assessment of the tolerance to the procedure.

One of the nursing challenges in the care of the child with CF is encouraging compliance with the therapeutic medication regimen, which often involves a significant number of medications—pancreatic enzymes; vitamins A, D, E, and K; oral antifungals for *Candida* infection; antihistamines; antiinflammatory agents; and oral antibiotics. This may be overwhelming to the child. Factor in multiple inhaled bronchodilators, ACTs and postural and aerosol treatments, blood glucose monitoring and insulin administration, various other medications, and increased mucus production during the acute phase, and it is common for the child with CF to rebel and be noncompliant with this regimen. Gentle coaxing, positive reinforcement, and frank negotiation may be required to enlist cooperation for effective medication compliance.

The diet for the child with CF represents another challenge; careful planning with a pediatric dietitian and the child's input may help decrease the loss of appetite and weight loss that are often part of the condition. Children in the early stages of CF often have a good appetite. With infection and increased lung involvement, their appetite diminishes, and eventually it becomes a challenge to tempt failing appetites. When dietary intake fails to meet the child's needs for growth, enteral feedings or supplements may be considered. These feedings may be administered via a gastrostomy tube during the night to minimize the disruption of daily activities, including school. A skin-level feeding gastrostomy affords the child few activity restrictions and minimal disruption of body image compared with a nasogastric tube or conventional gastrostomy tube. The child and parents are encouraged to not perceive this therapy as a last-ditch effort but as an adjunct therapy to maintain optimum growth and prevent excessive weight loss. Some children have a nasogastric tube placed before bedtime and receive enteral feeds overnight, removing the tube in the morning so that it does not interfere with regular activities.

The child or adolescent needs support during the many treatments and tests that are a part of the hospitalization. IV fluids, IV antibiotics and antifungals, PICC line placement or port accessing, and blood tests are almost always a part of the acute care treatment, and the child soon associates hospitalization with these stress-provoking procedures.

Depression, anxiety, and disturbed self-image may occur in children and adolescents with CF; older adolescents and young adults with severe symptoms may be especially prone to depression as a result of the realization of the poor prognosis and the reality of unmet life expectations and goals.

Providing support to both the child and the family is essential. Skilled nursing care and sympathetic attention to the emotional needs of the child and family help them cope with the stresses associated with repeated respiratory tract infections and hospitalizations.

The care of the child or adolescent who is immobilized as a result of CF requires the same care and attention as the child with immobility from any other chronic or acute illness, including skin care, bowel management, passive range of motion, and positioning.

Home Care. Most children and adolescents with CF can be managed at home. The goals of care include normalization and daily activities, including school and peer involvement. The care plan should be flexible so that family activities are disrupted as little as possible. Parents may initially require assistance finding and contacting durable medical equipment companies that will provide home care equipment. They also need opportunities to learn how to use the equipment and to solve problems they may encounter while delivering therapy at home. A home health care provider may be required for assistance with the many medications required for maintenance of the condition, and total parenteral nutrition may also be provided through a home health care provider. Care coordination is an important nursing role in the care of

the child and adolescent with CF; as adolescents transition to adulthood, the primary care by one physician may cease to exist and the individual may have to consult multiple specialists to deal with the multiorgan problems often experienced; the care coordinator has an important role in assisting the adolescent and family with this aspect of care.

Patients and family members need education about the preferred diet of nutritious meals with tolerated fat, increased protein and carbohydrate, and the administration of pancreatic enzymes. For infants and young children, the enzymes can be mixed with pureed fruit, such as applesauce, and fed with a spoon. Capsules are usually suitable for older children. It is important to stress to parents that the enzymes, in the amount regulated to the child's needs, should be administered at the beginning of all meals and snacks. For enteral feeds administered overnight, enzymes are generally administered at the start and finish of the feeds.

One of the most important aspects of educating parents for home care is teaching techniques for the removal of mucus (ACT, vest, forced expiration) and breathing exercises. The success of a therapy program depends on conscientious performance of these treatments regularly as prescribed. The number of times these therapies are performed each day is determined on an individual basis, and often parents readily learn to adjust the number and intensity of the treatments to the child's needs. For pulmonary infection, home IV antibiotics may be prescribed pending verification of insurance coverage and availability of an agency with adequate staff to perform multiple daily home antibiotic infusions. With use of the venous access devices, such as PICC lines, and implanted ports, the parents and child can be taught the technique of direct administration into the IV line.

Families also need information about medications and possible side effects. Children receiving multiple antibiotics may require serum drug levels to ensure therapeutic dosing.

If the child has CFRD, education on SBGM, insulin therapy, diet control, and possible complications related to this is needed. Follow-up with a pediatric endocrinologist is recommended.

Children and adolescents with CF should receive routine primary care with special attention to diet, growth and development, and immunizations. Primary care providers should be alert to any weight loss or flattening in the growth curve associated with loss of appetite, which could indicate a pulmonary exacerbation in children with CF. Anticipatory guidance concerning issues of discipline, how to incorporate aspects of the treatment regimen into the school environment, and delayed pubertal development are also important considerations for the primary care provider.

Home palliative care for the child or adolescent with CF who is in the terminal stages may be carried out with the assistance of palliative care or hospice as appropriate (see Chapter 36).

The nurse can assist the family in contacting resources that provide help to families with affected children. Various special child health services, many local clinics, private agencies, service clubs, and other community groups often offer equipment and medications either free or at reduced rates. The Cystic Fibrosis Foundation*

---

*6931 Arlington Road, Bethesda, MD 20814-3205; 301-951-4422 or 800-FIGHT CF; www.cff.org. In Canada: Canadian Cystic Fibrosis Foundation, 2221 Yonge St., Suite 601, Toronto, Ontario, Canada M4S 2B4; 800-378-2233 (toll free in Canada only); www.cysticfibrosis.ca. For information about specialized medications, especially dornase alfa, and equipment for CF and other pulmonary diseases, contact the Cystic Fibrosis Services Pharmacy, 6931 Arlington Road, 2nd floor, Bethesda, MD; 800-541-4959; www.cfservicespharmacy.com.

has chapters throughout the United States that provide education and services to families and professionals.

Family Support. One of the most challenging aspects of providing care for the family of a child or adolescent with CF is meeting the emotional needs of the child and family. The diagnosis, treatment, and prognosis for CF are often associated with many problems and frustrations. The diagnosis can evoke feelings of guilt and self-recrimination in parents.

The long-range problems for an infant, child, or adolescent with CF are those encountered in any chronic illness (see Chapter 36). Both the child and the family must make many adjustments, the success of which depends on their ability to cope and on the quality and quantity of support they receive from outside sources. It is often the nurse who assesses the home situation, organizes and coordinates these services, and collects the data needed to evaluate the effectiveness of the services.

The persistent need for treatment several times a day places tremendous strain on the family. When the child is young, a family member must perform postural drainage and other ACTs. Children often balk at these treatments, and the parents are placed in the position of insisting on adherence. The stress and anxiety related to this routine may produce feelings of resentment in both the child and the family members. When possible, occasional trusted respite care should be available to allow parents to leave the situation for short periods without undue anxiety about the child's welfare.

The affected child or adolescent may become resentful about the disease, its relentless routine of therapy, and the necessary curtailment it places on activities and relationships. The child's activities are interrupted or built around treatments, medications, and diet. This imposes hardships and influences the child's quality of life. The child should be encouraged to attend school, seek employment when old enough, and join age-appropriate peer groups to foster a life that is as normal and productive as possible. Sports are often an important part of the child's and adolescent's life; interaction with peers includes valuable life experiences, especially to adolescents. The child or adolescent with CF should be encouraged to participate in sports activities in as much as physical and pulmonary health allows. Exercise is encouraged to increase pulmonary vital capacity, promote muscle development, and enhance cardiovascular function.

As the disease progresses, however, family stress should be expected and the patient may become angry and may resist medical therapy. It is important for the nurse to recognize the family's changing needs and the grief they may experience as the CF worsens. Families should be made aware of resources for counseling. Patients need to be guided into activities that enable them to express anger, sorrow, and fear without guilt.

Transition to Adulthood. As life expectancy continues to rise for children and adolescents with CF, issues related to marriage, sexuality, childbearing, and career choice become more pressing. Male patients must be informed at some point that they will often be unable to produce offspring. It is important that the distinction be made between sterility and impotence. Normal sexual relationships can be expected. Female patients may be able to bear children but should be informed of the possible deleterious effects on the respiratory system created by the burden of pregnancy. They also need to know that their children will be carriers of the CF gene. Adolescent females may need counseling concerning the use of oral contraceptives and other contraceptive options (Hazle, 2010).

Adolescents with CF are encouraged to take personal ownership and management of the illness to maximize their life's potential.

Many adolescents and young persons with the illness enroll in college or vocational and technical training school and complete degrees either by distance learning or by attending a local school. Young people are encouraged to set life goals and live normal lives to the extent their illness allows.

Anticipatory grieving and other aspects related to care of a child with a terminal illness are also part of nursing care. For example, it is important to prepare the child and family members for end-of-life decisions and care when appropriate.

Obstructive Sleep-Disordered Breathing

Pediatric obstructive sleep-disordered breathing reportedly affects between 10% and 12% of children ages 2 to 8 years; obstructive sleep apnea syndrome (OSAS) may occur in as many as 2% of all children (Benninger and Walner, 2007b). Others report OSAS incidence of 1.2% in elementary school–age children (Bixler, Vgontzas, Lin, et al., 2009). Obstructive sleep-disordered breathing is said to form a continuum of sleep-disordered breathing ranging from partial obstruction of the upper airway to continuous episodes of complete upper airway obstruction, with the most severe form being OSAS (Benninger and Walner, 2007b). OSAS is defined by the American Thoracic Society (1996) as a disorder of breathing during sleep with prolonged partial upper airway obstruction or complete obstruction that disrupts normal respiration during sleep and normal sleep patterns. Common symptoms include habitual snoring, interrupted or disturbed sleep patterns, enuresis, and daytime neurobehavioral problems (AAP, 2012). OSAS is to be distinguished from primary snoring, which is snoring without obstructive apnea, frequent sleep arousals, or abnormalities in gas exchange. Children with OSAS usually do not exhibit daytime sleepiness as do adults, with the possible exception of obese children. If left untreated, obstructive sleep-disordered breathing may result in complications such as failure to thrive, cardiovascular problems, hypertension, poor learning, and neurobehavioral problems such as attention deficit hyperactivity disorder (AAP, 2012).

The diagnosis of obstructive sleep-disordered breathing is made by an overnight in-laboratory sleep study (polysomnography), which provides evidence of sleep disturbance, respiratory pauses, and changes in oxygenation. The six-channel polysomnography can be performed in children of all ages with videotaping or audiotaping, and abbreviated (vs. full night sleep study) polysomnography, nocturnal oximetry, or daytime nap polysomnography may be useful; however, these latter methods do not predict the severity of OSAS (AAP, 2012). Polysomnography can distinguish between OSAS and primary snoring (Owens, 2011).

The most recent AAP clinical practice guideline recommends adenotonsillectomy for OSAS as long as the child has no contraindications for surgery (AAP, 2012). Evidence indicates that tonsillectomy or adenoidectomy alone may not be sufficient to resolve OSAS because residual lymphoid tissue may contribute to continual obstruction (AAP, 2012). Complications of these surgical interventions are discussed previously in this chapter. The AAP (2012) recommends that high risk patients undergoing adenotonsillectomy be monitored as inpatients postoperatively for complications. CPAP may be helpful in older children with sleep-disordered breathing whose condition persists after surgical intervention. CPAP is a long-term therapy with frequent assessments to evaluate the required amount of pressure and the overall effectiveness of the intervention. The most recent AAP guidelines (2012) also recommend the use of topical intranasal corticosteroids for children with mild OSAS (defined as an apnea hypopnea index [AHI] of less than 5 per hour).

Surgical interventions such as tracheotomy may be required for children with craniofacial syndromes, such as Goldenhar, Pierre Robin, Apert, and Crouzon syndromes, in which there is partial or complete upper airway obstruction.

Nursing care of the child with sleep-disordered breathing involves early detection by observation of the infant's or child's sleep patterns and active participation in the diagnostic polysomnography. Important nursing roles are inserting the pH probe into the esophagus, ensuring accurate placement by radiography, and monitoring the sleep study and the patient's response to diagnostic therapy. Counseling families of children with sleep-disordered breathing may involve dietary counseling for exercise programs and weight management, use of the CPAP equipment, and direct postoperative care after the surgical intervention of tonsillectomy or adenoidectomy. Some children may resist wearing CPAP devices and will need encouragement to do this. The nurse can be instrumental in helping the child and family cope with the chronic illness diagnosis if intervention such as CPAP is required.

RESPIRATORY EMERGENCY

Respiratory Failure

Effective pulmonary gas exchange requires clear airways, normal lungs and chest wall, and adequate pulmonary circulation. Anything that affects these functions or their relationships can compromise respiration. In general, the term respiratory insufficiency is applied to two situations: (1) when there is increased work of breathing but gas exchange function is near normal; and (2) when normal blood gas tensions cannot be maintained and hypoxemia and acidosis develop secondary to carbon dioxide retention.

Respiratory failure is defined as the inability of the respiratory apparatus to maintain adequate oxygenation of the blood with or without carbon dioxide retention. This process involves pulmonary dysfunction that generally results in impaired alveolar gas exchange, which can lead to hypoxemia or hypercapnia. Respiratory failure is the most common cause of cardiopulmonary arrest in children. Respiratory arrest is the complete cessation of respiration. Apnea is the cessation of breathing for more than 20 seconds or for a shorter period when associated with hypoxemia or bradycardia. Apnea can be (1) central, in which respiratory efforts are absent; (2) obstructive, in which respiratory efforts are present; and (3) mixed, in which both central and obstructive components are present (see Apparent Life-Threatening Event, Chapter 31) Respiratory dysfunction may have an abrupt or an insidious onset. Respiratory failure can occur as an emergency situation or may be preceded by gradual and progressive deterioration of respiratory function. Most clinical manifestations are nonspecific and are affected by variations among individual patients and differences in the severity and duration of inadequate gas exchange.

Diagnostic Evaluation

The diagnosis of respiratory failure is determined by the combined application of three sources of information:

1. Presence or history of a condition that might predispose the patient to respiratory failure
2. Observation of respiratory failure
3. Measurement of ABGs and pH

Nursing observation and judgment are vital to the recognition and early management of respiratory failure. Nurses must be able to assess a situation and initiate appropriate action within moments. Signs of respiratory failure are listed in Box 40-17.

> **BOX 40-17** **CLINICAL MANIFESTATIONS OF RESPIRATORY FAILURE**
>
> **Cardinal Signs**
> - Restlessness
> - Tachypnea
> - Tachycardia
> - Diaphoresis (except in neonates)
>
> **Early But Less Obvious Signs**
> - Mood changes such as euphoria or depression
> - Headache
> - Altered depth and pattern of respirations
> - Hypertension
> - Exertional dyspnea
> - Anorexia
> - Increased cardiac output and renal output
> - Central nervous system symptoms (decreased efficiency, impaired judgment, anxiety, confusion, restlessness, irritability, depressed level of consciousness)
> - Nasal flaring
> - Chest wall retractions
> - Expiratory grunt
> - Wheezing or prolonged expiration
>
> **Signs of More Severe Hypoxia**
> - Hypotension or hypertension
> - Dimness of vision
> - Somnolence
> - Stupor
> - Coma
> - Dyspnea
> - Depressed respirations
> - Bradycardia
> - Cyanosis, peripheral or central

Therapeutic Management

The interventions used in the management of respiratory failure are often dramatic, requiring special skills and emergency procedures. If respiratory arrest occurs, the primary objectives are to recognize the situation and immediately initiate resuscitative measures, such as airway positioning, administration of oxygen, cardiopulmonary resuscitation (CPR), suctioning, CPAP or BiPAP, or intubation. When the situation is not an arrest, the suspicion of respiratory failure is confirmed by assessment; the severity may be defined by ABG analysis. Interventions such as administering supplemental oxygen, positioning, stimulation, suctioning, and early intubation may avert an arrest. When the severity is established, an attempt is made to determine the underlying cause by thorough evaluation.

The principles of management are to (1) maintain ventilation and maximize oxygen delivery, (2) correct hypoxemia and hypercapnia, (3) treat the underlying cause, (4) minimize extrapulmonary organ failure, (5) apply specific and nonspecific therapy to control oxygen demands, and (6) anticipate complications. Monitoring the patient's condition closely is critical.

CARE MANAGEMENT

For families whose child has a respiratory arrest, support is aimed at keeping the family informed of the child's status and helping them cope with a near-death experience or an actual death (see Chapter 36). Knowing that their child requires CPR is a frightening and often overwhelming experience for parents. Uncertainty regarding the outcome—both mortality and morbidity—is a primary concern. Traditionally, family members are not allowed to be present during resuscitation efforts in the ED. However, studies indicate that family presence during emergencies alleviates the family's anger about being separated from the patient during a crisis, reduces their anxiety, eliminates doubts about what was done to help the patient, and facilitates the grieving process if the patient dies (Mangurten, Scott, Guzzetta, et al., 2006).

Regardless of whether an institution permits parental presence during CPR, nurses must consider the needs, fears, and concerns of family members during this situation. If family presence is not permitted, nurses should arrange for someone to remain with the family during CPR. After the child's recovery or death, the family will continue to need support and thorough medical information regarding lifesaving measures, the prognosis if the child survives, and the cause of death if the child dies.

KEY POINTS

- Acute infection of the respiratory tract is the most common cause of illness in infancy and childhood.
- The incidence and severity of respiratory tract infections are influenced by the infectious agents involved, the child's age, and the child's natural defenses.
- Common respiratory tract infections of childhood include nasopharyngitis, pharyngitis (including tonsillitis), influenza, infectious mononucleosis, and AOM.
- Croup syndromes involve acute inflammation and variable degrees of obstruction of the epiglottis, larynx, or trachea.
- The primary goals in the care of children with croup are observation for signs of respiratory distress and relief of laryngeal inflammation.
- Common infections of the lower airways are bacterial tracheitis, bronchitis, and RSV-bronchiolitis.
- Pneumonias are classified according to site (lobar, bronchial, or interstitial) or by etiologic agent (viral, bacterial, or mycoplasmal) or are associated with aspiration of foreign material.

- In TB, susceptibility to the bacillus can be influenced by heredity, age, stress, poor nutrition, and intercurrent infection.
- Secondhand smoke exposure is a major environmental pollutant contributing to respiratory illness in children.
- Asthma is the leading cause of chronic illness in children.
- General therapeutic management of asthma includes assessment of asthma severity, allergen control, drug therapy, symptom management, and sometimes hyposensitization.
- Support for the family of the child with asthma includes education about the disease and its therapy and facilitation of self-management.
- CF is the most common inherited disease in children.
- The diagnosis of CF is based on newborn screening finding of elevated IRT, DNA analysis showing a CFTR mutation, and a positive sweat chloride test (increased sweat electrolyte content).

REFERENCES

Akinbami LJ, Moorman JE, Garbe PL, et al: Status of childhood asthma in the United States, 1980–2007, *Pediatrics* 123(Suppl 3):S131–S145, 2009.

Albuali WH, Singh RN, Fraser DD, et al: Have changes in ventilation practice improved outcome in children with acute lung injury? *Pediatr Crit Care Med* 8(4):324–330, 2007.

American Academy of Otolaryngology—Head and Neck Surgery: Clinical practice guideline: tonsillectomy in children, *Bulletin* 19(6), 2011.

American Academy of Pediatrics (AAP): Clinical practice guideline: diagnosis and management of acute otitis media, *Pediatrics* 113(5):1451–1465, 2004a.

American Academy of Pediatrics (AAP): Clinical practice guideline: otitis media with effusion, *Pediatrics* 113(5):1412–1429, 2004b.

American Academy of Pediatrics (AAP): Clinical practice guideline: diagnosis and management of bronchiolitis, *Pediatrics* 118(4):1774–1793, 2006.

American Academy of Pediatrics (AAP): Clinical practice guideline: diagnosis and management of childhood obstructive sleep apnea syndrome, *Pediatrics* 130(3):576–584, 2012.

American Academy of Pediatrics (AAP) Committee on Infectious Diseases, Pickering L, editor: *Red book: 2012 report of the Committee on Infectious Diseases*, ed 29, Elk Grove Village, IL, 2012, Author.

American Academy of Pediatrics (AAP) Committee on Nutrition and the Council on Sports Medicine and Fitness: Clinical report—sports drinks and energy drinks for children and adolescents: are they appropriate? *Pediatrics* 127(6):1182–1189, 2011.

American Academy of Pediatrics (AAP) Task Force on Sudden Infant Death Syndrome: The changing concept of sudden infant death syndrome: diagnostic coding shifts, controversies regarding the sleeping environment, and new variables to consider in reducing risk, *Pediatrics* 116(5):1245–1255, 2005.

American Thoracic Society: Standards and indications for cardiopulmonary sleep studies in children, *Am J Respir Crit Care Med* 153(2):866–878, 1996.

Antoon AY, Donovan MK: Burn injuries. In Kliegman RM, Stanton BF, St. Geme JW, et al, editors: *Nelson textbook of pediatrics*, ed 19, Philadelphia, 2011, Saunders.

Bell EA, Tunkel DE: Over-the-counter cough and cold medications in children: are they helpful? *Otolaryngol Head Neck Surg* 142(5):647–650, 2010.

Benninger M, Walner D: Coblation: improving outcomes for children following adenotonsillectomy, *Clin Cornerstone* 9(Suppl 1):S13–S23, 2007a.

Benninger M, Walner D: Obstructive sleep-disordered breathing in children, *Clin Cornerstone* 9(Suppl 1):S6–S12, 2007b.

Bernard GR, Artigas A, Brigham KL, et al: Report of the American-European consensus conference on ARDS: definitions, mechanisms, relevant outcomes and clinical trial coordination. The Consensus Committee, *Intensive Care Med* 20(3):225–232, 1994.

Bixler EO, Vgontzas AN, Lin HM, et al: Sleep disordered breathing in children in a general population sample: prevalence and risk factors, *Sleep* 32(6):731–736, 2009.

Borowitz D, Baker RD, Stallings V: Consensus report on nutrition for pediatric patients with cystic fibrosis, *J Pediatr Gastroenterol Nutr* 35(3):246–259, 2002.

Burkhart PV, Rayens MK, Revelette WR, et al: Improved health outcomes with peak flow monitoring for children with asthma, *J Asthma* 44(2):137–142, 2007.

Centers for Disease Control and Prevention (CDC): Licensure of a 13-valent pneumococcal conjugate vaccine (PCV13) and recommendations for use among children—Advisory Committee on Immunization Practices (ACIP), 2010, *MMWR Morb Mortal Wkly Rep* 59(9):258–261, 2010.

Centers for Disease Control and Prevention (CDC): Prevention and control of influenza with vaccines: recommendations of the Advisory Committee on Immunization Practices (ACIP)—United States, 2012–2013 influenza season, *MMWR Morb Mortal Wkly Rep* 61(32):613–618, 2012.

Chávez-Bueno S, Mejías A, Jafri H, et al: Respiratory syncytial virus: old challenges and new approaches, *Pediatr Ann* 34(1):62–68, 2005.

Checchia P: Identification and management of severe respiratory syncytial virus, *Am J Health-Syst Pharm* 65(1 Suppl 8):S7–S12, 2008.

Chen CM, Tischer C, Schnappinger M, et al: The role of cats and dogs in asthma and allergy: a systematic review, *Int J Hyg Environm Health* 213(1):1–31, 2010.

Cystic Fibrosis Foundation: *Frequently asked questions*, Bethesda, MD, 2011, Author, www.cff.org/AboutCF/Faqs/.

Egan M: Cystic fibrosis. In Kliegman RM, Stanton BF, St. Geme JW, et al, editors: *Nelson textbook of pediatrics*, ed 19, Philadelphia, 2011, Saunders.

Flume PA, Robinson KA, O'Sullivan BP, et al: Cystic fibrosis pulmonary guidelines: airway clearance therapies, *Respir Care* 54(4):522–537, 2009.

Food and Drug Administration (FDA): *Early communication about an ongoing safety review of omalizumab (marketed as Xolair)*, 2009, www.fda.gov/Drugs/DrugSafety/PostmarketDrugSafetyInformationfor PatientsandProviders/DrugSafety InformationforHeathcareProfessionals/ ucm172218.htm.

Food and Drug Administration (FDA): Long-acting beta-agonists (LABAs): new safe use requirements, 2011, http://www.fda.gov/Safety/MedWatch/SafetyInformation/SafetyAlertsforHumanMedicalProducts/ucm201003.htm.

Food and Drug Administration (FDA): Post-surgery codeine puts kids at risk, 2013, http://www.fda.gov/ForConsumers/ConsumerUpdates/ucm315497.htm.

Goldstein NA, Mandel EM, Kurs-Lasky M, et al: Water precautions and tympanostomy tubes: a randomized, controlled trial, *Laryngoscope* 115(2):324–330, 2005.

Hazle LA: Cystic fibrosis. In Allen PJ, Vessey JA, Schapiro NA, editors, *Primary care of the child with a chronic condition*, ed 5, St Louis, 2010, Mosby.

Heinrich J: Influence of indoor factors in dwellings on the development of childhood asthma, *Int J Hyg Environm Health* 214(1):1–25, 2011.

Hopkins A, Lahiri T, Salerno R, et al: Changing epidemiology of life-threatening upper airway infections: the reemergence of bacterial tracheitis, *Pediatrics* 118(4):1418–1421, 2006.

Kinyon Munch K: What do you tell parents when their child is sick with the common cold? *J Spec Pediatr Nurs* 16(1):8–15, 2010.

Li YF, Langholz B, Salam MT, et al: Maternal and grandmaternal smoking patterns are associated with early childhood asthma, *Chest* 127(4):1232–1241, 2005.

Lieberthal AS, Carroll AE, Chonmaitree T, et al: Clinical Practice Guideline: the diagnosis and management of acute otitis media, *Pediatrics* 131(3):e964–e994, 2013.

Liu AH, Covar RA, Spahn JD, et al: Childhood asthma. In Kliegman RM, Stanton BF, St. Geme JW, et al, editors: *Nelson textbook of pediatrics*, ed 19, Philadelphia, 2011, Saunders.

Mangurten J, Scott SH, Guzzetta CE, et al: Effects of family presence during resuscitation and invasive procedures in a pediatric emergency department, *J Emerg Nurs* 32(3):225–233, 2006.

Mazor R, Green TP: Pulmonary edema. In Kliegman RM, Stanton BF, St. Geme JW, et al, editors: *Nelson textbook of pediatrics*, ed 19, Philadelphia, 2011, Saunders.

Meissner HC, Bocchini JA: Reducing RSV hospitalizations: AAP modifies recommendation for use of palivizumab in high-risk infants, young children, *AAP News* 30(7):1–2, 2009.

Michel SH, Maqbool A, Hanna MD, et al: Nutrition management of pediatric patients who have cystic fibrosis, *Pediatr Clin North Am* 56(5):1123–1141, 2009.

Moore M, Little P: Humidified air inhalation for treating croup: a systematic review and meta-analysis, *Fam Pract* 24(4):295–301, 2007.

Moran A, Brunzell C, Cohen RC, et al: Clinical care guidelines for cystic fibrosis-related diabetes: a position statement of the American Diabetes Association and a clinical practice guideline of the Cystic Fibrosis Foundation endorsed by the Pediatric Endocrine Society, *Diabetes Care* 33(12):2697–2708, 2010.

National Asthma Education and Prevention Program: *Guidelines for the diagnosis and management of asthma*, August 2007, www.nhlbi.nih.gov/guidelines/asthma/index.htm.

National Newborn Screening and Genetics Resource Center: National Newborn Screening Status Report, National Newborn Screening and Genetics Resource Center, UTHSCSA, 2013, Austin, TX, http://genes-r-us.uthscsa.edu/sites/genes-r-us/files/nbsdisorders.pdf.

Newton TJ: Respiratory care of the hospitalized patient with cystic fibrosis, *Respir Care* 54(6):769–775, 2009.

O'Riordan SMP, Dattani MT, Hindmarsh PC: Cystic fibrosis-related diabetes in childhood, *Horm Res Paediatr* 73(1):15–24, 2010.

Owens JA: Sleep medicine. In Kliegman RM, Stanton BF, St. Geme JW, et al, editors: *Nelson textbook of pediatrics*, ed 19, Philadelphia, 2011, Saunders.

Perez-Velez CM: Pediatric tuberculosis: new guidelines and recommendations, *Curr Opin Pediatr* 24(3):319–328, 2012.

Pettit RS: Cystic fibrosis transmembrane conductance regulator–modifying medications: the future of cystic fibrosis treatment, *Ann Pharmacother* 46(7–8):1065–1075, 2012.

Pratter MR: Cough and the common cold: ACCP evidence-based clinical practice guidelines, *Chest* 129(Suppl):S72–S74, 2006.

Rafei K, Lichenstein R: Airway infectious disease emergencies, *Pediatr Clin North Am* 53(2):215–242, 2006.

Randolph AG: Management of acute lung injury and acute respiratory distress syndrome in children, *Crit Care Med* 37(8):2448–2454, 2009.

Ranganathan SC, Sonnappa S: Pneumonia and other respiratory infections, *Pediatr Clin North Am* 56(1):135–156, 2009.

Redding GJ: Bronchiectasis in children, *Pediatr Clin North Am* 56(1):157–171, 2009.

Ren CL, Morgan WJ, Konstan KW, et al: Presence of methicillin-resistant *Staphylococcus aureus* in respiratory cultures from cystic fibrosis patients is associated with lower lung function, *Pediatr Pulmonol* 42(6):513–518, 2007.

Rimsza ME, Newberry S: Unexpected infant deaths associated with use of cough and cold medications, *Pediatrics* 122(2):e318–e322, 2008.

Rodgers GL, Klugman KP: The future of pneumococcal disease prevention, *Vaccine* 29(Suppl 3):C43–C48, 2011.

Roosevelt GE: Bacterial tracheitis. In Kliegman RM, Stanton BF, St. Geme JW, et al, editors: *Nelson textbook of pediatrics*, ed 19, Philadelphia, 2011, Saunders.

Roque Figuls M, Gine-Garriga M, Granados Rugeles C, et al: Chest physiotherapy for acute bronchiolitis in paediatric patients between 0 and 24 months old, *Cochrane Database Syst Rev* 2:CD004873, 2012.

Ryan T, Brewer M, Small L: Over-the-counter cough and cold medication use in young children, *Pediatr Nurs* 34(2):174–180, 184, 2008.

Sandora TJ, Sectish TC: Community-acquired pneumonia. In Kliegman RM, Stanton BF,

St. Geme JW, et al, editors: *Nelson textbook of pediatrics*, ed 19, Philadelphia, 2011, Saunders.

Sheahan SL, Free TA: Counseling parents to quit smoking, *Pediatr Nurs* 31(2):98–108, 2005.

Sicherer SH, Wood RA, AAP Section on Allergy and Immunology: Allergy testing in childhood: using allergen-specific IgE tests, *Pediatrics* 129(1): 193–197, 2012.

Siegel JD, Rhinehart J, Jackson M, et al: *2007 guidelines for isolation precautions: preventing transmission of infectious agents in healthcare settings*, Centers for Disease Control and Prevention, 2007, Atlanta, http://www.cdc.gov/hicpac/2007ip /2007isolationprecautions.html.

Sovari AA, Ooi HH: Cardiogenic pulmonary edema, 2008, http://emedicine.medscape. com/article/157452-overview#a0104.

Thomson NC, Chaudhuri R: Omalizumab: clinical use for the management of asthma, *Clin Med Insights Circ Respir Pulm Med* 6:27–40, 2012.

Vassilev ZP, Kabadi S, Villa R: Safety and efficacy of over-the-counter cough and cold medicines for use in children, *Expert Opin Drug Saf* 9(2):233–242, 2010.

Ventre K, Randolph AG: Ribavirin for respiratory syncytial virus infection of the lower respiratory tract in infants and young children, *Cochrane Database Syst Rev* 24(1):CD000181, 2007.

Volpe DI, Smith MF, Sultan K: Managing pediatric asthma exacerbations in the ED, *Am J Nurs* 111(2):48–53, 2011.

Watts KD, Goodman DM: Wheezing in infants: bronchiolitis. In Kliegman RM, Stanton BF, St. Geme JW, et al, editors: *Nelson textbook of pediatrics*, ed 19, Philadelphia, 2011, Saunders.

Wessels MR: Streptococcal pharyngitis, *NEJM* 364(7):648–655, 2011.

World Health Organization (WHO): *Global Alert and Response (GAR): pandemic preparedness*, 2011, www.who.int/csr/disease/ influenza/pandemic/en/.

Wright M, Piedimonte G: Respiratory syncytial virus prevention and therapy: past, present, and future, *Pediatr Pulmonology* 46(4):324– 347, 2011.

Wu P, Hartert TV: Evidence for a causal relationship between respiratory syncytial virus infection and asthma, *Expert Rev Anti Infect Ther* 9(9):731–745, 2011.

Zhang K, Wang X: Maternal smoking and increased risk of sudden infant death syndrome: a meta-analysis, *Leg Med (Tokyo)* 15(3):115–121, 2012.

Zoorob R, Sidani M, Murray J: Croup: an overview, *Am Fam Physician* 83(9):1067– 1073, 2011.

41

Gastrointestinal Dysfunction

David Wilson

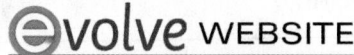 **WEBSITE**

http://evolve.elsevier.com/Perry/maternal

LEARNING OBJECTIVES

On completion of this chapter, the reader will be able to:

- Identify children at increased risk of developing nutritional disorders.
- Outline a nutritional counseling plan for vitamin or mineral deficiency or excess.
- Describe the characteristics of infants and small children that affect their ability to adapt to fluid loss or gain.
- Formulate a plan of care for the infant with acute diarrhea.
- Compare and contrast the inflammatory bowel diseases.
- Identify the routes of transmission for hepatitis A, B, and C.
- Describe the nursing care of the child with hepatitis.
- Formulate a plan for teaching parents preoperative and postoperative care of the child with a cleft lip, cleft palate, or both.

- Formulate a plan of care for the child with an obstructive gastrointestinal disorder.
- Identify nutritional therapies for the child with a malabsorption syndrome.
- Outline a teaching plan designed to prevent transmission of intestinal parasites.
- Identify the principles in the emergency treatment of accidental poisoning.
- Name four sources of lead in the environment.
- Describe the nursing care of the child with lead poisoning.
- Describe the nursing care of the child with appendicitis.

NUTRITIONAL DISORDERS

Reports of severe nutritional disorders in childhood in most developed countries are uncommon, yet small numbers of children who may experience a nutritional deficiency of some type often exist. The 2008 Feeding Infants and Toddlers Study (FITS) found that usual nutrient intake of infants, toddlers, and preschoolers (ages 0 to 47 months) met or exceeded energy and protein requirements based on the Dietary Reference Intakes (DRIs) and the 2005 Dietary Guidelines for Americans (Butte, Fox, Briefel, et al., 2010). According to the study, a small but significant number of infants were at risk for inadequate intake of iron and zinc. Dietary fiber intakes in toddlers and preschoolers were low, and saturated fat intakes exceeded recommendations for the majority of preschoolers (Butte, Fox, Briefel, et al., 2010). There are reports of an increased dependence on fortified foods and supplements in toddlers to meet nutritional requirements rather than meeting such needs with a wide variety of fruits, vegetables, and whole grains (Fox, Reidy, Novak, et al., 2006).

The findings of these studies and other similar reports are important for nurses who work with infants and children. Nurses must work to promote healthy nutrition habits early in children's lives through proper education of families and children about healthy lifestyle habits, including diet and exercise for health promotion and prevention of morbidities associated with poor micronutrient intake and sedentary lifestyle.

Vitamin Imbalances

Although true vitamin deficiencies are rare in the United States, subclinical deficiencies are commonly seen in population subgroups in which either maternal or child dietary intake is imbalanced and contains inadequate amounts of vitamins. Vitamin D–deficiency rickets, once rarely seen because of the widespread commercial availability of vitamin D–fortified milk, increased before the turn of the century. Populations at risk include the following:

- Children who are breastfed exclusively by mothers with an inadequate intake of vitamin D or breastfed exclusively longer than 6 months without adequate maternal vitamin D intake or supplementation
- Children with dark skin pigmentation who are exposed to minimal sunlight because of socioeconomic, religious, or

cultural beliefs or housing in urban areas with high levels of pollution

- Children with diets that are low in sources of vitamin D and calcium
- Individuals who use milk products not supplemented with vitamin D (e.g., yogurt,* raw cow's milk) as the primary source of milk

The American Academy of Pediatrics (AAP) (2008) recommends that infants who are breastfed exclusively receive 400 IU of vitamin D beginning shortly after birth to prevent rickets and vitamin D deficiency. Vitamin D supplementation should continue until the infant is consuming at least 1 L/day (or 1 quart/day) of vitamin D–fortified formula (AAP, 2008). Nonbreastfed infants who are taking less than 1 L/day of vitamin D–fortified formula should also receive a daily vitamin D supplement of 400 IU. Inadequate maternal ingestion of cobalamin (vitamin B_{12}) may contribute to infant neurologic impairment when exclusive breastfeeding (past 6 months) is the only source of the infant's nutrition. A correlation between the incidence of childhood upper respiratory infections and vitamin D deficiency has been found, but the implications of the findings have yet to be completely understood (Taylor and Camargo, 2011; Walker and Modlin, 2009).

Children may also be at risk for vitamin deficiencies secondary to disorders or their treatment. For example, vitamin deficiencies of the fat-soluble vitamins A and D may occur in malabsorptive disorders such as cystic fibrosis and short bowel syndrome. Preterm infants may develop rickets in the second month of life as a result of inadequate intake of vitamin D, calcium, and phosphorus. Children receiving high doses of salicylates may have impaired vitamin C storage. Environmental tobacco smoke exposure has been implicated in decreased concentrations of ascorbate in children; therefore increased intake of sources of vitamin C should be encouraged even in children minimally exposed to environmental tobacco smoke (Preston, Rodriguez, and Rivera, 2003). Children with chronic illnesses resulting in anorexia, decreased food intake, or possible nutrient malabsorption as a result of multiple medications should be evaluated carefully for adequate vitamin and mineral intake in some form (parenteral or enteral).

Children with sickle cell disease are reported to have suboptimal intakes (according to DRI recommendations) of vitamins E and D, folate, calcium, and fiber, which decrease significantly with increasing age. Poor dietary intake was a significant factor in the findings of the study (Kawchak, Schall, Zemel, et al., 2007). One study found that children with intestinal failure who were being transitioned from parenteral to enteral nutrition had at least one vitamin and mineral deficiency; vitamin D was the most common deficiency identified, and zinc and iron were the most common minerals identified as being deficient (Yang, Duro, Zurakowski, et al., 2011).

Vitamin A deficiency has been reported with increased morbidity and mortality in children with measles. However, a Cochrane review of studies wherein a single dose of vitamin A was administered to children with measles found no decrease in mortality. Children with measles younger than the age of 2 years who received two doses of vitamin A (200,000 IU) on consecutive days did have decreased mortality rates and a reduced rate of pneumonia-specific mortality (Huiming, Chaomin, and Meng, 2005). Complications from diarrhea and infections are often increased in infants and children with vitamin A deficiency. Although scurvy (caused by a deficiency of vitamin C) is rare in developed countries, cases have been reported in children who were fed an organic diet deficient in vegetables and fruits (Burk and Molodow, 2007).

An excessive dose of a vitamin is generally defined as 10 or more times the Recommended Dietary Allowance (RDA), although the fat-soluble vitamins, especially vitamins A and D, tend to cause toxic reactions at lower doses. With the addition of vitamins to commercially prepared foods, the potential for hypervitaminosis has increased, especially when combined with the excessive use of vitamin supplements. Hypervitaminosis of vitamins A and D presents the greatest problems because these fat-soluble vitamins are stored in the body. High intakes of vitamin A have been linked to physeal growth arrest, which can lead to osteoporosis, fracture, and metaphyseal irregularity (Saltzman and King, 2007). Chronic hypervitaminosis A may result in signs and symptoms of headache; vomiting; dry, itching desquamating skin; anorexia; fissures at the corner of the mouth; weight loss; bulging fontanels; and neurologic signs such as irritability and stupor (Zile, 2011). An excessive intake of vitamin A in pregnant women has also been linked to fetal defects (Zile, 2011). Vitamin D is the most likely of all vitamins to cause toxic reactions in relatively small overdoses. The water-soluble vitamins, primarily niacin, B_6, and C, can also cause toxicity. Poor outcomes in infants (e.g., fatal hypermagnesemia) have been associated with megavitamin therapy with high doses of magnesium oxide, and severe anemia and thrombocytopenia have resulted from megadoses of vitamin A.

One vitamin supplement that is recommended for all women of childbearing age is a daily dose of 0.4 mg of folic acid, the usual RDA. Folic acid taken before conception and during early pregnancy can reduce the risk of neural tube defects such as spina bifida by as much as 70%. Drugs such as oral contraceptives and antidepressants may decrease folic acid absorption; thus adolescent girls taking such medications should consider supplementation. (See Spina Bifida (Myelomeningocele, Chapter 49.)

Mineral Imbalances

A number of minerals are essential nutrients. The macrominerals refer to those with daily requirements greater than 100 mg and include calcium, phosphorus, magnesium, sodium, potassium, chloride, and sulfur. Microminerals, or trace elements, have daily requirements of less than 100 mg and include several essential minerals and those in which the exact role in nutrition is still unclear. The greatest concern with minerals is deficiency, especially iron deficiency anemia (see Chapter 43). However, other minerals that may be inadequate in children's diets, even with supplementation, include calcium, phosphorus, magnesium, and zinc. Low levels of zinc can cause nutritional growth failure (failure to thrive [FTT]). Some of the macrominerals may be overlooked inadvertently when a child with intestinal failure or recent surgery is making the transition from total parenteral to enteral intake.

An imbalance in the intake of calcium and phosphorous may occur in infants who are given whole cow's milk instead of infant formula; neonatal tetany may be observed in such cases. Whole cow's milk is also a poor source of iron, and inadequate intake of iron from other food sources such as iron-fortified cereal may cause iron deficiency anemia.

The regulation of mineral balance in the body is a complex process. Dietary extremes of mineral intake can cause a number of mineral-mineral interactions that could result in unexpected deficiencies or excesses. For example, excessive amounts of one mineral such as zinc can result in a deficiency of another mineral such as copper even if sufficient amounts of copper are ingested. Thus

---

*Yogurt does not contain adequate amounts of vitamins A and D (unless specifically fortified with these vitamins) but is an acceptable source of calcium and phosphorus.

megadose intake of one mineral may cause an inadvertent deficiency of another essential mineral by blocking its absorption in the blood or intestinal wall or competing with binding sites on protein carriers needed for metabolism.

Deficiencies can also occur when various substances in the diet interact with minerals. For example, iron, zinc, and calcium can form insoluble complexes with phytates or oxalates (substances found in plant proteins), which impair the bioavailability of the mineral. This type of interaction is important in vegetarian diets because plant foods such as soy are high in phytates. Contrary to popular opinion, spinach is not an ideal source of iron or calcium because of its high oxalate content. Factors that affect iron absorption are listed in Chapter 32.

Children with certain illnesses are at greater risk for growth failure, especially in relation to bone mineral deficiency as a result of the treatment of the disease, decreased nutrient intake, or decreased absorption of necessary minerals. Those at risk for such deficiencies include children who are receiving or have received radiation and chemotherapy for cancer; children with human immunodeficiency virus (HIV), sickle cell disease, cystic fibrosis, gastrointestinal (GI) malabsorption, or nephrosis; and extremely low–birth-weight (ELBW) and very low–birth-weight (VLBW) preterm infants.

CARE MANAGEMENT

Identification of adequacy of nutrient intake is the initial nursing goal and requires assessment based on a dietary history and physical examination for signs of deficiency or excess (see Nutrition, Chapter 32, and Nutritional Assessment, Chapter 29). After assessment data are collected, this information is evaluated against standard intakes to identify areas of concern. DRIs are one source of standard nutrient intakes (see Chapter 32, Dietary Guidelines).

Standardized growth reference charts should be used in infants, children, and adolescents to compare and assess growth parameters such as height and head circumference with the percentile distribution of other children at the same ages. The World Health Organization (WHO) growth chart is a standardized growth reference now recommended for infants and toddlers up to 24 months of age. This growth chart includes head circumference, height, and weight references that were derived from healthy children in six different countries around the world. These growth standards are based on the growth of healthy breastfed infants throughout the first year of life. The Centers for Disease Control and Prevention (CDC) growth charts are now recommended for children 2 to 19 years of age (Grummer-Strawn, Reinold, Krebs, et al., 2010).

Infants should be breastfed for the first 6 months and preferably for 1 year, be introduced to some solid foods after about 4 to 6 months, and receive iron-fortified cereal for at least 18 months (see Chapter 31). Vitamin B_{12} supplementation is recommended if the breastfeeding mother's intake of the vitamin is inadequate or if she is not taking vitamin supplements (Dunham and Kollar, 2006). If the infant is being breastfed exclusively after 4 months (when fetal iron stores are depleted), iron supplementation (1 mg/kg/day) is recommended until appropriate iron-containing complementary foods such as iron-fortified cereal are introduced (Baker, Greer, and AAP Committee on Nutrition, 2010). The introduction of solids for vegetarian infants may occur using the same guidelines as for other children (see Chapter 32). A variety of foods should be introduced during the early years to ensure a well-balanced intake. Infants who are identified as having particular nutritional deficits should be identified; a multidisciplinary approach should be taken for identifying the deficit and the etiology, and a plan established with the caregiver to promote adequate growth and development.

Protein-Energy Malnutrition (Severe Childhood Undernutrition)

Malnutrition continues to be a major health problem in the world today, particularly in children younger than 5 years of age. However, lack of food is not always the primary cause of malnutrition. In many developing and underdeveloped nations, diarrhea (gastroenteritis) is a major factor. Additional factors are bottle-feeding (in poor sanitary conditions), inadequate knowledge of proper child care practices, parental illiteracy, economic and political factors, climate conditions, cultural and religious food preferences, and simply a lack of adequate food. Müller and Krawinkel (2005) point out that poverty is the underlying cause of malnutrition. The most extreme forms, or protein-energy malnutrition (PEM), are kwashiorkor and marasmus. Some authorities suggest that severe malnutrition encompasses more than protein-energy deficits and thus prefer the term *severe childhood undernutrition (SCU)*. Another term used is *severe acute malnutrition (SAM)*. Entities such as the WHO continue to use the term *protein-energy malnutrition*. SCU may also be subdivided into edematous (kwashiorkor) and nonedematous (marasmus) types.

In the United States milder forms of PEM are seen as a result of primary malnutrition, although the classic cases of marasmus and kwashiorkor may also occur. Unlike in developing countries, where the main reason for PEM is inadequate food, in the United States PEM occurs despite ample dietary supplies (see Failure to Thrive, Chapter 31). It may also be seen in people with chronic health problems such as cystic fibrosis, renal dialysis, cancer, and GI malabsorption; in elderly adults who have chronic malnutrition; and in people with acute illnesses such as prolonged, untreated anorexia nervosa. Kwashiorkor has been reported in the United States in children fed only a rice beverage diet (Rice Dream) and few solid foods and in infants who were fed nonstandard infant diets such as flour water, corn porridge, molasses, and nondairy creamer (Katz, Mahlberg, Honig, et al., 2005; Tierney, Sage, and Shwayder, 2010). Kwashiorkor has also been reported in the United States when infants have been fed inappropriate food as a result of parental (caretaker) nutritional ignorance, a perceived cow's milk–based formula intolerance, family social chaos, or cow's milk intolerance. Therefore it is important that health care workers not assume that PEM cannot occur in developed countries; a comprehensive dietary history should be obtained in any child with clinical features resembling PEM.

Kwashiorkor

Kwashiorkor has been defined primarily as a deficiency of protein with an adequate supply of calories. A diet consisting mainly of starch grains or tubers provides adequate calories in the form of carbohydrates but an inadequate amount of high-quality proteins. However, some evidence supports a multifactorial etiology, including cultural, psychologic, and infective factors, that may interact to place the child at risk for kwashiorkor. Some experts suggest that kwashiorkor may result from the interplay of nutrient deprivation, response to infection and oxidative stress, and environmental stresses, which combined produce an imbalanced response to such insults (Penny, 2008). It often occurs subsequent to an infectious outbreak of measles and dysentery. There is further evidence that oxidative stress occurs in children with kwashiorkor, resulting in free radical damage, which may precipitate cellular changes, resulting in edema and muscle wasting. The role of the essential fatty acid arachidonic acid in lipid metabolism, altered leukotriene production, and oxidative stress in kwashiorkor has yet to be fully understood, but abnormal essential fatty acid metabolism seems to have an interactive role in its development (Penny, 2008).

Taken from the Ga language (Ghana), the word *kwashiorkor* means "the sickness the older child gets when the next baby is born" and aptly describes the syndrome that develops in the first child, usually between 1 and 4 years of age, when weaned from the breast after the second child is born.

The child with kwashiorkor has thin, wasted extremities and a prominent abdomen from edema (ascites). The edema often masks severe muscular atrophy, making the child appear less debilitated than he or she actually is. The skin is scaly and dry and has areas of depigmentation. Several dermatoses may be evident, partly resulting from the vitamin deficiencies. Permanent blindness often results from the severe lack of vitamin A. Mineral deficiencies especially iron, calcium, and zinc, are common. Acute zinc deficiency is a common complication of severe PEM and results in skin rashes, loss of hair, impaired immune response and susceptibility to infections, digestive problems, night blindness, changes in affective behavior, defective wound healing, and impaired growth. Its depressant effect on appetite further limits food intake. The hair is thin, dry, coarse, and dull. Depigmentation is common, and patchy alopecia may occur.

Diarrhea (persistent diarrhea malnutrition syndrome) commonly occurs from a lowered resistance to infection and further complicates the electrolyte imbalance. Low levels of cytokines (protein cells involved in the primary response to infection) have been reported in children with kwashiorkor, suggesting that such children have a blunted immune response to infection. A large number of deaths in children with kwashiorkor occur in those who develop HIV infection. GI disturbances such as fatty infiltration of the liver and atrophy of the acini cells of the pancreas occur. Anemia is also a common finding in malnourished children. Protein deficiency increases the child's susceptibility to infection, which eventually results in death. Fatal deterioration may be caused by diarrhea and infection or by circulatory failure.

Marasmus

Marasmus results from general malnutrition of both calories and protein. It is common in underdeveloped countries during times of drought, especially in cultures where adults eat first; the remaining food is often insufficient in quality and quantity for the children.

Marasmus is usually a syndrome of physical and emotional deprivation and is not confined to geographic areas where food supplies are inadequate. It may be seen in children with growth failure in whom the cause is not solely nutritional but primarily emotional. Marasmus may be seen in infants as young as 3 months of age if breastfeeding is not successful and there are no suitable alternatives. Marasmic kwashiorkor is a form of PEM in which clinical findings of both kwashiorkor and marasmus are evident; the child has edema, severe wasting, and stunted growth. In marasmic kwashiorkor the child has inadequate nutrient intake and superimposed infection. Fluid and electrolyte disturbances, hypothermia, and hypoglycemia are associated with a poor prognosis.

Marasmus is characterized by gradual wasting and atrophy of body tissues, especially of subcutaneous fat. The child appears to be very old, with loose and wrinkled skin, unlike the child with kwashiorkor, who appears more rounded from the edema. Fat metabolism is less impaired than in kwashiorkor; thus deficiency of

fat-soluble vitamins is usually minimal or absent. In general the clinical manifestations of marasmus are similar to those seen in kwashiorkor with the following exceptions: with marasmus there is no edema from hypoalbuminemia or sodium retention, which contributes to a severely emaciated appearance; no dermatoses caused by vitamin deficiencies; little or no depigmentation of hair or skin; moderately normal fat metabolism and lipid absorption; and a smaller head size and slower recovery after treatment. There is also an abnormal regulation of the sodium-potassium pump, resulting in an increase in intracellular sodium and a decrease in potassium (Penny, 2008).

The child is fretful, apathetic, withdrawn, and so lethargic that prostration frequently occurs. Intercurrent infection with debilitating diseases such as tuberculosis, parasitosis, HIV, and dysentery is common.

Therapeutic Management

The treatment of PEM includes providing a diet with high-quality proteins, carbohydrates, vitamins, and minerals. When PEM occurs as a result of persistent diarrhea, three management goals are identified:

1. Rehydration with an oral rehydration solution (ORS) that also replaces electrolytes
2. Administration of antibiotics to prevent intercurrent infections
3. Provision of adequate (energy intake) nutrition by either breastfeeding or a proper weaning diet

Local protocols are used in developing countries to deal with PEM. Penny (2008) and Alderman and Shekar (2011) recommend a three-phase treatment protocol: (1) acute or initial phase in the first 2 to 10 days involving initiation of treatment for oral rehydration, diarrhea, and intestinal parasites; prevention of hypoglycemia and hypothermia; and subsequent dietary management; (2) recovery or rehabilitation (2 to 6 weeks) focusing on increasing dietary intake, iron fortification, and weight gain; and (3) follow-up phase, focusing on care after discharge in an outpatient setting to prevent relapse and promote weight gain, provide developmental stimulation, and evaluate cognitive and motor deficits. In the acute phase care is taken to prevent fluid overload; the child is observed closely for signs of food or fluid intolerance. The refeeding syndrome may occur if intake progresses too rapidly; cardiac failure may cause sudden death in a child who has been malnourished and refed too rapidly (Grover and Ee, 2009). Severe hypophosphatemia may develop during the first week of initiating feedings and is considered to be the hallmark of refeeding syndrome (Alderman and Shekar, 2011). Signs and symptoms include weakness, arrhythmias, altered levels of consciousness, seizures, cardiorespiratory failure, and sudden death.

Vitamin and mineral supplementation is required in most cases of PEM; vitamin A, zinc, and copper are recommended; iron supplementation is not recommended until the child is able to tolerate a steady food source. In addition, the child is observed for signs of skin breakdown, which should be treated to prevent infection. Breastfeeding is encouraged if the mother and child are able to do so effectively; in some cases partial supplementation with a modified cow's milk–based formula may be necessary.

The WHO (2006) issued a statement recognizing the importance of breastfeeding for the first 6 months in developing countries where HIV is prevalent among childbearing women and children. It recognizes that appropriate sources of food and water for infants may not be available after the 6 months are concluded and that the risk for malnutrition is greater among such children than the theoretic risk of HIV. However, the organization does recommend that breastfeeding continue after 6 months with the introduction of complementary foods, provided they are safe for child consumption. In severely malnourished children a modest energy food source is given initially, followed by a high-protein and energy food source; severely malnourished children do not tolerate a high-energy and high-protein source initially. A number of food sources may be provided to treat PEM. They include ORSs (ReSoMal), amino acid–based elemental food, and ready-to-feed foods that do not require the addition of water (to minimize contaminated water consumption); parenteral and oral antibiotics are often part of the standard treatment for PEM (Amadi, Mwiya, Chomba, et al., 2005; Ciliberto, Sandige, Ndekha, et al., 2005).

CARE MANAGEMENT

Because PEM appears early in childhood, primarily in children 6 months to 2 years of age, and is associated with early weaning, a low-protein diet, delayed introduction of complementary foods, and frequent infections (Grover and Ee, 2009; Müller and Krawinkel, 2005), it is essential that nursing care focus on *prevention* of PEM through parent education about feeding practices during this crucial period. Prevention should also focus on the nutritional health of pregnant women because this directly impacts the health of their unborn children. Breastfeeding is the optimal method of feeding for the first 6 months. The immune properties naturally found in breast milk not only nourish infants but also help prevent opportunistic infections, which may contribute to PEM. Providing for essential physiologic needs such as appropriate nutrient intake, protection from infection, adequate hydration, skin care, and restoration of physiologic integrity is paramount. Additional nursing care focuses on education about and administration of childhood vaccinations to prevent illness, promotion of nutrition and well-being for the lactating mother, encouragement and participation in well-child visits for infants and toddlers, appropriate food sources for children being weaned from breastfeeding, and education regarding sanitation practices to prevent childhood GI diseases.

Poor skin integrity further increases the chance of infections, hypothermia, water loss, and skin breakdown. Tube feedings may be required for infants too weak to breastfeed or bottle-feed. Oral rehydration with an approved ORS is commonly used in cases of PEM in which diarrhea and infection are not immediately life threatening.

One approach that has gained acceptance for treating childhood malnutrition in developing countries is the home-based use of ready-to-use therapeutic food (RUTF). RUTF is a paste based on peanut butter and dried skim milk with vitamins and minerals; it requires no mixing with water or milk. The packaged RUTF can be stored without refrigeration. Studies have demonstrated improved survival rates in malnourished children (Amthor, Cole, and Manary, 2009; Ciliberto, Sandige, Ndehka, et al., 2005). Some of the reported advantages of home-based (community-based) treatment include that children are not exposed to hospital-acquired infections and may receive the RUTF from village health aides (Kapil, 2009).

It is imperative that nurses be at the forefront in educating and reinforcing healthy nutrition habits in parents of small children to prevent malnutrition. Because children with marasmus may experience emotional starvation as well, care should be consistent with that for children with FTT.

The WHO has published guidelines for the treatment and management of children with severe acute malnutrition (Ashworth, Khanum, Jackson, et al., 2003; Grover and Ee, 2009). These guidelines include a two-phase program with a 10-step guide to treating the child with malnutrition.

Food Allergy

In late 2010 the National Institute of Allergy and Infectious Diseases (NIAID), working with 34 other professional organizations, published new evidence-based guidelines for the diagnosis and management of food allergy. A food allergy is defined by the NIAID as "an adverse health effect arising from a specific immune response that occurs reproducibly on exposure to a given food" (Boyce, Assa'ad, Burks, et al., 2010, p. 1108). Food allergens are defined as specific components of food or ingredients in food such as a protein that are recognized by allergen-specific immune cells eliciting an immune reaction that results in the characteristic symptoms (Boyce, Assa'ad, Burks, et al., 2010). A food intolerance is said to exist when a food or food component elicits a reproducible adverse reaction but does not have an established or likely immunologic mechanism (Boyce, Assa'ad, Burks, et al., 2010). The example given suggests that a person may have an immune-mediated allergy to cow's milk protein, but the person who is unable to digest the lactose in cow's milk is considered to be intolerant, not allergic, to it. The NIAID guidelines classify food allergy according to the following: food-induced anaphylaxis, GI food allergies, and specific syndromes; cutaneous reactions to foods; respiratory manifestation; and Heiner syndrome (Boyce, Assa'ad, Burks, et al., 2010). The exact prevalence of food allergies in children is reported to be much lower than that which parents report. Approximately 6% of children may experience food allergic reactions in the first 2 to 3 years of life; 1.5% will have an allergy to eggs, 2.5% to cow's milk, and 1% to peanuts (Sampson and Leung, 2011). Seafood allergies in children are reported to be low in the United States: 0.2% for fish and 0.5% for crustaceans (Boyce, Assa'ad, Burks, et al., 2010). Diagnosed allergy to milk and eggs was found to be 2.2% in a Danish study and 1.6% in a Norwegian study. The NIAID report further points out that most children will eventually be able to tolerate milk, eggs, soy, and wheat; far fewer will ever tolerate tree nut and peanuts (Boyce, Assa'ad, Burks, et al., 2010). The NIAID report indicates that 50% to 90% of all presumed food allergies are not actually allergies. The NIAID's (Boyce, Assa'ad, Burks, et al., 2010) guidelines also recommend the following:

- Infants should be breastfed exclusively until 4 to 6 months of age.
- Soy formula is not recommended to prevent the development of food allergy.
- Introduction of complementary foods should not be delayed beyond 6 months of age.
- Hydrolyzed formula (versus cow's milk) may be used in at-risk infants to prevent or modify food allergy.
- Maternal diet during pregnancy or lactation should not be restricted to prevent food allergy.
- Children should be vaccinated with the measles, mumps, and rubella (MMR) and measles, mumps, rubella, and varicella (MMRV) vaccines (even with egg allergy [unless severe reaction occurred]).
- Patients with severe egg allergy reactions should not receive the influenza vaccine without consulting the primary practitioner for an analysis of the risks versus benefits.

A summary of the NIAID guidelines is provided by McBride (2011).

The clinical manifestations of food allergy may be divided as follows (AAP, 2009):

Systemic—Anaphylactic, growth failure

GI—Abdominal pain, vomiting, cramping, diarrhea

Respiratory—Cough, wheezing, rhinitis, infiltrates

Cutaneous—Urticaria, rash, atopic dermatitis

Food allergies usually occur either as an immunoglobulin E (IgE)–mediated or non–IgE-mediated immune response; some toxic reactions may occur as a result of a toxin found within the food. Food allergy is caused by exposure to allergens, usually proteins (but not the smaller amino acids), that are capable of inducing IgE antibody formation (sensitization) when ingested. Sensitization refers to the initial exposure of an individual to an allergen, resulting in an immune response; subsequent exposure induces a much stronger response that is clinically apparent. Consequently food allergy typically occurs after the food has been ingested one or more times. The NIAID report (Boyce, Assa'ad, Burks, et al., 2010) indicates that sensitization alone is not sufficient to classify as a food allergy; rather an immune-mediated response *and* manifestation of specific sign and symptoms are necessary to categorize an individual as having a food allergy. The most common food allergens are listed in Box 41-1.

Oral allergy syndrome occurs when a food allergen (commonly fruits and vegetables) is ingested and there is subsequent edema and pruritus involving the lips, tongue, palate, and throat. Recovery from symptoms is usually rapid. Immediate GI hypersensitivity is an IgE-mediated reaction to a food allergen; reactions include nausea, abdominal pain, cramping, diarrhea, vomiting, anaphylaxis, or all of these. Additional food allergies seen in young children include allergic eosinophilic esophagitis, allergic eosinophilic gastroenteritis, food protein–induced proctocolitis, and food protein–induced enterocolitis.

Food allergy or hypersensitivity may also be classified according to the interval between ingestion and the manifestation of symp-toms: immediate (within minutes to hours) or delayed (2 to 48 hours) (AAP, 2009).

Food allergies can occur at any time but are common during infancy because the immature intestinal tract is more permeable to proteins than the mature intestinal tract, thus increasing the likelihood of an immune response. Allergies in general demonstrate a genetic component: children who have one parent with an allergy have a 50% or greater risk of developing one; children who have both parents with an allergy have up to a 100% risk of developing one. Allergy with a hereditary tendency is referred to as *atopy*. Some infants with atopy can be identified at birth from elevated levels of IgE in umbilical cord blood.

Deaths have been reported in children who experienced an anaphylactic reaction to food. Onset of the reactions occurred shortly after ingestion (5 to 30 minutes). In most of the children the reactions did not begin with skin signs such as hives, red rash, and flushing but rather mimicked an acute asthma attack (wheezing, decreased air movement in airways, dyspnea). Watch children with food anaphylaxis closely because a biphasic response has been recorded in a number of cases in which there is an immediate response, apparent recovery, and acute recurrence of symptoms (Simons, 2009) (see Nursing Alert and Emergency box). Children with extremely sensitive food allergies should wear a medical identification bracelet and have an injectable epinephrine cartridge (EpiPen) readily available. (See Anaphylaxis, Chapter 42.) Any child with a history of food allergy or previous severe reaction to food should have a written emergency treatment plan and an EpiPen. Note that Benadryl and cetirizine are effective for cutaneous and nasal manifestations but not for airway manifestations (Keet, 2011).

Although the reason is unknown, many children "outgrow" their food allergies, especially to milk and eggs. Approximately 50% of all infants who are intolerant to cow's milk usually develop tolerance by 3 to 5 years of age (Sampson and Leung, 2011). More than half (60%) of infants have an IgE-mediated reaction to cow's milk, and 25% retain sensitivity until the second decade of life. Children who are allergic to more than one food may develop tolerance to each food at a different time. The most common allergens such as peanuts are outgrown less readily than other food allergens. Because of the tendency to lose the hypersensitivity, allergenic foods should be reintroduced into the diet after a period of abstinence (usually ≥1 year) to evaluate whether the food can safely be added to the diet. However, foods that are associated with severe anaphylactic reactions continue to present a lifelong risk and must be avoided.

BOX 41-1   COMMON ALLERGENIC FOODS AND SOURCES

Nuts*—Some chocolates, candy, baked goods, cherry soda (may be flavored with a nut extract), walnut oil

Eggs*—Mayonnaise, creamy salad dressing, baked goods, egg noodles, some cake icing, meringue, custard, pancakes, French toast, root beer

Wheat*—Almost all baked goods, wieners, bologna, pressed or chopped cold cuts, gravy, pasta, some canned soups

Legumes—Peanuts,* peanut butter or oil, beans, peas, lentils

Fish or shellfish*—Cod liver oil, pizza with anchovies, Caesar salad dressing, any food fried in same oil as fish

Soy*—Soy sauce, teriyaki or Worcestershire sauce, tofu, baked goods using soy flour or oil, soy nuts, soy infant formulas or milk, soybean paste, tuna packed in vegetable oil, many margarines

Chocolate—Cola beverages, cocoa, chocolate-flavored drinks

Milk—Ice cream, butter, margarine (if it contains dairy products), yogurt, cheese, pudding, baked goods, wieners, bologna, canned creamed soups, instant breakfast drinks, powdered milk drinks, milk chocolate

Buckwheat—Some cereals, pancakes

Pork, chicken—Bacon, wieners, sausage, pork fat, chicken broth

Strawberries, melon, pineapple—Gelatin, syrups

Corn—Popcorn, cereal, muffins, cornstarch, corn meal, corn bread, corn tortillas, corn syrup

Citrus fruits—Orange, lemon, lime, grapefruit; any of these in drinks, gelatin, juice, or medicines

Tomatoes—Juice, some vegetable soups, spaghetti, pizza sauce, catsup

Spices—Chili, pepper, vinegar, cinnamon

*Most common allergens.

➕ EMERGENCY

*Emergency Management of Anaphylaxis**

Drug—Epinephrine 0.001 mg/kg up to maximum of 0.3 mg

Dose—EpiPen Jr (0.15 mg) intramuscularly (IM) for child weighing 8 to 25 kg (17.5-55 lbs)

EpiPen (0.3 mg) IM for child weighing 25 kg (55 lbs) or more

Observe for adverse reactions: tachycardia, hypertension, irritability, headaches, nausea, and tremors.

*Data from Keet C: Recognition and management of food-induced anaphylaxis, *Pediatr Clin North Am* 58(2):377-388, 2011; Sampson HA, Leung DYM: Adverse reactions to foods. In Kliegman RM, Stanton BF, St Geme JW, et al., editors: *Nelson textbook of pediatrics,* ed 19, Philadelphia, 2011, Saunders.

Indications for the administration of *intramuscular* epinephrine in a child with a life-threatening anaphylactic reaction or one who is experiencing severe symptoms include any one of the following (Wang and Sampson, 2007):

- Itching sensation or tightness in throat; hoarseness
- "Barky" cough
- Difficulty swallowing; dyspnea
- Wheezing
- Cyanosis
- Respiratory arrest; mild dysrhythmia or mild hypotension
- Severe bradycardia, hypotension, or cardiac arrest; loss of consciousness

Diagnosis and Therapeutic Management

The diagnosis of food allergy is made based on a number of factors, including the occurrence of anaphylaxis or any combination of 37 symptoms listed in the NIAID guidelines within minutes to hours of ingesting food or if such symptoms have occurred after the ingestion of a specific food on one or more occasions. The gold standard is the double-blind, placebo-controlled food challenge; the skin prick test and serum IgE (sIgE) measurements may be used as an adjunct to diagnose food allergy but singly should not be used for the diagnosis. The atopy patch test, intradermal test, and sIgE test are not recommended for establishing a diagnosis. A single oral food challenge may be used in certain circumstances (Boyce, Assa'ad, Burks, et al., 2010). The management of food allergy consists of avoiding the specific food or ingredient that causes the manifestations. Because children with food allergies (usually two or more) are at risk for inadequate nutrient intake and growth failure, it is recommended that they have an annual nutritional assessment to prevent such problems.

CARE MANAGEMENT

Nursing care of children with potential food allergy consists of helping to collect vital health assessment data for the establishment of a diagnosis and helping with diagnostic tests. It is important for nurses to be informed about food allergy and provide parents, caregivers, and older children with accurate information regarding food allergy.

Educate parents, teachers, and day care workers regarding signs and symptoms of food allergy and reactions. People with food allergy should avoid unfamiliar foods and restaurants that do not disclose food ingredients. New labeling guidelines require that food additives such as spices and flavoring be labeled clearly on commercially sold, store-bought foods. Hidden ingredients in prepared foods are also potential sources of food allergy.

Children with a history of food allergy may spend a considerable amount of time in day care; therefore people working in day care centers and other children's settings need to be educated properly regarding recognition and management of severe anaphylactic reactions (see Critical Thinking Case Study).

Breastfeeding is now considered a primary strategy for avoiding atopy in families with known food allergies; however, there is no evidence that maternal avoidance (during pregnancy or lactation) of cow's milk protein or other dietary products known to cause food allergy prevents food allergy in children (AAP, 2009; Boyce, Assa'ad, Burks, et al., 2010). Researchers indicate that delaying the introduction of highly allergenic foods past 4 to 6 months of age may not be

Food Allergy Anaphylaxis

A group of nursing students is holding a health promotion fair at a local elementary school for first, second, and third graders. The nursing students have several booths set up in the school cafeteria. Three second-grade boys are horseplaying in front of one of the booths when one of the boys, Jason, an 8-year-old child, suddenly starts coughing and clutching his throat. The students also observe that he is developing red splotches on his face, neck, and throat and that he is scratching. Jason says, "I can't breathe!" The school nurse is nearby and comes over to see what's causing the commotion. One of the boys with Jason says, "We didn't mean any harm; we were just goofing around when we put peanuts in his trail mix." One of the student nurses says, "He's in obvious distress. What should we do?"

1. Evidence—Is there sufficient evidence to draw any conclusions at this time about Jason's condition?
2. Assumptions—Describe some underlying assumptions about the following:
   a. Clinical manifestations of food allergy
   b. The emergency treatment of a food allergy "reaction," or anaphylaxis
   c. Which one of the following interventions would have highest immediate priority?
      (1) Call Jason's parents and ask them to come pick him up from school.
      (2) Call Jason's family practitioner to obtain orders for medication.
      (3) Promptly administer an intramuscular dose of epinephrine.
      (4) Call 911 and wait for the emergency response personnel to arrive.
3. What implication for nursing care exists in this situation after an intervention in the previous question has been chosen and implemented?
4. Describe the potential results of taking a "Let's observe Jason for a few minutes before we do anything" stance in this scenario.
5. Is there evidence to support your immediate and secondary nursing interventions? Provide objective evidence to support your decisions for action.

as protective for food allergy as previously believed (Greer, Sicherer, Burks, et al., 2008). Likewise studies have shown that soy formula does not prevent allergic disease in infants and children (AAP, 2009).*

Cow's Milk Allergy

Cow's milk allergy (CMA) is a multifaceted disorder representing adverse systemic and local GI reactions to cow's milk protein. Approximately 2.5% of infants develop cow's milk hypersensitivity, with 60% of these being IgE mediated. It is estimated that 50% of these children may outgrow the hypersensitivity by 3 to 4 years of age (Sampson and Leung, 2011). Some studies suggest that milk allergy may persist and some children may not be able to tolerate

---

*Additional information for parents of infants with food allergies is available from the American Academy of Allergy, Asthma and Immunology, 555 E. Wells St., Suite 1100, Milwaukee, WI 53202, 414-272-6071, www.aaaai.org. Additional helpful websites for information on food allergy include MedlinePlus (sponsored by U.S. National Library of Medicine and National Institutes of Health), www.nlm.nih.gov/medlineplus; Food Allergy and Anaphylaxis Network, 800-929-4040, www.foodallergy.org; and NIAID, www.niaid.nih.gov/Pages/default.aspx and www.allergicchild.com.

BOX 41-2   COMMON CLINICAL MANIFESTATIONS OF COW'S MILK ALLERGY

Gastrointestinal
- Diarrhea
- Vomiting
- Colic (controversial)
- Abdominal pain
- Nausea and vomiting
- Oral itching
- Constipation (controversial)
- Gastroesophageal reflux (controversial)
- Blood streaked mucous, loose stools (protein-induced allergic enterocolitis)

Respiratory
- Rhinitis
- Conjunctivitis
- Bronchitis
- Asthma
- Wheezing
- Sneezing
- Coughing
- Chronic nasal discharge
- Asthma exacerbation
- Laryngeal edema

Cutaneous
- Urticaria
- Atopic dermatitis

Systemic
- Anaphylaxis

Other Signs and Symptoms
- Eczema
- Excessive crying
- Pallor (from anemia secondary to chronic blood loss in gastrointestinal tract)

2009). In breastfed infants cow milk protein products should be eliminated (by the mother) to improve the diagnostic results (Kattan, Cocco, and Järvinen, 2011).

The most definitive diagnostic strategy is elimination of milk in the diet followed by challenge testing after improvement of symptoms. A clinical diagnosis is made when symptoms improve after removal of milk from the diet and two or more challenge tests produce symptoms (Ewing and Allen, 2005; Kattan, Cocco, and Järvinen, 2011). Challenge testing involves reintroducing small quantities of milk in the diet to detect resurgence of symptoms; at times it involves the use of a placebo so the parent is unaware of (or "blind" to) the timing of allergen ingestion. A double-blind, placebo-controlled food challenge is the gold standard for diagnosing food allergies such as CMA, yet it may not be used often for diagnosing CMA because of the expense, time involved, and risk for further exposure and anaphylactic reaction (Ewing and Allen, 2005). Careful observation of the child is required during a challenge test because of the possibility of anaphylactic reaction.

Therapeutic Management. Treatment of CMA is elimination of cow's milk–based formula and all other dairy products. For infants fed cow's milk–based formula, this primarily involves changing the formula to a casein hydrolysate milk formula (Pregestimil, Nutramigen, or Alimentum) in which the protein has been broken down into its amino acids through enzymatic hydrolysis. Although the AAP (2009) recommends the use of extensively hydrolyzed formulas for CMA, many practitioners may start a soy formula instead because of the expense of the hydrolyzed formulas. Approximately 50% of infants who are sensitive to cow's milk protein also demonstrate sensitivity to soy, but soy is less expensive than protein hydrolysate formula. Other choices for children who are intolerant to cow's milk–based formula are the amino acid–based formulas Neocate or EleCare, but their cost is a major consideration. Goat's milk (raw) is not an acceptable substitute because it cross-reacts with cow's milk protein, is deficient in folic acid, has a high sodium and protein content, and is unsuitable as the only source of calories. Some suggest that goat's milk infant formula may be a suitable substitute for cow's milk formula (Basnet, Schneider, Gazit, et al., 2010). Infants usually remain on the milk-free diet for 12 months, after which time small quantities of milk are reintroduced.

Children who have CMA may tolerate extensively heated cow's milk (Nowak-Wegrzyn, Bloom, Sicherer, et al., 2008). One study reports that these children became tolerant to uncooked milk products over time after consuming baked milk products (Kim, Nowak-Wegrzyn, Sicherer, et al., 2011).

CARE MANAGEMENT

The principal nursing objectives are identification of potential CMA and appropriate counseling of parents regarding substitute formulas. Parents often interpret GI symptoms such as spitting up and loose stools or fussiness as indications that the infant is allergic to cow's milk and switch the infant to a variety of formulas in an attempt to resolve the problem.

Parents need much reassurance regarding the needs of nonverbal infants with such an array of symptoms. Endless nights of lost sleep and a crying infant may promote feelings of parenting inadequacy and role conflict, thus aggravating the situation. Nurses can reassure parents that many of these symptoms are common and the reasons are often never found, yet the child does achieve appropriate growth and development. Report acute symptoms to the practitioner for further evaluation. Parents need reassurance that the infant will

milk until they are 16 years of age (AAP, 2009). (This discussion centers on cow's milk protein contained in commercial infant formulas; whole milk is not recommended for infants younger than 12 months of age.) The allergy may be manifested within the first 4 months of life through a variety of signs and symptoms that may appear within 45 minutes of milk ingestion or after several days (Box 41-2). The diagnosis initially may be made from the history, although the history alone is not diagnostic. The timing and diversity of clinical manifestations vary greatly. For example, CMA may be manifested as colic (see Chapter 31), diarrhea, vomiting, GI bleeding, gastroesophageal reflux (GER), chronic constipation, or sleeplessness in an otherwise healthy infant.

Diagnostic Evaluation. A number of diagnostic tests may be performed, including stool analysis for blood, eosinophils, and leukocytes (both frank and occult bleeding can occur from the colitis); sIgE levels; skin-prick or scratch testing; and radioallergosorbent test (RAST) (measures IgE antibodies to specific allergens in serum by radioimmunoassay). Both skin testing and RAST may help identify the offending food, but the results are not always conclusive. No single diagnostic test is considered definitive for the diagnosis (AAP,

receive complete nutrition from the new formula and will have no ill effects from the absence of cow's milk.

When solid foods are started, parents need guidance in avoiding milk product. Carefully reading all food labels helps avoid exposure to prepared foods containing milk products. Although labeled as nondairy, milk, cream, and butter substitutes may contain cow's milk protein (Kattan, Cocco, Järvinen, et al., 2011).

Lactose Intolerance

Lactose intolerance refers to at least four different entities that involve a deficiency of the enzyme lactase, which is needed for the hydrolysis or digestion of lactose in the small intestine; lactose is hydrolyzed into glucose and galactose. Congenital lactase deficiency occurs soon after birth after the newborn has consumed lactose-containing milk (human milk or commercial formula). This inborn error of metabolism involves the complete absence or severely reduced presence of lactase, is extremely rare, and requires a lifelong lactose-free or extremely reduced lactose diet.

Primary lactase deficiency, sometimes referred to as late-onset lactase deficiency, is the most common type of lactose intolerance and is manifested usually after 4 or 5 years of age, although the time of onset is variable. Ethnic groups with a high incidence of lactase deficiency include Asians, southern Europeans, Arabs, Israelis, and African-Americans; Scandinavians tend to have the lowest incidence. Lactose malabsorption manifests as lactose intolerance and is characterized by an imbalance between the ability for lactase to hydrolyze the ingested lactose and the amount of lactose ingested (Heyman and AAP Committee on Nutrition, 2006).

Secondary lactase deficiency may occur secondary to damage of the intestinal lumen, which decreases or destroys the enzyme lactase. Cystic fibrosis; sprue; celiac disease; kwashiorkor; and infections such as giardiasis, HIV, or rotavirus may cause a temporary or permanent lactose intolerance.

Developmental lactase deficiency refers to the relative lactase deficiency observed in preterm infants of less than 34 weeks of gestation (Heyman and AAP Committee on Nutrition, 2006).

The primary symptoms of lactose intolerance include abdominal pain, bloating, flatulence, and diarrhea after the ingestion of lactose. The onset of symptoms occurs within 30 minutes to several hours of lactose consumption. Lactose intolerance is often perceived as an allergy; and, in several studies with reports of acute GI symptoms ascribed to lactose intolerance, measurement of lactase activity is normal.

Lactose intolerance may be diagnosed on the basis of the history and improvement with a lactose-reduced diet. The breath hydrogen test is used to positively diagnose the condition. Breath samples in lactose-deficient individuals yield a higher percentage of hydrogen ($\geq$20 parts per million [ppm] above baseline). In infants lactose malabsorption may be diagnosed by evaluating fecal pH and reducing substances; fecal pH in infants is usually lower than in older children, but an acidic pH may indicate malabsorption (Heyman and AAP Committee on Pediatrics, 2006).

Treatment of lactose intolerance is elimination of offending dairy products; however, some advocate decreasing amounts of dairy products rather than total elimination, especially in small children (Heyman and AAP Committee on Nutrition, 2006). In infants lactose-free or low-lactose formula offers no special advantages over lactose-containing formula except in those who are severely malnourished (Heyman and AAP Committee on Pediatrics, 2006).

One concern is that dairy avoidance in children and adolescents with lactose intolerance contributes to reduced bone mineral density and osteoporosis (AAP, 2009; Suchy, Brannon, Carpenter, et al.,

2010). Evidence indicates that dietary lactose enhances calcium absorption and that lactose-free diets may negatively affect bone mineralization (Heyman and AAP Committee on Nutrition, 2006). It is recommended that individuals with lactose maldigestion who do not experience lactose intolerance symptoms continue to consume small amounts of dairy products with meals to prevent reduced bone mass density and subsequent osteoporosis. Some evidence indicates that probiotics (food preparations containing microorganisms such as *Lactobacillus*, which alter the GI microflora and thus are beneficial to the host) improve lactose intolerance when live cultures are fermented in dairy products (de Vrese and Schrezenmeir, 2008). The positive attributes of probiotics for those with lactose maldigestion include delayed GI transit (slower than milk), positive effects on intestinal and colonic microflora, and a reduction of maldigestion symptoms.

Most people are able to tolerate small amounts of lactose ($\approx$1 cup of milk per day) even in the presence of deficient lactase activity (Heyman and AAP Committee on Nutrition, 2006; Suchy, Brannon, Carpenter, et al., 2010) and should be encouraged to continue their intake of dairy products in small amounts to obtain much-needed nutrients. Milk taken at meals may be better tolerated than when taken alone (see Family-Centered Care box). Pretreated milk (with microbial-derived lactase) is reported to be effective in improving lactose absorption. Because dairy products are a major source of calcium and vitamin D, supplementation of these nutrients is needed to prevent deficiency. Yogurt contains inactive lactase enzyme, which is activated by the temperature and pH of the duodenum; this lactase activity substitutes for the lack of endogenous lactase. Fresh, plain yogurt may be tolerated better than frozen or flavored yogurt; hard cheeses, lactase-treated dairy products, and lactase tablets taken with dairy products are also viable options. An important distinction between lactose intolerance and food allergy is that lactose intolerance does not manifest as an anaphylactic-type reaction.

CARE MANAGEMENT

Nursing care is similar to the interventions discussed for CMA in this chapter and includes explaining the dietary restrictions to the family; identifying alternate sources of calcium such as yogurt and calcium supplementation; explaining the importance of

---

FAMILY-CENTERED CARE
Controlling Symptoms of Lactose Intolerance

- In infants substitute lactose-free or soy-based formula for cow's milk–based formula or human milk (only after a diagnosis of congenital lactase deficiency or secondary lactase intolerance is made).
- Limit milk consumption to one to two glasses per day.
- Drink milk with other foods rather than alone.
- Eat hard cheese, cottage cheese, or yogurt instead of drinking milk.
- Use enzyme tablets (Lactaid, Lactrase, Dairy Ease) to metabolize the lactose in milk or supplement the lactase in the body (add tablets to milk or sprinkle on dairy products such as ice cream).
- Eat small amounts of dairy foods daily to help colonic bacteria adapt to ingested lactose.
- Include a probiotic (yogurt or cultured [fermented] milk) in meal or as a snack that has *Lactobacillus* or *Bifidobacterium* organisms.
- Take a calcium supplement if unable to consume any dairy products such as cheese.

supplementation; and discussing sources of lactose, especially hidden sources such as its use as a bulk agent in certain medications, and ways of controlling the symptoms (see Family-Centered Care box). Parents are advised to check with the pharmacist regarding this possibility when obtaining medication.

GASTROINTESTINAL DYSFUNCTION

The extensive surface area of the GI tract and its digestive function represent the major means of exchange between the human organism and the environment. Disorders that impair the functional integrity of the GI system have the potential to cause serious alterations in fluid and electrolyte balance. Disorders that involve GI losses of large amounts of fluid, absorption disorders, inflammatory disorders, and decreased or excessive water intake have the potential to cause fluid and electrolyte imbalance in infants and children.

Clinical observations often provide clues to specific GI problems (Box 41-3). In any disorder that involves GI losses of large amounts of fluid, dehydration poses a serious threat to life and demands immediate attention.

Dehydration

Dehydration is a common body fluid disturbance in infants and children and occurs whenever the total output of fluid exceeds the total intake, regardless of the cause. It may result from a number of diseases that cause insensible fluid losses through the skin and respiratory tract, through increased renal excretion, and through the GI tract. Although dehydration can result from impaired oral intake, it is often a result of abnormal losses such as those that occur in vomiting or diarrhea when oral intake only partially compensates for the abnormal losses. Other significant causes of dehydration include diabetic ketoacidosis and burns.

Types of Dehydration

The pathophysiology of dehydration is understood by recognizing that the distribution of water between the extracellular fluid (ECF) and intracellular fluid (ICF) spaces depends on active transport of potassium into and sodium out of cells by energy-requiring processes. Sodium is the chief solute in ECF and the primary determinant of ECF volume. It is considered a unique electrolyte in that water balance determines sodium concentration; when water is lost and sodium concentration becomes elevated, compensatory mechanisms in the kidney stop ADH secretion so water is retained. The thirst mechanism (not fully functional in infants) is also stimulated so water is replaced, thus increasing the total body water content and returning sodium to a normal level (Greenbaum, 2011). Potassium is found primarily inside the cell (intracellular), but small amounts are also found in ECF. Sodium depletion in diarrhea occurs in two ways: out of the body in stool and into the ICF compartment to replace potassium to maintain electrolyte equilibrium.

Dehydration is classified into three categories on the basis of osmolality and depends primarily on the serum sodium concentration: (1) isotonic, (2) hypotonic, and (3) hypertonic.

Isotonic (isosmotic or isonatremic) dehydration, the primary form of dehydration in children, occurs in conditions in which electrolyte and water deficits are present in approximately balanced proportions. Water and sodium are lost in approximately equal amounts. The observable fluid losses are not necessarily isotonic because losses from other avenues make adjustments so the sum of all losses, or the net loss, is isotonic. There is no osmotic force between the ICF and the ECF; thus the major loss is sustained from the ECF compartment. This significantly reduces the plasma volume and the circulating blood volume, which affects the skin, muscles, and kidneys. Shock is the greatest threat to life, and children with isotonic dehydration display symptoms characteristic of hypovolemic shock. Plasma sodium remains within normal limits, between 130 and 150 mEq/L.

Hypotonic (hyposmotic or hyponatremic) dehydration occurs when the electrolyte deficit exceeds the water deficit, leaving the

---

BOX 41-3   CLINICAL MANIFESTATIONS OF GASTROINTESTINAL DYSFUNCTION IN CHILDREN

Growth failure—Weight consistently below the third percentile, body mass index below the fifth percentile, or a decrease from established growth pattern

Spitting up or regurgitation—Passive transfer of gastric contents into the esophagus or mouth

Vomiting—Forceful ejection of gastric contents; involves a complex process under central nervous system control that causes salivation, pallor, sweating, and tachycardia; usually accompanied by nausea
   Projectile vomiting—Vomiting accompanied by vigorous peristaltic waves and typically associated with pyloric stenosis or pylorospasm

Nausea—Unpleasant sensation vaguely referred to the throat or abdomen with an inclination to vomit

Constipation—Delay or difficulty with the passage of stools that is present for 2 weeks or longer; associated with symptoms that may include blood-streaked stools and abdominal discomfort

Encopresis—Involuntary overflow of incontinent stool causing soiling or incontinence secondary to fecal retention or impaction

Diarrhea—Increase in the number of stools with increased water content as a result of alterations of water and electrolyte transport by the gastrointestinal (GI) tract; may be acute or chronic

Hypoactive, hyperactive, or absent bowel sounds—Evidence of intestinal motility problems that may be caused by inflammation or obstruction

Abdominal distention—Protuberant contour of the abdomen that may be caused by delayed gastric emptying, accumulation of gas or stool, inflammation, or obstruction

Abdominal pain—Pain associated with the abdomen that may be localized or diffuse, acute or chronic; often caused by inflammation, obstruction, or hemorrhage

Gastrointestinal bleeding—May be from an upper or lower GI source and may be acute or chronic
   Hematemesis—Vomiting of bright red or denatured blood that results from bleeding in the upper GI tract or from swallowed blood from the nose or oropharynx
   Hematochezia—Passage of bright red blood per rectum, usually indicating lower GI tract bleeding
   Melena—Passage of dark-colored, "tarry" stools resulting from denatured blood, suggesting upper GI tract bleeding or bleeding from the right colon

Jaundice—Yellow coloration of the skin and sclerae associated with liver dysfunction in infants and children over 4 weeks of age

Dysphagia—Difficulty swallowing caused by abnormalities in the neuromuscular function of the pharynx or upper esophageal sphincter or by disorders of the esophagus

Dysfunctional swallowing—Impaired swallowing caused by central nervous system defects or structural defects of the oral cavity, pharynx, or esophagus; can cause feeding problems or aspiration

Fever—Common manifestation of illness in children with GI disorders; usually associated with dehydration, infection, or inflammation

serum hypotonic. Because ICF is more concentrated than ECF in hypotonic dehydration, water moves from the ECF to the ICF to establish osmotic equilibrium. This movement further increases the ECF volume loss, and shock is a frequent finding. Because there is a greater proportional loss of ECF in hypotonic dehydration, the physical signs tend to be more severe with smaller fluid losses than with isotonic or hypertonic dehydration. Serum sodium concentration is less than 130 mEq/L.

Hypertonic (hyperosmotic or hypernatremic) dehydration results from water loss in excess of electrolyte loss and is usually caused by a proportionately larger loss of water or a larger intake of electrolytes. This type of dehydration is the most dangerous and requires more specific fluid therapy. Hypertonic dehydration may occur in infants who are given fluids by mouth that contain large amounts of solute or in children who receive high-protein nasogastric (NG) tube feedings that place an excessive solute load on the kidneys. In hypertonic dehydration fluid shifts from the lesser concentration of the ICF to the ECF. Plasma sodium concentration is greater than 150 mEq/L.

Because the ECF volume is proportionately larger, hypertonic dehydration consists of a greater degree of water loss for the same intensity of physical signs. Shock is less apparent. However, central nervous system (CNS) disturbances, including alterations in consciousness, poor ability to focus attention, lethargy, increased muscle tone with hyperreflexia, and hyperirritability to stimuli, are more likely to occur. CNS changes are serious and may result in permanent damage.

Degree of Dehydration

Diagnosis of the type and degree of dehydration is necessary to develop an effective plan of therapy. The degree of dehydration has been described as a percentage of body weight dehydrated: mild—less than 3% in older children or less than 5% in infants; moderate—5% to 10% in infants and 3% to 6% in older children;

and severe—more than 10% in infants and more than 6% in older children (Greenbaum, 2011). Water constitutes only 60% to 70% of an infant's weight. However, adipose tissue contains little water and is highly variable in individual infants and children. A more accurate means of describing dehydration is to reflect acute loss (time frame of ≤48 hours) in milliliters per kilogram of body weight. For example, a loss of 50 mL/kg is considered to be a mild fluid loss, but a loss of 100 mL/kg produces severe dehydration. Weight is the most important determinant of the percent of total body fluid loss in infants and younger children. However, often the preillness weight is unknown. Other predictors of fluid loss include a changing level of consciousness (irritability to lethargy), altered response to stimuli, decreased skin elasticity and turgor, prolonged capillary refill (>2 sec), increased heart rate, and sunken eyes and fontanels. There is evidence that the clinical signs of abnormal capillary refill, abnormal skin turgor, and abnormal respiratory pattern are the most useful in predicting dehydration of 5% or more in children (Colletti, Brown, Sharieff, et al., 2010; Emond, 2009; Steiner, DeWalt, and Byerly, 2004).

Clinical signs provide clues to the extent of dehydration (Table 41-1). The earliest detectable sign usually is tachycardia followed by dry skin and mucous membranes, sunken fontanels, signs of circulatory failure (coolness and mottling of extremities), loss of skin elasticity, and prolonged capillary filling time (Table 41-2).

Compensatory mechanisms attempt to maintain fluid volume by adjusting to these losses. Interstitial fluid moves into the vascular compartment to maintain the blood volume in response to hemoconcentration and hypovolemia, and vasoconstriction of peripheral arterioles helps maintain pumping pressure. When fluid losses exceed the ability of the body to sustain blood volume and blood pressure, circulation is seriously compromised, and the blood pressure falls. This results in tissue hypoxia with accumulation of lactic acid, pyruvate, and other acid metabolites, which contribute to the development of metabolic acidosis.

TABLE 41-1	**EVALUATING EXTENT OF DEHYDRATION**		
	LEVEL OF DEHYDRATION		
CLINICAL SIGNS	**MILD**	**MODERATE**	**SEVERE**
Weight loss—infants	3%-5%	6%-9%	≥10%
Weight loss—children	3%-4%	6%-8%	10%
Pulse	Normal	Slightly increased	Very increased
Respiratory rate	Normal	Slight tachypnea (rapid)	Hyperpnea (deep and rapid)
Blood pressure	Normal	Normal to orthostatic (>10 mm Hg change)	Orthostatic to shock
Behavior	Normal	Irritable, more thirsty	Hyperirritable to lethargic
Thirst	Slight	Moderate	Intense
Mucous membranes*	Normal	Dry	Parched
Tears	Present	Decreased	Absent, sunken eyes
Anterior fontanel	Normal	Normal to sunken	Sunken
External jugular vein	Visible when supine	Not visible except with supraclavicular pressure	Not visible even with supraclavicular pressure
Skin*	Capillary refill >2 sec	Slowed capillary refill (2-4 sec [decreased turgor])	Very delayed capillary refill (>4 sec) and tenting; skin cool, acrocyanotic or mottled
Urine specific gravity	>1.020	>1.020; oliguria	Oliguria or anuria

Data from Jospe N, Forbes G: Fluids and electrolytes—clinical aspects, *Pediatr Rev* 17(11):395–403, 1996; and Steiner MJ, DeWalt DA, Byerly JS: Is this child dehydrated? *JAMA* 291(22):2746–2754, 2004.
*These signs are less prominent in patients who have hypernatremia.

Renal compensation is impaired by reduced blood flow through the kidneys, and little urine is formed. Increased serum osmolality stimulates the secretion of antidiuretic hormone (ADH) to conserve fluid and initiates the renin-angiotensin mechanisms in the kidney, causing further vasoconstriction. Aldosterone is released to promote sodium retention and conserve water in the kidneys. If dehydration increases in severity, urine formation is greatly diminished, and metabolites and hydrogen ions that are normally excreted by this route are retained.

Shock, a common manifestation of severe depletion of ECF volume, is preceded by tachycardia and signs of poor perfusion and tissue oxygenation (by pulse oximeter readings). Peripheral circulation is poor as a result of reduced blood volume; therefore the skin is cool and mottled, with decreased capillary filling after blanching. Impaired kidney circulation often leads to oliguria and azotemia. Although low blood pressure may accompany other symptoms of shock, in infants and young children it is usually a late sign and may herald the onset of cardiovascular collapse.

Diagnostic Evaluation

To initiate a therapeutic plan, several factors must be determined:
* The degree of dehydration based on physical assessment
* The type of dehydration based on the pathophysiology of the specific illness responsible for the dehydrated state
* Specific physical signs other than general signs
* Initial plasma sodium concentrations
* Serum bicarbonate concentration
* Any associated electrolyte (especially serum potassium) and acid-base imbalances (as indicated)

Initial and regular ongoing evaluations assess the patient's progress toward equilibrium and the effectiveness of therapy.

In the examination of an infant or younger child, one of the most important determinants of the extent of dehydration is body weight because this can help to determine the percentage of total body fluid lost; however, because the preillness weight is often unknown, clinical manifestations must be evaluated. Important clinical manifestations include changing sensorium (irritability to lethargy), decreased response to stimuli, integumentary changes (decreased elasticity and

turgor), prolonged capillary refill, increased heart rate, sunken eyes, and in infants sunken fontanels. Using multiple predictors increases the sensitivity of assessing the fluid deficit, and early studies have shown a reasonably high degree of agreement between experienced observers in assessment of the level of dehydration. Objective signs of dehydration are present at a fluid deficit of less than 5%.

Laboratory data are said to be useful only when results are significantly abnormal (Emond, 2009). Urine specific gravity, urine ketones, and urinary output during rehydration reportedly are unreliable assessments for determining dehydration in children (Steiner, Nager, and Wang, 2007). Shock, tachycardia, and very low blood pressure are common features of severe depletion of ECF volume (see Shock, Chapter 42).

Therapeutic Management

Medical management is directed at correcting the fluid loss or deficit and treating the underlying cause. When the child is alert, awake, and not in danger, correction of dehydration may be attempted with oral fluid administration. Mild cases of dehydration can be managed at home by this method. Several commercial rehydration fluids are available for use (Table 41-3). Oral rehydration management consists of replacement of fluid loss over 4 to 6 hours, replacement of continuing losses, and provision for maintenance fluid requirements. In general a mildly dehydrated child may be given 50 mL/kg of ORS, and a child with moderate dehydration may be given 100 mL/kg of ORS. A child with fluid losses from diarrhea may be given 10 mL/kg for each stool. Amounts and rates are determined from body weight and the severity of dehydration and are increased if rehydration is incomplete or if excess losses continue until the child is well hydrated and the basic problem is under control (Box 41-4).

Enhance the flavor of an ORS such as Pedialyte (unflavored) by adding 1 tsp of unsweetened powder Kool-Aid to each 60 to 90 mL of ORS. Older children may take a small Popsicle orally instead of fluids that require drinking. Many commercially available Popsicles are relatively inexpensive and contain small amounts of sucrose and approximately 40 to 50 mL of fluid. Frozen oral hydration may be accepted by some children when conventional ORS is rejected.

TABLE 41-2	CLINICAL MANIFESTATIONS OF DEHYDRATION		
MANIFESTATION	ISOTONIC (LOSS OF WATER AND SODIUM)	HYPOTONIC (LOSS OF SODIUM IN EXCESS OF WATER)	HYPERTONIC (LOSS OF WATER IN EXCESS OF SODIUM)
Skin			
Color	Gray	Gray	Gray
Temperature	Cold	Cold	Cold or hot
Turgor	Poor	Very poor	Fair
Feel	Dry	Clammy	Thickened, doughy
Mucous membranes	Dry	Slightly moist	Parched
Tearing and salivation	Absent	Absent	Absent
Eyeball	Sunken	Sunken	Sunken
Fontanel	Sunken	Sunken	Sunken
Body temperature	Subnormal or elevated	Subnormal or elevated	Subnormal or elevated
Pulse	Rapid	Very rapid	Moderately rapid
Respirations	Rapid	Rapid	Rapid
Behavior	Irritable to lethargic	Lethargic or comatose; seizures	Marked lethargy with extreme hyperirritability on stimulation

TABLE 41-3 COMPOSITION OF SOME ORAL REHYDRATION SOLUTIONS

FORMULA	NA (mEq/L)	K (mEq /L)	CL (mEq /L)	BASE (mEq /L)	GLUCOSE (g/L)
Pedialyte (Abbott)*	45	20	35	30 (citrate)	25
Rehydralyte (Abbott)	75	20	65	30 (citrate)	25
Infalyte (Mead Johnson)	50	25	45	34 (citrate)	30
World Health Organization†	75§	30	65	10 (bicarbonate)	13.5

Cl, Chloride; *K*, potassium; *Na*, sodium.
*Note that many generic products are available with compositions identical to Pedialyte.
†Must be reconstituted with 1 L water.
§Reduced osmolarity 224 mmol/L formulation.

BOX 41-4 MODEL FOR REHYDRATION

- Rehydration solution should consist of 75 to 90 mEq/L of sodium (Na⁺).
- Give 40 to 50 mL/kg of rehydration solution over 4 hours.
- Replacement and maintenance solution should consist of 40 to 60 mEq/L of Na⁺.
- Reevaluate the need for further rehydration; initiate maintenance therapy using maintenance formulations, with daily volumes not to exceed 150 mL/kg/day.
- In children with diarrhea without significant dehydration, the maintenance phase may be initiated without the need for rehydration solution.
- If additional fluids are needed, use low-salt fluids such as breast milk or water.

Modified from Centers for Disease Control and Prevention: Managing acute gastroenteritis among children: oral rehydration, maintenance, and nutritional therapy, *MMWR Recommend Rep* 52(RR-16):1–16, 2003.

TABLE 41-4 DAILY MAINTENANCE FLUID REQUIREMENTS*

BODY WEIGHT (kg)	AMOUNT OF FLUID PER DAY
1-10	100 mL/kg
11-20	1000 mL plus 50 mL/kg for each kg >10 kg
>20	1500 mL plus 20 mL/kg for each kg >20 kg

*Not appropriate for neonatal use.

The child may not be thirsty even though dehydrated and may refuse oral fluids initially for fear of continued emesis (if occurring) or because of decreased strength, oral stomatitis, or thrush. In such children rehydration may proceed by administering 2 to 5 mL of ORS by a syringe or small medication cup every 2 to 3 minutes until the child is able to tolerate larger amounts; if the child has emesis, administering small amounts (5 to 10 mL) of ORS approximately every 5 minutes may help overcome fluid deficit, and the emesis often lessens over time. Evidence indicates that oral administration of ondansetron (Zofran) to children with acute gastroenteritis and vomiting reduces emesis and increases time to oral rehydration, thus preventing intravenous (IV) therapy (Carter and Fedorowicz, 2012). Oral rehydration therapy (ORT) is effective for treating mild or moderate dehydration in children, is less expensive, and involves fewer complications than therapy (AAP, 2009).

Parenteral Fluid Therapy. Parenteral fluid therapy is initiated whenever the child is unable to ingest sufficient amounts of fluid and electrolytes to (1) meet ongoing daily physiologic losses, (2) replace previous deficits, and (3) replace ongoing abnormal losses. Patients who usually require IV fluids are those with severe dehydration, with uncontrollable vomiting, who are unable to drink for any reason (e.g., extreme fatigue, coma), and with severe gastric distention.

Because dehydration constitutes a great threat to life, the first priority is the restoration of circulation by rapid expansion of the ECF volume to treat or prevent shock. IV administration of fluid begins immediately, although the exact nature of the dehydration and the serum electrolyte values may not be known initially. The solution selected is based on what is known regarding the probable type and cause of the dehydration. This usually involves an isotonic solution such as 0.9% sodium chloride or lactated Ringer's solution, both of which are close to the body's serum osmolality of 285 to 300 mOsm/kg and do not contain dextrose (which is contraindicated in the early treatment stages of diabetic ketoacidosis).

Parenteral rehydration therapy has three phases. The initial therapy is used to expand ECF volume quickly and improve circulatory and renal function. During initial therapy an isotonic solution is used at a rate of 20 mL/kg given as an IV bolus over 20 minutes and repeated as necessary after assessment of the child's response to therapy (Ford, 2009; Friedman, 2010). Subsequent therapy is used to replace deficits, meet maintenance water and electrolyte requirements, and catch up with ongoing losses. Table 41-4 lists daily maintenance fluid requirements for children. Water and sodium requirements for the deficit, maintenance, and ongoing losses are calculated at 8-hour intervals, taking into consideration the amount of fluids given with the initial boluses and the amount administered during the first 24-hour period. With improved circulation during this phase, water and electrolyte deficits can be evaluated, and acid-base status can be corrected either directly through the administration of fluids or indirectly through improved renal function. Potassium is withheld until kidney function is restored and assessed and circulation has improved.

The final phase of therapy allows the patient to return to normal and begin oral feedings, with a gradual correction of total body deficits. The potassium loss in ICF is replaced slowly by way of the ECF. The body fat and protein stores are replaced through diet. If the child is unable to eat or if feeding aggravates a chronic condition, IV maintenance fluids are provided.

Although the initial phase of fluid replacement is rapid in both isotonic and hypotonic dehydration, it is contraindicated in hypertonic dehydration because of the risk of water intoxication, especially in the brain cells, specifically the central pontine cells. Central pontine myelinolysis may occur with an overcorrection of fluid deficit and an overly rapid correction of serum sodium concentration. There is an apparent lag time for sodium to reach a steady state when diffusing in and out of brain cells, but water diffuses almost instantaneously. Consequently rapid administration of fluid causes equally rapid diffusion of water into the dehydrated brain cells, causing marked cerebral edema. Because ECF volume is maintained relatively well in hypertonic as opposed to the other types of dehydration, shock is not a usual manifestation.

CARE MANAGEMENT

Nursing observation and intervention are essential for detection and therapeutic management of dehydration. A variety of circumstances cause fluid losses in infants and small children, and changes can take place quickly. An important nursing responsibility is observing for signs of dehydration. Nursing assessment should begin with observing general appearance and proceed to more specific observations. Conditions in which dehydration may develop quickly include diarrhea; vomiting; sweating; fever; disorders such as diabetic ketoacidosis, renal disease, and cardiac anomalies; administration of certain drugs (e.g., diuretics and steroids); and trauma (major surgery, burns, and other extensive injury).

Whether the child is at home, in the practitioner's office or clinic, or in the hospital, nursing assessment is an essential part of the nursing care plan. The assessment of suspected or potential fluid and electrolyte disturbance begins with the observation of general appearance. Ill children usually have drawn expressions, have dry mucous membranes and lips, and "look sick." Loss of appetite is one of the first behaviors observed in most childhood illnesses, and the infant's or child's activity level is diminished from baseline or usual activities. The cry of an ill infant is less vigorous, often whining, and higher pitched than usual. The child is irritable, seeks the parent's comfort and attention, and displays purposeless movements and inappropriate responses to people and familiar objects. In some cases he or she may not protest advances by the health care worker and procedures such as taking vital signs or starting an IV infusion. These are signs that the child truly feels bad and that the condition is serious and immediate intervention is necessary. As the child's illness and level of dehydration become more severe, irritability progresses to lethargy and even unconsciousness.

Assess capillary filling time by pinching the abdominal skin, chest, arm, or leg and estimating the time it takes for the blood to return. Capillary filling time in mild dehydration is less than 2 seconds, increasing to more than 4 seconds in severe dehydration. The technique is effective in children of all ages. However, it can be altered in the presence of heart failure, which affects circulation time, and hypertonic dehydration, in which fluid loss is primarily intracellular. Additional clinical signs observed in children with dehydration include cool mottled extremities, sunken eyes, tachypnea, and changes in sensorium.

When caring for the ill child, assess the vital signs as often as every 15 to 30 minutes and record fluid intake and output and body weight frequently during the initial phase of therapy. It is important to use the same scale each time the child is weighed and predetermine the weight of any equipment or devices that must remain attached during the weighing process, including elbow restraints, and any clothing the child might be wearing. Obtain routine weights at the same time each day using the same scales.

Accurate measurements of fluid intake and output are vital to the assessment of dehydration. This includes oral and parenteral intake and losses from urine, stools, vomiting, fistulas, NG suction, sweat, and wound drainage:

Urine—Frequency, color, consistency, and volume (when weighing diapers, ≈1 g of wet diaper weight equals 1 mL of urine)

Stools—Frequency, volume, and consistency

Vomitus—Volume, frequency, and type

Sweating—Can only be estimated from frequency of clothing and linen changes

In addition to fluid intake and output, the following observations help to assess dehydration:

Vital signs—Temperature (normal, elevated, or lowered depending on degree of dehydration), pulse (tachycardia), respirations (hyperpnea), and blood pressure (hypotension)

Skin—Color, temperature, turgor, presence or absence of edema, and capillary refill

Mucous membranes—Moisture, color, and presence and consistency of secretions

Body weight—Decreased in relation to degree of dehydration

Fontanel (infants)—Sunken, soft, or normal

Sensory alterations—Presence of thirst (only in older child)

It is important to measure and record all intake, oral and parenteral, and output from all sources, including urine, stool, emesis, drainage tubes, fistulas, and wounds from which appreciable amounts of fluid are lost. At home advise parents to observe the number of times and how much the child voids. A newborn may be expected to void at least once in the first 24 hours, 2 or 3 times in the second 24 hours of life, 3 or 4 times in the third and fourth days of life, and a minimum of 5 or 6 times by the fifth and sixth days; if intake is adequate, an infant 5 to 6 days old and older may be expected to have a minimum of six to eight voidings per day (AAP, 2009). Infants younger than 1 year of age may void every 1 to 2 hours; toddlers urinate approximately every 3 hours. As children get older they void less frequently. Instruct the parents to notify the nurse or clinician if the child appears to be voiding an insufficient amount or persistently losing fluid through vomiting or diarrhea.

For nursing interventions see discussion under specific disorders in this chapter.

DISORDERS OF MOTILITY

Diarrhea

Diarrhea is a symptom that results from disorders involving digestive, absorptive, and secretory functions. It is caused by abnormal intestinal water and electrolyte transport. Worldwide there are an estimated 1.7 billion episodes of diarrhea each year (WHO, 2013). Approximately 19% of all deaths in children living in developing countries are related to diarrhea and dehydration (Boschi-Pinto, Velebit, and Shibuya, 2008). Most children living in developed countries who have gastroenteritis have mild forms. However, in the United States approximately 200,000 children younger than 5 years of age are hospitalized, and approximately 200 children younger than 5 years die of diarrhea and dehydration each year (Malek, Curns, Holman, et al., 2006; Staat, 2006).

Diarrheal disturbances involve the stomach and intestines (gastroenteritis), the small intestine (enteritis), the colon (colitis), or the colon and intestines (enterocolitis). Diarrhea is classified as acute or chronic.

Acute diarrhea, a leading cause of illness in children younger than 5 years of age, is defined as a sudden increase in frequency and a change in consistency of stools, often caused by an infectious agent in the GI tract. It may be associated with upper respiratory or urinary tract infections, antibiotic therapy, or laxative use. Acute diarrhea is usually self-limited (<14 days' duration) and subsides without specific treatment if dehydration does not occur. Acute infectious diarrhea (infectious gastroenteritis) is caused by a variety of viral, bacterial, and parasitic pathogens (Table 41-5).

TABLE 41-5   INFECTIOUS CAUSES OF ACUTE DIARRHEA

ORGANISM	PATHOLOGY	CHARACTERISTICS	COMMENTS
Viral Agents			
Rotavirus Incubation: 48 hr Diagnosis: enzyme immunoassay (EIA) and latex agglutination assay	Fecal-oral transmission Seven groups (A-G): Most group A virus replicates in mature villous epithelial cells of small intestine; leads to (1) imbalance in ratio of intestinal fluid absorption to secretion, and (2) malabsorption of complex carbohydrates	Mild-to-moderate fever Vomiting followed by the onset of watery stools Fever and vomiting generally abate in approximately 2 days, but diarrhea persists 5-7 days Adult contacts in household may develop symptomatic infection	Most common cause of diarrhea in children <5 yr of age Infants 6-12 mo are most vulnerable Peak occurrences in winter months; important cause of hospital-acquired infections Affects all ages; usually milder in children >3 yr of age; immune-compromised children at greater risk for complications Virus can live on toys and hard surfaces (sinks, countertops) Vaccine available for infants
Noroviruses (formerly Norwalk-like) **Caliciviruses** Incubation: 12-48 hr Diagnosis: EIA, reverse-transcriptase polymerase chain reaction (RT-PCR)	Fecal-oral; contaminated food or water Pathology similar to rotavirus Affects villous epithelial cells of small intestine Leads to (1) imbalance in ratio of intestinal fluid absorption to secretion, and (2) malabsorption of complex carbohydrates	Abdominal cramps; nausea, vomiting, malaise, low-grade fever, watery diarrhea without blood; duration brief, 2-3 days; tends to resemble so-called food poisoning symptoms with nausea predominating	Affects all ages Multiple strains often named for location of outbreak (e.g., Norwalk, Sapporo, Snow Mountain, Montgomery) Common in closed populations such as day care and cruise ships
Bacterial Agents			
Escherichia coli Incubation: 3-4 days Variable, depending on strain Diagnosis: sorbitol MacConkey agar (SMAC agar) + for blood, but fecal leukocytes are absent or rare	Five *E. coli* strains produce diarrhea as a result of enterotoxin production, adherence, or invasion: enterotoxigenic-producing (ETEC), enteroaggregative (EAEC), Shiga toxin–producing (STEC), enteropathogenic (EPEC), and enteroinvasive *E. coli* (EIEC)	Watery diarrhea 1-2 days; then severe abdominal cramping and bloody diarrhea STEC can progress to hemolytic uremic syndrome (HUS) and postdiarrheal thrombotic thrombocytopenia (TTP); 50% require dialysis and 3%-5% die	Foodborne pathogen Traveler's diarrhea Highest incidence in summer Cause of nursery epidemics Symptomatic treatment Antibiotics may worsen course, but meta-analysis shows no harm or benefit from antibiotic therapy (AAP Committee on Infectious Diseases and Pickering, 2012) Antimotility agents and opioids should be avoided
Salmonella groups (nontyphoidal; gram-negative rods, nonencapsulated, nonsporulating) Incubation 6-72 hr Diagnosis: gram-stained stool culture	Invasion of mucosa in small and large intestine; edema of lamina propria; focal acute inflammation with disruption of mucosa and microabscesses	Nausea, vomiting, colicky abdominal pain, bloody diarrhea, fever; symptoms variable: mild to severe May have headache, cerebral manifestations (e.g., drowsiness, confusion, meningismus, seizures) Infants may be afebrile and nontoxic May result in life-threatening septicemia and meningitis Nausea/vomiting typically short duration; diarrhea may persist as long as 2-3 wk Typically shed virus for average of 5 wk; cases reported up to 1 yr	Incidence highest in warm months: July to November Foodborne outbreaks common Usually transmitted person to person but may transmit via undercooked meats, poultry Poultry and poultry products cause about half the cases In children: pets (e.g., dogs, cats, hamsters, turtles) Communicable as long as organisms are excreted Antibiotics not recommended in uncomplicated cases Antimotility agents also not recommended—prolong transit time and carrier state Incidence decreasing over past 10 yr

TABLE 41-5   INFECTIOUS CAUSES OF ACUTE DIARRHEA—cont'd

ORGANISM	PATHOLOGY	CHARACTERISTICS	COMMENTS
Salmonella typhi Produces enteric fever—systemic syndrome Incubation: Usually 7-14 days but could be 3-30 days, depending on size of inoculum Diagnosis: positive blood cultures; also sometimes positive stool and urine Late stage: positive bone marrow culture	Bloodstream invasion; after ingestion organism attaches to microvilli of ileal brush borders, and bacteria invade intestinal epithelium via Peyer's patches; is then transported to intestinal lymph nodes and enters bloodstream via thoracic ducts; circulating organisms reach reticuloendothelial cells, causing bacteremia	Manifestations depend on age Abdominal pain; diarrhea; nausea, vomiting, high fever, lethargy Must be treated with antibiotics	Incidence is much lower in developed countries; United States has about 400 cases/yr 65% of U.S. cases acquired via international cases Ingestion of food/water contaminated with human feces is most common mode of transmission Congenital and intrapartum transmission can occur Three vaccines are available
Shigella species Gram-negative organisms Nonmotile Anaerobic bacilli Incubation: 1-7 days Diagnosis: stool culture Loaded with polymorphonuclear leukocytes	Enterotoxins: invade epithelium with superficial mucosal ulcerations	Patients appear sick Symptoms begin with fever, fatigue, anorexia Crampy abdominal pain precedes watery or bloody diarrhea Symptoms usually subside in 5-10 days	Most cases in children younger than 9 yr with about one third of cases in children ages 1-4 wk Antibiotics shorten illness and lower mortality risk All patients are at risk for dehydration Acute symptoms may persist for 1 wk or more Antidiarrheal medications not recommended; may predispose to toxic megacolon
Yersinia enterocolitica Incubation period: dose dependent, 1-3 wk Diagnosis: stool culture serology; enzyme-linked immunosorbent assay (ELISA) Patients have leukocytosis; elevated sedimentation rate	Pathology poorly understood; possible production of enterotoxin	Mucoid diarrhea, sometimes bloody; abdominal pain suggestive of appendicitis; fever, vomiting	Seen more frequently in winter months Transmitted by pets and contaminated food, especially raw or poorly cooked meat; rarely person-to-person Antibiotics usually do not alter clinical course in uncomplicated cases; should be used in complicated infections and compromised hosts
Campylobacter jejuni and **Campylobacter coli** Microaerophilic, motile, gram-negative bacilli Incubation period: 1-7 days Ability to cause illness appears dose related Diagnosis by stool culture, sometimes in blood Commonly found in gastrointestinal (GI) tract of wild or domestic animals	Not fully understood; possibly (1) adherence to intestinal mucosa by toxin; (2) invasion of mucosa in terminal ileum and colon; (3) translocation, in which organisms penetrate mucosa and replicate in lamina propria	Fever, abdominal pain, diarrhea, can be bloody; vomiting Watery, profuse, foul-smelling diarrhea Clinically similar to *Salmonella* or *Shigella* Fecal-oral transmission	Most infections in humans relate to consumption of contaminated foods or water; undercooked meats, particularly chicken; unpasteurized milk Also acquired from contaminated household pets (e.g., dogs, cats, hamsters) Bimodal peaks in infants >1 yr and again at ages 15-29 mo Antibiotics do not prolong carriage of bacteria and may eliminate organism more quickly Erythromycin and azithromycin drugs of choice (5-7 days) Antimotility agents not recommended and tend to prolong symptoms
Vibrio cholerae Gram-negative, motile, curved bacillus living in bodies of salt water Incubation period: 1-3 days Diagnosis by stool culture	Enters via oral route in contaminated food or water; if survives acid stomach environment, travels to small intestine, adheres to mucosa, and produces toxin	Onset abrupt; vomiting, watery diarrhea without cramping or tenesmus Dehydration can occur quickly	More prevalent in developing countries Rehydration most important treatment Antibiotics can shorten diarrhea Despite continued efforts, still no vaccine

Continued

TABLE 41-5   INFECTIOUS CAUSES OF ACUTE DIARRHEA—cont'd

ORGANISM	PATHOLOGY	CHARACTERISTICS	COMMENTS
Clostridium difficile Gram-positive anaerobic bacillus Diagnosis by detecting *C. difficile* toxin in stool culture	Produces two important toxins (A and B) Toxin binds to enterocyte surface receptor, resulting in alteration of permeability, protein synthesis, and direct cytotoxicity	Most cases: mild, watery diarrhea lasting few days Some cases: prolonged diarrhea and illness May cause pseudomembranous colitis Some individuals are extremely ill with high fever, leukocytosis, hypoalbuminemia	Associated with alteration of normal intestinal flora by antibiotics More common in hospitalized persons Adults tend to have more severe symptoms than children Treatment with antibiotics in symptomatic patients; and metronidazole Resistant strains have developed Relapse common
Clostridium perfringens Incubation period: 8-24 hr; anaerobic, gram-positive, spore-producing bacilli	Toxins produced in intestine after ingestion of organism	Acute onset: watery diarrhea, crampy abdominal pain Fever, nausea and vomiting rare Duration of illness usually 24 hr	Transmitted by contaminated food products, most often meats and poultry Usually self-limiting and medical intervention not needed Oral rehydration usually sufficient Antibiotics serve no purpose and should not be used
Clostridium botulinum Incubation period: 12-26 hr (range, 6 hr to 8 days) Gram-positive, anaerobic, spore-producing bacilli Blood and stool culture should be obtained and transmitted to special laboratory (usually state health department) to detect toxin	Botulism caused by binding of toxin to neuromuscular junction	Clinical presentation related to age and strain of botulism Abdominal pain, cramping, and diarrhea Other strains: respiratory compromise, central nervous system symptoms	Transmitted in contaminated food products Can be acquired via wound infection Treatment involves supportive care and neutralization of toxin See Infant Botulism, Chapter 49
Staphylococcus (food poisoning) Incubation period: generally short, 1-8 hr Gram-positive, nonmotile, aerobic, or facultative anaerobic bacteria Diagnosis by identifying organism in food, blood, pus, aspirate	Direct tissue invasion and production of toxin	Clinical presentation depends on site of entry In food poisoning: profuse diarrhea, nausea and vomiting Low-grade fever and hypothermia may occur	GI illness transmitted in inadequately cooked or refrigerated foods Self-limiting in GI illness Symptomatic treatment Antibiotics not recommended

Chronic diarrhea is defined as an increase in stool frequency and increased water content with a duration of more than 14 days. It is often caused by chronic conditions such as malabsorption syndromes, inflammatory bowel disease (IBD), immunodeficiency, food allergy, lactose intolerance, or chronic nonspecific diarrhea or as a result of inadequate management of acute diarrhea.

Intractable diarrhea of infancy is a syndrome that occurs in the first few months of life, persists for more than 2 weeks with no recognized pathogens, and is refractory to treatment. The most common cause is inadequately managed acute infectious diarrhea.

Chronic nonspecific diarrhea (CNSD), also known as irritable colon of childhood and toddlers' diarrhea, is a common cause of chronic diarrhea in children 6 to 54 months of age. These children have loose stools, often with undigested food particles, and diarrhea lasting more than 2 weeks. Children with CNSD grow normally and have no evidence of malnutrition, no blood in their stool, and no enteric infection. Dietary indiscretions and food sensitivities have been linked to chronic diarrhea. The excessive intake of juices and artificial sweeteners such as sorbitol, a substance found in many commercially prepared beverages and foods, may be a factor.

Etiology

Most pathogens that cause diarrhea are spread by the fecal-oral route through contaminated food or water or are from person to person where there is close contact (e.g., day care centers). Lack of clean water, crowding, poor hygiene, nutritional deficiency, and poor sanitation are major risk factors, especially for bacterial or parasitic pathogens. The increased frequency and severity of diarrheal disease in infants is also related to age-specific alterations in susceptibility to pathogens. For example, the immune systems of infants have not been exposed to many pathogens and have not acquired protective antibodies. Worldwide the most common causes of acute gastroenteritis are infectious agents, viruses, bacteria, and parasites. In developed nations viruses, primarily rotavirus, cause 70% to 80% of infectious diarrhea.

Rotavirus is the most important cause of serious gastroenteritis among children and a significant nosocomial (hospital-acquired) pathogen, accounting for 55,000 to 70,000 hospitalizations annually (AAP Committee on Infectious Diseases, 2012; CDC, 2009). However, population-based surveys in three U.S. counties indicate that hospitalizations among children younger than 36 months old decreased by as much as 87% among 6 to 11 month olds, 96% among children ages 12 to 23 months, and 92% among those 24 to 35 months of age after introduction of the rotavirus vaccine in 2006 (Payne, Staat, Edwards, et al., 2011). Rotavirus disease is most severe in children 3 to 24 months of age. Children younger than 3 months of age have some protection from the disease because of maternally acquired antibodies. Approximately 25% of severe cases of rotavirus occur in older children.

Salmonella, Shigella, and *Campylobacter* organisms are the most frequently isolated bacterial pathogens. *Salmonella* has the highest occurrence in infants; *Giardia* and *Shigella* have the highest incidence among toddlers. *Shigella* infection is uncommon in the United States, accounting for fewer than 5% of diarrheal illnesses in infants and toddlers. *Campylobacter* infection has a bimodal presentation (highest in children younger than 12 months of age with a second rise in incidence at age 15 to 19 years). *Giardia* and *Cryptosporidium* organisms are parasites. *Giardia* infection represents 15% of nondysenteric illness in the United States; *Cryptosporidium* infection is often associated with outbreaks in young children in day care centers; an increase in infections has been seen in association with outdoor swimming (pools, lakes, splash fountains) in the summer and early fall (AAP Committee on Infectious Diseases, 2012). *Plesiomonas shigelloides* is frequently responsible for causing traveler's diarrhea. (See also Intestinal Parasitic Diseases, p. 1272.)

Antibiotic administration is frequently associated with diarrhea because antibiotics alter the normal intestinal flora, resulting in an overgrowth of other bacteria such as *Clostridium difficile.* National rates of *C. difficile* have more than doubled since 2000 (Richards, 2006), and it has become more virulent with a high rate of recurrence and treatment failure (Bakken, 2009; DuPont, 2011). Antibiotic-associated diarrhea can also be caused by *Salmonella* organisms, *Clostridium porringers* type A, and *Staphylococcus aureus* pathogens.

Pathophysiology

Invasion of the GI tract by pathogens results in increased intestinal secretion as a result of enterotoxins, cytotoxic mediators, or decreased intestinal absorption secondary to intestinal damage or inflammation. Enteric pathogens attach to the mucosal cells and form a cuplike pedestal on which the bacteria rest. The pathogenesis of the diarrhea depends on whether the organism remains attached to the cell surface, resulting in a secretory toxin (noninvasive, toxin-producing, noninflammatory type diarrhea) or penetrates the mucosa (systemic diarrhea). Noninflammatory diarrhea is the most common diarrheal illness, resulting from the action of enterotoxin that is released after attachment to the mucosa. The most serious and immediate physiologic disturbances associated with severe diarrheal disease are (1) dehydration, (2) acid-base imbalance with acidosis, and (3) shock that occurs when dehydration progresses to the point that circulatory status is seriously impaired.

Diagnostic Evaluation

Evaluation of a child with acute gastroenteritis begins with a careful history that seeks to discover the possible cause of diarrhea, assess the severity of symptoms and the risk of complications, and elicit information about current symptoms indicating other treatable illnesses that could be causing the diarrhea. The history should include questions about recent travel, exposure to untreated drinking or washing water sources, contact with animals or birds, day care center attendance, recent treatment with antibiotics, or recent diet changes. History questions should also explore the presence or absence of other symptoms such as fever and vomiting, frequency and character of stools (e.g., watery, bloody), urinary output, dietary habits, and recent food intake.

Extensive laboratory evaluation is not indicated in children who have uncomplicated diarrhea and no evidence of dehydration because most diarrheal illnesses are self-limiting. Laboratory tests are indicated for children who are severely dehydrated and receiving IV therapy. Watery, explosive stools suggest glucose intolerance; foul-smelling, greasy, bulky stools suggest fat malabsorption. Diarrhea that develops after the introduction of cow's milk, fruits, or cereal may be related to enzyme deficiency or protein intolerance. Neutrophils or red blood cells in the stool indicate bacterial gastroenteritis or IBD. The presence of eosinophils suggests protein intolerance or parasitic infection. Stool cultures should be performed only when blood, mucus, or polymorphonuclear leukocytes are present in the stool; when symptoms are severe; when there is a history of travel to a developing country; and when a specific pathogen is suspected. Gross or occult blood may indicate pathogens such as *Shigella, Campylobacter,* or hemorrhagic *Escherichia coli* strains. An enzyme-linked immunosorbent assay (ELISA) may be used to confirm the presence of rotavirus or *Giardia* organisms. If there is a history of recent antibiotic use, the stool should be tested for *C. difficile* toxin. When bacterial and viral culture results are negative and diarrhea persists for more than a few days, stools should be examined for ova and parasites. A stool specimen with a pH of less than 6.0 and the presence of reducing substances may indicate carbohydrate malabsorption or secondary lactase deficiency. Stool electrolyte measurements may help identify children with secretory diarrhea.

The serum bicarbonate (CO_2) may be useful when combined with other clinical signs. In the presence of metabolic acidosis an anion gap may be helpful to distinguish between types of metabolic imbalance. Obtain a complete blood count (CBC), serum electrolytes, creatinine, and blood urea nitrogen (BUN) in the child who has moderate-to-severe dehydration or who requires hospitalization. The hemoglobin, hematocrit, creatinine, and BUN levels are usually elevated in acute diarrhea and should normalize with rehydration.

Therapeutic Management

The major goals in the management of acute diarrhea include (1) assessment of fluid and electrolyte imbalance, (2) rehydration, (3) maintenance fluid therapy, and (4) reintroduction of an adequate diet. Infants and children with acute diarrhea and dehydration should be treated first with oral rehydration therapy (ORT). ORT is one of the major worldwide health care advances. It is more effective, safer, less painful, and less costly than IV rehydration. The AAP, WHO, and CDC recommend ORT as the treatment of choice for most cases of dehydration caused by diarrhea (CDC, 2003) (see Box 41-4). Oral rehydration solutions (ORSs) enhance and promote the resorption of sodium and water; studies indicate that these solutions greatly reduce vomiting, volume loss from diarrhea, and the duration of the illness. ORSs, including reduced-osmolarity ORS, are available in the United States as commercially prepared solutions and are successful in treating the majority of infants with dehydration. Guidelines for rehydration recommended by the AAP are included in Table 41-6.

After rehydration ORS may be used during maintenance fluid therapy by alternating the solution with a low-sodium fluid such as

TABLE 41-6	**TREATMENT OF ACUTE DIARRHEA**			
DEGREE OF DEHYDRATION	**SIGNS AND SYMPTOMS**	**REHYDRATION THERAPY***	**REPLACEMENT OF STOOL LOSSES**	**MAINTENANCE THERAPY**
Minimal	Increased thirst Slightly dry buccal mucous membranes	ORS, 50 mL/kg over 4 hr ORS, give 5-10 mL every 2-3 minutes	<10 kg: 60-120 mL per vomiting or diarrheal episode >10 kg:120-140 mL ORS per episode of vomiting or diarrhea	Breastfeeding, if established, should continue; give regular infant formula if tolerated. If lactose intolerance suspected, give undiluted lactose-free formula (or half-strength lactose-containing formula for brief period only); infants and children who receive solid food should continue their usual diet.
Mild to Moderate	Loss of skin turgor, dry buccal mucous membranes, sunken eyes, sunken fontanel	ORS, 100 mL/kg within 4 hr	Same as for Minimal	
Severe	Signs of moderate dehydration plus one of following: rapid, thready pulse; cyanosis; rapid breathing; lethargy; or coma	IV fluids (Ringer's lactate; 0.9 NS), 20 mL/kg bolus over 30 minutes and repeat until pulse and state of consciousness return to normal; then maintenance fluids with dextrose and 0.45 NS; add K+ after renal function adequate; give 50-100 mL/ kg or ORS	Same as for Minimal	

Modified from Centers for Disease Control and Prevention: Managing acute gastroenteritis among children: oral rehydration, maintenance, and nutritional therapy, *MMWR Recommend Rep* 52(RR-16):1–16, 2003.
IV, Intravenous; *NS*, normal saline; *ORS*, oral rehydration solution.
*If no signs of dehydration are present, rehydration therapy is not necessary. Proceed with maintenance therapy and replacement of stool losses.

breast milk or commercial infant formula. In older children ORS can be given, and a regular diet continued. Ongoing stool losses should be replaced on a 1:1 basis with ORS. If the stool volume is not known, approximately 10 mL/kg (4 to 8 oz) of ORS should be given for each diarrheal stool.

The WHO and UNICEF (United Nations Children's Fund) recommend the addition of zinc to ORS for the treatment of diarrheal disease in children (Granado-Villar, Cunill-de Sautu, and Granados, 2012). Zinc supplementation has been shown to decrease the frequency of stools in acute gastroenteritis (Atia and Buchman, 2009). Liquids such as sports drinks, tea, juices, or carbonated beverages are not appropriate for ORT in small children.

Solutions for oral hydration are useful in most cases of dehydration, and vomiting is not a contraindication. A child who is vomiting should be given an ORS at frequent intervals and in small amounts. For young children the caregiver may give the fluid with a spoon or small syringe in 5- to 10-mL increments every 1 to 5 minutes. An ORS may also be given via NG or gastrostomy tube infusion. Infants without clinical signs of dehydration do not need ORT. However, they should receive the same fluids recommended for infants with signs of dehydration in the maintenance phase and for ongoing stool losses. The use of probiotics in tandem with rehydration therapy reduces the duration and stool frequency in acute infectious diarrhea (Allen, Martinez, Gregorio, et al., 2010).

Early reintroduction of nutrients is desirable and is gaining more widespread acceptance. Continued feeding or early reintroduction

> **! NURSING ALERT**
>
> Diarrhea is not managed by encouraging intake of clear fluids by mouth such as fruit juices, carbonated soft drinks, and gelatin. These fluids usually have a high carbohydrate content, a very low electrolyte content, and a high osmolality. Caffeinated soda is avoided because caffeine is a mild diuretic and may lead to increased loss of water and sodium. Chicken or beef broth is not given because it contains excessive sodium and inadequate carbohydrate. A BRAT diet (bananas, rice, applesauce, and toast or tea) is contraindicated for children and especially for infants with acute diarrhea because it has little nutritional value (low in energy and protein), is high in carbohydrates, and is low in electrolytes (AAP, 2009).

of a normal diet has no adverse effects and actually lessens the severity and duration of the illness and improves weight gain compared with the gradual reintroduction of foods (AAP, 2009; Bhutta, 2011). Infants who are breastfeeding should continue to do so, and ORS should be used to replace ongoing losses in these infants. Formula-fed infants should resume their formula; if it is not tolerated, a lactose-free formula may be used for a few days. In older children a regular diet, including milk, generally can be offered after rehydration has been achieved. In toddlers there is no contraindication to continuing soft or pureed foods. A diet of easily digestible foods such as cereals, cooked vegetables, and meats is adequate for older children.

In cases of severe dehydration and shock, IV fluids are initiated whenever the child is unable to ingest sufficient amounts of fluid and electrolytes to (1) meet ongoing daily physiologic losses, (2) replace previous deficits, and (3) replace ongoing abnormal losses. Patients who usually require IV fluids are those with severe dehydration, with uncontrollable vomiting, who are unable to drink for any reason (e.g., extreme fatigue, coma), and with severe gastric distention.

The IV solution for fluid replacement is selected based on what is known regarding the probable type and cause of the dehydration—usually a saline solution (0.9 normal saline [NS] or lactated Ringer's solution for rapid volume replacement (see Parenteral Fluid Therapy, p. 1258).

After the severe effects of dehydration are under control, specific diagnostic and therapeutic measures are begun to detect and treat the cause of the diarrhea. The use of antibiotic therapy in children with acute gastroenteritis is controversial. Antibiotics may shorten the course of some diarrheal illnesses (e.g., those caused by *Shigella* organisms). However, most bacterial diarrheas are self-limiting, and the diarrhea often resolves before the causative organism can be determined. Antibiotics may prolong the carrier period for bacteria such as *Salmonella* spp. However, they may be considered in patients with immunosuppression, severe symptoms, or persistent disease and in patients who have had transplantation. Antimotility drugs such as loperamide are not recommended in children, and antiemetic drugs such as the phenothiazines are not recommended because of their side effects. Because of the self-limiting nature of vomiting and its tendency to improve when dehydration is corrected, historically the use of antiemetic agents has not been recommended; however, ondansetron has few side effects and may be administered if vomiting persists and interferes with ORT (Bhutta, 2011).

The treatment of relapsing *Clostridium difficile* with antibiotics has met partial success, but relapses are common. Recently a novel therapy has been used widely in adults (Mellow and Kanatzar, 2011) and on a limited basis in children to colonize the gut with donor fecal bacteria in order to stop diarrhea associated with *C. difficile*. The fecal bacteriotherapy resulted in a resolution of symptoms within 36 hours of treatment (Russell, Kaplan, Ferraro, et al., 2010).

Prevention. Two rotavirus vaccines are now available for children. Human-bovine reassortant rotavirus vaccine (RotaTeq), which became available in 2006, and live-attenuated human rotavirus vaccine (Rotarix) may be used to prevent this infectious diarrheal disease. Infants should receive three doses of RotaTeq oral vaccine at 2, 4, and 6 months of age. Two doses of Rotarix induce protective immunity and may be administered at 2 and 4 months of age (AAP Committee on Infectious Diseases and Pickering, 2012) (see Chapter 31, Immunizations). Population-based studies show a reduction of diarrhea-associated hospitalizations by as much as 87% to 96% in the years after rotavirus vaccination (Payne, Staat, Edwards, et al., 2011). Breastfeeding during the first 6 months of life has been found to have a protective effect against rotavirus infection (Plenge-Bönig, Soto-Ramirez, Karmaus, et al., 2010).

CARE MANAGEMENT

The management of most cases of acute diarrhea takes place in the home with education of the caregiver. Caregivers are taught to monitor for signs of dehydration (especially the number of wet diapers or voidings) and the amount of fluids taken by mouth and to assess the frequency and amount of stool losses. Education

CRITICAL THINKING CASE STUDY

Diarrhea

A mother brings her 8-month-old infant, Mary, to the primary care clinic. The mother reports that Mary has had a "cold" for about 2 days and this morning she began to vomit and has had diarrhea for the past 8 hours. The mother states that Mary is still breastfeeding but that she is not taking as much milk as usual and she is having 3 times as many stools as usual (the stools are watery in consistency). When the nurse practitioner examines Mary, she notes that her temperature is 38° C (100.4° F), her pulse and blood pressure are in the normal range, her mucous membranes are moist, and she has tears when she cries. The nurse practitioner also notes that Mary's weight has not changed from what it was when she was seen in the clinic 2 weeks ago for her well-child visit.

1. Evidence—Is there sufficient evidence for the nurse practitioner to draw any conclusions for her initial plan of management?
2. Assumptions—Describe some underlying assumptions about the following:
   a. Clinical manifestations of various levels of dehydration
   b. Management of acute diarrhea
   c. Breastfeeding and the management of acute diarrhea
   d. Use of antidiarrheal medications for acute diarrhea
3. Which nursing interventions should the nurse practitioner implement at this time?
4. Does the evidence support the nurse practitioner's conclusion?

relating to ORT, including the administration of maintenance fluids and replacement of ongoing losses, is important (see Critical Thinking Case Study). ORS should be administered in small quantities at frequent intervals. Vomiting is not a contraindication to ORT unless it is severe. Information concerning the introduction of a normal diet is essential. Parents need to know that a slightly higher stool output initially occurs with continuation of a normal diet and with ongoing replacement of stool losses. The benefits of a better nutritional outcome with fewer complications and a shorter duration of illness outweigh the potential increase in stool frequency. Parents' concerns should be addressed to ensure adherence to the treatment plan.

If the child with acute diarrhea and dehydration is hospitalized, an accurate weight must be obtained, and fluid intake and output carefully monitored. The child may be placed on parenteral fluid therapy with nothing by mouth (NPO) for 12 to 48 hours, but the trend is to start small amounts of oral fluids to tolerance unless there are other illness factors that preclude ORT. Monitoring the IV infusion is an important nursing function. The nurse must ensure that the correct fluid and electrolyte concentration is infused, the flow rate is adjusted to deliver the desired volume in a given time, and the IV site is maintained.

Accurate measurement of output is essential to determine whether renal blood flow is sufficient to permit the addition of potassium to the IV fluids. The nurse is responsible for examination of stools and collection of specimens for laboratory examination (see Collection of Specimens, Chapter 39). Care should be taken when obtaining and transporting stools to prevent possible spread of infection. Stool specimens should be transported to the laboratory in appropriate containers and media.

Diarrheal stools are highly irritating to the perianal skin, and extra care is needed to protect the skin of the diaper region from excoriation (see Diaper Dermatitis, Chapter 47). Taking the temperature rectally is usually avoided because it stimulates the bowel, increasing the passage of stool and causing mucosal irritation.

Support for the child and family involves the same care and consideration given to all hospitalized children (see Chapter 38). Parents are kept informed of the child's progress and instructed in the use of frequent and proper hand washing and the disposal of soiled diapers, clothes, and bed linens. Everyone caring for the child must be aware of "clean" and "dirty" areas, especially in the hospital, where the sink in the child's room is used for many purposes. Soiled diapers and linens should be discarded in receptacles close to the bedside.

Prevention. The best intervention for diarrhea is prevention. The fecal-oral route spreads most infections, and parents need information about preventive measures such as personal hygiene, protection of the water supply from contamination, and careful food preparation.

! NURSING ALERT

To reduce the risk of bacteria transmitted via food, encourage parents to:
- Quickly freeze or refrigerate all ground meat and other perishable foods.
- Never thaw food on the counter or let it sit out of the refrigerator for more than 2 hours.
- Wash hands, utensils, and work areas with hot, soapy water after contact with raw meat to keep bacteria from spreading.
- Check ground meat with a fork to make certain that no pink is showing before taking a bite.
- Cook all dishes made with ground meat until brown or gray inside or to an internal temperature of 71° C (160° F).
- Use soap or a weak chlorine bleach solution to wash all fruits and vegetables that are unable to be peeled.

Meticulous attention to perianal hygiene, disposal of soiled diapers, proper hand washing, and isolation of infected people also minimize the transmission of infection (see Infection Control, Chapter 39).

Parents need information about preventing diarrhea while traveling. They are cautioned against giving their children adult medications that are used to prevent traveler's diarrhea. Until vaccines or other prophylactic measures are proved to be safe for children, the best measure during travel to areas where water may be contaminated is to allow children to drink only bottled water and carbonated beverages. Tap water, ice, unpasteurized dairy products, raw vegetables, unpeeled fruits, meats, and seafood should also be avoided.

Constipation

Constipation is an alteration in the frequency, consistency, or ease of passing stool. It is defined as a decrease in bowel movement frequency or trouble defecating for more than 2 weeks (Philichi, 2008). It is an alteration in the frequency, consistency, or ease of passing stool. Parents often define constipation as passing less than three stools per week. It may also be defined as painful bowel movements, which are often blood streaked or include the retention of stool, with or without soiling, even with a stool frequency of more than three stools per week (Loening-Baucke and Pashankar, 2006). However, the frequency of bowel movements is not considered a diagnostic criterion because it varies widely among children. Having extremely long intervals between defecation is obstipation. Constipation with fecal soiling is encopresis.

Constipation may arise secondary to a variety of organic disorders or in association with a wide range of systemic disorders.

Structural disorders of the intestine such as strictures, ectopic anus, and Hirschsprung disease (HD), may be associated with constipation. Systemic disorders associated with constipation include hypothyroidism, hypercalcemia resulting from hyperparathyroidism or vitamin D excess, and chronic lead poisoning. Constipation may be associated with use of drugs such as antacids, diuretics, antiepileptics, antihistamines, opioids, and iron supplementation. Spinal cord lesions may be associated with loss of rectal tone and sensation. Affected children are prone to chronic fecal retention and overflow incontinence.

The majority of children have idiopathic or functional constipation because no underlying cause can be identified. Chronic constipation may occur as a result of environmental or psychosocial factors or a combination of both. Transient illness, stool withholding and avoidance secondary to painful or negative experiences with stooling, and dietary intake with decreased fluid and fiber all play a role in the etiology of constipation.

Newborn Period

Normally newborn infants pass a first meconium stool within 24 to 36 hours of birth. Any infant who does not do so should be assessed for evidence of intestinal atresia or stenosis, HD, hypothyroidism, meconium plug, or meconium ileus. Meconium plug is caused by meconium that has reduced water content and is usually evacuated after digital examination but may require irrigations with a hypertonic solution or contrast medium.

Meconium ileus, the initial manifestation of cystic fibrosis, is the luminal obstruction of the distal small intestine by abnormal meconium. Treatment is the same as for a meconium plug; early surgical intervention may be needed to evacuate the small intestine.

Infancy

The onset of constipation frequently occurs during infancy and may result from organic causes such as HD, hypothyroidism, and strictures. It is important to differentiate these conditions from functional constipation. Constipation in infancy is often related to dietary practices. It is less common in breastfed infants, who have softer stools than bottle-fed infants. Breastfed infants may also have decreased stools because of more complete digestion of breast milk with little residue. When constipation occurs with a change from human milk or modified cow's milk to whole cow's milk (12 months old and older), simple measures such as adding or increasing the amount of cereal, vegetables, and fruit in the infant's diet usually correct the problem. When a bottle-fed infant passes a hard stool that results in an anal fissure, stool-withholding behaviors may develop in response to pain on defecation (see Critical Thinking Case Study).

Childhood

Most constipation in early childhood is attributable to environmental changes or normal development when a child begins to attain control over bodily functions. A child who has experienced discomfort during bowel movements may deliberately try to withhold stool. Over time the rectum accommodates to the accumulation of stool, and the urge to defecate passes. When the bowel contents ultimately are evacuated, the accumulated feces are passed with pain, thus reinforcing the desire to withhold stool.

Constipation in school-age children may represent an ongoing problem or a first-time event. The onset of constipation at this age is often the result of environmental changes, stresses, and changes in toileting patterns. A common cause of new-onset constipation at school entry is fear of using the school bathrooms, which are noted

? CRITICAL THINKING CASE STUDY

Constipation

Harry, an 8-month-old infant, is seen by the pediatric nurse practitioner for his well-child visit. Harry's mother states that he usually has one hard stool every 4 or 5 days, which causes discomfort when the stool is passed. He has also had one episode of diarrhea and two episodes of ribbonlike stools. Abdominal distention and vomiting have not accompanied the constipation, and Harry's growth has been appropriate for his age. Currently his diet consists of formula only. Harry's mother reports that the infrequent passage of hard stools began approximately 6 weeks ago when she stopped breastfeeding.

1. Evidence—Is there sufficient evidence for the nurse practitioner to draw any conclusions about the management of Harry's problem?
2. Assumptions—Describe some underlying assumptions about the following:
   a. Causes of constipation in infants
   b. Factors associated with functional constipation in infants
   c. Management of functional constipation in infants
3. Which interventions should the nurse practitioner implement at this time?
4. Does the evidence support these interventions?

for their lack of privacy. Early and hurried departure for school immediately after breakfast may also impede bathroom use.

The management of simple constipation consists of a plan to promote regular bowel movements. Often this is as simple as changing the diet to provide more fiber and fluids, eliminating foods known to be constipating, and establishing a bowel routine that allows for regular passage of stool. An increase in dietary fiber is recommended as a treatment for constipation in the healthy child. The amount of fiber for children of different ages varies by various authorities, but the formula of "age + 5 g" daily intake of fiber is recommended for children 3 years old and older (Kranz, Brauchla, Slavin et al., 2012). The DRI average intake (AI) for children 4 to 8 years old is 25 g of fiber daily. AI dietary fiber intake recommendations for children 9 to 13 years (boys) are 31 g/day and 26 g/day for girls of the same age and up to age 18 years. For boys ages 14 to 18 years the AI for fiber intake is 38 g/day.

Stool-softening agents such as docusate or lactulose may also be helpful. Polyethylene glycol (PEG) 3350 without electrolytes (Miralax) is a chemically inert polymer that has been introduced as a new laxative in recent years. It is usually tolerated well by children because it can be mixed in a beverage of choice. If other symptoms such as vomiting, abdominal distention, or pain and evidence of growth failure are associated with the constipation, the condition should be investigated further.

CARE MANAGEMENT

Constipation tends to be self-perpetuating. A child who has difficulty or discomfort when attempting to evacuate the bowels has a tendency to retain the bowel contents, and this may initiate a vicious cycle. Nursing assessment begins with an accurate history of bowel habits; diet; events associated with the onset of constipation; drugs or other substances that the child may be taking; and the consistency, color, frequency, and other characteristics of the stool. If there is no evidence of a pathologic condition, the major task is to educate the parents regarding normal stool patterns and participate in the education and treatment of the child.

TABLE 41-7 FIBER CONTENT OF SELECT FOODS

FOOD	SERVING SIZE	GRAMS OF FIBER
Apple, raw, with skin	1 apple	3.3
Bananas, ripe, raw		3.1
Beans, baked, canned	1 cup	10.4
Beans, pinto, mature seeds*	1 cup	15.4
Beets*	1 cup	3.4
Blackberries, raw	1 cup	7.6
Blueberries, raw	1 cup	3.5
Bread, mixed grain (includes whole grain)	1 slice	1.6
Broccoli*	1 cup	5.1
Brussel sprouts*	1 cup	4.1
Carrots*	1 cup	4.7
Cereals, ready-to-eat, General Mills, Cheerios	1 cup	3.6
Cereals, ready-to-eat, General Mills, Raisin nut bran	1 cup	5.1
Cereals, ready-to-eat, Kellogg's All Bran, original	½ cup	8.8
Cereals, ready-to-eat, Kellogg's Raisin Bran	1 cup	7.3
Collards*	1 cup	5.3
Dates, daglet noor	1 cup	14.2
Lentils, mature seeds*	1 cup	15.6
Lima beans, large, mature*	1 cup	13.2
Oat bran, cooked	1 cup	5.7
Oranges, raw	1 orange	3.1
Pears, raw	1 pear	5.1
Peas, green, frozen*	1 cup	8.8
Raisins, seedless	1 cup	5.4
Spinach*	1 cup	4.3
Vegetables, mixed, frozen*	1 cup	8.0
Wheat flour, whole grain	1 cup	14.6
Wheat flour, white, all-purpose, enriched	1 cup	3.5

Modified from USDA National Nutrient Database for Standard Reference, Release 17, Fiber, total dietary content of selected foods per common measure, sorted alphabetically, http://www.nal.usda.gov/fnic/foodcomp/Data/SR17/wtrank/sr17a291.pdf.
*Cooked, boiled, drained, no salt.

Dietary modifications are essential in preventing constipation. Lactulose (1 to 3 mL/kg/day) and glycerin suppositories are safe and effective in infants, whereas the addition of other ingredients to formula is not recommended (Rowan-Legg and Canadian Paediatric Society, 2011). During childhood the diet should contain increased amounts of fiber and fluid. Parents benefit from guidance in selecting foods that facilitate bowel movements (Table 41-7). They need reassurance concerning the benign nature of the condition. It is also important to discuss their attitudes and expectations regarding toilet habits.

When constipation persists despite dietary intervention, more aggressive management may be necessary. It is important to differentiate an acute episode of constipation from chronic functional constipation, which can result from chronic stool-withholding behavior. As the rectal vault becomes distended over time, further complications such as fecal impaction and encopresis may develop (see Chapter 34).

Hirschsprung Disease

HD is a congenital anomaly that results in mechanical obstruction from inadequate motility of part of the intestine. It accounts for about one fourth of all cases of neonatal intestinal obstruction. The incidence is 1 in 5000 live births. It is 4 times more common in males than in females and follows a familial pattern in a small number of cases. Mutations in the *RET* protooncogene have been found in 17% to 38% of children with short-segment HD and in 70% to 80% of those with long-segment involvement (Dasgupta and Langer, 2004). In more than 80% of cases the aganglionosis is restricted to the internal sphincter, rectum, and a few centimeters of the sigmoid colon and is termed *short-segment disease* (Theocharatos and Kenny, 2008).

Pathophysiology

The pathology of HD relates to the absence of ganglion cells in the affected areas of the intestine, resulting in a loss of the rectosphincteric reflex and an abnormal microenvironment of the cells of the affected intestine (Theocharatos and Kenny, 2008). The term *congenital aganglionic megacolon* describes the primary defect, which is the absence of ganglion cells in the myenteric plexus of Auerbach and the submucosal plexus of Meissner (Fig. 41-1).

The absence of ganglion cells in the affected bowel results in a lack of enteric nervous system stimulation, which decreases the ability of the internal sphincter to relax. Unopposed sympathetic stimulation of the intestine results in increased intestinal tone. In addition to the contraction of the abnormal bowel and the resulting lack of peristalsis, there is a loss of the rectosphincteric reflex. Normally, when a stool bolus enters the rectum, the internal sphincter relaxes, and the stool is evacuated. In HD the internal sphincter does not relax. In most cases the aganglionic segment includes the rectum and some portion of the distal colon. However, the entire colon or

part of the small intestine may be involved (long-segment disease). Occasionally skip segments or total intestinal aganglionosis may occur.

Diagnostic Evaluation

Most children with HD are diagnosed in the first few months of life. Clinical manifestations vary according to the age when symptoms are recognized and the presence of complications, such as enterocolitis (Box 41-5). A neonate usually is seen with distended abdomen, feeding intolerance with bilious vomiting, and delay in the passage of meconium. Typically 95% of normal term infants pass meconium in the first 24 hours of life, but fewer than 10% of infants with HD do so. In older children a careful history is helpful. Radiographs, an unprepped contrast enema, and anorectal manometric examinations assist in the differential diagnosis, which is confirmed by a full-thickness rectal biopsy demonstrating the absence of ganglion cells in the myenteric and submucosal plexuses.

Therapeutic Management

The majority of children with HD require surgery rather than medical therapy with frequent enemas (Levitt, Martin, Olesevich, et al., 2009). After the child is stabilized with fluid and electrolyte replacement if needed, surgery is performed with a high rate of success. Surgical management consists primarily of the removal of the aganglionic portion of the bowel to relieve obstruction, restore normal motility, and preserve the function of the external anal sphincter. The majority of children with HD require one of the following operative procedures: a Soave transanal pull-through procedure, the Swenson procedure, or the Duhamel procedure (Gourlay, 2013). With earlier diagnosis the proximal bowel may not be extremely distended, thus allowing for a primary pull-through or one-stage procedure and eliminating the need for a temporary colostomy. Simpler operations such as an anorectal myomectomy may be indicated in very short–segment disease.

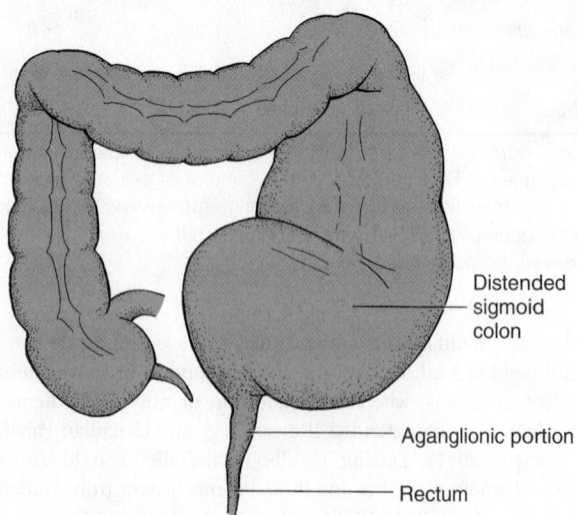

FIG 41-1 Hirschsprung disease.

Distended sigmoid colon

Aganglionic portion

Rectum

| BOX 41-5 | CLINICAL MANIFESTATIONS OF HIRSCHSPRUNG DISEASE |

Newborn Period
- Failure to pass meconium within 24 to 48 hours after birth
- Refusal to feed
- Bilious vomiting
- Abdominal distention

Infancy
- Growth failure
- Constipation
- Abdominal distention
- Episodes of diarrhea and vomiting
- Signs of enterocolitis
- Explosive, watery diarrhea
- Fever
- Appears significantly ill

Childhood (Symptoms Appear More Chronic)
- Constipation
- Ribbonlike, foul-smelling stools
- Abdominal distention
- Visible peristalsis
- Easily palpable fecal mass
- Undernourished, anemic appearance

Prognosis. After the pull-through procedure, anal stricture and incontinence may occur and require further therapy, including dilations or bowel retraining therapy. Constipation and fecal incontinence are chronic problems in a small proportion of patients after surgical correction for HD (Fiorino and Liacouras, 2011). As these children grow older, this can significantly affect their quality of life (Mills, Konkin, Milner, et al., 2008).

CARE MANAGEMENT

The nursing concerns depend on the child's age and the type of treatment. If the disorder is diagnosed during the neonatal period, the main objectives are to (1) help the parents adjust to a congenital defect in their child, (2) foster infant-parent bonding, (3) prepare them for the medical-surgical intervention, and (4) assist them in colostomy care after discharge (as applicable).

Preoperative Care. The child's preoperative care depends on age and clinical condition. A child who is malnourished may not be able to withstand surgery until his or her physical status improves. Often this involves symptomatic treatment with enemas; a low-fiber, high-calorie, and high-protein diet; and in severe situations the use of total parenteral nutrition (TPN).

Physical preoperative preparation includes the same measures that are common to any surgery (see Surgical Procedures, Chapter 39). In newborns whose bowels are relatively sterile, no additional preparation may be necessary. However, in other children preparation for the pull-through procedure involves emptying the bowels with saline enemas and decreasing bacterial flora with oral or systemic antibiotics and colonic irrigations using antibiotic solution. Enterocolitis is the most serious complication of HD. Emergency preoperative care includes frequent monitoring of vital signs and blood pressure for signs of shock; monitoring fluid and electrolyte replacements and plasma or other blood derivatives; and observing for symptoms of bowel perforation such as fever, increasing abdominal distention, vomiting, increased tenderness, irritability, dyspnea, and cyanosis.

The child's age dictates the type and extent of psychologic preparation. When a colostomy is performed, the child who is of preschool age is told about the procedure in concrete terms with the use of visual aids (see Chapter 39). It is important to time explanations appropriately to prevent the anxiety and confusion that could result from too much information. It is also important to stress to parents and older children that the colostomy for HD is temporary unless so much bowel is involved that a permanent ileostomy must be performed. In most instances the extent of bowel resection is known before surgery, although the nurse should be aware of cases when doubt exists concerning repair. The nurse should remember that, although a temporary colostomy is favorable in terms of future health and adjustment, it requires additional surgery, which may be stressful to parents and children.

Postoperative Care. Postoperative care is the same as that for any child or infant with abdominal surgery (see Surgical Procedures, Chapter 39). When a colostomy is part of the corrective procedure, skin and stomal care is a major nursing task (see Ostomies, Chapter 39). To prevent contamination of an infant's abdominal wound with urine, the diaper should be placed below the dressing.

Discharge Care. After surgery parents need instruction concerning colostomy care (as applicable) and establishment of a bowel training program (age appropriate). Even a preschooler can be included in the care by handing articles to the parent, rolling up the colostomy pouch after it is emptied, or applying barrier preparations to the surrounding skin. Although the diagnosis of HD is less frequent in school-age children and adolescents, children this age can often be involved in colostomy care to the point of total responsibility.

An enterostomal therapy nurse can provide expert assistance in planning home care. If families require financial assistance and psychologic support, referral to a social worker, home health care agency, or community health nurse provides continuity of care.

Vomiting

Vomiting is the forceful ejection of gastric contents through the mouth. It is a well-defined, complex, coordinated process that is under CNS control and is often accompanied by nausea and retching. Vomiting may be divided into two categories: nonbilious and bilious. Some small intestinal reflux is common in all vomiting. In nonbilious vomiting the majority of bile drains into the more distal portions of the intestine. If an obstruction is present, nonbilious vomiting suggests a more proximal obstruction. Bilious vomiting implies a disorder of motility or distal physical blockage. Causes of nonbilious vomiting include infectious, inflammatory, metabolic or endocrinologic, neurologic, and psychologic causes and obstructive lesions such as pyloric stenosis. Causes of bilious vomiting include intestinal atresia and stenosis, malrotation with or without volvulus, ileus, intussusception, intestinal duplication, mass lesions, incarcerated inguinal hernia, and appendicitis. Vomiting may also be associated with other processes, including acute infectious diseases, increased intracranial pressure, toxic ingestion, food intolerance and allergies, mechanical obstruction of the GI tract, metabolic disorders, and psychogenic problems. Vomiting is common in childhood, is usually self-limiting, and requires no specific treatment. However, complications may occur, including acute fluid volume loss (dehydration) and electrolyte disturbances, malnutrition, aspiration, and Mallory-Weiss syndrome (small tears in the distal esophageal mucosa).

Vomiting is a well-recognized response to psychologic stress. During stress adrenaline levels rise and may stimulate the chemoreceptor trigger zone. Nausea and vomiting are likely a protective mechanism to remove toxins from the system. Vomiting may follow GI infection or toxic ingestion, or it can be a learned behavioral response.

Cyclic vomiting syndrome is a rare disorder characterized by bouts of vomiting that can last from hours to several days (McRonald and Fleisher, 2005). The cause of this syndrome is unknown (Bullard and Page, 2005).

Therapeutic Management

Management is directed toward detection and treatment of the cause of the vomiting and prevention of complications from the loss of fluid. Fluids are administered in the same manner and in an electrolyte composition similar to those administered for diarrhea. Although most children respond to these measures, antiemetic drugs may be needed. Antiemetics such as ondansetron (Zofran) and trimethobenzamide (Tigan) block receptors in the chemoreceptor trigger zone; others such as metoclopramide (Reglan) enhance gastroduodenal peristalsis; still others such as promethazine (Phenergan) compete for H_1-receptor sites. For children who are prone to motion sickness, it is helpful to administer an appropriate dose of dimenhydrinate (Dramamine) before a trip.

CARE MANAGEMENT

The major focus of nursing care is observing and reporting vomiting behavior and associated symptoms and implementing measures to reduce the vomiting. Accurate assessment of the type of vomiting, the appearance of the vomitus, and the child's behavior in association with the vomiting helps to establish a diagnosis.

Nursing interventions are determined by the cause of the vomiting. When it is a manifestation of improper feeding methods, establishing proper techniques through teaching and example usually corrects the situation. If vomiting is believed to be an indication of obstruction, food is usually withheld or special feeding techniques are implemented. In situations in which vomiting is related to concurrent infection, dietary indiscretion, or emotional factors, efforts are directed toward maintaining hydration or preventing dehydration.

The thirst mechanism is the most sensitive guide to fluid needs, and *ad libitum* administration of an oral rehydration solution to an alert child restores water and electrolytes satisfactorily. It is important to include carbohydrate to spare body protein and avoid ketosis resulting from exhaustion of glycogen stores. Small, frequent feedings of fluids or foods are preferred. After vomiting has stopped, more liberal amounts of fluids are offered followed by gradual resumption of the regular diet.

The vomiting infant or child is positioned on the side or semi-reclining to prevent aspiration and observed for evidence of dehydration. It is important to emphasize the need for the child to brush the teeth or rinse the mouth after vomiting to dilute hydrochloric acid that comes in contact with the teeth. A flavored mouthwash or toothbrushing freshens the mouth. Careful monitoring of fluid and electrolyte status is necessary to prevent an electrolyte disturbance.

Gastroesophageal Reflux

GER is defined as the transfer of gastric contents into the esophagus. This phenomenon is physiologic, occurring throughout the day, most frequently after meals and at night; therefore it is important to differentiate GER from gastroesophageal reflux disease (GERD). GERD represents symptoms or tissue damage that result from GER. Approximately 50% of infants younger than 2 months old are reported to have GER (Suwandhi, Ton, and Schwarz, 2006). This "physiologic" GER usually resolves spontaneously by 1 year of age (Blanco, Davenport, and Kane, 2012).

Certain conditions predispose children to a high prevalence of GERD, including neurologic impairment, hiatal hernia, repaired esophageal atresia (EA), and morbid obesity (Suwandhi, Ton, and Schwarz, 2006). *Sandifer syndrome* is an uncommon condition, usually occurring in young children and characterized by repetitive stretching and arching of the head and neck that can be mistaken for a seizure (Blanco, Davenport, and Kane, 2012). This maneuver likely represents a physiologic neuromuscular response attempting to prevent acid refluxate from reaching the upper portion of the esophagus (Cavataio and Guandalini, 2005).

Infants who are prone to develop GER include preterm infants and those with bronchopulmonary dysplasia. Children who have had tracheoesophageal or EA repairs, extracorporeal membrane oxygenation (ECMO), neurologic disorders, scoliosis, asthma, cystic fibrosis, cerebral palsy, or other neuromuscular conditions are also prone to developing GER. The clinical manifestations of GER are listed in Box 41-6.

Pathophysiology

Although the pathogenesis of GER is multifactorial, its primary causative mechanism likely involves inappropriate transient relaxation of the lower esophageal sphincter (LES) (Suwandhi, Ton, and Schwarz, 2006). Factors that increase abdominal pressure such as coughing and sneezing, scoliosis, and overeating may contribute to

GERD. Esophageal symptoms are caused by inflammation from the acid in the gastric refluxate, but *reactive airway disease (RAD)* may result from stimulation of airway reflexes by the acid refluxate.

Diagnostic Evaluation

The history and physical examination are usually sufficiently reliable to help establish the diagnosis of GER, but many experts suggest that a combination of tests is required for a definitive diagnosis (Blanco, Davenport, and Kane, 2012). The upper GI series is helpful in evaluating the presence of anatomic abnormalities (e.g., pyloric stenosis, malrotation, annular pancreas, hiatal hernia, esophageal stricture). The 24-hour intraesophageal pH monitoring study is the gold standard in the diagnosis of GER (Blanco, Davenport, and Kane, 2012; Suwandhi, Ton, and Schwarz, 2006). Endoscopy with biopsy may be helpful to assess the presence and severity of esophagitis, strictures, and Barrett esophagus and to exclude other disorders such as Crohn's disease (CD). Scintigraphy (gastroesophageal) detects radioactive substances in the esophagus after a feeding of the compound and assesses gastric emptying. It can differentiate between aspiration of gastric contents from reflux versus aspiration from poor oropharyngeal muscle coordination. A modified barium swallow study with video fluoroscopy may also be used as a diagnostic tool for this condition.

Therapeutic Management

Therapeutic management of GER depends on its severity. No therapy is needed for the infant who is growing and has no respiratory complications. Avoidance of certain foods that exacerbate acid reflux (e.g., caffeine, citrus, tomatoes, alcohol, peppermint, spicy or fried foods), lifestyle modifications in older children (e.g., weight control if indicated; small, more frequent meals; smoking cessation), and feeding maneuvers in infants (e.g., thickened feedings) can improve mild GER symptoms. Thickened feedings do not improve

---

BOX 41-6 | **CLINICAL MANIFESTATIONS OF GASTROESOPHAGEAL REFLUX**

Infants
- Spitting up, regurgitation, vomiting (may be forceful)
- Excessive crying, irritability, arching of the back with neck extension, stiffening
- May be "silent" (no clinical signs observed)
- Weight loss, failure to grow (thrive)
- Respiratory problems (cough, wheeze, stridor, gagging, choking with feedings)
- Hematemesis
- Feeding refusal
- Apnea or ALTE

Children
- Heartburn
- Dyspepsia
- Abdominal pain
- Noncardiac chest pain
- Chronic cough
- Dysphagia
- Nocturnal bronchospasm and asthma
- Recurrent pneumonia, pneumonitis

ALTE, Apparent life-threatening event.

pH scores on 24-hour intraesophageal monitoring but may decrease the number of vomiting episodes. Feedings thickened with 1 tsp to 1 Tbsp of rice cereal per ounce of formula may be recommended. This may benefit infants who are underweight as a result of GERD. NG feedings may be necessary for infants with severe reflux and growth failure until surgery can be performed. Elevating the head of the bed 30 degrees or placing the infant in an infant seat elevated 30 degrees for 1 hour after feedings may decrease GER. Prone positioning of infants also decreases episodes of GER but is recommended only with extreme caution when the risk of GERD complications exceeds the risk of sudden infant death syndrome (Cavataio and Guandalini, 2005). The AAP Task Force on Sudden Infant Death Syndrome (2011) recommends supine positioning for sleep (see Chapter 31). If the prone position is used, parents need to be cautioned to avoid soft bedding. If cow's milk protein sensitivity is suspected, a brief trial of extensively hydrolyzed formula may alleviate reflux symptoms; however, changes in formula should occur under medical supervision. A weight loss program may be necessary for children with GERD symptoms that occur as a result of obesity.

Pharmacologic therapy may be used to treat infants and children with GERD. Both H$_2$-receptor antagonists (H$_2$-RAs) (cimetidine [Tagamet], ranitidine [Zantac], or famotidine [Pepcid]) and proton pump inhibitors (PPIs) (esomeprazole [Nexium], lansoprazole [Prevacid], omeprazole [Prilosec], pantoprazole [Protonix], and rabeprazole [Aciphex]) reduce gastric hydrochloric acid secretion and may stimulate some increase in LES tone. Use of available prokinetic drugs (e.g., bethanechol [Urecholine] and metoclopramide) remains controversial. Published clinical practice guidelines for the management of GER in infants and children recommend the use of PPIs over H$_2$RAs for relieving symptoms and healing esophagitis (Vandenplas, Rudolph, Di Lorenzo, et al., 2009).

Surgical management of GER is reserved for children with severe complications such as recurrent aspiration pneumonia, apnea, severe esophagitis, or FTT and for children who have failed to respond to medical therapy. The Nissen fundoplication (Fig. 41-2) is the most common surgical procedure, which is commonly performed laparoscopically with outcomes of decreased time to

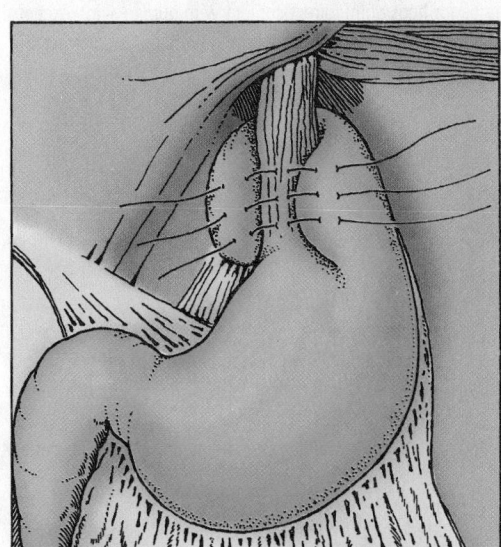

FIG 41-2 Nissen fundoplication sutures passing through esophageal musculature. (Redrawn from Campbell A, Ferrara B: *AORN J* 57:671-679, 1993.)

feedings, better cosmetic results, less pain, and fewer complications (Kane, 2009). This surgery involves passage of the gastric fundus behind the esophagus to encircle the distal esophagus. Long-term complications from fundoplication include breakdown of the wrap, small bowel obstruction, gas-bloat syndrome, infection, retching, and dumping syndrome.

CARE MANAGEMENT

Nursing care is directed at (1) identifying children with symptoms suggestive of GER; (2) educating parents regarding home care, including feeding, positioning, and medications when indicated; and (3) caring for the child undergoing surgical intervention. For the majority of infants parental reassurance of the benign nature of the condition and its relationship to physiologic maturity is the most important intervention. To help parents cope with the inconvenience of dealing with a child who spits up or regurgitates frequently, simple tips such as using bibs and protective clothes during feeding and prone positioning when holding the infant after feeding are beneficial.

It is important to educate and reassure parents about positioning. In the past recommendations encouraged upright positioning during sleeping for both infants and older children. The supine position for sleeping continues to be recommended by the AAP Task Force on Sudden Infant Death Syndrome (2011). Parents should not place infants on their sides as an alternative to fully supine sleeping, and avoiding soft bedding and soft objects in the bed is important. Infant sleep positioners have been associated with 13 infant deaths since 1997 and should not be used to position infants on their sides for GER (Lawrence, Gantt, Samuels-Reid, et al., 2012). Rescheduling of the family's routine may be required to accommodate more frequent feeding times. If parents thicken formula with cereal, they should also enlarge the nipple opening for easier sucking. Usually breastfeeding may continue, and the mother may provide more frequent feeding times or express the milk for thickening with rice cereal. Parents should avoid feeding the child spicy foods or any foods that they find aggravate symptoms in general and avoid caffeine, chocolate, tobacco smoke, and alcohol when breastfeeding. Other practical advice includes advising the parents to avoid vigorous play after feedings and feeding just before bedtime.

When regurgitation is severe and growth is restricted, continuous NG tube or gastrostomy feedings may be considered; these feedings decrease the amount of emesis and provide constant buffering of gastric acid. Special preparation of caregivers is required when this type of nutritional therapy is indicated.

The nurse can support the family by providing information about all aspects of treatment. Parents often require specific information about the medications given for GER. PPIs are most effective when administered 30 minutes before breakfast so the peak plasma concentrations occur with mealtime. If they are given twice a day, the second best time for administration is 30 minutes before the evening meal. Parents need to be reassured because it takes several days of administration to achieve a steady state of acid suppression. They may not see the results that they expect right away. A number of new formulations available in PPIs allow for more efficient administration. Some preparations are available in dissolvable pills. Powder and granule preparations are available as well. Many pharmacies compound the medication in a liquid form for administration.

Postoperative nursing care after the Nissen fundoplication is similar to that for other types of laparoscopic or open abdominal surgery.

INTESTINAL PARASITIC DISEASES

Intestinal parasitic diseases, including helminths (worms) and protozoa, constitute the most frequent infections in the world. In the United States the incidence of intestinal parasitic disease, especially giardiasis, has increased among young children who attend day care centers. Young children are especially at risk because of typical hand-mouth activity and uncontrolled fecal activity.

Intestinal parasitic diseases in humans are caused by various infecting organisms. This discussion is limited to the two most common parasitic infections among children in the United States: giardiasis and pinworms. Table 41-8 describes the outstanding features of selected helminths that belong to the family of nematodes.

General Nursing Care Management

Nursing responsibilities related to intestinal parasitic infections involve helping to identify the parasite, treat the infection, and prevent initial infection or reinfection. Identification of the organism is accomplished by laboratory examination of substances containing the worm, its larvae, or ova. Most are identified by examining fecal smears from the stools of persons suspected of harboring the parasite. Fresh specimens are best for revealing parasites or larvae; therefore collected specimens should be taken directly to the laboratory for examination. If this is not feasible, the specimen is placed in a container with a preservative. Parents need clear instructions on obtaining an adequate sample and the number of samples required (see Stool Specimens, Chapter 39). In most parasitic infections examination of other family members, especially children, may be carried out to identify those who are similarly affected.

Once the diagnosis is confirmed and appropriate treatment is planned, parents need further explanation and reinforcement. Compliance in terms of drug therapy and other measures such as thorough hand washing is essential for eradication of the parasite. The family needs to understand the nature of transmission and that in some cases the medication must be repeated in 2 weeks to 1 month to kill organisms hatched since initial treatment.

TABLE 41-8   SELECTED INTESTINAL PARASITES

CLINICAL MANIFESTATIONS	COMMENTS
Ascariasis—*Ascaris lumbricoides* (Common Roundworm)	
Light infections: asymptomatic	Transferred to mouth by way of contaminated food, fingers, or toys
Heavy infections: anorexia, irritability, nervousness, enlarged abdomen, weight loss, fever, intestinal colic	Largest of the intestinal helminths
	Affects principally young children 1-4 yr of age
Severe infections: intestinal obstruction, appendicitis, perforation of intestine with peritonitis, obstructive jaundice, lung involvement—pneumonitis	Prevalent in warm climates
Hookworm Disease—*Necator americanus*	
Light infections in well-nourished individuals: no problems	Transmitted by discharging eggs on the soil, which are picked up, causing infection from direct skin contact with contaminated soil
Heavier infections: mild-to-severe anemia, malnutrition	
May be itching and burning followed by erythema and a papular eruption in areas to which the organism migrates	Wearing shoes is recommended, although children playing in contaminated soil expose many skin surfaces
Strongyloidiasis—*Strongyloides stercoralis* (Threadworm)	
Light infection: asymptomatic	Transmission is same as for hookworm (direct contact with human skin), except that autoinfection (organism can complete its life cycle in humans) is common
Heavy infection: respiratory signs and symptoms; abdominal pain, distention; nausea and vomiting; diarrhea—large, pale stools, often with mucus	Older children and adults affected more often than young children
Threat to life in children with weakened immunologic defenses	Severe infections may lead to severe nutritional deficiency
Elevated eosinophils may be the only manifestation	Prevalent in warm climates
Visceral Larva Migrans—*Toxocara canis* (Dogs); Intestinal Toxocariasis—*Toxocara cati* (Cats)	
Depends on reactivity of infected individual	Transmitted by ingestion of or contact with soil containing eggs from feces of infected dog or cat
May be asymptomatic except for eosinophilia	Dogs and cats should be kept away from areas where children play; sandboxes are especially common transmission areas
Specific diagnosis difficult	More prevalent in hot, humid environments where eggs remain in soil
	Periodic deworming of diagnosed dogs and cats
	Control of dog and cat population
	Continued education and laws to prevent indiscriminate canine and feline defecation
Trichuriasis—*Trichuris trichiura* (Whipworm)	
Light infections: asymptomatic	Transmitted from contaminated soil or vegetables grown in soil where eggs are present
Heavy infections: abdominal pain and distention, diarrhea	Most frequent in warm, moist climates
	Occurs most often in undernourished children living in unsanitary conditions

The nurse's most important function is preventive education of children and families regarding hygiene and health habits. Thorough hand washing before eating or handling food and after using the toilet is the most important precautionary method.

Giardiasis

Giardiasis is caused by the protozoan *Giardia lamblia* (also called *Giardia intestinalis, Giardia duodenalis,* and *Lamblia intestinalis*). It is the most common intestinal parasitic pathogen in the United States. Child care centers and institutions providing care for persons with developmental disabilities are common sites for urban giardiasis, and children may pass cysts for months. Giardiasis should also be considered in those with a history of recent travel to an endemic area (Shields, Gleim, and Beach, 2008; Yoder and Beach, 2010).

The potential for transmission is great because the cysts (i.e., the nonmotile stage of the protozoa) can survive in the environment for months. Chief modes of transmission are person to person; contaminated water, especially in mountain lakes and streams and swimming or wading pools frequented by diapered infants (who have the condition); food; and animals, especially puppies. In children person-to-person transmission is the most likely cause and is commonly seen in day care centers and institutions where staff or family become infected. Recent studies indicate swimming pool filters and interactive water fountains to be sites of contamination (Eisenstein, Bodager, and Ginzl, 2008; Shields, Gleim, and Beach, 2008).

Although individuals infected with giardiasis may be asymptomatic, common symptoms include abdominal cramps and diarrhea (Box 41-7).

Diagnosis of giardiasis may be made by microscopic examination of stool specimens or duodenal fluid or identification of *G. lamblia* antigens in these specimens by techniques such as enzyme immunoassay (EIA). Because the *Giardia* organisms live in the upper intestine and are excreted in a highly variable pattern, repeated microscopic examination of stool specimens may be required to identify *trophozoites* (active parasites) or cysts. Duodenal specimens are obtained by direct aspiration, biopsy, or the *string* test. In the string test the child swallows a gelatin capsule with a nylon string attached. Several hours later the string is withdrawn, and the contents are sent for laboratory analysis. With the availability of EIA techniques to identify *Giardia* antigens in stool specimens, other tests are being used less often.

Therapeutic Management

The drugs of choice for treatment of giardiasis are metronidazole (Flagyl), tinidazole (Tindamax), and nitazoxanide (Alinia). Tinidazole is said to have an 80% to 100% cure rate after a single dose and has fewer side effects than metronidazole (AAP Committee on Infectious Diseases and Pickering, 2012). Metronidazole and tinidazole have a metallic taste and GI side effects, including nausea and vomiting; nitazoxanide has no bitter taste and should be taken with food to avoid GI symptoms. Albendazole is also used to treat the disease and reportedly has fewer side effects than metronidazole (AAP Committee on Infectious Diseases and Pickering, 2012).

CARE MANAGEMENT

The most important nursing considerations are preventing giardiasis and educating parents, child care center staff, and those who are entrusted with the daily care of small children. Attention to meticulous sanitary practices, especially during diaper changes, is essential (Fig. 41-3). Nurses can play an important role in educating parents of small children and day care staff regarding appropriate sanitation practices. In addition, young children who are infected or who have diarrhea should be discouraged from swimming in community or private pools until they are infection free. Lakes and streams may contain high numbers of *Giardia* spore cysts, which can be swallowed in the water. Discourage children from swimming in stagnant bodies of water or water where children who are known to be infected are swimming when there is a high chance of swallowing water. *Giardia* organisms are said to be resistant to chlorine (Eisenstein, Bodager, and Ginzl, 2008). Parents are encouraged to take small children to the restroom frequently when swimming, to avoid

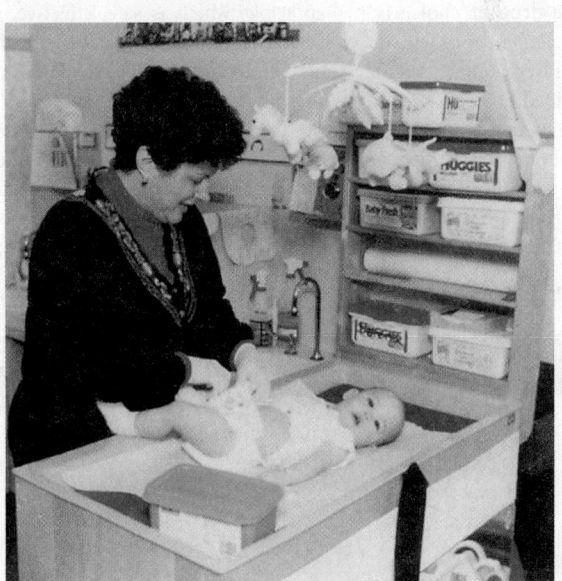

FIG 41-3 Prevention of giardiasis, especially in day care centers, requires sanitary practices during diaper changes such as discarding paper diapers in a covered receptacle, changing paper covers on the diaper-changing surface, and having facilities for hand washing nearby. NOTE: Soiled cloth diapers and clothing should be stored in a plastic bag for transport home.

BOX 41-7   CLINICAL MANIFESTATIONS OF GIARDIASIS

- Infants and young children:
  - Diarrhea
  - Vomiting
  - Anorexia
  - Growth failure
- Children older than 5 years of age:
  - Abdominal cramps
  - Intermittent loose stools
  - Constipation
  - Stools may be malodorous, watery, pale, and greasy
- Most infections resolve spontaneously in 4 to 6 weeks
- Rarely chronic form occurs:
  - Intermittent loose, foul-smelling stools
  - Possibility of abdominal bloating, flatulence, sulfur-tasting belches, epigastric pain, vomiting, headache, and weight loss

letting children in diapers in swimming areas, and to change diapers away from the water source (see also CDC information on recreational water illnesses [www.cdc.gov/healthywater/swimming]). After children are infected, family education regarding drug administration is essential.

Enterobiasis (Pinworms)

Enterobiasis, or pinworms, caused by the nematode *Enterobius vermicularis,* is the most common helminthic infection in the United States. It is universally present in temperate climatic zones and may infect more than 30% of all children at any one time. Crowded conditions such as in classrooms and day care centers favor transmission.

Infection begins when the eggs are ingested or inhaled (they float in the air). The eggs hatch in the upper intestine and then mature and migrate through the intestine. After mating adult females migrate out the anus and lay eggs. The movement of the worms on skin and mucous membrane surfaces causes intense itching. As the child scratches, eggs are deposited on the hands and underneath the fingernails. The typical hand-to-mouth activity of youngsters makes them especially prone to reinfection. Pinworm eggs persist in the indoor environment for 2 to 3 weeks, contaminating anything they contact such as toilet seats, doorknobs, bed linen, underwear, and food. Except for the intense rectal itching associated with pinworms, the clinical manifestations are nonspecific (Box 41-8).

Diagnostic Evaluation

Diagnosis is most commonly made from the tape test (see Care Management). Repeated tests to collect eggs may be necessary; and, if there is a possibility that other family members may be infected, a tape test should be performed on them.

Therapeutic Management

The drugs available for treatment of pinworms include mebendazole (Vermox), pyrantel pamoate (Pin-Rid, Antiminth), and albendazole. The drug of choice is mebendazole, which is safe, effective, and convenient with few side effects; however, it is not recommended for children younger than 2 years of age. If pyrvinium pamoate is prescribed, advise parents that the drug stains stool, vomitus, and clothing or skin with which it comes in contact bright red; it is available without prescription and should not be used in children under 2 years without consulting the primary practitioner. Because pinworms are transmitted easily, all household members should be treated. The dose of antiparasitic medication should be repeated

in 2 weeks to completely eradicate the parasite and prevent reinfection.

CARE MANAGEMENT

Nursing care is directed at identifying the parasite, eradicating the organism, and preventing reinfection. Parents need clear, detailed instructions for the *tape test*. A loop of transparent (not "frosted" or "magic") tape, sticky side out, is placed around the end of a tongue depressor, which is then firmly pressed against the child's perianal area. A convenient, commercially prepared tape is also available for this purpose. Pinworm specimens are collected in the morning as soon as the child awakens and *before* he or she has a bowel movement or bathes. The procedure may need to be performed on 3 or more consecutive days before eggs are collected. Parents are instructed to place the tongue blade in a glass jar or loosely in a plastic bag so it can be brought in for microscopic examination. For specimens collected in the hospital, practitioner's office, or clinic, the tape is placed smoothly on a glass slide, sticky side down, for examination.

Adherence to the drug regimen is usually excellent because the duration of treatment is typically only one dose. However, the family is reminded of the need to take a second dose in 2 weeks to ensure eradication of the eggs.

To prevent reinfection washing all clothes and bed linens in hot water and vacuuming the house may be recommended. However, there is little documentation about the effectiveness of these measures because pinworms survive on many surfaces. Helpful suggestions include hand washing after toileting and before eating, keeping the child's fingernails short to minimize the chance of ova collecting under the nails, dressing children in one-piece sleeping outfits, and daily showering rather than tub bathing. Families should be informed that recurrence is common. Repeated infections should be treated in the same manner as the first one.

INFLAMMATORY DISORDERS

Acute Appendicitis

Appendicitis, inflammation of the vermiform appendix (blind sac at the end of the cecum), is the most common cause of emergency abdominal surgery in childhood. In the United States, 60,000 to 80,000 cases are diagnosed each year. The peak incidence is between the ages of 12 and 18 years of age, with boys and girls equally affected before puberty; more cases occur in the fall and winter. Classically the first symptom of appendicitis is periumbilical pain followed by nausea, right lower quadrant pain, and later vomiting with fever; however, more than 50% of children may have an atypical presentation (Aiken and Oldham, 2011). Perforation of the appendix can occur within approximately 48 hours of the initial complaint of pain. At the time of initial presentation, about one third of all cases involve an already perforated appendix. Complications from appendiceal perforation include major abscess, phlegmon, enterocutaneous fistula, peritonitis, and partial bowel obstruction. A phlegmon is an acute suppurative inflammation of subcutaneous connective tissue that spreads.

Etiology

The cause of appendicitis is obstruction of the lumen of the appendix, usually by hardened fecal material (*fecalith*). Swollen lymphoid tissue, frequently occurring after a viral infection, can also obstruct the appendix. Another rare cause of obstruction is a parasite such as *Enterobius vermicularis,* or pinworms, which can obstruct the appendiceal lumen.

BOX 41-8 **CLINICAL MANIFESTATIONS OF PINWORMS**

- Intense perianal itching (principal symptom); evidence of itching in young children includes the following:
  - General irritability
  - Restlessness
  - Poor sleep
  - Bed-wetting
  - Distractibility
  - Short attention span
- Perianal dermatitis and excoriation secondary to itching
- If worms migrate, possible vaginal (vulvovaginitis) and urethral infection

Pathophysiology

With acute obstruction the outflow of mucus secretions is blocked; pressure builds within the lumen, resulting in compression of blood vessels. The resulting ischemia is followed by ulceration of the epithelial lining and bacterial invasion. Subsequent necrosis causes perforation or rupture with fecal and bacterial contamination of the peritoneal cavity. The resulting inflammation spreads rapidly throughout the abdomen *(peritonitis)*, especially in young children who are unable to localize infection. Progressive peritoneal inflammation results in functional intestinal obstruction of the small bowel *(ileus)* because intense GI reflexes severely inhibit bowel motility. Because the peritoneum represents a major portion of total body surface, the loss of ECF to the peritoneal cavity leads to electrolyte imbalance and hypovolemic shock.

Diagnostic Evaluation

Diagnosis is not always straightforward. Fever, vomiting, abdominal pain, and an elevated white blood cell (WBC) count are associated with appendicitis but are also seen in IBD, pelvic inflammatory disease, gastroenteritis, urinary tract infection, right lower lobe pneumonia, mesenteric adenitis, Meckel diverticulum, and intussusception. Prolonged symptoms and delayed diagnosis often occur in younger children, in whom the risk of perforation is greatest because of their inability to verbalize their complaints.

The diagnosis is based primarily on the history and physical examination (Box 41-9). Pain, the cardinal feature, initially is generalized (usually periumbilical); however, it usually descends to the lower right quadrant. The most intense site of pain may be at McBurney point, located at a point midway between the anterior superior iliac crest and the umbilicus. Rebound tenderness is not a reliable sign and is extremely painful to the child. Referred pain, elicited by light percussion around the perimeter of the abdomen, indicates peritoneal irritation. Movement such as riding over bumps in an automobile or stretcher aggravates the pain. In addition to pain, significant clinical manifestations include fever, a change in behavior, anorexia, and vomiting.

Laboratory studies usually include a CBC, urinalysis (to rule out a urinary tract infection), and in adolescent females serum human chorionic gonadotropin (to rule out an ectopic pregnancy). A WBC count greater than $10,000/mm^3$ and an elevated C-reactive protein (CRP) are common but not necessarily specific for appendicitis. An elevated percentage of bands (often referred to as *a shift to the left*) may indicate an inflammatory process. CRP is an acute-phase reactant that rises within 12 hours of the onset of infection.

BOX 41-9 CLINICAL MANIFESTATIONS OF APPENDICITIS

- Right lower quadrant abdominal pain
- Fever
- Rigid abdomen
- Decreased or absent bowel sounds
- Vomiting (typically follows onset of pain)
- Constipation or diarrhea may be present
- Anorexia
- Tachycardia; rapid, shallow breathing
- Pallor
- Lethargy
- Irritability
- Stooped posture (guarding)

Computed tomography (CT) has become the imaging technique of choice, although ultrasonography may also be helpful in diagnosing appendicitis. Ultrasonography is preferred by many because of the decreased radiation exposure in comparison to CT scan (Pepper, Stanfill, and Pearl, 2012). A CT scan result is considered positive in the presence of enlarged appendiceal diameter; appendiceal wall thickening; and periappendiceal inflammatory changes, including fat streaks, phlegmon, and fluid collection (Aiken and Oldham, 2011; Vissers and Lennarz, 2010).

> **! NURSING ALERT**
>
> In addition to fever, signs of peritonitis include sudden relief from pain after perforation; a subsequent increase in pain (usually diffuse and accompanied by rigid guarding of the abdomen); progressive abdominal distention; tachycardia; rapid, shallow breathing; pallor; chills; and irritability.

Therapeutic Management

Treatment of appendicitis before perforation includes rehydration, antibiotics, and surgical removal of the appendix (appendectomy). Laparoscopic surgery is now commonly used to treat nonperforated acute appendicitis (Aiken and Oldham, 2011); however, this approach may also be used for perforated cases by some surgeons. Recovery is rapid, and if no complications occur the hospital stay is short. A one-time dose of antibiotics may be administered intravenously before surgery.

Ruptured Appendix. Management of the child diagnosed with peritonitis caused by a ruptured appendix often begins before surgery with IV administration of fluid and electrolytes, systemic antibiotics, and NG decompression. Postoperative management includes IV fluids, continued administration of antibiotics, and NG suction for abdominal decompression until intestinal activity returns. Sometimes surgeons close the wound after irrigation of the peritoneal cavity. At other times the wound is left open (delayed closure) to prevent wound infection. A Penrose drain may be used to permit transperitoneal drainage.

Prognosis. Complications are uncommon after a simple appendectomy. The mortality rate for perforating appendicitis has improved from nearly certain death a century ago to 0.3% or less at present (Aiken and Oldham, 2011). Early recognition of the illness is essential to prevent complications.

CARE MANAGEMENT

Because abdominal pain is the most common childhood complaint with appendicitis, it is important to assess the severity of pain (see Pain Assessment, Chapter 30). One of the most reliable estimates is the degree of change in behavior. Younger, nonverbal children assume a rigid, motionless, side-lying posture with the knees flexed on the abdomen, and there is decreased range of motion of the right hip. Older children may exhibit all of these behaviors while complaining of abdominal pain. They can always indicate a point at which the pain is worse than at any other location.

> **! NURSING ALERT**
>
> Whenever appendicitis is suspected, be aware of the danger of administering laxatives or enemas or applying heat to the area. Such measures stimulate bowel motility and increase the risk of perforation.

Postoperative Care. Postoperative care for the nonperforated appendix is the same as for most abdominal procedures. Care of the child with a ruptured appendix and peritonitis involves more complex care, and the course of recovery is considerably longer. The child is maintained on IV fluids, NPO, and the NG tube is kept on low continuous gastric decompression until there is evidence of intestinal activity. Listening for bowel sounds and observing for other signs of bowel activity (e.g., passage of flatus or stool) are part of the routine assessment. Management of IV therapy is the same as for any child receiving fluids and parenteral antibiotics. A drain may be placed in the wound during surgery, and frequent dressing changes with meticulous skin care are essential to prevent excoriation of the area surrounding the surgical site. Wound care includes irrigation with antibacterial solution or saline. Montgomery straps or a wound binder may be used when the wound is left open after surgery to facilitate dressing changes and prevent frequent placement and removal of tape on sensitive skin.

Management of pain from the incision and repeated dressing changes and irrigations are an essential part of the child's care. Psychologic care of the child and parents is similar to that used in other emergency situations (see Emergency Admission, Chapter 38). Parents and older children need to express their feelings and concerns regarding the events surrounding the illness and hospitalization. The nurse can provide education and psychosocial support to promote adequate coping and alleviate anxiety for both the child and the family (see Nursing Care Plan).

Meckel Diverticulum

Meckel diverticulum is a remnant of the fetal omphalomesenteric duct, which connects the yolk sac with the primitive midgut during fetal life (Olson, Kim, and Donnelly, 2009). Normally the structure is obliterated by the seventh to eighth week of gestation, when the placenta replaces the yolk sac as the source of nutrition for the fetus. Failure of obliteration may result in an omphalomesenteric fistula (a fibrous band connecting the small intestine to the umbilicus), known as *Meckel diverticulum.*

Meckel diverticulum is a true diverticulum because it arises from the antimesenteric border of the small intestine and includes all layers of the intestinal wall. The position of the diverticulum varies, but it is usually found within 40 to 50 cm (16 to 20 inches) of the ileocecal valve.

Meckel diverticulum is the most common congenital malformation of the GI tract and is present in 2% to 4% of the population, with more frequent occurrence in boys than girls (Menezes, Tareen, Saeed, et al., 2008; Pepper, Stanfill, and Pearl, 2012). Often it exists without ever causing symptoms.

Pathophysiology

Bleeding, obstruction, or inflammation causes the symptomatic complications of Meckel diverticulum. Gastric mucosa is the most common ectopic tissue found. Bleeding, which is the most common problem in children, is caused by peptic ulceration or perforation because of the unbuffered acidic secretion. Several mechanisms may cause obstruction (Olson, Kim, and Donnelly, 2009). Intussusception may be led by Meckel diverticulum. Obstruction may also be caused by entanglement of the small intestine around a fibrous cord, trapping of a loop of intestine under the band, incarceration within a hernia sac, or volvulus of the intestinal segment containing the diverticulum. Diverticulitis occurs when peptic ulceration or obstruction leads to inflammation.

BOX 41-10 **CLINICAL MANIFESTATIONS OF MECKEL DIVERTICULUM**

Abdominal Pain
- Similar to appendicitis
- May be vague and recurrent

Bloody Stools*
- Painless
- Bright or dark red with mucus ("currant jelly" stool)
- In infants bleeding may be accompanied by pain

Sometimes
- Severe anemia
- Shock

*Often an initial sign.

Diagnostic Evaluation

Diagnosis is usually based on the history, physical examination, and radiographic studies. Meckel diverticulum is often a diagnostic challenge. Radionucleotide scintigraphy (Meckel scan) is most often used but is less reliable in the presence of bleeding (Menezes, Tareen, Saeed, et al., 2008). CT scan, wireless capsule endoscopy, and mesenteric angiography may be used to investigate complications of Meckel diverticulum (Thurley, Halliday, Somers, et al., 2009). Laboratory studies are usually part of the general workup to rule out any bleeding disorder and evaluate the severity of the anemia.

The most common clinical presentation in children includes painless rectal bleeding, abdominal pain, or signs of intestinal obstruction (Box 41-10). Bleeding, which may be mild or profuse, often appears as dark red or "currant jelly" stools; it may be significant enough to cause hypotension.

Therapeutic Management

The standard treatment is surgical removal of the diverticulum. When severe hemorrhage increases the surgical risk, interventions to correct hypovolemic shock such as blood replacement, IV fluids, and oxygen may be necessary. Antibiotics may be used before surgery to control infection. If intestinal obstruction has occurred, appropriate preoperative measures are used to reverse electrolyte imbalances and prevent abdominal distention.

Prognosis. If this condition is diagnosed and treated early, full recovery is likely. The mortality rate of untreated Meckel diverticulum ranges from 2.5% to 15%. Complications of untreated Meckel diverticulum include GI hemorrhage and bowel obstruction.

CARE MANAGEMENT

Nursing care is the same as for any child undergoing abdominal surgery (see Chapter 38). When intestinal bleeding is present, specific preoperative considerations include frequent monitoring of vital signs, including blood pressure; recording the approximate amount of blood lost in stools; and reassuring the child and parents of the surgical success. Pain management is essential to preoperative and postoperative care of the child with this condition.

After surgery the child requires IV fluids and an NG tube for decompression and evacuation of gastric secretions; laparoscopic surgery may avoid the necessity for an NG tube. Signs of return of normal bowel function should be monitored in the postoperative

⊚ NURSING CARE PLAN

The Child with Appendicitis

NURSING DIAGNOSIS	EXPECTED OUTCOMES	NURSING INTERVENTIONS	RATIONALE
Acute Pain related to inflamed appendix (tissue trauma) **Child's or Family's Defining Characteristics** *(Subjective and Objective Data)* Crying Guarding abdomen Limited movement Withdrawal Refusal to eat or drink Fever Increased pulse	The child will have no pain, or pain will be reduced to a level acceptable to child.	Allow child to choose position most comfortable (usually legs flexed). Provide small pillow or stuffed animal for abdomen. Administer analgesia on ATC basis in the first 24 hours after surgery. Teach child (as age appropriate) use of PCA pump	To promote the most comfortable position To splint the abdomen To provide pain relief To minimize breakthrough pain
Risk for Infection related to possibility of rupture before surgery and open wound after surgery (if open procedure is performed) **Child's or Family's Defining Characteristics** *(Subjective and Objective Data)* Abdominal pain Fever Rebound tenderness Nausea and vomiting Anorexia Increased WBC count Fluid around the appendix visualized on ultrasound imaging	Child will be free of signs and symptoms of peritonitis. Signs of peritonitis will be recognized early.	Monitor wound status and integrity and type of dressing (e.g., dressing dry, intact; saline or antiseptic solution irrigation or soaks [wet-to-dry] required for open wound]); specify interval for dressing change Monitor vital signs, including temperature, pulse oximeter, and blood pressure at least every 4 hours in stable child and more often in child with rupture Monitor bowel function, including bowel sounds, passage of flatus Monitor wound drain(s) in relation to proper function, amount, and character of drainage (specify time interval) Encourage early ambulation after surgery with assistance after administration of analgesia Sit in bedside chair at least twice a day For child on lengthy bed rest, place antiembolism devices For child with NG tube, monitor status of NG and suction apparatus to ensure proper function and skin care where anchored Administer antibiotics as prescribed Ensure adequacy and function of IV fluid infusion Provide dietary instructions for foods that provide sufficient calories and protein for growth (once able to eat)	To detect infection and plan interventions To prevent infection at surgical site To promote tissue healing To detect fever or hemodynamic instability and plan necessary intervention To evaluate bowel status and function after surgery To evaluate wound status and healing To decrease accumulation of flatus and abdominal distention and promote early return of proper bowel function To improve circulation, decrease flatus, and promote bowel function To prevent DVT To prevent nausea and vomiting; to promote drainage of GI secretions and acid To prevent wound infection To promote appropriate fluid intake To support an appropriate diet that can increase wound healing
Risk for Deficient Fluid Volume related to decreased fluid intake and fluid losses secondary to loss of appetite, vomiting **Child's or Family's Defining Characteristics** *(Subjective and Objective Data)* Dry mucous membranes Loss of skin turgor Sunken eyes, sunken fontanel Rapid thready pulse, rapid breathing Lethargy	Child will receive sufficient fluids to replace losses. Child will exhibit signs of adequate hydration (specify).	Maintain NPO status as prescribed For child with uncomplicated appendectomy (nonperforation), encourage intake of small amounts of ice chips and progress to clear fluids as prescribed Maintain integrity of infusion site for IV fluids Administer IV fluids and electrolytes as prescribed Monitor fluid intake and output	To minimize fluid losses through vomiting and minimize abdominal distention To promote fluid intake and bowel function To infuse fluids and electrolytes To replace fluid losses To assess hydration status and renal function

Continued

NURSING CARE PLAN

The Child with Appendicitis—cont'd

NURSING DIAGNOSIS	EXPECTED OUTCOMES	NURSING INTERVENTIONS	RATIONALE
Surgical Recovery, Delayed because of absence of bowel motility **Child's or Family's Defining Characteristics** **(Subjective and Objective Data)** Abdominal distention Nausea and vomiting Absence of bowel sounds Abdominal tenderness No passage of stools	Child will not experience abdominal distention or vomiting caused by delayed bowel mobility.	Maintain NPO status in early postoperative period Maintain NG tube decompression as necessary (if used) Assess abdomen for distention, tenderness, flatus, and presence of bowel sounds Monitor passage of flatus and stool Ambulate in room and sit in chair a minimum of 3 times daily	To prevent abdominal distention and vomiting To remove gastric acid and secretions To assess presence of peristalsis (bowel function) To assess for an indicator of bowel motility To increase movement, systemic circulation, and peristalsis

ATC, Around the clock; *DVT,* deep venous thrombosis; *GI,* gastrointestinal; *IV,* intravenous; *NG,* nasogastric; *NPO,* nothing by mouth; *PCA,* patient-controlled analgesia.

TABLE 41-9	CLINICAL MANIFESTATIONS OF INFLAMMATORY BOWEL DISEASES	
CHARACTERISTICS	**ULCERATIVE COLITIS**	**CROHN DISEASE**
Rectal bleeding	Common	Uncommon
Diarrhea	Often severe	Moderate to severe
Pain	Less frequent	Common
Anorexia	Mild or moderate	May be severe
Weight loss	Moderate	May be severe
Growth delay	Usually mild	May be severe
Anal and perianal lesions	Rare	Common
Fistulas and strictures	Rare	Common
Rashes	Mild	Mild
Joint pain	Mild to moderate	Mild to moderate

period. Because the onset of illness is usually rapid, psychologic support is important as in other acute conditions such as appendicitis. It is important to remember that rectal bleeding is usually traumatic to both the child and the parents and may significantly affect their emotional reaction to hospitalization and surgery.

Inflammatory Bowel Disease

Inflammatory bowel disease (IBD) is a term used to refer to two major forms of chronic intestinal inflammation: Crohn disease (CD) and ulcerative colitis (UC). CD and UC have similar epidemiologic, immunologic, and clinical features, but they are distinct disorders (Table 41-9).

In addition to GI symptoms, both CD and UC are characterized by extraintestinal and systemic inflammatory responses. Exacerbations and remissions without complete resolution are also characteristics of IBD. Growth failure, which is particularly common in CD, is an important problem unique to the pediatric population.

CD is also more disabling, has more serious complications and is often less amenable to medical and surgical treatment than is UC. Because UC is confined to the colon, theoretically it may be cured by a colectomy.

The prevalence of IBD is between 12 and 40 per 100,000 people, with 25% of these individuals being diagnosed before 20 years of age (Wong, Clark, Garnett, et al., 2009). Over the past 30 years the incidence of CD has risen, but the incidence of UC in children has remained stable. Children 6 to 17 years of age with CD appear to have a more complicated disease course compared with that of 0- to 5-year-old children (Gupta, Bostrom, Kirschner, et al., 2008).

Etiology

Despite decades of research, the etiology of IBD is not completely understood, and there is no known cure. There is evidence to indicate a multifactorial etiology. Research is focused on theories of defective immunoregulation of the inflammatory response to bacteria or viruses in the GI tract in individuals with a genetic predisposition (Silbermintz and Markowitz, 2006). In CD the chronic immune process is characterized by a T–helper 1 cytokine profile; in UC the response is more humoral and mediated by T–helper 2 cells (Silbermintz and Markowitz, 2006).

Development of IBD has a genetic influence. Several IBD susceptibility genes have now been identified through family and twin studies. Family-based genetic studies have linked chromosome 6 in UC and the *NOD2* gene in CD (Sauer and Kugathasan, 2010).

Pathophysiology of Ulcerative Colitis

The inflammation found with UC is limited to the colon and rectum, with the distal colon and rectum the most severely affected. Inflammation affects the mucosa and submucosa and involves continuous segments along the length of the bowel with varying degrees of ulceration, bleeding, and edema. Thickening of the bowel wall and fibrosis are unusual, but long-standing disease can result in shortening of the colon and strictures. Extraintestinal manifestations are less common in UC than in CD. Toxic megacolon is the most dangerous form of severe colitis.

Pathophysiology of Crohn Disease

The chronic inflammatory process of CD involves any part of the GI tract from the mouth to the anus but most often affects the terminal ileum. The disease involves all layers of the bowel wall (transmural) in a discontinuous fashion, meaning that between areas of intact mucosa there are areas of affected mucosa (skip lesions). The inflammation may result in ulcerations; fibrosis; adhesions; stiffening of the bowel wall; stricture formation; and fistulas to other loops of bowel, bladder, vagina, or skin.

Diagnostic Evaluation

The diagnosis of UC and CD comes from the history, physical examination, laboratory evaluation, and other diagnostic procedures. Laboratory tests include a CBC to evaluate anemia and an erythrocyte sedimentation rate (ESR) or CRP to assess the systemic reaction to the inflammatory process. Levels of total protein, albumin, iron, zinc, magnesium, vitamin B_{12}, and fat-soluble vitamins may be low in children with CD. Stools are examined for blood, leukocytes, and infectious organisms. A serologic panel is often used in combination with clinical findings to diagnose IBD and differentiate between CD and UC. Observational studies on the use of blood tests to detect perinuclear antineutrophilic cytoplasmic antibodies (pANCA) and anti–*Saccharomyces cerevisiae* antibodies (ASCA) showed that the combination is specific but not sensitive for diagnosing UC (Reese, Constantinides, Simillis, et al., 2006).

In patients with CD an upper GI series with small-bowel follow-through assists in assessing the existence, location, and extent of disease. Upper endoscopy and colonoscopy with biopsies are an integral part of diagnosing IBD (Langan, Gotsch, Krafczyk, et al., 2007). Endoscopy allows direct visualization of the surface of the GI tract so the extent of inflammation and narrowing can be evaluated. CT and ultrasonography also may be used to identify bowel wall inflammation, intraabdominal abscesses, and fistulas. CD lesions may pierce the walls of the small intestine and colon, creating tracts called *fistulas* between the intestine and adjacent structures such as the bladder, anus, vagina, or skin.

Therapeutic Management

The natural history of the disease continues to be unpredictable and characterized by recurrent flare-ups that can severely impair patients' physical and social functioning (Vernier-Massouille, Balde, Salleron, et al., 2008). The goals of therapy are to (1) control the inflammatory process to reduce or eliminate the symptoms, (2) obtain long-term remission, (3) promote normal growth and development, and (4) allow as normal a lifestyle as possible. Treatment is individualized and managed according to the type and the severity of the disease, its location, and the response to therapy.

Medical Treatment. The goal of any treatment regimen is first to induce remission of acute symptoms and then to maintain remission over time. 5-Aminosalicylates (5-ASAs) are effective in the induction and maintenance of remission in mild-to-moderate UC. Mesalamine, olsalazine, and balsalazide are now preferred over sulfasalazine because of reduced side effects (headache, nausea, vomiting, neutropenia, and oligospermia). Suppository and enema preparations of mesalamine are used to treat left-sided colitis. These drugs decrease inflammation by inhibiting prostaglandin synthesis. 5-ASAs can be used to induce remission in mild CD. Corticosteroids such as prednisone and prednisolone are indicated in induction therapy in children with moderate-to-severe UC and CD. These drugs inhibit the production of adhesion molecules, cytokines, and leukotrienes. Although they reduce the acute symptoms of IBD, they have side effects that relate to long-term use, including growth suppression (adrenal suppression), weight gain, and decreased bone density. High doses of IV corticosteroids may be administered in acute episodes and tapered according to clinical response.

Budesonide, a synthetic corticosteroid, is designed for controlled release in the ileum and indicated for ileal and right-sided colitis; budesonide has fewer side effects than prednisone and prednisolone (Silbermintz and Markowitz, 2006). Rectal steroid therapy (enemas and foam-based preparations) are available for both induction and maintenance therapy in left-sided colitis.

Immunomodulators such as azathioprine and its metabolite 6-mercaptopurine (6-MP) are used to induce and maintain remission in children with IBD who are steroid resistant or steroid dependent and to treat chronic draining fistulas. They block the synthesis of purine, thus inhibiting the ability of deoxyribonucleic acid (DNA) and ribonucleic acid (RNA) to hinder lymphocyte function, especially that of T-cells. Side effects include infection, pancreatitis, hepatitis, bone marrow toxicity, arthralgia, and malignancy. Methotrexate is also useful in inducing and maintaining remission in CD patients unresponsive to standard therapies. Cyclosporine and tacrolimus have both been effective in inducing remission in severe steroid-dependent UC. 6-MP or azathioprine is then used to maintain remission. Patients taking immunomodulating medications require regular monitoring of their CBC and differential to assess for changes that reflect suppression of the immune system because many of the side effects can be prevented or managed by dose reduction or discontinuation of medication.

Antibiotics such as metronidazole and ciprofloxacin may be used as an adjunctive therapy to treat complications such as perianal disease or small-bowel bacterial overgrowth in CD. Side effects of these drugs are peripheral neuropathy, nausea, and a metallic taste.

Biologic therapies act to regulate inflammatory and antiinflammatory cytokines. With the emergence of the biologic agents, specifically the use of antitumor necrosis factor (TNF-α) agents such as adalimumab and infliximab, progress has been made in targeting specific pathogenetic mechanisms and achieving a more prolonged clinical response (Bradley and Oliva-Hemker, 2012; Hyams and Markowitz, 2005; Ricart, García-Bosch, Ordás, et al., 2008). TNF-α is believed to influence active inflammation.

Nutritional Support. Nutritional support is important in the treatment of patients with IBD. Growth failure is a common serious complication, especially in CD. It is characterized by weight loss, alteration in body composition, restricted height, and delayed sexual maturation. Malnutrition causes the growth failure, and its etiology is multifactorial. Malnutrition occurs as a result of inadequate dietary intake, excessive GI losses, malabsorption, drug-nutrient interaction, and increased nutritional requirements. Inadequate dietary intake occurs with anorexia and episodes of increased disease activity. Excessive loss of nutrients (protein, blood, electrolytes, and minerals) occurs secondary to intestinal inflammation and diarrhea. Carbohydrate, lactose, fat, vitamin, and mineral malabsorption and vitamin B_{12} and folic acid deficiencies occur with disease episodes, with drug administration, and when the terminal ileum is resected. Finally nutritional requirements are increased with inflammation, fever, fistulas, and periods of rapid growth (e.g., adolescence).

The goals of nutritional support include (1) correction of nutrient deficits and replacement of ongoing losses, (2) provision of adequate energy and protein for healing, and (3) provision of adequate nutrients to promote normal growth. Nutritional support includes both enteral and parenteral nutrition (PN). A well-balanced, high-protein, high-calorie diet is recommended for children whose symptoms do not prohibit an adequate oral intake. There is little evidence that avoiding specific foods influences the severity of the disease. Supplementation with multivitamins, iron, and folic acid is recommended.

Special enteral formulas given either by mouth or continuous NG infusion (often at night) may be required. Elemental formulas are completely absorbed in the small intestine with almost no residue. A diet consisting only of elemental formula not only improves nutritional status but also induces disease remission, either without steroids or with a diminished dosage of steroids required. An elemental diet is a safe and potentially effective primary therapy for patients with CD. Unfortunately remission is not sustained when NG feedings are discontinued unless maintenance medications are added to the treatment regimen.

TPN has also improved nutritional status in patients with IBD. Short-term remissions have been achieved after TPN, although complete bowel rest has not reduced inflammation or added to the benefits of improved nutrition by TPN. Nutritional support is less likely to induce a remission in UC than in CD. However, improvement of nutritional status is important in preventing deterioration of the patient's health status and preparing the patient for surgery.

Surgical Treatment. Surgery is indicated for UC when medical and nutritional therapies fail to prevent complications. Surgical options include a subtotal colectomy and ileostomy that leaves a rectal stump as a blind pouch. A reservoir pouch is created in the configuration of a J or S to help improve continence after surgery. An ileoanal pull-through preserves the normal pathway for defecation. *Pouchitis*, an inflammation of the surgically created pouch, is the most common late complication of this procedure and had been reported to occur in up to 50% of cases. In many cases UC can be cured with a total colectomy.

Surgery may be required in children with CD when complications cannot be controlled by medical and nutritional therapy. Segmental intestinal resections are performed for small-bowel obstructions, strictures, or fistulas. Partial colonic resection is not curative, and the disease often recurs.

Prognosis. IBD is a chronic disease. Relatively long periods of quiescent disease may follow exacerbations. The outcome is influenced by the regions and severity of involvement and appropriate therapeutic management. Malnutrition, growth failure, and bleeding are serious complications. The overall prognosis for UC is good.

The development of colorectal cancer (CRC) is a long-term complication of IBD. In UC the cumulative incidence of CRC is 2.5% after 20 years, increasing to 10.8% after 30 years (Rutter, Saunders, Wilkinson, et al., 2006). Surveillance colonoscopy with multiple biopsies should begin approximately 10 years after diagnosis of UC or Crohn's colitis and continue every 1 to 2 years (Rubin and Kavitt, 2006). Removal of the diseased colon prevents development of CRC. However, in CD surgical removal of the affected colon does not prevent cancer from developing elsewhere in the GI tract.

CARE MANAGEMENT

The nursing considerations in the management of patients with IBD extend beyond the immediate period of hospitalization. These interventions involve continued guidance of families in terms of (1) managing diet; (2) coping with factors that increase stress and emotional lability; (3) adjusting to a disease of remissions and exacerbations; and (4) when indicated, preparing the child and parents for the possibility of diversionary bowel surgery.

Because nutritional support is an essential part of therapy, encouraging the anorexic child to consume enough food is often a challenge. Successful interventions include involving the child in

meal planning; encouraging small, frequent meals or snacks rather than three large meals a day; serving meals around medication schedules when diarrhea, mouth pain, and intestinal spasm are controlled; and preparing high-protein, high-calorie foods such as eggnog, milkshakes, cream soups, puddings, or custard (if lactose is tolerated). (See Feeding the Sick Child, Chapter 39.) Using bran or a high-fiber diet for active IBD is questionable. Bran, even in small amounts, has been shown to worsen the condition. Occasionally the occurrence of *aphthous stomatitis* further complicates adherence to dietary management. Mouth care before eating and the selection of bland foods help relieve the discomfort of mouth sores.

When NG feedings or TPN is indicated, nurses play an important role in explaining the purpose and expected outcomes of this therapy. The nurse should acknowledge the anxieties of the child and family members and give them adequate time to demonstrate the skills necessary to continue the therapy at home if needed (see Critical Thinking Case Study).

The importance of continued drug therapy despite remission of symptoms must be stressed to the child and family members. Failure to adhere to the pharmacologic regimen can result in exacerbation of the disease (see Compliance, Chapter 39). Unfortunately exacerbation of IBD can occur even if the child and family are compliant with the treatment regimen, and it is difficult for the child and family to cope.

Family Support. The nurse should attend to the emotional components of the disease and assess any sources of stress. Frequently she or he can help children adjust to problems of growth restriction, delayed sexual maturation, dietary restrictions, feelings of being "different" or "sickly," inability to compete with peers, and necessary absence from school during exacerbations of the illness (see Impact of the Child's Chronic Illness, Chapter 36).

If a permanent colectomy-ileostomy is required, the nurse can teach the child and family how to care for the ileostomy. The nurse

---

? CRITICAL THINKING CASE STUDY

Inflammatory Bowel Disease

Susan, a 13-year-old girl, was admitted to the hospital because of bloody diarrhea, abdominal pain, and weight loss. After a thorough evaluation, including laboratory tests, radiographic studies, and gastrointestinal endoscopy procedures, the diagnosis of Crohn disease (CD) was made. Medical treatment, including corticosteroid drugs and nutritional support, was implemented during this hospitalization.

Susan has improved considerably and is to be discharged home this week. Enteral formula administered by continuous nighttime gastrostomy infusion will be continued at home, and both Susan and her family are eager to learn how to perform these feedings. You are the nurse who is responsible for Susan's discharge planning.

1. Evidence—Are there sufficient data to formulate any specific interventions for discharge?
2. Assumptions—Describe some underlying assumptions about the following:
   a. The goals of nutritional support for children with CD
   b. Teaching required by an adolescent or family member who is administering gastrostomy tube feedings at home
   c. Psychosocial issues related to CD
3. What are the priorities for discharge planning at this time?
4. Does the evidence support your conclusion?

can also emphasize the positive aspects of the surgery, particularly accelerated growth and sexual development, permanent recovery, the eliminated risk of colonic cancer in UC, and the normality of life despite bowel diversion. Introducing the child and parents to other ostomy patients, especially those who are the same age, can be effective in fostering eventual acceptance. Whenever possible continent ostomies should be offered as options to the child, although they are not performed in all centers in the United States.

Because of the chronic and often lifelong nature of the disease, families benefit from the educational services provided by organizations such as the Crohn's and Colitis Foundation of America (CCFA).* If diversionary bowel surgery is indicated, the United Ostomy Associations of America (UOAA)† and the Wound, Ostomy and Continence Nurses Society‡ are available to assist with ileostomy care and provide important psychologic support through their self-help groups. Adolescents often benefit by participating in peer-support groups, which are sponsored by the CCFA.

Peptic Ulcer Disease

Peptic ulcers may be classified as acute or chronic, and peptic ulcer disease (PUD) is a chronic condition that affects the stomach or duodenum. Ulcers are described as gastric or duodenal and as primary or secondary. A gastric ulcer involves the mucosa of the stomach; a duodenal ulcer involves the pylorus or duodenum. Most primary ulcers occur in the absence of a predisposing factor and tend to be chronic, occurring more frequently in the duodenum. Secondary or *stress ulcers* result from the stress of a severe underlying disease or injury (e.g., severe burns, sepsis, increased intracranial pressure, severe trauma, multisystem organ failure) and are more frequently acute and gastric.

About 1.7% of children in general pediatric practices have PUD, and the disease represents about 3.4% per 10,000 of pediatric hospital admissions. Primary ulcers are more common in children older than 6 years, and stress ulcers are more common in infants younger than 6 months. Except for very young children, the incidence is 2 to 3 times greater in boys than in girls.

Etiology

The exact cause of PUD is unknown, although infectious, genetic, and environmental factors are important. There is an increased familial incidence, and the disease is increased in people with blood group O.

There is a significant relationship between the bacterium *Helicobacter pylori* and ulcers. *H. pylori* is a microaerophilic, gram-negative, slow-growing, spiral-shaped, and flagellated bacterium known to colonize the gastric mucosa in about half of the population of the world (Sung, Kuipers, and El-Serag, 2009). *H. pylori* synthesizes the enzyme urease, which hydrolyses urea to form ammonia and carbon dioxide. Ammonia then absorbs acid to form ammonium, thus raising the gastric pH. *H. pylori* may cause ulcers by weakening the gastric mucosal barrier and allowing acid to damage the mucosa. It

is believed that it is acquired via the fecal-oral route, and this hypothesis is supported by finding viable *H. pylori* in feces.

In addition to ulcerogenic drugs, both alcohol and smoking contribute to ulcer formation. There is no conclusive evidence to implicate particular foods such as caffeine-containing beverages or spicy foods, but polyunsaturated fats and fiber may play a role in ulcer formation. Psychologic factors may play a role in the development of PUD, and stressful life events, dependency, passiveness, and hostility have all been implicated as contributing factors.

Pathophysiology

Most likely the pathology is caused by an imbalance between the destructive (cytotoxic) factors and defensive (cytoprotective) factors in the GI tract. The toxic mechanisms include acid, pepsin, medications such as aspirin and nonsteroidal antiinflammatory drugs (NSAIDs), bile acids, and infection with *H. pylori*. The defensive factors include the mucus layer, local bicarbonate secretion, epithelial cell renewal, and mucosal blood flow. Prostaglandins play a role in mucosal defense because they stimulate both mucus and alkali secretion. The primary mechanism that prevents the development of peptic ulcer is the secretion of mucus by the epithelial and mucous glands throughout the stomach. The thick mucus layer acts to diffuse acid from the lumen to the gastric mucosal surface, thus protecting the gastric epithelium. The stomach and the duodenum produce bicarbonate, decreasing acidity on the epithelial cells and thereby minimizing the effects of the low pH. When abnormalities in the protective barrier exist, the mucosa is vulnerable to damage by acid and pepsin. Exogenous factors such as aspirin and NSAIDs cause gastric ulcers by inhibition of prostaglandin synthesis.

Zollinger-Ellison syndrome may occur in children who have multiple, large, or recurrent ulcers. This syndrome is characterized by hypersecretion of gastric acid, intractable ulcer disease, and intestinal malabsorption caused by a gastrin-secreting tumor of the pancreas.

Diagnostic Evaluation

Diagnosis is based on the history of symptoms, physical examination, and diagnostic testing. The focus is on symptoms such as epigastric abdominal pain, nocturnal pain, oral regurgitation, heartburn, weight loss, hematemesis, and melena (Box 41-11). History should include questions relating to the use of potentially causative substances such as NSAIDs, corticosteroids, alcohol, and tobacco. Frequently a history of epigastric and periumbilical pain accompanies PUD. However, children often find it difficult to describe the location of their pain and often indicate the location by moving their hand in circular movement all around the stomach area. Asking the child to take one finger and point to the area where it hurts the most often helps to identify the location of the pain. Pain may also be elicited during the examination with palpation. Laboratory studies may include a CBC to detect anemia, stool analysis for occult blood, liver function tests (LFTs), ESR, or CRP to evaluate IBD; amylase and lipase to evaluate pancreatitis; and gastric acid measurements to identify hypersecretion. A lactose breath test may be performed to detect lactose intolerance.

Radiographic studies such as an upper GI series may be performed to evaluate obstruction or malrotation. An endoscopy of the esophagus, stomach, and duodenum is the most reliable procedure to diagnose PUD. A biopsy can determine the presence of *H. pylori*. A blood test can also identify the presence of the antigen to this organism. The ^{13}C-urea breath test measures bacterial

*386 Park Ave. South, 17th Floor, New York, NY 10016, 800-932-2423, www.ccfa.org. In Canada: Crohn's and Colitis Foundation of Canada, www.ccfc.ca.
†UOAA, PO Box 512, Northfield, MN 55057-0512, 800-826-0826, www.ostomy.org. In Canada: United Ostomy Association of Canada, 344 Bloor Street West, Suite 501, Toronto, Ontario, Canada M5S3A7, 416-595-5452, fax: 888-969-9698, 416-595-9924, www.ostomycanada.ca.
‡15000 Commerce Pkwy, Suite C, Mt. Laurel, NJ, 888-224-9626, www.wocn.org.

BOX 41-11 **CHARACTERISTICS OF PEPTIC ULCER**

Neonates
- Usually gastric and secondary to stress or critical illness
- Commonly has a history of preterm birth, respiratory distress, sepsis, hypoglycemia, or an intraventricular hemorrhage
- Perforation may be first sign of an ulcer
- Hematemesis, feeding difficulty, crying episodes, or melena

Infants to 3-Year-Old Children
- Most likely to have a secondary ulcer located equally in the stomach or duodenum
- Primary ulcers less common and usually located in stomach
- Likely to occur in relation to illness, surgery, or trauma
- Hematemesis, melena, or perforation

2- to 6-Year-Old Children
- Primary or secondary ulcers
- Located equally in stomach and duodenum
- Perforation more likely in secondary ulcers
- Periumbilical pain, poor eating, vomiting, irritability, nighttime waking, hematemesis, melena

Children 6 Years and Older
- Usually primary and most often duodenal
- More typical of adult type
- Chance of recurrence greater
- Often associated with *Helicobacter pylori*
- Epigastric or vague abdominal pain
- Possibly nighttime waking, hematemesis, melena, and anemia

colonization in the gastric mucosa. This test may be used to screen for *H. pylori* in adults and children. Polyclonal and monoclonal stool antigen tests are an accurate, noninvasive method for both the initial diagnosis of *H. pylori* and the confirmation of its eradication after treatment (Gisbert, de la Morena, and Abraira, 2006). In children, however, an initial upper endoscopy is recommended to evaluate and confirm H. pylori disease (Blanchard and Czinn, 2011).

Therapeutic Management

The major goals of therapy for children with PUD are to relieve discomfort, promote healing, prevent complications, and prevent recurrence. Management is primarily medical and consists of administration of medications to treat the infection and reduce or neutralize gastric acid secretion.

- Antacids are beneficial medications to neutralize gastric acid.
- Histamine (H2) receptor antagonists (antisecretory drugs) act to suppress gastric acid production. Cimetidine (Tagamet), ranitidine (Zantac), and famotidine (Pepcid) are examples of these medications. These medications have few side effects, although cimetidine has multiple drug interactions and therefore should be used with caution.
- PPIs such as omeprazole and lansoprazole act to inhibit the hydrogen ion pump in the parietal cells, thus blocking the production of acid. These agents have been shown to be effective in children and adolescents but not in infants (van der Pol, Smits, van Wijk, et al., 2011). Long-term side effects are not fully known but may include decreased bone density with

long-term use because of reduced gastric absorption of calcium and hypergastrinemia of unknown significance (Hassall, Owen, Kerr, et al., 2011). With short-term use these agents appear to be well tolerated and have infrequent side effects (e.g., headache, diarrhea, nausea and vomiting).

- Mucosal protective agents such as sucralfate and bismuth-containing preparations may be prescribed for PUD. Sucralfate is an aluminum-containing agent that forms a protective barrier over ulcerated mucosa to protect against acid and pepsin. Sucralfate is available in both pill and liquid forms. Because sucralfate blocks the absorption of other medications, it should be given separately from them.
- Bismuth compounds are sometimes prescribed for the relief of ulcers, but they are used less frequently than PPIs. Although these compounds inhibit the growth of microorganisms, the mechanism of their activity is poorly understood. In combination with antibiotics, bismuth is effective against *H. pylori*. Although concern has been expressed about the use of bismuth salts in children because of potential side effects, none of these side effects has been reported when these compounds have been used in the treatment of *H. pylori* infection.

Triple-drug therapy is the standard first-line treatment regimen for *H. pylori* (O'Connor, Gisbert, and O'Morain, 2009). Combination therapy has demonstrated 90% effectiveness in eradication of *H. pylori* compared with antibiotic monotherapy. Examples of drug combinations used in triple therapy are (1) bismuth, clarithromycin, and metronidazole; (2) lansoprazole, amoxicillin, and clarithromycin; and (3) metronidazole, clarithromycin, and omeprazole. Recently, however, there has been an increase in resistance to metronidazole and clarithromycin, with resulting treatment failure, and a 10- to 14-day course of bismuth-based quadruple therapy has been proposed (Luther, Chey, and Saad, 2011). The benefits on the use of probiotics as an adjunct to treatment remain unclear, with conflicting literature on their effect on eradication and minimizing side effects (O'Connor, Gisbert, and O'Morain, 2009).

Common side effects of medications include diarrhea and nausea and vomiting. In addition to medications, children with PUD should have a nutritious diet and avoid caffeine. Warn adolescents about gastric irritation associated with alcohol use and smoking.

Children with an acute ulcer who have developed complications such as significant hemorrhage require emergency care. The administration of IV fluids, blood, or plasma depends on the amount of blood loss. Replacement with whole blood or packed cells may be necessary for significant loss.

Surgical intervention may be required for complications such as hemorrhage, perforation, or gastric outlet obstruction. Ligation of the source of bleeding or closure of a perforation is performed. A vagotomy and pyloroplasty may be indicated in children with recurring ulcers despite aggressive medical treatment.

Prognosis. The long-term prognosis for PUD is variable. Many ulcers are successfully treated with medical therapy; however, primary duodenal peptic ulcers often recur. Complications such as GI bleeding can occur and extend into adult life. The effect of maintenance drug therapy on long-term morbidity remains to be established with further studies.

CARE MANAGEMENT

The primary nursing goal is to promote healing of the ulcer through compliance with the medication regimen. If an analgesic-antipyretic is needed, acetaminophen, not aspirin or NSAIDs, is used. Critically ill neonates, infants, and children in intensive care units (ICUs) should receive H_2 blockers to prevent stress ulcers.

 MEDICATION ALERT

Critically ill children receiving IV H_2 blockers should have their gastric pH values checked at frequent intervals.

For nonhospitalized children with chronic illnesses, consider the role stress plays. In children many ulcers occur secondary to other conditions, and the nurse should be aware of family and environmental conditions that may aggravate or precipitate ulcers. Children may benefit from psychologic counseling and from learning how to cope constructively with stress.

HEPATIC DISORDERS

Acute Hepatitis

Etiology

Hepatitis is an acute or chronic inflammation of the liver that can result from several different causes. One cause is infection. Many types of hepatitis are caused by viruses such as the hepatitis viruses, Epstein-Barr virus (EBV), cytomegalovirus (CMV), and HIV. Other causes of hepatitis are nonviral (abscess, amebiasis), autoimmune, metabolic, chemical, neoplastic, anatomic (choledochal duct cyst and biliary atresia [BA]), hemodynamic (shock, congestive heart failure), and idiopathic (sclerosing cholangitis and Reye syndrome). The following six viruses cause 90% of cases of viral hepatitis (Table 41-10):

1. Hepatitis A virus (HAV)
2. Hepatitis B virus (HBV)
3. Hepatitis C virus (HCV)
4. Hepatitis D virus (HDV)
5. Hepatitis E virus (HEV)
6. Hepatitis G virus (HGV)

Hepatitis A. Hepatitis A incidence in the United States has declined 92%, from 12 cases per 100,000 population in 1995 to one case per 100,000 population in 2007, the lowest rate ever recorded. Declines were greatest among children and in states where routine vaccination of children was recommended beginning in 1999 (Daniels, Grytdal, Wasley, et al., 2009). The virus is spread directly or indirectly by the fecal-oral route by ingestion of contaminated foods, direct exposure to infected fecal material, or close contact with an infected person. The virus is particularly prevalent in developing countries with poor living conditions, inadequate sanitation, crowding, and poor personal hygiene practices. The spread of HAV has been associated with improper food handling and high-risk areas such as households with infected persons, residential centers for people with disabilities, and day care centers. The average incubation period is about 4 weeks, with a range of 15 to 50 days. Fecal shedding of the virus can occur for 2 to 3 weeks before and for 1 week after the onset of jaundice. During this time, although the individual is asymptomatic, the virus is most likely to be transmitted. Infants with HAV infection are likely to be asymptomatic (*anicteric hepatitis*). Children often have diarrhea, and their symptoms are frequently attributed to gastroenteritis. Only one in 12 young children develops jaundice. Most adults develop clinical signs with *icteric hepatitis*. The

prognosis of HAV infection is usually good, and complications are rare.

Hepatitis B. Hepatitis B can be an acute or chronic infection, ranging from an asymptomatic, limited infection to fatal, fulminant (rapid and severe) hepatitis. There are no environmental or animal reservoirs for HBV. Humans are the main source of infections. HBV may be transmitted parenterally, percutaneously, or transmucosally. Hepatitis B surface antigen (HBsAg) has been found in all body fluids, including feces, bile, breast milk, sweat, tears, vaginal secretions, and urine; but only blood, semen, and saliva have been found to contain infectious HBV particles. HBV infection from human bites has been documented, but transmission from feces has not. HBV has been acquired after blood transfusion, but the likelihood of this has been reduced through blood product screening procedures. Adults whose occupations are associated with considerable exposure to blood or blood products such as health care workers are at an increased risk of contracting HBV.

Most HBV infection in children is acquired perinatally. Transmission from mother to infant during the perinatal period (e.g., blood exposure during delivery) results in chronic infection in 70% to 90% of infants if the mother is positive for HBsAg and HBeAg (AAP Committee on Infectious Diseases and Pickering, 2012). Perinatal infection occurs during the birthing process when the infant comes in contact with maternal body fluids, most likely blood. It is still not known if the virus enters infants via mucosal membranes, the intestinal tract, or skin abrasions. HBsAg has been detected in breast milk, but it is not clear whether HBV infection is transmitted through ingested breast milk or from swallowed maternal blood from injured nipples (Tran, 2009). Infants and children who are not infected during the perinatal period remain at high risk for acquiring person-to-person transmission from their mothers during the first 5 years of life.

Hepatitis B virus infection occurs in children and adolescents in specific high-risk groups, which are (1) individuals with hemophilia or other disorders who have received multiple transfusions, (2) children and adolescents involved in IV drug abuse, (3) institutionalized children, (4) preschool children in endemic areas, and (5) individuals engaged in heterosexual activity or sexual activity with homosexual men. The incubation period for HBV infection ranges from 45 to 160 days with an average of 120 days (AAP Committee on Infectious Diseases and Pickering, 2012). HBV infection can cause a carrier state and lead to chronic hepatitis with eventual cirrhosis or hepatocellular carcinoma in adulthood.

Hepatitis C. Hepatitis C virus is transmitted parenterally through exposure to blood and blood products from HCV-infected people (AAP Committee on Infectious Diseases and Pickering, 2012). The most common risk factors associated with HCV acquisition are injections, drug use, having received a blood product before 1992 (e.g., hemophilia), and having multiple sex partners. Recent improvements in donor screening and inactivation procedures for blood products such as the factor concentrates used for patients with hemophilia have significantly reduced the risk of transmission through blood products. The mechanism of nonparenteral or nonpercutaneous transmission of HCV is uncertain. Sexual transmission among monogamous couples and among family contacts is rare. Maternal co-infection with HIV has been associated with increased risk of perinatal transmission of HCV and may depend on the HCV genotype and the serum titer of maternal HCV-RNA. All persons with HCV antibody or HCV-RNA in their blood are considered to be infectious (AAP Committee on Infectious Diseases and Pickering, 2012).

TABLE 41-10   COMPARISON OF TYPES A, B, AND C HEPATITIS

CHARACTERISTICS	TYPE A	TYPE B	TYPE C
Incubation period	15-50 days; average 25-30 days	30-180 days; average 50 days	2 weeks-6 months; average, 6-7 weeks
Period of communicability	Believed to be latter half of incubation period to first week after onset of clinical illness	Variable Virus in blood or other body fluids during late incubation period and acute stage of disease; may persist in carrier state for years to lifetime	Begins before onset of symptoms May persist in carrier state for years
Mode of transmission	Principal route—fecal-oral Rarely—parenteral	Principal route—parenteral Less frequent route—oral, sexual, any body fluid Perinatal transfer—transplacental blood (last trimester); at delivery; or during breastfeeding, especially if mother has cracked nipples	Principal route—parenteral Nonparenteral spread possible
Clinical features			
Onset	Usually rapid, acute	More insidious	Usually insidious
Fever	Common and early	Less frequent	Less frequent
Anorexia	Common	Mild to moderate	Mild to moderate
Nausea and vomiting	Common	Sometimes present	Mild to moderate
Rash	Rare	Common	Sometimes present
Arthralgia	Rare	Common	Rare
Pruritus	Rare	Sometimes present	Sometimes present
Jaundice	Present (however, many cases anicteric)	Present	Present
Immunity	Present after one attack; no crossover to type B or C	Present after one attack; no crossover to type A or C	Present after one attack; no crossover to type A or B
Carrier state	No	Yes	Yes
Chronic infection	No	Yes	Yes
Prophylaxis			
IG	Passive immunity Successful, especially in early incubation period and preexposure prophylaxis	Passive immunity Inconsistent benefits; probably of no use	Not currently recommended by CDC
HAV vaccine	Two inactivated vaccines approved for children ages 12 months to 18 years: Havrix and Vaqta; given in a two-dose schedule (6-12 months between doses); TWINRIX contains both HAV and HBV (for patients 18 years old and older)		
HBV immunoglobulin (HBIG)	No benefit	Passive immunity	No benefit
HBV vaccine	No benefit	Postexposure protection possible if given immediately after definite exposure Provides active immunity Universal vaccination recommended for all newborns (see also Chapter 31)	No benefit
Mortality rate	0.1%-0.2%	0.5%-2% in uncomplicated cases; may be higher in complicated cases	1%-2% in uncomplicated cases; may be higher in complicated cases

CDC, Centers for Disease Control and Prevention; *HAV,* hepatitis A virus; *HBIG,* hepatitis B immunoglobulin; *HBV,* hepatitis B virus; *IG,* immunoglobulin.

The clinical course varies. The incubation period for HCV ranges from 14 to 180 days with an average of 45 days. The natural history of the disease in children is not well defined. Some children may be asymptomatic, but hepatitis C can become a chronic condition and can cause cirrhosis and hepatocellular carcinoma. About 60% to 70% of individuals infected with HCV develop chronic disease. Infection with HCV is the leading reason for liver transplantation in the United States (AAP Committee on Infectious Diseases and Pickering, 2012).

Hepatitis D. Hepatitis D occurs in children already infected with HBV. HDV is a defective RNA virus that requires the helper function of HBV. The incubation period is from 2 to 8 weeks. Both acute and chronic forms of hepatitis D tend to be more severe than hepatitis B and can lead to cirrhosis. HDV infection occurs mostly in drug abusers, individuals with hemophilia, and people immigrating from endemic areas.

Hepatitis E. Hepatitis E is enterically transmitted non-A, non-B hepatitis. Transmission may occur through the fecal-oral route or from contaminated water. The incubation period is 2 to 9 weeks. This illness is uncommon in children, does not cause chronic liver disease, is not a chronic condition, and has no carrier state. However, it can be a devastating disease among pregnant women, with an unusually high case-fatality rate (10%) (AAP Committee on Infectious Diseases and Pickering, 2012).

Hepatitis G. Hepatitis G virus is a bloodborne virus that may also be transmitted by organ transplantation. High-risk groups include transfusion recipients, IV drug users, and individuals infected with HCV. Individuals with the virus are often asymptomatic, and most infections are chronic. The incubation period is unknown.

Pathophysiology

Pathologic changes occur primarily in the parenchymal cells of the liver and result in variable degrees of swelling; infiltration of liver cells by mononuclear cells; and subsequent degeneration, necrosis, and fibrosis. Structural changes within the hepatocyte account for altered liver functions such as impaired bile excretion, elevated transaminase levels, and decreased albumin synthesis. The disorder may be self-limiting with regeneration of liver cells without scarring, leading to a complete recovery. However, some forms of hepatitis do not result in complete return of liver function. These include fulminant hepatitis, which is characterized by a severe, acute course with massive destruction of the liver tissue causing liver failure and high mortality within 1 to 2 weeks; and subacute or chronic active hepatitis, which is characterized by progressive liver destruction, uncertain regeneration, scarring, and potential cirrhosis.

The progression of liver disease is characterized according to histopathology by Ludwig's classification of four stages: (1) stage 1 is characterized by mononuclear inflammatory cells surrounding small bile ducts; (2) in stage 2 there is proliferation of small bile ductules; (3) stage 3 is characterized by fibrosis or scarring; and (4) stage 4 is cirrhosis (Angulo and Lindor, 2010).

Clinical Manifestations

The clinical manifestations and course of uncomplicated acute viral hepatitis are similar for most of the hepatitis viruses. Usually the prodromal, or anicteric, phase (absence of jaundice) lasts 5 to 7 days. Anorexia, malaise, lethargy, and easy fatigability are the most common symptoms. Fever may be present, especially in adolescents. Nausea, vomiting, and epigastric or right upper quadrant abdominal pain or tenderness may occur. Arthralgia and skin rashes may occur and are more likely in children with hepatitis B than those with hepatitis A. The transaminases rather than bilirubin are often elevated in acute hepatitis, and hepatomegaly may be present. Some mild cases of acute viral hepatitis do not cause symptoms or can be mistaken for influenza.

In young children most of the prodromal symptoms disappear with the onset of jaundice, or the icteric phase. However, many children with acute viral hepatitis never develop jaundice. If jaundice occurs, it is often accompanied by dark urine and pale stools. Pruritus may accompany jaundice and can be bothersome for children.

Children with chronic active hepatitis may be asymptomatic but more commonly have nonspecific symptoms of malaise, fatigue, lethargy, weight loss, or vague abdominal pain. Hepatomegaly may be present, and the transaminases are often very high, with mild-to-severe hyperbilirubinemia (conjugated [direct]).

Fulminant hepatitis is primarily caused by HBV or HCV. Many children with fulminant hepatitis develop characteristic clinical symptoms and rapidly develop manifestations of liver failure, including encephalopathy, coagulation defects, ascites, deepening jaundice, and an increasing WBC count. Changes in mental status or personality indicate impending liver failure. Although children with acute hepatitis may have hepatomegaly, a rapid decrease in the size of the liver (indicating loss of tissue caused by necrosis) is a serious sign of fulminant hepatitis. Complications of fulminant hepatitis include GI bleeding, sepsis, renal failure, and disseminated coagulopathy.

Diagnostic Evaluation

Diagnosis is based on the history; physical examination; and serologic markers for hepatitis A, B, and C. No LFT is specific for hepatitis, but serum aspartate (AST) and serum aminotransferase (ALT) levels are markedly elevated. Serum bilirubin levels peak 5 to 10 days after clinical jaundice appears. Histologic evidence from liver biopsy may be required to establish the diagnosis and assess the severity of the liver disease. Serologic markers indicate the antibodies or antigens formed in response to the specific virus and confirm the diagnosis. Serum immunologic tests are not available to detect HAV antigen, but there are two HAV antibody tests: anti-HAV immunoglobulin G (IgG) and immunoglobulin M (IgM). Anti-HAV antibodies are present at the onset of the disease and persist for life. A positive anti-HAV antibody test result indicates acute infection, immunity from past infection, passive antibody acquisition (e.g., from transfusion, serum immunoglobulin infusion), or immunization. To diagnose an acute or recent HAV infection, a positive anti-HAV IgM test result that is present with the onset of the disease and that persists for only 2 or 3 days is required.

Diagnosis of hepatitis B is confirmed by the detection of various hepatitis virus antigens and the antibodies that are produced in response to the infection. These antibodies and antigens and their significance include the following:

HBsAg—HBsAg (found on the surface of the virus), indicating ongoing infection or carrier state

Anti-HBs—Antibody to surface antigen HbsAg, indicating resolving or past infection

HBcAg—Hepatitis B core antigen (found on the inner core of the virus), detected only in the liver

Anti-HBc—Antibody to core antigen HbcAg, indicating ongoing or past infection

HBeAg—Hepatitis Be antigen (another component of the HBV core), indicating active infection

Anti-HBe—Antibody to HBeAg, indicating resolving or past infection

IgM anti-HBc—IgM antibody to core antigen

Tests are available for detection of all the HBV antigens and antibodies except HBcAg. HBsAg is detectable during acute infection. The presence of HBsAg indicates that the individual has been infected with the hepatitis virus. If the infection is self-limiting, HBsAg disappears in most patients before serum anti-HBs can be detected (termed the *window phase of infection*). IgM anti-HBc is highly specific in establishing the diagnosis of acute infection and during the window phase in older children and adults. However, IgM anti-HBc usually is not present in perinatal HBV infection (AAP Committee on Infectious Diseases and Pickering, 2012). Neonatal infection is most likely to occur in infants born to mothers who are HBeAg positive. In contrast, hepatitis B is much less likely to occur in infants whose mothers are HbsAg positive but HBeAg negative and who have antibodies to HBeAg.

Clinical improvement is usually associated with a decrease in or disappearance of these antigens followed by the appearance of their antibodies. For example, anti-HBc of the IgM class often occurs early in the disease followed by a rise in anti-HBc of the IgG class. Because the antibodies persist indefinitely, they are used to identify the carrier state (individuals with HBV who have no clinical disease but are able to transmit the organism). People with chronic HBV infection have circulating HBsAg and anti-HBc, and on rare occasions anti-HBsAg is present. Both anti-HBs and anti-HBc are detected in people with resolved infection, but anti-HBs alone is present in individuals who have been immunized with the HBV vaccine.

Hepatitis C virus RNA is the earliest serologic marker for HCV. HCV-RNA can be detected during the incubation period before symptoms of HCV disease are expressed. A positive HCV-RNA result indicates active infection, and persistence of HCV-RNA indicates chronic infection. A negative test result correlates with resolution of the disease. HCV-RNA is also used to determine patient response to antiviral therapy for HCV.

The history of all patients should include questions to seek evidence of (1) contact with a person known to have hepatitis, especially a family member; (2) unsafe sanitation practices such as contaminated drinking water; (3) ingestion of certain foods such as clams or oysters (especially from polluted water); (4) multiple blood transfusions; (5) ingestion of hepatotoxic drugs such as salicylates, sulfonamides, antineoplastic agents, acetaminophen, and anticonvulsants; and (6) parenteral administration of illicit drugs or sexual contact with a person who uses these drugs.

Therapeutic Management

Treatment options for viral hepatitis are limited in children and adolescents. The goals of management include early detection, prevention of further viral replication, support and monitoring of the disease, recognition of chronic liver disease, and prevention of spread of the disease. Special high-protein, high-carbohydrate, low-fat diets are generally not of value. The use of corticosteroids alone or with immunosuppressive drugs is not advocated in the treatment of chronic viral hepatitis. However, steroids have been used to treat chronic autoimmune hepatitis. Hospitalization is required in the event of coagulopathy or fulminant hepatitis. Human interferon-α has been used in the treatment of chronic hepatitis B and C in adults and is being used to treat these infections in children. Therapy for hepatitis depends on the severity of inflammation and the cause of the disorder.

A number of antiviral medications are being used currently to treat HBV and HCV (Degertekin and Lok, 2009; Yazigi and Balistreri, 2011). Telbivudine is more potent than lamivudine but is associated with a high rate of antiviral resistance compared with entecavir or tenofovir. Combined therapy with lamivudine and adefovir reduces the rate of antiviral resistance compared with lamivudine monotherapy. Interferon-α-2b (IFN-α-2b) has both immunomodulatory and antiviral effects but has drawbacks of subcutaneous administration; a 24-week treatment; and side effects of retinal changes, marrow suppression, and autoimmune disorders (Yazigi and Balistreri, 2011). Individualizing dose and duration of pegylated interferon-α (PEG-IFN-α) and oral ribavirin according to on-treatment virologic response may improve sustained virologic response rates in children with HCV (Mack, Gonzalez-Peralta, Gupta, et al., 2012). Several specifically targeted antiviral therapies, notably protease and polymerase inhibitors, are promising but must be used in combination with PEG-IFN-α and ribavirin; recently these have been approved only for use in adults. These agents have multiple side effects, and patients require regular monitoring and support. Many products are under current investigation in clinical trials, largely with adult patients.

Prevention. Proper hand washing and Standard Precautions prevent the spread of viral hepatitis. Prophylactic use of standard immunoglobulin is effective in preventing hepatitis A in situations of preexposure (e.g., anticipated travel to areas where HAV is prevalent) or within 2 weeks of exposure.

Hepatitis B immunoglobulin (HBIG) is effective in preventing HBV infection after 1-time exposures such as accidental needle punctures or other contact of contaminated material with mucous membranes and should be given to newborns whose mothers are HbsAg positive. It is prepared from plasma that contains high titers of antibodies against HBV. HBIG should be given within 72 hours of exposure.

Vaccines have been developed to prevent HAV and HBV infection (see Table 41-10). HBV vaccination is recommended for all newborns and for high-risk groups. HAV vaccination is recommended for infants starting at 12 months of age. (See Immunizations, Chapter 31.) In addition, the AAP (AAP Committee on Infectious Diseases and Pickering, 2012) recommends universal immunization of all adolescents with the HBV vaccine. Because HDV cannot be transmitted in the absence of HBV infection, it is possible to prevent HDV infection by preventing HBV infection. Routine serologic testing for anti-HCV of children born to women previously identified as being infected with HCV is also recommended (AAP Committee on Infectious Diseases and Pickering, 2012).

Prognosis. The prognosis for children with hepatitis varies and depends on the type of virus and the child's age and immunocompetence. Hepatitis A and E are usually mild, brief illnesses with no carrier state. Hepatitis B can cause a wide spectrum of acute and chronic illness. Infants are more likely than older children to develop chronic hepatitis. Hepatocellular carcinoma during adulthood is a potentially fatal complication of chronic HBV infection. Hepatitis C frequently becomes chronic, and cirrhosis may develop in these children; however, a small percentage of children go into spontaneous remission; approximately 25% of children infected develop chronic hepatitis C and cirrhosis, liver failure, and possibly hepatocellular carcinoma (Yazigi and Balistreri, 2011). Limited data concerning hepatitis G suggest that the rate of progression to cirrhosis with this virus may be very low. The highest mortality occurs in hepatitis D. Viral hepatitis causes approximately 50% of the cases of fulminant hepatic failure. The mechanism by which fulminant hepatic failure occurs is not well understood, and survival varies.

CARE MANAGEMENT

Nursing care depends largely on the severity of the hepatitis, the medical treatment, and factors influencing the control and transmission of the disease. Because children with mild viral hepatitis are frequently cared for at home, it is often the nurse's responsibility to explain any medical therapies and infection control measures. When further assistance is needed for parents to comply with instructions, a community health nursing referral is necessary.

Encourage a well-balanced diet and a schedule of rest and activity adjusted to the child's condition. Because the child with HAV is not infectious within 1 week after the onset of jaundice, he or she may feel well enough to resume school shortly thereafter. Caution parents about administering any medication to the child because normal doses of many drugs may become dangerous because of the inability of the liver to detoxify and excrete them.

Standard Precautions should be followed when children are hospitalized. However, these children are not usually isolated in a separate room unless they are fecally incontinent or their toys and other personal items are likely to become contaminated with feces. Discourage children from sharing their toys.

Hand washing is the single most effective measure in prevention and control of hepatitis in any setting. Parents and children need an explanation of the usual ways in which HAV (fecal-oral route) and HBV (parenteral route) are spread. Parents should also be aware of the recommendation for universal vaccination against HBV for newborns and adolescents (see Chapter 31).

The nurse has the responsibility of helping young people with HBV infection who have a known or suspected history of illicit drug use realize the associated dangers of drug abuse, stressing the parenteral mode of transmission of hepatitis, and encouraging them to seek counseling through a drug program.

Cirrhosis

Cirrhosis occurs at the end stage of many chronic liver diseases, including BA and chronic hepatitis. It can also result from infectious, autoimmune, or toxic factors and from chronic diseases such as hemophilia and cystic fibrosis. A cirrhotic liver is irreversibly damaged.

Clinical manifestations of cirrhosis include jaundice, poor growth, anorexia, muscle weakness, and lethargy. Ascites, edema, GI bleeding, anemia, and abdominal pain may be present in children with impaired intrahepatic blood flow. Pulmonary function may be impaired because of pressure against the diaphragm caused by hepatosplenomegaly and ascites. Dyspnea and cyanosis may occur, especially on exertion. Intrapulmonary arteriovenous shunts may develop, which can also cause hypoxemia. Spider angiomas and prominent blood vessels on the upper torso are often present.

Therapeutic Management

There is no successful treatment to arrest the progression of cirrhosis. The goals of management include monitoring liver function and managing specific complications such as esophageal varices and malnutrition. Assessment of the child's degree of liver dysfunction is important so the child can be evaluated for transplantation at the appropriate time.

Liver transplantation has improved the prognosis substantially for many children with cirrhosis. The combination of new immunosuppressive medications and new surgical techniques has resulted in 83% to 91% 1-year survival rates in many large hospital centers and 5-year survival rates of 82% to 83% (Kamath and Olthoff, 2010). The policy governing the allocation of livers for transplantation by the United Network for Organ Sharing allows patients with acute fulminant liver failure plus those with failed liver grafts and the sickest pediatric patients to be placed at the top of the network transplantation lists. Although this change has benefited many pediatric patients, the shortage of available donors for children continues to dictate transplantation decisions, and many children continue to die while waiting for a suitable donor.

Nutritional support is an important therapy for children with cirrhosis and malnutrition. Supplements of fat-soluble vitamins are often required, and mineral supplements may be indicated. In some instances aggressive nutritional support in the form of continuous tube feedings or PN may be necessary.

Esophageal and gastric varices are life-threatening complications of portal hypertension. Acute hemorrhage is managed with IV fluids, blood products, vasopressin, and gastric lavage. Balloon tamponade with a Sengstaken-Blakemore tube may be indicated. Endoscopic sclerotherapy and endoscopic banding ligation are also effective therapies for esophageal and gastric varices.

Ascites can be managed by sodium restriction and diuretics. Severe ascites with respiratory compromise can be managed with administration of albumin or by paracentesis.

Although the full mechanism of hepatic encephalopathy is unknown, failure of the damaged liver to remove endogenous toxins such as ammonia plays a role. Treatment is directed at limiting the ammonia formation and absorption that occur in the bowel, especially with the drugs neomycin and lactulose. Because ammonia is formed in the bowel by the action of bacteria on ingested protein, neomycin reduces the number of intestinal bacteria so less ammonia is produced. The fermentation of lactulose by colonic bacteria produces short-chain fatty acids, which lower the colonic pH, thereby inhibiting bacterial metabolism. This decreases the formation of ammonia from bacterial metabolism of protein.

Prognosis. The success of liver transplantation has revolutionized the approach to liver cirrhosis. Liver failure and cirrhosis are indications for transplantation. Retransplantation occurs in 10% to 30% of recipients because of primary nonfunction or hepatic artery thrombosis; rejection of the transplanted graft is seen in approximately 60% of children who have a liver transplant (Kamath and Olthoff, 2010). About 20% of infants who undergo portoenterostomy survive into adulthood with their native liver; more than half of patients undergoing portoenterostomy normalize their bilirubin within 6 months, and 5-year survival rates after portoenterostomy (with native liver) are reported to be about 60% (Pakarinen and Rintala, 2011). Careful monitoring of the child's condition and quality of life is necessary to evaluate the need for and timing of transplantation (see Family-Centered Care box).

CARE MANAGEMENT

Several factors influence nursing care of the child with cirrhosis, including the cause of the cirrhosis, the severity of complications, and the prognosis. The prognosis is often poor unless successful liver transplantation occurs. Therefore nursing care of the child is similar to that for any child with a life-threatening illness (see Chapter 36). Hospitalization is required when complications such as hemorrhage, severe malnutrition, or hepatic failure occur. Nursing assessments are directed at monitoring the child's condition, and interventions

BOX 41-12   CLINICAL MANIFESTATIONS OF BILIARY ATRESIA

- Jaundice
  - Earliest manifestation and most striking feature of disorder
  - First observed in sclera
  - May be present at birth but usually not apparent until age 2 to 3 weeks
- Urine dark
- Stools lighter than expected or white or tan
- Hepatomegaly and abdominal distention common
- Splenomegaly occurs later
- Poor fat metabolism results in:
  - Poor weight gain
  - General growth failure
- Pruritus
- Irritability; difficulty comforting infant

are aimed at treatment of specific complications. If liver transplantation is an option, the family needs support and assistance to cope.

Biliary Atresia

Biliary atresia, or extrahepatic biliary atresia (EHBA), is a progressive inflammatory process that causes both intrahepatic and extrahepatic bile duct fibrosis, resulting in eventual ductal obstruction. The incidence of BA is approximately one in 10,000 to 15,000 live births (A-Kader and Balistreri, 2011; Kelly and Davenport, 2007). Associated malformations include polysplenia, intestinal atresia, and malrotation of the intestine. If untreated, BA usually leads to cirrhosis, liver failure, and death in the first 2 years of life.

Etiology and Pathophysiology

The exact cause of BA is unknown, although immune mechanisms or viral injury may be responsible for the progressive process that results in complete obliteration of the bile ducts. BA is not seen in fetuses or stillborn or newborn infants. This suggests that BA is acquired late in gestation or in the perinatal period and is manifested a few weeks after birth. The majority of cases of BA (85%) have a complete obliteration of the extrahepatic biliary tree at or above the porta hepatitis (A-Kader and Balistreri, 2011).

Jaundice, manifesting with yellow discoloration of the skin or sclerae, is the most common early symptom of BA. Jaundice, indicating cholestasis (the accumulation of compounds that cannot be excreted because of occlusion or obstruction of the biliary tree), can be visible at a total serum bilirubin concentration as low as 5 mg/dL. An abnormal direct bilirubin has been designated as greater than 1 mg/dL if the total bilirubin is less than 5 mg/dL or a value of direct bilirubin that represents more than 20% of the total bilirubin if it is greater than 5 mg/dL. Direct hyperbilirubinemia first appears after the resolution of physiologic jaundice (see Chapter 24). Jaundice is often associated with pale stool and dark urine. Histologic study demonstrates bile duct remnants and a progressive inflammatory process. In the fetal embryonic form of BA, which represents 10% to 35% of cases, there is a congenital absence of biliary ductal patency and an absence of bile duct remnants. Many infants have associated congenital anomalies. Varying degrees of cholestasis occur, resulting in retention of irritants and toxins. Injury to the liver occurs as a result of the inflammation caused by the cholestasis.

Diagnostic Evaluation

Early diagnosis is the key to the survival of children with BA. Infants who undergo surgery in the first 60 days of life have an 80% chance of establishing bile flow. Between 60 to 90 days of life the chance of reestablishing flow drops to 50%, and after 90 days to 10% (Chen,

Chang, Du, et al., 2006). The typical infant is thriving, appears well, and has only very mild jaundice during the first 6 to 8 weeks (Emerick and Whitington, 2006) but soon begins failing to grow. Several clinical signs may indicate the presence of BA (Box 41-12). Blood tests should include a CBC, electrolytes, bilirubin, and liver enzymes. Additional laboratory analyses, including α_1-antitrypsin level, TORCH titers (see Maternal Infections, Chapter 25), hepatitis serology, α-fetoprotein, urine CMV, and a sweat chloride test, are indicated to rule out other conditions that cause persistent cholestasis and jaundice. Abdominal ultrasonography allows inspection of the liver and biliary system. Hepatobiliary scintigraphy demonstrates biliary patency but does not provide diagnostic certainty. Endoscopic retrograde cholangiopancreatography is performed in very young infants. This procedure, which is done using general anesthesia, has an 80% reported diagnostic accuracy. Percutaneous liver biopsy is highly reliable when the biopsy contains specimens from a number of portal areas. Definitive diagnosis of BA is obtained during surgical laparotomy and an intraoperative cholangiogram.

Therapeutic Management

The primary treatment of BA is *hepatic portoenterostomy* (Kasai procedure) in which a segment of intestine is anastomosed to the resected porta hepatis to attempt bile drainage. A Roux-en-Y jejunal limb is then anastomosed to the porta hepatis (a Y-shaped anastomosis performed to provide bile drainage without reflux). This procedure has several variations. Bile drainage is achieved in approximately 80% to 90% of infants who undergo surgery when younger than 8 weeks of age (A-Kader and Balistreri, 2011). However, progressive cirrhosis still occurs in many children, necessitating liver transplantation. Prophylactic antibiotics are given after the Kasai procedure to minimize the risk of ascending cholangitis.

Medical management of BA is primarily supportive. It includes nutritional support with infant formulas that contain medium-chain triglycerides and essential fatty acids. Supplementation with fat-soluble vitamins (A, D, E, K); a multivitamin; and minerals, including iron, zinc, and selenium, is usually required. Aggressive nutritional support in the form of continuous gastrostomy feedings or TPN may be indicated for moderate-to-severe growth failure; the enteral solution should be low in sodium. Phenobarbital may be prescribed after hepatic portoenterostomy to stimulate bile flow, and

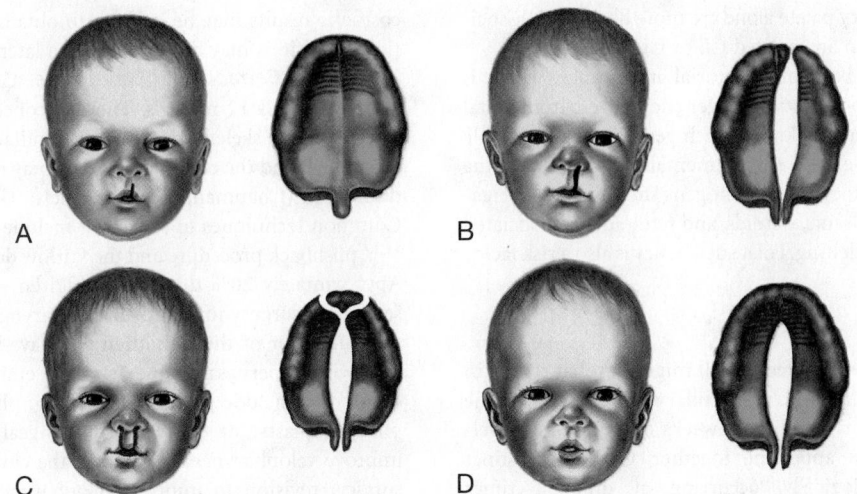

FIG 41-4 Variations in clefts of lip and palate at birth. **A,** Notch in vermilion border. **B,** Unilateral cleft lip and cleft palate. **C,** Bilateral cleft lip and cleft palate. **D,** Cleft palate.

ursodeoxycholic acid may be used to decrease cholestasis and the intense pruritus from jaundice. In cases of advanced liver dysfunction management is the same as in infants with cirrhosis.

Prognosis. Untreated BA results in progressive cirrhosis and death in most children by 2 years of age. The Kasai procedure improves the prognosis but is not a cure. Biliary drainage can often be achieved if the surgery is done before the intrahepatic bile ducts are destroyed. Long-term survival has been reported in children who receive the Kasai procedure; however, even with successful bile drainage, many children ultimately develop liver failure.

Advances in surgical techniques and the use of immunosuppressive and antifungal drugs have improved the success of transplantation. The major obstacle continues to be a shortage of donor livers. Reduced-size, split-liver transplantation, retransplantation, and increased public awareness may improve donor organ availability in the future.

CARE MANAGEMENT

Nursing interventions for the child with BA include support of the family before, during, and after surgical procedures and education regarding the treatment plan. In the postoperative period of a portoenterostomy, nursing care is similar to that after major abdominal surgery. Teaching includes the proper administration of medications. Administration of nutritional therapy, including special formulas, vitamin and mineral supplements, gastrostomy feedings, or PN, is an essential nursing responsibility. Growth failure in such infants is common, and increased metabolic needs combined with ascites, pruritus, and nutritional anorexia constitute a challenge for care. The nurse teaches caregivers how to monitor and administer nutritional therapy in the home. Pruritus may be a significant problem that is addressed by drug therapy and comfort measures such as baths in colloidal oatmeal compounds and trimming of fingernails. The risk of complications of BA such as cholangitis, portal hypertension, GI bleeding, and ascites should be explained to the caregivers.

Children and their families also need psychosocial support. The uncertain prognosis, discomfort, and waiting for transplantation produce stress; and hospitalizations, pharmacologic therapy, and nutritional therapy impose financial burdens on the family. Families can receive help from the Children's Liver Association for Support

Services,* an organization that provides educational materials, programs, and support systems, and the American Liver Foundation.†

STRUCTURAL DEFECTS

Cleft Lip and Cleft Palate

Clefts of the lip (CL) and palate (CP) are facial malformations that occur during embryonic development and are the most common congenital deformities in the United States. They may appear separately or more often together. CL results from failure of the maxillary and median nasal processes to fuse; CP is a midline fissure of the palate that results from failure of the two palatal processes to fuse.

The palate can be divided into the primary and secondary palates. The primary palate consists of the medial portion of the upper lip and the portion of the alveolar ridge that contains the central and lateral incisors. The secondary palate consists of the remaining portion of the hard palate and all of the soft palate. CL may vary from a small notch in the upper lip to a complete cleft extending into the base of the nose, including the lip and the alveolar ridge (Fig. 41-4). CL can be unilateral or bilateral. Deformed dental structures are associated with CL. Isolated CP occurs in the midline of the secondary palate and may also vary from a bifid uvula (the mildest form of CP) to a complete cleft extending from the soft to the hard palate.

Cleft lip and palate (CL/P) is more common than CP alone and varies by ethnicity. The occurrence is one in 1000 births in Caucasians, 1.7 per 1000 in Asians, 3.6 per 1000 in Native Americans and one in 2000 in African-Americans (Moller and Glaze, 2009). CP occurs alone in only one in 2500 cases and does not display variation by ethnicity (Wilkins-Haug, 2010). CL/P tends to be more common in boys, and isolated CP occurs more frequently in girls.

Etiology

Cleft deformities may be an isolated anomaly, or they may occur with a recognized syndrome. CL/P and CP are distinct from isolated

*25379 Wayne Mills Place, Suite 143, Valencia, CA 91355, 877-679-8256, www.classkids.org.
†75 Maiden Lane, Suite 603, New York, NY 10038, 212-668-1000, www.liverfoundation.org/education/info/biliaryatresia.

CP. Clefts of the secondary palate alone are more likely to be associated with syndromes than are isolated CL or CL/P.

Most cases of CL/P have multifactorial inheritance, which is generally caused by a combination of genetic and environmental factors. Researchers do not yet know which gene(s) are responsible for clefting or to what extent environmental factors impact the developing structures. Exposure to teratogens such as alcohol, cigarette smoking, anticonvulsants, steroids, and retinoids are associated with higher rates of oral clefting. Folate deficiency is also a risk factor for clefting.

Pathophysiology

Cleft deformities represent a defect in cell migration that results in a failure of the maxillary and premaxillary processes to come together between the fourth and tenth weeks of embryonic development. Although often appearing together, CL/P are distinct malformations embryologically, occurring at different times during the developmental process. Merging of the primary palate (upper lip and alveolus bilaterally) is completed by the seventh week of gestation. Fusion of the secondary palate (hard and soft palate) takes place later, between the seventh and tenth weeks of gestation. In the process of migrating to a horizontal position, the palates are separated by the tongue for a short time. If there is delay in this movement or if the tongue fails to descend soon enough, the remainder of development proceeds, but the palate never fuses.

Diagnostic Evaluation

Cleft lip and CL/P are apparent at birth. The defect may elicit severe emotional reactions in parents. CP is less obvious than CL and may not be detected immediately without a thorough assessment of the oropharynx. CP is identified through visual examination of the oropharynx or when the examiner places a gloved finger directly on the palate. Clefts of the hard and soft palate form a continuous opening between the mouth and the nasal cavity. The severity of the CP has an impact on feeding; the infant is unable to create suction in the oral cavity that is necessary for feeding. However, in most cases the infant's ability to swallow is normal.

Prenatal diagnosis with fetal ultrasonography is not reliable until the soft tissues of the fetal face can be visualized at 13 to 14 weeks. About 20% to 30% of infants with CL and CL/P are prenatally diagnosed through ultrasonography (Robbins, Damiano, Druschel, et al., 2010), although infants with CP only are rarely diagnosed prenatally.

Therapeutic Management

Treatment of the child with CL/P involves the cooperative efforts of a cleft/craniofacial multidisciplinary health care team, including pediatrics, plastic surgery, orthodontics, otolaryngology, speech/language pathology, audiology, nursing, and social work. Management is directed toward closure of the cleft(s), prevention of complications, and facilitation of normal growth and development in the child.

Surgical Correction of Cleft Lip. CL repair typically occurs at most centers between 2 and 3 months of age. Common procedures for repair of CL include the Tennison-Randall triangular flap (Z-plasty), the Fisher technique, and the Millard rotational advancement technique. Improved surgical techniques have minimized scar retraction, and in the absence of infection or trauma healing occurs with little scar formation. Nasoalveolar molding (NAM) may also be used to bring the cleft segments closer together before definitive CL repair, reducing the need for CL revision. However, optimal cosmetic results may be difficult to obtain in severe defects. Additional revisions may be necessary at a later age.

Surgical Correction of Cleft Palate. CP repair typically occurs between 6 and 12 months. There is concern that early CP repair interferes with skeletal growth of the midface, but postponing palate closure beyond the child's first words may result in increased speech disorders (Chapman, Hardin-Jones, Goldstein, et al., 2008). Common techniques to repair CP include the Veau-Wardill-Kilner V-Y pushback procedure and the Furlow double-opposing Z-plasty. Approximately 20% to 30% of children with repaired CP need a secondary surgery to improve velopharyngeal closure for speech. A small number of these children will have velopharyngeal dysfunction with hypernasality and nasal air emission. Secondary procedures may include palatal lengthening, pharyngeal flap, sphincter pharyngoplasty, or posterior pharyngeal wall augmentation to improve velopharyngeal closure. If the child is not a candidate for surgical revision to improve velopharyngeal function, prosthetic management may be considered.

> ### ! NURSING ALERT
> Avoid the use of suction or other objects in the mouth such as tongue depressors, thermometers, pacifiers, spoons, or straws following a palatoplasty to maintain the integrity of the surgically repaired palate.

Prognosis. Children with CL may require multiple surgeries to achieve optimal aesthetic outcomes but are not at risk for increased speech problems. Although some children with CP and CL/P do not require speech therapy, many have some degree of speech impairment that requires speech therapy at some point throughout childhood. Articulation errors result from a history of velopharyngeal dysfunction, incorrect articulatory placement, improper tooth alignment, and varying degrees of hearing loss. Improper drainage of the middle ear as a result of inefficient function of the eustachian tube relating to the history of CP contributes to recurrent otitis media, which leads to conductive hearing loss in many children with CP. As a prophylactic measure, many children with palatal clefts have pressure-equalization tubes placed. Extensive orthodontics and prosthodontics may be needed to correct malposition of the teeth and maxillary arches. Academic achievement, social adjustment, and behavior should be monitored, particularly in children with syndromic cleft conditions.

CARE MANAGEMENT

The immediate nursing problems for an infant with CL/P deformities are related to feeding. Parents of newborns with clefts place high priority on learning how to feed their infants and identify when they are sick, but they also express interest in learning about the infant's "normal" features. Whenever possible, they should be referred to a comprehensive CP team.

Feeding. Feeding the infant with a cleft presents a challenge to nurses and parents. Growth failure in infants with CL/P or CP has been attributed to preoperative feeding difficulties. After surgical repair most infants who have isolated CL, CP, or CL/P with no associated syndromes gain weight or achieve adequate weight and height for age.

CL may interfere with an infant's ability to achieve an adequate anterior lip seal. An infant with an isolated CL typically has no difficulty breastfeeding because the breast tissue is able to conform to the cleft. Cheek support (squeezing the cheeks together to decrease the width of the cleft) may be useful in improving lip seal during feeding.

Infants with CP and CL/P are often unable to feed using conventional methods before surgical management. CP reduces the infant's ability to suck, which interferes with breastfeeding and traditional bottle-feeding. Modifications to positioning, bottle selection, and feeder supportive techniques can help infants with CP feed efficiently. Begin by positioning an infant with CP in an upright position with the head supported by the caregiver's hand or cradled in the arm; this position allows gravity to assist with the flow of the liquid so it is swallowed instead of resulting in a loss of liquid through the nose.

Suction is almost certainly impaired in infants with CP because the velum is unable to elevate and separate the oral nasal cavities while generating adequate negative intraoral pressure. Several types of bottles work well with infants unable to generate adequate suction, including the Special Needs Feeder (formerly Haberman), the Pigeon bottle, and the Mead-Johnson Cleft Palate Nurser. The Special Needs Feeder and the Pigeon bottles use a one-way flow valve that allows the infant to feed successfully by compressing the nipple with the intact segments of the palate and the mandible or tongue. With the one-way flow valve in place, the liquid flows into the oral cavity rather than back into the bottle chamber when the nipple is compressed. The Special Needs Feeder also has a large nipple chamber that allows the feeder to provide extra assistance by squeezing the chamber if needed. The tip has a slit cut, which allows the feeder to control the flow of liquid by positioning the slit vertically or horizontally within the mouth, which can reduce choking and gagging. The Pigeon bottle has a bulbous tip that fits naturally into the oral cavity with a Y-cut nipple that increases the flow of liquid. The third bottle, the Mead Johnson Cleft Palate Nurser, is a squeezable bottle with a long, thin X-cut nipple; this bottle requires the feeder to pulse the bottle throughout the feeding and does not require the infant to actively compress the nipple during the feeding.

Infants with clefts tend to swallow excessive air during feedings; thus it is important to pause during feedings and burp the infant. Some CP specialists advocate for the use of feeding obturators to help with feeding; these devices may increase compression surfaces within the oral cavity but do not improve feeding efficiency or growth within the first year of life (Masarei, Wade, Mars, et al., 2007).

Regardless of the feeding method used, the mother should begin feeding the infant as soon as possible, preferably after the initial nursery feeding. When maternal feeding is initiated early, the mother can help to determine the method best suited to her, and the infant and can become adept in the technique before discharge from the hospital.

Preoperative Care. In preparation for surgical repair, parents may be taught to use alternative feeding systems (e.g., syringes) several days before surgery.

Postoperative Care. The major efforts in the postoperative period are directed toward protecting the operative site. For CL parents may be advised to apply petroleum jelly to the operative site for several days after surgery. For CL, CP, or CL/P, elbow immobilizers may be used to prevent the infant from rubbing or disturbing the suture line; they are applied immediately after surgery and may be used for 7 to 10 days. Some centers advocate using a syringe for feeding for 7 to 10 days after CL or CP repair. Adequate analgesia is required to relieve postoperative pain and prevent restlessness. Feeding is resumed when tolerated. An upright or infant seat position is helpful in the immediate postoperative period (especially for infants who have difficulty handling secretions). Avoid the use of suction or other objects in the mouth such as tongue depressors, thermometers, pacifiers, spoons, and straws.

The older infant or child may be discharged on a blenderized or soft diet, and parents are instructed to continue the diet until the surgeon directs them otherwise. Parents are cautioned against allowing the child to eat hard items (e.g., toast, hard cookies, and potato chips) that can damage the repaired palate.

Long-Term Care. Children with CL/P often require a variety of services during recovery. Family members need support and encouragement by health professionals and guidance in activities that facilitate a normal outcome for their child. Parents frequently cite financial stress as a difficult issue. With the combined efforts of the family and the health team, most children achieve a satisfactory outcome. Many children with CL/P have surgical correction that creates a near normal–appearing lip and permits good function of the palate for speech and feeding. Parents need to understand the function of speech therapy. the purpose and care of all orthodontic appliances, and the importance of establishing good mouth care and proper brushing habits.

Throughout the child's development, an important goal is the development of a healthy personality and self-esteem. Many communities have CP parents' groups that offer help and support to families. Agencies that provide services and information for children with CL/P and their families include the American Cleft Palate–Craniofacial Association (www.acpa-cpf.org), the Cleft Palate Foundation (www.cleftline.org), Cleft Advocate (www.cleftadvocate.org), the March of Dimes (www.marchforbabies.org), and various state children's medical services.

Esophageal Atresia and Tracheoesophageal Fistula

Congenital EA and tracheoesophageal fistula (TEF) are rare malformations that represent a failure of the esophagus to develop as a continuous passage and a failure of the trachea and esophagus to separate into distinct structures. These defects may occur as separate entities or in combination; without early diagnosis and treatment they pose a serious threat to the infant's well-being.

Etiology

EA with or without an associated TEF is the most common esophageal malformation, occurring in approximately 90% of the one in 4000 affected neonates (Khan and Orenstein, 2011). There appears to be an equal sex incidence; but the birth weight of most affected infants is significantly lower than average, and the incidence of preterm birth is high. A history of maternal polyhydramnios is present in approximately 50% of infants with the defect.

Approximately 50% of the cases of EA/TEF are a component of VATER or VACTERL association, acronyms used to describe associated anomalies (VATER for *v*ertebral defects, imperforate *a*nus, tracheoesophageal fistula, and *r*adial and *r*enal dysplasia; and VACTERL for *v*ertebral, *a*nal, *c*ardiac, *t*racheal, *e*sophageal, *r*enal, and *l*imb) (Khan and Orenstein, 2011). Other associated conditions include DiGeorge syndrome, Down syndrome, Pierre-Robin sequence, Fanconi syndrome, and CHARGE syndrome (coloboma, heart defects, choanal atresia, developmental restriction, genital hypoplasia, and ear deformities) (Guidry and McGahren, 2012).

Pathophysiology

The cause of EA/TEF is unknown. In the most frequently encountered form of EA and TEF (80% to 95% of cases), the proximal esophageal segment terminates in a blind pouch, and the distal segment is connected to the trachea or primary bronchus by a short fistula at or near the bifurcation. The second most common variety

BOX 41-13   CLINICAL MANIFESTATIONS OF TRACHEOESOPHAGEAL FISTULA

- Excessive salivation and drooling
- Three *C's* of tracheoesophageal fistula:
  - *C*oughing
  - *C*hoking
  - *C*yanosis
- Apnea
- Increased respiratory distress during and after feeding
- Abdominal distention

(5% to 8%) consists of a blind pouch at each end, widely separated and with no communication to the trachea. An H-type EA refers to an otherwise normal trachea and esophagus connected by a fistula (4% to 5%). Extremely rare anomalies involve a fistula from the trachea to the upper esophageal segment (0.8%) or to both the upper and lower segments (0.7% to 6%).

Diagnostic Evaluation

The disorder is suspected on the basis of clinical manifestations (Box 41-13). EA should also be suspected in cases of maternal polyhydramnios. Although the diagnosis is established on the basis of clinical signs and symptoms, the exact type of anomaly is determined by radiographic studies. A radiopaque catheter is inserted into the hypopharynx and advanced until it encounters an obstruction. Chest radiographs are taken to ascertain esophageal patency or the presence and level of a blind pouch. Sometimes fistulas are not patent, which makes them more difficult to diagnose. The presence of gas in the stomach or small bowel indicates a coexisting TEF. Prenatal diagnosis is possible with ultrasonography or MRI, and delivery at a tertiary care center is desired (Guidry and McGahren, 2012).

Therapeutic Management

The treatment of patients with EA and TEF includes maintenance of a patent airway, prevention of pneumonia, gastric or blind pouch decompression, supportive therapy, and surgical repair of the anomaly.

When EA with a TEF is suspected, the infant is immediately deprived of oral intake, IV fluids are initiated, and the infant is positioned prone or semi-upright to facilitate drainage of secretions and decrease the likelihood of aspiration. Accumulated secretions are suctioned frequently from the mouth and pharynx. A double-lumen catheter should be placed into the upper esophageal pouch and attached to intermittent or continuous low suction. The infant's head is kept upright to facilitate removal of fluid collected in the pouch and prevent aspiration of gastric contents. Broad-spectrum antibiotic therapy is often instituted if there is a concern about aspiration of gastric contents.

Most malformations can be corrected surgically in one operation or in two or more staged procedures. The success depends on early diagnosis before complications occur and on the presence and severity of associated anomalies and illness factors, including preterm birth. With measures instituted to prevent aspiration pneumonia and ensure adequate hydration and nutrition, surgery may be postponed to allow for more effective treatment of pneumonia and physiologic stabilization so the infant can better withstand the complex surgery. The delay also offers an opportunity for further evaluation and assessment to rule out any associated anomalies and optimize respiratory support.

The surgery consists of a thoracotomy with division and ligation of the TEF and an end-to-end or end-to-side anastomosis of the esophagus. A chest tube may be inserted to drain intrapleural air and fluid. For infants who are not stable enough to undergo definitive repair or those with a lengthy gap between the proximal and distal esophagus, a staged operation is preferred that involves gastrostomy, ligation of the TEF, and constant drainage of the esophageal pouch. A delayed esophageal anastomosis is usually attempted after several weeks to months. Thoracoscopic repair of EA/TEF is being used successfully, thus negating the need for a thoracotomy and minimizing associated postoperative complications and morbidities (Guidry and McGahren, 2012; MacKinlay, 2009; Rothenberg, 2009).

If an esophageal anastomosis cannot be accomplished, a gastrostomy is recommended; a cervical esophagostomy (to allow drainage of saliva through a stoma in the neck) was performed in cases of a long gap atresia but this is no longer recommended because it makes subsequent surgical repair more difficult (Kunisaki and Foker, 2012).

A primary anastomosis may be impossible because of insufficient length of the two segments of esophagus. This occurs if the distance between the two segments is 3 to 4 cm (1.2 to 1.6 inches) or greater; this is often referred to as *long-gap EA* (Khan and Orenstein, 2011). In these cases an esophageal replacement procedure using a part of the colon or gastric tube interposition may be necessary to bridge the missing esophageal segment. An esophageal growth induction procedure may also be used; this is described in the Kunisaki and Foker (2012) reference.

Tracheomalacia may occur as a result of weakness in the tracheal wall that exists when a dilated proximal pouch compresses the trachea early in fetal life. It may also occur as a result of inadequate intratracheal pressure causing abnormal tracheal development. Clinical signs of tracheomalacia include a barking cough, stridor, wheezing, recurrent respiratory tract infections, cyanosis, and sometimes apnea. Tracheomalacia may occur in up to 75% of children with EA/TEF but may be clinically significant in only 10% to 20% of infants with EA/TEF; surgical intervention is required in severe cases (Achildi and Grewal, 2007).

Prognosis. The survival rate is nearly 100% in otherwise healthy children. Most deaths are the result of extreme prematurity or other lethal associated anomalies. Potential complications after the surgical repair of EA and TEF depend on the type of defect and surgical correction. Complications of repair include an anastomotic leak, strictures caused by tension or ischemia, esophageal motility disorders causing dysphagia, respiratory compromise, scoliosis, chest wall deformity, and GER. Anastomotic esophageal strictures may cause dysphagia, choking, and respiratory distress. The strictures are often treated with routine esophageal dilation. Feeding difficulties are often present for months or years after surgery, and the infant must be monitored closely to ensure adequate weight gain, growth, and development. In some cases laparoscopic fundoplication may be required. At times the infant must be fed via gastrostomy or jejunostomy to provide adequate caloric intake.

CARE MANAGEMENT

Nursing responsibility for detection of this serious malformation begins immediately after birth. For an infant with the classic signs and symptoms of EA, the major concern is the establishment of a patent airway and prevention of further respiratory compromise. Cyanosis is usually a result of laryngeal spasm caused by overflow of saliva into the larynx from the proximal esophageal pouch or aspiration; it normally resolves after removal of the secretions from the oropharynx by suctioning. The passage of a small-gauge orogastric feeding tube via the mouth into the stomach during the initial nursing physical assessment is helpful to rule out EA or other obstructive defects.

> ### ❗ NURSING ALERT
>
> Any infant who has an excessive amount of frothy saliva in the mouth or difficulty with secretions and unexplained episodes of apnea, cyanosis, or oxygen desaturation should be suspected of having an EA or TEF and referred immediately for medical evaluation.

Preoperative Care. The nurse carefully suctions the mouth and nasopharynx and places the infant in an optimum position to facilitate drainage and avoid aspiration. The most desirable position for a newborn who is suspected of having the typical EA with a TEF (e.g., type C) is supine (or sometimes prone) with the head elevated on an inclined plane of at least 30 degrees. This positioning minimizes the reflux of gastric secretions at the distal esophagus into the trachea and bronchi, especially when intraabdominal pressure is elevated.

It is imperative to immediately remove any secretions that can be aspirated. Until surgery the blind pouch is kept empty by intermittent or continuous suction through an indwelling double-lumen or Replogle catheter passed orally or nasally to the end of the pouch. In some cases a percutaneous gastrostomy tube is inserted and left open so any air entering the stomach through the fistula can escape, thus minimizing the danger of gastric contents being regurgitated into the trachea. The gastrostomy tube is emptied by gravity drainage. Feedings through the gastrostomy tube and irrigations with fluid are contraindicated before surgery in an infant with a distal TEF.

Nursing interventions include respiratory assessment, airway management, thermoregulation, fluid and electrolyte management, and PN support.

Often the infant must be transferred to a hospital with a specialized care unit and pediatric surgical team. The nurse advises the parents of the infant's condition and provides them with necessary support and information.

Postoperative Care. Postoperative care for these infants is the same as for any high-risk newborn. The infant is returned to a radiant warmer or isolette, the double-lumen NG catheter is attached to low-suction or gravity drainage, PN is provided, and the gastrostomy tube (if applicable) is returned to gravity drainage until feedings are tolerated. If a thoracotomy is performed and a chest tube is inserted, attention to the appropriate function of the closed drainage system is imperative. Pain management in the postoperative period is important even if only a thoracoscopic approach is used. In the first 24 to 36 hours the nurse should provide pain management for the neonate just as for an adult undergoing a similar surgical procedure. Tracheal suction should only be done using a premeasured catheter and with extreme caution to avoid injury to the suture line.

If tolerated, gastrostomy feedings may be initiated and continued until the esophageal anastomosis is healed. Before oral feedings are initiated and the chest tube is removed a contrast study or esophagram will verify the integrity of the esophageal anastomosis.

The nurse must observe the initial attempt at oral feeding carefully to make certain the infant is able to swallow without choking. Until the infant is able to take a sufficient amount by mouth, oral intake may need to be supplemented by bolus or continuous gastrostomy feedings. Ordinarily infants are not discharged until they can take oral fluids well. The gastrostomy tube may be removed before discharge or maintained for supplemental feedings at home.

Special Problems. Upper respiratory tract complications are a threat to life in both the preoperative and postoperative periods. In addition to pneumonia, there is a constant danger of respiratory distress resulting from atelectasis, pneumothorax, and laryngeal edema. Any persistent respiratory difficulty after removal of secretions is reported to the surgeon immediately. The infant is monitored for anastomotic leaks, as evidenced by purulent chest tube drainage, increased WBC count, and temperature instability.

For an infant who requires esophageal replacement, nonnutritive sucking is provided by a pacifier. Other appropriate oral stimulation prevents feeding aversion. Infants who remain NPO for an extended period or who have not received oral stimulation have difficulty eating by mouth after corrective surgery and may develop oral hypersensitivity and food aversion. They require patient, firm guidance to learn how to take food into the mouth and swallow after repair. A referral to a multidisciplinary feeding behavior program is recommended.

Some infants and children with EA/TEF may require periodic esophageal dilations on an outpatient basis. Discharge education should include instructions about feeding techniques in the child with a repaired esophagus, including a semi-upright feeding position, small feedings, and observation for adequacy of swallowing (regurgitation, cyanosis, choking). *Tracheomalacia* is often a complication; and parents are educated regarding the signs and symptoms of this condition, which include a barking cough, stridor, wheezing, recurrent respiratory tract infections, cyanosis, and sometimes apnea. GER may also occur when feedings resume and may contribute to reactive airway disease with wheezing and labored respirations as the prominent clinical manifestations. Problems with thriving and gaining weight may occur in the first 5 years of life in the child with EA/TEF, especially if the infant is born preterm; the nurse should be alert to the achievement of developmental milestones that indicate a need for early intervention and multidisciplinary referral.

As with any congenital anomaly, parents need support in adjusting to the child's condition (see Chapter 36). One difficulty is the immediate transfer of the sick newborn to the ICU and the length of hospitalization. Encouraging parents to visit the infant, participate in care when appropriate, and express their feelings regarding his or her condition facilitates the attachment process. The nurse in the ICU should assume responsibility for ensuring that the parents are kept fully informed of the infant's progress.

Preparing parents for discharge involves teaching them skills they will need at home. Parents are taught to observe for behaviors that indicate the need for suctioning and signs of respiratory distress and constriction of the esophagus (e.g., poor feeding, dysphagia, drooling, regurgitation of undigested food). Discharge planning also includes obtaining the necessary equipment and home nursing services to provide home care.

Hernias

A hernia is a protrusion of a portion of an organ or organs through an abnormal opening. The danger from herniation arises when the organ protruding through the opening is constricted to the extent that circulation is impaired or when the protruding organs encroach on and impair the function of other structures. An inguinal hernia that cannot be reduced easily is called an *incarcerated hernia*. A *strangulated inguinal hernia* is one in which the blood supply to the herniated organ is impaired. The herniations of concern are those that protrude through the diaphragm, the abdominal wall, or the inguinal canal. The hernias of significance to the pediatric age-groups are outlined in Table 41-11. The abdominal wall defects gastroschisis and omphalocele are considered separately in Table 41-12.

OBSTRUCTIVE DISORDERS

Obstruction in the GI tract occurs when the passage of nutrients and secretions is impeded by a constricted or occluded lumen or when there is impaired motility *(paralytic ileus)*. Obstructions may be congenital or acquired. Many congenital obstructions such as atresia, imperforate anus, meconium plug, and meconium ileus usually appear in the neonatal period. Other obstructions of congenital etiology such as malrotation, HD, pyloric stenosis, volvulus, incarcerated hernia, and Meckel diverticulum appear after the first few weeks of life. Intestinal obstruction from acquired causes such as intussusception and tumors may occur in infancy or childhood. Intestinal obstructions from any cause are characterized by similar signs and symptoms (Box 41-14).

Hypertrophic Pyloric Stenosis

Hypertrophic pyloric stenosis (HPS) occurs when the circumferential muscle of the pyloric sphincter becomes thickened, resulting in elongation and narrowing of the pyloric channel. This produces an outlet obstruction and compensatory dilation, hypertrophy, and hyperperistalsis of the stomach. This condition usually develops in the first 2 to 5 weeks of life, causing projectile nonbilious vomiting, dehydration, metabolic alkalosis, and growth failure if detection is delayed. The precise etiology is unknown. The reported incidence is one to three per 1000 live births with a male-to-female ratio of 4 to 6:1. There is a genetic predisposition, and siblings and offspring of affected persons are at increased risk of developing HPS. It is more common in full-term than in preterm infants and is seen less frequently in African-American and Asian infants than in white infants.

Pathophysiology

The circular muscle of the pylorus thickens as a result of hypertrophy (increased size) and hyperplasia (increased mass). This produces severe narrowing of the pyloric canal between the stomach and the duodenum, causing partial obstruction of the lumen (Fig. 41-5, *A*). Over time inflammation and edema further reduce the size of the opening, resulting in complete obstruction. The hypertrophied pylorus may be palpable as an olivelike mass in the upper abdomen. Pyloric stenosis is not a congenital disorder. Substantial evidence supports decreased expression of neuronal nitric oxide synthase in the nerve fibers of the pyloric circular muscle in infants with HPS (Hunter and Liacouras, 2011). In most cases HPS is an isolated lesion; however, it may be associated with intestinal malrotation, esophageal and duodenal atresia, and anorectal anomalies. HPS has also been linked to the administration of erythromycin in the first few weeks of life as well as eosinophilic gastroenteritis, Apert syndrome, Cornelia de Lange syndrome, Zellweger syndrome, trisomy 18, and Smith-Lemli-Opitz syndrome (Hunter and Liacouras, 2011).

Diagnostic Evaluation

The diagnosis of HPS is often made after the history and physical examination. The olivelike mass is palpated easily when the stomach is empty, the infant is quiet, and the abdominal muscles are relaxed. Vomiting usually occurs 30 to 60 minutes after feeding and becomes projectile as the obstruction progresses. Emesis is nonbilious, usually consisting of stale milk. These infants may become dehydrated and appear malnourished if an early diagnosis is not established.

If the diagnosis is inconclusive from the history and physical signs (Box 41-15), ultrasonography demonstrates an elongated, sausage-shaped mass with an elongated pyloric channel. If ultrasonography fails to demonstrate a hypertrophied pylorus, an upper GI radiography should be done to rule out other causes of vomiting. Laboratory findings reflect the metabolic alterations (hypochloremic, hypokalemic metabolic alkalosis) created by severe depletion of both fluid and electrolytes from extensive and prolonged vomiting. Hyperbilirubinemia (unconjugated) may also be present and often resolves after surgical correction of the obstruction occurs (Hunter and Liacouras, 2011).

Therapeutic Management

Surgical relief of the pyloric obstruction by pyloromyotomy is the standard therapy for this disorder. Before surgery the infant must be rehydrated, and metabolic alkalosis corrected with parenteral fluid and electrolyte administration. Replacement fluid therapy may delay surgery for 24 to 48 hours. The stomach is decompressed with an NG tube. In infants with no evidence of fluid and electrolyte imbalance, surgery is performed without delay.

The surgical procedure is often performed by laparoscope and consists of a longitudinal incision through the circular muscle fibers of the pylorus down to, but not including, the submucosa (pyloromyotomy, sometimes called *Fredet-Ramstedt procedure*) (see Fig. 41-5, *B*). The procedure has a high success rate. Laparoscopic surgery through a single small incision often results in a shorter surgical time, more rapid postoperative feeding, and shorter hospital stay (Sola and Neville, 2009).

Feedings are usually begun 3 to 6 hours after surgery, beginning with small, frequent feedings of an electrolyte solution such as Pedialyte or sterile water. If clear fluids are retained, formula or breast feedings are initiated to the infant's tolerance. The amount and the interval between feedings are gradually increased until a full feeding schedule is reinstated, which usually takes about 24 to 48 hours.

Prognosis. Most infants recover completely and rapidly after pyloromyotomy. Postoperative complications include persistent pyloric obstruction and rarely wound dehiscence.

CARE MANAGEMENT

The diagnosis of HPS is considered in very young infants who appear alert but fail to gain weight and have a history of vomiting after feedings. Assessment is based on observation of eating behaviors and evidence of other characteristic clinical manifestations.

Preoperative Care. Before surgery the emphasis is placed on restoring hydration and electrolyte balance. Infants are usually made NPO and receive IV fluids with dextrose and electrolyte replacement based on laboratory serum electrolyte values and clinical appearance.

Observations also include assessment of vital signs, particularly those that might indicate fluid or electrolyte imbalances. These

TABLE 41-11 SUMMARY OUTLINE OF HERNIAS

MANIFESTATIONS AND TYPE	DIAGNOSTIC EVALUATION	NURSING CARE MANAGEMENT
Congenital Diaphragmatic Protrusion of abdominal organs through opening in diaphragm, commonly on left side, causing severe respiratory compromise and inability to adequately expand affected lung, which may be hypoplastic	**Symptoms**—Commonly severe respiratory distress at birth or within a few hours; tachypnea, cyanosis, dyspnea, a scaphoid abdomen; absent breath sounds on affected side; impaired cardiac output; possible symptoms of shock, severe acidosis Milder cases may be seen after birth without severe respiratory distress. **Diagnosis**—Suspected on basis of symptoms, confirmed by radiographic study; often diagnosed prenatally as early as 25th week of gestation	**Therapeutic:** Provide prompt recognition, resuscitation, and stabilization. Avoid bag and mask ventilation in diagnosed or suspected CDH because this fills stomach with air and further compromises respiratory function. Provide supportive treatment of respiratory distress and correction of pulmonary hypertension and persistence of fetal circulation; correct acidosis*; endotracheal intubation, GI decompression. Additional treatments to reverse pulmonary hypertension may involve administration of inhaled nitric oxide, use of high-frequency oscillation, sildenafil, or ECMO. Administer prophylactic antibiotics. Perform surgical reduction of hernia and repair of defect after respiratory status is stable (corrected acidosis*; pulmonary hypertension). **Nursing:** *Preoperative:* Monitor respiratory status; provide supplemental oxygen; assist with and monitor mechanical ventilation. Monitor cardiovascular status; support with inotropes may be necessary. Reduce stimulation—environmental and nursing care activities (cluster care to prevent constant interruptions). Maintain NG suction, oxygen, and IV fluids. Administer medications: sedation, muscular paralysis, inotropes, sildenafil (to reverse pulmonary hypertension). *Postoperative:* Carry out routine postoperative care and observation for acutely ill infant. Relieve pain and provide comfort. Support family because this is a critical illness.
Hiatal **Sliding**—Protrusion of an abdominal structure (usually stomach) through esophageal hiatus	**Symptoms**—Dysphagia, failure to thrive, vomiting, neck contortions, frequent unexplained respiratory problems, bleeding; usually associated with GER; may cause gastric volvulus and obstruction **Diagnosis**—Made by fluoroscopy	**Therapeutic:** Manage GER symptoms; provide patient positioning, pharmacologic treatment, and dietary management. Surgical treatment is necessary when complications are related to GER despite medical management. **Nursing:** Be alert to significant signs and carry out routine postoperative care.
Abdominal **Umbilical**—Weakness in abdominal wall around umbilicus; incomplete closure of abdominal wall, allowing intestinal contents to protrude through opening	**Symptoms**—Noted by inspection and palpation of the abdomen High incidence in preterm and African-American infants Usually closes spontaneously by 1-2 years of age	**Therapeutic:** No treatment is necessary for small defects. Provide operative repair if persists to ages 4-6 years or if defect is >1.5-2 cm by age 2 years. Strangulation requires immediate attention. **Nursing:** Discourage use of home remedies (e.g., belly bands, coins). Reassure parents.

*Some advocate for permissive hypercapnia and mild acidosis during acute phase of illness.
CDH, Congenital diaphragmatic hernia; *ECMO,* extracorporeal membrane oxygenation; *GER,* gastroesophageal reflux; *GI,* gastrointestinal; *IV,* intravenous; *NG,* nasogastric.

TABLE 41-12   ABDOMINAL WALL DEFECTS

DEFECT	SYMPTOMS	NURSING MANAGEMENT
Omphalocele—Protrusion of intraabdominal viscera into base of umbilical cord; sac covered with peritoneum without skin	Usually obvious on inspection; however, small omphalocele may appear to be a hematoma in umbilical cord Observe for associated malformations	**Therapeutic:** Surgical repair of defect **Nursing:** *Preoperative:* Protect defect from trauma or drying. Keep sac or viscera moist with saline-soaked dressings. Maintain thermoregulation. Carry out routine care of IV fluids and line. Administer prophylactic antibiotics as prescribed. Provide nasogastric suction for gastric decompression. Keep patient NPO. Assess for associated birth defects such as CL or CP. *Postoperative:* Monitor vital signs and BP. Assess for and manage pain Bowel decompression—NG tube IV fluid intake Monitor return of bowel function.
Gastroschisis—Protrusion of intraabdominal contents through defect in abdominal wall lateral to umbilical ring; no peritoneal sac covering the exposed bowel	Defect obvious at delivery if not detected prenatally by ultrasonography	**Therapeutic:** Surgical repair of defect. For large lesions provide gradual reduction of abdominal contents via Siloh pouch before surgical closure. **Nursing:** *Preoperative:* Keep sac covered with a bowel bag to prevent trauma, drying of viscera. NG decompression. Maintain thermoregulation. Administer IV fluids. Administer antibiotics. Observe exposed bowel for signs of necrosis or constriction at exit site. *Postoperative:* Monitor vital signs and BP. Bowel decompression with NG tube. Administer IV fluids. Assess for and manage pain. Monitor surgical closure site for infection. Monitor lower extremities for pulses and circulation (in case of vena cava compression by large bowel in small abdominal cavity). Monitor for return of bowel function and peristalsis. In event of Siloh pouch, nursing care should also include monitoring vital signs, keeping pouch clean, and aseptic technique with dressing changes (if not done by surgeon). Monitor lower extremities for circulation (as noted previously). Provide emotional support for parents. Long-term problems associated with feeding and weight gain for gastroschisis and large omphalocele.

BP, Blood pressure; *CL,* cleft lip; *CP,* cleft palate; *IV,* intravenous; *NG,* nasogastric; *NPO,* nothing by mouth.

infants are prone to metabolic alkalosis from loss of hydrogen ions and to potassium, sodium, and chloride depletion. The skin, mucous membranes, and daily weight are assessed for alterations in hydration status and water gain or loss.

If stomach decompression and gastric lavage are used before surgery, the nurse is responsible for ensuring that the tube is patent and functioning properly and for measuring and recording the type and amount of drainage. Parental involvement is encouraged and promoted.

Postoperative Care. Postoperative vomiting is common, and even with successful surgery most infants exhibit some vomiting during the first 24 to 48 hours. IV fluids are administered until the infant is taking and retaining adequate amounts by mouth. Much of the same care that was instituted before surgery is continued after surgery, including observation of vital signs, monitoring of IV fluids, and careful monitoring of fluid intake and output. In addition, the infant is observed for responses to the stress of surgery and evidence of pain. Appropriate analgesics should be given around the clock

BOX 41-14 CLINICAL MANIFESTATIONS OF MECHANICAL/PARALYTIC INTESTINAL OBSTRUCTION

Colicky abdominal pain—From peristalsis attempting to overcome the obstruction

Abdominal distention—As a result of accumulation of gas and fluid above the level of the obstruction

Vomiting—Often the earliest sign of a high obstruction; a later sign of lower obstruction (may be bilious or feculent)

Constipation and obstipation—Early signs of low obstructions; later signs of higher obstructions

Dehydration—From losses of large quantities of fluid and electrolytes into the intestine

Rigid and boardlike abdomen—From increased distention and infection (peritonitis)

Bowel sounds—Gradually diminish and cease

Respiratory distress—Occurs as the diaphragm is pushed up into the pleural cavity

Shock—Plasma volume diminishes as fluids and electrolytes are lost from the bloodstream into the intestinal lumen (third spacing)

Sepsis—Caused by bacterial proliferation with invasion into the circulation

BOX 41-15 CLINICAL MANIFESTATIONS OF HYPERTROPHIC PYLORIC STENOSIS

- Projectile vomiting
  - May be ejected 3 to 4 feet from the child when in a side-lying position, 1 foot or more when in a back-lying position
  - Occurs shortly after a feeding (may not occur for several hours)
  - May follow each feeding or appear intermittently
  - Nonbilious vomitus; may be blood tinged
- Infant hungry, avid nurser; eagerly accepts a second feeding after vomiting episode
- No evidence of pain or discomfort except that of chronic hunger
- Weight loss
- Signs of dehydration
- Distended upper abdomen
- Readily palpable olive-shaped tumor in the epigastrium just to the right of the umbilicus
- Visible gastric peristaltic waves that move from left to right across the epigastrium

because pain is continuous. The surgical incision(s) is inspected for drainage or erythema, and any signs of infection are reported to the surgeon. A surgical adhesive may be used for incision closure, and parents are instructed regarding the care of the incision and any dressings before discharge. With laparoscopic surgery, the infant may have one to three small incisions.

Feedings are usually instituted soon after surgery, beginning with clear liquids and advancing to formula or breast milk as tolerated. Observation and recording of feedings and the infant's responses to feedings are a vital part of postoperative care. Care of the operative site consists of observation for any drainage or signs of inflammation and care of the incision.

Parents are encouraged to remain with their child and become involved in the child's care. Vomiting of a projectile nature is frightening to parents, and they often believe that they may have done something wrong or that surgery was not successful. Most parents need support and reassurance that the condition is caused by a structural problem and is in no way a reflection on their parenting skills and capacities.

Intussusception

Intussusception is the most common cause of intestinal obstruction in children between the ages of 3 months and 3 years (Pepper, Stanfill, and Pearl, 2012; Waseem and Rosenberg, 2008). Intussusception is more common in boys than in girls. Although specific intestinal lesions occur in a small percentage of the children, generally the cause is not known. More than 90% of intussusceptions do not have a pathologic lead point such as a polyp, lymphoma, or Meckel diverticulum. The idiopathic cases may be caused by hypertrophy of intestinal lymphoid tissue secondary to viral infection

Pathophysiology

Intussusception occurs when a proximal segment of the bowel invaginates into the distal segment, pulling the mesentery with it

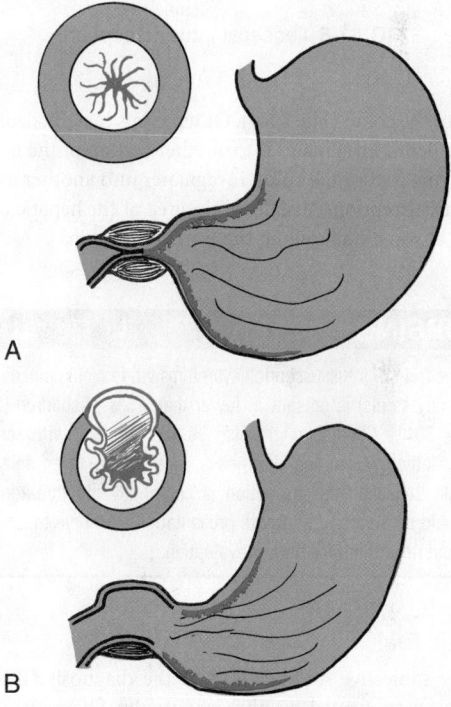

FIG 41-5 Hypertrophic pyloric stenosis. **A,** Enlarged muscular area nearly obliterates pyloric channel. **B,** Longitudinal surgical division of muscle down to submucosa establishes adequate passageway.

(Pepper, Stanfill, and Pearl, 2012). The mesentery is compressed and angled, resulting in lymphatic and venous obstruction. As the edema from the obstruction increases, pressure within the area of intussusception increases. When the pressure equals the arterial pressure, arterial blood flow stops, resulting in ischemia and the pouring of mucus into the intestine. Venous engorgement also leads to leaking of blood and mucus into the intestinal lumen, forming the classic currant jelly–like stools. The most common site is the ileocecal valve (ileocolic), where the ileum invaginates into the cecum and then

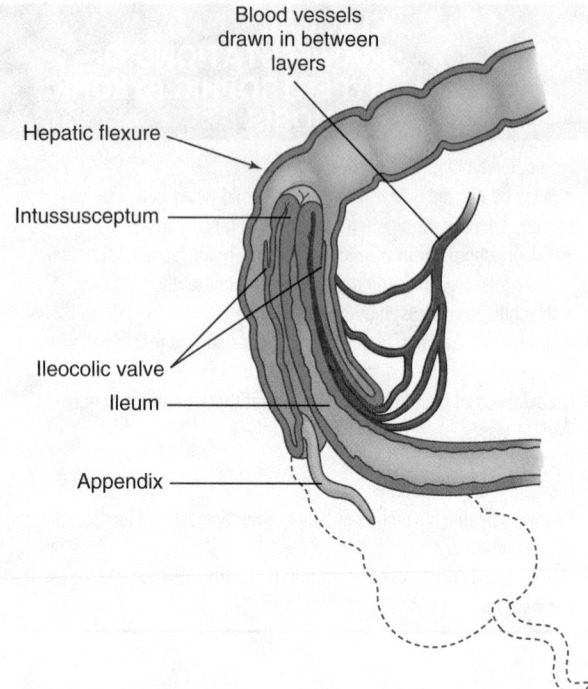

FIG 41-6 Ileocecal intussusception.

involves manually reducing the invagination and, when indicated, resecting any nonviable intestine.

Prognosis. Nonoperative reduction is successful in approximately 80% of cases (Huppertz, Soriano-Gabarro, Grimprel, et al., 2006). Surgery is required for patients in whom the hydrostatic enema is unsuccessful. With early diagnosis and treatment, serious complications and death are uncommon.

CARE MANAGEMENT

The nurse can help establish a diagnosis by listening to the parent's description of the child's physical and behavioral symptoms. It is not unusual for parents to state that they thought something was seriously wrong before others shared their concerns. The description of the child's severe colicky abdominal pain combined with vomiting is a significant sign of intussusception.

As soon as a possible diagnosis of intussusception is made, the nurse prepares the parents for the immediate need for hospitalization, the nonsurgical technique of hydrostatic reduction, and the possibility of surgery. It is important to explain the basic defect of intussusception. A model of the defect is demonstrated easily by pushing the end of a finger on a rubber glove back into itself or using the example of a telescoping rod. The principle of reduction by hydrostatic pressure can be simulated by filling the glove with water, which pushes the "finger" into a fully extended position.

Physical care of the child does not differ from that for any child undergoing abdominal surgery. Even though nonsurgical intervention may be successful, the usual preoperative procedures such as maintenance of NPO status, routine laboratory testing (CBC and urinalysis), signed parental consent, and preanesthetic sedation, are performed. For the child with signs of electrolyte imbalance, hemorrhage, or peritonitis, additional preparation such as replacement fluids, whole blood or plasma, and NG suctioning may be needed. Before surgery the nurse monitors all stools.

further into the colon (Fig. 41-6). Other forms include ileoileal (one part of the ileum invaginates into another section of the ileum) and colocolic (one part of the colon invaginates into another area of the colon) intussusceptions, usually in the area of the hepatic or splenic flexure or at some point along the transverse colon.

> **! NURSING ALERT**
>
> The classic triad of intussusception symptoms (abdominal pain, abdominal mass, bloody stools) is present in fewer than 15% of children (Chu and Liacouras, 2011). Children might also be seen initially with screaming, irritability, lethargy, vomiting, diarrhea or constipation, fever, dehydration, and shock. Because intussusception is potentially life threatening, the nurse should be aware of alternate presentations, observe these children closely, and refer them for further evaluation.

Diagnostic Evaluation

Frequently subjective findings lead to the diagnosis (Box 41-16), which can be confirmed by ultrasonography. Spontaneous reduction occurs in up to 10% of patients.

Therapeutic Management

Conservative treatment consists of radiologist-guided pneumoenema (air enema) with or without water-soluble contrast or ultrasound-guided hydrostatic (saline) enema; the advantage of the latter is that no ionizing radiation is needed (Pepper, Stanfill, and Pearl, 2012). Recurrence of intussusception after conservative treatment is rare. Herwig, Brenkert, and Losek (2009) found that hospitalized children needed minimal interventions after undergoing enema-reduced intussusception.

IV fluids, NG decompression, and antibiotic therapy may be used before hydrostatic reduction is attempted. If these procedures are not successful, the child may require surgical intervention. Surgery

> **! NURSING ALERT**
>
> Passage of a normal brown stool usually indicates that the intussusception has reduced itself. This is reported to the practitioner immediately, who may choose to alter the diagnostic and therapeutic care plan.

Postprocedural care includes observations of vital signs, blood pressure, intact sutures and dressing, and the return of bowel sounds. After spontaneous or hydrostatic reduction, the nurse observes for passage of water-soluble contrast material (if used) and the stool patterns because the intussusception may recur. Children may be admitted to the hospital or monitored on an outpatient basis. A recurrence of intussusception is treated with the conservative reduction techniques described previously, but a laparotomy is considered for multiple recurrences.

Because hospitalization may be the child's first separation from the parents, it is important to preserve the parent-child relationship by encouraging rooming-in or extended visiting. It may be the parents' first experience with hospitalization, necessitating their preparation for procedures such as IV therapy, frequent vital sign and blood pressure monitoring, dressings, and NPO status. More commonly the child may be seen in the emergency department, and treatment initiated there with eventual discharge home in uncomplicated cases (Gilmore, Reed, and Tenenbein, 2011). Because of the rapidity of the onset, diagnosis, and treatment, parents may feel stunned or numb. They may ask few questions; or they may make inquiries constantly, sometimes the same ones several times. Because of the circumstances surrounding this condition, be accepting and understanding of the parents' reactions.

Malrotation and Volvulus

Malrotation of the intestine is caused by the abnormal rotation of the intestine around the superior mesenteric artery during embryologic development. It may manifest in utero or may be asymptomatic throughout life. Infants may have intermittent bilious vomiting, recurrent abdominal pain, distention, or lower GI bleeding. Malrotation is the most serious type of intestinal obstruction because, if the intestine undergoes complete volvulus (the intestine twisting around itself), compromise of the blood supply results in intestinal necrosis, peritonitis, perforation, and death.

Diagnostic Evaluation

It is imperative that malrotation and volvulus be diagnosed promptly and surgical treatment instituted quickly. An upper GI series is the definitive procedure to diagnose this condition.

Therapeutic Management

Surgery is indicated to remove the affected area. Because of the extensive nature of some lesions, short-gut syndrome is a postoperative complication.

CARE MANAGEMENT

Before surgery the nursing care is the same as that provided to an infant or child with intestinal obstruction. After surgery, the nursing care is similar to that provided to the infant or child who has undergone abdominal surgery.

Anorectal Malformations

Anorectal malformations are among the more common congenital malformations caused by abnormal development, with an incidence of approximately one in 5000 births (Levitt and Peña, 2007). These malformations may range from simple imperforate anus to include other associated complex anomalies of genitourinary (GU) and pelvic organs, which may require extensive treatment for fecal, urinary, and sexual function. Anorectal malformations may occur in isolation or as a part of the VACTERL association (see p. 1291). These anomalies are classified according to the newborn's gender and abnormal anatomic features, including GU defects.

The anus and rectum originate from an embryologic structure called the cloaca. Lateral growth of the cloaca forms the urorectal septum that separates the rectum dorsally from the urinary tract ventrally. The rectum and urinary tract separate completely by the seventh week of gestation. Anomalies that occur reflect the stage of development of these processes.

Rectal atresia and stenosis occur when the anal opening appears normal, there is a midline intergluteal groove, and usually no fistula exists between the rectum and urinary tract. *Rectal atresia* is a complete obstruction (inability to pass stool) and requires immediate surgical intervention. *Rectal stenosis* may not become apparent until later in infancy when the infant has a history of difficult stooling, abdominal distention, and ribbonlike stools.

A *persistent cloaca* is a complex anorectal malformation in which the rectum, vagina, and urethra drain into a common channel opening into the perineum (Fig. 41-7, A).

Imperforate anus includes several forms of malformation without an obvious opening (see Fig. 41-7, B). Frequently a *fistula* (an abnormal communication) leads from the distal rectum to the perineum or GU system (see Fig. 41-7, A to C). The fistula may be evidenced when meconium is evacuated through the vaginal opening, the perineum below the vagina, the male urethra, or the perineum under the scrotum. The presence of meconium on the perineum does not indicate anal patency. A fistula may not be apparent at birth, but as peristalsis increases, meconium is forced through the fistula into the urethra or onto the newborn's perineum.

Anorectal anomalies are classified according to gender and abnormal anatomic features, including GU and associated pelvic anomalies (Box 41-17). The classification of high, intermediate, and low may also be used; the level of rectal descent is determined by

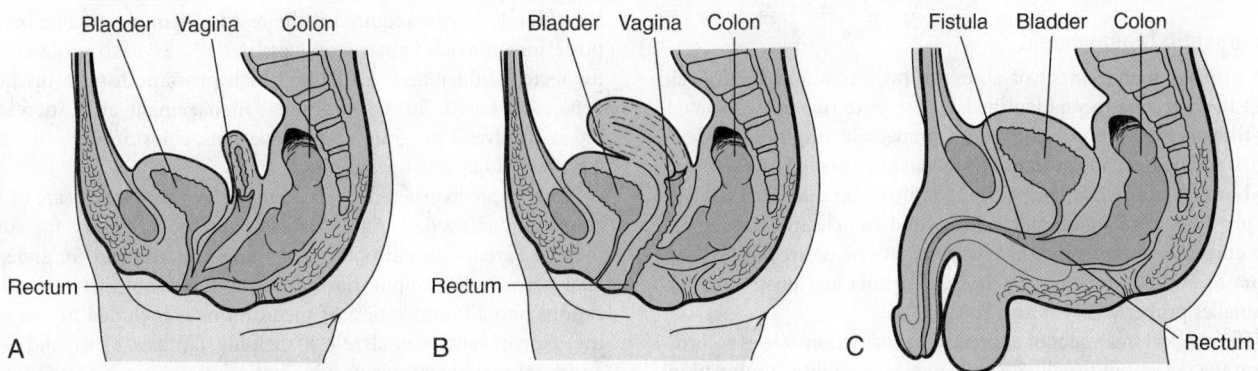

FIG 41-7 Anorectal malformations. **A,** Typical cloaca (female). **B,** Low rectovaginal fistula (female). **C,** Rectourethral bulbar fistula (male).

BOX 41-17	CLASSIFICATION OF ANORECTAL MALFORMATIONS

Male Defects
- Perineal fistula
- Rectourethral bulbar fistula
- Rectourethral prostatic fistula
- Rectovesicular (bladder neck) fistula
- Imperforate anus without fistula
- Rectal atresia and stenosis

Female Defects
- Perineal fistula
- Vestibular fistula
- Imperforate anus without fistula
- Rectal atresia and stenosis
- Cloaca

From Peña A, Hong A: Advances in the management of anorectal malformations, *Am J Surg* 180(5):370–376, 2000.

the relationship of the termination of the bowel to the puborectalis sling of the levator ani musculature. About 50% of children with anorectal anomalies have a urologic problem.

Diagnostic Evaluation

The diagnosis of an anorectal malformation is based on the physical finding of an absent anal opening. Other symptoms may include abdominal distention, vomiting, absence of meconium passage, or presence of meconium in the urine. Additional physical findings with an anorectal malformation are a flat perineum and the absence of a midline intergluteal groove. The appearance of the perineum alone does not predict the extent of the defect and associated anomalies accurately. GU and spinal-vertebral anomalies associated with anorectal malformations should be considered when an anomaly is noted. EA with or without TEF, cardiac defects, and neural tube defects or vertebral anomalies may occur in association with anorectal malformations; the infant should be carefully evaluated for the presence of these and other anomalies.

A perineal fistula (see Box 41-17) may be diagnosed by clinical observation. The presence of a prominent anal dimple and a band of skin tissue commonly known as a *bucket handle* indicates a perineal fistula (Levitt and Peña, 2007). Abdominal and pelvic ultrasonography is performed to further evaluate the infant's anatomic malformation. An IV pyelogram and a voiding cystourethrogram are performed to evaluate associated anomalies involving the urinary tract. Other diagnostic examinations that may be performed include pelvic magnetic resonance imaging, radiography, ultrasonography, and fluoroscopic examination of pelvic anatomic contents and lower spinal anatomy.

Therapeutic Management

The primary management of anorectal malformations is surgical. After the defect has been identified, take steps to rule out associated life-threatening defects, which need immediate surgical intervention. Provided no immediate life-threatening problems exist, the newborn is stabilized and kept NPO for further evaluation. IV fluids are provided to maintain glucose and fluid and electrolyte balance. The current recommendation is that surgery be delayed at least 24 hours to evaluate for the presence of a fistula and possibly other anomalies properly (Levitt and Peña, 2007).

The surgical treatment of anorectal malformations varies according to the defect but usually involves one or possibly a combination of several of the following procedures: anoplasty, colostomy, *posterior sagittal anorectoplasty (PSARP)* or other pull-through with colostomy, and colostomy (take-down) closure. The Care Management discussion that follows outlines some aspects of preoperative and postoperative care.

A primary laparoscopic repair (without colostomy) of anorectal malformations is being performed successfully in some centers. This minimizes surgical risks, associated morbidity, and postoperative pain management.

CARE MANAGEMENT

The first nursing responsibility is helping to identify anorectal malformations. A newborn who does not pass stool within 24 hours after birth or has meconium that appears at a location other than the anal opening requires further assessment. Preoperative care includes diagnostic evaluation, GI decompression, bowel preparation, and IV fluids.

For the newborn with a perineal fistula an *anoplasty* is performed, which involves moving the fistula opening to the center of the sphincter and enlarging the rectal opening. Postoperative nursing care after anoplasty is primarily directed toward healing the surgical site without other complications. A program of anal dilations is usually initiated when the child returns for the 2-week check-up. Feedings are started soon after surgical repair, and breastfeeding is encouraged because it causes less constipation.

In neonates with anomalies such as cloaca (girls), rectourethral prostatic fistula (boys), and vestibular fistula (girls), a descending colostomy may be performed to allow fecal elimination and avoid fecal contamination of the distal imperforate section and subsequent urinary tract infection in infants with urorectal fistulas. With a colostomy postoperative nursing care is directed toward maintaining appropriate skin care at the stoma sites (both distal and proximal), managing postoperative pain, and administering IV fluids and antibiotics. Postoperative NG decompression may be required with laparotomy, and nursing care focuses on maintenance of appropriate drainage. (See Chapter 39 for colostomy care.)

The PSARP is a common surgical procedure for the repair of anorectal malformations in infants approximately 1 to 2 months after the initial colostomy. Preoperative PSARP care often involves irrigation of the distal stoma to prevent fecal contamination of the operative site. During this time parents must be given accurate yet simple information regarding the infant's appearance after surgery and expectations as to their level of involvement in the child's care.

In the PSARP procedure the repair is made via a posterior midline sacral approach to dissect the different muscle groups involved without damaging strategic innervation of pelvic structures so optimum postoperative bowel continence is achieved. A laparotomy may be required if the rectum is unidentifiable by the posterior approach. Laparoscopic-assisted PSARP has been described for recto–bladder neck fistula and high prostatic fistula (Bischoff, Peña, and Levitt, 2013). Additional management after successful repair involves a program of anal dilations, colostomy closure, and a bowel management program.

Parents are instructed in perineal and wound care or care of the colostomy as needed. Anal dilations may be necessary for some infants. Parents should observe stooling patterns and for signs of anal stricture or complications. Information about dietary modifications and administration of medications is included in counseling. Nurses have a vital role in helping families of a child with anorectal malformations provide optimum care so bowel management is successful and quality of life enhanced for the child and family.

Family Support, Discharge Planning, and Home Care. Long-term follow-up is important for children with complex malformations. After the definitive pull-through procedure, toilet training is delayed, and complete continence is seldom achieved at the usual age of 2 to 3 years. Prevention of constipation is important, and breastfeeding is encouraged after surgery. If a cow's milk–based formula is used, a mild laxative may be prescribed. Bowel habit training, diet modification, and administration of stool softeners or fiber are important aspects of bowel management. Optimum bowel function may not be achieved until late childhood or adolescence. Support and reassurance are important during the slow progression to normal function.

Parents are instructed in perineal and wound care or care of the colostomy. Anal dilations may be necessary for some infants. Parents are advised to observe stooling patterns and notify the health care provider if there are any signs of anal stricture or complications.

MALABSORPTION SYNDROMES

Chronic diarrhea and malabsorption of nutrients characterize malabsorption syndromes. An important complication of malabsorption syndromes in children is growth failure. Most cases are classified according to the location of the supposed anatomic or biochemical defect. The term celiac disease is often used to describe a symptom complex with four characteristics: (1) steatorrhea (fatty, foul, frothy, bulky stools), (2) general malnutrition, (3) abdominal distention, and (4) secondary vitamin deficiencies.

Digestive defects are conditions in which the enzymes necessary for digestion are diminished or absent, such as (1) cystic fibrosis, in which pancreatic enzymes are absent; (2) biliary or liver disease, in which bile flow is affected; or (3) lactase deficiency, in which there is congenital or secondary lactose intolerance.

Absorptive defects are conditions in which the intestinal mucosal transport system is impaired. This may occur because of a primary defect (e.g., celiac disease) or secondary to inflammatory disease of the bowel that results in impaired absorption because bowel motility is accelerated (e.g., UC). Obstructive disorders (e.g., HD) also cause secondary malabsorption from enterocolitis.

Anatomic defects such as extensive resection of the bowel or short-bowel syndrome (SBS) affect digestion by decreasing the transit time of substances and affect absorption by severely compromising the absorptive surface.

Celiac Disease (Gluten-Sensitive Enteropathy)

Celiac disease, also known as *gluten-induced enteropathy, gluten-sensitive enteropathy,* and *celiac sprue,* is a permanent intestinal intolerance to dietary wheat gliadin and related proteins that produces mucosal lesions in genetically susceptible individuals. It is second only to cystic fibrosis as a cause of malabsorption in children.

The incidence varies and has been reported in one in 3000 to one in 4000 people. More recently the incidence has been shown to be closer to one in 266 as a result of improved screening tests (McCabe, Toughill, Parkhill, et al., 2012). The disease is seen more frequently in Europe than in the United States. It is more prevalent in women than men and is rarely reported in Asians or African-Americans. Although the exact cause is unknown, it is now generally accepted that celiac disease is a T-cell–mediated autoimmune and genetic small intestine enteropathy (McCabe, Toughill, Parkhill, et al., 2012). The mucosal lesions contain features that suggest both humoral and cell-mediated immunologic overstimulation.

Infant feeding practices, including breastfeeding for at least 4 months and gradual introduction of gluten in the infant's diet, may play a role in the prevention of celiac disease. Infectious diseases in infancy, specifically rotavirus, have been noted to increase the incidence of this condition (Branski and Troncone, 2011; Ivarsson, Myléus, Norström, et al., 2013).

Pathophysiology

Celiac disease is characterized by villous atrophy in the small bowel in response to the protein gluten. Gluten is found in wheat, barley, rye, and oat grains. When individuals are unable to digest the gliadin component of gluten, an accumulation of a toxic substance that is damaging to the mucosal cells occurs. Damage to the mucosa of the small intestine leads to villous atrophy, hyperplasia of the crypts, and infiltration of the epithelial cells with lymphocytes. Villous atrophy leads to malabsorption caused by the reduced absorptive surface area.

Genetic predisposition is an essential factor in the development of celiac disease. Membrane receptors involved in preferential antigen presentation to CD4+ T-cells play a crucial role in the immune response characteristic of celiac disease. Genes located on the human leukocyte antigen (HLA) region of chromosome 6 (i.e., *HLA-DQ2* or *HLA-DQ8)* are found in almost 100% of those affected with celiac disease (Murdock and Johnston, 2005). When the inflammatory reaction is activated by gluten, CD4+ T-cells produce cytokines, which are likely to contribute to the intestinal damage. The damage consists of infiltration of the lamina propria, crypt hyperplasia, and villous atrophy and flattening. With sufficient villous atrophy, malabsorption occurs.

Classic symptoms of celiac disease are GI manifestations usually noted several months after the introduction of gluten-containing grains into the diet, typically between the ages of 6 months and 2 years (Box 41-18). Typically children are seen with impaired growth, chronic diarrhea, abdominal distention, muscle wasting with hypotonia, poor appetite, and lack of energy. The clinical manifestations are usually insidious and chronic. The first evidence may be growth failure and diarrhea. Less typical presentation has been observed in children ages 5 to 7 years who have abdominal pain; nausea; vomiting; bloating; constipation; or extraintestinal manifestations, including iron deficiency anemia, short stature, pubertal delay, dental enamel defects, alopecia, and abnormal LFT results. Older children have been found to have osteoporosis. Untreated celiac disease can evolve into celiac crisis, characterized by abdominal distention, explosive watery diarrhea, and dehydration with electrolyte imbalance, leading to hypotensive shock and lethargy.

Diagnostic Evaluation

The diagnosis of celiac disease is based on a biopsy of the small intestine demonstrating the characteristic changes of villous atrophy with hyperplasia of the crypts and abnormal surface epithelium while the individual is eating adequate amounts of gluten and a full clinical remission after gluten is withdrawn (Branski and Troncone, 2011). Within 1 or 2 days of instituting the diet, most children with celiac disease demonstrate a favorable response, including weight gain and improved appetite. Within a few weeks there is resolution of the diarrhea and steatorrhea.

Genetic testing for the HLA genes associated with celiac disease may help in ruling out the disease in individuals at high risk for the condition. A negative test indicates the individual does not have the condition; a positive test indicates there is an increased likelihood of having the condition, and antibody screening should be considered (University of Chicago Celiac Disease Center, 2013).

BOX 41-18 **CLINICAL MANIFESTATIONS OF CELIAC DISEASE**

Classic Celiac Disease
- Diarrhea
- Abdominal distention
- Failure to thrive, or weight loss
- Positive serology, HLA, and villous atrophy

Atypical Celiac Disease
- Iron deficiency anemia
- Osteoporosis
- Short stature
- Arthritis
- Infertility
- Peripheral neuropathy
- Abnormal LFTs, positive serology, HLA, and varying degrees of villous atrophy

Silent Celiac Disease
- Asymptomatic but with positive serology, HLA, and villous atrophy

Latent Celiac Disease
- Variation in expression between atypical and asymptomatic
- Positive or negative serology, HLA, and no villous atrophy

Modified from Scanlon SA, Murray JA: Update on celiac disease—etiology, differential diagnosis, drug tests, and management advances, *Clin Exp Gastroenterol* 4:297–311, 2011.
HLA, Human leukocyte antigen; *LFT*, liver function test.

Commercially available serologic tests for celiac disease include antigliadin antibodies of both the immunoglobulin A and G classes (IgA and IgG); antiendomysium IgA; and antitissue transglutaminase IgA (anti-TTG) and IgG antibodies for screening first-degree relatives of known celiac disease patients and those with known celiac disease–associated disorders such as type 1 diabetes, thyroiditis, arthritis, primary biliary cirrhosis, Down syndrome, Turner syndrome, Williams syndrome, and osteopenia or osteoporosis. False-positive results are likely when only one serologic test is used because patients with these disorders can also test positive for these antibodies. Use of more than one test increases diagnostic accuracy (Gelfond and Fasano, 2006). Ruling out total IgA deficiency is necessary to minimize false-negative results.

Therapeutic Management

Treatment of patients with chronic celiac disease is primarily dietary and consists of strict adherence to a gluten-free diet. Because gluten is found primarily in the grains of wheat and rye but also in smaller quantities in barley and oats, these four foods are eliminated. Corn and rice become substitute grain foods.

Children with untreated celiac disease may have lactose intolerance, especially if their mucosal lesions are extensive. Lactose intolerance usually improves as the mucosa heals with gluten withdrawal. Specific nutritional deficiencies such as iron, folic acid, and fat-soluble vitamin deficiencies are treated with appropriate supplements. Some patients may not respond to the gluten-free diet and exhibit refractory celiac disease; such individuals continue to have diarrhea and malabsorption and may need to rely on PN and immunosuppressants (McCabe, Toughill, Parkhill, et al., 2012).

Prognosis. Celiac disease is regarded as a chronic disease. The most severe symptoms usually occur in early childhood and again in adult life. Strict dietary avoidance of gluten prevents symptoms and may minimize the risk of developing lymphoma, especially of the small intestine, the most serious complication of the disease.

CARE MANAGEMENT

The main nursing consideration is helping the child adhere to the dietary regimen. This requires a wheat-, barley-, and rye-free diet. Oats may be safe for most patients, but contamination with other gluten products may occur in harvesting; therefore caution should be exercised with oats. Children who have silent celiac disease, without clinical manifestations should also adhere to a strict gluten-free diet (Branski and Troncone, 2011). Considerable time is involved in explaining the disease process to the child and parents, the specific role of gluten in aggravating the disorder, and the foods that must be restricted. It is difficult to maintain a diet indefinitely when the child has no symptoms and temporary transgressions result in no difficulties. However, most individuals who relax their diet experience a relapse of their disease and possibly exhibit growth restriction, iron deficiency anemia, or osteomalacia. There is also the risk of developing malignant T-cell lymphoma of the small intestine or other GI malignancies.

Although the chief sources of gluten are cereal and baked goods, grains are frequently added to processed foods as thickeners or fillers. To compound the difficulty, gluten is added to many foods as hydrolyzed vegetable protein, which is derived from cereal grains. The nurse must advise parents of the necessity of reading all label ingredients carefully to avoid hidden sources of gluten.

Many of children's favorite foods contain gluten, including bread, cake, cookies, crackers, donuts, pies, spaghetti, pizza, prepared soups, some processed ice cream, many types of chocolate candy, milk preparations such as malts, hot dogs, luncheon meats, meat gravy, and some prepared hamburgers. Many of these products can be eliminated from an infant's or young child's diet fairly easily, but monitoring the diet of a school-age child or adolescent is more difficult. Luncheon preparation away from home is particularly difficult because bread, luncheon meats, and instant soups are not allowed. For families on restricted food budgets, the diet adds an additional financial burden because many inexpensive and convenient foods cannot be used.

In addition to restricting gluten, other dietary alterations may be necessary. For example, in some children who have more severe mucosal damage, the digestion of disaccharides is impaired, especially in relation to lactose. Therefore these children often need a temporarily lactose-free diet, which necessitates eliminating all milk products. In general dietary management includes a diet high in calories and proteins with simple carbohydrates such as fruits and vegetables but low in fats. Because the bowel is inflamed as a result of the pathologic processes in absorption, the child must avoid high-fiber foods such as nuts, raisins, raw vegetables, and raw fruits with skin until inflammation has subsided.

It is important to stress long-range complications and remind parents of the child's physical status before dietary treatment and the dramatic improvement after treatment. The nurse can be instrumental in allowing the child to express concerns and frustration while focusing on ways in which he or she can still feel normal. Encourage the child and parents to find new recipes using suitable ingredients such as Mexican or Chinese dishes that use corn or rice.

Consult a clinical dietician to provide children and their families with detailed dietary instructions and education.*

Several resources are available to help children and parents in all aspects of coping with celiac disease. The Celiac Sprue Association/United States of America† provides support and guidance to families and supplies educational materials concerning a gluten-free diet, food sources, recipes, and travel information.

Short-Bowel Syndrome

SBS is a malabsorptive disorder that occurs as a result of decreased mucosal surface area, usually because of extensive resection of the small intestine. Malabsorption may be exacerbated by other factors such as bacterial overgrowth and dysmotility. The most common causes of SBS in children are necrotizing enterocolitis, volvulus, jejunal atresias, and gastroschisis. Other causes include midgut volvulus and diffuse small-bowel CD in older children. Less frequent causes include trauma to the GI tract and Hirschprung disease (HD) with extension into the small bowel.

The definition of SBS includes two important findings: (1) decreased intestinal surface area for absorption of fluid, electrolytes, and nutrients; and (2) a need for PN (Goday, 2009). The prognosis for infants with SBS has improved dramatically in the past 20 to 30 years as a result of advances in PN and enteral feeding.

Therapeutic Management

The goals of therapy for infants and children with SBS include: (1) preserve as much length of bowel as possible during surgery; (2) maintain optimum nutritional status, growth, and development while intestinal adaptation occurs; (3) stimulate intestinal adaptation with enteral feeding; and (4) minimize complications related to the disease process and therapy (Goday, 2009).

Nutritional support is the long-term focus of care for children with SBS (Sadlier, 2008). The initial phase of therapy includes PN as the primary source of nutrition. The second phase is the introduction of enteral feeding, which usually begins as soon as possible after surgery. Elemental formulas containing glucose, sucrose and glucose polymers, hydrolyzed proteins, and medium-chain triglycerides facilitate absorption. Usually these formulas are given by continuous infusion through an NG or gastrostomy tube. As the enteral feedings are advanced, the PN solution is decreased in terms of calories, amount of fluid, and total hours of infusion per day.

The final phase of nutritional support occurs when growth and development are sustained exclusively by enteral feedings. When PN is discontinued, there is a risk of nutritional deficiency secondary to malabsorption of fat-soluble vitamins (A, D, E, and K) and trace minerals (iron, selenium, and zinc). Obtain serum vitamin and mineral levels and require enteral supplementation of vitamins and minerals. Pharmacologic agents have been used to reduce secretory losses. H_2 blockers, PPIs, and octreotide inhibit gastric or pancreatic secretion. Cholestyramine is often prescribed to improve diarrhea that is associated with bile salt malabsorption. Growth factors have also been used to hasten adaptation and enhance mucosal growth, but these uses are still experimental.

Numerous complications are associated with SBS and long-term PN. Infectious, metabolic, and technical complications can occur. Catheter sepsis can occur after improper care of the catheter. The GI tract can also be a source of microbial seeding of the catheter. Bowel atrophy may foster increased intestinal permeability of bacteria. A lack of adequate sites for central lines may become a significant problem for the child in need of long-term PN. Hepatic dysfunction, hepatomegaly with abnormal LFTs, and cholestasis may also occur (Diamond, Sterescu, Pencharz, et al., 2009).

Bacterial overgrowth is likely to occur when the ileocecal valve is absent or when stasis exists as a result of a partial obstruction or a dilated segment of bowel with poor motility. Alternating cycles of broad-spectrum antibiotics are used to reduce bacterial overgrowth. This treatment may also decrease the risk of bacterial translocation and subsequent central venous catheter infections. Other complications of bacterial overgrowth and malabsorption include metabolic acidosis and gastric hypersecretion.

Many surgical interventions, including intestinal valves, tapering enteroplasty or stricturoplasty, intestinal lengthening, and interposed segments, have been used to slow intestinal transit, reduce bacterial overgrowth, or increase mucosal surface area. Intestinal transplantation has been performed successfully in children. Only children with a permanent dependence on PN or severe complications of long-term PN are candidates for transplantation.

Prognosis. The prognosis for infants with SBS has improved with advances in PN and with the understanding of the importance of intraluminal nutrition. Improved surgical techniques for the management of therapy-related problems and the development of more specific immunosuppressive medications for transplantation have all contributed to improved management. The prognosis depends in part on the length of the residual small intestine. An intact ileocecal valve also improves the prognosis. Infants and children with SBS die from PN-related problems such as fulminant sepsis or severe PN cholestasis.

CARE MANAGEMENT

The most important components of nursing care are administering and monitoring nutritional therapy. During TPN therapy care must be taken to minimize the risk of complications related to the central venous access device (i.e., catheter infections, occlusions, dislodgment, or accidental removal). Care of enteral feeding tubes and monitoring of enteral feeding tolerance are also important nursing responsibilities.

When long-term PN is required, preparing the family for home care is a major nursing responsibility that should be initiated early to prevent a lengthy hospitalization with subsequent problems such as family dysfunction and developmental delays. Many infants and children can be cared for at home successfully with enteral nutrition and PN when the family is prepared and provided with adequate support services. Follow-up by a multidisciplinary nutritional support team is essential. The nurse plays an active and important role in the success of a home nutrition program. Home infusion companies provide portable infusion equipment, which enables the child and family to maintain a more normal lifestyle.

Many infants with SBS have an intestinal ostomy performed at the time of the initial bowel resection. Routine ostomy care is another important nursing responsibility. Because infants and children with SBS have chronic diarrhea, perineal skin irritation is often a problem after ostomy closure. Frequent diaper changes, gentle perineal cleansing, and protective skin barriers help prevent skin breakdown.

---

*A booklet, *Pointers for Parents: Coping with Celiac Sprue*, provides information on shopping, cooking, and living with an affected child and is available from the Clinical Dietetics Department, Children's Memorial Hospital, 2300 Children's Plaza, Chicago, IL 60614, 773-880-4793.

†PO Box 31700, Omaha, NE 68131-0700, 877-CSA-4CSA or 402-558-0600, www.csaceliacs.org. In Canada: Canadian Celiac Association, 5025 Orbitor Dr., Suite 400, Mississauga, Ontario, Canada L4W 4Y5, 800-363-7296, 905-507-6208, www.celiac.ca.

When hospitalization is prolonged, the child's developmental and emotional needs must be met. This often requires special planning to promote normal family adjustment and adaptation of the hospital routines. Care of hospitalized children is discussed in Chapter 38.

INGESTION OF INJURIOUS AGENTS

Since the passage of the Poison Prevention Packaging Act of 1970, which requires that certain potentially hazardous drugs and household products be sold in child-resistant containers, the incidence of poisonings in children has decreased dramatically. However, despite these advances poisoning remains a significant health concern, with most cases (48.9% in 2009) occurring in children younger than 6 years of age (Bronstein, Spyker, Cantilena, et al., 2012). The home environment lends itself to injury in this vulnerable age-group of children (Dessypris, Dikalioti, Skalkidis, et al., 2009). Although pharmaceuticals such as analgesics, cough and cold preparations, topical preparations, antibiotics, vitamins, GI preparations, hormones, and antihistamines are frequently the agents of poisonings, a variety of other substances can also poison children. According to the 2011 report of the American Association of Poison Control Centers, the highest number of exposure fatalities in children age 5 years or less were attributed to analgesics (21.1%) (Bronstein, Spyker, Cantilena, et al., 2012). The type of analgesic was unspecified, but in past years acetaminophen has been associated with a large number of accidental poisonings in children under 5 years of age and intentional poisoning in adolescents. The most frequently ingested poisons include (Bronstein, Spyker, Cantilena, et al., 2012; Franklin and Rodgers, 2008):*

- Cosmetics and personal care products (perfume, cologne, aftershave)
- Cleaning products (hypochlorite [household] bleach, pine oil disinfectants)
- Plants (nontoxic GI irritants, oxalates)
- Foreign bodies, toys, and miscellaneous substances (desiccants, thermometers, bubble-blowing solutions)

Disk or button battery ingestion has recently emerged as the primary cause of fatal ingestions in children younger than 5 years of age; lithium batteries are reported to cause the most harm (CDC, 2012; Panella, Kirse, Pranikoff, et al., 2013; Sharpe, Rochette, and Smith, 2012). Esophageal perforation and liquefaction necrosis may result in serious harm, and emergent removal is recommended (Ikenberry, Jue, Anderson, et al., 2011).

Children are exposed to toxic substances more frequently than any other age-group (Eldridge, Van Eyk, and Kornegay, 2007). Many poisonings reflect the ready accessibility of the products in the home, where more than 90% of poisonings occur. A significant number of poisonings take place elsewhere such as in a grandparent's or friend's home, school, or health care facility.

The developmental characteristics of young children predispose them to poisoning by ingestion. Infants and toddlers explore their environment through oral experimentation. Because their sense of taste is not discriminating at this age, they ingest many unpalatable substances. In addition, toddlers and preschoolers are developing autonomy and initiative, which increase their curiosity and noncompliant behavior. Imitation is also a powerful motivator, especially when combined with a lack of awareness of danger.

---

*The most common substances in each category are in parentheses. Substances ingested are not necessarily the most toxic but often are readily available.

EMERGENCY

Poisoning

1. Assess the victim:
   - Initiate cardiorespiratory support if needed (airway, breathing, circulation).
   - Take vital signs; reevaluate routinely.
   - Treat associated complications.
2. Terminate exposure:
   - Empty mouth of pills, plant parts, or other material.
   - Flush eyes continuously with normal saline (or room-temperature tap water at home) for 15 to 20 minutes.
   - Flush skin and wash with soap and a soft cloth; remove contaminated clothes, especially if a pesticide, acid, alkali, or hydrocarbon is involved.
   - Bring victim of an inhalation poisoning into fresh air.
3. Identify the poison:
   - Question the victim and witnesses.
   - Look for environmental clues (empty container, nearby spill, odor on breath) and save all evidence of poison (container, vomitus, urine).
   - In absence of other evidence, be alert to signs and symptoms of potential poisoning in the absence of other evidence, including symptoms of ocular or dermal exposure.
   - Call the *poison control center* or other competent emergency facility for immediate advice regarding treatment.
4. Prevent poison absorption:
   - Place the child in a side-lying, sitting, or kneeling position with the head below the chest to prevent aspiration.
   - Administer activated charcoal if ordered (unless used repeatedly, usual dose is 1 g/kg unless the amount of toxin is known), administer drug antidote, or perform gastric lavage.

This section is concerned primarily with the immediate emergency treatment of ingestion of injurious agents. Box 41-19 summarizes specific management of corrosive, hydrocarbon, acetaminophen, salicylate, iron, and plant poisoning. Because of the importance of lead poisoning among young children, ingestion of lead is discussed separately.

Principles of Emergency Treatment

A poisoning may or may not require emergency intervention, but in every instance medical evaluation is necessary to initiate appropriate action. Advise parents to call the poison control center (PCC) *before* initiating any intervention (after terminating exposure [see Emergency box]). Parents should post the local PCC telephone number (usually listed in the front of the telephone directory) near each phone in the house* (see Emergency box).

! NURSING ALERT

The national number for the PCC is 800-222-1222; or online at American Association of Poison Control Centers, www.aapcc.org.

Based on the initial telephone assessment, the PCC counsels the parents to begin treatment at home or to take the child to an emergency facility. When a call is taken, the name and telephone number of the caller are recorded to reestablish contact if the connection is interrupted. Because most poisonings are managed in the home, expert advice is essential to minimize adverse effects. When the exact

---

*Also available by calling 800-222-1222 or online at American Association of Poison Control Centers, www.aapcc.org.

BOX 41-19   SELECTED ACCIDENTAL POISONINGS IN CHILDREN

Corrosives (Strong Acids or Alkali)

- Drain, toilet, or oven cleaners
- Electric dishwasher detergent (liquid, because of higher pH, is more hazardous than granular)
- Mildew remover
- Batteries (disk or button)—lithium
- Clinitest tablets
- Denture cleaners
- Bleach

Clinical Manifestations

- Severe burning pain in mouth, throat, and stomach
- White, swollen mucous membranes; edema of lips, tongue, and pharynx (respiratory obstruction)
- Violent vomiting (hemoptysis)
- Drooling and inability to clear secretions
- Signs of shock
- Anxiety and agitation

Comments

- Household bleach is a frequently ingested corrosive but rarely causes serious damage.
- Liquid corrosives cause more damage than granular preparations.

Treatment

- Assess child's breathing and level of consciousness.
- Contact poison control center (800-222-1222) for advice.
- Inducing emesis is contraindicated (vomiting redamages the mucosa).
- Dilute corrosive with water or milk (usually no more than 120 mL [4 oz]).
- *Do not neutralize.* Neutralization can cause an exothermic reaction (which produces heat and causes increased symptoms or produces both a thermal and a chemical burn).
- Maintain patent airway as needed.
- Administer analgesics (under medical supervision).
- Do not allow oral intake.
- Esophageal stricture may require repeated dilations or surgery.

Hydrocarbons

- Gasoline
- Kerosene
- Lamp oil
- Mineral seal oil (found in furniture polish)
- Lighter fluid
- Turpentine
- Paint thinner and remover (some types)

Clinical Manifestations

- Gagging, choking, and coughing
- Nausea
- Vomiting
- Alterations in sensorium such as lethargy
- Weakness
- Respiratory symptoms of pulmonary involvement
  - Tachypnea
  - Cyanosis
  - Retractions
  - Grunting

Comments

- Immediate danger is aspiration (even small amounts can cause bronchitis and chemical pneumonia).
- Gasoline, kerosene, lighter fluid, mineral seal oil, and turpentine cause severe pneumonia.

Treatment

- Contact poison control center (800-222-1222).
- Inducing emesis is generally contraindicated.
- Gastric decontamination and emptying are questionable, even when the hydrocarbon contains a heavy metal or pesticide; if gastric lavage must be performed, a cuffed endotracheal tube should be in place before lavage because of a high risk of aspiration.
- Symptomatic treatment of chemical pneumonia includes high humidity, oxygen, hydration, and antibiotics for secondary infection.

Acetaminophen

Clinical Manifestations

Occurs in four stages:

1. Initial period (2 to 4 hours after ingestion)
   - Nausea
   - Vomiting
   - Sweating
   - Pallor
2. Latent period (24 to 36 hours)
   - Patient improves
3. Hepatic involvement (may last up to 7 days and be permanent)
   - Pain in right upper quadrant
   - Jaundice
   - Confusion
   - Stupor
   - Coagulation abnormalities
4. Patients who do not die in hepatic stage gradually recover.

Comments

- It is the most common drug poisoning in children.
- It occurs from acute ingestion.
- Toxic dose is 150 mg/kg or greater in children.
- Because of multiple formulations and concentrations, chronic acetaminophen toxicity is a significant problem.
- Parents should be counseled to read product packaging carefully and consult a health care professional to avoid inappropriate dosing.

Treatment

- Antidote *N*-acetylcysteine (Mucomyst) can usually be given orally but is first diluted in fruit juice or soda because of the antidote's offensive odor.
- It is given as 1 loading dose and usually 17 maintenance doses in different dosages.
- It may be given intravenously, but use is investigational.

Aspirin (Acetylsalicylic Acid [ASA])

Clinical Manifestations

- Acute poisoning
  - Nausea
  - Disorientation
  - Vomiting
  - Dehydration

Continued

BOX 41-19	**SELECTED ACCIDENTAL POISONINGS IN CHILDREN—cont'd**

- Diaphoresis
- Hyperpnea
- Hyperpyrexia
- Oliguria
- Tinnitus
- Coma
- Convulsions
- Chronic poisoning
  - Same as for acute poisoning but subtle onset (often mistaken for viral illness)
  - Dehydration, coma, and seizures may be more severe
  - Bleeding tendencies

Comments
- It may be caused by acute ingestion (severe toxicity occurs with 300 to 500 mg/kg).
- It may be caused by chronic ingestion (i.e., more than 100 mg/kg/day for 2 or more days) and can be more serious than acute ingestion.
- Time to peak serum salicylate level can vary with enteric aspirin or the presence of concretions (bezoars).

Treatment
- Hospitalization is required for severe toxicity.
- Emesis, lavage, activated charcoal, or cathartic measures may be used.
- Lavage will not remove concretions of ASA.
- Activated charcoal is important early in ASA toxicity.
- Sodium bicarbonate (intravenous) to correct metabolic acidosis and urinary alkalinization may be effective in enhancing elimination; urinary alkalinization is very difficult to achieve.
- Be aware of the risk for fluid overload and pulmonary edema.
- Prescribe:
  - External cooling for hyperpyrexia.
  - Anticonvulsants.
  - Oxygen and ventilation for respiratory depression.
  - Vitamin K for bleeding.
- In severe cases hemodialysis (not peritoneal dialysis) may be used.

Iron
- Mineral supplement or vitamin containing iron

Clinical Manifestations
Occurs in five stages:
1. Initial period (0.5 to 6 hours after ingestion) (if child does not develop gastrointestinal symptoms in 6 hours, toxicity is unlikely)
   - Vomiting
   - Hematemesis
   - Diarrhea
   - Hematochezia (bloody stools)
   - Gastric pain
2. Latency (2 to 12 hours)
   - Patient improves

3. Systemic toxicity (4 to 24 hours after ingestion)
   - Metabolic acidosis
   - Fever
   - Hyperglycemia
   - Bleeding
   - Shock
   - Death (may occur)
4. Hepatic injury (48 to 96 hours)
   - Seizures
   - Coma
5. Rarely pyloric stenosis develops at 2 to 5 weeks

Comments
- Factors related to frequency of iron poisoning:
  - Widespread availability
  - Packaging of large quantities in individual containers
  - Lack of parental awareness of iron toxicity
  - Resemblance of iron tablets to candy (e.g., M&M's)
- Toxic dose is based on the amount of elemental iron in various salts (sulfate, gluconate, fumarate), which ranges from 20% to 33%; ingestions of 60 mg/kg are considered dangerous.

Treatment
- Emesis or lavage may be used.
- For toxic doses lavage may be necessary for all chewable tablets or liquids if spontaneous vomiting has not occurred.
- Chelation therapy with deferoxamine is used in severe intoxication (may turn urine a red to orange color).
- If intravenous deferoxamine is given too rapidly, hypotension, facial flushing, rash, urticaria, tachycardia, and shock may occur; stop the infusion, maintain the intravenous line with normal saline, and notify the practitioner immediately.

Plants
Clinical Manifestations
- Depends on type of plant ingested
- May cause local irritation of oropharynx and entire gastrointestinal tract
- May cause respiratory, renal, and central nervous system symptoms
- Topical contact with plants can cause dermatitis

Comments
- Plants are some of the most frequently ingested substances.
- Plant ingestions rarely cause serious problems, although some can be fatal.
- Plants can also cause choking and allergic reactions.

Treatment
- Induce emesis.
- Wash from skin or eyes.
- Supportive care as needed.

quantity or type of ingested toxin is not known, admission to a health care facility with pediatric emergency treatment services for laboratory evaluation and surveillance during the time after ingestion is critical.

Assessment

The first and most important principle in dealing with a poisoning is to treat the child first, not the poison. This requires an immediate concern for life support. Vital signs are taken, and respiratory or circulatory support is instituted as needed. The child's condition is reevaluated routinely. Because shock is a complication of several types of household poisons, particularly corrosives, measures to reduce the effects of shock are important, beginning with the ABCs (airway, breathing, and circulation). Establishing and maintaining vascular access for rapid intravascular volume expansion is vital in the treatment of pediatric shock.

The emergency department nurse's responsibility is to be prepared for immediate intervention with all of the necessary equipment. Because time and speed are critical factors in recovery from serious poisonings, anticipation of potential problems and complications may mean the difference between life and death.

Gastric Decontamination

Although pediatric poison ingestions are common, they rarely result in significant morbidity or mortality (Albertson, Owen, Sutter, et al., 2011; Bronstein, Spyker, Cantilena, et al., 2012; Greene, Harris, and Singer, 2008). Consider using *GI decontamination (GID)* only after careful evaluation of the potential toxicity of the poison and the risks versus benefits. When GID is needed, the immediate treatment is to remove the ingested poison by adsorbing the toxin with activated charcoal (AC), performing gastric lavage, or increasing bowel motility (catharsis). Because of continuing controversy regarding the use of these methods, treat each toxic ingestion individually (Albertson, Owen, Sutter, et al., 2011; Eldridge, Van Eyk, and Kornegay, 2007; Madden, 2008). Specific antidotes may be administered for certain poisonings.

Syrup of ipecac, an emetic that exerts its action through irritation of the gastric mucosa and by stimulation of the vomiting center, is no longer recommended for routine treatment of poison ingestion (Criddle, 2007; Greene, Harris, and Singer, 2008; McGregor, Parkar, and Rao, 2009; Sheffield and Serwint, 2008).

> **! NURSING ALERT**
>
> Ipecac is not recommended for routine poison treatment intervention in the home because it induces vomiting. Once the ingested poison has been neutralized, the goal of treatment is to hydrate the victim with oral fluids; ipecac prevents adequate intake of oral fluids because of its emetic properties.

Medications such as calcium channel blockers and benzodiazepines either produce a rapid onset of adverse symptoms (e.g., sedation, seizures, coma) or exaggerate the vagal response induced by gagging, which can lead to significant bradycardia. Under either circumstance uncontrolled vomiting becomes an undesirable and unsafe event.

A commonly used method of GID is the use of *activated charcoal* (AC), an odorless, tasteless, fine black powder that adsorbs many compounds, creating a stable complex (Frithsen and Simpson, 2010; Sheffield and Serwint, 2008). AC is mixed with water or a saline cathartic to form slurry. Slurries are neither gritty nor distasteful but resemble black mud. To increase the child's acceptance of AC, the nurse should mix it with diet soda and serve it through a straw in an opaque container with a cover (e.g., a disposable coffee cup and lid) or an ordinary cup covered with aluminum foil or placed inside a small paper bag. For small children an NG tube may be required to administer AC (Greene, Harris, and Singer, 2008). However, recent data indicate that, except in cases of severe poisoning, the use of AC has not significantly improved clinical outcomes (Albertson, Owen, Sutter, et al., 2011). Best results are achieved when AC is administered within 30 to 60 minutes of a poison ingestion.

There is discussion about the use of AC in the home for pediatric poison ingestion. The evidence is not clear regarding the risk versus benefit of home AC administration (Eldridge, Van Eyk, and Kornegay, 2007). Potential complications from the use of AC include aspiration (usually in patients with impaired gag reflexes), constipation, and intestinal obstruction (in multiple doses) (Sheffield and Serwint, 2008). Superactivated charcoal products for gastric

decontamination are often more palatable and just as effective (Criddle, 2007).

If the child is admitted to an emergency facility, gastric lavage may be performed to empty the stomach of the toxic agent; however, this procedure can be associated with serious complications (GI perforation, hypoxia, aspiration), and it is no longer recommended in all cases of ingestion. There is no conclusive evidence that gastric lavage decreases morbidity (Criddle, 2007; Greene, Harris, and Singer, 2008; Sheffield and Serwint, 2008). In addition, gastric lavage may be of little benefit if used later than 1 hour after ingestion (Frithsen and Simpson, 2010; Greene, Harris, and Singer, 2008). Conditions that may be appropriate for the use of gastric lavage include presentation within 1 hour of ingestion of a toxin, ingestion in patient who has decreased GI motility, the ingestion of a toxic amount of sustained-release medication, and a massive or life-threatening amount of poison (Criddle, 2007; Madden, 2008). When gastric lavage is used, the patient requires a protected airway, possible sedation, and the largest diameter tube that can be inserted to facilitate passage of gastric contents.

In a minority of poisonings, specific antidotes are available to counteract the poison. They are highly effective and should be available in all emergency facilities. The supply of antidotes should be checked routinely and replaced as used or according to expiration dates. Antidotes available to treat toxin ingestion include *N*-acetylcysteine for acetaminophen poisoning, oxygen for carbon monoxide inhalation, naloxone for opioid overdose, flumazenil (Romazicon) for benzodiazepines (diazepam [Valium], midazolam [Versed]) overdose, digoxin immune Fab (Digibind) for digoxin toxicity, amyl nitrate for cyanide, and antivenin for certain poisonous bites.

Prevention of Recurrence

The ultimate objective is to prevent poisonings from occurring or recurring. Home safety education improves poison prevention practices (Kendrick, Smith, Sutton, et al., 2008). Research supports the effectiveness of parent education on preventing unintentional injuries (Kendrick, Barlow, Hampshire, et al., 2007; Kendrick, Coupland, Mulvaney, et al., 2007). One effective counseling method is first to discuss the difficulties of constantly watching and safeguarding young children (see Family-Centered Care box). In this way the challenging task of raising children can lead to a discussion of injury prevention as part of the parental role. This approach also incorporates contributory causes for the incident such as inadequate support systems; marital discord; discipline techniques (especially use of physical punishment); and any disruption in the family or family activities such as vacations, moves, visitors, illnesses, or births. A visit to the home, especially after repeat poisonings, is recommended as part of the follow-up care to assess hazards, including family factors, and to evaluate appropriate injury-proofing measures. One method of identifying risk areas is to ask specific questions or have the parent complete a questionnaire designed to isolate factors that predispose children to poisoning. Another approach is to encourage parents to bend down to the child's eye level and survey the home environment for potential hazards. Have the parents try to open cabinets and reach shelves to access poisons.

Passive measures (those that do not require active participation) have been the most successful in preventing poisoning and include using child-resistant closures and limiting the number of tablets in one container. However, these measures alone are not sufficient to prevent poisoning because most toxic agents in the home do not have safety closures. Therefore active measures (those that require

FAMILY-CENTERED CARE

Accidental Poisoning

An accidental poisoning is more than a physical emergency for the child; it usually represents an emotional crisis for the parents, particularly in terms of guilt, self-reproach, and insecurity in the parenting role. The emergency department is no place to admonish the family for negligence, lack of appropriate supervision, or failure to injury-proof the home. Rather it is a time to calm and support the child and parents while unaccusingly exploring the circumstances of the injury. If the nurse prematurely attempts to discuss ways of preventing such an incident from recurring, the parents' anxiety will block out any suggestions or offered guidance. Therefore it is preferable for the nurse to delay the discussion until the child's condition is stabilized or, if the child is discharged immediately after emergency treatment, to make a public health referral or send a packet of information.

GUIDELINES

Poison Prevention

- Assess possible contributing factors in occurrence of injury such as discipline, parent-child relationship, developmental ability, environmental factors, and behavior problems.
- Institute anticipatory guidance for possible future injuries based on child's age and maturational level.
- Refer to visiting nurse agency to evaluate home environment and need for injury-proofing measures.
- Provide assistance with environmental manipulation such as lead removal when necessary.
- Educate parents regarding safe storage of toxic substances.
- Advise parents to take drugs out of sight of children.
- Teach children the hazards of ingesting nonfood items.
- Advise parents against using plants for teas or medicine.
- Discuss problems of discipline and children's noncompliance and offer strategies for effective discipline.
- Instruct parents regarding correct administration of drugs for therapeutic purposes and discontinuation of drug if there is evidence of mild toxicity.
- Advise parents to contact the poison control center or practitioner immediately when a poisoning occurs.
- Post number of regional poison control center (800-222-1222) with emergency phone list by telephone.
- Include by the telephone the home address with nearest cross street in case an ambulance is needed. (In an emergency family members may not remember the house address, and baby-sitters may not be aware of the information.)

participation) are essential. The Guidelines box lists the guidelines for preventing the occurrence or recurrence of a poisoning.

Heavy Metal Poisoning

Heavy metal poisoning can occur from the ingestion of a variety of substances, the most common being lead. Other sources that are important in terms of children are iron and mercury. Mercury toxicity, a rare form of heavy metal poisoning, has occurred in children from a variety of sources such as broken thermometers or thermostats, broken fluorescent light bulbs, disk batteries, topical medications, gas regulators, cathartics, and interior latex house paint (Bose-O'Reilly, McCarthy, Steckling, et al., 2010; Clifton, 2007).

Elemental mercury (also called *metallic mercury* or *quicksilver*) is nontoxic if ingested and if the GI tract is healthy (e.g., has no fistulas). However, mercury is volatile at room temperature and enters the bloodstream after it is inhaled, causing toxicity (tremors, memory loss, insomnia, gingivitis, diarrhea, anorexia, weight loss). The classic form of mercury poisoning is called acrodynia (or "painful extremities").

! NURSING ALERT

Mercury thermometers are no longer recommended because if they are broken the inhaled vapors can cause toxicity. To prevent inhalation clean up spilled mercury quickly, using disposable towels and rubber gloves and washing the hands well afterward.

Heavy metals have an affinity for certain essential tissue chemicals, which must remain free for adequate cell functioning. When metals are bound to these substances, cellular enzyme systems are inactivated. Treatment involves *chelation,* use of a chemical compound that combines with the metal for rapid and safe excretion.

Lead Poisoning

Poisoning from lead has been a problem throughout history and throughout the world. In the United States the problem became apparent in the early 1900s when white lead was added to paints and tetraethyl lead was added to gasoline as an antiknock compound. Lead content in paint was decreased in 1950, and in 1978 the use of lead in household paint was banned. The use of lead in paint and leaded gasoline has been banned in the United States. After this change in policy, the average blood lead level (BLL) in the United States for people ages 1 to 74 years dropped from 12.8 mcg/dL in 1980 to 1.9 mcg/dL in 1999 (AAP Committee on Environmental Health, 2005). However, children continue to be exposed to lead; an estimated 1.6% of U.S. children had BLLs of more than 10 mcg/dL in 2002, and almost 14% had BLLs of 5 to 9 mcg/dL (Levin, Brown, Kashtock, et al., 2008). Therefore the CDC recently issued a recommendation that the BLL of 10 mcg no longer be considered a "level of concern" but that a reference value of 97.5 percentile of BLL among children ages 1 to 5 years be used to guide treatment; the 97.5 percentile (based on the most recent NHANES data) currently represents a BLL of 5 mcg/dL, but this would be subject to review within 4 years (CDC Advisory Committee on Childhood Lead Poisoning Prevention, 2012). This recommendation further emphasizes that there is currently no safe level of blood lead at which children may not experience adverse health effects.

Causes of Lead Poisoning

Although there are numerous sources of lead (Box 41-20), in most instances of acute childhood lead poisoning the source is nonintact lead-based paint in an older home or lead-contaminated bare soil in the yard. Microparticles of lead gain entrance into a child's body through ingestion or inhalation and, in the case of an exposed pregnant woman, by placental transfer. When measured, a mother's lead level is nearly the same as that of her unborn child. However, although the level of lead may not be harmful to adult women, it can be harmful to fetuses.

Inhalation exposure usually occurs during renovation and remodeling activities in the home, but ingestion happens during normal day-to-day play and mouthing activities. Sometimes a child actually swallows loose chips of lead-based paint because it has a sweet taste. Water and food may also be contaminated with lead. A

BOX 41-20 SOURCES OF LEAD*

- Lead-based paint in deteriorating condition
- Lead solder
- Lead crystal
- Battery casings
- Lead fishing sinkers
- Lead curtain weights
- Lead bullets
- The following may contain lead:
  - Ceramic ware
  - Water
  - Pottery
  - Pewter
  - Dyes
  - Industrial factories
  - Vinyl miniblinds
  - Playground equipment
  - Collectible toys
  - Artists' paints
  - Pool cue chalk
  - Some imported toys or children's metal jewelry
- Occupations and hobbies involving lead:
  - Battery and aircraft manufacturing
  - Lead smelting
  - Brass foundry work
  - Radiator repair
  - Construction work
  - Bridge repair work
  - Painting contracting
  - Mining
  - Ceramics work
  - Stained-glass making
  - Jewelry making

*The U.S. Consumer Product Safety Commission issues alerts and recalls for products that contain lead and that may unexpectedly pose a hazard to young children.

CULTURAL COMPETENCE

Sources of Lead

In some cultures the use of traditional ethnic remedies that contain lead may increase children's risk of lead poisoning. These remedies include the following:

Azarcon (Mexico)—For digestive problems; a bright orange powder; usual dose is 0.25 to 1 tsp, often mixed with oil, milk, or sugar or sometimes given as a tea; sometimes a pinch is added to a baby bottle or tortilla dough for preventive purposes

Greta (Mexico)—Yellow-orange powder used in the same way as azarcon

Paylooah (Southeast Asia)—Used for rash or fever; an orange-red powder given as 0.5 tsp straight or in a tea

Surma (India)—Black powder applied to the inner lower eyelid that is used as a cosmetic to improve eyesight

Unknown ayurvedic (Tibet)—Small, gray-brown balls used to improve slow development; two balls are given orally 3 times a day

Tamarindo jellied, fruit candy (Mexico)—Fruit candy packaged in paper wrappers that contain high lead levels

Lozeena (Iraq)—Bright orange powder used to color meat and rice

Modified from Centers for Disease Control and Prevention: Lead poisoning associated with use of traditional ethnic remedies—California, 1991-1992, *MMWR Morb Mortal Wkly Rep* 42(27):521–524, 1993; Centers for Disease Control and Prevention: Lead poisoning associated with imported candy and powdered food coloring—California and Michigan, *MMWR Morb Mortal Wkly Rep* 47(48):1041–1043, 1998; Centers for Disease Control and Prevention: Childhood lead poisoning associated with tamarind candy and folk remedies—California, 1992-2000, *MMWR Morb Mortal Wkly Rep* 51(31):684–686, 2002.

child does not need to eat loose paint chips to be exposed to the toxin; normal hand-to-mouth behavior, coupled with the presence of lead dust in the environment that has settled over decades, is the usual method of poisoning (AAP Committee on Environmental Health, 2005; Bose-O'Reilly, McCarthy, Steckling, et al., 2010; Erickson and Thompson, 2005; Frazer, 2008).

Because of family, cultural, or ethnic traditions, a source of lead may be a routine part of life for a child. Nurses must educate themselves about the practices of their patients and identify when such products may be a source of lead. The use of pottery or dishes containing lead may be an issue, as may the use of folk remedies for stomachaches or the use of some cosmetics (see Cultural Competence box). Children of immigrants and internationally adopted children may have been exposed to sources of lead before arrival in the United States and should also be carefully evaluated for lead exposure (Woolf, Goldman, and Bellinger, 2007). Other risk factors for having an elevated BLL include living in poverty, being younger than 6 years of age, dwelling in urban areas, and living in older rental homes where lead decontamination may not be a priority. Nurses are often in a position to observe or elicit information about these practices and educate families about their potential harm.

Pathophysiology and Clinical Manifestations

Lead can affect any part of the body, including the renal, hematologic, and neurologic systems (Fig. 41-8). Of most concern for young children is the developing brain and nervous system, which are more vulnerable than those of older children and adults. Lead in the body moves via an equilibration process between the blood, the soft tissues and organs, and the bones and teeth. It ultimately settles in the bones and teeth, where it remains inert and in storage. This makes up the largest portion of the body burden, approximately 75% to 90%. At the cellular level it competes with molecules of calcium, interfering with the regulating action of calcium. In the

brain lead disrupts the biochemical processes and may have a direct effect on the release of neurotransmitters, may cause alterations in the blood-brain barrier, and may interfere with the regulation of synaptic activity (Lidsky and Schneider, 2006).

There is a relationship between anemia and lead poisoning. Children who are iron deficient absorb lead more readily than those with sufficient iron stores. Lead can interfere with the binding of iron onto the heme molecule. This sometimes creates a picture of anemia even though the child is not iron deficient. Lead toxicity to the erythrocytes leads to the release of the enzyme erythrocyte protoporphyrin (EP). Because EP is not sensitive to BLLs of less than approximately 16 to 25 mcg/dL, it is no longer used as a screening test. Therefore the BLL test is currently used for screening and diagnosis. However, elevation of the EP level (>35 mcg/dL of whole blood) is a good indicator of toxicity from lead and reflects the length of exposure and body burden of lead in an individual child.

Although adults have been shown to experience adverse renal effects from occupational lead exposure, few studies document renal effects in children except at extremely high lead levels. One can hypothesize that lead can affect the renal integrity of both children and adults. Therefore the renal system of a child is still considered a potential target for the harmful effects of lead.

The lead levels identified in children have declined since the initiation of screening for children at risk for lead poisoning. With earlier intervention the most prevalent effects have changed. Since the late 1960s children have rarely died of lead poisoning, and seizures or cognitive impairment have become less likely. However, even mild and moderate lead poisoning can cause a number of cognitive and behavioral problems in young children, including aggression, hyperactivity, impulsivity, delinquency, disinterest, and

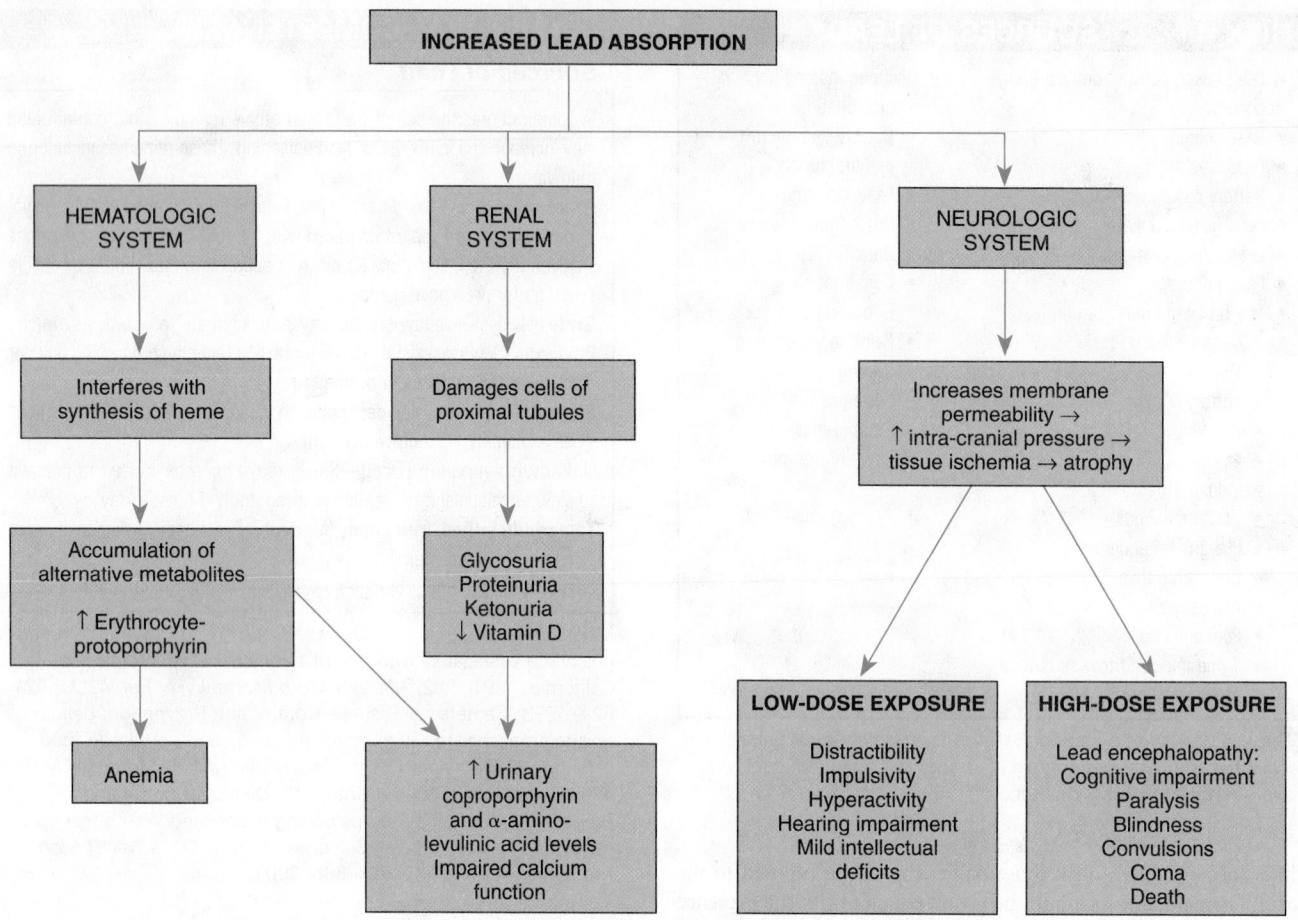

FIG 41-8 Main effects of lead on body systems.

withdrawal. Long-term neurocognitive signs of lead poisoning include developmental delays, lowered intelligence quotient (IQ), reading skill deficits, visual-spatial problems, visual-motor problems, learning disabilities, and lower academic success. Chronic lead toxicity may also affect physical growth and reproductive efficiency (Woolf, Goldman, and Bellinger, 2007).

> **❗ NURSING ALERT**
>
> Acute signs of lead poisoning include nausea, vomiting, constipation, anorexia, and abdominal pain. Additional clinical manifestations are hypophosphatemia, glycosuria, and aminoaciduria (Erickson and Thompson, 2005).

Diagnostic Evaluation

Children with lead poisoning rarely have symptoms, even at levels requiring chelation therapy. A diagnosis of lead poisoning is based only on the lead testing of a venous blood specimen from a venipuncture. The collection process is important. Blood must be collected carefully to avoid contamination by lead on the skin. As noted on p. 1308, a BLL of concern is now considered a BLL in the 97.5 percentile, which is currently 5 mcg/dL in children 1 to 5 years of age.

Anticipatory Guidance

Anticipatory guidance lends support to primary prevention efforts. The CDC (2005) recommends that the following information be made available to families beginning during prenatal care, at 3 to 6 months, and at 1 year of age:

- Hazards of lead-based paint in older housing
- Ways to control lead hazards safely
- How to choose safe toys
- Hazards accompanying repainting and renovating homes built before 1978
- Other exposure sources such as traditional remedies that might be relevant for a family

There has been recent concern regarding toys and other imported items with which children play that were found to contain lead. Parents should carefully evaluate the source of the toy (manufacturer) or item with which the child may play and not assume that it is safe because it is sold in a U.S. market. The U.S. Consumer Product Safety Commission (www.cpsc.gov) is an excellent resource for parents and caregivers concerned about the safety of a given toy or product that may be harmful.

Screening for Lead Poisoning

When primary prevention fails, secondary prevention screening efforts for elevated BLLs can identify children much earlier than in the past. Guidelines recommend universal or targeted screening (Levin, Brown, Kashtock, et al., 2008). This need is established using blood lead surveillance and other risk factor data collected over time to establish the status and risk of children throughout the state. In areas without available data, universal screening is recommended.

Universal screening should be done at ages 1 and 2 years. Any child between the ages of 3 and 6 years who has not been screened previously should also be tested. All children with risk factors should be screened more often.

Targeted screening is acceptable when an area has been determined by existing data to have less risk. Children should be screened when they live in a high-risk geographic area or are members of a group determined to be at risk (e.g., Medicaid recipients) or if their family cannot answer "no" to the following personal risk questions:

- Does your child live in or regularly visit a house that was built before 1950?
- Does your child live in or regularly visit a house built before 1978 with recent or ongoing renovations or remodeling within the past 6 months?
- Does your child have a sibling or playmate who has or had lead poisoning?

Therapeutic Management

The degree of concern, urgency, and need for medical intervention change as the lead level increases. Education is one of the most important elements of the treatment process. Several areas that the nurse needs to discuss with the family of every child who has an elevated BLL (≥5 mcg/dL) include (Heavey, 2008; Levin, Brown, Kashtock, et al., 2008):

- The child's BLL and what it means
- Potential adverse health effects of an elevated BLL
- Sources of lead exposure and suggestions on how to reduce exposure such as the importance of wet cleaning to remove lead dust on floors, windowsills, and other surfaces
- Importance of proper nutrition in reducing the absorption and effects of lead; for people with poor nutritional patterns, adequate intake of calcium and iron and importance of regular meals
- Need for follow-up testing to monitor the child's BLL
- Results of an environmental investigation if applicable
- Hazards of improper removal of lead paint (dry sanding, scraping, or open-flame burning)

Treatment actions vary, depending on the child's BLL. Based on a diagnosis from a venous BLL test, the CDC Advisory Committee on Childhood Lead Poisoning Prevention (2012) recommends that a BLL of 45 mcg/dL entails consideration of chelation therapy. Additional guidelines are expected to appear in publication in relation to the new recommendation that children ages 1 to 5 years with BLLs of 5 mcg/dL or more receive education and guidance for decreasing BLLs.

Chelation Therapy. Chelation is the term used for removing lead from circulating blood and theoretically some lead from organs and tissues. It is unclear whether chelation affects lead stores in bones. Although not an antidote in the truest sense, it does serve a similar purpose in that the toxic substance or poison is removed from the body. However, chelation does not counteract any effects of the lead.

Historically, two chelating agents have been used consistently: calcium disodium edetate (CaNa$_2$EDTA, or calcium EDTA) and succimer (Chemet, *meso*-2,3-dimercaptosuccinic acid [DMSA]). British antilewisite (BAL, dimercaprol, dimercaptopropanol) is used in conjunction with EDTA. All of the agents have potential toxic side effects and contraindications. Renal, hepatic, and hematologic parameters should be monitored.

Because of the equilibration process between blood, soft tissues, and other sites in the body, there is often a rebound of the BLL after chelation. After the body burden of lead is reduced enough to stabilize the BLL, rebound ceases. Multiple chelation treatments may be necessary. Adequate hydration is essential during therapy because the chelates are excreted via the kidneys.

BAL must not be used in the presence of a glucose 6-phosphate dehydrogenase deficiency or peanut allergy, nor should it be given in conjunction with iron. It is never used as a single-agent therapy, only in conjunction with EDTA. BAL must be given only at a deep intramuscular site. EDTA should be given intravenously over several hours or may be given intramuscularly when necessary to restrict fluids.

Succimer is given orally over a 19-day course of treatment. The capsule is opened and sprinkled on a small amount of food or may be swallowed whole. Adverse effects include nausea, vomiting, diarrhea, loss of appetite, rash, elevated LFTs, and neutropenia.

An oral chelating agent, D-penicillamine, is sometimes used to treat lead poisoning, but low doses should be used in children. Monitoring renal function and blood counts during administration is essential (Woolf, Goldman, and Bellinger, 2007).

Prognosis. Although most of the pathophysiologic effects of lead are reversible, the most serious consequences of both high and low lead exposure are the effects on the CNS. In children with lead encephalopathy, permanent brain damage can result in cognitive impairment, behavior changes, possible paralysis, and seizures. However, moderate- to low-dose exposure may also cause permanent neurologic deficits. Increased distractibility, short attention span, impulsivity, reading disabilities, and school failure have been associated with lead exposure. Some evidence indicates that treatment of moderate levels of lead poisoning can result in cognitive improvement (AAP Committee on Environmental Health, 2005; CDC Advisory Committee on Childhood Lead Poisoning Prevention, 2007).

CARE MANAGEMENT

The primary nursing goal in lead poisoning is to prevent the child's initial or further exposure to lead. For children with low-level exposure, this requires identifying the sources of lead in the environment. Careful history taking is the most useful and most valuable tool and should concentrate on the personal risk questions listed at left. Suggestions for reducing lead in the child's environment are listed in the Community Focus box.

The nurse prepares children who undergo chelation therapy for the injections and makes all efforts to reduce injection pain. Chelating agents are administered deeply into a large muscle mass. To lessen the pain from EDTA, the local anesthetic procaine is injected with the drug. Rotation of sites is essential to prevent the formation of painful areas of fibrotic tissue. Because EDTA and lead are toxic to the kidneys, keep records of fluid intake and output and assess the results of urinalysis to monitor renal functioning.

> ### ! NURSING ALERT
>
> Calcium EDTA is only administered when there is adequate urinary output. Children receiving the drug intramuscularly must be able to maintain adequate oral intake of fluids.

Discharge planning for children with lead poisoning must include thorough education of families regarding safety from lead

Reducing Blood Lead Levels

- Make sure that child does not have access to peeling paint or chewable surfaces painted with lead-based paint, especially window sills and wells.
- If a house was built before 1960 (possibly before 1980) and has hard-surface floors, wet mop them at least once per week. Wipe other hard surfaces (e.g., window sills, baseboards). If there are loose paint chips in an area such as a window well, use a wet disposable cloth to pick up and discard them. Do not vacuum hard-surfaced floors or windowsills or wells because this spreads dust. Use vacuum cleaners with agitators to remove dust from rugs rather than vacuum cleaners with suction only. If a rug is known to contain lead dust and cannot be washed, it should be discarded.
- Wash and dry child's hands and face frequently, especially before eating.
- Wash toys and pacifiers frequently.
- If soil around home is or is likely to be contaminated with lead (e.g., if home was built before 1960 or is near a major highway), plant grass or other ground cover; plant bushes around outside of house so child cannot play there.
- During remodeling of older homes be sure to follow correct procedures. Be certain that children and pregnant women are not in the home, day or night, until process is completed. After deleading thoroughly clean house using cleaning solution to damp mop and dust before inhabitants return.
- In areas where lead content of water exceeds the drinking water standard and a particular faucet has not been used for 6 hours or more, "flush" the cold-water pipes by running the water until it becomes as cold as it will

get (30 seconds to more than 2 minutes). The more time water has been sitting in pipes, the more lead it may contain.*
- *Use only cold water* for consumption (drinking, cooking, and especially for making infant formula).
- Hot water dissolves lead more quickly than cold water and thus contains higher levels of lead. First-flush water may be used for nonconsumption uses.
- Have water tested by a competent laboratory. This action is especially important for apartment dwellers; flushing may not be effective in high-rise buildings or other buildings with lead-soldered central piping.
- Do not store food in open cans, particularly if cans are imported.
- Do not use pottery or ceramic ware that was inadequately fired or is meant for decorative use for food storage or service. Do not store drinks or food in lead crystal.
- Avoid folk remedies or cosmetics that contain lead.
- Make sure that home exposure is not occurring from parental occupations or hobbies. Household members employed in occupations such as lead smelting should shower and change into clean clothing before leaving work. Construction and lead abatement workers may also bring home lead contaminants.
- Make sure that child eats regular meals because more lead is absorbed on an empty stomach.
- Make sure that child's diet contains sufficient iron and calcium and not excessive fat.

*For more information, contact the county or state department of health or environment for information on local water quality. For general information on lead, call the EPA Safe Drinking Water Hotline, 800-426-4791, www.epa.gov; National Lead Information Center, 422 S. Clinton Ave., Rochester, NY 14620, 800-424-LEAD (5323), www.epa.gov/lead/pubs/nlic.htm; Water Quality Association, 630-505-0160, www.wqa.org; or NSF International, 877-867-3435, www.nsf.org.

hazards, clear instructions regarding medication administration and follow-up, and confirmation that the child will be discharged to a home without lead hazards. Although the nurse must use caution to avoid alarming parents unnecessarily, it is important that they know the risk implications for their child's behavior and cognitive functions. Nurses should observe the development and behavior of children who are hospitalized. Thoroughly evaluate any concerns

that are identified. Referral to a child development or speech and language specialist may be necessary.

As in any situational crisis, parents need support and understanding if their child is treated for lead poisoning. Many families at the highest risk for lead poisoning have the fewest resources to comply with measures such as relocation or removal of lead from the environment where the child experiences exposure.

KEY POINTS

- Common nutritional disorders of infancy and early childhood may result from vitamin and mineral deficiency or excess, some types of vegetarian diets, PEM, and food intolerance.
- Food consumption varies among vegetarians; therefore a detailed dietary intake is essential for planning adequate intakes, particularly in children and pregnant and lactating women.
- PEM may occur as a complication of underlying disease, lack of parental education about infant nutrition, inappropriate management of food allergy, or incorrect preparation of formula.
- Food intolerance encompasses food allergies and food sensitivities, which can have a number of systemic and local clinical manifestations. CMA and lactose intolerance may occur in some children.
- Infants are subject to fluid depletion because of their greater surface area relative to body mass, high rate of metabolism, and immature kidney function.
- Dehydration can be classified as isotonic, hypotonic, and hypertonic.

- Vomiting and diarrhea account for significant fluid depletion, especially in infants and small children.
- The amount, frequency, and characteristics of stool and vomitus are important nursing observations.
- Diarrhea can be caused by an inflammatory process of infectious origin, a toxic reaction to ingestion of poisonous substances, dietary indiscretions, or infections outside the alimentary tract. The primary treatment of diarrhea is the use of an oral rehydrating solution.
- Structural disorders of the GI tract include CL, CP, EA with TEF, anorectal malformations, and BA.
- CL/P, the most common facial malformation, may involve nutritional, dental, and speech problems.
- Hernias related to the GI tract can be minor (umbilical) or life-threatening (diaphragmatic, gastroschisis, omphalocele).
- HD requires surgical removal of aganglionic segments of bowel.
- Postoperative care of the child with abdominal surgery involves assessing the abdomen and providing hydration and nutrition,

IV fluids, proper positioning, wound care, and psychologic support.

- Nursing care of GER is aimed at identifying children with suggestive symptoms, helping parents with home care feeding and possibly regurgitation, and caring for the child undergoing surgical intervention, if indicated.
- Although the cause of appendicitis is poorly understood, it is typically a result of obstruction of the lumen, usually by a fecalith. Common signs and symptoms are right lower quadrant abdominal pain, tenderness, and fever.
- Meckel diverticulum is a congenital malformation of the GI tract characterized by bloody stools.
- IBD refers to UC and CD.
- Peptic ulcers are poorly understood, but contributing factors include interference with the normal protective mechanisms of the mucosal lining and the presence of *Helicobacter pylori*.
- Viral hepatitis is caused by six types of virus: HAV, HBV, HCV, HDV, HEV, and HGV.
- HAV is spread by the fecal-oral route, whereas HBV and HCV are transmitted primarily by the parenteral route. The most effective measure in prevention and control of hepatitis in any setting is hand washing.
- BA is a serious condition, often causing progressive liver failure, which is an indication for liver transplantation.
- General signs of intestinal obstruction include colicky abdominal pain, nausea and vomiting, abdominal distention, and decreased stool output.
- HPS is recognized by characteristic projectile vomiting, malnutrition, dehydration, and sometimes a palpable mass in the epigastrium and is relieved by pyloromyotomy.
- Intussusception is one of the most common causes of intestinal obstruction during infancy and is characterized by abdominal pain and blood in stools. Treatment is either nonsurgical enema reduction or surgical reduction.

- Malabsorption syndromes are disorders associated with some degree of impaired digestion or absorption. They include digestive, absorptive, and anatomic defects.
- Celiac disease is characterized by an intolerance to gluten. The postulated causes include genetic, environmental, and immune factors that result in significant malabsorption.
- SBS is characterized by a loss of intestine resulting in a diminished ability to absorb a regular diet normally. Specialized enteral and parenteral nutrition is a major element of care for these children.
- Intestinal parasitic diseases constitute the most common infections in the world; giardiasis and enterobiasis are the most widespread parasitic infections among children in the United States.
- Although the incidence of poisoning has decreased in the past 30 years as a result of more stringent packaging regulations, accidental childhood poisoning remains a serious health concern.
- The major principles of treatment for poisoning include assessment and the ABCs (airway, breathing and measures to support circulation); minimization of poison absorption, prevention of complications, family support, and prevention of recurrence.
- Communication with the area PCC is essential in the treatment of any poisoning.
- The most important factor contributing to lead poisoning is its availability in the child's environment. Lead-based paint is the most toxic source of lead.
- Because of increasing awareness of the detrimental effects of low levels of lead on the developing nervous system, acceptable BLLs have been decreasing; but children with cognitive and health effects are still seen. The latest guidelines recommend using a BLL reference value of 97.5 percentile which is roughly 5 mcg/dL to guide treatment.

REFERENCES

Achildi A, Grewal H: Congenital anomalies of the esophagus, *Otolaryngol Clin North Am* 40(1):219–244, 2007.

Aiken JJ, Oldham KT: Acute appendicitis. In Kliegman RM, et al, editors: *Nelson textbook of pediatrics*, ed 19, Philadelphia, 2011, Saunders.

A-Kader HH, Balistreri WF: Neonatal cholestasis. In Kliegman RM, Stanton BF, St Geme JW, et al, editors: *Nelson textbook of pediatrics*, ed 19, Philadelphia, 2011, Saunders.

Albertson TE, Owen KP, Sutter ME, et al: Gastrointestinal decontamination in the acutely poisoned patient, *Int J Emerg Med* 4(1):65, 2011.

Alderman H, Shekar M: Nutrition, food security, and health. In Kliegman RM, Stanton BF, St Geme JW, et al, editors: *Nelson textbook of pediatrics*, ed 19, Philadelphia, 2011, Saunders.

Allen SJ, Martinez EG, Gregorio GV, et al: Probiotics for treating acute infectious diarrhea, *Cochrane Database Syst Rev* 10(11):CD003048, 2010.

Amadi B, Mwiya M, Chomba E, et al: Improved nutritional recovery on an elemental diet in

Zambian children with persistent diarrhoea and malnutrition, *J Trop Pediatr* 51(1):5–10, 2005.

American Academy of Pediatrics (AAP): Prevention of rickets and vitamin D deficiency in infants, children, and adolescents, *Pediatrics* 122(5):1142–1148, 2008.

American Academy of Pediatrics (AAP): *Pediatric nutrition handbook*, ed 6, Elk Grove Village, Ill, 2009, The Academy.

American Academy of Pediatrics (AAP) Committee on Environmental Health: Lead exposure in children: prevention, detection, and management, *Pediatrics* 116(4):1036–1046, 2005.

American Academy of Pediatrics (AAP) Committee on Infectious Diseases: Prevention of rotavirus disease: updated guidelines for use of rotavirus vaccine, *Pediatrics* 123(5):1412–1420, 2009.

American Academy of Pediatrics (AAP) Committee on Infectious Diseases, Pickering L, editor: *Red book: report of the Committee on Infectious Diseases*, ed 29, Elk Grove Village, Ill, 2012, Author.

American Academy of Pediatrics, Task Force on Sudden Infant Death Syndrome: SIDS and other sleep-related infant deaths: expansion of recommendations for a safe infant sleeping environment, *Pediatrics* 128(5):1030–1038, 2011.

Amthor RE, Cole SM, Manary MJ: The use of home-based therapy with ready-to-use therapeutic food to treat malnutrition in a rural area during a food crisis, *J Am Diet Assoc* 109(3):464–467, 2009.

Angulo P, Lindor KD: Primary biliary cirrhosis. In Feldman M, Friedman LS, Brandt LJ, editors: *Sleisenger and Fordtran's gastrointestinal and liver disease*, ed 9, Philadelphia, 2010, Saunders.

Ashworth A, Khanum S, Jackson A, et al: Guidelines for the inpatient treatment of severely malnourished children, Geneva, 2003, www.who.int/nutrition/publications/severemalnutrition/9241546093_eng.pdf.

Atia AN, Buchman AL: Oral rehydration solutions in non-cholera diarrhea: a review, *Am J Gastroenterol* 104(10):2596–2604, 2009.

Baker RD, Greer FR, American Academy of Pediatrics Committee on Nutrition: Clinical report—diagnosis and prevention of iron deficiency and iron-deficiency anemia in infants and young children (0-3 years of age), *Pediatrics* 126(5):1040–1050, 2010.

Bakken JS: Fecal bacteriotherapy for *Clostridium difficile* infection, *Anaerobe* 15(6):285–289, 2009.

Basnet S, Schneider M, Gazit A, et al: Fresh goat's milk for infants: myths and realities—a review, *Pediatrics* 125(4):e973–e977, 2010.

Bhutta ZA: Acute gastroenteritis in children. In Kliegman RM, Stanton BF, St Geme JW, et al, editors: *Nelson textbook of pediatrics*, ed 19, Philadelphia, 2011, Saunders.

Bischoff A, Peña A, Levitt MA: Laparoscopic-assisted PSARP: the advantage of combining both techniques for the treatment of anorectal malformations with recto-bladder neck or high prostatic fistulas, *J Pediatr Surg* 48(2):367–371, 2013.

Blanchard SS, Czinn SJ: Peptic ulcer disease in children. In Kliegman RM, Stanton BF, St Geme JW, et al, editors: *Nelson textbook of pediatrics*, ed 19, Philadelphia, 2011, Saunders.

Blanco FC, Davenport KP, Kane TD: Pediatric gastroesophageal reflux disease, *Surg Clin North Am* 92(3):541–558, 2012.

Bose-O'Reilly S, McCarthy KM, Steckling N, et al: Mercury exposure and children's health, *Curr Probl Pediatr Adolesc Health Care* 40(8):186–215, 2010.

Boshi-Pinto C, Velebit L, Shibuya K: Estimating child mortality due to diarrhoea in developing countries, *Bull World Health Organ* 86(9):710–717, 2008.

Boyce JA, Assa'ad A, Burks AW, et al: Guideline for the diagnosis and management of food allergy in the United States: summary of the NIAID-sponsored expert panel report, *J Allergy Clin Immunol* 126(6):1005–1118, 2010.

Bradley GM, Oliva-Hemker M: Infliximab for the treatment of pediatric ulcerative colitis, *Expert Rev Gastroenterol Hepatol* 6(6):659–665, 2012.

Branski D, Troncone R: Gluten-sensitive enteropathy (celiac disease). In Kliegman RM, Stanton BF, St Geme JW, et al, editors: *Nelson textbook of pediatrics*, ed 19, Philadelphia, 2011, Saunders.

Bronstein AC, Spyker DA, Cantilena LR Jr, et al: 2011 Annual report of the American Association of Poison Control Centers' National Poison Data System (NPDS): 29th annual report, *Clin Toxicol (Phila)* 50(10):911–1161, 2012.

Bullard J, Page NE: Cyclic vomiting syndrome: a disease in disguise, *Pediatr Nurs* 31(1):27–29, 2005.

Burk CJ, Molodow R: Infantile scurvy: an old diagnosis revisited with a modern dietary twist, *Am J Clin Dermatol* 8(2):103–106, 2007.

Butte NF, Fox MK, Briefel RR, et al: Nutrient intakes of US infants, toddlers, and preschoolers meet or exceed dietary reference intakes, *J Am Diet Assoc* 110(12 suppl):S27–S37, 2010.

Cavataio F, Guandalini S: Gastroesophageal reflux. In Guandalini S, editor: *Essential pediatric gastroenterology and nutrition*, New York, 2005, McGraw-Hill.

Carter B, Fedorowicz Z: Antiemetic treatment for acute gastroenteritis in children: an updated Cochrane systematic review with meta-analysis and mixed treatment comparison in a Bayesian framework, *BMJ Open* 2(4):e000622, 2012.

Centers for Disease Control and Prevention: Injuries from batteries among children aged <13 years—United States, 1995-2010, *MMWR Weekly Rep* 61(34):661–666, 2012.

Centers for Disease Control and Prevention (CDC): *Statewide plan for childhood blood lead screening*, Atlanta, Ga, 2005, Author.

Centers for Diseases Control and Prevention (CDC): Prevention of rotavirus gastroenteritis among infants and children: recommendations of the Advisory Committee on Immunization Practices (ACIP), *MMWR Rec Rep* 58(RR02):1–25, 2009.

Centers for Disease Control and Prevention: Managing acute gastroenteritis among children: oral rehydration, maintenance, and nutritional therapy, *MMWR Recommend Rep* 52(RR-16):1–16, 2003.

Centers for Disease Control and Prevention (CDC) Advisory Committee on Childhood Lead Poisoning Prevention: Interpreting and managing blood lead levels <10 μg/dL in children and reducing childhood exposures to lead, *MMWR Morb Mortal Wkly Rep* 56(47):1241, 2007.

Centers for Disease Control and Prevention (CDC), Advisory Committee on Childhood Lead Poisoning Prevention: *Low-level lead exposure harms children: a renewed call for primary prevention*, Atlanta, Ga, 2012, Author, www.cdc.gov/nceh/lead/ACCLPP/Final_Document_030712.pdf.

Chapman, KL, Hardin-Jones, MA, Goldstein JA, et al: Timing of palatal surgery and speech outcome, *Cleft Palate Craniofac J* 45(3):297–308, 2008.

Chen S-M, Chang M-H, Du J-C, et al: Screening for biliary atresia by infant stool color card in Taiwan, *Pediatrics* 117(4):1147–1154, 2006.

Chu A, Liacouras CA: Ileus, adhesions, intussusceptions, and closed-loop obstructions. In Kliegman RM, Stanton BF, St Geme JW, et al, editors: *Nelson textbook of pediatrics*, ed 19, Philadelphia, 2011, Saunders.

Ciliberto MA, Sandige H, Ndekha MJ, et al: Comparison of a home-based therapy with ready-to-use therapeutic food with standard therapy in the treatment of malnourished Malawin children: a controlled, clinical effectiveness trial, *Am J Clin Nutr* 81(4):864–870, 2005.

Clifton JC: Mercury exposure and public health, *Pediatr Clin North Am* 54(2):237–269, 2007.

Colletti JE, Brown KM, Sharieff GQ, et al: The management of children with gastroenteritis and dehydration in the emergency department, *J Emerg Med* 38(5):686–698, 2010.

Criddle LM: An overview of pediatric poisonings, *AACN Adv Crit Care* 18(2):109–118, 2007.

Daniels D, Grytdal S, Wasley A, et al: Surveillance for acute viral hepatitis—United States, 2007, *MMWR Surveill Summ* 58(3):1–27, 2009.

Dasgupta R, Langer JC: Hirschsprung disease, *Curr Probl Surg* 41(12):949–988, 2004.

de Vrese M, Schrezenmeir J: Probiotics, prebiotics, and synbiotics, *Adv Biochem Eng Biotechnol* 111:1–66, 2008.

Degertekin B, Lok AS: Update on viral hepatitis: 2008, *Curr Opin Gastroenterol* 25(3):180–185, 2009.

Dessypris N, Dikalioti SK, Skalkidis I, et al: Combating unintentional injury in the United States: lessons learned from the ICD-10 classification period, *J Trauma* 66(2):519–525, 2009.

Diamond IR, Sterescu A, Pencharz PB, et al: Changing the paradigm: omegaven for the treatment of liver failure in pediatric short bowel syndrome, *J Pediatr Gastroenterol Nutr* 48(2):209–215, 2009.

Dunham L, Kollar L: Vegetarian eating for children and adolescents, *J Pediatr Health Care* 20(1):27–34, 2006.

DuPont HL: The search for effective treatment of *Clostridium difficile* infection, *N Engl J Med* 364(5):473–475, 2011.

Eisenstein L, Bodager D, Ginzl D: Outbreak of giardiasis and cryptosporidiosis associated with a neighborhood interactive water fountain—Florida, 2006, *J Environ Health* 71(3):18–22, 2008.

Eldridge DL, Van Eyk J, Kornegay C: Pediatric toxicology, *Emerg Med Clin North Am* 25(2):283–308, 2007.

Emerick KM, Whitington PF: Neonatal liver disease, *Pediatr Ann* 35(4):281–286, 2006.

Emond S: Dehydration in infants and young children, *Ann Emerg Med* 53(3):395–397, 2009.

Erickson L, Thompson T: A review of a preventable poison: pediatric lead poisoning, *J Soc Pediatr Nurs* 10(4):171–182, 2005.

Ewing WM, Allen PJ: The diagnosis and management of cow milk protein intolerance in the primary care setting, *Pediatr Nurs* 31(6):486–492, 2005.

Fiorino K, Liacouras CA: Congenital aganglionic megacolon (Hirschprung disease). In Kliegman RM, Stanton BF, St Geme JW, et al, editors: *Nelson textbook of pediatrics*, ed 19, Philadelphia, 2011, Saunders.

Ford DM: Fluid, electrolyte, and acid-base disorders. In Hay WW, Levin MJ, Sondheimer JM, et al, editors: *Current diagnosis and treatment*, ed 19, Philadelphia, 2009, McGraw Hill.

Fox M, Reidy K, Novak T, et al: Sources of energy and nutrients in the diets of infants and toddlers, *J Am Diet Assoc* 106(1 suppl 1):S28–S42, 2006.

Franklin RL, Rodgers GB: Unintentional child poisonings treated in United States hospital emergency departments: national estimates of incident cases, population-based poisoning rates, and product involvement, *Pediatrics* 122(6):1244–1251, 2008.

Frazer L: Soil in the city: a prime source of lead, *Environ Health Perspect* 116(12):A522, 2008.

Friedman A: Fluid and electrolyte therapy: a primer, *Pediatr Nephrol* 25(5):843–846, 2010.

Frithsen I, Simpson W: Recognition and management of acute medication poisoning, *Am Fam Physician* 81(3):316–323, 2010.

Gelfond D, Fasano A: Celiac disease in the pediatric population, *Pediatr Ann* 35(4):275–279, 2006.

Gilmore AW, Reed M, Tenenbein M: Management of childhood intussusceptions after reduction by enema, *Am J Emerg Med* 29(9):1136–1140, 2011.

Gisbert JP, de la Morena F, Abraira V: Accuracy of monoclonal stool antigen test for the diagnosis of *H. pylori* infection: a systematic review and meta-analysis, *Am J Gastroenterol* 101(8):1921–1930, 2006.

Goday PS: Short bowel syndrome: how short is too short? *Clin Perinatol* 36(1):101–110, 2009.

Gourlay DM: Colorectal considerations in pediatric patients, *Surg Clin North Am* 93(2):251–272, 2013.

Granado-Villar D, Cunill-de Sautu B, Granados A: Acute gastroenteritis, *Pediatr Rev* 33(11):487–494, 2012.

Greenbaum LA: Electrolyte and acid-base disorders. In Kliegman RM, Stanton BF, St Geme JW, et al, editors: *Nelson textbook of pediatrics*, ed 19, Philadelphia, 2011, Saunders.

Greene S, Harris C, Singer J: Gastrointestinal decontamination of the poisoned patient, *Pediatr Emerg Care* 24(3):176–189, 2008.

Greer FR, Sicherer SH, Burks AW, et al: Effects of early nutritional interventions on the development of atopic disease in infants and children: the role of maternal dietary restriction, breastfeeding, timing of introduction of complementary foods, and hydrolyzed formulas, *Pediatrics* 121(1):183–191, 2008.

Grover Z, Ee LC: Protein energy malnutrition, *Pediatr Clin North Am* 56(5):1055–1068, 2009.

Grummer-Strawn LM, Reinold C, Krebs NF, et al: Use of World Health Organization and CDC growth charts for children aged 0-59 months in the United States, *MMWR Recomm Rep* 59(RR-9):1–15, 2010.

Guidry C, McGahren ED: Pediatric chest I: developmental and physiologic conditions for the surgeon, *Surg Clin N Am* 92(3):615–643, 2012.

Gupta N, Bostrom AG, Kirschner BS, et al: Presentation and disease course in early- compared to later-onset pediatric Crohn's disease, *Am J Gastroenterol* 103(8):2092–2098, 2008.

Hassall E, Owen D, Kerr W, et al: Gastric histology in children treated with proton pump inhibitors long term, with emphasis on enterochromaffin cell-like hyperplasia, *Aliment Pharmacol Ther* 4(33):829–836, 2011.

Heavey E: Lead poisoning in children: still a threat, *Nursing* 38(12):17–18, 2008.

Herwig K, Brenkert T, Losek JD: Enema-reduced intussusception management: is hospitalization necessary? *Pediatr Emerg Care* 25(2):74–77, 2009.

Heyman MB, American Academy of Pediatrics (AAP) Committee on Nutrition: Lactose intolerance in infants, children, and adolescents, *Pediatrics* 118(3):1279–1286, 2006.

Huiming Y, Chaomin W, Meng M: Vitamin A for treating measles in children, *Cochrane Database Syst Rev* (4):CD001479, 2005.

Hunter AK, Liacouras CA: Pyloric stenosis and other congenital anomalies of the stomach. In Kliegman RM, Stanton BF, St Geme JW, et al, editors: *Nelson textbook of pediatrics*, ed 19, Philadelphia, 2011, Saunders.

Huppertz H-I, Soriano-Gabarro M, Grimprel E, et al: Intussusception among young children in Europe, *Pediatr Infect Dis J* 25(1):S22–S29, 2006.

Hyams JS, Markowitz JR: Can we alter the natural history of Crohn disease in children? *J Pediatr Gastroenterol Nutr* 40(3):262–272, 2005.

Ikenberry SO, Jue TL, Anderson MA, et al: Management of ingested foreign bodies and food impactions, *Gastrointest Endosc* 73(6):1085–1091, 2011.

Ivarsson A, Myléus A, Norström F, et al: Prevalence of childhood celiac disease and changes in infant feeding, *Pediatrics* 131(3):e687–e694, 2013.

Kamath BM, Olthoff KM: Liver transplantation in children: update 2010, *Pediatr Clin North Am* 57(2):401–414, 2010.

Kane TD: Laparoscopic Nissen fundoplication, *Minerva Chir* 64(2):147–157, 2009.

Kapil U: Ready to use therapeutic food (RUTF) in the management of severe acute malnutrition in India, *Indian Pediatr* 46(5):381–382, 2009.

Kattan JD, Cocco RR, Järvinen KM: Milk and soy allergy, *Pediatr Clin North Am* 58(2):407–426, 2011.

Katz KA, Mahlberg MA, Honig PJ, et al: Rice nightmare: kwashiorkor in two Philadelphia-area infants fed Rice Dream beverage, *J Am Acad Dermatol* 52(5 suppl 1):S69–S72, 2005.

Kawchak DA, Schall JI, Zemel BS, et al: Adequacy of dietary intake declines with age in children with sickle cell disease, *J Am Diet Assoc* 107(5):843–848, 2007.

Keet C: Recognition and management of food-induced anaphylaxis, *Pediatr Clin North Am* 58(2):377–388, 2011.

Kelly DA, Davenport M: Current management of biliary atresia, *Arch Dis Child* 92(12):1132–1135, 2007.

Kendrick D, Barlow J, Hampshire A, et al: Parenting interventions for the prevention of unintentional injuries in childhood, *Cochrane Database Syst Rev* 17(4):CD006020, 2007.

Kendrick D, Coupland C, Mulvaney C, et al: Home safety education and provision of safety equipment for injury prevention, *Cochrane Database Syst Rev* 24(1):CD005014, 2007.

Kendrick D, Smith S, Sutton A, et al: Effect of education and safety equipment on poisoning-prevention practices and poisoning: systematic review, meta-analysis and meta-regression, *Arch Dis Child* 93(7):599–608, 2008.

Khan S, Orenstein SR: Esophageal atresia and tracheoesophageal fistula. In Kliegman RM, Stanton BF, St Geme JW, et al, editors: *Nelson textbook of pediatrics*, ed 19, Philadelphia, 2011, Saunders.

Kim JS, Nowak-Wegrzyn A, Sichere SH, et al: Dietary baked milk accelerates the resolution of cow's milk allergy in children, *J Allergy Clin Immunol* 128(1):125–131.e2, 2011.

Kranz S, Brauchla M, Slavin JL, et al: What do we know about dietary fiber intake in children and health? The effects of fiber intake on constipation, obesity, and diabetes in children, *Adv Nutr* 3(1):47–53, 2012.

Kunisaki SM, Foker JE: Surgical advances in the fetus and neonate: esophageal atresia, *Clin Perinatol* 39(2):349–361, 2012.

Langan RC, Gotsch PB, Krafczyk MA, et al: Ulcerative colitis: diagnosis and treatment, *Am Fam Physician* 76:1323–1330, 2007.

Lawrence B, Gantt G, Samuels-Reid J, et al: Suffocation deaths associated with use of infant sleep positioners—United States, 1997-2011, *MMWR Morb Mortal Wkly Rep* 61(46):933–937, 2012.

Levin R, Brown MJ, Kashtock ME, et al: Lead exposures in U.S. children, 2008: implications for prevention, *Environ Health Perspect* 116(10):1285–1293, 2008, www.ncbi.nlm.nih.gov/pmc/articles/PMC2569084/?tool=pubmed.

Levitt MA, Martin CA, Olesevich M, et al: Hirschsprung disease and fecal incontinence: diagnostic and management strategies, *J Pediatr Surg* 44(1):271–277, 2009.

Levitt MA, Peña A: Anorectal malformations, *Orphanet J Rare Dis* 2:33, 2007.

Lidsky TI, Schneider JS: Adverse effects of childhood lead poisoning: the clinical neuropsychological perspective, *Environ Res* 100(1):284–293, 2006.

Loening-Baucke V, Pashankar DS: A randomized, prospective, comparison study of polyethylene glycole 3350 without electrolytes and milk of magnesia for children with constipation and fecal incontinence, *Pediatrics* 118(2):528–535, 2006.

Luther J, Chey WD, Saad RJ: A clinician's guide to salvage therapy for persistent *Helicobacter pylori* infection, *Hospital Pract* 39(1):133–140, 2011.

Mack CL, Gonzalez-Peralta RP, Gupta N, et al: NASPGHAN Practice Guidelines: diagnosis and management of hepatitis C infection in infants, children, and adolescents, *JPGN* 54(6):838–855, 2012.

MacKinlay GA: Esophageal atresia surgery in the 21st century, *Semin Pediatr Surg* 18(1):20–22, 2009.

Madden MA: Responding to pediatric poisoning, *Nursing* 38(8):52–55, 2008.

Malek MA, Curns AT, Holman RC, et al: Diarrhea- and rotavirus-associated hospitalizations among children less than 5 years of age: United States, 1997 and 2000, *Pediatrics* 117(6):1887–1892, 2006.

Masarei AG, Wade A, Mars M, et al: A randomized control trial investigating the effect of presurgical orthopedics on feeding in infants with cleft lip and/or cleft palate, *Cleft Palate Craniofac J* 44(2):182–193, 2007.

McBride DL: New food allergy guidelines, *J Pediatr Nurs* 26(3):262–263, 2011.

McCabe MA, Toughill EH, Parkhill AM, et al: Celiac disease: a medical puzzle, *Am J Nurs* 112(10):34–44, 2012.

McGregor T, Parkar M, Rao S: Evaluation and management of common childhood poisonings, *Am Fam Physician* 79(5):397–403, 2009.

McRonald FE, Fleisher DR: Anticipatory nausea in cyclical vomiting, *BMC Pediatr* 5(1):3, 2005.

Mellow MH, Kanatzar A: Colonoscopic fecal bacteriotherapy in the treatment of recurrent *Clostridium difficile* infection: results and follow-up, *J Okla Stat Medical Assoc* 104(3):89–91, 2011.

Menezes M, Tareen F, Saeed A, et al: Symptomatic Meckel's diverticulum in children: a 16-year review, *Pediatr Surg Int* 24(5):575–577, 2008.

Mills JLA, Konkin DE, Milner R, et al: Long-term bowel function and quality of life in children with Hirschsprung's disease, *J Pediatr Surg* 43(5):899–905, 2008.

Moller KT, Glaze LE, editors: *Cleft lip and palate: interdisciplinary issues and treatment*, Austin, TX, 2009, Pro-Ed.

Müller O, Krawinkel M: Malnutrition and health in developing countries, *CMAJ* 173(3):279–286, 2005.

Murdock AM, Johnston SD: Diagnostic criteria for coeliac disease: time for change? *Eur J Gastroenterol Hepatol* 17(1):41–43, 2005.

Nowak-Wegrzyn A, Bloom KA, Sicherer SH, et al: Tolerance to extensively heated milk in children with cow's milk allergy, *J Allergy Clin Immunol* 122(2):342–347, 2008.

O'Connor A, Gisbert J, O'Morain C: Treatment of *Helicobacter pylori* infection, *Helicobacter* 14(suppl 1):46–51, 2009.

Olson DE, Kim YW, Donnelly LF: CT findings in children with Meckel's diverticulum, *Pediatr Radiol* 39(7):659–663, 2009.

Pakarinen MP, Rintala RJ: Surgery of biliary atresia, *Scand J Surg* 100(1):49–53, 2011.

Panella NJ, Kirse DJ, Pranikoff T, et al: Disk battery ingestion: case series with assessment of clinical and financial impact of a preventable disease, *Pediatr Emerg Care* 29(2):165–169, 2013.

Payne DC, Staat MA, Edwards KM, et al: Direct and indirect effects of rotavirus vaccination upon childhood hospitalizations in 3 US counties, 2-6-2009, *Clin Infect Dis* 53(3):245–253, 2011.

Penny ME: Protein-energy malnutrition: pathophysiology, clinical consequences, and treatment. In Duggan C, Watkins JB, Walker WA, editors: *Nutrition in pediatrics, Basic science: clinical applications*, ed 4, Hamilton, Ontario, 2008, Decker.

Pepper VK, Stanfill AB, Pearl RH: Diagnosis and management of pediatric appendicitis, intussusceptions, and Meckel's diverticulum, *Surg Clin North Am* 92(3):505–526, 2012.

Philichi L: When the going gets tough: pediatric constipation and encopresis, *Gastroenterol Nurs* 31(2):121–130, 2008.

Plenge-Bönig A, Soto-Ramirez N, Karmaus W, et al: Breastfeeding protects against gastroenteritis due to rotavirus in infants, *Eur J Pediatr* 169(12):1471–1476, 2010.

Preston AM, Rodriguez C, Rivera C, et al: Influence of environmental tobacco smoke on vitamin C status in children, *Am J Clin Nutr* 77(1):167–172, 2003.

Reese GE, Constantinides VA, Simillis C, et al: Diagnostic precision of anti–*Saccharomyces cerevisiae* antibodies and perinuclear antineutrophil cytoplasmic antibodies in inflammatory bowel disease, *Am J Gastroenterol* 101:2410–2422, 2006.

Ricart E, García-Bosch O, Ordás I, et al: Are we giving biologics too late? The case for early versus late use, *World J Gastroenterol* 14(36):5523–5527, 2008.

Richards CA: *C. difficile* epidemic continuing to spread, *Infect Dis Children* 19(9):39–41, 2006.

Robbins JM, Damiano P, Druschel, et al: Prenatal diagnosis of orofacial clefts: association with maternal satisfaction, team care, and treatment outcomes, *Cleft Palate Craniofac J* 47(5):476–481, 2010.

Rothenberg SS: Experience with thoracoscopic tracheal surgery in infants and children, *J Laparoendosc Adv Surg Tech A* 19(5):671–674, 2009.

Rowan-Legg A, Canadian Paediatric Society: Managing functional constipation in children, *Paediatr Child Health* 16(10):661–665, 2011.

Rubin DT, Kavitt RT: Surveillance for cancer and dysplasia in inflammatory bowel disease, *Gastroenterol Clin North Am* 35(3):581–604, 2006.

Russell G, Kaplan J, Ferraro MJ, et al: Fecal bacteriotherapy for relapsing *Clostridium difficile* infection in a child: a proposed treatment protocol, *Pediatrics* 126(1):e239–e242, 2010.

Rutter MD, Saunders BP, Wilkinson KH, et al: Thirty-year analysis of colonoscopic surveillance program for neoplasia in ulcerative colitis, *Gastroenterology* 130(4):1030–1038, 2006.

Sadlier C: Intestinal failure and long-term parenteral nutrition in children, *Paediatr Nurs* 20(10):37–43, 2008.

Saltzman MD, King EC: Central physeal arrests as a manifestation of hypervitaminosis A, *J Pediatr Orthop* 27(3):351–353, 2007.

Sampson HA, Leung DYM: Adverse reactions to foods. In Kliegman RM, Stanton BF, St Geme JW, et al, editors: *Nelson textbook of pediatrics*, ed 19, Philadelphia, 2011, Saunders.

Sauer CG, Kugathasan S: Pediatric inflammatory bowel disease: highlighting pediatric differences in IBD, *Med Clin North Am* 94(1):35–52, 2010.

Sharpe SJ, Rochette LM, Smith GA: Pediatric battery-related emergency department visits in the United States, 1990-2009, *Pediatrics* 129(6):1111–1117, 2012.

Sheffield P, Serwint JR: Emetics, cathartics, and gastric lavage, *Pediatr Rev* 29(6):214–215, 2008.

Shields JM, Gleim ER, Beach MJ: Prevalence of *Cryptosporidium* spp. and *Giardia intestinalis* in swimming pools, Atlanta, *Emerg Infect Dis* 14(6):948–950, 2008.

Silbermintz A, Markowitz J: Inflammatory bowel diseases, *Pediatr Ann* 35(4):268–274, 2006.

Simons FE: Anaphylaxis: recent advances in assessment and treatment, *J Allergy Clin Immunol* 124(4):625–636, 2009.

Sola JE, Neville HL: Laparoscopic vs open pyloromyotomy: a systematic review and meta-analysis, *J Pediatr Surg* 44(8):1631–1637, 2009.

Staat MA: What is the disease burden associated with rotavirus? In *The management and prevention of rotavirus*, Thorofare, NJ, 2006, Vindico Medical Education.

Steiner MJ, DeWalt D, Byerly JS: Is this child dehydrated? *JAMA* 291(22):2746–2754, 2004.

Steiner MJ, Nager AL, Wang VJ: Urine specific gravity and other urinary indices: inaccurate tests for dehydration, *Pediatr Emerg Care* 23(5):298–303, 2007.

Suchy FJ, Brannon PM, Carpenter TO, et al: National Institutes of Health consensus development conference: lactose intolerance and health, *Ann Intern Med* 152(12):792–796, 2010, consensus.nih.gov/2010/lactose.htm.

Sung JJ, Kuipers EJ, El-Serag HB: Systematic review: the global incidence and prevalence of peptic ulcer disease, *Aliment Pharmacol Ther* 29(9):938–946, 2009.

Suwandhi E, Ton MN, Schwarz SM: Gastroesophageal reflux in infancy and childhood, *Pediatr Ann* 35(4):259–266, 2006.

Taylor CE, Camargo CA: Impact of micronutrients on respiratory infections, *Nutr Rev* 69(5):259–269, 2011.

Theocharatos S, Kenny SE: Hirschsprung's disease: current management and prospects for transplantation of enteric nervous system progenitor cells, *Early Hum Dev* 84(12):801–804, 2008.

Thurley PD, Halliday KE, Somers JM, et al: Radiological features of Meckel's diverticulum and its complications, *Clin Radiol* 64(2):109–118, 2009.

Tierney EP, Sage RJ, Shwayder T: Kwashiorkor from a severe dietary restriction in an 8-month infant in suburban Detroit, Michigan: case report and review of the literature, *Int J Dermatol* 49(5):500–506, 2010.

Tran TT: Management of hepatitis B in pregnancy: weighing the options, *Cleve Clin J Med* 76(suppl 3):S25–S29, 2009.

University of Chicago Celiac Disease Center: *Fact Sheet: genetic screening for celiac disease*, 2013, University of Chicago, http://www.cureceliacdisease.org/living-with-celiac/guide/fact-sheets.

Vandenplas Y, Rudolph CD, Di Lorenzo C, et al: Pediatric gastroesophageal reflux clinical practice guidelines: joint recommendations of the North American Society for Pediatric Gastroenterology, Hepatology, and Nutrition (NASPGHAN) and the European Society for Pediatric Gastroenterology, Hepatology, and Nutrition (ESPGHAN), *J Pediatr Gastroenterol Nutr* 49(4):498–547, 2009.

van der Pol RJ, Smits MJ, van Wijk MP et al: Efficacy of proton pump inhibitors in children with gastroesophageal reflux disease: a systematic review, *Pediatrics* 127(5):925–935, 2011.

Vernier-Massouille G, Balde M, Salleron J, et al: Natural history of pediatric Crohn's disease: a population-based cohort study, *Gastroenterology* 135(4):1106–1113, 2008.

Vissers RJ, Lennarz WB: Pitfalls in appendicitis, *Emerg Med Clin North Am* 28(1):103–118, 2010.

Walker VP, Modlin RL: The vitamin D connection to pediatric infections and immune function, *Pediatr Res* 65(5 Pt 2):106R–113R, 2009.

Wang J, Sampson HA: Food anaphylaxis, *Clin Exp Allergy* 37(5):651–660, 2007.

Waseem M, Rosenberg HK: Intussusception, *Pediatr Emerg Care* 24(11):793–800, 2008.

Wilkins-Haug L: Prenatal diagnosis of orofacial clefts, *UptoDate*, September 29, 2010, /www.uptodate.com.

Wong AP, Clark AL, Garnett EA, et al: Use of complementary medicine in pediatric patients with inflammatory bowel disease: results from a multicenter survey, *J Pediatr Gastroenterol Nutr* 48(1):55–60, 2009.

Woolf AD, Goldman R, Bellinger DC: Update on clinical management of childhood lead poisoning, *Pediatr Clin North Am* 54(2):271–294, 2007.

World Health Organization (WHO): *HIV and infant feeding update*, Geneva, 2006, Author.

World Health Organization (WHO): *Fact Sheet: Diarrhoeal disease*, Geneva, 2013, Author, http://www.who.int/mediacentre/factsheets/fs330/en/.

Yang CF, Duro D, Zurakowski D, et al: High prevalence of multiple micronutrient deficiencies in children with intestinal failure: a longitudinal study, *J Pediatr* 159(1):39–44, 2011.

Yazigi N, Balistreri WF: Viral hepatitis. In Kliegman RM, Stanton BF, St Geme JW, et al, editors: *Nelson textbook of pediatrics*, ed 19, Philadelphia, 2011, Saunders.

Yoder JS, Beach MJ: Centers for Disease Control and Prevention (CDC): Giardiasis surveillance—United States, 2006-2008, *MMWR Surveill Summ* 59(SS06):15–25, 2010.

Zile MH: Vitamin A: deficiencies and excess. In Kliegman RM, Stanton BF, St Geme JW, et al, editors: *Nelson textbook of pediatrics*, ed 19, Philadelphia, 2011, Saunders.

Cardiovascular Dysfunction

Marilyn J. Hockenberry

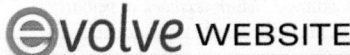 WEBSITE

http://evolve.elsevier.com/Perry/maternal

LEARNING OBJECTIVES

On completion of this chapter, the reader will be able to:

- Design a plan for assisting children during cardiac diagnostic procedures.
- Demonstrate an understanding of the hemodynamics, distinctive manifestations, and therapeutic management of congenital heart disease.
- Outline a care plan for an infant or child with heart failure.
- Describe the care for a child who has hypoxia.
- Describe the care for an infant or a child with a congenital heart defect and its surgical repair.

- Discuss the nurse's role in helping the child and family cope with congenital heart disease.
- Differentiate between rheumatic fever and rheumatic heart disease.
- List the criteria for selected cholesterol screening of children.
- Discuss the assessment and management of hypertension in children and adolescents.
- Outline a care plan for a child with Kawasaki disease.
- Describe the emergency treatment for shock, including anaphylaxis.

CARDIOVASCULAR DYSFUNCTION

Cardiovascular disorders in children are divided into two major groups—congenital heart disease and acquired heart disorders. Congenital heart disease (CHD) includes primarily anatomic abnormalities present at birth that result in abnormal cardiac function. The clinical consequences of congenital heart defects fall into two broad categories—heart failure (HF) and hypoxemia. Acquired cardiac disorders are disease processes or abnormalities that occur after birth and can be seen in the normal heart or in the presence of congenital heart defects. They result from various factors, including infection, autoimmune responses, environmental factors, and familial tendencies. The pathophysiology review found in Fig. 42-1 describes the flow of blood through the heart.

History and Physical Examination

Taking an accurate health history is an important first step in assessing an infant or child for possible heart disease. Parents may have specific concerns, such as an infant with poor feeding or fast breathing or a 7-year-old who can no longer keep up with friends on the soccer field. Others may not realize that their child has a medical problem because their baby has always been pale and fussy.

Asking details about the mother's health history, pregnancy, and birth history is important in assessing infants. Mothers with chronic health conditions, such as diabetes or lupus, are more likely to have infants with heart disease. Some medications, such as phenytoin (Dilantin), are teratogenic to fetuses. Maternal alcohol use or illicit drug use increases the risk for congenital heart defects. Exposures to infections, such as rubella, early in pregnancy may result in congenital anomalies. Infants with low birth weight resulting from intrauterine growth restriction are more likely to have congenital anomalies. High-birth-weight infants have an increased incidence of heart disease.

A detailed family history is also important. There is an increased incidence of congenital cardiac defects if either parent or a sibling has a heart defect. Some diseases, such as Marfan syndrome, and some cardiomyopathies are hereditary. A family history of frequent fetal loss, sudden infant death, and sudden death in adults may indicate heart disease. Congenital heart defects are seen in many syndromes such as Down and Turner syndromes.

The physical assessment of suspected cardiac disease begins with observation of general appearance and then proceeds with more specific observations. The following are supplementary to the general assessment techniques described for physical examination of the chest and heart in Chapter 29:

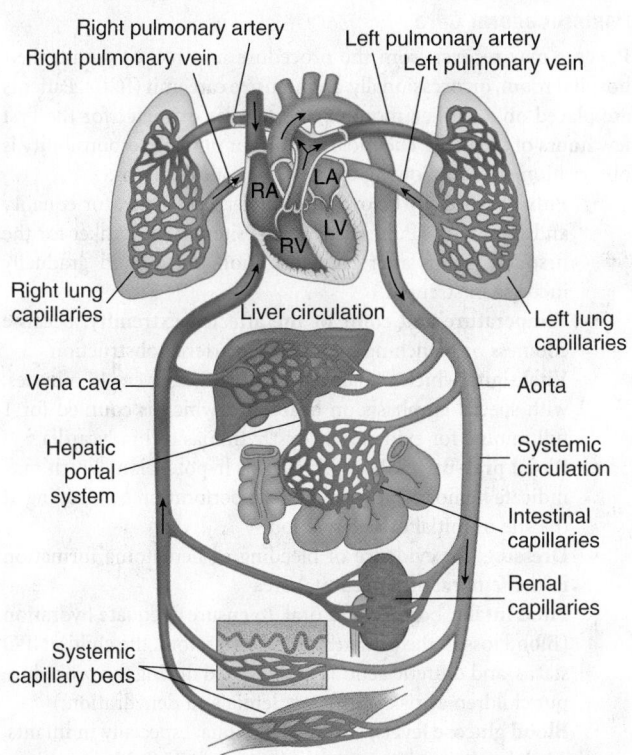

FIG 42-1 Diagram showing serially connected pulmonary and systemic circulatory systems and how to trace the flow of blood. Right heart chambers propel unoxygenated blood through the systemic circulation. *LA,* Left atrium; *LV,* left ventricle; *RA,* right atrium; *RV,* right ventricle. (From McCance KL, Heuther SE: *Pathophysiology: the biological basis for disease in adults and children,* ed 6, St Louis, 2010, Mosby.)

Inspection

Nutritional state—Failure to thrive or poor weight gain is associated with heart disease.

Color—Cyanosis is a common feature of CHD, and pallor is associated with poor perfusion.

Chest deformities—An enlarged heart sometimes distorts the chest configuration.

Unusual pulsations—Visible pulsations of the neck veins are seen in some patients.

Respiratory excursion—This refers to the ease or difficulty of respiration (e.g., tachypnea, dyspnea, expiratory grunt).

Clubbing of fingers—This is associated with cyanosis.

Palpation and Percussion

Chest—These maneuvers help discern heart size and other characteristics (e.g., thrills) associated with heart disease.

Abdomen—Hepatomegaly or splenomegaly may be evident.

Peripheral pulses—Rate, regularity, and amplitude (strength) may reveal discrepancies.

Auscultation

Heart rate and rhythm—Listen for fast heart rates (tachycardia), slow heart rates (bradycardia), and irregular rhythms.

Character of heart sounds—Listen for distinct or muffled sounds, murmurs, and additional heart sounds.

Diagnostic Evaluation

A variety of invasive and noninvasive tests may be used in the diagnosis of heart disease. Some of the more common diagnostic tools that require nursing assessment and intervention are described here.

Electrocardiogram

Bedside cardiac monitoring with the electrocardiogram (ECG) is commonly used in pediatrics, especially in the care of children with heart disease. The bedside monitor provides valuable information about heart rate and rhythm through a graphic display of the ECG tracing and a digital display. An alarm can be set with parameters for individual patient requirements and will sound if the heart rate is above or below the set parameters. Gelfoam electrodes are commonly placed on the right side of the chest (above the level of the heart) and on the left side of the chest, and a ground electrode is placed on the abdomen. Electrodes should be changed every 1 or 2 days because they irritate the skin. Bedside monitors are an adjunct to patient care and should never be substituted for direct assessment and auscultation of heart sounds. The nurse should assess the patient, not the monitor.

> **! NURSING ALERT**
>
> Electrodes for cardiac monitoring are often color coded: white for right, green (or red) for ground, and black for left. Always check to ensure that these colors are placed correctly.

Echocardiography

Echocardiography is one of the most frequently used tests for detecting cardiac dysfunction in children. Recent improvements in echocardiographic techniques have made it increasingly possible to confirm the diagnosis without resorting to cardiac catheterization. In more and more cases, a prenatal diagnosis of CHD can be made by fetal echocardiography.

Echocardiography involves the use of ultra-high-frequency sound waves to produce an image of the heart's structure. A transducer placed directly on the chest wall delivers repetitive pulses of ultrasound and processes the returned signals (echoes).

Although the test is noninvasive, painless, and associated with no known side effects, it can be stressful for children. The child must lie quietly in the standard echocardiographic positions; crying, nursing, or sitting up often leads to diagnostic errors or omissions. Therefore infants and young children may need a mild sedative; older children benefit from psychologic preparation for the test. The distraction of a video or movie is often helpful.

Cardiac Catheterization

Cardiac catheterization is an invasive diagnostic procedure in which a radiopaque catheter is inserted through a peripheral blood vessel into the heart. The catheter is usually introduced through percutaneous technique, in which the catheter is threaded through a large-bore needle that is inserted into the vein. The catheter is guided through the heart with the aid of fluoroscopy. After the tip of the catheter is within a heart chamber, contrast material is injected and films are taken of the dilution and circulation of the material (angiography). Types of cardiac catheterizations include:

Diagnostic catheterizations—These studies are used to diagnose congenital cardiac defects, particularly in symptomatic infants and before surgical repair. They are divided into (1) right-sided catheterizations, in which the catheter is introduced through a vein (usually the femoral vein) and threaded to the right atrium (most common); and (2) left-sided catheterizations, in which the catheter is threaded through an artery into the aorta and into the heart.

Interventional catheterizations (therapeutic catheterizations)— A balloon catheter or other device is used to alter the cardiac anatomy. Examples include dilating stenotic valves or vessels or closing abnormal connections.

Electrophysiology studies—Catheters with tiny electrodes that record the impulses of the heart directly from the conduction system are used to evaluate dysrhythmias and sometimes destroy accessory pathways that cause some tachydysrhythmias.

CARE MANAGEMENT

Cardiac catheterization has become a routine diagnostic procedure and may be done on an outpatient basis. However, it is not without risks, especially in neonates and seriously ill infants and children. Possible complications include acute hemorrhage from the entry site (more likely with interventional procedures because larger catheters are used), low-grade fever, nausea, vomiting, loss of pulse in the catheterized extremity (usually transient, resulting from a clot, hematoma, or intimal tear), and transient dysrhythmias (generally catheter induced) (Uzark, 2001). Rare risks include stroke, seizures, tamponade, and death.

Preprocedural Care

A complete nursing assessment is necessary to ensure a safe procedure with minimum complications. This assessment should include accurate height (essential for correct catheter selection) and weight. Obtaining a history of allergic reactions is important because some of the contrast agents are iodine based. Specific attention to signs and symptoms of infection is crucial. Severe diaper rash may be a reason to cancel the procedure if femoral access is required. Because assessment of pedal pulses is important after catheterization, the nurse should assess and mark the pulses (dorsalis pedis, posterior tibial) before the child goes to the catheterization room. The presence and quality of pulses in both feet are clearly documented. Baseline oxygen saturation using pulse oximetry in children with cyanosis is also recorded.

Preparing the child and family for the procedure is the joint responsibility of the patient care team. School-age children and adolescents benefit from a description of the catheterization laboratory and a chronologic explanation of the procedure, emphasizing what they will see, feel, and hear. Older children and adolescents may bring earphones and favorite music so they can listen during the catheterization procedure. Preparation materials such as picture books, videotapes, or tours of the catheterization laboratory may be helpful. Preparation should be geared to the child's developmental level. The child's caregivers often benefit from the same explanations. Additional information, such as the expected length of the catheterization, description of the child's appearance after catheterization, and usual postprocedure care, should be outlined. (See also Prepare the Child and Family for Invasive Procedures, p. 1341.)

Methods of sedation vary among institutions and may include oral or intravenous (IV) medications. The child's age, heart defect, clinical status, and type of catheterization procedure planned are considered when sedation is determined. General anesthesia may be needed for some interventional procedures. Children are allowed nothing by mouth (NPO) for 4 to 6 hours or more before the procedure according to institutional guidelines. Infants and patients with polycythemia may need IV fluids to prevent dehydration and hypoglycemia.

Postprocedural Care

Patients may recover from the procedure in a recovery unit, their hospital room, or, occasionally, an intensive care unit (ICU). Patients are placed on a cardiac monitor and a pulse oximeter for the first few hours of recovery. The most important nursing responsibility is observation of the following for signs of complications:

- **Pulses**, especially below the catheterization site, for equality and symmetry (Pulse distal to the site may be weaker for the first few hours after catheterization but should gradually increase in strength.)
- **Temperature and color of the affected extremity**, because coolness or blanching may indicate arterial obstruction
- **Vital signs**, which are taken as frequently as every 15 minutes, with special emphasis on heart rate, which is counted for 1 full minute for evidence of dysrhythmias or bradycardia
- **Blood pressure (BP)**, especially for hypotension, which may indicate hemorrhage from cardiac perforation or bleeding at the site of initial catheterization
- **Dressing**, for evidence of bleeding or hematoma formation in the femoral or antecubital area
- **Fluid intake**, both IV and oral, to ensure adequate hydration (Blood loss in the catheterization laboratory, the child's NPO status, and diuretic actions of dyes used during the procedure put children at risk for hypovolemia and dehydration.)
- **Blood glucose levels**, for hypoglycemia, especially in infants, who should receive dextrose-containing IV fluids

> **! NURSING ALERT**
>
> If bleeding occurs, direct continuous pressure is applied 2.5 cm (1 inch) above the percutaneous skin site to localize pressure over the vessel puncture.

Depending on hospital policy, the child may be kept in bed with the affected extremity maintained straight for 4 to 6 hours after venous catheterization and 6 to 8 hours after arterial catheterization to facilitate healing of the cannulated vessel. If younger children have difficulty complying, they can be held in the parent's lap with the leg maintained in the correct position. The child's usual diet can be resumed as soon as tolerated, beginning with sips of clear liquids and advancing as the condition allows. The child is encouraged to void to clear the contrast material from the blood. Generally, there is only slight discomfort at the percutaneous site. To prevent infection, the catheterization area is protected from possible contamination. If the child wears diapers, the dressing can be kept dry by covering it with a piece of plastic film and sealing the edges of the film to the skin with tape. However, the nurse must be careful to continue observing the site for any evidence of bleeding (see Family-Centered Care box and Critical Thinking Case Study).

CONGENITAL HEART DISEASE

The incidence of CHD in children is approximately 5 to 8 per 1000 live births (Park, 2008). About 2 or 3 in 1000 infants will be symptomatic during the first year of life with significant heart disease that requires treatment (Hoffman and Kaplan, 2002). CHD is the major cause of death (other than prematurity) in the first year of life. Although there are more than 35 well-recognized cardiac defects, the most common heart anomaly is ventricular septal defect (VSD).

The exact cause of most congenital cardiac defects is unknown. Most are thought to be a result of multiple factors, including a

FAMILY-CENTERED CARE

After Cardiac Catheterization

- Remove pressure dressing the day after catheterization. Cover site with an adhesive bandage strip for several days.
- Keep site clean and dry. Avoid tub baths for several days; patient may shower.
- Observe site for redness, swelling, drainage, and bleeding. Monitor for fever. Notify health care practitioner if these occur.
- Avoid strenuous exercise for several days; patient may attend school.
- Resume regular diet without restrictions.
- Use acetaminophen or ibuprofen for pain.
- Keep follow-up appointments per health care practitioner's instruction.

Adapted from Children's Hospital (Boston) Cardiovascular Program, 1996.

? CRITICAL THINKING CASE STUDY

Cardiac Catheterization

Tommy, a 3-year-old boy with tetralogy of Fallot, has just returned to his hospital room from the cardiac catheterization recovery room. His mother calls you to the bedside to tell you that he is vomiting and bleeding. You arrive to find Tommy anxious, pale, crying, and sitting in a puddle of blood.

1. Evidence—Is there sufficient evidence to draw conclusions about Tommy's situation?
2. Assumptions—Describe an underlying assumption about each of the following:
   a. Risks of cardiac catheterization
   b. Association between vomiting and bleeding after cardiac catheterization
   c. Concerns related to acute blood loss
3. What priorities for nursing care should be established for Tommy?
4. Does the evidence support your nursing interventions?

complex interaction of genetic and environmental influences. Some risk factors are known to be associated with increased incidence of congenital heart defects. Maternal risk factors include chronic illnesses such as diabetes or poorly controlled phenylketonuria, alcohol consumption, and exposure to environmental toxins and infections. Family history of a cardiac defect in a parent or sibling increases the likelihood of a cardiac anomaly. The risk for CHD increases if a first-degree relative (parent or sibling) is affected. The familial risk is higher with left-sided obstructive lesions.

Congenital heart anomalies are often associated with chromosomal abnormalities, specific syndromes, or congenital defects in other body systems. Down syndrome (trisomy 21) and trisomies 13 and 18 are highly correlated with congenital heart defects. Syndromes associated with heart defects include DiGeorge syndrome, a syndrome characterized by deletion of part of chromosome 22q11 (interrupted aortic arch, truncus arteriosus, tetralogy of Fallot, and posterior malaligned VSDs), Noonan syndrome (pulmonic valve anomalies and cardiomyopathy), Williams syndrome (aortic and pulmonic stenosis), and Holt-Oram syndrome (upper limb anomalies and atrial septal defect [ASD]). Extracardiac defects such as tracheoesophageal fistula, renal abnormalities, and diaphragmatic hernia are seen in association with heart anomalies.

Altered Hemodynamics

To appreciate the physiology of heart defects, it is necessary to understand the role of pressure gradients, flow, and resistance within the circulation. As blood is pumped through the heart, it (1) flows from an area of high pressure to one of low pressure and (2) takes the path of least resistance. In general, the higher the pressure gradient, the faster the rate of flow; the higher the resistance, the slower the rate of flow.

Normally, the pressure on the right side of the heart is lower than that on the left side and the resistance in the pulmonary circulation is less than that in the systemic circulation. Vessels entering or exiting these chambers have corresponding pressures. Therefore, if an abnormal connection exists between the heart chambers (e.g., a septal defect), blood will necessarily flow from an area of higher pressure (left side) to one of lower pressure (right side). Such a flow of blood is termed a left-to-right shunt. Anomalies resulting in cyanosis may result from a change in pressure so that the blood is shunted from the right to the left side of the heart (right-to-left shunt) because of either increased pulmonary vascular resistance or obstruction to blood flow through the pulmonic valve and artery. Cyanosis may also result from a defect that allows mixing of oxygenated and deoxygenated blood within the heart chambers or great arteries, such as occurs in truncus arteriosus.

Classification of Defects

There are typically two classification systems used to categorize congenital heart defects. Traditionally, cyanosis, a physical characteristic, has been used as the distinguishing feature, dividing anomalies into acyanotic defects and cyanotic defects (Fig. 42-2). In clinical practice, this system is problematic because children with acyanotic defects may develop cyanosis. Also, more often, those with cyanotic defects may appear pink and have more clinical signs of HF.

A more useful classification system is based on hemodynamic characteristics (blood flow patterns within the heart). These blood flow patterns are (1) increased pulmonary blood flow; (2) decreased pulmonary blood flow; (3) obstruction to blood flow out of the heart; and (4) mixed blood flow, in which saturated and desaturated blood mix within the heart or great arteries. As a comparison, Fig. 42-3 outlines both classification systems. With the hemodynamic classification system, the clinical manifestations of each group are more uniform and predictable. Defects that allow blood flow from the higher-pressure left side of the heart to the lower-pressure right side (left-to-right shunt) result in increased pulmonary blood flow and cause heart failure (HF). Obstructive defects impede blood flow out of the ventricles; whereas obstruction on the left side of the heart results in HF, severe obstruction on the right side causes cyanosis. Defects that cause decreased pulmonary blood flow result in cyanosis. Mixed lesions present a variable clinical picture based on the degree of mixing and amount of pulmonary blood flow; hypoxemia (with or without cyanosis) and HF usually occur together. Using this classification system, the clinical presentation and management of the most common defects are outlined in the following sections and Box 42-1.

The outcomes of surgical treatment for patients with moderate to severe disease are variable. Patient risk factors for increased morbidity and mortality include prematurity or low birth weight, a genetic syndrome, multiple cardiac defects, a noncardiac congenital anomaly, and age at time of surgery (neonates are a higher risk group). For example, aortic stenosis or coarctation manifesting in the first week of life is more severe and carries a higher mortality than if it becomes apparent at 1 year of age. Outcomes for surgical repair of similar congenital heart defects also vary among treatment centers. In general, the outcomes of surgical procedures have steadily improved in the past decade, with mortality rates for many severe

BOX 42-1   DEFECTS WITH INCREASED PULMONARY BLOOD FLOW

Atrial Septal Defect

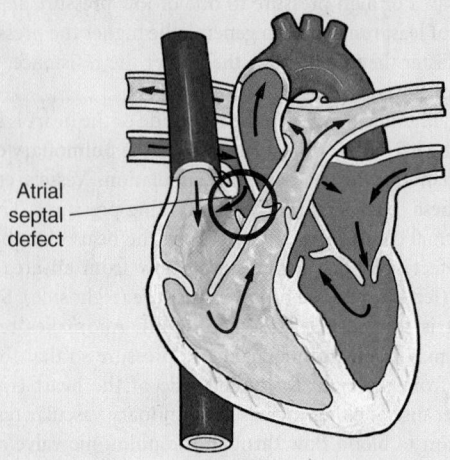

Atrial septal defect

Ventricular Septal Defect

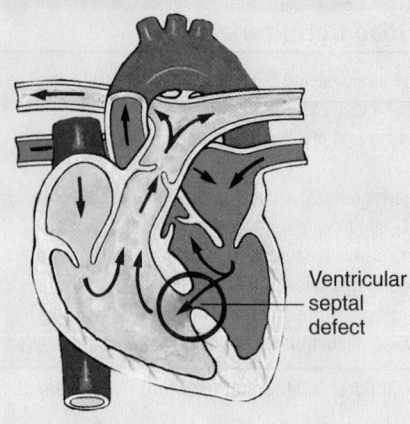

Ventricular septal defect

Description—Abnormal opening between the atria, allowing blood from the higher-pressure left atrium to flow into the lower-pressure right atrium. There are three types of ASD:

- *Ostium primum (ASD 1)*—Opening at lower end of septum; may be associated with mitral valve abnormalities
- *Ostium secundum (ASD 2)*—Opening near center of septum
- *Sinus venosus defect*—Opening near junction of superior vena cava and right atrium; may be associated with partial anomalous pulmonary venous connection

Pathophysiology—Because left atrial pressure slightly exceeds right atrial pressure, blood flows from the left to the right atrium, causing an increased flow of oxygenated blood into the right side of the heart. Despite the low pressure difference, a high rate of flow can still occur because of low pulmonary vascular resistance and the greater distensibility of the right atrium, which further reduces flow resistance. This volume is well tolerated by the right ventricle because it is delivered under much lower pressure than with a VSD. Although there is right atrial and ventricular enlargement, cardiac failure is unusual in an uncomplicated ASD. Pulmonary vascular changes usually occur only after several decades if the defect is left unrepaired.

Clinical manifestations—Patients may be asymptomatic. They may develop HF. There is a characteristic systolic murmur with a fixed split second heart sound. There may also be a diastolic murmur. Patients are at risk for atrial dysrhythmias (probably caused by atrial enlargement and stretching of conduction fibers) and pulmonary vascular obstructive disease and emboli formation later in life from chronically increased pulmonary blood flow.

Surgical treatment—Surgical patch closure (pericardial patch or Dacron patch) is done for moderate to large defects. Open repair with cardiopulmonary bypass is usually performed before school age. In addition, the sinus venosus defect requires patch placement, so the anomalous right pulmonary venous return is directed to the left atrium with a baffle. ASD 1 type may require mitral valve repair or, rarely, replacement of the mitral valve.

Nonsurgical treatment—ASD 2 closure with a device during cardiac catheterization is becoming commonplace and can be done as an outpatient procedure. The Amplatzer Septal Occluder is most commonly used. Smaller defects that have a rim around them for attachment of the device can be closed with a device; large, irregular defects without a rim require surgical closure. Successful closure in appropriately selected patients yields results similar to those from surgery but involves shorter hospital stays and fewer complications. Patients receive low-dose aspirin for 6 months (Rome and Kreutzer, 2004).

Prognosis—Operative mortality is very low (<1%).

Description—Abnormal opening between the right and left ventricles. May be classified according to location: membranous (accounting for 80%); or muscular. May vary in size from a small pinhole to absence of the septum, which results in a common ventricle. VSDs are frequently associated with other defects, such as pulmonary stenosis, transposition of the great vessels, PDA, atrial defects, and COA. Many VSDs (20%-60%) close spontaneously. Spontaneous closure is most likely to occur during the first year of life in children having small or moderate defects. A left-to-right shunt is caused by the flow of blood from the higher-pressure left ventricle to the lower-pressure right ventricle.

Pathophysiology—Because of the higher pressure within the left ventricle and because the systemic arterial circulation offers more resistance than the pulmonary circulation, blood flows through the defect into the pulmonary artery. The increased blood volume is pumped into the lungs, which may eventually result in increased pulmonary vascular resistance. Increased pressure in the right ventricle as a result of left-to-right shunting and pulmonary resistance causes the muscle to hypertrophy. If the right ventricle is unable to accommodate the increased workload, the right atrium may also enlarge as it attempts to overcome the resistance offered by incomplete right ventricular emptying.

Clinical manifestations—HF is common. There is a characteristic loud holosystolic murmur heard best at the left sternal border. Patients are at risk for BE and pulmonary vascular obstructive disease.

Surgical Treatment

- *Palliative*—Pulmonary artery banding (placement of a band around the main pulmonary artery to decrease pulmonary blood flow) may be done in infants with multiple muscular VSDs or complex anatomy. Improvements in surgical techniques and postoperative care make complete repair in infancy the preferred approach.
- *Complete repair (procedure of choice)*—Small defects are repaired with sutures. Large defects usually require that a knitted Dacron patch be sewn over the opening. CPB is used for both procedures. The approach for the repair is generally through the right atrium and the tricuspid valve. Postoperative complications include residual VSD and conduction disturbances.

Nonsurgical treatment—Device closure during cardiac catheterization is being performed in some centers under investigational protocols. One device has been approved for closure of muscular defects, and another is in clinical trials. Early results are encouraging, with successful defect closure and few complications (Rome and Kreutzer, 2004).

Prognosis—Risks depend on the location of the defect, the number of defects, and the presence of other associated cardiac defects. Single-membranous defects are associated with low mortality (<2%); multiple muscular defects can carry a higher risk (Jacobs, Mavroudis, Jacobs, et al., 2004).

BOX 42-1   DEFECTS WITH INCREASED PULMONARY BLOOD FLOW—cont'd

Atrioventricular Canal Defect

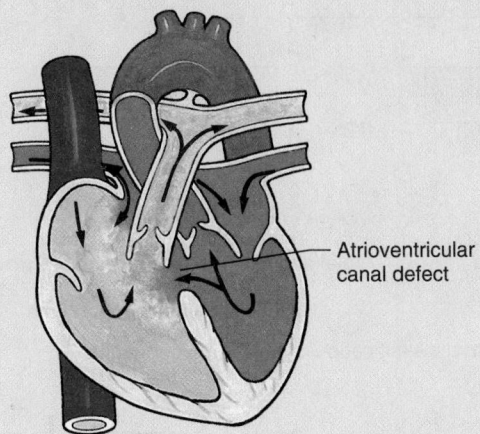

Atrioventricular canal defect

Patent Ductus Arteriosus

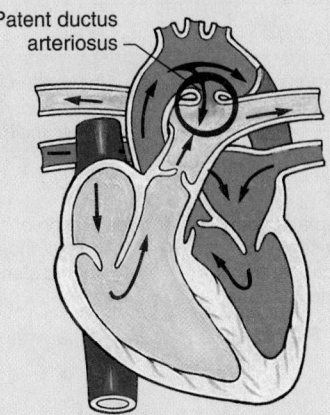

Patent ductus arteriosus

Description—Incomplete fusion of the endocardial cushions. Consists of a low ASD that is continuous with a high VSD and clefts of the mitral and tricuspid valves, which create a large central AV valve that allows blood to flow between all four chambers of the heart. The directions and pathways of flow are determined by pulmonary and systemic resistance, left and right ventricular pressures, and the compliance of each chamber, although flow is generally from left to right. It is the most common cardiac defect in children with Down syndrome.

Pathophysiology—The alterations in hemodynamics depend on the severity of the defect and the child's pulmonary vascular resistance. Immediately after birth, while the newborn's pulmonary vascular resistance is high, there is minimum shunting of blood through the defect. When this resistance falls, left-to-right shunting occurs and pulmonary blood flow increases. The resultant pulmonary vascular engorgement predisposes the child to development of HF.

Clinical manifestations—Patients usually have moderate to severe HF. There is a loud systolic murmur. There may be mild cyanosis that increases with crying. Patients are at high risk for developing pulmonary vascular obstructive disease.

Surgical Treatment

- *Palliative*—Pulmonary artery banding is occasionally done in small infants with severe symptoms. Complete repair in infancy is most common.
- *Complete repair*—Surgical repair consists of patch closure of the septal defects and reconstruction of the AV valve tissue (either repair of the mitral valve cleft or fashioning of two AV valves). Postoperative complications include heart block, HF, mitral regurgitation, dysrhythmias, and pulmonary hypertension.

Prognosis—Operative mortality is less than 5% (Jacobs, Mavroudis, Jacobs, et al., 2004). A potential later problem is mitral regurgitation, which may require valve replacement.

Description—Failure of the fetal ductus arteriosus (artery connecting the aorta and pulmonary artery) to close within the first weeks of life. The continued patency of this vessel allows blood to flow from the higher-pressure aorta to the lower-pressure pulmonary artery, which causes a left-to-right shunt.

Pathophysiology—The hemodynamic consequences of PDA depend on the size of the ductus and the pulmonary vascular resistance. At birth, the resistance in the pulmonary and systemic circulations is almost identical, so that the resistance in the aorta and pulmonary artery is equalized. As the systemic pressure comes to exceed the pulmonary pressure, blood begins to shunt from the aorta across the duct to the pulmonary artery (left-to-right shunt). The additional blood is recirculated through the lungs and returned to the left atrium and left ventricle. The effects of this altered circulation are increased workload on the left side of the heart, increased pulmonary vascular congestion and possibly resistance, and potentially increased right ventricular pressure and hypertrophy.

Clinical manifestations—Patients may be asymptomatic or show signs of HF. There is a characteristic machinery-like murmur. A widened pulse pressure and bounding pulses result from runoff of blood from the aorta to the pulmonary artery. Patients are at risk for BE and pulmonary vascular obstructive disease in later life from chronic excessive pulmonary blood flow.

Medical management—Administration of indomethacin (a prostaglandin inhibitor) has proved successful in closing a PDA in preterm infants and some newborns.

Surgical treatment—Surgical division or ligation of the patent vessel is performed via a left thoracotomy. In a newer technique, video-assisted thoracoscopic surgery, a thoracoscope and instruments are inserted through three small incisions on the left side of the chest to place a clip on the ductus. The technique is used in some centers and eliminates the need for a thoracotomy, thereby speeding postoperative recovery.

Nonsurgical treatment—Coils to occlude the PDA are placed in the catheterization laboratory in many centers. Preterm or small infants (with small-diameter femoral arteries) and patients with large or unusual PDAs may require surgery.

Prognosis—Both surgical and nonsurgical procedures can be done at low risk with less than 1% mortality. PDA closure in very preterm infants has a higher mortality rate because of the additional significant medical problems.

ASD, Atrial septal defect; *AV*, atrioventricular; *BE*, bacterial endocarditis; *COA*, coarctation of the aorta; *CPB*, cardiopulmonary bypass; *HF*, heart failure; *PDA*, patent ductus arteriosus; *VSD*, ventricular septal defect.

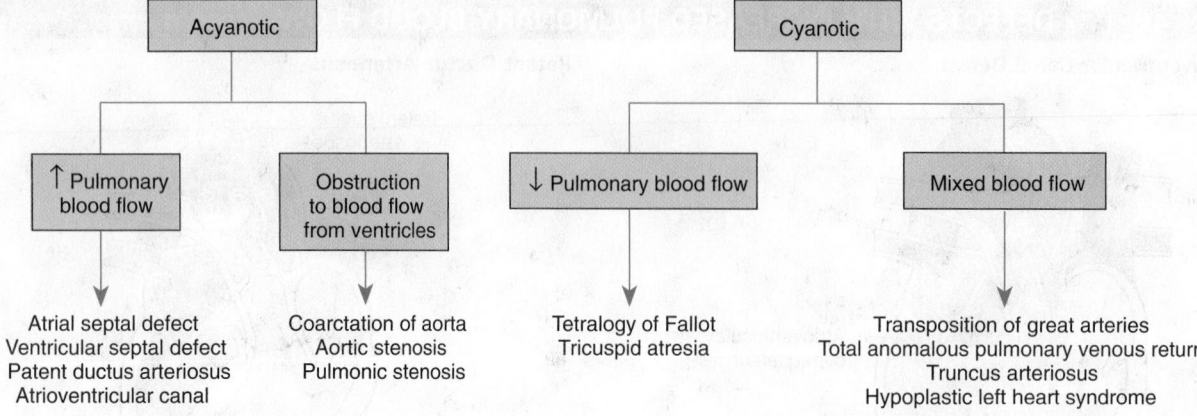

FIG 42-2 Comparison of acyanotic-cyanotic and hemodynamic classification systems of congenital heart disease.

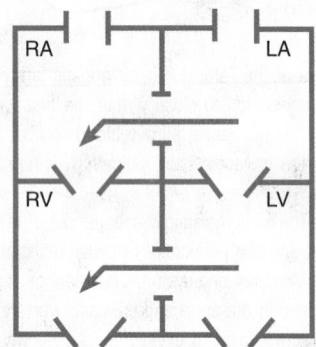

FIG 42-3 Hemodynamics in defects with increased pulmonary blood flow. *LA,* Left atrium; *LV,* left ventricle; *RA,* right atrium; *RV,* right ventricle.

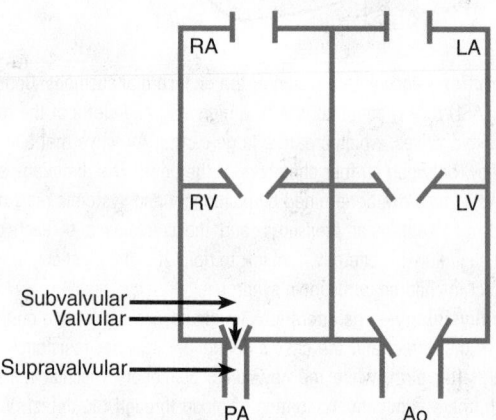

FIG 42-4 Obstruction to ventricular ejection can occur at the valvular level *(shown),* below the valve (subvalvular), or above the valve (supravalvular). Pulmonary stenosis is shown here. *Ao,* Aorta; *LA,* left atrium; *LV,* left ventricle; *PA,* pulmonary artery; *RA,* right atrium; *RV,* right ventricle.

defects below 10% and a decrease in the incidence of complications and length of hospital stay.

Defects with Increased Pulmonary Blood Flow

In this group of cardiac defects, intracardiac communications along the septum or an abnormal connection between the great arteries allows blood to flow from the higher pressure left side of the heart to the lower pressure right side of the heart. Increased blood volume on the right side of the heart increases pulmonary blood flow at the expense of systemic blood flow. Clinically, patients demonstrate signs and symptoms of HF. ASD, VSD, and patent ductus arteriosus are typical anomalies in this group (see Box 42-1).

Obstructive Defects

Obstructive defects are those in which blood exiting the heart meets an area of anatomic narrowing (stenosis), causing obstruction to blood flow. The pressure in the ventricle and in the great artery before the obstruction is increased, and the pressure in the area beyond the obstruction is decreased. The location of the narrowing is usually near the valve (Fig. 42-4), as follows:

- **Valvular**—At the site of the valve itself
- **Subvalvular**—Narrowing in the ventricle below the valve (also referred to as the ventricular outflow tract)
- **Supravalvular**—Narrowing in the great artery above the valve

Coarctation of the aorta (narrowing of the aortic arch), aortic stenosis, and pulmonic stenosis are typical defects in this group (Box 42-2). Hemodynamically, there is a pressure load on the ventricle and decreased cardiac output. Clinically, infants and children exhibit

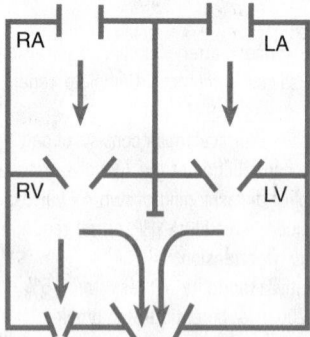

FIG 42-5 Hemodynamic defects with decreased pulmonary blood flow. *LA,* Left atrium; *LV,* left ventricle; *RA,* right atrium; *RV,* right ventricle.

signs of HF. Children with mild obstruction may be asymptomatic. Rarely, as in severe pulmonic stenosis, hypoxemia may be seen.

Defects with Decreased Pulmonary Blood Flow

In this group of defects, there is obstruction of pulmonary blood flow and an anatomic defect (ASD or VSD) between the right and left sides of the heart (Fig. 42-5). Because blood has difficulty exiting the right side of the heart via the pulmonary artery, pressure on the right side increases, exceeding left-sided pressure. This allows

BOX 42-2   OBSTRUCTIVE DEFECTS

Coarctation of the Aorta

Description—Localized narrowing near the insertion of the ductus arteriosus, which results in increased pressure proximal to the defect (head and upper extremities) and decreased pressure distal to the obstruction (body and lower extremities).

Pathophysiology—The effect of a narrowing within the aorta is increased pressure proximal to the defect (upper extremities) and decreased pressure distal to it (lower extremities).

Clinical manifestations—The patient may have high blood pressure and bounding pulses in the arms, weak or absent femoral pulses, and cool lower extremities with lower blood pressure. There are signs of HF in infants. In infants with critical coarctation, the hemodynamic condition may deteriorate rapidly with severe acidosis and hypotension. Mechanical ventilation and inotropic support are often necessary before surgery. Older children may experience dizziness, headaches, fainting, and epistaxis resulting from hypertension. Patients are at risk for hypertension, ruptured aorta, aortic aneurysm, and stroke.

Surgical treatment—Surgical repair is the treatment of choice for infants younger than 6 months and for patients with long-segment stenosis or complex anatomy; it may be performed for all patients with coarctation. Repair is by resection of the coarctated portion with an end-to-end anastomosis of the aorta or enlargement of the constricted section using a graft of prosthetic material or a portion of the left subclavian artery. Because this defect is outside the heart and pericardium, cardiopulmonary bypass is not required and a thoracotomy incision is used. Postoperative hypertension is treated with intravenous sodium nitroprusside, esmolol, or milrinone followed by oral medications, such as ACE inhibitors or beta blockers. Residual permanent hypertension after repair of COA seems to be related to age and time of repair. To prevent both hypertension at rest and exercise-provoked systemic hypertension after repair, elective surgery for COA is advised within the first 2 years of life. There is a 15% to 30% risk

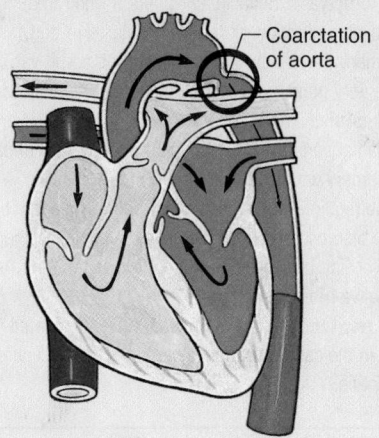

Coarctation of aorta

for recurrence in patients who underwent surgical repair as infants (Beekman, 2001). Percutaneous balloon angioplasty techniques have proved to be effective in relieving residual postoperative coarctation gradients.

Nonsurgical treatment—Balloon angioplasty is being performed as a primary intervention for COA in older infants and children. In adolescents, stents may be placed in the aorta to maintain patency. Recent studies have demonstrated that balloon angioplasty is effective in children and that aneurysm formation is rare. The high restenosis rate in young infants limits its application in this group (Rome and Kreutzer, 2004).

Prognosis—Mortality is less than 5% in patients with isolated coarctation; the risk is increased in infants with other complex cardiac defects (Jacobs, Mavroudis, Jacobs, et al., 2004).

Aortic Stenosis

Description—Narrowing or stricture of the aortic valve, causing resistance to blood flow in the left ventricle, decreased cardiac output, left ventricular hypertrophy, and pulmonary vascular congestion. The prominent anatomic consequence of AS is the hypertrophy of the left ventricular wall, which eventually leads to increased end-diastolic pressure, resulting in pulmonary venous and pulmonary arterial hypertension. Left ventricular hypertrophy also interferes with coronary artery perfusion and may result in myocardial infarction or scarring of the papillary muscles of the left ventricle, which causes mitral insufficiency. Valvular stenosis, the most common type, is usually caused by malformed cusps that result in a bicuspid rather than tricuspid valve or fusion of the cusps. Subvalvular stenosis is a stricture caused by a fibrous ring below a normal valve; supravalvular stenosis occurs infrequently. Valvular AS is a serious defect for the following reasons: (1) the obstruction tends to be progressive; (2) sudden episodes of myocardial ischemia, or low cardiac output, can result in sudden death; and (3) surgical repair rarely results in a normal valve. This is one of the rare instances in which strenuous physical activity may be curtailed because of the cardiac condition.

Pathophysiology—A stricture in the aortic outflow tract causes resistance to ejection of blood from the left ventricle. The extra workload on the left ventricle causes hypertrophy. If left ventricular failure develops, left atrial pressure will increase; this causes increased pressure in the pulmonary veins, which results in pulmonary vascular congestion (pulmonary edema).

Clinical manifestations—Newborns with critical AS demonstrate signs of decreased cardiac output with faint pulses, hypotension, tachycardia, and

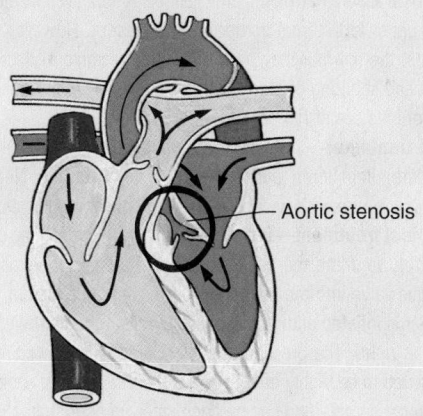

Aortic stenosis

poor feeding. Children show signs of exercise intolerance, chest pain, and dizziness when standing for a long period. A systolic ejection murmur may or may not be present. Patients are at risk for BE, coronary insufficiency, and ventricular dysfunction.

Valvular Aortic Stenosis

Surgical treatment—Aortic valvotomy is performed under inflow occlusion. Used rarely because balloon dilation in the catheterization laboratory is the first-line procedure. Newborns with critical AS and small left-sided structures may undergo a stage 1 Norwood procedure (see Hypoplastic Left Heart Syndrome, Box 42-4).

Continued

BOX 42-2   OBSTRUCTIVE DEFECTS—cont'd

Prognosis—Aortic valve replacement offers a good treatment option and may lead to normalization of left ventricular size and function (Arnold, Ley-Zaporozhan, Ley, et al., 2008). Results of aortic valvotomy in older children are very good, with mortality and morbidity close to 0% (Shanmugam, MacArthur, and Pollock, 2005). However, aortic valvotomy remains a palliative procedure and approximately 25% of patients require additional surgery within 10 years for recurrent stenosis. A valve replacement may be required at the second procedure. An aortic homograft with a valve may also be used (extended aortic root replacement), or the pulmonary valve may be moved to the aortic position and replaced with a homograft valve (Ross procedure).

Nonsurgical treatment—The narrowed valve is dilated using balloon angioplasty in the catheterization laboratory. This procedure is usually the first intervention.

Prognosis—Complications include aortic insufficiency or valvular regurgitation, tearing of the valve leaflets, and loss of pulse in the catheterized limb.

Subvalvular Aortic Stenosis

Surgical treatment—Procedure may involve incising a membrane if one exists or cutting the fibromuscular ring. If the obstruction results from narrowing of the left ventricular outflow tract and a small aortic valve annulus, a patch may be required to enlarge the entire left ventricular outflow tract and annulus and replace the aortic valve; this is known as the *Konno procedure.*

Prognosis—Mortality from surgical repairs of subvalvular AS is less than 5% in major centers; however, about 20% of these patients develop recurrent subaortic stenosis and require additional surgery (Freed, 2001).

Pulmonic Stenosis

Description—Narrowing at the entrance to the pulmonary artery. Resistance to blood flow causes right ventricular hypertrophy and decreased pulmonary blood flow. Pulmonary atresia is the extreme form of PS in that there is total fusion of the commissures and no blood flows to the lungs. The right ventricle may be hypoplastic.

Pathophysiology—When PS is present, resistance to blood flow causes right ventricular hypertrophy. If right ventricular failure develops, right atrial pressure will increase and this may result in reopening of the foramen ovale, shunting of unoxygenated blood into the left atrium, and systemic cyanosis. If PS is severe, HF occurs and systemic venous engorgement will be noted. An associated defect such as a PDA partially compensates for the obstruction by shunting blood from the aorta to the pulmonary artery and into the lungs.

Clinical manifestations—Patients may be asymptomatic; some have mild cyanosis or HF. Progressive narrowing causes increased symptoms. Newborns with severe narrowing are cyanotic. A loud systolic ejection murmur at the upper left sternal border may be present. However, in severely ill patients, the murmur may be much softer because of decreased cardiac output and shunting of blood. Cardiomegaly is evident on chest radiography. Patients are at risk for BE.

Surgical treatment—In infants, transventricular (closed) valvotomy (Brock procedure). In children, pulmonary valvotomy with CPB. Need for surgical treatment is rare with widespread use of balloon angioplasty techniques.

Nonsurgical treatment—Balloon angioplasty in the cardiac catheterization laboratory to dilate the valve. A catheter is inserted across the stenotic pulmonic valve into the pulmonary artery, and a balloon at the end of the catheter is inflated and rapidly passed through the narrowed opening (see figure at right). The procedure is associated with few complications and has proved to be highly effective. It is the treatment of choice for discrete PS in most centers and can be done safely in neonates.

Prognosis—The risk is low for both surgical and nonsurgical procedures; mortality is lower than 1% and slightly higher in neonates (Latson, 2001). Both balloon dilation and surgical valvotomy leave the pulmonic valve incompetent because they involve opening the fused valve leaflets; however, these patients are clinically asymptomatic. Long-term problems with restenosis or valve incompetence may occur.

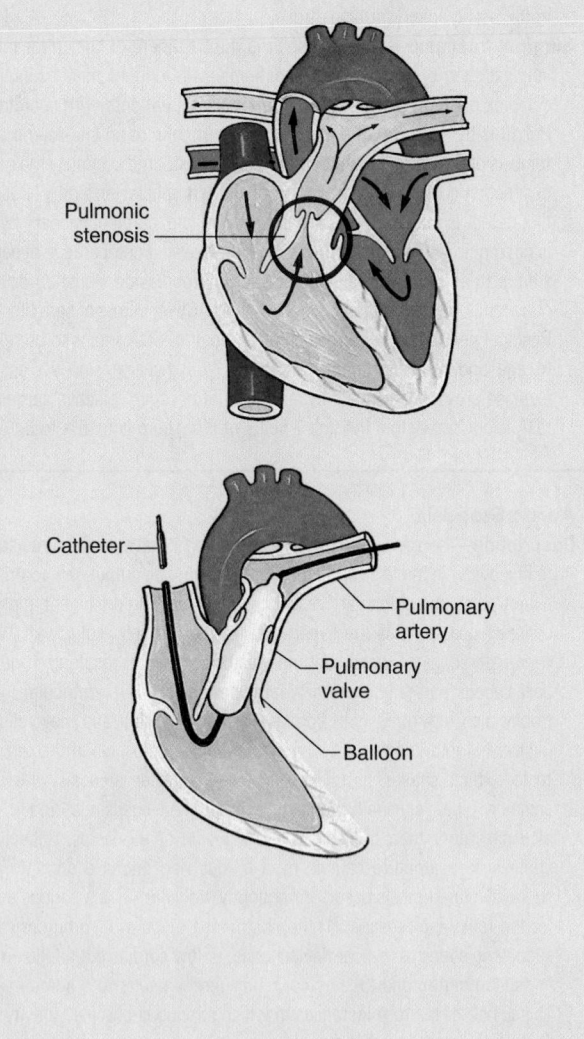

Pulmonic stenosis

Catheter

Pulmonary artery

Pulmonary valve

Balloon

ACE, Angiotensin-converting enzyme; *AS,* aortic stenosis; *BE,* bacterial endocarditis; *COA,* coarctation of the aorta; *CPB,* cardiopulmonary bypass; *HF,* heart failure; *PDA,* patent ductus arteriosus; *PS,* pulmonic stenosis.

desaturated blood to shunt right to left, causing desaturation in the left side of the heart and in the systemic circulation. Clinically, these patients have hypoxemia and usually appear cyanotic. Tetralogy of Fallot and tricuspid atresia are the most common defects in this group (Box 42-3).

Mixed Defects

Many complex cardiac anomalies are classified together in the **mixed** category (Box 42-4) because survival in the postnatal period depends on mixing of blood from the pulmonary and systemic circulations within the heart chambers. Hemodynamically, fully saturated systemic blood flow mixes with the desaturated pulmonary blood flow, causing a relative desaturation of the systemic blood flow. Pulmonary congestion occurs because the differences in pulmonary artery pressure and aortic pressure favor pulmonary blood flow. Cardiac output decreases because of a volume load on the ventricle. Clinically, these patients have a variable picture that combines some degree of desaturation (although cyanosis is not always visible) and

---

BOX 42-3   DEFECTS WITH DECREASED PULMONARY BLOOD FLOW

Tetralogy of Fallot

Description—The classic form includes four defects: (1) VSD, (2) PS, (3) overriding aorta, and (4) right ventricular hypertrophy.

Pathophysiology—The alteration in hemodynamics varies widely, depending primarily on the degree of PS but also on the size of the VSD and the pulmonary and systemic resistance to flow. Because the VSD is usually large, pressures may be equal in the right and left ventricles. Therefore the shunt direction depends on the difference between pulmonary and systemic vascular resistance. If pulmonary vascular resistance is higher than systemic resistance, the shunt is from right to left. If systemic resistance is higher than pulmonary resistance, the shunt is from left to right. PS decreases blood flow to the lungs and consequently the amount of oxygenated blood that returns to the left side of the heart. Depending on the position of the aorta, blood from both ventricles may be distributed systemically.

Clinical manifestations—Some infants may be acutely cyanotic at birth; others have mild cyanosis that progresses over the first year of life as the PS worsens. There is a characteristic systolic murmur that is often moderate in intensity. There may be acute episodes of cyanosis and hypoxia, called *blue spells* or *tet spells* (see p. 1337). Anoxic spells occur when the infant's oxygen requirements exceed the blood supply, usually during crying or after feeding. Patients are at risk for emboli, seizures, and loss of consciousness or sudden death after an anoxic spell.

Surgical Treatment

- *Palliative shunt*—In infants who cannot undergo primary repair, a palliative procedure to increase pulmonary blood flow and increase oxygen saturation may be performed. The preferred procedure is a modified Blalock-Taussig shunt operation, which provides blood flow to the pulmonary arteries from the left or right subclavian artery via a tube graft (see Table 42-2). In general, however, shunts are avoided because they may result in pulmonary artery distortion.

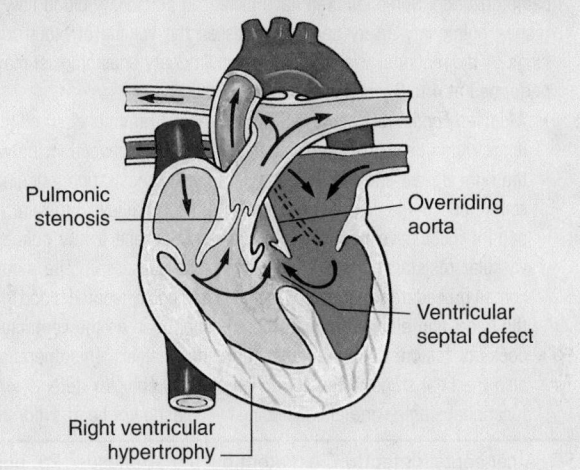

Pulmonic stenosis

Overriding aorta

Ventricular septal defect

Right ventricular hypertrophy

- *Complete repair*—Elective repair is usually performed in the first year of life. Indications for repair include increasing cyanosis and the development of hypercyanotic spells. Complete repair involves closure of the VSD and resection of the infundibular stenosis, with placement of a pericardial patch to enlarge the RVOT. In some repairs, the patch may extend across the pulmonary valve annulus (transannular patch), making the pulmonary valve incompetent. The procedure requires a median sternotomy and the use of cardiopulmonary bypass.

Prognosis—The operative mortality for total correction of tetralogy of Fallot is less than 3% (Jacobs, Mavroudis, Jacobs, et al., 2004). With improved surgical techniques, there is a lower incidence of dysrhythmias and sudden death; surgical heart block is rare. Heart failure may occur postoperatively.

Tricuspid Atresia

Description—The tricuspid valve fails to develop; consequently there is no communication from the right atrium to the right ventricle. Blood flows through an ASD or a patent foramen ovale to the left side of the heart and through a VSD to the right ventricle and out to the lungs. The condition is often associated with PS and TGA. There is complete mixing of unoxygenated and oxygenated blood in the left side of the heart, which results in systemic desaturation, and varying amounts of pulmonary obstruction, which causes decreased pulmonary blood flow.

Pathophysiology—At birth, the presence of a patent foramen ovale (or other atrial septal opening) is required to permit blood flow across the septum into the left atrium; the PDA allows blood flow to the pulmonary artery into the lungs for oxygenation. A VSD allows a modest amount of blood to enter the right ventricle and pulmonary artery for oxygenation. Pulmonary blood flow usually is diminished.

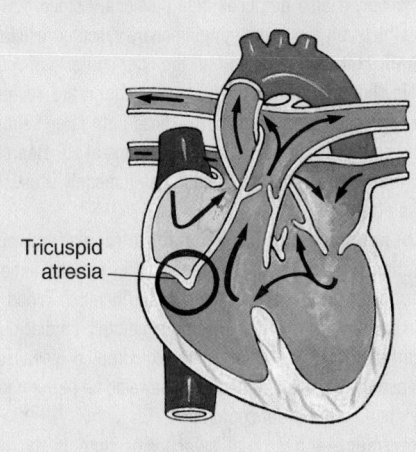

Tricuspid atresia

Continued

BOX 42-3   DEFECTS WITH DECREASED PULMONARY BLOOD FLOW—cont'd

Clinical manifestations—Cyanosis is usually seen in the newborn period. There may be tachycardia and dyspnea. Older children have signs of chronic hypoxemia with clubbing.

Therapeutic management—For neonates whose pulmonary blood flow depends on the patency of the ductus arteriosus, a continuous infusion of prostaglandin E_1 is started at 0.1 mcg/kg/min until surgical intervention can be arranged.

Surgical treatment—Palliative treatment is the placement of a shunt (pulmonary-to-systemic artery anastomosis) to increase blood flow to the lungs. If the ASD is small, an atrial septostomy is performed during cardiac catheterization. Some children have increased pulmonary blood flow and require pulmonary artery banding to lessen the volume of blood to the lungs. A bidirectional Glenn shunt (cavopulmonary anastomosis) may be performed at 4 to 9 months as a second stage.

- *Modified Fontan procedure*—Systemic venous return is directed to the lungs without a ventricular pump through surgical connections between the right atrium and the pulmonary artery. A fenestration (opening) is sometimes made in the right atrial baffle to relieve pressure. The patient must have normal ventricular function and a low pulmonary vascular resistance for the procedure to be successful. The modified Fontan procedure separates oxygenated and unoxygenated blood inside the heart and eliminates the excess volume load on the ventricle but does not restore normal anatomy or hemodynamics. This operation is also the final stage in the correction of many complex defects with a functional single ventricle, including hypoplastic left heart syndrome.

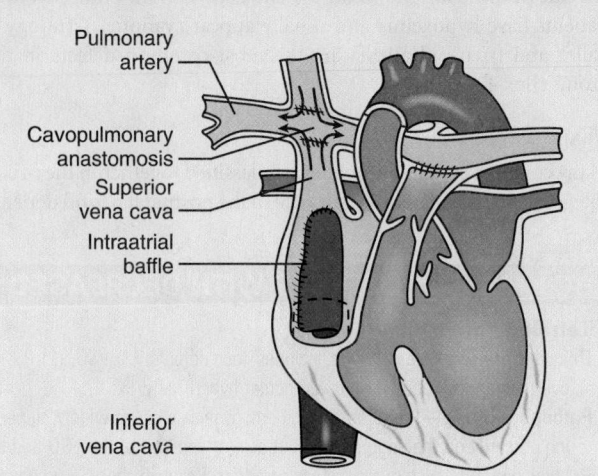

Prognosis—Surgical mortality is less than 5% (Jacobs, Mavroudis, Jacobs, et al., 2004); the rate increases when the anatomy is more complex and other risk factors are present. Postoperative complications include dysrhythmias, systemic venous hypertension, pleural and pericardial effusions, and ventricular dysfunction. Long-term concerns are the development of protein-losing enteropathy, atrial dysrhythmias, late ventricular dysfunction, and developmental delays.

ASD, Atrial septal defect; *PDA,* patent ductus arteriosus; *PS,* pulmonic stenosis; *RVOT,* right ventricular outflow tract; *TGA,* transposition of the great arteries; *VSD,* ventricular septal defect.

BOX 42-4   MIXED DEFECTS

Transposition of the Great Arteries, or Transposition of the Great Vessels

Description—The pulmonary artery leaves the left ventricle, and the aorta exits from the right ventricle with no communication between the systemic and pulmonary circulations.

Pathophysiology—Associated defects such as septal defects or PDA must be present to permit blood to enter the systemic circulation or the pulmonary circulation for mixing of saturated and desaturated blood. The most common defect associated with TGA is a patent foramen ovale. At birth, there is also a PDA, although in most instances, this closes after the neonatal period. Another associated defect may be a VSD. The presence of a VSD increases the risk for HF because it permits blood to flow from the right to left ventricle, into the pulmonary artery, and finally to the lungs. However, it also produces high pulmonary blood flow under high pressure, which can result in high pulmonary vascular resistance.

Clinical manifestations—Depend on the type and size of the associated defects. Newborns with minimum communication are severely cyanotic and have depressed function at birth. Those with large septal defects or a PDA may be less cyanotic but have symptoms of HF. Heart sounds vary according to the type of defect present. Cardiomegaly is usually evident a few weeks after birth.

Therapeutic management (to provide intracardiac mixing)—The administration of intravenous prostaglandin E_1 may be initiated to keep the ductus arteriosus open to temporarily increase blood mixing and provide an oxygen saturation of 75% or to maintain cardiac output. During cardiac catheterization or under echocardiographic guidance, a balloon atrial septostomy (Rashkind procedure) may also be performed to increase mixing by opening the atrial septum.

Surgical treatment—An arterial switch procedure is the procedure of choice performed in the first weeks of life. It involves transecting the great

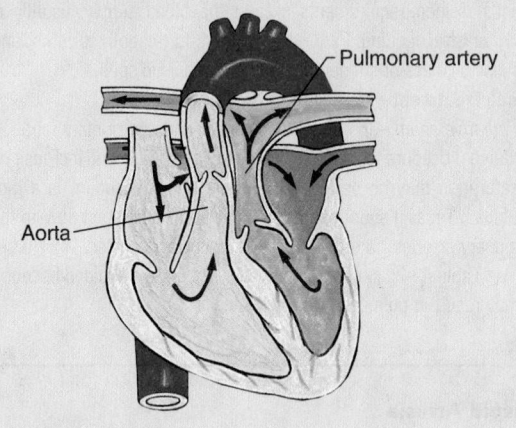

arteries and anastomosing the main pulmonary artery to the proximal aorta (just above the aortic valve) and anastomosing the ascending aorta to the proximal pulmonary artery. The coronary arteries are switched from the proximal aorta to the proximal pulmonary artery to create a new aorta. Reimplantation of the coronary arteries is critical to the infant's survival, and they must be reattached without torsion or kinking to provide the heart with its supply of oxygen. The advantage of the arterial switch procedure is the reestablishment of normal circulation, with the left ventricle acting as the systemic pump. Potential complications of the arterial switch include narrowing at the great artery anastomoses and coronary artery insufficiency.

- *Intraatrial baffle repairs*—Intraatrial baffle repairs are rarely performed, although many adolescents and adults survive today with repairs that were done more than 15 years ago. An intraatrial baffle is created to

BOX 42-4 MIXED DEFECTS—cont'd

divert venous blood to the mitral valve and pulmonary venous blood to the tricuspid valve using the patient's atrial septum (Senning procedure) or a prosthetic material (Mustard procedure). A disadvantage is the continuing role of the right ventricle as the systemic pump and the late development of right ventricular failure and rhythm disturbances. Other potential postoperative complications include loss of normal sinus rhythm, baffle leaks, and ventricular dysfunction.

- *Rastelli procedure*—This procedure is the operative choice in infants with TGA, VSD, and severe PS. It involves closure of the VSD with a baffle, so that left ventricular blood is directed through the VSD into the aorta. The pulmonic valve is then closed, and a conduit is placed from the right ventricle to the pulmonary artery to create a physiologically normal circulation. Unfortunately, this procedure requires multiple conduit replacements as the child grows.

Prognosis—Operative mortality is less than 2% (Jacobs, Mavroudis, Jacobs, et al., 2004). Potential long-term problems include suprapulmonic stenosis and neoaortal dilation and regurgitation.

Total Anomalous Pulmonary Venous Connection

Description—Rare defect characterized by failure of the pulmonary veins to join the left atrium. Instead, the pulmonary veins are abnormally connected to the systemic venous circuit via the right atrium or various veins draining toward the right atrium, such as the SVC. The abnormal attachment results in mixed blood being returned to the right atrium and shunted from the right to the left through an ASD. TAPVC (also called *total anomalous pulmonary venous return* or *total anomalous pulmonary venous drainage*) is classified according to the pulmonary venous point of attachment as follows:

- *Supracardiac*—Attachment above the diaphragm, such as to the SVC (most common form)
- *Cardiac*—Direct attachment to the heart, such as to the right atrium or coronary sinus
- *Infradiaphragmatic*—Attachment below the diaphragm, such as to the IVC (most severe form)

Pathophysiology—The right atrium receives all the blood that normally would flow into the left atrium. As a result, whereas the right side of the heart hypertrophies, the left side, especially the left atrium, may remain small. An associated ASD or patent foramen ovale allows systemic venous blood to shunt from the higher-pressure right atrium to the left atrium and into the left side of the heart. As a result, the oxygen saturation of the blood in both sides of the heart (and ultimately in the systemic arterial circulation) is the same. If the pulmonary blood flow is large, pulmonary venous return is also large and the amount of saturated blood is relatively high. However, if there is obstruction to pulmonary venous drainage, pulmonary venous return is impeded, pulmonary venous pressure rises, and pulmonary interstitial edema develops and eventually contributes to HF. Infradiaphragmatic TAPVC is often associated with obstruction to pulmonary venous drainage and is a surgical emergency.

Clinical manifestations—Most infants develop cyanosis early in life. The degree of cyanosis is inversely related to the amount of pulmonary blood flow—the more pulmonary blood, the less cyanosis. Children with unobstructed TAPVC may be asymptomatic until pulmonary vascular resistance decreases during infancy, increasing pulmonary blood flow with resulting

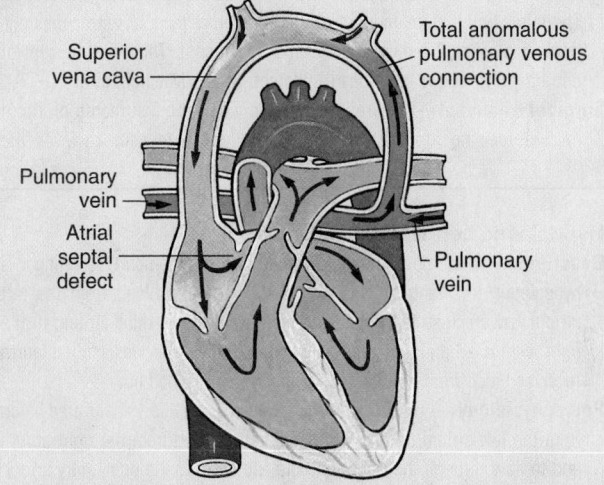

signs of HF. Cyanosis becomes worse with pulmonary vein obstruction; when obstruction occurs, the infant's condition usually deteriorates rapidly. Without intervention, cardiac failure will progress to death.

Surgical treatment—Corrective repair is performed in early infancy. The surgical approach varies with the anatomic defect. In general, however, the common pulmonary vein is anastomosed to the back of the left atrium, the ASD is closed, and the anomalous pulmonary venous connection is ligated. The cardiac type is most easily repaired; the infradiaphragmatic type carries the highest morbidity and mortality because of the higher incidence of pulmonary vein obstruction. Potential postoperative complications include reobstruction; bleeding; dysrhythmias, particularly heart block; pulmonary artery hypertension; and persistent heart failure.

Prognosis—Mortality for all types is less than 10% (Jacobs, Mavroudis, Jacobs, et al., 2004) and is lowest for the cardiac type; morbidity increases with the presence of pulmonary vein obstruction.

Truncus Arteriosus

Description—Failure of normal septation and division of the embryonic bulbar trunk into the pulmonary artery and the aorta, which results in development of a single vessel that overrides both ventricles. Blood from both ventricles mixes in the common great artery, which leads to desaturation and hypoxemia. Blood ejected from the heart flows preferentially to the lower-pressure pulmonary arteries, so that pulmonary blood flow is increased and systemic blood flow is reduced. There are three types:

- *Type I*—A single pulmonary trunk arises near the base of the truncus and divides into the left and right pulmonary arteries.
- *Type II*—The left and right pulmonary arteries arise separately but in close proximity and at the same level from the back of the truncus.
- *Type III*—The pulmonary arteries arise independently from the sides of the truncus.

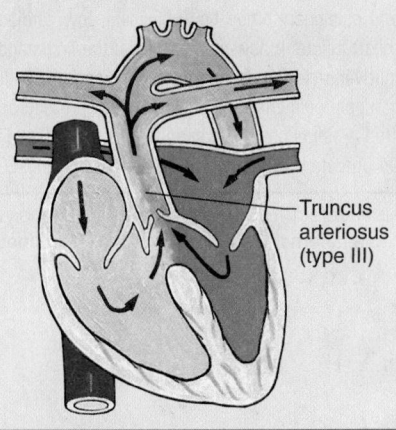

Continued

BOX 42-4 MIXED DEFECTS—cont'd

Pathophysiology—Blood ejected from the left and right ventricles enters the common trunk so that pulmonary and systemic circulations are mixed. Blood flow is distributed to the pulmonary and systemic circulations according to the relative resistances of each system. The amount of pulmonary blood flow depends on the size of the pulmonary arteries and the pulmonary vascular resistance. Generally, resistance to pulmonary blood flow is less than systemic vascular resistance, which results in preferential blood flow to the lungs. Pulmonary vascular disease develops at an early age in patients with truncus arteriosus.

Clinical manifestations—Most infants are symptomatic with moderate to severe HF and variable cyanosis, poor growth, and activity intolerance. There is a holosystolic murmur at the left sternal murmur with a diastolic murmur present if truncal regurgitation is present. Thirty-five percent of patients have 22q11 deletions (Goldmuntz, Clark, Mitchell, et al., 1998).

Surgical treatment—Early repair is performed in the first month of life. It involves closing the VSD so that the truncus arteriosus receives the outflow from the left ventricle and excising the pulmonary arteries from the aorta and attaching them to the right ventricle by means of a homograft. Currently, homografts (segments of cadaver aorta and pulmonary artery that are treated with antibiotics and cryopreserved) are preferred over synthetic conduits to establish continuity between the right ventricle and pulmonary artery. Homografts are more flexible and easier to use during the procedure and appear less prone to obstruction. Postoperative complications include persistent heart failure, bleeding, pulmonary artery hypertension, dysrhythmias, and residual VSD. Because conduits are not living tissue, they will not grow along with the child and may also become narrowed with calcifications. One or more conduit replacements will be needed in childhood.

Prognosis—Mortality is greater than 10%; future operations are required to replace the conduits.

Hypoplastic Left Heart Syndrome

Description—Underdevelopment of the left side of the heart, resulting in a hypoplastic left ventricle and aortic atresia. Most blood from the left atrium flows across the patent foramen ovale to the right atrium, to the right ventricle, and out the pulmonary artery. The descending aorta receives blood from the PDA supplying systemic blood flow.

Pathophysiology—An ASD or patent foramen ovale allows saturated blood from the left atrium to mix with desaturated blood from the right atrium and to flow through the right ventricle and out into the pulmonary artery. From the pulmonary artery, the blood flows both to the lungs and through the ductus arteriosus into the aorta and out to the body. The amount of blood flow to the pulmonary and systemic circulations depends on the relationship between the pulmonary and systemic vascular resistances. The coronary and cerebral vessels receive blood by retrograde flow through the hypoplastic ascending aorta.

Clinical manifestations—The patient has mild cyanosis and signs of HF until the PDA closes and then progressive deterioration with cyanosis and decreased cardiac output, leading to cardiovascular collapse. The condition is usually fatal in the first months of life without intervention.

Therapeutic management—Neonates require stabilization with mechanical ventilation and inotropic support preoperatively. A prostaglandin E_1 infusion is needed to maintain ductal patency and ensure adequate systemic blood flow.

Surgical treatment—A multiple-stage approach is used. The first stage is a Norwood procedure, which involves an anastomosis of the main pulmonary artery to the aorta to create a new aorta, shunting to provide pulmonary blood flow (usually with a modified Blalock-Taussig shunt), and creation of a large ASD. Postoperative complications include imbalance of systemic and pulmonary blood flow, bleeding, low cardiac output, and persistent heart failure. A new modification of the first-stage repair is the use of a right ventricle-to-pulmonary artery homograft conduit instead of a shunt to supply pulmonary blood flow (Sano procedure). The second stage is often a bidirectional Glenn shunt procedure (see Fig. 42-8) or a hemi-Fontan operation. Both involve anastomosing the SVC to the right

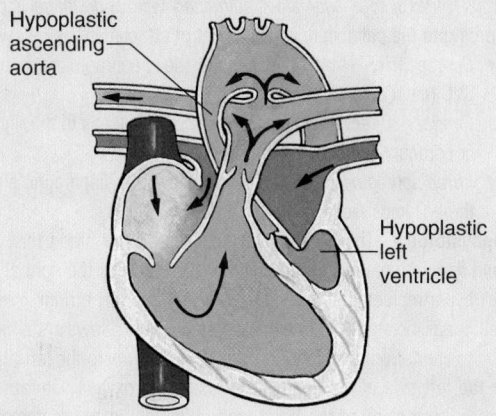

Hypoplastic ascending aorta

Hypoplastic left ventricle

pulmonary artery so SVC flow bypasses the right atrium and flows directly to the lungs. The procedure is usually done at 3 to 6 months of age to relieve cyanosis and reduce the volume load on the right ventricle. The final repair is a modified Fontan procedure (see Tricuspid Atresia, Box 42-3).

Transplantation—Heart transplantation in the newborn period is another option for these infants. Problems include the shortage of newborn organ donors, risk for rejection, long-term problems with chronic immunosuppression, and infection (see Heart Transplantation, p. 1351).

Prognosis—For the first-stage repair, survival rates vary widely in different centers. Much progress has been made, and some experienced centers are reporting mortality rates of about 10% (Tweddell, Hoffman, Mussatto, et al., 2002), but a large multicenter series reports a mortality rate of about 30% (Jacobs, Mavroudis, Jacobs, et al., 2004). Long-term problems with repair include worsening ventricular function, tricuspid regurgitation, recurrent aortic arch narrowing, dysrhythmias, and developmental delays. There is a risk for mortality between surgical procedures. The mortality for the later two operations is less than 5%.

ASD, Atrial septal defect; *HF*, heart failure; *IVC*, inferior vena cava; *PDA*, patent ductus arteriosus; *PS*, pulmonic stenosis; *SVC*, superior vena cava; *TAPVC*, total anomalous pulmonary venous connection; *TGA*, transposition of the great arteries; *VSD*, ventricular septal defect.

signs of HF. Some defects, such as transposition of the great arteries, cause severe cyanosis in the first days of life and later cause HF. Others, such as truncus arteriosus, cause severe HF in the first weeks of life and mild desaturation.

CLINICAL CONSEQUENCES OF CONGENITAL HEART DISEASE

Heart Failure

HF is the inability of the heart to pump an adequate amount of blood to the systemic circulation at normal filling pressures to meet the body's metabolic demands. In children, HF most frequently occurs secondary to structural abnormalities (e.g., septal defects) that result in increased blood volume and pressure within the heart. It can also result from myocardial failure in which the contractility of the ventricle is impaired. This can occur with cardiomyopathy, dysrhythmias, or severe electrolyte disturbances. HF can also occur because of excessive demands on a normal heart muscle, such as sepsis or severe anemia.

Pathophysiology

Heart failure is often separated into two categories—right-sided failure and left-sided failure. In right-sided failure, the right ven-

tricle is unable to pump blood effectively into the pulmonary artery, resulting in increased pressure in the right atrium and systemic venous circulation. Systemic venous hypertension causes hepatosplenomegaly and occasionally edema. In left-sided failure, the left ventricle is unable to pump blood into the systemic circulation, resulting in increased pressure in the left atrium and pulmonary veins. The lungs become congested with blood, causing elevated pulmonary pressures and pulmonary edema.

Although each type of HF produces different signs and symptoms, clinically, it is unusual to observe solely right- or left-sided failure in children. Because each side of the heart depends on adequate function of the other side, failure of one chamber causes a reciprocal change in the opposite chamber.

If the abnormalities precipitating HF are not corrected, the heart muscle becomes damaged. Despite compensatory mechanisms, the heart is unable to maintain an adequate cardiac output. Decreased blood flow to the kidneys continues to stimulate sodium and water reabsorption, leading to fluid overload, increased workload on the heart, and congestion in the pulmonary and systemic circulations (Fig. 42-6).

Clinical Manifestations

The signs and symptoms of HF can be divided into three groups: (1) impaired myocardial function, (2) pulmonary congestion, and

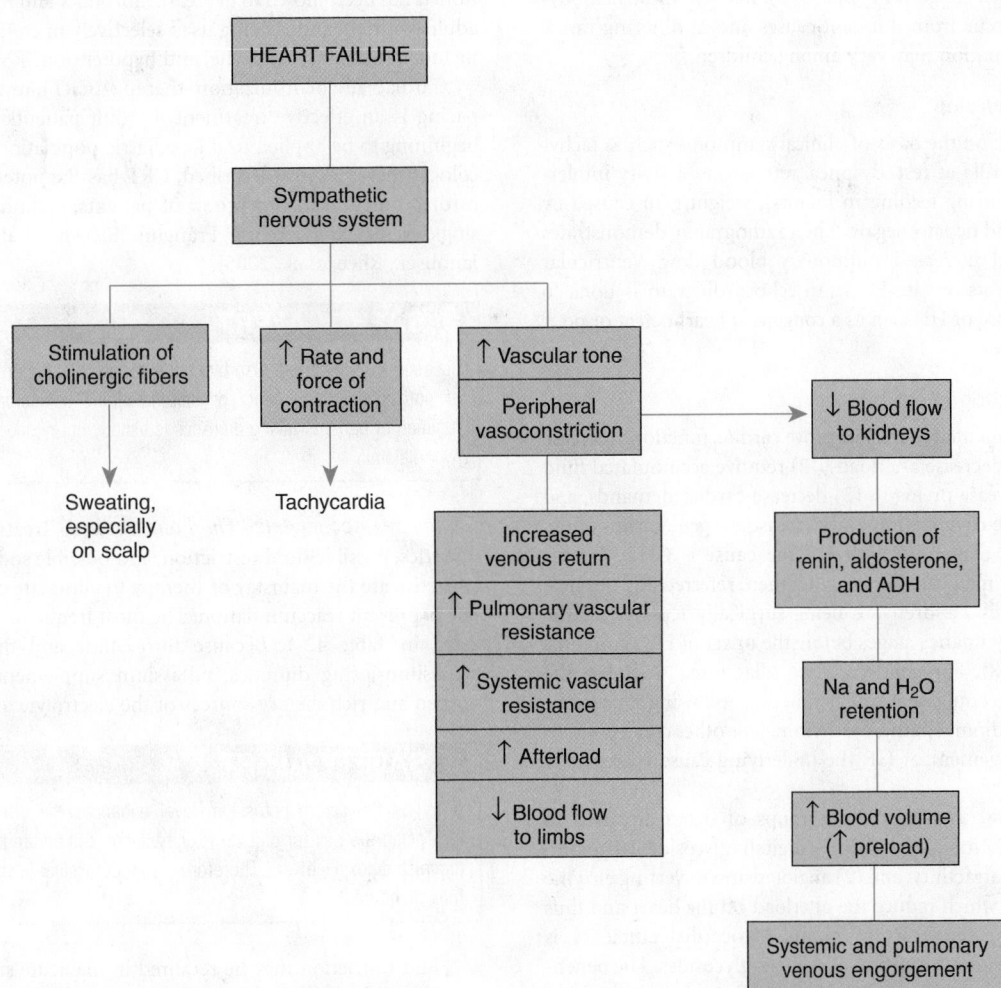

FIG 42-6 Pathophysiology of heart failure. *ADH,* Antidiuretic hormone; *Na,* sodium.

(3) systemic venous congestion (Box 42-5). Because these hemodynamic changes occur from different causes and at differing times, the clinical presentation may vary among children.

Diagnostic Evaluation

Diagnosis is made on the basis of clinical symptoms such as tachypnea and tachycardia at rest, dyspnea, retractions, activity intolerance (especially during feeding in infants), weight gain caused by fluid retention, and hepatomegaly. Chest radiography demonstrates cardiomegaly and increased pulmonary blood flow. Ventricular hypertrophy appears on the ECG. An echocardiogram is done to determine the cause of HF such as a congenital heart defect or poor ventricular function.

Therapeutic Management

The goals of treatment are to (1) improve cardiac function (increase contractility and decrease afterload), (2) remove accumulated fluid and sodium (decrease preload), (3) decrease cardiac demands, and (4) improve tissue oxygenation and decrease oxygen consumption. For most infants diagnosed with HF, the cause is CHD. Infants are stabilized on medical therapy and then referred for surgical repair. Today many children are being surgically repaired in the neonatal and early infancy stages before the onset of HF symptoms (Margossian, 2008). For children newly diagnosed with HF, the cause may be worsening ventricular function following a previous cardiac repair, cardiomyopathy, dysrhythmia, or other conditions. In addition to management of HF, the underlying cause is treated if possible.

Improve Cardiac Function. Two groups of drugs are used to enhance myocardial function in HF: (1) digitalis glycosides (digoxin), which improve contractility; and (2) angiotensin-converting enzyme (ACE) inhibitors, which reduce the afterload on the heart and thus make it easier for the heart to pump. Myocardial efficiency is improved through administration of digitalis glycosides. The beneficial effects are increased cardiac output, decreased heart size, decreased venous pressure, and relief of edema. In children, digoxin

(Lanoxin) is used almost exclusively because of its more rapid onset. It is available as an elixir (0.05 mg/mL) for oral administration. For infants, the dose is calculated in micrograms (1000 mcg = 1 mg).

Treatment consists of (1) a digitalizing dosage, given orally or intravenously in divided doses over 24 hours to produce optimal cardiac effects, and (2) a maintenance dosage, given orally twice a day to maintain blood levels. During digitalization, the child is monitored by means of an ECG to observe for the desired effects (prolonged PR interval and reduced ventricular rate) and detect side effects, especially dysrhythmias.

Another group of drugs used in the treatment of HF, the ACE inhibitors, inhibit the normal function of the renin-angiotensin system in the kidney. The ACE inhibitors block the conversion of angiotensin I to angiotensin II so that, instead of vasoconstriction, vasodilation occurs. Vasodilation results in decreased pulmonary and systemic vascular resistance, decreased BP, and a reduction in afterload. It also reduces the secretion of aldosterone, which reduces preload by preventing volume expansion from fluid retention and decreases the risk for hypokalemia. Common medications used in children are captopril (Capoten), enalapril (Vasotec), and lisinopril. The principal side effects of ACE inhibitors are hypotension, cough, and renal dysfunction.

β-Blockers, specifically metoprolol and carvedilol (Coreg), are the newest medications to be added to the treatment of some children with chronic HF. The α- and β-adrenergic receptors are blocked, causing decreased heart rate, decreased BP, and vasodilation. It has been shown to decrease morbidity and mortality in some adults with HF and is being used selectively in children. Side effects included dizziness, headache, and hypotension.

Cardiac resynchronization therapy (CRT) using biventricular pacing is an effective treatment in adult patients with HF and is beginning to be applied in the pediatric population. With pharmacologic therapies just described, CRT has the potential to improve cardiac function in this group of patients, including those with a single ventricle (Cecchin, Frangini, Brown, et al., 2009; Dubin, Janousek, Rhee, et al., 2005).

> ⚡ **SAFETY ALERT**
>
> Because ACE inhibitors also block the action of aldosterone, the addition of potassium supplements or spironolactone (Aldactone) to the drug regimen of patients taking diuretics is usually not needed and may cause hyperkalemia.

Remove Accumulated Fluid and Sodium. Treatment consists of diuretics, possible fluid restriction, and possible sodium restriction. Diuretics are the mainstay of therapy to eliminate excess water and salt to prevent reaccumulation. The most frequently used agents are listed in Table 42-1. Because furosemide and the thiazides are potassium-losing diuretics, potassium supplements may be prescribed and rich dietary sources of the electrolyte are encouraged.

> ⚡ **SAFETY ALERT**
>
> A fall in the serum potassium level enhances the effects of digitalis, increasing the risk for digoxin toxicity. Increased serum potassium levels diminish digoxin's effect. Therefore serum potassium levels must be carefully monitored.

Fluid restriction may be required in the acute stages of HF and must be carefully calculated to avoid dehydrating the child, especially if cyanotic CHD and significant polycythemia are present.

TABLE 42-1 DIURETICS USED IN HEART FAILURE

ACTIONS	COMMENTS	NURSING CARE MANAGEMENT
Furosemide (Lasix)—Blocks reabsorption of sodium and water in proximal renal tubule and interferes with reabsorption of sodium	Drug of choice in severe HF Causes excretion of chloride and potassium (hypokalemia may precipitate digitalis toxicity)	Begin to record output as soon as drug is given. Observe for dehydration caused by profound diuresis. Observe for side effects (nausea and vomiting, diarrhea, ototoxicity, hypokalemia, dermatitis, postural hypotension). Encourage foods high in potassium, or give potassium supplements. Monitor chloride and acid-base balance with long-term therapy. Observe for signs of digoxin toxicity.
Chlorothiazide (Diuril)—Acts directly on distal tubules to decrease sodium, water, potassium, chloride, and bicarbonate absorption	Less frequently used drug Causes hypokalemia, acidosis from large doses	Observe for side effects (nausea, weakness, dizziness, paresthesia, muscle cramps, skin eruptions, hypokalemia, acidosis). Encourage foods high in potassium, or give potassium supplements.
Spironolactone (Aldactone)—Blocks action of aldosterone, which promotes retention of sodium and excretion of potassium	Weak diuretic Has potassium-sparing effect; frequently used with thiazides, furosemide Poorly absorbed from GI tract Takes several days to achieve maximum actions	Observe for side effects (skin rash, drowsiness, ataxia, hyperkalemia). Do not administer potassium supplements.

GI, Gastrointestinal; *HF,* heart failure.

Infants rarely need fluid restrictions because HF makes feeding so difficult that they struggle to take maintenance fluids.

Sodium-restricted diets are used less often in children than in adults to control HF because of their potential negative effects on the child's appetite and ultimate growth. If salt intake is restricted, additional table salt and highly salted foods are avoided.

Decrease Cardiac Demands. To lessen the workload on the heart, metabolic needs are minimized by (1) providing a neutral thermal environment to prevent cold stress in infants, (2) treating any existing infections, (3) reducing the effort of breathing (by placement in semi-Fowler position), (4) using medication to sedate an irritable child, and (5) providing for rest and decreasing environmental stimuli.

Improve Tissue Oxygenation. The preceding measures serve to increase tissue oxygenation, either by improving myocardial function or by lessening tissue oxygen demands. In addition, supplemental cool humidified oxygen may be administered to increase the amount of available oxygen during inspiration. Oxygen administration is especially helpful in patients with pulmonary edema, intercurrent respiratory tract infections, and increased pulmonary vascular resistance (oxygen is a vasodilator that decreases pulmonary vascular resistance).

MEDICATION ALERT

Oxygen is a drug and is administered only with an appropriate order. There are some uncommon circumstances in patients with complex hemodynamics in which oxygen can be detrimental.

An oxygen hood, nasal cannula, or face tent is used to deliver oxygen. Nasal cannulas are ideal for long-term oxygen administration because the child can be ambulatory and can easily eat and drink. Cool humidification is necessary to counteract the drying effect of oxygen. The amount of cool humidity is carefully regulated to prevent chilling.

CARE MANAGEMENT

The infant or child with HF may be acutely ill, and some may require intensive care until the symptoms improve. Expert nursing care is essential to reduce the cardiac demands that strain the failing heart muscle. During this time, the child and family require emotional support. Although the objectives of nursing care are the same, interventions differ depending on the child's age (see Nursing Care Plan).

Assist in Measures to Improve Cardiac Function. The nurse's responsibility in administering digoxin includes calculating and administering the correct dosage, observing for signs of toxicity, and instituting parental teaching regarding drug administration at home. The child's apical pulse is always checked before administering digoxin. As a general rule, the drug is not given if the pulse is below 90 to 110 beats/min in infants and young children or below 70 beats/min in older children (the cutoff point for adults is 60 beats/min). However, because the pulse rate varies in children in different age-groups, the written drug order should specify at what heart rate the drug is withheld. The nurse should also use judgment in evaluating the pulse rate. If it is significantly lower than the previous recording, the dose should be withheld until the health care practitioner is notified.

The apical rate is taken because a pulse deficit (radial pulse rate lower than apical) may be present with decreased cardiac output. It is auscultated for 1 full minute to evaluate alterations in rhythm. If the child is monitored by means of an ECG, a rhythm strip is obtained and attached to the chart for rate and rhythm analysis, such as abnormal lengthening of the PR interval (>50% increase over predigitalization interval) and dysrhythmias.

Digoxin is a potentially dangerous drug because of its narrow margin of safety of therapeutic, toxic, and lethal doses. Many toxic responses are extensions of its therapeutic effects. Therefore the nurse must maintain a high index of suspicion for signs of toxicity when administering digoxin (Box 42-6).

Because digoxin toxicity can occur from accidental overdose, great care must be taken in properly calculating and measuring the dosage. When converting milligrams to micrograms to milliliters, the nurse carefully checks the placement of the decimal point because an error causes a significant change in dosage. For example, 0.1 mg is 10 times the dosage of 0.01 mg.

⚕ MEDICATION ALERT

Infants rarely receive more than 1 mL (50 mcg or 0.05 mg) of digoxin in one dose; a higher dose is an immediate warning of a dosage error. To ensure safety, compare the calculation with another staff member's calculation before giving the drug.

These same principles are taught to parents in preparation for discharge, although the correct dose in milliliters is usually specified on the container, thus reducing potential errors in calculation. The nurse watches the parent measure the elixir in the dropper and stresses the level mark as the meniscus of the fluid that is observed at eye level.

Parents are also advised of the signs of toxicity. According to the health care practitioner's preference, they may be taught to take the pulse before giving the drug. A return demonstration of the procedure from the parents or another principal caregiver is included as part of the teaching plan. Their level of anxiety in counting the pulse is assessed because overconcern about the heart rate may result in excessive withholding of the drug.

Monitor Afterload Reduction. For patients receiving ACE inhibitors for afterload reduction, the nurse should carefully monitor BP before and after dose administration, observe for symptoms of hypotension, and notify the health care practitioner if BP is low. Numerous medications affecting the kidney can potentiate renal dysfunction, so children taking multiple diuretics and an ACE inhibitor require careful assessment of serum electrolytes and renal function.

◎ NURSING CARE PLAN

The Child with Heart Failure

NURSING DIAGNOSIS	EXPECTED OUTCOMES	NURSING INTERVENTIONS	RATIONALES
Decreased Cardiac Output related to structural defect, myocardial dysfunction, altered hemodynamics	Child will have adequate cardiac output as evidenced by:	Assess and record heart rate, respiratory rate, blood pressure, and any signs or symptoms of decreased cardiac output (listed under Defining Characteristics) every 2 to 4 hr and as necessary	To detect change in vital signs and child's physical status that reflect altered cardiac output
Child's or Family's Defining Characteristics (Subjective and Objective Data)	• Heart rate within acceptable range (state specific range) • Respiratory rate within acceptable range (state specific range) • Skin warm to touch	Administer cardiac drugs on schedule; assess and record any side effects or any signs and symptoms of toxicity; follow hospital protocol for administration	To avoid dangers inherent in failure to administer cardiac drugs as prescribed and to perform careful assessment before administration
Tachycardia	• Strong and equal peripheral pulses		
Tachypnea	• Blood pressure normal for age		
Ineffective peripheral circulation, cool extremities	• Brisk capillary refill within 2 or 3 seconds	Keep accurate record of intake and output	To detect HF, which causes decreased urinary output
Hypotension	• Lack of distended neck veins • Normal sinus rhythm	Weigh child or infant on same scale at same time of day as previously; document results and compare with previous weight	To monitor for weight increases, which may indicate excess fluid accumulation
Rapid, weak peripheral pulses	• Lack of edema • Adequate urinary output (state specific; 1-2 mL/kg/hr)		
Prolonged capillary refill, longer than 2 or 3 seconds	• Age-appropriate weight gain on standardized growth curve • Successful feeding	Administer diuretics on schedule; assess and record effectiveness and any side effects noted	To eliminate excess water and salt because fluid retention commonly occurs with HF
Narrow pulse pressure	Child or family will be able to state at least four characteristics of heart failure such as:	Elevate head of bed at a 30- to 45-degree angle	To promote maximum chest expansion
Distended neck veins in older children	• Rapid heart rate	Offer small, frequent feedings to infant's or child's tolerance	To increase caloric intake and compensate for fatigue during feeding and increased metabolic rate because of poor cardiac function
Cardiomegaly revealed on chest radiograph	• Fast breathing		
Gallop rhythm	• Cool extremities		
Edema	• Puffiness (edema)		
Rapid weight gain	• Fussiness	Organize nursing care to allow child or infant uninterrupted rest	To allow adequate rest because poor cardiac output decreases energy level and lowers tolerance to activity
Feeding difficulty	• Decreased appetite		
Irritability	Child or family will be able to state knowledge of care regarding:		
	• Medication administration	Educate child and family about characteristics of HF; assess and record teaching session	To promote measures to improve cardiac function and decrease demands
	• Head elevated positioning		
	• Sufficient rest periods		
	• Monitoring of intake and output	Educate child and family about care such as medication administration; assess and record results and family's participation in care	To promote safety and minimize medication side effects
	• When to contact health care provider		

◎ NURSING CARE PLAN

The Child with Heart Failure—cont'd

NURSING DIAGNOSIS	EXPECTED OUTCOMES	NURSING INTERVENTIONS	RATIONALES
Ineffective Breathing Pattern related to pulmonary congestion, decreased cardiac output **Child's or Family's Defining Characteristics (Subjective and Objective Data)** Tachypnea Dyspnea Retractions Crackles Shortness of breath Cyanosis Pallor Mottling Nasal flaring Grunting Head bobbing Cough Use of accessory muscles Activity intolerance	Child will have effective breathing pattern as evidenced by: • Respiratory rate within acceptable range (state specific range) • Clear and equal breath sounds bilaterally anteriorly and posteriorly • Pink or tan color • Absence of nasal flaring, retractions, cough, and head bobbing • Unlabored breath sounds • Tolerance of activities appropriate for age Child or family will be able to state four characteristics of ineffective breathing pattern such as: • Color change from pink or tan to pale, dusky, or blue • Fast breathing • Change in amount or characteristics of secretions • Retractions, head bobbing • Ineffective cough • Decreased or altered activity level Child or family will be able to state knowledge of care regarding: • Positioning to facilitate respiratory effort • Oxygen administration • When to contact health care provider	Assess and record respiratory rate, breath sounds, and any signs or symptoms of ineffective pattern (listed under Defining Characteristics) every 2 to 4 hr and as needed Administer humidified oxygen in correct amount and route of delivery Record percent of oxygen and route of delivery Assess and record child's response to therapy Keep head of bed elevated at a 30- to 45-degree angle Suction if child has ineffective cough or is unable to manage secretions; assess and record amount and characteristics of secretions Assess and record oxygen saturation every 2 to 4 hr and as needed Educate child and family about characteristics of ineffective breathing pattern; assess and record results Educate child and family about care; assess and record results and family participation in care	To detect indicators of worsening HF To reduce respiratory distress by easing respiratory effort To promote maximum chest expansion To maintain patent airway to promote respiratory expansion To evaluate pulmonary effectiveness To promote measures to improve breathing effort

HF, heart failure; *NIC*, Nursing Intervention Classification; *NOC*, Nursing Outcomes Classification.

BOX 42-6	COMMON SIGNS OF DIGOXIN TOXICITY IN CHILDREN
Gastrointestinal	**Cardiac**
• Nausea	• Bradycardia
• Vomiting	• Dysrhythmias
• Anorexia	

Decrease Cardiac Demands. The infant requires rest and conservation of energy for feeding. Every effort is made to organize nursing activities to allow for uninterrupted periods of sleep. Whenever possible, parents are encouraged to stay with their infant to provide the holding, rocking, and cuddling that help children sleep more soundly. To minimize disturbing the infant, changing bed linens and complete bathing are done only when necessary. Feeding is planned to accommodate the infant's sleep and wake patterns. The child is fed at the first sign of hunger, such as when sucking on fists, rather than waiting until he or she cries for a bottle because the stress of crying exhausts the limited energy supply. Because infants with HF tire easily and may sleep through feedings, smaller feedings every 3 hours may be helpful. Gavage feedings may be instituted to provide adequate nutrition and allow the infant to rest.

Every effort is made to minimize unnecessary stress. Older children need an explanation of what is happening to them to decrease anxiety about their illness and necessary treatments such as cardiac monitoring, oxygen administration, and medications. Outlining a plan for the day, preparing the child for tests and procedures, providing quiet activities, and providing adequate rest periods are all helpful interventions with older children. Some infants and children require sedation during the acute phase of illness to allow them to rest.

Temperature is carefully monitored because hyperthermia or hypothermia increases the need for oxygen. Febrile states are reported to the physician because infection must be promptly treated. Maintaining body temperature is of special importance in children who are receiving cool, humidified oxygen and in infants, who tend to be diaphoretic and lose heat by way of evaporation.

Skin breakdown from edema is prevented with a change of position every 2 hours (from side to side while in semi-Fowler position) and use of a pressure-relieving mattress or bed. The skin, especially over the sacrum, is checked for evidence of redness from pressure.

Reduce Respiratory Distress. Careful assessment, positioning, and oxygen administration can reduce respiratory distress. Respirations are counted for 1 full minute during a resting state. Any evidence of increased respiratory distress is reported because this may indicate worsening HF.

Infants are positioned to encourage maximum chest expansion, with the head of the bed elevated; they should sit up in an infant seat or be held at a 45-degree angle. Children prefer to sleep on several pillows and remain in a semi-Fowler or high-Fowler position during waking hours. Safety restraints, such as those used with infant seats, are applied low on the abdomen and loosely enough to provide both safety and maximum expansion.

The infant or child is often given humidified supplemental oxygen via oxygen hood or tent, nasal cannula, or mask. The child's response to oxygen therapy is carefully evaluated by noting respiratory rate, ease of respiration, color, and especially oxygen saturation as measured by oximetry.

Respiratory tract infections can exacerbate HF and should be appropriately treated and prevented if possible. The child should be protected from persons with respiratory tract infections and have a noninfectious roommate. Good hand washing is practiced before and after caring for any hospitalized child. Antibiotics may be given to combat respiratory tract infection. The nurse ensures that the drug is given at equally divided times over a 24-hour schedule to maintain high blood levels of the antibiotic.

Maintain Nutritional Status. Meeting the nutritional needs of infants with HF or serious cardiac defects is a nursing challenge. The metabolic rate of these infants is greater because of poor cardiac function and increased heart and respiratory rates. Their caloric needs are greater than those of the average infant because of their increased metabolic rate, yet their ability to take in adequate calories is hampered by their fatigue. Feeding for a fragile infant with serious CHD is similar to exercising for an adult, and these infants often do not have the energy or cardiac reserve to do extra work. The nurse seeks measures to enable the infant to feed easily without excess fatigue and to increase the caloric density of the formula.

The infant should be well rested before feeding and fed soon after awakening so as not to expend energy on crying. A 3-hour feeding schedule works well for many infants. (Feeding every 2 hours does not provide enough rest between feedings, and a 4-hour schedule requires an increased volume of feeding, which many infants are unable to take.) The feeding schedule should be individualized to the infant's needs. A feeding goal of 150 mL/kg/day and at least 120 kcal/kg/day is common for newborns with significant heart disease (Stetzler, Rudd, and Pick, 2005). A soft preemie nipple or a slit in a regular nipple to enlarge the opening decreases the infant's energy expenditure while sucking. Infants should be well supported and fed in a semiupright position. Infants may need to rest frequently and may need to have the jaw and cheeks stroked to encourage sucking. Generally, giving an infant about a half-hour to complete a feeding is reasonable. Prolonging the feeding time can exhaust the infant and decrease the rest period between feedings.

Infants with feeding difficulties are often gavage-fed using a nasogastric tube to supplement their oral intake and ensure adequate calories. If they are very stressed and fatigued, in respiratory distress, or tachypneic to 80 to 100 breaths/min, oral feedings may be withheld and all nutrition given by gavage feedings. Gavage feedings are usually a temporary measure until the infant's medical status improves and nutritional needs can be met through oral feedings. Some infants with severe HF, neurologic deficits, or significant gastroesophageal reflux may need placement of a gastrostomy tube to allow adequate nutrition.

The caloric density of formulas is frequently increased by concentration and then adding Polycose, medium-chain triglyceride oil, or corn oil. Infant formulas provide 20 kcal/oz, and the use of additives can increase the calories to 30 kcal/oz or more. This allows the infant to obtain more calories despite a smaller volume intake of formula. The caloric density of the formula needs to be increased slowly (by 2 kcal/oz/day) to prevent diarrhea or formula intolerance. Breastfeeding mothers are encouraged to provide the infant with alternating feedings of breast milk and high-calorie formulas. Some lactating mothers prefer to feed the child expressed breast milk that

has been fortified with Similac or Enfamil powder, Polycose, or corn oil to increase caloric intake. A diet plan specific to the individual infant's needs is calculated and prescribed by the nutritionist in collaboration with the other health care personnel. The nurse needs to reinforce this information with the parents as necessary.

Assist in Measures to Promote Fluid Loss. When diuretics are given, the nurse records fluid intake and output and monitors body weight at the same time each day to evaluate benefit from the drug. Because profound diuresis may cause dehydration and electrolyte imbalance (loss of sodium, potassium, chloride, bicarbonate), the nurse observes for signs indicating either complication, as well as signs and symptoms suggesting reactions to the drugs. Diuretics should be given early in the day to children who are toilet trained to avoid the need to urinate at night. If potassium-losing diuretics are given, the nurse encourages foods high in potassium, such as bananas, oranges, whole grains, legumes, and leafy vegetables and administers prescribed supplements. Serum potassium levels are checked frequently.

💊 MEDICATION ALERT

Mix the elixir with fruit juice (red punch or grape juice works well) to disguise the bitter taste and to prevent intestinal irritation from a concentrated solution.

Fluid restriction is rarely necessary in infants because of their difficulty in feeding. However, if fluids are restricted, the nurse plans fluid intake schedules for a 24-hour period, allowing for most fluids during waking hours. Toddlers and preschoolers should be given small amounts of liquid in small cups so the containers appear full. Older children's cooperation is gained by placing them in charge of recording their fluid intake.

If salt is limited, the nurse discusses food sources of sodium with the family and discourages their bringing salt-containing treats to the child. At mealtimes, the child's tray is checked to make sure the appropriate diet is given.

Support Child and Family. HF is a serious complication of heart disease. Parents and older children are usually acutely aware of the critical nature of the condition. Because stress places additional demands on cardiac function, the nurse should focus on reducing anxiety through anticipatory preparation, frequent communication with the parent regarding the child's progress, and constant reassurance that everything possible is being done.

The nurse teaches the family about the medications that need to be administered and alerts them to the signs of worsening HF that require medical attention, such as increased sweating, decreased urinary output (noted in fewer wet diapers or infrequent use of the toilet), or poor feeding. Every effort is made to improve the family's adherence to the medication schedule by adapting the schedule to their usual home routines, avoiding medications during the night, making it as simple as possible, and using charts or visual aids to remember when to give medications. Written instructions regarding correct administration of digoxin are essential.

Hypoxemia

Hypoxemia refers to an arterial oxygen tension (or pressure, Pao$_2$) that is less than normal and can be identified by a decreased arterial saturation or a decreased Pao$_2$. Hypoxia is a reduction in tissue oxygenation that results from low oxygen saturations and Pao$_2$ and results in impaired cellular processes. Cyanosis is a blue discoloration in the mucous membranes, skin, and nail beds of the child with reduced oxygen saturation. It results from the presence of deoxygenated hemoglobin (hemoglobin not bound to oxygen) in a concentration of 5 g/dL of blood. Cyanosis is usually apparent when arterial oxygen saturations are 80% to 85%. Determination of cyanosis is subjective. It can vary depending on skin pigment, quality of light, color of the room, or clothing worn by the child. The presence of cyanosis may not accurately reflect arterial hypoxemia because both oxygen saturation and the amount of circulating hemoglobin are involved. Children with severe anemia may not be cyanotic despite severe hypoxemia because the hemoglobin level may be too low to produce the characteristic blue color. Conversely, patients with polycythemia may appear cyanotic despite a near-normal Pao_2. Heart defects that cause hypoxemia and cyanosis result from desaturated venous blood (blue blood) entering the systemic circulation without passing through the lungs.

Clinical Manifestations

Over time, two physiologic changes occur in the body in response to chronic hypoxemia—polycythemia and clubbing. Polycythemia, an increased number of red blood cells, increases the oxygen-carrying capacity of the blood. However, anemia may result if iron is not readily available for the formation of hemoglobin. Polycythemia increases the viscosity of the blood and increases the risk for blood clot formation. Clubbing, a thickening and flattening of the tips of the fingers and toes, is thought to occur because of chronic tissue hypoxemia and polycythemia (Fig. 42-7). Infants with mild hypoxemia may be asymptomatic except for cyanosis and exhibit near-normal growth and development. Those with more severe hypoxemia may exhibit fatigue with feeding, poor weight gain, tachypnea, and dyspnea. Severe hypoxemia resulting in tissue hypoxia is manifested by clinical deterioration and signs of poor perfusion.

Hypercyanotic spells, also referred to as blue spells or tet spells because they are often seen in infants with tetralogy of Fallot, may occur in any child whose heart defect includes obstruction to pulmonary blood flow and communication between the ventricles. The infant becomes acutely cyanotic and hyperpneic because sudden infundibular spasm decreases pulmonary blood flow and increases right-to-left shunting (the proposed mechanism in tetralogy of Fallot). Spells, rarely seen before 2 months of age, occur most frequently in the first year of life. They occur more often in the morning and may be preceded by feeding, crying, defecation, or stressful procedures. Because profound hypoxemia causes cerebral hypoxia, hypercyanotic spells require prompt assessment and treatment to prevent brain damage or possibly death.

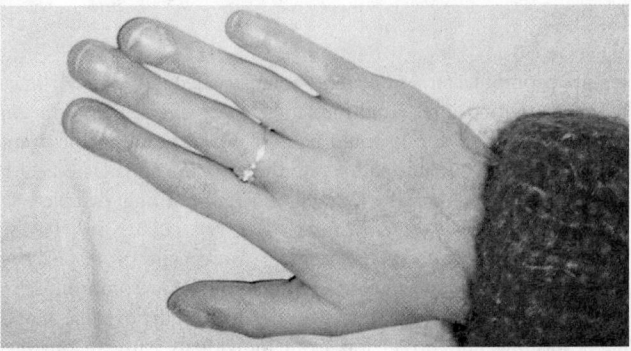

FIG 42-7 Clubbing of the fingers.

Persistent cyanosis as a result of cyanotic heart defects places the child at risk for significant neurologic complications. Cerebrovascular accident (CVA, stroke), brain abscess, and developmental delays (especially in motor and cognitive development) may result from chronic hypoxia.

Diagnostic Evaluation

Cyanosis in a newborn can be the result of cardiac, pulmonary, metabolic, or hematologic disease, although cardiac and pulmonary causes occur most often. To distinguish between the two, a hyperoxia test is helpful. The infant is placed in a 100% oxygen environment, and blood parameters are monitored. A Pao_2 of 100 mm Hg or higher suggests lung disease, and a Pao_2 lower than 100 mm Hg suggests cardiac disease (Park, 2008). An accurate history, a chest radiograph, and especially an echocardiogram contribute to the diagnosis of cyanotic heart disease.

Therapeutic Management

Newborns generally exhibit cyanosis within the first few days of life as the ductus arteriosus, which provided pulmonary blood flow, begins to close. Prostaglandin E_1, which causes vasodilation and smooth muscle relaxation, thus increasing dilation and patency of the ductus arteriosus, is administered intravenously to reestablish pulmonary blood flow. The use of prostaglandins has been lifesaving for infants with ductus-dependent cardiac defects. The increase in oxygenation allows the infant to be stabilized and have a complete diagnostic evaluation performed before further treatment is needed.

Hypercyanotic spells occur suddenly, and prompt recognition and treatment are essential. In the hospital setting, spells are often seen during blood drawing or IV insertion, when the child is highly agitated, or after cardiac catheterization. Treatment of a hypercyanotic spell is outlined in the Guidelines box. Morphine, administered subcutaneously or through an existing IV line, helps reduce infundibular spasm. A spell indicates the need for prompt surgical treatment if possible. In infants with defects not amenable to surgical repair, a shunt may be created surgically to increase blood flow to the lungs. Several commonly used shunt procedures are described in Table 42-2 and Fig. 42-8.

The cyanotic infant and child are well hydrated to keep the hematocrit and blood viscosity within acceptable limits to reduce the risk for CVAs. The infant is monitored closely for anemia because of the risk for CVAs and the reduced arterial oxygen-carrying capacity that occurs. Iron supplementation and possibly blood transfusion are used as needed.

Respiratory tract infections or reduced pulmonary function from any cause can worsen hypoxemia in the cyanotic child. Aggressive pulmonary hygiene, chest physical therapy, administration of antibiotics, and use of oxygen to improve arterial saturations are important interventions.

CARE MANAGEMENT

The general appearance of infants and children with significant cyanosis poses unique concerns. Blue lips and fingernails are obvious signs of their hidden cardiac defect. Clubbing and small, thin stature in older children further indicate severe heart disease. Adolescents are especially concerned about their body image; children with cyanosis are often teased about their appearance and singled out as different. Many children, when asked what surgery will do, reply, "Make me pink." Their joy and excitement after surgery are evident when they see their pink fingers. Parents are often fearful of their child's bluish color because cyanosis is usually associated with lack

TABLE 42-2 SELECTED SHUNT PROCEDURES FOR CHILDREN WITH CARDIAC DEFECTS

SHUNT TYPE	COMMENTS
Modified Blalock-Taussig shunt—Subclavian artery to pulmonary artery using GORE-TEX or IMPRA tube graft	Shunt flow sometimes excessive, requiring use of diuretics Possibility of thrombosis; aspirin usually prescribed postoperatively Easy to ligate at time of definitive correction Shunt size fixed and may become too small as child grows
Sano Modification—Right ventricular to pulmonary artery using GORE-TEX	Prevents diastolic runoff of systemic blood into the pulmonary arteries Provides a higher diastolic blood pressure and seemingly better coronary perfusion Used in place of the modified Blalock-Taussig shunt in the Norwood procedure
Central shunt—Ascending aorta to main pulmonary artery using GORE-TEX graft	Length of shunt acts to restrict blood flow; possibility of symptoms of HF; diuretic therapy sometimes required Uncommon; used when modified Blalock-Taussig shunt cannot be used Easy to insert and remove at time of repair Possibility of thrombosis; aspirin usually prescribed postoperatively
Biderectional Glenn shunt (cavopulmonary anastomosis)—SVC to side of right pulmonary artery; blood flow to both lungs	Done as a second shunt; often used as a staging step to a Fontan procedure Can be incorporated into eventual modified Fontan procedure Relieves severe cyanosis and decreases volume overload on ventricle Carries risk for embolic events (mixing defect); aspirin often prescribed Pulmonary arteriovenous fistulas may occur months or years later, causing desaturation (uncommon finding)

HF, Heart failure; *SVC,* superior vena cava.

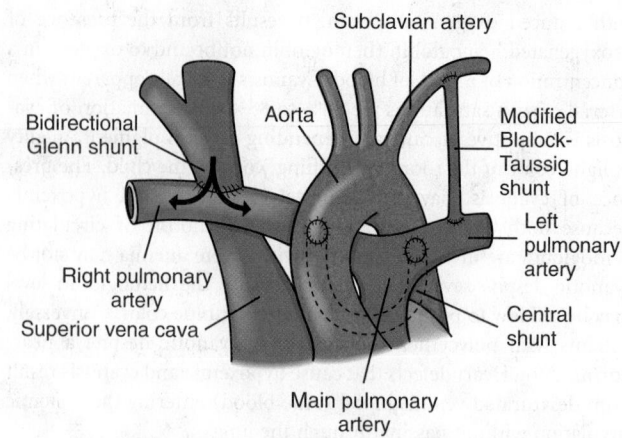

FIG 42-8 Schematic diagram of cardiac shunts.

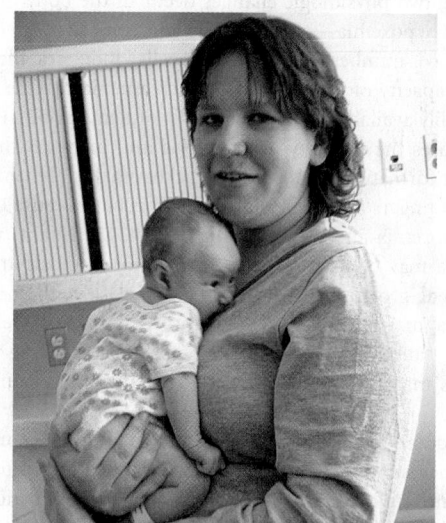

FIG 42-9 Infant held in a knee-chest position.

📋 GUIDELINES

Treating Hypercyanotic Spells

- Place infant in knee-chest position (Fig. 42-9).
- Use a calm, comforting approach.
- Administer 100% oxygen by blow-by.
- Give morphine subcutaneously or through an existing IV line.
- Begin IV fluid replacement and volume expansion if needed.
- Repeat morphine administration.

IV, Intravenous.

of oxygen and severe illness. They also must deal with comments from relatives, friends, and strangers about their child's abnormal color. They need a simple explanation of hypoxemia and cyanosis and reassurance that cyanosis does not imply a lack of oxygen to the brain. Their questions and fears need to be addressed in a calm, supportive manner, and positive aspects of their child's growth and development are emphasized. They are taught the treatment for hypercyanotic spells (see Guidelines box).

Dehydration must be prevented in children with hypoxemia because it potentiates the risk for CVAs. Fluid status is carefully monitored, with accurate intake and output and daily weight measurements. Maintenance fluid therapy is the minimum requirement, supplemental fluids should be readily available, and gavage feeding or IV hydration is given to children unable to take adequate oral fluids. Fever, vomiting, and diarrhea can cause dehydration and

require prompt treatment. Parents are instructed in the importance of adequate fluid intake and measures to prevent dehydration. An oral electrolyte solution should be available at home in the event that the infant is unable to tolerate the usual formula. The health care practitioner should be notified of fever, vomiting, diarrhea, or other problems.

Preventive measures and accurate assessment of respiratory infection are important nursing considerations. Any compromise in pulmonary function will increase the infant's hypoxemia. Good hand washing and protection from individuals with an obvious respiratory tract infection are important. Aggressive pulmonary hygiene, treatment with antibiotics or antiviral agents as indicated, and supplemental oxygen to decrease hypoxemia are necessary measures. Infants may need to be gavage fed or given parenteral hydration if respiratory distress prevents oral feeding.

> ## ! NURSING ALERT
>
> Intracardiac shunting of blood from the right side (desaturated) to the left side of the heart allows air in the venous system to go directly to the brain, resulting in an air embolism. Therefore all IV lines should have filters in place to prevent air from entering the system, the entire tubing should be checked for air, all connections should be taped securely, and any air should be removed.

NURSING CARE OF THE FAMILY AND CHILD WITH CONGENITAL HEART DISEASE

When a child is born with a severe cardiac anomaly, the parents are faced with the immense psychologic and physical tasks of adjusting to the birth of a child with special needs. The following discussion is directed primarily (1) toward the family of an infant who has a serious heart defect and requires home care before definitive repair and (2) toward preparation and care of the child and family when invasive procedures (catheterization and surgery) are performed. For nursing care related to the child with hypoxemia and HF, the reader should refer to earlier discussions of these topics.

Nursing care of the child with a congenital heart defect begins as soon as the diagnosis is suspected. Prenatal diagnosis of congenital heart defects is becoming increasingly frequent. New demands are being placed on nurses to counsel and support families as they prepare for the birth of these infants.

Help the Family Adjust to the Disorder

When parents learn of the heart defect, they are initially in a period of shock followed by high anxiety and fear that the child will die. The family needs time to grieve before they can assimilate the meaning of the defect. Unfortunately, the demands for medical treatment may not allow this, instead necessitating that the parents immediately give informed consent for diagnostic-therapeutic procedures. The nurse can be instrumental in supporting parents in their loss, assessing their level of understanding, supplying information as needed, and helping other members of the health care team understand the parents' reactions (see Family-Centered Care box).

The effect of a child with a serious heart defect on the family is complex. No member, regardless of the degree of positive adjustment, is unaffected. Mothers frequently feel inadequate in their mothering ability because of the more complex care infants with congenital heart defects require. They often feel exhausted from the pressures of caring for these children and the other family members. Fathers and siblings may feel neglected and resentful, a reaction similar to the feelings toward family members with other chronic conditions (see Chapter 36). Often, parents do not feel confident leaving the child in another person's care. This often sets up a trap for parents, especially mothers, who become locked into the child's care with no relief. Although the fears are justified, they can be minimized by gradually teaching someone (a reliable relative or neighbor) how to care for the child.

The need to maintain discipline and set consistent limits can be difficult for parents. Using behavior modification techniques, in the form of either concrete awards (e.g., a favorite activity) or social reinforcement (e.g., approval), can be effective. However, it is most

> ## 👪 FAMILY-CENTERED CARE
> ### Diagnosis of Heart Disease
>
> Remember, we don't have your experience. We don't see children every day who have heart disease. We would have been upset finding out our child had to have his tonsils out. How could we ever be prepared for this? Please remember, we only know people who have trivial heart murmurs. How could we ever expect this to happen? And to us, this is the worst problem we've ever heard of.
>
> We still fear most what we don't know and understand. Be honest with us. If you don't know either, tell us. But at least don't leave us wondering about what you know and we don't. Not knowing anything really can be worse than knowing something bad. Be honest but don't strip us of hope ...
>
> Please, remember we are trying to learn complex information in a moment of time. And trying to learn it in a context of great pain and emotional investment. This is our lives you're talking about. Please be thorough but keep it simple. Tell us again, maybe even again and again, when we can hear better.

From Schrey C, Schrey M: A parent's perspective: our needs and our message, *Crit Care Nurs Clin North Am* 6(1):113-119, 1994.

beneficial if used *before* the child learns to control the family. To prevent later problems, it is necessary to begin discussions with parents while the child is in infancy regarding the need for discipline as the child gets older.

Another issue that may develop within family relationships is the child's overdependency. This is often the result of parental fear that the child may die. Parents need guidance to recognize the eventual hazards of continuing dependency and protectiveness as the child grows older, and the nurse can assist parents in learning ways to foster optimum development. Unless parents are shown what activities the child can do, they may focus on physical limitations and encourage dependency.

The child also needs opportunities for normal social interaction with peers. These children do not need to be prevented from playing with other children because of concern regarding overexertion. Children usually limit their activities if allowed to set their own pace. A child with CHD may constitute a long-term family crisis. Frequently, the continuing unremitting stresses of care—physical exhaustion, financial costs, emotional upset, fear of death, and concern for the child's future—are not fully appreciated by those caring for the family. Even when the child's condition is stabilized or corrected, the family may need to make adjustments in their lifestyle. Introducing them to other families with similarly affected children can help them adjust to the daily stresses.

Educate the Family About the Disorder

When parents are ready to hear about the heart condition, they require a clear explanation based on their level of understanding. A review of the basic structure and function of the heart is helpful before describing the defect. A simple diagram, pictures, or a model of the heart can help parents visualize the heart and the congenital defect. Parents appreciate receiving written information about the specific condition.[*] Health care professionals should take advantage

---

[*]American Heart Association, 7272 Greenville Ave., Dallas, TX 75231; 800-242-8721; www.americanheart.org.
Kids with Heart National Association for Children's Heart Disorders, 1578 Careful Dr, Green Bay, WI 54307; 800-538-5390; http:kidswithheart.org.
Little Hearts, Inc., PO Box 171, Cromwell, CT 06416; 860-635-0006, 866-435-4673; www.littlehearts.org.

of subsequent encounters to assess parental understanding of the condition and clarify information as needed.

Increasingly, families are using the Internet as a source of information about heart disease in children. They are also finding support through contacts with other parents and parent groups.* It is important for parents to realize that not all websites offer medically accurate information and that information from other parents might not be applicable to their own situation. Some children with rare, complex heart defects require individualized treatment plans, and general information on the Internet or in books may not apply to their child. Parents should use their health care team, in particular their cardiologist, to discuss information they have received from other sources.

Information given to the child must be tailored to the child's developmental age. As the child matures, the level of information is revised to meet the child's new cognitive level. Preschoolers need basic information about what they will experience more than what is actually occurring physiologically. School-age children benefit from a concrete explanation of the defect. Preadolescents and adolescents often appreciate a more detailed description of how the defect affects their heart. Children of all ages need to express their feelings concerning the diagnosis.

Help the Family Manage the Illness at Home

Parents are the child's principal caregivers and need to develop a positive, supportive working relationship with the health care team. Because most children spend the majority of their time at home with episodic trips to the hospital, parents manage their child's illness on a daily basis. They monitor for signs of illness, give medications and treatments, bring their child to appointments, work with a variety of caregivers, and alert the team about problems. Successful relationships are partnerships between parents and caregivers that is built on mutual trust and respect. Good communication among the family, the cardiology specialists, and the primary care practitioner is essential. As children reach adolescence, they begin to take a larger role in managing their illness and making decisions about their care.

Parents should be aware of the symptoms of their child's cardiac condition and signs of worsening clinical status. Parents of children who may develop HF should be familiar with the symptoms (see Box 42-5) and know when to contact the health care practitioner. Parents of children with cyanosis should be informed about fluid management and hypercyanotic spells (see p. 1337). Parents should have an information sheet with their child's diagnosis, significant treatments such as surgical procedures, allergies, other health care problems, current medications, and health care providers' contact numbers available in case of emergencies and to share with other caregivers such as teachers, babysitters, and day care providers.

The family also needs to be knowledgeable regarding the therapeutic management of the disorder and the role that surgery, other procedures, medications, and a healthy lifestyle plays in maintaining good health. Medications play a critical role in managing some cardiac conditions such as dysrhythmias, severe HF, anticoagulation for artificial valves, and antirejection medications after heart transplantation. Some patients must take multiple medications daily for their lifetime. Many medications can be dangerous if taken incorrectly and require close monitoring. Parents are taught the correct procedure for giving medications and cautioned to keep them in a safe area to prevent accidental ingestion.

Another area of parental concern is the child's level of physical activity. Most children do not need to restrict activity, and the best approach is to treat the child normally and allow self-limited activity. Exceptions to self-determined activity primarily involve strenuous recreational and competitive sports in children with specific cardiac problems. Activities and exercise restrictions should be discussed with the child's cardiologist. Deliberately attempting to prevent crying should be avoided because it can establish a maladaptive parental pattern of relating to the infant.

Infants and children with CHD require good nutrition. Breastfeeding should be possible for many infants with CHD. Providing adequate nutrition to infants with HF or complex congenital defects is especially difficult because of their high caloric requirements and inability to suck effectively because of fatigue and tachypnea. Instructing parents in feeding methods that decrease the infant's work and giving high-calorie formula are important interventions (see p. 1336 for a discussion on feeding the infant with HF). Children with severe cardiac defects are often anorexic. Encouraging them to eat can be a tremendous challenge. Consultation with a dietitian is often helpful. The child should be given a choice of available high-nutrient foods.

Infants with heart disease should be immunized according to the current guidelines. Immunization schedules may need to be modified around times of acute illness or surgical procedures (Smith, 2001). Infants and children younger than 2 years with unrepaired heart defects, cyanotic lesions, pulmonary hypertension, or history of prematurity should receive the vaccine for respiratory syncytial virus (RSV) monthly during RSV season (November to April in North America) for a total of five doses (American Academy of Pediatrics [AAP] Committee on Infectious Diseases, 2009).

Infants and children who have serious heart disease are at risk for developmental delays. Multiple factors can influence neurodevelopmental outcomes, including genetics (chromosomal abnormalities and microdeletions), family background (parental intelligence quotient [IQ] and socioeconomic status), preoperative factors (including prematurity, cyanosis, shock), intraoperative factors (use of cardiopulmonary bypass, deep hypothermic circulatory arrest), and postoperative factors (hemodynamic instability, hypoxia, acidosis, cardiac arrest, stroke, ischemic events).

Research in the past decade has begun to identify specific risk factors and common developmental concerns for CHD. Bellinger, Wypij, duPlessis, et al. (2003) found an association between longer periods of deep hypothermic circulatory arrest and the presence of postoperative seizures, delayed motor development, and a downward trend in full-scale IQ. At 8 years of age, more than one third of the study patients had received remedial services in school. Shillingford, Glanzman, Ittenbach, et al. (2008) also found that a significant proportion of children with complex CHD were at risk for inattention and hyperactivity and nearly half were using remedial school services. In another longitudinal study, Limperopoulos, Majnemer, Shevell, et al. (2002) found that preoperative and early postoperative neurologic status, microcephaly, type of cardiac lesions, length of deep hypothermic circulatory arrest, age at surgery, and length of ICU stay were predictors of developmental delay.

Recent efforts to limit the time of deep hypothermic circulatory arrest and provide better neuroprotection during infant surgery may improve outcomes in the future. Although most children with serious heart disease are within the normal range for IQ, there is a higher incidence of neurodevelopmental deficits in children after

---

*The Congenital Heart Information Network, http://tchin.org; Heart Rhythm Society (information on arrhythmias), www.hrsonline.org; Adult Congenital Heart Association, www.achaheart.org; Congenital Heart Defects, www.congenitalheartdefects.com; Children's Heart Foundation, www.childrensheartfoundation.com. Many major medical centers that perform pediatric heart surgery also have information on their websites.

heart surgery than in the normal population, specifically in speech and language, fine motor skills, and cognitive processes (Majnemer and Limperopoulos, 1999). Severe neurologic problems such as cerebral palsy, epilepsy, and intellectual disability are uncommon.

Prepare the Child and Family for Invasive Procedures

Chapter 39 provides an extensive discussion of the principles for preparing children for invasive procedures. The American Heart Association published a scientific statement "Recommendations for Preparing Children and Adolescents for Invasive Cardiac Procedures" (LeRoy, Elixson, O'Brien, et al., 2003), which addresses issues specific to the child with heart disease. The following discussion highlights some important aspects of preparation for cardiac catheterization and cardiac surgery.

The expected outcomes for preprocedure preparation include reducing anxiety, improving patient cooperation with procedures, enhancing recovery, developing trust with caregivers, and improving long-term emotional and behavioral adjustments after procedures (LeRoy, Elixson, O'Brien, et al., 2003). Important factors to consider in planning preparation strategies are the child's cognitive development, previous hospital experiences, the child's temperament and coping style, the timing of preparation, and the involvement of the parents. The most beneficial preparation strategies usually combine information giving and coping-skills training such as conscious breathing exercises, distraction techniques, guided imagery, or other behavioral interventions.

Outpatient preoperative and precatheterization workups are common for most elective procedures. Children are then admitted on the morning of the procedure. Preprocedure teaching is often done in the clinic setting or at home and may include a tour of the ICU and inpatient facilities. Children of different ages and developmental levels require different amounts of information and different approaches. Whereas young children should be prepared close in time to the event, older children and adolescents may benefit from teaching several weeks in advance. Parents should be included in the preparation session to support their child and learn about upcoming events.

Topics to include in preoperative or precatheterization preparation include information on the environment, equipment, and procedures that the child will encounter during and after the procedure. Many information-giving techniques can be used such as verbal and written information, hospital tours, preoperative classes, picture books, or videos. Information about what the child will see, hear, and feel should be included, especially for older children and adolescents. Some of the sensory experiences of being in an ICU or catheterization laboratory include sights (monitors, many people, much equipment), sounds (beeping noises, alarms, voices), and sensations (lines and dressings, tape, discomfort, thirst). Familiar aspects of the environment, such as BP cuffs, stethoscopes, or oximeter probes, are reviewed, and new equipment, such as monitors, IV lines, and oxygen masks, is described. Comforting aspects of the environment, such as play areas, chairs for parents, and televisions, are emphasized. Many patients who will be sedated during catheterization or receiving narcotic pain relievers after surgery will have minimal recall of that period and will not need detailed information about the equipment or procedures used. Information should be specific to the planned procedure for each patient.

A discussion of ways the child can cope with the experience should be included. For a young child, bringing a familiar stuffed animal or comfort object will help relieve anxiety, and advising an older child to bring headphones and favorite music to the catheterization laboratory will help distract him or her during the procedure. Recovery topics after catheterization include lying still to prevent bleeding at the catheter site, advancing diet, controlling pain, and monitoring. After surgery, the nurse reviews the importance of ambulation, coughing, deep breathing, drinking, and eating and describes pain management and monitoring routines. Simple coping strategies for use during painful procedures should be reviewed; these include distraction techniques such as counting, blowing, singing, and telling stories.

Children and their families should have a choice about an ICU tour. Exposure to the ICU environment can actually increase anxiety in some children, particularly young children, those with previous hospital experiences, and those who are highly anxious (LeRoy, Elixson, O'Brien, et al., 2003). Usually the day before the procedure is ample time to allow the child to ask questions and to prevent undue fantasizing about the experience. The child should be protected from the frightening sights in the unit; equipment not in view postoperatively, such as equipment located behind or below the bed, needs less attention. The child and parents are encouraged to ask questions or to explore further any equipment in the room, but they should not be pushed to assimilate more information than they are able.

Preoperative physical care differs little, if any, from that for any other surgery and is discussed in Chapter 39. The child should be assured that the parents will be there when the child wakes up; parents should be allowed to accompany their child as far as possible to the operating suite (see Surgical Procedures, p. 1136). After all of the equipment and procedures have been explained, it is important to talk about "getting well" and going home.

Provide Postoperative Care

Immediate postoperative care is usually provided by specially trained nurses in ICUs. Many of the procedures, such as arterial pressure and central venous pressure (CVP) monitoring, and the observations related to vital functions require advanced educational training (readers should refer to critical care texts for further information). However, nurses caring for the child before surgery and during the convalescent period need to be familiar with the major principles of care. Selected complications that may occur postoperatively are described in Box 42-7.

Observe Vital Signs

Vital signs and BP are recorded frequently until stable. Heart rate and respirations are counted for 1 full minute, compared with the ECG monitor, and recorded with activity. The heart rate is normally increased after surgery. The nurse observes cardiac rhythm and notifies the health care practitioner of any changes in regularity. Dysrhythmias may occur postoperatively secondary to anesthetics, acid-base and electrolyte imbalance, hypoxia, surgical intervention, or trauma to conduction pathways (p. 1347).

At least hourly, the lungs are auscultated for breath sounds. Diminished or absent sounds may indicate an area of atelectasis or a pleural effusion or pneumothorax, which necessitates further medical assessment. Temperature changes are typical during the early postoperative period. Hypothermia is expected immediately after surgery from hypothermia procedures, effects of anesthesia, and loss of body heat to the cool environment. During this period, the child is kept warm to prevent additional heat loss. Infants may be placed under radiant heat warmers. During the next 24 to 48 hours, the body temperature may rise to 37.7° C (100° F) or slightly higher as part of the inflammatory response to tissue trauma. After this period, an elevated temperature is most likely a sign of infection and warrants immediate investigation for probable cause.

BOX 42-7 **SELECTED COMPLICATIONS AFTER CARDIAC SURGERY AND TREATMENT APPROACHES**

Cardiac

Heart failure—Digoxin, diuretics (see p. 1332)

Low cardiac output—Intravenous inotropes (see Shock, p. 1355)

Dysrhythmias—Identification, drug treatment, possible pacing, cardioversion (see p. 1349)

Tamponade (blood or fluid in the pericardial space constricting the heart)—Prompt removal of fluid by pericardiocentesis

Respiratory

Atelectasis—Chest physical therapy, coughing, deep breathing, ambulation

Pulmonary edema—Diuretics

Pleural effusions—Diuretics, possible chest tube drainage

Pneumothorax—Possible chest tube drainage

Neurologic

Seizures—Assessment, antiepileptic drugs

Cerebrovascular accident (stroke), cerebral edema, neurologic deficits—Assessment and treatment

Infectious Disease

Infections (especially wound, pneumonia, otitis media, and sepsis)—Antibiotics

Hematologic

Anemia—Iron supplementation, possible transfusion

Postoperative bleeding—Initially, clotting factors, blood products; may need repeat surgery to locate and ligate source of bleeding

Other

Postpericardiotomy syndrome (syndrome of fever, leukocytosis, friction rub, pericardial and pleural effusions, and lethargy seen about 7 to 21 days after cardiac surgery; possible viral or autoimmune etiologies)—Antipyretics, diuretics, antiinflammatory medications

Intraarterial monitoring of BP is commonly done after openheart surgery. A catheter is passed into the radial artery or other artery, and the other end is attached to an electronic monitoring system, which provides a continuous recording of the BP. The intraarterial line is maintained with a low-rate, constant infusion of heparinized saline to prevent clotting.

Several IV lines are inserted preoperatively, including a peripheral IV line to give fluids and medications and a central venous line, usually in a large vessel in the neck, to measure CVP. Additional intracardiac monitoring lines are sometimes placed intraoperatively in the right atrium, left atrium, or pulmonary artery. Intracardiac lines allow assessment of pressures inside the cardiac chambers, providing vital information about volume status, cardiac output, and ventricular function. All lines must be cared for using strict aseptic technique, and patients must be carefully assessed for bleeding at the time of line removal.

Maintain Respiratory Status

Infants usually require mechanical ventilation in the immediate postoperative period. Early extubation in the operating room or early postoperative period is becoming more common. Children, especially those not requiring cardiopulmonary bypass, may be extubated in the operating room or in the first few postoperative hours. Suctioning is performed only as needed and performed carefully to avoid vagal stimulation (which can trigger cardiac dysrhythmias) and laryngospasm, especially in infants. Suctioning is intermittent and maintained for no more than 5 seconds at a time to avoid depleting the oxygen supply. Supplemental oxygen is administered with a manual resuscitation bag before and after the procedure to prevent hypoxia. The heart rate is monitored after suctioning to detect changes in rhythm or rate, especially bradycardia. The child should always be positioned facing the nurse to permit assessment of the child's color and tolerance of the procedure.

When weaning and extubation are completed, humidified oxygen is delivered by mask, hood, or nasal cannula to prevent drying of mucosa. The child is encouraged to turn and deep breathe at least hourly. Measures are used to enhance ventilation and decrease pain, such as splinting of the operative site and use of analgesics. Chest tubes are inserted into the pleural or mediastinal space during surgery or in the immediate postoperative period to remove secretions and air to allow reexpansion of the lung. Drainage is checked hourly for color and quantity. Immediately after surgery, the drainage may be bright red, but afterward, it should be serous. The largest volume of drainage occurs in the first 12 to 24 hours and is greater in extensive heart surgery.

> **! NURSING ALERT**
>
> Chest tube drainage greater than 3 mL/kg/hr for more than 3 consecutive hours or 5 to 10 mL/kg in any 1 hour is excessive and may indicate postoperative hemorrhage. The surgeon should be notified immediately because cardiac tamponade can develop rapidly and is life threatening.

Chest tubes are usually removed on the first to third postoperative day. Removal of chest tubes is a painful, frightening experience. Analgesics such as morphine sulfate, often combined with midazolam (Versed), should be given before the procedure. Older children are forewarned that they will feel a sharp, momentary pain. After the suture is cut, the tubes are quickly pulled out at the end of full inspiration in the extubated patient to prevent intake of air into the pleural cavity. (In the intubated patient, the tubes are pulled out on inspiration because the lungs are stented open with the positive-pressure ventilation.) A purse-string suture (placed when the tubes were inserted) is pulled tight to close the opening. A petrolatum-covered gauze dressing is immediately applied over the wound and securely taped on all four sides to the skin so that an airtight seal is formed. It is left on for 1 or 2 days. Breath sounds are checked to assess for a pneumothorax—a possible complication of chest tube removal. A chest radiograph is usually obtained after removal to evaluate for possible pneumothorax or pleural effusion.

Monitor Fluids

Intake and output of all fluids must be accurately calculated. Intake is primarily IV fluids; however, a record of fluid used to flush the arterial and CVP lines or to dilute medications is also kept. Output includes hourly recordings of urine (usually a Foley catheter is inserted and attached to a closed collecting device), drainage from chest and nasogastric tubes, and blood drawn for analysis. Renal failure is a potential risk from a transient period of low cardiac output.

Fluids are restricted during the immediate postoperative period to prevent hypervolemia, which places additional demands on the myocardium, predisposing the patient to cardiac failure. If the child is to be extubated within the first 24 to 48 hours, fluids are provided primarily intravenously. If the child is to be intubated longer, fluids may be given via a nasogastric or nasojejunal tube to optimize nutrition and gut motility. Approximately 4 hours after extubation, enteral fluids may be reinitiated in the setting of a stable hemodynamic and respiratory status. To monitor fluid retention, the child is weighed daily, and the same scale is used at approximately the same time each day to avoid errors in measurement. Fluid restriction may be imposed even when oral fluids are given. The nurse calculates the distribution over a 24-hour period based on the child's preoperative weight and drinking habits. The distribution should allow for most fluid to be given during the child's most wakeful and active periods.

Provide Rest and Progressive Activity

After heart surgery, rest should be provided to decrease the workload of the heart and promote healing. The simplest way to ensure individualized, efficient, high-quality care is to plan at the beginning of the shift the nursing procedures to be done, with periods of rest identified. The schedule should be shared with parents to allow them to visit at the most advantageous times, such as after a rest period when no special treatments are anticipated.

A progressive schedule of ambulation and activity is planned, based on the child's preoperative activity patterns and postoperative cardiovascular and pulmonary function. Ambulation is initiated early, usually by the second postoperative day, when chest tubes, arterial lines, and assisted ventilatory equipment have been removed. Activity progresses from sitting on the edge of the bed and dangling the legs to standing up and sitting in a chair. Heart rate and respirations are carefully monitored to assess the degree of cardiac demand imposed by each activity. Tachycardia, dyspnea, cyanosis, desaturation, progressive fatigue, and dysrhythmias indicate the need to limit further energy expenditure.

Provide Comfort and Emotional Support

Heart surgery is both painful and frightening for children, and comfort is a primary nursing concern. Several types of incisions are used by the cardiac surgeon. A median sternotomy is most common, following the sternum down the center of the chest. A ministernotomy opens the lower sternum. A thoracotomy incision is most uncomfortable because it goes through muscle tissue. It allows access to the side of the chest through an incision from under the arm around the back to the scapula.

Most patients need IV analgesics for pain control during the immediate postoperative period. Patient-controlled analgesia may be used with children old enough to understand the concept. Nonsteroidal antiinflammatory drugs (NSAIDs) such as ketorolac (Toradol) may be used intravenously. Paralyzing agents may also be used with the analgesics for children who are hemodynamically unstable.

After extubation and removal of lines and tubes, pain can be satisfactorily controlled with oral medications such as ibuprofen, codeine with acetaminophen (Tylenol No. 3), or oxycodone and acetaminophen. Acetaminophen alone provides adequate pain relief for most children at discharge. Sternotomy incisions are usually well tolerated, with some discomfort when walking and coughing. Thoracotomy incisions are usually more painful because the incision is through muscle; a more aggressive pain management plan with around-the-clock medications for several days is often necessary to allow for adequate rest, ambulation, and pulmonary hygiene.

In addition to pharmacologic pain control, every effort is made to minimize the discomfort of procedures, such as using a firm pillow or favorite stuffed animal placed against the chest incision during movement and performing treatments *after* pain medication is given, preferably at a time that coincides with the drug's peak effect. Nonpharmacologic measures are used to lessen the perception of pain, and parents are encouraged to comfort their child as much as possible. (See also Pain Assessment; Pain Management, Chapter 30.)

Children may become depressed after surgery. This is thought to be caused by preoperative anxiety, postoperative psychologic and physiologic stress, and sensory overstimulation. Typically, the child's disposition improves on leaving the ICU.

Children may also be angry and uncooperative after surgery as a response to the physical pain and to the loss of control imposed by the surgery and treatments. They need an opportunity to express feelings, either verbally or through activity. Children often regress in their behavior during the stress of surgery and hospitalization. They also may express feelings of anger or rejection toward their parents. The nurse can support the parents by being available for information and explaining all of the procedures to them. The first few postoperative days are particularly difficult because parents see their child in pain and realize the potential risks from surgery. They often are overwhelmed by the physical environment of the ICU and feel useless because they can do so little for their child. The nurse can minimize such feelings by including parents in caregiving activities and comfort and play activities, providing information about the child's condition, and being sensitive to their emotional and physical needs. The importance of their presence in making the child feel more secure is stressed even if they do not provide physical care.

Plan for Discharge and Home Care

Ideally, discharge planning begins on admission for cardiac surgery and includes an assessment of the parents' adjustment to the child's altered state of health. Neonates need additional screening tests (e.g., newborn metabolic screen and hearing tests) and may need immunizations before discharge (Dodds and Merle, 2005). The family will need both verbal and written instructions on medication, nutrition, activity restrictions, subacute bacterial endocarditis (SBE), return to school, wound care, and signs and symptoms of infection or complications (see Family-Centered Care box). Referrals to community agencies may be warranted to assist parents in the transition from the hospital to home and to reinforce the teaching.

The parents will also need clear instructions on when to seek medical care for complications and how to contact the health care provider. Follow-up with the cardiologist and primary care provider is also arranged before discharge. Parents should have a summary, including their child's medical condition, medications, and health care providers available for emergencies. Appropriate identification, such as a MedicAlert device, is indicated for children with a pacemaker or a heart transplant and for those receiving anticoagulation therapy or antidysrhythmic medication.

Although surgical correction of heart defects has improved dramatically, it is still not possible to completely repair many of the complex anomalies. For many children, repeat procedures are

FAMILY-CENTERED CARE

Topics to Include in Discharge Teaching After Cardiac Surgery

- Medication teaching
- Activity restrictions
- Diet and nutrition
- Wound care (including dressings, if any; suture removal; bathing)
- Bacterial (infective) endocarditis prophylaxis (see Box 42-9)
- Follow-up appointments (cardiologist, primary care provider)
- Community agencies as needed (visiting nurse service, early developmental intervention)
- When to call health care practitioner; signs and symptoms of postoperative problems
- Review of cardiac defect and surgical repair

BOX 42-8   CLINICAL MANIFESTATIONS OF INFECTIVE ENDOCARDITIS

- Onset usually insidious
- Unexplained fever (low grade and intermittent)
- Anorexia
- Malaise
- Weight loss
- Characteristic findings caused by extracardiac emboli formation:
  - Splinter hemorrhages (thin black lines) under the nails
  - Osler nodes (red, painful intradermal nodes found on pads of phalanges)
  - Janeway lesions (painless hemorrhagic areas on palms and soles)
  - Petechiae on oral mucous membranes
- May be present:
  - Heart failure
  - Cardiac dysrhythmias
  - New murmur or change in previously existing one

required to replace conduits or grafts or to manage complications such as restenosis. Consequently, the long-term prognosis is uncertain and full recovery is not always possible. For these families, medical follow-up and continued emotional support are essential. The nurse can often serve as an important primary health care professional and as a resource for referrals when needed.

ACQUIRED CARDIOVASCULAR DISORDERS

Bacterial (Infective) Endocarditis

Bacterial endocarditis (BE), or subacute bacterial endocarditis (SBE), is now commonly referred to as infective endocarditis (IE). IE is an infection of the inner lining of the heart (endocardium), generally involving the valves. Although it can occur without underlying heart disease, it is most often a sequela of bacteremia in children with acquired or congenital anomalies of the heart or great vessels. It especially affects children with valvular abnormalities, prosthetic valves, shunts, recent cardiac surgery with invasive lines, and rheumatic heart disease with valve involvement. The most common causative agents are *Staphylococcus aureus* and *Streptococcus viridans;* other causative agents include gram-negative bacteria and fungi such as *Candida albicans.*

Pathophysiology

Organisms may enter the bloodstream from any site of localized infection. In the past, endocarditis was believed to be highly associated with invasive procedures; however, endocarditis is most likely to occur from routine exposure to bacteremia associated with usual daily activities, although it can also occur after procedures such as dental work (*S. viridans*); after invasive procedures involving the gastrointestinal and genitourinary tracts; after cardiac surgery, especially if synthetic material is used (valves, patches, conduits); or from long-term indwelling catheters. The microorganisms grow on the endocardium, forming vegetations (verrucae), deposits of fibrin, and platelet thrombi. The lesion may invade adjacent tissues, such as the aortic and mitral valves, and may break off and embolize elsewhere, especially in the spleen, kidney, and central nervous system (CNS).

Diagnostic Evaluation

The diagnosis of IE is suspected on the basis of clinical manifestations (Box 42-8). The most commonly used guidelines for diagnosis use the revised Duke criteria, which outline major and minor criteria consistent with IE (Li, Sexton, Mick, et al., 2000). Several laboratory findings may suggest IE (e.g., ECG changes [prolonged PR interval], radiographic evidence of cardiomegaly, anemia, elevated erythrocyte sedimentation rate [ESR], leukocytosis, microscopic hematuria). Vegetations on the valve and abnormal valve function can often be visualized by echocardiography. Definitive diagnosis rests on growth and identification of the causative agent in the blood. A diagnosis of culture-negative IE is made when the patient has echocardiographic or clinical evidence of IE but no organism can be cultured (Ferrieri, 2002).

Therapeutic Management

Treatment should be instituted immediately and consists of administration of high doses of appropriate antibiotics intravenously for 2 to 8 weeks. Blood cultures are taken periodically to evaluate the response to antibiotic therapy.

Prevention involves administration of prophylactic antibiotic therapy 1 hour before certain procedures that are associated with the risk for entry of organisms in very high risk patients. Recent guidelines recommend prophylaxis only in patients with the highest risk for poor outcome if they develop endocarditis (Box 42-9). Drugs of choice for prophylaxis include amoxicillin, ampicillin, clindamycin, cephalexin, cefadroxil, azithromycin, and clarithromycin.

CARE MANAGEMENT

Ideally, the objective of nursing care is to counsel parents of high risk children concerning the signs and symptoms of endocarditis and, in certain cases, the need for prophylactic antibiotic therapy before procedures such as dental work. The family's dentist should be advised of the child's cardiac diagnosis as an added precaution to ensure preventive treatment. SBE prophylaxis is now reserved for very high risk patients. Many patients who met criteria established in the past may not require prophylaxis under the new guidelines (Wilson, Taubert, Gewitz, et al., 2007) (see Box 42-9). Parents should be counseled regarding the rationale for discontinuing prophylaxis and should be educated as to the fact that their child is still at higher risk for IE than the general population. It is important that all children with congenital or acquired heart disease maintain the highest level of oral health to reduce the chance of bacteremia from oral infections.

BOX 42-9 CARDIAC CONDITIONS ASSOCIATED WITH THE HIGHEST RISK FOR ADVERSE OUTCOME FROM ENDOCARDITIS

- Prophylaxis with dental procedures recommended for*:
  - Previous episode of infective endocarditis
  - Prosthetic cardiac valve
- CHD, including only:
  - Unrepaired cyanotic CHD, including palliative shunts and conduits
  - Completely repaired congenital heart defect with prosthetic material or device, whether placed by surgery or by catheter intervention, during the first 6 months after the procedure
- Repaired CHD with residual defects at the site or adjacent to the site of a prosthetic patch or prosthetic device (which inhibit endothelialization)
- Cardiac transplantation recipients who develop cardiac valvulopathy

Adapted from Wilson W, Taubert K, Gewitz M, et al: Prevention of infective endocarditis: guidelines from the American Heart Association, *Circulation* 116(15):1736-1754, 2007.
CHD, Congenital heart disease.
*Except for the conditions listed, antibiotic prophylaxis is no longer recommended for any other form of CHD.

Parents should also have a high index of suspicion regarding potential infections. Without unduly alarming them, the nurse stresses that any unexplained fever, weight loss, or change in behavior (lethargy, malaise, anorexia) must be brought to the health care practitioner's attention. Such symptoms should not be self-diagnosed as a cold or flu. Early diagnosis and treatment are important in preventing further cardiac damage, embolic complications, and growth of resistant organisms.

Treatment of endocarditis requires long-term parenteral drug therapy. In many cases, IV antibiotics may be administered at home with nursing supervision. Nursing goals during this period are (1) preparation of the child for IV infusion, usually with an intermittent-infusion device and several venipunctures for blood cultures; (2) observation for side effects of antibiotics, especially inflammation along venipuncture sites; (3) observation for complications, including embolism and HF; and (4) education regarding the importance of follow-up visits for cardiac evaluation, echocardiographic monitoring, and blood cultures.

Rheumatic Fever

Rheumatic fever (RF) is a poorly understood inflammatory disease that occurs after infection with group A β-hemolytic streptococcal (GABHS) pharyngitis. It occurs most often in late school-age children and adolescents and is rare in adults. It is a self-limited illness that involves the joints, skin, brain, serous surfaces, and heart. Cardiac valve damage (referred to as rheumatic heart disease) is the most significant complication of RF. The mitral valve is most often affected. In developed countries, RF and rheumatic heart disease have become uncommon. However, RF remains a devastating problem in developing countries.

Etiology

Strong evidence supports a relationship between upper respiratory tract infection with GABHS and subsequent development of RF (usually within 2 to 6 weeks). In almost all cases of RF, a previous infection with GABHS can be documented by laboratory evidence of rising antibody titers. Prevention or treatment of GABHS infection prevents RF.

Diagnostic Evaluation

Diagnosis continues to be based on a set of guidelines known as the *modified Jones criteria* (Guidelines for the diagnosis of rheumatic fever, 1992). These guidelines were reviewed and again endorsed by the American Heart Association in 2002 and continue to be used to this date (Ferrieri, 2002). The updated Jones criteria suggest that the presence of two major manifestations or one major and two minor manifestations, with supportive evidence of recent streptococcal infection, indicates a high probability of RF.

Children suspected of having RF are tested for streptococcal antibodies. The most reliable and best standardized test is an elevated or rising antistreptolysin O (ASO or ASLO) titer, which occurs in 80% of children with RF. Additional antistreptococcal antibody titers may be sent if ASO titers are negative. Acute-phase reactants, ESR, and C-reactive protein (CRP) are usually elevated as well.

Therapeutic Management

The goals of medical management are (1) eradication of hemolytic streptococci, (2) prevention of permanent cardiac damage, (3) palliation of the other symptoms, and (4) prevention of recurrences of RF. Penicillin is the drug of choice or an alternative in penicillin-sensitive children (Gerber, Baltimore, Eaton, et al., 2009). Salicylates are used to control the inflammatory process, especially in the joints, and reduce the fever and discomfort. Bed rest is recommended during the acute febrile phase but need not be strict.

Children who have had acute RF are susceptible to recurrent RF for the rest of their lives and should be followed medically because repeated infections are likely to result in rheumatic heart disease.

Prophylactic treatment against recurrence of RF (secondary prevention) is started after the acute therapy and involves monthly intramuscular injections of benzathine penicillin G (1.2 million units), two daily oral doses of penicillin (200,000 units), or one daily dose of sulfadiazine (1 g). The current American Heart Association guidelines recommend secondary prophylaxis for all patients diagnosed with RF. The exact length of secondary prophylaxis is based on whether or not a patient has residual heart disease. In RF with carditis, prophylaxis is recommended for 5 years or until age 21 years. In the setting of carditis, prophylaxis is recommended for 10 years or until 21 years old. In the setting of RF with carditis and residual heart disease, prophylaxis can continue until the age of 40 years and may be indicated indefinitely depending on the individual's risk (Gerber, Baltimore, Eaton, et al., 2009).

CARE MANAGEMENT

The objectives of nursing care for the child with RF are to (1) encourage compliance with drug regimens, (2) facilitate recovery from the illness, (3) provide emotional support, and (4) prevent the disease. Because compliance is a major concern in long-term drug therapy, every effort is made to encourage adherence to the therapeutic plan (see Compliance, Chapter 39). When compliance is poor, monthly injections may be substituted for daily oral administration of antibiotics and children need preparation for this often-dreaded procedure.

Interventions during home care are concerned primarily with providing rest and adequate nutrition. Usually, after the febrile stage is over, children can resume moderate activity and their appetite improves. If carditis is present, the family must be aware of any activity restrictions and may need help in choosing less strenuous activities for the child.

One of the most disturbing and frustrating manifestations of the disease is chorea. The onset is gradual and may occur weeks to months after the illness; it sometimes even occurs in children who have not been diagnosed with RF. It may be mistaken for nervousness, clumsiness, behavioral changes, inattentiveness, and learning disability. It is usually a source of great frustration to the child because the movements, incoordination, and weakness severely limit physical ability. Of utmost importance is stressing to parents and schoolteachers the involuntary, sudden nature of the movements; that the chorea is transitory; and that all manifestations eventually disappear.

Nurses also have a role in prevention, primarily in screening school-age children for sore throats caused by GABHS. This may involve actively participating in throat culture screening programs or in referring children with a possible streptococcal infection for testing.

Hyperlipidemia (Hypercholesterolemia)

Hyperlipidemia is a general term for excessive lipids (fat and fatlike substances); hypercholesterolemia refers to excessive cholesterol in the blood. Dyslipidemia is a term used to describe all abnormalities in lipid metabolism, including low levels of high-density lipoprotein (HDL) or "good" cholesterol. High lipid or cholesterol levels play an important role in producing atherosclerosis (fatty plaque on the arteries), which eventually can lead to coronary artery disease—a primary cause of morbidity and mortality in the adult population. A presymptomatic phase of atherosclerosis can begin in childhood. Preventive cardiology focuses on the screening and management of lipid levels in childhood. The goal is to identify children at high risk and intervene early.

Cholesterol is part of the lipoprotein complex in plasma that is essential for cellular metabolism. Triglycerides, natural fats synthesized from carbohydrates, are used for energy. Both are major lipids transported on lipoproteins, a combination of lipids and proteins, which include:

- Low-density lipoproteins (LDLs)—These contain low concentrations of triglycerides, high levels of cholesterol, and moderate levels of protein. LDL is the major carrier of cholesterol to the cells. Cells use cholesterol for synthesis of membranes and steroid production. Elevated circulating LDL is a strong risk factor in cardiovascular disease.
- High-density lipoproteins (HDLs)—These contain very low concentrations of triglycerides, relatively little cholesterol, and high levels of protein. They transport free cholesterol to the liver for excretion in the bile. High levels of HDL are thought to protect against cardiovascular disease.

Diagnostic Evaluation

Hyperlipidemia is diagnosed on the basis of analysis of blood for a full lipid profile, drawn after a 12-hour fast. Hyperlipidemia can have a genetic basis or a lifestyle component or can be caused by secondary problems, such as hypothyroidism. In children with elevated cholesterol levels, a screening thyroid-stimulating hormone is also measured once to rule out hypothyroidism as a cause of secondary hypercholesterolemia. Additional blood work is individualized based on other risk factors. In overweight children, a fasting glucose level may be obtained to assess for risk factors associated with metabolic syndrome, which is a combination of multiple symptoms that are associated with increased cardiovascular risk in adults. Blood samples should be collected after having the child sit for 5 minutes,

TABLE 42-3	CLASSIFICATION OF CHOLESTEROL LEVELS IN CHILDREN FROM FAMILIES WITH A HISTORY OF HEART DISEASE	
CATEGORY	**TOTAL CHOLESTEROL (MG/DL)**	**LDL CHOLESTEROL (MG/DL)**
Acceptable	<170	<110
Borderline	170-199	110-129
High	≥200	≥130

From Daniels SR, Greer FR, Committee on Nutrition: Lipid screening and cardiovascular health in childhood, *Pediatrics* 122(1):198-208, 2008.
LDL, Low-density lipoprotein.

and the tourniquet should be applied immediately before the needle puncture because posture and vascular stasis may affect results. Diagnostic values for acceptable, borderline, and high total cholesterol and LDL cholesterol levels are listed in Table 42-3.

The National Heart, Lung, and Blood Institute (NHLBI) (NHLBI, 2011) recently issued a recommendation for universal lipid (nonfasting or fasting) screening of all children and adolescents between the ages of 9 and 11 years and again between the ages of 17 and 21 years. LDL cholesterol–lowering drug therapy is recommended for children and adolescents 10 years of age and older whose LDL remains elevated after 6 months to 1 year on a restricted fat diet, lifestyle modification (exercise), and weight management (NHLBI, 2011). Additional information and practice guidelines for monitoring cholesterol levels and initiation of cholesterol-lowering medication as well as specific dietary modifications are found in the 2011 NHLBI summary report at www.nhlbi.nih.gov/guidelines/cvd_ped/summary.htm#chap5.

Therapeutic Management

The first step in the treatment of high cholesterol is oriented to lifestyle modification. The American Academy of Pediatrics (AAP) (Daniels, Greer, and Committee on Nutrition, 2008) guidelines continue to advocate the benefits of a heart-healthy diet for all children. Children with known elevated cholesterol should have individual nutritional counseling by a nutritionist with expertise in pediatric lipids.

Research continues to support the benefit of diets low in saturated fats. Current thinking favors a "Mediterranean"-type diet. Whole grains, fruits, and vegetables form the foundation of this diet. In addition, this diet allows the use of monounsaturated fats, such as olive oil and canola oil, which have beneficial effects on HDL cholesterol values. The use of these fats also makes the diet more realistic. Patients who have elevated triglycerides, especially in the setting of an elevated body mass index (BMI), should receive targeted counseling related to decreasing their intake of simple carbohydrates. Aerobic exercise of at least 60 minutes a day 5 days a week is also recommended for children with high cholesterol. In addition, patients and parents should be counseled regarding the negative effects of smoking (both firsthand and secondhand).

For children with severe hypercholesterolemia who fail to respond to dietary modifications, drug therapy may be necessary. Pharmacologic therapy is recommended for children older than 8 years who have LDL cholesterol greater than 190 mg/dL without other risk factors or over 160 mg/dL in patients with two or more other risk factors. In young people with other risk factors, such as diabetes, medication can be considered when LDL values are greater than 130 mg/dL. The use of medication in young people needs to be a cooperative decision with the parents. Parents should understand what data are available about statin use in young people because long-term evidence-based practice is not practical or available for this population. In the past, bile acid–binding resins were the only class of drugs recommended for treatment of younger children. This class of drug acts by binding bile acids in the intestinal lumen. Because they are not absorbed by the intestine, resin binders do not produce systemic toxicity and are safe for children. Both cholestyramine (Questran) and colestipol (Colestid) are powders that are mixed with water or juice just before ingestion. Unfortunately, the vast majority of patients do not get adequate reduction in LDL cholesterol from bile acid–binding resins. Many cannot tolerate the medication because of the taste; gritty texture; and side effects, the most significant being constipation, abdominal pain, gastrointestinal bloating, flatulence, and nausea. The most recent guidelines on lipid abnormalities in children give the option for treatment with statins if pharmacologic therapy is indicated using the previously outlined guidelines for treatment (Daniels, Greer, and Committee on Nutrition, 2008; McCrindle, Urbina, Dennison, et al., 2007). Statins are much more effective than other drugs at lowering LDL cholesterol. To a lesser degree, they also help lower triglycerides levels and can raise HDL cholesterol. Statins work by inhibiting the enzyme necessary for cholesterol synthesis. Statins are most effective when taken in the evening and are started at the lowest possible dose in young people. Blood work should be followed closely in children and adolescents and usually includes a fasting lipid profile, liver function tests, and creatinine kinase repeated at 4- and 8-week intervals initially and with dosage changes.

Patients beginning therapy with a statin should be counseled regarding rare but potentially serious side effects such as rhabdomyolysis, elevated transaminases, and elevated creatinine kinase. Patients should discontinue their medication and contact their practitioner if they develop dark urine or new muscle aches. Last, statin medications are not safe during pregnancy; therefore sexually active adolescents need to take adequate birth control measures. Very long–term studies are unlikely to be available over decades; however, in the shorter-term studies that have been completed, statins seem to have a similar safety profile for children as they do for adults (McCrindle, Urbina, Dennison, et al., 2007).

CARE MANAGEMENT

Nurses play an important role in the screening, education, and support of children with lipid abnormalities and their families. When a child is referred to a preventive cardiology clinic, it is essential that the family be adequately prepared for the first visit. Generally, the parents will be asked to keep a dietary history of the child before this visit. Sometimes they will need to complete a questionnaire regarding the child's normal dietary habits during the preceding year. Families should be instructed to keep their child fasting for at least 12 hours before screening. Last, parents should be aware that lipids should not be drawn within 3 weeks of a febrile illness because doing so can affect cholesterol values. It is important to schedule the blood test early in the morning and to arrange for nourishment immediately thereafter. At the visit, a full family history should be taken, including the health of both parents and all first-degree relatives. Specific questions should be asked regarding early heart disease, hypertension, strokes (CVAs), sudden death, hyperlipidemia, diabetes, and endocrine abnormalities.

Parents and extended families should be educated about cholesterol and lipid abnormalities. This education should include a brief introduction of the different lipoprotein categories, including cholesterol, HDL, LDL, and triglycerides. Also, behavioral risk factors for heart disease, such as smoking and exercise, should be reviewed. For management to be effective, parents and patients need to understand that the rationale for dietary or pharmacologic intervention is prevention of future cardiovascular disease.

Stringent dietary guidelines may become an issue of control and a source of great stress for many families. A child with a lipid disorder should not be viewed as having a disease. Rather, the positive aspects of healthy eating, regularly exercising, and avoiding smoking should be emphasized. Basic dietary changes should be encouraged for the whole family so the affected child is not singled out. Cultural differences must be considered and recommendations individualized. Substitution rather than elimination needs to be emphasized. Visual aids (e.g., test tubes depicting the amount of fat in a hot dog or the number or packs of sugar in a glass of juice) are often helpful, especially for children. Diets should be flexible and individually tailored by a nutritionist who is experienced in lipid disorders. Dietary recommendations need to meet the nutritional demands of growing children while providing benefit to the overall profile. Parents are encouraged to participate in dietary and educational sessions, ask questions, and share ideas and experiences.

Parents often feel guilty about the hereditary component of hyperlipidemia. Many also believe they have failed if the diet alone is not making a significant difference in their child's lipid profile. They need to be reassured that a dietary approach alone is often not sufficient, especially for children with significantly elevated values.

Parents of children who require pharmacologic therapy need to understand the purpose, dosage, and possible side effects of the various drugs. Medication schedules should remain flexible and should not interfere with the child's daily activities. Follow-up phone calls by the nurse between visits allow parents to discuss their concerns and ask any questions that have arisen (see Evidence-Based Practice box).

Cardiac Dysrhythmias

Dysrhythmias, or abnormal heart rhythms, can occur in children with structurally normal hearts, as features of some congenital heart defects, and in patients after surgical repair of congenital heart defects. They are also seen in patients with cardiomyopathy and with cardiac tumors. They can occur secondary to metabolic and electrolyte imbalances. They can be classified in several ways, including by heart rate characteristics (bradycardia and tachycardia) and by the origin of the dysrhythmia in the atria or ventricles. Some dysrhythmias are well tolerated and self-limiting. Others may cause decreased cardiac output with associated symptoms. Some dysrhythmias can cause sudden death. Treatment depends on the cause of the dysrhythmia and its severity.

Many advances have been made in the diagnosis and treatment of pediatric dysrhythmias in the past decade. Improvements in technology have allowed better diagnosis, the development of ablation techniques, and the expansion of pacemaker capabilities. New antidysrhythmic medications have proven safe and effective in children. Radiofrequency ablation has offered a cure for some dysrhythmias. Pediatric electrophysiology has become a highly specialized field, and students should consult more detailed sources for an in-depth discussion. The following sections address diagnostic studies and

Cholesterol Screening for Children

Ask the Question
Should cholesterol screening be performed in children?

Search for the Evidence
Search Strategies
The literature was searched to locate clinical research studies related to this issue. Selection criteria included English-language publications, research-based articles (level 3 or lower), and infant and child populations.

Databases Used
PubMed, Cochrane Collaboration, MD Consult, Joanna Briggs Institute, National Guidelines Clearinghouse (AHRQ), TRIP Database Plus, PedsCCM, BestBETs

Critically Analyze the Evidence
- In late 2011, an expert panel of the National Heart, Lung, and Blood Institute (NHLBI) made a recommendation that lipid screening be performed on all children ages 9 to 11 years; this recommendation was based on evidence that as many as 30% to 60% of children with dyslipidemia might be missed when screening is performed by family history alone (National Heart, Lung, and Blood Institute, 2011). The expert panel's guidelines also include comprehensive screening and treatment guidelines for children with cardiovascular disease risk factors.
- Diagnosis of obesity is paramount in enhancing care of obese pediatric patients. Current laboratory (cholesterol or glucose) screening rates (10%) are inadequate in the outpatient setting (Patel, Madsen, Maselli, et al., 2010).
- Testing for cardiovascular risk factors: HDL cholesterol, LDL cholesterol, fasting glucose, blood pressure, OGTT, thyrotropin, and ALT should be considered in pediatric patients with increased waist circumference and even normal BMI (l'Allemand-Jander, 2010).
- In obese children, LDL cholesterol, HDL cholesterol, total cholesterol, and triglycerides are significantly different from those of subjects who are not obese (Simsek, Balta, Balta, et al., 2010).
- Serum triglyceride levels are a predictive risk factor of carotid intima-media thickness (Simsek, Balta, Balta, et al., 2010).
- In children and adolescents (12-19 years old) fasting non-HDL cholesterol levels were strongly associated with metabolic syndrome. A non-HDL cholesterol threshold of 120 mg/dL indicated borderline risk for metabolic syndrome, and a threshold of 145 mg/dL indicated high metabolic syndrome risk (Li, Ford, McBride, et al., 2011).
- Cholesterol levels in childhood are a major population predictor for adult cholesterol levels (Daniels, Greer, Committee on Nutrition, 2008).
- Precursors of atherosclerosis are present in young people. The atherosclerotic process begins early in life with early phases characterized by the development of fatty streaks in the vessels (PDAY study) (Enos, Holmes, Beyer, 1953; Strong, Malcom, McMahan, et al., 1999).
- Atherosclerosis is related to the presence and degree of cardiovascular risk factors in adults (Berenson, Srinivasan, Bao, et al., 1998).
- Most severely affected children come from families with a high incidence of early heart disease. Children whose genetic family history is unknown should also be screened (AAP Committee on Nutrition, 1998).
- Universal cholesterol screening in children would identify all individuals with dyslipidemia. Using solely the family history to identify subjects for cholesterol screening missed individuals with moderate dyslipidemia and those with potentially genetic dyslipidemia (Ritchie, Murphy, Ice, et al., 2010).

Apply the Evidence: Nursing Implications
There are strong recommendations (Guyatt, Oxman, Vist, et al., 2008) that lipid screening should be performed on all children 9 to 11 years of age. The NHLBI guidelines have been endorsed by the American Academy of Pediatrics (AAP, 2011).

Quality and Safety Competencies: Evidence-Based Practice*
Knowledge
Differentiate clinical opinion from research and evidence-based summaries.
Describe use of cholesterol screening in children.

Skills
Base individualized care plan on patient values, clinical expertise, and evidence.
Integrate evidence into practice by using cholesterol screening in children.

Attitudes
Value the concept of evidence-based practice as integral to determining best clinical practice.
Appreciate strengths and weakness of evidence for using cholesterol screening in children.

References
American Academy of Pediatrics (AAP): Expert panel on integrated guidelines for cardiovascular health and risk reduction in children and adolescents: summary report, *Pediatrics* 128(Suppl 5):S213–S256, 2011.

American Academy of Pediatrics (AAP) Committee on Nutrition: Cholesterol in childhood, *Pediatrics* 101(1 Part 1):141–147, 1998.

Berenson GS, Srinivasan SR, Bao W, et al: Association between multiple cardiovascular risk factors and atherosclerosis in children and young adults, *N Engl J Med* 338(23):1650–1656, 1998.

Daniels SR, Greer FR, Committee on Nutrition: Lipid screening and cardiovascular health in childhood, *Pediatrics* 122(1):198–208, 2008.

Enos WF, Holmes RH, Beyer J: Coronary disease among United States soldiers killed in action in Korea, *JAMA* 152(12):1090–1093, 1953.

Guyatt GH, Oxman AD, Vist GE, et al: GRADE: an emerging consensus on rating quality of evidence and strength of recommendations, *BMJ* 336(7650):924–926, 2008.

l'Allemand-Jander D: Clinical diagnosis of metabolic and cardiovascular risk in overweight children: early development of chronic diseases in the obese child, *Int J Obes* 34(Suppl 2):S32–S36, 2010.

Li C, Ford ES, McBride PE, et al: Non-high-density lipoprotein cholesterol concentration is associated with the metabolic syndrome among U.S. youth aged 12-19 years, *J Pediatr* 158(2):201–207, 2011.

National Heart, Lung, and Blood Institute: *Expert panel on integrated guidelines for cardiovascular health and risk reduction in children and adolescents,* November 2011, www.nhlbi.nih.gov/guidelines/cvd_ped/.

Patel AI, Madsen KA, Maselli JH, et al: Underdiagnosis of pediatric obesity during outpatient preventive care visits, *Acad Pediatr* 10(6):406–409, 2010.

Ritchie SK, Murphy EC, Ice C, et al: Universal versus targeted blood cholesterol screening among youth: the CARDIAC project, *Pediatrics* 126(2):260–265, 2010.

Simsek E, Balta H, Balta Z, et al: Childhood obesity-related cardiovascular risk factors and carotid intima-media thickness, *Turk J Pediatr* 52(6):602–611, 2010.

Strong JP, Malcom GT, McMahan CA, et al: Prevalence and extent of atherosclerosis in adolescents and young adults: implications for prevention from the Pathobiological Determinants of Atherosclerosis in Youth Study, *JAMA* 281(8):727–735, 1999.

Updated by Olga A. Taylor

*Adapted from QSEN at www.qsen.org.
ALT, Alanine aminotransferase; *BMI,* body mass index; *HDL,* high-density lipoprotein; *LDL,* low-density lipoprotein; *OGTT,* oral glucose tolerance test; *PDAY,* Pathobiological Determinants of Atherosclerosis in Youth.

provide a general discussion of the most common tachycardia (**supraventricular tachycardia [SVT]**) and the most common bradycardia (complete heart block) that require treatment in the pediatric population.

Diagnostic Evaluation

Nurses must be familiar with the standards of normal heart rate for the particular age-group (see Appendix C). An initial nursing responsibility is recognition of an abnormal heartbeat, either in rate or rhythm. When a dysrhythmia is suspected, the apical rate is counted for 1 full minute and compared with the radial rate, which may be lower because not all of the apical beats are felt. Consistently high or low heart rates should be regarded as suspicious. The patient should be placed on a cardiac monitor with recording capabilities. A 12-lead ECG yields more information than the monitor recording and should be done as soon as possible.

The basic diagnostic procedure is the ECG, including 24-hour Holter monitoring. Electrophysiologic cardiac catheterization allows for identification of the conduction disturbance and immediate investigation of drugs that may control the dysrhythmia. Another procedure that may be used is transesophageal recording. An electrode catheter is passed to the lower esophagus and, when in position at a point proximal to the heart, is used to stimulate and record dysrhythmias.

Dysrhythmias can be classified according to various criteria, such as effect on heart rate and rhythm, as follows:

- **Bradydysrhythmias**—Abnormally slow rate
- **Tachydysrhythmias**—Abnormally rapid rate
- **Conduction disturbances**—Irregular heart rate

Bradydysrhythmias. Sinus bradycardia (slower than normal rate) in children can be attributed to the influence of the autonomic nervous system, as with hypervagal tone, or in response to hypoxia and hypotension. Sinus bradycardias are also known to develop after some complex cardiac surgical repairs involving extensive atrial suture lines such as atrial baffle repairs (Mustard and Senning repairs) and the Fontan procedure.

Complete atrioventricular (AV) block is also referred to as complete heart block. This can be either congenital (occurring in children with structurally normal hearts) or acquired after surgery to repair cardiac defects. AV blocks are most often related to edema around the conduction system and resolve without treatment. Temporary epicardial wires are placed in most patients at surgery; if a rhythm disturbance occurs, temporary pacing can be used. Several days after surgery, the health care practitioner removes the wires by pulling slowly and deliberately down on them from the site of insertion.

Some children may need a permanent pacemaker. The pacemaker takes over or assists in the heart's conduction function. The implantation of a pacemaker, in the operating room or possibly the catheterization laboratory, is usually a low risk procedure. The pacemaker is made up of two basic parts, the pulse generator and the lead. The pulse generator is composed of the battery and the electronic circuitry. The lead is an insulated, flexible wire that conducts the electrical impulse from the pulse generator to the heart. Two types of leads are available—transvenous and epicardial. After the lead has been attached to the heart, a small incision is made and a pocket is formed under the muscle to house and protect the generator. Continuous ECG monitoring is necessary during the recovery phase to assess pacemaker function. The nurse should be aware of the programmed rate and expected individual generator variations. The pacemaker insertion site is monitored for signs of infection. Analgesics are given for pain.

Pacemaker functions have become more sophisticated, and some models can adjust the heart rate to activity demands or be programmed for overdrive pacing or cardioversion.

Discharge teaching includes information about the signs and symptoms of infection, general wound care, and activity restrictions. Parents, and patients if they are old enough, should be taught to take a pulse and know the settings of the pacemaker. If the patient's low rate is set at 80 beats/min and the heart rate is only 68 beats/min, there is a possible problem with the pacemaker that needs to be investigated. Instructions for telephone transmission of ECG readings are also given. Telephone transmission can be used to transmit ECG strips and to monitor battery life and pacemaker function. The pacemaker generator will have to be replaced periodically because of battery depletion. Children with pacemakers should wear a MedicAlert device, and their parents should have a paper identification card with specific pacer data in case of an emergency. Cardiopulmonary resuscitation (CPR) instruction is suggested for parents.

Tachydysrhythmias. Sinus tachycardia (an abnormally fast heart rate) secondary to fever, anxiety, pain, anemia, dehydration, or any other etiologic factor requiring increased cardiac output should be ruled out before diagnosing an increased heart rate as pathologic. SVT is the most common tachydysrhythmia found in children and refers to a rapid regular heart rate of 200 to 300 beats/min. As many as one in 250 children experience SVT (Schlente, Boramanand, and Funk, 2008). The onset of SVT is often sudden, the duration is variable, and the rhythm may end abruptly and convert back to a normal sinus rhythm. Clinical signs in infants and young children are poor feeding, extreme irritability, and pallor. Children may experience palpitations, dizziness, chest pain, and diaphoresis. If SVT is sustained, signs of HF may be seen.

The treatment of SVT depends on the degree of compromise imposed by the dysrhythmia (see Critical Thinking Case Study). In some cases, vagal maneuvers, such as applying ice to the face, massaging the carotid artery (on one side of the neck only), or having an older child perform a Valsalva maneuver (e.g., exhaling against a closed glottis, blowing on a thumb as if it were a trumpet for 30 to 60 seconds), have terminated SVT. If vagal maneuvers fail or the child is hemodynamically unstable, adenosine (a drug that impairs AV conduction) may be used. Adenosine is given by rapid IV push with a saline bolus immediately after the drug because of its very short half-life. If this is unsuccessful or cardiac output is compromised, esophageal overdrive pacing or synchronized cardioversion (delivering an electrical shock to the heart) can be used in the intensive care setting. Sedation is needed for both procedures. Cardioversion should never be done in a conscious patient. More long-term pharmacologic treatment includes digoxin or possibly propranolol (Inderal) or amiodarone for severe or recurrent SVT.

A primary focus of nursing care is education of the family regarding the symptoms of SVT and its treatment. SVT may occur again despite therapy. Parents should be taught to take a radial pulse for a full minute. If medication is prescribed, instructions regarding accurate dosage and the importance of administering the correct dose at specified intervals are stressed.

Radiofrequency ablation has become first-line therapy for some types of SVT. The procedure is done in the cardiac catheterization laboratory and begins with mapping of the conduction system to identify the dysrhythmia focus. A catheter delivering radiofrequency current is directed at the site, and the area is heated to destroy the tissue in the area. These are lengthy procedures, often lasting 6 to 8 hours, and sedation or general anesthesia is required. Preparation is similar to that for cardiac catheterization. Another procedure,

CRITICAL THINKING CASE STUDY

Supraventricular Tachycardia

You are working in the emergency department when a father comes through the doors, crying, carrying his 1-month-old infant. The infant is awake and very irritable. The father reports that the infant has not been feeding well for the past 6 hours, and the father has noticed sweating (diaphoresis) with attempted feeds. No history of fever is noted. Further assessment reveals a diaphoretic, crying infant with a respiratory rate of 60 breaths/min, BP of 60/40 mm Hg, and heart rate that is too fast to count by auscultation. When the infant is attached to the cardiorespiratory monitor, the heart rate is 220 beats/min, nonvariable, with an oxygen saturation of 97%. Capillary refill time is slightly prolonged at 3 seconds, and femoral pulses are palpable but weak.

1. Evidence—Is there sufficient evidence to draw conclusions about this infant?
2. Assumptions—Describe an underlying assumption about each of the following:
   a. Symptoms associated with heart failure
   b. An infant younger than 3 months with poor feeding
   c. Tachydysrhythmias in infants
3. What priorities for nursing care should be established?
4. Does the evidence support your nursing interventions?

BP, Blood pressure.

cryoablation, is also used in treatment of SVT. Liquid nitrous oxide is used to cool a catheter to subfreezing temperatures, which then destroys the tissue of target by freezing.

Pulmonary Artery Hypertension

Pulmonary artery hypertension (PAH) describes a group of rare disorders that result in an elevation of pulmonary artery pressure above 25 mm Hg at rest after the neonatal period (Barst, 1999). These disorders are poorly understood, and until recently, there was no treatment beyond supportive care. PAH is a progressive, eventually fatal disease for which there is no known cure. It can be difficult to diagnose in the early stages. Often when patients become symptomatic and a diagnosis is made, their disease is rapidly progressing, treatment is unsuccessful, and death occurs within several years. There is now evidence of a genetic basis for some PAH; some mutations localized to chromosome 2 have been identified in about half of patients with familial PAH (Lane, Machado, Pauciulo, et al., 2000).

Pulmonary artery hypertension affects the small pulmonary arteries and is characterized by vascular narrowing leading to an increase in pulmonary vascular resistance. Generally, these abnormalities result in remodeling of the pulmonary circulation, characterized by occlusion of the lumen in medium and small pulmonary arteries because of cellular proliferation (Michelakis, Wilkins, and Rabinovitch, 2008). Why some children develop the disease and others do not is unclear. There are many possible causes of PAH. Cardiac causes occur primarily in patients with a large left-to-right shunt producing increased pulmonary blood flow. If these defects are not repaired early, the high pulmonary flow will cause changes in the pulmonary artery vessels and the vessels will lose their elasticity. Other causes of PAH include hypoxic lung diseases, thromboembolic diseases causing pulmonary vascular obstruction, collagen vascular diseases, and exposure to toxic substances. Many of the patients have no identifiable cause for PAH and have primary or idiopathic PAH.

Clinical Manifestations

The clinical manifestations include dyspnea with exercise, chest pain, and syncope. Dyspnea is the most common symptom and is caused by impaired oxygen delivery. Chest pain is the result of coronary ischemia in the right ventricle from severe hypertrophy. Syncope reflects a limited cardiac output leading to decreased cerebral blood flow. Right-sided heart dysfunction is steadily progressive, and when symptoms of venous congestion and edema are present, the prognosis is poor.

Therapeutic Management

Although no cure is known, several therapies have shown promise in slowing the progression of the disease and improving quality of life. In general, situations that may exacerbate the disease and cause hypoxia, such as exercise and high altitudes, are avoided. Supplemental oxygen, especially at night while sleeping, is commonly used to relieve hypoxia. Patients are at risk for thromboembolic events leading to pulmonary emboli, so anticoagulation with warfarin (Coumadin) is often prescribed.

Vasodilator therapy (which relaxes vascular smooth muscle and reduces pulmonary artery pressure) can prolong survival of patients with PAH. Oral calcium channel blockers have been successful in some children. Now available for patients who are nonresponders in vasodilator testing is a new oral drug, bosentan, an endothelin-receptor antagonist, that reduces pulmonary artery pressure and resistance and is safe and well tolerated in children (Barst, Ivy, Dingemanse, et al., 2003). It has been used in combination with IV prostacyclin.

Continuous IV prostacyclin has been used with some success in children who did not respond to oral therapy. Both of these therapies, although promising, have been used in only small numbers of patients and are expensive. Lung transplantation may be another treatment option.

Cardiomyopathy

Cardiomyopathy refers to abnormalities of the myocardium in which the cardiac muscle's ability to contract is impaired. Cardiomyopathies are relatively rare in children. Possible etiologic factors include familial or genetic causes, infection, deficiency states, metabolic abnormalities, and collagen vascular diseases. Most cardiomyopathies in children are considered primary or idiopathic, in which the cause is unknown and the cardiac dysfunction is not associated with systemic disease. Some of the known causes of secondary cardiomyopathy are anthracycline toxicity (the antineoplastic agents *doxorubicin* [Adriamycin] and *daunomycin*), hemochromatosis (from excessive iron storage), Duchenne muscular dystrophy, Kawasaki disease (KD), collagen diseases, and thyroid dysfunction.

Cardiomyopathies can be divided into three broad clinical categories according to the type of abnormal structure and dysfunction present: dilated cardiomyopathy, hypertrophic cardiomyopathy, and restrictive cardiomyopathy.

Dilated cardiomyopathy is characterized by ventricular dilation and greatly decreased contractility, resulting in symptoms of HF. This is the most common type of cardiomyopathy in children. Its cause is often unknown. The clinical findings are of HF with tachycardia, dyspnea, hepatosplenomegaly, fatigue, and poor growth. Dysrhythmias may be present and may be more difficult to control with worsening HF.

Hypertrophic cardiomyopathy is characterized by an increase in heart muscle mass without an increase in cavity size, usually occurring in the left ventricle and associated with abnormal diastolic filling. It is a familial autosomal dominant genetic abnormality in most cases and is probably the most common genetically transmitted cardiovascular disease (Maron, 2001). The expression of clinical disease varies greatly among patients. Clinical symptoms usually appear in the school-age period or adolescence and may include anginal chest pain, dysrhythmias, and syncope. One recent study confirmed that unexplained syncope in the childhood age-group (younger than 18 years) with known hypertrophic cardiomyopathy had a 60% cumulative risk for sudden death within 5 years of the syncopal event (Spirito, Autore, Rapezzi, et al., 2009). Presentation in infancy includes signs of HF and has a poor prognosis. The ECG demonstrates left ventricular hypertrophy, often with ST-T changes. The echocardiogram is most helpful and demonstrates asymmetric septal hypertrophy and an increase in left ventricular wall thickness, with a small left ventricle cavity.

Restrictive cardiomyopathy, which is rare in children, describes a restriction to ventricular filling caused by endocardial or myocardial disease or both. It is characterized by diastolic dysfunction and absence of ventricular dilation or hypertrophy. Symptoms are similar to those of HF (see p. 1331).

Therapeutic Management

Treatment is directed toward correcting the underlying cause whenever feasible. However, in most affected children, this is not possible and treatment is aimed at managing HF (p. 1332) and dysrhythmias. Digoxin, diuretics, and aggressive use of afterload reduction agents have been found to be helpful in managing symptoms in those with dilated cardiomyopathy. Practice guidelines for the management of HF in children have recently been outlined and provide an in-depth review of available therapies (Rosenthal, Chrisant, Edens, et al., 2004). Digoxin and inotropic agents are usually not helpful in the other forms of cardiomyopathy because increasing the force of contraction may exacerbate the muscular obstruction and actually impair ventricular ejection. β-Blockers such as propranolol and calcium channel blockers such as verapamil (Calan) have been used to reduce left ventricular outflow obstruction and improve diastolic filling in those with hypertrophic cardiomyopathy.

Careful monitoring and treatment of dysrhythmias are essential. The placement of an automatic implantable cardioverter defibrillator (AICD) should be considered for patients at high risk for sudden death because of ventricular dysrhythmias. Anticoagulants may be given to reduce the risk for thromboemboli, a complication of the sluggish circulation through the heart. For worsening HF and signs of poor perfusion, IV inotropic or vasodilating drugs may be needed. Severely ill children may require mechanical ventilation, oxygen administration, and IV medications. Heart transplantation may be a treatment option for patients who have worsening symptoms despite maximum medical therapy.

CARE MANAGEMENT

Because of the poor prognosis in many children with cardiomyopathy, nursing care is consistent with that for any child with a life-threatening disorder (see Chapter 36). One of the most difficult adjustments for the child (especially normally active youngsters with hypertrophic cardiomyopathy) may be the realization of failing health and the need for restricted activity. The child should be included in decisions regarding activity and allowed to discuss feelings, particularly if the disease follows a progressively fatal course. After symptoms of HF or dysrhythmias develop, the same nursing interventions are implemented as discussed on p. 1333. If heart transplantation is considered, the needs of the child and family are great in terms of psychologic preparation and postoperative care.

The nurse plays an important role in assessing the family's understanding of the procedure and long-term consequences. Children of school age and older should be fully informed to give their assent to the procedure (see Informed Consent, Chapter 39).

HEART TRANSPLANTATION

Heart transplantation has become a treatment option for infants and children with worsening HF and a limited life expectancy despite maximum medical and surgical management. Indications for heart transplantation in children are cardiomyopathy and end-stage CHD. It is also an option for patients with some forms of complex congenital cardiac defects, such as hypoplastic left heart syndrome, for whom conventional surgical approaches have a high mortality rate.

The heart transplant procedure may be orthotopic or heterotopic. Orthotopic heart transplantation refers to removing the recipient's own heart and implanting a new heart from a donor who has had brain death but a healthy heart. The donor and recipient are matched by weight and blood type. Heterotopic heart transplantation refers to leaving the recipient's own heart in place and implanting a new heart to act as an additional pump, or "piggyback" heart; this type of transplant is rarely done in children.

Before transplantation, potential recipients undergo a careful cardiac evaluation to determine if there are any other medical or surgical options to improve the patient's cardiac status. Other organ systems are assessed to identify problems that might increase the risk of or preclude transplantation. A psychosocial evaluation of the patient and family is done to assess family function, support systems, and ability to comply with the complex medical regimen after the transplant. Support services to help the family successfully care for their child are provided when possible. Parents and older adolescents need extensive education about the risks and benefits of transplantation so they can make an informed decision. Patients are listed on a national computer network organized by the United Network for Organ Sharing to match donors and recipients. (See also Organ or Tissue Donation and Autopsy, Chapter 36.)

According to the Scientific Registry of Transplant Recipients, the number of pediatric candidates active on the waiting list was 134 in 2009, (SRTR, 2011). The 1-year graft survival rate for pediatric heart transplants performed in 2008 was 87.5% (SRTR, 2011).

Waiting list mortality remains high, particularly in the smallest children. Recent progress in suitable ventricular assist devices for use in children as a bridge to transplantation has made outcomes to survival for cardiac transplantation more successful (Blume, Naftel, Bastardi, et al., 2006). A multicenter study using the U.S. Scientific Registry of Transplant Recipients was recently conducted (Almond, Thiagarajian, Piercy, et al., 2009). Among 3098 children listed for a heart transplant between 1999 and 2006, the median age was 2 years. Of those children, 60% were listed as a top status (30% ventilated and 18% on supportive measures), and of those children, 17% died, 63% received transplants, 8% recovered, and 12% remained listed. These numbers concluded that waiting time in the United States remains high in the current era and high risk groups in these categories could benefit from emerging cardiac assist devices, such as extracorporeal membrane oxygenation and ventricular assist devices.

The posttransplant course is complex. Although heart function is greatly improved or normal after transplantation, the risk for rejection is serious. The leading cause of death in the first 3 years after heart transplantation is rejection, with the greatest risk in the first 6 months (Blume, 2003). Rejection of the heart is diagnosed primarily by endomyocardial biopsy in older children. Serial echocardiograms are often used in infants and young children to reduce the need for invasive biopsies. Immunosuppressants must be taken for life and have many systemic side effects. Triple-drug therapy for immunosuppression with a calcineurin inhibitor (cyclosporine or tacrolimus), steroids, and azathioprine is most commonly used in pediatric patients, although mycophenolate mofetil is being used more frequently and replacing azathioprine. Steroids are weaned in the first year and may be discontinued in some patients.

Infection is always a risk. Potential long-term problems that may limit survival include chronic rejection, causing coronary artery disease; renal dysfunction and hypertension resulting from cyclosporine administration; lymphoma; and infection. Coronary artery disease is the leading cause of death among late survivors of heart transplantation (Boucek, Aurora, Edwards, et al., 2007). In the short term, after successful transplantation, children are able to return to full participation in age-appropriate activities and appear to adapt well to their new lifestyle. Transplantation is not a cure because patients must live with the lifetime consequences of chronic immunosuppression.

CARE MANAGEMENT

Successfully caring for a child after a heart transplant requires the expertise and dedication of many members of the health care team. Nurses play vital roles in assessment, coordination of care, psychosocial support, and patient and family education. The heart transplant recipient must be carefully monitored for signs of rejection, infection, and the side effects of the immunosuppressant medications. The patient's and family's psychosocial well-being also need to be assessed to identify issues such as increased family stress, depression, substance abuse, and school problems. Noncompliance with an intense medication regimen, especially during adolescence, can lead to serious medical problems and can be fatal.

The first 6 months to 1 year after the transplant are most intense because the risk for complications is greatest and the patient and family are adjusting to a new lifestyle. Patients are monitored closely by the health care team, with frequent visits and laboratory tests. Care is usually shared between local health care providers and the transplant center. Many patients are able to return to school and other age-appropriate activities within 2 to 3 months after the transplant.

VASCULAR DYSFUNCTION

Systemic Hypertension

Hypertension is defined as the consistent elevation of BP beyond values considered to be the upper limits of normal. The two major categories are essential hypertension (no identifiable cause) and secondary hypertension (subsequent to an identifiable cause). In recent years, there has been increasing interest in this disorder in adolescents and children. Hypertension in children and adolescents is defined as having a systolic or diastolic BP that consistently falls at or over the 95th percentile. This group is further delineated as follows:

- **Stage 1 hypertension** includes patients who have BP readings between the 95th and 99th percentiles.
- **Stage 2 hypertension** includes patients with BP readings over the 99th percentile plus 5 mm Hg.

An additional group includes children and adolescents who have prehypertension (or high-normal BP). This prehypertensive group includes those with BP readings that fall consistently between the 90th and 95th percentiles. The *Fourth Report on the Diagnosis, Evaluation, and Treatment of High Blood Pressure in Children and Adolescents* outlines in detail the identification, testing, and treatment recommendations for young people with high BP (National High Blood Pressure Education Program Working Group on High Blood Pressure in Children and Adolescents, 2004).

Etiology

Most instances of hypertension observed in young children occur secondary to a structural abnormality or an underlying pathologic process, although this is being challenged by screening programs of relatively healthy children. The most common cause of secondary hypertension is renal disease, followed by cardiovascular, endocrine, and some neurologic disorders. As a rule, the younger the child and the more severe the hypertension, the more likely it is to be secondary.

The causes of essential hypertension are undetermined, but evidence indicates that both genetic and environmental factors play a role. The incidence of hypertension has been shown to be higher in children whose parents are hypertensive. African Americans have a higher incidence of hypertension than Caucasians; in African Americans, it develops earlier, is frequently more severe, and results in death at an earlier age. Environmental factors that contribute to the risk for developing hypertension include obesity, salt ingestion, smoking, and stress.

Diagnostic Evaluation

Because of the increasing numbers of hypertensive or potentially hypertensive children and adolescents being identified, a BP determination should be a routine part of annual assessment in healthy children older than 3 years. BP readings should be done in children younger than 3 years who have high risk family histories or those with individual risk factors, including CHD, kidney disease, malignancy, transplant, certain neurologic problems, or systemic illnesses known to cause hypertension. Although clinical manifestations associated with hypertension depend largely on the underlying cause, some observations can provide clues to the examiner that an elevated BP may be a factor (Box 42-10). In infants and very young children who cannot communicate symptoms, observation of behavior provides clues, although gross behavioral changes may not be apparent until complications are present.

No definitive cutoff values are used in the diagnosis of hypertension in the pediatric patient. The *Fourth Report on the Diagnosis, Evaluation, and Treatment of High Blood Pressure in Children and Adolescents* (National High Blood Pressure Education Program Working Group on High Blood Pressure in Children and Adolescents, 2004) provides normative data for children (see Appendix C). BP tables now include the 50th, 90th, 95th, and 99th percentiles for BP readings based on age, gender, and height percentiles.

BOX 42-10	CLINICAL MANIFESTATIONS OF HYPERTENSION	
Adolescents and Older Children	**Infants or Young Children**
• Frequent headaches	• Irritability
• Dizziness	• Head banging or head rubbing
• Changes in vision	• Waking up screaming in the night

These guidelines are based on auscultatory readings, and therefore this is currently the preferred method of assessment. These charts take into account differences in body height. It is therefore important to note that a child who is large for his or her age may normally have a higher BP than a child of average size. Before a diagnosis is made, BP should be measured on at least three separate occasions. An ambulatory BP monitor may be ordered if "white-coat hypertension" is suspected. These are useful in that they provide BP readings over a 24-hour period. There are different normative values for ambulatory BP readings (Urbina, Alpert, Flynn, et al., 2008).

A careful medical history and family history should be obtained to screen for other relatives with hypertension or other cardiovascular risk factors. In children with suspected hypertension, initial laboratory data include a urinalysis, renal function studies such as creatinine and blood urea nitrogen, a lipid profile, complete blood count, and electrolytes. Depending on the severity of hypertension, additional testing may be indicated. Testing may include a retinal examination, renal ultrasonography to measure kidney size and Doppler flow to detect the possibility of a renal causes, and an ECG and an echocardiogram to evaluate the presence of end-organ involvement such as left ventricular hypertrophy. Further testing for a secondary cause may be indicated based on individual circumstances, especially in children with significant hypertension and normal initial screening test findings.

Therapeutic Management

Therapy for secondary hypertension involves diagnosis and treatment of the underlying cause. Children and adolescents with consistently elevated BP readings from no known cause or those with secondary hypertension not amenable to surgical correction may be treated with a combination of nonpharmacologic and pharmacologic interventions. Dietary practices and lifestyle changes are important in the control of hypertension both for children and for adults. Nonpharmacologic measures, such as weight control in overweight patients, increased exercise, limited salt intake, and avoidance of stress and smoking, carry no risk and should be instituted as first-line therapy except in severe cases in which pharmacologic therapy may be indicated as well.

Drug therapy is instituted with caution in children with significant elevations of BP resistant to nonpharmacologic intervention. The treatment should begin with one drug and should add other drugs if control is not obtained. The oral antihypertensive drugs used in children include the β-blockers, ACE inhibitors, calcium channel blockers, angiotensin-receptor blockers, and diuretics. The goal is to achieve a normotensive state throughout the day without accompanying drug side effects.

CARE MANAGEMENT

Blood pressure measurement should always be a part of the routine assessment of children older than 3 years and patients younger than 3 years who are considered to be at high risk for hypertension. To obtain an accurate reading, care is taken to quiet the child or relax the adolescent while the measurement is recorded to avoid false readings caused by excitement. BP should be measured in the sitting position with the arm at the level of the heart. Initial evaluation should also include four extremity pressures (in the supine position) to rule out coarctation of the aorta. The chief cause of falsely elevated BP readings is the use of improperly fitting, narrow cuffs. Therefore attention to correct measurement technique is essential (see Blood Pressure, Chapter 29).

Home BP measurements can facilitate surveillance in youngsters with chronic hypertension and can document the effectiveness of therapy. A family member can be instructed in how to take and record accurate BP measurements, thus decreasing the number of trips to a health care facility. This individual needs to understand when to contact the health care practitioner regarding elevated values. The school nurse can often be a valuable resource in monitoring BP. The nurse plays an important role in assessing individual families and providing targeted information regarding nonpharmacologic modes of intervention, such as diet, weight loss, smoking cessation, and exercise programs. If extensive dietary counseling is required, the child should be referred to a nutritionist with expertise in working with children and adolescents. Exercise regimens should be individualized but should emphasize the benefits of regular aerobic exercise. Schoolchildren and young adolescents generally prefer team sports rather than individual training, which they may view as a burden rather than an enjoyable activity. If peers and family members can be encouraged to participate in any of the management strategies, the child's compliance is likely to be greater.

If drug therapy is prescribed, the nurse needs to provide information to the family regarding the reasons for it, how the drug works, and possible side effects. General instructions for antihypertensive drugs include:

- Rise slowly from a horizontal position, and avoid sudden position changes.
- Take drugs as prescribed.
- Maintain adequate hydration.
- Notify the health care practitioner if unpleasant side effects occur, but do not discontinue the drug.
- Avoid alcohol, and stay on the prescribed diet.

The need for follow-up is stressed, especially because antihypertensive therapy can sometimes be safely discontinued if BP remains under control over time.

Kawasaki Disease (Mucocutaneous Lymph Node Syndrome)

Kawasaki disease is an acute systemic vasculitis of unknown cause. It is seen in every racial group, and about 75% of the cases occur in children younger than 5 years, with peak incidence in the toddler age-group. The acute disease is self-limited; however, without treatment, approximately 20% of children develop coronary artery dilation or aneurysm formation. Infants younger than 1 year are most seriously affected by KD and are at the greatest risk for heart involvement, although an increased incidence has also been reported in older children, perhaps because of later diagnosis in many.

The etiology of KD is unknown. It is not spread by person-to-person contact; however, several factors support infectious etiologic factors. It is often seen in geographic and seasonal outbreaks, with most cases reported in the late winter and early spring (Newburger, Takahashi, Gerber, et al., 2004).

Pathophysiology

The principal area of concern in KD is the cardiovascular system. During the initial stage of the illness, extensive inflammation of the arterioles, venules, and capillaries occurs, causing many of the clinical symptoms. In addition, segmental damage to the medium-size muscular arteries, mainly the coronary arteries, can occur, resulting in the formation of coronary artery aneurysms in some children. When death occurs, which is very rare (in <0.17% of cases), it is usually the result of myocardial ischemia from coronary thrombosis or, years later, from severe scar formation and stenosis in coronary aneurysms (Wilder, Palinkas, Kao, et al., 2007).

BOX 42-11   DIAGNOSTIC CRITERIA FOR KAWASAKI DISEASE

Child must have fever for more than 5 days along with four of five clinical criteria (diagnosis may be made on day 4 by an experienced clinician if child has all the clinical criteria):

1. Changes in the extremities: in the acute phase, edema, erythema of the palms and soles; in the subacute phase, periungual desquamation (peeling) of the hands and feet
2. Bilateral conjunctival injection (inflammation) without exudation
3. Changes in the oral mucous membranes, such as erythema of the lips, oropharyngeal reddening; or "strawberry tongue" (large papillae are exposed)
4. Polymorphous rash
5. Cervical lymphadenopathy (one lymph node >1.5 cm)

NOTE: Kawasaki disease can be diagnosed with fewer clinical criteria when coronary artery changes are noted.

Clinical Manifestations

Because no specific diagnostic test exists for KD, the diagnosis is established on the basis of clinical findings and associated laboratory results (Box 42-11). These criteria should be used as guidelines. It is important to note that many children with KD do not fulfill standard diagnostic criteria and infants often have an incomplete presentation. It is therefore important to consider KD as a possible diagnosis in any infant or child with prolonged elevated temperature that is unresponsive to antibiotics and is not attributable to another cause.

Kawasaki disease manifests in three phases: acute, subacute, and convalescent. The acute phase begins with the abrupt onset of a high fever that is unresponsive to antibiotics and antipyretics. The child then develops the remaining diagnostic symptoms. Symptoms may come and go and are not always present simultaneously, although the fever is persistent throughout. During this stage, the child is typically *very* irritable. The subacute phase begins with resolution of the fever and lasts until all clinical signs of KD have disappeared. During this phase, the child is at greatest risk for the development of coronary artery aneurysms. Echocardiograms are used to monitor myocardial and coronary artery status. A baseline echocardiogram should be obtained at the time of diagnosis for comparison with future studies. Irritability persists during this phase. In the convalescent phase, all of the clinical signs of KD have resolved but the laboratory values have not returned to normal. This phase is complete when all blood values are normal (6-8 weeks after onset). At the end of this stage, the child has regained his or her usual temperament, energy, and appetite.

Cardiac Involvement. Long-term complications of KD include the development of coronary artery aneurysms, disrupting blood flow. Children with larger aneurysms have the potential for myocardial infarction, which can result from thrombotic occlusion of a coronary aneurysm. Affected coronary arteries dilate progressively, reaching their maximum diameter approximately 1 month from the onset of fever. Over time, as the damaged vessel tries to heal, stenosis of the aneurysm may develop and may lead to myocardial ischemia. Most of the morbidity and mortality occur in children affected with the largest aneurysms (giant aneurysms >8 mm or z-score >10). Symptoms of acute myocardial infarction in children are often confusing and may include abdominal pain, vomiting, restlessness, inconsolable crying, pallor, and shock, as well as chest pain or pressure (noted less in younger children). In the initial phase of the illness, children with KD may have signs or symptoms related to inflammation of the myocardium, including myocarditis, valvulitis, or dysrhythmias.

Therapeutic Management

The current treatment of children with KD includes high-dose IV gamma globulin (IVGG) along with salicylate therapy. IVIG has been demonstrated to be effective at reducing the incidence of coronary artery abnormalities when given within the first 10 days of the illness and ideally in the first 7 days of illness. A single, large infusion of 2 g/kg over 10 to 12 hours is recommended. Retreatment with IV gamma globulin is indicated in patients who continue with fever after treatment.

Aspirin is given initially in an antiinflammatory dose (80-100 mg/kg/day in divided doses every 6 hours) to control fever and symptoms of inflammation. After fever has subsided, aspirin is continued at an antiplatelet dose (3-5 mg/kg/day). Low-dose aspirin is continued in patients without echocardiographic evidence of coronary abnormalities until the platelet count has returned to normal (6-8 weeks). If the child develops coronary abnormalities, salicylate therapy is continued indefinitely. Additional anticoagulation (e.g., clopidogrel [Plavix], enoxaparin [Lovenox], or warfarin) may be indicated in children who have medium-size or giant coronary artery aneurysms.

Prognosis. Most children with KD recover fully after treatment. However, when cardiovascular complications occur, serious morbidity may result. The prognosis for patients is strongly related to the extent of coronary damage, with patients who have giant aneurysms being at the highest risk for complications.

CARE MANAGEMENT

In the initial phase, the nurse must monitor the child's cardiac status carefully. Intake and output and daily weight measurements are recorded. Although the child may be reluctant to eat and therefore may be partially dehydrated, fluids need to be administered with care because of the usual finding of myocarditis. The child should be assessed frequently for signs of HF, including decreased urinary output, gallop rhythm (an additional heart sound), tachycardia, and respiratory distress.

Administration of IVIG should follow the same guidelines as for any blood product, with frequent monitoring of vital signs. Patients must be watched for allergic reactions. Cardiac status must be monitored because of the large volume being administered to patients who may have diminished left ventricular function.

The majority of nursing care focuses on symptomatic relief. To minimize skin discomfort, cool cloths, unscented lotions, and soft, loose clothing are helpful. During the acute phase, mouth care, including lubricating ointment to the lips, is important for mucosal inflammation. Clear liquids and soft foods can be offered.

Patient irritability is perhaps the most challenging problem. These children need a quiet environment that promotes adequate rest. Their parents need to be supported in their efforts to comfort an often inconsolable child. They may need time away from their child, and nurses can often provide respite care for the family. Parents need to understand that irritability is a hallmark of KD and that they need not feel guilty or embarrassed about their child's behavior.

Discharge Teaching. Parents need accurate information about the progression of KD, including the importance of follow-up monitoring and when they should contact their health care practitioner. Irritability is likely to persist for up to 2 months after the onset of symptoms. Periungual desquamation (peeling of the hands and feet) begins in the second and third weeks. Usually the fingers peel first, followed by the feet. The peeling is painless, but the new skin may be tender. Arthritis, especially of the larger weight-bearing joints, may occur and persist for several weeks, although it is temporary. Children are typically most stiff in the mornings, during cold weather, and after naps. Passive range-of-motion exercises in the bathtub are often helpful in increasing flexibility. Any live immunizations (e.g., measles, mumps, and rubella; varicella) should be deferred for 11 months after the administration of gamma globulin because the body might not produce the appropriate amount of antibodies to provide lifelong immunity. The decision to give the varicella (chickenpox) vaccine while the child is receiving aspirin therapy is made individually by the health care practitioner. Temperature should be recorded after discharge, and the occurrence of fever should be communicated to the health care provider.

Parents of children with large aneurysms should be educated as to the unlikely but real possibility of myocardial infarction, as well as the signs and symptoms of cardiac ischemia in a child. At discharge, the ultimate cardiac sequelae are generally not fully known because vessels do not reach their maximum diameter until 4 to 6 weeks after the onset of KD. CPR should be taught to parents of children with known severe coronary artery sequelae.

Long-Term Follow-up. The frequency and type of follow-up are based on the presence or absence of coronary damage. The long-term outlook for children without aneurysms is promising. After more than 30 years of follow-up, an increased incidence of early heart disease is not being seen in this population. However, the literature regarding subtle effects of inflammation on the vessels is conflicting, and it is recommended that these children be screened and treated for the presence of coronary risk factors as they grow older. They should have a cholesterol screen performed, BP monitored, and education recommending a heart-healthy lifestyle, including exercise, a heart-healthy diet, and avoidance of smoking. This group of patients is seen at infrequent intervals—approximately every 5 years depending on the institution. In patients with aneurysms, follow-up focuses on the prevention and early detection of coronary ischemia in patients. Noninvasive modalities of coronary imaging, such as cardiac computed tomography angiography, magnetic resonance imaging, echocardiography, and stress testing, are used as much as possible. Patients with coronary aneurysms may require long-term antiplatelet or anticoagulation and possibly β-blocker therapy or other therapies, depending on the severity of coronary involvement.

Shock

Shock, or circulatory failure, is a complex clinical syndrome characterized by inadequate tissue perfusion to meet the metabolic demands of the body, resulting in cellular dysfunction and eventual organ failure. Although the causes are different, the physiologic consequences are the same and include hypotension, tissue hypoxia, and metabolic acidosis. Circulatory failure in children is a result of hypovolemia, altered peripheral vascular resistance, or pump failure. Types of shock are listed in Box 42-12.

Pathophysiology

A healthy child's circulatory system is able to transport oxygen and metabolic substrates to body tissues, which require a constant source for these essential needs. The cardiac output and distribution to the various body tissues can change rapidly in response to intrinsic (myocardial and intravascular) or extrinsic (neuronal) control

---

BOX 42-12 TYPES OF SHOCK

Hypovolemic

Characteristics
- Reduction in size of vascular compartment
- Falling blood pressure
- Poor capillary filling
- Low CVP

Most Frequent Causes
- Blood loss (hemorrhagic shock)—Trauma, gastrointestinal bleeding, intracranial hemorrhage
- Plasma loss—Increased capillary permeability associated with sepsis and acidosis, hypoproteinemia, burns, peritonitis
- Extracellular fluid loss—Vomiting, diarrhea, glycosuric diuresis, sunstroke

Distributive

Characteristics
- Reduction in peripheral vascular resistance
- Profound inadequacies in tissue perfusion
- Increased venous capacity and pooling
- Acute reduction in return blood flow to the heart
- Diminished cardiac output

Most Frequent Causes
- Anaphylaxis (anaphylactic shock)—Extreme allergy or hypersensitivity to a foreign substance
- Sepsis (septic shock, bacteremic shock, endotoxic shock)—Overwhelming sepsis and circulating bacterial toxins
- Loss of neuronal control (neurogenic shock)—Interruption of neuronal transmission (spinal cord injury)
- Myocardial depression and peripheral dilation—Exposure to anesthesia or ingestion of barbiturates, tranquilizers, opioids, antihypertensive agents, or ganglionic blocking agents

Cardiogenic

Characteristic
- Decreased cardiac output

Most Frequent Causes
- After surgery for congenital heart disease
- Primary pump failure—Myocarditis, myocardial trauma, biochemical derangements, heart failure
- Dysrhythmias—Supraventricular tachycardia, atrioventricular block, and ventricular dysrhythmias; secondary to myocarditis or biochemical abnormalities (occasionally)

CVP, Central venous pressure.

---

mechanisms. In shock states, these mechanisms are altered or challenged.

Reduced blood flow, as in hypovolemic shock, causes diminished venous return to the heart, low CVP, low cardiac output, and hypotension. Vasomotor centers in the medulla are signaled, causing a compensatory increase in the force and rate of cardiac contraction and constriction of arterioles and veins, thereby increasing peripheral vascular resistance. Simultaneously, the lowered blood volume leads to the release of large amounts of catecholamines, antidiuretic hormone, adrenocorticosteroids, and aldosterone in an effort to conserve body fluids. This causes reduced blood flow to the skin, kidneys, muscles, and viscera to shunt the available blood to the brain and heart. Consequently, the skin feels cold and clammy, there is poor capillary filling, and glomerular filtration rate and urinary output are significantly reduced.

As a result of impaired perfusion, oxygen is depleted in the tissue cells, causing them to revert to anaerobic metabolism, producing lactic acidosis. The acidosis places an extra burden on the lungs as they attempt to compensate for the metabolic acidosis by increasing the respiratory rate to remove excess carbon dioxide. Prolonged vasoconstriction results in fatigue and atony of the peripheral arterioles, which leads to vessel dilation. Venules, which are less sensitive to vasodilator substances, remain constricted for a time, causing massive pooling in the capillary and venular beds, which further depletes blood volume.

Complications of shock create further hazards. CNS hypoperfusion may eventually lead to cerebral edema, cortical infarction, or intraventricular hemorrhage. Renal hypoperfusion causes renal ischemia with possible tubular or glomerular necrosis and renal vein thrombosis. Reduced blood flow to the lungs can interfere with surfactant secretion and result in acute respiratory distress syndrome, which is characterized by sudden pulmonary congestion and atelectasis with formation of a hyaline membrane. Gastrointestinal tract bleeding and perforation are always possibilities after splanchnic ischemia and necrosis of intestinal mucosa. Metabolic complications of shock may include hypoglycemia, hypocalcemia, and other electrolyte disturbances.

Diagnostic Evaluation

The etiology of shock can be discerned from the history and the physical examination. The severity of the shock is determined by measurements of vital signs, including CVP and capillary filling (Box 42-13). Shock can be regarded as a form of compensation for circulatory failure. Because of the progressive nature of shock, it can be divided into the following three stages or phases:

1. **Compensated shock**—Vital organ function is maintained by intrinsic compensatory mechanisms; blood flow is usually normal or increased but generally uneven or maldistributed in the microcirculation.
2. **Decompensated shock**—Efficiency of the cardiovascular system gradually diminishes until perfusion in the microcirculation becomes marginal despite compensatory adjustments. The outcomes of circulatory failure that progress

beyond the limits of compensation are tissue hypoxia, metabolic acidosis, and eventual dysfunction of all organ systems.

3. **Irreversible, or terminal, shock**—Damage to vital organs, such as the heart or brain, is of such magnitude that the entire organism will be disrupted regardless of therapeutic intervention. Death occurs even if cardiovascular measurements return to normal levels with therapy.

At all stages, the principal differentiating signs are observed in the (1) degree of tachycardia and perfusion to the extremities, (2) level of consciousness, and (3) BP. Additional signs or modifications of these more universal signs may be present depending on the type and cause of the shock. Initially, the child's ability to compensate is effective; therefore early signs are subtle. As the shock state advances, signs are more obvious and indicate early decompensation.

Additional signs may be present, depending on the type and cause of the shock. In early septic shock, there are chills, fever, and vasodilation, with increased cardiac output that results in warm, flushed skin (hyperdynamic, or "hot," shock). A later and ominous development is disseminated intravascular coagulation (DIC) (see Chapter 43)—the major hematologic complication of septic shock. Anaphylactic shock is frequently accompanied by urticaria and angioneurotic edema, which is life threatening when it involves the respiratory passages (see Anaphylaxis, below).

Laboratory tests that assist in assessment are blood gas measurements, pH, and sometimes liver function tests. Coagulation tests are evaluated when there is evidence of bleeding, such as oozing from a venipuncture site, bleeding from any orifice, or petechiae. Cultures of blood and other sites are indicated when there is a high suspicion of sepsis. Renal function tests are performed when impaired renal function is evident.

Therapeutic Management

Treatment of shock consists of three major interventions: (1) ventilation, (2) fluid administration, and (3) improvement of the pumping action of the heart (vasopressor support). The first priority is to establish an airway and administer oxygen. After the airway is ensured, circulatory stabilization is the major concern. Establishment of adequate IV access, ideally with multilumen central lines, is essential to deliver fluids and medications.

Ventilatory Support. The lung is the organ that is most sensitive to shock. Decreased distribution or redistribution of blood flow to respiratory muscles plus the increased work of breathing can rapidly lead to respiratory failure. Critically ill patients are unable to maintain an adequate airway. To place the lung at rest and improve ventilation, tracheal intubation is initiated early with positive-pressure ventilation. Supplemental oxygen is always given as soon as possible. Blood gases and pH are monitored frequently.

Increased extravascular lung water caused by edema contributes to the development of respiratory complications. Therapy is directed toward maintaining normal arterial blood gas measurements, normal acid-base balance, and circulation. Efforts are made to remove fluid and prevent its accumulation with the use of diuretics.

Cardiovascular Support. In most cases, rapid restoration of blood volume is all that is needed for resuscitation of the child in shock. An isotonic crystalloid solution (normal saline or lactated Ringer's) is the fluid of choice; colloids such as albumin are also used. Successful resuscitation is reflected by an increase in BP and a reduction in heart rate; increased cardiac output results in improved capillary circulation and skin color. CVP measurements of right atrial pressure help guide fluid therapy, and urinary output measurement is an important indicator of adequacy of circulation.

BOX 42-13   CLINICAL MANIFESTATIONS OF SHOCK

Compensated
- Apprehensiveness
- Irritability
- Unexplained tachycardia
- Normal blood pressure
- Narrowing pulse pressure
- Thirst
- Pallor
- Diminished urinary output
- Reduced perfusion of extremities

Decompensated
- Confusion and somnolence
- Tachypnea
- Moderate metabolic acidosis
- Oliguria
- Cool, pale extremities
- Decreased skin turgor
- Poor capillary filling

Irreversible
- Thready, weak pulse
- Hypotension
- Periodic breathing or apnea
- Anuria
- Stupor or coma

Correction of acidosis, hypoxemia, hypoglycemia, hypothermia, and any metabolic derangements is mandatory.

Temporary pharmacologic support may be required to enhance myocardial contractility, reverse metabolic or respiratory acidosis, and maintain arterial pressure. The principal agents used to improve cardiac output and circulation are catecholamines, such as dopamine (Intropin) and epinephrine (Adrenalin). Vasodilators that are sometimes used include nitroprusside (Nipride) and milrinone.

CARE MANAGEMENT

The child who is in shock requires intensive observation and care. *The initial action is to ensure adequate tissue oxygenation.* The nurse should be prepared to administer oxygen by the appropriate route and to assist with any intubation and ventilatory procedures indicated. Other procedures and activities that require immediate attention are establishing an IV line, weighing the child, obtaining baseline vital signs, placing an indwelling catheter, obtaining blood gases and other measurements, and administering medications as indicated. The child is best positioned flat with the legs elevated.

> ### ! NURSING ALERT
>
> Early clinical signs of shock include apprehension, irritability, normal BP, narrowing pulse pressure (difference between diastolic and systolic BP), thirst, pallor, diminished urinary output, unexplained mild tachycardia, and decreased perfusion of the hands and feet.

The nurse's responsibilities are to monitor the IV infusion, intake and output, vital signs (including CVP), and general systems assessments on a routine basis. IV medications are titrated according to patient responses, and vital signs are taken every 15 minutes during the critical periods and thereafter as needed. Urinary output is measured hourly; blood gases, hematocrit, pH, and electrolytes are monitored frequently to assess the child's status and the efficacy of therapy. An apnea and cardiac monitor is attached and monitored continuously. In the initial stages of acute shock, more than one nurse is often needed to manage all of the necessary activities that must be carried out simultaneously (see Emergency box).

Throughout the intense activity, support for the family must not be overlooked. Someone should contact family members at frequent intervals to inform them about what is being done and whether

> ### ✚ EMERGENCY
>
> #### *Shock*
>
> **Ventilation**
> - Establish airway; be prepared for intubation.
> - Administer oxygen, usually 100% by mask.
>
> **Fluid Administration**
> - Restore fluid volume as ordered.
>
> **Cardiovascular Support**
> - Administer vasopressors (epinephrine 1:1000, 0.01 mg/kg subcutaneously; maximum dose of 0.5 mg; may repeat if needed).
>
> **General Support**
> - Keep child flat with legs raised above level of heart.
> - Keep child warm and calm.

there is any progress. Ideally, someone should remain with the parents to serve as a liaison between them and the intensive care team. However, this is not always feasible in such a critical situation. As soon as possible, the family should be allowed to see the child. A member of the clergy or a social worker may be called to help provide comfort and support.

Anaphylaxis

Anaphylaxis is the acute clinical syndrome resulting from the interaction of an allergen and a patient who is hypersensitive to that allergen. When the antigen enters the circulatory system, a generalized reaction rapidly takes place. Vasoactive amines (principally histamine or a histamine-like substance) are released and cause vasodilation, bronchoconstriction, and increased capillary permeability.

Severe reactions are immediate in onset; are often life threatening; and frequently involve multiple systems, primarily the cardiovascular, respiratory, gastrointestinal, and integumentary systems. Exposure to the antigen can be by ingestion, inhalation, skin contact, or injection. Examples of common allergens associated with anaphylaxis include drugs (e.g., antibiotics, chemotherapeutic agents, radiologic contrast media), latex, foods, venom from bees or snakes, and biologic agents (antisera, enzymes, hormones, blood products).

> ### ⚡ SAFETY ALERT
>
> Penicillin allergy is associated with immediate onset (within 1 hour of administration) or accelerated onset (1-72 hours after administration) of skin eruption, especially a urticarial rash, or more serious symptoms such as laryngeal edema or anaphylactic shock.

Clinical Manifestations

The onset of clinical symptoms usually occurs within seconds or minutes of exposure to the antigen, and the rapidity of the reaction is directly related to its intensity: the sooner the onset, the more severe the reaction. The reaction may be preceded by symptoms of uneasiness, restlessness, irritability, severe anxiety, headache, dizziness, paresthesia, and disorientation. The patient may lose consciousness. Cutaneous signs of flushing and urticaria are common early signs, followed by angioedema, most notable in the eyelids, lips, tongue, hands, feet, and genitalia.

Bronchiolar constriction may follow, causing narrowing of the airway; pulmonary edema and hemorrhage also may occur. Laryngeal edema with severe acute upper airway obstruction may be life threatening and requires rapid intervention. Shock occurs as a result of mediator-induced vasodilation, which causes capillary permeability and loss of intravascular fluid into the interstitial space. Sudden hypotension and impaired cardiac output with poor perfusion are seen.

Therapeutic Management

Successful outcome of anaphylactic reactions depends on rapid recognition and institution of treatment. The goals of treatment are to provide ventilation, restore adequate circulation, and prevent further exposure by identifying and removing the cause when possible.

A mild reaction with no evidence of respiratory distress or cardiovascular compromise can be managed with subcutaneous administration of antihistamines, such as diphenhydramine (Benadryl) and epinephrine.

Moderate or severe distress presents a potentially life-threatening emergency. Establishing an airway is the first concern, as with all shock states. Epinephrine is given subcutaneously or intravenously as an antihistamine and to support the cardiovascular system and increase BP. Other routes for giving epinephrine are intramuscular and via the airway, either nebulized or injected through an endotracheal tube. In severe anaphylaxis, epinephrine by any route is better than none. Fluids are given to restore blood volume. Additional vasopressors may be given to improve cardiac output.

Prevention of a reaction is preferable. Preventing exposure is more easily accomplished in children known to be at risk, including those with (1) a history of previous allergic reaction to a specific antigen; (2) a history of atopy; (3) a history of severe reactions in immediate family members; and (4) a reaction to a skin test, although skin tests are not available for all allergens. Desensitization may be recommended in certain cases.

CARE MANAGEMENT

When an anaphylactic reaction is suspected, both immediate intervention and preparation for medical therapy are nursing responsibilities. Ventilation is ensured by placing the child in a head-elevated position, unless contraindicated by hypotension, to facilitate breathing and administer oxygen. If the child is not breathing, CPR is initiated and emergency medical services are summoned.

If the cause can be determined, measures are implemented to slow the spread of the offending substance. An IV infusion is established immediately. Emergency medications are given intravenously whenever possible; however, epinephrine may be given subcutaneously (see Emergency box). Vital signs and urinary output are monitored frequently. Medications are administered as prescribed, with regular assessment to monitor effectiveness and to detect signs of side effects of medication and fluid overload.

To prevent an anaphylactic reaction, parents are always asked about possible allergic responses to foods, latex, medications, and environmental conditions. These are displayed prominently on the patient's chart. The specific allergen is noted, as are the type and severity of the reaction. Parents are excellent historians, especially when the child has displayed a pronounced reaction to a substance. Drugs, including related drugs (e.g., penicillin, nafcillin), and other items, such as latex, that have produced a reaction previously are *never* used. If the child is allergic to insect venom, the family is instructed to purchase an emergency kit to be kept with the child at all times. Both the family and the child, if the child is old enough, are taught how to use the equipment. The patient should carry medical identification at all times.

Septic Shock

Sepsis and septic shock are caused by an infectious organism (Maar, 2004). Normally, an infection triggers an inflammatory response in a local area, which results in vasodilation, increased capillary permeability, and eventually elimination of the infectious agent. The widespread activation and systemic release of inflammatory mediators is called the systemic inflammatory response syndrome (SIRS). Box 42-14 provides the exact definitions for SIRS, infection, sepsis, and severe sepsis. SIRS can occur in response to both infectious and noninfectious (e.g., trauma, burns) causes. When caused by infection, it is called sepsis. Septic shock is defined as sepsis with organ dysfunction and hypotension.

Most of the physiologic effects of shock occur because the exaggerated immune response triggers more than 30 different mediators that result in diffuse vasodilation, increased capillary permeability, and maldistribution of blood flow. This impairs oxygen and nutrient delivery to the cells, resulting in cellular dysfunction. If the process

---

> **BOX 42-14** **DEFINITIONS OF SYSTEMIC INFLAMMATORY RESPONSE SYNDROME, INFECTION, SEPSIS, AND SEVERE SEPSIS**
>
> **SIRS**—The presence of at least two of the following four criteria, one of which must be abnormal temperature or leukocyte count:
>
> 1. Core temperature of more than 38.5° C (101.3° F) or less than 36° C (96.8° F)
> 2. *Tachycardia*, defined as a mean heart rate more than 2 SD above normal for age in the absence of external stimulus, chronic drugs, or painful stimuli; or otherwise unexplained persistent elevation over a 0.5- to 4-hour period; or, for children younger than 1 year: *bradycardia*, defined as a mean heart rate less than the 10th percentile for age in the absence of external vagal stimulus, β-blocker drugs, or congenital heart disease; or otherwise unexplained persistent depression over a 0.5-hour period.
> 3. Mean respiratory rate more than 2 SD above normal for age or mechanical ventilation for an acute process not related to underlying neuromuscular disease or the receipt of general anesthesia.
> 4. Leukocyte count elevated or depressed for age (not secondary to chemotherapy-induced leukopenia) or more than 10% immature neutrophils.
>
> **Infection**—A suspected or proven (by positive culture, tissue stain, or PCR test) infection caused by any pathogen; or a clinical syndrome associated with a high probability of infection. Evidence of infection includes positive findings on clinical examination, imaging, or laboratory tests (e.g., white blood cells in a normally sterile body fluid, perforated viscus, chest radiograph consistent with pneumonia, petechial or purpuric rash, or purpura fulminans).
>
> **Sepsis**—SIRS in the presence of or as a result of suspected or proven infection.
>
> **Severe sepsis**—Sepsis plus cardiovascular organ dysfunction or ARDS or two or more other organ dysfunctions.

From Goldstein B, Giroir B, Randolph A, et al: International Pediatric Sepsis Consensus Conference: definitions for sepsis and organ dysfunction in pediatrics, *Pediatr Crit Care Med* 6(1):2-8, 2005.

ARDS, Acute respiratory distress syndrome; *PCR,* polymerase chain reaction; *SD,* standard deviation; *SIRS,* systemic inflammatory response syndrome.

---

continues, multiple-organ dysfunction occurs and may result in death. Table 42-4 includes the age-specific vital signs and laboratory values reflective of septic shock in children.

The incidence of septic shock is increasing in adults and children (Arnal and Stein, 2003), possibly as a result of greater numbers of immunosuppressed patients, more widespread use of invasive devices in seriously ill patients, increased awareness of the diagnosis, and a growing number of resistant microorganisms.

Three stages have been identified in septic shock. In early septic shock, the patient has chills, fever, and vasodilation with increased cardiac output, which results in warm, flushed skin that reflects vascular tone abnormalities and hyperdynamic, warm, or hyperdynamic-compensated responses. BP and urinary output are normal. The patient has the best chance for survival in this stage. The second stage—the normodynamic, cool, or hyperdynamic-decompensated stage—lasts only a few hours. The skin is cool, but pulses and BP are still normal. Urinary output diminishes, and the mental state becomes depressed. With advancing disease, certain

TABLE 42-4	AGE-SPECIFIC VITAL SIGNS AND LABORATORY VARIABLES IN SEPTIC SHOCK*				
	HEART RATE (BEATS/MIN)		**RESPIRATORY RATE (BREATHS/MIN)**	**LEUKOCYTE COUNT (LEUKOCYTES × 103/MM³)**	**SYSTOLIC BLOOD PRESSURE (MM HG)**
AGE-GROUP	**TACHYCARDIA**	**BRADYCARDIA**			
0 days-1 week	>180	<100	>50	>34	<65
1 week-1 month	>180	<100	>40	>19.5 or <5	<75
1 month-1 year	>180	<90	>34	>17.5 or <5	<100
2-5 years	>140	N/A	>22	>15.5 or <6	<94
6-12 years	>130	N/A	>8	>13.50 or <4.5	<105
13-<18 years	>110	N/A	>4	>11 or <4.5	<117

From Goldstein B, Giroir B, Randolph A, et al: International pediatric sepsis consensus conference: definitions for sepsis and organ dysfunction in pediatrics, *Pediatr Crit Care Med* 6(1):2-8, 2005.
N/A, Not applicable.
*Lower values for heart rate, leukocyte count, and systolic blood pressure are for 5th percentile, and upper values for heart rate, respiratory rate, or leukocyte count are for 95th percentile.

signs of circulatory decompensation that deteriorate to signs of circulatory collapse are indistinguishable from late shock of any cause. In the hypodynamic, or cold, stage of shock, cardiovascular function progressively deteriorates even with aggressive therapy. The patient has hypothermia, cold extremities, weak pulses, hypotension, and oliguria or anuria. Patients are severely lethargic or comatose. Multiorgan failure is common. This is the most dangerous stage of shock.

Management of septic shock involves measures to provide hemodynamic stability and adequate oxygenation to the tissues and the use of antimicrobials to treat the infectious organism. As with other forms of shock, hemodynamic stability is achieved with fluid volume resuscitation and inotropic agents as needed. Providing adequate oxygenation often requires intubation and mechanical ventilation, supplemental oxygen, sedation, and paralysis to decrease the work of breathing. Septic shock involves activation of complement proteins that promote clumping of the granulocytes in the lung. The granulocytes can release chemicals that can cause direct lung injury to the pulmonary capillary endothelium. This causes a fluid leak into the alveoli, which causes stiff, noncompliant lungs. DIC and multiorgan dysfunction may also occur and require prompt assessment and management.

Newer therapies are being developed to modify the host immune response by attempting to block various mediators, thereby interrupting the inflammatory cascade.

Early identification of the symptoms of septic shock is critical to patient survival. A high index of suspicion is required in all critically ill patients who are at greater risk for sepsis because of multiple invasive lines and devices, poor nutrition, and impaired immune function. Subtle alterations in tissue perfusion and unexplained tachypnea and tachycardia often are early warning signs. Identification of the infectious agent and prompt treatment are also critical to patient survival. Broad-spectrum antibiotics should be given, and the site of infection should be removed if possible (e.g., drain abscesses, remove indwelling lines). Patients should be managed in an ICU in which continuous monitoring and sophisticated cardiac and respiratory support are available. Multidisciplinary collaboration is essential in managing these critically ill patients.

KEY POINTS

- CHD is the most common form of cardiac disease in children.
- Major categories to investigate in the cardiac history are poor weight gain, poor feeding habits, and fatigue during feeding; frequent respiratory tract infections and difficulties; and evidence of exercise intolerance.
- The most common tests used in assessing cardiac function are radiography, ECG, echocardiography, and cardiac catheterization.
- Cardiac catheterization procedures can be divided into three groups: (1) diagnostic procedures, including angiography, that measure pressures and saturations to establish cardiac diagnosis; (2) interventional procedures, in which catheters or balloon devices are used to correct cardiac defects; and (3) electrophysiology studies, in which catheters with electrodes are used to evaluate dysrhythmias.
- Diagnostic cardiac catheterization provides important information about oxygen saturation of blood within the chambers and great vessels, pressure changes, changes in cardiac output or stroke volume, and anatomic abnormalities.
- Several prenatal factors may predispose children to CHD; these include maternal rubella during pregnancy, maternal alcoholism, maternal age older than 40 years, and maternal type 1 diabetes.
- Congenital heart defects can be divided into four main groups, as determined by hemodynamic patterns: (1) defects that result in increased pulmonary blood flow, (2) obstructive defects, (3) defects that result in decreased pulmonary blood flow, and (4) mixed defects.
- Clinical consequences of congenital heart defects include HF and hypoxemia. A child can have both hypoxemia and HF, although usually they occur independently.
- Clinical manifestations of HF are impaired myocardial function (tachycardia, cardiomegaly), pulmonary congestion (dyspnea, tachypnea, orthopnea, cyanosis), and systemic congestion (hepatosplenomegaly, edema, distended veins).
- Nursing measures in the care of a child with HF are to assist in improving cardiac function, decrease cardiac demands, reduce respiratory distress, maintain nutritional status, promote fluid loss, and provide family support.

- Clinical manifestations of hypoxemia are cyanosis, polycythemia, clubbing, and delayed growth and development. The child is at increased risk for hypercyanotic spells, CVAs, brain abscess, and BE.
- Caring for the child with CHD and the family requires helping them adjust to the disorder and cope with the effects of the defect and fostering growth-promoting family relationships.
- Preoperative care of the child with a congenital heart defect involves introducing the child and family to the hospital and preparing them for preoperative and postoperative procedures.
- Providing postoperative care includes observing vital signs and arterial and venous pressures, maintaining respiratory status, allowing maximum rest, providing comfort, monitoring fluids, planning for progressive activities, giving emotional support, observing for complications of surgery, and planning for discharge and home care.
- Acquired cardiovascular disorders include BE, RF, hyperlipidemia (hypercholesterolemia), KD, and cardiac dysrhythmias.
- Prevention of BE in certain children with CHD involves administration of prophylactic antibiotics when specific procedures are performed.
- Acute RF is a systemic inflammatory disease that can damage the cardiac valves and is associated with previous GABHS infection. Its incidence has increased in some areas of the United States.
- Cholesterol screening in children is controversial; currently, children with known risk factors for hyperlipidemia are screened and treated as needed. The influence of childhood cholesterol levels on later development of coronary artery disease is under investigation.
- Common dysrhythmias in children include slow rhythms (bradycardias, heart block) and fast rhythms (sinus tachycardia, SVT).
- Heart transplantation has been extended to infants and children with cardiomyopathy and complex congenital heart defects involving ventricular dysfunction, such as hypoplastic left heart syndrome.
- Education of the child with hypertension and the family focuses on drug therapy, diet control, and appropriate exercise.
- KD is an extensive inflammation of small vessels and capillaries that may progress to involve the coronary arteries, causing aneurysm formation. The administration of gamma globulin is an important aspect of treatment.
- Emergency treatment for shock includes ensuring ventilation; administering vasopressors, fluids, blood, and antibiotics as needed; and providing supportive measures such as correct positioning, warmth, and psychologic reassurance to the child and family.
- Persons at risk for anaphylaxis may be identified by a history of previous allergic reaction, history of atopy, history of severe reactions in family, and positive skin test to the allergen.

REFERENCES

Almond C, Thiagarajian RR, Piercy GE, et al: Waiting list mortality among children listed for heart transplantation in the United States, *Circulation* 119(5):717–727, 2009.

American Academy of Pediatrics (AAP) Committee on Infectious Diseases, Pickering L, editor: *2009 Red book: report of the Committee on Infectious Diseases*, ed 28, Elk Grove Village, IL, 2009, Author.

Arnal LE, Stein F: Pediatric septic shock: why has mortality decreased? The utility of goal-directed therapy, *Semin Pediatr Infect Dis* 14(2):165–172, 2003.

Arnold R, Ley-Zaporozhan J, Ley S, et al: Outcome after mechanical aortic valve replacement in children and young adults, *Ann Thorac Surg* 85(2):604–610, 2008.

Barst RJ: Recent advances in the treatment of pediatric pulmonary artery hypertension, *Pediatr Clin North Am* 46(2):333–345, 1999.

Barst RJ, Ivy D, Dingemanse J, et al: Pharmacokinetics, safety, and efficacy of bosentan in pediatric patients with pulmonary artery hypertension, *Clin Pharmacol Ther* 73(4):372–382, 2003.

Beekman RH: Coarctation of the aorta. In Allen HD, Driscoll DJ, Shaddy RE, et al, editors: *Moss and Adams' heart disease in infants, children and adolescents*, ed 6, Philadelphia, 2001, Lippincott Williams & Wilkins.

Bellinger DC, Wypij D, duPlessis AJ, et al: Neurodevelopmental status at eight years in children with dextro-transposition of the great arteries: the Boston Circulatory Arrest Trial, *J Thorac Cardiovasc Surg* 126(5):1385–1396, 2003.

Blume ED: Current status of heart transplantation in children: update 2003, *Pediatr Clin North Am* 50(6):1375–1391, 2003.

Blume ED, Naftel DC, Bastardi HJ, et al: Outcomes of children bridged to heart transplantation with ventricular assist devices: a multi-institutional study, *Circulation* 113(19):2313–2319, 2006.

Boucek MM, Aurora P, Edwards LB, et al: The Registry of the International Society for Heart and Lung Transplantation: tenth official pediatric heart transplantation report—2007, *J Heart Lung Transplant* 26(8):796–807, 2007.

Cecchin F, Frangini PA, Brown DW, et al: Cardiac resynchronization therapy (and multisite pacing) in pediatrics and congenital heart disease: five years experience in a single institution, *J Cardiovasc Electrophysiol* 20(1):58–65, 2009.

Daniels SR, Greer FR, Committee on Nutrition: Lipid screening and cardiovascular health in childhood, *Pediatrics* 122(1):198–208, 2008.

Dodds KM, Merle C: Discharging neonates with congenital heart disease after cardiac surgery: a practical approach, *Clin Perinatol* 32(4):1031–1042, 2005.

Dubin AM, Janousek J, Rhee E, et al: Resynchronization therapy in pediatric and congenital heart disease patients, *J Am Coll Cardiol* 46(12):2277–2283, 2005.

Ferrieri P: Jones Criteria Working Group: proceedings of the Jones Criteria Workshop, *Circulation* 106(19):2521–2523, 2002.

Freed MD: Aortic stenosis. In Allen HD, Driscoll DJ, Shaddy RE, et al, editors: *Moss and Adams' heart disease in infants, children, and adolescents*, ed 6, Philadelphia, 2001, Lippincott Williams & Wilkins.

Gerber MA, Baltimore RS, Eaton CB, et al: Prevention of rheumatic fever and diagnosis and treatment of acute streptococcal pharyngitis: a scientific statement from the American Heart Association, *Circulation* 119(11):1541–1551, 2009.

Goldmuntz E, Clark BJ, Mitchell LE, et al: Frequency of 22q11 deletion in patients with conotruncal defects, *J Am Coll Cardiol* 32(2):492–498, 1998.

Guidelines for the diagnosis of rheumatic fever: Jones criteria, 1992 update, Special Writing Group of the Committee on Rheumatic Fever, Endocarditis, and Kawasaki Disease of the Council on Cardiovascular Disease in the Young of the American Heart Association, *JAMA* 268(15):2069–2073, 1992.

Hoffman JIE, Kaplan S: The incidence of congenital heart disease, *J Am Coll Cardiol* 39(12):1890–1900, 2002.

Jacobs JP, Mavroudis C, Jacobs ML, et al: Lessons learned from the data analysis of the second harvest (1998-2001) of the Society of Thoracic Surgeons (STS) Congenital Heart Surgery Database, *Eur J Cardiothorac Surg* 26(1):18–37, 2004.

Lane KB, Machado RD, Pauciulo MW, et al: Heterozygous germline mutations in BMPR2 encoding a TGF-beta receptor, causing familial primary pulmonary hypertension:

the International PPH Consortium, *Nat Genet* 26(1):81–84, 2000.

Latson LA: Critical pulmonic stenosis, *J Intervent Cardiol* 14(3):345–350, 2001.

LeRoy S, Elixson EM, O'Brien P, et al: Recommendations for preparing children and adolescents for invasive cardiac procedures: AHA Scientific Statement, *Circulation* 108(20):2550–2564, 2003.

Li JS, Sexton DJ, Mick N, et al: Proposed modifications to the Duke criteria for the diagnosis of infective endocarditis, *Clin Infect Dis* 30(4):633–638, 2000.

Limperopoulos C, Majnemer A, Shevell MI, et al: Predictors of developmental disabilities after open heart surgery in young children with congenital heart defects, *J Pediatr* 141(1):51–58, 2002.

Maar SP: Emergency care in pediatric septic shock, *Pediatr Emerg Care* 20(9):617–624, 2004.

Majnemer A, Limperopoulos C: Developmental progress of children with congenital heart defects requiring open heart surgery, *Semin Pediatr Neurol* 6(1):12–19, 1999.

Margossian R: Contemporary management of pediatric heart failure, *Expert Rev Cardiovasc Ther* 6(2):187–197, 2008.

Maron BJ: Hypertrophic cardiomyopathy. In Allen HD, Driscoll DJ, Shaddy RE, et al, editors: *Moss and Adams' heart disease in infants, children, and adolescents*, ed 6, Philadelphia, 2001, Lippincott Williams & Wilkins.

McCrindle BW, Urbina EM, Dennison BA, et al: Drug therapy of high-risk lipid abnormalities in children and adolescents: a scientific statement from the American Heart Association Atherosclerosis, Hypertension, and Obesity in Youth Committee, Council of Cardiovascular Disease in the Young, with the Council on Cardiovascular Nursing, *Circulation* 115(14):1948–1967, 2007.

Michelakis ED, Wilkins MR, Rabinovitch M: Emerging concepts and translational priorities in pulmonary arterial hypertension, *Circulation* 118(14):1486–1495, 2008.

National Heart, Lung, and Blood Institute (NHLBI): *Expert panel on integrated guidelines for cardiovascular health and risk reduction in children and adolescents: Summary report*, Bethesda, MD, 2011, U.S. Department of Health and Human Services, NHLBI, www.nhlbi.nih.gov/guidelines/cvd_ped/summary.htm#chap5.

National High Blood Pressure Education Program Working Group on High Blood Pressure in Children and Adolescents: The fourth report on the diagnosis, evaluation, and treatment of high blood pressure in children and adolescents, *Pediatrics* 114(2):555–576, 2004.

Newburger JW, Takahashi M, Gerber MA, et al: Diagnosis, treatment, and long-term management of Kawasaki disease: a statement for health professionals from the Committee on Rheumatic Fever, Endocarditis and Kawasaki Disease, Council on Cardiovascular Disease in the Young, American Heart Association, *Circulation* 110(17):2747–2771, 2004.

Park MK: *Pediatric cardiology handbook*, ed 5, Philadelphia, 2008, Mosby.

Rome JJ, Kreutzer J: Pediatric interventional catheterization: reasonable expectations and outcomes, *Pediatr Clin North Am* 51(6):1589–1610, 2004.

Rosenthal D, Chrisant MR, Edens E, et al: International Society for Heart and Lung Transplantation: practice guidelines for management of heart failure in children, *J Heart Lung Transplant* 23(12):1313–1333, 2004.

Schlente EA, Boramanand N, Funk MF: Supraventricular tachycardia in the pediatric primary care setting: age-related presentation, diagnosis, and management, *J Pediatr Health Care* 22(5):289–299, 2008.

Scientific Registry of Transplant Recipients (SRTR): *OPTN/SRTR 2010 Annual Data Report*, Rockville, MD, 2011, Department of Health and Human Services, Health Resources and Services Administration, Healthcare Systems Bureau, Division of Transplantation.

Shanmugam G, MacArthur K, Pollock J: Mechanical aortic valve replacement: long-term outcomes in children, *J Heart Valve Dis* 14(2):166–171, 2005.

Shillingford AJ, Glanzman MM, Ittenbach RF, et al: Inattention, hyperactivity, and school performance in a population of school-age children with complex congenital heart disease, *Pediatrics* 121(4):e759–e767, 2008

Smith P: Primary care in children with congenital heart disease, *J Pediatr Nurs* 16(5):308–319, 2001.

Spirito P, Autore C, Rapezzi C, et al: Syncope and risk of sudden death in hypertrophic cardiomyopathy, *Circulation* 119(13):1703–1710, 2009.

Steltzer M, Rudd N, Pick B: Nutrition care for newborns with congenital heart disease, *Clin Perinatol* 32(4):1017–1030, 2005.

Tweddell JS, Hoffman GM, Mussatto KA, et al: Improved survival of patients undergoing palliation of hypoplastic left heart syndrome: lessons learned from 115 consecutive patients, *Circulation* 106(12 suppl 1):182–189, 2002.

Urbina E, Alpert B, Flynn J, et al: Ambulatory blood pressure monitoring in children and adolescents: recommendations for standard assessment—a scientific statement from the American Heart Association Atherosclerosis, Hypertension, and Obesity in Youth Committee of the Council on Cardiovascular Disease in the Young and the Council for High Blood Pressure Research, *Hypertension* 52(3):433–451, 2008.

Uzark K: Therapeutic cardiac catheterization for congenital heart disease: a new era in pediatric care, *J Pediatr Nurs* 16(5):300–307, 2001.

Wilder M, Palinkas L, Kao A, et al: Delayed diagnosis by physicians contributes to the development of coronary artery aneurysms in children with Kawasaki syndrome, *Pediatr Infect Dis* 26(3):256–260, 2007.

Wilson W, Taubert KA, Gewitz M, et al: Prevention of infective endocarditis: guidelines from the American Heart Association, *Circulation* 116(15):1736–1754, 2007.

Hematologic and Immunologic Dysfunction

Marilyn J. Hockenberry

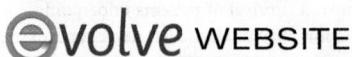

http://evolve.elsevier.com/Perry/maternal

LEARNING OBJECTIVES

On completion of this chapter, the reader will be able to:
- Distinguish among the various categories of anemia.
- Describe the prevention of iron deficiency anemia and the care of the child with iron deficiency anemia.
- Compare sickle cell anemia and β-thalassemia major in relation to pathophysiology and nursing care.
- Describe the mechanisms of inheritance and nursing care of the child with hemophilia.
- Relate the pathophysiology and clinical manifestations of leukemia.

- Demonstrate an understanding of the rationale of therapies for neoplastic disease.
- Outline a care plan for the child with neoplastic disease and the family.
- Contrast the pathophysiology and management of the immunodeficiency disorders.
- List nursing precautions and responsibilities during blood transfusion.
- Describe the types of hematopoietic stem cell transplants.

HEMATOLOGIC DYSFUNCTION

Several tests can be performed to assess hematologic function, including additional procedures to identify the cause of the dysfunction. The following discussion is limited to a description of the most common and one of the most valuable tests, the complete blood cell count (CBC). Other procedures, such as those related to iron, coagulation, and immune status, are discussed throughout the chapter as appropriate. The nurse should be familiar with the significance of the findings from the CBC (Table 43-1) and be aware of normal values for age, which are listed in Appendix B.

As with any disorder, the history and physical examination are essential to identify hematologic dysfunction, and the nurse is often the first person to suspect a problem based on information from these sources. Comments by the parent regarding the child's lack of energy, food diary of poor sources of iron, frequent infections, and bleeding that is difficult to control offer clues to the more common disorders affecting the blood. A careful physical appraisal, especially of the skin, can reveal findings (e.g., pallor, petechiae, bruising) that may indicate minor or serious hematologic conditions. Nurses need to be aware of the clinical manifestations of blood diseases to assist in recognizing symptoms and establishing a diagnosis.

> **! NURSING ALERT**
>
> A common term used in describing an abnormal CBC is *shift to the left*, which refers to the presence of immature neutrophils in the peripheral blood from hyperfunction of the bone marrow, as seen during a bacterial infection.

RED BLOOD CELL DISORDERS

Anemia

The term anemia describes a condition in which the number of red blood cells (RBCs) or the hemoglobin (Hgb or Hb) concentration is reduced below normal values for age. This diminishes the oxygen-carrying capacity of the blood, causing a reduction in the oxygen available to the tissues. Anemia is the most common hematologic disorder of infancy and childhood and is not a disease itself but an indication or manifestation of an underlying pathologic process.

Classification

Anemias are classified in relation to (1) etiology or physiology, manifested by erythrocyte or Hgb depletion, and (2) morphology,

TABLE 43-1 TESTS PERFORMED AS PART OF A COMPLETE BLOOD COUNT

TEST (AVERAGE VALUE)*	DESCRIPTION, COMMENTS
RBC count (4.5-5.5 million/mm³)	Number of RBCs/mm³ of blood Indirectly estimates Hgb content of blood Reflects function of bone marrow
Hgb determination (11.5-15.5 g/dL)	Amount of Hgb (g)/dL of whole blood Total blood Hgb depends primarily on number of circulating RBCs but also on amount of Hgb in each cell
Hct (35%-45%)	Percent volume of packed RBCs in whole blood Indirectly measures Hgb content Is approximately 3 times Hgb content
RBC Indices MCV (77-95 fL)	Average or mean volume (size) of a single RBC MCV values are expressed as femtoliters (fL) or cubic microns (mm³)
MCH (25-33 pg/cell)	Average or mean quantity (weight) of Hgb in a single RBC MCH values are expressed as picograms (pg) or micromicrograms (mmcg) Whereas MCV and MCH depend on accurate counts of RBCs, MCHC does not; therefore MCHC is often more reliable All indices depend on average cell measurements and do not show individual RBC variations (anisocytosis)
MCHC (31%-37% Hgb [g]/dL RBC)	Average concentration of Hgb in a single RBC MCHC values are expressed as percent Hgb (g)/cell or Hgb (g)/dL RBC
RBC volume distribution width (13.4% ± 1.2%)	Average size of RBCs Differentiates some types of anemia
Reticulocyte count (0.5%-1.5% erythrocytes)	Percent reticulocytes in RBCs Index of production of mature RBCs by bone marrow Decreased count indicates depressed bone marrow function Increased count indicates erythrogenesis in response to some stimulus When reticulocyte count is extremely high, other forms of immature RBCs (normoblasts, even erythroblasts) may be present Indirectly estimates hypochromic anemia Usually elevated in patients with chronic hemolytic anemia
WBC count (4.5-13.5 × 10³ cells/mm³)	Number of WBCs/mm³ of blood Total number of WBCs less important than differential count
Differential WBC count	Inspection and quantification of WBC types present in peripheral blood Values are expressed as percentages; to obtain absolute number of any type of WBC, multiply its respective percentage by total number of WBCs
Neutrophils (polys) (54%-62%) (3-5.8 × 10³ cells/mm³)	Primary defense in bacterial infection; capable of phagocytizing and killing bacteria
Bands (3%-5%) (0.15-0.4 × 10³ cells/mm³)	Immature neutrophil Increased numbers in bacterial infection Also capable of phagocytosis and killing
Eosinophils (1%-3%) (0.05-0.25 × 10³ cells/mm³)	Named for their staining characteristics with eosin dye Increased in allergic disorders, parasitic diseases, certain neoplasms, and other diseases
Basophils (0.075%) (0.015-0.030 × 10³ cells/mm³)	Named for their characteristic basophilic stippling Contain histamine, heparin, and serotonin; believed to cause increased blood flow to injured tissues while preventing excessive clotting
Lymphocytes (25%-33%) (1.5-3.0 × 10³ cells/mm³)	Involved in development of antibody and delayed hypersensitivity
Monocytes (3%-7%)	Large phagocytic cells that are involved in early stage of inflammatory reaction
ANC (>1000/mm³)	Percent neutrophils/bands times WBC count Indicates body's capability to handle bacterial infections
Platelet count (150-400 × 10³/mm³)	Number of platelets/mm³ of blood Cellular fragments that are necessary for clotting to occur
Stained peripheral blood smear	Visual estimation of amount of Hgb in RBCs and overall size, shape, and structure of RBCs Various staining properties of RBC structures may be evidence of immature forms of erythrocytes Shows variation in size and shape of RBCs: microcytic, macrocytic, poikilocytic (variable shapes)

ANC, Absolute neutrophil count; Hct, hematocrit; Hgb, hemoglobin; MCH, mean corpuscular hemoglobin; MCHC, mean corpuscular hemoglobin concentration; MCV, mean corpuscular volume; RBC, red blood cell; WBC, white blood cell.

*See Appendix B for normal values according to age.

the characteristic changes in RBC size, shape, or color (Box 43-1). Although the morphologic classification is more useful in terms of laboratory evaluation of anemia, the etiologic approach provides direction for planning nursing care. For example, anemia with reduced Hgb concentration may be caused by a dietary depletion of iron and the principal intervention is replenishing iron stores. The classification of anemias is found in Fig. 43-1.

Consequences of Anemia

The basic physiologic defect caused by anemia is a decrease in the oxygen-carrying capacity of blood and consequently a reduction in the amount of oxygen available to the cells. When the anemia

has developed slowly, the child usually adapts to the declining Hgb level.

The effects of anemia on the circulatory system can be profound. Because the viscosity of blood depends almost entirely on the concentration of RBCs, the resulting hemodilution of severe anemia decreases peripheral resistance, causing greater quantities of blood to return to the heart. The increased circulation and turbulence within the heart may produce a murmur. Because the cardiac workload is greatly increased, especially during exercise, infection, or emotional stress, cardiac failure may ensue.

Children seem to have a remarkable ability to function well despite low levels of Hgb. Cyanosis (the result of the quantity of deoxygenated Hgb in arterial blood) is typically not evident. Growth retardation, resulting from decreased cellular metabolism and coexisting anorexia, is a common finding in chronic severe anemia and is frequently accompanied by delayed sexual maturation in the older child.

Diagnostic Evaluation

In general, anemia may be suspected based on findings on the history and physical examination, such as a lack of energy, easy fatigability, and pallor, but unless the anemia is severe, the first clue to the disorder may be alterations in the CBC, such as decreased RBCs, and decreased Hgb and hematocrit (Hct) levels (see Fig. 43-1). Although anemia is sometimes defined as an Hgb level below 10 or 11 g/dL, this arbitrary cutoff is inappropriate for all children because Hgb levels normally vary with age (see Table 43-1 and Appendix B).

Other tests specific to a particular type of anemia are used to determine the underlying cause of anemia. These are discussed in relation to the particular disorder.

Therapeutic Management

The objective of medical management is to reverse the anemia by treating the underlying cause and to make up for any deficiency of

---

BOX 43-1	RED BLOOD CELL MORPHOLOGY

Size (Cell Size)
Variation in RBC sizes (anisocytosis)
- Normocytes (normal cell size)
- Microcytes (smaller than normal cell size)
- Macrocytes (larger than normal cell size)

Shape (Cell Shape)
Variation in RBC shapes (poikilocytosis)
- Spherocytes (globular cells)
- Drepanocytes (sickle-shaped cells)
- Numerous other irregularly shaped cells

Color (Cell Staining Characteristics)
Variation in hemoglobin concentration in the RBC
- Normochromic (sufficient or normal amount of hemoglobin per RBC)
- Hypochromic (reduced amount of hemoglobin per RBC)
- Hyperchromic (increased amount of hemoglobin per RBC)

RBC, Red blood cell.

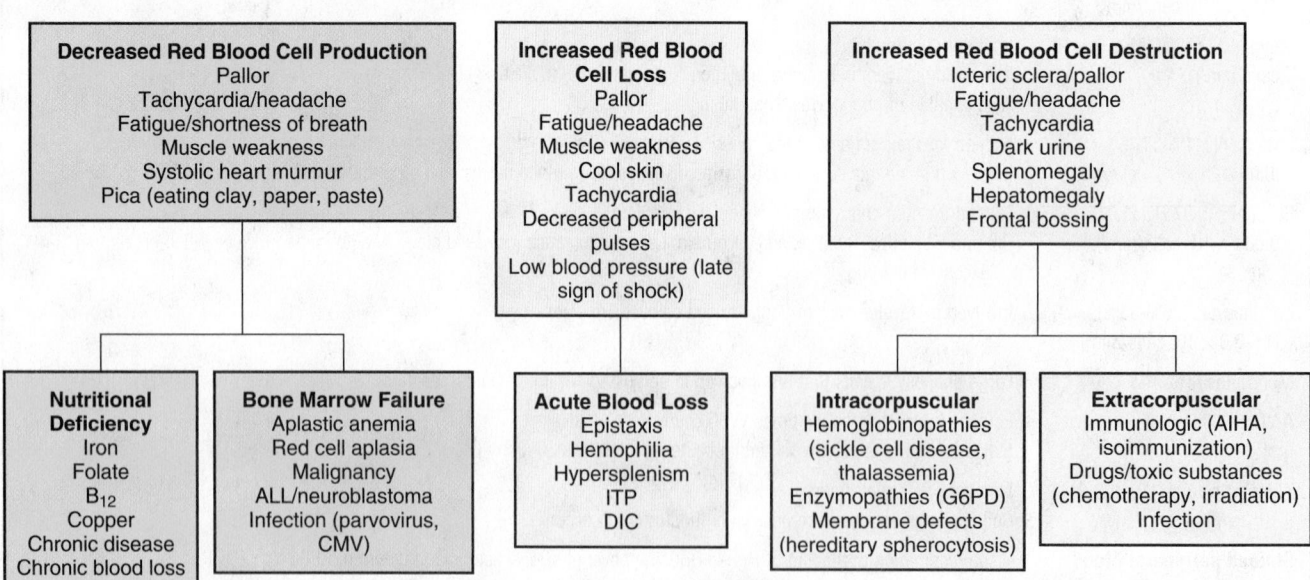

FIG **43-1** Classifications of anemias. *AIHA,* Autoimmune hemolytic anemia; *ALL,* acute lymphoid leukemia; *CMV,* cytomegalovirus; *DIC,* disseminated intravascular coagulation; *G6PD,* glucose-6-phosphate dehydrogenase; *ITP,* idiopathic thrombocytopenic purpura; *RBC,* red blood cell; *SCD,* sickle cell disease.

blood, blood component, or substance the blood needs for normal functioning. For example, blood or blood cells are replaced after hemorrhage; in nutritional anemias, the specific deficiency is replaced.

In patients with severe anemia, supportive medical care may include oxygen therapy, bed rest, and replacement of intravascular volume with intravenous (IV) fluids. The prognosis for anemia depends on the correction of the cause.

CARE MANAGEMENT

The assessment of anemia includes the basic techniques that are applicable to any condition. The age of the infant or child provides some clues regarding the possible etiology of the anemia. For example, iron deficiency anemia occurs more frequently in toddlers between 12 and 36 months of age and during the growth spurt of adolescence.

Racial or ethnic background is significant. For example, the anemias related to abnormal Hgb levels are found in Southeast Asians and persons of African or Mediterranean ancestry. These same groups may be genetically deficient in the enzyme *lactase* after the period of infancy. Affected individuals are unable to tolerate lactose in the diet, with consequent intestinal irritation and chronic blood loss.

Special emphasis is placed on a careful history to elicit any information that might help identify the cause of the anemia. For example, a statement such as: "My child drinks lots of milk" is a frequent finding in toddlers with iron deficiency anemia. An episode of diarrhea may have precipitated temporary lactose intolerance in a young child.

Stool examination for occult (microscopic) blood (Hemoccult test) can identify chronic intestinal bleeding that results from a primary or secondary lactase deficiency. It is also important to understand the significance of various blood tests (see Table 43-1).

Prepare the Child and Family for Laboratory Tests. Usually, several blood tests are ordered, but because they are generally done sequentially rather than at one time, the child is subjected to multiple finger or heel punctures or venipunctures. Laboratory technicians frequently are not aware of the trauma that repeated punctures represent to a child. However, these invasive procedures need not be painful (see Blood Specimens, Chapter 39). For example, the topical application of EMLA (an eutectic mix of lidocaine and prilocaine) or 4% lidocaine (Ela-Max or LMX) before needle punctures can eliminate pain (see Pain Management, Chapter 30). Therefore the nurse is responsible for preparing the child and family for the tests by:

- Explaining the significance of each test, particularly why the tests are not all done at one time
- Encouraging parents or another supportive person to be with the child during the procedure
- Allowing the child to play with the equipment on a doll or participate in the actual procedure (e.g., by cleansing the finger with an alcohol swab)

Older children may appreciate the opportunity to observe the blood cells under a microscope or in photographs. This experience is especially important if a serious blood disorder, such as leukemia, is suspected because it serves as a foundation for explaining the pathophysiology of the disorder.

Bone marrow aspiration is not a routine hematologic test but is essential for definitive diagnosis of the leukemias, lymphomas, and certain anemias.

> ### ! NURSING ALERT
>
> The following are suggested explanations for teaching children about blood components:
>
> - **Red blood cells**—Carry the oxygen you breathe from your lungs to all parts of your body
> - **White blood cells**—Help keep germs from causing infection
> - **Platelets**—Small parts of cells that help make bleeding stop by forming a clot (scab) over the hurt area
> - **Plasma**—The liquid portion of blood, which has clotting factors that help make bleeding stop

Decrease Tissue Oxygen Needs. Because the basic pathologic process in anemia is a decrease in oxygen-carrying capacity, an important nursing responsibility is to assess the child's energy level and minimize excess demands. The child's level of tolerance for activities of daily living and play is assessed, and adjustments are made to allow as much self-care as possible without undue exertion. During periods of rest, the nurse takes vital signs and observes behavior to establish a baseline of nonexertion energy expenditure. During periods of activity, the nurse repeats these measurements and observations to compare them with resting values.

> ### ! NURSING ALERT
>
> Signs of exertion include tachycardia, palpitations, tachypnea, dyspnea, shortness of breath, hyperpnea, breathlessness, dizziness, lightheadedness, diaphoresis, and change in skin color. The child looks fatigued (sagging, limp posture; slow, strained movements; inability to tolerate additional activity; difficulty sucking in infants).

Prevent Complications. Children who are so severely anemic that they are hospitalized may require oxygen to prevent or reduce tissue hypoxia. Because these children are susceptible to infection, every effort is expended to prevent exposure to infectious agents. All of the usual precautions are taken to prevent infection, such as practicing thorough hand washing, selecting an appropriate room in a noninfectious area, restricting visitors or hospital personnel with active infection, and maintaining adequate nutrition. The nurse also observes for signs of infection, particularly temperature elevation and leukocytosis.

Iron Deficiency Anemia

Anemia caused by an inadequate supply of dietary iron is the most prevalent nutritional disorder in the United States and the most preventable mineral disturbance. The prevalence of iron deficiency anemia has decreased during infancy in the United States, probably in part because of families' participation in the Women, Infants, and Children (WIC) program, which provides iron-fortified formula for the first year of life and routine screening of Hgb levels during early childhood (Baker, Greer, and Committee on Nutrition American Academy of Pediatrics [AAP], 2010; Cusick, Mei, Freedman, et al., 2008). Preterm infants are especially at risk because of their reduced fetal iron supply. Children 12 to 36 months of age are at risk for anemia as a result of primarily cow's milk intake and not eating an adequate amount of iron-containing food (Andrews, Ullrich, and Fleming, 2009; Baker, Greer, and Committee on Nutrition AAP, 2010; Richardson, 2007). Adolescents are also at risk because of their rapid growth rate combined with poor eating habits, menses, obesity, or strenuous activities.

Pathophysiology

Iron deficiency anemia can be caused by any number of factors that decrease the supply of iron, impair its absorption, increase the body's need for iron, or affect the synthesis of Hgb. Although the clinical manifestations and diagnostic evaluation are similar regardless of the cause, the therapeutic and nursing care management depend on the specific reason for the iron deficiency. The following discussion is limited to iron deficiency anemia resulting from inadequate iron in the diet.

During the last trimester of pregnancy, iron is transferred from the mother to the fetus. Most of the iron is stored in the circulating erythrocytes of the fetus, with the remainder stored in the fetal liver, spleen, and bone marrow. These iron stores are usually adequate for the first 5 to 6 months in a full-term infant but for only 2 to 3 months in preterm infants and multiple births. If dietary iron is not supplied to meet the infant's growth demands after the fetal iron stores are depleted, iron deficiency anemia results. Physiologic anemia should not be confused with iron deficiency anemia resulting from nutritional causes.

Although most toddlers with iron deficiency anemia are underweight, many infants are overweight because of excessive milk ingestion (known as milk babies). These children become anemic for two reasons: milk, a poor source of iron, is given almost to the exclusion of solid foods; and 50% of iron deficient infants fed cow's milk have an increased fecal loss of blood.

Therapeutic Management

After the diagnosis of iron deficiency anemia is made, therapeutic management focuses on increasing the amount of supplemental iron the child receives. This is usually done through dietary counseling and the administration of oral iron supplements.

In formula-fed infants, the most convenient and best sources of supplemental iron are iron-fortified commercial formula and iron-fortified infant cereal. Iron-fortified formula provides a relatively constant and predictable amount of iron and is not associated with an increased incidence of gastrointestinal (GI) symptoms, such as colic, diarrhea, or constipation. Infants younger than 12 months should *not* be given fresh cow's milk because it may increase the risk for GI blood loss occurring from exposure to a heat-labile protein in cow's milk or cow's milk–induced GI mucosal damage resulting from a lack of cytochrome iron (heme protein) (Glader, 2007; Richardson, 2007). If GI bleeding is suspected, the child's stool should be guaiac tested on at least four or five occasions to identify any intermittent blood loss.

Dietary addition of iron-rich foods is usually inadequate as the sole treatment of iron deficiency anemia because the iron is poorly absorbed and thus provides insufficient supplemental quantities of iron. If dietary sources of iron cannot replace body stores, oral iron supplements are prescribed for approximately 3 months. Ferrous iron, more readily absorbed than ferric iron, results in higher Hgb levels. Ascorbic acid (vitamin C) appears to facilitate absorption of iron and may be given as vitamin C–enriched foods and juices with the iron preparation.

If the Hgb level fails to rise after 1 month of oral therapy, it is important to assess for persistent bleeding, iron malabsorption, noncompliance, improper iron administration, or other causes of the anemia. Parenteral (IV or intramuscular [IM]) iron administration is safe and effective but painful, expensive, and occasionally associated with regional lymphadenopathy, transient arthralgias, or serious allergic reaction (Andrews, Ullrich, and Fleming, 2009; Glader, 2007; McKenzie, 2004). Therefore parenteral iron is reserved for children who have iron malabsorption or chronic

hemoglobinuria. Transfusions are indicated for the most severe anemia and in cases of serious infection, cardiac dysfunction, or surgical emergency when anesthesia is required. Packed RBCs (2-3 mL/kg), not whole blood, are used to minimize the chance of circulatory overload. Supplemental oxygen is administered when tissue hypoxia is severe.

Prognosis. The prognosis for a child with this condition is very good. However, some evidence indicates that if the iron deficiency anemia is severe and longstanding, cognitive, behavioral, and motor impairment may result (Andrews, Ullrich, and Fleming, 2009; Lokeshwar, Mehta, Mehta, et al., 2011; McCann and Ames, 2007).

CARE MANAGEMENT

An essential nursing responsibility is instructing parents in the administration of iron. Oral iron should be given as prescribed in two divided doses between meals, when the presence of free hydrochloric acid is greatest, because more iron is absorbed in the acidic environment of the upper GI tract. A citrus fruit or juice taken with the medication aids in absorption.

> ### 💊 MEDICATION ALERT
>
> Cow's milk contains substances that bind the iron and interfere with absorption. Iron supplements should not be administered with milk or milk products (Carley, 2003).

An adequate dosage of oral iron turns the stools a tarry green color. The nurse advises parents of this normally expected change and inquires about its occurrence on follow-up visits. Absence of the greenish black stool may be a clue to poor administration of iron, either in schedule or in dosage. Vomiting or diarrhea can occur with iron therapy. If the parents report these symptoms, the iron can be given with meals and the dosage reduced and then gradually increased until tolerated.

> ### 💊 MEDICATION ALERT
>
> Liquid preparations of iron may temporarily stain the teeth. If possible, the medication should be taken through a straw or given through a syringe or medicine dropper placed toward the back of the mouth. Brushing the teeth after administration of the drug lessens the discoloration. Because iron ingestion in excessive quantities is toxic or even fatal, parents should be instructed to keep no more than a month's supply in the home and store it safely away from the reach of children.

If parenteral iron preparations are prescribed, iron dextran must be injected deeply into a large muscle mass using the Z-track method. The injection site is *not* massaged after injection to minimize skin staining and irritation. Because no more than 1 mL should be given in one site, the IV route should be considered to avoid multiple injections. Careful observation is required because of the risk for adverse reactions, such as anaphylaxis, with IV administration. A test dose is recommended before routine use. Recently, a new IV iron preparation (ferumoxytol) was approved in the United States that shows promise in complete replacement of iron with little toxicity (Auerbach, 2011).

Diet. A primary nursing objective is to prevent nutritional anemia through family education. Because breast milk is a low iron source, the nurse must reinforce the importance of administering iron supplementation to exclusively breastfed infants by 4 months of age (Baker, Greer, and Committee on Nutrition AAP, 2010; Lokeshwar, Mehta, Mehta, et al., 2011). The American Academy of Pediatrics (AAP) recommends preterm, marginally low–birth-weight and low-birth-weight infants or infants with inadequate iron stores at birth receive iron supplements at approximately 2 months of age (Berglund, Westrup, and Domellof, 2010).

In formula-fed infants, the nurse discusses with parents the importance of using iron-fortified formula and introducing solid foods at the appropriate age during the first year of life. Traditionally, cereals are one of the first semisolid foods to be introduced into the infant's diet at approximately 6 months of age (Baker, Greer, and Committee on Nutrition AAP, 2010; Glader, 2007; Lokeshwar, Mehta, Mehta, et al., 2011). The best solid-food source of iron is commercial iron-fortified cereals. It may be difficult at first to teach the infant to accept foods other than milk. The same principles are applied as those for introducing new foods (see Nutrition, Chapter 31), especially feeding the solid food before the milk. Predominantly milk-fed infants rebel against solid foods, and parents are cautioned about this and the need to be firm in not relinquishing control to the child. It may require intense problem solving on the part of both the family and the nurse to overcome the child's resistance.

A difficulty encountered in discouraging the parents from feeding milk to the exclusion of other foods is dispelling the popular myth that milk is a "perfect food." Many parents believe that milk is best for infants and equate weight gain with a "healthy child" and "good mothering." The nurse can also stress that overweight is not synonymous with good health.

Diet education of teenagers is especially difficult, especially because teenage girls are particularly prone to following weight-reduction diets. Emphasizing the effect of anemia on appearance (pallor) and energy level (difficulty maintaining popular activities) may be useful.

Sickle Cell Anemia

Sickle cell anemia (SCA) is one of a group of diseases collectively termed hemoglobinopathies in which normal adult Hgb (Hgb A [HbA]) is partly or completely replaced by abnormal sickle Hgb (HbS). Sickle cell disease (SCD) includes all those hereditary disorders whose clinical, hematologic, and pathologic features are related to the presence of HbS. Even though the term *SCD* is sometimes used to refer to SCA, this use is incorrect. Other correct terms for SCA are SS and homozygous SCD.

The following are the most common forms of SCD in the United States:

- SCA, the homozygous form of the disease (HbSS or SS)
- Sickle cell–C disease, a heterozygous variant of SCD, including both HbS and HbC (SC)
- Sickle cell–hemoglobin E disease, a variant of SCD in which glutamic acid has been substituted for lysine in the number 26 position of the β-chain (SE)
- Sickle thalassemia disease, a combination of sickle cell trait and β-thalassemia trait (Sβthal). β+ refers to the ability to still produce some normal HbA. β0 indicates that there is no ability to produce HbA.

Of the SCDs, SCA is the most common form in African-Americans, followed by sickle cell–C disease and sickle thalassemia. Sickle syndromes exist when the HbS is paired with other mutant globins.

Sickle cell disease is one of the most common genetic diseases worldwide. SCD affects approximately 90,000 Americans, primarily African-American, followed by Hispanics, with a lower incidence in the other ethnic groups (Driscoll, 2007). The incidence of the disease varies in different geographic locations. Among African-Americans, the incidence of sickle cell trait is about 9%. In West Africa, the incidence is reported to be as high as 40% among native Africans. The high incidence of sickle cell trait in West Africans is believed by some to be the result of selective protection afforded trait carriers against one type of malaria.

The gene that determines the production of HbS is situated on an autosome and, when present, is always detectable and therefore dominant. Heterozygous persons who have both normal HbA and abnormal HbS are said to have sickle cell trait. Persons who are homozygous have predominantly HbS and have SCA. The inheritance pattern is essentially that of an autosomal recessive disorder. Therefore, when both parents have sickle cell trait, there is a 25% chance with each pregnancy of producing an offspring with SCA.

Although the defect is inherited, the sickling phenomenon is usually not apparent until later in infancy because of the presence of fetal Hbg (HbF). As long as the child has predominantly HbF, sickling does not occur because there is less HbS. Newborns with SCA are generally asymptomatic because of the protective effect of HbF (60%-80% HbF), but this rapidly decreases during the first year, so these children are at risk for sickle cell–related complications (Driscoll, 2007; Heeney and Dover, 2009).

Pathophysiology

The clinical features of SCA are primarily the result of (1) obstruction caused by the sickled RBCs, (2) vascular inflammation, and (3) increased RBC destruction (Fig. 43-2). The abnormal adhesion, entanglement, and enmeshing of rigid sickle-shaped cells accompanied by the inflammatory process intermittently block the microcirculation, causing vasoocclusion (Fig. 43-3). The resultant absence of blood flow to adjacent tissues causes local hypoxia, leading to tissue ischemia and infarction (cellular death). Most of the complications seen in SCA can be traced to this process and its impact on various organs of the body (Box 43-2).

The clinical manifestations of SCA vary greatly in severity and frequency. The most acute symptoms of the disease occur during periods of exacerbation called crises. There are several types of episodic crises, including vasoocclusive, acute splenic sequestration, aplastic, hyperhemolytic, cerebrovascular accident, chest syndrome, and infection. The crises may occur individually or concomitantly with one or more other crises. The vasoocclusive crisis (VOC), preferably called a "painful episode," is characterized by ischemia causing mild to severe pain that may last from minutes to days. Sequestration crisis is a pooling of a large amount of blood—usually in the spleen and infrequently in the liver—that causes a decreased blood volume and ultimately shock. Aplastic crisis is diminished RBC production usually caused by viral infection that may result in profound anemia. Hyperhemolytic crisis is an accelerated rate of RBC destruction characterized by anemia, jaundice, and reticulocytosis.

Another serious complication is acute chest syndrome (ACS), which is clinically similar to pneumonia. It is the presence of a new pulmonary infiltrate and may be associated with chest pain, fever, cough, tachypnea, wheezing, and hypoxia. A cerebrovascular accident (CVA, stroke) is a sudden and severe complication, often with no related illnesses. Sickled cells block the major blood vessels in the brain, resulting in cerebral infarction, which causes variable degrees of neurologic impairment. The current treatment for SCD children who have experienced a stroke is chronic transfusion therapy. Repeat CVAs causing progressively greater brain damage occur in

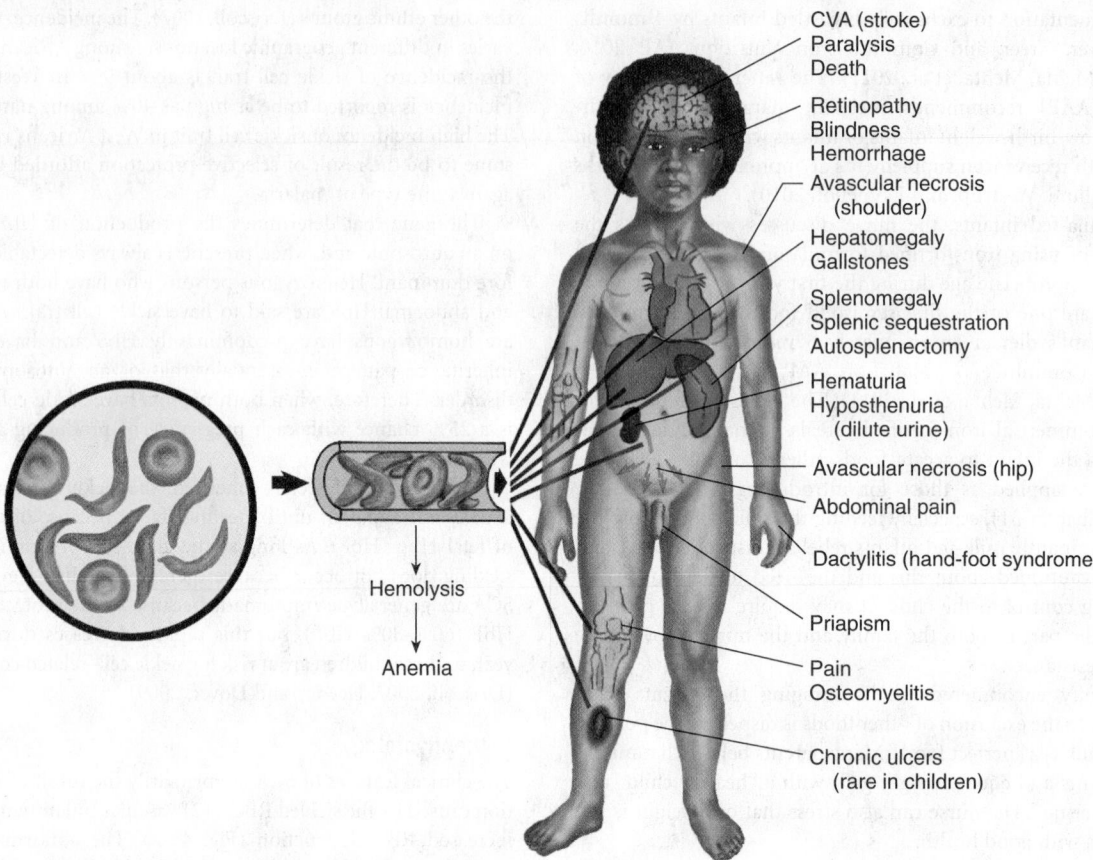

CVA (stroke)
Paralysis
Death

Retinopathy
Blindness
Hemorrhage

Avascular necrosis
(shoulder)

Hepatomegaly
Gallstones

Splenomegaly
Splenic sequestration
Autosplenectomy

Hematuria
Hyposthenuria
(dilute urine)

Avascular necrosis (hip)

Abdominal pain

Dactylitis (hand-foot syndrome)

Priapism

Pain
Osteomyelitis

Chronic ulcers
(rare in children)

Hemolysis

Anemia

FIG 43-2 Clinical features of sickle cell anemia from red blood cell obstruction and destruction. *CVA,* Cerebrovascular accident.

approximately 70% of untreated children who have experienced one stroke (Heeney and Dover, 2009).

Diagnostic Evaluation

Newborn screening for SCA is mandatory in most of the United States so that infants can be identified before symptoms occur. At birth, infants have up to 80% of HbF, which does not carry the defect. Because levels of HbS are low at birth, Hgb electrophoresis or other tests that measure Hgb concentrations are indicated. Early diagnosis (before 3 months of age) enables initiation of appropriate interventions to minimize complications. The family is taught to administer prophylactic antibiotics and identify early signs of infection and to seek medical therapy as soon as possible.

If SCA is not diagnosed in early infancy, it is likely to manifest symptoms during the toddler and preschool years. SCA is occasionally first diagnosed during a crisis that follows an acute respiratory tract or GI infection. Routine hematologic tests are done to evaluate the anemia. Several specific tests detect the presence of the abnormal Hgb in the heterozygote or the homozygote. For screening purposes, the sickle-turbidity test (Sickledex) is frequently used because it can be performed on blood from a fingerstick and yields accurate results in 3 minutes. However, if the test result is positive, Hgb electrophoresis is necessary to distinguish between children with the trait and those with the disease. Hemoglobin electrophoresis ("fingerprinting" of the protein) is an accurate, rapid, and specific test for detecting the homozygous and heterozygous forms of the disease, as well as the percentages of the various types of Hgb.

Therapeutic Management

The aims of therapy are to (1) prevent the sickling phenomena, which are responsible for the pathologic sequelae, and (2) treat the medical emergencies of sickle cell crisis. The successful achievement of the aims depends on prompt nursing interventions, medical therapies, patient and family preventive measures, and use of innovative treatments.

Medical management of a crisis is usually directed toward supportive and symptomatic treatment. The main objectives are to provide (1) rest to minimize energy expenditure and to improve oxygen utilization; (2) hydration through oral and IV therapy; (3) electrolyte replacement because hypoxia results in metabolic acidosis, which also promotes sickling; (4) analgesia for the severe pain from vasoocclusion; (5) blood replacement to treat anemia and to reduce the viscosity of the sickled blood; and (6) antibiotics to treat any existing infection.

Administration of pneumococcal and meningococcal vaccines is recommended for these children because of their susceptibility to infection as a result of functional asplenia. In addition to routine immunizations, children with SCD should receive a yearly influenza vaccination (see Immunizations, Chapter 31). Oral penicillin prophylaxis is also recommended by 2 months of age to reduce the chance of pneumococcal sepsis (see Evidence-Based Practice box) (AAP Committee on Infectious Diseases, 2009; Hirst and Owusu-Ofori, 2010; National Institutes of Health, 2002; Pack-Mabien and Haynes, 2009).

Oxygen therapy is of little therapeutic value unless the patient has hypoxia (Heeney and Dover, 2009). Severe hypoxia must be

Normal red blood cells

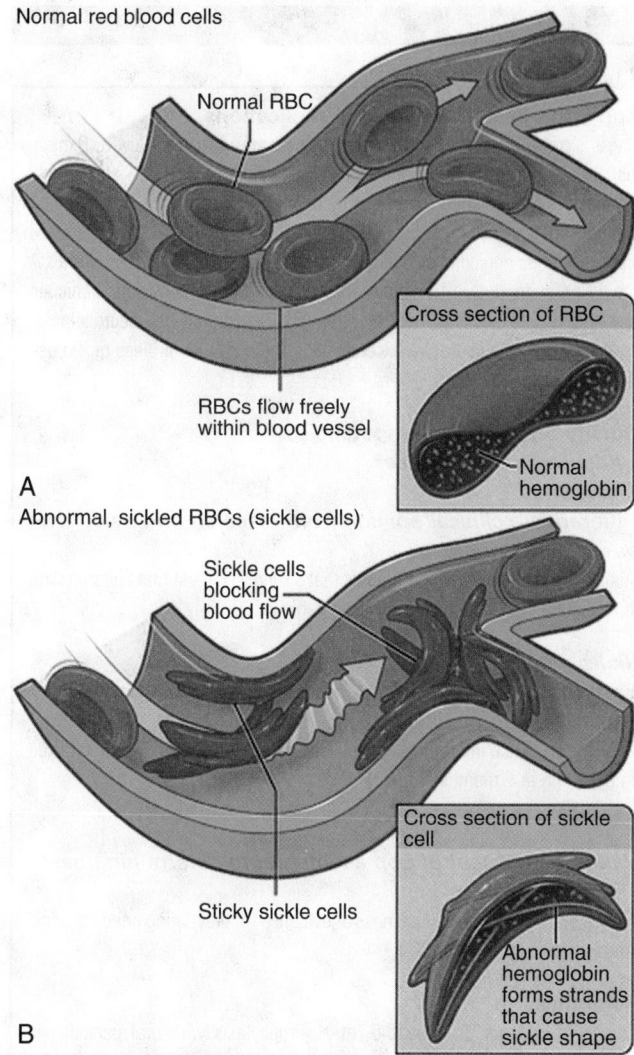

A

Abnormal, sickled RBCs (sickle cells)

B

FIG 43-3 A, Normal red blood cells (RBCs) flowing freely in a blood vessel. The *inset* shows a cross section of a normal RBC with normal hemoglobin. **B,** Abnormal, sickled RBCs clumping and blocking blood flow in a blood vessel. (Other cells also may play a role in this clumping process.) The *inset* shows a cross section of a sickle cell with abnormal hemoglobin. (From National Heart, Lung, and Blood Institute: *What is sickle cell anemia?* Bethesda, MD, August 2008, Author.)

| BOX 43-2 | **CLINICAL MANIFESTATIONS OF SICKLE CELL ANEMIA** |

General
- Possible growth retardation
- Chronic anemia (hemoglobin level of 6-9 g/dL)
- Possible delayed sexual maturation
- Marked susceptibility to sepsis

Vasoocclusive Crisis
- Pain in area(s) of involvement
- Manifestations related to ischemia of involved areas
  Extremities—Painful swelling of hands and feet (sickle cell dactylitis, or hand-foot syndrome), painful joints
  Abdomen—Severe pain resembling acute surgical condition
  Cerebrum—Stroke, visual disturbances
  Chest—Symptoms resembling pneumonia, protracted episodes of pulmonary disease
  Liver—Obstructive jaundice, hepatic coma
  Kidney—Hematuria
  Genitalia—Priapism (painful penile erection)

Sequestration Crisis
- Pooling of large amounts of blood
  - Hepatomegaly
  - Splenomegaly
  - Circulatory collapse

Effects of Chronic Vasoocclusive Phenomena
Heart—Cardiomegaly, systolic murmurs
Lungs—Altered pulmonary function, susceptibility to infections, pulmonary insufficiency
Kidneys—Inability to concentrate urine, enuresis, progressive renal failure
Liver—Hepatomegaly, cirrhosis, intrahepatic cholestasis
Spleen—Splenomegaly, susceptibility to infection, functional reduction in splenic activity progressing to autosplenectomy
Eyes—Intraocular abnormalities with visual disturbances; sometimes progressive retinal detachment and blindness
Extremities—Avascular necrosis of hip or shoulder; skeletal deformities, especially lordosis and kyphosis; chronic leg ulcers; susceptibility to osteomyelitis
Central nervous system—Hemiparesis, seizures

EVIDENCE-BASED PRACTICE

Sickle Cell Anemia and Penicillin Prophylaxis

Ask the Question
In children with SCA, does prophylaxis with penicillin reduce the risk for pneumococcal infection?

Search for Evidence
Search Strategies
Search selection criteria included English language, publication within the past 30 years, research-based articles (level 3 or lower), and child populations.

Databases Used
PubMed, Cochrane Collaboration, MD Consult

Critically Analyze the Evidence
- Hirst and Owusu-Ofori (2010) conducted an updated systematic Cochrane review of three trials that showed a reduced rate of infection in children with SCD receiving penicillin preventatively. Two trials looked at whether treatment was effective. The third trial followed from one of the early trials and looked at when it was safe to stop treatment. Adverse drug effects were rare and minor. Penicillin given preventatively reduces the rate of pneumococcal infections in children with SCD younger than 5 years.
- Researchers combined the clinical experiences of three sickle cell programs in the eastern United States in an attempt to determine the age and disease-specific risk for *Streptococcus pneumoniae* bacteremia and meningitis in children with SCD at a time when penicillin prophylaxis was

Continued

EVIDENCE-BASED PRACTICE

Sickle Cell Anemia and Penicillin Prophylaxis—cont'd

routine. Forty-seven pneumococcal infections (44 bacteremia; 3 meningitis) among 40 patients with SCD were observed. Most children in whom infections developed were taking prophylactic penicillin and received Pneumovax at 24 months of age. The observed severe pneumococcal infection rate in HgbSS children younger than 5 years was less than that reported before penicillin prophylaxis in this specific population (Hord, Byrd, Stowe, et al., 2002).

- Administration of oral prophylactic penicillin was compared with the 14-valent pneumococcal vaccine in preventing pneumococcal infection in 242 children between the ages of 6 months and 3 years with HgbSS. In the first 5 years of the trial, there were 11 pneumococcal infections in the pneumococcal vaccine group and higher infection rates in those given the vaccine before 1 year of age. No pneumococcal isolates were found in the group receiving penicillin, although 4 pneumococcal isolates were found in this group within 1 year of stopping the penicillin prophylaxis at age 3 years. This study supported the use of penicillin prophylaxis to prevent pneumococcal infection in children younger than 3 years (John, Ramlal, Jackson, et al., 1984).

- In a multicenter, randomized, double-blind, placebo-controlled clinical trial, 105 children received penicillin twice daily; a control group of 110 children received a placebo twice daily. The trial was terminated 8 months early when an 84% reduction in the incidence of pneumococcal infections was observed in the group treated with penicillin compared with the placebo group. There were no deaths in the penicillin group, but three deaths from infection occurred in the placebo group. Researchers stressed the importance of screening children during the neonatal period and prescribing prophylactic penicillin to decrease the morbidity and mortality associated with pneumococcal infection (Gaston, Verter, Woods, et al., 1986).

- Zarkowsky, Gallagher, Gill, et al. (1986) conducted a retrospective analysis of 178 episodes of bacteremia in children with sickle hemoglobinopathies that occurred during 13,771 patient-years of follow-up (n = 3451). The predominant pathogen in patients younger than 6 years was *S. pneumoniae* (66%), and gram-negative organisms were responsible for 50% of the bacteremias in patients 6 years and older. The incidence of pneumococcal bacteremia in children with SCA younger than 3 years was 6.1 events per 100 patient-years. The results of this study supported prophylactic administration of penicillin for prevention of pneumococcal bacteremia in children younger than 3 years.

- A cohort study of 315 patients with HgbSS who lived in Jamaica was conducted between June 1973 and December 1981. The patients were divided into three groups to determine whether interventions such as penicillin prophylaxis, parental education in early diagnosis of acute splenic sequestration, and close monitoring in a sickle cell clinic improved survival. A significant decline in deaths from acute splenic sequestration and pneumococcal septicemia and meningitis was found. The research indicated that early detection of SCD and prophylactic measures could significantly reduce deaths associated with HgbSS (Lee, Thomas, Cupidore, et al., 1995).

- Riddington and Owusu-Ofori (2002) conducted a systematic review of randomized controlled trials evaluating the effectiveness of prophylactic antibiotic administration in preventing pneumococcal infection in children with SCD. The review of published research found that penicillin prophylaxis significantly reduced the risk for pneumococcal infection in children with HgbSS with minimal adverse reactions.

Apply the Evidence: Nursing Implications

There is **good evidence with strong recommendations** (Guyatt, Oxman, Vist, et al., 2008) that demonstrates that penicillin prophylaxis significantly reduces the risk for pneumococcal infection in children with SCA. The epidemiologic studies strongly suggest that all children with SCA should be started on prophylactic penicillin at 2 months of age. Parents and children with SCA should be instructed in the importance of taking the prophylactic penicillin twice daily and seeking medical attention immediately for acute illness, especially if the temperature exceeds 38.3° C (101° F), regardless of the use of prophylaxis.

Quality and Safety Competencies: Evidence-Based Practice*

Knowledge

Differentiate clinical opinion from research and evidence-based summaries.

Summarize the epidemiologic studies that strongly suggest that children with SCA should be started on prophylactic penicillin.

Skills

Base individualized care plan on patient values, clinical expertise, and evidence.

Integrate evidence into practice by making sure infants with SCD are started on penicillin at 2 months of age.

Attitudes

Value the concept of Ebp as integral to determining best clinical practice.

Appreciate strengths and weakness of evidence for preventing pneumococcal infection in children with SCD.

References

Gaston MH, Verter JI, Woods G, et al: Prophylaxis with oral penicillin in children with sickle cell anemia: a randomized trial, *N Engl J Med* 314(25):1593–1599, 1986.

Guyatt GH, Oxman AD, Vist GE, et al: GRADE: an emerging consensus on rating quality of evidence and strength of recommendations, *BMJ* 336(7650):924–926, 2008.

Hirst C, Owusu-Ofori S: Prophylactic antibiotics for preventing pneumococcal infection in children with sickle cell disease, *Cochrane Database Syst Rev* (11):CD003427, 2010.

Hord J, Byrd R, Stowe L, et al: *Streptococcus pneumoniae* sepsis and meningitis during the penicillin prophylaxis era in children with sickle cell disease, *J Pediatr Hematol Oncol* 24(6):470–472, 2002.

John AB, Ramlal A, Jackson H, et al: Prevention of pneumococcal infection in children with homozygous sickle cell disease, *BMJ* 288(6430):1567–1570, 1984.

Lee A, Thomas P, Cupidore L, et al: Improved survival in homozygous sickle cell disease: lessons from cohort study, *BMJ* 311(7020):1600–1602, 1995.

Riddington C, Owusu-Ofori S: Prophylactic antibiotics for preventing pneumococcal infection in children with sickle cell disease, *Cochrane Database Syst Rev* (3):CD003427, 2002.

Zarkowsky HS, Gallagher D, Gill FM, et al: Bacteremia in sickle hemoglobinopathies, *J Pediatr* 109(4):579–585, 1986.

EBP, Evidence-based practice; *HgbSS*, homozygous sickle cell disease; *SCA*, sickle cell anemia; *SCD*, sickle cell disease.
*Adapted from the QSEN at www.qsen.org.

prevented because it causes massive systemic sickling that can be fatal. Oxygen administration is usually not effective in reversing sickling or reducing pain because the oxygen is unable to reach the enmeshed sickled erythrocytes in clogged vessels (Chiocca, 1996). In addition, prolonged administration of oxygen can depress bone marrow, further aggravating the anemia (Khoury and Grimsley, 1995).

Another important component of care is the use of blood transfusions. Exchange RBC transfusion (erythrocytapheresis) is the replacement of sickle cells with normal RBCs. Exchange transfusion is a successful, rapid method of reducing the number of circulating sickle cells and therefore slowing down the vicious circle of hypoxia, thrombosis, tissue ischemia, and injury. The procedure is advocated as a possible technique in preventing reoccurrence of ACS and CVA (Velasquez, Mariscalco, Goldstein, et al., 2009). A transcranial Doppler (TCD) test identifies the child with SCD who is at high risk for developing a CVA by monitoring the intracranial vascular flow (Driscoll, 2007; Kwiatkowski, Yim, Miller, et al., 2011). The TCD test is performed yearly for children from 2 to 16 years of age. The recommended treatment for children with confirmed abnormal TCD is chronic transfusion therapy (Armstrong-Wells, Grimes, Sidney, et al., 2009; Driscoll, 2007; Kwiatkowski, Yim, Miller, et al., 2011). Multiple transfusions carry the risk for transmission of viral infection, hyperviscosity, transfusion reactions, alloimmunization, and hemosiderosis (Driscoll, 2007; Heeney and Dover, 2009). After a CVA, blood transfusions are usually given every 3 to 4 weeks to help prevent a repeat stroke. To reduce iron overload from chronic transfusion therapy, chelation therapy may be started (see p. 1311).

In children with recurrent life-threatening splenic sequestration, splenectomy may be a lifesaving measure. However, the spleen usually atrophies on its own through progressive fibrotic changes (functional asplenia) by 6 years of age in children with SCA. Prophylactic penicillin and pneumococcal vaccines have decreased the incidence of pneumococcal sepsis. Packed RBC transfusions are recommended for treatment of splenic sequestration and stroke and are used preoperatively accompanied with maintenance IV hydration for most surgical procedures in children with SCD.

The most common and debilitating symptom experienced by patients with SCD is VOC, which is accompanied by increasing heath care cost because of prolonged hospitalization associated with pulmonary and GI complications (Driscoll, 2007; Raphael, Mei, Mueller, et al., 2012). The chronic nature of this pain can greatly affect the child's development. A multidisciplinary team (e.g., physician, psychologist, family, nurse, social worker) approach is best for vasoocclusive pain management that includes pharmacologic treatment, hydration, physical therapy, and complementary treatment (e.g., prayer, spiritual healing, massage, herbs, relaxation, acupuncture, and biofeedback) (Brandow, Weisman, and Panepinto, 2011; Redding-Lallinger and Knoll, 2006). When mild to moderate VOC is reported, nonsteroidal antiinflammatory medication (e.g., ibuprofen, ketorolac) or acetaminophen (Tylenol) is used initially. If these drugs are not effective alone, codeine can be added. The dosages of both drugs are titrated (adjusted) to a therapeutic level. Opioids such as immediate- and sustained-release morphine, oxycodone, hydromorphone (Dilaudid), and methadone are administered intravenously or orally for severe pain and are given around the clock. In conjunction with the opioid, IV ketorolac for a maximum of a 5-day course is commonly used to enhance the pain management effect. Patient-controlled analgesia (PCA) has been used successfully for sickle cell–related pain. PCA reinforces the patient's role and responsibility in managing the pain and provides

flexibility in dealing with pain, which may vary in severity over time (see Pain Management, Chapter 30).

🔔 MEDICATION ALERT

Meperidine (Demerol) is not recommended. Normeperidine, a metabolite of meperidine, is a central nervous system (CNS) stimulant that produces anxiety, tremors, myoclonus, and generalized seizures when it accumulates with repetitive dosing. Patients with SCD are particularly at risk for normeperidine-induced seizures (Howard and Davies, 2007; National Institutes of Health, 2002).

Prognosis. The prognosis varies, but most patients live into the fifth decade. Most of the time, children are without symptoms and participate in normal activities without restrictions. The greatest risk is usually in children younger than 5 years, and the majority of deaths in these children are caused by overwhelming infection. Consequently, SCA is a chronic illness with a potentially terminal outcome. Physical and sexual maturation are delayed in adolescents with SCA. Although adults achieve normal height, weight, and sexual function, the delay may present problems to adolescents (Heeney and Dover, 2009; Redding-Lallinger and Knoll, 2006).

Individuals with SCD who have higher levels of HbF tend to have a milder disease with fewer complications than those with lower levels (Anderson, 2006; Driscoll, 2007). Hydroxyurea is a U.S. Food and Drug Administration–approved medication that increases the production of HbF, reduces endothelial adhesion of sickle cells, improves the sickle cell hydration, increases nitric oxide production (a vasodilator), and lowers leukocyte and reticulocyte counts (McGann and Ware, 2011; National Institutes of Health, 2002). Long-term follow-up of patients taking hydroxyurea alone revealed a 40% reduction in mortality and decreased frequency of VOC, ACS, hospital admissions, and need for transfusions, thus making SCD crises milder (Anderson, 2006; Strouse, Lanzkron, Beach, et al., 2008). Pediatric studies have shown that hydroxyurea can be safely used in children (Wang, Ware, Miller, et al., 2011; Zimmerman, Schultz, Davis, et al., 2004).

Hematopoietic stem cell transplantation (HSCT) offers a curative approach for some children with SCD with event-free survival of 95% (Driscoll, 2007; Haining, Duncan, and Lehmann, 2009) (see p. 1389).

CARE MANAGEMENT

Educate the Family and Child. Family education begins with an explanation of the disease and its consequences. After this explanation, the most important issues to teach the family are to (1) seek early intervention for problems, such as fever of 38.5° C (101.3° F) or greater; (2) give penicillin as ordered; (3) recognize signs and symptoms of splenic sequestration, as well as respiratory problems that can lead to hypoxia; and (4) treat the child normally. The nurse tells the family that the child is normal but can get sick in ways that other children cannot.

The nurse emphasizes the importance of adequate hydration to prevent sickling and to delay the adhesion-stasis-thrombosis-ischemia cycle. It is not sufficient to advise parents to "force fluids" or "encourage drinking." They need specific instructions on how many glasses or bottles of fluid are required daily. Many foods are also a source of fluid, particularly soups, flavored ice pops, ice cream, sherbet, gelatin, and puddings.

Increased fluids combined with impaired kidney function result in the problem of enuresis. Parents who are unaware of this fact

FAMILY-CENTERED CARE

Fear of Addiction

Although the pain during a sickle cell crisis is usually severe and opioids are needed, many families fear that their child will become addicted to the narcotic. Unfortunately, misinformed health care professionals may foster this unfounded fear, which results in needless suffering. Extremely few children who receive opioids for severe pain become behaviorally addicted to the drug (American Pain Society, 1999; Howard and Davies, 2007; National Institutes of Health, 2002). Families and older children, especially adolescents, need to be reassured that opioids are medically indicated, high doses may be needed, and children rarely become addicted.

frequently use the usual measures to discourage bedwetting, such as limiting fluids at night, and may resort to punishment and shame to force bladder control. To alleviate parental pressure on the child, enuresis should be considered a complication of the disease just as joint pain or some other symptom is regarded.

Promote Supportive Therapies During Crises. The success of many of the medical therapies relies heavily on nursing implementation. Management of pain is an especially difficult problem and often involves experimenting with various analgesics, including opioids, and schedules before relief is achieved. Unfortunately, these children tend to be undermedicated, resulting in their "clock watching" and demands for additional doses sooner than might be expected. Often this incorrectly raises suspicions of drug addiction, when in fact the problem is one of improper dosage (see Family-Centered Care box). In choosing and scheduling analgesics, the goal should be *prevention* of pain.

! NURSING ALERT

Advise parents to be particularly alert to situations in which dehydration may be a possibility, such as hot weather, and to recognize early signs of reduced intake, such as decreased urinary output (e.g., fewer wet diapers) and increased thirst.

Any pain program should be combined with psychologic support to help the child deal with the depression, anxiety, and fear that may accompany the disease. This includes regular visits with the child to discuss any concerns during the hospitalization and positive reinforcement of coping skills, such as successful methods of dealing with the pain and compliance with treatment prescriptions. To reduce the negative connotation associated with the term *crisis*, it is best to say *pain episode.*

If blood transfusions or exchange transfusions are given, the nurse has the responsibility of observing for signs of transfusion reaction. Because hypervolemia from too-rapid transfusion can increase the workload of the heart, the nurse also is alert to signs of cardiac failure.

In splenic sequestration, the size of the spleen is gently measured by abdominal palpation (see Abdomen, Chapter 29). The nurse should be aware of spleen size because increasing splenomegaly is an ominous sign. A decreasing spleen size denotes response to therapy. Vital signs and blood pressure are also closely monitored for impending shock. Anemia is typically not a presenting complication in vasoocclusive crises but is a critical problem in other types of crises. The nurse monitors for evidence of increasing anemia and institutes appropriate nursing interventions. Oxygen is not

beneficial in vasoocclusive episodes unless hypoxemia is present (Heeney and Dover, 2009). It does not reverse sickled RBCs, and if used in a nonhypoxic patient, it will decrease erythropoiesis (Vichinsky and Styles, 1996). Because prolonged use of oxygen can aggravate the anemia, signs of lack of therapeutic benefit, such as restlessness, increased pallor, and continued pain, are reported.

Record intake, especially of IV fluids, and output. The child's weight should be taken on admission to serve as a baseline for evaluating hydration. Because diuresis can result in electrolyte loss, the nurse also observes for signs of hypokalemia and should be familiar with normal serum electrolyte values to report changes.

Recognize Other Complications. Nurses also need to be aware of the signs of ACS and CVA, both potentially fatal complications.

! NURSING ALERT

Report signs of the following immediately:
- ACS:
  - Severe chest, back, or abdominal pain
  - Fever of 38.5° C (101.3° F) or higher
  - Cough
  - Dyspnea, tachypnea
  - Retractions
  - Declining oxygen saturation (oximetry)
- CVA:
  - Severe, unrelieved headaches
  - Severe vomiting
  - Jerking or twitching of the face, legs, or arms
  - Seizures
  - Strange, abnormal behavior
  - Inability to move an arm or leg
  - Stagger or an unsteady walk
  - Stutter or slurred speech
  - Weakness in the hands, feet, or legs
  - Changes in vision

Support the Family. Families need the opportunity to discuss their feelings regarding transmitting a potentially fatal, chronic illness to their child. Because of the widely publicized prognosis for children with SCA, many parents express their prevalent fear of the child's death. Three manifestations of SCD that may appear in the first 2 years of life (dactylitis, severe anemia, leukocytosis) can be predictors of disease severity (DeBaun and Vichinsky, 2007; Ohls and Christensen, 2007). The nurse should care for the family as for any family with a child who has a chronic and life-threatening illness and consider the siblings' reactions, the stress on the marital relationship, and the childrearing attitudes displayed toward the child. Several resources are available to families with a sickling disorder.*

*Sickle Cell Disease Association of America, Inc., 231 E. Baltimore St., Suite 800, Baltimore, MD 21202; 410-528-1555, 800-421-8453; fax: 410-528-1495; e-mail: scdaa@sicklecelldisease.org; www.sicklecelldisease.org.
National Heart, Lung, and Blood Institute, PO Box 30105, Bethesda, MD 20824-0105; 301-592-8573, fax: 240-629-3246; www.nhlbi.nih.gov.
Sickle cell disease in newborns and infants: a guide for parents, Pub No AHCPR 93-0564. Available from the AHCPR Publications Clearinghouse, PO Box 8547, Silver Spring, MD 20907-8547; 800-358-9295; www.ahcpr.gov.
Guideline for the management of acute and chronic pain in sickle-cell disease is available from the American Pain Society, 4700 W. Lake Ave., Glenview, IL 60025-1485; 847-375-4715; fax: 866-574-2654; e-mail: info@ampainsoc.org; www.ampainsoc.org.

The nurse advises parents to inform all treating personnel of the child's condition. The use of medical identification, such as a bracelet, is another way of ensuring awareness of the disease.

If family members have the SCD trait or SCA, genetic counseling is necessary. A primary consideration in genetic counseling is informing parents of the 25% chance with each pregnancy of having a child with the disease when both parents carry the trait.

β-Thalassemia (Cooley Anemia)

Worldwide, thalassemia is a common genetic disorder, affecting as many as 15 million people (Yaish, 2010). The term thalassemia, which is derived from the Greek word *thalassa*, meaning "sea," is applied to a variety of inherited blood disorders characterized by deficiencies in the rate of production of specific globin chains in Hgb. The name appropriately refers to descendants of or people living near the Mediterranean Sea, who have the highest incidence of the disease, namely Italians, Greeks, and Syrians. Evidence suggests that the high incidence of the disorders among these groups is a result of the selective advantage the trait confers in relation to malaria, as is postulated in SCD. However, the disorder has a wide geographic distribution, probably as a result of genetic migration through intermarriage or possibly as a result of spontaneous mutation.

β-Thalassemia is the most common of the thalassemias and occurs in four forms:

- Two heterozygous forms, thalassemia minor, an asymptomatic silent carrier; and thalassemia trait, which produces a mild microcytic anemia
- Thalassemia intermedia, which is manifested as splenomegaly and moderate to severe anemia
- A homozygous form, thalassemia major (also known as Cooley anemia), which results in a severe anemia that would lead to cardiac failure and death in early childhood without transfusion support

Pathophysiology

Normal postnatal Hgb is composed of two α– and two β–polypeptide chains. In β-thalassemia, there is a partial or complete deficiency in the synthesis of the β-chain of the Hgb molecule. Consequently, there is a compensatory increase in the synthesis of α-chains, and γ-chain production remains activated, resulting in defective Hgb formation. This unbalanced polypeptide unit is very unstable; when it disintegrates, it damages RBCs, causing severe anemia.

To compensate for the hemolytic process, an overabundance of erythrocytes is formed unless the bone marrow is suppressed by transfusion therapy. Excess iron from hemolysis of supplemental RBCs in transfusions and from the rapid destruction of defective cells is stored in various organs (hemosiderosis).

Diagnostic Evaluation

The onset of thalassemia major may be insidious and not recognized until the latter half of infancy. The clinical effects of thalassemia major are primarily attributable to (1) defective synthesis of HbA, (2) structurally impaired RBCs, and (3) shortened life span of erythrocytes (Box 43-3).

Hematologic studies reveal the characteristic changes in RBCs (i.e., microcytosis, hypochromia, anisocytosis, poikilocytosis, target cells, and basophilic stippling of various stages). Low Hgb and Hct levels are seen in severe anemia, although they are typically lower than the reduction in RBC count because of the proliferation of immature erythrocytes. Hgb electrophoresis confirms the

---

BOX 43-3   CLINICAL MANIFESTATIONS OF β-THALASSEMIA

Anemia (Before Diagnosis)
- Pallor
- Unexplained fever
- Poor feeding
- Enlarged spleen or liver

Progressive Anemia
- Signs of chronic hypoxia
  - Headache
  - Precordial and bone pain
  - Decreased exercise tolerance
- Listlessness
- Anorexia

Other Features
- Small stature
- Delayed sexual maturation
- Bronzed, freckled complexion (if not receiving chelation therapy)

Bone Changes (Older Children If Untreated)
- Enlarged head
- Prominent frontal and parietal bossing
- Prominent malar eminences
- Flat or depressed bridge of the nose
- Enlarged maxilla
- Protrusion of the lip and upper central incisors and eventual malocclusion
- Generalized osteoporosis

---

diagnosis, and radiographs of involved bones reveal characteristic findings.

Therapeutic Management

The objectives of supportive therapy are to maintain sufficient Hgb levels to prevent bone marrow expansion and the resulting bony deformities and to provide sufficient RBCs to support normal growth and normal physical activity. Transfusions are the foundation of medical management with the goal of maintaining the Hgb level above 9.5 g/dL, an aim that may require transfusions as often as every 3 to 5 weeks. The advantages of this therapy include (1) improved physical and psychologic well-being because of the ability to participate in normal activities, (2) decreased cardiomegaly and hepatosplenomegaly, (3) fewer bone changes, (4) normal or near-normal growth and development until puberty, and (5) fewer infections.

One of the potential complications of frequent blood transfusions is iron overload (hemosiderosis). Because the body has no effective means of eliminating the excess iron, the mineral is deposited in body tissues. To minimize the development of hemosiderosis, the oral iron chelator *deferasirox* has been shown to be a safe equivalent to deferoxamine (Desferal), a parenteral iron-chelating agent, and more tolerable by patients and families (Cappellini, Porter, El-Beshlawy, et al., 2010; Vichinsky, Bernaudin, Forni, et al., 2011; Vichinsky, Onyekwere, Porter, et al., 2007).

In some children with severe splenomegaly who require repeated transfusions, a splenectomy may be necessary to decrease the disabling effects of abdominal pressure and to increase the life span of supplemental RBCs. Over time, the spleen may accelerate the rate of RBC destruction and thus increase transfusion requirements. After a splenectomy, children generally require fewer transfusions, although the basic defect in Hgb synthesis remains unaffected. A major postsplenectomy complication is severe and overwhelming infection. Therefore these children continue to receive prophylactic antibiotics with close medical supervision for many years and should receive the pneumococcal and meningococcal vaccines in addition to the regularly scheduled immunizations (see Immunizations, Chapter 31).

> **⚠ NURSING ALERT**
>
> Ensure that the family and patient understand the need to notify the health care professional of all fevers of 38.5° C (101.3° F) or greater because of the risk for sepsis in a child with asplenia.

Prognosis. Most children treated with blood transfusion and early chelation therapy survive well into adulthood. The most common causes of death are heart disease, postsplenectomy sepsis, and multiple-organ failure secondary to hemochromatosis (Cunningham, Sankaran, Nathan, et al., 2009). A curative treatment for some children is HSCT. Children younger than 16 years who undergo allogeneic HSCT have a high rate of complication-free survival; approximately 80% of these children are cured (Lucarelli and Gaziev, 2008).

CARE MANAGEMENT

The objectives of nursing care are to (1) promote compliance with transfusion and chelation therapy, (2) assist the child in coping with the anxiety-provoking treatments and the effects of the illness, (3) foster the child's and family's adjustment to a chronic illness, and (4) observe for complications of multiple blood transfusions. Basic to each of these goals is explaining to parents and older children the defect responsible for the disorder, its effect on RBCs, and the potential effects of untreated iron overload (e.g., diabetes and heart disease). Because the prevalence of this condition is high among families of Mediterranean descent, the nurse also inquires about the family's previous knowledge about thalassemia. All families with a child with thalassemia should be tested for the trait and referred for genetic counseling.

As with any chronic illness, the family's needs must be met for optimal adjustment to the stresses imposed by the disorder (see Chapter 36). Sources of information for the family include the Cooley's Anemia Foundation* and the Northern California Comprehensive Thalassemia Center.† Genetic counseling for the parents and fertile offspring is mandatory, and both prenatal diagnosis using amniocentesis at 20 weeks' gestation or fetal blood sampling at 10 weeks and screening for thalassemia trait are available.

Aplastic Anemia

Aplastic anemia (AA) refers to a bone marrow failure condition in which the formed elements of the blood are simultaneously depressed. The peripheral blood smear demonstrates pancytopenia or the triad of profound anemia, leukopenia, and thrombocytopenia. Hypoplastic anemia is characterized by a profound depression of RBCs but normal or slightly decreased white blood cells (WBCs) and platelets.

Etiology

Aplastic anemia can be primary (congenital, or present at birth) or secondary (acquired). The best-known congenital disorder of which AA is an outstanding feature is Fanconi syndrome, a rare hereditary disorder characterized by pancytopenia, hypoplasia of the bone marrow, and patchy brown discoloration of the skin resulting from the deposit of melanin and associated with multiple congenital

*330 Seventh Ave., No. 200, New York, NY 10001; 800-522-7222; fax: 212-279-5999; www.thalassemia.org.
†747 52nd St., Oakland, CA 94609; 510-428-3885, ext. 5427; http://hemonc.cho.org/thalassemia.

> **BOX 43-4   COMMON CAUSES OF ACQUIRED APLASTIC ANEMIA**
>
> - Human parvovirus infection, hepatitis, or overwhelming infection
> - Irradiation
> - Immune disorders such as hypoimmunoglobulinemia and eosinophilic fasciitis
> - Drugs such as certain chemotherapeutic agents, anticonvulsants, and antibiotics
> - Industrial and household chemicals, including benzene and its derivatives, which are found in petroleum products, dyes, paint remover, shellac, and lacquers
> - Infiltration and replacement of myeloid elements, such as in leukemia or the lymphomas
> - Idiopathic (In most cases, no identifiable precipitating cause can be found.)

anomalies of the musculoskeletal and genitourinary systems. The syndrome appears to be inherited as an autosomal recessive trait with varying penetrance; therefore affected siblings may demonstrate several different combinations of defects.

Several etiologic factors contribute to the development of acquired hypoplastic anemia; however, most of the cases are considered idiopathic (Box 43-4). Acquired AA is classified as either *severe acquired AA* or *moderate acquired AA*. The following discussion focuses on severe acquired AA, which carries a poorer prognosis and follows a more rapidly fatal course than the primary types.

Diagnostic Evaluation

The onset of clinical manifestations, which include anemia, leukopenia, and decreased platelet count, is usually insidious. Definitive diagnosis is determined from bone marrow examination, which demonstrates the conversion of red bone marrow to yellow, fatty bone marrow. Severe AA is defined as less than 25% bone marrow cellularity with at least two of the following findings: absolute granulocyte count less than 500/mm^3, platelet count less than 20,000/mm^3, and absolute reticulocyte count less than 40,000/mm^3 (Hord, 2007; Passweg and Marsh, 2010). Moderate AA is defined as more than 25% bone marrow cellularity with the presence of mild or moderate cytopenia (Shimamura and Guinan, 2009).

Therapeutic Management

The objectives of treatment are based on the recognition that the underlying disease process is failure of the bone marrow to carry out its hematopoietic functions. Therefore therapy is directed at restoring function to the marrow and involves two main approaches: (1) immunosuppressive therapy to remove the presumed immunologic functions that prolong aplasia; or (2) replacement of the bone marrow through transplantation. Bone marrow transplantation is the treatment of choice for severe AA when a suitable donor exists (see p. 1389).

Antilymphocyte globulin (ALG) or antithymocyte globulin (ATG) is the principal drug treatment used for AA. The rationale for using ATG is based on the theory that AA may be a result of autoimmunity. ATG and cyclosporine suppress T cell–dependent autoimmune responses but do not cause bone marrow suppression. Cyclosporine is administered orally for several weeks to months. ATG usually is administered intravenously over 12 to 16 hours for 4 days after a test dose to check for hypersensitivity. A course may be repeated, depending on the reduction in circulating lymphocytes and the patient's response. Because of the hypersensitivity response associated with ATG (i.e., fever, chills, myalgias), methylprednisolone is given intravenously to prevent these side effects. Colony-stimulating factor (CSF) and granulocyte-macrophage colony-stimulating factor (GM-CSF), given parenterally, may be used to enhance bone marrow production. Androgens may be used with ATG to stimulate erythropoiesis if the AA is unresponsive to initial therapies.

Hematopoietic stem cell transplantation should be considered early in the course of the disease if a compatible donor can be found. Transplantation is more successful when performed before multiple transfusions have sensitized the child to leukocyte and human leukocyte antigens (HLAs). HSCT is associated with an approximately 90% survival rate in patients who receive a bone marrow transplant from an HLA-identical sibling (Hord, 2007; Marsh, 2005; Trigg, 2004).

CARE MANAGEMENT

The care of the child with AA is similar to that of the child with leukemia (see p. 1380) and includes preparing the child and family for the diagnostic and therapeutic procedures, preventing complications from the severe pancytopenia, and emotionally supporting them in the face of a potentially fatal outcome. Information and support are available from the Aplastic Anemia and MDS International Foundation, Inc.*

Because the aspects of nursing care are discussed in the section on leukemia, only the exceptions are presented here. The drug *ATG* is usually administered by way of a central vein. If not, vigilant care must be directed to the IV infusion to prevent extravasation. Meticulous care of the venous access is essential because of the child's susceptibility to infection. CSFs are usually given by subcutaneous injection over several days. Chemotherapeutic agents have been reported in the treatment of relapsed patients with AA after ATG and CSF therapy. Many of the side effects associated with chemotherapy such as nausea and vomiting, alopecia, and mucositis are experienced by children receiving treatment for AA. Specialized care is required for children who have HSCT (see p. 1389).

DEFECTS IN HEMOSTASIS

Hemostasis is the process that stops bleeding when a blood vessel is injured. Vascular and plasma clotting factors, as well as platelets, are required. A complex system of clotting, anticlotting, and clot breakdown (fibrinolysis) mechanisms exists in equilibrium to ensure clot formation only in the presence of blood vessel injury and to limit the clotting process to the site of vessel wall injury. Dysfunction in these systems leads to bleeding or abnormal clotting. Although the coagulation process is complex, clotting depends on three factors: (1) vascular influence, (2) platelet role, and (3) clotting factors.

Hemophilia

The term hemophilia refers to a group of bleeding disorders in which there is a deficiency of one of the factors (proteins) necessary for coagulation of the blood. Although the symptomatology is similar regardless of which clotting factor is deficient, the

identification of specific factor deficiencies allows definitive treatment with replacement agents.

In about 80% of all cases of hemophilia, the inheritance pattern is demonstrated as X-linked recessive. The two most common forms of the disorder are factor VIII deficiency (hemophilia A, or classic hemophilia) and factor IX deficiency (hemophilia B, or Christmas disease). Von Willebrand disease (vWD) is another hereditary bleeding disorder characterized by a deficiency, abnormality, or absence of the protein called *von Willebrand factor (vWF)* and a deficiency of factor VIII. Unlike hemophilia, vWD affects both males and females. The following discussion is concerned primarily with factor VIII deficiency, which accounts for 80% of all hemophilia cases.

Pathophysiology

The basic defect of hemophilia A is a deficiency of factor VIII (antihemophilic factor [AHF]). AHF is produced by the liver and is necessary for the formation of thromboplastin in phase I of blood coagulation (Fig. 43-4). The less AHF found in the blood, the more severe the disease. Individuals with hemophilia have two of the three factors required for coagulation: vascular influence and platelets. Therefore they may bleed for longer periods but not at a faster rate.

Bleeding into subcutaneous and IM tissue is common. Hemarthrosis, which is bleeding into a joint space, is the most frequent type of internal bleeding. Bony changes and crippling deformities occur after repeated bleeding episodes over several years. Signs of hemarthrosis are swelling, warmth, redness, pain, and loss of movement. Bleeding in the neck, mouth, or thorax is serious because the airway can become obstructed. Intracranial hemorrhage can have fatal consequences and is one of the major causes of death. Hemorrhage anywhere along the GI tract can lead to anemia, and bleeding into the retroperitoneal cavity is especially hazardous because of the large space for blood to accumulate. Hematomas in the spinal cord can cause paralysis.

Diagnostic Evaluation

Overt, prolonged hemorrhage is readily apparent; bleeding into tissues is less apparent (Box 43-5). The diagnosis is usually made from a history of bleeding episodes, evidence of X-linked inheritance (only one third of the cases are new mutations), and laboratory findings. The tests specific for hemophilia plasma depend on specific factors for a reaction to occur, such as the partial thromboplastin time (PTT). Specific determination of factor deficiencies requires assay procedures normally performed in specialized laboratories. Carrier detection is possible in classic hemophilia using DNA testing and is an important consideration in families in whom female offspring may have inherited the trait.

Therapeutic Management

The primary therapy for hemophilia is replacement of the missing clotting factor. The products available are factor VIII concentrates, either produced through genetically engineering (recombinant) or derived from pooled plasma, which are reconstituted with sterile water immediately before use. A synthetic form of vasopressin, 1-deamino-8-D-arginine vasopressin (DDAVP), increases plasma factor VIII activity and is the treatment of choice in mild hemophilia and certain types of vWD if the child shows an appropriate response. DDAVP is not effective in the treatment of severe hemophilia A, severe vWD, or any form of hemophilia B. Aggressive factor concentrate replacement therapy is initiated to prevent chronic crippling effects from joint bleeding.

Other drugs may be included in the therapy plan, depending on the source of the hemorrhage. Corticosteroids are given for

*100 Park Ave., Suite 108, Rockville, MD 20850; 800-747-2820, 301-279-7202; fax: 301-279-7205; e-mail: help@aamds.org; www.aamds.org.

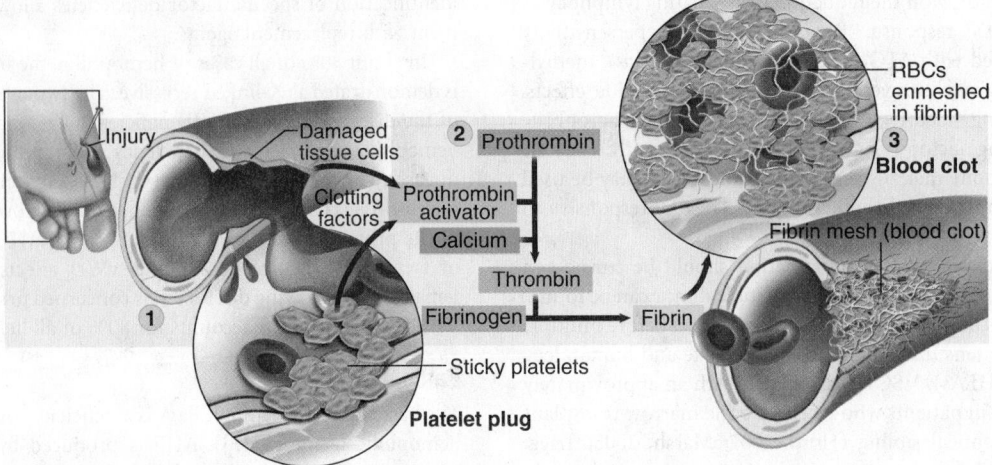

FIG 43-4 Blood clotting. The extremely complex clotting mechanism can be distilled into three basic steps: *(1)* release of clotting factors from both injured tissue cells and sticky platelets at the injury site (which form a temporary platelet plug); *(2)* a series of chemical reactions that eventually result in the formation of thrombin; and *(3)* formation of fibrin and trapping of red blood cells (RBCs) to form a clot. (From Thibodeau GA: *The human body in health and disease,* ed 5, St Louis, Mosby, 2010.)

BOX 43-5 CLINICAL MANIFESTATIONS OF HEMOPHILIA

- Prolonged bleeding anywhere from or in the body
- Hemorrhage from any trauma—loss of deciduous teeth, circumcision, cuts, epistaxis, injections
- Excessive bruising, even from a slight injury, such as a fall
- Subcutaneous and intramuscular hemorrhages
- Hemarthrosis (bleeding into the joint cavities), especially the knees, ankles, and elbows
- Hematomas—pain, swelling, and limited motion
- Spontaneous hematuria

---

hematuria, acute hemarthrosis, and chronic synovitis. Nonsteroidal antiinflammatory drugs (NSAIDs), such as ibuprofen, are effective in relieving pain caused by synovitis; however, they are occasionally used with caution because they inhibit platelet function (Curry, 2004). Oral administration of ε-aminocaproic acid (Amicar) prevents clot destruction. Its use is limited to mouth or trauma surgery with a dose of factor concentrate given first.

A regular program of exercise and physical therapy is an important aspect of management. Physical activity within reasonable limits strengthens muscles around joints and may decrease the number of spontaneous bleeding episodes.

Treatment without delay results in more rapid recovery and a decreased likelihood of complications; therefore most children are treated at home. The family is taught the technique of venipuncture and to administer the AHF to children older than 2 to 3 years. The child learns the procedure for self-administration at 8 to 12 years of age. Home treatment is highly successful, and the rewards, in addition to the immediacy, are less disruption of family life, fewer school or work days missed, and enhancement of the child's self-esteem and independence.

Primary prophylaxis in hemophilia patients has proved to be effective in preventing bleeding complications by administrating periodic factor replacement. Primary prophylaxis involves the infusion of factor VIII concentrate on a regular basis before the onset of joint damage. Secondary prophylaxis involves the infusion of factor VIII concentrate on a regular basis after the child experiences his or her first joint bleed. The infusions are given 3 times a week. Aggressive or on-demand factor replacement may be a cost-effective alternative to primary prophylaxis, but prophylaxis decreases the development of joint disease compared with on-demand factor replacement treatment (Manco-Johnson, Abshire, Shapiro, et al., 2007). Prompt appropriate treatment of hemorrhage and prophylactic therapy are key to excellent care and prevention of long-term morbidity in patients with hemophilia (Montgomery, Gill, and DiPaola, 2009; Sharathkumar and Pipe, 2008).

Prognosis. Although there is no cure for hemophilia, its symptoms can be controlled and its potentially crippling deformities greatly reduced or even avoided. Today many children with hemophilia function with minimal or no joint damage. They are normal children with an average life expectancy in every respect but one: they have a tendency to bleed, which is a significant inconvenience but not necessarily a life-threatening event.

Gene therapy may prove to be a treatment option in the future. This therapy involves introducing a working copy of the factor VIII gene into a patient who has a flawed copy of the gene. Problems exist with appropriate selection of the vector, identification of the cell for gene expression, and control of side effects (Matrai, Chuah, and VandenDriessche, 2010; Montgomery, Gill, and DiPaola, 2009).

CARE MANAGEMENT

The earlier a bleeding episode is recognized, the more effectively it can be treated. Signs that indicate internal bleeding are especially important to recognize. Children are aware of internal bleeding and are reliable in telling the examiner where an internal bleed is. In addition to the manifestations described (see Box 43-5), the nurse maintains a high level of suspicion when a child with hemophilia demonstrates signs such as headache, slurred speech, loss of consciousness (from cerebral bleeding), and black tarry stools (from GI bleeding).

Prevent Bleeding. The goal of prevention of bleeding episodes is directed toward decreasing the risk for injury. Prevention of bleeding episodes is geared mostly toward appropriate exercises to strengthen muscles and joints and to allow age-appropriate activity.

During infancy and toddlerhood, the normal acquisition of motor skills creates innumerable opportunities for falls, bruises, and minor wounds. Restraining the child from mastering motor development can foster more serious long-term problems than allowing the behavior. However, the environment should be made as safe as possible, with close supervision during playtime to minimize incidental injuries.

For older children, the family usually needs assistance in preparing for school. A nurse who knows the family can be instrumental in discussing the situation with the school nurse and in jointly planning an appropriate activity schedule. Because almost all persons with hemophilia are boys, the physical limitations in regard to active sports may be a difficult adjustment and activity restrictions must be tempered with sensitivity to the child's emotional and physical needs. Use of protective equipment, such as padding and helmets, is particularly important, and noncontact sports, especially swimming, walking, jogging, tennis, golf, fishing, and bowling, are encouraged (National Hemophilia Foundation, 2006). However, the use of prophylaxis to prevent joint hemorrhage or overuse during low-impact athletic participation remains unknown (Ross, Goldenberg, Hund, et al., 2009).

To prevent oral bleeding, some readjustment in terms of dental hygiene may be needed to minimize trauma to the gums, such as use of a water irrigating device, softening the toothbrush in warm water before brushing, or using a sponge-tipped disposable toothbrush. A regular toothbrush should be soft bristled and small.

Because any trauma can lead to a bleeding episode, all persons caring for these children must be aware of their disorder. These children should wear medical identification, and older children should be encouraged to recognize situations in which disclosing their condition is important, such as during dental extraction or injections. Health care personnel need to take special precautions to prevent the use of procedures that may cause bleeding, such as IM injections. The subcutaneous route is substituted for IM injections whenever possible. Venipunctures for blood samples are usually preferred for these children. There is usually less bleeding after the venipuncture than after finger or heel punctures. Neither aspirin nor any aspirin-containing compound should be used. Acetaminophen is a suitable aspirin substitute, especially for controlling pain at home.

Recognize and Control Bleeding. As noted, the earlier a bleeding episode is recognized, the more effectively it can be treated. Factor replacement therapy should be instituted according to established medical protocol, and supportive measures may be implemented, such as RICE, which stands for *r*est, *i*ce, *c*ompression, and *e*levation. When parents and older children are taught such measures beforehand, they can be prepared to initiate immediate treatment. Plastic bags of ice or cold packs should be kept in the freezer for such emergencies. However, such measures do not take the place of factor replacement.

Prevent Crippling Effects of Bleeding. As a result of repeated episodes of hemarthrosis, incompletely absorbed blood in the joints, and limitation of motion, bone and muscle changes occur that result in flexion contractures and joint fixation. During bleeding episodes, the joint is elevated and immobilized. Active range-of-motion exercises are usually instituted after the acute episode. This allows the child to control the degree of exercise and discomfort. If an exercise program is instituted in the home, a physical therapist or home health nurse may need to supervise compliance with the regimen. Rarely, orthopedic intervention, such as casting, application of traction, or aspiration of blood, may be necessary to preserve joint function. Diet is also an important consideration because excessive body weight can increase the strain on affected joints, especially the knees, and predispose the child to hemarthrosis. Consequently, calorie intake should be balanced in accordance with energy requirements.

Support the Family and Prepare for Home Care. Genetic counseling is essential as soon as possible after diagnosis. Unlike many other disorders in which both parents carry the trait, the feeling of responsibility for this condition usually rests with the mother. Without an opportunity to discuss her feelings, the marital relationship can suffer. Technology is now available to identify carriers in approximately 80% of cases and may reduce the anxiety regarding childbearing in women who may be at risk of carrying the defective gene, such as sisters or maternal aunts of an affected boy. Factor concentrates have greatly changed the outlook for these children by minimizing bleeding and allowing the child to live a normal, unrestricted life. Children are taught to take responsibility for their disease at an early age. They learn their limitations, other preventive measures, and self-administration of the prophylactic AHF.

The needs of families who have children with hemophilia are best met through a comprehensive team approach of physicians (pediatrician, hematologist, orthopedist), nurse practitioner, nurse, social worker, and physical therapist. Parent-group discussions are beneficial in meeting the needs that are often best met by similarly affected families. For example, with the improved prognosis for these children, parents and adolescents with hemophilia face vocational and financial problems in addition to concern over future childbearing. After children reach 21 years of age, many insurance companies will no longer carry them. This can be disastrous in terms of the cost of treatment. Financial support is particularly important. A person with severe hemophilia may require factor replacement therapy and other medical treatments that cost in excess of $100,000 a year. The National Hemophilia Foundation* and the Canadian Hemophilia Society† provide numerous services and publications for both health care providers and families.

Children who have become infected with HIV through transfusions and factor replacement products are faced with the consequences of this dreaded disease. Consequently, they need the support of health care professionals, especially in the areas of safe sexual practices to avoid disease transmission and public education regarding acquired immunodeficiency syndrome (AIDS) and ways to deal with public reactions to persons who have AIDS (see p. 1387).

Immune Thrombocytopenia (Idiopathic Thrombocytopenic Purpura)

Idiopathic or immune thrombocytopenic purpura, as a formerly used term because purpura is an infrequent sign at presentation, is now referred to as *immune thrombocytopenia* (ITP) (Rodeghiero, Stasi, Gernsheimer, et al., 2009). ITP is an acquired hemorrhagic disorder characterized by (1) thrombocytopenia, (2) absence or minimal signs of bleeding (easy bruising, mucosal bleeding, petechiae) in most childhood cases, and (3) normal bone marrow with normal or increased number of immature platelets (megakaryocytes) and eosinophils. Although all causes of ITP are not known, it is understood that ITP involves the evolution of antibodies against multiple platelet antigens, leading to reduced platelet survival and impaired platelet production (Consolini, 2011; McCrae, 2011). It is the most frequently occurring thrombocytopenia of

*116 W. 32nd St., 11th Floor, New York, NY 10001; 800-42-HANDI, 212-328-3700; fax: 212-328-3777; e-mail: handi@hemophilia.org; www.hemophilia.org.
†400-1255 University Street, Montreal, Quebec, Canada H3B 3B6; 800-668-2686, 514-848-0503; fax: 514-848-9661; e-mail: chs@hemophilia.ca; www.hemophilia.ca.

childhood. The greatest frequency of occurrence is in children younger than 10 years with the peak incidence at age 2 to 5 years (Consolini, 2011; McCrae, 2011; Wilson, 2009).

The disease occurs in one of two forms: an acute, self-limiting course; or a chronic condition (>12 months' duration). The acute form is most often seen after upper respiratory tract infections; after the childhood diseases *measles, rubella, mumps,* and *chickenpox;* or after infection with parvovirus B19.

Diagnostic Evaluation

The diagnosis is suspected on the basis of clinical manifestations (Box 43-6). In ITP, the platelet count is reduced to below 20,000/mm³; therefore tests that depend on platelet function, such as the tourniquet test, bleeding time, and clot retraction, have abnormal results. Although there is no definitive test on which to establish a diagnosis of ITP, several tests are usually performed to rule out other disorders in which thrombocytopenia is a manifestation, such as systemic lupus erythematosus, lymphoma, or leukemia.

Therapeutic Management

Management of ITP is primarily supportive because the course of the disease is self-limited in the majority of cases. Activity is restricted at the onset while the platelet count is low and while active bleeding or progression of lesions is occurring. Treatment for acute presentation is symptomatic and has included prednisone, IV immune globulin (IVGG), and anti-D antibody. These are not curative therapies. Anti-D antibody is a relatively new therapy for ITP. Infusion of anti-D antibody causes a transient hemolytic anemia in the patient. Along with the clearance of antibody-coated RBCs, there is prolonged survival of platelets resulting from the blockade of the Fc receptors of the reticuloendothelial cells. The platelet count does not increase until 48 hours after an infusion of anti-D antibody; therefore it is not appropriate therapy for patients who are actively bleeding. The benefits of choosing anti-D antibody therapy over prednisone or IVIG is that anti-D antibody can be given in one dose over 5 to 10 minutes and is significantly less expensive than IVIG. Historically, patients who are treated with prednisone may first undergo a bone marrow examination to rule out leukemia, which is controversial because leukemia rarely manifests with low platelet

count alone (Scott and Montgomery, 2007; Wilson, 2009). Therefore the use of anti-D antibody and IVIG alleviates the need for a bone marrow examination. Before receiving the initial dose of anti-D antibody, patients must meet certain criteria (Box 43-7). Premedication with acetaminophen 5 to 10 minutes before the infusion is recommended.

> **! NURSING ALERT**
>
> After administration of anti-D antibody, observe the child for a minimum of 1 hour and maintain a patent IV line. Obtain baseline vital signs before the infusion and again 5, 20, and 60 minutes after beginning the infusion. Fever, chills, and headache may occur during or shortly after the infusion. If so, diphenhydramine (Benadryl) and hydrocortisone (Solu-Cortef) should be given and the patient observed for an additional hour.

Splenectomy is for patients who have chronic ITP that is not responsive to pharmacologic management and have increased risk for severe hemorrhage. It is the useful option associated with long-term remission for the majority of these children and reduces the risk for hemorrhage (McCrae, 2011; Scott and Montgomery, 2007; Wilson, 2009). Before splenectomy is considered, waiting until the child is older than 5 years is generally recommended because of the increased risk for bacterial infection. Pneumococcal and meningococcal vaccines are recommended before splenectomy (see Immunizations, Chapter 31). The child also receives penicillin prophylaxis after splenectomy. The length of prophylactic therapy is controversial, but in general, a minimum of 3 years is recommended.

Prognosis. The majority of children have a self-limited course without major complications. Some children may develop chronic ITP and require ongoing therapy. A splenectomy may modify the disease process, and the child will be asymptomatic.

CARE MANAGEMENT

Nursing care is largely supportive and should include teaching regarding possible side effects of therapy and limitation in activities while the child's platelet count is less than 50,000/mm³ (Consolini, 2011). Children with ITP should not participate in *any* contact sports, bike riding, skateboarding, in-line skating, gymnastics, climbing, or running. Parents are encouraged to engage their children in quiet activities and to prevent any injuries to the child's head. The harmful effects of using aspirin and NSAIDs to control pain are critical for these children; therefore salicylate substitutes (e.g., acetaminophen) are always used. As in any condition with an uncertain outcome, the family needs emotional support.

Disseminated Intravascular Coagulation

Disseminated intravascular coagulation (DIC), also known as consumption coagulopathy, is characterized by diffuse fibrin deposition in the microvasculature, consumption of coagulation factors, and endogenous generation of thrombin and plasmin. DIC is a secondary disorder of coagulation that occurs as a complication of a number of pathologic processes, such as hypoxia, acidosis, shock, and endothelial damage. It can result from many severe systemic diseases, such as congenital heart disease, necrotizing enterocolitis, gram-negative bacterial sepsis, rickettsial infections, and some severe viral infections.

Pathophysiology

DIC occurs when the first stage of the coagulation process is abnormally stimulated. Although no well-defined sequence of events occurs, two distinct phases can be identified. First, when the clotting mechanism is triggered in the circulation, thrombin is generated in greater amounts than can be neutralized by the body. Consequently, there is rapid conversion of fibrinogen to fibrin, with aggregation and destruction of platelets. If local and widespread fibrin deposition in blood vessels takes place, obstruction and eventual necrosis of tissues occur. Second, the fibrinolytic mechanism is activated, causing extensive destruction of clotting factors. With a deficiency of clotting factors, the child is vulnerable to uncontrollable hemorrhage into vital organs. An additional complication is damage and hemolysis of RBCs.

Diagnostic Evaluation

DIC is suspected when the patient has an increased tendency to bleed (Box 43-8). Hematologic findings include prolonged prothrombin time, PTT, and thrombin time. There is a profoundly depressed platelet count, fragmented RBCs, and depleted fibrinogen.

Therapeutic Management

Treatment of DIC is directed toward control of the underlying or initiating cause, which in most instances stops the coagulation problem spontaneously. Platelets and fresh-frozen plasma may be needed to replace lost plasma components, especially in children whose underlying disease remains uncontrolled. Extremely ill newborn infants may require exchange transfusion with fresh blood. The IV administration of heparin to inhibit thrombin formation is most often restricted to patients who have not responded to treatment of the underlying disease or replacement of coagulation factors and platelets.

CARE MANAGEMENT

The goals of nursing care are to be aware of the possibility of DIC in severely ill children and to recognize signs that might indicate its presence. The skills needed to monitor IV infusion and blood transfusions and to administer heparin are the same as for any child receiving these therapies (see p. 1388). (See Chapter 36 for care of children with life-threatening illnesses.)

Epistaxis (Nosebleeding)

Isolated and transient episodes of epistaxis, or nosebleeding, are common in childhood. The nose, especially the septum, is a highly vascular structure, and bleeding usually results from direct trauma, including blows to the nose, foreign bodies, and nose picking, or from mucosal inflammation associated with allergic rhinitis and upper respiratory tract infections. The bleeding ordinarily stops spontaneously or with minimal pressure and requires no medical evaluation or therapy.

Recurrent epistaxis and severe bleeding may indicate an underlying disease, particularly vascular abnormalities, leukemia, thrombocytopenia, and clotting factor deficiency diseases (e.g., hemophilia, vWD). Nosebleeds are sometimes associated with administration of aspirin, even in normal amounts. Persistent episodes of epistaxis require medical evaluation.

CARE MANAGEMENT

In the event of a nosebleed, an essential intervention is to remain calm. Otherwise, the child will become more agitated, the blood pressure will increase, and the child will not cooperate. Although in most instances a nosebleed is not serious, it can be upsetting to family members as well. They need reassurance that the loss of blood is not serious and that the bleeding usually stops in less than 10 minutes with nasal pressure.

To control the bleeding, the child is instructed to sit up and lean forward (not to lie down) to avoid aspiration of blood. Most of the nosebleeding originates in the anterior part of the nasal septum and can be controlled by applying pressure to the soft lower portion of the nose with the thumb and forefinger (see Emergency box). During this time, the child breathes through the mouth.

In the event that hemorrhage continues, the child should be evaluated by a health care practitioner, who may pack the nose with epinephrine-soaked gauze. After a nosebleed, petroleum or water-soluble jelly can be inserted into each nostril to prevent crusting of old blood and to lessen the likelihood of the child's picking at the nose and restarting the hemorrhage. If a child has numerous nosebleeds, factors believed to increase the likelihood of bleeds are eliminated, such as discouraging nose picking or altering the household humidity by placing a cool-mist humidifier in the child's room.

BOX 43-8   CLINICAL MANIFESTATIONS OF DISSEMINATED INTRAVASCULAR COAGULATION

- Petechiae
- Purpura
- Bleeding from openings in the skin
  - Venipuncture site
  - Surgical incision
- Bleeding from umbilicus, trachea (newborn)
- Evidence of gastrointestinal bleeding
- Hypotension
- Organ dysfunction from infarction and ischemia

✚ EMERGENCY

Epistaxis

- Have child sit up and lean forward (not lie down).
- Apply continuous pressure to nose with thumb and forefinger for at least 10 minutes.
- Insert cotton or wadded tissue into each nostril and apply ice or cold cloth to bridge of nose if bleeding persists.
- Keep child calm and quiet.

Repeated bleeding episodes lasting longer than 30 minutes may be an indication to refer the child for evaluation for the possibility of a bleeding disorder.

NEOPLASTIC DISORDERS

Neoplastic disorders are the leading cause of death from disease in children past infancy, and almost half of all childhood cancers involve the blood or blood-forming organs. Leukemias and lymphomas are discussed here. Malignant solid tumors of childhood are discussed elsewhere in relation to the tissues or organs involved.

Leukemias

Leukemia, cancer of the blood-forming tissues, is the most common form of childhood cancer. The annual incidence is 3 to 4 cases per 100,000 Caucasian children (Jemal, Siegel, Ward, et al., 2009). It is more common in boys and Caucasians, with the peak onset between 2 and 5 years of age (Hutter, 2010; Margolin, Rabin, Steuber, et al., 2011; Pui, Relling, and Downing, 2004). It is one of the forms of cancer that has demonstrated dramatic improvements in survival rates. Whereas current long-term disease-free survival for children with acute lymphoid leukemia approaches 80% (Margolin, Rabin, Steuber, et al., 2011; Pui, Relling, and Downing, 2004), acute non-lymphoid leukemia has a 50% to 65% survival rate (Kaspers and Creutzig, 2005; Pearce and Sills, 2005). (See also Prognosis, p. 1381.)

Classification

Leukemia is a broad term given to a group of malignant diseases of the bone marrow and lymphatic system. Research has revealed that it is a complex disease of varying heterogeneity. Consequently, classification has become increasingly complex, sophisticated, and essential because identification of the subtype of leukemia has therapeutic and prognostic implications. The following is a brief overview of the major classification systems currently being used.

Morphology. Two forms are generally recognized in children—acute lymphoid leukemia (ALL) and acute nonlymphoid (myelogenous) leukemia (ANLL or AML). Synonyms for ALL include *lymphatic, lymphocytic, lymphoblastic,* and *lymphoblastoid leukemia.* Usually the terms stem cell or blast cell leukemia also refer to the lymphoid type. Synonyms for the AML type include *granulocytic, myelocytic, monocytic, myelogenous, monoblastic,* and *monomyeloblastic.*

- **Cytochemical markers**—Several chemical stains (e.g., terminal deoxynucleotidyl transferase [TdT]) aid in differentiation between ALL and ANLL.
- **Chromosome studies**—Chromosome analysis has become an important tool in the diagnosis of ALL. For example, children with trisomy 21 have 20 times the risk of other children for developing ALL. Children with more than 50 chromosomes on the leukemic cells (hyperdiploid) have the best prognosis (Margolin, Rabin, Steuber, et al., 2011). Translocations of chromosomes also found on the leukemic cells can denote good prognosis, as in the trisomies 4 and 10, or a poor prognosis, as in the t(9:22) or Philadelphia chromosome.
- **Cell-surface immunologic markers**—Cell-surface antigens have permitted differentiation of ALL into three broad classes: B-cell ALL; T-cell ALL; and common ALL antigen (CALLA or CD 10+) formally known as *non-T, non-B ALL,* which is actually of early B-cell lineage (Margolin, Rabin, Steuber, et al., 2011). Children with the common ALL antigen on their cell surfaces have the more favorable prognosis (Margolin, Rabin, Steuber, et al., 2011).

Pathophysiology

Leukemia is an unrestricted proliferation of immature WBCs in the blood-forming tissues of the body. Although not a "tumor" as such, the leukemic cells demonstrate the same neoplastic properties as solid cancers. Therefore the resulting pathologic condition and clinical manifestations are caused by infiltration and replacement of any tissue of the body with nonfunctional leukemic cells. Highly vascular organs, such as the spleen and liver, are the most severely affected.

To understand the pathophysiology of the leukemic process, it is important to clarify two common misconceptions. First, although leukemia is an overproduction of WBCs, most often in the acute form, the leukocyte count is low (thus the term *leukemia*). Second, these immature cells do not deliberately attack and destroy the normal blood cells or vascular tissues. Cellular destruction takes place by infiltration and subsequent competition for metabolic elements.

In all types of leukemia, the proliferating cells depress the production of formed elements of the blood in bone marrow by competing for and depriving the normal cells of the essential nutrients for metabolism. The most frequent presenting signs and symptoms of leukemia are a result of infiltration of the bone marrow. The three main consequences are (1) anemia from decreased RBCs, (2) infection from neutropenia, and (3) bleeding from decreased platelet production. The invasion of the bone marrow with leukemic cells gradually causes a weakening of the bone and a tendency toward fractures. As leukemic cells invade the periosteum, increasing pressure causes severe pain.

The spleen, liver, and lymph glands demonstrate marked infiltration, enlargement, and eventually fibrosis. Hepatosplenomegaly is typically more common than lymphadenopathy. The next most important site of involvement is the central nervous system (CNS) secondary to leukemic infiltration, which may cause increased intracranial pressure (see Box 45-1).

Leukemic cells may also invade the testes, kidneys, prostate, ovaries, GI tract, and lungs. With long-term survivors becoming more common, such sites of leukemia invasion, especially the testes, are becoming more important clinically.

Diagnostic Evaluation

Leukemia is usually suspected based on the history and physical presentation that often includes fever, signs and symptoms of low blood counts, lymph node enlargement, and an enlarged liver and spleen. Peripheral blood smear may reveal immature forms of leukocytes, frequently combined with low blood counts. Definitive diagnosis is based on bone marrow aspiration or biopsy. Flow cytometry identifies the specific type of blast cell. Typically, the bone marrow is hypercellular, with primarily blast cells. After the diagnosis is confirmed, a lumbar puncture is performed to determine whether there is any CNS involvement. A few children will have CNS involvement at diagnosis, although most are asymptomatic.

Therapeutic Management

Treatment of leukemia involves the use of chemotherapeutic agents, with or without cranial irradiation, in four phases: (1) induction therapy, which achieves a complete remission or less than 5% leukemic cells in the bone marrow; (2) CNS prophylactic therapy, which prevents leukemic cells from invading the CNS; (3) intensification therapy (consolidation), which eradicates residual leukemia cells, followed by delayed intensification, which prevents emergence of resistant leukemic clones; and (4) maintenance therapy, which serves to maintain the remission phase.

Hematopoietic Stem Cell Transplantation. Hematopoietic stem cell transplantation has been used successfully for treating children who have ALL and AML. HSCT is *not* recommended for children with ALL during the first remission because of the excellent results possible with chemotherapy. In the United States, patients with intermediate risk and high risk AML with a suitable donor available are recommended for transplant during the first clinical remission (Bollard, Krance, and Heslop, 2011).

Hematopoietic stem cell transplantation may be not only from antigen-matched related donors but also from matched unrelated donors or mismatched donors. Peripheral blood stem cell transplants are capable of differentiating into specialized cells of the hematologic system and can be obtained from related or unrelated donors or from umbilical cord blood. Regardless of the type of transplant, it is accompanied by significant morbidity and mortality, including graft-versus-host disease (GVHD), overwhelming infection, or severe organ damage.

Prognosis. The most important prognostic factors for determining long-term survival for children with ALL (in addition to treatment) are (1) the initial WBC count, (2) the child's age at the time of diagnosis, (3) the type of cell involved, (4) the sex of the child, and (5) karyotype analysis. Children with a normal or low WBC count who are CALLA positive have a much better prognosis than those with a high count or other cell types. Children diagnosed between 2 and 9 years of age have consistently demonstrated a better outlook than those diagnosed before 2 or after 10 years of age, and girls appear to have a more favorable prognosis than boys. Children with more than 50 chromosomes indicated by a DNA index greater than 1.16 (hyperdiploid) have a better prognosis. Similarly, patients with ALL and trisomies of chromosomes 4 and 10 have a good prognosis with a low risk for treatment failure (Margolin, Rabin, Steuber, et al., 2011).

Late Effects of Treatment

Although vigorous treatment of childhood cancers has resulted in dramatically improved survival rates, increasing concern surrounds late effects—adverse changes related to treatment modalities—and recurrence of the disease process. Almost no organ is exempt, and almost every antineoplastic agent, especially irradiation, is responsible for some adverse effect.

The most devastating late effect is development of a second malignancy. Children who received cranial irradiation at age 5 years or younger are most susceptible to developing brain tumors and increase risk for developing cognitive defects that can affect school performance (Bhatia, 2004; Hutter, 2010). Treatment with an anthracycline is associated with cardiomyopathy; cranial irradiation and intrathecal chemotherapy are associated with cognitive and neuropsychologic deficits, which are just a few of the long-term sequelae. Consequently, close monitoring for late effects is essential, especially with the advent of additional clinical trials.

CARE MANAGEMENT

Nursing care of the child with leukemia is directly related to the therapeutic regimen. General psychologic interventions during each phase of therapy are discussed in Chapter 36.

Prepare the Child and Family for Diagnostic and Therapeutic Procedures. From the time before diagnosis to cessation of therapy, children must undergo several tests; the most traumatic are bone marrow aspiration, bone marrow biopsy, and lumbar punctures. Multiple fingersticks and venipunctures for blood analysis and drug infusion are common occurrences. Therefore the child needs an explanation of each procedure and what can be expected. In addition, effective pharmacologic measures, including conscious and unconscious sedation, and nonpharmacologic strategies are used to reduce discomfort associated with these painful procedures.

Relieve Pain. The effective use of analgesia is especially important when the malignant process is uncontrolled and causes acute pain. Dosages of opioids (narcotics) are adjusted, or *titrated*, to the child's needs and administered *around the clock* for optimal pain control. Nonpharmacologic strategies should be implemented as needed but are not substitutes for pharmacologic management. Readers are encouraged to review the principles of pain assessment and management presented in Chapter 30 and Preparation for Diagnostic and Therapeutic Procedures, Chapter 39, when caring for a child with leukemia.

Prevent Complications of Myelosuppression. The leukemic process and most of the chemotherapeutic agents cause myelosuppression. The reduced numbers of blood cells result in secondary problems of infection, bleeding tendencies, and anemia. Supportive care involves both medical and nursing management. Because these are so closely linked, they are discussed together.

Infection. A frequent complication of treatment for childhood cancer is overwhelming infection secondary to neutropenia. The child is most susceptible to overwhelming infection during three phases of the disease: (1) at the time of diagnosis and relapse when the leukemic process has replaced normal leukocytes; (2) during immunosuppressive therapy; and (3) after prolonged antibiotic therapy, which predisposes the child to the growth of resistant organisms. However, the use of granulocyte colony-stimulating factor (GCSF) has reduced the incidence and duration of infection in children receiving treatment for cancer.

The first defense against infection is prevention. When the child is hospitalized, the nurse uses all measures to control transfer of infection. These typically include the use of a private room, restriction of all visitors and health care personnel with active infection, and strict hand washing technique with an antiseptic solution. In some research centers, special germ-free environments are available during complete myelosuppression from intensive chemotherapy or for bone marrow transplant. The nurse should be aware of these guidelines and educate patients and families.

> ### ! NURSING ALERT
>
> The child is not immunized against live viral vaccines (measles, rubella, mumps) until the immune system is capable of responding appropriately to the vaccine (AAP Committee on Infectious Diseases, 2009; Koh and Pizzo, 2011). Most institutions have individual guidelines regarding vaccinations in children undergoing immunosuppressive therapy.

The child is evaluated for potential sites of infection (e.g., mucosal ulceration; skin abrasion; skin tear, such as a hangnail) and observed for any elevation in temperature. To identify the source of infection, chest radiographs and blood, stool, urine, and nasopharyngeal cultures are taken. IV antibiotics are administered, and if this therapy is prolonged, a venous access device, such as a peripherally inserted central catheter or intermittent infusion device (saline lock or PRN [as-needed] adaptor), is used to maintain IV access.

Prevention of infection continues to be a priority after discharge from the hospital. Ordinarily, the child is allowed to return to school when the WBC count is at a satisfactory level—usually an absolute neutrophil count greater than 500/mm³ (see Guidelines box). At all times, family members are encouraged to practice good hand washing to prevent introducing pathogens into the home. The child

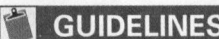

GUIDELINES

Calculating the Absolute Neutrophil Count

Determine the total percent of neutrophils ("polys," or "segs," and bands). Multiply WBC count by percent of neutrophils.

Example:

WBC = 1000; neutrophils = 7%; nonsegmented neutrophils (bands) = 7%

Step 1: 7% + 7% = 14%

Step 2: 0.14 × 1000 = 140 ANC

ANC, Absolute neutrophil count; *WBC,* white blood cell.

may need to be isolated from school contacts in the event of an outbreak of a childhood disease, especially chickenpox.

Nutrition is another important component of infection prevention. An adequate protein-caloric intake provides the child with better host defenses against infection and increased tolerance to chemotherapy and irradiation. However, providing optimal nutrition during periods of anorexia and vomiting from chemotherapy is a tremendous challenge (see Feeding the Sick Child, Chapter 39).

Hemorrhage. Before the use of transfused platelets, hemorrhage was a leading cause of death in patients with leukemia. Now most bleeding episodes can be prevented or controlled with the administration of platelet concentrates or platelet-rich plasma.

Skin punctures are avoided whenever possible because bleeding sites can become easily infected. When fingersticks, venipunctures, IM injections, and bone marrow aspirations are performed, aseptic technique must be used along with continued observation for bleeding. Meticulous mouth care is essential because gingival bleeding with resultant mucositis is a frequent problem. Because the rectal area is prone to ulceration from various drugs, feces and urine are removed immediately and the perianal area is washed. Using rectal temperatures is avoided to prevent trauma. Children are advised to avoid activities that might cause injury or bleeding, such as riding bicycles and skateboards, climbing trees and playground equipment, and playing contact sports.

Platelet transfusions are generally reserved for active bleeding episodes that do not respond to local treatment and that may occur during induction or relapse therapy. Epistaxis and gingival bleeding are the most common. The nurse teaches parents and older children measures to control nosebleeding (see p. 1379). Pressure at the site without disturbing clot formation is the general rule.

During bleeding episodes, the parents and child need much emotional support. Often parents request a platelet transfusion, unaware of the need for trying local measures first. The nurse can be instrumental in allaying anxiety by acknowledging the feelings of the child and family and explaining the reason for delaying a platelet transfusion until absolutely necessary.

Anemia. Initially, anemia may be profound from complete replacement of the bone marrow by leukemic cells. During induction therapy, blood transfusions may be necessary. The usual precautions in caring for the child with anemia are instituted (see p. 1365).

Use Precautions in Administering and Handling Chemotherapeutic Agents. In addition to the nurse's many responsibilities in regard to the child and family, nurses must also use safeguards to protect themselves. Handling chemotherapeutic agents may present risks to handlers and to their offspring, although the exact degree of risk is not known. Many chemotherapeutic agents are vesicants

(sclerosing agents) that can cause severe cellular damage if even minute amounts of the drug infiltrate surrounding tissue. Only nurses experienced with chemotherapeutic agents should administer vesicants. Guidelines are available* and must be followed exactly to prevent tissue damage to patients. Interventions for extravasation vary, but each nurse should be aware of the institution's policies and implement them at once.

In addition to extravasation, a potentially fatal complication is anaphylaxis, especially from L-asparaginase, teniposide (VM-26), etoposide (VP-16), bleomycin, and cisplatin. Nursing responsibilities include prevention of, recognition of, and preparation for serious reactions. Prevention begins with a careful history for known allergies.

Most children with cancer have a venous access device, which facilitates administration of IV drugs. During treatment and remission, many drugs are taken orally at home. Compliance with the medication schedule is essential, and nurses play an important role in educating the family about the drugs and encouraging adherence to the plan.

! NURSING ALERT

Chemotherapeutic drugs must be given through a free-flowing IV line. The infusion is stopped immediately if any sign of infiltration (pain, stinging, swelling, or redness at the cannulation site) occurs. When chemotherapeutic and immunologic agents are given, the child must be observed for 20 minutes after the infusion for signs of anaphylaxis (cyanosis, hypotension, wheezing, severe urticaria). Emergency equipment (especially blood pressure monitor and bag-valve-mask) and emergency drugs (especially oxygen, epinephrine, antihistamine, aminophylline, corticosteroids, and vasopressors) must be available. If a reaction is suspected, the drug is discontinued, the IV line is flushed with saline, and the child's vital signs and subsequent responses are monitored.

Manage Problems of Drug Toxicity. Chemotherapy presents several nursing challenges. The complexity of the treatment protocols is often overwhelming to families. In addition, each therapy is associated with a number of predictable side effects. Nurses must be aware of these side effects and use judgment in recognizing reactions, as well as toxicities.†

Nausea and Vomiting. The nausea and vomiting that occur shortly after administration of several of the drugs and from cranial or abdominal radiation can be profound. The serotonin-receptor antagonists (e.g., ondansetron, granisetron, palonosetron) are effective in the control of nausea and vomiting occurring after emetogenic chemotherapy and radiotherapy. When combined with dexamethasone, these agents are the treatment of choice in the prevention of delayed emesis (Lindley, Goodin, McCune, et al., 2005; Saito, Aogi, Sekine, et al., 2009).

The most beneficial regimen for antiemetic control has been the administration of the antiemetic *before* chemotherapy begins. The goal is to prevent the child from ever experiencing nausea or vomiting, thus preventing development of anticipatory symptoms (the conditioned response of developing nausea and vomiting before receiving the drug).

Cancer Chemotherapy Guidelines can be obtained from the Oncology Nursing Society, 125 Enterprise Drive, Pittsburgh, PA 15275; 866-257-4ONS, 412-859-6100; fax: 877-369-5497; e-mail: customer.service@ons.org; www.ons.org.

†Detailed chemotherapeutic agents are outlined in Wilson D, Hockenberry MJ: *Wong's clinical manual of pediatric nursing,* ed 8, St Louis, 2012, Mosby.

Anorexia. Loss of appetite is a direct consequence of the chemotherapy or irradiation. It is a major problem for parents because it is the one area they feel responsible for, particularly when so many other facets of care are outside their control. There are no universally successful techniques for encouraging a sick child to eat. However, the guidelines in Chapter 39 can be helpful during the anorexic period and can prevent additional problems during the remission.

Some children still do not eat despite these approaches. When loss of appetite and weight persist, the nurse should investigate the family situation to determine whether any factors (e.g., conditioned aversion to food, environmental stress related to eating, controlling behavior, anger) might be contributing to the problem. Nasogastric tube feedings or total parenteral nutrition may be implemented for children with significant nutritional problems.

Mucosal Ulceration. One of the most distressing side effects of several drugs is GI mucosal cell damage, which can produce ulcers anywhere along the alimentary tract. Oral ulcers greatly compound anorexia because eating is extremely uncomfortable, but the following interventions may be helpful:

- Provide a bland, moist, soft diet appropriate for the child's age and preferences.
- Use a soft sponge toothbrush (Toothette) or cotton-tipped applicator.
- Provide frequent mouthwashes with normal saline (using a solution of 1 tsp of table salt in 1 pt of water) or sodium bicarbonate mouth rinses (using a solution of 1 tsp of baking soda in 1 qt of water).
- Use local anesthetics (e.g., Chloraseptic lozenges) or nonprescription preparations without alcohol (e.g., hydrocortisone dental paste [Orabase], antiseptic mouth rinse [UlcerEase], diphenhydramine [Benadryl], and aluminum and magnesium hydroxide [Maalox] solution). Although local anesthetics are effective in temporarily relieving the pain, many children dislike the taste and numb feeling they produce.

Other preparations that may be used to prevent or treat mucositis include chlorhexidine gluconate (Peridex) because of its dual effectiveness against candidal and bacterial infections, antifungal troches (lozenges) or mouthwash, and lip balm (e.g., Aquaphor) to keep the lips moist. Agents that should not be used include lemon glycerin swabs (irritate eroded tissue and can decay teeth), hydrogen peroxide (delays healing by breaking down protein), and milk of magnesia (dries mucosa).

Stomatitis may cause such difficulty with eating that the child may require hospitalization for hydration, parenteral nutrition, and pain control (often with IV morphine). The child will usually choose the foods that are best tolerated, and the nurse should encourage parents to relax any eating pressures. Because the stomatitis is a temporary condition, the child can resume good food habits after the ulcers heal. Dental hygiene can become a serious problem for children with orthodontic appliances. Sometimes it may be necessary to remove the braces to allow chemotherapy to continue.

Rectal ulcers are managed by meticulous toilet hygiene, warm sitz baths after each bowel movement, and use of an occlusive ointment or dressing applied to the ulcerated area to promote epithelialization. Stool softeners are necessary to prevent further discomfort. Parents are advised to record bowel movements because the child may voluntarily avoid defecation to prevent discomfort. Rectal thermometers and suppositories are contraindicated because insertion may further traumatize the area.

Neuropathy. Vincristine and, to a lesser extent, vinblastine can cause various neurotoxic effects. Nursing interventions for management of these effects include:

- Administering stool softeners or laxatives for severe constipation caused by decreased bowel innervation
- Maintaining good body alignment and, if patient is on bed rest, using a footboard or high-top shoes to minimize or prevent footdrop
- Carrying out safety measures during ambulation because of weakness and numbing of the extremities, which may cause difficulty in walking or fine hand movement
- Providing a soft or liquid diet for severe jaw pain

Hemorrhagic Cystitis. Sterile hemorrhagic cystitis, a side effect of chemical irritation to the bladder from cyclophosphamide, can be decreased and often prevented by (1) promoting a liberal fluid intake (at least 1½ times the recommended daily fluid requirement); (2) frequent voiding immediately after feeling the urge, before bed, and after arising; (3) administering the drug early in the day to allow for sufficient oral intake and voiding; and (4) administering mesna (an agent that provides protection to the bladder) as ordered. If oral home administration is prescribed, the family needs *specific* instructions regarding exactly how much fluid the child must have.

Alopecia. Hair loss is a common side effect of several chemotherapeutic drugs and cranial irradiation, although not all children lose their hair during drug therapy. It is better to warn children and parents of this side effect than to allow them to think that it is only a remote possibility. A soft cotton cap is the most comfortable headwear for children. Polyester increases perspiration and causes itching. Other options include scarves, hats, or a wig.

The nurse should also inform the family that hair regrows in 3 to 6 months and may be of a different color and texture. Frequently, the hair is darker, thicker, and curlier than before. If the child chooses not to wear a wig, attention to some type of head covering, especially in cold climates and during exposure to sun, and scalp hygiene are important. The scalp should be washed like any other body part.

Moon Face. Short-term steroid therapy produces no acute toxicities and produces two beneficial reactions: increased appetite and a sense of well-being. However, it does produce alterations in appearance, which, although not clinically significant, can be extremely distressing to older children. One of these is *moon face*, in which the child's face becomes rounded and puffy. It is helpful to reassure the child that after cessation of the drug, the facial shape will return to normal. Unlike hair loss, little can be done to camouflage this obvious change. If the child resumes activity early in the course of treatment, the change may be less noticeable to peers than after a long absence.

Mood Changes. Shortly after beginning steroid therapy, children experience a number of mood changes that range from feelings of well-being and euphoria to depression and irritability. If parents are unaware of these drug-induced changes, they may become unduly concerned. The nurse should warn them of the reactions and encourage them to discuss the behavioral changes with each other and the child.

Provide Emotional Support. An important aspect of continued emotional support involves the prognosis. Although leukemia is no longer invariably fatal, it must be remembered that survival statistics are only average estimates and apply to those children treated with the latest protocols since diagnosis. For low risk children, the chances may be better, but for high risk children, they may be significantly poorer. Of those who do survive after discontinuing therapy, some will relapse. Therefore, at present, only the passage of time is positive confirmation of the child's being ultimately "cured" of the disease. Remission, even in excess of 5 years, cannot be equated with a cure.

With increasing concern regarding late effects of treatment, continued surveillance of the child's health status is needed. The nurse who is working with family members must individualize information regarding the "numbers" and the potential risks. An understanding of each member's emotional needs, as well as competent care of physical ones, is essential to the positive, growth-promoting support of the family. Comprehensive emotional support for the family of the child with a potentially fatal illness is discussed in Chapter 36.

Lymphomas

Pediatric lymphomas are the third most common group of malignancies in children and adolescents. The lymphomas, a group of neoplastic diseases that arise from the lymphoid and hematopoietic systems, are divided into Hodgkin lymphoma (HL) and non-Hodgkin lymphoma (NHL). These diseases are further subdivided according to tissue type and extent of disease. Whereas NHL is more prevalent in children younger than 14 years, HL is prevalent in adolescence and the young adult period, with a striking increase between ages 15 and 19 years.

Hodgkin Lymphoma

Hodgkin lymphoma is a neoplastic disease that originates in the lymphoid system and primarily involves the lymph nodes. It predictably metastasizes to nonnodal or extralymphatic sites, especially the spleen, liver, bone marrow, and lungs, although no tissue is exempt from involvement (Fig. 43-5). It is classified according to four histologic types: (1) lymphocytic predominance, (2) nodular sclerosis, (3) mixed cellularity, and (4) lymphocytic depletion. Accurate staging of the extent of disease is the basis for treatment protocols and expected prognoses.

The Ann Arbor staging system assigns a stage based on the number of sites of lymph node involvement, presence of extranodal disease, and history of any symptoms. Patients are classified as *A* if asymptomatic and as *B* if they have the following symptoms: temperature of 38°C (100.4°F) or higher for 3 consecutive days, drenching night sweats, or unexplained loss of body weight (≥10%) over the preceding 6 months. Nonspecific systemic symptoms include

fatigue, anorexia, mild to severe pruritus, and slight weight loss (Metzger, Krasin, Hudson, et al., 2011).

Asymptomatic enlarged cervical or supraclavicular lymphadenopathy is the most common presentation of HL. Other systemic symptoms may be manifested, including cough, abdominal discomfort, and anorexia. Because multiple organs may be involved, diagnosis is based on several tests and the extent of metastatic disease. Tests include a CBC, erythrocyte sedimentation rate, serum copper, ferritin level, fibrinogen, immunoglobulins, uric acid level, liver function tests, T-cell function studies, and urinalysis. Radiographic tests include chest radiography and computed tomography (CT) of the neck and chest; CT and magnetic resonance imaging of the abdomen and pelvis; and positron emission tomography (PET), which is replacing the gallium scan and bone scan to identify metastatic disease.

A lymph node biopsy is essential to establish histologic diagnosis and staging. The presence of Reed-Sternberg cells is characteristic of HL. These large cells, which are multilobed and nucleated with abundant cytoplasm and a typically halolike clear zone around the nucleolus, are often described as having an "owl's eyes" appearance (Metzger, Krasin, Hudson, et al., 2011). A bone marrow aspiration and biopsy is usually performed in patient with advanced disease, B symptoms, or disease recurrence (Metzger, Krasin, Hudson, et al., 2011). With the advent of CT and PET scans to identify metastatic disease and multiagent therapy to eradicate metastatic disease, surgical staging involving a laparotomy with splenectomy is no longer performed.

Therapeutic Management. The primary modalities of therapy are radiation and chemotherapy. Each may be used alone or in combination based on the clinical staging. Radiation may involve only the involved field (IF), an extended field (EF) (involved areas plus adjacent nodes), or total nodal irradiation (TNI), depending on the extent of involvement.

An effective combination of chemotherapy widely used is MOPP (mechlorethamine, vincristine [Oncovin], procarbazine, prednisone) or ABVD (Adriamycin, bleomycin, vinblastine, dacarbazine). However, this therapy combination has caused severe late effects, especially secondary malignancies. Other drug combinations such as COPP (cyclophosphamide, vincristine, prednisone, procarbazine) as a substitute for MOPP have minimized late effects.

Follow-up care of children no longer receiving therapy is essential to identify relapse and secondary cancers. In children with splenic irradiation, prophylactic antibiotics are administered for an indefinite period. Also, immunizations against pneumococci and meningococci are recommended.

Prognosis. Long-term survival for all stages of HL is excellent. The goal for pediatric HL's curative treatment is to provide minimal morbidity with the highest quality of life (Metzger, Krasin, Hudson, et al., 2011).

CARE MANAGEMENT

Nursing care involves the same objectives as for patients with other types of cancer, specifically: (1) preparation for diagnostic and operative procedures, (2) explanation of treatment side effects, and (3) child and family support (see Chapter 36). Because this is most often a disease of adolescents and young adults, the nurse must have an appreciation of their psychologic needs and reactions during the diagnostic and treatment phases.

The most common side effect of irradiation is fatigue. This is particularly difficult for active, outgoing school-age children and adolescents because it prevents them from keeping up with their

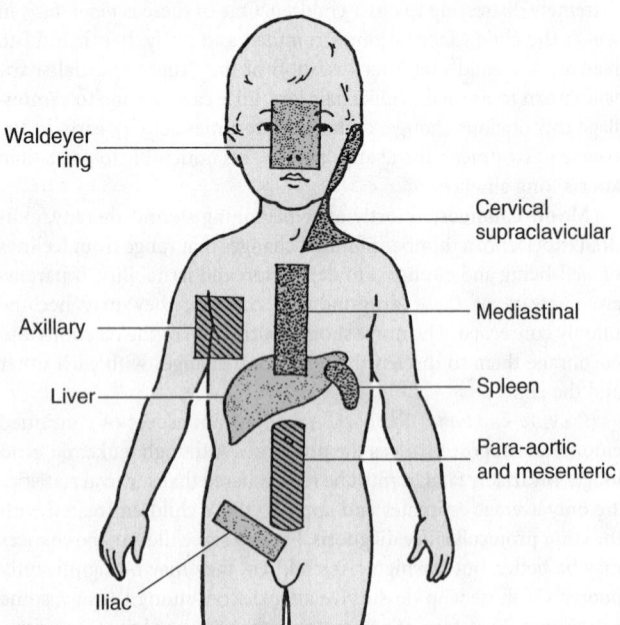

FIG 43-5 Main areas of lymphadenopathy and organ involvement in Hodgkin lymphoma.

Waldeyer ring

Cervical supraclavicular

Axillary

Mediastinal

Liver

Spleen

Para-aortic and mesenteric

Iliac

peers. Sometimes adolescents will push themselves to the point of physical exhaustion rather than admit and succumb to the decreased activity tolerance. The nurse cautions parents to observe for behavior such as extreme fatigue at the end of the day, falling asleep at the dinner table, inability to concentrate on homework, or an increased susceptibility to infection. A regular bedtime and scheduled rest periods are important for these children, especially during chemotherapy, when myelosuppression increases the risk for infection and debilitation. Before discharge, the nurse should discuss a feasible school schedule with the parents and child.

An area of concern for adolescents is the high risk for sterility from irradiation and chemotherapy. Both drugs, particularly procarbazine and alkylating agents, and irradiation to the gonads can lead to infertility. Adolescents should be informed of these side effects early in the course of the diagnosis and treatment. Sperm banking is now offered at many cancer centers before the initiation of treatment in adolescent boys. Sexual function is not altered, although the appearance of secondary sexual characteristics and menstruation may be delayed in pubescent children. Delayed sexual maturation may be an extremely sensitive and stressful issue for children (see Chapter 35).

Non-Hodgkin Lymphoma

Non-Hodgkin lymphoma occurs more frequently in children than HL. Histologic classification of childhood NHL is strikingly different from that of HL, as demonstrated in the following statements:

- The disease is usually diffuse rather than nodular.
- The cell type is either undifferentiated or poorly differentiated.
- Dissemination occurs early, more often, and rapidly.
- Mediastinal involvement and invasion of meninges are common.

NHL exhibits a variety of morphologic, cytochemical, and immunologic features, similar to the diversity seen in leukemia. Classification is based on the histologic pattern: (1) lymphoblastic, (2) Burkitt or non-Burkitt, or (3) large cell. Immunologically, these cells are also classified as T cells; B cells; or non-T, non-B cells (lacking immunologic properties). The clinical staging system used in HL is of little value in NHL, although it has been modified, and other systems have been developed.

Diagnostic Evaluation. Because the clinical presentation of most children with NHL is widespread disseminated disease, thorough pathologic staging is unnecessary. Clinical manifestations depend on the anatomic site and extent of involvement. These manifestations include many of those seen in Hodgkin disease and leukemia, as well as organ symptoms related to pressure from enlargement of adjacent lymph nodes, such as intestinal or airway obstruction, cranial nerve palsies, and spinal paralysis.

Recommendations for staging include a surgical biopsy of an enlarged node, histopathologic confirmation of disease with cytochemical and immunologic evaluation, bone marrow examination, radiographic studies (especially tomograms of the lungs and GI organs), and lumbar puncture.

Therapeutic Management. The treatment protocols for NHL include aggressive use of irradiation and chemotherapy. Similar to leukemic therapy, the protocols include induction, consolidation, and maintenance phases, some with intrathecal chemotherapy. Several antineoplastic agents used in the treatment of NHL include vincristine, prednisone, L-asparaginase, methotrexate, 6-mercaptopurine, cytarabine, cyclophosphamide, anthracyclines, and teniposide or etoposide. Chemotherapy is the main component of treatment for NHL in children (Gross and Perkins, 2011).

Prognosis. The prognosis is excellent for children with NHL. In developed countries, more than 80% of children with NHL are now cured with modern therapy, even patients with widely disseminated disease (Gross and Perkins, 2011).

CARE MANAGEMENT

Nursing care of children with NHL is similar to that required for children with leukemia. Many of the same drugs are used, although the schedules differ. Because of the intense chemotherapy, nursing care is directed primarily toward managing the side effects of these agents and providing supportive care to the child and family.

IMMUNOLOGIC DEFICIENCY DISORDERS

A number of disorders can cause profound, often life-threatening alterations within the body's immune system. The most serious are those conditions that completely depress immunity, such as severe combined immunodeficiency disease (SCID). However, the one disorder that generates the most anxiety, within both the family and the community at large, is human immunodeficiency virus (HIV) infection/AIDS.

Several classifications of immune dysfunction exist. AIDS, SCID, and Wiskott-Aldrich syndrome (WAS) are syndromes wherein the body is unable to mount an immune response. The immune response can also be misdirected. In autoimmune disorders, antibodies, macrophages, and lymphocytes attack healthy cells.

Human Immunodeficiency Virus Infection and Acquired Immunodeficiency Syndrome

Since the first cases of AIDS were identified in the early 1980s, HIV infection has generated intense medical investigation. Research has led to early diagnosis of and improved medical treatments for HIV infection, changing this disease from a rapidly fatal one to a chronic disease.

Epidemiology

The first AIDS cases in the pediatric population in the United States were identified in children born to HIV-infected mothers and in children who received blood products. More than 90% of these children acquired the disease perinatally from their mothers. Smaller numbers of children were infected through the transfusion of contaminated blood or blood products before 1985 or were infected through sexual abuse. Currently, the principal modes of HIV transmission to the pediatric population are mother-to-child transmission and adolescent risky behaviors such as sexual activity and IV drug use (Simpkins, Siberry, and Hutton, 2009).

The estimated number of children with perinatally acquired AIDS peaked in 1992; subsequent years have seen significant declines. This trend is a result of implementation of recommended HIV counseling and voluntary testing practices and the use of highly active antiretroviral therapy (HAART) to prevent perinatal transmission. HAART, typically a combination of two nucleoside analog reverse transcriptase inhibitors and a protease inhibitor, is the current standard in the United States for the treatment of HIV-infected pregnant women, and it has significantly reduced the transmission of HIV (Perinatal HIV Guidelines Working Group, 2007; Simpkins, Siberry, and Hutton, 2009). Routine HIV counseling and voluntary testing using the opt-out approach (right of refusal) is the recommended standard of care for pregnant women in the United States (AAP Committee on Pediatric AIDS, 2008; Centers for Disease Control and Prevention [CDC], 2007; Simpkins, Siberry, and Hutton, 2009).

Etiology

Human immunodeficiency virus is a retrovirus that is transmitted by lymphocytes and monocytes. It is found in the blood, semen, vaginal secretions, and breast milk. It has an incubation or latency period of months to years (Yogev and Chadwick, 2007). There are different strains of HIV. Whereas HIV-2 is prevalent in Africa, HIV-1 is the dominant strain in the United States and elsewhere. Horizontal transmission of HIV occurs through intimate sexual contact or parenteral exposure to blood or body fluids containing visible blood. Perinatal (vertical) transmission occurs when an HIV-infected pregnant woman passes the infection to her infant. There is no evidence that *casual* contact between infected and uninfected individuals can spread the virus.

Pathophysiology

The HIV virus primarily infects a specific subset of T lymphocytes, the CD_4^+ T cells. The virus takes over the machinery of the CD_4^+ lymphocyte, using it to replicate itself, rendering the CD_4^+ cell dysfunctional. The CD_4^+ lymphocyte count gradually decreases over time, leading to progressive immunodeficiency. The count eventually reaches a critical level below which there is substantial risk for opportunistic illnesses, followed by death.

Clinical Manifestations

Common clinical manifestations of HIV infection in children are varied (Box 43-9). The diagnosis of AIDS is associated with certain illnesses or conditions. The most common AIDS-defining conditions observed among American children are listed in Box 43-10. Other problems in these children may include short stature, malnutrition, and cardiomyopathy. CNS abnormalities resulting from HIV infection may include neuropsychologic deficits, developmental disabilities, and deficits in motor skills, communication, and behavioral functioning.

BOX 43-9   COMMON CLINICAL MANIFESTATIONS OF HUMAN IMMUNODEFICIENCY VIRUS INFECTION IN CHILDREN

- Lymphadenopathy
- Hepatosplenomegaly
- Oral candidiasis
- Chronic or recurrent diarrhea
- Failure to thrive
- Developmental delay
- Parotitis

BOX 43-10   COMMON DEFINING CONDITIONS FOR ACQUIRED IMMUNODEFICIENCY SYNDROME IN CHILDREN

- *Pneumocystis carinii* pneumonia
- Lymphoid interstitial pneumonitis
- Recurrent bacterial infections
- Wasting syndrome
- Candidal esophagitis
- Human immunodeficiency virus encephalopathy
- Cytomegalovirus disease
- *Mycobacterium avium-intracellulare* complex infection
- Pulmonary candidiasis
- Herpes simplex disease
- Cryptosporidiosis

Diagnostic Evaluation

For children 18 months of age and older, the HIV enzyme-linked immunosorbent assay (ELISA) and Western blot immunoassay are performed to determine HIV infection. In infants born to HIV-infected mothers, these assays will be positive because of the presence of maternal antibodies derived transplacentally. Maternal antibodies may persist in the infant up to 18 months of age. Therefore other diagnostic tests are used, most commonly the HIV polymerase chain reaction for detection of proviral DNA. With this technique, almost all infected infants can be diagnosed between 1 and 6 months of age (Goldschmidt and Fogler, 2006; Yogev and Chadwick, 2007).

The Centers for Disease Control and Prevention (CDC) (CDC, 1994) has developed a classification system to describe the spectrum of HIV disease in children (Table 43-2). The system indicates the severity of clinical signs and symptoms and the degree of immunosuppression. Mild signs and symptoms include lymphadenopathy, parotitis, hepatosplenomegaly, and recurrent or persistent sinusitis or otitis media. Moderate signs and symptoms include lymphoid interstitial pneumonitis (LIP) and a variety of organ-specific dysfunctions or infections. Severe signs and symptoms include AIDS-defining illnesses with the exception of LIP. Children with LIP have a better prognosis than those with other AIDS-defining illnesses. In children whose HIV infection is not yet confirmed, the letter *E* (vertically exposed) is placed in front of the classification. The immune categories are based on CD_4^+ lymphocyte counts and percentages. Age adjustment of these numbers is necessary because normal counts, which are relatively high in infants, decline steadily until 6 years of age, when they reach adult norms.

Therapeutic Management

The goals of therapy for HIV infection include slowing the growth of the virus, preventing and treating opportunistic infections, and providing nutritional support and symptomatic treatment. Antiretroviral drugs work at various stages of the HIV life cycle to prevent reproduction of functional new virus particles. Although not a cure, these drugs can suppress viral replication, preventing further deterioration of the immune system, and thus delay disease progression. Classes of antiretroviral agents include nucleoside reverse transcriptase inhibitors (e.g., zidovudine, didanosine, stavudine, lamivudine, abacavir), nonnucleoside reverse transcriptase inhibitors (e.g., nevirapine, delavirdine, efavirenz), nucleotide reverse transcriptase inhibitors (e.g., adefovir), protease inhibitors (e.g., indinavir, saquinavir, ritonavir, nelfinavir, amprenavir), and adjunctive antiretrovirals (e.g., hydroxyurea). Combinations of antiretroviral drugs are used to stall the emergence of drug resistance. Antiretroviral therapy regimens and guidelines are continually evolving. Therapy is lifelong, making adherence difficult. Laboratory markers (CD_4^+ lymphocyte count, viral load) assist in monitoring both disease progression and response to therapy.

Pneumocystis carinii pneumonia (PCP) is the most common opportunistic infection of children infected with HIV. It occurs most frequently between 3 and 6 months of age. All infants born to HIV-infected women should receive prophylaxis until HIV infection is reasonably excluded (AAP Committee on Pediatric AIDS, 2000a; Havens, Mofenson, and AAP Committee on Pediatric AIDS, 2009; Simpkins, Siberry, and Hutton, 2009). Trimethoprim-sulfamethoxazole (TMP-SMZ) is the agent of choice. If adverse effects are experienced with TMP-SMZ, dapsone or pentamidine can be used.

Prophylaxis is often employed for other opportunistic infections, such as disseminated *Mycobacterium avium-intracellulare* complex, candidiasis, or herpes simplex. IVIG has been helpful in preventing recurrent or serious bacterial infections in some HIV-infected children.

Immunization against common childhood illnesses, including the pneumococcal and influenza vaccines, is recommended for all children exposed to and infected with HIV (AAP Committee on Pediatric AIDS, 2000b; Simpkins, Siberry, and Hutton, 2009). Varicella (chickenpox) vaccine and measles, mumps, and rubella (MMR) vaccine can be administered if there is no evidence of severe immunocompromise. Because antibody production to vaccines may be poor or decrease over time, immediate prophylaxis after exposure to several vaccine-preventable diseases (e.g., measles, varicella) is warranted. It should be recognized that children receiving IV gamma globulin (IVGG) prophylaxis may not respond to the MMR vaccine if given in close proximity to the IVGG dose (Allen, 2007; CDC, 2003).

HIV infection often leads to marked failure to thrive and multiple nutritional deficiencies. Nutritional management may be difficult because of recurrent illness, diarrhea, and other physical problems. Intensive nutritional interventions should be instituted when the child's growth begins to slow or weight begins to decrease.

Prognosis. Early recognition and improved medical care have changed HIV disease from a rapidly fatal illness to a chronic disease. After the introduction of combination antiretroviral therapy, the numbers of new AIDS cases and deaths declined substantially. In the United States, the annual number of AIDS cases affecting children younger than 13 years had a sharp, steady decline since the early 1990s (Klause and Johnson, 2007; Simpkins, Siberry, and Hutton, 2009). In contrast, adolescents and young adults (13 to 24 years of age) with AIDS that represent a minority of U.S. cases (≈5%) constitute one of the fastest growing groups of newly infected persons in the country (Simpkins, Siberry, and Hutton, 2009; Yogev and Chadwick, 2007).

CARE MANAGEMENT

Education concerning transmission and control of infectious diseases, including HIV infection, is essential for individuals with HIV infection and anyone involved in their care. The basic tenets of Standard Precautions should be presented in an age-appropriate manner, with careful consideration of the educational levels of the individuals (see Infection Control, Chapter 39). Safety issues, including appropriate storage of special medications and equipment (e.g., needles and syringes), are emphasized.

Unfortunately, relatives, friends, and others in the general public may be fearful of contracting HIV infection, and criticism and ostracism of the child and family may occur. In an effort to protect the child, the family may limit the child's activities outside the home. Although certain precautions are justified in limiting exposure to sources of infections, they must be tempered with concern for the child's normal developmental needs. Both the family and the community need ongoing education about HIV to dispel many of the myths that have been perpetuated by uninformed persons.*

Prevention is a key component of HIV education. Educating adolescents about HIV is essential in preventing HIV infection in this age-group. Education should include the routes of transmission, the hazards of IV and other recreational drug use, and the value of sexual abstinence and safe sex practices. Such education should be a part of anticipatory guidance provided to all adolescent patients. Nurses can also encourage adolescents at risk to undergo HIV counseling and testing. In addition to identifying infected teenagers and getting them into care, such counseling affords adolescents an opportunity to learn about and possibly change their risky behaviors.

The multiple complications associated with HIV disease are potentially painful (Ezekowitz, 2009). Aggressive pain management is essential for these children to have an acceptable quality of life. Their pain may be caused by infections (e.g., otitis media, dental abscess), encephalopathy (e.g., spasticity), adverse effects of medications (e.g., peripheral neuropathy), or an unknown source (e.g., deep musculoskeletal pain). Pain is related not only to the disease processes but also to various treatments these children often undergo, including venipunctures, lumbar punctures, biopsies, and endoscopies. Ongoing assessment of pain is crucial and is most easily accomplished in older children who are able to communicate. Nonverbal and developmentally delayed children are more difficult to assess. The nurse should be alert for signs of pain such as emotional detachment, lack of interactive play, irritability, and depression. Effective pain management depends on the appropriate use of pharmacologic agents, including EMLA or LMX cream, acetaminophen, NSAIDs, muscle relaxants, and opioids. Tolerance to opioids may indicate increased dosing; monitored use ensures safety. Nonpharmacologic interventions (e.g., guided imagery, hypnosis, relaxation, and distraction techniques) are useful adjuncts.

Common psychosocial concerns include disclosing the diagnosis to the child, making custody plans when the parent is infected, and anticipating the loss of a family member. Other stressors may include financial difficulties, HIV-associated stigma, efforts to keep the diagnosis secret, other infected family members, and the

---

*Additional information is available from the National HIV/AIDS Hotline: 800-448-0440; outside the United States: 301-315-2816.

TABLE 43-2	**PEDIATRIC HUMAN IMMUNODEFICIENCY VIRUS INFECTION CLASSIFICATION***			
IMMUNOLOGIC CATEGORY	**N: NO SIGNS OR SYMPTOMS**	**A: MILD SIGNS OR SYMPTOMS**	**B: MODERATE SIGNS OR SYMPTOMS†**	**C: SEVERE SIGNS OR SYMPTOMS†**
No evidence of suppression	N1	A1	B1	C1
Evidence of moderate suppression	N2	A2	B2	C2
Severe suppression	N3	A3	B3	C3

From Centers for Disease Control and Prevention (CDC): 1994 Revised classification system for human immunodeficiency virus infection in children less than 13 years of age, *MMWR Recomm Rep* 43(RR-12):1–10, 1994.
*Children whose human immunodeficiency virus infection status is not confirmed are classified by using this table with the letter *E* (for perinatally exposed) placed before the appropriate classification code (e.g., EN2).
†Both category C and lymphoid interstitial pneumonitis in category B are reportable to state and local health departments as acquired immunodeficiency syndrome.

multiple losses associated with HIV. Many mothers of these children are single mothers who are also HIV infected. As primary caregivers, they often attend to the needs of their child first, neglecting their own health in the process. The nurse is an integral part of the multidisciplinary team necessary for the successful management of the complex medical and social problems of these families.

Children with HIV infection attend day care centers and schools. It is well established that the risk for HIV transmission in these settings is minimal. These institutions are required to follow CDC and Occupational Safety and Health Administration (OSHA) guidelines for infection control measures. Standard Precautions describing proper management of blood and body fluids should also be followed. It is recommended that school personnel receive current HIV information and include it in the health education curriculum for kindergarten through twelfth grade (AAP Committee on Pediatric AIDS and Committee on Infectious Diseases, 1999; AAP Committee on Pediatric AIDS, 2000a). School nurses play a vital role in educating the school staff, students, and parents. They are also invaluable in monitoring the needs of known affected children.

Confidentiality is another major issue in day care or school attendance. Parents and legal guardians have the right to decide whether they inform the day care or school of their child's HIV diagnosis. Unfortunately, myths about HIV infection continue to exist, and the family often wishes to avoid any potential criticism or ostracism of the child.

Severe Combined Immunodeficiency Disease

Severe combined immunodeficiency disease is a defect characterized by absence of both humoral and cell-mediated immunity. The terms Swiss-type lymphopenic agammaglobulinemia (an autosomal recessive form of the disease) and X-linked lymphopenic agammaglobulinemia have been used to describe this disorder, which, as the names imply, can follow either mode of inheritance.

Susceptibility to infection occurs early in life, most often in the first month of life. The child has chronic infections, fails to completely recover from infections, is frequently reinfected, and is infected with unusual agents. Failure to thrive is a consequence of the persistent illnesses.

Diagnosis is usually based on a history of recurrent, severe infections from early infancy; a familial history of the disorder; and specific laboratory findings, which include lymphopenia, lack of lymphocyte response to antigens, and absence of plasma cells in the bone marrow. Documentation of immunoglobulin deficiency is difficult during infancy because of the normally delayed response of infants in producing their own immunoglobulins and material transfer of immunoglobulin G (IgG).

Therapeutic Management
The definitive treatment for SCID is HSCT from a histocompatible donor, a haplo-identical donor (usually a parent), or a matched unrelated donor. IVIG infusions and PCP prophylaxis are used to augment the humoral immunity until the transplant is performed. Several investigators are attempting gene therapy with some success, offering hope that gene therapy may eventually be the treatment of choice for cases of SCID (Bonilla and Geha, 2009; Buckley, 2007).

CARE MANAGEMENT

Nursing care focuses on preventing infection and supporting the child and family. The care is consistent with that needed for HSCT for any condition (see p. 1389). Because the prognosis for SCID is very poor if a compatible bone marrow donor is not available,

nursing care is directed at supporting the family in caring for a child with a life-threatening illness (see Chapter 36). Genetic counseling is essential because of the modes of transmission in either form of the disorder.

Wiskott-Aldrich Syndrome

Wiskott-Aldrich syndrome is an X-linked recessive disorder characterized by a triad of abnormalities: (1) thrombocytopenia, (2) eczema, and (3) immunodeficiency of selective functions of B lymphocytes and T lymphocytes. An abnormal gene has been identified on the proximal arm of the X chromosome and designated the *WAS protein* (Bonilla and Geha, 2009; Buckley, 2007). At birth, the presenting feature may be bleeding such as bloody diarrhea as a result of thrombocytopenia. As the child grows older, recurrent infection and eczema become more severe and the bleeding becomes less frequent.

Eczema is typical of the allergic type and readily becomes superinfected. Chronic infection with herpes simplex is a frequent problem and may lead to chronic keratitis of the eye with loss of vision. Chronic pulmonary disease, sinusitis, and otitis media result from repeated infections. In children who survive the bleeding episodes and overwhelming infections, malignancy presents an additional risk to survival. Medical treatment involves:

- Counteracting the bleeding tendencies with platelet transfusions
- Administering IVIG to provide passive immunity
- Administering prophylactic antibiotics to prevent and control infection.
- Providing aggressive local therapy for the eczema

WAS can be cured with HSCT (Albert, Notarangelo, and Ochs, 2011; Buckley, 2007). Several clinical trials focused on replacing the normal WAS gene are being conducted to determine the most effective vector (Albert, Notarangelo, and Ochs, 2011).

CARE MANAGEMENT

Because of the poor prognosis for these children, the main nursing consideration is supporting the family in the care of a fatally ill child (see Chapter 36). Physical care is directed at controlling the problems imposed by the disorder. The measures used to control bleeding are similar to those for hemophilia and vWD (see previous discussions). Another major goal is prevention or control of infection. Because eczema is a troublesome problem, nursing measures specific to this condition are especially important (see Chapter 47). The genetic implications of this X-linked recessive disorder differ little from those of any other X-linked disorder.

TECHNOLOGIC MANAGEMENT OF HEMATOLOGIC AND IMMUNOLOGIC DISORDERS

Blood Transfusion Therapy

Technologic advances in blood banking and transfusion medicine enable the administration of only the blood component needed by the child, such as packed RBCs for anemia or platelets for bleeding disorders. However, regardless of the blood component infused, all transfusions have some risks. Nurses need to be aware of the possible complications and the appropriate interventions. General guidelines that apply to all transfusions include:

- Take vital signs, including blood pressure, *before* administering blood to establish baseline data for intratransfusion and posttransfusion comparison; 15 minutes after initiation;

hourly while blood is infusing; and on completion of transfusion.

- Check the identification of the recipient with the donor's blood group and type regardless of the blood product being used.
- Administer the first 50 mL of blood or 20% of the volume (whichever is smaller) *slowly,* and stay with the child.
- Administer with normal saline on a piggyback setup, or have normal saline available.
- Administer blood through an appropriate filter to eliminate particles in the blood and prevent the precipitation of formed elements; gently shake the container frequently.
- Use blood within 30 minutes of its arrival from the blood bank; if it is not used, return it to the blood bank—do not store it in the regular unit refrigerator.
- Infuse a unit of blood (or the specified amount) within 4 hours. If the infusion will exceed this time, the blood should be divided into appropriate-size quantities by the blood bank and the unused portion refrigerated under controlled conditions.
- If a reaction of any type is suspected, stop the transfusion, take vital signs, maintain a patent IV line with normal saline and new tubing, notify the health care practitioner, and do not restart the transfusion until the child's condition has been medically evaluated.

Although hemolytic reactions are rare, ABO incompatibility remains the most common cause of death from blood transfusion, and human error (administration of the wrong type to the patient or mislabeling of the blood product) is usually responsible (Bell, 2007; Tondon, Pandey, Mickey, et al., 2010). Hemolysis can also cause the release of large quantities of phospholipids, which are capable of stimulating DIC (see p. 1379). Acute kidney shutdown and eventual renal failure are a result of renal vasoconstriction from antigen-antibody complexes derived from the RBC surface.

Blood is usually administered to children by infusion pump; therefore the usual precautions and management related to pumps apply. When the blood is started with a standard transfusion set, the filter chamber is filled to allow the total filter to be used. The drip chamber is partially filled with blood to permit counting of the drops. In adjusting the flow rate, it is important to remember that blood administration sets do not use microdrops (60 drops/mL) but, instead, regular drops (usually 10-15 drops/mL). The nurse must consider this when calculating the flow rate.

Hematopoietic Stem Cell Transplantation

Hematopoietic stem cell transplantation is used to establish healthy hematopoiesis in both malignant and nonmalignant disease. Candidates for transplantation are children who have disorders that are unlikely to be cured by other means. The most common conditioning allogenic regimens use intensive ablative therapy consisting of high-dose combination chemotherapy with or without total-body irradiation (Bollard, Krance, and Heslop, 2011). After the immune system is suppressed to prevent rejection of the transplanted marrow, the stem cells are harvested from the bone marrow, peripheral blood, or the umbilical vein of the placenta and given to the patient by IV transfusion. The newly transfused stem cells will begin to repopulate the ablative bone marrow. In essence, the recipient will accept a new blood-forming organ.

The selection process for a suitable donor and the potential complications in transplantation are related to the HLA system complex. Some of the major HLA antigens are A, B, C, D, and DR. There is a wide diversity for each of these HLA loci. There are more than 20

different HLA-A antigens that can be inherited and more than 40 different HLA-B antigens.

The genes are inherited as a single unit or haplotype. A child inherits one unit from each parent; thus a child and each parent have one identical and one nonidentical haplotype. Because the possible haplotype combinations among siblings follow the laws of mendelian genetics, there is a one-in-four chance that two siblings have two identical haplotypes and are perfectly matched at the HLA loci.

The importance of HLA matching is to prevent the serious complication known as GVHD. Because the child's immune system is essentially rendered nonfunctional, there is little difficulty with bone marrow rejection by the recipient. However, the donor's marrow may contain antigens not matched to the recipient's antigens, which begin attacking body cells. The more closely the HLA systems match, the less likely GVHD is to develop. However, for patients with low risk disease, the increase risk for chronic GVHD needs to be balanced against the risk for relapse (Bollard, Krance, and Heslop, 2011).

Different types of HSCT are now performed. Allogeneic HSCT involves matching a histocompatible donor with the recipient. However, allogeneic HSCT is limited by the presence of a suitable marrow donor.

Because of the limited numbers of patients having HLA-identical siblings, other types of allogeneic transplants have evolved. Umbilical cord blood stem cell transplantation is an established rich source of hematopoietic stem cells. Because stem cells can be found with high frequency in the circulation of newborns, cord blood transplantation has become an alternative for some children. The benefit of using umbilical cord blood is the blood's relative immunodeficiency at birth because of naivety of cord T cells, which have a lower risk for GVHD-related problems (Bollard, Krance, and Heslop, 2011).

Autologous HSCTs use the patient's own marrow that was collected from disease-free tissue, frozen, and sometimes treated to remove malignant cells. Children with solid tumors such as neuroblastoma, lymphomas, rhabdomyosarcoma, Ewing sarcoma, and Wilms tumor have been treated with autologous HSCTs.

Peripheral stem cell transplants (PSCTs) are also used in children with cancer. PSCT, a type of autologous transplant, differs in the way stem cells are collected from the patient. CSF is first given to stimulate the production of peripheral blood stem cells (PBSCs) as an alternative to marrow as source of stem cells (Bollard, Krance, and Heslop, 2011). After the WBC count is high enough, the stem cells are collected by an apheresis machine. This machine filters out peripheral stem cells from whole blood, returning the remainder of the blood cells and plasma to the child. The peripheral stem cells are then frozen until the patient is ready for the PSCT.

CARE MANAGEMENT

The care of children undergoing HSCT is similar to that of any child receiving chemotherapy and radiotherapy. These children are usually hospitalized for several weeks after HSCT. Because of the risk for infection, the unit may use such measures as strict hand washing, screening visitors, laminar airflow rooms, and institutional isolation policies. Throughout this long ordeal, the family is concerned with successful engraftment and fear of fatal complications (see Family-Centered Care box). Consequently, nurses need to provide sensitive care and maintain a supportive attitude during the many crises that may arise. If the procedure is not successful, the families need care consistent with that required by the family of any child with a life-threatening disorder (see Chapter 36).

The Decision for a Hematopoietic Stem Cell Transplant

A family's decision for a child to undergo HSCT may be fraught with challenges. Often the child is facing certain death from the malignancy. The preparation of the child for the transplant also places the patient at great medical risk.

When the preparatory regimen is begun and the child's immune system is destroyed, there is no turning back. Unlike kidney transplantation, HSCT does not have a "rescue" procedure, such as dialysis, for supportive therapy. If the donor is a sibling, the issue of his or her marrow "saving" the brother or sister can be a concern, especially if the transplant fails. Parents often must leave the home to stay at the transplant center and encounter additional stressors such as arranging child care, taking a leave from work, and managing finances. The patient faces the greatest stress—fear of HSCT failure or life-threatening complications.

HSCT, Hematopoietic stem cell transplantation.

Apheresis

Apheresis is the removal of blood from an individual, separation of the blood into its components, retention of one or more of these components, and reinfusion of the remainder of the blood into the individual. Apheresis is most often used to remove large quantities of platelets from healthy adult donors. These transfusion products have greatly prolonged the survival of patients with hematologic and oncologic diseases.

This technique is used to remove PBSCs from children before they receive HSCT or high-dose chemotherapy or radiotherapy, which is severely toxic to the bone marrow. These PBSCs can then be used to restore the child's bone marrow. Apheresis is also used as a therapeutic modality. The blood component that is diseased or toxic is separated from the blood, and the remainder is returned to the individual. Therapeutic apheresis is considered part of standard therapy for many diseases. Plasma is selectively removed from individuals with hyperviscosity, life-threatening complications of myasthenia gravis, Guillain-Barré syndrome, thrombotic thrombocytopenic purpura, and certain drug overdoses. WBCs are removed from individuals with high-WBC-count leukemia.

CARE MANAGEMENT

Difficult venous access and small blood volume can limit the ability to use this therapy in infants and young children. Education of the family and child includes the purposes of the therapy and the technology.

Specially trained individuals perform the apheresis procedure. Attention focuses on the rate of removal, blood component separation, and reinfusion of blood into the child. Vital signs are monitored, and the child is continuously observed for any adverse reactions secondary to the circulatory volume changes and the anticoagulant used.

When apheresis components are infused, nursing measures differ depending on whether the product is autologous (blood component from the child) or allogeneic (blood component from another individual). Autologous components are the child's own blood; therefore a major precaution is proper identification to ensure the correct component. The rate of infusion should be adjusted to the child's tolerance. If the product is allogeneic, all precautions for blood transfusions apply.

KEY POINTS

- Anemia is defined as reduction of RBCs or Hgb concentration to levels below normal for age; disorders are classified by etiology and physiology or morphology.
- The nurse's role in treatment of anemia is to assist in establishing a diagnosis, prepare the child for laboratory tests, administer prescribed medications, decrease tissue oxygen needs, implement safety precautions, and observe for complications.
- The main nursing goal in prevention of nutritional anemia is parent education regarding correct feeding practices.
- SCA is a hereditary hemoglobinopathy caused by normal adult HbA being partly or completely replaced by sickle HbS.
- Nursing care of the child with SCA focuses on teaching the family how to prevent and recognize sickle cell problems; managing pain during crises; and helping the child and parents adjust to a lifelong, chronic disease.
- Nursing care of the child with β-thalassemia includes observing for complications of multiple blood transfusions, assisting the child in coping with the effects of illness, and fostering parent-child adjustment to long-term illness.
- Causes of acquired AA include irradiation, drugs, industrial and household chemicals, infections, and infiltration and replacement of myeloid elements; however, the majority of cases are idiopathic.
- Clotting depends on three processes: vascular spasm, platelet aggregation, and coagulation and clot formation.

- Nursing care of the child with hemophilia involves preventing bleeding by decreasing the risk for injury, recognizing and managing bleeding with factor replacement, preventing the crippling effects of joint degeneration, and preparing and supporting the child and family for home care.
- Goals in the care of the child with leukemia are to prepare the family for diagnostic and therapeutic procedures, prevent complications of myelosuppression, manage problems of irradiation and drug toxicity, and provide continued emotional support.
- The lymphomas include HL and NHL and are disorders involving the lymphoid system.
- Immunodeficiency disorders render the affected individual unable to fight infectious organisms.
- HIV infection is primarily acquired in infancy from a HIV-infected parent and in adolescence from engaging in high risk behaviors.
- Blood transfusions supply needed blood components.
- HSCT replaces the diseased or malfunctioning bone marrow with viable blood stem cells.
- Apheresis is the selective removal of a blood component. It can be used to supply cellular elements needed for therapy (i.e., platelets or stem cells) or to remove diseased components.

REFERENCES

Albert MH, Notarangelo LD, Ochs HD: Clinical spectrum, pathophysiology and treatment of Wiskott-Aldrich syndrome, *Curr Opin Hematol* 18(1):42–48, 2011.

Allen UD: Immunizations for children with cancer, *Pediatr Blood Cancer* 49(7 suppl):1102–1108, 2007.

American Academy of Pediatrics (AAP) Committee on Infectious Diseases, Pickering L, editor: *Red Book: report of the Committee on Infectious Diseases*, ed 28, Elk Grove Village, IL, 2009, Author.

American Academy of Pediatrics (AAP) Committee on Pediatric AIDS: Identification and care of HIV-exposed and HIV-infected infants, children, and adolescents in foster care, *Pediatrics* 106(1):149–153, 2000a.

American Academy of Pediatrics (AAP) Committee on Pediatric AIDS: Technical report: perinatal human immunodeficiency virus testing and prevention of transmission, *Pediatrics* 106(6):1–12, 2000b.

American Academy of Pediatrics (AAP) Committee on Pediatric AIDS: HIV testing and prophylaxis to prevent mother-to-child transmission in the United States, *Pediatrics* 122(5):1127–1134, 2008.

American Academy of Pediatrics (AAP) Committee on Pediatric AIDS and Committee on Infectious Diseases: Issues related to human immunodeficiency virus transmission in schools, child care, medical settings, the home, and community, *Pediatrics* 104(2):318–324, 1999.

American Pain Society: *Guidelines for the management of acute and chronic pain in sickle-cell disease*, Glenview, IL, 1999, Author.

Anderson N: Hydroxyurea therapy: improving the lives of patients with sickle cell disease, *Pediatr Nurs* 32(6):541–543, 2006.

Andrews NC, Ullrich CK, Fleming MD: Disorders of iron metabolism and sideroblastic anemia. In Orkin SH, Nathan D, Ginsburg D, et al, editors: *Nathan and Oski's hematology of infancy and childhood*, ed 7, Philadelphia, 2009, Saunders.

Armstrong-Wells J, Grimes S, Sidney D, et al: Utilization of TCD screening for primary stroke prevention in children with sickle cell disease, *Neurology* 72(15):1316–1321, 2009.

Auerbach M: Should intravenous iron be upfront therapy for iron deficiency anemia? *Pediatr Blood Cancer* 56(4):511–512, 2011.

Baker RD, Greer FR, Committee on Nutrition American Academy of Pediatrics (AAP): Diagnosis and prevention of iron deficiency and iron-deficiency anemia in infants and young children (0-3 years of age), *Pediatrics* 126(5):1040–1050, 2010.

Bell MD: Red blood cell transfusions, *Pediatr Rev* 28(8):299–304, 2007.

Berglund S, Westrup B, Domellof M: Iron supplements reduce the risk of iron deficiency anemia in marginally low birth weight infants, *Pediatrics* 126(4):e874–e883, 2010.

Bhatia S: Epidemiology. In Wallace WHB, Green DM, editors: *Late effects of childhood cancer*, London, 2004, Arnold.

Bollard CM, Krance RA, Heslop HE: Hematopoietic stem cell transplantation in pediatric oncology. In Pizzo PA, Poplack DG, editors: *Principles and practice of pediatric oncology*, ed 6, Philadelphia, 2011, Lippincott.

Bonilla FA, Geha RS: Primary immunodeficiency diseases. In Orkin SH, Nathan D, Ginsburg D, et al, editors: *Nathan and Oski's hematology of infancy and childhood*, ed 7, Philadelphia, 2009, Saunders.

Brandow AM, Weisman SJ, Panepinto JA: The impact of a multidisciplinary pain management model on sickle cell disease pain hospitalizations, *Pediatr Blood Cancer* 56(5):789–793, 2011.

Buckley RH: Evaluation of the immune system. In Behrman RE, Kliegman RM, Jenson HTS, et al, editors: *Nelson textbook of pediatrics*, ed 18, Philadelphia, 2007, Saunders.

Cappellini MD, Porter JB, El-Beshlawy A, et al: Tailoring iron chelation by iron intake and serum ferritin trends: the prospective multicenter EPIC study of deferasirox in 1744 patients with various transfusion-dependent anemias, *Haematologica* 95(4):557–566, 2010.

Carley A: Anemia: when is it iron deficiency? *Pediatr Nurs* 29(2):127–133, 2003.

Centers for Disease Control and Prevention (CDC): 1992 Revised classified system for human immunodeficiency virus infection in children less than 13 years of age, *MMWR Recomm Rep* 43(RR-12):1–10, 1994.

Centers for Disease Control and Prevention (CDC): Advancing HIV prevention: new strategies for a changing epidemic—United States, *MMWR Morb Mortal Wkly Rep* 52(15):329–332, 2003.

Centers for Disease Control and Prevention (CDC): *Mother-to-child (perinatal) HIV transmission and prevention*, Atlanta Department of Health and Human Services, 2007, www.cdc.gov/hiv/topics/perinatal/resources/factsheets/perinatal.htm#2.

Chiocca EM: Sickle cell crisis: severe pain and potential tissue necrosis are the major concerns, *Am J Nurs* 96(9):49, 1996.

Consolini DM: Thrombocytopenia in infants and children, *Pediatr Rev* 32(4):135–151, 2011.

Cunningham MJ, Sankaran VG, Nathan DG, et al: The thalassemias. In Orkin SH, Nathan DG, Ginsburg D, et al, editors: *Nathan and Oski's hematology of infancy and childhood*, ed 7, Philadelphia, 2009, Saunders.

Curry H: Bleeding disorder basics, *Pediatr Nurs* 30(5):402–405, 2004.

Cusick SE, Mei Z, Freedman DS, et al: Unexplained decline in the prevalence of anemia among U.S. children and women between 1988-1994 and 1999-2002, *Am J Clin Nutr* 88(6):1611–1617, 2008.

DeBaun MR, Vichinsky E: Hemoglobinopathies. In Kliegman RM, Jenson HB, Behrman RE, et al, editors: *Nelson textbook of pediatrics*, ed 18, Philadelphia, 2007, Saunders.

Driscoll MC: Sickle cell disease, *Pediatr Rev* 28(7):259–267, 2007.

Ezekowitz RAB: Hematologic manifestations of systemic diseases. In Orkin SH, Nathan DG, Ginsburg D, et al, editors: *Nathan and Oski's hematology of infancy and childhood*, ed 7, Philadelphia, 2009, Saunders.

Glader B: Anemias of inadequate production. In Behrman RE, Kliegman RM, Jenson HTS, et al, editors: *Nelson textbook of pediatrics*, ed 18, Philadelphia, 2007, Saunders.

Goldschmidt RH, Fogler JA: Opportunities to prevent HIV transmission to newborns, *Pediatrics* 117(1):208–209, 2006.

Gross TG, Perkins SL: Malignant non-Hodgkin lymphomas in children. In Pizzo PA, Poplack DG, editors: *Principles and practice of pediatric oncology*, ed 6, Philadelphia, 2011, Lippincott.

Haining, WN, Duncan C, Lehmann LE: Principles of bone marrow and stem cell transplantation. In Orkin SH, Nathan DG, Ginsburg D, et al, editors: *Nathan and Oski's hematology of infancy and childhood*, ed 7, Philadelphia, 2009, Saunders.

Havens PL, Mofenson LM, AAP Committee on Pediatric AIDS: Evaluation and management of the infant exposed to HIV-1 in the United States, *Pediatrics* 123(1):175–187, 2009.

Heeney M, Dover GJ: Sickle cell disease. In Orkin SH, Nathan DG, Ginsburg D, et al, editors: *Nathan and Oski's hematology of infancy and childhood*, ed 7, Philadelphia, 2009, Saunders.

Hirst C, Owusu-Ofori S: Prophylactic antibiotics for preventing pneumococcal infection in children with sickle cell disease, *Cochrane Database Syst Rev* (11):CD003427, 2010.

Hord JD: The acquired pancytopenia. In Behrman RE, Kliegman RM, Jenson HTS, et al, editors: *Nelson textbook of pediatrics*, ed 18, Philadelphia, 2007, Saunders.

Howard J, Davies SC: Sickle cell disease in North Europe, *Scand J Clin Lab Invest* 67(1):27–38, 2007.

Hutter JJ: Childhood leukemia, *Pediatr Rev* 31(6):234–241, 2010.

Jemal A, Siegel R, Ward E, et al: Cancer statistics, 2009, *CA Cancer J Clin* 59(4):225–249, 2009.

Kaspers GJ, Creutzig U: Pediatric acute myeloid leukemia: international progress and future directions, *Leukemia* 19(12):2025–2029, 2005.

Khoury H, Grimsley E: Oxygen inhalation in nonhypoxic sickle cell patients during vaso-occlusive crisis, *Blood* 86(10):3998, 1995.

Klause BD, Johnson M: Paradigm shift: new testing guidelines for HIV, *Adv Nurse Pract* 15(3):59–93, 2007.

Koh AY, Pizzo PA: Infectious complications in pediatric cancer patients. In Pizzo PA,

Poplack DG, editors: *Principles and practice of pediatric oncology*, ed 6, Philadelphia, 2011, Lippincott.

Kwiatkowski JL, Yim E, Miller S, et al; for the STOP 2 study investigators: Effect of transfusion therapy on transcranial Doppler ultrasonography velocities in children with sickle cell disease, *Pediatr Blood Cancer* 56(5):777–782, 2011.

Lindley C, Goodin S, McCune J, et al: Prevention of delayed chemotherapy-induced nausea and vomiting after moderately high to highly emetogenic chemotherapy, *Am J Clin Oncol* 28(3):270–276, 2005.

Lokeshwar MR, Mehta M, Mehta N, et al: Prevention of iron deficiency anemia (IDA): how far have we reached? *Indian J Pediatr* 78(5):593–602, 2011.

Lucarelli G, Gaziev J: Advances in the allogeneic transplantation for thalassemia, *Blood Rev* 22(2):53–63, 2008.

Manco-Johnson MJ, Abshire TC, Shapiro AD, et al: Prophylaxis versus episodic treatment to prevent joint disease in boys with severe hemophilia, *N Engl J Med* 357:535–544, 2007.

Margolin JF, Rabin KR, Steuber CP, et al: Acute lymphoblastic leukemia. In Pizzo PA, Poplack DG, editors: *Principles and practice of pediatric oncology*, ed 6, Philadelphia, 2011, Lippincott.

Marsh JCW: Management of acquired aplastic anemia, *Blood Rev* 19(3):143–151, 2005.

Matrai J, Chuah MKL, VandenDriessche T: Preclinical and clinical progress in hemophilia gene therapy, *Curr Opin Hematol* 17(5):387–392, 2010.

McCann JC, Ames BN: An overview of evidence for a causal relation between iron deficiency during development and deficits in cognitive or behavioral function, *Am J Clin Nurs* 85(4):931–945, 2007.

McCrae K: Immune thrombocytopenia: no longer "'idiopathic," *Cleve Clin J Med* 78(6):358–373, 2011.

McGann PT, Ware RE: Hydroxyurea for sickle cell anemia: what have we learned and what questions remain? *Curr Opin Hematol* 18(3):158–165, 2011.

McKenzie SB: Anemias of disordered iron metabolism and heme synthesis. In McKenzie SB, editor: *Clinical laboratory hematology*, Upper Saddle River, NJ, 2004, Pearson Prentice Hall.

Metzger M, Krasin MJ, Hudson MM, et al: Hodgkin lymphoma. In Pizzo PA, Poplack DG, editors: *Principles and practice of pediatric oncology*, ed 6, Philadelphia, 2011, Lippincott.

Montgomery RR, Gill JC, DiPaola J: Hemophilia and von Willebrand disease. In Orkin SH, Nathan D, Ginsburg D, et al, editors: *Nathan and Oski's hematology of infancy and childhood*, ed 7, Philadelphia, 2009, Saunders.

National Hemophilia Foundation, Bleeding Disorders Information Center: *Newly*

diagnosed: parents FAQ, 2006, www.hemophilia.org/bdi/bdi_newly7c.htm.

National Institutes of Health, National Heart, Lung, and Blood Institute, Division of Blood Disease and Resources: *The management of sickle cell disease*, NIH Pub No 02-2117, Bethesda, MD, 2002, NHLBI Health Information Network.

Ohls R, Christensen RD: Hemoglobin disorders. In Behrman RE, Kliegman RM, Jenson HTS, et al, editors: *Nelson textbook of pediatrics*, ed 18, Philadelphia, 2007, Saunders.

Pack-Mabien A, Haynes J: A primary care provider's guide to prevention and acute care management of adults and children with sickle cell disease, *J Am Acad Nurse Pract* 21(5):250–257, 2009.

Passweg JR, Marsh JCW: Aplastic anemia: first-line treatment by immunosuppression and sibling marrow transplantation, *Hematol Am Soc Hematol Educ Program* 2010:36–42, 2010.

Pearce JM, Sills RH: Childhood leukemia, *Pediatr Rev* 26(3):96–104, 2005.

Perinatal HIV Guidelines Working Group, Public Health Service Task Force: *Recommendations for use of antiretroviral drugs in pregnant HIV-infected women for maternal health and interventions to reduce perinatal HIV transmission in the United States*, 2007, www.aidsinfo.nih.gov/ContentFiles/PerinatalGL.pdf.

Pui CH, Relling MV, Downing JR: Acute lymphoblastic leukemia, *N Engl J Med* 350(15):1535–1548, 2004.

Raphael JL, Mei M, Mueller BU, et al: High resource hospitalizations among children with vaso-occlusive crises in sickle cell disease, *Pediatr Blood Cancer* 58(4):584–590, 2012.

Redding-Lallinger R, Knoll C: Sickle cell disease: pathophysiology and treatment, *Curr Probl Pediatr Adolesc Health Care* 36(10):346–376, 2006.

Richardson M: Microcytic anemia, *Pediatr Rev* 28(1):5–13, 2007.

Rodeghiero F, Stasi R, Gernsheimer T, et al: Standardization of terminology, definitions, and outcome criteria in immune thrombocytopenic purpura of adults and children: report from an international working group, *Blood* 113(11):2386–2393, 2009.

Ross C, Goldenberg NA, Hund D, et al: Athletic participation in severe hemophilia: bleeding and joint outcomes in children on prophylaxis, *Pediatrics* 124(5):1267–1272, 2009.

Saito M, Aogi K, Sekine I, et al: Palonosetron plus dexamethasone versus granisetron plus dexamethasone for prevention of nausea and vomiting during chemotherapy: a double-blind, double-dummy, randomised, comparative phase III trial, *Lancet Oncol* 10(2):115–124, 2009.

Scott JP, Montgomery RR: Platelet and blood vessel disorder. In Behrman RE, Kliegman RM, Jenson HTS, et al, editors: *Nelson*

textbook of pediatrics, ed 18, Philadelphia, 2007, Saunders.

Sharathkumar AA, Pipe SW: Post-thrombotic syndrome in children: a single center experience, *J Pediatr Hematol Oncol* 30(4):261–266, 2008.

Shimamura A, Guinan EC: Acquired aplastic anemia. In Orkin SH, Nathan D, Ginsburg D, et al, editors: *Nathan and Oski's hematology of infancy and childhood*, ed 7, Philadelphia, 2009, Saunders.

Simpkins EP, Siberry GK, Hutton N: Thinking about HIV infection, *Pediatr Rev* 30(9):337–349, 2009.

Strouse JJ, Lanzkron S, Beach MC, et al: Hydroxyurea for sickle cell disease: a systematic review for efficacy and toxicity in children, *Pediatrics* 122(6):1332–1342, 2008.

Tondon R, Pandey P, Mickey KB, et al: Errors reported in cross match laboratory: a prospective data analysis, *Transfus Aphers Sci* 43(3):309–314, 2010.

Trigg M: Hematopoietic stem cells, *Pediatrics* 113(4):1051–1057, 2004.

Velasquez MP, Mariscalco MM, Goldstein Sl, et al: Erythrocytapheresis in children with sickle cell disease and acute chest syndrome, *Pediatr Blood Cancer* 53(6):1060–1063, 2009.

Vichinsky E, Bernaudin F, Forni GL, et al: Long-term safety and efficacy of deferasirox (Exjade) for up to 5 years in transfusional iron-overloaded patients with sickle cell disease, *Br J Haematol* 154(3):387–397, 2011.

Vichinsky E, Onyekwere O, Porter J, et al: A randomized comparison of deferasirox versus deferoxamine for the treatment of transfusional iron overload in sickle cell disease, *Br J Haematol* 136(3):501–508, 2007.

Vichinsky E, Styles L: Sickle cell disease: pulmonary complications, *Hematol Oncol Clin North Am* 10(6):1275–1286, 1996.

Wang WC, Ware RE, Miller ST, et al: Hydroxycarbamide in very young children with sickle-cell anaemia: a multicentre, randomized, controlled trial (BABY HUG), *Lancet* 377(9778):1663–1672, 2011.

Wilson DB: Acquired platelet defects. In Orkin SH, Nathan DG, Ginsburg D, et al, editors: *Nathan and Oski's hematology of infancy and childhood*, ed 7, Philadelphia, 2009, Saunders.

Yaish HM: Pediatric thalassemia, *Medscape* 2010, http://emedicine.medscape.com/article/958850-overview#a0199.

Yogev R, Chadwick EG: Acquired immunodeficiency syndrome (human immunodeficiency virus). In Kliegman RM, Jenson HB, Behrman RE, et al, editors: *Nelson textbook of pediatrics*, ed 18, Philadelphia, 2007, Saunders.

Zimmerman S, Schultz W, Davis J, et al: Sustained long-term hematologic efficacy of hydroxyurea at maximum tolerated dose in children with sickle cell disease, *Blood* 103(6):2039–2045, 2004.

Genitourinary Dysfunction

Marilyn J. Hockenberry

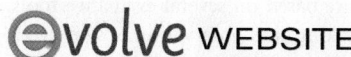 WEBSITE

http://evolve.elsevier.com/Perry/maternal

LEARNING OBJECTIVES

On completion of this chapter, the reader will be able to:

- Describe the various aspects of enuresis.
- Describe the various factors that contribute to urinary tract infections in infants and children.
- Discuss the preoperative preparation of the child and parents when the child has a structural defect of the genitourinary tract.
- Demonstrate an understanding of the causes and mechanisms of edema formation in nephrotic syndrome.

- Outline a nursing care plan for a child with nephrotic syndrome.
- Compare the child with minimal-change nephrotic syndrome and the child with acute glomerulonephritis in terms of clinical manifestations and nursing care.
- Contrast the causes, complications, and management of acute and chronic renal failure.
- List the types of renal dialysis.
- Recognize signs of kidney transplant rejection.

PROBLEMS RELATED TO ELIMINATION

Enuresis

Enuresis (bedwetting), or nocturnal enuresis, is a common and troublesome disorder that is defined as the intentional or involuntary passage of urine into the bed (usually at night) in children who are beyond the age when voluntary bladder control should normally have been acquired. The inappropriate voiding of urine must occur at least twice a week for at least 3 months, and the chronologic or developmental age of the child must be at least 5 years. The predominant symptom is urgency that is immediate and is accompanied by acute discomfort, restlessness, and urinary frequency. In addition, the urinary incontinence must not be related to the direct physiologic effects of a substance (e.g., diuretics) or a general medical condition (e.g., diabetes mellitus or diabetes insipidus, spina bifida, seizure disorder, or sickle cell disease).

Enuresis is more common in boys; nocturnal bedwetting usually ceases between 6 and 8 years of age. Enuresis can also be defined as primary (bedwetting in children who have never been dry for extended periods) or secondary (the onset of wetting after a period of established urinary continence). The passage of urine may be monosymptomatic and occur only during nighttime sleep, with the child remaining dry during the day; or it may be polysymptomatic, in which the child has daytime urinary urgency and an occasional daytime accident in conjunction with other conditions such as sleep

apnea, urinary tract infection, neurologic impairment, constipation, or emotional stressors (Berry, 2006; Katz and DeMaso, 2011). The nocturnal, monosymptomatic type is most common. The condition may be particularly distressing to adolescents, who may refuse therapy. Although enuresis may occur during the daytime, the following discussion primarily focuses on nocturnal enuresis.

Before psychogenic factors are considered, organic causes that may be related to enuresis should be ruled out. These include structural disorders of the urinary tract; urinary tract infection; neurologic deficits; disorders that increase the normal output of urine, such as diabetes; and disorders that impair the concentrating ability of the kidneys, such as chronic renal failure or sickle cell disease. A bladder volume of 300 to 350 mL (10 to 12 oz) is sufficient to hold a night's urine. Normal bladder capacity (in ounces) is the child's age plus 2 (up to age 14 years). In other cases, enuresis is influenced by emotional factors, although it is doubtful that they are causative factors. Parents report that these children sleep more soundly than other children, but the depth of sleep has not been identified as the cause of nocturnal enuresis (Berry, 2006; Elder, 2011). Nocturnal enuresis has a strong familial tendency.

Therapeutic techniques used to manage nocturnal enuresis include medications, complementary and alternative medicine techniques (such as hypnotherapy), restriction or elimination of fluids after the evening meal, avoidance of caffeinated and sugar-containing beverages after 4 PM, purposeful interruption of sleep to void, motivational therapy, and various devices designed to establish a conditioned reflex response to waken the child at the initiation of voiding (alarms).

Drug therapy is increasingly being prescribed to treat enuresis. Three types of drugs are used: tricyclic antidepressants (TCAs), antidiuretics, and antispasmodics. The drug used depends on the interpretation of the cause. The most commonly used drug is the TCA imipramine (Tofranil), which exerts an anticholinergic action in the bladder to inhibit urination. The dosage and time of administration are individualized, and the drug is given in amounts sufficient to lighten sleep but not to cause wakefulness. Some practitioners prescribe low doses, which reduces bedwetting in two thirds of children. However, it is important to note that almost all children relapse when the medication is stopped. The suggested length of treatment is 6 to 8 weeks followed by gradual withdrawal over 4 weeks. Because overdosage of this drug is especially dangerous, caution parents about the safe use of this drug and the need to keep supplies of the drug out of the reach of children.

Anticholinergic drugs, especially oxybutynin, reduce uninhibited bladder contractions and may be helpful for children with daytime urinary frequency. Success has also been achieved with desmopressin acetate (DDAVP) nasal spray, an analog of vasopressin, which reduces nighttime urinary output to a volume less than functional bladder capacity. Typically, the child receives two sprays before bedtime. The medication is generally well tolerated but may cause nasal irritation or, rarely, headache or nausea. A preparation of desmopressin acetate is also available in tablet form. This preparation is as effective and safe as the nasal spray but avoids the problem of nasal irritation.

These drugs are considered second-line management, and parents should be cautioned not to think these agents will cure the condition; parents are also advised of the side effects of these drugs (Katz and DeMaso, 2011; Sethi, Bhargava, and Shipra, 2005).

▌CARE MANAGEMENT

No matter which techniques are used, the nurse can help both children and parents understand the problem of enuresis, the treatment plan, and the difficulties they may encounter in the process. Essential to the success of any method is the supportive management of parents and their children. Both need encouragement and patience. The problem is discussed with both the parent and the child because all treatments involve and require the child's active participation. In some treatment interventions, the child is in charge of the intervention; therefore parents must learn to support the child rather than intervene themselves. For example, children can strip their wet covers, limit fluids, and use the toilet before bedtime. Parents should encourage the child to maintain a regular bowel evacuation regimen; constipation can contribute to nocturnal enuresis (Katz and DeMaso, 2011). A calendar with wet and dry nights may be helpful to motivate the child to stay dry and maintain a positive perspective on the problem; positive rewards are also helpful.

Parents need to understand that punishment such as scolding, shaming, and threatening is contraindicated because of its negative emotional impact and limited success in reducing the behavior. Positive reinforcement of the desired behavior may be beneficial. Children need to believe they are helping themselves, and they need to sustain feelings of confidence and hope. Many parents believe enuresis is caused by an emotional disturbance and fear that they have somehow produced the situation by improper childrearing practices. They need reassurance that bedwetting is not a manifestation of an emotional disturbance and does not represent willful

misbehavior. Encourage parents to be patient and understanding and to communicate love and support to the child.

Communication with children is directed toward eliminating the emotional impact of the problem, relieving feelings of shame and guilt and the burden of parental disapproval, building self-confidence, and motivating children toward independent control. More important, the nurse can provide consistent support and encouragement to help children through the inconsistent and unpredictable treatment process. Children need to believe they are helping themselves and need to maintain feelings of confidence and hope.

Parents should also be taught to observe for side effects of any medications used. All children with primary enuresis should be encouraged to void before bedtime, and diapering should be avoided.

GENITOURINARY DYSFUNCTION

Assessment of kidney and urinary tract integrity and diagnosis of renal or urinary tract disease are based on several evaluative tools. Physical examination, history taking, and observation of symptoms are the initial procedures. In suspected urinary tract diseases or disorders, further assessment by laboratory, radiologic, and other evaluative methods is carried out. Fig. 44-1 provides a review of the kidney and nephron structures.

Clinical Manifestations

As in most disorders of childhood, the incidence and type of kidney or urinary tract dysfunction change with the age and maturation of the child. In addition, the presenting complaints and the their significance vary with maturation. For example, a complaint of enuresis has greater significance at age 8 years than at age 4 years. In newborns urinary tract disorders are associated with a number of obvious malformations of other body systems, including the curious and unexplained but frequent association between malformed or low-set ears and urinary tract anomalies.

Many of the clinical manifestations of renal disease are common to a variety of childhood disorders, but their presence is an indication to obtain further information from the child's history, family history, and laboratory studies as part of a complete physical examination. Suspected renal disease can be evaluated further by means of radiographic studies and renal biopsy (Table 44-1).

Laboratory Tests

Both urine and blood studies contribute vital information for detection of renal problems. The single most important test is probably routine urinalysis. Specific urine and blood tests provide additional information. Because nurses are usually the people who collect the specimens for examination and who often perform many of the screening tests, they should be familiar with the test, its function, and factors that can alter or distort the results of the test. The major urine and blood tests are outlined in Tables 44-2 and 44-3.

▌CARE MANAGEMENT

Nursing responsibilities in the assessment of genitourinary disorders or diseases begin with observation of the child for any manifestations that might indicate dysfunction. Many conditions have specific characteristics that distinguish them from other disorders. These are discussed as appropriate throughout the chapter.

The nurse is generally the one who is responsible for preparing infants, children, and parents for tests and collection of urine and (sometimes) blood specimens for observation and laboratory

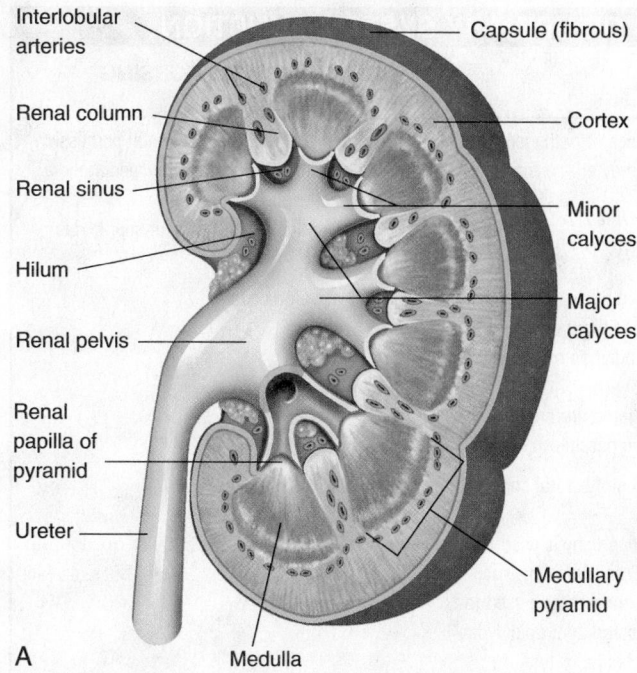

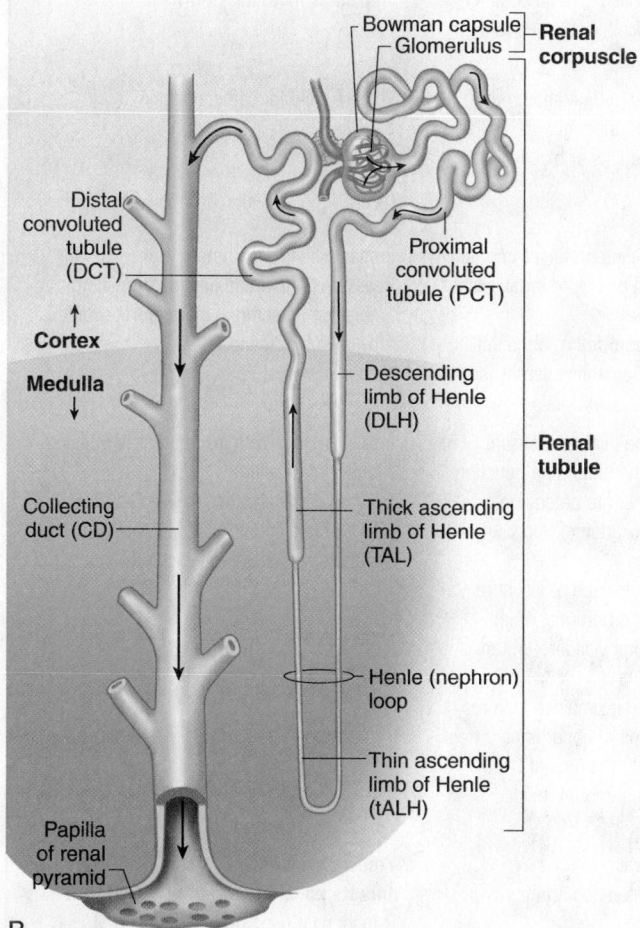

FIG 44-1 A, Kidney structure. **B,** Components of the nephron. (From Patton KT, Thibodeau GA: *Anatomy and physiology,* ed 7, St Louis, 2010, Mosby.)

analysis (see Preparation for Diagnostic and Therapeutic Procedures and Collection of Specimens, Chapter 39). An important nursing responsibility is to maintain careful intake and output measurements and blood pressure for most children with genitourinary dysfunction and those who might be at risk for developing renal complications (e.g., children in shock, postoperative patients). For example, any significant degree of renal disease can diminish the glomerular filtration rate (GFR), a measure of the amount of plasma from which a given substance is totally cleared in 1 minute. A number of substances can be used, but the most useful clinical estimation of glomerular filtration is the clearance of creatinine, an end product of protein metabolism in muscle and a substance that is filtered freely by the glomerulus and secreted by renal tubular cells. The nurse's responsibility in this test is collection of urine, usually a 12- or 24-hour specimen.

GENITOURINARY TRACT DISORDERS AND DEFECTS

Urinary Tract Infection

Infection of the genitourinary tract is one of the most common conditions of childhood. As many as 10% of children will have a febrile urinary tract infection (UTI) during the first 2 years of life (Kanellopoulos, Salakos, Spiliopoulou, et al., 2006). Among febrile boys circumcision status is important in determining the risk for UTI. Uncircumcised male infants younger than 3 months of age had the highest prevalence of UTI (20.1%) of any group, male or female (Shaikh, Morone, Bost, et al., 2008). Circumcision status should be assessed in male infants with unexplained fever. UTI may involve the urethra and bladder (lower urinary tract) or the ureters, renal pelvis, calyces, and renal parenchyma (upper urinary tract). Because it is often impossible to localize the infection, the broad designation UTI is applied to the presence of significant numbers of microorganisms anywhere within the urinary tract except the distal third of the urethra, which is usually colonized with bacteria.

Classification

Infection of the urinary tract may be present with or without clinical symptoms. As a result, the site of infection is often difficult to pinpoint with any degree of accuracy. Various terms used to describe urinary tract disorders include:

Bacteriuria—Presence of bacteria in the urine

Asymptomatic bacteriuria—Significant bacteriuria (usually defined as >100,000 colony-forming units [CFUs]) with no evidence of clinical infection

Symptomatic bacteriuria—Bacteriuria accompanied by physical signs of UTI (dysuria, suprapubic discomfort, hematuria, fever)

Recurrent UTI—Repeated episode of bacteriuria or symptomatic UTI

Persistent UTI—Persistence of bacteriuria despite antibiotic treatment

Febrile UTI—Bacteriuria accompanied by fever and other physical signs of UTI; presence of a fever typically implies pyelonephritis

Cystitis—Inflammation of the bladder

Urethritis—Inflammation of the urethra

Pyelonephritis—Inflammation of the upper urinary tract and kidneys

Urosepsis—Febrile UTI coexisting with systemic signs of bacterial illness; blood culture reveals presence of urinary pathogen

TABLE 44-1   RADIOLOGIC AND OTHER TESTS OF URINARY SYSTEM FUNCTION

TEST	PROCEDURE	PURPOSE	COMMENTS AND NURSING RESPONSIBILITIES
Urine culture and sensitivity	Collection of sterile specimen	Determines presence of pathogens and drugs to which they are sensitive	Does not require specific parental permission Send specimen to laboratory immediately after collection Catheterization, clean-catch, or suprapubic specimen
Renal and bladder ultrasonography	Transmission of ultrasonic waves through renal parenchyma, along ureteral course, and over bladder	Allows visualization of renal parenchyma and renal pelvis without exposure to external-beam radiation or radioactive isotopes Visualization of dilated ureters and bladder wall also possible	Noninvasive procedure
Testicular (scrotal) ultrasonography	Transmission of ultrasonic waves through scrotal contents and testis	Allows visualization of scrotal contents, including testis Testicular ultrasonography is used to identify masses, and Doppler-enhanced ultrasonography is used to differentiate hyperemia of epididymo-orchitis from ischemia or torsion	Noninvasive procedure
Scout film	Flat plate radiograph of abdomen and pelvis for KUB	Detects and establishes renal outlines, presence of calculi, or opaque foreign bodies in bladder	Prepare as for routine x-ray film
Voiding cystourethrography	Contrast medium injected into bladder through urethral catheter until bladder is full; films taken before, during, and after voiding	Visualizes bladder outline and urethra, reveals reflux of urine into ureters, and shows complications of bladder emptying	Prepare child for catheterization
Radionuclide (nuclear) cystogram	Radionuclide-containing fluid injected through urethral catheter until bladder is full; images generated before, during, and after voiding	Alternative to voiding cystourethrography in children with allergy to intravesical contrast material Allows evaluation of reflux, although visualization of anatomic details is relatively poor	Prepare child for catheterization Reassure patient and parents that allergic response to contrast materials is avoided by use of radionuclide
Radioisotope imaging studies	Contrast medium injected intravenously; computer analysis to measure uptake or washout (excretion) for analysis of organ function	DTPA radioisotope used to measure GFR; estimate of differential renal function and renal washout to determine presence and location of upper urinary tract obstruction DMSA radioisotope used to visualize renal scars and differential renal function; does not visualize ureters and bladder MAG3 radioisotope combines features of DTPA (evaluation of upper urinary tract obstruction) with features of DMSA radioisotope (differential renal function)	Insert or assist with insertion of IV infusion Monitor IV infusion Urethral catheterization may accompany DTPA radioisotope scan; prepare child for catheterization when indicated
IVP (IV urography; excretory urography)	IV injection of a contrast medium Medium secreted and concentrated by tubules X-ray films made 5, 10, and 15 minutes after injection; delayed films (30, 60 minutes, and so on) are obtained if obstruction suspected	Defines urinary tract Provides information about integrity of KUB Retroperitoneal masses visualized when they shift position of ureters	Preparation for test: **Infants up to 2 years of age**—no solid food; omit one bottle on morning of examination; perform studies early to avoid withholding of fluids **Children ages 2-14 years of age**—give cathartic evening before examination, nothing orally after midnight, enema (soapsuds) morning of examination

TABLE 44-1	RADIOLOGIC AND OTHER TESTS OF URINARY SYSTEM FUNCTION—cont'd		
TEST	**PROCEDURE**	**PURPOSE**	**COMMENTS AND NURSING RESPONSIBILITIES**
CT	Narrow-beam x-ray films and computer analysis provide precise reconstruction of area	Visualizes vertical or horizontal cross section of kidney Especially valuable to distinguish tumors and cysts	Noncontrast scan is noninvasive Contrast-enhanced CT scan preparation similar to that for IVP
Cystoscopy	Direct visualization of bladder and lower urinary tract through small scope inserted via urethra	Investigation of bladder and lower tract lesions; visualizes ureteral openings, bladder wall, trigone, and urethra	Give nothing orally after midnight Carry out preoperative preparations Prepare child for cystoscopy
Retrograde pyelography	Contrast medium injected through ureteral catheter	Visualizes pelvic calyces, ureters, and bladder	Give cathartic if ordered Give preoperative medication if ordered Observe for reaction to contrast medium Monitor vital signs after procedure
Renal angiography	Contrast medium injected directly into renal artery via catheter placed in femoral artery (or umbilical artery in newborn) and advanced to renal artery	Visualizes renal vascular system, especially for renal arterial stenosis	Prepare child for insertion of spinal needle or perfusion catheter in renal pelvis (anesthetic often required)
Whitaker perfusion test	Injection of contrast material through renal pelvis and ureters Measures pressures in renal pelvis and urinary bladder	Determine presence of obstruction causing upper urinary tract dilation	
Renal biopsy	Removal of kidney tissue by open or percutaneous technique for study by light, electron, or immunofluorescent microscopy	Yields histologic and microscopic information about glomeruli and tubules; helps distinguish among types of nephritic syndromes Distinguishes other renal disorders	Nothing orally 4-6 hours before test Premedicate as ordered Prepare setup for procedure Assist with procedure Take vital signs Apply pressure to area with pressure dressing and, if feasible, a sandbag Bed rest for 24 hours Observe for abdominal pain, tenderness Monitor input and output Surgical incision may be required in infants
Urodynamics	Set of tests designed to measure bladder filling, storage, and evacuation functions **Uroflowmetry**—Test to determine efficiency of urination **Cystometrography**—Graphic comparison of bladder pressure as a function of volume **Voiding pressure study**— Comparison of detrusor contraction pressure, sphincter electromyelogram, and urinary flow	Determine characteristic of voiding dysfunction Used to identify type (cause) of incontinence or urinary retention Especially valuable for voiding dysfunction complicated by urinary infection, urinary retention, or neurogenic bladder dysfunction	Prepare child for urinary catheterization Bladder will be filled with saline solution, and filling pressures will be recorded; child may experience fullness, coolness from saline fluid, and urine leakage during study Insertion of needles may be required for sphincter EMG

CT, Computed tomography; *DMSA*, dimercaptosuccinic acid; *DTPA*, diethylenetriamine pentaacetic acid; *EMG*, electromyography; *GFR*, glomerular filtration rate; *IV*, intravenous; *IVP*, intravenous pyelography; *KUB*, kidney, ureters, and bladder; *MAG3*, mercaptoacetyltriglycine.

TABLE 44-2	URINE TESTS OF RENAL FUNCTION		
TEST	**NORMAL RANGE**	**DEVIATIONS**	**SIGNIFICANCE OF DEVIATIONS**
Physical Tests			

Volume	Age related
	Newborn—30-60 mL
	Children—Bladder capacity (oz) =
	  Age (years) + 2
		Polyuria
		Oliguria
		
		Anuria
			Osmotic factors (urinary glucose level in diabetes mellitus)
			Retention caused by obstructive disease
			Inadequate bladder emptying caused by neurogenic bladder
			  or obstructive disorder
			Obstruction of urinary tract; ARF

Specific gravity	With normal fluid intake—1.016-
	  1.022
	Newborn—1.001-1.020
	Others—1.001-1.030
		High
		
		Low
			Dehydration
			Presence of protein or glucose
			Presence of radiopaque contrast medium after radiologic
			  examinations
			Excessive fluid intake
			Distal tubular dysfunction
			Insufficient ADH
			Diuresis

Osmolality	Newborn—50-600 mOsm/L Thereafter—50-1400 mOsm/L	Fixed at 1.010 High or low	Chronic glomerular disease Same as for specific gravity More sensitive index than specific gravity
Appearance	Clear pale yellow to deep gold	Cloudy Cloudy reddish-pink to reddish-brown Light Dark Red	Contains sediment Blood from trauma or disease Myoglobin after severe muscle destruction Dilute Concentrated Trauma
Chemical Tests			

pH	Newborn—5-7
	Thereafter—4.8-7.8
	Average—6
		Weak acid or neutral
		
		Alkaline
			If associated with metabolic acidosis, suggests tubular
			  acidosis
			If associated with metabolic alkalosis, suggests potassium
			  deficiency
			Urinary infection
			Metabolic alkalosis

Protein level	Absent	Present	Abnormal glomerular permeability (e.g., glomerular disease, changes in blood pressure) Most kidney disease Orthostatic in some individuals
Glucose level	Absent	Present	Diabetes mellitus Infusion of concentrated glucose-containing fluids Glomerulonephritis Impaired tubular reabsorption
Ketone levels	Absent	Present	Conditions of acute metabolic demand (stress) Diabetic ketoacidosis
Leukocyte esterase	Absent	Present	Can identify both lysed and intact WBCs via enzyme detection
Nitrites	Absent	Present	Most species of bacteria convert nitrates to nitrites in urine
Microscopic Tests			
WBC count	<1 or 2	>5 polymorphonuclear leukocytes/field Lymphocytes	Urinary tract inflammatory process Allograft rejection Malignancy
RBC count	<1 or 2	4-6/field in centrifuged specimen	Trauma Stones Glomerular injury Infection Neoplasms

TABLE 44-2	**URINE TESTS OF RENAL FUNCTION—cont'd**		
TEST	**NORMAL RANGE**	**DEVIATIONS**	**SIGNIFICANCE OF DEVIATIONS**
Presence of bacteria	Absent to a few	>100,000 organisms/ mL in centrifuged specimen	UTI
Presence of casts	Occasional	Granular casts	Tubular or glomerular disorders Degenerative process in advanced renal disease
		Cellular casts	Pyelonephritis
		WBC	Glomerulonephritis
		RBC	Proteinuria; usually transient
		Hyaline casts	

ADH, Antidiuretic hormone; *ARF,* acute renal failure; *RBC,* red blood cell; *UTI,* urinary tract infection; *WBC,* white blood cell.

TABLE 44-3	**BLOOD TESTS OF RENAL FUNCTION**		
TEST	**NORMAL RANGE (MG/DL)**	**DEVIATIONS**	**SIGNIFICANCE OF DEVIATIONS**
BUN	Newborn—4-18 Infant, child— 5-18	Elevated	Renal disease— acute or chronic (the higher the BUN, the more severe the disease) Increased protein catabolism Dehydration Hemorrhage High protein intake Corticosteroid therapy
Uric acid	Child—2.0-5.5	Increased	Severe renal disease
Creatinine	Infant—0.2-0.4 Child—0.3-0.7 Adolescent— 0.5-1	Increased	Renal impairment

BUN, Blood urea nitrogen.

Etiology

A variety of organisms can be responsible for UTI. *Escherichia coli* (80% of cases) and other gram-negative enteric organisms are most frequently implicated; these organisms are usually found in the anal and perineal region. Other organisms associated with UTI include *Proteus, Pseudomonas, Klebsiella,* and *Haemophilus* spp.; *Staphylococcus aureus;* and coagulase-negative *Staphylococcus* organisms. Several factors contribute to the development of UTI in childhood.

Anatomic and Physical Factors. The structure of the lower urinary tract is believed to account for the increased incidence of bacteriuria in females (Rosenthal, 2004). The short urethra, which measures about 2 cm (0.75 inch) in young girls and 4 cm (1.6 inches) in mature women, provides a ready pathway for invasion of organisms. In addition, the closure of the urethra at the end of micturition may return contaminated bacteria to the bladder. The longer male urethra (as long as 20 cm [8 inches] in an adult) and the antibacterial properties of prostatic secretions inhibit the entry and growth of pathogens.

The single most important host factor influencing the occurrence of UTI is urinary stasis. Ordinarily urine is sterile, but at 37° C (98.6° F) it provides an excellent culture medium. Under normal conditions the act of completely and repeatedly emptying the bladder flushes away any organisms before they have an opportunity to multiply and invade surrounding tissue. However, urine that remains in the bladder allows bacteria from the urethra to rapidly become established in the rich medium. Incomplete bladder emptying (stasis) may result from reflux (see Vesicoureteral Reflux, p. 1400), anatomic abnormalities (especially those involving the ureters), dysfunction of the voiding mechanism, or extrinsic ureteral or bladder compression that may be caused by constipation. The key to preventing UTI is to maintain adequate blood supply to the bladder wall by avoiding overdistention and high bladder pressure.

Altered Urine and Bladder Chemistry. Several mechanical and chemical characteristics of the urine and bladder mucosa help maintain urinary sterility. Increased fluid intake promotes flushing of the normal bladder and lowers the concentration of organisms in the infected bladder. Diuresis also seems to enhance the antibacterial properties of the renal medulla.

Most pathogens favor an alkaline medium. Normally urine is slightly acidic with a median pH of 6.0. A urine pH of about 5.0 hampers but does not eliminate bacterial multiplication. Much has been reported about the use of cranberry products to increase urine acidity in an effort to prevent UTI. Recent review of the literature in adult subjects supports the use of cranberry products in reducing the incidence of UTI in women (Jepson, Mihaljevic, and Craig, 2008). Results of one study in children suggests that daily consumption of concentrated cranberry juice can prevent recurrence of symptomatic UTIs (Ferrara, Romaniello, Vitelli, et al., 2009). Further research that controls for type of cranberry product used, dosing regimens, and patient selection based on age and underlying medical condition is required to clarify unanswered questions before recommendations can be made regarding the use of this supplement, especially in the pediatric population.

BOX 44-1	CLINICAL MANIFESTATIONS OF URINARY TRACT DISORDERS OR DISEASE

Neonatal Period (Birth-1 Month)
- Poor feeding
- Vomiting
- Failure to gain weight
- Rapid respiration (acidosis)
- Respiratory distress
- Spontaneous pneumothorax or pneumomediastinum
- Frequent urination
- Screaming on urination
- Poor urine stream
- Jaundice
- Seizures
- Dehydration
- Other anomalies or stigmata
- Enlarged kidneys or bladder

Infancy (1-24 Months)
- Poor feeding
- Vomiting
- Failure to gain weight
- Excessive thirst
- Frequent urination
- Straining or screaming on urination
- Foul-smelling urine
- Pallor
- Fever
- Persistent diaper rash
- Seizures (with or without fever)
- Dehydration
- Enlarged kidneys or bladder

Childhood (2-14 Years)
- Poor appetite
- Vomiting
- Growth failure
- Excessive thirst
- Enuresis, incontinence, frequent urination
- Painful urination
- Swelling of face
- Seizures
- Pallor
- Fatigue
- Blood in urine
- Abdominal or back pain
- Edema
- Hypertension
- Tetany

Diagnostic Evaluation

The clinical manifestations of UTI depend on the child's age (Box 44-1). Diagnosis is confirmed by detection of bacteriuria in urine culture; but urine collection is often difficult, especially in infants and very small children. Several factors may alter a urine specimen, and contamination of a specimen by organisms from sources other than the urine such as perineal and perianal flora in bag specimens is the most frequent cause of false-positive results. Unless the specimen is a first morning sample, a recent high fluid intake may indicate a falsely low organism count. Therefore children should not be encouraged to drink large volumes of water in an attempt to obtain a specimen quickly.

> ! **NURSING ALERT**
>
> A child who exhibits the following should be evaluated for UTI:
> - Incontinence in a toilet-trained child
> - Strong-smelling urine
> - Frequency or urgency

More accurate estimates of bacterial content are obtained from suprapubic aspiration (in children younger than 2 years of age) and properly performed bladder catheterization (as long as the first few milliliters are excluded from collection). The specimen should be taken directly to the laboratory for immediate culture.

Tests to detect bacteriuria are being used with increased frequency in screening for UTI. The dipstick tests for leukocyte esterase or nitrite are quick and inexpensive methods for detecting infection before obtaining final culture results.

Localization of the infection site may involve more specific tests, including percutaneous kidney taps and bladder washout procedures. Other tests such as ultrasonography, voiding cystourethrogram (VCUG), intravenous pyelogram (IVP), and dimercaptosuccinic acid (DMSA) scan, may be performed after the infection subsides to identify anatomic abnormalities contributing to the development of infection and existing kidney changes from recurrent infection.

Therapeutic Management

The objectives of treatment of children with UTI are to (1) eliminate current infection, (2) identify contributing factors to reduce the risk of recurrence, (3) prevent systemic spread of the infection, and (4) preserve renal function. Antibiotic therapy should be initiated on the basis of identification of the pathogen, the child's history of antibiotic use, and the location of the infection. Several antimicrobial drugs are available for treating UTI, but all of them can be ineffective occasionally because of resistance of organisms. Common antiinfective agents used for UTI include the penicillins, sulfonamide (including trimethoprim and sulfisoxazole in combination), the cephalosporins, and nitrofurantoin.

If anatomic defects such as primary reflux or bladder neck obstruction are present, surgical correction of these abnormalities may be necessary to prevent recurrent infection. Follow-up study is an important component of medical management because the relapse rate is high and infection tends to recur 1 to 2 months after termination of treatment. The aim of therapy and careful follow-up is to reduce the chance of renal scarring. However, recurrent infection of the urinary bladder predisposes the individual to transient episodes of vesicoureteral reflux (VUR).

Vesicoureteral Reflux. VUR refers to the abnormal retrograde flow of bladder urine into the ureters. During voiding urine is swept up the ureters and then flows back into the empty bladder, where it acts as a reservoir for bacterial growth until the next void. Primary reflux results from congenitally abnormal insertion of ureters into the bladder; secondary reflux occurs as a result of an acquired condition.

It is not clear that reflux necessarily causes infections. What is clear is that it is more likely to be associated with recurring kidney infections rather than simple bladder infections (cystitis). In the presence of reflux, infected urine (bacteria) from the bladder has access to the kidney, resulting in kidney infections (pyelonephritis). These children are usually very symptomatic with high fevers, vomiting, and chills. When reflux is associated with UTI, it is the most common cause of renal scarring in children. Renal scarring may occur with the first episode of febrile UTI. Reflux in the presence of sterile urine does not cause renal damage. Therefore the most important concept in managing VUR is preventing bacteria from reaching the kidneys. VUR is managed conservatively with daily low-dose antibiotic therapy. A urine culture should be done every 2 to 3 months and any time the child has a fever. This method of management requires a motivated, reliable, and cooperative family. Many children outgrow the reflux over a period of years. An annual VCUG is done to assess the status of the reflux.

For children with mild-to-moderate reflux, a minimally invasive endoscopic option (subtrigonal injection or STING) is an alternative to daily antibiotics or open surgical intervention. A bulking agent—dextranomer–hyaluronic acid polymer (Deflux)—is injected into the mucous membrane of the ureter, making retrograde flow of urine more difficult. Overall cure rates relate to degree of reflux and range from 67.4% to 88.3%, although more than one injection may be needed to achieve resolution (Chen, Yeh, and Chou, 2010).

Indications for open surgical intervention include significant anatomic abnormality at the ureterovesical junction, recurrent UTIs, severe forms of VUR, noncompliance with medical therapy, intolerance to antibiotics, and VUR after puberty in women.

Prognosis. With prompt and adequate treatment at the time of diagnosis, the long-term prognosis for UTI is usually excellent. However, the hazard of progressive renal injury is greatest when infection occurs in young children (especially those younger than 2 years of age) and is associated with congenital renal malformations and reflux. Therefore early diagnosis of children at risk is particularly important.

CARE MANAGEMENT

Nurses should instruct parents to observe regularly for clues suggesting UTI. Unfortunately the signs of UTI are not as evident as those of upper respiratory tract infection. Therefore many cases go undetected because no one thought to investigate this very common problem.

Because infants and young children often are unable to express their feelings and sensations verbally, it is difficult to detect discomfort that they may be experiencing from dysuria. A careful history regarding voiding habits, stooling pattern, and episodes of unexplained irritability may help to detect less obvious cases of UTI. Consequently parents should be cautioned to observe for specific clues of UTI in suspected cases.

> **! NURSING ALERT**
>
> Check the diaper every half hour. This increases the opportunity for observing the stream for such findings as straining or fretting before voiding begins, signs of discomfort before and during urinating, starting and stopping the stream intermittently, and frequent dripping of small amounts of urine.

When infection is suspected, collecting an appropriate specimen is essential. It is the nurse's responsibility to take every precaution to obtain acceptable clean-voided specimens to avoid the use of other more invasive collecting procedures except when absolutely indicated. Because of the unreliability of a specimen obtained via a urine collection bag, suprapubic aspiration of urine or sterile catheterization should be done in infants and young children who are seen with fever.

Frequently additional tests are performed to detect anatomic defects. Children are prepared for these tests as appropriate for their age. This includes an explanation of the procedure, its purpose, and what the children will experience (see Preparation for Diagnostic and Therapeutic Procedures, Chapter 39). Sometimes a simple description of the urinary system is helpful. Especially for preschool children, the nurse must clarify that the urinary tract is separate from any sexual function and that the test is for a problem that they did not cause. Children may associate blame for perceived wrongdoing (e.g., masturbation) or unacceptable thoughts with the reason for the illness or the tests. For children younger than 3 to 4 years of

> **GUIDELINES**
>
> *Prevention of Urinary Tract Infection*
>
> **Factors Predisposing to Development**
> - Short female urethra close to vagina and anus
> - Incomplete emptying (reflux) and overdistention of bladder
> - Concentrated urine
> - Constipation
>
> **Measures of Prevention**
> - Practice perineal hygiene: wipe from front to back.
> - Avoid tight clothing or diapers; wear cotton panties rather than nylon.
> - Check for vaginitis or pinworms, especially if child scratches between legs.
> - Avoid "holding" urine; encourage child to void frequently, especially before long trips or other circumstances in which toilet facilities are not available.
> - Empty bladder completely with each void. Have child "double void" (void, wait a few minutes, and void again). Severe cases may require clean, intermittent catheterization or biofeedback instruction.
> - Avoid straining during defecation and avoid constipation.
> - Encourage generous fluid intake.

age, the procedure can be explained on a doll. For those who are older, a simple drawing of the bladder, urethra, ureters, and kidneys makes the procedure more understandable.

Handling actual equipment when feasible can help to allay anxiety in children of all ages. Anticipatory instruction on distraction techniques such as deep breathing, storytelling, and imagery may help the child relax and be more cooperative during the actual procedures. If surgery is indicated, facts and understanding of the procedure help decrease the child's fear and anxiety concerning more extensive medical-surgical intervention.

Because antibacterial drugs are indicated in UTI, the nurse advises parents of proper dosage and administration. When antiseptics such as nitrofurantoin are used for prolonged therapy to maintain urine sterility, parents need an explanation of the continued need for the drug when no signs of infection are present. For all children an adequate or increased fluid intake is encouraged.

Prevention. Prevention is the most important goal in both primary and recurrent infection, and most preventive measures are simple hygienic habits that should be a routine part of daily care (see Guidelines box). For example, parents are taught to cleanse their infant's genital areas from front to back to avoid contaminating the urethral area with fecal organisms. Girls are taught to wipe from front to back after voiding and defecating. Children should void as soon as they feel the urge (see Critical Thinking Case Study).

Sexually active female adolescents are advised to urinate as soon as possible after they have intercourse to flush out bacteria introduced during the activity. Children who have recurrent UTIs or neurogenic bladder are frequently maintained on daily low-dose antibiotics. Giving the dose at bedtime allows the drug to remain in the bladder overnight. The nurse should reinforce the importance of compliance to parents and older children.

Obstructive Uropathy

Structural or functional abnormalities of the urinary system that obstruct the normal flow of urine can produce renal disorders. When there is interference with urine flow, the backup of urine

? CRITICAL THINKING CASE STUDY

Urinary Tract Infection and Constipation

During your assessment of Lisa, a 5-year-old girl admitted to the hospital for a severe UTI, her mother tells you that Lisa has bowel movements every third or fourth day. They are usually large, hard-formed stools, and Lisa sometimes has trouble evacuating the stool.

1. Evidence—Is there sufficient evidence to draw a conclusion about Lisa's UTI and constipation?
2. Assumptions—Describe an underlying assumption about each of the following:
   a. UTIs and girls
   b. Normal bowel patterns for 4-year-old children
   c. Association between UTIs and constipation
3. Which priorities for nursing care should be established for Lisa?
4. Does the evidence support your nursing intervention?

UTI, Urinary tract infection.

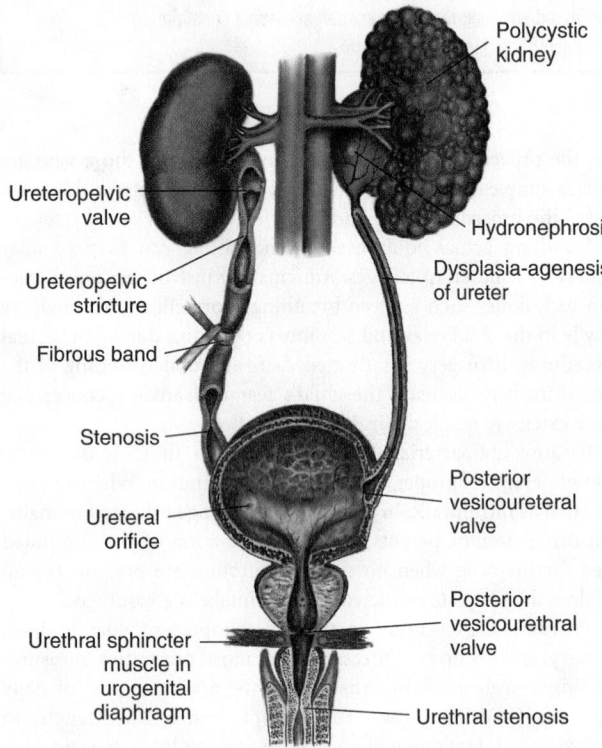

FIG 44-2 Major sites of urinary tract obstruction.

above the obstruction causes hydronephrosis (dilation of the renal pelvis from distention) with eventual pressure destruction of renal parenchyma, although the dilating ureters form a reservoir that reduces the effect on the kidneys for a long time.

Obstruction may be congenital or acquired, unilateral or bilateral, and complete or incomplete with acute or chronic manifestations. The obstruction can occur at any level of the upper or lower urinary tract (Fig. 44-2). Partial obstruction may not be symptomatic unless there is a water or solute diuresis. Boys are affected more frequently than girls, and malformations should be suspected when patients have some other congenital defects (e.g., prune belly syndrome, chromosome anomalies, anorectal malformations, defects of the pinna of the ear).

Damage to distal nephrons in chronic uropathy alters the ability to concentrate urine, contributing to increased urine flow and metabolic acidosis occurring from decreased excretion of acid secondary to impaired ability of the distal nephron to secrete hydrogen ions. Partial obstruction results in progressive loss of renal function as a result of irreversible damage to the nephrons. Pooled urine serves as a medium for bacterial growth; therefore UTIs further increase the extent of renal damage.

Early diagnosis and surgical correction or procedures that divert the flow of urine to bypass the obstruction such as placement of a temporary percutaneous nephrostomy tube or cutaneous ureterostomy are essential to prevent progressive renal damage. Medical complications of acute or chronic renal failure (CRF) or infection are managed as described for those disorders.

CARE MANAGEMENT

Nursing goals in urinary tract obstruction include helping to identify cases, assisting with diagnostic procedures, and caring for children with complications (described elsewhere). Preparing parents and children for procedures is a major nursing responsibility. Preparation for urinary diversion procedures is of special importance (see Preparation for Diagnostic and Therapeutic Procedures, Chapter 39).

Parents and children need emotional support and counseling during the lengthy management of these disorders. Many children are discharged with ureteral drainage systems in place that must be protected from damage, and the danger of infection is a constant concern. Parents are taught to care for the equipment and recognize the signs of possible obstruction or infection within the system. Maintaining adequate urine flow is imperative. Fluids should be encouraged. The tube should be observed frequently for indications of obstruction resulting from sediment, small blood clots, or kinking. The health care provider should inspect any drainage from around the tube.

Children with external diversional systems need psychologic support and guidance, especially as they reach adolescence and body image concerns assume more prominence. Those with progressive renal deterioration may face the prospect of dialysis or transplantation and the emotions that accompany these procedures.

External Defects

Defects of the external genitourinary tract are serious conditions primarily because of the psychologic impact on the child. Satisfactory surgical repair is successful for the more common disorders and is carried out or initiated as early as possible. The major anomalies of the lower genitourinary tract, their description, and their management are outlined in Table 44-4.

Psychologic Problems Related to Genital Surgery

Surgery involving sexual organs can be particularly disruptive to children, especially preschoolers fearing punishment, retaliation, body mutilation, or castration. Some of the problems of hospitalization, separation, and anxiety can be eased by hospital practices that are sensitive to the child's needs (see Chapter 38).

A child's body image is largely derived as a result of feedback from the primary caregivers, and parental anxiety regarding an acceptable physical appearance and adequate future sexual competency is readily communicated to an affected child. Therefore children with birth defects are at risk for developing a distorted body image that reflects the caregiver's subtly communicated evaluation of their bodies. The trend toward repair of visible genital defects is

TABLE 44-4   DEFECTS OF THE GENITOURINARY TRACT

DEFECT	THERAPEUTIC MANAGEMENT
Inguinal hernia—Protrusion of abdominal contents through inguinal canal into scrotum	Detected as painless inguinal swelling of variable size Surgical closure of inguinal defect
Hydrocele—Fluid in scrotum	Surgical repair indicated if spontaneous resolution not accomplished in 1 year
Phimosis—Narrowing or stenosis of preputial opening of foreskin	**Mild cases**—Manual retraction of foreskin and proper cleansing of area **Severe cases**—Circumcision or vertical division and transverse suturing of foreskin
Hypospadias—Urethral opening located behind glans penis or anywhere along ventral surface of penile shaft	Objectives of surgical correction: Enable child to void in standing position and direct stream voluntarily in usual manner Improve physical appearance of genitalia Produce a sexually adequate organ
Chordee—Ventral curvature of penis, often associated with hypospadias	Surgical release of fibrous band causing deformity
Epispadias—Meatal opening located on dorsal surface of penis	Surgical correction, usually including penile and urethral lengthening and bladder neck reconstruction (if necessary)

Cryptorchidism—Failure of one or both testes to descend normally through inguinal canal	Detected by inability to palpate testes within scrotum
	Medical—Administration of human chorionic gonadotropin (older child)
	Surgical—Orchiopexy
	Objectives of therapy:
	    Prevent damage to undescended testicle
	    Decrease incidence of malignant tumor formation
	    Avoid trauma and torsion
	    Close inguinal canal
	    Prevent cosmetic and psychologic disability from empty scrotum

Exstrophy of bladder—Eversion of posterior bladder through anterior bladder wall and lower abdominal wall; associated with open pubic arch (severe defect)	Potential objectives of surgical correction:
	    Preserve renal function
	    Attain urinary control
	    Provide adequate reconstructive repair
	    Improve sexual function (especially in males)

Disorders of Sexual Differentiation	
Masculinized female (female pseudohermaphrodite)	Assign gender as female; assign gender while avoiding irreversible surgery, realizing that some children may change gender later in life; family participation essential
Incompletely masculinized male (male pseudohermaphrodite)	Assign gender while avoiding irreversible surgery, realizing that some children may change gender later in life; family participation essential
True hermaphrodite (both ovaries and testes)	Assign gender while avoiding irreversible surgery, realizing that some children may change gender later in life; gender assignment depends on predominant characteristics; family participation essential
Mixed gonadal dysgenesis	Assign gender while avoiding irreversible surgery, realizing that some children may change gender later in life; gender assignment depends on predominant characteristics; family participation essential

based in large part on these psychologic variables. The earlier a repair can be achieved, the more likely it is that the child will develop a normal body image.

During the years from ages 3 to 6 (i.e., the phallic-oedipal period), children show a strong interest and concern about the genital area, sex differences, and genital normality or its lack. It is also a time when children are frightened of what they perceive to be threats to their body and bodily function. They also view any untoward happening as a punishment for real or imagined wrongdoing or unacceptable sexual feelings such as masturbation, sex play, or erotic feelings. Surgical repair is recommended before these fears and anxieties develop.

After extensive review of the emotional, cognitive, and body image problems that may occur in children undergoing surgical reconstruction of a genital deformity, Kass (1996) recommended that surgery be accomplished between the ages of 6 and 15 months to minimize the psychologic effects of surgery and anesthesia.

CARE MANAGEMENT

Preparing children and their families for diagnostic and surgical procedures (see Preparation for Diagnostic and Therapeutic Procedures, Chapter 39) and for home care is a major nursing function. Most postoperative care involves care of the surgical site. Tub baths are discouraged for 1 week after simple surgeries. The surgical site is kept clean and otherwise protected from infection and inspected for signs of infection. Dressings, if any, are inspected regularly. More complex surgeries require additional care and observation (e.g., catheter care for urethral reconstruction and care of urinary diversion stomas and collection devices).

Some older children's activities such as pushing, lifting, playing with straddle toys or in sandboxes, swimming, and rough activities may be restricted after some types of surgical repairs. Precise restrictions depend on the specific type of surgery. Activities of infants and toddlers are not limited.

In most cases the results of surgery are satisfactory. However, in some of the more severe defects such as exstrophy and those that require stomas, additional emotional interventions may be needed. A major concern of parents and children is related to surgery affecting the genitalia directly. Concerns about penis size, appearance of the genitalia, potential ability to procreate, and rejection by peers (especially the opposite sex) are potential fears that require psychologic adjustment, particularly during adolescence.

GLOMERULAR DISEASE

Nephrotic Syndrome

Nephrotic syndrome is a clinical state that includes massive proteinuria, hypoalbuminemia, hyperlipidemia, and edema. The disorder can occur as (1) a primary disease known as idiopathic nephrosis, childhood nephrosis, or minimal-change nephrotic syndrome (MCNS); (2) a secondary disorder that occurs as a clinical manifestation after or in association with glomerular damage that has a known or presumed cause; or (3) a congenital form inherited as an autosomal recessive disorder. The disorder is characterized by increased glomerular permeability to plasma protein, which results in massive urinary protein loss. The glomerulus is responsible for the initial step in the formation of urine, and the filtration rate depends on an intact glomerular membrane. This discussion is devoted to MCNS because it constitutes 80% of nephrotic syndrome cases.

Pathophysiology

The onset of MCNS can occur at any age but predominantly occurs in children between 2 and 7 years of age. It is rare in children younger than 6 months of age, uncommon in infants younger than 1 year of age, and unusual after the age of 8 years. Patients with MCNS are twice as likely to be male.

The pathogenesis of MCNS is not fully understood. There may be a metabolic, biochemical, physiochemical, or immune-mediated disturbance that causes the basement membrane of the glomeruli to become increasingly permeable to protein; but the cause and mechanisms are only speculative.

The glomerular membrane, normally impermeable to albumin and other proteins, becomes permeable to proteins, especially albumin, that leak through the membrane and are lost in urine (hyperalbuminuria). This reduces the serum albumin level (hypoalbuminemia), decreasing the colloidal osmotic pressure in the capillaries. As a result the vascular hydrostatic pressure exceeds the pull of the colloidal osmotic pressure, causing fluid to accumulate in the interstitial spaces (edema) and body cavities, particularly in the abdominal cavity (ascites). The shift of fluid from the plasma to the interstitial spaces reduces the vascular fluid volume (hypovolemia), which in turn stimulates the renin-angiotensin system and the secretion of antidiuretic hormone and aldosterone. Tubular reabsorption of sodium and water is increased in an attempt to increase intravascular volume. The elevation of serum lipids is not fully understood. The sequence of events in nephrotic syndrome is diagrammed in Fig. 44-3.

Diagnostic Evaluation

The disease is suspected on the basis of clinical manifestations (Box 44-2), especially when weight gain in a previously well child increases slowly over days or weeks. The generalized edema may develop rapidly or gradually but eventually prompts the family to seek medical attention. Parents usually give a history of the child being well but steadily gaining weight; appearing edematous; and then becoming anorexic, irritable, and less active.

The diagnosis of MCNS is suspected on the basis of the history and clinical manifestations (edema, proteinuria, hypoalbuminemia, and hypercholesterolemia in the absence of hematuria and hypertension) in children between the ages of 2 and 8 years. The hallmark of MCNS is massive proteinuria (higher than 2+ on urine dipstick). Hyaline casts, oval fat bodies, and a few red blood cells (RBCs) can be found in the urine of some affected children, although there is seldom gross hematuria. The GFR is usually normal or high.

Total serum protein concentration is low, with the serum albumin significantly reduced and plasma lipids elevated. Hemoglobin and hematocrit are usually normal or elevated as a result of hemoconcentration. The platelet count may be elevated. Serum sodium concentration may be low. If the patient does not respond to a 4- to 8-week course of steroids, a renal biopsy may be needed to distinguish among other types of nephrotic syndrome. The biopsy results of children with MCNS are remarkable for effacement of the foot processes of the epithelial cells lining the basement membrane, but otherwise the kidney tissue is normal.

Therapeutic Management

Objectives of therapeutic management include (1) reducing excretion of urinary protein, (2) reducing fluid retention in the tissues, (3) preventing infection, and (4) minimizing complications related to therapies. Dietary restrictions include a low-salt diet and in more severe cases fluid restriction. If complications of edema develop, diuretic therapy may be initiated to provide temporary relief. Sometimes infusions of 25% albumin are used. Acute infections are treated with appropriate antibiotics.

Corticosteroids are the first line of therapy for MCNS. The starting dosage for prednisone is usually 2 mg/kg of body weight per day for 6 weeks followed by 1.5 mg/kg every other day for 6 weeks (Gipson, Massengill, Yao, et al., 2009). Approximately two thirds of children with MCNS have a relapse, heralded first by increased urine protein. Relapses can be diagnosed early if parents are taught routine home monitoring of urine protein by dipstick. They are treated with a repeated, but usually shorter, course of high-dose steroid therapy. Side effects of the steroids include weight gain, rounding of the face, behavior changes, and increased appetite. Long-term therapy may result in hirsutism, growth retardation, cataracts, hypertension, gastrointestinal bleeding, bone demineralization, infection, and hyperglycemia. Children who do not respond to steroid therapy, those who have frequent relapses, and those in whom the side effects threaten their growth and general health may be considered for a course of therapy using other immunosuppressant medications (cyclophosphamide, chlorambucil, or cyclosporine).

Episodes of MCNS, both the first episode and relapse, often happen in conjunction with a viral or bacterial infection. Relapses can also be triggered by allergies and immunizations. Relapses in children with MCNS may continue over many years.

Complications of nephrotic syndrome include infection, circulatory insufficiency secondary to hypovolemia, and thromboembolism. Infections that may be seen in children with nephrotic syndrome include peritonitis, cellulitis, and pneumonia and require

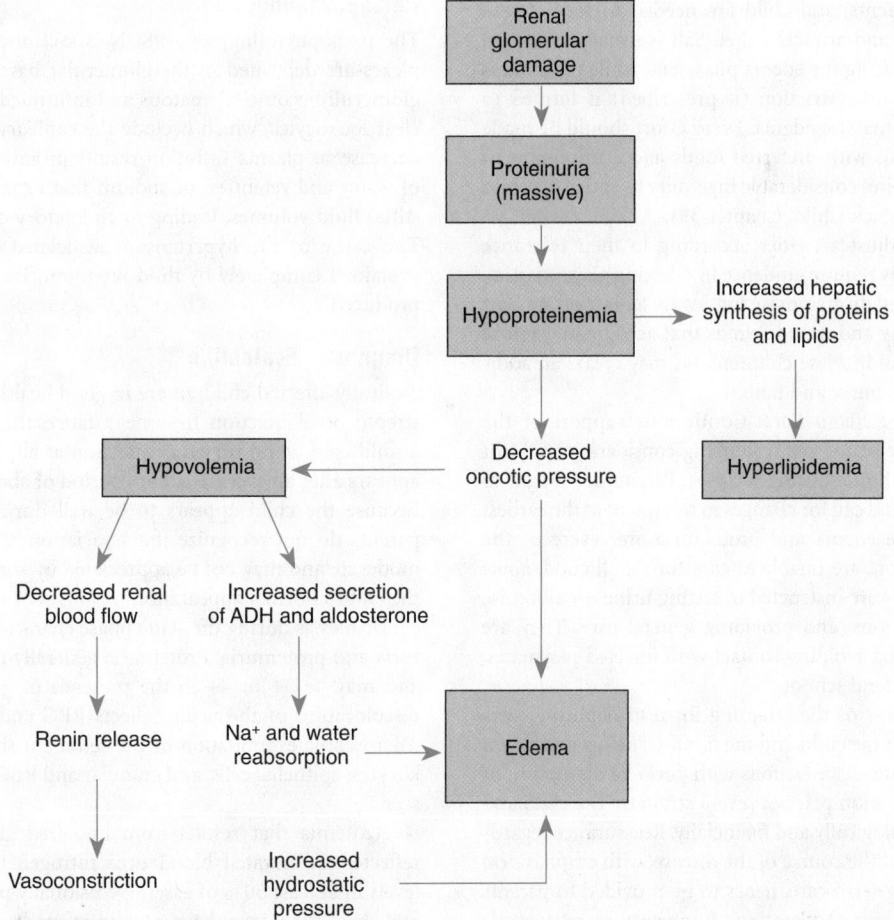

FIG 44-3 Sequence of events in nephrotic syndrome. *ADH,* Antidiuretic hormone.

prompt recognition and vigorous treatment with appropriate antibiotic therapy.

Prognosis. The prognosis for ultimate recovery in most cases is good. It is a self-limiting disease, and in children who respond to steroid therapy the tendency to relapse decreases with time. With early detection and prompt implementation of therapy to eradicate proteinuria, progressive basement membrane damage is minimized so that, when the tendency to relapse is past, renal function is usually normal or near normal. It is estimated that approximately 80% of affected children have this favorable prognosis.

CARE MANAGEMENT

Continuous monitoring of fluid retention or excretion is an important nursing function. Strict intake and output records are essential but may be difficult to obtain from very young children. Application of collection bags is irritating to edematous skin that is readily subject to breakdown. Applying diapers or weighing wet pads may be necessary.

Other methods of monitoring progress include urine examination for albumin, daily weight, and measurement of abdominal girth. Assessment of edema (e.g., increased or decreased swelling around the eyes and dependent areas), the degree of pitting, and the color and texture of skin are part of nursing care. Vital signs are monitored to detect any early signs of complications such as shock or an infective process.

Infection is a constant source of danger to edematous children and those receiving corticosteroid therapy. These children are particularly vulnerable to upper respiratory tract infection; therefore they must be kept warm and dry, active, and protected from contact with infected individuals (e.g., roommates, visitors, and personnel). Vital signs are monitored to detect any early signs of an infective process.

Loss of appetite accompanying active nephrosis creates a perplexing problem for nurses. During this time the combined efforts of nurse, dietitian, parents, and child are needed to formulate a nutritionally adequate and attractive diet. Salt is usually restricted (but not eliminated) during the edema phase and while the child is on steroid therapy. Fluid restriction (if prescribed) is limited to short-term use during massive edema. Every effort should be made to serve attractive meals with preferred foods and a minimum of fuss, but it usually requires considerable ingenuity to entice the child to eat (see Feeding the Sick Child, Chapter 39).

Children usually adjust activities according to their tolerance level. However, they may require guidance in selecting play activities. Suitable recreational and diversional activities are an important part of their care. Irritability and mood swings that accompany steroid therapy are not unusual in these children and may create an additional challenge for the nurse and family.

Family Support and Home Care. Continuous support of the child and family is one of the major nursing considerations. Most children are treated at home during relapses. Parents are taught to detect signs of relapse and call for changes in treatment at the earliest indications. Unless the edema and proteinuria are severe or the parents, for some reason, are unable to care for the ill child, *home care is preferred.* Parents are instructed in testing urine for albumin, administering medications, and providing general care. They are also instructed regarding avoiding contact with infected playmates, but the child should attend school.

The prolonged course of the relapsing form of nephrotic syndrome is taxing to both the child and the family. The up-and-down course of remissions and exacerbations with periodic disruption of family life by hospitalization places a severe strain on the child and the family, both psychologically and financially. Reassurance regarding this characteristic of the course of the disease, with emphasis on the importance of long-term care, needs to be provided to parents and children to gain their cooperation. A satisfactory response is more likely when relapses are detected and therapy is instituted early, and remissions are prolonged when instructions are carried out faithfully. Continuous support of the child and family is one of the major nursing considerations (see Chapter 36).

Acute Glomerulonephritis

Acute glomerulonephritis (AGN) may be a primary event or a manifestation of a systemic disorder that can range from minimal to severe. Common features include oliguria, edema, hypertension and circulatory congestion, hematuria, and proteinuria. Most cases are postinfectious and have been associated with pneumococcal, streptococcal, and viral infections. Acute poststreptococcal glomerulonephritis (APSGN) is the most common of the postinfectious renal diseases in childhood and the one for which a cause can be established in the majority of cases. It can occur at any age but affects primarily early school-age children, with a peak age of onset of 6 to 7 years. It is uncommon in children younger than 2 years of age, and boys outnumber girls two to one.

Etiology

APSGN is an immune-complex disease that occurs after an antecedent streptococcal infection with certain strains of the group A β-hemolytic streptococcus. Most streptococcal infections *do not* cause APSGN. A latent period of 10 to 21 days occurs between the streptococcal infection and the onset of clinical manifestations. Disease secondary to streptococcal pharyngitis is more common in the winter or spring; however, when APSGN is associated with pyoderma (principally impetigo), it may be more prevalent in later summer or early fall, especially in warmer climates. Second episodes of AGN are rare.

Pathophysiology

The pathophysiology of APSGN is still uncertain. Immune complexes are deposited in the glomerular basement membrane. The glomeruli become edematous and infiltrated with polymorphonuclear leukocytes, which occlude the capillary lumen. The resulting decrease in plasma filtration results in an excessive accumulation of water and retention of sodium that expands plasma and interstitial fluid volumes, leading to circulatory congestion and edema. The cause of the hypertension associated with AGN cannot be explained completely by fluid retention. Excess renin may also be produced.

Diagnostic Evaluation

Typically affected children are in good health until they experience streptococcal infection. In some instances they have a history of only a mild cold or no previous infection at all. The onset of nephritis appears after an average latency period of about 10 days (Box 44-3). Because the child appears to be well during the latency period, parents do not recognize the association. The edema is relatively moderate and may not be appreciated by someone unfamiliar with the child's normal appearance.

Urinalysis during the acute phase characteristically shows hematuria and proteinuria. Proteinuria generally parallels the hematuria and may be 3+ or 4+ in the presence of gross hematuria. Gross discoloration of the urine reflects RBC and hemoglobin content. Microscopic examination of the sediment shows many RBCs, leukocytes, epithelial cells, and granular and RBC casts. Bacteria are not seen.

Azotemia that results from impaired glomerular filtration is reflected in elevated blood urea nitrogen (BUN) and creatinine levels in at least 50% of cases. Occasionally proteinuria is excessive, and the patient may have nephrotic syndrome (i.e., hypoproteinemia and hyperlipidemia).

Cultures of the pharynx are rarely positive for streptococci because the renal disease occurs weeks after the infection.

BOX 44-3 **CLINICAL MANIFESTATIONS OF ACUTE POSTSTREPTOCOCCAL GLOMERULONEPHRITIS**

- Edema:
  - Especially periorbital
  - Facial edema more prominent in the morning
  - Spreads during the day to involve extremities and abdomen
- Anorexia
- Urine:
  - Cloudy, smoky brown (resembles tea or cola)
  - Severely reduced volume
- Pallor
- Irritability
- Lethargy
- Child appearing ill
- Child seldom expresses specific complaints
- Older children complaining of the following:
  - Headaches
  - Abdominal discomfort
  - Dysuria
- Vomiting possible
- Mildly to severely elevated blood pressure

Some serologic tests are necessary to make the diagnosis of AGN. Circulating serum antibodies to streptococci indicate the presence of a previous infection. The antistreptolysin O (ASO) titer is the most familiar and readily available test for streptococcal infection. Other antibodies that may aid in diagnosis are elevated antihyaluronidase (AHase), antideoxyribonuclease B (ADNase-B), and streptozyme.

All patients with APSGN have reduced serum complement (C3) activity in the early stages of the disease. Rising C3 levels are used as a guide to indicate improvement of the disease and should be normal in almost all patients 8 weeks after the disease onset.

Studies that may be useful include chest x-ray film examination, which generally shows cardiac enlargement, pulmonary congestion, or pleural effusion during the edematous phase of acute disease. Renal biopsy for diagnostic purposes is seldom required but may be useful in the diagnosis of atypical cases.

Therapeutic Management

Management consists of general supportive measures and early recognition and treatment of complications. Children who have normal blood pressure and a satisfactory urinary output can generally be treated at home. Those with substantial edema, hypertension, gross hematuria, or significant oliguria should be hospitalized because of the unpredictability of complications.

Dietary restrictions depend on the stage and severity of the disease, especially the extent of edema. Moderate sodium restriction and even fluid restriction may be instituted for children with hypertension and edema. Foods with substantial amounts of potassium are generally restricted during the period of oliguria.

Regular measurement of vital signs, body weight, and intake and output is essential to monitor the progress of the disease and detect complications that may appear at any time during its course. *A record of daily weight is the most useful means for assessing fluid balance.* Rarely children with AGN develop acute renal failure (ARF) with oliguria that significantly alters the fluid and electrolyte balance (resulting in hyperkalemia, acidosis, hypocalcemia, or hyperphosphatemia). These children require careful management. Peritoneal dialysis or hemodialysis is seldom needed.

Acute hypertension must be anticipated and identified early. Blood pressure measurements are taken every 4 to 6 hours. A variety of antihypertensive medications and diuretics are used to control hypertension. Antibiotic therapy is indicated only for children with evidence of persistent streptococcal infections. It is used to prevent transmission of nephritogenic streptococci to other family members.

Prognosis. Almost all children correctly diagnosed as having APSGN recover completely, and specific immunity is conferred; thus subsequent recurrences are uncommon. Some of these children have been reported to develop chronic disease, but most of these cases are now believed to be different glomerular diseases misdiagnosed as poststreptococcal disease.

CARE MANAGEMENT

Nursing care of the child with glomerulonephritis involves careful assessment of the disease status, with regular monitoring of vital signs (including frequent measurement of blood pressure), fluid balance, and behavior.

Vital signs provide clues to the severity of the disease and early signs of complications. They are carefully measured, and any deviations are reported and recorded. The volume and character of urine are noted, and the child is weighed daily. Children with restricted fluid intake, especially those who are not severely edematous or those who have lost weight, are observed for signs of dehydration.

Assessment of the child's appearance for signs of cerebral complications is an important nursing function because the severity of the acute phase is variable and unpredictable. The child with edema, hypertension, and gross hematuria may be subject to complications; anticipatory preparations such as seizure precautions and intravenous (IV) equipment are included in the nursing care plan.

For most children a regular diet is allowed, but it should contain no added salt. Foods high in sodium and salted treats are eliminated, and parents and friends are advised not to bring snacks such as potato chips or pretzels. However, the total amount of salt ingested is usually less than prescribed because of the child's poor appetite. Fluid restriction, if prescribed, is more difficult, and the amount permitted should be divided evenly throughout the waking hours. Meal preparation and service require special attention because the child is indifferent to meals during the acute phase. Again collaboration with parents and the dietitian and special consideration for food preferences facilitate meal planning.

During the acute phase children are generally content to lie in bed. As they begin to feel better and their symptoms subside, they want to be up and about. Activities should be planned to allow for frequent rest periods and avoidance of fatigue. Children who have mild edema and no hypertension and convalescent children who are being treated at home need follow-up care. Parents are instructed regarding general measures, including diet and prevention of infection.

Health supervision is continued with weekly followed by monthly visits for evaluation and urinalysis. Parent education and support in preparation for discharge and home care include education in home management and the need for follow-up care and health supervision.

MISCELLANEOUS RENAL DISORDERS

Hemolytic Uremic Syndrome

Hemolytic uremic syndrome (HUS) is an uncommon, acute renal disease that occurs primarily in infants and small children between the ages of 6 months and 5 years. It is one of the most frequent causes of acquired ARF in children (Duzova, Bakkaloglu, Kalyoncu, et al., 2010). The clinical features of the disease include acquired hemolytic anemia, thrombocytopenia, renal injury, and central nervous system (CNS) symptoms. The etiology of HUS is thought to be associated with bacterial toxins, chemicals, and viruses. The appearance of the disease has been associated with *Rickettsia* organisms, viruses (especially coxsackievirus, echovirus, and adenovirus), *E. coli,* pneumococci, shigellae, and salmonellae and may represent an unusual response to these infections. Multiple cases of HUS caused by enteric infection of the *E. coli* O157:H7 serotype have been traced to undercooked meat, especially ground beef. Other sources are unpasteurized milk or fruit juice, especially apple; alfalfa sprouts; lettuce; and salami. Drinking or swimming in sewage-contaminated water can also cause infection. The clinical presentation is usually a history of a prodromal illness (most often gastroenteritis or an upper respiratory tract infection) followed by the sudden onset of hemolysis and renal failure.

Pathophysiology

The primary site of injury appears to be the endothelial lining of the small glomerular arterioles, which become swollen and occluded with deposits of platelets and fibrin clots (intravascular coagulation). RBCs are damaged as they attempt to move through the

BOX 44-4	CLINICAL MANIFESTATIONS OF HEMOLYTIC UREMIC SYNDROME

- Vomiting
- Irritability
- Lethargy
- Marked pallor
- Hemorrhagic manifestations:
  - Bruising
  - Petechiae
  - Jaundice
  - Bloody diarrhea
- Oliguria or anuria
- CNS involvement:
  - Seizures
  - Stupor or coma
- Signs of acute heart failure (sometimes)

CNS, Central nervous system.

BOX 44-5	CLINICAL MANIFESTATIONS OF WILMS' TUMOR

- Abdominal swelling or mass:
  - Firm
  - Nontender
  - Confined to one side
- Hematuria (less than one fourth of cases)
- Fatigue and malaise
- Hypertension (occasionally)
- Weight loss
- Fever
- Manifestations resulting from compression of tumor mass
- Secondary metabolic alterations from tumor or metastasis
- If metastasis, symptoms of lung involvement:
  - Dyspnea
  - Cough
  - Shortness of breath
  - Chest pain (sometimes)

partially occluded blood vessels. These damaged cells are removed by the spleen, causing acute hemolytic anemia. The platelet aggregation within the damaged blood vessels or the damage and removal of platelets produce the characteristic thrombocytopenia.

Diagnostic Evaluation

The triad of anemia, thrombocytopenia, and renal failure is sufficient for diagnosis (Box 44-4). Renal involvement is evidenced by proteinuria, hematuria, and urinary casts; BUN and serum creatinine levels are elevated. A low hemoglobin and hematocrit and a high reticulocyte count confirm the hemolytic nature of the anemia.

Therapeutic Management

The goals of therapy are early diagnosis and aggressive, supportive care of the ARF and hemolytic anemia. The most consistently effective treatment of HUS is hemodialysis or peritoneal dialysis, which is instituted in any child who has been anuric for 24 hours or who demonstrates oliguria with uremia or hypertension and seizures. Other treatments include use of pharmacologic agents, fresh-frozen plasma, and plasmapheresis. Blood transfusions with fresh, washed packed cells are administered for severe anemia but are used with caution to prevent circulatory overload from added volume.

Prognosis. With prompt treatment, the recovery rate is about 95%, but residual renal impairment ranges from 10% to 50%. Long-term complications include CRF, hypertension, and CNS disorders. Death is usually caused by residual renal impairment or CNS injury.

CARE MANAGEMENT

Nursing care is the same as that provided in ARF and, for children with continued impairment, includes management of chronic disease. Because of the sudden and life-threatening nature of the disorder in a previously well child, parents are often ill prepared for the impact of hospitalization and treatment. Therefore support and understanding are especially important aspects of care.

Wilms' Tumor

Wilms' tumor, or nephroblastoma, is the most common malignant renal and intraabdominal tumor of childhood. The incidence is estimated to be eight cases per million children. Approximately 500 new cases are diagnosed each year in the United States, with 6% involving both kidneys (Cendron and Gomez, 2010).Wilms' tumor occurs about 3 times more often in African-Americans than in East Asians in the United States. The peak age at diagnosis is approximately 3 years, and occurrence is slightly more frequent in boys than

in girls. The majority of patients with Wilms' tumor are diagnosed at younger than 5 years of age, with 1% to 2.5% having a familial origin. Unfortunately there is no method of identifying gene carriers at this time.

Etiology

Wilms' tumor probably arises from a malignant, undifferentiated cluster of primordial cells capable of initiating the regeneration of an abnormal structure. Its occurrence slightly favors the left kidney, which is advantageous because surgically this kidney is easier to manipulate and remove. In about 10% of cases both kidneys are involved. Studies have shown that development of Wilms' tumor is frequently associated with aniridia, hemihypertrophy, Beckwith-Wiedemann syndrome, or genitourinary anomalies (Cendron and Gomez, 2010; Dome, Perlman, Ritchey, et al., 2006).

Diagnostic Evaluation

In a child suspected of having Wilms' tumor, special emphasis is placed on the history and physical examination for the presence of congenital anomalies, a family history of cancer, and signs of malignancy (e.g., weight loss, size of liver and spleen, indications of anemia, lymphadenopathy). Most children with Wilms' tumor are brought to the practitioner because of abdominal swelling or an abdominal mass (Box 44-5). Specific tests include radiographic studies, including abdominal ultrasonography and abdominal and chest computed tomography scan; hematologic studies; biochemical studies; and urinalysis. Studies to demonstrate the relationship of the tumor to the ipsilateral kidney and the presence of a normal, functioning kidney on the contralateral side are essential. If a large tumor is present, an inferior venacavogram is necessary to demonstrate possible tumor involvement adjacent to the vena cava. A bone marrow aspiration may be performed to rule out metastasis, which is rare in children with Wilms' tumor.

!	NURSING ALERT

To reinforce the need for caution, it may be necessary to post a sign on the bed that reads, "DO NOT PALPATE ABDOMEN." Careful bathing and handling are also important in preventing trauma to the tumor site.

Therapeutic Management

Combined treatment with surgery and chemotherapy with or without radiation is based on the histologic pattern and clinical stage.

Surgery is scheduled as soon as possible after confirmation of a renal mass, usually within 24 to 48 hours of admission. A large transabdominal incision is performed for optimal visualization of the abdominal cavity. The tumor, affected kidney, and adjacent adrenal gland are removed. Great care is taken to keep the encapsulated tumor intact because rupture can seed cancer cells throughout the abdomen, lymph channel, and bloodstream. The contralateral kidney is inspected carefully for evidence of disease or dysfunction. Regional lymph nodes are inspected, and a biopsy is performed when indicated. Any involved structures such as part of the colon, diaphragm, or vena cava are removed. Metal clips are placed around the tumor site for exact marking during radiotherapy.

If both kidneys are involved, the child may be treated with radiotherapy or chemotherapy before surgery to decrease the size of the tumor, allowing more conservative surgery. It may be possible to perform a partial nephrectomy on the less affected kidney, with a total nephrectomy on the opposite side. When a transplant is feasible such as from a twin, sibling, or parent, bilateral nephrectomy is considered as a last resort.

Postoperative radiotherapy is indicated for children with large tumors, metastasis, residual postoperative disease, unfavorable histologic characteristics, or recurrence. Chemotherapy is indicated for all stages. The most effective agents for treating Wilms' tumor are actinomycin D (dactinomycin), vincristine, and Adriamycin, with the addition of cyclophosphamide for unfavorable histology or advanced disease (Cendron and Gomez, 2010; Dome, Perlman, Ritchey, et al., 2006). The duration of therapy ranges from 6 to 15 months.

Prognosis. Survival rates for Wilms' tumor are the highest among all childhood cancers. Children with localized tumor (stages I and II) have a 90% chance of cure with multimodal therapy. Factors that favorably affect the success of further therapy include initial treatment with only vincristine and dactinomycin, relapse to the lungs only, relapse in the abdomen of a patient who received no prior abdominal irradiation, and relapse more than 12 months after diagnosis. Wilms' tumor may recur, especially in the lungs. Both chemotherapy and radiotherapy can induce second malignancies, usually in areas that have been irradiated (Cendron and Gomez, 2010; Dome, Perlman, Ritchey, et al., 2006).

CARE MANAGEMENT

Nursing care of the child with Wilms' tumor is similar to that of children with other cancers treated with surgery, irradiation, and chemotherapy. However, there are some significant differences; these are discussed for each phase of nursing intervention.

Preoperative Care. The preoperative period is one of swift diagnosis. The nurse faces the challenge of preparing the child and parents for all laboratory and operative procedures within 24 to 48 hours of admission. Because of the minimal preparatory time, explanations should be simple, repetitive, and focused on the child's actual experiences. In addition to the usual preoperative observations, blood pressure is monitored because hypertension from excess renin production is a possibility.

There are several special preoperative concerns, the most important of which is that the *tumor is not palpated unless absolutely necessary* because manipulation of the mass may cause dissemination of cancer cells to adjacent and distant sites.

Because radiotherapy and chemotherapy are usually begun immediately after surgery, parents need an explanation of what to expect such as major benefits and side effects. The timing of the information should be considered to avoid overwhelming the family. Ideally the nurse should be present during physician-parent conferences to answer questions as they arise. It is usually better to postpone telling the child about these side effects until after surgery. Alopecia, usually of most concern to older children, does not occur until approximately 2 weeks after the initial treatment regimen. Therefore the child can be prepared for the hair loss after surgery.

Postoperative Care. Despite the extensive surgical intervention necessary in many children with Wilms' tumor, the recovery is usually rapid. The major nursing responsibilities are the same as those after any abdominal surgery (see Surgical Procedures, Chapter 39). Because these children are at risk for intestinal obstruction from vincristine-induced ileus, radiation-induced edema, and postsurgical adhesion formation, the nurse carefully monitors gastrointestinal activity such as bowel movements, bowel sounds, distention, vomiting, and pain. She or he also monitors blood pressure, urinary output, and signs of infection and institutes pulmonary hygiene to prevent postoperative pulmonary complications.

Family Support. The postoperative period is frequently difficult for parents. The shock of seeing their child immediately after surgery may be the first realization of the seriousness of the diagnosis. It also marks the confirmation of the stage of the tumor. During this period the nurse should be with the parents to assure them of the child's recovery after surgery and assess their understanding of the total experience. They need an opportunity to express their feelings and need to be provided the same emotional care discussed in Chapter 36 for families who have a child with a life-threatening disorder.

> **! NURSING ALERT**
>
> Prompt detection and treatment of any genitourinary signs or symptoms are mandatory. Children with a solitary kidney should be assessed and advised about the need for protective equipment before engaging in contact, collision, or limited contact activities (Rice and Council on Sports Medicine and Fitness, 2008).

Older children need an opportunity to deal with their feelings concerning the many procedures to which they have been subjected in rapid succession. Play therapy with dolls or puppets or through drawing can be extremely beneficial in helping them adjust. It is not unusual for children to feel angry because of the extent of surgery, the need for additional therapy, or the seriousness of the disorder.

RENAL FAILURE

Renal failure is the inability of the kidneys to excrete waste material, concentrate urine, and conserve electrolytes. It can occur suddenly (acute renal failure [ARF]) in response to inadequate perfusion, kidney disease, or urinary tract obstruction; or it can develop slowly (chronic renal failure [CRF]) as a result of longstanding kidney disease or an anomaly.

Azotemia and *uremia* are terms often used in relation to renal failure. Azotemia is the accumulation of nitrogenous waste within the blood. Uremia is a more advanced condition in which retention of nitrogenous products produces toxic symptoms. Azotemia is not life threatening, but uremia is a serious condition that often involves other body systems.

Acute Renal Failure

ARF is said to exist when the kidneys suddenly are unable to regulate the volume and composition of urine appropriately in response to food and fluid intake and the needs of the organism. The principal feature of ARF is oliguria* associated with azotemia, metabolic acidosis, and diverse electrolyte disturbances. ARF is not common in childhood; but the outcome depends on the cause, associated findings, and prompt recognition and treatment.

The pathologic conditions that produce ARF caused by glomerulonephritis and HUS are discussed in relation to those disorders. ARF can also develop as a result of a large number of related or unrelated clinical conditions: poor renal perfusion; urinary tract obstruction; acute renal injury; or the final expression of chronic, irreversible renal disease. The most common cause in children is transient renal failure resulting from severe dehydration or other causes of poor perfusion that may respond to restoration of fluid volume.

Pathophysiology

ARF is usually reversible, but the deviations of physiologic function can be extreme, and mortality in the pediatric age-group remains high. There is severe reduction in the GFR, an elevated BUN level, and a significant reduction in renal blood flow.

The clinical course varies and depends on the cause. In reversible ARF there is a period of severe oliguria, or a low-output phase, followed by an abrupt onset of diuresis, or a high-output phase, and then a gradual return to (or toward) normal urine volumes.

Diagnostic Evaluation

In many instances of ARF, the infant or child is already critically ill with the precipitating disorder, and the explanation for development of oliguria may or may not be readily apparent (Box 44-6). When a previously well child develops ARF without an obvious cause, a careful history is taken to reveal symptoms that may be related to glomerulonephritis, obstructive uropathy, or exposure to nephrotoxic chemicals (e.g., ingestion of heavy metals, inhalation of carbon tetrachloride or other organic solvents, or medications such as nonsteroidal antiinflammatory drugs [Patzer, 2008] known to be toxic to the kidneys). Significant laboratory measurements during renal shutdown that serve as a guide for therapy are BUN, serum creatinine, pH, sodium, potassium, and calcium.

> **! NURSING ALERT**
>
> Diminished urinary output and lethargy in a child who is dehydrated, is in shock, or has recently undergone surgery should be evaluated for possible ARF.

> **! NURSING ALERT**
>
> Any of the following signs of hyperkalemia constitute an emergency and are reported immediately:
> - Serum potassium concentrations in excess of 7 mEq/L
> - Presence of electrocardiographic abnormalities, such as prolonged QRS complex, depressed ST segment, high peaked T waves, bradycardia, or heart block

*The definition of oliguria varies extensively in the literature, from 1.8 to 4 dL/m^2/24 hr.

BOX 44-6   CLINICAL MANIFESTATIONS OF ACUTE RENAL FAILURE

- Specific:
  - Oliguria
  - Anuria uncommon (except in obstructive disorders)
- Nonspecific (may develop):
  - Nausea
  - Vomiting
  - Drowsiness
  - Edema
  - Hypertension
- Manifestations of underlying disorder or pathologic condition

---

Therapeutic Management

Treatment of ARF is directed toward (1) treatment of the underlying cause, (2) management of the complications of renal failure, and (3) provision of supportive therapy within the constraints imposed by the renal failure.

Treatment of poor perfusion resulting from dehydration consists of volume restoration, as described in Chapter 41 in treatment of dehydration. If oliguria persists after restoration of fluid volume or if the renal failure is caused by intrinsic renal damage, the physiologic and biochemical abnormalities that have resulted from kidney dysfunction must be corrected or controlled. Initially a Foley catheter is inserted to rule out urine retention, collect available urine for analysis, and monitor results of diuretic administration. The catheter may or may not be removed during the oliguric phase.

The amount of exogenous water provided should not exceed the amount needed to maintain zero water balance. It is calculated on the basis of estimated endogenous water formation and losses from sensible (primarily gastrointestinal) and insensible sources. No allotment is calculated for urine as long as oliguria persists.

When the output begins to increase, either spontaneously or in response to diuretic therapy, the intake of fluid, potassium, and sodium must be monitored, and adequate replacement provided to prevent depletion and its consequences. Some patients pass enormous amounts of electrolyte-rich urine.

Complications. The child with ARF has a tendency to develop water intoxication and hyponatremia, which makes it difficult to provide calories in sufficient amounts to meet his or her needs and reduce tissue catabolism, metabolic acidosis, hyperkalemia, and uremia. If the child is able to tolerate oral foods, food sources high in concentrated carbohydrate and fat but low in protein, potassium, and sodium may be provided. However, many children have functional disturbances of the gastrointestinal tract such as nausea and vomiting; therefore the IV route generally is preferred and usually consists of essential amino acids or a combination of essential and nonessential amino acids administered by the central venous route.

Control of water balance in these patients requires careful monitoring of feedback information such as accurate intake and output, body weight, and electrolyte measurements. In general, during the oliguric phase no sodium, chloride, or potassium is given unless there are other large, ongoing losses. Regular measurement of plasma electrolyte, pH, BUN, and creatinine levels is required to assess the adequacy of fluid therapy and anticipate complications that require specific treatment.

Hyperkalemia is the most immediate threat to the life of the child with ARF. It can be minimized and sometimes avoided by eliminating potassium from all food and fluid, reducing tissue catabolism, and correcting acidosis. Measures used for the reduction of serum potassium levels are oral or rectal administration of an ion-exchange resin such as sodium polystyrene sulfonate (Kayexalate) and peritoneal dialysis or hemodialysis (see p. 1414). The resin produces its effect by exchange of its sodium for the potassium, thus binding potassium for removal from the body. This increased sodium concentration may contribute to fluid overload, hypertension, and cardiac failure. Dialysis removes potassium and other waste products from the serum by diffusion through a semipermeable membrane.

Hypertension is a frequent and serious complication of ARF; to detect it early, blood pressure measurements are made every 4 to 6 hours. The most common cause of hypertension in ARF is overexpansion of extracellular fluid and plasma volume together with activation of the renin-angiotensin system. Hypertension is controlled with antihypertensive drugs. Other measures that may be used include limiting fluids and salt.

Anemia is frequently associated with ARF, but transfusion is not recommended unless the hemoglobin drops below 6 g/dL. Transfusions, if used, consist of fresh, packed RBCs given slowly to reduce the likelihood of increasing blood volume, hypertension, and hyperkalemia.

Seizures occur often when renal failure progresses to uremia and are also related to hypertension, hyponatremia, and hypocalcemia. Treatment is directed to the specific cause when known. More obscure causes are managed with antiepileptic drugs.

Cardiac failure with pulmonary edema is almost always associated with hypervolemia. Treatment is directed toward reduction of fluid volume, with water and sodium restriction and administration of diuretics.

Prognosis. The prognosis of ARF depends largely on the nature and severity of the causative factor or precipitating event and the promptness and competence of management. The outcome is least favorable in children with rapidly progressive nephritis and cortical necrosis. Children in whom ARF is a result of HUS or AGN may recover completely, but residual renal impairment or hypertension is more often the rule. Complete recovery is usually expected in children whose renal failure is a result of dehydration, nephrotoxins, or ischemia. ARF after cardiac surgery is less favorable. It is often impossible to assess the extent of recovery for several months.

CARE MANAGEMENT

Meticulous attention to fluid intake and output is mandatory and includes all of the physical measurements discussed previously in relation to problems of fluid balance. Monitoring fluid balance and vital signs is a continuous process, and observers are constantly on the alert for signs of complications so appropriate interventions can be implemented. Because these children require intensive observation and often specialized treatment such as dialysis, they are usually admitted to an intensive care unit in which needed equipment and trained personnel are available.

Limiting fluid intake requires ingenuity on the part of caregivers to cope with the child who is thirsty. Rationing the daily intake in small amounts of fluid served in containers that give the impression of larger volumes is one strategy. Older children who understand the rationale of fluid limits can help determine how their daily ration should be distributed.

Meeting nutritional needs is sometimes a problem. The child may be nauseated, and encouraging concentrated foods without fluids may be difficult. When nourishment is provided by the IV route, careful monitoring is essential to prevent fluid overload. In addition, nursing measures such as maintaining an optimal thermal environment, reducing any elevation of body temperature, and reducing restlessness and anxiety are used to decrease the rate of tissue catabolism.

The nurse must be continually alert for changes in behavior that indicate the onset of complications. Infection from reduced resistance, anemia, and general morbidity is a constant threat. Fluid overload and electrolyte disturbances can precipitate cardiovascular complications such as hypertension and cardiac failure. Fluid and electrolyte imbalances, acidosis, and accumulation of nitrogenous waste products can produce neurologic involvement manifested by coma, seizures, or alterations in sensorium.

Although children with ARF are usually quite ill and voluntarily diminish their activity, infants may become restless and irritable, and children are often anxious and frightened. Frequent, painful, and stress-producing treatments and tests must be performed. A supportive, empathetic nurse can provide comfort and stability in a threatening and unnatural environment.

Family Support. Providing support and reassurance to parents are among the major nursing responsibilities. The seriousness of ARF and its emergency nature are stressful to parents; and most feel some degree of guilt regarding the child's condition, especially when the illness is a result of ingestion of a toxic substance, dehydration, or a genetic disease. They need reassurance and a sympathetic listener. They also need to be kept informed of the child's progress and provided explanations regarding the therapeutic regimen. The equipment and the child's behavior are sometimes frightening and anxiety provoking. Nurses can do much to help parents comprehend and deal with the stresses of the situation.

Chronic Renal Failure

The kidneys are able to maintain the chemical composition of fluids within normal limits until more than 50% of functional renal capacity is destroyed by disease or injury. Chronic renal insufficiency or failure begins when the diseased kidneys can no longer maintain the normal chemical structure of body fluids under normal conditions. Progressive deterioration over months or years produces a variety of clinical and biochemical disturbances that eventually culminate in the clinical syndrome known as uremia.

A variety of diseases and disorders can result in CRF. The most frequent causes are congenital renal and urinary tract malformations, VUR associated with recurrent UTI, chronic pyelonephritis, hereditary disorders, chronic glomerulonephritis, and glomerulonephropathy associated with systemic diseases such as anaphylactoid purpura and lupus erythematosus.

Pathophysiology

Early in the course of progressive nephrotic destruction, the child remains asymptomatic with only minimal biochemical abnormalities. Unless the presence of CRF is detected in the process of routine assessment, signs and symptoms that indicate advanced renal damage frequently emerge only late in the course of the disease. Midway in the disease process, as increasing numbers of nephrons are totally destroyed and most others are damaged to varying degrees, the few that remain intact are hypertrophied but functional. These few normal nephrons are able to make sufficient adjustments to stresses to maintain reasonable degrees of fluid and electrolyte balance. Definitive biochemical examination at this time reveals restricted tolerance to excesses or restrictions. As the disease progresses to the end stage, because of a severe reduction in the number of functioning nephrons, the kidneys are no longer able to maintain fluid and electrolyte balance, and the features of uremic syndrome appear.

The accumulation of various biochemical substances in the blood resulting from diminished renal function produces complications such as the following:

- Retention of waste products, especially BUN and creatinine
- Water and sodium retention, which contributes to edema and vascular congestion
- Hyperkalemia of dangerous levels
- Metabolic acidosis of a sustained nature because of continual hydrogen ion retention and bicarbonate loss
- Calcium and phosphorus disturbances, resulting in altered bone metabolism, which in turn causes growth arrest or retardation, bone pain, and deformities known as renal osteodystrophy
- Anemia caused by hematologic dysfunction, including a shortened life span of RBCs, impaired RBC production related to decreased production of erythropoietin, prolonged bleeding time, and nutritional anemia
- Growth disturbance, probably caused by such factors as renal osteodystrophy, poor nutrition associated with dietary restrictions and loss of appetite, and biochemical abnormalities

Children with CRF seem to be more susceptible to infection, especially pneumonia, UTI, and septicemia, although the reason for this is unclear. These children become extraordinarily sensitive to changes in vascular volume that may cause pulmonary overload, CNS symptoms, hypertension, and cardiac failure.

Diagnostic Evaluation

The diagnosis of CRF is usually suspected on the basis of any number of clinical manifestations, a history of prior renal disease, or biochemical findings. The onset is usually gradual, and the initial signs and symptoms are vague and nonspecific (Box 44-7).

Laboratory and other diagnostic tools and tests are of value in assessing the extent of renal damage, biochemical disturbances, and related physical dysfunction (see Tables 44-1 to 44-3). Often they can help establish the nature of the underlying disease and differentiate among other disease processes and the pathologic consequences of renal dysfunction.

Therapeutic Management

In irreversible renal failure the goals of medical management are to (1) promote maximum renal function, (2) maintain body fluid and electrolyte balance within safe biochemical limits, (3) treat systemic complications, and (4) promote as active and normal a life as possible for the child for as long as possible. The child is allowed unrestricted activity and to set his or her own limits regarding rest and extent of exertion. School attendance is encouraged as long as the child is able. When the effort is too great, home tutoring is arranged.

Diet regulation is the most effective means, short of dialysis, of reducing the quantity of materials that require renal excretion. The goals of diet management in renal failure are to provide sufficient calories and protein for growth while limiting the excretory demands made on the kidneys, to minimize metabolic bone disease (osteodystrophy), and to minimize fluid and electrolyte disturbances. Dietary protein intake is limited only to the reference daily intake (RDI) for the child's age. Restriction of protein intake below the RDI is believed to negatively affect growth and neurodevelopment. Malnutrition may develop in patients with CRF even before they need dialysis (Sylvestre, Fonseca, Stinghen, et al., 2007).

BOX 44-7   CLINICAL MANIFESTATIONS OF CHRONIC RENAL FAILURE

- Early signs:
  - Loss of normal energy
  - Increased fatigue on exertion
  - Pallor, subtle (may not be noticed)
  - Elevated blood pressure (sometimes)
- As the disease progresses:
  - Decreased appetite (especially at breakfast)
  - Less interest in normal activities
  - Increased or decreased urinary output with compensatory intake of fluid
  - Pallor more evident
  - Sallow, muddy appearance of skin
- Child may complain of:
  - Headache
  - Muscle cramps
  - Nausea
- Other signs and symptoms:
  - Weight loss
  - Facial edema
  - Malaise
  - Bone or joint pain
  - Growth retardation
  - Dryness or itching of the skin
  - Bruised skin
  - Sensory or motor loss (sometimes)
  - Amenorrhea (common in adolescent girls)
- Uremic syndrome (untreated):
- Gastrointestinal symptoms:
  - Anorexia
  - Nausea and vomiting
- Bleeding tendencies:
  - Bruises
  - Bloody diarrheal stools
  - Stomatitis
  - Bleeding from lips and mouth
- Intractable itching
- Uremic frost (deposits of urea crystals on skin)
- Unpleasant "uremic" breath odor
- Deep respirations
- Hypertension
- Congestive heart failure
- Pulmonary edema
- Neurologic involvement:
  - Progressive confusion
  - Dulled sensorium
  - Coma (ultimately)
  - Tremors
  - Muscular twitching
  - Seizures

Sodium and water are not usually limited unless there is evidence of edema or hypertension, and potassium is not usually restricted. However, restrictions of any or all three may be imposed in later stages or at any time that abnormal serum concentrations are evident.

Dietary phosphorus is controlled through reduction of protein and milk intake to prevent or correct the calcium-phosphorus imbalance. Phosphorus levels can be reduced further by oral administration of calcium carbonate preparations or other phosphate-binding agents that combine with the phosphorus to decrease gastrointestinal absorption and thus the serum levels of phosphate. Treatment with 25-OH vitamin D is begun to increase calcium absorption and suppress elevated parathyroid hormone levels.

Metabolic acidosis is alleviated through administration of alkalizing agents such as sodium bicarbonate or a combination of sodium and potassium citrate.

Growth failure is one major consequence of CRF, especially in preadolescents. These children grow poorly both before and after the initiation of hemodialysis. The use of recombinant human growth hormone to accelerate growth in children with growth retardation secondary to CRF has been successful (Vimalachandra,

Hodson, Willis, et al., 2006). Osseous deformities that result from renal osteodystrophy, especially those related to ambulation, are troublesome and require correction if they occur. Dental defects are common in children with CRF; the earlier the onset of the disease, the more severe are the dental manifestations (including hypoplasia, hypomineralization, tooth discoloration, alteration in size and shape of teeth, malocclusion, and ulcerative stomatitis). Therefore regular dental care is important in these children.

Anemia in children with CRF is related to decreased production of erythropoietin. Recombinant human erythropoietin (rHuEPO) is being offered to these children as thrice-weekly or weekly subcutaneous injections and is replacing the need for frequent blood transfusions. The drug corrects the anemia and in turn increases appetite, activity, and general well-being in the children who receive it.

Hypertension may be managed initially by cautious use of a low-sodium diet, fluid restriction, and perhaps diuretics such as hydrochlorothiazide or furosemide. Severe hypertension requires the use of antihypertensive agents singly or in combination.

Intercurrent infections are treated with appropriate antimicrobials at the first sign of infection; however, any drug eliminated through the kidneys is administered with caution. Other complications are treated symptomatically (e.g., central-acting antiemetics for nausea, antiepileptics for seizures, and diphenhydramine [Benadryl] for pruritus).

When evidence of end-stage renal disease (ESRD) appears in a child, the disease runs its relentless course and results in death in a few weeks unless waste products and toxins are removed from body fluids by dialysis or kidney transplantation. These techniques have been adapted for infants and small children and are implemented in most cases of renal failure after conservative management is no longer effective (see Technologic Management of Renal Failure, p. 1414).

Prognosis. Dialysis and transplantation are the only treatments currently available for children with ESRD. Although they may survive on dialysis, it is not an ideal long-term modality. Complications include infection of access sites, growth failure, and disruption of normal socialization. Many pediatric centers encourage families of children with ESRD to consider kidney transplantation. The North American Pediatric Renal Trials and Collaborative Studies' annual transplant report (2010) documents graft survival of 96% at 1 year and 84% at 5 years for living donor kidneys and 95% at 1 year and 78% at 5 years for deceased donor kidneys.

Posttransplant complications include infection, hypertension, steroid toxicity, hyperlipidemia, aseptic necrosis, malignancy, and growth retardation (Dharnidharka and Araya, 2009). Long-term graft survival is not guaranteed, and many children require a second or third transplant. Successful kidney transplantation does improve rehabilitation of children with CRF, both educationally and psychologically. Increasing use of primary or preemptive kidney transplants is becoming the optimal form of renal replacement therapy, leading to substantial improvement in quality of life (Goldstein, Graham, Burwinkle, et al., 2006).

CARE MANAGEMENT

The multiple complications of ESRD are managed according to medical protocols such as the evidence-based clinical practice guidelines of the National Kidney Foundation Kidney Disease Outcomes Quality Initiative (www.kidney.org/professionals/kdoqi). However, progressive disease places a number of stresses on the child and family, including those of a potentially fatal illness (see Chapter 36).

There is a continuing need for repeated examinations that often entail painful procedures, side effects, and frequent hospitalizations. Diet therapy becomes progressively more restricted and intense, and the child is required to take a variety of medications. Ever present in all aspects of the treatment regimen is the agonizing realization that without treatment death is inevitable.

Some specific stresses related to ESRD and its treatment are predictable. When it first becomes apparent that ESRD is inevitable, both parents and child experience depression and anxiety. Acceptance is particularly difficult if renal failure progresses rapidly after diagnosis. Denial and disbelief are usually pronounced, especially among the parents. After renal failure is established and symptoms become progressively more distressing, the initiation of dialysis is usually perceived as a positive experience; after experiencing initial concerns regarding the treatment, the child begins to feel better, and parental anxiety is relieved for a time.

Initiating a dialysis regimen is a traumatic and anxiety-provoking experience for most children because it involves surgery for implantation of a graft, fistula, or peritoneal catheter. The initial experience with the dialysis procedure is frightening to most children. They need reassurance about the nature of the preparations for dialysis and the conduct of the treatment.

Both the graft and the fistula require needle insertions at each dialysis. The goal is to perform pain-free venipuncture. Using buffered lidocaine with a small-gauge needle (30 gauge) to anesthetize the area before venipuncture of the graft or fistula is one method. Using an anesthetizing topical preparation such as EMLA (eutectic mixture of local anesthetics [lidocaine and prilocaine]) 1 hour before venipuncture is another approach (see Pain Management, Chapter 30). External dual-lumen venous access devices eliminate the need for needles but are more prone to infection and other central line complications.

Adolescents, with their increased need for independence and their urge for rebellion, usually adapt less well than younger children. They resent the control and enforced dependence imposed by the rigorous and unrelenting therapy program. They resent being dependent on hemodialysis technology, their parents, and the professional staff. Depression or hostility is common in adolescents undergoing hemodialysis.

The availability of home peritoneal dialysis has offered a greater degree of freedom for people undergoing long-term dialysis. The nurse is responsible for teaching the family about (1) the disease, its implications, and the therapeutic plan; (2) the possible psychologic effects of the disease and the treatment; and (3) the technical aspects of the procedure. The family learns to manage the various aspects of the dialysis procedure, how to maintain accurate records, and how to observe for signs of complications that need to be reported to the proper persons.

Body changes related to the disease process such as pale or ashen skin color, growth retardation, and lack of sexual maturation are stress provoking. Dietary restrictions are particularly burdensome for both children and parents. Children feel deprived when they are unable to eat foods previously enjoyed and that are unrestricted for other family members. Consequently they may fail to cooperate. Diet restrictions may be interpreted as punishment. Some children who are unable to understand fully the purpose of restrictions sneak forbidden food items at every opportunity. Allowing children, especially adolescents, maximum participation in and responsibility for their own treatment program is helpful.

After months or years of dialysis, the parents and child feel anxiety associated with the prognosis and continued pressures of the treatment. The relentless need for treatment interferes with family

FAMILY-CENTERED CARE

Family Priorities

Families who have children with long-term chronic illnesses such as end-stage renal disease spend much time in hospitals, outpatient clinics, and primary health care facilities. When they miss appointments or respond less quickly than anticipated, sometimes they are quickly labeled "noncompliant." It is important to remember that families have to develop priorities for the unit as a whole. Sometimes they may decide that it is more important for the parent to go to work or attend a sibling's school performance than to attend an appointment scheduled for them by health care personnel. The chronically ill child cannot and should not always be the number one priority for the family. The professional staff who work with the family can help the parents prioritize the needs of the ill child within the needs of the family constellation.

Teresa Hall, MS, RN
Hathaway Children's Services
Sylmar, CA

plans. The time spent in transportation to and from the dialysis unit and the time spent undergoing dialysis treatments cut into time for outside activities, including school. Graft and fistula problems and peritoneal catheter exit site infections may develop and present a common source of aggravation (see Family-Centered Care box).

The possibility of kidney transplantation often provides hope for relief from the rigors of hemodialysis and peritoneal dialysis. Most children and families respond well to a kidney transplant, and most children can be rehabilitated successfully.

The National Kidney Foundation* and other agencies provide a number of services and information for families of children with renal disease.

TECHNOLOGIC MANAGEMENT OF RENAL FAILURE

Dialysis

Dialysis is the process of separating colloids and crystalline substances in solution by the difference in their rate of diffusion through a semipermeable membrane. Methods of dialysis currently available for clinical management of renal failure are peritoneal dialysis, wherein the abdominal cavity acts as a semipermeable membrane through which water and solutes of small molecular size move by osmosis and diffusion according to their respective concentrations on either side of the membrane; and hemodialysis, in which blood is circulated outside the body through artificial membranes that permit a similar passage of water and solutes. A third type of dialysis is hemofiltration, in which blood filtrate is circulated outside the body by hydrostatic pressure exerted across a semipermeable membrane with simultaneous infusion of a replacement solution. Types of hemofiltration include continuous venovenous hemofiltration, continuous venovenous hemodialysis, and continuous venovenous hemodiafiltration. These continuous renal replacement therapies are used in ARF, severe fluid overload, and inborn errors of metabolism or after bone marrow transplant.

*30 E. 33rd St., New York, NY 10016, 212-889-2210, 800-622-9010, www.kidney.org. In Canada: Kidney Foundation of Canada, 300-5165 Sherbrooke St. West, Montreal, Canada QC H4A 1T6, 514-369-4806, 800-361-7494, www.kidney.ca.

Peritoneal dialysis is the preferred form of dialysis for infants, children, and parents who wish to remain independent; families who live a long distance from the medical center; and children who prefer fewer dietary restrictions and a gentler form of dialysis. Chronic peritoneal dialysis is most often performed at home. The two types of peritoneal dialysis are continuous ambulatory peritoneal dialysis and continuous cycling peritoneal dialysis. In both methods commercially available sterile dialysis solution is instilled into the peritoneal cavity through a surgically implanted indwelling catheter tunneled subcutaneously and sutured into place. The warmed solution is allowed to enter the peritoneal cavity by gravity and remains a variable length of time according to the rate of solute removal and glucose absorption in individual patients. The care and management of the procedure are the responsibility of the parents of young children. Some centers have initiated use of home health nurses to give parents respite from care. Older children and adolescents can carry out the procedure themselves, which provides them with some control and less dependency. This is especially important for adolescents.

! NURSING ALERT

Observe for changes in the color of the dialysate draining from the child. The spent solution should be clear. If the color is cloudy, notify the practitioner immediately (Schaefer, 2003).

Hemodialysis requires the creation of a vascular access and the use of special dialysis equipment (i.e., the hemodialyzer, or so-called *artificial kidney*). Vascular access may be one of three types: fistulas, grafts, or external vascular access devices. An arteriovenous fistula is an access in which a vein and artery are connected surgically. The preferred site is the radial artery and a forearm vein that produces dilation and thickening of the superficial vessels of the forearm to provide easy access for repeated venipuncture. An alternative is the creation of a subcutaneous (internal) arteriovenous graft by anastomosing artery and vein, with a synthetic prosthetic graft for circulatory access. The most commonly used material is expanded polytetrafluoroethylene (ePTFE). Both the graft and the fistula require needle insertions with each dialysis treatment.

For external vascular access devices, percutaneous catheters are inserted in the femoral, subclavian, or internal jugular veins, even in very small children. A more permanent form of external access is available via a central catheter inserted surgically into the internal jugular vein. This catheter has a dual lumen, which allows a larger volume of blood flow with minimum recirculation. Catheters eliminate the need for skin punctures but may require some home care.

Hemodialysis is best suited to children who do not have someone in the family able to perform home peritoneal dialysis and to those who live close to a dialysis center. The procedure is usually performed 3 times per week for 4 to 6 hours, depending on the child's size. It achieves rapid correction of fluid and electrolyte abnormalities but can cause problems in association with this rapid change such as muscle cramping and hypotension. Disadvantages include school absence during dialysis and strict fluid and dietary restrictions between dialysis sessions. Boredom for the child and family is often a problem during dialysis, and planned activities should be introduced (Fig. 44-4).

Most children show rapid clinical improvement with the implementation of dialysis, although it is directly related to the duration of uremia before dialysis and good nutrition. Growth rate and skeletal maturation improve, but recovery of normal growth is

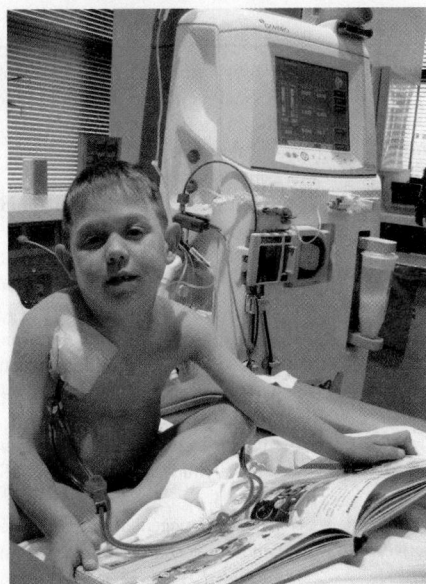

FIG 44-4 Diversional activities help lessen the boredom that children can experience during hemodialysis.

infrequent. In many cases sexual development, although delayed, progresses to completion.

Transplantation

Kidney transplantation is an acceptable and effective means of therapy in the pediatric age-group. Although peritoneal dialysis and hemodialysis are life preserving, both require major alterations in lifestyle. Transplantation offers the opportunity for a relatively normal life and is the preferred form of treatment for children with ESRD. Primary or preemptive transplants maintain the greatest amount of normalcy in the family's life.

Kidneys for transplant are available from two sources: a living related donor, usually a parent or a sibling, or a cadaver donor,

wherein the family of a dead or brain-dead patient consents to donation of a healthy kidney. Retransplantation may be required.

The primary goal in transplantation is the long-term survival of grafted tissue by securing tissue that is antigenically similar to that of the recipient and suppressing the recipient's immune mechanism. The immunosuppressant therapy of choice has been corticosteroids (prednisone) in conjunction with cyclosporine or tacrolimus and mycophenolate mofetil. Other therapies include antilymphoblast globulin or monoclonal antibodies. New immunosuppressant medications and early withdrawal of steroids or steroid-free protocols are rapidly coming into clinical trials and use in large transplant centers (Grenda and Webb, 2010). It is important for the nurse to learn about the medications used in the antirejection protocol(s) and their side effects. Because the immunosuppressant medications are taken indefinitely, transplant patients experience many side effects of the drugs, including hypertension, growth retardation, cataracts, risk of infection, obesity, characteristics of Cushing syndrome, and hirsutism (McDonald, 2011).

> **! NURSING ALERT**
>
> The child with a kidney transplant who exhibits any of the following should be evaluated immediately for possible rejection:
> - Fever
> - Swelling and tenderness over graft area
> - Diminished urinary output
> - Elevated blood pressure
> - Elevated serum creatinine

Rejection of the transplanted kidney is the most common cause of transplant failure. Rejection is treated aggressively with immunosuppressant medications and can often be reversed. Some patients do not respond to treatment of acute rejection or develop chronic rejection and must eventually return to dialysis or undergo another kidney transplant.

▌ KEY POINTS

- Common inflammatory disorders of the genitourinary tract include UTI, nephrotic syndrome, and AGN.
- Management of UTIs is directed at eliminating infection, detecting and correcting functional or anatomic abnormalities, preventing recurrences, and preserving renal function.
- VUR is the retrograde flow of bladder urine into the ureters.
- Obstructive uropathy is a result of structural or functional abnormalities of the urinary system that obstruct the normal flow of urine.
- The more common defects of the genitourinary tract include phimosis, cryptorchidism, inguinal hernia, hydrocele, and hypospadias.
- Body image concerns and castration anxiety are particularly intense in children with defects in the genital area.
- Nephrotic syndrome is characterized by increased glomerular permeability to protein, with massive urinary loss of protein resulting in hypoproteinemia and edema.
- Management of nephrotic syndrome is aimed at reducing excretion of protein, reducing or preventing fluid retention by tissues, and preventing infection and other complications.
- Common features of AGN are oliguria, edema, hypertension, circulatory congestion, hematuria, and proteinuria.

- Therapeutic management of AGN involves maintenance of fluid balance, treatment of hypertension, and antibiotic therapy.
- Management of HUS is aimed at control of complications and hematologic manifestations of renal failure.
- Wilms' tumor is the most common malignant neoplasm of the kidney in infants and children.
- In ARF management is directed at determining treatment of the underlying cause, managing complications of renal failure, and providing supportive therapy.
- Abnormalities in CRF are waste product retention, water and sodium retention, hyperkalemia, acidosis, calcium and phosphorus disturbance, anemia, and growth disturbances.
- The types of dialysis used in ESRD are peritoneal dialysis and hemodialysis.
- When the child needs home dialysis, the nurse educates the family about the disease, its implications, the therapeutic plan, possible psychologic effects of the disease, and the treatment and technical aspects of the procedure.
- The major concerns in kidney transplantation are tissue matching and prevention of rejection; psychologic concerns involve self-image as related to possible body changes as a result of the effects of corticosteroid therapy.

REFERENCES

American Academy of Pediatrics Task Force on Circumcision: Circumcision policy statement, *Pediatrics* 103(3):686–693, 1999.

Berry AD: Helping children with nocturnal enuresis: the wait-and-see approach may not be in everyone's interest, *Am J Nurs* 106(8):56–63, 2006.

Cendron M, Gomez P: *Wilms tumor*, 2010, emedicine.medscape.com/article/453076-overview.

Chen HC, Yeh CM, Chou CM: Endoscopic treatment of vesicoureteral reflux in children with dextranomer/hyaluronic acid—a single surgeon's 6 year experience, *Diagn Ther Endosc Epub* 2010, DOI 10.1155/2010/278012.

Dharnidharka VR, Araya CE: Complications of renal transplantation. In Avner ED, Harmon WE, Niaudet P, et al, editors: *Pediatric nephrology*, ed 6, Berlin Heidelberg, 2009, Springer-Verlag.

Dome JS, Perlman EJ, Ritchey ML, et al: Renal tumors. In Pizzo PA, Poplack DP, editors: *Principles and practices of pediatric oncology*, ed 5, Philadelphia, 2006, Lippincott.

Duzova A, Bakkaloglu A, Kalyoncu M, et al: Etiology and outcome of acute kidney injury in children, *Pediatr Nephrol* 25(8):1453–1461, 2010.

Elder JS: Voiding dysfunction. In Kliegman RM, Stanton BE, St. Geme JW, et al, editors. *Nelson textbook of pediatrics*, ed 19, Philadelphia, 2011, Saunders.

Ferrara P, Romaniello L, Vitelli O, et al: Cranberry juice for the prevention of recurrent urinary tract infections: a randomized controlled trial in children, *Scan J Urol Nephrol* 43:369–372, 2009.

Gipson DS, Massengill SF, Yao L, et al: Management of childhood onset nephrotic syndrome, *Pediatrics* 124(2):747–757, 2009.

Goldstein SL, Graham N, Burwinkle T, et al: Health-related quality of life in pediatric patients with ESRD, *Pediatr Nephrol* 21(6):846–850, 2006.

Grenda R, Webb NJ: Steroid minimization in pediatric renal transplantation: early withdrawal or avoidance? *Pediatr Transplantation* 14(8):961–967, 2010.

Jepson RG, Mihaljevic L, Craig J: Cranberries for preventing urinary tract infections, *Cochrane Database Syst Rev* (2):CD001321, 2008.

Kanellopoulos TA, Salakos C, Spiliopoulou I, et al: First urinary tract infection in neonates, infants and young children: a comparative study, *Pediatr Nephrol* 21(8):1131–1137, 2006.

Kass E: Timing of elective surgery on the genitalia of male children with particular reference to the risks, benefits, and psychological effects of surgery and anesthesia, *Pediatrics* 97(4):590–594, 1996.

Katz ER, DeMaso D: Enureis (bed-wetting). In Kliegman RM, Stanton BF, St. Geme JW, et al, editors. *Nelson textbook of pediatrics*, ed 19, Philadelphia, 2011, Saunders.

McDonald RA: Immunosuppression in renal transplantation in children, *UpToDate* 2011, www.uptodate.com.

National Kidney Foundation: *The National Kidney Foundation kidney disease outcomes quality initiative, (NKF KDOQI)*, 2013. www.kidney.org/professionals/kdoqi.

North American Pediatric Renal Trials and Collaborative Studies: *NAPRTCS 2010 annual transplant report*, 2010, web.emmes.com/study/ped/annlrept/2010_Report.pdf.

Patzer L: Nephrotoxicity as a cause of acute kidney injury in children, *Pediatr Nephrol* 23(12):2159–2173, 2008.

Rice SG, Council on Sports Medicine and Fitness: Medical conditions affecting sports participation, *Pediatrics* 121(4):841–848, 2008.

Rosenthal M: Current concept in managing UTIs in children, *Infect Dis Child* 17(3):30–31, 2004.

Schaefer F: Management of peritonitis in children receiving chronic peritoneal dialysis, *Paediatr Drugs* 5(5):315–325, 2003.

Sethi S, Bhargava S, Shipra PM: Nocturnal enuresis: a review, *J Pediatr Neurol* 3(1):11–18, 2005.

Shaikh N, Morone NE, Bost JE, et al: Prevalence of urinary tract infection in childhood: a meta-analysis, *Pediatr Infect Dis J* 27(4):302–308, 2008.

Sylvestre LC, Fonseca K, Stinghen A, et al: The malnutrition and inflammation axis in pediatric patients with chronic kidney disease, *Pediatr Nephrol* 22(6):864–873, 2007.

Vimalachandra D, Hodson EM, Willis NS, et al: Growth hormone for children with chronic kidney disease, *Cochrane Database Syst Rev* (3):CD003264, 2006.

Cerebral Dysfunction

Marilyn J. Hockenberry

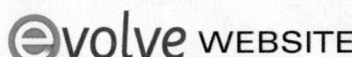

LEARNING OBJECTIVES

On completion of this chapter, the reader will be able to:
- Describe the various modalities for assessment of cerebral function.
- Differentiate among the stages of consciousness.
- Formulate a care plan for the unconscious child.
- Distinguish among the types of head injuries and the serious complications.
- Describe the nursing care of a child with a tumor of the central nervous system.

- Outline a care plan for the child with bacterial meningitis.
- Differentiate between the various types of seizure disorders.
- Demonstrate an understanding of the manifestations of a seizure disorder and the management of a child with such a disorder.
- Describe the preoperative and postoperative care of a child with hydrocephalus.

CEREBRAL DYSFUNCTION

Most of the information about the status of the brain is obtained by indirect measurements. Some of these measurements are discussed elsewhere in relation to numerous aspects of child care (e.g., as part of assessments of health [Chapter 29], newborn status [Chapter 24], intellectual disability [Chapter 37], hypoxic injury [cerebral palsy, Chapter 49], and attainment of developmental milestones at each stage of development). Because increased intracranial pressure (ICP) and altered states of consciousness have such prominent places in neurologic dysfunction, they are described here, followed by techniques for neurologic assessment and diagnostic tests.

Increased Intracranial Pressure

The brain, tightly enclosed in the solid bony cranium, is well protected but highly vulnerable to pressure that may accumulate within the enclosure (Fig. 45-1). The total volume of the cranium—brain (80%), cerebrospinal fluid (CSF) (10%), and blood (10%)—must remain approximately the same at all times. A change in the proportional volume of one of these components (e.g., increase or decrease in intracranial blood) must be accompanied by a compensatory change in another. In this way the volume and pressure normally remain constant. Examples of compensatory changes are reduction in blood volume, decrease in CSF production, increase in CSF

absorption, or shrinkage of brain mass by displacement of intracellular and extracellular fluid. Children with open fontanels compensate by skull expansion and widened sutures. However, at any age the capacity for spatial compensation is limited. An increase in ICP may be caused by tumors or other space-occupying lesions, accumulation of fluid within the ventricular system, bleeding, or edema of cerebral tissues. When compensation is exhausted, any further increase in the volume of the cranium results in a rapid rise in ICP.

Early signs and symptoms of increased ICP are often subtle and assume many patterns (Box 45-1). As pressure increases, signs and symptoms become more pronounced, and the level of consciousness (LOC) deteriorates.

Altered States of Consciousness

Consciousness implies awareness (i.e., the ability to respond to sensory stimuli and have subjective experiences). There are two components of consciousness: alertness, an arousal-waking state, including the ability to respond to stimuli; and cognitive power, including the ability to process stimuli and produce verbal and motor responses.

An altered state of consciousness usually refers to varying states of unconsciousness that may be momentary or extend for hours, for days, or indefinitely. Unconsciousness is depressed cerebral function (i.e., the inability to respond to sensory stimuli and have subjective

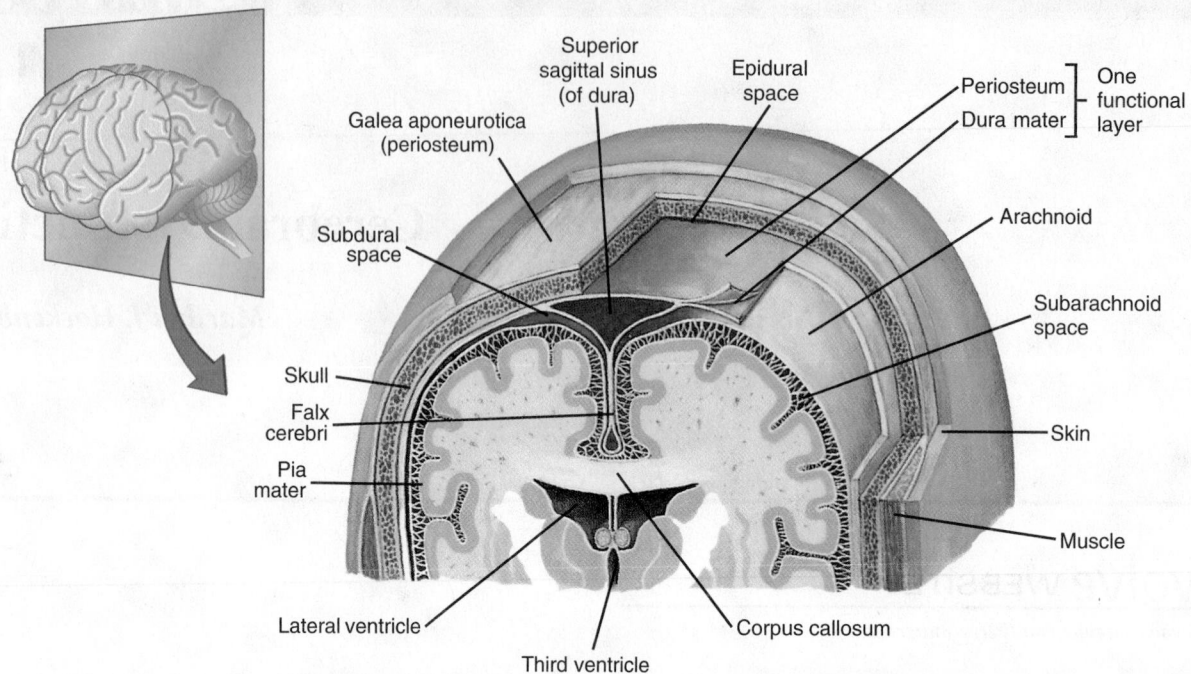

FIG 45-1 Coronal section of the top of the head showing meningeal layers. (From Patton KT, Thibodeau GA: *Anatomy and physiology,* ed 7, St Louis, 2010, Mosby.)

BOX 45-1	CLINICAL MANIFESTATIONS OF INCREASED INTRACRANIAL PRESSURE IN INFANTS AND CHILDREN

Infants
- Tense, bulging fontanel
- Separated cranial sutures
- Macewen (cracked-pot) sign
- Irritability and restlessness
- Drowsiness
- Increased sleeping
- High-pitched cry
- Increased fronto-occipital circumference
- Distended scalp veins
- Poor feeding
- Crying when disturbed
- Setting-sun sign

Children
- Headache
- Nausea
- Forceful vomiting
- Diplopia, blurred vision

- Seizures
- Indifference, drowsiness
- Decline in school performance
- Diminished physical activity and motor performance
- Increased sleeping
- Inability to follow simple commands
- Lethargy

Late Signs in Infants and Children
- Bradycardia
- Decreased motor response to command
- Decreased sensory response to painful stimuli
- Alterations in pupil size and reactivity
- Extension or flexion posturing
- Cheyne-Stokes respirations
- Papilledema
- Decreased consciousness
- Coma

---

experiences). Coma is defined as a state of unconsciousness from which the patient cannot be aroused even with powerful stimuli.

Levels of Consciousness

Assessment of LOC remains the earliest indicator of improvement or deterioration in neurologic status. LOC is determined by observations of the child's responses to the environment. When it is being assessed in young children, it is often useful to have a parent present to help elicit a desired response. An infant or child may not respond in an unfamiliar environment or to unfamiliar voices. Children

older than 3 years of age should be able to give their name, although they may not be cognizant of place or time. Other diagnostic tests such as motor activity, reflexes, and vital signs vary more and do not necessarily directly parallel the depth of the comatose state. The most consistently used terms are described in Box 45-2.

Coma Assessment

Several scales have been devised in an attempt to standardize the description and interpretation of the degree of depressed consciousness. The most popular of these is the Glasgow Coma Scale (GCS),

BOX 45-2 LEVELS OF CONSCIOUSNESS

Full consciousness—Awake and alert, orientated to time, place, and person; behavior appropriate for age

Confusion—Impaired decision making

Disorientation—Confusion regarding time, place; decreased LOC

Lethargy—Limited spontaneous movement, sluggish speech, drowsy, falling asleep quickly

Obtundation—Arousable with stimulation

Stupor—Remaining in a deep sleep, slow response to vigorous and repeated stimulation or moaning responses to stimuli

Coma—No motor or verbal response or extension posturing to noxious (painful) stimuli

Persistent vegetative state—Permanently lost function of the cerebral cortex. Eyes follow objects only by reflex or when attracted to the direction of loud sounds; all four limbs are spastic but can withdraw from painful stimuli; hands show reflexive grasping and groping; the face can grimace, some food may be swallowed, and the child may groan or cry but utter no words.

LOC, Level of consciousness.

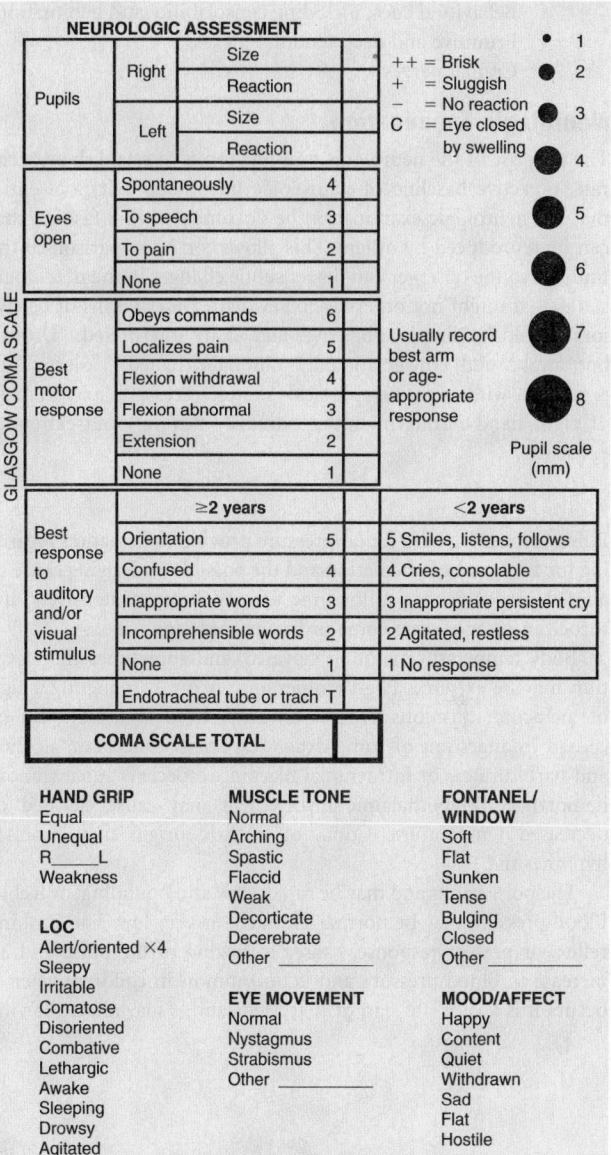

FIG 45-2 Pediatric coma scale.

which consists of a three-part assessment: eye opening, verbal response, and motor response (Fig. 45-2). Numeric values of 1 through 5 are assigned to the levels of response in each category. The sum of these numeric values provides an objective measure of the patient's LOC. A person with an unaltered LOC would score the highest, 15; a score of 8 or below is generally accepted as a definition of coma; and the lowest score, 3, indicates deep coma. A decrease in the GCS score indicates a deterioration of the patient's condition. In 1987 major medical and legal societies developed specific guidelines for the determination of brain death among children of all ages (Mathur, Peterson, Stadtier, et al., 2008).

General Aspects

Children younger than 2 years of age require special evaluation because they are unable to respond to directions designed to elicit specific neurologic responses. Early neurologic responses in infants are primarily reflexive; these responses are gradually replaced by meaningful movement in the characteristic cephalocaudal direction of development. This evidence of progressive maturation reflects more extensive myelinization and changes in neurochemical and electrophysiologic properties.

Most information about infants and small children is gained by observing their spontaneous and elicited reflex responses as they develop increasingly complex motor skills and by eliciting progressively sophisticated communicative and adaptive behaviors. Delay or deviation from expected milestones helps identify high-risk children. Persistence or reappearance of reflexes that normally disappear indicates a pathologic condition. In evaluating an infant or young child, it is also important to obtain the pregnancy and delivery history to determine the possible impact of intrauterine environmental influences known to affect the orderly maturation of the central nervous system (CNS). These influences include maternal infections, cigarette or alcohol consumption, drug use, toxin exposure, trauma, and metabolic insults.

General aspects of assessment that provide clues to the etiology of dysfunction include the following:

Family history—Sometimes offers clues regarding possible genetic disorders with neurologic manifestations.

Health history—May provide valuable clues regarding the cause of dysfunction. Information should include Apgar scores, age of developmental milestones, trauma or injuries, acute and chronic illnesses, encounters with animals or insects, and ingestion or inhalation of neurotoxic substances.

Physical evaluation of infants—Includes assessment of:
- Level of alertness.
- Size and shape of the head, including presence of fontanels.
- Sensory responses.
- Motor function, including posture, tone, and muscle strength.
- Motility, including symmetry of movements and involuntary movements.
- Respirations, including signs of prolonged apnea, ataxic breathing, paradoxical chest movement, or hyperventilation.
- Dysmorphic facial features.

- Behavioral cues, including consolability and habituation.
- Primitive and deep tendon reflexes.
- Cranial nerves.

Neurologic Examination

The purpose of the neurologic examination is to establish an accurate, objective baseline of neurologic information. It is essential that the neurologic examination be documented in a fashion that can be reproduced by others. This allows for a comparison of the findings so the observer can detect subtle changes in the neurologic status that might not otherwise be evident. Descriptions of behaviors should be simple, objective, and easily interpreted: "Drowsy but awake and conversationally rational/oriented"; "Sleepy but arousable with vigorous physical stimuli. Pressure to nail base of right hand results in upper-extremity flexion/lower-extremity extension."

Vital Signs

Pulse, respiration, and blood pressure provide information regarding the adequacy of circulation and the possible underlying cause of altered consciousness. Autonomic activity is most intensively disturbed in cases of deep coma or brainstem lesions.

Body temperature is often elevated, and sometimes the elevation may be extreme. High temperature is most frequently a sign of an acute infectious process or heat stroke but may also be caused by ingestion of some drugs (especially salicylates, alcohol, and barbiturates) or intracranial bleeding, especially subarachnoid hemorrhage. Hypothalamic involvement may cause elevated or decreased temperature. Coma of a toxic origin may produce hypothermia.

The pulse varies and may be rapid, slow and bounding, or feeble. Blood pressure may be normal, elevated, or very low. The Cushing reflex, or pressor response, causes a slowing of the pulse and an increase in blood pressure and is uncommon in children; when it occurs it is a very late sign of ICP. Medications may affect the vital

signs. For assessment purposes actual *changes* in pulse and blood pressure are more important than the direction of the change.

Respirations are often slow, deep, and irregular. Slow, deep breathing is often seen in the heavy sleep caused by sedatives, after seizures, or in cerebral infections. Slow, shallow breathing may result from sedatives or opioids (narcotics). Hyperventilation (deep and rapid respirations) is usually a result of metabolic acidosis or abnormal stimulation of the respiratory center in the medulla caused by salicylate poisoning, hepatic coma, or Reye's syndrome (RS).

Breathing patterns have been described with a number of terms (e.g., *apneustic, cluster, ataxic, Cheyne-Stokes*). However, it is better to describe what is being observed rather than placing a label on it because the traditional terms are often used and interpreted incorrectly. Periodic or irregular breathing is an ominous sign of brainstem (especially medullary) dysfunction that often precedes complete apnea. The odor of the breath may provide additional clues (e.g., the fruity, acetone odor of ketosis; the foul odor of uremia; the fetid odor of hepatic failure; or the odor of alcohol).

Skin

The skin may offer clues to the cause of unconsciousness. The head should be examined for trauma such as lacerations, ecchymosis, or hematoma; the body surface should be examined for signs of injury, needle marks, petechiae, bites, and ticks. Evidence of toxic substances may be found on the hands, face, mouth, and clothing, especially in small children.

Eyes

Pupil size and reactivity are assessed (Fig. 45-3; see also Fig. 45-2). Pinpoint pupils are commonly observed in poisoning such as opiate or barbiturate poisoning and in brainstem dysfunction. Widely dilated and reactive pupils are often seen after seizures and may involve only one side. Dilated pupils may also be caused by eye trauma. Widely dilated and fixed pupils suggest paralysis of cranial nerve III secondary to pressure from herniation of the brain through

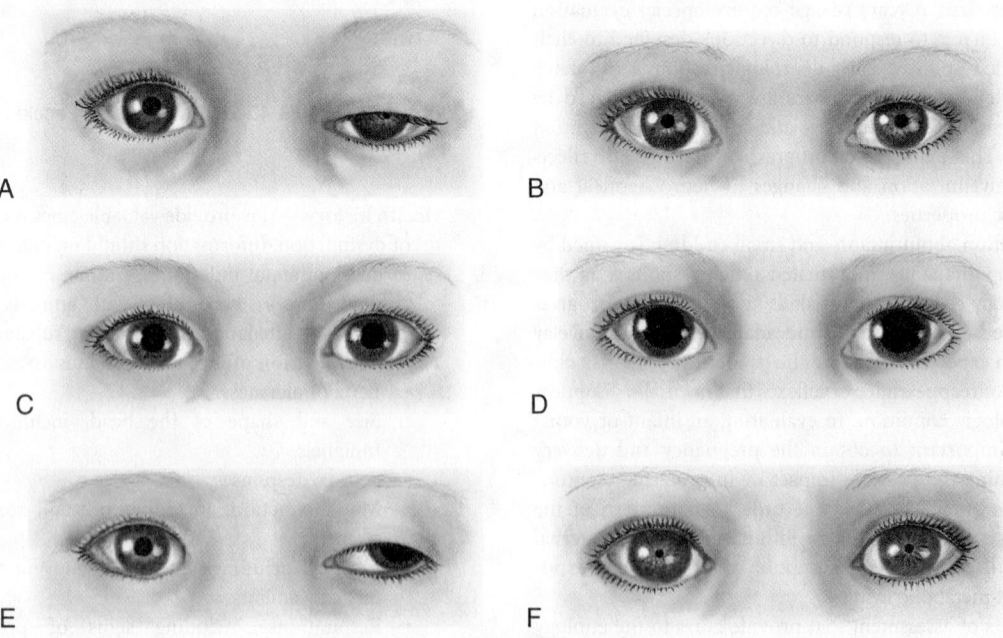

FIG 45-3 Variations in pupil size with altered states of consciousness. **A,** Ipsilateral pupillary constriction with slight ptosis. **B,** Bilateral small pupils. **C,** Midposition, light fixed to all stimuli. **D,** Bilateral dilated and fixed pupils. **E,** Dilated pupils, left eye abducted with ptosis. **F,** Pinpoint pupils.

the tentorium. A unilateral fixed pupil usually suggests a lesion on the same side. If pupils are fixed bilaterally for more than 5 minutes, brainstem damage is usually implied. Dilated and nonreactive pupils are also seen in hypothermia, anoxia, ischemia, poisoning with atropine-like substances, or prior instillation of mydriatic drugs.

> ### ! NURSING ALERT
>
> The sudden appearance of a fixed and dilated pupil(s) is a neurologic emergency.

The description of eye movements should indicate whether one or both eyes are involved and how the reaction was elicited. The parents should be asked about preexisting strabismus, which causes the eyes to appear normal under compromise. Posttraumatic strabismus indicates cranial nerve VI damage.

Special tests, usually performed by qualified persons, include:

- Doll's head maneuver–Elicited by rotating the child's head quickly to one side and then to the other. Conjugate (paired or working together) movement of the eyes in the direction opposite to the head rotation is normal. Absence of this response suggests dysfunction of the brainstem or oculomotor nerve (cranial nerve III).

> ### ! NURSING ALERT
>
> Any tests that require head movement are not attempted until after cervical spine injury has been ruled out.

- Caloric test, or oculovestibular response (RS)—Elicited with the child's head up (head of bed is elevated 30 degrees) by irrigating the external auditory canal with 10 mL of ice water for 20 seconds, which normally causes conjugate movement of the eyes toward the side of stimulation. This movement is lost when the pontine centers are impaired, thus providing important information in assessment of the comatose patient.

> ### ! NURSING ALERT
>
> The caloric test is painful and is never performed on a child who is awake or an individual with a ruptured tympanic membrane.

- Funduscopic examination—Reveals additional clues. Papilledema is not evident early in the course of unconsciousness because it takes 24 to 48 hours to develop, if it develops at all. It is characterized by optic disc swelling, indistinct optic disc margins, hemorrhage, tortuosity of vessels, and absence of venous pulsations. The presence of preretinal (subhyaloid) hemorrhages in children is almost invariably a result of acute trauma with intracranial bleeding, usually subarachnoid or subdural hemorrhage.

Motor Function

Observing spontaneous activity, gait, and response to painful stimuli provides clues to the location and extent of cerebral dysfunction. Even subtle movements (e.g., the outward rotation of a hip) should be noted, and the child observed for other signs. Asymmetric movements of the limbs or absence of movement suggests paralysis. In hemiplegia the affected limb lies in external rotation and falls

uncontrollably when lifted and allowed to drop. In patients with cerebellum abnormalities heel-to-toe walking is difficult. Patients with cerebellar ataxia have an unsteady, broad-based gait. All motor functions should be described rather than labeled.

In the deeper comatose states there is little or no spontaneous movement, and the musculature tends to be flaccid. There is considerable variability in the motor behavior in lesser degrees of coma. For example, the child may be relatively immobile or restless and hyperkinetic; muscle tone may be increased or decreased. Tremors, twitching, and spasms of muscles are common observations. The patient may display purposeless movements. Combative or negativistic behavior is common. Hyperactivity is more common in toxic states than in cases of increased ICP. Seizures are common in children and may be present from any cause. Any repetitive or seizure movements should be described precisely.

Posturing

Primitive postural reflexes emerge as cortical control over motor function is lost in brain dysfunction. These reflexes are evident in posturing and motor movements directly related to the area of the brain involved. Posturing reflects a balance between the lower exciting and the higher inhibiting influences and strong muscles overcoming weaker ones. Decorticate or flexion posturing (Fig. 45-4, A) is seen with severe dysfunction of the cerebral cortex or lesions to corticospinal tracts above the brainstem. Typical posturing includes rigid flexion with the arms held tightly to the body; flexed elbows, wrists, and fingers; plantar flexed feet; legs extended and internally rotated; and possibly the presence of fine tremors or intense stiffness. Decerebrate posture or extension posturing (see Fig. 45-4, B) is a sign of dysfunction at the level of the midbrain or lesions to the brainstem. It is characterized by rigid extension and pronation of the arms and legs, flexed wrists and fingers, a clenched jaw, an extended neck, and possibly an arched back. Unilateral decerebrate posture is often caused by tentorial herniation.

Posturing may not be evident when the child is quiet but can usually be elicited by applying painful stimuli such as a blunt object pressed on the base of the nail. Nurses should avoid applying thumb pressure to the supraorbital region of the frontal bone (risk of orbital damage). Noxious stimuli (e.g., suctioning) elicits a response,

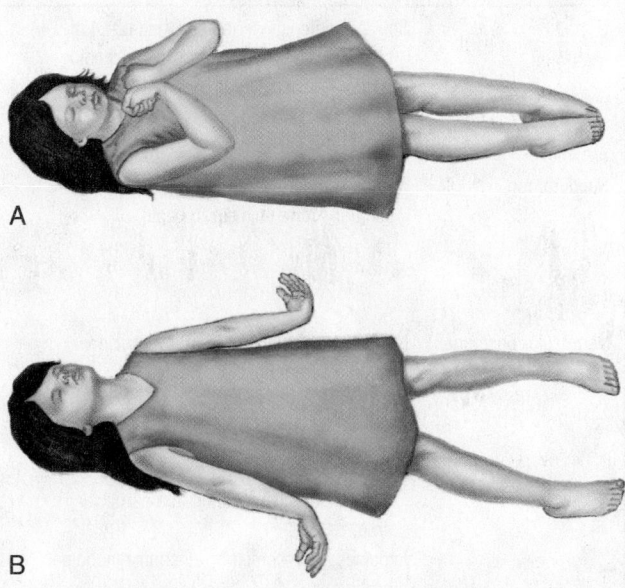

A

B

FIG 45-4 A, Flexion posturing. **B,** Extension posturing.

as may turning or touching. When the nurse is describing posturing, the stimulus needed to provoke the response is as important as the reaction.

Reflexes

Testing of some reflexes may be of limited value. In general the corneal, pupillary, muscle-stretch, superficial, and plantar reflexes tend to be absent in deep coma. The state of reflexes varies in lighter grades of unconsciousness and depends on the underlying pathologic process and the location of the lesion. Absence of corneal reflexes and presence of a tonic neck reflex are associated with severe brain damage. The Babinski reflex (see Extremities, Chapter 29) may be of value if it is found to be present consistently in children older than 18 months. A positive Babinski reflex is significant in assessment of pyramidal tract lesions when it is unilateral and associated with other pyramidal signs.

> **! NURSING ALERT**
>
> Three key reflexes that demonstrate neurologic health in young infants are the Moro, tonic neck, and withdrawal reflexes.

Special Diagnostic Procedures

Numerous diagnostic procedures are used for the assessment of cerebral function. Laboratory tests that may help delineate the cause of unconsciousness include blood glucose, urea nitrogen, and electrolyte (pH, sodium, potassium, chloride, calcium, and bicarbonate) tests; blood ammonia levels; clotting studies, hematocrit, and a complete blood count; liver function tests; blood cultures if there is fever; and urine toxicology screen and blood lead levels if clinically indicated.

An electroencephalogram (EEG) may provide important information. For example, generalized random, slow activity suggests suppressed cortical function; and localized slow activity suggests a space-occupying issue such as a hematoma, tumor, or infectious process. A flat tracing is one of the criteria used as evidence of brain death.

Examination of spinal fluid is performed when toxic encephalopathy or infection is suspected. Lumbar puncture ordinarily is delayed if intracranial hemorrhage is suspected and is contraindicated in the presence of ICP because of the potential for tentorial herniation.

Auditory and visual evoked potentials are sometimes used in neurologic evaluation of infants and very young children. Visual evoked potentials are useful in evaluating visual abnormalities from the retina to the visual cortex, and brainstem auditory evoked potentials are useful for assessing hearing acuity and brainstem function. Both are particularly useful for detecting demyelinating disease and neoplasms.

Highly sophisticated tests are carried out with specialized equipment. Two imaging techniques, computed tomography (CT) and magnetic resonance imaging (MRI), assist in diagnosis by scanning both soft tissues and solid matter. Most of these tests are outlined in Table 45-1. Because such tests can be threatening to children, the nurse needs to prepare patients for them and provide support and reassurance during them (see Preparation for Diagnostic and Therapeutic Procedures, Chapter 39). Children who are old enough to understand require careful explanation of the procedure, reason for it, what they will experience, and how they can help. School-age children usually appreciate a more detailed description of why contrast material is injected. The importance of lying still for tests needs to be stressed. Children unfamiliar with the machines can be shown a picture beforehand.

Although radiographic examinations are not painful, the appearance of the machinery is often so frightening that the child protests because of anxiety. This is especially true of CT and MRI, both of which require that the child's head be placed within a special immobilizing device. Chin and cheek pads are sometimes used to prevent the slightest head movement, and straps are applied to the body to prevent a slight change in body position. The nurse can explain these events to a frightened child by comparing them to an astronaut's

TABLE 45-1   NEUROLOGIC DIAGNOSTIC PROCEDURES

TEST	DESCRIPTION	PURPOSE	COMMENTS
LP	Spinal needle is inserted between L3-L4 or L4-L5 vertebral spaces into subarachnoid space; CSF pressure is measured, and sample is collected.	Diagnostic—Measures spinal fluid pressure, obtains CSF for laboratory analysis Therapeutic—Injection of medication	Contraindicated in patients with increased ICP or infected skin over puncture site.
Subdural tap	Needle is inserted into anterior fontanel or coronal suture (midline to pupil).	Helps rule out subdural effusions Removes CSF to relieve pressure	Place infant in semi-erect position after subdural tap to minimize leakage from site; prevent child from crying if possible. Check site frequently for evidence of leakage.
Ventricular puncture	Needle is inserted into lateral ventricle via coronal suture (midline to pupil).	Removes CSF to relieve pressure	Risk of intracerebral or ventricular hemorrhage.
EEG	EEG records changes in electrical potential of brain. Electrodes are placed at various points to assess electrical function in a particular area. Impulses are recorded by electromagnetic pen or digitally.	Detects spikes, or bursts of electrical activity that indicate the potential for seizures Used to determine brain death	Patient should remain quiet during procedure; may require sedation. Minimize external stimuli during procedure.

TABLE 45-1   NEUROLOGIC DIAGNOSTIC PROCEDURES—cont'd

TEST	DESCRIPTION	PURPOSE	COMMENTS
Nuclear brain scan	Radioisotope is injected intravenously and then counted and recorded after fixed time intervals. Radioisotope accumulates in areas where blood-brain barrier is defective.	Identifies focal brain lesions (e.g., tumors, abscesses) Positive uptake of material with encephalitis and subdural hematoma Visualizes CSF pathways	Requires IV access; patient may require sedation. In normal children or noncommunicating hydrocephalus, no retrograde filling of ventricles occurs. Areas of concentrated uptake of material are termed *hot spots*.
Endocephalography	Pulses of ultrasonic waves are beamed through head; echoes from reflecting surfaces are recorded graphically.	Identifies shifts in midline structures from their normal positions as a result of intracranial lesions May show ventricular dilation	Simple, safe, rapid procedure. Fontanel must be patent.
RTUS	Similar to CT but uses ultrasound instead of ionizing radiation.	Allows high-resolution anatomic visualization in variety of imaging planes	Produces images similar to CT scan. Especially useful in neonatal CNS problems. Anterior fontanel must be patent.
Radiography	Skull films are taken from different views—lateral, posterolateral, axial (submentoventricular), half-axial.	Shows fractures, dislocations, spreading suture lines, craniosynostosis Shows degenerative changes, bone erosion, calcifications	Simple, noninvasive procedure.
CT scan	Pinpoint x-ray beam is directed on horizontal or vertical plane to provide series of images that are fed into computer and assembled in image displayed on video screen. CT uses ionizing radiation.	Visualizes horizontal and vertical cross section of brain in three planes (axial, coronal, sagittal) Distinguishes density of various intracranial tissues and structures—congenital abnormalities, hemorrhage, tumors, demyelinating and inflammatory processes, calcification	Requires IV access if contrast agent is used. Patient may require sedation. Rapid.
MRI	MRI produces radiofrequency emissions from elements (e.g., hydrogen, phosphorus), which are converted to visual images by computer.	Permits visualization of morphologic feature of target structures Permits tissue discrimination unavailable with many techniques	MRI is noninvasive procedure except when IV contrast agent is used. No exposure to radiation occurs. Patient may require sedation. Parent or attendant can remain in room with child. MRI does not visualize bone detail or calcifications. No metal can be present in scanner.
PET	PET involves IV injection of positron-emitting radionucleotide; local concentrations are detected and transformed into visual display by computer.	Detects and measures blood volume and flow in brain, metabolic activity, and biochemical changes within tissue	Requires lengthy period of immobility. Minimum exposure to radiation occurs. Patient may require sedation.
DSA	Contrast dye is injected intravenously; computer "subtracts" all tissues without contrast medium, leaving clear image of contrast medium in vessels studied.	Visualizes vasculature of target tissue Visualizes finite vascular abnormalities	Safe alternative to angiography. Patient must remain still during procedure; may require sedation.
SPECT	Involves IV injection of photon-emitting radionuclide; radionuclides are absorbed by healthy tissue at different rate than by diseased or necrotic tissue; data are transferred to computer that converts image to film.	Provides information regarding blood flow to tissues; analyzing blood flow to organ may help determine how well it is functioning	Requires lengthy period of immobility. Minimum exposure to radiation occurs. Patient may require sedation.

CNS, Central nervous system; *CSF*, cerebrospinal fluid; *CT*, computed tomography; *DSA*, digital subtraction angiography; *EEG*, electroencephalography; *ICP*, intracranial pressure; *IV*, intravenous; *LP*, lumbar puncture; *MRI*, magnetic resonance imaging; *PET*, positron emission tomography; *RTUS*, real-time ultrasonography; *SPECT*, single-photon emission computed tomography.

preparation for a space flight. It is important to emphasize to the child that at no time is the procedure painful.

The nurse should not expect cooperation from a young child. Sedation may be required. Many different agents are currently used for sedation of children undergoing neurologic diagnostic procedures. Chloral hydrate, pentobarbital, or benzodiazepines have been used for decades as short-term sedative agents and remain safe methods of pediatric outpatient sedation (Mason, 2008). Chloral hydrate and pentobarbital have no analgesic proprieties but can provide successful sedation for nonpainful procedures such as CT and MRI (Mason, 2008). In recent years propofol has been used as a sedation agent for diagnostic procedures because of its short induction and recovery time, but this medication should be used with caution because it can cause respiratory depression and apnea with little warning (Machata, Willschke, Kabon, et al., 2008; Mason, 2008). (See Pain Management, Chapter 30.)

Physical preparation for the diagnostic test may involve administration of a sedative. If so, children should be helped through the preparation and administration and assured that someone will remain with them (if possible). Children need continual support and reinforcement during procedures in which they remain conscious. Vital signs and physiologic responses to the procedure are monitored throughout. Many diagnostic procedures performed on an outpatient basis require sedation, and children need recovery time and observation. The nurse should review written instructions with parents if the child is discharged after a procedure. Children who have undergone a procedure with a general anesthetic require postanesthesia care, including positioning, to prevent aspiration of secretions and frequent assessment of the vital signs and LOC. In addition, other neurologic functions such as pupillary responses, motor strength, and movement are tested at regular intervals. Any surgical wound resulting from the test is checked for bleeding, CSF leakage, and other complications. Children who undergo repeated subdural taps should have their hematocrit monitored to detect excessive blood loss from the procedure.

NURSING CARE OF THE UNCONSCIOUS CHILD

The unconscious child requires nursing attention, with observation, recording, and evaluation of changes in objective signs. These observations provide valuable information regarding the patient's progress. Often they serve as a guide to the diagnosis and treatment. Therefore careful and detailed observations are essential for the patient's welfare. In addition, vital functions must be maintained, and complications prevented through conscientious and meticulous nursing care. The outcome of unconsciousness may be early and complete recovery, death within a few hours or days, persistent and permanent unconsciousness, or recovery with varying degrees of residual mental or physical disability. The outcome and recovery of the unconscious child may depend on the level of nursing care and observational skills.

Emergency measures are directed toward ensuring a patent airway, breathing, and circulation; stabilizing the spine when indicated; treating shock; and reducing ICP if present. Delayed treatment often leads to increased damage. As soon as emergency measures have been implemented, and in many cases concurrently, therapies for specific causes are begun. Because nursing care is closely related to medical management, both are considered here.

Continual observation of LOC, pupillary reaction, and vital signs is essential to manage CNS disorders. Regular assessment of neurologic status is an essential part of nursing comatose children. The assessment frequency depends on the cause of unconsciousness, the

LOC, and the progression of cerebral involvement. Intervals may be as short as every 15 minutes or as long as every 2 hours. Significant alterations must be reported immediately.

Vital signs provide important information about the status of the unconscious child. Hypothalamic and brainstem disorders may affect the patient's thermoregulation; thus frequent monitoring is needed. The temperature is taken every 2 to 4 hours, depending on the patient's condition. Hypothermia is defined as a core body temperature less than 35°C (95°F). EEG slowing is noted at 30°C, and loss of pupillary light reflex is lost at 28°C (Young, 2009). Hyperthermia is defined as a core body temperature greater than 38.5°C (101.3°F); and temperatures greater than 42°C can cause EEG slowing, seizures, and encephalopathy (Young, 2009).

The neurologic examination is performed periodically and includes evaluating pupillary abnormalities, brainstem function, LOC, and motor response (Sharma, Kochar, Sankhyan, et al., 2010). Pupils are observed for their size, symmetry, and reaction to light. Signs of meningeal irritation such as nuchal rigidity are also assessed. The presence of the oculovestibular response, corneal (blink) response, and cough and gag reflexes is evaluated. Aspects of LOC assessment include response to vocal commands, resistance to care, and response to painful stimuli. Spontaneous movement, changes in muscle tone or strength, and body position are noted. Seizure activity is described according to the duration and body areas involved.

Pain management for the comatose child requires astute nursing observation and management. Responses to pain include motor reactions such as increased agitation or posturing; facial changes such as grimaces; and physiologic reactions such as tachycardia, tachypnea, diaphoresis, or hypertension (Schnakers and Zasler, 2007). Because these findings may not be specific for pain, the nurse should observe for their appearance during times of induced or suspected pain and their disappearance after the end of the inciting procedure or the administration of analgesia. A pain assessment record should be used to document indications of pain and the effectiveness of interventions (see Pain Assessment, Chapter 30).

The use of opioids such as morphine to relieve pain is controversial because they may mask signs of altered consciousness or depress respirations. However, unrelieved pain activates the stress response, which can elevate ICP. To block the stress response, some authorities advocate the use of analgesics; sedatives; and in some cases paralyzing agents via continuous intravenous (IV) infusion. A frequently used combination is fentanyl, midazolam, and vecuronium (Norcuron). If there are concerns about assessing the LOC or respiratory depression, naloxone (Narcan) can be used to reverse the opioid effects. Regardless of which drugs are used, adequate dosage and regular administration are essential to provide optimal pain relief (see Pain Management, Chapter 30).

Other measures to relieve discomfort include providing a quiet, dimly lit environment; limiting visitors; preventing any sudden, jarring movement such as banging into the bed; and preventing an increase in ICP. The last is most effectively achieved by proper positioning and prevention of straining such as during coughing, vomiting, suctioning, and defecating.

💊 MEDICATION ALERT

When opioids are used, bowel elimination must be monitored closely because of the potential constipating effect. Stool softeners should be given with laxatives as needed to prevent constipation.

Respiratory Management

Respiratory effectiveness is the primary concern in the care of the unconscious child, and establishing an adequate airway is *always* the first priority. Carbon dioxide has a potent vasodilating effect and increases cerebral blood flow (CBF) and ICP. Cerebral hypoxia that lasts longer than 4 minutes nearly always causes irreversible brain damage.

Children in lighter states of coma may be able to cough and swallow; but those in deeper states are unable to handle secretions, which tend to pool in the throat and pharynx. Dysfunction of cranial nerves IX and X places the child at risk for aspiration and cardiac arrest; therefore the child is positioned to prevent aspiration of secretions, and the stomach is emptied to reduce the likelihood of vomiting. In infants blockage of air passages from secretions can happen in seconds. In addition, upper airway obstruction from laryngospasm is a frequent complication in comatose children.

An oral airway can be used for children who have a temporary loss of consciousness such as after a contusion, seizure, or anesthesia. For children who remain unconscious for a longer time, a nasotracheal or orotracheal tube is inserted to maintain the open airway and facilitate removal of secretions. Endotracheal intubation should be considered in children with a GCS score of less than 8, evidence of herniation, apnea, or inability to maintain an airway (Sankhyan, Raju, Sharma, et al., 2010). A tracheostomy is performed in cases in which laryngoscopy for introduction of an endotracheal tube would be difficult or for a child who needs long-term ventilatory support. Suctioning is used only as needed to clear the airway, exerting care to prevent increasing ICP. Respiratory status is observed and evaluated regularly. Signs of respiratory distress may be an indication for ventilatory assistance.

When the respiratory center is involved, mechanical ventilation is usually indicated (see Chapter 39). Blood gas analysis is performed regularly, and oxygen is administered as indicated. Moderately severe hypoxia and respiratory acidosis are often present but not always evident from clinical manifestations. Hyperventilation frequently accompanies unconsciousness and may lead to respiratory alkalosis, or it may represent the attempt by the body to compensate for metabolic acidosis. Therefore blood gas and pH determinations are essential guides for therapy. Chest physiotherapy is carried out on a regular basis, and the child's position is changed at least every 2 hours to prevent pulmonary complications.

Intracranial Pressure Monitoring

An acute rise in ICP can cause secondary brain injury (Singhi and Tiwari, 2009), and management of the child with increased ICP is a complex and important task. ICP monitoring is used to guide therapy to reduce ICP and provides information on intracranial compliance, cerebrovascular status, and cerebral perfusion (Sankhyan, Raju, Sharma, et al., 2010). Nonetheless ICP monitoring is an invasive procedure that has associated risks, including infection, hemorrhage, malfunction, and obstruction (Singhi and Tiwari, 2009). Indications for inserting an ICP monitor are as follows:

- GCS evaluation of less than 8:
  - Traumatic brain injury with an abnormal head CT scan
  - Deterioration of condition
- Subjective judgment regarding clinical appearance and response

Four major types of ICP monitors are:

1. Intraventricular catheter with fibroscopic sensors attached to a monitoring system
2. Subarachnoid bolt (Richmond screw)
3. Epidural sensor
4. Anterior fontanel pressure monitor.

Direct ventricular pressure measurement with an intraventricular catheter remains the gold standard of ICP monitoring (Singhi and Tiwari, 2009). Subarachnoid and epidural monitoring can be used when a catheter cannot be cannulated in the ventricle, but they often must be replaced after several days because of measurement drift (Singhi and Tiwari, 2009). Transducers for both ventricular and subarachnoid monitoring should be set up without the use of a flush device.

Placement of the intraventricular catheter and subarachnoid bolt occurs through a burr hole in the skull. The intraventricular method involves introduction of a catheter into the lateral ventricle on the nondominant side, if known. The subarachnoid bolt involves placement of a bolt in the subarachnoid space, and the epidural sensor involves placement of a sensor between the dura and the skull. The intraventricular catheter has the advantage of providing a means for recalibration when measurement drift occurs, but both the catheter and the bolt can be used for therapeutic CSF drainage to reduce pressure. A drainage bag attached to the system is kept at the level of the ventricles and can be lowered to decrease ICP (see Critical Thinking Case Study).

! NURSING ALERT

If the external ventricular drain is unclamped for CSF drainage, carefully monitor the level of the collection container. If the container is too low, improper CSF decompression could lower ICP too rapidly, causing bleeding and pain.

! NURSING ALERT

The bolt is stabilized with dressings, and these are not changed or disturbed, even to check the site.

? CRITICAL THINKING CASE STUDY

Hydrocephalus

Three-year-old Emma had a posterior fossa tumor removed 5 days ago. Although an EVD was placed to treat her hydrocephalus, she continues to demonstrate signs of increased ICP, including holding the back of her head, anorexia, crying when moved or when strangers enter the room, and intermittent lethargy. On examination fluid drainage is noted on the mother's clothes, and Emma is experiencing repetitive, rapid eyelid blinking.

1. Evidence—Is there sufficient evidence to draw conclusions about Emma's behavior, physical assessment findings, and ICP?
2. Assumptions—Describe any underlying assumption about each of the following:
   a. A preschool-age child who had a posterior fossa tumor removed 5 days ago
   b. A preschool-age child who has an EVD placed to treat the hydrocephalus
   c. A preschool-age child with an EVD who continues to demonstrate physical signs associated with increased ICP after recent surgery
3. What priorities for nursing care should be established?
4. Does the evidence support your nursing intervention?

EVD, External ventricular drain; *ICP*, intracranial pressure.

Placement of the subarachnoid bolt is not adjusted by anyone except the neurosurgeon who placed the device. The neurosurgeon is notified if a satisfactory waveform on the ICP monitoring is not observed.

An epidural sensor provides a readout of the ICP with a stopcock assembly and transducer. Although less invasive, ICP measurements may be inconsistent. In infants a fontanel transducer can be used to detect impulses from a pressure sensor and convert them to electrical energy. The electrical energy is then converted to visible waves or numeric readings on an oscilloscope. ICP measurement from the anterior fontanel is noninvasive but may prove to be inaccurate if the equipment is poorly placed or recalibrated inconsistently.

ICP can be increased by instilling solutions; therefore antibiotics are administered systemically if a positive CSF culture is obtained. CSF is a body fluid; therefore Standard Precautions are implemented according to hospital policy (see Infection Control, Chapter 39).

Nurses caring for patients with intracranial monitoring devices must be acquainted with the system, assist with insertion, interpret the monitor readings, and be able to distinguish between danger signals and mechanical dysfunction.

For sustained ICP elevations greater than 20 to 25 mm Hg, several medical measures are available. Osmotic diuretics may provide rapid relief in emergency situations. Although their effect is transient, lasting only about 6 hours, they can be lifesaving in emergencies. These substances are rapidly excreted by the kidneys and carry with them large quantities of sodium and water. Mannitol (or sometimes urea) administered intravenously is the drug most frequently used for rapid reduction and can lower ICP in 1 to 5 minutes. The infusion is generally given slowly but may be pushed rapidly in cases of herniation or impending herniation. Hypertonic saline in concentrations of 3% to 23% has been shown to reduce ICP by its osmotic force and can be beneficial for hypovolemic and hypotensive patients by increasing intravascular volume and blood pressure (Singhi and Tiwari, 2009). Adrenocorticosteroids are not recommended for cerebral edema secondary to head trauma. $Paco_2$ should be maintained at 25 to 30 mm Hg to produce vasoconstriction, which reduces CSF, thereby decreasing ICP; but this effect is sustained only 11 to 20 hours because the CSF equilibrates to the new $PaCO_2$ level (Singhi and Tiwari, 2009).

Nursing Activities

In cases of high levels of increased ICP, procedures tend to trigger reactive pressure waves in many patients. For example, increased intrathoracic or abdominal pressure is transmitted to the cranium. Particular care should be taken in positioning these patients to avoid neck vein compression, which may further increase ICP by interfering with venous return.

The child can be propped to one side or the other, and the use of an alternating-pressure mattress reduces the chance of prolonged pressure to vulnerable areas. Frequent clinical assessment of the child cannot be replaced by an ICP monitoring device.

! NURSING ALERT

The head of the bed is elevated to 30 degrees, and the child is positioned so the head is maintained in midline to facilitate venous drainage and avoid jugular compression (Sankhyan, Raju, Sharma, et al., 2010). Turning side to side is contraindicated because of the risk of jugular compression.

It is important to avoid activities that may increase ICP by causing pain or emotional stress. Gentle range-of-motion exercises can be carried out but should not be performed vigorously. Nontherapeutic touch can cause an increase in ICP. Any disturbing procedures to be performed should be scheduled to take advantage of therapies such as osmotherapy and sedation that reduce ICP. Efforts are taken to minimize or eliminate environmental noise. Assessment and intervention to relieve pain are important nursing functions to decrease ICP. Individualizing nursing activities and minimizing environmental stimuli by decreasing elective procedures help control ICP (Sankhyan, Raju, Sharma, et al., 2010).

Suctioning

Suctioning and percussion are poorly tolerated and therefore are contraindicated unless concurrent respiratory problems exist. Hypoxia and the Valsalva maneuver associated with cough both acutely elevate ICP. Vibration, which does not increase ICP, accomplishes excellent results and should be tried first if treatment is needed. If suctioning is necessary, it should be brief and proceeded by hyperventilation with 100% oxygen, which can be monitored during suctioning with a pulse oxygen sensor reading to determine oxygen saturation.

Nutrition and Hydration

In the unconscious child fluids and calories are supplied initially by the IV route (see Chapter 39). An IV infusion is started early, and the type of fluid administered is determined by the patient's general condition. Fluid therapy requires careful monitoring and adjustment based on neurologic signs and electrolyte determinations. The goal of fluid therapy is euvolemia. Often comatose children are unable to cope with the same amounts of fluid they can tolerate when they are healthy, and overhydration must be avoided to prevent fatal cerebral edema. When cerebral edema is a threat, fluids may be restricted to reduce the chance of fluid overload. Skin and mucous membranes are examined for signs of dehydration. Observation for signs of altered fluid balance related to abnormal pituitary secretions is a part of nursing care.

Long-term nutrition is provided with a balanced formula via a nasogastric or gastrostomy tube. Most children have continuous feedings; but, if bolus feedings are used, the tube is rinsed with water after each feeding. Avoid overfeeding to prevent vomiting and the risk of aspiration.

Altered Pituitary Secretion

An altered ability to handle fluid loads is attributed in part to the syndrome of inappropriate antidiuretic hormone secretion (SIADH) and diabetes insipidus (DI) resulting from hypothalamic dysfunction (see Chapter 46). SIADH frequently accompanies CNS diseases such as head injury, meningitis, encephalitis, brain abscess, brain tumor, and subarachnoid hemorrhage. In patients with SIADH, scant quantities of urine are excreted, electrolyte analysis reveals hyponatremia and hyposmolality, and manifestations of overhydration are evident. It is important to evaluate all parameters because the reduced urinary output might be erroneously interpreted as a sign of dehydration. The treatment of SIADH consists of restriction of fluids until serum electrolytes and osmolality return to normal levels.

DI may occur after intracranial trauma. In DI there are large amounts of diluted urine and the accompanying danger of dehydration. Adequate replacement of fluids is essential, and observation of electrolyte balance is necessary to detect signs of hypernatremia and hyperosmolality. Exogenous vasopressin may be administered.

Medications

The cause of unconsciousness determines specific drug therapies. Children with infectious processes are given antibiotics appropriate to the disease and the infecting organism. Corticosteroids are prescribed for inflammatory conditions and edema. Cerebral edema is an indication for osmotherapy. Sedatives or antiepileptics are prescribed for seizure activity (see p. 1449).

MEDICATION ALERT

Sedation in the combative child provides amnesic and anxiolytic properties in conjunction with a paralytic agent. The combination decreases ICP and allows treatment of cerebral edema. Usual drugs include morphine, midazolam, and pancuronium (Pavulon). Midazolam is appealing because of its short half-life. Prolonged use of propofol should be avoided in children because of the risk of metabolic acidosis (Orliaguet, Meyer, and Baugnon, 2008).

Deep coma induced by administration of barbiturates is controversial in the management of ICP. Barbiturates are currently reserved for the reduction of increased ICP when all else has failed. They decrease the cerebral metabolic rate for oxygen and protect the brain during times of reduced cerebral perfusion pressure. Barbiturate coma requires extensive monitoring, cardiovascular and respiratory support, and ICP monitoring to assess response to therapy. Paralyzing agents such as pancuronium also may be needed to aid in performing diagnostic tests, improving effectiveness of therapy, and reducing risks of secondary complications. Elevation of ICP or heart rate of patients who are being given paralyzing agents or are under sedation may indicate the need for another dose of either or both medications.

Thermoregulation

Hyperthermia often accompanies cerebral dysfunction; if it is present, measures are implemented to reduce the temperature to prevent brain damage and reduce metabolic demands generated by the increased body temperature. Antipyretic agents are usually ineffective with hyperthermia as a result of traumatic brain injury; therefore external cooling should be used (Badjatia, 2009). External cooling consists of evaporation (sponge baths), conduction (ice packs, cooling blankets), convection (fans), and radiation (skin exposure) (Badjatia, 2009). Laboratory tests and other methods are used in an attempt to determine the cause of the hyperthermia.

Elimination

A urinary catheter is usually inserted in the acute phase, although diapers may be used and weighed to record urinary output. The child who formerly had bowel and bladder control is generally incontinent. If the child remains comatose for a long period, the indwelling catheter may be removed, and periodic bladder emptying can be accomplished by intermittent catheterization. Stool softeners are usually sufficient to maintain bowel function, but suppositories or enemas may be needed occasionally for adequate elimination and to prevent fecal impaction. The passage of liquid stool after a period of no bowel activity is usually a sign of an impaction. To avoid this preventable problem, daily recording of bowel activity is essential.

Hygienic Care

Routine measures for cleansing and maintaining skin integrity are an integral part of nursing care of the unconscious child (see Maintaining Healthy Skin, Chapter 39).

Mouth care is performed at least twice daily because the mouth tends to become dry or coated with mucus. The teeth are brushed carefully with a soft toothbrush or cleaned with gauze saturated with saline. Commercially prepared cleansing devices such as Toothettes are convenient for cleansing the mouth and teeth. Lips are coated with ointment or other preparations to protect them from drying, cracking, or blistering.

Unconscious children are susceptible to eye irritation. The corneal reflexes are absent; therefore the eyes are easily irritated or damaged by linen, dust, or other substances that may come in contact with them. Excessive dryness results from incomplete closure of the eyes or decreased secretions, especially if the child is undergoing osmotherapy to reduce or prevent cerebral edema.

NURSING ALERT

The eyes should be examined regularly and carefully for early signs of irritation or inflammation. Artificial tears or a lubricating ointment is placed in the eyes every 1 to 2 hours. Eye dressings may be necessary to protect the eyes from possible damage.

Positioning and Exercise

The unconscious child is positioned to minimize ICP and prevent aspiration of saliva, nasogastric secretions, and vomitus. The head of the bed is elevated, and the child is placed in a side-lying or semiprone position. A small, firm pillow is placed under the head, and the uppermost limbs are flexed and supported with pillows. The weight of the body should not rest on the dependent arm. In the semiprone position the child lies with the dependent arm at the side behind the body, the opposite side supported on pillows, and the uppermost arm and leg flexed and resting on the pillows. This position prevents undue pressure on the dependent extremities. The dependent position of the face encourages drainage of secretions and prevents the flaccid tongue from obstructing the airway.

Normal range-of-motion exercises help maintain function and prevent contractures of joints. Exercises should be performed gently and with full range of motion. A small rolled pad can be placed in the palms to help maintain proper position of fingers; footboards or high-top shoes can help prevent footdrop; and splinting may be needed to prevent severe contractures of the wrist, knee, or ankle in decerebrate children.

Stimulation

Sensory stimulation is important in the care of the unconscious child. It helps arouse a temporarily unconscious or semiconscious child to the conscious state and orient him or her to time and place. Auditory and tactile stimulation are especially valuable. Tactile stimulation is not appropriate for children in whom it may elicit an undesirable response. However, for other children it often has a relaxing and calming effect. When the child's condition permits, holding or rocking has a soothing effect and provides the body contact needed by young children. Involving family members with the sensory stimulation can create a positive effect on the child and allows the family to participate in the care (Abbasi, Mohammadi, and Rezayi, 2009).

The auditory sense is often intact in a state of coma. Hearing is the last sense to be lost and the first one to be regained; therefore the child should be spoken to as any other child. Conversation around the child should not include thoughtless or derogatory remarks. Soft music is used frequently to provide auditory stimulation. Singing the child's favorite songs or reading a favorite story is a tactic used to maintain the child's contact with a familiar world. Playing songs or stories recorded in the parents' voices can provide a continuous source of familiar stimulation.

Regaining Consciousness

Awakening from a coma is a gradual process; however, sometimes children regain consciousness within a short time. Regaining orientation involves knowing person, place, and time in that order.

Certain behaviors have been observed when children awaken from the unconscious state. The stress and anxiety they appear to feel in a strange and unfamiliar environment can be expressed in silent, withdrawn behavior. They respond to basic questioning but usually do not display their prehospitalization personality and social behavior until they are transferred from the critical care area.

Family Support

Helping the parents of an unconscious child cope with the situation is especially difficult. They may demonstrate all of the guilt, fear, hostility, and anxiety of any parent of a seriously ill child (see Chapter 38). In addition, these parents are faced with the uncertain outcome of the cerebral dysfunction. The fear of death, intellectual disability, or other permanent disability is present. Nursing intervention with parents depends on the nature of the pathologic condition, the parents' personality, and the parent-child relationship before the injury or illness. Parents need the most intensive nursing intervention during the period of crisis and uncertainty. Throughout the treatment and recovery phase the nurse provides parents with information and encourages them to become involved in the child's care.

Probably the most difficult situations involve children who never regain consciousness. Family members often attempt to construct a representation of the child by bringing items that belong to him or her such as favorite toys or music. This is interpreted as an attempt to provide stimulation for the child in the hope of eliciting a response, to let the hospital staff know the child as the unique individual that he or she was, and to reconstitute an image of the child "lost" to them and for whom they mourn. Unlike losing a child through death, these situations lack finality, which often leaves family members in a state of prolonged grief and searching for signs of hope. An awareness of these behaviors and coping mechanisms provides nurses with the understanding that helps them support the parents in their grief process.

Superimposed on the process of grieving for the "lost" child, parents may be faced with difficult decisions. When the child's brain is so severely damaged that vital functions must be maintained by artificial means, the parents along with guidance from the health care team must make the final decision of whether to remove life-support systems. Nurses continue to provide specialty care during this time that maintains the patient's physiologic status while addressing informational and psychologic needs of the family (Ashwal and Serna-Fonseca, 2006). This decision is difficult for parents, but having an open and honest dialog about the child's medical condition and prognosis can help make patient-centered conclusions (Young, 2009). Parents' cultural, religious, and language needs along with their intellectual level, decision-making preferences, and emotional state are considered during the discussions (Truog, Campbell, Curtis, et al., 2008). Sometimes parents may choose to refuse or not initiate treatment if they believe it to be best for the child and the family (informed dissent). At other times they request that "everything possible" be done for the child.

When the child has survived the cerebral insult and is not comatose but physical or mental capacity is limited either minimally or severely, families must cope with the long and tedious rehabilitation process and the uncertain outcome. The drain on financial, emotional, and social resources can be enormous.

For parents who choose to care for their child at home, planning for home care begins early in the recovery process. The family should become involved with the child's care as soon as they indicate an interest and ability to do so. They need education and support in learning to care for the child, regular follow-up observation and assessment of the home management, and planning for some respite care of the child. Parents need to understand that it is important to plan for periodic relief from the continual care of the child (see Preparing for Discharge and Home Care, Chapter 38).

CEREBRAL TRAUMA

Head Injury

Head injury is a pathologic process involving the scalp, skull, meninges, or brain as a result of trauma. According to national statistics and Safe Kids Worldwide,* unintentional injuries are the number one health risk for children and the leading cause of death in children older than 1 year of age. Annually one in eight children in the United States will sustain an injury serious enough to require medical attention. Tragically 5100 children ages 1 to 14 years are killed every year by injuries (Safe Kids, 2009). It has been estimated that 500,000 children per year sustain a traumatic brain injury and that 2170 children per year die as a result of the brain injury (Faul, Xu, Wald, et al., 2010). Evidence demonstrates that a previous head injury increases a child's risk of having a subsequent head injury (Swaine, Tremblay, Platt, et al., 2007).

Etiology

The three major causes of brain damage in childhood, in order of importance, are falls, motor vehicle injuries, and bicycle or sports-related injuries. Neurologic injury accounts for the highest mortality rate, with boys affected twice as often as girls. In motor vehicle accidents children younger than 2 years of age are almost exclusively injured as passengers, but older children may also be injured as pedestrians or cyclists. The majority of deaths from brain trauma caused by bicycle injuries occur between the ages of 5 and 14 years. Bicycle helmet laws have been effective in reducing the risk of head injury by 85% and brain injury by 88% (Rivara and Grossman, 2011).

The exposed nature of the head renders it particularly vulnerable to trauma, and many of the physical characteristics of children predispose them to craniocerebral trauma. For example, infants can be left unattended on beds, in high chairs, and in other places from which they can fall. Because the head of an infant or toddler is proportionately larger and heavier in relation to other body parts, it is the most likely to be injured. Incomplete motor development contributes to falls at young ages, and the natural curiosity and exuberance of children also increase their risk of injury.

Pathophysiology

The pathology of brain injury is directly related to the force of impact. Intracranial contents (brain, blood, CSF) are damaged because the force is too great to be absorbed by the skull and

---

*1301 Pennsylvania Ave., NW, Suite 1000, Washington, DC 20004-1707, 202-662-0600, www.safekids.org.

musculoligamentous support of the head. Although nervous tissue is delicate, it usually requires a severe blow to cause significant damage.

Primary head injuries are those that occur at the time of trauma and include skull fracture, contusions, intracranial hematoma, and diffuse injury. Subsequent complications include hypoxic brain damage, increased ICP, infection, and cerebral edema. The predominant feature of a child's brain injury is the amount of diffuse swelling that occurs. Hypoxia and hypercapnia threaten the energy requirements of the brain and increase CBF. The added volume across the blood-brain barrier, along with the loss of autoregulation, exacerbates cerebral edema. Pressure inside the skull that is greater than arterial pressure results in inadequate perfusion.

A child's response to head injury is different from that of an adult. The larger head size and insufficient musculoskeletal support render the very young child particularly vulnerable to head injuries. Physical forces act on the head through acceleration, deceleration, or deformation. Acceleration or deceleration is responsible for most head injuries. When the stationary head receives a blow, the sudden acceleration causes deformation of the skull and mass movement of the brain. Continued movement of the intracranial contents allows the brain to strike parts of the skull (e.g., the sharp edges of the sphenoid or the irregular surface of the anterior fossa) or the edges of the tentorium. Sudden deceleration such as takes place during a fall causes the greatest cerebral injury at the point of impact.

Although the brain volume remains unchanged, significant distortion takes place as the brain changes shape in response to the force of impact to the skull. This movement can cause bruising at the point of impact (coup) or at a distance as the brain collides with the unyielding surfaces far removed from the point of impact (contrecoup) (Fig. 45-5). Thus a blow to the occipital region can cause severe injury to the frontal and temporal areas of the brain. Children with an acceleration-deceleration injury demonstrate diffuse

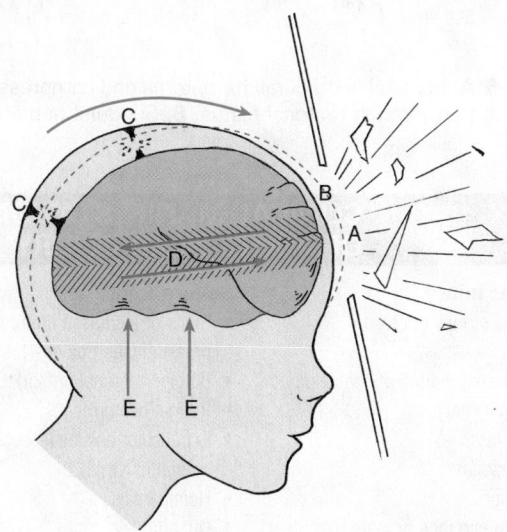

FIG 45-5 Mechanical distortion of the cranium during a closed head injury. **A,** Preinjury contour of the skull. **B,** Immediate postinjury contour of the skull. **C,** Torn subdural vessels. **D,** Shearing forces. **E,** Trauma from contact with the floor of the cranium. (Redrawn from Grubb RL, Coxe WS: Central nervous system trauma: cranial. In Eliasson SG, Presky AL, Hardin Jr WB, editors: *Neurological pathophysiology,* New York, 1974, Oxford University Press.)

generalized cerebral swelling produced by increased blood volume or a redistribution of cerebral blood volume (cerebral hyperemia) rather than by increased water content (edema) as seen in adults.

Another effect of brain movement is shearing stresses, which may tear small arteries and cause subdural hemorrhages. Damage can also occur when severe compression of the skull causes the brain to be forced through the tentorial opening. This can produce irreparable damage to the brainstem (see Fig. 45-6).

Concussion. The most common head injury is concussion, an alteration in neurologic or cognitive function with or without loss of consciousness, which occurs immediately after a head injury (Landry, 2011). Confusion and amnesia after head injury are the hallmarks of concussion; however, loss of consciousness is not an accurate indicator for the presence of a concussion (Meehan and Mannix, 2010). Concussions usually resolve in 7 to 10 days without complications; however, some individuals may require several months to recover (Lee, 2007).

The pathogenesis of concussion is still unclear but may be a result of shearing forces that cause stretching, compression, and tearing of nerve fibers, particularly in the area of the central brainstem, the seat of the reticular activating system. It has also been suggested that the anatomic alterations of nerve fibers cause the release of large quantities of acetylcholine into the CSF and a reduction in oxygen consumption with increased lactate production.

Contusion and Laceration. The terms contusion and laceration are used to describe visible bruising and tearing of cerebral tissue. Contusions represent petechial hemorrhages or localized bruising along the superficial aspects of the brain at the site of impact (coup injury) or a lesion remote from the site of direct trauma (contrecoup injury). In serious accidents there may be multiple sites of injury.

The major areas of the brain susceptible to contusion or laceration are the occipital, frontal, and temporal lobes. In addition, the irregular surfaces of the anterior and middle fossae at the base of the skull are capable of producing bruises or lacerations on forceful impact. Contusions may cause focal disturbances in strength, sensation, or visual awareness. The degree of brain damage in the contused areas varies according to the extent of vascular injury. Signs vary from mild, transient weakness of a limb to prolonged unconsciousness and paralysis. However, the signs and symptoms may be clinically indistinguishable from those of concussion.

The lower incidence of cerebral contusion in infancy has been attributed to infants' pliable skulls with less convolutional markings of the inner space between brain tissue and bone. However, infants who are shaken roughly (shaken baby syndrome) can sustain profound neurologic impairment, seizures, retinal hemorrhages, intracranial subarachnoid or subdural hemorrhages, high cervical spinal cord hemorrhages, and contusions (Walls, 2006).

Cerebral lacerations are generally associated with penetrating or depressed skull fractures. However, they may occur without fracture in small children. When brain tissue is actually torn, with bleeding into and around the tear, more severe and prolonged unconsciousness and paralysis occur, leaving permanent scarring and some degree of disability.

Fractures. Because of its flexibility, the immature skull is able to sustain a greater degree of deformation than the adult skull before it incurs a fracture. A great deal of force is required to produce a fracture in an infant's skull.

The types of skull fractures that occur are linear, depressed, comminuted, basilar, open, and growing. As a rule the faster the blow, the greater the likelihood of a depressed fracture; a low-velocity impact tends to produce a linear fracture.

A linear fracture is a single fracture line that starts at the point of maximum impact but does not cross suture lines. Linear fractures constitute the majority of childhood skull fractures. Most are associated with an overlying hematoma or soft-tissue swelling (Erlichman, Blumfield, Rajpathak, et al., 2010).

Depressed fractures are those in which the bone is broken locally, usually into several irregular fragments that are pushed inward, causing pressure on the brain. Depressed skull fractures may be associated with direct underlying parenchymal damage and should be suspected when a child's head appears misshapen. Surgery may be needed to elevate the depressed bone fragment if there is an associated intracranial hematoma or pressure.

Comminuted fractures consist of multiple associated linear fractures. They usually result from intense impact. These types of fractures often result from repeated blows against an object and may suggest child abuse.

Basilar fractures involve the basilar portion of the frontal, ethmoid, sphenoid, temporal, or occipital bones. Because of the proximity of the fracture line to structures surrounding the brainstem, a basal skull fracture is a serious head injury. Approximately 80% of the cases may include clinical features such as subcutaneous bleeding in the posterior neck area and over the mastoid process (battle sign), bleeding around the eyes (raccoon eyes), bleeding behind the tympanic membrane (hemotympanum), or CSF leakage from the nose or ear (Perheentupa, Kinnunen, Grénman, et al., 2010).

Open fractures cause communication between the skull and the scalp or the mucosa of the upper respiratory tract. Open fractures increase the risk of CNS infection when the fracture creates an opening in the paranasal sinuses or middle ear that causes CSF leakage. They may have a skin laceration overlying the bone fracture called a *compound fracture*. Antibiotics are recommended to prevent osteomyelitis.

Growing fractures are skull fractures associated with an underlying dural tear that may be caused by a leptomeningeal cyst, dilated ventricles, or a herniated brain. Ninety percent of all growing fractures occur before the age of 3 years (Vignes, Jeelani, Jeelani, et al., 2007). Physical examination reveals a pulsatile mass or sunken skull defect; symptoms include headaches, seizures, or both.

Complications

The major complications of trauma to the head are hemorrhage, infection, edema, and herniation through the brainstem. Infection is always a hazard in open injuries, and edema is related to tissue trauma. Vascular rupture may occur even in minor head injuries, causing hemorrhage between the skull and cerebral surfaces. Compression of the underlying brain produces effects that can be rapidly fatal or insidiously progressive.

Epidural Hemorrhage. An epidural hemorrhage is bleeding between the dura and the skull to form a hematoma. This bleeding causes the dura to be stripped from bone, forcing the underlying brain contents downward and inward as the brain expands (Fig. 45-6, *A*). Because bleeding is generally arterial, brain compression occurs rapidly. Most often the expanding hematoma is located in the parietal and temporal regions, although it can occur in the frontal or occipital posterior fossa (Case, 2008). The lower incidence of epidural hematoma in childhood has been attributed to the fact that the middle meningeal artery is not embedded in the bone surface of the skull until approximately 2 years of age. Therefore a fracture of the temporal bone is less likely to lacerate the artery. Second, the dura closely adheres to the inner table of the skull, especially at the level of the sutures, making separation from bleeding less likely.

However, a child's skull can be indented with sufficient force to tear the middle meningeal artery and rebound intact without causing a fracture. Hemorrhage can also derive from dural veins or the dural sinuses, especially in infants and small children in whom fracture is less likely to occur. In 20% to 40% of children a skull fracture is not detectable. The classic clinical picture of epidural hemorrhage (momentary unconsciousness followed by a normal period and then lethargy or coma) can be less evident in children (see Box 45-3 for

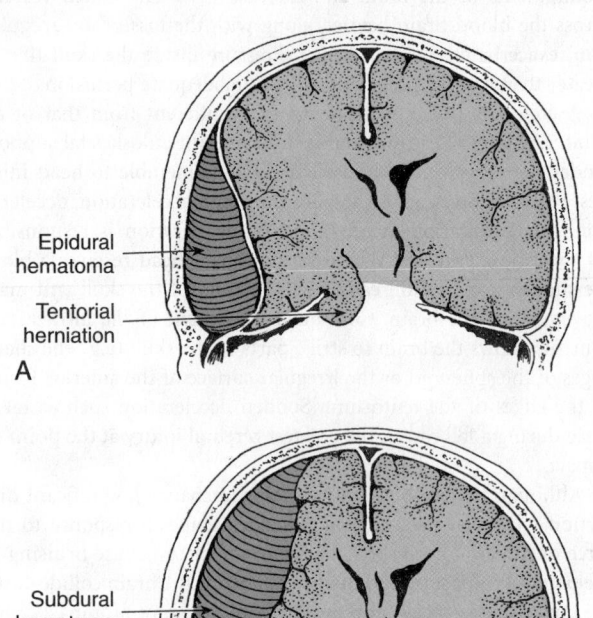

FIG 45-6 A, Epidural (extradural) hematoma and compression of temporal lobe through tentorial hiatus. **B,** Subdural hematoma.

BOX 45-3 CLINICAL MANIFESTATIONS OF ACUTE HEAD INJURY

Minor Injury
- May or may not lose consciousness
- Transient period of confusion
- Somnolence
- Listlessness
- Irritability
- Pallor
- Vomiting (one or more episodes)

Signs of Progression
- Altered mental status (e.g., difficulty arousing child)
- Mounting agitation
- Development of focal lateral neurologic signs
- Marked changes in vital signs

Severe Injury
- Signs of increased intracranial pressure (see Box 45-1)
- Bulging fontanel (infant)
- Retinal hemorrhages
- Extraocular palsies (especially cranial nerve III)
- Hemiparesis
- Quadriplegia
- Elevated temperature
- Unsteady gait
- Papilledema

Associated Signs
- Scalp trauma
- Other injuries (e.g., to extremities)

clinical manifestations). Frequently the period of impaired consciousness is lacking; and the symptom-free period is atypical because of nonspecific symptoms such as irritability, headache, and vomiting. Physical findings can include pallor with anemia and cephalhematoma, with infants exhibiting hypotonia and a bulging fontanel. If the severity of the child's signs and symptoms is not recognized, herniation and death will occur.

Subdural Hemorrhage. A subdural hemorrhage is bleeding between the dura and the arachnoid membrane, usually as a result of rupture of cortical veins that bridge the subdural space (see Fig. 45-6, *B*). Subdural hematomas are more common than epidural hematomas, occurring most often in infancy.

Unlike epidural hemorrhage, which develops inwardly against the less resistant brain tissue, subdural hemorrhage tends to develop more slowly and spreads thinly and widely until it is limited by the dural barriers (i.e., the falx and tentorium). Subdural hematomas are fairly common in infants, frequently as a result of birth trauma, falls, assaults, or violent shaking. Presenting signs can include irritability, vomiting, increased head circumference, bulging fontanels in infants, lethargy, or seizures. The small subdural space and dura firmly attached to the skull in this area are highly vulnerable to increased ICP. Hemiparesis, hemiplegia, and unequal pupils are signs of brainstem compression and increased ICP.

> **! NURSING ALERT**
>
> Children with a subdural hematoma and retinal hemorrhages should be evaluated for the possibility of child abuse, especially shaken baby syndrome.

Subdural taps often provide relief in the infant, as revealed by follow-up CT scans, improved neurologic status, and a flat anterior fontanel. The need for surgical evacuation of the hematoma depends on the physical examination, size of the hematoma, and CT scan abnormalities.

Cerebral Edema. Some degree of brain edema is expected, especially 24 to 72 hours after craniocerebral trauma. Cerebral edema associated with traumatic brain injury may be caused by direct cellular injury leading to intracellular swelling or vascular injury leading to increased intracellular fluid. Either mechanism can result in increased ICP as a result of the increased intracranial volume and changes in CBF.

Diagnostic Evaluation

A detailed health history, both past and present, is essential in evaluating the child with a craniocerebral trauma. Certain disorders such as drug allergies, hemophilia, diabetes mellitus, or epilepsy may produce similar symptoms. Even minor traumatic injury can aggravate a preexisting disease process, thereby producing neurologic signs out of proportion to the injury. It must be determined whether the infant or child exhibited alterations in consciousness, and any other signs and behaviors exhibited by the child must be noted. Because head injuries are frequently accompanied by injuries in other areas, the examination is performed with care to avoid further damage.

> **! NURSING ALERT**
>
> Stabilize a child's spine after head injury until a spinal cord injury is ruled out.

Initial Assessment. Priorities in the initial stabilization phase of a child with a head injury include assessment of the ABCs (airway, breathing, circulation); evaluation for shock; a neurologic examination focusing on mental status, pupillary responses, and motor responses; and assessment for spinal cord injury. The assessment is carried out quickly in relation to vital signs (see Emergency box).

> **! NURSING ALERT**
>
> Deep, rapid, periodic, or intermittent and gasping respirations; wide fluctuations or noticeable slowing of the pulse; and widening pulse pressure or extreme fluctuations in blood pressure are signs of brainstem involvement. Note that marked hypotension may represent internal injuries.

> **✚ EMERGENCY**
>
> ### Head Injury
>
> 1. Assess child:
>   - **A**—Airway
>   - **B**—Bleeding
>   - **C**—Circulation
>   - Neurologic and thermoregulatory status
> 2. Stabilize neck and spine immediately. Use jaw thrust, not chin lift, to open airway.
> 3. Clean any abrasions with soap and water.
>   - Apply clean dressing.
>   - If bleeding, apply pressure and then ice to relieve pain and swelling.
> 4. Keep NPO until instructed otherwise.
> 5. Assess pain but do not give analgesics or sedatives.
> 6. Check pupil reaction every 4 hours (including twice during night) for 48 hours.
> 7. Awaken twice during the night to check LOC.
> 8. Seek medical attention if any of the following apply:
>   - Injury sustained:
>   - At high speed (e.g., automobile)
>   - From fall from a significant distance (e.g., height greater than that of the child)
>   - From great force (e.g., baseball bat)
>   - Under suspicious circumstances
>   - Loss of consciousness
>   - Amnesia
>   - Discomfort (crying) more than 10 minutes after injury
>   - Headache that is severe, worsening, interferes with sleep, or lasts more than 24 hours
>   - Fluid leak from ears or nose; blackened eyes
>   - Vomiting 3 or more times, beginning after injury, or continuing 4 to 6 hours after injury
>   - Swelling in front of or above earlobe or swelling that increases in size
>   - Confusion or abnormal behaving
>   - Difficulty arousing child from sleep
>   - Difficulty speaking
>   - Blurred vision or diplopia
>   - Unsteady gait
>   - Difficulty using extremities, weakness, or incoordination
>   - Neck pain or stiffness
>   - Pupils dilated, unequal, or fixed
>   - Infant with bulging fontanel
>   - Seizures
>
> *LOC,* Level of consciousness; *NPO,* nothing by mouth.

Ocular signs such as fixed, dilated, and unequal pupils; fixed and constricted pupils; and pupils that are poorly reactive or nonreactive to light and accommodation indicate increased ICP or brainstem involvement. It is important to remain with the child who demonstrates fixed and dilated pupils because these are ominous signs with a high probability of respiratory arrest. Dilated, nonpulsating blood vessels indicate increased ICP before the appearance of papilledema. Retinal hemorrhages are seen in acute head injuries, including shaken baby syndrome.

> ### ! NURSING ALERT
>
> Observation of asymmetric pupils or one dilated, nonreactive pupil in a comatose child is a neurologic emergency.

Less urgent but important additional assessments include examination of the scalp for lacerations and palpation for other abnormalities. A significant amount of blood loss can occur from scalp lacerations. An underlying skull fracture should be ruled out by CT scan.

> ### ! NURSING ALERT
>
> Bleeding from the nose or ears needs further evaluation, and a watery discharge from the nose (rhinorrhea) that is positive for glucose (as tested with Dextrostix) suggests leaking of CSF from a skull fracture.

An accurate assessment of clinical signs provides baseline information. Serial evaluations, preferably by a single observer, help to detect changes in the neurologic status. Alterations in mental status, evidenced by increased difficulty in rousing the child, mounting agitation, development of focal lateral neurologic signs, or marked changes in vital signs, usually indicate extension or progression of the basic pathologic process.

Special Tests. After a thorough clinical examination a variety of diagnostic tests are helpful in providing a more definitive diagnosis of the type and extent of the trauma. The severity of a head injury may not be apparent on clinical examination of a child but is detectable on a CT scan. Whenever the child has a history consistent with a serious head injury (unrestrained occupant in a severe motor vehicle accident or a fall from a significant height), it is important to perform a diagnostic scan even if the child initially appears alert and oriented. All children with head injuries who have any alteration of consciousness, headache, vomiting, skull fracture, seizure, or a predisposing medical condition should undergo CT scanning.

After early head injury MRI may be useful in evaluating cerebral edema or structural brain abnormalities, and neurobehavioral assessment can document any cognitive impairments. Skull radiographs are of little benefit in diagnosing skull fractures. EEG is not helpful for diagnosis of head injury but is useful for defining seizure activity. Lumbar puncture is rarely used in craniocerebral trauma and is contraindicated in the presence of increased ICP because of the possibility of herniation.

Posttraumatic Syndromes. Posttraumatic syndromes include postconcussion syndrome, posttraumatic seizures, and structural complications after a head injury.

Postconcussion syndrome is a common sequela to brain injury with or without loss of consciousness. Symptoms can develop within hours to days after a mild head injury but can also occur after moderate-to-severe head injury. The manifestations vary with the child's age and include nausea, dizziness, headache, diplopia, disorientation, and other mental status changes. The duration of manifestations can vary from several days to several months. Death from concussion is preventable unless overwhelming secondary brain injury has occurred (Blinman, Houseknecht, Snyder, et al., 2009).

Posttraumatic seizures occur in a number of children who survive a head injury and are more common in children than in adults (Boran, Boran, Barut, et al., 2006). Seizures are more likely to occur within the first few days after a severe head injury.

Structural complications (e.g., hydrocephalus) may occur as a result of head injuries. Clinical sequelae include cognitive deterioration, motor deficits, optic atrophy, cranial nerve palsies, or aphasia. The type of residual effect depends on the location and nature of the trauma.

Therapeutic Management

The majority of children with mild traumatic brain injury who have not lost consciousness can be cared for and observed at home after a careful examination reveals no serious intracranial injury. Nurses should provide parents with verbal and written instructions of signs and symptoms that warrant concern and the need for medical reevaluation (see Family-Centered Care box).

Parents are instructed to check the child every 2 hours to determine any changes in responsiveness. The sleeping child should be wakened to see if he or she can be roused normally. Parents are advised to maintain contact with the health care provider, who typically examines the child again in 1 or 2 days. The manifestations of epidural hematoma in children do not generally appear until 24 hours or more after injury.

Children with severe injuries, those who have lost consciousness for more than a few minutes, and those with prolonged and continued seizures or other focal or diffuse neurologic signs must be hospitalized until their condition is stable and their neurologic signs have diminished. The child is maintained on NPO status (nothing by mouth) or restricted to clear liquids until it is determined that vomiting will not occur. IV fluids are indicated in the child who is comatose, displays dulled sensorium, or is vomiting persistently. Fluid balance is monitored closely by daily weights; accurate intake and output measurements; and serum osmolality to detect early signs of water retention, excessive dehydration, and states of hypertonicity or hypotonicity.

The volume of IV fluid is monitored carefully to minimize the possibility of overhydration in cases of SIADH and cerebral edema. However, damage to the hypothalamus or pituitary gland may produce DI with its accompanying hypertonicity and dehydration.

> ### 👪 FAMILY-CENTERED CARE
> #### *Maintaining Contact*
>
> Maintaining contact with parents for continued observation and reevaluation of the child, when indicated, facilitates early diagnosis and treatment of possible complications from head injury such as hematoma, hydrocephalus, and posttraumatic seizures. Children are generally hospitalized for 24 to 48 hours of observation if their family lives far from medical facilities or lacks transportation or a telephone that would provide access to immediate help. Other circumstances such as language or other communication barriers or even emotional trauma may hinder learning and make it difficult for families to feel confident in caring for their child at home.

Surgical Therapy. Scalp lacerations are sutured after the underlying bone is carefully examined. Depressed fractures require surgical reduction and removal of bone fragments. Torn dura is sutured. Ping-Pong–ball skull fractures in very young infants ordinarily correct themselves within a few weeks; however, some may require surgical intervention.

Prognosis. The outcome of craniocerebral trauma depends on the extent of injury and complications. In general the prognosis is more favorable for children than for adults. More than 90% of children with concussions or simple linear fractures recover without symptoms after the initial period. Outcomes in children with brain injuries are focused increasingly on long-term cognitive, emotional, and mental problems. The vulnerability of young children's developing brains can result in detrimental disruptions after significant brain injury (Bonnier, Marique, Van Hout, et al., 2007).

True coma (not obeying commands, eyes closed, and not speaking) usually does not last more than 2 weeks. A child's eventual outcome can range from brain death to a persistent vegetative state to complete recovery. However, even the best recovery after a coma may be associated with personality changes, including mood lability and loss of confidence, impaired short-term memory, headaches, and subtle cognitive impairments. Many children are left with significant disabilities after head injury that appear months later as learning difficulties, behavioral changes, or emotional disturbances (Bonnier, Marique, Van Hout, et al., 2007).

CARE MANAGEMENT

The hospitalized child requires careful neurologic assessment and evaluation that are repeated at frequent intervals to establish a correct diagnosis, identify signs and symptoms of increased ICP, determine clinical management, and prevent many complications.

The child is placed on bed rest, usually with the head of the bed elevated slightly and the head in midline position. Appropriate safety measures such as side rails kept up and seizure precautions are implemented. Children may be restless and irritable, but often their reaction is to fall asleep when left undisturbed. A quiet environment helps reduce restlessness and irritability. For extremely restless children hard surfaces may need to be padded, and restraint used to prevent the possibility of further injury. Care is individualized according to the child's specific needs. Shining bright lights directly into the child's face is irritating and makes assessment of ocular responses difficult.

Frequent examinations of vital signs, neurologic signs, and LOC are extremely important nursing observations. When possible, they should be performed by a single observer to better detect subtle changes that may indicate worsening neurologic status. Pupils are checked for size, equality, reaction to light, and accommodation. After the initial elevations usually seen after injury, the vital signs generally return to normal unless there is brainstem involvement.

The most important nursing observation is assessment of the child's LOC. Alterations in consciousness appear earlier in the progression of an injury than alterations of vital signs or focal neurologic signs. Some expected responses may be misinterpreted as deviations from the normal. Frequent examinations of alertness are fatiguing to the child; therefore he or she often desires to fall asleep, which may be confused with depressed consciousness. It is common to observe ocular divergence through the partially closed eyelids.

A key nursing role is to provide sedation and analgesia for the child. The conflict between the need to promote comfort and relieve anxiety in the child versus the need to assess for neurologic changes presents a dilemma. Both goals can be achieved with close observation of the child's LOC and response to analgesics, use of a pain assessment record, and effective communication with the practitioner. Decreasing restlessness after administration of an analgesic most likely reflects pain control rather than a declining LOC.

Observations of position and movement provide additional information. Any abnormal posturing and whether it occurs continuously or intermittently are noted. Questions nurses might consider include:

- Are the child's handgrips strong and equal in strength?
- Are there any signs of flexion or extension posturing?
- What is the child's response to stimulation?
- Is movement purposeful, random, or absent?
- Are movement and sensation equal on both sides or restricted to one side only?

The child may complain of headache or other discomfort. A child who is too young to describe a headache may be fussy and resist being handled. A child who has vertigo often assumes a position of comfort and vigorously resists efforts to be moved. Forcible movement causes the child to vomit and display spontaneous nystagmus. Seizures are relatively common in children with head trauma and may be of any type. Carefully observe, record, and report in detail any seizure activity. Children in postictal (postseizure) states are lethargic with sluggish pupils.

Document drainage from any orifice. Bleeding from the ear suggests the possibility of a basal skull fracture. Clear nasal drainage suggests an anterior basal skull fracture. The amount and characteristics of the drainage should be observed, recorded, and reported.

Head trauma is frequently accompanied by other undetected injuries; therefore any bruises, lacerations, or evidence of internal injuries or fractures of the extremities is noted and reported. Associated injuries are evaluated and treated appropriately.

The child with normal LOC is usually allowed clear liquids unless fluid is restricted. If the child has an IV infusion, it is maintained as prescribed. The diet is advanced to that appropriate for the child's age as soon as the condition permits. Intake and output are measured and recorded, and any incontinence of bowel or bladder is noted if the child has been toilet trained.

Observe the child for any unusual behavior, but behavior should be interpreted in relation to the child's normal behavior. For example, urinary incontinence during sleep would be of no consequence in a child who routinely wets the bed but would be highly significant for one who is always dry. Parents are valuable resources in evaluating objective behavior of their child. Information obtained from parents at or shortly after admission is helpful in evaluating the child's behavior (e.g., the ease with which the child is roused normally, the usual sleeping position and patterns, motor activities [rolling over, sitting up, climbing], hearing and visual acuity, appetite, and manner of eating [spoon, bottle, cup]).

Family Support. The emotional and educational support of the family presents a challenging aspect to nursing care. Witnessing the parents' grief and helplessness on seeing their child in an altered state, connected to monitoring equipment, and in an intensive care unit evokes empathy. The nurse can encourage the family to be involved in the child's care, bring in familiar belongings, or make a tape recording of familiar voices and sounds. Parents may need a demonstration on how to touch or cuddle their child and may want to talk about their grief. The nurse can listen attentively, reinforce what is being done to help the child, and direct parents toward signs and symptoms of recovery to instill hope without promises. Honesty and kindness along with competent care can help families through this difficult time.

When the child is discharged, the parents are advised of probable posttraumatic symptoms that may be expected. They should understand necessary monitoring and how to contact health care providers in case the child develops any unusual signs or symptoms. The importance of follow-up evaluation should be emphasized.

Rehabilitation. Rehabilitation and management of the child with permanent brain injury are essential aspects of care. Rehabilitation begins as soon as feasible and usually involves the family and a rehabilitation team. Careful assessment of the child's capabilities, limitations, and probable potential is made as early as possible; and appropriate interventions are implemented to maximize the residual capacities. The Brain Injury Association of America* provides information and listings of rehabilitation services and support groups throughout the country.

Pediatric trauma rehabilitation is a national concern. Coordinating care and services for early rehabilitation involves identifying the child's and family's response to the traumatic injury and disability, securing available resources, and recognizing the parental role in the process.

Children with disabilities resulting from head trauma require assessment on a physical, cognitive, emotional, and social level. These children have experienced separation, pain, sensory deprivation and overload, changes in circadian cycle, and fear of the unknown. Recovery and transition require new coping strategies at the same time that regressive and acting-out behavior may start. Parents and children need honest communication for decision making. Rehabilitation is advocated when the child has progressed beyond what can be provided in a hospital setting. The Rancho Los Amigos Scale provides a systematic assessment of the possible progress a child may achieve after a severe head injury.

Prevention. Tremendous strides have been taken to prevent cerebral damage after head injury in children. New developments are directed toward the prevention of cellular injury or the primary insult. Nurses can exert a valuable influence on prevention of children's head injuries through education. Preventable head injuries occur because unnecessary risks go unchecked. Inadequate supervision combined with children's natural sense of indestructibility and exploration can lead to lethal results. Nurses are in the unique position of influencing caregivers in terms of growth and development risks. Banning the use of infant walkers is an example. This equipment does not help develop motor skills and places infants at risk

for head and neck injuries from falls, especially down steps. Public education coupled with legislative support can prevent childhood injuries.

Submersion Injury

Submersion injury is a major cause of accidental death in children older than 1 year of age. The term submersion injury has replaced *near-drowning* to include any person who experiences distress from submersion or immersion in liquid that results either in death (drowning) or survival at least 24 hours after submersion (near-drowning) (Weiss and American Academy of Pediatrics [AAP] Committee on Injury, Violence, and Poison Prevention, 2010). Most cases of submersion are accidental, usually involving children who are helpless in water such as inadequately attended children in or near swimming pools or infants in bathtubs; small children who fall into ponds, streams, and flooded excavations; occupants of pleasure boats who fail to wear life preservers; children who have diving accidents; and children who are able to swim but overestimate their endurance. Accidental drowning occurs more commonly in toddlers, boys, and African-Americans (Nasrullah and Muazzam, 2011). Drowning can take place in any body of liquid, and sites of drowning are important to consider for preventive education. Children younger than 1 year old are most likely to drown in a bathtub, and buckets filled with fluid cause a risk of drowning to top-heavy toddlers who can fall head first into the buckets (Hon and Leung, 2010). Preschoolers are at risk for drowning in swimming pools; and drowning in school-age children and adolescents most commonly occurs in natural bodies of water such as lakes, ponds, and rivers (Shephard and Quan, 2011). The suction created at the outlet of pools, hot tubs, or whirlpool spas is strong enough to trap any child, even larger children, underwater. Drowning as a form of fatal child abuse has also been recognized as a problem.

Pathophysiology

Hypoxia is the primary cause of injury when submersion occurs and can cause damage to the brain, lungs, heart, kidneys, liver, and gastrointestinal system. Cerebral hypoxia is the major component of morbidity and mortality with submersion events. Within minutes of a submersion, a lack of oxygen leads to coma and ultimately cardiac arrest (Shephard and Quan, 2011). Recovery depends on the timeliness and effectiveness of initial resuscitation and subsequent supportive care measures.

Pathophysiologic features in submersion injuries are hypoxia, aspiration, and hypothermia.

Hypoxia is related to the duration of anoxia and asphyxia. Different cells tolerate variable lengths of anoxia, causing variations of cell damage. Neurons, especially cerebral cells, sustain irreversible damage after 4 to 6 minutes of submersion; but the heart and lungs can survive up to 30 minutes. Regardless of the amount of water aspirated, there is arterial hypoxemia (resulting from atelectasis with shunting of blood through the nonventilated alveoli) and a combined respiratory acidosis (resulting from retained carbon dioxide) and metabolic acidosis (caused by buildup of acid metabolites from anaerobic metabolism). Approximately 10% of drowning victims die without aspirating fluid but succumb from acute asphyxia as a result of prolonged reflex laryngospasm.

Aspiration of fluid is quickly absorbed in the pulmonary circulation, resulting in pulmonary edema, atelectasis, and airway spasm, which aggravates the hypoxia. No clinical or physiologic difference, therapy, or outcome has been noted among human survivors in the submersion of salt water versus fresh water (Shephard and Quan, 2011).

---

*1608 Spring Hill Road, Suite 110, Vienna, VA 22182, 703-761-0750, fax: 703-761-0755, www.biausa.org.

Hypothermia is common after submersion; children are at an increased risk of hypothermia because of their large surface area relative to body mass, decreased subcutaneous fat, and limited thermoregulation (Shephard and Quan, 2011). The temperature of the liquid plays an important role in developing hypoxemia. Cold water decreases metabolic demands and activates the diving reflex, which causes blood to be shunted away from the periphery and concentrated to the brain and heart. However, prolonged submersion in cold liquids can impair cognition, coordination, and muscle strength, ultimately resulting in a loss of consciousness, decreased cardiac output, and cardiac arrest (Shephard and Quan, 2011).

Therapeutic Management

The outcome of children after a submersion event depends on the circumstances and duration of the submersion and the speed and effectiveness of resuscitation efforts (Shephard and Quan, 2011). Resuscitative measures should begin at the scene of a drowning, and the victim should be transported to the hospital with maximal ventilatory and circulatory support. In the hospital intensive care is implemented and continued according to the patient's needs.

In general the management of the victims with submersion injuries is based on the degree of cerebral insult. The first priority is to restore oxygen delivery to the cells and prevent further hypoxic damage. A spontaneously breathing child does well in an oxygen-enriched atmosphere; a more severely affected child requires endotracheal intubation and mechanical ventilation. Blood gases and pH are monitored frequently as a guide to oxygen, fluid, and electrolyte therapies.

> ### ! NURSING ALERT
>
> All children who have a submersion injury should be hospitalized for observation. Almost half of asymptomatic or minimally symptomatic alert children experience complications (e.g., respiratory compromise, cerebral edema) during the first 24 hours after the incident (Shephard and Quan, 2011).

Aspiration pneumonia is a frequent complication that occurs about 48 to 72 hours after the episode. Bronchospasm, alveolocapillary membrane damage, atelectasis, abscess formation, and acute respiratory distress syndrome are other complications that occur after aspiration of fluid.

Prognosis. The best predictors of a good outcome are length of submersion less than 5 minutes and the presence of sinus rhythm, reactive pupils, and neurologic responsiveness at the scene. The worst prognoses—for death or severe neurologic impairment—are children submerged for more than 10 minutes and not responding to advanced life support within 25 minutes. All children without purposeful movement and normal brainstem function 24 hours after a submersion injury have sustained severe neurologic deficits or death (Shephard and Quan, 2011). (See Guidelines box.)

CARE MANAGEMENT

Nursing care depends on the child's condition. A child who survives may need intensive respiratory nursing care with attention to vital signs, mechanical ventilation, or tracheostomy, blood gas determination, chest physiotherapy, and IV infusion. Frequently a child who has sustained a submersion injury requires the same care as an unconscious child. A difficult aspect in the care of the child victim of submersion injury is helping the parents cope with severe

> ### 📋 GUIDELINES
>
> #### Establishing Brain Death in Children
>
> 1. Coma and apnea must coexist. Child must exhibit complete loss of consciousness, vocalization, and volitional activity.
> 2. Brainstem function must be absent, as defined by:
>   a. Midposition or fully dilated pupils that do not respond to light. Drugs may influence and invalidate pupillary assessment.
>   b. Absence of spontaneous eye movements and those induced by oculocephalic and caloric (oculovestibular) testing.
>   c. Absence of movement of bulbar musculature, corneal, gag, cough, sucking, and rooting reflexes.
>   d. Absence of respiratory movements with standardized methods for testing apnea.
> 3. Child must not be hypothermic or hypotensive for age.
> 4. Flaccid tone and absence of spontaneous or induced movements, excluding activity mediated at the spinal cord level.
> 5. Examination should remain consistent with brain death throughout the observation and testing period.
> 6. Observation periods according to age:
>   **Seven days to 2 months**—Two separate examinations and two EEGs separated by at least 48 hours
>   **Two months to 1 year**—Two separate examinations and two EEGs separated by at least 24 hours
>   **Over 1 year**—Two separate examinations separated by at least 12 hours

Modified from Ashwal S, Serna-Fonseca T: Brain death in infants and children, *Crit Care Nurse* 26:117–128, 2006.
EEG, Electroencephalogram.

guilt reactions. Given the magnitude of the event, parents need repeated assurance that everything possible is being done to treat the child.

The parents of the child who is saved from death face the anxiety of not knowing the final outcome. The situation generates such intense feelings of loneliness and guilt that it is important for families to know that they are not alone. They should be reminded frequently that people are available to help them during the crisis. Additional sources of support include psychiatric and social work consultants, community services, and religious support. Self-help groups may be beneficial if these are available in the community.

Nurses often have difficulty relating to the parents if obvious neglect has precipitated the accident and subsequent problems; therefore it is important for those who care for these children and their families to assess their own feelings about the situation in addition to assessing the family's coping abilities and resources. Caring for victims of a submersion injury and their families requires nurses to be sensitive to the needs of the child and family and recognize their own reactions and emotions.

Prevention. Most submersion injuries are preventable. The most common cause of submersion injury of infants and young children is inadequate adult supervision, including a momentary lapse of supervision (Weiss and AAP Committee on Injury, Violence, and Poison Prevention, 2010). Close adult supervision of infants and children around any body of water is essential and should include the adult not engaging in any distracting activities. Other strategies include environmental prevention strategies such as pool fencing; pool covers; water-entry alarms; and lifeguard and individual prevention such as swimming and survival skills, cardiopulmonary resuscitation training, and the use of personal flotation devices

(Weiss and AAP Committee on Injury, Violence, and Poison Prevention, 2010).

NERVOUS SYSTEM TUMORS

CNS tumors account for approximately 20% of all childhood cancers, with an estimated annual incidence of 3.1 cases per 100,000 children younger than 15 years of age (Howlader, Noone, Krapcho, et al., 2011).

Brain Tumors

Brain tumors are the most common solid tumor in children and the second most common childhood cancer. In children the use of reference terms *benign* or *malignant* is generally avoided because any tumor, despite its nature, can be fatal or associated with significant morbidities in the developing brain of a child.

CNS tumors can arise from any cell within the brain or spinal cord. The cell origin provides a histologic classification. For instance, astrocytes (cells that form the supportive tissue for neurons) may form a common glial tumor called an astrocytoma. A specific type of tumor called *ependymoma* typically arises within or adjacent to the ependymal lining of the ventricular system. CNS tumors in children are typically glial or neuronal in origin, located in the infratentorium, and generally sensitive to radiation and adjuvant chemotherapy (Merchant, Pollack, and Loeffler, 2010). Infratentorial brain tumors occur in the area of the brain below the tentorium cerebelli involving the cerebellum or brainstem. Types of infratentorial tumors include medulloblastoma, ependymoma, cerebellar astrocytoma, and brainstem glioma. Tumors above the tentorium are referred to as supratentorial and may include astrocytoma, primitive neuroectodermal tumor, craniopharyngioma, and optic pathway glioma. The suprasellar and pineal regions of the brain often are the location of germ cell tumors.

Diagnostic Evaluation

The signs and symptoms of brain tumors are directly related to their anatomic location and size and, to some extent, the child's age. Supratentorial tumors can cause symptoms that include seizures, contralateral hemiparesis, memory loss, personality and behavioral changes, decline in school performance, and vision loss. Infratentorial tumors often cause the obstruction of normal CSF flow, resulting in signs and symptoms of increased ICP. Tumors involving the brainstem may cause cranial neuropathies, difficulty in micturition (if the pontine micturition center is affected), weakness, hypertonicity, and changes in respiratory pattern. Cerebellar tumors often cause ataxia, dysmetria, or nystagmus. In infants and very young children whose cranial sutures are still open, initial signs and symptoms of increased ICP (headache, vomiting, and lethargy) may not be evident, and symptoms may include irritability, failure to thrive, and loss of developmental milestones. Brain tumors involving the pineal gland or suprasellar region often present with endocrinopathies, which include growth failure, precocious puberty, DI, and adrenal insufficiency.

Diagnosis of a brain tumor is based subjectively on presenting clinical signs, objectively on neurologic tests, and surgical confirmation of the histologic diagnosis. A number of tests may be used in the neurologic evaluation, but the most common diagnostic procedure is MRI, which determines the location and extent of the tumor. Other tests that may be used include CT, angiography, EEG, and lumbar puncture. CT or MRI is routinely performed before a lumbar puncture procedure to identify intracranial abnormalities that may cause a contraindication to the procedure (Lin and Safdieh, 2010).

Lumbar puncture is dangerous in the presence of increased ICP because of the possibility of brainstem herniation after a sudden release of pressure. The definitive diagnosis of a brain tumor is based on brain tissue specimens obtained during surgery.

Therapeutic Management

Treatment may involve the use of surgery, radiotherapy, and chemotherapy or a combination of these treatment modalities. The optimum treatment is complete surgical resection of the primary tumor with preservation of adequate neurologic function. Radiation therapy is an integral part of treatment for many brain tumors but can cause significant neurocognitive side effects and endocrinopathies. Because rapid brain development occurs during the first 3 years of life, radiation therapy, particularly craniospinal radiation, is avoided in children younger than 3 years of age. Chemotherapy may be used as primary treatment or in an effort to delay radiation therapy until patients are older and may experience fewer neurocognitive side effects. One of the challenges in using chemotherapy for CNS tumors is the blood-brain barrier, which is a natural barrier that significantly influences the penetration of substances into the CNS. Commonly used chemotherapy agents for treatment of brain tumors in children include vincristine, cisplatin, carboplatin, cyclophosphamide, etoposide, lomustine, and temozolomide (Blaney, Haas-Kogan, Young Poussaint, et al., 2011).

Prognosis. The prognosis for a child with a brain tumor varies greatly and depends on the type of brain tumor, the size of the tumor, the extent of the disease, age, and surgical resectability. Recent advances in surgical instrumentation allowing aggressive surgical intervention, modifications in radiation, and use of chemotherapy have increased the long-term survival rates for many children with brain tumors. Currently the overall survival rate for CNS tumors in children younger than 15 years of age is approximately 75% (Howlader, Noone, Krapcho, et al., 2011). Despite an improvement in overall survival, children with brain tumors, particularly those who are very young at diagnosis, may have significant physical, cognitive, and endocrinologic sequelae because of their tumor and associated treatment (Shaw, 2009).

CARE MANAGEMENT

If a brain tumor is suspected in a child admitted to the hospital for cerebral dysfunction, establishing baseline data with which to compare preoperative and postoperative changes is an essential step. It also allows the nurse to assess the degree of physical incapacity and the family's emotional reaction to the diagnosis.

Vital signs, including blood pressure and pulse pressure (the difference between systolic and diastolic pressures), are taken routinely and more often when any change is noted. Any sudden variations are reported immediately. Observation for symptoms of Cushing triad (i.e., a hallmark sign of increased ICP, which includes bradycardia, hypertension, and irregular respirations) is a crucial role of the nurse. It is also important to note a change in vital signs during or after diagnostic procedures. A routine neurologic assessment is performed at the same time as vital signs, and head circumference should be measured for infants and very young children. The child is observed for evidence of headache, vomiting, and any seizure activity. The location, severity, and duration of the headache and its relationship to activity, time of day, and any associated factors are noted. Behaviors such as lying flat and facing away from light or refusing to engage in play are clues to discomfort in nonverbal children. The child's gait is observed at least once daily. Head tilt while talking or performing an activity and other changes in posturing should always be documented.

Prevent Postoperative Complications. Usually the surgeon prescribes specific orders for vital signs, neurologic checks, positioning, fluid regulation, and medication. These vary somewhat, depending on the location of the craniotomy. The following are general principles of care for infratentorial or supratentorial surgery. Additional aspects of care that are discussed elsewhere may include care of the child with seizures and neurologic assessment of the unconscious child.

Vital signs are taken as frequently as every 15 to 30 minutes until the child is stable. Temperature measurement is particularly important because of hyperthermia resulting from surgical intervention in the hypothalamus or brainstem and from some types of general anesthesia. To prepare for this reaction, a cooling blanket is often placed on the bed *before* the child returns to the unit so it is ready for use when needed. The temperature is monitored carefully when any cooling measures are taken because hypothermia can occur suddenly. Recognizing signs of other complications such as increased ICP, meningitis, and respiratory tract infection is imperative.

Neurologic checks are an essential aspect of care and include pupillary reaction to light, LOC, sleep patterns, and response to stimuli. Although children may be less responsive for a few days after surgery, when they regain full consciousness there should be a steady increase in alertness. Regression to a lethargic, irritable state indicates increasing ICP, possibly caused by hemorrhage, cerebral edema, or meningitis.

> **! NURSING ALERT**
>
> Sluggish, dilated, or unequal pupils are reported immediately because they may indicate increased ICP and potential brainstem herniation, a medical emergency.

Observations for function are not instituted until the child regains consciousness. However, as soon as possible the nurse should begin testing reflexes, hand grip, and functioning of the cranial nerves. Muscle strength is usually diminished as a result of general weakness after surgery but should improve daily. Ataxia may be significantly worse with cerebellar intervention but will improve slowly. Edema near the cranial nerves may depress important functions such as the gag, blink, or swallowing reflex.

Dressings are observed for evidence of drainage. If soiled, the dressing is not removed but is reinforced with dry sterile gauze. The approximate amount of drainage is estimated and recorded. A drain may be placed in the operative site.

> **! NURSING ALERT**
>
> To keep an accurate account of drainage, the soiled area is circled with a pen approximately every hour. In this way continuous bleeding is easily recognized. The presence of colorless drainage is reported immediately because it most likely is CSF from the incisional area. A foul odor from the dressing may indicate an infection. This should be reported immediately, and the nurse should anticipate cultures to be taken from the site.

Correct positioning after surgery is critical to prevent pressure against the operative site, reduce ICP, and avoid the danger of aspiration. If a large tumor was removed, the child is not placed on the operative side because the brain may suddenly shift to that cavity, causing trauma to the blood vessels, linings, and the brain itself. The nurse confers with the surgeon to be certain of the correct position, including degree of neck flexion. The first 24 to 48 hours after brain surgery are critical. If the child's position is restricted, notice of this is posted above the head of the bed. When the child is turned, every precaution is used to prevent jarring or malalignment to prevent undue strain on the sutures. Two nurses are needed—one supporting the head and the other supporting the body. The use of a turning sheet may facilitate turning a heavy child.

The child with an infratentorial procedure is usually positioned on either side with the bed flat. When a supratentorial craniotomy is performed, the head of bed is elevated 20 to 30 degrees with the child on either side or on the back. In a supratentorial craniotomy the head elevation facilitates CSF drainage and decreases excessive blood flow to the brain to prevent hemorrhage. Pillows should be placed against the child's back, not head, to maintain the desired position. Ordinarily the head and neck are kept in midline with the body, and the neck should not be flexed to support venous drainage (Christie, 2008).

> **! NURSING ALERT**
>
> The Trendelenburg position is contraindicated in both infratentorial and supratentorial surgeries because it increases ICP and the risk of hemorrhage. If shock is impending, the practitioner is notified immediately before the head is lowered.

With an infratentorial craniotomy the child is kept NPO for at least 24 hours or longer if the gag and swallowing reflexes are depressed or the child is comatose. With a supratentorial operation cranial neuropathy is less likely, and clear fluids may be resumed soon after the child is alert, sometimes within 24 hours. If the child vomits, oral liquids are stopped. Vomiting not only predisposes the child to aspiration but also increases ICP and the potential for incisional rupture.

The child should be fed to conserve energy and minimize movement. If there is any sign of cranial nerve deficits, he or she is fed slowly to prevent choking and aspiration. Thickening agents can be used if the patient experiences dysphagia with thin liquids. Sometimes enteral feeding is necessary when body functions are too depressed to permit safe oral feedings or when the child refuses to eat or drink. IV fluids are continued until oral fluids are well tolerated or a method of enteral feeding is established. Because of the postoperative cerebral edema and danger of increased ICP, fluid status is monitored carefully.

Headache may be severe and is largely a result of cerebral edema. Measures to relieve some of the discomfort include providing a quiet, dimly lit environment; restricting visitors; preventing any sudden jarring movement such as banging into the bed; and preventing an increase in ICP. Avoiding increased ICP is most effectively achieved by proper positioning and prevention of straining such as during coughing, vomiting, or defecating. The use of opioids such as morphine to relieve pain is controversial because it is thought that they may mask signs of altered consciousness or depress respirations. However, opioids can be given safely because naloxone can be used to reverse their effects (e.g., as sedation or respiratory depression). Acetaminophen and codeine are also effective analgesics for mild-to-moderate pain. When giving medication such as acetaminophen for pain, the nurse should be aware that this medication may also mask the presence of a fever, which could indicate postoperative infection. Regardless of the drugs used, adequate dosage and regular administration are essential to providing optimal pain relief (see also Pain Assessment; Pain Management, Chapter 30). Placing an ice bag on the forehead may also provide some headache relief, especially if facial edema is severe. Constipation is a common postoperative issue because of anesthesia and immobility. It is important to note that the use of narcotics for pain control may further contribute to constipation. Patients should be given a bowel regimen during the postoperative period until normal bowel function returns.

Support the Child and Family. The family's emotional needs are immense when the diagnosis is a brain tumor; feelings are influenced by the extent of surgery, any neurologic deficits, the expected prognosis, and possible additional therapy. Because few definitive answers can be given before surgery, the surgeon's report after surgery is a significant finding that can vary from a low-grade, completely resected neoplasm to a highly malignant, invasive, and only partially removed tumor. Although parents often try to prepare themselves for the worst possible scenario, being given the news that their child has a potentially fatal tumor or may have significant neurologic impairment from the necessary treatment is always devastating.

Parents should be encouraged to verbalize their feelings about the diagnosis. Often they express tremendous guilt for viewing the insidious onset of symptoms such as ataxia, visual difficulty, or headache, as "minor complaints" by the child. In retrospect many parents feel guilt that they did not associate their child's decline in school performance with an actual medical problem. The nurse needs to exercise particular care not to make any comments that insinuate that the parents should have sought medical advice sooner because this only compounds any feelings of guilt that already exist. During this period the nurse should also discuss with the parents what they plan to tell the child. If the child was prepared honestly, the diagnosis can be expressed in a similar age-appropriate manner. During recovery the child needs additional explanation about the treatment and the reason for any residual neurologic effects such as ataxia or blindness. The increasing availability of child life specialists has served as a tremendous resource in explaining diagnoses such as brain tumors to children, helping them cope with hospitalization and necessary treatment, and helping them understand physical sequelae they may experience (Reynolds and Boyd, 2010).

Neuroblastoma

Neuroblastomas are the most common malignant extracranial solid tumors in children, accounting for 8% to 10% of all childhood cancers (Mullassery, Dominici, Jesudason, et al., 2009). They occur in about one per 7000 live births, with a slightly higher incidence in boys (Brodeur, Hogarty, Mosse, et al., 2011). Approximately 95% of children with neuroblastoma manifest the disease before 10 years of age, with the median age of occurrence at 23 months (Park, Eggert, and Caron, 2010). These tumors originate from embryonic neural crest cells that normally give rise to the adrenal medulla and the sympathetic ganglia. Consequently the majority of tumors develop in the abdomen along the adrenal gland or the retroperitoneal sympathetic chain. Other sites may be in the head, neck, chest, or pelvis.

The signs and symptoms of neuroblastoma depend on the location and stage of the disease. Neuroblastoma is a commonly referred to as a "silent" tumor because approximately half of the patients present with localized disease and display few symptoms. However, children with advanced disease are ill appearing with symptoms of periorbital ecchymoses, proptosis, bone pain, and irritability caused by extensive tumor metastasis, usually in the lymph nodes, bone marrow, skeletal system, skin, or liver (Park, Eggert, and Caron, 2010).

Diagnostic Evaluation

The objective of diagnosis is to locate the primary site and areas of metastasis. Skeletal survey; skull, neck, chest, abdominal, and bone CT scans; and bilateral bone marrow aspirations and biopsies are used to locate a tumor mass and metastasis. A metaiodobenzylguanidine (MIBG) scan is used to determine involvement of bone, bone marrow, and soft tissue involvement.

Urinary excretion of catecholamines is detected in approximately 95% of children with adrenal or sympathetic tumors. Analyzing the breakdown products excreted in the urine (i.e., vanillylmandelic acid, homovanillic acid, dopamine, and norepinephrine) permits detection of suspected tumor before and after medical-surgical intervention (Mullassery, Dominici, Jesudason, et al., 2009). Amplification of proto-oncogene, known as the *MYCN gene,* and chromosome abnormalities correlate strongly with advanced-stage disease, rapid tumor progression, and a poor prognosis (Brodeur, Hogarty, Mosse, et al., 2011).

Therapeutic Management

Accurate clinical staging is important for establishing initial treatment. Therefore surgery is used both to remove as much of the tumor as possible and to obtain biopsies. In early stages complete surgical removal of the tumor is the treatment of choice. If the tumor is large, partial resection is attempted, with a course of irradiation after surgery to shrink it in the hope of complete removal at a later date. Surgery is usually limited to biopsy in stages III and IV because of the extensive metastasis, although the use of additional surgery to assess tumor regression or remove a regressed tumor is not unlikely.

Because radiotherapy can cause vertebral damage and growth arrest, it is contraindicated with intraspinal tumors; however, it can be used for emergency management of a massive neuroblastoma that is causing spinal cord compression (Mullassery, Dominici, Jesudason, et al., 2009). Radiotherapy also offers palliation for metastatic lesions in the bones, lung, liver, or brain.

Chemotherapy is the mainstay of therapy for extensive local or disseminated disease. Agents used in various combinations include cyclophosphamide, doxorubicin, cisplatin, etoposide, vincristine, ifosfamide, carboplatin, topotecan, and teniposide. In children with high-risk or recurrent disease, retinoic acid, radiotherapy, and myeloablative chemotherapy with peripheral stem cell rescue may be used to obtain a longer remission even though a poor overall survival rate is seen (Brodeur, Hogarty, Mosse, et al., 2011).

Prognosis. If all stages are grouped together, the 5-year disease-free survival rates range from 95% for children in the low-risk stage to only 30% in children in the high-risk stage (Park, Eggert, and Caron, 2010). Generally the younger the child at diagnosis (especially younger than 1 year of age), the better the survival rate. Neuroblastoma is one of the few tumors demonstrating spontaneous regression (especially stage IV-S), possibly as a result of maturity of the embryonic cell or the development of an active immune system.

CARE MANAGEMENT

Nursing considerations are similar to those discussed for leukemia and brain tumors, including psychologic and physical preparation for diagnostic and operative procedures; prevention of postoperative complications for abdominal, thoracic, or cranial surgery; and explanation of chemotherapy, radiotherapy, and their side effects.

Because this tumor carries a poor prognosis for many children, every consideration must be given to the family in terms of coping with a life-threatening illness (see Chapter 38). Because of the high degree of metastasis at the time of diagnosis, many parents experience substantial guilt for not having recognized signs earlier. Parents need much support in dealing with these feelings and expressing them to the appropriate people.

INTRACRANIAL INFECTIONS

The nervous system is subject to infection by the same organisms that affect other organs of the body. However, it is limited in the ways in which it responds to injury. Laboratory studies are needed to identify the causative agent. The inflammatory process can affect the meninges (meningitis) or brain (encephalitis).

Meningitis can be caused by a variety of organisms, but the three main types are (1) bacterial, or pyogenic, caused by pus-forming bacteria, especially meningococci, pneumococci, and *Haemophilus* organisms; (2) viral, or aseptic, caused by a wide variety of viral agents; and (3) tuberculous, caused by the tuberculin bacillus. The majority of children with acute febrile intracranial infections have either bacterial meningitis or viral meningitis as the underlying cause. Bacterial meningitis is considered much more serious than viral meningitis. Compared with viral meningitis, which typically is short lived, self-limiting, and followed by complete recovery, complications from bacterial meningitis can be quite severe and include shock, coma, seizures, intellectual deficits, hearing loss, vision loss, and death (Somand and Meurer, 2009).

Bacterial Meningitis

Bacterial meningitis is an acute inflammation of the meninges and CSF. Suspected bacterial meningitis is a medical emergency, and immediate action must be taken to identify the causative organism and to initiate prompt treatment.

The advent of antimicrobial therapy has had a significant effect on the overall clinical course and prognosis of children with bacterial meningitis. However, the introduction of vaccines has made the most significant impact on the incidence of this disease. After the introduction of the *Haemophilus* influenza type b (Hib) vaccine in 1990 and the pneumococcal conjugate vaccines in 2000, the incidence of bacterial meningitis declined in all age-groups except children younger than 2 months of age. The incidence of bacterial meningitis caused by *Haemophilus influenzae, Streptococcus pneumoniae, Neisseria meningitidis*, group B streptococcus (GBS), and *Listeria monocytogenes* in children from 2 months of age to 17 years decreased from approximately 17 cases per 100,000 in 1998 to approximately eight cases per 100,000 in 2007 (Thigpen, Whitney, Messonnier, et al., 2011).

Although it is encouraging to recognize the dramatic decline in the incidence of bacterial meningitis, this disease still results in death with the fatality rate of approximately 6.9% in children. The incidence is highest for patients younger than 2 months of age, and GBS is the most common causative organism in these patients. In children older than 2 months of age *S. pneumoniae* and *N. meningitidis* are the most common etiologies for bacterial meningitis (Thigpen, Whitney, Messonnier, et al., 2011). Other causative organisms include β-hemolytic streptococci, *Staphylococcus aureus*, and *Escherichia coli*. The leading causes of neonatal meningitis are GBS, *E. coli*, and *L. monocytogenes*. *E. coli* infection is seldom seen beyond infancy. Meningococcal meningitis occurs in epidemic form and is the only type readily transmitted by droplet infection from nasopharyngeal secretions. Although this condition may develop at any age, the risk of meningococcal infection increases with the number of contacts; therefore it occurs predominantly in school-age children and adolescents. College students, especially those living in dormitory residences, are at moderately increased risk for meningococcal disease compared with other people their age. The meningococcal conjugate vaccine should be given to all people ages 11 to 18 years with a booster dose administered 5 years later (Granoff and Gilsdorf, 2011).

There appear to be some seasonal variations with the organisms. Meningitis caused by *H. influenzae* primarily occurs in autumn or early winter. Pneumococcal and meningococcal infections can occur at any time but are more common in later winter and early spring.

Pathophysiology

The most common route of infection is vascular dissemination from a focus of infection elsewhere. For example, organisms from the nasopharynx invade the underlying blood vessels and enter the cerebral blood supply or form local thromboemboli that release septic emboli into the bloodstream. Invasion by direct extension from infections in the paranasal and mastoid sinuses is less common. Organisms also gain entry by direct implantation after penetrating wounds, skull fractures that provide an opening into the skin or sinuses, lumbar puncture or surgical procedures, anatomic abnormalities such as spina bifida, or foreign bodies such as an internal ventricular shunt or an external ventricular device. After implanting, the organisms spread into the CSF, by which the infection spreads throughout the subarachnoid space.

The infective process is similar to that seen in any bacterial infection and includes inflammation, exudation, white blood cell accumulation, and varying degrees of tissue damage. The brain becomes hyperemic and edematous, and the entire surface of the brain is covered by a layer of purulent exudate that varies with the type of organism. For example, meningococcal exudate is most evident over the parietal, occipital, and cerebellar regions; the thick, fibrinous exudate of pneumococcal infection is confined chiefly to the surface of the brain, particularly the anterior lobes; and the exudate of streptococcal infections is similar to that of pneumococcal infections but thinner. As infection extends to the ventricles, thick pus, fibrin, or adhesions may occlude the narrow passages and obstruct the flow of CSF.

Clinical Manifestations

Patients with bacterial meningitis may present with fever and signs of meningeal irritation, including nausea, vomiting, irritability, anorexia, headache, photophobia, confusion, back pain, and nuchal rigidity. A history of an upper respiratory infection often precedes these symptoms. See Box 45-4 for clinical manifestations of bacterial meningitis. Nuchal rigidity is manifested by inability to flex neck and place chin on chest and presence of Kernig and Brudzinski signs. The Kernig sign is present if the patient, in the supine position with the hip and knee flexed at 90 degrees, cannot extend the knee more than 135 degrees and pain is felt in the hamstrings. Flexion of the opposite knee may also occur. The Brudzinski sign is present if the patient, while in the supine position, flexes the lower extremities if passive flexion of the neck is attempted (Feigin and Cutrer, 2009).

> **! NURSING ALERT**
>
> Any child who is ill and develops a purpuric or petechial rash may have (overwhelming) meningococcemia and must receive medical attention immediately.

BOX 45-4   CLINICAL MANIFESTATIONS OF BACTERIAL MENINGITIS

Children and Adolescents
- Usually abrupt onset
- Fever
- Chills
- Headache
- Vomiting
- Alterations in sensorium
- Seizures (often the initial sign)
- Irritability
- Agitation
- May develop:
  - Photophobia
  - Delirium
  - Hallucinations
  - Aggressive behavior
  - Drowsiness
  - Stupor
  - Coma
- Nuchal rigidity; may progress to opisthotonos
- Positive Kernig and Brudzinski signs
- Hyperactivity but variable reflex responses
- Signs and symptoms peculiar to individual organisms:
  - Petechial or purpuric rashes (meningococcal infection), especially when associated with a shocklike state
  - Joint involvement (meningococcal and *Haemophilus influenzae* infection)
  - Chronically draining ear (pneumococcal meningitis)

Infants and Young Children
- Classic presentation in children (above) is rarely seen in children between 3 months and 2 years of age
- Fever
- Poor feeding

- Vomiting
- Marked irritability
- Frequent seizures (often accompanied by a high-pitched cry)
- Bulging fontanel
- Nuchal rigidity possible
- Brudzinski and Kernig signs not helpful in diagnosis
- Difficult to elicit and evaluate in this age-group
- Subdural empyema (*H. influenzae* infection)

Neonates
Specific Signs
- Extremely difficult to diagnose
- Manifestations vague and nonspecific
- Child well at birth but within a few days begins to look and behave poorly
- Refuses feedings
- Poor sucking ability
- Vomiting or diarrhea
- Poor tone
- Lack of movement
- Weak cry
- Full, tense, and bulging fontanel may appear late in course of illness
- Neck usually supple

Nonspecific Signs That May Be Present
- Hypothermia or fever (depending on infant's maturity)
- Jaundice
- Irritability
- Drowsiness
- Seizures
- Respiratory irregularities or apnea
- Cyanosis
- Weight loss

Diagnostic Evaluation

A lumbar puncture is the definitive diagnostic test for meningitis. The fluid pressure is measured; and samples are obtained for culture, Gram stain, blood cell count, and determination of glucose and protein content. These findings are usually diagnostic. Culture and sensitivity testing are needed to identify the causative organism. Spinal fluid pressure is usually elevated, but interpretation is often difficult when the child is crying. Sedation with fentanyl and midazolam can alleviate the child's pain and fear associated with this procedure. If there is evidence or suspicion of increased ICP (papilledema, focal neurologic deficits, bulging fontanel), a CT scan of the head is warranted before the procedure. Lumbar puncture is contraindicated in any patient with imaging to suggest that the procedure is not safe (e.g., midline shift, mass effect, transependymal migration of CSF). However, a "normal" CT does not always mean that a lumbar puncture is safe in the case of bacterial meningitis. It is important to take the clinical status into careful consideration. Clinical signs, including recent seizure, deteriorating LOC, or brainstem signs (posturing, pupillary changes, respiratory pattern changes), are clinical predictors of when a lumbar puncture should be delayed (Joffe, 2007).

The patient with meningitis generally has an elevated white blood cell count, often predominantly polymorphonuclear leukocytes. Typically in bacterial meningitis the CSF glucose level is reduced, generally in proportion to the duration and severity of the infection. It is a common misconception that the CSF glucose is low because of bacterial consumption of glucose. However, CNS infections may alter glucose transport across the blood-CSF barrier, resulting in a low CSF glucose value. The CSF glucose value in viral meningitis is usually normal (Logan and MacMahon, 2008). The protein concentration is usually increased.

A blood culture is advisable for all children suspected of having meningitis and occasionally is positive when CSF culture is negative. Nose and throat cultures may provide helpful information in some cases.

Therapeutic Management

Acute bacterial meningitis is a medical emergency that requires early recognition and immediate institution of therapy to prevent death or residual disabilities. The initial therapeutic management includes the following:

- Isolation precautions
- Initiation of antimicrobial therapy
- Restrict hydration
- Maintenance of ventilation
- Reduction of increased ICP
- Management of systemic shock
- Control of seizures
- Control of temperature
- Treatment of complications

The child is isolated from other children, usually in an intensive care unit for close observation. An IV infusion is started to facilitate the administration of antimicrobial agents, fluids, antiepileptic drugs, and blood, if needed. The child is placed on a cardiac monitor and in respiratory isolation.

Drugs. Until the causative organism is identified, the choice of antibiotic is based on the known sensitivity of the organism most likely to be the infective agent. After identification of the organism, antimicrobial agents are adjusted accordingly.

> ### 🔹 MEDICATION ALERT
>
> Dexamethasone may play a role in the initial management of increased ICP and cerebral herniation, but its ability to reduce long-term complications of bacterial meningitis remains controversial. Evidence indicates that dexamethasone therapy decreases the risk of neurologic sequelae in children with Hib meningitis, but data regarding the benefits in other types of bacterial meningitis are inconclusive (Prober and Dyner, 2011a). It is not recommended to be used if aseptic or nonbacterial meningitis is suspected (Granoff and Gilsdorf, 2011).

Signs of gastrointestinal hemorrhage or secondary infection may complicate steroid administration. Antibiotic treatment with cephalosporins demonstrates superiority for promptly sterilizing the CSF and reducing the incidence of severe hearing impairment.

Nonspecific Measures. Maintaining hydration is a prime concern, and the type and amount of IV fluids are determined by the patient's condition. Children with bacterial meningitis must be monitored closely for electrolyte and fluid abnormalities. The optimum hydration involves correction of any fluid deficits followed by fluid restriction until normal serum sodium levels and no signs of increased ICP are present. If needed, measures to decrease ICP are implemented (see p. 1425). Long-term fluid restriction is not the standard of care because a lack of adequate fluid volume can reduce blood pressure and cerebral perfusion pressure, causing CNS ischemia (Prober and Dyner, 2011a).

Complications such as aspiration of subdural effusion in infants and disseminated intravascular coagulation syndrome are treated appropriately. Shock is managed by restoration of circulating blood volume and maintenance of electrolyte balance. Seizures can occur during the first few days of treatment. These are controlled with the appropriate antiepileptic drug. Hearing loss is common. The patient should undergo auditory evaluation 6 months after the illness has resolved.

Lumbar puncture is carried out as needed to determine the effectiveness of therapy. The patient is evaluated neurologically during the convalescent period.

Prognosis. Fewer than 10% of cases of bacterial meningitis in children are fatal (Thigpen, Whitney, Messonnier, et al., 2011). The child's age, duration of illness before antibiotic therapy, rapidity of diagnosis after onset, type of organism, and adequacy of therapy are important in the prognosis of bacterial meningitis. Survivors can experience significant physical and neurologic sequelae. The most common sequelae in children include hearing loss, intellectual disability, spasticity or paresis, and seizure disorder. Approximately half of the survivors of pediatric bacterial meningitis will have at least one sequela at a 5-year follow-up time point (Chandran, Herbert, Misurski, et al., 2011).

Clinical features that are associated with an increased risk of developing neurologic complications include young age, infection with *S. pneumoniae*, CSF with more than 10^7 colony-forming units/

mL or low CSF glucose content, delay in antimicrobial therapy for longer than 2 days, prolonged or complicated seizures, focal neurologic deficits, and adequacy of response to infection (Chandran, Herbert, Misurski, et al., 2011). The residual deficits in infants are primarily a result of communicating hydrocephalus and the greater effects of cerebritis on the immature brain. In older children they are related to the inflammatory process itself or result from vasculitis associated with the disease.

Prevention. Vaccines are available for types A, C, Y, and W-135 meningococci and Hib. Meningococcal polysaccharide vaccination is given routinely to children 11 years of age or older; however, children ages 2 to 11 years may be given the vaccine if they are at increased risk for meningococcal disease (Granoff and Gilsdorf, 2011). Routine vaccinations for Hib are recommended for all children beginning at 2 months of age. Pneumococcal conjugate vaccine is now recommended for all children beginning at 2 months of age (Prober and Dyner, 2011a) (see Evidence-Based Practice box).

> ### ❗ NURSING ALERT
>
> A major priority of nursing care of a child suspected of having meningitis is to administer antibiotics as soon as they are ordered. The child is placed on respiratory isolation for at least 24 hours after initiation of antimicrobial therapy.

CARE MANAGEMENT

The room is kept as quiet as possible, and environmental stimuli are kept to a minimum because most children with meningitis are sensitive to noise, bright lights, and other external stimuli. Most children are more comfortable without a pillow and with the head of the bed slightly elevated. A side-lying position is more often assumed because of nuchal rigidity. The nurse should avoid actions that cause pain or increase discomfort such as lifting the child's head. Evaluating the child for pain and implementing appropriate relief measures are important during the initial 24 to 72 hours. Acetaminophen with codeine is often used. The nurse should be cautious to evaluate if a patient is febrile before giving acetaminophen or ibuprofen because either of these medications may mask a fever, which is an important clinical indication of infection.

The nursing care of the child with meningitis is determined by the child's symptoms and treatment. Observation of vital signs, neurologic signs, LOC, urinary output, and other pertinent data is carried out at frequent intervals. The child who is unconscious is managed as described previously (see p. 1424); and all children are observed carefully for signs of the complications just described, especially increased ICP, shock, or respiratory distress. Frequent assessment of the open fontanels is needed in the infant because subdural effusions and obstructive hydrocephalus can develop as a complication of meningitis.

Fluids and nourishment are determined by the child's status. The child with dulled sensorium is usually kept NPO. Other children are allowed clear liquids initially and, if these are tolerated, progress to a diet suitable for their age. Careful monitoring and recording of intake and output are needed to determine deviations that might indicate impending shock or increasing fluid accumulation such as cerebral edema or subdural effusion.

One of the most difficult problems in the nursing care of children with meningitis is maintaining IV infusion for the length of time needed to provide adequate antimicrobial therapy (usually 10 days). Because continuous IV fluids are usually not necessary, an

EVIDENCE-BASED PRACTICE

Children with Bacterial Meningitis and Preventive Vaccines

Ask the Question

In children and adolescents with bacterial meningitis, has the administration of Hib, pneumococcal, and meningococcal preventive vaccines reduced the incidence and mortality associated with bacterial meningitis?

Search for Evidence
Search Strategies

Search selection criteria included English, publications within past 10 years, research-based articles (level 3 or lower), children and adult populations.

Databases Used

PubMed and Cochrane Collaboration

Critically Analyze the Evidence

- Laval, Pimenta, de Andrade, et al. (2003) conducted a systematic review of studies done in developed and developing countries that compared the effect of the conjugate of the Hib vaccine in the early 1990s with the more recent use of the heptavalent pneumococcal and the serogroup C meningococcal vaccines. The researchers concluded that all the vaccines mentioned have contributed directly to the decline in acute bacterial meningitis.
- Data trends on *Streptococcus pneumoniae* infections from the Bacterial Core Surveillance of the Centers for Disease Control and Prevention were evaluated during 1998 to 2001. After being licensed in early 2000, the pneumococcal conjugate vaccine significantly reduced the number of invasive pneumococcal cases, with the largest decline in young children younger than 2 years of age (Whitney, Farley, Hadler, et al., 2003).
- Haddy, Perry, Chacko, et al. (2005) compared the incidence of *S. pneumoniae* disease before and after the introduction of conjugated pneumococcal vaccine from 1999 to 2002. The trend in the rates of invasive pneumococcal disease cases showed significant declines during the study period for all ages after the introduction of the heptavalent *S. pneumoniae* protein conjugate vaccine.
- Children's Hospital of Pittsburgh reported the occurrence of bacterial meningitis before and after the licensure of the Hib conjugate vaccine. A total of 221 children, ages 1 month to 18 years, diagnosed with bacterial meningitis were identified from 1988 to 1998. *Haemophilus influenzae* was the organism responsible for approximately 58% of cases of bacterial meningitis. The absolute number of cases of bacterial meningitis caused by *H. influenzae* declined to 2.5 cases per year after the introduction of the Hib conjugate vaccine (Neuman and Wald, 2001).
- Watt, Wolfson, O'Brien, et al. (2009) performed a literature review with studies evaluating Hib disease incidence, fatality ratios, and the effect of Hib vaccine. In 2000 there were 173,000 cases of Hib meningitis and 78,300 deaths among children younger than the age of 5 years worldwide. Expanded use of Hib vaccine can reduce the incidence and mortality of Hib-related disease.
- A recent Cochrane review determined the effect, duration of protection, and age-specific effects of polysaccharide SgAV to prevent meningococcal meningitis in children. The vaccine had a 95% protective effect during the first year in children older than 5 years of age, but its efficacy after the first year could not be determined. Children ages 1 to 5 years in low-income countries were also protected, but the exact efficacy could not be determined (Patel and Lee, 2010).

Apply the Evidence: Nursing Implications

There is *good evidence with strong recommendations* (Guyatt, Oxman, Vist, et al., 2008) to suggest that all children should be immunized against the most common organisms responsible for bacterial meningitis (i.e., Hib, *S. pneumoniae*, and *Neisseria meningitidis*) as preventive vaccines to decrease the incidence of bacterial meningitis. The nurse should stress to the parents, children, adolescents, and young adults the importance of adhering to the immunization schedule to protect the child against serious childhood diseases.

Quality and Safety Competencies:
Evidence-Based Practice*
Knowledge

Differentiate clinical opinion from research and evidence-based summaries.

Describe the rationale for using vaccines to prevent bacterial meningitis.

Skills

Base individualized care plan on patient values, clinical expertise, and evidence.

Integrate evidence into practice by determining whether a patient needs Hib, pneumococcal, or meningococcal preventive vaccines.

Attitudes

Value the concept of evidence-based practice as integral to determining best clinical practice.

Appreciate the strengths and weakness of evidence for preventive vaccination in children.

References

Guyatt GH, Oxman AD, Vist GE, et al: GRADE: An emerging consensus on rating quality of evidence and strength of recommendations, *BMJ* 336:924–926, 2008.

Haddy RI, Perry K, Chacko CE, et al: Comparison of incidence in invasive *Streptococcus pneumoniae* disease among children before and after introduction of conjugated pneumococcal vaccine, *Pediatr Infect Dis J* 24(4):320–330, 2005.

Laval CA, Pimenta FC, de Andrade JG, et al: Progress towards meningitis prevention in the conjugate vaccines era, *Braz J Infect Dis* 7(5):315–324, 2003.

Neuman HB, Wald ER: Bacterial meningitis in childhood at the Children's Hospital of Pittsburgh: 1988–1998, *Clin Pediatr (Phila)* 40(11):595–600, 2001.

Patel M, Lee CK: Polysaccharide vaccines for preventing serogroup A meningococcal meningitis, *Cochrane Database Syst Rev* (1):CD001093, 2010.

Watt JP, Wolfson LJ, O'Brien KL, et al: Burden of disease caused by *Haemophilus influenzae* type b in children younger than 5 years, *Lancet* 374:903–911, 2009.

Whitney CG, Farley MM, Hadler J, et al: Decline in invasive pneumococcal disease after the introduction of protein-polysaccharide conjugate vaccine, *N Engl J Med* 348(18):1737–1746, 2003.

Hib, Haemophilus influenzae type b; *SgAV,* serogroup A vaccine.
*Adapted from the QSEN at www.quen.org.

intermittent infusion device is used. In some cases children who are recovering uneventfully are sent home with the device, and the parents are taught IV drug administration.

Family Support. The sudden nature of the illness makes emotional support of the child and parents extremely important. Parents are upset and concerned about their child's condition and often feel guilty for not having suspected the seriousness of the illness sooner. They need much reassurance that the natural onset of meningitis is sudden and that they acted responsibly in seeking medical assistance when they did. The nurse encourages the parents to openly discuss their feelings to minimize blame and guilt. They also are kept informed of the child's progress and of all procedures, results, and treatments. In the event that the child's condition worsens, they need the same psychologic supportive care as parents who face the possible death of their child (see Chapter 36).

Nonbacterial (Aseptic) Meningitis

Aseptic meningitis is caused by many different viruses, including arbovirus, herpes simplex virus (HSV), cytomegalovirus, adenovirus, and HIV. Enteroviruses are the most common cause of viral meningitis (Prober and Dyner, 2011b). The term *aseptic meningitis* refers to the onset of meningeal symptoms, fever, and pleocytosis without bacterial growth from CSF cultures. Viral meningitis can occur at any age but is most common in very young children. It has many of the same presenting signs and symptoms as bacterial meningitis, including headache, fever, photophobia, and nuchal rigidity. It can also be accompanied by cutaneous and mucosal manifestations of enterovirus, including hand, foot, and mouth syndrome; herpangina; and maculopapular rash. The clinical course of viral meningitis is much shorter and typically without any significant complications (Logan and MacMahon, 2008).

Diagnosis is based on clinical features and CSF findings. Variations in CSF values in bacterial and viral meningitis are listed in Table 45-2. It is important to differentiate this self-limiting disorder from the more serious forms of meningitis.

Treatment is primarily symptomatic such as acetaminophen for headache and muscle pain, maintenance of hydration, and positioning for comfort. Until a definitive diagnosis is made, antimicrobial agents may be administered, and isolation enforced as a precaution against the possibility that the disease might be of bacterial origin.

TABLE 45-2	VARIATION OF CEREBROSPINAL FLUID ANALYSIS IN BACTERIAL AND VIRAL MENINGITIS	
MANIFESTATIONS	**BACTERIAL***	**VIRAL**
WBC count	Elevated; increased polys	Slightly elevated; increased lymphs
Protein content	Elevated	Normal or slightly increased
Glucose content	Decreased	Normal
Gram stain; bacteria culture	Positive	Negative
Color	Cloudy	Clear

WBC, White blood cell.
*Results may vary in the neonate.

Nursing care is similar to the care of the child with bacterial meningitis.

Encephalitis

Encephalitis is an inflammatory process of the CNS resulting in inflammation of the brain parenchyma itself and is caused by a variety of organisms, including bacteria, spirochetes, fungi, protozoa, helminths, and viruses. Most infections are associated with viruses, and this discussion is limited to these agents.

Etiology

Encephalitis can occur as a result of (1) direct invasion of the CNS by a virus, or (2) postinfectious involvement of the CNS after a viral disease. Often the specific type of encephalitis may not be identified. The cause of more than half of the cases reported in the United States is unknown. The majority of cases of known etiology are associated with the childhood diseases of measles, mumps, varicella, and rubella and, less often, with the enteroviruses, herpesviruses, and West Nile virus.

Herpes simplex encephalitis is an uncommon disease, but 30% of cases involve children. The initial clinical findings are nonspecific (fever, altered mental status), but most cases evolve to demonstrate focal neurologic signs and symptoms. Children may experience focal seizures. The CSF is abnormal in most cases. Because of a rise in the number of children with HSV encephalitis, suspected cases require prompt attention, especially because the diagnosis can be difficult. CSF polymerase chain reaction testing can confirm the clinical diagnosis rapidly. The early use of IV acyclovir reduces mortality and morbidity. Empiric therapy with acyclovir is given before precise virologic diagnosis has been established. Approximately two thirds of children with HSV encephalitis have residual neurologic deficits (James, Kimberlin, and Whitley, 2009).

The multiplicity of causes of viral encephalitis makes diagnosis difficult. Most are those involved with arthropod vectors (togaviruses and bunyaviruses) and those associated with hemorrhagic fevers (arenaviruses, filoviruses, and Hantaviruses). In the United States the vector reservoir for most agents pathogenic for humans is the mosquito (St. Louis or West Nile encephalitis); therefore most cases of encephalitis appear during the hot summer months and subside during the autumn.

The clinical features of encephalitis are similar regardless of the agent involved. Manifestations can range from a mild benign form that resembles aseptic meningitis, lasts a few days, and is followed by rapid and complete recovery to a fulminating encephalitis with severe CNS involvement. The onset may be sudden or gradual with malaise, fever, headache, dizziness, apathy, nuchal rigidity, nausea and vomiting, ataxia, tremors, hyperactivity, and speech difficulties (Box 45-5). In severe cases the patient has a high fever, stupor, seizures, disorientation, spasticity, and coma that may proceed to death. Ocular palsies and paralysis also may occur.

Diagnostic Evaluation

The diagnosis is made on the basis of clinical findings and, when possible, identification of the specific virus. Early in the course of encephalitis, CT scan results may be normal. Later hemorrhagic areas in the frontotemporal region may be seen. Togaviruses (some of which were formerly labeled arboviruses) are rarely detected in the blood or spinal fluid; but viruses of herpes, mumps, measles, and enteroviruses may be found in the CSF. Serologic testing may be required. The first blood sample should be drawn as soon as possible after onset, with the second sample drawn 2 or 3 weeks later. There are a number of characteristic EEG findings in encephalitis,

BOX 45-5	CLINICAL MANIFESTATIONS OF ENCEPHALITIS

Onset
- Malaise
- Fever
- Headache
- Dizziness
- Apathy
- Lethargy
- Nuchal rigidity

Severe Cases
- High fever
- Stupor
- Seizures
- Disorientation
- Nausea and vomiting
- Ataxia
- Tremors
- Hyperactivity
- Speech difficulties—mutism
- Altered mental status
- Spasticity
- Coma (may proceed to death)
- Ocular palsies
- Paralysis

particularly in HSV encephalitis, and an EEG is often part of the diagnostic evaluation (Somand and Meurer, 2009).

Therapeutic Management

Patients suspected of having encephalitis are hospitalized promptly for observation. Only HSV encephalitis has specific treatment available. In other cases treatment is primarily supportive and includes conscientious nursing care, control of cerebral manifestations, and adequate nutrition and hydration, with observation and management as for other cerebral disorders. Viral encephalitis can cause devastating neurologic injury. Cerebral edema, seizures, abnormal fluid and electrolyte balances, aspiration, and cardiac or respiratory arrest occur in severe viral encephalitis; and close monitoring is needed (Prober and Dyner, 2011b).

The prognosis for the child with encephalitis depends on his or her age, the type of organism, and residual neurologic damage. Long-term outcomes of HSV encephalitis in children can be serious; deficits include visual, auditory, motor, and psychiatric (Prober and Dyner, 2011b). Very young children (younger than 2 years of age) may exhibit increased neurologic disabilities, including learning difficulties and seizure disorders. Follow-up care with periodic reevaluation is important because symptoms are often subtle, and rehabilitation is essential for patients who develop residual effects of the disease.

CARE MANAGEMENT

Nursing care of the child with encephalitis is the same as for any unconscious child and for children with meningitis. Additional nursing interventions include observation for deterioration in consciousness. Isolation of the child is not necessary; however, good hand washing technique must be followed. A main focus of nursing management is the control of rapidly rising ICP. Neurologic monitoring, administration of medications, and support of the child and parents are the major aspects of care.

Rabies

Rabies is an acute infection of the nervous system caused by a virus that is almost invariably fatal if left untreated. It is transmitted to humans by the saliva of an infected mammal and is introduced through a bite or skin abrasion. After entry into a new host, the virus multiplies in muscle cells and is spread through neural pathways without stimulating a protective host immune response.

Approximately 92% of rabies cases are transmitted by wild animals, and the remainder from domestic animals (Blanton, Palmer, and Rupprecht, 2010). Wild animals such as skunks, raccoons, foxes, and bats are the animals most often infected with rabies and the cause of most indigenous cases of human rabies in the United States. The likelihood of human exposure to a rabid domestic animal has decreased greatly. In 2009 only four cases of human rabies were reported in the United States (Blanton, Palmer, and Rupprecht, 2010).

The circumstances of a biting incident are important. An unprovoked attack is more likely than a provoked attack to indicate a rabid animal. Bites inflicted on a child attempting to feed or handle an apparently healthy animal can generally be regarded as provoked. Any child bitten by a wild animal is assumed to be exposed to rabies.

Although rabies is common among wildlife species, human rabies is rarely acquired. Modern-day prophylaxis is nearly 100% successful. The highest incidence occurs in children younger than age 15 years. The incubation period usually ranges from 1 to 3 months but may be as short as 5 days or as long as 8 months (Willoughby, 2011). Only 10% to 15% of persons bitten develop the disease; but, when symptoms are present, rabies progresses to a fatal outcome. In the United States human fatalities associated with rabies occur in people who fail to seek medical attention, usually because they are unaware of their exposure.

The disease is characterized by a period of nonspecific symptoms, including general malaise, fever, headache, and weakness, followed by typical symptoms of severe encephalitis, including agitation, changes in LOC, and seizures. Attempts at swallowing may cause such severe spasm of the pharynx, neck, and diaphragm muscles that apnea, cyanosis, and anoxia (i.e., the characteristics from which the term *hydrophobia* was derived) are produced.

Diagnosis is made on the basis of history and clinical features. Hydrophobia is a cardinal sign of a rabies diagnosis.

Therapeutic Management

Treatment is of little avail after symptoms appear, but the long incubation period allows time for the induction of active and passive immunity before the onset of illness. Two types of immunizing products are available for use in humans: (1) the inactivated rabies vaccines, which induce an active immune response, and (2) the globulins, which contain preformed antibodies. The two types of products should be used concurrently for rabies postexposure treatment when prophylaxis is indicated; however, they are contraindicated after rabies symptoms develop (Willoughby, 2011).

The current therapy for a rabid animal bite consists of thoroughly cleansing the wound with soap and water and administering antibiotics as indicated. Suturing the wound should be avoided whenever possible. Passive immunization with human rabies immunoglobulin should be administered as soon as possible after exposure to provide rapid, short-term passive immunity (Manning, Rupprecht, Fishbein, et al., 2008).

Postexposure active immunity is conferred by administration of the human diploid cell rabies vaccine. The first intramuscular injection of the vaccine is given at the same time as the immunoglobulin (day 0) and is followed by injections at 3, 7, 14, and 28 days after the first dose (Manning, Rupprecht, Fishbein, et al., 2008). Before antirabies prophylaxis is initiated, the local or state health department should be consulted.

CARE MANAGEMENT

Parents and children are frightened by the urgency and seriousness of the situation. They need anticipatory guidance for the therapy and support and reassurance regarding the efficacy of the preventive measures for this dreaded disease. The vaccine is well tolerated by children, although they need preparation for the series of injections. Mass immunization is unnecessary and unlikely to be implemented. In areas where rabies is rare, the schedule given is sufficient. However, certain circumstances may warrant preexposure vaccination such as when a child is being taken to an area of the world where rabies in stray dogs is still a problem.

Reye's Syndrome

RS is a disorder defined as acute encephalopathy associated with other characteristic organ involvement. It is characterized by fever, profoundly impaired consciousness, and disordered hepatic function.

The etiology of RS is not well understood, but most cases follow a common viral illness, typically influenza or varicella. It is a condition characterized pathologically by cerebral edema and fatty changes of the liver. The onset is notable for profuse effortless vomiting and varying degrees of neurologic impairment, including personality changes, seizures, and coma, that lead to increased ICP, herniation, and death (Carey and Balistreri, 2011). The cause of RS is abnormal mitochondrial function induced by various viruses, drugs, exogenous toxins, and genetic factors. Elevated serum ammonia levels tend to correlate with the clinical manifestations and prognosis.

Definitive diagnosis is established by liver biopsy. The staging criteria for RS are based on liver dysfunction and neurologic signs that range from lethargy to coma. As a result of improved diagnostic techniques, children who in the past would have been diagnosed with RS are now diagnosed with other illnesses such as viral or metabolic diseases. Cases of unrecognized, drug-induced encephalopathy by antiemetics given to children during viral illnesses have symptoms similar to those of RS.

The potential association between aspirin therapy for the treatment of fever in children with varicella or influenza and the development of RS precludes its use in these patients. However, by the time the Food and Drug Administration required aspirin product labeling in 1986, most of the decline in RS incidence had already occurred.

CARE MANAGEMENT

The most important aspect of successful management of a child with RS is early diagnosis and aggressive supportive therapy. Rapid progression to coma and high peak ammonia concentrations are associated with a more serious prognosis. Cerebral edema with increased ICP represents the most immediate threat to life.

Care and observations are implemented as for any child with an altered state of consciousness (see p. 1424) and increasing ICP. Accurate and frequent monitoring of intake and output is essential for adjusting fluid volumes to prevent both dehydration and cerebral edema. Because of related liver dysfunction, laboratory studies to determine impaired coagulation such as prolonged bleeding time should be monitored.

Parents of children with RS need to be kept informed of the child's progress, have diagnostic procedures and therapeutic management explained, and be given concerned and sympathetic support. Families need to be aware that salicylate, the alleged offending ingredient in aspirin, is contained in other products (e.g., Pepto-Bismol). They should refrain from administering any product for influenza-like symptoms without first checking the label for "hidden" salicylates.

Prognosis. Recovery from RS is rapid and usually without sequelae if the diagnosis is determined early and therapy is initiated promptly. Patients who survive have full liver function recovery; however, approximately one third may have subtle neuropsychologic deficits (Carey and Balistreri, 2011; Pugliese, Beltramo, and Torre, 2008).

SEIZURE DISORDERS

Seizures are the most common pediatric neurologic disorder. Approximately 4% of children will have at least one seizure by the age of 15 years, with half of those episodes being febrile seizures (Friedman and Ghazala, 2006). Seizures are caused by excessive and disorderly neuronal discharges in the brain. The manifestation of seizures depends on the region of the brain in which they originate and may include unconsciousness or altered consciousness; involuntary movements; and changes in perception, behaviors, sensations, and posture.

Seizures are a symptom of an underlying disease process. Causes may be infectious, neurologic, metabolic, traumatic, or related to ingestion of toxins (Friedman and Ghazala, 2006). Epilepsy is a condition characterized by two or more unprovoked seizures and can be caused by a variety of pathologic processes in the brain. A single seizure event should not be classified as epilepsy and is generally not treated with long-term antiepileptic drugs. Some seizures may result from an acute medical or neurologic illness and cease after the illness is treated. In other cases children may have a single seizure without the cause ever being known.

After it is determined that the child has had a seizure, it is important to classify it according to the International Classification of Epileptic Seizures and assign it to the appropriate epilepsy syndrome, according to the International Classification of Epilepsies and Epileptic Syndromes. Optimum treatment and prognosis require an accurate diagnosis and a determination of the cause whenever possible.

Etiology

Seizures in children have many different causes. They are classified not only according to type but also according to etiology. Acute symptomatic seizures are associated with an acute insult such as head trauma or meningitis. Remote symptomatic seizures are those without an immediate cause but with an identifiable prior brain injury such as major head trauma, meningitis or encephalitis, hypoxia, stroke, or a static encephalopathy such as cognitive impairment or cerebral palsy. Cryptogenic seizures are those occurring with no clear cause. Idiopathic seizures are genetic in origin. A partial list of causative factors is presented in Box 45-6.

Pathophysiology

Regardless of the etiologic factor or type of seizure, the basic mechanism is the same. Abnormal electrical discharges (1) may arise from central areas in the brain that affect consciousness; (2) may be restricted to one area of the cerebral cortex, producing manifestations characteristic of that particular anatomic focus; or (3) may begin in a localized area of the cortex and spread to other portions of the brain and, if sufficiently extensive, produce generalized seizure activity.

Seizure activity begins with a group of neurons in the CNS that, because of excessive excitation and loss of inhibition, amplify their

BOX 45-6 ETIOLOGY OF SEIZURES IN CHILDREN

Nonrecurrent (Acute)
- Febrile episodes
- Intracranial infection
- Intracranial hemorrhage
- Space-occupying lesions (cyst, tumor)
- Acute cerebral edema
- Anoxia
- Toxins
- Drugs
- Tetanus
- Lead encephalopathy
- *Shigella* or *Salmonella* organisms
- Metabolic alterations:
  - Hypocalcemia
  - Hypoglycemia
  - Hyponatremia or hypernatremia
  - Hypomagnesemia
  - Alkalosis
  - Disorders of amino acid metabolism
  - Deficiency states
  - Hyperbilirubinemia

Recurrent (Chronic)
- Idiopathic epilepsy
- Epilepsy secondary to:
  - Trauma
  - Hemorrhage
  - Anoxia
  - Infections
  - Toxins
  - Degenerative phenomena
  - Congenital defects
  - Parasitic brain disease
  - Hypoglycemia injury
- Epilepsy—sensory stimulus
- Epilepsy-stimulating states
  - Narcolepsy and cataplexy
  - Psychogenic
  - Tetany from hypocalcemia, alkalosis
- Hypoglycemic states
  - Hyperinsulinism
  - Hypopituitarism
  - Adrenocortical insufficiency
  - Hepatic disorders
- Uremia
- Allergy
- Cardiovascular dysfunction or syncopal episodes
- Migraine

discharge simultaneously. In response to physiologic stimuli such as cellular dehydration, severe hypoglycemia, electrolyte imbalance, sleep deprivation, emotional stress, and endocrine changes, these hyperexcitable cells activate normal cells in surrounding areas and in distant, synaptically related cells. A generalized seizure develops when the neuronal excitation from the epileptogenic focus spreads to the brainstem, particularly the midbrain and reticular formation. These centers within the brainstem, known as the centrencephalic system, are responsible for the spread of the epileptic potentials. The discharges can originate spontaneously in the centrencephalic system or be triggered by a focal area in the cortex. On the basis of these characteristic neuronal discharges (as recorded by the EEG), seizures are designated as partial, generalized, and unclassified epileptic seizures.

Hallmark early systemic clinical changes during a generalized seizure include tachycardia, hypertension, hyperglycemia, and hypoxemia. Brief seizures rarely produce significant durable side effects. In contrast, prolonged seizures can lead to lactic acidosis, rhabdomyolysis, hyperkalemia, hyperthermia, and hypoglycemia. All of these changes can cause long-term neurologic damage (Friedman and Ghazala, 2006).

Seizure Classification and Clinical Manifestations

There are many different types of seizures, and each has unique clinical manifestations. Seizures are classified into three major categories:
- Partial seizures, which have a local onset and involve a relatively small location in the brain

- Generalized seizures, which involve both hemispheres of the brain and are without local onset
- Unclassified epileptic seizures

Descriptions of the different types of seizures are found in Box 45-7 and Table 45-3.

Diagnostic Evaluation

Establishing a diagnosis is critical for establishing a prognosis and planning the proper treatment. The process of diagnosis in a child suspected of having epilepsy includes (1) determining whether epilepsy or seizures exist rather than an alternative diagnosis, and (2) defining the underlying cause if possible. The assessment and diagnosis rely heavily on a thorough history, skilled observation, and several diagnostic tests.

It is especially important to differentiate epilepsy from other brief alterations in consciousness or behavior. Clinical entities that mimic seizures include migraine headaches, toxic effects of drugs, syncope (fainting), breath-holding spells in infants and young children, movement disorders (tics, tremor, chorea), prolonged QT syndrome, sleep disturbances (night terrors), psychogenic seizures, rage attacks, and transient ischemic attacks (rare in children) (Friedman and Ghazala, 2006). Cocaine intoxication should be considered in the differential diagnosis of new-onset seizure activity in a newborn infant.

The history of the seizure should be detailed, including the type of seizure or description of the child's behavior during the event, the age at onset, and the time at which the seizure occurs (e.g., early morning, before meals, while awake, or during sleep). Any factors that may have precipitated the seizure are important, including fever, infection, head trauma, anxiety, fatigue, sleep deprivation, menstrual cycle, alcohol, and activity (e.g., hyperventilation or exposure to strong stimuli such as bright flashing light or loud noises). Record any sensory phenomena that the child can describe. The duration and progression of the seizure (if any) and the postictal feelings and behavior (e.g., confusion, inability to speak, amnesia, headache, and sleep) should also be recorded. It is important to determine whether more than one seizure type exists. It is often more informative to ask the parents to mime the seizure rather than relying on their oral description. Miming often reveals features such as head turning that would otherwise go unrecognized. Some seizures are overlooked by parents. For example, some parents may not identify brief head nods or brief single jerks as seizures unless specifically asked whether their child has these symptoms. The family history should include whether other family members have had a seizure, cognitive impairments, cerebral palsy, or other neurologic disorders. A family history can offer clues to paroxysmal disorders such as migraine headaches, breath-holding spells, febrile seizures, or neurologic diseases.

A complete physical and neurologic examination, including developmental assessment of language, learning, behavior, and motor abilities, may provide clues to the cause of the seizures. A number of laboratory and neuroimaging tests may be ordered, depending on the child's age, whether it is a new-onset seizure, characteristics of the seizure, and the history. Laboratory studies that may prove to be of value include a venous lead level if the history warrants or white blood cell count (for signs of infection). Blood glucose measurements may give evidence of hypoglycemic episodes; and serum electrolytes, blood urea nitrogen, calcium, serum amino acids, lactate, ammonia, and urine organic acids may indicate metabolic disturbances. Blood for chromosome analysis may also be tested if a genetic etiology is suspected. A toxic screen should be performed if alcohol or drug ingestion is suspected. Lumbar puncture can confirm a suspected diagnosis of meningitis.

BOX 45-7   CLASSIFICATION AND CLINICAL MANIFESTATIONS OF SEIZURES

Partial Seizures

Simple Partial Seizures with Motor Signs

- Characterized by:
  - Localized motor symptoms
  - Somatosensory, psychic, autonomic symptoms
  - Combination of these
  - Abnormal discharges remaining unilateral
- Manifestations
  - Aversive seizure (most common motor seizure in children)—eye or eyes and head turn away from the side of the focus; awareness of movement or loss of consciousness
  - Rolandic (Sylvan) seizure—tonic-clonic movements involving the face, salivation, arrested speech; most common during sleep
  - Jacksonian march (rare in children)—orderly, sequential progression of clonic movements beginning in a foot, hand, or face and moving, or "marching," to adjacent body parts

Simple Partial Seizures with Sensory Signs

- Uncommon in children younger than 8 years of age
- Characterized by various sensations, including:
  - Numbness, tingling, prickling, paresthesia, or pain originating in one area (e.g., face or extremities) and spreading to other parts of the body
  - Visual sensations or formed images
  - Motor phenomena such as posturing or hypertonia

Complex Partial Seizures (Psychomotor Seizures)

- Observed more often in children from 3 years through adolescence
- Characterized by:
  - Period of altered behavior
  - Amnesia for event (no recollection of behavior)
  - Inability to respond to environment
  - Impaired consciousness during event
  - Drowsiness or sleep usually following seizure
  - Confusion and amnesia possibly prolonged
  - Complex sensory phenomena (aura)—most frequent sensation is strange feeling in the pit of the stomach that rises toward the throat and is often accompanied by odd or unpleasant odors or tastes; complex auditory or visual hallucinations; ill-defined feelings of elation or strangeness (e.g., déjà vu, a feeling of familiarity in a strange environment); strong feelings of fear and anxiety; a distorted sense of time and self; and in small children emission of a cry or attempt to run for help
- Patterns of motor behavior:
  - Stereotypic
  - Similar with each subsequent seizure
  - May suddenly cease activity, appear dazed, stare into space, become confused and apathetic, and become limp or stiff or display some form of posturing
  - May be confused
  - May perform purposeless, complicated activities in a repetitive manner (automatisms) such as walking, running, kicking, laughing, or speaking incoherently, most often followed by postictal confusion or sleep; may exhibit oropharyngeal activities such as smacking, chewing, drooling, swallowing, and nausea or abdominal pain followed by stiffness, a fall, and postictal sleep; rarely manifests actions such as rage or temper tantrums; aggressive acts uncommon during seizure

Generalized Seizures

Tonic-Clonic Seizures (Formerly Known As Grand Mal)

- Most common and dramatic of all seizure manifestations
- Occur without warning
- Tonic phase lasts approximately 10 to 20 seconds
- Manifestations:
  - Eyes roll upward
  - Immediate loss of consciousness
  - If standing, falls to floor or ground
  - Stiffens in generalized, symmetric tonic contraction of entire body musculature
  - Arms usually flexed
  - Legs, head, and neck extended
  - May utter a peculiar piercing cry
  - Apneic, may become cyanotic
  - Increased salivation and loss of swallowing reflex
- Clonic phase: lasts about 30 seconds but can vary from only a few seconds to a half hour or longer
- Manifestations:
  - Violent jerking movements as the trunk and extremities undergo rhythmic contraction and relaxation
  - May foam at the mouth
  - May be incontinent of urine and feces
- As event ends, movements less intense, occurring at longer intervals and then ceasing entirely
- Status epilepticus—series of seizures at intervals too brief to allow the child to regain consciousness between the time one event ends and the next begins
  - Requires emergency intervention
  - Can lead to exhaustion, respiratory failure, and death
- Postictal state:
  - Appears to relax
  - May remain semiconscious and difficult to arouse
  - May awaken in a few minutes
  - Remains confused for several hours
  - Poor coordination
  - Mild impairment of fine motor movements
  - May have visual and speech difficulties
  - May vomit or complain of severe headache
  - When left alone, usually sleeps for several hours
  - On awakening is fully conscious
  - Usually feels tired and complains of sore muscles and headache
  - No recollection of entire event

Absence Seizures (Formerly Called Petit Mal or Lapses)

- Characterized by:
  - Onset usually between 4 and 12 years of age
  - More common in girls than boys
  - Usually cease at puberty
  - Brief loss of consciousness
  - Minimum or no alteration in muscle tone
  - May go unrecognized because of little change in child's behavior
  - Abrupt onset; suddenly develops 20 or more attacks daily
  - Event often mistaken for inattentiveness or daydreaming
  - Events possibly precipitated by hyperventilation, hypoglycemia, stresses (emotional and physiologic), fatigue, or sleeplessness

Continued

BOX 45-7   CLASSIFICATION AND CLINICAL MANIFESTATIONS OF SEIZURES—cont'd

- Manifestations:
  - Brief loss of consciousness
  - Appear without warning or aura
  - Usually last about 5 to 10 seconds
  - Slight loss of muscle tone may cause child to drop objects
  - Ability to maintain postural control; seldom falls
  - Minor movements such as lip smacking, twitching of eyelids or face, or slight hand movements
  - Not accompanied by incontinence
  - Amnesia for episode
  - May need to reorient self to previous activity

Atonic and Akinetic Seizures (Also Known As Drop Attacks)

- Characterized by:
  - Onset usually between 2 and 5 years of age
  - Sudden, momentary loss of muscle tone and postural control
  - Events recurring frequently during the day, particularly in the morning hours and shortly after awakening
- Manifestations:
  - Loss of tone causing child to fall to the floor violently
  - Unable to break fall by putting out hand
  - May incur serious injury to face, head, or shoulder
  - Loss of consciousness only momentary

Myoclonic Seizures

- Variety of seizure episodes
- May be isolated as benign essential myoclonus
- May occur in association with other seizure forms

- Characterized by:
  - Sudden, brief contractures of a muscle or group of muscles
  - Occur singly or repetitively
  - No postictal state
  - May or may not be symmetric
  - May or may not include loss of consciousness

Infantile Spasms

- Also called *infantile myoclonus, massive spasms, hypsarrhythmia, salaam episodes,* or *infantile myoclonic spasms*
- Most commonly occur during the first 6 to 8 months of life
- Twice as common in boys as girls
- Numerous seizures during the day without postictal drowsiness or sleep
- Poor outlook for normal intelligence
- Manifestations:
  - Possible series of sudden, brief, symmetric, muscular contractions
  - Head flexed, arms extended, and legs drawn up
  - Eyes sometimes rolling upward or inward
  - May be preceded or followed by a cry or giggling
  - May or may not include loss of consciousness
  - Sometimes flushing, pallor, or cyanosis
- Infants who are able to sit but not stand:
  - Sudden dropping forward of head and neck with trunk flexed forward and knees drawn up—the *salaam* or *jackknife* seizure
- Less often: alternate clinical forms
  - Extensor spasms rather than flexion of arms, legs, and trunk, and head nodding
  - Lightning events involving a single, momentary, shocklike contraction of the entire body

TABLE 45-3   COMPARISON OF SIMPLE PARTIAL, COMPLEX PARTIAL, AND ABSENCE SEIZURES

CLINICAL MANIFESTATIONS	SIMPLE PARTIAL	COMPLEX PARTIAL	ABSENCE
Age of onset	Any age	Uncommon before age 3 years	Uncommon before age 3 years
Frequency (per day)	Variable	Rarely over one or two times	Multiple
Duration	Usually <30 sec	Usually >60 sec, rarely <10 sec	Usually >10 sec, rarely >30 sec
Aura	May be sole manifestation of seizure	Frequent	Never
Impaired consciousness	Never	Always	Always; brief loss of consciousness
Automatisms	Never	Frequent	Frequent
Clonic movements	Frequent	Occasional	Occasional
Postictal impairment	Rare	Frequent	Never
Mental disorientation	Rare	Common	Unusual

CT may be done to detect a cerebral hemorrhage, infarctions, and gross malformations. MRI provides greater anatomic detail and is used to detect developmental malformations, tumors, and cortical dysplasias.

An EEG is obtained for most children with seizures and is the most useful tool for evaluating a seizure disorder. It confirms the presence of abnormal electrical discharges and provides information on the seizure type and the focus. The EEG is carried out under varying conditions (e.g., with the child asleep, awake, awake with provocative stimulation [flashing lights, noise], and hyperventilation). Stimulation may elicit abnormal electrical activity, which is recorded on the EEG. Various seizure types produce characteristic EEG patterns: high-voltage spike discharges are seen in tonic-clonic seizures, with abnormal patterns in the intervals between seizures; a three-per-second spike and wave pattern is observed in an absence seizure; and absence of electrical activity in an area suggests a large lesion such as an abscess or subdural collection of fluid.

A normal EEG does not rule out seizures because the EEG is only a surface recording. It only represents approximately 1 hour of time and therefore may show normal interictal activity. If there is concern about whether a child has seizures or the seizure type cannot be determined, a long-term video EEG may be done to record the child during wakefulness and sleep. The full-body image is recorded on video, with selected EEG channels displayed on the same screen for simultaneous recording and viewing. EEG monitoring is also available in digital EEG and digital video imaging, which allows for greater selection of EEG channels and is available in both routine and long-term EEGs. Although the EEG is very valuable, it should not be used alone to determine the type of seizure. Rather the EEG interpretation along with a thorough clinical description of the patient's behavior during the seizure episode guides to the correct classification of the seizure and the appropriate treatment choice.

Therapeutic Management

The goal of treatment of seizure disorders is to control the seizures or reduce their frequency and severity, discover and correct the cause when possible, and help the child live as normal a life as possible. If the seizure activity is a manifestation of an infectious, traumatic, or metabolic process, the seizure therapy is instituted as part of the general therapeutic regimen and may only be necessary for a certain period of time if the underlying cause is corrected. Management of epilepsy has four treatment options: drug therapy, the ketogenic diet, vagus nerve stimulation (VNS), and epilepsy surgery.

Drug Therapy. It is known that people predisposed to epilepsy have seizures when their basal level of neuronal excitability exceeds a critical point; no event occurs if the excitability is maintained below this threshold. The administration of antiepileptic drugs serves to raise this threshold and prevent seizures. Consequently the primary therapy for seizure disorders is the administration of the appropriate antiepileptic drug or combination of drugs in a dosage that provides the desired effect without causing undesirable side effects or toxic reactions. Antiepileptic drugs are believed to exert their effect primarily by reducing the responsiveness of normal neurons to the sudden, high-frequency nerve impulses that arise in the epileptogenic focus. Thus the seizure is effectively suppressed; however, the abnormal brain waves may or may not be altered. Complete control of seizures can be achieved in 70% to 80% of children (Curatolo, Moavero, Lo Castro, et al., 2009; Lozsadi, Von Oertzen, and Cock, 2010).

The initiation of anticonvulsant therapy is based on several factors, including the child's age, type of seizure, risk of recurrence, and other comorbid or predisposing medical issues. For children who develop recurrent seizures or epilepsy, treatment is begun with a single drug known to be effective and have the lowest toxicity (i.e., the safest side effect profile for the child's particular type of seizure). The dosage is gradually increased until the seizures are controlled or the child develops side effects. If the drug is effective but does not control the seizures sufficiently, a second drug is added in gradually increasing doses. When seizures are controlled, the first drug may be tapered to reduce the potential adverse effects and drug interactions of polytherapy. Monotherapy remains the treatment method of choice for epilepsy, but a combination of medications may be a viable alternative for children who cannot attain seizure control with only one medication (Mikati, 2011).

Measurement of blood levels of the drug is important if the seizures continue when the child is on a therapeutic dose of medication, to adjust the dosage, and to help determine which medication may be causing the side effects if the child is on multiple antiepileptic medications. Some possible causes of low serum blood concentrations are noncompliance, poor absorption, and drug interactions. The dosage needs to be increased as the child grows. Blood cell counts, urinalysis, and liver function tests are obtained at frequent intervals in children receiving particular antiepileptic medications that can affect organ function.

If complete seizure control is maintained on an anticonvulsant drug for 2 years, it is safe to discontinue the drug for patients with no risk factors. Risk factors include children older than 12 years of age at onset, history of neonatal seizures, numerous seizures before control is achieved, and the presence of a neurologic dysfunction (e.g., motor or cognitive impairment). Up to 40% of children whose medications are discontinued experience seizure recurrence. Recurrence occurs most frequently within 6 months of discontinuation (Sillanpää and Schmidt, 2006).

When seizure medications are discontinued, the dosage is decreased gradually over several weeks. Sudden withdrawal of a drug is not recommended because it can cause an increase in the number and severity of seizures.

🔔 MEDICATION ALERT

Fosphenytoin is often used to treat seizures instead of IV phenytoin because of possible complications and drug interactions associated with IV phenytoin. If IV phenytoin is used, it should be administered via slow IV push at a rate that does not exceed 50 mg/min. Because phenytoin precipitates when mixed with glucose, only normal saline is used to flush the tubing or catheter. Fosphenytoin may be given in saline or glucose solutions at a rate of up to 150 mg phenytoin equivalent (PE)/min, and it may be given intramuscularly if necessary.

Ketogenic Diet. The ketogenic diet is a high-fat, low-carbohydrate, and adequate protein diet (Freeman, Kossoff, and Hartman, 2007). Consumption of such a diet forces the body to shift from using glucose as the primary energy source to using fat, and the individual develops a state of ketosis. The diet is rigorous. All foods and liquids that the child consumes must be carefully weighed and measured. The diet is deficient in vitamins and minerals; therefore vitamin supplements are necessary. Early side effects of the diet are diarrhea, hypoglycemia, dehydration, acidosis, and lethargy; long-term side effects include dyslipidemia, kidney stones, and poor growth (Freeman, Kossoff, and Hartman, 2007).

The ketogenic diet has been shown to be an efficacious and tolerable treatment for medically refractory seizures (Freeman, Kossoff, and Hartman, 2007). Studies have shown that as many as 56% of children on the diet had greater than a 50% reduction in seizure episodes (Hartman and Vining, 2007).

Vagus Nerve Stimulation. VNS uses an implantable device that reduces seizures in individuals who have not had effective control with drug therapy. It is currently indicated as adjunct therapy in patients 12 years and older with partial-onset seizures (with or without secondary generalization) who are refractory to antiepileptic drugs (Elliott, Rodgers, Bassani, et al., 2011). A programmable signal generator is implanted subcutaneously in the chest. Electrodes tunneled underneath the skin deliver electrical impulses to the left vagus nerve (cranial nerve X). The device is programmed noninvasively to deliver a precise pattern of stimulation to the left vagus nerve. The patient or caregiver can activate the device using a magnet at the onset of a seizure. No long-term adverse effects have been reported with VNS; but dysphonia, throat or neck pain, and cough can occur during stimulation. Studies show that approximately one third to one half of patients have a reduction in seizures after 1 year of therapy (Elliott, Rodgers, Bassani, et al., 2011).

Surgical Therapy. When seizures are determined to be caused by a hematoma, tumor, or other cerebral lesion, surgical removal is the treatment. In children with epilepsy, surgery is reserved for those who have incapacitating, refractory seizures. Refractory seizures are usually defined as the persistence of seizures despite adequate trials of three antiepileptic medications, alone or in combination (Mikati, 2011). An extensive medical (e.g., invasive EEG monitoring), psychosocial, and psychoneurologic evaluation is required before surgery. There are several types of surgical interventions. Focal resection entails removal of the epileptogenic zone, and hemispherectomy involves removing all or most of one hemisphere in patients with catastrophic hemispheric epilepsy (Mikati, 2011). Corpus callosotomy consists of the separation of the connections between the two hemispheres in the brain to prevent seizure activity by blocking epileptic discharges (Spencer and Huh, 2008). Patients undergoing surgical resection can experience a decrease in the frequency and severity of seizures, a decrease in antiepileptic medication requirements, and an improvement in their quality of life (Spencer and Huh, 2008).

Status Epilepticus. Status epilepticus is a continuous seizure that lasts more than 30 minutes or a series of seizures from which the child does not regain a premorbid LOC (Huff and Fountain, 2011). It has been suggested that the term *impending status epilepticus* be used for a continuous seizure or series of seizures lasting between 5 to 30 minutes (Mikati, 2011). The initial treatment is directed toward support and maintenance of vital functions (i.e., the ABCs of life support, administering oxygen, and gaining IV access) immediately followed by IV administration of antiepileptic agents.

MEDICATION ALERT

Buccal midazolam and rectal diazepam are quick, effective, and safe treatments for home or prehospital treatment of status epilepticus (Shorvon, 2011). Cessation of seizure occurred in 8 minutes with buccal midazolam and 15 minutes with rectal diazepam (Shorvon, 2011). Respiratory depression is a potential side effect of both medications, and patients should be monitored closely after administration (Mikati, 2011).

For in-hospital management of status epilepticus, IV diazepam or lorazepam (Ativan) is the first-line drug of choice (Mikati, 2011). Lorazepam is the preferred agent because of its rapid onset (2 to 5 minutes) and long half-life (12 to 24 hours). The child must be monitored closely during administration to detect early alterations in vital signs that may indicate impending respiratory depression. When a benzodiazepine (diazepam or lorazepam) is ineffective, fosphenytoin followed by phenobarbital is given as the next line of treatment. This combination of therapy places the child at high risk for apnea; therefore respiratory support is generally necessary. Children may also receive an antiepileptic medication, IV valproate, which does not cause respiratory compromise (Mikati, 2011). Children who continue to have seizures despite this drug treatment may require general anesthesia with a continuous infusion of midazolam, propofol, or pentobarbital (Shorvon, 2011). In this situation the patient may need to be intubated, and continuous EEG monitoring is typically done to monitor for and treat electrographic seizures (Friedman and Ghazala, 2006).

MEDICATION ALERT

Diazepam is incompatible with many drugs. To give it intravenously, inject it slowly and directly into the vein or through tubing as close as possible to the vein insertion site.

Nursing care of a child with status epilepticus includes, in addition to the ABCs of life support, monitoring blood pressure and body temperature. During the first 30 to 45 minutes of the seizure, the blood pressure may be elevated. Thereafter it typically returns to normal but may be decreased, depending on the medications being administered for seizure control. Hyperthermia requiring treatment may occur as a result of increased motor activity.

Prognosis. Most children who experience a second seizure experience additional seizures, with as many as 72% of children having additional seizures within 5 years after the second seizure (Berg, 2008). Therefore a history of two seizures is sufficient to diagnose epilepsy. Epidemiologic studies using population- or community-based cohorts show that the underlying etiology of the child's epilepsy is the most important factor affecting prognosis (Nei and Bagla, 2007). Children with epilepsy and severe neurologic disorders were 22 times more likely to die than children with epilepsy and a normal neurologic status (Nei and Bagla, 2007). Mortality is also associated with the severity and frequency of the child's seizures. It does not significantly increase in children who are seizure free but can be as high as 46% in patients with status epilepticus (Nei and Bagla, 2007).

CARE MANAGEMENT

An important nursing responsibility is to observe the seizure episode and accurately document the events. Any alterations in behavior preceding the seizure and the characteristics of the episode such as sensory-hallucinatory phenomena (e.g., an aura), motor effects (e.g., eye movements, muscular contractions), alterations in consciousness, and postictal state are noted and recorded (Box 45-8). The nurse should describe only what is observed rather than trying to label a seizure type. Note the duration of the seizure with start and stop times.

Based on a thorough assessment, several nursing diagnoses are identified. The more common diagnoses for the child with a seizure disorder are included in the Nursing Care Plan.

The child must be protected from injury during the seizure. Nursing observations made during the event provide valuable information for diagnosis and management of the disorder (see Emergency box on p. 1453).

It is impossible to halt a seizure after it has begun, and no attempt should be made to do so. The nurse must remain calm, stay with the child, and prevent her or him from sustaining any harm during the seizure. If possible, the child should be isolated from the view of others by closing a door or pulling screens. A seizure can be upsetting to the child, other visitors, and their families. If other people are present, they should be assured that everything is being done for the child. After the seizure they can be given a simple explanation about the event as needed.

If the nurse is able to reach the child in time, a child who is standing or seated in a chair (including a wheelchair) is eased to the floor immediately. During (and sometimes after) the tonic-clonic seizure, the swallowing reflex is lost, salivation increases, and the tongue is hypotonic. Therefore the child is at risk for aspiration and airway occlusion. Placing the child on the side facilitates drainage

BOX 45-8 GENERAL OBSERVATIONS: THE CHILD DURING A SEIZURE

Observations During Seizure
Describe
- Order of events (before, during, and after)
- Duration of seizure
  - Tonic-clonic—from first signs of event until jerking stops
  - Absence—from loss of consciousness until consciousness is regained
  - Complex partial—from first sign of unresponsiveness, motor activity, and automatisms until there are signs of responsiveness to environment

Onset
- Time of onset
- Significant precipitating events—missed medication dosage, illness, stress, sleep deprivation, menses

Behavior
- Change in facial expression
- Cry or other sound
- Stereotypic or automatous movements
- Random activity (wandering)
- Position of eyes, head, body, extremities
- Unilateral or bilateral posturing of one or more extremities

Movement
- Change of position, if any
- Site of commencement—hand, thumb, mouth, generalized
- Tonic phase—length, parts of body involved
- Clonic phase—twitching or jerking movements, parts of body involved, sequence of parts involved, generalized, change in character of movements
- Lack of movement or muscle tone of body part or entire body

Face
- Color change—pallor, cyanosis, flushing
- Perspiration
- Mouth—position, deviating to one side, teeth clenched, tongue bitten, frothing at mouth, flecks of blood or bleeding
- Lack of expression
- Asymmetric expression

Eyes
- Position—straight ahead, deviation upward or outward, conjugate or divergent gaze
- Pupils—change in size, equality, reaction to light

Respiratory Effort
- Presence and length of apnea

Other
- Incontinence

Postictal Observations
- Duration of postictal period
- State of consciousness
- Orientation
- Arousability
- Motor ability
  - Any change in motor function
  - Ability to move all extremities
  - Paresis or weakness
- Speech
- Sensations
  - Complaint of discomfort or pain
  - Any sensory impairment
  - Recollection of preseizure sensations or aura

and helps maintain a patent airway. Suctioning the oral cavity and posterior oropharynx may be necessary. Take vital signs and allow the child to rest if at school or away from home. When feasible he or she is integrated into the environment as soon as possible. Sending a child with a chronic seizure disorder home from school is not necessary unless requested by the parents.

Seizure precautions are required for children who are known to have seizures or who are under observation for them. The extent of these measures depends on the type and frequency of the seizure (Box 45-9).

! NURSING ALERT

Do not move or forcefully restrain the child during a tonic-clonic seizure and do not place a solid object between the teeth.

Long-Term Care. Care of the child with a recurrent seizure disorder involves physical care and instruction regarding the importance of the drug therapy and, probably more significant, the problems related to the emotional aspects of the disorder. Few diseases generate as much anxiety among relatives as epilepsy. Fears and misconceptions about the disease and its treatment are common. For many it represents the archetype of severe hereditary affliction. Nursing care is directed toward educating the child and family about epilepsy and helping them develop strategies to cope with the psychologic and sociologic problems related to it.

BOX 45-9 SEIZURE PRECAUTIONS

- The extent of precautions depends on type, severity, and frequency of seizures. They may include the following:
  - Side rails raised when child is sleeping or resting
  - Side rails and other hard objects padded
  - Waterproof mattress or pad on bed or crib
- Appropriate precautions during potentially hazardous activities may include the following:
  - Swimming with a companion
  - Showers preferred; bathing only with close supervision
  - Use of protective helmet and padding during bicycle riding, skateboarding, in-line skating
  - Supervision during use of hazardous machinery or equipment
- Have child carry or wear medical identification.
- Alert other caregivers to need for any special precautions.
- Child may not drive or operate hazardous machinery or equipment unless seizure free for designated period (varies by state).

Children with epilepsy are prescribed antiepileptic medications. These medications are administered at regular intervals to maintain adequate levels in the blood. The nurse can help the parents plan the administration of the medication at convenient times to avoid disruptions of family routines as much as possible. It is important to impress on the family the necessity of giving the antiepileptic

⊚ NURSING CARE PLAN

The Child with Seizures

NURSING DIAGNOSIS	EXPECTED OUTCOMES	NURSING INTERVENTIONS	RATIONALE
Risk for Injury related to CNS dysfunction and inability to control self (motor) secondary to type of seizure	Child will not experience physical injury as a result of seizure activity.	Administer AEDs	To prevent seizure activity
Child's or Family's Defining Characteristics		Teach family and child, as appropriate, the purpose of AEDs, expected response and action, potential side effects, timing, dosage, route of administration, and how to monitor effects	To promote understanding of chronic condition To prevent seizure activity and encourage self-care
(Subjective and Objective Data)		Monitor for side effects of AEDs and therapeutic levels according to child's growth, illness factors that affect metabolism, and effects of drug	To prevent secondary effects of AEDs and prevent seizures from occurring because of subtherapeutic drug levels
Change in LOC Disorientation			
Clonic movements		Stress importance of adherence to medication regimen even if child has no evidence of seizure activity	To prevent seizure activity
Automatisms		Teach patient and family to identify and avoid situations that are known to precipitate a seizure (e.g., blinking lights, sleep deprivation, excess activity or exercise, physical factors)	To prevent seizure activity
Aura			
Postictal impairment (dependent on type of seizure)			
		Initiate seizure precautions in the hospital: • Pad side rails of bed, crib, or wheelchair • Keep bed relatively free of objects • Set up suction and oxygen in room	To prevent physical harm
		Educate family to initiate seizure precautions at home: • Bathroom safety includes taking showers instead of baths to prevent drowning; use shower seat if falls occur during typical seizure; leave bathroom door unlocked • Kitchen safety includes cooking when someone else is nearby, using back burners of the stove to prevent accidental burns, and using shatterproof containers as much as possible • Sports safety includes wearing protective equipment, having others nearby, not climbing higher than 10 feet without special equipment	To prevent physical harm
		Teach family seizure first aid: • If child is at risk of falling at beginning of episode, ease child to floor • Loosen tight or restrictive clothing • Turn child to side-lying position • Prevent child from hitting head on objects • Time seizure • Allow seizure to end spontaneously • Reassure child when awakening from seizure • Do not put anything in child's mouth • Do not attempt to restrain child or use force • Call EMS (see Emergency box, p. 1453) if seizure persists more than 5 minutes, for repeated seizures, or if child does not wake up after movements have stopped	To prepare family for emergencies
		Counsel women of childbearing age about contraception and birth defects associated with AEDs	To prevent birth defects
Risk for Aspiration and Ineffective Breathing Pattern related to impaired motor activity, LOC, and loss of airway protection (tonic-clonic seizure)	Child's airway will remain patent. Child will have effective ventilation.	In the event of a seizure, place child in side-lying position on flat surface such as floor or bed	To prevent aspiration and choking
		Remain with patient.	To protect airway
		Remove secretions, food, and liquids from mouth when seizure subsides	To prevent aspiration
Child's or Family's Defining Characteristics		In postictal state monitor oxygenation status	To determine need for oxygen
(Subjective and Objective Data)		Administer oxygen as necessary	To prevent hypoxia
		Administer rescue breaths if spontaneous respirations do not resume shortly after seizure subsides.	To prevent hypoxia
Decreased LOC Depressed cough reflex Apnea Decreased inspiratory pressure		Administer medications intended to stop seizure longer than 5 minutes (rectal diazepam, IV Dilantin, IV lorazepam)	To prevent continued seizure activity

◎ NURSING CARE PLAN

The Child with Seizures—cont'd

NURSING DIAGNOSIS	EXPECTED OUTCOMES	NURSING INTERVENTIONS	RATIONALE
Anxiety/Fear, Parent, related to child having life-threatening and incapacitating seizure activity*	Parent will cope with child's condition and receive adequate support.	Allow parent to remain with child during seizure	To decrease fear of unknown and allow parent to see measures taken to protect child
Child's or Family's Defining Characteristics *(Subjective and Objective Data)*		Instruct parent on proper protection interventions during child's seizure activity, including positioning, safety, airway maintenance, reassurance techniques, and emergency medication administration	To promote parent participation and foster sense of control over situation
Anguish		Provide information regarding nature (type) of seizure, therapeutic interventions, and lifestyle modifications	To promote knowledge of condition, parental intervention, and sense of control
Fear			
Feelings of inadequacy and hopelessness			
Worry, apprehension		Encourage family involvement in daily care of child with goal of normalization and promotion of optimum growth and development	To provide hope
Report of apprehension			
Panic			
Excitement		Involve parents in discussion of fears, anxieties, and resources and support options available to family	To promote family functioning and coping

AED, Antiepileptic drug; *CNS,* central nervous system; *EMS,* emergency medical services; *IV,* intravenous; *LOC,* level of consciousness.
*Nursing diagnosis may also apply to child in the postictal phase, depending on the type of seizure and the child's understanding and cognition level.

➕ EMERGENCY

Seizures

Tonic-Clonic Seizure
During the Seizure
- Remain calm.
- Time seizure episode.
- If child is standing or seated, ease child down to floor.
- Place pillow or folded blanket under child's head.
- Loosen restrictive clothing.
- Remove eyeglasses.
- Clear area of any hazards or hard objects.
- Allow seizure to end without interference.
- If vomiting occurs, turn child to one side.
- Do not:
  - Attempt to restrain child or use force.
  - Put anything in child's mouth.
  - Give any food or liquids.

After the Seizure
- Time postictal period.
- Check for breathing. Check position of head and tongue.
- Reposition if head is hyperextended. If child is not breathing, give rescue breathing and call EMS.
- Keep child on side.
- Remain with child.
- Do not give food or liquids until child is fully alert and swallowing reflex has returned.
- Call EMS when necessary.
- Look for medical identification and determine which factors occurred before onset of seizure that may have been triggering factors.

- Check head and body for possible injuries.
- Check inside of mouth to see if tongue or lips have been bitten.

Complex Partial Seizure
During the Seizure
- Do not restrain.
- Remove harmful objects from area.
- Redirect to safe area.
- Do not agitate; instead, talk in calm, reassuring manner.
- Do not expect child to follow instructions.
- Watch to see if seizure generalizes.

After the Seizure
- Stay with child and reassure until fully conscious.

Call Emergency Medical Services If:
- Child stops breathing.
- There is evidence of injury or child has diabetes or is pregnant.
- Seizure lasts for more than 5 minutes (unless duration of seizure is typically longer than 5 minutes) and written medical order is present.
- Status epilepticus occurs.
- Pupils are not equal after seizure.
- Child vomits continuously 30 minutes after seizure has ended (sign of possible acute problem).
- Child cannot be awakened and is unresponsive to pain after seizure has ended.
- Seizure occurs in water.
- This is child's first seizure.

Modified from *Seizure recognition and first aid,* 2001, Epilepsy Foundation, www.epilepsyfoundation.org.
EMS, Emergency medical services.

medication regularly and for as long as required. In general antiepileptic medications are continued until the child has been seizure free for 2 years (Johnston and Smith, 2007). The medication is then slowly tapered over a period of weeks to avoid the possibility of precipitating a seizure. It is sometimes easy to skip doses or omit them for a variety of reasons, especially when the child is free of seizures most of the time. This is particularly so when the child is older and assumes responsibility for his or her medication. The seizure threshold may be lowered during any illness but particularly with fever. Therefore parents should be aware that, if their child has an illness, he or she is at increased risk for seizures. They should contact their health care provider if the child misses medications during an illness because of vomiting.

Rectal preparations of some antiepileptic medications are highly effective when a child is unable to take oral medications because of repeated vomiting, gastrointestinal surgery, or status epilepticus. Parents can learn to administer rectal antiepileptic medication for home treatment. Buccal midazolam or rectal diazepam is a useful adjunctive home treatment for children at risk for prolonged seizures or clusters of seizures and can minimize the need for hospitalization while enhancing parental confidence.

⬥ MEDICATION ALERT

Children taking phenobarbital or phenytoin should receive adequate vitamin D and folic acid because deficiencies of both have been associated with these drugs. Phenytoin should not be taken with milk.

Nurses should educate the child and parents about the possible adverse reactions to the medications used to treat seizures. Parents should understand the common side effects and be encouraged to report their observations to their health care provider. They should understand that the child needs periodic physical assessment and laboratory studies. Possible adverse effects on the hematopoietic system, liver, and kidneys may be reflected in symptoms such as fever, sore throat, enlarged lymph nodes, jaundice, and bleeding (e.g., easy bruising, petechiae, ecchymoses, epistaxis). A common factor in status epilepticus is inadequate blood levels of antiepileptic drugs.

Although children with epilepsy are at increased risk for injury, few limitations should be placed on activities. The degree to which activities are restricted is individualized for each child and depends on the type, frequency, and severity of the seizures; the child's response to therapy; and the length of time the seizures have been controlled. To prevent head injuries children should always wear appropriate safety devices such as helmets and avoid activities involving heights. Although bike riding is safe for most children, children with frequent seizures and impairment of consciousness should avoid it. Skating, in-line skating, and skateboarding should be restricted only in children with frequent seizures. Helmets must be worn while participating in these activities.

Children with epilepsy are at higher risk for submersion injury than children without epilepsy. Young children should never be left alone in the bathtub, even for a few seconds. Older children and adolescents should be encouraged to use a shower and reminded not to lock the bathroom door when showering. They should never swim unsupervised.

Because the child is encouraged to attend school, camp, and other normal activities, the school nurse and teachers should be made aware of his or her condition and therapy. They can help ensure regularity of medication administration and provision of any

special care the child might need. Teachers, child care providers, camp counselors, youth organization leaders, coaches, and other adults who assume responsibility for children should be instructed regarding care of the child during a seizure so they can act calmly for the child's welfare and influence the attitude of her or his peers.

Triggering Factors. Careful and detailed documentation of seizures over time may indicate a pattern. In the general population as many as 90% of individuals with epilepsy can recognize at least one trigger for their seizures (Haut and Lipton, 2009). When this occurs, the child, nurse, or responsible adult can intervene to make changes in the lifestyle or environment that may prevent seizures or decrease their frequency. Often the necessary changes are simple but can make an enormous difference in the lives of the child and family.

The most common factors that may trigger seizures in children include emotional stress, sleep deprivation, fatigue, and fever, and illness (Nakken, Solaas, Kjeldsen, et al., 2005). Other precipitating factors include flickering lights, menstrual cycle, and alcohol (Haut and Lipton, 2009). Some individuals have pattern- or photo-sensitive epilepsy (i.e., seizures precipitated by changes in dark-light patterns such as those that occur with a flash on a camera, automobile headlights, reflections of light on snow or water, or rotating blades on a fan). Most of these individuals have absence, myoclonic, or generalized tonic-clonic seizures. Some children have seizures while playing video games. Although the actual incidence of video game–induced epilepsy is unknown, it most commonly affects children between the ages of 9 and 15 years (Shoja, Tubbs, Malekian, et al., 2007). These children are sensitive to intermittent photic stimulation, usually more than three flashes per second, that can trigger an epileptic episode (Shoja, Tubbs, Malekian, et al., 2007). The prognosis for pattern- or photo-epilepsy is good. Prevention techniques such as keeping a distance greater than 2 m from the television or computer screen, using a smaller screen, and taking frequent breaks can reduce the incidence (Shoja, Tubbs, Malekian, et al., 2007).

Febrile Seizures

Febrile seizures are one of the most common neurologic conditions of childhood, affecting approximately 2% to 5% of children between the ages of 6 and 60 months (Steering Committee on Quality Improvement and Management, Subcommittee on Febrile Seizures AAP, 2008). They are classified as simple or complex. Simple febrile seizures occur in children between the ages of 6 months and 5 years with no preexisting neurologic abnormality and consist of a general tonic-clonic seizure that occurs with a fever (>38.0° C) and resolves within 15 minutes with a return to alert mental status after the seizure and with no further seizure occurring within a 24-hour period (Hampers and Spina, 2011). On the other hand, complex febrile seizures can occur in children of any age usually with a previous neurologic impairment and consist of a prolonged seizure lasting more than 15 minutes that can recur within 24 hours and result in neurologic deficits after the seizure (Fetveit, 2008). Most febrile seizures occur between 6 months and 5 years of age, with the peak incidence occurring at 18 months of age (Østergaard, 2009).

The cause of febrile seizures is still uncertain. Risk factors for simple febrile seizures include viral infections and a family history of febrile seizures (Fetveit, 2008). Associations with chromosome mutations, premature birth, and developmental delay have been evaluated but have not demonstrated any conclusive evidence (Fetveit, 2008). Most febrile seizures have stopped by the time the child is taken to a medical facility and require no treatment. However, if the seizure continues, treatment consists of controlling it with IV or rectal diazepam and reducing the temperature with acetaminophen or ibuprofen (Hampers and Spina, 2011). Antiepileptic prophylaxis usually is not indicated. Antipyretic therapy may lower the child's temperature and provide symptomatic relief but will not prevent a seizure (Steering Committee on Quality Improvement and Management, Subcommittee on Febrile Seizures AAP, 2008). Tepid sponge baths are not recommended for several reasons: they are ineffective in significantly lowering the temperature, the shivering effect further increases metabolic output, and cooling causes discomfort to the child. Parental education and emotional support are important interventions, and information may need to be repeated, depending on the parents' anxiety and education level. Parents need reassurance regarding the benign nature of simple febrile seizures. Several large studies show no difference in neurologic deficits, cognitive functioning, or memory impairments in children with simple or complex febrile seizures compared with population control participants (Fetveit, 2008).

Long-term antiepileptic therapy is usually not required for children with simple febrile seizures. These children have only a 1% risk of developing epilepsy, but children with a complex febrile seizure along with a preexisting neurologic abnormality and a family history of afebrile seizure have a 10% risk of developing epilepsy (Hampers and Spina, 2011).

! NURSING ALERT

If a febrile seizure lasts more than 5 minutes, parents should seek medical attention right away. They should call for emergency assistance (911) and not place the child who is actively having a seizure in the car.

CEREBRAL MALFORMATIONS

Cranial Deformities

In a normal newborn the cranial sutures are separated by membranous seams several millimeters wide. Up to 2 days after birth the cranial bones are highly mobile, which allows them to mold and slide over one another, adjusting the circumference of the head to accommodate to the changing shape and character of the birth canal. The principal sutures in the infant's skull are the sagittal, coronal, and lambdoidal sutures; and the major soft areas at the juncture of these sutures are the anterior and posterior fontanels (see Fig. 13-1).

After birth, growth of the skull bones occurs in a direction perpendicular to the line of the suture, and normal closure occurs in a regular and predictable order. Although there are wide variations in the age at which closure takes place in individual children, normally all sutures and fontanels are ossified by the following ages:

Eight weeks—Posterior fontanel closed
Six months—Fibrous union of suture lines and interlocking of serrated edges
Eighteen months—Anterior fontanel closed
After 12 years—Sutures unable to be separated by increased ICP
Solid union of all sutures is not completed until late childhood. Craniosynostosis (i.e., closure of a suture before the expected time) inhibits the perpendicular growth. Because normal increase in brain volume requires expansion, the skull is forced to grow in a direction *parallel* to the fused suture. This alteration in skull growth always produces a distortion of the head shape when the underlying brain growth is normal. A small head with a closed and normal shape is a result of deficient brain growth; the suture closure is secondary to this brain growth failure. Failure of brain growth is not secondary to suture closure.

Various types of cranial deformities are encountered in early infancy. These include an enlarged head with frontal protrusion (bossing; characteristic of hydrocephalus), parietal bossing that is seen in chronic subdural hematoma, a small head, and a variety of skull deformities. Some occur during prenatal development; in others head circumference is usually within normal limits at birth, and the deviation from normal development becomes apparent with advancing age.

Prognosis. The majority of infants with craniosynostosis have normal brain development. The exceptions are those with genetic disorders that involve brain pathologic conditions.

■ CARE MANAGEMENT

Nursing care of families in which there is a child with a cranial defect involves identifying children with deformities and referring them for evaluation. Because no therapy is available for children with microcephaly, nursing care is directed toward helping parents adjust to caring for a child with brain damage (see Chapter 37).

Infants who benefit from surgery require special emphasis on observation for signs of anemia because of the large blood loss during surgery (see Family Centered-Care box). Nursing care includes observation for signs of hemorrhage, infection, pain, and swelling and parental education for suture care and safety. Surgical sutures should remain dry and intact. Parents need to observe for any signs of redness, drainage, or swelling and report any temperature greater than 38.4°C (101°F).

Hydrocephalus

Hydrocephalus is a condition caused by an imbalance in the production and absorption of CSF in the ventricular system. When production is greater than absorption, CSF accumulates within the ventricular system, usually under increased pressure, producing passive dilation of the ventricles.

Pathophysiology

The causes of hydrocephalus are varied, but the result is either (1) impaired absorption of CSF fluid within the subarachnoid space, obliteration of the subarachnoid cisterns, or malfunction of the arachnoid villi (nonobstructive or communicating hydrocephalus); or (2) obstruction to the flow of CSF through the ventricular system (obstructive or noncommunicating hydrocephalus) (Kinsman and Johnston, 2011). Any imbalance of secretion and absorption causes an increased accumulation of CSF in the ventricles, which become dilated (ventriculomegaly) and compress the brain substance against the surrounding rigid bony cranium. When this occurs before fusion of the cranial sutures, it causes enlargement of the skull and dilation of the ventricles (Fig. 45-7). In children younger than 10 to 12 years

---

👪 FAMILY-CENTERED CARE

Blood Donation

Parents may wish to provide a compatible blood donor for their infant undergoing a planned surgical correction for craniosynostosis. Nurses need to inform and guide parents through the blood bank procedure.

Early surgical management of craniosynostosis in children ages 3 to 9 months allows proper expansion of the brain and the creation of an acceptable appearance (Ursitti, Fadda, Papetti, et al., 2011). Parents require special support and education during this time, especially from the health care team.

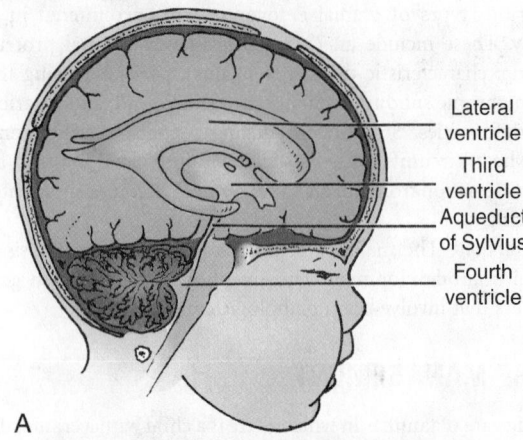

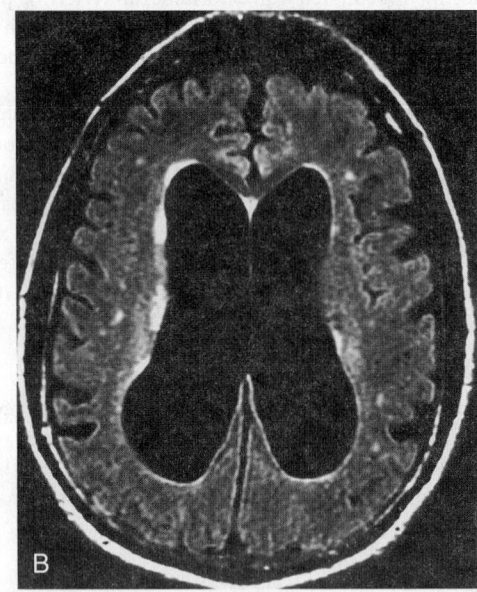

Lateral ventricle

Third ventricle

Aqueduct of Sylvius

Fourth ventricle

A

B

FIG 45-7 Hydrocephalus: a block in flow of cerebrospinal fluid (CSF). **A,** Patent CSF circulation. **B,** Normal-pressure hydrocephalus. (*B* From Grossman RI, Yousem DM: *Neuroradiology,* ed 2, St Louis, 2003.)

of age, partially closed suture lines, especially the sagittal suture, may become diastatic or opened. After 12 years of age the sutures are fused and will not open.

Most cases of noncommunicating hydrocephalus are a result of developmental malformations. Although the defect usually is apparent in early infancy, it may become evident at any time from the prenatal period to late childhood or early adulthood. Other causes include neoplasms, infections, and trauma. An obstruction to the normal flow can occur at any point in the CSF pathway to produce increased pressure and dilation of the pathways proximal to the site of obstruction.

Developmental defects (e.g., Arnold-Chiari malformations, aqueduct stenosis, aqueduct gliosis, and atresia of the foramina of Luschka and Magendie [Dandy-Walker syndrome]) account for most cases of hydrocephalus from birth to 2 years of age. It is so often associated with myelomeningocele that all such infants should be observed for its development. In the remainder of cases there is a history of intrauterine infection, hemorrhage, and neonatal meningoencephalitis. In older children hydrocephalus is most often a result of intracranial masses, intracranial infections, hemorrhage,

preexisting developmental defects (e.g., aqueduct stenosis, Arnold-Chiari malformation), or trauma.

Clinical Manifestations

The factors that influence the clinical picture in hydrocephalus are the time of onset, acuity of onset, and associated structural malformations. In infancy before closure of the cranial sutures, head enlargement is the predominant sign; but in older infants and children the lesions responsible for hydrocephalus produce other neurologic signs through pressure on adjacent structures before causing CSF obstruction (Box 45-10).

In infants with hydrocephalus the head grows at an abnormal rate; fontanels are bulging and nonpulsatile; scalp veins are dilated, especially when the infant cries; and skull bones are thin with separated sutures, causing a cracked-pot sound (Macewen sign) when palpated. In severe cases infants display frontal protrusion (frontal bossing), eyes depressed and rotated downward (setting-sun sign), and sluggish pupils. The signs and symptoms in early-to-late childhood are caused by increased ICP, and specific manifestations are related to the focal lesion. Most commonly resulting from posterior fossa neoplasms and aqueduct stenosis, the clinical manifestations are primarily those associated with space-occupying lesions (e.g., headaches on awakening with improvement after emesis or being in an upright position, strabismus, ataxia).

Diagnostic Evaluation

Hydrocephalus in infants is based on head circumference that crosses at least one percentile line on the head measurement chart within 2 to 4 weeks. In evaluation of a preterm infant specially adapted head circumference charts are consulted to distinguish abnormal head growth from normal rapid head growth. The primary diagnostic tools to detect hydrocephalus in older infants and children are CT and MRI. Diagnostic evaluation of children who have symptoms of hydrocephalus after infancy is similar to that used in those with suspected intracranial tumor. In neonates echoencephalography is useful in comparing the ratio of lateral ventricle to cortex.

Therapeutic Management

The treatment of hydrocephalus is directed toward relief of the hydrocephalus, treatment of the cause, treatment of associated complications, and management of problems related to the effect of the disorder on psychomotor development. With few exceptions the treatment is surgical. This is accomplished by direct removal of an obstruction (e.g., a tumor) or placement of a shunt that provides primary drainage of the CSF from the ventricles to an extracranial compartment, usually the peritoneum (ventriculoperitoneal [VP] shunt) (Fig. 45-8).

Most shunt systems consist of a ventricular catheter, a flush pump, a unidirectional flow valve, and a distal catheter. In all models the valves are designed to open at a predetermined intraventricular pressure and close when the pressure falls below that level, thus preventing backflow of secretions.

The major complications of VP shunts are malfunction and infection. All shunts are subject to mechanical difficulties such as kinking, plugging, or separation or migration of the tubing. Malfunction is most often caused by mechanical obstruction either within the ventricles from particulate matter (tissue or exudate) or at the distal end from thrombosis or displacement as a result of growth. Revisions are needed when signs of malfunction appear. The child with a shunt obstruction is often first seen in an emergency

BOX 45-10   CLINICAL MANIFESTATIONS OF HYDROCEPHALUS

Infancy (Early)
- Abnormally rapid head growth
- Bulging fontanels (especially anterior) sometimes without head enlargement:
  - Tense
  - Nonpulsatile
- Dilated scalp veins
- Separated sutures
- Macewen sign (cracked-pot sound on percussion)
- Thinning of skull bones

Infancy (Later)
- Frontal enlargement, or bossing
- Depressed eyes
- Setting-sun sign (sclera visible above iris)
- Pupils sluggish with unequal response to light

Infancy (General)
- Irritability
- Lethargy
- Infant cries when picked up or rocked and quiets when allowed to lie still
- Early infantile reflex acts may persist
- Normally expected responses fail to appear
- May display:
  - Change in LOC
  - Opisthotonos (often extreme)
  - Lower-extremity spasticity
  - Vomiting
- Advanced cases:
  - Difficulty in sucking and feeding
  - Shrill, brief, high-pitched cry
  - Cardiopulmonary embarrassment

Childhood
- Headache on awakening; improvement after emesis or upright posture
- Papilledema
- Strabismus
- Extrapyramidal tract signs (e.g., ataxia)
- Irritability
- Lethargy
- Apathy
- Confusion
- Incoherence
- Vomiting

LOC, Level of consciousness.

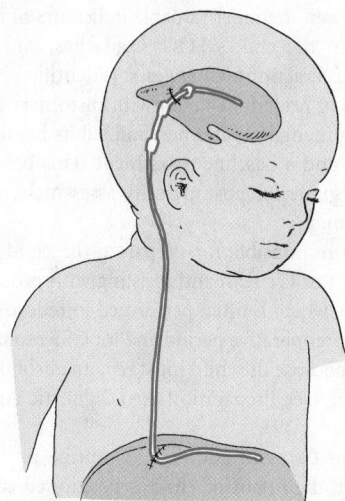

FIG 45-8 Ventriculoperitoneal shunt. The catheter is threaded beneath the skin.

administered intravenously or intrathecally for a minimum of 7 to 10 days. A persistent infection requires removal of the shunt until the infection is controlled. External ventricular drainage (EVD) is used until CSF is sterile. The EVD allows for removal of CSF through a tube that is placed in the child's ventricle and flows by gravity into a collection device.

An alternative to shunt placement is the endoscopic third ventriculostomy in children with noncommunicating hydrocephalus. In this procedure a small opening is made in the floor of the third ventricle that allows the CSF to flow freely through the previously blocked ventricle. Complications include CSF leak, intraventricular hemorrhage, meningitis, cranial nerve injury, obstruction, and hypothalamic injury (Hader, Walker, Myles, et al., 2008).

Prognosis. The prognosis for children with treated hydrocephalus depends largely on the rate at which it develops, the duration of increased ICP, the frequency of complications, and the cause of the hydrocephalus. For example, children with malignant tumors may have a high mortality rate regardless of other complicating factors.

Surgically treated hydrocephalus with continued neurosurgical and medical management has a survival rate of about 80%, with the highest incidence of mortality occurring within the first year of treatment (Paulsen, Lundar, and Lindegaard, 2010). Of the surviving children, approximately 60% were reported to have normal intellectual ability, but only 30% had an IQ above 90 (Gupta, Park, Solomon, et al., 2007). Although most children with a history of hydrocephalus are good-natured and friendly, some can have aggressive or delinquent behavior and may be depressed (Gupta, Park, Solomon, et al., 2007; Kinsman and Johnston, 2011).

CARE MANAGEMENT

An infant with diagnosed or suspected hydrocephalus is observed carefully for signs of increasing ventricular size and increasing ICP. In infants the head is measured daily at the largest point, the occipitofrontal circumference (see Head Circumference, Chapter 29, for technique). Fontanels and suture lines are palpated for size, signs of bulging, tenseness, and separation. Irritability, lethargy, or seizure activity and altered vital signs and feeding behavior may indicate an advancing pathologic condition.

department with clinical manifestations of increased ICP, frequently accompanied by worsening neurologic status.

The most serious complication, shunt infection, can occur at any time, but the period of greatest risk is 1 to 2 months after placement. The infection is generally a result of intercurrent infections at the time of shunt placement. Infections include septicemia, bacterial endocarditis, wound infection, shunt nephritis, meningitis, and ventriculitis. Meningitis and ventriculitis are of greatest concern because any complicating CNS infection is a significant predictor of poor intellectual outcome. Infection is treated with antibiotics

In older children the most valuable indicators of increasing ICP are alterations in the child's LOC, headaches, and changes with environmental interactions. Changes are identified by observation and comparison of present behavior with customary behavior, sleep patterns, developmental capabilities, and habits obtained through a detailed history and a baseline assessment. This baseline information serves as a guide for postoperative assessment and evaluation of shunt function.

The nurse is responsible for preparing the child for diagnostic tests such as MRI or CT scan and assisting with procedures such as a ventricular tap, which is often performed to relieve excessive pressure during the preoperative period and for CSF examination. Sedation is required because the child must remain absolutely still during diagnostic testing (see Preparation for Diagnostic and Therapeutic Procedures, Chapter 39).

Postoperative Care. In addition to routine postoperative care and observation, the infant or child is positioned carefully on the unoperated side to prevent pressure on the shunt valve. She or he is kept flat to avoid complications resulting from too-rapid reduction of intracranial fluid. The surgeon indicates the position to be maintained and the extent of activity allowed. Pain management can be achieved with acetaminophen with or without codeine for mild-to-moderate pain and opioids for severe pain (see Pain Management, Chapter 30).

Observation is continued for signs of increased ICP, which indicates obstruction of the shunt. Neurologic assessment includes evaluation of pupillary dilation (pressure causes compression or stretching of the oculomotor nerve, producing dilation on the same side as the pressure) and blood pressure (hypoxia to the brainstem causes variability in these vital signs). If there is increased ICP, the surgeon prescribes elevation of the head of the bed and allows the child to sit up to enhance gravity flow through the shunt.

> **! NURSING ALERT**
>
> Arbitrary pumping of the shunt may cause obstruction or other problems and should not be performed unless indicated by a neurosurgeon.

Because infection is the greatest hazard of the postoperative period, nurses are continually on the alert for the usual manifestations of CSF infection such as elevated temperature, poor feeding, vomiting, decreased responsiveness, and seizure activity. There may be signs of local inflammation at the operative sites and along the shunt tract. The child is also observed for abdominal distention because CSF may cause peritonitis or a postoperative ileus as a complication of distal catheter placement. Antibiotics are administered by the IV route as ordered, and the nurse may also need to assist with intraventricular instillation. The incision site is inspected for leakage, and any suspected drainage is tested for glucose, an indication of CSF.

Family Support. Specific needs and concerns of parents during periods of hospitalization are related to the reason for the child's hospitalization (shunt revision, infection, diagnosis) and the diagnostic and surgical procedures to which the child is subjected. Parents may have little understanding of anatomy; therefore they need further exploration and reinforcement of information that was given to them by the physician and neurosurgeon, including information about what to expect. They are especially frightened of any procedure that involves the brain, and the fear of intellectual disability or brain damage is real and pervasive. Nurses can calm their anxiety with explanations of the rationale underlying the various nursing and medical activities such as positioning or testing and by simply being available and willing to listen to their concerns.

To prepare for the child's discharge and home care, the parents are instructed on how to recognize signs that indicate shunt malfunction or infection. Active children may have injuries such as a fall that can damage the shunt, and the tubing may pull out of the distal insertion site or become disconnected during normal growth. Contact sports should be avoided, and a helmet should be worn when outside play is vigorous.

The management of hydrocephalus in a child is a demanding task for both family and health care providers, and helping a family cope with the child's difficulties is an important nursing responsibility. Children with hydrocephalus have lifelong special health care needs and require evaluation on a regular basis. The overall aim is to establish realistic goals and an appropriate educational program that will help the child to achieve his or her optimal potential.

Families can be referred to community agencies for support and guidance. The National Hydrocephalus Foundation* and the Hydrocephalus Association† provide information on the condition for families and help interested groups establish local organizations.

---

*12413 Centralia Road, Lakewood, CA 90715-1653, 562-924-6666, 888-857-3434, www.nhfonline.org.
†4340 East West Highway, Suite 905, Bethesda, MD 20814, 301-202-3811, 888-598-3789, www.hydroassoc.org.

KEY POINTS

- LOC is the most important indicator of neurologic health; altered levels include full consciousness, confusion, disorientation, lethargy, obtundation, stupor, coma, and a persistent vegetative state.

- Complete neurologic examination includes LOC; posture; motor, sensory, cranial nerve, and reflex testing; and vital signs.

- Nursing care of the unconscious child focuses on ensuring respiratory management; performing neurologic assessment; monitoring ICP; supplying adequate nutrition and hydration; providing drug therapy; promoting elimination, hygienic care, proper positioning, exercise, and stimulation; and providing family support.

- Fractures resulting from head injuries may be classified as linear, depressed, comminuted, basilar, open, and growing.

- Primary head injury involves features that occur at the time of trauma, including fractured skull, contusions, intracranial hematoma, and diffuse injury. Secondary complications include hypoxic brain damage, increased ICP, infection, cerebral edema, and posttraumatic syndromes.

- The young child's response to head injury is different because of the following features: larger head size, expandable skull, larger blood volume to the brain, and small subdural spaces.

- Problems resulting from submersion injury include hypoxia, asphyxiation, aspiration, and hypothermia.

- Nursing care of the child with a brain tumor includes observing for signs and symptoms related to the tumor, preparing the child and family for diagnostic tests and operative procedures, preventing postoperative complications, planning for discharge, and promoting a return to optimal health.

- Nursing care of the child with meningitis includes administering antibiotics, taking isolation precautions, removing environmental stimuli, ensuring correct positioning, monitoring vital signs, administering IV therapy, promoting adequate fluid and nutritional status, and providing supportive care to the family.

- Routine immunization of infants with Hib and pneumococcal conjugate vaccines has reduced the incidence of bacterial meningitis.

- Encephalitis may result from direct invasion of the CNS by a virus or from involvement of the CNS after viral disease.

- A seizure is a symptom of an underlying pathologic condition and may be manifested by sensory-hallucinatory phenomena, motor effects, sensorimotor effects, or loss of consciousness.

- Partial seizures are categorized as simple (without associated impairment of consciousness) or complex (with impaired consciousness); both types may become generalized.

- Generalized seizures are categorized as tonic, clonic, tonic-clonic, absence, atonic, and myoclonic.

- Long-term care of a child with recurrent seizure disorders includes physical care and education regarding the importance of drug therapy and problems related to emotional aspects of the disorder.

- Febrile seizures are the most common type of childhood seizure.

- Many cranial deformities are amenable to surgical correction.

- Hydrocephalus is a symptom of underlying brain pathologic condition demonstrated by impaired absorption of CSF or obstruction to the flow of CSF within the ventricles.

- Therapy for hydrocephalus involves relief of the hydrocephalus, treatment of the underlying brain disorder if possible, prevention or treatment of complications, and management of problems related to development.

REFERENCES

Abbasi M, Mohammadi E, Rezayi S: Effect of a regular family visiting program as an affective, auditory, and tactile stimulation on the consciousness level of comatose patients with a head injury, *Jpn J Nurs Sci* 6:21–26, 2009.

Ashwal S, Serna-Fonseca T: Brain deaths in infants and children, *Crit Care Nurse* 26(2):117–128, 2006.

Badjatia N: Hyperthermia and fever control in brain injury, *Crit Care Med* 37(7 suppl): S250–S255, 2009.

Berg AT: Risk of recurrence after a first unprovoked seizure, *Epilepsia* 49(suppl 1): 13–18, 2008.

Blaney SM, Haas-Kogan D, Young Poussaint T, et al: Gliomas, ependymomas, and other nonembryonal tumors of the central nervous system. In Pizzo PA, Poplack DG, editors: *Principles and practice of pediatric oncology*, ed 6, Philadelphia, 2011, Lippincott Williams & Wilkins.

Blanton JD, Palmer D, Rupprecht CE: Rabies surveillance in the United States during 2009, *J Am Vet Med Assoc* 237(6):646–657, 2010.

Blinman TA, Houseknecht E, Snyder C, et al: Postconcussive symptoms in hospitalized pediatric patients after mild traumatic brain injury, *J Pediatr Surg* 44:1223–1228, 2009.

Bonnier C, Marique P, Van Hout A, et al: Neurodevelopmental outcome after severe traumatic brain injury in very young children, *J Child Neurol* 22:519–529, 2007.

Boran BO, Boran P, Barut N, et al: Evaluation of mild head injury in a pediatric population, *Pediatr Neurosurg* 42:203–207, 2006.

Brodeur GM, Hogarty MD, Mosse YP, et al: Neuroblastoma. In Pizzo PA, Poplack DG, editors: *Principles and practice of pediatric oncology*, ed 6, Philadelphia, 2011, Lippincott Williams & Wilkins.

Carey RG, Balistreri WF: Mitochondrial hepatopathies. In Kliegman RM, Stanton BF, St Geme JW, et al, editors: *Nelson textbook of*

pediatrics, ed 19, Philadelphia, 2011, Saunders.

Case ME: Accidental traumatic head injury in infants and young children, *Brain Pathol* 18:583–589, 2008.

Chandran A, Herbert H, Misurski D, et al: Long-term sequelae of childhood bacterial meningitis: an underappreciated problem, *Pediatr Infect Dis J* 30(1):3–6, 2011.

Christie RJ: Therapeutic positioning of the multiply-injured trauma patient in ICU, *Br J Nurs* 17(10):638–642, 2008.

Curatolo P, Moavero R, Lo Castro A, et al: Pharmacotherapy of idiopathic generalized epilepsies, *Expert Opin Pharmacother* 10(1):5–17, 2009.

Erlichman DB, Blumfield E, Rajpathak S, et al: Association between linear skull fractures and intracranial hemorrhage in children with minor head trauma, *Pediatr Radiol* 40:1375–1379, 2010.

Elliott RE, Rodgers SD, Bassani L, et al: Vagus nerve stimulation for children with treatment resistant epilepsy, *J Neurosurg Pediatr* 7:491–500, 2011.

Faul M, Xu L, Wald MM, et al: *Traumatic brain injury in the United States*, 2010, Centers for Disease Control and Prevention, www.cdc.gov/traumaticbraininjury/pdf/tbi_blue_book_age.pdf.

Feigin RD, Cutrer WB: Bacterial meningitis beyond the neonatal period. In Feigin RD, Cherry JD, Demmler-Harrison GJ, et al, editors: *Textbook of pediatric infectious diseases*, ed 6, Philadelphia, 2009, Saunders.

Fetveit A: Assessment of febrile seizures in children, *Eur J Pediatr* 167:17–27, 2008.

Freeman JM, Kossoff EH, Hartman AL: The ketogenic diet: one decade later, *Pediatrics* 119(3):535–543, 2007.

Friedman MJ, Ghazala SQ: Seizures in children, *Pediatr Clin North Am* 53:257–277, 2006.

Granoff DM, Gilsdorf, JR: *Neisseria* meningitis. In Kliegman RM, Stanton BF, St Geme JW,

et al, editors: *Nelson textbook of pediatrics*, ed 19, Philadelphia, 2011, Saunders.

Gupta N, Park J, Solomon C, et al: Long-term outcomes in patients with treated childhood hydrocephalus, *J Neurosurg* 106:334–339, 2007.

Hader WJ, Walker RL, Myles ST, et al: Complications of endoscopic third ventriculostomy in previously shunted patients, *Neurosurgery* 63:168–175, 2008.

Hampers LC, Spina LA: Evaluation and management of pediatric febrile seizures in the emergency department, *Emerg Med Clin North Am* 29(1):83–93, 2011.

Hartman AL, Vining EP: Clinical aspects of the ketogenic diet, *Epilepsia* 48(1):31–42, 2007.

Haut SR, Lipton RB: Predicting seizures: a behavioral approach, *Neurol Clin* 27:925–940, 2009.

Hon KE, Leung AK: Childhood accidents: injuries and poisoning, *Adv Pediatr* 57:33–62, 2010.

Howlader N, Noone AM, Krapcho M, et al: *SEER cancer statistics review 1975–2008*, 2011, National Cancer Institute, seer.cancer.gov/csr/1975_2008/.

Huff JS, Fountain NB: Pathophysiology and definitions of seizures and status epilepticus, *Emerg Med Clin North Am* 29(1):1–13, 2011.

James SH, Kimberlin DW, Whitley RJ: Antiviral therapy for herpesvirus central nervous system infections, *Antiviral Res* 83:207–213, 2009.

Joffe AR: Lumbar puncture and brain herniation in acute bacterial meningitis: a review, *J Intensive Care Med* 22(4):194–207, 2007.

Johnston A, Smith P: Sudden unexpected death in epilepsy, *Expert Rev Neurother* 7(12):1751–1761, 2007.

Kinsman SL, Johnston MV: Hydrocephalus. In Kliegman RM, Stanton BF, St Geme JW, et al, editors: *Nelson textbook of pediatrics*, ed 19, Philadelphia, 2011, Saunders.

Landry GL: Head and neck injuries. In Kliegman RM, Stanton BF, St Geme JW, et al, editors:

Nelson textbook of pediatrics, ed 19, Philadelphia, 2011, Saunders.

Lee LK: Controversies in the sequelae of pediatric mild traumatic brain injury, *Pediatr Emerg Care* 23:580–583, 2007.

Lin AL, Safdieh JE: The evaluation and management of bacterial meningitis, current practice and emerging developments, *Neurologist* 16(3):143–151, 2010.

Logan SA, MacMahon E: Viral meningitis, *BMJ* 336:36–40, 2008.

Lozsadi DA, Von Oertzen J, Cock HR: Epilepsy: recent advances, *J Neurol* 257:1946–1951, 2010.

Machata AM, Willschke H, Kabon B, et al: Propofol-based sedation regimen for infants and children undergoing ambulatory magnetic resonance imaging, *Br J Anaesth* 101(2):239–243, 2008.

Manning SE, Rupprecht CE, Fishbein D, et al: CDC, *Human rabies prevention—United States 2008*, Centers for Disease Control, *MMWR* 57(No. RR-3), 2008, www.cdc.gov/mmwr/preview/mmwrhtml/rr57e507a1.htm.

Mason KP: The pediatric sedation service: who is appropriate to sedate, which medications should I use, who should prescribe the drugs, how do I bill, *Pediatr Radiol* 38(suppl):S218–S224, 2008.

Mathur M, Peterson L, Stadtier M, et al: Variability in pediatric brain death determination and documentation in Southern California, *Pediatrics* 121(5):988–993, 2008.

Meehan WP, Mannix R: Pediatric concussions in United States Emergency Departments in the Years 2002 to 2006, *J Pediatr* 157(6):889–893, 2010.

Merchant TE, Pollack IF, Loeffler JS: Brain tumors across the age spectrum: biology, therapy and late effects, *Semin Radiat Oncol* 20(1):58–66, 2010.

Mikati MA: Treatment of seizures and epilepsy. In Kliegman RM, Stanton BF, St Geme JW, et al, editors: *Nelson textbook of pediatrics*, ed 19, Philadelphia, 2011, Saunders.

Mullassery D, Dominici D, Jesudason EC, et al: Neuroblastoma: contemporary management, *Arch Dis Child Educ Pract Ed* 94:177–185, 2009.

Nakken KO, Solaas MH, Kjeldsen MJ, et al: Which seizure-precipitating factors do patients with epilepsy most frequently report? *Epilepsy Behav* 6:85–89, 2005.

Nasrullah M, Muazzam S: Drowning mortality in the United States 1999–2006, *J Commun Health* 36:69–75, 2011.

Nei M, Bagla R: Seizure-related injury and death, *Curr Neurol Neurosci Rep* 7:335–341, 2007.

Orliaguet G, Meyer PG, Baugnon T: Management of critically ill children with traumatic brain injury, *Pediatr Anesth* 18:455–461, 2008.

Østergaard JR: Febrile seizures, *Acta Paediatr* 98:771–773, 2009.

Park JR, Eggert A, Caron H: Neuroblastoma: biology, prognosis, and treatment, *Hematol Oncol Clin North Am* 24(1):65–86, 2010.

Paulsen AH, Lundar T, Lindegaard KF: Twenty-year outcome in young adults with childhood hydrocephalus: assessment of surgical outcome, work participation, and health-related quality of life, *J Neurosurg Pediatr* 6:527–535, 2010.

Perheentupa U, Kinnunen I, Grénman R, et al: Management and outcome of pediatric skull base fractures, *Int J Pediatr Otorhinolaryngol* 74:1245–1250, 2010.

Prober CG, Dyner L: Acute bacterial meningitis beyond the neonatal period. In Kliegman RM, Stanton BF, St Geme JW, et al, editors: *Nelson textbook of pediatrics*, ed 19, Philadelphia, 2011a, Saunders

Prober CG, Dyner L: Viral meningoencephalitis. In Kliegman RM, Stanton BF, St Geme JW, et al, editors: *Nelson textbook of pediatrics*, ed 19, Philadelphia, 2011b, Saunders.

Pugliese A, Beltramo T, Torre D: Reye's and Reye's-like syndromes, *Cell Biochem Funct* 26(7):741–746, 2008.

Reynolds D, Boyd M: Child life specialists and nurses working together, *Imprint* 57(1):22–25, 2010.

Rivara FP, Grossman DC: Injury control. In Kliegman RM, Stanton BF, St Geme JW, et al, editors: *Nelson textbook of pediatrics*, ed 19, Philadelphia, 2011, Saunders.

Safe Kids: Report to the nation: *Trends in unintentional childhood injury mortality and parental views on child safety, 2008*, Safe Kids Worldwide 2009, www.safekids.org/assets/docs/ourwork/research/research-report-safe-kids-week-2008.pdf.

Sankhyan N, Raju KN, Sharma S, et al: Management of raised intracranial pressure, *Indian J Pediatr* 77:1409–1416, 2010.

Schnakers C, Zasler ND: Pain assessment and management in disorders of consciousness, *Curr Opin Neurol* 20:620–626, 2007.

Sharma S, Kochar GS, Sankhyan N, et al: Approach to the child with coma, *Indian J Pediatr* 77:1279–1287, 2010.

Shaw S: Endocrine late effects in survivors of pediatric brain tumors, *J Pediatr Oncol Nurs* 26(5):295–302, 2009.

Shephard E, Quan L: Drowning and submersion injury. In Kliegman RM, Stanton BF, St Geme JW, et al, editors: *Nelson textbook of pediatrics*, ed 19, Philadelphia, 2011, Saunders.

Shoja MM, Tubbs RS, Malekian A, et al: Video game epilepsy in the twentieth century: a review, *Childs Nerv Syst* 23:265–267, 2007.

Shorvon S: The treatment of status epilepticus, *Curr Opin Neurol* 24:165–170, 2011.

Sillanpää M, Schmidt D: Prognosis of seizure recurrence after stopping antiepileptic drugs in seizure-free patients: a long term population-based study of childhood-onset epilepsy, *Epilepsy Behav* 8(4):713, 2006.

Singhi SC, Tiwari L: Management of intracranial hypertension, *Indian J Pediatr* 76:519–529, 2009.

Somand D, Meurer W: Central nervous system infections, *Emerg Med Clin North Am* 27:89–100, 2009.

Spencer S, Huh L: Outcomes of epilepsy surgery in adults and children, *Lancet Neurol* 7:525–537, 2008.

Steering Committee on Quality Improvement and Management, Subcommittee on Febrile Seizures American Academy of Pediatrics: Febrile seizures: clinical practice guideline for the long-term management of the child with simple febrile seizures, *Pediatrics* 121(6):1281–1286, 2008.

Swaine BR, Tremblay C, Platt RW, et al: Previous head injury is a risk factor for subsequent head injury in children: a longitudinal cohort study, *Pediatrics* 119(4):749–758, 2007.

Thigpen MC, Whitney CG, Messonnier NE, et al: Bacterial meningitis in the United States 1998–2007, *N Engl J Med* 364(21):2016–2025, 2011.

Truog RD, Campbell ML, Curtis JR, et al: Recommendations for end-of-life care in the intensive care unit, *Crit Care Med* 36(3):953–963, 2008.

Ursitti F, Fadda T, Papetti L, et al: Evaluation and management of nonsyndromic craniosynostosis, *Acta Paediatr* 100(9):1185–1194, 2011.

Vignes JR, Jeelani NU, Jeelani A, et al: Growing skull fracture after minor closed-head injury, *J Pediatr* 151:316–318, 2007.

Walls C: Shaken baby syndrome education: A role for nurse practitioners working with families of small children, *J Pediatr Health Care* 20(5):304–310, 2006.

Weiss J, American Academy of Pediatrics Committee on Injury, Violence, and Poison Prevention: Prevention of drowning, *Pediatrics* 126:e253–e262, 2010.

Willoughby RE Jr: Rabies. In Kliegman RM, Stanton BF, St Geme JW, et al, editors: *Nelson textbook of pediatrics*, ed 19, Philadelphia, 2011, Saunders.

Young GB: Coma, *Ann NY Acad Sci* 1157:32–47, 2009.

Endocrine Dysfunction

Marilyn J. Hockenberry

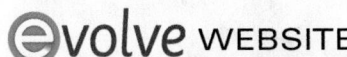 WEBSITE

http://evolve.elsevier.com/Perry/maternal

LEARNING OBJECTIVES

On completion of this chapter, the reader will be able to:

- Differentiate between the disorders caused by hypopituitary and hyperpituitary dysfunction.
- Describe the manifestations of thyroid hypofunction and hyperfunction and the management of children with the disorders.
- Distinguish between the manifestations of adrenal hypofunction and hyperfunction.

- Differentiate among the various categories of diabetes mellitus.
- Discuss the management and nursing care of the child with diabetes mellitus in the acute care setting.
- Distinguish between a hypoglycemic and a hyperglycemic reaction.
- Formulate a teaching plan for instructing the parents of a child with diabetes mellitus.

THE ENDOCRINE SYSTEM

The endocrine system consists of three components: (1) the cells, which send chemical messages by means of hormones; (2) the target cells, or end organs, which receive the chemical messages; and (3) the environment through which the chemicals are transported (blood, lymph, extracellular fluids) from the sites of synthesis to the sites of cellular action. The endocrine system controls or regulates metabolic processes governing energy production, growth, fluid and electrolyte balance, response to stress, and sexual reproduction (Baxter and Ribeiro, 2004). The pathophysiology review in Fig. 46-1 provides a summary of the principal pituitary hormones and their target organs.

Hormones

A hormone is a complex chemical substance produced and secreted into body fluids by a cell or group of cells that exerts a physiologic controlling effect on other cells (Kliegman, Stanton, St. Geme, et al., 2011). These effects may be local or distant and may affect either most cells of the body or specific "target" tissues. Hormones are released by the endocrine glands into the bloodstream, and production is regulated by a feedback mechanism. The master gland of the endocrine system is the anterior pituitary, which is in turn controlled by the hypothalamus. Some hormones, such as insulin, are regulated by other mechanisms.

DISORDERS OF PITUITARY FUNCTION

The pituitary gland is divided into two lobes—the anterior and the posterior lobe. Each lobe is responsible for different hormones. Disorders of the anterior pituitary hormones may be attributable to organic defects or have an idiopathic etiology and may occur as a single hormonal problem or in combination with other hormonal disorders. The clinical manifestations depend on the hormones involved and the age of onset. Panhypopituitarism is often defined clinically as the loss of all anterior pituitary hormones, leaving only posterior function intact (Toogood and Stewart, 2008).

> **! NURSING ALERT**
>
> Children with panhypopituitarism should wear medical identification, such as a bracelet.

Hypopituitarism

Hypopituitarism is diminished or deficient secretion of pituitary hormones. The consequences of the condition depend on the degree of dysfunction and can lead to gonadotropin deficiency with absence or regression of secondary sex characteristics; growth hormone (GH) deficiency, in which children display slowed somatic growth;

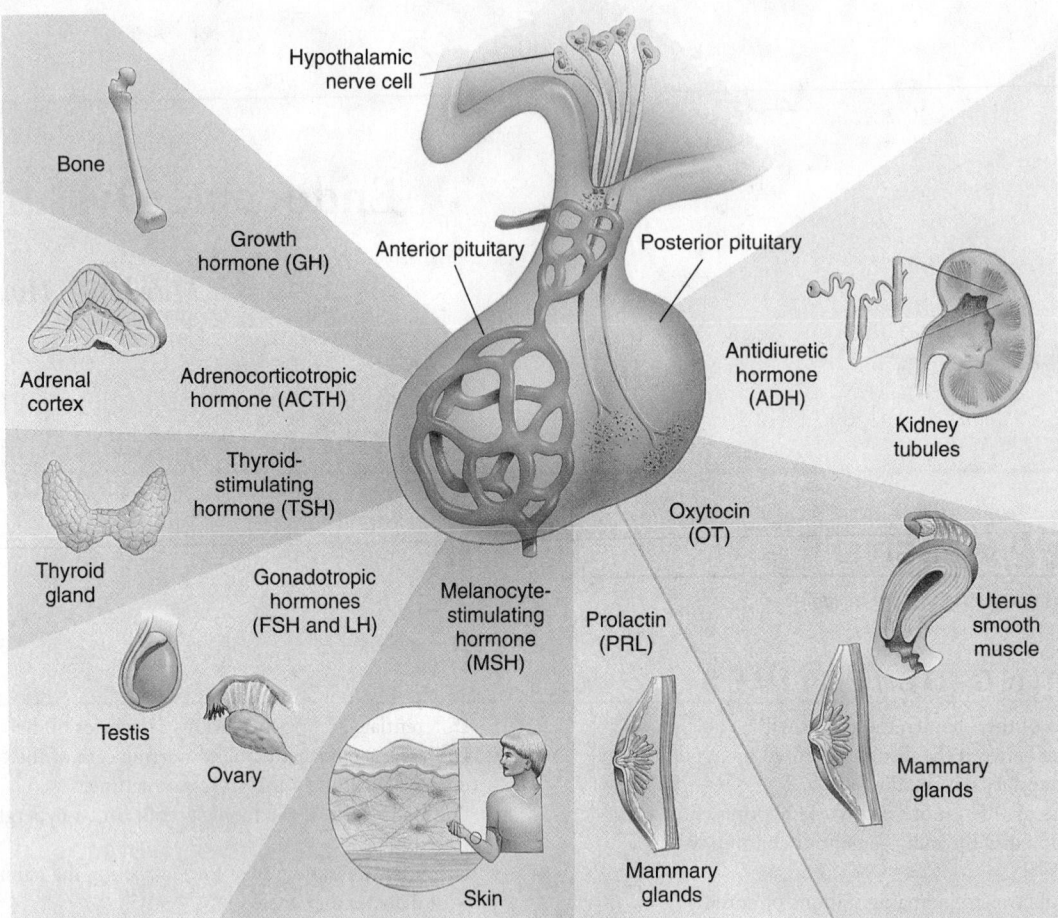

FIG 46-1 Principal anterior and posterior pituitary hormones and their target organs. *FSH,* Follicle-stimulating hormone; *LH,* luteinizing hormone. (From Patton KT, Thibodeau GA: *Anatomy and physiology,* ed 8, St Louis, 2013, Mosby.)

thyroid-stimulating hormone (TSH) deficiency, which produces hypothyroidism; and corticotropin deficiency, which results in manifestations of adrenal hypofunction. Hypopituitarism can result from any of the conditions listed in Box 46-1. The most common organic cause of pituitary undersecretion is tumors in the pituitary or hypothalamic region, especially the craniopharyngiomas. Congenital hypopituitarism can be seen in newborn infants, often as a result of birth trauma. Symptoms of hypoglycemia and seizure activity often manifest within the first 24 hours after birth (Toogood and Stewart, 2008).

Idiopathic hypopituitarism, or idiopathic pituitary growth failure, is usually related to GH deficiency, which inhibits somatic growth in all cells of the body (Miller and Zimmerman, 2004). Growth failure is defined as an absolute height of less than −2 standard deviation (SD) for age or a linear growth velocity consistently less than −1 SD for age. When this occurs without the presence of hypothyroidism, systemic disease, or malnutrition, an abnormality of the GH–insulin-like growth factor (IGF-I) axis should be considered (Richmond and Rogol, 2008). Not all children with short stature have GH deficiency. In most instances, the cause is either familial short stature or constitutional growth delay. Familial short stature refers to otherwise healthy children who have ancestors with adult height in the lower percentiles. Constitutional growth delay refers to individuals (usually boys) with delayed linear growth,

generally beginning as a toddler, and skeletal and sexual maturation that is behind that of age mates (Halac and Zimmerman, 2004; Miller and Zimmerman, 2004). Typically, these children will reach normal adult height. Often there is a history of a similar pattern of growth in one of the child's parents or other family members. The untreated child will proceed through normal changes as expected on the basis of bone age. Although treatment with GH is not usually indicated, its use has become controversial, especially in relation to parental and child requests for treatment to accelerate growth.

Clinical Manifestations

Children with hypopituitarism generally grow normally during the first year and then follow a slowed growth curve that is below the third percentile. Skeletal proportions and weight are normal for the age, but these children may appear younger than their chronologic age. Dentition is delayed, and teeth may be overcrowded and malpositioned because of the undeveloped jaw. Sexual development is usually delayed but is otherwise normal unless the gonadotropin hormones are deficient. Growth may extend into the third or fourth decade of life, but permanent height is usually diminished if the disorder is left untreated. Symptoms such as headache and vision changes may indicate the presence of a tumor. Clinical manifestations of panhypopituitarism are listed in Box 46-1.

BOX 46-1 **CLINICAL MANIFESTATIONS OF PANHYPOPITUITARISM**

Growth Hormone
- Short stature but proportional height and weight
- Delayed epiphyseal closure
- Delayed bone age proportional to height
- Premature aging common in later life
- Increased insulin sensitivity

Thyroid-Stimulating Hormone
- Short stature with infantile proportions
- Dry, coarse skin; yellow discoloration, pallor
- Cold intolerance
- Constipation
- Somnolence
- Bradycardia
- Dyspnea on exertion
- Delayed dentition, loss of teeth

Gonadotropins
- Absence of sexual maturation or loss of secondary sexual characteristics
- Atrophy of genitalia, prostate gland, breasts
- Amenorrhea without menopausal symptoms
- Decreased spermatogenesis

Adrenocorticotropic Hormone
- Severe anorexia, weight loss
- Hypoglycemia
- Hypotension
- Hyponatremia, hyperkalemia
- Adrenal apoplexy, especially in response to stress
- Circulatory collapse

Antidiuretic Hormone
- Polyuria
- Polydipsia
- Dehydration

Melanocyte-Stimulating Hormone
- Decreased pigmentation

BOX 46-2 **EVALUATING THE GROWTH CURVE**

Ensure reliability of measurements. Accurately obtain and plot height and weight measurements.

Determine absolute height. The child's absolute height bears some relationship to the likelihood of a pathologic condition. However, the majority of children who have a height below the lowest percentile (either the third or fifth percentile on the height curve) do not have a pathologic growth problem.

Assess height velocity. The most important aspect of a growth evaluation is the observation of a child's height over time, or height velocity. Accurate determination of height velocity requires at least 4 and preferably 6 months of observation. A substantial deceleration in height velocity (crossing several percentiles) between 3 and 12 or 13 years of age indicates a pathologic condition until proven otherwise.

Determine weight-to-height relationship. Determination of the weight-to-height ratio has some diagnostic value in ascertaining the cause of growth delay in a short child.

Project target height. The height of a child can be judged inappropriately short only in the context of his or her genetic potential. Determine the target height of the child with the formula:

$$[\text{Father's height (cm)} + \text{Mother's height (cm)}] + 13\tfrac{1}{2} \text{ for boys}$$
$$\text{or}$$
$$[\text{Father's height (cm)} + \text{Mother's height (cm)}] - 13\tfrac{1}{2} \text{ for girls}$$

Most children achieve an adult stature within approximately 10 cm (4 inches) of the target height.

Adapted from Vogiatzi MG, Copeland KC: The short child, *Pediatr Rev* 19(3):92–99, 1998.

BOX 46-3 **BONE AGE FOR EVALUATING GROWTH DISORDERS**

Bone age refers to a method of assessing skeletal maturity by comparing the appearance of representative epiphyseal centers obtained on x-ray examination with age-appropriate published standards.

Most conditions that cause poor linear growth also cause a delay in skeletal maturation and a delayed bone age. Observation of even a profoundly delayed bone age is never diagnostic or even indicative of a specific diagnosis. A delayed bone age merely indicates that the associated short stature is to some extent "partially reversible" because linear growth will continue until epiphyseal fusion is complete. In comparison, a bone age that is not delayed in a short child is of much greater concern and may, in fact, be of some diagnostic value under certain circumstances.

Adapted from Vogiatzi MG, Copeland KC: The short child, *Pediatr Rev* 19(3):92–99, 1998.

Diagnostic Evaluation

Only a small number of children with delayed growth or short stature have hypopituitary dwarfism. In the majority of instances, the cause is constitutional delay. Diagnostic evaluation is aimed at isolating organic causes, which, in addition to GH deficiency, may include hypothyroidism, oversecretion of cortisol, gonadal aplasia, chronic illness, nutritional inadequacy, Russell-Silver dwarfism, or hypochondroplasia.

A complete diagnostic evaluation should include a family history, a history of the child's growth patterns and previous health status, physical examination, psychosocial evaluation, radiographic surveys, and endocrine studies. Accurate measurement of height (using a calibrated stadiometer) and weight and comparison with standard growth charts are essential. Multiple height measures reflect a more accurate assessment of abnormal growth patterns (Box 46-2) (Hall, 2000). Parental height and familial patterns of growth are important clues to diagnosis.

A skeletal survey in children younger than 3 years and radiographic examination of the hand-wrist for centers of ossification (bone age) (Box 46-3) in older children are important in evaluating growth.

Definitive diagnosis is based on absent or subnormal reserves of pituitary GH. Because GH levels are variable in children, GH stimulation testing is usually required for diagnosis. Initial assessment of the serum IGF-I and IGF binding protein 3 (IGFBP3) indicates a need for further evaluation of GH dysfunction if levels are less than −1 SD below the mean for age. It is recommended that GH stimulation tests be reserved for children with low serum IGF-I and IGFBP3 levels and poor growth who do not have other causes for short stature (Richmond and Rogol, 2008). GH stimulation testing involves the use of pharmacologic agents such as levodopa, clonidine, arginine, insulin, propranolol, or glucagon to provoke the release of GH (Kliegman, Stanton, St. Geme, et al., 2011). Children with poor linear growth, delayed bone age, and abnormal GH stimulation tests are considered GH deficient.

Therapeutic Management

Treatment of GH deficiency caused by organic lesions is directed toward correction of the underlying disease process (e.g., surgical removal or irradiation of a tumor). The definitive treatment of GH deficiency is replacement of GH, which is successful in 80% of affected children. Biosynthetic GH is administered subcutaneously on a daily basis. Growth velocity increases in the first year and then declines in subsequent years. Final height is likely to remain less than normal (Bryant, Baxter, Cave, et al., 2007), and early diagnosis and intervention are essential (Leschek, Rose, Yanovski, et al., 2004).

The decision to stop GH therapy is made jointly by the child, family, and health care team. Growth rates of less than 1 inch per year and a bone age of more than 14 years in girls and more than 16 years in boys are often used as criteria to stop GH therapy (Kliegman, Stanton, St. Geme, et al., 2011). Children with other hormone deficiencies require replacement therapy to correct the specific disorders.

CARE MANAGEMENT

The principal nursing consideration is identifying children with growth problems. Even though the majority of growth problems are not a result of organic causes, any delay in normal growth and sexual development poses special emotional adjustments for these children.

The nurse may be a key person in helping establish a diagnosis. For example, if serial height and weight records are not available, the nurse can question parents about the child's growth compared with that of siblings, peers, or relatives. Preparation of the child and family for diagnostic testing is especially important if a number of tests are being performed, and the child requires particular attention during provocative testing. Blood samples are usually taken every 30 minutes for a 3-hour period. Children also have difficulty overcoming hypoglycemia generated by tests with insulin so they must be observed carefully for signs of hypoglycemia, but those receiving glucagon are at risk for nausea and vomiting. Clonidine may cause hypotension, requiring administration of intravenous (IV) fluids.

Child and Family Support. Children undergoing hormone replacement require additional support. The nurse should provide education for patient self-management during the school-age years. Nursing functions include family education concerning medication preparation and storage, injection sites, injection technique, and syringe disposal (see Chapter 39). Administration of GH is facilitated by family routines that include a specific time of day for the injection. Younger children may enjoy using a calendar and colorful stickers to designate received injections.

! NURSING ALERT

Optimum dosing is often achieved when GH is administered at bedtime. Physiologic release is more normally stimulated as a result of pituitary release of GH during the first 45 to 90 minutes after the onset of sleep.

Even when hormone replacement is successful, these children attain their eventual adult height at a slower rate than their peers; therefore they need assistance in setting realistic expectations regarding improvement. Because these children appear younger than their chronologic age, others frequently relate to them in infantile or childish ways. Parents and teachers benefit from guidance directed toward setting realistic expectations for the child based on age and abilities. For example, in the home, such children should have the same age-appropriate responsibilities as their siblings. As they approach adolescence, they should be encouraged to participate in group activities with peers. If abilities and strengths are emphasized rather than physical size, such children are more likely to develop a positive self-image.

Professionals and families can find resources for research, education, support, and advocacy from the Human Growth Foundation.* The treatment is expensive, but the cost is often partially covered by insurance if the child has a documented deficiency. Children with panhypopituitarism should be advised to wear medical identification at all times.

Pituitary Hyperfunction

Excess GH before closure of the epiphyseal shafts results in proportional overgrowth of the long bones until the individual reaches a height of 2.4 m (8 ft) or more. Vertical growth is accompanied by rapid and increased development of muscles and viscera. Weight is increased but is usually in proportion to height. Proportional enlargement of head circumference also occurs and may result in delayed closure of the fontanels in young children. Children with a pituitary-secreting tumor may also demonstrate signs of increasing intracranial pressure, especially headache.

If oversecretion of GH occurs after epiphyseal closure, growth is in the transverse direction, producing a condition known as acromegaly. Typical facial features include overgrowth of the head, lips, nose, tongue, jaw, and paranasal and mastoid sinuses; separation and malocclusion of the teeth in the enlarged jaw; disproportion of the face to the cerebral division of the skull; increased facial hair; thickened, deeply creased skin; and an increased tendency toward hyperglycemia and diabetes mellitus (DM). Acromegaly can develop slowly, leading to delays in diagnosis and treatment.

Diagnostic Evaluation

Diagnosis is based on a history of excessive growth during childhood and evidence of increased levels of GH. Radiographic studies may reveal a tumor in an enlarged sella turcica, normal bone age, enlargement of bones (e.g., the paranasal sinuses), and evidence of joint changes. Endocrine studies to confirm excess of other hormones, specifically thyroid, cortisol, and sex hormones, should also be included in the differential diagnosis.

Therapeutic Management

If a lesion is present, surgery is performed to remove the tumor when feasible. Other therapies aimed at destroying pituitary tissue include external irradiation and radioactive implants. New pharmacologic agents have evolved and may be used in combination with other therapies (Natchtigall, Delgado, Swearingen, et al., 2008). Depending on the extent of surgical extirpation and degree of pituitary insufficiency, hormone replacement with thyroid extract, cortisone, and sex hormones may be necessary.

---

*997 Glen Cove Ave., Suite 5, Glen Head, NY 11545; 800-451-6434; e-mail: hgf1@hgfound.org; www.hgfound.org.

CARE MANAGEMENT

The primary nursing consideration is early identification of children with excessive growth rates. Although medical management cannot reduce growth already attained, further growth can be delayed. The earlier the treatment, the more control there is in predetermining a normal adult height. Nurses should also observe for signs of a tumor, especially headache, and evidence of concurrent hormonal excesses, particularly the gonadotropins, which cause sexual precocity. Children with excessive growth rates require as much emotional support as those with short stature.

Precocious Puberty

Manifestations of sexual development before age 9 years in boys or age 8 years in girls have traditionally been considered precocious development, and these children were recommended for further evaluation (Kempers and Otten, 2002; Midyett, Moore, and Jacobson, 2003). Recent examination of the age limit for defining when puberty is precocious reveals that the onset of puberty in girls is occurring earlier than previous studies have documented (Biro, Huang, Crawford, et al., 2006; Slyper, 2006). The mean onset of puberty is 10.2 years in Caucasian girls and 9.6 years in African-American girls. Based on these findings, precocious puberty evaluation for a pathologic cause should be performed for Caucasian girls younger than 7 years or for African-American girls younger than 6 years. No change in the guidelines for evaluation of precocious puberty in boys is recommended. However, recent data suggest that boys may be beginning maturation earlier as well (Herman-Giddens, 2006; Slyper, 2006).

Normally, the hypothalamic-releasing factors stimulate secretion of the gonadotropic hormones from the anterior pituitary at the time of puberty. In boys, interstitial cell–stimulating hormone stimulates Leydig cells of the testes to secrete testosterone; in girls, follicle-stimulating hormone (FSH) and luteinizing hormone (LH) stimulate the ovarian follicles to secrete estrogens (Nebesio and Eugster, 2007). This sequence of events is known as the hypothalamic-pituitary-gonadal axis. If for some reason the cycle undergoes premature activation, the child will display evidence of advanced or precocious puberty. Causes of precocious puberty are found in Box 46-4.

Isosexual precocious puberty is more common among girls than boys. Approximately 80% of children with precocious puberty have central precocious puberty (CPP), in which pubertal development is activated by the hypothalamic gonadotropin-releasing hormone (GnRH) (Greiner and Kerrigan, 2006). This produces early maturation and development of the gonads with secretion of sex hormones, development of secondary sex characteristics, and sometimes production of mature sperm and ova (Lee, Houk, Ahmed, et al., 2006; Root, 2000). CPP may be the result of congenital anomalies; infectious, neoplastic, or traumatic insults to the central nervous system (CNS); or treatment of longstanding sex hormone exposure (Trivin, Couto-Silva, Sainte-Rose, et al., 2006). CPP occurs more frequently in girls and is usually idiopathic, with 95% demonstrating no causative factor (Greiner and Kerrigan, 2006; Nebesio and Eugster, 2007; Root, 2000). A CNS insult or structural abnormality is found in more than 90% of boys with CPP (Root, 2000).

Peripheral precocious puberty (PPP) includes early puberty resulting from hormone stimulation other than the hypothalamic GnRH–stimulated pituitary gonadotropin release. Isolated manifestations that are usually associated with puberty may be seen as variations in normal sexual development (Greiner and Kerrigan,

---

BOX 46-4	CAUSES OF PRECOCIOUS PUBERTY

Central Precocious Puberty
- Idiopathic, with or without hypothalamic hamartoma
- Secondary:
  - Congenital anomalies
  - Postinflammatory—Encephalitis, meningitis, abscess, granulomatous disease
  - Radiotherapy
  - Trauma
  - Neoplasms
- After effective treatment of longstanding pseudosexual precocity

Peripheral Precocious Puberty
- Familial male-limited precocious puberty
- Albright syndrome
- Gonadal or extragonadal tumors
- Adrenal:
  - Congenital adrenal hyperplasia
  - Adenoma, carcinoma
  - Glucocorticoid resistance
- Exogenous sex hormones
- Primary hypothyroidism

Incomplete Precocious Puberty
- Premature thelarche
- Premature menarche
- Premature pubarche or adrenarche

Adapted from Root AW: Precocious puberty, *Pediatr Rev* 21(1):10–19, 2000.

2006). They appear without other signs of pubescence and are caused by excess secretion of sex hormones through the gonads or adrenal glands and may be isosexual or contrasexual. Included are premature thelarche (development of breasts in prepubertal girls), premature pubarche (premature adrenarche, early development of sexual hair), and premature menarche (isolated menses without other evidence of sexual development).

Therapeutic Management

Treatment of precocious puberty is directed toward the specific cause when known. In 50% of cases, precocious pubertal development regresses or stops advancing without any treatment (Carel and Leger, 2008). If needed, precocious puberty of central (hypothalamic-pituitary) origin is managed with monthly injections of a synthetic analog of luteinizing hormone–releasing hormone, which regulates pituitary secretions (Greiner and Kerrigan, 2006; Muir, 2006). The available preparation, leuprolide acetate (Lupron Depot), is given in a dosage of 0.2 to 0.3 mg/kg intramuscularly once every 4 weeks. Longer-acting formulations have recently been developed as well. Breast development regresses or does not advance, and growth returns to normal rates, enhancing predicted height. Studies suggest that not all patients attain adult targeted heights, and the addition of GH therapy may be warranted (Carel and Leger, 2008). Treatment is discontinued at a chronologically appropriate time, allowing pubertal changes to resume. Psychologic management of the patient and family is an important aspect of care. Both parents and the affected child should be taught the injection procedure.

CARE MANAGEMENT

Psychologic support and guidance of the child and family are the most important aspects of management. Parents need anticipatory guidance, support and information resources, and reassurance of the benign nature of the condition (Greiner and Kerrigan, 2006; O'Sullivan and O'Sullivan, 2002). Dress and activities for the physically precocious child should be appropriate to the chronologic age. Sexual interest is not usually advanced beyond the child's chronologic age, and parents need to understand that the child's mental age is congruent with the chronologic age.

Diabetes Insipidus

The principal disorder of posterior pituitary hypofunction is diabetes insipidus (DI), also known as neurogenic DI, resulting from undersecretion of antidiuretic hormone (ADH), or vasopressin (Pitressin), and producing a state of uncontrolled diuresis (Makaryus and McFarlane, 2006). This disorder is not to be confused with nephrogenic DI, a rare hereditary disorder affecting primarily males and caused by unresponsiveness of the renal tubules to the hormone.

Neurogenic DI may result from a number of different causes. Primary causes are familial or idiopathic; of the total cases, approximately 45% to 50% are idiopathic. Secondary causes include trauma (accidental or surgical), tumors, granulomatous disease, infections (meningitis or encephalitis), and vascular anomalies (aneurysm). Certain drugs, such as alcohol and phenytoin (diphenylhydantoin), can cause a transient polyuria. DI may be an early sign of an evolving cerebral process (De Buyst, Massa, Christophe, et al., 2007).

The cardinal signs of DI are polyuria and polydipsia. In older children, signs such as excessive urination accompanied by a compensatory insatiable thirst may be so intense that the child does little more than go to the toilet and drink fluids (Cheetham and Baylis, 2002). Frequently, the first sign is enuresis. In infants, the initial symptom is irritability that is relieved with feedings of water but not milk. These infants are also prone to dehydration, electrolyte imbalance, hyperthermia, azotemia, and potential circulatory collapse.

Dehydration is usually not a serious problem in older children, who are able to drink larger quantities of water. However, any period of unconsciousness, such as after trauma or anesthesia, may be life threatening because the voluntary demand for fluid is absent. During such instances, careful monitoring of urine volumes, blood concentration, and IV fluid replacement is essential to prevent dehydration.

> **! NURSING ALERT**
>
> Children with DI complicated by congenital absence of the thirst center must be encouraged to drink sufficient quantities of liquid to prevent electrolyte imbalance.

Diagnostic Evaluation

The simplest test used to diagnose this condition is restriction of oral fluids and observation of consequent changes in urine volume and concentration. Normally, reducing fluids results in concentrated urine and diminished volume. In DI, fluid restriction has little or no effect on urine formation but causes weight loss from dehydration. Accurate results from this procedure require strict monitoring of fluid intake and urinary output, measurement of urine concentration (specific gravity or osmolality), and frequent weight checks. A weight loss between 3% and 5% indicates significant dehydration and requires termination of the fluid restriction.

> **! NURSING ALERT**
>
> Small children require close observation during fluid deprivation to prevent them from drinking, even from toilet bowls, flower vases, and other unlikely sources of fluid.

If this test result is positive, the child should be given a test dose of injected aqueous vasopressin, which should alleviate the polyuria and polydipsia. Unresponsiveness to exogenous vasopressin usually indicates nephrogenic DI. An important diagnostic consideration is to differentiate DI from other causes of polyuria and polydipsia, especially DM. DI may be the early sign of an evolving cerebral process (De Buyst, Massa, Christophe, et al., 2007).

Therapeutic Management

The usual treatment is hormone replacement, either with an intramuscular or subcutaneous injection of vasopressin tannate in peanut oil or with a nasal spray of aqueous lysine vasopressin (Makaryus and McFarlane, 2006; Verbalis, 2003). The injectable form has the advantage of lasting 48 to 72 hours, which affords the child a full night's sleep. However, it has the disadvantage of requiring frequent injections and proper preparation of the drug.

> **! NURSING ALERT**
>
> To be effective, vasopressin must be thoroughly resuspended in the oil by being held under warm running water for 10 to 15 minutes and shaken vigorously before being drawn into the syringe. If this is not done, the oil may be injected minus the ADH. Small brown particles, which indicate drug dispersion, must be seen in the suspension.

CARE MANAGEMENT

The initial objective is identification of the disorder. Because an early sign may be sudden enuresis in a child who is toilet trained, excessive thirst with bedwetting is an indication for further investigation. Another clue is persistent irritability and crying in an infant that is relieved only by bottle feedings of water. After head trauma or certain neurosurgical procedures, the development of DI can be anticipated; therefore these patients must be closely monitored.

Assessment includes measurement of body weight, serum electrolytes, blood urea nitrogen (BUN), hematocrit, and urine specific gravity. Fluid intake and output should be carefully measured and recorded. Alert patients are able to adjust intake to urine losses, but unconscious or very young patients require closer fluid observation. In children who are not toilet trained, collection of urine specimens may require application of a urine-collecting device.

After confirmation of the diagnosis, parents need a thorough explanation regarding the condition with specific clarification that DI is a different condition from DM. They must realize that treatment is lifelong. Caregivers should be taught the correct procedure for preparation and administration of the injectable form of the drug. When children are old enough, they should be encouraged to assume full responsibility for their care.

For emergency purposes, these children should wear medical alert identification. Older children should carry the nasal spray with them for temporary relief of symptoms. School personnel need to be aware of the problem so they can grant children unrestricted use of the lavatory.

Syndrome of Inappropriate Antidiuretic Hormone

The disorder that results from hypersecretion of ADH from the posterior pituitary hormone is known as *syndrome of inappropriate ADH secretion (SIADH)*. It is observed with increased frequency in a variety of conditions, especially those involving infections, tumors, or other CNS disease or trauma, and is the most common cause of hyponatremia in the pediatric population (Lin, Liu, and Lim, 2005, Rivkees, 2008).

The manifestations are directly related to fluid retention and hypotonicity. Excess ADH causes most of the filtered water to be reabsorbed from the kidneys back into central circulation. Serum osmolality is low, and urine osmolality is inappropriately elevated. When serum sodium levels are diminished to 120 mEq/L, affected children may display anorexia, nausea (and sometimes vomiting), stomach cramps, irritability, and personality changes. With progressive reduction in sodium, other neurologic signs, stupor, and convulsions may be evident. The symptoms usually disappear when the underlying disorder is corrected.

The immediate management consists of restricting fluids. Subsequent management depends on the cause and severity. Fluids continue to be restricted to one-fourth to one-half maintenance. When there are no fluid abnormalities but SIADH can be anticipated, fluids are often restricted expectantly at two-thirds to three-fourths maintenance.

CARE MANAGEMENT

The first goal of nursing management is recognizing the presence of SIADH from symptoms described in patients at risk.

> ### ! NURSING ALERT
>
> Nausea, vomiting, and malaise may precede the onset of more severe stages such as disorientation, confusion, coma, and seizures (Majzoub and Muglia, 2003).

Accurately measuring intake and output, noting daily weight, and observing for signs of fluid overload are primary nursing functions, especially in children receiving IV fluids. Seizure precautions are implemented, and the child and family need education regarding the rationale for fluid restrictions. The rare child with chronic SIADH will be placed on long-term ADH-antagonizing medication, and the child and family will require instructions for its administration.

DISORDERS OF THYROID FUNCTION

The thyroid gland secretes two types of hormones: thyroid hormone (TH), which consists of the hormones thyroxine (T_4) and triiodothyronine (T_3), and calcitonin. The secretion of THs is controlled by TSH from the anterior pituitary, which in turn is regulated by thyrotropin-releasing factor (TRF) from the hypothalamus as a negative feedback response. Consequently, hypothyroidism or hyperthyroidism may result from a defect in the target gland or from a disturbance in the secretion of TSH or TRF. Because the functions of T_3 and T_4 are qualitatively the same, the term *thyroid hormone* is used throughout the discussion.

The synthesis of TH depends on available sources of dietary iodine and tyrosine. The thyroid is the only endocrine gland capable of storing excess amounts of hormones for release as needed. During circulation in the bloodstream, T_4 and T_3 are bound to carrier proteins (thyroxine-binding globulin). They must be unbound before they are able to exert their metabolic effect.

The main physiologic action of TH is to regulate the basal metabolic rate and thereby control the processes of growth and tissue differentiation. Unlike GH, TH is involved in many more diverse activities that influence the growth and development of body tissues. Therefore a deficiency of TH exerts a more profound effect on growth than that seen in hypopituitarism.

Calcitonin helps maintain blood calcium levels by decreasing the calcium concentration. Its effect is the opposite of parathyroid hormone (PTH) in that it inhibits skeletal demineralization and promotes calcium deposition in the bone.

Juvenile Hypothyroidism

Hypothyroidism is one of the most common endocrine problems of childhood. It may be either congenital or acquired and represents a deficiency in secretion of TH (Foley, 2001).

Beyond infancy, primary hypothyroidism may be caused by a number of defects. For example, a congenital hypoplastic thyroid gland may provide sufficient amounts of TH during the first year or two but be inadequate when rapid body growth increases demands on the gland. A partial or complete thyroidectomy for cancer or thyrotoxicosis can leave insufficient thyroid tissue to furnish hormones for body requirements. Radiotherapy for Hodgkin disease or other malignancies may lead to hypothyroidism (Pizzo and Poplack, 2010). Infectious processes may cause hypothyroidism. It can also occur when dietary iodine is deficient, although it is now rare in the United States because iodized salt is a readily available source of the nutrient.

Clinical manifestations depend on the extent of dysfunction and the child's age at onset. Primary congenital hypothyroidism is characterized by low levels of circulating THs and raised levels of TSH at birth (Macchia, 2000). If left untreated, congenital hypothyroidism causes decreased mental capacity. Improvements in newborn screening have led to earlier detection and prevention of complications (American Academy of Pediatrics [AAP], 2006). The GnRH test and baseline measurement of gonadotropin and sex hormone serum concentrations at 3 months of age are promising options for assessment of hypothalamic-pituitary-gonadal function in infants with congenital hypothyroidism (van Tijn, Schroor, Delemarre-van de Waal, et al., 2007). The presenting symptoms are decelerated growth from chronic deprivation of TH or thyromegaly. Impaired growth and development are less severe when hypothyroidism is acquired at a later age, and because brain growth is nearly complete by 2 to 3 years of age, intellectual disability and neurologic sequelae are not associated with juvenile hypothyroidism. Other manifestations are myxedematous skin changes (dry skin, puffiness around the eyes, sparse hair), constipation, lethargy, and mental decline (Box 46-5).

Therapy is TH replacement, the same as for hypothyroidism in infants, although the prompt treatment needed in infants is not required in children. L-thyroxine is administered over a period of 4 to 8 weeks to avoid symptoms of hyperthyroidism. Researchers have found that children treated early continue to have mild delays in reading, comprehension, and arithmetic but catch up by grade six (Rovet and Ehrlich, 2000). However, adolescents may demonstrate problems with memory, attention, and visuospatial processing.

CLINICAL MANIFESTATIONS OF JUVENILE HYPOTHYROIDISM

- Decelerated growth:
  - Less when acquired at later age
- Myxedematous skin changes:
  - Dry skin
  - Puffiness around eyes
  - Sparse hair
  - Constipation
  - Sleepiness
  - Mental decline

BOX 46-6 **CLINICAL MANIFESTATIONS OF LYMPHOCYTIC THYROIDITIS**

Enlarged Thyroid Gland
- Usually symmetric
- Firm
- Freely movable
- Nontender

Tracheal Compression
- Sense of fullness
- Hoarseness
- Dysphagia

Hyperthyroidism (Possible)
- Nervousness
- Irritability
- Increased sweating
- Hyperactivity

CARE MANAGEMENT

Growth cessation in a child whose growth has previously been normal should alert the health care provider to the possibility of hypothyroidism. After diagnosis and implementation of thyroxine therapy, the importance of compliance and periodic monitoring of response to therapy should be stressed to parents. Children should learn to take responsibility for their own health as soon as they are old enough, at about 9 or 10 years of age.

Goiter

A goiter is an enlargement or hypertrophy of the thyroid gland. It may occur with deficient (hypothyroid), excessive (hyperthyroid), or normal (euthyroid) TH secretion. It can be congenital or acquired. Congenital disease occurs as a result of maternal administration of antithyroid drugs or iodides during pregnancy or as an inborn error of TH production. Acquired disease can result from increased secretion of pituitary TSH in response to decreased circulating levels of TH or from infiltrative neoplastic or inflammatory processes. In most children, goiter is caused by chronic autoimmune thyroiditis (de Vries, Bulvik, and Phillip, 2009). In areas where dietary iodine (essential for TH production) is deficient, goiter can be endemic.

Enlargement of the thyroid gland may be mild and noticeable only when there is an increased demand for TH (e.g., during periods of rapid growth). Enlargement of the thyroid at birth can be sufficient to cause severe respiratory distress. Colloid goiters are diffuse and benign and occur more frequently in adolescent girls. Thyroid function is normal, and the gland will gradually decrease over several years without treatment. TH replacement may be necessary to treat the hypothyroidism and reverse the TSH effect on the gland.

CARE MANAGEMENT

Large goiters are identified by their obvious appearance. In older children, each lobe of the thyroid should be approximately the same as the terminal phalanx of the child's thumb (de Vries, Bulvik, and Phillip, 2009). Smaller nodules may be evident only on palpation. Benign enlargement of the thyroid gland may occur during adolescence and should not be confused with pathologic states. Nodules rarely are caused by a cancerous tumor but always require evaluation. Questions regarding exposure to radiation should be included in the assessment.

Immediate surgery to remove part of the gland may be lifesaving in infants born with a goiter. When thyroid replacement is necessary,

parents have the same needs regarding its administration as discussed for the parents of children who have hypothyroidism.

Lymphocytic Thyroiditis

Lymphocytic thyroiditis (Hashimoto disease, chronic autoimmune thyroiditis) is the most common cause of thyroid disease in children and adolescents and accounts for the largest percentage of juvenile hypothyroidism (Szymborska and Staroszczyk, 2000). It accounts for many of the enlarged thyroid glands formerly designated *thyroid hyperplasia of adolescence* or *adolescent goiter*. Although it can occur during the first 3 years of life, it occurs more frequently after age 6 years. It reaches a peak incidence during adolescence, and there is evidence that the disease is self-limiting. The presence of a goiter and elevated thyroglobulin antibody with progressive increase in both thyroid peroxidase antibody and TSH may be predictive factors for future development of hypothyroidism (Radetti, Gottardi, Bona, et al., 2006).

The presence of the enlarged thyroid gland is usually detected during a routine examination, although it may be noted by parents when the child swallows. In most children, the entire gland is enlarged symmetrically (although it may be asymmetric) and is firm, freely movable, and nontender. There may be manifestations of moderate tracheal compression (sense of fullness, hoarseness, and dysphagia), but it is extremely rare for a nontoxic diffuse goiter to enlarge to the extent that it causes mechanical obstruction. Most children are euthyroid, but some display symptoms of hypothyroidism, including delayed growth and puberty and declining school performance. Other signs suggestive of thyroiditis are found in Box 46-6.

Diagnostic Evaluation

Thyroid function test results are usually normal, although TSH levels may be slightly or moderately elevated. With progressive disease, the T_4 decreases followed by a decrease in T_3 levels and an increase in TSH. The majority of children have antithyroid antibody titers. However, levels in children are lower than in adults; therefore repeated measurements may be needed in doubtful cases because titers may increase later in the disease.

Therapeutic Management

In many cases, the goiter is transient and asymptomatic and regresses spontaneously within a year or two. Therapy of a nontoxic diffuse goiter is usually simple, uncomplicated, and effective. Oral administration of TH decreases the size of the gland significantly and provides the feedback needed to suppress TSH stimulation, and the hyperplastic thyroid gland gradually regresses in size. TSH levels should be monitored, with the goal of restoring normal growth and development. Surgery is contraindicated in this disorder. Untreated patients should be evaluated periodically.

CARE MANAGEMENT

Nursing care consists of identifying the child with thyroid enlargement, reassuring the child that the condition is probably only temporary, and reinforcing instructions for thyroid therapy.

Hyperthyroidism

The largest percentage of hyperthyroidism in childhood is caused by Graves disease, which is usually associated with an enlarged thyroid gland and exophthalmos (Ma, Xie, Kuang, et al., 2006; Streetman and Khanderia, 2004; Thompson, 2002). Most cases of Graves disease in children occur between ages 6 and 15 years, with a peak incidence at 12 to 14 years of age, but the disease may be present at birth in children of thyrotoxic mothers. The incidence is 5 times higher in girls than in boys.

The hyperthyroidism of Graves disease is apparently caused by an autoimmune response to TSH receptors, but no specific etiology has been identified. There is definitive evidence for familial association, with a high concordance incidence in twins. Patients with Graves disease possess the histocompatibility antigens *A1*, *B8*, and *DR3* (Dallas and Foley, 2003; Simmonds, Howson, Heward, et al., 2005). There may be an association with other autoimmune diseases such as rheumatoid arthritis and lupus.

The development of manifestations is highly variable. Signs and symptoms develop gradually, with an interval between onset and diagnosis of approximately 6 to 12 months. The principal clinical features are excessive motion, including irritability, hyperactivity, short attention span, tremors, insomnia, and emotional lability. Clinical manifestations are presented in Box 46-7.

Exophthalmos (protruding eyeballs), which is observed in many children, is accompanied by a wide-eyed staring expression, increased blinking, eyelid lag, lack of convergence, and absence of wrinkling of the forehead when looking upward. As protrusion of the eyeball increases, the child may not be able to completely cover the cornea with the eyelid. Visual disturbances may include blurred vision and loss of visual acuity. Ophthalmopathy can develop long before or after the onset of hyperthyroidism. A consistent pathogenic link between them has not been identified. It is now thought that Graves ophthalmopathy is a disorder of autoimmune origin caused by a complex interplay of endogenous and environmental factors (Bartalena, Tanda, Piantanida, et al., 2003).

Diagnostic Evaluation

The presence of a thyroid mass in a child requires a thorough history, including inquiry into prior irradiation to the head and neck and exposure to a goitrogen. The diagnosis is established on the basis of increased levels of T_4 and T_3. TSH is suppressed to unmeasurable levels (Ma, Xie, Kuang, et al., 2006). Graves disease is confirmed by measurement of thyroid-stimulating immunoglobulin.

Therapeutic Management

Therapy for hyperthyroidism is controversial, but all methods are directed toward slowing the rate of hormone secretion. The three acceptable modes available are antithyroid drugs (methimazole), which interferes with the biosynthesis of TH; subtotal thyroidectomy; and ablation with radioiodine (^{131}I iodide) (Rivkees and Cornelius, 2003; Streetman and Khanderia, 2004). Each is effective, but each has advantages and disadvantages. Pharmacologic therapy

---

BOX 46-7   CLINICAL MANIFESTATIONS OF HYPERTHYROIDISM (GRAVES DISEASE)

Cardinal Signs
- Emotional lability
- Physical restlessness, characteristically at rest
- Decelerated school performance
- Voracious appetite with weight loss in 50% of cases
- Fatigue

Physical Signs
- Tachycardia
- Widened pulse pressure
- Dyspnea on exertion
- Exophthalmos (protruding eyeballs)
- Wide-eyed, staring expression with eyelid lag
- Tremor
- Goiter (hypertrophy and hyperplasia)
- Warm, moist skin
- Accelerated linear growth
- Heat intolerance (may be severe)
- Hair fine and unable to hold a curl
- Systolic murmurs

Thyroid Storm
- Acute onset:
  - Severe irritability and restlessness
  - Vomiting
  - Diarrhea
  - Hyperthermia
  - Hypertension
  - Severe tachycardia
  - Prostration
- May progress rapidly to:
  - Delirium
  - Coma
  - Death

---

may induce a remission, and treatment may be discontinued. However, relapse may occur. Radioactive iodine ablation is usually effective but response may be slower, and there have been concerns about a possible link to thyroid cancer in younger children. Surgery is often used when other treatments are not effective. These children require lifelong monitoring.

When affected children exhibit signs and symptoms of hyperthyroidism (e.g., increased weight loss, pulse, pulse pressure, and blood pressure), their activity should be limited to classwork only. Vigorous exercise is restricted until thyroid levels are decreased to normal or near-normal values.

Thyrotoxicosis (thyroid "crisis" or thyroid "storm") may occur from sudden release of the hormone. Although thyrotoxicosis is unusual in children, a crisis can be life threatening. These "storms" are evidenced by the acute onset of severe irritability and restlessness, vomiting, diarrhea, hyperthermia, hypertension, severe tachycardia, and prostration. There may be rapid progression to delirium, coma, and even death. A crisis may be precipitated by acute infection, surgical emergencies, or discontinuation of antithyroid therapy. Treatment, in addition to antithyroid drugs, is administration of β-adrenergic blocking agents (propranolol), which provide relief from the adrenergic hyperresponsiveness that produces the disturbing side effects of the reaction. Therapy is usually required for 2 to 3 weeks.

The American Thyroid Association* has an extensive website with information related to prevention, treatment, and cure of thyroid disease.

CARE MANAGEMENT

The initial nursing objective is identification of children with hyperthyroidism. Because the clinical manifestations often appear gradually, the goiter and ophthalmic changes may not be noticed and the excessive activity may be attributed to behavioral problems. Nurses in ambulatory settings, particularly schools, need to be alert to signs that suggest this disorder, especially weight loss despite an excellent appetite, academic difficulties resulting from a short attention span and inability to sit still, unexplained fatigue and sleeplessness, and difficulty with fine motor skills such as writing. Exophthalmos may develop long before the onset of signs and symptoms of hyperthyroidism and may be the only presenting sign (Thompson, 2002). Exophthalmos is less common in adults than in children (Jospe, 2001).

Much of these children's care is related to treating physical symptoms before a response to drug therapy is achieved. A regular routine is beneficial in providing frequent rest periods, minimizing the stress of coping with unexpected demands, and meeting the children's needs promptly. Physical activity is restricted. Mood swings and irritability can disrupt interpersonal relationships, creating difficulties within and outside the home. The child and parents should be encouraged to express feelings about the behavior and its effect on others. Heat intolerance may be minimized by the use of light cotton clothing, good ventilation, air conditioning or fans, frequent baths, and adequate hydration. Dietary requirements should be adjusted to meet the child's increased metabolic rate. Rather than three large meals, the child's appetite may be better satisfied by five or six moderate meals throughout the day.

> ### ! NURSING ALERT
>
> Children being treated with methimazole must be carefully monitored for side effects of the drug. Because sore throat and fever accompany the grave complication of leukopenia, these children should be seen by a health care practitioner if such symptoms occur. Parents and children should be taught to recognize and report symptoms immediately.

> ### ! NURSING ALERT
>
> The earliest indication of hypoparathyroidism may be anxiety and mental depression followed by paresthesia and evidence of heightened neuromuscular excitability, such as:
>
> * **Chvostek sign**—facial muscle spasm elicited by tapping the facial nerve in the region of the parotid gland
> * **Trousseau sign**—carpal spasm elicited by pressure applied to nerves of the upper arm
> * **Tetany**—Carpopedal spasm (sharp flexion of wrist and ankle joints), muscle twitching, cramps, seizures, and stridor

*6066 Leesburg Pike, Suite 550, Falls Church, VA 22041; 800-THYROID; e-mail: thyroid@thyroid.org; www.thyroid.org.

DISORDERS OF PARATHYROID FUNCTION

The parathyroid glands secrete PTH, the main function of which, along with vitamin D and calcitonin, is homeostasis of serum calcium concentration (Perheentupa, 2003). The effect of PTH on calcium is opposite that of calcitonin. The net result of the integrated action of PTH and vitamin D is maintenance of serum calcium levels within a narrow normal range and the mineralization of bone. Secretion of PTH is controlled by a negative feedback system involving the serum calcium ion concentration. Low ionized calcium levels stimulate PTH secretion, causing absorption of calcium by the target tissues; high ionized calcium concentrations suppress PTH.

Hypoparathyroidism

Hypoparathyroidism is a spectrum of disorders that result in deficient PTH. Congenital hypoparathyroidism may be caused by a specific defect in the synthesis or cellular processing of PTH or by aplasia or hypoplasia of the gland (Perheentupa, 2003).

Hypoparathyroidism can also occur secondary to other causes, including infection and autoimmune syndromes. Postoperative hypoparathyroidism may follow thyroidectomy with acute or gradual onset and be transient or permanent. Two forms of transient hypoparathyroidism may be present in newborns, both of which are the result of a relative PTH deficiency. One type is caused by maternal hyperparathyroidism or maternal DM. A more common, later form appears almost exclusively in infants fed a milk formula with a high phosphate-to-calcium ratio.

Pseudohypoparathyroidism occurs when there is a genetic defect in the cellular receptors to PTH. The result is normal parathyroid gland and elevated PTH levels. Abnormal calcium and phosphorus levels are not affected by administration of PTH. These children typically have a short, stocky build; a round face; and abnormally shaped hands and fingers. Other endocrine dysfunction may be found concurrently (Shoback, 2008).

Clinical signs of hypoparathyroidism are found in Box 46-8. Muscle cramps are an early symptom, progressing to numbness, stiffness, and tingling in the hands and feet. A positive Chvostek or Trousseau sign or laryngeal spasms may be present. Convulsions with loss of consciousness may occur. These episodes may be preceded by abdominal discomfort, tonic rigidity, head retraction, and cyanosis. Headaches and vomiting with increased intracranial pressure and papilledema may occur and may suggest a brain tumor (Kliegman, Stanton, St. Geme, et al., 2011).

Diagnostic Evaluation

The diagnosis of hypoparathyroidism is made on the basis of clinical manifestations associated with decreased serum calcium and increased serum phosphorus. Levels of plasma PTH are low in idiopathic hypoparathyroidism but high in pseudohypoparathyroidism. End-organ responsiveness is tested by the administration of PTH with measurement of urinary cyclic adenosine monophosphate (cAMP). Kidney function tests are included in the differential diagnosis to rule out renal insufficiency. Magnesium levels should also be tested. Although bone radiograph findings are usually normal, they may demonstrate increased bone density and suppressed growth.

Therapeutic Management

The objective of treatment is to maintain normal serum calcium and phosphate levels with minimal complications. Acute or severe tetany is corrected immediately by IV and oral administration of calcium

BOX 46-8	CLINICAL MANIFESTATIONS OF HYPOPARATHYROIDISM

Pseudohypoparathyroidism

- Short stature
- Round face
- Short, thick neck
- Short, stubby fingers and toes
- Dimpling of skin over knuckles
- Subcutaneous soft tissue calcifications
- Intellectual disability a prominent feature

Idiopathic Hypoparathyroidism

- None of the above physical characteristics observed
- May include papilledema
- May have intellectual disability

Both Types

- Dry, scaly, coarse skin with eruptions
- Hair often brittle
- Nails thin and brittle with characteristic transverse grooves
- Dental and enamel hypoplasia
- Muscle contractions:
  - Tetany
  - Carpopedal spasm
  - Laryngospasm (laryngeal stridor)
  - Muscle cramps and twitching
  - Positive Chvostek sign or Trousseau sign (see Nursing Alert on p. 1470)
- Neurologic:
  - Headache
  - Seizures (generalized, absence, or focal)
  - Swings of emotion
  - Loss of memory
  - Depression
  - Confusion possible
  - Paresthesias, tingling
- Gastrointestinal:
  - Muscle cramps
  - Diarrhea
  - Vomiting
- Delayed skeletal growth

BOX 46-9	CLINICAL MANIFESTATIONS OF HYPERPARATHYROIDISM

Gastrointestinal

- Nausea
- Vomiting
- Abdominal discomfort
- Constipation

Central Nervous System

- Delusions
- Confusion
- Hallucinations
- Impaired memory
- Lack of interest and initiative
- Depression
- Varying levels of consciousness

Neuromuscular

- Weakness
- Easy fatigability
- Muscle atrophy (especially proximal muscles of lower limbs)
- Tongue twitching
- Paresthesias in extremities

Skeletal

- Vague bone pain
- Subperiosteal resorption of phalanges
- Spontaneous fractures
- Absence of lamina dura around teeth

Renal

- Polyuria
- Polydipsia
- Renal colic
- Hypertension

CARE MANAGEMENT

The initial objective is recognition of hypocalcemia. Unexplained convulsions, irritability (especially to external stimuli), gastrointestinal symptoms (diarrhea, vomiting, cramping), and positive signs of tetany should lead the nurse to suspect this disorder. Much of the initial nursing care is related to the physical manifestations and includes institution of seizure and safety precautions; reduction of environmental stimuli; and observation for signs of laryngospasm such as stridor, hoarseness, and a feeling of tightness in the throat. A tracheostomy set and injectable calcium gluconate should be available for emergency use. The administration of calcium gluconate requires precautions against extravasation of the drug and tissue destruction.

After initiating treatment, the nurse discusses with the parents the need for continuous daily administration of calcium salts and vitamin D. Because vitamin D toxicity can be a serious consequence of therapy, parents are advised to watch for signs that include weakness, fatigue, lassitude, headache, nausea, vomiting, and diarrhea. Early renal impairment is manifested by polyuria, polydipsia, and nocturia.

Hyperparathyroidism

Hyperparathyroidism is rare in childhood but can be primary or secondary. The most common cause of primary hyperparathyroidism is adenoma of the gland (Kliegman, Stanton, St. Geme, et al., 2011). The most common causes of secondary hyperparathyroidism are chronic renal disease, renal osteodystrophy, and congenital anomalies of the urinary tract. The common factor is hypercalcemia. The clinical signs of hyperparathyroidism are listed in Box 46-9.

Diagnostic Evaluation

Blood studies to identify elevated calcium and decreased phosphorus levels are routinely performed. Measurement of PTH, as well as several tests to isolate the cause of the hypercalcemia, such as renal function studies, should be included. Other procedures used to sub-

gluconate and follow-up daily doses to achieve normal levels. Twice-daily serum calcium measurements are taken to monitor the efficacy of therapy and prevent hypercalcemia. When diagnosis is confirmed, vitamin D therapy is begun. Vitamin D therapy is somewhat difficult to regulate because the drug has a prolonged onset and a long half-life. Some authorities advocate beginning with a lower dose with stepwise increases and careful monitoring of serum calcium until stable levels are achieved. Others prefer rapid induction with higher doses and rapid reduction to lower maintenance levels (Cooper and Gittoes, 2008; Kliegman, Stanton, St. Geme, et al., 2011).

Long-term management usually consists of vitamin D and oral calcium supplementation. Blood calcium and phosphorus are monitored frequently until the levels have stabilized and then routinely thereafter. Renal function, blood pressure, and serum vitamin D levels are measured every 6 months. Serum magnesium levels are measured to permit detection of hypomagnesemia, which may raise the requirement for vitamin D.

stantiate the physiologic consequences of the disorder include electrocardiography and radiographic bone surveys.

Therapeutic Management

Treatment depends on the cause of hyperparathyroidism. The treatment of primary hyperparathyroidism is surgical removal of the tumor or hyperplastic tissue. Treatment of secondary hyperparathyroidism is directed at the underlying contributing cause, which subsequently restores the serum calcium balance. However, in some instances, such as in chronic renal failure, the underlying disorder is irreversible. In this case, treatment is aimed at raising serum calcium levels to inhibit the stimulatory effect of low levels on the parathyroids. This includes oral administration of calcium salts, high doses of vitamin D to enhance calcium absorption, a low-phosphorus diet, and administration of a phosphorus-mobilizing aluminum hydroxide to reduce phosphate absorption.

▌CARE MANAGEMENT

The initial nursing objective is recognition of the disorder. Because secondary hyperparathyroidism is a consequence of chronic renal failure, the nurse is always alert to signs that suggest this complication, especially bone pain and fractures. Because urinary symptoms are the earliest indication, assessment of other body systems for evidence of high calcium levels is indicated when polyuria and polydipsia coexist. Clues to the possibility of hyperparathyroidism include change in behavior, especially inactivity; unexplained gastrointestinal symptoms; and cardiac irregularities.

DISORDERS OF ADRENAL FUNCTION

The adrenal cortex secretes three main groups of hormones collectively called steroids and classified according to their biologic activity: (1) glucocorticoids (cortisol, corticosterone); (2) mineralocorticoids (aldosterone); and (3) sex steroids (androgens, estrogens, and progestins). Alterations in the levels of these hormones produce significant dysfunction in a variety of body tissues and organs. Because the adrenocortical cells are capable of producing any of the steroids, pathologic conditions may result in a deficiency or an excess of more than one type of hormone. However, most are rare in children.

The adrenal medulla secretes the catecholamines epinephrine and norepinephrine. Both hormones have essentially the same effects on various organs as those caused by direct sympathetic stimulation except that the hormonal effects last several times longer. Catecholamine-secreting tumors are the primary cause of adrenal medullary hyperfunction.

Acute Adrenocortical Insufficiency

The acute form of adrenocortical insufficiency (adrenal crisis) may have a number of causes during childhood. Although a rare disorder, some of the more common etiologic factors include hemorrhage into the gland from trauma, which may be caused by a prolonged, difficult labor; fulminating infections, such as meningococcemia, which result in hemorrhage and necrosis (Waterhouse-Friderichsen syndrome); abrupt withdrawal of exogenous sources of cortisone or failure to increase exogenous supplies during stress; or congenital adrenogenital hyperplasia of the salt-losing type.

Early symptoms of adrenocortical insufficiency include increased irritability, headache, diffuse abdominal pain, weakness, nausea and vomiting, and diarrhea. Other clinical signs are found in Box 46-10. In newborns, adrenal crisis is accompanied by extreme hyperpyrexia

---

BOX 46-10 CLINICAL MANIFESTATIONS OF ACUTE ADRENOCORTICAL INSUFFICIENCY

Early Symptoms
- Increased irritability
- Headache
- Diffuse abdominal pain
- Weakness
- Nausea and vomiting
- Diarrhea

Generalized Hemorrhagic Manifestations (Waterhouse-Friderichsen Syndrome)
- Fever (increases as condition worsens)
- Central nervous system signs:
  - Nuchal rigidity
  - Seizures
  - Stupor
  - Coma

Shocklike State
- Weak, rapid pulse
- Decreased blood pressure
- Shallow respirations
- Cold, clammy skin
- Cyanosis
- Circulatory collapse (terminal event)

Newborn
- Hyperpyrexia
- Tachypnea
- Cyanosis
- Seizures
- Gland evident as palpable retroperitoneal mass (hemorrhagic)

(high temperature), tachypnea, cyanosis, and seizures. Usually there is no evidence of infection or purpura. However, hemorrhage into the adrenal gland may be evident as a palpable retroperitoneal mass.

Diagnostic Evaluation

There is no rapid, definitive test for confirmation of acute adrenocortical insufficiency. Routine procedures such as measurement of plasma cortisol levels are too time consuming to be practical. Therefore diagnosis is usually made based on clinical presentation, especially when a fulminating sepsis is accompanied by hemorrhagic manifestations and signs of circulatory collapse despite adequate antibiotic therapy. Because there is no real danger in administering a cortisol preparation for a short period, treatment should be instituted immediately. Improvement with cortisol therapy confirms the diagnosis.

Therapeutic Management

Treatment involves replacement of cortisol, replacement of body fluids to combat dehydration and hypovolemia, administration of glucose solutions to correct hypoglycemia, and specific antibiotic therapy in the presence of infection. Initially, IV hydrocortisone (Solu-Cortef) is administered. Normal saline containing 5% glucose is given parenterally to replace lost fluid, electrolytes, and glucose. If hemorrhage has been severe, whole blood may be replaced. In the event that these measures do not reverse the circulatory collapse, vasopressors are used for immediate vasoconstriction and elevation of blood pressure.

After the child's condition has been stabilized, oral doses of cortisone, fluids, and salt are given, similar to the regimen used for chronic adrenal insufficiency. To maintain sodium retention, aldosterone is replaced by synthetic salt-retaining steroids.

▌CARE MANAGEMENT

Because of the abrupt onset and potentially fatal outcome of this condition, prompt recognition is essential. Vital signs, including blood pressure, are taken every 15 minutes to monitor the hyperpyrexia and shocklike state. Seizure precautions are instituted because convulsions from the elevated temperature are not uncommon. As soon as therapy is instituted, the nurse should monitor the child's response to fluid and cortisol replacement. Whereas too rapid administration of fluids can precipitate cardiac failure, overdosage with cortisol produces hypotension and a sudden fall in temperature.

When the acute phase is over and the hypovolemia has been corrected, the child is given oral fluids, such as small quantities of ginger ale, fruit juice, or salted broth. Too rapid ingestion of oral fluids may induce vomiting, which increases dehydration. Therefore the nurse should plan a gradual schedule for reintroducing liquids.

> **! NURSING ALERT**
>
> Monitor serum electrolyte levels and observe for signs of hypokalemia or hyperkalemia (e.g., weakness, poor muscle control, paralysis, cardiac dysrhythmias, and apnea). The condition is rapidly corrected with IV or oral potassium replacement.

> **! NURSING ALERT**
>
> When an oral potassium preparation is given, it should be mixed with a small amount of strongly flavored fruit juice to disguise its bitter taste.

The sudden, severe nature of this disorder necessitates a great deal of emotional support for the child and family. The child may be placed in an intensive care unit where the surroundings are strange and frightening. Despite the need for emergency intervention, the nurse must be sensitive to the family's psychologic needs and prepare them for each procedure even if this is a brief statement such as "The IV infusion is necessary to replace fluid that your child is losing." Because recovery within 24 hours is often dramatic, the nurse should keep the parents apprised of the child's condition, emphasizing signs of improvement such as a lowered temperature and improved blood pressure.

Chronic Adrenocortical Insufficiency (Addison Disease)

Chronic adrenocortical insufficiency is rare in children. Causes include infections, destructive lesion of the adrenal gland or neoplasms, autoimmune processes, or idiopathic. Formerly, generalized tuberculosis was the leading cause of adrenal gland destruction.

Evidence of this disorder is usually gradual in onset because 90% of adrenal tissue must be nonfunctional before signs of insufficiency are manifested. However, during periods of stress, when demands for additional cortisol are increased, symptoms of acute insufficiency may appear in a previously well child (Box 46-11).

Definitive diagnosis is based on measurements of functional cortisol reserve. The fasting serum cortisol and urinary 17-hydroxycorticosteroid levels are low and fail to rise, and plasma adrenocorticotropic hormone (ACTH) levels are elevated with corticotropin (ACTH) stimulation, the definitive test for the disease.

Therapeutic Management

Treatment involves replacement of glucocorticoids (cortisol) and mineralocorticoids (aldosterone). Some children are able to be maintained solely on oral supplements of cortisol (cortisone or hydrocortisone preparations) with a liberal intake of salt. During

> ### BOX 46-11   CLINICAL MANIFESTATIONS OF CHRONIC ADRENOCORTICAL INSUFFICIENCY
>
> **Neurologic Symptoms**
> - Muscular weakness
> - Mental fatigue
> - Irritability, apathy, and negativism
> - Increased sleeping, listlessness
>
> **Pigmentary Changes**
> - Previous scars
> - Palmar creases
> - Mucous membranes
> - Hair
> - Hyperpigmentation over pressure points (elbows, knees, or waist)
> - Less frequently, vitiligo (loss of pigmentation)
>
> **Gastrointestinal Symptoms**
> - Dehydration
> - Anorexia
> - Weight loss
>
> **Circulatory Symptoms**
> - Hypotension
> - Small heart size
> - Dizziness
> - Syncopal (fainting) attacks
>
> **Hypoglycemia**
> - Headache
> - Hunger
> - Weakness
> - Trembling
> - Sweating
>
> **Other Signs (Seen in Some Children)**
> - Recurrent, unexplained seizures
> - Intense craving for salt
> - Acute abdominal pain
> - Electrolyte imbalances

stressful situations, such as fever, infection, emotional upset, or surgery, the dosage must be tripled to accommodate the body's increased need for glucocorticoids. Failure to meet this requirement will precipitate an acute crisis. Overdosage produces appearance of cushingoid signs.

Children with more severe states of chronic adrenal insufficiency require mineralocorticoid replacement to maintain fluid and electrolyte balance. Other forms of therapy include monthly injections of desoxycorticosterone acetate or implantation of desoxycorticosterone acetate pellets subcutaneously every 9 to 12 months.

CARE MANAGEMENT

After the disorder is diagnosed, parents need guidance concerning drug therapy. They must be aware of the continuous need for cortisol replacement. Sudden termination of the drug because of inadequate supplies or inability to ingest the oral form because of vomiting places the child in danger of an acute adrenal crisis. Therefore parents should always have a spare supply of the medication in the home. Ideally, they will have a prefilled syringe of hydrocortisone and be instructed in proper technique for intramuscular administration of the drug in case of crisis. Unnecessary administration of cortisone will not harm the child, but if it is needed, it may be lifesaving. Any evidence of acute insufficiency should be reported to the health care practitioner immediately.

Parents also need to be aware of side effects of the drugs. Undesirable side effects of cortisone include gastric irritation, which is minimized by ingestion with food or the use of an antacid; increased excitability and sleeplessness; weight gain, which may require dietary management to prevent obesity; and, rarely, behavioral changes,

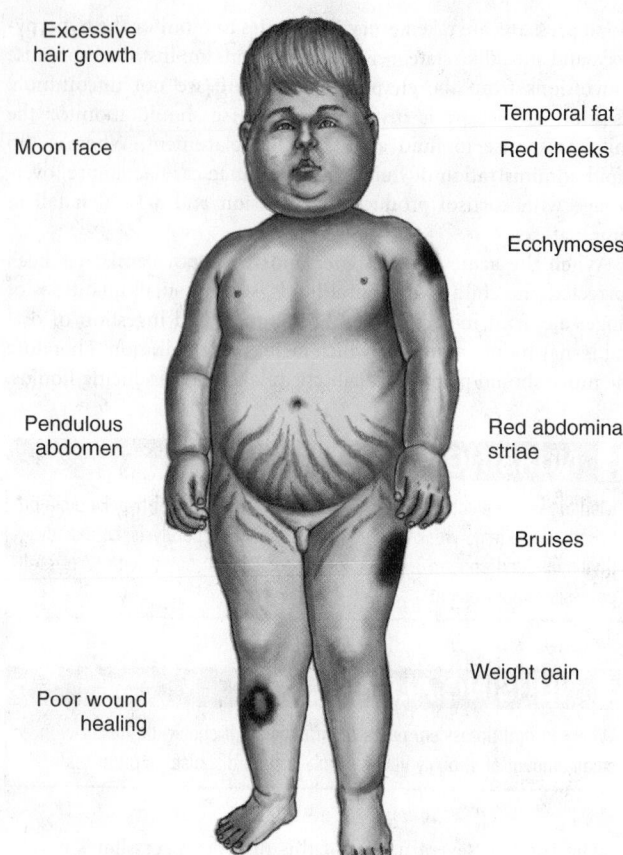

FIG 46-2 Characteristics of Cushing syndrome.

Labels: Excessive hair growth · Moon face · Pendulous abdomen · Poor wound healing · Temporal fat · Red cheeks · Ecchymoses · Red abdominal striae · Bruises · Weight gain

BOX 46-12 · ETIOLOGY OF CUSHING SYNDROME

Pituitary—Cushing syndrome with adrenal hyperplasia, usually attributed to an excess of ACTH

Adrenal—Cushing syndrome with hypersecretion of glucocorticoids, generally a result of adrenocortical neoplasms

Ectopic—Cushing syndrome with autonomous secretion of ACTH, most often caused by extrapituitary neoplasms

Iatrogenic—Cushing syndrome frequently a result of administration of large amounts of exogenous corticosteroids

Food dependent—Inappropriate sensitivity of adrenal glands to normal postprandial increases in secretion of gastric inhibitory polypeptide

Adapted from Magiakou MA, Mastorakos G, Oldfield EH, et al: Cushing's syndrome in children and adolescents: presentation, diagnosis, and therapy, *N Engl J Med* 331(10):629–636, 1994. *ACTH*, Adrenocorticotropic hormone.

including depression or euphoria. Parents should be aware of signs of overdose and report these to the health care practitioner. In addition, the drug has a bitter taste, which creates a challenge for nurses and parents in its administration.

Because the body cannot supply endogenous sources of cortical hormones during times of stress, the home environment should be stable and relatively free of stress. Parents need to be aware that during periods of emotional or physical crisis, the child requires additional hormone replacement. The child should wear medical identification, such as a bracelet, to permit medical personnel to adjust requirements during emergency care.

Cushing Syndrome

Cushing syndrome is a characteristic group of manifestations caused by excessive circulating free cortisol. It can result from a variety of causes, which generally fall into one of five categories (Box 46-12). Cushing syndrome in young children may be caused by an adrenal tumor (Moshang, 2003).

Cushing syndrome is uncommon in children. When seen, it is often caused by excessive or prolonged steroid therapy that produces a cushingoid appearance (Fig. 46-2). This condition is reversible after the steroids are gradually discontinued. Abrupt withdrawal will precipitate acute adrenal insufficiency. Gradual withdrawal of exogenous supplies is necessary to allow the anterior pituitary an opportunity to secrete increasing amounts of ACTH to stimulate the adrenals to produce cortisol.

Clinical Manifestations

Because the actions of cortisol are widespread, clinical manifestations are equally profound and diverse. The symptoms that produce changes in physical appearance occur early in the disorder and are of considerable concern to school-age and older children. The physiologic disturbances, such as hyperglycemia, susceptibility to infection, hypertension, and hypokalemia, may have life-threatening consequences unless recognized early and treated successfully. Children with short stature may be responding to increased cortisol levels, resulting in Cushing syndrome. Cortisol inhibits the action of GH.

Diagnostic Evaluation

Several tests are helpful in confirming excess Cushing syndrome. Serum cortisol levels should be measured at midnight and in the morning along with corticotropin hormone, urinary free cortisol,

fasting blood glucose levels for hyperglycemia, serum electrolyte levels for hypokalemia and alkalosis, and 24-hour urinary levels of elevated 17-hydroxycorticoids and 17-ketosteroids. Imaging of the pituitary and adrenal glands to assess for tumors, bone density studies for evidence of osteoporosis, and skull radiographs to determine enlargement of the sella turcica may also aid in the diagnosis. Another procedure used to establish a more definitive diagnosis is the dexamethasone (cortisone) suppression test (Nieman and Ilias, 2005). Administration of an exogenous supply of cortisone normally suppresses ACTH production. However, in individuals with Cushing syndrome, cortisol levels remain elevated. This test is helpful in differentiating between children who are obese and those who appear to have cushingoid features.

Therapeutic Management

Treatment depends on the cause. In most cases, surgical intervention involves bilateral adrenalectomy and postoperative replacement of the cortical hormones (the therapy for this is the same as that outlined for chronic adrenal insufficiency). If a pituitary tumor is found, surgical extirpation or irradiation may be chosen. In either of these instances, treatment of panhypopituitarism with replacement of GH, thyroid extract, ADH, gonadotropins, and steroids may be necessary for an indefinite period (Nieman and Ilias, 2005).

CARE MANAGEMENT

Nursing care also depends on the cause. When cushingoid features are caused by steroid therapy, the effects may be lessened with administration of the drug early in the morning and on an alternate-day basis. Giving the drug early in the day maintains the normal diurnal pattern of cortisol secretion. If given during the evening, it is more likely to produce symptoms because endogenous cortisol levels are already low and the additional supply exerts more pronounced effects. An alternate-day schedule allows the anterior pituitary an opportunity to maintain more normal hypothalamic-pituitary-adrenal control mechanisms.

If an organic cause is found, nursing care is related to the treatment regimen. Although a bilateral adrenalectomy permanently solves one condition, it reciprocally produces another syndrome. Before surgery, parents need to be adequately informed of the operative benefits and disadvantages. Postoperative teaching regarding drug replacement is the same as discussed in the previous section.

> **! NURSING ALERT**
>
> Postoperative complications of adrenalectomy are related to the sudden withdrawal of cortisol. Observe for shocklike symptoms (e.g., hypotension, hyperpyrexia).

Anorexia and nausea and vomiting are common and may be improved with the use of nasogastric decompression. Muscle and joint pain may be severe, requiring use of analgesics. The psychologic depression can be profound and may not improve for months. Parents should be aware of the physiologic reasons behind these symptoms in order to be supportive of the child.

Congenital Adrenal Hyperplasia

Congenital adrenal hyperplasia (CAH) is a family of disorders caused by decreased enzyme activity required for cortisol production in the adrenal cortex. The adrenal gland produces excessive amounts of cortisol precursors and androgens to compensate. The most common defect is 21-hydroxylase deficiency, which constitutes more than 90% of all cases of CAH (AAP, 2000). This deficiency is an autosomal recessive disorder that results in improper steroid hormone synthesis. It occurs in approximately 1 in 12,000 to 15,000 births and can be life threatening in its most severe form (Glatt, Garzon, and Popovic, 2005).

Excessive androgens cause masculinization of the urogenital system at approximately the tenth week of fetal development. The most pronounced abnormalities occur in girls, who are born with varying degrees of ambiguous genitalia. Masculinization of external genitalia causes the clitoris to enlarge so that it appears as a small phallus. Fusion of the labia produces a saclike structure resembling the scrotum without testes. However, no abnormal changes occur in the internal sexual organs, although the vaginal orifice is usually closed by the fused labia. The label *ambiguous genitalia* should be applied to any infant with hypospadias or micropenis and no palpable gonads, and a diagnostic evaluation for CAH should be contemplated. Males do not display genital abnormalities at birth (New and Ghizzoni, 2003).

Increased pigmentation of skin creases and genitalia caused by increased ACTH may be a subtle sign of adrenal insufficiency. A salt-wasting crisis frequently occurs, usually within the first few weeks of life (Kliegman, Stanton, St. Geme, et al., 2011). Infants fail to gain weight, and hyponatremia and hyperkalemia may be significant. Cardiac arrest can occur.

Untreated CAH results in early sexual maturation, with enlargement of the external sexual organs; development of axillary, pubic, and facial hair; deepening of the voice; acne; and a marked increase in musculature with changes toward an adult male physique.

However, in contrast to precocious puberty, breasts do not develop in girls and they remain amenorrheic and infertile. In boys, the testes remain small and spermatogenesis does not occur. In both sexes, linear growth is accelerated and epiphyseal closure is premature, resulting in short stature by the end of puberty.

Diagnostic Evaluation

Clinical diagnosis is initially based on congenital abnormalities that lead to difficulty in assigning sex to the newborn and on signs and symptoms of adrenal insufficiency. Newborn screening is currently done in all 50 U.S. states by measurement of the cortisol precursor *17-hydroxyprogesterone*. Definitive diagnosis is confirmed by evidence of increased 17-ketosteroid levels in most types of CAH (AAP, 2000). In complete 21-hydroxylase deficiency, blood electrolytes demonstrate loss of sodium and chloride and elevation of potassium. In older children, bone age is advanced and linear growth is increased. DNA analysis for positive sex determination and to rule out any other genetic abnormality (e.g., Turner syndrome) is always done in any case of ambiguous genitalia.

Another test that can be used to visualize the presence of pelvic structures is ultrasonography, a noninvasive, painless imaging technique that does not require anesthesia or sedation. It is especially useful in CAH because it readily identifies the absence or presence of female reproductive organs or male testes in a newborn or child with ambiguous genitalia. Because ultrasonography yields immediate results, it has the advantage of determining the child's sex long before the more complex laboratory results for chromosome analysis or steroid levels are available.

Therapeutic Management

After diagnosis is confirmed, medical management includes administration of glucocorticoids to suppress the abnormally high secretions of ACTH and adrenal androgens (Glatt, Garzon, and Popovic, 2005). If cortisone is begun early enough, it is very effective. Cortisone depresses the secretion of ACTH by the adenohypophysis, which in turn inhibits the secretion of adrenocorticosteroids, which stems the progressive virilization. The signs and symptoms of masculinization in girls gradually disappear, and excessive early linear growth is slowed. Puberty occurs normally at the appropriate age.

The recommended oral dosage is divided to simulate the normal diurnal pattern of ACTH secretion. Because these children are unable to produce cortisol in response to stress, it is necessary to increase the dosage during episodes of infection, fever, surgery, or other stresses. Acute emergencies require immediate IV or intramuscular administration. Children with the salt-losing type of CAH require aldosterone replacement, as outlined in the discussion of chronic adrenal insufficiency, and supplementary dietary salt. Frequent laboratory tests are conducted to assess the effects on electrolytes, hormonal profiles, and renin levels. The frequency of testing is individualized to the child.

Gender assignment and surgical intervention in the newborn with ambiguous genitalia is complex and controversial. It is a significant stress for families, who need support from a multidisciplinary team of experienced specialists. Factors that influence gender assignment include genetic diagnosis, genitalia appearance, surgical options, fertility, and family and cultural preferences. Generally, genetically female (46,XX) infants should be raised as girls. Early reconstructive surgery should be considered only in the case of severe virilization (Lee, Houk, Ahmed, et al., 2006). Emphasis is on functional rather than cosmetic outcomes, and surgery can often be delayed. Reports concerning sexual satisfaction after partial clitoridectomy indicate that the capacity for orgasm and sexual gratification is not necessarily impaired. Male infants may require phallic reconstruction by an experienced surgeon.

Unfortunately, not all children with CAH are diagnosed at birth and raised in accordance with their genetic sex. Particularly in the case of affected females, masculinization of the external genitalia may have led to gender assignment as a male. In males, diagnosis is usually delayed until early childhood, when signs of virilism appear. In these situations, it is advisable to continue rearing the child as a male in accordance with assigned gender and phenotype. Hormone replacement may be required to permit linear growth and to initiate male pubertal changes. Surgery is usually indicated to remove the female organs and reconstruct the phallus for satisfactory sexual relations. These individuals are not fertile.

CARE MANAGEMENT

Of major importance is recognition of ambiguous genitalia and diagnostic confirmation in newborns. Parents need assistance in understanding and accepting the condition and time to grieve for the loss of perfection in their newborn child. As soon as the gender is determined, parents should be informed of the findings and encouraged to choose an appropriate name, and the child should be identified as a male or female with no reference to ambiguous gender.

In general, rearing a genetically female child as a girl is preferred because of the success of surgical intervention and the satisfactory results with hormones in reversing virilism and providing a prospect of normal puberty and the ability to conceive. This is in contrast to the choice of rearing the child as a boy, in which case the child is sterile and may never be able to function satisfactorily in heterosexual relationships. If the parents persist in their decision to assign a male gender to a genetically female child, a psychologic consultation should be requested to explore their motivations and ensure their understanding of the future consequences for the child.

Nursing care management regarding cortisol and aldosterone replacement are the same as those discussed for chronic adrenocortical insufficiency. Because infants are especially prone to dehydration and salt-losing crises, parents need to be aware of signs of dehydration and the urgency of immediate medical intervention to stabilize the child's condition. Parents should have injectable hydrocortisone available and know how to prepare and administer the intramuscular injection (see Chapter 39).

In the unfortunate situation in which the gender is erroneously assigned and the correct gender determined later, parents need a great deal of help in understanding the reason for the incorrect gender identification and the options for gender reassignment or medical-surgical intervention.

Parents should be referred for genetic counseling before they conceive another child because CAH is an autosomal recessive disorder. Prenatal diagnosis and treatment are available.

> ⚠ **NURSING ALERT**
>
> The parents should be advised that there is no physical harm in treating for suspected adrenal insufficiency that is not present, but the consequence of not treating acute adrenal insufficiency can be fatal.

Pheochromocytoma

Pheochromocytoma is a rare tumor characterized by secretion of catecholamines. The tumor most commonly arises from the chromaffin cells of the adrenal medulla but may occur wherever these cells are found, such as along the paraganglia of the aorta or thoracolumbar sympathetic chain (Pacak, Eisenhofer, Ahlman, et al., 2007). Approximately 10% of these tumors are located in extraadrenal sites. In children, they are frequently bilateral or multiple and are generally benign. Often there is a familial transmission of the condition as an autosomal dominant trait (Kliegman, Stanton, St. Geme, et al., 2011).

The clinical manifestations of pheochromocytoma are caused by an increased production of catecholamines, producing hypertension, tachycardia, headache, decreased gastrointestinal activity with resultant constipation, increased metabolism with anorexia, weight loss, hyperglycemia, polyuria, polydipsia, hyperventilation, nervousness, heat intolerance, and diaphoresis. In severe cases, signs of congestive heart failure are evident.

Diagnostic Evaluation

The clinical manifestations mimic those of other disorders, such as hyperthyroidism or DM. Usually the tumor is identified by computed tomography (CT) scan or magnetic resonance imaging (MRI). Definitive tests include 24-hour measurement of urinary levels of the catecholamine metabolites, histamine stimulation, and α-adrenergic blocking agents.

Therapeutic Management

Definitive treatment consists of surgical removal of the tumor. In children, the tumors may be bilateral, requiring a bilateral adrenalectomy and lifelong glucocorticoid and mineralocorticoid therapy. The major complications that can occur during surgery are severe hypertension, tachydysrhythmias, and hypotension. The first two are caused by excessive release of catecholamines during manipulation of the tumor, and the latter results from catecholamine withdrawal and hypovolemic shock.

Preoperative medication to inhibit the effects of catecholamines is begun 1 to 3 weeks before surgery to prevent these complications. The major group of drugs used is the α-adrenergic blocking agents with or without β-adrenergic blocking agents. The most commonly used β-adrenergic blocker is phenoxybenzamine (Dibenzyline), a long-acting medication given orally every 12 hours. The shorter-acting phentolamine (Regitine) is equally effective but less satisfactory for long-term use, although it is useful for acute hypertension. The importance of meticulous preoperative conditioning with alpha-blockers cannot be overemphasized. This intervention is largely responsible for the improvement in outcomes. In select cases, beta-blockers (medications that slow the heart rate) may be added after adequate alpha-blockade has been established.

Success of therapy is judged by lowering of blood pressure to normal, absence of hypertensive attacks (flushing or blanching, fainting, headache, palpitations, tachycardia, nausea and vomiting, profuse sweating), heat tolerance, a decrease in perspiration, and disappearance of hyperglycemia. A disadvantage of these drugs is their inability to block the effects of catecholamines on beta receptors.

CARE MANAGEMENT

An initial nursing objective is identification of children with this disorder. Outstanding clues are hypertension and hypertensive attacks. Because of behavioral changes (nervousness, excitability, overactivity, and even psychosis), increased cardiac and respiratory activity may appear to be related to an acute anxiety attack. Therefore a careful history of the onset of symptoms and association with stressful events is helpful in distinguishing between an organic and a psychologic cause for the symptoms.

Preoperative nursing care involves frequent monitoring of vital signs and observation for evidence of hypertensive attacks and congestive heart failure. Therapeutic effects are evidenced by normal vital signs and absence of glycosuria. Daily blood glucose levels, urine acetone, and any signs of hyperglycemia are noted and reported immediately.

> **! NURSING ALERT**
>
> Do not palpate the mass. Preoperative palpation of the mass releases catecholamines, which can stimulate severe hypertension and tachydysrhythmias.

The environment is made conducive to rest and free of emotional stress. This requires adequate preparation during hospital admission and before surgery. Parents are encouraged to room-in with their child and to participate in care. Play activities need to be tailored to the child's energy level without being overly strenuous or challenging because these can increase metabolic rate and promote frustration and anxiety.

After surgery, the child is observed for signs of shock from removal of excess catecholamines. If a bilateral adrenalectomy was performed, the nursing interventions are those discussed for chronic adrenocortical insufficiency.

DISORDERS OF PANCREATIC HORMONE SECRETION

Diabetes Mellitus

Diabetes mellitus is a chronic disorder of metabolism characterized by a partial or complete deficiency of the hormone insulin. It is the most common metabolic disease, resulting in metabolic adjustment or physiologic change in almost all areas of the body. In the United States, approximately 215,000 individuals younger than 20 years have either type 1 or type 2 diabetes (Centers for Disease Control and Prevention [CDC], 2012). The odds are higher for African-American and Hispanic children—nearly 50% of them will develop diabetes (Urrutia-Rojas and Menchaca, 2006). DM in children can occur at any age but has a peak incidence between ages 10 and 15 years, with 75% diagnosed before 18 years of age. The incidence in boys is slightly higher than in girls (1:1 to 1.2:1).

Traditionally, DM had been classified according to the type of treatment needed. The former categories were insulin-dependent diabetes mellitus (IDDM), or type I, and non–insulin-dependent diabetes mellitus (NIDDM), or type II. In 1997, these terms were eliminated because treatment can vary (some people with NIDDM require insulin) and because the terms do not indicate the underlying problem. The new terms are *type 1* and *type 2,* using Arabic symbols to avoid confusion (e.g., *type II* could be read as *type eleven*) (American Diabetes Association, 2001). The characteristics of type 1 DM and type 2 DM are outlined in Table 46-1.

In the age-group younger than 10 years, most diabetes cases are type 1 and occur most frequently in non-Hispanic whites. In the age-group 10 to 19 years, type 1 diabetes is more prominent in non-Hispanic whites followed by African-Americans and then Hispanics; the lowest prevalence is among Native Americans. In type 2 diabetes, Native Americans have the highest incidence followed by African-Americans, Asian Pacific individuals, and Hispanics; the lowest

prevalence is in non-Hispanic whites (CDC, 2011). The Pima Indian Tribe reports a greater than 51% incidence of type 2 DM.

Type 1 diabetes is characterized by destruction of the pancreatic β cells, which produce insulin; this usually leads to absolute insulin deficiency. Type 1 diabetes has two forms. Immune-mediated DM results from an autoimmune destruction of the β cells; it typically starts in children or young adults who are slim, but it can arise in adults of any age. Idiopathic type 1 refers to rare forms of the disease that have no known cause.

Type 2 diabetes usually arises because of insulin resistance in which the body fails to use insulin properly combined with relative (rather than absolute) insulin deficiency. People with type 2 can range from predominantly insulin resistant with relative insulin deficiency to predominantly deficient in insulin secretion with some insulin resistance. It typically occurs in those who are older that 45

TABLE 46-1	CHARACTERISTICS OF TYPE 1 AND TYPE 2 DIABETES MELLITUS	
CHARACTERISTIC	**TYPE 1**	**TYPE 2**
Age at onset	<20 years	Increasingly occurring in younger children
Type of onset	Abrupt	Gradual
Sex ratio	Affects males slightly more than females	Females outnumber males
Percentage of diabetic population	5%-8%	85%-90%
Heredity:		
Family history	Sometimes	Frequently
Human leukocyte antigen	Associations	No association
Twin concordance	25%-50%	90%-100%
Ethnic distribution	Primarily Caucasians	Increased incidence in Native Americans, Hispanics, African-Americans
Presenting symptoms	3 P's common: polyuria, polydipsia, polyphagia	May be related to long-term complications
Nutritional status	Underweight	Overweight
Insulin (natural):		
Pancreatic content	Usually none	>50% normal
Serum insulin	Low to absent	High or low
Primary resistance	Minimum	Marked
Islet cell antibodies	80%-85%	<5%
Therapy:		
Insulin	Always	20%-30% of patients
Oral agents	Ineffective	Often effective
Diet only	Ineffective	Often effective
Chronic complications	>80%	Variable
Ketoacidosis	Common	Infrequent

BOX 46-13	**CLINICAL MANIFESTATIONS OF TYPE 1 DIABETES MELLITUS**

- Polyphagia
- Polyuria
- Polydipsia
- Weight loss
- Enuresis or nocturia
- Irritability; "not himself" or "herself"
- Shortened attention span
- Lowered frustration tolerance
- Dry skin
- Blurred vision
- Poor wound healing
- Fatigue
- Flushed skin
- Headache
- Frequent infections
- Hyperglycemia:
  - Elevated blood glucose levels
  - Glucosuria
- Diabetic ketosis:
  - Ketones and glucose in urine
  - Dehydration in some cases
- Diabetic ketoacidosis:
  - Dehydration
  - Electrolyte imbalance
  - Acidosis
  - Deep, rapid breathing (Kussmaul respirations)

years, are overweight and sedentary, and have a family history of diabetes.

The symptomatology of diabetes is more readily recognizable in children than in adults, so it is surprising that the diagnosis may sometimes be missed or delayed. Diabetes is a great imitator; influenza, gastroenteritis, and appendicitis are the conditions most often diagnosed when it turns out that the disease is really diabetes (Box 46-13).

Pathophysiology

Insulin is needed to support the metabolism of carbohydrates, fats, and proteins, primarily by facilitating the entry of these substances into the cells. Insulin is needed for the entry of glucose into the muscle and fat cells, prevention of mobilization of fats from fat cells, and storage of glucose as glycogen in the cells of liver and muscle. Insulin is not needed for the entry of glucose into nerve cells or vascular tissue. The chemical composition and molecular structure of insulin are such that it fits into receptor sites on the cell membrane. Here it initiates a sequence of poorly defined chemical reactions that alter the cell membrane to facilitate the entry of glucose into the cell and stimulate enzymatic systems outside the cell that metabolize the glucose for energy production.

With a deficiency of insulin, glucose is unable to enter the cells and its concentration in the bloodstream increases. The increased concentration of glucose (hyperglycemia) produces an osmotic gradient that causes the movement of body fluid from the intracellular space to the interstitial space and then to the extracellular space and into the glomerular filtrate to "dilute" the hyperosmolar filtrate. Normally, the renal tubular capacity to transport glucose is adequate to reabsorb all the glucose in the glomerular filtrate. When the glucose concentration in the glomerular filtrate exceeds the renal threshold (≤ 180 mg/dL), glucose spills into the urine (glycosuria) along with an osmotic diversion of water (polyuria), a cardinal sign of diabetes. The urinary fluid losses cause the excessive thirst (polydipsia) observed in diabetes. This water "washout" results in a depletion of other essential chemicals, especially potassium.

Protein is also wasted during insulin deficiency. Because glucose is unable to enter the cells, protein is broken down and converted to glucose by the liver (glucogenesis); this glucose then contributes to the hyperglycemia. These mechanisms are similar to those seen in starvation when substrate (glucose) is absent. The body is actually in a state of starvation during insulin deficiency. Without the use of carbohydrates for energy, fat and protein stores are depleted as the body attempts to meet its energy needs. The hunger mechanism is triggered, but increased food intake (polyphagia) enhances the problem by further elevating blood glucose.

Ketoacidosis. When insulin is absent or insulin sensitivity is altered, glucose is unavailable for cellular metabolism and the body chooses alternate sources of energy, principally fat. Consequently, fats break down into fatty acids and glycerol in the fat cells is converted by the liver to ketone bodies (β-hydroxybutyric acid, acetoacetic acid, acetone). Any excess is eliminated in the urine (ketonuria) or the lungs (acetone breath). The ketone bodies in the blood (ketonemia) are strong acids that lower serum pH, producing ketoacidosis.

Ketones are organic acids that readily produce excessive quantities of free hydrogen ions, causing a fall in plasma pH. Then chemical buffers in the plasma, principally bicarbonate, combine with the hydrogen ions to form carbonic acid, which readily dissociates into water and carbon dioxide. The respiratory system attempts to eliminate the excess carbon dioxide by increased depth and rate (Kussmaul respirations, or the hyperventilation characteristic of metabolic acidosis). The ketones are buffered by sodium and potassium in the plasma. The kidneys attempt to compensate for the increased pH by increasing tubular secretion of hydrogen and ammonium ions in exchange for fixed base, thus depleting the base buffer concentration.

With cellular death, potassium is released from the cells (intracellular fluid) into the bloodstream (extracellular fluid) and excreted by the kidneys, where the loss is accelerated by osmotic diuresis. The total body potassium is then decreased even though the serum potassium level may be elevated as a result of the decreased fluid volume in which it circulates. Alteration in serum and tissue potassium can lead to cardiac arrest.

If these conditions are not reversed by insulin therapy in combination with correction of the fluid deficiency and electrolyte imbalance, progressive deterioration occurs, with dehydration, electrolyte imbalance, acidosis, coma, and death. Diabetic ketoacidosis (DKA) should be diagnosed promptly in a seriously ill patient and therapy instituted in an intensive care unit.

Long-Term Complications. Long-term complications of diabetes involve both the microvasculature and the macrovasculature. The principal microvascular complications are nephropathy, retinopathy, and neuropathy. Microvascular disease develops during the first 30 years of diabetes, beginning in the first 10 to 15 years after puberty, with renal involvement evidenced by proteinuria and clinically apparent retinopathy. Macrovascular disease develops after 25 years of diabetes and creates the predominant problems in patients with type 2 DM. The process appears to be one of glycosylation, wherein proteins from the blood become deposited in the walls of small vessels (e.g., glomeruli), where they become trapped by "sticky" glucose compounds (glycosyl radicals). The buildup of these substances over time causes narrowing of the vessels, with subsequent interference with microcirculation to the affected areas (Rosenson and Herman, 2008).

With poor diabetic control, vascular changes can appear as early as $2\frac{1}{2}$ to 3 years after diagnosis; however, with good to excellent control, changes can be postponed for 20 or more years. Intensive insulin therapy appears to delay the onset and slow the progression of retinopathy, nephropathy, and neuropathy. Hypertension and atherosclerotic cardiovascular disease are also major causes of morbidity and mortality in patients with DM (Karnik, Fields, and Shannon, 2007).

Other complications have been observed in children with type 1 DM. Hyperglycemia appears to influence thyroid function, and altered function is frequently observed at the time of diagnosis and in poorly controlled diabetes. Limited mobility of small joints of the hand occurs in 30% of 7- to 18-year-old children with type 1 DM and appears to be related to changes in the skin and soft tissues surrounding the joint as a result of glycosylation.

> **! NURSING ALERT**
>
> Recurrent vaginal and urinary tract infections, especially with *Candida albicans*, are often an early sign of type 2 DM, especially in adolescents.

Diagnostic Evaluation

Three groups of children who should be considered as candidates for diabetes are (1) children who have glycosuria, polyuria, and a history of weight loss or failure to gain despite a voracious appetite; (2) those with transient or persistent glycosuria; and (3) those who display manifestations of metabolic acidosis, with or without stupor or coma. In every case, diabetes must be considered if there is glycosuria, with or without ketonuria, and unexplained hyperglycemia.

Glycosuria by itself is not diagnostic of diabetes. Other sugars, such as galactose, can produce a positive result with certain test strips, and a mild degree of glycosuria can be caused by other conditions, such as infection, trauma, emotional or physical stress, hyperalimentation, and some renal or endocrine diseases.

An 8-hour fasting blood glucose level of 126 mg/dL or more, a random blood glucose value of 200 mg/dL or more accompanied by classic signs of diabetes, or an oral glucose tolerance test (OGTT) finding of 200 mg/dL or more in the 2-hour sample is almost certain to indicate diabetes (Silverstein, Klingensmith, Copeland, et al., 2005). Postprandial blood glucose determinations and the traditional OGTTs have yielded low detection rates in children and are not usually necessary for establishing a diagnosis. Serum insulin levels may be normal or moderately elevated at the onset of diabetes; delayed insulin response to glucose indicates impaired glucose tolerance.

Ketoacidosis must be differentiated from other causes of acidosis or coma, including hypoglycemia, uremia, gastroenteritis with metabolic acidosis, salicylate intoxication encephalitis, and other intracranial lesions. DKA is a state of relative insulin insufficiency and may include the presence of hyperglycemia (blood glucose level ≥200 mg/dL), ketonemia (strongly positive), acidosis (pH <7.30 and bicarbonate <15 mmol/L), glycosuria, and ketonuria (Wolsdorf, Craig, Daneman, et al., 2009). Tests used to determine glycosuria and ketonuria are the glucose oxidase tapes (Keto-Diastix).

Therapeutic Management

The management of the child with type 1 DM consists of a multidisciplinary approach involving the family; the child (when appropriate); and professionals, including a pediatric endocrinologist, diabetes nurse educator, nutritionist, and exercise physiologist. Often psychologic support from a mental health professional is also needed. Communication among the team members is essential and extends to other individuals in the child's life, such as teachers, school nurse, school guidance counselor, and coach.

The definitive treatment is replacement of insulin that the child is unable to produce. However, insulin needs are also affected by emotions, nutritional intake, activity, and other life events such as illnesses and puberty. The complexity of the disease and its management require that the child and family incorporate diabetes needs into their lifestyle. Medical and nutritional guidance are primary, but management also includes continuing diabetes education, family guidance, and emotional support.

Insulin Therapy. Insulin replacement is the cornerstone of management of type 1 DM. Insulin dosage is tailored to each child based on home blood glucose monitoring. The goal of insulin therapy is maintaining near-normal blood glucose values while avoiding too frequent episodes of hypoglycemia. The goals of treatment are to maintain near-normal glucose levels of less than 126 mg/dL and glycosylated hemoglobin (hemoglobin A_{1c}) of 7% or less (Hannon, Gungor, and Arslanian, 2006). Glycemic control decreases the likelihood of long-term complications in patients with DM (Petitti, Imperatore, Palla, et al., 2007). Insulin is administered as two or more injections per day or as continuous subcutaneous infusion using a portable insulin pump.

Healthy pancreatic cells secrete insulin at a low but steady basal rate with superimposed bursts of increased secretion that coincide with intake of nutrients. Consequently, insulin levels in the blood increase and decrease coincidentally with rises and falls in blood glucose levels. In addition, insulin is secreted directly into the portal circulation; therefore the liver, which is the major site of glucose disposal, receives the largest concentration of insulin. No matter which method of insulin replacement is used, this normal pattern cannot be duplicated. Subcutaneous injection results in absorption of the drug into the general circulation, thus reducing the concentrations of insulin to which the liver is exposed.

Insulin Preparations. Insulin is available in highly purified pork preparations and in human insulin biosynthesized by and extracted from bacterial or yeast cultures. Most clinicians suggest human insulin as the treatment of choice. Insulin is available in rapid-, intermediate-, and long-acting preparations, and all are packaged in the strength of 100 units/mL. Some insulins are available as premixed insulins, such as 70/30 and 50/50 ratios, the first number indicating the percentage of intermediate-acting insulin and the second number the percentage of rapid-acting insulin. The different types of insulin are found in Box 46-14.

> **! NURSING ALERT**
>
> The human insulins from various manufacturers may be interchangeable, but human insulin and pork insulin or pure pork insulin should never be substituted for one another.

Dosage. Conventional management has consisted of a twice-daily insulin regimen of a combination of rapid-acting and intermediate-acting insulin drawn up into the same syringe and injected before breakfast and before the evening meal. The amount of morning regular insulin is determined by patterns in the late morning and lunchtime blood glucose values. The morning intermediate-acting dosage is determined by patterns in the late afternoon and supper blood glucose values. Fasting blood glucose patterns at breakfast help determine the evening dose of intermediate-acting insulin, and the blood glucose patterns at bedtime help determine the evening dose of rapid-acting (regular) insulin. For some children, better morning glucose control is achieved by a later (bedtime) injection of intermediate-acting insulin.

Regular insulin is best administered at least 30 minutes before meals. This allows sufficient time for absorption and results in a significantly greater reduction in the postprandial rise in blood glucose than if the meal were eaten immediately after the insulin injection. Intensive therapy consists of multiple injections throughout the day with a once- or twice-daily dose of long-acting (Ultralente) insulin to simulate the basal insulin secretion and injections of rapid-acting insulin before each meal. A multiple daily injection program reduces microvascular complications of diabetes in young, healthy patients who have type 1 DM.

The precise dose of insulin needed cannot be predicted. Therefore the total dosage and percentage of regular- to intermediate-acting insulin should be determined empirically for each child. Usually 60% to 75% of the total daily dose is given before breakfast

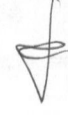

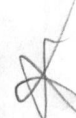

BOX 46-14   TYPES OF INSULIN

- There are four types of insulin, based on the following criteria:
  - How soon the insulin starts working (onset)
  - When the insulin works the hardest (peak time)
  - How long the insulin lasts in the body (duration)
- However, each person responds to insulin in his or her own way. That is why onset, peak time, and duration are given as ranges.

  Rapid-acting insulin (e.g., NovoLog) reaches the blood within 15 minutes after injection. The insulin peaks 30 to 90 minutes later and may last as long as 5 hours.

  Short-acting (regular) insulin (e.g., Novolin R) usually reaches the blood within 30 minutes after injection. The insulin peaks 2 to 4 hours later and stays in the blood for about 4 to 8 hours.

  Intermediate-acting insulins (e.g., Novolin N) reach the blood 2 to 6 hours after injection. The insulins peak 4 to 14 hours later and stay in the blood for about 14 to 20 hours.

  Long-acting insulin (e.g., Lantus) takes 6 to 14 hours to start working. It has no peak or a very small peak 10 to 16 hours after injection. The insulin stays in the blood between 20 and 24 hours.

- Some insulins come mixed together (e.g., Novolin 70/30). For example, you can buy regular insulin and NPH insulins already mixed in one bottle, which makes it easier to inject two kinds of insulin at the same time. However, you cannot adjust the amount of one insulin without also changing how much you get of the other insulin.

Adapted from American Diabetes Association: *Resource guide 2005*, www.diabetes.org/rg2005/insulin.jsp.
NPH, Neutral protamine Hagedorn.

---

and the remainder is given before the evening meal. Furthermore, insulin requirements do not remain constant but change continuously during growth and development; the need varies according to the child's activity level and pubertal status. For example, less insulin is required during spring and summer months when children are more active. Illness also alters insulin requirements. Some children require more frequent insulin administration. This includes children with difficult-to-control diabetes and children during the adolescent growth spurt.

Methods of Administration. Daily insulin is administered subcutaneously by twice-daily injections, by multiple-dose injections, or by means of an insulin infusion pump. The insulin pump is an electromechanical device designed to deliver fixed amounts of regular or lispro insulin continuously (basal rate), thereby more closely imitating the release of the hormone by the islet cells (Phillip, Battelino, Rodriguez, et al., 2007). Although the pump delivers a programmed amount of basal insulin, the child or parent must program a dose for the pump to deliver before each meal.

The system consists of a syringe to hold the insulin, a plunger, and a computerized mechanism to drive the plunger. The insulin flows from the syringe through a catheter to a needle inserted into subcutaneous tissue (the abdomen or thigh), and the lightweight device is worn on a belt or a shoulder holster. The needle and catheter are changed every 48 to 72 hours by the child or parent using aseptic technique and then taped in place.

Although the pump provides more consistent insulin delivery, it has certain disadvantages. Pump therapy is expensive and requires commitment from the parent and child. A certain level of math skills is required to calculate infusion rates. It should also not be removed for more than 1 hour at a time, which may limit some activities. Skin infections are common, and as with any other mechanical device, it is subject to malfunction. However, the pumps are equipped with alarms that signal problems, such as a depleted battery, an occluded needle or tubing, or a microprocessor malfunction.

Monitoring. Daily monitoring of blood glucose levels is an essential aspect of appropriate DM management. Plasma blood glucose and hemoglobin A_{1c} goal ranges are found in Table 46-2.

Blood Glucose. Self-monitoring of blood glucose (SMBG) has improved diabetes management and is used successfully by children from the onset of their diabetes. By testing their own blood, children are able to change their insulin regimen to maintain their glucose level in the euglycemic (normal) range of 80 to 120 mg/dL. Diabetes

---

TABLE 46-2   PLASMA BLOOD GLUCOSE AND HEMOGLOBIN A_{1c} GOALS FOR TYPE 1 DIABETES MELLITUS BY AGE-GROUP

AGE	VALUE* BEFORE MEALS (mg/dL)	VALUE* AT BEDTIME/ OVERNIGHT (mg/dL)	HEMOGLOBIN A_{1c} (%)	IMPLICATIONS
Toddlers and preschoolers (<6 years)	100-180	110-200	≤8.5% (but ≥7.5%)	High risk and vulnerability to hypoglycemia
School age (6-12 years)	90-180	100-180	<8%	Risks for hypoglycemia and relatively low risk for complications before puberty
Adolescents (>12 years) and young adults	90-130	90-150	<7.5%	Risk for hypoglycemia Developmental and psychologic issues

Adapted from American Diabetes Association: Standards of medical care in diabetes, *Diabetes Care* 28(Suppl):S4–36, 2005.
*Plasma blood glucose goal range.

management depends to a great extent on SMBG. In general, children tolerate the testing well.

Glycosylated Hemoglobin. The measurement of glycosylated hemoglobin (hemoglobin A_{1c}) levels is a satisfactory method for assessing control of the diabetes. As red blood cells circulate in the bloodstream, glucose molecules gradually attach to the hemoglobin A molecules and remain there for the lifetime of the red blood cell, approximately 120 days. The attachment is not reversible; therefore this glycosylated hemoglobin reflects the average blood glucose levels over the previous 2 to 3 months. The test is a satisfactory method for assessing control, detecting incorrect testing, monitoring the effectiveness of changes in treatment, defining patients' goals, and detecting nonadherence. Nondiabetic hemoglobin A_{1c} values are generally between 4% and 6% but can vary by laboratory. Diabetes control for children depends on age, with hemoglobin A_{1c} levels of 6.5% to 8% indicating a slightly elevated but acceptable range (Silverstein, Klingensmith, Copeland, et al., 2005). Hemoglobin A_{1c} levels of less than 7% are a well-established goal at most care centers.

Urine. Urine testing for glucose is no longer used for diabetes management; there is poor correlation between simultaneous glycosuria and blood glucose concentrations. However, urine testing can be carried out to detect evidence of ketonuria.

> **! NURSING ALERT**
>
> It is recommended that urine be tested for ketones every 3 hours during an illness or whenever the blood glucose level is over 240 mg/dL when illness is not present.

Nutrition. Essentially, the nutritional needs of children with diabetes are no different from those of healthy children. Children with diabetes need no special foods or supplements. They need sufficient calories to balance daily expenditure for energy and to satisfy the requirement for growth and development. Unlike children without diabetes, whose insulin is secreted in response to food intake, insulin injected subcutaneously has a relatively predictable time of onset, peak effect, duration of action, and absorption rate depending on the type of insulin used. Consequently, the timing of food consumption must be regulated to correspond to the timing and action of the insulin prescribed.

Meals and snacks must be eaten according to peak insulin action, and the total number of calories and proportions of basic nutrients must be consistent from day to day. The constant release of insulin into the circulation makes the child prone to hypoglycemia between the three daily meals unless a snack is provided between meals and at bedtime. The distribution of calories should be calculated to fit the activity pattern of each child. For example, a child who is more active in the afternoon will need a larger snack at that time. This larger snack might also be split to allow some food at school and some food after school. Food intake should be altered to balance food, insulin, and exercise. Extra food is needed for increased activity.

Concentrated sweets are discouraged, and because of the increased risk for atherosclerosis in persons with DM, fat is reduced to 30% or less of the total caloric requirement. Dietary fiber has become increasingly important in dietary planning because of its influence on digestion, absorption, and metabolism of many nutrients. It has been found to diminish the rise in blood glucose after meals.

For growing children, food restriction should never be used for diabetes control, although caloric restrictions may be imposed for weight control if the child is overweight. In general, the child's appetite should be the guide for the amount of calories needed, with the total caloric intake adjusted to appetite and activity.

Exercise. Exercise is encouraged and never restricted unless indicated by other health conditions. Exercise lowers blood glucose levels, depending on the intensity and duration of the activity. Consequently, exercise should be included as part of diabetes management, and the type and amount of exercise should be planned around the child's interests and capabilities. However, in most instances, children's activities are unplanned, and the resulting decrease in blood glucose can be compensated for by providing extra snacks before and, if the exercise is prolonged, during the activity. In addition to a feeling of well-being, regular exercise aids in utilization of food and often results in a reduction of insulin requirements.

Hypoglycemia. Occasional episodes of hypoglycemia are an integral part of insulin therapy, and an objective of diabetes management is to achieve the best possible glycemic control while minimizing the frequency and severity of hypoglycemia. Even with good control, a child may frequently experience mild symptoms of hypoglycemia. If the signs and symptoms are recognized early and promptly relieved by appropriate therapy, the child's activity should be interrupted for no more than a few minutes.

> **! NURSING ALERT**
>
> Hypoglycemic episodes most commonly occur before meals or when the insulin effect is peaking.

The signs and symptoms of hypoglycemia are caused by both increased adrenergic activity and impaired brain function. The increased adrenergic nervous system activity plus increased secretion of catecholamines produce nervousness, pallor, tremulousness, palpitations, sweating, and hunger (Cryer, 2008). Weakness, dizziness, headache, drowsiness, irritability, loss of coordination, seizures, and coma are more severe responses and reflect CNS glucose deprivation and the body's attempts to elevate the serum glucose levels.

It is often difficult to distinguish between hyperglycemia and a hypoglycemic reaction (Table 46-3). Because the symptoms are similar and usually begin with changes in behavior, the simplest way to differentiate between the two is to test the blood glucose level. The blood glucose level is low in hypoglycemia, but in hyperglycemia, the glucose level is significantly elevated. Urinary ketones may be present after hypoglycemia as a result of starvation ketone production. In doubtful situations, it is safer to give the child some simple carbohydrate. This will help alleviate the symptoms in the case of hypoglycemia but will do little harm if the child is hyperglycemic.

Children are usually able to detect the onset of hypoglycemia, but some are too young to implement treatment. Parents should become adept at recognizing the onset of symptoms—for example, a change in a child's behavior, such as tearfulness or euphoria. In the majority of cases, 10 to 15 g of simple carbohydrate, such as 1 Tbsp of table sugar, will elevate the blood glucose level and alleviate the symptoms. The simpler the carbohydrate, the more rapidly it will be absorbed (8 oz of milk equals 15 g of carbohydrate). The rapidly releasing sugar is followed by a complex carbohydrate such as a slice of bread or a cracker and by a protein such as peanut butter or milk.

For a mild reaction, milk or fruit juice is a good food to use in children. Milk supplies them with lactose or milk sugar, as well as a

TABLE 46-3	COMPARISON OF MANIFESTATIONS OF HYPOGLYCEMIA AND HYPERGLYCEMIA	
VARIABLE	**HYPOGLYCEMIA**	**HYPERGLYCEMIA**
Onset	Rapid (minutes)	Gradual (days)
Mood	Labile, irritable, nervous, weepy	Lethargic
Mental status	Difficulty concentrating, speaking, focusing, coordinating Nightmares	Dulled sensorium Confusion
Inward feeling	Shaky feeling Hunger Headache Dizziness	Thirst Weakness Nausea and vomiting Abdominal pain
Skin	Pallor Sweating	Flushed Signs of dehydration
Mucous membranes	Normal	Dry, crusty
Respirations	Shallow, normal	Deep, rapid (Kussmaul)
Pulse	Tachycardia, palpitations	Less rapid, weak
Breath odor	Normal	Fruity, acetone
Neurologic	Tremors	Diminished reflexes Paresthesia
Ominous signs	Late—Hyperreflexia, dilated pupils, seizure Shock, coma	Acidosis, coma
Blood:		
Glucose	Low: <60 mg/dL	High: ≥250 mg/dL
Ketones	Negative	High, large
Osmolarity	Normal	High
pH	Normal	Low (≤7.25)
Hematocrit	Normal	High
Bicarbonate	Normal	<20 mEq/L
Urine:		
Output	Normal	Polyuria (early) to oliguria (late)
Glucose	Negative	Enuresis, nocturia
Ketones	Negative or trace	High
Vision	Diplopia	Blurred vision

more prolonged action from the protein and fat (aids in decreased absorption). Other glucose sources include Insta-Glucose (cherry-flavored glucose), carbonated drinks (not sugarless), sherbet, gelatin, or cake icing. All children with diabetes should carry with them glucose tabs, Insta-Glucose, sugar cubes, or sugar-containing candy such as LifeSavers or Charms. A difficulty with candies or icing is that the child may learn to fake a reaction to get the sweets; therefore commercial treatment products such as Insta-Glucose or glucose tabs may be preferred.

Glucagon is sometimes prescribed for home treatment of hypoglycemia. It is available as an emergency kit that must be mixed at the time of use and is administered intramuscularly or subcutaneously. Glucagon functions by releasing stored glycogen from the liver and requires about 15 to 20 minutes to elevate the blood glucose level.

> **! NURSING ALERT**
>
> Vomiting may occur after administration of glucagon; therefore precautions against aspiration must be taken (e.g., placing the child on the side) because the child often becomes unconscious.

When the child is responsive, the lost glycogen stores are replaced by small amounts of sugar-containing fluid administered frequently until the child feels comfortable trying solid foods.

Morning Hyperglycemia. The management of elevated morning blood glucose levels depends on whether the increase is a true dawn phenomenon (insulin waning), or a rebound hyperglycemia (the Somogyi effect). Insulin waning is a progressive rise in blood glucose levels from bedtime to morning. It is treated by increasing the nocturnal insulin dose. The true dawn phenomenon shows relatively normal blood glucose level until about 3 AM, when the level begins to rise. The Somogyi effect may occur at any time but often entails an elevated blood glucose level at bedtime and a drop at 2 AM with a rebound rise following. The treatment for this phenomenon is decreasing the nocturnal insulin dose to prevent the 2 AM hypoglycemia. The rebound rise in the blood glucose level is a result of counterregulatory hormones (epinephrine, GH, and corticosteroids), which are stimulated by hypoglycemia. More frequent blood monitoring (especially at times of anticipated peak insulin action) will usually identify these conditions. Trace amounts of urinary ketones aid in identifying undetected hypoglycemia.

Illness Management. Illness alters diabetes management, and maintaining control is usually related to the seriousness of the illness. In a well-controlled child, an illness will run its course as it does in unaffected children. The goals during an illness are to restore euglycemia, treat urinary ketones, and maintain hydration. Blood glucose levels and urinary ketones should be monitored every 3 hours. Some hyperglycemia and ketonuria are expected in most illnesses, even with diminished food intake, and are an indication for increased insulin. Insulin should never be omitted during an illness, although dosage requirements may increase, decrease, or remain unchanged, depending on the severity of the illness and the child's appetite. Often the child will need supplemental insulin between usual dose times. If the child vomits more than once, if blood glucose levels remain above 240 mg/dL, or if urinary ketones remain high, the health care practitioner should be notified. Simple carbohydrates may be substituted for carbohydrate-containing exchanges in the meal plan. Although insulin and diet are important tools in sick-day care, fluids are the most important intervention. Fluids must be encouraged to prevent dehydration and to flush out ketones.

Therapeutic Management of Diabetic Ketoacidosis

Diabetic ketoacidosis, the most complete state of insulin deficiency, is a life-threatening situation. Management consists of rapid assessment, adequate insulin to reduce the elevated blood glucose level, fluids to overcome dehydration, and electrolyte replacement (especially potassium).

Because DKA constitutes an emergency situation, the child should be admitted to an intensive care facility for management. The priority is to obtain a venous access for administration of fluids, electrolytes, and insulin. The child should be weighed, measured, and placed on a cardiac monitor. Blood glucose and ketone levels are determined at the bedside, and samples are obtained for laboratory measurement of glucose, electrolytes, BUN, arterial pH, Po_2, Pco_2, hemoglobin, hematocrit, white blood cell count and differential, calcium, and phosphorus.

Oxygen may be administered to patients who are cyanotic and in whom arterial oxygen is less than 80%. Gastric suction is applied to unconscious children to avoid the possibility of pulmonary aspiration. Antibiotics may be administered to febrile children after appropriate specimens are obtained for culture. A Foley catheter may or may not be inserted for urine samples and measurement. Unless the child is unconscious, a collection bag is usually sufficient for accurate assessments.

Fluid and Electrolyte Therapy. All patients with DKA experience dehydration (10% of total body weight in severe ketoacidosis) because of the osmotic diuresis, accompanied by depletion of electrolytes, sodium, potassium, chloride, phosphate, and magnesium. Serum pH and bicarbonate reflect the degree of acidosis. Prompt and adequate fluid therapy restores tissue perfusion and suppresses the elevated levels of stress hormones.

The initial hydrating solution is 0.9% saline solution. Traditionally, deficits have been replaced at a rate of 50% over the first 8 to 12 hours and the remaining 50% over the next 16 to 24 hours. Current trends suggest more cautious fluid management to reduce the risk for cerebral edema. The fluid deficit is replaced evenly over a period of 36 to 48 hours (Cooke and Plotnick, 2008).

> **! NURSING ALERT**
>
> Potassium must never be given until the serum potassium level is known to be normal or low and urinary voiding is observed. All maintenance IV fluids should include 20 to 40 mEq/L of potassium. Never give potassium as a rapid IV bolus, or cardiac arrest may result.

Serum potassium levels may be normal on admission, but after fluid and insulin administration, the rapid return of potassium to the cells can seriously deplete serum levels, with the attendant risk for cardiac dysrhythmias. As soon as the child has established renal function (is voiding at least 25 mL/hr) and insulin has been given, vigorous potassium replacement is implemented. The cardiac monitor is used as a guide to therapy, and configuration of T waves should be observed every 30 to 60 minutes to determine changes that might indicate alterations in potassium concentration (widening of the QT interval and the appearance of a U wave following a flattened T wave indicate hypokalemia; an elevated and spreading T wave and shortening of the QT interval indicate hyperkalemia).

Insulin should not be given until urinary ketones and a blood glucose level have been obtained. Continuous IV regular insulin is given at a dosage of 0.1 units/kg/hr. Insulin therapy should be started after the initial rehydration bolus because serum glucose levels fall rapidly after volume expansion. Blood glucose levels should decrease by 50 to 100 mg/dL/hr. When blood glucose levels fall to 250 to 300 mg/dL, dextrose is added to the IV solution. The goal is to maintain blood glucose levels between 120 and 240 mg/dL by adding 5% to 10% dextrose. Sodium bicarbonate is used conservatively; it is used for pH less than 7.0, severe hyperkalemia, or cardiac instability. Because sodium bicarbonate has been associated with an increased risk for cerebral edema, children receiving this substance must be carefully monitored for changes in level of consciousness (Brown, 2004).

When the critical period is over, the task of regulating the insulin dosage in relation to diet and activity is started. Children should be actively involved in their own care and are given responsibility according to their ability and the guidance of the nurse.

> **! NURSING ALERT**
>
> Because insulin can chemically bind to plastic tubing and in-line filters, thereby reducing the amount of medication reaching the systemic circulation, an insulin mixture is run through the tubing to saturate the insulin-binding sites before the infusion is started.

CARE MANAGEMENT

Children with DM may be admitted to the hospital at the time of their initial diagnosis; during illness or surgery; or for episodes of ketoacidosis, which may be precipitated by any of a variety of factors. Many children are able to keep the disease under control with periodic assessment and adjustment of insulin, diet, and activity as needed under the supervision of a health care practitioner. Under most circumstances, these children can be managed well at home and require hospitalization only for serious illnesses or upsets.

However, a small number of children with diabetes exhibit a degree of metabolic lability and have repeated episodes of DKA that require hospitalization, which interferes with their education and social development. These children appear to display a characteristic personality structure. They tend to be unusually passive and nonassertive and to come from families that are inclined to smooth over conflicts without resolution. Children in this type of setting experience emotional arousal with little, if any, opportunity or ability to resolve it. Other children from psychosocially dysfunctional families display behavioral and personality problems. This emotional stress causes an increased production of endogenous catecholamines, which stimulate fat breakdown, leading to ketonemia and ketonuria.

Hospital Management. Children with DKA require intensive nursing care. Vital signs should be observed and recorded frequently. Hypotension caused by the contracted blood volume of the dehydrated state may cause decreased peripheral blood flow, which can be particularly hazardous to the heart, lungs, and kidneys. An elevated temperature may indicate infection and should be reported so that treatment can be implemented immediately.

Careful and accurate records should be maintained, including vital signs (pulse, respiration, temperature, blood pressure), weight, IV fluids, electrolytes, insulin, blood glucose level, and intake and output. A urine collection device or retention catheter is used to obtain the urine measurements, which include volume, specific gravity, and glucose and ketone values. The volume relative to the glucose content is important because 5% glucose in a 300-mL sample is a significantly greater amount than a similar reading from a 75-mL sample. A diabetic flow sheet maintained at the bedside provides an ongoing record of the vital signs, urine and blood tests, amount of insulin given, and intake and output. The level of consciousness is assessed and recorded at frequent intervals. The comatose child generally regains consciousness fairly soon after initiation of therapy but is managed like any unconscious child until then.

When the critical period is over, the task of regulating insulin dosage to diet and activity is begun. The same meticulous records of intake and output, urine glucose and acetone levels, and insulin administration are maintained. Capable children should be actively involved in their own care and are given responsibility for keeping the intake and output record; testing the blood and urine; and, when appropriate, administering their own insulin—all under the supervision and guidance of the nurse (see Nursing Care Plan).

Child and Family Education. Several organizations are prepared to assist with education and dissemination of knowledge about diabetes. The American Diabetes Association,* Canadian Diabetes Association,† Juvenile Diabetes Research Foundation International,‡ and American Association of Diabetes Educators§ are valuable resources for a wide variety of educational materials. The

*1701 N. Beauregard St., Alexandria, VA 22311; 800-342-2383; www.diabetes.org.
†1400-522 University Ave., Toronto, Ontario, Canada M5G 2R5; 800-226-8464; www.diabetes.ca.
‡26 Broadway, 14th Floor, New York, NY 10004; 800-533-CURE; www.jdrf.org.
§200 W. Madison St., Suite 800, Chicago, IL 60606; 800-338-3633; e-mail: education@aadenet.org; www.diabeteseducator.org.

National Institute of Diabetes and Digestive and Kidney Diseases* publishes a number of comprehensive annotated bibliographies, including "Educational Materials for and About Young People with Diabetes," a compilation of resource materials for children, siblings, parents, teachers, and health care professionals, and "Sports and Exercise for People with Diabetes."

Medical Identification. One of the first things the nurse should call to the parents' attention is the need for the child to wear some means of medical identification. Usually recommended is the MedicAlert identification, a stainless steel or silver- or gold-plated

*Office of Communications and Public Liaison, NIDDK, NIH, Building 31, Room 9A06, 31 Center Drive, MSC 2560, Bethesda, MD 20892-2560; 301-496-3583; www.niddk.nih.gov.

◎ NURSING CARE PLAN

The Child with Diabetes Mellitus

NURSING DIAGNOSIS	EXPECTED OUTCOMES	NURSING INTERVENTIONS	RATIONALES
Risk for Injury related to insulin deficiency	Child will demonstrate normal blood glucose levels.	Obtain blood glucose level	To determine most appropriate dosage of insulin
Child's or Family's Defining Characteristics		Administer insulin as prescribed	To maintain normal blood glucose level
(Subjective and Objective Data)		Understand action of insulin, including differences in composition, time of onset, and duration of action for various preparations	To ensure accurate insulin administration
Polyphagia			
Polydipsia		Use aseptic techniques when preparing and administering insulin	To prevent infection
Polyuria			
Weight loss		Rotate sites	To enhance absorption of insulin
Enuresis or nocturia			
Abnormal blood profile— glucose, insulin			
Irritability			
Shortened attention span			
Fatigue			
Dry skin			
Blurred vision			
Headache			
Frequent infections			
Hyperglycemia			
Flushed skin			
Risk for Injury related to hypoglycemia	Child will exhibit no evidence of hypoglycemia.	Recognize signs of hypoglycemia early; be alert at times when blood glucose levels are lowest (before meals and snacks; 2-4 AM; after bursts of physical activity without additional food; or with delayed, omitted, or incompletely consumed meal or snack)	To prevent hypoglycemia
Child's or Family's Defining Characteristics			
(Subjective and Objective Data)		Test blood glucose	To evaluate glucose level
Shaky feeling		Offer 10-15 g of readily absorbed carbohydrates, such as orange juice, hard candy, or milk	To elevate blood glucose level and alleviate symptoms of hypoglycemia
Hunger			
Headache			
Dizziness		Follow with complex carbohydrate and protein, such as bread or cracker spread with peanut butter or cheese	To maintain blood glucose level
Difficulty concentrating, speaking, or focusing		Administer glucagons to unconscious or combative child; position child to minimize risk of aspiration because vomiting may occur	To elevate blood glucose level
Tremors			
Tachycardia			
Shallow respirations			
Can lead to convulsion, shock, and coma			

NURSING CARE PLAN

The Child with Diabetes Mellitus—cont'd

NURSING DIAGNOSIS	EXPECTED OUTCOMES	NURSING INTERVENTIONS	RATIONALES
Deficient Knowledge (Diabetes Management) related to care of child with newly diagnosed diabetes mellitus	Child and family will have attitude conducive to learning.	Select methods, vocabulary, and content appropriate to learner's level	To maximize learning
		Allow time for family and child to begin to adjust to initial impact of diagnosis	To allow child and family to set pace
Child's or Family's Defining Characteristics		Select environment conducive to learning	To promote learning
(Subjective and Objective		Involve all senses and use variety of teaching strategies, especially participation	To promote effective learning
Data)		Provide pamphlets or other supplementary materials	To promote learning
Lack of understanding	Child and family will demonstrate understanding of meal planning.	Emphasize relationship between normal nutritional needs and disease	To encourage sense of normalcy
Inability to prepare and administer insulin		Become familiar with family's culture and food preferences	To include culture preferences in meal planning
Inability to follow meal planning guidelines		Teach or reinforce learners' understanding of basic food groups and prescribed meal plan	To reinforce existing knowledge base
Difficulty describing treatment plan		Help child and family estimate portion sizes by volume	To provide more practical method than weighing food
		Suggest low-carbohydrate snack items	To promote appropriate food choices
		Guide family in assessing labels of food products for carbohydrate content	To reinforce that consistency in carbohydrate portions is essential
	Child and family will demonstrate knowledge of and ability to administer insulin.	Teach child and family characteristics of insulins prescribed	To increase understanding that there are several insulin preparations
		Teach proper mixing of insulins	To prevent contaminating vials
		Teach injection procedure	To promote appropriate administration
		Teach basic techniques using orange or similar item	To build confidence
		Use demonstration and return demonstration techniques on another adult before injecting child	To minimize stress for child
		Help family and child work out set rotational pattern	To ensure maximum absorption of insulin and prevent hypertrophy at injection site
		Teach proper care of insulin and equipment	To prevent contamination and minimize complications
	Child and family will demonstrate ability to test blood glucose level.	Teach family and child, if old enough, blood glucose monitoring or use of equipment, interpretation of results, and care and maintenance of equipment	To ensure that child and family learn how to adjust insulin based on blood glucose level
	Child and family will demonstrate knowledge of management of hyperglycemia and hypoglycemia.	Instruct learners in how to recognize signs of hyperglycemia and hypoglycemia	To prevent delay of treatment
		Explain relationship of insulin needs to illness, activity, and intense emotion	To ensure appropriate treatment
		Teach how to adjust food, activity, and insulin at times of illness and during other situations that alter blood glucose levels	To ensure appropriate treatment
		Suggest carrying source of carbohydrate, such as sugar cubes or hard candy, in pocket	To prevent delay in treatment
		Instruct parents and child in how to treat hypoglycemia with food, simple sugars, or glucagons	To establish health practices that last a lifetime
	Child and family will demonstrate understanding of proper hygiene.	Emphasize importance of personal hygiene	To promote child's general health
		Encourage regular dental care and yearly ophthalmologic examinations	To minimize risk of infection
		Teach proper care of cuts and scratches; teach proper foot care	To prevent infection

identification bracelet that is visible and immediately recognizable. It contains a collect telephone number that medical personnel can call around the clock for medical records and personal information.

Nature of Diabetes. The better the parents understand the pathophysiology of diabetes and the function and action of insulin and glucagon in relation to caloric intake and exercise, the better they will understand the disease and its effects on the child. Parents need answers to a number of questions (voiced or unvoiced) to increase their confidence in coping with the disease. For example, they may want to know about the various procedures performed on their child and treatment rationale, such as what is being put in the IV fluid and the expected effect.

Meal Planning. Normal nutrition is a major aspect of the family education program. Diet instruction is usually conducted by the nutritionist, with reinforcement and guidance from the nurse. The emphasis is on adequate intake for age, consistent menus, complex carbohydrates, and consistent eating times. The family is taught how the meal plan relates to the requirements of growth and development, the disease process, and the insulin regimen. Meals and snacks are modified based on the child's preferences and current menu, preserving cultural patterns and preferences as much as possible. Extensive exchange lists are available that include foods compatible with most lifestyles.

Learning about foods within specific food groups helps in making choices. Weights and measures of foods are used as eye-training devices for defining serving sizes and should be practiced for about 3 months, with gradual progression to estimation of food portions. Even when the child and family become competent in estimating portion sizes, reassessment should take place weekly or monthly and when there is any change of brands.

Family members should also be guided in reading labels for the nutritional value of foods and food content. They need to become familiar with the carbohydrate content of food groups. Substitution with foods of equal carbohydrate content is the skill needed for successful carbohydrate counting. Substitution might be necessary if a food is not available in sufficient quantity or for the teenager who wishes to eat fast food with peers. The use of a multiple daily injection program lends flexibility to the timing of meals.

Lists of popular fast-food items and items served at the major fast-food chains can be obtained from the restaurants to help guide food selections. It is important that the child know the nutritional value of these items (the major chains are remarkably uniform), but the child should be cautioned to avoid high-fat and high-sugar/high-carbohydrate items; for example, the child could choose a plain hamburger instead of a double cheeseburger.

Children should use sugar substitutes in moderation in items such as soft drinks. Artificial sweeteners have been shown to be safe, but if there is any question about amounts, the physician, dietitian, or nurse specialist can provide guidelines based on body weight. Sugar-free chewing gum and candies made with sorbitol may be used in moderation by children with DM. Although sorbitol is less cariogenic than other varieties of sugar substitutes, it is an alcohol sugar that is metabolized to fructose and then to glucose. Furthermore, large amounts can cause osmotic diarrhea. Most dietetic foods contain sorbitol. They are more expensive than regular foods. Also, although a product may be sugar free, it is not necessarily carbohydrate free.

Traveling. Traveling requires planning, especially when a trip involves crossing time zones. A number of tips are included in pamphlets available free of charge. Suggestions for traveling encompass what will be needed from the health care practitioner before leaving, what and how much to take along, needs in transit, what to consider at the destination, and planning for when the child returns home. Planning is needed no matter what type of travel is considered—automobile, plane, bus, or train.

Insulin. Families need to understand the treatment method and the insulin prescribed, including the effective duration, onset, and peak action. They also need to know the characteristics of the various types of insulins, the proper mixing and dilution of insulins, and how to substitute another type when their usual brand is not available (insulin is a nonprescription drug). Insulin need not be refrigerated but should be maintained at a temperature between 15° and 29.4°C (59° and 85°F). Freezing renders insulin inactive.

Insulin bottles that have been "opened" (i.e., the stopper has been punctured) should be stored at room temperature or refrigerated for up to 28 to 30 days. After 1 month, these vials should be discarded. Unopened vials should be refrigerated and are good until the expiration date on the label. Diabetic supplies should not be left in a hot environment.

Injection Procedure. Learning to give insulin injections is a source of anxiety for both parents and children. It is helpful for the learner to know that this important aspect of care will become as routine as brushing the teeth. First, the basic injection technique is taught using an orange or similar item and sterile normal saline for practice. To gain children's confidence, the nurse can demonstrate the technique by giving a skillful injection to the parent and then having the parent return the demonstration by giving the nurse an injection. With practice and confidence, the parents will soon be able to give the insulin injection to their children and their children will trust them. Another effective strategy is to instruct the children and then have them teach the technique to the parents while the nurse observes. Both parents should participate, and as little time as possible should elapse between instruction and the actual injection, especially with parents and teenage learners.

Insulin can be injected into any area in which there is adipose (fat) tissue over muscle; the drug is injected at a 90-degree angle. Newly diagnosed children may have lost adipose tissue, and care should be exerted not to inject intramuscularly. The pinch technique is the most effective method for tenting the skin to allow easy entrance of the needle to subcutaneous tissues in children. The site selected will sometimes depend on whether children or parents administer the insulin. The arms, thighs, hips, and abdomen are usual injection sites for insulin. The children can reach the thighs, abdomen, and part of the hip and arm easily but may require help to inject other sites. For example, a parent can pinch a loose fold of skin of the arm while the child injects the insulin.

The parents and child are helped to work out a rotation pattern to various areas of the body to enhance absorption because insulin absorption is slowed by fat pads that develop in overused injection areas. The most efficient rotation plan involves giving about four to six injections in one area (each injection about 2.5 cm [1 inch] apart, or the diameter of the insulin vial from the previous injection) and then moving to another area.

It is important to remember that the absorption rate varies in different parts of the body (Table 46-4). The methodical use of one anatomic area and then movement to another (as described in the previous paragraph) minimizes variations in absorption rates. However, absorption is also altered by vigorous exercise, which enhances absorption from exercised muscles; therefore it is recommended that a site be chosen other than the exercising extremity (e.g., avoiding legs and arms when playing in a tennis tournament).

TABLE 46-4	ONSET AND DURATION OF ACTION RELATED TO INJECTION SITE			
	SITE OF INJECTION			
	ABDOMEN	**ARM**	**LEG**	**BUTTOCK**
Rate	Very fast	Fast	Slow	Very slow
Duration	Very short	Short	Long	Very long

From Albisser AM, Sperlich M: Adjusting insulins, *Diabetes Educ* 18(3):211–218, 1992.

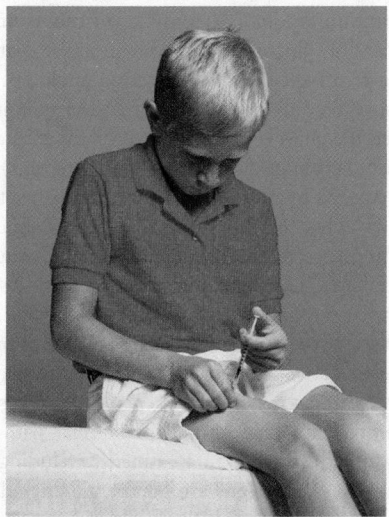

FIG 46-3 School-age children are able to administer their own insulin.

Injection sites for an entire month can be determined in advance on a simple chart. For example, a "paper doll" (body outline) can be constructed and insulin sites marked by the child. After injection, the child places the date on the appropriate site. To keep in practice, it is a good idea for the parent to give two or three injections a week in areas that are difficult for the child to reach. The same basic methodology is used when teaching children to give their own insulin injections (Fig. 46-3). They should practice first on an orange or a doll, building courage gradually. Other devices are available for insulin injection and may offer advantages to some children. Children who do not wish to give themselves injections can be taught to use a syringe-loaded injector (Inject-Ease). With the device, puncture is always automatic. Adolescents respond well to a self-contained and compact device resembling a fountain pen (NovoPen), which eliminates conventional vials and syringes. Preloaded pens may also cause less pain because the needle is not blunted by piercing the rubber top of the insulin vial (Rex, Jensen, and Lawton, 2006).

Continuous Subcutaneous Insulin Infusion. Some children are considered candidates for use of a portable insulin pump, and even some young children with unsatisfactory metabolic control can benefit from its use. The child and the parents are taught to operate the device, including the mechanics of the pump, battery changes, and alarm systems. A number of devices are on the market that vary in the basal rates they are able to deliver and in the cost of the equipment. Families can investigate the various devices and select the

ATRAUMATIC CARE
Minimizing Pain of Blood Glucose Monitoring

- To enhance blood flow to the finger, hold it under warm water for a few seconds before the puncture.
- When obtaining blood samples, use the ring finger or thumb (blood flows more easily to these areas) and puncture the finger just to the side of the finger pad (more blood vessels and fewer nerve endings).
- To prevent a deep puncture, press the platform of the lancet device lightly against the skin and avoid steadying the finger against a hard surface.
- Use lancet devices with adjustable-depth tips. Begin with the shallowest setting.
- Use glucose monitors that require small blood samples (e.g., Ascensia Elite) to avoid repeated punctures.

model that best suits their needs. Product information is available from pump manufacturers and distributors.*

Parents and children learn (1) the technical aspects of the pump and self-monitoring of blood glucose (SMBG); (2) prevention and treatment for hyperglycemia, sick-day management, and meal planning; (3) the effects of exercise, stress, and diet on blood glucose levels; and (4) decision-making strategies to evaluate blood glucose patterns and make adjustments in all aspects of the regimen.

Numerous blood glucose measurements (at least 4 times per day) are an essential part of infusion pump use. Intensive education and supervision are critical to obtaining maximum efficiency and control. This is particularly important if the family has been accustomed to a conventional insulin regimen. They must realize that simply wearing the pump will not normalize blood glucose. The pump is merely an insulin delivery device, and frequent, routine blood glucose determinations are necessary to adjust the insulin delivery rate.

The major problems with use of the insulin pump are inflammation from irritation and infection at the insertion site. The site should be cleaned thoroughly before the needle is inserted and then covered with a transparent dressing. The site is changed and rotated every 48 to 72 hours (this may vary) or at the first sign of inflammation. Nurses working where pumps are part of the therapeutic regimen should become familiar with the operation of the specific device being used and the protocol of disease management. Others should be aware of this management technique and be prepared to assist patients using the pump.

Monitoring. Nurses should also be prepared to teach and supervise blood glucose monitoring. SMBG is associated with few complications, and although it does not necessarily lead to improved metabolic control, it provides a more accurate assessment of blood glucose levels than can be obtained with the historical urine testing. Blood glucose monitoring has the added advantage that it can be performed anywhere (see Atraumatic Care box).

Blood for testing can be obtained by two different methods: manually or with a mechanical bloodletting device. A mechanical device is recommended for children, although the child and family should learn to use both methods in the event of mechanical failure. Several lancet devices are available, and each provides a means for obtaining a large drop of blood for testing (Fig. 46-4).

*Medtronic, www.medtronicdiabetes.com; Accu-Chek, www.accu-chek.com; Animas, www.animas.com.

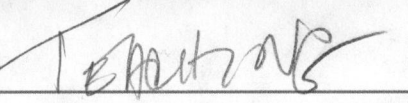

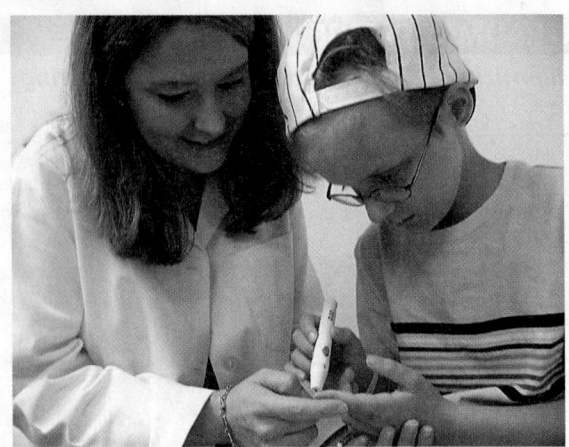

FIG 46-4 Child using a fingerstick device to obtain a blood sample.

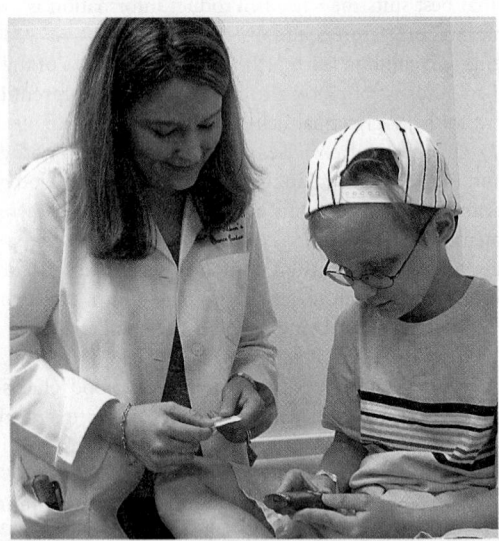

FIG 46-5 Child using a blood glucose monitor and reagent strips to test his blood for glucose.

! NURSING ALERT

Caution children not to allow anyone else to use their lancet because of the risk for contracting hepatitis B virus or human immunodeficiency virus infection.

The blood sample may be obtained from fingertips or alternate sites such as the forearm. Alternate site testing requires a meter that can test a small volume of blood. Not all meters are capable of this.

Signs of redness and soreness at the site of finger puncture should be examined by the health care practitioner. It may be evidence of poor technique, poor hygiene, or poor skin healing relative to poor control. Many types of blood-testing meters are available for home use. Newer technology has brought about improvements in meter size and ease of use. The family should be shown features of several meters, including advantages and disadvantages, and allowed to choose equipment that best meets their needs.

The least expensive testing method uses a reagent strip to which blood is applied (Fig. 46-5). After blotting, the color change is compared against a color scale for an estimation of the blood glucose level. The strips can be cut in half (although not all professionals recommend this) to obtain two readings per strip. This method is not accepted practice but may be necessary for some families or situations.

Urine Testing. Testing for urinary ketones is recommended during times of illness and when blood glucose values are elevated. Information on a specific ketone-testing product should include correct procedure, storage, and product expiration. Families need a clear understanding of home management of ketones (fluids and additional insulin as directed by the health care team).

Signs of Hyperglycemia. Severe hyperglycemia is most often caused by illness, growth, emotional upset, or missed insulin doses. Emotional stress from school finals or examinations and physical response to immunizations are examples of causes of hyperglycemia. With careful glucose monitoring, any elevation can be managed by adjustment of insulin or food intake. Parents should understand how to adjust food, activity, and insulin at the time of illness or when the child is treated for an illness with a medication known to raise the blood glucose level (e.g., steroids). The hyperglycemia is managed by increasing insulin soon after the increased glucose level is noted. Health care professionals should be aware that adolescent girls often become hyperglycemic around the time of their menses and should be advised to increase insulin dosages if necessary.

Signs of Hypoglycemia. Hypoglycemia is caused by imbalances of food intake, insulin, and activity. Ideally, hypoglycemia should be prevented, and parents need to be prepared to prevent, recognize, and treat the problem. They should be familiar with the signs of hypoglycemia and instructed in treatment, including care of the child with seizures. Early signs are adrenergic, including sweating and trembling, which help raise the blood glucose level, similar to the reaction when an individual is startled or anxious. The second set of symptoms that follow an untreated adrenergic reaction is neuroglycopenic (also called *brain hypoglycemia*). These symptoms typically include difficulty with balance, memory, attention, or concentration; dizziness or lightheadedness; and slurred speech. Severe and prolonged hypoglycemia leads to seizures, coma, and possible death (Cryer, 2008). Hypoglycemia can be managed effectively as outlined in the Emergency box.

It is advisable for parents to plan for anticipated excitement or exercise. In addition, gastroenteritis may decrease insulin needs slightly as a result of poor appetite, vomiting, or diarrhea. If the blood glucose level is low but urinary ketones are present, the family should be aware of the increased need for simple carbohydrates and liquids.

Hygiene. All aspects of personal hygiene should be emphasized for children with diabetes. Children should be cautioned against wearing shoes without socks, wearing sandals, and walking barefoot. Correct nail and extremity care tailored to the individual child (with the guidance of a podiatrist) can begin health practices that last a lifetime. These children's eyes should be checked once a year unless the child wears glasses and then as directed by the ophthalmologist. Regular dental care is emphasized, and cuts and scratches should be treated with plain soap and water unless otherwise indicated. Diaper rash in infants and candidal infections in teens may indicate poor diabetes control.

Exercise. Exercise is an important component of the treatment plan. If the child is more active at one time of the day than at another time, food or insulin can be altered to meet that activity pattern. Food should be increased in the summer, when children tend to be more active. Decreased activity on return to school may require a

✚ EMERGENCY

Hypoglycemia

Mild Reaction—Adrenergic Symptoms
- Give child 10 to 15 g of a simple, high-carbohydrate substance (preferably liquid (e.g., 3-6 oz of orange juice).
- Follow with starch-protein snack.

Moderate Reaction—Neuroglycopenic Symptoms
- Give child 10 to 15 g of a simple carbohydrate as above.
- Repeat in 10 to 15 minutes if symptoms persist.
- Follow with larger snack.
- Watch child closely.

Severe Reaction—Unresponsive, Unconscious, or Seizures
- Administer glucagon as prescribed.
- Follow with planned meal or snack when child is able to eat or add a snack of 10% of daily calories.

Nocturnal Reaction
- Give child 10 to 15 g of a simple carbohydrate.
- Follow with snack of 10% of daily calories.

decrease in food intake or increase in insulin dosage. Children who are active in team sports will need a snack about a half-hour before the anticipated activity. Races or other competition may call for a slightly higher food intake than at practice times.

Food intake will usually need to be repeated for prolonged activity periods, often as frequently as every 45 minutes to 1 hour. Families should be informed that if increased food is not tolerated, decreased insulin is the next course of action. If the timing of the exercise is changed so that the supper meal is delayed, the insulin in the second or third dose of the day may be moved back to precede the mealtime. Sugar may sometimes be needed during exercise periods for quick response. Elevated blood glucose levels after extreme activity may represent the body's adrenergic response to exercise. If the blood glucose level is elevated (>240 mg/dL) before planned exercise, urinary ketones should be checked and the activity may need be postponed until the blood glucose is controlled.

❗ NURSING ALERT

Ketonuria in the presence of hyperglycemia is an early sign of ketoacidosis and a contraindication to exercise.

Record Keeping. Home records are an invaluable aid to diabetes self-management. The nurse and family devise a method to chart insulin administered, blood glucose values, urine ketone results, and other factors and events that affect diabetes control. The child and family are encouraged to observe for patterns of blood glucose responses to events such as exercise. If lapses in management occur (e.g., eating a candy bar), the child should be encouraged to note this and not be criticized for the transgression.

Self-Management. Self-management is the key to close control. Being able to make changes when they are needed rather than waiting until the next contact with health care professionals is important for self-management and gives the individual and family

the feeling that they have control over the disease. Psychologically, this helps family members believe they are useful and participating members of the team. Allowing the child to learn to look at records objectively promotes independence in self-management support. As children grow and assume more responsibility for self-management, they develop confidence in their ability to manage their disease and confidence in themselves as persons. They learn to respond to the disease and to make more accurate interpretations and changes in treatment when they become adults.

Puberty is associated with decreased sensitivity to insulin that normally would be compensated for by an increased insulin secretion. Health care professionals should anticipate that pubertal patients will have more difficulty maintaining glycemic control. Insulin doses commonly need to be increased, often dramatically (Tfayli and Arsianian, 2007). Patients should be taught to give themselves additional doses of rapid-acting insulin (5% to 10% of their daily dose) when their blood glucose levels are increased. The use of supplemental rapid-acting insulin is preferred to withholding food in adolescents.

Child or Adolescent and Family Support. Just as the physiologic responses affect the child, the parents and other family members of the child with newly diagnosed DM experience various emotional responses to the crisis. Care in the acute setting is short but may create fears and frustrations. The prospect of a chronic illness in their child engenders all the feelings and concerns that are faced by parents of children with other chronic illnesses (see Chapter 36). The threat of complications and death is always present, as well as the continuing drain on emotional and financial resources.

Certain fears may develop as a result of past experiences with the disease. A severe insulin reaction with seizures can contribute to fear of repetition. If parents observe a seizure or the adolescent has one in a public place, the desire to maintain better control is reinforced. They must understand how to prevent problems and how to handle problems calmly and coolly if they occur, and they must understand the complexities of the body, the disease, and its complications. Young children usually adjust well to problems related to the disease. With toddlers and preschoolers, insulin injections and glucose testing may be difficult at first. However, they usually accept the procedures when the parents use a matter-of-fact approach, without calling attention to a "hurt," and treat the procedure like any other routine part of the child's life. After the injection, time with some special and positive attention, such as reading, talking, or another pleasant activity, is one way to convert children who initially refuse injections to those who accept them.

In the years before adolescence, children probably accept their condition most easily. They are able to understand the basic concepts related to their disease and its treatment. They are able to test blood glucose and urine, recognize food groups, give injections, keep records, and distinguish fear or excitement from hypoglycemia. They understand how to recognize, prevent, and treat hypoglycemia. However, they still need considerable parental involvement.

❗ NURSING ALERT

Ongoing motivation to adhere to a regimen is difficult. An older child and parent (or another caregiver) may enjoy negotiating a day off when the responsibility for testing and recording blood glucose is delegated from the child to the caregiver (or vice versa).

Adolescents appear to have the most difficulty adjusting. Adolescence is a time of stress in trying to be perfect and similar to one's peers, and no matter what others say, having diabetes is being different. Some adolescents are more upset about not being able to have a candy bar than about injections, diet, and other aspects of management. If children can accept the difference as a part of life—in other words, that each person is different in some way—then, with adequate parental support, they should be able to adjust well (see Critical Thinking Case Study).

Camping and other special group activities are useful. At diabetes camp, children learn that they are not alone. As a result, they become more independent and resourceful in other settings. Useful information about such camps and organizations can be obtained from the American Diabetes Association. A list of accredited camps specifically for children and teenagers with diabetes is also available from the American Camping Association.*

*5000 State Road 67 N., Martinsville, IN 46151; 765-342-8456, 800-428-2267; www.acacamps.org.

CRITICAL THINKING CASE STUDY

Type 1 Diabetes Mellitus

Shelly, a 14-year-old adolescent with a 3-year history of type 1 DM, has been admitted to the pediatric intensive care unit for treatment of DKA. This is her fifth hospital admission for DKA in the past year. Rebecca's parents are divorced, and she has four younger siblings, none of whom has diabetes. Shelly's mother has maintained two jobs for the past 5 years and frequently leaves Shelly in charge of the household. In anticipation of her discharge, you are planning a patient education program for Shelly and her mother. What important issues regarding Shelly's unstable diabetes management must you consider to plan the education program?

1. Evidence—Is there sufficient evidence to draw conclusions about Shelly's recurrent episodes of DKA?
2. Assumptions—Describe an underlying assumption about each of the following:
   a. Type 1 DM in adolescence
   b. Type 1 DM and menses
   c. Emotional stress and elevated blood glucose levels
   d. Blood glucose monitoring for insulin management
3. What priorities for nursing care should be established for Shelly?
4. Does the evidence support your nursing intervention?

DKA, Diabetic ketoacidosis; *DM,* diabetes mellitus.

KEY POINTS

- The endocrine system has three components: the cells, which send chemical messages via hormones; target cells, which receive the messages; and the environment through which the chemicals are transported from the sites of synthesis to the sites of cellular action.
- Pituitary dysfunction is manifested primarily by growth disturbance.
- The main physiologic action of TH is to regulate the basal metabolic rate and control the processes of growth and tissue differentiation.
- Disorders of thyroid function include hypothyroidism, autoimmune thyroiditis, goiter, and hyperthyroidism.
- Therapy for hyperthyroidism is directed at slowing the rate of hormone secretion and may include drug therapy, thyroidectomy, or radioiodine therapy.
- Classic forms of hypoparathyroidism in childhood are idiopathic (deficient production of PTH) and pseudohypoparathyroidism (increased PTH production with end-organ unresponsiveness to PTH).
- The adrenal cortex secretes three important groups of hormones: glucocorticoids, mineralocorticoids, and sex steroids.
- Disorders of adrenal function include acute adrenocortical insufficiency, chronic adrenocortical insufficiency, Cushing syndrome, and CAH.
- Five categories of Cushing syndrome are pituitary, adrenal, ectopic, iatrogenic, and food dependent.
- Management of CAH includes assignment of a gender according to genotype; administration of cortisone; and, possibly, reconstructive surgery.
- DM is categorized as type 1 diabetes and type 2 diabetes.
- The focus of type 1 DM is insulin replacement, diet, and exercise.
- Education of families includes explanation of diabetes, meal planning, administering insulin injections, monitoring general hygienic practices, promoting exercise, record keeping, and observing for complications.

REFERENCES
American Academy of Pediatrics (AAP) Section on Endocrinology and Committee on Genetics: Technical report: congenital adrenal hyperplasia, *Pediatrics* 106(6):1511–1518, 2000. Reaffirmation statement published 2005.

American Academy of Pediatrics (AAP), Rose SR, Section on Endocrinology and Committee on Genetics, American Thyroid Association, et al: Update of newborn screening and therapy for congenital hypothyroidism, *Pediatrics* 7(6):2290–2303, 2006.

American Diabetes Association: Report of the Expert Committee on the Diagnosis and Classification of Diabetes Mellitus, *Diabetes Care* 24(Suppl 1):S5–S20, 2001.

Bartalena L, Tanda ML, Piantanida E, et al: Oxidative stress and Graves' ophthalmopathy: in vitro studies and therapeutic implications, *Biofactors* 19(3–4):155–163, 2003.

Baxter JD, Ribeiro RCJ: Introduction to endocrinology. In Greenspan FS, Gardner DG, editors: *Basic and clinical endocrinology,*

ed 7, New York, 2004, Lange Medical Books/McGraw-Hill.

Biro FM, Huang B, Crawford PB, et al: Pubertal correlates in black and white girls, *J Pediatr* 148(2):234–240, 2006.

Brown TB: Cerebral edema in childhood diabetic ketoacidosis: is treatment a factor? *Emerg Med J* 21:141–144, 2004.

Bryant J, Baxter L, Cave CB, et al: Recombinant growth hormone for idiopathic short stature in children and adolescents, *Cochrane Database Syst Rev* 18(3):CD004440, 2007.

Carel JC, Léger J: Clinical practice. Precocious puberty, *N Engl J Med* 358(22):2366–2377, 2008.

Centers for Disease Control and Prevention: *Diabetes Report Card 2012*. Atlanta, GA, 2012, Centers for Disease Control and Prevention, US Department of Health and Human Services.

Centers for Disease Control and Prevention (CDC): *National Diabetes Fact Sheet 2011: national estimates and general information on diabetes and prediabetes in the U.S.*, 2011, US Department of Health and Human Services.

Cheetham T, Baylis PH: Diabetes insipidus in children: pathophysiology, diagnoses and management, *Paediatr Drugs* 4(12):785–796, 2002.

Cooke D, Plotnick L: Management of diabetic ketoacidosis in children and adolescents, *Pediatr Rev* 29:431–436, 2008.

Cooper MS, Gittoes NJ: Diagnosis and management of hypocalcemia, *BMJ* 336:1298–1302, 2008.

Cryer PE: The barriers of hypoglycemia in diabetes, *Diabetes* 57(12):3169–3176, 2008.

Dallas JS, Foley TP: Hyperthyroidism. In Lifshitz F, editor: *Pediatric endocrinology*, ed 4, New York, 2003, Marcel Dekker.

De Buyst J, Massa G, Christophe C, et al: Clinical, hormonal and imaging findings in 27 children with central diabetes insipidus, *Eur J Pediatr* 166(1):43–49, 2007.

de Vries L, Bulvik S, Phillip M: Chronic autoimmune thyroiditis in children and adolescents: at presentation and during long term follow up, *Arch Dis Child* 94(1):33–37, 2009.

Foley TP: Hypothyroidism. In Hoekelman RA, Adam HM, Nelson NM, et al, editors: *Primary pediatric care*, ed 4, St Louis, 2001, Mosby.

Glatt K, Garzon D, Popovic J: Congenital adrenal hyperplasia due to 21–hydroxylase deficiency, *Soc Pediatr Nurs* 10(3):104–114, 2005.

Greiner MV, Kerrigan JR: Puberty: timing is everything, *Pediatr Ann* 35(12):916–922, 2006.

Halac I, Zimmerman D: Evaluating short stature in children, *Pediatr Ann* 33(3):171–176, 2004.

Hall DMB: Growth monitoring, *Arch Dis Child* 82(1):10–15, 2000.

Hannon TS, Gungor N, Arslanian SA: Type 2 diabetes in children and adolescents: a review for the primary care provider, *Pediatr Ann* 35(12):880–887, 2006.

Herman-Giddens ME: Recent data on pubertal milestones in United States children: the secular trend toward earlier development, *Int J Androl* 29(1):241–246, 2006.

Jospe N: Hyperthyroidism. In Hoekelman RA, Adam HM, Nelson NM, et al, editors: *Primary pediatric care*, ed 4, St Louis, 2001, Mosby.

Karnik AA, Fields AV, Shannon RP: Diabetic cardiomyopathy, *Curr Hypertens Rep* 9(6):467–473, 2007.

Kempers MJ, Otten BJ: Idiopathic precocious puberty versus puberty in adopted children: auxological response to gonadotrophin-releasing hormone agonist treatment and final height, *Eur J Endocrinol* 147(5):609–616, 2002.

Kliegman RM, Stanton B, St. Geme J, et al: *Nelson textbook of pediatrics*, ed 19, Philadelphia, 2011, Saunders.

Lee PA, Houk CP, Ahmed SF, et al: Consensus statement on management of intersex disorders, *Pediatrics* 118(2):e488, 2006.

Leschek EW, Rose SR, Yanovski FA, et al: Effect of growth hormone treatment on adult height in peripubertal children with idiopathic short stature: a randomized, double blind, placebo-controlled trial, *J Clin Endocrino Metab* 89(7):3140–3148, 2004.

Lin M, Liu SJ, Lim IT: Disorders of water imbalance, *Emerg Med Clin North Am* 23(3):749–770, 2005.

Ma C, Xie JW, Kuang AR, et al: Radioiodine treatment for pediatric Grave's disease (protocol), *Cochrane Database Syst Rev* (4):CD006294, 2006.

Macchia PE: Recent advances in understanding the molecular basis of primary congenital hypothyroidism, *Mol Med Today* 6(1):36–42, 2000.

Majzoub JA, Muglia LJ: Disorders of water homeostasis. In Lifshitz F, editor: *Pediatric endocrinology*, ed 4, New York, 2003, Marcel Dekker.

Makaryus AN, McFarlane SI: Diabetes insipidus: diagnosis and treatment of a complex disease, *Cleve Clin J Med* 73(1):65–71, 2006.

Midyett LK, Moore WV, Jacobson JD: Are pubertal changes in girls before age 8 benign? *Pediatrics* 111(1):47–51, 2003.

Miller BS, Zimmerman D: Idiopathic short stature in children, *Pediatr Ann* 33(3):177–181, 2004.

Moshang T: Cushing's disease, 70 years later … and the beat goes on (editorial), *J Clin Endocrinol Metab* 88(1):31–33, 2003.

Muir A: Precocious puberty, *Pediatr Rev* 27(10):373–381, 2006.

Natchtigall L, Delgado A, Swearingen B, et al: Extensive clinical experience: changing patterns in diagnosis and therapy of acromegaly over two decades, *J Clin Endocrinol Metab* 93(6):2035–2041, 2008.

Nebesio TD, Eugster EA: Current concepts in normal and abnormal puberty, *Curr Prob Pediatr Adolesc Health Care* 37(2):50–72, 2007.

New MI, Ghizzoni L: Update on congenital adrenal hyperplasia. In Lifshitz F, editor: *Pediatric endocrinology*, ed 4, New York, 2003, Marcel Dekker.

Nieman LK, Ilias I: Evaluation and treatment of Cushing's syndrome, *Am J Med* 118(12):1340–1346, 2005.

O'Sullivan E, O'Sullivan M: Precocious puberty: a parent's perspective, *Arch Dis Childhood* 86:320–321, 2002.

Pacak K, Eisenhofer G, Ahlman H, et al: Pheochromocytoma: recommendations for clinical practice from the First International Symposium, *Nat Clin Pract Endocrinol Metab* 3(2):92–102, 2007.

Perheentupa J: Hypoparathyroidism and mineral homeostasis. In Lifshitz F, editor: *Pediatric endocrinology*, ed 4, New York, 2003, Marcel Dekker.

Petitti BD, Imperatore G, Palla SL, et al: Serum lipids and glucose control: the SEARCH for Diabetes in Youth study, *Arch Pediatr Adolesc Med* 161(2):159–165, 2007.

Phillip M, Battelino T, Rodriguez H, et al: Use of insulin pump therapy in the pediatric age group, *Diabetes Care* 30:1653–1662, 2007.

Pizzo PA, Poplack DG: *Principles and theories of pediatric oncology*, Philadelphia, 2010, Lippincott Williams & Wilkins.

Radetti G, Gottardi E, Bona G, et al: The natural history of euthyroid Hashimoto's thyroiditis in children, *J Pediatr* 149(6):827–832, 2006.

Rex J, Jensen KH, Lawton SA: A review of 20 years of experience with the NovoPen family of insulin injection devices, *Clin Drug Invest* 26(7):367–401, 2006.

Richmond EJ, Rogol AD: Growth hormone deficiency in children, *Pituitary* 71:115–120, 2008.

Rivkees SA: Differentiating appropriate antidiuretic hormone secretion, inappropriate antidiuretic hormone secretion and cerebral salt wasting: the common, uncommon and misnamed, *Curr Opin Pediatr* 20(4):448–452, 2008.

Rivkees SA, Cornelius EA: Influence of iodine-131 dose on the outcome of hyperthyroidism in children, *Pediatrics* 111(4):745–748, 2003.

Root AW: Precocious puberty, *Pediatr Rev* 21(1):10–19, 2000.

Rosenson RS, Herman WH: Glycated proteins and cardiovascular disease in glucose intolerance and type 11 diabetes, *Curr Cardiovascular Risk Rep* 2(1):43–46, 2008.

Rovet JF, Ehrlich R: Psychoeducational outcome in children with early-treated congenital hypothyroidism, *Pediatrics* 105(3):515–522, 2000.

Shoback D: Clinical practice: hypoparathyroidism, *N Engl J Med* 359(4):391–403, 2008.

Silverstein J, Klingensmith G, Copeland K, et al: Care of children and adolescents with type 1 diabetes: a statement of the American Diabetes Association, *Diabetes Care* 28(1):186–212, 2005.

Simmonds MJ, Howson JM, Heward JM, et al: Regression mapping of association between the human leukocyte antigen region and Graves disease, *Am J Hum Genet* 76(1):157–163, 2005.

Slyper AH: The pubertal timing controversy in the USA, and a review of possible causative factors for the advance in timing of onset of puberty, *Clin Endocrinol (Oxf)* 65(1):1–8, 2006.

Streetman DD, Khanderia U: Diagnosis and treatment of Graves disease, *Am J Nurse Pract* 8(1):27–36, 2004.

Szymborska M, Staroszczyk B: Thyroiditis in children, *Med Wieku Rozwoj* 4(4):383–391, 2000.

Tfayli H, Arsianian S: The challenge of adolescence: hormonal changes and sensitivity to insulin, *Diabetic Voice* 52:28–30, 2007.

Thompson GB: Surgical management in Graves' disease, *Panminerva Med* 44(4):287–293, 2002.

Toogood M, Stewart PM: Hypopituitarism: clinical features, diagnosis, and management, *Endocrino Metab Clin North Am* 37(1):235–261, 2008.

Trivin C, Couto-Silva AC, Sainte-Rose Z, et al: Presentation and evolution of organic central precocious puberty according to the type of CNS lesion, *Clin Endocrinol (Oxf)* 65(2):239–245, 2006.

Urrutia-Rojas X, Menchaca J: Prevalence of risk for type 2 diabetes in school children, *J Sch Health* 76(5):189–194, 2006.

van Tijn DA, Schroor EJ, Delemarre-van de Waal HA, et al: Early assessment of hypothalamic-pituitary-gonadal function in patients with congenital hypothyroidism of central origin, *J Clin Endocrinol Metab* 92(1):104–109, 2007.

Verbalis JG: Diabetes insipidus, *Rev Endocr Metab Disord* 4(2):177–185, 2003.

Wolsdorf J, Craig ME, Daneman D, et al: Diabetic ketoacidosis in children and adolescents with diabetes: ISPAD Clinical Practice Consensus Guidelines 2009 Compendium, *Pediatr Diabetes* 10(Suppl 12):118–133, 2009.

Integumentary Dysfunction

Marilyn J. Hockenberry

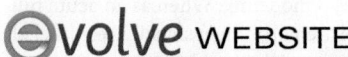

LEARNING OBJECTIVES

On completion of this chapter, the reader will be able to:
- Describe the distribution and configuration of various skin lesions.
- List the benefits of a moist environment for wound healing.
- Discuss the nursing care related to therapies for skin disorders.
- Contrast the manifestations of and therapies for bacterial, viral, and fungal infections of the skin.
- Compare the skin manifestations related to age in children.
- Outline a care plan to prevent and treat diaper dermatitis.
- Outline a care plan for a child with atopic dermatitis.
- Formulate a teaching plan for an adolescent with acne.
- Describe the methods for assessing a burn wound.
- Discuss the physical and emotional care of a child with a severe burn wound.

INTEGUMENTARY DYSFUNCTION

Skin Lesions

Lesions of the skin result from a variety of etiologic factors. Skin lesions originate from (1) contact with injurious agents (infective organisms, toxic chemicals, and physical trauma), (2) hereditary factors, (3) external factors (e.g., allergens), or (4) systemic diseases (e.g., measles, lupus erythematosus, nutritional deficiency diseases). Responses to these agents or factors are highly individualized. An agent that is harmless to one individual may be damaging to another, and a single agent may produce varying degrees of response.

An important factor in the etiology of skin manifestations is the child's age. Infants are subject to "birthmark" malformations and atopic dermatitis (AD) that appear early in life, school-age children are susceptible to ringworm of the scalp, and acne is a characteristic skin disorder of puberty. Contact dermatitis, such as poison ivy, is seen only when the noxious agent is found in the environment. Tension and anxiety may produce, modify, or prolong skin conditions.

Skin of Younger Children

The major skin layers arise from different embryologic origins. Early in the embryonic period, a single layer of epithelium forms from the ectoderm and simultaneously the corium develops from the mesenchyme. In infants and small children, the epidermis is loosely bound to the dermis. This poor adherence causes the layers to separate easily during an inflammatory process to form blisters. This is especially true in preterm infants, who have a propensity to blister formation and separation of the skin with minor trauma such as the removal of adhesive tape. In contrast, the skin of older children is thinner than that of younger children, and the cells of all the strata are more compressed.

Pathophysiology of Dermatitis

More than half of the dermatologic problems in children are forms of dermatitis. This implies a sequence of inflammatory changes in the skin that are grossly and microscopically similar but diverse in course and causation. Acute responses produce intercellular and intracellular edema, the formation of intradermal vesicles, and an initial infiltration of inflammatory cells into the epidermis. In the dermis, there is edema, vascular dilation, and early perivascular cellular infiltration. The location and manner of these reactions produce the lesions characteristic of each disorder. The changes are usually reversible, and the skin ordinarily recovers without blemish unless complicating factors such as ulceration from the primary irritant, scratching, and infection are introduced or underlying vascular disease develops. In chronic conditions, permanent effects are seen that vary according to the disorder, the general condition of the affected individual, and the available therapy.

Diagnostic Evaluation

Although the history and subjective symptoms of skin lesions are explored first, the obvious objective characteristics of the lesions are often noted simultaneously. Many skin lesions are easily diagnosed after careful inspection.

History and Subjective Symptoms. Many cutaneous lesions are associated with local symptoms. The most common local symptom is itching (pruritus), which varies in intensity. Pain or tenderness often accompanies some skin lesions. Other skin sensations such as burning, prickling, stinging, or crawling are also described. Alterations in local feeling include absence of sensation (anesthesia); excessive sensitiveness (hyperesthesia); diminished sensation (hypesthesia or hypoesthesia); or abnormal sensation, such as burning or prickling (paresthesia). These symptoms may remain localized or migrate; may be constant or intermittent; and may be aggravated by a specific activity, such as exposure to sunlight.

It is important to determine whether the child has an allergic condition such as asthma or hay fever or history of a previous skin disease. AD, often associated with allergies, frequently begins in infancy. Important questions for the parent include when the lesion or symptom first appeared; whether it occurred with ingestion of a food or other substance, including any medication; and whether the condition was related to activity such as contact with plants, insects, or chemicals.

Objective Findings. The distribution, size, morphology, and arrangement of skin lesions provide significant information. Extrinsic causes usually result from physical, chemical, or allergic irritants or from an infectious agent such as bacteria, fungi, viruses, or animal parasites. Skin manifestations are also produced by intrinsic causes such as an infection (measles or chickenpox), drug sensitization, or other allergic phenomenon.

Types of Lesions. Skin lesions assume distinct characteristics that are related to the pathologic process. Nurses should become familiar with the common terms that are applied to skin lesions because these terms are used in the processes of record keeping and communication. These terms include:

- Erythema—A reddened area caused by increased amounts of oxygenated blood in the dermal vasculature
- Ecchymoses (bruises)—Localized red or purple discolorations caused by extravasation of blood into dermis and subcutaneous tissues
- Petechiae—Pinpoint, tiny, and sharp circumscribed spots in the superficial layers of the epidermis
- Primary lesions—Skin changes produced by a causative factor; common primary lesions in pediatric skin disorders are macules, papules, and vesicles
- Secondary lesions—Changes that result from alteration in the primary lesions, such as those caused by rubbing, scratching, medication, or involution and healing
- Distribution pattern—The pattern in which lesions are distributed over the body, whether local or generalized, and the specific areas associated with the lesions
- Configuration and arrangement—The size, shape, and arrangement of a lesion or groups of lesions (e.g., discrete, clustered, diffuse, or confluent)

Laboratory Studies. If a skin problem is related to a systemic disease (e.g., collagen or immunodeficiency disease), laboratory studies are performed to identify these conditions. Diagnostic techniques include microscopic examination, cultures, skin scrapings or biopsy, cytodiagnosis, patch testing, Wood light examination, allergic skin testing, and other laboratory tests such as blood count and sedimentation rate.

Wounds

Wounds are structural or physiologic disruptions of the skin that activate normal or abnormal tissue repair responses. Wounds are classified as acute or chronic. Acute wounds are those that heal uneventfully within 2 to 3 weeks. Chronic wounds are those that do not heal in the expected time frame or are associated with complications. Cofactors that disrupt or delay wound healing include compromised perfusion, malnutrition, and infection. In children, most wounds are acute and can be prevented from becoming chronic wounds through appropriate nursing care. Wounds are also classified as surgical and nonsurgical and then further classified in the same manner as burns: superficial, partial thickness, or full thickness (complex wounds that include muscle or bone).

Factors That Influence Healing

Wound care management has shifted from interventions aimed at maintaining a dry environment to those that promote a moist, crust-free environment that enhances the migration of epithelial cells across the wound and facilitates remodeling. Whereas an acute full-thickness wound kept in a moist environment usually reepithelializes in 12 to 15 days, the same wound when kept open to the air heals in about 25 to 30 days.

Numerous factors can delay healing (Table 47-1). For example, traditional practices, such as the use of antiseptics (hydrogen peroxide and povidone-iodine [Betadine] solutions), which were once thought to prevent infection, are now known to have a cytotoxic effect on healthy cells and minimal effect on controlling infections. Povidone-iodine may also be absorbed through the skin in neonates and young children.

General Therapeutic Management

Some skin disorders demand aggressive therapy, but by and large, the major aim of treatment is to prevent further damage, eliminate the cause, prevent complications, and provide relief from discomfort while tissues undergo healing (McCord and Levy, 2006). Factors that contribute to the development of dermatitis and that prolong the course of the disease should be eliminated when possible. The most common causative agents of dermatitis in infants, children, and adolescents are environmental factors (e.g., soaps, bubble baths, shampoos, rough or tight clothing, wet diapers, blankets, and toys) and the natural elements (e.g., dirt, sand, heat, cold, moisture, and wind). Dermatitis may also result from home remedies and medications.

Dressings

No one dressing meets the needs of all wounds. The traditional dry gauze dressing should not be used on open wounds because it allows the wound surface to dry, does little to prevent bacterial invasion, and adheres to the dried scab so that removal disturbs the newly regenerating epithelial cells. In most instances, traditional gauze dressings have been replaced by dressings that promote moist wound healing. Moist wound healing increases the rate of collagen synthesis and reepithelialization and decreases pain and inflammation. It also creates an environment for autolytic débridement of necrotic tissue, which creates a clean wound bed and enhances granulation. However, a balance must be achieved between creating a moist wound bed and maintaining a dry periwound area that protects the skin and wound from maceration. The dressing type and frequency of dressing changes help achieve this balance. The frequency of dressing changes is based on the presence of infection, the type of dressing, the location of the wound, and the amount of drainage. Dressings should always be changed when they are loose or soiled.

TABLE 47-1	FACTORS THAT DELAY WOUND HEALING
FACTOR	**EFFECT ON HEALING**
Dry wound environment	Allows epithelial cells to dry out and die; impairs migration of epithelial cells across wound surface
Nutritional deficiencies	
Vitamin A	Results in inadequate inflammatory response
Vitamin B₁	Results in decreased collagen formation
Vitamin C	Inhibits formation of collagen fibers and capillary development
Protein	Reduces supply of amino acids for tissue repair
Zinc	Impairs epithelialization
Immunocompromise	Results in inadequate or delayed inflammatory response
Impaired circulation	Inhibits inflammatory response and removal of debris from wound area
	Reduces supply of nutrients to wound area
Stress (pain, poor sleep)	Releases catecholamines that cause vasoconstriction
Antiseptics	
Hydrogen peroxide	Toxic to fibroblasts; can cause subcutaneous gas formation (mimics gas-forming infection)
Povidone-iodine	Toxic to white and red blood cells and fibroblasts
Chlorhexidine	Toxic to white blood cells
Medications	
Corticosteroids	Impair phagocytosis
	Inhibit fibroblast proliferation
	Depress formation of granulation tissue
	Inhibit wound contraction
Chemotherapy	Interrupts the cell cycle; damages DNA or prevents DNA repair
Antiinflammatory drugs	Decrease the inflammatory phase
Foreign bodies	Increase inflammatory response
	Inhibit wound closure
Infection	Increases inflammatory response
	Increases tissue destruction
Mechanical friction	Damages or destroys granulation tissue
Fluid accumulation	Accumulation in area inhibits tissues from approximating
Radiation	Inhibits fibroblastic activity and capillary formation
	May cause tissue necrosis
Diseases	
Diabetes mellitus	Inhibits collagen synthesis
	Impairs circulation and capillary growth
	Hyperglycemia impairs phagocytosis
Anemia	Reduces oxygen supply to tissues
Peripheral vascular disease	Reduces oxygen supply to wounds
Uremia	Decreases collagen and granulation tissue

They should be changed more frequently in areas where contamination is likely (e.g., the sacral area, the buttocks, the tracheal area) or when wound infection is suspected or present.

Topical Therapy

Several agents and methods are available for treatment. In selecting a therapeutic regimen, the practitioner considers (1) the choice of active ingredient, (2) the proper vehicle or base, (3) the cosmetic effect, (4) the cost, and (5) instructions for use. Several basic concepts must also be considered. Overtreatment is avoided. For example, when dermatitis is acute, topical applications should be mild and bland to avoid further irritation. Broken or inflamed skin, especially in children, is more absorbent than intact skin, and chemicals that are nonirritating to intact skin may be quite irritating to inflamed skin.

Topical applications may be applied to treat the disorder, reduce itching, decrease external stimuli, or apply external heat or cold. The emollient action of soaks, baths, and lotions provides a soothing film over the skin surface that reduces external stimuli. Ordinarily, lukewarm or cool applications offer the greatest relief.

> **! NURSING ALERT**
>
> Application of heat tends to aggravate most conditions, and its use is usually reserved for reducing specific inflammatory processes, such as folliculitis and cellulitis.

Ointments in a petrolatum base provide protection from moisture. Therefore this type of ointment is indicated around gastrostomy tubes, in skinfolds, and in the diaper area. Creams are absorbed by the skin and are used for areas where a nongreasy "feel" is desired (e.g., face, hands).

Topical Corticosteroid Therapy. Glucocorticoids are the therapeutic agents used most frequently for skin disorders. Their local antiinflammatory effects are merely palliative, so the medication must be applied until the condition undergoes a remission or the causative agent is eliminated. Corticosteroids are applied directly to the affected area, are essentially nonsensitizing, and have only minor side effects. As with the use of any steroids, their use in large amounts may mask signs of infection and symptoms may be exacerbated after termination of the drug. Families are cautioned that the medication cannot be used for all skin disorders. The concentrations available without prescription are not adequate for stubborn skin conditions (e.g., psoriasis) and may further aggravate inflammation caused by fungi or bacteria. Most parents and children apply too much topical hydrocortisone; therefore they should be counseled that it is both effective and economical to apply only a thin film and to massage it into the skin. Parents and children should also be advised to use the application for no more than 5 to 7 days because these agents may cause depigmentation and other changes in the skin.

Other Topical Therapies. Other topical treatments include chemical cautery (especially useful for warts), cryosurgery, electrodesiccation (chiefly used for warts, granulomas, and nevi), ultraviolet (UV) therapy (primarily used in psoriasis and acne), laser therapy (especially for birthmarks), and acne therapies such as dermabrasion and chemical peels. New drugs called topical immunomodulators are effective in reducing the itching of AD (eczema) and preventing the recurrence of "flares."

Systemic Therapy. Systemic drugs may be used as an adjunct to topical therapy in some dermatologic disorders. The drugs most frequently used are corticosteroids, antibiotics, and antifungal agents. Corticosteroids are valuable because of their capacity to inhibit inflammatory and allergic reactions. The dosage is carefully adjusted and gradually tapered to the minimum dosage that is effective and tolerated. In infants and children, the dosage is larger than is usually calculated from body weight ratios. However, prolonged use may temporarily suppress growth.

Antibiotics are used in severe or widespread skin infections. However, because these drugs tend to produce hypersensitivity in some patients, they are used with caution. Antifungal agents are the only means for treating systemic fungal infections.

CARE MANAGEMENT

The child's subjective symptoms and the parent's history provide valuable information to help establish a diagnosis. Older children often describe the condition as painful, itching, or tingling or in other descriptive terms. However, much can be determined by also observing the younger child's behavior. Does the child scratch? Is the child restless or irritable? Does the child favor or avoid using a body part? A careful history provides important clues. Has the child had access to chemicals or been in the woods or around a woodpile? Has the child eaten a new food? Is the child taking medication? Has the child any known allergy? Do siblings or playmates have similar lesions? What soap or bubble bath is used for bathing?

It is important for nurses to not only describe but also assess skin lesions and wounds. The color, shape, and distribution of lesions and wounds are important. Individual lesions are described according to standard terminology. Sometimes two descriptors are used for a particular characteristic (e.g., maculopapular rash). To confirm or amplify the findings made by inspection, the nurse may gently palpate the skin to detect characteristics such as temperature, moisture, texture, elasticity, and edema. Wounds are assessed for depth of tissue damage, evidence of healing, and signs of infection.

> ! **NURSING ALERT**
>
> Signs of wound infection are:
> - Increased erythema, especially beyond the wound margin
> - Edema
> - Purulent exudate
> - Pain
> - Increased temperature

The frequency of wound assessment depends on the severity and complexity of the wound. For example, simple or chronic wounds are assessed weekly; infected or complex wounds are assessed daily. Wounds are measured at least weekly (height, width, and depth). The wound bed is assessed for color, drainage, odor, necrosis, granulation tissue, fibrin slough, undermining and condition of the wound edges, and the color and condition of the surrounding skin (Butler, 2007).

Therapeutic programs are designed to include general measures such as rest, protection, and relief of discomfort and specific treatments such as medication and physical techniques. Only a few skin diseases are contagious; therefore it is usually not necessary to isolate the affected child except from persons in danger of acquiring a secondary infection (e.g., a child receiving large doses of corticosteroids or other immunosuppressant drugs or a child with an immunologic deficiency disorder). However, if the skin manifestation is caused by a viral exanthema, such as measles or chickenpox, the child is prevented from exposing other susceptible children.

Wound Care

Parents can generally manage small skin lesions or wounds at home. The parents are instructed to wash their hands and then wash the wound gently with mild soap and water or normal saline. They are cautioned to avoid povidone-iodine, alcohol, and hydrogen peroxide because these products are toxic to wounds.

> ! **NURSING ALERT**
>
> Do not put anything in a wound that you would not put in the eye. The safest solution is normal saline.

Open wounds are covered with a dressing, such as a commercial adhesive bandage, although larger wounds may benefit from the use of occlusive dressings. If occlusive dressings are applied, parents should learn how to apply and remove the dressings correctly. For example, hydrocolloid dressings adhere best if a wide margin is left around the wound and the dressing is pressed against intact skin until it adheres. If a dressing needs to be secured, a nonalcohol skin barrier can be applied to protect the skin or the wound can be "picture framed" with hydrocolloid dressing and dressing tape can be secured to the hydrocolloid. This method of securing the dressing protects the skin when the tape is removed. Montgomery straps or stretch netting can also be used to secure dressings and to avoid the use of tape.

> ! **NURSING ALERT**
>
> Advise parents that the yellow gel forming under hydrocolloid dressings may look like pus and has a distinct odor (somewhat fruity) but is normal leakage.

Dressings are removed carefully to protect intact skin and the epithelial surface of the wound. When removing transparent or hydrocolloid dressings, the nurse or parent should raise one edge of the dressing and pull *parallel* to the skin to loosen the adhesive. The longer the dressings are left on, the easier they are to remove. Less frequent dressing changes decrease wound contamination.

Lacerations present a special challenge. The injured child and family are usually distressed by the bleeding. In particular, scalp lacerations tend to bleed profusely. Parental guilt and shock usually accompany the injury. The initial nursing intervention is to apply pressure to the area and to attempt to calm the child before further examination. Unless there is bleeding from a severed artery, the wound is cleansed with a forced jet of sterile tepid water or saline (via syringe) and examined for extent, depth, and presence of foreign material such as dirt, glass, or fabric fragments.

The location of the wound facilitates assessment. Wounds over bony areas may contain bone chips, and clear fluid seeping from severe head wounds may indicate cerebrospinal fluid. A pressure dressing is applied for transfer to medical care. After the child is in a medical facility, he or she is prepared for suturing.

Puncture wounds that do not require a tetanus booster are soaked in warm water and soap for several minutes. Causing the wound to rebleed may be helpful. An adhesive bandage can be applied if desired. Puncture wounds of the head, chest, or abdomen or those that could still contain a portion of the puncturing object must be evaluated carefully.

Parents are cautioned against opening blisters or kissing a wound "to make it better." The wound can easily become contaminated from germs in the human mouth. If scabs form, they are allowed to slough off without assistance; picking or early removal may cause scarring and secondary infection. Parents are advised to seek medical help if there is evidence of infection.

Relief of Symptoms

Most therapeutic regimens for skin lesions are directed toward relief of pruritus, the most common subjective complaint. Cooling the affected area and increasing the skin pH with cool baths or compresses and alkaline applications (e.g., baking soda baths) help reduce the itching. Clothing and bed linens should be soft and lightweight to decrease the irritation from friction and stimulation.

During treatment, both the affected and unaffected skin are protected from damage and secondary infection. Preventing scratching is important. Older children can cooperate, although they may need to be reminded to stop scratching or rubbing. However, small or uncooperative children may require the use of devices such as mittens (especially during sleep) or special coverings. Keeping fingernails clean, short, and trimmed reduces the risk for secondary infection.

Antipruritic medications, such as diphenhydramine (Benadryl) or hydroxyzine (Atarax), may be prescribed for severe itching, especially if it disturbs the child's rest. Pain and discomfort are usually managed with nonpharmacologic measures and mild analgesia. Severe pain requires more potent medication. Occlusive dressings over wounds reduce pain. For suturing wounds, a topical anesthetic or intradermal buffered lidocaine should be used (see Pain Management, Chapter 30).

Topical Therapy

The specific type of topical therapy and the mode of application depend on the nature and location of the lesion. It is especially important to wash the hands before and after application of any topical therapy. The skin is assessed before the application and reassessed after treatment. Any observed changes are noted and described.

Wet compresses or dressings cool the skin by evaporation, relieve itching and inflammation, and cleanse the area by loosening and removing crusts and debris. A variety of ingredients, such as plain water or Burow solution (available without a prescription), can be applied on Kerlix gauze; plain gauze; or (preferably) soft cotton cloths such as freshly laundered handkerchiefs or strips from diaper, sheeting, or pillowcase material.

Dressings immersed in the desired solution are wrung out slightly and applied to the affected area wet but not dripping. They are applied flat and smooth in such a way that motion is not totally restricted—fingers are wrapped separately, and arms and legs are wrapped so that elbows and knees can bend. Dressings are held in place by Kerlix or other cotton wrap, tubular stockinette, mittens, and socks (two pairs—one to hold the dressings in place and the other to protect from movement). When evaporation begins to dry them, the dressings are removed, rewet in the solution, and reapplied using aseptic technique. The solution is *not* poured or applied with a syringe directly over the dressings. As fluid evaporates, the solution becomes more concentrated, and this could damage sensitive lesions.

Fresh solution at room temperature is applied at 2-, 3-, or 4-hour intervals and allowed to remain on the lesion for 20 to 90 minutes. Wet dressings are seldom continued after about 48 hours. The child is protected against chilling during treatment, and no more than 20% of the body is covered with a dressing at one time to avoid the risk for hypothermia. After treatment, the skin is dried thoroughly by patting with a towel. Lotion or other medication (if prescribed) is applied at this time.

When children are uncooperative in the use of wet dressings, soaks are often used for removal of crusts and for their mild astringent action. The same solutions are used as for wet compresses. Gaining young children's cooperation for hand or foot soaks is difficult unless the procedure is accompanied by play. Older infants and toddlers delight in playing with brightly colored objects or poker chips scattered over the bottom of the receptacle, and preschoolers can be challenged to hold a floating item beneath the water's surface. However, these activities require supervision; infants and small children place items in their mouths, and children easily lose control with water play. Washing dishes, cars, dolls, or doll clothes will also occupy time during soaks.

Although older children can cooperate, they, too, need something to do during the procedure, such as listening to music or a story or watching television. Placing the solution and the extremity in a plastic sealable bag is an effective method to soak a hand or foot.

Baths are useful in the treatment of widespread dermatitis by evenly distributing the soothing antipruritic and antiinflammatory effects of the solution, usually oatmeal or mineral oil preparations. The solution is added to a tub of lukewarm water. The temperature of the bath is tepid, and the treatment usually lasts 15 to 30 minutes. Therapeutic baths are more interesting when toy boats or other items for water play accompany the procedure.

Topical applications are applied to skin lesions to ease discomfort, prevent further injury, and facilitate healing. A thin application of the ointment or cream may be covered with a plastic film and anchored with adhesive, covered with a commercial transparent dressing, or wrapped in Kerlix gauze and held in place by a stretchy net dressing. Topical preparations are applied systematically with the contour of the body surface (not simply up and down). Children love to be "painted," and lotion applications can be fun when an ordinary paintbrush is used. Regardless of the type of preparation used, parents need detailed information on how to apply it and how long the preparation should remain on the skin.

> ## ! NURSING ALERT
>
> Provide written instructions and demonstrate to parents the correct amount of topical medication to apply (e.g., size of a pea, thin film to cover). If more than one preparation is applied, mark the containers with numbers so the parents remember the correct order of application. Stress that more is not necessarily better with some medications, such as steroids.

Home Care and Family Support

Dermatologic conditions always involve the family, but few situations require hospitalization and most care is delivered at home. Because the family members must carry out the treatment plan, their cooperation is essential. Regimens that are simple to accomplish in the clinic, hospital, or primary care provider's office may be frustrating and baffling at home. The family may also need assistance in adapting equipment available for home therapy.

It is important that the child and family be given as detailed explanations as possible about both the expected and unexpected results of treatment, including any ill effects that might occur. If unexplained reactions develop, the family is directed to discontinue treatment and report the reactions to the appropriate person. The use of over-the-counter medicines is discouraged unless the preparations have been discussed with and approved by the health care provider.

Because the skin is the most visible portion of the body, defects in its surface alter its appearance and distress the child. Skin problems may also result in rejection by others. Parents of other children may fear that their children will "catch" the disorder. Occasionally, the affected child's own family members reduce their interaction or physical contact with the child. This is seldom a problem with dermatitis of short duration, but chronic conditions can frequently create problems and affect the child's self-esteem.

INFECTIONS OF THE SKIN

Bacterial Infections

Normally, the skin harbors a variety of bacterial flora, including the major pathogenic varieties of staphylococci and streptococci. The degree of pathogenicity of the organism depends on its invasiveness and toxicity, the integrity of the skin, and the immune and cellular defenses of the host. Children with congenital or acquired immunodeficiency disorders (e.g., acquired immunodeficiency syndrome [AIDS]), those in a debilitated condition, those receiving immunosuppressant therapy, and those with a generalized malignancy such as leukemia or lymphoma are at risk for developing bacterial infections.

Because of the characteristic "walling-off" process of the inflammatory reaction (abscess formation), staphylococci are more difficult to treat and the local infected area is associated with an increase in bacteria all over the skin surface that serves as a source of continuing infection. In previous years, methicillin-resistant *Staphylococcus aureus* (MRSA) infections were seen primarily in nursing homes and hospitals. In recent years, the number of MRSA community-acquired infections has risen (Kaplan, 2006). All of these factors underline the importance of careful hand washing and cleanliness when caring for infected children and their lesions to prevent the spread of infection and as an essential prophylactic measure when caring for infants and small children. Common bacterial skin disorders are outlined in Table 47-2.

❚ CARE MANAGEMENT

The major nursing functions related to bacterial skin infections are to prevent the spread of infection and to prevent complications. Impetigo contagiosa and MRSA infection can easily spread by self-inoculation; therefore caution the child against touching the involved area. Hand washing is mandatory before and after contact with an affected child. Also emphasize hand washing to both the child and the family. Many children with AD are colonized with MRSA in the nares and under the fingernails (Rosenthal, 2004). For many bacterial infections and for MRSA infection in particular, the child should be provided with washcloths and towels separate from those of other family members. The child's pajamas, underwear, and other clothes should be changed daily and washed in hot water. Razors used for shaving should be discarded after each use and not shared. To prevent recurrence, some infectious disease specialists recommend bathing in a chlorine bath once or twice weekly. A 5-minute soak of 2.5 mL of bleach diluted in 13 gallons of water or $\frac{1}{2}$ cup of bleach diluted in a standard 50-gallon tub one-fourth filled with water could decrease community-acquired MRSA colonies by more than 99.9% (Fisher, Chain, Hair, et al., 2008; Kaplan, 2008). In addition, mupirocin can be applied to the nares of patients and families twice daily for 2 to 4 weeks to prevent reinfection (Dohil and Eichenfield, 2005).

Children and parents are often tempted to squeeze follicular lesions. They must be warned that squeezing will not hasten the resolution of the infection and that there is a risk for making the lesion worse or spreading the infection. No attempt should be made

to puncture the surface of the pustule with a needle or sharp instrument. A child with a sty may waken with the eyelids of the affected eye sealed shut with exudate. The child or the parents are instructed to gently wipe the eyelid from the inner to the outer edge with warm water and a clean washcloth until the exudate is removed.

The child with limited cellulitis of an extremity is usually managed at home on a regimen of oral antibiotics and warm compresses. The parents are taught the procedures and instructed in administration of the medication. Children with more extensive cellulitis, especially around a joint with lymphadenitis or on the face, are usually admitted to the hospital for parenteral antibiotics with continued treatment at home. Nurses are responsible for teaching the family to administer the medication and apply compresses.

Viral Infections

Viruses are intracellular parasites that produce their effect by using the intracellular substances of the host cells. Composed of only a DNA or ribonucleic acid (RNA) core enclosed in an antigenic protein shell, viruses are unable to provide for their own metabolic needs or to reproduce themselves. After a virus penetrates a cell of the host organism, it sheds the outer shell and disappears within the cell, where the nucleic acid core stimulates the host cell to form more virus material from its intracellular substance. In a viral infection, the epidermal cells react with inflammation and vesiculation (as in herpes simplex) or by proliferating to form growths (warts).

Many of the communicable viral diseases of childhood are associated with rashes, and each rash is characteristic. The type of lesion and the configuration of rubeola, rubella, and chickenpox are described in Table 33-2. Other common viral disorders of the skin are outlined in Table 47-3.

Dermatophytoses (Fungal Infections)

The dermatophytoses (ringworm) are infections caused by a group of closely related filamentous fungi that invade primarily the stratum corneum, hair, and nails. These are superficial infections that live on, not in, the skin. They are confined to the dead keratin layers and are unable to survive in the deeper layers. Because the keratin is desquamated constantly, the fungus must multiply at a rate that equals the rate of keratin production to maintain itself; otherwise, the infection would be shed with the discarded skin cells. Common dermatophytoses are outlined in Table 47-4.

Dermatophytoses are designated by the Latin word *tinea*, with further designation related to the area of the body where they are found (e.g., tinea capitis [ringworm of the scalp]). Dermatophyte infections are most often transmitted from one person to another or from infected animals to humans. Diagnosis is made from microscopic examination of scrapings taken from the advancing periphery of the lesion, which almost always produces a scale.

❚ CARE MANAGEMENT

When teaching families how to care for ringworm, the nurse should emphasize good health and hygiene. Because of the infectious nature of the disease, affected children should not exchange grooming items, headgear, scarves, or other articles of apparel that have been in proximity to the infected area with other children. Affected children are provided with their own towels and directed to wear a protective cap at night to avoid transmitting the fungus to bedding, especially if they sleep with another person. Because the infection can be acquired by animal-to-human transmission, all household

TABLE 47-2   BACTERIAL INFECTIONS

DISORDER AND ORGANISM	MANIFESTATIONS	MANAGEMENT	COMMENTS
Impetigo contagiosa (Fig. 47-1)— *Staphylococcus*	Begins as a reddish macule Becomes vesicular Ruptures easily, leaving superficial, moist erosion Tends to spread peripherally in sharply marginated irregular outlines Exudate dries to form heavy, honey-colored crusts Pruritus common *Systemic effects*—Minimal or asymptomatic	Careful removal of undermined skin, crusts, and debris by softening with 1:20 Burow solution compresses Topical application of bactericidal ointment Systemic administration of oral or parenteral antibiotics (penicillin) in severe or extensive lesions	Tends to heal without scarring unless secondary infection Autoinoculable and contagious Common in toddlers and preschoolers May be superimposed on eczema
Pyoderma— *Staphylococcus, Streptococcus*	Deeper extension of infection into dermis Tissue reaction more severe *Systemic effects*—Fever, lymphangitis	Soap and water cleansing Wet compresses Bathing with antibacterial soap as prescribed Do not share washcloths or towels Mupirocin to nares and lesions as prescribed Systemic antibiotics	Autoinoculable and contagious May heal with or without scarring
Folliculitis (pimple), furuncle (boil), carbuncle (multiple boils)— *Staphylococcus aureus*	Folliculitis—Infection of hair follicle Furuncle—Larger lesion with more redness and swelling at a single follicle Carbuncle—More extensive lesion with widespread inflammation and "pointing" at several follicular orifices *Systemic effects*—Malaise if severe	Skin cleanliness Local warm, moist compresses Topical application of antibiotic agents Systemic antibiotics in severe cases Incision and drainage of severe lesions followed by wound irrigations with antibiotics or suitable drain implantation	Autoinoculable and contagious Furuncle and carbuncle tend to heal with scar formation Never squeeze a lesion
Cellulitis— *Streptococcus, Staphylococcus, Haemophilus influenzae* (Fig. 47-2)	Inflammation of skin and subcutaneous tissues with intense redness, swelling, and firm infiltration Lymphangitis "streaking" frequently seen Involvement of regional lymph nodes common May progress to abscess formation *Systemic effects*—Fever, malaise	Oral or parenteral antibiotics Rest and immobilization of both affected area and child Hot, moist compresses to area	Hospitalization may be necessary for child with systemic symptoms Otitis media may be associated with facial cellulitis
Staphylococcal scalded skin syndrome—*S. aureus*	Macular erythema with "sandpaper" texture of involved skin Epidermis becoming wrinkled (in ≤2 days), and large bullae appearing	Systemic administration of antibiotics Gentle cleansing with saline, Burow solution, or 0.25% silver nitrate compresses	Infants subject to fluid loss; impaired body temperature regulation; and secondary infection, such as pneumonia, cellulitis, and septicemia Heals without scarring

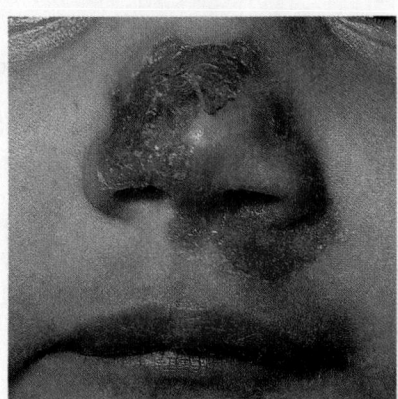

FIG 47-1 Impetigo contagiosa. (From Weston WL, Lane AT: *Color textbook of pediatric dermatology*, ed 4, St Louis, 2007, Mosby.)

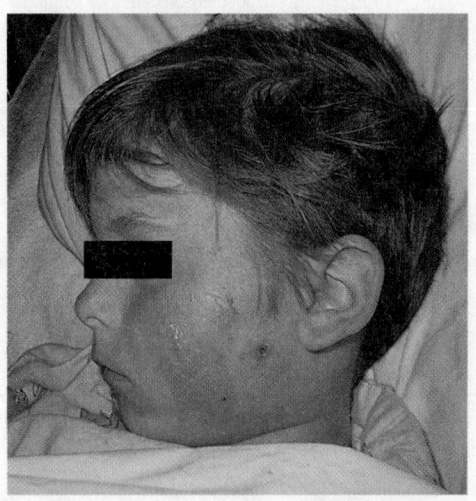

FIG 47-2 Cellulitis of cheek from a puncture wound. (From Weston WL, Lane AT: *Color textbook of pediatric dermatology*, ed 4, St Louis, 2007, Mosby.)

TABLE 47-3 VIRAL INFECTIONS

INFECTION	MANIFESTATIONS	MANAGEMENT	COMMENTS
Verruca (warts) *Cause*—Human papillomavirus (various types)	Usually well-circumscribed, gray or brown, elevated, firm papules with a roughened, finely papillomatous texture Occur anywhere but usually appear on exposed areas such as fingers, hands, face, and soles May be single or multiple Asymptomatic	Not uniformly successful Local destructive therapy, individualized according to location, type, and number—surgical removal, electrocautery, curettage, cryotherapy (liquid nitrogen), caustic solutions (lactic acid and salicylic acid in flexible collodion, retinoic acid, salicylic acid plasters), x-ray treatment, laser	Common in children Tend to disappear spontaneously Course unpredictable Most destructive techniques tend to leave scars Autoinoculable Repeated irritation will cause to enlarge Apply topical anesthetic *EMLA*
Verruca plantaris (plantar wart)	Located on plantar surface of feet and, because of pressure, are practically flat; may be surrounded by a collar of hyperkeratosis	Apply caustic solution to wart and wear foam insole with hole cut to relieve pressure on wart; soak 20 minutes after 2-3 days; repeat until wart comes out	Destructive techniques tend to leave scars, which may cause problems with walking Apply topical anesthetic *EMLA*
Herpes simplex virus Type I (cold sore, fever blister) Type II (genital)	Grouped, burning, and itching vesicles on inflammatory base, usually on or near mucocutaneous junctions (lips, nose, genitalia, buttocks) Vesicles dry, forming a crust followed by exfoliation and spontaneous healing in 8-10 days May be accompanied by regional lymphadenopathy	Avoidance of secondary infection Burow solution compresses during weeping stages Topical therapy (penciclovir) to shorten duration of cold sores Oral antiviral (acyclovir) for initial infection or to reduce severity in recurrence Valacyclovir (Valtrex), an oral antiviral, used for episodic treatment of recurrent genital herpes; reduces pain, stops viral shedding, and has a more convenient administration schedule than acyclovir	Heal without scarring unless secondary infection Type I cold sores prevented by using sunscreens protecting against UVA and UVB light to prevent lip blisters Aggravated by corticosteroids Positive psychologic effect from treatment May be fatal in children with depressed immunity
Varicella-zoster virus (herpes zoster; shingles)	Caused by same virus that causes varicella (chickenpox) Virus has affinity for posterior root ganglia, posterior horn of spinal cord, and skin; crops of vesicles usually confined to dermatome following along course of affected nerve Usually preceded by neuralgic pain, hyperesthesias, or itching May be accompanied by constitutional symptoms	Symptomatic Analgesics for pain Mild sedation sometimes helpful Local moist compresses Drying lotions sometimes helpful Ophthalmic variety: use systemic corticotropin (ACTH) or corticosteroids Acyclovir Lidocaine (Lidoderm) topical anesthetic	Pain in children usually minimal Postherpetic pain does not occur in children Chickenpox may follow exposure; isolate affected child from other children in a hospital or school May occur in children with depressed immunity; can be fatal
Molluscum contagiosum *Cause*—Pox virus Small, benign tumors	Flesh-colored papules with a central caseous plug (umbilicated) Usually asymptomatic	Cases in well children resolve spontaneously in about 18 months Treatment reserved for troublesome cases Apply topical anesthetic *EMLA* and remove with curette Use tretinoin gel 0.01% or cantharidin (Cantharone) liquid* Curettage or cryotherapy	Common in school-age children Spread by skin-to-skin contact, including autoinoculation and fomite-to-skin contact

ACTH, Adrenocorticotropic hormone; *EMLA*, eutectic mixture of lidocaine and prilocaine; *UVA*, ultraviolet A; *UVB*, ultraviolet B.
*Not available in the United States but can be purchased in Canada.

TABLE 47-4   DERMATOPHYTOSES (FUNGAL INFECTIONS)

DISEASE AND ORGANISM	MANIFESTATIONS	MANAGEMENT	COMMENTS
Tinea capitis— *Trichophyton tonsurans,* *Microsporum audouinii,* *Microsporum canis* (Fig. 47-3, *A*)	Lesions in scalp but may extend to hairline or neck Characteristic configuration of scaly, circumscribed patches or patchy, scaling areas of alopecia Generally asymptomatic but severe, deep inflammatory reaction may occur that manifests as boggy, encrusted lesions (kerions) Pruritic Microscopic examination of scales is diagnostic	Oral griseofulvin Oral ketoconazole for difficult cases Selenium sulfide shampoos Topical antifungal agents (e.g., clotrimazole, haloprogin, miconazole)	Person-to-person transmission Animal-to-person transmission Rarely, permanent loss of hair *M. audouinii* transmitted from one human being to another directly or from personal items; *M. canis* usually contracted from household pets, especially cats Atopic individuals more susceptible
Tinea corporis— *Trichophyton rubrum,* *Trichophyton mentagrophytes, M. canis, Epidermophyton* (see Fig. 47-3, *B*)	Generally round or oval, erythematous scaling patch that spreads peripherally and clears centrally; may involve nails (tinea unguium) *Diagnosis*—Direct microscopic examination of scales Usually unilateral	Oral griseofulvin Local application of antifungal preparation such as tolnaftate, haloprogin, miconazole, clotrimazole; apply 1 inch beyond periphery of lesion; continual application 1-2 weeks after no sign of lesion	Usually of animal origin from infected pets Majority of infections in children caused by *M. canis* and *M. audouinii*
Tinea cruris ("jock itch")—*Epidermophyton floccosum, T. rubrum, T. mentagrophytes*	Skin response similar to tinea corporis Localized to medial proximal aspect of thigh and crural fold; may involve scrotum in boys Pruritic *Diagnosis*—Same as for tinea corporis	Local application of tolnaftate liquid Wet compresses or sitz baths may be soothing	Rare in preadolescent children Health education regarding personal hygiene

Tinea pedis ("athlete's foot")—*T. rubrum, Trichophyton interdigitale, E. floccosum*	On intertriginous areas between toes or on plantar surface of feet
	Lesions vary:
	   Maceration and fissuring between toes
	   Patches with pinhead-size vesicles on plantar surface
	Pruritic
	Diagnosis—Direct microscopic examination of scrapings
		Oral griseofulvin
		Local applications of tolnaftate liquid and antifungal powder containing tolnaftate
		Acute infections—Compresses or soaks followed by application of glucocorticoid cream
		Elimination of conditions of heat and perspiration by clean, light socks and well-ventilated shoes; avoidance of occlusive shoes
			Most frequent in adolescents and adults; rare in children, but occurrence increases with wearing of plastic shoes
			Transmission to other individuals rare despite general opinion to contrary
			Ointments not successful

Candidiasis (moniliasis)— *Candida albicans*	Grows in chronically moist areas Inflamed areas with white exudate, peeling, and easy bleeding Pruritic *Diagnosis*—Characteristic appearance	Amphotericin B, nystatin ointment, or other antifungal preparations to affected areas	Common form of diaper dermatitis (see Fig. 47-8) Oral form common in infants Vaginal form in older girls May be disseminated in immunosuppressed children

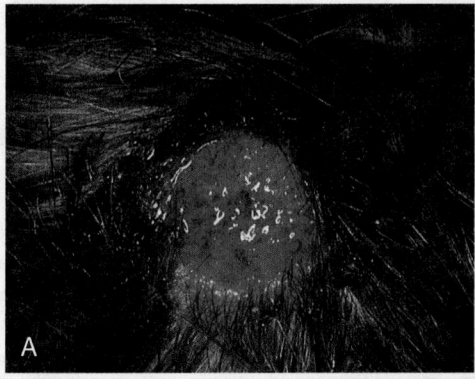
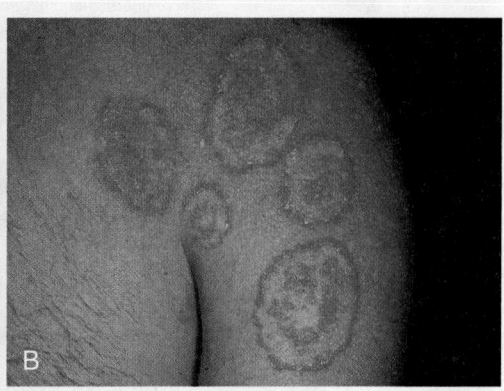

FIG 47-3 A, Tinea capitis. **B,** Tinea corporis. Both infections are caused by *Microsporum canis,* the "kitten" or "puppy" fungus. (From Habif TP: *Clinical dermatology: a color guide to diagnosis and therapy,* ed 4, St Louis, 2004, Mosby.)

pets should be examined for the disorder. Other sources of infection are seats with headrests (theater seats), seats in public transportation vehicles, helmets, and gymnasium mats.

Both 2% ketoconazole and 1% selenium sulfide shampoos may reduce colony counts of dermatophytes. These shampoos can be used in combination with oral therapy to reduce the transmission of disease to others. The shampoo should be applied to the scalp for 5 to 10 minutes at least 3 times per week. The child may return to school after the therapy is initiated.

Alternately, if the child is treated with the drug *griseofulvin,* the therapy frequently continues for weeks or months, and because subjective symptoms subside, children or parents may be tempted to decrease or discontinue the drug. The nurse should emphasize to family members the importance of maintaining the prescribed dosage schedule and of taking the medication with high-fat foods for best absorption. They are also instructed regarding possible drug side effects, such as headache, gastrointestinal upset, fatigue, insomnia, and photosensitivity. For children who take the drug over many months, periodic testing is required to monitor for leukopenia and assess liver and renal function. Newer antifungal medications such as terbinafine, itraconazole, and fluconazole may be used when there are adverse reactions to griseofulvin. These drugs are being studied to determine their efficacy and safety in treating tinea capitis in children but are not approved by the U.S. Food and Drug Administration (FDA) for this indication.

Systemic Mycotic (Fungal) Infections

Mycotic (systemic or deep fungal) infections have the capacity to invade the viscera, as well as the skin. The most common infections are the lung diseases, which are usually acquired by inhalation of fungal spores. These fungi produce a variable spectrum of disease, and some are common in certain geographic areas. They are not transmitted from person to person but appear to reside in the soil, from which their spores are airborne. The cutaneous lesions caused by deep fungal infections are granulomatous and appear as ulcers, plaques, nodules, fungating masses, and abscesses. The course of deep fungal diseases is chronic with slow progression that favors sensitization (Table 47-5).

TABLE 47-5	**SYSTEMIC MYCOSES**			
DISORDER AND ORGANISM	**SKIN MANIFESTATIONS**	**SYSTEMIC MANIFESTATIONS**	**MANAGEMENT**	**COMMENTS**
North American blastomycosis— *Blastomyces dermatitidis*	Chronic granulomatous lesions and microabscesses in any part of body Initial lesion is a papule; undergoes ulceration and peripheral spread	Pulmonary symptoms, such as cough, chest pain, weakness, and weight loss May have skeletal involvement, with bone destruction and formation of cutaneous abscesses	IV administration of amphotericin B	Usual portal of entry is lungs Source of infection unknown Noninfectious Pulmonary infections may be mild and self-limiting and require no treatment Progressive disease often fatal
Cryptococcosis— *Cryptococcus neoformans (Torula histolytica)*	Usually on face; acneiform, firm, nodular, painless eruption	CNS *manifestations*— Headache, dizziness, stiff neck, and signs of increased intracranial pressure Low-grade fever, mild cough, lung infiltration	IV amphotericin B; may be administered intrathecally for CNS involvement 5-Fluorocytosine for meningitis Excision and drainage of local lesions	Acquired by inhalation of dust but may enter through skin Prognosis serious Noninfectious Increased incidence in persons receiving corticosteroids with lymphoreticular malignancies or type 2 diabetes
Histoplasmosis— *Histoplasma capsulatum*	Not distinctive or uniform but most appear as punched-out or granulomatous ulcers	General systemic symptoms may include pallor, diarrhea, vomiting, irregular spiking temperature, hepatosplenomegaly, and pulmonary symptoms Any tissue of body may be involved with related symptoms	IV amphotericin B for severe cases Oral ketoconazole	Organism cultured from soil, especially where contaminated with fowl droppings Fungus enters through skin or mucous membranes of mouth and respiratory tract Endemic in Mississippi and Ohio River valleys Disseminated diseases most common in infants and children
Coccidioidomycosis (valley fever)— *Coccidioides immitis*	Erythema nodosum Erythema multiforme Erythematous maculopapular rash	Primary lung disease usually asymptomatic May be sign of acute febrile illness Disseminated disease is serious	IV amphotericin B IV miconazole (synthetic imidazole) Intraventricular miconazole plus oral ketoconazole for CNS involvement Surgical resection of persistent pulmonary cavities	Inhalation of aerospores from soil Endemic in southwestern United States Usually resolves spontaneously Increased incidence in dark-skinned races (Filipino, African-American, Mexican, Asian)

CNS, Central nervous system; *IV,* intravenous.

SKIN DISORDERS RELATED TO CHEMICAL OR PHYSICAL CONTACTS

Contact Dermatitis

Contact dermatitis is an inflammatory reaction of the skin to chemical substances, natural or synthetic, that evoke a hypersensitivity response or direct irritation. The initial reaction occurs in an exposed region, most commonly the face and neck, backs of the hands, forearms, male genitalia, and lower legs. Early in the reaction, there is usually a sharp delineation between inflamed and normal skin that ranges from a faint, transient erythema to massive bullae on an erythematous swollen base. Itching is a constant symptom.

The cause may be a primary irritant or a sensitizing agent. A primary irritant is one that irritates any skin. A sensitizing agent produces an irritation on those individuals who have met the irritant or something chemically related to it, have undergone an immunologic change, and have become sensitized. Prior exposure is not necessarily a factor in the reaction. A sensitizer irritates in relatively low concentrations only persons who are allergic to it.

In infants, contact dermatitis occurs on the convex surfaces of the diaper area (see Diaper Dermatitis, p. 1511). Other agents that produce contact dermatitis include plants (poison ivy, oak, and sumac), animal irritants (wool, feathers, and furs), metal (nickel found in jewelry and the snaps on sleepers and denim), vegetable irritants (oleoresins, oils, and turpentine), synthetic fabrics (e.g., shoe components), dyes, cosmetics, perfumes, and soaps (including bubble baths). The list is endless.

The major goal in treatment is to prevent further exposure of the skin to the offending substance. Provided there is no further irritation, the skin's normal recuperative powers will often produce healing without treatment. Otherwise, treatment of contact dermatitis is based on severity. Mild cases are treated with topical steroids. Mild to moderately severe cases may require a 2-week course of strong topical corticosteroids. Very severe cases require systemic corticosteroids.

CARE MANAGEMENT

Nurses frequently detect evidence of contact dermatitis during routine physical assessments. Skin manifestations in specific areas suggest limited contact, such as around the eyes (mascara), areas of the body covered by clothing but not protected by undergarments (wool), or areas of the body not covered by clothing (UV injury). Generalized involvement is more likely to be caused by bubble bath or soap. Often nurses can determine the offending agent and counsel families regarding management. However, if the lesions persist, are extensive, or show evidence of infection, medical evaluation is indicated.

Poison Ivy, Oak, and Sumac

Contact with the dry or succulent portions of any of three poisonous plants (ivy, oak, and sumac) produces localized, streaked or spotty, oozing, and painful impetiginous lesions. The offending substance in these plants is an oil, urushiol, that is extremely potent. Sensitivity to urushiol is not inborn but is developed after one or two exposures and may change over a lifetime. All parts of the plants contain the oil, including dried leaves and stems (Fig. 47-4, A). Even smoke from burning brush piles can produce a reaction.

Animals do not seem to be affected by the oil; however, dogs or other animals that have run or played in the plants may carry the sap on their fur, and animals that eat the plants can transfer the oil

in their saliva. Shoes, tools, and toys can transfer the oil. Golf balls that have been in the rough are another source of contact.

Urushiol takes effect as soon as it touches the skin. It penetrates through the epidermis and bonds with the dermal layer, where it initiates an immune response. The full-blown reaction is evident after about 2 days, with redness, swelling, and itching at the site of contact. Several days later, streaked or spotty blisters oozing serum from damaged cells produce the characteristic impetiginous lesions (Fig. 47-4, B). The lesions dry and heal spontaneously, and itching stops by 10 to 14 days.

Therapeutic Management

As soon as an exposure is realized, there is no time to waste. The earlier the skin is cleansed, the greater the chance of removing the urushiol before it attaches to the skin. The exposed skin can be cleansed with isopropyl alcohol followed by water. A shower with soap and warm water should follow. Clothes, tools, shoes, and any other objects that had contact with the plants should be cleaned with alcohol and then water.

Treatment of the lesions includes calamine lotion, soothing Burow solution compresses, or Aveeno baths to relieve discomfort. Topical corticosteroid gel is effective for prevention or relief of inflammation, especially when applied before blisters form. Oral corticosteroids may be needed for severe reactions, and a sedative such as diphenhydramine may be ordered.

CARE MANAGEMENT

When it is known that the child has made contact with the plant, the area is immediately flushed (preferably within 15 minutes) with *cold* running water to neutralize the urushiol not yet bonded to the skin. If there is a stream nearby, an effective method is to have the child enter the water (clothes and all) and allow the water to rinse the oil from both skin and clothing. Harsh soap is contraindicated because it removes protective skin oils and dilutes the urushiol, allowing it to spread; hard scrubbing irritates the skin. All clothing that has come in contact with the plant is removed with care and thoroughly laundered in hot water and detergent. Every effort is made to prevent the child from scratching the lesions. Although the lesions do not spread by contact with the blister serum or from scratching, they can become secondarily infected.

Prevention. Prevention is best accomplished by avoiding contact and removing the plant from the environment. All children, especially those known to be sensitive, should be taught to recognize the plant. Information regarding means for destroying plants can be obtained from the U.S. Department of Agriculture or U.S. Forestry Service. Home garden sprays that kill broad-leaf plants or all vegetation (e.g., Roundup or Spectracide) are ineffective. If poisonous plants are growing in a public community area, the local authorities should be contacted to remove the plants. A cream that protects exposed skin from poison oak and ivy is Ivy Block.

Drug Reactions

Adverse reactions to drugs are seen more often in the skin than in any other organ, although any organ of the body can be affected. The reaction may be a result of toxicity related to drug concentration, individual intolerance to the average dosage of the drug, or an allergic or idiosyncratic response. The manifestations may be associated with side effects or secondary effects of a drug, either of which are unrelated to its primary pharmacologic actions.

Although any drug is capable of producing a reaction in the susceptible individual, some drugs have a tendency to produce a

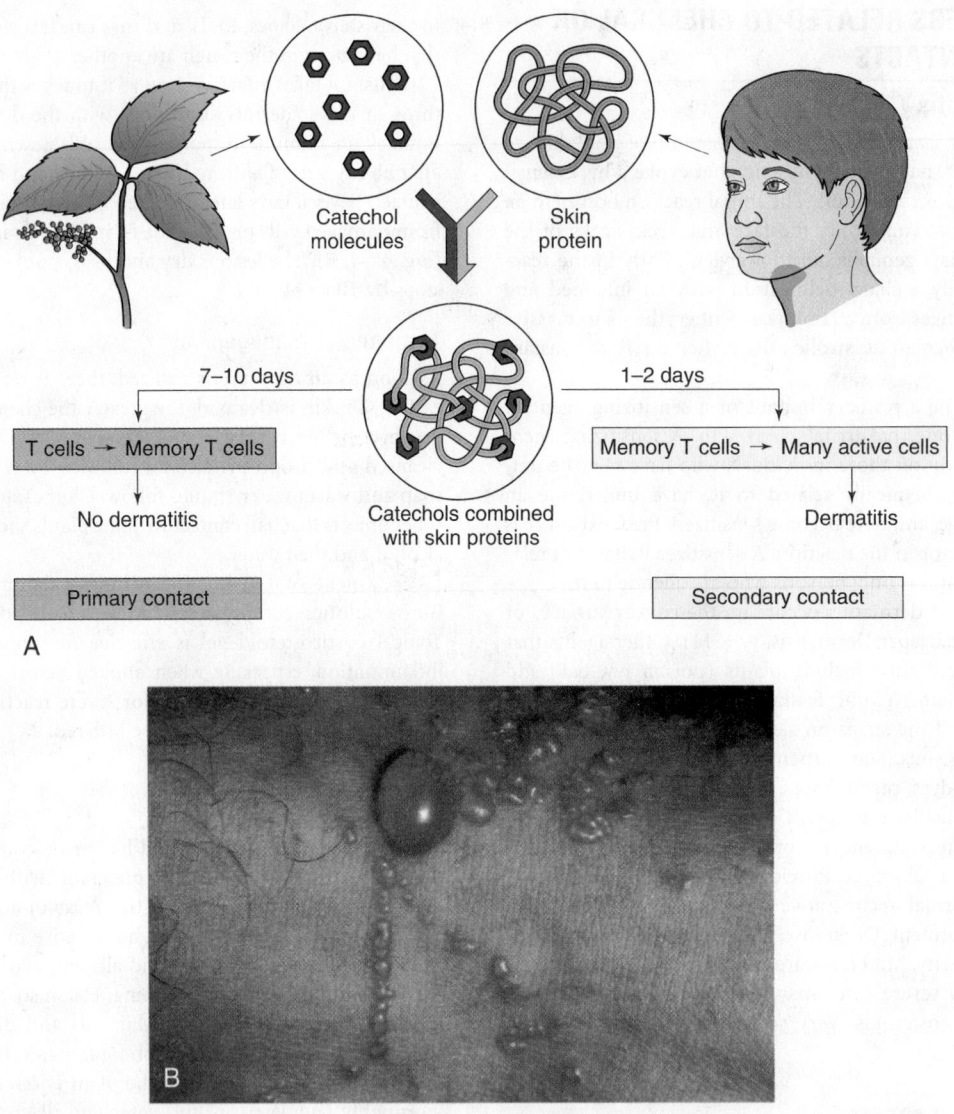

FIG 47-4 A, Development of allergic contact dermatitis. **B,** Poison ivy lesions; note the "streaked" blisters surrounding one large blister. (*A,* From McCance K, Huether S: *Pathophysiology: the biological basis for disease in adults and children,* ed 6, St Louis, 2010, Mosby. *B,* From Habif TP: *Clinical dermatology: a color guide to diagnosis and therapy,* ed 5, St Louis, 2010, Mosby.)

particular reaction consistently and others are more likely to produce an untoward effect. Many are allergenic responses that occur after a previous administration of the drug, even a topical application. Other factors influence a drug response in a particular individual. For example, the incidence increases with the amount and number of drugs given.

> **⚠ NURSING ALERT**
>
> Intravenous (IV) drugs are more likely to cause a reaction than oral drugs. Stop the drug but maintain the infusion with normal saline.

Manifestations of drug reactions may be delayed or immediate. A period of 7 days is usually required for a child to develop sensitivity to a drug that has never been administered previously. With prior sensitivity, the manifestations appear almost immediately. Rashes are the most common manifestation of adverse drug reactions in children. However, individual drug reactions may vary from a single lesion to extensive, generalized epidermal necrosis such as that seen in Stevens-Johnson syndrome (see Table 47-8). Cutaneous manifestations can resemble almost any skin disease and can be seen in almost any degree of severity. With few exceptions, the distribution of a drug eruption is widespread because it results from a circulating agent; appears as an inflammatory response with itching; is sudden in onset; and may be associated with constitutional symptoms such as fever, malaise, gastrointestinal upsets, anemia, or liver and kidney damage.

In most cases, treatment for simple cutaneous reactions consists of discontinuing the drug. Sometimes a decision is made to continue the drug (e.g., an antibiotic in an infant or small child) until the cause of the rash is clearly indicated. In urticarial-type eruptions, antihistamines may be ordered, and for widespread and severe lesions, corticosteroids are beneficial. Severe anaphylactic reactions are a medical emergency (see Anaphylaxis, Chapter 42).

CARE MANAGEMENT

The most effective means of management is prevention. Parents always remember a severe reaction. A careful history will elicit evidence of a previous drug reaction. The history should include the name of the drug, nature of the reaction, drug dosage, and how soon after administration the reaction occurred (see Chapter 29).

Nurses who suspect that a rash is caused by a medication should withhold any further dose and report the eruption to the health care practitioner. Frequent offenders in drug reactions are penicillin and sulfonamides, and nurses must be alert to this possibility. However, even common drugs, including aspirin, barbiturates, chemical agents in some foods, flavoring agents, and preservatives, are capable of producing an undesired response. Persons who have severe reactions should wear a medical identification bracelet or necklace in case of emergency or inadvertent administration of the offending drug.

Foreign Bodies

Parents can remove small wooden splinters with a needle and tweezers that have been sterilized with alcohol or a flame. The area around the sliver is washed with soap and water before removal is attempted. The sliver is exposed with the needle and then grasped firmly by the tweezers and pulled out. Some foreign bodies, such as a fishhook, pieces of glass, a difficult-to-see object, or a deeply embedded object (e.g., a needle in a foot or near a joint), require medical evaluation.

Small cactus prickles or spines are troublesome to remove, but the following methods may prove helpful:

- Apply a thin layer of water-soluble household glue and cover it with gauze; when the glue dries, peel off the gauze.
- Apply hair removal wax or body sugar, let it dry, and remove.
- Place cellophane tape, sticky side down, over the spines and lift it off.

SKIN DISORDERS RELATED TO ANIMAL CONTACTS

ARTHROPOD BITES AND STINGS

Bites and stings account for a significant amount of mild to moderate discomfort in children. Most bites and stings are managed by simple symptomatic measures, such as compresses, calamine lotion, and prevention of secondary infection. Arthropods include insects and arachnids, such as mites, ticks, spiders, and scorpions. Most arthropods in the United States, including tarantulas, are relatively harmless. Although all spiders produce venom that is injected via fangs, some are unable to pierce the skin and others produce venom that is insufficiently toxic to be harmful. Only scorpions and two spiders—the brown recluse and the black widow—inject venom deadly enough to require immediate attention. Children bitten by these arachnids must receive medical attention as soon as possible. Major offending creatures, their manifestations, and management are outlined in Table 47-6.

When a hymenopteran (bees in particular) stings, its barbed stinger penetrates the skin. As long as the stinger remains in the skin, the muscles push the stinger deeper and the venom is pumped into the wound. The best approach is to remove the stinger as quickly as possible and to get away from the vicinity of other insects to prevent further injury. Children who have become sensitized to hymenopteran bites may demonstrate a severe systemic response that can be life threatening. One sting can produce generalized urticaria, respiratory difficulty (from laryngeal edema), hypotension, and death. Intramuscular administration of epinephrine provides immediate relief and must be available for emergency use.

Hypersensitive children should wear a medical identification bracelet. They should also have a kit that contains epinephrine and a hypodermic syringe. Families are reminded to check the expiration date on the kit and to replace an outdated one. They should determine whether a nurse is available at the school and find out what the school policy is regarding administration of drugs. If a school nurse is not present, someone at the school should be designated to inject the epinephrine in case of an emergency.

Scabies

Scabies is an endemic infestation caused by the scabies mite, *Sarcoptes scabiei*. Lesions are created as the impregnated female burrows into the stratum corneum of the epidermis (never into living tissue) to deposit her eggs and feces. The inflammatory response and intense itching occur after the host becomes sensitized to the mite, approximately 30 to 60 days after initial contact. If the person has been previously sensitized to the mite, the response occurs within 48 hours after exposure. After this time, the areas over which the mite has traveled will begin to itch and develop the characteristic eruption (Box 47-1). Consequently, mites will not necessarily be located at all sites of eruption.

There is great variability in the type of lesions. Infants often develop an eczematous eruption; therefore the observer must look for discrete papules, burrows, or vesicles.

CARE MANAGEMENT

The treatment of scabies is the application of a scabicide. The drug of choice in children and infants older than 2 months is permethrin 5% cream (Elimite). Alternative drugs are 10% crotamiton, ivermectin, or 1% lindane cream or lotion. Lindane can be neurotoxic and is contraindicated in several age-groups. Lindane should be reserved for treatment of patients who fail to respond to other preparations (American Academy of Pediatrics [AAP], 2009).

Ivermectin, an oral medication, may be used to treat scabies in patients with secondary excoriations for whom topical scabicides are irritating and not well tolerated or whose infestation is refractory (AAP, 2009). However, the safety and efficacy of ivermectin for children younger than 5 years or children weighing less than 15 kg (33 lb) have not been established.

Because of the length of time between infestation and physical symptoms (30-60 days), all persons who were in close contact

---

BOX 47-1	CLINICAL MANIFESTATIONS OF SCABIES

Lesion

Children—Minute grayish brown, threadlike (mite burrows), pruritic
  Black dot at end of burrow (mite)
Infants—Eczematous eruption, pruritic

Distribution

Generally in intertriginous areas—Interdigital, axillary-cubital, popliteal, inguinal
Children older than 2 years—Primarily hands and wrists
Children younger than 2 years—Primarily feet and ankles

TABLE 47-6   SKIN LESIONS CAUSED BY ARTHROPODS

MECHANISM AND CHARACTERISTIC	MANIFESTATIONS	MANAGEMENT
Insect Bites—Flies, Gnats, Mosquitoes, Fleas		
Mechanism Foreign protein in insects' saliva introduced when skin is penetrated for a blood-sucking meal	Hypersensitivity reaction Papular urticaria Firm papules; may be capped by vesicles or excoriated Little or no reaction in nonsensitized person	*Treatment* Use antipruritic agents and baths. Administer antihistamines. Prevent secondary infection.
Distribution Almost everywhere—Fleas, mosquitoes, ants Suburbs and rural areas—Bees Urban areas—Hornets, wasps, yellow jackets		*Prevention* Avoid contact. Remove focus, such as treating furniture, mattresses, carpets, and pets, where insects may live. Apply insect repellent when exposure is anticipated.
Chiggers—Harvest Mites		
Mechanism Attach with claws and secrete a digestive substance that liquefies the host's epidermis	Same as insect bites Favor warm areas of body, especially intertriginous areas and areas covered with clothing	Avoid contact, especially in areas of tall grass and underbrush. Apply insect repellant when exposure is anticipated. Administer systemic steroids for extensive bites.
Manifestations Erythematous papules Intense itching		
Hymenopterans—Bees, Wasps, Hornets, Yellow Jackets, Fire Ants		
Mechanism Injection of venom through stinging apparatus Venom contains histamine; allergenic proteins; and often a spreading factor, hyaluronidase Severe reactions caused by hypersensitivity or multiple stings	*Local reaction*—Small red area, wheal, itching, and heat *Systemic reactions*—May be mild to severe, including generalized edema, pain, nausea and vomiting, confusion, respiratory embarrassment, and shock	*Treatment* Carefully scrape off stinger or pull out stinger as quickly as possible. Cleanse with soap and water. Apply cool compresses. Apply common household product (e.g., lemon juice, paste made with aspirin or baking soda). Administer antihistamines. *Severe reactions*—Administer epinephrine, corticosteroids; treat for shock.
		Prevention Teach child to wear shoes; to avoid wearing bright clothing, flowery prints, shiny jewelry, or perfumed grooming products (cologne, scented hairspray), which might attract the insect; and to avoid places where the insect may be contacted. Hypersensitive children should wear medical identification to indicate allergy and therapy needed; family should keep emergency medication and be taught its administration.
Black Widow Spider		
Mechanism Venom injected through a clawlike appendage; has neurotoxic action	Mild sting at time of bite Area becomes swollen, painful, and erythematous Dizziness, weakness, and abdominal pain May produce delirium, paralysis, seizures, and (if large amount of venom absorbed) death	*Treatment* Cleanse wound with antiseptic. Apply cool compresses. Administer antivenin. Administer muscle relaxant, such as calcium gluconate; analgesics or sedatives; hydrocortisone or diazepam intravenously.
Characteristics Shiny black spider, with a body about 1.25 cm (0.5 inch) long and a red or orange hourglass-shaped marking on underside Avoids light and bites in self-defense		*Prevention* Teach children to avoid places that harbor the spider (e.g., woodpiles).

TABLE 47-6	SKIN LESIONS CAUSED BY ARTHROPODS—cont'd	
MECHANISM AND CHARACTERISTIC	**MANIFESTATIONS**	**MANAGEMENT**
Brown Recluse Spider ***Mechanism*** Venom injected via fangs Venom contains powerful necrotoxin ***Characteristics*** Slender spider, with long legs and body length of 1-2 cm (0.4-0.8 inch); color is fawn to dark brown; recognized by fiddle-shaped mark on head Shy; bites only when annoyed or surprised Prefers dark areas where seldom disturbed	Mild sting at time of bite Transient erythema followed by bleb or blister; mild to severe pain in 2-8 hours; purple, star-shaped area in 3-4 days; necrotic ulceration in 7-14 days (Fig. 47-5) Systemic reactions may include fever, malaise, restlessness, nausea, vomiting, and joint pain Generalized petechial eruption Wounds heal with scar formation	***Treatment*** Apply cool compresses locally. Administer antibiotics, corticosteroids. Relieve pain. Wound may require skin graft. ***Prevention*** Teach children to avoid possible nesting sites.
Scorpions ***Mechanism*** Sting by means of a hooked caudal stinger that discharges venom Venom of more venomous species contains hemolysins, endotheliolysins, and neurotoxins ***Characteristics*** Usual habitat southwestern United States	Intense local pain, erythema, numbness, burning, restlessness, vomiting Ascending motor paralysis with seizures, weakness, rapid pulse, excessive salivation, thirst, dysuria, pulmonary edema, coma, and death Some species produce only local tissue reaction with swelling at puncture site (distinctive) Symptoms subside in a few hours Deaths occur among children younger than 4 years, usually in first 24 hours	***Treatment*** Delay absorption of venom by keeping child quiet; place involved area in dependent position. Administer antivenin. Relieve pain. Admit to pediatric intensive care unit for surveillance. ***Prevention*** Teach children to avoid possible nesting sites.
Ticks ***Mechanism*** In process of sucking blood, head and mouth parts are buried in skin ***Characteristics*** Feed on blood of mammals Significant in humans because of pathologic organism carried May be vectors of various infectious diseases, such as Rocky Mountain spotted fever, Q fever, tularemia, relapsing fever, Lyme disease, tick paralysis Must attach and feed for 1-2 hours to transmit disease Usual habitat is wooded area	Tick usually attached to skin, head embedded Produce firm, discrete, intensely pruritic nodules at site of attachment May cause urticaria or persistent localized edema	***Treatment*** Grasp tick with tweezers (forceps) as close as possible to point of attachment. Pull straight up with steady, even pressure; if using bare hands, use a tissue to touch tick during removal; wash hands thoroughly with soap and water. Remove any remaining part (e.g., head) with sterile needle. Cleanse wounds with soap and disinfectant. ***Prevention*** Teach children to avoid areas where prevalent. Inspect skin (especially scalp) after being in wooded areas. (See discussion on p. 1510.)

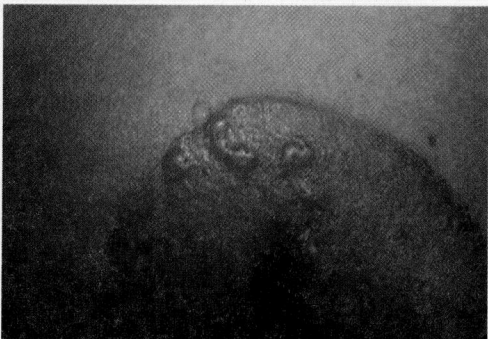

FIG 47-5 Brown recluse spider bite. Note central necrosis surrounded by purplish area and blisters. (From Weston WL, Lane AT: *Color textbook of pediatric dermatology,* ed 4, St Louis, 2007, Mosby.)

with the affected child need treatment. This may include boyfriends or girlfriends, babysitters, grandparents, and immediate family members. The objective is to treat as thoroughly as possible the first time. Enough medication for the entire family should be prescribed, with 2 oz allowed for each adult and 1 oz for each child.

Pediculosis Capitis

Pediculosis capitis (head lice) is an infestation of the scalp by *Pediculus humanus capitis,* a common parasite in school-age children. The adult louse lives only about 48 hours when away from a human host, and the life span of the average female is 1 month. The female lays her eggs at night at the junction of a hair shaft and close to the skin because the eggs need a warm environment. The nits, or eggs, hatch in approximately 7 to 10 days. Itching is usually the only symptom.

Common areas involved are the occipital area, behind the ears, and the nape of the neck (Box 47-2).

Diagnostic Evaluation

Diagnosis is made by observation of the white eggs (nits) firmly attached to the hair shafts (Fig. 47-6). Because of their brief life span and mobility, adult lice are more difficult to locate. Nits must be differentiated from dandruff, lint, hair spray, and other items of similar size and shape. Scratch marks or inflammatory papules, caused by secondary infection, may also be found on the scalp in the vulnerable areas.

Therapeutic Management

Treatment consists of the application of pediculicides and manual removal of nit cases. The drug of choice for infants and children is permethrin 1% cream rinse (Nix), which kills adult lice and nits. This product and preparations of pyrethrin with piperonyl butoxide (RID or A-200 Pyrinate) can be obtained without a prescription and are more effective and safer than lindane (Strong and Johnstone, 2008). Most experts advise a second treatment at 7 to 10 days to ensure a cure (AAP, 2009). However, pyrethrin products are contraindicated for individuals with contact allergy to ragweed or turpentine. If neither permethrin nor pyrethrin products are effective, the prescription drug *0.5% malathion,* which has been approved for treatment of head lice, can be used. However, malathion contains flammable alcohol, must remain in contact with the scalp for 8 to 12 hours, and is not recommended for children younger than 2 years.

Because of concerns that head lice may be developing resistance to chemical shampoos and that repeated exposure of children to

strong chemicals on the scalp may be unwise, effective nonchemical control measures are essential. Removal of nits from the child's hair with a metal nit comb at least every 2 or 3 days is a control measure following treatment with a pediculicide (Mumcuoglu, Barker, Burgess, et al., 2007).

CARE MANAGEMENT

An important nursing role is educating the parents about pediculosis. Nurses should emphasize that *anyone* can get pediculosis; it has no respect for age, socioeconomic level, or cleanliness. Lice do not jump or fly, but they can be transmitted from one person to another on personal items. Lice are more likely to infest Caucasian children, those with straight hair, and girls. Children are cautioned against sharing combs, hair ornaments, hats, caps, scarves, coats, and other items used on or near the hair. Children who share lockers are more likely to become infested, and slumber parties place children at risk. Lice are not carried or transmitted by pets.

Nurses or parents should carefully inspect children who scratch their heads more than usual for bite marks, redness, and nits. The hair is systematically spread with two flat-sided sticks or tongue depressors, and the scalp is observed for any movement that indicates a louse. Nurses should wear gloves when examining the hair. Lice are small and grayish tan, have no wings, and are visible to the naked eye. The nits, or eggs, appear as tiny whitish oval specks adhering to the hair shaft about 6 mm (0.25 inch) from the scalp. The adherent nature of the nits distinguishes them from dandruff, which falls off readily. Empty nit cases, indicating hatched lice, are translucent rather than white and are located more than 6 mm from the scalp (see Fig. 47-6).

If evidence of infestation is found, it is important to treat the child according to the directions on the label of the pediculicide. Parents are advised to read the directions carefully before beginning treatment. The child is made as comfortable as possible during the application process because the pediculicide must remain on the scalp and hair for several minutes. Playing "beauty parlor" while shampooing is a useful strategy. The child lies supine with the head over a sink or basin and covers the eyes with a dry towel or washcloth. This prevents medication, which can cause chemical conjunctivitis, from splashing into the eyes. If eye irritation occurs, the eyes must be flushed well with tepid water. It is not necessary to remove the nits after treatment because only live lice cause infestation. However, because none of the pediculicides is 100% effective in killing all the eggs, the makers of some pediculicides recommend manual removal of the nits after treatment. An extra-fine-tooth comb that is included in many commercial pediculicides or is available at community pharmacies facilitates manual removal. If the comb is ineffective in removing the nit cases, the examiner should remove them by scraping them off the strands of hair with his or her fingernails.

Live lice survive for up to 48 hours away from the host, but nits are shed into the environment and are capable of hatching in 7 to 10 days; retreatment may be required. Therefore measures must be taken to prevent further infestation (see Community Focus box). Spraying with insecticide is not recommended because of the danger to children and animals. Families should also be advised that the pediculicide is relatively expensive, especially when several members of the household require treatment. Families may be inclined to try home remedies such as vinegar or petroleum jelly to treat the lice, but most are ineffective. A study by Pearlman (2004) showed that dry-on pediculicide lotions may effectively treat lice without the use

---

BOX 47-2   CLINICAL MANIFESTATIONS OF PEDICULOSIS

- Pruritus (caused by crawling insects and insect saliva on skin)
- Nits observable on hair shaft (see Fig. 47-6)

Distribution
- Occipital area
- Behind ears
- Nape of neck
- Eyebrows and eyelashes (occasionally) (caused by pubic lice)

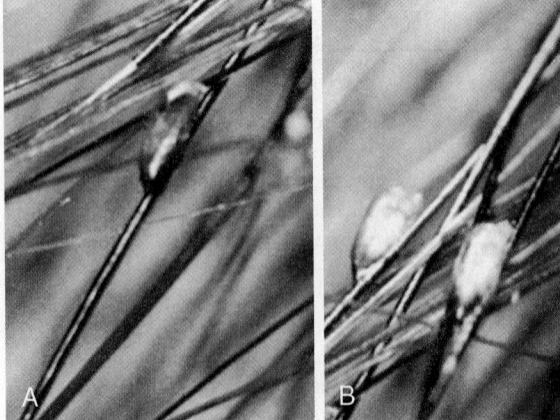

FIG 47-6 A, Empty nit case. **B,** Viable nits. (From *The contemporary approach to the control of head lice in schools and communities,* Pittsburgh, 1991, SmithKline Beecham.)

of current shampoos with neurotoxins, nit removal, or extensive housecleaning.

Prevention. The increasing incidence of pediculosis in schoolchildren is a serious concern for school nurses, parents, and community health agencies. However, school head lice screening programs have not proven to have a significant effect on the incidence of head lice in the school setting; parent education programs may be more helpful in the management of head lice. Children with head lice should be allowed to return to school after proper treatment. Both the American Academy of Pediatrics (AAP) and the National Association of School Nurses discourage a "no nit" policy for schools.

RICKETTSIAL DISEASES

The organisms responsible for a number of disorders are transmitted to human beings via arthropods (Table 47-7). Mammals become infected only through the bites of infected lice, fleas, ticks, and mites, all of which serve as both infectors and reservoirs. Rickettsiae are intracellular parasites, similar in size to bacteria that inhabit the alimentary tract of a wide range of natural hosts. Rickettsial diseases are more common in temperate and tropical climates where humans live in association with arthropods. Infection in humans is incidental (except epidemic typhus) and not necessary for the survival of the rickettsial species. However, after the organism invades a human, it causes a disease that varies in intensity from a benign, self-limiting illness to a disease that is fulminating and fatal.

🏠 COMMUNITY FOCUS

Preventing the Spread and Recurrence of Pediculosis

- Machine wash all washable clothing, towels, and bed linens in hot water and dry them in a hot dryer for at least 20 minutes. Dry-clean nonwashable items.
- Thoroughly vacuum carpets, car seats, pillows, stuffed animals, rugs, mattresses, and upholstered furniture.
- Seal nonwashable items in plastic bags for 14 days if unable to dry-clean or vacuum.
- Soak combs, brushes, and hair accessories in lice-killing products for 1 hour or in boiling water for 10 minutes.
- In day-care centers, store children's clothing items such as hats and scarves and other headgear in separate cubicles.
- Discourage the sharing of items such as hats, scarves, hair accessories, combs, and brushes among children in group settings such as day-care centers.
- Avoid physical contact with infested individuals and their belongings, especially clothing and bedding.
- Inspect children in a group setting regularly for head lice.
- Provide educational programs on the transmission of pediculosis, its detection, and treatment.

Adapted from Chin J, editor: *Control of communicable diseases manual,* Washington, DC, 2000, American Public Health Association.

TABLE 47-7	ERUPTIONS CAUSED BY RICKETTSIAE		
DISORDER, ORGANISM, AND HOST	**MANIFESTATIONS**	**MANAGEMENT**	**COMMENTS**
Rocky Mountain spotted fever—*Rickettsia rickettsii* Arthropod—Tick Transmission—Tick Mammal source—Wild rodents, dogs	*Gradual onset*—Fever, malaise, anorexia, myalgia *Abrupt onset*—Rapid temperature elevation, chills, vomiting, myalgia, severe headache Maculopapular or petechial rash primarily on extremities (ankles and wrists) but may spread to other areas, characteristically on palms and soles	*Control* Protection from tick bite by wearing proper apparel, tick repellent Tetracycline or chloramphenicol Vigorous supportive therapy	Usually self-limiting in children Onset in children may resemble any infectious disease Severe disease rare in children Inspect children and dogs regularly if they play in wooded areas See Table 47-6 for management of ticks
Epidemic typhus— *R. prowazekii* Arthropod—Body louse Transmission—Infected feces into broken skin Mammal source—Humans	Abrupt onset of chills, fever, diffuse myalgia, headache, malaise Maculopapular rash becoming petechial 4-7 days later, spreading from trunk outward	*Control* Immediate destruction of vectors Tetracycline or chloramphenicol Supportive treatment	Patient should be isolated until deloused See discussion on p. 1508 for management of pediculosis Excreta from infected lice also in dust; disinfect patient's clothing, bedding, and possessions and wash in hot water
Endemic typhus—*R. typhi* Arthropod—Rat fleas or lice Transmission—Flea bite; inhaling or ingesting flea excreta Mammal source—Rats	Headache, arthralgia, backache followed by fever; may last 9-14 days Maculopapular rash after 1-8 days of fever; begins in trunk and spreads to periphery; rarely involves face, palms, soles	*Control* Eliminate rat reservoir, insect vectors, or both Tetracycline or chloramphenicol Supportive treatment	Fairly common in United States Shorter duration than epidemic typhus Mild, seldom fatal illness Difficult to distinguish from epidemic typhus
Rickettsialpox—*R. akari* Arthropod—Mouse mite Transmission—Mite Mammal source—House mouse	Maculopapular rash after primary lesion; eschar at site of bite; fever, chills, headache	*Control* Eradication of rodent reservoir and mite vector Tetracycline or chloramphenicol Supportive treatment	Self-limiting nonfatal disease Endemic in New York City Found in many cities in United States

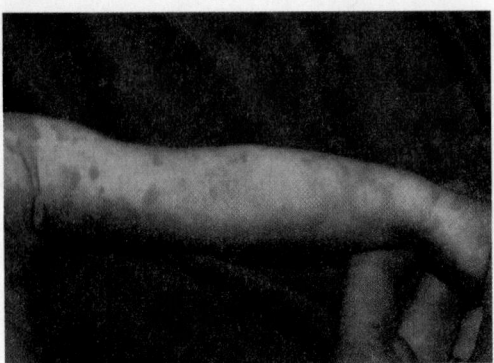

FIG 47-7 Lyme disease. Note annular red rings in erythema chronicum migrans. (From Weston WL, Lane AT: *Color textbook of pediatric dermatology,* ed 4, St Louis, 2007, Mosby.)

Lyme Disease

Lyme disease is the most common tickborne disorder in the United States. It is caused by the spirochete *Borrelia burgdorferi,* which enters the skin and bloodstream through the saliva and feces of ticks, especially the deer tick (Moreno, 2011). Most cases of Lyme disease are reported in the Northeast from southern Maine to northern Virginia. The disease may initially appear in any of three stages:

- **Stage 1** consists of the tick bite at the time of inoculation, followed in 3 to 31 days by the development of erythema migrans at the site of the bite (Fig. 47-7).
- **Stage 2,** the most serious stage of the disease, is characterized by systemic involvement of neurologic, cardiac, and musculoskeletal systems that appears several weeks after the cutaneous phase is completed.
- **Stage 3,** or the late stage, includes musculoskeletal pain that involves the tendons, bursae, muscles, and synovia. Arthritis may occur, and late neurologic problems include deafness and chronic encephalopathy.

Diagnostic Evaluation

Diagnosis is best made clinically during the early stages by recognizing the characteristic rash, erythema migrans. Serologic testing may be used to establish the diagnosis in later stages of the disease.

Therapeutic Management

Early and appropriate treatment is essential to prevent complications. Children older than 8 years are treated with oral doxycycline; amoxicillin is recommended for children younger than 8 years (Centers for Disease Control and Prevention [CDC], 2009). For patients who are allergic to penicillin, alternative drugs include cefuroxime or erythromycin. Most experts treat individuals with early Lyme disease for 14 to 21 days. Persons who have removed ticks from themselves should be monitored closely for signs and symptoms of tickborne diseases for 30 days; in particular, they should be monitored for erythema migrans, a red expanding skin lesion at the site of the tick bite that may suggest Lyme disease. People who develop a skin lesion or viral infection–like illness within 1 month of an attached tick should seek prompt medical attention (Wormser, Dattwyler, Shapiro, et al., 2006). Treatment of erythema migrans most often prevents development of later stages of Lyme disease.

CARE MANAGEMENT

The major thrust of nursing care should be educating parents to protect their children from exposure to ticks. Children should avoid tick-infested areas or wear light-colored clothing so that ticks can be spotted easily, tuck pant legs into socks, and wear a long-sleeved shirt tucked into pants when in wooded areas. Parents and children need to perform regular tick checks when they are in infested areas (with special attention to the scalp, neck, armpits, and groin areas) (Network to Reduce Lyme Disease in School-Aged Children, 2010). Parents should also be alert for signs of the skin lesion, especially if their children have been in tick-infested areas. Insect repellents containing diethyltoluamide (DEET) and permethrin can protect against ticks, but parents should use these chemicals cautiously. Although there have been reports of serious neurologic complications in children resulting from frequent and excessive application of DEET repellants, the risk is low when they are used properly. Products with DEET should be applied sparingly according to label instructions and not applied to a child's face, hands, or any areas of irritated skin. After the child returns indoors, treated skin should be washed with soap and water. Information about Lyme disease can be obtained from the American Lyme Disease Foundation, Inc.*

PET AND WILD ANIMAL BITES

Animal bites are common in childhood. However, children are bitten more often by animals belonging to the family or to neighbors than by stray animals. The majority of victims of dog bites are boys between the ages of 5 and 9 years (CDC, 2003). Most dog or cat injuries are to the upper extremities. Small children are likely to be bitten or scratched on the head, face, and neck because they tend to put their heads near the animal's head and flail their arms rather than protecting their heads (Kaye, Belz, and Kirschner, 2009). Animal bites are potentially serious because of the likelihood of significant infection. Injuries vary in intensity from small puncture wounds to complete evulsion of tissue that is associated with significant crush injury.

Therapeutic Management

General wound care consists of rinsing the wound with copious amounts of saline or lactated Ringer solution under pressure via a large syringe and of washing the surrounding skin with mild soap. A clean pressure dressing is applied, and the extremity is elevated if the wound is bleeding. Medical evaluation is advised because of the danger of tetanus and rabies, although dogs in most urban areas must be immunized against rabies. Bites from wild animals, such as squirrels, bats, raccoons, foxes, and skunks, are also dangerous.

Prophylactic antibiotics are indicated for puncture wounds and wounds in areas that may prove to be cosmetically or functionally impaired if infected. Extensive lacerations are débrided and loosely sutured to allow drainage in the event of infection. Tetanus toxoid is administered according to standard guidelines (see Immunizations, Chapter 31), and rabies protocol is followed (see Rabies, Chapter 45). Injuries to poorly vascularized areas, such as the hands, are more likely to become infected than those in more vascularized areas, such as the face; puncture wounds are more likely to become infected than lacerations.

CARE MANAGEMENT

The most important aspect related to animal bites is prevention. Children should understand animal behavior and develop respect for animals (see Community Focus box). Parents should monitor their children's behavior with dogs and instruct them not to tease

---

*PO Box 466, Lyme, CT 06371; e-mail: inquire@aldf.com; www.aldf.com.

or surprise dogs, invade their territory, interfere with their feeding or sleeping, take their toys, or interact with sick or injured dogs or dogs with pups. Parents who are considering getting a pet, especially a dog, for themselves or their children should select a dog that has a high level of sociability with and is unlikely to be a danger to children.

Human Bites

Children often acquire lacerations from the teeth of other humans in rough play, during fights, or as victims of child abuse. Many preschool children bite others out of frustration or anger. Because human dental plaque and gingiva harbor pathogenic organisms, all human bites should receive attention. Delayed treatment increases the risk for infection.

If the laceration is less than 6 mm (0.25 inch) in length, the wound can be treated at home. The wound is washed vigorously with soap and water, and a pressure dressing is applied to stop bleeding. Ice applications minimize discomfort and swelling. Increased pain or redness at the wound site is an indication that the child should receive medical attention for antibiotic therapy. Tetanus toxoid is needed if the child is insufficiently immunized. Wounds larger than 6 mm should receive medical attention.

Cat Scratch Disease

Cat scratch disease is the most common cause of regional lymphadenitis in children and adolescents. It usually follows the scratch or bite of an animal (a cat or kitten in 99% of cases). The disease is usually a benign, self-limiting illness that resolves spontaneously in about 2 to 4 months. Diagnosis is made on the basis of (1) history of contact with a cat or kitten, (2) the presence of regional lymphadenopathy for several days, and (3) serologic identification of the causative organism by indirect fluorescent antibody assay or polymerase chain reaction test. The disease may persist for several months before gradual resolution. In some children, especially those who are immunocompromised, the adenitis may progress to suppuration and serious complications. Treatment is primarily supportive, but antibiotic therapy may hasten the resolution of adenopathy in the disease (CDC, 2002).

MISCELLANEOUS SKIN DISORDERS

A number of miscellaneous skin lesions occur in children. Some occur as a result of congenital disorders and are inherited as an autosomal dominant trait (Table 47-8). Ichthyoses are a heterogeneous group of disorders characterized by scaling that create challenging problems in treatment. These disorders are not discussed in detail here because of their wide variability.

SKIN DISORDERS ASSOCIATED WITH SPECIFIC AGE-GROUPS

Several common dermatologic conditions are confined to children in specific age-groups. These conditions include diaper, atopic, and seborrheic dermatitis, which occur predominantly in infants, and acne, which is most common in adolescence.

Diaper Dermatitis

Diaper dermatitis is common in infants and one of several acute inflammatory skin disorders caused either directly or indirectly by wearing diapers. The peak age of occurrence is 9 to 12 months, and the incidence is greater in bottle-fed infants than in breastfed infants.

Pathophysiology and Clinical Manifestations

Diaper dermatitis is caused by prolonged and repetitive contact with an irritant (e.g., urine, feces, soaps, detergents, ointments, friction). Although the irritant in the majority of cases is urine and feces, a combination of factors contributes to irritation.

Prolonged contact of the skin with diaper wetness produces higher friction, greater abrasion damage, increased transepidermal permeability, and increased microbial counts. Healthy skin is less resistant to potential irritants.

Although ammonia was once thought to cause diaper rash because of the association between the strong odor on diapers and dermatitis, ammonia alone is not sufficient. The irritant quality of urine is related to an increase in pH from the breakdown of urea in the presence of fecal urease. The increased pH promotes the activity of fecal enzymes, principally the proteases and lipases, which act as

TABLE 47-8   MISCELLANEOUS SKIN DISORDERS

DISEASE AND CAUSATIVE AGENT	LOCAL MANIFESTATIONS	MANAGEMENT	COMMENTS
Urticaria—Usually allergic response to drugs or infection	Development of wheals Vary in size and configuration and tend to appear quickly, spread irregularly, and fade within a few hours May be constant or intermittent, sparse or profuse, small or large, discrete or confluent May be acute, chronic, or recurrent in acute attacks	Local soothing and antipruritic applications Antihistamines Epinephrine or ephedrine Cortisone in severe cases Severe upper respiratory tract involvement may require tracheostomy	Known etiologic agents should be avoided May be accompanied by malaise, fever, lymphadenopathy Severe cases may involve mucous membranes, internal organs, and joints Obstruction to air passages constitutes medical emergency (see Chapter 40)
Intertrigo—Mechanical trauma and aggravating factors of excessive heat, moisture, and sweat retention	Red, inflamed, moist, partially denuded, marginated areas, the shape of which is determined by location Appears where opposing skin surfaces rub together, such as intergluteal folds, groin, neck, and axilla Excessive moisture and obesity are often factors	Affected areas kept clean and dry Skinfolds kept separated with a generous supply of nonmedicated powder Expose to air and light Remove excess clothing	A form of diaper irritation Prevent recurrence by keeping susceptible areas clean and dry Frequently associated with overheating from too much clothing; common in tracheostomy patients with short necks and copious secretions
Psoriasis—Unknown; hereditary predisposition; may be triggered by stress	Round, thick, dry, reddish patches covered with coarse, silvery scales over trunk and extremities; first lesions commonly appear in scalp; facial lesions more common in children than in adults Affected cells proliferate at a much more rapid rate than normal cells	Tar preparations in combination with UVB light or natural sunlight Topical corticosteroids Topical vitamin D analog *calcipotriene* Phenol and saline solutions followed by a tar shampoo to remove scales Keratolytic agents (salicylic acid) Acitretin Emollients may provide relief	Uncommon in children younger than 6 years Patients are otherwise healthy Coal tar acts synergistically with UVB light Keratolytic agents enhance absorption of corticosteroids Humidifiers may help in winter
Alopecia*			
Alopecia areata	Sudden onset of asymptomatic, noninflammatory, round, bald patches in hairy parts of body	Psychologic support Inducement of allergic contact dermatitis to stimulate growth of hair Minoxidil (peripheral vasodilator)	Family history in 10%-26% of cases Some concern regarding drug therapy safety Refer to support groups*
Traumatic alopecia	Traction alopecia around scalp margins from tight hair styles (e.g., braids, pony tails, corn rows)	Counseling regarding hair styling, use of hair cosmetics, hot combs, rollers	More prevalent in African-American children and adolescents Prolonged traction can produce fibrosis of hair root and permanent loss
Trichotillomania	Compulsive hair pulling	Determine and treat cause	Chronic hair pulling may require psychologic therapy
Tinea capitis	See Table 47-4	See Table 47-4	See Table 47-4
Erythema multiforme (Stevens-Johnson syndrome)—Unknown; associated with ingestion of some drugs; often follows upper respiratory tract infection	Erythematous papular rash Lesions enlarge by peripheral expansion, develop central vesicle Involves most skin surfaces except scalp May extend to mucous membranes, especially oral, ocular, and urethral	Symptomatic and supportive Maintain adequate intake of fluids (oral or intravenous), calories, and protein Moist wound care, hydrogels such as CarraGauze, Vaseline, or Aquaphor Appropriate treatment of complications Diligent monitoring of urine volume and specific gravity, hemoglobin and hematocrit, serum electrolyte levels, total body weight	Rash often preceded by fever and malaise Complications include renal failure and severe eye disease Respiratory involvement in a number of cases Self-limiting, but recovery may extend for weeks; skin lesions may subside without scarring; mucous membrane lesions may persist for months Recurrence rate, 20%; mortality rate as high as 10% High mutation rate
Neurofibromatosis—Inherited disorder; autosomal dominant inheritance pattern	Café-au-lait spots, pigmented nevi, axillary freckling Slow-growing cutaneous and subcutaneous neurofibromas	Symptomatic treatment of associated manifestations (e.g., speech defects, seizures, skeletal defects [scoliosis, kyphosis], learning disabilities) Surgical removal of troublesome tumors	Refer to support groups† Family needs to know about genetic implications

UVB, Ultraviolet B.

*National Alopecia Areata Foundation, 14 Mitchell Blvd., San Rafael, CA 94903; 415-472-3780; fax: 415-472-5343; e-mail: info@naaf.org; www.naaf.org.

†Children's Tumor Foundation, 95 Pine St., 16th Floor, New York, NY 10005; 800-323-7938 or 212-344-6633; fax: 212-747-0004; e-mail: info@ctf.org; www.ctf.org.

irritants. Fecal enzymes also increase the permeability of skin to bile salts, another potential irritant in feces.

The eruption of diaper dermatitis is manifested primarily on convex surfaces or in folds. The lesions represent a variety of types and configurations. Eruptions involving the skin in most intimate contact with the diaper (e.g., the convex surfaces of buttocks, inner thighs, mons pubis, scrotum) but sparing the folds are likely to be caused by chemical irritants, especially from urine and feces (Fig. 47-8). Other causes are detergents or soaps from inadequately rinsed cloth diapers or the chemicals in disposable wipes. Perianal involvement is usually the result of chemical irritation from feces, especially diarrheal stools. *Candida albicans* infection produces perianal inflammation and a maculopapular rash with satellite lesions that may cross the inguinal fold (Fig. 47-9). It is seen in up to 90% of

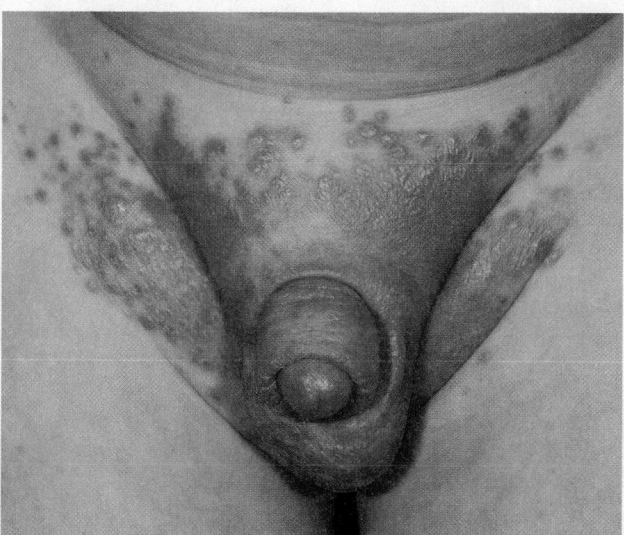

FIG 47-8 Irritant diaper dermatitis. Note the sharply demarcated edges. (From Habif TP: *Clinical dermatology: a color guide to diagnosis and therapy*, ed 5, St Louis, 2010, Mosby.)

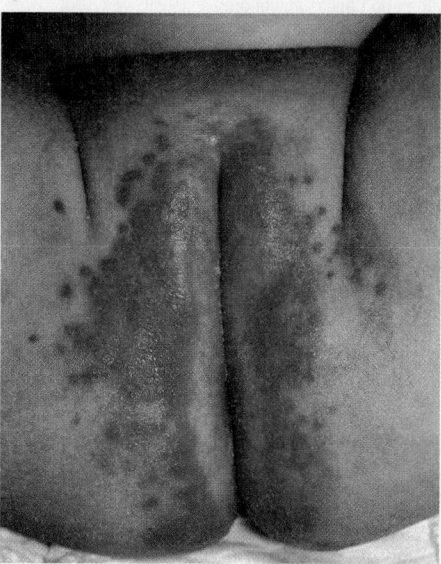

FIG 47-9 Candidiasis of diaper area. Note the beefy red central erythema with satellite pustules. (From Paller AS, Mancini AJ: *Hurwitz clinical pediatric dermatology*, ed 4, St Louis, 2011, Saunders.)

infants with chronic diaper dermatitis and should be considered in diaper rashes that are recalcitrant to treatment.

CARE MANAGEMENT

Nursing interventions are aimed at altering the three factors that produce dermatitis: wetness, pH, and fecal irritants. The most significant factor amenable to intervention is the moist environment created in the diaper area. Changing the diaper as soon as it becomes wet eliminates a large part of the problem, and removing the diaper to expose healthy skin to air facilitates drying. The use of a hair dryer or heat lamp is not recommended because these devices can cause burns.

Diaper construction has a significant impact on the incidence and severity of diaper dermatitis. Superabsorbent disposable paper diapers reduce diaper dermatitis. They contain an absorbent gelling material that binds water tightly to decrease skin wetness, maintains pH control by providing a buffering capacity, and decreases skin irritation by preventing mixing of urine and feces in the diaper. Another advance in diapers is the addition of an inner layer or top sheet that is impregnated with petrolatum (as in Pampers Swaddler with Absorb-Away Liner).

Guidelines for controlling diaper rash are presented in the Family-Centered Care box. A common misconception about using cornstarch on skin is that it promotes the growth of *C. albicans*. Neither cornstarch nor talc promotes the growth of fungi under conditions normally found in the diaper area. Cornstarch is more effective in reducing friction and tends to cake less than talc when the skin is wet. On the basis of these properties and its safety in terms of inhalation injury, cornstarch is the preferred product. Talc should not be used.

FAMILY-CENTERED CARE

Controlling Diaper Rash

- Keep skin dry*:
  - Use superabsorbent disposable diapers to reduce skin wetness.
  - If using cloth diapers, use only overwraps that allow air to circulate; avoid rubber pants.
  - Change diapers as soon as soiled—especially with stool—whenever possible, preferably once during the night.
  - Expose healthy or only slightly irritated skin to air, not heat, to dry completely.
- Apply ointment, such as zinc oxide or petrolatum, to protect skin, especially if skin is very red or has moist, open areas:
  - Avoid removing skin barrier cream with each diaper change; remove waste material and reapply skin barrier cream.
  - To completely remove ointment, especially zinc oxide, use mineral oil; do not wash vigorously.
- Avoid overwashing the skin, especially with perfumed soaps or commercial wipes, which may be irritating:
  - May use a moisturizer or nonsoap cleanser, such as cold cream or Cetaphil, to wipe urine from skin.
  - Gently wipe stool from skin using water and mild soap, such as Dove.
  - When traveling, fill an old baby wipe container with soft paper towels and warm water.

*Powder helps keep the skin dry, but talc is dangerous if breathed into the lungs. Plain cornstarch or cornstarch-based powder is safer. When using any powder product, first shake it into your hand and then apply it to the diaper area. Store the container away from the infant's reach; keep the container closed when not in use.

Atopic Dermatitis (Eczema)

Eczema or eczematous inflammation of the skin refers to a descriptive category of dermatologic diseases and not to a specific etiology. AD is a type of pruritic eczema that usually begins during infancy and is associated with an allergic contact dermatitis with a hereditary tendency (atopy) (Jacob, Yang, Herro, et al., 2010). AD manifests in three forms based on the child's age and the distribution of lesions:

1. Infantile (infantile eczema)—Usually begins at 2 to 6 months of age; generally undergoes spontaneous remission by 3 years of age
2. Childhood—May follow the infantile form; occurs at 2 to 3 years of age; 90% of children have manifestations by age 5 years
3. Preadolescent and adolescent—Begins at about 12 years of age; may continue into the early adult years or indefinitely

The diagnosis of AD is based on a combination of history and morphologic findings (Box 47-3). Children with AD have a lower threshold for cutaneous itching compared with children who do not have AD, and many authorities believe the dermatologic manifestations appear subsequent to scratching from the intense pruritus (Alanne, Nermes, Soderlund, et al., 2011). For example, infants rub their faces against bed linen, and their crawling (a form of scratching) results in irritation of knees and elbows. Lesions disappear if the scratching is stopped.

The majority of children with infantile AD have a family history of eczema, asthma, food allergies, or allergic rhinitis, which strongly supports a genetic predisposition. The cause is unknown but appears to be related to abnormal function of the skin, including alterations in perspiration, peripheral vascular function, and heat tolerance. Manifestations of the chronic disease improve in humid climates and get worse in the fall and winter, when homes are heated and environmental humidity is lower. The disorder can be controlled but not cured. A recent study of 134 infants with AD showed that itching and scratching and sleep disturbance were specific features detracting from quality of life in these young children (Alanne, Nermes, Soderlund, et al., 2011).

Therapeutic Management

The major goals of management are to (1) hydrate the skin, (2) relieve pruritus, (3) reduce flare-ups or inflammation, and (4) prevent and control secondary infection. The general measures for managing AD focus on reducing pruritus and other aspects of the disease. Management strategies include avoiding exposure to skin irritants or allergens; avoiding overheating; and administrating medications such as antihistamines, topical immunomodulators, topical steroids, and (sometimes) mild sedatives as indicated.

Enhancing skin hydration and preventing dry, flaky skin are accomplished in a number of ways, depending on the child's skin characteristics and individual needs. A tepid bath with a mild soap (Dove or Neutrogena), no soap, or an emulsifying oil followed immediately by application of an emollient (within 3 minutes) assists in trapping moisture and preventing its loss. Bubble baths and harsh soaps should be avoided. The bath may need to be repeated once or twice daily, depending on the child's status; excessive bathing without emollient application only dries out the skin. Some lotions are not effective, and emollients should be chosen carefully to prevent excessive skin drying. Aquaphor, Cetaphil, and Eucerin are acceptable lotions for skin hydration. A nighttime bath followed by emollient application and dressing in soft cotton pajamas may help alleviate most nighttime pruritus.

BOX 47-3 CLINICAL MANIFESTATIONS OF ATOPIC DERMATITIS

Distribution of Lesions

Infantile form—Generalized, especially cheeks, scalp, trunk, and extensor surfaces of extremities (Fig. 47-10)

Childhood form—Flexural areas (antecubital and popliteal fossae, neck), wrists, ankles, and feet

Preadolescent and adolescent form—Face, sides of neck, hands, feet, and antecubital and popliteal fossae (to a lesser extent)

Appearance of Lesions

Infantile Form
- Erythema
- Vesicles
- Papules
- Weeping
- Oozing
- Crusting
- Scaling
- Often symmetric

Childhood Form
- Symmetric involvement
- Clusters of small erythematous or flesh-colored papules or minimally scaling patches
- Dry and may be hyperpigmented
- Lichenification (thickened skin with accentuation of creases)
- Keratosis pilaris (follicular hyperkeratosis) common

Adolescent or Adult Form
- Same as childhood manifestations
- Dry, thick lesions (lichenified plaques) common
- Confluent papules

Other Physical Manifestations
- Intense itching
- Unaffected skin dry and rough
- African-American children likely to exhibit more papular or follicular lesions than do Caucasian children
- May exhibit one or more of the following:
  - Lymphadenopathy, especially near affected sites
  - Increased palmar creases (many cases)
  - Atopic pleats (extra line or groove of lower eyelid)
  - Prone to cold hands
  - Pityriasis alba (small, poorly defined areas of hypopigmentation)
  - Facial pallor (especially around nose, mouth, and ears)
  - Bluish discoloration beneath eyes ("allergic shiners")
  - Increased susceptibility to unusual cutaneous infections (especially viral)

Sometimes colloid baths, such as the addition of 2 cups of cornstarch to a tub of warm water, provide temporary relief of itching and may help the child sleep if given before bedtime. Cool wet compresses are soothing to the skin and provide antiseptic protection.

Oral antihistamine drugs such as hydroxyzine or diphenhydramine usually relieve moderate or severe pruritus. Nonsedating antihistamines such as loratadine (Claritin) or fexofenadine (Allegra) may be preferred for daytime pruritus relief. Because pruritus increases at night, a mildly sedating antihistamine may be needed.

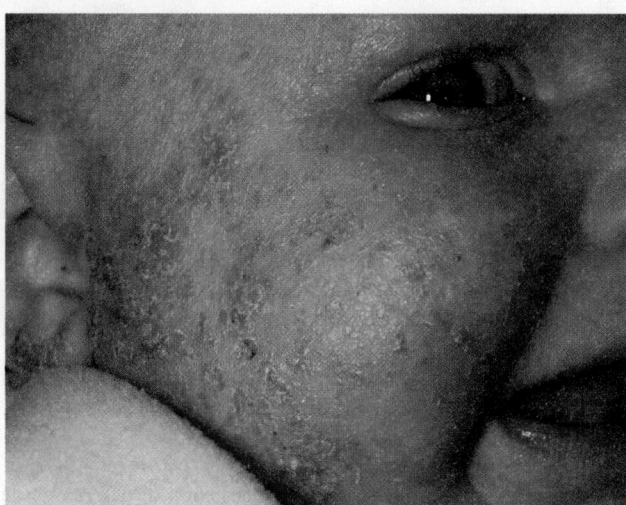

FIG 47-10 Atopic dermatitis. (From Habif TP: *Clinical dermatology: a color guide to diagnosis and therapy,* ed 5, St Louis, 2010, Mosby.)

Occasional flare-ups require the use of topical steroids to diminish inflammation. Low-, moderate-, or high-potency topical corticosteroids are prescribed, depending on the degree of involvement, the area of the body to be treated, the child's age, the potential for local side effects (striae, skin atrophy, and pigment changes), and the type of vehicle to be used (e.g., cream, lotion, ointment). Patients receiving topical corticosteroid therapy for chronic conditions should be evaluated for risk factors for suboptimal linear growth and reduced bone density. Topical immunomodulators, a new nonsteroidal treatment for AD, are best used at the beginning of a "flare-up" just as the skin becomes red and itches. Two newer immunomodulator medications used in children with AD are tacrolimus and pimecrolimus (Walling and Swick, 2010). Tacrolimus is available in two ointment strengths (0.03% and 0.1%); the 0.03% concentration has been approved for use in children 2 years of age and older (Doss, Kamoun, Dubertret, et al., 2010). Pimecrolimus is available in a 1% cream that has no systemic accumulation or effects. This drug is approved for use in children with mild to moderate AD. Both drugs can be used freely on the face without worrying about steroid side effects.

If secondary skin infections occur in children with AD, these infections are managed with appropriate systemic antibiotics. In a subgroup of patient with moderate to severe AD, the disease may require systemic treatment (Ricci, Dondi, Patrizi, et al., 2009).

CARE MANAGEMENT

Assessment of the child with AD includes a family history for evidence of atopy, a history of previous involvement, and any environmental or dietary factors associated with the present and previous exacerbations. The skin lesions are examined for type, distribution, and evidence of secondary infection. Parents are interviewed regarding the child's behavior, especially in relation to scratching, irritability, and sleeping patterns. Exploration of the family's feelings and methods of coping is also important.

The nursing care of the child with AD is challenging. Controlling the intense pruritus is imperative if the disorder is to be successfully managed because scratching leads to new lesions and may cause secondary infection. In addition to the medical regimen, other measures can be taken to prevent or minimize the scratching. Fingernails and toenails are cut short, kept clean, and filed frequently to prevent sharp edges. Gloves or cotton stockings can be placed over the hands and pinned to shirtsleeves. One-piece outfits with long sleeves and long pants also decrease direct contact with the skin. If gloves or socks are used, the child needs time to be free from such restrictions. An excellent time to remove gloves, socks, or other protective devices is during the bath or after receiving sedative or antipruritic medication.

Conditions that increase itching are eliminated when possible. Woolen clothes or blankets, rough fabrics, and furry stuffed animals are removed from the child's environment. Because heat and humidity cause perspiration (which intensifies itching), proper dress for climatic conditions is essential. Pruritus is often precipitated by exposure to the irritant effects of certain components of common products such as soaps, detergents, fabric softeners, perfumes, and powders. Most children experience less itching when soft cotton fabrics are worn next to the skin. During cold months, synthetic fabrics (not wool) should be used for overcoats, hats, gloves, and snowsuits. Exposure to latex products, such as gloves and balloons, should also be avoided.

Clothes and sheets are laundered in a mild detergent and rinsed thoroughly in clear water (without fabric softeners or antistatic chemicals). Putting the clothes through a second complete wash cycle without using detergent reduces the amount of residue remaining in the fabric.

Preventing infection is usually accomplished by preventing scratching. Baths are given as prescribed; the water is kept tepid; and soaps (except as indicated), bubble baths, oils, and powders are avoided. Skinfolds and diaper areas need frequent cleansing with plain water. A room humidifier or vaporizer may benefit children with extremely dry skin. The skin lesions are examined for signs of infection—usually honey-colored crusts or pustules with surrounding erythema. Any signs of infection are reported to the health care practitioner.

Wet soaks and compresses are applied and medications for pruritus or infection are administered as directed. The family is given explicit instructions on the preparation and use of soaks, special baths, and topical medications, including the order of application if more than one is prescribed. It is important to emphasize that one thick application of topical medication is *not* equivalent to several thin applications and that excessive use of an agent (particularly steroids) can be hazardous. If children have difficulty remaining still for a 10- or 15-minute soak, bath, or dressing application, these can be carried out at naptime or when the child is engrossed in watching television, listening to a story, or playing with tub toys.

Diet modification is another source of frustration to parents. When a hypoallergenic diet is prescribed, parents need help to understand the reason for the diet and the guidelines for avoiding hyperallergenic foods (see Guidelines box). Because hypoallergenic diets take time before visible effects are apparent, parents need reassurance that results may not be seen immediately. If airborne allergens make eczema worse, the family is counseled about "allergy proofing" the home (see Asthma, Chapter 40).

Family Support. Parents are assured that the lesions will not produce scarring (unless secondarily infected) and that the disease is not contagious. However, the child may have repeated exacerbations and remissions. Spontaneous and permanent remission takes place at approximately 2 to 3 years of age in most children with the infantile disorder.

During acute phases, emotional stress can become intense for the family. They need time to discuss negative feelings and to be reassured that these feelings are normal. Stress tends to aggravate the

GUIDELINES

Preventing Atopy in Children

Identify Children at Risk
- Family history of allergy
- Increased immunoglobulin E in cord blood and postnatal serum
- Dry, flaky skin

Prenatal Precautions (Last Trimester)
- Avoid any known food allergens
- Avoid milk and other dairy products, peanuts, and eggs
- Minimize ingestion of other hyperallergenic foods

Postnatal Precautions
- Breast milk or casein-whey hydrolysate formula (e.g., Nutramigen, Pregestimil, Alimentum) exclusively for at least 6 months
- No solid food for first 6 months
- No cow's milk or soy formula for 12 months
- No eggs, fish, corn, citrus, peanuts, nuts, or chocolate for 12 to 18 months
- One new food added at 5- to 7-day intervals to identify possible reaction

Environmental Control
- Limited exposure to dust, molds, furry animals, and cigarette smoke

Data from Johnstone D: Strategy for intervention of food allergy in infants, *Int Pediatr* 4(4):319–325, 1989; Wood RA: Prospects for the prevention of allergy in children, *Curr Opin Pediatr* 8(6):601–605, 1995; Zeiger R, Heller S, Mellon M, et al: Effectiveness of dietary manipulation in the prevention of food allergy in infants, part II, *J Allergy Clin Immunol* 78(1 Pt 2):224–238, 1986.

severity of the condition. Therefore efforts to relieve as much anxiety as possible in both the parents and the child have a beneficial emotional and physical effect.

Seborrheic Dermatitis

Seborrheic dermatitis is a chronic, recurrent, inflammatory reaction of the skin. It occurs most commonly on the scalp (cradle cap) but may involve the eyelids (blepharitis), external ear canal (otitis externa), nasolabial folds, and inguinal region. The cause is unknown, although it is more common in early infancy, when sebum production is increased. The lesions are characteristically thick, adherent, yellowish, scaly, oily patches that may or may not be mildly pruritic. Unlike AD, seborrheic dermatitis is not associated with a positive family history for allergy and is common in infants shortly after birth and in adolescents after puberty. Diagnosis is made primarily on the basis of the appearance and the location of the crusts or scales.

CARE MANAGEMENT

Cradle cap may be prevented with adequate scalp hygiene. Frequently, parents omit shampooing the infant's hair for fear of damaging the "soft spots," or fontanels. The nurse should discuss how to shampoo the infant's hair and emphasize that the fontanel is similar to skin anywhere else on the body—it does not puncture or tear with mild pressure.

When seborrheic lesions are present, the treatment is directed at removing the crusts. Parents are taught the appropriate procedure to clean the scalp. Education may need to include a demonstration.

Shampooing should be done daily with a mild soap or commercial baby shampoo; medicated shampoos are not necessary, but an anti-seborrheic shampoo containing sulfur and salicylic acid may be used. Shampoo is applied to the scalp and allowed to remain on the scalp until the crusts soften. Then the scalp is thoroughly rinsed. A fine-tooth comb or a soft facial brush helps remove the loosened crusts from the strands of hair after shampooing.

Acne

Acne vulgaris is the most common skin problem treated by physicians during patients' adolescence. Acne is not caused by dirt but by testosterone, a hormone present in boys and girls that increases during puberty. It stimulates the sebaceous glands of the skin to enlarge, or produce oil, and plug the pores. Whiteheads, blackheads, and pimples are present in teenage acne.

Half of the adolescent population experience acne by the end of the teenage years. Although the disorder can appear before the age of 10 years, the peak incidence occurs in middle to late adolescence (age 16 to 17 years in girls and 17 to 18 years in boys). It is more common in boys than in girls. The degree to which an individual is affected may range from nothing more than a few isolated comedones to a severe inflammatory reaction. Although the disease is self-limiting and not life threatening, it has great significance to adolescents. Health care professionals should not underestimate the impact that acne has on teens.

Numerous factors affect the development and course of acne. Its distribution in families and a high degree of concordance in identical twins suggest hereditary factors. Premenstrual flare-ups of acne occur in nearly 70% of adolescent girls, suggesting a hormonal cause. Studies do not indicate a clear association between stress and acne, but adolescents commonly cite stress as a cause for acne outbreaks. Cosmetics containing lanolin, petrolatum, vegetable oils, lauryl alcohol, butyl stearate, and oleic acid can increase comedone production. Exposure to oils in cooking grease can be a precursor in adolescents who work over fast-food restaurant hot oils. There is no known link between dietary intake and the development or worsening of acne.

Pathophysiology

Contributors to acne development include sebum secretion, abnormal desquamation of follicles, bacterial growth, and inflammation (Kim and Armstrong, 2011). Comedogenesis (formation of comedones) results in a noninflammatory lesion that may be either an open comedone ("blackhead") or a closed comedone ("whitehead"). Inflammation occurs with the proliferation of *Propionibacterium acnes*, which draws in neutrophils, causing inflammatory papules, pustules, nodules, and cysts (Fig. 47-11).

Therapeutic Management

Successful management of acne depends on a cooperative effort among the health care provider, the adolescent, and the parents. Unlike many other dermatologic conditions, acne lesions resolve slowly and improvement may not be apparent for at least 6 weeks. Individual comedones can take several weeks to months to resolve, and papules and pustules usually resolve in about 1 week. The multifactorial causes of acne necessitate a combined approach for successful treatment. Treatment consists of general measures of care and specific treatments determined by the type of lesions involved.

General Measures. Improvement of the adolescent's overall health status is part of the general management. Adequate rest, moderate exercise, a well-balanced diet, reduction of emotional

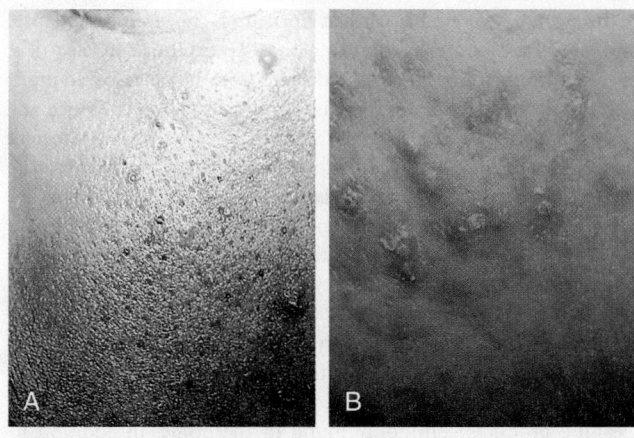

FIG 47-11 Acne vulgaris. **A,** Acne vulgaris. **B,** Comedones with a few inflammatory pustules. (From Zitelli BJ, McIntire SC, Nowalk AJ: *Zitelli and Davis' atlas of pediatric physical diagnosis*, ed 6, St Louis, 2012, Saunders.)

stress, and elimination of any foci of infection are all part of general health promotion.

Cleansing. Dirt or oil on the surface of the skin does not cause acne. Gentle cleansing with a mild cleanser once or twice daily is usually sufficient. Antibacterial soaps are ineffective and may be too drying when used in combination with topical acne medications. For some adolescents, hygiene of the hair and scalp appears to be related to the clinical activity of the acne. Acne on the forehead may improve with brushing the hair away from the forehead and more frequent shampooing.

Medications. Treatment success depends on commitment from the adolescent. Before prescribing treatment, the health care practitioner should determine the adolescent's level of comfort and readiness to begin treatment.

Tretinoin (Retin-A) is the only drug that effectively interrupts the abnormal follicular keratinization that produces microcomedones—the invisible precursors of the visible comedones. Tretinoin alone is usually sufficient for management of comedonal acne (Kim and Armstrong, 2011). Tretinoin is available as a cream, gel, or liquid. This drug can be extremely irritating to the skin and requires careful patient education for optimal usage. The patient should be instructed to begin with a pea-size dot of medication, which is divided into the three main areas of the face and then gently rubbed into each area. The medication should not be applied for at least 20 to 30 minutes after washing to decrease the burning sensation. The avoidance of the sun and the daily use of sunscreen must be emphasized because sun exposure can result in severe sunburn. Adolescents should be advised to apply the medication at night and to use a sunscreen with a sun protection factor (SPF) of at least 15 in the daytime.

Topical benzoyl peroxide is an antibacterial agent that inhibits the growth of *P. acnes* organisms. It is effective against both inflammatory and noninflammatory acne and is an effective first-line agent. This medication is available as a cream, lotion, gel, or wash. The patient should be informed that the medication may have a bleaching effect on sheets, bedclothes, and towels. The adolescent can be reassured that skin bleaching will not occur. Accommodation to the medication can be gained with a gradual increase in the strength and frequency of application.

When inflammatory lesions accompany the comedones, a topical antibacterial agent may be prescribed. These agents are used to prevent new lesions and to treat preexisting acne. Clindamycin, erythromycin, metronidazole, azelaic acid, and the combination of either benzoyl peroxide and erythromycin (Benzamycin) or benzoyl peroxide and glycolic acid are all choices for topical antibacterial therapy. The combination of 5% benzoyl peroxide and 3% erythromycin is especially beneficial, although the exact mechanism of action is not understood (Kim and Armstrong, 2011).

Systemic antibiotic therapy is used when moderate to severe acne does not respond to topical treatments. Oral antibiotics such as tetracycline, erythromycin, minocycline, and doxycycline are considered safe to use (Fanelli, Kupperman, Lautenbach, et al., 2011; Leyden and Del Rosso, 2011).

Young women with mild to moderate acne may respond well to topical treatment and the addition of an oral contraceptive pill (OCP). OCPs reduce the endogenous androgen production and decrease the bioavailability of the woman's circulating androgens. Both of these actions result in decreased acne.

Isotretinoin, 13-cis-retinoic acid (Accutane), is a potent and effective oral agent that is reserved for severe cystic acne that has not responded to other treatments. Isotretinoin is the only agent available that affects factors involved in the development of acne. However, treatment with isotretinoin should be managed *only* by a dermatologist. Adolescents with multiple, active, deep dermal or subcutaneous cystic and nodular acne lesions are treated for 20 weeks. Multiple side effects can occur, including dry skin and mucous membranes, nasal irritation, dry eyes, decreased night vision, photosensitivity, arthralgia, headaches, mood changes, aggressive or violent behaviors, depression, and suicidal ideation. Adolescents taking this drug should be monitored for depression, depressive symptoms, and suicidal ideation (Misery, 2011). The drug should be given only at the recommended doses for no longer than the recommended duration. The most significant side effects of this drug are the teratogenic effects. Isotretinoin is absolutely contraindicated in pregnant women. Sexually active young women must use an effective contraceptive method during treatment and for 1 month after treatment. Patients receiving isotretinoin should also be monitored for elevated cholesterol and triglyceride levels. Significant elevation may require discontinuation of the medication.

CARE MANAGEMENT

Because acne is so common and its appearance may seem so mild, the health care provider may underestimate the relative importance of the disease to the adolescent. The nurse should assess the individual adolescent's level of distress, current management, and perceived success of any regimen before initiating a referral. If adolescents do not perceive the acne to be a problem, they may lack motivation to follow the treatment plan.

The nurse can provide ongoing support for the adolescent when a treatment plan is initiated. The family is also encouraged to support the adolescent in his or her efforts. Use of medications and basic skin care information should be discussed in detail with the adolescent. Written instructions should accompany the verbal discussion. Information to dispel myths regarding the use of abrasive cleansing products can prevent unnecessary costs and trauma to the skin.

Teenagers need education about the factors that aggravate and damage the skin, such as too vigorous scrubbing. In addition, picking, squeezing, and manual expression with fingernails break down the ductal walls of lesions and cause the acne to worsen. Mechanical irritation, such as vinyl helmet straps that rub areas predisposed to acne, can also cause the development of lesions.

THERMAL INJURY

Burns

Burn injuries are usually attributed to extreme heat sources but may also result from exposure to cold, chemicals, electricity, or radiation. Most burns are relatively minor and do not require definitive medical treatment. However, burns involving a large body surface area, critical body parts, or the geriatric or pediatric population often benefit from treatment in specialized burn centers. The American Burn Association has established criteria to guide decisions regarding the severity of injury and the need for transfer for specialized care.*

When burns are categorized according to the patient's age and type of injury, the following patterns become apparent: (1) hot-water scalds are most frequent in toddlers; (2) flame-related burns are more common in older children; (3) 10% to 20% of documented cases of child abuse include burn injuries (Herndon, 2007); and (4) children playing with matches or lighters account for 1 in 10 house fires.

The extent of tissue destruction is determined by the intensity of the heat source, the duration of contact or exposure, the conductivity of the tissue involved, and the rate at which the heat energy is dissipated by the skin. A brief exposure to high-intensity heat from a flame can produce burn injuries similar to those induced by long exposure to less intense heat in hot water.

Characteristics of Burn Injury

The physiologic responses, treatment modalities, prognosis, and disposition of the injured child are all directly related to the *amount of tissue destroyed*. Therefore the severity of the burn injury is assessed on the basis of the percentage of total body surface area (TBSA) burned and depth of the burn. Among children in the school-age group or younger age-groups, a burn that is 10% TBSA can be life threatening if not treated correctly. Other important factors in determining the seriousness of the injury are the location of the wounds, the child's age and general health, the causative agent, the presence of respiratory involvement, and any associated injury or condition.

Type of Injury. The majority of burns result from contact with thermal agents such as a flame, hot surfaces, or hot liquids. Electrical injuries caused by household current have the greatest incidence in young children, who insert conductive objects into electrical outlets and bite or suck on connected electrical cords (Herndon, 2007). These burns occur most commonly during the spring and summer months and are also associated with risk-taking behaviors in boys. Direct contact with high- or low-voltage current, as well as lightning strikes, is the most frequent mechanism of injury. The resistance of the tissue and the path of the electric current are responsible for the damage incurred. Electric current travels through the body following the path of least resistance, which involves the tissues, fluid, blood vessels, and nerves. A more localized burn is produced if skin resistance is high at the area of contact, and a more systemic pattern of injury is produced if skin resistance is low. Often compared with a crush injury, serious electrical trauma results from current passing through vital organs, muscle compartments, and nerve or vascular

pathways. Loss of limbs, cardiac fibrillation, respiratory collapse, and burns are common occurrences after exposure to electrical energy. Criteria for admission, as derived from evidence-based practice for electrical burn injuries, includes a history of loss of consciousness, electrocardiographic (ECG) changes, 10% TBSA affected, or the need for monitoring an affected extremity. Cardiac monitoring is therefore included in standard burn care when ECG changes are identified on admission (Arnoldo, Klein, and Gibran, 2006).

Chemical burns are seen in the pediatric population and can cause extensive injury. The severity of injury is related to the chemical agent (acid, alkali, or organic compound) and the duration of contact. The mechanism of injury differs from that in other burns in that there is a chemical disruption and alteration of the physical properties of the exposed body area. Noxious agents exist in many cleaning products commonly found in the home. In addition to concern for localized damage, the potential for systemic toxicity must be addressed. Of particular concern is the exposure of the eyes to chemical agents, the ingestion of caustic substances, and inhalation of toxic gases produced from chemicals.

Extent of Injury. The extent of a burn is expressed as a percentage of the TBSA. This is most accurately estimated by using specially designed age-related charts (Fig. 47-12). It is more efficient to use a chart designed to assign body proportions to children of different ages.

Depth of Injury. A thermal injury is a three-dimensional wound that is also assessed in relation to depth of injury. Traditionally, the terms *first*, *second*, and *third degree* have been used to describe the depth of tissue injury. However, with the current emphasis on wound healing, these have been replaced by more descriptive terms based on the extent of destruction to the epithelializing elements of the skin (Fig. 47-13).

Superficial (first-degree) burns are usually of minor significance. This type of injury involves the epidermal layer only. There is often a latent period followed by erythema. Tissue damage is minimal, and there is no blistering. The protective functions of the skin remain intact, and systemic effects are rare. Pain is the predominant symptom, and the burn heals in 5 to 10 days without scarring. A mild sunburn is an example of a superficial burn.

Partial-thickness (second-degree) burns involve the epidermis and varying degrees of the dermal layer. These wounds are painful, moist, red, and blistered. With superficial partial-thickness burns, dermal elements are intact and the wound should heal in approximately 14 to 21 days with variable amounts of scarring (Fig. 47-14). The wound is extremely sensitive to temperature changes, exposure to air, and light touch. Although classified as second-degree or partial-thickness burn, deep dermal burns resemble full-thickness injuries in many respects except that sweat glands and hair follicles remain intact. The burn may appear mottled, with pink, red, or waxy white areas exhibiting blisters and edema formation. Systemic effects are similar to those encountered with full-thickness burns. Although many of these wounds heal spontaneously, healing time may be extended beyond 21 days. These burn wounds often heal with extensive scarring.

Full-thickness (third-degree) burns are serious injuries that involve the entire epidermis and dermis and extend into subcutaneous tissue (Fig. 47-15). Nerve endings, sweat glands, and hair follicles are destroyed. The burn varies in color from red to tan, waxy white, brown, or black and is distinguished by a dry, leathery appearance (Fig. 47-16). Normally, full-thickness burns lack sensation in the area of injury because of the destruction of nerve endings. However, most full-thickness burns have superficial and partial-thickness burned areas at the periphery of the burn, where nerve

---

*The American Burn Association offers an Advanced Burn Life Support Program; www.ameriburn.org/ablsnow.php.

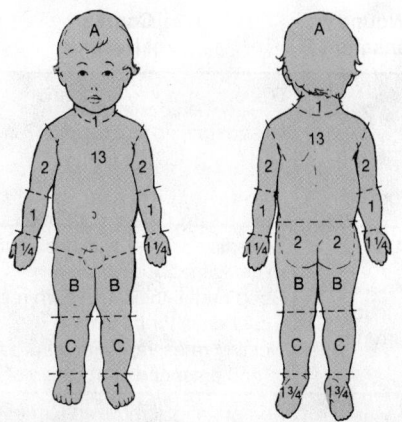

RELATIVE PERCENTAGES OF AREAS AFFECTED BY GROWTH

AREA	BIRTH	AGE 1 YR	AGE 5 YR
A = ½ of head	9½	8½	6½
B = ½ of one thigh	2¾	3¼	4
C = ½ of one leg	2½	2½	2¾

A

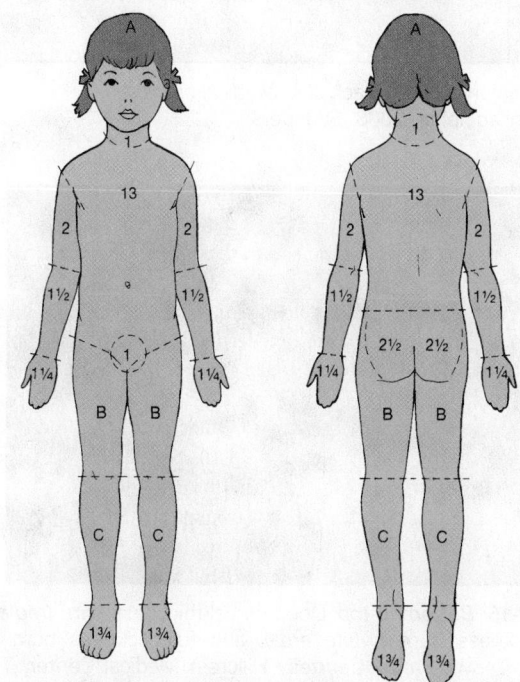

RELATIVE PERCENTAGES OF AREAS AFFECTED BY GROWTH

AREA	AGE 10 YR	AGE 15 YR	ADULT
A = ½ of head	5½	4½	3½
B = ½ of one thigh	4½	4½	4¾
C = ½ of one leg	3	3¼	3½

B

FIG 47-12 Estimation of distribution of burns in children. **A,** Children from birth to age 5 years. **B,** Older children.

endings are intact and exposed. As the peripheral fibers regenerate, painful sensations return. Consequently, children often experience severe pain related to the size and depth of the burn. Full-thickness wounds are not capable of reepithelialization and require surgical excision and grafting to close the wound.

Fourth-degree burns are full-thickness burns that involve underlying structures such as muscle, fascia, and bone. The wound appears dull and dry, and ligaments, tendons, and bone may be exposed (see Fig. 47-16).

TABLE 47-9	SEVERITY GRADING SYSTEM ADOPTED BY THE AMERICAN BURN ASSOCIATION		
	MINOR*	**MODERATE**	**MAJOR**
Partial-thickness burns (% TBSA)	<10	10-20	>20
Full-thickness burns			All
Treatment	Usually outpatient; may require 1-day to 2-day admission	Admission to hospital, preferably one with expertise in burn care	Admission to a burn center

From Vaccaro P, Trofino RB: Care of the patient with minor to moderate burns. In Trofino RB, editor: *Nursing care of the burn-injured patient,* Philadelphia, 1991, FA Davis.
TBSA, Total body surface area.
*Minor burns exclude any burn involving the face, hands, feet, perineum, or crossing joints; electrical burns; any injury complicated by the presence of inhalation injury or concomitant trauma; and children with psychosocial factors affecting the injury.

Severity of Injury. Burns are classified as minor, moderate, or major, which is useful in determining the disposition of the patient for treatment. Burn patients are categorized as (1) those with a major burn injury, who require the services and facilities of a specialized burn center; (2) those with a moderate burn, who may be treated in a hospital with expertise in burn care; and (3) those with minor injuries, who may be treated on an outpatient basis. The extent and depth of the burn (Table 47-9), the causative agent, the body area involved, the patient's age, and concomitant injuries and illnesses determine the severity of the injury.

Because the skin of infants is so thin, they are likely to sustain deeper injuries compared with older children. Children younger than 2 years, especially 6 months or younger, have a significantly higher mortality rate than older children with burns of similar magnitude. Acute or chronic illnesses or superimposed injuries also complicate burn care and response to treatment.

Inhalation Injury. Trauma to the tracheobronchial tree often follows inhalation of heated gases and toxic chemicals produced during combustion. Although direct thermal injury to the upper airway may occur, heat damage below the vocal cords is rare. Inspired heated air is cooled in the upper airway before reaching the trachea. Reflex closure of the cords and laryngospasm also prevent full inhalation. However, evidence of direct thermal injury to the upper airway includes burns of the face and lips, singed nasal hairs, and laryngeal edema. Clinical manifestations may be delayed as long as 24 to 48 hours. Wheezing, increasing secretions, hoarseness, wet rales, and carbonaceous secretions are signs of respiratory tract involvement. Upper airway obstruction is often associated with burn shock and fluid resuscitation. In such situations, endotracheal intubation may also be necessary to preserve a patent airway.

Inhalation of carbon monoxide is suspected when the injury has occurred in an enclosed space. Mucosal erythema and edema followed by sloughing of the mucosa are manifestations of respiratory

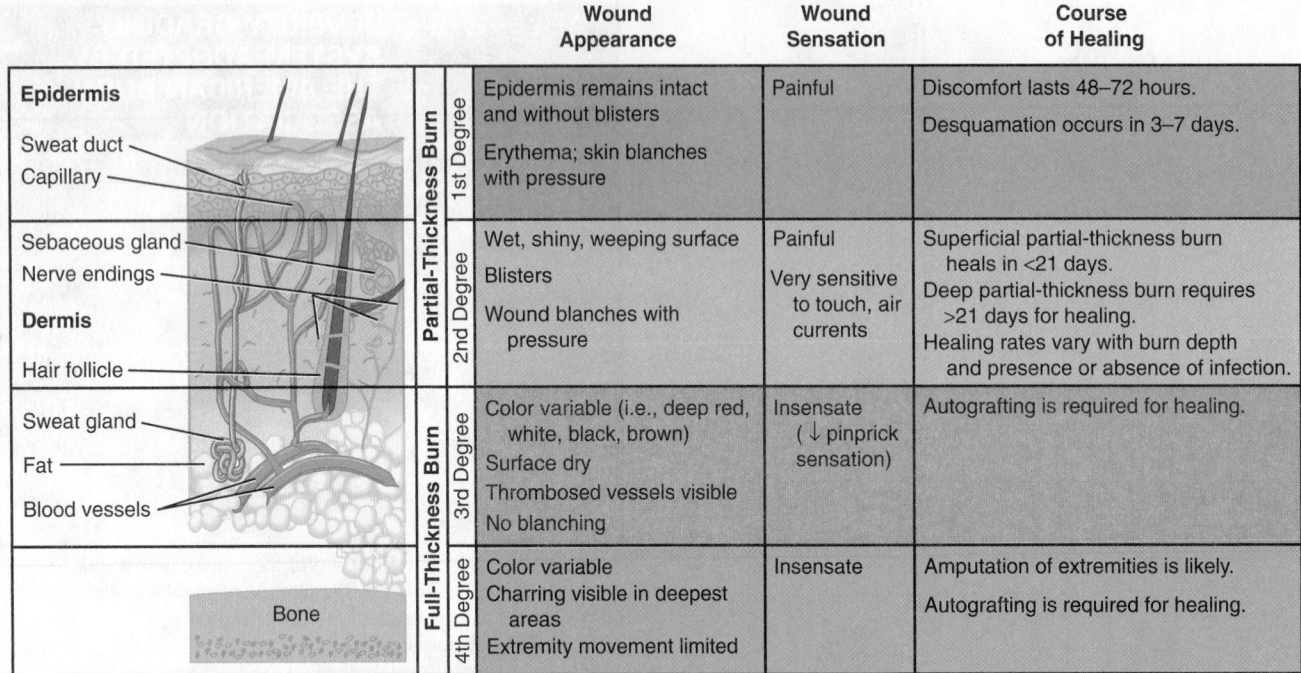

			Wound Appearance	Wound Sensation	Course of Healing
Epidermis Sweat duct Capillary Sebaceous gland Nerve endings Dermis Hair follicle Sweat gland Fat Blood vessels Bone	Partial-Thickness Burn	1st Degree	Epidermis remains intact and without blisters Erythema; skin blanches with pressure	Painful	Discomfort lasts 48–72 hours. Desquamation occurs in 3–7 days.
		2nd Degree	Wet, shiny, weeping surface Blisters Wound blanches with pressure	Painful Very sensitive to touch, air currents	Superficial partial-thickness burn heals in <21 days. Deep partial-thickness burn requires >21 days for healing. Healing rates vary with burn depth and presence or absence of infection.
	Full-Thickness Burn	3rd Degree	Color variable (i.e., deep red, white, black, brown) Surface dry Thrombosed vessels visible No blanching	Insensate (↓ pinprick sensation)	Autografting is required for healing.
		4th Degree	Color variable Charring visible in deepest areas Extremity movement limited	Insensate	Amputation of extremities is likely. Autografting is required for healing.

FIG 47-13 Classification of burn depth according to depth of injury. (From Black JM: *Medical-surgical nursing: clinical management for positive outcomes,* ed 8, Philadelphia, 2008, Saunders.)

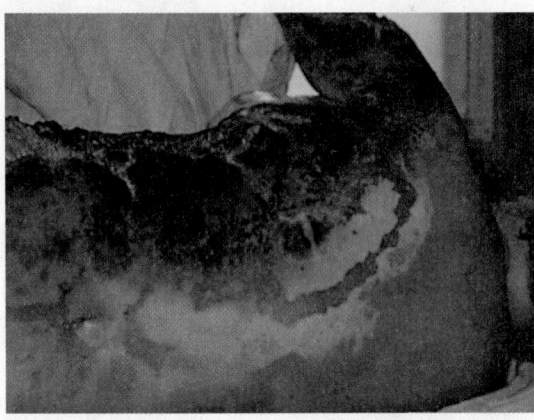

FIG 47-15 *Bottom* to *top:* Deep partial-thickness burn *(red area),* full-thickness burn *(white area),* and full-thickness burn with eschar *(brown area).* (Courtesy Hillcrest Medical Center, Tulsa, OK.)

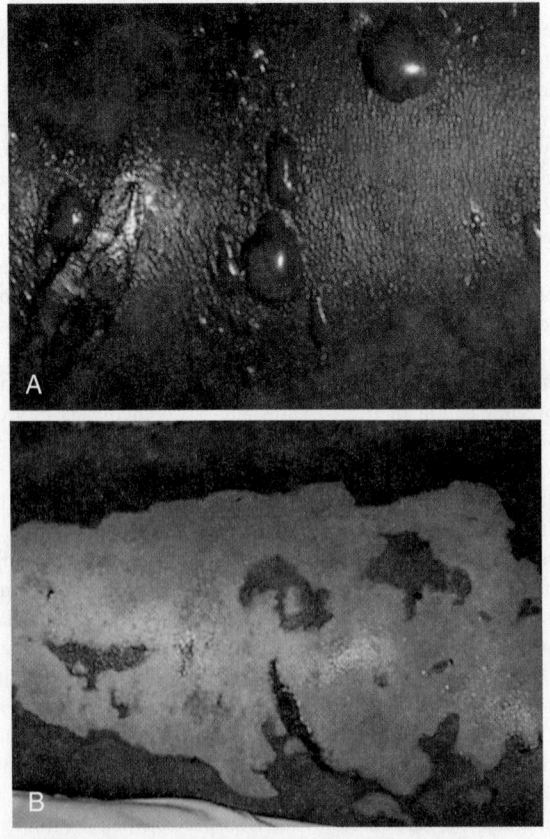

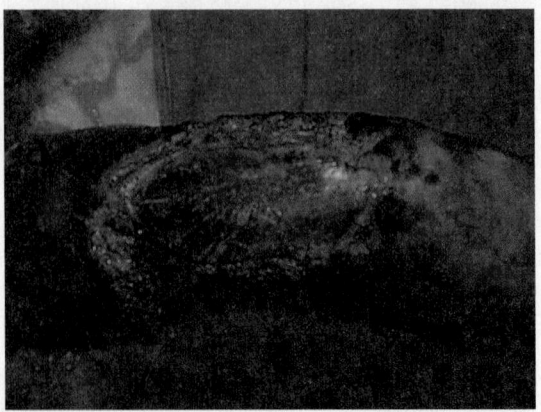

FIG 47-14 Superficial partial-thickness burns on an African-American child. **A,** Blisters intact. **B,** Blisters removed. (Courtesy Hillcrest Medical Center, Tulsa, OK.)

FIG 47-16 Full-thickness burn with muscle and fascia involved. (Courtesy Hillcrest Medical Center, Tulsa, OK.)

tract injury. A mucopurulent membrane replaces the mucosal lining and seriously compromises respiration and ventilation. A significant increase in mortality has been observed when inhalation injury and pneumonia are both present. Deep burns, especially those encircling the thorax, may cause restriction of chest excursion as a result of edema and inelastic eschar formation. Young children are particularly at risk because of the pliability of the skeletal structure.

Pathophysiology

Thermal injuries produce both local and systemic effects that are related to the extent of tissue destruction. In superficial burns, the tissue damage is minimal. In partial-thickness burns, there is considerable edema and more severe capillary damage. With a major burn greater than 30% TBSA, there is a systemic response involving an increase in capillary permeability, allowing plasma proteins, fluids, and electrolytes to be lost. Maximum edema formation in a small wound occurs about 8 to 12 hours after injury. After a larger injury, hypovolemia, associated with this phenomenon, will slow the rate of edema formation, with maximum effect at 18 to 24 hours.

Another systemic response is anemia, caused by direct heat destruction of red blood cells (RBCs), hemolysis of injured RBCs, and trapping of RBCs in the microvascular thrombi of damaged cells. A long-term decrease in the number of RBCs may occur as a result of increased RBC fragility. Initially, there is an increased blood flow to the heart, brain, and kidneys, with decreased blood flow to the gastrointestinal tract. There is an increase in metabolism to maintain body heat, providing for the increased energy needs of the body.

Complications. Thermally injured children are subject to a number of serious complications, both from the wound and from systemic alterations resulting from the injury. The immediate threat to life is related to airway compromise and profound shock. During healing, infection—both local and systemic sepsis—is the primary complication. Mortality associated with thermal trauma in children increases with the severity of injury and decreases as age advances. In children older than 3 years, the mortality rate is similar to that of adults. Below this age, the survival rate with burns and their associated complications lessens considerably.

A less apparent respiratory tract injury is inhalation of carbon monoxide. Carbon monoxide has a greater affinity for hemoglobin than does oxygen, thereby depriving peripheral tissues and oxygen-dependent organs (e.g., the heart and brain) of the oxygen needed for survival. Treatment for either of these two problems is 100% oxygen, which reverses the situation rapidly.

Pulmonary problems are a major cause of fatality in children with either thermal burns or complications in the respiratory tract. Early in the postburn period, most pulmonary infections result from nosocomial exposure, immobility, and abdominal distention. The hematogenous variety occurs later and is related to the septic burn wound or other foci, such as phlebitis at the site of an invasive intravenous (IV) line. Respiratory problems include inhalation injuries, aspiration in unconscious patients, bacterial pneumonia, pulmonary edema, pulmonary embolus, post-traumatic pulmonary insufficiency, and atelectasis. The most common cause of respiratory failure in the pediatric age-group is bacterial pneumonia, which requires prolonged intubation and sometimes a tracheostomy. Tracheostomies increase the incidence of serious complications and are performed only in extreme cases.

A less common complication is pulmonary edema resulting from fluid overload or acute respiratory distress syndrome (ARDS) in association with gram-negative sepsis. ARDS results from pulmonary capillary damage and leakage of fluid into the interstitial spaces

of the lung. A loss of compliance and interference with oxygenation are the consequences of pulmonary insufficiency in conjunction with systemic sepsis.

Wound Sepsis. Sepsis is a critical problem in the treatment of burns and an ever-present threat after the shock phase. Decreased level of consciousness and lethargy are early signs of sepsis. Initially, burn wounds are relatively pathogen free unless they are contaminated with potentially infectious material, such as dirt or polluted water. However, dead tissue and exudate provide a fertile field for bacterial growth. On approximately the third postburn day, early colonization of the wound surface by a preponderance of gram-positive organisms (primarily staphylococci) changes to predominantly gram-negative opportunistic organisms, particularly *Pseudomonas aeruginosa*. By the fifth postburn day, bacterial invasion is well under way beneath the surface of the burn wound. Early surgical excision of eschar together with placement of autograft reduces the incidence of sepsis.

Therapeutic Management

Emergency Care. The initial management of the burn patient begins at the scene of injury. The first priority is to stop the burning process (see Emergency box). The child should then be transported immediately to the nearest medical facility for treatment and evaluation. The child and the family are usually extremely frightened and anxious; sensitivity to their emotional state and reassurance should be provided during the transport process.

Stop the Burning Process. The chief aim of rescue in flame burns is to smother the fire, not fan it. Children tend to panic and run, which spreads the flames and makes assistance more difficult. The injured child should be placed in a horizontal position and rolled in a blanket, rug, or similar article, with care taken not to cover the head and face because of the danger of inhalation of toxic fumes. If nothing is available, the victim should lie down and roll over

---

✚ EMERGENCY

Burns

Minor Burns
- Stop the burning process:
  - Apply cool water to the burn or hold the burned area under cool running water.
  - Do not use ice.
- Do not disturb any blisters that form unless the injury is from a chemical substance.
- Do not apply anything to the wound.
- Cover with a clean cloth if risk for damage or contamination.
- Remove burned clothing and jewelry.

Major Burns
- Stop the burning process:
  - Flame burns—smother the fire.
  - Place victim in the horizontal position.
  - Roll victim in a blanket or similar object; avoid covering the head.
- Assess for an adequate airway and breathing.
- If child is not breathing, begin mouth-to-mouth resuscitation.
- Remove burned clothing and jewelry.
- Cover wound with a clean cloth.
- Keep victim warm.
- Transport to medical aid.
- Begin intravenous and oxygen therapy as prescribed.

slowly to extinguish the flames. Remaining in the vertical position may cause the hair to ignite or the inhalation of flames, heat, or smoke.

Major burns with large amounts of denuded skin should not be cooled. Heat is rapidly lost from burned areas, and additional cooling leads to a drop in core body temperature and potential circulatory collapse. Wet dressings also promote vasoconstriction because of cooling, resulting in impaired circulation to the burned area and increased tissue damage. Chemical burns require continuous flushing with large amounts of water before transport to a medical facility. The use of neutralizing agents on the skin is contraindicated because a chemical reaction is initiated and further injury may result. If the chemical is in powder form, the addition of water may spread the caustic agent. The powder should be brushed off if possible before flushing the area.

Burned clothing is removed to prevent further damage from smoldering fabric and hot beads of melted synthetic materials. Jewelry is removed to eliminate the transfer of heat from the metal and constriction resulting from edema formation. This also provides access to the wound and prevents painful removal later.

Assess the Victim's Condition. As soon as the flames are extinguished, the child is assessed. Airway, breathing, and circulation are the primary concerns. Cardiopulmonary complications may result from exposure to electric current, inhalation of toxic fumes and smoke, hypovolemia, and shock. Emergency measures are instituted as appropriate.

Cover the Burn. The burn wound should be covered with a clean dry cloth to prevent contamination, decrease pain by eliminating air contact, and prevent hypothermia. No attempt should be made to treat the burn. Application of topical ointments, oils, or other home remedies is contraindicated.

Transport the Child to Medical Aid. The child with an extensive burn is not given anything by mouth to avoid aspiration in the presence of paralytic ileus and upper airway edema and to prevent water intoxication. The child is transported to the nearest medical facility. If this cannot be accomplished within a relatively short period, IV access should be established, if possible, with a large-bore catheter. Oxygen is administered, if available, at 100%. A report of the initial assessment, associated trauma, and any interventions implemented is given to the medical facility assuming care of the child.

Provide Reassurance. Providing reassurance and psychologic support to both the family and the child helps immeasurably during the period of postinjury crisis. Reducing anxiety conserves energy the family and child will need to cope with the physiologic and emotional stress of injury.

Minor Burns. Treatment of burns classified as minor can usually be managed adequately on an outpatient basis when it is determined that the parent can be relied on to carry out instructions for care and observation. Patients with less-than-optimum circumstances may require close follow-up to ensure adherence with treatment.

The wound is cleansed with a mild soap and tepid water. Débridement of the wound includes removal of any embedded debris, chemicals, and devitalized tissue. Removal of intact blisters remains controversial. Some authorities argue that blisters provide a barrier against infection; others maintain that blister fluid is an effective medium for the growth of microorganisms. However, blisters should be broken if the injury is from a chemical agent to control absorption. Most health care practitioners favor covering the wound with an antimicrobial ointment to reduce the risk for infection and to provide some form of pain relief. The dressing consists of nonadherent fine-mesh gauze placed over the ointment and a

light wrap of gauze dressing that avoids interference with movement. This helps keep the wound clean and protect it from trauma. The caregiver is instructed to wash the wound, reapply the dressing, and return the child to the office or clinic as directed for wound observation. The frequency of dressing changes may vary from every other day to once a day.

Some health care practitioners prefer an occlusive dressing, such as a hydrocolloid, which is placed over the wound after cleansing. Hydrogel dressings, which are soothing and nonadherent, may also be used. The dressing is changed when leakage occurs—at regular intervals or at least weekly. This method eliminates the discomfort associated with frequent dressing changes but limits visualization of the wound surface.

If there is a high probability of infection or other complications or if there is doubt about the ability to carry out instructions, the caregiver may be directed to bring the patient in daily for dressing changes and inspection. Another option is have a nurse make a home visit to inspect the wound and change the dressing. Frequent removal of the dressing is an effective mode of débridement. Soaking the dressing in tepid water or normal saline before removal helps loosen the dressing and debris and reduce discomfort. Burns of the face are usually treated by an open method. The wound is washed and débrided in the same manner, and a thin film of antimicrobial ointment is applied.

A tetanus history is obtained on admission. If there is no history of immunization or if more than 5 years have passed since the last immunization, tetanus prophylaxis is administered. A mild analgesic such as acetaminophen is usually sufficient to relieve discomfort; the antipyretic effect of the drug also alleviates the sensation of heat.

Most minor burns heal without difficulty; however, hospitalization is indicated if the wound margin becomes erythematous, gross purulence is noted, or the child develops evidence of systemic reaction, such as fever or tachycardia. The child should also be evaluated for functional impairment, and the caregiver should be instructed in the exercise and ambulation program. After wound healing, an evaluation of scar maturation and range of motion will indicate any need for further therapy.

Major Burns. The first priority is airway maintenance. The inhalation of noxious agents or respiratory burns is suggested when there is a history of injury in an enclosed space; edema of the oral and nasal membranes; thermal injury to the face, nares, and upper torso; hyperemia; and blisters or evidence of trauma to the upper respiratory passages. When respiratory involvement is suspected or evident, 100% oxygen is administered and blood gas values, including carbon monoxide levels, are determined.

If the child exhibits changes in sensorium, air hunger, or other signs of respiratory distress, an endotracheal tube is inserted to maintain the airway. When severe edema of the face and neck is anticipated, intubation is performed before swelling makes intubation difficult or impossible. Controlled intubation is preferred to an emergency intubation. Intubation allows for the delivery of humidified oxygen, the removal of secretions from respiratory passages, and the provision of ventilatory support. When full-thickness burns encircle the chest, constricting eschar may limit chest wall excursion and ventilation of the child becomes more difficult. Escharotomy of the chest relieves this constriction and improves ventilation.

Fluid Replacement Therapy. The objectives of fluid therapy are to (1) compensate for water and sodium lost to traumatized areas and interstitial spaces, (2) reestablish sodium balance, (3) restore circulating volume, (4) provide adequate perfusion, (5) correct acidosis, and (6) improve renal function.

Fluid replacement is required during the first 24 hours because of fluid shifts that occur after the injury. Various formulas are used to calculate fluid needs, and the one adopted depends on the preference of the health care practitioner. Crystalloid solutions are used during this initial phase of therapy. Parameters such as vital signs (especially heart rate), urinary output volume, adequacy of capillary filling, and state of sensorium determine adequacy of fluid resuscitation.

After the initial 24-hour period, theoretically there is a capillary seal and capillary permeability is restored. Colloid solutions such as albumin, Plasma-Lyte, or fresh-frozen plasma are useful in maintaining plasma volume. However, children with burn injuries usually require fluids in excess of their calculated maintenance and replacement volume. Reasons for this may include underestimation of burn size (particularly in pediatric patients), pulmonary injury that sequesters resuscitation fluid in the lung, electrical injury with greater tissue destruction than that which is visible, and a delay in the initiation of fluid resuscitation. Irreversible burn shock that persists despite aggressive fluid resuscitation remains a significant cause of death in the immediate postburn period. Fluid balance may continue to be a problem throughout the course of treatment, especially during periods in which there may be considerable evaporative loss from the wound.

Nutrition. The enhanced metabolic requirements and catabolism in severe burns make nutritional needs of paramount importance and often difficult to satisfy. To avoid protein breakdown, the diet must provide sufficient calories to meet the increased metabolic needs and enough protein. Hypoglycemia can result from the stress of the burn injury because the liver glycogen stores are rapidly depleted.

A high-protein, high-calorie diet is encouraged. Many children have poor appetites and are unable to meet energy requirements solely by oral feeding. Oral feedings are encouraged unless the child is intubated or paralytic ileus persists. Most children with burns in excess of 25% TBSA require supplementation with tube feeding. Early and continued nutritional support is an important part of therapy for seriously burned patients. Enteral feeding provides direct nourishment to the gastrointestinal tract and helps reverse the defective gut barrier that accompanies burn shock (Purdue, 2007). Children who require enteral supplementation must be monitored for feeding intolerance and tube malposition. The nurse should also monitor and report any abdominal distention, diarrhea, or electrolyte and metabolic deviations. If nutritional requirements cannot be met entirely by the enteral route, parenteral hyperalimentation is used to supplement intake. However, enteral feeding increases blood flow in the intestinal tract, preserves gastrointestinal function, and minimizes bacterial translocation by decreasing mucosal atrophy of the intestines. These factors make enteral feeding the preferred route of nutritional support (Herndon, 2007).

To facilitate growth and proliferation of epithelial cells, administration of vitamins A and C is begun early in the postburn period. Zinc is also supplemented because of its important role in wound healing and epithelialization.

Medication. Antibiotics are usually not administered prophylactically. The administration of systemic antibiotics to control wound colonization is not indicated because decreased circulation to the injured area prevents delivery of the medication to areas of deepest injury. Surveillance cultures and monitoring of the clinical course provide the most reliable indicators of developing infection. Appropriate antibiotics are instituted to treat the specific identified organism. Otitis media should not be overlooked as a source of fever in the pediatric population (Herndon, 2007).

Some form of sedation and analgesia is required in the care of burned children. Morphine sulfate is the drug of choice for severe burn injuries. Morphine has extensive distribution but is metabolized rapidly; continuous infusion or frequent administration is needed for pain management in burns. Morphine is administered intravenously and titrated to individual needs. The unstable circulatory status and edema formation preclude intramuscular or subcutaneous administration. When combined, midazolam (Versed) and fentanyl (Sublimaze) also provide excellent IV sedation and analgesia to control procedural pain in children with burns (Herndon, 2007). The oral form of fentanyl, Oralet, provides effective analgesia in a convenient form that children can suck. Dosage monitoring is important because tolerance to opioids may develop. IV analgesics are most effective when they are administered just before the onset of procedural pain.

The use of short-acting anesthetic agents, such as propofol (Diprivan) and nitrous oxide, has proved beneficial in eliminating procedural pain. Pharyngeal reflexes remain intact, thus ensuring a patent airway. Propofol is an IV sedative hypnotic agent that produces sedation in less than 1 minute and lasts only a few minutes. Nitrous oxide is a useful short-term analgesic when given in a mixture of gases on a fixed ratio of 50% nitrous oxide and 50% oxygen (Annequin, Carbajal, Chauvin, et al., 2000). Initiation of action is approximately 1 minute, with peak effect reached in 3 to 5 minutes. Nitrous oxide is useful to alleviate anxiety and raise the threshold of pain during procedures. The child may self-administer the nitrous oxide mixture with assistance. For any conscious or unconscious sedation, the child must be monitored continuously during the procedure (see Preoperative Care, Chapter 39; and Pain Assessment and Pain Management, Chapter 30).

Management of the Burn Wound. After the initial period of shock and the restoration of fluid balance, the primary concern is the burn wound. The objectives of wound management include prevention of infection, removal of devitalized tissue, and closure of the wound. The application of dressings and topical antimicrobial therapy reduce pain by minimizing the exposure to air.

Primary Excision. In children with large, full-thickness burn wounds, excision is performed as soon as the patient is hemodynamically stable after initial resuscitation. Because the burn wound precipitates an exaggerated physiologic response, many complications do not resolve until the eschar is excised and the wound is closed. Early excision of deep partial- and full-thickness burns reduces the incidence of infection and the threat of sepsis.

Débridement. Partial-thickness wounds require débridement of devitalized tissue to promote healing. Débridement is painful and requires analgesia and a sedative before the procedure. Medications given for pain need to be readily available during this procedure and may need to be titrated up during the procedure. Hydroxyzine and diphenhydramine are often needed for itching that occurs after whirlpool and débridement. The itching becomes particularly bothersome as the burns heal.

Hydrotherapy is used to cleanse the wound and involves soaking in a tub or showering at least once a day for no more than 20 minutes. The water acts to loosen and remove sloughing tissue, exudate, and topical medications. Hydrotherapy helps cleanse not only the wound but also the entire body and aids in maintenance of range of motion. Mesh gauze serves to entrap the exudative slough and is readily removed during hydrotherapy. Any loose tissue is carefully trimmed away before the wound is redressed.

Topical Antimicrobial Agents. Methods used for managing the burn wound include:

- Exposure—Wounds are left open to air; crust forms on partial-thickness wounds, and eschar forms on full-thickness burns.
- Open—Topical antimicrobial agent is applied directly to the wound surface, and the wound is left uncovered.
- Modified—Antimicrobial agent is applied directly or impregnated into thin gauze and applied to the wound; gauze or net secures the area.
- Occlusive—Antimicrobial agent is impregnated in gauze or applied directly to the wound; multiple layers of bulky gauze are placed over the primary layer and secured with gauze or net.

All of these methods provide wound coverage and use some type of topical agent. Topical agents do not eliminate organisms from the wound but can effectively inhibit bacterial growth. To be effective, a topical application must be nontoxic, capable of diffusing through eschar, harmless to viable tissue, inexpensive, and easy to apply. A topical ointment should not encourage the development of resistant strains of bacteria and should produce minimal electrolyte derangement. A variety of specific agents are available; examples include Bacitracin, silver sulfadiazine (Thermazene), collagenase (Santyl), and mafenide acetate (Sulfamylon). Some topical agents are packaged and prepared on a fine-meshed gauze that allows ease of application. The gauze provides necessary protection for the wound, maximizes patient comfort, increases rate of healing, decreases the necessity for frequent dressing changes, and is cost effective. Examples include a nanocrystalline film of pure silver (Acticoat), a hydrofiber with ionic silver (Aquacel Ag), a flexible nylon mesh matrix with oat-beta glucan and silver (Glucan Silver Matrix), and a silicone foam dressing with silver (Mepilex Ag).

Biologic Skin Coverings. Permanent coverage of extensive burns is a prolonged process that requires repeated operative procedures using general anesthesia for atraumatic care in débridement and grafting. Early closure shortens the period of metabolic stress and decreases the likelihood of burn wound sepsis. In the acute phase, biologic dressings cover and protect the wound from contamination, reduce fluid and protein loss, increase the rate of epithelialization, reduce pain, and facilitate movement of joints to retain range of motion.

Allograft (homograft) skin is obtained from human cadavers that are screened for communicable diseases. Allograft is particularly useful in the coverage of surgically excised deep partial- and full-thickness wounds in extensive burns when available donor sites are limited. Severe immunosuppression occurs in massively burned children, and the allograft becomes adherent. The allograft can remain in place until suitable donor sites become available. Typically, rejection is seen approximately 3 to 4 weeks after application (Herndon, 2007). The availability of tissue banks and a supply of suitable donors limit the use of allografts.

Xenograft from a variety of species, most notably pigs, is commercially available. In large burns, the porcine xenograft is commonly applied when extensive early débridement is indicated to cover a partial-thickness burn; this provides a temporary covering for the wound until an available autograft can be applied to the full-thickness areas (Herndon, 2007). Pigskin dressings are replaced every 1 to 3 days. They are particularly effective in children with partial-thickness scald burns of the hands and face because they allow relatively pain-free movement, which reduces contracture formation and has the added benefit of improving appetite and morale.

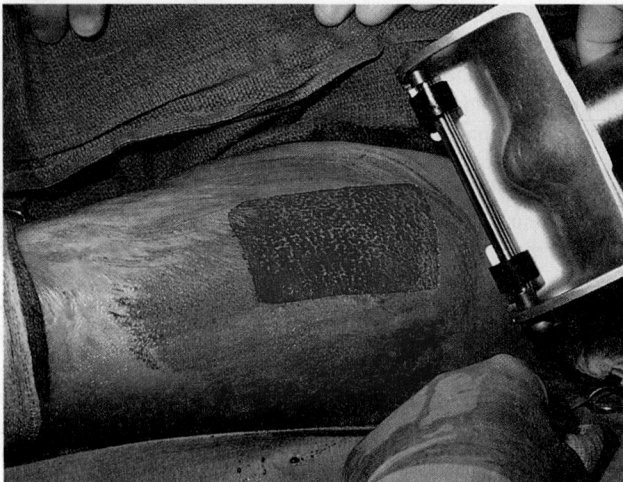

FIG 47-17 Removal of split-thickness skin graft with a dermatome.

When applied early to a superficial partial-thickness injury, biologic dressings stimulate epithelial growth and faster wound healing. However, biologic dressings must be applied to clean wounds. If the dressing covers areas of heavy microbial contamination, infection occurs beneath the dressing. In the case of partial-thickness burns, such infection may convert the wound to a full-thickness injury.

Synthetic skin coverings are available for the management of partial-thickness burn wounds. Ideally, the dressing should provide the properties of human skin, including adherence, elasticity, durability, and hemostasis. Synthetic skin substitutes are readily available, have an indefinite shelf life, and are relatively inexpensive.

Synthetic dressings are composed of a variety of materials and can be used successfully in the management of superficial partial-thickness burns and donor sites. Examples include adherent elastic films; hydroactive materials; or colloidal suspensions that are usually permeable to air, vapor, and fluids.

Biobrane is a flexible silicone-nylon membrane bonded to collagenous peptides of porcine skin. Calcium alginate is another treatment for donor sites. As with biologic dressings, it is important that the wound be free of debris before the dressing is applied. Body temperature elevation or evidence of purulence, erythema, or cellulitis around the wound edges may indicate that the wound has become infected beneath the dressing. If this occurs, prompt discontinuance of the synthetic dressing is indicated. All synthetic dressings are reputed to hasten wound healing and reduce discomfort.

Permanent Skin Coverings. Permanent coverage of deep partial- and full-thickness burns is usually accomplished with a split-thickness skin graft. This graft consists of the epidermis and a portion of the dermis removed from an intact area of skin by a special instrument, the dermatome (Fig. 47-17). With extensive burns, it is often difficult to find enough viable skin to cover the wounds; therefore available donor sites and special techniques are used. Split-thickness skin grafts may be sheet graft or mesh graft.

Sheet Graft. A sheet of skin removed from the donor site is placed intact over the recipient site and sutured in place; this is used in areas where cosmetic results are most visible (Fig. 47-18).

Mesh Graft. A sheet of skin is removed from the donor site and passed through a mesher, which produces tiny slits in the skin that allow the skin to cover 1.5 to 9 times the area of the sheet graft; this results in a less desirable cosmetic and functional outcome (Fig. 47-19).

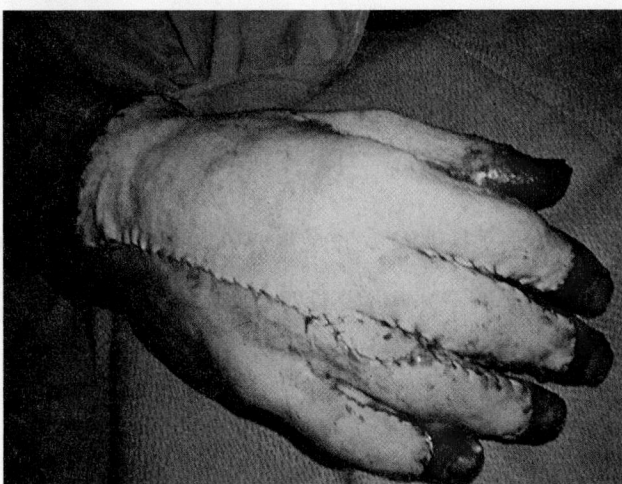

FIG 47-18 Sheet graft.

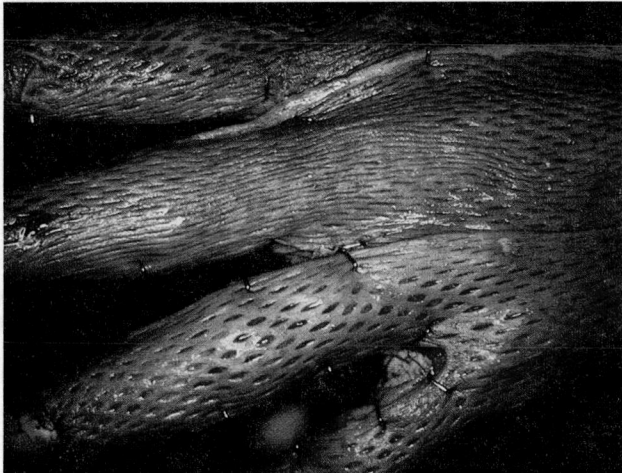

FIG 47-19 Mesh graft.

The donor site is dressed with synthetic wound coverings or fine-mesh gauze until the dressing separates at 10 to 14 days when the wound is healed. Dressings are not changed on donor sites to avoid damage to newly healed, delicate epithelium. Healed donor sites are available for reharvesting in patients with extensive burns and limited undamaged skin, but the quality of skin is decreased when multiple grafts are taken.

Artificial Skin. The development of Integra, a product that allows the dermis to regenerate, has produced significant improvement in burn wound healing and decreased scar formation. It is applied to partial- and full-thickness burns. The two-layer membrane is made of collagen (a fibrous protein from animal tendons and cartilage) and silicone rubber (i.e., Silastic). The Silastic layer is peeled off after the dermis is formed. The application of artificial skin does not replace the grafting procedure, but it prepares the burn wound to accept an ultrathin autograft. Advantages include faster healing of the burn wound when integrity of the dermis is restored, faster healing of donor sites with the use of ultrathin grafts, and restoration of sweat glands and hair follicles. A disadvantage is its high cost.

Cultured Epithelium. When burns are extensive and donor sites for split-thickness skin grafting are limited, it is possible to culture cells from a full-thickness skin biopsy and produce coherent sheets that can be applied to clean, excised full-thickness wounds. Epithelial cell culture grafts offer the possibility of an unlimited source of autografts in patients with extensive burns. Cultured epithelial autografts are effective in early wound closure. The child's own skin is fractionated and cultured in a porcine media to form a thin epithelial layer that is applied to the burn wound. This technique offers an improved rate of survival in patients with extensive burns and limited donor sites.

Prognosis. Children differ from adults in their responses to thermal injury, and the mortality rates in young children are significantly higher than those in older children and adults. Mortality is greatest for children younger than 48 months. Many children who do survive have long-term functional and cosmetic impairments.

CARE MANAGEMENT

Because the care of burned children encompasses a broad range of skills, nursing care has been divided into segments that correspond with the major phases of burn treatment. The acute phase, also referred to as the *emergent* or *resuscitative phase,* involves the first 24 to 48 hours. The management phase extends from the completion of adequate resuscitation through wound coverage. The rehabilitative phase begins when the majority of the wounds have healed and rehabilitation has become the predominant focus of the care plan. This phase continues until all reconstructive procedures and corrective measures are accomplished (often a period of months or years).

Acute Phase. The primary emphasis during the emergent phase is the treatment of burn shock and the management of pulmonary status. Monitoring vital signs, output, fluid infusion, and respiratory parameters are ongoing activities in the hours immediately after injury. IV infusion is begun immediately and is regulated to maintain a urinary output of at least 1 to 2 mL/kg in children weighing less than 30 kg (66 lb); an output of 30 to 50 mL/hr is expected in children weighing more than 30 kg. Urinary output and specific gravity, vital signs, laboratory data, and objective signs of adequate hydration guide the rate of fluid administration.

Children who are hospitalized with burns require constant observation and assessment for complications. Alterations in electrolyte balance produce clinical symptoms of confusion, weakness, cardiac irregularities, and seizures. Changes in respiratory function and gas exchange are reflected clinically by restlessness, irritability, increased work of breathing, and alterations in blood gas values. The loss of protective function of the skin exposes burned children to increased risk for hypothermia. Edema formation and circulatory impairment result in the loss of sensation and deep, throbbing pain.

> **! NURSING ALERT**
>
> Evaluate the burned extremity and check the pulse every hour. If unable to palpate, use Doppler to ascertain loss of circulation and pulse. If the pulse is lost, escharotomy may be necessary to relieve the edema causing pressure on blood vessels to restore adequate circulation.

Burn centers maintain a pictorial record of wounds to record progress and for legal purposes (if child abuse is suspected). Burn wounds are treated according to the protocol of the specific burn center. The burn team monitors infection control procedures and ensures that staff and visitors comply with established protocols to prevent cross-contamination in the burn unit.

Throughout the acute phase of care, the psychosocial needs of the children and their families should not be overlooked. The child is frightened, uncomfortable, and often confused. Children may be isolated from familiar persons and surroundings; the overwhelming physical needs at this time are the primary focus of the staff and parents. In addition to feeling concern for their child, the family experiences guilt, which may be related to the fact that the parents did not or could not protect their child from injury. Consistency in the information presented and in the attitude of the staff creates a sense of familiarity and stability during the acute phase of care. Consistent caregivers can also help decrease the patient's and family's anxiety and provide coordination of care. For example, when many teams of consultants and specialists are involved in the child's care, appointing a burn team "spokesperson" decreases the confusion and enhances communication regarding the child's care.

Management and Rehabilitative Phases. After the patient's condition is stabilized, the management phase begins. The multidisciplinary team concentrates on preventing wound infections, closing the wound as quickly as possible, and managing the numerous complications. Although the rehabilitative phase begins when permanent wound closure has been achieved, rehabilitation issues are identified on admission and are included in the care plan throughout the hospital course.

> **! NURSING ALERT**
>
> In a pediatric burn patient, a decreased level of consciousness, increased restlessness, and lethargy are some of the first signs of overwhelming sepsis and may indicate inadequate hydration. Assessment of capillary refill and pulses is another important indicator of the adequacy of hydration. With inadequate hydration, a spiking fever and diminished bowel sounds accompanied by paralytic ileus are noted and progressively increase over 48 to 72 hours, after which the temperature falls to subnormal limits. At this time, the wound deteriorates, the white blood cell count is depressed, and septic shock becomes manifest.

Comfort Management. The severe pain of the wound and resultant therapies, the anxiety generated by these experiences, sleep deprivation, itching related to wound healing, and the conscious and unconscious interpretations of traumatic events contribute to the psychologic behaviors commonly observed in children with burns. It is always difficult to deal with a child in pain, and inflicting pain on a helpless child is contrary to the empathic nature of nursing. Interventions to promote comfort may include medications (including IV morphine, fentanyl, or midazolam and short-term anesthetics such as propofol), relaxation techniques, distraction therapy, behavioral techniques, operant conditioning (e.g., tokens, star chart), and family participation.

Children need age-appropriate explanations before all procedures. When children appear to accept pain with little or no response, psychologic consultation may be needed. Consistency in caregivers is important. If this is not possible, a carefully developed multidisciplinary care plan is necessary to provide consistency.

Care of the Burn Wound. The nurse has a major responsibility for cleansing, débriding, and applying topical medications and dressings to the burn wound. Pain medication should be administered so that the peak effect of the drug coincides with the procedure. Children who have an understanding of the procedure to be performed and some perceived control demonstrate less maladaptive behavior. Children also respond well to participating in decisions (see Atraumatic Care box).

Outer dressings are removed. Any dressings that have adhered to the wound can be more easily removed by applying tepid water or normal saline. Loose or easily detached tissue is débrided during the

cleansing process. In dressing the wound, it is important that all areas be clean, that medication be amply applied, and that no two burned surfaces touch each other (e.g., fingers or toes; ears touching the side of the head). If they are touching, the burned surfaces will heal together, causing deformity or dysfunction.

Topical medications may be applied directly to the wound with a tongue blade or gloved hand as well as using impregnated fine-mesh gauze. Dressings are then applied to assist in exudate absorption, wound débridement, and increased patient comfort. All dressings applied circumferentially should be wrapped in a distal-to-proximal manner. The dressing is applied with sufficient tension to remain in place but not so tightly as to impair circulation or limit motion. An elastic net is then applied to secure the dressing in place. A stable dressing is especially important when the child is ambulatory.

Standard Precautions, including the use of protective garb and barrier techniques, should be followed when caring for patients with burns. Frequent hand and forearm washing is the single most important element of the infection control program. Strict policies for cleaning the environment and patient care equipment should be implemented to minimize the risk for cross-contamination. All visitors and members of other departments should be oriented to the infection control policies, including the importance of hand and forearm washing and use of protective garb. Visitors should be screened for infection and contagious diseases before patient contact.

Prevention of Complications

Acute Care. The maintenance of body temperature is important to children with burns. Core body temperature is supported when energy is conserved with an environmental temperature of 28° to 33°C (82.4° to 91.4°F). Large areas of the body should not be exposed simultaneously during dressing changes. Warmed solutions, linens, occlusive dressings, heat shields, a radiant warmer, and warming blankets assist in preventing hypothermia.

The chief danger during acute care is infection—wound infection, generalized sepsis, or bacterial pneumonia. Accurate and ongoing assessments of all parameters that provide clues to the early diagnosis and treatment of infection are essential. Symptoms of sepsis include a decreased level of consciousness, a rising or falling white blood cell count, hyperthermia progressing to hypothermia, increasing fluid requirements, hypoactive or absent bowel sounds, a rising or falling blood glucose level, tachycardia, tachypnea, and thrombocytopenia. Infection delays the progress of wound healing.

Children are reluctant to move if movement causes pain, and they are likely to assume a position of comfort. Unfortunately, the most comfortable position often encourages the formation

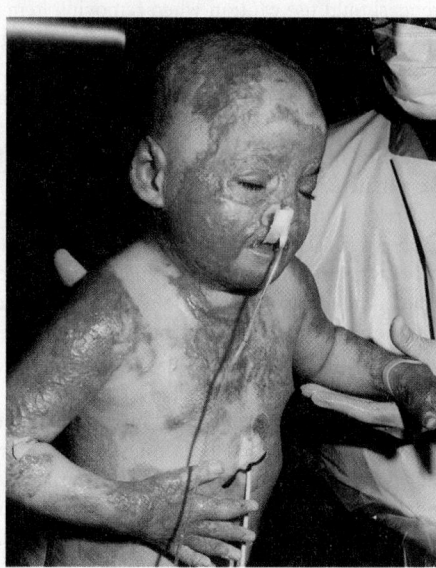

FIG 47-20 Extensive scars from a flame burn. (Courtesy The Paul and Carol David Foundation Burn Institute, Akron, OH.)

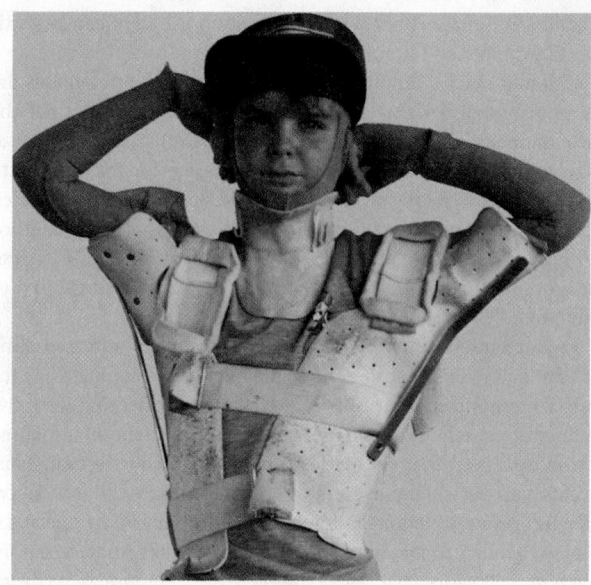

FIG. 47-21 Child in an elasticized (Jobst) garment and "airplane" splints.

of contractures and loss of function. Ongoing efforts to prevent contractures include maintaining proper body alignment, positioning and splinting involved extremities in extension, providing active and passive physical therapy, and encouraging spontaneous movement when feasible. Frequent position changes are important to promote adequate bronchopulmonary hygiene and capillary perfusion to common pressure areas. Low–air loss beds are beneficial for morbidly obese children or children with posterior grafts. Special attention should be given to areas at risk for increased pressure, such as the posterior scalp, heels, sacrum, and areas exposed to mechanical irritation from splints and dressings.

Long-Term Care. When the burn heals, the rehabilitative phase of care begins. Scar formation becomes a major problem as burn wounds heal (Fig. 47-20). Contractile properties of the scar tissue can result in disabling contractures, deformity, and disfigurement.

Uniform pressure applied to the scar decreases the blood supply. When pressure is removed, blood supply to the scar is immediately increased; therefore periods without pressure should be brief to avoid nourishment of the hypertrophic tissue. Continuous pressure to areas of scarring can be achieved by elastic bandages or commercially available pressure garments. Because these custom-made garments are often worn for months, revisions may be required as the child grows. It is much easier to prevent scarring and contracture of the wound than to resolve an existing problem. Splints and appliances may also be needed until wound maturation is achieved (Fig. 47-21).

Scar tissue has certain significant properties, particularly for growing children. Intense itching occurs in healing burn wounds and scar tissue until the scar is no longer active. Itching is usually treated with a combination of H_1 and H_2 antagonists such as cetirizine (Zyrtec) and cimetidine (Tagamet) (Baker, Zeller, Klein, et al., 2001); an H_1 antagonist alone; and frequent applications of a moisturizer, such as Vaseline Intensive Care Rescue, Aveeno Baby, Alpha Keri, or Eucerin. Massage therapy during the application of moisturizers is also beneficial to stretch scar tissue and aid in contracture prevention. Scar tissue has no sweat glands, and children with extensive scarring may experience difficulty during hot weather. Caregivers should be alerted to this possibility and be prepared to institute alternate methods of cooling when necessary.

Scar tissue does not grow and expand as does normal tissue, which may create difficulties, especially in functional areas such as on the hands and over joints. Additional surgery is sometimes required to allow independent functioning in daily activities, to improve cosmetic appearance, or to restore anatomic integrity.

The nursing activities in the rehabilitative phase of treatment focus on the child's and family's adaptation to the burn injury and their ability to reintegrate into the community. The psychologic pain and sequelae of severe burn injury are as intense as the physical trauma. The impact of severe burns taxes the coping mechanisms at all ages. Very young children, who suffer acutely from separation anxiety, and adolescents, who are developing an identity, are probably the most affected psychologically. Toddlers cannot understand why the parents they love and who have protected them can leave them in such a frightening and unfamiliar place. Adolescents, in the process of achieving independence from the family, find themselves in a dependent role with a damaged body. Being different from others at a time when conformity with peers is so important is difficult to accept.

Anticipation of the return to school can be overwhelming and frightening. It is essential that health care professionals recognize the importance of preparing teachers and classmates for the child's return. Teachers need to be provided with information to assist the child and family and to promote the child's optimal adjustment. Hospital-sponsored school reentry programs use a variety of methods to provide education and information about the implications of the injury, the garments and appliances, and the need for support and acceptance. Telephone calls, videotapes, information packets, and visits by members of the health care team offer opportunities to help with reintegration into the school environment—a focal point of the child's life.

Psychosocial Support of the Child. Children should begin early to do as much for themselves as possible and to be active participants in their care. Loss of control and perceived helplessness may result in acting-out behaviors. During illness, children can regress to a previous developmental level that allows them to deal with stress. As children begin to participate in their care, they gain confidence and self-esteem. Fears and anxieties diminish with accomplishment and self-confidence. If the child demonstrates nonadherence in the rehabilitative phase, a behavior modification program can be initiated to promote or reward the child's accomplishment in care.

Children need to know that their injury and the treatments are not punishment for real or imagined transgressions and that the nurse understands their fear, anger, and discomfort. They also need body contact. This is often difficult to arrange for the child with massive burns. Stroking areas of unburned skin is comforting. Even older children enjoy sitting on the parent's lap and being cuddled and hugged. This can be a reward or a comfort in times of stress, but most of all it should be kept in mind that it is a natural part of childhood.

Psychosocial Support of the Family. Recognizing and respecting each family's strengths, differences, and methods of coping allow the nurse to respond to their unique needs by implementing a family-centered approach to care. In the acute phase, all attention is focused on the child and the parents feel powerless and ineffectual. Most parents feel overwhelming guilt, whether or not the guilt is justified. They feel responsible for the injury. These feelings may impede the child's rehabilitation. Parents may indulge the child and allow non-adherent behaviors that affect physical and emotional recovery. Parents need to be informed of the child's progress and helped to cope with their feelings while providing support to their child. The nurse can help them understand that it is not selfish to look after themselves and their own needs to meet their child's needs. It is important to recognize the parents' need to grieve the change in their child's normal appearance as part of the grieving process. Definitive professional help may be needed for parents whose response to the injury is severe or whose response to stress is manifested in destructive behavior.

The parents are members of the multidisciplinary team and participate in the development of the care plan. It is important to facilitate their input; to consider all aspects of the physical, emotional, social, and cultural factors affecting the child and family; and to establish a realistic home therapy program. The family's willingness to assume responsibility for care and their ability to implement the therapeutic regimen are assessed. Home, school, and other environmental factors are explored; financial concerns and available community resources are discussed; and a specific care plan for the child, with an anticipated follow-up program, is developed.

Prevention of Burn Injury. The best intervention is to prevent burns from occurring. Hot liquids in the kitchen and bathroom most commonly injure infants and toddlers. Hot liquids should be kept out of reach; tablecloths and dangling appliance cords are often pulled by toddlers, who spill hot grease and liquids on themselves. Electrical cords and outlets represent a potential risk to small children, who may chew on accessible cords and insert objects into outlets.

The Consumer Product Safety Commission recommends a reduction of water heater thermostats to a maximum of 48.9°C (120°F). The "dial-down" recommendation has been suggested by utility companies, burn treatment centers, medical personnel, and others interested in public safety. However, many water heaters continue to remain set at levels well above the safe level. Small children are especially at risk for scald injuries from hot tap water because of their decreased reaction time and agility, their curiosity, and the thermal sensitivity of their skin. Caregivers should never leave a child unattended in a bath and without adult supervision. Water should always be tested before a child is placed in the tub or shower.

The increased use of microwave ovens has resulted in burn injuries from the extremely hot internal temperatures generated in heated items. Baby formula, jelly-filled pastries, and hot liquids and dishes may result in cutaneous scalds or the ingestion of overheated liquids. Parents should use caution when removing items from the microwave oven and should always test the food before giving it to children.

As children mature, risk-taking behaviors increase. Matches and lighters are dangerous in the hands of children. Adults must remember to keep potentially hazardous items out of the reach of children; a lighter, like a match, is a tool for adult use.

Education related to fire safety and survival should begin with very young children. They can practice "stop, drop, and roll" to extinguish a fire. The fire escape route, including a safe meeting place away from the home in case of fire, also should be practiced. Additional information on burn care and prevention can be obtained from the American Burn Association* and the National Safety Council†.

Community activities are also helpful in supporting burn survivors and preventing burns. The Aluminum Cans for Burned Children (ACBC) is an exemplary effort based at the Paul and Carol David Foundation Burn Institute in Akron, Ohio‡. Activities funded by ACBC include a Burn Survivors Support Group, Burn Camp, and meetings of Juvenile Firestoppers (for children with fire-setting behavior). Adult weekend retreats and school and family education sessions are a part of this program. The burn center and fire department provide the personnel to present programs.

Sunburn

Sunburn is a common skin injury caused by overexposure to ultraviolet radiation (UVR). The sun emits a continuous spectrum of visible and nonvisible light rays that range in length from very short to very long. The shorter, higher-frequency waves are more damaging than longer wavelengths, but much of the light is filtered out as it travels through the atmosphere. Of the light that does filter through, ultraviolet A (UVA) waves are the longest and cause only minimum burning, but they play a significant role in photosensitive and photoallergic reactions. They are also responsible for premature aging of the skin and potentiate the effects of ultraviolet B (UVB) waves. UVB waves are shorter and are responsible for tanning, burning, and most of the harmful effects attributed to sunlight, especially skin cancer.

Numerous factors influence the amount of UVR exposure. Maximum exposure occurs at midday (10 AM–4 PM), when the distance from the sun to a given spot on the earth is shortest. There is more exposure at higher altitudes and near the equator and less when the sky is hazy (although the amount of UVR that does penetrate is easily underestimated). Window glass effectively screens out UVB but not UVA rays. Fresh snow, water, and sand reflect UVR, especially when the sun is directly overhead.

Sunburn is usually an epidermal burn, although severe sunburn can be a partial-thickness burn with blister formation. Treatment of sunburn involves stopping the burning process, decreasing the inflammatory response, and rehydrating the skin. Local application of cool tap water soaks or immersion in a tepid-water bath (temperature slightly below 36.7°C [98°F]) for 20 minutes or until the skin is cool limits tissue destruction and relieves the discomfort. After the cool applications, a bland oil-in-water moisturizing lotion

*311 S Wacker Drive, Suite 4150, Chicago, IL 60606; 312-642-9260; fax: 312-642-9130; e-mail: info@ameriburn.org; www.ameriburn.org.
†1121 Spring Lake Drive, Itasca, IL 60143-3201; 630-285-1121, 800-621-7615; e-mail: info@nsc.org; www.nsc.org.
‡Akron Children's Hospital, One Perkins Square, Akron, OH 44308-1062; 330-543-1000; fax: 330-543-9998; www.akronchildrens.org.

can be applied. Partial-thickness burns are treated the same as those from any heat source (see earlier discussion on burns).

CARE MANAGEMENT

Protection from sunburn is the major goal of management, and the harmful effects of the sun on the delicate skin of infants and children are currently receiving increased attention. To protect skin exposed to the sun for extended periods, skin should be covered with clothing and FDA-approved sun protection agents should be applied.

Two types of products are available for sun protection: topical sunscreens, which partially absorb UVR; and sun blockers, which block out UVR by reflecting sunlight. The most frequently recommended sun blockers are zinc oxide and titanium dioxide ointments. Sunscreens are products containing a sun protection factor (SPF) based on evaluation of effectiveness against UVR. For example, if individuals normally burn in 10 minutes without a sunscreen, use of a sunscreen with SPF 15 allows them to remain in the sun 15 times 10, or 150, minutes (2½ hours), before acquiring the same degree of burns. The most effective sunscreens against UVB are *p*-aminobenzoic acid (PABA) and PABA-esters. However, many individuals are allergic to PABA, and sunscreens without PABA are encouraged to prevent these reactions in children.

Sunscreens are applied evenly to all exposed areas, with special attention to skinfolds and areas that might become exposed as clothing shifts. Avoid eye contact. Parents are directed to read labels of sunscreen products carefully for the SPF and follow the manufacturer's directions for application.

> **! NURSING ALERT**
>
> Sunscreens are not recommended for infants younger than 6 months. However, infants younger than 6 months may have sunscreen applied over small areas of skin such as the back of hands that may not be adequately covered by clothing when they are in the sun. Infants should be kept out of the sun or physically shaded from it. Fabric with a tight weave, such as cotton, offers good protection.

Individuals who work in the community, such as teachers, day-care workers, coaches, and youth group leaders, as well as relatives, should all be made aware of sun safety for children. Sunscreens must be applied *liberally and frequently*.

Cold Injury

In cold injuries the nature of the heat-regulating mechanisms of the body are such that the inner portion of the body, or core, produces heat and the periphery, or outer area, conserves or dissipates heat. When the body attempts to conserve heat, the outer tissues are subjected to low temperatures and local trauma may result.

Chilblain (redness and swelling of the skin) occurs when extremities, usually the hands, are exposed to cold temperatures and moisture. The response may vary but is characterized by intense vasodilation that increases the temperature of involved tissues above that of unaffected tissue and produces edematous, reddish blue patches that itch and burn. As warming takes place, the sensations become more intense, but ordinarily they subside in a few days.

Frostbite is the term used to describe tissue damage caused when excessive heat loss to local tissues allows ice crystals to form in tissues. The frostbitten part appears white or blanched, feels solid, and is without sensation. Rapid rewarming is associated with less tissue necrosis than slow thawing. It restores blood flow and shortens the period of cellular damage. Rewarming produces a flush (sometimes deep purple) and a return of sensation, which is extremely painful. Large blisters may appear in 24 to 48 hours after rewarming and begin to reabsorb within 5 to 10 days followed by the formation of a hard black eschar. Superficial injury often heals without incident. Rewarming is accomplished by immersing the part in well-agitated water at 37.8° to 42.2°C (100° to 108°F). Discomfort is managed with analgesics and sedatives. Care of blistered skin is similar to that described for burns. It is seldom possible to estimate the extent of tissue loss until new skin layers are revealed after the eschar layer separates.

KEY POINTS

- A variety of factors can produce lesions of the skin.
- It is important for nurses to be able to describe skin lesions accurately.
- The process of wound healing consists of hemostasis, inflammation, proliferation, and remodeling.
- A moist environment promotes wound healing.
- Bacterial, viral, and fungal infections are common in childhood.
- Some skin diseases are transmitted by arthropod vectors, especially ticks.
- The most common skin infestations of childhood—scabies and pediculosis capitis—affect children of any age and from any social class.
- Contact dermatitis may involve a primary irritant or a sensitizing agent.
- Adverse reactions to drugs are manifested more often in the skin than in any other body organ.
- The most common skin disorders of infancy are diaper dermatitis, seborrheic dermatitis, and AD.
- Acne, a disorder affecting many adolescents, is related to hormonal fluctuation, stimulation of the sebaceous glands, excessive sebum production, the formation of comedones, and the overgrowth of the *P. acnes* organism.
- Medication and gentle facial cleansing are the treatments of choice for acne.
- Burns are caused by thermal, chemical, electric, or radioactive agents.
- Burns are assessed on the extent, depth, and severity of the wound.
- Essentials of emergency care of burn injury include stopping the burning process, covering the burn, transporting the injured child to medical aid, and providing reassurance to the child and family.
- Management of minor burns consists of facilitating wound healing, relieving discomfort, and preventing complications.
- Management of major burns consists of facilitating wound healing, relieving discomfort, replacing destroyed skin, preventing or treating complications, and providing rehabilitation.
- Sunscreen is recommended for use when the skin is exposed to the damaging effects of the sun's rays.
- Thermal injuries to the skin can result from exposure to extreme cold.

REFERENCES

Alanne S, Nermes M, Soderlund R, et al: Quality of life in infants with atopic dermatitis and healthy infants: a follow-up from birth to 24 months, *Acta Pediatr* 100(8):e65–e70, 2011.

American Academy of Pediatrics (AAP) Committee on Infectious Diseases, Pickering LK, editor: *Red Book: report of the Committee on Infectious Diseases*, ed 28, Elk Grove Village, IL, 2009, Author.

Annequin D, Carbajal R, Chauvin P, et al: Fixed 50% nitrous oxide oxygen mixture for painful procedures: a French survey, *Pediatrics* 105(4):E47, 2000.

Arnoldo B, Klein M, Gibran NS: Practice guidelines for the management of electrical injuries, *J Burn Care Res* 27(4):439–447, 2006.

Baker RAU, Zeller RA, Klein RL, et al: Burn wound itch control using H$_1$ and H$_2$ antagonists, *J Burn Care Rehabil* 22(4):263–268, 2001.

Butler C: Pediatric skin care: guidelines for assessment, prevention, and treatment, *Dermatol Nurs* 19(5):471–485, 2007.

Centers for Disease Control and Prevention (CDC): Cat-scratch disease in children: Texas, September 2000–August 2001, *MMWR Morb Mortal Wkly Rep* 51(10):212–214, 2002.

Centers for Disease Control and Prevention (CDC): Nonfatal dog bite–related injuries treated in hospital emergency departments—United States, 2001, *MMWR Morb Mortal Wkly Rep* 52(26):605–610, 2003.

Centers for Disease Control and Prevention (CDC): *Lyme disease*, 2009, www.cdc.gov/ncidod/dvbid/lyme/index.htm.

Dohil MA, Eichenfield LF: A treatment approach for atopic dermatitis, *Pediatr Ann* 34(3):201–210, 2005.

Doss N, Kamoun MR, Dubertret L, et al: Efficacy of tacrolimus 0.03% ointment as second-line treatment for children with moderate-to-severe atopic dermatitis, *Pediatr Allergy Immunol* 21(2 pt 1):321–329, 2010.

Fanelli M, Kupperman E, Lautenbach E, et al: Antibiotics, acne and *Staphylococcus aureus* colonization, *Arch Dermatol* 147(8):917–921, 2011.

Fisher RG, Chain RL, Hair PS, et al: Hypochlorite killing of community-acquired methicillin-resistant *Staphylococcus aureus*, *Pediatr Infect Dis J* 27(10):934–935, 2008.

Herndon DN, editor: *Total burn care*, ed 3, London, 2007, Saunders.

Jacob SE, Yang A, Herro E, et al: Contact allergens in a pediatric population, *J Clin Aesthet Derm* 3(101):29–35, 2010.

Kaplan SL: Community-acquired methicillin-resistant *Staphylococcus aureus* infections in children, *Semin Pediatr Infect Dis* 17(3):113–119, 2006.

Kaplan SL: Commentary: prevention of recurrent staphylococcal infections, *Pediatr Infect Dis J* 27(10):935–937, 2008.

Kaye AE, Belz JM, Kirschner RE: Pediatric dog bite injuries: a 4-year review of experience at the Children's Hospital of Philadelphia, *Plast Reconstr Surg* 124(2):551–558, 2009.

Kim RH, Armstrong AQ: Current state of acne treatment: highlighting lasers, photodynamic therapy, and chemical peels, *Dermatol Online J* 17(3):1–13, 2011.

Leyden JJ, Del Rosso JQ: Oral antibiotic therapy for acne vulgaris, *Clin Aesthet Derm* 4(2):40–47, 2011.

McCord SS, Levy ML: Practical guide to pediatric wound care, *Semin Plast Surg* 20(3):92–199, 2006.

Misery L: Consequences of psychological distress in adolescents with acne, *J Invest Derm* 131(2):290–292, 2011.

Moreno MA: Lyme disease in children and adolescents, *Arch Pediatr Adolesc Med* 165(1):96, 2011.

Mumcuoglu KY, Barker SC, Burgess IE, et al: International guidelines for effective control of head louse infestations, *J Drugs Dermatol* 6(4):409–414, 2007.

Network to Reduce Lyme Disease in School-Aged Children: You can make a difference to a child by reducing risk of Lyme disease, *NASN School Nurse* 25(3):110–113, 2010.

Pearlman DL: A simple treatment for head lice: dry on, suffocation based pediculicide, *Pediatrics* 114(3):e275–e279, 2004.

Purdue GF: American Burn Association presidential address 2006 on nutrition: yesterday, today, and tomorrow, *J Burn Care Res* 28(1):1–5, 2007.

Ricci G, Dondi A, Patrizi A, et al: Systemic therapy of atopic dermatitis in children, *Drugs* 69(3):297–306, 2009.

Rosenthal M: Bacterial colonization, hyperresponsive immune systems conspire in eczema: diagnosing dermatological disorders, *Infect Dis Child* 17(3):47–48, 2004.

Strong M, Johnstone PW: Interventions for treating scabies, *Cochrane Database Syst Rev* (3):CD000320, 2008.

Walling HW, Swick BL: Update on the management of chronic eczema: new approaches and emerging treatment options, *Clin Cosmet Invest Derm* 3:99–117, 2010.

Wormser GP, Dattwyler RJ, Shapiro ED, et al: The clinical assessment, treatment, and prevention of Lyme disease, human granulocytic anaplasmosis, and babesiosis: clinical practice guidelines by the Infections Diseases Society of America, *Clin Infect Dis* 43(9):1089–1134, 2006.

Musculoskeletal or Articular Dysfunction

David Wilson

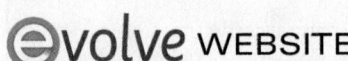 WEBSITE

http://evolve.elsevier.com/Perry/maternal

LEARNING OBJECTIVES

On completion of this chapter, the reader will be able to:
- Outline a care plan for a child immobilized with an injury or a debilitating condition.
- Formulate a teaching plan for the parents of a child in a cast.
- Explain the functions of the various types of traction.
- Differentiate among the various congenital skeletal defects.
- Design a teaching plan for the parents of a child with a congenital skeletal deformity.

- Describe the therapies and nursing care of a child with scoliosis.
- Outline a plan of care for a child with osteomyelitis.
- Differentiate between osteosarcoma and Ewing sarcoma.
- Describe the nursing care of a child with juvenile arthritis.
- Demonstrate an understanding of the management of systemic lupus erythematosus.

THE IMMOBILIZED CHILD

One of the most difficult aspects of illness in children is the immobility it imposes. Children by nature are usually active; and immobility, however temporary, may have lasting effects on the child's developmental progress. The most frequent reasons for immobility are congenital defects (e.g., spina bifida); degenerative disorders (e.g., muscular dystrophy); and infections or injuries that impair the integumentary system (severe burns), the musculoskeletal system (e.g., multiple fractures, osteomyelitis), or the neurologic system (e.g., spinal cord injury, Guillain-Barré syndrome, traumatic brain injury). At times therapies such as traction and spinal fusion are responsible for prolonged immobilization, although the increasing trends in health care are early mobilization and discharge and outpatient treatment.

Physiologic Effects of Immobilization

Many clinical studies, including space program research, have documented predictable consequences that occur after immobilization and the absence of gravitational force. Functional and metabolic responses to restricted movement can be noted in most of the body systems. Each has a direct influence on the child's growth and development because homeostatic mechanisms thrive on normal use and need feedback to maintain dynamic equilibrium. Inactivity leads to a decrease in the functional capabilities of the whole body as dramatically as the lack of physical exercise leads to muscle weakness.

Disuse from illness, injury, or a sedentary lifestyle can limit function and potentially delay age-appropriate milestones. Most of the pathologic changes that occur during immobilization arise from decreased muscle strength and mass, decreased metabolism, and bone demineralization, which are closely interrelated, with one change leading to or affecting the other. Some results of immobilization are primary and produce a direct effect; other pathophysiologic consequences occur frequently but seem to be more indirect and therefore are secondary effects. Many pathophysiologic changes affect more than one body system, with the primary or secondary effect being demonstrated in both systems.

The major effects of immobilization are outlined briefly in Table 48-1 and are related directly or indirectly to decreased muscle activity, which produces numerous primary changes in the musculoskeletal system with secondary alterations in the cardiovascular, respiratory, metabolic, and renal systems. The musculoskeletal changes that occur during disuse are a result of alterations in gravity and stress on the muscles, joints, and bones. Muscle disuse leads to tissue breakdown and loss of muscle mass (atrophy). Muscle atrophy causes decreased strength and endurance, which may take weeks or months to restore.

During immobilization a joint contracture begins when the arrangement of collagen, the main structural protein of connective tissues, is altered, resulting in a denser tissue that does not glide as easily. Eventually muscles, tendons, and ligaments can shorten and reduce joint movement, ultimately producing contractures that

TABLE 48-1	SUMMARY OF PHYSICAL EFFECTS OF IMMOBILIZATION WITH NURSING INTERVENTIONS*	
PRIMARY EFFECTS	**SECONDARY EFFECTS**	**NURSING CONSIDERATIONS**
Muscular System		
Decreased muscle strength, tone, and endurance	Decreased venous return and decreased cardiac output	Use antiembolism stockings or intermittent compression devices to promote venous return (monitor circulatory and neurovascular status of extremities when such devices are used).
	Decreased metabolism and need for oxygen	Plan play activities to use uninvolved extremities.
	Decreased exercise tolerance	Place in upright posture when possible.
	Bone demineralization	Perform passive range-of-motion exercises.
Disuse atrophy and loss of muscle mass	Catabolism Loss of strength	Have patient perform range-of-motion, active, passive, and stretching exercises.
Loss of joint mobility	Contractures, ankylosis of joints	Maintain correct body alignment. Use joint splints as indicated to prevent further deformity. Maintain range of motion.
Weak back muscles	Secondary spinal deformities	Maintain body alignment.
Weak abdominal muscles	Impaired respiration	See nursing considerations for respiratory system.
Skeletal System		
Bone demineralization— osteoporosis, hypercalcemia	Negative bone calcium uptake Pathologic fractures Calcium deposits Extraosseous bone formation, especially at hip, knee, elbow, and shoulder Renal calculi	With paralysis use upright posture on tilt table. Handle extremities carefully when turning and positioning. Administer calcium-mobilizing drugs (diphosphonates) and normal saline infusions as ordered. Ensure adequate intake of fluid; monitor output. Acidify urine. Promptly treat urinary tract infections.
Negative bone calcium uptake	Life-threatening electrolyte imbalance	Monitor serum calcium levels. Provide electrolyte replacement as indicated.
Metabolism		
Decreased metabolic rate	Slowing of all systems Decreased food intake	Mobilize as soon as possible. Have patient perform active and passive resistance and deep-breathing exercises. Ensure adequate food intake. Provide a high-protein diet.
Negative nitrogen balance	Decline in nutritional state Impaired healing	Encourage small, frequent feedings with protein and preferred foods. Monitor for and prevent pressure areas.
Hypercalcemia	Electrolyte imbalance	See nursing consideration for skeletal system.
Decreased production of stress hormones	Decreased physical and emotional coping capacity	Identify causes of stress. Implement appropriate interventions to lower physical and psychosocial stresses.
Cardiovascular System		
Decreased efficiency of orthostatic neurovascular reflexes	Inability to adapt readily to upright position (orthostatic intolerance) Pooling of blood in extremities in upright posture	Monitor peripheral pulses and skin temperature changes. Use antiembolism stockings or intermittent compression devices to decrease pooling when upright.
Diminished vasopressor mechanism	Orthostatic intolerance with syncope, hypertension, deceased cerebral blood flow, tachycardia	Provide abdominal support. In severe cases use antigravitational pants. Position horizontally.
Altered distribution of blood volume	Increased cardiac workload Decreased exercise tolerance	Monitor hydration, blood pressure, and urinary output.

TABLE 48-1	SUMMARY OF PHYSICAL EFFECTS OF IMMOBILIZATION WITH NURSING INTERVENTIONS—cont'd	
PRIMARY EFFECTS	**SECONDARY EFFECTS**	**NURSING CONSIDERATIONS**
Venous stasis	Pulmonary emboli or thrombi	Encourage and assist with frequent position changes. Elevate extremities without knee flexion. Ensure adequate fluid intake. Have patient perform active or passive exercises or movement as needed. Prescribe routine wearing of antiembolism stockings or intermittent compression devices. Monitor for signs of *pulmonary embolism*—sudden dyspnea, chest pain, respiratory arrest. Promptly intervene to maintain adequate oxygenation if signs and symptoms of pulmonary emboli are noted. Measure circumference of extremities periodically. Give anticoagulant drugs as prescribed.
Dependent edema	Tissue breakdown and susceptibility to infection	Administer skin care. Turn every 2-4 hr. Monitor skin color, temperature, and integrity. Use pressure-reduction surface as necessary to prevent skin breakdown. (See Chapter 47.)
Respiratory System		
Decreased need for oxygen	Altered oxygen–carbon dioxide exchange and metabolism	Promote exercise as tolerated. Encourage deep-breathing exercises.
Decreased chest expansion and diminished vital capacity	Diminished oxygen intake Dyspnea and inadequate arterial oxygen saturation; acidosis	Position for optimum chest expansion. Semi-Fowler position may assist in lung expansion if patient can tolerate. Use prone positioning without pressure on abdomen to allow gravity to aid in diaphragmatic excursion. Ensure that patient maintains proper alignment when sitting to prevent pressure on respiratory mechanism.
Poor abdominal tone and distention	Interference with diaphragmatic excursion	Avoid restriction of chest and abdominal musculature. Supply torso support to promote chest expansion.
Mechanical or biochemical secretion retention	Hypostatic pneumonia Bacterial and viral pneumonia Atelectasis	Change position frequently. Carry out percussion, vibration, and drainage (or suctioning) as necessary. Use incentive spirometer. Monitor breath sounds.
Loss of respiratory muscle strength	Poor cough	Encourage coughing and deep breathing. Support chest wall by splinting with pillow when patient coughs. Use incentive spirometer. Observe for signs of respiratory distress with pulse oximetry or blood gas measurement as necessary.
	Upper respiratory tract infection	Prevent contact with infected persons. Provide adequate hydration. Administer immunizations as necessary (pneumococcal, meningococcal).
Gastrointestinal System		
Distention caused by poor abdominal muscle tone	Interference with respiratory movements Difficulty in feeding in prone position	Monitor bowel sounds. Encourage small, frequent feedings. Have patient sit in upright position in bedside chair if possible.
No specific primary effect	Possible constipation caused by gravitational effect on feces through ascending colon or weakened smooth muscle tone Anorexia	Carry out bowel training program with hydration, stool softeners, increased fiber intake, and mild laxatives if necessary. Stimulate appetite with favored foods.

Continued

TABLE 48-1	SUMMARY OF PHYSICAL EFFECTS OF IMMOBILIZATION WITH NURSING INTERVENTIONS—cont'd	
PRIMARY EFFECTS	**SECONDARY EFFECTS**	**NURSING CONSIDERATIONS**
Urinary System		
Alteration of gravitational force	Difficulty in voiding in prone or supine position	Position as upright as possible to void.
Impaired ureteral peristalsis	Urinary retention in calyces and bladder Infection Renal calculi	Hydrate to ensure adequate urinary output for age. Stimulate bladder emptying with warm running water as necessary. Catheterize only for severe urinary retention. Administer antibiotics as indicated.
Integumentary System		
Altered tissue integrity	Decreased circulation and pressure leading to tissue injury	Turn and reposition at least every 2-4 hr. Frequently inspect total skin surface. Eliminate mechanical factors causing pressure, friction, moisture, or irritation. Place on pressure-relief mattress.
	Difficulty with personal hygiene	Assess ability to perform self-care and assist with bathing, grooming, and toileting as needed. Encourage self-care to potential ability. Ensure adequate intake of protein, vitamins, and minerals.

*Individualize care according to child's needs; interventions may vary in different institutions.

restrict function. The daily stresses on bone created by motion and weight bearing maintain the balance between bone formation (osteoblastic activity) and bone resorption (osteoclastic activity). During immobilization increased calcium leaves the bone, causing osteopenia (demineralization of the bones), which may predispose bone to pathologic fractures.

The major musculoskeletal consequences of immobilization are as follows:

- Significant decrease in muscle size, strength, and endurance
- Bone demineralization leading to osteoporosis
- Contractures and decreased joint mobility.

Circulatory stasis combined with hypercoagulability of the blood, which results from factors such as damage to the endothelium of blood vessels (Virchow triad), can lead to thrombus and embolus formation. *Deep vein thrombosis (DVT)* involves the formation of a thrombus in a deep vein such as the iliac and femoral veins and can cause significant morbidity if it remains undetected and untreated. The larger the portion of the body immobilized and the longer the immobilization, the greater the risks of consequences of immobility.

Psychologic Effects of Immobilization

For children one of the most difficult aspects of illness is immobilization. Throughout childhood physical activity is an integral part of daily life and is essential for physical growth and development. The activity helps children deal with a variety of feelings and impulses and provides a mechanism by which they can exert control over inner tensions. Children respond to anxiety with increased activity. Removal of this power deprives them of necessary input and a natural outlet for their feelings and fantasies.

When children are immobilized by disease or as part of a treatment regimen, they experience diminished environmental stimuli with a loss of tactile input and an altered perception of themselves and their environment. Sudden or gradual immobilization narrows the amount and variety of environmental stimuli that children receive by means of all of their senses: touch; sight; hearing; taste; smell; and proprioception, or the feeling of where they are in their environment. This sensory deprivation commonly leads to feelings of isolation and boredom and of being forgotten, especially by peers.

Physical interference with the activity of young children makes them feel frustrated and helpless. Even speech and language skills require sensorimotor activity and experience. For the toddler exploration and imitative behaviors are essential to developing a sense of autonomy; the preschooler's expression of initiative is evidenced by the need for vigorous physical activity; the school-age child's development is strongly influenced by physical achievement and competition; and the adolescent relies on mobility to achieve independence and self-identity. The quest for mastery at every stage of development is related to mobility.

The monotony of immobilization may lead to sluggish intellectual and psychomotor responses, decreased communication skills, increased fantasizing, and rarely hallucinations and disorientation. Children are likely to become depressed over loss of ability to function or the marked changes in body image. They may regress to earlier developmental behaviors such as wanting to be fed, bedwetting, and baby talk.

Children may react to immobility by active protest, anger, and aggressive behavior; or they may become quiet, passive, and submissive. They may believe that the immobilization is a justified punishment for misbehavior. Children should be allowed to display their anger, but it should be within the limits of safety to their self-esteem and not damaging to the integrity of others. When children are unable to express anger, aggression is often displayed inappropriately through regressive behavior and outbursts of crying or temper tantrums.

Effect on Families

Even brief periods of immobilization may disrupt family function, and sudden catastrophic illness or chronic disability may severely tax their resources and coping abilities.

The family's needs often must be met by the services of a multidisciplinary team, and nurses play a key role in anticipating the services they will need and coordinating conferences to plan care. In preparation for discharge home visits are advisable, and home management is commonly planned weeks in advance of the actual discharge. Such planning includes special considerations for cultural, economic, physical, and psychologic needs. A child with a severe disability is very dependent, and caregivers need rest periods to revitalize themselves (respite). Individual and group counseling is beneficial for solving problems in advance and provides an emotional support system. Parent groups may also be helpful and often allow nonthreatening social contact. The families of children with permanent disabilities need long-term resources because some of the most difficult problems arise as they try to sustain high-quality care for many years (see Chapter 36).

CARE MANAGEMENT

Physical assessment of the child who is immobilized for any number of reasons (e.g., injury or illness) includes a focus not only on the injured part (e.g., fracture) but also on the functioning of other systems that may be affected secondarily (i.e., the circulatory, renal, respiratory, muscular, and gastrointestinal systems). With long-term immobilization there may also be neurologic impairment and changes in electrolytes (especially calcium), nitrogen balance, and the general metabolic rate. The psychologic impact of immobilization should also be assessed.

Children who require prolonged total immobility and are unable to move themselves in bed should be placed on a pressure-reduction mattress to prevent skin breakdown. Frequent position changes also help prevent dependent edema and stimulate circulation, respiratory function, gastrointestinal motility, and neurologic sensation. Children at greater risk for skin breakdown include those with prolonged immobilization; mechanical ventilation; orthotic and prosthetic devices, including wheelchairs; and casts. Additional risk factors include poor nutrition, friction (from bed linen with traction), and moist skin (from urine or perspiration). Nursing care of children at risk includes strategies for preventing skin breakdown when such conditions are present. The Braden Q Scale is a reliable, objective tool that may be used in the assessment for pressure ulcer development in children who are acutely ill or at risk for skin breakdown from neurologic conditions and immobilization (Noonan, Quigley, and Curley, 2011) (see also Maintaining Healthy Skin, Chapter 39).

The use of antiembolism stockings or intermittent compression devices prevents circulatory stasis and dependent edema in the lower extremities and the development of DVT. Anticoagulant therapy may also be implemented with low-molecular-weight heparin, vitamin K antagonists, or unfractionated heparin. The child should be allowed as much activity as possible within the limitations of the illness or treatment. Any functional mobility, however minimal, is preferred to total immobility. High-protein, high-calorie foods are encouraged to prevent negative nitrogen balance, which may be difficult to correct by diet, especially if there is anorexia as a result of immobility and decreased gastrointestinal function (decreased motility and possibly constipation). Stimulating the appetite with small servings of attractively arranged, preferred foods may be sufficient. Sometimes supplementary nasogastric or gastrostomy feedings or intravenous (IV) fluids may be needed, but these are reserved for serious disability in which oral intake is impossible.

Adequate hydration and, when possible, an upright position and remobilization promote bowel and kidney function and help prevent complications in these systems. Children are encouraged to be as active as their condition and restrictive devices allow. This poses few problems for children, whose innate ingenuity and natural inclination toward mobility provide them with the impetus for physical activity. They need the opportunity, the materials or objects to stimulate activity, and the encouragement and participation of others. Those who are unable to move benefit from passive exercise and movement in consultation with a physical therapist.

Whenever possible, transporting the child outside the confines of the room increases environmental stimuli and allows social contact with others. Specially designed wheelchairs for increased mobility and independence are available. While hospitalized, children benefit from same-age visitors, computers, books, interactive video games, and other items brought from their own room at home, all of which help them to function in a more normal way. They also benefit from frequent visitors, accessibility of clocks and calendars, and a program of diversional therapy to help them function more normally. A child life specialist should be consulted for recreational planning. An activity center or slanting tray can be helpful for the child with limited mobility to use for drawing, coloring, writing, and playing with small toys such as trucks and cars. Children are able to express frustration, displeasure, and anger through play activities (see Chapter 38), which are helpful in the child's recovery. Hospitalized children should be allowed to wear their own clothes (street clothes, especially for preadolescent and adolescent girls) and resume school and preinjury activities. A parent or siblings should be allowed to stay overnight and room in with the hospitalized child to prevent the effects of family disruption caused by hospitalization. All efforts should be made to minimize this disruption. Although most of the suggestions discussed relate to hospital care, the same consultations (physical therapist, occupational therapist, child life specialist, speech therapist) and environment may also be considered in the home to help the child and family achieve independence and normalization.

Using dolls, stuffed animals, or puppets to illustrate and explain the immobilization method (e.g., traction, cast) is a valuable tool for small children. Placing a cast, tubing, or other restraining equipment on the doll offers the child a nonthreatening opportunity to express, through the doll, feelings about the restrictions, the nurse, and other health care providers. The doll or puppet may also be used for teaching the child and family procedures such as IV therapy, procedural sedation, and general anesthesia.

One of the most useful interventions to help children cope with immobility is participation in their own care. Self-care to the maximum extent is usually well received by children. They can help plan their daily routine; select their diet; and choose "street clothes," including innovative adornment such as a baseball cap or brightly colored socks to express their autonomy and individuality. They are encouraged to do as much for themselves as they are able to keep their muscles active and their interest alive.

Visits from significant people such as family members and friends offer occasions for emotional support and also provide opportunities for learning how to care for the child. Privacy is necessary, especially for adolescents.

For a child with greatly restricted movement (e.g., child with a large bilateral hip spica cast), nursing care is often a challenge. These situations require long-term care either in the hospital or at home; but, wherever the care occurs, consistent planning and coordination of activities with other health care workers and significant others are vital nursing functions.

With the increased trend toward early mobilization, early discharge, and home health care, many children are discharged home within a few days of hospitalization. Follow-up treatment may take place in the home setting or an outpatient ambulatory facility.

Family Support and Home Care

The needs of a child with severe disabilities can be complex, and family members require time to assimilate the teachings and demonstrations needed to understand the child's situation and care. Even a child who is confined on a short-term basis can be a challenge for the family, who are usually unprepared for the problems imposed by the child's special needs. Home modification is usually needed for facilitating care, especially when it involves traction, a large cast, or extended confinement. Suitable child care may be needed for times when all family members work.

Just as in the hospital, the child at home is encouraged to be as independent as possible and follow a schedule that approximates his or her normal lifestyle as nearly as possible such as continuing school lessons, regular bedtime, and suitable recreational activities.

TRAUMATIC INJURY

Soft-Tissue Injury

Injuries to the muscles, ligaments, and tendons are common in children (Fig. 48-1). In young children soft-tissue injury usually results from mishaps during play. In older children and adolescents, participation in sports is the more common cause.

Contusions

A *contusion* is damage to the soft tissue, subcutaneous structures, and muscle. The tearing of these tissues and small blood vessels and the inflammatory response lead to hemorrhage, edema, and associated pain when the child attempts to move the injured part. The escape of blood into the tissues is observed as *ecchymosis,* a black-and-blue discoloration.

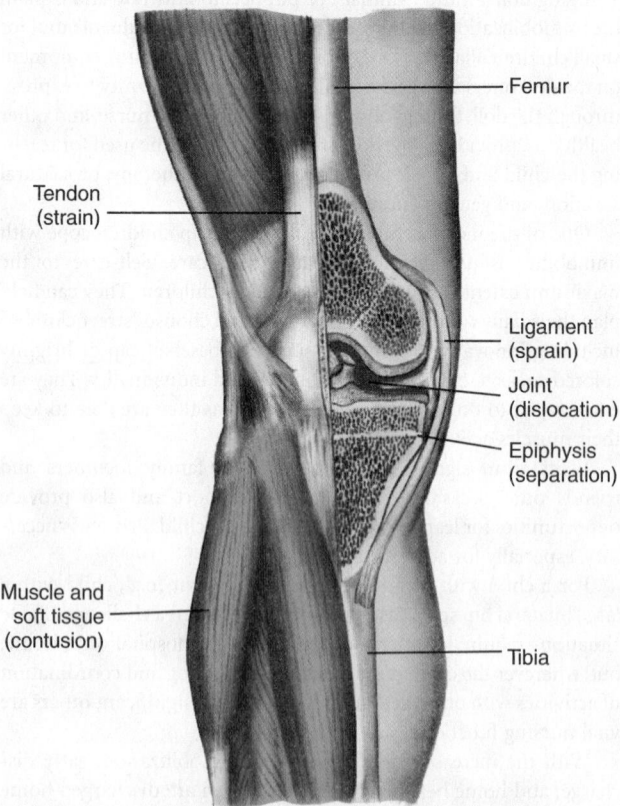

FIG 48-1 Sites of injuries to bones, joints, and soft tissues.

Femur

Tendon (strain)

Ligament (sprain)

Joint (dislocation)

Epiphysis (separation)

Muscle and soft tissue (contusion)

Tibia

Large contusions cause gross swelling, pain, and disability; those sustained while the child is participating in sports usually receive immediate attention from health personnel. The less spectacular, smaller injuries may go unnoticed, allowing continued participation; however, they can become disabling after rest because of pain and muscle spasm. The young athlete is commonly instructed to "walk it off" or disregard the pain. Instead of this approach, first a qualified health care worker or certified athletic trainer should carry out an assessment of the affected area because further damage to the site may result if the area is severely traumatized. Immediate treatment consists of cold application, as described in the section on sprains. Return to participation is allowed when the strength and range of motion of the affected extremity are equal to those of the opposite extremity. *Myositis ossificans* may occur from deep contusions to the biceps or quadriceps muscles; this condition may result in a restriction of flexibility of the affected limb.

Contusions are crush injuries that occur in children when they slam their fingers (in doors, folding chairs, or equipment) or hit them (as when hammering a nail). A severe crush injury involves the bone, with swelling and bleeding beneath the nail (subungual) and sometimes laceration of the pulp of the distal phalanx. The *subungual hematoma* can be released by creating a hole at the proximal end of the nail with a battery-operated microcautery device or a heated sterile 18-gauge needle.

Dislocations

Long bones are held in approximation to one another at the joint by ligaments. A dislocation occurs when the force of stress on the ligament is so great as to displace the normal position of the opposing bone ends or the bone end from its socket. The predominant symptom is pain that increases with attempted passive or active movement of the extremity. In dislocations there may be an obvious deformity and inability to move the joint. Dislocation of the phalanges is the most common type seen in children, followed by elbow dislocation. One of the most common injuries in young children is subluxation of the annular ligament, also called *pulled elbow* or *nursemaid elbow.* With this injury the annular ligament slips proximally off the radial head into the joint between the radial head and ulna, causing immediate pain and limited supination (Carrigan, 2011). In the majority of cases the injury occurs in a child younger than 5 years who receives a sudden longitudinal pull or traction at the wrist while the arm is fully extended and the forearm pronated. It usually occurs when an adult or older sibling who is holding the child by the hand or wrist gives a sudden pull or jerk to prevent a fall or attempts to lift the child by pulling the wrist or when the child pulls away by dropping to the floor or ground. The child often cries, appears anxious, and refuses to use the affected limb; there is an absence of swelling. The practitioner manipulates the arm by applying firm finger pressure to the head of the radius, then supinates and flexes the forearm to return the ligament to its place. A click or clunk may be heard or felt, and functional use of the arm returns within minutes. However, the longer the subluxation is present, the longer it takes for the child to recover mobility after treatment. Usually no anesthetic is required, but a mild pain reliever such as acetaminophen may be given. In an older child severe elbow injury or dislocation should be carefully evaluated by a practitioner immediately; likewise a traumatic elbow injury in the younger child that is not a subluxation should be evaluated carefully.

In children younger than 5 years of age the hip can be dislocated by a fall. The greatest risk after this injury is the potential loss of blood supply to the head of the femur. Relocation of the hip within

60 minutes after the injury provides the best chance for preventing damage to the femoral head.

Shoulder dislocations occur most often in older adolescents and are often sports related. Temporary restriction of the joint with a sling or bandage that secures the arm to the chest in a shoulder dislocation can provide sufficient comfort and immobilization until medical attention is received.

Simple dislocations should be reduced as soon as possible with the child under mild (procedural) sedation and often local anesthesia. Anesthetics such as IV ketamine (Ketalar), midazolam (Versed), IV propofol (Diprivan), or fentanyl (Sublimaze) can be used to produce partial or complete analgesia. Nitrous oxide in concentrations of 50% to 70% has been shown to be safe for relatively short periods (15 to 20 minutes) in children ages 1 year and above (Babl, Oakley, Seaman, et al., 2008; Zier and Liu, 2011) An unreduced dislocation is complicated by increased swelling, making reduction difficult and increasing the risk of neurovascular problems. Treatment depends on the severity of the injury.

Sprains

A sprain occurs when trauma to a joint is so severe that a ligament is partially or completely torn or stretched by the force created as a joint is twisted or wrenched, often accompanied by damage to associated blood vessels, muscles, tendons, and nerves.

The presence of joint laxity is the most valid indicator of the severity of a sprain. In a severe injury the child complains of the joint "feeling loose" or as if "something is coming apart," and may describe hearing a "snap," "pop," or "tearing." Pain is seldom the principal subjective symptom. There is a rapid onset with swelling (often diffuse), accompanied by immediate disability and appreciable reluctance to use the injured joint.

Strains

A strain is a microscopic tear to the musculotendinous unit and has features in common with sprains. The area is painful to touch and swollen. Most strains are incurred over time rather than suddenly, and the rapidity of the appearance provides clues regarding severity. In general the more rapidly the strain occurs, the more severe the injury. When the strain involves the muscular portion, there is more bleeding, often palpable soon after injury and before edema obscures the hematoma.

Therapeutic Management

The first minutes to 12 hours are the most critical period for virtually all soft-tissue injuries. Basic principles of managing sprains and other soft-tissue injuries are summarized in the acronyms *RICE* and *ICES*:

R—Rest	**I**—Ice
I—Ice	**C**—Compression
C—Compression	**E**—Elevation
E—Elevation	**S**—Support

Soft-tissue injuries should be iced immediately. This is best accomplished with crushed ice wrapped in a towel or encased in a screw-top ice bag or resealable storage bag. A wet elastic wrap, which transfers cold better than dry wrap, is applied to provide compression and keep the ice pack in place. Chemical-activated ice packs are also effective for immediate treatment but are not reusable and must be monitored closely for leakage. A cloth barrier should be used between the ice container and the skin to prevent trauma to the tissues. Ice has a rapid cooling effect on tissues and reduces the pain threshold. However, it should never be applied for more than 30 minutes at a time because of the homeostatic response of the body to cold, which may trigger a decrease in vascularization at the injury site. A plastic bag of frozen vegetables such as peas serves as a convenient ice pack for soft-tissue injuries. It is clean, watertight, and easily molded to the injured part. When available, snow placed in a plastic bag may serve as an ice bag.

Elevating the extremity uses gravity to facilitate venous return and reduce edema formation in the damaged area. The point of injury should be kept several inches above the level of the heart for therapy to be effective. Several pillows can be used for elevation. Allowing the extremity to be dependent causes excessive fluid accumulation in the area of injury, delaying healing and causing painful swelling.

Torn ligaments, especially those in the knee, are usually treated by immobilization with a knee immobilizer or range-of-motion brace until the child is able to walk without a limp. Crutches are used for mobility to rest the affected extremity. Passive leg exercises, gradually increased to active ones, are begun as soon as sufficient healing has taken place. Parents and children are cautioned against using any form of liniment or other heat-producing preparation before examination. If the injury requires casting or splinting, the heat generated in the enclosed space can cause extreme discomfort and even tissue damage. In many cases torn knee ligaments are managed with arthroscopy and ligament repair or reconstruction as necessary, depending on the extent of the tear, the ligaments involved, and the child's age. Surgical reconstruction of the anterior cruciate ligament may be performed in young athletes who wish to continue in active sports (Sarwark, 2010).

Fractures

Bone fractures occur when the resistance of bone against the stress being exerted yields to the stress force. Fractures are a common injury at any age but are more likely to occur in children and older adults. Because childhood is a time of rapid bone growth, the pattern of fractures, problems of diagnosis, and methods of treatment differ in the child and the adult. In children fractures heal much faster than in adults. Consequently children may not require as long a period of immobilization of the affected extremity as an adult with a fracture.

Fracture injuries in children are most often a result of traumatic incidents at home, at school, in a motor vehicle, or in association with recreational activities. Children's everyday activities include vigorous play that predisposes them to injury (i.e., climbing, falling down, running into immovable objects, skateboarding, and receiving blows to any part of their bodies).

Aside from automobile accidents or falls from heights, true injuries that cause fractures rarely occur in infancy; therefore bone injury in children of that age-group warrants further investigation. In any small child, especially under the age of 12 months, radiographic evidence of fractures at various stages of healing is, with few exceptions, a result of *nonaccidental trauma* (child abuse). Any investigation of fractures in infants, particularly multiple fractures, should include consideration of *osteogenesis imperfecta*.

Fractures in school-age children are often a result of playground falls or bicycle-automobile or skateboard injuries. Adolescents are vulnerable to multiple and severe trauma because they are mobile on bicycles, all-terrain vehicles, skateboards, skis, snowboards, trampolines, and motorcycles and are active in sports.

A distal forearm (radius, ulna, or both) injury is the most common fracture in children. The clavicle is also a common fracture sustained in childhood, with approximately half of clavicle fractures occurring in children younger than 10 years of age. Common mechanisms of injury include a fall with an outstretched hand or direct trauma to the bone. In neonates a fractured clavicle may occur with a large newborn and a small maternal pelvis. This may be noted in the first few days after birth by a unilateral Moro reflex or at the 2-week well-child check, when a fracture callus is palpated on the infant's healing clavicle.

Types of Fractures

A fractured bone consists of fragments—the fragment closer to the midline, or the proximal fragment; and the fragment farther from the midline, or the distal fragment. When fracture fragments are separated the fracture is complete; when fragments remain attached the fracture is incomplete. The fracture line can be any of the following:

- Transverse—Crosswise at right angles to the long axis of the bone
- Oblique—Slanting but straight between a horizontal and perpendicular direction
- Spiral—Slanting and circular, twisting around the bone shaft

The twisting of an extremity while the bone is breaking results in a spiral break. If the fracture does not produce a break in the skin, it is a simple, or closed, fracture. Open, or compound, fractures are those with an open wound through which the bone protrudes. If the bone fragments cause damage to other organs or tissues (e.g., the lung, liver), the injury is said to be a complicated fracture. When small fragments of bone are broken from the fractured shaft and lie in the surrounding tissue, the injury is a comminuted fracture. This type of fracture is rare in children. The types of fractures that are seen most often in children are described in Box 48-1 and Fig. 48-2.

Growth Plate (Physeal) Injuries

The weakest point of long bones is the cartilage growth plate, or the physis. Consequently this is a frequent site of damage of childhood trauma. Growth plate fractures are classified with the Salter-Harris classification system (Fig. 48-3). Detection of physeal injuries is sometimes difficult but critical. Close monitoring and early treatment, if indicated, are essential to prevent longitudinal or angular growth deformities (or both). Treatment of these fractures may

include surgical open reduction and internal fixation to prevent or reduce growth disturbances.

Immediately after a fracture occurs, the muscles contract and physiologically splint the injured area. This phenomenon accounts for the muscle tightness observed over a fracture site and the deformity that is produced as the muscles pull the bone ends out of alignment. This muscle response must be overcome by traction or complete muscle relaxation (e.g., anesthesia) to realign the distal bone fragment to the proximal bone fragment.

Bone Healing and Remodeling

Bone healing is rapid in growing children because of the thickened periosteum and generous blood supply. When there is a break in the continuity of bone, the osteoblasts are stimulated to maximal

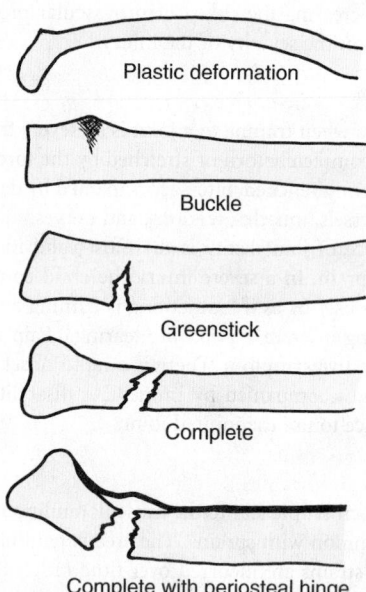

FIG 48-2 Types of fractures in children.

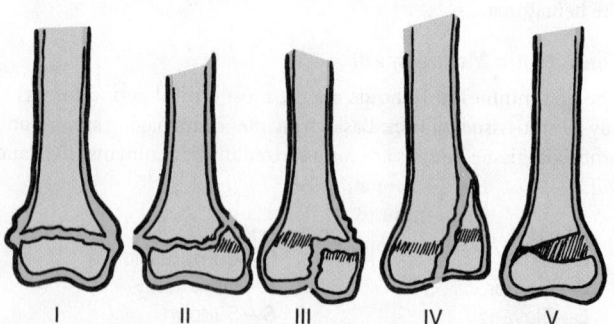

FIG 48-3 Salter Harris fracture classification. Types of epiphyseal injury in order of increasing risk. The injuries are classified as follows: type I, separation or slip of growth plate without fracture of the bone; type II, separation of growth plate and breaking off of section of metaphysis; type III, fracture of epiphysis extending through joint surface; type IV, fracture of growth plate, epiphysis, and metaphysis; and type V, crushing injury of epiphysis (can be diagnosed only in retrospect). This classification of epiphyseal injuries was developed by orthopedists RB Salter and WR Harris. (First published in Salter RB, Harris WR: Injuries involving the physeal plate, *J Bone Joint Surg Am* 45[3]:587-622, 1963.)

BOX 48-1 TYPES OF FRACTURES IN CHILDREN

Plastic deformation—Occurs when the bone is bent but not broken. A child's flexible bone can be bent 45 degrees or more before breaking. However, if bent, the bone will straighten slowly, but not completely, to produce some deformity but without the angulation seen when the bone breaks. Bends occur most commonly in the ulna and fibula, often in association with fractures of the radius and tibia.

Buckle, or torus, fracture—Produced by compression of the porous bone; appears as a raised or bulging projection at the fracture site. These fractures occur in the most porous portion of the bone near the metaphysis (the portion of the bone shaft adjacent to the epiphysis) and are more common in young children.

Greenstick fracture—Occurs when a bone is angulated beyond the limits of bending. The compressed side bends, and the tension side fails, causing an incomplete fracture similar to the break observed when a green stick is broken.

Complete fracture—Divides the bone fragments. These fragments often remain attached by a periosteal hinge, which can aid or hinder reduction.

activity. New bone cells are formed in immense numbers almost immediately after the injury and in time are evidenced by a bulging growth of new bone tissue between the fractured bone fragments. This is followed by deposition of calcium salts to form a *callus*. Remodeling is a process that occurs in the healing of long bone fractures in growing children. The irregularities produced by the fracture become indistinct as the angles and bone overgrowth are smoothed out, giving the bone a straighter appearance. A general rule of thumb is that an angulated fracture in a growing child remodels by one degree per month (Green and Swiontkowski, 2008).

Fractures heal in less time in children than in adults. The approximate healing times for a femoral shaft are as follows:

- Neonatal period—2 to 3 weeks
- Early childhood—4 weeks
- Later childhood—6 to 8 weeks
- Adolescence—8 to 12 weeks

Diagnostic Evaluation

A history of the injury may be lacking in some childhood injuries. Infants and toddlers are unable to communicate, and older children may not volunteer information (even under direct questioning) when the injury occurred during forbidden activities. Whenever possible it is helpful to obtain information from someone who witnessed the injury. In cases of nonaccidental trauma providers may give false information to protect themselves or family members.

The child may exhibit the same manifestations seen in adults (Box 48-2). However, often a fracture is remarkably stable because of intact periosteum. The child may even be able to use an affected arm or walk on a fractured leg. Because bones are highly vascular, a soft, pliable hematoma may be felt around the fracture site.

Radiographic examination is the most useful diagnostic tool for assessing skeletal trauma. The calcium deposits in bone make the entire structure radiopaque. Radiographic films are taken after fracture reduction and in some cases during the healing process to determine satisfactory progress.

> **! NURSING ALERT**
>
> A fracture should be strongly suspected in a mobile small child who refuses to walk or crawl.

Therapeutic Management

The goals of fracture management are as follows:

- To regain alignment and length of the bony fragments (reduction)
- To retain alignment and length (immobilization)
- To restore function to the injured parts
- To prevent further injury and deformity

> **BOX 48-2   CLINICAL MANIFESTATIONS OF A FRACTURE**
>
> - Signs of injury:
>   - Generalized swelling
>   - Pain or tenderness
>   - Diminished functional use of affected part
> - May be:
>   - Bruising
>   - Severe muscular rigidity
>   - Crepitus (grating sensation at fracture site)

Most children's fractures heal well, and nonunion is rare. Fractures are splinted or casted to immobilize and protect the injured extremity. Children with displaced fractures may have immediate surgical reduction and fixation (internal or external) rather than being immobilized by traction. This practice is more common and holds true for all types of fractures, including femur fractures, although there is variation based on provider preference and institutional practice. Some conditions, including open fractures, compartment syndrome, fractures associated with vascular or nerve injury, and joint dislocations that are unresponsive to reduction maneuvers, require immediate medical attention.

In children immobilization is used until adequate callus is formed. The position of the bone fragments in relation to one another influences the rapidity of healing and residual deformity. Weight bearing and active movement for the purpose of regaining function may begin after the fracture site is determined to be stable by the medical provider. The child's natural tendency to be active is usually sufficient to restore normal mobility, and physical or occupational therapy is rarely indicated.

Children are most frequently hospitalized for fractures of the femur and supracondylar area of the distal humerus. If simple reduction cannot be achieved or a neurovascular problem is detected after the injury, observation in a hospital setting may be indicated. The trend is to avoid hospitalization. The major methods for immobilizing a fracture (i.e., casting and traction) are described later.

CARE MANAGEMENT

Nurses are frequently the people who make the initial assessment of a child with a suspected fracture (see Emergency box). The child and parents may be frightened and upset, and the child is often in pain. Therefore, if the child is alert and there is no evidence of hemorrhage, the initial nursing interventions are directed toward calming and reassuring the child and parents so a more extensive assessment can be more easily accomplished.

> **✚ EMERGENCY**
>
> ### Fracture
>
> - Assess the extent of injury—Six *P*s:
>   1. *P*ain and point of tenderness
>   2. *P*ulses—Distal to fracture site
>   3. *P*allor
>   4. *P*aresthesia—Sensation distal to fracture site
>   5. *P*aralysis—Movement distal to fracture site
>   6. *P*ressure
> - Determine the mechanism of injury.
> - Move the injured part as little as possible.
> - Cover open wounds with a sterile or clean dressing.
> - Immobilize the limb, including joints above and below the fracture site; do not attempt to reduce the fracture or push protruding bone under the skin.
>   - Soft splint (pillow or folded towel)
>   - Rigid splint (rolled newspaper or magazine)
>   - Uninjured leg can serve as a splint for a leg fracture if no splint available
> - Reassess neurovascular status.
> - Apply traction if circulatory compromise is present.
> - Elevate the injured limb if possible.
> - Apply cold to the injured area.
> - Call emergency medical services or transport to medical facility.

While remaining calm and speaking in a quiet voice, the nurse can ask the parents and older child to describe what happened. The child may arrive with the limb supported in some manner; if not, careful support or immobilization may be provided to the affected site. In the event that the limb is supported or immobilized, it may be best not to touch the child but to ask him or her to point to the painful area and wiggle the fingers or toes. By this time the child may feel relatively safe and will allow someone to gently touch the area just enough to feel the pulses and test for sensation. A child's anxiety is greatly influenced by previous experiences with injury and with health care providers. However, he or she needs to be told what will happen and what to do to help. The affected limb need not be palpated, and it should not be moved unless properly splinted. If the child is at home or the practitioner is not present to examine her or him, some type of splint is applied carefully for transport to the medical facility. Parental anxiety may be heightened by the child's pain reaction and fear and possibly by other events surrounding the accident. It is important to communicate to the parent that the child will receive the necessary care, including pain management.

> **! NURSING ALERT**
>
> **Compartment syndrome** is a serious complication that results from compression of nerves, blood vessels, and muscle inside a closed space. This injury may be devastating, resulting in tissue death, and thus requires emergency treatment (fasciotomy). The six *P*s of ischemia from a vascular, soft tissue, nerve, or bone injury should be included in an assessment of any injury (Box 48-3):
> 1. *P*ain
> 2. *P*allor
> 3. *P*ulselessness
> 4. *P*aresthesia
> 5. *P*aralysis
> 6. *P*ressure

The Child in a Cast

The completeness of the fracture, the type of bone involved, and the amount of weight bearing influence how much of the extremity must be included in the cast to immobilize the fracture site completely. In most cases the joints above and below the fracture are immobilized to eliminate the possibility of movement that might cause displacement at the fracture site. Four major categories of casts are used for fractures: *upper extremity* to immobilize the wrist or elbow, *lower extremity* to immobilize the ankle or knee, *spinal* and

---

> **BOX 48-3 COMPARTMENT SYNDROME EVALUATION**
>
> Assess the extent of injury—6 *P*s:
> 1. **Pain:** Severe pain that is not relieved by analgesics or elevation of the limb; movement that increases pain
> 2. **Pulse:** Inability to palpate a pulse distal to the fracture or compartment
> 3. **Pallor:** Pale-appearing skin, poor perfusion, capillary refill greater than 3 seconds
> 4. **Paresthesia:** Tingling or burning sensations
> 5. **Paralysis:** Inability to move extremity or digits
> 6. **Pressure:** Involved limb or digits may feel tense and warm; skin tight, shiny; pressure within the compartment elevated

---

cervical for immobilization of the spine, and *spica* to immobilize the hip and knee.

The Cast

Casts are constructed from gauze strips and bandages impregnated with plaster of Paris or more commonly from synthetic lighter-weight and water-resistant materials (e.g., waterproof liners, fiberglass and polyurethane resin).

Both types of casting produce heat from chemical reaction activated by water immediately after application. Plaster casts mold closely to the body part, take 10 to 72 hours to dry, have a smooth exterior, and are inexpensive. The newer synthetic casting material is lightweight, dries in 5 to 20 minutes, permits earlier weight bearing, and is water resistant when applied with a waterproof liner. It is always desirable to give children choices, and synthetic casting materials come in a variety of colors. The disadvantages of synthetic casting are its inability to mold closely to body parts; rough exterior, which may scratch surfaces; and increased cost. It is also difficult to write on synthetic casts; a waterproof marker or color markers may be used.

Cast Application. The child's developmental age should be considered before the cast is applied. For preschoolers who fear bodily harm and fantasize about the loss of an extremity, it may be helpful to use a plastic doll or stuffed animal to explain the procedure beforehand. Toddlers and preschoolers do not have easily defined body boundaries; if an extremity is wrapped in a bandage, cast, or splint, to the young child the extremity ceases to function or exist. It is also helpful to explain that some synthetic cast material will become warm during application but will not burn. During the application of the cast various distraction methods can be used, including discussing favorite pets or activities at school and blowing bubbles. In this age-group explanations such as, "This will help your arm get better" are futile because the child has no concept of causality.

Before the cast is applied, the extremities are checked for any abrasions, cuts, or other alterations in the skin surface and for the presence of rings or other items that might cause constriction from swelling; such objects are removed. A tube of cloth stockinette or Gore-Tex liner is stretched over the area to be casted, and bony prominences are padded with soft cotton sheeting. Dry rolls of casting material are immersed in a pail of water. The wet rolls are put on in a bandage fashion and molded to the extremity. During application of the cast the underlying stockinette is pulled over the rough edges of the cast and secured with casting material to form a padded edge to protect the skin.

■ CARE MANAGEMENT

The complete evaporation of the water from a hip spica cast can take 24 to 48 hours when older types of plaster materials are used. Drying occurs within minutes with fiberglass cast material. The cast must remain uncovered to allow it to dry from the inside out. Turning the child in a plaster cast at least every 2 hours helps to dry a body cast evenly and prevents complications related to immobility. A regular fan or cool-air hair dryer to circulate air may be helpful when the humidity is high.

> **! NURSING ALERT**
>
> Heated fans or dryers are not used because they cause the cast to dry on the outside and remain wet beneath or cause burns from heat conduction by way of the cast to the underlying tissue.

A wet plaster cast should be supported by a pillow that is covered with plastic. The cast should be handled by the palms of the hands instead of the fingertips to prevent indenting the cast, which can create pressure areas. A dry plaster-of-Paris cast produces a hollow sound when it is tapped with the finger. After it has dried "hot spots" felt on the cast surface or a foul-smelling odor may indicate an infection. This should be reported for further evaluation; if concern continues, an opening, or a "window," could be exposed over the area of concern to evaluate the site.

During the first few hours after a cast is applied, the chief concern is that the extremity may continue to swell to the extent that the cast becomes a tourniquet, shutting off circulation and producing neurovascular complications (compartment syndrome) (see Box 48-3). To reduce the likelihood of this potential problem, the body part should be elevated, thereby increasing venous return. If edema is excessive, casts are *bivalved* (i.e., cut to make anterior and posterior halves that are held together with an elastic bandage). The cast and the involved extremity are observed frequently for neurovascular integrity and any signs of compromise. Permanent muscle and tissue damage can occur within a few hours.

> ### ! NURSING ALERT
>
> Observations such as pain (unrelieved by pain medication 1 hour after administration, especially with passive range of motion), swelling, discoloration (pallor or cyanosis) of the exposed portions, decreased pulses, decreased temperature, paresthesia, or the inability to move the distal exposed part(s) should be reported immediately. Pallor, paralysis, and pulselessness are late signs (see Box 48-3).

When an extremity that has sustained an open fracture is casted, a window is often left over the wound area to allow for observation and dressing of the wound. For the first few hours after surgery substantial bleeding may soak through the cast. Periodically the circumscribed bloodstained area should be outlined with a waterproof marker, and the time indicated to provide a guide for assessing the amount of bleeding.

Appropriate cast care guidelines for the child's caregiver are necessary before discharge. Instructions are also given for checking for signs and symptoms that indicate that the cast is too tight (see Patient Teaching box). Parents should also be told to take the child to the health care provider for attention if the cast becomes too loose because a loose cast no longer serves its purpose.

Nurses can help families adapt the child's home environment to meet the temporary encumbrance of a large cast or one that restricts the child's mobility (e.g., a long-leg or spica cast [Fig. 48-4]). Commonplace situations become problematic (e.g., transporting a child safely and comfortably in a car). Standard seat belts and car seats may not be readily adapted for use by children in some casts. Specially designed car seats and restraints are available that meet safety requirements.* Alterations to standard car seats to accommodate the cast are not recommended because the structure may be adversely

altered and fail to properly restrain the child. A bedside commode or rental wheelchair may be necessary equipment for a child who is nonambulatory.

Parents are taught the proper care of the cast or brace and helped to devise means for maintaining cleanliness. A superabsorbent

---

PATIENT TEACHING

Cast Care

- Keep the casted extremity elevated on pillows or similar support for the first day or as directed by the health care provider.
- Avoid denting the plaster cast with fingertips (use palms of hand to handle) while it is still wet to avoid creating pressure points.
- Observe the extremities (fingers or toes) for any evidence of swelling or discoloration (darker or lighter than a comparable extremity) and contact the health care provider if noted.
- Check movement and sensation of the visible extremities frequently.
- Follow health care provider's orders regarding any restriction of activities.
- Restrict strenuous activities for the first few days.
  - Engage in quiet activities but encourage use of muscles.
  - Move the joints above and below the cast on the affected extremity.
- Encourage frequent rest for a few days, keeping the injured extremity elevated while resting.
- Avoid allowing the affected limb to hang in a dependent position for any length of time.
  - Keep an injured upper extremity elevated (e.g., in a sling) while upright.
  - Elevate a lower limb when sitting and avoid standing for too long.
- Do not allow the child to put anything inside the cast. Keep small items that might be placed inside the cast away from small children.
- Keep a clear path for ambulation. Remove toys, hazardous floor rugs, pets, or other items over which the child might stumble.
- Use crutches appropriately if lower-limb fracture requires nonweight bearing on affected extremity.
- The crutches should fit properly, have a soft rubber tip to prevent slipping, and be well padded at the axilla.
- With crutch walking the child's body weight is supported on the hand grips, not the axilla.

---

*For information on specially adapted molded-plastic chairs for children who have spica casts, contact Snug Seat at 800-336-7684, www.snugseat.com/en-US/Welcome-to-Snug-Seat.aspx. The E-Z-On vest is a special safety harness for larger children with poor trunk control. Additional safety restraints and a listing of distributors are available from SafetyBeltSafe USA, www.carseat.org. Another resource is the National Center for the Safe Transportation of Children with Special Health Care Needs, 800-543-6227, www.preventinjury.org/specNeeds.asp.

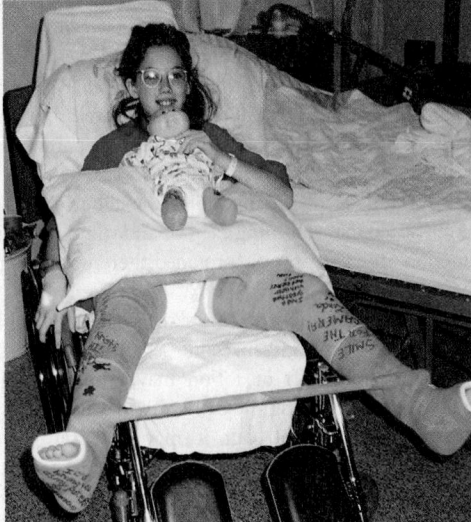

FIG 48-4 Spica cast with hip abductor. Note casts on doll as well.

disposable diaper is tucked beneath the entire perineal opening of the cast. A larger diaper can be applied and fastened over the small diaper and cast to hold the smaller diaper in place. In the event that the larger diaper becomes wet or soiled, it is likely that the cast is as well.

For tightly fitting casts transparent film dressings can be cut into strips as for petaling, with one edge applied to the cast edge and the other directly to the perineum; this forms a continuous waterproof bridge between the perineum and the cast to prevent leakage. An additional advantage to the use of this transparent dressing is that it keeps both the skin and the cast dry while allowing for observation of skin beneath the dressing.

Older infants and small children may stuff bits of food, small toys, or other items under the cast; parents should be alerted to this possibility so they can initiate suitable preventive measures.

Feeding an infant in a hip spica cast offers problems in positioning. Very young infants can be fed in the supine position with the head elevated. With the infant's hips and legs supported on a pillow at the side, the parent can cuddle the infant in his or her arms during feeding. A somewhat similar position can be used for breastfeeding (i.e., with the infant supported on pillows or held in a "football" hold facing the mother with the legs behind her). An alternate position is to hold the infant upright on the caregiver's lap with the legs of the infant astride the adult's leg.

Children in spica casts usually find the prone position easier for self-feeding from a small table placed next to the dining table; alternatively they may manage a semisitting position in bed or a wheelchair (see Fig. 48-4). The use of a conventional toilet is almost impossible. A bedside toilet can be adapted for use. Small bedpans or other containers offer alternatives for elimination. The nurse may suggest waterproofing methods by devising plastic wraps for elimination and showers. Baths are possible only if the plaster cast is kept out of the water and covered to prevent it from becoming wet.

Cast Removal. Cutting the cast to remove it or relieve tightness is frequently a frightening experience for children. They fear the sound of the cast cutter and are terrified that both their flesh and the cast will be cut. The oscillating blade vibrates rapidly back and forth and will not cut when placed *lightly* on the skin. Children have described it as producing a "tickly" sensation. The vibration also generates heat that the child may feel. Both of these feelings should be explained.

Preparation for the procedure helps reduce anxiety, especially if a trusting relationship has been established between the child and the nurse. Many young children come to regard the cast as part of themselves, which intensifies their fear of removal (Fig. 48-5). They need continual reassurance that all is going well and that their behavior is accepted. After the cast is removed, the parents and child should be given the option of keeping it. If the cast has been in place for a lengthy period, decreased muscle mass will be noted. The child should be reassured that resuming exercise and routine activities will return function and appearance (provided there was no significant trauma beforehand).

After the cast is removed, the skin surface will be caked with desquamated skin and sebaceous secretions. Application of mineral oil (e.g., baby oil) or lotion may remove the particles and provide comfort. Soaking the extremity in a bathtub is usually sufficient for their removal, but it may take several days to eliminate the accumulation completely. The parents and child should be instructed not to pull or forcibly remove this material with vigorous scrubbing because it may cause excoriation and bleeding.

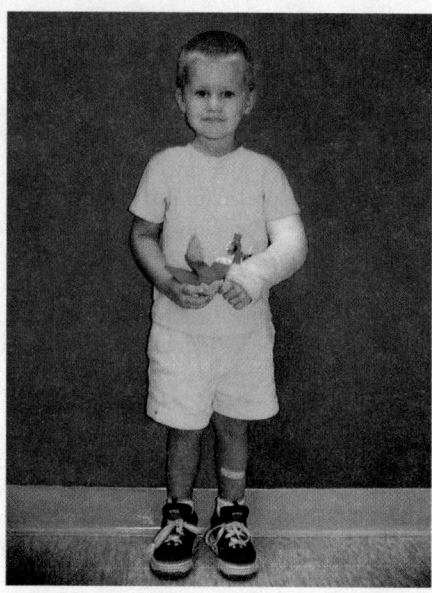

FIG 48-5 Young children usually adapt well to a cast but often fear the removal.

The Child in Traction

The ever-changing health care arena has witnessed the demise of many long-term treatments involving lengthy hospitalization; one such change is in the area of traction. Most balanced skeletal traction is applied in children after a severe or complex injury to allow physiologic stability, align bone fragments, and permit closer evaluation of the injured site. Newer technology has produced orthopedic fixation devices that allow partial or full mobility, thus preventing long-term immobilization and its consequences. In many situations surgical intervention may be carried out within a matter of days; therefore skeletal traction devices described herein may be used infrequently in pediatrics.

Purposes of Traction

The six primary purposes of traction areas are
1. To fatigue the involved muscles and reduce muscle spasm so bones can be realigned.
2. To position the distal and proximal bone ends in desired realignment to promote satisfactory bone healing.
3. To immobilize the fracture site until realignment has been achieved and sufficient healing has taken place to permit casting or splinting.
4. To help prevent or improve contracture deformity.
5. To provide immobilization of specific areas of the body.
6. To reduce muscle spasms (rare in children).

The three essential components of traction management are traction, counter traction, and friction (Fig. 48-6). To reduce or realign a fracture site, traction (forward force) is produced by attaching weight to the distal bone fragment. Body weight provides counter traction (backward force), and the patient's contact with the bed constitutes the frictional force. These forces are used to align the distal and proximal bone fragments by adjusting the line of pull upward or downward and adducting or abducting the extremity.

To attain equilibrium the amount of forward force is adjusted by adding weight to or subtracting weight from the traction; or counter traction can be increased by elevating the foot of the bed to create a greater gravitational pull to the backward force.

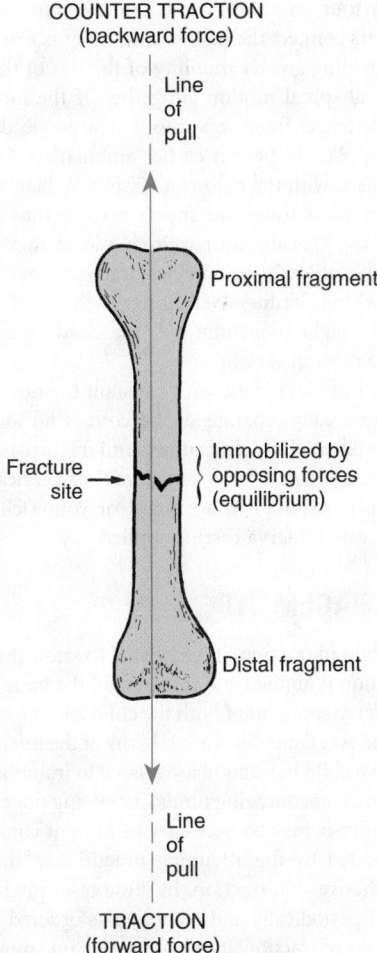

FIG 48-6 Application of traction to maintain bone alignment.

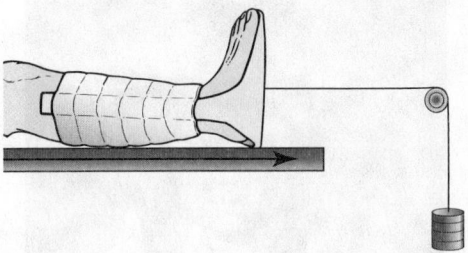

FIG 48-7 Buck extension traction. (From Lewis SL, Heitkemper MM, Dirksen S, et al, editors: *Medical-surgical nursing: assessment and management of clinical problems*, ed 8, St Louis, 2011, Mosby.)

BOX 48-4   TYPES OF TRACTION

Manual traction—Applied to the body part by the hands placed distal to the fracture site. Manual traction may be provided during application of a cast but more commonly when a closed reduction is performed.

Skin traction—Applied directly to the skin surface and indirectly to the skeletal structures. The pulling mechanism is attached to the skin with adhesive material or an elastic bandage. Both types are applied over soft, foam-backed traction straps to distribute the traction pull.

Skeletal traction—Applied directly to the skeletal structure by a pin, wire, or tongs inserted into or through the diameter of the bone distal to the fracture.

The all-or-none law, characteristic of muscle contractibility, influences the complete relaxation. When muscles are stretched, muscle spasm ceases, which permits the realignment of the bone ends. The continuous maintenance of traction is important during this phase because releasing the traction allows the normal contracting ability of the muscle to again cause a malpositioning of the bone ends.

The realignment of the fragments is a gradual process that is achieved more rapidly in infants, who have limited muscle tone, than in muscular teenagers. The desired vector force and callus formation are checked periodically by radiographic examination. The traction pull to some degree immobilizes the fracture site; however, adjunctive immobilizing devices such as splints or casts are sometimes used with skeletal traction. Immobilization with traction is maintained until the bone ends are in satisfactory realignment or muscle fatigue is achieved, after which a less confining type of immobilization (i.e., a cast, pins, or external stabilization device) is applied.

Types of Traction (General)

The pull needed for traction can be applied to the distal bone fragment in several ways (Box 48-4). The type of traction applied is determined primarily by the child's age, the condition of the soft tissues, and the type and degree of displacement of the fracture. Fractures most commonly treated by application of traction are those involving the femur and vertebrae. The major types of traction for specific fractures are discussed briefly in the following sections.

The use of upper-extremity traction in children is uncommon. Newer surgical techniques allow for early mobilization and optimal results without traction. Nursing care of the child with upper-extremity traction is the same as that for lower-extremity traction, which is discussed in the following paragraphs.

The frequent site for a femoral fracture is in the middle third of the shaft. With this fracture there may be significant overriding but minimal displacement. In a fracture in the lower third of the shaft, the pull of the gastrocnemius muscle causes the distal fragment to become downwardly displaced.

Fractures of the femur can often be reduced with immediate application of a hip spica cast in young children. When traction is required, several types may be used based on the initial assessment.

Bryant traction is a type of running traction in which the pull is in only one direction. Skin traction is applied to the legs, which are flexed at a 90-degree angle at the hips. The child's trunk (with the buttocks raised slightly off the bed) provides counter traction. Bryant traction may be used to treat a femoral shaft fracture in young children.

Buck extension traction (Fig. 48-7) is a type of traction with the legs in an extended position. Except for fracture cases turning from side to side with care is permitted to maintain the involved leg in alignment. Buck extension traction is used primarily for short-term immobilization such as preoperative management of a child with a dislocated hip or correction of contractures or bone deformities such as in Legg-Calvé-Perthes disease. Buck traction may be accomplished with either skin straps or a special foam boot designed for traction.

Russell traction uses skin traction on the lower leg and a padded sling under the knee. Two lines of pull, one along the longitudinal

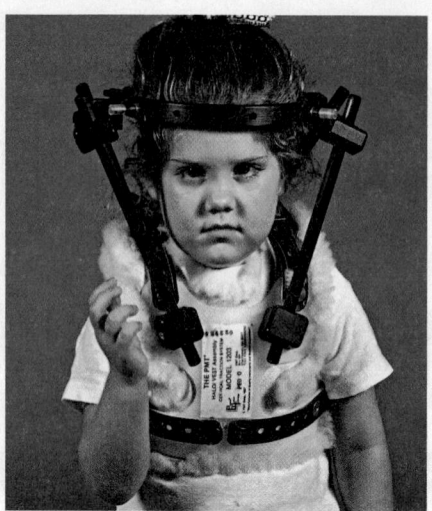

FIG 48-8 Halo vest. (From Herring JA: *Tachdjian's pediatric orthopaedics*, ed 4, Philadelphia, 2008, Saunders.)

line of the lower leg and one perpendicular to the leg, are produced. This combination of pulls allows realignment of the lower extremity and immobilizes the hip and knee in a flexed position. The hip flexion must be kept at the prescribed angle to prevent fracture malalignment because there is no direct support under the fracture and the skin traction may slip. Special nursing measures include carefully checking the position of the traction so the amount of desired hip flexion is maintained and damage to the common peroneal nerve under the knee does not produce footdrop.

A common skeletal traction is 90-degree–90-degree traction (90-90 traction). The lower leg is supported by a boot cast or calf sling, and a skeletal Steinmann pin or Kirschner wire is placed in the distal fragment of the femur, resulting in a 90-degree angle at both the hip and the knee. From a nursing standpoint this traction facilitates position changes, toileting, and prevention of complications related to traction.

Balanced suspension traction may be used with or without skin or skeletal traction. Unless used with another traction, the balanced suspension merely suspends the leg in a desired flexed position to relax the hip and hamstring muscles and does not exert any traction directly on a body part. A Thomas splint extends from the groin to midair above the foot, and a Pearson attachment supports the lower leg. Towels or pieces of felt covered with stockinette are clipped or pinned to the splints for leg support. When the child is lifted off the bed, the traction lifts with the child without loss of alignment. This traction requires careful checking of splints and ropes to make certain that no slippage or fraying has occurred. The traction is of great value in an older and heavier child when it is essential to lift the patient for care.

The cervical area is a vulnerable site for flexion or extension injuries to muscle, vertebrae, or the spinal cord. Cervical muscle trauma without other complications is treated with a cervical hard collar to relieve the weight of the head from the fracture site. When a child displaces or fractures a cervical vertebra, it may be necessary to reduce and immobilize the site with cervical skeletal traction. The spinal cord runs through the intravertebral canal, and dislocation or fracture of the vertebrae can also cause spinal cord injury. Nursing assessment of neurologic function is essential to prevent further injury during the application and use of cervical skeletal traction. Most cervical traction is accomplished with the use of a halo brace or halo vest (Fig. 48-8). This device consists of a steel halo attached to the head by four screws (or pins) inserted into the outer skull; several rigid bars connect the halo to a vest that is worn around the chest, thus providing greater mobility of the rest of the body while avoiding cervical spinal motion altogether. If the injury has been limited to a vertebral fracture without neurologic deficit, a halo brace can be applied to permit earlier ambulation. Gardner-Wells tongs may be used with the halo vest (Fisher, Williams, and Levine, 2008). Gardner-Wells tongs are spring loaded; thus making burr holes and shaving hair are not required; a local anesthetic may be used during application. In-line cervical traction may also be accomplished by attaching Gardner-Wells tongs to the child's head, with a 3- to 4-pound weight (depending on the child's weight) exerting traction on the cervical vertebrae.

As the neck muscles fatigue with constant traction pull, the vertebral bodies gradually separate so the cord is no longer pinched between the vertebrae. Immobilization until fracture healing or surgical fixation can occur is an essential goal of cervical traction. If immobilization is required in an infant or young child, a special cervical spine cast (Minerva cast) is applied.

CARE MANAGEMENT

To assess the child in traction, it is essential to know the purpose for which the traction is applied and understand the basic principles of traction. Regular assessment of both the child and the traction apparatus is required (see Guidelines box). Many of the nursing problems associated with a child in traction are related to immobility. Modifying the child's diet, encouraging fluids, increasing fiber, and offering a mild stool softener may be necessary to prevent constipation.

When indicated by the attending practitioner, the nurse may remove nonadhesive skin traction. In these cases intermittent traction is released periodically and reapplied as ordered. A child may have several types of traction at one time; each one must be assessed separately to avoid problems.

> **! NURSING ALERT**
>
> Skeletal traction is never released by the nurse (except under direct supervision by the practitioner). This precaution includes not lifting the weights that are applying traction (e.g., for moving the child in bed, for repositioning).

In addition to routine skin observation and care, the child in skeletal traction needs special skin care at the pin site according to hospital policy or practitioner preference. Pin sites should be frequently assessed and cleaned to prevent infection; after the first 48 to 72 hours pin site care may be performed once daily or weekly for mechanically stable pins (Holmes, Brown, and Pin Site Care Expert Panel, 2005). Use of a 2-mg/mL chlorhexidine solution has been proposed as best practice care for skeletal pin sites by the National Association of Orthopaedic Nurses (Holmes, Brown, and Pin Site Care Expert Panel, 2005). A pressure-reduction device such as a special air mattress decreases the chance of skin breakdown. A small hand mirror facilitates visualization of inaccessible skin areas.

When the child is first placed in traction, increased discomfort is common as a result of the traction pull fatiguing the muscle. It has been determined that orthopedic conditions are associated with a higher-than-average number of painful events and a higher percentage of bodily symptoms than other common conditions. Analgesics, including IV opioids and muscle relaxants, help during this phase of care and should be administered liberally.

GUIDELINES

Traction Care

Understand Therapy
- Understand purposes of traction.
- Understand function of traction in each specific situation.

Maintain Traction
- Check desired line of pull and relationship of distal fragment to proximal fragment. Check whether fragment is being directed upward, adducted, or abducted.
- Check function of each component.
  - Position of bandages, frames, splints, specialized boot
  - Ropes—In center track of pulley, taut, no fraying, knots tied securely
  - Pulleys—In original position on attachment bar; have not been displaced from original site
  - Wheels freely moveable
  - Weights—Correct amount of weight, hanging freely, in safe location
- Check bed position; head or foot should be elevated as directed for desired amount of pull and counter traction.
- Do not remove skeletal traction or adhesive traction straps on skin traction.

Maintain Alignment
- Observe for correct body alignment with emphasis on alignment of shoulder, hip, and leg.
- Check after child has moved.
- Maintain correct angles at joints.

Skin Traction
- Replace nonadhesive straps and/or elastic bandage on skin traction *when permitted* and/or absolutely necessary, but make certain that traction on limb is maintained by someone during procedure.
- Assess straps or bandages to ascertain whether they are applied correctly (diagonal or spiral), not too loose or too tight, which could cause slippage and malalignment of traction.
- Assess traction boot to ensure that it has not slipped and is not causing compression of the foot, thus impairing the circulation.

Skeletal Traction
- Check pin sites frequently for signs of bleeding, inflammation, or infection.
- Cleanse and dress pin sites per evidence-based guidelines or institution protocol.
- Apply topical antiseptic or antibiotic to pin sites daily as ordered.

- Cover ends of pins with protective rubber or padding to prevent child's being scratched by pin.
- Note pull of traction on pin; pull should be even.
- Check pin screws to be certain that screws are tight in metal clamp that attaches traction apparatus to pin.

Prevent Skin Breakdown
- Provide foam overlay or alternating-pressure mattress underneath hips and back.
- Make total-body skin checks for redness or breakdown, especially over areas that receive greatest pressure.
- Wash and dry skin at least daily.
- Inspect pressure points daily or more often if risk of breakdown is observed.
- Use a skin breakdown assessment scale such as Modified Braden Q.
- Stimulate circulation with gentle massage over pressure areas.
- Change position at least every 2 hours to relieve pressure.
- Encourage increased intake of oral fluids.
- Provide and encourage patient to eat a balanced diet, including vegetables and fruits.

Prevent Complications
- Check pulses in affected area and compare with pulses in contralateral site.
- Assess circular dressings for excessive tightness.
- Assess restrictive bandages or devices used to maintain traction on affected limb.
  - Make certain that they are not too loose or too tight.
  - Remove periodically and check for pressure areas.
- Encourage deep breathing exercises. Note any neurovascular changes such as the following:
  - Changes in color in skin and nail beds
  - Alterations in sensation, increased pain
  - Alterations in motor ability
- Take immediate action to correct problem or report to practitioner if neurovascular changes are found.
- Record findings of neurovascular changes.
- Carry out passive, active, or active-with-resistance exercises of uninvolved joints.
- Note if any tightness, weakness, edema, or contractures are developing in uninvolved joints and muscles.
- Take measures to correct or prevent further development of weakness such as applying footboard or foot orthoses to prevent footdrop.

! NURSING ALERT

For skeletal traction to be effective, ensure that the weights are hanging freely at all times. The specific nursing responsibilities for the patient in traction are outlined in the Guidelines box above.

Distraction

Unlike traction, which helps bones realign and fuse properly, distraction is the process of separating opposing bone to encourage regeneration of new bone in the created space. Distraction can also be used when limbs are of unequal lengths and new bone is needed to elongate the shorter limb.

External Fixation

Monolateral, Taylor Spatial Frame, and Ilizarov external fixators (IEFs) are common external fixation devices. The IEF uses a system of wires, rings, and telescoping rods that permits limb lengthening to occur by manual distraction (Fig. 48-9). In addition to lengthening bones, the device can be used to correct angular or rotational defects or immobilize fractures. It is attached surgically by securing a series of external full or half rings to the bone with wires. External telescoping rods connect the rings to one another. Manual distraction is accomplished by manipulating the rods to increase the distance between the rings. A percutaneous osteotomy is performed when the device is applied to create a "false" growth plate. A special osteotomy or corticotomy involves cutting only the cortex of the

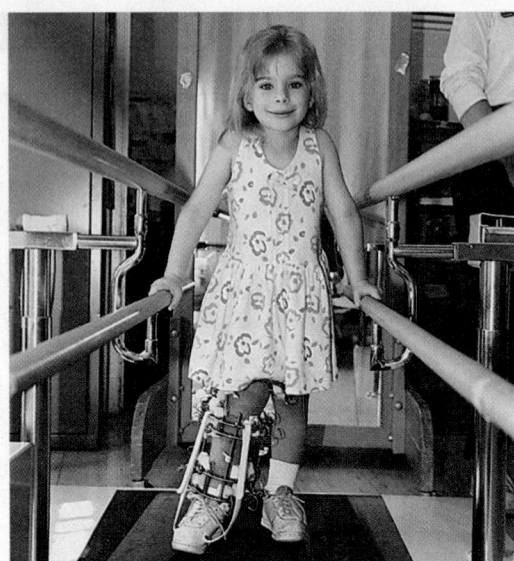

FIG 48-9 Child with Ilizarov external fixator (right leg) during physical therapy on parallel bars.

bone while preserving its blood supply, bone marrow, endosteum, and periosteum. Capillary blood flow to the transected area is essential for proper bone growth. Cut bone ends typically grow at a rate of 1 cm (0.4 inches) per month. The IEF can result in up to a 15-cm (6-inch) gain in length.

CARE MANAGEMENT

Success of the external fixation devices depends on the child's and family's cooperation; therefore before surgery they must be fully informed of the appearance of the device and how it accomplishes bone growth and limits bone mobility, alterations in activities, and home and follow-up care. Children are involved in learning to adjust the device to accomplish distraction. Children and parents should be instructed in pin care, including observation for infection and loosening of the pins. Cleaning routines for the pin sites vary among practitioners but should not traumatize the skin.

Children who participate actively in their care report less discomfort. Because the device is external, the child and family need to be prepared for the reactions of others and helped to camouflage it with appropriate apparel such as wide-legged pants that close with self-adhering fasteners around it. A loose sock or stockinette may also be used over the device to decrease public awareness. Partial weight bearing is allowed, and the child learns to walk with crutches. Alterations in activity include modifications at school and in physical education. Full weight bearing is not allowed until the distraction is completed and bone consolidation has occurred. Follow-up care is essential to maintain appropriate distraction until the desired limb length is achieved. The device is removed surgically after the bone has consolidated, and the child may need to use crutches or have a cast for 4 to 6 weeks after removal to reduce the risk of fracture.

Amputation

A child may be born with the congenital absence of an extremity, have a traumatic loss of an extremity, or need a surgical amputation for a pathologic condition such as osteosarcoma (see p. 1561). With today's surgical technology and the quick thinking of bystanders who save a traumatically amputated body part, some children have had fingers and arms sewn back on with variable degrees of functional use regained.

Surgical amputation or the surgical repair of a permanently severed limb focuses on constructing an adequately nourished residual limb. A smooth, healthy, padded stump, free of nerve endings, is important in prosthesis fitting and subsequent ambulation. In some situations in which there is no vascular or neurologic deficit, a cast is applied to the stump immediately after the procedure; and a pylon, metal extension, and artificial foot are attached so the patient can walk on the temporary prosthesis within a few hours.

CARE MANAGEMENT

Stump shaping is done after surgery with special elastic bandaging using a figure-eight bandage, which applies pressure in a cone-shaped fashion. This technique decreases stump edema, controls hemorrhage, and aids in developing desired contours so the child will bear weight on the posterior aspect of the skin flap rather than on the end of the stump. Stump elevation may be used during the first 24 hours, but after this time the extremity should not be left in this position because contractures in the proximal joint will develop and seriously hamper ambulation.

> ### ! NURSING ALERT
>
> For an amputated limb or body part that may be reattached, do the following:
> 1. Rinse limb gently with normal saline.
> 2. Loosely wrap limb in sterile gauze.
> 3. Place wrapped limb in a watertight bag.
> 4. Cool (without freezing) bag in ice water (do not pack in ice because this may harm tissue).
> 5. Label with child's name, date, and time and transport with the child to the hospital.

For older children and adolescents, arm exercises, bed pushups, and prosthesis-training programs using parallel bars help build up the arm muscles necessary for walking with crutches. Full range-of-motion exercises of joints above the amputation must be performed several times daily using active and isotonic exercises. Young children are often spontaneously active and require little encouragement.

Depending on the child's age, children or their parents will need to learn hygiene, including carefully washing with soap and water every day and checking for skin irritation, breakdown, and infection. A tube of stockinette or powder is used to slide the prosthesis on more easily. Skin must be checked carefully every time the prosthesis is removed, and prosthesis tolerance time must be adjusted to prevent skin breakdown.

For children who have had an amputation, *phantom limb sensation* is an expected experience because the nerve-brain connections are still present. Gradually these sensations fade, although in many people who have had amputations they persist for years. Preoperative discussion of this phenomenon helps a child understand these "unusual feelings" and not to hide the experiences from others. Limb pain, especially pain that increases with ambulation, should be evaluated for the possibility of a neuroma at the free nerve endings in the stump or other problems such as a poorly fitting prosthesis or joint instability.

SPORTS PARTICIPATION AND INJURY

Every sport has the potential for injury to participants, whether an adolescent engages in serious competition or participates for enjoyment. Serious injury occurs most often during rough contact sports or to people who are not physically prepared for the activity. Injuries also occur when the children's or adolescents' bodies are not suited to the sport, when their muscles and body systems (respiratory and cardiovascular) are not conditioned to endure physical stress, or when they lack the insight and judgment to recognize that an activity exceeds their physical abilities. Rapidly growing bones, muscles, joints, and tendons are especially vulnerable to unusual strain. In general more injuries occur during recreational sports participation than during organized athletic competition.

The environment and the sports or recreational equipment can also present risks. Children and adolescents who participate in physical activity or sports do so in many different environments, including indoors and outdoors, on floors, on the ground and snow, on or beneath water surfaces, and sometimes in free air space. Most of these activities also involve equipment, which children and adolescents may not be physically mature enough to manage safely. A common example is skateboarding when the child or adolescent does not take safety precautions and perceives increased risk taking as a part of the sport.

Acute overload injuries are those that occur suddenly during an activity and produce immediate symptoms. A blow or overstretching, twisting, or sudden stress to tissues can cause these injuries. For descriptions and management of traumatic injuries see p. 1536.

Overuse Injury

To excel in sports young athletes are forced to train longer, harder, and earlier in life than previously. The rewards are an increased level of fitness, better performance, faster times, and the satisfaction of attaining a personal goal. However, risks are associated when young people overtrain; these risks include recurrent upper-respiratory infections, sleep and mood disturbances, loss of appetite, decreased interest in training and competition, and inability to concentrate (Winsley and Matos, 2011). Growing numbers of young people participate in organized sports, resulting in an increase in overuse injuries. Nearly half of all injuries evaluated in pediatric sports medicine are overuse injuries (Biber and Gregory, 2010). Evidence-based recommendations for prevention and identification of risk factors for overuse injuries in older children and adolescents have been published elsewhere (Valovich McLeod, Decoster, Loud, et al., 2012).

The risk of overuse injury is always present and can be related to several factors, including training errors, muscle-tendon imbalance, anatomic malalignment (e.g., femoral anteversion, excessive lumbar lordosis, tibial torsion), incorrect footwear or playing surface, an associated disease state, and growth (growth cartilage is less resistant to microtrauma). Chronic pain in athletes is often associated with overuse injury, which can occur at any level of athletic participation. The common feature in overuse injuries is the *repetitive microtrauma* that occurs to a particular anatomic structure. Performing the same movements repeatedly can cause several types of injury:

- Frictional, or rubbing of one structure against another
- Tractional, or repeated pull on a ligament or tendon
- Cyclic, or repetitive loading of impact forces (stress fractures)

The end result is inflammation of the involved structure with complaints of pain, tenderness, swelling, and disability.

Stress Fractures

Stress fractures are a consequence of repetitive, excessive stress on the bone that causes microfractures within the bone. Continued stress to the bone can lead to spread of the microfracture and eventual macrofracture. The pathogenesis of stress injury to the bone is multifactorial and includes everything from the footwear to the fitness level of the athlete. Stress fractures occur most commonly in the lower extremities, particularly the tibia. Track and field athletes have the highest incidence of stress fractures (Patel, 2010).

The most common symptom of stress fracture is a sharp, persistent, progressive pain or a deep, persistent dull ache located over the bone. Sometimes there is pain on impact (heel strike), but the most important clinical sign is pain over the involved bony surface. Diagnosis is based on clinical observation and history. Plain radiographs are rarely diagnostic of stress fractures during the initial few weeks because callus formation is not yet evident. Magnetic resonance imaging (MRI) is used when other causes of pain must be excluded.

Therapeutic Management

Development of inflammation is common to all overuse injuries; therefore management involves rest or alteration of activities, physical therapy, and medication. Rest is the primary therapy, usually interpreted as reduced activity and the use of alternative exercise—not bed rest or immobilization with casting. The main purpose is to alleviate the repetitive stress that initiated the symptoms. It is important to keep the adolescent mobile, and training can be continued. Alternative exercise is selected that maintains conditioning without aggravating the injury. For example, pool running (treading water in the deep end of a pool) can use the same movements as running but without the weight bearing; bicycling, swimming, and rowing are viable alternatives.

Other modalities include cryotherapy and cold whirlpool baths. Sometimes taping, bracing, splinting, and other orthoses are used, depending on the injury. Nonsteroidal antiinflammatory drugs (NSAIDs) are often prescribed to reduce inflammation and pain. Topical medications are of questionable value.

Nurse's Role in Sports for Children and Adolescents

Nurses are often involved in sports activities in the areas of preparation and evaluation for activities, prevention of injury, treatment of injuries, and rehabilitation after injury. Selecting an appropriate sport for both recreation and competition is a joint effort of the adolescent, parents, and health care providers. The best approach to counseling children, adolescents, and parents regarding sports participation is to encourage activities that are most likely to provide pleasure and physical benefits throughout childhood and into adulthood. Exposure to a variety of activities is better for young children than limiting them to one sport. Parents should be cautioned against overcommitting children to sports activities so they have time for other activities.

When children sustain athletic injuries, nurses are often responsible for instructions regarding care. Instructions (e.g., schedule for appointments, application of ice, any restrictions in activity) should be clear and accompanied by written directions. Nurses should emphasize the importance of taking medications as prescribed, especially if they are needed for an extended period and if adherence is an issue. Antiinflammatory medications given an hour before practice or competition may help children continue their activities.

Prevention of sports injuries is the most important aspect of athletic programs. Children should be suited to the activity, and the

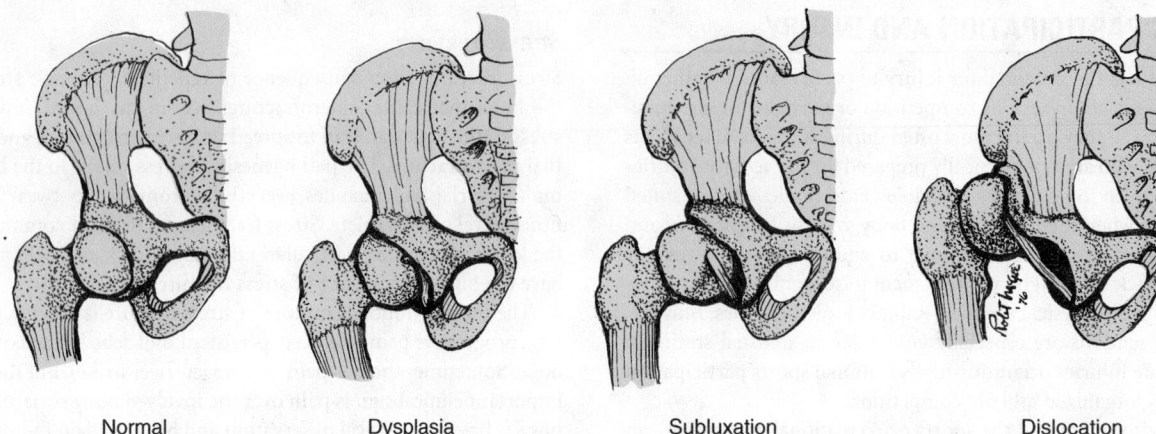

Normal Dysplasia Subluxation Dislocation

FIG 48-10 Configuration and relationship of structures in developmental dysplasia of the hip.

environment and the equipment must be safe. Children should be prepared for the sport, especially if it requires strenuous or continuous physical exertion. Nurses, coaches, and athletic trainers must collaborate to ensure that safety measures are implemented. Stretching exercises, warm-up and cool-down activities, and appropriate training are requirements for safe participation. Protective measures such as pads, taping, and wrapping are also important to prevent injury. Finally nurses must be aware of environmental safety risks.

BIRTH AND DEVELOPMENTAL DEFECTS

Some skeletal defects may be diagnosed at birth or within days, weeks, or months after birth. In other cases the deviation may be difficult to detect without careful inspection Therefore it is imperative that nurses become acquainted with signs of these defects and understand the principles of therapy to direct others in the care and management of these children.

Developmental Dysplasia of the Hip

The broad term developmental dysplasia of the hip (DDH) describes a spectrum of disorders related to abnormal development of the hip that may occur at any time during fetal life, infancy, or childhood. A change in terminology from *congenital hip dysplasia* and *congenital dislocation of the hip* to DDH more properly reflects a variety of hip abnormalities in which there is a shallow acetabulum, subluxation, or dislocation.

The incidence of hip instability is approximately 1.5 per 1000 live births, and approximately 15% to 50% of infants with DDH are born breech. Girls are affected more commonly (80%), and there is a positive family history in approximately 12% to 33% of affected individuals (Sankar, Horn, Wells, et al., 2011a). Two published meta-analyses have identified the following risk factors: breech birth, female gender, family history of DDH, left hip, first-born child, and positive clicking hips with clinical examination (de Hundt, Vlemmix, Bais, et al., 2012; Ortiz-Neira, Paolucci and Donnon, 2012).

Pathophysiology

The cause of DDH is unknown, but certain factors such as gender, birth order, family history, intrauterine position, delivery type, joint laxity, and postnatal positioning are believed to affect the risk of DDH. Predisposing factors associated with it may be divided into three broad categories: (1) physiologic factors, which include

maternal hormone secretion and intrauterine positioning; (2) mechanical factors, which involve breech presentation, multiple fetus, oligohydramnios, and large infant size (other mechanical factors may include continued maintenance of the hips in adduction and extension that will in time cause a dislocation); and (3) genetic factors, which entail a higher incidence of DDH in siblings of affected infants and an even greater incidence of recurrence if a sibling and one parent were affected.

Some experts categorize DDH into two major groups: (1) idiopathic, in which the infant is neurologically intact; and (2) teratologic, which involves a neuromuscular defect such as arthrogryposis or spina bifida. The teratologic forms usually occur in utero and are much less common.

Three degrees of DDH are illustrated in Fig. 48-10:
1. *Acetabular dysplasia*—This is the mildest form of DDH, in which there is neither subluxation nor dislocation. There is a delay in acetabular development evidenced by osseous hypoplasia of the acetabular roof that is oblique and shallow, although the cartilaginous roof is comparatively intact. The femoral head remains in the acetabulum.
2. *Subluxation*—The largest percentage of DDH, subluxation, implies incomplete dislocation of the hip and is sometimes regarded as an intermediate state in the development from primary dysplasia to complete dislocation. The femoral head remains in contact with the acetabulum, but a stretched capsule and ligamentum teres cause the head of the femur to be partially displaced. Pressure on the cartilaginous roof inhibits ossification and produces a flattening of the socket.
3. *Dislocation*—The femoral head loses contact with the acetabulum and is displaced posteriorly and superiorly over the fibrocartilaginous rim. The ligamentum teres is elongated and taut.

Factors related to infant handling are indicated in the Cultural Competence box.

Recently several prominent orthopedic specialty organizations recommended that infants' hips be placed in slight flexion and abduction during swaddling. It was further recommended that their knees be maintained in slight flexion and that forced or sustained passive hip extension in the first few months should be avoided (Price and Schwend, 2011). These recommendations were supported by evidence that demonstrated a significant relationship between tight swaddling and hip dysplasia and are aimed at decreasing the incidence of hip dysplasia in infants.

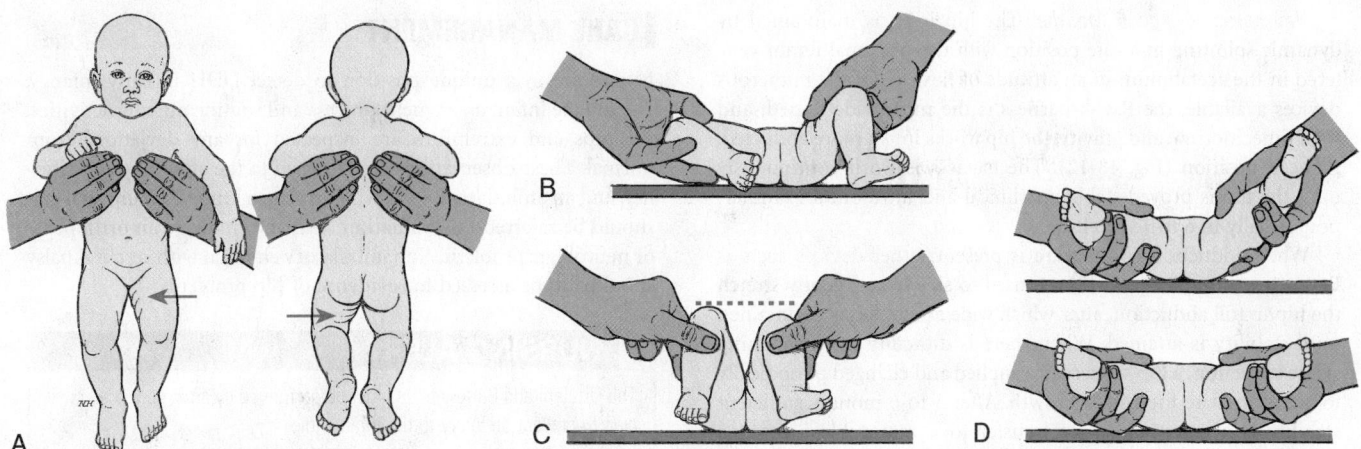

FIG 48-11 Signs of developmental dysplasia of the hip. **A,** Asymmetry of gluteal and thigh folds. **B,** Limited hip abduction as seen in flexion. **C,** Apparent shortening of the femur as indicated by the level of the knees in flexion. **D,** Ortolani maneuver clunk elicited (in infants <4 weeks of age).

🌐 CULTURAL COMPETENCE

Developmental Dysplasia of the Hip

A striking relationship exists between the development of the dislocation and methods of handling infants. Among the cultures with the highest incidence of dislocation, newly born infants are tightly wrapped in blankets or other swaddling material or strapped to cradle boards. In cultures such as the Far East, where mothers traditionally carry infants on their backs or hips in the widely abducted straddle position, the disorder is virtually unknown.

Diagnostic Evaluation

DDH is often not detected at the initial examination after birth; thus all infants should be carefully monitored for hip dysplasia at follow-up visits throughout the first year of life and routine well-child checks. In the newborn period hip dysplasia usually appears as hip joint laxity rather than outright dislocation (Fig. 48-11). Subluxation and the tendency to dislocate can be demonstrated by the Ortolani or Barlow tests (see Fig. 48-11, *B* to *D*). The Ortolani and Barlow tests are most reliable from birth to 4 weeks of age. With the Barlow test the thighs are adducted; the Ortolani test involves abducting the thighs to test for hip subluxation or dislocation (Seidel, Ball, Dains, et al., 2006). Other signs of DDH are shortening of the limb on the affected side (see Fig. 48-11, *C*), asymmetric thigh and gluteal folds (see Fig. 48-11, *A*), broadening of the perineum (in bilateral dislocation) (Box 48-5), and decreased hip abduction on the affected side.

Radiographic examination in early infancy is not reliable because ossification of the femoral head does not normally take place until the fourth to sixth month of life. However, the cartilaginous head can be visualized directly by ultrasonography. Universal newborn screening with ultrasonography has been proposed in the United States; however, numerous studies reveal that this approach has a high rate of false-positive results and subsequent overtreatment. Therefore ultrasonography is recommended as an adjunct to other diagnostic procedures (AAP Committee on Quality Improvement, 2000; Sankar, Horn, Wells, et al., 2011a). Radiographic examination is useful in confirming the diagnosis in infants older than age 4 months and children. An upward slope in the roof of the acetabulum

BOX 48-5 CLINICAL MANIFESTATIONS OF DEVELOPMENTAL DYSPLASIA OF THE HIP

Infants
- Shortening of limb on affected side (Galeazzi sign)
- Restricted abduction of hip on affected side
- Unequal gluteal folds (best visualized with infant prone)
- Positive Ortolani test (hip reduced by abduction)
- Positive Barlow test (hip dislocated by adduction)

Older Infants and Children
- Affected leg appears shorter than the other
- Telescoping or piston mobility of joint—Head of femur felt to move up and down in buttock when extended thigh is pushed first toward child's head and then pulled distally
- Trendelenburg sign—When child stands first on one foot and then on the other (holding onto a chair, rail, or someone's hands) bearing weight on affected hip, pelvis tilts downward on normal side instead of upward, as it would with normal stability
- Greater trochanter prominent and appearing above a line from antero-superior iliac spine to tuberosity of ischium
- Marked lordosis and waddling gait (bilateral hip dislocation)

(the acetabular angle) greater than 30 degrees with upward and outward displacement of the femoral head is a frequent finding in older children. Computed tomography (CT) may be useful to assess the position of the femoral head relative to the acetabulum after closed reduction and casting. The AAP (2000) has published extensive clinical guidelines for screening and early detection of DDH.

Therapeutic Management

Treatment is begun as soon as the condition is recognized because early intervention is more favorable to the restoration of normal bony architecture and function. The longer treatment is delayed, the more severe the deformity, the more difficult the treatment, and the less favorable the prognosis. The treatment varies with the child's age and the extent of the dysplasia. The goal of treatment is to obtain and maintain a safe, congruent position of the hip joint to promote normal hip joint development.

Newborns to Age 6 Months. The hip joint is maintained by dynamic splinting in a safe position with the proximal femur centered in the acetabulum in an attitude of flexion. Of the numerous devices available, the Pavlik harness is the most widely used; and with time, motion, and gravity, the hip works into a more abducted, reduced position (Fig. 48-12). The harness is worn continuously until the hip is proved stable on clinical and ultrasound examination, usually in 6 to 12 weeks.

When adduction contracture is present, other devices such as Bryant traction (see p. 1543) are used to slowly and gently stretch the hip to full abduction, after which wide abduction is maintained until stability is attained. When there is difficulty in maintaining stable reduction, a hip spica cast is applied and changed periodically to accommodate the child's growth. After 3 to 6 months sufficient stability is acquired to allow transfer to a removable protective abduction brace. The duration of treatment depends on development of the acetabulum but is usually accomplished within the first year.

Ages 6 to 24 Months. In this age-group the dislocation may not be recognized until the child begins to stand and walk, when attendant shortening of the limb and contractures of hip adductor and flexor muscles become apparent (DDH hip radiograph). A surgical closed reduction is performed, and the child is placed in a spica cast for approximately 12 weeks. An abduction orthosis may be used instead of a hip spica cast. In the event that the hip remains unstable, an open reduction is performed (Sankar, Horn, Wells, et al., 2011a).

Older Children. Correction of the hip deformity in older children is inherently more difficult than in the preceding age-groups because secondary adaptive changes and other etiologic factors (e.g., juvenile arthritis or nonambulatory cerebral palsy) complicate the condition. Operative reduction, which may involve preoperative traction, tenotomy of contracted muscles, and any one of several innominate osteotomy procedures designed to construct an acetabular roof, often combined with proximal femoral osteotomy, is usually required. After cast removal range-of-motion exercises help restore movement. Successful reduction and reconstruction become increasingly difficult after the age of 4 years and are usually impossible or inadvisable in children older than 6 years of age because of severe shortening and contracture of muscles and deformity of the femoral and acetabular structures.

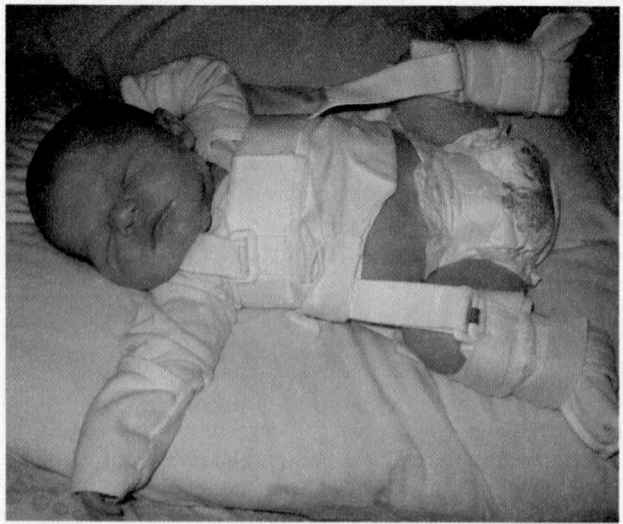

FIG 48-12 Child in Pavlik harness. (Courtesy Amanda Politte, St Louis, MO.)

CARE MANAGEMENT

Nurses are in a unique position to detect DDH in early infancy. During the infant assessment process and routine nursing activities, the hips and extremities are inspected for any deviations from normal. These observations are reported to the attending practitioner, and an ambulatory child who displays a limp or an unusual gait should be referred for evaluation. This may indicate an orthopedic or neurologic problem. Nonambulatory children with cerebral palsy should also be assessed for evidence of hip problems.

> ### ! NURSING ALERT
> The Ortolani and Barlow tests must be performed by an experienced clinician to prevent an injury to the infant's hip.

The major nursing problems in the care of an infant or child in a cast or other device are related to maintenance of the device and adaptation of nurturing activities to meet the patient's needs. Generally treatment and follow-up care of these children are carried out in an outpatient setting.

The primary nursing goal is teaching parents to apply and maintain the reduction device. The Pavlik harness allows for easy handling of the infant and usually produces less apprehension in the parent than heavy braces and casts. Because of infants' rapid growth, the straps should be checked in the beginning of therapy and every 1 to 2 weeks for adjustments (Hart, Albright, Rebello, et al., 2006). It is important that parents understand the correct use of the appliance, which may or may not allow for its removal during bathing. Removing the harness is determined individually on the basis of the provider's recommendation, the family's level of understanding, and the degree of hip deformity. Parents are instructed to not adjust the harness. The child should be examined by the practitioner before any adjustment is attempted to make certain that the hips are in correct placement.

> ### ! NURSING ALERT
> The former practice of double or triple diapering for DDH is not recommended because there is no evidence to support its efficacy.

Skin care is an important aspect of the care of an infant in a harness. The following instructions for preventing skin breakdown are stressed:

- Always put an undershirt (or a shirt with extensions that close at the crotch) under the chest straps and put knee socks under the foot and leg pieces to prevent the straps from rubbing the skin.
- Check frequently (at least 2 or 3 times a day) for red areas under the straps and clothing.
- Gently massage healthy skin under the straps once a day to stimulate circulation. In general avoid lotions and powders because they can cake and irritate the skin.
- Always place the diaper under the straps.

Parents are encouraged to hold the infant with a harness and continue care and nurturing activities. The nurse can assist by being available for parents' questions about the necessary adaptations to daily care to decrease their anxiety and possible feelings about the child being hurt by routine caring.

Casts and orthotic devices (braces) offer more challenging nursing and caregiver problems because they cannot be removed for routine care, although sometimes a brace may be removed for bathing. Care of an infant or a small child with a cast requires nursing innovation to reduce irritation and maintain cleanliness of both the child and the cast, particularly in the diaper area. (See p. 1540 for care of the child in a cast.)

It is important for nurses, parents, and other caregivers to understand that children in corrective devices need to be involved in all of the activities of any child in the same age-group. Confinement in a cast or appliance should not exclude children from family (or unit) activities. They can be held astride the lap for comfort and transported to areas of activity. The child may be allowed to walk in a cast or orthotic device. An adapted wheelchair, stroller, or scooter can offer mobility to an older infant or child.

Clubfoot

Clubfoot is a complex deformity of the ankle and foot that includes forefoot adduction, midfoot supination, hindfoot varus, and ankle equinus. Deformities of the foot and ankle are described according to the position of the ankle and foot. The more common positions involve the following variations:

- *Talipes varus*—An inversion, or bending inward
- *Talipes valgus*—An eversion, or bending outward
- *Talipes equinus*—Plantar flexion, in which the toes are lower than the heel
- *Talipes calcaneus*—Dorsiflexion, in which the toes are higher than the heel
- *Talipes equinovarus*—Toes lower than the heel and facing inward

Most cases of clubfoot are a combination of these positions, and the most frequently occurring type of clubfoot (≈95% of cases) is the composite deformity talipes equinovarus (TEV), in which the foot is pointed downward (plantar flexed) and inward in varying degrees of severity (Fig. 48-13). Clubfoot may occur as an isolated deformity or in association with other disorders or syndromes such as chromosome abnormalities, arthrogryposis, cerebral palsy, or spina bifida.

The incidence of clubfoot in the general population is approximately one per 1000 live births, with boys affected twice as often as girls. Bilateral clubfeet occur in 50% of the cases (Hosalkar, Spiegel, and Davidson, 2011). The precise cause of clubfoot is unknown. Some authorities attribute the defect to abnormal positioning and restricted movement in utero, although the evidence is not conclusive. Other experts implicate arrested or abnormal embryonic development. Arrested development during this early stage tends to result in a rigid deformity; however, mechanical pressures from intrauterine positioning are likely causes of more flexible deformities (Shyy, Wang, Sheffield, et al., 2010).

Classification

Clubfoot may be further divided into three categories: (1) positional clubfoot (also called *transitional, mild,* or *postural clubfoot*), which is believed to occur primarily from intrauterine crowding and responds to simple stretching and casting; (2) *syndromic* (or teratologic) clubfoot, which is associated with other congenital anomalies such as myelomeningocele or arthrogryposis and is a more severe form of clubfoot that is often resistant to treatment; and (3) *congenital* clubfoot, also referred to as *idiopathic,* which may occur in an otherwise normal child and has a wide range of rigidity and prognosis.

The mild, or postural, clubfoot may correct spontaneously or may require passive exercise or serial casting. There is no bony abnormality, but there may be tightness and shortening of the soft tissues medially and posteriorly. The teratologic clubfoot usually requires surgical correction and has a high incidence of recurrence. The congenital idiopathic clubfoot, or "true clubfoot," almost always requires surgical intervention because there is bony abnormality.

Diagnostic Evaluation

The deformity is readily apparent and easily detected prenatally through ultrasonography or at birth. However, it must be differentiated from some positional deformities that can be corrected passively or overcorrected. Paralytic changes in the lower extremity of children with neuromuscular involvement often produce equinovarus deformity. An increased risk of hip dysplasia is associated with clubfoot deformities.

Therapeutic Management

The goal of treatment for clubfoot is to achieve a painless, plantigrade, and stable foot. Treatment of clubfoot involves three stages: (1) correction of the deformity, (2) maintenance of the correction until normal muscle balance is regained, and (3) follow-up observation to avert possible recurrence of the deformity. Some feet respond to treatment readily; some respond only to prolonged, vigorous, and sustained efforts; and the improvement in others remains disappointing even with maximal effort on the part of all concerned.

A common approach to clubfoot management is the Ponseti method (Ponseti, 1996). Serial casting is begun shortly after birth. Weekly gentle manipulation and serial long-leg casts allow for gradual repositioning of the foot (Fig. 48-14). The extremity or extremities are casted until maximum correction is achieved, usually within 6 to 10 weeks. Most of the time a percutaneous heel cord tenotomy is performed at the end of the serial casting to correct the equinus. After the tenotomy, a long-leg cast is applied and left in place for 3 weeks. A Denis Browne bar with Ponseti sandals or straight-laced shoes placed in abduction is then fitted to prevent recurrence. Inability to achieve normal foot alignment after casting and tenotomy indicates the need for surgical intervention.

CARE MANAGEMENT

Nursing care of the child with clubfoot is the same as for any child who has a cast (see p. 1540). Because the child will spend considerable time in a corrective device, nursing care plans include both long- and short-term goals. Conscientious observation of the skin and circulation is particularly important in young infants because

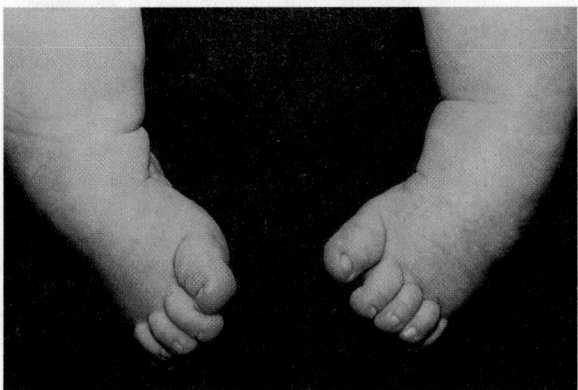

FIG 48-13 Bilateral congenital talipes equinovarus (congenital clubfoot) in 2-month-old infant. (From Zitelli BJ, Davis HW: *Atlas of pediatric physical diagnosis,* ed 4, St Louis, 2002, Mosby.)

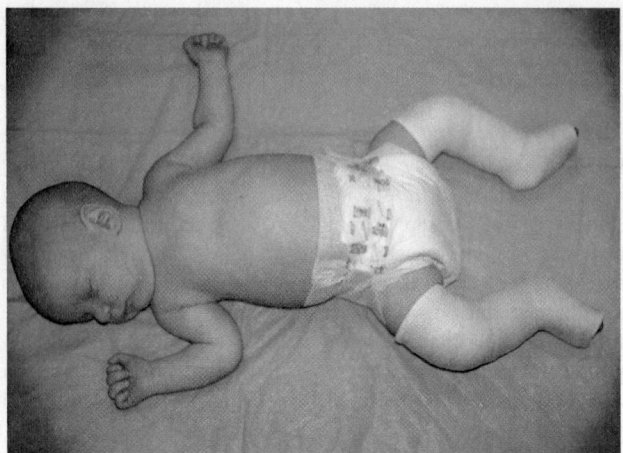

FIG 48-14 Feet casted for correction of bilateral congenital talipes equinovarus.

of their rapid growth rate. Because treatment and follow-up care are handled in the orthopedist's office, clinic, or outpatient department, parent education and support are important in nursing care of these children.

It is important for parents to understand the overall treatment program, the importance of regular cast changes, and the role they play in the long-term effectiveness of the therapy. Reinforcing and clarifying the orthopedist's explanations and instructions, teaching parents about care of the cast or appliance (including vigilant observation for potential problems), and encouraging parents to facilitate normal development within the limitations imposed by the deformity or therapy are all part of nursing responsibilities.

Metatarsus Adductus (Varus)

Metatarsus adductus, or metatarsus varus, is probably the most common congenital foot deformity. In most instances, it is a result of abnormal intrauterine positioning, particularly in a firstborn child, and is usually detected at birth. The deformity is characterized by medial adduction of the toes and forefoot, frequently in association with inversion, and by convexity of the lateral border of the foot. Metatarsus adductus may be divided into three categories: type I, in which the forefoot is flexible and corrects easily with manipulation; type II, in which there is only partial flexibility in the forefoot, and it corrects passively past neutral position but only to neutral position with active manipulation; and type III, in which the forefoot is rigid and will not stretch to neutral position with manipulation. Unlike TEV, with which it is often confused, the angulation occurs at the tarsometatarsal joint, but the heel and ankle remain in a neutral position. Ankle range of motion is normal. This deformity often causes a pigeon-toed gait in the child.

Management depends on the rigidity and type of the deformity. With types I and II correction can usually be accomplished by gentle manipulation and passive stretching of the foot, which the parent is taught to perform. Repeated and consistent stretching is continued for the first 6 weeks, after which the treatment is based on the flexibility of the foot. With type III the child usually requires serial manipulation and casting to correct the defect. Casting is performed every 1 to 2 weeks for 6 to 8 weeks, after which a corrective shoe or orthosis may be used. Surgical correction is rarely required for the condition but may be performed in children 4 to 6 years of age who have considerable pain on ambulation or are unable to wear certain

kinds of shoes as a result of the defect (Hosalkar, Spiegel, and Davidson, 2011).

CARE MANAGEMENT

The nursing role primarily involves identifying the defect so early therapy and instruction of the parents can be initiated. The nurse teaches the parents how to hold the heel firmly and stretch only the forefoot; otherwise undue force on the heel may produce a valgus deformity. If casting or an orthosis is required, the nurse instructs the parents in cast care and observation of the corrective device (see p. 1540).

Skeletal Limb Deficiency

Congenital limb deficiencies, or reduction malformations, are manifested by a variety of degrees of loss of functional capacity. They are characterized by underdevelopment of skeletal elements of the extremities. The range of malformation can extend from minor defects of the digits to serious abnormalities such as *amelia*, absence of an entire extremity; or *meromelia*, partial absence of an extremity, which includes *phocomelia* (seal limbs), the interposed deficiency of long bones with relatively good development of hands and feet attached at or near the shoulder or the hips. Most reduction defects are primary defects of development of the limb, but prenatal destruction of the limb such as full or partial amputation of a limb in utero from constriction of an *amniotic band* (amniotic band syndrome) can occur. Neonates with congenital limb deficiencies often have associated malformations and should be thoroughly investigated for cardiovascular, central nervous system (CNS), renal, and digestive abnormalities (Stoll, Alembik, Dott, et al., 2010).

Pathophysiology

Limb deficiencies can be attributed to both heredity and environment and can originate at any stage of limb development. Formation of limbs may be suppressed at the time of limb bud formation, or there may be interference in later stages of differentiation and growth. Heredity appears to play a prominent role, and prenatal environmental insults have been implicated in a number of cases such as the well-publicized thalidomide tragedy of the 1950s and early 1960s, which demonstrated a clear relationship between the time of exposure of the pregnant woman to the antiemetic drug and the presence and type of limb deformity in the newborn. There still are many drugs that may have similar teratogenic effects in the first trimester of pregnancy; therefore medication administration during this period should be evaluated carefully by the practitioner. Deletion or shortening of digits or limbs may also be associated with chorionic villus sampling, especially before 10 to 12 weeks of gestation; however, the incidence and relationship remain uncertain.

Therapeutic Management

Children with congenital limb deficiencies should be fitted with prosthetic devices whenever possible, and the devices should be applied at the earliest possible stage of development in an attempt to match the infant's motor readiness. This favors natural progression of prosthetic use. For example, an infant with an upper-extremity deficiency is fitted with a simple passive device such as a mitten prosthesis to encourage limb exploration, sitting (with the extremities needed for support), and bilateral hand activities.

Lower-limb prostheses are applied when the infant begins sitting up and can maintain balance. In preparation for prosthetic devices, surgical modification may be necessary to ensure the most favorable use of the device because severe deformity can interfere with its effective use. Phocomelic digits are preserved for controlling switches of externally powered appliances in the upper extremities. Digits (in both the upper and lower extremities) provide the child with surfaces for tactile exploration and stimulation. Prostheses are replaced to accommodate the child's growth and increasing capabilities.

CARE MANAGEMENT

Prosthetic application training and habilitation are most successfully carried out in a center that specializes in meeting the special needs of these children, especially very young children and those with amputations or missing limbs. Management involves a prosthetist who specializes in the development, fitting, and maintenance of prosthetic limbs and other health care workers such as physical and occupational therapists. Parents need special attention and support and are encouraged to help the child make age-commensurate adjustments to the environment. Although these children need assistance, overprotection may produce overdependence, with later maladjustment to school and other situations.

Osteogenesis Imperfecta

Osteogenesis imperfecta (OI) is the most common osteoporosis syndrome in childhood. However, it is very rare. OI is a heterogeneous, autosomal dominant disorder characterized by fractures and bone deformity. There are at least eight described types of OI, which accounts for significant disease variability. Clinical features may include varying degrees of bone fragility, deformity, and fracture; blue sclerae; hearing loss; and *dentinogenesis imperfecta* (hypoplastic discolored teeth). Although inheritance follows an autosomal dominant pattern in most cases, rare autosomal recessive inheritance exists primarily in populations with consanguineous marriages (Marini, 2011).

Most types of OI have defects in the *COL1A1* or *COL1A2* genes, which code for polypeptide chains in type 1 procollagen, a precursor of type 1 collagen, a major structural component of bone. The error results in faulty bone mineralization, abnormal bone architecture, and increased susceptibility to fracture. Additional autosomal recessive genes linked to OI have been identified and help explain bone biology and pathogenetic mechanisms in OI (Aglan, Hosny, El-Houssini, et al., 2012).

OI has several classifications based on clinical features and patterns of inheritance (Box 48-6). Clinically type I is the most common, with wide variability of bone fragility; some affected family members have significant deformity and disability, but others lead agile, active lives. Type II variants are the most severe and are considered lethal in infancy. Type III OI is characterized by multiple fractures; bone deformity; and severe disability, including scoliosis and vertebral compression; affected individuals rarely live to 30 years of age. Growth failure and short stature are common. Type IV is similar to type I with blue or white sclerae. Another variant, or type V, has been described in which those affected have a hyperplastic callus, a radiodense metaphyseal band, and calcification of the interosseous membrane of the forearm; no collagen mutations are noted in this group (Marini, 2011). A type VI has been described with a characteristic mineralization defect, which does not respond to pamidronate therapy as do types I to V (Land, Rauch, Travers, et al., 2007). However, a small group of children with type VI responded favorably to denosumab, a RANK ligand inhibitor (Semler, Netzer, Hoyer-Kuhn, et al., 2012). Children affected with this type have no dental involvement and normal sclerae; a bone biopsy is the only way to establish a diagnosis because of the similarities to other types. Types VII and VIII overlap types II and III in relation to clinical features; but these types who survive have white sclerae, a normal-to-small head circumference, short stature, and rhizomelia (Marini, 2011).

Therapeutic Management

The treatment for OI is primarily supportive, although patients and families are optimistic about new research advances. The use of bisphosphonate therapy with IV pamidronate to promote increased bone density and prevent fractures has become standard therapy for many children with OI; however, long bones are weakened by prolonged treatment. One of the advantages of bisphosphonate therapy is the decrease in vertebral compression and scoliosis (Marini, 2011).

The goals of a rehabilitative approach to management are directed toward preventing (1) positional contractures and deformities, (2) muscle weakness and osteoporosis, and (3) malalignment of lower-extremity joints prohibiting weight bearing.

Lightweight braces and splints help support limbs, prevent fractures, and aid in ambulation. Physical therapy helps prevent disuse osteoporosis and strengthens muscles, which in turn improve bone density.

Surgery is sometimes used to help treat the manifestations of the disease. Surgical techniques are used to correct deformities that interfere with bracing, standing, or walking. For a child with

---

BOX 48-6   CLASSIFICATION OF OSTEOGENESIS IMPERFECTA†

Type I*

A—Mild bone fragility; blue sclerae; normal teeth; hearing loss (occurs between ages 20 and 30 years); autosomal dominant inheritance

B—Same as A except dentinogenesis imperfecta instead of normal teeth

C—Same as B but no bone fragility

Type II—Lethal; stillborn or die in early infancy; severe bone fragility; multiple fractures at birth; 10% of cases of OI; autosomal recessive inheritance

Type III—Severe bone fragility leading to severe progressive deformities; normal sclerae; marked growth failure; most autosomal recessive inheritance; few autosomal dominant inheritance

Type IV

A—Mild-to-moderate bone fragility; normal sclerae; normal teeth; short stature; variable deformity; autosomal dominant inheritance

B—Same as A except dentinogenesis imperfecta instead of normal teeth; approximately 6% of cases of OI

Type V—Clinically similar to type IV; hyperplastic callus; collagen mutation negative

Type VI—Sclerae and dentition normal; moderate-to-severe bone fragility; diagnosis by bone biopsy because of similarities to other types (Land, Rauch, Travers, et al., 2007)

Types VII and VIII (recessive form)—Clinically overlap types II and III but have white sclerae, rhizomelia, and small-to-normal head circumference; severe osteochondroplasia and short stature in survivors (Marini, 2011)

OI, Osteogenesis imperfecta.

*Two thirds of cases are type I.

†This classification is based on that proposed by Sillence DO, Senn A, Danks DM: Genetic heterogeneity in osteogenesis imperfecta, *J Med Genet* 16(2):101-116, 1979; which originally included OI type I-IV. Additional types have been described but are not included herein.

recurrent fractures, inserting an intramedullary rod provides stability to bones.

CARE MANAGEMENT

Infants and children with this disorder require careful handling to prevent fractures. They must be supported when they are being turned, positioned, moved, and held. Even changing a diaper may cause a fracture in severely affected infants. These children should never be held by the ankles when being diapered but should be gently lifted by the buttocks or supported with pillows.

Both parents and the affected child need education regarding the child's limitations and guidelines in planning suitable activities that promote optimal development and protect the child from harm. Realistic occupational planning and genetic counseling are part of the long-term goals of care. Educational materials and information can be obtained from the Osteogenesis Imperfecta Foundation,* which also has a network that can put a family in contact with other families with a similar problem.

OI is a differential diagnosis that must be ruled out in the event of multiple fractures that could be attributed to nonaccidental injury (child abuse). A detailed history, no evidence of associated soft-tissue injury, and the presence of other symptoms related to OI help to determine the diagnosis.

> ### ! NURSING ALERT
>
> Children with multiple fractures should be screened for OI. The possibility that nonaccidental trauma is the cause of fractures in children must be evaluated carefully by a multidisciplinary team.

ACQUIRED DEFECTS

Legg-Calvé-Perthes Disease

Legg-Calvé-Perthes disease, sometimes called *coxa plana* or *osteochondritis deformans juvenilis*, is a self-limiting disorder in which there is aseptic necrosis of the femoral head. The disease affects children ages 2 to 12 years, but most cases occur in boys between 4 and 8 years of age as an isolated event. In approximately 10% of cases the involvement is bilateral; most of the affected children have a skeletal age significantly below their chronologic age (Sankar, Horn, Wells, et al., 2011b). The male-to-female ratio is 4:1 or 5:1. Caucasian children are affected 10 times more frequently than African-American children.

Pathophysiology

The cause of the disease is unknown, but a disturbance of circulation to the femoral capital epiphysis produces an ischemic aseptic necrosis of the femoral head. During middle childhood circulation to the femoral epiphysis is more tenuous than at other ages and can become obstructed by trauma, inflammation, coagulation defects, and a variety of other causes. The pathologic events seem to take place in four stages (Box 48-7). The entire process may encompass as little as 18 months or continue for several years. The reformed femoral head may be severely altered or appear entirely normal.

Clinical Manifestations and Diagnostic Evaluation

The onset of Legg-Calvé-Perthes disease is usually insidious, and the history may reveal only intermittent appearance of a limp on the

*804 W. Diamond Ave., Suite 210, Gaithersburg, MD 20878, 800-981-2663, www.oif.org.

affected side or a symptom complex, including hip soreness, ache, or stiffness, which can be constant or intermittent. The parents may report seeing the child limping, and the limp becomes more pronounced with increased activity. The pain may be experienced in the hip, along the entire thigh, or in the vicinity of the knee joint. The pain and limp are usually most evident on arising and at the end of a long day of activities. The pain is usually accompanied by joint dysfunction and limited range of motion. There may be a vague history of trauma. The diagnosis is established by history, examination, radiographs, and rarely MRI.

Therapeutic Management

Because deformity occurs early in the disease process, the aims of treatment are to eliminate hip instability; restore and maintain adequate range of hip motion; prevent capital femoral epiphyseal collapse, extrusion, or subluxation; and ensure a well-rounded femoral head at the time of healing. Treatment varies according to the child's age at the time of diagnosis and the appearance of the femoral head vasculature and position within the acetabulum. Nonsurgical containment of the femoral head may be accomplished with abduction casts, immobilization, and NSAIDs; and a pelvic or proximal femoral osteotomy may be used to contain the femoral head. Activity causes microfractures of the soft ischemic epiphysis, which tend to induce synovitis, stiffness, and adductor contracture. The initial therapy is rest and nonweight bearing, which helps reduce inflammation and restore motion. Later active motion is encouraged. In some cases traction is applied to stretch tight adductor muscles.

Containment can be accomplished in several ways. One is the use of nonweight-bearing devices such as an abduction brace (e.g., Atlanta Scottish Rite orthosis), leg casts, or a leather harness sling, which prevent weight bearing on the affected limb. Another includes the use of various weight-bearing appliances such as abduction-ambulation braces or casts after a period of bed rest and traction. A third option consists of surgical reconstruction and containment procedures. Conservative therapy must be continued for 2 to 4 years, although braces constructed from lightweight materials allow the child to maintain a nearly normal activity level. Although surgical correction subjects the child to additional risks (e.g., from anesthesia, infection, blood transfusion), it returns him or her to normal activities in 3 to 4 months. The use of home traction has also been explored.

> ### BOX 48-7 RADIOGRAPHIC STAGES OF LEGG-CALVÉ-PERTHES DISEASE
>
> **Stage I: initial** or **avascular stage**—Aseptic necrosis or infarction of the capital femoral epiphysis with degenerative changes producing flattening of the upper surface of the femoral head
>
> **Stage II: fragmentation** or **revascularization stage**—Capital bone resorption and revascularization with fragmentation (vascular resorption of the epiphysis) that gives a mottled appearance on radiographs
>
> **Stage III: reossification** or **reparative stage**—New bone formation, which is represented on radiographs as calcification and ossification or increased density in the areas of radiolucency. This filling-in process appears to take place from the periphery of the head centrally
>
> **Stage IV: residual** or **regenerative stage**—Gradual reformation of the head of the femur without radiolucency and, it is hoped, to a spherical form

Another surgical option is hip resurfacing; in this procedure the hip joint is replaced with a metal cup in the acetabulum that interfaces with a capped bearing located on the femoral head. Hip resurfacing decreases the risk of dislocation and is more bone conserving than hip arthroplasty (Costa, Johnson, Naziri, et al., 2011). Total hip arthroplasty may be offered to adolescents and young adults with Legg-Calvé-Perthes when other surgical methods have failed to provide a stable hip joint or when conditions such as femoral acetabular impingement or avascular necrosis are present (Shrader, 2012).

The disease is self-limiting, but the ultimate outcome of therapy depends on early and efficient treatment and the child's age at the onset of the disorder. Younger children (5 years and younger) whose epiphyses are more cartilaginous have the best prognosis for complete recovery. Children 10 years and older have a significant risk for degenerative arthritis, especially with femoral head deformity at the time of diagnosis. The later the diagnosis is made, the more femoral damage will have occurred before treatment is implemented. In most cases, with good patient compliance with the prescribed regimen, the prognosis is excellent.

CARE MANAGEMENT

Nurses may be the first health care providers to identify affected children and refer them for medical evaluation. They are also people on whom the child and the family can rely to help them understand and adjust to the therapeutic measures. Because most of the child's care is conducted on an outpatient basis, the major emphasis of nursing care is teaching the family the care and management of the corrective appliance selected for therapy. The family must learn the purpose, function, application, and care of the corrective device and the importance of compliance to achieve the desired outcome (see Family-Centered Care).

One of the most difficult aspects associated with the disorder is coping with a normally active child who feels well but must remain relatively inactive during periods when nonweight bearing is required. Suitable activities must be devised to meet the needs of a child in the process of developing a sense of initiative or industry. Activities that meet the creative urges are well received.

👪 FAMILY-CENTERED CARE

Legg-Calvé–Perthes Disease

A family with five healthy children was one day startled to learn that their 2-year-old son could no longer walk. He was diagnosed with Legg-Calvé-Perthes disease. Through several years of prosthetic devices and numerous physician visits, hospitalizations, and surgeries, this family turned a potentially devastating experience into one with cherished memories.

Today the parents reflect on how their family coped with the reality of a debilitating disease. It was difficult for the parents to observe an eager, energetic child watch other children riding bicycles, running, or playing outdoor games. But they are warmed by memories of watching their other children make the difference for their sibling. They all developed a strong bond through caring and sharing with one another. Coping as a family was an easy adjustment and, most of all, therapeutic. Today, more than 20 years later, the parents believe that each family member has grown with feelings of faith and trust. The experience proved to them that life will go on and that life is what you make it!

—Shona Swenson Lenss, MS, RN, FNP
Cheyenne, WY

Slipped Capital Femoral Epiphysis

Slipped capital femoral epiphysis (SCFE) refers to the spontaneous displacement of the proximal femoral epiphysis in a posterior and inferior direction. It develops most frequently shortly before or during accelerated growth and the onset of puberty (children between the ages of 9 and 16 years; median age 13 years for boys and 12 years for girls) and is most frequently observed in boys and obese children. The incidence is 11 cases per 100,000 children. Bilateral involvement occurs in up to 40% to 60% of cases (Lehmann, Aarons, Loder, et al., 2006; Sankar, Horn, Wells, et al., 2011c).

Pathophysiology

Most cases of SCFE are idiopathic, although it can be associated with endocrine disorders, growth hormone therapy, renal osteodystrophy, and radiotherapy. The cause of idiopathic SCFE is multifactorial and includes obesity, physeal architecture and orientation, and pubertal hormone changes that affect physeal strength. Although obesity stresses the physeal plate, SCFE can also occur in children who are not obese. Radiographs show medial displacement of the epiphysis and uncovered upper portion of the femoral neck adjacent to the physis. There is a widened growth plate and irregular metaphysis. The capital femoral epiphysis remains in the acetabulum, but the femoral neck slips, deforming the femoral head and stretching blood vessels to the epiphysis.

Diagnostic Evaluation

The disorder is suspected when an adolescent or preadolescent displays clinical signs or complains of hip, groin, thigh, or knee pain (Box 48-8). The diagnosis is confirmed by anteroposterior and frog-leg radiographic examination that reflects a change in position of the proximal femoral epiphysis.

Therapeutic Management

The treatment goals of SCFE are to (1) prevent further slipping until physeal closure, (2) avoid further complication such as avascular necrosis, and (3) maintain adequate hip function (Loder, 2006; Sankar, Horn, Wells, et al., 2011c). After the diagnosis has been established, the child should be nonweight bearing to prevent further slippage. Some surgeons prefer to take the child to surgery within 24 hours of the onset of acute symptoms and avoid further risk for avascular necrosis (Loder, 2006). Surgical treatment varies with the degree of displacement. Surgical pinning in situ involves the placement of a single pin or multiple pins and screws through the femoral neck into the proximal femoral epiphysis to prevent further slippage. An osteotomy for deformity is seldom needed in the acute setting. Hip arthroscopy performed before in situ pinning has been shown to be effective in decreasing hip pain and allowing

BOX 48-8 CLINICAL MANIFESTATIONS OF SLIPPED CAPITAL FEMORAL EPIPHYSIS

- Limp on affected side
- Pain in hip
  - Continuous or intermittent
  - Frequently referred to groin, anteromedial aspect of thigh, or knee
- Restricted internal rotation on adduction with external rotation deformity
- Loss of abduction and internal rotation as severity increases
- Shortening of lower extremity

early hip movement in some children with SCFE (Jayakumar, Ramachandran, Youm, et al., 2012). Total hip arthroplasty may also be used in adolescents and young adults (Shrader, 2012). Postsurgical care includes nonweight bearing with crutch ambulation until acceptable, painless range of motion is achieved. SCFE is an emergency and requires early diagnosis and treatment to increase the likelihood of an acceptable outcome.

CARE MANAGEMENT

Nursing care is the same as that for a child in a cast or in traction, as discussed earlier in this chapter. Postoperative care involves hemodynamic stabilization and assessment for complications.

> ## ! NURSING ALERT
>
> Children with hip issues such as Legg-Calvé-Perthes or SCFE often present with groin, thigh, or knee pain. This is often because of referred pain and is anatomically related to the obturator nerve. Any time a child presents with groin, thigh, or knee pain, a complete hip examination is paramount to rule out underlying hip pathology.

Kyphosis and Lordosis

The spine, consisting of numerous segments, can acquire deformity curves of three types, kyphosis, lordosis, and scoliosis (Fig. 48-15). Kyphosis is an abnormally increased lateral angulation in the convex curvature of the spine (see Fig. 48-15, *B*). It can occur secondary to disease processes such as tuberculosis (TB), chronic arthritis, osteodystrophy, or compression fractures of the thoracic spine. The most common form of kyphosis is postural. Children are prone to exaggeration of a normal kyphosis, especially when skeletal growth outpaces growth of muscle. They assume abnormal sitting and standing positions. *Scheuermann kyphosis* is a thoracic curve greater than 45 degrees with wedging greater than 5 degrees of at least three adjacent vertebral bodies and vertebral irregularity.

Postural (flexible) kyphosis is almost always accompanied by a compensatory postural lordosis (i.e., an abnormally exaggerated concave lumbar curvature). Treatment of kyphosis consists of exercises to strengthen shoulder and abdominal muscles and bracing for more marked deformity. With adolescents who are self-conscious about their appearance, the best approach is to emphasize the cosmetic value of corrective therapy and place the responsibility on the adolescent for carrying out an exercise program at home with regular visits to and assessments by a therapist. Treatment with a brace may be indicated until skeletal maturity, and surgical fusion may be considered for severe, painful, or progressive thoracic curves such as Scheuermann kyphosis.

Lordosis is an accentuation of the cervical or lumbar curvature beyond physiologic limits (see Fig. 48-15, *C*). It may be a secondary complication of a disease process, a result of trauma, or idiopathic. It is often seen in association with flexion contractures of the hip, scoliosis, obesity, DDH, and SCFE. During the pubertal growth spurt lordosis of varying degrees is observed in teenagers, especially girls. In obese children the weight of the abdominal fat alters the center of gravity, causing a compensatory lordosis. Unlike kyphosis, severe lordosis is usually accompanied by pain.

Treatment involves management of the predisposing cause (e.g., weight loss and correction of deformities) when possible. Postural exercises or support garments are helpful in relieving symptoms in some cases; however, these do not usually effect a permanent cure.

Idiopathic Scoliosis

Idiopathic *scoliosis* is a complex spinal deformity in three planes, usually involving lateral curvature, spinal rotation causing rib asymmetry, and thoracic hypokyphosis. It is the most common spinal deformity and can be further classified according to age of onset: infantile, at birth or up to 3 years of age; childhood or juvenile, which develops during childhood (4 to 10 years); or most commonly adolescent (diagnosed at age 10 years or later), which develops during the growth spurt of early adolescence.

Scoliosis can be caused by a number of conditions and may occur alone or in association with other diseases, particularly neuromuscular conditions. However, in most cases there is no apparent cause; hence the name *idiopathic scoliosis*. There appears to be a genetic component to the etiology of idiopathic scoliosis;

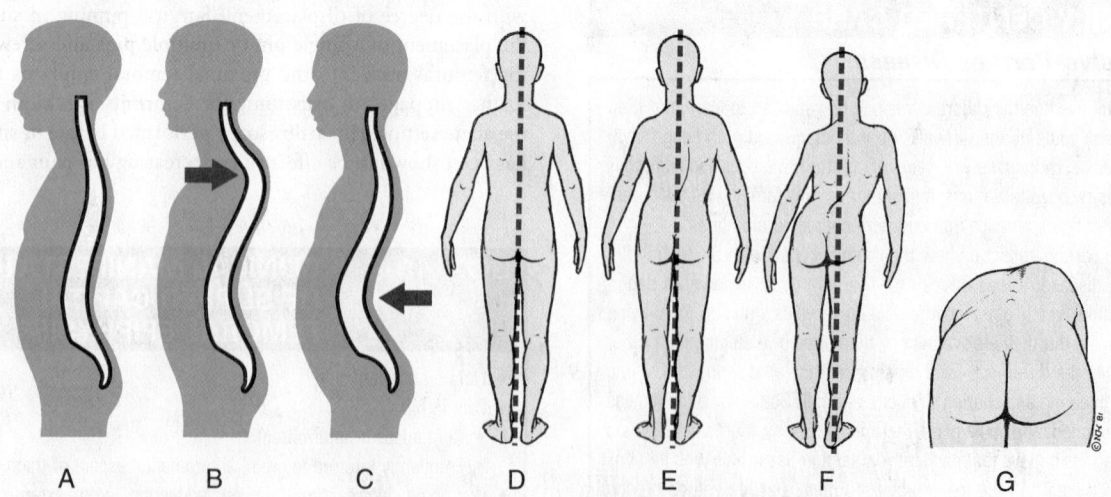

FIG 48-15 Spinal column curvatures. **A,** Normal spine. **B,** Kyphosis. **C,** Lordosis. **D,** Normal spine in balance. **E,** Mild scoliosis in balance. **F,** Severe scoliosis not in balance. **G,** Rib hump and flank asymmetry seen in flexion caused by rotary component. (Redrawn from Hilt NE, Schmitt EW: *Pediatric orthopedic nursing*, St Louis, 1975, Mosby.)

however, the exact relationship has yet to be established. The following section is limited to a discussion of adolescent idiopathic scoliosis.

Idiopathic scoliosis is most noticeable during the preadolescent growth spurt. Parents frequently bring a child for follow-up on an abnormal school scoliosis screening or because of ill-fitting clothes such as poorly fitting slacks. School screening is somewhat controversial because no controlled studies have demonstrated improved outcomes, and a reported number of false-positive results lead to referrals. The American Academy of Orthopaedic Surgeons and the AAP published a joint statement favoring scoliosis screening for preadolescents and adolescents either in the school, health care provider's office, or nurses' clinic (Richards and Vitale, 2008). According to the American Academy of Orthopaedic Surgeons (Richards and Vitale, 2008), girls should be screened at ages 10 and 12 years, and boys should be screened once at either age 13 or 14 years. The benefits of early detection, referral, and medical treatment are considered to be significant, but the people performing the screenings must be educated in the detection of spinal deformity.

Diagnostic Evaluation

Observation is performed behind an undressed (in undergarments), standing child, noting shoulder height, scapular or flank shape, and hip height and alignment. When the child bends forward at the waist (the Adams forward bend test) with hanging arms, asymmetry of the ribs and flanks may be noted. A scoliometer is also used in the initial screening to measure the angle of truncal rotation. Often a primary and a compensatory curve place the head in alignment with the gluteal cleft. However, in the uncompensated curve the head and hips are not aligned (see Fig. 48-15, *E* and *F*). (See Spine, Chapter 29, for additional information.) Definitive diagnosis is made by radiographs of the child in the standing position and use of the Cobb technique that establishes the degree of curvature. The Risser scale is used to evaluate skeletal maturity on the radiographs; the scale helps to make a determination of the likely progression of the spinal angulature based on growth potential. Radiographic curves need to measure at least 10 degrees for diagnosis. Curves of less than 25 degrees are mild and require observation during growth.

> **! NURSING ALERT**
>
> Intraspinal conditions or other disease processes that can cause scoliosis must be ruled out. The presence of pain, sacral dimpling or hairy patches, cutaneous vascular changes, absent or abnormal reflexes, bowel or bladder incontinence, or left thoracic curve may indicate an intraspinal abnormality such as syringomyelia, diastematomyelia, or tethered cord syndrome. An MRI scan should be obtained for evaluation.

Therapeutic Management

Current management options include observation with regular clinical and radiographic evaluation, orthotic intervention (bracing), and surgical spinal fusion. Treatment decisions are based on the magnitude, location, and type of curve; the child's age and skeletal maturity; and any underlying or contributing disease process.

Bracing and Exercise. For many curves in growing children and adolescents, bracing may be the treatment of choice. It is important to understand that *bracing is not curative* but that it may slow the progression of the curvature to allow skeletal growth and maturity. The two most common types of bracing are (1) the Boston and Wilmington braces, which are underarm orthoses customized from prefabricated plastic shells, with corrective forces for each patient using lateral pads and decreasing lumbar lordosis; and (2) a TLSO (thoracolumbosacral orthosis), which is an underarm orthosis made of plastic that is custom molded to the body and then shaped to correct or hold the deformity (Fig. 48-16). The Milwaukee brace, or CTLSO (cervical thoracolumbosacral orthosis), which is an individually adapted brace that includes a neck ring, is rarely used in scoliosis but is sometimes used in the treatment of kyphosis. The Charleston nighttime bending brace is worn only when the child is in bed because it prevents walking because of the severity of the trunk bend. Compliance in wearing the brace is difficult because of the child's age and preoccupation with body image and appearance. Bracing is the standard treatment for moderate curvatures in growing children (Sponseller, 2011).

Exercises, transcutaneous electrical stimulation, and chiropractic treatment are rarely of value for managing scoliosis. Exercises are beneficial when used in conjunction with bracing to maintain and strengthen spinal and abdominal muscles during treatment.

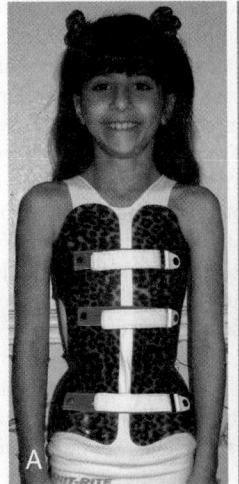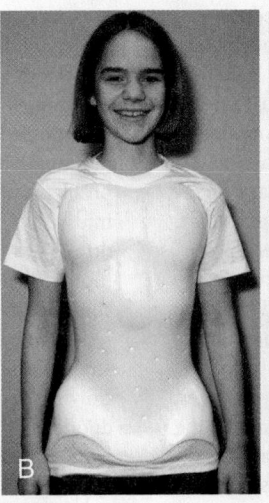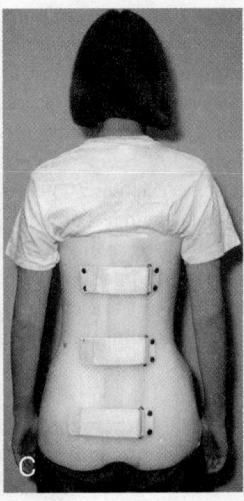

FIG 48-16 A, Standard thoracolumbosacral orthosis (TLSO) brace for idiopathic scoliosis. Note the color and design incorporated into the brace to make it more acceptable to children and adolescents. **B,** Variation of a standard TLSO that fastens in the back **(C)** to provide needed support for the spine curvature.

Surgical Management. Surgical intervention may be required for treatment of severe curves, which are typically greater than 45 degrees. The degree of curvature, its behavior, the etiology, and the symptoms guide the decision for surgery. Bracing is ineffective in managing curves greater than 45 degrees. Progressive curves that do not respond to bracing and progressive congenital and neuromuscular curves require surgical intervention.

The surgical technique of spinal fusion consists of realignment with internal fixation and instrumentation combined with bony fusion (*arthrodesis*) of the realigned spine. Bone from the iliac crest or donor bone is used to fuse the spine. The goals of surgical intervention are to improve the curvatures on the sagittal and coronal planes and have a solid, pain-free fusion in a well-balanced torso, with maximum mobility of the remaining spinal segments. Surgical approaches may be posterior, anterior, or both.

Many instrumentation systems are available, including Dwyer, Zielke, Luque, Cotrel-Dubousset, Isola, TSRH (Texas Scottish Rite Hospital), and Moss Miami. Selection of the system is individualized according to the patient's needs and surgeon's preference. Combinations of rods, hooks, wires, and pedicle screws may be used.

The Luque-rod segmental spinal instrumentation provides segmental stability with the use of wires and L-shaped rods. By way of a posterior approach, the wires are threaded beneath the lamina of each vertebra and tightened around the rods resting along the transverse processes to stabilize the spine. The advantage of this method is that the patient can be mobile within a few days and requires no postoperative immobilization. A higher risk of nerve damage has been reported.

The Cotrel-Dubousset instrumentation is a newer generation of spinal instrumentation and implements bilateral rods and hooks at many sites. Anterior approaches using the Dwyer or Zielke instrumentation involve screws into the vertebral bodies connected by a cable or rod. These systems require postoperative immobilization with a custom-fitted plastic jacket.

CARE MANAGEMENT

Treatment for scoliosis extends over a significant portion of the affected child's period of growth. In adolescents this period is the one in which their identity, both physical and psychologic, is formed. The identification of scoliosis as a "deformity," in combination with unattractive appliances and a significant surgical procedure, can have a negative effect on the already fragile adolescent body image. The adolescent and family require excellent nursing care not only for physical needs to be met but also for psychologic needs associated with the diagnosis, surgery, postoperative recovery, and eventual rehabilitation. Although adolescents with scoliosis are encouraged to participate in most peer activities, necessary therapeutic modifications are likely to make them feel different and apart. Nursing care of the adolescent who is facing scoliosis surgery, potential social isolation, pain, and uncertainty, in addition to misunderstood emotions and body image issues, must be evaluated from the adolescent's perspective to be successful in meeting the individual's needs (Napierkowski, 2007).

When a child or adolescent first faces the prospect of a prolonged period in a brace or other device, the therapy program and the nature of the device must be explained thoroughly to both the child and the parents so they understand the anticipated results, how the appliance corrects the defect, the freedoms and constraints imposed by the device, and what they can do to help achieve the desired goal. Management involves the skills and services of a team of specialists, including the orthopedist, neurosurgeon, physical therapist,

orthotist (a specialist in fitting orthopedic braces), nurse, social worker, and sometimes a thoracic or pulmonary specialist.

It is difficult for a child or adolescent to be restricted at any phase of development; but adolescents need continual positive reinforcement, encouragement, and as much independence as can be safely assumed during this time. They appreciate guidance and assistance regarding anticipated problems such as selection of clothing and participation in social activities. Socialization with peers is strongly encouraged, and every effort is expended to help the adolescent feel attractive and worthwhile.

Preoperative Care. The preoperative workup usually involves a radiographic series, including bending and traction films, pulmonary function studies, and laboratory studies (including prothrombin, partial thromboplastin, and platelet function test; blood count; electrolyte levels; urinalysis and urine culture; and blood levels of any medications). Because spinal surgery usually involves considerable blood loss, several options are considered before surgery to maintain or replace blood volume. These options include autologous blood donations obtained from the patient before the surgery; intraoperative blood salvage; intraoperative hemodilution; erythropoietin administration; and controlled induced hypotension, which must be monitored carefully at all times to prevent physiologic instability (Newton and Wenger, 2005).

Surgery for spinal fusion is complex; and often adolescents who require the procedure because of idiopathic scoliosis are not familiar with medical terms, procedures, or experiences. Preoperative teaching is critical for the adolescent to be able to cooperate and participate in his or her treatment and recovery. Because the surgery is extensive, the patient is taught how to manage his or her own patient-controlled analgesia (PCA) pump, how to log roll, and the use and function of other equipment such as a chest tube (for anterior repair) and Foley catheter. It is recommended that the child or adolescent bring a favorite toy (age dependent) or personal items such as a favorite stuffed animal, laptop computer (with Internet access), cell phone or iPod, or movie player for postoperative use. Meeting with a peer who has undergone a similar surgery may also be valuable.

Postoperative Care. After surgery patients are monitored in an acute care setting and log rolled when changing position to prevent damage to the fusion and instrumentation. Skin care is important, and pressure-relieving mattresses or beds may be needed to prevent pressure wounds (see Maintaining Healthy Skin, Chapter 39).

In addition to the usual postoperative assessments of wound, circulation, and vital signs, the neurologic status of the patient's extremities requires special attention. Prompt recognition of any neurologic impairment is imperative because delayed paralysis may develop that requires surgical intervention. Common postoperative problems after spinal fusion include neurologic or spinal cord injury, hypotension from acute blood loss, wound infection, syndrome of inappropriate antidiuretic hormone, atelectasis, pneumothorax, ileus, delayed neurologic injury, and implanted hardware complications (Freeman, 2007; Newton and Wenger, 2005). *Superior mesenteric artery syndrome* may occur several days after spinal surgery; this involves duodenal compression by the aorta and superior mesenteric artery and may result in acute partial or complete duodenal obstruction. Clinical manifestations include epigastric pain, nausea, copious vomiting, and eructation; symptoms are aggravated in the supine position and often relieved with the patient in a left lateral decubitus or prone position.

The child usually has considerable pain for the first few days after surgery and requires frequent administration of pain medication, preferably IV opioids administered on a regular schedule. For children able to understand the concept, PCA is recommended (see Pain Assessment; Pain Management, Chapter 30).

In most cases the patient begins ambulation as soon as possible, depending on the instrumentation used—generally by the second or third postoperative day. The patient is discharged by 1 week, depending on the surgical approach. In addition to pain management, she or he is evaluated for skin integrity, adequate urinary output, fluid and electrolyte balance, and ileus. Discharge planning should include a timetable for follow-up with the practitioner and resumption of regular activities.

The patient may start physical therapy as soon as he or she is able, beginning with range-of-motion exercises on the first postoperative day and many of the activities of daily living in the following days. Self-care such as washing and eating is always encouraged. Throughout the hospitalization age-appropriate activities and contact with family and friends are important parts of nursing care and planning (see The Immobilized Child, p. 1531).

The family is encouraged to become involved in the patient's care to facilitate the transition from hospital to home management. An organization that provides education and services to both families and professionals is the National Scoliosis Foundation.* The American Academy of Orthopaedic Surgeons† and Scoliosis Research Society,‡ an organization of physicians and scientists, have published an excellent book, *Scoliosis;* and the Scoliosis Research Society has educational information available on its website.

INFECTIONS OF BONES AND JOINTS

Osteomyelitis

Osteomyelitis, an infectious process in the bone, can occur at any age but most frequently is seen in children 10 years of age or younger. Boys are more commonly affected than girls, and the median age of diagnosis is 5 to 6 years of age. The limbs most commonly affected include the foot, femur, tibia, and pelvis. It is estimated that one in 5000 children younger than the age of 13 years is diagnosed each year with this condition (Zaoutis, Localio, Leckerman, et al., 2009). *Staphylococcus aureus* is the most common causative organism. Neonates are also likely to have osteomyelitis caused by group B streptococci. Children with sickle cell disease may develop osteomyelitis from *Salmonella* organisms and *S. aureus*. *Neisseria gonorrhoeae* is a potential causative organism in sexually active adolescents. *Kingella kingae* has been reported as one of the most causative organisms in children younger than age 5 years (Kaplan, 2011a).

Acute hematogenous osteomyelitis results when a bloodborne bacterium causes an infection in the bone. Common foci include infected lesions, upper respiratory tract infections, otitis media, tonsillitis, abscessed teeth, pyelonephritis, and infected burns. Exogenous osteomyelitis is acquired from direct inoculation of the bone from a puncture wound, open fracture, surgical contamination, or adjacent tissue infection. Subacute osteomyelitis has a longer course and may be caused by less virulent microbes with a walled-off abscess or Brodie abscess, typically in the proximal or distal tibia. Chronic osteomyelitis is a progression of acute osteomyelitis and is characterized by dead bone, bone loss, and drainage and sinus tracts.

Generally healthy bone is not likely to become infected. Factors that contribute to infection include inoculation with a large number

*Five Cabot Place, Stoughton, MA 02072, 800-673-6922, www.scoliosis.org.
†6300 N. River Road, Rosemont, IL 60018-4262, 847-823-7186, www.aaos.org.
‡555 E. Wells St, Suite 1100, Milwaukee, WI 53202, 414-289-9107, www.srs.org/about/contact.

BOX 48-9	CLINICAL MANIFESTATIONS OF ACUTE OSTEOMYELITIS

General Manifestations
- History of trauma to affected bone (frequent)
- Child appears very ill
- Irritability
- Elevated temperature
- Restlessness
- Rapid pulse
- Dehydration

Local Manifestations
- Tenderness
- Increased warmth
- Diffuse swelling over involved bone
- Involved extremity painful, especially on movement
- Involved extremity held in semiflexion
- Surrounding muscles tense and resistant to passive movement

of organisms, presence of a foreign body, bone injury, high virulence of an organism, immunosuppression, and malnutrition; certain types and locations of bone are also more vulnerable to infection.

Typically children with acute hematogenous osteomyelitis are seen with a 2- to 7-day history of pain, warmth, tenderness, and decreased range of motion in the affected limb along with systemic symptoms of fever, irritability, and lethargy (Box 48-9). Infants may have an adjacent joint effusion as well. Symptoms often resemble those observed in other diseases involving bones such as arthritis, leukemia, or sarcoma.

Pathophysiology

In acute osteomyelitis bacteria adhere to bone, causing a suppurative infection with inflammatory cells, edema, vascular congestion, and small-vessel thrombosis; the result is bone destruction, abscess formation, and dead bone (sequestra). Infection within the bone can rupture through the cortex into the subperiosteal space, stripping loose periosteum and forming an abscess. As dead bone is resorbed, new bone is formed along the live bone and infection borders. This surrounding sheath of live bone is called an *involucrum*. Sinus tracts from perforations in the involucrum may drain pus through soft tissue to the skin.

The pathology of osteomyelitis is different in infants, children older than 1 year of age, and adults. In infants blood vessels cross the growth plate into the epiphysis and joint space, which allows infection to spread into the joint. In children the infection is contained by the growth plate, and joint infection is less likely (unless the infection is intracapsular). In older adolescents (with a closed growth plate) the infection is poorly contained, and the joint is compromised. Adult periosteum is attached to bone; consequently rupture through the periosteum and sinus drainage are more common in adults.

Diagnostic Evaluation

Organism identification and antibiotic susceptibility testing are essential for effective therapy. Cultures of aspirated purulent drainage along with cultures of blood, joint fluid, and infected skin samples should be obtained. Bone biopsy is indicated if blood culture results and radiographic findings are not consistent with osteomyelitis. Supporting evidence for osteomyelitis includes leukocytosis and elevated erythrocyte sedimentation rate (ESR) and

C-reactive protein (CRP). Radiographic signs, except for soft-tissue swelling, are evident only after 2 to 3 weeks. A three-phase technetium bone scan can show areas of increased blood flow such as occurs in early stages in infected bone and is useful in locating multiple sites; however, it is not a diagnostic test. CT can detect bone destruction, and MRI provides anatomic details useful in delineating the area of involvement, especially if surgical intervention is planned. MRI is reported to be the most sensitive diagnostic radiologic tool for diagnosing osteomyelitis (Kaplan, 2011a). Sometimes the osteomyelitis may be unrecognized if it occurs as a complication of a severe toxic and debilitating disease. Neonates may not present with clinical manifestations other than limited mobility of the affected extremity; fever may or may not be present, and the neonate may not appear to be sick (Kaplan, 2011a).

Therapeutic Management

After culture specimens are obtained, empiric therapy is started with IV antibiotics covering the mostly likely organisms. For *S. aureus* nafcillin or clindamycin is generally used. Consideration should be given to the increased rates of *community-acquired methicillin-resistant S. aureus (CA-MRSA)* in the selection of first-line antibiotic therapy; MRSA may require vancomycin, or in some cases clindamycin may be appropriate. In one study children with MRSA osteomyelitis had an increased length of hospitalization, longer antibiotic course, and a greater number of complications (Saavedra-Lozano, Mejías, Ahmad, et al., 2008). When the infectious agent is identified, administration of the appropriate antibiotic is initiated and continued for at least 3 to 4 weeks; but the length of therapy is determined by the duration of the symptoms, the response to treatment, and the sensitivity of the organism; 6 weeks to 4 months may be required in some cases (Kaplan, 2011a). In selected cases oral antibiotic therapy may follow the IV treatment. Because of the prolonged duration of high-dose antibiotic therapy, it is important to monitor for hematologic, renal, hepatic, ototoxic, and other potential side effects. To prevent antibiotic-associated diarrhea in some children, administration of a probiotic may be considered.

Surgery may be indicated if there is no response to specific antibiotic therapy, a penetrating injury, persistent soft-tissue abscess is seen, or the infection spreads to the joint. Opinions differ regarding surgical intervention, but many advocate sequestrectomy and surgical drainage to decompress the metaphyseal space before purulent fluid erupts and spreads to the subperiosteal space, forming abscesses that strip the periosteum from bone or form draining sinuses. When these complications occur, a chronic infection usually persists, which may require antibiotic therapy for several months.

CARE MANAGEMENT

During the acute phase of illness movement of the affected limb causes discomfort; therefore the child is positioned comfortably with the affected limb supported. A temporary splint or cast may be applied. Weight bearing is avoided in the acute phase, and moving and turning are carried out carefully to minimize pain. The child may require long-term pain medication to deal with the bone pain. After surgery pain medication should be considered as with any other surgical procedure.

Antibiotic therapy requires careful observation and monitoring of the IV equipment and site. A peripherally inserted central catheter (PICC) may be inserted for long-term antibiotic therapy. Antibiotic therapy is often continued at home or through an outpatient infusion clinic.

Standard Precautions are implemented for all children with osteomyelitis. If there is an open wound, it is managed according to standard wound care precautions. If a PICC line or central venous catheter (CVC) is inserted, meticulous care should be taken to prevent catheter-related infection.

Providing diversional and constructive activities becomes an important nursing intervention. Children are usually confined to bed for some time during the acute phase but may be allowed to move about on a stretcher or in a wheelchair if isolation is not necessary.

As the infection subsides, physical therapy is instituted to ensure restoration of optimum function. The child may eventually be transitioned to a regimen of oral antibiotics, and progress is followed closely for some time.

Septic Arthritis

Septic arthritis is a bacterial infection in the joint. It usually results from hematogenous spread or direct extension of an adjacent cellulitis or osteomyelitis. Direct inoculation from trauma accounts for 15% to 20% of septic arthritis cases. The most common causative organism is *S. aureus*. Community-acquired MRSA is commonly a cause of septic arthritis. In addition to *S. aureus*, pathogens seen in neonates include group B streptococci, *Escherichia coli*, and *Candida albicans*. In children 2 months to 5 years of age, *S. aureus*, *Streptococcus pyogenes*, *Streptococcus pneumoniae*, and *K. kingae* are the primary organisms causing infection. Children older than 5 years are more likely to be infected by *S. aureus* and *S. pyogenes*, and sexually active adolescents may be infected by *N. gonorrhoeae* (Gutierrez, 2005; Kaplan, 2011b).

The knees, hips, ankles, and elbows are the most common joints affected. Clinical manifestations include severe joint pain, swelling, warmth of overlying tissue, and occasionally erythema. However, an infection involving the hip is considered a surgical emergency to prevent compromised blood supply to the head of the femur (Kaplan, 2011b).

The child is resistant to any joint movement. Features of systemic illness such as fever, malaise, headache, nausea, vomiting, and irritability may also be present.

THERAPEUTIC MANAGEMENT AND CARE MANAGEMENT

The affected joint is aspirated; and the specimen evaluated by Gram stain, cultures (including separate cultures for *Haemophilus influenzae* and *N. gonorrhoeae*), and determination of leukocyte count. In addition, blood cultures are performed, and a complete blood count with differential and ESR or CRP level is obtained. Early radiographic findings are limited to soft-tissue swelling but may reveal a foreign body, and such films always provide a baseline for comparison. Technetium scans reveal areas of increased blood flow but do not differentiate between sites. MRI and CT scans provide more detailed images of cartilage loss, joint narrowing, erosions, and ankylosis of progressive disease. Ultrasonography is helpful in the detection of joint effusions and fluid in the soft tissue and subperiosteum (Kaplan, 2011b).

Treatment is IV antibiotic therapy based on Gram stain results and the clinical presentation. The benefits of serial aspirations to demonstrate sterility of synovium fluid and reduce pressure or pain are controversial. Pain management is an important aspect of nursing care, particularly with involvement of a large joint such as the hip. Surgical intervention may also be required if there was a penetrating wound or a foreign object was possibly involved.

Physical therapy may be initiated for the child who is immobilized to prevent flexion contractures. Additional nursing care is the same as for osteomyelitis.

Skeletal Tuberculosis

In children tubercular infection of the bones and joints is acquired by lymphohematogenous spread at the time of primary infection. Occasionally it is from chronic pulmonary TB. Skeletal tubercular infection is not common in the United States but should be considered in communities with high TB case rates. The condition is a late manifestation of TB and is most likely to involve the vertebrae, causing tubercular spondylitis. If the infection is progressive, it causes Pott disease with destruction of the vertebral bodies and results in kyphosis and spinal malalignment. Symptoms are insidious. The child may report persistent or intermittent pain. Other findings include joint swelling and stiffness; fever and weight loss are not common. Tubercular arthritis can also affect single joints such as a knee or hip and tends to cause severe destruction of adjacent bone. Infection in the fingers causes spina ventosa, a tuberculous dactylitis.

As with pulmonary TB, the index case should be located. A family and environmental history needs to be obtained, and tuberculin skin tests (TSTs) performed. Results of TSTs are positive for the majority of children with tuberculous arthritis; however, the results are not diagnostic, and the clinical and laboratory features do not differentiate tubercular arthritis from a nontubercular septic arthritis. Diagnosis requires isolation of *Mycobacterium tuberculosis* from the site. Patients with the susceptible organism start treatment with combined antituberculosis chemotherapy (isoniazid, rifampin, and pyrazinamide); directly observed therapy (DOT) is preferred. (See also Chapter 40.)

CARE MANAGEMENT

Nursing care depends on the site and extent of infection. Tuberculous spondylitis and hip infection may require immobilization, casting, and surgical fusion. Nursing care is individualized but is generally the same as for osteomyelitis and septic arthritis.

BONE AND SOFT-TISSUE TUMORS

General Concepts: Bone Tumors

Bone tumors account for approximately 6% of all malignant neoplasms in children. Approximately 90% of all primary malignant bone tumors in children are either osteogenic sarcoma or Ewing sarcoma; osteosarcoma, the most common, occurs in 56% of all cases. The peak age for pediatric bone tumors is 15 years, and they occur more often in boys.

Most malignant bone tumors produce localized pain in the affected site, which may be severe or dull and may be attributed to trauma or the vague complaint of "growing pains." The pain is often relieved by a flexed position, which relaxes the muscles overlying the stretched periosteum. Frequently it draws attention when the child limps, curtails physical activity, or is unable to hold heavy objects (Box 48-10). A palpable mass is also a common manifestation of bone tumors, but systemic symptoms such as fever and other clinical symptoms such as spinal cord compression and respiratory distress are more frequent in patients with Ewing sarcoma.

Diagnostic Evaluation

Diagnosis begins with a thorough history and physical examination. A primary objective is to rule out causes such as trauma or infection.

BOX 48-10	**CLINICAL MANIFESTATIONS OF BONE TUMORS**

- Pain localized at affected site
  - May be severe or dull
  - Often relieved by position of flexion
- Frequently brought to attention when child:
  - Limps
  - Curtails own physical activity
  - Is unable to hold heavy objects

Careful questioning regarding pain is essential in attempting to determine the duration and rate of tumor growth. Physical assessment focuses on functional status of the affected area; signs of inflammation; size of the mass; and any systemic indication of generalized malignancy such as anemia, weight loss, and frequent infection.

Definitive diagnosis is based on radiologic studies such as plain films and CT or MRI of the primary site, CT of the chest, and radioisotope bone scans to evaluate metastasis and bone marrow examination in patients with Ewing sarcoma. A needle or surgical biopsy is necessary to establish the diagnosis. Ewing sarcoma most commonly involves the pelvis, long bones of the lower extremities, and chest wall and radiographically involves the diaphysis with detachment of the periosteum from the bone (Codman triangle). In osteosarcoma lesions are most commonly located in the metaphyseal region of the bone, often involving the long bones. Radial ossification in the soft tissue gives the tumor a "sunburst" appearance on plain radiograph.

Osteosarcoma

Osteosarcoma (osteogenic sarcoma) is the most common bone cancer in children and most commonly affects patients in the second decade of life during their growth spurt. It presumably arises from bone-forming mesenchyme, which gives rise to malignant osteoid tissue. Most primary tumor sites are in the diametaphyseal region (wider part of the shaft, adjacent to the epiphyseal growth plate) of long bones, especially in the lower extremities. More than half occur in the femur, particularly the distal portion, with the rest involving the humerus, tibia, pelvis, jaw, and phalanges.

Therapeutic Management

Optimum treatment of osteosarcoma includes surgery and chemotherapy. The surgical approach consists of surgical biopsy followed by either *limb salvage* or amputation. To ensure local control, all gross and microscopic tumors must be resected. A limb salvage procedure involves en bloc resection of the primary tumor with prosthetic replacement of the involved bone. For example, with osteosarcoma of the distal femur, a total femur and joint replacement are performed. Frequently children undergoing a limb salvage procedure receive preoperative chemotherapy in an attempt to decrease the tumor size and make surgery more manageable (Gorlick, Bielack, Teot, et al., 2011; Lanzkowsky, 2010).

Chemotherapy plays a vital role in treatment of osteosarcoma. Antineoplastic drugs such as high-dose methotrexate with citrovorum factor rescue, doxorubicin, cisplatin, ifosfamide, and etoposide may be administered singly or in combination and may be used either before or after surgical resection of the tumor. The use of postoperative chemotherapy after amputation has comparable results to trials using preoperative chemotherapy followed by limb salvage surgery. Preoperative chemotherapy allows for examination of the surgical specimen at the time of definitive surgery, which predicts clinical outcome. When pulmonary metastases are found, thoracotomy and chemotherapy have resulted in prolonged survival and potential cure. These combined-modality approaches have significantly improved the prognosis in osteosarcoma to approximately 78% for nonmetastatic patients (Lanzkowsky, 2010). Ongoing trials are evaluating the use of muramyl tripeptide phosphatidylethanolamine (Mifamurtide) to eradicate micrometastases by stimulating macrophages to kill tumor cells not eliminated by chemotherapy (Lanzkowsky, 2010). This drug has been used successfully in patients with nonmetastatic osteosarcoma (Anderson, Tomaras, and McConnell, 2010).

CARE MANAGEMENT

Nursing care depends on the type of surgical approach. Obviously the family may have more difficulty adjusting to an amputation than a limb salvage procedure. In either instance preparation of the child and family is critical. Straightforward honesty is essential in gaining the child's cooperation and trust. The diagnosis of cancer should not be disguised with falsehoods such as "infection." To accept the need for radical surgery, the child must be aware of the lack of alternatives for treatment. Although the responsibility of telling the child is generally left to the physician, the nurse should be present at the discussion or be aware of exactly what is said. The child should be told a few days before surgery to allow him or her time to think about the diagnosis and consequent treatment and ask questions. (See Nursing Care Plan: The Child with a Bone Tumor.*)

Sometimes children have many questions about the prosthesis, limitations on physical ability, and prognosis in terms of cure. At other times they react with silence or a calm manner that belies their concern and fear. Either response must be accepted because it is part of the grieving process of a loss. For those who desire information, it may be helpful to introduce them to another person who has had an amputation before surgery or to show them pictures of the prosthesis.† However, the nurse must be careful not to overwhelm children with information. A sound approach is to answer questions without offering additional information. For those who do not pursue additional information, the nurse expresses a willingness to talk.

The child is also informed of the need for chemotherapy and its side effects before surgery. Exercise caution about offering too much information at one time. When discussing hair loss, emphasize positive aspects such as wearing a wig. Because bone tumors affect adolescents and young adults, it is not unusual for them to become angry over all of the radical body alterations.

If an amputation is performed, the child is usually fitted with a temporary prosthesis immediately after surgery, which permits early functioning and fosters psychologic adjustment. If this is not done, the child requires stump care, which is the same as for any person with an amputation. A permanent prosthesis is usually fitted within 6 to 8 weeks. During hospitalization the child begins physical therapy to become proficient in the use and care of the device.

Phantom limb pain may develop after amputation. This symptom is characterized by sensations such as tingling, itching, and more frequently pain felt in the amputated limb. The child and family need to know that the sensations are real, not imagined. Amitriptyline (Elavil) has been used successfully in children to decrease the pain. In addition, an epidural is often used before surgery as a nerve block in an effort to decrease or eliminate the occurrence of phantom limb pain. Much research is needed to further delineate the best care for these patients (Ong, Arneja, and Ong, 2006).

Discharge planning must begin early in the postoperative period. After the child has begun physical therapy, the nurse should consult with the therapist and practitioner to evaluate his or her physical and emotional readiness to reenter school. It is an opportune time to involve a community nurse in the child's home care. Every effort is made to promote normalcy and gradual resumption of realistic preamputation activities.* Role-playing in anticipation of such experiences is beneficial in preparing the child for the inevitable confrontation by others. Environmental barriers such as stairs are assessed in terms of the accessibility in the school and home, especially because the child may need to use crutches or a wheelchair before complete healing and prosthetic competency are achieved.

The nurse encourages the child to select clothing that best camouflages the prosthesis such as pants or long-sleeved shirts. Well-fitted prostheses are so natural looking that girls can usually wear sheer stockings without revealing the device. Emphasizing feminine or masculine apparel helps the child regain a feeling of self-identity. Even during the postoperative period, encouraging the child to wear blue jeans and a T-shirt may distract attention from the deformity and focus it on familiar aspects of appearance.

The family and child need much support in adjusting not only to a life-threatening diagnosis but also to alteration in body form and function. Because loss of a limb entails a grieving process, those caring for the child need to recognize that the reactions of anger and depression are normal and necessary. Often parents view the anger as a direct affront to them for allowing the amputation to occur, or they see the depression as rejection. These are not personal attacks but the child's attempts to cope with a loss.

Ewing Sarcoma (Primitive Neuroectodermal Tumor)

Ewing sarcomas, or the Ewing sarcoma family of tumors, which includes primitive neuroectodermal tumor of the bone, are the second most common malignant bone tumor (after osteosarcoma) in childhood (Lanzkowsky, 2010). Ewing sarcoma arises in the marrow spaces of the bone rather than from osseous tissue. The tumor originates in the shaft of long and trunk bones, most often affecting the pelvis, femur, tibia, fibula, humerus, ulna, vertebra, scapula, ribs, and skull. It occurs almost exclusively in individuals younger than age 30 and affects Caucasians much more often than other races.

Therapeutic Management

Limb salvage procedures might be feasible in extremity lesions, and amputation may be considered if the results of radiotherapy render the extremity useless or deformed (e.g., from restricted growth in young children). The treatment of choice for the majority of lesions is involved field radiotherapy and chemotherapy. A widely used drug regimen includes vincristine, doxorubicin, cyclophosphamide alternating with ifosfamide, and etoposide. The addition of ifosfamide and etoposide has increased the 3-year survival rate to 78% for patients with localized disease (Lanzkowsky, 2010).

---

*In Wilson D, Hockenberry MJ: *Wong's clinical manual of pediatric nursing,* ed 8, St Louis, 2012, Mosby.

†Information about prostheses can be obtained from the National Amputation Foundation, 40 Church St, Malverne, NY 11565, 516-887-3600, www.nationalamputation.org.

---

*Information about special programs for children with amputations is available from the Candlelighters Childhood Cancer Foundation, 8323 Southwest Freeway, Suite 435, Houston, TX 77074, 713-270-4700, www.candle.org.

CARE MANAGEMENT

The psychologic adjustment to Ewing sarcoma is typically less traumatic than it is to osteosarcoma because of the preservation of the affected limb. Many families accept the diagnosis with a sense of relief in knowing that this type of bone cancer does not necessitate amputation, and initially they may not be aware of the damaging effects on the irradiated site. Consequently they need preparation for the various diagnostic tests, including bone marrow aspiration and surgical biopsy, and adequate explanation of the treatment regimen. High-dose radiotherapy often causes a skin reaction of dry or moist desquamation followed by hyperpigmentation. The child should wear loose-fitting clothes over the irradiated area to minimize additional skin irritation. Because of increased sensitivity, the area should be protected from sunlight and sudden changes in temperature such as from heating pads or ice packs. Encourage the child to use the extremity as tolerated. Occasionally the physical therapist may plan an active exercise program to preserve maximum function.

The child needs the same considerations for adjusting to the effects of chemotherapy as any other patient with cancer. The drug regimen usually results in hair loss, severe nausea and vomiting, peripheral neuropathy, and possibly cardiotoxicity. Make every effort to outline a treatment plan that allows the child maximum resumption of a normal lifestyle and activities. (See Nursing Care Plan: The Child with Cancer.*)

Rhabdomyosarcoma

Rhabdomyosarcoma (*rhabdo*, striated) is the most common soft-tissue sarcoma in children. Striated (skeletal) muscle is found almost anywhere in the body; thus these tumors occur in many sites, the most common of which are the head and neck, especially the orbit. The disease occurs in children in all age-groups but is most common in children younger than 5 years of age. Its incidence is approximately 8.5 per 1 million for Caucasian children but only 4 per 1 million for African-American children in the age-group from 2 to 19 years (Lanzkowsky, 2010).

Rhabdomyosarcoma arises from embryonic mesenchyme. Three subtypes are recognized: embryonal, alveolar, and pleomorphic. Soft-tissue sarcomas are the fourth most common type of solid tumors in children. These malignant neoplasms originate from undifferentiated mesenchymal cells in muscles, tendons, bursae, and fascia or in fibrous, connective, lymphatic, or vascular tissue. They derive their name from the specific tissue(s) of origin such as myosarcoma (*myo*, muscle).

The initial signs and symptoms are related to the site of the tumor and compression of adjacent organs (Table 48-2). Some tumor locations such as the orbit manifest early in the course of the illness. Other tumors such as those of the retroperitoneal area only produce symptoms when they are relatively large and compress adjacent organs. Unfortunately many of the signs and symptoms attributable to rhabdomyosarcoma are vague and frequently suggest a common childhood illness such as "earache" or "runny nose." In rare instances the site of the primary tumor site is never identified.

Diagnostic Evaluation

Diagnosis begins with a careful history and physical examination. Radiographic studies to delineate the primary tumor site should

---

*In Wilson D, Hockenberry MJ: *Wong's clinical manual of pediatric nursing*, ed 8, St Louis, 2012, Mosby.

TABLE 48-2	CLINICAL MANIFESTATIONS OF RHABDOMYOSARCOMA ACCORDING TO TUMOR SITE
LOCATION	**SIGNS AND SYMPTOMS**
Orbit	Rapidly developing unilateral proptosis Ecchymosis of conjunctiva Loss of extraocular movements (strabismus)
Nasopharynx	Stuffy nose (earliest sign) Nasal obstruction—dysphagia, nasal voice (obstruction of posterior nasal conches), otitis media with effusion (obstruction of eustachian tube) Pain (sore throat and ear) Epistaxis Palpable neck nodes Visible mass in oropharynx (late sign)
Paranasal sinuses	Nasal obstruction Local pain Discharge Sinusitis Swelling
Middle ear	Signs of chronic serous otitis media with effusion (OME) Pain Sanguinopurulent drainage Facial nerve palsy
Retroperitoneal area (usually a "silent" tumor)	Abdominal mass Pain Signs of intestinal or genitourinary obstruction
Perineum	Visible superficial mass Bowel or bladder dysfunction (from tumor compression)

BOX 48-11	STAGING OF RHABDOMYOSARCOMA

Group I—Localized disease; tumor completely resected, and regional nodes not involved
Group II—Localized disease with microscopic residual, or regional disease with no residual or with microscopic residual
Group III—Incomplete resection or biopsy with gross residual disease
Group IV—Metastatic disease present at diagnosis

include CT or MRI. Metastatic evaluation should include a CT of the chest, bone scan, and bilateral bone marrow aspirates and biopsies. For patients with tumors in the parameningeal area, a lumbar puncture should be done to examine the spinal fluid. When possible, an excisional biopsy or surgical resection of the tumor is done to confirm the diagnosis.

Careful staging is extremely important for planning treatment and determining the prognosis. The Intergroup Rhabdomyosarcoma Study has developed a surgicopathologic staging system, shown in Box 48-11 (Helman, 2011; Lanzkowsky, 2010).

With the use of contemporary multimodal therapy, more than 80% of patients with nonmetastatic disease are expected to survive

(Helman, 2011; Lanzkowsky, 2010). If relapse occurs, the prognosis for long-term survival is poor.

Therapeutic Management

All rhabdomyosarcomas are high-grade tumors with the potential for metastases. Therefore multimodal therapy is recommended for all patients. Complete removal of the primary tumor is advocated whenever possible. However, because the tumor is chemosensitive, radical procedures with high morbidity should be avoided. In most cases a biopsy is followed by chemotherapy, irradiation, or both. Patients with embryonal tumors and group I disease can be treated with chemotherapy alone, but all others require chemotherapy and radiotherapy. Drugs that are used most often for the treatment of rhabdomyosarcoma include vincristine, actinomycin D, cyclophosphamide (VAC); ifosfamide; topotecan; irinotecan; and doxorubicin, which are administered for about 1 year (Lanzkowsky, 2010).

CARE MANAGEMENT

The nursing responsibilities are similar to those for other types of cancer, especially the solid tumors when surgery is used. Specific objectives include (1) careful assessment for signs of the tumor, especially during well-child examinations; (2) preparation of the child and family for the multiple diagnostic tests; and (3) supportive care during each stage of multimodal therapy (see also Chapter 43).

DISORDERS OF JOINTS

Juvenile Idiopathic Arthritis

Juvenile idiopathic arthritis (JIA) is a new name replacing *juvenile rheumatoid arthritis (JRA)* in the research literature and now in clinical practice. The JRA nomenclature revision to JIA was partly attributable to the minimally applicable reference to "rheumatoid" in JRA. Only a small percentage of children have a positive rheumatoid factor, yet the name burdens the family with images of adult disfiguring rheumatoid arthritis, a distinctly different disease. Furthermore the JRA classification system focused more on disease at onset versus disease progression, which is more important.

Semantics aside, JIA is a chronic autoimmune inflammatory disease causing inflammation of joints and other tissue with an unknown cause. It starts before age 16, with a peak onset between 1 and 3 years of age. Twice as many girls as boys are affected. The reported incidence of chronic childhood arthritis varies from one to 20 cases per 100,000 children with a prevalence of 10 to 400 per 100,000 (Cassidy and Petty, 2011). The cause is unknown, but two factors are hypothesized: immunogenic susceptibility and an environmental or external trigger such as a virus (e.g., rubella, Epstein-Barr virus, parvovirus B19). There are a few known genetic risk factors, including HLA class I and class II genes, the *PTPN22* gene, and the *IL2RA/CD 25* gene; however, the genetic contribution is complicated and still not well understood.

Pathophysiology

The disease process is characterized by chronic inflammation of the synovium with joint effusion and eventual erosion, destruction, and fibrosis of the articular cartilage. Adhesions between joint surfaces and ankylosis of joints occur if the inflammatory process persists.

Clinical Manifestations

The outcome of JIA is variable and unpredictable. Even in severe forms the disease is rarely life threatening but can cause significant disability. The arthritis tends to wax and wane; however, patterns of clinical remission indicate that approximately 25% will obtain clinical remission off medication for a follow-up duration of at least 4 years. Children with arthritis in four or fewer joints had the greatest likelihood for a sustained remission. Children with extensive arthritis and a positive rheumatoid factor were less likely to have a sustained remission (Wallace, Huang, and Bandeira, 2005). Their arthritis can cause significant joint deformity and functional disability, requiring medication, physical therapy, and perhaps future joint replacement. Chronic and acute uveitis can cause permanent vision loss if undiagnosed and not aggressively treated.

Classification of Juvenile Idiopathic Arthritis

JIA is not a single disease but a heterogeneous group of diseases. The universal Durban classification of JIA, revised and published in 1998, lists several disease categories, each with its own set of criteria and exclusions, which continue to be revised (Petty, Southwood, Manners, et al., 2004):

- *Systemic arthritis* is arthritis in one or more joints associated with at least 2 weeks of quotidian fever, rash, lymphadenopathy, hepatosplenomegaly, and serositis.
- *Oligoarthritis* is arthritis in one to four joints for the first 6 months of disease. It is subdivided to *persistent oligoarthritis* if it remains in four joints or fewer or becomes *extended oligoarthritis* if it involves more than four joints after 6 months.
- *Polyarthritis rheumatoid factor negative* affects five or more joints in the first 6 months with a negative rheumatoid factor.
- *Polyarthritis rheumatoid factor positive* also affects five or more joints in the first 6 months, but these children have a positive rheumatoid factor.
- Psoriatic arthritis is arthritis with psoriasis or an associated dactylitis, nail pitting, or onycholysis or psoriasis in a first-degree relative.
- *Enthesitis-related arthritis* is arthritis or enthesitis associated with at least two of the following: sacroiliac or lumbosacral pain, HLA-B27 antigen, arthritis in a boy older than 6 years, acute anterior uveitis, inflammatory bowel disease, Reiter syndrome, or acute anterior uveitis in a first-degree relative.
- *Undifferentiated arthritis* fits none of the previous categories or fits more than one category.

Diagnostic Evaluation

JIA is a diagnosis of exclusion; there are no definitive tests. Classifications are based on the clinical criteria of age of onset before age 16 years, arthritis in one or more joints for 6 weeks or longer, and exclusion of other causes. Laboratory tests may provide supporting evidence of disease. The ESR may or may not be elevated. Leukocytosis is present frequently during exacerbations of systemic JIA. Antinuclear antibodies are common in JIA but are not specific for arthritis; however, they help identify children who are at greater risk for uveitis. Plain radiographs are the best initial imaging studies and may show soft-tissue swelling and joint space widening from increased synovial fluid in the joint. Later films can reveal osteoporosis, narrow joint space, erosions, subluxation, and ankylosis. A slit-lamp eye examination is necessary to diagnosis uveitis (i.e., inflammation in the anterior chamber of the eye), which is most common in antinuclear antibody–positive young girls with oligoarthritis. Routine examinations are necessary for early diagnosis and treatment to avoid or minimize sight-threatening disease (Qian and Acharya, 2010).

Therapeutic Management

There is no cure for JIA. The major goals of therapy are to control pain, preserve joint range of motion and function, minimize effects of inflammation such as joint deformity, and promote normal growth and development. Outpatient care is the mainstay of therapy; lengthy hospitalizations are infrequent in this era of managed care. The treatment plan can be exhaustive and intrusive for the child and family, including medications, physical and occupational therapy, ophthalmologic slit-lamp examinations, splints, comfort measures, dietary management, school modifications, and psychosocial support.

Medications. Many arthritis medications are available, and most are effective in suppressing the inflammatory process and relieving pain. These drugs may be given alone or in combination and are prescribed in a stepwise manner dependent on arthritis severity.

NSAIDs are the first drugs used. Naproxen, ibuprofen, tolmetin, indomethacin, celecoxib, meloxicam, and aspirin are approved for use in children. They are effective with few common side effects other than gastrointestinal irritation and bruising; with naproxen skin fragility is a possible side effect. NSAIDs must be taken with food. Aspirin, once the drug of choice, has been replaced by other NSAIDs because they have fewer side effects and easier administration schedules.

Methotrexate is the second-line medication used in children who have failed with NSAIDs alone. It is started in combination with an NSAID. It is effective, with acceptable toxicity, which requires monitoring of complete blood cell counts and liver functions. Patient education about possible side effects, including discussions with teens about birth defects and avoiding alcohol, is essential.

Corticosteroids are potent immunosuppressives used for life-threatening complications, incapacitating arthritis, and uveitis. They are administered at the lowest effective dosage for the briefest period and discontinued on a tapering schedule. They may be administered orally, as intraarticular joint injections, as IV infusions, or in eyedrop form for uveitis. A single intraarticular injection may provide effective relief for children with pauciarticular disease unresponsive to NSAIDs. Prolonged use of systemic steroids is associated with significant side effects, including Cushing syndrome, osteoporosis, increased infection risk, glucose intolerance, cataracts, and growth suppression.

Biologic agents that work by several mechanisms to interrupt and minimize the inflammatory process are used in children with severe or progressive arthritis. They may be used in combination with methotrexate. The Food and Drug Administration (FDA) has approved etanercept, adalimumab, and abatacept use in children with JIA. Etanercept is a tumor necrosis factor-α (TNF-α) receptor blocker and an effective drug for children with JIA unresponsive to methotrexate (Lovell, Giannini, Reiff, et al., 2003). It is given once or twice a week via subcutaneous injections. The long-term safety and efficacy of etanercept have been confirmed (Giannini, Ilowite, Lovell, et al., 2009; Kerensky, Gottlieb, Yaniv, et al., 2012). Adalimumab is a monoclonal antibody that also inhibits TNF, thereby reducing inflammation; it is a subcutaneous injection given every 2 weeks (Lovell, Ruperto, and Goodman, 2008). Abatacept reduces inflammation by inhibiting T cells and is given intravenously every 4 weeks. Possible side effects of biologics include an increased infection risk, rare reports of demyelinating disease and pancytopenia, and allergic reactions. Because of the infection risk, children should be evaluated for TB exposure before starting these medications. Live vaccines should be avoided while taking them. There is a reported potential increased risk of malignancy with anti-TNF agents etanercept, adalimumab, and infliximab at high doses (FDA, 2011). Parents and patients should be informed that biologic drugs are new therapies and more will be learned about potential side effects in the postmarketing period.

Physical and Occupational Therapy. Programs of physical management are individualized for each child and designed to reach the ultimate goal: preserving function or preventing deformity. Physical therapy is directed toward specific joints, focusing on strengthening muscles, mobilizing restricted joint motion, and preventing or correcting deformities. Occupational therapy assumes responsibility for generalized mobility and performance of activities of daily living.

General treatment or maintenance programs vary; physical therapists may be involved several times weekly to monthly in management of a home program; or their visits may be limited to infrequent review of the home program for compliance, effectiveness, and need. Normal activities of daily living and the child's natural tendency to be active are usually sufficient to maintain muscle strength and joint mobility.

Exercising in a pool is excellent therapy because it allows freedom of movement with support and minimal gravitational pull. If there is pain on motion, a hot pack or warm bath before therapy may help.

Practitioners may recommend nighttime splinting to help minimize pain and reduce flexion deformity. Joints most frequently splinted are the knees, wrists, and hands. Loss of extension in the knee, hip, and wrist causes special problems and requires vigilance to detect the earliest signs of involvement and vigorous attention to prevent deformity with specialized passive stretching, positioning, and resting splints.

CARE MANAGEMENT

Nursing the child with JIA involves assessment of the child's general health, the status of involved joints, and the child's emotional response to all ramifications of the disease (i.e., discomfort, physical restrictions, therapies, and self-concept) (see Nursing Care Plan).

The effects of JIA are manifest in every aspect of the child's life, including physical activities, social experiences, and personality development. Nursing interventions to support the parents may foster successful adaptation for the entire family. Parental concerns about the disease prognosis, financial and insurance issues, spouse and sibling relationships, and job and schedule conflicts must all be addressed. Referral to social workers, counselors, or support groups may be needed.

Relieve Pain. The pain of JIA is related to several aspects of the disease, including disease severity, functional status, individual pain threshold, family variables, and psychologic adjustment. The aim is to provide as much relief as possible with medication and other therapies to help children tolerate the pain and cope as effectively as possible. Nonpharmacologic modalities such as behavioral therapy and relaxation techniques have proved effective in modifying pain perception (see Pain Management, Chapter 30) and activities that aggravate pain. Opioid analgesics typically are avoided in juvenile arthritis; however, for children immobilized with refractory pain, short-term opioid analgesics can be part of a comprehensive plan that uses multiple pain-relief techniques (Connelly and Schanberg, 2006).

Promote General Health. The child's general health must be considered. A well-balanced diet with sufficient calories to maintain growth is essential. If the child is relatively inactive, caloric intake needs to match energy needs to avoid excessive weight gain, which places additional stress on affected joints. Sleep and rest are essential for children with JIA. Some children require rest during

NURSING CARE PLAN

The Child with Arthritis

NURSING DIAGNOSIS	EXPECTED OUTCOME	NURSING INTERVENTIONS	RATIONALE
Chronic Pain related to joint inflammation	Child is able to move (joints) and complete activities of daily living with no or minimal discomfort.	Use pain-rating scale to evaluate pain (discomfort) level	To provide objective assessment of pain level
Child's/Family's Defining Characteristics (Subjective and Objective Data)		Administer antiinflammatory medications (nonsteroidal antiinflammatory drugs [NSAIDs]) promptly on report of pain and around the clock when discomfort is acute	To manage pain and prevent breakthrough pain
Verbal report of pain		Administer other drugs such as methotrexate or biologic agents such as etanercept	To provide relief from inflammation
Guarding behavior			
Change in sleep pattern		Schedule routine rest periods throughout the day	
		Encourage child to eat a well-balanced diet and exercise daily	To prevent obesity and promote wellness
		Help child set up a routine of daily exercise	To prevent further joint stiffness
		Encourage nonpharmacologic pain-relief remedies such as use of heat pad, moist heat, and pool therapy	To promote mobility of joints and relieve painful stiff joints
			To prevent excessive weight gain
		Encourage child to discuss effect of pain on lifestyle and activities	To provide outlet for emotions such as anger, frustration, depression at having a chronic illness
Impaired Physical Mobility related to pain and swelling in joints	Child engages in activities of daily living.	Encourage ambulation and performance of activities of daily living to maximum potential every day	To keep joints limber and prevent disuse contractures
Child's/Family's Defining Characteristics (Subjective and Objective Data)		Assist with range-of-motion exercises for child who is severely limited	To promote muscle movement and keep joints limber
Limited ability to perform fine and gross motor skills		Encourage child to be as active as tolerated	To promote independence
		Help with planning and encourage rest periods during the day	To prevent fatigue
Limited range of motion		Encourage taking pain medication such as NSAIDs before ambulation and activity	To promote activity with minimum pain
Verbal report of pain		Use nonpharmacologic pain adjuncts such as heat pad and hydrotherapy	To decrease pain and encourage mobility of joints
Measurable pain on pain scale		Encourage child to be active in self-care activities to maximum potential	To enhance self-worth and independence

the day; however, daytime napping that interferes with nighttime sleepiness should be avoided. A bedtime routine that involves comfort measures can help induce sleep. A firm mattress, electric blanket, or sleeping bag helps provide warmth, comfort, and rest. Nighttime splints needed to maintain range of motion initially might be a source of bedtime conflict. The family needs to be instructed on how to use the splint appropriately; it should not be painful or impede sleep. Behavior modification programs that reward splint and exercise compliance may be helpful in reducing adherence barriers. Well-child care to assess growth, development, and immunization requirements needs to be coordinated between the primary care provider and the rheumatologist. Common childhood illnesses such as upper respiratory tract infections may cause arthritis to worsen; consequently medical attention must be sought quickly for relatively minor illness to prevent arthritis flares. Effective communication among the family, the primary care provider, and the rheumatology team is essential for care coordination.

Children are encouraged to attend school even on days when they have some pain or discomfort. The school nurse's assistance is enlisted so a child is permitted to take the prescribed medication at school and arrange for rest in the nurse's office during the day. Split days or half days may help a child remain involved in school. Permitting the child to come to school late allows time to gain joint movement and reduces the time at school to avoid exhaustion. It is important that the child attend school to learn skills and engage in social interaction, especially if the JIA continues to limit physical skills. Arranging for two sets of textbooks eliminates the need to carry books to and from school, thus reducing discomfort and difficulty walking. A formal school hearing may be necessary to obtain an Individualized Education Program, ensured by public law, which includes intensive school modifications.

Facilitate Adherence. The child and family are involved in the therapeutic plan. They need to know the purpose and correct use of any splints and appliances and the medication regimen. The family is instructed regarding administration of medications and the value of a regular schedule of administration to maintain a satisfactory drug level in the body. They need to know that NSAIDs should not be given on an empty stomach and to be alert for signs of medication toxicity. If evidence of drug toxicity is noted, the family is instructed to notify the health care provider and follow that person's instructions.

Encourage Heat and Exercise. Heat has been shown to be beneficial to children with arthritis. Moist heat is best for relieving pain and stiffness, and the most efficient and practical method is in the bathtub with warm water. In some cases a daily whirlpool bath, paraffin bath, or hot packs may be used as needed for temporary relief of acute swelling and pain. Hot packs are easily applied using a bath towel wrung out after being immersed in hot water or heated in a microwave oven, applied to the area, and covered with plastic for 20 minutes. Commercial pads that warm in only a few minutes in the microwave are also available. Painful hands or feet can be immersed in a pan of warm water for 10 minutes 2 or 3 times daily in addition to tub baths.

Pool therapy is the easiest method for exercising a large number of joints. Swimming activities strengthen muscles and maintain mobility in larger joints. Very small children who are frightened of the water can carry out their exercises in the bathtub. Small children love to splash, kick, and throw things in the water. Remember that adult supervision is necessary for all water activities.

Activities of daily living provide satisfactory exercise for older children to maintain maximal mobility with minimal pain. These children are encouraged in their efforts to be independent and patiently allowed to dress and groom themselves, assume daily tasks, and care for their belongings. It is often difficult for children to manipulate buttons, comb or brush their hair, and turn faucets; but, unless there is an acute flare, parents and other caregivers should not offer assistance. In addition, children should learn and understand why others do not help them. Many helpful devices such as self-adhering fasteners, tongs for manipulating difficult items, and grab bars installed in bathrooms for safety can be used to facilitate tasks. A raised (higher) toilet seat often makes the difference between dependent and independent toileting because weak quadriceps muscles and sore knees inhibit the ability to raise the body from a low sitting position.

A child's natural affinity for play offers many opportunities for incorporating therapeutic exercises. Throwing or kicking a ball and riding a tricycle (with the seat raised to achieve maximum leg extension) are excellent moving and stretching exercises for a very young child whose daily living activities are physically limited.

An effective approach to beginning the day's activities is to awaken children early to give them their medication and then to allow them to sleep for an hour. On arising children take a hot bath (or shower) and perform a simple ritual of limbering-up exercises, after which they commence the activities of the day such as going to school. Exercise, heat, and rest are spaced throughout the remainder of the day according to the child's individual needs and schedules. Parents are instructed in exercises that meet the child's needs.

The Arthritis Foundation and the American Juvenile Arthritis Alliance* (an organization within the Arthritis Foundation) provide information and services for both parents and professionals, and nurses can refer families to these agencies as an added resource.

Support Child and Family. JIA affects every aspect of life for the child and family. Physical limitations may interfere with self-care, school participation, and recreational activities. The intensive treatment plan, including multiple medications, physical therapy, comfort measures, and medical appointments, is intrusive and

disruptive to the parents' work schedule and the family routine. To prevent isolation and foster independence, the family is encouraged to pursue their normal activities. Unfortunately the adaptations necessary to make that occur take resourcefulness and commitment from all family members. At diagnosis and throughout the span of JIA it is essential to recognize signs of stress and counterproductive coping and provide the necessary support to maximize adaptation. The problems and needs of these families are discussed in Chapter 36, and readers are directed to that chapter for guidance in planning care.

Systemic Lupus Erythematosus

Systemic lupus erythematosus (SLE) is a chronic, multisystem, autoimmune disease of the connective tissues and blood vessels characterized by inflammation in potentially any body tissue. Its course and symptoms are variable and unpredictable, with mild to life-threatening complications. In addition to SLE, there are other forms of lupus such as *neonatal lupus,* which occurs when maternal autoantibodies cross the placenta and cause transient lupuslike symptoms in a newborn, with the potential serious complication of heart block. The remaining discussion focuses on SLE.

A recent review of the Indianapolis Pediatric Rheumatology Disease Registry indicates that survival rates in children with SLE have improved significantly; 5-year survival rates were 99.6%, and 10-year survival rates are 98.2% (Hashkes, Wright, Lauer, et al., 2010). SLE is more common in females, with an approximate 5 : 1 female-to-male ratio before puberty and a 9 : 1 ratio during reproductive years; it typically occurs between the ages of 10 and 19 years and rarely before the age of 5, however, some cases may be diagnosed in infancy (Ardoin and Schanberg, 2011; Zulian, Pluchinotta, Martini, et al., 2008). There is a familial tendency, although many newly diagnosed patients are unaware of other affected family members. SLE has been reported in all cultures, but within the United States there has been a disproportionately higher incidence in African-American, Asian, and Hispanic children.

The cause of SLE is not known. It appears to result from a complex interaction of genetics with an unidentified trigger that activates the disease. Suspected triggers include exposure to ultraviolet light, estrogen, pregnancy, infections, and drugs. Genetic predisposition to SLE is evidenced in an increased concordance rate in twins (10-fold), increased incidence within family members (10% to 16%), and increased frequency of certain gene alleles in population-based studies.

Clinical Manifestations and Diagnostic Evaluation

The child with SLE may have any clinical manifestation with mild to life-threatening severity (Box 48-12). The diagnosis is established when four of the 11 diagnostic criteria are met (Box 48-13). Kidney involvement heralds progressive disease and the need for rigorous therapeutic management.

Therapeutic Management

The goal of treatment is to ensure the child's health by balancing the medications necessary to avoid exacerbation and complications while preventing or minimizing treatment-associated morbidity. Therapy involves the use of specific medications and general supportive care. The drugs used to control inflammation are corticosteroids administered in doses sufficient to control inflammation and then tapered to the lowest suppressive dose. Other drugs include antimalarial preparations, which are useful for rash and arthritis; NSAIDs, which relieve muscle and joint inflammation; and immunosuppressive agents such as cyclophosphamide for renal and CNS

---

*PO Box 7669, Atlanta, GA 30357, 800-283-7800, www.arthritis.org. In Canada: The Arthritis Society, 393 University Ave., Suite 1700, Toronto, Ontario, Canada M5G 1E6, 416-979-7228, fax: 416-979-8366, www.arthritis.ca.

> ### BOX 48-12   CLINICAL MANIFESTATIONS OF SYSTEMIC LUPUS ERYTHEMATOSUS RELATED TO TISSUES INVOLVED
>
> **Constitutional**—Fever, fatigue, weight loss, anorexia
>
> **Cutaneous**—Erythematous butterfly rash over bridge of nose and across cheeks, discoid rash, photosensitivity, mucocutaneous ulceration, alopecia, periungual telangiectasias
>
> **Musculoskeletal**—Arthritis, arthralgia, myositis, myalgia, tenosynovitis
>
> **Neurologic**—Headache, seizure, forgetfulness, behavior change, change in school performance, psychosis, chorea, stroke, cranial and peripheral neuropathy, pseudotumor cerebri
>
> **Pulmonary and cardiac**—Pleuritis, basilar pneumonitis, atelectasis, pericarditis, myocarditis, endocarditis
>
> **Renal**—Glomerulonephritis, nephrotic syndrome, hypertension
>
> **Gastrointestinal**—Abdominal pain, nausea, vomiting, blood in stool, abdominal crisis, esophageal dysfunction, colitis
>
> **Hepatic, splenic, and nodal**—Hepatomegaly, splenomegaly, lymphadenopathy
>
> **Hematologic**—Anemia, cytopenia
>
> **Ophthalmologic**—Cotton wool spots, papilledema, retinopathy
>
> **Vascular**—Raynaud's phenomenon, thrombophlebitis, livedo reticularis

> ### BOX 48-13   CLASSIFICATION CRITERIA FOR SYSTEMIC LUPUS ERYTHEMATOSUS
>
> Four of the following 11 criteria must be met for diagnosis:
> 1. Malar rash—Fixed malar erythema
> 2. Discoid rash—Patchy erythematous lesions
> 3. Photosensitivity—Rash with sun exposure
> 4. Oral ulcers—Painless ulcers in mouth, nose
> 5. Arthritis—Swelling, tenderness, or effusion in two or more peripheral joints (nonerosive)
> 6. Serositis—Pleuritis, pericarditis
> 7. Renal disorder—Proteinuria, casts
> 8. Neurologic disorder—Psychosis, seizures
> 9. Hematologic disorder—Hemolytic anemia, thrombocytopenia, leukopenia, lymphopenia
> 10. Immunologic disorder—Anti-dsDNA, anti-SM, antiphospholipid antibodies, lupus anticoagulant, false-positive syphilis test (RPR [rapid plasma reagin])
> 11. Antinuclear antibody

disease. Mycophenolate, azathioprine, and methotrexate are effective immunosuppressive drugs that may be used to control SLE and allow steroids to be reduced. Antihypertensives, aspirin, and antibiotics are just a few of the additional drugs that may be necessary to treat or avoid complications.

General supportive care includes sufficient nutrition, sleep and rest, and exercise. Exposure to the sun and ultraviolet B (UVB) light is limited because of its association with SLE exacerbation.

CARE MANAGEMENT

The principal nursing goal is to help the child and family positively adjust to the disease and therapy. The child and family must learn to recognize subtle signs of disease exacerbation and potential complications of medication therapy and communicate these concerns to their care provider. Consequently patient and family education is an ongoing process initiated at diagnosis and tailored to the patient's individual needs. Referral to a social worker, psychologist, or support group may help the child and family make a successful adjustment. Support groups are associated with the Lupus Foundation of America* and the Arthritis Foundation.†

Key issues include therapy compliance; body-image problems associated with rash, hair loss, and steroid therapy; school attendance; vocational activities; social relationships; sexual activity; and pregnancy. (See Chapter 36 for a discussion on adjusting to a chronic illness.) Specific instructions for avoiding exposure to the sun and UVB light such as using sunscreens, wearing sun-resistant clothing, and altering outdoor activities must be provided with great sensitivity to ensure compliance while minimizing the associated feeling of being different from peers (see Sunburn, Chapter 47). Patients need to be instructed to maintain regular medical supervision and seek attention quickly during illness or before elective surgical procedures such as dental extraction because of potential needs for increased steroids or prophylactic antibiotics. People with SLE should carry medical identification for their disease and steroid dependence.

---

*2000 L St. NW, Suite 710, Washington, DC 20036, 202-349-1155, 800-558-0121, www.lupus.org/newsite.
†PO Box 7669, Atlanta, GA 30357-0669, 800-283-7800; www.arthritis.org/index.php. In Canada the Arthritis Society may be contacted for locations of all local Canadian province offices: www.arthritis.ca.

KEY POINTS

- Immobility has a profound effect on all aspects of growth and development.
- The major physical consequences of immobilization are loss of muscle strength, endurance, and muscle mass; bone demineralization; loss of joint mobility; and contractures.
- Features of children's fractures not observed in the adult include presence of growth plate, thicker and stronger periosteum, bone porosity, more rapid healing, and less joint stiffness.
- The goals of fracture management are to regain alignment and length of bony fragments, retain alignment and length, and restore function to injured parts.
- The method of fracture reduction is determined by the child's age, degree of displacement, amount of overriding, amount of edema, condition of the skin and soft tissues, sensation, and circulation distal to the fracture.
- The primary purposes of traction are to fatigue involved muscles and reduce muscle spasm, position bone ends in desired realignment, and immobilize the fracture site until realignment has been achieved to permit casting or splinting.
- The etiology of DDH appears to be related to intrauterine, genetic, and cultural factors.
- Treatment of clubfoot consists of manipulation and casting to correct the deformity, maintenance of the correction, and prevention of possible recurrence of the deformity.
- Acquired hip deformities are managed with nonweight-bearing devices (Legg-Calvé-Perthes disease) or surgical stabilization (SCFE).

- Observation for idiopathic scoliosis is an important part of an adolescent's routine physical assessment.
- Idiopathic scoliosis is managed by observation, bracing, and exercise or surgical correction.
- Bone infections are managed with vigorous antibiotic therapy, immobilization of the affected part, and (sometimes) surgical drainage.
- Osteosarcoma is a neoplasm of bone-forming tissues; Ewing sarcoma is a neoplasm that arises from bone marrow spaces.

- Rhabdomyosarcoma may occur almost anywhere in the body, but the most common sites are the head and neck.
- Nursing care of the child with juvenile arthritis consists of promoting general health, relieving discomfort, preventing deformity, and preserving function.
- SLE is a chronic autoimmune disorder that affects the collagen tissues of the body.

REFERENCES

Aglan MS, Hosny L, El-Houssini R, et al: A scoring system for the assessment of clinical severity in osteogenesis imperfecta, *J Child Othrop* 6(1):29–35, 2012.

American Academy of Pediatrics (AAP) Committee on Quality Improvement and Subcommittee on Developmental Dysplasia of the Hip: Clinical practice guideline: early detection of developmental dysplasia of the hip, *Pediatrics* 105(4):896–905, 2000.

Anderson PM, Tomaras M, McConnell K: Mifamurtide in osteosarcoma—a practical review, *Drugs Today (Barc)* 46(5):327–337, 2010.

Ardoin SP, Schanberg LE: Systemic lupus erythematosus. In Kliegman RM, Stanton BF, St Geme JW, et al, editors: *Nelson textbook of pediatrics*, ed 19, Philadelphia, 2011, Saunders.

Babl FE, Oakley E, Seaman C, et al: High-concentration nitrous oxide for procedural sedation in children: adverse events and depth of sedation, *Pediatrics* 121(3):e528–e532, 2008.

Biber R, Gregory A: Overuse injuries in youth sports: is there such a thing as too much sports? *Pediatr Ann* 39(5):286–292, 2010.

Carrigan RB: The upper limb. In Kliegman RM, Stanton BF, St Geme JW, et al, editors: *Nelson textbook of pediatrics*, ed 19, Philadelphia, 2011, Saunders.

Cassidy JT, Petty RE: Chronic arthritis in childhood. In Cassidy JT, Petty RE, Laxer RM, et al, editors: *Textbook of pediatric rheumatology*, ed 6, Philadelphia, 2011, Saunders.

Connelly M, Schanberg L: Opioid therapy for the treatment of refractory pain in children with juvenile rheumatoid arthritis, *Natl Clin Pract Rheumatol* 2(12):636–637, 2006.

Costa CR, Johnson AJ, Naziri Q, et al: Review of total hip resurfacing and total hip arthroplasy in young patients who had Legg-Calvé-Perthes disease, *Orthop Clin North Am* 42(3):419–422, 2011.

de Hundt M, Vlemmix F, Bais JM, et al: Risk factors for developmental dysplasia of the hip: a meta-analysis, *Eur J Obstet Gynecol Reprod Biol* 165(1):8–17, 2012.

Fisher TJ, Williams SL, Levine AM: Spinal orthosis. In Browner BD, Jupiter JB, Levine AM, et al, editors: *Skeletal trauma: basic science, management, and reconstruction*, ed 4, Philadelphia, 2008, Saunders.

Food and Drug Administration: *FDA Drug Safety Communication: UPDATE on tumor necrosis factor (TNF) blockers and risk for pediatric malignancy*, 2011, Food and Drug Administration, www.fda.gov/Drugs/DrugSafety/ucm278267.htm.

Freeman BL III: Scoliosis and kyphosis. In Canale ST, Beaty JH, editors: *Campbell's operative orthopaedics*, ed 11, Philadelphia, 2007, Mosby.

Giannini EH, Ilowite NT, Lovell DJ, et al: Long-term safety and effectiveness of etanercept in children with selected categories of juvenile idiopathic arthritis, *Arthritis Rheum* 60(9):2794–2804, 2009.

Gorlick R, Bielack S, Teot L, et al: Osteosarcoma: biology, diagnosis, treatment and remaining challenges. In Pizzo PA, Poplack DG, editors: *Principles and practices of pediatric oncology*, ed 6, Philadelphia, 2011, Lippincott.

Green NE, Swiontkowski MF: *Skeletal trauma in children*, ed 4, Philadelphia, 2008, Saunders.

Gutierrez K: Bone and joint infections in children, *Pediatr Clin North Am* 52(3):779–794, 2005.

Hart ES, Albright MB, Rebello GN, et al: Developmental dysplasia of the hip: nursing implications and anticipatory guidance for parents, *Orthop Nurs* 25(2):100–109, 2006.

Hashkes PJ, Wright BM, Lauer MS, et al: Mortality outcomes in pediatric rheumatology in the US, *Arthritis Rheum* 62(2):599–608, 2010.

Helman LJ: Rhabdomyosarcoma and the undifferentiated sarcomas of childhood. In Pizzo PA, Poplack DG, editors: *Principles and practices of pediatric oncology*, ed 6, Philadelphia, 2011, Lippincott.

Holmes SB, Brown SJ: Pin Site Care Expert Panel: skeletal pin site care: National Association of Orthopaedic Nurses guidelines for orthopaedic nursing, *Orthop Nurs* 24(2):99–107, 2005.

Hosalkar HS, Spiegel DA, Davidson RS: Talipes equinovarus (clubfoot). In Kliegman RM, Stanton BF, St Geme JW, et al, editors: *Nelson textbook of pediatrics*, ed 19, Philadelphia, 2011, Saunders.

Jayakumar P, Ramachandran M, Youm T, et al: Arthroscopy of the hip for paediatric and adolescent disorders, *J Bone Joint Surg* 94(3):290–296, 2012.

Kaplan SL: Osteomyelitis. In Kliegman RM, Stanton BF, St Geme JW, et al, editors:

Nelson textbook of pediatrics, ed 19, Philadelphia, 2011a, Saunders.

Kaplan SL: Septic arthritis. In Kliegman RM, Stanton BF, St Geme JW, et al, editors: *Nelson textbook of pediatrics*, ed 19, Philadelphia, 2011b, Saunders.

Kerensky TA, Gottlieb AB, Yaniv S, et al: Etanercept: efficacy and safety for approved indication, *Expert Opin Drug Saf* 11(1):121–139, 2012.

Land C, Rauch F, Travers R, et al: Osteogenesis imperfecta type VI in childhood and adolescence: effects of cyclical intravenous pamidronate treatment, *Bone* 40(3):638–644, 2007.

Lanzkowsky P: *Manual of pediatric hematology and oncology*, ed 5, San Diego, 2010, Academic Press.

Lehmann, CL, Aarons, RR, Loder, RT, et al: The epidemiology of slipped capital femoral epiphysis: an update, *J Pediatr Orthop* 26(3) 286–290, 2006.

Loder RT: Controversies in slipped capital femoral epiphysis, *Orthop Clin North Am* 37(2):211–221, 2006.

Lovell DJ, Giannini EH, Reiff A, et al: Long-term efficacy and safety of etanercept in children with polyarticular-course juvenile rheumatoid arthritis: interim results from an ongoing multicenter, open-label, extended-treatment trial, *Arthritis Rheum* 48(1):218–226, 2003.

Lovell DJ, Ruperto N, Goodman S, et al: Adalimumab with or without methotrexate in juvenile rheumatoid arthritis, *N Engl J Med* 359(8):810–820, 2008.

Marini JC: Osteogenesis imperfect. In Kliegman RM, Stanton BF, St Geme JW, et al, editors: *Nelson textbook of pediatrics*, ed 19, Philadelphia, 2011, Saunders.

Napierkowski DB: Scoliosis: a case study in an adolescent boy, *Orthop Nurs* 26(3):147–153, 2007.

Newton PO, Wenger DR: Idiopathic scoliosis. In Morrissy RT, Weinstein SL, editors: *Lovell and Winter's pediatric orthopaedics*, Philadelphia, 2005, Williams & Wilkins.

Noonan C, Quigley S, Curley MA: Using the Braden Q Scale to predict pressure ulcer risk in pediatric patients, *J Pediatr Nurs* 26(6):566–575, 2011.

Ong BY, Arneja A, Ong EW: Effects of anesthesia on pain after lower-limb amputation, *J Clin Anesth* 18(8):600–604, 2006.

Ortiz-Neira CL, Paolucci EO, Donnon T: A meta-analysis of common risk factors associated with the diagnosis of developmental dysplasia of the hip in newborns, *Eur J Radiol* 81(3):e344–e351, 2012.

Patel DR: Stress fractures: diagnosis and management in the primary care setting, *Pediatr Clin North Am* 57(3):819–827, 2010.

Petty RE, Southwood TR, Manners P, et al: International League of Associations for Rheumatology classification of juvenile idiopathic arthritis: second revision, Edmonton, 2001, *J Rheumatol* 31(2):390–392, 2004.

Ponseti IV: *Congenital clubfoot: Fundamentals of treatment*, Oxford, 1996, Oxford University Press.

Price CT, Schwend RM: Improper swaddling a risk factor for developmental dysplasia of hip, *AAP News* 32(9):11–12, 2011.

Qian Y, Acharya NR: Juvenile idiopathic arthritis-associated uveitis, *Curr Opin Ophthalmol* 21(6):468–472, 2010.

Richards BS, Vitale MG: Screening for idiopathic scoliosis in adolescents: an information statement, *J Bone Joint Surg* 90(1):195–198, 2008.

Saavedra-Lozano J, Mejías A, Ahmad N, et al: Changing trends in acute osteomyelitis in children: impact of methicillin-resistant *Staphylococcus aureus* infections, *J Pediatr Orthop* 28(5):569–575, 2008.

Sankar WN, Horn D, Wells, L, et al: Developmental dysplasia of the hip. In Kliegman RM, Stanton BF, St Geme JW, et al, editors: *Nelson textbook of pediatrics*, ed 19, Philadelphia, 2011a, Saunders.

Sankar WN, Horn D, Wells, L, et al: Legg-Calvé-Perthes disease. In Kliegman RM, Stanton BF, St Geme JW, et al, editors: *Nelson textbook of pediatrics*, ed 19, Philadelphia, 2011b, Saunders.

Sankar WN, Horn D, Wells, L, et al: Slipped capital femoral epiphysis. In Kliegman RM, Stanton BF, St Geme JW, et al, editors: *Nelson textbook of pediatrics*, ed 19, Philadelphia, 2011c, Saunders.

Sarwark JF, editor: *Essentials of musculoskeletal care*, ed 4, Rosemont, Ill, 2010, American Academy of Orthopaedic Surgeons.

Seidel HM, Ball JW, Dains JE, et al: *Mosby's guide to physical examination*, ed 5, St Louis, 2006, Mosby.

Semler O, Netzer C, Hoyer-Kuhn H, et al: First use of the RANKL antibody denosumab in osteogenesis imperfecta type VI, *J Musculoskelet Neuronal Interact* 12(3):183–188, 2012.

Shrader MW: Total hip arthroplasty and hip resurfacing arthroplasty in the very young patient, *Orthop Clin N Am* 43(3):359–367, 2012.

Shyy W, Wang K, Sheffield VC, et al: Evaluation of embryonic and perinatal myosin gene mutations and the etiology of congenital idiopathic clubfoot, *J Pediatr Orthop* 30(3):231–234, 2010.

Sponseller PD: Bracing for adolescent idiopathic scoliosis in practice today, *J Pediatr Orthop* 31(suppl 1):S53–S60, 2011.

Stoll C, Alembik Y, Dott B, et al: Associated malformations in patients with limb reduction deficiencies, *Eur J Med Genet* 53(5):286–290, 2010.

Valovich McLeod TC, Decoster LC, Loud KJ, et al: National Athletic Trainers' Association position statement: Prevention of pediatric overuse injuries, *J Athletic Train* 46(2):206–220, 2012.

Wallace C, Huang B, Bandeira M, et al: Patterns of clinical remission in select categories of juvenile idiopathic arthritis, *Arthritis Rheum* 52(11):3554–3562, 2005.

Winsley R, Matos N: Overtraining and elite young athletes, *Med Sport Sci* 56:97–105, 2011.

Zaoutis T, Localio AR, Leckerman K, et al: Prolonged intravenous therapy versus early transition to oral antimicrobial therapy for acute osteomyelitis in children, *Pediatrics* 123(2):636–642, 2009.

Zier JL, Liu M: Safety of high-concentration nitrous oxide by nasal mask for pediatric procedural sedation: experience with 7802 cases, *Pediatr Emerg Care* 27(12):1107–1112, 2011.

Zulian F, Pluchinotta F, Martini G, et al: Severe clinical course of systemic lupus erythematosus in the first year of life, *Lupus* 17(9):780–786, 2008.

Neuromuscular or Muscular Dysfunction

David Wilson

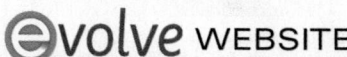

LEARNING OBJECTIVES

On completion of this chapter, the reader will be able to:

- Discuss the nursing role in helping parents care for the child with cerebral palsy.
- Formulate a nursing care plan for the preoperative and postoperative care of a child with myelomeningocele (spina bifida).
- Outline a plan of care for a child with Duchenne or Becker muscular dystrophy.

- Discuss the prevention and treatment of tetanus.
- Identify the causes of botulism in infants and children.
- List three causes of spinal cord injury in children.
- Discuss the emergent nursing care of the child or adolescent with a spinal cord injury.

CONGENITAL NEUROMUSCULAR OR MUSCULAR DISORDERS

Cerebral Palsy

Cerebral palsy (CP) has been defined as a "group of permanent disorders of the development of movement and posture, causing activity limitation, that are attributed to nonprogressive disturbances that occurred in the developing fetal or infant brain" (Rosenbaum, Paneth, Leviton, et al., 2007). In addition to motor disorders, the condition often involves disturbances of sensation, perception, communication, cognition, and behavior; secondary musculoskeletal problems; and epilepsy (Rosenbaum, Paneth, Leviton, et al., 2007). The etiology, clinical features, and course vary and are characterized by abnormal muscle tone and coordination as the primary disturbances. CP is the most common permanent physical disability of childhood, and the incidence is reported to be between 2.4 and 3.6 per every 1000 live births in the United States (Hirtz, Thurman, Gwinn-Hardy, et al., 2007; Yeargin-Allsopp, Van Naarden Braun, Doernberg, et al., 2008). Prevalence of CP among extremely low-birth-weight infants (less than 28 weeks' gestation) is said to be nearly 100 times the rate in term infants; however, these rates reportedly have declined in recent years (O'Shea, 2008).

CP is currently believed to result more often from existing prenatal brain abnormalities; the exact cause of these abnormalities remains elusive but may include genetic factors, including clotting disorders as well as brain malformations. It has been estimated that as many as 80% of CP cases are attributable to unidentified prenatal factors (Johnston, 2011; Krigger, 2006). Intrauterine exposure to maternal chorioamnionitis is associated with an increased risk for CP in infants of normal birth weight and preterm infants (Hermansen and Hermansen, 2006); however, not all term infants exposed to chorioamnionitis develop CP (Grether, Nelson, Walsh, et al., 2003; Wu, Escobar, Grether, et al., 2003). Perinatal ischemic stroke is also associated with a later diagnosis of CP (Golomb, Saha, Garg, et al., 2007). One study found a higher risk for CP occurring among infants born at 42 weeks' gestation or later than among those born at 37 or 38 weeks' gestation (Moster, Wilcox, Vollset, et al., 2010). Additional factors that may contribute to the development of CP postnatally include bacterial meningitis, multiple births, viral encephalitis, motor vehicle crashes (MVCs), and child abuse (shaken baby syndrome [traumatic brain injury]). A significant percentage (15% to 60%) of children with CP also have epilepsy. In summary, as many as 80% of the total cases of CP may be linked to a perinatal or neonatal brain lesion or brain maldevelopment, regardless of the cause (Krageloh-Mann and Cans, 2009).

Pathophysiology

It is difficult to establish a precise location of neurologic lesions on the basis of etiology or clinical signs because there is no characteristic pathologic picture. In some cases, there are gross malformations of the brain. In others, there may be evidence of vascular occlusion, atrophy, loss of neurons, and laminar degeneration that produce narrower gyri, wider sulci, and low brain weight. Anoxia appears to play the most significant role in the pathologic state of brain damage, which is often secondary to other causative mechanisms.

There are a few exceptions. In some cases, the manifestations or etiology is related to anatomic areas. For example, CP associated with preterm birth is usually spastic diplegia caused by hypoxic infarction or hemorrhage with periventricular leukomalacia in the area adjacent to the lateral ventricles. The athetoid (extrapyramidal) type of CP is most likely to be associated with birth asphyxia but can also be caused by kernicterus and metabolic genetic disorders such as mitochondrial disorders and glutaricaciduria (Johnston, 2011). Hemiplegic (hemiparetic) CP is often associated with a focal cerebral infarction (stroke) secondary to an intrauterine or perinatal thromboembolism, usually a result of maternal thrombosis or hereditary clotting disorder (Johnston, 2011). Cerebral hypoplasia and sometimes severe neonatal hypoglycemia are related to ataxic CP. Generalized cortical and cerebral atrophy often cause severe quadriparesis with cognitive impairment and microcephaly.

Clinical Classification

A revision of the Winter classification was proposed in 2005 to reflect the child's actual clinical problems and their severity, an assessment of the child's physical and quality-of-life status across time, and long-term support needs (Bax, Goldstein, Rosenbaum, et al., 2005; Nehring, 2010). The proposed new definition has four major dimensions of classification (Bax, Goldstein, Rosenbaum, et al., 2005):

Motor abnormalities—Nature and typology of the motor disorder; functional motor abilities

Associated impairments—Seizures; hearing or vision impairment; attentional, behavioral, communicative, or cognitive deficits; oral motor and speech function

Anatomic and radiologic findings—Anatomic distribution or parts of the body affected by motor impairments or limitations; radiologic findings sometimes including white matter lesions or brain anomaly noted on computed tomography (CT) or magnetic resonance imaging (MRI)

Causation and timing—Identification of a clearly identified cause such as a postnatal event (e.g., meningitis, traumatic brain injury)

Cerebral palsy has four primary types of movement disorders: spastic, dyskinetic, ataxic, and mixed (Nehring, 2010). The most common clinical type, spastic CP, represents an upper motor neuron muscular weakness (Box 49-1). The reflex arc is intact, and the characteristic physical signs are increased stretch reflexes, increased muscle tone, and (often) weakness. Early neurologic manifestations are usually generalized hypotonia or decreased tone that lasts for a few weeks or may extend for months or even as long as 1 year.

Diagnostic Evaluation

Infants at risk according to known etiologic factors associated with CP warrant careful assessment during early infancy to identify the signs of neuromotor dysfunction as soon as possible. The neurologic examination and history are the primary means for diagnosis. Neuroimaging of the child with suspected brain abnormality and CP is now recommended for diagnostic assessment, with MRI preferred to CT scan. Metabolic and genetic testing is recommended if no structural abnormality is identified by neuroimaging; laboratory tests are no longer recommended in the diagnostic process for CP.

BOX 49-1   CLINICAL CLASSIFICATION OF CEREBRAL PALSY

Spastic (Pyramidal)

- Characterized by persistent primitive reflexes, positive Babinski reflex, ankle clonus, exaggerated stretch reflexes, eventual development of contractures
  - Seventy percent to 80% of all cases of CP
  - Diplegia—All extremities affected; lower more than upper (30%-40% of spastic CP)
  - Tetraplegia—All four extremities involved: legs and trunk, mouth, pharynx, and tongue (10%-15% of spastic CP)
  - Triplegia—Three limbs involved
  - Monoplegia—Only one limb involved
  - Hemiplegia—Motor dysfunction on one side of the body; upper extremity more affected than lower (20%-30% of spastic CP)
- Other features:
  - Hypertonicity with poor control of posture, balance, and coordinated motion
  - Impairment of fine and gross motor skills

Dyskinetic (Nonspastic, Extrapyramidal)

- Athetoid—Chorea (involuntary, irregular, jerking movements); characterized by slow, wormlike, writhing movements that usually involve the extremities, trunk, neck, facial muscles, and tongue
- Dystonic—Slow, twisting movements of the trunk or extremities; abnormal posture
- Involvement of the pharyngeal, laryngeal, and oral muscles causing drooling and dysarthria (imperfect speech articulation)

Ataxic (Nonspastic, Extrapyramidal)

- Wide-based gait
- Rapid, repetitive movements performed poorly
- Disintegration of movements of the upper extremities when the child reaches for objects

Mixed Type

- Combination of spastic CP and dyskinetic CP
- May be labeled *mixed* when no specific motor pattern is dominant; however, this term is losing favor to more precise descriptions of motor function and affected area of brain involved (Rosenbaum, Paneth, Leviton, et al., 2007)

Data from Nehring W: Cerebral palsy. In Allen PJ, Vessey JA, Schapiro NA, editors: *Primary care of the child with a chronic condition*, ed 5, St Louis, 2010, Mosby; Jones MW, Morgan E, Shelton JE, et al: Cerebral palsy: introduction and diagnosis, part 1, *J Pediatr Health Care* 21(3):146–152, 2007; and National Institute of Neurologic Disorders and Stroke: *Cerebral palsy: hope through research*, 2006, www.ninds.nih.gov/disorders/cerebral_palsy/detail_cerebral_palsy.htm.
CP, Cerebral palsy.

Early recognition is made more difficult by the lack of reliable neonatal neurologic signs. However, nurses should monitor infants with known etiologic risk factors and evaluate them closely in the first 2 years of life. Because cortical control of movement does not occur until later in infancy, motor impairment associated with voluntary control is usually not apparent until after 2 to 4 months of age at the earliest. More often, the diagnosis cannot be confirmed until the age of 2 years because motor tone abnormalities may be indicative of another neuromuscular illness. In addition, some children who show signs consistent with CP before 2 years do not demonstrate such signs after 2 years (Nehring, 2010). However, there is no consensus regarding an age cut-off for the onset of symptoms. Clinical manifestations of CP at the time of diagnosis are listed in Box 49-2; early warning signs are listed in Box 49-3, but these are not considered diagnostic.

Establishing a diagnosis may be easier with the persistence of primitive reflexes: (1) either the asymmetric tonic neck reflex or persistent Moro reflex (beyond 4 months of age); and (2) the crossed extensor reflex. The tonic neck reflex normally disappears between 4 and 6 months of age. An obligatory response is considered abnormal. This is elicited by turning the infant's head to one side and holding it there for 20 seconds. When a crying infant is unable to move from the asymmetric posturing of the tonic neck reflex when crying, it is considered obligatory and an abnormal response. The crossed extensor reflex, which normally disappears by 4 months, is elicited by applying a noxious stimulus to the sole of one foot with the knee extended. Normally, the contralateral foot responds with extensor, abduction, and then adduction movements. The possibility of CP is suggested if these reflexes occur after 4 months.

A number of assessment instruments are now available to evaluate muscle spasticity: functional independence in self-care, mobility, and cognition; self-initiated movements over time; and capability and performance of functional activities in self-care, mobility, and social function.

Therapeutic Management

The goals of therapy for children with CP are early recognition and promotion of optimal development to enable affected children to attain normalization and their potential within the limits of their existing health problems. The disorder is permanent, and therapy is primarily preventive and symptomatic.

Therapy has five broad aims:
1. To establish locomotion, communication, and self-help skills
2. To gain optimal appearance and integration of motor functions
3. To correct associated defects as effectively as possible
4. To provide educational opportunities adapted to the child's needs and capabilities
5. To promote socialization experiences with other affected and unaffected children

Each child is evaluated and managed on an individual basis. The scope of the child's needs requires multidisciplinary planning and care coordination among health care professionals and the child's family. The outcome for the child and family with CP is normalization and promotion of self-care activities that empower the child and family to achieve maximum potential.

Ankle-foot orthoses (AFOs, braces) are worn by many children with CP and are used to help prevent or reduce deformity, increase the energy efficiency of gait, and control alignment. Wheeled go-carts that provide sitting balance may serve as early "wheelchair" experience for young children. Manual or powered wheelchairs allow for more independent mobility (Figs. 49-1 and 49-2). Strollers can be equipped with custom seats for dependent mobilization.

Orthopedic surgery may be required between the ages of 5 and 7 years to correct contracture or spastic deformities, to provide stability for an uncontrollable joint, and to provide balanced muscle power. This includes tendon-lengthening procedures, release of spastic muscles, and correction of hip and adductor muscle spasticity or contracture to improve locomotion. Hip dislocation often occurs in children with CP. Spinal fusion may be done for scoliosis. Computerized motion analysis, radiographs, and clinical findings are used to make decisions about orthopedic surgery. *Selective*

BOX 49-2   CLINICAL MANIFESTATIONS OF CEREBRAL PALSY (AT TIME OF DIAGNOSIS)

Delayed Gross Motor Development
- A universal manifestation
- Delay in all motor accomplishments
- Increases as growth advances
- Delays more obvious as growth advances

Abnormal Motor Performance
- Very early preferential unilateral hand preference
- Abnormal and asymmetric crawl
- Standing or walking on toes
- Uncoordinated or involuntary movements
- Poor sucking
- Feeding difficulties
- Persistent tongue thrust

Alterations of Muscle Tone
- Increased or decreased resistance to passive movements
- Opisthotonic posturing (arching of back)
- Feels stiff on handling or dressing
- Difficulty in diapering
- Rigid and unbending at the hip and knee joints when pulled to sitting position (early sign)

Abnormal Postures
- Maintains hips higher than trunk in prone position with legs and arms flexed or drawn under the body
- Scissoring and extension of legs with feet plantar flexed in supine position
- Persistent infantile resting and sleeping position
- Arms abducted at shoulders
- Elbows flexed
- Hands fisted

Reflex Abnormalities
- Persistence of primitive infantile reflexes
- Obligatory tonic neck reflex at any age
- Nonpersistence beyond 6 months of age
- Persistence or hyperactivity of the Moro, plantar, and palmar grasp reflexes
- Hyperreflexia, ankle clonus, and stretch reflexes elicited in many muscle groups on fast, passive movements

Associated Disabilities*
- Altered learning and reasoning
- Seizures
- Impaired behavioral and interpersonal relationships
- Sensory impairment (vision, hearing)

From Nehring WM: Cerebral palsy. In Allen PJ, Vessey JA, Schapiro NA, editors: *Primary care of the child with a chronic condition*, ed 5, St Louis, 2010, Mosby. Adapted from Jones MW, Morgan E, Shelton JE: Primary care of the child with cerebral palsy: a review of systems (part II), *J Pediatr Health Care* 21(4):226–237, 2007.
*May or may not be present.

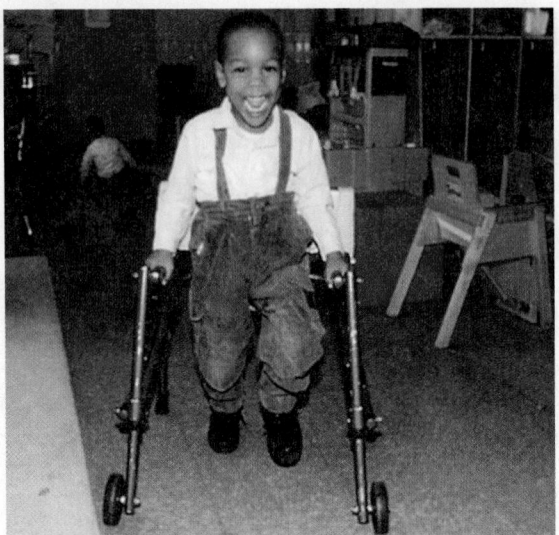

FIG 49-1 Mobilization device for child.

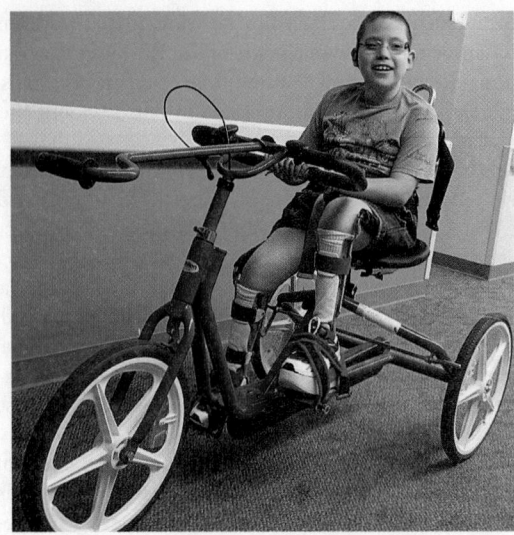

FIG 49-2 Bike walker used to provide mobility and to enhance leg muscle strength. (Courtesy Texas Children's Hospital, Houston, TX.)

BOX 49-3   EARLY WARNING SIGNS OF CEREBRAL PALSY

- Failure to meet any developmental milestones such as rolling over, raising head, sitting up, crawling
- Persistent primitive reflexes such as Moro, asymmetric tonic neck reflex
- Poor head control (head lag) and clenched fists after 3 months of age
- Stiff or rigid arms or legs; scissoring legs
- Pushing away or arching back; stiff posture
- Floppy or limp body posture, especially while sleeping
- Inability to sit up without support by 8 months
- Using only one side of the body or only the arms to crawl
- Feeding difficulties
  - Persistent gagging or choking when fed
  - After 6 months of age, tongue pushing soft food out of the mouth
- Extreme irritability or crying
- Failure to smile by 3 months
- Lack of interest in surroundings

Data from Pathways Awareness Foundation: *Parents ... if you see any of these warning signs ... don't delay,* Chicago, 1991, Author; Nehring W: Cerebral palsy. In Allen PJ, Vessey JA, editors: *Primary care of the child with a chronic condition,* St Louis, 2004, Mosby; and Jones MW, Morgan E, Shelton JE, et al: Cerebral palsy: introduction and diagnosis (part 1), *J Pediatr Health Care* 21(3): 146–152, 2007.

dorsal rhizotomy provides marked improvement in some children with CP. The procedure involves selectively cutting dorsal column sensory rootlets that have an abnormal response to electrical stimulation. Achieving the benefits from the surgery requires intensive physical therapy and family commitment. Because the procedure results in flaccid muscles, the child must be retaught to sit, stand, and walk.

Surgical intervention is usually reserved for children who do not respond to the more conservative measures such as bracing, but it is also indicated for children whose spasticity causes progressive deformities. Surgery is used primarily to improve function and enable proper sitting, standing, and walking rather than for cosmetic purposes and is followed by physical therapy.

Intense pain may occur with muscle spasms in patients with CP. Pharmacologic agents given orally (dantrolene sodium, baclofen [Lioresal], and diazepam [Valium]) have had little effectiveness in improving muscle coordination in children with CP; however, they are effective in decreasing overall spasticity. The most common side effects of these agents include hepatotoxicity (dantrolene), drowsiness, fatigue, and muscle weakness; less commonly, diaphoresis and constipation may be seen with baclofen.

Botulinum toxin A (Botox) is also used to reduce spasticity in targeted muscles, primarily those of the upper and lower extremities. Botulinum toxin A is injected into a selected muscle (commonly the quadriceps, gastrocnemius, or medial hamstrings) after a topical anesthetic is applied. The drug acts to inhibit the release of acetylcholine into a specific muscle group, thereby preventing muscle movement. When it is administered early in the course of the condition, affected muscle contractures may be minimized, particularly in lower extremities, thus avoiding surgical procedures with possible adverse effects. The goal is to allow stretching of the muscle as it relaxes and permit ambulation with an AFO. The major reported adverse effects of botulinum toxin A injection are pain at the injection site and temporary weakness (Lukban, Rosales, and Dressler, 2009). Prime candidates for botulinum toxin A injections are children with spasticity confined to the lower extremities; the drug weakens spasticity so the muscles can be stretched and the child may walk with or without orthoses. The onset of action occurs within 24 to 72 hours, with a peak effect observed at 2 weeks and a duration of action of 3 to 6 months. Diazepam has proved effective on a short-term basis in reducing spasticity in children with CP (Delgado, Hirtz, Aisen, et al., 2010).

Children with CP may also experience pain as a result of surgical procedures intended to reduce contracture deformities, position and gastroesophageal reflux, and physical therapy. Therefore pain management is an important aspect of care of children with CP.

The neurosurgical and pharmacologic approach to relieving the spasticity associated with CP involves the implantation of a pump to infuse baclofen directly into the intrathecal space surrounding the spinal cord. Intrathecal baclofen therapy is best suited for children with severe spasticity that interferes with activities of daily living (ADLs) and ambulation; however, this drug and method of administration (intrathecal) have had a significant number of adverse or side effects (Delgado, Hirtz, Aisen, et al., 2010). Patients may be screened before pump placement by the infusion of a "test dose" of intrathecal baclofen delivered via a lumbar puncture, followed by close monitoring for side effects (hypotonia, somnolence, seizures, nausea, vomiting, headache). Relief of spasticity occurs for several hours after the infusion. If a positive effect is noted, the patient is considered a candidate for pump placement. The implantation procedure is done in the operating room by a neurosurgeon. The pump, which is approximately the size of a hockey puck, is placed in the subcutaneous space of the midabdomen. An intrathecal catheter is tunneled from the lumbar area to the abdomen and connected to the pump. The pump is filled with baclofen and programmed to provide a set dose using a telemetry wand and a computer. Benefits of intrathecal baclofen include fewer systemic side effects than oral baclofen, dosage titration for maximizing effects, and reversibility of therapy with removal of the pump if so desired. The patient may remain hospitalized for 3 to 7 days to adjust the dosage and ensure proper healing. Outpatient visits to refill the pump and make dosage adjustments occur about every 3 to 6 months, depending on the patient's response to the treatment. This procedure is most suited for a multidisciplinary setting where rehabilitation specialists are readily available and consistently involved in the patient's ongoing care. Abrupt withdrawal of intrathecal baclofen may result in adverse effects such as rebound spasticity, pruritus, hyperthermia, rhabdomyolysis, disseminated intravascular coagulation, multiorgan failure, and death; in some cases, intrathecal baclofen withdrawal may mimic sepsis.

Oral baclofen has also been widely used in children with CP to treat spasticity; however, side effects are common and include systemic toxicity, drowsiness, and sedation (Delgado, Hirtz, Aisen, et al., 2010).

Antiepileptic drugs (AEDs) such as carbamazepine (Tegretol) and divalproex (valproate sodium and valproic acid; Depakote) are prescribed routinely for children who have seizures. Gabapentin (Neurontin) has been used in adults with spinal cord injury (SCI) to decrease spasticity with success; no studies are available on the effectiveness of the drug in children. The α_2-adrenergic agonists *clonidine* (Catapres) and *tizanidine* (Zanaflex) have been used to decrease spasticity in adults with SCI and multiple sclerosis. The use of oral tizanidine in children has been limited, and only a few small studies have been conducted in children with CP specifically evaluating the reduction of spasticity (Delgado, Hirtz, Aisen, et al., 2010). Oral tizanidine given in conjunction with botulinum type A has been reported to be more effective than oral baclofen and botulinum type A in one study of children with CP (Dai, Wasay, and Awan, 2008). All medications should be monitored for maintenance of therapeutic levels and avoidance of subtherapeutic or toxic levels. Other medications include levodopa to treat dystonia; Artane for treating dystonia and for increasing the use of upper extremities and vocalizations; and reserpine for hyperkinetic movement disorders such as chorea or athetosis (Johnston, 2011).

Dental hygiene is especially important. Regular visits to the dentist and prophylaxis, including brushing, fluoride, and flossing, should be instituted as soon as the teeth erupt. Dental care is especially important for children being given phenytoin, since they often develop gum hyperplasia. Additional problems common among children with CP include constipation caused by neurologic deficits and lack of exercise, poor bladder control and urinary retention, chronic respiratory tract infections, problems with airway clearance, and aspiration pneumonia. These occur as a result of gastroesophageal reflux, abnormal muscle tone, immobility, and altered positioning, and skin problems may occur as a result of altered positioning, poor nutrition, and immobility.

A wide variety of technical aids are available to improve the functioning of children with CP. These include electromechanical toys that employ the concept of biofeedback and operate from a head unit. The toy is manipulated only when the head and trunk are in correct alignment. Eye-hand coordination can also be enhanced by computerized toys and games. Microcomputers combined with voice synthesizers help children with speech difficulties to "speak." These and other devices print messages onto screen monitors and paper.

Many other electronic devices allow independent functioning. Sensors can be activated and deactivated by using a head-stick or tongue or other voluntary muscle movement over which the child has control. Voice-activated computer technology may also allow increased mobility and ambulation with specially designed equipment such as wheelchairs. The application of this technology makes it possible for persons with CP to function eventually in their own residences and can be extended into the workplace.

There is some evidence that *neuromuscular electrical stimulation (NMES)* in addition to dynamic splinting may result in increased muscle strength, range of motion, and function of upper limbs in children with CP. Further studies are needed in children with CP to support the use of botulinum toxin A in conjunction with NMES to decrease muscle spasticity and improve function (Wright, Durham, Ewins, et al., 2012).

Behavior problems may occur and often interfere with the child's development. Attention deficit hyperactivity disorder and other learning problems require professional attention. In addition, children with CP may have vision difficulties such as strabismus, nystagmus, and optic atrophy (Johnston, 2011). Speech-language therapy involves the services of a speech-language pathologist who may also assist with feeding problems.

Physical therapy is one of the most frequently used conservative treatment modalities. It requires the specialized skills of a qualified therapist with an extensive repertoire of exercise methods who can design a program to stimulate each child to achieve his or her functional goals.

An active therapy program involves the family, the physical therapist, and often other members of the health care team, including the nurse. The most common approach uses traditional types of therapeutic exercises that consist of stretching, passive, active, and resistive movements applied to specific muscle groups or joints to maintain or increase range of motion, strength, or endurance.

Prognosis. The prognosis for the child with CP depends largely on the type and severity of the condition. Children with mild to moderate involvement (85%) have the capability of achieving ambulation between the ages of 2 and 7 years (Berker and Yalçin, 2008). If the child does not achieve independent ambulation by this time, chances are poor for ambulation and independence. Approximately 30% to 50% of individuals with CP have significant cognitive impairments, and an even higher percentage have mild cognitive and learning deficits. However, many children with severe spastic tetraplegic CP have normal intelligence. Growth is affected in children with spastic tetraplegia, and many children remain below the 5th percentile for age and gender.

Vocational rehabilitation and higher education are possible for adults with CP. Children with severe CP mobility impairment and feeding problems often succumb to respiratory tract infection in childhood (Liptak, Murphy, and Council on Children with Disabilities, 2011). The few survival rate studies on children and adults with CP show that survival is influenced by existing comorbidities (Nehring, 2010).

Neurorehabilitation involves rehabilitating and stimulating nerves (that control muscle movement) that have been damaged to improve brain development; *brain plasticity* is being examined closely as a possible avenue for reorganizing traditionally damaged neural pathways to function optimally for children with CP. Children with CP or SCI may benefit from therapies such as *constraint-induced movement* therapy wherein a stronger extremity is constrained to force the weaker extremity to function; these treatments have shown improvement in some children with CP (Aisen, Kerkovich, Mast, et al., 2011).

Prevention of CP in many children may become a reality in the near future. Studies indicate that early neuroprotection in term infants with the use of *therapeutic hypothermia* (head cooling or whole-body cooling) within 6 hours of birth improved survival without CP by approximately 40% (Johnston, Fatemi, Wilson, et al., 2011). More recent studies have found lower death rates and less severe disability with the use of therapeutic hypothermia, but overall intelligence quotient (IQ) scores at 6 to 7 years of age were not statistically significant in those receiving hypothermia (as compared with those receiving conventional treatment) (Shankaran, Pappas, McDonald, et al., 2012).

CARE MANAGEMENT

Because children with CP are being identified and treated at an earlier age, parents are participating earlier in treatment programs for their children with disabilities. They are taught the proper handling and home care of young children with CP and need a carefully planned program so that their change of role from parent to caregiver can be melded into the already established relationship. Close work with other multidisciplinary team members is essential. Nurses reinforce the therapeutic plan and assist the family in devising and modifying equipment and activities to continue the therapy program in the home. The nursing process in the care of the child with CP is outlined in the Nursing Care Plan.

◎ NURSING CARE PLAN

The Child with Cerebral Palsy

NURSING DIAGNOSIS	EXPECTED OUTCOMES	NURSING INTERVENTIONS	RATIONALES
Impaired Physical Mobility related to neuromuscular impairment **Child's or Family's Defining Characteristics** ***(Subjective and Objective Data)*** Postural instability during performance of routine ADLs Limited ability to perform gross motor skills Limited range of motion Limited ability to perform fine motor skills Gait changes Movement-induced tremor Persistence of primitive reflexes	Infant or toddler will demonstrate active muscle movement. Child will have adequate mobility to perform ADLs to maximum potential.	Carry out and teach family to perform stretching exercises on affected muscles Use assistive devices such as wheelchair, AFOs, and wrist splints Administer medications (specify) intended to decrease muscle spasticity Encourage and teach parent(s) to use jaw control during feedings Position child semiupright during feedings Encourage play exercises that involve joint movement and promote fine and gross motor skill acquisition and repetition	To prevent muscle contractures To increase mobility and prevent contractures To minimize pain and decrease muscle spasticity To facilitate eating To decrease chance of aspiration and facilitate mobilization of food and fluids through esophagus To promote joint movement To promote achievement of developmental milestones

Risk for Injury related to mobility limitation, neuromuscular impairment, and perception and cognition impairment
Child's or Family's Defining Characteristics
(Subjective and Objective Data)
Physical factors:
  Altered mobility
  Limited ability to chew food and swallow food particles
Neuromuscular factors:
Limited perception of danger
Uncontrollable muscular movements
	Child will remain injury free.
	Home physical environment will be safe.
		Educate family regarding child's physical limitations that place him or her at greater risk for injury
		Instruct family in steps to avoid injury, including padded furniture, lowered bed or side rails as appropriate, gates on stairs, avoidance of throw rugs, thick carpeting
		Position child in semiupright position after feedings
		Assess child's ability to manage (chewing and swallowing) oral feedings
		Use jaw support as needed during feedings
		Use appropriate mobilization devices and ensure they are safe for child's age
		Encourage mobilization and play activities that stretch muscles
		Teach child which ADLs are safe and appropriate to perform without assistance of another person
			To prevent accidental injury during mobilization
			To promote family involvement in injury prevention
			To prevent aspiration
			To determine appropriate feeding method and prevent aspiration
			To prevent choking and possible aspiration
			To prevent muscle contractures
			To promote personal safety
			To promote self-care

◎ NURSING CARE PLAN

The Child with Cerebral Palsy—cont'd

NURSING DIAGNOSIS	EXPECTED OUTCOMES	NURSING INTERVENTIONS	RATIONALES
Chronic Pain related to involuntary muscle movements (spasticity) and treatments for muscle spasticity	Child's optimum comfort level will be maintained.	Administer medications to control spasticity (specify)	To prevent muscle spasm pain
Child's or Family's Defining Characteristics		Perform stretching exercises after pain medication has been administered (60 minutes for oral medications)	To manage pain impulses during exercises
(Subjective and Objective Data)		Administer pain medications (specify) such as NSAIDs	To minimize pain
Observed evidence of guarded behavior, grimace, crying, restlessness, irritability		For treatments such as botulinum toxin A (Botox) injections, assist with administration of appropriate pain medications and monitoring child for pain sensation (specify)	To decrease pain of injection at site
Atrophy of involved muscle group			
Altered ability to continue previous ADLs		For postoperative pain, administer pain medications on around-the-clock schedule for 48 to 72 hours; use PCA pump as child's cognitive and motor skills allow	To promote personal physical comfort
		Use objective pain scale to assess pain level	To provide objective measure of pain for intervention
		Encourage child to verbalize effects of pain on ADLs	To provide outlet for frustration related to chronic pain experience
		Use assistive devices such as AFOs or KAFOs	To decrease muscle spasticity and contractures
		Teach parent(s) and child appropriate positions to assume while sitting and recumbent to minimize effects of muscle spasticity	To promote self-care

ADLs, Activities of daily living; *AFO,* ankle-foot orthosis; *KAFO,* knee-ankle-foot orthoses; *NSAID,* nonsteroidal antiinflammatory drug; *PCA,* patient-controlled analgesia.

Because children with CP expend so much energy in their efforts to accomplish ADLs, more frequent rest periods should be arranged to avoid fatigue. The diet should be tailored to the child's activity and metabolic needs. Gastrostomy feedings may be necessary to supplement regular feedings and ensure adequate weight gain, particularly in children at risk for growth failure and chronic malnutrition, those with severe CP and subsequent oral feeding difficulties, and children whose well-being is affected by illness and decreased fluid or medication intake. Oral feedings may be continued to maintain oral motor skills. Weight gain is perceived as an important measure of adequate oral feeding efficiency.

A skin-level gastrostomy is particularly suited for children with CP. Parents may need assistance and advice with medication administration through a gastrostomy tube to prevent clogging. Because jaw control is often compromised, more normal control can be achieved if the feeder provides stability of the oral mechanism from the side or front of the face. When directed from the front, the middle finger of the nonfeeding hand is placed posterior to the body portion of the chin, the thumb is placed below the bottom lip, and the index finger is placed parallel to the child's mandible (Fig. 49-3). Manual jaw control from the side assists with head control, correction of neck and trunk hyperextension, and jaw stabilization. The middle finger of the nonfeeding hand is placed posterior to the bony portion of the chin, the index finger is placed on the chin below the lower lip, and the thumb

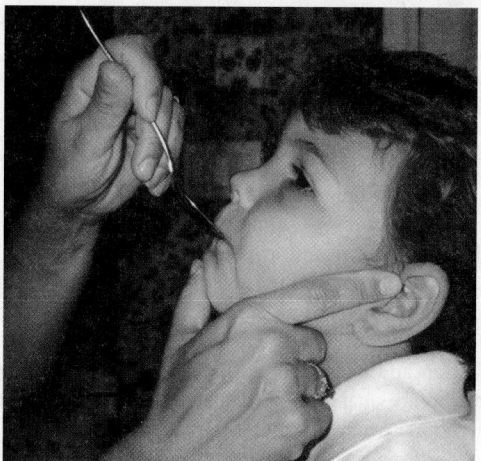

FIG 49-3 Manual jaw control provided anteriorly.

is placed obliquely across the cheek to provide lateral jaw stability (Fig. 49-4).

Safety precautions are implemented, such as having children wear protective helmets if they are subject to falls or capable of injuring their heads on hard objects. Because children with CP are at risk for altered proprioception and subsequent falls, the home and

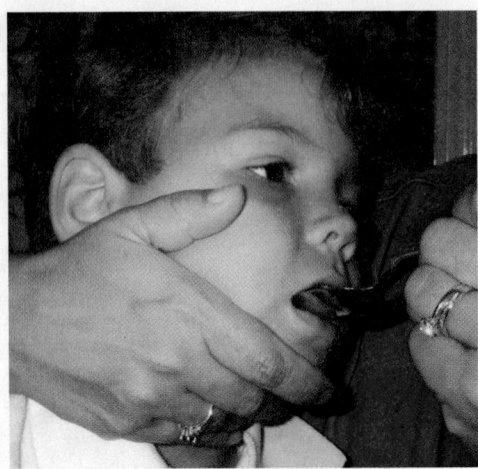

FIG 49-4 Manual jaw control provided from the side.

play environment should be adapted to their needs to prevent bodily harm. Appropriate immunizations should be administered to prevent childhood illnesses and protect against respiratory tract infections such as influenza and pneumonia. Dental problems may be more common in children with CP, which creates a need for meticulous attention to all aspects of dental care. Transportation of the child with motor problems and restricted mobility may be especially challenging for the family and child. Attention must be given to the child's safety when riding in a motor vehicle; a federally approved safety restraint should be used at all times. It is recommended that children with CP ride in a rear-facing position as long as possible because of their poor head, neck, and trunk control (Lovette, 2008). Car restraints especially designated for children with poor head and neck control are available and should be used.*

The involvement of physical therapy, speech therapy, and occupational therapy is particularly important in establishment and maintenance of muscle function, development of adequate speech and phonation, and identification of modifications necessary for the child's environment so that ADLs can be performed to the child's satisfaction.

As in all aspects of care, educational requirements are determined by the child's needs and potential. Children with mild to moderate cognitive involvement are generally able to participate in regular classes. Resource rooms are available in most schools to provide more individualized attention. Integration of children with CP into regular classrooms should be the initial goal. For those who are unable to benefit from formal education, a vocational training program may be appropriate. At adolescence, prevocational and vocational counseling and guidance are arranged. At any phase or in any setting, education is geared toward the child's assets.

Recreation and after-school activities should be considered for children who are unable to participate in the regular athletic programs and other peer activities. Some children can compete in athletic and artistic endeavors, and many games and pastimes are suited

to their capabilities. Competitive sports are also becoming increasingly available to children with disabilities and offer an added dimension to physical activities. Recreational activities serve to stimulate children's interest and curiosity, help them adjust to their disability, improve their functional abilities, and build self-esteem. Any accomplishment that helps children approach a normal way of life enhances their self-concept.

Support the Family. Probably the nursing interventions most valuable to the family are support and help in coping with the emotional aspects of the disorder, many of which are discussed in relation to the child with a disability (see Chapter 36). Initially, the parents need supportive counseling directed toward understanding the meaning of the diagnosis and all of the feelings that it engenders. Later, they need clarification regarding what they can expect from the child and from health care professionals. Educating families in the principles of family-centered care and parent-professional collaboration is essential. The family may require help in modifying the home environment for care of the child. Home modifications to facilitate the use of a wheelchair may be necessary. The child or adolescent should be encouraged to be as independent as possible; making necessary home modifications to facilitate the child's independence is strongly encouraged. Transportation to the health care practitioner's office and other health care agencies also requires special arrangements. The home health care nurse should be consulted for assistance in making the home environment accessible to the child or adolescent with CP.

Care coordination for the child and family with CP is an important nursing role. The home health care nurse or care manager has an important role in the support and encouragement for families who assume the primary care of a child with CP. Having a child with CP implies numerous challenges of daily management and changes in family life, and the nurse can help with education, assessment, and mobilization of resources.

The nurse needs to support the parents in their frustration, problem solving, concerns, approaches to helping the child, and the positive approaches they use. Parents and other family members may need support and counseling. Siblings of a child with a disability are affected and may respond to the child's presence with overt or less evident behavioral issues. The family needs a relationship with nurses who can provide continued contact, support, and encouragement through the long process of habilitation.

Parents may also find help and comfort from parent groups, with whom they can share challenges and concerns and from whom they can derive comfort and practical information. Parent support groups are most helpful through sharing experiences and accomplishments. For example, parents can learn from others what it is like to have a child with CP, which is generally not possible from professionals (see Family-Centered Care box). The national organization *United Cerebral Palsy** has branches in most communities. The association provides a variety of services for children and families. A number of excellent books also are available to guide parents and nurses who work with children with CP.

Support the Hospitalized Child. Cerebral palsy is not a disorder that requires ongoing hospitalization; therefore, when children with CP are hospitalized, they are usually admitted for illness or corrective surgery. Nursing care of the child with CP is similar to that of any child with a disability, and children with CP should be approached as would any child in the hospital. Speech impairment

---

*For information on specially adapted molded-plastic chairs for children with CP, contact Snug Seat at 800-336-7684; www.snugseat.com/en-US/Welcome-to-Snug-Seat.aspx. The E-Z-On vest is a special safety harness for larger children with poor trunk control. Additional safety restraints and a listing of distributors are available from SafetyBeltSafe U.S.A., www.carseat.org. Another resource is National Center for the Safe Transportation of Children with Special Health Care Needs; 800-543-6227; www.preventinjury.org/specNeeds.asp.

*1660 L St., NW, Suite 700, Washington, DC 20036; 800-872-5827; fax: 202-776-0414; e-mail: info@ucp.org; www.ucp.org. The website also has links to each state's United Cerebral Palsy organization.

is common in children with CP, but this may not correlate with their ability to understand. Therapy programs should be continued, when appropriate, during the time they are hospitalized. Encouraging the parent to room-in and actively participate in the child's care helps promote family-centered care. However, it is also important to remember that hospitalization may be the first time a parent can defer care to a nurse and not be the primary caregiver. Discuss this with the family to find the right level of involvement for them.

Spina Bifida (Myelomeningocele)

Abnormalities that derive from the embryonic neural tube (neural tube defects [NTDs]) constitute the largest group of congenital anomalies that are consistent with multifactorial inheritance. Normally, the spinal cord and cauda equina are encased in a protective sheath of bone and meninges (Fig. 49-5, A). Failure of neural tube closure produces defects of varying degrees (Box 49-4). They may involve the entire length of the neural tube or may be restricted to a small area.

In the United States, rates of NTDs have declined from 1.3 per 1000 births in 1970 to 0.3 per 1000 births after the introduction of mandatory food fortification with folic acid in 1998. One concern is that NTD rates have not decreased among Hispanic and non-Hispanic Caucasian mothers since 1999 (Centers for Disease Control and Prevention [CDC], 2009). In 2005, the rates for spina bifida were estimated by the CDC to be 17.96 per 100,000 live births, thus making this one of the most common birth defects in the United States (Matthews, 2009; Wolff, Witkop, Miller, et al., 2009). Increased use of prenatal diagnostic techniques and termination of pregnancies have also affected the overall incidence of NTDs (see also Prevention, p. 1582).

Anencephaly, the most serious NTD, is a congenital malformation in which both cerebral hemispheres are absent. The condition

---

FAMILY-CENTERED CARE

The Reality of Acceptance of Cerebral Palsy

Acceptance is rarely achieved in the length of time implied in the literature.

In the first place, what is it? To me, it is the end of comparing my son with every other child I see. I focus on *his* gains, not society's expectations.

It is also being able to laugh periodically *at* his "clumsiness." It is "gallows humor" as he achieves adulthood; jokes about CP can be funny now.

The bitterness is gone; I am now happy for people who have children without CP.

I no longer feel sorry for my son, but rather for the people who cannot see him for the great person he is; the CP does *not* come first.

He is now a young man of 25 years and I am learning to accept his independence.

It is a "never-ending story."

—Elaine A. Dunham, RN, Shriners Hospitals for Children
Springfield, MA

BOX 49-4 NEURAL TUBE DEFECTS

Cranioschisis—A skull defect through which various tissues protrude

Exencephaly—Brain totally exposed or extruded through an associated skull defect; fetus usually aborted

Anencephaly—If fetus with exencephaly survives, degeneration of the brain to a spongiform mass with no bony covering; incompatible with life usually beyond a few days or, rarely, weeks

Encephalocele—Herniation of brain and meninges through a defect in the skull producing a fluid-filled sac

Rachischisis or spina bifida—Fissure in the spinal column that leaves the meninges and spinal cord exposed

Meningocele—Hernial protrusion of a saclike cyst of meninges filled with spinal fluid (see Fig. 49-5, *C*)

Myelomeningocele (meningomyelocele)—Hernial protrusion of a saclike cyst containing meninges, spinal fluid, and a portion of the spinal cord with its nerves (see Fig. 49-5, *D*)

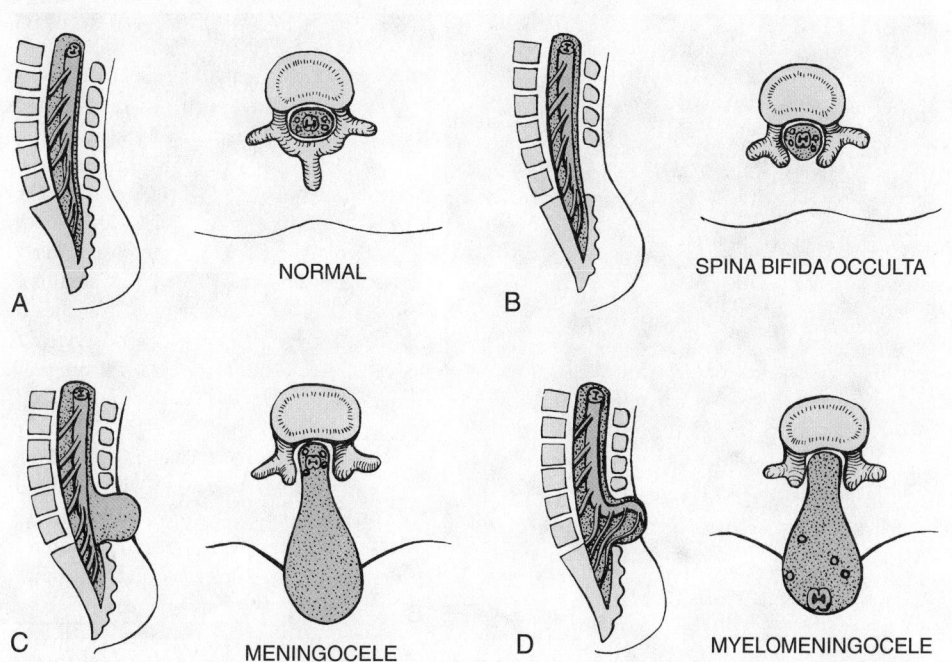

A — NORMAL
B — SPINA BIFIDA OCCULTA
C — MENINGOCELE
D — MYELOMENINGOCELE

FIG 49-5 A through **D,** Midline defects of osseous spine with varying degrees of neural herniations.

is incompatible with life, and many affected infants are stillborn. For those who survive, no specific treatment is available. The infants have a portion of the brainstem and are able to maintain vital functions (e.g., temperature regulation and cardiac and respiratory function) for a few hours to several weeks but eventually die of respiratory failure.

Myelodysplasia refers broadly to any malformation of the spinal canal and cord. Midline defects involving failure of the osseous (bony) spine to close are called spina bifida (SB), the most common defect of the central nervous system (CNS). SB is categorized into two types—SB occulta and SB cystica.

Spina bifida occulta refers to a defect that is not visible externally. It occurs most frequently in the lumbosacral area (L5 and S1) (see Fig. 49-5, *B*). SB occulta may not be apparent unless there are associated cutaneous manifestations or neuromuscular disturbances.

Spina bifida cystica refers to a visible defect with an external saclike protrusion. The two major forms of SB cystica are meningocele, which encases meninges and spinal fluid but no neural elements (see Fig. 49-5, *C*), and myelomeningocele (MMC) (or meningomyelocele), which contains meninges, spinal fluid, and nerves (see Fig. 49-5, *D*). Meningocele is not associated with neurologic deficit, which occurs in varying, often serious, degrees in myelomeningocele. Clinically, the term *spina bifida* is used to refer to myelomeningocele.

Pathophysiology

The pathophysiology of SB is best understood when related to the normal formative stages of the nervous system. At approximately 20 days of gestation, a dedicated depression, the neural groove, appears in the dorsal ectoderm of the embryo. During the fourth week of gestation, the groove deepens rapidly and its elevated margins develop laterally and fuse dorsally to form the neural tube. Neural tube formation begins in the cervical region near the center of the embryo and advances in both directions—caudally and cephalically—until by the end of the fourth week of gestation, the ends of the neural tube, the anterior and posterior neuropores, close.

Most experts believe the primary defect in neural tube malformations is a failure of neural tube closure. However, some evidence indicates that the defects are a result of splitting of the already closed neural tube as a result of an abnormal increase in cerebrospinal fluid (CSF) pressure during the first trimester.

There is evidence of a multifactorial etiology, including drugs, radiation, maternal malnutrition, chemicals, and possibly a genetic mutation in folate pathways in some cases, which may result in abnormal development. There is also evidence of a genetic component in the development of SB; myelomeningocele may occur in association with syndromes such as trisomy 18, PHAVER (limb **p**terygia, congenital **h**eart **a**nomalies, **v**ertebral defects, **e**ar anomalies, and **r**adial defects) syndrome, and Meckel-Gruber syndrome (Shaer, Chescheir, and Schulkin, 2007). Additional factors predisposing children to an increased risk for NTDs include prepregnancy maternal obesity, maternal diabetes mellitus, low maternal vitamin B$_{12}$ status, maternal hyperthermia, and the use of AEDs in pregnancy. The genetic predisposition is supported by evidence of the risk for recurrence after one affected child (3%-4%) and a 10% risk for recurrence with two previously affected children (Kinsman and Johnston, 2011).

The degree of neurologic dysfunction depends on where the sac protrudes through the vertebrae, the anatomic level of the defect, and the amount of nerve tissue involved. The majority of myelomeningoceles (75%) involve the lumbar or lumbosacral area (Fig. 49-6). Hydrocephalus is a frequently associated anomaly in 80% to 90% of the children. About 80% of patients with myelomeningocele develop a type II Chiari malformation (Kinsman and Johnston, 2011). There is some evidence that prolonged exposure of the MMC sac to amniotic fluid predisposes an infant to the development of hindbrain herniation and Chiari II malformation (Adzick, 2013).

Diagnostic Evaluation

The diagnosis of SB is made on the basis of clinical manifestations (Box 49-5) and examination of the meningeal sac (see Fig. 49-6, *A*).

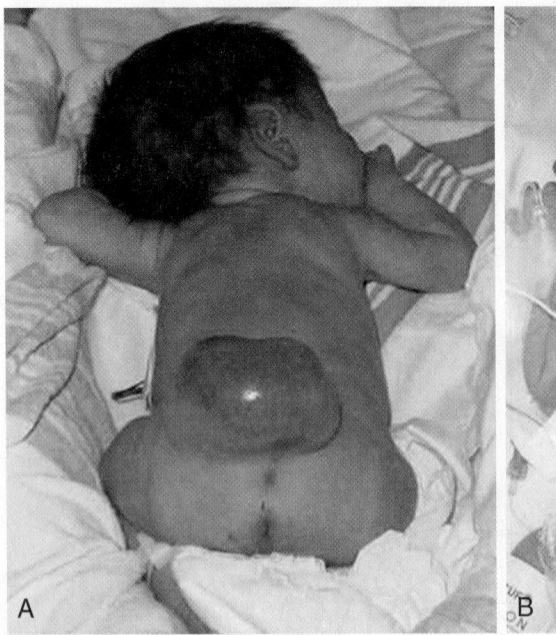
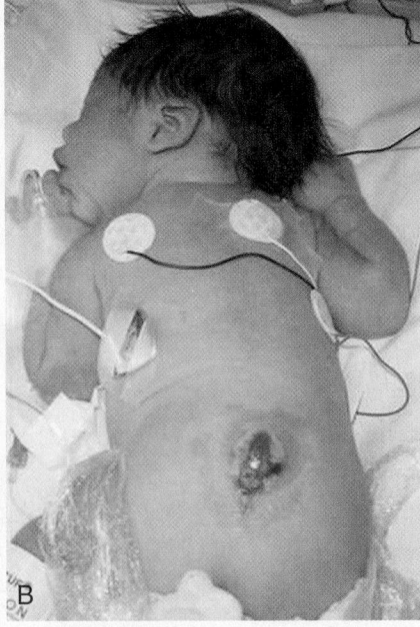

FIG 49-6 A, Myelomeningocele with intact sac. **B,** Myelomeningocele with ruptured sac. (Courtesy Dr. Robert C. Dauser, Neurosurgery, Baylor College of Medicine, Houston, TX.)

Diagnostic measures used to evaluate the brain and spinal cord include MRI, ultrasonography, and CT. A neurologic evaluation will determine the extent of involvement of bowel and bladder function as well as lower extremity neuromuscular involvement. Flaccid paralysis of the lower extremities is a common finding with absent deep tendon reflexes.

Prenatal Detection. It is possible to determine the presence of some major open NTDs prenatally. Ultrasonographic scanning of the uterus and elevated maternal concentrations of α-fetoprotein (AFP, or MS-AFP), a fetal-specific γ_{-1}-globulin, in amniotic fluid may indicate anencephaly or myelomeningocele. The optimum time for performing these diagnostic tests is between 16 and 18 weeks of gestation before AFP concentrations normally diminish and in sufficient time to permit a therapeutic abortion. It is recommended that such diagnostic procedures and genetic counseling be considered for all mothers who have borne an affected child, and testing is offered to all pregnant women (American College of Obstetrics and Gynecology [ACOG], 2007). Chorionic villus sampling is also a method for prenatal diagnosis of NTDs; however, it carries certain risks (skeletal limb depletion) and is not recommended before 10 weeks of gestation (Simpson, Richards, Otaño, et al., 2012).

Therapeutic Management

Management of the child who has a myelomeningocele requires a multidisciplinary team approach involving the specialties of neurology, neurosurgery, pediatrics, urology, orthopedics, rehabilitation, physical therapy, occupational therapy, and social services, as well as intensive nursing care in a variety of specialty areas. The collaborative efforts of these specialists focus on:

- The myelomeningocele and the problems associated with the defect—hydrocephalus, paralysis, orthopedic deformities (e.g., developmental dysplasia of the hip, clubfoot), and genitourinary abnormalities

---

BOX 49-5 CLINICAL MANIFESTATIONS OF SPINA BIFIDA

Spina Bifida Cystica
- Sensory disturbances usually parallel to motor dysfunction:
  - Below second lumbar vertebra—Flaccid, partial paralysis of lower extremities, varying degrees of sensory deficit, overflow incontinence with constant dribbling of urine, lack of bowel control, rectal prolapse (sometimes)
  - Below third sacral vertebra—No motor impairment, may have saddle anesthesia with bladder and anal sphincter paralysis
- Associated deformities (sometimes produced in utero):
  - Talipes valgus or varus contractures
  - Kyphosis
  - Lumbosacral scoliosis
  - Hip dislocation or subluxation

Spina Bifida Occulta
- Frequently no observable manifestations
- May be associated with one or more cutaneous manifestations:
  - Skin depression or dimple
  - Port-wine angiomatous nevi
  - Dark tufts of hair
  - Soft, subcutaneous lipomas
- May have neuromuscular disturbances:
  - Progressive disturbance of gait with foot weakness
  - Bowel and bladder sphincter disturbances

- Possible acquired problems that may or may not be associated, such as Chiari II malformation, meningitis, seizures, hypoxia, and hemorrhage
- Other abnormalities, such as cardiac or gastrointestinal (GI) malformations

Many hospitals have routine outpatient care by multidisciplinary teams to provide the complex follow-up care needed for children and families with myelodysplasia.

Many authorities believe that early closure, within the first 24 to 72 hours, offers the most favorable outcome. Surgical closure within the first 24 hours is recommended if the sac is leaking CSF (Kinsman and Johnston, 2011).

A variety of neurosurgical and plastic surgical procedures are used for skin closure without disturbing the neural elements or removing any portion of the sac. The objective is satisfactory skin coverage of the lesion and meticulous closure. Wide excision of the large membranous covering may damage functioning neural tissue.

Associated problems are assessed and managed by appropriate surgical and supportive measures. Shunt procedures provide relief from imminent or progressive hydrocephalus (see Chapter 45). When diagnosed, ventriculitis, meningitis, urinary tract infection, and pneumonia are treated with vigorous antibiotic therapy and supportive measures. Surgical intervention for Chiari II malformation is indicated only when the child is symptomatic (i.e., high-pitched crowing cry, stridor, respiratory difficulties, oral-motor difficulties, upper extremity spasticity).

Early surgical closure of the myelomeningocele sac through fetal surgery has been evaluated in relation to prevention of injury to the exposed spinal cord tissue and the improvement of neurologic and urologic outcomes in the affected child. The Management of Myelomeningocele Study, a clinical trial supported by the National Institutes of Health, found that prenatal surgery for myelomeningocele reduced the need for shunting (for hydrocephalus) as evaluated at 12 months and also decreased the incidence of hindbrain herniation. In addition, there was an improvement in mental and motor function scores at 30 months in the children who had prenatal surgery (compared with children who had postnatal surgery) (Adzick, Thom, Spong, et al., 2011). However, the surgery is not without risks to the fetus and mother, and premature delivery is common. Outcome data for urologic and bowel function, motor function, cognition, and spina bifida–associated outcomes are being gathered in the MOMS2 study, which is expected to end in late 2013 (Clinical Trials, 2013).

Postnatal Care. Initial care of the newborn involves preventing infection; performing a neurologic assessment, including observing for associated anomalies; and dealing with the impact of the anomaly on the family. Although meningoceles are repaired early, especially if there is danger of rupture of the sac, the philosophy regarding skin closure of myelomeningocele varies. Most authorities believe that early closure, within the first 24 to 72 hours, offers the most favorable outcome. Early closure, preferably in the first 12 to 18 hours, not only prevents local infection and trauma to the exposed tissues but also avoids stretching of other nerve roots (which may occur as the meningeal sac expands during the first hours after birth), thus preventing further motor impairment. Broad-spectrum antibiotics are initiated, and neurotoxic substances such as povidone-iodine are avoided at the malformation.

Associated problems are assessed and managed by appropriate surgical and supportive measures. Shunt procedures provide relief from imminent or progressive hydrocephalus (see Chapter 45). Improved surgical techniques do not alter the major physical disability and deformity or chronic urinary tract and pulmonary infections that affect the quality of life for these children. Superimposed on these physical problems are the disorder's effects on family life and finances and on school and hospital services.

Musculoskeletal Considerations. According to most orthopedists, musculoskeletal problems that will affect later locomotion should be evaluated early, and treatment, when indicated, should be instituted without delay. Neurologic assessment will determine the neurosegmental level of the lesion and enable recognition of spasticity and progressive paralysis, potential for deformity, and functional expectations. Orthopedic management includes prevention of joint contractures, correction of the existing deformity, prevention or minimization of the effects of motor and sensory deficits, prevention of skin breakdown, and acquisition of the best possible function of affected lower extremities. Common orthopedic problems requiring attention in SB include deformities of the knees, hips, feet, and spine; fractures and insensate skin further complicate orthopedic care. Other problems that may occur later include kyphosis and scoliosis (Lazzaretti and Pearson, 2010). Because children with this condition often have decreased sensitivity in their lower extremities, preventive skin care is important. A high percentage (60%) of children seen in a wound clinic for skin breakdown had myelomeningocele. The status of the neurologic deficit remains the most important factor in determining the child's ultimate functional abilities.

With technologic advances, a variety of lightweight orthoses, including braces, special "walking" devices, and custom-built wheelchairs, are available to provide mobility to children with spinal cord lesions (see also Chapter 36). Early in infancy, intervention with passive range-of-motion exercises, positioning, and stretching exercises may help decrease the incidence of muscle contractures. Corrective surgical procedures, when indicated, are best initiated at an early age so the child will not lag significantly behind age mates in developmental progress. When there is little hope for lower extremity functioning, surgery is seldom recommended unless it will improve sitting position in a wheelchair and function for ADLs and mobility.

Management of Genitourinary Function. Myelomeningocele is one of the most common causes of neuropathic (neurogenic) bladder dysfunction among children. In infants, the goal of treatment is to preserve renal function. In older children, the goal is to preserve renal function and achieve optimal urinary continence. Urinary incontinence is a chronic, often debilitating problem for the child. In addition, the neuropathic bladder may produce urinary system distress, characterized by symptomatic urinary tract infections, ureterohydronephrosis, and vesicoureteral reflux or renal insufficiency. The characteristics of bladder dysfunction in children vary according to the level of the neurologic lesion and the influence of bony growth and development on the spine. Therefore ongoing urologic monitoring is essential. Evidence is growing that early intervention, based on evaluation during the neonatal period and before complications occur, serves to improve bladder function, reduces the risk for subsequent urinary system distress, and decreases the need for reconstructive surgery of the lower urinary tract (Snodgrass and Gargollo, 2010; Tarcan, Onol, Ilker, et al., 2006).

Treatment of renal problems includes:
- Regular urologic care with prompt and vigorous treatment of infections
- A method of regular emptying of the bladder, such as clean intermittent catheterization (CIC) taught to and performed by parents and self-catheterization taught to children
- Medications to improve bladder storage and continence, such as oxybutynin chloride (Ditropan) and tolterodine (Detrol)

- Surgical procedures such as *vesicostomy* (bladder surgically brought out to the abdominal wall, allowing continuous urinary drainage) and *augmentation enterocystoplasty* (using a segment of bowel or stomach to increase bladder capacity, thereby reducing high bladder pressures)

However, despite the combined efforts of CIC, medication, and surgical intervention, some children with myelodysplasia may continue to experience debilitating urinary incontinence. Many of these children are able to attain social continence with a continent urinary diversion commonly referred to as a *Mitrofanoff procedure.* In this procedure, a catheterizable channel is surgically created from appendix, ureter, or tapered bowel. The proximal end of the channel is connected to the bladder with the distal end brought out as a small stoma on the abdominal wall, usually near the umbilicus. The bladder neck may be sutured to prevent urinary leakage from the urethra. CIC through the easily accessible abdominal route fosters greater independence in children, especially in those unable to transfer from wheelchair to toilet to perform CIC.

Bowel Control. Some degree of fecal continence can be achieved in most children with myelomeningocele with diet modification, regular toilet habits, and prevention of constipation and impaction. It is frequently a lengthy process. Dietary fiber supplements (recommended age of child in years + 5 = g/day of fiber), laxatives, suppositories, or enemas aid in producing regular evacuation. Older children and adolescents seeking more independence may attain bowel continence and higher quality of life after undergoing an *antegrade continence enema (ACE)* procedure (Doolin, 2006). In a procedure similar to the Mitrofanoff, the appendix or ileum is used to create a catheterizable channel with attachment of the proximal end to the colon. The distal end of the channel exits through a small abdominal stoma. Every 1 or 2 days, a catheter is passed through the stoma, allowing enema solution to be instilled directly into the colon. After administration of the enema solution, the child sits on the toilet for 30 to 60 minutes as stool is flushed out through the rectum. The frequency of enemas and volume of solution used to completely evacuate the bowel vary among individuals.

Prognosis. The early prognosis for the child with myelomeningocele depends on the neurologic deficit present at birth, including motor ability, bladder innervation, and associated neurologic anomalies. Early surgical repair of the spinal defect, antibiotic therapy to reduce the incidence of meningitis and ventriculitis, prevention of urinary system dysfunction, and early detection and correction of hydrocephalus have significantly increased the survival rate and quality of life in such children. Children with spina bifida have normal intelligence. Many children with SB achieve partial independent living and gainful employment. Reports of survival rates vary, and many include adults who were born before medical advances and surgical techniques seen in the past 25 years. Coordinated care for adults with SB is essential; however, multidisciplinary adult care is often inadequate (Lazzaretti and Pearson, 2010). In children and adolescents with SB, the achievement of urinary continence is associated with improved self-concept and esteem, especially among girls (Moore, Kogan, and Parekh, 2004). This chronic condition has an array of associated complications, including hydrocephalus and shunt malfunctions, Chiari II development, scoliosis, bowel and bladder management issues, latex allergy, and epilepsy. However, based on current medical knowledge and ethical considerations, aggressive, early management is favored for the child with myelomeningocele.

Prevention. The Centers for Disease Control and Prevention (CDC) (2009) continues to affirm that 50% to 70% of NTDs can be prevented by daily consumption of 0.4 mg of folic acid by women of childbearing age. The data indicate that serum folate concentrations among women of childbearing age decreased 16% from 2003 to 2004 in all ethnic groups studied. Lowest serum folate levels were seen in non-Hispanic Caucasians in 2003 to 2004; however, overall serum folate levels remained below recommended levels in non-Hispanic African-Americans during all three periods studied (CDC, 2007). These results indicate that nurses and other health care workers have an important task in disseminating information that may decrease the incidence of birth defects in children by promoting maternal consumption of folic acid.*

To ensure adequate daily intake of the recommended amount of folic acid, women must take a folic acid supplement, eat a fortified breakfast cereal containing 100% of the recommended dietary allowance of folic acid (e.g., Kellogg's Product 19, General Mills Total, Multigrain Cheerios Plus), or increase their consumption of fortified foods (cereal, bread, rice, grits, pasta) and foods naturally rich in folate (green leafy vegetables and citrus fruits). For women who have had a previous pregnancy affected by NTDs, folic acid intake is increased to 4 mg/day under the supervision of a health care practitioner beginning 1 month before a planned pregnancy and continuing through the first trimester. Supplementation of 4 mg of folate should not be given solely in multivitamin preparations because of the risk for overdose of other vitamins. Drugs that affect folic acid metabolism and increase the risk for myelomeningocele should be avoided before pregnancy (if plans are to become pregnant in the near future) and during pregnancy; these include trimethoprim and the AEDs *carbamazepine, phenytoin, phenobarbital, valproic acid,* and *primidone* (Kinsman and Johnston, 2011).

CARE MANAGEMENT

At birth, an examination is performed to assess the intactness of the membranous cyst. During transport to the nursery, every effort is made to prevent trauma to this protective covering. In addition to the routine assessment of the newborn (see Chapter 23), the infant is assessed for the level of neurologic involvement. Movement of extremities or skin response, especially an anal reflex that might provide clues to the degree of motor or sensory impairment, is noted. It is important to observe the infant's behavior in conjunction with the stimulus because limb movements can be induced in response to spinal cord reflex activity that has no connection with the higher centers. Observation of urinary output, especially if a diaper remains dry, may reveal urinary retention. Abdominal assessment revealing bladder distention, even with a wet diaper, may indicate urinary overflow in a retentive bladder. The head circumference is measured daily (see Chapter 23), and the fontanels are examined for signs of tension or bulging.

> **! NURSING ALERT**
>
> Avoid measuring rectal temperatures in infants with SB. Because bowel sphincter function is frequently affected, the thermometer can cause irritation and rectal prolapse.

---

*Information is available from CDC, National Center on Birth Defects and Developmental Disabilities, Division of Birth Defects and Developmental Disabilities, 1600 Clifton Road NE, MS E-86, Atlanta, GA 30333; 800-CDC-INFO; e-mail: cdcinfo@cdc.gov; www.cdc.gov/ncbddd/folicacid; and from the March of Dimes Resource Center, 1275 Mamaroneck Ave., White Plains, NY 10605; www.marchofdimes.com.

Care of the Myelomeningocele Sac. The infant is usually placed in an incubator or warmer so temperature can be maintained without clothing or covers that might irritate the spinal lesion. Before surgical closure, the myelomeningocele is prevented from drying by the application of a sterile, moist, nonadherent dressing over the defect. The moistening solution is usually sterile normal saline. When an overhead warmer is used, the dressings over the defect require more frequent moistening because of the drying effect of the radiant heat.

Dressings are changed frequently (every 2-4 hours), and the sac is closely inspected for leaks, abrasions, irritation, and any signs of infection. The sac must be carefully cleansed if it becomes soiled or contaminated. Sometimes the sac ruptures during delivery or transport, and any opening in the sac greatly increases the risk for infection to the CNS.

> **! NURSING ALERT**
>
> Observe for early signs of infection, such as temperature instability (axillary), irritability, and lethargy, and for signs of increased intracranial pressure, which might indicate developing hydrocephalus.

One of the most important and challenging aspects in the early care of the infant with myelomeningocele is positioning. Before surgery, the infant is kept in the prone position to minimize tension on the sac and the risk for trauma. The prone position allows for optimal positioning of the legs, especially in cases of associated hip dysplasia. The infant is placed prone with the hips slightly flexed and supported to reduce tension on the defect. The legs are maintained in abduction with a pad between the knees to counteract hip subluxation, and a small roll is placed under the ankles to maintain a neutral foot position. A variety of aids, including diaper rolls, small foam pads, or specially designed frames and appliances, can be used to maintain the desired position.

Prevent Complications. The prone position affects other aspects of the infant's care. For example, in this position, the infant is more difficult to keep clean, pressure areas are a constant threat, and feeding becomes a problem. The infant's head is turned to one side for feeding. Fortunately, most defects are repaired early, and the infant can be held for feeding soon after surgery. Special care must be taken to avoid pressure on the operative site.

Diapering the infant may be contraindicated until the defect has been repaired and healing is well advanced or epithelialization has taken place. The padding beneath the diaper area is changed as needed to keep the skin dry and free of irritation. When urinary retention is detected, CIC is used. Because the bowel sphincter is frequently affected, there is continual passage of stool, often misinterpreted as diarrhea, which is a constant irritant to the skin and a potential source of infection to the spinal lesion.

Areas of sensory and motor impairment are subject to skin breakdown and therefore require meticulous care. Placing the infant on a special mattress or mattress overlay reduces pressure on the knees and ankles. Periodic cleansing, application of lotion, and gentle massage aid circulation.

Gentle range-of-motion exercises are carried out to prevent contractures, and stretching of contractures is performed when indicated. However, these exercises may be restricted to the foot, ankle, and knee joints. When the hip joints are unstable, stretching against tight hip flexors or adductor muscles, which act much like bowstrings, may aggravate a tendency toward subluxation. Consultation with a physical therapist is an important aspect of the short- and long-term management of infants with myelomeningocele.

Cuddling infants with unrepaired myelomeningocele may be contraindicated depending on the status of the lesion. Their need for tactile stimulation is met by caressing, stroking, and other comfort measures. Individualized developmental care with age-appropriate stimulation is provided (see Developmental Outcome, Chapter 25).

Provide Postoperative Care. Postoperative care of the infant with myelomeningocele involves the same basic care as that of any postsurgical infant and includes monitoring vital signs, monitoring intake and output, providing nourishment, observing for signs of infection, and managing pain as needed. Care of the operative site is carried out under the direction of the surgeon and includes close observation for signs of leakage of CSF. General care is continued as preoperatively.

The prone position is maintained after surgical closure, although many neurosurgeons allow a side-lying or partial side-lying position unless it aggravates a coexisting hip dysplasia or permits undesirable hip flexion. This offers an opportunity for position changes, which reduces the risk for pressure sores and facilitates feeding. If permitted, the infant can be held upright against the body, with care taken to avoid pressure on the operative site. After the effects of anesthesia have subsided and the infant is alert, feedings may be resumed unless there are other anomalies or associated complications.

Support Family and Educate About Home Care. As soon as the parents are able to cope with the infant's condition, they are encouraged to become involved in care. They need to learn how to continue at home the care that has been initiated in the hospital, including positioning, feeding, skin care, and range-of-motion exercises when appropriate. They are taught CIC technique when it is prescribed. Parents also need to know the signs of complications (urinary, neurologic, orthopedic) and how to obtain assistance when needed.

The mother who wishes to breastfeed the infant is encouraged to do so because this will be beneficial. Shortly after birth, the mother is started on a program of pumping to initiate and maintain milk supply until the infant is stable enough to begin breastfeeding (Hurtekant and Spatz, 2007). This process may require considerable support from nurses, physicians, and family members because of separation from the infant for surgical care and recovery.

The long-range planning with and support of the parents and newborn begins in the hospital and continues throughout childhood and even into young adulthood. The life expectancy of children with SB extends well into adulthood; therefore planning should involve long-term goals and plans for optimum function as an adult. Discussion about aspects of adulthood such as receiving educational or vocational training and education, living independently, having a mate, having sexual relationships, and bearing and rearing children is important and should not be overlooked. The unique service needs of adolescents with SB as they attempt to gain independence from family and establish lives of their own have not been adequately addressed in the literature (Sawyer and Macnee, 2010). Betz, Linroth, Butler, et al. (2010) interviewed young people with SB making the transition to adulthood. Some common themes that emerged among these young people were (1) challenges in preparation for self-management, (2) limited social relationships, (3) awareness of their cognitive challenges, and (4) the cost of independence. Nurses assume an important role as central members of the health care team. As a health care manager and coordinator, nurses review information with the family, take responsibility for family teaching, and act as a liaison between inpatient and outpatient services. The child may need numerous hospitalizations over the years, and each one will be a source of stress to which the younger child is especially vulnerable (see Chapter 36 for a discussion of care of the child with a disability).

BOX 49-6	MEDICAL CONDITIONS ASSOCIATED WITH RISK FOR LATEX ALLERGY

- Spina bifida
- Urogenital anomalies
- Imperforate anus
- Tracheoesophageal fistula
- VATER association (**v**ertebral defects, imperforate **a**nus, **t**racheo**e**sophageal fistula, and **r**adial and **r**enal dysplasia)
- Preterm infants
- Ventriculoperitoneal shunt
- Cognitive impairment
- Cerebral palsy
- Tetraplegia
- Multiple surgeries
- Atopy

Habilitation involves not only solving problems of self-help and locomotion but also solving the most distressing challenge of urinary or bowel incontinence, which threatens the child's social acceptability. Assistance in preparing the child and the school regarding the child's special needs helps provide a better initial adjustment to this broader social experience.

A Life Course Model has been developed for patients, families, caregivers, teachers, and clinicians to facilitate, through a developmental approach, the care of the child and young person with SB; this program has been made into a web-based tool that can be used to assist in the transition to adulthood (Dicianno, Fairman, Juengst, et al., 2010). Additional information regarding this program is available through the Spina Bifida Association's website at www.sbpreparations.org.

The Spina Bifida Association of America* is organized to provide services and support for families of children with spinal lesions.

Latex Allergy

Latex allergy, or latex hypersensitivity, was identified as being a serious health hazard when a report linked intraoperative anaphylaxis with latex in children with SB. Latex, a natural product derived from the rubber tree, is used in combination with other chemicals to give elasticity, strength, and durability to many products. Children with SB are at high risk for developing latex allergy because of repeated exposure to latex products during surgery and procedures. Therefore such children should not be exposed to latex products from birth onward to minimize the occurrence of latex hypersensitivity. Allergic reactions range from urticaria, wheezing, watery eyes, and rashes to anaphylactic shock. More severe reactions tend to occur when latex comes in contact with mucous membranes, wet skin, the bloodstream, or an airway. There also can be cross-reactions to a number of foods (e.g., banana, avocado, kiwi, chestnut).

Allergic reactions to latex protein can also occur when the substance is transferred to food by food handlers wearing latex gloves, prompting several states to pass legislation that prohibits the use of latex gloves in food service. In addition to patients with SB, high-risk populations include patients with urogenital anomalies or multiple surgeries as well as health care workers. See Box 49-6 for medical conditions associated with the risk for latex allergy.

The most important goals are prevention of latex sensitivity and identification of children with a known hypersensitivity (see Guidelines box). High risk and latex-allergic individuals must be managed in a latex-free environment. Take care that they do not come in

---

*4590 McArthur Blvd., NW, Suite 250, Washington, DC 20007-4226; 202-944-3285, 800-621-3141; fax: 202-944-3295; www.sbaa.org.

direct or secondary contact with products or equipment containing latex at *any time* during medical treatment. Allergy testing can identify latex sensitivity with varying success. Skin prick testing and provocation testing carry the risk for allergic reaction or anaphylaxis. Several commercially available assays can be useful in confirming latex sensitivity. To date, none of these tests demonstrates complete diagnostic reliability, and they should not be the sole determinant of the presence or absence of an allergic response to latex.

Because children who have SB are prone to develop sensitivity to latex, reducing exposure from birth on may decrease the chance of allergy development. Nonlatex products lists are available to parents and health care workers; these products may be substituted for those containing latex. In the health care arena, it is important to use products with the lowest potential risk for sensitizing patients and staff members.*

The identification of those sensitive to latex is best accomplished through careful screening of all patients. During the health interview with the parent or child, ask *all* patients, not only those at risk, about sensitivity to latex. Be certain this is a routine part of all preoperative and preprocedural histories. Stress the importance of the allergy history to all personnel (e.g., phlebotomists, respiratory therapists). (See Guidelines box for questions related to latex allergy.) Children with latex hypersensitivity should carry some form of allergy identification, such as a MedicAlert bracelet. Education programs regarding latex hypersensitivity are aimed at those who care for high risk groups, such as children with SB, and may include relatives, school nurses, teachers, child care workers, and babysitters. In addition to educating caregivers about the child's exposure to medical products that contain latex, nurses need to inform them of common nonmedical latex objects such as water toys, pacifiers, and plastic storage bags.† Items brought to the hospital, such as floral bouquets, should also be screened for latex toys and balloons. Parents should also receive literature explaining signs and symptoms of latex

hypersensitivity and appropriate emergency treatment. (See Anaphylaxis, Chapter 42.)

Spinal Muscular Atrophy Type 1 (Werdnig-Hoffmann Disease)

Spinal muscular atrophy (SMA) type 1 (Werdnig-Hoffmann disease) is a disorder characterized by progressive weakness and wasting of skeletal muscles caused by degeneration of anterior horn cells. It is inherited as an autosomal recessive trait and is the most common paralytic form of the *floppy infant syndrome* (congenital hypotonia). The sites of the pathologic condition are the anterior horn cells of the spinal cord and the motor nuclei of the brainstem, but the primary effect is atrophy of skeletal muscles. The age of onset is variable, but the earlier the onset, the more disseminated and severe the motor weakness. The disorder may be manifested early—often at birth—and almost always before 2 years of age; death may occur as a result of respiratory failure by age 2 years (Iannaccone and Burghes, 2002; Lunn and Wang, 2008). The manifestations (Box 49-7) and prognosis are categorized according to the age of onset, severity of weakness, and clinical course; some children may fluctuate between exhibiting symptoms of types 1 and 2 or types 2 and 3 in regard to clinical function (Sarnat, 2011c). Some experts also categorize SMA according to the highest level of motor function (Lunn and Wang, 2008); type 1 includes "nonsitters," type 2 includes "sitters," and type 3 includes "walkers" (Iannaccone, 2007). A severe rare fetal form of SMA, classified as *type 0*, is reported to be quite lethal in the perinatal period; motor neuron degeneration may be noted as early as midgestation in type 0 (Sarnat, 2011c). Type 4 may present between 20 and 30 years of age and may be referred to as *proximal adult type SMA* (Prior, 2010).

Diagnostic Evaluation and Therapeutic Management

The diagnosis is based on the molecular genetic marker for the *SMN* (survival motor neuron) gene, which is located on chromosome *5q13*. Prenatal diagnosis may be made by genetic analysis of circulating fetal cells in maternal blood or circulating fetal cells in amniotic fluid. The risk for subsequent affected offspring in carriers of the mutant gene or in families with known cases of SMA may also be evaluated genetically. Further diagnostic studies include muscle electromyography (EMG), which demonstrates a denervation pattern, and muscle biopsy; however, the genetic analysis has become the gold standard for diagnosis of the condition.

There is no cure for the disease, and treatment is symptomatic and preventive, primarily preventing joint contractures and treating orthopedic problems, the most serious of which is scoliosis. Hip subluxation and dislocation may also occur. Many children benefit from powered wheelchairs, lifts, special pressure-adjustable mattresses, and accessible environmental controls. Muscle and joint contractures require careful attention and care to prevent further complications. Nutritional growth failure may occur in infants and toddlers as a result of poor feeding; supplemental gastrostomy feedings may be required to maintain adequate nutritional status and maintain weight gain. The use of lower extremity orthoses may assist with ambulation, but eventually, the child may be confined to a wheelchair as muscle atrophy progresses. Restrictive lung disease is the most serious complication of SMA (Iannaccone, 2007). Upper respiratory tract infections often occur and are treated with antibiotic therapy; they are the cause of death in many children. Rapid eye movement (REM)–related sleep-disordered breathing is common in children with SMA type 1; this progresses to sleep-disordered breathing during REM and non-REM sleep followed by respiratory failure, which often requires nocturnal

---

*For a list of latex products and alternative products, see the SBAA National Resource Center and the Latex List on the Spina Bifida Association's home page, www.spinabifidaassociation.org.

†Latex-free product lists are available from the American Latex Allergy Association's online resource manual, available at www.latexallergyresources.org/ResourceManual/section1/index.cfm. American Latex Allergy Association, PO Box 198, Slinger, WI 53086; 888-972-5378; www.latexallergyresources.org.

BOX 49-7 CLINICAL MANIFESTATIONS OF SPINAL MUSCULAR ATROPHY

Type 1 (Werdnig-Hoffmann Disease)
- Disease acquired in utero or during first 2 months of life
- Hypotonia and inactivity most prominent features
- Infant lying in the frog position with legs externally rotated, abducted, and flexed at knees
- Weakness
- Absent deep tendon reflexes
- Limited movements of shoulder and arm muscles
- Active movement usually limited to fingers and toes
- Diaphragmatic breathing with intercostal retractions (diaphragmatic paralysis may occur)
- Abnormal tongue movements
- Weak cry and cough (may be absent)
- Secretions tending to pool in oropharynx
- Alert facies
- Normal sensation and intellect
- Tiring quickly during feedings (if breastfed, may lose weight before noticeable)
- Affected infants failing to progress to sitting alone, rolling over, or walking
- Early death (usually by 2 years of age) from respiratory failure or infection

Type 2 (Intermediate Spinal Muscular Atrophy)
- Symptoms manifest between 2 and 12 months of age:
  - **Early**—Weakness confined to arms and legs
  - **Later**—Weakness becomes generalized
- Legs usually involved to greater extent than arms
- Prominent pectus excavatum
- Movements absent during complete relaxation or sleep
- Some infants able to sit if placed in position
- Failure to walk is common
- Life span varies from 7 months to 7 years or even longer in some cases

Type 3 (Kugelberg-Welander Disease)
- Onset of symptoms in late childhood or adolescence (may be initially misdiagnosed as muscular dystrophy [limb-girdle])
- Normal head control and ability to sit unassisted by 6 to 8 months of age
- Thigh and hip muscles weak
- In those who manage to walk:
  - Lumbar lordosis
  - Waddling gait
  - Genu recurvatum
  - Protuberant abdomen
  - Ambulation increasingly difficult
  - Age of onset influences ambulatory difficulty—the later (after 2 years) the onset, the better the prognosis
  - Confined to a wheelchair by second decade (may vary)
- Deep tendon reflexes may be present early but disappear
- Scoliosis common

NOTE: These classifications are general, and experts suggest there may be variations in life span and other characteristics (Iannaccone and Burghes, 2002; Russman, 1996; Russman, Iannaccone, Buncher, et al., 1992).

noninvasive mechanical ventilation (Schroth, 2009). Noninvasive ventilation methods such as bilevel positive airway pressure (BiPAP) have decreased the morbidity and increased the survival rate of children with SMA types 1 and 2. Children with SMA type 1 who undergo tracheotomy and invasive ventilation often remain ventilator dependent for the rest of their lives; some families choose to withdraw support when invasive ventilation becomes necessary (Mercuri, Bertini, and Iannaccone, 2012). *Palliative care* is an important aspect of care for families of children with SMA type 1. A decreased ability to cough and clear secretions may be managed with airway clearance therapies such as the cough-assist machine and manual cough assistance. Guidelines for the standardization of respiratory care for patients with SMA have been published elsewhere (Schroth, 2009).

Prognosis. Prognosis varies according to the age of onset or group as described in Box 49-7. Individuals with SMA type 1 may succumb to respiratory infections or failure between 1 and 24 months of age (Iannaccone and Burghes, 2002; Sarnat, 2011c); however, some may live longer with enteral feeding and noninvasive mechanical ventilation techniques (Mercuri, Bertini, and Iannaccone, 2012). A significant number of infants with SMA require a tracheotomy, and associated medical conditions in survivors include gastroesophageal reflux, scoliosis, early-onset puberty, hip dysplasia, and recurrent oral candidiasis (Bach, 2007). Drug therapy with riluzole, valproic acid, gabapentin, and oral phenylbutyrate has been shown to slow the progression of the condition, but none has demonstrated significant overall benefits (Bosboom, Vrancken, van den Berg, et al., 2009; Sarnat, 2011c).

CARE MANAGEMENT

An infant or small child with progressive muscle weakness requires nursing care similar to that of an immobilized patient (see Chapter 48). However, the underlying goal of treatment should be to assist the child and family in dealing with the illness while progressing toward a life of normalization within the child's capabilities. Special attention should be directed to preventing muscle and joint contractures, promoting independence in performance of ADLs, and becoming incorporated into the mainstream of school when possible. In addition, parents need support and resources to be able to provide for the child and remain an intact family. Because children with neuromuscular disease have abnormal breathing patterns that often contribute to early death, it is important to assess adequate oxygenation, especially during the sleep phase when shallow breathing occurs and hypoxemia may develop. Home pulse oximetry may be used to assess the child during sleep and provide noninvasive mechanical ventilation as necessary (Bush, Fraser, Jardine, et al., 2005; Young, Lowe, Fitzgerald, et al., 2007) (see Duchenne [Pseudohypertrophic] Muscular Dystrophy on p. 1588 for respiratory management). Supportive care also includes management of orthoses and other orthopedic equipment as required. Because children with SMA are intellectually normal, verbal, tactile, and auditory stimulation are important aspects of developmental care. Supporting them so they can see the activities around them and transporting them in appropriate equipment (e.g., wagon, power wheelchair) for a change of environment provide stimulation and a broader scope of contacts.

Children who are able to sit require proper support and attention to alignment to prevent deformities and other complications. Children who survive beyond infancy need attention to educational needs and opportunities for social interaction with other children. The parents of a child who is chronically ill require much support

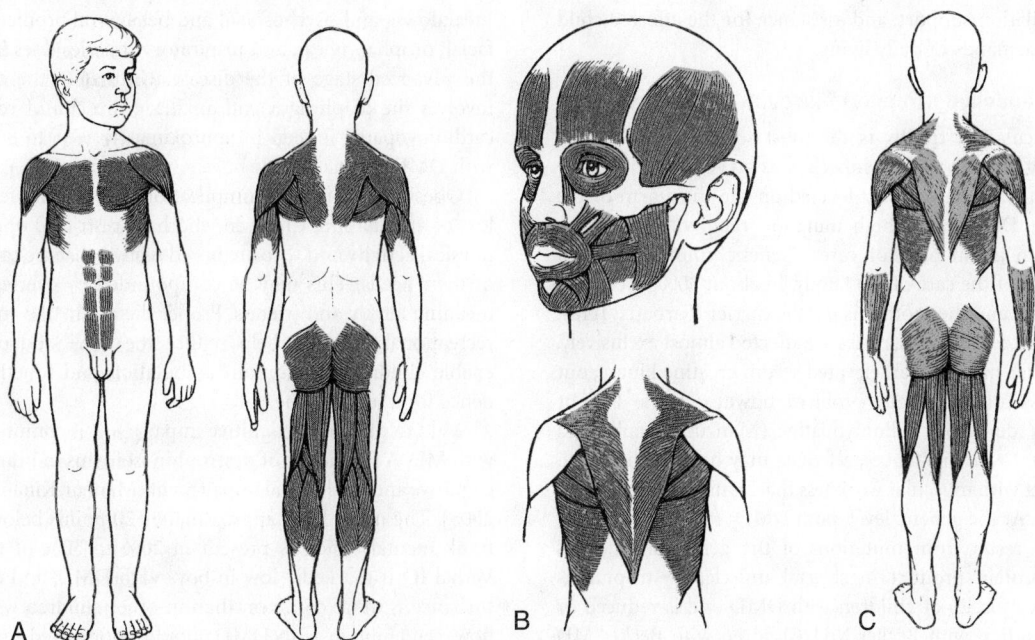

FIG 49-7 Initial muscle groups involved in muscular dystrophies. **A,** Pseudohypertrophic. **B,** Facioscapulohumeral. **C,** Limb-girdle.

and encouragement* (see Chapter 38). Parents who have not sought genetic counseling should be encouraged to do so to evaluate further risk potential.

Spinal Muscular Atrophy Type 3 (Kugelberg-Welander Disease)

Spinal muscular atrophy type 3 (Kugelberg-Welander disease) is a result of anterior horn cell and motor nerve degeneration. The disease is characterized by a pattern of muscular weakness similar to that of infantile SMA (see Box 49-7). Several modes of inheritance have been reported for the disease: autosomal recessive, autosomal dominant, and X-linked recessive.

The onset occurs from younger than 1 year of age into adulthood, with symptoms resembling type 3 SMA. Proximal muscle weakness (especially of the lower limbs) and muscular atrophy are the predominant features. The disease runs a slowly progressive course. Some children lose the ability to walk 8 to 9 years after the onset of symptoms, but many can still walk after 30 years or more. One source notes that approximately one half of all children with SMA type 3 lose ambulation by age 14 years and may require a wheelchair for times when falls are more frequent (Mercuri, Bertini, and Iannaccone, 2012). Many affected persons have a normal life expectancy (Lunn and Wang, 2008).

THERAPEUTIC MANAGEMENT AND CARE MANAGEMENT

The management is primarily symptomatic and supportive and is related to maintaining mobility as long as possible, preventing

---

*Family resources include Families of SMA, 925 Busse Road, Elk Grove Village, IL 60007; 800-886-1762; www.fsma.org; and Muscular Dystrophy Association—USA, 3300 E. Sunrise Drive, Tucson, AZ 85718; 800-572-1717; www.mda.org. In Canada: Families of Spinal Muscular Atrophy Canada, 103-7134 Vedder Rd., Chilliwack, British Columbia, Canada V2R 4G4; toll free 855-824-1266; www.curesma.ca.

complications such as skin breakdown, optimizing and maintaining respiratory function, and providing support to the child and family. The discussion of family support in the section for Duchenne muscular dystrophy is also applicable to families of children with SMA.

Muscular Dystrophies

Muscular dystrophies (MDs) constitute the largest and most important single group of muscle diseases of childhood. The MDs have a genetic origin in which there is gradual degeneration of muscle fibers, and they are characterized by progressive weakness and wasting of symmetric groups of skeletal muscles, with increasing disability and deformity. In all forms of MD, there is an insidious loss of strength, but each type differs in regard to the muscle groups affected (Fig. 49-7), age of onset, rate of progression, and inheritance pattern. The most common form, Duchenne muscular dystrophy (DMD), is discussed separately in the next section.

Facioscapulohumeral (Landouzy-Dejerine) *muscular dystrophy* is inherited as an autosomal dominant disorder with onset in early adolescence. It is characterized by difficulty in raising the arms over the head, lack of facial mobility, and a forward slope of the shoulders. The progression is slow, and the life span is usually unaffected.

Limb-girdle muscular dystrophy (LGMD) is a heterogenous group of disorders with autosomal dominant and recessive inheritance whose clinical manifestations often appear in later childhood, adolescence, or early adulthood with variable but usually slow progression (Quan, 2011). All types of LGMD are characterized by weakness of proximal muscles of the pelvic and shoulder girdles. Other forms of MD include myotonic dystrophy, scapulohumeral MD (Emery-Dreifuss MD), fascioscapulohumeral MD (Landouzy-Dejerine disease), and congenital MD; these forms consist of subtypes of MD and are discussed at length elsewhere (see Sarnat, 2011a).

Treatment of the MDs consists mainly of supportive measures, including physical therapy, orthopedic procedures to minimize deformity, ventilation support, and assistance for the affected child in meeting the demands of daily living.

Duchenne (Pseudohypertrophic) Muscular Dystrophy

Duchenne muscular dystrophy is the most severe and the most common MD of childhood. It is inherited as an X-linked recessive trait, and the single-gene defect is located on the short arm of the X chromosome. DMD has a high mutation rate, with a positive family history in about 65% of cases. Genetic counseling is an important aspect of the care of the family. In about 30% of cases, it is a new mutation and the mother is *not* the carrier (Sarnat, 2011a).

As in all X-linked disorders, males are affected almost exclusively. The female carrier may have an elevated serum creatine kinase, but muscle weakness is usually not a problem; however, about 10% of female carriers develop cardiomyopathy (Manzur, Kinali, and Muntoni, 2008). In rare instances, a female may be identified with DMD disease yet with muscular weakness that is milder than in boys (Sarnat, 2011a). At the genetic level, both DMD and Becker MD (a milder variant) result from mutations of the gene that encodes *dystrophin*, a protein product in skeletal muscle. Dystrophin is absent from the muscles of children with DMD and is reduced or abnormal in children with Becker MD. Children with Becker MD have a later onset of symptoms, which are usually not as severe as those seen in DMD. The incidence is approximately 1 in 3600 male births for the Duchenne form and approximately 1 in 30,000 live births for the Becker type (Sarnat, 2007, 2011a). Box 49-8 describes the characteristics of DMD.

Most children with DMD reach the appropriate developmental milestones early in life, although they may have mild, subtle delays. Evidence of muscle weakness usually appears during the third to seventh year, although there may have been a history of delay in motor development, particularly walking. Difficulties in running, riding a bicycle, and climbing stairs are usually the first symptoms noted. Typically, affected boys have a waddling gait and lordosis, fall frequently, and develop a characteristic manner of rising from a squatting or sitting position on the floor (Gower sign). Lordosis occurs as a result of weakened pelvic muscles, and the waddling gait is a result of weakness in the gluteus medius and maximus muscles (Battista, 2010). In the early years, rapid developmental gains may mask the progression of the disease.

Muscles, especially in the calves, thighs, and upper arms, become enlarged from fatty infiltration and feel unusually firm or woody on palpation (Box 49-9). The term pseudohypertrophy is derived from this muscular enlargement. Profound muscular atrophy occurs in the later stages; contractures and deformities involving large and small joints are common complications as the disease progresses. Ambulation usually becomes impossible by 12 years of age. The loss of mobilization further increases the spectrum of complications, which may include osteoporosis, fractures, constipation, skin breakdown, and psychosocial and behavioral problems. Atrophy of facial, oropharyngeal, and respiratory muscles does not occur until the advanced stage of the disease. Ultimately, the disease process involves the diaphragm and auxiliary muscles of respiration, and cardiomyopathy is seen in approximately 50% to 80% of patients with DMD (Sarnat, 2011a).

Obesity is a common complication that contributes to premature loss of ambulation. Children who have restricted opportunities for physical activity and who are bored easily consume calories in excess of their needs. This may be compounded by overfeeding by well-meaning family and friends. Proper dietary intake and a diversified recreational program help reduce the likelihood of obesity and enable children to maintain ambulation and functional independence for a longer time.

Mild to moderate cognitive impairment is commonly associated with MD. A deficiency of dystrophin isoforms in brain tissue causes cognitive and intellectual impairment (Manzur, Kinali, and Muntoni, 2008). The mean IQ is approximately 20 points below normal, and frank mental deficit is present in 20% to 30% of these children. Verbal IQ is markedly low in boys with DMD, and emotional disturbance is more common than in other children with disabilities; however, children with DMD should be involved in early learning programs and eventually moved into regular classrooms as much as possible. Patients with Becker MD present later in life than those with DMD, but they often do not survive past the middle of the second decade, with few patients living into their 40s (Sarnat, 2011a).

Diagnostic Evaluation. The diagnosis of DMD is primarily established by blood polymerase chain reaction (PCR) for the dystrophin gene mutation (Sarnat, 2011a). Prenatal diagnosis is also possible as early as 12 weeks of gestation. Serum enzyme measurement, muscle biopsy, and EMG may also be used in establishing the diagnosis. Serum creatine kinase (CK) levels are extremely high in the first 2 years of life before the onset of clinical weakness. If the child demonstrates the usual characteristics, has a positive family history for DMD, and the PCR result is positive, the muscle biopsy may be deferred.

Therapeutic Management. No effective treatment exists for childhood MD. The use of the corticosteroids *prednisone* and

---

BOX 49-8   CHARACTERISTICS OF DUCHENNE MUSCULAR DYSTROPHY

- Early onset, usually between 3 and 5 years of age
- Progressive muscular weakness, wasting, and contractures
- Calf muscle hypertrophy in most patients
- Loss of independent ambulation by 9 to 11 years of age
- Slowly progressive, generalized weakness during teenage years
- Relentless progression until death from respiratory or cardiac failure

---

BOX 49-9   CLINICAL MANIFESTATIONS OF DUCHENNE MUSCULAR DYSTROPHY

- Waddling gait
- Lordosis
- Frequent falls
- Gower sign (child turning onto side or abdomen, flexing knees to assume a kneeling position, then with knees extended gradually pushing torso to an upright position by "walking" the hands up the legs)
- Enlarged muscles (especially thighs and upper arms); feel unusually firm or woody on palpation
- Later stages: profound muscular atrophy
- Cognitive impairment (common):
  - Mild (about 20 IQ points below normal)
  - Cognitive impairment present in 25% to 30% of patients
- Complications:
  - Contracture deformities of hips, knees, and ankles
  - Disuse atrophy
  - Obesity

deflazacort has been evaluated as a treatment for DMD. Several clinical trials demonstrated increased muscle strength and improved performance and pulmonary function, with significant decrease in the progression of weakness, when prednisone was administered for 6 months to 2 years (Manzur, Kuntzer, Pike, et al., 2008). The American Academy of Neurology has published a practice parameter for the administration of corticosteroids in the treatment of DMD (Moxley, Ashwal, Pandya, et al., 2005). Major side effects in these studies included weight gain and a cushingoid facial appearance.

Maintaining optimal function in all muscles for as long as possible is the primary goal; secondary is the prevention of contractures. Children with DMD who remain as active as possible are able to avoid wheelchair confinement for a longer time. Maintenance of function often involves stretching exercises, strength and muscle training, breathing exercises to increase and maintain vital lung capacity, range-of-motion exercises, surgery to release contracture deformities, bracing, and performance of ADLs.

Parents should always be involved in making decisions about the child's care, and teaching regarding home safety and prevention of falls is important as well. Parents should also be encouraged to have the child keep follow-up appointments for medical care and physical and occupational therapy. Because respiratory tract infections are most troublesome in these children, influenza and pneumococcal vaccines are encouraged and contact with persons with respiratory tract infections should be avoided. Action plans for prompt treatment of respiratory illness are important.

Eventually, respiratory and cardiac problems become the central focus of the debilitating illness. Children with neuromuscular disease develop abnormal breathing patterns, and hypoxia may occur as a result of inadequate oxygenation. The child and parents should be involved in a discussion of long-term ventilation options. Cardiac and respiratory assessment during wake-sleep cycles is imperative. Respiratory care for children with neuromuscular conditions such as SMA and DMD may involve the use of noninvasive ventilation with BiPAP on a temporary or full-time basis, mechanically assisted coughing (MAC), or tracheostomy and relief of airway obstruction with coughing and suctioning devices; the tracheostomy, however, is associated with more complications (Simonds, 2006; Young, Lowe, Fitzgerald, et al., 2007). Home pulse oximetry may be used to monitor oxygenation during sleep or to aid in decision making regarding the use of MAC to clear the airways.

Several devices are available for children with neuromuscular disease to assist in clearing the airway when the cough reflex is ineffective or diminished. The mechanical cough in-exsufflator (MIE; also referred to as *cough assist*) has been found to be safe and effective in the daily management of respiratory function (Kravitz, 2009; Miske, Hickey, Kolb, et al., 2004). The MIE delivers positive inspiratory pressures at a set rate followed by negative pressure exsufflation coordinated with the patient's own breathing rhythm. The exsufflation is designed to mimic a cough reflex so mucus can be effectively cleared. Airway suctioning after exsufflation is accomplished as necessary to clear the airways. In children, the MIE device may be connected directly to a tracheostomy or used with a mouthpiece or face mask. The Boitano (2009) reference contains a variety of equipment options, including various masks that can be used to deliver noninvasive positive pressure.

Manual cough-assisting techniques include glossopharyngeal breathing or air stacking (frog breathing); the abdominal thrust, which is similar to the Heimlich maneuver (Kravitz, 2009); and manual hyperinflation with a self-inflating resuscitation bag (without oxygen) and a mouthpiece. Hyperinflation may be used in conjunction with abdominal thrusts to improve peak cough flows (Boitano, 2009).

The use of routine chest physiotherapy (postural drainage) for DMD has not been adequately evaluated for its effectiveness in clearing the airway of mucus except when there is focal atelectasis and mucus plugging the airways (Kravitz, 2009).

Survival in individuals with DMD may be prolonged several years with the use of noninvasive ventilation and MAC as alternatives to tracheostomy and airway suctioning (Simonds, 2006). The American Thoracic Society (2004) has published extensive guidelines for respiratory monitoring and care of children and adults with DMD.

The American Academy of Pediatrics (AAP, 2005) recommends an extensive cardiac evaluation of the child diagnosed with either DMD or Becker MD. Patients with neuromuscular conditions may not be seen with the typical signs and symptoms of cardiac dysfunction. Therefore symptoms such as weight loss, nausea and vomiting, cough, increased fatigue on performance of ADLs, and orthopnea should be carefully evaluated to detect early signs of cardiomyopathy.

Genetic counseling is recommended for parents, sisters, and maternal aunts and their daughters. Long-term care, end-of-life care, and palliative care options are issues that the health care team must discuss with the child and family affected by MD (Finder, 2009). Professional counseling is necessary in some cases to allow frank discussion of these issues, and referrals should be made as appropriate.

CARE MANAGEMENT

The care and management of a child with MD involve the combined efforts of a multidisciplinary health care team. Nurses can help clarify the roles of these health care professionals to family and others. The major emphasis of nursing care is to help the child and family cope with a chronic, progressive, incapacitating disease; to help design a program that will afford maximal independence and reduce the predictable and preventable disabilities associated with the disorder; and to help the child and family deal constructively with the limitations the disease imposes on their daily lives. Because of advances in technology, children with MD may live into early adulthood; therefore the goals of care should also involve decisions regarding quality of life, achievement of independence, and transition to adulthood.

Working closely with other team members, nurses assist the family in developing the child's self-help skills to give the child the satisfaction of being as independent as possible for as long as possible. This requires continual evaluation of the child's capabilities, which are often difficult to assess. Fortunately, most children with MD instinctively recognize the need to become as independent as possible and strive to do so.

Practical difficulties faced by families are physical limitations of housing and mobility. Some families live in houses or apartments that are unsuited to wheelchairs. Transportation may also be a barrier for families of children with MD. Assisting with these challenges requires team problem solving. Diet, nutritional needs, and nutrition modification are discussed according to the needs of the individual child and family.

Children with MD tend to become socially isolated as their physical condition deteriorates to the point that they can no longer keep up with their friends and classmates. Their physical capabilities diminish, and their dependency increases at the age at which most children are expanding their range of interests and relationships. To gain peer associations, they often learn and use behaviors that bring them the rewards of other children's company. These friends are often children who have been rejected by more able-bodied classmates.

The parents' social activities are also restricted, and the family's activities must be continually modified to accommodate the needs of the affected child. When the child becomes increasingly incapacitated, the family may consider home-based care, an assisted living facility, or respite care. Unless the child is severely incapacitated, he should also be involved in the decisions regarding such care. Nurses can assist with decision making by exploring all available options and resources and support the child and family in the decision. Older boys with MD may also need psychiatric or psychologic counseling to deal with issues such as depression, anger, and quality of life. Parents also need to be encouraged to become involved in support groups because evidence indicates that adequate social support from family, community, and other parents is crucial to appropriate coping in families with children with chronic illness.

Regardless of how successful the program or how well the family adapts to the disorder, superimposed on the physical and emotional problems associated with a child with a long-term disability is the constant knowledge of the ultimate outcome of the disease. All of the manifestations seen in the child with a chronic fatal illness are encountered in these families (see Chapter 38).

Nurses are especially valuable health care professionals as they come to know the family and the family's problems. Nurses can be alert to the family's problems and needs and make necessary referrals when supplementary services are indicated. The Muscular Dystrophy Association—USA* has branches in most communities to assist families who have a member with MD.

ACQUIRED NEUROMUSCULAR DISORDERS

Guillain-Barré Syndrome (Infectious Polyneuritis)

Guillain-Barré syndrome (GBS), also known as *infectious polyneuritis*, is an uncommon acute demyelinating polyneuropathy with a progressive, usually ascending flaccid paralysis. The hallmark of GBS is acute peripheral motor weakness. The paralysis usually occurs approximately 10 days after a nonspecific viral infection; GBS has also been reported after administration of certain vaccines (rabies, influenza, polio, and meningococcal) (Sarnat, 2011b). Several subtypes of GBS include acute inflammatory demyelinating neuropathy, acute motor axonal neuropathy, acute motor sensory axonal neuropathy, and Miller Fisher syndrome. Children are less often affected than adults; among children, those between ages 4 and 10 years have higher susceptibility. The male-to-female ratio is reported to be 1.5 to 1. Two peak periods with an increased incidence of GBS have been identified: late adolescence and young adulthood.

Chronic inflammatory demyelinating polyradiculoneuropathies (CIDPs) are chronic types of GBS that recur intermittently or do not improve over a period of months to years (Sarnat, 2011b). The following discussion focuses on GBS.

Congenital GBS is rare yet may occur in the neonatal period and consists of hypotonia, weakness, and decreased or absent reflexes. Maternal neuromuscular disease may or may not be present. Diagnosis is established by the same criteria as in older children, but the

*3300 E. Sunrise Drive, Tucson, AZ 85718; 800-572-1717; e-mail: mda@mdausa.org; www.mda.org. In Canada: Muscular Dystrophy Canada, 2345 Yonge St., Suite 900, Toronto, Ontario, Canada M4P 2E5; 866-MUSCLE-8; fax: 416-488-7523; www.muscle.ca/national/home.html.

symptoms gradually subside over the first few months of life and disappear by 12 months (Sarnat, 2011b).

Pathophysiology

Guillain-Barré syndrome is an immune-mediated disease often associated with a number of viral or bacterial infections or the administration of certain vaccines. It has been associated with infectious mononucleosis, measles, mumps, *Campylobacter jejuni* (gastroenteritis), cytomegalovirus, *Borrelia burgdorferi* (Lyme disease), Epstein-Barr virus, *Helicobacter pylori*, and *Mycoplasma* and *Pneumocystis* infections. Onset of GBS symptoms usually occurs within 10 days of the primary infection. Pathologic changes in spinal and cranial nerves consist of inflammation and edema with rapid, segmented demyelination and compression of nerve roots within the dural sheath. Nerve conduction is impaired, producing ascending partial or complete paralysis of muscles innervated by the involved nerves. GBS has three phases:

1. **Acute**—Phase starts when symptoms begin and continues until new symptoms stop appearing or deterioration ceases; it may last as long as 4 weeks.
2. **Plateau**—Symptoms remain constant without further deterioration; it may last from days to weeks.
3. **Recovery**—Patient begins to improve and progress to optimal recovery; it usually lasts a few weeks to months depending on the deficits incurred by the illness.

Diagnostic Evaluation

The diagnosis of GBS is based on clinical manifestations (Box 49-10), CSF analysis, and EMG findings. CSF analysis reveals an abnormally elevated protein concentration, normal glucose, and fewer than 10 white blood cells (WBCs)/mm^3 (Sarnat, 2011b). EMG shows evidence of acute muscle denervation, but other laboratory studies are usually noncontributory. The symmetric nature of the

---

BOX 49-10   CLINICAL MANIFESTATIONS OF GUILLAIN-BARRÉ SYNDROME

Initial Symptoms
- Muscle tenderness
- Paresthesia and cramps (sometimes)
- Proximal symmetric muscle weakness

Paralysis
- Ascending bilateral paralysis from lower extremities
- Frequent involvement of muscles of trunk and upper extremities and those supplied by cranial nerves (especially facial)
- Flaccid paralysis with loss of reflexes
- May involve facial, extraocular, labial, lingual, pharyngeal, and laryngeal muscles
- Intercostal and phrenic nerves:
  - Breathlessness in vocalizations
  - Shallow, irregular respirations

Other Manifestations
- Tendon reflexes depressed or absent
- Variable degrees of sensory impairment
- Muscle tenderness or sensitivity to slight pressure
- Urinary incontinence or retention and constipation

paralysis helps differentiate this disorder from spinal paralytic poliomyelitis, which usually affects sporadic muscles.

Therapeutic Management

Treatment of GBS is primarily supportive. In the acute phase, patients are hospitalized because respiratory and pharyngeal involvement may require assisted ventilation, sometimes with a temporary tracheostomy. Treatment modalities include aggressive ventilatory support in the event of respiratory compromise, intravenous (IV) administration of immunoglobulin (IVIG), and sometimes steroids; plasmapheresis and immunosuppressive drugs may also be used. Plasmapheresis has been shown to decrease the length of recovery in patients with severe GBS; however, it is expensive, and side effects include hypotension, fever, bleeding disorders, chills, urticaria, and bradycardia. Further evidence reports equal benefits to treatment of GBS with IVIG administration or plasmapheresis; both sped up recovery time in studies reviewed (Hughes and Cornblath, 2005). There is evidence, however, of significant improvement in children with high-dose IVIG therapy (versus supportive treatment alone) (Hughes, Swan, and van Doorn, 2010). IVIG is now recommended as the primary treatment of GBS when administered within 2 weeks of disease onset (Hughes, 2008). Corticosteroids alone do not decrease the symptoms or shorten the duration of the disease.

Medications that may be administered during the acute phase include a low-molecular-weight heparin to prevent deep vein thrombosis (DVT), a mild laxative or stool softener to prevent constipation, pain medication such as acetaminophen, and a histamine-antagonist to prevent stress ulcer formation. Chronic neuropathic pain after GBS may be treated with gabapentin, which is reported to be more effective than carbamazepine (Sarnat, 2011b).

Rehabilitation after the acute phase may involve physical therapy, occupational therapy, and speech therapy. Additional consideration should be given to problems of general weakness and retraining for toileting and feeding (Lyons, 2008).

Course and Prognosis. Better outcomes are associated with younger age, no requirement for mechanical respiratory assistance, slower progression of disease, normal peripheral nerve function on EMG, and treatment with either IVIG or plasmapheresis. Recovery usually begins within 2 to 3 weeks, and most patients regain full muscle strength. The recovery of muscle strength progresses in the reverse order of onset of paralysis, with lower extremity strength being the last to recover. Poor prognosis with subsequent residual effects in children is reportedly associated with cranial nerve involvement, extensive disability at time of presentation, and intubation.

Most deaths associated with GBS are caused by respiratory failure; therefore early diagnosis and access to respiratory support are especially important. The rate of recovery is usually related to the degree of involvement and may extend from a few weeks to months. The greater the degree of paralysis, the longer the recovery phase.

CARE MANAGEMENT

Nursing care is primarily supportive and is the same as that required for children with immobilization and respiratory compromise. The emphasis of care is on close observation to assess the extent of paralysis and on prevention of complications, including aspiration, ventilator-associated pneumonia (VAP), atelectasis, DVT, pressure ulcer, fear and anxiety, autonomic dysfunction, and pain.

During the acute phase of the disease, the nurse should carefully observe the child's condition for possible difficulty in swallowing and respiratory involvement. The child's respiratory function is closely monitored, and oxygen source, appropriate-size insufflation bag and mask, endotracheal intubation and suctioning equipment, tracheotomy tray, and vasoconstrictor drugs are kept available. Vital signs are monitored frequently along with neurologic signs and level of consciousness. For children who develop respiratory impairment, the care is the same as that for any child with respiratory distress requiring mechanical ventilation.

Respiratory care, if intubation is required, requires close monitoring of oxygenation status (usually by pulse oximetry and sometimes arterial blood gases), maintenance of an open airway with suctioning, and postural changes to prevent pneumonia. Consideration should be given to preventing opportunistic infections such as VAP; meticulous oral care and hypopharynx suctioning, elevation of the head of bed 30 degrees, and strict asepsis with suctioning equipment (including catheters, a Yankauer device, or both) should be implemented to prevent VAP. Children with oral and pharyngeal involvement may be fed via a nasogastric or gastrostomy tube to ensure adequate feeding. It is also important to consider the possibility of stress ulcers in such patients and to administer a proton pump inhibitor. Immobilization, which occurs with GBS, decreases GI function; therefore problems such as decreased gastric emptying, constipation, and feeding residuals require nursing assessment and appropriate collaborative interventions. Temporary urinary catheterization may be required; urinary retention is common, and appropriate assessment of urinary output is vital. Sensory impairment and paralysis in the lower extremities make the child susceptible to skin breakdown; therefore attention should be given to meticulous skin care. Passive range-of-motion exercises and application of orthoses to prevent muscle contractures are important when paralysis is present. Prevention of DVT is accomplished with pneumatic compression (antiembolism) devices, administration of a low-molecular-weight heparin, and early mobilization and ambulation. Autonomic dysfunction may be life threatening; thus close monitoring of vital signs in the acute phase is essential.

A key to recovery in the child with GBS is the prevention of muscle and joint contractures, so passive range-of-motion exercises must be carried out routinely to maintain vital function. Although the child may have a generalized paralysis, cognitive function remains intact; therefore it is important for nursing care to involve communication with the child or adolescent regarding procedures and treatments that may be frightening, especially if mechanical ventilation is required. Encourage parents to talk to the child and make eye and physical contact and to reassure the child during this phase of the illness.

Pain management is crucial in the care of children with GBS. Although neuromuscular impairment may make pain perception more difficult to accurately evaluate, objective pain scales should be used. Gabapentin and carbamazepine may be used to manage neuropathic pain in patients with GBS.

Physical therapy may be limited to passive range-of-motion exercises during the evolving phase of the disease. Later, as the disease stabilizes and recovery begins, an active physical therapy program is implemented to prevent contracture deformities and facilitate muscle recovery. This may include active exercise, gait training, and bracing.

Throughout the course of the illness, child and parent support are paramount. The usual rapidity of the paralysis and the long recovery period greatly tax the emotional reserves of all family members. The parents and child benefit from repeated reassurance that recovery is occurring and from realistic information regarding the possibility of permanent disability. In the event of a residual disability, the family needs assistance in accepting and adjusting to the loss of function. (See Chapter 38.) The GBS/CIDP Foundation International* is a nonprofit organization devoted to support, education, and research. It provides families with support from recovered persons, publishes informational literature and a newsletter, and maintains a list of health care practitioners experienced with the disease.

Tetanus

Tetanus, or lockjaw, is an acute, preventable, but often fatal disease caused by an exotoxin produced by the anaerobic spore-forming, gram-positive bacillus *Clostridium tetani*. It is characterized by painful muscular rigidity primarily involving the masseter and neck muscles. There are four requirements for the development of tetanus: (1) presence of tetanus spores or vegetative forms of the bacillus, (2) injury to the tissues, (3) wound conditions that encourage multiplication of the organism, and (4) a susceptible host.

Tetanus spores are found in soil, dust, and the intestinal tracts of humans and animals, especially herbivorous animals. The organisms are more prevalent in rural areas but are readily carried to urban areas by the wind. The organisms are not invasive but enter the body by way of wounds, particularly a puncture wound, burn, or crushed area. They may enter through a minor, unnoticed break in the skin, such as a thorn or needle prick, bee sting, or scratch. In newborns, infection may occur through the umbilical cord, usually in situations in which infants are delivered in severely contaminated surroundings or the mother is not adequately immunized. The disease has the greatest incidence in months when persons are more involved in outdoor activities.

Pathophysiology

When prevention efforts are not effective and conditions are favorable, the organisms proliferate and form potent exotoxins, one of which is *tetanospasmin*. Tetanospasmin affects the CNS to produce the clinical manifestations of the disease. The ideal conditions for the organisms' growth are devitalized tissues without access to air, such as wounds that have not been washed or kept clean and those that have crusted over, trapping pus beneath. The exotoxin appears to reach the CNS by way of either the neuron axons or the vascular system. The toxin becomes fixed on nerve cells of the anterior horn of the spinal cord and the brainstem. The toxin acts at the myoneural junction to produce muscular stiffness and lower the threshold for reflex excitability.

The incubation period for tetanus varies from 2 days to months and averages 8 days; most cases occur within 14 days. In neonates, it is usually 5 to 14 days. Shorter incubation periods have been associated with more heavily contaminated wounds, more severe disease, and a worse prognosis (AAP, 2012).

The manner of onset varies, but the initial symptoms are usually a progressive stiffness and tenderness of the muscles in the neck and jaw. Eventually, all voluntary muscles are affected (Box 49-11). As the child recovers from the disease, the paroxysms become less frequent and gradually subside. Survival beyond 4 days usually indicates recovery, but complete recovery may require weeks.

Therapeutic Management

Primary prevention is key and occurs through immunization and boosters (AAP, 2012). After an injury has occurred, further

---

BOX 49-11 CLINICAL MANIFESTATIONS OF TETANUS

Initial Symptoms
- Progressive stiffness and tenderness of muscles in neck and jaw
- Characteristic difficulty in opening the mouth *(trismus)*
- *Risus sardonicus* (sardonic smile) caused by facial muscle spasm

Progressive Involvement
- **Opisthotonic** positioning (severe back arching)
- Boardlike rigidity of abdominal and limb muscles
- Difficulty swallowing
- High sensitivity to external stimuli (slight noise, gentle touch, or bright light):
  - Trigger paroxysmal muscular contractions that last seconds to minutes
  - Contractions recur with increased frequency until almost continuous (sustained tetanic)
- Laryngospasm and tetany of respiratory muscles:
  - Accumulated secretions
  - Respiratory arrest
  - Atelectasis
  - Pneumonia

Other Aspects
- Mentation unaffected; patient alert
- Pain and distress are reflected in:
  - Rapid pulse
  - Sweating
  - Anxious expression
- Fever usually absent or only mild

---

preventive measures are based on the child's immune status and the nature of the injury. Specific prophylactic therapy after trauma is administration of tetanus toxoid (note that equine tetanus antitoxin [TAT] is not available in the United States) (see Immunizations, Chapter 31, for age-specific recommendations).

An unprotected or inadequately immunized child who sustains a "tetanus-prone" wound (including wounds contaminated with dirt, feces, soil, and saliva; puncture wounds; avulsions; and wounds resulting from missiles, crushing, burns, and frostbite) should receive tetanus immunoglobulin (TIG). Concurrent administration of both TIG and tetanus toxoid at separate sites is recommended both to provide protection and to initiate the active immune process.

After the individual has received primary tetanus immunization, antitoxin is believed to provide protection for at least 10 years and for a longer period after booster immunization (AAP, 2012). Recently, the Advisory Committee on Immunization Practices (CDC, 2011) recommended no specific time intervals between the administration of a tetanus- or diphtheria-toxoid containing vaccine and Tdap (tetanus, diphtheria, and pertussis) to provide protection against pertussis; other than a localized pain reaction, no other side effects were noted in persons who received the tetanus and diphtheria (Td) and Tdap at intervals as short as 18 months. Completion of active immunization is carried out according to the usual pattern. Antibiotic treatment with penicillin G (or erythromycin or tetracycline in older children with allergy to penicillin) is important in the management of tetanus as an adjunct against clostridia; metronidazole is a viable alternative (Arnon, 2011b).

MEDICATION ALERT

TIG and tetanus toxoid are always administered via the intramuscular route in separate syringes and at separate sites; they are never administered by the intravenous route.

Aggressive supportive care is necessary to treat tetanus in the acute phase. Acutely ill children are best treated in an intensive care facility where close and constant observation and equipment for monitoring and respiratory support are readily available. A quiet environment is preferred to reduce external stimuli.

General supportive care is indicated, including maintaining an adequate airway and fluid and electrolyte balance, managing pain, and ensuring adequate caloric intake. Indwelling NG or tube feedings may be required to maintain adequate fluid and caloric intake; continued laryngospasm may necessitate total parenteral nutrition or gastrostomy feeding. Severe or recurrent laryngospasm or excessive secretions may require advanced airway management such as endotracheal intubation or tracheotomy.

Tetanus immunoglobulin therapy to neutralize toxins is the most specific therapy for tetanus. Local care of the wound by surgical debridement and cleansing helps reduce the numbers of proliferating organisms at the site of injury. The cleansing should be repeated several times during the first 48 hours, and deep, infected lacerations are usually exposed and debrided. Infiltration of the wound with TIG is no longer considered necessary (AAP, 2012).

Diazepam is the drug of choice for seizure control and muscle relaxation (Arnon, 2011b), but lorazepam (Ativan) may be used in some cases. Intrathecal baclofen, IV magnesium sulfate, dantrolene sodium, and midazolam may also be used in the management of muscle spasticity associated with tetanus. Patients with severe tetanus and those who do not respond to other muscle relaxants may require the administration of a neuromuscular blocking agent, such as rocuronium or vecuronium; intrathecal baclofen may be used as a muscle relaxant but only in the intensive care unit because it often induces apnea. Because of their paralytic effect on respiratory muscles, use of these drugs requires mechanical ventilation with endotracheal intubation or tracheotomy and constant cardiopulmonary monitoring. Endotracheal tube insertion or tracheotomy is often indicated and should be performed before severe respiratory distress develops. Despite the absence of pain manifestation with these drugs, it is important to provide adequate analgesia. The administration of corticosteroids has met with success in some cases.

CARE MANAGEMENT

The care of the child with tetanus requires supportive management with particular attention to airway and breathing. Respiratory status is carefully evaluated for any signs of distress, and appropriate emergency equipment is kept available at all times. The location, extent, and severity of muscle spasms are important nursing observations. Muscle relaxants, opioids, and sedatives that may be prescribed can also cause respiratory depression; therefore the child should be assessed for excessive CNS depression. Attention to hydration and nutrition involves monitoring an IV infusion, monitoring nasogastric or gastrostomy feedings, and suctioning oropharyngeal secretions when indicated.

In caring for a child with tetanus during the acute phase, every effort should be made to control or eliminate stimulation from sound, light, and touch. Although a darkened room is ideal, sufficient light is essential so that the child can be carefully observed; light appears to be less irritating than vibratory or auditory stimuli. The infant or child is handled as little as possible, and extra effort is expended to avoid any sudden or loud noise to prevent seizures.

If a potent muscle relaxant such as vecuronium is used, the total paralysis makes oral communication impossible. The drug is not a sedative, however, and anxiety should be considered in children who are intubated. Therefore all the child's needs must be anticipated and procedures carefully explained beforehand. Additional care is focused on preventing the complications associated with prolonged immobility, including decreased bowel and bladder tone and subsequent constipation, anorexia, DVT, pneumonia, and skin breakdown.

Botulism

Botulism is an acute flaccid paralysis caused by the preformed toxin produced by the anaerobic bacillus *Clostridium botulinum*. In classic, or foodborne, botulism, the most common source of the toxin is a contaminated food source. The disease has a wide variation in severity, from constipation to progressive sequential loss of neurologic function and respiratory failure. The most common source of the toxin is improperly sterilized home-canned foods. CNS symptoms appear abruptly approximately 12 to 36 hours after ingestion of contaminated food and may or may not be preceded by acute digestive disturbance (Box 49-12).

Human botulism is caused by neurotoxins A, B, E, and, rarely, F (AAP, 2012). In addition to foodborne botulism, other forms include wound botulism; infant botulism; and artificial botulism, usually a result of bioterrorism.

Treatment consists of IV administration of botulism antitoxin and general supportive measures, primarily respiratory and nutritional. Toxins vary in protein-binding capacity. Some have a relatively short half-life and do not bind to tissues firmly; therefore therapy is continued until paralysis subsides. Other toxins appear to bind irreversibly to nerve endings and are therefore not amenable to neutralization.

Infant Botulism

Infant botulism, unlike foodborne botulism in older persons, is caused by ingestion of spores or vegetative cells of *C. botulinum* and

BOX 49-12   CLINICAL MANIFESTATIONS OF BOTULISM

General Signs
- Weakness
- Dizziness
- Headache
- Difficulty talking and speaking
- Diplopia
- Vomiting
- Progressive, life-threatening respiratory paralysis

Infant Botulism*
- Constipation (a common symptom)
- Generalized weakness
- Decrease in spontaneous movements
- Diminished or absent deep tendon reflexes
- Loss of head control
- Difficulty feeding
- Weak cry
- Reduced gag reflex
- Progressive respiratory paralysis

*Most commonly diagnosed as a "rule out sepsis" in the acute phase because of clinical presentation.

the subsequent release of the toxin from organisms colonizing the GI tract. *C. botulinum* types A and B are the most common causative strains of infant botulism. This form of botulism has become more prevalent than any other form. Many cases of infant botulism occur in breastfed infants who are being introduced to nonhuman milk substances (AAP, 2012). There appears to be no common food or drug source of the organisms; however, the *C. botulinum* organisms have been found in honey. Botulism may occur in infants as young as 1 week of age up to 12 months of age with peak incidence between 2 and 4 months of age.

The severity of the disease varies widely, from mild constipation to progressive sequential loss of neurologic function and respiratory failure (see Box 49-12). The affected infant is usually well before the onset of symptoms. Constipation is a common presenting symptom, and almost all infants exhibit generalized weakness and a decrease in spontaneous movements. Deep tendon reflexes are usually diminished or absent. Cranial nerve deficits are common, as evidenced by loss of head control, difficulty in feeding, weak cry, and reduced gag reflex. SMA type 1 and metabolic disorders are often mistaken for infant botulism in the initial diagnostic phase because of the similarities in clinical manifestations of hypotonia, lethargy, and poor feeding (Arnon, 2011a). Presenting clinical signs also often mimic those of sepsis in young infants. Botulism toxin exerts its effect by inhibiting the release of acetylcholine at the myoneural junction, thereby impairing motor activity of muscles innervated by affected nerves.

Diagnosis is made on the basis of the clinical history, physical examination, and laboratory detection of the organism in the patient's stool and, less commonly, blood. However, isolation of the organism may take several days; therefore suspicion of botulism by clinical presentation should require emergent treatment (Arnon, 2011a). EMG may be helpful in establishing the diagnosis; however, results may be normal early in the course of the illness.

Treatment consists of immediate administration of botulism immune globulin intravenously (BIG-IV) (Arnon, 2011b) without delaying for laboratory diagnosis. Early administration of BIG-IV neutralizes the toxin and stops the progression of the disease. The human-derived botulism antitoxin (BIG-IV) has been evaluated and is now available nationwide for use only in infant botulism. Infants treated with BIG-IV usually have a shortened hospital stay from approximately 6 weeks to 2 weeks, reportedly as a result of decreased requirements for mechanical ventilation and intensive care (Arnon, 2011a). Approximately 50% of affected infants require intubation and mechanical ventilation; therefore respiratory support is crucial, as is nutritional support because theses infants are unable to feed. Trivalent equine botulinum antitoxin and bivalent antitoxin, used in adults and older children, are *not* administered to infants. Antibiotic therapy is not part of the management because the botulinum toxin is an intracellular molecule and antibiotics would not be effective; aminoglycosides in particular should not be administered because they may potentiate the blocking effects of the neurotoxin (Arnon, 2011a).

The prognosis is generally good if the patient is adequately treated, although recovery may be slow, requiring a few weeks after severe illness. Untreated patients may require a longer hospitalization.

> ### ! NURSING ALERT
>
> Although the precise source of *C. botulinum* spores has not been identified as originating from honey in many cases of infant botulism, it is still recommended that honey not be given to infants younger than 12 months because the spores have been found in honey (CDC, 2010).

CARE MANAGEMENT

Nursing responsibilities include observing, recognizing, and reporting signs of poor feeding, constipation, and muscle impairment in the infant with botulism and providing intensive nursing care when an infant is hospitalized. (See Care Management for the infant with SMA, p. 1586, and Nursing Care of High Risk Newborns, Chapter 25.) Parental support and reassurance are important. Most infants recover when the disorder is recognized and BIG-IV therapy is implemented. Nursing care of the infant on mechanical ventilation requires observation of oxygenation status and vigilance for any complications. Parents should be aware that during recovery, infants fatigue easily when muscular action is sustained. This has important implications for timing the resumption of feedings because of the risk for aspiration. Parents should also be advised that normal bowel activity may not return for several weeks. Therefore a stool softener can be beneficial.

Spinal Cord Injuries

Spinal cord injuries (SCIs) with major neurologic involvement traditionally have not been a common cause of physical disability in children. However, a sufficient number of children with these injuries are admitted to major medical centers, and because of the increased survival rate as a result of improved management, nurses are often involved in the care and rehabilitation of children with SCI.

Mechanisms of Injury

The most common cause of serious spinal cord damage in children is trauma involving motor vehicle crashes (MVCs) (including automobile-bicycle, all-terrain vehicles, and snowmobiles), sports injuries (especially from diving, trampoline activities, gymnastics, and football), birth trauma, and nonaccidental trauma. MVCs accounted for 56% of SCIs in children and adolescents, and falls and firearm injury caused 14% and 9% of SCIs. The children injured (SCI) in MVCs were not properly restrained in 67.7% of the cases (Vitale, Goss, Matsumoto, et al., 2006). The increased use of recreational activities involving motorized vehicles such as jet water skis, all-terrain vehicles, and motorcycles has also increased the incidence of SCIs in children. Congenital defects of the spine such as *myelomeningocele* also may in some cases produce the effects of SCI.

Transverse myelitis (inflammation of the spinal cord) may be caused by illness and has also been reported to develop from inadvertent intraarterial administration of long-acting penicillin injected into the buttocks. Damage can be extensive enough to result in paraplegia or even lower limb amputation.

In MVCs, most SCIs in children are a result of indirect trauma caused by sudden hyperflexion or hyperextension of the neck, often combined with a rotational force. Trauma to the spinal cord without evidence of vertebral fracture or dislocation (SCI without radiographic abnormality, or SCIWORA) is particularly likely to occur in an MVC when proper safety restraints are not used. An unrestrained child becomes a projectile during sudden deceleration and is subject to injury from contact with a variety of objects inside and outside the vehicle. Individuals who use only a lap seat belt restraint are at greater risk for SCI than those who use a combination lap and shoulder restraint. High cervical spine injuries have been reported in children younger than 2 years who are improperly restrained in forward-facing car seats. Infants who are improperly restrained in an infant car seat may experience cervical trauma in a car crash. Small children may also be severely injured by deploying front seat air bags.

Falling from heights occurs less often in children than in adults, but vertebral compression from blows to the head or buttocks can occur in water sports (diving and surfing), falls from horses, or other athletic activities. Birth injuries may occur in breech births from traction force on the spinal cord during birth of the head and shoulders. When shaken, infants commonly sustain cervical cord damage, as well as subdural hematoma and retinal hemorrhage; cognitive impairment and death may occur subsequent to the traumatic event. Infants have weak neck muscles, and during vigorous shaking, their large and heavy heads rapidly wobble back and forth. A significant number of adolescents receive SCIs secondary to gunshot wounds, stabbings, and other violent inflicted injury.

Because of the marked mobility of the neck, fracture or sublux-ation (partial dislocation) is the most common immediate cause of SCI, particularly in the lower cervical region. Although unusual in adults, SCI without fracture is common in children, whose spines are supple, weaker, and more mobile than those of adults. Therefore the force is more easily dissipated over a larger number of segments. In infants and small children younger than 5 years, upper cervical spine fractures and spinal compression are more common, but adolescents tend to have lower cervical and thoracolumbar fracture dislocations (Retake, 2011).

The severity of the force, the mechanisms of the injury, and the degree of the individual's muscular relaxation at the time of the injury greatly influence the extent of the trauma. SCIs are classified as either *complete* or *incomplete*. In a complete injury, there is no motor or sensory function more than three segments below the neurologic level of the injury (Mathison, Kadom, and Krug, 2008). Incomplete lesions have several typical characteristics (Mathison, Kadom, and Krug, 2008):

- **Central cord syndrome**—Central gray matter destruction and preservation of peripheral tracts; tetraplegia with sacral sparing common; some motor recovery gained
- **Anterior cord syndrome**—Complete motor and sensory loss with trunk and lower extremity proprioception and sensation of pressure
- **Posterior cord syndrome**—Loss of sensation, pain, and proprioception with normal cord function, including motor function; able to move extremities but have difficulty controlling such movements
- **Brown-Séquard syndrome**—Unilateral cord lesion with a motor deficit on the opposite side of the body from the primary insult; absence of pain and temperature sensation on the opposite side from the injury
- **Spinal cord concussion**—Transient loss of neural function below the level of the acute spinal cord lesion, resulting in flaccid paralysis and loss of tendon, autonomic, and cutaneous reflex activity; may last hours to weeks

The American Spinal Injury Association (ASIA) International Standards for Neurological Classification of Spinal Cord Injury worksheet (2011) is available online at http://www.asia-spinalinjury.org/elearning/ISNCSCI_Exam_Sheet_r4.pdf. The ASIA Impairment Scale (Box 49-13) combines motor and sensory function and is used to determine the severity of impairment from the injury (complete or incomplete). It may also be used to measure neurologic changes and functional goals for rehabilitation (Mathison, Kadom, and Krug, 2008).

The injury sustained can affect any of the spinal nerves, and the higher the injury, the more extensive the damage. The child can be left with complete or partial paralysis of the lower extremities (para-plegia) or with damage at a higher level and without functional use of any of the four extremities (tetraplegia). A high cervical cord

---

BOX 49-13 AMERICAN SPINAL INJURY ASSOCIATION IMPAIRMENT SCALE

A—Complete: No motor or sensory function is preserved in the sacral segments S4-S5.

B—Sensory Incomplete: Sensory but not motor function is preserved below the neurologic level and includes the sacral segments S4-S5, AND no motor function is preserved more than 3 levels below the motor level on either side of the body.

C—Motor Incomplete: Motor function is preserved below the neurologic level, and more than half of key muscle functions below the single neurologic level of injury have a muscle grade less than 3.

D—Motor Incomplete: Motor function is preserved below the neurologic level, and at least half (or more) of key muscles below the neurologic level have a muscle grade of 3 or more.

E—Normal: If sensation and motor function as tested with the ISNCSCI are graded as normal in all segments and the patient had prior deficits, then the AIS grade is E.

For further details and instructions, see the online page at http://www.asia-spinalinjury.org/elearning/ISNCSCI_Exam_Sheet_r4.pdf. Used with permission, American Spinal Injury Association, 2011.

---

injury that affects the phrenic nerve paralyzes the diaphragm and leaves the child dependent on mechanical ventilation.

A mild but equally frightening form of cord trauma is spinal cord compression, a temporary neural dysfunction without visible damage to the cord. Complete quadriplegia can result but initially may not be differentiated from serious cord injury.

Clinical Manifestations

It is often difficult to determine the extent and severity of damage at first. Immediate loss of function is caused by both anatomic and impaired physiologic function, and improved function may not be evident for weeks or even months. Manifestation of the initial response to acute SCI is flaccid paralysis below the level of the damage. This stage is often referred to as spinal shock syndrome and is caused by the sudden disruption of central and autonomic pathways. Local effects of cord edema and ischemia produce a physiologic transection with or without an anatomic severance. Most children with an SCI experience some spinal shock. Manifestations include the absence of reflexes at or below the cord lesion, with flaccidity or limpness of the involved muscles, loss of sensation and motor function, and autonomic dysfunction (symptoms of hypotension, low or high body temperature, loss of bladder and bowel control, and autonomic dysreflexia).

Autonomic paralysis also affects thermoregulatory functions. Afferent impulses from temperature receptors in the skin are not integrated; therefore the patient is subject to temperature increases or decreases in response to alterations in environmental temperature. Hyperthermia can result from excessive ambient temperature, such as too many covers.

Except in the situations previously mentioned, flaccid paralysis is replaced by spinal reflex activity and increasing spasticity or, in incomplete lesions, greater or lesser degree of neurologic recovery.

The paralytic nature of autonomic function is replaced by autonomic dysreflexia, especially when the lesions are above the midthoracic level. This autonomic phenomenon is caused by visceral distention or irritation, particularly of the bowel or bladder. Sensory impulses are triggered and travel to the cord lesion, where they are blocked, which causes activation of sympathetic reflex action with disturbed central inhibitory control. Excessive sympathetic activity is manifested by a flushing face, sweating forehead, pupillary constriction, marked hypertension, headache, and bradycardia. The precipitating stimulus may be merely a full bladder or rectum or other internal or external sensory input. It can be a catastrophic event unless the irritation is relieved.

Additional clinical findings of SCI may include numbness, tingling, or burning; priapism; weakness; and loss of bowel and bladder control (Hayes and Arriola, 2005).

Neurogenic shock occurs as a result of a disruption in the descending sympathetic pathways with loss of vasomotor tone and sympathetic innervations to the cardiovascular system (Hayes and Arriola, 2005). Hypotension, bradycardia, and peripheral vasodilation occur as a result of neurogenic shock.

Children with suspected SCI may have suffered multiple injuries (e.g., head injury); therefore multiple clinical manifestations may occur that may mask those of an SCI.

Therapeutic Management

Initial care begins at the scene of the accident with proper immobilization of the cervical, thoracic, and lumbar spine. Because of the complexity of these injuries, it is usually recommended that these persons be transported to a spinal injury center for care by specially trained health care personnel as soon as possible after the injury for appropriate diagnostic evaluation and intervention.

The initial management of the child with a suspected SCI should begin with an assessment of the ABCs: **a**irway, **b**reathing, and **c**irculation. The airway should be opened using the jaw-thrust technique to minimize damage to the cervical spine. The child is monitored for cardiovascular instability, and measures are taken to support systemic blood pressure and maintain optimal cardiac output. Because MVCs and other trauma in children may involve internal organ damage and potential bleeding, abdominal distention and other signs are acted on immediately to prevent further systemic shock. After the child is stabilized and transported to a regional trauma center, a thorough evaluation of neurologic status and any other associated trauma is carried out by the multidisciplinary team. In the emergency department, spinal immobilization should be maintained until a thorough neurologic assessment is completed and spinal cord injury is ruled out; in children, this typically involves a CT scan and possibly an MRI. Additional interventions are discussed in the Care Management section.

Spinal cord injury management guidelines and standards of care have been published for adult and pediatric patients with SCIs by the American Association of Neurological Surgeons and the Congress of Neurological Surgeons. However, there are no evidence-based guidelines for the management of SCI in children (Mathison, Kadom, and Krug, 2008).

Intravenous methylprednisone may be started within the first 12 hours after the injury to decrease inflammation and minimize further injury; however, its use in small children is controversial.

A number of progressive rehabilitation modalities have been developed in recent years that have the potential for increasing the quality of life for children with SCI. One treatment is functional electrical stimulation (FES), also referred to as *functional neuromuscular stimulation,* or *neuromuscular electrical stimulation.* With this treatment, an electrical stimulator is surgically implanted under the skin in the abdomen and electrode leads are tunneled to paralyzed leg muscles, enabling the child to sit, stand, and walk with the aid of crutches, a walker, or other orthoses. The stimulator can also be used to elicit a voluntary grasp and release with the hand. Before the latter can be accomplished, a number of surgical tendon transfers may be required for elbow extension, wrist extension, and finger and thumb flexion. In addition, FES has therapeutic benefits, which include increased muscle strength, improved gait function, and increased cardiovascular fitness (Thrasher and Popovic, 2008). Tendon transfers have been shown to be successful in enhancing hand and arm function, increasing pinch force, and facilitating independence in ADLs (Hosalkar, Pandya, Hsu, et al., 2009). Restoration of hand and arm function enables children with SCI to perform self-catheterization and achieve greater independence in personal hygiene.

Exercise is considered an integral part of SCI rehabilitation; exercise may enhance neuroplasticity and decrease further muscle atrophy. Examples of exercise modalities in SCI patients include upper body strength training and hand cycling (Hosalkar, Pandya, Hsu, et al., 2009).

Administration of pharmacologic agents such as clonidine hydrochloride may improve ambulation in patients with partial SCIs, and exercise therapy through interactive locomotor training has helped some individuals with SCI regain ambulatory function.

A number of orthoses or ambulation aids such as braces may still be necessary to achieve upright mobility, yet as robotic technology advances, so do the chances for improved mobilization in children with SCI. Mechanical or robotic orthoses may be used in conjunction with FES to enable ambulation in persons with SCI (To, Kirsch, Kobetic, et al., 2005). Gait training may be achieved with a number of different modalities, including a stationary cycle; however, no specific method has proved superior to the others. FES has also been effective in reducing complications from bladder and bowel incontinence and in assisting males in achieving penile erection. Ambulation is an important part of rehabilitation in SCI; retrospective studies found that ambulation was dependent on age at injury and extent of neurologic injury (as measured by ASIA motor scales) (Vogel, Mendoza, Schottler, et al., 2007). Knee-ankle-foot orthosis and reciprocating gait orthosis may also be used to assist with early rehabilitation and ambulation (Vogel, Betz, and Mulcahey, 2012).

Surgical interventions for SCI include early cord decompression (decompression laminectomy) and cervical or thoracic fusion. Crutchfield, Vinke, or Gardner-Wells tongs and skeletal traction may be used for early cervical vertebral stabilization. A halo vest may be suited for ambulation after the acute phase. (See also Cervical Traction, Chapter 48.) After cervical spinal fusion, a hard cervical collar or sterno-occipital-mandibular immobilizer brace may be worn until the fusion is solidified. When SCI occurs in young children and preteens, scoliosis develops over time and often requires surgical consideration (Parent, Mac-Thiong, Roy-Beaudry, et al., 2011).

CARE MANAGEMENT

The nursing care of the child affected by SCI is complex and challenging. A multidisciplinary SCI team is equipped to manage the acute phase of the injury, and some members, including the nurse, may follow the patient to eventual recovery. Nursing management is concerned with ensuring adequate initial stabilization of the entire spinal column with a rigid cervical collar with supportive blocks on a rigid backboard. The traumatic event causing the injury may or may not be recalled if the child lost consciousness; such events are extremely frightening to the child. The young child may also be frightened by the immobilization process and the inability to move the extremities; therefore it is important to reassure and comfort the child during this process.

During the acute phase of the injury, it is imperative that airway patency be ensured, complications prevented, and function maintained. Evaluate the extent of the neurologic damage early to establish a baseline for neurologic function. Continual assessment of sensory and motor function should occur to prevent further deterioration of neurologic status as a result of spinal cord edema. The ASIA Impairment Scale can be used to assess neurologic function on a routine basis during the patient's recovery. After the patient is admitted, further evaluation of his or her ability to perform ADLs and need for assistance during recovery can be made with the Functional Independence Measure scale.

Nursing care during the acute phase should also focus on frequent monitoring of neurologic signs to determine any changes in neurologic function that require further intervention (e.g., level of consciousness using the Glasgow Coma Scale). In addition to airway maintenance, the nurse should monitor for changes in hemodynamic status that may require immediate medical attention. Neurogenic shock consists of hypotension, bradycardia, and vasodilation. Inotropic medications may be required to maintain adequate perfusion. Renal function is closely monitored by measuring urinary output and fluids administered.

The child with a head injury may experience elevated intracranial pressure; therefore changes in neurologic status are reported to the health care practitioner. Fluid restriction may be required if intracranial pressure is elevated, so fluid intake should be closely monitored.

The nursing care of the child with an SCI is, in most respects, the same as that of any immobilized child (see The Immobilized Child, Chapter 48). Additional aspects of care that should be addressed on an individual basis include hypercalcemia in adolescent boys, DVT, latex sensitization, pain, spasticity, autonomic dysreflexia, and sleep-disordered breathing (Vogel, Hickey, Klaas, et al., 2004; Vogel, Betz, and Mulcahey 2012).

Respiratory care often focuses on maintaining an adequate airway and effective ventilation. The child with a high-level cervical injury (C3 and above) requires continuous ventilatory assistance. In most instances, a tracheostomy is the method of choice for greater ease in clearing secretions and for less trauma to tissues during long-term ventilatory dependence. In some children, breathing pacemaker devices (phrenic nerve stimulators) are implanted to stimulate the phrenic nerve and produce diaphragmatic contractions and lung expansion without assisted ventilation. In the child who does not require mechanical ventilation, special attention to clearance of secretions is vital because of decreased pulmonary function. In addition to percussion and postural drainage, the child may require a cough-assist device to clear secretions effectively (see Duchenne Muscular Dystrophy: Therapeutic Management).

Temperature is often poorly regulated in children with SCI; therefore body temperature must be monitored closely for fluctuations. Response to environmental temperature changes may be slow or absent, and the ability to dissipate heat through the process of shivering may be compromised.

Children with SCI have unique needs in relation to skin care. Because of decreased sensation and impaired mobility, they depend on others to assess and assist in the management of intact skin. Skin care practices are the same as those for any child who is immobilized. A skin score scale such as the Braden Q Scale should be used to objectively evaluate risks for skin breakdown and skin conditions (Noonan, Quigley, and Curley, 2011). An alternating-pressure mattress or other pressure relief or reduction device is kept underneath the child, and the skin is thoroughly inspected at least once a day (or more often if there is increased risk) for signs of pressure and breakdown, especially over bony prominences. Children and adolescents confined to a wheelchair also require meticulous skin care to prevent skin breakdown on insensate areas; frequent position changes and air or gel cushions are helpful but do not eliminate the need for close observation of skin status (McCaskey, Kirk, and Gerdes, 2011).

Bowel and bladder function are often affected in the child with SCI. CIC may be required to regularly empty the neurogenic bladder and prevent urinary tract infections. A regular bowel management program is tailored to the child's needs.

Pain management is vital in children and adolescents with SCI. In children with upper motor neuron involvement, the spasticity that develops may require administration of an antispasmodic medication such as diazepam. Baclofen is considered the drug of choice for reducing muscle spasticity. Gabapentin may be used to treat neuropathic pain. Botulinum toxin type A and α_2-adrenergic agonists may be used in older children with SCI to decrease muscle spasticity.

All adaptive devices help children increase their mobility, function, and endurance. Children with some lower extremity function progress to parallel bars and then to a walker; children with tetraplegia learn to use a wheelchair—among the most valuable aids available to children with SCIs (Fig. 49-8). The wheelchair should be selected carefully in relation to where it will be used, the architectural barriers, and the child's functional capacity. For children with severe upper extremity paralysis, a variety of motorized wheelchairs are used; however, the more complex they are, the greater their cost, weight, and tendency to break down. Wheelchair tolerance is gained over time and is accompanied by measures to prevent orthostatic hypotension and pressure ulcers.

A variety of orthoses and other appliances can be adapted for use by many children. The primary purpose of lower extremity bracing in children with SCIs is for ambulation.

During the recovery and rehabilitation phase, patients with SCI must be carefully monitored for complications of immobility such as DVT and pulmonary embolus. Children with high-level lesions

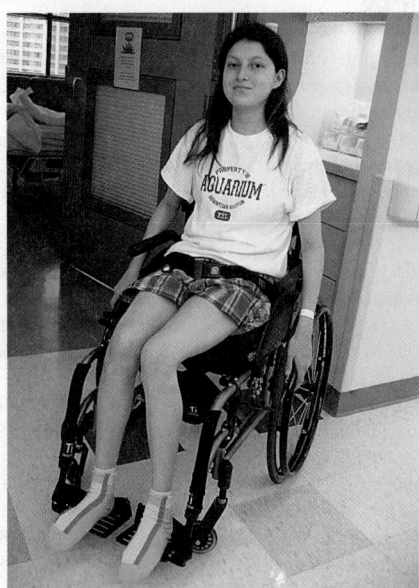

FIG 49-8 Wheelchair allows adolescent mobility and independence. (Courtesy Texas Children's Hospital, Houston, TX.)

are susceptible to the development of autonomic dysreflexia, which requires prompt action to prevent encephalopathy and shock. Clinical manifestations of autonomic dysreflexia include a drastic increase in systemic blood pressure, headache, bradycardia, profuse diaphoresis, cardiac dysrhythmias, flushing, piloerection, blurred vision, nasal congestion, anxiety, spots on the visual field, or absent or minimum symptoms (Vogel, Hickey, Klaas, et al., 2004). Small children who are unable to verbalize may only become irritable. Early recognition of autonomic dysreflexia by caregivers is essential, especially in small children who are unable to verbalize their feelings. Medications such as nitropaste, nifedipine, prazosin, or terazosin may be administered to counteract the effects of the condition depending on the child's response to interventions (Vogel, Betz, and Mulcahey, 2012).

The child and family with SCI are prepared for the eventual discharge from the acute care facility to a rehabilitation center. The major aims of physical rehabilitation are to prepare the child and family to achieve normalization and resume life at home and in the community. Additional goals of rehabilitation in children with SCI are to promote independence in mobility and self-care skills, academic achievement, independent living, and employment.

The nurse is a crucial member of the health care team in relation to helping the family cope with the magnitude of the injury and disability, understand the extent of the disability, verbalize expected outcomes, and move toward eventual rehabilitation and normalization within the child's capabilities. The goals of rehabilitation include preparing the child and family to live at home and function as independently as possible.

KEY POINTS

- Clinical manifestations of CP include delayed gross motor development; abnormal motor performance; alterations of muscle tone; abnormal postures; reflex abnormalities; and associated disabilities such as cognitive impairment, seizures, and sensory impairment.
- Therapy for CP takes into account the nature of the physical disability, defects associated with the disorder, and interpersonal and social influences encountered by the affected child.
- Care of the infant and child with myelomeningocele is directed toward protecting the meningeal sac, preventing infection and skin breakdown, observing for signs of urologic and bowel complications, and planning appropriate interventions to optimize the child's development.
- SMA is characterized by progressive weakness and wasting of skeletal muscles caused by degeneration of anterior horn cells of the spinal cord.
- MDs are the greatest and most important cause of muscular dysfunction of childhood.

- Major complications of DMD include joint contractures, disuse atrophy, obesity, and respiratory and cardiac problems.
- Nursing care of the child with GBS consists of monitoring vital signs, providing respiratory support and physical therapy, providing reassurance, and providing support to the child and family.
- Tetanus occurs when tetanus spores or vegetative bacilli enter a wound and multiply in a susceptible host.
- Infant botulism results from the release of toxins from *C. botulinum* colonizing the gastrointestinal tract.
- Therapeutic management of SCI is directed toward immobilizing the entire spinal column at the scene of the traumatic event, safely transporting the patient by health care personnel trained to transport possible spinal trauma victims, evaluating neurologic damage, preventing further neurologic damage, and implementing an aggressive rehabilitation program designed to help achieve independence and movement.

REFERENCES

Adzick NS: Fetal surgery for spina bifida: past, present, future, *Semin Pediatr Surg* 22(1):10–17, 2013.

Adzick NS, Thom EA, Spong CY, et al: A randomized trial of prenatal versus postnatal repair of myelomeningocele, *N Engl J Med* 364(11):993–1104, 2011.

Aisen ML, Kerkovich D, Mast J, et al: Cerebral palsy: clinical care and neurological rehabilitation, *Lancet Neurol* 10(9):844–852, 2011.

American Academy of Pediatrics (AAP) Committee on Infectious Diseases, Pickering L, editor: *2012 Red Book: report of the Committee on Infectious Diseases*, ed 29, Elk Grove Village, IL, 2012, Author.

American Academy of Pediatrics (AAP) Section on Cardiology and Cardiac Surgery: Cardiovascular health supervision for individuals affected by Duchenne or Becker muscular dystrophy, *Pediatrics* 116(6):1569–1573, 2005.

American College of Obstetrics and Gynecology (ACOG): ACOG Practice Bulletin No. 77: screening for fetal chromosomal abnormalities, *Obstet Gynecol* 109(1):217–227, 2007.

American Spinal Injury Association (ASIA): *International standards for neurological classification of spinal cord injury*, 2011, Author, http://www.asia-spinalinjury.org/elearning/ISNCSCI_Exam_Sheet_r4.pdf.

American Thoracic Society: Respiratory care of the patient with Duchenne muscular dystrophy, *Am J Respir Crit Care Med* 170(4):456–465, 2004.

Arnon SS: Anaerobic bacterial infections: botulism (*Clostridium botulinum*). In Kliegman RM, Stanton BF, St. Geme JW, et al, editors: *Nelson textbook of pediatrics*, ed 19, Philadelphia, 2011a, Saunders.

Arnon SS: Tetanus (*Clostridium tetani*). In Kliegman RM, Stanton BF, St. Geme JW, et al, editors: *Nelson textbook of pediatrics*, ed 19, Philadelphia, 2011b, Saunders.

Bach JR: Medical considerations of long-term survival of Werdnig-Hoffmann disease, *Am J Phys Med Rehabil* 86(5): 349–355, 2007.

Battista V: Muscular dystrophy, Duchenne. In Jackson PL, Vessey JA, Schapiro NA: *Primary care of the child with a chronic illness*, ed 5, St Louis, 2010, Mosby.

Bax M, Goldstein M, Rosenbaum P, et al: Proposed definition and classification of cerebral palsy, *Dev Med Child Neurol* 47(8):571–576, 2005.

Berker AN, Yalçin MS: Cerebral palsy: orthopedic aspects and rehabilitation, *Pediatr Clin North Am* 55(5):1209–1225, 2008.

Betz C, Linroth R, Butler C, et al: Spina bifida: what we learned from consumers, *Pediatr Clin North Am* 57(4):935–944, 2010.

Boitano LJ: Equipment options for cough augmentation, ventilation, and noninvasive interfaces in neuromuscular respiratory management, *Pediatrics* 123(Suppl 4):S226–S230, 2009.

Bosboom WM, Vrancken AF, van den Berg LH, et al: Drug treatment for spinal muscular atrophy type I, *Cochrane Database Syst Rev* (1):CD006281, 2009.

Bush A, Fraser J, Jardine E, et al: Respiratory management of the infant with type 1 spinal muscular atrophy, *Arch Dis Child* 90(7):709–711, 2005.

Centers for Disease Control and Prevention (CDC): Folate status in women of childbearing age, by race/ethnicity—United States, 1999-2000, 2001-2002, and 2003-2004, *MMWR Morb Mortal Wkly Rep* 55(51):1377–1380, 2007.

Centers for Disease Control and Prevention (CDC): Racial/ethnic differences in the birth prevalence of spina bifida—United States, 1995-2005, *MMWR Morb Mortal Wkly Rep* 57(53):1409–1413, 2009.

Centers for Disease Control and Prevention (CDC): *Botulism: general information— frequently asked questions*, 2010, www.cdc.gov/nczved/divisions/dfbmd/ diseases/botulism.

Centers for Disease Control and Prevention (CDC): Updated recommendation for use of tetanus toxoid, reduced diphtheria toxoid and acellular pertussis (Tdap) vaccine from the Advisory Committee on Immunization Practices, 2010, *MMWR Morb Mortal Wkly Rep* 60(01):13–15, 2011.

Clinical Trials: *Management of myelomeningocele study (MOMS)*, Washington, DC, 2013, US National Institute of Child Health and Human Development, http:// clinicaltrials.gov/show/NCT00060606 (accessed May 13, 2013).

Dai AI, Wasay M, Awan S: Botulinum toxin type A with oral baclofen versus oral tizanidine: a randomized pilot comparison in patients with cerebral palsy and equines foot deformity, *J Child Neurol* 23(12):1464–1466, 2008.

Delgado MR, Hirtz D, Aisen M, et al: Practice parameter: pharmacologic treatment of spasticity in children and adolescents with cerebral palsy (an evidence-based review), *Neurology* 74(1):336–343, 2010.

Dicianno BE, Fairman AD, Juengst SB, et al: Using the spina bifida Life Course Model in clinical practice: an interdisciplinary approach, *Pediatr Clin North Am* 57(4):945–957, 2010.

Doolin E: Bowel management for patients with myelodysplasia, *Surg Clin North Am* 86(2):505–514, 2006.

Finder JD: A 2009 perspective on the 2004 American Thoracic Society statement, "Respiratory care of the patient with Duchenne muscular dystrophy," *Pediatrics* 123(Suppl 4):S239–S241, 2009.

Golomb MR, Saha C, Garg BP, et al: Association of cerebral palsy with other disabilities in children with perinatal arterial ischemic stroke, *Pediatr Neurol* 37(4):245–249, 2007.

Grether JK, Nelson, KB, Walsh E, et al: Intrauterine exposure to infection and risk of cerebral palsy in very preterm infants, *Arch Pediatr Adolesc Med* 157(1):26–32, 2003.

Hayes JS, Arriola T: Pediatric spinal injuries, *Pediatr Nurs* 31(6):464–467, 2005.

Hermansen MC, Hermansen MG: Perinatal infections and cerebral palsy, *Clin Perinatol* 33(2):315–333, 2006.

Hirtz D, Thurman DJ, Gwinn-Hardy K, et al: How common are the "common" neurological disorders? *Neurology* 68(5):326–337, 2007.

Hosalkar H, Pandya NK, Hsu J, et al: Specialty update: what's new in orthopaedic rehabilitation, *J Bone Joint Surg Am* 91(9):2296–2310, 2009.

Hughes R: The role of IVIG in autoimmune neuropathies: the latest evidence, *J Neuro* 255(Suppl 3):7–11, 2008.

Hughes RA, Cornblath DR: Guillain-Barré syndrome, *Lancet* 366(9497):1653–1666, 2005.

Hughes RA, Swan AV, van Doorn PA: Intravenous immunoglobulin for Guillain-Barré syndrome, *Cochrane Database Syst Rev* (6):CD002063, 2010.

Hurtekant KM, Spatz DL: Special considerations for breastfeeding the infant with spina bifida, *J Perinat Neonatal Nurs* 21(1):69–75, 2007.

Iannaccone ST: Modern management of spinal muscular atrophy, *J Child Neurol* 22(8):974–978, 2007.

Iannaccone ST, Burghes A: Spinal muscular atrophies, *Adv Neurol* 88:83–98, 2002.

Johnston MV: Cerebral palsy. In Kliegman RM, Stanton BF, St. Geme JW, et al, editors: *Nelson textbook of pediatrics*, ed 19, Philadelphia, 2011, Saunders.

Johnston MV, Fatemi A, Wilson MA, et al: Treatment advances in neonatal neuroprotection and neurointensive care, *Lancet Neurol* 10(4):372–382, 2011.

Kinsman SL, Johnston MV: Myelomeningocele. In Kliegman RM, Stanton BF, St. Geme JW, et al, editors: *Nelson textbook of pediatrics*, ed 19, Philadelphia, 2011, Saunders.

Krageloh-Mann I, Cans C: Cerebral palsy update, *Brain Dev* 31(7):537–544, 2009.

Kravitz RM: Airway clearance in Duchenne muscular dystrophy, *Pediatrics* 123(Suppl 4):S231–S235, 2009.

Krigger KW: Cerebral palsy: an overview, *Am Fam Physician* 73(1):91–102, 2006.

Lazzaretti CC, Pearson C: Myelodysplasia. In Allen PJ, Vessey JA, editors: *Primary care of the child with a chronic condition*, ed 5, St Louis, 2010, Mosby.

Liptak GS, Murphy NA, AAP Council on Children with Disabilities: Providing a primary care medical home for children and youth with cerebral palsy, *Pediatrics* 128(5):e1321–e1329, 2011.

Lovette B: Safe transportation for children with special needs, *J Pediatr Health Care* 22(5):323–328, 2008.

Lukban MB, Rosales RL, Dressler D: Effectiveness of botulinum toxin A for upper and lower limb spasticity in children with cerebral palsy: a summary of evidence, *J Neural Transm* 116(3):319–331, 2009.

Lunn MR, Wang CH: Spina muscular atrophy, *Lancet* 371(9630):2120–2133, 2008.

Lyons R: Elusive belly pain and Guillain-Barré syndrome, *J Pediatr Health Care* 22(5):310–314, 2008.

Manzur AY, Kinali M, Muntoni F: Update on the management of Duchenne muscular dystrophy, *Arch Dis Child* 93(11):986–990, 2008.

Manzur AY, Kuntzer T, Pike M, et al: Glucocorticoid corticosteroids for Duchenne muscular dystrophy, *Cochrane Database Syst Rev* (1):CD003725, 2008.

Mathison DJ, Kadom N, Krug SE: Spinal cord injury in the pediatric patient, *Clin Pediatr Emerg Med* 9(2):106–123, 2008.

Matthews TJ: *Trends in spina bifida and anencephalus in the United States, 1991-2006*, Hyattsville, MD, 2009, National Center on Health Statistics, www.cdc.gov/nchs/ products/pubs/pubd/hestats/spine_anen.pdf.

McCaskey MS, Kirk L, Gerdes C: Preventing skin breakdown in the immobile child in the home care setting, *Home Healthcare Nurse* 29(4):248–255, 2011.

Mercuri E, Bertini E, Iannaccone ST: Childhood spinal muscular atrophy: controversies and challenges, *Lancet Neurol* 11(5):443–452, 2012.

Miske LJ, Hickey EM, Kolb SM, et al: Use of the mechanical in-exsufflator in pediatric patients with neuromuscular disease and impaired cough, *Chest* 125(4):1406–1412, 2004.

Moore C, Kogan BA, Parekh A: Impact of urinary incontinence on self-concept in children with spina bifida, *J Urol* 171(4):1659–1662, 2004.

Moster D, Wilcox AJ, Vollset SE, et al: Cerebral palsy among term and postterm births, *JAMA* 304(9):976–982, 2010.

Moxley RT, Ashwal S, Pandya S, et al: Practice parameter: corticosteroid treatment of Duchenne dystrophy, *Neurology* 64(1):13–20, 2005.

Nehring WM: Cerebral palsy. In Jackson PL, Vessey JA, Schapiro NA, editors: *Primary care of the child with a chronic illness*, ed 5, St Louis, 2010, Mosby.

Noonan C, Quigley S, Curley MA: Using the Braden Q Scale to predict pressure ulcer risk in pediatric patients, *J Pediatr Nurs* 26(6):566–575, 2011.

O'Shea TM: Diagnosis, treatment, and prevention of cerebral palsy in near term/ term infants, *Clin Obstet Gynecol* 51(4):816–828, 2008.

Parent S, Mac-Thiong JM, Roy-Beaudry M, et al: Spinal cord injury in the pediatric population: a systematic review of the literature, *J Neurotrauma* 28(8):1515–1524, 2011.

Prior TW: Spinal muscular atrophy: newborn and carrier screening, *Obstet Gynecol Clin North Am* 37(1):23–26, 2010.

Quan D: Muscular dystrophies and neurologic diseases that present as myopathy, *Rheum Dis Clin North Am* 37(2):233–244, 2011.

Retake HL: Spinal cord injuries in children. In Kliegman RM, Stanton BF, St. Geme JW, et al, editors: *Nelson textbook of pediatrics*, ed 19, Philadelphia, 2011, Saunders.

Rosenbaum P, Paneth N, Leviton A, et al: A report: the definition and classification of cerebral palsy April 2006, *Dev Med Child Neurol* 49(S109):1–44, 2007.

Russman BS: Function changes in spinal muscular atrophy II and III: the DCN/SMA group, *Neurology* 47(4):973–976, 1996.

Russman BS, Iannaccone ST, Buncher CR, et al: Spinal muscular atrophy: new thoughts on the pathogenesis and classification schema, *J Child Neurol* 7(4):347–353, 1992.

Sarnat HB: Neuromuscular disorders. In Kliegman RM, Behrman RE, Jenson HB and others, editors: *Nelson textbook of pediatrics*, ed 18, Philadelphia, 2007, Saunders.

Sarnat HB: Guillain-Barré syndrome. In Kliegman RM, Stanton BF, St. Geme JW, et al, editors: *Nelson textbook of pediatrics*, ed 19, Philadelphia, 2011a, Saunders.

Sarnat HB: Muscular dystrophies. In Kliegman RM, Stanton BF, St. Geme JW, et al, editors: *Nelson textbook of pediatrics*, ed 19, Philadelphia, 2011b, Saunders.

Sarnat HB: Spinal muscular atrophies. In Kliegman RM, Stanton BF, St. Geme JW, et al, editors: *Nelson textbook of pediatrics*, ed 19, Philadelphia, 2011c, Saunders.

Sawyer SM, Macnee S: Transition to adult health care for adolescents with spina bifida: research issues, *Dev Disabil Res Rev* 16(1):60–65, 2010.

Schroth MK: Special considerations in the respiratory management of spinal muscular atrophy, *Pediatrics* 123(Suppl 4):S245–S249, 2009.

Shaer CM, Chescheir N, Schulkin J: Myelomeningocele: a review of the epidemiology, genetics, risk factors for conception, prenatal diagnosis, and prognosis for affected individuals, *Obstet Gynecol Surv* 62(7):471–479, 2007.

Shankaran S, Pappas A, McDonald SA, et al: Childhood outcomes after hypothermia for neonatal encephalopathy, *N Engl J Med* 366(22):2085–2092, 2012.

Simonds AK: Recent advances in respiratory care for neuromuscular disease, *Chest* 130(6):1879–1886, 2006.

Simpson JL, Richards DS, Otaño L: Prenatal genetic diagnosis. In Gabbe SG, Niebyl JR, Simpson JL, et al, editors: *Obstetrics: normal and problem pregnancies*, ed 6, Philadelphia, 2012, Saunders.

Snodgrass WT, Gargollo PC: Urologic care of the neurogenic bladder in children, *Urol Clin North Am* 37(2):207–214, 2010.

Tarcan T, Onol FF, Ilker Y, et al: The timing of primary neurosurgical repair significantly affects neurogenic bladder prognosis in children with myelomeningocele, *J Urol* 176(3):1161–1165, 2006.

Thrasher TA, Popovic MR: Functional electrical stimulation of walking: function, exercise and rehabilitation, *Ann Readapt Med Phys* 51(6):452–460, 2008.

To CS, Kirsch RF, Kobetic R, et al: Simulation of a functional neuromuscular stimulation powered mechanical gait orthosis with coordinated joint locking, *IEEE Trans Neural Syst Rehabil Eng* 13(2):227–235, 2005.

Vitale MG, Goss JM, Matsumoto H, et al: Epidemiology of pediatric spinal cord injury in the United States: years 1997 and 2000, *J Pediatr Orthop* 26(6):745–749, 2006.

Vogel LC, Hickey KJ, Klaas SJ, et al: Unique issues in pediatric spinal cord injury, *Orthop Nurs* 23(5):300–308, 2004.

Vogel LC, Mendoza MM, Schottler JC, et al: Ambulation in children and youth with spinal cord injuries, *J Spinal Cord Med* 30(Suppl 1):S158–S164, 2007.

Vogel LC, Betz RR, Mulcahey MJ: Spinal cord injuries in children and adolescents. In Verhaagen J, McDonald JW, editors, *Handbook of clinical neurology*, 109:131–148, Philadelphia, 2012, Elsevier.

Wolff T, Witkop CT, Miller T, et al: Folic acid supplementation for the prevention of neural tube defects: an update of the evidence for the U.S. Preventive Services Task Force, *Ann Intern Med* 150(9):632–639, W112–W115, 2009.

Wright PA, Durham S, Ewins DJ, et al: Neuromuscular electrical stimulation for children with cerebral palsy: a review, *Arch Dis Child* 97(4):364–371, 2012.

Wu YW, Escobar GJ, Grether JK, et al: Chorioamnionitis and cerebral palsy in term and near-term infants, *JAMA* 290(20):2677–2684, 2003.

Yeargin-Allsopp M, Van Naarden Braun K, Doernberg NS, et al: Prevalence of cerebral palsy in 8-year-old children in three areas of the United States in 2002: a multisite collaboration, *Pediatrics* 121(3):547–554, 2008.

Young HK, Lowe A, Fitzgerald DA, et al: Outcome of noninvasive ventilation in children with neuromuscular disease, *Neurology* 68(3):198–201, 2007.

Growth Measurements

HEIGHT AND WEIGHT MEASUREMENTS FOR BOYS

	HEIGHT BY PERCENTILES						WEIGHT BY PERCENTILES					
	5		**50**		**95**		**5**		**50**		**95**	
AGE*	cm	inches	cm	inches	cm	inches	kg	lb	kg	lb	kg	lb
Birth	46.4	18¼	50.5	20	54.4	21½	2.54	5½	3.27	7¼	4.15	9¼
3 mo	56.7	22¼	61.1	24	65.4	25¾	4.43	9¾	5.98	13¼	7.37	16¼
6 mo	63.4	25	67.8	26¾	72.3	28½	6.20	13¾	7.85	17¼	9.46	20¾
9 mo	68.0	26¾	72.3	28½	77.1	30¼	7.52	16½	9.18	20¼	10.93	24
1	71.7	28¼	76.1	30	81.2	32	8.43	18½	10.15	22½	11.99	26½
1½	77.5	30½	82.4	32½	88.1	34¾	9.59	21¼	11.47	25¼	13.44	29½
2†	82.5	32½	86.8	34¼	94.4	37¼	10.49	23¼	12.34	27¼	15.50	34¼
2½†	85.4	33½	90.4	35½	97.8	38½	11.27	24¾	13.52	29¾	16.61	36½
3	89.0	35	94.9	37¼	102.0	40¼	12.05	26½	14.62	32¼	17.77	39¼
3½	92.5	36½	99.1	39	106.1	41¾	12.84	28¼	15.68	34½	18.98	41¾
4	95.8	37¾	102.9	40½	109.9	43¼	13.64	30	16.69	36¾	20.27	44¾
4½	98.9	39	106.6	42	113.5	44¾	14.45	31¾	17.69	39	21.63	47¾
5	102.0	40¼	109.9	43¼	117.0	46	15.27	33¾	18.67	41¼	23.09	51
6	107.7	42½	116.1	45¾	123.5	48½	16.93	37¼	20.69	45½	26.34	58
7	113.0	44½	121.7	48	129.7	51	18.64	41	22.85	50¼	30.12	66½
8	118.1	46½	127.0	50	135.7	53½	20.40	45	25.30	55¾	34.51	76
9	122.9	48½	132.2	52	141.8	55¾	22.25	49	28.13	62	39.58	87¼
10	127.7	50¼	137.5	54¼	148.1	58¼	24.33	53¾	31.44	69¼	45.27	99¾
11	132.6	52¼	143.3	56½	154.9	61	26.80	59	35.30	77¾	51.47	113½
12	137.6	54¼	149.7	59	162.3	64	29.85	65¾	39.78	87¾	58.09	128
13	142.9	56¼	156.5	61½	169.8	66¾	33.64	74¼	44.95	99	65.02	143¼
14	148.8	58½	163.1	64¼	176.7	69½	38.22	84¼	50.77	112	72.13	159
15	155.2	61	169.0	66½	181.9	71½	43.11	95	56.71	125	79.12	174½
16	161.1	63½	173.5	68¼	185.4	73	47.74	105¼	62.10	137	85.62	188¾
17	164.9	65	176.2	69¼	187.3	73¾	51.50	113½	66.31	146¼	91.31	201¼
18	165.7	65¼	176.8	69½	187.6	73¾	53.97	119	68.88	151¾	95.76	211

Modified from National Center for Health Statistics, Health Resources Administration, Department of Health, Education and Welfare, Hyattsville, MD.

Conversion of metric data to approximate inches and pounds by Ross Laboratories.

*Years unless otherwise indicated.

†Height data include some recumbent length measurements, which make values slightly higher than if all measurements had been of stature (standing height).

HEIGHT AND WEIGHT MEASUREMENTS FOR GIRLS

| | HEIGHT BY PERCENTILES | | | | | | WEIGHT BY PERCENTILES | | | | | |
| | 5 | | 50 | | 95 | | 5 | | 50 | | 95 | |
AGE*	cm	inches	cm	inches	cm	inches	kg	lb	kg	lb	kg	lb
Birth	45.4	17¾	49.9	19¾	52.9	20¾	2.36	5¼	3.23	7	3.81	8½
3 mo	55.4	21¾	59.5	23½	63.4	25	4.18	9¼	5.4	12	6.74	14¾
6 mo	61.8	24¼	65.9	26	70.2	27¾	5.79	12¾	7.21	16	8.73	19¼
9 mo	66.1	26	70.4	27¾	75.0	29½	7.0	15½	8.56	18¾	10.17	22½
1	69.8	2½	74.3	29¼	79.1	31¼	7.84	17¼	9.53	21	11.24	24¾
1½	76.0	30	80.9	31¾	86.1	34	8.92	19¾	10.82	23¾	12.76	28¼
2†	81.6	32¼	86.8	34¼	93.6	36¾	9.95	22	11.8	26	14.15	31¼
2½†	84.6	33¼	90.0	35½	96.6	38	10.8	23¾	13.03	28¾	15.76	34¾
3	88.3	34¾	94.1	37	100.6	39½	11.61	25½	14.1	31	17.22	38
3½	91.7	36	97.9	38½	104.5	41¼	12.37	27¼	15.07	33¼	18.59	41
4	95.0	37½	101.6	40	108.3	42¾	13.11	29	15.96	35¼	19.91	44
4½	98.1	38½	105.0	41¼	112.0	44	13.83	30½	16.81	37	21.24	46¾
5	101.1	39¾	108.4	42¾	115.6	45½	14.55	32	17.66	39	22.62	49¾
6	106.6	42	114.6	45	122.7	48¼	16.05	35½	19.52	43	25.75	56¾
7	111.8	44	120.6	47½	129.5	51	17.71	39	21.84	48¼	29.68	65½
8	116.9	46	126.4	49¾	136.2	53½	19.62	43¼	24.84	54¾	34.71	76½
9	122.1	48	132.2	52	142.9	56¼	21.82	48	28.46	62¾	40.64	89½
10	127.5	50¼	138.3	54½	149.5	58¾	24.36	53¾	32.55	71¾	47.17	104
11	133.5	52½	144.8	57	156.2	61½	27.24	60	36.95	81½	54.0	119
12	139.8	55	151.5	59¾	162.7	64	30.52	67¼	41.53	91½	60.81	134
13	145.2	57¼	157.1	61¾	168.1	66¼	34.14	75¼	46.1	101¾	67.3	148¼
14	148.7	58½	160.4	63¼	171.3	67½	37.76	83¼	50.28	110¾	73.08	161
15	150.5	59½	161.8	63¾	172.8	68	40.99	90¼	53.68	118¼	77.78	171½
16	151.6	59¾	162.4	64	173.3	68¼	43.41	95¾	55.89	123¼	80.99	178½
17	152.7	60	163.1	64¼	173.5	68¼	44.74	98¾	56.69	125	82.46	181¾
18	153.6	60½	163.7	64½	173.6	68¼	45.26	99¾	56.62	124¾	82.47	181¾

Modified from National Center for Health Statistics, Health Resources Administration, Department of Health, Education and Welfare, Hyattsville, MD.

Conversion of metric data to approximate inches and pounds by Ross Laboratories.

*Years unless otherwise indicated.

†Height data include some recumbent length measurements, which make values slightly higher than if all measurements had been of stature.

Common Laboratory Tests and Test Results*

	AGE/GENDER/	NORMAL RANGES			
TEST/SPECIMEN	REFERENCE	CONVENTIONAL UNITS		INTERNATIONAL UNITS (SI)	
Acetaminophen					
Serum or plasma	Therap. conc.	10-30 mcg/mL		66-200 µmol/L	
	Toxic conc.	>200 mcg/mL		>1300 µmol/L	
Ammonia nitrogen					
Plasma or serum	Newborn	90-150 mcg/dL		64-107 µmol/L	
	0-2 wk	79-129 mcg/dL		56-92 µmol/L	
	>1 mo	29-70 mcg/dL		21-50 µmol/L	
	Thereafter	0-50 mcg/dL		0-35.7 µmol/L	
Antistreptolysin O titer (ASO)					
Serum	2-4 yr	<160 Todd units			
	School-age children	170-330 Todd units			
Base excess					
Whole blood	Newborn	(−10)-(−2) mEq/L		(−10)-(−2) mmol/L	
	Infant	(−7)-(−1) mEq/L		(−7)-(−1) mmol/L	
	Child	(−4)-(+2) mEq/L		(−4)-(+2) mmol/L	
	Thereafter	(−3)-(+3) mEq/L		(−3)-(+3) mmol/L	
Bicarbonate (HCO_3)					
Serum	Arterial	21-28 mEq/L		21-28 mmol/L	
	Venous	22-29 mEq/L		22-29 mmol/L	
Bilirubin, total		**Premature** (mg/dL)	**Full term** (mg/dL)	**Premature** (µmol/L)	**Full term** (µmol/L)
Serum	Cord	<2.0	<2.0	<34	<34
	0-1 d	<8.0	<6.0	<137	<103
	1-2 d	<12.0	<8.0	<205	<137
	2-5 d	<16.0	<12.0	<274	<205
	Thereafter	<20.0	<10.0	<340	<171
Bilirubin, direct (conjugated)					
Serum		0.0-0.2 mg/dL		0-3.4 µmol/L	
Bleeding time					
Blood from skin puncture					
Ivy	Normal	2-7 min		2-7 min	
	Borderline	7-11 min		7-11 min	
Simplate (G-D)		2.75-8 min		2.75-8 min	
Blood volume					
Whole blood	Male	52-83 mL/kg		0.052-0.083 L/kg	
	Female	50-75 mL/kg		0.050-0.075 L/kg	
C-reactive protein (CRP)					
Serum	Cord	52-1330 ng/mL		52-1330 mcg/L	
	2-12 yr	67-1800 ng/mL		67-1800 mcg/L	

Continued

TEST/SPECIMEN	AGE/GENDER/ REFERENCE	NORMAL RANGES	
		CONVENTIONAL UNITS	INTERNATIONAL UNITS (SI)
Calcium, ionized			
Serum, plasma, or whole	Cord	5.0-6.0 mg/dL	1.25-1.50 mmol/L
blood	Newborn, 3-24 hr	4.3-5.1 mg/dL	1.07-1.27 mmol/L
	24-48 hr	4.0-4.7 mg/dL	1.00-1.17 mmol/L
	Thereafter	4.8-4.92 mg/dL or 2.24-2.46 mEq/L	1.12-1.23 mmol/L
Calcium, total			
Serum	Cord	9.0-11.5 mg/dL	2.25-2.88 mmol/L
	Newborn, 3-24 hr	9.0-10.6 mg/dL	2.3-2.65 mmol/L
	24-48 hr	7.0-12.0 mg/dL	1.75-3.0 mmol/L
	4-7 d	9.0-10.9 mg/dL	2.25-2.73 mmol/L
	Child	8.8-10.8 mg/dL	2.2-2.70 mmol/L
	Thereafter	8.4-10.2 mg/dL	2.1-2.55 mmol/L
Carbon dioxide, partial pressure (PCO_2)			
Whole blood, arterial	Newborn	27-40 mm Hg	3.6-5.3 kPa
	Infant	27-41 mm Hg	3.6-5.5 kPa
	Thereafter:		
	Male	35-48 mm Hg	4.7-6.4 kPa
	Female	32-45 mm Hg	4.3-6.0 kPa
Carbon dioxide, total (tCO_2)			
Serum or plasma	Cord	14-22 mEq/L	14-22 mmol/L
	Premature (1 wk)	14-27 mEq/L	14-27 mmol/L
	Newborn	13-22 mEq/L	13-22 mmol/L
	Infant, child	20-28 mEq/L	20-28 mmol/L
	Thereafter	23-30 mEq/L	23-30 mmol/L
Cerebrospinal fluid (CSF)			
Pressure		70-180 mm H_2O	70-180 mm H_2O
Volume	Child	60-100 mL	0.06-0.10 L
	Adult	100-160 mL	0.10-0.16 L
Chloride			
Serum or plasma	Cord	96-104 mEq/L	96-104 mmol/L
	Newborn	97-110 mEq/L	97-110 mmol/L
	Thereafter	98-106 mEq/L	98-106 mmol/L
Sweat	Normal (homozygote)	<40 mEq/L	<40 mmol/L
	Marginal (e.g., asthma, Addison disease, malnutrition)	45-60 mEq/L	45-60 mmol/L
	Cystic fibrosis	>60 mEq/L	>60 mmol/L
Cholesterol, total			
Serum or plasma†	Acceptable	<170 mg/dL	<4.4 mmol/L
	Borderline	170-199 mg/dL	4.4-5.1 mmol/L
	High	≥200 mg/dL	≥5.2 mmol/L
Clotting time (Lee-White)			
Whole blood		5-8 min (glass tubes)	5-8 min
		5-15 min (room temp)	5-15 min
		30 min (silicone tube)	30 min
Creatine kinase (CK, CPK)			
Serum	Cord	70-380 U/L	70-380 U/L
	5-8 hr	214-1175 U/L	214-1175 U/L
	24-33 hr	130-1200 U/L	130-1200 U/L
	72-100 hr	87-725 U/L	87-725 U/L
	Adult	5-130 U/L	5-130 U/L

TEST/SPECIMEN	AGE/GENDER/ REFERENCE	NORMAL RANGES	
		CONVENTIONAL UNITS	**INTERNATIONAL UNITS (SI)**
Creatinine			
Serum	Cord	0.6-1.2 mg/dL	53-106 μmol/L
	Newborn	0.3-1.0 mg/dL	27-88 μmol/L
	Infant	0.2-0.4 mg/d	18-35 μmol/L
	Child	0.3-0.7 mg/dL	27-62 μmol/L
	Adolescent	0.5-1.0 mg/dL	44-88 μmol/L
	Adult:		
	Male	0.6-1.2 mg/dL	53-106 μmol/L
	Female	0.5-1.1 mg/dL	44-97 μmol/L
Urine, 24 hr	Premature	8.1-15.0 mg/kg/24 hr	72-133 μmol/kg/24 hr
	Full term	10.4-19.7 mg/kg/24 hr	92-174 μmol/kg/24 hr
	1.5-7 yr	10-15 mg/kg/24 hr	88-133 μmol/kg/24 hr
	7-15 yr	5.2-41 mg/kg/24 hr	46-362 μmol/kg/24 hr
Creatinine clearance (endogenous)			
Serum or plasma and urine	Newborn	40-65 mL/min/1.73 m^2	
	<40 yr:		
	Male	97-137 mL/min/1.73 m^2	
	Female	88-128 mL/min/1.73 m^2	
Digoxin			
Serum, plasma; collect at least 12 hr after dose	Therap. conc.		
	CHF	0.8-1.5 ng/mL	1.0-1.9 nmol/L
	Arrhythmias	1.5-2.0 ng/mL	1.9-2.6 nmol/L
	Toxic conc.		
	Child	>2.5 ng/mL	>3.2 nmol/L
	Adult	>3.0 ng/mL	>3.8 nmol/L
Eosinophil count			
Whole blood, capillary blood		50-250 cells/mm^3 (μL)	50-250 × 10^6 cells/L
Erythrocyte (RBC) count			
Whole blood	Cord	3.9-5.5 million/mm^3	3.9-5.5 × 10^{12} cells/L
	1-3 d	4.0-6.6 million/mm^3	4.0-6.6 × 10^{12} cells/L
	1 wk	3.9-6.3 million/mm^3	3.9-6.3 × 10^{12} cells/L
	2 wk	3.6-6.2 million/mm^3	3.6-6.2 × 10^{12} cells/L
	1 mo	3.0-5.4 million/mm^3	3.0-5.4 × 10^{12} cells/L
	2 mo	2.7-4.9 million/mm^3	2.7-4.9 × 10^{12} cells/L
	3-6 mo	3.1-4.5 million/mm^3	3.1-4.5 × 10^{12} cells/L
	0.5-2 yr	3.7-5.3 million/mm^3	3.7-5.3 × 10^{12} cells/L
	2-6 yr	3.9-5.3 million/mm^3	3.9-5.3 × 10^{12} cells/L
	6-12 yr	4.0-5.2 million/mm^3	4.0-5.2 × 10^{12} cells/L
	12-18 yr:		
	Male	4.5-5.3 million/mm^3	4.5-5.3 × 10^{12} cells/L
	Female	4.1-5.1 million/mm^3	4.1-5.1 × 10^{12} cells/L
Erythrocyte sedimentation rate (ESR)			
Whole blood			
Westergren (modified)	Child	0-10 mm/hr	0-10 mm/hr
	<50 yr:		
	Male	0-15 mm/hr	0-15 mm/hr
	Female	0-20 mm/hr	0-20 mm/hr
Wintrobe	Child	0-13 mm/hr	0-13 mm/hr
	Adult:		
	Male	0-9 mm/hr	0-9 mm/hr
	Female	0-20 mm/hr	0-20 mm/hr

Continued

TEST/SPECIMEN	AGE/GENDER/ REFERENCE	NORMAL RANGES			
		CONVENTIONAL UNITS		INTERNATIONAL UNITS (SI)	
Fibrinogen					
Plasma	Newborn	125-300 mg/dL		1.25-3.00 g/L	
	Thereafter	200-400 mg/dL		2.00-4.00 g/L	
Galactose					
Serum	Newborn	0-20 mg/dL		0-1.11 mmol/L	
	Thereafter	<5 mg/dL		<0.28 mmol/L	
Urine	Newborn	≤60 mg/dL		≤3.33 mmol/L	
	Thereafter	<14 mg/24 hr		<0.08 mmol/d	
Glucose					
Serum	Cord	45-96 mg/dL		2.5-5.3 mmol/L	
	Newborn, 1 d	40-60 mg/dL		2.2-3.3 mmol/L	
	Newborn, >1 d	50-90 mg/dL		2.8-5.0 mmol/L	
	Child	60-100 mg/dL		3.3-5.5 mmol/L	
	Thereafter	70-105 mg/dL		3.9-5.8 mmol/L	
Whole blood	Adult	65-95 mg/dL		3.6-5.3 mmol/L	
CSF	Adult	40-70 mg/dL		2.2-3.9 mmol/L	
Urine (quantitative)		<0.5 g/d		<2.8 mmol/d	
Urine (qualitative)		Negative		Negative	
Glucose tolerance test (GTT), oral					
Serum					
Dosages		**Normal**	**Diabetic**	**Normal**	**Diabetic**
Adult: 75 g	Fasting	70-105 mg/dL	≥126 mg/dL	3.9-5.8 mmol/L	≥7.0 mmol/L
Child: 1.75 g/kg of ideal	60 min	120-170 mg/dL	≥200 mg/dL	6.7-9.4 mmol/L	≥11 mmol/L
weight up to maximum	90 min	100-140 mg/dL	≥200 mg/dL	5.6-7.8 mmol/L	≥11 mmol/L
of 75 g	120 min	70-120 mg/dL	≥200 mg/dL	3.9-6.7 mmol/L	≥11 mmol/L
Growth hormone (GH, somatotropin)					
Plasma	1 d	5-53 ng/mL		5-53 mcg/L	
	1 wk	5-27 ng/mL		5-27 mcg/L	
	1-12 mo	2-10 ng/mL		2-10 mcg/L	
	Fasting child/adult	<0.7-6.0 ng/mL		<0.7-6.0 mcg/L	
Hematocrit (HCT, Hct)					
Whole blood	1 d (cap)	48%-69%		0.48-0.69 vol fraction	
	2 d	48%-75%		0.48-0.75 vol fraction	
	3 d	44%-72%		0.44-0.72 vol fraction	
	2 mo	28%-42%		0.28-0.42 vol fraction	
	6-12 yr	35%-45%		0.35-0.45 vol fraction	
	12-18 yr:				
	Male	37%-49%		0.37-0.49 vol fraction	
	Female	36%-46%		0.36-0.46 vol fraction	
Hemoglobin (Hb)					
Whole blood	1-3 d (cap)	14.5-22.5 g/dL		2.25-3.49 mmol/L	
	2 mo	9.0-14.0 g/dL		1.40-2.17 mmol/L	
	6-12 yr	11.5-15.5 g/dL		1.78-2.40 mmol/L	
	12-18 yr:				
	Male	13.0-16.0 g/dL		2.02-2.48 mmol/L	
	Female	12.0-16.0 g/dL		1.86-2.48 mmol/L	
Hemoglobin A					
Whole blood		>95% of total		>0.95 fraction of Hb	
Hemoglobin F					
Whole blood	1 d	63%-92% HbF		0.63-0.92 mass fraction HbF	
	5 d	65%-88% HbF		0.65-0.88 mass fraction HbF	
	3 wk	55%-85% HbF		0.55-0.85 mass fraction HbF	
	6-9 wk	31%-75% HbF		0.31-0.75 mass fraction HbF	
	3-4 mo	<2%-59% HbF		<0.02-0.59 mass fraction HbF	
	6 mo	<2%-9% HbF		<0.02-0.09 mass fraction HbF	
	Adult	<2.0% HbF		<0.02 mass fraction HbF	

TEST/SPECIMEN	AGE/GENDER/ REFERENCE	NORMAL RANGES	
		CONVENTIONAL UNITS	INTERNATIONAL UNITS (SI)
Immunoglobulin A (IgA)			
Serum	Cord	1.4-3.6 mg/dL	14-36 mg/L
	1-3 mo	1.3-53 mg/dL	13-530 mg/L
	4-6 mo	4.4-84 mg/dL	44-840 mg/L
	7-12 mo	11-106 mg/dL	110-1060 mg/L
	2-5 yr	14-159 mg/dL	140-1590 mg/L
	6-10 yr	33-236 mg/dL	330-2360 mg/L
	Adult	70-312 mg/dL	700-3120 mg/L
Immunoglobulin D (IgD)			
Serum	Newborn	None detected	None detected
	Thereafter	0-8 mg/dL	0-80 mg/L
Immunoglobulin E (IgE)			
Serum	Male	0-230 IU/mL	0-230 kIU/L
	Female	0-170 IU/mL	0-170 kIU/L
Immunoglobulin G (IgG)			
Serum	Cord	636-1606 mg/dL	6.36-16.06 g/L
	1 mo	251-906 mg/dL	2.51-9.06 g/L
	2-4 mo	176-601 mg/dL	1.76-6.01 g/L
	5-12 mo	172-1069 mg/dL	1.72-10.69 g/L
	1-5 yr	345-1236 mg/dL	3.45-12.36 g/L
	6-10 yr	608-1572 mg/dL	6.08-15.72 g/L
	Adult	639-1349 mg/dL	6.39-13.49 g/L
Immunoglobulin M (IgM)			
Serum	Cord	6.3-25 mg/dL	63-250 mg/L
	1-4 mo	17-105 mg/dL	170-1050 mg/L
	5-9 mo	33-126 mg/dL	330-1260 mg/L
	10-12 mo	41-173 mg/dL	410-1730 mg/L
	2-8 yr	43-207 mg/dL	430-2070 mg/L
	9-10 yr	52-242 mg/dL	520-2420 mg/L
	Adult	56-352 mg/dL	560-3520 mg/L
Iron			
Serum	Newborn	100-250 mcg/dL	18-45 μmol/L
	Infant	40-100 mcg/dL	7-18 μmol/L
	Child	50-120 mcg/dL	9-22 μmol/L
	Thereafter:		
	Male	65-170 mcg/dL	12-30 μmol/L
	Female	50-170 mcg/dL	9-30 μmol/L
	Intoxicated child	280-2550 mcg/dL	50.12-456.5 μmol/L
	Fatally poisoned child	>1800 mcg/dL	>322.2 μmol/L
Iron-binding capacity, total (TIBC)			
Serum	Infant	100-400 mcg/dL	17.90-71.60 μmol/L
	Thereafter	250-400 mcg/dL	44.75-71.60 μmol/L
Lead			
Whole blood	Child	<10 mcg/dL	<0.48 μmol/L
Urine, 24 hr		<80 mcg/L	<0.39 μmol/L
Leukocyte count (WBC count)			
Whole blood		×1000 cells/mm^3 (μL)	×10^9 cells/L
	Birth	9.0-30.0	9.0-30.0
	24 hr	9.4-34.0	9.4-34.0
	1 mo	5.0-19.5	5.0-19.5
	1-3 yr	6.0-17.5	6.0-17.5
	4-7 yr	5.5-15.5	5.5-15.5
	8-13 yr	4.5-13.5	4.5-13.5
	Adult	4.5-11.0	4.5-11.0

Continued

TEST/SPECIMEN	AGE/GENDER/ REFERENCE	NORMAL RANGES		INTERNATIONAL UNITS (SI)
		CONVENTIONAL UNITS		INTERNATIONAL UNITS (SI)
CSF (cell count)		$\times$1000 cells/mm^3 (μL)		$\times$10^6 cells/L
	Premature	0-25 mononuclear		0-25
		0-10 polymorphonuclear		0-10
		0-1000 RBC		0-1000
	Newborn	0-20 mononuclear		0-20
		0-10 polymorphonuclear		0-10
		0-800 RBC		0-800
	Neonate	0-5 mononuclear		0-5
		0-10 polymorphonuclear		0-10
		0-50 RBC		0-50
	Thereafter	0-5 mononuclear		0-5
Leukocyte differential count				
Whole blood	Myelocytes	0%	0 cells/mm^3 (μL)	Number fraction 0
	Neutrophils— "bands"	3%-5%	150-400 cells/ mm^3 (μL)	Number fraction 0.03-0.05
	Neutrophils— "segs"	54%-62%	3000-5800 cells/ mm^3 (μL)	Number fraction 0.54-0.62
	Lymphocytes	25%-33%	1500-3000 cells/ mm^3 (μL)	Number fraction 0.25-0.33
	Monocytes	3%-7%	285-500 cells/ mm^3 (μL)	Number fraction 0.03-0.07
	Eosinophils	1%-3%	50-250 cells/mm^3 (μL)	Number fraction 0.01-0.03
	Basophils	0%-0.75%	15-50 cells/mm^3 (μL)	Number fraction 0-0.0075
Mean corpuscular hemoglobin (MCH)				
Whole blood	Birth	31-37 pg/cell		0.48-0.57 fmol/cell
	1-3 d (cap)	31-37 pg/cell		0.48-0.57 fmol/cell
	1 wk-1 mo	28-40 pg/cell		0.43-0.62 fmol/cell
	2 mo	26-34 pg/cell		0.40-0.53 fmol/cell
	3-6 mo	25-35 pg/cell		0.39-0.54 fmol/cell
	0.5-2 yr	23-31 pg/cell		0.36-0.48 fmol/cell
	2-6 yr	24-30 pg/cell		0.37-0.47 fmol/cell
	6-12 yr	25-33 pg/cell		0.39-0.51 fmol/cell
	12-18 yr	25-35 pg/cell		0.39-0.54 fmol/cell
	18-49 yr	26-34 pg/cell		0.40-0.53 fmol/cell
Mean corpuscular hemoglobin concentration (MCHC)				
Whole blood	Birth	30%-36% Hb/cell or g Hb/dL RBC		4.65-5.58 mmol Hb/L RBC
	1-3 d (cap)	29%-37% Hb/cell or g Hb/dL RBC		4.50-5.74 mmol Hb/L RBC
	1-2 wk	28%-38% Hb/cell or g Hb/dL RBC		4.34-5.89 mmol Hb/L RBC
	1-2 mo	29%-37% Hb/cell or g Hb/dL RBC		4.50-5.74 mmol Hb/L RBC
	3 mo-2 yr	30%-36% Hb/cell or g Hb/dL RBC		4.65-5.58 mmol Hb/L RBC
	2-18 yr	31%-37% Hb/cell or g Hb/dL RBC		4.81-5.74 mmol Hb/L RBC
	>18 yr	31%-37% Hb/cell or g Hb/dL RBC		4.81-5.74 mmol Hb/L RBC
Mean corpuscular volume (MCV)				
Whole blood	1-3 d (cap)	95-121 μm^3		95-121 fl
	0.5-2 yr	70-86 μm^3		70-86 fl
	6-12 yr	77-95 μm^3		77-95 fl
	12-18 yr:			
	Male	78-98 μm^3		78-98 fl
	Female	78-102 μm^3		78-102 fl
Osmolality				
Serum	Child, adult	275-295 mOsm/kg H$_2$O		
Urine, random		50-1400 mOsm/kg H$_2$O, depending on fluid intake; after 12-hr fluid restriction: >850 mOsm/kg H$_2$O		
Urine, 24 hr		$\cong$300-900 mOsm/kg H$_2$O		

	AGE/GENDER/	NORMAL RANGES	
TEST/SPECIMEN	REFERENCE	CONVENTIONAL UNITS	INTERNATIONAL UNITS (SI)
Oxygen, partial pressure (PO$_2$)			
Whole blood, arterial	Birth	8-24 mm Hg	1.1-3.2 kPa
	5-10 min	33-75 mm Hg	4.4-10.0 kPa
	30 min	31-85 mm Hg	4.1-11.3 kPa
	>1 hr	55-80 mm Hg	7.3-10.6 kPa
	1 d	54-95 mm Hg	7.2-12.6 kPa
	Thereafter (decreased with age)	83-108 mm Hg	11-14.4 kPa
Oxygen saturation (SaO$_2$)			
Whole blood, arterial	Newborn	85%-90%	Fraction saturated 0.85-0.90
	Thereafter	95%-99%	Fraction saturated 0.95-0.99
Partial thromboplastin time (PTT)			
Whole blood (Na citrate)			
Nonactivated		60-85 s (Platelin)	60-85 s
Activated		25-35 s (differs with method)	25-35 s
pH			H$^+$ concentration
Whole blood, arterial (must be corrected for body temperature)	Premature (48 hr)	7.35-7.50	31-44 nmol/L
	Birth, full term	7.11-7.36	43-77 nmol/L
	5-10 min	7.09-7.30	50-81 nmol/L
	30 min	7.21-7.38	41-61 nmol/L
	>1 hr	7.26-7.49	32-54 nmol/L
	1 d	7.29-7.45	35-51 nmol/L
	Thereafter	7.35-7.45	35-44 nmol/L
Urine, random	Newborn/neonate	5-7	0.1-10 µmol/L
	Thereafter	4.5-8 (average ≅6)	0.01-32 µmol/L (average ≅1.0 µmol/L)
Stool		7.0-7.5	31-100 nmol/L
Phenylalanine			
Serum	Premature	2.0-7.5 mg/dL	120-450 µmol/L
	Newborn	1.2-3.4 mg/dL	70-210 µmol/L
	Thereafter	0.8-1.8 mg/dL	50-110 µmol/L
Urine, 24 hr	10 d-2 wk	1-2 mg/d	6-12 µmol/d
	3-12 yr	4-18 mg/d	24-110 µmol/d
	Thereafter	Trace—17 mg/d	Trace—103 µmol/d
Plasma volume			
Plasma	Male	25-43 mL/kg	0.025-0.043 L/kg
	Female	28-45 mL/kg	0.028-0.045 L/kg
Platelet count (thrombocyte count)			
Whole blood (EDTA)	Newborn (after 1 wk, same as adult)	84-478 × 10^3/mm^3 (µL)	84-478 × 10^9/L
	Adult	150-400 × 10^3/mm^3 (µL)	150-400 × 10^9/L
Potassium			
Serum	Newborn	3.0-6.0 mEq/L	3.0-6.0 mmol/L
	Thereafter	3.5-5.0 mEq/L	3.5-5.0 mmol/L
Plasma (heparin)		3.4-4.5 mEq/L	3.4-4.5 mmol/L
Urine, 24 hr		2.5-125 mEq/d (varies with diet)	2.5-125 mmol/L
Protein			
Serum, total	Premature	4.3-7.6 g/dL	43-76 g/L
	Newborn	4.6-7.4 g/dL	46-74 g/L
	1-7 yr	6.1-7.9 g/dL	61-79 g/L
	8-12 yr	6.4-8.1 g/dL	64-81 g/L
	13-19 yr	6.6-8.2 g/dL	66-82 g/L
Total			
Urine, 24 hr		1-14 mg/dL	10-140 mg/L
		50-80 mg/d (at rest)	50-80 mg/d
		<250 mg/d (after intense exercise)	<250 mg/d (after intense exercise)
CSF		Lumbar: 8-32 mg/dL	80-320 mg/L

Continued

TEST/SPECIMEN	AGE/GENDER/ REFERENCE	NORMAL RANGES	
		CONVENTIONAL UNITS	INTERNATIONAL UNITS (SI)
Prothrombin time (PT)			
One-stage (Quick)			
Whole blood (Na citrate)	In general	11-15 s (varies with type of thromboplastin)	11-15 s
	Newborn	Prolonged by 2-3 s	Prolonged by 2-3 s
Two-stage modified (Ware and Seegers)			
Whole blood (sodium citrate)		18-22 s	18-22 s
RBC count: see Erythrocyte (RBC) count			
Red blood cell volume			
Whole blood	Male	20-36 mL/kg	0.020-0.036 L/kg
	Female	19-31 mL/kg	0.019-0.031 L/kg
Reticulocyte count			
Whole blood	Adults	0.5%-1.5% of erythrocytes or 25,000-75,000/mm³ (µL)	0.005-0.015 (number fraction) or 25,000-75,000 × 10^6/L
Capillary	1 d	0.4%-6.0%	0.004-0.060 (number fraction)
	7 d	<0.1%-1.3%	<0.001-0.013 (number fraction)
	1-4 wk	<0.1%-1.2%	<0.001-0.012 (number fraction)
	5-6 wk	<0.1%-2.4%	<0.001-0.024 (number fraction)
	7-8 wk	0.1%-2.9%	0.001-0.029 (number fraction)
	9-10 wk	<0.1%-2.6%	<0.001-0.026 (number fraction)
	11-12 wk	0.1%-1.3%	0.001-0.013 (number fraction)
Salicylates			
Serum, plasma	Therap. conc.	15-30 mg/dL	1.1-2.2 mmol/L
	Toxic conc.	>30 mg/dL	>18.5 mmol/L
Sedimentation rate: see Erythrocyte sedimentation rate (ESR)			
Sodium			
Serum or plasma	Newborn	134-146 mEq/L	134-146 mmol/L
	Infant	139-146 mEq/L	139-146 mmol/L
	Child	138-145 mEq/L	138-145 mmol/L
	Thereafter	136-146 mEq/L	136-146 mmol/L
Urine, 24 hr		40-220 mEq/L (diet dependent)	40-220 mmol/L
Sweat	Normal	<40 mEq/L	<40 mmol/L
	Indeterminate	45-60 mEq/L	45-60 mmol/L
	Cystic fibrosis	>60 mEq/L	>60 mmol/L
Specific gravity			
Urine, random	Adult	1.002-1.030	1.002-1.030
	After 12-hr fluid restriction	>1.025	>1.025
Urine, 24 hr		1.015-1.025	
Theophylline			
Serum, plasma	Therap. conc.		
	Bronchodilator	10-20 mcg/mL	56-110 µmol/L
	Premature apnea	5-10 mcg/mL	28-56 µmol/L
	Toxic conc.	>20 mcg/mL	>110 µmol/L
Thrombin time			
Whole blood (Na citrate)		Control time ±2 s when control is 9-13 s	Control time ±2 s when control is 9-13 s
Thyroxine, total (T_4)			
Serum	Cord	8-13 mcg/dL	103-168 nmol/L
	Newborn	11.5-24 mcg/dL (lower in low-birth-weight infants)	148-310 nmol/L
	Neonate	9-18 mcg/dL	116-232 nmol/L
	Infant	7-15 mcg/dL	90-194 nmol/L
	1-5 yr	7.3-15 mcg/dL	94-194 nmol/L
	5-10 yr	6.4-13.3 mcg/dL	83-172 nmol/L
	Thereafter	5-12 mcg/dL	65-155 nmol/L
	Newborn screen (filter paper)	6.2-22 mcg/dL	80-284 nmol/L

TEST/SPECIMEN	AGE/GENDER/ REFERENCE	NORMAL RANGES			
		CONVENTIONAL UNITS		INTERNATIONAL UNITS (SI)	
Triglycerides (TG)		**Male** (mg/dL)	**Female** (mg/dL)	**Male** (g/L)	**Female** (g/L)
Serum, after ≥2-hr fast	Cord	10-98	10-98	0.10-0.98	0.10-0.98
	0-5 yr	30-86	32-99	0.30-0.86	0.32-0.99
	6-11 yr	31-108	35-114	0.31-1.08	0.35-1.14
	12-15 yr	36-138	41-138	0.36-1.38	0.41-1.38
	16-19 yr	40-163	40-128	0.40-1.63	0.40-1.28
Triiodothyronine (T$_3$), free					
Serum	Cord	20-240 pg/dL		0.3-3.7 pmol/L	
	1-3 d	200-610 pg/dL		3.1-9.4 pmol/L	
	6 wk	240-560 pg/dL		3.7-8.6 pmol/L	
	Adults (20-50 yr)	230-660 pg/dL		3.5-10.0 pmol/L	
Triiodothyronine, total (T$_3$-RIA)					
Serum	Cord	30-70 ng/dL		0.46-1.08 nmol/L	
	Newborn	72-260 ng/dL		1.16-4 nmol/L	
	1-5 yr	100-260 ng/dL		1.54-4 nmol/L	
	5-10 yr	90-240 ng/dL		1.39-3.70 nmol/L	
	10-15 yr	80-210 ng/dL		1.23-3.23 nmol/L	
	Thereafter	115-190 ng/dL		1.77-2.93 nmol/L	
Urea nitrogen					
Serum or plasma	Cord	21-40 mg/dL		7.5-14.3 mmol/L	
	Premature (1 wk)	3-25 mg/dL		1.1-9 mmol/L	
	Newborn	3-12 mg/dL		1.1-4.3 mmol/L	
	Infant/child	5-18 mg/dL		1.8-6.4 mmol/L	
	Thereafter	7-18 mg/dL		2.5-6.4 mmol/L	
Urine volume					
Urine, 24 hr	Newborn	50-300 mL/d		0.05-0.3 L/d	
	Infant	350-550 mL/d		0.35-0.5 L/d	
	Child	500-1000 mL/d		0.5-1 L/d	
	Adolescent	700-1400 mL/d		0.7-1.4 L/d	
	Thereafter:				
	Male	800-1800 mL/d		0.8-1.8 L/d	
	Female	600-1600 mL/d (varies with intake and other factors)		0.6-1.6 L/d	

WBC: see Leukocyte count (WBC count)

Modified from Kliegman RM, Behrman RE, Jenson HB, et al, editors: *Nelson textbook of pediatrics*, ed 18, Philadelphia, 2007, Saunders; McMillan JA, Deangelis CD, Feigin RD, et al, editors: *Oski's pediatrics: principles and practice*, ed 3, Philadelphia, 1999, Lippincott Williams & Wilkins; and Fischbach F: *A manual of laboratory and diagnostic tests*, ed 6, Philadelphia, 2000, Lippincott Williams & Wilkins.
*For a description of abbreviations, see p. 1612.
†From National Cholesterol Education Program: Report of the expert panel on blood cholesterol levels in children and adolescents, *Pediatrics* 89(3 pt 2):527, 1992.

ABBREVIATIONS USED IN LABORATORY TESTS

ABBREVIATION	TERM	ABBREVIATION	TERM
cap	capillary	mo	month
CHF	congestive heart failure	mol	mole
conc.	concentration	mOsm	milliosmole
CSF	cerebrospinal fluid	Na	sodium
d	day; diem	Pa	pascal
EDTA	ethylenediaminetetraacetate	RBC	red blood cells
g	gram	s	second
H^+	hydrogen ion	temp	temperature
H_2O	water	therap.	therapeutic
Hb	hemoglobin	U	International unit of enzyme activity
HbF	fetal hemoglobin	vol	volume
hr	hour	WBC	white blood cells
IU	International unit	wk	week
L	liter	yr	year
m	meter	>	greater than
mEq	milliequivalent	≥	greater than or equal to
min	minute	<	less than
mm	millimeter	≤	less than or equal to
mm Hg	millimeters of mercury	±	plus/minus
mm H_2O	millimeters of water	≅	approximately equal to
mm^3	cubic millimeter		

PREFIXES DENOTING DECIMAL FACTORS

PREFIX	SYMBOL	AMOUNT
kilo	k	one thousand (10^3)
deci	d	one tenth (10^{-1})
centi	c	one hundredth (10^{-2})
milli	m	one thousandth (10^{-3})
micro	mc, μ	one millionth (10^{-6})
nano	n	one billionth (10^{-9})
pico	p	one trillionth (10^{-12})
femto	f	one quadrillionth (10^{-15})

Pediatric Vital Signs and Parameters

CENTIGRADE-TO-FAHRENHEIT TEMPERATURE CONVERSIONS

°C	°F	°C	°F	°C	°F
35.0	95.0	37.0	98.6	39.0	102.2
35.2	95.4	37.2	99.0	39.2	102.6
35.4	95.7	37.4	99.3	39.4	102.9
35.6	96.1	37.6	99.7	39.6	103.3
35.8	96.4	37.8	100.0	39.8	103.6
36.0	**96.8**	**38.0**	**100.4**	**40.0**	**104.0**
36.2	97.2	38.2	100.8	40.2	104.4
36.4	97.5	38.4	101.1	40.4	104.7
36.6	97.9	38.6	101.5	40.6	105.1
36.8	98.2	38.8	101.8	40.8	105.4
				41.0	**105.8**

Conversion formulas:
°F = (°C × ⅘) + 32 or (°C × 1.8) + 32
°C = (°F − 32) + ⅝ or (°F − 32) + 0.556

NORMAL HEART RATES FOR INFANTS AND CHILDREN

AGE	RATE (beats/min)		
	RESTING (AWAKE)	RESTING (SLEEPING)	EXERCISE (FEVER)
Newborn	100-180	80-160	Up to 220
1 week to 3 months	100-220	80-200	Up to 220
3 months to 2 years	80-150	70-120	Up to 200
2 years to 10 years	70-110	60-90	Up to 200
10 years to adult	55-90	50-90	Up to 200

From Gillette PC: Dysrhythmias. In Adams FH, Emmanoulides GC, Riemenschneider TA, editors: *Moss' heart disease in infants, children, and adolescents*, ed 4, Baltimore, 1989, Williams & Wilkins.

NORMAL TEMPERATURES IN CHILDREN

AGE	TEMPERATURE	
	°F	°C
3 months	99.4	37.5
6 months	99.5	37.5
1 year	99.7	37.7
3 years	99.0	37.2
5 years	98.6	37.0
7 years	98.3	36.8
9 years	98.1	36.7
11 years	98.0	36.7
13 years	97.8	36.6

Adapted from Lowrey GH: *Growth and development of children*, ed 8, St Louis, 1986, Mosby.

NORMAL RESPIRATORY RATES FOR CHILDREN

AGE	RATE (BREATHS/MIN)
Newborn	35
1 to 11 months	30
2 years	25
4 years	23
6 years	21
8 years	20
10 years	19
12 years	19
14 years	18
16 years	17
18 years	16-18

BLOOD PRESSURE (BP) LEVELS FOR BOYS BY AGE AND HEIGHT PERCENTILE

AGE (yr)	BP PERCENTILE	SYSTOLIC BP (mm Hg) PERCENTILE OF HEIGHT							DIASTOLIC BP (mm Hg) PERCENTILE OF HEIGHT						
		5TH	10TH	25TH	50TH	75TH	90TH	95TH	5TH	10TH	25TH	50TH	75TH	90TH	95TH
1	50th	80	81	83	85	87	88	89	34	35	36	37	38	39	39
	90th	94	95	97	99	100	102	103	49	50	51	52	53	53	54
	95th	98	99	101	103	104	106	106	54	54	55	56	57	58	58
	99th	105	106	108	110	112	113	114	61	62	63	64	65	66	66
2	50th	84	85	87	88	90	92	92	39	40	41	42	43	44	44
	90th	97	99	100	102	104	105	106	54	55	56	57	58	58	59
	95th	101	102	104	106	108	109	110	59	59	60	61	62	63	63
	99th	109	110	111	113	115	117	117	66	67	68	69	70	71	71
3	50th	86	87	89	91	93	94	95	44	44	45	46	47	48	48
	90th	100	101	103	105	107	108	109	59	59	60	61	62	63	63
	95th	104	105	107	109	110	112	113	63	63	64	65	66	67	67
	99th	111	112	114	116	118	119	120	71	71	72	73	74	75	75
4	50th	88	89	91	93	95	96	97	47	48	49	50	51	51	52
	90th	102	103	105	107	109	110	111	62	63	64	65	66	66	67
	95th	106	107	109	111	112	114	115	66	67	68	69	70	71	71
	99th	113	114	116	118	120	121	122	74	75	76	77	78	78	79
5	50th	90	91	93	95	96	98	98	50	51	52	53	54	55	55
	90th	104	105	106	108	110	111	112	65	66	67	68	69	69	70
	95th	108	109	110	112	114	115	116	69	70	71	72	73	74	74
	99th	115	116	118	120	121	123	123	77	78	79	80	81	81	82
6	50th	91	92	94	96	98	99	100	53	53	54	55	56	57	57
	90th	105	106	108	110	111	113	113	68	68	69	70	71	72	72
	95th	109	110	112	114	115	117	117	72	72	73	74	75	76	76
	99th	116	117	119	121	123	124	125	80	80	81	82	83	84	84
7	50th	92	94	95	97	99	100	101	55	55	56	57	58	59	59
	90th	106	107	109	111	113	114	115	70	70	71	72	73	74	74
	95th	110	111	113	115	117	118	119	74	74	75	76	77	78	78
	99th	117	118	120	122	124	125	126	82	82	83	84	85	86	86
8	50th	94	95	97	99	100	102	102	56	57	58	59	60	60	61
	90th	107	109	110	112	114	115	116	71	72	72	73	74	75	76
	95th	111	112	114	116	118	119	120	75	76	77	78	79	79	80
	99th	119	120	122	123	125	127	127	83	84	85	86	87	87	88
9	50th	95	96	98	100	102	103	104	57	58	59	60	61	61	62
	90th	109	110	112	114	115	117	118	72	73	74	75	76	76	77
	95th	113	114	116	118	119	121	121	76	77	78	79	80	81	81
	99th	120	121	123	125	127	128	129	84	85	86	87	88	88	89
10	50th	97	98	100	102	103	105	106	58	59	60	61	61	62	63
	90th	111	112	114	115	117	119	119	73	73	74	75	76	77	78
	95th	115	116	117	119	121	122	123	77	78	79	80	81	81	82
	99th	122	123	125	127	128	130	130	85	86	86	88	88	89	90
11	50th	99	100	102	104	105	107	107	59	59	60	61	62	63	63
	90th	113	114	115	117	119	120	121	74	74	75	76	77	78	78
	95th	117	118	119	121	123	124	125	78	78	79	80	81	82	82
	99th	124	125	127	129	130	132	132	86	86	87	88	89	90	90
12	50th	101	102	104	106	108	109	110	59	60	61	62	63	63	64
	90th	115	116	118	120	121	123	123	74	75	75	76	77	78	79
	95th	119	120	122	123	125	127	127	78	79	80	81	82	82	83
	99th	126	127	129	131	133	134	135	86	87	88	89	90	90	91
13	50th	104	105	106	108	110	111	112	60	60	61	62	63	64	64
	90th	117	118	120	122	124	125	126	75	75	76	77	78	79	79
	95th	121	122	124	126	128	129	130	79	79	80	81	82	83	83
	99th	128	130	131	133	135	136	137	87	87	88	89	90	91	91
14	50th	106	107	109	111	113	114	115	60	61	62	63	64	65	65
	90th	120	121	123	125	126	128	128	75	76	77	78	79	79	80
	95th	124	125	127	128	130	132	132	80	80	81	82	83	84	84
	99th	131	132	134	136	138	139	140	87	88	89	90	91	92	92

BLOOD PRESSURE (BP) LEVELS FOR BOYS BY AGE AND HEIGHT PERCENTILE—cont'd

AGE (yr)	BP PERCENTILE	SYSTOLIC BP (mm Hg) PERCENTILE OF HEIGHT							DIASTOLIC BP (mm Hg) PERCENTILE OF HEIGHT						
		5TH	10TH	25TH	50TH	75TH	90TH	95TH	5TH	10TH	25TH	50TH	75TH	90TH	95TH
15	50th	109	110	112	113	115	117	117	61	62	63	64	65	66	66
	90th	122	124	125	127	129	130	131	76	77	78	79	80	80	81
	95th	126	127	129	131	133	134	135	81	81	82	83	84	85	85
	99th	134	135	136	138	140	142	142	88	89	90	91	92	93	93
16	50th	111	112	114	116	118	119	120	63	63	64	65	66	67	67
	90th	125	126	128	130	131	133	134	78	78	79	80	81	82	82
	95th	129	130	132	134	135	137	137	82	83	83	84	85	86	87
	99th	136	137	139	141	143	144	145	90	90	91	92	93	94	94
17	50th	114	115	116	118	120	121	122	65	66	66	67	68	69	70
	90th	127	128	130	132	134	135	136	80	80	81	82	83	84	84
	95th	131	132	134	136	138	139	140	84	85	86	87	87	88	89
	99th	139	140	141	143	145	146	147	92	93	93	94	95	96	97

The 90th percentile is 1.28 SD, the 95th percentile is 1.645 SD, and the 99th percentile is 2.326 SD over the mean.
From www.nhlbi.nih.gov/guidelines/hypertension/child_tbl.pdf.

BLOOD PRESSURE (BP) LEVELS FOR GIRLS BY AGE AND HEIGHT PERCENTILE

AGE (yr)	BP PERCENTILE	SYSTOLIC BP (mm Hg) PERCENTILE OF HEIGHT							DIASTOLIC BP (mm Hg) PERCENTILE OF HEIGHT						
		5TH	10TH	25TH	50TH	75TH	90TH	95TH	5TH	10TH	25TH	50TH	75TH	90TH	95TH
1	50th	83	84	85	86	88	89	90	38	39	39	40	41	41	42
	90th	97	97	98	100	101	102	103	52	53	53	54	55	55	56
	95th	100	101	102	104	105	106	107	56	57	57	58	59	59	60
	99th	108	108	109	111	112	113	114	64	64	65	65	66	67	67
2	50th	85	85	87	88	89	91	91	43	44	44	45	46	46	47
	90th	98	99	100	101	103	104	105	57	58	58	59	60	61	61
	95th	102	103	104	105	107	108	109	61	62	62	63	64	65	65
	99th	109	110	111	112	114	115	116	69	69	70	70	71	72	72
3	50th	86	87	88	89	91	92	93	47	48	48	49	50	50	51
	90th	100	100	102	103	104	106	106	61	62	62	63	64	64	65
	95th	104	104	105	107	108	109	110	65	66	66	67	68	68	69
	99th	111	111	113	114	115	116	117	73	73	74	74	75	76	76
4	50th	88	88	90	91	92	94	94	50	50	51	52	52	53	54
	90th	101	102	103	104	106	107	108	64	64	65	66	67	67	68
	95th	105	106	107	108	110	111	112	68	68	69	70	71	71	72
	99th	112	113	114	115	117	118	119	76	76	76	77	78	79	79
5	50th	89	90	91	93	94	95	96	52	53	53	54	55	55	56
	90th	103	103	105	106	107	109	109	66	67	67	68	69	69	70
	95th	107	107	108	110	111	112	113	70	71	71	72	73	73	74
	99th	114	114	116	117	118	120	120	78	78	79	79	80	81	81
6	50th	91	92	93	94	96	97	98	54	54	55	56	56	57	58
	90th	104	105	106	108	109	110	111	68	68	69	70	70	71	72
	95th	108	109	110	111	113	114	115	72	72	73	74	74	75	76
	99th	115	116	117	119	120	121	122	80	80	80	81	82	83	83
7	50th	93	93	95	96	97	99	99	55	56	56	57	58	58	59
	90th	106	107	108	109	111	112	113	69	70	70	71	72	72	73
	95th	110	111	112	113	115	116	116	73	74	74	75	76	76	77
	99th	117	118	119	120	122	123	124	81	81	82	82	83	84	84
8	50th	95	95	96	98	99	100	101	57	57	57	58	59	60	60
	90th	108	109	110	111	113	114	114	71	71	71	72	73	74	74
	95th	112	112	114	115	116	118	118	75	75	75	76	77	78	78
	99th	119	120	121	122	123	125	125	82	82	83	83	84	85	86

Continued

BLOOD PRESSURE (BP) LEVELS FOR GIRLS BY AGE AND HEIGHT PERCENTILE—cont'd

AGE (yr)	BP PERCENTILE	SYSTOLIC BP (mm Hg) PERCENTILE OF HEIGHT							DIASTOLIC BP (mm Hg) PERCENTILE OF HEIGHT						
		5TH	10TH	25TH	50TH	75TH	90TH	95TH	5TH	10TH	25TH	50TH	75TH	90TH	95TH
9	50th	96	97	98	100	101	102	103	58	58	58	59	60	61	61
	90th	110	110	112	113	114	116	116	72	72	72	73	74	75	75
	95th	114	114	115	117	118	119	120	76	76	76	77	78	79	79
	99th	121	121	123	124	125	127	127	83	83	84	84	85	86	87
10	50th	98	99	100	102	103	104	105	59	59	59	60	61	62	62
	90th	112	112	114	115	116	118	118	73	73	73	74	75	76	76
	95th	116	116	117	119	120	121	122	77	77	77	78	79	80	80
	99th	123	123	125	126	127	129	129	84	84	85	86	86	87	88
11	50th	100	101	102	103	105	106	107	60	60	60	61	62	63	63
	90th	114	114	116	117	118	119	120	74	74	74	75	76	77	77
	95th	118	118	119	121	122	123	124	78	78	78	79	80	81	81
	99th	125	125	126	128	129	130	131	85	85	86	87	87	88	89
12	50th	102	103	104	105	107	108	109	61	61	61	62	63	64	64
	90th	116	116	117	119	120	121	122	75	75	75	76	77	78	78
	95th	119	120	121	123	124	125	126	79	79	79	80	81	82	82
	99th	127	127	128	130	131	132	133	86	86	87	88	88	89	90
13	50th	104	105	106	107	109	110	110	62	62	62	63	64	65	65
	90th	117	118	119	121	122	123	124	76	76	76	77	78	79	79
	95th	121	122	123	124	126	127	128	80	80	80	81	82	83	83
	99th	128	129	130	132	133	134	135	87	87	88	89	89	90	91
14	50th	106	106	107	109	110	111	112	63	63	63	64	65	66	66
	90th	119	120	121	122	124	125	125	77	77	77	78	79	80	80
	95th	123	123	125	126	127	129	129	81	81	81	82	83	84	84
	99th	130	131	132	133	135	136	136	88	88	89	90	90	91	92
15	50th	107	108	109	110	111	113	113	64	64	64	65	66	67	67
	90th	120	121	122	123	125	126	127	78	78	78	79	80	81	81
	95th	124	125	126	127	129	130	131	82	82	82	83	84	85	85
	99th	131	132	133	134	136	137	138	89	89	90	91	91	92	93
16	50th	108	108	110	111	112	114	114	64	64	65	66	66	67	68
	90th	121	122	123	124	126	127	128	78	78	79	80	81	81	82
	95th	125	126	127	128	130	131	132	82	82	83	84	85	85	86
	99th	132	133	134	135	137	138	139	90	90	90	91	92	93	93
17	50th	108	109	110	111	113	114	115	64	65	65	66	67	67	68
	90th	122	122	123	125	126	127	128	78	79	79	80	81	81	82
	95th	125	126	127	129	130	131	132	82	83	83	84	85	85	86
	99th	133	133	134	136	137	138	139	90	90	91	91	92	93	93

The 90th percentile is 1.28 SD, the 95th percentile is 1.645 SD, and the 99th percentile is 2.326 SD over the mean.
From www.nhlbi.nih.gov/guidelines/hypertension/child_tbl.pdf.

S

Special Features

Special Features (cont'd)